Neonatology

Giuseppe Buonocore • Rodolfo Bracci
Michael Weindling
Editors

Neonatology

A Practical Approach to Neonatal Diseases

Second Edition

Volume 1

With 568 Figures and 386 Tables

Springer

Editors
Giuseppe Buonocore
Department of Pediatrics
Obstetrics and Reproductive Medicine
University of Siena
Siena, Italy

Rodolfo Bracci
Department of Pediatrics
Obstetrics and Reproductive Medicine
University of Siena
Siena, Italy

Michael Weindling
Liverpool Women's Hospital Neonatal Unit
Liverpool, UK

ISBN 978-3-319-29487-2 ISBN 978-3-319-29489-6 (eBook)
ISBN 978-3-319-29488-9 (print and electronic bundle)
https://doi.org/10.1007/978-3-319-29489-6

Library of Congress Control Number: 2018940273

Printed on acid-free paper

This Springer imprint is published by the registered company Springer International Publishing AG part of Springer Nature.
The registered company address is: Gewerbestrasse 11, 6330 Cham, Switzerland

Introduction

Neonatology is a science in rapid evolution. The speed of this evolution may cause some to doubt what a traditional textbook is able to achieve in bringing the most up-to-date developments to a reader's attention. Although the interested reader will use other electronic means to access current information, this is not always possible. We firmly believe that, through their own experience, experts are able to bring their own perspective and interest to a subject and act as a guide to the interested and committed reader. We therefore believe that this textbook should act as a conduit of reliable information from the expert to the clinician. We have tried to make this textbook into a genuine guide to the best and most up-to-date answers for neonatologists who are striving to give the best and highest quality care to sick babies.

All practicing clinicians work within their own culture and resources. Each has to make judgments about the best and most appropriate application of available resources to the care of their small sick patients. We hope that this textbook will support the dedicated clinician by providing the best evidence available in the various sub-specialisms of neonatology, particularly when the issue of best treatment continues to be debated. The reader who needs rapid and comprehensive information about a topic requires that the information provided should be synthetized intelligently, exhaustively, and clearly. Subjects should be updated as much as possible. We have endeavored to meet these requirements. We think that the aim of a modern textbook should be to describe the present state of the science, suggesting ways in which this might be improved, and to provide a sound understanding of pathophysiology and diagnostic and therapeutic procedures. Our overall aim is to support and optimize the care of the newborn. In this way, our approach is "practical" and aims to assist neonatologists in their daily work.

In this second edition, the text has been largely revised by experts who contributed to the previous volume. They have added new information, some of it through short- and long term follow-up, to support the evidence that underpins good clinical practice. Some chapters are completely new.

We are grateful to all the authors for their time and contributions. We would also like to thank Andrew Spencer, Tina Shelton, Vasowati Shome, and the publication team of Springer for their great efforts in publishing this book.

We sincerely hope that this volume has built on the success of its predecessor and continues to support clinicians in a readily accessible and useful way.

Contents

Volume 1

About the Editors

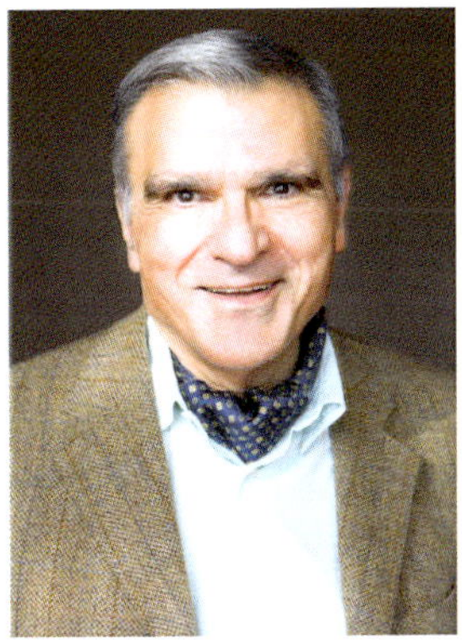

Giuseppe Buonocore is an Italian pediatrician, who is internationally recognized for his research on neonatal diseases, oxidative stress, and early identification of the newborn at high risk of brain damage. He is a full Professor of Pediatrics, Department of Molecular and Developmental Medicine, University of Siena, Italy, and Director of the Division of Pediatric-Neonatology, Azienda Ospedaliera-Universitaria of Siena, Italy. He is Chairman of Pediatrics at the School of Specialization in Pediatrics and Neonatology, University of Siena, Italy.

He is the President and Coordinator of European scientific network EURope Against Infant Brain Injury (EURAIBI). He has been a Visiting Professor at the University of Pennsylvania, the University of Florida, the University Hospitals of New York, as well as at the University of Oulu, Finland, at Taipei Medical University, and at Chang Gung Memorial Hospital at Linkou, Taiwan.

He is also the past President of ESPR and UENPS and currently President of the National College of University Full Professors of Pediatrics. He is involved in the coordination of numerous pan-European clinical trials as well as American and Australian. He has received many scientific awards: including the Seventh annual Dr. Donald V Eitzman lectures "Iron homeostasis metabolism and toxicity," University of Florida (2000), and the "Goccia d'oro 2010" for the efforts and results in the scientific research in the field of

Prenatal, Perinatal, and Neonatal Brain Damage. He also holds the patent of a scientific invention: the "Machine for automatic assessment of pain in neonates."

Dr. Buonocore has supervised more than 200 M.D./Ph.D. students (1994/2018) in Medicine and Surgery, Pediatrics, and Diagnostic Biochemistry. His current research interests are in the mechanisms of cell damage in the neonatal brain, with special reference to hypoxia, and the role of oxidant radicals in neonatal diseases and in babies with birth asphyxia. Additional research interest fields are ethics in perinatology and fetal and neonatal pain prevention. His research team is funded by several agencies including the Italian Ministry of University and Scientific Research as well as the European Community. Prof. Buonocore is author of more than 900 publications: 3 books and 27 book chapters, 300 peer-reviewed articles, and more than 617 presentations at international conferences and national meetings. He is currently Editor-in Chief of *Current Pediatric Reviews*, Associate Editor of *Journal of Pineal Research*, and on the editorial board of several international scientific journals. He has organized more than 20 European conferences and has been the scientific coordinator or participant in several national and international clinical trials.

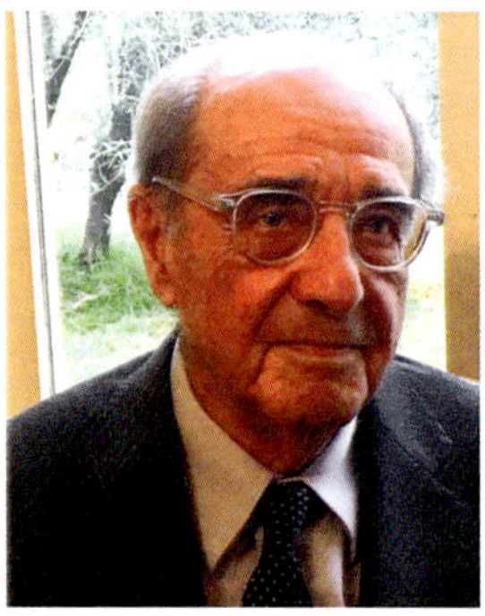

Rodolfo Bracci was born in Siena (Italy) in 1931. After graduating in Medicine and Surgery from the University of Siena Medical School in 1955, he became Assistant Professor of Pediatrics in the University of Siena. He was Post doctoral Trainee at the Albert Einstein College of Medicine, New York (1964–1965). At that time, working under the direction of Professor Ruth Gross, he made the first experiences on the antioxidant properties of the red cells of newborn. After his return to Italy, he became Assistant Professor of Pediatrics at the University of Florence and later at the University of Siena. He continued to be involved in the field of oxygen toxicity of the erythrocyte of newborn, and in 1967, he demonstrated that the red cells of newborn may have not only a low protection against reacting oxygen species but also an increased production of them.

Professor of Neonatology of the University of Siena and Director of the Neonatal Intensive Care Unit of the Siena Hospital, he was leading a staff of researchers involved in the physiopathology of the neonate, particularly in the calcium homeostasis, in the opioids metabolism, and especially in the

problems of oxygen toxicity in the red cells as well as in various organs. More than a hundred papers were published in important international journals by the doctors working under the guidance of Rodolfo Bracci. He was invited speaker in many international congresses and seminars in various cities in Europe and in America.

He has been member of the European Society of Pediatric Hematology and Immunology, the European Society for Pediatric Research, the European Society for Perinatal Medicine, the Neonatal Intensive Care Collegium, the Italian Society of Pediatrics, and the Italian Society of Neonatology.

Retired from University of Siena in 2001, he continued to publish papers, mainly together with Professor G. Buonocore.

Michael Weindling is Emeritus Professor of Perinatal Medicine at the University of Liverpool and Honorary Consultant Neonatologist at Liverpool Women's Hospital, where he was responsible for the care of newborn babies in a tertiary neonatal intensive care unit until he retired from clinical work in 2013. He is an Associate Editor of *Acta Paediatrica*. He continues with his research interest into the maintenance of appropriate brain oxygenation, cerebral hemodynamics, and the prevention of acquired damage of the developing brain.

He studied medicine at Guy's Hospital in London and qualified in 1973. His training in London included a period at the Great Ormond Street Hospital for Sick Children and then as research fellow at the University of Oxford, where he studied the cerebral hemodynamics of the developing brain. Michael Weindling was appointed a Senior Lecturer and consultant in Liverpool in 1985. During his early years as a consultant, he undertook a master's degree in medical ethics at the University of Keele with a dissertation into the changing moral status of the developing human from conceptus to neonate. He was promoted to Professor in 1996 with a personal chair entitled Professor of Perinatal Medicine, a title chosen to reflect his interest into the rapidly changing requirements of the developing brain. He has a considerable interest in medical education and for several years was Head of the School of Paediatrics in Merseyside.

Contributors

Steven H. Abman University of Colorado Denver – Anschutz Medical Campus, Denver, CO, USA

Massimo Agosti Neonatology and NICU – Maternal and Child Department, Ospedale "F del Ponte", Varese, Italy

Rocco Agostino Ethics Committee, Pediatric Hospital Bambino Gesù, Rome, Italy

Carlo Agostoni Pediatric Clinic, Department of Clinical Sciences and Community Health, University of Milan Fondazione, IRCCS Ca Granda, Ospedale Maggiore Policlinico, Milano, Italy

Munir Ahmed Division of Asthma, Allergy and Lung Biology, MRC Centre for Allergic Mechanisms of Asthma, King's College London, London, UK

Uma Sankari Ali Nephrology Division and PICU, BJ Wadia Hospital for Children, Mumbai, India

Karel Allegaert Neonatal Intensive Care Unit, University Hospitals Leuven, Leuven, Belgium

Department of Development and Regeneration, KU Leuven, Leuven, Belgium

Intensive Care and Department of Pediatric Surgery, Erasmus MC – Sophia Children's Hospital, Rotterdam, The Netherlands

Ruben E. Alvaro Department of Pediatrics, WR004 Women's Hospital, University of Manitoba, Winnipeg, MB, Canada

Gina Ancora Neonatology and Neonatal Intensive Care Unit, Ospedale Infermi, Rimini, Italy

Endla K. Anday Department of Pediatrics, Drexel University College of Medicine, St. Christopher's Hospital for Children, Neonatal-Perinatal Medicine, Philadelphia, PA, USA

Generoso Andria Department of Translational Medicine, Section of Pediatrics, Federico II University of Naples, Naples, Italy

Rajesh K. Aneja Departments of Critical Care Medicine and Pediatrics, University of Pittsburgh School of Medicine, Children's Hospital of Pittsburgh, Pittsburgh, PA, USA

Ruby V. Aneja Division of Neonatology, Temple University, West Penn Hospital, Pittsburgh, PA, USA

Molinari Angelo Claudio Thrombosis and Hemostasis Unit, Giannina Gaslini Children's Hospital, Genova, Italy

Rossella Angotti Department of Pediatrics, Obstetrics and Reproductive Medicine, Section of Pediatric Surgery, University of Siena, Siena, Italy

Carmelo Arcidiacono Department of Pediatric Cardiology, IRCCS Policlinico San Donato, San Siro, Milan, Italy

Domenico Arduini Department of Obstetrics and Gynecology, University of Rome Tor Vergata, Rome, Italy

Roberto Aufieri Division of Neonatology and Neonatal Intensive Care, Casilino General Hospital, Rome, Italy

Franco Bagnoli Department of Pediatrics, Obstetrics and Reproductive Medicine, University of Siena, Siena, Italy

Milica Bajcetic Institute of Pharmacology, Clinical Pharmacology and Toxicology, Medical Faculty, University of Belgrade, Belgrade, Serbia

Clinical Pharmacology Unit, University Children's Hospital, Belgrade, Serbia

Sarah Bajorek Department of Pediatrics, Division of Neonatology, University of Florida, College of Medicine, Gainesville, FL, USA

Antonio Balsamo Department of Medical and Surgical Sciences, Pediatric Unit, Center for Rare Endocrine Diseases (CARENDO BO), S.Orsola Malpighi University Hospital, Bologna, Italy

Jane E. Barthell Children's Hospitals and Clinics of Minnesota, Minneapolis, MN, USA

Francesco Bazzini Department of Molecular and Developmental Medicine, University of Siena, Siena, Italy

Roberto Bellù NICU, Ospedale Manzoni, Lecco, Italy

Franca Fossati-Bellani Pediatric Oncology Department, Fondazione IRCCS Istituto Nazionale dei Tumori, Milan, Italy

Carlo V. Bellieni Neonatal Intensive Care Unit, Siena University Hospital, Siena, Italy

Simonetta Bellone Department of Health Sciences, Division of Pediatrics, University of Piemonte Orientale, Novara, Italy

Elisa Belvisi Department of Molecular and Developmental Medicine, University of Siena, Siena, Italy

Britney Benoit School of Nursing, Centre for Pediatric Pain Research, Maternal-Newborn Program, Dalhousie University, IWK Health Centre, Halifax, Canada

Silvano Bertelloni Adolescent Medicine Unit, Division of Pediatrics, S. Chiara Hospital, University of Pisa, Pisa, Italy

Giovanna Bertini Neonatal Intensive Care Unit, Careggi University Hospital, Florence, Italy

Enrico Bertino Neonatal Unit, University of Turin, Turin, Italy

Natascia Bertoncelli Neonatal Intensive Care Unit, Department of Medical and Surgical Sciences of the Mother, Children and Adults, University Hospital of Modena, Modena, Italy

Giulio Bevilacqua Department of Pediatrics and Neonatology, Eastern Liguria Hospital, La Spezia, Italy

Stefania Bezzio Department of Pediatrics, University of Turin, Turin, Italy

Vineet Bhandari Neonatology/Pediatrics, St. Christopher's Hospital for Children/Drexel University College of Medicine, Philadelphia, PA, USA

Drexel University, Philadelphia, PA, USA

Paolo Biban Azienda Ospedaliera Universitaria Integrata Verona, Verona, Italy

Roberta Bilenchi Department of Medical, Surgical and Neurological Sciences, Dermatology Section, University of Siena, Siena, Italy

Caterina Bocchi Obstetrics and Gynecology, Department of Molecular and Developmental Medicine, University of Siena, Siena, Italy

Antonio Boldrini Department of Clinical and Experimental Medicine, Division of Neonatology and Neonatal Intensive Care Unit, Santa Chiara University Hospital, Pisa, Italy

Maria Elena Bolis Neonatology and NICU – Maternal and Child Department, Ospedale "F del Ponte", Varese, Italy

Gianni Bona Department of Health Sciences, Division of Pediatrics, University of Piemonte Orientale, Novara, Italy

Rachele Bonfiglio Department of Anesthesia, Pediatric and Neonatal Intensive Care, Istituto Giannina Gaslini, Genoa, Italy

Alessandro Borghesi Neonatal Intensive Care Unit, Fondazione IRCCS Policlinico 'San Matteo', Pavia, Italy

Giulio Bosco Sapienza Università di Roma, Policlinico Umberto I di Roma, Rome, Italy

Farid Boubred Division of Neonatology, La Conception Hospital, Marseille, France

Rodolfo Bracci University of Siena, Siena, Italy

Nicola Brunetti-Pierri Department of Translational Medicine, Section of Pediatrics, Federico II University of Naples, Naples, Italy

Jenny Bua Division of Neonatology, Institute for Maternal and Child Health IRCCS 'Burlo Garofolo', Trieste, Italy

Wilma Buffolano Heading Coordinating Centre for Perinatal Infection-Campania Region, Translational Medicine Department, Federico II Medical School, Naples, Italy

Giuseppe Buonocore University of Siena, Siena, Italy

Marsha Campbell-Yeo Departments of Pediatrics, Psychology and Neuroscience, Dalhousie University School of Nursing, Halifax, Canada

Letizia Capasso Division of Neonatology, Department of Translational Medical Sciences, Università "Federico II" di Napoli, Naples, Italy

Joseph A. Carcillo Departments of Critical Care Medicine and Pediatrics, University of Pittsburgh School of Medicine, Children's Hospital of Pittsburgh, Pittsburgh, PA, USA

Mario Carminati Department of Pediatric Cardiology, IRCCS Policlinico San Donato, San Siro, Milan, Italy

Virgilio P. Carnielli Division of Neonatology, Salesi Hospital, Polytechnic University of Marche, Ancona, Italy

Elisa della Casa Neonatal Intensive Care Unit, Department of Medical and Surgical Sciences of the Mother, Children and Adults, University Hospital of Modena, Modena, Italy

Alessandra Cassio Department of Medical and Surgical Sciences, Pediatric Endocrinology Unit, S. Orsola-Malpighi University Hospital, Bologna, Italy

Serena Catania Pediatric Oncology Department, Fondazione IRCCS Istituto Nazionale dei Tumori, Milan, Italy

Paolo Cavarzere Pediatric Unit, Department of Mother and Child, University Hospital of Verona, Verona, Italy

Sylvain Chemtob Departments of Pediatrics, Ophthalmology and Pharmacology, Centre Hospitalier, Universitaire Sainte-Justine, Research Center, Montréal, QC, Canada

Department of Ophthalmology, Maisonneuve-Rosemont Hospital Research Center, Montréal, QC, Canada

Stefano Chiaravalli Pediatric Oncology Department, Fondazione IRCCS Istituto Nazionale dei Tumori, Milan, Italy

Gaetano Chirico Neonatology and Intensive Neonatal Therapy Unit, Spedali Civili of Brescia, Brescia, Italy

Robert D. Christensen Divisions of Neonatology and Hematology, Department of Pediatrics, University of Utah School of Medicine, Intermountain Healthcare, Salt Lake City, UT, USA

Massimiliano Ciantelli Department of Clinical and Experimental Medicine, Division of Neonatology and Neonatal Intensive Care Unit, S. Chiara University Hospital, Pisa, Italy

Azienda Ospedaliero-Universitaria Pisana, Pisa, Italy

Elena Ciarmoli Neonatologia e Terapia Intensiva Neonatale, Fondazione MBBM, ASST-Ospedale San Gerardo-Monza, Monza, Italy

Alessandro Cicognani Department of Medical and Surgical Sciences, Pediatric Unit, Center for Rare Endocrine Diseases (CARENDO BO), S.Orsola Malpighi University Hospital, Bologna, Italy

Giovanni Cioni IRCCS Stella Maris, Department of Developmental Neuroscience, Pisa, Italy

University of Pisa, Department of Clinical and Experimental Neuroscience, Pisa, Italy

Olivier Claris Department of Neonatology, Hôpital Femme Mère Enfant, Bron, France

Hospices Civils de Lyon and Université Claude Bernard, Lyon, France

Paola E. Cogo Division of Pediatrics, Department of Medicine, S. Maria della Misericordia University Hospital, University of Udine, Udine, Italy

Richard J. Cooke Department of Pediatrics, University of Tennessee Health Science Center, Memphis, TN, USA

Giovanni Corsello Department of Sciences for Health Promotion and Mother and Child Care, University of Palermo, Palermo, Italy

Alessandra Coscia Neonatal Unit, University of Turin, Turin, Italy

Frans J. C. Cuperus Department of Gastroenterology and Hepatology, University Medical Center Groningen, Groningen, The Netherlands

Tore Curstedt Department of Molecular Medicine and Surgery, Karolinska Institutet, Karolinska University Hospital, Stockholm, Sweden

Mario De Curtis Dipartimento Materno-Infantile, Università "La Sapienza", Rome, Italy

Carlo Dani Neonatal Intensive Care Unit, Careggi University Hospital, Florence, Italy

Università degli Studi di Firenze, Florence, Italy

Riccardo Davanzo Department of Mother and Child Health, Madonna delle Grazie Hospital, Matera, Italy

Franco D'Alberton Department of Medical and Surgical Sciences, Pediatric Unit, Center for Rare Endocrine Diseases (CARENDO BO), S.Orsola Malpighi University Hospital, Bologna, Italy

Andrea De Luca Department of Medical Biotechnologies, University of Siena, Siena, Italy

UOC Malattie Infettive Universitarie, Azienda Ospedaliera Universitaria Senese, Siena, Italy

Linda S. de Vries Department of Neonatology, Wilhelmina Children's Hospital, University Medical Center, Utrecht, The Netherlands

Antonio Del Vecchio Department of Women's and Children's Health, Neonatal Intensive Care Unit, Di Venere Hospital, ASL Bari, Bari, Italy

Maria Delivoria-Papadopoulos Department of Pediatrics, Drexel University College of Medicine, St. Christopher's Hospital for Children, Neonatal-Perinatal Medicine, Philadelphia, PA, USA

Marco Della Monaca Sapienza Università di Roma, Policlinico Umberto I di Roma, Rome, Italy

Paola Di Nicola Neonatal Unit, University of Turin, Turin, Italy

Petr H. Dijk Beatrix Children's Hospital, University Medical Center Groningen, Groningen, The Netherlands

Carmelita D'Ippolito Pediatric Oncohematology and Bone Marrow Transplant, Spedali Civili Hospital, Brescia, Italy

Timothy Disher Centre for Pediatric Pain Research, Dalhousie University School of Nursing and IWK Health Centre, Halifax, Canada

Nicola Disma Department of Anesthesia, Pediatric and Neonatal Intensive Care, Istituto Giannina Gaslini, Genoa, Italy

Marcello Dòmini U.O. di Chirurgia pediatrica – Ospedale S.Orsola, Università degli Studi – Alma Mater Studiorum, di Bologna, Italy

Allison Dorfman Department of Ophthalmology/Neurology, McGill University-Montreal Children's Hospital Research Institute, Montreal, QC, Canada

Elsa Duchemin-Kermorvant INSERM UMRS1138, Centre de Recherche des Cordeliers, Paris, France

Jennifer M. Duchon Division of Neonatology, St. Joseph's Regional Medical Center, Paterson, NJ, USA

Jeroen Dudink Neonatology, Sophia Children's Hospital, Erasmus MC Rotterdam, Rotterdam, Zuid-Holland, The Netherlands

Claudio Fabris Neonatal Unit, University of Turin, Turin, Italy

Maria Teresa Fadda Sapienza Università di Roma, Policlinico Umberto I di Roma, Rome, Italy

Avroy A. Fanaroff Case Western Reserve University School of Medicine Rainbow Babies and Children's Hospital, Cleveland, OH, USA

Jonathan M. Fanaroff Case Western Reserve University School of Medicine Rainbow Babies and Children's Hospital, Cleveland, OH, USA

Vassilios Fanos Department of Surgery, Neonatal Intensive Care Unit, Neonatal Pathology and Neonatal Section, AOU and University of Cagliari, Cagliari, Italy

Maria Grazia Faticato Department of Pediatric Surgery, University of Genoa, Genoa, Italy

Giannina Gaslini Institute, Genoa, Italy

Silvia Ferranti Department of Molecular Medicine and Development, University of Siena, Siena, Italy,

Fabrizio Ferrari Neonatal Intensive Care Unit, Department of Medical and Surgical Sciences of the Mother, Children and Adults, University of Modena and Reggio Emilia, Modena, Italy

Enrico Ferrazzi Prenatal Diagnosis and Fetal Surgery Unit, Dept. of Woman, Mother and Neonate, Buzzi Children's Hospital Department of Clinical Sciences, University of Milan, Milan, Italy

Michele Fimiani Dipartimento di Medicina Clinica e Scienze Immunologiche – Sezione di Dermatologia, Università degli Studi di Siena, Policlinico "Santa Maria alle Scotte", Siena, Italy

Department of Medical, Surgical and Neurological Sciences, Dermatology Section, University of Siena, Siena, Italy

Vittorio Fineschi Department of Anatomical, Histological, Forensic Medicine and Orthopaedic Sciences, "Sapienza" University of Rome, Rome, Italy

Bobbi Fleiss UMR1141, Insem-Paris Diderot University, Hôpital Robert Debré, Paris, France

Centre for the Developing Brain, Department of Perinatal Imaging and Health, Division of Imaging Sciences and Biomedical Engineering, King's College London, King's Health Partners, St. Thomas' Hospital, London, UK

Monica Fumagalli NICU, Department of Clinical Sciences and Community Health, Fondazione IRCCS Ca' Granda Ospedale Maggiore Policlinico Milano, Università degli Studi di Milano, Milan, Italy

Clara Gabiano Department of Pediatrics, University of Turin, Turin, Italy

Silvia Garazzino Department of Pediatrics, University of Turin, Regina Margherita Childrens Hospital, AOU Città della Salute e della Scienza di Torino, Turin, Italy

Elisabetta Garetti Neonatal Intensive Care Unit, Department of Medical and Surgical Sciences of the Mother, Children and Adults, University of Modena and Reggio Emilia, Modena, Italy

Alfredo Garzi Department of Pediatrics, Obstetrics and Reproductive Medicine, Section of Pediatric Surgery, University of Siena, Siena, Italy

Università degli Studi di Salerno, Fisciano, Italy

Diego Gazzolo Neonatal Intensive Care Unit, Department of Maternal, Fetal and Neonatal Medicine, S. Arrigo Children's Hospital, Alessandria, Italy

Giulia Genoni Department of Health Sciences, Division of Pediatrics, University of Piemonte Orientale, Novara, Italy

Maurizio Gente Department of Pediatrics and Infant Neuropsychiatry, Neonatal Emergency Transport Service, Sapienza University of Rome, Rome, Italy

Michael K. Georgieff Division of Neonatology, Department of Pediatrics Center for Neurobehavioral Development, University of Minnesota, Minneapolis, MN, USA

Paolo Ghirri Department of Clinical and Experimental Medicine, Division of Neonatology and Neonatal Intensive Care Unit, Santa Chiara University Hospital, Pisa, Italy

Daniela Gianotti Department of Pediatrics and Neonatology, Eastern Liguria Hospital, La Spezia, Italy

Jason Gien University of Colorado Denver, Denver, CO, USA

Enza Giglione Department of Health Sciences, Division of Pediatrics, University of Piemonte Orientale, Novara, Italy

Mario Giuffrè Department of Sciences for Health Promotion and Mother and Child Care, University of Palermo, Palermo, Italy

Francesca Giuliani Neonatal Unit, University of Turin, Turin, Italy

Kirsten Glaser University Children's Hospital, University of Würzburg, Würzburg, Germany

Peter D. Gluckman Liggins Institute, University of Auckland, Auckland, New Zealand

Sergio Golombek New York Medical College, New York, USA

Misty Good Division of Neonatology, University of Pittsburgh School of Medicine, Children's Hospital of Pittsburgh, Pittsburgh, PA, USA

Glenn R. Gourley Department of Pediatrics, University of Minnesota, Minneapolis, USA

Paul P. Govaert Neonatology, Sophia Children's Hospital, Erasmus MC Rotterdam, Rotterdam, Zuid-Holland, The Netherlands

Anne Greenough Division of Asthma, Allergy and Lung Biology, MRC Centre for Allergic Mechanisms of Asthma, King's College London, London, UK

NIHR Biomedical Centre at Guy's and St Thomas NHS Foundation Trust and King's College London, London, UK

NICU, King's College Hospital, London, UK

Pierre Gressens UMR1141, Insem-Paris Diderot University, Hôpital Robert Debré, Paris, France

Centre for the Developing Brain, Department of Perinatal Imaging and Health, Division of Imaging Sciences and Biomedical Engineering, King's College London, King's Health Partners, St. Thomas' Hospital, London, UK

Floris Groenendaal Department of Neonatology, Wilhelmina Children's Hospital, University Medical Center Utrecht, Utrecht, The Netherlands

Salvatore Grosso Department of Molecular Medicine and Development, University of Siena, Siena, Italy,

Renzo Guerrini Pediatric Neurology and Neurogenetics Unit and Laboratories, Neuroscience Department, A. Meyer Children's Hospital – University of Florence, Florence, Italy

Isotta Guidotti Neonatal Intensive Care Unit, Department of Medical and Surgical Sciences of the Mother, Children and Adults, University Hospital of Modena, Modena, Italy

Jean-Pierre Guignard Lausanne University Medical School, Lausanne, Switzerland

Andrea Guzzetta IRCCS Stella Maris, Department of Developmental Neuroscience, Pisa, Italy

University of Pisa, Department of Clinical and Experimental Neuroscience, Pisa, Italy

Henrik Hagberg Perinatal Center, Department of Obstetrics and Gynecology, Sahlgrenska Academy, University of Gothenburg, Goteborg, Sweden

Centre for the Developing Brain, Division of Imaging Sciences and Biomedical Engineering, King's College London, King's Health Partners, St. Thomas' Hospital, London, UK

Nigel J. Hall University Surgery Unit, Faculty of Medicine, University of Southampton, Southampton, UK

Henry L. Halliday Formerly Regional Neonatal Unit, Royal Maternity Hospital, Belfast, UK

Formerly Department of Child Health, Queen's University Belfast, Belfast, UK

Mikko Hallman Department of Children and Adolescents, Oulu University Hospital, and PEDEGO Research Unit, Medical Research Center Oulu, University of Oulu, Oulu, Finland

Dominique Haumont Department of Neonatology, Saint – Pierre University Hospital, Brussels, Belgium

Axel Heep Department of Neonatology, Southmead Hospital, North Bristol NHS Trust, Bristol, UK

Lena K. Hellström-Westas Department of Women's and Children's Health, Uppsala University and University Hospital, Uppsala, Sweden

Martin J. Herman Department of Orthopaedic Surgery, Drexel University College of Medicine, St. Christopher's Hospital for Children, Philadelphia, PA, USA

Christian V. Hulzebos Beatrix Children's Hospital, University Medical Center Groningen, Groningen, The Netherlands

Petra S. Hüppi Division of Neonatology, Giannina Gaslini Children's Hospital, Genoa, Italy

Giorgio Iannetti Università degli Studi di Siena, Policlinico S. Maria alle Scotte, Siena, Italy

Sapienza Università di Roma, Policlinico Umberto I di Roma, Rome, Italy

Vincenzo Jasonni Department of Pediatric Surgery, University of Genoa, Genoa, Italy

Giannina Gaslini Institute, Genoa, Italy

Kathryn Johnson Centre for Newborn Care, Leeds Teaching Hospitals Trust, Leeds, UK

Celeste Johnston School of Nursing, McGill University, Montreal, Canada

Michael Kaplan Department of Neonatology, Shaare Zedek Medical Center, Jerusalem, Israel

The Faculty of Medicine, Hebrew University, Jerusalem, Israel,

Nandini Kataria Department of Pediatrics, University of Minnesota, Long Beach, California, USA

Tuula Kaukola Department of Children and Adolescents, Oulu University Hospital, and PEDEGO Research Center, MRC Oulu, University of Oulu, Oulu, Finland

Hirokazu Kimura Infectious Diseases Surveillance Center, National Institute of Infectious Diseases, Tokyo, Japan

John P. Kinsella University of Denver, Denver, CO, USA

Panagiotis Kratimenos Neonatologist, Children's National Medical Center, Center for Research in Neuroscience, George Washington University School of Medicine and Health Sciences, Washington, DC, USA

Edmund F. La Gamma Division of Newborn Medicine, Maria Fareri Children's Hospital, Westchester Medical Center – New York Medical College, Valhalla, NY, USA

Arianna Lamberti Department of Medical, Surgical and Neurological Sciences, Dermatology Section, University of Siena, Siena, Italy

Mariano Lanna Prenatal Diagnosis and Fetal Surgery Unit, Dept. of Woman, Mother and Neonate, Buzzi Children's Hospital Department of Clinical Sciences, University of Milan, Milan, Italy

Malcolm Levene Academic Unit of Paediatrics and Child Health, University of Leeds, Leeds, UK

Department of Neonatal Medicine, Leeds Teaching Hospitals Trust, Leeds, UK

Isabelle Ligi Division of Neonatology, La Conception Hospital, Marseille, France

Otwin Linderkamp Division of Neonatology, Department of Pediatrics, University of Heidelberg, Heidelberg, Germany

Gianluca Lista Neonatology and Neonatal Intensive Care Unit, Ospedale dei Bambini V. Buzzi, Milan, Italy

Mariangela Longini Department of Molecular and Developmental Medicine, University of Siena, Siena, Italy

Alessandra Del Longo Department of Pediatric Ophthalmology, Niguarda Ca' Granda Hospital, Milan, Italy

Vassilios Lougaris Pediatrics Clinic, Department of Clinical and Experimental Sciences, University of Brescia and Spedali Civili of Brescia, Brescia, Italy

Felicia M. Low Liggins Institute, University of Auckland, Auckland, New Zealand

Laura Lucaccioni Neonatal Intensive Care Unit, Department of Medical and Surgical Sciences of the Mother, Children and Adults, University Hospital of Modena, Modena, Italy

Licia Lugli Neonatal Intensive Care Unit, Department of Medical and Surgical Sciences of the Mother, Children and Adults, University Hospital of Modena, Modena, Italy

Giuseppe Maggiore Department of Medical Sciences-Pediatrics, University of Ferrara, University Hospital Arcispedale Sant Anna di Cona, CONA (Ferrara), Italy

Francesca Maglietta Department of Legal Medicine, University of Foggia, Foggia, Italy

Akhil Maheshwari Division of Neonatology, University of South Florida, Tampa, FL, USA

Liam Mahoney Academic Department of Paediatrics, Royal Alexandra Children's Hospital, Brighton, UK

M. Jeffrey Maisels Department of Pediatrics, Oakland University William Beaumont School of Medicine, Beaumont Children's Hospital, Royal Oak, MI, USA

Carina Mallard Department of Physiology, Institute of Neuroscience and Physiology, Sahlgrenska Academy, University of Gothenburg, Gothenburg, Sweden

Leila Mameli Department of Anesthesia, Pediatric and Neonatal Intensive Care, Istituto Giannina Gaslini, Genoa, Italy

Filomena Mandato Department of Medical, Surgical and Neurological Sciences, Dermatology Section, University of Siena, Siena, Italy

Paolo Manzoni Division of Neonatology, Department of Obstetrics and Neonatology, AOU Città della Salute e della Scienza, Turin, Italy

Viviana Marchi IRCCS Stella Maris, Department of Developmental Neuroscience, Pisa, Italy

University of Pisa, Department of Clinical and Experimental Neuroscience, Pisa, Italy

Neil Marlow Institute for Women's Health, University College London, London, UK

Richard J. Martin Rainbow Babies and Children's Hospital, Division of Neonatology, Case Western Reserve University School of Medicine, Cleveland, OH, USA

Maura Massimino Pediatric Oncology Department, Fondazione IRCCS Istituto Nazionale dei Tumori, Milan, Italy

Girolamo Mattioli Department of Pediatric Surgery, University of Genoa, Genoa, Italy

Giannina Gaslini Institute, Genoa, Italy

Liz McKechnie Centre for Newborn Care, Leeds Teaching Hospitals Trust, Leeds, UK

Stefania Mei Department of Medical, Surgical and Neurological Sciences, Dermatology Section, University of Siena, Siena, Italy

Mario Messina Department of Pediatrics, Obstetrics and Reproductive Medicine, Section of Pediatric Surgery, Policlinico "Le Scotte", University of Siena, Siena, Italy

Department of Medical, Surgical and Neurological Sciences, Section of Pediatric Surgery, University of Siena, Siena, Italy

Angelo Micheletti Department of Pediatric Cardiology, IRCCS Policlinico San Donato, San Siro, Milan, Italy

Fiorella Migliaro Division of Neonatology, Department of Translational Medical Sciences, Università "Federico II" di Napoli, Naples, Italy

Federica Mignone Department of Pediatrics, University of Turin, Regina Margherita Childrens Hospital, AOU Città della Salute e della Scienza di Torino, Turin, Italy

Francesco Molinaro Department of Pediatrics, Obstetrics and Reproductive Medicine, Section of Pediatric Surgery, Policlinico "Le Scotte", University of Siena, Siena, Italy

Department of Medical, Surgical and Neurological Sciences, Section of Pediatric Surgery, University of Siena, Siena, Italy

Davide Montin Division of Neonatology, Department of Obstetrics and Neonatology, AOU Città della Salute e della Scienza, Turin, Italy

Department of Pediatrics, University of Turin, Turin, Italy

Alice Monzani Department of Health Sciences, Division of Pediatrics, University of Piemonte Orientale, Novara, Italy

Corrado Moretti Università degli Studi di Roma "La Sapienza", Rome, Italy

Colin Morley Dept Obstetrics and Gynecology, University of Cambridge at Rosie Maternity Hospital, Cambridge, UK

Fabio A. Mosca NICU, Department of Clinical Sciences and Community Health, Fondazione IRCCS Ca' Granda Ospedale Maggiore Policlinico Milano, Università degli Studi di Milano, Milan, Italy

Michele Mussap Laboratory Medicine, Ospedale Policlinico San Martino, Genoa, Italy

Niccolò Nami Department of Medical, Surgical and Neurological Sciences, Dermatology Section, University of Siena, Siena, Italy

Diana Negura Department of Pediatric Cardiology, IRCCS Policlinico San Donato, San Siro, Milan, Italy

Josef Neu Department of Pediatrics, Division of Neonatology, University of Florida, College of Medicine, Gainesville, FL, USA

Giovanni Nigro Maternal-Infant Department, University of L'Aquila, L'Aquila, Italy

Akira Nishida Department of Neonatology, Tokyo Metropolitan Children's Medical Center, Tokyo, Japan

Giovanna Oggè Maternal-Fetal Medicine Unit, University of Turin, Turin, Italy

Robin K. Ohls Department of Pediatrics, Division of Neonatology, University of New Mexico, Albuquerque, NM, USA

Kaoru Okazaki Department of Neonatology, Tokyo Metropolitan Children's Medical Center, Tokyo, Japan

Luca Ori Neonatal Intensive Care Unit, Department of Medical and Surgical Sciences of the Mother, Children and Adults, University Hospital of Modena, Modena, Italy

Luis H. Ospina Departments of Pediatrics, Ophthalmology and Pharmacology, Centre Hospitalier, Universitaire Sainte-Justine, Research Center, Montréal, QC, Canada

Erin A. Osterholm Division of Neonatology, Department of Pediatrics Center for Neurobehavioral Development, University of Minnesota, Minneapolis, MN, USA

Roberto Paludetto Translational Medical Sciences, Università "Federico II" di Napoli, Naples, Italy

Niovi Papalexopoulou Division of Asthma, Allergy and Lung Biology, MRC Centre for Allergic Mechanisms of Asthma, King's College London, London, UK

Paola Papoff Pediatric Intensive Care Unit, Sapienza University of Rome, Rome, Italy

Giancarlo Parenti Department of Translational Medicine, Section of Pediatrics, Federico II University of Naples, Naples, Italy

Stefano Parmigiani Department of Pediatrics and Neonatology, Eastern Liguria Hospital, La Spezia, Italy

Elena Parrini Pediatric Neurology and Neurogenetics Unit and Laboratories, Neuroscience Department, A. Meyer Children's Hospital – University of Florence, Florence, Italy

Gaia Pasquali Department of Obstetrics and Gynecology, University of Rome Tor Vergata, Rome, Italy

Mary Elaine Patrinos Case Western Reserve University School of Medicine, Cleveland, OH, USA

Pierluigi Pedersini National Center for Surgical Treatment of Pediatric Hepatobiliary Malformations, Pediatric Surgery, University of Brescia, Brescia, Italy

Serafina Perrone Department of Molecular and Developmental Medicine, University Hospital of Siena, Siena, Italy

Felice Petraglia Obstetrics and Gynecology, Department of Molecular and Developmental Medicine, University of Siena, Siena, Italy

Luciane Piazza Department of Pediatric Cardiology, IRCCS Policlinico San Donato, San Siro, Milan, Italy

Catherine Pieltain Department of Neonatology, University of Liège, CHR de la Citadelle, Liège, Belgium

Agostino Pierro Division of General and Thoracic Surgery, The Hospital for Sick Children, Toronto, Canada

Alessio Pini Prato Giannina Gaslini Institute, Genoa, Italy

Elena Piozzi Department of Pediatric Ophthalmology, Niguarda Ca' Granda Hospital, Milan, Italy

Peter D. Pizzutillo Section of Orthopaedic Surgery, St. Christopher's Hospital for Children, Philadelphia, PA, USA

Tenet Healthcare, Dallas, TX, USA

Alessandro Plebani Pediatrics Clinic, Department of Clinical and Experimental Sciences, University of Brescia and Spedali Civili of Brescia, Brescia, Italy

Francesca R. Pluchinotta Department of Pediatric Cardiology, IRCCS Policlinico San Donato, San Siro, Milan, Italy

Christian F. Poets Department of Neonatology, Tübingen University Hospital, Tübingen, Germany

Simone Pratesi Neonatal Intensive Care Unit, Careggi University Hospital, Florence, Italy

Flavia Prodam Department of Health Sciences, Division of Pediatrics, University of Piemonte Orientale, Novara, Italy

Fabrizio Proietti Department of Molecular and Developmental Medicine, University of Siena, Siena, Italy

Marisa Pugliese Neonatal Intensive Care Unit, Department of Medical and Surgical Sciences of the Mother, Children and Adults, University of Modena and Reggio Emilia, Modena, Italy

Guy Putet Department of Neonatology, Hopital de la Croix-Rousse, Hospices Civils de Lyon and Universite Claude Bernard, Lyon, France

Heike Rabe Academic Department of Paediatrics, Royal Alexandra Children's Hospital, Brighton, UK

Francesco Raimondi Division of Neonatology, Department of Translational Medical Sciences, Università "Federico II" di Napoli, Naples, Italy

Luca A. Ramenghi Division of Neonatology, Giannina Gaslini Children's Hospital, Genoa, Italy

Tara M. Randis Department of Pediatrics, New York University School of Medicine, New York, NY, USA

Roberta Ricotti Department of Health Sciences, Division of Pediatrics, University of Piemonte Orientale, Novara, Italy

Henrique Rigatto Department of Pediatrics, WR004 Women's Hospital, University of Manitoba, Winnipeg, MB, Canada

Jacques Rigo Department of Neonatology, University of Liège, CHR de la Citadelle, Liège, Belgium

Arieh Riskin Department of Neonatology, Bnai Zion Medical Center, Rappaport Faculty of Medicine, Technion, Israel Institute of Technology, Haifa, Israel

Francesco Risso Neonatal Intensive Care Unit, Department of Emergency Medicine, G. Gaslini Children's Hospital, Genoa, Italy

Silvia Riva Pediatric Hepatology and Liver Transplant Unit, IRCCS-ISMETT - University of Pittsburgh Medical Center (UPMC), Palermo, Italy

José Carlos Rivera Departments of Pediatrics, Ophthalmology and Pharmacology, Centre Hospitalier, Universitaire Sainte-Justine, Research Center, Montréal, QC, Canada

Department of Ophthalmology, Maisonneuve-Rosemont Hospital Research Center, Montréal, QC, Canada

Rodney P. A. Rivers Section of Paediatrics, Department of Medicine, Imperial College, London, UK

Hector Rojas-Anaya Academic Department of Paediatrics, Royal Alexandra Children's Hospital, Brighton, UK

Maria Angela Rustico Prenatal Diagnosis and Fetal Surgery Unit, Dept. of Woman, Mother and Neonate, Buzzi Children's Hospital Department of Clinical Sciences, University of Milan, Milan, Italy

Karin Sävman Department of Pediatrics, Sahlgrenska Academy, University of Gothenburg, Gothenburg, Sweden

Timo Saarela Department of Children and Adolescents, Oulu University Hospital, Oulu, Finland

Elie Saliba Department of Neonatology and Pediatric Intensive Care, Université François Rabelais and CHRU de Tours, Tours, France

Inserm U930, France, Université François Rabelais and CHRU de Tours, Tours, France

Janko Samardzic Department of Paediatric Pharmacology, University Children's Hospital Basel, Basel, Switzerland

Institute of Pharmacology, Clinical Pharmacology and Toxicology, Medical Faculty, University of Belgrade, Belgrade, Serbia

Fabrizio Sandri Neonatology and Neonatal Intensive Care Unit, Ospedale Maggiore, Bologna, Italy

Andrea Sannia Neonatal Intensive Care Unit, Department of Emergency Medicine, G. Gaslini Children's Hospital, Genoa, Italy

Javier Fernandez Sarabia Department of Pediatric Cardiology, IRCCS Policlinico San Donato, San Siro, Milan, Italy

Paola Saracco Pediatric Hematology, Department of Pediatrics, University Hospital Città della Salute e della Scienza, Torino, Italy

Antonio Saracino Department of Pediatric Cardiology, IRCCS Policlinico San Donato, San Siro, Milan, Italy

Ola D. Saugstad Department of Pediatric Research, Rikshospitalet, Oslo University Hospital, University of Oslo, Oslo, Norway

Rosa T. Scaramuzzo Neonatology and Neonatal Intensive Care Unit, Santa Chiara University Hospital, Pisa, Italy

Kurt R. Schibler Perinatal Institute, Cincinnati Children's Hospital Medical Center, Cincinnati, OH, USA

Marco Sciveres Pediatric Hepatology and Liver Transplant Unit, IRCCS-ISMETT - University of Pittsburgh Medical Center (UPMC), Palermo, Italy

Carlo Scolfaro Department of Pediatrics, University of Turin, Regina Margherita Childrens Hospital, AOU Città della Salute e della Scienza di Torino, Turin, Italy

Gunnar Sedin Department of Women's and Children's Health, University Children's Hospital, Uppsala, Sweden

Thibault Senterre Department of Neonatology, University of Liège, CHR de la Citadelle, Liège, Belgium

Filiberto Maria Severi Obstetrics and Gynecology, Department of Molecular and Developmental Medicine, University of Siena, Siena, Italy

Raanan Shamir Institute of Gastroenterology Nutrition and Liver Diseases, Schneider Children's Medical Center, Sackler Faculty of Medicine, Tel-Aviv University, Petach-Tikva, Israel

Davide Silvagni Azienda Ospedaliera Universitaria Integrata Verona, Verona, Italy

Umberto Simeoni Division of Pediatrics, CHUV and UNIL, Lausanne, Vaud, Switzerland

Adam P. R. Smith Division of Asthma, Allergy and Lung Biology, MRC Centre for Allergic Mechanisms of Asthma, King's College London, London, UK

Augusto Sola Ibero American Society of Neonatology (SIBEN), Wellington, FL, USA

Michael Spear Department of Pediatrics, Drexel University College of Medicine, St. Christopher's Hospital for Children, Philadelphia, PA, USA

Christian P. Speer University Children's Hospital, University of Würzburg, Würzburg, Germany

David K. Stevenson Department of Pediatrics, Stanford University School of Medicine, Medical School Office Building, Stanford, CA, USA

Rosa Maria Strangi Department of Medical, Surgical and Neurological Sciences, Dermatology Section, University of Siena, Siena, Italy

Mauro Stronati Neonatal Intensive Care Unit, Fondazione IRCCS Policlinico 'San Matteo', Pavia, Italy

Veena Supramaniam Perinatal Imaging Group, Robert Steiner MR Unit, MRC Clinical Sciences Centre and Wigglesworth Perinatal Pathology Services, Hammersmith Hospital, Imperial College, London, UK

Paolo Tagliabue Neonatologia e Terapia Intensiva Neonatale, Fondazione MBBM, ASST-Ospedale San Gerardo-Monza, Monza, Italy

Sophie Tardieu Medical Evaluation Department, Public Health Department, La Conception Hospital, Marseille, France

Elena Tavella Division of Neonatology, Department of Obstetrics and Neonatology, AOU Città della Salute e della Scienza, Turin, Italy

Claire Thornton Centre for the Developing Brain, Department of Perinatal Imaging and Health, Division of Imaging Sciences and Biomedical Engineering, King's College London, King's Health Partners, St. Thomas' Hospital, London, UK

Claudio Tiribelli Liver Research Centre, University of Trieste, Trieste, Italy

Tullia Todros Maternal-Fetal Medicine Unit, University of Turin, Turin, Italy

Michela Torricelli Obstetrics and Gynecology, Department of Molecular and Developmental Medicine, University of Siena, Siena, Italy

Pier Angelo Tovo Department of Pediatrics, University of Turin, Regina Margherita Childrens Hospital, AOU Città della Salute e della Scienza di Torino, Turin, Italy

Alberto E. Tozzi Multifactorial and Complex Diseases Research Area, Bambino Gesù Children's Hospital, Rome, Italy

Laura Travan Division of Neonatology, Institute for Maternal and Child Health IRCCS 'Burlo Garofolo', Trieste, Italy

Daniele Trevisanuto Department of Women's and Children's Health, Azienda Ospedaliere di Padova, University of Padua, Padua, Italy

Pietro Tuo Department of Anesthesia, Pediatric and Neonatal Intensive Care, Istituto Giannina Gaslini, Genoa, Italy

Emanuela Turillazzi Department of Legal Medicine, University of Foggia, Foggia, Italy

Alberto G. Ugazio Institute of Child and Adolescent Health, Bambino Gesù Children's Hospital, Rome, Italy

Frank van Bel Department of Neonatology, Wilhelmina Children's Hospital, University Medical Center Utrecht, Utrecht, The Netherlands

John N. van den Anker Division of Pediatric Clinical Pharmacology, Children's National Health System, Washington, DC, USA

Departments of Pediatrics, Integrative Systems Biology, Pharmacology and Physiology, George Washington University, School of Medicine and Health Sciences, Washington, DC, USA

Intensive Care and Department of Pediatric Surgery, Erasmus MC – Sophia Children's Hospital, Rotterdam, The Netherlands

Johannes B. (Hans) van Goudoever Department of Pediatrics, Emma Children's Hospital – AMC and VU University Medical Center, Amsterdam, The Netherlands

Tim van Mieghem Department of Development and Regeneration, KU Leuven, Leuven, Belgium

Obstetrics and Gynecology, University Hospitals Leuven, Leuven, Belgium

Bart Van Overmeire Neonatology Service, Erasmus Hospital Université Libre de Bruxelles, Brussels, Belgium

Silvia Vannuccini Obstetrics and Gynecology, Department of Molecular and Developmental Medicine, University of Siena, Siena, Italy

Maximo Vento Neonatal Research Unit, Health Research Institute Hospital La Fe, University and Polytechnic Hospital La Fe, Valencia, Spain

Gennaro Vetrano U.O.C. Pediatria/Neonatologia/UTIN, Osp. "Sacro Cuore di Gesù", Benevento, Italy

Renaud Viellevoye Department of Neonatology, University of Liège, CHR de la Citadelle, Liège, Belgium

Betty R. Vohr Department of Pediatrics, The Warren Alpert Medical School of Brown University, Providence, RI, USA

Women and Infants Hospital, Providence, RI, USA

Jon F. Watchko Division of Newborn Medicine, Department of Pediatrics, University of Pittsburgh School of Medicine, Pittsburgh, PA, USA

Ronald J. Wong Department of Pediatrics, Stanford University School of Medicine, Stanford, CA, USA

Marco Zaffanello Department of Surgical Sciences, Dentistry, Gynecology and Pediatrics, University of Verona, Verona, Italy

Department of Life and Reproduction Sciences Pediatric Section, University of Verona, Verona, Italy

Department of Surgery, University of Cagliari, Cagliari, Italy

Clelia Zanaboni Department of Anesthesia, Pediatric and Neonatal Intensive Care, Istituto Giannina Gaslini, Genoa, Italy

Giacomo Zanelli Department of Medical Biotechnologies, University of Siena, Siena, Italy

Rinaldo Zanini NICU, Ospedale Manzoni, Lecco, Italy

Tianwei Ellen Zhou Departments of Pediatrics, Ophthalmology and Pharmacology, Centre Hospitalier, Universitaire Sainte-Justine, Research Center, Montréal, QC, Canada

Ekhard E. Ziegler Department of Pediatrics, University of Iowa, Iowa City, IA, USA

Luc J. I. Zimmermann Department of Pediatrics and Neonatology, School for Oncology and Developmental Biology (GROW), Maastricht University Medical Center, Maastricht, The Netherlands

Part I

Epidemiology and Fetal Neonatal Medicine

Development and General Characteristics of Preterm and Term Newborn

1

Domenico Arduini, Gaia Pasquali, Stefano Parmigiani, Daniela Gianotti, and Giulio Bevilacqua

Contents

Abstract

The embryonic phase is a critical stage of development. Fetal growth is mostly influenced by maternal, uteroplacental factors, as well as genetic and environmental factors. During pregnancy, noninvasive screening tests are used to evaluate a baby's health. Severe acute or chronic intrauterine hypoxic stress in utero are responsible for compromised circulation, organ dysfunction, and threaten survival or intact survival. The objective of modern obstetrics is the accurate detection of suboptimal fetal growth. Currently, sonography plays a critical role in providing a reliable estimate of fetal biometry, thus confirming the clinical suspicion of growth restriction and substantially influencing pregnancy management. Preterm birth, defined as birth at less than 37 weeks of gestation, is the main determinant of adverse infant outcome in terms of both survival and quality of life: the more preterm these infants are, the more serious are the complications. Because of advances in the care of these very vulnerable infants, survival at the earliest gestation is continuosly improving.

D. Arduini (✉) · G. Pasquali
Department of Obstetrics and Gynecology, University of Rome Tor Vergata, Rome, Italy
e-mail: nico.arduini@gmail.com; gaia.pasquali@gmail.com

S. Parmigiani · D. Gianotti · G. Bevilacqua
Department of Pediatrics and Neonatology, Eastern Liguria Hospital, La Spezia, Italy
e-mail: steparmi@inwind.it; drdanig@gmail.com; giulbevi@gmail.com

G. Buonocore et al. (eds.), *Neonatology*,
https://doi.org/10.1007/978-3-319-29489-6_150

1.1 Salient Points

- Fetal hemoglobin has a higher affinity for oxygen than adult hemoglobin, which facilitates diffusion of oxygen from the maternal circulation to the fetus.
- A continuous placental supply of glucose provides the substrate for energy metabolism to the fetus, and this converts after birth to intermittent feeding.
- Individual characteristics based on the race, obstetric history, and the constitution of the parents, especially of the mother, should be taken into account to improve diagnostic accuracy and the construction of customized fetal growth charts and for the antenatal detection of the true small fetus, whose risk of adverse perinatal outcomes is substantially increased.
- Hypoxemia produces various circulatory adaptations in the fetus that enhance fetal survival, including the development of tachycardia, hypertension, redistribution of blood flow toward the brain, myocardium and adrenals, and depression of fetal breathing and skeletal muscle activity.
- The goal in the management of the preterm fetus is to deliver the most mature fetus possible, at least at 32–34 weeks, in the best possible condition by improving fetal and maternal monitoring.
- The history of family, pregnancy, and delivery together with the first examination at birth has a pivotal role on assessing neonatal well-being.
- A baby's well-being is determined by periconceptional events.
- Signs of immaturity should be recognized and a favorable environment should be created.

1.2 Part 1 The Development from Fetus to Newborn

1.2.1 Developmental Phases of the Fetus

The embryonic phase is a critical stage of development, when systems undergo important basic development.

The third week after conception marks the beginning of the embryonic period. It ends at the end of the tenth week, when the embryo comprises three layers from which all organs will develop.

The second fetal phase begins after the tenth week and continues until the end of pregnancy. During this phase, organs (liver, kidneys) begin to function.

From the 16th to 20th weeks, the fetus undergoes a rapid growth spurt. Fat develops under a thin skin. Cardiac output increases. Meconium accumulates in the bowel. The fetus hiccups and spends time awake and asleep.

Fetal development slows down between the 21st and 24th weeks. By the 24th week, the fetus weighs approximately 1.3 pounds (600 g).

Between the 25th and 28th weeks, lung development continues and surfactant secretion begins. By the 28th week, 90% of fetuses will survive *ex utero* with appropriate support.

From the 29th to the 40th weeks, the amount of body fat rapidly increases. Thalamic brain connections, which mediate sensory input, form. Bones are fully developed. Most of the major systems and organs are complete. The immune system develops.

By weeks 35–40, the fetus is sufficiently developed for life outside the uterus without any more support than that which would be required by any newborn baby delivered at term. At 37 weeks, the fetus will continue to add approximately one ounce (28 g) per day to its body weight and it will be 48–53 cm (19–21 inches) in length at birth.

1.2.2 Fetal Constitutional Characteristics

1.2.2.1 The Central Nervous System (CNS)

The CNS is formed by four subdivisions of the neural tube that develop into distinct regions of the central nervous system.

The neural tube is initially open both cranially and caudally. These openings close during the fourth week. Failure of closure of these neuropores can result in neural tube defects such as anencephaly or spina bifida.

The dorsal part of the neural tube comprises the alar plate, which is primarily associated with sensation. The ventral part of the neural tube comprises the basal plate, which is primarily associated with motor control.

The spinal cord is a long, thin, tubular bundle of nervous tissue and supports cells that extend from the brain. The brain and spinal cord together make up the central nervous system. The spinal cord functions primarily for the transmission of neural signals between the brain and the rest of the body but also contains neural circuits that independently control numerous reflexes and central pattern generators.

1.2.2.2 The Fetal Circulation

The essential difference between the circulatory system of a fetus and that of the baby after birth is that the lungs are not in use: the fetus obtains oxygen and nutrients from the mother through the placenta and the umbilical cord. Blood from the placenta is carried to the fetus by the umbilical vein. A large proportion enters the fetal ductus venosus and passes to the inferior vena cava, while the remainder enters the liver from vessels on its inferior border. The branch of the umbilical vein that supplies the right lobe of the liver joins the portal vein and blood then passes to the right atrium. In the fetus, there is an opening between the right and left atria (the foramen ovale), and most of the blood flows from the right into the left atrium, thus bypassing pulmonary circulation. The majority of blood flow is then into the left ventricle from where it is pumped through the aorta to supply the various organs. Blood then flows from the aorta through the internal iliac arteries to the umbilical arteries and reenters the placenta, where carbon dioxide and other waste products from the fetus are taken up and enter the maternal circulation. A small proportion (about 4%) of the blood from the right atrium does not enter the left atrium but enters the right ventricle and is pumped into the pulmonary artery. In the fetus, a connection between the pulmonary artery and the aorta, called the ductus arteriosus, directs most of the blood away from the lungs (which are not being used for respiration at this point, as the fetus is suspended in amniotic fluid).

An important concept of the fetal circulation is that fetal hemoglobin has a higher affinity for oxygen than adult hemoglobin, which facilitates diffusion of oxygen from the maternal circulation to the fetus. The circulatory system of the mother is not directly connected to that of the fetus, so gas exchange takes place at the placenta. Oxygen diffuses from the placenta to the chorionic villus, an alveolus-like structure, from which it is then carried to the umbilical vein. Fetal hemoglobin enhances the fetal ability to draw oxygen from the placenta because the oxygen dissociation curve is shifted to the left, which has the effect of oxygen being taken up at a lower concentration than by adult hemoglobin. This enables fetal hemoglobin to take up oxygen from adult hemoglobin in the placenta, which has a lower partial pressure of oxygen than at the lungs after birth.

A developing fetus is highly susceptible to anomalies of growth and metabolism, increasing the risk of birth defects.

1.2.2.3 Fetal Metabolism

A continuous placental supply of glucose provides the substrate for energy metabolism to the fetus, and this converts after birth to intermittent feeding. While the fetus is dependent on maternal glucose as the main source of energy, it can also use lactate, free-fatty acids, and ketone bodies under some conditions (e.g., starvation or hypoxia). Fetal glucose utilization is augmented by insulin produced by the developing fetal pancreas in increasing amounts as gestation proceeds; this enhances glucose utilization in insulin-sensitive tissues (skeletal muscle, liver, heart, adipose tissue), which increase in mass and thus glucose requirement during late gestation. Glucose-stimulated insulin secretion increases with gestation. Glycogen stores are maximal at term, but even the term fetus only has sufficient glycogen available to meet energy needs for 8–10 h, and this store can be depleted even more quickly if demand is high. At 27 weeks' gestation, only 1% of a fetus's body weight is fat; this increases to 16% at 40 weeks. Inadequate glucose substrate can lead to hypoglycemia and fetal growth restriction. In cases of intrauterine growth restriction, fetal weight-specific tissue-glucose uptake rates and glucose transporters are maintained or increased, while synthesis of amino acids into protein and corresponding insulin-like growth factor (IGF) signal transduction proteins are decreased. These observations demonstrate the mixed phenotype of the intrauterine growth restriction (IUGR) fetus that has an enhanced capacity for glucose utilization, but a diminished capacity for protein synthesis and growth. Excess substrate can also lead to problems, as with infants of diabetic mothers (IDM). Thus, the normal fetus has a considerable capacity to adapt to changes in glucose supply (Way 2006).

1.2.2.4 Regulation of Fetal Growth

Fetal growth depends on many different aspects, mostly influenced by maternal and uteroplacental factors.

Role of the Mother in Fetal Growth Regulation

Fetal growth and development are influenced by genetic as well as environmental factors. Maternal genes have an important specific influence on fetal growth; for example, maternal height is a major determinant of fetal size, representing uterine capacity and the potential for growth.

In fact, the individual characteristic based on the race, obstetric history, and constitutional characteristics of the parents, especially of the mother, could be taken into account to improve diagnostic accuracy construction of customized fetal growth and for antenatal detection of the true small fetuses, whose risk of adverse perinatal outcomes is substantially increased (Ghi et al. 2016).

Although the birth weights of siblings are similar and correlate, environmental influences are also important in determining growth. Maternal constraint refers to the limited capacity of the uterus to support fetal growth and is important in limiting fetal overgrowth and subsequent dystocia, to ensure the mother's capacity for future successful pregnancies (Picciano 2003).

Maternal Nutrient Intake

The mother is the supplier of oxygen and essential nutrients to the fetus via the placenta. Maternal diet, caloric intake, and metabolic function have an important role in supplying nutrients to the fetus. Increased caloric intake is necessary during the second and third trimesters to allow for fetal and placental growth (Christian et al. 2003). A Cochrane systematic review of six randomized controlled trials found that balanced protein-energy supplementation reduced the risk of small for gestational age (SGA) neonates by approximately 30% (Kramer and Kakuma 2003). Glucose is an important nutrient in the control of fetal growth. Studies of diabetic women have shown that low blood glucose levels during pregnancy as a result of excessively tight glycemic control lead to a greater incidence of SGA neonates, whereas high blood glucose levels increase the likelihood of macrosomia (Leguizamon and von Stecher 2003).

Maternal Uterine Artery Blood Flow

Increased uterine blood flow is essential to meet the metabolic demands of the growing uterus as well those of the placenta and fetus (Kliman 2000). Uterine artery blood flow increases by more than threefold during pregnancy, partly influenced by an increased artery diameter and reduced resistance to flow. In addition to increased uterine blood flow during normal pregnancy, new blood vessels develop in the uterus, promoted by the placental hormones human chorionic gonadotropin (hCG) (Zygmunt et al. 2002) and IGF-II (Zygmunt et al. 2003). Using Doppler assessment of uterine arterial flow at 23 weeks' gestation, Albaiges et al. (2000) found that increased uterine artery blood flow resistance was associated with an increased risk of an SGA baby. In the clinical practice, women with an abnormal uterine artery Doppler at 20–24 weeks (defined as a pulsatility index >95th centile) and women who have one major risk factor for SGA (maternal age > 40 years; chronic hypertension; diabetes with vascular disease; renal impairment; antiphospholipid syndrome; smoker >11cigarettes per day; cocaine; maternal or paternal SGA; previous SGA baby; previous still-birth; intensive exercise; previous pre-eclampsia; pregnancy interval <6 months; pregnancy interval >60 months; heavy bleeding similar to menses; PAPP-A < 0,4 MoM on first trimester screening) should be referred for serial ultrasound measurement of fetal size and assessment of well-being with umbilical artery Doppler commencing at 26–28 weeks of pregnancy (RCOG 2014).

Maternal Smoking and Drug Use

Maternal cigarette smoking is associated with reduced birth weight. Early reports suggested a doubling of the rate of low birth weight in babies of smokers compared with those of nonsmokers and a dose-dependent effect with increasing number of cigarettes smoked. More recent studies demonstrated a 3.5-fold increased risk of SGA infants in women who smoked during pregnancy (Bamberg and Kalache 2004; Rich-Edwards et al. 2003), with a greater effect on low birth weight with increasing maternal age (Krampl et al. 2000). Growth restriction is usually symmetrical with reduced weight, head circumference, and abdominal circumference. The use of drugs, such as cocaine and marijuana, also has significant negative effects on fetal growth. Cocaine use contributes to an increased rate of low birth weight and a reduction in mean birth weight of at least 100 g.

Maternal Hypoxia

Maternal hypoxia influences fetal growth. Its effect is independent of socioeconomic status, prematurity, maternal smoking, pregnancy-induced hypertension, and parity. The combination of hypoxia and pregnancy appears to be important in altering maternal physiology, including changes in immune pathways (Clapp 2003). Maternal hypoxia affects placental and uterine blood flow, which contribute to reduced nutrient transport to the fetus (Skomsvoll et al. 2002).

Maternal Inflammatory Diseases

The presence of maternal inflammatory disease may contribute to reduced fetal growth. Several inflammatory diseases are associated with reduced fetal growth, including rheumatoid arthritis (McGaw 2002), inflammatory bowel disease, systemic lupus erythematosus, and periodontal disease (Bowden et al. 2001). Women with active inflammatory arthritis during pregnancy have smaller babies compared with healthy women or women whose disease is in remission (Xiao et al. 2003), suggesting that active inflammation during pregnancy may contribute to reduced fetal growth. Maternal health influences the maternal state during pregnancy with implications for fetal growth. In addition to inflammatory diseases, many other maternal factors, including preeclampsia (Allen 2001), anemia (Fowden and Forhead 2004), infections, and alcohol consumption, influence fetal growth via changes in placental function.

Role of the Placenta in Fetal Growth Regulation

The placenta receives and transmits endocrine signals between the mother and fetus and is the site of nutrient and waste exchange.

During human pregnancy, the placenta is an important endocrine organ. It produces hormones, including estrogens and progesterone, hCG, human growth hormone (GH) variant, and human placental lactogen. Some of these play a role in the regulation of fetal growth. Fetal insulin promotes growth of the fetus, acting as a signal of nutrient availability (Ferrazzi et al. 2000). Insulin deficiency results in reduced fetal growth, as the fetal tissues decrease their uptake and utilization of nutrients. There is also a relationship between increased insulin production and increased fetal growth. It has been proposed that the fetus increases its own production of insulin in response to maternal hyperglycemia and that this increase in fetal insulin is responsible for the increased growth and macrosomia observed in diabetic pregnancies.

Adequate placental growth is essential for adequate fetal growth. Several aspects of placental function are critical for human fetal growth and development, including adequate trophoblast invasion, an increase in uteroplacental blood flow during gestation, transport of nutrients such as glucose and amino acids from mother to fetus, and the production and transfer of growth-regulating hormones. Increased blood flow during pregnancy increases the flow of nutrients from mother to fetus, and uteroplacental blood flow has been shown to be reduced by up to 50% in women with preeclampsia (ACOG 2012). Doppler velocimetry is used to detect increased vascular resistance in the uterine arteries, which occurs as a result of abnormal trophoblast invasion of the spiral arteries. In addition, examination of the fetal circulation, particularly umbilical artery waveforms, may reflect placental insufficiency (ACOG 2012). Umbilical vein blood flow, measured by Doppler ultrasound, is decreased in IUGR fetuses, representing reduced perfusion of the fetal tissues.

1.2.3 Diagnosis of Fetal Well-being

During pregnancy, women are generally offered noninvasive screening tests, such as blood tests, ultrasound, and cardiotocography (CTG) to evaluate the baby's health. Alternatively, more invasive tests, such as chorionic villous sampling (CVS) or amniocentesis, may be performed.

1.2.3.1 Ultrasound

Obstetric ultrasound is usually used to:

- Diagnose pregnancy
- Assess possible risks to the mother (miscarriage or molar pregnancy)
- Check for fetal malformation
- Determine intrauterine growth restriction
- Note the development of fetal body parts
- Check the amniotic fluid and the umbilical cord

Generally an ultrasound examination is ordered whenever an abnormality is suspected or following a schedule similar to that outlined below:

7 weeks: Confirm pregnancy
11–13 weeks: Determine expected date of delivery and screening for aneuploidy
20–22 weeks: Perform a scan to assess anatomic integrity
32 weeks: Evaluate fetal growth, verify the position of the placenta, and perform the Doppler study to establish fetal well-being

Three-dimensional (3-D) and four-dimensional (4-D) ultrasound techniques are used to provide additional imaging of fetal structures. Today 3-D ultrasound is most commonly performed for the visualization of the baby's face (Fig. 1). However, it has the potential to become part of routine care and many hospitals use the 3-D ultrasound to detect fetal anomalies, especially of the heart and of the CNS (Figs. 2 and 3).

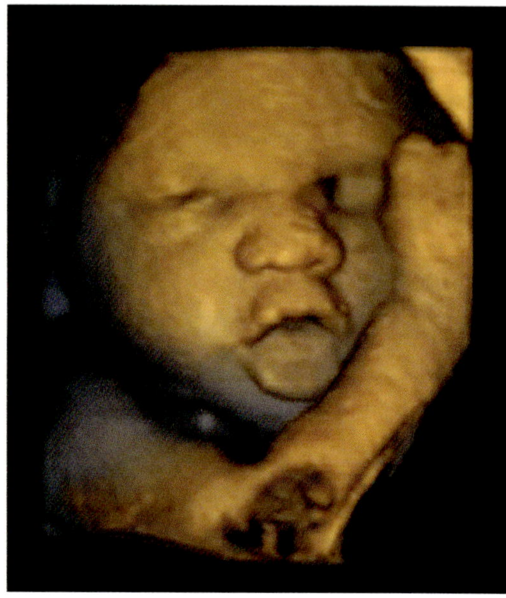

Fig. 1 Reconstructed 3-D imaging of fetal face (Image courtesy of G. Rizzo)

1.2.3.2 Screening Tests for Aneuploidy

Women should be offered prenatal assessment for aneuploidy by screening or diagnostic testing regardless of maternal age or other risk factors (Practice Bulletin No. 162 2016).

Prenatal genetic diagnostic testing is intended to determine, with as much certainty as possible, whether a specific genetic disorder or condition is present in the fetus. In contrast, prenatal genetic screening is designed to assess whether a patient is at increased risk of having a fetus affected by a genetic disorder (Spencer et al. 1999).

Two methods are currently available in the screening for aneuploidy:

1. At 11–13 weeks' gestation, combination of maternal age, fetal nuchal translucency

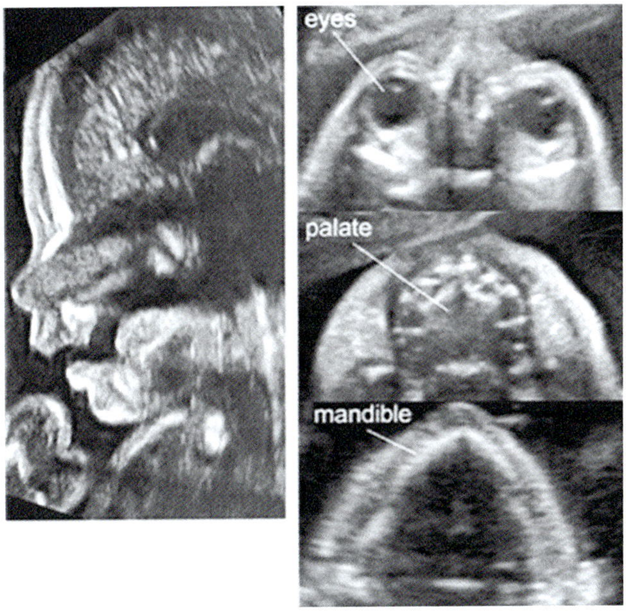

Fig. 2 Reconstructed 3 D imaging of the eyes, palate, and mandible from the fetal profile

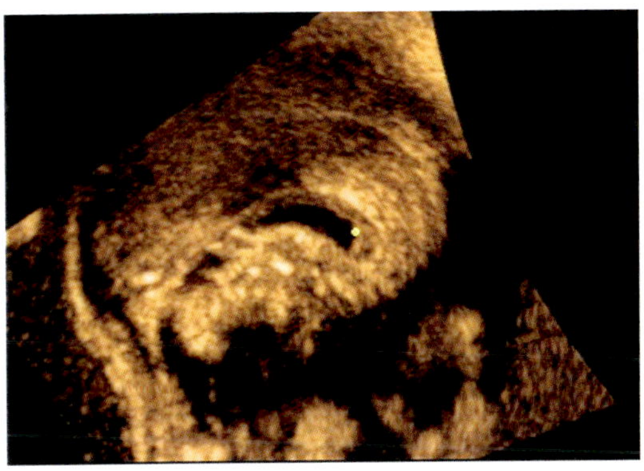

Fig. 3 Reconstructed 3-D imaging of the corpus callosum (Image courtesy of G. Rizzo)

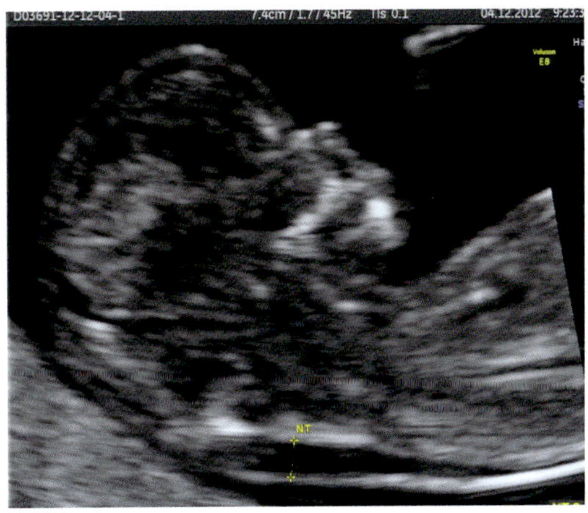

Fig. 4 Fetal profile at 12 weeks of gestation showing nuchal translucency (Image courtesy of G. Rizzo)

thickness measured by ultrasound (Fig. 4) and maternal serum concentration of free β-human chorionic gonadotropin and pregnancy-associated plasma protein-A could assess the risk for trisomy 21, trisomy 18, and trisomy 13 (Nicolaides 2004; Palomaki et al. 2011).

The incidence of fetal trisomies is directly related to maternal age. The risk of having a child with Down syndrome increases in a gradual, linear trend until about age 30 and increases exponentially thereafter.

Nuchal translucency (NT) is the sonographic appearance of a collection of fluid under the skin behind the fetal neck in the first-trimester of pregnancy. NT normally increases with gestation. Increased NT thickness over the normal range for gestational age is related to chromosomal defects, especially trisomy 21, but is also associated with major abnormalities of the heart and great arteries and a wide range of genetic syndromes.

The level of free b-hCG in maternal blood normally decreases with gestation. In trisomy 21 pregnancies, free b-hCG is increased. The level of PAPP-A in maternal blood normally increases with gestation, and in trisomy 21 pregnancies the level is decreased.

Some studies demonstrated that the detection rate of this test can increase to about 95% by also examining the nasal bone (absent or hypoplastic in a high proportion of fetuses with trisomy 21 and other chromosomal abnormalities), ductus venosus flow (a-wave absent or reversed in fetal aneuploidies or in fetal cardiac defects), and tricuspid flow (tricuspid regurgitation is a common finding in fetuses with trisomy 21, 18, and 13 and in those with major cardiac defects).

2. From the 10th week of gestation, analysis of cell-free DNA in maternal blood. Circulating cell-free DNA in the plasma of pregnant women is a mixture of genomic DNA fragments of maternal and fetal (placental) origin that could be extracted and analyzed (Sparks et al. 2012; Zimmermann et al. 2012; Canick et al. 2013; Botto et al. 1996). Screening for fetal aneuploidy in pregnant women using cell-free DNA has demonstrated high sensitivity and specificity to screen for common aneuploidies in high-risk populations. Recently, this method started to include microdeletion screening and whole genome screening.

1.2.3.3 Invasive Tests

After an abnormal first-trimester ultrasound examination or screening test, it is necessary to confirm the diagnosis with an invasive procedure, chorionic villous sampling, or amniocentesis. The earlier CVS results allow for more management options, although amniocentesis also is an option for diagnosis (Spencer et al. 1999).

Chorionic Villous Sampling

Chorionic villus sampling for prenatal genetic diagnosis generally is performed between 10 and 13 weeks of gestation. In fact, before 10 weeks there is a risk of limb-reduction defects (Akolekar et al. 2015).

The primary advantage of CVS over amniocentesis is that the procedure can be performed earlier in pregnancy and the viable cells obtained by CVS for analysis allow for shorter specimen processing time (5–7 days versus 7–14 days), so the results are available earlier in pregnancy.

The most recent meta-analysis of studies calculated a procedure-related loss rate of 0.22% (Alfirevic et al. 2003).

The incidence of culture failure, amniotic fluid leakage, or infection after CVS is less than 0.5% (Winsor et al. 1999).

Amniocentesis

Amniocentesis for the purpose of genetic diagnosis usually is performed between 15 weeks and 20 weeks of gestation, but it can be performed at any later gestational age. An amniotic fluid sample of 20–30 ml is obtained from a pocket free of fetal parts and umbilical cord.

The most recent meta-analysis of studies calculated a procedure-related loss rate of 0.11% (Alfirevic et al. 2003).

The incidence of culture failure is approximately 0.1% of samples (Winsor et al. 1999).

1.2.3.4 Cardiotocography

Cardiotocography is a technique of surveillance of fetal well-being useful first of all during labor to identify the fetus compromise. When the risk of antepartum fetal demise is increased (e.g., pregestational and gestational diabetes mellitus; hypertension; gestational hypertension; preeclampsia; systemic lupus erythematosus; chronic renal disease; antiphospholipid syndrome; hyperthyroidism; hemoglobinopathies; heart disease; decreased fetal movement; oligohydramnios; fetal growth restriction; late-term or postterm pregnancy; isoimmunization; previous fetal demise; monochorionic multiple gestation), it may be necessary to monitor fetal activity during pregnancy with a nonstress test (NST) to identify some degree of uteroplacental compromise (Liston et al. 2007). The NST is based on the premise that the heart rate of a fetus that is not acidotic or neurologically depressed will temporarily accelerate with fetal movement. Heart rate reactivity is thought to be a good indicator of normal fetal autonomic function. Loss of reactivity may result from any cause of central nervous system depression, including fetal acidemia. Attention is required for the preterm fetuses; in fact, the NST of the normal preterm fetus is frequently nonreactive: from 24 weeks to 28 weeks of gestation, up to 50% of NSTs may not be reactive (Bishop 1981), and from 28 weeks to 32 weeks of gestation, 15% of NSTs are not reactive (Macones et al. 2008). For this reason, starting fetal monitoring after 32 weeks of gestation is appropriate for most at-risk patients. However, in pregnancies with very high-risk conditions, testing might begin at a gestational age when delivery would be considered for perinatal benefit (ACOG 2014).

1.2.4 Fetal Injuries

It is important during fetal development to maintain good fetal oxygen delivery to avoid irreversible fetal compromise. Fetal hypoxia from any cause leads to conversion from aerobic to anaerobic metabolism, which produces less energy and more acid. If the oxygen supply is not restored, the fetus dies. Hypoxia may be classified as follows:

- *Hypoxemic hypoxia*: reduced placental perfusion with maternal blood and consequent decrease in fetal arterial blood oxygen content due to low pO_2
- *Anemic hypoxia*: reduced arterial blood oxygen content due to low fetal hemoglobin concentration
- *Ischemic hypoxia*: reduced blood flow to the fetal tissues

Making this diagnose can be difficult, and some episodes of hypoxia before and during birth may pass unnoticed at the time but may affect the central nervous system and not become evident until much later in life.

1.2.4.1 Causes of Hypoxia

Two major categories of neurological injury can be observed in the full-term infant: (1) hypoxic-ischemic encephalopathy (HIE) and (2) intracranial hemorrhage (ICH). Brain hypoxia and ischemia due to systemic hypoxemia, reduced cerebral blood flow (CBF), or both are the primary pathophysiological processes that lead to a hypoxic-ischemic encephalopathy.

The first compensatory adjustment to a hypoxic-ischemic (asphyxic) event is an increase in CBF due to hypoxia and hypercapnia. This is associated with a redistribution of cardiac output so that the brain receives an increased proportion of the cardiac output. This is followed by a slight increase in systemic blood pressure (BP) due to increased release of epinephrine. In the fetus suffering from acute asphyxia (hypoxic ischemia), if early compensatory adjustments fail, cerebral blood flow (CBF) may become pressure passive, and brain perfusion becomes dependent on systemic BP. As BP falls, CBF falls below critical levels, and a diminished blood supply in the brain leads to insufficient oxygen to meet its needs and intracellular energy failure.

Neuronal injury in hypoxic ischemia is an evolving process. During the early phases of brain injury, brain temperature drops, and there is local release of neurotransmitters, such as g-aminobutyric acid transaminase (GABA). The magnitude of the final neuronal damage depends on both the severity of the initial insult and damage due to energy failure, injury during reperfusion, and apoptosis. The extent, nature, severity, and duration of the primary injury are all important in determining the magnitude of the residual neurological damage.

Intracranial hemorrhage in the full-term infant can be intraventricular, subarachnoid, subdural, or intracerebellar. There is often ventilatory disturbance and hypoxia because of varying neurological depression. Intraventricular hemorrhage (IVH), which is unusual in term infants, may be associated with evidence of intrapartum asphyxia but may also be clinically silent and underdiagnosed, causing later deficits or hydrocephalus (Rohan and Golombek 2009).

Approximately 20% of neonatal HIE is primarily related to antepartum events that lead to hypoxic ischemia. Maternal conditions such as hypotension, placental vasculopathy, and insulin-dependent diabetes mellitus may predispose the fetus to intrapartum hypoxic ischemia because there is little reserve to compensate for the stresses of labor (Volpe 2008). Intrapartum events such as prolapsed cord, abruptio placentae, and traumatic delivery have been linked to 35% of cases of HIE. Because of the limitations in determining the actual timing of the insult, it may be difficult to identify the antepartum contribution separately from the intrapartum. Other events besides intrapartum hypoxia may be responsible for HIE or CP, as less than 25% of these infants have symptoms of hypoxic ischemia at birth (Task Force on Neonatal Encephalopathy and Cerebral Palsy Staff American College of Obstetricians and Gynecologists with American Academy of Pediatrics Staff 2014).

The true incidence of intracranial hemorrhage (ICH) in utero has not been determined. Significant subarachnoid hemorrhage can occur with intrapartum hypoxia or may result from trauma at delivery. It can be isolated or associated with subdural bleeding and cerebral contusion. The presentation is variable but generally includes CNS depression, irritability, and seizures. When subarachnoid hemorrhage is associated with other signs of physical injury and is caused by a difficult delivery, outcome is frequently poor.

1.2.5 Fetal Response to Injury

During normal development, cardiovascular and circulatory functions progress from fetal life, which is characterized by low PaO_2 (20–24 mmHg; 2.66–3.19 kPa) through transition at birth, to normoxemia after birth (PaO_2 70–80 mmHg; 9.31–10.64 kPa); the fetus and newborn are clearly able to thrive despite their "hypoxic" environment. Adaptive responses by the cardiovascular, metabolic, and endocrine systems allow fairly severe intrauterine hypoxic stress to be tolerated, with the fetus having relatively normal growth and development. However, severe acute or chronic intrauterine hypoxic stress in utero can cause compromised circulation, organ dysfunction, and threaten survival or intact survival. At the time of transition to extrauterine life, signs of a depressed circulatory system because of intrauterine hypoxia may become apparent because of the increased metabolic demands at birth and loss of placental gas exchange (Anderson et al. 2004).

The fetal heart also has a greater capacity for anaerobic metabolism than the adult heart (Philipps 2004).

Renal impairment is commonly reported following a generalized hypoxic-ischemic insult at birth. The degree of insult varies in effect from oliguria with minor electrolyte abnormality and minimally elevated creatinine to complete renal failure requiring dialysis.

An elevated blood concentration of liver enzymes, as a marker of hepatocellular injury due to perinatal hypoxia, is also common after acute hypoxia, but irreversible liver damage is rare.

Fetal cardiovascular and endocrine responses may be altered, both in acute and in chronic hypoxia. Recurrence of mild hypoxia may occur in pregnancies where the blood flow to placenta, uterus, and fetus is repeatedly compromised by physiological and environmental influences. In chronic hypoxia, fetal growth restriction is not uncommon, and depression of growth factors during hypoxia has an important protective effect in conserving fetal substrate for energy as opposed to growth needs (Noori et al. 2004; Seri and Evens 2001). The full-term infant, while more likely to survive a severe hypoxic-ischemic insult at birth than a preterm infant (approximately 70% vs. 30%), is also more likely to have significant long-term morbidity (Cressens and Huppi 2006). In umbilical venous blood, mild hypoxemia may be manifest through an absence of hypercapnia or acidemia. In severe uteroplacental insufficiency, the fetus cannot compensate hemodynamically, and hypercapnia and acidemia increase exponentially (Bastek et al. 2008). Hypoxemic growth-restricted fetuses also demonstrate a range of hematological and metabolic abnormalities, including erythroblastosis, thrombocytopenia, hypoglycemia, deficiency in essential amino acids, hypertriglyceridemia, hypoinsulinemia, and hypothyroidism. Low birth weight increases the risk for perinatal mortality (death shortly after birth), asphyxia, hypothermia, polycythemia, hypocalcemia, immune dysfunction, neurologic abnormalities, and other long-term health problems (Petrini et al. 2009).

1.2.5.1 Fetal Hemodynamic Aspects

Acute hypoxemia produces various circulatory adaptations in the fetus that enhance fetal survival, including the development of tachycardia, hypertension, redistribution of blood flow toward the brain, myocardium and adrenals, and depression of fetal breathing and skeletal muscle activity.

This results in an increased blood supply to the brain, myocardium, and adrenal glands and reduced perfusion of the kidneys, gastrointestinal tract, and the lower extremities. There is preferential delivery of nutrients and oxygen to vital organs, compensating for a diminished placental supply (Sheridan 2005).

This compensation is manifest as cerebral vasodilatation and there is a decrease in the pulsatility index (PI) in cerebral vessels (Figs. 5 and 6). The PI index is an arterial blood-flow velocity waveform index designed to quantify the pulsatility or oscillations of the waveform. It is calculated by the formula PI = (Vmax − Vmin)/Vmax mean, where Vmax is the peak systolic velocity, Vmin is the minimum forward diastolic velocity in unidirectional flow or the maximum negative velocity in diastolic flow reversal, and Vmax mean is the maximum velocity averaged over one cardiac cycle. Cerebral vasodilatation produces a decrease in left ventricular afterload, while increased placental and systemic resistance result in an increased right ventricular afterload.

In severe hypoxemia, there is also redistribution of umbilical venous blood towards the ductus venosus. Consequently, blood flow in the umbilical vein, which contributes to the fetal cardiac output, is increased. In contrast, a reduced afterload is associated with an increase in peak diastolic forward flow, indicating that fetal systemic vascular resistance has a major influence on venous return and filling patterns of the right heart. Increased placental resistance and peripheral vasoconstriction cause an increase in right ventricular afterload, and thus ventricular end-diastolic pressure increases. This may result in highly pulsatile venous blood flow waveforms and umbilical venous pulsations due to the transmission of atrial pressure waves through the ductus venosus.

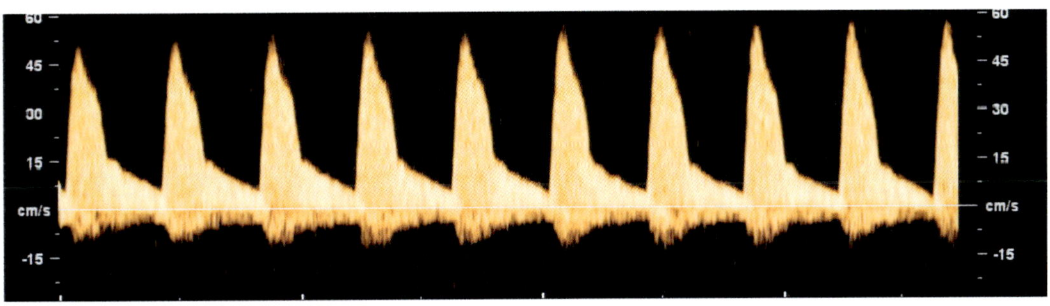

Fig. 5 Flow velocity waveforms from the middle cerebral artery in a normal fetus (Image courtesy of G. Rizzo)

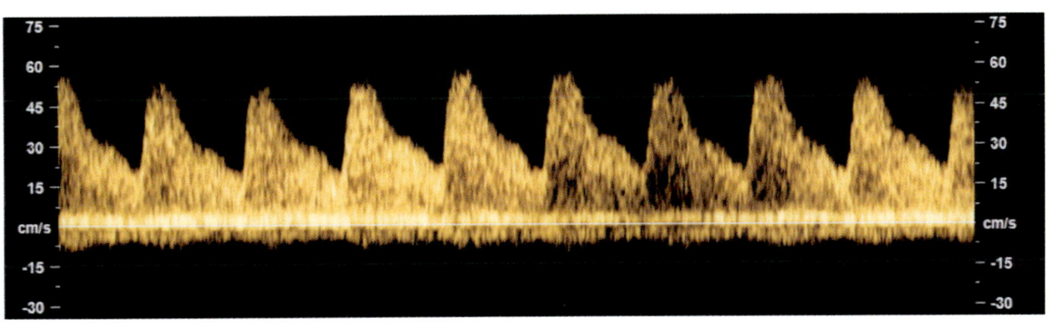

Fig. 6 Flow velocity waveforms from the middle cerebral artery in a growth-restricted fetus (Image courtesy of G. Rizzo)

Investigations of the venous vascular system have become increasingly important in the assessment of fetal myocardial function, and different indices are used to evaluate the blood flow velocity during the different phases of the cardiac cycle in the ductus venosus. Reference values for ductus venosus flow velocities are represented by ventricular systole (S wave) and diastole (D wave), the lowest forward velocity during atrial contraction (A wave) (Fig. 7). Different indices are calculated, e.g., the S/A ratio. The most important parameter which represents the final stage of disease is the abnormal reversal of blood flow velocities in the ductus venosus, inducing an increase in the S/A ratio, mainly due to a reduced A component of the velocity waveforms (Fig. 8). Reference values should be used for ductus venosus flow velocities during ventricular systole (S wave) and diastole (D wave), the lowest forward velocity during atrial contraction (A wave) and different calculated indices as the S/A.

In the inferior vena cava, there is an increase of reverse flow during atrial contraction with progressive fetal deterioration, suggesting a higher pressure gradient in the right atrium. (Figs. 9 and 10). A high venous pressure induces a reduced velocity at end-diastole in the umbilical vein, causing typical end-diastolic pulsations. The development of these pulsations is close to the onset of abnormal fetal heart rate patterns and is frequently associated with acidemia and fetal endocrine changes. At this stage, there may be an increased coronary blood flow velocity compared with that seen in normally grown third-trimester fetuses and, if the affected fetus is not delivered, intrauterine death may occur within a few days.

1.2.5.2 Fetal Growing Aspects

Accurate detection of suboptimal fetal growth is among the objectives of modern obstetrics. To achieve this result, sonography plays a critical role in providing a reliable estimate of fetal biometry, thus confirming the clinical suspicion of growth restriction and substantially influencing pregnancy management. An approach based on customized charts has proved to be more accurate than traditional population-based charts for antenatal detection of the true small fetuses, whose risk of adverse perinatal outcomes is substantially increased (Ghi et al. 2016).

The term small for gestational age (SGA) describes a condition in which the fetus is smaller than expected for the number of weeks of pregnancy (below the tenth percentile) and is unable to achieve its genetically determined potential size; when a SGA fetus shows also signs of placental insufficiency, it is defined an intrauterine growth restriction (IUGR) fetus. IUGR is not synonymous with SGA. Some, but not all, growth-restricted fetuses/infants are SGA, while 50–70% of SGA fetuses are constitutionally small, with fetal growth appropriate for maternal size and ethnicity.

This functional definition is useful to identify a population of fetuses at risk of poor outcome. The clinician's challenge is to distinguish between these two conditions and identify IUGR fetuses whose health is endangered in utero because of a hostile intrauterine environment and consequently to monitor and intervene appropriately.

In fact, data support the notion that long-term consequences of IUGR last well into adulthood. These individuals are predisposed to the development of a metabolic syndrome later in life, manifesting as obesity, hypertension, hypercholesterolemia, cardiovascular disease, and type 2 diabetes. Several hypotheses suggest that intrauterine malnutrition results in insulin resistance, loss of pancreatic beta-cell mass, and an adult predisposition to type 2 diabetes. Although the causative pathophysiology is uncertain, the risk of a metabolic syndrome in adulthood is increased among individuals who were IUGR at birth (Engle et al. 2007). In addition to an increased risk for physical sequelae, mental health problems have been found more commonly in children with growth restriction.

1.2.5.3 Diagnosis

Fetal arterial Doppler studies are useful in the differential diagnosis of SGA and IUGR fetuses. In normal pregnancies, umbilical artery (UA) resistance shows a continuous decline as the pregnancy progresses (Fig. 11), but this does not occur in fetuses with uteroplacental insufficiency.

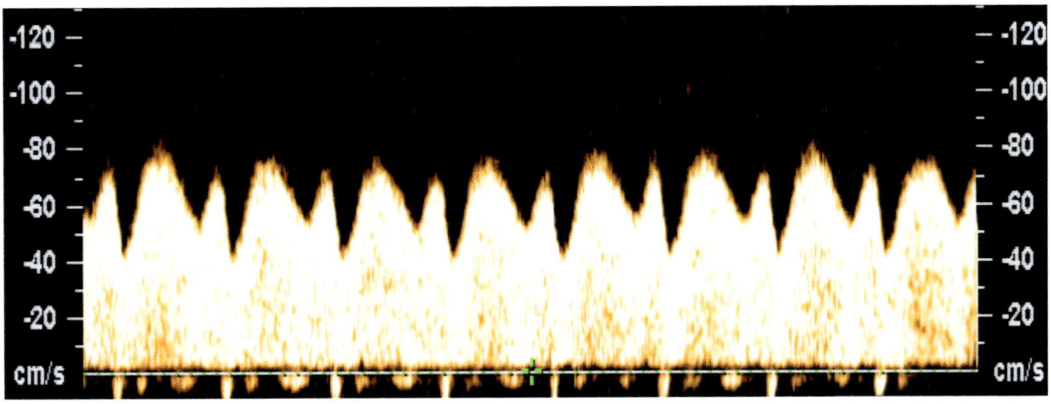

Fig. 7 Color Doppler examination of the ductus venosus with normal flow velocity waveforms (Image courtesy of G. Rizzo)

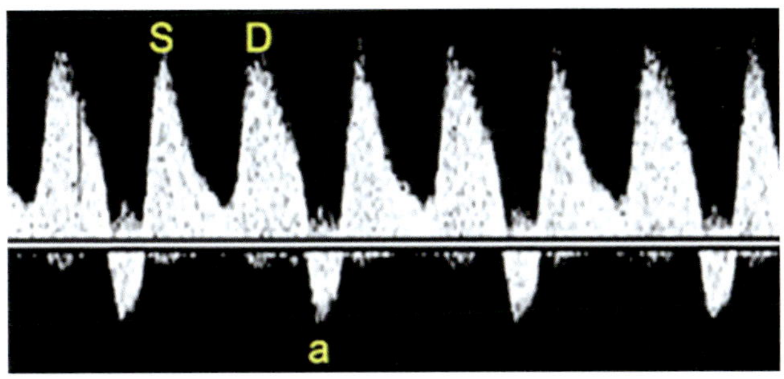

Fig. 8 Abnormal DV waveform with reversal of flow during atrial contraction and markedly increased pulsatility systole (*S*), diastole (*D*), atrial contraction (*a*)

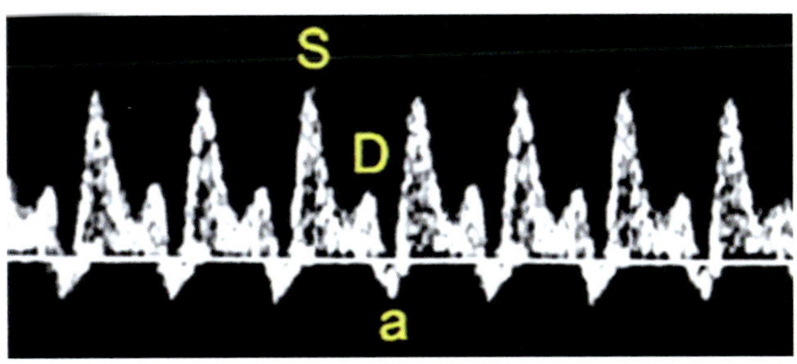

Fig. 9 Doppler examination of the inferior vena cava with normal flow velocity waveforms

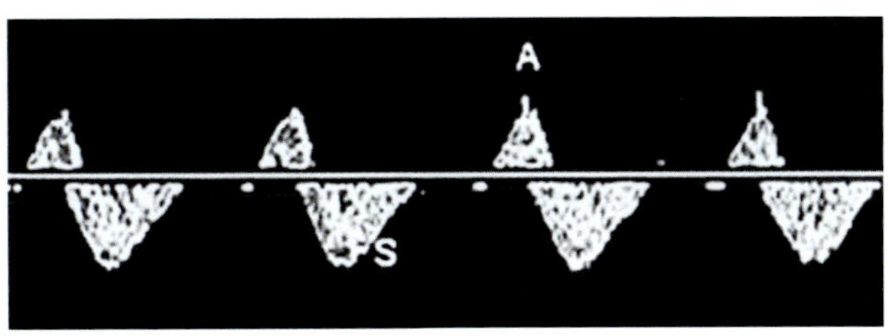

Fig. 10 Abnormal waveform with increase in reversed flow during atrial contraction in a growth-restricted fetus

The most commonly used measure of gestational age-specific UA resistance is the systolic-to-diastolic ratio of flow, the Pulsatility Index (PI), which increases with worsening disease. As the insufficiency progresses, end-diastolic velocity is lost and eventually reversed (Fig. 12). The status of UA blood flow supports the diagnosis of IUGR and provides early evidence of circulatory abnormalities in the fetus, helping clinicians to identify these high-risk fetuses. UA Doppler measurements may help the clinician decide whether a small fetus is truly growth restricted and to identify a small fetus at risk of chronic hypoxemia, but IUGR diagnosis is challenging and cannot only be based only on umbilical artery Doppler (Cruz-Martínez et al. 2011).

In hypoxemic fetuses with impaired placental perfusion, the PI in the umbilical artery is increased and the fetal middle cerebral artery PI is decreased; consequently, the PI ratio of the middle cerebral artery to umbilical artery (MCA/UA), defined as cerebroplacental ratio, (CPR) is decreased.

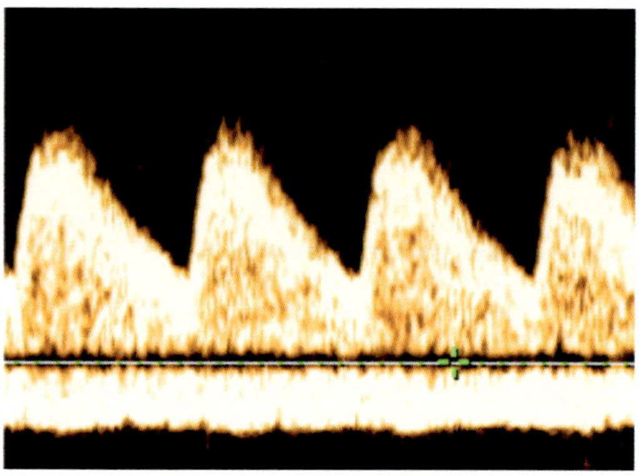

Fig. 11 Color Doppler of the umbilical artery with normal flow velocity waveforms (Image courtesy of G. Rizzo)

The CPR is emerging as an important predictor of adverse outcome not only for IUGR fetuses but also for SGA and appropriate for gestational age (AGA) fetuses close to term (DeVore 2015).

Recent evidence suggests that a proportion of these SGA fetuses have milder forms of late-onset intrauterine growth restriction as suggested by an increased risk of adverse perinatal outcome (McCowan et al. 2000; Doctor et al. 2001; Figueras et al. 2008a), abnormal neonatal neurobehavioral performance (Figueras et al. 2009), and suboptimal neurodevelopment in childhood (McCowan et al. 2002; Figueras et al. 2008b). These findings add to the body of evidence suggesting that the diagnostic category of SGA includes a proportion of cases with true growth restriction and mild placental insufficiency, which is not reflected in the umbilical artery Doppler. Recent studies suggest that the risk of adverse outcome in these fetuses is best established by means of brain Doppler examination. Thus, brain sparing as measured by the middle cerebral artery Doppler is associated with poorer perinatal outcome, higher risk of cesarean delivery for nonreassuring fetal status (Severi et al. 2002), and increased risk of abnormal neurodevelopmental tests at birth (Oros et al. 2010) and at 2 years of age (Eixarch et al. 2008).

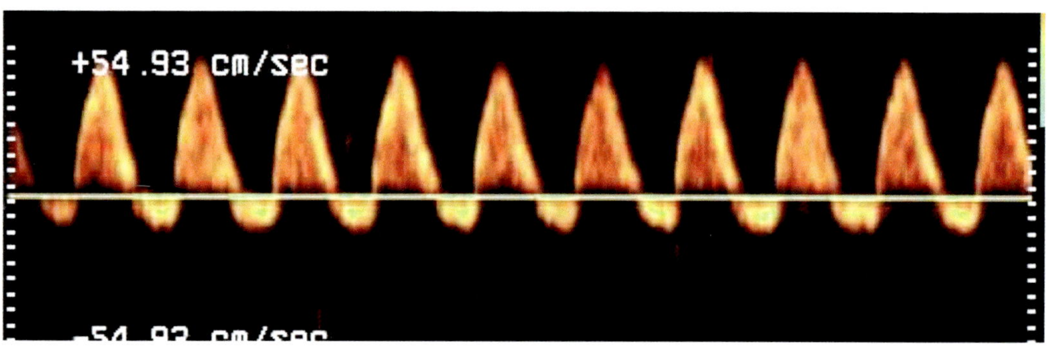

Fig. 12 Color Doppler of the umbilical artery with reversed flow (Image courtesy of G. Rizzo)

1.2.5.4 Timing of Delivery and Management

In the past, the period from 3 weeks before until 2 weeks after the estimated date of delivery was considered "term," with the expectation that neonatal outcomes from deliveries in this interval were uniform and good. Increasingly, however, research has shown that neonatal outcomes, especially respiratory morbidity, vary depending on the timing of delivery within this 5-week gestational age range. To address this lack of uniformity, The American College of Obstetricians and Gynecologists and the Society for Maternal-Fetal Medicine recommended that the label "term" be replaced with the designations below (ACOG 2013):

- Early term (37 0/7 weeks of gestation through 38 6/7 weeks of gestation)
- Full term (39 0/7 weeks of gestation through 40 6/7 weeks of gestation)
- Late term (41 0/7 weeks of gestation through 41 6/7 weeks of gestation)
- Postterm (42 0/7 weeks of gestation and beyond)

Preterm birth, defined as birth at less than 37 + 0 weeks of gestation, is the most important single determinant of adverse infant outcome in terms of both survival and quality of life (Saigal and Doyle 2008).

An useful pragmatic definition for a "premature" infant is one who has not yet reached the level of fetal development that generally allows life outside the womb. In the normal human fetus, several organ systems mature between 34 and 37 weeks, and the fetus reaches adequate maturity by the end of this period. One of the main organs greatly affected by premature birth is the lung.

In Europe and many developed countries, the preterm birth rate is generally 5–9%, and in the USA, it has risen to 12–13% in the last decades. There are three categories of preterm birth: (1) spontaneous preterm births are the 40–45% preterm births that follow preterm labor of spontaneous (i.e., idiopathic) onset; (2) 25–30% preterm births occur after premature rupture of the membranes; (3) the remaining 30–35% are preterm births that are induced for obstetric reasons.

Babies born just a few weeks earlier than full-term usually do not experience any problems related to their slight prematurity. However, the more premature these infants are, the more serious are the complications.

Although there are recommendations that term IUGR fetuses should be monitored during delivery as high-risk pregnancies (Royal College of Obstetricians and Gynaecologists 2002), there is no consensus about the best strategy for delivery.

The Lancet published data on brain development in survivors of the multicenter Growth Restriction Intervention Trial (GRIT) (Thornton et al. 2004). The aim of this study was to identify compromised fetuses between 24 and 36 weeks' gestation and answer the question of whether it was safer to deliver them immediately or to delay until there was no clinical doubt that delivery was necessary. In the GRIT study, the 24 week gestation babies were very different from those at 36 weeks. In the absence of severe congenital abnormalities, the current infant mortality after 32 weeks' gestation is low: the causes of this rare event include asphyxia, necrotising enterocolitis, and infection; respiratory distress syndrome is rare in this group. By contrast, before 32 weeks, and particularly in the extreme preterm fetus, there is a much higher mortality, and the levels of morbidity were also emphasized by the EPICure Study, in which 49% of surviving infants born at less than 26 weeks' gestation had some disability at 30 months of age and 19% were severely disabled (Wood et al. 2000). The EPICure study reached some important conclusions. It demonstrated that 44% of infants born at 25 weeks' gestation survived to discharge, whereas delivery at 22 weeks almost invariably resulted in neonatal death.

Neonatologists, obstetricians, and parents must increasingly recognize that infants born less than 25 weeks' gestation who survive are at risk of disability at school age. In the EPICure study, only 20% were totally free of disability at school age and so the prognosis must be guarded. Disability was classified as follows:

1. *Severe*: The child was likely to be highly dependent on care-givers, e.g., non-ambulant cerebral palsy, profound hearing loss, or blindness.

2. *Moderate*: Children who were likely to be reasonably independent, e.g., ambulant cerebral palsy, some hearing loss, or some visual impairment.
3. *Mild*: Children with neurological signs with minimal functional consequences.

In the EPICure study, over half of the survivors had moderate disability or no disability at school age. In addition, some of the 24% with moderate disability were improved with spectacles and hearing aids.

There is uncertainty about whether iatrogenic delivery of the very preterm (before 33 weeks of gestation) growth-restricted fetus should be undertaken before the development of signs of severe hypoxemia, with a consequent risk of prematurity-related neonatal complications, or whether delivery should be delayed, incurring risks of prolonged exposure to hypoxia and malnutrition imposed by the hostile intrauterine environment (Walter et al. 2009). With every week that passes, there is a decreasing risk of complications including intraventricular hemorrhage, retinopathy of prematurity, and sepsis. However, delay may expose the growth-restricted fetus to ischemic injury of the brain, resulting in asphyxia, periventricular leukomalacia, and intraventricular hemorrhage, as well as a significant risk of intrauterine death. It is important to weigh the risks and benefits of early interventions. This is a dynamic process, in which advancements in both fetal and neonatal medicine are of crucial importance for the appropriate counseling of parents and the management of these pregnancies.

The GRIT study showed a small increase in fetal death if the obstetrician delayed delivery, and a small increase in neonatal death if early delivery was chosen. Thus the monitoring of fetal health is particularly important if there is growth restriction. Such fetuses have few metabolic reserves, and sudden death during pregnancy may occur. Labor is an intermittently hypoxic event, and anaerobic metabolism may not be an option when there are inadequate stores of fat and glycogen.

In recent years, placental and fetal arterial Doppler flow-velocity waveforms have guided the timing of delivery. Doppler has been particularly effective in assessing the growth-restricted pregnancy and has been a useful adjunct for the assessment of the very preterm fetus, when cardiotocographical monitoring is unhelpful. However, in the growth-restricted hypoxemic fetus, redistribution of well-oxygenated blood to vital organs, such as the brain, heart, and adrenals, represents a compensatory mechanism to prevent fetal damage, and when the reserve capacities of the circulatory redistribution reach their limits, fetal deterioration may occur rapidly. In clinical practice, serial Doppler investigations estimate the duration and degree of fetal blood flow redistribution. The onset of an abnormal venous Doppler recording indicates deterioration in the fetal condition and iatrogenic delivery should be considered.

Delivery of IUGR fetuses remain a challenging problem for clinicians not only for preterm but also for fetuses near term. In practice, term pregnancies are often delivered, and the delivery of the late preterm (34 + 0–36 + 6 weeks) or early term (37 weeks) growth-restricted fetus is also recommended if there are additional risk factors for adverse outcome, such as maternal medical/obstetrical disorders, arrest of growth over a 3–4 week interval, and/ or absence or reversal Doppler flow in the umbilical artery (Spong et al. 2011).

A recent multicenter clinical trial, the Disproportionate Intrauterine Growth Intervention Trial At Term (DIGITAT), failed to demonstrate differences in perinatal outcome between expectant management compared with induction of labor in fetuses beyond 36 weeks' gestation (Boers et al. 2010; Tajik et al. 2014).

The study confirms that the relatively favorable neonatal outcomes in both study groups could reflect the fact that participants and clinicians were more alert to possible complications and monitoring was intensified.

In conclusion, the goal in the management of the preterm fetus is to deliver the most mature fetus possible, at least at 32–34 weeks, in the best condition possible increasing fetal and maternal monitoring (Table 1).

Table 1 Suggested management of the preterm fetus

What to do	Perform parental counseling
	Share any type of decisions with the neonatologist, the anesthesiologist, and the couple, personalizing the specific situation
	Fill the informed consent as much detailed as it is possible
Considering	Short-term consequences: RDS, NEC, IVH, PVL, pulmonary dysplasia, sepsis
	Long-term consequences: cerebral palsy, mental impairment, attention disorders
	Pregnancy age and prognosis age
	Etiology of the preterm labor (maternal causes, fetal causes)
	Maternal mortality related to the type of delivery
	Fetal presentation
	Obstetric anamnesis of the patient
	Combination of the multiple factors
When	Better after 26 weeks
	Using corticosteroids between 48 h and 7 days before delivery
Where	Any hospital with NICU
How	Trying to reduce the effects of the hypoxia
	Balance maternal and fetal morbidity
	Preterm delivery is not itself an indication of cesarean section unless associated with maternal or fetal consequences

1.3 Part 2 General Characteristics of Preterm and Term Newborn

1.3.1 History

A full family history is essential. This should include a full medical and social history. Note should be taken of alcohol ingestion and of any drugs (prescribed or recreational). It should enquire about the possibility of consanguinity – the question, "Are your families related?" to both parents is one way of approaching this often delicate subject. Enquiry should be made about the presence of possible transmissible and inheritable diseases in the families of both parents. Tall or short stature can generate a search for specific undiagnosed diseases in the parents (e.g., Marfan syndrome, gluten intolerance, achondroplasia). Anemia in the parents can be a marker of a hematological defect (e.g., thalassemia), as well as the place of origin and ethnicity of the parents (e.g., G6PD deficiency).

1.3.1.1 History of the Pregnancy and Delivery

A baby's well-being is determined by periconceptional events. The mother's medical history is important, including the possibility of maternal diabetes mellitus and other illnesses and her immune status (HBV, HCV, HIV, CMV, toxoplasmosis, rubella, HSV-HZV, and syphilis). The possibility of seroconversion during pregnancy should be considered. Enquiry should be made about the course of the pregnancy. Account should be taken of the time of booking for antenatal care (late booking may be a sign of a disorganized life style and associated problems).

The results of antenatal checks should be noted: fetal growth and ultrasound results, amniotic fluid volume, maternal anemia, urine results and maternal diabetes mellitus, and pregnancy-induced hypertension or pre-eclampsia. The results of vaginal and anal bacterial swabs within the month before delivery should be noted (group B streptococci or *Listeria monocytogenes*) and whether the mother was given appropriate intrapartum antibiotic prophylaxis.

A history of the pregnancy should include note of drugs taken during the pregnancy and their indications. Consider evidence of infectious illnesses or fever close to the time of delivery and take note of the timing of membrane rupturing and the quantity and color (blood or meconium staining) of the amniotic fluid.

Details of the delivery should be noted, i.e., whether vaginal, operative (forceps of vacuum extraction), cesarean section (planned or emergency, before or during the labor), and evidence of fetal distress.

The baby's presentation should be noted because abnormal limb position may be due to a breech presentation. The possibility of birth trauma (e.g., cephalohematoma, fracture of the clavicle) should be considered.

Adaptation to postnatal life should be considered, bearing in mind that during the first hours after birth the baby is in a transitional period, passing from intra- to extrauterine life.

A baby's condition during the minutes just after birth is described by the Apgar score, usually recorded at 1 and 5 min (see Table 2). Although the Apgar score may be criticized (it is subjective on the part of the observer, often recorded some time after delivery), in its favor, it is almost universally recorded. The score was described in 1953 by Dr. Virginia Apgar, a North American pediatric anesthetist. She intended it to indicate whether or not resuscitation was needed. Although imperfect, there is no doubt that a low score (0 or 1, signifying an absent or slowly beating heart) indicates a baby who is barely alive at the time of birth, and a score of 8 or more indicates an individual whose general condition is good. However, the Apgar score is an imperfect indicator of subsequent progress or outcome. A baby who has a high initial score may develop difficulties with gas exchange in the minutes that follow, even if these problems are transient.

More recent researches have shown that the great majority of normal term infants reach transcutaneous pre-ductal values of oxygen saturation ≥90% after 10 min from birth and that premature infants <32 weeks' gestation can require a longer time to reach the same target (Wychoff et al. 2015; Parmigiani and Corona 2016).

Table 2 Apgar score

Sign	0	1	2
Appearance (color)	Blue or pale	Pink body with blue extremities	Completely pink
Pulse (heart rate)	Absent or <60 beats/min	≥60– <100 beats/min	>100 beats/min
Grimace (reflex irritability)	No response	Grimace	Cough or sneeze
Activity (muscle tone)	Limp	Some flexion	Active movements
Respiration	Absent	Slow, irregular	Good, crying

Another new approach is to start the resuscitation of term babies with room air, adding oxygen after 30–60 s preferably under pulsoximeter guidance. In fact, it has been shown that asphyxiated infants resuscitated with room air started regular breathing significantly before than those resuscitated with 100% oxygen (Rabi et al. 2011).

Another important topic related to assistance at birth is if delayed cord clamping can improve cardio-circulatory adaptation after birth. Some data seem in favor of retarded cord clamping after 1 min or after first breath in term infants; however, this is still controversial and not yet well understood under the physiopathologic aspect (Parmigiani and Corona 2016; Hooper et al. 2016).

Most healthy babies are inclined to breastfeed during the first hour of life, and babies recognize their mother's smell. This is the best moment to favor mother-infant bonding and breastfeeding.

A baby's size is an indicator of intrauterine development and nutrition. Intrauterine growth restriction can be a consequence of poor placental function (e.g., due to diseases such as pregnancy-induced hypertension, systemic lupus erythematosus, cocaine ingestion, or infection) and congenital disease, chromosomopathy, or fetal alcohol syndrome.

Observation of a baby's movements, when undressed and preferably in the presence of one or both parents, allows for observation of the quality of movements (whether symmetrical, coordinate, and smooth).

Eyes may be difficult to examine at birth because there is often some eyelid edema, but they must be checked later to note the presence of a red reflex. In the case of babies who are discharged early from hospital, this may need to be done at home by the family doctor or community midwifery team.

Lips, gums, and palate must be examined to exclude the presence of a cleft or other malformation.

The hips should be examined to exclude congenital dislocation. During the immediate neonatal period, the ability to achieve full abduction is a useful sign. It may only be possible to elicit a positive Ortolani sign, an index of hip luxation/subluxation, later during the first week.

Arms, legs, fingers, and toes should be examined to identify any abnormality (e.g., webbing, number, length). Examination of the chest should note any asymmetry during respiration, subcostal or intercostal retraction, and ancillary nipples. The skin may show areas of hypo- or hyperpigmentation, scars, blisters, pustules, petechiae, or evidence of birth trauma (cuts, bruises). The diaper area should be examined to look for anomalies of the external genitalia, an imperforate or anterior anus, and hairy tufts or dimples over the sacrum.

1.3.1.2 Clinical Aspects of CNS Development

Motor and sensory functions mature during pregnancy and are already in great part developed by the middle of the second trimester of pregnancy and the process continues after birth. Ultrasound, particularly so-called 4D ultrasound, allows for the identification and classification of fetal movements, and natural fetal behavior has been studied. Sporadic, irregular ("vermiform") movements are seen between 6 and 7 weeks' gestation, involving the whole body. Generalized, brief movements from the legs to the neck and head (such as "startle") are observed at 8 weeks' gestation. At 9 weeks, flexor movements of the cranial and caudal poles towards the centre appear, interspersed with jerks that allow small movements within the amniotic liquid and partial rotation of the head. At the tenth week, hand-to-head movements, mouth opening with tongue protrusion, swallowing, rotation along the longitudinal axis, and independent movements of limb flexion and extension can be observed (Ianniruberto and Tajani 1981; Kurjak et al. 2008).

The maturation of the central nervous system (CNS) determines an infant's response and tolerance to various sensory inputs. A premature infant may demonstrate signs of immaturity (Holditch-Davis et al. 2003) such as:

Diffuse and indeterminate sleep or waking states with frequent whimpering, facial twitches, or apparent smiling

Abrupt transitions between states

Periods of fussiness or crying

Low-level alertness, characterized by a dull, glassy-eyed look

Hyperalertness, characterized by wide-open eyes with a panicked, worried look; an appearance of extreme vigilance

Uncoordinated eye movements: roving or floating eyes

Immature tone, posture, and general coordination

The five senses can be altered by prematurity:

1. The earliest response to auditory stimulation has been recorded at 19 weeks' gestation but consistent responsiveness is established by 25 weeks. Deafness is a complication of intraventricular hemorrhage or periventricular leukomalacia affecting 5–10% of preterm infants. It may also be the result of a cytomegalovirus infection, which may have caused preterm delivery. The ambient noise of a NICU is rarely less than 40 dB (as in the womb), and more often around 70–100 dB (American Academy of Pediatrics. Committee on Environmental Health 1997).
2. Functional maturation of the visual system starts at around 5 months and it is still immature at term (Graven 2004). Retinopathy of prematurity (ROP), formerly known as retrolental fibroplasia and affecting premature babies exposed to excessive oxygen, is nowadays largely preventable: oxygen delivery is monitored carefully and all infants below 32 weeks' gestation have regular examination of the retina following a generally accepted international protocol. Advanced stages of ROP are treated by cryo- or laser therapy. However, decreased visual acuity or strabismus may follow. Nowadays, total blindness is infrequent.
3. Taste develops under the influence of amniotic fluid flavonoids and odorants transmitted from the maternal diet from as early as 14 weeks' gestation. Taste after birth can be disturbed by drugs, by the late introduction of oral feeding, or by the impaired development of taste centers.
4. The sensory system starts to develop at 8 weeks and is functional by 12 weeks' gestation. Being touched may be uncomfortable

even for full-term infants who have not developed all the receptors and pathways, and perception may also be disturbed by drugs, e.g., maternal cocaine use. In the preterm infant, touch may be a powerful stressor. Touch should be gentle and combined with the stimulation of other senses, for example, speaking to the baby. Touching for no good reason should similarly be avoided. Parents should be taught to touch gently and about "kangaroo care".

5. The olfactory tract is part of the primitive encephalon and a baby at term is able to recognize its mother's odor. The olfactory system is fully functional by 14 weeks' gestation. Strong odors can be stressful for preterm babies who are unable to communicate this to their carer.

These signs of immaturity should be recognized and a favorable environment should be created, avoiding overstimulation. Woolf (1959, 1966), Brazelton (1984), and Prechtl (1974) described different states of behavior. The Brazelton scale assesses neonatal behavior in six states: quiet sleep, active sleep, drowsiness, alert inactivity, active awake, and crying (Table 3). The baby should be observed in a state of quiet wakefulness.

Table 3 Neonatal states classification scale

State	Characteristics
Quiet sleep	Regular breathing, eyes closed. Spontaneous activity confined to startle and jerky movements at regular intervals.
	Responses to external stimuli are partially inhibited, and any response is likely to be delayed. No eye movements, and state changes are less likely after stimuli or startles than in other states.
Active sleep	Irregular breathing patterns, sucking movements, eyes closed but rapid eye movements can be detected underneath the closed lids. Infants also have some low-level and irregular motor activity. Startles occur in response to external stimuli and can produce a change in state.
Drowsiness	While the newborn is semi-dosing, eyes may be open or closed; eyelids often flutter; activity level variable and interspersed with mild startles. Drowsy newborns are responsive to sensory stimuli but with some delay, and state change frequently follows stimulation.
Alert inactivity	A bright alert look, with attention focused on sources of auditory or visual stimuli; motor activity is inhibited while attending to stimuli.
Active awake	Eyes open, considerable motor activity, thrusting movements of extremities, and occasional startles set off by activity; reactive to external stimulation with an increase in startles or motor activity. Discrete responses are difficult to distinguish due to general high activity level.
Crying	Intense irritability in the form of sustained crying and jerky limb movement. This state is difficult to break through with stimulation.

Data from (Brazelton 1984)

1.3.1.3 The Preterm Infant

Maturity is determined by the length of gestation, and the severity of problems related to prematurity is directly related to gestation.

Weeks of gestation are generally considered as completed weeks. The World Health Organization has defined preterm infants as those with gestational age less than 37 weeks. Recently, the term "late preterm infants" (instead of "near-term") has been used for those infants that are born at a gestational age between 34 weeks and 36 weeks and 6 days. These infants have a rather higher morbidity and mortality than term infants (gestational age ≥37 weeks), even though they are of similar size (Woolf 1959, 1966; Brazelton 1984; Prechtl 1974). Some North American authors have also used the terms "premies" and "micropremies" to describe very immature babies.

Classification by birth weight is as follows:

- *Low birth weight* (LBW), 1501–2500 g
- *Very low birth weight* (VLBW), 1001–1500 g
- *Extremely low birth weight* (ELBW), ≤1000 g

Because of the survival of very light and premature babies, the term "incredibly low birth weight" has been used to refer to babies weighing less than 750 g.

A fundamental problem for all preterm infants is their poor ability to maintain body temperature because of reduced glycogen stores (depending on gestational age) and thinner skin, with the most immature lacking the ability to shiver. Thus a primary aim is to avoid heat loss (and insensible water losses) by drying, heating, and covering the baby. This also decreases glucose consumption, reducing the risk of hypoglycemia. Plastic wrapping of body and head (apart the face) immediately after birth is advisable for babies <32 weeks'gestation to maintain temperature between 36.5 °C and 37.5 °C (Wychoff et al. 2015).

The preterm baby often experiences delayed respiratory adaptation. Depending on the degree of immaturity, the lungs are morphologically immature and lack surfactant. Such babies may require the endotracheal administration of exogenous surfactant and mechanical ventilation. Bronchopulmonary dysplasia (chronic lung disease with O_2 dependency) is a complication of severe prematurity, which may continue to cause problems during subsequent years.

Premature infants have reduced immune defenses. Furthermore, infection may be the primary cause of preterm delivery, sometimes affecting the baby before birth. Such infections, in combination with lung and brain immaturity, increase the risk of later disability (see ▶ Chap. 14, "Follow-Up Outcomes of High-Risk Infants").

The gastrointestinal tract is not yet adapted to enteral feeds, posing considerable challenges to those responsible for their care. Early nonnutritive feeding should be considered. Milk, preferably from the mother or a human milk bank, may be started early but cautiously, particularly for the most immature infant. Careful note should be taken of early signs of gastrointestinal intolerance, e.g., increased volume or bile-staining of gastric aspirates or abdominal swelling. The most immature infants require parenteral nutrition (partial or total) to provide adequate nutrients and calories for growth, and this may need to be continued for several weeks. This practice requires a central, indwelling catheter, increasing the risk of infection.

Because of advances in the care of these very vulnerable infants, survival at the earliest gestation is improving.

Survival at early gestation and the associated risks of neurodevelopmental impairment are considered elsewhere (see ▶ Chap. 17, "Cerebral Plasticity and Functional Reorganization in Children with Congenital Brain Lesions").

Not only babies at extremely low gestation but also those born late preterm are at risk.

Various evidence points to the environment being of major importance for appropriate development. Although neonatologists strive to recreate an extrauterine environment that is similar to that of the womb, there are many differences.

Light, painful interventions, development in air instead of surrounded by amniotic fluid, noise, stress, sleep-wake cycles interrupted by nursing procedures, continuous intravenous nutrition (without the intermittent glycemic peaks of normal feeding and maternal ingestion), fluctuations in oxygen delivery, carbon dioxide, pH levels, and blood pressure may all interfere with normal brain development. A high tech/soft touch approach may be beneficial and a mother's touch and breastfeeding should be encouraged even for very tiny babies.

In some units, parents are supported by a psychologist to help with attachment. In spite of the best endeavors of staff, having a baby in a neonatal unit, often for several months, is undoubtedly stressful, giving rise to feelings of inadequacy on the part of the mother, who may feel a biological failure, and anxiety on the part of the father, who is no longer in control of the situation.

References

ACOG (2012) Committee Opinion 545 Noninvasive Prenatal Testing for Fetal Aneuploidy

ACOG (2013) Committee Opinion No 579: definition of term pregnancy. Obstet Gynecol 122(5):1139–1140

ACOG (2014) Antepartum fetal surveillance. Obstet Gynecol 124:1

Akolekar R et al (2015) Procedure-related risk of miscarriage following amniocentesis and chorionic villus sampling: a systematic review and meta-analysis. Ultrasound Obstet Gynecol 45:16–26

Albaiges G, Missfelder-Lobos H, Lees C et al (2000) One-stage screening for pregnancy complications by color Doppler assessment of the uterine arteries at 23 weeks' gestation. Obstet Gynecol 96:559–564

Alfirevic Z, Mujezinovic F, Sundberg K (2003) Amniocentesis and chorionic villus sampling for prenatal diagnosis. Cochrane Database Syst Rev Issue 3. Art. No.: CD003252.

Allen LH (2001) Biological mechanisms that might underlie iron's effects on fetal growth and preterm birth. J Nutr 131:S581–S589

American Academy of Pediatrics. Committee on Environmental Health (1997) Noise: a hazard for the fetus and the newborn. Pediatrics 100:724–727

Anderson P, Kleiman C, Lister G, Telner N (2004) Cardiovascular function during development and response to hypoxia. In: Polin R, Fox W, Abman S (eds) Fetal and neonatal physiology. Saunders, Philadelphia, pp 645–669

Bamberg C, Kalache KD (2004) Prenatal diagnosis of fetal growth restriction. Semin Fetal Neonatal Med 9:387–394

Bastek LA, Sammel MD, Paré E et al (2008) Adverse neonatal outcomes: examining the risk between preterm, late preterm, and term infants. Am J Obstet Gynecol 199:367.e1–367.e8

Bishop EH (1981) Fetal acceleration test. Am J Obstet Gynecol 141:905–909

Boers KE et al (2010) Induction versus expectant monitoring for intrauterine growth restriction at term: randomised equivalence trial (DIGITAT). BMJ 341:c7087

Botto LD, Olney RS et al (1996) Chorionic villus sampling and transverse digital deficiencies: evidence for anatomic and gestational-age specificity of the digital deficiencies in two studies. Am J Med Genet 62:173–178

Bowden AP, Barrett JH, Fallow W, Silman AJ (2001) Women with inflammatory polyarthritis have babies of lower birth weight. J Rheumatol 28:355–359

Brazelton TB (1984) Neonatal behavioral assesment scale, 2nd edn. Heinemann, London

Canick JA et al (2013) The impact of maternal plasma DNA fetal fraction on next generation sequencing tests for common fetal aneuploidies. Prenatal Diagnosis 33:667–674

Christian P, Khatry SK, Katz J et al (2003) Effects of alternative maternal micronutrient supplements on low birth weight in rural Nepal: double blind randomised community trial. BMJ 326:571

Clapp JF (2003) The effects of maternal exercise on fetal oxygenation and feto-placental growth. Eur J Obstet Gynecol Reprod Biol 110(Suppl 1):S80–S85

Cressens P, Huppi PS (2006) The CNS: hypoxic ischemic encephalopathy. In: Fanaroff AA, Martin R, Walsh MC (eds) Neonatal-perinatal medicine. Mosby, St Louis

Cruz-Martínez R et al. (2011) Fetal brain doppler to predict cesarean delivery for nonreassuring fetal status in term small-for-gestational-age fetuses. Obstet Gynecol 117(3):618–26

DeVore GR (2015) The importance of the cerebroplacental ratio in the evaluation of fetal well-being in SGA and AGA foetuses. Am J Obstet Gynecol 213(1):5–15

Doctor BA et al (2001) Perinatal correlates and neonatal outcomes of small for gestational age infants born at term gestation. Am J Obstet Gynecol 185:652–659

Eixarch E et al (2008) Neurodevelopmental outcome in 2-year-old infants who were small-for-gestational age term fetuses with cerebral blood flow redistribution. Ultrasound Obstet Gynecol 32:894–899

Engle A, Tomashek KM, Wallman C, Committee on Fetus and Newborn (2007) 'Late preterm' infants: a population at risk. Pediatrics 120:1390–1401

Ferrazzi E, Rigano S, Bozzo M et al (2000) Umbilical vein blood flow in growth-restricted fetuses. Ultrasound Obstet Gynecol 16:432–438

Figueras F, Eixarch E, Gratacos E, Gardosi J (2008a) Predictiveness of antenatal umbilical artery Doppler for adverse pregnancy outcome in small-for-gestational-age babies according to customised birthweight centiles: population-based study. BJOG 115:590–594

Figueras F et al (2008b) Small-for-gestational-age fetuses with normal umbilical artery Doppler have suboptimal perinatal and neurodevelopmental outcome. Eur J Obstet Gynecol Reprod Biol 136:34–38

Figueras F et al (2009) Neurobehavior in term, small-forgestational age infants with normal placental function. Pediatrics 124:e934–e941

Fowden AL, Forhead AJ (2004) Endocrine mechanisms of intrauterine programming. Reproduction 127:515–526

Ghi T et al (2016) Customized fetal growth charts for parents' characteristics, race, and parity by quantile regression analysis. J Ultrasound Med 35:e35–e44

Graven SN (2004) Early neurosensory visual development of the fetus and newborn. Clin Perinatol 31:199–216

Holditch-Davis D, Blackburn ST, Vandenberg K (2003) Newborn and infant neurobehavioural development. In: Kenner C, Wright Lott J (eds) Comprehensive neonatal nursing: a physiological perspective, 3rd edn. WB Saunders, St Louis, pp 236–284

Hooper SB, Binder-Heschl C, Polglase GR et al (2016) The timing of umbilical cord clamping at birth: physiological considerations. Maternal Health Neonatol Perinatol 2:4

Ianniruberto A, Tajani E (1981) Ultrasonographic study of fetal movements. Semin perinatol 5:175–181

Kliman HJ (2000) Uteroplacental blood flow. The story of decidualization, menstruation, and trophoblast invasion. Am J Pathol 157:1759–1768

Kramer MS, Kakuma R (2003) Energy and protein intake in pregnancy. Cochrane Database Syst Rev CD000032

Krampl E, Lees C, Bland JM et al (2000) Fetal biometry at 4300 m compared to sea level in Peru. Ultrasound Obstet Gynecol 16:9–18

Kurjak A, Tikvica A, Stanojevic M et al (2008) The assessment of fetal neurobehavior by three-dimensional and four-dimensional ultrasound. J Matern Fetal Neonatal Med 21:675–684

Leguizamon G, von Stecher F (2003) Third trimester glycemic profiles and fetal growth. Curr Diab Rep 3:323–326

Liston R, Sawchuck D, Young D (2007) Fetal health surveillance: antepartum and intrapartum consensus guideline. J Obstet Gynaecol Can 29:909

Macones GA, Hankins GD, Spong CY, Hauth J, Moore T (2008) The 2008 National Institute of Child Health and Human Development workshop report on electronic

fetal monitoring: update on definitions, interpretation, and research guidelines. Obstet Gynecol 112:661–666
McCowan LM, Harding JE, Stewart AW (2000) Umbilical artery Doppler studies in small for gestational age babies reflect disease severity. BJOG 107:916–925
McCowan LM, Pryor J, Harding JE (2002) Perinatal predictors of neurodevelopmental outcome in small-for-gestational-age children at 18 months of age. Am J Obstet Gynecol 186:1069–1075
McGaw T (2002) Periodontal disease and preterm delivery of low-birth-weight infants. J Can Dent Assoc 68:165–169
Nicolaides KH (2004) Nuchal translucency and other first-trimester sonographic markers of chromosomal abnormalities. Am J Obstet Gynecol 191:45–67
Noori S, Friedlich P, Seri I (2004) Pathophysiology of shock in the fetus and newborn. In: Polin R, Fox W, Abman S (eds) Fetal and neonatal physiology. Saunders, Philadelphia, pp 772–781
Oros D et al (2010) Middle versus anterior cerebral artery Doppler for the prediction of perinatal outcome and neonatal neurobehavior in term small-for-gestational-age fetuses with normal umbilical artery Doppler. Ultrasound Obstet Gynecol 35:456–461
Palomaki GE et al (2011) DNA sequencing of maternal plasma to detect down syndrome: an international clinical validation study. Genet Med 13:913–920
Parmigiani S, Corona MF (2016) Capitolo 28. Promozione dell'allattamento al seno. In: Felis S, Parmigiani S (eds) Il parto. Edi-Ermes Publisher, Milan, pp 359–372
Petrini JR, Dias T, Mc Cormick MC et al (2009) Increased risk of adverse neurological development for late preterm infants. J Pediatr 154:169–176
Philipps A (2004) Oxygen consumption and general carbohydrate metabolism of the fetus. In: Polin R, Fox W, Abman S (eds) Fetal and neonatal physiology. Saunders, Philadelphia, pp 465–478
Picciano MF (2003) Pregnancy and lactation: physiological adjustments, nutritional requirements and the role of dietary supplements. J Nutr 133:1997S–2002S
Practice Bulletin No. 162 (2016 May) Prenatal diagnostic testing for genetic disorders. Obstet Gynecol 127(5): e108–e122
Prechtl HFR (1974) The behavioral states of the newborn infant: a review. Brain Res 76:1304–1311
Rabi Y, Singhal N, Nettel-Aguirre A (2011) Room-air versus oxygen administration for resuscitation of preterm infants: the ROAR study. Pediatrics 128: e374–e381
RCOG (2014) The investigation and management of the small-for-gestational-age fetus. Green top guideline 31 Jan 2014
Rich-Edwards JW, Buka SL, Brennan RT, Earls F (2003) Diverging associations of maternal age with low birthweight for black and white mothers. Int J Epidemiol 32:83–90
Rohan AJ, Golombek SG (2009) Hypoxia in the term newborn: part three – sepsis and hypotension, neurologic, metabolic and hematologic disorders. MCN Am J Matern Child Nurs 34:224–233
Royal College of Obstetricians and Gynaecologists (2002) The investigation and management of the small-for-gestational-age fetus. Evidence-based clinical guideline no. 31. RCOG, London, pp 1–16
Saigal S, Doyle LW (2008) An overview of mortality and sequelae of preterm birth from infancy to adulthood. Lancet 371:261–269
Seri I, Evens J (2001) Controversies in the diagnosis and management of hypotension in the newborn infant. Curr Opin Pediatr 13:116–123
Severi FM et al (2002) Uterine and fetal cerebral Doppler predict the outcome of third-trimester small-for-gestational age fetuses with normal umbilical artery Doppler. Ultrasound Obstet Gynecol 19:225–228
Sheridan C (2005) Intrauterine growth restriction. Aust Fam Physic 34:717–723
Skomsvoll JF, Baste V, Irgens LM, Ostensen M (2002) The recurrence risk of adverse outcome in the second pregnancy in women with rheumatic disease. Obstet Gynecol 100:1196–1202
Sparks AB et al (2012) Noninvasive prenatal detection and selective analysis of cell-free DNA obtained from maternal blood: evaluation for trisomy 21 and trisomy 18. Am J Obstet Gynecol 206:319 e311–319 e319
Spencer K, Souter V, Tul N, Snijders R, Nicolaides KH (1999) A screening program for trisomy 21 at 10–14 weeks using fetal nuchal translucency, maternal serum free b-human chorionic gonadotropin and pregnancy-associated plasma protein-A. Ultrasound Obstet Gynecol 13:231–237
Spong CY, Mercer BM, D'alton M, Kilpatrick S, Blackwell S, Saade G (2011) Timing of indicated late-preterm and early-term birth. Obstet Gynecol 118:323–333
Tajik P et al (2014) Which intrauterine growth restricted fetuses at term benefit from early labour induction? A secondary analysis of the DIGITAT randomised trial. Eur J Obstet Gynecol Reprod Biol 172:20–25
Task Force on Neonatal Encephalopathy and Cerebral Palsy Staff American College of Obstetricians and Gynecologists with American Academy of Pediatrics Staff (2014) Neonatal Encephalopathy and Neurologic Outcome, Second Edition. Obstetrics & Gynecology 123(4): 896–901
Thornton JG, Hornbuckle J, Vail A et al (2004) Infant wellbeing at 2 years of age in the Growth Restriction Intervention Trial (GRIT): multicentred randomized controlled trial. Lancet 364:513–520
Volpe JJ (2008) Hypoxic-ischemic encephalopathy: clinical aspects. In: Volpe JJ (ed) Neurology of the newborn. Elsevier Saunders, Philadelphia, pp 400–480
Walter EC, Ehlenbach WJ, Hotchkin DL et al (2009) Low birth weight and respiratory disease in adulthood. A population-based case-control study. Am J Respir Crit Care Med 180:176–180
Way W (2006) Recent observations on the regulation of the fetal metabolism of glucose. J Physiol 572:17–24
Winsor EJ et al (1999) Cytogenetic aspects of the Canadian early and mid-trimester amniotic fluid trial (CEMAT). Prenat Diagn 19:620–627

Wolff PH (1959) Observations on newborn infants. Psychosom Med 21:110–118

Wolff PH (1966) The causes, controls and organization of behaviour in the neonate. Psychol Issues 5:1–105

Wood NS, Marlow N, Costeloe K et al (2000) Neurologic and developmental disability after extremely preterm birth. N Engl J Med 343:378–384. comment 343:429–430

Wychoff MH, Aziz K, Escobedo M et al (2015) Part 13: neonatal resuscitation. 2015 American Heart Association guidelines update for cardiopulmonary resuscitation and emergency cardiovascular care. Circulation 132(Suppl 2):S543–S560

Xiao R, Sorensen TK, Williams MA, Luthy DA (2003) Influence of pre-eclampsia on fetal growth. J Matern Fetal Neonatal Med 13:157–162

Zimmermann B et al (2012) Noninvasive prenatal aneuploidy testing of chromosomes 13, 18, 21, X, and Y, using targeted sequencing of polymorphic loci. Prenat Diagn 32:1233–1241

Zygmunt M, Herr F, Keller-Schoenwetter S et al (2002) Characterization of human chorionic gonadotropin as a novel angiogenic factor. J Clin Endocrinol Metab 87:5290–5296

Zygmunt M, Herr F, Munstedt K et al (2003) Angiogenesis and vasculogenesis in pregnancy. Eur J Obstet Gynecol Reprod Biol 110(Suppl 1):S10–S18

Risk Factors for Gestational Diseases

2

Silvia Vannuccini, Michela Torricelli, Filiberto Maria Severi, and Felice Petraglia

Contents

Abstract

Preterm birth (PTB) and preeclampsia (PE) are severe pathologies that may affect and compromise the course of pregnancy, with a high perinatal morbidity and mortality. They represent the main "obstetric syndromes," caused by multiple conditions and characterized by complex pathogenesis. The knowledge of the pathogenetic mechanisms leading to these conditions is very important in order to recognize women at risk and to perform the strategies for preventing their onset and reducing associated morbidity and mortality.

S. Vannuccini · M. Torricelli · F. M. Severi · F. Petraglia (✉)
Obstetrics and Gynecology, Department of Molecular and Developmental Medicine, University of Siena, Siena, Italy
e-mail: felice.petraglia@unisi.it

2.1 Salient Points

- Preterm birth (PTB) and preeclampsia (PE) are severe pathologies that may affect and compromise the course of pregnancy, with a high perinatal morbidity and mortality.
- Knowledge of the pathogenic mechanisms that lead to preterm birth and preeclampsia is needed for the recognition of women at risk, their prevention, and reduction of associated morbidity and mortality.
- Preterm birth is a syndrome initiated by various conditions, such as inflammation/infection, uteroplacental ischemia or hemorrhage, uterine overdistension, cervical disease, stress and endocrine disorders, and other immunologically mediated processes.
- Preeclampsia (PE) is defined as persistent blood pressure elevation, edema, and proteinuria first diagnosed after 20 weeks of gestation. Maternal risk factor profiles of early onset PE

G. Buonocore et al. (eds.), *Neonatology*,
https://doi.org/10.1007/978-3-319-29489-6_151

(<32 weeks) and late onset PE differ, suggesting that early and late PE may be different diseases.

2.2 Introduction

Preterm birth (PTB) and preeclampsia (PE) are severe pathologies that may affect and compromise the course of pregnancy, with a high perinatal morbidity and mortality (Plunkett et al. 2008). They represent the main "obstetric syndromes," caused by multiple conditions and characterized by complex pathogenesis. Nonetheless, recent evidences attest that deregulation of the immune system and exaggeration of inflammatory processes, taking place in the fetoplacental unit, represent common central mechanisms occurring in both diseases (Torricelli et al. 2012).

The knowledge of the pathogenetic mechanisms leading to these conditions is very important in order to recognize women at risk and to perform the strategies for reducing perinatal morbidity and mortality. Interventions can be classified as primary (detected in all women before or during pregnancy to prevent and reduce risk), secondary (aimed at eliminating or reducing risk in women with known risk factors), or tertiary (initiated after disease has developed, with a goal of preventing delivery or improving outcomes for infants). Most obstetric interventions are intended to reduce the burden of prematurity-related illness, but the primary prevention is a desirable goal (Iams et al. 2008).

2.3 Preterm Birth

PTB, defined as birth before 37 weeks' gestational age, occurs with an incidence of 5–18% (Beck et al. 2010), and it is the leading cause of neonatal death and the second cause of childhood death below the age of 5 years (Liu et al. 2010). Neonates born preterm are at an increased risk of short-term complications attributed to immaturity of multiple organ systems as well as neurodevelopmental disorders, such as cerebral palsy, intellectual disabilities, and vision and hearing impairments (Mwaniki et al. 2012). Two-thirds of preterm births occur after the spontaneous onset of labor, whereas the remainder is medically indicated because of maternal or fetal complications, such as preeclampsia or intrauterine growth restriction (Goldenberg et al. 2012). The condition merely describes an event that occurs before its due time and is not a diagnosis in itself. There are many pathways leading to preterm birth, and the prevention of each requires different types of scientific inquiry and clinical strategies (Newnham et al. 2014). Despite the high global burden of PTB on childhood mortality, morbidity, and healthcare expenditure, few strategies are available to effectively detect women at risk and prevent preterm delivery (Rubens et al. 2014).

The risk factors associated with spontaneous preterm births (sPTB) seem to vary by gestational age, social, and environment factors. However, more than 50% them have no causal factor identified (Menon 2008; Lockwood 2002). Preterm and term labor shared the same clinical events of increased uterine contractility, cervical dilatation, and rupture of the chorioamniotic membranes. The common pathway is activated physiologically in the case of labor at term, whereas in preterm labor several disease processes activate one or more of the components. In fact, PTB is considered a syndrome initiated by various conditions, such as inflammation/infection, uteroplacental ischemia or hemorrhage, uterine overdistension, cervical disease, stress and endocrine disorders, and other immunologically mediated processes (Petraglia et al. 2012; Romero et al. 2014a).

2.3.1 Risk Factors of Preterm Birth

Multiple risk factors increase a woman's risk of PTB (Rubens et al. 2014; Institute of Medicine (US) Committee on Understanding Premature Birth and Assuring Healthy Outcomes et al. 2007), and they may be identified before pregnancy, at conception, or during pregnancy (Iams 2014). These include maternal genetics and demography (e.g., age, ethnicity, poor socioeconomic status), poor nutritional status, pregnancy history, external factors (e.g., smoking, alcohol ingestion, drugs of abuse), characteristics of the present pregnancy, and associated conditions (infection, uterine contractions, and cervical length shortening) (Table 1). However, the biological basis for many of these risk factors and the underlying mechanisms remain poorly understood. Although some of these risk factors are not modifiable, others represent potential targets for treatment and risk reduction (Goldenberg et al. 2005, 2008).

Table 1 Risk factors for preterm birth

Preconceptional
Genetics
Ethnicity
Age
Nutritional status
Socioeconomic status
Obstetric history
Interval between pregnancies
Previous preterm birth
Maternal disorders
Systemic diseases
Hypertension
Diabetes
Asthma
Thyroid diseases
Local or systemic infections
Reproductive disorders
PCOS
Endometriosis/adenomyosis
Uterine fibroids
Previous cervical surgery
External factors
Stress
Smoking
Drugs and substances of abuse
Pregnancy-associated risk factors
ART conception
Multiple pregnancy
Intrauterine infection and bacterial vaginosis
Vaginal bleeding
Short cervix and cervical insufficiency
Biochemical markers
fFN, phIGFBP1
Biophysical markers
TVS cervical length

2.3.1.1 Preconceptional Factors

- *Genetics*: Genetic factors are thought to be important causal components (Plunkett and Muglia 2008), as both maternal and fetal genomes have been shown to influence the risk of sPTB (Haataja et al. 2011). Epidemiological analyses of large, population-based cohorts have revealed increased risk of PTB if the mother herself was born preterm or has sisters that have had preterm children (Boyd et al. 2009). More formal genetic studies in offspring of twins and segregation analysis of traits in families consistently demonstrated that 30–40% of the variation in birth timing is due to genetic factors (Bezold et al. 2013). However, recent evidence showed that a maternal effect accounts for 15.2% of the variance of gestational age at birth, while the remaining 60.3% is contributed by individual environmental effects (Wu et al. 2015).
- *Ethnicity*: Women classified as black, African-American, and Afro-Caribbean are three times more likely to have a very early PTB than women from other ethnic groups. The racial disparity persists after adjustment for social, educational, economic, and medical risk factors (Healy et al. 2006; Smith et al. 2007a).
- *Age*: Low and high maternal age are associated with PTB. Age $\geq$40 is associated with signif icantly higher rates of preterm birth (8% vs 16%). Similarly, prematurity is more likely in adolescents (Auger et al. 2013).
- *Nutritional status*: A low pregnancy body mass index (BMI) is associated with high risk of spontaneous PTB. Women with low serum concentrations of iron, folate, or zinc have more PTB than those with measurements within the normal range (Bloomfield 2011). The risk of PTB is increased in obese and overweight women as well (Cnattingius et al. 2013; Lynch et al. 2014; McDonald et al. 2010).
- *Socioeconomic status*: Low socioeconomic status is an important risk factor for preterm birth. Socioeconomic disadvantage is associated with unhealthy or risky behaviors,

exposure to stress, and psychological reactions that influence gestation negatively. Indeed, behavioral risk factors, such as cigarette smoking, alcohol and drug use, sexually transmitted infections, poor food intake, and obesity, are all associated with preterm birth (Kramer et al. 2001).

- *Obstetric history*:
  - *Interval between pregnancies*: An interpregnancy interval of less than 6 months confers a greater than twofold increased risk of PTB (Smith et al. 2003). Indeed, Caesarean delivery in the first pregnancy and short interpregnancy interval <18 months are significant risk factors for term-preterm sequence (Wong et al. 2015). Furthermore, women whose first birth was preterm are far more likely to have a short interval than women who had a term first birth, thus compounding the risk.
  - *Previous PTB*: The recurrence risk in women with a previous PTB ranges from 15% to 50%, depending on the number and gestational age of previous deliveries (Kazemier et al. 2014). The number, sequence, and weeks of gestation of previous births all affect the risk of recurrence, which ranges from less than 15% among women with one preterm birth after 32 weeks of gestation followed by a term delivery to nearly 60% among women with a history of two or more preterm births (Goldenberg et al. 2006). Based on the clinical presentation of a prior spontaneous preterm birth, patients with a history of advanced cervical dilatation are at an increased risk of having recurrent preterm birth and cervical shortening in a subsequent pregnancy compared with women with prior preterm birth associated PPROM or preterm labor (Drassinower et al. 2015). Spontaneous preterm births are also more common among women with a history of giving birth between 16 and 20 weeks of gestation or with a history of stillbirth before 24 weeks of gestation (McManemy et al. 2007; Edlow et al. 2007).

2.3.1.2 Maternal Disorders

- *Systemic diseases*: Thyroid diseases, asthma, diabetes, and hypertension are associated with increased rates of PTB (Czeizel and Bánhidy 2011; Bramham et al. 2014; American College of Obstetricians and Gynecologists 2015; Gage et al. 2015).
- *Local or systemic infections*: Infections, such as pyelonephritis and asymptomatic bacteriuria, pneumonia, and appendicitis, are associated with PTB (Wing et al. 2014). Periodontal disease appears to cause an inflammatory condition, predisposing to increased risk of PTB (Horton and Boggess 2012).
- *Reproductive disorders*: Women with uterine fibroids, endometriosis, adenomyosis, and polycystic ovary syndrome (PCOS) have an increased risk of poor obstetric outcome, including preterm birth (Conti et al. 2013, 2015; Naver et al. 2014; Palomba et al. 2015; Juang et al. 2007). Inflammatory, endocrine, and metabolic aberrations associated with these disorders are implicated in the pathogenesis of obstetric complications (Vannuccini et al. 2016). Infertility and subfertility itself are also risk factors for preterm birth (DoPierala et al. 2015; Stern et al. 2015).
- *Previous cervical surgery*: Cervical surgery is associated with spontaneous preterm birth; however, it is unclear whether this increased risk is due to the surgery itself or to the cervical intraepithelial neoplasia underlying the surgery (Bruinsma and Quinn 2011). Women who attend colposcopy for precancerous changes in cervix are at a higher risk of a subsequent preterm birth (regardless of whether or not they are treated) (Castanon et al. 2012, 2015). The risk is greater still among those who receive an excisional treatment (biopsy sample or loop electrocautery excision), and it is particularly high when the depth of the tissue excised is ≥15 mm (Castanon et al. 2014).

2.3.1.3 External Factors

- *Stress*: Mothers experiencing psychological stress are at increased risk of PTB (Dole et al. 2003). Although the mechanism underlying the link between psychological or social stress and increased risk of PTB is unknown, a role has been proposed for corticotrophin-releasing hormone (Voltolini and Petraglia 2014; Ruiz et al. 2015). Moreover, exposure to two or more adverse childhood experiences was associated with a twofold risk of preterm birth in adulthood, demonstrating that stressors throughout life can have a significant effect on pregnancy outcomes (Christiaens et al. 2015).

- *Smoking*: Tobacco use increases the risk of PTB. Both nicotine and carbon monoxide are powerful vasoconstrictors and are associated with placental damage and decreased uteroplacental blood flow, leading to fetal growth restriction and PTB (Shah and Bracken 2000; Ko et al. 2014; Ion et al. 2015).
- *Drugs and substances of abuse*: Several maternal drugs affect the developing fetus, and the baby after birth may manifest signs attributable to withdrawal. Maternal cocaine, opiate, and diazepam use are particularly relevant, as a history of excessive alcohol ingestion, especially binge drinking (Bonello et al. 2014).

2.3.1.4 Pregnancy-Associated Risk Factors

- *Assisted reproductive technologies (ART)*: Pregnancies from assisted conception are at increased risk of both spontaneous and indicated preterm births than those with natural conception. In vitro techniques, ovarian stimulation, culture media, and possibly additional freezing or vitrification procedures, together with infertility itself, seem to play a role in the pathogenesis of adverse obstetric outcome in ART pregnancies (Pinborg et al. 2013; Messerlian et al. 2013; Dunietz et al. 2015).
- *Multiple pregnancy*: Multiple gestations carry a risk of PTB and result in 15–20% of all PTB. Uterine overdistension, resulting in contractions and PPROM, is believed to be the causative mechanism for the rate of increased spontaneous PTB (Voltolini et al. 2013).
- *Bacterial vaginosis (BV) and intrauterine infection*: Inflammation, whether or not related to infection, is one of the best-studied pathways in humans and animal models of PTB. Infection commonly ascends from the vagina and cervix into the choriodecidual space, affecting the myometrium, fetal membranes, and amniotic fluid. Ascending bacterial infection is implicated in about 40–50% of preterm births. Infection may infrequently enter the uterus by the hematogenous route, through retrograde seeding via the fallopian tube (Witkin 2015). Intrauterine infection is an important mechanism leading to PTB through the activation of the innate immune system. Microbial endotoxins and proinflammatory cytokines stimulate the production of prostaglandins and matrix-degrading enzymes. Prostaglandins stimulate uterine contractility, whereas degradation of the extracellular matrix in the fetal membranes leads to PPROM (Kemp 2014). Recent studies have examined the role of the vaginal, gastrointestinal, and oral microbiome and possible associations with PTB. Advances in DNA sequencing technology have dramatically improved our understanding of the maternal microbiome and its impact on pregnancy and PTB, far beyond what traditional culture-based technology has done to date (Fox and Eichelberger 2015). Metagenomic studies have begun to characterize the healthy vaginal and gut microbiomes in the nongravid and gravid state, as well as the rich diverse placental microbiome. It has been proposed that the increased stability of the vaginal microbiome during pregnancy may play a protective role in the prevention of ascending vaginal infection by means of the dominance of lactobacilli (Romero et al. 2014b). Disturbances in lactobacilli in the vaginal microbiome often lead to dysbiosis and bacterial vaginosis (BV), a known risk factor for preterm delivery. Common bacterial species identified in PTB-associated infections include *Ureaplasma urealyticum*, *Mycoplasma hominis*, *Bacteroides* spp., *Gardnerella vaginalis*, and *Fusobacterium nucleatum*. These organisms typically display low virulence unless they reach the intrauterine environment (Mysorekar and Cao 2014; Petricevic et al. 2014).
- *Vaginal bleeding*: Uterine contractions and PTB can be instigated by bleeding between the chorion and decidua at the placental bed, causing overt or subclinical separation of the

placenta from the implantation site at the uterine wall, clinically known as abruption (Norman et al. 2010). The plasma protease thrombin plays a central role in the signaling cascade that is initiated by blood in the subchorionic space. Vaginal bleeding caused by placental abruption is associated with a very high risk of PTB. Similarly, placental implantation abnormalities such as placenta previa, placenta accreta, and vasa previa are associated with increased risk of preterm birth (Vahanian et al. 2015). However, bleeding in the first and second trimesters, that is not associated with either placental abruption or placental abnormalities, is also associated with subsequent PTB (Krupa et al. 2006).

- *Short cervix and cervical insufficiency*: At the beginning of pregnancy, the etiology of a short cervix differs from what occurs in the middle and at the end of pregnancy. A cervix that starts to diminish at the beginning of pregnancy may be a sign of previous damage to the cervix, such as through surgery (conization or excision using a LEEP loop) or due to uterine malformations (Vaisbuch et al. 2010; Poon et al. 2012; Miller et al. 2015). In the second trimester of pregnancy, isthmocervical incompetence is the most important cause of cervical shortening, thereby causing late abortions and spontaneous preterm delivery. This may be congenital (primary) or be acquired (secondary) through trauma to the isthmocervical region, such as untimely cervical dilatation, application of a high forceps, or amputation. However, distinguishing cervical insufficiency from cervical shortening attributable to other causes has proven difficult, and the exact contribution to preterm birth is unknown. Short cervical length (i.e., values below the tenth percentile for gestational age), as measured with the use of transvaginal ultrasonography at 18–24 weeks of gestation, is a consistent predictor of an increased risk of preterm delivery, regardless of other factors. The risk increases as cervical length decreases in the second trimester; the risk associated with a cervical length below the tenth percentile (25 mm) is 25–30%, and the risk associated with a cervical length at or below the third percentile (15 mm) is 50% (Hughes et al. 2015).

2.3.1.5 Biochemical Markers

Biological fluids (amniotic fluid, urine, cervical mucus, vaginal secretions, serum or plasma, and saliva) have been used to assess the value of biomarkers for the prediction of PTB. These body fluids provide rich sources of proteins and metabolites that vary in concentration in response to pregnancy and adverse pregnancy states. With the development of genomic and proteomic technologies over the past two decades, the simultaneous screening of thousands of genes and gene products from small samples of tissue or body fluid has become possible. Hormones and inflammatory and angiogenic mediators are implicated in PTB pathogenesis. However, it has becoming evident that single biomarker approaches for the early detection of preterm birth may never achieve the desired diagnostic efficiency (Klein et al. 2014; De Bonis et al. 2012).

There are two commonly used clinical biomarker tests for the prediction of preterm labor, namely, fetal fibronectin (fFN) and phosphorylated insulin-like growth factor binding protein-1 (phIGFBP1). The most useful biochemical PTB predictor is fetal fibronectin, a glycoprotein that when present in cervicovaginal fluid is a marker of choriodecidual disruption (Goldenberg et al. 1996). Although fetal fibronectin is normally absent from cervicovaginal secretions from 24 weeks until term, 3–4% of women undergoing routine screening at 24–26 weeks are positive and at increased risk of PTB. Owing to its high negative predictive value, a negative fFN result has been shown to reduce unnecessary interventions, change patient management, and reduce healthcare costs, by allowing early reassurance and return to normal care pathways, while care can be concentrated on those at risk. Indeed, the fFN test appears to be more informative in predicting spontaneous preterm birth within the 7–14 days in women presenting with threatened preterm labor, due to its generally poor positive predictive value (Foster and Shennan 2014).

phIGFBP1 is secreted by decidual cells and leaks into cervical secretions when fetal membranes detach from decidua. It has been used to clinically assess cervical maturation. Clinical diagnostic trials indicate that, like fFN, phIGFBP1 is a good negative predictor of preterm birth (92% specificity) but lacks suitable sensitivity and positive predictive value in asymptomatic women (Conde-Agudelo and Romero 2015).

2.3.1.6 Biophysical Markers

Ultrasound measurement of uterine cervical length can be useful in evaluating the likelihood of early labor in those women known to be at increased risk for prematurity (Hughes et al. 2015). A statistically significant inverse relationship between cervical length seen on transvaginal ultrasonography in the second trimester and the risk of preterm delivery has been demonstrated in both low-risk asymptomatic single pregnancies and high-risk patients, including those with previous preterm delivery. The risk of preterm delivery varies as a function of the gestational age at the time of diagnosing the cervical shortening. Almost two-thirds of the women diagnosed with a short cervix before the 20th week of pregnancy will deliver at the threshold of viability (<24 weeks of gestation), and less than one quarter of them will still be pregnant when the 28th week of gestation is completed. Between 22 and 30 weeks, the tenth percentile for cervical length is 25 mm, and a length less than this measurement is significantly associated with preterm birth. Women with a history of preterm birth and a cervical length less than 25 mm are 3.3–4.5 times more likely to experience preterm birth than the general population (Iams et al. 1996; Hibbard et al. 2000).

2.4 Preeclampsia

PE is defined as persistent blood pressure elevation, edema, and proteinuria first diagnosed after 20 weeks of gestation. The minimal criteria for the diagnosis of PE are proteinuria, defined as 300 mg or more of urinary protein excretion per 24 h, and hypertension, defined as blood pressure of 140/90 mmHg or higher (Sibai et al. 2005). PE affects 5–7% of all pregnancies and is responsible for 7–15% of maternal mortality. Severe and/or early-onset PE is an important cause of fetal and maternal morbidity and mortality. Neonatal outcomes are directly related to iatrogenic prematurity, although uteroplacental insufficiency may also be associated with the disease. The only known cure is cessation of pregnancy, although temporizing measures are often undertaken (Sibai 2005; Steegers et al. 2010). In general, the maternal risk factor profiles vary between early-onset PE (<32 weeks) and late-onset PE. This has led to the view that early and late PE may be different diseases. An alternative view is that PE is a spectrum disorder, the degree of which is reflected in gestational age at the time of delivery (Poon and Nicolaides 2014).

The exact cause of preeclampsia is currently unknown, but there is a consensus that the placenta plays a cardinal role in the pathogenesis of preeclampsia because delivery of the placenta resolves the clinical symptoms. Changes in the oxygenation levels of the placenta due to failure of spiral artery transformation are thought to be responsible for the underlying pathology of preeclampsia. This syndrome is thought to occur in two stages with abnormal placentation leading to a maternal inflammatory response. In preeclampsia, cytotrophoblast invasion of the interstitial uterine compartment is frequently shallow, and in many locations spiral artery invasion is incomplete. There are many fewer endovascular cytotrophoblasts, and some vessels retain portions of their endothelial lining with relatively intact muscular coats, showing deficits in the differentiation program that enables cytotrophoblast invasion of the uterine wall (Fisher 2015).

Recent discoveries of an imbalance in antiangiogenic factors and loss of cytoprotective mechanisms in preeclamptic placentas have provided new insights into the pathophysiology of PE. Systemic maternal vascular dysfunction seems to be a major phenotype of pregnancies with preeclampsia, contributing to increased peripheral vascular resistance, maternal hypertension, and proteinuria. The mechanisms of systemic vascular dysfunction in preeclamptic pregnancies involve an imbalance in the production of constrictors and dilators in vascular cells, hyperresponsiveness to constrictor stimuli, reduced endothelium-dependent dilation, and oxidative stress (Goulopoulou and Davidge 2015).

2.4.1 Risk Factors for Preeclampsia

Early identification of women at risk for preeclampsia (before 13 weeks) is a core tenet of management. Several studies identified risk factors for early detection of high risk women (Table 2) (Dekker and Sibai 2001; Duckitt and Harrington 2005).

2.4.1.1 Preconceptional Factors

- *Age*: The risk of preeclampsia increases by 30% for every additional year of age past 34. Women aged ≥40 had approximately twice the risk of developing preeclampsia (Lamminpää et al. 2012).
- *Nulliparity*: Nulliparous women have almost three times the risk for preeclampsia, as consequence of an abnormal response to paternal antigens in fetoplacental unit (Bdolah et al. 2014).
- *A family history of preeclampsia*: Severe PE and eclampsia have a familial occurrence. A family history of PE is associated with a threefold increased risk of PE and a fourfold increased risk of severe PE (North et al. 2011).

Table 2 Risk factors for preeclampsia

Preconceptional
Age
Nulliparity
Previous preeclampsia
Family history
Maternal disorders
Chronic hypertension and renal diseases
Obesity
Insulin resistance and diabetes
PCOS
Thrombophilic disorders
External factors
Stress
Pregnancy-associated risk factors
Oocyte donation
Multiple pregnancy
Congenital and chromosomal anomalies
Biophysical markers
Uterine artery Doppler study
Biochemical markers
hCG, activin A, inhibin A, PIGF, VEGF, sFlt-1, PAPP-A

- *Previous preeclampsia*: Mothers who had PE in their first pregnancy are at higher risk for the development of PE in a subsequent pregnancy, especially when PE is severe, occurs early during the pregnancy, or is associated with a low birth weight (Duckitt and Harrington 2005).
- *Time between pregnancies*: The association between risk of preeclampsia and interval is more significant than the association between risk and change of partner. The risk in a second or third pregnancy was directly related to the time elapsed since the previous delivery. When the interval was 10 years or more, the risk of preeclampsia was about the same as that in nulliparous women (Skjaerven et al. 2002).

2.4.1.2 Maternal Disorders

- *Chronic hypertension and renal disease*: The risk of developing superimposed PE is particularly increased in women with severe hypertension and in those with cardiovascular or renal disease. The incidence of superimposed PE increases in patients with chronic renal disease, especially if there is coexisting hypertension (Bramham et al. 2014).
- *Obesity, insulin resistance, PCOS, and diabetes*: Obesity, insulin resistance, and glucose intolerance are strongly associated with nonpregnant hypertension and PCOS. Essential hypertension is an insulin-resistant state itself. Obesity is probably the most common cause of insulin resistance and represents a risk factor for developing pregnancy-induced hypertension as well as PE (Bhattacharya et al. 2007; Spradley et al. 2015). In women with PCOS, the prevalence of gestational hypertension and preeclampsia is estimated at 10–30% and 8–15%, respectively. This prevalence may be even higher when PCOS women are obese and hyperinsulinemic (Petraglia et al. 2015). There is a certain degree of insulin resistance and hyperinsulinemia in preeclamptic women during pregnancy. The insulin resistance appears to be based on a higher mean body mass index in women with PE. Overt type 1 diabetes mellitus is associated with an increased incidence of PE (Colatrella et al. 2010).

- *Thrombophilic disorders*: Patients with severe early-onset PE often have hemostatic or metabolic abnormalities, which are associated with a tendency to vascular thrombosis. There is an increased incidence of activated protein C (aPC) resistance or factor V Leiden mutation in women with a history of PE and/or adverse perinatal outcome. Thus, women with familial thrombophilia are at increased risk not only of PE but also of fetal loss. Protein S deficiency and aPC resistance both result in an impaired aPC pathway. This impairment appears to be associated with a more aggressive course of the pathologic changes (thrombosis, acute atherosis) in the spiral arteries. Classic homocystinuria is the homozygous form of the autosomal recessively inherited cystathionine β-synthase deficiency. The incidence of hyperhomocysteinemia increases the risk for preeclampsia, mainly for severe early-onset PE (Berks et al. 2015).

2.4.1.3 External Factors

- *Stress*: Working women have 2.3 times the risk of developing PE compared with nonworking women (Klonoff-Cohen et al. 1996), even if more recent studies reported controversial results (Vollebregt et al. 2008).

2.4.1.4 Pregnancy-Associated Risk Factors

- *Oocyte donation*: The risk of preeclampsia is higher in oocyte donation pregnancies compared to other methods of assisted reproductive technology or natural conception (Masoudian et al. 2016).
- *Multiple pregnancy*: The incidence and severity of PE, the incidence of eclampsia, and the incidence of early-onset PE are significantly increased in patients with twin pregnancies, who have a fourfold increased risk of PE (Fox et al. 2014).
- *Congenital and chromosomal anomalies*: Malformations of the male genital apparatus should be considered as risk factors for PE (Vesce et al. 1997). There is also an increased incidence of preeclampsia in cases of fetal hydrops. Preeclampsia was significantly associated with noncritical heart defects in offspring, while PE before 34 weeks was associated with critical heart defects (Auger et al. 2015).

2.4.1.5 Biophysical Markers

Reduced uteroplacental blood flow and placental ischemia leads to the release of placental factors with detrimental effects on the maternal vascular endothelium, leading to a rise in blood pressure and changes in the uterine artery flow velocities. In the early days, the most important predictors of PE were those related to the early recognition of raised blood pressure in the mother (Wright et al. 2015); more recently, there has been detection of impaired uterine artery blood velocities and particularly their wave forms by uterine artery Doppler sonography (notch). Assessed during midtrimester, such abnormal Doppler findings indicate a substantially increased risk for the development of PE. Uterine artery Doppler sonography more accurately predicted PE than intrauterine growth retardation, and the most powerful Doppler index for predicting PE was an increased pulsatility with notching in the second trimester (Akolekar et al. 2013).

2.4.1.6 Biochemical Markers

Trophoblastic abnormalities play a central role in the development of PE and precede the appearance of clinical signs and symptoms; some placental hormones change in the maternal circulation, indicating altered placental function. The levels of several placental hormones are elevated in maternal serum before the diagnosis of PE, and these may be considered preclinical manifestations of the earlier stages of the disease. Such hormones have therefore been proposed as early predictive markers of PE (Anderson et al. 2012).

Women with PE in the third trimester have increased maternal serum human chorionic gonadotropin (hCG) levels. Maternal hCG levels are already increased in the second trimester in pregnancies that subsequently develop PE (Kalinderis et al. 2011; Bahado-Singh et al. 1998). Maternal serum activin A and inhibin A levels are increased in the presence of hypertensive disorders. Because activin A is involved in the control of trophoblast cell differentiation in the first trimester, altered expression of this protein may affect placental invasiveness, resembling the pathogenesis of PE. Inhibin A is elevated several weeks before the onset of clinical signs of PE. However, when both proteins are measured at 15–19 weeks, inhibin A appears to be more sensitive than activin A in predicting early-onset PE culminating with delivery before 34 weeks (Florio et al. 2001, 2002; Muttukrishna et al. 2000).

Phosphatidylinositol-glycan biosynthesis class F (PlGF) and vascular endothelial growth factor (VEGF) are potent angiogenic factors, inhibited by the soluble form of the vascular endothelial growth factor receptor-1 (sVEGFR-1), also known as soluble fms-like tyrosine kinase-1 (sFlt-1), which may be considered the most important candidate for preventing of PE and also targets placental growth factor. PlGF and VEGF-A are expressed by trophoblasts and show altered expression patterns in PE, and particularly lower PlGF. sFLT-1 serum concentrations are also increased in PE and correlate with the severity of the disease (Cooper et al. 1996; Andraweera et al. 2012; Smith et al. 2007b). Pregnancy-associated plasma protein A (PAPP-A) is a large glycoprotein complex, which is predominantly produced by the placenta. PAPP-A cleaves insulin-like growth factor binding protein (IGFBP)-4 and -5 and, thereby, modulates the activity of insulin-like growth factor (IGF)-1 and -2. Moreover, PAPP-A has been suggested to play a role in human implantation. Its circulating levels were found to be elevated after the onset of PE and lower in women who subsequently developed PE (Spencer et al. 2006, 2008).

In pregnancies that experienced preeclampsia, the values of uterine artery pulsatility index and mean arterial pressure were increased, and the values of serum pregnancy-associated plasma protein-A and placental growth factor were decreased. For all biomarkers, the deviation from normal was greater for early than late preeclampsia; therefore, the performance of screening was related inversely to the gestational age at which delivery became necessary for maternal and/or fetal indications. Combined screening by maternal factors, uterine artery pulsatility index, mean arterial pressure, and placental growth factor predicted 75% of PE (O'Gorman et al. 2016).

References

Akolekar R, Syngelaki A, Poon L et al (2013) Competing risks model in early screening for preeclampsia by biophysical and biochemical markers. Fetal Diagn Ther 33:8–15

American College of Obstetricians and Gynecologists (2015) Practice bulletin no. 148: thyroid disease in pregnancy. Obstet Gynecol 125:996–1005

Anderson UD, Olsson MG, Kristensen KH et al (2012) Review: biochemical markers to predict preeclampsia. Placenta 33(Suppl):S42–S47

Andraweera PH, Dekker GA, Laurence JA et al (2012) Placental expression of VEGF family mRNA in adverse pregnancy outcomes. Placenta 33:467–472

Auger N, Hansen AV, Mortensen L (2013) Contribution of maternal age to preterm birth rates in Denmark and Quebec, 1981–2008. Am J Public Health 103:e33–e38

Auger N, Fraser WD, Healy-Profitós J et al (2015) Association between preeclampsia and congenital heart defects. JAMA 314:1588–1598

Bahado-Singh RO, Oz U, Isozaki T et al (1998) Midtrimester urine human chorionic gonadotropin beta-subunit core fragment levels and the subsequent development of pre-eclampsia. Am J Obstet Gynecol 179:738–741

Bdolah Y, Elchalal U, Natanson-Yaron S, Yechiam H et al (2014) Relationship between nulliparity and preeclampsia may be explained by altered circulating soluble fms-like tyrosine kinase 1. Hypertens Pregnancy 33:250–259

Beck S, Wojdyla D, Say L et al (2010) The worldwide incidence of preterm birth: a systematic review of maternal mortality and morbidity. Bull World Health Organ 88:31–38

Berks D, Duvekot JJ, Basalan H et al (2015) Associations between phenotypes of preeclampsia and thrombophilia. Eur J Obstet Gynecol Reprod Biol 194:199–205

Bezold KY, Karjalainen MK, Hallman M et al (2013) The genomics of preterm birth: from animal models to human studies. Genome Med 5:34

Bhattacharya S, Campbell DM, Liston WA et al (2007) Effect of Body Mass Index on pregnancy outcomes in nulliparous women delivering singleton babies. BMC Public Health 7:168

Bloomfield FH (2011) How is maternal nutrition related to preterm birth? Annu Rev Nutr 31:235–261

Bonello MR, Xu F, Li Z et al (2014) Mental and behavioral disorders due to substance abuse and perinatal outcomes: a study based on linked population data in New South Wales, Australia. Int J Environ Res Public Health 11:4991–5005

Boyd HA, Poulsen G, Wohlfahrt J et al (2009) Maternal contributions to preterm delivery. Am J Epidemiol 170:1358–1364
Bramham K, Parnell B, Nelson-Piercy C, Seed PT et al (2014) Chronic hypertension and pregnancy outcomes: systematic review and meta-analysis. BMJ 348: g2301
Bruinsma FJ, Quinn MA (2011) The risk of preterm birth following treatment for precancerous changes in the cervix: a systematic review and meta-analysis. BJOG 118:1031–1041
Castanon A, Brocklehurst P, Evans H et al (2012) Risk of preterm birth after treatment for cervical intraepithelial neoplasia among women attending colposcopy in England: retrospective-prospective cohort study. BMJ 345:e5174
Castanon A, Landy R, Brocklehurst P et al (2014) Risk of preterm delivery with increasing depth of excision for cervical intraepithelial neoplasia in England: nested case–control study. BMJ 349:g6223
Castañon A, Landy R, Brocklehurst P, PaCT Study Group et al (2015) Is the increased risk of preterm birth following excision for cervical intraepithelial neoplasia restricted to the first birth post treatment? BJOG 122:1191–1199
Christiaens I, Hegadoren K, Olson DM (2015) Adverse childhood experiences are associated with spontaneous preterm birth: a case-control study. BMC Med 13:124
Cnattingius S, Villamor E, Johansson S et al (2013) Maternal obesity and risk of preterm delivery. JAMA 309:2362–2370
Colatrella A, Loguercio V, Mattei L et al (2010) Hypertension in diabetic pregnancy: impact and long-term outlook. Best Pract Res Clin Endocrinol Metab 24:635–651
Conde-Agudelo A, Romero R (2015) Cervical phosphorylated insulin-like growth factor binding protein-1 test for the prediction of preterm birth: a systematic review and metaanalysis. Am J Obstet Gynecol 214:57–73
Conti N, Tosti C, Pinzauti S et al (2013) Uterine fibroids affect pregnancy outcome in women over 30 years old: role of other risk factors. J Matern Fetal Neonatal Med 26:584–587
Conti N, Cevenini G, Vannuccini S et al (2015) Women with endometriosis at first pregnancy have an increased risk of adverse obstetric outcome. J Matern Fetal Neonatal Med 28:1795–1798
Cooper JC, Sharkey AM, Charnock-Jones DS et al (1996) VEGF mRNA levels in placentae from pregnancies complicated by pre-eclampsia. Br J Obstet Gynaecol 103:1191–1196
Czeizel AE, Bánhidy F (2011) Chronic hypertension in pregnancy. Curr Opin Obstet Gynecol 23:76–81
De Bonis M, Vellucci FL, Di Tommaso M et al (2012) Clinical use of placental hormones in pregnancy management. J Endocrinol Invest 8:776–781
Dekker G, Sibai B (2001) Primary, secondary, and tertiary prevention of pre-eclampsia. Lancet 357:209–215
Dole N, Savitz DA, Hertz-Picciotto I et al (2003) Maternal stress and preterm birth. Am J Epidemiol 157:14–24
DoPierala AL, Bhatta S, Raja EA et al (2015) Obstetric consequences of subfertility: a retrospective cohort study. BJOG 123:1320–8
Drassinower D, Običan SG, Siddiq Z et al (2015) Does the clinical presentation of a prior preterm birth predict risk in a subsequent pregnancy? Am J Obstet Gynecol 213:686.e1–686.e7
Duckitt K, Harrington D (2005) Risk factors for pre-eclampsia at antenatal booking: systematic review of controlled studies. BMJ 330:565
Dunietz GL, Holzman C, McKane P et al (2015) Assisted reproductive technology and the risk of preterm birth among primiparas. Fertil Steril 103:974–979
Edlow AG, Srinivas SK, Elovitz MA (2007) Second trimester loss and subsequent pregnancy outcomes: what is the real risk? Am J Obstet Gynecol 197:581.e1–581.e6
Fisher SJ (2015) Why is placentation abnormal in preeclampsia? Am J Obstet Gynecol 213(4 Suppl): S115–S122
Florio P, Cobellis L, Luisi S et al (2001) Changes in inhibins and activin secretion in healthy and pathological pregnancies. Mol Cell Endocrinol 180:123–130
Florio P, Ciarmela P, Luisi S et al (2002) Pre-eclampsia with fetal growth restriction: placental and serum activin A and inhibin A levels. Gynecol Endocrinol 16:365–372
Foster C, Shennan AH (2014) Fetal fibronectin as a biomarker of preterm labor: a review of the literature and advances in its clinical use. Biomark Med 8:471–484
Fox C, Eichelberger K (2015) Maternal microbiome and pregnancy outcomes. Fertil Steril 104:1358–1363
Fox NS, Roman AS, Saltzman DH et al (2014) Risk factors for preeclampsia in twin pregnancies. Am J Perinatol 31:163–166
Gage S, Kan P, Lee HC et al (2015) Maternal asthma, preterm birth, and risk of bronchopulmonary dysplasia. J Pediatr 167:875–880
Goldenberg RL, Mercer BM, Meis PJ et al (1996) The preterm prediction study: fetal fibronectin testing and spontaneous preterm birth. Obstet Gynecol 87:643–648
Goldenberg RL, Goepfert AR, Ramsey PS (2005) Biochemical markers for the prediction of preterm birth. Am J Obstet Gynecol 192:36–46
Goldenberg RL, Andrews WW, Faye O et al (2006) The Alabama preterm birth project: placental histology in recurrent spontaneous and indicated preterm birth. Am J Obstet Gynecol 195:792–796
Goldenberg RL, Culhane JF, Iams JD, Romero R (2008) Epidemiology and causes of preterm birth. Lancet 371:75–84
Goldenberg RL, Gravett MG, Iams J et al (2012) The preterm birth syndrome: issues to consider in creating a classification system. Am J Obstet Gynecol 206:113–118
Goulopoulou S, Davidge ST (2015) Molecular mechanisms of maternal vascular dysfunction in preeclampsia. Trends Mol Med 21:88–97

Haataja R, Karjalainen MK, Luukkonen A et al (2011) Mapping a new spontaneous preterm birth susceptibility gene, IGF1R, using linkage, haplotype sharing, and association analysis. PLoS Genet 7:e1001293

Healy AJ, Malone FD, Sullivan LM et al (2006) Early access to prenatal care: implications for racial disparity in perinatal mortality. Obstet Gynecol 107:625–631

Hibbard JU, Tart M, Moawad AH (2000) Cervical length at 16–22 weeks' gestation and risk for preterm delivery. Obstet Gynecol 96:972–978

Horton AL, Boggess KA (2012) Periodontal disease and preterm birth. Obstet Gynecol Clin N Am 39:17–23

Hughes K, Kane SC, Araujo Júnior E et al (2015) Cervical length as a predictor of spontaneous preterm birth in high-risk singleton pregnancy – current knowledge. Ultrasound Obstet Gynecol 48:7–15

Iams JD (2014) Prevention of preterm parturition. N Engl J Med 370:1861

Iams JD, Goldenberg RL, Meis PJ et al (1996) The length of the cervix and the risk of spontaneous premature delivery. N Engl J Med 334:567–572

Iams JD, Romero R, Culhane JF, Goldenberg RL (2008) Primary, secondary, and tertiary interventions to reduce the morbidity and mortality of preterm birth. Lancet 371:164–175

Institute of Medicine (US) Committee on Understanding Premature Birth and Assuring Healthy Outcomes, Behrman RE, Butler AS (eds) (2007) Preterm birth: causes, consequences, and prevention. National Academies Press, Washington, DC

Ion RC, Wills AK, Bernal AL (2015) Environmental tobacco smoke exposure in pregnancy is associated with earlier delivery and reduced birth weight. Reprod Sci 22:1603–1611

Juang CM, Chou P, Yen MS et al (2007) Adenomyosis and risk of preterm delivery. BJOG 114:165–169

Kalinderis M, Papanikolaou A, Kalinderi K et al (2011) Elevated serum levels of interleukin-6, interleukin-1β and human chorionic gonadotropin in pre-eclampsia. Am J Reprod Immunol 66:468–475

Kazemier BM, Buijs PE, Mignini L et al (2014) Impact of obstetric history on the risk of spontaneous preterm birth in singleton and multiple pregnancies: a systematic review. BJOG 121:1197–1208

Kemp MW (2014) Preterm birth, intrauterine infection, and fetal inflammation. Front Immunol 5:574

Klein J, Buffin-Meyer B, Mullen W et al (2014) Clinical proteomics in obstetrics and neonatology. Expert Rev Proteomics 11:75–89

Klonoff-Cohen HS, Cross JL, Pieper CF (1996) Job stress and preeclampsia. Epidemiology 7:245–249

Ko TJ, Tsai LY, Chu LC et al (2014) Parental smoking during pregnancy and its association with low birth weight, small for gestational age, and preterm birth offspring: a birth cohort study. Pediatr Neonatol 55:20–27

Kramer MS, Goulet L, Lydon J et al (2001) Socio-economic disparities in preterm birth: causal pathways and mechanisms. Paed Perinat Epidemiol 15:104–123

Krupa FG, Faltin D, Cecatti JG et al (2006) Predictors of preterm birth. Int J Gynaecol Obstet 94:5–11

Lamminpää R, Vehviläinen-Julkunen K, Gissler M et al (2012) Preeclampsia complicated by advanced maternal age: a registry-based study on primiparous women in Finland 1997–2008. BMC Pregnancy Childbirth 12:47

Liu L, Johnson HL, Cousens S, Child Health Epidemiology Reference Group of WHO and UNICEF et al (2010) Global, regional, and national causes of child mortality: an updated systematic analysis for 2010 with time trends since 2000. Lancet 380:1308

Lockwood CJ (2002) Predicting premature delivery-no easy task. N Engl J Med 346:282–284

Lynch AM, Hart JE, Agwu OC et al (2014) Association of extremes of prepregnancy BMI with the clinical presentations of preterm birth. Am J Obstet Gynecol 210: e19, 428

Masoudian P, Nasr A, De Nanassy J et al (2016) Oocyte donation pregnancies and the risk of preeclampsia or gestational hypertension: a systematic review and meta-analysis. Am J Obstet Gynecol 214:328–39

McDonald SD, Han Z, Mulla S, Knowledge Synthesis Group et al (2010) Overweight and obesity in mothers and risk of preterm birth and low birth weight infants: systematic review and meta-analyses. BMJ 341:c3428

McManemy J, Cooke E, Amon E et al (2007) Recurrence risk for preterm delivery. Am J Obstet Gynecol 196:576.e1–576.e6

Menon R (2008) Spontaneous preterm birth, a clinical dilemma: aetiological, pathophysiological and genetic heterogeneities and racial disparity. Acta Obstet Gynecol Scand 87:590–600

Messerlian C, Maclagan L, Basso O (2013) Infertility and the risk of adverse pregnancy outcomes: a systematic review and meta-analysis. Hum Reprod 28:125–137

Miller ES, Sakowicz A, Grobman WA (2015) The association between cervical dysplasia, a short cervix, and preterm birth. Am J Obstet Gynecol 213:543.e1–543.e4

Muttukrishna S, North RA, Morris J et al (2000) Serum inhibin A and activin A are elevated prior to the onset of pre-eclampsia. Hum Reprod 15:1640–1645

Mwaniki MK, Atieno M, Lawn JE et al (2012) Long-term neurodevelopmental outcomes after intrauterine and neonatal insults: a systematic review. Lancet 379:445–452

Mysorekar I, Cao B (2014) Microbiome in parturition and preterm birth. Semin Reprod Med 32:50–55

Naver KV, Grinsted J, Larsen SO et al (2014) Increased risk of preterm delivery and pre-eclampsia in women with polycystic ovary syndrome and hyperandrogenaemia. BJOG 121:575–581

Newnham JP, Dickinson JE, Hart RJ et al (2014) Strategies to prevent preterm birth. Front Immunol 5:584

Norman SM, Odibo AO, Macones GA et al (2010) Ultrasound detected subchorionic hemorrhage and the obstetric implications. Obstet Gynecol 116:311–315

North RA, McCowan LM, Dekker GA et al (2011) Clinical risk prediction for pre-eclampsia in nulliparous women: development of model in international prospective cohort. BMJ 342:d1875

O'Gorman N, Wright D, Syngelaki A et al (2016) Competing risks model in screening for preeclampsia by maternal factors and biomarkers at 11–13 weeks gestation. Am J Obstet Gynecol 214:103.e1–103.e12

Palomba S, de Wilde MA, Falbo A et al (2015) Pregnancy complications in women with polycystic ovary syndrome. Hum Reprod Update 21:575–592

Petraglia F, Arcuri F, de Ziegler D et al (2012) Inflammation: a link between endometriosis and preterm birth. Fertil Steril 98:36–40

Petraglia F, Orlandini C, Vannuccini S et al (2015) PCOS and pregnancy: impact of endocrine and metabolic factors. In: Ferrazzi E, Sears B (eds) Metabolic syndrome and complications of pregnancy. Springer International Publishing, Cham, pp 91–102

Petricevic L, Domig K, Nierscher F et al (2014) Characterisation of the vaginal Lactobacillus microbiota associated with preterm delivery. Sci Rep 4:5136

Pinborg A, Wennerholm UB, Romundstad LB et al (2013) Why do singletons conceived after assisted reproduction technology have adverse perinatal outcome? Systematic review and meta-analysis. Hum Reprod Update 19:87–104

Plunkett J, Muglia LJ (2008) Genetic contributions to preterm birth: implications from epidemiological and genetic association studies. Ann Med 40:167–195

Plunkett J, Borecki I, Morgan T et al (2008) Population-based estimate of sibling risk for preterm birth, preterm premature rupture of membranes, placental abruption and pre-eclampsia. BMC Genet 9:44

Poon LC, Nicolaides KH (2014) Early prediction of pre-eclampsia. Obstet Gynecol Int 2014:297397

Poon LC, Savvas M, Zamblera D et al (2012) Large loop excision of transformation zone and cervical length in the prediction of spontaneous preterm delivery. BJOG 119:692–698

Romero R, Dey SK, Fisher SJ (2014a) Preterm labor: one syndrome, many causes. Science 345:760–765

Romero R, Hassan S, Gajer P et al (2014b) The vaginal microbiota of pregnant women who subsequently have spontaneous preterm labor and delivery and those with a normal delivery at term. Microbiome 2:18

Rubens CE, Sadovsky Y, Muglia L et al (2014) Prevention of preterm birth: harnessing science to address the global epidemic. Sci Transl Med 6:262sr5

Ruiz RJ, Dwivedi AK, Mallawaarachichi I et al (2015) Psychological, cultural and neuroendocrine profiles of risk for preterm birth. BMC Pregnancy Childbirth 15:204

Shah NR, Bracken MB (2000) A systematic review and meta-analysis of prospective studies on the association between maternal cigarette smoking and preterm delivery. Am J Obstet Gynecol 182:465–472

Sibai BM (2005) Diagnosis, prevention, and management of eclampsia. Obstet Gynecol 105:402–410

Sibai M, Dekker G, Kupferminc M (2005) Pre-eclampsia. Lancet 365:785–799

Skjaerven R, Wilcox AJ, Lie RT (2002) The interval between pregnancies and the risk of preeclampsia. N Engl J Med 346:33–38

Smith GC, Pell JP, Dobbie R (2003) Interpregnancy interval and risk of preterm birth and neonatal death: retrospective cohort study. BMJ 327:313

Smith LK, Draper ES, Manktelow BN et al (2007a) Socioeconomic inequalities in very preterm birth rates. Arch Dis Child Fetal Neonatal Ed 92:F11–F14

Smith GC, Crossley JA, Aitken DA et al (2007b) Circulating angiogenic factors in early pregnancy and the risk of preeclampsia, intrauterine growth restriction, spontaneous preterm birth, and stillbirth. Obstet Gynecol 109:1316–1324

Spencer K, Yu CK, Savvidou M et al (2006) Prediction of pre-eclampsia by uterine artery Doppler ultrasonography and maternal serum pregnancy-associated plasma protein-A, free beta-human chorionic gonadotropin, activin A and inhibin A at 22 + 0 to 24 + 6 weeks' gestation. Ultrasound Obstet Gynecol 27:658–663

Spencer K, Cowans NJ, Nicolaides KH (2008) Low levels of maternal serum PAPP-A in the first trimester and the risk of pre-eclampsia. Prenat Diagn 28:7–10

Spradley FT, Palei AC, Granger JP (2015) Immune mechanisms linking obesity and preeclampsia. Biomolecules 5:3142–3176

Steegers EA, von Dadelszen P, Duvekot JJ et al (2010) Pre-eclampsia. Lancet 376:631–644

Stern JE, Luke B, Tobias M et al (2015) Adverse pregnancy and birth outcomes associated with underlying diagnosis with and without assisted reproductive technology treatment. Fertil Steril 103:1438–1445

Torricelli M, Voltolini C, De Bonis M et al (2012) The identification of high risk pregnancy: a new challenge in obstetrics. J Matern Fetal Neonatal Med 25(Suppl 1):2–5

Vahanian SA, Lavery JA, Ananth CV et al (2015) Placental implantation abnormalities and risk of preterm delivery: a systematic review and metaanalysis. Am J Obstet Gynecol 213(4 Suppl):S78–S90

Vaisbuch E, Romero R, Erez O et al (2010) Clinical significance of early (<20 weeks) vs. late (20–24 weeks) detection of sonographic short cervix in asymptomatic women in the mid-trimester. Ultrasound Obstet Gynecol 36:471–481

Vannuccini S, Clifton VL, Fraser IS et al (2016) Infertility and reproductive disorders: impact of hormonal and inflammatory mechanisms on pregnancy outcome. Hum Reprod Update 22:104–115

Vesce F, Farina A, Giorgetti M et al (1997) Increased incidence of pre-eclampsia in pregnancies complicated by fetal malformations. Gynecol Obstet Invest 44:107–111

Vollebregt KC, van der Wal MF, Wolf H et al (2008) Is psychosocial stress in first ongoing pregnancies associated with pre-eclampsia and gestational hypertension? BJOG 115:607–615

Voltolini C, Petraglia F (2014) Neuroendocrinology of pregnancy and parturition. Handb Clin Neurol 124:17–36

Voltolini C, Torricelli M, Conti N et al (2013) Understanding spontaneous preterm birth: from underlying mechanisms to predictive and preventive interventions. Reprod Sci 20:1274–1292

Wing DA, Fassett MJ, Getahun D (2014) Acute pyelonephritis in pregnancy: an 18-year retrospective analysis. Am J Obstet Gynecol 210:219.e1–219.e6

Witkin SS (2015) The vaginal microbiome, vaginal antimicrobial defence mechanisms and the clinical challenge of reducing infection-related preterm birth. BJOG 122:213–218

Wong LF, Wilkes J, Korgenski K et al (2015) Risk factors associated with preterm birth after a prior term delivery. BJOG 2015:28

Wright A, Wright D, Ispas CA et al (2015) Mean arterial pressure in the three trimesters of pregnancy: effects of maternal characteristics and medical history. Ultrasound Obstet Gynecol 45:698–706

Wu W, Witherspoon DJ, Fraser A et al (2015) The heritability of gestational age in a two-million member cohort: implications for spontaneous preterm birth. Hum Genet 134:803–808

Epigenetic Mechanisms

3

Felicia M. Low and Peter D. Gluckman

Contents

Abstract

Epidemiological and experimental studies have provided considerable evidence that early environmental cues may influence an individual's susceptibility to disease in later life. Organisms have evolved with the capacity for developmental plasticity in order to match their developmental trajectory to the environment, and this adaptive response is driven in part by epigenetic mechanisms. However, a mismatch between the induced phenotype and mature environment contributes to an increased propensity toward developing chronic noncommunicable disease. In this chapter we describe several epigenetic mechanisms and some diseases that arise from non-environmentally induced epigenetic errors. We also provide an overview of the evidence that early-life environmental variations alter predisposition to chronic metabolic and cardiovascular disease at maturity and that this is mediated by epigenetic processes. The potential for reversibility of developmentally induced epigenetic changes is discussed.

The authors would like to thank Emilia Tng for assistance with research.

F. M. Low · P. D. Gluckman (✉)
Liggins Institute, University of Auckland, Auckland, New Zealand
e-mail: pd.gluckman@auckland.ac.nz

G. Buonocore et al. (eds.), *Neonatology*,
https://doi.org/10.1007/978-3-319-29489-6_152

3.1 Salient Points

- Early environmental cues may modulate disease risk in later life.
- Epigenetic mechanisms have been implicated in the development of cardiometabolic diseases and imprinting disorders.
- Epigenetic mechanisms include modification of histone proteins, DNA methylation, and noncoding RNA activity.
- Emerging evidence suggests that developmentally induced epigenetic changes may be reversed.

3.2 Introduction

While phenotypic variation such as disease vulnerability has traditionally been viewed as being determined by the interaction between genes and the environment, it is now clear that this is oversimplistic. *Developmental plasticity* describes the phenomenon whereby development of the phenotype from a given genotype is influenced by developmental experiences, and phenotypic variation in turn influences how the individual interacts with its mature environment, thus affecting disease risk. It is now recognized that developmental plasticity is underpinned at least in part by epigenetic processes (Low et al. 2011). These are the environmentally induced changes in patterns and regulation of gene expression brought about by a set of modifications in DNA and DNA-associated molecules, without changes in the base sequence. Epigenetic processes are phylogenetically old, and the mechanisms involved modulate both gene dosage and the conditions under which genes are expressed. Developmental plasticity is but one of several processes which are mediated by epigenetic mechanisms; in mammals other processes include transposable element suppression, cell differentiation, X-chromosome inactivation in females, and genomic imprinting.

This chapter describes several of the most extensively studied epigenetic mechanisms to date. Their involvement in the development of metabolic and cardiovascular diseases that stem from maladaptive fetal responses, and in imprinting disorders, which result from defects in the establishment or erasure of specific epigenetic marks, is discussed.

3.3 Epigenetic Mechanisms

Epigenetics, as used in the context of this chapter, refers to the molecular mechanisms that give rise to stable, mitotically heritable changes in gene function without a corresponding change in the DNA sequence. They include chromatin remodeling through histone modifications, DNA methylation, and posttranscriptional control by noncoding RNAs. The mammalian epigenome in early life appears susceptible to a range of physiological and pathophysiological cues that can have persistent effects on structure and function (Low et al. 2014).

3.3.1 Histone Modifications

In eukaryotes, DNA is wound around an octameric complex of histone proteins – two subunits each of the histones H2A, H2B, H3, and H4 – forming the nucleosome (Fig. 1a). Chromatin is formed when nucleosomes are packaged closely, strung together by double-stranded DNA (Fig. 1b). Therefore, certain covalent modifications such as acetylation, methylation, phosphorylation, sumoylation, ADP ribosylation, and glycosylation at specific amino acid residues on histone proteins can cause higher-order structural changes. This remodeling of chromatin can influence gene expression depending on whether the modifications result in chromatin condensation or unwinding and the subsequent accessibility of DNA to transcription factors (specific proteins which facilitate DNA recognition by RNA polymerases) and other DNA-associated complexes (Beaujean 2014).

Histone modifications occur on residues at the amino termini of histone tails via activity of enzymes such as histone acetyltransferases (HAT), histone deacetylases (HDAC), methyltransferases, kinases, and ubiquitilases. Some of the most common modifications include acetylation, which involves addition of CH_3OH in a reaction catalyzed

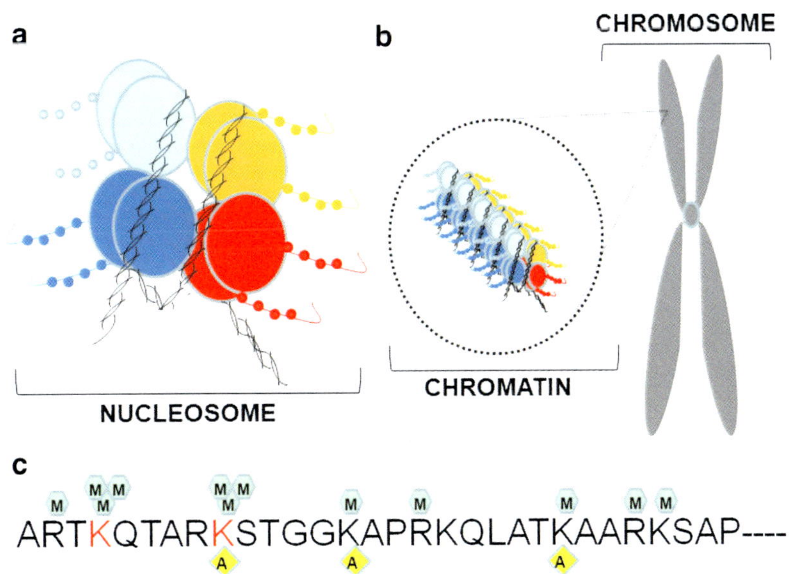

Fig. 1 (**a**) DNA is wound around an octameric complex of histones to form the nucleosome. The amino-terminal histone tails may be amenable to posttranslational modification. (**b**) Chromatin consists of multiple nucleosome units strung together by double-stranded DNA. (**c**) Schematic representation of known modifications of the first 30 amino acids at the amino-terminal tail of H3. The lysine residues at positions 4 and 9 are indicated in red. *M* methylation, *A* acetylation

by HAT, and methylation, which involves addition of CH_3 (Fig. 1c). The impact of each type of modification on chromatin configuration varies and often in a context-dependent manner (Bowman and Poirier 2015). Generally, increased acetylation leads to an increase in transcriptional activity (so-called active chromatin; see Fig. 3), whereas deacetylation, catalyzed by HDAC, leads to transcriptional repression (inactive chromatin) (Galvani and Thiriet 2015). Some histone marks may have opposing effects on gene expression depending on the residue modified; trimethylation of the ninth lysine residue on histone H3 (H3K9me3) favors gene silencing while that on the fourth residue (H3K4me3) promotes gene expression.

3.3.2 DNA Methylation

In mammals, DNA methylation involves the addition of a methyl group on the C5 position of cytosine residues in a process mediated by DNA methyltransferases (Schubeler 2015). This usually occurs in the context of CpG dinucleotides (cytosine linked to guanine by a phosphate group); non-CpG methylation has been observed in the mammalian brain and skeletal muscle, but its functional significance remains unclear. Genomic regions with an enrichment of CpG dinucleotides are called CpG islands, which are usually found at the promoter regions of many genes and are normally unmethylated.

DNA methylation exerts a regulatory effect in a combination of ways: modifying the binding affinity of transcription factors to their target sites on DNA and inhibiting RNA polymerase activity, recruiting methyl-CpG-binding proteins such as MeCP1 and MeCP2 that in turn attract associated proteins that cause the nucleosome to condense, thereby inhibiting transcription, and modulating the transcription of noncoding RNAs (Figs. 2 and 3). DNA methylation is commonly associated with gene silencing, although there is increasing evidence that this may be dependent on other factors such as the site of modification and CpG density. An individual's DNA methylome is established during embryogenesis and generally persists through the life course. However during early life, when levels of developmental plasticity tend to be highest, environmental cues may lead to persistent alteration of specific epigenetic marks with long-term phenotypic consequences (Low et al. 2014). Acute challenges later in life, such as those involving dietary or exercise challenges, may induce transient and reversible changes in methylation state.

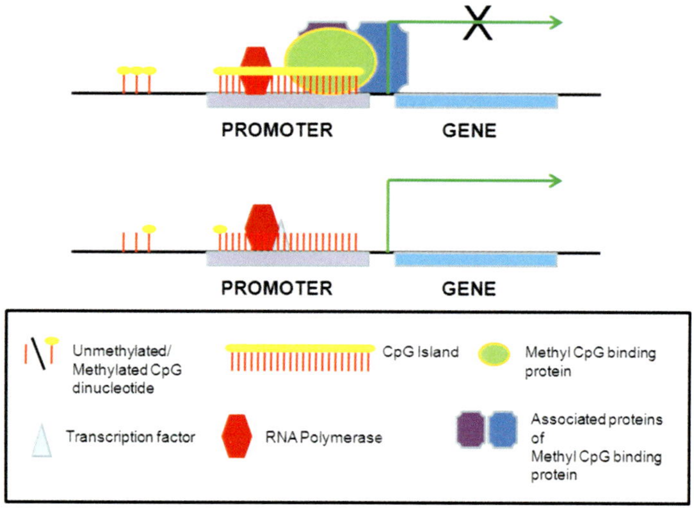

Fig. 2 Gene expression is modulated by nearby DNA sequences called promoters, which often include CpG islands. Methylated DNA (*top*) recruits methyl-CpG-binding proteins that in turn attract associated proteins to inhibit transcription. In contrast, unmethylated CpG islands (*bottom*) allow binding of RNA polymerase and transcription factors for initiation of transcription

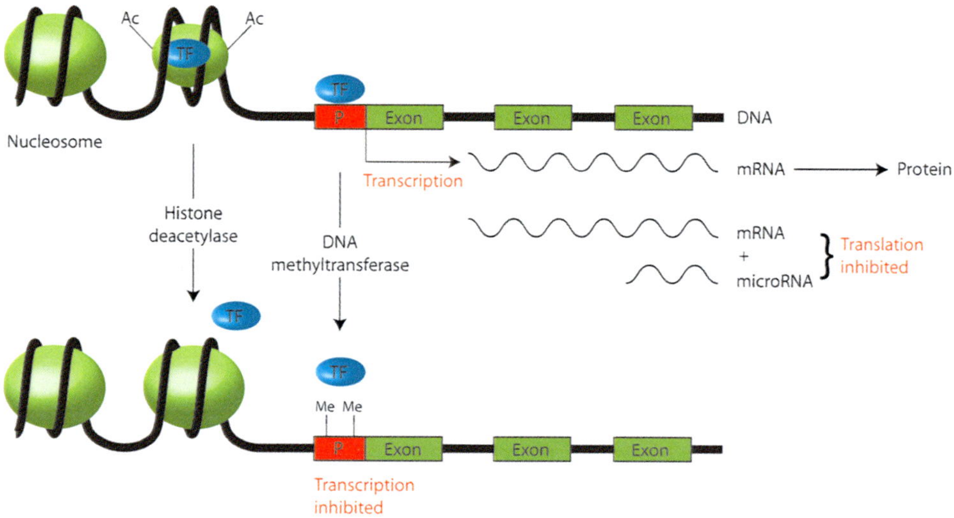

Fig. 3 In transcriptionally active chromatin (*top*), acetyl groups (Ac) on specific lysine residues of core histones in the nucleosome decrease their binding to DNA. The resulting "open" chromatin structure, coupled with the unmethylated state of CpG sequences in promoter regions of actively transcribed genes, facilitates access of transcription factors to DNA. Conversely, transcriptionally inactive chromatin (*bottom*) is characterized by histone deacetylation and promoter CpG methylation (Me) and hence decreased binding of transcriptional factors. miRNA molecules are among the ncRNAs that provide posttranscriptional epigenetic control, in this case by binding to complementary sequences at the 3′ end of mRNA, thus reducing the rate of protein synthesis (Modified from Gluckman et al. 2008, with permission)

3.3.3 Noncoding RNAs

The regulatory role of RNA began to emerge upon the discovery of RNAs that are not translated into proteins. These so-called noncoding RNAs (ncRNAs) are highly involved in myriad aspects of the regulation of cell differentiation and development through modulation of chromatin (Meller et al. 2015) and are further classified based on their length and mechanism of action. For example, microRNAs (miRNAs), which are approximately 22 nucleotides long, form base pairs with their target messenger RNA (mRNA) and promote its destabilization through the recruitment of effector proteins (Iwakawa and Tomari 2015). Gene expression can therefore be regulated at the post-transcriptional level (Fig. 3). Small nucleolar RNAs (snoRNAs), which range from about 60–140 nucleotides in length, regulate ribosome biogenesis as well as the alternative splicing and posttranscriptional modification of mRNA. SnoRNAs have been implicated in physiological functions that regulate feeding and growth and in pathological conditions such as the Prader-Willi and Angelman syndromes (see later) and cancer (Stepanov et al. 2015). The long noncoding RNAs (lncRNAs; >200 nucleotides in length) participate in numerous biological functions as diverse as genomic imprinting, protein assembly, and regulation of enzyme activity (Quinn and Chang 2016).

3.4 Genomic Imprinting

Some mammalian genes are expressed from only the maternal or paternal allele in a phenomenon known as genomic imprinting (Adalsteinsson and Ferguson-Smith 2014). Many imprinted genes play major roles in fetal growth and nutrition as they are required for the formation of a functional placenta. The first genes shown to be imprinted were the fetal growth factor *IGF2* and its receptor *IGF2R*. More than 100 imprinted genes have been identified to date in mice and humans, with a majority of them located in clusters throughout the genome. These clusters usually contain a few protein-coding genes and at least one ncRNA gene. Each gene cluster is regulated by a cis-acting element called an imprinting control region (ICR). Between them, the ICRs of the chromosome pair acquire different levels of methylation; this determines which allele is silent or active, thereby enabling imprinting control of all the genes within the cluster. The regulation of the imprinted mouse gene *Igf2r*, which encodes a growth suppressor, is shown in Fig. 4.

A consequence of genomic imprinting is that viable embryos must receive two haploid genome complements from each parent. Parent-specific imprinting marks are established during gametogenesis. Deletions, duplications, mutations, or alterations of imprinting of the only active allele, or loss of imprinting of the inactive allele, lead to an imbalance in the dosage of the gene product. The loss or gain of function of imprinted genes may then have phenotypic consequences.

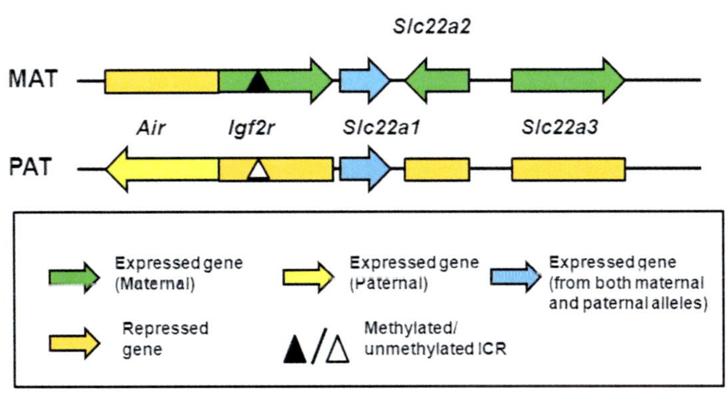

Fig. 4 The *Igf2r*/*Air* imprinted region. *Igf2r*, *Slc22a2*, and *Slc22a3* are maternally expressed protein-coding genes. *Slc22a1* is a biallelically expressed gene (expressed from both maternal and paternal alleles). *Air* is paternally expressed and encodes an ncRNA. The ICR contains the *Air* promoter and is methylated on the maternal allele. When the *Air* transcript is truncated, biallelic expression of *Igf2r*, *Slc22a2*, and *Slc22a3* is acquired, indicating a role for the *Air* ncRNA in the repression of the paternal alleles (Regha et al. 2006)

3.5 Developmental Plasticity, Epigenetics, and Disease Risk

The influence of the fetal environment on later-life susceptibility to chronic noncommunicable disease has been demonstrated by a multitude of epidemiological and experimental studies. In humans, in utero exposure to adverse conditions such as maternal undernutrition has been associated with hypertension, ischemic heart disease, glucose intolerance, insulin resistance, type 2 diabetes mellitus, obesity, and reproductive disorders in adulthood (Hanson and Gluckman 2014). In rodent studies used to simulate human pathology, manipulation of maternal nutrition (e.g., food intake or protein restriction), stress (e.g., via glucocorticoid administration), or physical condition (e.g., ligation of uterine arteries to reduce uteroplacental blood flow, thus inducing intrauterine growth restriction) can induce slowed fetal growth and permanent changes in cardiovascular and metabolic function in the offspring. The fetus' ability to respond to challenging environmental cues and adjust its developmental trajectory to match its environment reflects the processes of developmental plasticity. Although these responses are adaptive and aimed at promoting fitness later in life, a mismatch between the eventual phenotypic outcome and the later environment may manifest as chronic noncommunicable disease, and this is the basis for the "developmental origins of health and disease" paradigm (Gluckman et al. 2015). Indeed, there is growing evidence that developmental plasticity can account, at least in part, for a broad array of diseases.

The mechanistic basis of the effect of early environmental cues on subsequent susceptibility to metabolic disease has been extensively investigated in animals. For example, offspring of pregnant rats fed a low-protein diet during pregnancy developed hypertension and endothelial dysfunction. Concomitant changes were detected at the epigenetic and gene expression levels, including gene promoter hypomethylation, and accordingly protein over-expression, of the hepatic glucocorticoid receptor (*GR*) and peroxisome proliferator-activated receptor-α (*PPARα*) (Lillycrop et al. 2005). In sheep, exposure to periconceptional maternal undernutrition had effects on the epigenetic state of hypothalamic *GR* through alterations in promoter methylation, histone acetylation, and histone methylation (Begum et al. 2013). There is also increasing evidence for the role of epigenetic mechanisms in modulating clinically relevant traits in humans. For example, a 2011 study reported a graded association between neonatal methylation levels at a specific CpG site in the *RXRA* gene promoter and childhood fat mass; the effect size was large, with at least 25% of the variation in adiposity being attributed to methylation levels (Godfrey et al. 2011).

The epigenetic mechanisms underlying several imprinting disorders are well established. Human chromosome 15q11-q13 contains an imprinted cluster called the Prader-Willi/Angelman syndrome (PWS/AS) region. Incorrect establishment of imprinting in this region results in two distinct neurological disorders, Prader-Willi syndrome (PWS) and Angelman syndrome (AS). PWS is characterized by multiple symptoms including hypotonia, hyperphagia, obesity, and short stature. Psychomotor development is mildly affected and behavioral problems are evident. Patients with AS show a completely different phenotype characterized by severe mental retardation, absent speech, autistic-like behavior, severe epilepsy, and postnatal microcephaly. PWS is caused by the loss of the normal paternal contribution of gene expression, whereas AS is caused by the loss of the normal maternal contribution (Kalsner and Chamberlain 2015).

Other imprinting disorders include Silver-Russell syndrome and Beckwith-Wiedemann syndrome, which arise from imprinting defects in human chromosome imprinted region 11p15.

Rett syndrome is a devastating X-linked neurological disease that affects mostly females. Girls with this condition initially exhibit normal growth but show signs of deteriorating motor and cognitive function such as repetitive teeth-grinding, hand-wringing, and autistic-like behaviors sometime between the age of 6 and 18 months. This eventually culminates in severe intellectual disability. Rett syndrome is associated with loss of function mutations in *MECP2* (Liyanage and

Rastegar 2014). Absence of MeCP2 interferes with transcriptional regulation of the maternally imprinted *DLX5* through the loss of a silent chromatin-associated loop and the activation of additional neighboring chromatin (Horike et al. 2005). Mouse studies have also implicated aberrant lncRNA transcriptional patterns in the pathology of Rett syndrome. This disease thus illustrates how different epigenetic mechanisms – in this case loss of imprinting, chromatin remodeling, and ncRNA transcriptome dysregulation – can act in concert to cause various perturbations in gene expression, ultimately leading to a disease phenotype.

3.6 Reversibility of Developmentally Induced Epigenetic Changes

The "plastic" responses demonstrated by the developing fetus to cope with an adverse prenatal environment may not be irreversible. Numerous animal studies have demonstrated that maternal or postnatal dietary supplementation, and postnatal pharmacological interventions, may reverse the phenotypic fates induced in early development (reviewed in Vickers and Sloboda 2012). For example, offspring of undernourished rats develop obesity, hyperinsulinemia, and hyperleptinemia in adulthood, especially in the presence of a high-fat diet. Intervention by way of neonatal leptin administration to primed rat pups normalized weight gain, insulin levels, and leptin concentrations (Vickers et al. 2005). The corrective effects on phenotype were accompanied by normalized promoter methylation and expression of *PPARα*, reflecting an epigenetic basis for the physiological mechanisms that lead to either phenotype (Gluckman et al. 2007). Dietary supplements as varied as methyl donors, antioxidants, taurine, and n-3 fatty acids have been reported to ameliorate the adverse effects of a primed phenotype.

In the rat, variations in postnatal maternal care stably alter the development of behavioral and endocrine responses to stress in the offspring (Anacker et al. 2014). High levels of maternal care over the first week of postnatal life are associated with reduced fearfulness and a dampened hypothalamic-pituitary-adrenal axis response when exposed to stress. Interestingly, pharmacological intervention in adulthood may alter these behavioral responses by changing the epigenetic status of relevant genes, in particular the hippocampal *GR*. The administration of the HDAC inhibitor trichostatin A in stress-challenged offspring that had received lower maternal care induces behavior more similar to that of offspring exposed to high levels of maternal care (Weaver et al. 2004). The methyl donor L-methionine induces the opposite effect, with adult offspring exposed to high maternal care exhibiting a potentiated behavioral response to stress. The effects of these interventions have been linked to methylation and expression levels of hippocampal GR.

At present, the prevention or reversibility of developmentally induced epigenetic changes has only been investigated in animals. Nevertheless, the contribution of epigenetic mechanisms to the elucidation of developmental pathways to human disease is now well recognized. Emerging evidence from the clinical and epidemiological domains increasingly supports the notion that specific epigenetic marks can serve as biomarkers of later-life disease risk (García-Giménez 2016). The clinical implications of such prognostics are clear – by identifying individuals with increased susceptibility to chronic disease in later life, appropriate nutritional, pharmacological, or educational interventions could be then employed as preventative measures. Adopting a life-course approach with a particular focus on the prenatal and early postnatal periods appears to be prudent (Low et al. 2016).

References

Adalsteinsson BT, Ferguson-Smith AC (2014) Epigenetic control of the genome—lessons from genomic imprinting. Genes 5:635–655

Anacker C, O'Donnell KJ, Meaney MJ (2014) Early life adversity and the epigenetic programming of hypothalamic-pituitary-adrenal function. Dialogues Clin Neurosci 16(3):321–333

Beaujean N (2014) Histone post-translational modifications in preimplantation mouse embryos and their role in nuclear architecture. Mol Reprod Dev 81(2):100–112

Begum G, Davies A, Stevens A, Oliver M, Jaquiery A, Challis J et al (2013) Maternal undernutrition programs tissue-specific epigenetic changes in the glucocorticoid receptor in adult offspring. Endocrinology 154(12):4560–4569

Bowman GD, Poirier MG (2015) Post-translational modifications of histones that influence nucleosome dynamics. Chem Rev 115(6):2274–2295

Galvani A, Thiriet C (2015) Nucleosome dancing at the tempo of histone tail acetylation. Genes 6:607–621

García-Giménez JL (ed) (2016) Epigenetic biomarkers and diagnostics. Academic, London

Gluckman PD, Lillycrop KA, Vickers MH, Pleasants AB, Phillips ES, Beedle AS et al (2007) Metabolic plasticity during mammalian development is directionally dependent on early nutritional status. Proc Natl Acad Sci USA 104(31):12796–12800

Gluckman PD, Hanson MA, Cooper C, Thornburg KL (2008) Effect of in utero and early-life conditions on adult health and disease. N Engl J Med 359(1):61–73

Gluckman PD, Buklijas T, Hanson MA (2015) The developmental origins of health and disease (DOHaD) concept: past, present, and future. In: Rosenfeld CS (ed) The epigenome and developmental origins of health and disease. Academic, London, pp 1–13

Godfrey KM, Sheppard A, Gluckman PD, Lillycrop KA, Burdge GC, McLean C et al (2011) Epigenetic gene promoter methylation at birth is associated with child's later adiposity. Diabetes 60:1528–1534

Hanson MA, Gluckman PD (2014) Early developmental conditioning of later health and disease: physiology or pathophysiology? Physiol Rev 94:1027–1076

Horike S-i, Cai S, Miyano M, Cheng J-F, Kohwi-Shigematsu T (2005) Loss of silent-chromatin looping and impaired imprinting of *DLX5* in Rett syndrome. Nat Genet 37(1):31–40

Iwakawa H-o, Tomari Y (2015) The functions of MicroRNAs: mRNA decay and translational repression. Trends Cell Biol 25(11):651–665

Kalsner L, Chamberlain SJ (2015) Prader-Willi, Angelman, and 15q11-q13 duplication syndromes. Pediatr Clin North Am 62(3):587–606

Lillycrop KA, Phillips ES, Jackson AA, Hanson MA, Burdge GC (2005) Dietary protein restriction of pregnant rats induces and folic acid supplementation prevents epigenetic modification of hepatic gene expression in the offspring. J Nutr 135:1382–1386

Liyanage VRB, Rastegar M (2014) Rett syndrome and MeCP2. Neuromol Med 16:231–264

Low FM, Gluckman PD, Hanson MA (2011) Developmental plasticity and epigenetic mechanisms underpinning metabolic and cardiovascular diseases. Epigenomics 3(3):279–294

Low FM, Gluckman PD, Hanson MA (2014) Epigenetic and developmental basis of risk of obesity and metabolic disease. In: Ulloa-Aguirre A, Conn PM (eds) Cellular endocrinology in health and disease. Elsevier, London, pp 111–132

Low FM, Gluckman PD, Hanson MA (2016) A life course approach to public health: why early life matters. In: van den Bosch M, Bird W (eds) Oxford textbook of nature and public health. Oxford University Press, Oxford

Meller VH, Joshi SS, Deshpande N (2015) Modulation of chromatin by noncoding RNA. Annu Rev Genet 49:673–695

Quinn JJ, Chang HY (2016) Unique features of long non-coding RNA biogenesis and function. Nat Rev Genet 17(1):47–62

Regha K, Latos PA, Spahn L (2006) The imprinted mouse *Igf2r/Air* cluster – a model maternal imprinting system. Cytogenet Genome Res 113(1–4):165–177

Schubeler D (2015) Function and information content of DNA methylation. Nature 517(7534):321–326

Stepanov GA, Filippova JA, Komissarov AB, Kuligina EV, Richter VA, Semenov DV (2015) Regulatory role of small nucleolar RNAs in human diseases. BioMed Res Int 2015:10

Vickers MH, Sloboda DM (2012) Strategies for reversing the effects of metabolic disorders induced as a consequence of developmental programming. Front Physiol 3:242

Vickers MH, Gluckman PD, Coveny AH, Hofman PL, Cutfield WS, Gertler A et al (2005) Neonatal leptin treatment reverses developmental programming. Endocrinology 146:4211–4216

Weaver ICG, Cervoni N, Champagne FA, D'Alessio AC, Sharma S, Seckl JR et al (2004) Epigenetic programming by maternal behavior. Nat Neurosci 7(8):847–854

Congenital Malformations and Syndromes: Early Diagnosis and Prognosis in Neonatal Medicine

4

Giovanni Corsello and Mario Giuffrè

Contents

G. Corsello (✉) · M. Giuffrè
Department of Sciences for Health Promotion and Mother and Child Care, University of Palermo, Palermo, Italy
e-mail: Giocors@alice.it; mario.giuffre@unipa.it

G. Buonocore et al. (eds.), *Neonatology*,
https://doi.org/10.1007/978-3-319-29489-6_153

Abstract

Congenital malformations are defects of the morphogenesis of organs or body regions identified during intrauterine development or at birth. They may be isolated and single or multiple. Their global birth prevalence is about 2–3%. Congenital defects may be caused by genetic and/or environmental factors, acting singly or in combination. A deep knowledge of the family and pregnancy histories, of the congenital anomalies and/or dysmorphic features' classification, as well as of the most appropriate cytogenetic and/or molecular genetic tests may facilitate the neonatologist to the newborn's correct assessment and management.

4.1 Salient Points

- Congenital malformations are defects of the morphogenesis that can be classified based on clinical, etiological, or pathogenetic criteria.
- The clinical and instrumental approach to congenital malformations and syndromes is a complex, long-lasting, and stressful process for both patients and their families.
- Diagnosis, treatment, and follow-up of congenital defects require the involvement of a multidisciplinary team of different specialists.
- Improvement in diagnostic and therapeutic resources has determined an increase in survival and quality of life for many conditions with congenital defects.
- Congenital malformations and syndromes are a major issue for health services in terms of costs and resources.

4.2 Introduction

The genetic counseling has been recently defined as a unique combination of intense science, critical thinking, and empathic process. This multidimensional definition contains all domains for a correct approach to a newborn with congenital malformations, but at the same time, it highlights several critical issues for the clinician who needs to start an early approach soon after birth or even prenatally. Modern diagnostic tools and therapeutic resources have allowed better identification of congenital malformations and have reduced long-term morbidity and mortality in affected patients. Because of increased life expectancy, congenital malformations today represent a major issue in health care because of the resources needed for multidisciplinary care.

4.3 Classifications

Based on clinical criteria, *major malformations* are defined as defects causing functional impairment and therefore needing medical or surgical treatment. Defects that do not produce functional impairment and do not require medical intervention are termed *minor malformations* if their prevalence at birth is less than 4% and *phenotypic variants* when the birth prevalence is higher. Major and/or minor congenital malformations are frequently associated; apparently isolated defects may be associated with malformations that are not clinically evident at birth.

On the basis of etiological criteria, it is possible to distinguish primary malformations, secondary malformations (disruptions), and deformations

Table 1 Etiologic classification of congenital malformations

Primary (genetic)	Secondary (environmental)
Chromosomal abnormalities	Biologic agents
Numeric	Viruses
Polyploidy	Cytomegalovirus
Polysomy	Rubella
Monosomy	Herpesviruses
Structural	Bacteria
Deletions	*Treponema pallidum*
Duplications	Parasites
Insertions	*Toxoplasma gondii*
Translocations	Chemical agents
Monogenic	Drugs
Point mutations	Antiblastics
Nonsense	Anticonvulsants
Missense	Antibiotics
Frameshift	Abuse substances
Dynamic mutations	Alcohol
Triplet amplification	Smoke
Epigenetic regulation	Cocaine
Imprinting defects	Opiates
Uniparental disomy	Metabolic conditions
Polygenic	Hyperglycemia, hyperinsulinemia
Oligohydramnios	Hyperphenylalaninemia
Uterine malformations	Hyperandrogenism
	Physical agents
	Ionizing radiation
	Electromagnetic radiation
	Vascular disruptions
	Subclavian artery vascular disruption
	Twin-twin disruption sequence
	Mechanical causes (deformations)
	Amniotic bands
	Twinning
	Uterine tumors

(Table 1). *Primary malformations* are morphogenic defects arising from an intrinsic error of development with a genetic origin. *Disruptions* occur when an environmental factor interferes with an otherwise normal developmental process, causing global impairment or specific damage affecting a single developmental region. The causes of secondary malformations may be biological, chemical, metabolic, or physical. *Deformations* arise from extrinsic mechanical compression of one or more regions of the body during fetal development. The most common causes of deformations are amniotic bands, twinning, uterine malformations, and masses.

Patients with multiple malformations can be classified as having syndromes, sequences, associations, or dysplasias. *Syndromes* are conditions where all the structural defects arise from a single etiological factor, which may be genetic or environmental. *Sequences* are characterized by a cascade of dysmorphic processes, linked by a cause/effect relationship with a single initiating event. Thus, a primary defect may induce several secondary defects, which are chronologically and pathogenetically related. *Associations* are sporadic events with different defects being present more frequently than would be expected if they were random events, without evidence of any etiological or pathogenetic relationship. In recent years, some associations have been recognized as disorders of blastogenesis, which are caused by genetic or environmental factors that interfere with early development when the embryo is a single developmental field, and producing defects in apparently unrelated organs and body regions. Blastogenesis is the first 4 weeks after conception and is characterized by processes that determine the midline and body axes, symmetry and lateralization, neurulation, and somite formation. Some associations are identified by an acronym of the defects, such as VACTERLS (vertebral defects, anorectal atresia, cardiac anomalies, tracheoesophageal fistula, esophageal atresia, renal anomalies, limb defects, single umbilical artery) and MURCS (Mullerian duct aplasia, renal dysplasia, cervical somite anomalies). *Dysplasias* are structural defects involving specific tissues where a single gene mutation may determine the abolition or reduction of protein synthesis as well as the production of defective proteins.

4.4 Clinical Considerations

The birth of a baby with congenital malformations is the starting point of a clinical process that is aimed at making a precise diagnosis (Wiedemann et al. 1992; Twining et al. 2000). This leads to appropriate clinical planning and definition of prognosis and counseling of the parents. Different causal pathways may lead to a similar phenotype (Donnai and Winter 1995; Jones 1997), and the diagnostic process may be long and difficult, requiring follow-up to establish the natural history of the disorder. The diagnostic process includes an accurate history and description of the phenotype, with appropriate imaging and laboratory tests. Improvements in informatics have led to the development of computerized systems to improve diagnostic accuracy. The history should include consideration of the whole family with the definition of a genealogical tree and the identification of risk factors (consanguinity, multiple abortions, stillbirths, advanced maternal and/or paternal age), the preconceptional period and environmental factors (infections, maternal metabolic diseases, diabetes mellitus, drugs, alcohol), and the pregnancy. Analysis of the phenotype is aimed at the identification and description (with photographic documentation) of structural defects (isolated and multiple, major and minor) and should include a description of clinical associations with genetic syndromes, such as developmental delay, growth restriction, disorders of sexual differentiation, or pubertal development.

4.5 Genetic Counseling and Prenatal Diagnosis

Genetic counseling has been recently defined as unique combination of intense science, critical thinking, and empathy counseling (Barry 2015). It consists in a nondirective process of communicating with and giving information to a family (usually the parents) to enable the making of decisions relating to patients with genetic diseases that are considered, responsible, and rational. It is important that genetic counselors have (a) a confirmed diagnosis for the index patient, (b) an up-to-date knowledge of the natural history of the disease, (c) an understanding of its prognostic and therapeutic implications, (d) knowledge of its pattern of inheritance, and (e) an awareness of the possibilities for early (prenatal) diagnosis. The main factors that determine a need for genetic counseling are the presence of an index case with a congenital malformation or of genetic disease in the family as well as the presence of parental risk factors (consanguinity, advanced maternal age, recurrent abortions, mutation carrier). If the disease is multifactorial (due to a combination of genetic and environmental factors), a recurrence risk may be given only on the basis of an empirical approach that takes account of the prevalence in a certain population or at a certain maternal age, number of affected subjects, and consanguinity within the family. In the case of monogenic diseases with Mendelian inheritance (autosomal dominant, autosomal recessive, X-linked), the relative recurrence risk must be explained to the family, who must also be informed about available opportunities for early diagnosis (preconceptional, prenatal, neonatal). The recent identification of complex genetic mechanisms (genomic imprinting, uniparental disomy, triplet amplification) has increased the number of diseases in which it is possible to give helpful genetic counseling.

4.6 Associations

Associations are usually sporadic conditions with a low recurrence risk. Environmental factors (alcohol, drugs, maternal diabetes) as well as chromosomal and single gene disorders may interfere with the blastogenic processes. A genetic background may also increase an individual's susceptibility to environmental factors.

4.6.1 VACTERLS Association

VACTERLS association is characterized by the manifestation of some or all of the defects summarized by the acronym: *v*ertebral defects, *a*norectal atresia, *c*ardiac anomalies, *t*racheoesophageal fistula, *e*sophageal atresia, *r*enal anomalies, *l*imb defects, *s*ingle umbilical artery. Tracheoesophageal and anorectal defects require early surgery during the neonatal period. The most frequent heart defects affect the ventricular septum. Limb defects include radial ray abnormalities (radial hypoplasia, thumb aplasia, or hypoplasia as well as its duplication), polydactyly, and syndactyly. Other features may be prenatal and postnatal growth restriction and ear and external genitalia abnormalities. VACTERLS association is often sporadic with a low recurrence risk. It is more frequent in the offspring of diabetic mothers. In some patients with associated obstructive hydrocephalus, gene mutations with autosomal recessive (AR) inheritance have been documented. Antenatal diagnosis can be challenging, as certain features can be difficult to ascertain prior to birth. Management typically centers around surgical correction of the specific congenital anomalies (typically anal atresia, esophageal atresia, and certain types of cardiac malformations) in the immediate postnatal period, followed by long-term medical management of sequelae of the congenital malformations. If optimal surgical correction is achievable, the prognosis can be relatively good, though some patients will continue to be affected by their congenital malformations throughout life (Solomon 2011; Shaw-Smith 2006). Most patients have normal cognition, although they may present as failure to thrive and with neuromotor disabilities.

4.6.2 Infants of Diabetic Mothers

Congenital malformations in the offspring of diabetic mothers are clinically heterogeneous. Their frequency is two- to fourfold higher than in the general population. The relative risk for malformations is much higher in newborns of women with type 1 insulin-dependent diabetes mellitus and is inversely correlated with the effectiveness of maternal glycemic control, particularly during the periconceptional period. Several factors are involved in the pathogenesis of such defects: hyperglycemia, hyperglycosylation of proteins involved in differentiation, chronic hypoxia, polycythemia/hyperviscosity, and lactic acidosis (Mitanchez et al. 2015). All these factors may interact and interfere with blastogenesis, inducing abnormalities of the midline structures and symmetric organs. All types of malformations (skeletal, cardiac, renal, gastrointestinal, CNS) are more common in the infants of diabetic mothers. Some are specific, such as caudal dysgenesis, characterized by defects of vertebral, urogenital, and intestinal structures arising from the caudal mesoderm, with a wide spectrum of expression including sirenomelia, in which there is also a complex vascular defect. The fetus may be macrosomic because of fetal hyperinsulinemia, although a placental microangiopathy may also cause intrauterine growth restriction.

4.7 Sequences

Malformation sequences may be caused by genetic as well as environmental factors. Several organs and systems may be involved in malformation sequences (Table 2).

4.7.1 Holoprosencephalic Sequence

Holoprosencephalic sequence presents at birth with a wide spectrum of defects of the encephalon and the median craniofacial areas due to a developmental defect of the median subdivision of the prosencephalic vesicle and surrounding mesoderm.

Three anatomical variants (alobar, semilobar, and lobar) and four clinical variants (cyclopia, ethmocephaly, cebocephaly, and premaxillar agenesis) have been described. Clinical evaluation must include CNS imaging to define the full phenotype. The severity of CNS defects is the main reason for the high and early lethality of the condition. If the phenotype is only partially expressed, longer survival is possible, frequently associated with relevant neurologic problems. The parents and relatives of patients must be investigated for minor signs of the sequence (hypotelorism, single median incisor) in order to recognize a possible autosomal dominant (AD) inheritance (Dubourg et al. 2011; Lami et al. 2013).

Table 2 Main malformation sequences

Name	Developmental field and organs involved
Holoprosencephaly	Precordial mesoderm, prosencephalic vesicle, rhinencephalon, orbits, nose, premaxilla
Septo-optic dysplasia	Optic chiasm, hypophysis
Pierre Robin	Jaw bone, oropharyngeal region
Poland	Pectoral muscle, superior limb
Klippel-Feil	Spine
Potter	Kidneys, urinary tract, lungs, limbs, facies
Prune belly	Urinary tract, abdominal wall
Bladder-cloacal exstrophy	Periumbilical mesoderm
Rokitansky	Muller ducts
Sirenomelia	Caudal mesoderm
Caudal regression	Caudal mesoderm
Premature rupture of amnion	Median axis, limb deformations, facial clefts
Fetal akinesia	Multiple body regions
Twin-twin disruption sequence	Multiple body regions

The etiology is very heterogeneous: from chromosomal abnormalities (such as trisomy 13), known syndromes (such as Smith-Lemli-Opitz syndrome, CHARGE syndrome) to environmental factors (maternal diabetes or hypocholesterolemia during gestation). In nonchromosomal non-syndromic holoprosencephalic sequence, at least 14 genes have been implicated: four major genes *SHH*, *ZIC2*, *SIX3*, and *TGIF* and ten minor genes. Molecular analyses of the four main genes are routinely performed with a mutation detection rate of 25%. Array-CGH (comparative genomic hybridization) analysis shows 22% microrearrangements in HPE (Winter et al. 2015). However, the underlying genetic complexity is to be clarified yet; most cases are supposed to be multifactorial and the recurrence risk for families with a sporadic case is estimated at around 6%.

4.7.2 Pierre Robin Sequence

Pierre Robin sequence is a developmental defect of the mandible and surrounding oropharyngeal region. It is characterized by microretrognathia, cleft palate, and functional disturbances (swallowing deficit, respiratory distress). A deficiency of mesoderm induction may cause a primary cleft palate (V-shape). Alternatively, the cleft palate may be secondary to jaw arch hypoplasia, which leads to the position of the tongue being fixed between the palatine processes, causing a defect of fusion of the secondary palate in the midline (U-shape). Respiratory obstruction is caused by the tongue falling backwards and by a primitive pharyngeal stenosis (secondary to a migration deficit of neural crest cells). The sequence may present with a wide phenotypical spectrum, either in isolation or as part of a more complex syndrome (del 18q, Stickler syndrome, del 22q11, etc.). All these variables influence the prognosis (Thouvenin et al. 2013). Newborns may require prolonged respiratory and/or nutritional support and long-term hospitalization and follow-up. In the most severely affected cases, surgery to the jaw distraction may improve the outcome.

4.7.3 Potter Sequence

The Potter sequence is caused by absent or severely reduced fetal urine output from the first trimester. It may be secondary to bilateral renal agenesis (a differentiation defect of the metanephric blastema) or to other renal and urinary tract malformations. The cascade mechanism starts with diminished urine production by the fetus; this leads to a reduced volume of amniotic fluid (anhydramnios or oligohydramnios), which gives rise to pulmonary hypoplasia, leading to respiratory distress at birth, facial dysmorphism (prominent nose and flat profile), and diminished fetal movements with multiple postural deformations particularly of the lower limbs. When the phenotype is fully expressed, the severe renal and pulmonary damage is responsible for the high perinatal mortality (Shastry et al. 2012). Prenatal diagnosis by ultrasound reveals the kidney defect, oligohydramnios, and other associated malformations. The sequence is often sporadic, with etiological heterogeneity and a recurrence risk of about 3%. It may occasionally be associated with other defects in a more complex syndrome (Meckel-Gruber syndrome: occipital encephalocele, renal cystic disease, polydactyly, and an autosomal recessive inheritance).

4.7.4 Prune Belly Sequence

This sequence was named because of the characteristic appearance of the abdomen (wrinkled skin, also referred to as "flabby abdomen") in the affected newborns. The sequence may be related to various defects of the genitourinary tract, involving the proximal urethra (urethral agenesis, cloacal persistence, urethral stenosis, posterior urethral valves in males) (Smolkin et al. 2008). Urethral obstruction is responsible for oligohydramnios (and possible secondary Potter sequence) and accumulation of urine in the proximal renal tract, leading to parenchymal damage (bladder dilatation, bilateral ureteric dilatation, and hydronephrosis). Bladder hypertrophy and dilatation may interfere with development of the abdominal wall muscles and diaphragm and testicular migration in the scrotum in males (cryptorchidism). Abdominal wall muscle hypoplasia is responsible for the prune belly appearance because of visible intestinal loops through the thin abdominal wall. Diaphragmatic defects and oligohydramnios cause lung hypoplasia and severe respiratory distress at birth. Although early prenatal diagnosis by ultrasonography is possible, the differential diagnosis between isolated renal cystic conditions and obstructive uropathies may be difficult. Prenatal bladder catheterization allows urine to flow into the amniotic cavity and must be followed by surgical correction after birth.

4.8 Syndromes

4.8.1 Chromosomal Abnormalities

The overall incidence of chromosomal anomalies is estimated at about 1:170 live births. Their prevalence at conception is much higher, giving rise to a spontaneous abortion or fetal death because of developmental impairment. About 50% of spontaneous abortions have an abnormal chromosomal structure. Chromosomal aberrations may affect *autosomes* and/or *sex chromosomes* and may involve their number or structure. *Numeric aberrations* have a prezygotic origin (meiotic nondisjunction, frequently related to advanced maternal age). They may also arise from a postzygotic error when they are present only in a variable proportion of cells (mosaics). *Structural aberrations* may occur de novo from a meiotic rearrangement or may be inherited from one parent, who carries a balanced non-symptomatic chromosomal translocation.

4.8.1.1 Down Syndrome (Trisomy 21)

Down syndrome is the most frequent chromosomal aberration at birth (about 1:700). It is determined by a trisomy of chromosome 21. In most (95%) cases, trisomy 21 is secondary to a maternal meiotic nondisjunction of homologous chromosomes 21; more rarely there may be a Robertsonian translocation or a postzygotic mitotic nondisjunction (mosaic with milder phenotype). The incidence is related to maternal age at conception (1/1,500 at 20 years and 1/28 at 45 years). The overall recurrence risk is low (about 1%), although it significantly increases when one of the parents carries a balanced translocation. The phenotype at birth is characteristic: main facial features are Brushfield spots (gray spots in the median zone of the iris), upslanting palpebral fissures, epicanthal folds, small nose, small mouth with prominent tongue, flat facial profile, brachycephaly with a flat occipital bone, small low-set ears, and short neck with redundant skin folds. Newborn babies are hypotonic with lax joints. A single palmar crease and clinodactyly of the little finger are frequent. Organ involvement includes congenital heart defects (atrioventricular canal, ventricular septal defects, tetralogy of Fallot), duodenal atresia or stenosis, Hirschsprung's disease, hypothyroidism, and urinary tract malformations. Long-term follow-up is required because of developmental delay, intellectual disability, growth retardation, occurrence of autoimmune diseases, immunodeficiencies, and leukemia (Karmiloff-Smith et al. 2016). Survival rates and the quality of life have improved significantly with educational and screening programs and the development of multidisciplinary follow-up.

4.8.1.2 Edwards Syndrome (Trisomy 18)

Edwards syndrome is determined by trisomy of chromosome 18, sometimes as a mosaic or in association with other chromosomal abnormalities. Its birth prevalence is about 1:8,000 because most affected fetuses abort spontaneously. Newborns show severe prenatal growth restriction, dolichocephaly with prominent occiput and low-set dysplastic external ears, jaw hypoplasia, flexed hands with the index finger overlapping the middle finger, single palmar crease, and talipes with rocker-bottom feet. There are frequently associated malformations (heart, renal, intestinal, CNS), which are responsible for the very grave prognosis and high neonatal mortality (Wu et al. 2013).

4.8.1.3 Patau Syndrome (Trisomy 13)

Patau syndrome is determined by trisomy of chromosome 13, sometimes with chromosomal translocation or rarely as mosaic. Its birth prevalence is about 1/10,000. Newborns show prenatal growth restriction, a small trigonocephalic skull, areas of aplasia cutis on the scalp, cleft lip and palate, microphthalmia, variable hypotelorism up to cyclopia (i.e., expression of an associated holoprosencephalic sequence), postaxial polydactyly and/or syndactyly, forced flexion of the fingers, single palmar crease, plantar convexity, and cryptorchidism. Other organs are frequently involved (heart, kidneys). Patients with fully expressed phenotype usually die during the first month of life; those with milder signs (mosaics) may survive with severe developmental deficits (Wu et al. 2013; Barry et al. 2015).

4.8.1.4 Wolf-Hirschhorn Syndrome (4p-)

This is a rare condition determined by deletion of the distal part of the short arm of chromosome 4. Newborns present with prenatal growth restriction, hypotonia, severe microcephaly with brachycephaly, prominent nose, downturned corners of the mouth, arched palate, jaw hypoplasia, hypertelorism, downslanting palpebral fissures, iris coloboma, and large low-set external ears. Heart, renal, and skeletal defects are frequent. The degree of extension of the chromosomal deletion influences the severity of phenotype and neonatal mortality rate. Surviving patients show severe postnatal growth retardation and psychomotor developmental delay.

4.8.1.5 Cri du chat Syndrome (5p-)

Cri du chat syndrome is due to a variable deletion of the short arm of chromosome 5, named because of the characteristic high-pitched catlike cry of affected newborns caused by hypoplasia of laryngeal cartilages, which disappears after the first months of life (Rodríguez-Caballero et al. 2012). Other phenotypical features are microcephaly, round face, hypertelorism, micrognathia, epicanthal folds, and low-set ears. At birth there is generalized hypotonia. Later there is limb hypertonia and severe developmental delay.

4.8.1.6 Mosaic 8 Chromosome Trisomy

The full trisomy of chromosome 8 is extremely rare in humans. It is more common as a mosaic. The phenotype of mosaic trisomy 8 includes scaphocephaly, ankylosed large joints, clubfoot, absent or hypoplastic patellae, arachnodactyly, and brachydactyly. Deep grooves in the palms and soles (Fig. 1) are virtually diagnostic in infancy but become less prominent with age (Biesecker and Spinner 2013). The face is

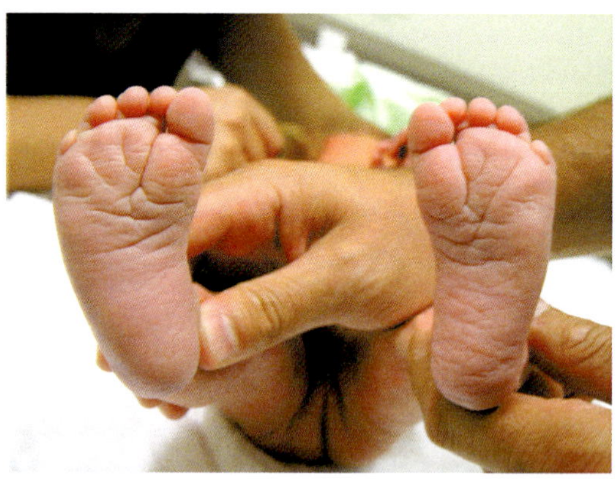

Fig. 1 Deep plantar grooves in a newborn with mosaic 8 chromosome trisomy

characterized by a prominent pouting lower lip and small jaw. Intellectual disability may be present but is often mild and may remain undetected.

4.8.1.7 Turner Syndrome

Turner syndrome is the most frequent aneuploidy of sex chromosomes with a birth prevalence of 1/2,500. It is determined by a monosomy of chromosome X, which may be complete (50%) or partial (20%); it frequently presents as a mosaic with a milder phenotype (30%). During the neonatal period, the diagnosis is suspected because of lymphedema of the hands and feet (Fig. 2), nail dysplasia, neck pterygium, a large mouth with downturned corners, dysplastic external ears, and left heart output defects (aortic coarctation, left heart hypoplasia). In addition, there may be a prenatal history of cystic hygroma. The clinical phenotype changes with age when other features become evident: short stature, short neck, low posterior hairline, restricted thorax, cubitus valgus, shortness of the fourth metacarpal bone, primary amenorrhea, absence of secondary sexual signs, and an endocrine profile of gonadal dysgenesis. Life expectancy is not reduced, but long-term follow-up is required and appropriate hormonal therapy (growth hormone in the first decade and estrogen-progesterone after puberty must be given in order to improve height and induce the menstrual cycle) (Blum et al. 2013).

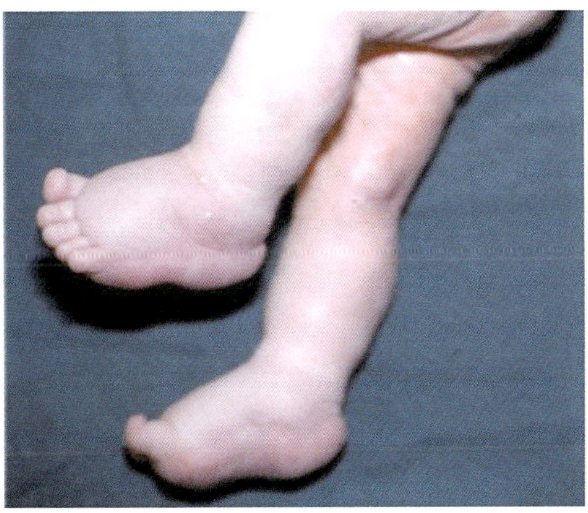

Fig. 2 Foot lymphedema in a baby with Turner syndrome

4.8.1.8 DiGeorge Syndrome

DiGeorge syndrome, also noted as 22q11.2 deletion syndrome, is a chromosomal disorder whose common features include cardiac defects, palatal anomalies, facial dysmorphism, developmental delay, and immune deficiency (McDonald-McGinn and Sullivan 2011; Botto et al. 2003). This condition has been previously reported with the acronym CATCH 22 (Cardiac abnormality, Abnormal face, Thymic hypoplasia, Cleft palate, Hypoparathyroidism, chromosome 22 microdeletion).

Heart defects are conotruncal (aortic arch interruption, common arterial trunk, tetralogy of Fallot). When the brachial structures are involved, there is dysfunction of the immune system (T-cell deficiency) and parathyroidal abnormalities with low serum calcium levels. During the neonatal period, the full expression of the phenotype results in hypocalcemia and craniofacial dysmorphism (micrognathia, cleft palate, anteverted nares, low-set external ears) with a conotruncal heart defect and absent thymic shadow at chest X-ray delineating the phenotype with full expressivity. In most cases, the syndrome is due to a 3 Mb deletion on the chromosomal region 22q11.2; there are also atypical deletions which are nested within the DiGeorge critical region. Some of them include the *TBX1* gene that has been shown to be implicated in cardiac, parathyroid, thymus, and facial structure development. The variable expression of the 22q11.2 phenotype is thought to be due to genetic modifiers on either the other 22q11.2 allele or on other chromosomes. Diagnosis is suspected upon clinical examination and detection of anomalies but needs to be confirmed by detection of the 22q11.2 deletion, using fluorescence in situ hybridization (FISH), MLPA, aCGH, or genome-wide SNP (single nucleotide polymorphism) microarrays (Hacıhamdioğlu et al. 2015).

4.8.2 Monogenic Disorders

Monogenic disorders are single gene mutations with a Mendelian mode of inheritance. The genotype-phenotype correlation remains undefined for many conditions. Each syndrome may be due to different mutations in the same gene or in different genes (genetic heterogeneity). The same mutation may determine different phenotypes (phenotypical variability) in the same family and appears to depend on interference by other genetic and/or environmental factors. In addition, epigenetic factors (e.g., DNA methylation) may act during the differentiation processes to modify gene expression and may depend on the parental origin of the gene (genomic imprinting).

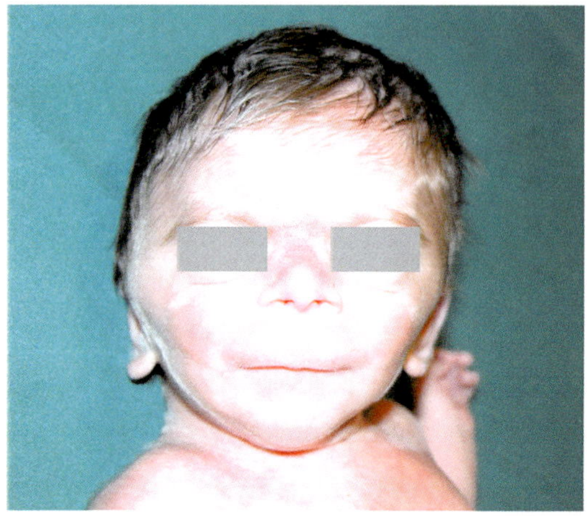

Fig. 3 Typical facial appearance of a newborn baby with Cornelia de Lange syndrome, showing synophrys, a depressed nasal bridge, anteverted nares, long philtrum, and carp mouth

4.8.2.1 Cornelia de Lange Syndrome (CdLS)

CdLS affects 1/10,000 newborns and is usually sporadic. Causative mutations in genes involved in chromosomal cohesion (cohesin complex) have been identified. The *NIPBL* gene (locus at 5p13.1) is mutated in approximately 50% of patients and is the major gene involved in the syndrome. Mutations in *SMC3*, *RAD21*, *SMC1A*, and *HDAC8* have recently been described with an autosomal dominant or an X-linked dominant pathways of inheritance. Newborns show a typical facial appearance (microbrachycephaly, low anterior and posterior hairline, synophrys, small nose with a depressed nasal bridge, anteverted nares, long philtrum, "carp" mouth, maxillary prognathism, low-set ears, Fig. 3), with intrauterine and postnatal growth retardation, hypertrichosis, and upper limb anomalies (small limbs, reduction defects including phocomelia, limited elbow extension, single palmar crease, oligosyndactyly) (Bhuiyan et al. 2006; Ramos et al. 2015).

Urogenital, heart, and intestinal malformations may also be present. Most patients show developmental delay and growth retardation. Infections, feeding difficulties, and neurologic disturbances (seizures, motor and speech retardation) require long-term multidisciplinary follow-up and family support.

4.8.2.2 Rubinstein-Taybi Syndrome (RSTS)

RSTS is a rare malformation syndrome characterized by intellectual disability, facial abnormalities, and broad thumbs and toes. Chromosome abnormalities are occasionally observed on routine cytogenetic testing. *CREBBP* and *EP300* are the only genes currently known to be associated with RSTS. FISH analysis of *CREBBP* detects microdeletions in approximately 10% of individuals with RSTS. Sequence analysis detects *CREBBP* pathogenic variants in another 40–50% of affected individuals. Pathogenic variants in *EP300* are identified in approximately 3–8% of individuals with RSTS (Schorry et al. 2008; Pagon et al. 1993). Familial cases with autosomal dominant inheritance have been described.

The diagnosis of RSTS is primarily based on clinical features. The main craniofacial features (Fig. 4) are microcephaly, frontal bossing, large anterior fontanelle, downslanting palpebral fissures, broad nasal bridge, beaked nose, epicanthal folds, strabismus, maxillary hypoplasia, high-arched palate, and external ear abnormalities. There is hand and foot involvement (broad distal phalanges of thumbs and halluces with medial deviation, clinodactyly, or duplication). There may also be hirsutism and abnormalities of the skeleton (spinal, pelvic), heart (septal defects, patent ductus arteriosus), and urogenital tract (hypospadias, cryptorchidism). Growth retardation, skeletal maturation delay, and severe intellectual

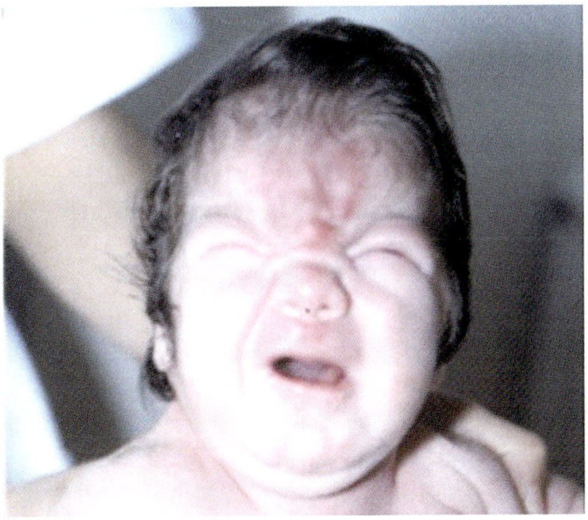

Fig. 4 Newborn with Rubinstein-Taybi syndrome showing microcephaly, frontal bossing, downslanting palpebral fissures, broad nasal bridge, beaked nose, epicanthus, and maxillary hypoplasia

disability are more common with increasing age (Pagon et al. 1993).

4.8.2.3 Marfan Syndrome (MS)

MS is characterized by several congenital defect of the connective tissue involving the skeleton, eye, and cardiovascular system. It is determined by heterozygous mutations in the *FBN1* gene (15q21.1) encoding for fibrillin-1 protein, which is a component of collagen (Tiecke et al. 2001). Frontier forms have been identified, secondary to mutations in the *TGFBR2* gene located on chromosome 3 which encodes for a TGF-beta receptor. It is inherited as an autosomal dominant with variable clinical expression; about 25% of cases are sporadic, due to de novo mutations correlated with advanced paternal age. Newborns show arachnodactyly, long and thin limbs, increased length joint laxity and hypermobility, muscular hypotonia, hernias, and pectus carinatum or excavatum. Cardiac abnormalities comprise mitral valve prolapse and aortic defects (aortic root dilatation and aortic aneurysm). Patients with most severe neonatal phenotype (neonatal Marfan syndrome) have high early mortality rates. Skeletal and cardiac problems usually evolve with growth (kyphoscoliosis, progressive aortic dilatation, aortic dissection) and ocular signs develop (ectopia lentis, early glaucoma) (Loeys et al. 2010).

4.8.2.4 Noonan Syndrome (NS)

NS is a relatively frequent (1/2,000) condition with some phenotypic features similar to those of Turner syndrome (male Turner, pseudo-Turner). In approximately 50% of cases, the disease is caused by missense mutations in the *PTPN11* gene (12q24.1), resulting in a gain of function of the non-receptor protein tyrosine phosphatase SHP-2 protein. Recently, mutations in other genes from the RAS-MAPK pathway (*KRAS*, *SOS1*, and *RAF1*) have been identified in a small portion of patients with NS. Mutation analysis can be carried out on blood samples and should be recommended for any subject with a suspected diagnosis of NS. However, the diagnosis cannot be excluded on a molecular basis, as the sensitivity of combined screening of all known genes allows confirmation in less than 75% of patients, with sporadic as well as familial cases (Roberts et al. 2013). The inheritance is autosomal dominant and parents must be always investigated for mild clinical signs.

Newborns show hypertelorism, upslanting palpebral fissures, low-set posteriorly rotated ears, neck pterygium, a shield chest with deformation of the sternum, and lymphedema (Fig. 5). Cardiac

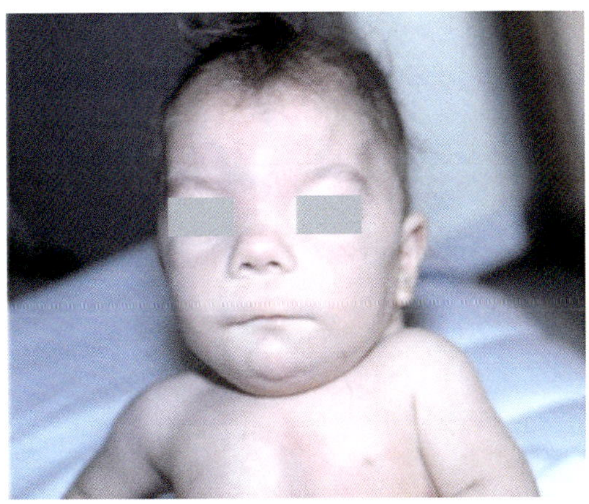

Fig. 5 A patient with Noonan syndrome with hypertelorism, upslanting palpebral fissures, and shield chest

involvement is mainly of the pulmonary outflow tract (pulmonary valve dysplasia and stenosis, cuspid thickening, and hypomobility). Other possible features are cryptorchidism in males and a bleeding tendency, due to thrombocytopenia and partial deficiency of coagulation factors. Later in infancy, other signs become evident: postnatal growth retardation (with short stature and retarded bone age), triangular face, mild psychomotor, and intellectual delay (Ferrero et al. 2008). The differential diagnosis should include Turner syndrome, cardiofaciocutaneous syndrome, Costello syndrome, neurofibromatosis type 1, and LEOPARD syndrome. Life expectancy depends exclusively on the severity of heart defects.

4.8.2.5 Prader-Willi Syndrome (PWS)

Prader-Willi syndrome is determined by the failure of expression of genes of paternal origin in the 15q11-q13 region. These genes are normally subjected to maternal imprinting (DNA methylation) which avoids maternal copy transcription and determines a functional gene monosomy (only the paternal copy is expressed). This condition may arise from microdeletions of paternal chromosome 15 (70–75%), maternal uniparental disomy (25–30%), or imprinting center defects (1%). Methylation testing identifies almost all patients; FISH and microsatellite DNA analysis may reveal microdeletions and maternal UPD. PWS newborns (Fig. 6) present with congenital hypotonia, a prenatal history of reduced fetal movements, poverty of facial expression, dolichocephaly with reduced bitemporal diameter, almond-shaped eyes with upslanting palpebral fissures, a small mouth with downturned corners and thin upper lip, small hands and feet, and genital hypoplasia with cryptorchidism in males (Gunay-Aygun et al. 2001). Hypotonia of the respiratory, orofacial, and pharyngoesophageal muscles causes variable degrees of respiratory and feeding difficulties (poor suction and swallowing), which are present from birth and tend to improve after the neonatal period. After the first year of life, the phenotype modifies and is characterized by hyperphagia, obesity, sleep disturbances, short stature, hypogonadotropic hypogonadism, mild to moderate mental retardation, and speech delay. Treatment with growth hormone (GH) is possible and good clinical results have been reported (Wolfgram et al. 2013).

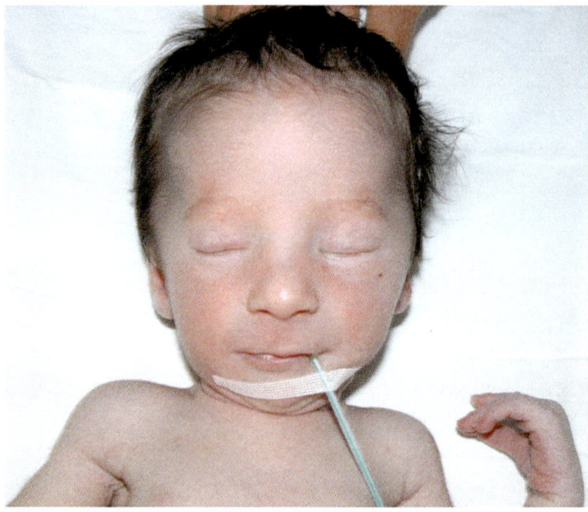

Fig. 6 The neonatal phenotype of Prader-Willi syndrome: hypomimic face, reduced bitemporal diameter, almond-shaped eyes, small mouth with downturned corners, and thin upper lip

4.8.2.6 Beckwith-Wiedemann Syndrome (BWS)

Beckwith-Wiedemann syndrome is a sporadic condition determined by an altered balance between cooperating genes in the region 11p15. The genetic mechanism is complex and involves imprinted genes encoding for several important growth factors and receptors. Various genotypic abnormalities have been described in BWS patients, e.g., microduplication of paternal region 11p15, microdeletion of the maternal region, and mutations and paternal uniparental disomy of chromosome 11. Molecular subgroups are associated with different recurrence risks and different clinical findings (e.g., tumor risks) (Weksberg et al. 2010).

The main neonatal clinical features (Fig. 7) are exomphalos, macroglossia, and gigantism (EMG syndrome). Other features are visceromegaly, adrenocortical cytomegaly, dysplasia of the renal medulla, typical linear indentations of the helix and the auricular lobe of the ear, hypoglycemia during the first days of life, and limb hemihypertrophy.

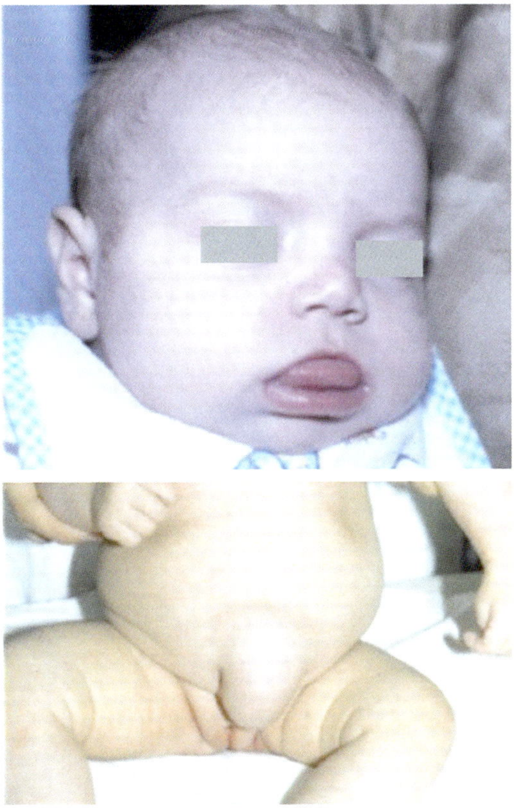

Fig. 7 Exomphalos, macroglossia, and gigantism

Prenatal diagnosis may be because of exomphalos and generalized overgrowth seen on ultrasound scanning. The neonatal diagnosis is based on clinical findings, although careful molecular cytogenetic analysis of the 11p15 region is recommended. Overgrowth and macroglossia tend to become less evident with age, but there is an increased risk of malignant tumors (Wilms' tumor, adrenal carcinoma, hepatoblastoma).

4.8.2.7 Silver-Russell Syndrome

Silver-Russell syndrome is a sporadic condition with genetic heterogeneity. Most cases are sporadic. Maternal uniparental disomy of chromosome 7 is observed in 10% of patients. Approximately 30% of the cases show hypomethylation of the *H19* gene, located in the 11p15 imprinted region. Hypomethylation results in most cases from an epigenetic mechanism or a genomic micro-rearrangement, such as a maternal microduplication of the region. Diagnosis is mainly clinical, as there is no specific biological test, but it can be confirmed by the detection of the underlying molecular anomaly with methylation-specific PCR, microsatellite typing, methylation-specific MLPA, and/or array CGH (Abu-Amero et al. 2008; Eggermann et al. 2011). The neonatal phenotype is characterized by severe intrauterine growth restriction with normal development of the skull (pseudohydrocephalic appearance), poor postnatal growth, craniofacial features (triangular-shaped face and broad forehead), body asymmetry, and a variety of minor malformations (clinodactyly and syndactyly of the little finger). The phenotypic expression changes during childhood and adolescence, with the facial features and asymmetry usually becoming more subtle with age. GH therapy should be considered to improve final height.

4.8.2.8 Goldenhar Syndrome (GS)

GS is a spectrum of malformations involving the eye, ear, and vertebrae with heterogeneous etiology and a highly variable phenotype (Gorlin et al. 1990). Its prevalence at birth is about 1/5,000. Most cases are sporadic, although some families with autosomal dominant inheritance have been described. GS originates from a vascular disruption of the first and second branchial arches, with consequent malformations of related organs and tissues. Defects are more often unilateral and an increased incidence has been reported in the offspring of diabetic mothers, as have other disorders of blastogenesis. GS newborns show multiple craniofacial anomalies (Fig. 8): hemifacial microsomia, ipsilateral deformity of the external ear (preauricular tags, atresia of the external auditory canal, anomalies in size and shape of the external auricle), epibulbar dermoid, and coloboma of the upper eyelid. In addition, defects of the cervical vertebrae (hemivertebrae, fusions, segmental agenesis), cleft palate, choanal atresia, heart, kidney, and CNS defects may be found. Auditory function must be assessed early to preserve speech and cognitive development (Paludetti et al. 2012).

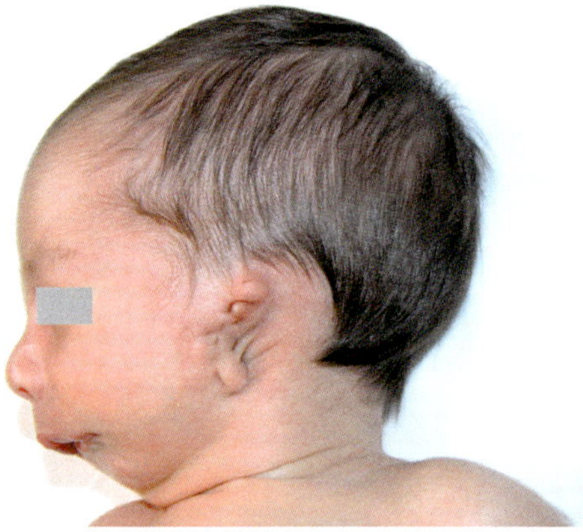

Fig. 8 Hemifacial microsomia and atresia of the external auricle in a baby with Goldenhar syndrome

4.8.2.9 Smith-Lemli-Opitz Syndrome (SLOS)

SLOS is a rare (1/30,000) autosomal recessive condition, caused by mutations in the *DHCR7* gene (11q13.4) leading to deficiency of the enzyme 3 beta-hydroxysterol-delta 7-reductase that converts 7-dehydrocholesterol (7DHC) to cholesterol (Wassif et al. 1998; Porter 2008). The enzyme deficiency causes a severe deficit of endogenous cholesterol production and its derivative compounds (sexual steroids, components of the myelin and cellular membranes), starting from intrauterine life. SLOS newborns show intrauterine growth restriction, severe hypotonia, microdolichocephaly, high forehead, palpebral ptosis, anteverted nares, and micrognathia. There may be other features, such as agenesis of the corpus callosum, cleft palate, syndactyly of the second and third toes, congenital heart defects, and liver dysfunction. Male patients usually have hypospadias, micropenis, cryptorchidism, and sometimes various degrees of ambiguous genitalia, because of the prenatal androgen deficiency. Diagnosis is based on the detection of low cholesterol and elevated 7DHC levels in plasma or tissues and confirmed due *DHCR7* sequence analysis, which allows confirmation of the prenatal diagnosis for at-risk couples. Failure to thrive worsens with age and there is always severe psychomotor delay. Management is symptomatic and most patients are treated with dietary cholesterol supplementation. Treatment trials are underway investigating combined treatment with cholesterol supplementation and a HMG-CoA reductase inhibitor. Surgery is proposed in case of secondary problems due to malformations (Porter 2008).

4.9 Disruptions

Some congenital malformations can be related to exogenous factors, which act during intrauterine life, inducing abnormalities of developmental and differentiation processes. The most susceptible period is the first trimester of pregnancy in which the identification of developmental fields, organogenesis, and differentiation take place. Biological, chemical, metabolic, physical and mechanical agents (Table 1) may cause defects of morphogenesis. The etiologic identification is important for effective genetic counseling and reducing the risk of recurrence in an affected family.

4.9.1 Biologic Agents

Most morphogenetic defects determined by biological agents are pathogenetically and clinically characterized. A high IgM level soon after birth is strongly suggestive of a prenatal infection of the fetus, although only 30% of these newborns show clinical consequences. The earlier the timing of intrauterine infection (particularly during the first trimester of gestation), the more severe is the effect of morphogenetic defects due to viral and bacterial agents, and there is usually associated intrauterine growth restriction. The most common embryofetopathies due to biologic agents are described in Table 3.

4.9.2 Chemical Agents

Any substance introduced to the human organism can be considered as a chemical agent. They may be drugs or foods associated with flawed lifestyle choices (alcohol consumption, cigarette smoking,

Table 3 Main disruptions determined by biologic agents

Biologic agent	Phenotype
Cytomegalovirus	Microcephaly, intracranial calcifications, psychomotor delay, sensorineural hearing loss, chorioretinitis, hepatosplenomegaly, thrombocytopenia, virus presence in secretions and biologic fluids (urine)
Rubella virus	Microcephaly, psychomotor delay, congenital cataract, sensorineural hearing loss, heart defects, hematologic alterations (anemia, thrombocytopenia)
Varicella-zoster virus	Mental retardation, cortical atrophy, seizures, chorioretinitis, skin scars
Treponema pallidum	Palmoplantar pemphigus, exanthema with skin scars, anemia, thrombocytopenia, hepatosplenomegaly, myocarditis, chorioretinitis, muco-hematic rhinitis, skeletal alterations (lacunae, caput quadratum, metaphyseal ossification defects, osteochondritis, and secondary pseudoparalysis)
Toxoplasma gondii	Hydrops, hydrocephalus, intracranial calcifications, chorioretinitis, cataract, seizures, hepatosplenomegaly, skin rush

ingestion of substances of abuse) or produced by maternal metabolism in specific situations. Some drugs and single molecules, which are well tolerated by an adult, may be seriously dangerous for the development of the embryo and fetus. Drug testing in human pregnancy is difficult and all drugs have therefore to be considered potentially harmful, requiring careful risk/benefit evaluation. Substances may cross the placenta and reach the fetus and placental function may reduce or increase their effects. Individual metabolism may influence the clinical effects, dosage, and timing of administration. The most frequent disruptions by chemical agents are reported in Table 4.

4.9.3 Vascular Disruptions

Any vascular accident during early embryonic and fetal development may determine subsequent

Table 4 Main disruptions determined by chemical agents

Chemical agent	Phenotype
Anticonvulsant drugs	Cleft lip and palate, neural tube defects, congenital heart defects
	Hydantoin (microcephaly, mental retardation, CNS abnormalities, small nose, facial bone hypoplasia, epicanthus, hypertelorism, strabismus, cleft lip and palate, micrognathia, short neck, heart defects)
	Trimethadione (microcephaly, facial bone hypoplasia, palpebral synophrys, epicanthus, external ear dysplasia, urogenital defects, heart defects)
	Valproic acid (trigonocephaly, reduced bitemporal diameter, facial bone hypoplasia, small nose, cleft lip and palate, urogenital and limb defects)
Alcohol	IUGR, peculiar face (microcephaly, short palpebral fissures, small nose with anteverted nares, hypoplastic nasal philtrum, microretrognathia), neurologic abnormalities (hypotonia, seizures, poor motor coordination, mental retardation)
Cocaine	Prematurity, IUGR, microcephaly, urogenital and skeletal malformations
Heroin	IUGR, low birth weight, congenital malformations
Maternal diabetes	Macrosomia, hypoglycemia, hypocalcemia, ventricular septal hypertrophy, caudal dysgenesis, any kind of congenital malformations (skeletal, cardiac, renal, intestinal, CNS, etc.)
Maternal	Defects of cellular proliferation and migration with myelinization delay (IUGR, severe microcephaly, hypotelorism)
Hyperphenylalaninemia	Prominent nose, low-set dysplastic external ears, mental retardation, cleft lip and palate, conotruncal heart defects

morphogenetic defects in the relevant body region.

Disruption of the subclavian artery includes a heterogeneous group of clinically and etiologically different conditions, characterized by alteration of different mesodermal structures supplied by the subclavian artery. Thus, the Poland sequence includes pectoral muscle agenesis and ipsilateral superior limb reduction defects. Kidney and urinary tract defects are frequently associated, expanding the phenotype toward an acro-pectoral-renal developmental field.

Twin-twin disruption sequence (TTDS) may involve various structures such as the brain, brachial arches, limbs, gut, and kidneys. It is caused by the intrauterine developmental impairment and subsequent death of a monozygotic twin. The presence of vascular placental anastomoses between the arterial supplies of twins and abnormal communicating flow allows the passage of thromboemboli to the surviving twin, with reduced or interrupted blood flow causing structural damage. The complex vascular interactions between monozygotic twins may result in other vascular disruptions (e.g., because of an acardiac twin) or a twin-twin transfusion sequence, which are particular features of monozygotic twins (Giuffrè et al. 2012).

4.10 Dysostoses

A heterogeneous group of birth defects with single or multiple involvement of skeletal segments (with no systemic cartilaginous tissue involvement), due to mutations of the genes involved in bone development. Dysostoses classification is based on phenotypic criteria and the body region most involved. In some instances, a genetic classification is now possible. Most syndromal craniosynostoses are determined by mutations in fibroblast growth factor receptor (*FGFR*) genes, with string evidence of genetic heterogeneity (the same condition being determined by different mutations in the same gene or in different *FGFR* genes) and genetic pleiotropism (the same mutation being responsible for different phenotypes). Genotype/phenotype correlation is not possible for all cases, and it can be influenced by other genes (epistatic) as well as other interactive cytoplasmic and environmental factors.

4.10.1 Craniofacial Dysostoses

Full fusion of all cranial sutures is normally achieved at about 25 years of age. Craniosynostoses depend on a precocious closure of one or more cranial sutures and may cause a restriction in the size of the cranium. The closure of a suture limits cranial growth at that site, and there is increased cranial growth at the other sutures, producing deformation of the skull (sometimes with brain growth restriction, hydrocephalus, and intracranial hypertension). Skull morphology depends on suture involvement (nature, timing, extension, and symmetry). The overall incidence of craniosynostoses is estimated to affect about 1/3,000 newborns. It may present in isolation or as part of a more complex syndrome.

4.10.1.1 Non-syndromal Craniosynostoses

Scaphocephaly depends on the premature fusion of the sagittal suture with consequent restriction of growth along the transverse axis and compensatory increased growth along the anteroposterior axis. *Plagiocephaly* depends on the premature fusion of a single coronal suture with consequent ipsilateral growth restriction and flattening of the frontal bone; the involvement of facial structures varies from simple deviation of nasal septum to severe asymmetry of the sphenoid and maxillary bones. *Brachycephaly* is due to premature fusion of both coronal sutures with consequent growth restriction along the anteroposterior axis and compensatory increase in skull height; hypoplasia of the frontal region is often present. Acrocephaly depends on the premature fusion of the coronal and sagittal sutures with consequent severe growth restriction along both anteroposterior and transverse axes and compensatory increased development of the frontal region. Intracranial hypertension is frequently present and requires early surgical correction to avoid severe CNS complications. *Trigonocephaly* is due to the premature fusion of the metopic suture, often evident because of a longitudinal bone crest in the median frontal region, giving the skull a triangular appearance with hypotelorism and flattening of the lateral frontal regions. *Cloverleaf skull* is due to the premature fusion of the coronal, sagittal, and lambdoidal sutures with excessive skull growth in height and to both sides, giving a trilobar appearance. Intracranial hypertension is consistently severe and gives rise to CNS complications.

4.10.1.2 Syndromal Craniosynostoses

Apert syndrome is a rare and serious phenotype described in newborns with acrocephaly and syndactyly of the hands and feet (Fig. 9). The premature fusion of both coronal sutures is responsible for acrocephaly, frontal bossing, flat occipital bone, and facial dysmorphic features (downslanting palpebral fissures, exophthalmus, hypertelorism, small upturned nose, maxillary hypoplasia, low-set ears). Hands and feet present a complete syndactyly (spoon-shaped hand) with bone and nail fusion. Synostosis may also be found in the carpal and tarsal bones and cervical vertebrae. Mental retardation may be present, as well as intracranial hypertension, particularly in the absence of early neurosurgical correction. A complex surgical program must be planned for the correction of multiple synostosis (skull remodeling, hand surgery). Apert syndrome is due to mutations in the exon 7 of the *FGFR2* gene (different mutations have been identified), with autosomal dominant inheritance and a high rate of de novo mutations correlated with advanced paternal age (Wilkie et al. 1995).

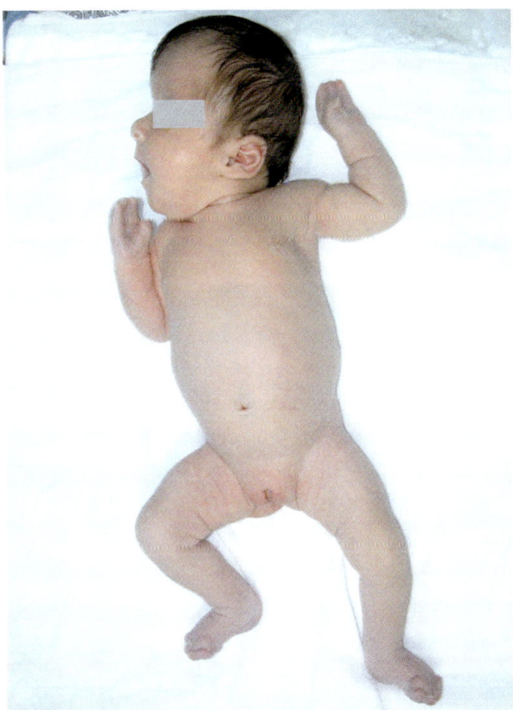

Fig. 9 Baby with Apert syndrome showing acrocephaly, frontal bossing, exophthalmus, small upturned nose, maxillary hypoplasia, and spoon-shaped hands

Crouzon syndrome is the most frequently reported syndromal craniosynostosis, characterized by acrocephaly with no hand and foot involvement. Premature fusion of the coronal sutures causes the acrocephaly, frontal bossing, and flat occipital bone. Looking at the face, there is hypoplasia of the midline structures, reduced orbital volume and ocular proptosis, strabismus, a small upturned nose, and maxillary hypoplasia. Fusions of cervical vertebrae and mild mental retardation may occur. Crouzon syndrome may be due to different mutations of the *FGFR2* gene with a wide range of phenotypical expression. It may be sporadic, due to a de novo mutation often related to advanced paternal age or familiar with autosomal dominant inheritance.

Muenke syndrome is a relatively frequent unilateral coronal craniosynostosis with brachydactyly. It is caused by a mutation (Pro250Arg) of the *FGFR3* gene, with autosomal dominant inheritance and variable clinical expression (Doherty et al. 2007). Most cases are familial, but unless there is an index case in the family, the diagnosis may be missed in newborns with a mild phenotype.

Pfeiffer syndrome is a rare acrocephalosyndactyly caused by several mutations in *FGFR1* and *FGFR2* genes, with autosomal dominant inheritance and variable clinical expressivity. Premature fusion of the coronal sutures causes acrocephaly, frontal bossing, and flat occipital bone. Concomitant synostosis of sagittal and lambdoidal sutures may cause a cloverleaf appearance of the skull. The face is characterized by downslanting palpebral fissures, ocular proptosis, strabismus, hypertelorism, maxillary hypoplasia, and low-set ears. Hands and feet usually show hypoplasia of the first ray (large first finger and toe, trapezoidal toe) and various degrees of postaxial syndactyly. There may be associated elbow ankylosis or synostosis and vertebral fusions. Most severely affected patients require early surgical correction to prevent CNS complications. The prognosis is related to the degree of phenotypical expression.

4.10.1.3 Treacher Collins Syndrome (Franceschetti Syndrome)

This syndrome is characterized by a developmental defect of the jaw and facial bones. There is wide variability. It is determined by several different mutations in the *TCOF1* gene (5q32) encoding the nucleolar phosphoprotein treacle, which has a key role in early craniofacial development, or in the *POLR1C* (6p21.1) or *POLR1D* (13q12.2) genes, encoding for RNA polymerase I and III subunits (Dixon 1996; Trainor et al. 2009). Neonatal features are downslanting palpebral fissures, palpebral coloboma, malar hypoplasia, macrostomia, micrognathia, external ear hypoplasia with atresia of the middle ear, and hearing loss. Cleft palate and choanal atresia may also be present. In the most severely affected patients, there may be impaired nutrition and respiratory function. Growth and psychomotor development are usually normal, but affected children need long-term multidisciplinary follow-up. Hearing loss requires early treatment to preserve speech development. Surgical treatment may correct bony defects and achieve useful functional and aesthetic advantages.

4.10.1.4 Nager Syndrome (Acrofacial Dysostosis Nager Type)

Nager syndrome is likely genetically heterogenous with confirmed autosomal dominant inheritance, but autosomal recessive inheritance is suspected based on sibling recurrence in consanguineous families. In approximately 50% of patients, NAFD has been associated with heterozygous mutations in the SF3B4 gene (1q21.2), coding for a component of the splicing machinery (Petit et al. 2014). Patients have a mandibulofacial dysostosis with associated preaxial limb abnormalities (Fig. 10). The mandibulofacial dysostosis is mainly characterized by microcephaly, severe micrognathia and malar hypoplasia, low-set posteriorly rotated ears, and external auditory canal atresia. The limb deformities consist of radial aplasia or hypoplasia, radioulnar synostosis with limitation of elbow extension, and hypoplasia or absence of the thumbs.

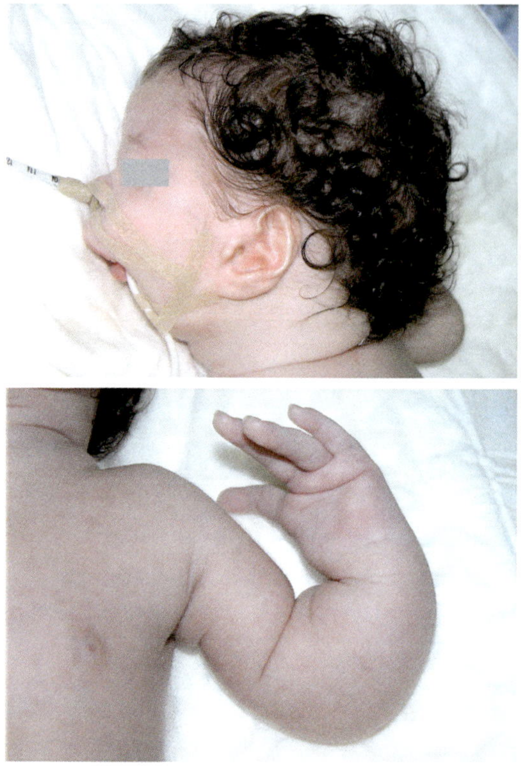

Fig. 10 Baby with Nager syndrome showing microcephaly, micrognathia, malar hypoplasia, and preaxial limb reduction defects

4.10.2 Thoraco-vertebral Dysostoses

Klippel-Feil malformation is a developmental defect of the spine, with possible changes at the cervical, thoracic, and/or lumbar level (short neck, pterygium, kyphosis, scoliosis). X-ray investigation of the spine is required to show vertebral changes (fusions, hemivertebrae, hemispondyls) and complete the diagnostic work-up; there are three clinical variants. It is more frequent in females. Its etiology is heterogeneous, with genetic and environmental (vascular disruptions) causes. It may also be part of a more complex phenotype (cervico-oculoacoustic syndrome, MURCS association).

4.10.3 Limb Dysostoses

Digital defects are caused by a differentiation defect of one or more contiguous bones. Digital development is determined by a complex genetic system, which is phylogenetically common to most vertebrates. Digital anomalies may be sporadic or familial with Mendelian inheritance and may be associated with other digital defects (polysyndactyly) and other syndromic defects.

Polydactyly may be defined as the presence of one or more supernumerary fingers or toes. It is termed as complete if it involves all phalanges, partial if it involves only distal phalanges (duplication). In the preaxial forms, the extra digit is related to the thumb; in the postaxial forms, it is related to the little finger.

Syndactyly is the fusion of two or more digits: it may involve only the skin and muscle or include the bones. In the most severe cases, it may affect all the fingers of the limb causing a "spoon" appearance. *Symphalangism* is the fusion of one or more phalanges in the same digit, with severe ankylosis of the interphalangeal joint.

Brachydactyly is the shortening of a digit due to developmental defect of one or more phalanges. It is often associated with metacarpal or meta tarsal hypoplasia.

Ectrodactyly is a severe developmental anomaly of the median axis of the hand or foot causing a "lobster-claw" appearance. It is usually caused by a genetic etiology and may be associated with other malformations (e.g., ectodermal defects and cleft palate in the ectrodactyly-ectodermal dysplasia-cleft syndrome [EEC syndrome]).

Oligodactyly is the absence or severe hypoplasia of one or more digital axes. It may be preaxial or postaxial and is frequently associated with other defects.

4.11 Osteochondrodysplasias

Osteochondrodysplasias are a wide and heterogeneous group of genetically determined conditions, involving the development and growth of bony and cartilaginous tissues. The bone involvement is often prenatally diagnosed, although some cases become evident after birth. The overall prevalence at birth is about 1/5,000. There has been a significant reduction in recent years because of ultrasonographic prenatal diagnosis of the most severe conditions. The classification of osteochondrodysplasias, based on phenotype, has recently been modified by advances in molecular genetics applied to genes involved in the synthesis of collagen and elastin, fibroblast growth factor receptors, cartilaginous proteins, vitamin D receptor complex, and lysosomal and peroxisomal enzymes.

Lethal osteochondrodysplasias are characterized by death during the perinatal period because of generalized involvement including long bones, spine, and cranial bones. Mortality is mainly related to respiratory failure (due to skeletal abnormalities and lung hypoplasia) and associated visceral and CNS malformations. Milder osteochondrodysplasias (with normal life expectancy, short stature, and abnormal bone development) may benefit from surgical bone elongation and other corrective surgery and rehabilitation programs.

4.11.1 Achondroplasia

This is the most common cause of disproportionate short stature with short limbs, determined by a heterozygous mutation (Gly380Arg) of the *FGFR3* gene at 4p16.3 which encodes a transmembrane receptor that is important in regulating linear bone growth,

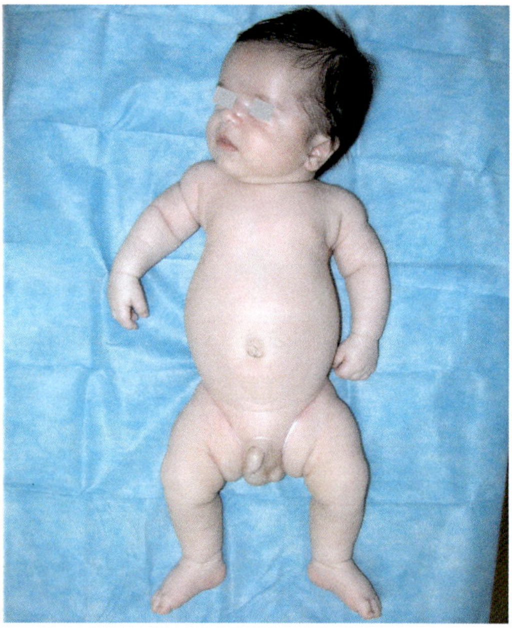

Fig. 11 Neonatal achondroplasia with rhizomelic short limb dwarfism, megalencephaly, frontal bossing, facial bone hypoplasia, and narrow thorax

among other functions. It is inherited as an autosomal dominant trait with a high rate of de novo mutations (80–90% of patients) and is related to advanced paternal age. The recurrence risk is low if parents are not affected. The phenotype at birth (Fig. 11) is characteristic: megalencephaly, frontal bossing, depressed nasal bridge, facial bone hypoplasia, prognathism, narrow thorax, rhizomelic short limb dwarfism, brachydactyly, trident hands, and hypotonia. Psychomotor development is normal. Patients frequently develop severe orthopedic complications (lumbar hyperlordosis). In some cases CNS complications, such as the cord compressions and hydrocephalus, may occur during childhood.

4.11.2 Thanatophoric Dysplasia

Thanatophoric dysplasia (TD) is a severe and generally lethal skeletal dysplasia. The phenotype is characterized by severe micromelic dwarfism with bowing and deformations of long bones, "telephone receiver" femurs, narrow thorax, severe platyspondyly (flattening of the vertebral bodies), facial bone hypoplasia, and craniosynostosis. TD includes two forms: TD, type 1 (TD1) and TD, type 2 (TD2) that can be differentiated from each other by femurs (bowed "telephone receiver" femurs in TD1) and skull shape (cloverleaf skull is main reported in TD2). All patients are sporadic and due to de novo autosomal dominant mutations in the FGFR3 gene (4p16.3) which cause overactivity of the FGFR3 protein, resulting in the disturbances in bone growth and other tissues that are characteristic of TD.

4.11.3 Campomelic Dysplasia

Campomelic dysplasia is a severe autosomal recessive bone dysplasia with high perinatal lethality and female prevalence, due to mutations in the *SOX9* gene at 17q24. The phenotype includes sex reversal (female external genitalia with male chromosomes), macrocephaly, large fontanelles, broad depressed nasal root, micrognathia, short neck, pectus carinatum, short limb dwarfism, talipes, anterior bowing of tibiae, and poor ossification signs (Mansour et al. 2002).

4.11.4 Diastrophic Dysplasia

Diastrophic dysplasia is a rare autosomal recessive condition due to mutations of the *SLC26A2* gene at 5q31-q34 which encodes a sulfate transporter that is predominantly expressed in the cartilage. Mutations in the same gene have been implicated in a moderate form of epiphyseal dysplasia and in several lethal disorders such as achondrogenesis type 1b and atelosteogenesis type 2. The distinct morphologic abnormality of the growth plate consists of an irregular distribution of degenerating chondrocytes in the resting cartilage with areas of intracartilaginous ossification. Patients have rhizomelic short limb dwarfism, bilateral clubbed foot, cystic lesions of the pinnae with calcification of the cartilage, premature calcification of the costal cartilages, kyphoscoliosis, hip contractures, and cleft palate. The "hitchhiker" thumb is particularly characteristic and is due to a deformity of the first metacarpal. Intelligence is normal. Short stature with skeletal abnormalities becomes more marked with advancing age.

4.11.5 Pseudodiastrophic Dysplasia

Pseudodiastrophic dysplasia is an autosomal recessive condition described by Burgio in patients with a phenotype similar to diastrophic dysplasia but with proximal phalangeal joint dislocation, normal first metacarpal, platyspondyly, tonguelike lumbar vertebral deformities, and marked lumbar lordosis without cystic deformity of the helix (Fischetto et al. 1997). The histologic appearance is different from diastrophic dysplasia and no *SLC26A2* mutations have been demonstrated. Most patients die during the first months of life.

4.11.6 Osteogenesis Imperfecta

Osteogenesis imperfecta is a genetically and phenotypically heterogeneous group of conditions characterized by increased bone fragility, low bone mass, and susceptibility to bone fractures with variable severity (Bodian et al. 2009). Most frequently affected genes are those encoding for type 1 collagen (*COL1A1* on 17q21-q22 and *COL1A2* on 7q22) with autosomal dominant (AD) and autosomal recessive (AR) inheritance. Five different clinical variants have been differentiated, but only type 2 and type 3 are present at birth with a severe phenotype and high perinatal lethality:

- Type 1: AD, triangular face, blue sclerae, otosclerosis with secondary hearing loss, mitral valve prolapse, macrocephaly, joint hyperlaxity, and possible dental abnormalities
- Type 2: AD/AR, ossification deficiency, craniotabes, pseudohydrocephalic skull, micrognathia, small nose, blue sclerae, cardiac valve degeneration, endocardic and aortic microcalcifications, and multiple dental abnormalities
- Type 3: AD/AR, blue sclerae, hydrocephalus, cortical atrophy, joint hyperlaxity, shortness and bowing of limbs, and possible dental abnormalities
- Type 4: AD, macrocephaly, frontal bossing, hearing loss, joint hyperlaxity, osteoporosis, mild long bone deformations, and possible dental abnormalities
- Type 5: AR, mild to moderate short stature, dislocation of the radial head, mineralized interosseous membranes, hyperplastic callus, white sclera, and no dental abnormalities

Other genetically different types have been observed (types 6–9) but they are not clinically different from types 2 to 4.

4.11.7 Osteodysplastic Primordial Dwarfism

Osteodysplastic primordial dwarfism is a group of brachymelic microcephalic dwarfisms with likely genetic heterogeneity and autosomal recessive inheritance. Different clinical variants have been described in patients with a prenatal onset of severe dwarfism (Fig. 12), microcephaly, delayed closure of fontanelles, prominent eyes and

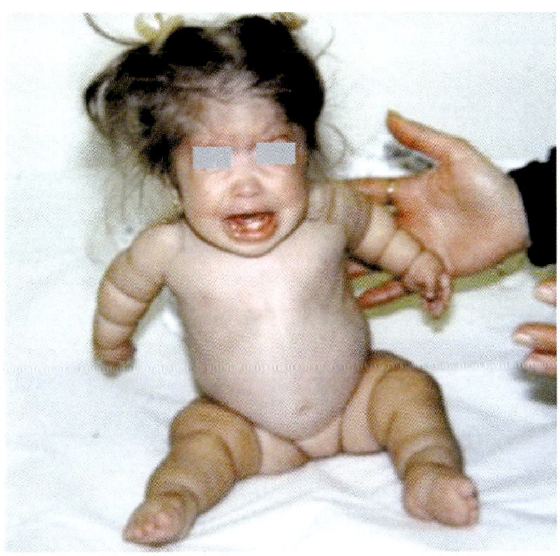

Fig. 12 Patient with osteodysplastic primordial dwarfism with microcephaly, severe shortness and deformations of long bones, and redundant skin folds at limbs

strabismus, microretrognathia, pointed nose, high-arched palate, oligodontia, small low-set dysplastic ears, sparse scalp hair, pectus carinatum, delayed bone age, severe osteoporosis, and multiple skeletal abnormalities (hip dislocation, coxa vara, joint contractures, short bowed long bones, small proximal femoral epiphyses, thin diaphyses of long bones, brachydactyly, talipes). Postnatal failure to thrive, mental retardation, sensory defects are consistently present during growth. Life expectancy is reduced.

References

Abu-Amero S, Monk D, Frost J et al (2008) The genetic aetiology of Silver-Russell syndrome. J Med Genet 45:193–199

Barry T (2015) Genetics counseling in the genomic era. https://www.jax.org. Accessed 6 Apr 2016

Barry SC, Walsh CA, Burke AL et al (2015) Natural history of fetal trisomy 13 after prenatal diagnosis. Am J Med Genet A 167(1):147–150

Bhuiyan ZA, Klein M, Hammond P et al (2006) Genotype-phenotype correlations of 39 patients with Cornelia de Lange syndrome: the Dutch experience. J Med Genet 43:568, 43:5

Biesecker LG, Spinner NB (2013) A genomic view of mosaicism and human disease. Nat Rev Genet 14 (5):307–320

Blum WF, Ross JL, Zimmermann AG et al (2013) GH treatment to final height produces similar height gains in patients with SHOX deficiency and Turner syndrome: results of a multicenter trial. J Clin Endocrinol Metab 98(8):E1383–E1392

Bodian DL, Chan T-F, Poon A et al (2009) Mutation and polymorphism spectrum in osteogenesis imperfecta type II: implications for genotype-phenotype relationships. Hum Mol Genet 18:463–471

Botto LD, May K, Fernhoff PM et al (2003) A population-based study of the 22q11.2 deletion: phenotype, incidence, and contribution to major birth defects in the population. Pediatrics 112:101–107

Dixon MJ (1996) Treacher Collins syndrome. Hum Mol Genet 1996:1391–1396

Doherty ES, Lacbawan F, Hadley DW (2007) Muenke syndrome (FGFR3-related craniosynostosis): expansion of the phenotype and review of the literature. Am J Med Genet 143A:3204–3215

Donnai D, Winter RM (1995) Congenital malformation syndromes. Chapman & Hall Medical, London

Dubourg C, David V, Gropman A et al (2011) Clinical utility gene card for: holoprosencephaly. Eur J Hum Genet 19(1):118, preceeding

Eggermann T, Buiting K, Temple IK (2011) Clinical utility gene card for: Silver-Russell syndrome. Eur J Human Genet 19(3):e1–e3

Ferrero GB, Baldassarre G, Delmonaco AG et al (2008) Clinical and molecular characterization of 40 patients with Noonan syndrome. Eur J Med Genet 51:566–572

Fischetto R, Causio F, Corso G et al (1997) Pseudodiastrophic dysplasia type Burgio in a newborn. Am J Med Genet 71(2):222–225

Giuffrè M, Piro E, Corsello G (2012) Prematurity and twinning. J Matern-Fetal Neonatal Med 25(sup3):6–10

Gorlin RJ, Cohen MM Jr, Levin LS (1990) Syndromes of the head and neck. Oxford University Press, New York

Gunay-Aygun M, Schwartz S, Heeger S et al (2001) The changing purpose of Prader-Willi syndrome clinical diagnostic criteria and proposed revised criteria. Pediatrics 108, e92

Hacıhamdioğlu B, Hacıhamdioğlu D, Delil K (2015) 22q11 deletion syndrome: current perspective. Appl Clin Genet 8:123

Jones KL (1997) Smith's recognizable patterns of human malformations. WB Saunders, Philadelphia

Karmiloff-Smith A, Al-Janabi T, D'Souza H, et al (2016) The importance of understanding individual differences in Down syndrome. F1000Research, 5

Lami F, Carli D, Ferrari P et al (2013) Holoprosencephaly: report of four cases and genotype–phenotype correlations. J Genet 92(1):97–101

Loeys BL, Dietz HC, Braverman AC et al (2010) The revised Ghent nosology for the Marfan syndrome. J Med Genet 47(7):476–485

Mansour S, Offiah AC, McDowall S et al (2002) The phenotype of survivors of campomelic dysplasia. J Med Genet 39:597–602

McDonald-McGinn DM, Sullivan KE (2011) Chromosome 22q11.2 deletion syndrome (DiGeorge syndrome/velocardiofacial syndrome). Medicine 90 (1):1–18

Mitanchez D, Yzydorczyk C, Siddeek B et al (2015) The offspring of the diabetic mother – short- and long-term implications. Best Pract Res Clin Obstet Gynaecol 29 (2):256–269

Paludetti G, Conti G, Di Nardo W et al (2012) Infant hearing loss: from diagnosis to therapy. Acta Otorhinolaryngol Ital 32:347–370

Petit F, Escande F, Jourdain AS et al (2014) Nager syndrome: confirmation of SF3B4 haploinsufficiency as the major cause. Clin Genet 86(3):246–251

Porter FD (2008) Smith–Lemli–Opitz syndrome: pathogenesis, diagnosis and management. Eur J Hum Genet 16(5):535–541

Ramos FJ, Puisac B, Baquero-Montoya C, et al (2015) Clinical utility gene card for: Cornelia de Lange syndrome. Eur J Hum Genet 23(10):e1–e4

Roberts AE, Allanson JE, Tartaglia M et al (2013) Noonan syndrome. Lancet 381(9863):333–342

Rodríguez-Caballero Á, Torres-Lagares D, Yáñez-Vico RM et al (2012) Assessment of orofacial characteristics and oral pathology associated with cri-du-chat syndrome. Oral Dis 18(2):191–197

Rubinstein-Taybi syndrome. In: Pagon RA, Adam MP, Ardinger HH, Wallace SE, Amemiya A, Bean LJH, Bird TD, Fong CT, Mefford HC, Smith RJH, Stephens K (eds). University of Washington, Seattle, GeneReviews®eneReviewsRJ Seattle. 1993–2016

Schorry EK, Keddache M, Lanphear N et al (2008) Genotype-phenotype correlations in Rubinstein-Taybi syndrome. Am J Med Genet 146A:2512–2519

Shastry SM, Kolte SS, Sanagapati PR (2012) Potter's sequence. J Clin Neonatol 1(3):157

Shaw-Smith C (2006) Oesophageal atresia, tracheo-oesophageal fistula, and the VACTERL association: review of genetics and epidemiology. J Med Genet 43 (7):545–554

Smolkin T, Soudack M, Goldstein I et al (2008) Prune belly syndrome: expanding the phenotype. Clin Dysmorphol 17:133–135

Solomon BD (2011) Vacterl/Vater association. Orphanet J Rare Dis 6(56):5

Thouvenin B, Djadi-Prat J, Chalouhi C et al (2013) Developmental outcome in Pierre Robin sequence: a longitudinal and prospective study of a consecutive series of severe phenotypes. Am J Med Genet A 161 (2):312–319

Tiecke F, Katzke S, Booms P et al (2001) Classic, atypically severe and neonatal Marfan syndrome: twelve mutations and genotype-phenotype correlations in FBN1 exons 24–40. Eur J Hum Genet 9:13, 9:1

Trainor PA, Dixon J, Dixon MJ (2009) Treacher Collins syndrome: etiology, pathogenesis and prevention. Eur J Hum Genet 17(3):275–283

Twining P, McHugo JM, Pilling DW (2000) Textbook of fetal abnormalities. Churchill Livingstone, London

Wassif CA, Maslen C, Kachilele-Linjewile S (1998) Mutations in the human sterol delta-7-reductase gene at 11q12-13 cause Smith-Lemli-Opitz syndrome. Am J Hum Genet 63:5555Ge

Weksberg R, Shuman C, Beckwith JB (2010) Beckwith–Wiedemann syndrome. Eur J Hum Genet 18(1):8–14

Wiedemann HR, Kunze J, Dibbern H (1992) An atlas of clinical syndromes. A visual aid to diagnosis, 2nd edn. Wolfe Publishing, London

Wilkie AOM, Slaney SF, Oldridge M et al (1995) Apert syndrome results from localized mutations of FGFR2 and is allelic with Crouzon syndrome. Nat Genet 9(165t 9):1

Winter TC, Kennedy AM, Woodward PJ (2015) Holoprosencephaly: a survey of the entity, with embryology and fetal imaging. Radiographics 35(1):275–290

Wolfgram PM, Carrel AL, Allen DB (2013) Long-term effects of recombinant human growth hormone therapy in children with Prader-Willi syndrome. Curr Opin Pediatr 25:509–514

Wu J, Springett A, Morris JK (2013) Survival of trisomy 18 (Edwards Syndrome) and trisomy 13 (Patau Syndrome) in England and Wales: 2004–2011. Am J Med Genet A 161(10):2512–2518

Prenatal and Postnatal Inflammatory Mechanisms

5

Kirsten Glaser and Christian P. Speer

Contents

Abstract

During the past 20 years, intrauterine infection and inflammation have been identified as significant risk factors in the development of fetal and neonatal morbidity and mortality, as well as adverse long-term outcome in very immature preterm infants. Besides severe infections, immature preterm infants are at high risk for syndromes of dysregulated inflammation including bronchopulmonary dysplasia (BPD), necrotizing enterocolitis

K. Glaser (✉) · C. P. Speer (✉)
University Children's Hospital, University of Würzburg, Würzburg, Germany
e-mail: Glaser_K@ukw.de; speer_c@ukw.de

G. Buonocore et al. (eds.), *Neonatology*,
https://doi.org/10.1007/978-3-319-29489-6_154

(NEC), and preterm cerebral white matter disease (WMD). Although pathogenesis is multifactorial, inflammation has been acknowledged as principle mechanism, being caused, sustained, and aggravated by multiple perinatal factors interacting in a multiple-hit sequence. An inflammatory state is presumed to be either initiated prenatally by chorioamnionitis or induced and sustained by pro-inflammatory postnatal conditions, such as oxygen toxicity, mechanical ventilation, and neonatal infection. Perturbation of pro- and anti-inflammatory central signaling pathways and subsequently imbalanced inflammatory responses may lead to severe organ injury affecting parenchymal development during a window of vulnerability. Maturation-dependent factors and genetic predisposition may underlie a particular vulnerability.

Abbreviations

BALF	Bronchoalveolar lavage fluid
BPD	Bronchopulmonary dysplasia
CA	Chorioamnionitis
CP	Cerebral palsy
CPAP	Continuous positive airway pressure
CSF	Cerebrospinal fluid
ELBW	Extremely low birth weight
EOS	Early-onset sepsis
FIRS	Fetal inflammatory response syndrome
ICAM	Intercellular adhesion molecules
IFN-γ	Interferon-y
IL	Interleukin
IL-1ra	IL-1 receptor antagonist
IRAK	IL-1 receptor-associated kinase
LOS	Late-onset sepsis
LPS	Lipopolysaccharide (endotoxin)
MCP	Monocyte chemoattractant protein
MIP	Macrophage inflammatory protein
MMP	Matrix metalloproteinase
MRI	Magnetic resonance imaging
NF-$_{K}$B	Nuclear transcription factor $_{K}$B
PCR	Polymerase chain reaction
PMNs	Polymorphonuclear cells
Pre-OLs	Pre-myelinating oligodendrocytes
PRR	Pattern recognition receptor
RDS	Respiratory distress syndrome
ROS	Reactive oxygen species
SP	Surfactant protein
TGF-β	Transforming growth factor-β
TLR	Toll-like receptor
TNF-α	Tumor necrosis factor-α
VCAM	Vascular cell adhesion molecules
VEGF	Vascular endothelial growth factor

5.1 Salient Points

- Inflammation is the final common mechanism through which many factors can affect fetal mortality and morbidity.
- Inflammation-promoting factors may be pre- or post-natal.
- Pre-natal factors may cause a "fetal systemic inflammatory response syndrome" – FIRS – in susceptible fetuses.
- Post-natal factors may act like a second hit, amplifying the damage.
- Brain and lung injury are the main expression of inflammation-induced damage.
- Many substances, such as cytokines, chemokines, oxygen radicals, and growth factors, may lead to an imbalance between pro- and anti-inflammatory factors.

5.2 Introduction

Various microorganisms residing in the maternal recto-vaginal tract may invade the chorioamniotic membranes and may induce an inflammatory response in the amniotic cavity, the fetus and the mother (Kim et al. 2015). Both ascending microbial infection and maternal bacteremia may initiate a similar sequence of inflammation in the placenta and the amniotic cavity, which is associated with an increased risk for the development of fetal systemic inflammatory response syndrome (FIRS) and adverse neonatal outcome (Khwaja and Volpe 2008; Speer 2011; Dammann and Leviton 2014; Garcia-Munoz Rodrigo et al. 2014; Korzeniewski et al. 2014; Thomas and Speer 2014). Activation of fetal inflammatory response may inversely correlate with gestational age, leaving very immature preterm infants at highest risk of long-term complications (Garcia-Munoz Rodrigo et al. 2014; Lee et al. 2015). However, clinical observations indicate that fetal exposure to severe chorioamnionitis (CA) might not necessarily result in an inflammatory response of an individual fetus. In contrast, a rather smoldering or nearly inapparent amniotic infection/inflammation might induce a severe fetal reaction (Thomas and Speer 2011). Since the underlying pathogenetic mechanisms are poorly understood, we are currently unable to identify a fetus at risk for developing serious sequelae following exposure to prenatal inflammation.

Acute fetal inflammatory response may promote secondary and tertiary damage mechanisms (Dammann and Leviton 2014; Korzeniewski et al. 2014; Thomas and Speer 2014; Viscardi 2012) and may result in subsequent neonatal inflammation-induced disorders, such as bronchopulmonary dysplasia (BPD) (Speer 2009), necrotizing enterocolitis (NEC) (Nanthakumar et al. 2011), and preterm cerebral white matter disease (WMD) (Khwaja and Volpe 2008) (Figs. 2 and 3). Moreover, respiratory distress syndrome (RDS) may be aggravated by an injurious inflammatory sequence inactivating the surfactant system and affecting the integrity of the immature lung (Speer 2011). Various adverse postnatal conditions such as oxygen toxicity, mechanical ventilation, and neonatal infection may act as a "second or third strike" amplifying or aggravating an injurious inflammatory response (Korzeniewski et al. 2014; Thomas and Speer 2014; Speer 2009; Reyburn et al. 2012; Bose et al. 2013). Cytokines, chemokines, oxygen radicals, growth factors, and other substances may orchestrate a complex interplay of sustained and dysregulated inflammation constituting neonatal inflammation-induced organ injury (Khwaja and Volpe 2008; Dammann and Leviton 2014; Viscardi 2012; Speer 2009; Reyburn et al. 2012; Bose et al. 2008). Immaturity and dysfunction of innate immune cells and impairments in the termination of inflammation may contribute to perpetuated inflammation (Dammann and Leviton 2014; Speer et al. 1988; Nguyen et al. 2010; Glaser and Speer 2013), subsequently affecting normal vascular and organ development (Thebaud and Abman 2007; Kaindl et al. 2009). The role of genetic predisposition has been subject of clinical studies and in vitro trials (Lal and Ambalavanan 2015). This chapter will try to summarize the current concepts of prenatal and postnatal inflammatory mechanisms in the human fetus and preterm infant with main emphasis on the pathogenetic role of inflammatory events in preterm lung and brain injury. Both aspects have been reasonably well studied and have been continuously discussed and updated (Khwaja and Volpe 2008; Dammann and Leviton 2014; Thomas and Speer 2014; Viscardi 2012; Speer 2009). BPD is the most common respiratory disease following preterm birth characterized by inflammation, apoptosis, and extensive extracellular matrix remodeling that significantly affects neonatal morbidity and mortality (Jobe 2011). Diffuse or focal preterm WMD, usually referred to as periventricular leukomalacia (PVL), is the most common form of brain injury in preterm infants of gestational ages less than 32 weeks, associated with a high risk of neurodevelopmental impairment (Khwaja and Volpe 2008). Although pathogenesis of preterm lung and brain injury is multifactorial, both infection-induced inflammation and nonspecific inflammation have been assumed principle underlying mechanisms.

5.3 Prenatal Inflammation

5.3.1 Chorioamnionitis

Intra-amniotic inflammation seems to be prevalent in about 30% of patients with preterm labor with intact membranes and in 50–80% of patients with preterm premature rupture of the membranes and spontaneous preterm birth (Kim et al. 2015). CA has been defined using histological, microbiological, clinical, and biochemical criteria (Fig. 1) (Kim et al. 2015). Histologic CA is an inflammatory condition of the placenta involving amnion, choriodecidua, and/or chorionic plate in response to microbial invasion or pathological processes (Kim et al. 2015). However, definition of CA may also refer to clinical data, such as fever,

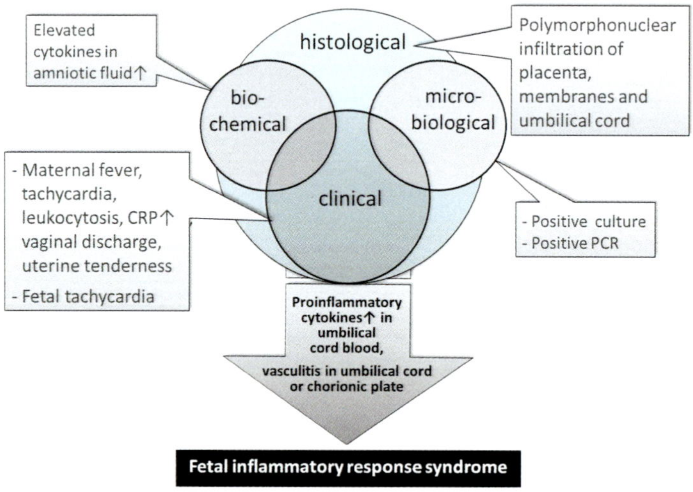

Fig. 1 Schematic illustration of different approaches to define chorioamnionitis (Modified from Thomas and Speer (2011)). The term "chorioamnionitis" is inconsistently used among clinicians and across epidemiologic studies. Definition of CA may refer to histologic examination, based on microscopic evidence of inflammation of the membranes, as well as clinical data, based on clinical manifestations of local or systemic inflammation (Kim et al. 2015). While acute chorioamnionitis is evidence of a maternal host response, funisitis and chorionic vasculitis represent fetal inflammatory response

tachycardia, elevated maternal inflammation parameters, uterine tenderness, foul-smelling vaginal discharge, and fetal tachycardia (Kim et al. 2015). Severity of CA may vary significantly and depend on the duration of in utero infection (Lee et al. 2015; Goldenberg et al. 2008). Most pathogens associated with CA are of low virulence implying subclinical courses in many cases. In general, anaerobic, aerobic, and atypical bacteria contribute to the list, such as *Ureaplasma* species (spp.), *Mycoplasma hominis*, *Fusobacterium* spp., *Streptococcus* spp., *Bacteroides* spp., and *Prevotella* spp. (Kim et al. 2015). *Ureaplasma*-induced intrauterine inflammation has been associated with increased risk of FIRS as well as perinatal lung and brain injury (Viscardi 2012, 2014; Goldenberg et al. 2008; Normann et al. 2009). In preterm infants who develop BPD, *Ureaplasma* spp. have been the most common microorganisms isolated from the amniotic fluid, cord blood, and respiratory tract (Viscardi 2012, 2014). In a mouse model of *Ureaplasma*-induced CA, fetal CNS inflammation is followed by significant disturbance of brain development (Normann et al. 2009). Incidence and prevalence of CA appear to be inversely related to gestational age with the highest risk in very immature preterm infants <28 weeks of gestation, contributing itself to prematurity-associated neonatal morbidities (Kim et al. 2015; Garcia-Munoz Rodrigo et al. 2014; Lee et al. 2015; Goldenberg et al. 2008; Hartling et al. 2012; Ericson and Laughon 2015). Attempts to assess a gestation-independent effect of CA on BPD and neonatal brain injury have presented inconclusive results (Khwaja and Volpe 2008; Thomas and Speer 2011; Viscardi 2012; Hartling et al. 2012; Ericson and Laughon 2015; Wu 2002). However, a relevant number of studies confirmed the impact of CA on preterm lung and brain injury in concert with adverse pro-inflammatory conditions, such as hyperoxia or hypoxia, mechanical ventilation, and postnatal infection (Reyburn et al. 2012; Bose et al. 2013; Kaindl et al. 2009; Inatomi et al. 2012). Correlation between CA and neonatal morbidities may be challenging due to a number of antenatal and postnatal confounding factors, such as imprecise diagnoses of CA, and diseases of prematurity, variability of study populations, higher prevalence of antenatal steroids and surfactant replacement therapy nowadays, polymicrobial immunomodulation and pathogen synergy, the individual fetal response, and contributing postnatal factors (Lee et al. 2015; Thomas and Speer 2011; Viscardi 2012; Hartling et al. 2012). CA clearly increases the likelihood of very premature preterm birth with the latter being the most important risk factor for the development of diseases of prematurity. Moreover, fetal exposure to prenatal inflammation may induce an adverse sequence of fetal inflammation that may directly affect the vulnerable immature lung and brain and, moreover, may confer a heightened susceptibility to postnatal adverse conditions. The latter – acting as "second or third strike" – may amplify inflammation-induced lung and white matter injury (Figs. 2 and 3).

5.3.1.1 Lung Injury

Clinical CA has been identified as an independent risk factor for RDS in preterm infants, whereas histological CA seems to confer a beneficial effect on the incidence of RDS. This maturational effect in turn seems to contribute to a heightened susceptibility of the lung to postnatal injury (Thomas and Speer 2011; Speer 2009). Data for histological CA are consistent with data of maturational effects in an animal model. However, in the same animal model, pulmonary maturation is followed by significantly disturbed structural development of the lung (Kramer et al. 2009). Attempts to correlate CA and BPD have presented inconclusive results (Thomas and Speer 2011, 2014). Various studies indicated an increased association of CA and BPD; others reported a decreased association or no effect of CA on neonatal respiratory outcome (Thomas and Speer 2011; Viscardi 2012).

5.3.1.2 Brain Injury

Attempts to assess a gestation-independent effect of CA on neonatal brain injury have not provided definite results. Controlling for gestational age

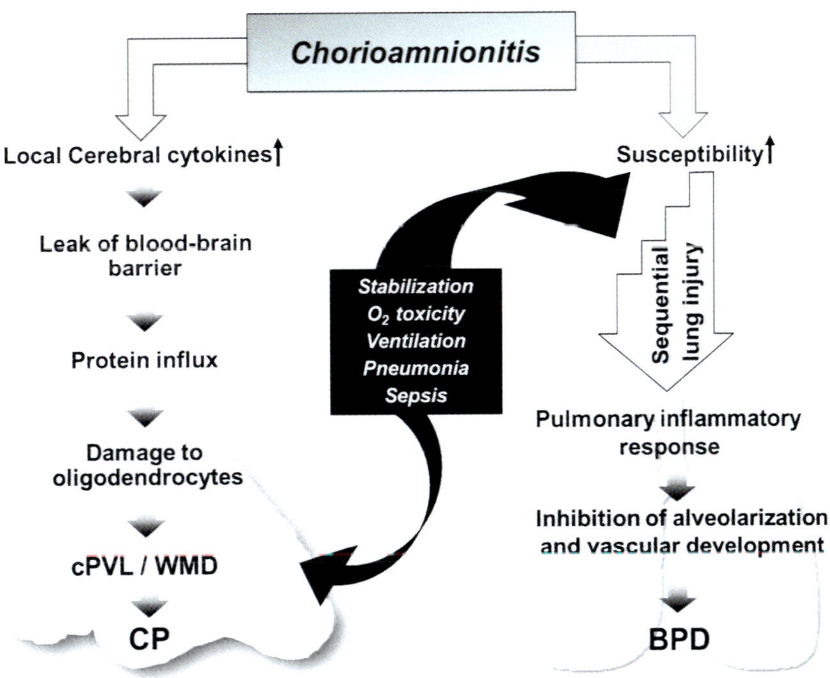

Fig. 2 Illustration of potential pathogenetic mechanisms linking chorioamnionitis and fetal inflammatory response with adverse sequences of neonatal lung and brain injury (Modified from Thomas and Speer (2011)). An inflammatory state is presumed to be either initiated prenatally by chorioamnionitis or induced and sustained by pro-inflammatory postnatal conditions, such as oxygen toxicity, mechanical ventilation, and neonatal infection

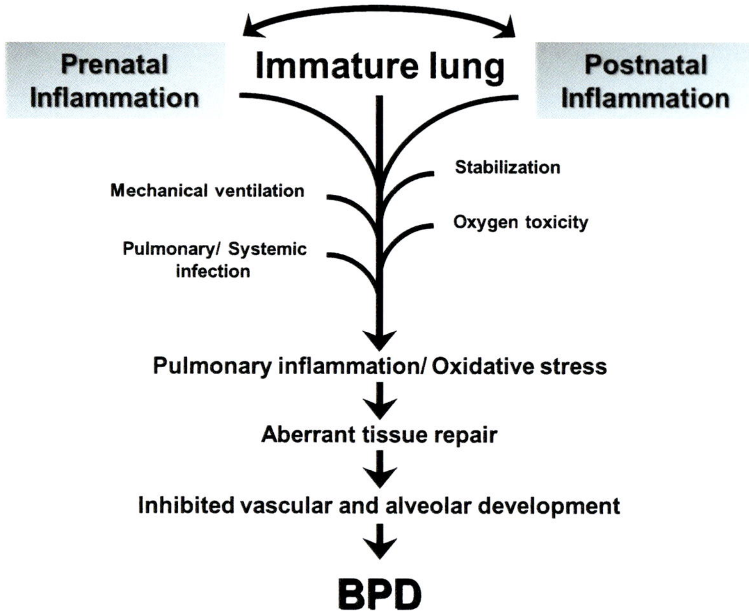

Fig. 3 Schematic illustration of the complex interplay of prenatal and postnatal pro-inflammatory conditions contributing to perpetuated adverse lung inflammation. BPD may result from inflammation-induced lung injury and impaired lung development during a window of vulnerability. Individual infants may be particularly susceptible to sustained lung inflammation due to predisposing genetic factors

reduced or abolished an association between CA and PVL in some studies (Thomas and Speer 2011; Wu 2002), while others confirmed an association of CA and WMD especially in very immature preterm infants (Khwaja and Volpe 2008; Thomas and Speer 2011; Leviton et al. 2010). CA has been associated with increased risk for arterial hypotension, which has been acknowledged as significant risk factor for WMD (Khwaja and Volpe 2008).

5.3.2 Fetal Inflammatory Response Syndrome

Intrauterine inflammation may induce a fetal inflammatory response, characterized histologically by funisitis with polymorphonuclear cell (PMN) infiltration and biochemically by elevated umbilical cord concentrations of pro-inflammatory cytokines, chemokines, matrix metalloproteinases (MMPs), and angiogenic factors such as vascular endothelial growth factor (VEGF) (Fig. 1) (Thomas and Speer 2011). Induction of cytokines and augmentation of deleterious effects, including free radical and excitatory amino acid release, have been implicated in the development of diseases of prematurity (Khwaja and Volpe 2008; Korzeniewski et al. 2014; Viscardi 2012; Viscardi et al. 2004). Increased levels of pro-inflammatory cytokines in fetal cord blood were identified as independent risk factors for BPD and adverse neurologic outcomes in preterm infants (Viscardi 2012; Speer 2009; Viscardi et al. 2004). Of note, fetal exposure to severe maternal chorioamnionitis might not necessarily result in an inflammatory response of an individual fetus, while a rather smoldering or nearly inapparent amniotic infection/inflammation might induce a severe fetal reaction (Thomas and Speer 2011).

5.3.2.1 Lung Injury

Pronounced infiltration of inflammatory cells, an increased expression of cytokines and markers of endothelial activation, and a large number of apoptotic airway cells were observed in lung tissues of human fetuses with funisitis (May et al. 2004).

5.3.2.2 Brain Injury

Experimental, epidemiological, and immunohistochemical data also confirm an association of FIRS and neonatal brain injury, documenting upregulation of cerebrospinal fluid (CSF) cytokines and augmentation of deleterious effects, such as free radical and excitatory amino acid release (Dammann and Leviton 2014; Viscardi 2014; Viscardi et al. 2004). Downstream pathogenetic mechanisms affecting the developing brain may comprise microglial activation, inhibition of oligodendrocyte differentiation, disturbances of apoptosis, impaired neurogenesis, and myelin degeneration (Khwaja and Volpe 2008; Kaindl et al. 2009).

5.4 Postnatal Inflammation

5.4.1 Infection

Bacteremia and neonatal sepsis are associated with considerable acute and long-term morbidity, especially in preterm infants, including death, chronic lung disease, and neurodevelopmental impairment (Stoll et al. 2011; Bersani and Speer 2012; Boghossian et al. 2013; Strunk et al. 2014). Early-onset sepsis (EOS), associated with acquisition of microorganisms by transplacental or ascending infection, is most commonly caused by *group B Streptococci* and *Escherichia coli* with decreasing incidence due to the implementation of a prenatal screening and treatment protocol for *group B Streptococci* (Stoll et al. 2011). Nosocomial late-onset sepsis (LOS) is mainly caused by bacterial infection from coagulase-negative *Staphylococci*, *S. aureus*, or gram-negative bacteria (Dong and Speer 2015). Highest incidence rates are documented in very immature preterm infants due to increased susceptibility and more frequent invasive procedures (Bersani and Speer 2012; Boghossian et al. 2013). Both EOS and LOS have been identified as individual risk factors of BPD and neonatal brain injury (Speer 2006a, 2009; Strunk et al. 2014). Conversely, both histological and clinical CA have been associated with increased risk of EOS in very immature preterm infants (Ericson and Laughon 2015; Strunk et al. 2012), underlying the pathogenetic role of intrauterine inflammation in the development of BPD and WMD.

5.4.1.1 Lung Injury

Priming of the fetal lung by endotoxin (lipopolysaccharide, LPS) may be a relevant orchestrating factor. Animal experiments indicate that LPS stimulation may initiate pulmonary inflammation reflected by increased expression of pro-inflammatory cytokines and chemokines, recruitment of PMNs and monocytes, and impaired alveolar and microvascular development (Kramer et al. 2009).

5.4.1.2 Brain Injury

In animal models of bacterial meningitis, elevated serum levels of pro-inflammatory mediators alter blood-brain barrier (BBB) integrity, promote BBB breakdown, and induce an adverse cascade of CNS inflammation involving perpetuated cytokine and chemokine synthesis, leukocyte activation, MMP and prostaglandin synthesis, and lipid peroxidation (Strunk et al. 2014; Kim 2003). Moreover, peripheral intravenous LPS stimulation was shown to result in CSF cytokine response and to exacerbate brain lesions similar to those found in human infants with cerebral palsy (CP) (Dommergues et al. 2000). LPS injected directly into the fetal brain of rats resulted in hypomyelination, loss of oligodendrocytes, cystic damage, and ventricular enlargement consistent with diffuse PVL and persistently impaired myelination in the long term (Cai et al. 2003). Of note, bacterial infection leads to a heightened susceptibility of the preterm brain to non-inflammatory insults, such as hypoxia (Strunk et al. 2014).

5.4.2 Mechanical Ventilation

Assisted ventilation may be the most common prolonged stimulus for systemic inflammation in preterm infants (Bose et al. 2013). Moreover, any kind of mechanical ventilation may be injurious to the airways and lung tissue, provoking a stretch-induced injurious cascade (Reyburn et al. 2012; Bose et al. 2013; Hillman et al. 2011) that is characterized by bronchial epithelial disruption and the release of pro-inflammatory mediators with subsequent leukocyte influx (Bose et al. 2013; Hillman et al. 2011). In animal models, the severity of inflammatory reaction was related to ventilation strategies characterized by high peak and lack of positive end expiratory pressure (Hillman et al. 2011). Current neonatal strategies attempt to minimize the need for endotracheal intubation and intermittent positive pressure ventilation and favor continuous positive airway pressure (CPAP)-based strategies (Morley 2010; Hallman et al. 2013). Lung volume recruitment and avoidance of high tidal volumes are key elements of current lung-protective ventilation strategies (Lozano and Newnam 2016). However, more and more extremely low birth weight (ELBW) infants exposed to no or minimal barotrauma and to relatively low levels of supplemental oxygen may develop respiratory deterioration at a postnatal age of 1–2 weeks (Martin and Fanaroff 2013).

5.4.2.1 Lung Injury

In a murine model of BPD, inflammation-induced alterations and structural lung damage were strongly related to developmental stages with the saccular stage of lung development being particularly vulnerable (Backstrom et al. 2011). Consistently, clinical studies documented that very immature preterm infants <28 weeks of gestation (saccular stage) are at highest risk for inflammation-induced BPD, whereas preterm infants born >32 weeks of gestation (early alveolar stage) are at much lower risk (Jobe 2011). In newborn rat lungs, even low tidal volume ventilation was shown to induce acute phase cytokines and CXC chemokines. This pro-inflammatory response was amplified by oxygen and oxygen combined with LPS pretreatment (Kroon et al. 2010). In a rat model of lung injury, LPS challenge resulted in significantly increased levels of pro-inflammatory cytokines in bronchoalveolar lavage fluid (BALF) despite "less injurious" ventilation strategies (Ricard et al. 2001). The latter data may underline the relevant pathogenetic role of pro-inflammatory priming on the downhill progression to BPD (Fig. 3).

5.4.2.2 Brain Injury

Irrespective of the strategy used, mechanical ventilation increased hemodynamic instability in neonatal lambs born with CA and, moreover, increased pro-inflammatory cytokine expression within the lungs and brains, contributing to CA-induced brain injury (Barton et al. 2014).

5.4.3 Hyperoxia and Hypoxia

Increased oxidative stress and imbalance of antioxidant enzymes may play a significant role in the pathogenesis of neonatal lung and brain injury. Reactive oxygen (ROS) and nitrogen species (RNS) are produced by several inflammatory cells. Profound deficiency in antioxidant enzyme activity may leave very immature preterm infants at high risk of suffering from hyperoxia-induced detrimental effects (Khwaja and Volpe 2008; Saugstad 2005). Transition from the fetal normotoxic in utero environment to postnatal room air represents a sudden exposure to a relatively "hyperoxic" environment. On the contrary, episodes of hypoxia or fluctuating oxygen saturations most often due to apnea of prematurity adversely affect lung and brain development, both directly and by iatrogenic oxygen supplementation (Bhandari 2010). Data from animal models demonstrate hypoxia-induced aggravation of LPS-induced inflammation in neonatal lung and brain tissue (Strunk et al. 2014; Vuichard et al. 2005; Girard et al. 2012).

5.4.3.1 Lung Injury

In animal models, hyperoxia has been shown to affect a complex orchestra of genes involved in inflammation, extracellular matrix turnover, coagulation, and other events and to induce influx of inflammatory cells in pulmonary tissue (Bhandari 2010; Wagenaar et al. 2004). Moreover, hyperoxia resulted in progressive lung disease demonstrating many features of the BPD phenotype (Wagenaar et al. 2004). A considerable number of studies confirmed injurious effects of perinatal supplemental oxygen administration on pulmonary development (Bhandari 2010). Subsequently, optimum target ranges of oxygen saturation in extremely premature preterm infants have been reassessed (Hallman et al. 2013).

5.4.3.2 Brain Injury

Experimental and clinical data suggest that both inflammation and elevated oxygen concentrations, by itself or in combination, may contribute to brain injury in preterm infants (Schmitz et al. 2011). In animal model, hyperoxia induced maturation-dependent cell death in oligodendroglia (Brehmer et al. 2012). Pro-inflammatory cytokines, induction of MMPs, and generation of ROS and RNS were shown to be involved in - hyperoxia-induced apoptosis (Brehmer et al. 2012).

However, beside inflammation, hypoxia-ischemia is the principle initiating mechanism in the pathogenesis of WMD, activating the adverse downstream mechanisms of excitotoxicity, referring to excessive glutamatergic activation, and free radical attack by ROS and RNS culminating in pre-OL injury (Khwaja and Volpe 2008). In animal model, systemic inflammation prior to an excitotoxic insult or oxidative stress significantly exacerbated white matter lesions, demonstrating a potentiating interaction between systemic inflammation and hypoxia-ischemia in the pathogenesis of neonatal brain injury (Khwaja and Volpe 2008; Kaindl et al. 2009).

5.5 Molecular Mechanisms of Adverse Inflammation

Inflammatory responses comprise initiation and resolution phases aiming at microbial clearance, remodeling, and tissue regeneration. Ideally, acute inflammation is self-limited and leads to complete resolution and restored homeostasis (Levy and Serhan 2014). This resolution of inflammation is tightly regulated by anti-inflammatory and pro-resolving proteins and a number of polyunsaturated fatty acid-derived pro-resolving mediators, potently reducing cytokine expression, terminating PMN invasion, and enhancing macrophage uptake (Dammann and Leviton 2014; Levy and Serhan 2014). Unresolved and perpetuated inflammation may lead to severe organ injury. In preterm infants, maturation-dependent impairments in inflammation-resolution mechanisms may contribute to the inflammatory state (Dammann and Leviton 2014; Speer et al. 1988; Nguyen et al. 2010; Levy and Serhan 2014).

5.5.1 Cellular and Humoral Mediators of Inflammation

Priming and activation of PMNs and mononuclear cells (peripheral blood mononuclear cells, PBMCs) are essential stages of the early immune response to invading microorganisms or tissue damage (Speer 2009; Nguyen et al. 2010). Circulating neutrophils and monocytes become rapidly activated within 1–3 h (Turunen et al. 2006), followed by adherence to the endothelium and initiation of pro-inflammatory events. Apoptosis of inflammatory neutrophils and their timely removal by resident macrophages is critical to resolution of inflammation. However, a relevant number of studies documented altered neonatal phagocyte function, a reduced phagocytosis of apoptotic tissue cells, and prolonged survival of neonatal PMNs, potentially contributing to prolonged and perpetuated inflammation (Speer et al. 1988; Nguyen et al. 2010).

5.5.1.1 Lung Injury

In BPD, several studies revealed significantly higher and persisting numbers of neutrophils and macrophages in BALFs and lung tissues of preterm infants affected compared to infants who did not develop chronic lung disease (Groneck et al. 1994; Murch et al. 1996a). Ventilation-induced influx of neutrophils and mononuclear cells has been associated with pulmonary edema formation reflecting injury to the alveolar-capillary unit (Groneck et al. 1994; Jaarsma et al. 2004). Neonatal neutrophils surviving spontaneous apoptosis were shown to exhibit augmented inflammatory function reflected by enhanced secretion of interleukin (IL)-8 and macrophage inflammatory protein (MIP)-1β (Nguyen et al. 2010). Besides, alveolar and pulmonary tissue macrophages have been shown to play a central role in lung inflammation by orchestrating the inflammatory response via cytokine release (Viscardi 2012; Bose et al. 2008).

5.5.1.2 Brain Injury

The neuropathologic hallmarks of preterm WMD are microglial activation and depletion of pre-myelinating oligodendroglia (Kaindl et al. 2009). Microglial cells are the main source of stimulus-induced cytokine synthesis as well as generation of ROS, RNS, and glutamate, thus playing a central role in the detrimental effects of a pro-inflammatory cytokine cascade on the neonatal brain. Neutrophils contribute to the release of cytotoxic factors, ROS, RNS, and lipid peroxidation (Khwaja and Volpe 2008). The maturation-dependent density of microglia throughout the white matter and a gestational age-dependent vulnerability of pre-OLs to toxic ROS and cytokine attack may underlie a particular vulnerability of the immature brain (Khwaja and Volpe 2008; Kaindl et al. 2009).

5.5.2 Cellular and Endothelial Interaction

A relevant number of adhesion molecules, such as intercellular adhesion molecules (ICAMs) and vascular cell adhesion molecules (VCAMs), promote attachment of inflammatory cells to the endothelium (Sarelius and Glading 2015).

5.5.2.1 Lung Injury

In infants with BPD, increased concentrations of selectins and ICAMs were detected in airway secretions and circulation, reflecting enhanced shedding in response to inflammation (D'Alquen et al. 2005). Moreover, significant upregulation of ICAM-1 on endothelial cord cells and increased serum levels of soluble ICAM-1 were shown in preterm infants exposed to CA (D'Alquen et al. 2005). These data may point to an effective recruitment of circulating neutrophils and monocytes into the airways and pulmonary tissue of preterm infants.

5.5.2.2 Brain Injury

In human brain microvascular endothelial cells, surface expression of both ICAM-1 and VCAM-1 has been found to be induced by pro-inflammatory stimuli, such as TNF-α and IL-1β, reflecting the inflammatory phenotype of human BBB (O'Carroll et al. 2015).

5.5.3 Chemotactic and Chemokinetic Factors

Recruitment of inflammatory cells is mainly promoted by chemokines (Baier et al. 2004). Chemokines are classified into four families (C, CC, CXC, and CX_3C) with the CC family being activators of monocytes and macrophages, lymphocytes, eosinophils, and basophils (Zlotnik and Yoshie 2012).

5.5.3.1 Lung Injury

IL-8 (CXCL8) may be the most important chemotactic factor for recruitment of monocytes and neutrophils to the site of inflammation (Garcia-Ramallo et al. 2002). Moreover, IL-8 plays a pivotal role in neutrophil activation by upregulation of neutrophil adhesion molecules, promotion of transendothelial migration, and stimulation of oxidative burst and lysosomal enzyme release (Garcia-Ramallo et al. 2002). A role for CC chemokines in the pathogenesis of acute and chronic lung disease was suggested by animal and clinical studies (Smith 1996). The application of a selective chemokine receptor antagonist was shown to inhibit neutrophil influx into the rat lung, to suppress pulmonary inflammation and to enhance lung growth (Yi et al. 2004). Increased concentrations of members of the CC family, monocyte chemoattractant protein (MCP)-1 and MIP-1α, were found in ventilated preterm infants suffering from acute lung injury and correlated with BPD (Murch et al. 1996a). Moreover, increased tracheal aspirate concentrations of MCP-1, MCP-2, MCP-3, and MIP-1β were identified as independent risk factors for RDS and BPD (Baier et al. 2004). Additional chemoattractants, such as C5a, IL-8, IL-16, lipoxygenase products, leukotriene B_4, elastin fragments, metalloproteases, and fibronectin, were also increased in infants with BPD compared to those who recovered from RDS (Speer 2006a, 2009).

5.5.3.2 Brain Injury

In infants diagnosed with inflammation-related WMD, levels of both pro-inflammatory cytokines and IL-8 are elevated in amniotic fluid, cord blood, CSF, and cerebral tissue (Strunk et al. 2014). Thus, beside other humoral mediators, IL-8 may be a key mediator in the pathogenesis of inflammation-induced neonatal brain injury (Dammann and Leviton 2014; Strunk et al. 2014).

5.5.4 Pro- and Anti-Inflammatory Cytokines

Pro-inflammatory cytokines, such as TNF-α, IL-1β and IL-6, play a crucial role in early inflammation, mediating up- and/or downregulation of genes and transcription factors (Bose et al. 2008). Pro-inflammatory cytokines are synthesized by various inflammatory cells, including PMNs; monocytes and macrophages; microglial and pulmonary cells, upon stimulation by LPS; other bacterial cell wall constituents; a wide range of endogenous ligands, hyperoxia, and hypoxia; and biophysical factors such as volutrauma and barotrauma (Khwaja and Volpe 2008; Speer 2006a). Innate and adaptive immune responses in term and especially preterm neonates exhibit quantitative and qualitative developmental particularities (Dammann and Leviton 2014; Speer et al. 1988; Nguyen et al. 2010; Glaser and Speer 2013). A propensity toward the pro-inflammatory state has been postulated (Kollmann et al. 2009; Levy and Wynn 2014). Experimental and clinical data indicate that the profound fetal pro-inflammatory response may, in part, be attributed to inadequate anti-inflammatory cytokine responses, involving IL-4, IL-10, IL-11, IL-12, IL-13, IL-18, or IL-1 receptor antagonist (IL-1ra) as well as pro-resolving proteins and a number of polyunsaturated fatty acid-derived pro-resolving mediators (Dammann and Leviton 2014; Viscardi 2012; Speer 2009; Brochu et al. 2011). Preterm infants appear to have a paucity of some of these proteins and mediators (Dammann and Leviton 2014).

5.5.4.1 Lung Injury

Macrophage-derived TNF-α is considered to contribute significantly to the pro-inflammatory reaction being a known trigger of various inflammatory mediators in alveolar cells (Speer 2009). IL-1β is a central pro-inflammatory cytokine found in the amniotic fluid in CA (Yoon et al. 1997) that has been shown to significantly disturb lung morphogenesis in a fetal mouse model (Hogmalm et al. 2014). Increased protein levels and high mRNA expression of pro-inflammatory TNF-α and IL-1β have been detected in respiratory fluids, in bronchoalveolar and pulmonary cells, and in the systemic circulation of preterm infants with RDS and evolving BPD pointing toward imbalance of pro- and anti-inflammatory factors (Speer 2006a, 2009; Bose et al. 2008). The influx of TNF-α-positive macrophages in pulmonary tissues of preterm infants who had died of severe RDS was found to be associated with severe destruction of pulmonary interstitium (Murch et al. 1996b). In a bi-transgenic mouse model, perinatal overexpression of IL-1β in pulmonary epithelial cells was shown to induce increased TNF-α and IL-6 expression and profound tissue injury similar to BPD (Hogmalm et al. 2014, Kolb et al. 2001). Both production of IL-1β and activation of nuclear transcription factor kappa (NF-$_k$B) in lung macrophages were found to significantly contribute to arrested lung development (Blackwell et al. 2011). IL-10 was undetectable in most airway samples of preterm infants with BPD, but regularly found in term infants with respiratory failure (Jones et al. 1996). Especially in preterm infants exposed to CA or affected by FIRS, insufficient inhibition of exaggerated fetal pro-inflammatory cytokine responses may increase the risk of BPD (Paananen et al. 2009). In surfactant-depleted rabbits, prophylactic treatment with aerosolized anti-inflammatory IL-1ra decreased inflammation in experimental lung injury (Narimanbekov and Rozycki 1995).

5.5.4.2 Brain Injury

Experimental, epidemiological, and immunohistochemical data support a *cytokine hypothesis* of brain injury considering microglial cytokine releases the major mediator of white matter damage (Dammann and Leviton 2014; Strunk et al. 2014; Girard et al. 2009). Several cytokines, such as TNF-α and IFN-γ, expressed in microglia and macrophages, have been detected in human PVL lesions (Khwaja and Volpe 2008). Pro-inflammatory cytokines may be released in response to infection and hypoxia-ischemia, both conditions mutually potentiating harmful effects (Khwaja and Volpe 2008). Injurious cytokine effects comprise inhibition of oligodendrocyte differentiation, generation of ROS, induction of glial apoptosis, and myelin degeneration (Khwaja and Volpe 2008; Berger et al. 2012). Moreover, TNF-α and IL-6 have been shown to increase BBB permeability and to disrupt BBB integrity (Berger et al. 2012). In a rat model of perinatal brain damage, neuroinflammatory response to LPS and hypoxia-ischemia was characterized by downregulated anti-inflammatory cytokines and predominance of IL-1β release in preterm-like brains, while term-like brains presented with stronger pro- and anti-inflammatory responses, including both Il-1β and TNF-α releases (Brochu et al. 2011). Of note, postnatal systemic administration of IL-1ra led to decreased long-term gliosis and myelin degeneration and protected against functional defects associated with perinatal brain injury (Girard et al. 2012). In neonatal rat and mouse model of inflammation-induced brain injury, administration of IL-10 reduced white matter damage following CA or neonatal sepsis (Mesples et al. 2003; Pang et al. 2005).

5.5.5 Pattern Recognition Receptors

Activation of PMNs and PBMCs is mediated by pattern recognition receptors (PRRs), which recognize structurally stable microbial membrane components (Takeuchi and Akira 2010). PRRs display a complex system of sentinel receptors including cell-associated receptors, such as TLRs (Takeuchi and Akira 2010). TLRs currently comprise ten human receptors, expressed either on the plasma membrane (TLR1, 2, 4, 5, 6) or intracellularly on endoplasmic reticulum and endosomal membranes (TLR3, 7, 8, 9, 10) (Glaser and Speer 2013; Takeuchi and Akira 2010; Akira 2006). Ligand binding is followed by recruitment of IL-1 receptor-associated kinases (IRAKs) or TNF receptor-associated factor (TRAF)-6 and subsequent activation of complex signaling cascades culminating in upregulation of pro-inflammatory cytokines, co-stimulatory molecules, and chemokines (Akira 2006; Yamamoto and Takeda 2010). Recognizing peptidoglycans and LPS, respectively, TLR2 and TLR4 provide an innate immune response against the most common pathogens involved in CA and neonatal sepsis and have been associated with inflammatory disorders of prematurity (Glaser and Speer 2013; O'Hare et al. 2013; Kemp 2014). In animal models of CA, LPS-induced cytokine synthesis directly correlated with TLR4 expression and subsequent activation of NF-$_{K}$B and enhanced secretion of TNF-α, IL-1β, IL-6, and IL-8 (Kramer et al. 2002; Harju et al. 2005). Animal models and in vitro data provide evidence of a gestational age-dependent expression of TLRs and TLR-related molecules on inflammatory as well as non-inflammatory cells (Glaser and Speer 2013; Harju et al. 2001; Hillman et al. 2008; Kollmann et al. 2012; Zhang et al. 2015). Maturation-dependent TLR activation and TLR signaling might render the immature lung and brain more susceptible to injurious exogenous and endogenous stimuli of pro-inflammation (Khwaja and Volpe 2008; Kollmann et al. 2012). TLR signaling is tightly controlled by a number of exo- and endogenous regulatory molecules (Akira 2006), including IL-1 receptor-associated kinase (IRAK)-M, which inhibits TLR-mediated NF-$_{K}$B activity, leading to significantly reduced LPS-induced TNF-α and IL-6 synthesis (Wesche et al. 1999).

5.5.5.1 Lung Injury

Maturation-dependent expression of TLR4 in lung tissue and lung fibroblasts has been demonstrated (Glaser and Speer 2013; Harju et al. 2001). In a mouse model of fetal lung development, activation of TLR2 and TLR4 inhibited expression of fibroblast growth factor (FGF)-10, leading to abnormal saccular airway morphogenesis demonstrating many features of the BPD phenotype (Benjamin et al. 2007). TLR4-mediated inflammatory response was associated with altered airway fibronectin expression, potentially inhibiting distal airway branching and alveolarization (Prince et al. 2005). In adult animal models, LPS-induced activation and overexpression of TLR4 was accompanied by heightened sensitivity to LPS and enhanced fibrosis (He et al. 2009). On the contrary, surfactant proteins (SP) A and D were shown to beneficially modulate TLR2 and TLR4 expression, to upregulate the regulatory protein IRAK-M and to inhibit NF-$_{\kappa}$B activation in experimental lung inflammation (Nguyen et al. 2012; Bersani et al. 2013).

5.5.5.2 Brain Injury

Activation of TLR2 and TLR4 has been shown to contribute to hypoxic-ischemic and LPS-induced neonatal brain injury (Eklind et al. 2005; Stridh et al. 2011). Moreover, TLRs seem to be involved in microglial activation and the subsequent generation of ROS and RNS toxic to pre-OLs (Khwaja and Volpe 2008). In fetal and neonatal rat model, administration of LPS induced cerebral expression of CD14 and TLR4, sensitizing the immature brain to a second hit, such as hypoxic-ischemic injury (Strunk et al. 2014). In neonatal mice, activation of the TLR1/2 complex was shown to induce choroid plexus transcription of TNF-α and influx of white blood cells into the CSF, potentially reflecting disturbances in choroid plexus barrier function (Stridh et al. 2013). A role for tissue-released endogenous TLR ligands has been discussed in the amplification of ischemic brain injury (Volpe 2008).

5.5.6 Oxygen Radicals and Proteolytic Mediators

Exposure to high inspiratory oxygen concentrations causes direct oxidative cell damage due to increased production of ROS released by neutrophils, macrophages, and microglia at sites of inflammation (Khwaja and Volpe 2008; Bhandari 2010). Moreover, ROS are generated upon hyperoxia or reoxygenation by free iron and the cell-bound xanthine-oxidase system. Very immature preterm infants are particularly susceptible to hyperoxia-induced organ damage due to a profound deficiency in antioxidant enzyme activity (Saugstad 2005). Animal experiments confirmed that oxidative stress may be a crucial event in the initiation of both pulmonary and brain inflammation (Khwaja and Volpe 2008; Kramer et al. 2002), with oxygen radicals exerting direct toxic effects on bronchoalveolar and brain parenchymal structures, such as lipid peroxidation, inactivation of protective antiproteases, upregulation of MMPs, and direct toxicity to pre-OLs (Khwaja and Volpe 2008; Saugstad 2005; Bhandari 2010; Gerber et al. 1999).

5.5.6.1 Lung Injury

Data from in vitro studies, animal experiments, and clinical observations indicate an imbalance of proteases and protease inhibitors contributing to preterm lung injury (Speer et al. 1993; Altiok et al. 2006). Following elastolytic damage, increased concentrations of various markers of tissue destruction were detected in airway secretions and urine of preterm infants (Speer 2006a, 2009). Of note, elastase and neutral proteases were shown to prime macrophages for increased release of toxic oxygen metabolites (Speer et al. 1984). At sites of inflammation, neutrophil and macrophage-released proteases, such as elastase, β-glucuronidase, myeloperoxidase, cathepsin, MMPs, and others, play an essential role in the destruction of the alveolar-capillary unit and in extracellular matrix remodeling (Bhandari 2010). Similarly, overexpression of MMPs might cause disruption of the extracellular matrix. High concentrations of MMPs were detected in airway secretions of infants with BPD (Cederqvist et al. 2001). Moreover, protective levels of tissue inhibitors of MMPs were rather low in infants with BPD (Cederqvist et al. 2001), and blocking of MMP-9 was shown to reduce hyperoxia-derived lung injury in fetal mice (Chetty et al. 2008). In the context of overexpression of IL-1β in a bi-transgenic mouse model, MMP-9 played a protective role, and MMP-9 deficiency, on the contrary, further exaggerated perturbation of lung morphogenesis (Lukkarinen et al. 2009).

5.5.6.2 Brain Injury

Oxidative stress is an important component of early injury to the neonatal brain. Human brain and experimental studies point to a maturation-dependent vulnerability of pre-OLs to ROS attack, presumably due to a delay in the development of enzymes of the superoxide dismutase complex (Khwaja and Volpe 2008). Aiming at reducing oxidative damage to the neonatal brain, a number of potential therapeutic strategies have been subject to research, including ROS scavengers, lipid peroxidation, and nitric oxide synthase inhibitors (Chew and DeBoy 2015).

5.5.7 Microvascular and Tissue Integrity

Inflammation and inflammatory mediators have detrimental effects on the microvascular integrity of the immature lung and on cytoarchitecture and tissue integrity of preterm white and gray matter (Speer 2009; Kaindl et al. 2009).

5.5.7.1 Lung Injury

Increased alveolar-capillary permeability is a pathognomonic feature of early stages of lung inflammation and has been associated with a deterioration of lung function (Speer 2006a, 2009). A variety of lipid mediators, such as leukotrienes, prostacyclin, platelet-derived factor, and endothelin-1, detected in airways of infants with BPD, seem to directly affect the alveolar-capillary unit (Speer 2006b). Within 1 h after initiation of mechanical ventilation, protein leakage into the alveoli and airways of preterm infants was documented (Jaarsma et al. 2004). Moreover, a drastic increase in albumin concentrations in airway secretions was reported at a postnatal age of 10–14 days in preterm infants who later developed BPD, significantly contributing to alveolar edema, inactivation of the surfactant system, and deterioration of lung function (Groneck et al. 1994). In magnetic resonance imaging (MRI) studies, infants with BPD showed an increased lung water content and were susceptible to gravity-induced collapse of the lung (Adams et al. 2004). In mechanically ventilated infants with RDS, a simultaneous activation of clotting, fibrinolysis, kinin-kallikrein system, and the complement system was observed (Speer 2006a), indicating that injury to the pulmonary vascular endothelium may subsequently promote neutrophil and platelet activation and may induce pulmonary as well as systemic inflammation and activation of the clotting system.

5.5.7.2 Brain Injury

Periventricular white matter injury, which is now the most common cause of brain injury in preterm infants, is characterized by microglial activation, axonal damage, damage to the developing subplate neurons, and disturbance of white matter fiber tracts (Kaindl et al. 2009). MRI-based techniques provide evidence of additional involvement of telencephalic gray matter and long tracts in perinatal brain injury, probably due to apoptotic transmigrating neurons (Kaindl et al. 2009).

5.5.8 Modulators of Angiogenesis and Growth Factors

Several key regulators of angiogenesis have been identified mediating vascular development and, thus, affecting parenchymal organ development. VEGF is a key regulator of angiogenesis (Hines and Sun 2014). It is essential and critical for vascular development and exists in high concentrations in heavily vascularized tissues (Thebaud and Abman 2007; Bhandari 2010).

5.5.8.1 Lung Injury

Alveolar simplification is the typical pathological finding in lung tissues from animal models and infants with BPD being caused by apoptosis of cells critical for alveolar and vessel formation (Jobe 2011). Increasing evidence suggests that pulmonary blood vessels actively promote normal alveolar development and contribute to the maintenance of alveolar structures (Thebaud and

Abman 2007). Perturbation of VEGF signaling has been implicated in impaired lung parenchymal development and long-term lung injury, demonstrating an essential role of intrapulmonary vascular structures on lung parenchymal development (Reyburn et al. 2012; Thebaud and Abman 2007; Kunig et al. 2006). While VEGF levels were shown to be significantly increased in newborn rabbits following exposure to prolonged hyperoxia, decreased VEGF levels and VEGF signaling were reported in the same setting in a premature fetal baboon model of BPD (Bhandari and Elias 2006). Significantly lower levels of VEGF were found in preterm infants, who developed BPD, compared to infants who recovered from ventilator- and hyperoxia-induced lung injury (D'Angio and Maniscalco 2002). Decreased VEGF signaling has been considered a potential mechanism in the pathogenesis of reduced pulmonary capillary volume and impaired alveolarization. In extremely preterm animals developing BPD, impaired expression of VEGF, its angiogenic receptors, and angiopoietin were shown to contribute to dysmorphic microvasculature and disrupted alveolarization (Thebaud et al. 2005; Thomas et al. 2008). In newborn rats, treatment with recombinant human VEGF as well as VEGF gene therapy promoted angiogenesis indicating a potential preventive strategy (Kunig et al. 2006; Thebaud et al. 2005). Adverse stimuli inhibiting pulmonary angiogenesis may significantly disturb and disrupt secondary septation characteristic of BPD (Thebaud and Abman 2007). In a rat model of neonatal lung injury, antenatal LPS administration resulted in arrest of alveolarization (Ueda et al. 2006). In preterm lambs a similar, time- and dose-dependent effect was observed (Kramer et al. 2001). Data from mouse model suggest that inflammation may induce abnormal angiogenesis in the developing preterm lung by upregulation of angiogenic CC chemokines, such as MIP-1α and MCP-1 (Miller et al. 2010). Of note, intra-amniotic LPS led to increased levels of the angiostatic chemoattractants IFN-γ -inducible protein (IP)-10 and monokine in preterm lamb lungs (Kallapur et al. 2003). Even inflammation in the absence of infection has been shown to result in structural remodeling of the lung, including altered extracellular matrix formation as well as impaired alveolarization and angiogenesis. Data from baboon, mouse, and rabbit models of neonatal lung injury confirmed potentiated airway inflammation and cytokine expression following a combination of hyperoxia and mechanical ventilation (Varughese et al. 2003; Wilson et al. 2005; Brew et al. 2011).

5.5.8.2 Brain Injury

VEGF has been shown to be expressed in the central nervous system after hypoxic-ischemic brain injury. It has been presumed a key modulator in the process of brain repair by regulating angiogenesis, neuronal cell proliferation, and migration (Fan et al. 2009; Guo et al. 2016). VEGF knockout mice showed severe impairments in vascularization, neuronal migration, and survival. On the contrary, VEGF overexpression seems to confer beneficial neuroprotective effects in mouse model, resulting from inhibition of apoptotic pathways (Chew and DeBoy 2015). In animal models, late administration of exogenous VEGF 48 h after hypoxia-ischemia resulted in enhanced angiogenesis and functional performance, while administration 1 h after insult enhanced BBB permeability and increased ischemic lesion (Chew and DeBoy 2015). The cytokine erythropoietin (EPO) has been shown to play a vital role in neural differentiation and neurogenesis in early brain development and to exert antiapoptotic and anti-inflammatory features in the central nervous system. It is expressed by neurons, glial cells, and cerebral endothelial cells (Chew and DeBoy 2015). In different animal models of neonatal brain injury, both treatment with EPO prior to hypoxic-ischemic injury and administration of EPO after hypoxia-ischemia attenuated injurious lesions (Chew and DeBoy 2015).

5.5.9 Repair Mechanisms

Inflammation-induced tissue injury may be followed by tissue repair which has only partially been studied in neonatal lung and brain injury.

5.5.9.1 Lung Injury

The inflammatory process seems to result in the induction of transforming growth factor (TGF)-β that limits inflammatory reactions and plays a key role in mediating tissue remodeling and repair (Bartram and Speer 2004). As a counter player to fibroblast growth factor-β and IL-1β, both lowering elastin mRNA in human lung fibroblasts, TGF-β seems to increase elastin by transcriptional and posttranscriptional mechanisms (Kuang et al. 2007). Hyperoxia-induced increased levels of TGF-β may contribute to impaired and simplified alveolarization characteristic of BPD (Zhao et al. 1997). In preterm animals, increased expression of TGF-β inhibited normal lung development and promoted fibrosis (Speer 2006a). A reduced expression of connective tissue growth factor (CTGF), which is responsible for various downstream actions of TGF-β and second important key mediator in the induction of pulmonary fibrosis, was found in a sheep model of BPD (Kunzmann et al. 2008). Moreover, low concentrations of hypoxic-inducible factor, keratinocyte and hepatocyte growth factors, all thought to participate in normal lung development and tissue regeneration after lung injury, were detected in infants with BPD (Danan et al. 2002; Lassus et al. 2003).

5.5.9.2 Brain Injury

PVL in preterm infants is characterized by loss of pre-OLs (Khwaja and Volpe 2008). Both the subventricular zone and the white matter are considered to be main sources of oligodendrocytes derived from endogenous glial progenitor cells (Curtis et al. 2007). The latter were shown to differentiate into mature glial cells and to migrate into injured white matter lesions for repair (Curtis et al. 2007). In a neonatal rat model of PVL, ischemia activated those endogenous self-repair mechanisms. However, repair capacity was found to be limited, and shortened survival of newly generated glial cells was observed (Li et al. 2015). Recently, UDP-glucose, an endogenous agonist of G protein-coupled receptor 17 (GPR17), the neurotrophic factor glial cell line-derived neurotrophic factor (GDNF), and blockade of glutamatergic receptor N-methyl-D-aspartate (NMDA) were shown to enhance ischemia-induced endogenous self-repair mechanisms by increasing survival rates and differentiation of newly generated pre-OLs into mature oligodendrocytes (Li et al. 2015).

5.5.10 Genetic Predisposition to Inflammation

Individual infants may be particularly susceptible to sustained inflammation. Genetic factors may significantly contribute to the variance in risk for disorders of prematurity. Genetic background of severe courses may be different from mild and moderate diseases, and associated genetic variations may vary by ethnicity. Twin concordance studies have pointed to a relevant impact of genetic risk, and current research has focused on identifying genetic factors contributing to heightened risk of intrauterine infection, preterm birth, and inflammatory disorders, such as BPD (Lal and Ambalavanan 2015). Genetic predisposition might comprise, e.g., variability in cytokine and chemokine response, imbalance toward exaggerated pro-inflammatory responses, and polymorphisms in key regulators of pro-inflammatory signaling, antioxidants, and modulators of angiogenesis (Lal and Ambalavanan 2015; Yu et al. 2016). Gene polymorphisms may confer an increased risk of altered vaginal flora, ascending infections and preterm birth (Genc and Onderdonk 2011). In BPD, however, candidate gene studies, genome-wide association studies, exome sequencing, integrative omics analysis, and pathway analysis did not identify genetic variations significantly and consistently associated with the disease (Yu et al. 2016; Huusko et al. 2014).

5.6 Conclusion

There is profound evidence that a complex interplay of pre- and postnatal pro-inflammatory conditions, primarily comprising oxygen toxicity, mechanical ventilation, and pre- and postnatal infection, initiates and perpetuates an adverse inflammation in the structural and functional immature organs of preterm infants. An initial injury, also referred to as "first hit," activates early immune responses directed to pathogen clearance and/or tissue repair. Functional immaturity in early and late immune responses, in antioxidant enzymes and protease system, in key regulators of homeostasis, in growth factors of angiogenesis, and in repair mechanisms may promote an injurious inflammatory response, characterized by rapid accumulation of neutrophils and macrophages or diffuse microglial activation, respectively. An arsenal of inflammatory mediators might subsequently affect tissue integrity with imbalance of pro-inflammatory and anti-inflammatory mechanisms favoring pro-inflammation. Adverse postnatal conditions may further aggravate the ongoing inflammation, as "second" or "third hit." Both neonatal lung and brain injury have been related to maturation-dependent factors underlying a particular vulnerability. As a devastating consequence, normal lung and brain development may be compromised with lifelong consequences. Seeking for strategies to prevent or ameliorate BPD and WMD in high-risk infants, we still need a deeper insight into the pathogenesis of inflammatory events. So far, we do not know whether, and to what extent, a preterm infant at risk will face the given sequence of adverse inflammation, since the orchestra of confounding pre- and postnatal factors, genetic susceptibility, and "window of vulnerability" may differ from infant to infant.

References

Adams EW, Harrison MC, Counsell SJ, Allsop JM, Kennea NL, Hajnal JV et al (2004) Increased lung water and tissue damage in bronchopulmonary dysplasia. J Pediatr 145:503–507

Akira S (2006) TLR signaling. Curr Top Microbiol Immunol 311:1–16

Altiok O, Yasumatsu R, Bingol-Karakoc G, Riese RJ, Stahlman MT, Dwyer W et al (2006) Imbalance between cysteine proteases and inhibitors in a baboon model of bronchopulmonary dysplasia. Am J Respir Crit Care Med 173:318–326

Backstrom E, Hogmalm A, Lappalainen U, Bry K (2011) Developmental stage is a major determinant of lung injury in a murine model of bronchopulmonary dysplasia. Pediatr Res 69:312–318

Baier RJ, Majid A, Parupia H, Loggins J, Kruger TE (2004) CC chemokine concentrations increase in respiratory distress syndrome and correlate with development of bronchopulmonary dysplasia. Pediatr Pulmonol 37:137–148

Barton SK, Moss TJ, Hooper SB, Crossley KJ, Gill AW, Kluckow M et al (2014) Protective ventilation of preterm lambs exposed to acute chorioamnionitis does not reduce ventilation-induced lung or brain injury. PLoS One 9:e112402

Bartram U, Speer CP (2004) The role of transforming growth factor beta in lung development and disease. Chest 125:754–765

Benjamin JT, Smith RJ, Halloran BA, Day TJ, Kelly DR, Prince LS (2007) FGF-10 is decreased in bronchopulmonary dysplasia and suppressed by Toll-like receptor activation. Am J Physiol Lung Cell Mol Physiol 292:L550–L558

Berger I, Peleg O, Ofek-Shlomai N (2012) Inflammation and early brain injury in term and preterm infants. Isr Med Assoc J 14:318–323

Bersani I, Speer CP (2012) Nosocomial sepsis in neonatal intensive care: inevitable or preventable? Z Geburtshilfe Neonatol 216:186–190

Bersani I, Kunzmann S, Speer CP (2013) Immunomodulatory properties of surfactant preparations. Expert Rev Anti Infect Ther 11:99–110

Bhandari V (2010) Hyperoxia-derived lung damage in preterm infants. Semin Fetal Neonatal Med 15:223–229

Bhandari V, Elias JA (2006) Cytokines in tolerance to hyperoxia-induced injury in the developing and adult lung. Free Radic Biol Med 41:4–18

Blackwell TS, Hipps AN, Yamamoto Y, Han W, Barham WJ, Ostrowski MC et al (2011) NF-kappaB signaling in fetal lung macrophages disrupts airway morphogenesis. J Immunol 187:2740–2747

Boghossian NS, Page GP, Bell EF, Stoll BJ, Murray JC, Cotten CM et al (2013) Late-onset sepsis in very low birth weight infants from singleton and multiple-gestation births. J Pediatr 162:1120–1124, 1124 e1121

Bose CL, Dammann CE, Laughon MM (2008) Bronchopulmonary dysplasia and inflammatory biomarkers in the premature neonate. Arch Dis Child Fetal Neonatal Ed 93:F455–F461

Bose CL, Laughon MM, Allred EN, O'Shea TM, Van Marter LJ, Ehrenkranz RA et al (2013) Systemic inflammation associated with mechanical ventilation among extremely preterm infants. Cytokine 61:315–322

Brehmer F, Bendix I, Prager S, van de Looij Y, Reinboth BS, Zimmermanns J et al (2012) Interaction of inflammation and hyperoxia in a rat model of neonatal white matter damage. PLoS One 7:e49023

Brew N, Hooper SB, Allison BJ, Wallace MJ, Harding R (2011) Injury and repair in the very immature lung following brief mechanical ventilation. Am J Physiol Lung Cell Mol Physiol 301:L917–L926

Brochu ME, Girard S, Lavoie K, Sebire G (2011) Developmental regulation of the neuroinflammatory responses to LPS and/or hypoxia-ischemia between preterm and term neonates: an experimental study. J Neuroinflammation 8:55

Cai Z, Pang Y, Lin S, Rhodes PG (2003) Differential roles of tumor necrosis factor-alpha and interleukin-1 beta in lipopolysaccharide-induced brain injury in the neonatal rat. Brain Res 975:37–47

Cederqvist K, Sorsa T, Tervahartiala T, Maisi P, Reunanen K, Lassus P et al (2001) Matrix metalloproteinases-2, -8, and -9 and TIMP-2 in tracheal aspirates from preterm infants with respiratory distress. Pediatrics 108:686–692

Chetty A, Cao GJ, Severgnini M, Simon A, Warburton R, Nielsen HC (2008) Role of matrix metalloprotease-9 in hyperoxic injury in developing lung. Am J Physiol Lung Cell Mol Physiol 295:L584–L592

Chew LJ, DeBoy CA (2015) Pharmacological approaches to intervention in hypomyelinating and demyelinating white matter pathology. Neurol. pii: S0028-3908(15)00266-X. https://doi.org/10.1016/j.neuropharm.2015.06.008. [Epub ahead of print]

Curtis MA, Kam M, Nannmark U, Anderson MF, Axell MZ, Wikkelso C et al (2007) Human neuroblasts migrate to the olfactory bulb via a lateral ventricular extension. Science 315:1243–1249

D'Alquen D, Kramer BW, Seidenspinner S, Marx A, Berg D, Groneck P et al (2005) Activation of umbilical cord endothelial cells and fetal inflammatory response in preterm infants with chorioamnionitis and funisitis. Pediatr Res 57:263–269

D'Angio CT, Maniscalco WM (2002) The role of vascular growth factors in hyperoxia-induced injury to the developing lung. Front Biosci 7:d1609–d1623

Dammann O, Leviton A (2014) Intermittent or sustained systemic inflammation and the preterm brain. Pediatr Res 75:376–380

Danan C, Franco ML, Jarreau PH, Dassieu G, Chailley-Heu B, Bourbon J et al (2002) High concentrations of keratinocyte growth factor in airways of premature infants predicted absence of bronchopulmonary dysplasia. Am J Respir Crit Care Med 165:1384–1387

Dommergues MA, Patkai J, Renauld JC, Evrard P, Gressens P (2000) Proinflammatory cytokines and interleukin-9 exacerbate excitotoxic lesions of the newborn murine neopallium. Ann Neurol 47:54–63

Dong Y, Speer CP (2015) Late-onset neonatal sepsis: recent developments. Arch Dis Child Fetal Neonatal Ed 100:F257–F263

Eklind S, Mallard C, Arvidsson P, Hagberg H (2005) Lipopolysaccharide induces both a primary and a secondary phase of sensitization in the developing rat brain. Pediatr Res 58:112–116

Ericson JE, Laughon MM (2015) Chorioamnionitis: implications for the neonate. Clin Perinatol 42:155–165, ix

Fan X, Heijnen CJ, van der Kooij MA, Groenendaal F, van Bel F (2009) The role and regulation of hypoxia-inducible factor-1alpha expression in brain development and neonatal hypoxic-ischemic brain injury. Brain Res Rev 62:99–108

Garcia-Munoz Rodrigo F, Galan Henriquez G, Figueras Aloy J, Garcia-Alix Perez A (2014) Outcomes of very-low-birth-weight infants exposed to maternal clinical chorioamnionitis: a multicentre study. Neonatology 106:229–234

Garcia-Ramallo E, Marques T, Prats N, Beleta J, Kunkel SL, Godessart N (2002) Resident cell chemokine expression serves as the major mechanism for leukocyte recruitment during local inflammation. J Immunol 169:6467–6473

Genc MR, Onderdonk A (2011) Endogenous bacterial flora in pregnant women and the influence of maternal genetic variation. BJOG 118:154–163

Gerber CE, Bruchelt G, Stegmann H, Schweinsberg F, Speer CP (1999) Presence of bleomycin-detectable free iron in the alveolar system of preterm infants. Biochem Biophys Res Commun 257:218–222

Girard S, Kadhim H, Roy M, Lavoie K, Brochu ME, Larouche A et al (2009) Role of perinatal inflammation in cerebral palsy. Pediatr Neurol 40:168–174

Girard S, Sebire H, Brochu ME, Briota S, Sarret P, Sebire G (2012) Postnatal administration of IL-1Ra exerts neuroprotective effects following perinatal inflammation and/or hypoxic-ischemic injuries. Brain Behav Immun 26:1331–1339

Glaser K, Speer CP (2013) Toll-like receptor signaling in neonatal sepsis and inflammation: a matter of orchestration and conditioning. Expert Rev Clin Immunol 9:1239–1252

Goldenberg RL, Andrews WW, Goepfert AR, Faye-Petersen O, Cliver SP, Carlo WA et al (2008) The Alabama Preterm Birth Study: umbilical cord blood *Ureaplasma urealyticum* and *Mycoplasma hominis* cultures in very preterm newborn infants. Am J Obstet Gynecol 198(43):e41–e45

Groneck P, Gotze-Speer B, Oppermann M, Eiffert H, Speer CP (1994) Association of pulmonary inflammation and increased microvascular permeability during the development of bronchopulmonary dysplasia: a sequential analysis of inflammatory mediators in respiratory fluids of high-risk preterm neonates. Pediatrics 93:712–718

Guo H, Zhou H, Lu J, Qu Y, Yu D, Tong Y (2016) Vascular endothelial growth factor: an attractive target in the treatment of hypoxic/ischemic brain injury. Neural Regen Res 11:174–179

Hallman M, Curstedt T, Halliday HL, Saugstad OD, Speer CP (2013) Better neonatal outcomes: oxygen, surfactant and drug delivery. Preface. Neonatology 103:316–319

Harju K, Glumoff V, Hallman M (2001) Ontogeny of toll-like receptors Tlr2 and Tlr4 in mice. Pediatr Res 49:81–83

Harju K, Ojaniemi M, Rounioja S, Glumoff V, Paananen R, Vuolteenaho R et al (2005) Expression of toll-like receptor 4 and endotoxin responsiveness in mice during perinatal period. Pediatr Res 57:644–648

Hartling L, Liang Y, Lacaze-Masmonteil T (2012) Chorioamnionitis as a risk factor for bronchopulmonary dysplasia: a systematic review and meta-analysis. Arch Dis Child Fetal Neonatal Ed 97:F8–F17

He Z, Zhu Y, Jiang H (2009) Inhibiting toll-like receptor 4 signaling ameliorates pulmonary fibrosis during acute lung injury induced by lipopolysaccharide: an experimental study. Respir Res 10:126

Hillman NH, Moss TJ, Nitsos I, Kramer BW, Bachurski CJ, Ikegami M et al (2008) Toll-like receptors and agonist responses in the developing fetal sheep lung. Pediatr Res 63:388–393

Hillman NH, Nitsos I, Berry C, Pillow JJ, Kallapur SG, Jobe AH (2011) Positive end-expiratory pressure and surfactant decrease lung injury during initiation of ventilation in fetal sheep. Am J Physiol Lung Cell Mol Physiol 301:L712–L720

Hines EA, Sun X (2014) Tissue crosstalk in lung development. J Cell Biochem 115:1469–1477

Hogmalm A, Bry M, Strandvik B, Bry K (2014) IL-1beta expression in the distal lung epithelium disrupts lung morphogenesis and epithelial cell differentiation in fetal mice. Am J Physiol Lung Cell Mol Physiol 306:L23–L34

Huusko JM, Karjalainen MK, Mahlman M, Haataja R, Kari MA, Andersson S et al (2014) A study of genes encoding cytokines (IL6, IL10, TNF), cytokine receptors (IL6R, IL6ST), and glucocorticoid receptor (NR3C1) and susceptibility to bronchopulmonary dysplasia. BMC Med Genet 15:120

Inatomi T, Oue S, Ogihara T, Hira S, Hasegawa M, Yamaoka S et al (2012) Antenatal exposure to *Ureaplasma* species exacerbates bronchopulmonary dysplasia synergistically with subsequent prolonged mechanical ventilation in preterm infants. Pediatr Res 71:267–273

Jaarsma AS, Braaksma MA, Geven WB, van Oeveren W, Bambang Oetomo S (2004) Activation of the inflammatory reaction within minutes after birth in ventilated preterm lambs with neonatal respiratory distress syndrome. Biol Neonate 86:1–5

Jobe AH (2011) The new bronchopulmonary dysplasia. Curr Opin Pediatr 23:167–172

Jones CA, Cayabyab RG, Kwong KY, Stotts C, Wong B, Hamdan H et al (1996) Undetectable interleukin (IL)-10 and persistent IL-8 expression early in hyaline membrane disease: a possible developmental basis for the predisposition to chronic lung inflammation in preterm newborns. Pediatr Res 39:966–975

Kaindl AM, Favrais G, Gressens P (2009) Molecular mechanisms involved in injury to the preterm brain. J Child Neurol 24:1112–1118

Kallapur SG, Jobe AH, Ikegami M, Bachurski CJ (2003) Increased IP-10 and MIG expression after intra-amniotic endotoxin in preterm lamb lung. Am J Respir Crit Care Med 167:779–786

Kemp MW (2014) Preterm birth, intrauterine infection, and fetal inflammation. Front Immunol 5:574

Khwaja O, Volpe JJ (2008) Pathogenesis of cerebral white matter injury of prematurity. Arch Dis Child Fetal Neonatal Ed 93:F153–F161

Kim KS (2003) Pathogenesis of bacterial meningitis: from bacteraemia to neuronal injury. Nat Rev Neurosci 4:376–385

Kim CJ, Romero R, Chaemsaithong P, Chaiyasit N, Yoon BH, Kim YM (2015) Acute chorioamnionitis and funisitis: definition, pathologic features, and clinical significance. Am J Obstet Gynecol 213:S29–S52

Kolb M, Margetts PJ, Anthony DC, Pitossi F, Gauldie J (2001) Transient expression of IL-1beta induces acute lung injury and chronic repair leading to pulmonary fibrosis. J Clin Invest 107:1529–1536

Kollmann TR, Crabtree J, Rein-Weston A, Blimkie D, Thommai F, Wang XY et al (2009) Neonatal innate TLR-mediated responses are distinct from those of adults. J Immunol 183:7150–7160

Kollmann TR, Levy O, Montgomery RR, Goriely S (2012) Innate immune function by Toll-like receptors: distinct responses in newborns and the elderly. Immunity 37:771–783

Korzeniewski SJ, Romero R, Cortez J, Pappas A, Schwartz AG, Kim CJ et al (2014) A "multi-hit" model of neonatal white matter injury: cumulative contributions of chronic placental inflammation, acute fetal inflammation and postnatal inflammatory events. J Perinat Med 42:731–743

Kramer BW, Moss TJ, Willet KE, Newnham JP, Sly PD, Kallapur SG et al (2001) Dose and time response after intraamniotic endotoxin in preterm lambs. Am J Respir Crit Care Med 164:982–988

Kramer BW, Kramer S, Ikegami M, Jobe AH (2002) Injury, inflammation, and remodeling in fetal sheep lung after intra-amniotic endotoxin. Am J Physiol Lung Cell Mol Physiol 283:L452–L459

Kramer BW, Ladenburger A, Kunzmann S, Speer CP, Been JV, van Iwaarden JF et al (2009) Intravenous lipopolysaccharide-induced pulmonary maturation and structural changes in fetal sheep. Am J Obstet Gynecol 200:195 e191 110

Kroon AA, Wang J, Huang Z, Cao L, Kuliszewski M, Post M (2010) Inflammatory response to oxygen and endotoxin in newborn rat lung ventilated with low tidal volume. Pediatr Res 68:63–69

Kuang PP, Zhang XH, Rich CB, Foster JA, Subramanian M, Goldstein RH (2007) Activation of elastin transcription by transforming growth factor-beta in human lung fibroblasts. Am J Physiol Lung Cell Mol Physiol 292:L944–L952

Kunig AM, Balasubramaniam V, Markham NE, Seedorf G, Gien J, Abman SH (2006) Recombinant human VEGF treatment transiently increases lung edema but enhances lung structure after neonatal hyperoxia. Am J Physiol Lung Cell Mol Physiol 291:L1068–L1078

Kunzmann S, Seher A, Kramer BW, Schenk R, Schutze N, Jakob F et al (2008) Connective tissue growth factor does not affect transforming growth factor-beta 1-induced Smad3 phosphorylation and T lymphocyte proliferation inhibition. Int Arch Allergy Immunol 147:152–160

Lal CV, Ambalavanan N (2015) Genetic predisposition to bronchopulmonary dysplasia. Semin Perinatol 39:584–591

Lassus P, Heikkila P, Andersson LC, von Boguslawski K, Andersson S (2003) Lower concentration of pulmonary hepatocyte growth factor is associated with more severe lung disease in preterm infants. J Pediatr 143:199–202

Lee Y, Kim HJ, Choi SJ, Oh SY, Kim JS, Roh CR et al (2015) Is there a stepwise increase in neonatal morbidities according to histological stage (or grade) of acute chorioamnionitis and funisitis?: effect of gestational age at delivery. J Perinat Med 43:259–267

Leviton A, Allred EN, Kuban KC, Hecht JL, Onderdonk AB, O'Shea TM et al (2010) Microbiologic and histologic characteristics of the extremely preterm infant's placenta predict white matter damage and later cerebral palsy. The ELGAN study. Pediatr Res 67:95–101

Levy BD, Serhan CN (2014) Resolution of acute inflammation in the lung. Annu Rev Physiol 76:467–492

Levy O, Wynn JL (2014) A prime time for trained immunity: innate immune memory in newborns and infants. Neonatology 105:136–141

Li WJ, Mao FX, Chen HJ, Qian LH, Buzby JS (2015) Treatment with UDP-glucose, GDNF, and memantine promotes SVZ and white matter self-repair by endogenous glial progenitor cells in neonatal rats with ischemic PVL. Neuroscience 284:444–458

Lozano SM, Newnam KM (2016) Modalities of mechanical ventilation: volume-targeted versus pressure-limited. Adv Neonatal Care 16:99–107

Lukkarinen H, Hogmalm A, Lappalainen U, Bry K (2009) Matrix metalloproteinase-9 deficiency worsens lung injury in a model of bronchopulmonary dysplasia. Am J Respir Cell Mol Biol 41:59–68

Martin RJ, Fanaroff AA (2013) The preterm lung and airway: past, present, and future. Pediatr Neonatol 54:228–234

May M, Marx A, Seidenspinner S, Speer CP (2004) Apoptosis and proliferation in lungs of human fetuses exposed to chorioamnionitis. Histopathology 45:283–290

Mesples B, Plaisant F, Gressens P (2003) Effects of interleukin-10 on neonatal excitotoxic brain lesions in mice. Brain Res Dev Brain Res 141:25–32

Miller JD, Benjamin JT, Kelly DR, Frank DB, Prince LS (2010) Chorioamnionitis stimulates angiogenesis in saccular stage fetal lungs via CC chemokines. Am J Physiol Lung Cell Mol Physiol 298:L637–L645

Morley CJ (2010) CPAP and low oxygen saturation for very preterm babies? N Engl J Med 362:2024–2026

Murch SH, Costeloe K, Klein NJ, MacDonald TT (1996a) Early production of macrophage inflammatory protein-1 alpha occurs in respiratory distress syndrome and is associated with poor outcome. Pediatr Res 40:490–497

Murch SH, Costeloe K, Klein NJ, Rees H, McIntosh N, Keeling JW et al (1996b) Mucosal tumor necrosis factor-alpha production and extensive disruption of sulfated glycosaminoglycans begin within hours of birth in neonatal respiratory distress syndrome. Pediatr Res 40:484–489

Nanthakumar N, Meng D, Goldstein AM, Zhu W, Lu L, Uauy R et al (2011) The mechanism of excessive intestinal inflammation in necrotizing enterocolitis: an immature innate immune response. PLoS One 6: e17776

Narimanbekov IO, Rozycki HJ (1995) Effect of IL-1 blockade on inflammatory manifestations of acute ventilator-induced lung injury in a rabbit model. Exp Lung Res 21:239–254

Nguyen CN, Schnulle PM, Chegini N, Luo X, Koenig JM (2010) Neonatal neutrophils with prolonged survival secrete mediators associated with chronic inflammation. Neonatology 98:341–347

Nguyen HA, Rajaram MV, Meyer DA, Schlesinger LS (2012) Pulmonary surfactant protein A and surfactant lipids upregulate IRAK-M, a negative regulator of TLR-mediated inflammation in human macrophages. Am J Physiol Lung Cell Mol Physiol 303:L608–L616

Normann E, Lacaze-Masmonteil T, Eaton F, Schwendimann L, Gressens P, Thebaud B (2009) A novel mouse model of *Ureaplasma*-induced perinatal inflammation: effects on lung and brain injury. Pediatr Res 65:430–436

O'Carroll SJ, Kho DT, Wiltshire R, Nelson V, Rotimi O, Johnson R et al (2015) Pro-inflammatory TNFalpha and IL-1beta differentially regulate the inflammatory phenotype of brain microvascular endothelial cells. J Neuroinflammation 12:131

O'Hare FM, William Watson R, Molloy EJ (2013) Toll-like receptors in neonatal sepsis. Acta Paediatr 102:572–578

Paananen R, Husa AK, Vuolteenaho R, Herva R, Kaukola T, Hallman M (2009) Blood cytokines during the perinatal period in very preterm infants: relationship of inflammatory response and bronchopulmonary dysplasia. J Pediatr 154:39–43 e33

Pang Y, Rodts-Palenik S, Cai Z, Bennett WA, Rhodes PG (2005) Suppression of glial activation is involved in the protection of IL-10 on maternal E. coli induced neonatal white matter injury. Brain Res Dev Brain Res 157:141–149

Prince LS, Dieperink HI, Okoh VO, Fierro-Perez GA, Lallone RL (2005) Toll-like receptor signaling inhibits structural development of the distal fetal mouse lung. Dev Dyn 233:553–561

Reyburn B, Martin RJ, Prakash YS, MacFarlane PM (2012) Mechanisms of injury to the preterm lung and airway: implications for long-term pulmonary outcome. Neonatology 101:345–352

Ricard JD, Dreyfuss D, Saumon G (2001) Production of inflammatory cytokines in ventilator-induced lung injury: a reappraisal. Am J Respir Crit Care Med 163:1176–1180

Sarelius IH, Glading AJ (2015) Control of vascular permeability by adhesion molecules. Tissue Barriers 3: e985954

Saugstad OD (2005) Oxidative stress in the newborn – a 30-year perspective. Biol Neonate 88:228–236

Schmitz T, Ritter J, Mueller S, Felderhoff-Mueser U, Chew LJ, Gallo V (2011) Cellular changes underlying hyperoxia-induced delay of white matter development. J Neurosci 31:4327–4344
Smith RE (1996) Chemotactic cytokines mediate leukocyte recruitment in fibrotic lung disease. Biol Signals 5:223–231
Speer CP (2006a) Inflammation and bronchopulmonary dysplasia: a continuing story. Semin Fetal Neonatal Med 11:354–362
Speer CP (2006b) Pulmonary inflammation and bronchopulmonary dysplasia. J Perinatol 26(Suppl 1): S57–S62; discussion S63–54
Speer CP (2009) Chorioamnionitis, postnatal factors and proinflammatory response in the pathogenetic sequence of bronchopulmonary dysplasia. Neonatology 95:353–361
Speer CP (2011) Neonatal respiratory distress syndrome: an inflammatory disease? Neonatology 99:316–319
Speer CP, Pabst MJ, Hedegaard HB, Rest RF, Johnston RB Jr (1984) Enhanced release of oxygen metabolites by monocyte-derived macrophages exposed to proteolytic enzymes: activity of neutrophil elastase and cathepsin G. J Immunol 133:2151–2156
Speer CP, Gahr M, Wieland M, Eber S (1988) Phagocytosis-associated functions in neonatal monocyte-derived macrophages. Pediatr Res 24:213–216
Speer CP, Ruess D, Harms K, Herting E, Gefeller O (1993) Neutrophil elastase and acute pulmonary damage in neonates with severe respiratory distress syndrome. Pediatrics 91:794–799
Stoll BJ, Hansen NI, Sanchez PJ, Faix RG, Poindexter BB, Van Meurs KP et al (2011) Early onset neonatal sepsis: the burden of group B Streptococcal and E. coli disease continues. Pediatrics 127:817–826
Stridh L, Smith PL, Naylor AS, Wang X, Mallard C (2011) Regulation of toll-like receptor 1 and -2 in neonatal mice brains after hypoxia-ischemia. J Neuroinflammation 8:45
Stridh L, Ek CJ, Wang X, Nilsson H, Mallard C (2013) Regulation of toll-like receptors in the choroid plexus in the immature brain after systemic inflammatory stimuli. Transl Stroke Res 4:220–227
Strunk T, Doherty D, Jacques A, Simmer K, Richmond P, Kohan R et al (2012) Histologic chorioamnionitis is associated with reduced risk of late-onset sepsis in preterm infants. Pediatrics 129:e134–e141
Strunk T, Inder T, Wang X, Burgner D, Mallard C, Levy O (2014) Infection-induced inflammation and cerebral injury in preterm infants. Lancet Infect Dis 14:751–762
Takeuchi O, Akira S (2010) Pattern recognition receptors and inflammation. Cell 140:805–820
Thebaud B, Abman SH (2007) Bronchopulmonary dysplasia: where have all the vessels gone? Roles of angiogenic growth factors in chronic lung disease. Am J Respir Crit Care Med 175:978–985
Thebaud B, Ladha F, Michelakis ED, Sawicka M, Thurston G, Eaton F et al (2005) Vascular endothelial growth factor gene therapy increases survival, promotes lung angiogenesis, and prevents alveolar damage in hyperoxia-induced lung injury: evidence that angiogenesis participates in alveolarization. Circulation 112:2477–2486
Thomas W, Speer CP (2011) Chorioamnionitis: important risk factor or innocent bystander for neonatal outcome? Neonatology 99:177–187
Thomas W, Speer CP (2014) Chorioamnionitis is essential in the evolution of bronchopulmonary dysplasia – the case in favour. Paediatr Respir Rev 15:49–52
Thomas W, Seidenspinner S, Kawczynska-Leda N, Kramer BW, Chmielnicka-Kopaczyk M, Marx A et al (2008) Systemic fetal inflammation and reduced concentrations of macrophage migration inhibitory factor in tracheobronchial aspirate fluid of extremely premature infants. Am J Obstet Gynecol 198(64):e61–e66
Turunen R, Nupponen I, Siitonen S, Repo H, Andersson S (2006) Onset of mechanical ventilation is associated with rapid activation of circulating phagocytes in preterm infants. Pediatrics 117:448–454
Ueda K, Cho K, Matsuda T, Okajima S, Uchida M, Kobayashi Y et al (2006) A rat model for arrest of alveolarization induced by antenatal endotoxin administration. Pediatr Res 59:396–400
Varughese R, Nayak JL, LoMonaco M, O'Reilly MA, Ryan RM, D'Angio CT (2003) Effects of hyperoxia on tumor necrosis factor alpha and Grobeta expression in newborn rabbit lungs. Lung 181:335–346
Viscardi RM (2012) Perinatal inflammation and lung injury. Semin Fetal Neonatal Med 17:30–35
Viscardi RM (2014) *Ureaplasma* species: role in neonatal morbidities and outcomes. Arch Dis Child Fetal Neonatal Ed 99:F87–F92
Viscardi RM, Muhumuza CK, Rodriguez A, Fairchild KD, Sun CC, Gross GW et al (2004) Inflammatory markers in intrauterine and fetal blood and cerebrospinal fluid compartments are associated with adverse pulmonary and neurologic outcomes in preterm infants. Pediatr Res 55:1009–1017
Volpe JJ (2008) Postnatal sepsis, necrotizing entercolitis, and the critical role of systemic inflammation in white matter injury in premature infants. J Pediatr 153:160–163
Vuichard D, Ganter MT, Schimmer RC, Suter D, Booy C, Reyes L et al (2005) Hypoxia aggravates lipopolysaccharide-induced lung injury. Clin Exp Immunol 141:248–260
Wagenaar GT, ter Horst SA, van Gastelen MA, Leijser LM, Mauad T, van der Velden PA et al (2004) Gene expression profile and histopathology of experimental bronchopulmonary dysplasia induced by prolonged oxidative stress. Free Radic Biol Med 36:782–801
Wesche H, Gao X, Li X, Kirschning CJ, Stark GR, Cao Z (1999) IRAK-M is a novel member of the Pelle/interleukin-1 receptor-associated kinase (IRAK) family. J Biol Chem 274:19403–19410
Wilson MR, Choudhury S, Takata M (2005) Pulmonary inflammation induced by high-stretch ventilation is mediated by tumor necrosis factor signaling in mice. Am J Physiol Lung Cell Mol Physiol 288:L599–L607

Wu YW (2002) Systematic review of chorioamnionitis and cerebral palsy. Ment Retard Dev Disabil Res Rev 8:25–29

Yamamoto M, Takeda K (2010) Current views of toll-like receptor signaling pathways. Gastroenterol Res Pract 2010:240365

Yi M, Jankov RP, Belcastro R, Humes D, Copland I, Shek S et al (2004) Opposing effects of 60% oxygen and neutrophil influx on alveologenesis in the neonatal rat. Am J Respir Crit Care Med 170:1188–1196

Yoon BH, Romero R, Jun JK, Park KH, Park JD, Ghezzi F et al (1997) Amniotic fluid cytokines (interleukin-6, tumor necrosis factor-alpha, interleukin-1 beta, and interleukin-8) and the risk for the development of bronchopulmonary dysplasia. Am J Obstet Gynecol 177:825–830

Yu KH, Li J, Snyder M, Shaw GM, O'Brodovich HM (2016) The genetic predisposition to bronchopulmonary dysplasia. Curr Opin Pediatr 28:318–323

Zhang J, Zhou J, Xu B, Chen C, Shi W (2015) Different expressions of TLRs and related factors in peripheral blood of preterm infants. Int J Clin Exp Med 8:4108–4114

Zhao Y, Gilmore BJ, Young SL (1997) Expression of transforming growth factor-beta receptors during hyperoxia-induced lung injury and repair. Am J Physiol 273:L355–L362

Zlotnik A, Yoshie O (2012) The chemokine superfamily revisited. Immunity 36:705–716

The Fetus at Risk: Chorioamnionitis

6

Mikko Hallman and Tuula Kaukola

Contents

Abstract

Histological chorioamnionitis (HCA) is common in extremely preterm births. HCA in very preterm births is associated with a low risk of respiratory distress syndrome (RDS) as the inflammatory stress in HCA promotes fetal maturity. Previous evidence on increased risk of respiratory distress, intraventricular hemorrhage (IVH), bronchopulmonary dysplasia (BPD), necrotizing enterocolitis (NEC), cerebral palsy (CP), and poor neurodevelopmental outcome, compared to gestation controls, has not been uniformly confirmed. Antenatal steroid that decreases the risk of RDS, IVH, NEC, and CP was rarely given in early studies. Clinical CA, defined on the basis of fever, leukocytosis, and local symptoms, represents 10–25% of all HCA cases. Clinical CA is associated with CP in near-term/term pregnancies and additional adverse outcomes in very preterm pregnancies. HCA combined with

M. Hallman (✉)
Department of Children and Adolescents, Oulu University Hospital, and PEDEGO Research Unit, Medical Research Center Oulu, University of Oulu, Oulu, Finland
e-mail: mikko.hallman@oulu.fi

T. Kaukola
Department of Children and Adolescents, Oulu University Hospital, and PEDEGO Research Center, MRC Oulu, University of Oulu, Oulu, Finland

G. Buonocore et al. (eds.), *Neonatology*,
https://doi.org/10.1007/978-3-319-29489-6_155

intrauterine growth restriction or placental perfusion defect strongly associates with neurological problems. Causes and consequences of HCA remain to be studied.

6.1 Salient Points

- Chorioamnionitis (CA) is a risk factor of spontaneous onset of very preterm birth. Only 10–25% of histologic CA (HCA) is presented as clinical CA, diagnosed on the basis fever, leukocytosis, and local signs of maternal infection.
- Microbes and inflammation from cervix, and also from fallopian tubes, endometrium, maternal blood, or via amniocentesis spread to chorioamnion. Cause-relationship between microbes and inflammation is not uniformly established.
- HCA promotes the host defense functions, decreasing the risk of respiratory distress syndrome (RDS). The benefits are balanced against severe potential adverse effects. The associated increases in the risks of bronchopulmonary dysplasia (BPD) and necrotizing enterocolitis (NEC) have not been lately confirmed.
- HCA may increase the risk of intraventricular hemorrhage (IVH), cerebral palsy (CP), and adverse cognitive consequences in children born very preterm. The adverse effects stand out in clinical CA, compound placental defects, and in intrauterine growth restriction.
- Antibiotics in preterm rupture of fetal membranes decrease the risk of CA, and antenatal glucocorticoid in threatened very preterm birth may decrease the risk of adverse consequences of HCA. Fetal-placental infections caused by specific microbes are often preventable.

6.2 Introduction

Infections and inflammatory injuries are the major threats during pregnancy. The extraembryonic tissues play important roles in protecting the fetus. From 10 to 12 days post conception (p.c.), yolk sack and allantois vessels provide nutrition to the embryo. By 20 days p.c. fetal vessels are discernible in developing placenta. They communicate with the embryo via a connecting stalk that later develops into the umbilical cord. By 40 days p.c. the embryo is completely surrounded by the amniotic cavity and attached via the umbilical cord to the hemomonochorial placenta (Benirschke et al. 2012). Upon complete adherence of the fetal membranes to the decidua at about 20 weeks of gestation, bacterial inflammation may still penetrate the chorioamnion and contaminate the amniotic fluid (Goldenberg and Culhane 2003; Gravett et al. 1986).

In high-risk pregnancies, the protective fetal chorioamnion and placental tissues are challenged in multiple ways. They respond by promoting inflammation that involves mediators with multiple functions, including defense against microbes, promoting the fetal maturity and the labor process. Oxidative and proteolytic effects of inflammation are obviously harmful to the developing organism. This chapter focuses on the consequences of chorioamnionitis (CA) in the fetus comparing the affected fetuses to the gestation controls.

6.3 Diagnosis and Incidence of Chorioamnionitis

Histologic chorioamnionitis (HCA) is characterized by mostly polymorphonuclear neutrophil (PMN) infiltration of the placenta, fetal membranes, and/or umbilical cord. Pathological exam of the placenta, fetal membranes, and umbilical cord defines CA (Benirschke et al. 2012; Salafia et al. 1989) (Fig. 1). In most cases HCA is a silent condition. It serves as a biomarker, indicating inflammatory activation at the feto-maternal interface that may have diverse consequences including the induction of labor. CA is a risk factor of spontaneous preterm birth (PTB).

Analysis of biochemical markers of PMNs in amniotic fluid provides accurate diagnosis of CA. Interleukin-6 (IL-6), IL-8, and other inflammatory cytokines also are elevated in the amniotic fluid (Hallman et al. 1989; Bracci and Buonocore 2003). However, amniocentesis is not indicated for diagnosis of CA. After birth, the inspection of the placenta, its vessels, and the fetal membranes helps to understand the pregnancy outcome (Fig. 1a). Placentas with severe CA reveal marginal hemorrhages, and

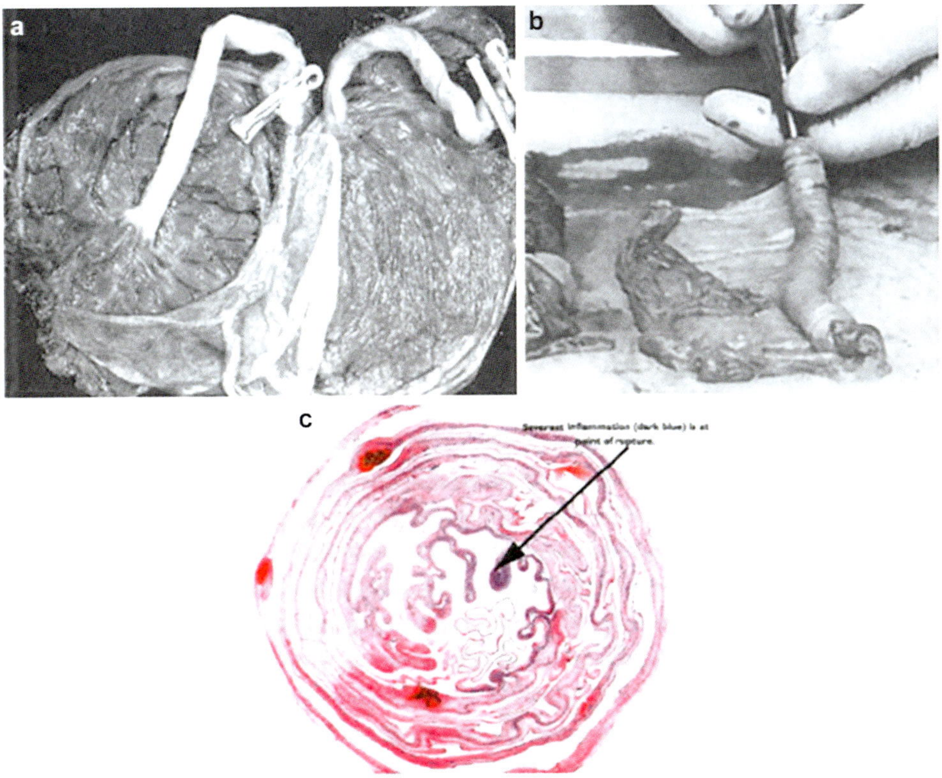

Fig. 1 Study of placenta and fetal membranes for diagnosis of chorioamnionitis. (**a**) Diamnionic, dichorionic twin placenta. Preterm placenta (single clamp), located in fundus, reveals vessels through visible membranes, suggesting no CA. Placenta with marginally inserted cord (two clamps) has cloudy appearance suggesting inflammation in fetal membranes. Presumptive diagnoses were confirmed by histology. (**b**) Rolling of fetal membranes is preferably started from the site of the rupture and proceeding towards the edge, with amnion inside. A segment of the well-rolled portion is fixed for a day. (**c**) Membrane roll of placenta with CA. Dark exudate is noted in the center near the site of rupture of fetal membranes (A. Page 558. Fig. 20.2. From Benirschke C, Burton GJ, Baegren RN. Pathology of human placenta. Springer-Verlag Berlin Heidelberg 2012. B. Page 4. Fig.1.3. Left segment. From Benirschke C, Burton GJ, Baegren RN. Pathology of human placenta. Springer Verlag Berlin Heidelberg 2012. C. Page 568. Fig 20.22. From Benirschke C, Burton GJ, Baegren RN. Pathology of human placenta. Springer-Verlag Berlin Heidelberg 2012)

the amniotic surfaces are covered with invisible white leukocyte-enriched film. Diagnostic specimens are recovered from three sites: chorionic plate, fetal membranes as a roll from the site of spontaneous membrane rupture, and segments of umbilical cord (Benirschke et al. 2012; Salafia et al. 1989). According to microscopy of fetal membranes, HCA is classified into three grades: (1) mild (5–10 neutrophils *per* high power field [HPF]), (2) moderate (11–30 neutrophils/HPF), and (3) severe (>30 neutrophils/HPF). All three sites are examined and CA is additionally defined on the basis of distribution of the inflammation in the three sites.

Clinical CA presents as fever, foul-smelling vaginal discharge, uterine tenderness, and laboratory findings, e.g., leukocytosis or elevated C-reactive protein. Two positive criteria (one clinical, one chemical/ laboratory) establish the diagnosis. In clinical CA, elective delivery is considered for fetal indication.

Prelabor rupture of fetal membranes (PROM) in preterm pregnancy exposes the intra-amniotic space to ascending infection and is associated with CA. PROM at term that proceeds to labor and delivery is one presentation of normal labor. In preterm PROM, labor mostly starts spontaneously. In other cases, pregnancy continues without concomitant induction of labor for weeks, and after delivery the study of placenta often reveals no HCA. In prolonged PROM, post-PROM pregnancy duration is at least one week. The cases of PROM that progress to preterm labor are often considered as clinical CA, although the diagnosis is not always confirmed by the histological exam, and typical maternal symptoms are absent. Unless the individual studies carefully describe the duration, symptoms, and histology associated with PROM, the comparison of the outcomes between different studies remains problematic.

Despite significant association between HCA and spontaneous PTB, neither the specificity nor the sensitivity of prediction is very high (Table 1). In late-preterm births due to spontaneous onset of labor, HCA is less frequent (10–25%) than in extremely preterm spontaneous births (40–60%). Although preterm labor and birth is often associated with bacterial colonization of fetal membranes and amniotic fluid, the dogma of sterile intrauterine environment during normal term pregnancy has been challenged. The new techniques allow identification and classification of genomes from various microbes. Even in elective term births without labor, genomes of commensal bacteria may be detectable in fetal compartment. The potential roles of normal and abnormal microbial colonization during later fetal development remain to be studied (Romano-Keeler and Weitkamp 2015).

Table 1 Prevalence of pregnancy conditions and the incidence of histological chorioamnionitis (HCA)

Pregnancy condition	Prevalence % of all births	HCA % in given pregnancy condition
Term	85–92	2–10
Postterm	1–5	5–15[a]
Preterm	5–13	15–25
Spontaneous onset	3–9	20–35
PROM	1.5–4	50–80
32–36 weeks	2–7	10–25
28–32 weeks	0.5–1.2	25–40
<28 weeks	0.3–0.6	40–60
No spontaneous onset	2–4	5–15

[a]Meconium in amniotic fluid (50 %) associates with green staining of chorioamnion that contains meconium-laden macrophages; associated chorioamnionitis suggests infection. The ranges of the incidence figures are based on population studies (Paananen et al. 2009; Andrews et al. 2008; McElrath et al. 2008)

Fetal inflammatory response syndrome (FIRS) is defined as an increase in IL-6 in cord blood in CA (Yoon et al. 2000). Funisitis is another diagnostic criterion associated with FIRS. Although FIRS is associated with an increased risk of early postnatal infection, in more recent reports most of the premature newborn affected by FIRS have negative blood cultures (>90%). According to a regional cohort of 163 preterm Finnish infants, born before 32 weeks of pregnancy, ~50% of HCA cases had FIRS on the basis of elevated levels of IL-6 in cord blood, <10% of infants had funisitis, and <5% revealed early sepsis.

6.4 Antenatal Findings in Chorioamnionitis

In term pregnancies, maturation and shortening of the cervix and rupture of fetal membranes expose the amniotic space to microbes. In the setting of spontaneous preterm labor, the inflammatory mediators appear to play a more prominent role in the activation of the labor process than in term labor. However, histological inflammation may persist for a long period during pregnancy as a condition with little consequence. HCA and microorganisms are present in at least 50% of second trimester pregnancy loss cases (Heller et al. 2003). It has been postulated that after mid-pregnancy when the expanding fetal membranes seal the endometrial cavity, the incidence of ascending infection becomes less common (Goldenberg et al. 2000).

Besides microbes and endotoxins, other triggering agents (factors decreasing the immune tolerance, meconium-induced HCA) may play a role in the etiology. In HCA, the amniotic fluid or fetal membranes reveal microbes that, however, may also be detected even in elective births without labor using molecular probes specific for bacteria (Bracci and Buonocore 2003; Romano-Keeler and Weitkamp 2015; Goldenberg et al. 2000). The most common microbe in HCA is *Ureaplasma urealyticum*

(20–40%). The traditional pathogens (Group B Streptococci or GBS, *E. coli*, Enterococci, *Listeria monocytogenes*) are less common (2–10%).

The ascending route is the most common in HCA, and bacterial vaginosis (BV) is a risk factor. In BV, the incidence of lactobacilli as a normal predominant colonization has decreased at the expense of other microbes, including *Gardnerella vaginalis*, *Mobiluncus* spp., anaerobic gram-negative rods, *M. hominis*, and *Ureaplasma urealyticum*. Most of microbes in BV have also been detected in fetal membranes and in amniotic fluid. However, BV predicts the risk of preterm birth with a low specificity (Goffinet 2005). Periodontitis is another proposed risk factor of spontaneous PTB (Sacco et al. 2008).

6.4.1 Specific Infections Associated with Chorioamnionitis

Placental villi are affected in infections causing intrauterine growth restriction (Benirschke et al. 2011). *Treponema pallidum* causes hypercellular villitis with mononuclear infiltration, sometimes necrotizing funicitis or plasma cell rich CA. Candida vaginitis is common during pregnancy and infections occasionally cause a serious placental and fetal disease. Intrauterine candidiasis is associated with clusters of characteristic structures, surrounded by inflammatory cells in umbilical cord, placenta, and fetal membranes (see ► Chap. 105, "Fetal Infections: Congenital Syphilis and Tuberculosis"). About 1% of women become infected with *Cytomegalovirus* (CMV) during pregnancy and nearly 50% of cases it is passed to her fetus. However, very few manifest congenital CMV, associated with characteristic chronic villitis and severe fetal disease. Typical placental findings of severe CMV infection include plasmacytic villitis, thrombosis of villous capillaries, necrosis of villous tissues, and inclusion-bearing cytomegalic cells. *Toxoplasma gondii* is associated with lymphoplasmacytic villitis and sclerosis, along with toxoplasma cysts in amnion/chorion. These findings and the risk of severe fetopathy are particularly evident during early pregnancy (see ► Chap. 106, "Toxoplasmosis in the Fetus and Newborn"). Enteroviruses, mumps, and rubella cause distinct placental inflammatory lesions.

Listeria monocytogenes from contaminated food or soil presents as severe necrotizing villitis with abscesses. The disease is associated with chorioamnionitis and generalized fetal infection that often leads to fetal death or to severe neonatal pneumonia or meningitis. Early-onset GBS causes CA, and amniotic fluid is a growth media of GBS: the reported incidences of CA and funicitis were 64% and 27%, respectively. The high-risk mothers are frequently heavily colonized with GBS (vaginal flora, urinary tract, breast milk). In these cases, the risk of early neonatal GBS is decreased by intrapartum administration of antibiotics. The recurrence rate of the carrier status is high (see Section X: Fetal and Neonatal Infections). A number of other pathogens have been associated with CA, including *Neisseria gonorrhoeae*, group A β-hemolytic streptococci, *Streptococcus penumoniae*, and *Hemophilus influenzae*. Gram-negative bacilli, particularly, *E. coli* is associated with CA and neonatal meningitis. *Salmonellae*, *Shigella*, *Clostridium*, *Fusobacterium*, *Bacterioides fragilis*, and *Gardnerella vaginalis* have been occasionally associated with chorioamnionitis and fetal pathology. *Clamydia* is a common cause of cervicitis. Conjuctivitis caused by gonococcus and *Chlamydia trachomatis* requires mostly local treatment. *Chlamydia pneumoniae* has been shown to infect extravillous trophoblasts.

Ureaplasma urealyticum is the most frequently isolated microbe in CA. Of other mycoplasma species, *Mycoplasma hominis* is associated with pelvic inflammatory diseases. *Ureaplasma* spp. may cause pneumonia and occasionally bactermia and meningitis in susceptible newborn infants. The infected infants are reported to have increased risk of BPD.

The causes of increased susceptibility in some pregnancies to CA and to specific infections causing characteristic feto-placental diseases remain to be studied. Genetic factors likely influence the individual susceptibility, as some alleles cause defects in innate immunity and others cause specific defects in acquired immunity. Environmental risk factors warrant further investigation.

6.4.2 Inflammation Without Microbes

Villitis of unknown etiology (VUE) is found in 5–15% of predominantly term placentas. It is associated with intrauterine growth restriction, fetal death, and perinatal asphyxia. In VUE, CD3-positive maternal T lymphocytes gain access to the villous stroma. Fetal antigen-presenting cells (Hofbauer cells) expand and express class II major histocompatibility complex molecules. Maternal monocyte-macrophages in the perivillous space likely amplify the immune response. VUE may represent a state combining maternal allograft rejection and graft versus host disease mechanisms (Kim et al. 2009; Redline 2007).

Meconium that is prevalent in postterm (20–70%) and term (5–15%) pregnancies associates with green staining of chorioamnion containing meconium-laden macrophages and often CA. Longstanding meconium may be associated with umbilical vascular myonecrosis; typical comorbidities include fetal distress and intrauterine growth restriction (Cimic and Baergen 2015).

6.5 Chorioamnionitis as a Risk Factor for Acute and Chronic Diseases

From chorioamnion the inflammation may spread transcellularly via amniotic fluid that is swallowed into GI tract and in part enters the airways by the fetal breathing movements. The umbilical cord is in direct contact with amniotic fluid and with chorionic plate in placenta. On the other hand, chorion is highly vascular and in generalized maternal infection her blood provides a direct source of infection/inflammation to placental structures, particularly the villae. In clinical CA, transplacental spreading to the fetus prevails. According to experimental studies and clinical observations, placental circulation is acutely affected as a result of transplacental inflammatory insult (Rounioja et al. 2005), whereas the transcellular spreading of inflammation acutely boosts the host defense (Bry et al. 1997; Jobe et al. 2000). The fetal consequences of CA are additionally dependent on severity and etiology of the inflammation, as well as multiple, poorly understood genetic and environmental risk factors. CA is traditionally diagnosed by histology. Characterization of the process biochemically (inflammatory cytokines), microbiologically, or by inspection provides additional information that is clinically useful when available shortly after birth (Thomas and Speer 2011).

6.5.1 Experimental Data

Introduction of bacterial endotoxin (LPS) or proinflammatory cytokine (IL-1) to amniotic fluid evokes an acute maturation of the surfactant system (Bry et al. 1997; Jobe et al. 2000). This cytokine-induced pulmonary epithelial differentiation enhances the capacity of premature neonatal respiratory adaptation. The cytokine effect on lung maturity is additive with that of glucocorticoid (Jobe et al. 2000). At the same time, LPS or the cytokine cascade induced by the inflammatory agent (e.g., IL-8) induces acute airway inflammation that is likely to spread to lung parenchyma and systemically (Thomas and Speer 2011). Antenatal glucocorticoid protects the preterm fetus affected by FIRS against vascular insults, stabilizing the blood pressure and strengthening endothelial and epithelial barriers after premature birth.

In pregnant rodents, a high dose of LPS to the maternal compartment induces an acute fetal perfusion defect, illustrated by increased resistance in placental villous perfusion and resulting in low-output fetal cardiac failure (Rounioja et al. 2005). According to animal data, acute transplacental inflammatory insult may result in brain injury, involving activation of pattern recognition receptors and subsequent innate immune response (Speer 1999). In addition hypoxemia-ischemia evokes an inflammatory response (Hagberg et al. 2015). Inflammatory mediators may gain access into the immature brain as specific chemokines serving as ligands for their receptors in the target tissue or promoting neutrophil-mediated breakdown of blood–brain barrier (Anthony et al. 1998). Intracerebral cytokine storm promotes free radical attack, failure in oxidative phosphorylation, necrosis, apoptosis, and brain injury. Immature oligodendrocytes are especially vulnerable (see ▶ Chap. 118, "Inflammation and Perinatal Brain Injury").

6.5.2 Pulmonary Consequences of CA

The reports of premature patients from the early 1990s associate CA with adverse outcomes. In these studies, clinical CA was overrepresented, antenatal glucocorticoid was rarely given, and advanced neonatal respiratory care practices were not available. Watterberg reported an association between CA and a low risk of RDS and a high risk of BPD as studied in 53 preterm infants (Watterberg et al. 1996). The risk of BPD is associated with increased tracheal IL-1β levels. Later reports representing the era of antenatal glucocorticoid and surfactant therapy confirm a HCA-associated substantial decrease in the risk of RDS and no increase in the risk of BPD (Kaukola et al. 2009; Paananen et al. 2009; Been and Zimmermann 2009) (Table 2).

Recent cohort studies with larger populations have additionally found that in very preterm infants the high levels of inflammatory cytokines detected in cord blood in HCA often *decrease* shortly after birth and do not associate with adverse pulmonary consequences (Paananen et al. 2009). This decrease is likely achieved by applying noninvasive, gentle ventilation techniques. In contrast, within 24 h after a very preterm birth, high levels of specific inflammatory cytokines are evident in non-CA pregnancies with RDS. Very high levels of cytokines, particularly IL-8, after birth associate with the risk of BPD (Kaukola et al. 2009; Paananen et al. 2009). Modest inflammatory response in CA may additionally be due to antenatal glucocorticoid treatment (Been and Zimmermann 2009; Kramer et al. 2009). Inappropriately low cytokines and transient immune paralysis occasionally complicate prolonged PROM cases that are born very preterm with severe respiratory distress (sometimes sepsis) and pulmonary hypertension (Aikio et al. 2012). Structural immaturity predisposes to "new" BPD (Thébaud and Abman 2007), suggesting that the respiratory adaptation after extremely preterm birth is harmful. It is possible that environmental factors, such as the inevitable increase in the oxygen tension after birth, still play important interactive roles in pathogenesis. In infants born after 30 weeks of pregnancy, the development of lung structure is more advanced and the risk of BPD is very low, despite neonatal respiratory distress.

6.5.3 Neurological Consequences

At least half of all children with CP are born at term (CP prevalence 1–1.5 per 1000 term born). The term-born cases mostly represent hemiplegia and quadriplegia, whereas among infants born very preterm, diplegia predominates and CP cases are fairly common in this population (4–8 per 100 very preterm) (Sellier et al. 2015;

Table 2 Fetal consequences of chorioamnionitis (CA) or CA with complicating event. Comparison of risk to infants born preterm with similar gestation and without evidence of CA

Postnatal morbidity	Histologic CA	+Fetal inflammation	+Clinical CA	+PROM
Infection	↑	↑	↑	↑
RDS	↓	~[a] or ↓	~[a] or ↓	~[a] or ↓
BPD	~[a]	~ or ↑[a]	~ or ↑[a]	~ or ↑[a]
Severe RDS	~[a] or ↓	~[a]	~[a]	↑
IVH	~ or ↑[a]	~ or ↑	↑	↑
CP	~or ↑[a]	~ or ↑	↑	↑
Adverse cognitive development	~[a]	~ or ↑	↑	~ or ↑

[a]Progress in antenatal and neonatal treatment practices (antenatal glucocorticoid and gentle neonatal cardiopulmonary treatment practices) has decreased the serious morbidity. Explanations: (~) no reported effect

Himmelmann and Uvebrant 2014). The pattern of cord blood immunoproteins predicting CP is different as compared between very preterm and term infants (Kaukola et al. 2004).

According to a large population-based cohorts, the incidence of CP among term and preterm infants has remained stable, or declined, since the 1970s, suggesting that advances in treatment practices influence the long-term outcomes (Sellier et al. 2015; Himmelmann and Uvebrant 2014).

6.5.3.1 Infants Born Very Preterm

In many but not all studies, CA is a risk factor of IVH among infants born very preterm (Kaukola et al. 2006; Andrews et al. 2006; Soraisham et al. 2009). Despite common use of antenatal glucocorticoid and more gentle neonatal treatment practices, decreasing the risk of IVH, CA has been linked to early IVH, emphasizing the role of immunological activation in fetus as a pathway to cerebral injury before birth. In populations mostly representing *clinical* CA, the risk of severe IVH is increased in preterm infants (Soraisham et al. 2009). There is also evidence of increased risk of CP and cognitive problems in children born preterm in clinical CA (Neufeld et al. 2005). Besides clinical CA, cases of "silent" CA with an additional defect in placental perfusion are associated with abnormal neurological outcome (Kaukola et al. 2006). According to other reports, infants born with HCA as a whole do not have a higher frequency of neurodevelopmental problems than the gestation controls (Andrews et al. 2008).

6.5.3.2 Infants Born Late-Preterm to Term

A case-control study of a cohort of 200,000 infants born at 36 weeks or later in gestation during the years 1991 and 1998 revealed CA or endometritis in 14% of CP cases and 4% of random controls, translating CA as an independent risk factor (OR 3.8, CI 1.4–9.3) of CP (Wu et al. 2003), consistent with other studies. Clinical CA and severe symptoms of infection are associated with increased risk.

The diagnosis of silent HCA covered only less than 25% of the CA population, and there was no detectable association between silent HCA and CP. In a meta-analysis, a significant association was found both between clinical CA and CP (RR 1.9, 95% CI 1.5–2.5) and between clinical CA and cystic periventricular leukomalacia (RR 2.6, 95% CI 1.7–3.9) (Wu 2002).

Quadriplegia as a separate trait in term and near-term neonates was associated with severe hypoxic-ischemic insult. In contrast, hemiplegia is associated with brain infarction, and one risk factor of brain infarction was preterm PROM (Lee et al. 2005; McElrath et al. 2008).

6.6 Prevention of Morbidity Associated with CA

HCA is diagnosed first after birth. However, symptoms of clinical CA strongly suggests HCA (sensitivity >80%), and preterm PROM suggests HCA (sensitivity ~50%). Inspection of fetal membranes by experienced observer enables the diagnosis of HCA with reasonable accuracy (Fig. 1). Stillbirths and spontaneous extremely preterm births (<28 weeks) are associated with HCA (sensitivity 40–80%). HCA and FIRS are prevalent in stillbirths at the extremes of gestation: <26 weeks and >40 weeks (Gordon et al. 2011).

Prevention of cause is the most effective approach. Vaccination programs against rubeola have virtually eradicated the virus. Development of vaccines against other pathogens, such as cytomegalovirus, would offer a tool for prevention. Prophylaxis programs against Listeriosis, group B Streptococci, Toxoplasma, and HIV have met with at least moderate success.

Meta-analysis of randomized controlled trials of prophylactic antibiotics in preterm PROM and particularly in prolonged (>7 days) PROM has revealed a decrease in HCA, a decrease preterm births within 48–168 h, and a decrease in invasive treatments (oxygen and surfactant therapies) of the preterm infants (Kenyon et al. 2013; Saccone and Berghella 2015). In addition, the treatment decreases the risk of abnormal head ultrasound before the discharge. In trials, the antibiotic often has been macrolide; choice of antibiotic depends on the resistance spectrum of individual centers. Co-amoxiclav has been associated with NEC.

Antibiotic prophylaxis in PROM at term has offered no detectable benefit. In imminent preterm birth the antibiotic treatment of parturient with vaginal GBS colonization significantly reduces the risk of serious pneumonia. In preterm labor without clear suspicion of bacterial infection, antibiotic treatment has no detectable benefit (Hutzal et al. 2008).

Treatment of the high-risk infants colonized by *Ureaplasma* has been suggested. Further randomized trials and studies on potential harmful effects of azithromycin and other macrolides are required to demonstrate that antimicrobial treatment eradicates *Ureaplasma* spp. and decreases the risk of BPD (Nair et al. 2014).

According to a number of observational studies of infants born very preterm, antenatal corticosteroid in HCA is associated with decreased neonatal deaths, lowered incidence of RDS, PDA, and IVH (all grades), periventricular leukomalacia, and neonatal seizures. In infants with same gestation and without HCA, the benefits associated with glucocorticoid were less striking. In clinical CA, antenatal corticosteroid was associated with a decrease in the risk of intracerebral complications (all grades of IVH and periventricular leukomalacia) (Hallman 2015).

According to a meta-analysis of randomized trials, magnesium sulfate decreases the risk of CP among preterm infants (Doyle et al. 2009). However, according to post hoc analysis of preterm infants born at week 24 or later with clinical CA, magnesium sulfate did not protect against CP, neurodevelopmental delay or deaths, or the risk of CP in the cohort of 396 children (Kamyar et al. 2015).

References

Aikio O, Metsola J, Vuolteenaho R et al (2012) Transient defect in nitric oxide generation after rupture of fetal membranes and responsiveness to inhaled nitric oxide in very preterm infants with hypoxic respiratory failure. J Pediatr 161:397–403

Andrews WW, Goldenberg RL, Faye-Petersen O et al (2006) The Alabama Preterm Birth study: polymorphonuclear and mononuclear cell placental infiltrations, other markers of inflammation, and outcomes in 23-to 32-week preterm newborn infants. J Obstet Gynecol 195:803–808

Andrews WW, Cliver SP, Biasini F et al (2008) Early preterm birth: association between in utero exposure to acute inflammation and severe neurodevelopmental disability at 6 years of age. Am J Obstet Gynecol 198:466.e1–466.e11

Anthony D, Dempster R, Fearn S et al (1998) CXC chemokines generate age-related increases in neutrophil-mediated brain inflammation and blood–brain barrier breakdown. Curr Biol 8:923–926

Been JV, Zimmermann LJ (2009) Histological chorioamnionitis and respiratory outcome in preterm infants. Arch Dis Child Fetal Neonatal Ed 94:F218–F225

Benirschke K, Burton GJ, Baergen RN (2011) Infectious diseases: specific microorganisms. In: Benirschke K, Burton GJ, Baergen RN (eds) Pathology of the human placenta. Springer, Berlin/Heidelberg, pp 575–655

Benirschke K, Burton GJ, Baergen RN (2012) Pathology of the human placenta, 6th edn. Springer, Berlin/Heidelberg, pp 27–39, 41–53, 180–190, 355–366

Bracci R, Buonocore G (2003) Chorioamnionitis: a risk factor for fetal and neonatal morbidity. Biol Neonate 83:85–96

Bry K, Lappalainen U, Hallman M (1997) Intraamniotic interleukin-1 accelerates surfactant protein synthesis in fetal rabbits and improves lung stability after premature birth. J Clin Invest 99:2992–2999

Cimic A, Baergen R (2015) Meconium-associated umbilical vascular myonecrosis: correlations with adverse outcome. Pediatr Dev Pathol. 2015 Oct 22. [Epub ahead of print]. https://doi.org/10.2350/15-06-1660-OA

Doyle LW1, Crowther CA, Middleton P et al (2009) Magnesium sulphate for women at risk of preterm birth for neuroprotection of the fetus. Cochrane Database Syst Rev CD004661. https://doi.org/10.1002/14651858.CD004661.pub3

Goffinet F (2005) Primary predictors of preterm labour. BJOG 112(Suppl 1):38 47

Goldenberg RL, Culhane JF (2003) Infection as a cause of preterm birth. Clin Perinatol 30:677–700

Goldenberg RL, Hauth JC, Andrews WW (2000) Intrauterine infection and preterm delivery. N Engl J Med 342:1500–1507

Gordon A, Lahra M, Raynes-Greenow C, Jeffery H (2011) Histological chorioamnionitis is increased at extremes of gestation in stillbirth: a population-based study. Infect Dis Obstet Gynecol 456728. https://doi.org/10.1155/2011/456728

Gravett MG, Hummel D, Eschenbach DA, Holmes KK (1986) Preterm labor associated with subclinical amniotic fluid infection and with bacterial vaginosis. Obstet Gynecol 67:229–237

Hagberg H, Mallard C, Ferriero DM et al (2015) The role of inflammation in perinatal brain injury. Nat Rev Neurol 11:192–208

Hallman M (2015) The story of antenatal steroid therapy before preterm birth. Neonatology 107:352–357

Hallman M, Bry K, PitkPitk O (1989) Ceramide lactoside in amniotic fluid: high concentration in chorioamnionitis and in preterm labor. Am J Obstet Gynecol 161:313–318

Heller DS, Moorehouse-Moore C, Skurnick J, Baergen RN (2003) Second-trimester pregnancy loss at an urban hospital. Infect Dis Obstet Gynecol 11:117–122

Himmelmann K, Uvebrant P (2014) The panorama of cerebral palsy in Sweden. XI. Changing patterns in the birth-year period 2003–2006. Acta Paediatr 103(6):618–624

Hutzal CE, Boyle EM, Kenyon SL et al (2008) Use of antibiotics for the treatment of preterm parturition and prevention of neonatal morbidity: a metaanalysis. Am J Obstet Gynecol 199:620.e1–620.e8

Jobe AH, Newnham JP, Willet KE et al (2000) Effects of antenatal endotoxin and glucocorticoids on the lungs of preterm lambs. Am J Obstet Gynecol 182:401–408

Kamyar M, Manuck TA, Stoddard GJ et al (2015) Magnesium sulfate, chorioamnionitis, and neurodevelopment after preterm birth. BJOG https://doi.org/10.1111/1471-0528.13460. [Epub ahead of print]

Kaukola T, Satyaraj E, Patel DD et al (2004) Cerebral palsy is characterized by protein mediators in cord serum. Ann Neurol 55:186–194

Kaukola T, Herva R, Perhomaa M et al (2006) Population cohort associating chorioamnionitis, cord inflammatory cytokines and neurologic outcome in very preterm, extremely low birth weight infants. Pediatr Res 59:478–483

Kaukola T, Tuimala J, Herva R et al (2009) Cord immunoproteins as predictors of respiratory outcome in preterm infants. Am J Obstet Gynecol 200:100.e1–100.e8

Kenyon S, Boulvain M, Neilson JP (2013) Antibiotics for preterm rupture of membranes. Cochrane Database Syst Rev 12, CD001058. https://doi.org/10.1002/14651858.CD001058.pub3

Kim MJ, Romero R, Kim CJ et al (2009) Villitis of unknown etiology is associated with a distinct pattern of chemokine up-regulation in the feto-maternal and placental compartments: implications for conjoint maternal allograft rejection and maternal antifetal graft-versus-host disease. J Immunol 182: 3919–3927

Kramer BW, Kallapur S, Newnham J, Jobe AH (2009) Prenatal inflammation and lung development. Semin Fetal Neonatal Med 14:2–7

Lee J, Croen LA, Backstrand KH et al (2005) Maternal and infant characteristics associated with perinatal arterial stroke in the infant. JAMA 293:723–729

McElrath TF, Hecht JL, Dammann O et al (2008) Pregnancy disorders that lead to delivery before the 28th week of gestation: an epidemiologic approach to classification. Am J Epidemiol 168:980–989

Nair V, Loganathan P, Soraisham AS (2014) Azithromycin and other macrolides for prevention of bronchopulmonary dysplasia: a systematic review and meta-analysis. Neonatology 106:337–347

Neufeld MD, Frigon C, Graham AS, Mueller BA (2005) Maternal infection and risk of cerebral palsy in term and preterm infants. J Perinatol 25:108–113

Paananen R, Husa AK, Vuolteenaho R et al (2009) Blood cytokines during the perinatal period in very preterm infants: relationship of inflammatory response and bronchopulmonary dysplasia. J Pediatr 154:39–43.e3

Redline RW (2007) Villitis of unknown etiology: noninfectious chronic villitis in the placenta. Hum Pathol 38:1439–1446

Romano-Keeler J, Weitkamp JH (2015) Maternal influences on fetal microbial colonization and immune development. Pediatr Res 77:189–195

Rounioja S, Räsänen J, Ojaniemi M et al (2005) Mechanism of acute fetal cardiovascular depression after maternal inflammatory challenge in mouse. Am J Pathol 166:1585–1592

Sacco G, Carmagnola D, Abati S et al (2008) Periodontal disease and preterm birth relationship: a review of the literature. Minerva Stomatol 57:233–246, 246–250

Saccone G, Berghella V (2015) Antibiotic prophylaxis for term or near-term premature rupture of membranes: metaanalysis of randomized trials. Am J Obstet Gynecol 212:627.e1–627.e9

Salafia CM, Weigl C, Silberman L (1989) The prevalence and distribution of acute placental inflammation in uncomplicated term pregnancies. Obstet Gynecol 73:383–389

Sellier E, Platt MJ, Andersen GL et al (2015) Surveillance of Cerebral Palsy Network. Decreasing prevalence in cerebral palsy: a multi-site European population-based study, 1980 to 2003. Dev Med Child Neurol. https://doi.org/10.1111/dmcn.12865. [Epub ahead of print]

Soraisham AS, Singhal N, McMillan DD, Sauve RS, Lee SK (2009) Canadian Neonatal Network. A multicenter study on the clinical outcome of chorioamnionitis in preterm infants. Am J Obstet Gynecol 200:372.e1–372.e6

Speer CP (1999) Inflammatory mechanisms in neonatal chronic lung disease. Eur J Pediatr 158(Suppl 1): S18–S22

Thébaud B, Abman SH (2007) Bronchopulmonary dysplasia: where have all the vessels gone? Roles of angiogenic growth factors in chronic lung disease. Am J Respir Crit Care Med 175:978–985

Thomas W, Speer CP (2011) Chorioamnionitis: important risk factor or innocent bystander for neonatal outcome? Neonatology 99:177–187

Watterberg KL, Demers LM, Scott SM, Murphy S (1996) Chorioamnionitis and early lung inflammation in infants in whom bronchopulmonary dysplasia develops. Pediatrics 97:210–215

Wu YW (2002) Systematic review of chorioamnionitis and cerebral palsy. Ment Retard Dev Disabil Res Rev 8:25–29

Wu YW, Escobar GJ, Grether JK et al (2003) Chorioamnionitis and cerebral palsy in term and near-term infants. JAMA 290:2677–2684

Yoon BH, Romero R, Park JS et al (2000) The relationship among inflammatory lesions of the umbilical cord (funisitis), umbilical cord plasma interleukin 6 concentration, amniotic fluid infection, and neonatal sepsis. Am J Obstet Gynecol 183:1124–1129

7 Diagnosis of Fetal Distress

Silvia Vannuccini, Caterina Bocchi, Filiberto Maria Severi, and Felice Petraglia

Contents

Abstract

Fetal distress is a very broad term, which can be used in many clinical situations. Although it is difficult to give a precise clinical definition, obstetricians usually use this term to indicate that the fetus is becoming hypoxic. Immediate delivery has to be considered, because neurological damage may occur when the fetal brain is deprived of oxygen. Antepartum fetal testing is used to assess hypoxia in high-risk pregnancies and monitoring during labor supplies information on the status of the fetus prior to birth. However, knowledge of the fetal responses to asphyxia, together with the known evolution of fetal heart rate patterns, should allow a more accurate definition of its onset and a more rational management and timing for intervention.

S. Vannuccini · C. Bocchi · F. M. Severi (✉) · F. Petraglia
Obstetrics and Gynecology, Department of Molecular and Developmental Medicine, University of Siena, Siena, Italy
e-mail: vannuccini6@student.unisi.it; caterina.bocchi@unisi.it; filiberto.severi@unisi.it; felice.petraglia@unisi.it

G. Buonocore et al. (eds.), *Neonatology*,
https://doi.org/10.1007/978-3-319-29489-6_156

7.1 Salient Points

- Fetal distress is a broad term used in many clinical situations. A precise clinical definition is difficult and usually indicates that the fetus is becoming hypoxic.
- Hypoxia may result from reduced placental perfusion due to low pO2 in maternal blood (hypoxemic hypoxia), reduced arterial blood oxygen content due to low fetal hemoglobin concentration (anemic hypoxia), or reduced blood flow to the fetal tissues (ischemic hypoxia).
- The identification of at-risk pregnancies and their surveillance are currently of high priority in obstetric practice. Fetal distress and antepartum death can be substantially reduced if fetal surveillance is aimed at the early detection of signs of fetal oxygen deprivation.
- Cardiotocography, Doppler examination of fetal and placental circulations, biophysical profile, and amniotic fluid evaluation are various antepartum tests that allow clinicians to evaluate fetal oxygenation and fetal well-being.

7.2 Fetal Distress

Fetal distress is a very broad term, which can be used in many clinical situations. Although it is difficult to give a precise clinical definition, obstetricians usually use this term to indicate that the fetus is becoming hypoxic (Cunningham et al. 2001). Low fetal oxygenation may lead to neonatal morbidity and mortality. Immediate delivery has to be considered, because neurological damage may occur when the fetal brain is deprived of oxygen (Weiner et al. 2015).

The diagnosis of fetal distress based upon heart rate is imprecise, because heart rate patterns are only a reflection of the efficiency of physiological mechanisms which depend on blood flow and oxygenation. Furthermore, activity of this control mechanism is influenced by the preexisting state of fetal oxygenation as with chronic placental insufficiency. In fact, fetal hypoxia can occur acutely, for instance, as a result of placental abruption, but more commonly from chronic deterioration of placental function (Everett and Peebles 2015).

Transfer of oxygen to the fetus during labor may be altered by various mechanisms, leading to hypoxic changes and acidosis, such as abnormal perfusion within the uteroplacental vasculature or compression of the spiral arteries or umbilical cord during contractions (Leung and Lao 2012). In addition, pregnancy complications, such as hypertensive disorders, diabetes mellitus (DM), inflammatory diseases, chorioamnionitis, preterm labor, and fetal growth restriction (FGR), all may further exaggerate the compromised blood supply to the fetus during labor. In an attempt to prevent hypoxic–ischemic morbidities to the neonate, non-reassuring fetal heart rate monitoring during labor is one of the major indications for prompt delivery by performing an emergent cesarean delivery.

However, the recognition of risk and the knowledge of the fetal responses to asphyxia, together with the known evolution of fetal heart rate patterns, should allow a more accurate definition of its onset and a more rational management and timing for intervention. Antepartum fetal testing is used to assess hypoxia in high-risk pregnancies and monitoring during labor supplies information on the status of the fetus prior to birth (Everett and Peebles 2015).

7.2.1 Fetal Oxygenation

7.2.1.1 Physiology

Oxygenation may be defined as the process of transporting molecular oxygen from air to the tissues of the body. In the fetus this first involves oxygen transfer across the placenta; then there is reversible binding of oxygen to fetal hemoglobin and transport in the fetal blood stream and, finally, oxygen consumption for growth and metabolism. Energy is derived from the combination of oxygen and glucose to form carbon dioxide and water. When there is inadequate oxygen supply, the Krebs cycle cannot operate and pyruvate is converted to lactic acid. This enters the blood and there is a systemic acidosis, unless it is either metabolized or excreted. Removal of carbon dioxide and protection against acidosis is the reverse mechanism of oxygen delivery through the rapid diffusion, high solubility, and volatility of carbon dioxide. In the adult, carbon dioxide is excreted in the lungs while bicarbonate and hydrogen ions are removed by the kidney. In the fetus, both these functions are carried out by the placenta (Cunningham et al. 2001).

Normal fetal metabolism results in the production of acids (carbonic and organic), and despite this, the extracellular pH is kept within a critical range due to the efficient buffer mechanisms of the blood system. This is because the functions of the various fetal organ systems, such as the central nervous system and the cardiovascular system, may be significantly affected by very small changes in pH. The major buffers utilized by the fetus for neutralizing hydrogen ion production are plasma bicarbonate and hemoglobin. Inorganic phosphates and erythrocyte bicarbonate are also potential buffers, although they play a lesser role in fetal acid–base hemostasis. The amount of oxygen bound to hemoglobin is not linearly related to oxygen tension (pO_2). Each type of hemoglobin has a characteristic oxygen dissociation curve which can be modified by various factors, such as pH and the concentration of 2,3-diphosphoglycerate (2,3-DPG). For example, when 2,3-DPG rises in response to anemia or hypoxia, it binds to and stabilizes the deoxygenated form of hemoglobin, resulting in a shift of the oxygen dissociation curve to the right and therefore release of oxygen to the tissues. Although, in vitro, both adult (HbA) and fetal (HbF) hemoglobins have the same oxygen dissociation curves, adult human blood has a lower affinity for oxygen than fetal blood because of its greater binding to 2,3-DPG. The higher affinity of fetal blood for oxygen helps the transplacental transfer of oxygen. Furthermore, since the P50 of fetal blood is similar to the umbilical arterial pO_2, the fetus operates over the steepest part of the hemoglobin oxygen dissociation curve, and, therefore, a relatively large amount of oxygen is released from the hemoglobin for any given drop in pO_2 (Cunningham et al. 2001).

7.2.1.2 Hypoxia

Fetal hypoxia is a condition characterized by oxygen deficiency in the tissues. Complete oxidative metabolism of carbohydrates to carbon dioxide (CO_2) and water is impaired and metabolism proceeds along an anaerobic pathway with production of organic acids, such as lactic acid, which are not readily excreted or metabolized. Accumulation of lactic acid can deplete the buffer system, resulting in metabolic acidosis (Martin 2008).

Hypoxia may result from:

1. Reduced placental perfusion with maternal blood and a consequent decrease in fetal arterial blood oxygen content due to low pO_2 (hypoxemic hypoxia)
2. Reduced arterial blood oxygen content due to low fetal hemoglobin concentration (anemic hypoxia)
3. Reduced blood flow to the fetal tissues (ischemic hypoxia) (Cunningham et al. 2001)

Reduced fetal oxygenation may result from a variety of sources (Table 1) (Regnault et al. 2007).

Table 1 Causes of reduced fetal oxygenation

Maternal	Respiratory insufficiency
	Hypotension
	Hypertension
	Shock
	Asthma/bronchospasm
	Diabetes
	Collagen/vascular disease
	Hematological disorders
	Hemolytic crisis
	Congenital heart diseases
Placental	Abruptio placentae
	Infarction
	Confined mosaicism
	Placenta previa
Uterine	Rupture
	Hyperstimulation
	Prolonged labor
Fetal	Arrhythmia
	Hydrops
	Myocarditis
	Congenital abnormality
Umbilical cord	Funicular loop
	Compression
	Prolapse
	Vasa previa bleeding

According to placenta role, hypoxic pregnancy conditions can be classified into three subtypes: (1) preplacental hypoxia, where both the mother and her fetus will be hypoxic (i.e., high-altitude and cyanotic maternal heart diseases); (2) uteroplacental hypoxia, where the maternal oxygenation is normal but the uteroplacental circulation is impaired (i.e., preeclampsia, placentar insufficiency, etc.); and (3) postplacental hypoxia, where only the fetus is hypoxic (Kingdom and Kaufmann 1997).

Predisposing conditions that may result in fetal acid–base status derangement might be classified as either acute or chronic clinical conditions of the mother, placenta, and/or fetus (Omo-Aghoja 2014).

Acute maternal conditions may include any clinical situation that causes hypotension or hypovolemia such as hemorrhage, a vasovagal attack, or epidural anesthesia, with a resultant reduction of maternal blood supply and therefore oxygen delivery to the uterus. Uterine contractions can also interrupt uterine blood flow by a pressure rise and if prolonged, as in hypertonus, may cause hypoxia and acidosis. Acute placental factors, on the other hand, include conditions such as abruption that usually result in the disruption of the uteroplacental circulation by separating and tearing the uterine spiral arteries from the placenta. Similarly, the blood flow from the placenta to the fetus is often affected during labor and delivery by the umbilical cord compression; this can sometimes happen before labor if there is reduced liquor or a true knot in the cord. However, there is significant reserve because the fetus can compensate by increased oxygen extraction, meaning blood flow to the fetus must be reduced by at least 50% to cause hypoxia (Omo-Aghoja 2014).

Chronic clinical conditions that have been associated with fetal acid–base derangement may also be maternal, placental, or fetal. Maternal causes of chronic fetal acidosis include reduced oxygenation of maternal blood, as in severe respiratory or cardiac disease, or reduced blood flow to the placenta, as in connective tissue diseases – for example, systemic lupus erythematosus – and preeclampsia. Chronic placental factors usually result from impairment of placental transfer of oxygen. This is thought to result from inadequate trophoblast invasion of the myometrium in early pregnancy, leading to reduced perfusion of the intervillous spaces. Finally, even with normal placental function, chronic conditions within the fetus can cause acidosis. Anemia from rhesus disease, parvovirus infection, thalassemia, or feto-maternal hemorrhage, when severe enough to reduce fetal hemoglobin concentrations below 40 g/l (equivalent to an oxygen content below 2 mmol/l), can lead to a fall in pH. Arteriovenous shunting in fetal tumors, serious cardiac structural abnormalities, or arrhythmias are other conditions which can lead to chronic acidosis by decreased oxygenation as a result of reduced feto-placental blood flow (Omo-Aghoja 2014) (Table 1).

Fetal Acid–Base Balance in Hypoxia

Hypoxia in fetuses is potentially very hazardous with an adverse outcome for the neonate because the fetus normally has a very low PaO_2 (approximately 35 mmHg in the umbilical vein) and high $PaCO_2$ (approximately 42 mmHg in the umbilical vein) (Pipkin 1999). The inherent response therefore is preferential redistribution of blood to vital organs, and hence in acute severe fetal hypoxemia, there is associated and sustained maintenance of blood flow to the brain, the adrenal gland, and the heart at the expense of other tissues. This results in activation of peripheral chemoreceptors, with an increase in sympathetic tone, and in later gestation there is also an increase in concentrations of circulating cortisol, catecholamines, angiotensin II, and vasopressin, with a resultant increase in peripheral resistance. Following severe hypoxia, there is a shift to anaerobic pathways of metabolism as the "deprived" tissues may not be able to maintain oxidative phosphorylation. Since the fetus has a lesser ability to cope with acid–base disturbances, lactic acidemia can rapidly develop. This shifts the oxyhemoglobin dissociation curve to the right, with a further reduction in blood O_2 content. Thus, the resulting vicious circle can quickly result in fetal death. The fetal oxyhemoglobin dissociation curve is left shifted in comparison with the mother's because fetal hemoglobin has a lower binding affinity for 2,3-diphosphoglycerate. The fetus has a high hemoglobin concentration (16 g/dl), which also contributes to the relatively high oxygen content. The low umbilical PaO_2 and fetal vasculature pO_2 means that although umbilical venous blood is approximately 85% saturated (compared with approximately 95% in the adult) and has a relatively high oxygen content, the steep dissociation curve allows adequate oxygen unloading to the tissues. The high fetal blood flow allows equivalent or higher oxygen deliveries compared with adults to most tissue beds. However, it appears that fetal PaO_2 varies inversely with oxygen consumption, as the capacity to increase oxygen uptake from the lungs is absent.

Fetal $PaCO_2$ is high with approximately 60% being carried as bicarbonate. As fetal blood is oxygenated, it releases hydrogen ions, which combine with bicarbonate and push the equilibrium toward CO_2 and H_2O which diffuse across the placenta, down the concentration gradient for CO_2.

During hypoxia, the fetal pCO_2 rises, increasing the level of H_2CO_3 in the fetal blood and giving rise to a respiratory acidosis and a fall in the blood pH. The combination of hypoxia, hypercapnia, and metabolic acidosis constitutes asphyxia. At any given level of oxygen depletion, the survival time of the hypoxic fetus will depend primarily on its glycogen reserve. Thus, the well-nourished fetus can be expected to withstand a standard hypoxic insult better than the growth-retarded fetus.

Hemodynamic Consequences to Hypoxia

At an initial stage, the human fetus may be able to adapt to hypoxia by increasing the blood supply to the brain, myocardium, and upper body and decreasing the perfusion of the kidneys, gastrointestinal tract, and lower extremities. This redistribution of blood allows preferential delivery of nutrients and oxygen to the most vital organs. Cerebral vasodilatation to spare the brain from hypoxic damage leads to a decrease in left ventricular afterload, while systemic arterial vasoconstriction of lower body vessels increases right ventricular afterload.

In fact, an increased middle cerebral artery blood flow and a shift of the cardiac output in favor of the left ventricle are shown. With further deterioration of the fetal oxygenation, this protective mechanism is overwhelmed by the decline in cardiac output and the emergence of fetal distress. The final stage is characterized by a decline in systolic and diastolic fetal cardiac function, secondary to myocardial ischemia. Moreover, raised atrial contraction results in the transmission of atrial pressure waves into the venous duct and umbilical vein, causing end-diastolic umbilical vein pulsation. At this stage, reduced or reversed end-diastolic flow velocity may also be found in pulmonary veins, and coronary blood flow may become visible with increased systo-diastolic flow velocities ("heart sparing"). If not delivered, intrauterine death occurs usually within a few days (Hutter et al. 2010).

7.3 Clinical Diagnosis of Fetal Distress

7.3.1 Antenatal Surveillance

7.3.1.1 Identification of a Fetus at High Risk of Distress

The identification of at-risk pregnancies and their surveillance are currently of high priority in obstetric practice. Fetal distress and antepartum death can be substantially reduced if fetal surveillance is aimed at the early detection of signs of fetal oxygen deprivation.

Comprehensive assessment of fetal well-being involves monitoring of fetal growth, placental function, central venous pressure, and cardiac function. Ultrasound evaluation of the fetus using 2D, color Doppler, and pulse-wave Doppler techniques forms the foundation of antenatal diagnosis of structural anomalies, rhythm abnormalities, and altered fetal circulation. Accurate and timely prenatal identification of the fetus at risk is critical for appropriate parental counseling, antenatal diagnostic testing, consideration for fetal intervention, perinatal planning, and coordination of postnatal care delivery (Pruetz et al. 2015).

Ultrasound imaging has helped with detection of the vulnerable fetus. The purposes of ultrasonography studies are (i) to have accurate pregnancy dating, to diagnose multiple pregnancies, and to detect fetal anomalies and (ii) to monitor fetal growth and to recognize small for gestational age (SGA) and growth-restricted (FGR) fetuses

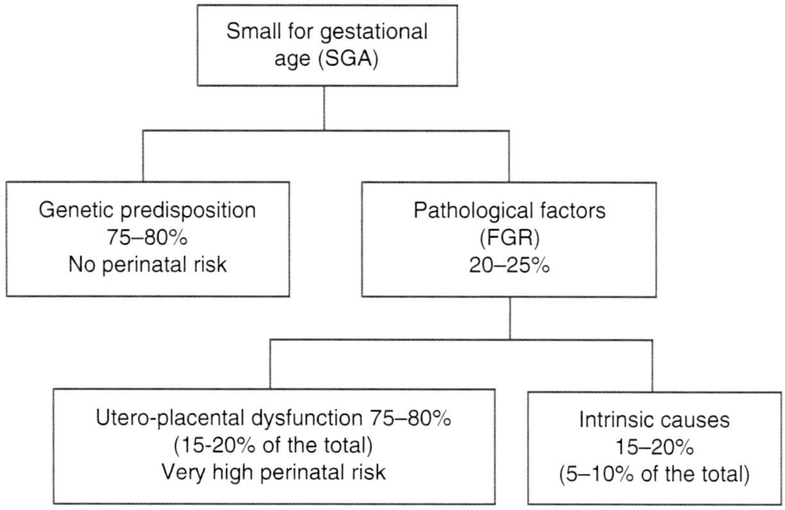

Fig. 1 Reduced fetal growth: etiopathogenesis

who may be more susceptible to the damaging effects of fetal hypoxia.

It is not always easy to decide whether a fetus is SGA as a result of genetic causes or if it suffers from placental insufficiency and malnutrition (fetal growth restriction [FGR]) (Fig. 1), but it is important to detect fetuses who did not reach their growth potential because these fetuses are at significant risk of hypoxia, acidosis, and death. This condition is also a common cause of premature delivery, is associated with increased perinatal mortality and morbidity, and is considered synonymous of "chronic fetal distress."

If FGR is suspected, it is important to perform an ultrasound biometric evaluation of the fetus as early as possible and then to follow fetal growth with serial and repeated (every 2 weeks) ultrasound investigations.

Before assessing fetal size, it is necessary to make an accurate assessment of gestational age.

Determination of Gestational Age and Assessment of Fetal Size

The accurate assessment of gestational age is very important in everyday clinical practice. Fetal body measurements reflect the gestational age of the fetus. This is particularly true in early gestation (first and early second trimester). In patients with an uncertain last menstrual period, biometric measurements must be made as early as possible to date the pregnancy accurately. The embryo crown–rump length (CRL) measured obtained by ultrasound has been shown as the best parameter during the first trimester (accuracy: ± 5–7 days). This measurement can be made between 6 and 13 weeks and gives a very accurate estimation of the gestational age.

Table 2 Second trimester: accuracy of multiple parameters in the determination of gestational age

Weeks	BPD	HC	FL
12–18	±1.19	±1.19	±1.38
19–24	±1.73	±1.48	±1.80
25–30	±2.18	±2.06	±2.08

The use of multiple parameters (biparietal diameter [BPD], head circumference [HC], transverse cerebellum diameter [TCD]) is generally recommended for the determination of gestational age in the second trimester (Table 2).

To assess if a fetus has normal growth, the following fetal biometry is used:

1. BPD and HC.
2. Abdominal circumference (AC), which is the most important measurement in the second half of pregnancy; it reflects fetal size and weight rather than age [3].
3. Femur length (FL), which reflects longitudinal growth of the fetus.

Repeated measurement of AC is considered the most sensitive parameter for following fetal growth (Table 3).

When the suspicion of FGR is confirmed, fetal surveillance, placental function, and fetal behavior measurements should be initiated, and fetal growth should be followed longitudinally with other diagnostic methods (see section "Antepartum Testing").

7.3.1.2 Identification of Fetal Distress

Fetal distress may be discovered in pregnancy ("antepartum testing") or during labor and delivery ("intrapartum testing") using different approaches.

7.4 Antepartum Testing

There are various tests that allow clinicians to evaluate fetal oxygenation and fetal well-being. These are described below.

Table 3 SGA: ultrasound diagnostic accuracy

Ultrasound parameters	Sensitivity (range) (%)	Specificity (range) (%)
Abdominal circumference	67–86	80–92
Ratio among biometrical parameters	62–82	80–93
Fetal weight estimation (FWE)	64–83	79–96

7.4.1 Biophysical Profile (BPP)

The biophysical profile (BPP) combines the use of CTG with the ultrasound assessment of fetal movement, fetal tone, fetal breathing movements, and amniotic fluid volume. Each parameter is scored 0 (abnormal) or 2 (normal) points, with a maximum total score of 10 (Table 4). A normal score (≥8) is reassuring and has a high negative predictive value and is associated with a low stillbirth rate (0.8%). A score below 6 is not reassuring and is considered borderline. The test may be repeated as often as daily until delivery, although most often it is a onetime event or a weekly event depending on the reason for the biophysical profile. The test is time consuming and labor intensive, but a modified BPP (deepest pool of amniotic fluid and CTG assessment) has been shown to have a similar negative predictive value as a full BPP (Lalor et al. 2012).

Described for the first time by Manning, the BPP is widely used for antepartum fetal surveillance (Manning 1999; Thompson et al. 2012). It can be done in the later stages of pregnancy from the beginning of the third trimester. The test is more frequently used in cases where the pregnancy is over 40 weeks to ensure fetal well-being; in some cases it is performed because of the presence of high-risk factors. However, a recent Cochrane review concluded that there is

Table 4 Fetal biophysical profile

Biophysical variable	Normal (score = 2)	Abnormal (score = 0)
Fetal tone	One or more episodes of active extension with return to flexion of fetal limb(s) or trunk (opening and closing of hand considered normal tone)	Slow extension with return to partial flexion, movement of limb in full extension, absent fetal movement, or partially open fetal hand
Gross body movements	Two or more discrete body/limb movements within 30 min (episodes of active continuous movement considered as a single movement)	<2 episodes of body/limb movements within 30 min
Fetal breathing movements	One or more episodes of ≥20 s within 30 min	Absent or no episode of ≥20 s within 30 min
Qualitative amniotic fluid volume	One or more pockets of fluid measuring ≥2 cm in vertical axis	Either no pockets or largest pocket <2 cm in vertical axis
Fetal heart rate (FHR)	Two or more episodes of acceleration of ≥15 bpm and of >15 s associated with fetal movement within 20 min	One or more episodes of acceleration of fetal heart rate or acceleration of <15 bpm within 20 min

Modified from Manning (1999)

insufficient evidence to support the use of BPP in high-risk pregnancies. The review also highlighted the possible risks of increased intervention (induction of labor and cesarean section) against the paucity of evidence of benefit in fetal or neonatal outcomes (Lalor et al. 2008).

7.4.1.1 Amniotic Fluid Evaluation

Amniotic fluid volume is an important parameter for the assessment of fetal well-being. It is a reflection of placental perfusion and normal fetal blood flow from the placenta and may be decreased when there are factors causing growth restriction (Chauhan et al. 2007).

Although an experienced examiner can assess the adequacy of the amniotic fluid volume, an amniotic fluid index (AFI) has been developed to standardize this assessment. This index is obtained by calculating the sum of deepest pocket of amniotic fluid in each of the four quadrants of the uterus. Another technique is the vertical measurement of the major pocket (Manning technique: cutoff 10 mm) (Manning 2009).

During the third trimester, normal amniotic fluid correlates with an AFI of 10–20 cm. Borderline values are 5–10 cm for decreased fluid and 20–24 cm for increased fluid depths (Hebbar et al. 2015). Pregnancies with decreased amniotic fluid volume are an indication for additional surveillance and assessment. For some authors, prospective evaluation of amniotic fluid index alone in low-risk pregnancies does not seem to be a good predictor of complications during a pregnancy or the perinatal period, but others consider that reduced amniotic fluid volume indicates chronic oxygen deficiency: perinatal mortality in pregnancies with oligohydramnios is 50 times higher than in pregnancies with normal AFI (Ott 2005; Morris et al. 2014).

7.4.1.2 Amnioscopy

At term, it is possible to visualize the amniotic fluid color using amnioscopy. If it is clear, the liquor is considered normal; if it is colored, there is a possibility of fetal distress because during fetal hypoxia there is an increase in fetal intestinal peristalsis with the release of meconium from the fetal rectum. This investigation is no longer used as often as it was in the past.

7.4.2 Cardiotocography

Cardiotocography (CTG) is the recording (-graphy) of the fetal heartbeat (cardio-) and the uterine contractions (-toco-). Recordings are done using two separate transducers, one for the measurement of the fetal heart rate and the other for measuring uterine contractions.

The CTG trace shows two lines: the upper shows the fetal heart rate in beats per minute; the lower is a recording of uterine contractions. Interpretation of the results of the monitoring is complex, and different patterns can be seen on a CTG (American College of Obstetricians and Gynecologists 2009).

1. *Baseline rate*. The baseline rate should be between 110 and 150 beats per minute (bpm) and is measured when the fetal heart rate is stable (i.e., without accelerations and decelerations). It should be taken over a period of 5–10 min. The rate may change over a period of time but normally remains fairly constant.
2. *Bradycardia*. This is defined as a baseline heart rate of less than 110 bpm. A suspicious bradycardia is defined as being between 110 and 100, whereas a pathological pattern is below 100. A steep sustained decrease in fetal heart rate is indicative of fetal distress.
3. *Tachycardia*. A suspicious tachycardia is defined when the FHR is between 150 and 170 bpm, whereas a pathological pattern is above 170 bpm. Tachycardias can be a response to fever, fetal infection, fetal movements, tocolytic drugs, and use of tea or coffee and occasionally a sign of fetal distress (in conjunction with other abnormalities). An epidural may also induce a tachycardia in the fetus.
4. *Baseline variations*. The short-term variations in the baseline should be between 10 and 15 bpm (except during fetal sleep, which should be no longer than 60 min). Prolonged reduced variability along with other abnormalities may indicate fetal distress.

5. *Accelerations*. This is a transient increase in the fetal heart rate of greater than 15 bpm for at least 15 s. Two accelerations in 20 min are required for the trace to be considered "reactive," i.e., normal. Accelerations are a good sign as they show fetal responsiveness and the integrity of mechanisms controlling the heart rate.
6. *Decelerations*. These may either be normal or pathological. Early decelerations occur at the same time as uterine contractions and are usually due to fetal head compression and therefore occur during the first and second stages of labor with descent of the head. They are normally benign. Late decelerations begin after the start of a contraction and persist after the end of a contraction and suggest fetal distress. Variable decelerations vary in timing and shape with respect to each other and may indicate hypoxia or cord compression.

The American College of Obstetricians and Gynecologists (ACOG) developed a new three-tiered classification of fetal heart rate abnormalities and a system for interpreting CTG abnormalities (American College of Obstetricians and Gynecologists 2010).

1. Category I FHR tracings are normal tracings which are not associated with fetal asphyxia. They include a baseline heart rate between 110 and 160, moderate variability defined as "fluctuations in the baseline heart rate that are irregular in amplitude and frequency of 6–25 bpm," no late or variable decelerations, possible early decelerations, and possible accelerations.
2. Category II FHR tracings are indeterminate and include a wide variety of possible tracings that do not fit in either Category I or Category III. The classification of Category II tracings includes the following: bradycardia with variability, tachycardia, minimal variability, no variability with no recurrent decelerations, marked variability, absence of induced accelerations even after fetal stimulation, recurrent variable decelerations with minimal or moderate baseline variability, prolonged decelerations lasting more than 2 min but less than 10 min, recurrent late decelerations with moderate variability, and variable decelerations with other characteristics such as slow return to baseline, overshooting the baseline, or "shoulders." Reduced FHR variability is the most reliable indicator of fetal compromise. A flat FHR tracing with no variability may reflect neurologic damage to the fetus that has already occurred.
3. Category III FHR tracings are abnormal and indicative of hypoxic risk to the fetus and possible acidemia. They include either no baseline variability or the presence of recurrent late decelerations, variable decelerations, bradycardia, or a sinusoidal pattern. According to a study by Jackson et al., Category I and Category II patterns are common in labor and Category III are unusual. Perinatal morbidity is associated with an increase in time in Category II during the last 2 h of labor.

7.4.2.1 Nonstress Test (NST)

Since its introduction during the 1970s, the nonstress test (NST) has remained one of the cornerstones of fetal surveillance. It is based on CTG and it reflects cardiorespiratory regulation of fetal heart: the monitor records fetal heart rate in conjunction with uterine activity.

The purpose of NTS is to try to identify potential fetal compromise as a result of placental insufficiency and hypoxia and to take corrective action (American College of Obstetricians and Gynecologists 2010). It is used to identify signs of fetal distress in all situations in which pregnancy complications may cause harm to the fetus. It can also be performed as a precaution when there have been problems complicating a previous pregnancy or in the presence of risk factors (e.g., diabetes, intrauterine growth restriction).

The test is more frequently done between 38 and 42 weeks' gestation; however, it can be used as early as the beginning of the third trimester.

A normal test is defined as a "reactive" pattern that requires a minimum of two accelerations

(15 bpm increase from the baseline during 15 s) during a 20 min test. A reactive trace after 10–20 min is generally regarded as sufficient for normality. A "nonreactive" result suggests the possibility of fetal distress, requiring further assessment (biophysical profile, a stress test).

The predictive value of a nonreactive NST is poor when outcome parameters such as fetal death and fetal distress during labor are used. A reactive test can be expected to impose a tenfold lower risk of intervention for fetal distress during labor than a pregnancy with a nonreactive test. There is a paucity of good-quality evidence regarding antenatal CTG monitoring. A Cochrane meta-analysis, including high-risk pregnancies, found no clear evidence that antenatal CTG improves perinatal outcome (Grivell et al. 2015).

Indeed, there are wide observer differences in the qualitative interpretation of the FHR trace, and agreement between observers is low, especially for decelerations, which are the most difficult pattern to interpret. For this reason, to eliminate observer variability and to increase the accuracy of CTG, a computerized analysis was developed by Dawes and coworkers (Dawes et al. 1995, 1996). Nowadays, the use of the computerized CTG has increased the predictive ability of NST for the diagnosis of fetal hypoxia during the antepartum period compared with the traditional CTG – compared to computer analysis, observers fail to identify 36% of FHR traces with at least one deceleration.

Computerized CTG monitoring can provide assessment of short-term variability (STV), which cannot be performed by visual assessment alone. STV has been shown to correlate with the fetal metabolic state, and significantly reduced STV is closely associated with fetal acidemia (Turan et al. 2007). In addition, computerized CTG has been shown to reduce perinatal mortality compared to traditional CTG in the high-risk population (Grivell et al. 2015).

The use of continuous intrapartum electronic fetal heart rate monitoring (EFM) using a cardiotocograph was developed to enable obstetricians and midwives to analyze the changes of fetal heart rate during labor so as to institute timely intervention to avoid intrapartum hypoxic–ischemic injury. Although CTG was initially developed as a screening tool to predict fetal hypoxia, its positive predictive value for intrapartum fetal hypoxia is approximately only 30%. Even though different international classifications have been developed with the aim of defining combinations of features that help predict intrapartum fetal hypoxia, the false-positive rate of the CTG is high (60%). Moreover, there has not been a demonstrable improvement in the rate of cerebral palsy or perinatal deaths since the introduction of CTG into clinical practice approximately 45 years ago. However, there has been a significant increase in intrapartum cesarean section and operative vaginal delivery rates. Unfortunately, existing guidelines employ the visual interpretation of CTG based on "pattern recognition," which is fraught with inter- and intra-observer variability. Therefore, clinicians need to understand the physiology behind fetal heart rate changes and to respond to them accordingly, instead of purely relying on guidelines for management. It is very likely that such a "physiology-based" approach would reduce unnecessary operative interventions and improve perinatal outcomes while reducing the need for "additional tests" of fetal well-being (Pinas and Chandraharan 2016).

7.4.2.2 Contraction Stress Test (CST)

The contraction stress test may be used after a nonreactive NST. This test monitors the response of fetal heart rate to uterine contractions. These contractions may occur on their own or following the administration of oxytocin.

A normal placenta has extra capacity for transporting oxygen, allowing large amounts of oxygen to pass easily from the maternal to the fetal circulation. If the placenta is damaged, less oxygen may cross. When there are contractions, the vessels feeding the placenta are squeezed, limiting the blood flow and oxygen delivery. If the oxygen passage across the placenta drops below a certain point, the fetus responds with a specific type of heart rate deceleration, which occurs after the peak of a contraction and which is known as a "late deceleration."

The contraction stress test is considered "positive" if there are regular late decelerations. When no late decelerations occur, the CST is negative, and this is considered reassuring. A positive CST is a sign that the placenta may not be delivering adequate amounts of oxygen to the fetus. Given a positive CST, a pregnancy at term should be delivered, although this is not necessarily appropriate for very premature pregnancies.

Because a contraction stress test takes more time to perform than a biophysical profile, it is seldom done these days.

7.4.3 Doppler Examination of Fetal and Placental Circulation

Doppler ultrasound provides a noninvasive method for the study of the fetus's hemodynamic status (Everett and Peebles 2015). The application of Doppler to obstetrical ultrasound provides new knowledge about fetal circulatory physiology in health as well as in those compromised by chronic hypoxia because of placental insufficiency. This functional assessment of fetal well-being is done by observing fetal movements, breathing, muscle tone, and heart rate. Additionally, the volume of amniotic fluid gives an indirect assessment of the pregnancy.

Investigation of the flow patterns of the uterine and umbilical arteries gives information on flow through the uteroplacental and feto-placental circulations, respectively. Doppler studies of fetal organs are used to detect the hemodynamic rearrangements that occur in response to fetal hypoxemia, in particular by insonnation of the middle cerebral arteries (MCA) and ductus venosus (DV).

The Doppler indices (Table 5) indirectly reflect the impedance of the circulation downstream to the point of insonnation, and there is a significant association between abnormal Doppler indices and fetal hypoxia, fetal acidosis, and adverse perinatal outcome.

Doppler ultrasonography is not routinely employed in low-risk pregnancies (Alfirevic et al. 2015), but has been extensively used for

Table 5 The most widely used indices used for studying uteroplacental, placental, and fetal arteries

Doppler indices	
Systolic/diastolic ratio	(S/D) Systolic peak/end-diastolic velocity
Resistance index	(RI) S-D/S
Pulsatility index	(PI) S-D/mean velocity

maternal–fetal evaluation in high-risk pregnancies, contributing to a reduction in perinatal mortality (Alfirevic et al. 2013a), especially in the management of IUGR. The jeopardized fetus seems to be at the highest risk of imminent demise when Doppler abnormalities are observed in the arterial and especially venous circulation (ductus venosus and umbilical vein). The temporal sequence of abnormal Doppler changes in the peripheral and central circulatory systems of the growth-restricted fetus has been described: early abnormal Doppler findings in the umbilical and middle cerebral arteries are followed by the reversal of flow in the ductus venosus or pulsatile umbilical venous flow.

For this reason the use of Doppler velocimetry is of great importance in high-risk pregnancies and in cases of non-reassuring test results.

7.4.3.1 Uteroplacental Vessels

Both the uterine and other uteroplacental vessels have been studied with Doppler sonography. Uterine arteries are two symmetrical vessels that bring the oxygenated blood of the mother to the placenta.

There are numerous Doppler studies on uterine and spiral arterial flow during normal first-trimester pregnancies which demonstrate a high vascular resistance that progressively disappears during the second trimester as a consequence of decreased resistance downstream. Decreasing vascular impedance with gestation (Fig. 2) is probably a consequence of dilatation of spiral arteries induced by trophoblast infiltration, hormonally mediated vasodilatation, and a decrease in maternal blood flow viscosity. Thus, changes in uterine blood flow are correlated with the development of complications in later pregnancy: if the process of trophoblastic invasion of the spiral arteries' muscular walls is incomplete, the arteries are still able to respond to vasoactive stimuli, which results

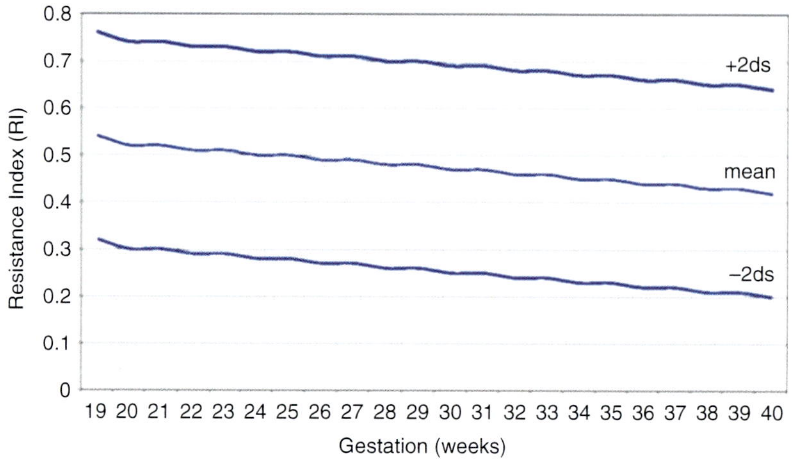

Fig. 2 Uterine artery resistance index

in vasoconstriction. In these pregnancies the uteroplacental circulation remains in a state of high resistance, which causes generalized endothelial cell injury, compromising vascular integrity and an atherosis-like process in the small arteries resulting in vessel occlusion, local ischemia, and necrosis. As a consequence of vasoconstriction, a chronic inadequate blood supply to the growing placenta leads to a poor outcome (spontaneous abortion, IUGR, stillbirth, or preeclampsia).

When an abnormal adaptation of pregnancy occurs, impedance to flow increases and Doppler examination often demonstrates the presence of a high-resistance index (RI) and/or the presence of an early mono- or bilateral diastolic notch (Becker and Vonk 2010). Adverse outcomes associated with abnormal uterine artery flow velocity include: preeclampsia and fetal growth restriction and its sequelae, mainly fetal distress (O'Gorman et al. 2016; Valiño et al. 2016; Savasan et al. 2014).

For this reason, in high-risk women, accurate uteroplacental investigation during the first and second trimester of pregnancy allows the clinician to identify, and therefore to monitor, fetuses at high risk of distress. Through the investigation of uterine artery flow in high-risk pregnancies, it has been shown that if the fetus has a normal umbilical flow, the compromise in growth will be mild, the risk of fetal distress slightly above normal, and the most common indication for intervention is maternal, not fetal. Present evidence does not support routine Doppler ultrasound for low-risk or unselected populations, which does not appear to benefit the mother or baby (Alfirevic et al. 2015).

Recent studies have shown that Doppler studies of the uterine arteries can be useful also during the third trimester of pregnancy: when both middle cerebral artery and uterine arteries show abnormal Doppler indices, the fetus has a significantly higher rate of poor outcome even in the presence of normal umbilical indices (Severi et al. 2002).

7.4.3.2 Feto-placental Vessels

The umbilical artery was the first fetal vessel to be evaluated by Doppler velocimetry, and Doppler velocimetry of the umbilical artery (UA) provides a noninvasive measure of the feto-placental hemodynamic state. In the Doppler assessment of fetal well-being, the UA is the most easily measured parameter and is the mainstay of assessment in small fetuses or those at risk of compromise (Everett and Peebles 2015; Berkley et al. 2012).

Umbilical arteries can be identified by Doppler ultrasound as early as 6–8 weeks, when the Doppler flow velocity profile shows only a systolic component. By 20 weeks, all fetuses should have end-diastolic flow in the umbilical vessels. As the pregnancy progresses, placental resistance shows a progressive decrease during gestation (Fig. 3), and there is an increasing diastolic flow velocity. A mature umbilical artery flow velocity waveform is usually achieved by 28–30 weeks, but some fetuses, e.g., twins, may show delayed

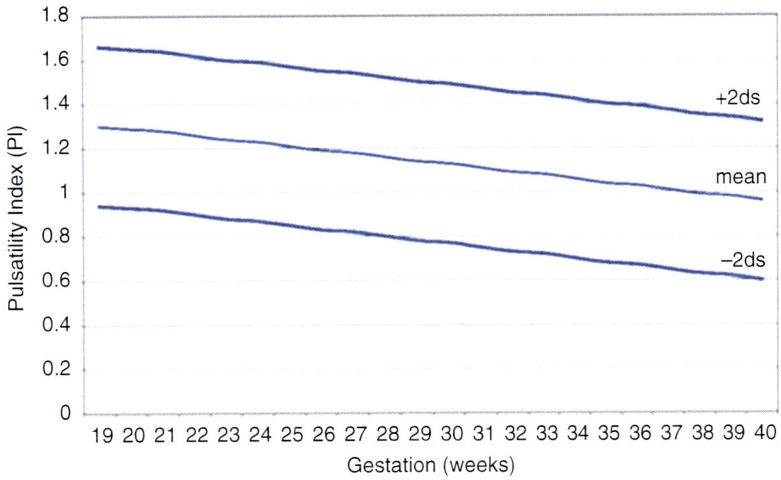

Fig. 3 Umbilical artery pulsatility index

maturation. Several studies have revealed a large standard deviation up to 26–28 weeks in the umbilical S/D ratio that reflects variations in placental development. Eighty percent of the flow velocity waveform is a reflection of the resistance beyond the point of measurement, but 20% can be a forward flow effect that is reduced in cardiac output changes, arrhythmias, and bradycardia.

Abnormality of the pulsatility index (PI) (the most significant quantitative parameter) has been correlated with feto-placental vascular maldevelopment. Changes in umbilical artery velocity waveforms reflect changes in the placental bed vascular resistance. Simply, increased resistance in the placenta results in reduced diastolic blood flow velocities. Initially, this is determined quantitatively through increasing PI values. As resistance further increases, qualitative changes in the waveform become evident, resulting in intermittently absent end-diastolic flow (EDF), progressing to persistently absent EDF and ultimately reversed EDF, which represents obliteration of >70% of placental tertiary villi. In fact, the primary and secondary branches of the umbilical circulation are in place after the first trimester, while in the next 3 months there is active proliferation of tertiary branches. Placental histology showed that growth-restricted fetuses with abnormal flow velocity have half as many tertiary arterioles as normal fetuses (Kingdom et al. 2000). Pathological studies have demonstrated that increased impedance in the umbilical arteries becomes evident only when at least 60% of the placental vascular bed is obliterated.

Although it may not be a separated entity, absent or reversed diastolic (ARED) flow in the umbilical artery has been the subject of a considerable body of literature. Clinical studies of umbilical arterial flow velocity waveforms in IUGR have reported a progressive increase in impedance to flow until end-diastolic flow becomes absent and, in extreme cases, reversed. This is associated with a high perinatal morbidity and mortality. In pregnancies with ARED flow, the capillary loops in terminal villi are decreased in number, longer, and with fewer branches than in normal pregnancies. For this reason, there is a strong association between the ARED velocity and hypoxia/acidosis (Gerber et al. 2006).

When there is reversed flow, it may be a clinical emergency because most of these fetuses will die within 2 weeks. The ARED flow, as a test for hypoxia, shows a high sensitivity, specificity, positive predictive value, and negative predictive value (Soregaroli et al. 2002). However, where flow is continuous throughout diastole, only a very high S/D ratio (greater than 4.5) is associated with hypoxia. Furthermore, the observation of ARED flow in the umbilical artery Doppler surveillance of pregnancies at risk for fetal distress has great clinical importance, especially in pregnancies associated with fetal growth restriction (Seyam et al. 2002). Umbilical artery Doppler applied to high-risk pregnancies significantly lowers perinatal mortality, the need for induction of delivery, and the emergency cesarean section rate (Morris et al. 2011). Conversely, the Doppler measurement of umbilical artery flow has repeatedly been shown not to be useful in a low-risk or unselected population (Alfirevic et al. 2015)

7.4.3.3 Fetal Vessels

Alteration in fetal vessel blood flow reflects an important hemodynamic modification that occurs in association with IUGR and fetal hypoxemia. The Doppler-detectable modifications in the fetal circulation associated with these conditions include increased resistance in both the umbilical artery (as described before) and fetal peripheral vessels, in association with decreased resistance in the fetal cerebral vessels.

Studies of other vascular beds in the fetus, including the cerebral circulation and the central arterial and venous systems, have increased the knowledge of compensatory and adaptive mechanisms and the time sequence of circulatory changes in the fetus subjected to hypoxia and severe growth restriction.

Arterial Compartment

The circle of Willis is an easy landmark to identify using ultrasound. Color flow makes it easy to see the common carotid and the anterior, middle, and posterior cerebral arteries.

Measurement by Doppler of the peak systolic flow velocity (PSV) of the fetal middle cerebral artery (MCA) is a predictor of moderate or severe fetal anemia (Mari 2005) in pregnancies complicated by red blood cell isoimmunization or in case of viral infections such as parvovirus B_{19}. However, if a raised PSV is detected in a woman without antibodies or recent viral infection, fetal anemia secondary to acute or chronic feto-maternal hemorrhage should be considered (Cosmi et al. 2012).

In fact, study of this vessel also yields important information for the detection of fetal distress. In some growth-restricted fetuses, the cerebral vessels are dilated. Usually these are fetuses with reduced umbilical artery flow velocity. This implies that fetuses with mild hypoxia will have dilated cerebral vessels as a compensatory response: this explains the so-called "brain-sparing" effect seen in FGR fetus. These changes occur early and may be present for weeks or even months before birth. In FGR fetuses the trend changes of the MCA-PI and MCA-PSV provide more clinical information than one single measurement. A high MCA-PSV predicts fetal distress and perinatal mortality better than a low MCA-PI. For this reason MCA-PSV might be valuable in the clinical assessment of IUGR fetuses that have abnormal UA Doppler (Mari et al. 2007; Fig. 4).

The value of MCA Doppler in the prediction of adverse fetal outcome and the assessment of the

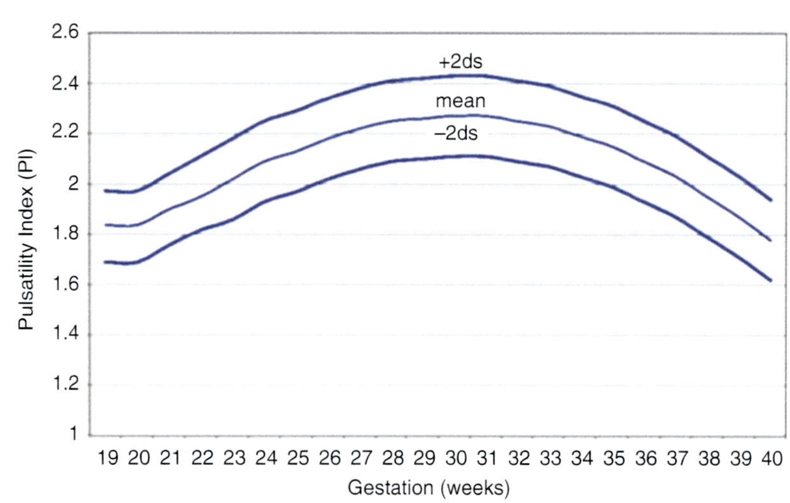

Fig. 4 Middle cerebral artery pulsatility index

"at-risk" fetus has been controversial. Some studies have suggested that the assessment of the MCA Doppler is a useful tool, whereas others have found poor predictive value. However, in a recent metanalysis low MCA-PI appears to be predictive of impaired fetal well-being assessed by either acidosis (pH < 7.20) at birth, 5 min Apgar score <7 or admission to a NICU. Abnormal MCA is also predictive of an overall composite measure of adverse perinatal outcome and perinatal mortality (Morris et al. 2012). Although these findings suggest that there is an association between abnormal MCA and adverse outcomes, the association is weak. In clinical practice, MCA alone has limited predictive value for compromised fetal or neonatal well-being.

Cerebroplacental Ratio

The cerebroplacental ratio (CPR) is emerging as an important predictor of adverse pregnancy outcome, and this has implications for the assessment of fetal well-being in fetuses diagnosed as small for gestational age (SGA) and those appropriate for gestational age close to term (DeVore 2015). Interest in this assessment tool has been rekindled because of recent reports associating an abnormal ratio with adverse perinatal events and associated postnatal neurological outcome. Fetuses with an abnormal CPR that are appropriate for gestational age or have late-onset SGA (>34 weeks of gestation) have a higher incidence of fetal distress in labor requiring emergency cesarean delivery, a lower cord pH, and an increased admission rate to the newborn intensive care unit when compared with fetuses with a normal CPR (Prior et al. 2013, 2015 Khalil et al. 2014; Morales-Rosello et al. 2015). Fetuses with early-onset SGA (<34 weeks of gestation) with an abnormal CPR have a higher incidence of the following when compared with fetuses with a normal CPR: (1) lower gestational age at birth, (2) lower mean birth weight, (3) lower birth weight centile, (4) birth weight less than the 10th centile, (5) higher rate of cesarean delivery for fetal distress in labor, (6) higher rate of Apgar scores less than 7 at 5 min, (7) an increased rate of neonatal acidosis, (8) an increased rate of newborn intensive care unit admissions, (9) higher rate of adverse neonatal outcome, and (10) a greater incidence of perinatal death (Figueras et al. 2015). Thus, the CPR should be considered as an assessment tool in fetuses undergoing third-trimester ultrasound examination, irrespective of the findings of the individual umbilical artery and middle cerebral artery measurements.

Fetal Arterial Blood Flow Redistribution

The "brain-sparing" effect is a phenomenon where fetuses that are hypoxic preferentially perfuse the brain, heart, and adrenals at the expense of the integument, viscera, gut, and kidneys.

Although knowledge of the factors governing circulatory rearrangements and their mechanism of action is incomplete, it appears that partial pressures of oxygen and carbon dioxide play a role, presumably through their action on chemoreceptors. This mechanism allows preferential delivery of nutrients and oxygen to vital organs, thereby compensating for diminished placental resources. However, compensation through cerebral vasodilatation is limited, and a plateau corresponding to a nadir of PI in cerebral vessels is reached at least 2 weeks before the onset of late fetal heart rate decelerations (Ferrazzi et al. 2002), and the development of the fetus is jeopardized. This suggests that maximal vascular adaptation to hypoxemia precedes the critical degree of impairment of fetal oxygenation, after which vascular dilatation may be suppressed by the development of cerebral edema. An alternative explanation may be that in severe hypoxemia, an increase in PI is the consequence of alterations in flow due to reduced cardiac contractility and to a fall in absolute cardiac output. Consequently, arterial vessels are not suitable for the longitudinal monitoring of growth-restricted fetuses, and cardiac and venous velocity waveforms give more information about fetal well-being or compromise.

Cardiac and Venous Compartment

Cardiac flow is influenced by the modifications of arterial impedance to flow. As long as the fetus is able to compensate for a reduced placental supply by arterial redistribution (a brain-sparing effect), there is preferential myocardial oxygenation, which delays the development of right heart failure despite an increasing afterload. Cerebral vasodilatation produces a decrease in left ventricular afterload, whereas increased placental and systemic resistance produce increased right ventricular afterload. At this stage, fetal Doppler measurements show high placental resistance and arterial redistribution in the presence of normal venous waveforms, and the majority of fetuses have normal, reactive heart rate traces and biophysical profiles. Progressive changes in the venous circulation may indicate failure of the compensatory mechanism and herald the development of right heart failure due to myocardial hypoxia (Baschat and Harman 2006).

Longitudinal studies of deteriorating growth-restricted fetuses have shown that PSV and cardiac output gradually decline, suggesting a progressive worsening in cardiac function. Similarly, there is a symmetrical decrease in ventricular ejection force at the level of both ventricles, despite the dramatically different hemodynamic conditions present downstream of the two ventricles (i.e., reduced cerebral resistances for the left ventricle and increased splanchnic and placental resistance for the right ventricle). This supports a pivotal role of the intrinsic myocardial function in the compensatory mechanism of the growth-restricted fetus following the establishment of the brain-sparing effect. Ventricular ejection force dramatically decreases in a short time interval (about 1 week), showing an impairment of ventricular force close to fetal distress. As a consequence, cardiac filling is also impaired (Severi et al. 2000; Baschat 2011).

Late Doppler changes generally accompany metabolic deterioration and are a result of declining cardiac function and abnormal organ autoregulation. Increasing venous Doppler indices are the hallmark of advancing circulatory deterioration since they indicate a decreasing ability of the heart to accommodate venous return. The ductus venosus (DV) waveform is sensitive to cardiac function, which in turn is adversely affected by chronic severe decrease in substrate/oxygen availability. In response to hypoxia, the DV becomes more dilated, and there is reduced flow during ventricular diastole, resulting in increased DV pulsatility index for veins (PIV), followed by increasingly retrograde flow during atrial systole, seen as absent or reversed a-wave (Baschat et al. 2006).

Fetal hypoxemia is associated with reduced umbilical venous blood flow, but, despite this decrease, a normal PSV in the ductus venosus is maintained. In the growth-restricted fetus, the percentage of umbilical venous blood passing through the ductus venosus is increased from about 40% (in normal fetuses) to about 60%. Thus, there is a redistribution of venous blood flow in favor of the ductus venosus at the expense of hepatic blood flow in growth-restricted fetuses. Unlike peak velocity during ventricular systole, flow velocities during atrial contraction are reduced or even reversed. One may speculate that increased end-diastolic right ventricular pressure would not influence ductus venosus blood flow velocities during atrial contraction, as flow is preferentially directed through the foramen ovale to the left atrium. However, the foramen ovale is closed during atrial contraction and blood flow velocity through the foramen ovale decreases to zero.

Altered venous flow velocity waveforms are more closely related to intrauterine fetal jeopardy than changes in arterial flow, which may occur quite early during the course of impaired placental function.

The degree of fetal acidemia can be estimated from Doppler measurements of pulsatility in both the arterial system and the ductus venosus. With moderate acidemia (pH between −2 and −4 standard deviations from the normal mean for gestational age), almost all fetuses have an MCA-PI below 2 standard deviations, whereas there is a wide scatter of individual results for the ductus venosus, with the majority of measurements being still within the reference ranges. With increasing severity of hypoxemia and acidemia, ductus venosus PI increases, and, in the most severe cases, velocities with atrial contraction were reduced to zero or even become negative. However, in severe fetal growth restriction, abnormal Doppler velocimetry of the ductus venosus is the only significant parameter associated with perinatal death and low 5 min Apgar scores (Baschat 2010; Baschat et al. 2003).

7.4.3.4 Doppler Findings and the Prediction of Perinatal Risks

Elevations of placental blood flow resistance and venous Doppler indices frequently progress in parallel. The recognition of venous Doppler changes has led to reexamination of the relationship between prenatal Doppler findings in growth-restricted fetuses and perinatal outcome.

Previously, delivery was recommended when umbilical artery Doppler end-diastolic velocities were absent or reversed. However, the Growth Restriction Intervention Trial (GRIT) (Thornton et al. 2004) showed that if there was early-onset IUGR, early and preterm delivery were independent risk factors for adverse neurodevelopment at 2 years of age. Safe prolongation of pregnancy in these fetuses is therefore critical. Daily biophysical profile scoring in fetuses with absent or reversed umbilical artery end-diastolic velocity with strict delivery criteria has been associated with good outcomes, suggesting that safe prolongation of these pregnancies is indeed possible. It is now apparent that prediction of perinatal risk based on umbilical artery alone, without accounting for venous circulatory changes, is inadequate. Prediction of stillbirth and acidemia is significantly enhanced by the addition of venous Doppler findings, irrespective of the umbilical arterial end-diastolic velocity. This rate increases when the arterial end-diastolic velocity is absent or reversed but venous Doppler indices are still normal and increases further when venous Doppler indices become abnormal (predominantly due to an increase in the rate of stillbirth). If the prevalence of stillbirth is 25%, abnormal venous Doppler findings have 65% sensitivity and 95% specificity for the prediction of stillbirth. Depending on the cutoff (2 vs. 3 SD) and the combination of veins examined, the sensitivity for acidemia ranges from 70% to 90% and specificity from 70% to 80%.

The TRUFFLE study has provided clarification of outcomes in the cases of IUGR prior to 32 weeks' gestation. In cases where delivery was determined by increased DV PIV or absent DV a-wave, perinatal mortality was 6% and 10%, respectively. However, neurologic impairment at 2 years of age was 9% and 5%, respectively. In those for whom delivery timing was based on reduced CTG STV, perinatal mortality and abnormal 2-year outcomes were 7% and 15%, respectively. Although the outcomes were not significantly different between the groups, the study suggests that delivery based on late Doppler changes, rather than on reduced CTG STV, may provide better long-term outcomes, possibly at the expense of a small increase in perinatal mortality (Lees et al. 2013, 2015).

7.5 During Labor Surveillance

7.5.1 Identification of Fetal Distress

Maternal blood flow to the placenta may be severely diminished by uterine contractions, so the potential for fetal hypoxia increases during labor. In the last century some asphyxiated fetuses were noted to have abnormally fast or slow heart rates, so heart auscultation evolved as a component of intrapartum care. However, the human ear is insensitive to subtle changes in rate, so electronic methods of recording have been developed. These methods generate paper traces that show features not obvious on auscultation, including the degree of variation of the heart rate and the shape of accelerations and decelerations in rate (the CTG).

Identification of fetal distress based on fetal heart rate patterns is imprecise, and intrapartum Doppler velocimetry was studied as a potential adjunct to conventional intrapartum fetal monitoring, but it was concluded that this technique was a poor predictor of adverse perinatal outcomes (Cunningham et al. 2001).

7.5.2 Monitoring of Fetal Heart Rate

The pattern of the fetal heartbeat during labor is often a good indicator of fetal well-being. The normal fetal heart rate (FHR) is 120–160 bpm. A normal heart rate suggests that the fetus is receiving enough oxygen from the mother's bloodstream. The typical fetal heart rate pattern is to slow somewhat during a contraction and increase again at the end of a contraction. Abnormal variations in heart rate can indicate decreased oxygen in the blood and tissues of the fetus that can potentially damage the fetus. The fetal heart can be monitored either intermittently by auscultation or continuously by CTG.

7.5.2.1 Auscultation with Fetal Stethoscope or Doppler Ultrasound Stethoscope

The fetal heartbeat and variability can be checked before, during, and after contractions, either using a Pinard fetal stethoscope or a Doppler ultrasound stethoscope, a small hand-held device which uses sound waves to monitor the heart beat. In low-risk births, the American College of Obstetricians and Gynecologists (American College of Obstetricians and Gynecologists 2009) suggests monitoring at least every 30 min during active labor and at least every 15 min during the second stage of labor. When risk factors are present, the fetal heart should be evaluated every 15 min and every 5 min in the second stage. The mother's abdomen may be also palpated to check for the strength of contractions.

7.5.2.2 Electronic External or Internal Monitoring

In last decade, approximately 85% of pregnancies were monitored in labor by continuous cardiotocography, also known as electronic fetal monitoring (EFM), making it the most commonly performed obstetric procedure.

A handheld Doppler ultrasound probe can be used to calculate and display, but not permanently record, the FHR. Electronic fetal monitors are used to both determine the FHR and continuously record it in graphical form. External measurement means taping or strapping the electrodes to the maternal abdominal wall, with a small Doppler ultrasound heart electrode overlying the fetal heart, and the contraction electrode measuring the tension of the abdominal wall, an indirect measure of the intrauterine pressure. Both electrodes are connected to video screens and a printer which produces graphs of the fetal heart rate and "intensity" of the contractions.

Internal measurement requires the cervix to be at least 2 cm dilated as it involves inserting a pressure catheter into the uterine cavity, as well as attaching a scalp electrode to the fetal head to adequately measure the heart rate. Membranes must be ruptured to place the electrodes. The electrode measures the fetal heart rate. It is used in some high-risk births if the external monitor shows suspicious results or if external monitoring is not generating an adequate trace. Internal monitoring offers better accuracy of readings than external monitoring, but there is an increased risk of infection after application of the electrode. The advantage of internal monitoring is that it is immediately apparent if the fetal heart rate slows down, stops, or is slow to recover from contractions. It can detect reduced oxygen flow due to cord compression (more common after rupture of the membranes), oxytocin-augmented contractions, or narcotic- and epidural-related changes in maternal blood pressure.

During the *first stage* of labor, a moderate fetal tachycardia may be considered a circulatory mechanism of adaptation against moderate fetal hypoxia. By contrast, a severe tachycardia is a clear sign of fetal hypoxia: it can be associated with high maternal temperature or fetal cardiac malformations or medications administered to the mother. The same is true for a bradycardia: a moderate bradycardia is considered without clinical significance, but a marked bradycardia is a sign of severe fetal hypoxia.

Similar considerations relating to the use of CTG apply during the antepartum period for what concerns *baseline variability*. Accelerations are, as before labor, an expression of normality. Early decelerations are not usually a sign of fetal distress. They are likely generated by vagal stimulation due to cephalic compression and are more frequent after rupture of the membranes.

Variable decelerations are usually due to umbilical cord compression. They may occur in association with fetal distress due to hemodynamic changes. However, late decelerations are a typical expression of fetal hypoxia. Their timing and shape are directly correlated with the severity of fetal hypoxia: the time elapsing between the contraction and the deceleration is directly proportional to the fetal partial oxygen pressure.

Obviously, in the presence of both late decelerations and baseline abnormalities, the prognosis is more serious.

Interpretation of the cardiotocogram is more difficult during the *second stage* of labor. In this period only a severe and persistent bradycardia is considered of serious prognostic significance, especially when associated with abnormalities in variability.

If the CTG is normal during labor, intermittent auscultation may be appropriate. It is considered normal if the FHR is between 120 and 160 bpm. It is also suggested that monitoring should be undertaken for 20–30 min every 2 h during labor.

Continuous cardiotocography during labor is associated with a reduction in neonatal seizures, but no significant differences in cerebral palsy, infant mortality, or other standard measures of neonatal well-being. However, continuous cardiotocography was associated with an increase in cesarean sections and instrumental vaginal births (Alfirevic et al. 2013b; Larma et al. 2007). For this reason, continuous electronic fetal monitoring should be reserved for high-risk pregnancies (Table 6).

7.5.3 Monitoring of Fetal Oxygenation

7.5.3.1 Pulse Oximetry

Fetal pulse oximetry has been advocated as a means of improving the specificity of CTG in intrapartum fetal surveillance. Fetal pulse oximetry was introduced into clinical practice about 30 years ago, but it has only recently been possible to use it as an additional measure to evaluate fetal well-being. It was developed as a less traumatic and invasive method of assessing fetal oxygenation than fetal scalp sampling. It allows for the real-time and continuous assessment of the fetus (Klauser et al. 2005; East et al. 2006; Bloom et al. 2006; Kühnert and Schmidt 2004). It uses a probe that sits inside the vagina during labor. It is possible only if the membranes are ruptured because the probe has to be placed on fetal skin.

Table 6 High-risk pregnancies

Abnormalities on intermittent auscultation or at CTG monitoring at the beginning of the labor
Discolored amniotic fluid
Oxytocin infusion
Fever during labor
Other conditions of pathological labor

Fetal oxygen saturation decreases between the first and the second stages of labor (from 60% to 53%): a value of 30% is considered pathological. A fetal oxygen saturation of 30% for 10 min is associated with acidosis and a poor fetal outcome. Low values of fetal oxygen saturation are associated with an abnormal CTG trace (low variability).

There are still controversies about the benefits of fetal pulse oximetry. Some authors have concluded that fetal pulse oximetry during active labor provides a more accurate assessment of fetal well-being and may reduce the need for interventions. Conversely, a recent Cochrane review showed that the addition of fetal pulse oximetry does not reduce overall cesarean section rates, providing limited support for the use of fetal pulse oximetry when used in the presence of a non-reassuring CTG. A better method for the evaluation of fetal well-being in labor is required (East et al. 2014).

7.5.3.2 Fetal Scalp Blood Sampling

A sample of blood from the fetal scalp may be tested during labor to determine the acidity of the blood. This test is called fetal scalp blood sampling (FSBS). If the fetus is not getting enough oxygen, the blood becomes highly acidic.

Fetal blood sampling is typically performed using a kit. An amnioscope with a light source is used to expose the fetal scalp. The blood is collected in long, heparinized capillary tubes. The test requires that the cervix be dilated at least 2–3 cm and can be difficult to perform.

Capillary blood collected from the fetal scalp usually has a pH lower than umbilical venous blood and correlates well with fetal arterial values. However, scalp edema can result in erroneous results. A scalp pH value of less than 7.20 has traditionally been used to represent the critical value for identifying fetal acidosis (Table 7). However, a scalp pH below 7.15 is more representative of the tenth percentile and is closer to the threshold currently used in umbilical cord blood analysis to define fetal acidemia associated with neurological deficits (Jørgensen and Weber 2014). In addition, when further testing to assess fetal well-being in labor is indicated, fetal scalp blood lactate estimation is more likely to be successfully undertaken than pH estimation. The smaller volume of blood required for this test, compared with the more traditional pH estimation, may improve sampling rates (East et al. 2015).

The accuracy of intermittent fetal scalp pH assessment for predicting neonatal acidosis with subsequent neurologic sequelae has been questioned. It is no longer used in many institutions, although its use can result in fewer cesarean deliveries performed for the indication of non-reassuring fetal status. FSBS was advocated as an "additional test" of fetal well-being to reduce the false-positive rate of CTG. The aim was to identify the presence of acidosis to differentiate at least 60% of fetuses who were not hypoxic from 40% of fetuses who were experiencing intrapartum hypoxia when the CTG was classified as "pathological," in order to avoid unnecessary operative interventions.

However, the test has poor sensitivity and positive predictive value (PPV) for predicting umbilical arterial pH <7.0 (sensitivity 35%, PPV 9%). The test also has poor sensitivity and PPV for identifying newborns with hypoxic–ischemic encephalopathy (sensitivity 50%, PPV 3%) (Allen et al. 2004).

Table 7 Recommended fetal management according to the pH value obtained by fetal scalp blood sampling

pH value	Management
pH > 7.25	Repeat test if CTG continues to deteriorate
pH 7.21–7.24	Repeat test in 30 min
pH < 7.20	Aim for delivery within 30 min

Indeed, the degree of technical skill required, cost, need for continuous availability of standardized equipment and trained personnel, and maternal discomfort have precluded the use of this modality in many labor and delivery units. Therefore, fetal scalp blood sampling had a historical importance, but currently there is very limited scientific evidence to support its use in modern obstetric practice (Chandraharan 2014).

7.5.3.3 Fetal Electrocardiography

A technical system, the fetal heart monitor, monitors the fetal electrocardiogram (ECG) during labor, as a reflection of fetal myocardial metabolism and acid–base balance. It can be used as an adjunct to continuous electronic FHR monitoring during labor. The rationale is that fetal acidemia is associated with fetal ECG ST-segment elevation and increased T-wave amplitude. The monitor's software automatically identifies and analyzes changes in the T wave and the ST segment of the fetal ECG, which is obtained via a spiral electrode attached to the fetal scalp.

The fetal heart monitor was approved by the United States Food and Drug Administration as an adjunct to the assessment of non-reassuring FHR tracings in pregnancies over 36 weeks of gestation, in labor, with vertex presentation and ruptured fetal membranes. Initial FDA approval was based primarily on European studies that suggested that fetal ST-segment analysis technology reduced the rates of fetal scalp sampling procedures and operative deliveries, with a significant reduction of neonatal academia and encephalopathy (Ojala et al. 2006; Amer-Wåhlin et al. 2001). Thus, this technique appeared to improve the clinician's ability to discriminate between fetuses in need of intervention and those who can be managed expectantly.

However, a recent Cochrane review showed that the modest benefits of fewer fetal scalp samplings during labor have to be considered against the disadvantages of needing to use an internal scalp electrode, after membrane rupture (Neilson 2015). Indeed, a recent large randomized, controlled trial showed no significant benefit of the adjunctive use of ST-segment analysis in reducing a composite of neonatal outcomes or in reducing cesarean or operative vaginal deliveries in a population undergoing conventional intrapartum continuous electronic fetal heart rate monitoring (Belfort et al. 2015).

References

Alfirevic Z, Stampalija T, Gyte GM (2013a) Fetal and umbilical Doppler ultrasound in high-risk pregnancies. Cochrane Database Syst Rev 11, CD007529

Alfirevic Z, Devane D, Gyte GM (2013b) Continuous cardiotocography (CTG) as a form of electronic fetal monitoring (EFM) for fetal assessment during labour. Cochrane Database Syst Rev 31(5), CD006066

Alfirevic Z, Stampalija T, Medley N (2015) Fetal and umbilical Doppler ultrasound in normal pregnancy. Cochrane Database Syst Rev 4, CD001450

Allen RM, Bowling FG, Oats JJ (2004) Determining the fetal scalp lactate level that indicates the need for intervention in labour. Aust N Z J Obstet Gynaecol 44:549–552

American College of Obstetricians and Gynecologists (2009) ACOG Practice Bulletin No. 106. Intrapartum fetal heart rate monitoring: nomenclature, interpretation, and general management principles. Obstet Gynecol 114:192–202

American College of Obstetricians and Gynecologists (2010) ACOG Practice Bulletin No. 116. Management of intrapartum fetal heart rate tracings. Reaffirmed 2015 Obstet Gynecol 116:1232–1240

Amer-Wåhlin I, Hellsten C, Norén H et al (2001) Cardiotocography only versus cardiotocography plus ST analysis of fetal electrocardiogram for intrapartum fetal monitoring: a Swedish randomised controlled trial. Lancet 358:534–538

Baschat AA (2010) Ductus venosus Doppler for fetal surveillance in high-risk pregnancies. Clin Obstet Gynecol 53:858e68

Baschat AA (2011) Examination of the fetal cardiovascular system. Semin Fetal Neonatal Med 16:2–12

Baschat AA, Harman CR (2006) Venous Doppler in the assessment of fetal cardiovascular status. Curr Opin Obstet Gynecol 18:156–163

Baschat AA, Gembruch U, Weiner CP et al (2003) Qualitative venous Doppler waveform analysis improves prediction of critical perinatal outcomes in premature growth-restricted fetuses. Ultrasound Obstet Gynecol 22:240e5

Baschat AA, Galan HL, Bhide A et al (2006) Doppler and biophysical assessment in growth restricted fetuses: distribution of test results. Ultrasound Obstet Gynecol 27:41e7

Becker R, Vonk R (2010) Doppler sonography of uterine arteries at 20–23 weeks: depth of notch gives information on probability of adverse pregnancy outcome and degree of fetal growth restriction in a low-risk population. Fetal Diagn Ther 27:78–86

Belfort MA, Saade GR, Thom E et al (2015) A randomized trial of intrapartum fetal ECG ST-segment analysis. N Engl J Med 373:632–641

Berkley E, Chauhan SP, Abuhamad A (2012) Doppler assessment of the fetus with intrauterine growth restriction. Am J Obstet Gynecol 206:300e8

Bloom SL, Spong CY, Thom E et al (2006) Fetal pulse oximetry and cesarean delivery. N Engl J Med 355:2195–2202

Chandraharan E (2014) Fetal scalp blood sampling during labour: is it a useful diagnostic test or a historical test that no longer has a place in modern clinical obstetrics? BJOG 121:1056–1062

Chauhan SP, Taylor M, Shields D et al (2007) Intrauterine growth restriction and oligohydramnios among high-risk patients. Am J Perinatol 24:215–221

Cosmi E, Rampon M, Saccardi C et al (2012) Middle cerebral artery peak systolic velocity in the diagnosis of fetomaternal hemorrhage. Int J Gynaecol Obstet 117:128e30

Cunningham FG, Gant NF, Leveno KJ et al (2001) Williams obstetrics, 21st edn. McGraw-Hill, New York

Dawes GS, Moulden M, Redman CW (1995) Computerized analysis of antepartum fetal heart rate. Am J Obstet Gynecol 173:1353–1354

Dawes GS, Moulden M, Redman CW (1996) Improvements in computerized fetal heart rate analysis antepartum. J Perinat Med 24:25–36

DeVore GR (2015) The importance of the cerebroplacental ratio in the evaluation of fetal well-being in SGA and AGA fetuses. Am J Obstet Gynecol 213:5–15

East CE, Brennecke SP, King JF et al (2006) The effect of intrapartum fetal pulse oximetry in the presence of a nonreassuring fetal heart pattern on operative delivery rates: a multicenter randomized controlled trial (the FOREMOST trial). Am J Obstet Gynecol 194:606.e1–606.e16

East CE, Begg L, Colditz PB et al (2014) Fetal pulse oximetry for fetal assessment in labour. Cochrane Database Syst Rev 10, CD004075

East CE, Leader LR, Sheehan P et al (2015) Intrapartum fetal scalp lactate sampling for fetal assessment in the presence of a non-reassuring fetal heart rate trace. Cochrane Database Syst Rev 5, CD006174

Everett TR, Peebles DM (2015) Antenatal tests of fetal wellbeing. Semin Fetal Neonatal Med 20:138–143

Ferrazzi E, Bozzo M, Rigano S et al (2002) Temporal sequence of abnormal Doppler changes in the peripheral and central circulatory systems of the severely growth-restricted fetus. Ultrasound Obstet Gynecol 19:140–146

Figueras F, Savchev S, Triunfo S et al (2015) An integrated model with classification criteria to predict small-for-gestational-age fetuses at risk of adverse perinatal outcome. Ultrasound Obstet Gynecol 45: 279–285

Gerber S, Hohlfeld P, Viquerat F et al (2006) Intrauterine growth restriction and absent or reverse end-diastolic blood flow in umbilical artery (Doppler class II or III): a retrospective study of short-and long-term fetal morbidity and mortality. Eur J Obstet Gynecol Reprod Biol 126:20–26

Grivell RM, Alfirevic Z, Gyte GM et al (2015) Antenatal cardiotocography for fetal assessment. Cochrane Database Syst Rev 9, CD007863

Hebbar S, Rai L, Adiga P et al (2015) Reference ranges of amniotic fluid index in late third trimester of pregnancy: what should the optimal interval between two ultrasound examinations be? J Pregnancy 2015:319204

Hutter D, Kingdom J, Jaeggi E (2010) Causes and mechanisms of intrauterine hypoxia and its impact on the fetal cardiovascular system: a review. Int J Pediatr 2010:401323

Jørgensen JS, Weber T (2014) Fetal scalp blood sampling in labor – a review. Acta Obstet Gynecol Scand 93:548–555

Khalil AA, Morales Rosello J, Morlando M et al (2014) Is fetal cerebroplacental ratio an independent predictor of intrapartum fetal compromise and neonatal unit admission? Am J Obstet Gynecol 213(54):e1–e10

Kingdom JCP, Kaufmann P (1997) Oxygen and placental villous development: origins of fetal hypoxia. Placenta 18:613–621

Kingdom J, Huppertz B, Seaward G, Kaufmann P (2000) Development of the placental villous tree and its consequences for fetal growth. Eur J Obstet Gynecol Reprod Biol 92:35–43

Klauser CK, Christensen EE, Chauhan SP et al (2005) Use of fetal pulse oximetry among high-risk women in labor: a randomized control trial. Am J Obstet Gynecol 192:1810–1817

Kühnert M, Schmidt S (2004) Intrapartum management of nonreassuring fetal heart rate patterns: a randomized controlled trial of fetal pulse oximetry. Am J Obstet Gynecol 191:1989–1995

Lalor JG, Fawole B, Alfirevic Z et al (2008) Biophysical profile for fetal assessment in high risk pregnancies. Cochrane Database Syst Rev 23, CD000038

Lalor JG, Fawole B, Alfirevic Z et al (2012) Biophysical profile for fetal assessment in high risk pregnancies. Wiley, Chichester

Larma JD, Silva AM, Holcroft CJ et al (2007) Intrapartum electronic fetal heart rate monitoring and the identification of metabolic acidosis and hypoxic-ischemic encephalopathy. Am J Obstet Gynecol 197:301.e1–301.e8

Lees C, Marlow N, Arabin B, TRUFFLE Group et al (2013) Perinatal morbidity and mortality in early-onset fetal growth restriction: cohort outcomes of the trial of randomized umbilical and fetal flow in Europe (TRUFFLE). Ultrasound Obstet Gynecol 42:400–408

Lees CC, Marlow N, van Wassenaer-Leemhuis A, TRUFFLE Study Group et al (2015) Two year neurodevelopmental and intermediate perinatal outcomes in infants with very preterm fetal growth restriction (TRUFFLE): a randomised trial. Lancet 385:2162–2172

Leung TY, Lao TT (2012) Timing of caesarean section according to urgency. Best Pract Res Clin Obstet Gynaecol 27:251–267

Manning FA (1999) Fetal biophysical profile. Obstet Gynecol Clin North Am 26:557–577

Manning FA (2009) Antepartum fetal testing: a critical appraisal. Curr Opin Obstet Gynecol 21:348–352

Mari G (2005) Middle cerebral artery peak systolic velocity: is it the standard of care for the diagnosis of fetal anemia? J Ultrasound Med 24:697–702

Mari G, Hanif F, Kruger M et al (2007) Middle cerebral artery peak systolic velocity: a new Doppler parameter in the assessment of growth-restricted fetuses. Ultrasound Obstet Gynecol 29:310–316

Martin CB Jr (2008) Normal fetal physiology and behavior, and adaptive responses in the fetus with hypoxemia. Semin Perinatol 32:239e42

Morales-Rosello J, Khalil A, Morlando M et al (2015) Poor neonatal acid-base status in term fetuses with low cerebroplacental ratio. Ultrasound Obstet Gynecol 45:156e61

Morris RK, Malin G, Robson SC, Kleijnen J et al (2011) Fetal umbilical artery Doppler to predict compromise of fetal/neonatal wellbeing in a high risk population: systematic review and bivariate meta-analysis. Ultrasound Obstet Gynecol 37:135e42

Morris RK, Say R, Robson SC et al (2012) Systematic review and meta-analysis of middle cerebral artery Doppler to predict perinatal wellbeing. Eur J Obstet Gynecol Reprod Biol 165:141e55

Morris RK, Meller CH, Tamblyn J et al (2014) Association and prediction of amniotic fluid measurements for adverse pregnancy outcome: systematic review and meta-analysis. BJOG 121:686–699

Neilson JP (2015) Fetal electrocardiogram (ECG) for fetal monitoring during labour. Cochrane Database Syst Rev 21(12), CD000116

O'Gorman N, Tampakoudis G, Wright A et al (2016) Uterine artery pulsutility index at 12, 22, 32 and 36 weeks' gestation in screening for preeclampsia. Ultrasound Obstet Gynecol 47:565–572

Ojala K, Vääräsmäki M, Mäkikallio K et al (2006) A comparison of intrapartum automated fetal electrocardiography and conventional cardiotocography: a randomised controlled study. BJOG 113:419–423

Omo-Aghoja L (2014) Maternal and fetal acid–base chemistry: a major determinant of perinatal outcome. Ann Med Health Sci Res 4:8–17

Ott WJ (2005) Reevaluation of the relationship between amniotic fluid volume and perinatal outcome. Am J Obstet Gynecol 192:1803–1809

Pinas A, Chandraharan E (2016) Continuous cardiotocography during labour: analysis, classification and management. Best Pract Res Clin Obstet Gynaecol 30:33–47

Pipkin FB (1999) Fetal growth and physiology. In: Edmonds KD (ed) Dewhurst's textbook of obstetrics and gynecology for postgraduates, 6th edn. Blackwell Science, Oxford, pp 104–112

Prior T, Mullins E, Bennett P et al (2013) Prediction of intrapartum fetal compromise using the cerebroumbilical ratio: a prospective observational study. Am J Obstet Gynecol 208:124.e1–124.e6

Prior T, Paramasivam G, Bennett P et al (2015) Are fetuses that fail to achieve their growth potential at increased risk of intrapartum compromise? Ultrasound Obstet Gynecol 46:460–464

Pruetz JD, Votava-Smith J, Miller DA (2015) Clinical relevance of fetal hemodynamic monitoring: perinatal implications. Semin Fetal Neonatal Med 20:217–224

Regnault TR, de Vrijer B, Galan HL et al (2007) Development and mechanisms of fetal hypoxia in severe fetal growth restriction. Placenta 28:714–723

Savasan ZA, Goncalves LF, Bahado-Singh RO (2014) Second- and third-trimester biochemical and ultrasound markers predictive of ischemic placental disease. Semin Perinatol 38:167–176

Severi FM, Rizzo G, Bocchi C et al (2000) Intrauterine growth retardation and fetal cardiac function. Fetal Diagn Ther 15:8–19

Severi FM, Bocchi C, Visentin A et al (2002) Uterine and fetal cerebral Doppler predict the outcome of third-trimester small-for-gestational age fetuses with normal umbilical artery Doppler. Ultrasound Obstet Gynecol 19:225–228

Seyam YS, Al-Mahmeid MS, Al-Tamimi HK (2002) Umbilical artery Doppler flow velocimetry in intrauterine growth restriction and its relation to perinatal outcome. Int J Gynecol Obstet 77:131–137

Soregaroli M, Bonera R, Danti L et al (2002) Prognostic role of umbilical artery Doppler velocimetry in growth-restricted fetuses. J Matern Fetal Neonatal Med 11:199–203

Thompson JL, Kuller JA, Rhee EH (2012) Antenatal surveillance of fetal growth restriction. Obstet Gynecol Surv 67:554e65

Thornton JG, Hornbuckle J, Vail A, GRIT Study Group et al (2004) Infant wellbeing at 2 years of age in the Growth Restriction Intervention Trial (GRIT): multicentred randomised controlled trial. Lancet 364:513–520

Turan S, Turan OM, Berg C et al (2007) Computerized fetal heart rate analysis, Doppler ultrasound and biophysical profile score in the prediction of acid-base status of growth-restricted fetuses. Ultrasound Obstet Gynecol 30:750e6

Valiño N, Giunta G, Gallo DM et al (2016) Uterine artery pulsatility index at 30–34 weeks' gestation in the prediction of adverse perinatal outcome. Ultrasound Obstet Gynecol 47:308–315

Weiner E, Bar J, Fainstein N et al (2015) Intraoperative findings, placental assessment and neonatal outcome in emergent cesarean deliveries for non-reassuring fetal heart rate. Eur J Obstet Gynecol Reprod Biol 185:103–107

In Vitro Fertilization and Multiple Pregnancies

8

Maria Angela Rustico, Mariano Lanna, and Enrico Ferrazzi

Contents

M. A. Rustico · M. Lanna · E. Ferrazzi (✉)
Prenatal Diagnosis and Fetal Surgery Unit, Dept. of Woman, Mother and Neonate, Buzzi Children's Hospital Department of Clinical Sciences, University of Milan, Milan, Italy
e-mail: enrico.ferrazzi@unimi.it

G. Buonocore et al. (eds.), *Neonatology*,
https://doi.org/10.1007/978-3-319-29489-6_157

Abstract

Multiple pregnancies may arise because of modified reproductive strategies (i.e., delayed parenthood) and the availability of assisted reproductive technologies. Dizygotic twinning rate is affected by different factors (race, genetic factors, seasonality, maternal age and parity, endogenous gonadotropins, fertility drugs, and sex of the embryo), while monozygotic twinning is largely determined by genetic mechanisms. Ultrasound techniques are very accurate (100% sensitivity and 99% specificity) for determining chorionicity and assessing the obstetric risk which is significantly different in dichorionic and monochorionic twins. The twin pregnancy is associated with an increased rate of fetal complications, such as miscarriage and fetal loss, intrauterine growth restriction (IUGR), and preterm birth. Twins present with an excess of structural anomalies compared to singletons. All monochorionic twin pregnancies are at risk of complications such as twin-twin transfusion syndrome, selective IUGR, and twin anemia-polycythemia sequence because of the presence of vascular anastomoses between the circulation of both twins on the shared placenta. The death of one twin, which occurs in about 6% of all MC twin pregnancies, puts the co-twin at greater risk of mortality and morbidity.

8.1 Salient Points

- Multiple pregnancies arise more frequently because of modified reproductive strategies and the availability of assisted reproductive technologies.
- The dizygotic twinning rate is affected by different factors (race, genetic factors, seasonality, maternal age and parity, endogenous gonadotropins, fertility drugs, and sex of the embryo), while monozygotic twinning is largely determined by genetic mechanisms.
- Ultrasound techniques are very accurate in determining chorionicity and assessing the obstetric risk which is significantly different in dichorionic and monochorionic twins.
- Twin pregnancy is always risky for the increased rate of fetal complications and structural anomalies compared to singletons. A monochorionic twin pregnancy may be complicated by twin-twin transfusion syndrome, selective IUGR, and twin anemia-polycythemia sequence.
- The death of one twin, which occurs in about 6% of all MC twin pregnancies, puts the co-twin at greater risk of mortality and morbidity.

8.2 Epidemiology of Natural Twinning

8.2.1 Actual Trend

The cultural modifications in women's reproductive strategies over the past 50 years have drastically influenced the demographic scenario. Higher levels of education and a desire for economic and social success, as well as difficulties in finding a permanent job, have played a major role in modifying the reproductive strategies, as evidenced by delayed parenthood and the reduction in family size (Astolfi et al. 2003). In addition to this expected twinning rate due to advancing maternal age, there is also evidence that natural twinning has increased in women who have been exposed to assisted reproduction technologies (Bortolus et al. 1999).

8.2.2 Dizygotic Twinning

In humans, multiple pregnancies arise more frequently from fertilization of two separate oocytes (1.2% of pregnancies). The incidence of excessive follicular recruitment is more or less 31% in mothers of dizygotic (DZ) twins. The DZ twinning rate is affected by race, genetic factors, seasonality, maternal age and parity, endogenous gonadotropins, fertility drugs, and sex of the embryo (ESHRE Capri Workshop Group 2000). The incidence of twin pregnancy also varies from country to country, the highest rates being reported in Nigeria (5%) and the lowest in Japan. In Italy the best estimate of DZ twinning is 1%. It has been suggested that genetic predisposition and malnutrition may play a role in this different frequency. Maternal age up to 35–39 years is linked with increasing twinning rates, and this pattern has been attributed to the rise in the level of gonadotropins with age (Bortolus et al. 1999). There is a slight tendency for twins to have been conceived during summer as compared with singletons; and this may reflect the effect of increased light during summer on the pineal gland, resulting in melatonin production, and consequent decreased inhibition of pituitary follicle-stimulating hormone (FSH) release (ESHRE Capri Workshop Group 2000).

8.2.3 Monozygotic Twinning

The constant frequency of monozygotic (MZ) pregnancies over time and in different areas, and the lack of association between maternal age and frequency of MZ twinning, suggests that MZ twins are largely determined by genetic mechanisms. In fact an excess of monozygotic twins occurs in mothers who are themselves one of monozygotic twins, whereas there is no evidence for a paternal effect on MZ twinning (Bortolus et al. 1999).

8.3 Epidemiology of Iatrogenic Twinning

There have always been some naturally, or spontaneously, occurring multiple pregnancies (with twins being more frequent than triplets, and quadruplets or even higher multiples being much rarer). However, the frequency has increased enormously since assisted reproductive technologies (ART) have become available. Because of the higher morbidity and mortality associated with twins and particularly triplets, every effort should be made to reduce the incidence (ESHRE Capri Workshop Group 2000). In Europe, the overall rate of multiple pregnancy in 2002 was 23% compared to 26% in 2000. This reduction has been determined by the transfer of fewer embryos, except in Italy where a controversial law obliged the transfer of three embryos until it was recently modified. A similar high prevalence of twinning in ART pregnancies was reported in 2006 in the USA (26%), where such a policy had not been universally adopted. In the USA, the proportion of multiple births attributable to ovulation induction or ART is 33%. In triplets and higher-order multiple pregnancies this rate must be even higher.

8.4 Placentation

8.4.1 Chorionicity and Zygosity

Two thirds of spontaneous twin pregnancies are dizygotic (DZ), resulting from the fertilization of two eggs by different spermatozoa, and are therefore dichorionic (DC). The DC twin placenta of DZ twins may be composed of separate disks or, alternatively, the two placental portions may be fused. Vascular communications are almost totally absent. The other third of spontaneous twin pregnancies are monozygotic (MZ), occurring when one single fertilized egg gives rise to two separate embryos. Of these MZ pregnancies, a third are DC. The other two thirds are monochorionic diamniotic (MCDA), meaning that a single placenta serves both embryos and that vascular communications connecting the twins are always present. Between 2% and 5% of monochorionic (MC) twins are monoamniotic (MCMA).

When twinning occurs after approximately 12 days from conception Siamese twins are generated.

Because of their placental angioarchitecture (Fig. 1), MC twins are more susceptible to additional complications than DC twins. In fact, the presence of vascular anastomoses, which mediates unidirectional or bidirectional flow between the two circulations, greatly influences intrauterine

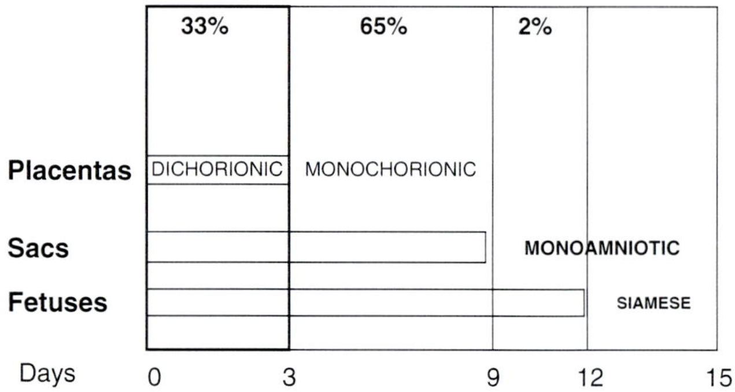

Fig. 1 Partition of placentas and chorion, amniotic sac, and fetuses as a function from days of conception in monozygotic twinning

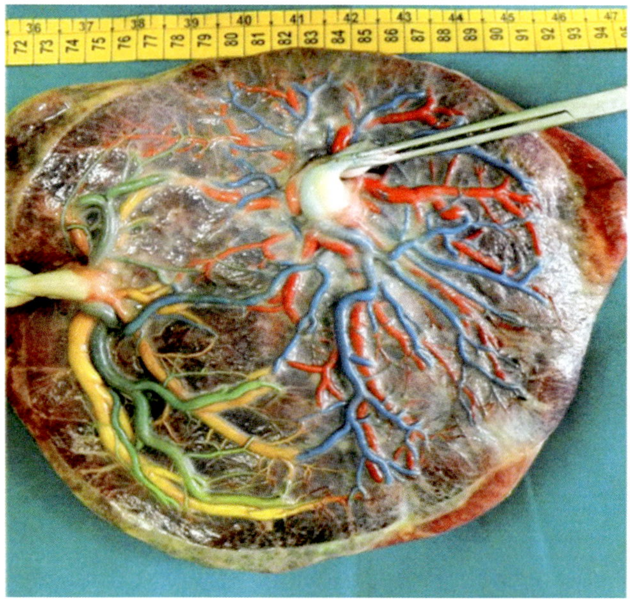

Fig. 2 Monochorionic placenta

development and plays a crucial role in causing those complications specific to MC twins, leading to a higher morbidity and mortality than in DC twins (Benirschke and Kaufmann 2000).

8.4.2 Monochorionic Placenta

In multiple pregnancies, ultrasound is a very accurate technique (100% sensitivity and 99% specificity) for determining chorionicity (Fig. 2). In twin pregnancies, in the first or early second trimester, ultrasound examination is mandatory to determine chorionicity in order to assess the obstetric risk which is significantly different in DC and MC twins (Fig. 3).

8.5 Fetal Complications of Twin Pregnancy

8.5.1 Miscarriage and Fetal Loss

8.5.1.1 Definitions

The World Health Organization in 2008 reported a consensus on definitions concerning miscarriage and fetal loss. Preclinical spontaneous miscarriage: a pregnancy diagnosed only by the detection of HCG in serum or urine, which does not develop into a clinical pregnancy. Spontaneous abortion/miscarriage: the spontaneous loss of a clinical pregnancy as diagnosed by ultrasound that occurs before 20 completed weeks of gestational age (18 weeks postfertilization) or, if

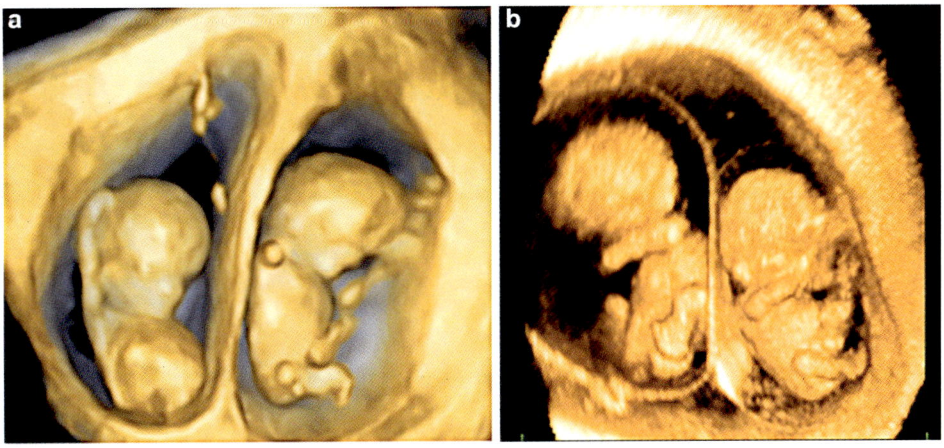

Fig. 3 (**a**) Dichorionic twins (*lambda sign*): chorion and decidua between the two sacs. (**b**) Monochorionic twins (T sign), only extraembryonic coelom between the two amniotic membranes

gestational age is unknown, the loss of an embryo/fetus of less than 400 g. Vanishing sac(s) or embryo(s): spontaneous disappearance of one or more gestational sacs or embryos in an ongoing pregnancy, documented by ultrasound.

8.5.1.2 Epidemiology

The "vanishing twin" phenomenon, which has been viewed as part of the general fetal wastage in human reproduction, suggests that while multiple conceptions are not rare events, multiple pregnancies are strongly selected against, especially during the early stages of embryonic development. The incidence of miscarriage during the first trimester is estimated to be between 10% and 20%. The true incidence of vanishing twins is difficult to assess. Landy and Keith (Landy and Neith 1998) reviewed the majority of pertinent studies, most of which described pregnancies conceived as a result of ART. Using these data, it was estimated that ~30% of these twins will ultimately result in singletons and <10% will end in a complete abortion.

8.5.1.3 Etiology

It is thought that intrinsic abnormalities within the embryo are the major reasons for failed conceptions or early fetal death. The most significant intrinsic factor contributing to embryonic loss is aberrations in the first meiotic division resulting in nondysjunction and aneuploidy. Trisomies 13, 15, 16, 18, and 21 account for the most common autosomal trisomies in spontaneous pregnancy losses. Some authors have observed an increased risk of fetal death, and in particular spontaneous abortion with increasing maternal age, and there is clear evidence from oocyte donation programs that this risk is associated with the aging of the oocytes (Andersen et al. 2005).

8.5.1.4 Diagnosis

The diagnosis of miscarriage is made by ultrasound (US) examination. A biochemical pregnancy is considered when implantation is revealed on day 16 by blood test, but there is a negative US scan result on day 23 (Simón et al. 1999).

8.5.2 Fetal Growth Restriction

8.5.2.1 Definition

Intrauterine growth restriction (IUGR) is a sonographic diagnosis consisting of either an estimated fetal weight below the 5th percentile of the intrauterine growth chart for gestational age, or declining abdominal fetal growth below the 5th percentile, or declining more than 40 centiles from midpregnancy to third trimester. Abnormal uterine Doppler velocimetry and/or an abnormal umbilical Doppler velocimetry are considered additional criteria of severity (Italian Society of Ultrasound in

Obstetrics and Gynecology). In a twin pregnancy, a growth discordance of more than 20% in estimated fetal weight is an index of selective growth restriction.

8.5.2.2 Epidemiology

Neonates from multiple gestations are overrepresented among preterm and low birth weight infants. Multiple pregnancies weigh less than their singleton counterparts. The prevalence of small for gestational age newborns in multiple pregnancy is higher than expected in singletons. Although many variables may influence the reference standard, the prevalence of small for gestational fetuses varies between 12% and 47%.

8.5.2.3 Etiology

For most of a pregnancy, twins grow at the same rate as singletons, regardless of chorionicity, up to at least 32 weeks' gestation. Thereafter, twins show a slower rate of growth (Kingdom et al. 2005). The decreased rate may be related to uteroplacental insufficiency. It is thought that, at some point in the third trimester, the placenta can no longer maintain the nutrient requirement of both fetuses. In patients with triplets or high-order multiples, this process occurs earlier.

When growth restricted fetuses are diagnosed in a twin pregnancy, one should keep in mind the diverse etiologies of IUGR (such as genetic/chromosomal problems, fetal anatomical anomalies, placental and cord abnormalities, maternal complications) rather than assuming that the cause is uteroplacental insufficiency, which is more frequent in twins than singletons. Although IUGR can complicate a pregnancy with growth discordance, the latter does not necessarily imply the former unless growth discordance is less than 20%. It is important to note that IUGR can affect both twins, leading to both twins being small but not discordant.

8.5.2.4 Diagnosis

Knowledge of chorionicity assessed during the first trimester or by gender discordance is paramount for managing patients with growth abnormalities. Since fetal growth is a dynamic process, serial ultrasound is helpful in the assessment of fetal growth in patients with multiple fetuses. In utero growth discordance is most often defined as the difference in sonographic estimated fetal weights expressed as a percentage of the larger twin's estimated fetal weight. Growth discrepancy may be mild (<15%), moderate (15–30%), or severe (>30%). This wide range (from 15% to 30%) is the consequence of clinical neonatal examination. It might help to note that a study by Naeye (Naeye and Letts 1964) in 1964 showed that the total number of organs and cells is not reduced until growth discrepancy is more than 25%. However, in less severe cases, weight discrepancy is determined by a smaller volume of cell cytoplasm. A clinical diagnosis of growth discordance is better achieved by adding information about fetoplacental conditions to biometric growth curves: for example, amniotic fluid index, Doppler examination of the umbilical artery and fetal vessels, computerized analysis of fetal heart rate, maternal complications that frequently cause placental insufficiency such as gestational hypertension and preeclampsia.

8.5.2.5 Consequences

IUGR has long been known to be associated with perinatal morbidity and mortality. Neonatal morbidity such as meconium aspiration syndrome, hypoglycemia, polycythemia, and pulmonary hemorrhage may affect up to 50% of IUGR neonates. The high prevalence of IUGR in twin pregnancies suggests that such patients should be included in protocols relating to the management of high-risk pregnancies.

8.6 Preterm Delivery

8.6.1 Definition

Preterm birth (PTB) is defined as a delivery at less than 37 completed weeks' gestation. This condition can be further divided into late preterm (33–37 weeks), moderate preterm (28–32 weeks), and severe preterm (20–27 weeks).

8.6.2 Epidemiology

There is a wide variation in preterm birth rates between countries, mostly because of different iatrogenic practices. In many states of the European Union, about half the children born following multiple births were preterm, accounting for between 18% and 25% of preterm birth in each country. The proportion of births before 37 weeks in twins ranges from 68.4% in Austria to 42.2% in the Republic of Ireland. This reflects different clinical protocols and the consideration of twin pregnancies being at high risk and providing parents with leave from work and other social maternal benefits.

8.6.3 Etiology

The etiology of preterm birth depends on multiple factors. The most investigated etiologies both in singletons and twins are infection and maternal stress. Twin pregnancy with its impact on cervical integrity is per se a risk factor for ascending infections. Twin pregnancy is also a risk factor for psychological and physical maternal stress. Other minor risk factors for preterm birth are: cervical incontinence, uterine malformations, infertility, previous preterm birth or intrauterine fetal death, low social status, and male fetal sex.

8.6.4 Diagnosis

High risk for PTB should induce clinicians to make a careful assessment of risk factors and to use appropriate diagnostic tests. Among these the evaluation of short cervical length by transvaginal sonography seems to be the best predictor of PTB. Infection and other possible direct causes of PTB should be excluded. Fetal fibronectin in vaginal secretions may add to the usefulness of cervical length measurements. A cervical length $\leq$25 mm at 18 weeks and $\leq$22 mm at 24 weeks seems the best predictors of preterm delivery.

8.6.5 Prevention

Cervical length measurement, the fibronectin test, and the assessment of uterine contractions might diagnose impending PTB but should not be confused with the cause of PTB. Efforts should be made to exclude intrauterine infections and subclinical chorioamnionitis. Blood and amniotic tests for infections and abnormalities of fetal heart rate should be taken into account. Tocolysis with Atosiban and bed rest may delay delivery by at least 48 h, permitting the administration of corticosteroids to improve fetal lung maturity. In cases of severe infection, delivery may well be the best option combined with antibiotic therapy. Opinions about cervical cerclage vary.

8.6.6 Fetal Complications

Prematurity is the main cause of low birth weight, perinatal mortality, and the most frequent determinant of neonatal and infant mortality and morbidity. The following diseases are frequently associated with prematurity: transient tachypnea of the newborn, respiratory distress syndrome, persistent pulmonary hypertension, respiratory failure, temperature instability, jaundice, feeding difficulties, intraventricular hemorrhage, necrotizing enterocolitis, and brain damage.

8.7 Monochorionic-Related Complications

A characteristic of all monochorionic twin pregnancy is the presence of vascular anastomoses between the circulation of both twins on the shared placenta (Benirschke 1995).

Three types of anastomoses are identifiable: two superficial ones, artero-arterial anastomoses (AAA) and veno-venous anastomoses (VVA), which mediate a bidirectional blood flow, and those that go deep in the cotyledon, artero-venous anastomoses (AVA), which allow unidirectional flow (Fig. 2).

The difference in type, position, and size of these anastomoses and the proportion of extension of each vascular territory contributes to bringing about certain complications typical of monochorionic twin pregnancies, including twin-twin transfusion syndrome (TTTS), selective intrauterine growth restriction (sIUGR), and twin anemia-polycythemia sequence (TAPS) (Lanna et al. 2015).

8.7.1 Twin-to-Twin Transfusion Syndrome

TTTS is the best-known complication of MC pregnancies, occurring in approximately 10% of cases (Lewi et al. 2008). Although hormonal and hemodynamic mechanisms may be involved, the current interpretation of TTTS is that it is caused by an imbalance in the blood exchange between one twin (the donor) and the other (the recipient) via placental anastomoses, due to a relative excess of unidirectional arterio-venous connections not compensated by reverse flow through other anastomoses. When a significant imbalance in blood flow occurs, the donor twin becomes hypovolemic and oliguric, develops severe oligohydramnios and Doppler signs of placental insufficiency. The recipient twin shows hypervolemia, polyuria, and polyhydramnios, with cardiac overload, leading in severe cases to hydrops (Galea et al. 2008). Without treatment, the prognosis is poor, with perinatal mortality as high as 90%. In survivors, preterm birth due to polyhydramnios is a major cause of mortality and morbidity. At 4 years follow-up, the incidence of cerebral palsy and abnormal neurologic development is 21% in surviving twins with TTTS (Lopriore et al. 2003).

The traditional neonatal criteria for diagnosing TTTS, based on an inter-twin hemoglobin difference (>5 g/100 mL) and weight discordance (>20%), do not apply in utero because similar discrepancies in hemoglobin and birthweight are also found in DC and in MC twins complicated by sIUGR and TAPS, without TTTS (Denbow et al. 1998).

The diagnosis of TTTS is only made by ultrasound (Fig. 4). In a twin pregnancy with a single placental mass, twins of the same gender, and a thin membrane dividing the twins, the crucial ultrasound sign for the diagnosis of TTTS is the combined presence of polyuric polyhydramnios in one sac (deepest vertical pocket >8 cm before 20 weeks' gestation, >10 cm after 20 weeks' gestation) and oligouric oligohydramnios in the other (deepest vertical pocket <2 cm) (Fig. 2) (Senat et al. 2004). TTTS is classified into five stages using the Quintero staging system, based on ultrasound criteria. Stages I or II are when the donor bladder is still either visible or empty, in association with the polyhydramnios-oligohydramnios sequence. Stage III is when Doppler findings are abnormal for either twin, while Stage IV and V are when there is congestive cardiac failure and hydrops in the recipient or the death of one or both twins (Quintero et al. 1999).

Considering the poor survival rate and the risk of neurological complications due to antenatal or postnatal injury, treatment should be offered in all cases.

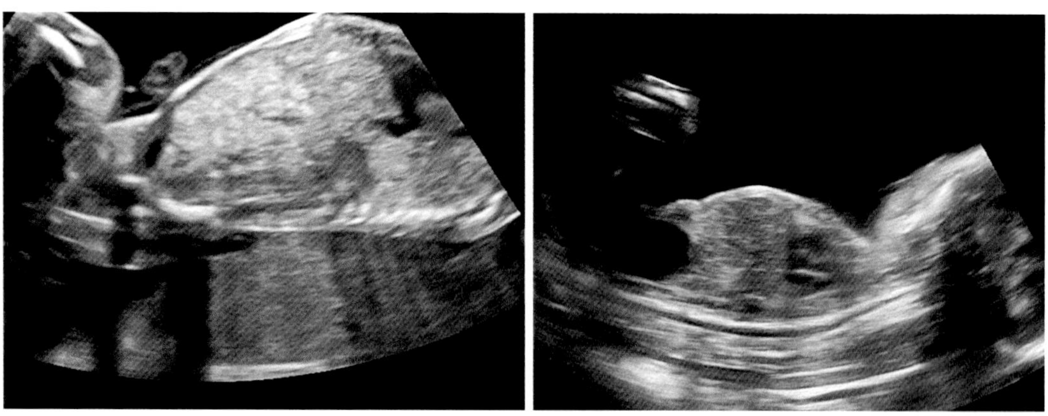

Fig. 4 Ultrasonographic evidence of TTTS: *on the left* the donor twin with anydramnios; *on the right* the recipient twin with polyhydramnios

In the past, the most common treatment for TTTS was serial amnioreduction (AR), which works by reducing the risk of preterm delivery secondary to uterine distension and possibly also by reopening compensatory placental vascular anastomoses. For MC twin pregnancies complicated by TTTS before 28 weeks, the International Amnioreduction Registry reported an overall survival rate at birth of 78%. In survivors, a central nervous system scan was abnormal in 25% of cases at 1 month of life (Mari et al. 2001).

In more recent years, endoscopic laser coagulation of the placental anastomoses, a procedure first described by De Lia in 1995, has been adopted as an effective treatment for TTTS because it severs the vascular connections which are thought to be responsible for the syndrome.

The Eurofetus randomized trial Senat et al. (2004) compared serial amnioreduction with laser coagulation and demonstrated that laser coagulation is the best first-line treatment for TTTS diagnosed before 26 weeks, with a better neurological outcome than serial amniotic reduction. The rate of periventricular leukomalacia in the laser group was 6% versus 14% in the AR group ($p = 0.002$).

8.7.1.1 Laser Treatment in Twin-to-Twin Transfusion Syndrome

This procedure is performed with fetoscopy under local anesthesia. A 3 mm cannula is introduced in the amniotic sac of the recipient twin under ultrasound guidance using a percutaneous approach. A 2 mm fiberscope is then passed through the cannula, so that the operator can explore the fetal surface of the placenta to identify the vascular connections and perform coagulation with a 400 μm laser fiber.

Two ways of performing the procedure have been compared: the nonselective technique, that requires coagulation of all vessels crossing the insertion of the inter-twin membrane, and the selective technique, that interrupts only those vessels involved in blood exchange between twins. The selective technique has proved to have a better outcome in terms of at least one survivor (Quintero et al. 2000).

Emerging evidence that the fetal complications (recurrence of TTTS and anemia – polycithemia sequence (TAPS)) occurring after selective or nonselective laser treatment were related to the persistence of residual small anastomoses found in almost 20% of treated placentas (Lewi et al. 2006) led to a new approach named the Solomon technique. Taking inspiration from the story of King Solomon, this procedure involves the coagulation of the entire territory between any anastomoses identified with the selective procedure, with the aim of obtaining complete dichorionization of the placenta (Fig. 5). The Solomon randomized trial (Slaghekke et al. 2014a) compared the two surgical approaches, selective and Solomon technique, and demonstrated better outcomes with the latter (Table 1).

Improvement of skills and technique lead to a better perinatal outcome. In our own experience, perinatal survival has improved from 52% (first 150 cases (Rustico et al. 2012) to 65.1% in the last 205 pregnancies treated, with a higher survival rate after the introduction of Solomon technique (77%).

Postnatal complications have been described both in ex-recipient and in ex-donor twin after laser therapy. The recipient twin, which is

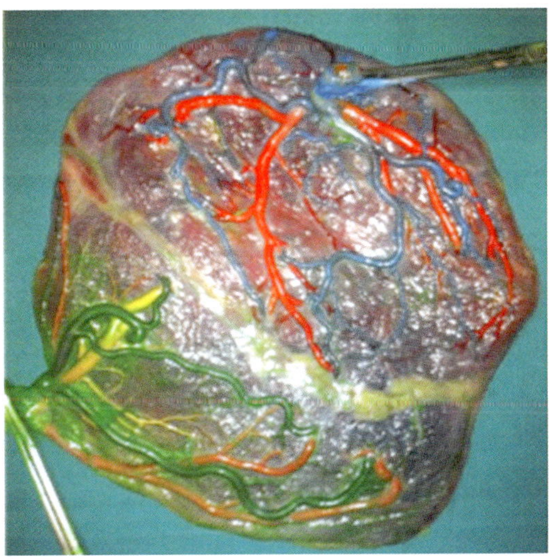

Fig. 5 Monochorionic placenta after laser coagulation of vascular anastomoses by Solomon technique. The complete dicorionization is evidenced by color dye injection of the vascular territories

Table 1 Comparison of different series consisting of more than 100 endoscopic laser coagulations of placental vessels, performed using different techniques

First author	N. cases	Median GA (weeks) at procedure	Median GA (weeks) at delivery	Overall survival rate (%)	Survivors (%)			
					2	1	≥1	0
Hecher et al. (2000)	127	20	34	68	54	27	81	19
Robyr et al. (2006)	101	21	32.1	76	66	22	88	12
Huber et al. (2006)	200	20	34.3	71	59	24	83	17
Quintero et al. (2000)	193	20	33.7	77	65	23	88	12
Middeldorp et al. (2007)	100	21	33	69	58	23	81	19
Stirnemann et al. (2008)	287	20	32.4	38	42	33	75	25
Cincotta et al. (2009)	100	21	31	75	66	19	85	15
Morris et al. (2010)	164	20.4	33.2	62	38	43	85	15
Rustico et al. (2012)	150	20.6	32.1	52	33	39	72	28
Valsky et al. (2012)	334	16–26 vs. >26	33	79	68	22	90	10
Baud et al. (2013)	325	>16 vs. >26	31	72	63	24	87	13
Baschat et al. (2013)	147	20	31.3	74	60	28	88	12
Ruano et al. (2013)	102	20	32	63	65	15	80	20
Slaghekke et al. (2014a)	272	20	32	73	62	23	85	15

hypervolemic, may develop right-heart hypertrophy with a tricuspid valve regurgitation leading to valvular pulmonary stenosis. This cardiac abnormality may persist after successful laser treatment because myocardial tissue may have been already damaged by persistent overload. In selected cases, pulmonary stenosis may be so severe that balloon valvuloplasty is required after birth (Stagnati et al. 2015). Similarly, severe hypovolemia may cause renal insufficiency. In this case, laser treatment can preserve kidney function in the surviving twin by establishing a normal circulating volume.

For both twins, neonatal morbidity is mainly related to neurological outcome. Most cerebral lesions result from hemorrhagic or ischemic injury. These lesions, which affect 10% of survivors after laser, are related to unbalanced blood flow and may occur before laser treatment of TTTS. Cerebral palsy affects nearly 6% of twins after laser; the risk of neurodevelopment impairment increases significantly with prematurity (van Klink et al. 2013). Neurological outcome worsens when laser treatment is performed at advanced gestational age and with a III/IV Quintero stage of TTTS.

8.7.2 Twin Anemia-Polycythemia Sequence (TAPS)

Postnatal evidence of significant hemoglobin discordance in some monochorionic twins at birth, in

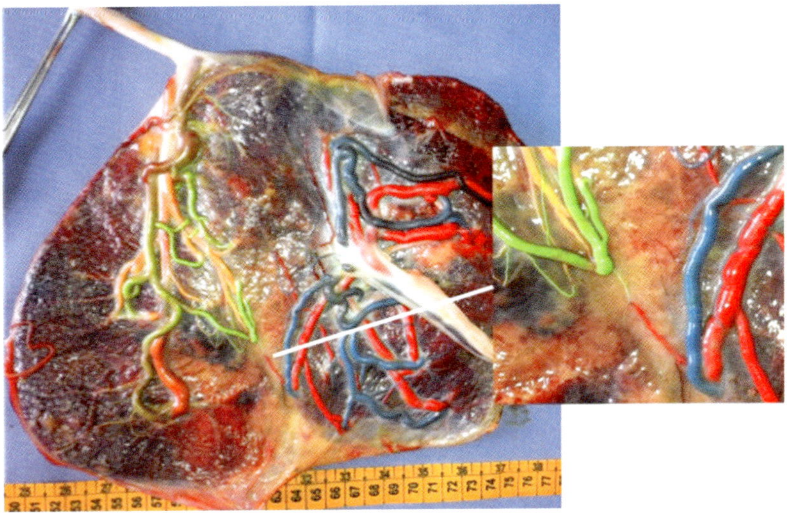

Fig. 6 Monochorionic placenta of a twin pregnancy complicated by twin anemia-polycythemia sequence (TAPS): in *blue* and *green* the arteries, in *red* and *yellow* the veins. In detail the small artero-venous anastomoses

absence of any prenatal sign of TTTS, indicates the presence of another complication typical of these pregnancies: the twin anemia-polycytemia sequence.

In recent years, the diagnostic criteria have been precisely defined, both during the prenatal and postnatal life of twins (Slaghekke et al. 2010).

In utero, Doppler velocimetry of the middle cerebral artery makes it possible to correlate the peak velocity value during systole with fetal hematocrit: prenatal TAPS is defined when a MCA-PV value is >1.55 MoM in one twin (indicative of anemia) and <0.8 MoM in the other twin (indicative of polycytemia).

Postnatal TAPS is defined by a hemoglobin discordance between twins >8.0 g /dL and at least one of the following: reticolocyte count ratio >1.7 or evidence of an artero-venous anastomoses <1 mm on placenta surface (Fig. 6). In this small anastomoses, the volume of bloodflow between twins cannot be as large as in TTTS, so the passage of only erythrocytes gives rise to TAPS.

On the basis of these criteria, TAPS complicates 3–13% of MC twins and can develop after laser treatment for TTTS, whenever a small anastomoses is left uncoagulated.

In some cases, spontaneous resolution of TAPS can be observed. Whenever there is a progression of sequence, both twins are at risk of death in utero or of neurologic sequelae (Slaghekke et al. 2014b). For that reason, tailored management is mandatory. The options for active management are selective feticide of the more compromised twin, laser coagulation of the residual anastomoses, or in utero fetal transfusion of the anemic twin.

8.7.3 Selective Intrauterine Growth Restriction of One Twin (sIUGR)

A typical complication of MC twin pregnancies is selective interauterine growth restriction of one twin (sIUGR) which is present in 10% of cases (Lewi et al. 2008).

Diagnosis is made in presence of a discordance in estimated fetal weight of twins ≥25% or by an estimated fetal weight in one twin ≤10° percentile, without the signs of TTTS described above.

The sIUGR worsens fetal and neonatal outcome, since it increases the risk of in utero fetal death of one or both twins and the risk of postnatal complications.

Prenatal surveillance of these pregnancies includes Doppler velocimetry of umbilical artery to gauge the severity of the condition and, in case of deterioration, to identify the best management option depending on gestational age and parental choice: either selective feticide of the IUGR twin or delivery of both twin.

Table 2 shows the postnatal outcome of a series of 140 cases managed at the Fetal Therapy Unit

Table 2 Neonatal/infant outcome in monochorionic diamniotic twin pregnancies complicated by sIUGR

	sIUGR twin N (%)	Large twin N (%)	Total N (%)	p-value
Neonatal death	*17/140 (12.1)*[a]	*9/140 (6.4)*	*26/280 (9.3)*	*n.s.*
Neonatal/infant outcome (N/217)[b]	97 (44.7)	120 (55.3)	217	
Healthy infants	75 (77.3)	107 (89.2)	182 (83.9)	0.03
Neonates/infants with complications	22 (22.7)	13 (10.8)	35 (16.1)	
Severe neurologic morbidity	5 (5.2)	6 (5.0)	11 (5.1)	n.s.
Spastic bilateral cerebral palsy	2	2	4	
Diplegia *Quadriplegia*	2	3	5	
Bilateral deafness	1	1	2	
Moderate neurologic morbidity	2 (2.1)	1 (0.8)	3 (1.4)	n.s.
Unilateral deafness	1	0	1	
Attention deficit Hyperactivity disorder	1	1	2	
Mild neurologic morbidity	6 (6.2)	1 (0.8)	7 (3.2)	0.05
Congenital heart disease	3 (3.1)[c]	2 (1.7)[d]	5 (2.3)	n.s.
Necrotizing enterocolitis	1 (1.0)	1 (0.8)	2 (0.9)	n.s.
Chronic lung disease	2 (2.1)	1 (0.8)	3 (1.3)	n.s.
ROP stage III	1 (1.0)	0 (0)	1 (0.5)	n.s.
Syndromes[e]	1 (1.0)	1 (0.8)	2 (0.9)	n.s.
Other (Intrahepatic bile ducts hypoplasia)	1 (1.0)	0	1 (0.5)	n.s

[a]Three neonatal deaths of sIUGR twin occurred from cardiac anomaly: Two aortic coarctation (after surgery), One complete AV block
[b]n.43 IUGR twins and 20 large twins were lost in utero
[c]One ventricular septal defect, One ostium secundum type atrial septal defect, One aortic coarctation
[d]One ventricular septal defect, One pulmonary valve stenosis. All babies had surgery before 1 year of life
[e]Neurofibromatosis, affecting both twins

"U. Nicolini" at the V. Buzzi Hospital, Milan (Rustico et al. 2016).

At follow-up, 13 IUGR and eight large neonates/infants (9.7% of survivors) showed neurologic morbidity. Even though the incidence of severe neurologic morbidity was similar between IUGR and large twins, the occurrence of mild neurodevelopmental impairment was higher in the IUGR infants ($p = 0.05$).

8.7.4 Single Intrauterine Death

In MC twin pregnancies, the death of one twin, which occurs in about 6% of these pregnancies, puts the co-twin at greater risk of mortality and morbidity. The mechanism for this adverse outcome is blood loss from the dying twin through placental vascular anastomoses. This leads to hypovolemia, which may cause the death of the co-twin from hypovolemic shock or parenchymal damage due to hypoperfusion (Fusi et al. 1991). Sequelae include ischemic cerebral lesions, periventricular leukomalacia, renal cortical necrosis, and small bowel atresia. A recent review of all published series on single IUFDs underlined how chorionicity makes the difference: MC survivor twins run a five times higher risk of dying (15%) than DC twins and a four times higher risk of neurological sequelae (26%) than DC twins (Shek et al. 2014). The risk of an adverse outcome for the surviving co-twin depends on the gestational age at the time of intrauterine death and the interval between death and delivery. In early pregnancy, the death of one twin frequently causes the death of the other fetus, but severe sequelae in the survivor are less common than at a more advanced gestation. Immediate delivery after a single intrauterine death only adds the risks of prematurity to the surviving twin. Indeed, damage may occur at the moment of death of the co-twin and therefore may not be preventable. Intrauterine transfusion can be a therapeutic solution but, if the critical moment preceding fetal death is missed, there is no treatment and conservative management is recommended (Nicolini and Poblete 1999). Dedicated ultrasonography of the fetal brain and magnetic resonance imaging (MRI) 2–3 weeks after an intrauterine fetal death may provide useful information for predicting neurodevelopmental outcome in the surviving twin.

Monochorionic twin survivors of a single IUFD after laser coagulation of placental anastomosis for treatment of TTTS, or after a selective feticide, are less exposed to neurological sequelae (O'Donoghue et al. 2009).

At the Fetal Therapy Unit "U Nicolini," at V. Buzzi Hospital, Milan, the rate of neurological sequelae in monochorionic twin survivors after spontaneous single IUFD was 16% (13 cases out of 79 pregnancies) higher than reported in single survivors after laser treatment for TTTS (8%, 9 out of 109 treated pregnancies with one survivor) or after selective feticide with bipolar cord coagulation (5%, 7 cases out of 128 pregnancies with a survivor twin). In 77% of all those cases, prenatal ultrasound and MRI detected the brain lesion; in the remaining cases, delivery of the baby occurred before MRI could be performed.

8.7.5 Twins Discordant for Fetal Anomalies

An excess of structural anomalies is observed in twins compared to singletons. While the frequency of malformations in a DZ pregnancy is similar to that for singletons (2–3%), it is two or three times higher than in a MZ pregnancy (Hall 2003). The reason is unknown, but it might be considered to be part of a teratogenic process during twinning.

MZ twins are considered identical, but recent observations have reported that this is not the rule, and a number of discordances have been observed for chromosomal anomalies (such as trisomy 21 and Turner syndrome), single gene disorders, X-linked diseases (such as Fragile-X, Aicardi's syndrome), and structural defects. These structural defects include malformations of the brain, abdominal wall anomalies, and cardiac disorders. The prevalence of cardiac defects has been reported as 2.3% in twins without TTTS, and 7% in those with TTTS, compared to 1% in the general population (Karatza et al. 2002).

Structural malformations which are not genetically determined may affect only one of the two MZ twins. It has been estimated that both twins are affected in less than 20% of cases, while in the majority of cases only one twin is involved. When a fetal anomaly affects only one fetus, clinicians face the dilemma of choosing between expectant management or selective termination of the anomalous fetus. The primary goal is to prevent the death of the normal twin. In monochorionic twin pregnancies, selective termination needs to be performed by ensuring complete and permanent occlusion of the umbilical cord of the abnormal twin, in order to avoid acute hemorrhage from the co-twin into the dying fetus, a process which may lead to death or organ damage (Rustico et al. 2005) Bipolar cord occlusion under ultrasound guidance is still considered the best method for selective feticide in these cases (Lanna et al. 2012).

Between 2004 and 2015, we observed 174 MC pregnancies with fetal anomaly (in a series of 1750 MC twin pregnancies). In this cohort, a discordant anomaly was detected in 159 (91.4%) cases. Figure 7 summarizes the type of anomalies observed.

8.7.6 Twin Reversed Arterial Perfusion (TRAP) Syndrome

Twin reversed arterial perfusion (TRAP) sequence, also known as acardiac twinning, is a rare complication of MC pregnancies which can lead to an unfavorable outcome for the normal co-twin. The reported incidence is 1 in 35,000 deliveries or 1% of MZ twins. In this condition, there is a twin without any functional cardiac tissue and variable developmental disruption (the acardiac twin). The acardiac twin is perfused by the normal twin (the pump twin) by arterial blood flowing in a retrograde fashion through a single superficial artery-to-artery placental anastomoses. Poorly oxygenated blood bypasses the placenta,

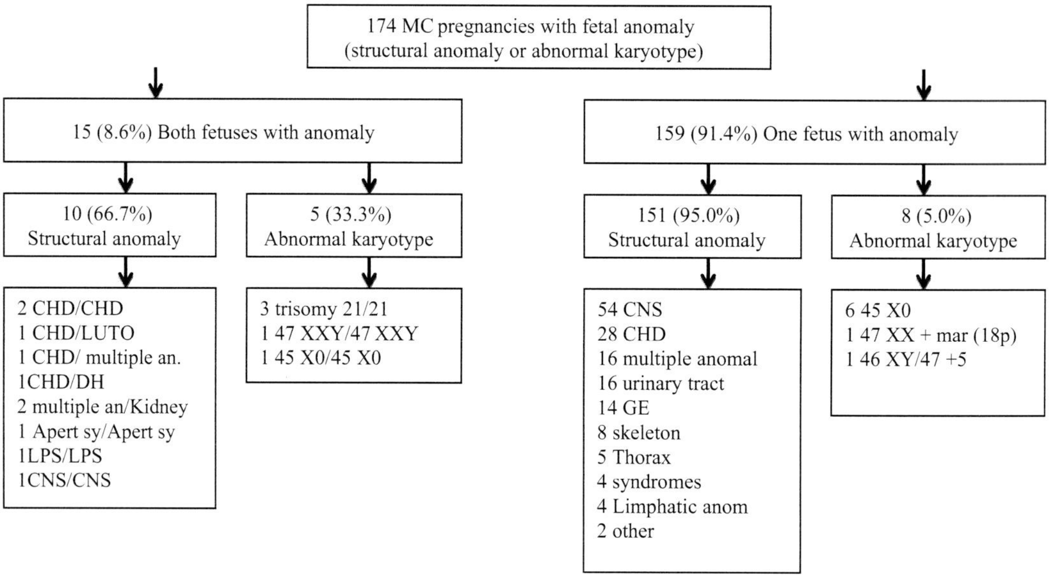

Fig. 7 Type of anomalies in a series of 174 MC twin pregnancies (personal experience)

enters the acardiac twin's circulation at low pressure, and preferentially perfuses its lower part. The blood flow returns to the pump twin via a single vein-to-vein connection (Benirschke and Kaufmann 2000). The acardiac twin acts as a parasite and space-occupying mass, being hemodynamically dependent on the other twin. Perinatal mortality rates reported for the pump twin range from 35% to 55%.

The primary causes leading to poor perinatal outcome are preterm delivery (because of the continuing growth of the acardiac fetus) and congestive heart failure (because of the volume of the acardiac twin's mass needing to be perfused by the normal heart). The deoxygenated blood circulating back to the pump may also cause chronic hypoxia, growth restriction, and hypoxic ischemic lesions.

In the case of rapid enlargement of the acardiac twin mass or signs of cardiac overload in the pump twin, blockade of the vascular supply to the parasitic twin is recommended. Possible treatments include intrafetal ablation procedures such as radiofrequency, interstitial laser, or cord occlusion of the acardiac twin. Although no single technique has been conclusively shown to be the best, some form of antenatal treatment seems to be beneficial, because there is a reported overall pump twin survival rate of 76%.

In a series of 46 cases of TRAP sequence during the period 2004–2013, 18 cases were managed expectantly. In four cases, intrauterine death of both twins occurred before 18 weeks. In three cases, there was a miscarriage. Eleven cases were delivered near term, with one neonatal death and one baby (where the acardiac fetus was very large, up to 1.5 kg) had a poor neurological outcome and periventricular leukomalacia.

In 28 cases, a cord occlusion of acardiac twin or interstitial laser was performed. Apart from complications related to the invasive procedures (8/28), 18 of the 28 cases (64%) who had in utero treatment are alive and well and free of neurological complications at postnatal follow-up.

8.8 Monoamniotic Twinning

Monoamniotic (MA) twinning is a rare condition, affecting 2% of all MZ pregnancies. MA twins share the same placenta and the amniotic sac and are at higher risk of structural anomalies, unexpected fetal death, and perinatal death (ranging from 30% to 70%), compared with MCDA twins. The excess fetal loss can be explained by umbilical cord entanglement (Fig. 8), and a crucial cofactor may be acute exsanguination across

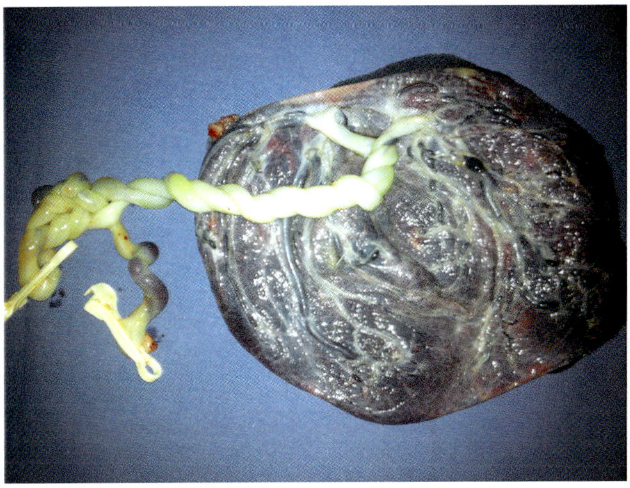

Fig. 8 Monoamniotic twin placenta with cord entaglement: twins were born at 32 weeks gestation

large placental anastomoses. Recent reviews compared the largest series reported and indicate an improvement in perinatal outcome over the years: the fetal loss is 11.4%, but in viable pregnancies after 24 weeks of gestational age mortality rate has been reported as 2% and is not correlated to the prenatal presence of cord entanglement (Ishii 2015; Rossi and Prefumo 2013). Based on the observation that the risk of neonatal death associated with preterm birth at 32 weeks is 1 in 100, the risk for MA twins at this gestational age appears to be four times lower.

8.9 Cord Occlusion in Monochorionic Twins

In some MC twin pregnancies complicated by TTTS, sIUGR, TRAP sequence, or TAPS the risk of IUD of one twin can be so high that selective termination of pregnancy (TOP) can be the last opportunity to save at least one fetus. In some other cases, parents require selective feticide for a severe discordant anomaly.

The presence of placental vascular anastomoses connecting the two fetal circulations makes it impossible to inject a drug for selective feticide, since there could be leakage into the normal co-twin's circulation, causing immediate death.

The feticide of a MC twin has to be performed with at least complete and permanent occlusion of both the arterial and venous blood flow in the umbilical cord of the affected twin. Numerous ways of achieving this have been described in the literature. Ligation of the umbilical cord by fetoscopy has been abandoned because of the complexity of the procedure and the lengthy operating time.

Fetoscopic laser coagulation has been performed as early as 16 weeks but is less effective at a more advanced gestational age or in presence of an edematous cord. The experience with radiofrequency ablation initially used for the treatment of TRAP sequence has recently been extended to non-TRAP fetuses. Ultrasound-guided bipolar cord coagulation (BCC) can be used at a later gestational age and in recent years has probably become the most common technique used for selective feticide in complicated MC pregnancies.

With a local anesthesia, a 3.3 mm cannula is introduced in the uterine cavity under ultrasound guidance. Coagulation is obtained by a power of 50 W for 30–40 s with the aim of reducing blood flow in the placenta of the selected fetus.

Whatever the technique, the risk of fetal loss is closely correlated to the gestational age at time of procedure: after 19 weeks gestational age, the risk of miscarriage and in utero fetal demise of the co-twin diminishes dramatically (Lanna et al. 2012).

Perinatal outcome in the surviving twin is dependent on gestational age at birth: risk of

Table 3 Cord occlusion in complicated monochorionic twin pregnancies: pregnancy outcome[a]

Indication	N. cases	GA (weeks) at procedure median	IUD n (%)	TOP n (%)	Ab n (%)	pPROM <24 weeks n (%)	PD <32 weeks n (%)	GA (weeks) at delivery median (range)	PND n (%)	Overall surv n (%)
TTTS	50	22.3	5 (10)	1 (2)	5 (10)	5 (10)	15 (30)	33 (25–40)	5 (10)	34 (68)
sIUGR	34	21.6	3 (9)	0	0	2 (6)	9 (26)	33.5 (23.5–40)	2 (6)	29 (85)
Anomaly	59	22.1	7(12)	0	5 (8)	5 (8)	9 (15)	37 (25–41)	4 (7)	43 (73)
TRAP s	6	22	2 (33)	0	1(16)	0	3 (50)	33 (30–37)	0	3 (50)
Total	149	22.1	17 (11)	1 (1)	11 (7)	12 (7)	36 (24)	34 (23.5–41)	11 (7)	109 (73)

TTTS twin-to-twin transfusion syndrome, *sIUGR* selective intrauterine growth restriction of one twin, *GA* gestational age, *IUD* intrauterine death, *TOP* termination of pregnancy, *Ab* abortion, *PD* premature delivery, *pPROM* premature rupture of membrane, *PND* perinatal death

[a]Fetal Medicine Unit, Buzzi Children's Hospital, Milan (1999–2014). First 118 cases are reported in reference Lanna et al. (2012)

premature delivery before 32 weeks is increased after selective feticide because of pPROM.

In a cohort of 149 pregnancies undergoing umbilical cord occlusion using bipolar coagulation, preterm delivery occurred in 33% of cases, with a procedure-to-delivery interval which varied from 1 to 22 weeks (median 11 weeks) (Table 3).

A review reported a prevalence of 4–7% of severe neurological lesions in surviving MC twins (Rossi and Prefumo 2013). This percentage is lower than expected if compared with neurological morbidity in surviving twins after the spontaneous IUD of the co-twin, which accounts for 22% of cases.

References

Andersen AN, Gianaroli L, Felberbaum R et al (2005) Assisted reproductive technology in Europe, 2001. Results generated from European registers by ESHRE. Hum Reprod 20:1158–1176

Astolfi P, Ulizzi L, Zonta LA (2003) Changes in twinning rate: Italy 1950–1996. Hum Reprod 18:207–211

Baschat AA, Barber J, Pedersen N et al (2013) Outcome after fetoscopic selective laser ablation of placental anastomoses vs equatorial laser dichorionization for the treatment of twin-to-twin transfusion syndrome. Am J Obstet Gynecol 209:234e.1–234e.8

Baud D, Windrim R, Keunen J et al (2013) Fetoscopic laser therapy for twin-twin transfusion syndrome before 17 and after 26 weeks' gestation. Am J Obstet Gynecol 208:197.e1–197.e7

Benirschke K (1995) The biology of the twinning process: how placentation influences outcome. Semin Perinatol 19:342–350

Benirschke K, Kaufmann P (eds) (2000) Pathology of the human placenta. Springer, New York

Bortolus R, Parazzini F, Chatenoud L et al (1999) The epidemiology of multiple births. Hum Reprod Update 5:179–187

Cincotta RB, Gray PH, Gardener G et al (2009) Selective fetoscopic laser ablation in 100 consecutive pregnancies with severe twin-twin transfusion syndrome. Aust N Z J Obstet Gynaecol 49:22–27

Denbow M, Fogliani R, Kyle P et al (1998) Haematological indices at fetal blood sampling in monochorionic pregnancies complicated by feto-fetal transfusion syndrome. Prenat Diagn 18:941–946

ESHRE Capri Workshop Group (2000) Multiple gestation pregnancy. Hum Reprod 15:1856–1864

Fusi L, McParland P, Fisk N et al (1991) Acute twin-to-twin transfusion: a possible mechanism for brain damaged survivors after intrauterine death of a monochorionic twin. Obstet Gynecol 78:517–520

Galea P, Barigye O, Wee L et al (2008) The placenta contributes to activation of the renin angiotensin system in twin-to-twin transfusion syndrome. Placenta 29:734–742

Hall JG (2003) Twinning. Lancet 362:735–743

Hecher K, Diehl W, Zikulnig L et al (2000) Endoscopic laser coagulation of placental anastomoses in 200 pregnancies with severe mid-trimester twin-to-twin transfusion syndrome. Eur J Obstet Gynecol Reprod Biol 92:135–139

Huber A, Diehl W, Bregenzer T (2006) Stage-related outcome in twin-twin transfusion syndrome treated by fetoscopic laser coagulation. Obstet Gynecol 108:333–337

Ishii K (2015) Prenatal diagnosis and management of monoamniotic twins. Curr Opin Obstet Gynecol 27:159–164

Karatza AA, Wolfenden JL, Taylor MJO et al (2002) Influence of twin-to-twin transfusion syndrome on fetal cardiovascular structure and function: prospective case–control study of 136 monochorionic twin pregnancies. Heart 88:271–277

Kingdom CP, Nevi O, Murphy KE (2005) Discordant growth in twins. Prenat Diag 25:759–765

Landy HJ, Neith LG (1998) The vanishing twin: a review. Hum Reprod Update 4:177–183

Lanna MM, Rustico MA, Dell'Avanzo M et al (2012) Bipolar cord coagulation for selective feticide in complicated monochorionic twin pregnancies: 118 consecutive cases at a single center. Ultrasound Obstet Gynecol 39:407–413

Lanna MM, Consonni D, Faiola S et al (2015) Color-dye injection of monochorionic placentas and correlation with pregnancy complications. Placenta 36:1095–1099

Lewi L, Jani J, Cannie M et al (2006) Intertwin anastomoses in monochorionic placentas after fetoscopic laser coagulation for twin-to-twin transfusion syndrome: is there more than meets the eye? Am J Obstet Gynecol 194:790–795

Lewi L, Jani J, Blickstein I et al (2008) The outcome of monochorionic diamniotic twin gestations in the era of invasive fetal therapy: a prospective cohort study. Am J Obstet Gynecol 199:514e1–514e8

Lopriore E, Nagel HT, Vandenbussche FP et al (2003) Long term neurodevelopmental outcome in twin-to-twin transfusion syndrome. Am J Obstet Gynecol 189.1314–1319

Mari G, Roberts A, Detti L et al (2001) Perinatal morbidity and mortality rates in severe twin-twin transfusion syndrome: results of the International Amnioreduction Registry. Am J Obstet Gynecol 185:708–715

Middeldorp JM, Sueters M, Lopriore E et al (2007) Fetoscopic laser surgery in 100 pregnancies with severe twin-to-twin transfusion syndrome in the Netherlands. Fetal Diagn Ther 22:190–194

Morris RK, Selman TJ, Harbidge A et al (2010) Fetoscopic laser coagulation for severe twin-to-twin transfusion syndrome: factors influencing perinatal outcome, learning curve of the procedure and lessons for new centres. BJOG 117:1350–1357

Naeye RL, Letts HW (1964) Body measurements of fetal and neonatal twins. Arch Pathol 77:393–396

Nicolini U, Poblete A (1999) Single intrauterine death in monochorionic twin pregnancies. Ultrasound Obstet Gynecol 14:297–301

O'Donoghue K, Rutherford MA, Engineer N et al (2009) Transfusional fetal complications after single intrauterine death in monochorionic multiple pregnancy are reduced but not prevented by vascular occlusion. BJOG 116:804–812

Quintero RA, Moeales WJ, Allen MH et al (1999) Staging of twin-to-twin transfusion syndrome. J Perinatol 19:550–555

Quintero RA, Comas C, Bornick PW et al (2000) Selective versus non-selective laser photocoagulation of placental vessels in twin-to-twin transfusion syndrome. Ultrasound Obstet Gynecol 16:230–236

Robyr R, Lewi L, Salomon LJ et al (2006) Prevalence and management of late fetal complications following successful selective laser coagulation of chorionic plate anastomoses in twin-to-twin transfusion syndrome. Am J Obstet Gynecol 194:796–803

Rossi AC, Prefumo F (2013) Impact of cord entanglement on perinatal outcome of monoamniotic twins: a systematic review of the literature. Ultrasound Obstet Gynecol 41:131–135

Ruano R, Rodo C, Peiro JL et al (2013) Fetoscopic laser ablation of placental anastomoses in twin-twin transfusion syndrome using 'Solomon technique'. Ultrasound Obstet Gynecol 42:434–439

Rustico MA, Baietti MG, Coviello D et al (2005) Managing twins discordant for fetal anomalies. Prenat Diagn 25:766–771

Rustico MA, Lanna MM, Faiola S et al (2012) Fetal and maternal complications after selective fetoscopic laser surgery for twin-to-twin transfusion syndrome: a single-center experience. Fetal Diagn Ther 31:170–178

Rustico MA, Consonni D, Lanna MM et al. (2016) Selective intrauterinbe growth restriction in monochorionic twins: changing pattern in umbilical artery Doppler flow and outcomes. Ultrasound Obstet Gynecol 8:45–56. https://doi.org/10.1002/uog.15933

Senat M, Deprest J, Bulvain M et al (2004) Endoscopic laser surgery versus serial amnioreduction for severe twin-to-twin transfusion syndrome. N Engl J Med 351:136–144

Shek NW, Hillman SC, Kilby MD (2014) Single-twin demise: pregnancy outcome. Best Pract Res Clin Obstet Gynaecol 28:249–263

Simón C, Landeras J, Zuzuarregui JL et al (1999) Early pregnancy losses in in vitro fertilization and oocyte donation. Fertil Steril 72:1061–1065

Slaghekke F, Kist WJ, Oepkes D et al (2010) Twin anemia-polycythemia sequence: diagnostic criteria, classification, perinatal management and outcome. Fetal Diagn Ther 27:181–190

Slaghekke F, Lopriore E, Lewi L et al (2014a) Fetoscopic laser coagulation of the vascular equator versus selective coagulation for twin-to-twin transfusion syndrome: an open-label randomised controlled trial. Lancet 383 (9935):2144–2151. https://doi.org/10.1016/S0140-6736(13)62419-8

Slaghekke F, van Klink JM, Koopman HM et al (2014b) Neurodevelopmental outcome in twin anemia-polycythemia sequence after laser surgery for twin-twin transfusion syndrome. Ultrasound Obstet Gynecol 44:316–321

Stagnati V, Chalouhi GE, Essaoui M et al (2015) Pulmonary stenosis in complicated monochorionic twin pregnancies: prevalence, management and outcome. Prenat Diagn 35:1085–1092

Stirnemann JJ, Nasr B, Quarello E et al (2008) A definition of selectivity in laser coagulation of chorionic plate anastomoses in twin-to-twin transfusion syndrome and its relationship to perinatal outcome. Am J Obstet Gynecol 198:62.e1–62.e6

Valsky DV, Eixarch E, Martinez-Crespo JM et al (2012) Fetoscopic laser surgery for twin-to-twin transfusion syndrome after 26 weeks of gestation. Fetal Diagn Ther 31:30–34

van Klink JM, Koopman HM, van Zwet EW et al (2013) Cerebral injury and neurodevelopmental impairment after amnioreduction versus laser surgery in twin-twin transfusion syndrome: a systematic review and meta-analysis. Fetal Diagn Ther 33:81–89

Intrauterine Growth Restriction: Obstetric and Neonatal Aspects. Intervention Strategies

9

Enrico Bertino, Giovanna Oggè, Paola Di Nicola, Francesca Giuliani, Alessandra Coscia, and Tullia Todros

Contents

E. Bertino (✉) · P. Di Nicola · F. Giuliani · A. Coscia
Neonatal Unit, University of Turin, Turin, Italy
e-mail: enrico.bertino@unito.it

G. Oggè · T. Todros
Maternal-Fetal Medicine Unit, University of Turin, Turin, Italy
e-mail: tullia.todros@unito.it

Abstract

Normal fetal growth can be altered by several pathological processes, including genetic diseases, infections, congenital anomalies, maternal hypoxia, and inadequate placental exchanges. The impossibility to reach the fetal genetic

G. Buonocore et al. (eds.), *Neonatology*,
https://doi.org/10.1007/978-3-319-29489-6_158

growth potential because of placental malfunction is defined *intrauterine growth restriction* (IUGR). IUGR causes slowing fetal growth, so that fetal biometry shifts from a higher to a significantly lower percentile during gestation, and it progressively leads to fetal hypoxia, acidemia, multiorgan damage, and death. Indeed, IUGR is associated with an excess of perinatal mortality and short- and long-term morbidity as well as metabolic syndrome in the adulthood. Prenatal diagnosis and appropriate timing of delivery improve neonatal outcomes.

When a fetus is found to be small for gestational age (SGA) at prenatal ultrasound, every effort has to be made to differentiate IUGR from other causes of impaired fetal growth. In case of IUGR, the clinical management is critically dependent on gestational age at onset. In early onset IUGR, the timing of delivery has to take into account the risks of prolonged intrauterine hypoxia versus the complications associated with preterm birth. In late onset IUGR, early induction of labor is probably the most cost-efficient method to prevent perinatal mortality and morbidity. In intermediate-onset IUGR there is a lack of clear evidence about the best tool to identify the fetuses that would benefit of timely delivery.

At birth, neonatal weight, length, and head circumference are indicators of the quality and quantity of intrauterine growth. SGA newborns, both preterm and term, have increased perinatal mortality risk and short-term complications such as birth asphyxia, infections, hypothermia, hypoglycemia, feeding difficulties, respiratory distress syndrome, bronchopulmonary dysplasia, retinopathy of prematurity, and necrotizing enterocolitis.

Even if most term children born SGA experience catch-up growth and achieve a normal adult height, approximately 10% of them remain shorter than peers born appropriate for gestational age. Preterm SGA infants can take four or more years to achieve heights in a normal range and the majority of them show a postnatal growth deficit at the time of hospital discharge (Extra Uterine Growth Restriction, EUGR).

Being born SGA is associated with long-term unfavorable outcomes such as learning difficulties, behavior problems, and development of metabolic syndrome.

The recognition of intrauterine malnutrition and the monitoring of early postnatal growth are of utmost importance for optimum survival and long-term outcomes of SGA infants.

List of Abbreviations

AGA	Appropriate for gestational age
BMI	Body mass index
BPD	Broncopulmonary displasia
EUGR	Extra uterine growth restriction
GA	Gestational age
GH	Growth hormone
INR	International mormalized ratio
IUGR	Intrauterine growth restriction
LGA	Large for gestational age
NEC	Necrotizing enterocolitis
PI	Ponderal index
PT	Protrombin time
RDS	Respiratory distress syndrome
ROP	Retinopathy of prematurity
SD	Standard deviation
SGA	Small for gestational age

9.1 Salient Points

- Normal fetal growth can be altered by several pathological processes, including inadequate placental exchanges determining intrauterine growth restriction (IUGR).
- IUGR leads to fetal hypoxia, acidemia, multiorgan damage and death that can only be prevented by elective delivery.
- At birth, weight, length and head circumference are indicators of the quality and quantity of intrauterine growth.
- Small for gestational age (SGA) newborns, both preterm and term, have an increased perinatal mortality risk and a number of unfavorable short and long term consequences.
- The recognition of any growth abnormalities and the monitoring of early postnatal growth are of utmost importance for optimum survival and long-term outcomes of SGA infants.

9.2 Normal and Abnormal Fetal Growth

Normal fetal growth is a complex process depending on cellular hyperplasia, prevailing during the first half of pregnancy, and cellular hypertrophy, being prevalent in the second half of pregnancy. Defects in fetal growth can therefore schematically be attributed to events that inhibit cellular mitosis (such as chromosomal or genetic diseases, infections or ischemia) or to events that restrict cellular metabolism (such as inadequate placental exchanges, maternal hypoxia due to respiratory, cardiac or hematologic diseases, maternal under-nutrition). The impossibility to reach the fetal genetic growth potential because of a pathologic event is defined *intrauterine growth restriction* (IUGR). In case of IUGR the limitation to maternal-fetal gas and metabolic exchanges progressively leads to fetal hypoxia and, when compensating mechanisms fail, to fetal acidemia, multi-organ damage and death. Such a cascade of events can only be interrupted by elective delivery of the fetus.

Based on the distribution of fetal and neonatal anthropometric parameters at each gestational age (GA) in the general population, every fetus and newborn can be defined as *small for gestational age* (SGA) if its biometric measures result below a pre-established threshold, *large for gestational age* (LGA) when they result above an upper threshold, or *appropriate for gestational age* (AGA) if they lay between these pre-defined limits of normality. However, a fetus that is SGA is not necessarily affected by IUGR, as it can be healthy but genetically determined to be smaller than the majority of the general population (*constitutional SGA*). On the contrary, an AGA fetus can actually be suffering from IUGR if its growth has slowed so that its biometry has shifted from a higher to a significantly lower percentile during gestation, but it has not fallen below the threshold of normality (Bardien et al. 2016) (Fig. 1).

IUGR is associated with a significant burden of perinatal mortality and neonatal morbidity (Garite et al. 2004; Aucott et al. 2004; Morsing et al. 2011) and impaired neurodevelopmental outcomes (Guellec et al. 2011), as well as the increased risk of hypertension, cardiovascular disease and type 2 diabetes in the adulthood (Barker and Osmond 1986; Barker 2006; Kanaka-Gantenbein 2010) due to epigenetic mechanisms influencing adaptation to the intrauterine environment (Hanson and Gluckman 2014). It has been demonstrated that prenatal identification of SGA fetuses (as a proxy of IUGR) improves neonatal outcomes (Lindqvist and Molin 2005), thus accurate diagnosis of IUGR is a primary goal of perinatal medicine.

Assessment of fetal growth in utero is performed by comparing fetal biometry with the normal value at that specific GA in the same population. To this purpose, three conditions are required:

1. *Exact knowledge of GA*, i.e., *accurate dating of pregnancy*. As the date of conception is usually unknown, the beginning of the last menstrual period (LMP) is conventionally adopted as a surrogate in clinical practice, assuming that ovulation and conception, occur 2 weeks after LMP and that pregnancy extends on average 280 days (40 weeks) from LMP (Baskett and Nagele 2000). However, many women are not able to reliably report the date of LMP and, moreover, the interval from the beginning of LMP and conception is subject to considerable biologic variation (Nakling et al. 2005). The introduction of ultrasound allowed a more accurate estimate of GA, based on the fact that the velocity of embryonic growth shows a high degree of uniformity during early pregnancy (particularly during the first trimester) (Blaas et al. 1998). Indeed, between 9 and 13 weeks' gestation, GA can be accurately estimated by the measure of crown-rump length (CRL) which growth is rapid and has a rather small inter individual variability. Later, biparietal diameter is typically used for dating, as CRL can no longer be measured owing to curling of the growing fetus; however, variation is greater, which results in less accurate assessment of GA. For this reason, first-trimester ultrasound estimation of GA is recommended in clinical practice (Kalish et al. 2004). However, it must be noted that

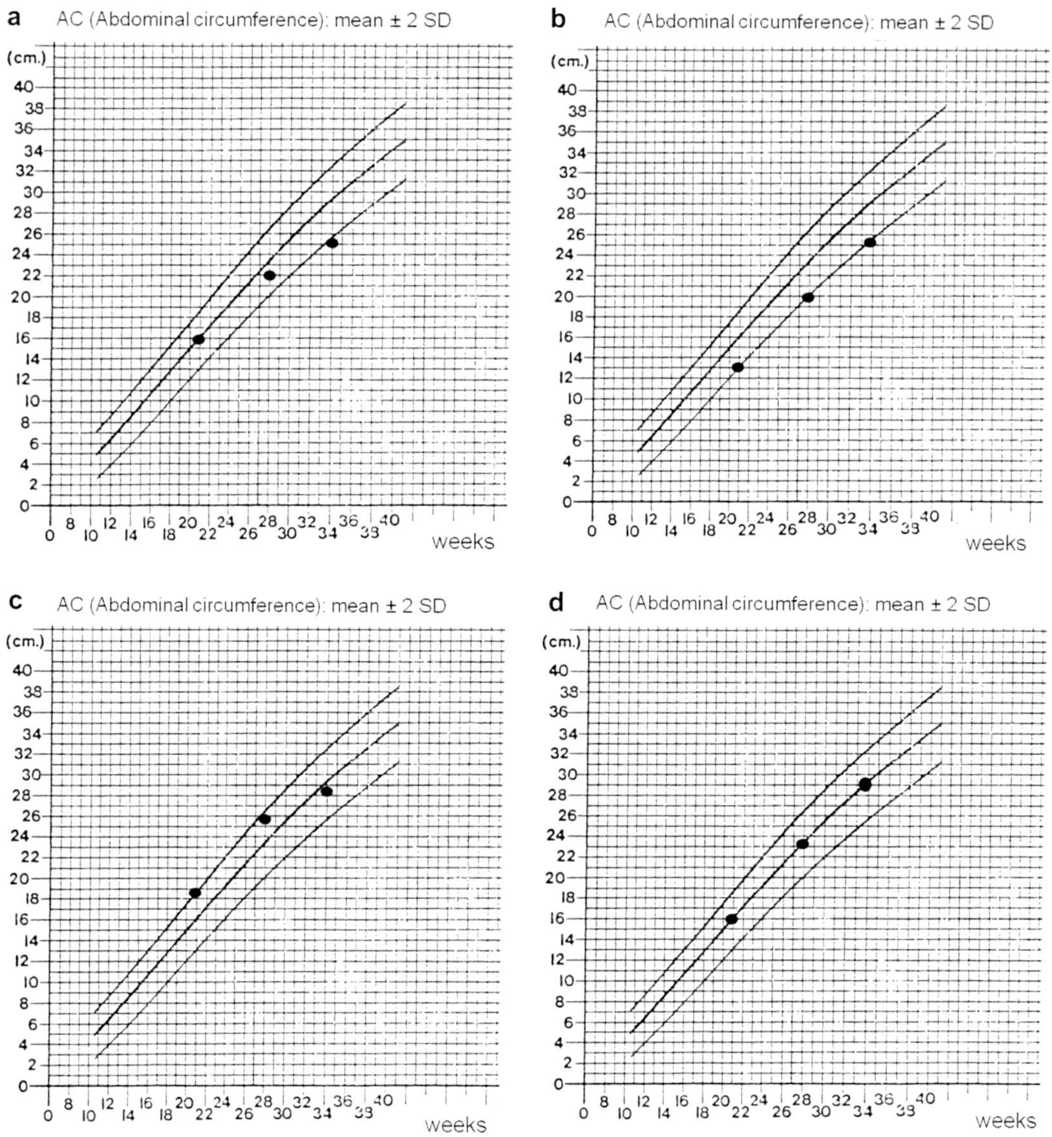

Fig. 1 Different patterns of fetal growth: (**a**) SGA fetus with IUGR: fetal abdominal circumference progressively shifts from the mean for GA to 2 standard deviations below the mean for GA, (**b**) SGA fetus without IUGR: fetal abdominal circumference is 2 standard deviations below the mean for GA, but it continues growing on the same trajectory throughout gestation; (**c**) AGA fetus with IUGR: fetal abdominal circumference progressively shifting from 2 standard deviations above the mean for GA to a lower percentile, without falling below the lower threshold of normality; (**d**) AGA fetus without IUGR: fetal abdominal circumference is between the limits of normality for GA and it continues growing on the same trajectory throughout gestation

pathologic processes can influence intrauterine growth even in its earliest stages, including very early forms of IUGR (Morin et al. 2005; Thorsell et al. 2008).

2. *Availability of an adequate fetal growth chart.* The classification of the biometry of an individual fetus as normal or abnormal for GA relies on the comparison with the normal value of each biometric variable at the same GA. Several charts have been published, including different populations and using different statistical methods; the choice of the

chart has consequences on the sensitivity and specificity of the diagnosis of IUGR. Growth charts can be constructed retrospectively or prospectively (in the latter case quality data is improved by strict pre-defined protocols); they can be cross-sectional (every fetus in the study population contributes with only one observation; these studies can provide references for fetal size, but not for fetal growth velocity) or longitudinal (every fetus is measured serially over time and its growth velocity is assessed); they can include only healthy individuals (therefore providing standards of how fetuses *should grow*), or they can comprehend the general population (therefore describing references of how fetuses *actually grow* in that specific setting). Recently, international standards for fetal growth were published based on a prospective, multicenter, population-based study including 4321 women in optimal health and nutritional status, with singleton pregnancy, without major obstetric complications, from eight countries (Papageorghiou et al. 2014). Such approach is based on the assumption that when adequate health and nutritional conditions are met, other genetic and environmental factors do not have significant influence on intrauterine growth. Conversely, customized growth charts are founded on the hypothesis that few genetic and environmental variables (namely ethnic group, maternal height and body mass index, fetal sex and parity) can physiologically modulate fetal growth, so that the same fetal weight at the same gestational age would represent a different percentile if the fetus is Caucasian or African, female or male etc. (De Jong et al. 2000; Kase et al. 2012; Rizzo et al. 2016). Which approach is more efficient for the diagnosis of IUGR is still debated.

3. *Accurate measurement of relevant fetal biometric parameters*.

   Ultrasonographic measurement of fetal biometry is considered the gold standard for prenatal diagnosis of IUGR. However, ultrasound accuracy is limited by several factors related to the operator's skills, technical characteristics of the ultrasound equipment, maternal body constitution, and dynamic nature of the pathology; under this regard, if ultrasound is performed late in pregnancy it has the potential to detect the majority of cases of abnormal growth, while it is going to miss a considerable proportion if it is performed earlier, when the deviation from normal growth is still mild or has not occurred yet. In a recent multicentric cohort study, universal ultrasound screening at 28 and 36 weeks of GA detected 57% of SGA fetuses with birthweight lower than the 10th percentile (vs. 20% of a policy of selective ultrasound when clinically indicated): even such an intensive protocol of monitoring (currently not feasible on the general population because of the limitation of resources even in high-income countries) is destined to miss nearly half of all SGA (Sovio et al. 2015). Not surprisingly, a series of papers from a prospective screening study in a single centre, found that ultrasonographic biometry, combined with maternal characteristics and medical history, can identify 44% of all SGA with birthweight lower than the 5th percentile born at term if it is performed at 19–24 weeks of GA, versus 58% if it is performed at 30–34 weeks of GA and 70% if it is performed at 35–37 weeks of GA (Lesmes et al. 2015; Bakalis et al. 2015; Fadigas et al. 2015). Of course, a program of screening by ultrasound late in pregnancy would miss the earliest and most severe cases.

9.3 Diagnosis of IUGR

As discussed above, every fetus can be defined as SGA if its biometric variables (usually abdominal circumference or estimated fetal weight) result below a pre-established lowest cut-off (e.g., 10th, 5th or 3rd percentile or 2 standard deviation below the mean for GA), LGA when they result above a highest cut-off (e.g., 90th, 95th, or 97th percentile or 2 standard deviation above the mean for GA), or AGA if they lay between the pre-defined limits of normality. However, such operation can only provide a cross-sectional measure of the size of the fetus: not all newborns falling below the cut-off are abnormally small because of growth restriction, as a proportion of them are representing the normal spectrum of fetal growth.

As growth is a dynamic process, the evaluation of fetal growth can only be obtained by a longitudinal sequence of biometric measurements during time. Accordingly, when fetal biometry shifts from a percentile to a significantly lower one, IUGR can be diagnosed, while the opposite passage, to a significantly higher percentile, allow the diagnosis of fetal growth acceleration.

However, ultrasound and Doppler velocimetry can provide several other clues to help differentiate a healthy, constitutional SGA fetus from one that is SGA because of IUGR, even when longitudinal assessment is not available:

(a) *Research for anatomical anomalies*. A careful assessment of fetal anatomy can identify signs of congenital malformations, chromosomal or genetic diseases and intrauterine infections. This is particularly important when an SGA biometry is detected during the first half of pregnancy, a time when placental inadequacy to supply for fetal requirements is unlikely, and therefore the etiology of the growth defect has to be searched elsewhere. When anatomical anomalies are suspected, moreover, amniocentesis is indicated, for karyotyping, research for specific genetic mutations, or infectivologic analyses.

(b) *Uterine artery Doppler velocimetry.* Doppler velocimetry tracings obtained from the uterine arteries reflect impedance to blood flow in the spiral arteries. These vessels are modified by trophoblastic invasion, producing vasodilatation, during the first half of pregnancy. Low resistance to flow and high diastolic velocities in the uterine arteries indicate normal trophoblastic invasion, while high resistance to flow and low diastolic velocities indicate shallow dilatation of the spiral arteries because of impaired placental invasion (Fig. 2). Therefore the finding of abnormally high resistance in the uterine arteries is

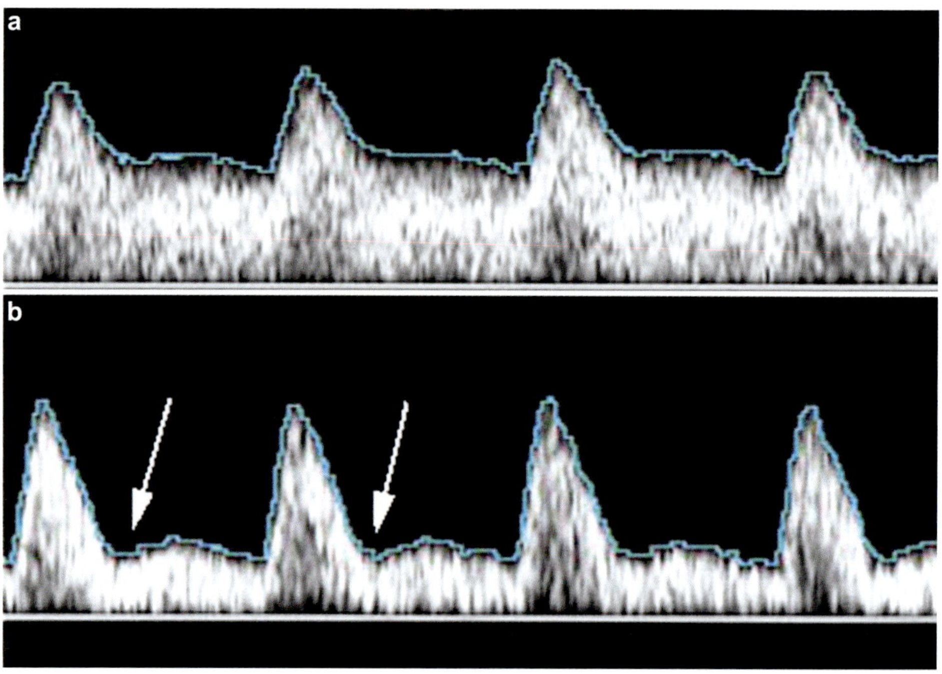

Fig. 2 Doppler velocimetry tracing of a uterine artery in the third trimester of pregnancy: (**a**) with normal resistance and high diastolic velocities; (**b**) with increased resistance and decreased early-diastolic velocities (*arrows*)

strongly suggestive for a placental etiology (Olofsson et al. 1993; Lyall et al. 2013; Figueras and Gratacos 2014) and is associated with cesarean section for fetal distress, neonatal acidosis and neonatal hospitalization (Cruz-Martinez et al. 2015).

(c) *Umbilical artery Doppler velocimetry.* Umbilical artery Doppler velocimetry reflects impedance to blood flow in the fetal side of placental circulation, i.e., in the villous tree. Abnormally high resistance in the umbilical arteries velocimetry are indicative of substantial placental pathology (McCowan et al. 1987; Todros et al. 1999). Indeed, elevated indices of resistance up to absent or reversed end-diastolic flow (ARED) in such vessels, correlate with worsening degrees of fetal hypoxia and acidosis and increased risk of perinatal mortality (Karsdorp et al. 1994; Nicolaides et al. 1988; Tyrrell et al. 1989) (Fig. 3). Hence the finding of elevated impedance in the umbilical arteries in an SGA fetus, is both diagnostic of IUGR of placental origin and prognostic, as its progression is indicative of worsening hypoxia, risk of fetal damage and intrauterine death and need for elective delivery.

(d) *Middle cerebral artery Doppler velocimetry.* Vasodilatation in the cerebral circulation (most easily assessed in the middle cerebral artery – Fig. 4) is a sign of fetal hemodynamic adaptation to chronic hypoxia, which is thought to secure oxygenation to the brain, to the expense of other organs (brain sparing). Decreased impedance in the middle cerebral artery is particularly useful for the identification of late-onset IUGR, a subgroup of fetuses in which umbilical artery flow can be only mildly altered or even normal, but are still at risk of fetal distress during labor and suboptimal neurobehavioral outcomes (Oros et al. 2011; Eixarch et al. 2008).

(e) *Estimated fetal weight.* Even when umbilical and middle cerebral artery Doppler assessment

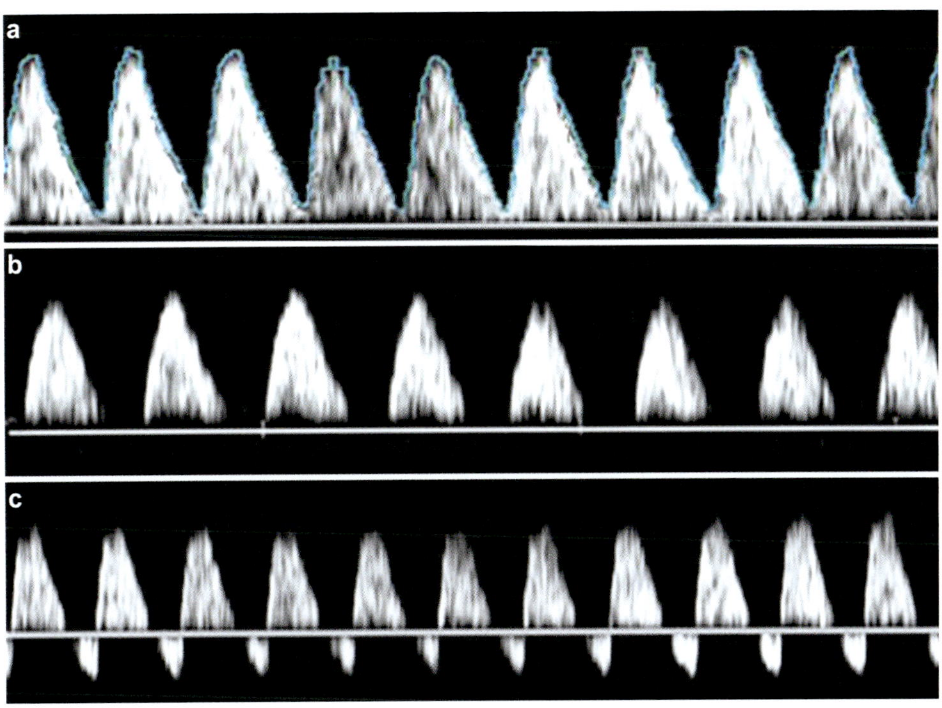

Fig. 3 Doppler velocimetry tracing of an umbilical artery in the third trimester of pregnancy with (**a**) increased resistance but present end-diastolic velocities; (**b**) increased resistance and absent end-diastolic velocities; (**c**) increased resistance and reversed end-diastolic velocities

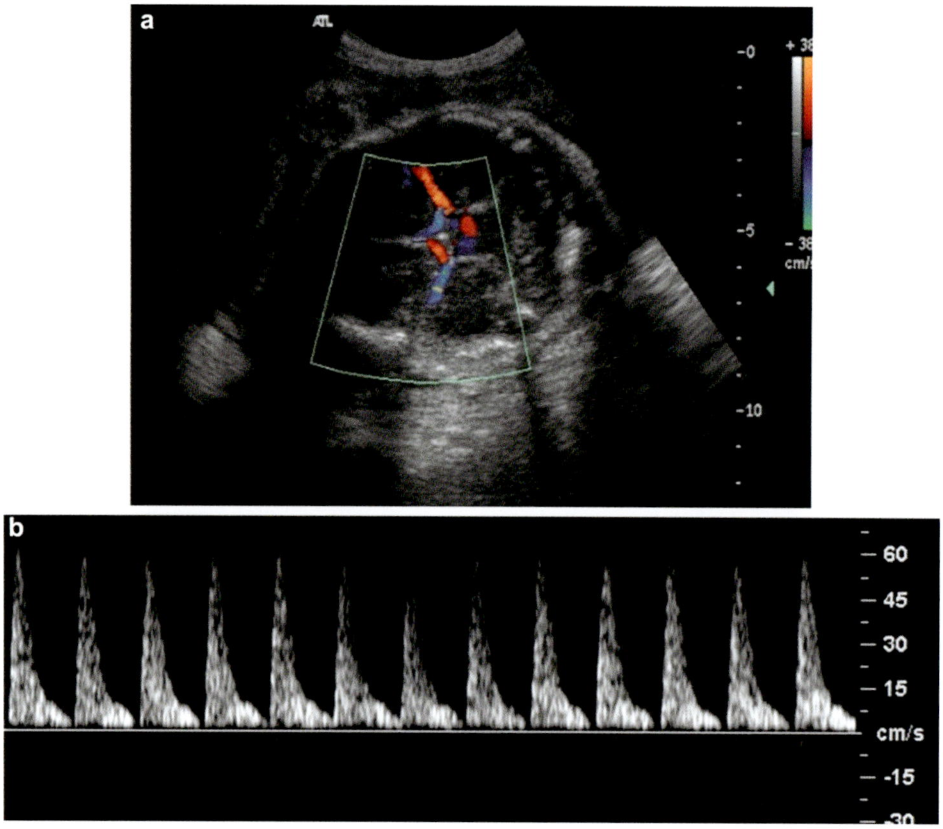

Fig. 4 Doppler velocimetry the middle cerebral artery; (**a**) visualization of the circle of Willisa with color Doppler; (**b**) Doppler velocimetry tracing of the middle cerebral artery

is normal, a very low estimated fetal weight (calculated by means of different algorithms on the basis of ultrasonographic biometry) is strongly predictive of adverse perinatal outcomes among SGA fetuses, and is therefore suggestive of IUGR (Savchev et al. 2012).

(f) *Pattern of growth*. Since the introduction of fetal ultrasonographic biometry, obstetricians classify SGA fetuses as symmetrical (proportionately small head circumference, abdominal circumference ad femur length) and asymmetrical (substantial reduction in abdominal circumference with relatively preserved head circumference and femur length) with the believing that IUGR fetuses tend to adopt an asymmetric pattern of growth as a consequence of brain sparing, while constitutional SGA and fetuses with aneuploidies, congenital infections and malformations are preferentially symmetrical (Campbell and Thoms 1977). In contrast with this assumption, it has been shown that all SGA fetuses show some degree of asymmetry although such pattern is more common among IUGR (Todros et al. 1996; David et al. 1995). However, newborns with low weight and preserved length (also referred to as *wasting*), corresponding to asymmetrical SGA fetuses, show a stronger association with poor neonatal outcomes including admission to neonatal intensive care unit, respiratory distress syndrome, transient tachypnea and difficulty in oral feeding, compared to newborns with low weight and short length (also referred as *stunting*), corresponding to symmetrical SGA fetuses (Victora 2015). Therefore asymmetrical SGA fetuses should be considered at high risk of intrauterine damage.

9.4 Monitoring, Timing and Mode of Delivery

Clinical management of IUGR is critically dependent on gestational age at its onset. Early onset IUGR is more easily diagnosed because it tends to rapidly touch extreme degrees of alterations in terms of fetal biometry and oxygenation and because of its frequent association with maternal hypertensive diseases. However, the only available therapeutic intervention, i.e., interruption of pregnancy, is a serious clinical dilemma because it exposes the fetus to the risks of severe preterm birth. On the other hand, late onset IUGR, which is much more frequent, is more easily missed by antenatal care, because deviation from normal fetal growth and hemodynamic function are more subtle, while, in this case, the risks of anticipating delivery appear to be a safer option; however, in light of the growing evidence on the perinatal risks of late preterm birth, solid criteria to choose the timing of delivery are lacking.

Early onset IUGR. Early-onset IUGR (occurring before 34 weeks of gestation) is associated with a risk of perinatal mortality as high as 41%, depending on definition, study population and GA (Mari et al. 2007). Neonatal short- and long-term prognosis is mainly determined by three variables: fetal cardiovascular status, birthweight, and GA at birth (Baschat et al. 2007, 2009; Torrance et al. 2010).

The fetal cardiovascular status, as indicated by Doppler velocimetry of arterial and venous vessels and by fetal heart rate tracing, is strictly related to the fetal acid–base status: hence serial testing with Doppler ultrasound and fetal heart rate tracings allows to follow the transition from fetal normal oxygenation to hypoxemia, hypoxia and acidemia, which in turn appears to be the nearest fetal antecedent of perinatal mortality and infant neurodevelopmental delay (Soothill et al. 1992).

Birthweight is the expression of both GA at birth and the severity of fetal malnutrition and correlates with major neonatal morbidity (Baschat et al. 2007) and abnormal neurodevelopment in infancy and childhood independently of Doppler parameters (Baschat et al. 2009; Torrance et al. 2010).

Prematurity (as a result of iatrogenic preterm delivery of fetuses considered to be at high risk of intrauterine acidemia and demise) is also an independent predictor of neonatal mortality and severe neonatal complications associated with abnormal neurodevelopmental outcomes in IUGR fetuses (Baschat et al. 2007, 2009; Torrance et al. 2010; Soothill et al. 1992; Lees et al. 2013). A multicenter cohort trial conducted between 2000 and 2006 in 12 centers of perinatal medicine in USA and Europe, reports neonatal outcomes of 604 singleton liveborn with IUGR delivered between 24 and 32 weeks + 6 days. Mortality within 28 days of life was 20% while incidence of severe morbidity was 36%; however, the rate of neonatal death decreased by 2% per each day of pregnancy prolongation between 24 and 27 weeks of GA. In contrast, after this threshold Doppler velocimetry of the venous circulation and arterial pH were the only independent variables predictive of neonatal mortality, while GA at delivery was not a determinant of neonatal survival. Similarly, GA was the main predictor of severe neonatal morbidity until 29 weeks, but it was replaced by venous Doppler between 29 and 33 weeks (Baschat et al. 2007).

More favorable data on neonatal mortality and morbidity are reported by the Trial of Umbilical and Fetal Flow in Europe (TRUFFLE). This is a randomized clinical trial conducted between 2005 and 2010 in 20 European centers, in which 503 fetuses with early-onset IUGR (diagnosed between 26 weeks and 31 weeks + 6 days of GA) were randomly allocated to be delivered according to one of three criteria: (1) fetal heart rate criteria (namely reduced short term variation); (2) early abnormalities in the Doppler velocimetry of the ductus venosus (reduced velocities during atrial contraction); (3) late abnormalities in the ductus venosus (absent or reversed velocities during atrial contraction) (Fig. 5). When the short-term outcomes of the whole cohort, regardless of the arm of randomization, were analyzed, neonatal mortality before discharge from hospital was 5.5% of all live born, and severe morbidity was 24%. Besides GA and birthweight, the major determinant of poor outcome was the occurrence

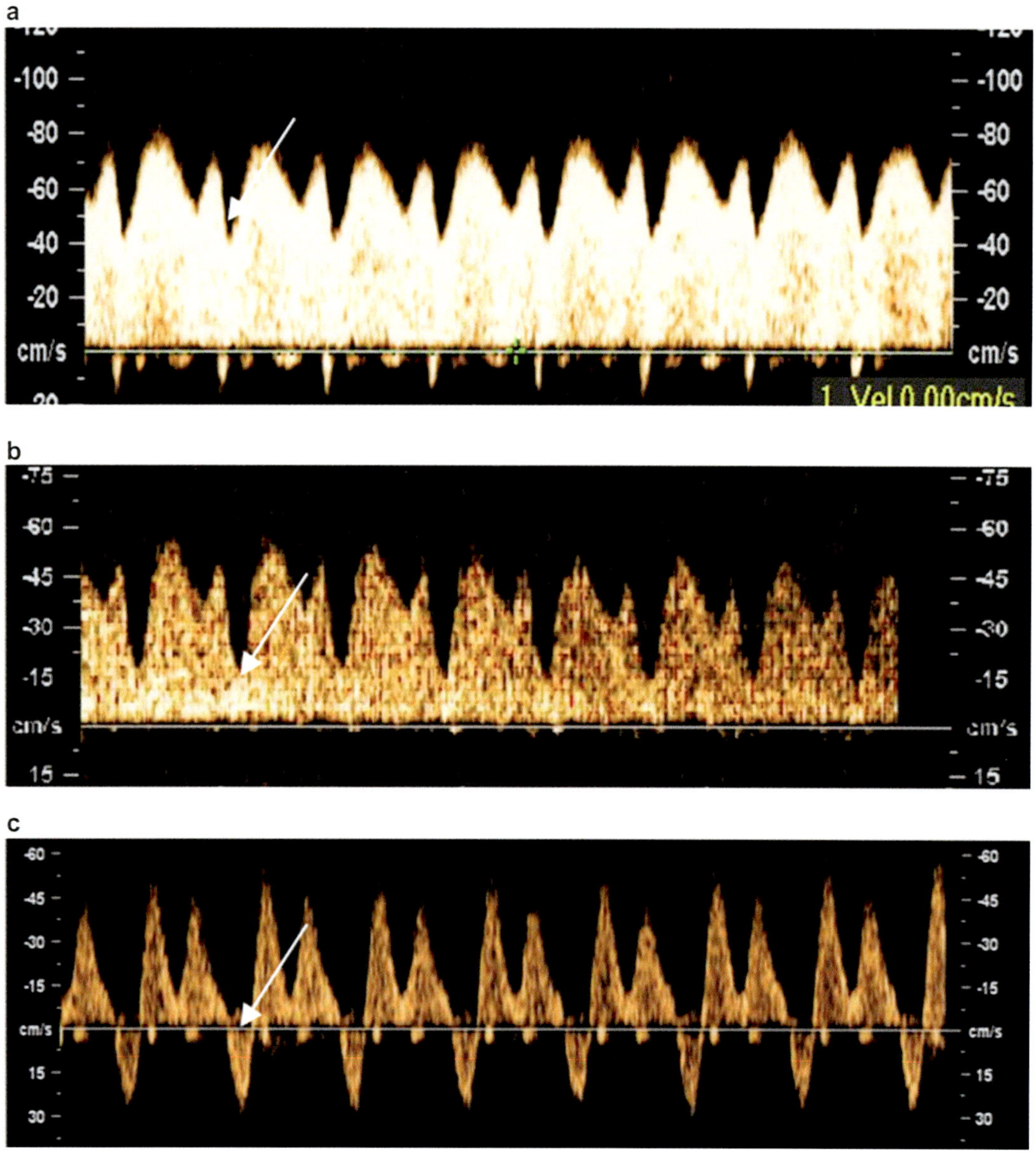

Fig. 5 Doppler velocimetry tracing of the ductus venosus in the third trimester of pregnancy with: (**a**) normal positive velocities during atrial contraction; (**b**) reduced velocities during atrial contraction; (**c**) reversed velocities during atrial contraction. *Arrows* indicate velocities during atrial contraction

of maternal hypertensive disease, which shortened the interval between diagnosis of IUGR and delivery (Lees et al. 2013).

In summary, the aim of clinical management of early-onset IUGR fetuses is focused on optimizing the timing of delivery in order to balance the risks of prolonged intrauterine hypoxia versus the complications associated with preterm birth. Unfortunately, there is no single test indicating the break point, in spite many tests reflecting fetal conditions and their deterioration have been developed in the last decades: fetal arterial and venous Doppler velocimetry, fetal heart rate tracing with computerized analysis of short term variability, ultrasound for assessment of fetal growth and amniotic fluid. The results of the TRUFFLE study recently demonstrated that the best neurodevelopmental outcome at 2 years in surviving fetuses is obtained when timing of delivery is based on the integration of results of ductus venosus Doppler and fetal heart rate (Lees et al. 2015).

Late onset IUGR. Late-onset IUGR is not a minor clinical issue, because most infants with intrauterine growth restriction are born at term (Clausson et al. 1998). Even when diagnosed late in gestation, IUGR is associated with increased risk of perinatal mortality and morbidity, such as fetal distress, hypoglycemia, seizures, behavioral problems, cerebral palsy, and cardiovascular disease (Jarvis et al. 2003; Pulver et al. 2009; Boulet et al. 2006; Dijxhoorn et al. 1987). Moreover growing evidence suggests that growth failure occurring around term is associated with a poorer mental and psychomotor development (Skuse et al. 1994). Early delivery by induction of labor might prevent the detrimental effects of inadequate nutrition and oxygenation, and indeed it is the common clinical practice; however, the excess of mortality and morbidity associated with late preterm (between 34 an 36 weeks) and early term (between 37 and 38 weeks) birth is increasingly recognized (Shapiro-Mendoza et al. 2008; Hansen et al. 2008; Engle 2011).

A multicenter randomized clinical trial (the Disproportionate Intrauterine Growth Intervention Trial At Term, DIGITAT) compared the effect of induction of labor and expectant management on a population of 650 women with prenatal diagnosis of IUGR after 36 weeks of GA and did not find any significant difference in terms of adverse neonatal outcomes (Boers et al. 2010, 2012), caesarean sections (Boers et al. 2010), and developmental and behavioral outcomes at two years of age (van Wyk et al. 2012). However, expectant management was associated with a higher chance of being born with severe IUGR, which is a major predicting factor for neurodevelopmental disturbances. On the other hand, early induction was associated with a higher rate of neonatal admission to intermediate care, but such excess of neonatal admissions seemed to be related to protocols of clinical management for late prematurity and not to specific neonatal complications (Boers et al. 2012). Evidence is still lacking regarding the best monitoring tool to identify those fetuses that would benefit from early induction of labor (Tajik et al. 2014). Therefore, in case of IUGR after 36 weeks of GA, it appears more reasonable to choose induction of labor in order to prevent fetal mortality and neonatal morbidity and in order to save the resources needed for intensive fetal monitoring.

Intermediate onset IUGR. The time interval between 34 and 36 weeks of GA is the source of the greatest uncertainty in the clinical management of pregnancies complicated by IUGR, as evidence is lacking about risks of chronic intrauterine hypoxia and preterm birth and the most efficient tools for identifying fetuses at highest risk of intrauterine compromise. As umbilical artery Doppler is frequently normal in this population, the middle cerebral artery velocimetry could be the best marker for impending fetal hypoxia and could be used for timing delivery. At the moment there is a need for clinical research on the subject.

9.5 Auxological Evaluation of the Newborn

Weight, length, and head circumference at birth are indicators of the quality and quantity of growth. These variables must be evaluated using standardized instruments and following the techniques required for accurate measurements as described by Cameron (2004).

In order to identify intrauterine malnutrition, some anthropometric indexes have been proposed. They compare variables, such as body length and head circumference, which are less influenced in cases of malnutrition, to those variables which are more compromised such as body weight.

The most well known is the Rörher ponderal index [PI = body weight (grams) × 100/length (centimeters)^3] whose normal value in a full-term newborn lies between 2.2 and 3 (3rd and 97th percentile) (Miller 1985). This neonatal body

Table 1 Suggested characteristics for a reliable neonatal anthropometric chart (Bertino et al. 2007)

Preplanned multicenter ad hoc study
Descriptive reference
Monoethnic population
Charts specific for gender
Charts specific for single or multiple pregnancy
Charts specific for parity
Reliable gestational age assessment
Reliable measuring techniques and instruments
Range of GA from 42 to 24 weeks or less

proportionality index corresponds to the Body Mass Index (BMI) used in children and adults [BMI= body weight (kg)/length $(m)^2$], and it is an indirect measure of soft tissue and inferentially of fat accumulation.

At birth, recognition of any growth abnormalities or intrauterine malnutrition is of utmost importance for prognostic purposes and in clinical practice. The so-called neonatal anthropometric charts or curves are used whereby graphs represent, at various gestational ages, either the percentile values or the mean and standard deviation of anthropometric variables considered which are computed on a reference population. A recent commentary defines the characteristics that a reliable anthropometric chart should possess to be of both epidemiological and clinical use (Table 1) (Bertino et al. 2007).

The neonatal anthropometric charts enable the classification of newborns at different gestational ages based on weight as follows:

- SGA – Small for Gestational Age: weight below the 10th centile for GA
- AGA – Appropriate for Gestational Age: weight between 10th and 90th centile for GA
- LGA – Large for Gestational Age: weight above 90th centile for GA

Some authors set down a cut-off of the 3rd and 97th centile among AGA, SGA, LGA newborns or equivalent limits of mean ± 2 SD (Clayton et al. 2007).

The American Academy of Pediatrics and the American College of Obstetricians and Gynecologists (The American Academy of Pediatrics and the American College of Obstetricians and Gynecologist 2007) recognize three groups of GA and define neonates as follows:

- Preterm: born before 37 completed weeks (less than 259 days)
- Full term: born between 37 and 41 weeks + 6 days (from 259 to 293 days)
- Postterm: born 42 weeks of GA (294 or more days)

As a consequence, nine different classes of newborns can be defined.

The definition of small, appropriate, and large newborn for GA is based on weight. However, similar classes may be defined considering body length and head circumference, so that at every GA, newborns can be defined as having small, appropriate, and large body length or head circumference.

Consideration of weight, body length, and head circumference traditionally allows identification, among the heterogeneous group of SGA newborns, those infants who are symmetrical (or proportionate) or asymmetrical (or disproportionate) (Brar and Rutherford 1988).

Symmetrical SGA newborns have reduced weight, body length, and head circumference. The insult leading to reduced growth occurs early in pregnancy, during the phase of growth primarily characterized by cellular hyperplasia, with consequent reduction in cell number (hypoplasia) that may limit the subsequent catch-up of organ and tissue growth (Vrachnis et al. 2006; Singer et al. 1991).

Asymmetrical SGA newborns have reduced weight, with normal or less reduced body length and head circumference. The insult, leading to reduced growth occurs later, interfering with the delivery of oxygen and nutrition during the phase of prevalent cellular hypertrophy, resulting in reduced cell size (hypotrophy), with the possibility of subsequent catch-up growth (Vrachnis et al. 2006; Singer et al. 1991). The weight deficit is principally due to a reduction in fat deposition, particularly during the third trimester of pregnancy. The disproportion is due to the redistribution of the blood flow, which occurs in these cases in the fetus, with preferential perfusion of the brain, heart, and adrenal glands to the detriment of other organs, such as the liver, spleen, kidneys, thymus, and adipose tissue, whose growth is more compromised not only as regards the brain but also body length (Barker and Hanson 2004). In the case of late noxa, the biggest reduction in fetal weight growth compared to body length may also be explained by the different dynamics of their intrauterine growth: the velocity peak of length growth, about the 20th week, occurs earlier than the peak of weight growth (Tanner 1989; Bertino et al. 1996). At six months of pregnancy the fetus reaches 70% of its full-term length but only 25% of its weight.

These newborns, once defined "dysmature," often seem to have clinical signs of intrauterine malnutrition, an "old man" appearance, wrinkled and hypoelastic skin, easily liftable and pliable skinfolds, poorly represented subcutaneous tissue, hypotrophic muscular mass, and thin umbilical cord. When meconium is passed in utero, there is a yellow-green staining of fingernails, skin, and umbilical cord (Fig. 6). Thanks to better prenatal diagnosis and management of fetal growth restriction, the newborns with all these features are uncommon nowadays. The main differences between symmetrical and asymmetrical SGA newborns are presented in Table 2.

Some studies have reassessed the distinction between proportionate and disproportionate SGA newborns. It has been suggested that these two classes represent a continuum rather than distinct classes (Todros et al. 1996; Kramer et al. 1989) and that both disproportionate and proportionate fetal growth restriction may start early in pregnancy (17–19 weeks of gestation) (Rasmussen et al. 2006). These observations lead to a partial reconsideration of causes, timing, and risk of symmetric or asymmetric IUGR. Of course recognizing specific underlying causes of reduced fetal growth may be more important than evaluating body proportionality at birth in predicting short- and long-term outcomes of SGA children.

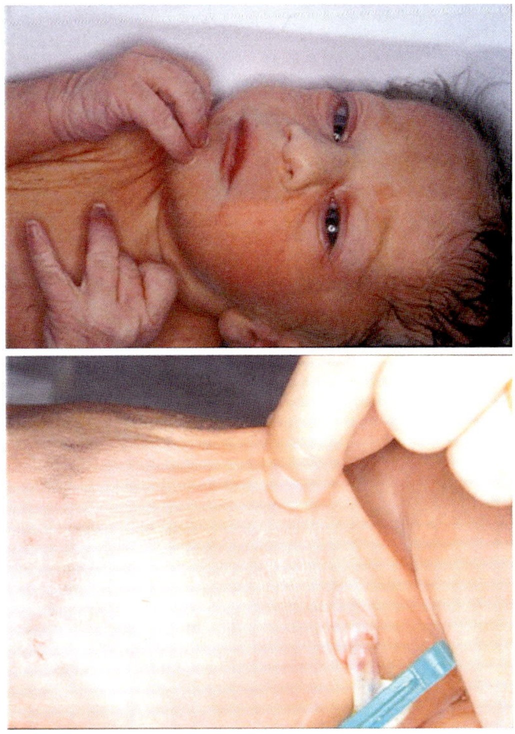

Fig. 6 Wrinkled and hypoelastic skin, easily liftable, and pliable skinfolds in a IUGR newborn

In contrast with the usual assessment based solely on weight, a recent paper suggests to classify newborns as proportionately or disproportionately developed and infants as stunted (short length for age, reflecting linear growth restriction) or wasted (low weight for length, or low BMI for age, often reflecting recent weight loss). Although newborn stunting and wasting share some common determinants, they are distinct phenotypes with their own risk factors and neonatal prognoses. This distinction could help to prioritize preventive interventions and focus the management of fetal undernutrition (Victora 2015).

Growth of the fetus relative to the placenta also seems to be important. Babies born small but with a relatively large placenta are less likely to show catch-up growth in the 18 months after birth and

Table 2 Symmetrical and asymmetrical SGA newborns (Sources: Vrachnis et al. (2006), Rosenberg (2008), Halliday (2009))

	Symmetric (20–30%)	Asymmetric (70–80%)
Onset of fetal growth restriction	Early in gestation	Late in gestation (late second trimester or third trimester)
Pathophysiology	Impaired cell hyperplasia Reduced cell number	Impaired cell hypertrophy Reduced cell size
Anthropometry	Small birth weight, length, and head circumference; normal ponderal index	Small birth weight, but relative sparing of length and head circumference growth; low ponderal index
Major clinical problems	Malformations, congenital infections, increased risk of postnatal neurological and growth impairment	Asphyxia, meconium aspiration syndrome, hypoglycemia, polycythemia. Increased risk of type 2 diabetes
Causes	• Genetic disorders and syndromes • Congenital infections • Teratogens exposure • Substance abuse, fetal alcohol syndrome • Constitutional healthy SGA without IUGR	• Impaired uteroplacental function (i.e., preeclampsia, chronic hypertension, long standing maternal diabetes) • Maternal disease (i.e., renal or heart disease, collagen vascular disease, anemia) • Maternal malnutrition • Environmental factors (i.e., high altitude) • Multiple pregnancy • Substance abuse

have an increased risk of hypertension in adult life (Casey 2008).

9.6 Neonatal Outcome

9.6.1 Mortality

Small for gestational age newborns, both preterm and term, have an increased perinatal mortality risk (Pallotto and Kilbride 2006; Vashevnik et al. 2007). A recent paper has demonstrated that the increased risk of neonatal and infant mortality observed in late preterm (34–36 weeks) and early term (37–38 weeks) SGA infants persists even when infants dying of congenital anomalies are excluded. In addition to congenital conditions, birth asphyxia and infections have a relevant role in neonatal mortality whereas sudden infant death syndrome contributes to infant mortality (Pulver et al. 2009). Some other data have indicated that birth weight is the predominant factor independently affecting neonatal mortality as well as risk for low Apgar score and neonatal sepsis during NICU stay (Mamopoulos et al. 2015).

A higher mortality rate is reported in SGA preterm infants with abnormal (absent or reversed end-diastolic flow) umbilical artery Doppler velocimetry (Shand et al. 2009).

9.6.2 Asphyxia

Transient diminished placental blood flow during labor is poorly tolerated by growth-restricted fetuses. Intrauterine chronic hypoxia and limited carbohydrate reserves as a consequence of placental insufficiency predispose to perinatal asphyxia SGA neonates more than AGA newborns. As a result, there is also an increased risk of all clinical sequelae of perinatal asphyxia (Rosenberg 2008).

9.6.3 Infections

Recent studies suggest possible interactions between immunological function and nutritional status. Thymic atrophy and prolonged impairment of cell immunity have been found in SGA infants and animal models of intrauterine growth retardation. These subjects also have a more pronounced hypogammaglobulinemia compared with AGA infants (Bartels et al. 2007). Neutropenia occurs frequently in infants born to mothers with preeclampsia (Snijders et al. 1993). In a recent paper, lower counts of leukocytes, total neutrophils, immature neutrophils, lymphocytes, and monocytes were detected in SGA infants not related to maternal preeclampsia (median birthweight 583 g) suggesting that IUGR may act as an independent factor for lower counts of different leukocytes in very immature preterm infants (Wirbelauer et al. 2010). All these aspects result in an increased risk of neonatal infections.

9.6.4 Coagulation Disorders

The hepatic dysfunction that results from chronic intrauterine hypoxia may lead to a reduction in vitamin-K dependent factors and thrombocytopenia. Such disorders are usually transient and easily corrected. Only occasionally severe bleeding, such as pulmonary hemorrhage, has been reported (Halliday 2009). In a recent study, prolonged PT and INR were observed in full-term healthy SGA neonates, indicating a predisposition to hemorrhagic events. However, the newborns included in the study did not appear to have any clinical symptoms of altered hemostasis (Mitsiakos et al. 2009).

9.6.5 Thermoregulation

SGA infants are at increased risk of hypothermia as a consequence of their higher brain weight and body surface area in relation to weight as well as to their lower subcutaneous adipose tissue stores, including depleted brown fat reserves (Yu and Upadhyay 2004).

9.6.6 Hypoglycemia

Reduced hepatic and skeleton muscle glycogen stores (the predominant source of glucose in the first hours after birth) and impaired glycogenolysis and gluconeogenesis are the main causes of hypoglycemia in IUGR infants. In addition, growth-restricted infants have limited fat stores and do not effectively oxidize free fatty acids and triglycerides (Sabel et al. 1982). The risk of hypoglycemia is greater during the first few days of life when the newborn must adapt to extrauterine life without the placental source of nutrients, but in some cases it may persist for weeks (Halliday 2009; Pallotto et al. 2004; Rozance 2014).

9.6.7 Polycytemia

Chronic fetal hypoxia results in increased erythropoietin production and release by the fetal kidney, with consequent excessive blood red cells production. Besides, a shift of blood from the placental compartment to the fetus during labour or a period of fetal asphyxia constitutes important causes of polycythemia in IUGR fetuses (Sarkar and Rosenkrantz 2008). Polycythemia contributes to the increased risk of pathologies such as hypoglycemia, hyperbilirubinemia, and NEC.

9.7 Respiratory Distress Syndrome (RDS) and Bronchopulmonary Dysplasia (BPD)

The common opinion that the intrauterine stress associated with IUGR enhances lung maturation has been challenged in some papers reporting that the incidence of RDS is inversely correlated with birth weight and gestational age (McIntire et al. 1999) and that growth-restricted infants may have the same (Piper et al. 1996) or a higher (McIntire et al. 1999; Bernstein et al. 2000; Peacock et al. 2013) incidence of RDS than AGA newborns of the same gestational age.

A higher BPD incidence has also been reported in IUGR preterm infants (Aucott et al. 2004; Gortner et al. 1999; Lal et al. 2003; Regev et al. 2003; Sharma et al. 2004; Soudée et al. 2014). BPD has a multifactorial etiology, and there are several hypotheses about its physiopathology in SGA including abnormal intrauterine lung development (Lal et al. 2003), oxidative injury in utero, more severe early lung disease with subsequent ventilator-induced lung injury, and fetal or neonatal systemic inflammatory response due to chronic hypoxia (Soudée et al. 2014; Kinsella et al. 2006).

9.7.1 Retinopathy of Prematurity (ROP)

It has been reported that SGA infants have an increased risk of developing ROP (Dhaliwal et al. 2009; Lundgren et al. 2014).

Changes in organ development due to fetal hypoxemia, nutrient restriction, and alterated endocrine environment can all contribute to the pathogenesis (McMillen et al. 2001). SGA infants are often sicker than their AGA peers, requiring more intensive and prolonged hospital care (Yu and Upadhyay 2004). They are therefore more likely to require supplementary oxygen, which is a well-documented risk factor for ROP. A lower serum concentration of insulin-like growth factor 1, documented in SGA infants, may as well play a role (Smith 2005).

9.7.2 Necrotizing Enterocolitis (NEC)

Infants who are growth-restricted in utero are considered as having a higher risk of developing NEC, especially if there has been antenatal detection of absent or reversed end-diastolic flow velocities in Doppler studies of fetal aorta or umbilical artery (Dorling et al. 2005; Ree et al. 2014). The underlying mechanism is unclear, but increasing thoracic aorta and umbilical artery resistance may be associated with alterations in blood flow in the viscera, particularly in the intestine and in the liver. Abnormalities of bowel blood flow persist postnatally, with some recovery during the first week of life, providing justification for a delayed and careful introduction of enteral feeding (Dorling et al. 2005). Early postnatal evaluation of superior mesenteric artery blood flow may also be used to identify infants at increased risk of developing NEC (Murdoch et al. 2006; Bora et al. 2009; Bozzetti et al. 2013).

It is common practice in neonatal intensive care units to delay enteral feeding administration for these infants. Recent trials, however, have shown that early enteral feeding in IUGR infants is safe and that human milk exerts a protective role against NEC.

9.8 Long-Term Outcome

9.8.1 Postnatal Growth Impairment

Most term children born SGA experience catch-up growth and achieve a normal adult height, above −2 SD. Approximately 10% of them remain shorter than peers born AGA (Clayton et al. 2007; Simon et al. 2008). Catch-up growth is typically an early postnatal process. Term SGA infants usually experience a period of accelerated linear growth during the first 12 months of life (Saenger et al. 2007) and in most cases catch-up growth is complete by two years of age (Clayton et al. 2007; Saenger et al. 2007). It is has been suggested that SGA children aged 2–4 years with no evidence of catch-up growth and heights less than −2.5 SD should be referred for endocrinological evaluation and could be eligible for GH treatment (Clayton et al. 2007). The preterm SGA infants can take 4 or more years to achieve heights in a normal range (Gibson et al. 2000).

The majority of preterm infants show a postnatal growth deficit at the time of hospital discharge, the so-called Extra Uterine Growth Restriction (EUGR). There is no consensus among neonatologists regarding the best way to define EUGR. At present, a definition based on the negative change of SDS from birth to term corrected age is probably the most appropriate because age at discharge could be biased by different discharge policies over time and between centers. The EUGR is largely due to inadequate postnatal nutrient intake as well as postnatal morbidities, and it increases with the decrease of gestational age at birth (Wit et al. 2006; Bertino et al. 2009). Studies demonstrate that premature infants with EUGR also have metabolic abnormalities similar to those observed in term SGA children and these occur irrespectively of whether they are SGA or AGA at birth (Hofman et al. 2006). Approximately 10% of very preterm children have heights below −2 SD at 4–5 years of age.

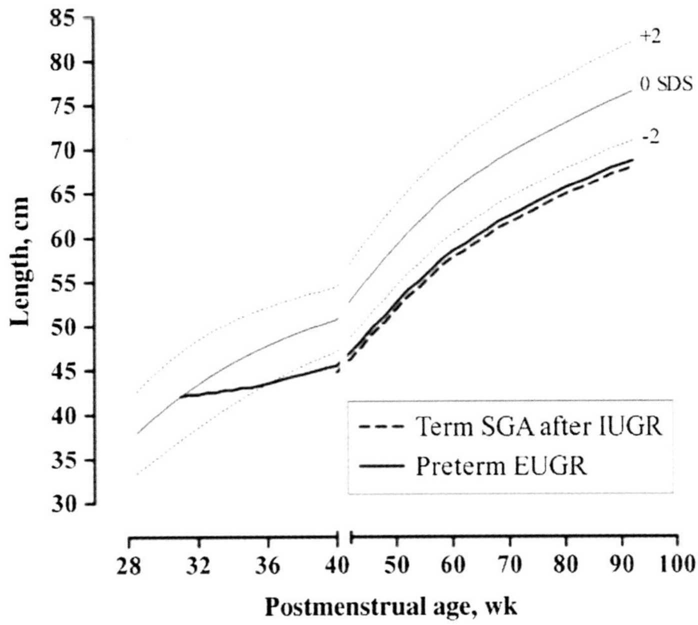

Fig. 7 Growth of a term SGA infant after IUGR and of a preterm AGA infant with EUGR (Reproduced with permission from "Pediatrics", Vol. 117, Pages e793-5, Copyright © 2006 by the AAP)

This percentage is similar to that of term SGA infants who do not show postnatal catch-up growth (Wit et al. 2006) (Fig. 7). SGA term infants suffer from an adverse fetal environment during the last trimester of pregnancy, whereas very preterm infants suffer from an adverse postnatal environment during the first three months, a time biologically equivalent to the third trimester of fetal life. Considering these similarities, an expert group has recently suggested that the indication of GH therapy should be expanded to preterm children with EUGR who failed to normalize over time (Wit et al. 2006). Several common comorbidities of prematurity are significantly associated with postnatal growth restriction including medical or surgical NEC, gastrointestinal perforation, and severe retinopathy of prematurity. These results should help clinicians to identify those infants at highest risk of adverse growth outcomes and work to further improve these outcomes (Griffin et al. 2015).

9.8.2 Neurological Outcome

There is an increasing evidence that being born SGA is independently associated with mild to moderate learning difficulties in childhood and adolescence, lower psychological and intellectual performance in young adulthood, low social competence and behavior problems when compared with AGA infants of the same gestational age (Lundgren and Tuvemo 2008; Walker and Marlow 2008; Levine et al. 2015).

A recent review suggests the association between cerebral redistribution based on middle cerebral artery Doppler indices and poorer neurodevelopmental outcome supporting the growing evidence that there is a need to reevaluate whether cerebral redistribution should be used as a criterion for delivering late preterm and term SGA or growth restricted babies, even in the absence of abnormal Umbilical artery Doppler (Meher et al. 2015). The most important predictor of subnormal performance is the absence of catch-up growth in height and/or head circumference (Clayton et al. 2007; Rosenberg 2008). SGA children who developed catch-up growth were shown to have completed successfully higher school grades and to get higher mean intelligence quotiens scores compared to those who fail to develop catch-up growth or to those with steady growth or to children with early catch-down (Varella and Moss 2015).

Long-term exclusive breastfeeding could help to prevent some of the neurological sequelae of being born SGA. Overfeeding with enriched formula could accelerate growth, but it does not seem to be an advantage for the intellectual development and could be a drawback in terms of metabolic and cardiovascular risks (Morley et al. 2004; Agostoni 2005). It has been suggested that GH treatment may improve IQ in short SGA children, but additional data are required (Clayton et al. 2007; Lundgren and Tuvemo 2008).

The association between cerebral palsy and IUGR which has been observed in both term and preterm infants may be due to placental insufficiency: reduced oxygen or nutrient delivery to the fetus may have adverse effects on brain development and differentiation (Halliday 2009; Lundgren and Tuvemo 2008).

9.8.3 Metabolic Risk

Since the late 1980s, epidemiological studies have shown that impaired intrauterine growth is associated with later development of the metabolic syndrome or one of its components (insulin resistance, hyperinsulinemia, impaired glucose tolerance or diabetes mellitus type 2, dyslipidemia, arterial hypertension, and obesity). Additionally, some other morbidities have been connected with the syndrome, such as hypercoagulability, nonalcoholic fatty liver disease, renal dysfunction (micro- or macroalbuminuria), polycystic ovary syndrome, endothelial dysfunction, and atherosclerosis leading to increased cardiovascular morbidity and mortality (Varda and Gregoric 2009).

A number of mechanisms for the development of metabolic syndrome have been proposed. One hypothesis is that the fetus adapts to an adverse intrauterine environment "reprogramming" the endocrine-metabolic status, with short-term survival benefits. This process consists mainly of insulin resistance and of reduced insulin secretion due to impaired development of beta cells. As a result, blood glucose concentration can be maintained for the benefit of brain development at the expense of less glucose transported to peripheral tissue (e.g., muscle and fat) (Barker et al. 2005). This reprogramming is adequate to maintaining gluco-homeostasis in the short term, when intrauterine nutrient supply is deficient, but it predisposes the child to metabolic syndrome in later life, when nutrient supplies are adequate (Halliday 2009; Saenger et al. 2007). Moreover, SGA newborns show postnatal accelerated growth with rapid weight gain, associated with later obesity, which is per se associated with the metabolic syndrome (Maiorana et al. 2007; Nobili et al. 2008). Overweight former SGA children have an increased risk of metabolic syndrome compared with overweight former AGA children (Reinehr et al. 2009). On the other hand, it is known that poor postnatal growth is associated with later poor neurocognitive outcome (Yeung 2006).

The challenge of neonatal nutrition is the achievement of a "healthy catch-up growth" of IUGR subjects, based on a nutritional strategy that improves neurodevelopmental outcome while minimizing long-term metabolic and cardiovascular adverse effects (Nobili et al. 2008).

9.8.4 Chronic Kidney Disease

As previously described, when resources in utero are restricted their allocation to the development of the kidney is restricted to guarantee appropriate development of the brain and heart (Barker and Hanson 2004). The result is a diminished number of nephrons which predisposes these subjects to albuminuria and to the risk of developing chronic kidney disease, as well as of hypertension. In parallel, metabolic syndrome and type 2 diabetes may contribute to renal complications (Koleganova et al. 2009).

9.8.5 Puberty and Reproductive Function

In girls born SGA most studies have shown an increased risk of earlier pubertal development or normal timing, but with rapid progression (Hernández and Mericq 2008). These aberrations may result in reduced adult stature. Today there are insufficient data to define the risk of ovarian dysfunction, reduced fertility, or early menopause in females born SGA. On the contrary, most boys born SGA have normal pubertal timing, but often heights below the target (Hernández and Mericq 2008) Information about the influence of fetal growth on gonadal function is scarce, but most studies have shown that low birth weight is a common risk factor for testicular cancer, hypospadia, and cryptorchidism (Main et al. 2006).

References

Agostoni C (2005) Small-for-gestational-age infants need dietary quality more than quantity for their development: the role of human milk. Acta Paediatr 94:827–829

Aucott SW, Donohue PK, Northington FJ (2004) Increased morbidity in severe early intrauterine growth restriction. J Perinatol 24:435–440

Bakalis S, Silva M, Akolekar R, Poon LC, Nicolaides KH (2015) Prediction of small-for-gestational-age neonates: screening by fetal biometry at 30–34 weeks. Ultrasound Obstet Gynecol 45:551–558

Bardien N, Whitehead CL, Tong S, Ugoni A, McDonald S, Walker SP (2016) Placental insufficiency in fetuses that slow in growth but are born appropriate for gestational age: a prospective longitudinal study. PLoS One 11:e0142788

Barker DJP (2006) Adult consequences of fetal growth restriction. Clin Obstet Gynecol 49:270–283

Barker DJ, Hanson MA (2004) Altered regional blood flow in the fetus: the origins of cardiovascular disease? Acta Paediatr 93:1559–1560

Barker DJ, Osmond C (1986) Infant mortality, childhood nutrition, and ischaemic heart disease in England and Wales. Lancet 1:1077–1081

Barker DJ, Osmond C, Forsén TJ, Kajantie E, Eriksson JG (2005) Trajectories of growth among children who have coronary events as adults. N Engl J Med 353:1802–1809

Bartels DB, Schwab F, Geffers C, Poets CF, Gastmeier P (2007) Nosocomial infection in small for gestational age newborns with birth weight <1500 g: a multicentre analysis. Arch Dis Child Fetal Neonatal Ed 92: F449–F453

Baschat AA, Cosmi E, Bilardo CM, Wolf H, Berg C, Rigano S, Germer U, Moyano D, Turan S, Hartung J, Bhide A, Müller T, Bower S, Nicolaides KH, Thilaganathan B, Gembruch U, Ferrazzi E, Hecher K, Galan HL, Harman CR (2007) Predictors of neonatal outcome in early-onset placental dysfunction. Obstet Gynecol 109:253–261

Baschat AA, Viscardi RM, Hussey-Gardner B, Hashmi N, Harman C (2009) Infant neurodevelopment following fetal growth restriction: relationship with antepartum surveillance parameters. Ultrasound Obstet Gynecol 33:44–50

Baskett TF, Nagele F (2000) Naegele's rule: a reappraisal. BJOG 107:1433–1435

Bernstein IM, Horbar JD, Badger GJ, Ohlsson A, Golan A (2000) Morbidity and mortality among very-low-birth-weight neonates with intrauterine growth restriction. The Vermont Oxford Network. Am J Obstet Gynecol 182:198e206

Bertino E, Di Battista E, Bossi A, Pagliano M, Fabris C, Aicardi G, Milani S (1996) Fetal growth velocity: kinetic, clinical, and biological aspects. Arch Dis Child 74:F10–F15

Bertino E, Milani S, Fabris C, De Curtis M (2007) Neonatal anthropometric charts: what they are, what they are not. Arch Dis Child Fetal Neonatal Ed 92:7–10

Bertino E, Coscia A, Boni L, Rossi C, Martano C, Giuliani F, Fabris C, Spada E, Zolin A, Milani S (2009) Weight growth velocity of very low birth weight infants: role of gender, gestational age and major morbidities. Early Hum Dev 85:339–347

Blaas HG, Eik-Nes SH, Bremnes JB (1998) The growth of the human embryo. A longitudinal biometric assessment from 7 to 12 weeks of gestation. Ultrasound Obstet Gynecol 12:346–354

Boers KE, Vijgen SM, Bijlenga D, van der Post JA, Bekedam DJ, Kwee A, van der Salm PC, van Pampus MG, Spaanderman ME, de Boer K, Duvekot JJ, Bremer HA, Hasaart TH, Delemarre FM, Bloemenkamp KW, van Meir CA, Willekes C, Wijnen EJ, Rijken M, le Cessie S, Roumen FJ, Thornton JG, van Lith JM, Mol BW, Scherjon SA, DIGITAT study group (2010) Induction versus expectant monitoring for intrauterine growth restriction at term: randomized equivalence trial (DIGITAT). BMJ 341:c7087

Boers KE, van Wyk L, van der Post JA, Kwee A, van Pampus MG, Spaanderdam ME, Duvekot JJ, Bremer HA, Delemarre FM, Bloemenkamp KW, de Groot CJ, Willekes C, Rijken M, Roumen FJ, Thornton JG, van Lith JM, Mol BW, le Cessie S, Scherjon SA, DIGITAT Study Group (2012) Neonatal morbidity after induction vs expectant monitoring in intrauterine growth restriction at term: a subanalysis of the DIGITAT RCT. Am J Obstet Gynecol 206:344 e1–344 e7

Bora R, Mukhopadhyay K, Saxena AK, Jain V, Narang A (2009) Prediction of feed intolerance and necrotizing enterocolitis in neonates with absent end diastolic flow in umbilical artery and the correlation of feed intolerance with postnatal superior mesenteric artery flow. J Matern Fetal Neonatal Med 22:1092–1096

Boulet SL, Alexander GR, Salihu HM, Kirby RS, Carlo WA (2006) Fetal growth risk curves: defining levels of fetal growth restriction by neonatal death risk. Am J Obstet Gynecol 195:1571–1577

Bozzetti V, Tagliabue PE, Visser GH, van Bel F, Gazzolo D (2013) Feeding issues in IUGR preterm infants. Early Hum Dev 89(S2):S21–S23

Brar HS, Rutherford SE (1988) Classification of intrauterine growth retardation. Semin Perinatol 12:2–10

Cameron N (2004) Measuring techniques and instruments. In: Nicoletti I, Benso L, Gilli G (eds) Physiological and pathological auxology. Edizioni Centro Studi Auxologici, Firenze, pp 117–159

Campbell S, Thoms A (1977) Ultrasound measurement of the fetal head to abdomen circumference ratio in the assessment of growth retardation. Br J Obstet Gynaecol 84:165–174

Casey PH (2008) Growth of low birth weight preterm children. Semin Perinatol 32:20–27

Clausson B, Cnattingius S, Axelsson O (1998) Preterm and term births of small for gestational age infants: a population-based study of risk factors among nulliparous women. Br J Obstet Gynaecol 105(9):1011–1017

Clayton PE, Cianfarani S, Czernichow P, Johannsson G, Rapaport R, Rogol A (2007) Management of the child born small for gestational age through to adulthood: a consensus statement of the International Societies of Pediatric ndocrinology and the Growth Hormone Research Society. J Clin Endocrinol Metab 92:804–810

Cruz-Martinez R, Savchev S, Cruz-Lemini M, Mendez A, Gratacos E, Figueras F (2015) Clinical utility of third-trimester uterine artery Doppler in the prediction of brain hemodynamic deterioration and adverse perinatal outcome in small-for-gestational-age fetuses. Ultrasound Obstet Gynecol 45:273–278

David C, Gabrielli S, Pilu G, Bovicelli L (1995) The head-to-abdomen circumference ratio: a reappraisal. Ultrasound Obstet Gynecol 5:256–259

De Jong CL, Francis A, Van Geijn HP, Gardosi J (2000) Customized fetal weight limits for antenatal detection of fetal growth restriction. Ultrasound Obstet Gynecol 15:36–40

Dhaliwal CA, Fleck BW, Wright E, Graham C, McIntosh N (2009) Retinopathy of premature in small- for gestational age infants compared with those of appropriate size for gestational age. Arch Dis Child Fetal Neonatal Ed 94:F193–F195

Dijxhoorn MJ, Visser GH, Touwen BC, Huisjes HJ (1987) Apgar score, meconium and acidaemia at birth in small-for-gestational age infants born at term, and their relation to neonatal neurological morbidity. Br J Obstet Gynaecol 94:873–879

Dorling J, Kempley S, Leaf A (2005) Feeding growth restricted preterm infants with abnormal antenatal Doppler results. Arch Dis Child Fetal Neonatal Ed 90: F359–F363

Eixarch E, Meler E, Iraola A, Illa M, Crispi F, Hernandez-Andrade E, Gratacos E, Figueras F (2008) Neurodevelopmental outcome in 2-year-old infants who were small-for-gestational-age term fetuses with cerebral blood flow redistribution. Ultrasound Obstet Gynecol 32:894–899

Engle WA (2011) Morbidity and mortality in late preterm and early term newborns: a continuum. Clin Perinatol 38:493–516

Fadigas C, Saiid Y, Gonzalez R, Poon LC, Nicolaides KH (2015) Prediction of small-for-gestational-age neonates: screening by fetal biometry at 35–37 weeks. Ultrasound Obstet Gynecol 45:559–565

Figueras F, Gratacos E (2014) Stage-based approach to the management of fetal growth restriction. Prenat Diagn 34:655–659

Garite TJ, Clark R, Thorp JA (2004) Intrauterine growth restriction increases morbidity and mortality among premature neonates. Am J Obstet Gynecol 191:481–487

Gibson AT, Carney S, Cavazzoni E, Wales JK (2000) Neonatal and postnatal growth. Horm Res 53:42–49

Gortner L, Wauer RR, Stock GJ, Reiter HL, Reiss I, Jorch G, Hentschel R, Hieronimi G (1999) Neonatal outcome in small for gestational age infants: do they really better? J Perinat Med 27:484e9

Griffin IJ, Tancredi DJ, Bertino E, Lee HC, Profit J (2015) Postnatal growth failure in very low birthweight infants born between 2005 and 2012. Arch Dis Child Fetal Neonatal Ed 101:F1–F6

Guellec I, Lapillonne A, Renolleau S, Charlaluk ML, Roze JC, Marret S, Vieux R, Monique K, Ancel PY, EPIPAGE Study Group (2011) Neurologic outcomes at school age in very preterm infants born with severe or mild growth restriction. Pediatrics 127:e883–e891

Halliday HL (2009) Neonatal management and long-term sequelae. Best Pract Res Clin Obstet Gynaecol 23:871–880

Hansen AK, Wisborg K, Uldbjerg N, Henriksen TB (2008) Risk of respiratory morbidity in term infants delivered by elective caesarean section: cohort study. BMJ 336:85–87

Hanson MA, Gluckman PD (2014) Early developmental conditioning of later health and disease: physiology or pathophysiology? Physiol Rev 94:1027–1076

Hernández MI, Mericq V (2008) Impact of being born small for gestational age on onset and progression of puberty. Best Pract Res Clin Endocrinol Metab 22:463–476

Hofman PL, Regan F, Cutfield WS (2006) Prematurity-another example of perinatal metabolic programming? Horm Res 66:33–39

Jarvis S, Glinianaia SV, Torrioli MG, Platt MJ, Miceli M, Jouk PS, Johnson A, Hutton J, Hemming K, Hagberg G, Dolk H, Chalmers J, Surveillance of Cerebral Palsy in Europe (SCPE) collaboration of European Cerebral Palsy Registers (2003) Cerebral palsy and intrauterine growth in single births: European collaborative study. Lancet 362:1106–1111

Kalish RB, Thaler HT, Chasen ST, Gupta M, Berman SJ, Rosenwaks Z, Chervenak FA (2004) First- and second-trimester ultrasound assessment of gestational age. Am J Obstet Gynecol 191:975–978

Kanaka-Gantenbein C (2010) Fetal origins of adult diabetes. Ann N Y Acad Sci 1205:99–105

Karsdorp VH, van Vugt JM, van Geijn HP, Kostense PJ, Arduini D, Montenegro N, Todros T (1994) Clinical significance of absent or reversed end-diastolic velocity waveforms in umbilical artery. Lancet 344:1664–1668

Kase BA, Carreno CA, Blackwell SC (2012) Customized estimated fetal weight: a novel antenatal tool to diagnose abnormal fetal growth. Am J Obstet Gynecol 207:218.e1–218.e5

Kinsella JP, Greenough A, Abman SH (2006) Bronchopulmonary dysplasia. Lancet 367:1421–1431

Koleganova N, Piecha G, Ritz E (2009) Prenatal causes of kidney disease. Blood Purif 27:48–52

Kramer MS, Mc Lean FH, Olivier M, Willis DM, Usher RH (1989) Body proportionality and head and length "sparing" in growth-retarded neonates: a critical reappraisal. Pediatrics 84:717–723

Lal MK, Manktelow BN, Draper ES, Field DJ (2003) Chronic lung disease of prematurity and intrauterine growth retardation: a population-based study. Pediatrics 111:483–487

Lees C, Marlow N, Arabin B, Bilardo CM, Brezinka C, Derks JB, Duvekot J, Frusca T, Diemert A, Ferrazzi E, Ganzevoort W, Hecher K, Martinelli P, Ostermayer E, Papageorghiou AT, Schlembach D, Schneider KT, Thilaganathan B, Todros T, van Wassenaer-Leemhuis-A, Valcamonico A, Visser GH, Wolf H, TRUFFLE Group (2013) Perinatal morbidity and mortality in early-onset fetal growth restriction: cohort outcomes of the trial of randomized umbilical and fetal flow in Europe (TRUFFLE). Ultrasound Obstet Gynecol 42:400–408

Lees C, Marlow N, van Wassenaer-Leemhuis A, Arabin B, Bilardo CM, Brezinka C, Calvert S, Derks JB, Diemert A, Duvekot JJ, Ferrazzi E, Frusca T, Ganzevoort W, Hecher K, Martinelli P, Ostermayer E, Papageorghiou AT, Schlembach D, Schneider KTM, Thilaganathan B, Todros T, Valcamonico A, Visser GHA, Wolf H, on behalf of the TRUFFLE Group (2015) The Trial of Randomized Umbilical and Fetal Flow in Europe (TRUFFLE) study: two year neurodevelopmental and intermediate perinatal outcomes. Lancet 385:2162–2172

Lesmes C, Gallo DM, Panaiotova J, Poon LC, Nicolaides KH (2015) Prediction of small-for-gestational-age neonates: screening by fetal biometry at 19–24 weeks. Ultrasound Obstet Gynecol 46:198–207

Levine TA, Grunau RE, McAuliffe FM, Pinnamaneni R, Foran A, Alderdice FA (2015) Early childhood neurodevelopment after intrauterine growth restriction: a systematic review. Pediatrics 135:126–141

Lindqvist PG, Molin J (2005) Does antenatal identification of small-for-gestational age fetuses significantly improve their outcome? Ultrasound Obstet Gynecol 25:258–264

Lundgren EM, Tuvemo T (2008) Effects of being born small for gestational age on long-term intellectual performance. Best Pract Res Clin Endocrinol Metab 22:477–488

Lundgren P, Kistner A, Andersson EM, Hansen Pupp I, Holmström G, Ley D, Niklasson A, Smith LE, Wu C, Hellström A, Löfqvist C (2014) Low birth weight is a risk factor for severe retinopathy of prematurity depending on gestational age. PLoS One 9:e109460

Lyall F, Robson SC, Bulmer JN (2013) Spiral artery remodeling and trophoblast invasion in preeclampsia and fetal growth restriction: relationship to clinical outcome. Hypertension 62:1046–1054

Main KM, Jensen RB, Asklund C, Høi-Hansen CE, Skakkebaek NE (2006) Low birth weight and male reproductive function. Horm Res 65:116–122

Maiorana A, Del Bianco C, Cianfarani S (2007) Adipose tissue: a metabolic regulator. Potential implications for the metabolic outcome of subjects born Small for Gestational Age (SGA). Rev Diabet Stud 4:134–146

Mamopoulos A, Petousis S, Tsimpanakos J, Masouridou S, Kountourelli K, Margioula-Siarkou C, Papouli M, Rousso D (2015) Birth weight independently affects morbidity and mortality of extremely preterm neonates. J Clin Med Res 7:511–516

Mari G, Hanif F, Treadwell MC, Kruger M (2007) Gestational age at delivery and Doppler waveforms in very preterm intrauterine growth-restricted fetuses as predictors of perinatal mortality. J Ultrasound Med 26:555–559

McCowan LM, Mullen BM, Ritchie K (1987) Umbilical artery flow velocity waveforms and the placental vascular bed. Am J Obstet Gynecol 157:900–902

McIntire DD, Bloom SL, Casey BM, Leveno KJ (1999) Birth weight in relation to morbidity and mortality among newborn infants. N Engl J Med 340:1234–1238

McMillen I, Adams M, Ross J, Coulter CL, Simonetta G, Owens JA, Robinson JS, Edwards LJ (2001) Fetal growth restriction: adaptation and consequences. Reproduction 122:195–204

Meher S, Hernandez-Andrade E, Basheer SN, Lees C (2015) Impact of cerebral redistribution on neurodevelopmental outcome in small for gestational age or growth restricted babies: a systematic review. Ultrasound Obstet Gynecol 46:398–404

Miller HC (1985) Prenatal factors affecting intrauterine growth retardation. Clin Perinatol 12:307–318

Mitsiakos G, Papaioannou G, Papadakis E, Chatziioannidis E, Giougi E, Karagianni P, Evdoridou J, Malindretos P, Athanasiou M, Athanassiadou F, Nikolaidis N (2009) Haemostatic profile of full-term, healthy, small for gestational age neonates. Thromb Res 124:288–291

Morin I, Morin L, Zhang X, Platt RW, Blondel B, Bréart G, Usher R, Kramer MS (2005) Determinants and consequences of discrepancies in menstrual and ultrasonographic gestational age estimates. BJOG 112:145–152

Morley R, Fewtrell MS, Abbott RA, Stephenson T, MacFadyen U, Lucas A (2004) Neurodevelopment in children born small for gestational age: a randomized trial of nutrient-enriched versus standard formula and comparison with a reference breastfed group. Pediatrics 113:515–521

Morsing E, Asard M, Ley D, Stjernqvist K, Marsál K (2011) Cognitive function after intrauterine growth restriction and very preterm birth. Pediatrics 127: e874–e882

Murdoch EM, Sinha AK, Shanmugalingam ST, Smith GC, Kempley ST (2006) Doppler flow velocimetry in the superior mesenteric artery on the first day of life in preterm infants and the risk of neonatal necrotizing enterocolitis. Pediatrics 118:1999–2003

Nakling J, Buhaug H, Backe B (2005) The biologic error in gestational length related to the use of the first day of last menstrual period as a proxy for the start of pregnancy. Early Hum Dev 81:833–839

Nicolaides KH, Bilardo CM, Soothill PW, Campbell S (1988) Absence of end diastolic frequencies in umbilical artery: a sign of fetal hypoxia and acidosis. BMJ 297:1026

Nobili V, Alisi A, Panera N, Agostoni C (2008) Low birth weight and catch-up-growth associated with metabolic syndrome: a ten year systematic review. Pediatr Endocrinol Rev 6:241–247

Olofsson P, Laurini RN, Marsál K (1993) A high uterine artery pulsatility index reflects a defective development of placental bed spiral arteries in pregnancies complicated by hypertension and fetal growth retardation. Eur J Obstet Gynecol Reprod Biol 49:161–168

Oros D, Figueras F, Cruz-Martinez R, Meler E, Munmany M, Gratacos E (2011) Longitudinal changes in uterine, umbilical and fetal cerebral Doppler indices in late-onset small-for-gestational age fetuses. Ultrasound Obstet Gynecol 37:191–195

Pallotto EK, Kilbride HW (2006) Perinatal outcome and later implications of intrauterine growth restriction. Clin Obstet Gynecol 49:257–269

Pallotto EK, Woelnerhanssen B, Putt M (2004) Incidence and risk factors for prolonged hypoglycemia in small for gestational age infants. Abstract, Society for Pediatric and Perinatal Epidemiology

Papageorghiou AT, Ohuma EO, Altman DG, Todros T, Cheikh Ismail L, Lambert A, Jaffer YA, Bertino E, Gravett MG, Purwar M, Noble JA, Pang R, Victora CG, Barros FC, Carvalho M, Salomon LJ, Bhutta ZA, Kennedy SH, Villar J, International Fetal and Newborn Growth Consortium for the 21st Century (INTERGROWTH-21st) (2014) International standards for fetal growth based on serial ultrasound measurements: the Fetal Growth Longitudinal Study of the INTERGROWTH-21st Project. Lancet 384:869–879

Peacock JL, Lo JW, D'Costa W, Calvert S, Marlow N, Greenough A (2013) Respiratory morbidity at follow-up of small-for-gestational age infants born very prematurely. Pediatr Res 73:457–463

Piper JM, Xenakis EM, McFarland M, Elliott BD, Berkus MD, Langer O (1996) Do growth-retarded premature infants have different rates of perinatal morbidity and mortality than appropriately grown premature infants? Obstet Gynecol 87:169–174

Pulver LS, Guest-Warnick G, Stoddard GJ, Byington CL, Young PC (2009) Weight for gestational age affects the mortality of late preterm infants. Pediatrics 123: e1072–e1077

Rasmussen S, Kiserud T, Albrechtsen S (2006) Foetal size and body proportion at 17–19 weeks of gestation and neonatal size, proportion, and outcome. Early Hum Dev 82:683–690

Ree IM, Smits-Wintjens VE, Rijntjes-Jacobs EG, Pelsma IC, Steggerda SJ, Walther FJ, Lopriore E (2014) Necrotizing enterocolitis in small-for-gestational-age neonates: a matched case–control study. Neonatology 105:74–78

Regev RH, Lusky A, Dolfin T, Litmanovitz I, Arnon S, Reichman B, Network IN (2003) Excess mortality and morbidity among small-for-gestational-age premature infants: a population-based study. J Pediatr 143:186–191

Reinehr T, Kleber M, Toschke AM (2009) Small for gestational age status is associated with metabolic syndrome in overweight children. Eur J Endocrinol 160:579–584

Rizzo G, Prefumo F, Ferrazzi E, Zanardini C, Di Martino D, Boito S, Aiello E, Ghi T, SIEOG working group on fetal biometric charts (2016) The effect of fetal sex on customized fetal growth charts. J Matern Fetal Neonatal Med 3:1–8

Rosenberg A (2008) The IUGR newborn. Semin Perinatol 32:219–224

Rozance PJ (2014) Update on neonatal hypoglycemia. Curr Opin Endocrinol Diabetes Obes 21:45–50

Sabel KG, Olegard R, Mellander M, Hildingsson K (1982) Interrelation between fatty acid oxidation and control of gluconeogenic substrates in small for gestational age (SGA) infants with hypoglycemia and with normoglycemia. Acta Paediatr Scand 71:53–61

Saenger P, Czernichow P, Hughes I, Reiter EO (2007) Small for gestational age: short stature and beyond. Endocr Rev 28:219–251

Sarkar S, Rosenkrantz TS (2008) Neonatal polycythemia and hyperviscosity. Semin Fetal Neonatal Med 13:248–255

Savchev S, Figueras F, Cruz-Martinez R, Illa M, Botet F, Gratacos E (2012) Estimated weight centile as a predictor of perinatal outcome in small-for-gestational-age pregnancies with normal fetal and maternal Doppler indices. Ultrasound Obstet Gynecol 39:299–303

Shand AW, Hornbuckle J, Nathan E, Dickinson JE, French NP (2009) Small for gestational age preterm infants and relationship of abnormal umbilical artery Doppler blood flow to perinatal mortality and neurodevelopmental outcomes. Aust N Z J Obstet Gynaecol 49:52–58

Shapiro-Mendoza CK, Tomashek KM, Kotelchuck M, Barfield W, Nannini A, Weiss J, Declercq E (2008) Effect of late-preterm birth and maternal medical conditions on newborn morbidity risk. Pediatrics 121: e223–e232

Sharma P, McKay K, Rosenkrantz TS, Hussain N (2004) Comparisons of mortality and pre-discharge respiratory outcomes in small-for-gestational-age and appropriate-for-gestational-age premature infants. BMC Pediatr 4:9

Simon D, Léger J, Carel JC (2008) Optimal use of growth hormone therapy for maximizing adult height in children born small for gestational age. Best Pract Res Clin Endocrinol Metab 22:525–537

Singer DB, Sung CJ, Wigglesworth JS (1991) Fetal growth and maturation with standards for body and organ development. In: Wigglesworth JS, Singer DB (eds) Textbook of fetal and perinatal pathology. Blackwell, London, pp 11–47

Skuse D, Pickles A, Wolke D, Reilly S (1994) Postnatal growth and mental development: evidence for a "sensitive period". J Child Psychol Psychiatry 35:521–545

Smith LE (2005) IGF-1 and retinopathy of prematurity in the preterm infant. Biol Neonate 88:237–244

Snijders RJ, Abbas A, Melby O, Ireland RM, Nicolaides KH (1993) Fetal plasma erythropoietin concentration in severe growth retardation. Am J Obstet Gynecol 168:615–619

Soothill PW, Ajayi RA, Campbell S, Ross EM, Candy DC, Snijders RM, Nicolaides KH (1992) Relationship between fetal acidemia at cordocentesis and subsequent neurodevelopment. Ultrasound Obstet Gynecol 2:80–83

Soudée S, Vuillemin L, Alberti C, Mohamed D, Becquet O, Farnoux C, Biran V, Baud O (2014) Fetal growth restriction is worse than extreme prematurity for the developing lung. Neonatology 106:304–310

Sovio U, White IR, Dacey A, Pasupathy D, Smith GC (2015) Screening for fetal growth restriction with universal third trimester ultrasonography in nulliparous women in the Pregnancy Outcome Prediction (POP) study: a prospective cohort study. Lancet 386:2089–2097

Tajik P, van Wyk L, Boers KE, le Cessie S, Zafarmand MH, Roumen F, van der Post JA, Porath M, van Pampus MG, Spaanderdam ME, Kwee A, Duvekot JJ, Bremer HA, Delemarre FM, Bloemenkamp KW, de Groot CJ, Willekes C, van Lith JM, Bossuyt PM, Mol BW, Scherjon SA, DIGITAT Study Group (2014) Which intrauterine growth restricted fetuses at term benefit from early labour induction? A secondary analysis of the DIGITAT randomised trial. Eur J Obstet Gynecol Reprod Biol 172:20–25

Tanner JM (1989) Foetus into man, 2nd edn. Castlemead Publication, Welwyn Garden City

The American Academy of Pediatrics and the American College of Obstetricians and Gynecologist (2007) Standard terminology for reporting of reproductive health statistics in the United States. In: Guideline for prenatal care. American Academy of Pediatrics, Elk Grove Village

Thorsell M, Kaijser M, Almström H, Andolf E (2008) Expected day of delivery from ultrasound dating versus last menstrual period–obstetric outcome when dates mismatch. BJOG 115:585–589

Todros T, Plazzotta C, Pastorin L (1996) Body proportionality of the small-for-date fetus: is it related to aetiological factors? Early Hum Dev 45:1–9

Todros T, Sciarrone A, Piccoli E, Guiot C, Kaufmann P, Kingdom J (1999) Umbilical Doppler waveforms and placental villous angiogenesis in pregnancies complicated by fetal growth restriction. Obstet Gynecol 93:499–503

Torrance HL, Bloemen MC, Mulder EJ, Nikkels PG, Derks JB, de Vries LS, Visser GH (2010) Predictors of outcome at 2 years of age after early intrauterine growth restriction. Ultrasound Obstet Gynecol 36:171–177

Tyrrell S, Obaid AH, Lilford RJ (1989) Umbilical artery Doppler velocimetry as a predictor of fetal hypoxia and acidosis at birth. Obstet Gynecol 74:332–337

van Wyk L, Boers KE, van der Post JA, van Pampus MG, van Wassenaer AG, van Baar AL, Spaanderdam ME, Becker JH, Kwee A, Duvekot JJ, Bremer HA, Delemarre FM, Bloemenkamp KW, de Groot CJ, Willekes C, Roumen FJ, van Lith JM, Mol BW, le Cessie S, Scherjon SA, DIGITAT Study Group (2012) Effects on (neuro developmental and behavioral outcome at 2 years of age of induced labor compared with expectant management in intrauterine growth-restricted infants: long-term outcomes of the DIGITAT trial. Am J Obstet Gynecol 206:406 e1–406 e7

Varda NM, Gregoric A (2009) Metabolic syndrome in the pediatric population: a short overview. Pediatric Rev 1:e1

Varella MH, Moss WJ (2015) Early growth patterns are associated with intelligence quotient scores in children born small-for-gestational age. Early Hum Dev 91:491–497

Vashevnik S, Walker S, Permezel M (2007) Stillbirths and neonatal deaths in appropriate, small and large birthweight for gestational age fetuses. Aust N Z J Obstet Gynaecol 47:302–306

Victora CG (2015) Anthropometric characterization of impaired fetal growth. Risk factors for and prognosis of newborns with stunting or wasting. JAMA Pediatr 169(7):e151431

Vrachnis N, Botsis D, Iliodromiti Z (2006) The fetus that is small for gestationel age. N Y Acad Sci 1092:304–309

Walker DM, Marlow N (2008) Neurocognitive outcome following fetal growth restriction. Arch Dis Child Fetal Neonatal Ed 93:F322–F325

Wirbelauer J, Thomas W, Rieger L, Speer CP (2010) Intrauterine growth retardation in preterm infants ≤32 weeks of gestation is associated with low white blood cell counts. Am J Perinatol 27(10):819–824

Wit JM, Finken MJ, Rijken M, de Zegher F (2006) Preterm growth restraint: a paradigm that unifies intrauterine growth retardation and preterm extrauterine growth retardation and has implications for the small-for-gestational-age indication in growth hormone therapy. Pediatrics 117:e793–e795

Yeung MY (2006) Postnatal growth, neurodevelopment and altered adiposity after preterm birth–from a clinical nutrition perspective. Acta Paediatr 95:909–917

Yu V, Upadhyay A (2004) Neonatal management of the growth-restricted infant. Semin Fetal Neonatal Med 9:403–409

10 Late Preterm Infants at Risk for Short-Term and Long-Term Morbidity and Mortality

Avroy A. Fanaroff

Contents

Abstract
Late preterm infants (LPIs) represent the largest subpopulation of preterm infants with significant short and long-term morbidity and even mortality compared to term infants. During birth hospitalization, the major causes of morbidity encountered in LPIs include

A. A. Fanaroff (✉)
Case Western Reserve University School of Medicine
Rainbow Babies and Children's Hospital, Cleveland, OH, USA
e-mail: avroy.fanaroff@uhhospitals.org

G. Buonocore et al. (eds.), *Neonatology*,
https://doi.org/10.1007/978-3-319-29489-6_159

transient tachypnea of the newborn, respiratory distress syndrome, persistent pulmonary hypertension of the newborn, respiratory failure, apnea, temperature instability, jaundice, hypoglycemia, and feeding difficulties, which result in a longer hospital stay and higher medical costs. In addition, LPIs have a higher prevalence of congenital malformations which may contribute to an increased mortality relative to term infants. There is a twofold risk of rehospitalization for LPIs compared with term infants. Hyperbilirubinemia, feeding difficulties, poor weight gain, dehydration, and apnea are the most common clinical conditions requiring hospital readmission during the first week of postnatal life. Respiratory and gastrointestinal disorders are the most common causes of late readmission during the first year of life. Evidence suggests that LPIs are at increased risk of adverse neurodevelopmental outcomes and academic difficulties up to 7 years of age in comparison to term infants.

10.1 Salient Points

- Late preterm infants are the commonest cause of prematurity and account for the bulk of preterm births
- Prevention of late preterm births provide the best opportunity to reduce the rates of preterm births
- Late preterm births have significant in hospital morbidity and a higher mortality when compared to term infants. The infant mortality rate for late preterm infants is at least threefold greater than that of term infants.
- Late preterm infants have significant cognitive and behavioral problems later in life. These problems are independent of maternal IQ, residential setting, and socio-demographics.
- Strategies to decrease the morbidity and mortality associated with late preterm infants in addition to prevention of late preterm delivery, include management to prevent and treat the associated complications of late preterm birth during birth hospitalization and post-birth discharge.

10.2 Introduction

Late preterm births were the first group of premature infants who neonatologists treated successfully. Over time with the very low birth weight infants surviving and demanding many resources, near-term infants were relatively ignored and unfortunately were no longer considered to be of high risk by many health care providers. The resurgence of interest in this group, and their renaming to late preterm resulted from the recognition that they were indeed the largest subpopulation of preterm infants, and had an increased mortality when compared to term infants and increased morbidity including transient tachypnea of newborn (TTNB), respiratory distress syndrome (RDS), persistent pulmonary hypertension (PPHN), respiratory failure, apnea, temperature instability, jaundice, hypoglycemia, feeding difficulties and a prolonged neonatal intensive care unit (NICU) stay (Raju et al. 2006; Engle et al. 2007; Jain 2007, 2008a; Ramachandrappa and Jain 2009; American College of Obstetricians and Gynecologists 2013). Furthermore, they have an increased prevalence of cognitive and neuro-developmental problems and a greater rate of readmission to hospital in the first weeks after discharge than term births. Escobar noted that many late preterm infants are never admitted to the NICU (Escobar et al. 2005). A possible explanation is that clinicians may be making clinical judgments based on infants' birth weight only rather than gestation and birth weight.

Preterm births are both emotionally and financially costly, taking a toll on the family and resulting in high direct health care costs due to longer hospital stays and hospital readmissions. Reducing the rate and toll from premature deliveries is both a national and international priority. Because late preterm deliveries, those between 34 and 37 weeks' gestation, account for about 70% of preterm births, they represent the low lying fruit, and are the logical initial target for prevention of prematurity.

10.3 The Late Preterm Infant

Until recently late preterm infants (those delivered between 34 weeks 0 days and 36 weeks plus 6 days) were regarded and treated as near-term infants. Consequently the considerable morbidity and mortality in this group of infants was largely unnoticed and disregarded. Recognizing that they indeed are the largest group of preterm infants with significant short and long-term morbidity and even mortality, the terminology has changed to emphasize the preterm birth, hence the terminology late preterm, and closer attention is being paid to this specific class of infant. As they account for over 70% of preterm births, utilize excessive resources and as many late preterm infants have no identifiable reasons for their early appearance, they present the best opportunity to substantially reduce the rate of preterm birth (Raju et al. 2006; Engle et al. 2007; Seikku et al. 2016; Spong et al. 2011; Hamilton et al. 2016)

10.3.1 Incidence and Prevention

In the US, premature births increased from 10.6% in 1990 to a high of 12.8% of all live births in 2006, declining to 12.7% in 2007 and 12.3% in 2008 (*Escobar et al.* 2005). *In 2013 in the USA, the preterm birth rate declined for the seventh straight year to 11.39%; the low birth weight (LBW) rate was essentially unchanged at 8.02%. The infant mortality rate was 5.96 infant deaths per 1000 live births in 2013, down 13% from 2005 (6.86). The age-adjusted death rate for 2013 was 7.3 deaths per 1000 population, unchanged from 2012. (Osterman et al. 2015) In 2015 there were 3.978 million births in the USA, down less than 1% from 2014. The cesarean delivery rate declined to 32.0% of births in 2015; the preterm birth rate rose slightly to 9.63% from 2014 to 2015* (Martin et al. 2016).

The rise of preterm births during the last three decades was primarily due to a rise in late preterm births from 7.3% to 9.1% of all live births in 2006 when there were 387,791 late preterm births in the USA. Indeed between 1996 and 2006, the rate of infants born late preterm in the US increased more than 18%. However, there was a slight decline of late preterm infants to 9% in 2007, perhaps reflecting progress in the prevention of late preterm delivery. Late preterm infants, more than 34 and less than 37 weeks' gestation, account for almost three quarters of preterm births (Fig. 1). Almost half of these deliveries are by elective cesarean section, for sound medical reasons and in the best interest of the mother and fetus.

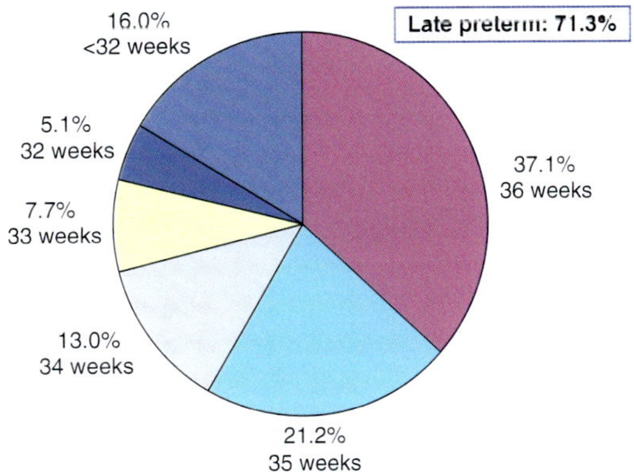

Fig. 1 Distribution of all preterm births, USA 2003

The American College of Obstetricians and Gynecologists has recommended that elective deliveries not be performed before 39 weeks of gestation (American College of Obstetricians and Gynecologists 1999).

Davidoff examined the changing epidemiology of gestational length among singleton births in the USA, from 1992 to 2002 (Davidoff et al. 2006). Analyzing gestational age by mode of delivery, the distribution of spontaneous births shifted to the left, with 39 weeks becoming the most common length of gestation in 2002, compared with 40 weeks in 1992 ($P < 0.001$). Deliveries at greater or equal to 40 weeks gestation markedly decreased, accompanied by an increase in those at 34–39 weeks. Singleton births with premature/prolonged rupture of the membranes or medical interventions had similar trends. Changes in the distribution of all singleton births differed by race/ethnicity, with non-Hispanic white infants having the largest increase in late preterm births.

To quantify the adverse neonatal and maternal outcomes associated with elective term delivery at less than 39 completed weeks of gestation, Clark et al. reviewed a cohort of 17,794 deliveries, including 14,955 (84%) at 37 weeks or greater. Remarkably, of these term deliveries, 6562 (44%) were planned, rather than spontaneous (Clark et al. 2009). Among the planned deliveries, 4645 (71%) were purely elective, and 17.8% of infants delivered electively without medical indication at 37–38 weeks and 8% of those delivered electively at 38–39 weeks required admission to a newborn special care unit compared with 4.6% of infants delivered at 39 weeks or beyond. Cesarean delivery rate in women undergoing induction of labor was not influenced by gestational age but was highly influenced by initial cervical dilatation and parity, ranging from 0% for parous women induced at 5 cm or greater to 50% for nulliparous women at 0 cm. They rightfully concluded that elective delivery before 39 weeks' gestation is associated with significant neonatal morbidity and is inappropriate.

Oshiro et al. (2009) reported that before initiation of a concerted system and multidisciplinary team effort (including information technology administrators as well as bedside care providers such as physicians and nurses) with the goal of reducing elective births before 39 weeks, 28% of elective deliveries were occurring before 39 completed weeks of gestation. Within 6 months of introducing the program, the rate was down to 10%, and 6 years later through continued education and a cultural change within the system, the rate is down to a very acceptable 3%.

Until 2007 the rate of preterm births has been increasing in the USA, especially for births at 34 weeks of gestation (late preterm). The causes for these trends remain unclear, but significant contributors to these large numbers of late preterm births are elective inductions and cesarean deliveries prior to 37 weeks' gestation. This is despite evidence and guidelines recommending against elective deliveries before 39 weeks without clinical indication (Seikku et al. 2016).

Reddy et al. (2009) characterized the delivery indications for late preterm births and their potential impact on neonatal and infant mortality rates. Using the 2001 US Birth Cohort Linked birth/death files which contained over three million singleton births, they categorized delivery indications as follows: (1) maternal medical conditions; (2) obstetric complications; (3) major congenital anomalies; (4) isolated spontaneous labor, vaginal delivery without induction and without associated medical/obstetric factors; and (5) no recorded indication. They noted that among 292,627 late preterm births, the first four categories (those with indications and isolated spontaneous labor) accounted for 77%. The remaining 23% (67,909) were classified as deliveries with no recorded indication. Factors significantly increasing the chance of no recorded indication were older maternal age, race, multiparity, or previous macrosomic infant of more than 4000 g birth weight. The neonatal and infant mortality rates were significantly higher among deliveries with no recorded indication compared with deliveries secondary to isolated spontaneous labor but not surprisingly lower compared with deliveries with an obstetric indication or congenital anomaly. These 23% of late preterm births with no recorded indication for delivery noted on birth certificates present a prime opportunity for preventing late preterm births.

The potential for success in this regard is documented by the Ohio Perinatal Quality Collaborative Writing Committee (Donovan et al. 2010). They sought to reduce scheduled births between 36(0/7)–38(6/7) weeks that lack appropriate medical indication. They collected baseline data for 60 days from 20 Ohio maternity units and then mandated recording of an indication for scheduled births between 36(0/7) and 38(6/7) weeks gestation. Deidentified birth data were analyzed centrally. Rates of scheduled births without a documented indication, birth certificate data, and implementation issues were shared regularly among sites. The rate of scheduled births between 36(0/7)–38(6/7) weeks without a documented medical indication declined significantly from 25% to less than 5% in participating hospitals. Birth certificate data showed inductions without an indication declined from a mean of 13–8%. Dating criteria were documented in 99% of charts.

Thus merely by establishing and applying dating criteria for gestational age and requiring documentation of the reasons for scheduled birth, the number of late preterm deliveries was substantially reduced. If we can accomplish this beyond 36 weeks, there is no reason to believe that it cannot be extrapolated to 34 weeks and beyond with a significant impact on reducing late preterm births. However, in order to sustain the success, it will be necessary for scheduled births to be a part of the culture of safety and for mothers to be better educated regarding the risks of late preterm delivery.

Bailit et al. (2010), utilizing electronic health records, sought to determine maternal and neonatal outcomes by labor onset type and gestational age. They reviewed 115,528 deliveries from 2002 through 2008 categorized by labor onset type (spontaneous, elective induction, indicated induction, unlabored cesarean). Neonatal and maternal outcomes were calculated by labor onset type and gestational age.

Neonatal intensive care unit admissions, the need for assisted ventilation, and sepsis improved with each week of gestational age until 39 weeks. The babies did better with elective induction, but there was increased risk of mothers requiring a hysterectomy in that group (Bailit et al. 2010).

10.4 Mortality

In 2002, the neonatal mortality rate (deaths among infants 0–27 days chronologic age) for late preterm infants was 4.6 times higher than the rate for term infants (4.1 vs. 0.9 per 1000 live births, respectively). This difference has actually widened when compared to 1995 data where there was a fourfold difference between late preterm and term infants (4.8 vs. 1.2 per 1000 live births, respectively). This relationship also carries over into infant mortality. In 2002, the infant mortality rate, deaths during the first year of life, for late preterm infants was also greater than the infant mortality rate for term infants (7.7 vs. 2.5 per 1000 live births, respectively) (Hamilton et al. 2016; Clark et al. 2009).

This is most notable for late preterm small for gestational age (SGA) infants who are 44 times more likely than term appropriate for gestational age (AGA) newborns to die in their first month and 22 times more likely to die in their first year. Even excluding deaths from congenital conditions, including birth defects, the differences in mortality rate ratios persisted for SGA infants, especially those born in the late preterm period.

Tomashek et al. (2007) observed that late preterm infants were particularly more likely to die in the early neonatal period compared with term infants from causes such as respiratory compromise, maternal complications of pregnancy, and congenital anomalies. They noted that infant mortality rates were three times higher in late preterm infants than term infants (7.9 vs. 2.4 deaths per 1000 live births) (Table 1). Because many of the deaths were caused by life-threatening congenital malformations, which may have precipitated the preterm delivery, the plea for prospective documentation of the indications for late preterm deliveries is timely and appropriate.

Kitsommart et al. (2009) compared data on 1193 late preterm, the majority of whom were 36 weeks (44%) followed by 35 weeks (29%) and 34 weeks (27%), respectively, and 8666 term infants. The prevalence of intensive care admission, respiratory support, pneumothorax, and mortality in late preterm infants was significantly higher compared with term infants. Although only 1% had positive cultures, almost 30% were treated with antibiotics. Despite a low

Table 1 Complications of prematurity in late preterm versus term infants

Complication	Frequency late preterm	Frequency term
Jaundice	54%	38%
Sepsis evaluation	37%	13%
Feeding difficulties	32%	7%
Receive IV fluids	27%	5%
Hypoglycemia	16%	5
Temp. instability	10%	<0.1%
Apnea	6%	<0.1%
Mechanical ventilation	3.4%	0.9
Mortality (2002)	7.9/1000 live births	2.4/1000 live births

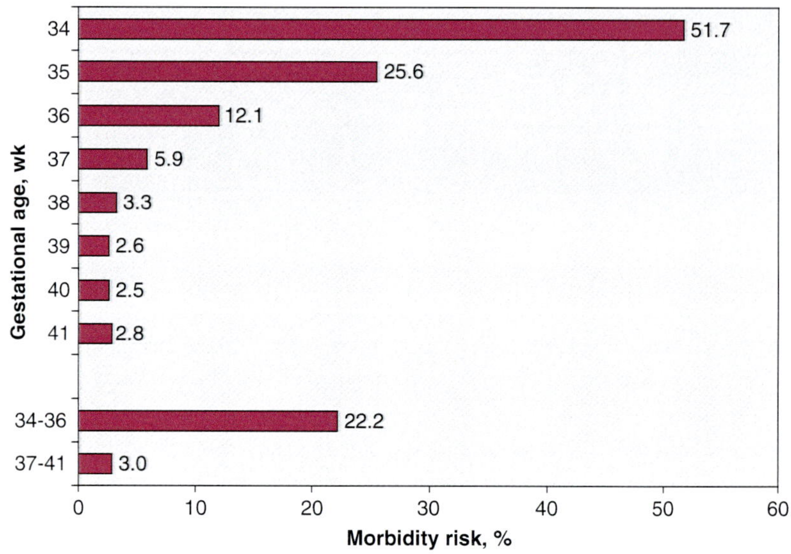

Fig. 2 Proportion with newborn morbidity during birth hospitalization according to gestational age (From (Shapiro-Mendoza et al. 2008), with permission)

overall mortality rate of 0.8%, the late preterm group had a 12-fold higher risk of death. The increased mortality and morbidity thus confirm the high-risk status of late preterm infants.

10.5 Morbidity

It is estimated that nearly 50% of infants born at 34 weeks' gestation require intensive care; this number drops to 15% at 35 weeks and 8% at 36 weeks gestation. In order to identify infants at the highest risk for life-threatening morbidity and those most likely to require specialized care, Shapiro-Mendoza et al. (2008) classified a newborn as having a morbid condition during initial hospitalization when at least one of the following three criteria was met: (1) newborn hospital stay of five nights and any morbidity diagnostic code considered life-threatening, (2) newborn hospital stay of five nights and transfer to a higher-level medical facility, and (3) infant death before hospital discharge. They reported that the risk for newborn morbidity increases twofold with each earlier week of gestation, beginning at 38 weeks' gestation until 34 weeks' gestation (Fig. 2). Late preterm infants are at greater risk for newborn morbidity than term infants, especially when maternal morbidity also is present. This risk seems to be particularly intensified when an infant has had prenatal maternal exposure to hypertensive disorders of pregnancy and antepartum hemorrhage.

Table 2 Risk for infant morbidity term versus late preterm (Clark et al. 2009)

Maternal condition	RR ratio LPT/term
Hypertensive disease	6.1
Diabetes	5.4
Antepartum hemorrhage	5.1
Acute or chronic lung disease	6.1
Maternal infection	4.4
Cardiac disease	5.7
Renal disease	4.6
Genital herpes	10.0

Late preterm infants were seven times more likely to have newborn morbidity than term infants (22 vs. 3%) (Fig. 2). Late preterm infants who were exposed to antepartum hemorrhage and hypertensive disorders of pregnancy (HDP) were especially vulnerable. Additionally HDP, diabetes, and asthma are associated with an increased risk for indicated or spontaneous preterm birth (Table 2).

Decisions regarding the delivery of late preterm infants take into account the risks and benefits to both mother and fetus of prolonging the pregnancy. Specific standards of care and protocols are necessary for late preterm infants rather than applying those developed for term infants. Furthermore better anticipation, recognition, and treatment of women with chronic and pregnancy-related health conditions may decrease the rates of newborn morbidity in all infants but especially in late preterm ones.

The major causes of morbidity encountered in late preterm infants include transient tachypnea of the newborn (TTNB), respiratory distress syndrome (RDS), persistent pulmonary hypertension of the newborn (PPHN), respiratory failure, apnea, temperature instability, jaundice, hypoglycemia, feeding difficulties, and a prolonged neonatal intensive care unit (NICU) stay. In addition they have a higher prevalence of congenital malformations which, as noted above, may contribute to an increased mortality relative to term infants. They are also more likely to develop bloodstream infections (Cohen-Wolkowiez et al. 2009) (Table 1).

10.6 Readmission

Escobar evaluated the large Kaiser Permanente database which included 33,276 survivors of neonatal intensive care with 862 (2.6%) < 34 weeks' gestation, 2153 (6.5%) between 34 and 36 weeks, and 30,261 (90.9%) of more than 37 weeks (American College of Obstetricians and Gynecologists 2013). Rehospitalization rates within 2 weeks after nursery discharge varied by gestational age range: 26/862 (3.0%) among babies <34 weeks, 94/2153 (4.4%) among babies 34–36 weeks, and 618/30261 (2.0%) among babies 37+ weeks. Hence there is a twofold risk of rehospitalization for late preterm infants compared with term infants, and jaundice was the major reason for readmission. These data are substantiated by McLaurin (24), who reported readmission rates over the first year of life for late preterm infants were 15%, compared to 8% in term infants (McLaurin et al. 2009). In particular, late preterm infants are three times more likely to be admitted within the first 15 days after discharge from the birth hospitalization (3.8 vs. 1.3%. The most common reasons for early readmission are jaundice, feeding difficulties, poor weight gain, dehydration, and apnea. Respiratory (including bronchiolitis) and gastrointestinal disorders are the most common diagnoses for late readmission ($\geq$ 15 days after the date of discharge) during the first year of life. Underwood et al. noted that the largest cohort of infants readmitted to the hospital at least once during the first month of life was infants born at 35 week's gestation, most commonly due to a respiratory illness (Underwood et al. 2007). The cost of hospital readmission for this cohort of infants approached 100 million dollars.

10.7 Thermal Instability

Whereas the late preterm infant is better equipped than the extremely low birth weight and premature infant, they are still vulnerable to cold exposure after delivery. Increasing amounts of fat are deposited in the final weeks of gestation so they have less white fat and brown fat accumulation and maturation, notably the controlling hormones surge at term. Late preterm infants often have temperature instability, which in turn leads to the consideration of sepsis, a sepsis evaluation, and often the initiation of antibiotic therapy (Wang et al. 2004).

10.8 Transient Tachypnea of the Newborn

A major respiratory disorder in late preterm infants is transient tachypnea of the newborn (TTNB). TTNB is best described as the consequence of delayed and inadequate lung liquid clearance. This self-limiting disease, characterized by an increase in respiratory rate, occurs more frequently in infants delivered by elective cesarean section and is thought to result from delayed activation of liquid clearance in infants not subjected to the stress of labor. Gowen and others showed that newborn infants with TTNB had a transient decrease in amiloride-sensitive nasal epithelial Na^+ transport compared with normal newborns, supporting the notion that suboptimal clearance of liquid is a cause of TTNB. Infants with TTNB were found to have low norepinephrine but normal epinephrine levels.

Lung ultrasound has been a very useful means of establishing the diagnosis of TTNB.

10.9 Respiratory Distress Syndrome

With more liberal use of antenatal corticosteroids commencing in 1994 and the introduction of surfactant in the early 1990s, infant deaths associated with respiratory distress syndrome decreased by 48% from 1989–1991 to 1995–1997 and then decreased by another 18% by 2002–2004 in the USA. The latter mortality reduction was evident at 28–32 weeks but not 33–36 weeks of gestation because these infants have not been optimally targeted to receive prenatal corticosteroid prophylaxis, despite evidence from randomized trials regarding the safety and efficacy of the treatment at this gestation. As corticosteroid use is infrequent beyond 33 weeks' gestation (15%), "addressing the knowledge practice gap in corticosteroid use at 33 and 34 weeks should reduce infant morbidity and mortality" (Gowen et al. 1988).

Extrapolating the data from infants born at 24–32 weeks gestation, Joseph et al. (Joseph et al. 2009) concluded that the number needed to treat estimates for 35 weeks (n = 21) and 36 weeks (n = 64) of gestation is sufficient to warrant additional attention in terms of future research addressing efficacy at these more advanced gestational ages. However meta-analyses reveal nonsignificant protective effects beyond 36 weeks.

Administration of betamethasone to women at risk for late preterm delivery significantly reduced the rate of neonatal respiratory complications. The primary outcome (the use of continuous positive airway pressure or high-flow nasal cannula for at least 2 h, supplemental oxygen with a fraction of inspired oxygen of at least 0.30 for at least 4 h, extracorporeal membrane oxygenation, or mechanical ventilation) or stillbirth or neonatal death within 72 h after delivery. occurred (11.6%) in the betamethasone group and(14.4%) in the placebo group (Gyamfi-Bannerman et al. 2016). Severe respiratory complications, transient tachypnea of the newborn, surfactant use, and bronchopulmonary dysplasia also occurred significantly less frequently in the betamethasone group. There were no significant between-group differences in the incidence of chorioamnionitis or neonatal sepsis. Neonatal hypoglycemia was more common in the betamethasone group than in the placebo group (24.0% vs. 15.0).

Dudell and Jain (2006) reviewed the ELSO neonatal registry to study the indications for and outcomes of late preterm infants requiring extracorporeal membrane oxygenation (ECMO). The cohort comprised 2258 late preterm infants, representing 14.5% of 15,590 registered neonates. The primary etiology of hypoxic respiratory failure in late preterm infants treated with ECMO was RDS or sepsis as compared to term infants who were more likely to have aspiration syndromes. The overall survival (74%) has not improved over time and was inferior for the late preterm infants as compared with 87% in the term population.

10.10 Apnea

Apnea occurs more frequently in late preterm infants (4–7%) than in term infants (1–2%) (Hunt 2006). In the Collaborative Home Infant Monitoring Evaluation (CHIME) study, the recorded rate of apnea (obstructive and central apnea) and bradycardia events was greater in late preterm infants versus term infants (Hunt 2006; Ramanathan et al. 2001). Late preterm infants may also be at increased risk for sudden infant death syndrome compared to term infants.

10.11 Feeding Difficulties

Late Preterm infants may have immature feeding mechanics with poor coordination of sucking and swallowing resulting in limited fluid intake and dehydration, often necessitating intravenous therapy. It is also more difficult to establish breast feeding, and there may also be accentuated gastroesophageal reflux in late preterm infants. The American Academy of Pediatrics (AAP) has recommended that prior to discharge, it is essential to establish successful feeding defined as coordinated sucking, swallowing, and breathing while feeding (Engle et al. 2007). Weight loss should not exceed 7% of birth weight during birth hospitalization. If the infant is breastfed, twice daily documented observation by trained caregivers of successful position, latch, and milk transfer after birth also should be performed.

10.12 Jaundice

Hyperbilirubinemia is the most common clinical condition requiring hospital readmission during the first week of postnatal life. Late preterm infants are at substantially higher risk for severe hyperbilirubinemia than infants born at term. Infants born at 36 weeks' gestation have almost an eightfold increased risk of developing a total serum bilirubin greater than 20 mg per 100 mL (5.2%) versus those born at 41 or 42 weeks gestation (0.7 and 0.6%, respectively) (Newman et al. 1999). Approximately 1 in 650–1000 infants >35 weeks' gestation develops, total serum bilirubin values greater than or equal to 25 mg per 100 mL, and 1 in 10,000 has levels greater than 30 mg per 100 mL.

The risk factors for readmission are documented in Table 3 and are dominated by gestational age and breast feeding (Maisels and Kring 1998). The jaundice may be attributed also to early discharge, inappropriate follow-up and monitoring, as well as diminished fluid intake related to poor feeding. Late preterm infants accounted for 40% of kernicterus in a large series reported by Bhutani and Johnson (2006). All were discharged early and breastfed.

Most vaginal deliveries, including the late preterm infants, are discharged by 48 h of life, well before the peak serum bilirubin that is observed in term infants on day 3–5 and later in preterm infants. The peak bilirubin thus occurs at home. It is therefore necessary to screen the bilirubin levels prior to discharge and arrange for early follow-up either at home or in the clinics to prevent catastrophic nonmonitored elevation of serum bilirubin. Decisions are made on the bilirubin levels according to age in hours and zones according to the Bhutani nomogram (Maisels and Kring 1998; Bhutani and Johnson 2006).

Table 3 Risk of being readmitted for phototherapy

Risk factor	Odds ratio (vs. 40 weeks)
35–36 weeks	13.2
37–38 weeks	7.
Breastfeeding	4.2
Jaundice in nursery	7.
Length of stay <72 h	3.

30,000 discharges from well-baby nursery 1988–1994; 4.2/1000 readmitted for phototherapy (Maisels and Kring 1998)

It has long been accepted that jaundice progresses in a cephalo-caudal fashion as the total serum bilirubin (TSB) level increases. Kramer provided the first systematic study of this process by dividing the body into five zones ranging from zone 1 (jaundice restricted to the head and neck) to zone 5 (jaundice in the hands and feet). As the jaundice progressed from the head to the extremities, the TSB levels increased, although there was a wide range of bilirubin values in each zone (Bhutani et al. 2008). To evaluate the visual assessment of jaundice, Keren et al. (Kramer 1969) utilized experienced well-baby nursery nurses to visually evaluate newborns for jaundice at a mean age of 47 h. The objective was to determine whether the pre discharge visual assessment would help to predict the subsequent risk of significant neonatal hyperbilirubinemia, defined as a bilirubin level that exceeded or came within 1 mg/dL of the AAP phototherapy treatment threshold (Keren et al. 2009). Those whose pre discharge jaundice was seen in zones 4 and 5 were five times more likely to develop significant hyperbilirubinemia than those with no jaundice or jaundice restricted to zone 1. Nevertheless, the correlation between cephalocaudal progression and the ability to predict the risk of hyperbilirubinemia was highly erratic. An exception was the complete absence of jaundice (zone 0), which was present in only 17% of the population but had a powerful negative predictive value of 99%. The conclusion is that it is dangerous to rely on visual assessment of jaundice and if there is clinical evidence of jaundice, then the bilirubin should be measured either chemically or by transcutaneous measurement. The AAP guidelines are directed at reducing the frequency of severe neonatal hyperbilirubinemia (levels >17 mg per 100 mL) and bilirubin encephalopathy, in addition to minimizing parental anxiety and discontinuation of breastfeeding and hoping to reduce costs. (American Academy of Pediatrics, Subcommittee on Hyperbilirubinemia 2004). The key elements of the guidelines are presented in Table 4.

Table 4 AAP Jaundice Guideline The 10 key elements (Maisels and Kring 1998)

1. Promote and support successful breastfeeding
2. Establish nursery protocols – include circumstances in which nurses can order a bilirubin
3. Measure TSB or TcB if jaundiced in the first 24 h
4. Visual estimation of jaundice can lead to errors, particularly in darkly pigmented infants
5. Interpret bilirubin levels according to the infant's age in hours
6. Infants <38 weeks particularly if breastfed are at high risk
7. Perform risk assessment prior to discharge
8. Give parents written and oral information
9. Provide appropriate follow-up based on time of discharge and risk assessment
10. Treat newborns when indicated with phototherapy or exchange transfusion

10.13 Long-Term Outcomes

Until recently, the assumption was that late preterm infants carry minimal risk for long-term morbidities. Morse et al. (2009) refuted these assumptions when they compared prekindergarten and kindergarten outcomes among healthy late preterm infants and healthy term infants. Outcomes were adjusted for 15 potential confounding maternal and infant variables. They observed that the risk for developmental delay or disability was 36% higher among late preterm infants compared with term infants. Furthermore the risk for retention and disability in kindergarten with need for special education was higher for late preterm infants. The assessment "not ready to start school" was borderline significant. Thus healthy late preterm infants compared with healthy term infants face a greater risk of developmental delay and school-related problems up through age 5 (Jain 2008b).

On the other hand, Gurka et al. (2010) applied 11 standard outcomes measuring cognition, achievement, social skills, and behavioral/emotional problems using the Woodcock-Johnson Psycho-Educational Battery-Revised and the Child Behavior Checklist, administered repeatedly through age 15 years. They detected no consistent significant differences between late preterm and full-term children for these standard measures from ages 4 to 15 years. They concluded that late preterm infants born otherwise healthy seem to have no real burdens regarding cognition, achievement, behavior, and socio-emotional development throughout childhood.

Shah et al. (2016) noted that late preterm infants demonstrate comparable developmental outcomes to full-term infants (early-term and full-term gestation) at 24 months, but demonstrate less optimal reading outcomes at preschool and kindergarten time points. Woyhuler et al. (2015) confirmed that late preterm infants continue to be delayed at kindergarten compared with full term infants (FTIs). However a child who tested within the normal range (>85) at 24 months had an excellent chance of testing in the normal range at kindergarten.

Taige (Talge et al. 2010) *observed that late* preterm birth was associated with an increased risk of full scale and performance (IQ scores below 85). Additionally late preterm birth was associated with higher levels of internalizing and attention problems. Late preterm birth is associated with behavioral problems and lower IQ at the age of 6, independent of maternal IQ, residential setting, and sociodemographics. It remains to be determined whether these findings relate to shorter gestational length in utero or ex utero (e.g., neonatal complications) factors marked by late preterm birth or some combination of these factors.

After a systematic review of 9 electronic data bases, examining early childhood outcomes in late preterm infants(LPI's), McGowan et al. (2011) concluded "Evidence suggests that LPIs are at increased risk of adverse developmental outcomes and academic difficulties up to 7 years of age in comparison to term infants. Of note, an infant control group matched for gestational age has not been used; thus, for LPIs, the effect of neonatal admission on longer-term outcomes has not been fully explored. Systematic measurement of early childhood outcomes is lacking, and focused long-term follow-up studies are needed to investigate early childhood development after late-preterm birth." There remain gaps in knowledge that urgently need to be addressed.

10.14 Discharge Planning

Clinicians who care for late preterm infants need to first recognize and establish that the infant is a late preterm infant. They must be aware of their increased risk for morbidity, mortality, and potential neuro-developmental problems. They must anticipate, screen for, and intervene in an appropriate and timely manner for the common problems encountered in these vulnerable infants. Prior to hospital discharge, parents need to be educated that their infant is at increased risk for jaundice, feeding difficulties, hypoglycemia, and dehydration. Parents must be taught to recognize these conditions and promptly seek appropriate care following hospital discharge.

The AAP has established the following guidelines for discharge criteria for late preterm infants (Engle et al. 2007):

Determine the accurate gestational age, and ensure that there are no abnormalities or medical condition (i.e., hyperbilirubinemia) that requires further hospitalization.

The infant demonstrates physiologic stability by demonstrating competency in the following:

Thermoregulation defined as an axillary temperature of 36.5–37.4°C in an open crib.

Cardiorespiratory control with stable vital signs of a respiratory rate less than 60 breaths per minute and a heart rate between 100 and 160 beats per minute and absence of medical illness

Passed at least one stool spontaneously

Completed other routine newborn care. This includes screening tests (i.e., hearing and disorders that are threatening to life or long-term health), vaccinations (i.e., hepatitis B vaccine), and prophylactic treatment (i.e., vitamin K prophylaxis).

Assessment of the family and home environment to identify any risk factors that may impact on the health of the infant.

Successful training of the parents who have demonstrated competency in the care of their infant and the ability to assess for hyperbilirubinemia, feeding difficulties, and dehydration.

A follow-up visit 24–48 h after discharge is scheduled with an identified primary care provider.

10.15 Summary and Recommendations

In the USA, late preterm infants, defined as infants with a gestational age between 34 and 36 weeks and 6 days, account for 9% of all births.

Late preterm infants have a reported sevenfold increased risk of morbidity compared to term infants during birth hospitalization, which results in a longer hospital stay and higher medical costs. The most common causes of morbidity include hypothermia, hypoglycemia, respiratory distress, apnea, hyperbilirubinemia, and feeding difficulties. Late preterm infants have a higher mortality than term infants. Readmission rates are two to three times greater for late preterm compared to term infants. Early readmission (within 15 days of discharge from birth hospitalization) includes hyperbilirubinemia, feeding difficulties, poor weight gain, dehydration, and apnea. During the first year of life, respiratory and gastrointestinal disorders are the most common diagnoses for late readmission. Late preterm infants also have more neurodevelopmental disabilities and school problems than their term-born peers.

References

American Academy of Pediatrics, Subcommittee on Hyperbilirubinemia (2004) Management of hyperbilirubinemia in the newborn infant 35 or more weeks of gestation. Pediatrics 114:297–316

American College of Obstetricians and Gynecologists (1999) Induction of labor. Practice bulletin, vol 10. ACOG, Washington, DC

American College of Obstetricians and Gynecologists (2013) ACOG committee opinion no. 560: medically indicated late-preterm and early-term deliveries. Obstet Gynecol 121:908

Bailit JL, Gregory KD, Reddy UM et al (2010) Maternal and neonatal outcomes by labor onset type and gestational age. Am J Obstet Gynecol 202:245.e1–245e12

Bhutani VK, Johnson L (2006) Kernicterus in late preterm infants cared for as term healthy infants. Semin Perinatol 30:89–97

Bhutani VK, Maisels MJ, Stark AR, Buonocore G (2008) Management of jaundice and prevention of severe neonatal hyperbilirubinemia in infants > or =35 weeks gestation. Neonatology 94:63–67

Clark SL, Miller DD, Belfort MA et al (2009) Neonatal and maternal outcomes associated with elective term delivery. Am J Obstet Gynecol 200:156.e1–156.e4

Cohen-Wolkowiez M, Moran C, Benjamin DK et al (2009) Early and late onset sepsis in late preterm infants. Pediatr Infect Dis J 28:1052–1056

Davidoff MJ, Dias T, Damus K et al (2006) Changes in the gestational age distribution among U.S. singleton births: impact on rates of late preterm birth, 1992 to 2002. Semin Perinatol 30:8–15

Donovan EF, Lannon C, Bailit J et al (2010) A statewide initiative to reduce inappropriate scheduled births at 36 (0/7)–38(6/7) weeks' gestation. Am J Obstet Gynecol 202:243.e1–243.e8

Dudell GG, Jain L (2006) Hypoxic respiratory failure in the late preterm infant. Clin Perinatol 33:803–830

Engle WA, Tomashek KM, Wallman C et al (2007) "late-preterm" infants: a population at risk. Pediatrics 120:1390–1401

Escobar GJ, Greene JD, Hulac P et al (2005) Rehospitalisation after birth hospitalisation: patterns among infants of all gestations. Arch Dis Child 90:125–131

Gowen CW Jr, Lawson EE, Gingras J et al (1988) Electrical potential difference and ion transport across nasal epithelium of term neonates: correlation with mode of delivery, transient tachypnea of the newborn, and respiratory rate. J Pediatr 113:121–127

Gurka MJ, LoCasale-Crouch J, Blackman JA (2010) Long-term cognition, achievement, socio-emotional, and behavioral development of healthy late-preterm infants. Arch Pediatr Adolesc Med 164:525–532

Gyamfi-Bannerman C, Thom EA, Blackwell SC et al (2016) NICHD maternal–fetal medicine units network. Antenatal betamethasone for women at risk for late preterm delivery. N Engl J Med 374(14):1311–1320

Hamilton BE, Martin JA, Osterman MJ (2016) Births: preliminary data for 2015. Natl Vital Stat Rep 65:1

Hunt CE (2006) Ontogeny of autonomic regulation in late preterm infants born at 34–37 weeks postmenstrual age. Semin Perinatol 30:73–76

Jain L (2007) Morbidity and mortality in late-preterm infants: more than just transient tachypnea! J Pediatr 151:445–446

Jain L (2008a) Respiratory morbidity in late-preterm infants: prevention is better than cure! Am J Perinatol 25:75–78

Jain L (2008b) School outcome in late preterm infants: a cause for concern. J Pediatr 153:5–6

Joseph KS, Nette F, Scott H, Vincer MJ (2009) Prenatal corticosteroid prophylaxis for women delivering at late preterm gestation. Pediatrics 124:e835–e843

Keren R, Teremont K, Luan X, Cnaan A (2009) Visual assessment of jaundice in term and late preterm infants. Arch Dis Child Fetal Neonatal Ed 94:F317–F322

Kitsommart R, Janes M, Mahajan V et al (2009) Outcomes of latepreterm infants: a retrospective, single-center, Canadian study. Clin Pediatr (Phila) 48:844–850

Kramer LI (1969) Advancement of dermal icterus in the jaundiced newborn. Am J Dis Child 118:454–458

Maisels MJ, Kring E (1998) Length of stay, jaundice and hospital readmission. Pediatrics 101:995–998

Martin JA, Hamilton BE, Osterman MJ (2016) Births in the United States, 2015. NCHS Data Brief 258:1–8

McGowan JE, Alderdice FA, Holmes VA, Johnston L (2011) Early childhood development of late-preterm infants: a systematic review. Pediatrics 127:1111

McLaurin KK, Hall CB, Jackson EA et al (2009) Persistence of morbidity and cost differences between late-preterm and term infants during the first year of life. Pediatrics 123:653–659

Morse SB, Zheng H, Tang Y, Roth J (2009) Early school-age outcomes of late preterm infants. Pediatrics 123: e622–e629

Newman TB, Escobar GJ, Gonzales VM et al (1999) Frequency of neonatal bilirubin testing and hyperbilirubinemia in a large health maintenance organization. Pediatrics 104:1198–1203

Oshiro BT, Henry E, Wilson J et al (2009) Decreasing elective deliveries before 39 weeks of gestation in an integrated health care system. Obstet Gynecol 113:804–811

Osterman MJ, Kochanek KD, MF MD, Strobino DM, Guyer B (2015) Annual summary of vital statistics: 2012–2013. Pediatrics 135(6):1115–1125

Raju TN, Higgins RD, Stark AR, Leveno KJ (2006) Optimizing care and outcome for late-preterm (near-term) infants: a summary of the workshop sponsored by the National Institute of Child Health and Human Development. Pediatrics 118:1207–1214

Ramachandrappa A, Jain L (2009) Health issues of the late preterm infant. Pediatr Clin N Am 56:565–577

Ramanathan R, Corwin MJ, Hunt CE et al (2001) Cardiorespiratory events recorded on home monitors: comparison of healthy infants with those at increased risk for SIDS. JAMA 285:2199–2207

Reddy UM, Ko CW, Raju TNK, Willinger M (2009) Delivery indications at late-preterm gestations and infant mortality rates in the United States. Pediatrics 124:234–240

Seikku L, Gissler M, Andersson S et al (2016) Asphyxia, neurologic morbidity, and perinatal mortality in early-term and postterm birth. Pediatrics 137(6): e20153334

Shah P, Kaciroti N, Richards B et al (2016) Developmental outcomes of late preterm infants from infancy to kindergarten. Pediatrics 138

Shapiro-Mendoza CK, Tomashek KM, Kotelchuck M et al (2008) Effect of late-preterm birth and maternal medical conditions on newborn morbidity risk. Pediatrics 121:e223–e232

Spong CY, Mercer BM, D'alton M et al (2011) Timing of indicated late-preterm and early-term birth. Obstet Gynecol 118:323

Talge NM, Holzman C, Wang J et al (2010) Late-preterm birth and its association with cognitive and socio-emotional outcomes at 6 years of age. Pediatrics 126:1124

Tomashek KM, Shapiro-Mendoza CK, Davidoff MJ, Petrini JR (2007) Differences in mortality between late-preterm and term singleton infants in the United States 1995–2002. J Pediatr 151:450–456

Underwood MA, Danielsen B, Gilbert WM (2007) Cost, causes and rates of rehospitalization of preterm infants. J Perinatol 27:614–619

Wang ML, Dorer DJ, Fleming MP, Catlin EA (2004) Clinical outcomes of near-term infants. Pediatrics 114:372–376

Woyhaler MCMC, Mao WY, Smith VC (2015) Late preterm infants and neurodevelopmental outcomes at kindergarten. Pediatrics 136:424

11 Ethical Problems in Neonatal Medicine

Otwin Linderkamp

Contents

O. Linderkamp (✉)
Division of Neonatology, Department of Pediatrics, University of Heidelberg, Heidelberg, Germany
e-mail: olinderkamp@yahoo.de

G. Buonocore et al. (eds.), *Neonatology*,
https://doi.org/10.1007/978-3-319-29489-6_160

Abstract
In perinatal and neonatal medicine, the Hippocratic Oath can be translated into the responsibility of the physicians to act in the "best interests" of the fetus and newborn infant and to avoid harming the fetus and infant and also the mother. This implies that the benefit of treatments should outweigh the harm and risks of the treatment for the patient. The decision-making process is extremely difficult for infants with uncertain prognosis such as extremely preterm infants. The knowledge of long-term outcome is essential for correct and complete antenatal and postnatal counseling of parents and for decision processes in the care of the high risk newborn. Laws and guidelines are necessary and available for care at the limit of viability, but there are different attitudes toward critically ill neonates in different countries, in different centers, and among caregivers in the same center. The decision-making process is articulated in at least three time points: care of mother and fetus before birth, initiation or withholding of resuscitation of the infant after birth, and continuation or withdrawal of neonatal intensive care. Knowledge of newborn and parental rights is the starting point for decisions by physicians from the antenatal until postnatal period.

11.1 Salient Points

- The knowledge of long-term outcome is of great importance for antenatal and postnatal counseling of parents and for decision processes in the care of high risk newborn.
- Several models have been developed that consider factors influencing the short- and long-term prognosis of high risk newborn and particularly of extremely preterm infants.
- Laws and guidelines are available for care at the limit of viability. However, attitudes toward critically sick neonates vary among different healthcare professions, countries, centers within a country, and caregivers in one center.
- The rights of newborn babies and parents have to be known in order to establish decision-making processes and withholding and withdrawal of intensive care.

11.2 Introduction

"I will prescribe regimens for the good of my patients according to my ability and my judgment and never do harm to anyone." The Hippocratic oath expressed beneficence and non-maleficence as basic principles of medical ethics more than 2000 years ago. Beneficence in perinatal and neonatal medicine refers to the responsibility of the physicians to act in the "best interests" of the fetus and newborn infant. Non-maleficence relates to the avoidance of harm to the fetus and infant but also to the mother. This implies that the benefit of treatments should outweigh the harm and risks of the treatment for the patient.

In the newborn infant, benefits are usefully defined as survival and the ability to live a self-determined life. For infants with no chance of survival, aggressive intensive care is not beneficial but harmful and futile, and is, therefore, generally assumed to be unethical. However, in infants with uncertain prognosis (i.e., high risk of survival with poor quality of life), the decision is extremely difficult and requires clear ethical guidelines.

A recent meta-analysis on decision-making in the best interests of the newborn demonstrated that prejudices play an important role in the attitudes (and hence decisions) of caregivers (Bellieni and Buonocore 2009). Janvier et al. (2008a) criticized that neonatal intensive care is usually far more scrutinized than intensive care of any older patient groups and that children and adults with a poor prognosis are more likely to be resuscitated than newborn infants with the same or a better prognosis. The authors explain the different attitudes by deficient knowledge about the actual outcomes or by irrational negative associations with low gestational ages. To avoid decision-making by prejudices and confirmation bias, evidence-based medical ethics applies research results (particularly epidemiology) in addition to ethical and legal principles to draw conclusions to ethical dilemmas in medicine.

Three groups of newborn infants are usually considered in end-of-life decisions: (1) infants at or below the gestational age limit of viability, (2) infants born with congenital anomalies incompatible with life, and (3) extremely ill preterm or full-term infants who might survive with severe damage of the brain or other vital organs after a long period of intensive care. This chapter focuses on the extremely preterm (EP) infant and reviews some of the important issues, such as outcome data, withdrawal and/or withholding life support, role of parents and health care providers, economics, and a framework for neonatal ethical issues.

11.3 Survival and Outcome of Extremely Preterm (EP) Infants

11.3.1 Survival of EP Infants

The knowledge of published survival and long-term outcome data is of great importance for antenatal and postnatal counseling of the parents and for the decision process in the care of EP infants. The prognosis depends on several factors such as gestational age, birth weight, gender, single or multiple births, prenatal and postnatal care, neonatal complications and morbidities, attitudes of the caregivers and parents, and on the individual maturity and resilience of the fetus and infant (Table 1).

Gestational age is accepted as a major prenatal predictor of the prognosis of EP infants (Levene 2004) since prenatal care (transfer to a perinatal center, corticosteroids) and antenatal counseling of the parents are mainly based on the gestational age. Most laws and guidelines on the limit of viability in EP infants use a defined gestational age as a limit. However, the estimated gestational age may deviate by ±7 days from the actual gestational age due to uncertain last menses and errors of prenatal ultrasonography, unless the time of (*in vitro*) fertilization is precisely known (Skupsi et al. 2010).

Table 1 Determinants of the outcome of extremely preterm (EP) infants

Fetal factors
Gestational age
Body weight
Gender
Single or multiple births
Social status and lifestyle of the mother
Individual maturity and resilience of the fetus
Antenatal and intrapartum care of the fetus
Maternal transfer to a level III center
Antenatal steroids, tocolysis, antibiotics, etc.
Cesarean section on fetal indication
Experience in "proactive care" of the mother and the EP fetus
Neonatal factors
Individual maturity, strength, and resilience of the infant
Sufficient maturity of vital organs for survival (lungs) and for intact survival (brain, eyes)
Condition of the EP infant at birth and response to resuscitation within 3–5–10 min.
Stability/instability in the first 12–24 postnatal hours
Extent and required time of intensive care
Neonatal complications and severe morbidities (IVH/PVL, ROPNEC, sepsis)
Neonatal and long-term care of EP infants
Experience in resuscitation and neonatal intensive care of EP infants
Availability of adequate equipment, resources, and experienced staff around the clock
Neonatal developmental care
Specialized long-term care
Socio-cognitive and learning support
Policies, attitudes, and individual decisions
Policies and guidelines concerning the care of EP infants
Attitudes of the obstetrical and neonatal staff toward the care of EP infants
Antenatal decisions of parents and caregivers (initiation and withholding of intensive care based on risk factors of death and long-term sequelae)
Postnatal decisions of parents and caretakers (withdrawal of intensive care if the prognosis of the infant deteriorates)

A recent review of 20 published studies on survival rates of EP infants born between 1985 and 2008 (Linderkamp 2012) shows that live-born preterm infants with a gestational age of 22 weeks had an overall survival rate of 8%

(145/1791) with no consistent trend to improvement with time. Survival rates ≥20% were noted in Japan (Nishida and Sakuma 2009; Kusuda et al. 2006; Itabashi et al. 2009) and in some single-center studies. In Japan, infants born at 22 weeks' gestation are principally considered viable and resuscitated. From 2004 to 2007, 1-year survival of infants born alive at 22–26 weeks of gestation in Sweden was 70% and ranged from 9.8% at 22 weeks to 85% at 26 weeks (Marsal and Express Group 2009). The overall survival rate of infants born at 23 weeks' gestation was 25% (1361/5383). Eight studies showed improvements, and six showed decreases in the survival rates with time. Survival rates above 50% were reported for Sweden (Marsal and Express Group 2009) and Japan (Nishida and Sakuma 2009; Kusuda et al. 2006; Itabashi et al. 2009).

Preterm infants born at 24 weeks' gestation showed an overall survival rate of 50% (3796/7555). A Japanese study on infants born in 2005 showed the highest survival rates in the whole-country studies (77%) (Itabashi et al. 2009), followed by Sweden in 2004–2007 (67%) (Marsal and Express Group 2009), England and Wales in 2005 (56%) (Moser et al. 2007), and Norway in 1999–2000 (55%) (Markestad et al. 2005). In 11 time-trend studies, a marked rise of the survival rates was observed with time. The overall survival rate of infants with 25 weeks' gestation was 68%. Japan, Sweden, Norway, and England and Wales reached again high survival rates of 85%, 81%, 77%, and 76%, respectively. Overall survival rates increased from 61% in infants born mainly in the 1990s to 74% in infants born mainly in the early 2000s. Infants born at 26 weeks' gestation had an overall survival rate of 80% (Linderkamp 2012).

11.3.2 Neonatal Morbidities and Long-Term Outcome in EP Infants

Seven recent studies on severe neonatal morbidity in surviving EP infants <27 weeks presenting week-by-week results have been reviewed elsewhere (Linderkamp 2012). At 23 weeks' gestation, the prevalence of intraventricular hemorrhage and/or periventricular leukomalacia ranged from 9% to 29%, at 24 weeks from 14% to 28%, and at 25 weeks from 7% to 15%. Infants with 23 weeks' gestation had a high risk of severe retinopathy (17–62%) requiring surgical treatment. Blindness resulting from retinopathy of prematurity (ROP) has, however, become rare due to modern laser coagulation techniques.

The high risk of EP infants for neurodevelopmental impairments, such as cerebral palsy and cognitive or sensory deficits, is of great concern to parents, caregivers, and society. Only few national and regional studies present week-by-week outcomes in EP infants (Linderkamp 2012). Severe disability was noted in 20–22%, 8–39%, and 11–27% of infants born at 23, 24, and 25 weeks' gestation, respectively. No disability was seen in 13–33%, 16–56%, and 17–52% in infants born at 23, 24, and 25 weeks' gestation, respectively. Two Japanese studies showed relatively low rates of neurodevelopmental disability in infants born at 23 weeks' gestation (32–35%) (Ikeda et al. 2006; Iijima et al. 2009). EP infants without visible disability in early years are at considerable risk for a variety of behavioral and educational deficits at school age.

There is concern that newly developed treatments and altered attitudes toward EP infants improve their survival rate, but that many of the additional surviving infants suffer from severe disability. A rising prevalence of long-term deficits such as cerebral palsy and poor cognitive outcome was indeed observed in several time-trend studies on EP infants born in the 1970s and 1980s and in some studies in the mid-1990s and the early 2000s (Linderkamp 2012; Wilson-Costello et al. 2007). Recent studies showed both increasing survival rates and decreases in the rates of short- and long-term neurodevelopmental disabilities in EP infants (Wilson-Costello et al. 2007). The recent improvements of short- and long-term outcomes are probably the result of a comprehensive antenatal and postnatal care philosophy including proactive antenatal care, optimal delivery procedure, competent neonatal care in the delivery room and the intensive care unit, better long-term care, and a positive attitude of more caretakers toward these patients (Hakansson et al. 2004).

11.3.3 Prediction of the Outcome of Individual EP Infants

The prognosis of EP infants depends on several factors in addition to the gestational age. Although it is difficult to consider all of these factors in counseling the parents and in decision-making, obstetricians and neonatologists should be aware of the complex risk profile in individual infants. Several models have been developed that consider some or several of the factors influencing the short- and long-term prognosis of EP infants. Several guidelines include the option of withholding treatment if the infant's condition appears poor immediately after birth. This agrees with the attitude of many neonatologists who want "to see what the infant looks like" if the infant is born at the limit of viability (Singh et al. 2007). However, several studies demonstrated that the infant's condition at birth (low Apgar scores and low heart rates at 1 min and 5 min, need of cardiopulmonary resuscitation) did not predict poor outcome in EP infants (Finer et al. 1999; Jankov et al. 2000). Thus, the condition at birth is an unreliable predictor of the prognosis of EP infants, unless resuscitation of more than 3–5 min is required to stabilize an EP infant.

Definitions of the limit of viability and of the "gray zone" in EP infants (Walter 2005; Seri and Evans 2008; Lagercrantz and Changeux 2009; Comitato Nazionale per la Bioetica 2008):

(a) Viability is defined as the possibility to live and survive outside the uterus independent of the risk for severe neurodevelopmental disability.
(b) Viability is determined as a reasonable chance to survive without "severe and unacceptable" morbidity (usually defined as severe neurodevelopmental disability).
(c) Viability is defined as the ability to grow and develop normally outside the uterus, the ability to communicate, and the ability to engage in meaningful relationships with others, to become a child and later achieve independent moral status and personhood.

The outcome of infants born at 22 weeks' gestation is actually extremely poor; infants born at 23–24 weeks' gestation have an uncertain prognosis, and infants born at 25 weeks' gestation have a reasonable chance to survive without severe disability. The lower limit of viability is currently set at 22–23 weeks and the "gray zone" at 23 0/7–24 6/7 weeks. Infants born in the "gray zone" have an uncertain prognosis with high risk of death or survival with severe long-term deficits, but the individual prognosis depends on a variety of biologic and individual (maturity, strength, and resilience), technologic, and general care factors (including antenatal proactive care, attitudes of staff, and developmental care in the NICU). The "gray zone" also considers the uncertainty of the assessment of gestational age by approximately ±7 days (Skupsi et al. 2010).

11.4 Laws and Guidelines for the Care at the Limit of Viability

The World Health Organization (WHO) defines a live birth as "a fetus, whatever its gestational age, exits the maternal body and subsequently shows any sign of life, such as voluntary movement, heartbeat, or pulsation of the umbilical cord, for however brief a time" (World Health Organization 1993). The term "live birth" was defined by the WHO mainly for public health, legal, and statistical purposes and should not be used synonymously with "viability." Signs of life may already be seen in extremely immature infants born at 20 weeks of gestation and no chance of survival.

The "Born-Alive Infant Protection Act" enacted by the US government in 2002 obliges the physician to "protect infants who are born alive at any stage of development." Enforcement guidelines to the law issued in 2005 requires the hospital and its medical staff "to perform a medical screening examination on that born-alive infant" and to treat the infant if signs of life are detected (Partridge and Dickey 2009). The legal conditions in the USA may explain that the guidelines of the American Academy of Pediatrics (MacDonald and American Academy of Pediatrics Committee on Fetus and Newborn 2002; American Academy of Pediatrics 2007) recommend withholding life support in infants with

22 weeks' gestation but do not give detailed recommendations for more mature infants. Similar guidelines have been issued in Spain (Pignotti and Donzelli 2008). In Italy, the National Bioethics Committee recommends resuscitation of all babies born alive when a possibility of survival exists (Turillazzi and Fineschi 2009).

Some national laws define the limit of viability to address primarily the limit of legal abortion (e.g., Japan and Italy, 22 weeks; the Netherlands, Singapore, and the UK, 24 weeks). In Japan the viability limit has been lowered from the previous 24 weeks' gestation to 22 completed weeks' gestation in 1991 (Motherhood Protection Act) based on surveys of survival rates in EP infants (Nishida and Sakuma 2009). As a result of the legislation in Japan, intensive care is provided to all EP infants born at ≥22 weeks' gestations (Iijima et al. 2009).

In most western countries, as well as in Japan and Australia, guidelines regarding the limit of viability have been established by medical organizations in agreement with national laws and court rulings (Nishida and Sakuma 2009; Comitato Nazionale per la Bioetica 2008; MacDonald and American Academy of Pediatrics Committee on Fetus and Newborn 2002; Pignotti and Donzelli 2008; Lui et al. 2006; Nuffield Council on Bioethics 2006; Wilkinson et al. 2009; Peerzada et al. 2006; Miljeteig et al. 2007; Rijken et al. 2007; Pohlandt 2008; Österreichische Gesellschaft für Kinder-und Jugendheilkunde 2005; Dehan et al. 2001; Fischer et al. 2009). The guidelines usually present recommendations for the care of infants with extremely poor, uncertain, and fairly good prognosis. No country recommends resuscitation of infants with gestational age below 22 weeks. For infants of 22 weeks' gestation, guidelines of five countries recommend "comfort care only" (MacDonald and American Academy of Pediatrics Committee on Fetus and Newborn 2002; Pignotti and Donzelli 2008; Lui et al. 2006; Peerzada et al. 2006; Rijken et al. 2007). The other guidelines propose individual decisions based on parental request or the infant's condition at birth. For infants with 23 weeks' gestation, three countries recommend "comfort care only" (Lui et al. 2006; Rijken et al. 2007; Dehan et al. 2001), while the other guidelines recommend individual decision or care according to parental request. At 24 weeks' gestation, four guidelines regard intensive care as due according with individual decisions (Wilkinson et al. 2009; Peerzada et al. 2006; Miljeteig et al. 2007; Fischer et al. 2009), four as generally indicated (Nishida and Sakuma 2009; Comitato Nazionale per la Bioetica 2008; Pohlandt 2008; Österreichische Gesellschaft für Kinder-und Jugendheilkunde 2005). At 25 weeks' gestation, most guidelines regard intensive care as "generally indicated." Resuscitation on the basis of gestational age has also been criticized (Fanaroff 2008): The likelihood of a favorable outcome with intensive care can be better estimated by considering four factors in addition to gestational age: sex, exposure to antenatal corticosteroids, single or multiple births, and birth weight (Tyson et al. 2008).

11.5 Quality of Life and the Best Interests of the Infant

Assessments of the quality of life, the harm/benefit ratio, and the best interests of the infant are often made to decide whether it is appropriate to begin or to continue intensive care. In the decision-making process, the estimated quality of life corresponds to the probable benefit resulting from medical care, and the best interests are deducted from the harm/benefit ratio. Parents and professional caregivers are particularly concerned with the risk of "brain damage" and what it means for the child. In the newborn infant, quality of life is usually related to the estimated future health and development. There are several concerns with the definition of the future quality of life in preterm and severely sick neonates:

The future quality of life is usually estimated from risk factors such as gestational age, birth weight, gender, signs of brain damage in ultrasound scans, and other complications during intensive care. Quality of life is thus estimated from individual factors that are compared with statistical data studied in a cohort of infants with similar risk factors. The epidemiological approach is objective but uncertain for the individual child.

The meaning of an estimated future quality of life in infants cannot be judged by the infants themselves but is estimated by the families, the caregivers, and the society. It includes effects of the health status on lifestyle in the children and their families, the quality of life probably experienced by the child, and the value placed by the public, the family, and the child on compromised health states.

The uncertainty of the estimation of the future quality of life is difficult to bear for many parents and caregivers, as the consequence of the judgment may be the death of the infant. This is admitted in some countries but cannot avoid the suspect of a conflict of interests: some parents can overestimate babies' future disability, or they cannot accept even a low-grade handicap that, on the other hand, the baby might bear.

Life-and-death decisions based on the judgment of the quality of life have been regarded discriminatory against handicapped persons. Many disabled persons might consider their quality of life as good or acceptable. Some can argue that the decision to withhold or withdraw intensive care is only made in infants with anticipated disability that will probably lead to intolerable suffering and burden and inability to interact with others, but some authors do not agree.

Several national laws, decrees, court rulings, and guidelines request that any decision made on behalf of a person lacking decision-making capacity must be in the person's "best interests." Three major interests of the premature or sick neonate have been defined (Hester 2007; Kopelman 2007; Chiswick 2008):

Interests in the neonate's health: reasonable care using recognized standards of care and appropriate individualized care measures have to be provided.

Immediate (short-term) interests of the infant: pain and suffering, harm, and indignity should be avoided by the selection of appropriate therapeutic measures (e.g., developmental care, pain treatment, comforting care).

Long-term or future potential interests of the infant: these are usually defined as good or acceptable long-term outcome.

In addition to the infant's interests, familial, communal, and public (moral and legal) interests play a role (Hester 2007; Kopelman 2007). The family members have their own interests and incorporate religious and cultural values. Communal or social interests consider cultural beliefs about the value of disabilities, concerns for dignity, and respect. Public interests include protection of citizens from abuse or neglect. Medical care of newborn infants has to be compatible with moral and legal duties to incapacitated individuals.

Pain and suffering from intensive care procedures (present quality of life) are related to the risk for long-term suffering and burden (future quality of life). If the infant has no chance of survival, intensive care will merely prolong pain and suffering, and natural death may be in the best interests of the baby. If the outcome of the infant is uncertain, but most likely associated with poor health and development, the best interests will be judged from both the present pain and suffering (intensive care) and the estimated future suffering and burden.

Financial considerations should not play a role in the judgment of the best interests of an infant with uncertain prognosis by the caregivers and the society. The best interest concept is mainly applied in uncertain situations but may be uncertain itself. What is the probability of survival of an individual infant? What is a reasonable, an acceptable, and an unacceptable long-term outcome? Kipnis (2007) defined three types of uncertainty in the estimation of the outcome: the vagueness of the definition of "intolerable deficits," the uncertainty of whether a baby will benefit from an intensive care intervention or be harmed by it, and the inability to determine the harm-to-benefit ratio of (sometimes aggressive and painful) intensive care measures. Moreover, the application of the best interest standards may be flawed by limited knowledge or lack of consensus about treatment choices, conflicts of interests, personal beliefs, bias and prejudice, lack of empathy, ignorance, or disregard of persons' rights and duties (Bellieni and Buonocore 2009; Kopelman 2007).

Critics of the "best interests" concept argue that it is vague, open to abuse, and permits decision-makers to do whatever they think is best. Decisions may be made in the interests of the parents and caregivers rather than in the best interests of the infant. To overcome the uncertainties of the best interests of an individual infant, it has been suggested that a best interests' standard should incorporate what a reasonable person of good will would want or consider acceptable in similar circumstances ("reasonable person standard" (Hester 2007; Kopelman 2007)). Physicians and other health professionals should be aware that in clinical practice, it is impossible to know the true best interests of an infant or to define the ideal best interests for an infant. The consideration of evidence-based facts, the clinical intuitions at predicting the outcome of an infant, has been found useful in one study (Meadow et al. 2002). In some countries the decision to withhold or withdraw intensive care in an infant is up to the parents. The best interests of the infant should be judged jointly by the parents and the physicians. The physicians do not make the final decision but rather provide the parents with all the information they need to make an explicit decision. This information includes the probable outcome, the necessary intensive care procedures to achieve this outcome, and the anticipated burden (including the social and financial burden).

Saigal and colleagues reported in a cohort of adults who were born extremely low birth weight, survivors had no difference in self-ratings of health-related quality of life (HRQOL) when compared with normal birth weight controls (Saigal et al. 2006; Wyatt 2007).

11.6 Attitudes Toward Extremely Preterm and Critically Sick Neonates

Attitudes of caregivers toward withholding and withdrawing intensive care of EP and critically sick infants with uncertain prognosis vary among different health professions, among different countries and regions, among various centers of a country or region, and among different caregivers in one center (Hakansson et al. 2004; Bilgen et al. 2007; Cuttini et al. 2009). Moreover, attitudes of caregivers and parents may deviate considerably. Attitudes of obstetricians and pediatricians were similar in most studies, while nurses in some countries tended to be more prone than physicians to withhold resuscitation in the delivery room and to consider parental opinion regarding subsequent treatment choices than physicians (Miljeteig et al. 2007; De Leeuw et al. 2000; Lavin et al. 2006). Nurses frequently underline the suffering of the newborn, whereas physicians often stress uncertainty in treatment outcome (van Zuuren and van Manen 2006).

The EURONIC study group revealed that most caregivers in seven European countries would limit intensive care in EP infants with fatal/terminal illness, but that 45–60% of the responders from Germany, Italy, and Spain would not set limits in case of poor neurological prognosis (Cuttini et al. 2009). Moreover, the attitude toward "explicit involvement" of parents in decision-making varied between 10% (France) and >90% (UK). If the physicians wished to discontinue intensive care of an infant with poor prognosis, approximately 50% would continue intensive care at parental request.

Bellieni and Buonocore (2009) reviewed attitudes of caregivers concerning the best interests of the newborn. They conclude that several aspects of the personal (age, gender, having own children, fear of litigation), social, religious, and professional background (position, experience, knowledge, number of cots) influence the attitudes of the caregivers. Religious convictions play an important role in the attitudes toward care of EP or severely critically infants independent of the denomination (Bilgen et al. 2007; Lam et al. 2009).

Janvier and colleagues demonstrated that attitudes toward the care of EP or critically sick newborn infants deviate markedly from the attitudes toward older children and adults with similar or worse prognosis (Janvier et al. 2008a, b). Asked if they would resuscitate patients with identical outcome (50% risk of death and 50%

risk of severe neurodevelopmental disability in survivors), 69% of the respondents would resuscitate an EP infant, 87% a full-term neonate, and 97% a two-month-old infant. The authors conclude that EP infants are considered "morally different from older children" (Janvier et al. 2007) and speculate that the majority of the respondents had either irrational negative associations with low gestational ages or they were unaware of actual outcomes (Janvier et al. 2008c).

Table 2 summarizes several indications that neonates, in particularly EP infants, are valued differently from older children and adults. A positive attitude of all prenatal and postnatal caregivers toward the care of a high-risk infant is an important determinant of the prognosis. If some physicians or nurses think that an EP or severely sick infant is not viable, they might treat the baby that way, resulting in self-fulfilling prophecy. Education of all staff involved in prenatal and postnatal care of high-risk infants about the actual outcomes using valid epidemiological data and elimination of irrational negative associations with low gestational age or other risk factors are important prerequisites for a good outcome of high-risk infants.

Table 2 Facts and causes of devaluation of the lives of preterm and full-term infants

- The fetus has almost no rights in utero but suddenly becomes a citizen after birth
- Termination of pregnancy is legal in many countries even after the limit of a preterm's viability
- The extremely preterm infant is frequently described as "living fetus" or "fetal infant," thereby implying the same lack of rights for the newborn infant as for the fetus
- Infants of older mothers or mothers conceived by in vitro fertilization are often called "precious" or "irreplaceable" children in contrast to apparently less precious other infants (e.g., of very young mothers). This relativity of the value of a preterm infant is unthinkable for a critically sick child
- Some ethicists believe that newborn infants lack "personhood" (personality) and consciousness and are thus comparable with an animal rather than with a human child or adult
- There is widespread belief that the bonding of infant and mother is less in newborn infants than in older infants and children and even less in premature infants
- Many caretakers are unaware of actual outcomes of extremely preterm infants and overestimate mortality and disability rates and the costs of care
- Irrational negative associations with low gestational ages are frequent in caregivers and the public. Confirmation bias results in the selection of arguments (and research results) that confirm the assumption of poor prognosis of extremely preterm infants
- Uncertainty of a prognosis (e.g., extreme prematurity, intracranial hemorrhage, severe asphyxia, or malformations) may justify withholding and withdrawal of treatment in a neonate but not in an older infant or child
- The informed decision process of the parents requires reliable information at a time when the caretakers themselves are still depending on subjective interpretation of benefits, risks, and burdens of the infant

11.7 The Rights of the Newborn and the Parents

Mercurio distinguishes three rights of the newborn, the right to life, the right to mercy, and the right to justice or fair treatment (Mercurio 2009). The right to life is part of many national constitutions and includes the right to appropriate medical treatment. He defined the right to mercy as "a right not to be subjected to pain or discomfort that is very unlikely to yield benefit." The right to justice or fair treatment includes the right to equal medical treatment independent of age, ethnicity, income, etc. Different attitudes to the care of preterm, full-term, and older infants (Janvier et al. 2008c) violate this right, if they influence the care. The right to justice and equal treatment includes the use of proper epidemiological data in the decision to treat or not to treat an EP infant.

Most countries grant parents the legal rights to decide on behalf of their minor children including the general upbringing, the education, the religion, and medical treatment decisions. The parents have the right to get all available information on the condition of their sick child and on therapeutic options for their child. After they have received all necessary information, the parents have the right to select from the therapeutic options but also to refuse treatment or to have the infant transferred to another hospital. It would be inappropriate to override parents' wishes, since they are usually motivated by their infant's best interest, have natural authority over their child, express religious views in their opinion, and bear the burden of treatment decisions (Dare 2009).

On the other hand, the parents do not have the right to refuse necessary and reasonable treatment. Thus, parents' rights are rebuttable when their decisions pose a significant risk to the life or well-being of the infant (Dare 2009). "Parents have a right to make martyrs of themselves, but not of their children" (Mercurio 2009). Moreover, parents have no right to demand treatment that is of no benefit to the child. Without perceived benefit to the child, the parental right to decide is outweighed by the child's right to mercy (Mercurio 2009). These limitations of parental authority in decision-making for their preterm or sick infants do not justify to bar parents from accurate information about the long-term prognosis, resuscitation, and treatment options. In many hospitals parents still have limited informed input, even if the infant is born in the "gray zone" of viability (Cuttini et al. 2009; Harrison 2008).

11.8 Informing and Counseling Parents

Guidelines in many countries give parents the major responsibility for the decision-making in EP infants in the gray zone. This responsibility requires comprehensive and accurate information on the prognosis of the infant and treatment options before and after birth.

The major purposes of antenatal and postnatal counseling are (Bellieni and Buonocore 2009) to inform the parents accurately about the condition, the reasonable treatment options, and the prognosis of the fetus or the newborn infant and (Janvier et al. 2008a) to assist the parents with decision-making (Walter 2005; Halamek 2003; Batton 2009). The consultations have to be honest, fair, compassionate, and sensitive to the culture and religion, the level of understanding, and the physical and psychological condition of the mother and the father. Translation services may be necessary for parents not proficient in the national language. Senior physicians together with other experienced staff should perform the consultations in a spirit of fairness and compassion. If the counseling physicians are sure that the parents have understood the information, options of care (inclusive withholding and withdrawing of intensive care) should be presented to the parents. Both parents should be present at the consultation, unless the father is legally or for other reasons not involved. In this case the mother should be given the possibility to have a confidant involved. If the mother is underage or incapacitated, the mother's parents may share the authority with their daughter (Ladd and Mercurio 2003).

Antenatal counseling may be necessary for women with a high risk of delivering an EP or critically sick infants within days or weeks and for women with imminent delivery of a high-risk baby. The prenatal consultation is a collaborative process that should involve obstetricians and midwives, neonatologists and neonatal nurses, and (if necessary) pediatric subspecialists, pediatric surgeons, and genetic counselors (Griswold and Fanaroff 2010). Communication among various specialists is of great importance to avoid inconsistent and contradictory information and counseling (Halamek 2003). A shared decision between parents and physicians requires a trusting relationship between parents and caregivers. The parents should be encouraged to consult their family doctor or other health professionals outside the hospital, discuss their situation with relatives and friends, and be offered support by clergy, psychologist, or social worker.

The first antenatal consultation is usually performed by the obstetrician and/or midwife and focuses on antenatal treatments (selection of hospital, tocolysis, corticosteroids, cesarean section). Parents should be given accurate information about the chance of their infant surviving and surviving without severe disability. Many physicians believe that the amount of specific medical information is too much for the parents. However, parents have the right to receive the same information as the physicians to make far-reaching decisions for their child. Framing of the information may influence the decision of the parents: Persons who were informed on the prognosis of an EP infant born at 23 weeks' gestation as having a chance of intact survival chose resuscitation of an EP infant more often than parents who were given prognosis as risk of death and disability (Hayward et al. 2008).

A neonatologist should become involved as early as possible to describe the anticipated immediate and long-term problems after birth, short-term and long-term prognosis, the expected extent of resuscitation, and subsequent intensive care. Current information on outcome data of EP infants should include the prognostic relevance of the gestational age, birth weight, gender, multiple births, and prenatal care (Tyson et al. 2008; Leversen et al. 2011). Moreover, the parents should be informed on local care possibilities and on local outcome data in comparison with referral centers. Statistical outcome data presented in counseling should include risk of death and risk of survival with severe/moderate/mild impairments (including their meanings). It should also be mentioned that "normal" surviving infants are at risk of a variety of behavioral and educational deficits. Financial obligations are of little importance in counseling and resuscitation in most countries (Martinez et al. 2006) but should be considered if the prognosis of the infant is poor and the financial costs for the family are high.

The anticipated quality of life, pain, and suffering of the infant from intensive treatments but also the burden for the family should be addressed. Moreover, the parents should be informed about the option to withdraw intensive care if the treatment becomes futile. During the consultation, the attitudes and preferences of the parents should be evaluated to assess the best interests of the infant as judged by the parents. An experienced neonatal nurse should explain nursing procedures in the NICU (including feeding of mother's milk, kangaroo care, developmental care) and (if possible) give the mother and/or the father a tour of the NICU. If possible, the consulting neonatologist(s) and neonatal nurse(s) should be part of the resuscitation team in the delivery room and the initial intensive care team for the infant. If this is not possible, the counselors have to make sure that the resuscitation team is informed on the decisions made before delivery and does not oppose to the decisions, unless the situation has changed considerably.

In countries where the decision is given to the parents, there is controversy as to whether counseling of parents should be directive or nondirective (Batton 2009). In nondirective counseling, information on outcome data is given (including the uncertainty of the data) without recommendation for the decision, and parents are asked to decide whether they want their infant resuscitated after birth. This gives the parents full authority but also the entire responsibility for a life-or-death decision. They might feel left alone with their decision, worries, and emotions and may later regret their decision and feel guilty. Kaempf et al. (2009) demonstrated that shared authority of the staff and parents using clear guidelines for counseling is well accepted by the parents.

For many parents detailed information on the prognosis and discussion of treatment options are less important than religion-, spirituality-, and hope-guided decision-making (Boss et al. 2008). These parents may be reluctant to make a decision but may prefer to leave "things in God's hands" and want everything done. Different moral and religious attitudes may be a source of conflicts between physicians and parents. Dunn (1990) proposed to ask five questions, particularly if the views and decisions of the parents do not agree with the medical staff:

Do the parents understand the clinical condition and prognosis of their child?
Do they wish or should they consult others before finally making up their minds?
Do they require more time?
Is their decision a loving, caring one made in the interests of their child?
Are they asking to pull life-saving treatment only for their baby's interest?
Is their decision a reasonable one in the interests of their child, and, if in doubt, is it so unreasonable as to request them to seek other medical advice or for me to take legal steps to take the child into care under the protection of the courts?

Breaking bad news is particularly challenging and requires the sensitivity and communication skills of the physician. If bad news is given with warmth and affection and parents are treated with respect and sensitivity, most parents will have positive memories and will be grateful to the staff involved (Henley and Judith Schot 2008).

11.9 Decision-Making in EP Infants

Decisions concerning the care of EP infants may be required at three times:

1. Care of the mother and the fetus before birth. Parents and physicians have to decide whether antenatal proactive care is provided (transfer of the mother to a perinatal center, tocolysis, antenatal corticosteroids, cesarean section on fetal indication).
2. Initiation or withholding of resuscitation of the infant after birth. The decision as to whether the infant will be resuscitated is made before birth but may be changed according to the infant's condition and the infant's response to resuscitation. The decision to provide proactive antenatal care is usually combined with the decision to resuscitate the infant and vice versa.
3. Continuation or withdrawal of neonatal intensive care. Reorientation of care may be considered if provisional care of an infant with assumed poor prognosis has been unsuccessful or if the prognosis deteriorated (e.g., large cerebral bleeding with inactive electric brain activity). The decision to withdraw intensive care in some countries should be made jointly by parents and staff.

The reasons for end-of-life decisions have to agree with national or hospital guidelines. Palliative care treatments (e.g., analgesic drugs) have to be compatible with national laws and court decisions. In most guidelines no or small chance of survival ("futility" of treatment) and no or small chance of survival without severe disability are recognized conditions. The entire team (including subspecialists as pediatric neurologists, etc.) and (as required) the Ethical Committee should become involved in the end-of-life decision.

If the prognosis is uncertain, the harm-to-benefit ratio (i.e., pain and suffering from intensive care, suffering and burden from long-term impairments in relation to probable long-term outcome) should be estimated and considered in decision-making. Most guidelines consider only severe disability leading to intolerable suffering and burden and/or inability to interact with others as justification for withholding and withdrawal of life-sustaining treatment. Whether suffering and burden resulting from intensive care and disability are intolerable has to be decided by the parents. However, the decision to withhold or withdraw intensive care is primarily a medical decision for which the doctor bears ultimate moral and legal responsibility.

The major concern of an end-of-life decision is that the outcome of an individual infant is estimated from statistical data determined in a group of (more or less) representative infants studied several years earlier. Because of the uncertainty of the prognosis, some authors are strictly against any end-of-life decision made before birth but rather opt for an individualistic approach based on the infant's clinical condition and initial response to intervention at birth (Turillazzi and Fineschi 2009). However, most authors agree that "extending intensive care to all of the most immature infants would entail considerable suffering, resource use, and cost in order to benefit only a small proportion of infants" (Leversen et al. 2011). This can be considered as a utilitarian viewpoint, but it is the logical consequence of dealing with an uncertain situation in which judgment and decision have to be made in the assumed best interests of the individual infant.

When parents are involved in end-of-life decision, the following scenarios may occur after birth in infants whose prognosis was uncertain before birth:

1. If a joint decision of parents and physicians has been made before birth to resuscitate the infant, resuscitation of the infant should usually be tried even when the condition of the infant is severely compromised at birth.
2. If a joint end-of-life decision of parents and physicians has been made before birth, resuscitation of the infant will usually not be attempted. If the infant appears viable (spontaneous

respiration), resuscitation should be started within 1–2 min to avoid severe hypoxia.

3. If no joint decision of parents and physicians has been made before birth because the mother was already in active labor when admitted to the hospital or because of other reasons (e.g., language), the neonatologist must decide on behalf of the infant and should in case of doubt resuscitate the baby until the parents can be involved in the decision.

Parents differ in their request to be supported in their decision by the staff. Some parents want staff to suggest to them what to do, while others wish to receive the necessary information but prefer to make decisions independently or with the support of family, friends, family doctor, or religious adviser (Henley and Judith Schot 2008). Although most parents wish support, the staff members have to avoid any devaluation of parental autonomy and self-worth. "Most parents want to feel guided, assisted and listened to, but not directed or controlled, and certainly not abandoned" (Henley and Judith Schot 2008). Parents will usually make concerned and loving decisions in their infant's interests.

In countries where the decision to withhold or withdraw intensive care is taken with the essential statement of the parents, the main causes of conflicts between parents and physicians are different opinions of the condition and best interests of the infant, insensitive behavior and communication of the team, and religious convictions of the parents that forbid withdrawal of life-sustaining treatment (Tripp and McGregor 2006; Verhagen et al. 2009a). Parents usually make concerned and loving decisions in their infant's interests. A Dutch analysis of disagreements in end-of-life decisions demonstrated that conflicts within the team occurred in 4% and between the team and the parents in 12% of the cases. All conflicts were resolved by postponing the end-of-life decision until consensus was achieved (Verhagen et al. 2009a). When treatment is clearly futile, the physicians can decide to stop intensive care without a decision of an Ethics Committee or court in some countries (Isaacs et al. 2006). In case of conflict between parents and neonatologists, that is, the parents request to withdraw treatment, while the team sees a realistic chance of survival without severe disability and wishes to continue intensive care, intensive care should generally be continued.

11.10 Withholding and Withdrawing of Intensive Care

11.10.1 Withholding Versus Withdrawing of Intensive Care

In various studies end-of-life decisions preceded death in 70–80% of dying newborn infants (Hentschel et al. 2006; Verhagen et al. 2009b). Principally three ways of ending or limiting intensive care are possible with the intention to shorten the life of a patient: (Bellieni and Buonocore 2009) withholding of resuscitation and intensive care after birth, (Janvier et al. 2008a) withdrawing of life support, and (Levene 2004) withholding of additional therapies (e.g., antibiotics, vasoactive drugs). The third way is preferred by many professionals and parents but may result in survival with additional damage (e.g., from sepsis, hypoxia). Although probably not uncommon, withholding of additional therapies is rarely mentioned in reports on end-of-life decisions (Hentschel et al. 2006).

Several guidelines see no moral or ethical difference between withholding and withdrawing intensive care (Walter 2005; American Academy of Pediatrics 2007; Nuffield Council on Bioethics 2006; Wilkinson et al. 2009; Fischer et al. 2009; Verhagen et al. 2009b). Some authors explicitly opt for withdrawal rather than withholding life support, since "provisional" treatment allows for evaluation of the clinical condition of the infant, including the actual gestational age and body weight, and the reaction to resuscitation and intensive care (Fischer et al. 2009; Verhagen et al. 2009b). Boyle (2004) describes the widespread American attitude: "If the treatment in question never is started, no one will benefit. If it is started, some may benefit, and it can be withdrawn from those whom it does not benefit." During "provisional" intensive care, a harm-to-benefit ratio can be estimated repeatedly to determine whether it is appropriate to continue or not. Some national guidelines (e.g., Swiss) recommend "provisional care" of EP infants born at a gestational age in the "gray zone" (Fischer et al. 2009).

However, some religious convictions allow withholding, but not withdrawing, of life support (Tripp and McGregor 2006). Furthermore, for many caregivers and parents, it is psychologically more difficult to withdraw than to withhold intensive care measures. The EURONIC study demonstrated that neonatologists in Italy, Spain, France, and Germany consider it more acceptable to withhold than to withdraw mechanical ventilation, whereas in the Netherlands, the UK, and Sweden, more than 93% of the neonatologists would withdraw intensive care in selected circumstances (Cuttini et al. 2009). Reasons for reluctance to withdraw intensive care include fear of legal consequences, increasing emotional attachment of parents and infants with time, and feeling of active life ending or even killing by extubation and application of pain- and stress-relieving drugs.

On the other hand, for some parents the death of their child may be more bearable if the neonatal team has "tried everything" and "gave him or her every chance" (Mercurio 2009). Moreover, a period of intensive care allows some time for the parents and siblings to meet the child, to perform baptism or other religious ceremonies, and to touch and cuddle the baby. The infant may die in the arms of the parents, and the family has time to grieve with their child and to mourn in dignity. Some parent-infant bonding may relief the mourning sorrow. These possible emotional benefits must be weighed against painful intensive care measures and the use of intensive care resources (Wyatt 1999).

11.10.2 Withholding Proactive Antenatal Care and Resuscitation After Birth

Proactive antenatal care (transfer to a center, corticosteroids, cesarean section on fetal indication) improves the prognosis of an EP infant to the level of a 1–2 weeks more mature infant (Itabashi et al. 2009; Hakansson et al. 2004; Fischer et al. 2009; Leversen et al. 2011). It is therefore reasonable to decide either for both active antenatal care and postnatal resuscitation or for neither of these active approaches, unless the postnatal condition of the infant requires reorientation of the decision made before birth. Some parents might prefer a passive approach before delivery but active life support when the infant appears viable after birth. Even for preterm infants with a gestational age below the limit of viability, an experienced neonatologist should be present or immediately available at birth to confirm or to reorient the medical decision made before birth. However, a joint decision of the parents and physicians made before delivery should not be reversed after birth without marked change in the expected clinical situation.

When resuscitation is futile, compassionate care must be provided as for babies whose intensive care is discontinued. The baby may be placed on the breast of the mother and die in peace. If the baby suffers, an analgesic and/or sedative drug should be given. An appropriate religious ceremony should be offered and organized.

Since EP infants requiring more than 3–5 min of resuscitation have a poor prognosis (Singh et al. 2007; Finer et al. 1999; Jankov et al. 2000; Janvier and Barrington 2005), the ILCOR guidelines (The International Liaison Committee on Resuscitation (ILCOR) 2006) suggest to stop resuscitation "if there are no signs of life after 10 min of continuous and adequate resuscitative efforts." In clinical practice 10 min may, however, be a rather brief resuscitation time, since ventilation and other resuscitation measures are not always adequate (The International Liaison Committee on Resuscitation (ILCOR) 2006). A framework of care of extremely preterm infants derived from various guidelines and personal experience of the author is shown in Table 3.

11.10.3 Withdrawing of Intensive Care

The decision to withdraw intensive care is usually made in several steps:

1. The medical decision of treatment futility or intolerable long-term suffering is made

Table 3 Framework of care of extremely preterm infants (<26 weeks' gestation)

General considerations
Extremely preterm infants deserve the best state-of-the-art care to attain the best possible outcomes. Withholding treatment because the hospital cannot provide the appropriate care is unacceptable. If experienced obstetricians and neonatologists are not available at the hospital, the mother has to be transferred to a specialized center. If a transport is not possible, the most experienced local staff should be involved and get advice from a specialized center
Accurate estimation of gestational age (as a major determinant of the prognosis) is extremely important. Moreover, body weight, gender, and multiple births influence the prognosis and should be considered in antenatal counseling of the parents
Parents' rights to comprehensive information and explicit involvement in decisions about antenatal care (transfer to level III center, tocolysis, corticosteroids, cesarean section) and postnatal care of their preterm infant born before or in the "gray zone" (23–24 weeks' gestation) have to be respected
A decision before birth not to resuscitate or to resuscitate may have to be reconsidered after birth due to inaccurate prenatal estimation of gestational age and individual variation of the maturity and viability of the infant. The heart rate response of the baby to ventilation within 3–5 (−10) min is a better indicator of the prognosis than the clinical condition at birth

collectively by the NICU team and other subspecialists (e.g., pediatric neurologist, cardiologist, or surgeon).

2. The parents are informed on the prognosis of their infant and explicitly involved in the judgment of the best interests of their infant. Moreover, the parents are informed about options to prevent pain and suffering when their baby dies, and they are involved in the decision of appropriate pain- and stress-relieving treatment. Parents are supported in seeking advice by medical professionals outside the hospital, friends, and religious advisers. In some countries parents are requested to take an active role in this decision.
3. If parents and caregivers agree on the decision to withdraw intensive care, a time is set for ending intensive care (usually assisted ventilation). The parents decide whether they wish baptism or other religious rituals in correspondence to their faith.
4. Intensive care is reoriented to compassionate and palliative care. If possible, the baby is cared for in a private family room. Invasive procedures, blood sampling, and any other painful or stressing interventions should be avoided or minimized. Maintaining dignity, warmth, skin contact (kangaroo care), and relief of pain and stress are basic elements of palliative care (Walter 2005; Carter 2004). A family-centered care philosophy is an optimal basis for neonatal intensive care and for the care of a dying infant. Family members and friends are given time and opportunity to stay with the infant, to touch, and cuddle the baby.
5. Withdrawal of life-sustaining treatment should take place in an unhurried, private, and dignified manner. In the presence of the parents, tubes and electrodes are removed, and the infant dies in the arms of the parents. Pain- and stress-relieving drugs should be given, and the bronchial and gastric tube should be sucked to avoid vomiting and choking (if possible, before the parents enter the room). A nurse and a physician (with a good relationship to the parents and the child) should be present until the infant has died and should see the family from time to time thereafter.
6. The staff shows empathy and supports the family in their grief. Mementos of the infant such as photos and video recordings, arm bands, the clothes, a footprint, and a strand of hair may be given to the parents. Parents should be supported with funeral arrangements and formalities such as death certificate. Some countries allow taking the dead baby home for some time before the funeral. Further consultations (outside the NICU!) should be offered. Information about bereavement and parent groups should be provided.

11.10.4 Pain- and Stress-Relieving Drugs

For intensively treated newborn infants with a good prognosis, indications and dosages of pain-reducing drugs are carefully adjusted to avoid serious side effects. After an end-of-life decision has been made, side effects are of little importance, and the dosages can be increased to reach complete elimination of pain and stress. Moreover, pain- and stress-relieving drugs are indicated to minimize pain and suffering resulting from the removal of tubes, lines, and electrodes and from dying itself. Several authors recommend administration of an adequate dose of opiate analgesia (morphine or analogues) together with a sedative (e.g., benzodiazepine) as part of humane care. Although the required high dosages of analgesics and sedatives may cause respiratory depression and shorten the life of the infant, their use is considered legal in most countries as long as the primary intention of the physicians is relief of pain and suffering and not shortening the life of the infant (Provost et al. 2004).

The administration of lethal dosages of drugs with the intention to hasten death is illegal in most countries. In the Netherlands, "non-voluntary euthanasia" is considered acceptable in selected infants for whom death appears to be in the infants' best interests but who are presently not dependent on life support. The Groningen Protocol for Euthanasia in Newborns gives detailed guidelines that are far more restricted than most guidelines and recommendations for withholding or withdrawing of intensive care (Verhagen and Sauer 2005). In fact, only 4% of infants with end-of-life decision (born in the Netherlands from 2005 to 2006) died from drugs given with the intention to hasten death (Verhagen and Sauer 2005).

11.11 Severe Asphyxia

Stillborn infants do not breathe and show no other evidence of life (such as beating of the heart, pulsation of the umbilical cord, definite movement of voluntary muscles). If the infant shows signs of maceration, the infant has died at least 12 h before birth. A fresh stillborn infant may have died hours or minutes before birth. If the fetal heartbeat was heard shortly before birth or fetal heartbeat was not monitored, resuscitation should be started.

Four studies on the outcome of infants with severe asphyxia defined by Apgar score 0 at 10 min following birth demonstrated that 69–98% died and all surviving infants developed severe (89–100%) or moderate neurodevelopmental disability (Byrne et al. 2008). This is why some justify cessation of resuscitation after 10 min (The International Liaison Committee on Resuscitation (ILCOR) 2006), unless resuscitation was not adequate. If a baby develops signs of severe hypoxic-ischemic encephalopathy with poor long-term prognosis, a decision (jointly made by the parents and physicians) to withdraw intensive care is justified by some authors (Boyle 2004).

11.12 Malformations

Malformation may justify withholding of postnatal resuscitation if the malformation is not compatible with life or if there is a high risk of death or if therapy burden is not bearable. The harm-to-benefit ratio (i.e., pain and suffering from early interventions in relation to the probable outcome) may be considered in the estimation of the best interests of the infant. Table 4 lists lethal malformations.

Termination of pregnancy for fetal malformation is liberally implemented in many countries. After birth the best interests of viable infants with malformations have to be judged individually for each infant, each malformation, and the probable long-term sequelae of the malformation. After birth, treatment decisions are primarily based on the best interests of the infant (and not primarily on the authority of the mother). This sudden change in authority is difficult to understand for many parents. Infants with Down syndrome pose particular dilemma for parents and physicians. On the one hand, the major purpose of prenatal screening is to detect trisomy 21 and to terminate pregnancy if the fetus suffers from

Table 4 Lethal malformations (according to the US American Birth Defect Center)

Trisomy 13
Trisomy 18
Anencephaly
Acranium
Bilateral renal agenesis (Potter syndrome)
Bart's hydrops fetalis

Down syndrome; on the other hand, there is general agreement that the diagnosis of Down syndrome is no indication for withholding resuscitation even if the infant suffers from severe cardiac or other malformations (Rennie and Leigh 2008).

References

American Academy of Pediatrics (2007) Noninitiation or withdrawal of intensive care for high-risk newborns. Pediatrics 119:401–403

Batton DG, Committee on Fetus and Newborn (2009) Clinical report—Antenatal counseling regarding resuscitation at an extremely low gestational age. Pediatrics 124:422–427

Bellieni CV, Buonocore G (2009) Flaws in the assessment of the best interests of the newborn. Acta Paediatr 98:613–617

Bilgen H, Topuzoglu A, Kuscu K et al (2007) End-of-life decisions in the newborn period: attitudes and practices of doctors and nurses. Turk J Pediatr 51:248–256

Boss RD, Hutton N, Sulpar LJ et al (2008) Values parents apply to decision-making regarding delivery room resuscitation for high-risk newborns. Pediatrics 122:583–589

Boyle RJ (2004) Ethical issues in the care of the neonate. NeoReviews 5:e471–e476

Byrne S, Szyld E, Kattwinkel J (2008) The ethics of delivery-room resuscitation. Semin Fetal Neonatal Med 13:440–447

Carter BS (2004) Comfort care principles for the high-risk newborn. NeoReviews 5:e484–e490

Chiswick M (2008) Infants at borderline viability: ethical and clinical consideration. Semin Fetal Neonatal Med 13:8–15

Comitato Nazionale per la Bioetica (2008) I grandi prematuri. Note bioetiche. [EP babies. Bioethical notes]. www.governo.it/bioetica

Cuttini M, Casotto V, Vonderweid U et al (2009) Neonatal end-of-life decisions and bioethical perspectives. Early Hum Dev 85:S21–S25

Dare T (2009) Parental rights and medical decisions. Pediatr Anesth 19:947–952

De Leeuw R, Cuttini M, Nadai M et al (2000) Treatment choices for extremely preterm infants: an international perspective. J Pediatr 137:608–616

Dehan M, Gold F, Grassin M et al (2001) Dilemmes éthiques de la période périnatale: recommendations pour les decisions de fin de vie. Arch Pediatr 8:407–419

Dunn PM (1990) Life saving intervention in the neonatal period: dilemmas and decisions. Arch Dis Child 65:557–558

Fanaroff AA (2008) Extremely low birthweight infants-the interplay between outcomes and ethics. Acta Paediatr 97:144–145

Finer NN, Tarin T, Vaucher YE et al (1999) Intact survival in extremely low birth weight infants after delivery room resuscitation. Pediatrics 104:e40

Fischer N, Steurer MA, Adams M et al (2009) Survival rates of extremely preterm infants (gestational age <26 weeks) in Switzerland: impact of the Swiss guidelines for the care of infants born at the limit of viability. Arch Dis Child Fetal Neonatal Ed 94:F407–F413

Griswold KJ, Fanaroff JM (2010) An evidence-based overview of prenatal consultation with a focus on infants born at the limits of viability. Pediatrics 125:e931–e937

Hakansson S, Farooqi A, Holmgren PA et al (2004) Proactive management promotes outcome in extremely preterm infants: a population-based comparison of two perinatal management strategies. Pediatrics 114:58–64

Halamek LP (2003) Prenatal consultation at the limits of viability. NeoReviews 4:e153–e156

Harrison HT (2008) The offer they can't refuse: parents and perinatal treatment decisions. Semin Fetal Neonatal Med 13:329–334

Hayward MF, Murphy RO, Lorenz JM (2008) Message framing and perinatal decisions. Pediatrics 122:109–118

Henley A, Judith Schot J (2008) The death of a baby before, during or shortly after birth: good practice from the parents' perspective. Semin Fetal Neonatal Med 13:325–328

Hentschel R, Lindner K, Krueger M, Reiter-Theil S (2006) Restriction of ongoing intensive care in neonates: a prospective study. Pediatrics 118:563–569

Hester DM (2007) Interests and neonates: there is more to the story than we explicitly acknowledge. Theor Med Bioeth 28:357–372

Iijima S, Arai H, Ozawa Y et al (2009) Clinical patterns in extremely preterm (22 to 24 weeks of gestation) infants in relation to survival time and prognosis. Am J Perinatol 26:399–406

Ikeda K, Hayashida S, Hokuto I (2006) International perspectives: recent outcomes of ultrapreterm and extremely low-birth weight infants. Neo Reviews 7: e511–e516

Isaacs D, Kilham H, Gordon A et al (2006) Withdrawal of neonatal mechanical ventilation against the parents' wishes. J Paediatr Child Health 42:311–315

Itabashi K, Horiuchi T, Kusuda S et al (2009) Mortality rates for extremely low birth weight infants born in Japan in 2005. Pediatrics 123:445–450

Jankov RP, Asztalos EV, Scidmore MB (2000) Favourable neurological outcomes following delivery room cardiopulmonary resuscitation of infants $\leq$750 g at birth. J Paediatr Child Health 36:19–22

Janvier A, Barrington KJ (2005) The ethics of neonatal resuscitation at the margins of viability: informed consent and outcomes. J Pediatr 147:579–585

Janvier A, Bauer KL, Lantos JD (2007) Are newborns morally different from older children? Theor Med Bioeth 28:413–425

Janvier A, Lantos J, Deschênes M et al (2008a) Caregivers attitudes for very premature infants: what if they knew? Acta Paediatr 97:276–279

Janvier A, Leblanc I, Barrington KJ (2008b) The best-interest standard is not applied for neonatal resuscitation decisions. Pediatrics 121:963–969

Janvier A, Leblanc I, Barrington KJ (2008c) Nobody likes premies: the relative value of patients' life. J Perinatol 28:821–826

Kaempf JW, Tomlinson MW, Campbell B et al (2009) Counseling pregnant women who may deliver extremely premature infants: medical care guidelines, family choices, and neonatal outcomes. Pediatrics 123:1509–1515

Kipnis K (2007) Harm and uncertainty in newborn intensive care. Theor Med Bioeth 28:393–412

Kopelman LM (2007) The best interests standard for incompetent or incapacitated persons of all ages. J Law Med Ethics 35:187–196

Kusuda S, Fujimura M, Sakuma I et al (2006) Morbidity and mortality of infants with very low birth weight in Japan. center variation. Pediatrics 118:e1131–e1139

Ladd RE, Mercurio MR (2003) Deciding for neonates: whose authority, whose interests? Semin Perinatol 27:488–494

Lagercrantz H, Changeux JP (2009) The emergence of human consciousness: from fetal to neonatal life. Pediatr Res 65:255–260

Lam HS, Wong SPS, Liu FYB et al (2009) Attitudes toward neonatal intensive care treatment of preterm infants with a high risk of developing long-term disabilities. Pediatrics 123:1501–1508

Lavin JP, Kantak A, Ohlinger J et al (2006) Attitudes of obstetric and pediatric health care providers toward resuscitation of infants who are born at the margins of viability. Pediatrics 118:S169–S176

Levene M (2004) Is intensive care for very immature babies justified? Acta Paediatr 93:149–152

Leversen KT, Sommerfelt K, Rønnestad A et al (2011) Prediction of neurodevelopmental and sensory outcome at 5 years in Norwegian children born extremely preterm. Pediatrics 127:e630–e638

Linderkamp O (2012) Survival and outcome of extremely preterm infants in the 90s and early 2000s. Acta Paediatr (in press)

Lui K, Bajuk B, Foster K et al (2006) Perinatal care at the borderlines of viability: a consensus statement based on a NSW and ACT consensus workshop. Med J Aust 185:495–500

MacDonald H, American Academy of Pediatrics Committee on Fetus and Newborn (2002) Perinatal care at the threshold of viability. Pediatrics 110:1024–1027

Markestad T, Kaaresen PI, Ronnestad A et al (2005) Early death, morbidity, and need of treatment among extremely premature infants. Pediatrics 15:1289–1298

Marsal K, Express Group (2009) Survival of extremely preterm infants after active perinatal care in Sweden. JAMA 301:2225–2233

Martinez AM, Partridge JC, Yu V et al (2006) Physician counselling practices and decision-making for extremely preterm infants in the Pacific Rim. J Paediatr Child Health 41:209–214

Meadow W, Frain L, Ren Y et al (2002) Serial assessment of mortality in the neonatal intensive care unit by algorithm and intuition: certainty, uncertainty, and informed consent. Pediatrics 109:878–886

Mercurio MR (2009) The ethics of newborn resuscitation. Semin Perinatol 33:354–363

Miljeteig I, Markestad T, Norheim OF (2007) Physicians' use of guidelines and attitudes to withholding and withdrawing treatment for extremely premature neonates in Norway. Acta Paediatr 96:825–829

Moser K, Macfarlane A, Chow YH et al (2007) Introducing new data on gestation-specific infant mortality among babies born in 2005 in England and Wales. Health Stat Q 35:13–27

Nishida H, Sakuma I (2009) Limit of viability in Japan: ethical consideration. J Perinat Med 37:457–460

Nuffield Council on Bioethics (2006) Critical care decisions in fetal and neonatal medicine: ethical issues, London. www.nuffieldbioethics.org/neonatal-medicine

Österreichische Gesellschaft für Kinder-und Jugendheilkunde (2005) Erstversorgung von Frühgeborenen an der Grenze der Lebensfähigkeit. Monatsschr Kinderheilkd 7:711–715

Partridge JC, Dickey BJ (2009) Decision-making in neonatal intensive care: interventions on behalf of preterm infants. NeoReviews 10:e270–e278

Peerzada JM, Schollin J, Håkansson S (2006) Delivery room decision-making for extremely preterm infants in Sweden. Pediatrics 117:1988–1995

Pignotti MS, Donzelli G (2008a) Perinatal care at the threshold of viability: an international comparison of practical guidelines for the treatment of extremely preterm births. Pediatrics 121:e193–e198

Pohlandt F (2008) Leitlinie zur Frühgeburt an der Grenze der Lebensfähigkeit des Kindes. Monatsschr Kinderheilkd 156:798–802

Provost V, Deliens L, Cools F et al (2004) A classification of end-of-life decisions in neonates and infants. Acta Paediatr 93:301–305

Rennie JM, Leigh B (2008) The legal framework for end-of-life decisions in the UK. Semin Fetal Neonatal Med 13:296–300

Rijken M, Veen S, Walther FJ (2007) Ethics of maintaining preterm infants. Pediatr Child Health 17:58–63

Saigal S, Stoskopf B, Pinelli J et al (2006) Transition of extremely low birthweight infants from adolescence to young adulthood. Pediatrics 118:1140–1148

Seri I, Evans J (2008) Limits of viability: definition of the gray zone. J Perinatol Suppl 1:S4–S8

Singh J, Fanaroff J, Andrews B et al (2007) Resuscitation in the "gray zone" of viability: determining physician preferences and predicting infant outcomes. Pediatrics 120:519–526

Skupsi DW, McCullough B, Levene M, Chervenak FA (2010) Improving obstetric estimation of outcomes of extremely premature infants: an evolving challenge. J Perinat Med 38:19–22

The International Liaison Committee on Resuscitation (ILCOR) (2006) Consensus on science with treatment recommendations for pediatric and neonatal patients. neonatal resuscitation. Pediatrics 117:e978–e988

Tripp J, McGregor D (2006) Withholding and withdrawing of life sustaining treatment in the newborn. Arch Dis Child Fetal Neonatal Ed 91:F67–F71

Turillazzi E, Fineschi V (2009) How old are you? Newborn gestational age discriminates neonatal resuscitation practices in the Italian debate. BMC Med Ethics 10:19

Tyson JE, Parikh NA, Langer J et al (2008) Intensive care for extreme prematurity-moving beyond gestational age. N Engl J Med 358:1672–1681

Verhagen E, Sauer PJJ (2005) The Groningen protocol-euthanasia in severely ill newborns. NEJM 352:959–992

Verhagen AAE, de Vos M, Dorscheidt JHHM et al (2009a) Conflicts about end-of-life decisions in NICUs in the Netherlands. Pediatrics 124:e112–e119

Verhagen AAE, Dorscheidt JHHM, Engels B et al (2009b) End-of-life decisions in Dutch neonatal intensive care units. Arch Pediatr Adolesc Med 163:895–901

Walter FJ (2005) Withholding treatment, withdrawing treatment, and palliative care in the neonatal intensive care unit. Early Hum Dev 81:865–872

Wilkinson AR, Ahluwalia J, Cole A et al (2009) Management of babies born extremely preterm at less than 25 weeks of gestation: a framework for clinical practices at the time of birth. Arch Dis Child Fetal Neonatal Ed 94:F2–F5

Wilson-Costello D, Friedman H, Minich N et al (2007) Improved neurodevelopmental outcomes for extremely low birth weight infants in 2000–2002. Pediatrics 119:37–45

World Health Organization (1993) International classification of diseases (ICD), vol 2, 10th rev edn. World Health Organization, Geneva, Switzerland

Wyatt JS (1999) Neonatal care: withholding or withdrawal of treatment in the newborn infant. Baillieres Best Pract Res Clin Obstet Gynaecol 13:503–511

Wyatt J (2007) End-of-life decisions, quality of life and the newborn. Acta Pædiatr 96:790–791

van Zuuren FJ, van Manen E (2006) Moral dilemmas in neonatology as experienced by health care practitioners: A qualitative approach. Med Health Care Philos 9:339–347

Care of Extremely Low-Birth-Weight Infants and Timing of Discharge. Information and Psychosocial Intervention in Neonatology

12

Fabio A. Mosca, Monica Fumagalli, Maria Elena Bolis, and Massimo Agosti

Contents

Abstract

The welcoming and assistance services of birth have evolved in the last decades. In western countries, birth at hospital went from a medical-sanitary assistance, aimed to guarantee the best security in hospital with more and more advanced and meticulous procedures and protocols, to a more humanitarian vision of the birth issue.

Prevention procedures have been established to promote attachment and bonding from the delivery room until discharge: the respect and promotion of birth physiology, the early and prolonged contact with the infant through the "skin to skin" technique immediately after birth, and the promotion of rooming-in practice, which is essential for the beginning of breastfeeding and bonding.

It has ever more clearly emerged the role of the emotional and psychological support of motherhood and the need to provide psychological services in the obstetric wards, in nurseries,

F. A. Mosca (✉) · M. Fumagalli
NICU, Department of Clinical Sciences and Community Health, Fondazione IRCCS Ca' Granda Ospedale Maggiore Policlinico Milano, Università degli Studi di Milano, Milan, Italy
e-mail: fabio.mosca@unimi.it

M. E. Bolis · M. Agosti
Neonatology and NICU – Maternal and Child Department, Ospedale "F del Ponte", Varese, Italy
e-mail: massimo.agosti@ospedale.varese.it

G. Buonocore et al. (eds.), *Neonatology*,
https://doi.org/10.1007/978-3-319-29489-6_161

and in all those "risky" contexts such as Neonatal Intensive Care Units (NICU), for extremely low birth weight infants (ELBW).

In fact ELBW infants are at high-risk for mortality, morbidities, and long-term complications. Optimizing perinatal and postnatal care is essential to improve their outcome and a better understanding of pathophysiological mechanisms involved in respiratory, cardiac, and cerebral injury is crucial to implement new preventive strategies.

Nevertheless an active and early involvement of parents in the infant's care is also greatly advisable. Specific guidelines to support the parents in these critical areas were created, in order to limit the traumatic effects connected to prematurity and pathologic births. NICU wards have increasingly promoted the early contact and involvement of parents, which allow the bonding not to be totally compromised by long separation, prolonged medicalization, and parental experiences.

Time of home discharge has to be carefully planned together with parents since ELBW infants are often discharged with some unresolved medical problems so an individualized, close, home-care plan has to be developed for these babies.

Long-term sequelae are mainly represented by neurodevelopmental disorders, neurosensory deficits, growth failure, and bronchopulmonary dysplasia. Long-term follow-up programs are recommended in order to early identify those babies who may benefit from intervention programs.

After hospital discharge, specific intervention models have been designed to support parenthood and to promote the parent's ability to take care of his own and his child's health.

In addition to psychological therapy, new types of services have been created as mutual self-help groups of parents and home visits service.

The diffusion of these intervention models has generated a significant improvement in the protection of parenthood and ELBW development.

12.1 Salient Points

- ELBW infants are at high risk for acute complications and long-term morbidities.
- Optimizing perinatal and postnatal care from the first minutes of life is essential to improve the outcome of ELBW infants.
- Timing of discharge has to be defined according to physiologic criteria and a safe home discharge plan has to be established with the family.
- Follow-up programs and early intervention strategies have to be implemented in order to improve long-term outcome.
- Prevention procedures have been established to promote attachment and bonding as much as possible.
- NICU wards have increasingly favored the early contact and involvement of parents, so that the bonding is not totally compromised by long separation, prolonged medicalization, and parental experiences.
- It has emerged ever more clearly the importance of the emotional and psychological support of parenthood and the need to provide psychological services.

12.2 Basic Approach to the Care of Extremely Low Birth Weight Infants: An Outline

Advances in perinatal and neonatal medicine have increased the survival rate of extremely low birth weight (ELBW) infants in the last decades (McCarthy 2015), but they are also at high-risk for morbidities and long-term sequelae. Optimizing perinatal and postnatal care is essential to improve their outcome.

ELBW infants represent an inhomogeneous population being constituted by two different groups of premature newborns with different underlying pathogenetic mechanisms: very premature babies and intrauterine growth restricted infants (IUGR) with higher gestational age but small for gestational age.

12.2.1 Delivery Room and First Hour of Life

The first hours of life of ELBW infants are crucial and several problems can arise in this time and develop at NICU admission, during the neonatal period and later in childhood.

At birth, careful attention to the maintenance of body temperature is essential. The most effective interventions seem to be gentle drying and occlusive wraps (polyethylene wraps or polyurethane bags), associated with hats. In spite of these procedures, low temperatures are common on admission and surveillance of temperatures in the delivery room and during transport should be identified as quality improvement initiatives (Laptook et al. 2009).

Most of ELBW infants need some kind of respiratory assistance in the delivery room to enhance lung fluid clearance, establish functional residual capacity (FRC), and maintain lung aeration (Hooper et al. 2016).

It is important to adequately tailor respiratory assistance in order to both prevent lung hyperinflation (avoiding excessively high pressure) and maintain an effective lung recruitment (applying positive end-expiratory pressure). The best respiratory strategy to support ELBW infants is still debated (Wiswell 2011).

The use of continuous positive airway pressure (CPAP) in spontaneously breathing infants seems to reduce the need of mechanical ventilation (Nowadzky et al. 2009); however, only marginal benefits have been shown in reducing the combined outcome of death or bronchopulmonary dysplasia (BPD) compared to intubation and endotracheal ventilation (Schmölzer et al. 2013).

Accurate monitoring of heart rate and oxygen saturation as soon after birth as practicable is recommended (Wyllie et al. 2015).

Delayed umbilical cord clamping has received increasing attention in the management of ELBW infants at birth as it seems to be beneficial and safe, being associated with improved hemodynamic stability, reduced need for red blood cell transfusion, and decreased rates of intraventricular hemorrhage (Oh et al. 2011).

12.2.2 Admission to NICU

On admission to NICU, body temperature and body weight should be measured to correct hypothermia or maintain normothermia and to optimize fluid management.

Sick ELBW infants need close monitoring of arterial blood pressure, blood gases, serum glucose, and electrolytes. Insertion of an umbilical arterial catheter is useful to avoid pain and discomfort. Arterial lines should be removed as soon as they are no longer necessary. The use of a double lumen umbilical venous catheter may be useful for the administration of fluid, drugs, and blood products. After the first week of life a percutaneous central venous catheter should be dedicated to infusion of parenteral nutrition (PN).

The skin of prematurely born ELBW infants is poorly effective as an epidermal barrier. Disturbances in temperature regulation and water balance, as well as infection can occur because of poor epidermal barrier function and the excessive use of adhesives. The routine prophylactic use of emollients is not recommended (Edwards et al. 2004).

In spite of progress in respiratory assistance due to new treatment options available and technological developments, respiratory distress syndrome (RDS) remains a significant problem for ELBW infants, being associated with a high number of complications, particularly BPD (Stoll et al. 2015).

The lung of preterm infants is biochemically immature and highly vulnerable to injury. For this reason the optimal respiratory approach should aim to gently open and ventilate the lung, preventing the damage due to barotrauma or atelectasis (Dargaville and Tingay 2012).

Different lung protective ventilation strategies have been suggested to minimize lung injury, including patient triggered or synchronized ventilation, volume targeted ventilation (VTV), INSURE strategy (INtubation, SURfactant Extubation to NCPAP), high frequency ventilation (HFV) (including both high frequency oscillatory ventilation (HFOV) and high frequency jet ventilation (HFJV)), and permissive hypercapnia (PH) (Reiterer et al. 2016).

Also a high number of noninvasive respiratory support options are now available both as primary treatment in infants with an adequate spontaneous breathing drive or for post-extubation (DeMauro et al. 2014).

The optimal timing for surfactant administration remains debated. A policy of early rescue surfactant should be standard in infants with RDS; however, there might be cases in which surfactant should be administered in delivery room such as in infants requiring urgent intubation for stabilization (Stevens et al. 2007).

INSURE might be considered in infants who fail NCPAP. Minimally invasive surfactant can be considered as an alternative to INSURE in unit with appropriate expertise (Dargaville et al. 2013; Kribs et al. 2015).

The most frequent cardiovascular problem in ELBW infants is represented by patent ductus arteriosus (PDA). PDA has been related to pulmonary function impairment, prolonged ventilator dependency, and development of BPD. However, definition (clinical and/or echocardiographic) of hemodynamically significant PDA, and timing and type of treatment are still debated (Hamrick and Hansmann 2010).

ELBW infants present a high risk to develop brain lesions and later neurodevelopmental disorders. Imaging the preterm brain of ELBW infants is part of clinical routine practice and sequential cranial ultrasound (cUS) scans from birth up to term corrected age (TCA) should be performed to detect the typical lesions occurring in preterm infants (germinal matrix-intraventricular hemorrhage, cystic periventricular leukomalacia) which correlate with adverse motor prognosis (de Vries et al. 2013).

Magnetic resonance imaging (MRI) has been demonstrated to be superior to cUS in identifying minor brain abnormalities occurring in the white matter and cerebellum, as well as minor degrees of germinal matrix-intraventricular hemorrhage undetected by cUS (Plaisier et al. 2015; Roelants-van Rijn et al. 2001).

However, indication to MRI at TEA in ELBW infants should be discussed with parents as there is no evidence that brain MRI at TCA ameliorates long-term outcomes, although it correlates with neurodevelopment (Ho et al. 2015).

After birth, water and electrolytes should be supplied to ELBW infants to avoid dehydration and hypertonicity. There should be close monitoring of body weight (every 12–24 h), urine output and osmolarity (every 12–24 h), and plasma electrolytes (mainly sodium and potassium). ELBW infants show limited nutritional reserves and immaturity of nutrient absorption in the face of high nutritional demands. For this reason, many ELBW infants experience postnatal growth retardation in spite of total PN and early enteral feeding. The main objectives of nutritional support are to maintain body stores and to assure adequate postnatal growth, avoiding metabolic complications and side effects. ELBW infants should receive glucose and amino acid infusion soon after birth to maintain normoglycemia and adequate protein levels. Within the second day of life, lipids and electrolytes may be administered. Total PN should be associated with early enteral feeding to limit complications associated with PN, mainly cholestasis and sepsis. Metabolic acidosis may become a problem with the progression of PN and its correction is still debated.

Structural and functional immaturity of the gastrointestinal tract may limit early enteral feeding. Minimal enteral feeding (trophic feeding at 10–20 mL/kg/day) should be started as soon as possible after achieving clinical stability to stimulate normal functional development of the gastrointestinal tract. Its progression will be determined by feeding tolerance, which is normally reduced in ELBW infants. Feeding strategies depend on the experience of caregivers and should be aimed at the establishment of enteral feeding, avoiding feeding intolerance and necrotizing enterocolitis. Enteral volume is increased gradually with close monitoring for abdominal distension, vomiting, or increased volume of gastric aspirates, especially if bile-stained or hemorrhagic. When feeding intolerance is diagnosed, enteral feeding should be reduced or stopped. Breast milk is preferred to premature formulae for both trophic and enteral feeding, but when it is insufficient to achieve normal postnatal growth, milk fortifiers should be added. Multicomponent fortification of human milk is associated with short-term improvements in weight gain, linear and head growth, but without evidence of long-term benefit (Dutta et al. 2015; Koletzko et al. 2014).

Infection is a major cause of mortality and morbidity for ELBW infants. The incidence of early-onset sepsis (EOS) (<72 h) is less than 5% with a mortality up to 50%, mainly for ELBW infants born after premature rupture of membranes and/or chorioamnionitis. Prenatal treatment of chorioamnionitis and prevention of group B streptococcal infection has changed the distribution of pathogens of EOS with an increasing rate of gram-negative bacterial sepsis (Stoll et al. 2011).

Taking a careful prenatal history, timely diagnosis (based on clinical signs, microbiological and biochemical tests) and therapy (empirical use of antibiotics) are important for the prevention and treatment of EOS and its complications.

Late-onset sepsis (LOS) affects 20–50% of ELBW infants and the mortality rate varies from 20% to 80%, depending on the causal pathogen (Stoll et al. 2010).

The main risk factors for LOS are the use of central lines, mechanical ventilation, and parenteral nutrition. The clinical diagnosis of LOS is more difficult in ELBW infants because of nonspecific clinical features and a lack of sensitive diagnostic tests. Thus, many of these infants receive several courses of antibiotics and antifungals during their hospital stay. Careful monitoring of a neonatal unit can help guide empirical antibiotic therapy and limit antibiotic resistance.

Strategies to prevent late-onset infections include hygiene measures, cautious use of indwelling devices, early human milk administration, the use of central line bundles, and antibiotic stewardship. Fluconazole prophylaxis may be indicated in ELBW infants hospitalized in NICUs with a high incidence of fungal infections. There is some medical evidence supporting the use of probiotics and prebiotics in the prevention of LOS in preterm infants, without adverse effects. However, clarifications regarding type of probiotic/prebiotic, dosing regimens for different weight classes, and long-term outcomes are still needed before recommending their use in clinical practice (Santos and Tristram 2015).

12.2.3 Long-Term Morbidities

ELBW infants are at high risk for neurodevelopmental impairment associated with acquired severe brain lesions. However, minor cognitive, behavioral, and academic developmental disorders have been observed also in children without overt brain injury at conventional neuroimaging performed during the neonatal period. Preterm infants, during their stay in the NICU, also face a period of stressful environment (exposure to pain, light and sounds, forced maternal separation), which may negatively impact early brain development and subsequent neurobehavioral outcomes. In this context, early intervention programs based on the concept of "individualized care" have proved to be effective in promoting brain maturation and neurodevelopmental outcome (Spittle et al. 2015).

A neurodevelopmental follow-up has to be established in order to early identify those babies who may benefit from long-term intervention programs.

ELBW infants may also develop neurosensorial deficits: hearing impairment is associated with illness and with the use of ototoxic drugs and a hearing screening program is mandatory in these babies. Retinopathy of prematurity (ROP) is a common morbidity in preterm infants and it is more severe in ELBW infants, potentially leading to blindness (Wallin and Eriksson 2009).

Although recent insights into pathogenesis and prevention, BPD continues to be one of the most common complications affecting ELBW infants.

12.3 Timing of Discharge and Problems of Home Care in ELBW Infants

ELBW infants are considered high-risk infants who are often discharged with unresolved medical problems requiring special care, respiratory and/or nutritional support after discharge.

At the time of discharge from NICU, parents of preterm infants often question their ability to care after babies without the support of NICU staff. An individualized home-care plan and a close follow-up have to be developed for these babies before discharge from NICU and programs that provide continuity of care at home need to be implemented, making the transition from hospital to home life safely.

12.3.1 Timing of Home Discharge

According to the guidelines of the American Academy of Pediatrics (Committee on Fetus and Newborn 2008) timing of home discharge should be based on physiologic criteria rather than body weight.

Physiologic stability and the acquisition of the following competencies are considered essential to allow home discharge: (1) respiratory control; (2) thermal stability in home environment; (3) competent oral feeding (by breast or bottle) for an appropriate growth.

12.3.1.1 Respiratory Control

Significant apneas of prematurity can persist up to 43 weeks' postmenstrual age (PMA). After stopping methylxanthines administration, babies who have experienced problematic apneas should have an event-free period of 5–7 days before discharge. It is known that the prone position improves oxygenation, while the nonprone position decreases the incidence of sudden infant death syndrome (SIDS) (Task Force on Sudden Infant Death Syndrome 2005; Blair et al. 2006). The association between prone sleeping and SIDS among ELBW infants is equal to or even stronger than the association among those born at term. Therefore, prior to discharge, babies should spend a period of weeks in the supine position monitoring the occurrence of desaturation events and mothers should be strongly advised by caregivers during hospitalization to maintain supine sleeping position once at home.

12.3.1.2 Immunization

Preterm infants should receive routine recommended vaccines at a chronological age consistent with the schedule recommended for full-term infants (Saari and Committee on Infectious Diseases 2003).

During the respiratory syncytial virus (RSV) season palivizumab should be given before discharge to high-risk neonates according to the national recommendations (American Academy of Pediatrics Subcommittee on Diagnosis and Management of Bronchiolitis 2006).

12.3.1.3 Neonatal Screening Programs

Newborn metabolic screening should be completed and reviewed before discharge.

Research data have shown that infants in the NICU are at highest risk of having neural hearing loss. Therefore, a hearing test should be performed before discharge in high-risk babies and a long-term careful monitoring for hearing loss, with subsequent appropriate audiological management, is essential after discharge.

12.3.1.4 Parental Education

An active program of parental involvement in the infant's care should be established by caregivers as soon as possible during the hospital stay in order to teach parents to handle the baby and let them acquire skills and competence needed to take care of their infant at home.

Breast milk should be strongly promoted as the optimal diet also for ELBW infants and soon after birth mothers should be encouraged to provide milk for their own infants. After discharge, mothers should be supported to continue breastfeeding or to give their own expressed milk; considerable psychological benefits of breastfeeding have been also described.

Before discharge a planned follow-up program should be offered to the parents by an identified primary care physician who will take the responsibility of the baby's care after discharge. Individualized discharge and follow-up plans are important to assure safe and effective care at home and to minimize avoidable hospital readmissions. In order to help parents to cope with the baby's needs at home additional support may be provided by home nursing care.

12.3.2 Special Care Needs

12.3.2.1 Ventilatory Suppor

Approximately 30% of surviving ELBW infants (Jensen et al. 2015) still need oxygen therapy beyond 36 weeks of postmenstrual age. Babies with BPD may require long-term oxygen supplementation or respiratory support to maintain oxygen saturation at an acceptable level (suggested range 93–95%) (Trzaski et al. 2012; Thoracic Society of Australia and New Zealand et al. 2008).

In order to shorten hospital stay, home respiratory support should be considered for these babies. Humidified high flow nasal cannulae (HHFNC) have been suggested as post-discharge ventilatory support although evidence of benefits compared to low-flow oxygen supplementation is still missing.

Some infants may require oxygen supplementation for months or even years and discontinuation should be considered when infants consistently maintain target saturation in room air; however, weaning from supplemental oxygen should be gradual to avoid worsening of pulmonary hypertension.

For infants who cannot be weaned from assisted ventilation home ventilation may be necessary. In this case a tracheostomy has to be performed before discharge and a special education for parents and qualified home care are needed. Respiratory support may range from CPAP, to fully ventilator-supported breathing. Both short and long term respiratory support requirements vary depending on the underlying disease and indication for tracheostomy.

High-risk newborns may require pulse oxymetry or apnea monitoring after discharge. Although criteria to home apnea monitoring vary widely among NICUs, recommendations for home monitoring include babies presenting mild episodes of apnea not requiring stimulation, having a feeding tube in situ, and requiring oxygen supplementation or ventilatory assistance.

The use of home monitoring is not indicated to prematurely discharge babies who do not demonstrate maturity of respiratory control.

12.3.2.2 Nutritional Support

Competent breast or bottle feeding supporting appropriate growth is advocated before discharge. Nevertheless, the use of a feeding tube at home may be considered when feeding is the last issue precluding home discharge. A safe home management of feeding tube can be assessed for a limited time period by well-trained parents; when the baby does not improve in oral feeding skills, a gastrostomy should be performed to guarantee safe and effective gastric nutrition. During gastrostomy feeding oral nutrition must be stimulated as removal of naso/orogastric tube reduces discomfort during suction and may improve oral feeding skills (Mills and Davies 2012; Abrams and American Academy of Pediatrics, Committee on Nutrition 2013).

Infants with short bowel syndrome due to pre- or postnatal damage of the gut require total PN when there is insufficient bowel length of sufficient quality for enteral independndcy, which, in turns, further depends also on the site of gut resected and the presence or absence of the ileocaecal valve. If total PN is likely to be needed long-term, home administration has to be planned to give these children a better quality of life. Home total PN requires medical devices and intense home nursing for surveillance of central venous catheter related problems until parents achieve competency and independency (Batra et al. 2013).

12.3.3 Rehospitalization

ELBW infants have a high rate of readmission in the first years of life (almost 50%), mainly due to respiratory illness, with the highest incidence in babies <25 weeks' gestation, with BPD, living with other children, first discharged during the RSV season or belonging to socially disadvantaged groups. The identification of associated risk factors can be useful to define high-risk groups of babies at discharge needing close follow-up and surveillance (Morris et al. 2005).

12.3.4 Safe Transportation

When positioned in a safety car seat premature babies and ELBW infants have an increased risk of airway obstruction (Bull and Engle 2009).

The potential risk of respiratory compromise is strictly related to anthropometric parameters (weight and length) and neurologic maturity as well as to the associated medical conditions, especially BPD. A car seat evaluation should be performed before discharge in newborns at risk for obstructive apnea, including babies with hypotonia (related to genetic or neuromuscular disorders), micrognathia or previous cardiac surgery. Parental education about the proper infant's position in the car seat is necessary to minimize the risk of respiratory impairment. A car bed may be indicated for infants who present apnea or decrease in oxygen saturation when positioned semi-reclined, unless evidence is not clear.

12.4 Information and Psychosocial Intervention

The welcoming and assistance services of birth have evolved in the last decades. In western countries, birth at hospital went from a medical-sanitary assistance, aimed to guarantee the best security in hospital with more and more advanced and meticulous procedures and protocols, to a more humanitarian vision of the birth issue (National Health Service, UK 2007). This evolution is witnessed by the spread of a different cultural approach to maternity, characterized by supportive methodologies for parents, methodologies that are adopted by obstetricians, neonatologists, and pediatricians (World Health Organization 2011).

In order to support mother and neonate, it is relevant to guarantee an intimate and prolonged contact to the couple since the very first moments of life in the delivery room, during hospital stay, and until discharge. Considering the birth as a multidimensional event attention moved to the perinatal period, which goes from pregnancy to the first months of life of the baby (Chalmers et al. 2001). It is important to stress the difficulties of the couples to cope with the changes imposed by the taking of the parental role: from the economic, working, organizational problems to the psychological issues related to the living conditions, the increased sense of solitude, the investments that changed because of the baby and the social pressures connected with the parental task. Besides the happiness and the satisfaction that every birth necessarily gives to the parents, it is frequent to find also the inconvenience, mostly by mothers, characterized by depression, anxiety, insecurity, fragility, and possibly by more serious psychopathologies (Song et al. 2015).

It has emerged in recent years the importance of the support of the emotional and sentimental sphere connected to the birth and it is essential to start psychological services in the obstetric wards, in nurseries, and in all those "risky" contexts such as Neonatal Intensive Care Units (NICU, see below) especially (Lassi et al. 2014). Specific guidelines to support the parents in these critical areas were created, in order to limit the traumatic effects connected to prematurity and pathologic births. NICU wards are working on the contact and on the involvement of parents, so that the bonding is not totally compromised by long separation, prolonged medicalization, and parental experiences (Shaw et al. 2013a). Latest scientific studies in various areas, such as neurology, psychology, and pedagogy, show more importance to the perinatal phase and to the first year of life. In the neuroscience field, it was clearly demonstrated that the first child's relational experiences, joined with the potential deriving from the genetic inheritance, are crucial to the architecture of the human brain and to his development (Newman et al. 2015). In the psychological field, researches and theories on attachment highlighted how the quality of the welcoming of birth and of the relationship between the baby and her/his parents are crucial for growth, deeply influencing the sentimental and emotional life, the construction of the sense of identity, and the development of the interactive capacities and of the cognitive competences (Bowlby 1969).

Many authors' studies (Stern and Bruschweiler-Stern 1998; Winnicott 1987) on *motherhood*, instead of maternity, underlined that the assumption of the parental identity does not coincide with the birth of the baby, but requires a long time to mature and for the woman it represents a moment of evolutional "crisis," characterized by a deep reorganization of her own psychic and emotional set. Lastly, researches in the socioeconomic field are significant as well: they showed how the preventive interventions during the early first infancy are cheaper than the following treatment interventions in social, educational, and therapeutic areas. Because of that, investing in quality services oriented to early infancy enables societies to save a lot of money in the long term (Weissbourd 1991).

This perspective led to increased interest in the safeguard of birth as "common good" and brought about a new awareness in operators, of their own role and responsibility in sustaining such an important and delicate process. In fact, there is plenty of evidence that the environment surrounding every woman – from the earliest moments of labor and delivery – influences and eases the development of parenthood and bonding. Recognizing women's need to engage with supportive and welcoming figures determined a change in considering assistance: assistance is *care*, taking care of the woman who "learns to take care of her own neonate." The newborn needs this kind of approach to face his entry into this world; the mother needs it too, in order to guarantee it. Therefore, prevention measures should be used to make attachment and bonding possible: the respect and promotion of physiology of birth, letting him come to the world instead of making him come to the world, fostering an early and prolonged contact with the baby, through the "skin to skin" technique since from the delivery room and through the *rooming in*, which is essential for the beginning of breastfeeding and bonding, providing parenthood with a support even after discharge. This kind of interventions cannot ignore the uniqueness of every single family unit, thinking of a one-to-one assistance and creating individualized programs aimed at promoting the mother's ability to take care of her own and her child's health, depending on their specific needs. In contrast to the rigid standardized procedures of traditional assistance to birth, it is extremely important to have flexibility and to offer a personalized response to every woman's, every child's, every family's specific needs, which may be different from each others because of their own personal stories, individual characteristics, social context, and culture of belonging (World Health Organization 2013). Moreover, considering the great sociocultural mutations in families, in which the father's role in western countries is becoming more important in child care, services to parents have changed in a new triadic perspective, welcoming not only the mothers' emotions but also the male need to find models of fatherhood, as the old ones are no longer suitable (Fivaz-Depeursinge and Corboz-Warnery 1999). New supportive methodologies to parenthood leave the old model (grounded on prescription and teaching the parents their duties) behind: they include father figures more and the keyword is *empowerment*, a concept which has become widespread in service terminology, referring to the task of helping parents to reinforce themselves. This type of intervention is founded on the idea that the transition to parenthood, the passage from maternity to *motherhood* is a process of personal maturation which cannot be taught nor prescribed: it can only be facilitated and protected from negative interferences. After hospital discharge, starting from the awareness of nowadays families' needs, a new kind of services is created among parents to offer support to each other. This opportunity promotes and facilitates the exchange between peers, the sharing of experiences and common problems, the exchange of practical solutions drawn from direct experience. In fact the absence of any kind of judgment allows to normalize one's own feelings, to give a meaning to one's own behavior, so that everyone can enrich his own inner world with others' experiences. This method has turned out to significantly improve parents' self-esteem, autonomy, expertise, and their perception to be active main characters of their own lives.

Offering *home care* to the new mother right after delivery is another particularly recommended supportive protocol to parenthood (Ammerman et al. 2012; Sweet and Appelbaum 2004); over the last years, it has been experienced by family consultants and local institutions in this field. A common element among new mothers is the acknowledge of difficulties faced during the postpartum, when physical and psychological tasks turn out to be arduous (such as regaining energy after delivery, reprocessing the experience, readjusting the body, beginning of breastfeeding, getting to know the baby, finding a new poise for the couple, reorganizing family life and its rhythms) because of the lacking of that function of protection, support, and help, once offered by the family and neighborhood.

Home care support has proved to be particularly effective in critical situations such as problematic families, in which a baby's arrival was not consciously chosen, in which either there is a social and psychological awkwardness (drug addicted parents, parents with psychiatric diseases, with personal stories of deprivation, single, underage, migrants, etc.) or a pathological birth occurred. For these mothers, for these parents, the perspective of raising a child in such conditions turns out to be strenuous and it can result in high psychopathological risks, affecting the formation of the bonding and child's growth, as a plentiful scientific literature shows. Home-care is thought in a wider project on the single family unit and it often combines with other sorts of intervention, which may be social, clinical, educational, in the knowledge that the needs of those families who have multidimensional problems cannot be faced with unidimensional action. Besides these home care services, clinical intervents with individual psychotherapies are synergically developing, with various goals, depending on the level of critical issues. One of the main focuses concerns consultations and psychological treatments offered to parents in the baby's first years, to either overcome difficult times or improve their well-being. These are the so-called *parent trainings*, strategies of intervention on parenthood with a therapeutic approach, though different from a real psychotherapy, as they are shorter (8–10 appointments); they are aimed at strengthening and enriching parents' abilities, at raising a different manner of "viewing things," at making them gain more awareness of their roles and learning new ways of engaging with their own children (Lundahl et al. 2006). A second group of interventions concerns clinical treatment of parent-child relationship at the earliest stages, since a maternal figure is utterly fundamental for the baby's mental health. A third group consists of preventive and supportive interventions in depression during pregnancy and after childbirth, based on international guidelines which classify their symptoms and give recommendations for both prevention and pharmacological-psychotherapic treatment.

In recent years the development of preventive and supportive intervention models for maternity, implemented especially in situations of increasing fragility and great "risk," has shown a significant effect in terms of preventing severe psychological issues and to protect and promote infant's growth.

12.4.1 Preterm Birth and Family Care

Even hospitalization of the premature infant in NICU is considered as a "psychological crisis" in the family, causing feelings of powerlessness and stress, especially for mothers (Woodward et al. 2014; Shaw et al. 2013b). Survival rates for small preterm infants have improved, especially those of very low birth weight infants (VLBW). Although the birth of an infant with VLBW poses a considerable challenge to parents, there is little information about how it affects family stress. For an event like preterm birth, different sources of parental stress have been identified. One of the most important is early separation of the mother and infant, which may adversely affect attachment between the mother-child dyad. Consequently, feelings of anxiety and depression are frequent in mothers of preterm infants and appear to be more intense during the hospitalization of the child in the neonatal intensive care unit. Maternal depression has been associated with impairment of child cognitive, emotional, and behavioral development. Early maternal depression or other psychological symptoms may have varying effects on preterm infants. The relationship of maternal mental health on parenting behavior is important for preterm populations because maternal psychological status and other social factors (e.g., socioeconomic status, maternal substance abuse, multiple birth, or other life stressors) have been found to correlate with childhood emotional and mental well-being in children of school age, who were of low birth weight or preterm. Signs of parental distress can emerge during hospitalization, which is why staff should adopt a holistic approach to understanding the uniqueness of each family and provide appropriate support.

If a problem is diagnosed during pregnancy, parents should be forewarned. If this does not occur, most women and their partners will not give serious consideration to the possibility of preterm delivery or illness in their newborn baby and admission to a neonatal unit. Parents are unfamiliar with the potentially complex problems their infant faces and there is uncertainty about the future. A lack of understanding and uncertainty are major sources of stress. In addition, maternal health is often compromised at this time. Mother and baby are separated when the infant is admitted to the neonatal unit, and this may last many months. Although in some hospitals a visit to the neonatal unit is a routine part of antenatal care, the neonatal unit is generally an alien environment for most parents. Units are often noisy, bright, and hot. They can be overcrowded and parts will be "high tech." Parents rarely know the neonatal unit staff before their baby is admitted, and the language and behaviors they encounter can contribute to an overwhelming feeling of isolation. The sickest preterm infants may be in hospital for many months, and visiting can be difficult, exhausting, and a financial drain for parents, especially as neonatal services become more centralized. All these factors put strain on the parents' relationship: a relationship is more likely to breakdown during the months after preterm delivery. Some couples, however, feel the experience makes their relationship closer, at least initially. Generally, stress and anxiety are higher in mothers than in fathers, and lessen with the passage of time. For some parents, the stress experienced is similar to that seen in adults diagnosed with post-traumatic stress disorder. High levels of stress may last beyond the first year of their infant's life, and the level and duration of stress may not be directly related to how preterm or how sick their baby was. In addition to high levels of stress and anxiety, these parents are more prone to clinical depression, which may be difficult to recognize.

Responses and feelings similar to those of a classic grief reaction can be encountered: shock, denial, anger, guilt, acceptance, and adjustment. Several models have explored how parents cope with having their baby in the neonatal unit. Various mechanisms are seen, however, and a single is not appropriate for all parents. Some coping strategies include trying to gain a deeper understanding of the problems, establishing a degree of control over the situation, seeking social support from other people, and escaping from or minimizing the apparent severity of the situation. These mechanisms are used to varying degrees by individual parents. There is a systematic difference between mothers and fathers. Mothers tend to look for support from others and to search for an explanation for what has happened, whereas fathers are more likely to try to minimize the situation, often by concentrating on supporting their partner.

A better understanding of the sources of stress and how parents try to cope allows appropriate interventions for the family. A complex network of structural, practical, social, and psychological interventions can promote acceptance by mothers and fathers of this challenging event (Morey and Gregory 2012; Kraljevic and Warnock 2013).

When designing neonatal units, great emphasis is placed on effective layout, lighting, and noise (Brumberg and Shah 2015) reduction. Facilities for families to stay close to their baby are usually provided, and rooms for parents allow mothers and fathers to relax and meet other parents. Play areas for siblings have been incorporated into some units. This more "family-orientated" approach to care is helped by less restrictive visiting policies in neonatal units (Welch et al. 2016; Cano Giménez and Sánchez-Luna 2015); most units allow parents and siblings open access if they comply with local infection control measures. Thus a more sensitive approach could affect faster bonding between mother and sick newborn (i.e., 24/24 open access to NICU, kangaroo mother-care, promotion of maternal/human milk).

Prenatal counseling is an aspect on which many units are currently engaged, especially if a prenatal diagnosis has been made. Members of the neonatal team meet with parents before the birth to discuss a likely admission and the approach that will be taken for the infant's problems. Parents are encouraged to visit the unit before their baby is born to familiarize themselves with the environment and the staff. After delivery, it is good practice to discuss medical and nursing issues in detail with parents to inform and, when possible, to involve them in decision making from an early stage. Parents should be informed as soon as possible about investigation results and any change in clinical condition. After overcoming their first moments of confusion and fear, parents can also help with the care of their preterm baby. This may extend beyond simple but important measures, including "skin-to-skin" contact (Mörelius et al. 2015), providing skilled care such as tube feeding, toileting practices, and joining intensive "developmental care" programs. Parents of other preterm babies can give support through "buddy" programs or informally. Counseling through external organizations or formal support can be helpful even for families whose babies are not critically ill. This can involve various professionals, such as psychologists, social services, religious advisers, and ethics committees. Written information about the neonatal unit, describing specific conditions or procedures may be useful. Routine contact between the neonatal unit and social services may allow financial support to be provided for the parents.

Despite intensive treatment and full medical support, patients in a neonatal unit may die. Although there are substantial differences between countries and cultures, a decision to limit active treatment may be considered because of the inevitability of death or a prognosis that indicates a very poor quality of life. Death, however it comes about, is a desperate time for affected families. In some cases, parents want to be involved in decision making at these times. They need full and frank information, given in a compassionate manner by experienced staff who know the family and their baby. In most cases, the decision to stop or limit treatment is made with senior medical and nursing staff. Family, friends, and external bodies (such as religious leaders and support groups) do not often have a substantial role in the decision to withdraw treatment but contribute to family support afterwards. Mothers and fathers may differ in the way they grieve and cope with their loss. Mementoes, formal contact with senior staff during the weeks after the death, and contact with a bereavement support worker or group may all help the process. Most families begin to come to terms with the death during the first year – not forgetting the child but adjusting to life without him or her. Bereaved parents often need factual information that may help explain why their baby has died. Without autopsy, important information can be missed, and in many neonatal units, postmortem examination is always considered and offered to the parents if appropriate. High pro- file cases where there have been procedural inadequacies and anxieties about organ retention have contributed to a decrease in the number of autopsies carried out. Additionally, there has been a natural reluctance by parents to authorize further "suffering" for their infant and a lack of awareness of the questions that remain unanswered.

Discharge home, although an exciting time for families, can also be a time of extreme anxiety, and so a formal approach to "discharge planning" is often adopted. Mothers "room in" with their baby to promote bonding, establish feeding, and learn practical skills that might be needed. Support for the family in the community once the infant is discharged can also be arranged, including specialist neonatal nurses, primary care health staff (e.g., health visitors, general practitioners), social workers, and national or local family support groups. Although managing the immediate stress of discharge home is important, it should be recognized that although practical issues may become easier with the passage of time, for some families considerable levels of stress and anxiety remain long after the discharge itself. Psychological support should be an integral part of neonatal follow-up programs.

Parents and families of babies who are admitted to a neonatal unit are exposed to a variety of stressors and may face extremely difficult decisions in unique and unfamiliar situations. Many studies suggest that current VLBW follow-up programs might benefit from the addition of psychological and family services to traditional neurodevelopmental assessment programs, particularly during the neonatal period and up to infant age of 2 years. Ten percent of mothers of infants with VLBW reported severe symptoms of psychological distress during the neonatal period, five times the rate for term mothers, while almost one third of mothers of infants with VLBW had clinically significant levels of depression and anxiety. For mothers of high-risk infants with VLBW, significant symptoms recurred when the child was 2 years old. The neonatal period affords an opportunity to identify mothers who are most at risk using standardized, simple screening techniques. Such identification and referral for treatment may prevent the development of more severe symptoms, which can interfere with effective parenting while the provision of social support may also effectively buffer distress. By targeting this support appropriately, staff on neonatal units can provide a more complete package of care.

References

Abrams SA, American Academy of Pediatrics, Committee on Nutrition (2013) Calcium and vitamin D requirements of enterally fed preterm infants. Pediatrics 131 (5):e1676–e1683

American Academy of Pediatrics Subcommittee on Diagnosis and Management of Bronchiolitis (2006) Diagnosis and management of bronchiolitis. Pediatrics 118:1774–1793

Ammerman RT, Putnam FW, Chard KM, Stevens J, Van Ginkel JB (2012) PTSD in depressed mothers in home visitation. Psychol Trauma

Batra A, Beattie RM (2013) Management of short bowel syndrome in infancy. Early Human Development 89:899–904

Blair PS, Ward Platt M, Smith IJ, Fleming PJ, CESDI SUDI Research Group (2006) Sudden infant death syndrome and sleeping position in pre-term and low birth weight infants: an opportunity for targeted intervention. Arch Dis Child 91:101–106

Bowlby J (1969) Attachment and loss, vol. I, attachment. Hogarth Press, London

Brumberg HL, Shah SI (2015) Born early and born poor: an eco-bio-developmental model for poverty and pretermbirth. J Neonatal Perinatal Med 8(3):179–187

Bull MJ, Engle WA (2009) Safe transportation of preterm and low birth weight infants at hospital discharge. Pediatrics 123:1424–1429

Cano Giménez E, Sánchez-Luna M (2015) Providing parents with individualised support in a neonatal intensive care unit reduced stress, anxiety and depression. Acta Paediatr 104(7):e300–e305

Chalmers B, Mangiaterra V, Porter R (2001) WHO principles of perinatal care: the essential antenatal, perinatal, and postpartum care course. Birth 28:202–207

Committee on Fetus and Newborn (2008) Hospital discharge of the high-risk neonate. Pediatrics 122:1119–1126

Dargaville PA, Tingay DG (2012) Lung protective ventilation in extremely preterm infants. J Paediatr Child Health 48(9):740–746

Dargaville PA, Aiyappan A, de Paoli AG, Kuschel CA, Kamlin CO, Carlin JB, Davis PG (2013) Minimally invasive surfactant therapy in preterm infants on continuous positive airway pressure. Arch Dis Child Fetal Neonatal Ed 98:F122–F126

DeMauro SB, Millar D, Kirpalani H (2014) Noninvasive respiratory support for neonates. Curr Opin Pediatr 26 (2):157–162

Dutta S, Singh B, Chessell L, Wilson J, Janes M, McDonald K, Shahid S, Gardner VA, Hjartarson A, Purcha M, Watson J, de Boer C, Gaal B, Fusch C (2015) Guidelines for feeding very low birth weight infants. Forum Nutr 7(1):423–442

Edwards WH, Conner JM, Soll RF (2004) The Effect of Prophylactic Ointment Therapy on Nosocomial Sepsis Rates and Skin Integrity in Infants With Birth Weights of 501 to 1000 g. Pediatrics 113(5):1195–1203

Fivaz-Depeursinge E, Corboz-Warnery A (1999) The primary triangle: a developmental systems view of mothers, fathers, and infants. Basic Books, New York

Hamrick SEG, Hansmann G (2010) Patent ductus arteriosus of the preterm infant. Pediatrics 125:1020–1030

Ho T, Dukhovny D, Zupancic JA, Goldmann DA, Horbar JD, Pursley DM (2015) Choosing wisely in newborn medicine: five opportunities to increase value. Pediatrics 136(2):e482–e489

Hooper SB, Te Pas AB, Kitchen MJ (2016) Respiratory transition in the newborn: a three-phase process. Arch Dis Child Fetal Neonatal Ed 101(3):266–271

Jensen EA, DeMauro SB, Kornhauser M, Aghai ZH, Greenspan JS, Dysart KC (2015) Effects of multiple ventilation courses and duration of mechanical ventilation on respiratory outcomes in extremely low-birth-weight infants. JAMA Pediatr 169(11):1011–1017

Koletzko B, Poindexeter B, Uauy R (eds) (2014) Nutritional care of preterm infants: scientific basis and practical guidelines. Karger, Basel

Kraljevic M, Warnock FF (2013) Early educational and behavioral RCT interventions to reduce maternal symptoms of psychological trauma following preterm birth: a systematic review. J Perinat Neonatal Nurs 27 (4):311–327

Kribs A, Roll C, Göpel W, Wieg C, Groneck P, Laux R, Teig N, Hoehn T, Böhm W, Welzing L, Vochem M, Hoppenz M, Bührer C, Mehler K, Stützer H, Franklin J, Stöhr A, Herting E, Roth B, NINSAPP Trial Investigators (2015) NonintubateLung-protective ventilatorytional therapy in extremely preterm infants: a randomized clinical trial. JAMA Pediatr 169:723–730

Laptook AR, Salhab W, Bhaskar B, Neonatal Research Network (2009) Admission temperature of low birth weight infants: predictors and associated morbidities. Pediatrics 119:e643–e649

Lassi ZS, Salam RA, Das JK, Bhutta ZA (2014) Essential interventions for maternal, newborn and child health:

background and methodology. Reprod Health 11(Suppl 1):S1
Lundahl BW, Risser HJ, Lovejoy MC (2006) A meta-analysis of parent training: moderators and follow-up effects. Clin Psychol Rev 26:86–104
McCarthy M (2015) Outcomes in extremely preterm US infants improve, study finds. BMJ 351:h4851
Mills RJ, Davies MW (2012) Enteral iron supplementation in preterm and low birth weight infants. Cochrane Database Syst Rev 3:CD005095
Mörelius E, Örtenstrand A, Theodorsson E, Frostell A (2015) A randomised trial of continuous skin-to-skin contact after preterm birth and the effects on salivary cortisol, parental stress, depression, and breastfeeding. Early Hum Dev 91(1):63–70
Morey JA, Gregory K (2012) Nurse-led education mitigates maternal stress and enhances knowledge in the NICU. MCN Am J Matern Child Nurs 37 (3):182–191
Morris BH, Gard CC, Kennedy K, For the NICHD Neonatal Research Network (2005) Rehospitalization of extremely low birth weight (ELBW)infants: are there racial/ethnic disparities? J Perinatol 25:656–663
National Health Service, UK (2007) Antenatal and postnatal mental health. Clinical management and service guidance, Nice Clinical Guideline 45, developed by The National Collaborating Centre for Mental Health
Newman L, Sivaratnam C, Komiti A (2015) Attachment and early brain development – neuroprotective interventions in infant–caregiver therapy. Transl Dev Psychiatry 3:28647
Nowadzky T, Pantoja A, Britton JR (2009) Bubble continuous positive airway pressure, a potentially better practice, reduces the use of mechanical ventilation among very low birth weight infants with respiratory distress syndrome. Pediatrics 123:1534–1540
Oh W, Fanaroff AA, Carlo WA, Donovan EF, McDonald SA, Poole WK, Eunice Kennedy Shriver National Institute of Child Health and Human Development Neonatal Research Network (2011) Effects of delayed cord clamping. J Perinatol 31(Suppl 1):S68–S71
Plaisier A, Raets MM, Ecury-Goossen GM, Govaert P, Feijen-Roon M, Reiss IK, Smit LS, Lequin MH, Dudink J (2015) Serial cranial ultrasonography or early MRI for detecting preterm brain injury? Arch Dis Child Fetal Neonatal Ed 100(4):F293–F300
Reiterer F, Schwaberger B, Freidl T, Schmölzer G, Pichler G, Urlesberger B (2016) Lung-protective ventilatory strategies in intubated preterm neonates with RDS. Paediatr Respir Rev S1526–0542(16)30121
Roelants-van Rijn AM, Groenendaal F, Beek FJ, Eken P, van Haastert IC, de Vries LS (2001) Parenchymal brain injury in the preterm infant: comparison of cranial ultrasound, MRI and neurodevelopmental outcome. Neuropediatrics 32(2):80–89
Saari TN and the Committee on Infectious Diseases (2003) Immunization of preterm and low birth weight infants. Pediatrics 112:193–198
Santos RP, Tristram D (2015) A practical guide to the diagnosis, treatment, and prevention of neonatal infections. Pediatr Clin N Am 62:491–508
Schmölzer GM, Kumar M, Pichler G, Aziz K, O'Reilly M, Cheung PY (2013) Non-invasive versus invasive respiratory support in preterm infants at birth: systematic review and meta-analysis. BMJ 347:f5980
Shaw RJ, Sweester CJ, St John N, Lilo E, Corcoran JB, Jo B, Howell SH, Benitz WE, Feinstein N, Melnyk B, Horwitz SM (2013a) Prevention of postpartum traumatic stress in mothers with preterm infants: manual development and evaluation. Issues Ment Health Nurs 34(8):578–586
Shaw RJ, St John N, Lilo EA, Jo B, Benitz W, Stevenson DK, Horwitz SM (2013b) Prevention of traumatic stress in mothers with preterm infants: a randomized controlled trial. Pediatrics 132(4):e886–e894
Song JE, Kim T, Ahn JA (2015) A systematic review of psychosocial interventions for women with postpartum stress. Joggn 44(2):183–192
Spittle A, Orton J, Anderson PJ, Boyd R, Doyle LW (2015) Early developmental intervention programmes provided post hospital discharge to prevent motor and cognitive impairment in preterm infants. Cochrane Database Syst Rev (11):CD005495
Stern, DN, Bruschweiler-Stern N (1998) The birth of a mother: how the motherhood experience changes you forever. Basic Books
Stevens TP, Harrington EW, Blennow M, Soll RF (2007) Early surfactant administration with brief ventilation vs selective surfactant and continued mechanical ventilation for preterm infants with or at risk for respiratory distress syndrome. Cochrane Database Syst Rev 4: CD003063
Stoll BJ, Hansen NI, Bell EF, Shankaran S, Laptook AR, Walsh MC, Hale EC, Newman NS, Schibler K, Carlo WA, Kennedy KA, Poindexter BB, Finer NN, Ehrenkranz RA, Duara S, Sánchez PJ, O'Shea TM, Goldberg RN, Van Meurs KP, Faix RG, Phelps DL, Frantz ID 3rd, Watterberg KL, Saha S, Das A, Higgins RD, Eunice Kennedy Shriver National Institute of Child Health and Human Development Neonatal Research Network (2010) Neonatal outcomes of extremely preterm infants from the NICHD neonatal Research network. Pediatrics 126:443–456
Stoll BJ, Hansen NI, Sánchez PJ, Faix RG, Poindexter BB, Van Meurs KP, Bizzarro MJ, Goldberg RN, Frantz ID 3rd, Hale EC, Shankaran S, Kennedy K, Carlo WA, Watterberg KL, Bell EF, Walsh MC, Schibler K, Laptook AR, Shane AL, Schrag SJ, Das A, Higgins RD, Eunice Kennedy Shriver National Institute of Child Health and Human Development Neonatal Research Network (2011) Early onset neonatal sepsis: the burden of group B streptococcal and *E. coli* disease continues. Pediatrics 127:817–826
Stoll BJ, Hansen NI, Bell EF, Walsh MC, Carlo WA, Shankaran S, Laptook AR, Sánchez PJ, Van Meurs KP, Wyckoff M, Das A, Hale EC, Ball MB, Newman NS, Schibler K, Poindexter BB, Kennedy KA, Cotten CM,

Watterberg KL, D'Angio CT, DeMauro SB, Truog WE, Devaskar U, Higgins RD, Eunice Kennedy Shriver National Institute of Child Health and Human Development Neonatal Research Network (2015) Trends in care practices, morbidity, and mortality of extremely preterm neonates, 1993–2012. JAMA 314:1039–1051

Sweet MA, Appelbaum MI (2004) Is home visiting an effective strategy? A meta-analytic review of home visiting programs for families with young children. Child Dev 75(5):1435–1456

Task Force on Sudden Infant Death Syndrome (2005) The changing concept of sudden infant death syndrome: diagnostic coding shifts, controversies regarding the sleeping environment, and new variables to consider in reducing risk. Pediatrics 116:1245–1255

Thoracic Society of Australia and New Zealand, Fitzgerald DA, Massie RJH, Nixon GM, Jaffe A, Wilson A, Landau LI, Twiss J, Smith G, Wainwright C, Harris M (2008) Infants with chronic neonatal lung disease: recommendations for the use of home oxygen therapy. Med J Aust 189(10):578–582

Trzaski JM, Hagadorn JI, Hussain N, Schwenn J, Wittenzellner C (2012) Predictors of successful discontinuation of supplemental oxygen in very low-birth-weight infants with bronchopulmonary dyplasia approaching neonatal intensive care unit discharge. Am J Perinatol 29(2):79–86

de Vries LS, Benders MJ, Groenendaal F (2013) Imaging the premature brain: ultrasound or MRI? Neuroradiology 55(Suppl 2):13–22

Wallin L, Eriksson M (2009) Newborn individual development care and assessment program (NIDCAP): a systematic review of the literature. Worldviews Evid-Based Nurs 6:54–69

Weissbourd B (1991) Family resource and support programs: changes and challenges in human services. Prev Hum Serv 69–85

Welch MG, Halperin MS, Austin J, Stark RI, Hofer MA, Hane AA, Myers MM (2016) Depression and anxiety symptoms of mothers of preterm infants are decreased at 4 months corrected age with family nurture intervention in the NICU. Arch Womens Ment Health 19 (1):51–61

Winnicott DW (1987) Babies and their mothers. Free Association Books/Addison-Wesley, London/Reading

Wiswell TE (2011) Resuscitation in the delivery room: lung protection from the first breath. Respir Care 56 (9):1360–1367

Woodward LJ, Bora S, Clark CA, Montgomery-Hönger A, Pritchard VE, Spencer C, Austin NC (2014) Very preterm birth: maternal experiences of the neonatal intensive care environment. J Perinatol 34(7): 555–561

World Health Organization (2011) A global review of the key interventions related to reproductive, maternal, newborn and child health. WHO-Partnership for Maternal, Newborn & Child Health, Geneve

World Health Organization (2013) WHO recommendations on postnatal care of the mother and newborn. WHO, Geneve

Wyllie J, Perlman JM, Kattwinkel J, Wyckoff MH, Aziz K, Guinsburg R, Kim HS, Liley HG, Mildenhall L, Simon WM, Szyld E, Tamura M, Velaphi S, Neonatal Resuscitation Chapter Collaborators (2015) Neonatal resuscitation: 2015 international consensus on cardiopulmonary resuscitation and emergency cardiovascular care science with treatment recommendations. Resuscitation 95:e169–e201

The Process of Decision-Making in Neonatology

13

Endla K. Anday and Michael Spear

Contents

Abstract

Advances in the field of neonatal–perinatal medicine over the past 40 years have resulted in marked improvement in survival and outcome of the prematurely born and critically ill infant. While the overall reduction in mortality and morbidity for infants is favorable, decisions regarding the care provided to newborns at the threshold of viability and those with complex medical, surgical, and potentially lethal congenital anomalies continue to present challenges to the families and healthcare providers. The dilemma surrounding the complexity of the decision-making process is based on a number of factors including the rights of the child as an individual, the values of the family and the healthcare personnel, the cultural influences, and the moral and ethical standards that impact the way physicians practice medicine and their approach to end-of-life decision-making. As an adjunct to help facilitate the process of decision-making, the role of neonatal palliative care has increased over the last few years. In fact, the field of pediatric palliative care and neonatal palliative care is relatively new and will provide added benefit to healthcare providers and families as they are confronted with difficult decisions.

E. K. Anday (✉) · M. Spear
Department of Pediatrics, Drexel University College of Medicine, St. Christopher's Hospital for Children, Philadelphia, PA, USA
e-mail: Endla.anday@drexelmed.edu; michael.spear@drexelemed.edu

G. Buonocore et al. (eds.), *Neonatology*,
https://doi.org/10.1007/978-3-319-29489-6_162

13.1 Salient Points

- Parents generally should be considered the spokesperson for determining the best interest of the child.
- A medical team should seek the opinions of parent(s), both prior to and following delivery of a child identified as extremely high risk for adverse outcome.
- Following birth, a period of transition to extra-uterine life should be offered to allow for the stabilization and evaluation of the infant to assess the degree of significant intervention likely to be required.
- Palliative care is a useful adjunct in counseling, before and after birth, parents of infants with potentially lethal anomalies. Palliative care teams should also support neonatologists in stressful clinical situations in perinatal period.
- The neonatal palliative care team can assist in resolving conflict resolution between the healthcare professionals and the family or between members of the healthcare team in a highly charged setting.

13.2 The Process of Decision-Making

When one prevents one's emotions from overtaking one's rationality it is called reason.
When one prevents one's rationality from overtaking one's emotions it is called compassion.
When one can do both it is called wisdom.
Ancient Chinese saying

13.3 Introduction

In the past 40 years, tremendous progress has occurred in the care of the neonatal patient. An in-depth understanding of fetal and neonatal physiology and the molecular basis of pathological processes, concurrent with advancements in biomedical technology, have impacted favorably upon the survival of the newborn. However, extremely premature infants at the threshold of viability; infants diagnosed with potentially lethal congenital malformations, including chromosomal abnormalities; and neonates suffering from profound intrapartum and postnatal insults present difficult moral, ethical, cultural, and social challenges for both families and caregivers in regard to providing or withholding life supportive measures. The decision to withhold or terminate treatment for an infant is based on defining the issues central to this process, including the values and rights of the infant as an individual, the values of the family and the medical caregivers, the cultural influences, and the societal values that shape the moral arguments that affect one's judgment. Part of the challenge resides in the complexity of defining *who is* or *should be* responsible for making difficult decisions resulting in the death of a newborn since fundamentally this type of decision is at odds with human nature even in situations where the end of life would mean no further suffering for the infant.

The goal of this chapter is to consider some of the issues confronting the clinician charged with practicing the art of medicine in the context of a certain degree of medical uncertainty and the implications for medical decision-making. The role of neonatal palliative care as an adjunct in counseling prospective parents or parents of infants with potentially lethal anomalies and/or for provision of care in under circumstances that are deemed futile has increased. In-depth discussions of ethical problems and guidelines for the care of the extremely low birth weight infant will be covered in other chapters of this book.

13.4 The Neuroscience of Decision-Making

Viner has stated that "Human behavior, in general is not under the constant and detailed guidance of careful and accurate hedonic calculations, but is the product of an unstable and irrational complex of reflex actions, impulses, instincts, habits, customs, fashion, and hysteria" (Viner 1925). Clearly, one would hope and expect that Viner's perspective of human behavior is not relevant to the process involved in making decisions to provide or withhold treatment for infants. Cognitive neuroscience supports that a variety of processes are essential to integrate novel incoming stimuli for decision-making in situations of uncertainty such as those pertaining to life-sustaining medical treatment. When considering options about incoming information, the key individuals involved must demonstrate flexibility to account for various outcomes, constantly monitor incoming information as it relates to the ultimate goal state or decision, and evaluate the risk–benefit ratio for various decision-making options (Gazzaniga et al. 2002). But medical decisions are not simply the rational calculation of benefit versus burden. The individuals involved often consider past experiences and values as well as future outcomes of their decisions as part of the basis for that choice. As such, a certain degree of individuality is defined that contributes to decision-making, particularly when one considers the emotional influences on this process.

In humans, emotions influence decision-making. Internal cues and external contextual information can positively or negatively impact the emotional state surrounding the decision-making process. The emotional evaluation of an action's consequences guides the individual who must be able to provide a basis for making certain choices (Bechara et al. 2000). Social neuroscience supports that the neuroanatomical substrate involved in complex decision-making in humans involves the integration of contextual social knowledge represented as event knowledge in the prefrontal cortex (PFC); social semantic knowledge, stored in the anterior and posterior temporal cortex; and motivational and basic emotional states, which depend on cortical–limbic circuits (Casebeer 2003a; Miller and Cohen 2001). While certain perceptual and emotional abilities have been shown to be shared by humans and other animals, morality and are a product of evolutionary pressures specific to the human species that have shaped social cognitive and motivational mechanisms into uniquely human forms of experience and behavior (Casebeer 2003b). Experiments using functional MRI in humans have identified that decision-making involving intelligence and complex resolution activates the ventral and medial aspect of the prefrontal cortex (VMPFC) (Greene et al. 2001). Activation of the VMPFC appears to signify that wisdom required in the decision-making process comes from categorizing and organizing past experiences from many situations and involves options for actions, deciding what actions to take and factual emotional outcomes (Damasio 2007).

Thus, the evolution of the human PFC is intimately related to the emergence of human morality, allowing for the motivational mechanisms to be integrated with an exceptional power to predict outcomes from a large repository of experiential wisdom. Coupled to semantic knowledge, cultural and situational factors become integrated into the neural substrate to weigh the motivational relevance of different behavioral choices in social situations. Clearly then, through a complex interaction of biological and cultural factors, the human moral mind emerges and integrates cognition to emotion and motivation, forming the framework for decision-making.

13.5 Steps in Decision-Making

13.5.1 Recognize the Moral Dimension

From a philosophical approach, neonatal medicine has been practiced to provide specialized and intensive care measures aimed at improving the health and survival of premature and critically ill newborns. But how are these goals affected when the curative model is inadequate such as with infants diagnosed with anencephaly or with the delivery of a 22-week gestational age infant; what do the goals become? And why is decision-making in this context so difficult? Consider the situation wherein prenatally a mother is diagnosed carrying a fetus with severe potentially lethal congenital anomalies; the physician is put into a unique situation in medicine in which he/she contemplates withholding support in a human being *that the physician has never even seen*! Or contemplate the situation of the 23-week gestational age infant with bilateral grade III intracranial bleeds and pneumoperitoneum trapped in NICU biomedical technology, hanging on to a thread of life and without reasonable expectation for improvement without incurring unnecessary pain and suffering; when is enough really enough? Compound the dilemma with both parental and physicians' attitudes toward life-saving technology and death, which have been shown in numerous studies to vary with race and ethnicity and are thought to result from complex interactions of factors including access to medical care, communication styles, family involvement in decision-making, trust in physicians, and religious background (Boss et al. 2008).

Each healthcare dilemma reminds caregivers of their limitations, including uncertainty, the human predicament, lack of knowledge, and decision-making abilities. All of these are tempered by the moral constraints under which we act. These are the difficult situations which, based on individual social, cultural, ethical, and moral differences, make it highly unlikely that we will all agree. Nevertheless, within the context of providing care to the high-risk neonate, the best interest of the child must be kept foremost in the minds of the caretakers and the professional staff and form the basis for decisions related to the care of that infant.

13.5.2 Recognize the Parties Involved

13.5.2.1 The Infant in His/Her Own Right as an Individual

The infant born at the threshold of viability or one who has potentially lethal congenital anomalies has no voice of its own; it depends on decisions made by a surrogate, most often its mother and/or family members to advocate on its behalf. Under ideal circumstances, prenatal diagnosis and counseling allow for effective communication between parents and physicians, and a reasonable approach to initiating or withholding resuscitation can be achieved based on the prognosis and risk versus benefit of treatment. During this decision-making process, the value of the infant's life is being judged. However, there may be disagreements between the medical care providers and surrogates where, in the opinion of the provider, the infant's best interest is not being served and in which the surrogate's decision should be overridden (American Academy of Pediatrics, Committee on Bioethics 1994). In 2001, the Senate and House of Representatives of the US Congress passed the "Born Alive Infant Protection Act." Specifically, the Act provides that any "member of the species homo sapiens ***at any stage of development*** that is expelled or extracted from the mother who then breathes or has a beating heart or movement of voluntary muscles is to be considered a person and granted full protection under the U.S. Constitution" (Born-Alive Infants Protection Act 2001). The Act provides that even a fertilized ovum, embryo, and fetus of any gestation are to be considered coequal with regard to protection from harm. While it was widely understood to be an antiabortion legislation, the Act altered the definition of the words, "person," "human being," "child," and "individual." Although the law did not impose a new standard of medical care upon physicians nor change existing law, it altered the physician's norm of deferring to parental discretion regarding the initiation or discontinuation of medical treatment for the extremely premature infant. However, the American Academy of Pediatrics (AAP) and the Neonatal Resuscitation Program Steering Committee issued an opinion that it would not affect day-to-day neonatal medical practice and standards. In fact, the Committee clearly stated that "decisions about withholding or discontinuing medical treatment that is considered futile may be considered by the medical care providers in conjunction with the parents… . Those newly born infants who are deemed appropriate to not resuscitate or to have medical support withdrawn should be treated with dignity and respect, and provided with "comfort care" measures" (Am Acad of Ped Neonatal Resuscitation Prog Steering Comm 2003).

Consider the Baby Doe Law, passed in 1984 in the United States, that sets forth specific guidelines for the treatment of seriously ill or disabled newborns and dictates what must be done for a child regardless of the wishes of the parents (Baby Doe Law 1984). Withholding treatment is considered neglectful unless an infant is irreversibly comatose or the treatment is futile in terms of the infant's survival, but "quality of life" is not a reason for withholding medical care. As a result of this law, hot lines were set up for anonymous reporting of alleged abuse such as withholding of medical care to seriously ill newborns leading to intrusions into the hospitals that were disruptive and ultimately found unwarranted. This Act was overturned in the Federal Courts in 1987.

Two laws, each illustrating potential conflicts between two or more values and the rights of the child as a distinct entity, contrasted to the rights of parental decision-making as the surrogate for the infant. Even more intriguing is the observation that, in spite of legal and ethical standards requiring resuscitation when it is considered to be in a patient's best interest, the newborn infant and particularly the preterm baby are devalued in comparison to older patients with comparable survival and morbidity outcomes (Janvier et al. 2008). In a questionnaire describing eight neurologically incompetent patients with potentially equivalent adverse neurological outcomes who required resuscitation (24-week preterm, term infant, 2-month-old infant, 7-year-old child, 14-year-old, 35-year-old, 50-year-old patient, and an 80-year-old subject), respondents were asked whether they would comply with the families' wishes if resuscitation was refused. The families' refusal of resuscitation was accepted most frequently for the 80-year-old subject and the 24-week-old premature infant, even though the majority of the respondents thought that resuscitation was indicated for the 24-week-old infant but not the 80-year-old patient. Since the decision was not made on the basis of outcome or what was perceived to be in the infant's best interest, there seems to be a different value placed on life at the extremes. While the root of this devaluation is not clear, it may be attributable to anthropologic, cultural, social, and evolutionary factors.

13.5.3 Parental Decision-Making

Regardless of the concept of provision of care, it is essential that parents understand the implications of the nature of aggressive care in situations where they "want everything done" for their infant, and physicians must be willing and prepared to recommend withdrawal of support in futile situations. Throughout this process, the infant must be afforded compassion and comfort. What is good for critically ill newborns and who determines this? The presence of numerous voices in deliberations about newborn patient care presses this question. What we as healthcare professionals think may be quite different than what the family or child might choose.

In the face of uncertainty and inability to predict outcome for an individual infant, there will usually be differences of opinion regarding outcome, viability, and treatment futility. Those who bear the ultimate burden of the decision ought to have the major role in the decision-making when outcomes are very uncertain. Simply put, once a physician has determined that an infant has no realistic expectation of survival based on the evidence at hand, parents should be informed and given the opportunity to withhold initiating treatment (e.g., prenatally diagnosed infant with trisomy 18 and complex congenital heart disease) or given the option of withdrawing the life-supporting interventions (e.g., 23-week gestational age ELBWI with bilateral grade IV IVH and necrotizing enterocolitis totalis). When faced with such a difficult moral decision, parents often will look to the physician for advice and counseling. The Committee on Bioethics of the American Academy of Pediatrics has advocated for a shared decision-making model whereby the physician has an ethical duty to seek and respect information regarding parental preferences and values in exchange for providing the parent with medical information (Leuthner 2001). A nondirective approach to counseling parents is advocated to allow parents to choose a course of action based on their own personal values. While the transfer of information from physician to parent should be unbiased, the manner in which information is communicated may have a framing effect on the parental decision. The recent study by Haward et al. examined message framing and perinatal decisions and demonstrated that the manner in which parents received prognostic information, i.e., framed as mortality data versus survival data, affected their treatment preference independent of religiousness, parental status, and beliefs regarding the sanctity of life (Haward et al. 2008). In subtle ways, framing bias can inadvertently affect the process of parental decision-making at a time when decisions dependent on moral values that deal with the consequences of life and death occur in close proximity to physician counseling.

However, for some parents noninitiation of or withholding life-sustaining treatment is a psychologically and morally impossible choice; they may want treatment withdrawn or not initiated so their child does not suffer but do not want the responsibility of making that decision because they do not want to give up hope. Under these circumstances, a "left unasked but not unaddressed" approach may allow transition of aggressive, futile care to care that is based upon medical indications (Paris et al. 2006). For example, instead of asking a parent if they want to initiate dopamine infusion for their infant with bilateral grade IV IVH and refractory hypotension, and giving them false hope, one can explain that everything reasonable has been done for their baby and that keeping their infant comfortable now and holding their baby is the best one can do at this time. In this manner, the parents are not tormented with decisions fraught with anguish, ambiguity, doubt, and guilt. There comes a time when "there is no need to compound the suffering of the patient by prolonging it, nor that of the parents by insisting they must make a decision as fate has already decreed" (Paris et al. 2006).

13.5.4 The Physician's Role

At the time of delivery of an extremely premature infant or one with potentially lethal congenital anomalies, it may be difficult for a physician to predict for parents what the outcome will be: possibilities range from death soon after delivery to survival with severe disabilities to intact survival. Similarly, an infant might have an initial postnatal course that would favor a reasonable outcome, only to suffer a devastating event in the NICU where the prognosis is poor. The physician is placed in a situation of weighing the benefits and burdens of ongoing support for the infant under conditions of medical uncertainty and communicating information in an effective manner to the parents, keeping in mind that the decision is in keeping with legal and organizational guidelines. The roles of authoritative statements, professional policies, and recommendations can be helpful in the decision-making process for the physician; however, most decisions are not based purely on a utilitarian approach.

During the course of refining the practice of neonatal medicine, a wealth of information relating to the care of the critically ill newborn has been accumulated, not only in the United States, but worldwide. A number of NICU guidelines and statements have been developed to establish norms and reference points in an effort to assist physicians in the day-to-day management of difficult situations including withholding or terminating life-sustaining therapy, but these may at times be of limited use in the discussion of risks, benefits, and other options with the parents and families (American Academy of Pediatrics (AAP) and American College of Obstetricians and Gynecologists (ACOG) 2012; Bell 2007). Although objective outcome data are available to many clinical populations, for a given infant and in many situations, the chance of a certain outcome may be either 0 or 100% (Watchko 1986; Pignotti and Donzelli 2008). The recommendations by the International Liaison Committee on Resuscitation for guidelines on neonatal resuscitation support the "do-not-resuscitate" order on evidence-based justification for the extremely low birth weight infant <23 weeks and <400 g and confirmed trisomies 13, 16, and 18 (International Liaison Committee on Resuscitation 2006). However, upon review of incorrect information, diagnosis, or prognosis about a specific situation, the guidelines provide for the opportunity of a trial of therapy with the option of subsequent withdrawal of support. The Groningen protocol wherein end-of-life decisions for newborns utilizing euthanasia under strict protocol are an acceptable choice in situations where there is severe and sustained suffering without relief is considered (Verhagen and Sauer 2005). Newborns are classified into three categories depending on the severity of their condition: Group 1 are infants who are expected to die in spite of invasive medical care and are actively removed from support to be held by the parent(s); Group 2 are infants who survive birth but are expected to have poor quality of life and who cannot survive without the assistance of invasive technology; and Group 3 are patients who could eventually survive without technology but who suffer severe, sustained pain and a life without hope of improvement. Of the three groups, Group 1 is least likely to present a dilemma. In Group 2 patients, quality-of-life issues form the basis for the decision-making, and in this situation, it is critical to maintain the best interest of the child in consideration and involve the opinion of the parent(s). However, the decision should not rest solely with the parent; discontinuation of support must be in concert with the physician together with the parent(s). At all times, the infant should be kept comfortable and without pain. The last Group presents the most difficult situation because it is a judgment call that death would be more humane than continuation of life. A passive approach to allowing "nature to take its course" and withholding creature comforts, such as nutrition, can lead to a period of severe suffering until death. Alternatively, deliberate termination of life or euthanasia with the use of medications to end the suffering is considered illegal. The article by Verhagen and Sauer (2005) discussed the Groningen protocol in regard to strict reporting and review of each case of proposed active termination of life to ensure that acceptance of this practice will not allow erosion of moral norms where other undesirable qualities in newborns can be used as justification to end their lives.

Physicians and parents may have different interpretations of what is discussed and what decisions are made during prenatal counseling, in the delivery room, and following the delivery of an infant. Studies support that it is the parents' perception that physicians do not always address values that parents consider important in the counseling they provide (Rebagliato et al. 2000; Lorenz 2005; Ishii et al. 2013; Stoll et al. 2010). Specific parental values such as hope, spirituality, and religion are often not incorporated in the discussions and may contribute to confusion about what has been discussed and what decisions have been made (Paris 2005; Curlin et al. 2007; Williams et al. 2009). To ignore these questions is to fail to recognize the significant influence that these values and cultural influences have had in shaping individual professional lives and human interactions.

13.5.4.1 Neonatal Palliative Care in the NICU: A New Role

The role of neonatal palliative care has increased over the last few years. In the field of pediatric palliative care, neonatal palliative care is relatively new. There are several clinicians in the medical and nursing field, however, who have been writing about this area for over a decade. The same resistance that is experienced in other areas of palliative care has also been seen in this patient population. Neonatologists, like other physician specialists, feel they have been doing this care without the services of a palliative care team and wonder about the added benefit. They feel they handle these difficult conversations well, and those that remain unenlightened are somewhat resistant.

Yet when neonatal palliative care is closely examined, it provides the same aid in decision-making and other services that it provides in the adult and pediatric arena. Mancini et al. define neonatal palliative care as "the active, total, holistic approach to care, focused on enhancing the quality of life for the baby and their family while recognizing potential or inevitable death" (Mancini 2013). The team can provide a multidisciplinary approach in decision making. Different perspectives can help in the decision-making process tremendously. The view of nursing and social work is incredibly valuable in this process, as those disciplines detect issues that physicians may be unaware of. Another key value the team possesses is time. The consultant can focus on the one or two families that need intensive support in decision-making. Some of the key questions they ask are to assess what the parents' current understanding of their infant's illness is, what they are hoping for, and what are they willing to do to achieve their goals. Then they help determine what is the most important to the family; is it prolongation of life at any cost, or providing the best quality of life, in a supportive but nonaggressive intervention strategy?

The other key component of neonatal palliative care includes the perinatal component of this care.

If the process of decision-making begins prior to the birth of an infant with potentially chronic or life-threatening diagnoses, the parents are more capable of acquiring the necessary understanding needed to make the difficult decisions ahead. They are empowered to participate in a less acute environment to develop a "birth plan" for the delivery room, and beyond, should the infant survive.

In particular, in delivery room primary palliative care has been found in one study to be inconsistent, and caregivers in that scenario often need high support during this stressful time. Primary palliative care given by the direct caregivers includes goals of care conversation, symptom management, and bereavement. Many of the staff in this situation feel ill prepared to handle this emotionally charged situation (Carter 2015). Given this study, this lends strength for the palliative care to begin in the perinatal period, long before delivery, so that staff and the patient's family are well prepared.

An additional role for the palliative care team has been described as "directive counseling" (Garten 2015). It is sometimes necessary for the caregivers to be more directive in guiding the family through the difficult decisions at end of life. Oftentimes, the parents may prefer more clear guidance through removal technology that is no longer effective. This decision can be tremendously difficult for parents, and there is supportive literature that some families may prefer this burden of choice be lifted from them.

Laing has discussed the importance of conflict resolution in the NICU regarding difficult decision-making (Garten 2015). He correctly sites that conflict can arise in this highly charged setting. This conflict can occur between the healthcare professionals and the family or between members of the healthcare team. One of the additional roles of a neonatal palliative care team is to help with this conflict resolution. By being somewhat outside the immediate conflict, the team can help understand each person's viewpoint and offer observation and clarification of the key issues, in order to move beyond the conflict.

Practically, in order to utilize a team effectively, the consultative model is most effective. The team is officially consulted, and they can either meet with the family in concert with the attending, by way of introduction, or meet separately. The key initial questions for the team to ask are:

1. What has your healthcare team told you about our role?
2. What is your understanding of your child's illness?
3. What are you most worried about?
4. What are you most hoping for?
5. What are you willing to do to achieve those goals?

These questions will align the team with the family's wishes and current thinking and will best yield a successful partnership. The team continues to meet with the family on a regular basis. The regularity is defined based on the family's needs. Contact can be daily, several times a week, or as needed by the family or medical team. The key to an effective consult is the understanding that the consultation is a process, not one visit. It takes time to build a successful alliance between the team and family. The stakes are often high and trust is not always instantaneous.

In summary, neonatal palliative care can provide an extra layer of support for families and staff as well, in facilitating the difficult decision-making needed during the perinatal period, extending through the NICU stay and beyond.

13.6 Summary

Ours is a global society in which one must be increasingly aware of the different value systems in multicultural societies across nations. While a deeper understanding of the cognitive and brain mechanisms that guide human behavior is of general interest, the moral and ethical decisions that are made regarding withholding or withdrawing care to an infant provoke anxiety and guilt that come with responsibility for making difficult decisions. When evidence-based guidelines are available as a frame of reference, one may choose to work within a set of guidelines; however, these must be individualized for each circumstance. Prognosis can change rapidly from the time of birth to the delivery room resuscitation; the likelihood of "reasonable outcome" should be reevaluated at each junction. Implicit in the decision-making is the assumption that parental counseling has occurred. Parental wishes regarding the extent of intervention initially should almost always be honored until further determination by the medical team supports the futility of further care. In the absence of a reasonable expectation of a steady improvement and in the presence of significant pain and suffering, withdrawal or withholding life-sustaining medical or surgical treatment is a decision that takes the best interest of the baby in consideration. In the end, the goal of care for the newborn must be focused upon the best interests of the child.

In the Hippocratic Corpus, medicine is defined as having three roles: "To do away with the suffering of the sick, to lessen the violence of their diseases, and to refuse to treat those overmastered by their diseases, realizing that in such cases medicine is powerless" (Hippocrates 1977). In the end, perhaps decision-making may best be summarized by the Jesuit ethicist, Father John Paris, "The best one can do is to make a human judgment based on probabilities" (personal communication).

References

Am Acad of Ped Neonatal Resuscitation Prog Steering Comm (2003) Born-alive infant protection act of 2001 public law no 107-207. Pediatric 111:680

American Academy of Pediatrics (AAP) and American College of Obstetricians and Gynecologists (ACOG) (2012) Guidelines for perinatal care, 7th edn. Elk Grove Village (IL)

American Academy of Pediatrics, Committee on Bioethics (1994) Guidelines on forgoing life-sustaining medical treatment. Pediatrica 93(3):532–536

Baby Doe Law (1984) USCA Title 42 Chapter 67 Sec 510a (http://frwebgate6.access.gpo.gov/cgi-bin/waisgate.cgi?)

Bechara A, Damasio H, Damasio AR (2000) Emotion, decision making and the orbitofrontal cortex. Cereb Cortex 10(3):295–307

Bell EF (2007) Noninitiation or withdrawal of intensive care for high-risk newborns. Pediatrica 119(2):401–403

Born-Alive Infants Protection Act (2001) 107th congress 1st session HR 2175. 1–38 http://thomas.loc.gov/

Boss RD, Hutton N, Sulpar LJ, West AM et al (2008) Values parents apply to decision-making regarding delivery room resuscitation for high-risk newborn. Pediatrica 122(3):583–589

Carter B (2015) End of life decision for newborns: an ethical and compassionate process? Arch Dis Child Fetal Neonatal Ed 101(2):F92–93. doi10.1136/archdischild - 2015.309380

Casebeer WD (2003a) Moral cognition and its neural constituents. Nat Rev Neurosci 4:840–846

Casebeer WD (2003b) Natural ethical facts: evolution, connectionism, and moral cognition. MIT Press, Cambridge, MA

Curlin FA, Lawrence RE, Chin MH, Lantos JD (2007) Religion, conscience, and controversial clinical practices. N Engl J Med 356(6):593–600

Damasio A (2007) Neuroscience and ethics: intersections. AJOB 7(1):3–10

Garten L (2015) Primary palliative care in the delivery room: patients' and medical personnel's perspectives. J Perinatol 35:1000–1005. IA L (2013) Conflict resolution in end-of-life decisions in the neonatal unit. Semin Fetal Neonatal Med 83–87

Gazzaniga RB, Ivry RB, Mangun GR (2002) Cognitive neuroscience: the biology of the mind, 2nd edn. Norton & Company, New York

Greene JD, Sommerville RB, Nystrom LE, Darley JM et al (2001) An fMRI investigation of emotional engagement in moral judgment. Science 293: 2105–2108

Haward MF, Murphy RO, Lorenz JM (2008) Message framing and perinatal decisions. Pediatrica 122:109–118

Hippocrates (1977) The art. In: Reiser SJ, Dyck AJ, Curran WJ (eds) Ethics in medicine: historical perspectives and contemporary concerns. MIT Press, Cambridge, MA, pp 6–7

International Liaison Committee on Resuscitation (2006) The International Liaison Committee on Resuscitation (ILCOR) consensus on science with treatment recommendations for pediatric and neonatal patients: neonatal resuscitation. Pediatrica 117(5):978

Ishii N, Kono Y, Yonemoto N et al (2013) Outcomes of infants born at 22 and 23 weeks' gestation. Pediatrica 132(1):62–71

Janvier A, Leblanc MD, Barrington KJ (2008) The best-interest standard is not applied for neonatal resuscitation decisions. Pediatrica 121(5):963–969

Leuthner S (2001) Decisions regarding resuscitation of the extremely premature infant and models of best interest. J Perinatol 21(3):193–198

Lorenz JM (2005) Prenatal counseling and resuscitation decisions at extremely premature gestation. J Pediatr 147(5):567–568

Mancini A (2013) Training neonatal staff for the future in neonatal palliative care. Semin Fetal Neonatal Med 18:111–115

Miller EK, Cohen JD (2001) An integrative theory of prefrontal cortex function. Annu Rev Neurosci 24:167–202

Paris JJ (2005) Resuscitation decisions for "fetal infants". Pediatrica 115(5):1415

Paris JJ, Graham N, Schreiber MD, Goodwin M (2006) Approaches to end-of-life decision-making in the

NICU: insights from Dostoevsky's *The Grand Inquisitor*. J Perinatol 26:389–391

Pignotti MS, Donzelli G (2008) Perinatal care at the threshold of viability: an international comparison of practical guidelines for the treatment of extremely preterm births 121(1);e193–198.

Rebagliato M, Cuttini M, Broggin L et al (2000) Neonatal end-of-life decision making: physicians' attitudes and relationship with self-reported practices in 10 European countries. JAMA 284(19):2451–2459

Stoll BJ, Hansen NI, Bell EF, Eunice Kennedy Shriver National Institute of Child Health and Human Development Neonatal Research Network et al (2010) Neonatal outcomes of extremely preterm infants from the NICHD Neonatal Research Network. Pediatrica 126(3):443–456

Verhagen AA, Sauer PJ (2005) End-of-life decisions in newborns: an approach from the Netherlands. Pediatrica 116:736–739

Viner J (1925) The utility concept in value theory and its critics. J Pol Econ 33:369–387

Watchko JF (1986) The tragic vision: acknowledging limits and uncertainty. J Perinatol 6(1):39–43

Williams C, Cairnie J, Fines V, Patey C et al (2009) Construction of a parent-derived questionnaire to measure end-of-life care after withdrawal of life-sustaining treatment in the neonatal intensive care unit. Pediatrica 123(1):e87–e95

Follow-Up Outcomes of High-Risk Infants

14

Neil Marlow

Contents

Abstract

Despite the emphasis on major disabling conditions, most survivors of very preterm or extremely preterm birth have mild or no impairments as they enter childhood. Alongside the major conditions discussed in ▶ Chap. 133, "Epidemiology of Adverse Cerebral Outcome of Newborns," a range of important cognitive, behavioral, and motor problems are now well recognized and persist into adult life. Alongside these are rarely considered important issues relating to lung function and cardiovascular health that also require consideration. This chapter will briefly review these areas and signpost further reading.

14.1 Salient Points

- The relationship between impaired outcome rises almost exponentially with decreasing gestational age, and the risk of problems becomes much greater as gestation falls below 32 weeks.
- Cognitive impairments may manifest as poor attainment at school. Infants born prematurely score lower in tests of reading and mathematics. Several executive processes plateau in middle childhood, and in these areas preterm

N. Marlow (✉)
Institute for Women's Health, University College London, London, UK
e-mail: n.marlow@ucl.ac.uk

G. Buonocore et al. (eds.), *Neonatology*,
https://doi.org/10.1007/978-3-319-29489-6_163

children may "catch up" with normally developing children, but at a later age.

- When children born prematurely reach school age, deficits in working memory and the speed of processing information have been reported. These appear to underpin a range of executive deficits, leading to poor school attainment and behavioral difficulties. These are specific areas targetting educational strategies, rather than using more general interventional strategies.
- Behavioral problems may put preterm infants at risk of bullying at school age, prompted by physical differences (small size, reduced lung function, etc.) and an internalized emotional phenotype. Bullying may be responsible for some emotional stress in early adolescence and should be enquired after.
- Multiple studies have demonstrated an excess of motor problems among very preterm children, in addition to a formal diagnosis of cerebral palsy.
- Excess cardiovascular risk with increased arterial blood pressure has been reported.
- Childhood growth may also be compromised, but the effect of the adolescent growth spurt requires further study.

14.2 Introduction

Initial research in the first half of the twentieth century seemed to point to there being no deficit from being born very preterm, but with large population studies and improving survival <34 weeks of gestation it became apparent that outcome was a continuum, with increasing problems being identified at the lowest gestations. The breakpoint at around 32 weeks identified by Wolke et al. (see ▸ Chap. 133, "Epidemiology of Adverse Cerebral Outcome of Newborns," Section 5) has been qualified in more recent database association studies, where the relationship between impaired outcome rises almost exponentially with decreasing gestational age, for example, in special educational needs (MacKay et al. 2010) (Fig. 1). Hence the risk of problems at more mature gestations, although elevated, is relatively small and becomes much greater as gestation falls below 32 weeks. The effect of brain injury and developmental changes found after very preterm birth is complex (Volpe 2009). Understanding the neuropsychological deficits that underpin this relationship may point to potential areas of intervention and allow better understanding of the pathways of abnormal development.

Other organ systems other than the brain are significantly affected by preterm birth. In particular lung function may be impaired, particularly in relation to gestational age, with superimposed lung injury following neonatal treatment. Understanding the relationship of treatment strategies to later outcomes and the implication of measured deficits in lung function to adult prognosis is only now becoming apparent. Similar issues in relationship to vascular function and cardiovascular risk to growth and final height pertain and will be discussed.

14.3 Cognition and Very Preterm Birth

General measures of intelligence are valuable indicators of attainment in childhood and adult life and are clearly related to prematurity as described above. IQ is a summative measure of general cognitive function, and many studies have shown increasing deficit with reducing gestational age (Fig. 2). Understanding the factors that lead to this deficit is important. "Cognition" comprises a series of executive processes that combine to produce the final IQ. Many groups have evaluated aspects of executive function and memory, which reveal more specific impairments (Mulder et al. 2009; Aarnoudse-Moens et al. 2009), which in turn can be evaluated against brain imaging and function to elucidate etiology and their role in generating neuropsychological outcomes more accurately than using a single global measure such as IQ.

Earlier studies revealed that very preterm children found sequential tasks easier in contrast to simultaneous tasks, indicating challenges with dealing with complex tasks that would be better processed as a series of tasks, a principle easily adapted into the classroom.

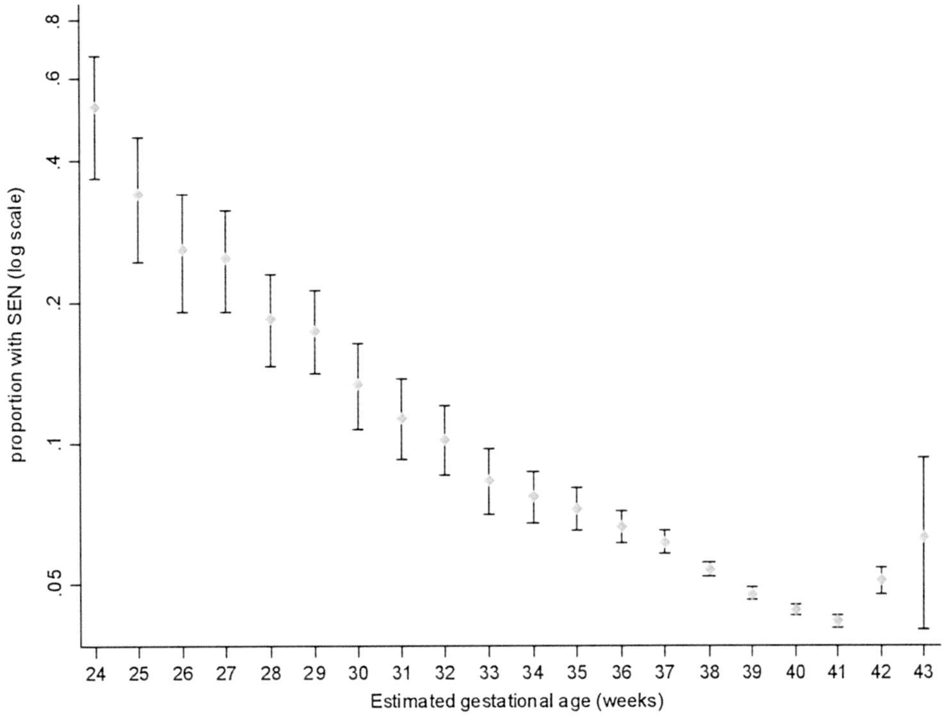

Fig. 1 Relationship between the risk of special educational needs and gestational age at birth (note "y" axis is a log scale) (MacKay et al. 2010) permission required (PLoS Medicine)

Several executive processes plateau in middle childhood, and in these areas preterm children may "catch up" with typically developing children, but at a later age. In contrast, other executive functions seem to diverge from typical development in preterm populations over late childhood/adolescence. Hence the pattern of differences seen is related to both the age of the child and the gestational age of the cohort, rendering comparative studies challenging (Mulder et al. 2009). This area is further complicated by the emergence and focusing of executive processes over the preschool years, such that early attempts to detail them before school age may not be entirely successful (Scherif 2010). More recently, critical deficits in working memory and the speed of processing of information at school age have been reported, which appear to underpin a range of executive deficits (Mulder et al. 2011a) and lead to poor school attainment (Mulder et al. 2010) and behavioral difficulties (Mulder et al. 2011b). It seems clear that these very specific areas may be prime areas at which to direct educational strategies, rather than seek more general interventional strategies.

Cognitive impairments may manifest as poor attainment at school. Educational tests of reading and mathematics, for example, demonstrate lower scores, particularly so in mathematics. Investigating the underlying causes for this has revealed that the same executive deficits, working memory/processing speed, rather than the educational concept of "dyscalculia" are indeed responsible for these (Simms et al. 2015). Hence it is not surprising that very preterm children have a higher rate of special needs at school (Fig. 1), resulting from impaired cognitive functioning, as well as the major disabling conditions described in ▶ Chap. 133, "Epidemiology of Adverse Cerebral Outcome of Newborns." In keeping with this, final school attainment may be at lower grades compared to children born at term. Within the Danish system the proportion failing to complete "basic schooling" rises in a similar fashion to that shown in Fig. 1 (Mathiasen et al. 2010).

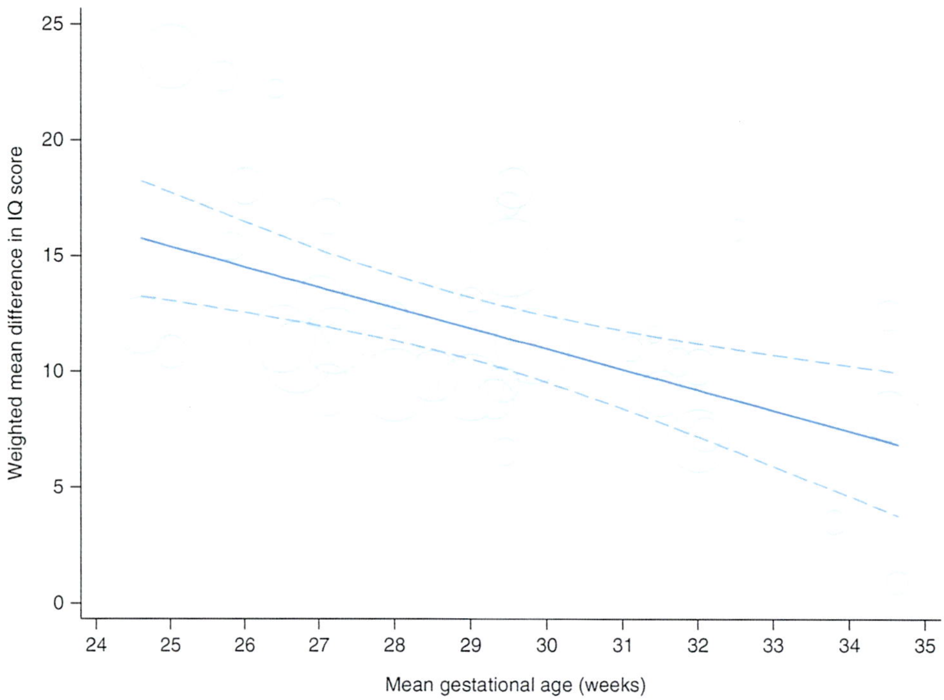

Fig. 2 Bubble plot of the relationship between IQ and gestational age at birth. The size of the bubble indicates relative study size and the position the mean gestation of the cohort (regression line and 95% confidence intervals shown) (Kerr-Wilson et al. 2012) permission required (J Public Health)

It must be emphasized that not all survivors of extremely or very preterm birth have such problems. Risk of impairment may be elevated over the relatively low rate seen in typically developing children, but a high proportion of very preterm children function normally. The challenge is to identify those who will go on to develop functional impairment and to provide effective interventions to enhance outcomes. Many studies in infancy have attempted to do this with varying effects, but few persist beyond early childhood (Spittle et al. 2015; Spittle 2015). At present, it seems unclear as to what should be the targets for such interventions, which ages are most susceptible to intervention, and what strategies are most effective. Part of the issue is the bias towards social disadvantage in populations of children entered into such trials. Risk factor profiles for poor cognitive outcomes include male sex, greater degrees of immaturity, and a range of markers of social disadvantage (Linsell et al. 2015), none of which suggest susceptibility to intervention. However, as neonatal care improves, general cognitive scores appear to have improved for extremely preterm children (Moore et al. 2012), suggesting that at least some of the answer lies in optimizing neonatal outcomes.

14.4 Behavioral Outcomes

Very preterm children are at risk of developing a broad series of behavioral problems, which has been characterized as the preterm behavioral phenotype. This is manifest as increased proportion of children with an internalized phenotype, namely inattentive-type ADHD, autistic symptoms, and emotional difficulties, such as anxiety (Johnson and Marlow 2011; Johnson and Wolke 2013). This contrasts with the predominance of externalized behaviors such as ADHD (combined and overactivity subtypes) in the general population. Many studies use the Child Behavior Checklist with results showing remarkable consistency across countries, particularly in the social, thought, and attention domains (Hille et al. 2001; Farooqi et al. 2013). This consistency between studies seems to confirm the phenotype. There is a general excess of symptoms among children in these specific areas, associated with increased numbers of children with disorders, and prevalence again rises with decreasing gestational age at birth. Many more children demonstrate increased symptom scores than present with disorders. Deficits in working memory and processing speed seem to explain the excess of behavioral problems in 10–11-year-old children (Mulder et al. 2011b), promoting speculation of different origins of disordered behavior among preterm populations, compared with the general population.

At least some of this behavioral profile may make such individuals at risk of bullying at school age, promoted by physical differences (small size, reduced lung function, etc) and the internalized emotional phenotype. Bullying may be responsible for some of the emotional distress in early adolescence (Wolke et al. 2015) and should be enquired about.

The key question remains as to how such childhood symptoms are manifest in adult life. Few studies have followed sufficient numbers into adult life to understand how the transition affects this spectrum. In database association studies there is evidence of increased prevalence of conditions and psychotrophic medication use, but these are somewhat difficult to interpret.

14.5 Motor Function

Multiple studies have demonstrated an excess of motor problems among very preterm children, setting aside a formal diagnosis of cerebral palsy. These are manifest by impaired scores on a range of motor competence and impairment scales. In a recent systematic review of childhood studies in very preterm or very low birthweight children, the odds of a score <5th percentile on the Movement-ABC were 6.3 (95% CI 4.4–9.1) and 5–15th percentile 8.7 (3.4–22) (Edwards et al. 2011). Developmental coordination disorder (DCD) should be identified early and children supported appropriately. In a recent study, neurological dysfunction (using Touwen's neurological examination), IQ, attention, and processing speed mediated the relationship between preterm birth and motor impairment (Van Hus et al. 2014), emphasizing the interrelationship between all neurocognitive and behavioral outcomes in these populations. Comprehensive psychometric assessment should always accompany motor assessment.

14.6 Somatic Outcomes

Alongside brain-based outcomes, key deficits in lung function appear to be the commonest adverse outcomes. Among extremely preterm children, BPD is common, but outcomes for those without moderate/severe neonatal BPD also appear impaired. At 11 years, scores for those without BPD showed on average a 0.5SD deficit and those with BPD showed 1.5SD deficit in FEV1 which did not completely correct after bronchodilator. This respiratory impairment is manifest in frequent hospitalizations over the first years of life and an increased risk of being assigned a diagnosis of asthma and receiving treatment (Lum et al. 2011). These findings are important as they indicate reduced performance in early adult life, on which the well-described age related decline in function is based. Maintaining good childhood respiratory health, promoting exercise, and avoiding cigarette smoke seem particularly important in this group of individuals (Fig. 3).

Alongside lung function deficits, very preterm children appear to be at excess cardiovascular risk, manifest as elevated group means of systolic and diastolic blood pressure consistently among studies in late childhood/early adolescence. We have also demonstrated increased augmentation pressures in central arteries, particularly related to lung function (Bolton et al. 2012) which suggests early emergence of cardiovascular risk may be related to combined cardiorespiratory factors, as a result of prematurity. The extent to which this is manifest in adult life as part of the metabolic syndrome is unclear and requires further study.

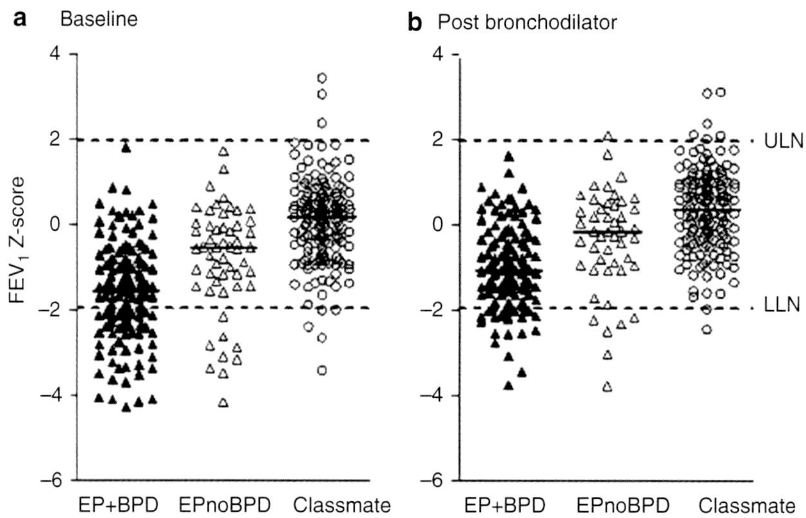

Fig. 3 Forced Expiratory Volume (FEV_1) with and without pretreatment with bronchodilator in 11-year-old children born before 26 weeks of gestation compared to controls using contemporary standards (Fawke et al. 2010). Permission required

Childhood growth may similarly be compromised, but the effect of the adolescent growth spurt does require some further study. Hack and colleagues demonstrated significant catch up growth for females between 8 and 20 years of age in their very low birthweight cohort, but not for males, in some part due to the excess of small for gestational age individuals in their birthweight defined cohort (Hack et al. 2003).

14.7 Adult Outcomes

As very preterm populations now reach early adult life, there is interest in the further progress of preterm populations across the range of areas of function described above. Poorer group performance at school may lead to reduced employment and earning potential, but the extent to which these findings are confounded by social disadvantage must be determined. In Hack's classic study (Hack et al. 2002), very low birthweight young adults at 20 years of age had reduced attainment but fewer adverse social consequences, such as cigarette, recreational drug, and alcohol use. This may be a manifestation of the relative poor socialization of this group of individuals. Other studies have identified persistence of many of the outcomes described above. In a cohort from Liverpool, UK, Cooke showed generally favorable outcomes for a well-characterized group of individuals who had a range of childhood problems (Cooke 2004), as did Saigal in her well-studied group from Hamilton, Ontario (Saigal et al. 2006). More recently Saigal has reported outcomes in the fourth decade for her group. There was an excess of reduced employment prospects, reduced earnings, and a greater need for social support compared to controls. They demonstrated fewer risk-taking behaviors, more health problems, and lower self-esteem (Saigal et al. 2016).

The challenges of neonatal care for this vulnerable group of individuals is thus apparent and emphasizes the critical need to provide ongoing data from more current cohorts exposed to modern neonatal intensive care, which is very different now than 30 years ago and may show signs that outcomes may not be as compromised for such a large proportion as it is appears to have been.

References

Aarnoudse-Moens CS, Weisglas-Kuperus N, van Goudoever JB et al (2009) Meta-analysis of neurobehavioral outcomes in very preterm and/or very low birth weight children. Pediatrics 124 (2):717–728

Bolton CE, Stocks J, Hennessy E et al (2012) The EPICure study: association between hemodynamics and lung function at 11 years after extremely preterm birth. J Pediatr 161(4):595–601 e2

Cooke RW (2004) Health, lifestyle, and quality of life for young adults born very preterm. Arch Dis Child 89 (3):201–206

Edwards J, Berube M, Erlandson K et al (2011) Developmental coordination disorder in school-aged children born very preterm and/or at very low birth weight: a systematic review. J Dev Behav Pediatr 32(9): 678–687

Farooqi A, Hagglof B, Serenius F (2013) Behaviours related to executive functions and learning skills at 11 years of age after extremely preterm birth: a Swedish national prospective follow-up study. Acta Paediatr 102 (6):625–634

Fawke J, Lum S, Kirkby J et al (2010) Lung function and respiratory symptoms at 11 years in children born extremely preterm: the EPICure study. Am J Respir Crit Care Med 182(2):237–245

Hack M, Flannery DJ, Schluchter M et al (2002) Outcomes in young adulthood for very-low-birth-weight infants. N Engl J Med 346(3):149–157

Hack M, Schluchter M, Cartar L et al (2003) Growth of very low birth weight infants to age 20 years. Pediatrics 112(1 Pt 1):e30–e38

Hille ET, den Ouden AL, Saigal S et al (2001) Behavioural problems in children who weigh 1000 g or less at birth in four countries. Lancet 357(9269):1641–1643

Johnson S, Marlow N (2011) Preterm birth and childhood psychiatric disorders. Pediatr Res 69(5 Pt 2):11R–18R

Johnson S, Wolke D (2013) Behavioural outcomes and psychopathology during adolescence. Early Hum Dev 89(4):199–207

Kerr-Wilson CO, Mackay DF, Smith GC et al (2012) Meta-analysis of the association between preterm delivery and intelligence. J Public Health 34(2):209–216

Linsell L, Malouf R, Morris J et al (2015) Prognostic factors for poor cognitive development in children born very preterm or with very low birth weight: A systematic review. JAMA Pediatr 169(12): 1162–1172

Lum S, Kirkby J, Welsh L et al (2011) Nature and severity of lung function abnormalities in extremely pre-term children at 11 years of age. Eur Respir J 37(5):1199–1207

MacKay DF, Smith GC, Dobbie R et al (2010) Gestational age at delivery and special educational need: retrospective cohort study of 407,503 schoolchildren. PLoS Med 7(6), e1000289

Mathiasen R, Hansen BM, Andersen AM et al (2010) Gestational age and basic school achievements: a national follow-up study in Denmark. Pediatrics 126 (6):e1553–e1561

Moore T, Hennessy EM, Myles J et al (2012) Neurological and developmental outcome in extremely preterm children born in England in 1995 and 2006: the EPICure studies. BMJ 345, e7961

Mulder H, Pitchford N, Hagger M et al (2009) Development of executive function and attention in preterm children: a systematic review. Develop Neuropsychol 34(4):393–421

Mulder H, Pitchford N, Marlow N (2010) Processing speed and working memory underlie academic attainment in very preterm children. Arch Dis Child Fetal Neonatal Ed 95:F267–F272

Mulder H, Pitchford NJ, Marlow N (2011a) Processing speed mediates executive function difficulties in very preterm children in middle childhood. J Int Neuropsychol Soc 17:1–10

Mulder H, Pitchford NJ, Marlow N (2011b) Inattentive behaviour is associated with poor working memory and slow processing speed in very pre-term children in middle childhood. Br J Educ Psychol 81 (Pt 1):147–160

Saigal S, Stoskopf B, Streiner D et al (2006) Transition of extremely low-birth-weight infants from adolescence to young adulthood: comparison with normal birth-weight controls. JAMA 295(6):667–675

Saigal S, Day KL, Van Lieshout RJ et al (2016) Health, wealth, social integration, and sexuality of extremely low-birth-weight prematurely born adults in the fourth decade of life. JAMA Pediatr 170(7):678–686

Scherif G (2010) Attention trajectories, mechanisms and outcomes: at the interface between developing cognition and environment. Dev Sci 13:805–812

Simms V, Gilmore C, Cragg L et al (2015) Nature and origins of mathematics difficulties in very preterm children: a different etiology than developmental dyscalculia. Pediatr Res 77(2):389–395

Spittle A (2015) Early intervention cognitive effects not sustained past preschool. J Pediatr 166(3):779

Spittle A, Orton J, Anderson PJ et al (2015) Early developmental intervention programmes provided post hospital discharge to prevent motor and cognitive impairment in preterm infants. Cochrane Database Syst Rev 11, CD005495

Van Hus JW, Potharst ES, Jeukens-Visser M et al (2014) Motor impairment in very preterm-born children: links with other developmental deficits at 5 years of age. Dev Med Child Neurol 56(6):587–594

Volpe JJ (2009) Brain injury in premature infants: a complex amalgam of destructive and developmental disturbances. Lancet Neurol 8(1):110–124

Wolke D, Baumann N, Strauss V et al (2015) Bullying of preterm children and emotional problems at school age: cross-culturally invariant effects. J Pediatr 166(6): 1417–1422

Early Markers of Poor Outcome in Neonatal Medicine

15

Fabrizio Ferrari, Licia Lugli, Elisabetta Garetti, Isotta Guidotti, Marisa Pugliese, and Laura Lucaccioni

Contents

Abstract

A major issue for neonatologists and developmental neurologists is the identification of those infants who are at risk of subsequent neurodevelopmental disability and who may benefit from neurological follow-up and early intervention strategies.

The incidence of major disabilities has decreased in very preterm and extremely preterm infants, although nearly half of the population suffers from minor disabilities as learning disabilities, cognitive defects, attention deficit/hyperactivity disorders, and behavioral problems, especially at school age. Neuroimaging needs to be accompanied by

F. Ferrari (✉) · L. Lugli · E. Garetti · I. Guidotti · M. Pugliese · L. Lucaccioni
Neonatal Intensive Care Unit, Department of Medical and Surgical Sciences of the Mother, Children and Adults, University of Modena and Reggio Emilia, Modena, Italy
e-mail: fabrizio.ferrari@unimore.it

G. Buonocore et al. (eds.), *Neonatology*,
https://doi.org/10.1007/978-3-319-29489-6_164

an accurate clinical assessment of the functional repertoire of the infant, which varies according to the stage of development.

15.1 Salient Points

- Poor outcomes comprise severe, moderate, and mild deficits.
- A variety of standardized examination tools have been developed to detect neurological abnormalities and determine their course during the neonatal period and later on during the first 2 years of life.
- General movements represent a reliable and sensitive method in the neonatal period and early infancy for predicting normal and abnormal motor outcome, particularly cerebral palsy.
- The use of MRI, both in preterm and term infants, is a powerful t ool with high prognostic value.
- The combination of MRI and neurodevelopmental assessments may increase the prognostic value of each tool, helping the identification of infants at risk for later neurological impairment.

15.2 Poor Outcome

Outcome can be categorized into severe and moderate-to-mild deficits. Severe deficits comprise CP, mental retardation (developmental quotient of less than 70), and severe visual or hearing impairment. Severe deficits can be detected within the first 2 years of life. Moderate-to-mild deficits, however, are often not detected until school age (Marlow et al. 2005).

15.2.1 Cerebral Palsy

Cerebral palsy (CP) is a major disability which is defined as a group of disorders of movement and postural control caused by a nonprogressive defect or lesion of the developing brain. The leading prenatal and perinatal risk factors for CP are birth weight and gestational age, but other risk factors include neonatal encephalopathy, multiple pregnancy, infection and inflammation, and a variety of genetic factors.

CP is in part a developmental diagnosis, and it is based on the description of motor signs that are disabling; such a clinical diagnosis is not easy to make, especially early in development. CP is divided into three major types to describe different movement impairments; this classification also reflects the areas of the brain that are damaged (Bax et al. 2005). The three major types are:

Spastic CP: Children with this type of CP are hypertonic and have a neuromuscular condition stemming from damage to the corticospinal tract or the motor cortex. Spastic CP is further classified by topography dependent on the region of the body affected: spastic hemiplegia with one side being affected, spastic diplegia with the lower extremities affected and less upper-body spasticity, and spastic tetraplegia with all four limbs affected equally. Monoplegia, paraplegia, and triplegia may be used to refer to specific manifestations of the spasticity.

Ataxic CP: Symptoms can be caused by damage to the cerebellum; some individuals have hypotonia and tremors, and motor skills might be affected, as well as balance, especially while walking.

Athetoid CP/dyskinetic: This is characterized by mixed tone and sometimes by hypotonia (hypotonia will usually occur before 1 year of age; the muscle tone will be increased with age and progress to hypertonia). People with athetoid CP have trouble holding themselves in an upright, steady position for sitting or walking and often show involuntary movements. The damage occurs to the extrapyramidal motor system and/or pyramidal tract and to the basal ganglia (BG) (Rosenbaum et al. 2005; Palisano et al. 1997).

In 2004, an international meeting on the definition and classification of CP was held in Bethesda. The major addition to the classic Bax and Mutch et al. (Rosenbaum et al. 2005) definitions involved emphasis on the accompanying developmental disturbances that accompany neurodevelopmental disabilities: these are often functionally more important than the developmental motor disorders that are, by definition, the hallmark of CP (Rosenbaum et al. 2005). The severity of CP is nowadays classified according to the Gross Motor Function Classification System (GMFCS) for cerebral palsy: it is a reliable and predictive internationally adopted method of scoring gross motor function in children with CP (Palisano et al. 1997).

The revised and expanded version of the GMFCS describes the movement ability of children with CP in one of five ordinal levels across five age bands, with emphasis on the child's typical performance in different settings. Children at level I perform the same activities as their age-matched peers but with some difficulty in speed, balance, and coordination, while children at level V have difficulty controlling their head and trunk posture in most positions and achieving any voluntary control of movement. The GMFCS has been incorporated recently into most CP registry data sets, so there are few studies comparing the distribution of GMFCS levels in CP population cohorts or assessing changes in levels over time (Palisano et al. 2008).

15.2.2 Mental Retardation

Mental retardation (MR) or intellectual disability is defined as a disability that involves significant limitations both in intellectual functioning and in adaptive behavior, which covers many everyday social and practical skills. This disability originates before the age of 18 years and encompasses a wide range of conditions, types, and levels.

15.2.2.1 Visual Disability and Hearing Impairment

Visual disability is the impairment of visual functioning even after treatment and/or standard refractive correction, with a visual acuity in the better eye of less than 6/18 for low vision and 3/60 for blindness or with a visual field of less than 10 degrees from the point of fixation (according to the WHO definition).

A hearing impairment or deafness is a full or partial decrease in the ability to detect or understand sounds. It can be classified as conductive or sensorineural hearing loss (Dubowitz et al. 1998; Romeo et al. 2009).

15.2.2.2 Minimal Neurological Dysfunction

Nearly half of very preterm (VP) and extremely preterm (EP) infants suffer from minor disabilities. The term "minor motor problems" indicates a wide spectrum of motor disorders other than CP; "minor" does not mean "minimal," as a relevant proportion of the preterm infants will develop academic and behavioral problems at school age. Early-onset disorders consist of abnormal general movements (GMs), transient dystonia, and postural instability; these conditions usually fade during the first months. They were underestimated in the past; recently, qualitative assessment of GMs using. Prechtl's method has become a major item of the neurological examination. Late-onset disorders include developmental coordination disorder (DCD) and/or minor neurological dysfunction (MND): both terms cover partly overlapping problems. Simple MND (MND-1) and complex MND (MND-2) can be identified, and MND-2 gives a higher risk for learning and behavioral disorders. A relationship between the qualities of GMs and MND in childhood has been recently described. The Touwen infant neurological examination (TINE) can reliably detect neurological signs of MND even in infancy. However, the prognostic value of these disorders requires further investigations. Anyway the high rate of MNDs and their association with an increased risk for learning difficulties justify their screening in case of (even moderate) prematurity. Moreover, children born extremely preterm are at high risk for intellectual disability (ID), learning disabilities (LD), executive dysfunction, and special educational needs (SEN), but little is understood about the comorbidity of intellectual and learning disabilities in this population. A recent study showed that extremely premature children with comorbid ID/LD had significantly poorer neuropsychological abilities and curriculum-based attainment than extremely premature children with an isolated disability or no disabilities. LD were associated with a three-times increased risk for SEN. Therefore, as extremely premature children are at high risk for comorbid intellectual and learning disabilities, education professionals should be aware of the complex nature of EP children's difficulties and the need for multi-domain assessments to guide intervention (Arnaud et al. 2007; Ferrari et al. 2012; Johnson et al. 2016).

15.3 Traditional Neurological Examination

A variety of standardized examination tools have been developed to estimate gestational age, detect neurological abnormalities, and determine their course during the neonatal period and later on during the first 2 years of life (Dubowitz et al. 1998). Infants at high risk of brain damage may be included in follow-up programs comprising serial neurological examinations in order to identify early indicators of abnormal neurological development. A simple and scorable neurological examination for infants between 2 and 24 months of age was developed in the Paediatric Department of the Hammersmith Hospital in London (the Hammersmith Infant Neurological Examination [HINE]) (Rosenbaum et al. 2005). The assessment consists of different items assessing cranial nerve function, posture, movements, tone, reflexes, the development of motor function, and the state of behavior (Dubowitz et al. 1998). For details, see ▶ Chap. 120, "Neurological Examination of the Newborn Infant."

The prognostic power of the HINE optimality score was explored in very preterm infants between 9 and 18 months of age: 48% had suboptimal scores; the scores were not associated with the degree of prematurity and had a very high accuracy to predict walking at 2 years. The scores were also not invariably associated with the pattern of ultrasonogram findings: cystic periventricular leukomalacia (PVL) was associated with low scores, and other ultrasonogram abnormalities with both optimal and suboptimal scores. This is not surprising because hemorrhages and periventricular densities can be associated with both normal and abnormal neurodevelopment. A high correlation between the HINE at 3 months and the developmental quotient at 24 months was found. The high predictive value of the HINE across the first year of life was probably granted by the effective combination of different groups of items for each age period. Indeed, although a number of items were found to be consistently among the most predictive ones (movement quality, quantity, and lateral tilting), other items changed across time. Tone items (ventral suspension, arm pronation/supination, and scarf sign) tended to be more predictive at 3 and 6 months post-term, while maturational items, such as arm protection, vertical suspension, and forward parachute, were highly predictive only after 9 months. Therefore these studies demonstrated that a standardized neurological examination performed from 3 to 12 months can be used reliably in very preterm infants to predict motor outcome (Romeo et al. 2009).

The predictive value of the HINE examination was also evaluated in infants with other neurodevelopmental risks, like infants with hypoxic-ischemic encephalopathy (HIE) (see ▶ Chap. 126, "Clinical Aspects and Treatment of the Hypoxic-Ischemic Syndrome").

Follow-up studies have demonstrated that the outcome cannot be always predicted by the severity of HIE. Although HIE stage 1 is usually associated with a normal outcome and HIE stage 3 with severe neurodevelopmental abnormalities, the outcome in infants with HIE stage 2 can be quite variable, ranging from normal to CP and severe MR. Several studies have reported that neurodevelopmental outcome is best predicted by the pattern of lesions observed on neonatal MRI (see ▶ Chap. 122, "Neuroimaging Studies"). The HINE was used in a group of infants with HIE at age 9–14 months to evaluate the correlation between the scores and early MRI findings and whether the scores can be used to predict locomotor function at 2 and 4 years. Approximately 40% of the infants had suboptimal scores on neurological examination, and the magnitude of the suboptimal scores was related to the pattern of the MRI lesion. Severe BG lesions, diffuse brain injuries, or both were associated with the most severe outcome (Romeo et al. 2009).

The use of the optimality score gave prognostic information on the severity of the functional motor outcome. Although neonatal MRI can identify early infants who will have CP, the neurological examination can provide information on the severity of the functional motor impairment and distinguish infants who will walk from those who will only sit or not even acquire the sitting posture. It is interesting, however, that few children who were able to walk without restrictions at 4 years had an abnormal gait, associated with a mild hemiplegia or with mild movement disorders, which suggested that mild neurological abnormalities can also occur in the absence of widespread lesions or severe abnormalities. Further studies evaluating follow-up at school age are required to evaluate whether these minor neurological abnormalities are related to any difficulty in everyday life (Ricci et al. 2006a).

15.4 Early Markers of Cerebral Palsy: The Role of General Movements

The types of brain injuries most frequently occurring in term infants are hypoxic-ischemic injury to the BGT and parasagittal injury, and in preterm infants PVL, intraventricular hemorrhages (IVH), and persistent flare.

CP occurs in 8–10% of very preterm babies and approximately 40% of all children with CP are born preterm. In preterm infants spastic diplegia prevails, followed by hemiplegia. In full-term infants, tetraplegia and hemiplegia are by far the most common forms; dyskinetic CP is more common in full-term infants (Marlow et al. 2005).

The early prediction of CP will lead to the child receiving neurological follow-up and earlier enrolment in rehabilitation program. It is generally reported that CP cannot be diagnosed before several months after birth or even before the age of 2 years. A so-called silent period, lasting up to few months, has also been described.

The neurological signs observed during the first months after birth in preterm infants who will develop CP are neither sensitive nor specific enough to allow for a reliable prognosis. Irritability, abnormal finger position, spontaneous Babinski reflex, weakness of the lower limbs, transient abnormalities of tone, and delay in achieving motor milestones are some of the neurological signs that have been described in these high-risk preterm infants. All of them may be encountered before the onset of CP or during transient dystonia, dissociated motor development, and other transient neurological disturbances that vanish during the first or second year of life.

In the last two decades, a technique for assessing spontaneous motor activity has been introduced and evaluated, namely, Prechtl's assessment of general movements (GMs). This approach, which involves observation of the infant without direct physical examination, has proved a reliable and sensitive method in the neonatal period and early infancy for predicting normal and abnormal motor outcome, particularly CP (Prechtl et al. 1997). It requires video recording of a few minutes of spontaneous motility and off-line observation of the quality of GMs. Serial assessments of GMs from preterm birth until 3–5 months post-term age define the developmental trajectory. Assessment based on developmental trajectory predicts CP at a much earlier age than other neurological assessment.

Recently, data evaluating the accuracy of multiple modalities used to predict a diagnosis of CP in high-risk patients showed how GMs present the highest predictive accuracy. Moreover, there were evidences to support the use of MRI at term-corrected age, neurological examination in the older infant, and, to a lesser extent, ultrasound in infants of preterm age (Bosanquet et al. 2013; Xie et al. 2015).

15.4.1 Diplegia and Tetraplegia

Early specific markers for spastic cerebral palsy are cramped-synchronized (CS) GMs and abnormal fidgety GMs. As far as CS GMs, the movements of limbs and trunk appear rigid and lack normal smooth and fluent character. The limb and trunk muscle contract and relax almost simultaneously. All infants who show consistent and prolonged CS GMs later develop CP. The earlier consistent CS GMs occur, the worse the later motor impairment of preterm infants. If the CS character is transient and followed by normal fidgety GMs, the infant may have a normal outcome (Ferrari et al. 2002); if the CS character is still present at 3 to 4 months of age, the infant will not develop fidgety movements (FMs) (Einspieler et al. 2015). The second specific marker for CP is absent FMs. Almost all infants who never had FMs developed CP. The absence of FMs can be preceded either by CS GMs or by poor repertoire (PR) GMs. Both abnormal qualities of GMs, i.e., CS GMs and absence of FMs, are seen within 3–5 months post-term, thus much earlier than with other neurological assessment (Ferrari et al. 2002). It was recently demonstrated by Einspieler et al. that infants with sporadic FMs and those with absent FMs (who developed CP) showed no difference with respect to their GMFCS levels 3 to 5 years later. However, sporadic FMs were linked to a slightly better (although not normal) concurrent movement repertoire (Einspieler et al. 2015).

15.4.2 Hemiplegia

Hemiplegia (HE) is usually due to focal one-sided lesions, either ischemic or hemorrhagic infarction, more rarely to cystic lesions due to focal or unilateral PVL. Brain US and MRI detect site and severity of the focal lesions: the neurological follow-up of these infants aims to detect (or exclude) early signs of HE. Traditional neonatal neurological examination is of low predictive value for such patients.

The studies carried on with the GM method have shown that all babies with a focal lesion have an abnormal quality of GMs (PR or CS) from term, and a silent window is not observed. Asymmetrical segmental movements can be recognized from as early as 3 months post-term in preterm infants and from 3–6 weeks post-term in full-term infants with neonatal cerebral infarction. Segmental movements are distinct wrist movements, occurring either in isolation or as a part of GMs.

In term infants who later develop HE asymmetry in wrist movements, a lower frequency of independent digit movements is seen as early as 12 weeks and predicts later HE. It is important to note that only infants with concomitant ipsilateral involvement of a cerebral hemisphere, BG, and the internal capsule on the MRI brain scan later develop HE. Early recognition of subtle motor asymmetries is not easy with unaided eyes; it is easier when video recording of spontaneous motor behavior is available (Guzzetta et al. 2003).

A more recent and accurate multicenter study in infants who later developed hemiplegia, conducted by the same research group but considering a new group of patients, confirmed the asymmetry and impoverishment of wrist segmental movements in the limb contralateral to the side of central focal lesion, but it also highlights new findings: hemiplegia can be predicted by an early reduction in the frequency of independent upper limb digit movements. In particular none of the infants with abnormal outcome showed more than one digit movement per minute (with one exception), whereas 10 out of the 13 infants with symmetrical wrist movements had normal motor development. It is important to note that the degree of impoverishment or asymmetry was not correlated with the severity of later motor impairment. All three of the infants with symmetrical wrist movements who had abnormal neurological outcome developed a very mild form of hemiplegia (Guzzetta et al. 2010).

15.4.3 Dyskinetic CP

Dyskinetic CP has a frequency of only 10–15% of all CP forms. The dyskinetic form of CP comprises two subtypes: a syndrome of choreoathetosis (infants showing mainly massive, purposeless involuntary movements) and a dystonic form, characterized by sudden shifts of muscle contraction and infantile reflex activity. This second subtype is more common. During the first 2 months, infants who will develop a dyskinetic form display a PR of GMs, arm movements in circles, and finger spreading. Abnormal arm and finger movements remain until at least 5 months and are associated with lack of arm and leg movements toward the midline (particularly foot-foot contact) and with lack of FMs. The abnormal unilateral or bilateral circular arm movements are monotonous, slow forward rotations from the shoulder. The monotony in speed and amplitude is the most characteristic quality of circular arm movements.

An early differential diagnosis of dyskinetic versus spastic later CP is not easy: later dyskinetic infants share the absence of FMs and antigravity movements, i.e., leg lifting in infants with later spastic form. Moreover, circular arm movements can be mistaken for windmilling arm movements seen during the first year of life and with cycling movements described in infants with HIE. Choreoathetoid movements are easy to recognize, but the sudden shifts of muscle contraction are difficult to differentiate from the abnormal muscle tone of spastic forms. Dystonic and spastic features are quite commonly mixed in the same infant (Einspieler et al. 2002).

15.5 Neuroimaging Predictors

Besides neurological assessment of the infant with neonatal brain injury or at risk for neurodevelopmental disturbances, neuroimaging can provide predictors of neurodevelopmental outcome. Two main imaging techniques have been used for the prediction of neurodevelopmental outcome in the neonatal period: US and MRI (see ▶ Chap. 122, "Neuroimaging Studies").

15.5.1 Cerebral Ultrasound

US is a simple bedside tool, and when used repeatedly, its sensitivity and specificity can be very high, especially in the preterm infant. US lesions can be detected in the majority of infants born below 32 weeks of gestation who develop CP. IVH grades III and IV, PVL, and focal infarctions are major cerebral lesions detected by US in the preterm population. Also infants with a grade I–II IVH are at an almost two times higher risk of developing neurodevelopmental impairments at 20 months compared with those without any hemorrhage. The degree of milder US findings (grade I or II PVL) and size of the corpus callosum are also related to neuromotor function in school-age children without CP. New techniques such as transmastoidal access have improved the representation of the cerebellum, a structure that can also be injured in very low birth weight (VLBW) infants. Cerebellar injuries may contribute to long-term neurocognitive disabilities, independent of associated supratentorial parenchymal lesions (Marlow et al. 2005).

Cerebral US is useful in the critically ill newborn who cannot be studied with MRI. During the first hours after asphyxia, US may give little information on the severity of lesions and prediction of outcome. Arterial Doppler studies (measurement of the pulsatility index) may better predict outcome, but in most cases it is still normal 6–12 h after the insult. The most frequent lesion observed by US in asphyxia is BGT hyper-echogenicity, while parasagittal ischemia is more difficult to detect, because the distance between brain lesions and the acoustic window is high.

15.5.2 MRI Abnormalities and Outcome

MRI of the preterm infant is best performed at term-equivalent age when the myelination of the posterior limb of the internal capsule (PLIC) may be used as a predictor of motor outcome. MRI lesions in the full-term infant are best seen after the first week.

In the preterm infant, MRI has been used to detect diffuse WM abnormalities and gray matter changes. Gray matter abnormalities are also associated with the same risks but to a lesser extent than WM abnormalities. WM abnormalities can be detected in more than 50% of VLBW children and are predictive of CP and psychomotor delay in early childhood and neurosensory impairment. A significant relationship between WM abnormalities on MRI and absent FMs in infants born at <30 weeks of gestation supports the idea that abnormal GMs reflect white matter injury (Spittle et al. 2008).

Recently it has been shown that HIE, typically described in full-term infants, can also be observed in preterm infants. These infants have a high incidence of severe BGT and brainstem involvement, and the lesions are associated with significant mortality and neurologic morbidity. Advanced MRI techniques such as volumetry and morphometry, diffusion tensor imaging, and tractography have been used to better determine the full spectrum of brain injury.

In infants born preterm and examined at term, abnormalities in the cortex and deep nuclear structures are related to the degree of immaturity at birth and concomitant WM injury. Volumetric changes in the sensorimotor, premotor, midtemporal, and parieto-occipital regions may be related to intellectual performance at school age. Brain volumes may be considered important markers for neurodevelopmental deficits in moderate and late preterm children. In fact, larger total brain tissue, WM, and cerebellar volumes at term-equivalent age are seen to be associated with better neurodevelopment in moderate and late preterm children (Cheong et al. 2016).

Recent findings indicate that the hippocampal volume may be reduced in preterm infants and that it is associated with reduced working memory and cognitive and motor performance at 2 years of age. Moreover, a small transcerebellar diameter and short corpus callosal length on brain MRI at term-equivalent age are related to adverse neurodevelopmental outcomes at a corrected age of 2 years and could be a useful adjunctive tool for counseling parents about future developmental outcomes. Biparietal width (BPW) and interhemispheric distance (ID) have recently been considered important MRI findings for brain development of preterm infants at term-equivalent age. It was found that decreased BPW and increased ID were independently associated with delayed cognitive development (Kidokoro et al. 2014). Cerebral cortical folding becomes dramatically more complex in the fetal brain during the third trimester of gestation; the process continues in a similar trend in children who are born prematurely. To quantify this morphological development, it is necessary to extract the interface between gray matter and white matter, which is particularly challenging due to changing tissue contrast during brain maturation. The prefrontal and temporal lobes exhibit most development during the preterm period, especially in the left hemisphere. Recent studies revealed impairment of cortical folding in extremely preterm newborns relative to late preterm newborns, demonstrating its potential to provide biomarkers of prematurity-related developmental outcome (Kim et al. 2016; Orasanu et al. 2016). However, MRI at term age by itself cannot predict the functional outcome with 100% accuracy: neurodevelopmental assessments, and in particular general movements, have an important role as they can identify infants at risk for later neurological impairment and may enhance the prognostic utility of MRI if used in combination (Olsen et al. 2016).

Brain injury in neonates following hypoxic-ischemic encephalopathy (HIE) prior to the introduction of neuroprotection with hypothermia was generally described in MRI studies as either WM injury extending to the cortical areas or deep gray nuclei injury in the BGT or involvement in both areas. In childhood, these areas of brain injury were associated with cognitive delays and motor impairment (Rutherford et al. 2006). HIE and BGT are often associated with abnormal signal intensity in the PLIC, brainstem, hippocampal region, and cortex, particularly around the central fissure and insula. Loss of the normal signal intensity from the PLIC is associated with adjacent BGT injury. The motor correlate is a spastic or dyskinetic CP. BGT lesions are the imaging signature of an acute and profound hypoxic-ischemic event. BGT lesions associated with severe WM damage, conversely, suggest a more prolonged hypoxic-ischemic insult. WM damage is proved by a loss of gray matter/WM differentiation, consistent with an overt infarction: in these infants a very poor outcome can be expected. When the predominant lesion involves the WM and cortex but spares the BG and PLIC, the pattern probably results from prolonged partial hypoxia-ischemia: the motor outcome is often good, but there may be cognitive and behavioral impairments that are proportionate to the extent of WM and cortical injury. Severe BGT lesions are associated with a high risk of developing CP and severe cognitive impairment regardless of the additional associated WM lesions (Rutherford et al. 1998). Hypothermia initiated within 6 h of age at 33–34 °C and continued for 72 h decreases death or disability at 18–24 months of age or increases the number of normal survivors. Rutherford et al. have reported MRI results of the "Total Body Hypothermia for Neonatal Encephalopathy Trial" demonstrating a reduction in lesions in the BGT, WM, and abnormal PLIC among cooled infants. The accuracy of prediction by MRI of death or disability to 18 months of age was 84% in the cooled group and 81% in the non-cooled group. The site and severity of brain lesions seen on MRI have been also correlated to the quality of general movements in term infants with HIE to and the prognostic value of MRI, and general movements for motor outcome have been compared. MRI scores for the basal ganglia and thalami, posterior limb of the internal capsule, white matter, and cortex and lesion patterns were correlated with 1-month and 3-month general movements and general movement trajectories; central gray matter scores were correlated most strongly with cramped-synchronized general movements and abnormal motor outcome. MRI scores were 100% sensitive and 72.2% specific for motor outcome, and cramped-synchronized general movements were 100% specific and 68.7% sensitive for motor outcome. Therefore, in term of infants with HIE, the site and severity of brain lesions seen on early MRI resulted highly correlated with general movements. Central gray matter damage leads to cramped-synchronized general movements and poor motor outcome. Early MRI scans and general movements are complementary tools for predicting motor outcome (Ferrari et al. 2011). The National Institute of Child Health and Human Development (NICHD) Neonatal Research Network (NRN) investigators described a decrease in areas of infarction in the watershed (WS) area among infants in the hypothermia group and described an MRI pattern of brain injury that correlated with death or disability at 18 months of age. The "Infant Cooling Evaluation trial group" showed that WM injury decreased among cooled infants compared with the non-cooled group, and PLIC and BGT injury were associated with death or disability at 24 months of age. Thus, the neonatal MRI assessment of brain injury appears to be a biomarker of 18- to 24-month outcome following hypothermia for neonatal HIE. The 6 to 7 year outcomes of trial participants in the NICHD trial and the Total Body Hypothermia for Neonatal Encephalopathy trial have recently been reported showing decreased mortality and better neurodevelopmental outcome in childhood in the cooled group. Shankaran et al. recently examined also the ability of MRI patterns of neonatal brain injury defined by NICHD to predict death or IQ at 6–7 years of age following hypothermia for neonatal encephalopathy. MRI pattern of neonatal brain injury resulted a marker of outcome at 6–7 years of age among neonates undergoing whole-body hypothermia or normothermia for neonatal HIE. It was demonstrated that pattern of neonatal brain injury with involvement of either BGT, PLIC, or area of infarction and additional cerebral lesions or cerebral hemispheric devastation has high predictive indices for death or IQ <70 at 6–7 years of age, and a normal MRI was also predictive of a normal outcome. Therefore, the neonatal MRI injury pattern may serve as a biomarker of brain injury and, along with follow-up, may be useful to evaluate response to future neuroprotective strategies (Shankaran et al. 2012; Azzopardi et al. 2014; Shankaran et al. 2015).

15.5.3 Cognitive Evaluation

The most widely used standardized developmental scales to assess mental development in the first two years after birth are the Bayley Scales of Infant Development (BSID) and the Griffiths Mental Developmental Scales.

The new Bayley Scales of Infant and Toddler Development, third edition, includes updated items and modernized stimulus materials and manipulatives and yields mental assessment results as separate cognitive and language scores rather than as separate scores for cognitive, language, and motor scales and separate scores for expressive and receptive communication and for fine and gross motor skills. The associated Adaptive-Behavior parent questionnaire is an excellent addition to the new Bayley scales, giving functional information that can be used to support a tested significant mental delay. On the other hand, the Griffiths Mental Development Scales for children from birth to

24 months, reviewed in 1996, comprises items to assess locomotor, personal-social, hearing and language, eye and hand coordination, and performance domain. Domain raw scores are obtained and converted to standardized sub-quotients, percentiles, and developmental age, the sum of which is the general quotient, a score for an overall developmental level.

The purpose of developmental standardized scales is to assess a child's development at the time of observation, to determine developmental delay or impairment, in order to implement early habilitation interventions. Despite the wide use of standardized scales to determine the extent of developmental delay or impairment, major concern remains about their accuracy in discriminating cognitive function. To evaluate specific cognitive deficits, it is essential to use neuropsychological tests and to continue cognitive follow-up at least until school age. Developmental scales are not intelligence tests, and developmental quotients (DQ) calculated in the first 2 years are not as reliable as the intelligence quotient (IQ) measurement, calculated after the first 3 years of life, nor do they have as good a predictive value for later IQ. However, in preterm populations, a score of two standard deviations (SD) below the normative mean has been used as a cutoff to identify abnormalities. Currently, following a consensus statement, many authors suggest that a cutoff of three SD is more appropriate and may be more predictive of later poor performance (Marlow et al. 2005).

Recent studies on preterm infants demonstrated that abnormal GMs also reflect impairment of brain areas involved in cognitive development. A systematic review by Einspieler et el. underlines that normal GMs associated with normal motor repertoire during the first months after term are markers for normal cognitive development until at least the age of 10 (Einspieler et al. 2016).

15.6 Visual Evaluation

Subcortical visual pathways have a major role in neonatal vision, while cortical visual modules progressively emerge during the first months of postnatal life. Abnormal visual function occurs in infants with brain lesions even in the absence of ocular abnormalities (cortical blindness). Blindness affects early motor development, especially self-initiated postures and locomotion.

Term infants with HIE can show visual abnormalities (reduction in visual acuity, fixation shift, or visual fields) in the first years of life. Occipital cortex and optic radiation injury have been found in infants with visual impairment, but cortical and WM lesions sparing the BG are not always associated with abnormal visual findings. Cortical and BG lesions are always associated with severe abnormalities of visual function during the first year of life, confirming the role of BG in human visual development. Poor acuity, weak stereopsis, and delayed visual maturation can occur in children with focal BG lesion (Mercuri et al. 1997).

VLBW infants are at risk of visual, visuocognitive, and visuomotor impairment. Vision loss for preterm infants is given as visual impairment with the best vision after correction of <20/60 or legal blindness with the best corrected vision of <20/200 (<6/60). Severe visual impairment occurs in 1–3% of ELBW and 2–6% in children with gestational ages below 27 weeks.

Retinopathy of prematurity (ROP) is one of the main causes of poor visual function and blindness; prevention is based on ophthalmic screening to identify cases requiring treatment. Less severe visual impairments include refractive errors, reduced visual acuity, strabismus, and nystagmus. IVH and PVL are other causes of visual impairment (Ricci et al. 2006b). Severity of visual impairment is also related to the extent of basal ganglia, lateral geniculate nuclei, and optic radiation involvement. Fractional anisotropy of the optic radiation was related to visual assessment scores, independent of WM maturation.

Assessment of visual function at term-corrected age includes ability to fix and follow a target, preferential looking, attention at distance, and color and stripe discrimination. Measures of early visual cortical function are orientation reversal visual event-related potentials (OR-VERP) and fixation shifts under competition. Both measures correlate with the severity of brain abnormalities and are sensitive predictors of neurodevelopmental outcome at 2 years.

Post-discharge eye examinations until preschool are useful to monitor refractive errors and to prevent amblyopia.

15.7 Hearing Evaluation

Hearing loss (HL) is one of the most common birth defects (3/1000) and is associated with language and perception disorders. Genetic factors, prematurity, low birth weight, hyperbilirubinemia, pharmacologic ototoxicity, and noise exposure are the main causes of HL. The introduction of universal screening resulted in a significant decrease of HL.

Otoacoustic emissions (OAE) and auditory brainstem response (ABR) are employed in newborn hearing screening programs. The OAE measures the inner ear response to sound by placing a microphone in the ear canal. The ABR records the brain's response to sound by placing electrodes on the head.

Auditory steady-state responses have been reported as a reliable and objective technique for evaluating the hearing threshold. ABR and auditory steady-state responses in infants with perinatal brain injury show a high sensitivity of auditory steady-state responses for detecting hearing impairment.

In term infants, much hearing impairment is due to specific gene abnormalities, including the connexin mutation. Some authors state that hypoxia-ischemia damages cochlear hair cells, causing hearing impairment. Infants carrying genetic mutations for hearing loss may coincidentally experience perinatal stress, but prevalence of hearing impairment in children born with HIE is not significantly increased.

In preterm infants, sensorineural HL has been associated with prolonged ventilation, ligation of patent ductus, hypotension and ototoxicity, infections, craniofacial abnormalities, and family history. All extremely low birth weight (ELBW) infants are considered at high risk for HL, and in most centers hearing testing is done prior to intensive care discharge, either as OAE or full diagnostic testing with ABR. Occasionally, this test defines auditory neuropathy with abnormal auditory brainstem function and a strong cochlear microphonic with normal OAE.

Although as many as 6% of children with gestational age below 26–27 weeks have severe to profound hearing impairment, many function well after the early placement of cochlear implants.

Children with undiagnosed HL can experience delays in the development of language, social, and academic skills. Besides the degree of hearing loss and age at onset of deafness, environmental factors (parental support and education methods) seem to play an important role in the cognitive development and academic success. As language development begins within the first months of life, it is important for parents to be aware of normal language and communication developmental milestones beginning when their baby is very young so that they can discuss development with their child's healthcare provider (Santiago-Rodriguez et al. 2005).

15.8 The International Classification of Functioning

The international classification of functioning describes "functioning" as the dynamic interaction among three dimensions: body function/structure, activity and participation, and environmental factors. Several authors have proposed "neuromotor" or "neurobehavioral" assessments that evaluate the dynamic and developing systems in order to identify the "emerging functions" and the skill of adaptability to different stimuli. The hypothesis is that this functional approach to neurodevelopmental evaluation may better relate to later outcomes and focus on the consequences rather than on the disease itself. The role of neurofunctional assessment has been emphasized by authors involved in rehabilitative fields: *neurodevelopmental treatment and bobathian practice* in the United Kingdom, *education therapeutique and evaluation factorielle* by Tardieu in France, and *pattern analysis and neurorehabilitative semeiotics* by Milani in Italy.

Identification of infants at higher risk of later negative developmental outcome remains a challenge for clinicians, especially in the preterm. This problem has been investigated mainly by using standard neurological assessments, which evaluate the relation between the nature and localization of brain lesions and related dysfunctions.

However, new approaches to disability are desirable considering the multidimensional nature of the problem. Neurofunctional assessment and study of emerging functions in premature infants relate to prognosis better than standard neurological examination.

Advances in obstetric and neonatal care have dramatically improved the survival rate of very low birth weight (VLBW; birth weight < 1500 g) infants over the last decade. As a result, questions arise about their long-term neurodevelopmental outcome. Cerebral palsy occurs in 10–15% of the VLBW population, with higher rates in infants of lower birth weight and gestational age. An increased incidence of minor neurological dysfunctions, such as learning disabilities, cognitive defects, attention deficit/hyperactivity disorders, and behavioral problems, has been reported, especially in school children of extremely low birth weight or gestational age.

Neurofunctional assessment is an additional method for evaluating neurodevelopmental disability in infants at high risk; the functional approach to pediatric and neontological fields is also recommended by the World Health Organization, as this approach allows early intervention and targeted follow-up, besides reassuring parents on integrity of function. In particular the International Classification of Functioning (ICF) for Children and Youth was proposed as instrument of global assessment of the child, the Alberta Infant Motor Scale (AIMS) for the evaluation of motor functions during the first 18 months of age, the Gross Motor Function Classification System (GMFCS) specific for severe mental retardations and cerebral palsy, and VINELAND for adaptive functions (World Health Organization 2001; Picciolini et al. 2006; Arpi and Ferrari 2013).

References

Arnaud C, Daubisse-Marliac L, White-Koning M, Pierrat V, Larroque B, Grandjean H, Alberge C, Marret S, Burguet A, Ancel PY, Supernant K, Kaminski M (2007) Prevalence and associated factors of minor neuromotor dysfunctions at age 5 years in prematurely born children: the EPIPAGE study. Arch Pediatr Adolesc Med 161:1053–1061

Arpi E, Ferrari F (2013) Preterm birth and behaviour problems in infants and preschool-age children: a review of the recent literature. Dev Med Child Neurol 55:788–796

Azzopardi D, Strohm B, Marlow N, Brocklehurst P, Deierl A, Eddama O et al (2014) Effects of hypothermia for perinatal asphyxia on childhood outcomes. N Engl J Med 371:140–149

Bax M, Goldstein M, Rosenbaum P et al (2005) Proposed definition and classification of cerebral palsy. Dev Med Child Neurol 47:571–576

Bosanquet M, Copeland L, Ware R, Boyd R (2013) A systematic review of tests to predict cerebral palsy in young children. Dev Med Child Neurol 55:418–426

Cheong JL, Thompson DK, Spittle AJ, Potter CR, Walsh JM, Burnett AC, Lee KJ, Chen J, Beare R, Matthews LG, Hunt RW, Anderson PJ, Doyle LW (2016) Brain Volumes at Term-Equivalent Age Are Associated with 2-Year Neurodevelopment in Moderate and Late Preterm Children. J Pediatr 174:91–97.e1

Dubowitz L, Mercuri E, Dubowitz V (1998) An optimality score for the neurologic examination of the term newborn. J Pediatr 133:406–416

Einspieler C, Cioni G, Paolicelli PB et al (2002) The early markers for later dyskinetic cerebral palsy are different from those for spastic cerebral palsy. Neuropediatrics 33:73–78

Einspieler C, Yang H, Bartl-Pokorny KD, Chi X, Zang FF, Marschik PB, Guzzetta A, Ferrari F, Bos AF, Cioni G (2015) Are sporadic fidgety movements as clinically relevant as is their absence? Early Hum Dev 91:247–252

Einspieler C, Bos AF, Libertus ME, Marschil PB (2016) The general movement assessment helps us to identify preterm infants at risk for cognitive dysfunction. Front Psychol 7:406

Ferrari F, Cioni G, Einspieler C et al (2002) Cramped synchronized general movements in preterm infants as an early marker for cerebral palsy. Arch Pediatr Adolesc Med 156:460–467

Ferrari F, Todeschini A, Guidotti I, Martinez-Biarge M, Roversi MF, Berardi A, Ranzi A, Cowan FM, Rutherford MA (2011) General movements in full-term infants with perinatal asphyxia are related to basal ganglia and thalamic lesions. J Pediatr 158:904–911

Ferrari F, Gallo C, Pugliese M, Guidotti I, Gavioli S, Coccolini E, Zagni P, Della Casa E, Rossi C, Lugli L, Todeschini A, Ori L, Bertoncelli N (2012) Preterm birth and developmental problems in the preschool age. Part I: minor motor problems. J Matern Fetal Neonatal Med 25:2154–2159. https://doi.org/10.3109/14767058.2012.696164

Guzzetta A, Mercuri E, Rapisardi G et al (2003) General movements detect early signs of hemiplegia in term infants with neonatal cerebral infarction. Neuropediatrics 34:61–66

Guzzetta A, Pizzardi A, Belmonti V, Boldrini A, Carotenuto M, D'Acunto G, Ferrari F, Fiori S,

Gallo C, Ghirri P, Mercuri E, Romeo D, Roversi MF, Cioni G (2010) Hand movements at 3 month predict later hemiplegia in term infants with neonatal cerebral infarction. Dev Med Child Neurol 52:767–772

Johnson S, Strauss V, Gilmore C, Jaekel J, Marlow N, Wolke D (2016) Learning disabilities among extremely preterm children without neurosensory impairment: comorbidity, neuropsychological profiles and scholastic outcomes. Early Hum Dev 103:69–75

Kidokoro H, Anderson PJ, Doyle LW, Woodward LJ, Neil JJ, Inder TE (2014) Brain injury and altered brain growth in preterm infants: predictors and prognosis. Pediatrics 134:e444–e453

Kim H, Lepage C, Maheshwary R, Jeon S, Evans AC, Hess CP, Barkovich AJ, Xu D (2016) NEOCIVET: towards accurate morphometry of neonatal gyrification and clinical applications in preterm newborns. NeuroImage 138:28–42

Marlow N, Wolke D, Bracewell MA et al (2005) Neurologic and developmental disability at six years of age after extremely preterm birth. N Engl J Med 352:9–19

Mercuri E, Atkinson J, Braddick O et al (1997) Basal ganglia damage and impaired visual function in the newborn infant. Arch Dis Child Fetal Neonatal Ed 77: F111–F114

Olsen JE, Brown NC, Eeles AL, Einspieler C, Lee KJ, Thompson DK, Anderson PJ, Cheong JL, Doyle LW, Spittle AJ (2016) Early general movements and brain magnetic resonance imaging at term-equivalent age in infants born <30 weeks' gestation. Early Hum Dev 101:63–68

Orasanu E, Melbourne A, Cardoso MJ, Lomabert H, Kendall GS, Robertson NJ, Marlow N, Ourselin S (2016) Cortical folding of the preterm brain: a longitudinal analysis of extremely preterm born neonates using spectral matching. Brain Behav 6:e00488

Palisano R, Rosenbaum P, Walter S et al (1997) Development and validation of a gross motor function classification system for children with cerebral palsy. Dev Med Child Neurol 39:214–223

Palisano RJ, Rosenbaum P, Bartlett D, Livingston MH (2008) Content validity of the expanded and revised gross motor function classification system. Dev Med Child Neurol 50:744–750

Picciolini O, Gianni ML, Vegni C, Fumagalli M, Mosca F (2006) Usefulness of an early neurofunctional assessment in predicting neurodevelopmental outcome in very low birthweight infants. Arch Dis Child Fetal Neonatal 91:F111–F117

Prechtl HF, Einspieler C, Cioni G et al (1997) An early marker for neurological deficits after perinatal brain lesions. Lancet 349:1361–1363

Ricci D, Guzzetta A, Cowan F et al (2006a) Sequential neurological examinations in infants with neonatal encephalopathy and low apgar scores: relationship with brain MRI. Neuropediatrics 37:148–153

Ricci D, Anker S, Cowan F et al (2006b) Thalamic atrophy in infants with PVL and cerebral visual impairment. Early Hum Dev 82:591–595

Romeo DM, Cioni M, Scoto M et al (2009) Prognostic value of a scorable neurological examination from 3 to 12 months post-term age in very preterm infants: a longitudinal study. Early Hum Dev 85:405–408

Rutherford MA, Pennock JM, Counsell SJ et al (1998) Abnormal magnetic resonance signal in the internal capsule predicts poor neurodevelopmental outcome in infants with hypoxic-ischemic encephalopathy. Pediatrics 102:323–328

Rutherford M, Srinivasan L, Dyet L, Ward P, Allsop J, Counsell S et al (2006) Magnetic resonance imaging in perinatal brain injury: clinical presentation, lesions and outcome. Pediatr Radiol 36:582–592

Santiago-Rodriguez E, Harmony T, Bernardino M et al (2005) Auditory steady-state responses in infants with perinatal brain injury. Pediatr Neurol 32:236–240

Shankaran S, Pappas A, McDonald SA, Vohr BR, Hintz SR, Yolton K et al (2012) Childhood outcomes after hypothermia for neonatal encephalopathy. N Engl J Med 366:2085–2092

Shankaran S, McDonald SA, Laptook AR, Hintz SR, Barnes PD, Das A, Pappas A, Higgins RD, on behalf of the Eunice Kennedy Shriver National Institute of Child Health and Human Development Neonatal Research Network (2015) Neonatal Magnetic Resonance Imaging Pattern of Brain Injury as a Biomarker of Childhood Outcomes following a Trial of Hypothermia for Neonatal Hypoxic Ischemic Encephalopathy. J Pediatr 167:987–993

Spittle AJ, Brown NC, Doyle LW, Boyd RN, Hunt RW, Bear M, Inder TE (2008) Quality of general movements is related to white matter pathology in very preterm infants. Pediatrics 121:e1184–e1189

World Health Organization (2001) International classification of functioning, disability and health. WHO, Geneva

Xie K, Zheng H, Li H, Zhang C, Li H, Jin H, Ma B (2015) The study of effect for general movements assessment in the diagnosis of neurological development disorders: a meta-analysis. Clin Pediatr (Phila) 55:36–43

Quality of Neonatal Intensive Care and Outcome for High-Risk Newborn Infants

16

Liz McKechnie and Kathryn Johnson

Contents

Abstract

It is generally accepted that neonatal outcome is related to the quality of care an infant receives, and therefore it should be closely monitored in order to improve outcome. Quality in neonatal care is a complex subject, but improving quality is a goal to which all neonatologists should aspire. Ongoing quality assessment needs to be implemented in order to improve care such as audit, benchmarking, and confidential enquiries, which are discussed below. Traditional measures of outcome such as death, neurodevelopmental status, and chronic lung disease are also discussed in detail later in this chapter. Improving quality of care can additionally be achieved by implementing modern, effective, evidence-based methods of knowledge translation in order to increase the use of evidence-based healthcare.

L. McKechnie (✉) · K. Johnson
Centre for Newborn Care, Leeds Teaching Hospitals Trust, Leeds, UK
e-mail: l.mckechnie@nhs.net; kathrynjohnson1@nhs.net

G. Buonocore et al. (eds.), *Neonatology*,
https://doi.org/10.1007/978-3-319-29489-6_165

16.1 Salient Points

- Neonatal outcome is closely related to quality of care.
- Defining quality allows development of standards of care or quality indicators.
- Which aspects of care to assess for quality depends on the audience it is aimed at.
- Audit is widely used to measure adherence to quality indicators.
- Benchmarking is popular with organizations such as the Vermont Oxford Network (VON).
- Quality improvement (QI) is enhanced by coordinated collaborative working.
- Improving quality of care should be the aspiration of every healthcare professional.

16.2 What Is Quality in Neonatal Care?

The quality of the care that we provide to all newborn babies has gained increasing prominence in the last decade or so.

Quality in healthcare has been defined in many different ways and by many different authors. The American Institute of Medicine defines six domains that should be assessed when looking to improve quality of care (Institute of Medicine (IOM) 2001):

- Safety: avoiding harm to patients when providing care.
- Effectiveness: providing evidence-based care only to the patients that will benefit from it.
- Patient-centeredness: ensuring care is respectful of a patient's (or families) beliefs and culture and that decision-making about clinical care is done in partnership with them.
- Timeliness: ensuring care is delivered when it is needed.
- Efficiency: ensuring care is not wasteful, e.g., equipment, time, etc.
- Equity: quality care is delivered regardless of differences, e.g., religion and race.

Many other institutions have developed their own definitions using similar domains.

Specific to neonatal care, quality is defined as providing an appropriate level of care to well newborn babies while providing a good quality of more specialized care to the few babies that need it. This should be done while obtaining the best medical neonatal outcome and satisfying parents and families as well as providers. This should be delivered in the context of sound managerial and financial performance and while developing perinatal services to further raise standards of care (Acolet 2008).

This definition clearly demonstrates the complexity of measuring quality in neonatal care; we need to consider the structures supporting the care that the baby has received and the processes and outcomes of that care. We also should consider the effect on the family, parents, and healthcare professionals surrounding that baby. Compounding these factors with the complexities of healthcare management and economics makes measurement of quality very difficult.

Defining quality of care within a specific field allows standards to be developed, i.e., quality indicators. Systems to assess quality of care can then be designed and where care does not reach the standard, improvements can be made.

16.2.1 Assessing Quality in Neonatal Healthcare

The assessment of quality in neonatal care is evolving, and the framework around which quality can be measured is that of clinical governance. This encompasses many different processes by which care can be measured.

Important to the choice of how to assess neonatal care is who the audience are: it may be for clinicians, politicians, families, etc. and so the choice of tool is important. The measurements that are used – otherwise known as quality indicators – should be clearly defined, valid, reliable, sensitive and specific, relevant, actionable, and evidence based (Mainz 2003).

When measuring quality it is important to recognize and differentiate the discrete aspects of healthcare – the structure or organization of care that is provided and the process of providing that care and the outcome of the care that has been provided. These different aspects may be assessed individually to measure quality.

In the past, outcome studies have been used for reflecting the quality of care, but more recently other methods have become more commonplace such as auditing, benchmarking, and confidential enquiries. These may be done locally; nationally, e.g., the National Neonatal Audit Project in the UK; or internationally, e.g., the Vermont Oxford Network.

16.2.2 Outcome Studies

In the past much of the neonatal literature has been focused on different aspects of care and their effect on outcome for a baby. Outcome can mean many different things, such as later neurodevelopmental attainment and the presence or absence of chronic lung disease. These outcome measures can be used as a proxy for the quality of care.

One of the problems with using studies reporting outcome as a marker for quality of care is that there are frequently differences in results between similarly designed studies. These differences can be in part accounted for by differences in clinical practice or in the demographics of the study populations. However, it has been shown that these differences in clinical practice and in demographics are not enough to explain the variation in results. It has been suggested that the differences may therefore be due to a difference in outcome in quality of care (Horbar 1999).

16.2.3 Audit

Clinical audit is a process whereby care is measured against predefined standards. It aims to improve patient care by logical review of care and subsequent implementation of change to improve quality of care. At this point audit can be repeated to measure the affect of the change made. It is a continuous circular process. Therefore, audit does not define what optimal care is, but whether perceived optimal care is actually provided.

In the UK, the National Neonatal Audit Programme (NNAP) uses the audit method to capture information on current practice measured against previously defined standards. The first annual report highlighted many of the problems encountered when auditing such a complex process as healthcare (McIntosh and Youle 2008). In light of the results of the first period, changes were made to the questionnaire and also to data ascertainment. The audit questions are adapted or changed annually in order to ensure that the correct data is being collected to answer a specific question.

The first report highlighted examples of difficulties in the analysis of data as a result of imprecise questions. One standard set by consensus of the NNAP Board was "of those receiving surfactant, 90% should receive it within 1 hour of birth." In answer to the audit question of whether this standard was achieved, there was data missing from 173/647 babies. Of all eligible babies, 64% received surfactant in the first hour (87% of babies with complete data) showing that the standard was not achieved. However, the question could not distinguish those babies who did not receive surfactant in the first hour because they were not intubated, following the increasingly common occurrence of babies of this gestation going directly onto nasal continuous positive airway pressure (nCPAP) after birth. Similar issues were highlighted with the remaining questions. However, despite the problems encountered, the quality of early surfactant administration is clearly not up to the expected standard, and so changes can be made to improve this.

Within Europe, the EuroNatal Study (Richardus et al. 2003) investigated differences in perinatal mortality rate by looking at quality of care in a geographical region within ten individual countries. Differences were demonstrated between different healthcare systems. Suboptimal care factors occurred significantly less in Finnish and Swedish regions than in the remaining participating regions (Spain, the Netherlands, Scotland, Belgium, Denmark, Norway, Greece, and England). An expert panel assessed 67% of neonatal deaths $\geq$ 34 weeks to have had suboptimal care factors that were likely or might have contributed to the fatal outcome. Clearly, this study showed that improvements in quality of care should be possible, but no reaudit has been carried out to date.

If, when auditing, the expected standard has not been met, change should be implemented to achieve that standard and improve quality. Reaudit is then imperative in order to demonstrate that change has been beneficial and the quality of care has improved.

16.2.4 Benchmarking

Benchmarking is a process whereby aspects of healthcare practice are evaluated against known best practice. It is a helpful way to compare activity and performance in different areas with other organizations and to provide an evidence base for further review and action planning. Benchmarking is a commonly used technique across a wide range of different sectors and industries to review and improve performance. It is one of the most widely applied management techniques used to improve organizational performance.

A useful definition of benchmarking is provided by the NHS Benchmarking Club (Productive Time Delivery and Benchmarking Club 2006), who define the process as "Making evidence-based comparisons of practice, drawing conclusions and implementing improvements."

Benchmarking has many benefits. It is an evidence-based quality improvement tool. It can provide the means to compare practice with similar organizations and thereby identify outliers from the standard of care, i.e., good and bad performers. It can assess whether current performance achieves practice standards and can provide the catalyst for organizational change to improve quality of care. Sharing benchmarking data can share good practice and motivate the need for change. The first large benchmarking collaboration in neonatal medicine was within the Vermont Oxford Network (VON) and now provides benchmarking data for participating units internationally. The UK Managed Clinical Networks (see below) can provide a group of similar units that can benchmark both internally and externally.

16.2.5 Confidential Enquiries

Standard methods of measurement (e.g., audit) may not be sufficiently powerful to capture the complexity of neonatal healthcare. A more focused approach may sometimes be needed such as that used in Project 27/28 (Confidential Enquiry into Stillbirths and Deaths in Infancy (CESDI) 2003), which was carried out in England, Wales, and Northern Ireland in the 2-year period between September 1998 and August 2000. The aim was to identify variations in the standards of care that might have contributed to the deaths of infants born at 27 and 28 weeks gestation during this period. Anonymized medical records were scrutinized by a panel of experts for deficiencies in the standards of care provided to the infants that died. Having highlighted consistent deficiencies in the standards of care, the working party published recommendations for changes to practice in order to improve the quality of care. Their main findings and recommendations were based upon early thermal, ventilatory, and cardiovascular care.

Confidential enquiries (CE) have been an ongoing method of quality improvement in the UK since the first report was published in 1952 looking at maternal deaths. Over time the body responsible for this has changed and is currently carried out by Mothers and Babies: Reducing Risk Through Audits and Confidential Enquiries Across the UK (MBRRACE-UK). They report into maternal and perinatal mortality as well as conducting CEs into specific conditions. In December 2014 a report into the CE of congenital diaphragmatic hernia was published (Field et al. 2014) with several recommendation for quality improvement.

16.3 How Can Quality Be Improved in Neonatal Care?

16.3.1 National and International Groups

Different groups whose aim is to improve quality within neonatal care have been set up. The largest organization is the Vermont Oxford Network (VON). This is an international collaborative of neonatal units with the objective of integrating research and clinical practice in order to improve the quality of neonatal care (Horbar 1995). Other organizations such as the Neonatal Survey (UK) and Australian and New Zealand Neonatal Network (ANZNN) collect data and use this to provide information on outcome. Contributors to these databases are then able to use the information provided for developing and enhancing their quality of care.

16.3.2 Managed Clinical Networks

Managed Clinical Networks are a way of delivering high-quality care to a population across a large geographical area. A Managed Clinical Network has been defined as:

Linked groups of health professionals from primary, secondary, and tertiary care, working in a coordinated manner, are unconstrained by existing professional and Trust/Health Authority boundaries, to ensure equitable provision of high-quality and clinically effective services (Baker and Lorimer 2000).

Managed Clinical Networks in the UK were set up after a government initiative called "The NHS Plan." The aim was to create a more effective and efficient service. The network should ensure appropriate access for patients to the right care delivered in the most relevant setting. Access to specialist knowledge and care should be streamlined and quality of care should be consistent (Cropper et al. 2002).

The network can play a central role in the maintenance of national standards for neonatal care but can also develop and implement local quality improvement measures such as taking a leading role in the development of education, audit, and guidelines (Marlow and Gill 2007). The networks can also provide support and advice for individual units about both clinical and nonclinical matters. All these network roles clearly can improve quality.

16.3.3 Education and Knowledge Translation

It is well described that there are major gaps between routine practice and what the evidence shows is optimal practice (Institute of Medicine 2001). An example of this is nicely demonstrated by the work done by Ligand in the early 1970s that showed the improvement in respiratory function of newborn premature lambs and later human preterm infants after antenatal maternal steroid administration. Although the benefit was clearly demonstrated, it took until the late 1990s to reach routine antenatal care.

Many barriers hamper translating audit and research findings into best practice and there are obstacles at all levels of care delivery. This has been addressed in several studies that show that using active methods of information dissemination (e.g., audit, feedback, multidimensional workshops, ongoing support) knowledge translation can be far more effective than traditional methods of learning such as lectures and seminars (Horbar et al. 2004; Acolet et al. 2008).

16.3.4 Quality Improvement

Quality improvement (QI) has been defined as the combined and unceasing efforts of everyone, healthcare professionals, patients and their families, researchers, payers, planners, and educators, to make the changes that will lead to better patient outcomes (health), better system performance (care), and better professional development (Batalden and Davidoff 2007). More succinctly, it is a formal approach to the analysis of performance and systematic efforts to improve it.

It is a fashionable method of improving care and can yield good results. There are several different models of QI, e.g., PDSA, Six Sigma, etc. The basis of QI is to embed a culture of quality improvement within the organization. This requires strong leadership and empowerment of the workforce. The goals of the QI project should be clear to all and have adequate resources to enable the work. The improvements made should be measurable and feedback to motivate the team is essential.

The largest neonatal organization using QI methodology is the Vermont Oxford Network. They have over 1000 neonatal units globally that can participate in collaborative efforts toward quality improvement. They have had many publications demonstrating positive effects on outcomes using this approach.

Although not a project with neonatal patients, a great example of the effectiveness of QI projects was demonstrated by Pronovost in 2006 (Provonost et al. 2006). He reported a collaborative cohort study that used five evidence-based interventions to reduce catheter-related bloodstream infections (CRBSIs) in adult intensive care. They reduced CRBSIs by 66% and sustained that over the 18 months of the project. This clearly had significant benefits in morbidity, mortality, and cost. This QI project has been replicated in many places with significant improvements to quality of care.

16.4 Short-Term and Long-Term Morbidity and Mortality in High-Risk Infants

Infants born prematurely are at significant risk of both increased morbidity and mortality compared with babies born at term and represent one of the leading causes of perinatal morbidity and mortality both in the developed and developing world (Ananth and Vintzileos 2008; Slattery and Morrison 2002; Hoyert et al. 2001). Of all early neonatal deaths (within 7 days) worldwide that are not related to congenital malformation, 28% are due to preterm birth (Beck et al. 2010).

Worldwide reported rates of preterm delivery (<37 weeks) are estimated at just less than 10% with 85% of the burden of preterm deliveries occurring in the developing world; in 2010 an estimated 14.9 million babies were born preterm (Beck et al. 2010). The highest morbidity and mortality not surprisingly are seen in the smallest, most premature infants (Slattery and Morrison 2002; El-Metwally et al. 2000; Fanaroff et al. 2007; Hack and Fanaroff 2005; Alexander et al. 2003; Markestad et al. 2005). Within the developing world, infants weighing less than 2000 g (corresponding generally to <32 weeks gestation) have little chance of survival. In contrast, the survival rate of infants born at 32 weeks in developed countries is similar to that of infants born at term (Beck et al. 2010).

Rates of premature delivery worldwide show no evidence of declining; there are many reports worldwide of increasing rates of preterm birth (Ananth and Vintzileos 2008; Slattery and Morrison 2002; Stoelhurst et al. 2005; Smith et al. 2007; Craig et al. 2002; Blencowe et al. 2012). A variety of factors have contributed to the increasing preterm birth rate, including increased use of assisted reproduction techniques and the associated increase in multiple births (Ananth and Vintzileos 2008; Slattery and Morrison 2002). Increases have also been seen in the rates of singleton preterm birth particularly among medically induced preterm births rather than those born following the spontaneous onset of labor (Ananth and Vintzileos 2008). In addition singletons born following assisted reproduction are more likely to be preterm than the spontaneously conceived counterparts. Socioeconomic status is well described to have a significant effect on preterm birth; however, this effect has been shown to be static over time (Smith et al. 2007). Racial origin also impacts on rates of preterm birth; changes in racial demographics over time may therefore have influenced rates of preterm birth (Alexander et al. 2003; Branum and Schoendorf 2002; Demissie et al. 2001). Reported rates of preterm birth may also have been influenced by changing attitudes in delivery units over time with more infants being classed as live births or offered resuscitation (Peerzada et al. 2006; Hakansson et al. 2004); in one large study, up to 22% of preterm infants born at 22 weeks were offered resuscitation (Rysavy et al. 2015).

Interventions to reduce preterm delivery may vary according to location with simple interventions being potentially much more effective in lower-income settings than in the developed world (Chang et al. 2013).

16.4.1 Mortality

Major advances in antenatal, delivery suite and neonatal management of preterm infants led to major advances in survival up until the mid- to late 1990s when compared with the 1980s or earlier (Fanaroff et al. 2007; Stoelhurst et al. 2005; The Victorian Infant Collaborative Study Group 1997; de Kleine et al. 2007; Horbar et al. 2002). Contributors to improved survival include the increasing and now widespread use of antenatal corticosteroids (Fanaroff et al. 2007; Markestad et al. 2005; Stoelhurst et al. 2005; Horbar et al. 2002), changes in attitude in delivery units to the management of extremely preterm infants, and widespread postnatal use of surfactant (Horbar et al. 2002; Costeloe et al. 2000). There is now a wide range of international data from the mid- to late 1990s following widespread introduction of antenatal corticosteroids and postnatal surfactant reporting mortality for the preterm infant for geographically based studies.

Survival data at the limits of viability are shown in the table below; not surprising there are large improvements in survival between gestational ages of 22 and 24 weeks; even within a single-week gestational age bracket, improved survival is seen toward the end of the completed week rather than at the beginning (Nguyen et al. 2012). Within the table major differences in survival will in part reflect both differing attitudes in the delivery suite to infants born at the threshold of viability and the denominator used.

Survival at limits of viability

	Survival at 22 + 0–22 + 6 weeks	Survival at 23 + 0–23 + 6 weeks	Survival at 24 + 0–24 + 6 weeks
USA (Rysavy et al. 2015)	(To discharge) 23.1% of infants who received active treatment	(To discharge) 33.3% of infants who received active treatment	(To discharge) 56.6% of infants who received active treatment
UK (Costeloe et al. 2012)	(To discharge) 16% of admitted infants	(To discharge) 30% of admitted infants	(To discharge) 47% of admitted infants
France (Ancel et al. 2015)	(To discharge) 0% of live-born infants	(To discharge) 1% of live-born infants	(To discharge) 58% of live-born infants

More recently into the twenty-first century, large studies in Europe, especially the UK, and North America describe survival in preterm infants over time (Costeloe et al. 2012; Ancel et al. 2015; Stoll et al. 2010). UK data shows significantly more infants are surviving at 24 and 25 weeks but not at 23 weeks as compared with their counterparts born 9 years previously (Costeloe et al. 2012), findings supported by European data (Berger et al. 2012).

16.4.1.1 Multiple Births

As a result of the well-described increase in multiple birth rates over recent decades, concerns have been raised regarding the potential for increased mortality and morbidity in such infants compared with their singleton counterparts. In a large retrospective study covering a time period spanning 1995–2009 of twins born at less than 27 weeks, mortality was significantly higher in multiples versus singletons although morbidity was comparable (Yeo et al. 2015), these findings supported by other studies looking at mortality in extremely preterm twins (Garg et al. 2010). At term multiples remain at high risk with increasing rates of cerebral palsy with increasing chronicity; the higher rates are explained, in the main, by increasing risks of prematurity (Topp et al. 2004). The death of a co-twin either prior to or shortly after birth has been shown in a large population-based study to result in the highest risk of cerebral palsy in this group.

16.4.1.2 Gender Effects

Male infants born extremely preterm are consistently shown to have a higher mortality than their female counterparts (Fanaroff et al. 2007; Costeloe et al. 2012), with some authors reporting females showing generally a week's additional maturity and a birth weight heavier by 100 g than their male counterparts (Taylor et al. 2000). This negative effect of male sex is pervasive into early childhood with higher rates of neurological and developmental disability when compared with females of the same age (Moore et al. 2012; Wood et al. 2005).

16.4.1.3 Geographical Variations

There are notable intercountry and interregional variations in overall mortality of extremely preterm infants. Frequent comparisons are made between different regions/countries, but such comparisons can be misleading. Crude perinatal mortality rate used alone will be significantly influenced by the rate of preterm birth which varies considerably between regions within Europe and worldwide (Draper et al. 2007; Zeitlin et al. 2008). Denominators vary for all infants including those terminated, to those admitted to the neonatal unit for ongoing care following delivery suite resuscitation.

16.4.2 Morbidity

As with mortality the smallest most immature infants are at highest risk of adverse outcome (Hack and Fanaroff 2005; Stoll et al. 2010). With the increased rate of survival seen in the 1990s following extremely preterm birth, it was anticipated that a significant increase in survivors with morbidity would be seen. Many authors have shown morbidity in survivors to be static over time rather than increasing, but with the increase in total numbers of survivors, the absolute numbers of those with morbidity will undoubtedly have increased (Fanaroff et al. 2007; Stoelhurst et al. 2005; Costeloe et al. 2012). The EPIPAGE study along with increased survival showed increased rates of survival without major morbidity although this was not seen below 25 weeks (Ancel et al. 2015).

When interpreting the wide range of studies examining morbidity in the preterm infant, one must be cautious with the interpretation of results, as the denominator used clearly will affect the results: the proportion of infants with a particular clinical condition may be a percentage of the total number of infants born, and the total number admitted for intensive care and for longer-term morbidities may be a percentage of the total survivors.

Morbidity in moderately preterm infants (30–36 weeks) is less than those born most preterm, but as these deliveries occur in much higher numbers than extremely preterm deliveries, absolute numbers are much higher, and therefore such infants do impact significantly on neonatal intensive care units. As infants then become more mature toward term, morbidities gradually decrease (Boyle et al. 2015).

16.4.2.1 Lung Disease

Respiratory distress syndrome (RDS) is a frequent early marker of respiratory morbidity in preterm infants. This may then evolve into chronic respiratory symptoms termed bronchopulmonary dysplasia (BPD) or chronic lung disease (CLD). Definitions of BPD/CLD generally define this as either oxygen dependence at 36 weeks' postmenstrual age (PMA) or at 28 days after birth. More recently definitions of BPD have been refined in order to provide more useful information and have been subclassified into mild, moderate, and severe BPD (Jobe and Bancalari 2001). Clear repeatable definitions of BPD/CLD are important; BPD/CLD at 36 weeks is frequently used as an outcome measure in studies of interventions designed to improve outcomes in high-risk infants; it must therefore be comparable from study to study.

As with mortality and other morbidities the highest rates of respiratory disease are seen in the smallest most immature infants. The widespread and routine use of antenatal steroids (ANS) has significantly reduced the risk of the need for respiratory support and respiratory distress syndrome in the premature infant (Roberts and Dalziel 2006). Postnatal surfactant therapy also improves survival and reduces risk of pneumothorax (Horbar et al. 2002). Despite this, RDS rates over time are frequently reported as static despite significant increase in the use of both ANS and surfactant. RDS however has a wide clinical phenotype, and it may be that cases over recent years following the widespread use of ANS and surfactant may be less severe. The use of European-wide consensus guidelines on the management of RDS should result in consistent best practice in management over a wide geographical area (Sweet et al. 2013) and may improve outcomes.

Rates of BPD/CLD across Europe and worldwide vary somewhat, with 40% of infants <28 weeks in the USA having BPD and 26% in a European cohort (Ancel et al. 2015; Stoll et al. 2010). Over two thirds of infants < 27 weeks in the UK EPICure II cohort had BPD.

Recent focus in reducing the risks of BPD has been on the avoidance of intubation both via the use of CPAP in the delivery suite, the use of the Intubate, Surfactant, Extubate (INSURE) technique, and the use of less invasive surfactant delivery techniques designed to avoid the need for intubation.

In a multicenter trial of CPAP versus intubation in infants <29 weeks, there was no difference in BPD or death in the two groups (Morley et al. 2008). The use of early CPAP rather than intubation and surfactant in a separate study was associated with less respiratory morbidity at toddler age (Stevens et al. 2014). A Cochrane review of the INSURE technique showed a reduction in significant BPD (Stevens et al. 2007). The technique of delivering surfactant is showing promise (Dargaville et al. 2011) which may translate into better long-term respiratory outcomes and less BPD (Kribs et al. 2015). Large multicenter trials on the technique are required to substantiate these findings.

BPD is known to act as a predictor of poor neurodevelopmental outcomes (Jobe 2011). At 2.5 years those infants with CLD have an odds ratio of >2 for cerebral palsy (Wood et al. 2005). These findings are supported by other studies showing an odds ratio of 2.5 for death or neurosensory impairment at 18 months if BPD is present at 26 weeks corrected gestational age (Schmidt et al. 2003).

16.4.2.2 Brain Pathology

Early neurodevelopmental morbidity can arguably be monitored by rates of intraventricular hemorrhage (IVH) and/or cystic periventricular leukomalacia (PVL) detected on cranial ultrasound scan (CUSS). The incidence of CUSS abnormalities varies significantly between countries and within regions of Europe (Zeitlin et al. 2008). In those infants with more severe IVH, intra-observer variability has been shown to be less when compared with minor abnormalities (Hintz et al. 2007). This intra-observer variability in the more minor abnormalities may explain some of the increases in less severe IVH described recently by some authors (Stoelhurst et al. 2005). Modern equipment with higher resolution may also influence detection rates of minor IVH detection.

Following improved perinatal care in recent decades and specifically the widespread introduction of antenatal steroids, a reduction in the rates of IVH has been reported (Genzel-Boroviczeny et al. 2006; Linder et al. 2003). Comparisons of individual data sets can be difficult as definitions of abnormality and inclusion criteria vary. Data from the UK shows a 13% rate of severe abnormality on last available CUSS in survivors born at 26 weeks or less, which is unchanged from 1995 (Costeloe et al. 2000; Costeloe et al. 2012) although rates of shunted hydrocephalus and seizures decreased. Multicenter French data from 2011 shows a comparable rate of nearly 13% of severe IVH (Grade 3 or 4) in the group 22–26 weeks with a rate of cystic PVL in the same gestational age group of 2.4% (Ancel et al. 2015).

In keeping with all morbidities associated with extreme prematurity, rates of IVH/PVL increase with decreasing gestational age. Those at the limits of viability with the lowest birth weights are most affected although absolute numbers are small (Costeloe et al. 2012; Ancel et al. 2015; Stoll et al. 2010).

The effect of early abnormalities seen on cranial ultrasound scan on long-term neurodevelopmental outcome is variable. A significantly abnormal final cranial ultrasound scan independently increased the risk of cerebral palsy (Wood et al. 2005). Follow-up of the large multicenter French cohort showed that 25% of those with white matter damage on CUSS had cerebral palsy at 2 years versus 4% of those with a normal CUSS. Conversely it is reported one third of children with cerebral palsy had a normal CUSS (Genzel-Boroviczeny et al. 2006).

16.4.3 Longer-Term Outcome

Increasing neurological and developmental morbidity data from discharge up into later childhood and adulthood is now available from large multicenter studies. The highest levels of poor long-term outcome are seen in those high-risk infants born the most preterm. Rates up to 59% of severe neurodisability have been described on short-term follow-up of some cohorts (Jarjour 2015), with rates at their highest in those born 22–23 weeks.

Challenges in complex cognition and learning are being increasingly recognized as the high-risk survivors of extreme prematurity grow up into school age and adulthood. Mathematics difficulties appear to be a particular challenge (Wolke et al. 2015). In the follow-up of the UK 2006 cohort, as compared with 1995, rates of cerebral palsy and severe disability remained unchanged although rates of disability-free survival increased (Berger et al. 2012). The original 1995 EPICure cohort is now being followed up into early adulthood, at 11 years; within this cohort, 50% were rated as having below-average attainment compared with 5% of classmates (Johnson et al. 2009).

High-risk infants born preterm may also have an increased risk of psychiatric disorders (Johnson and Marlow 2011).

Any disability pervasive into childhood and adulthood as a result of a high-risk preterm birth will have significant economic costs (Petrou et al. 2013).

Schools and providers of education need to be aware of these challenges in order to fully support the increasing numbers of high-risk preterm infants surviving the neonatal period.

16.4.3.1 Visual Disorders

Retinopathy of prematurity (ROP) is frequently used as a marker for morbidity in the high-risk preterm infant. It can be challenging to report comparable figures as studies report different outcomes including all ROP, severe ROP only, or treatment for ROP. As infants become more mature, rates of ROP reduce gradually with infants of higher gestations being very unlikely to develop severe ROP and hence require treatment (Ancel et al. 2015). Of infants born at less than 26 weeks, approximately one fifth had significant ROP (Grade 3 or above) with more than three quarters of these requiring laser treatment (Costeloe et al. 2012). Other studies report lower rates of severe ROP in similar gestational ages (Ancel et al. 2015).

Treatment for ROP in the two EPICure cohorts (1995 versus 2006) showed a significant increase from 13% to 21%, but it is likely that this increase represents a lower threshold for treatment rather than a true increase in morbidity (Costeloe et al. 2000; Costeloe et al. 2012). When ROP is combined with two other morbidities, BPD and brain injury, not surprisingly the three together were strongly predictive of death or neurosensory impairment at 18 months (Schmidt et al. 2003).

16.4.3.2 Other Outcome Measures

Significant additional morbidity is seen in preterm infants influencing both their short- and long-term clinical course and outcome. Necrotizing enterocolitis (NEC) continues to be a significant risk to the high-risk preterm infant; it is difficult to compare rates between cohorts as a variety of outcomes can be measured, all NEC, severe NEC, or NEC requiring surgery. Generally rates are highest in the most preterm infants with 12% of 23-week infants affected, as compared to 8% of those born at 28 weeks in one large American cohort (Stoll et al. 2010). With recent data showing less high-risk preterm infants dying of respiratory disease, the proportion dying from NEC (and sepsis) is increasing (Costeloe et al. 2012; Berrington et al. 2012).

Sepsis in the preterm also continues to be a significant source of morbidity and mortality. 60% of infants in the large UK cohort

<27 weeks had a positive blood culture during their stay (Costeloe et al. 2012). Data from the USA for the most high-risk infants (born at 28 weeks or less) shows an early-onset sepsis rate of 2%, with approximately one third of infants in the same group suffering from late-onset sepsis (Stoll et al. 2010). Again, as with all morbidities in the high-risk infant, rates were at their highest in the most extremely preterm. Rates of meningitis in the same cohort were 3%. Sepsis, meningitis, and NEC have all been shown to then increase the risk not only of death but also survival with neurosensory impairment (Bassler et al. 2009).

Given the increasing proportion of infants dying later in their neonatal stay from NEC and sepsis, much of the focus of research in recent years has focused on their prevention. The use of probiotics for prevention of NEC is controversial with the recent UK-wide multicenter trial showing no benefit (Costeloe et al. 2016). The increasing use of breast milk and donor breast milk may help to reduce NEC rates along with strategies to reduce late-onset infection that may result in future years in reduced morbidity and better long-term outcomes in high-risk preterm infants.

References

Acolet D (2008) Quality of neonatal care and outcome. Arch Dis Child Fetal Neonatal Ed 93:F69–F73

Acolet D, Allen E, Houston R, Elbourne D (2008) The Bliss Cluster randomised controlled trial of the effect of "active dissemination of information" on the standards of care for premature babies in England (BEADI). Perinatal Medicine Meeting, Harrogate, UK, June 2008

Alexander GR, Kogan M, Bader D et al (2003) US birth weight/gestational age-specific neonatal mortality: 1995–1997 rates for whites, hispanics and blacks. Pediatrics 111:e61–e66

Ananth C, Vintzileos A (2008) Epidemiology of preterm birth and its clinical subtypes. J Matern Fetal Neonatal Med 21:289–295

Ancel PY, Goffinet F, Kuhn P et al (2015) Survival and morbidity of preterm children born at 22 weeks through 34 weeks' gestation in France in 2011: results of the EPIPAGE-2 cohort study. JAMA Pediatr Mar 169(3):230–238

Baker CD, Lorimer AR (2000) Cardiology: the development of a managed clinical network. BMJ 321:1152–1153

Bassler D, Stoll BJ, Schmidt B et al (2009) Using a count of neonatal morbidities to predict poor outcome in extremely low birth weight infants: added role of neonatal infection. Pediatrics 123(1):313–318. https://doi.org/10.1542/peds.2008-0377

Batalden PB, Davidoff F (2007) What is "quality improvement" and how can it transform healthcare? Qual Saf Health Care 16:2–3

Beck S, Wojdyla D, Say L et al (2010) The worldwide incidence of preterm birth: a systematic review of maternal mortality and morbidity. Bulletin of the World Health Organization 88:31–38

Berger TM, Steurer MA, Woerner A et al (2012) Trends and centre-to-centre variability in survival rates of very preterm infants (<32 weeks) over a 10-year-period in Switzerland. Arch Dis Child Fetal Neonatal Ed 97(5): F323–F328

Berrington JE, Hearn RI, Bythell M et al (2012) Deaths in preterm infants: changing pathology over 2 decades. J Pediatr 160(1):49–53

Blencowe H, Cousens S, Oestergaard MZ et al (2012) National, regional, and worldwide estimates of preterm birth rates in the year 2010 with time trends since 1990 for selected countries: a systematic analysis and implications. Lancet 379(9832):2162–2172

Boyle EM, Johnson S, Manketlow B et al (2015) Neonatal outcomes and delivery of care for infants born late preterm or moderately preterm: a prospective population-based study. Arch Dis Child Fetal Neonatal Ed 100(6):F479–F485

Branum AM, Schoendorf KC (2002) Changing patterns of low birthweight and preterm birth in the United States, 1981–98. Paediatr Perinat Epidemiol 16:8–15

Chang HH, Larson J, Blencowe H et al (2013) Preventing preterm births: analysis of trends and potential reductions with interventions in 39 countries with very high human development index. Lancet 381(9862):223–234

Confidential Enquiry into Stillbirths and Deaths in Infancy (CESDI) (2003) Project 27/28. An enquiry into quality of care and its effect on the survival of babies born at 27–28 weeks. The Stationary Office, London

Costeloe K, Hennessy E, Gibson A et al (2000) The EPICure study: outcomes to discharge from hospital for infants born at the threshold of viability. Pediatrics 106:659–671

Costeloe LK, Hennessy EM, Haider S et al (2012) Short term outcomes after extreme preterm birth in England: comparison of two birth cohorts in 1995 and 2006 (the EPICure studies). BMJ 345, e7976

Costeloe K, Hardy P, Juszczak E et al (2016) Bifidobacterium breve BBG-001 in very preterm infants: a randomised controlled phase 3 trial. Lancet 387(10019):649–660

Craig ED, Thompson JMD, Mitchell EA et al (2002) Socioeconomic status and preterm birth: New Zealand trends, 1980 to 1999. Arch Dis Child Fetal Neonatal Ed 86:F142–F146

Cropper S, Hopper A, Spencer SA, Dodd K (2002) Managed clinical networks. Arch Dis Child 87:1–4

Dargaville PA, Aiyappan A, Cornelius A (2011) Preliminary evaluation of a new technique of minimally invasive surfactant therapy. Arch Dis Child Fetal Neonatal Ed 96:F243–F248

de Kleine MJ, Lya den Ouden AL, Kollée LA et al (2007) Lower mortality but higher neonatal morbidity over a decade in very preterm infants. Paediatr Perinat Epidemiol 21:15–25

Demissie K, Rhoads GG, Ananth CV et al (2001) Trends in preterm birth and neonatal mortality among blacks and whites in the United States from 1989 to 1997. Am J Epidemiol 154:307–315

Draper ES, Zeitlin J, Field DJ et al (2007) Mortality patterns among very preterm babies: a comparative analysis of two European regions in France and England. Arch Dis Child Fetal Neonatal Ed 92: 356–360

El-Metwally D, Vohr B, Tucker R (2000) Survival and neonatal morbidity at the limits of viability in the mid 1990s: 22 to 25 weeks. J Pediatr 137:616–622

Fanaroff AA, Stoll BJ, Wright LL et al (2007) Trends in neonatal morbidity and mortality for very low birthweight infants. Am J Obstet Gynecol 196:147. e1–e8

Field D, Hyman-Taylor P, Bacon C, Draper ES on behalf of MBRRACE-UK (2014) Perinatal confidential enquiry – congenital diaphragmatic hernia. The Infant Mortality and Morbidity Group, Department of Health Sciences, University of Leicester, Leicester

Garg P, Abdel-Latif ME, Bolisetty S et al (2010) Perinatal characteristics and outcome of preterm singleton, twin and triplet infants in NSW and the ACT, Australia (1994–2005). Arch Dis Child Fetal Neonatal Ed 95(1):F20–F24

Genzel-Boroviczeny O, Macwilliams S, Von Poblotzki M et al (2006) Mortality and major morbidity in premature infants less than 31 weeks gestational age in the decade after introduction of surfactant. Acta Obstet Gynecol Scand 85:68–73

Hack M, Fanaroff AA (2005) Outcomes of children of extremely low birthweight and gestational age in the 1990s. Semin Neonatol 5:89–106

Hakansson S, Farooqi A, Holmgren PA et al (2004) Proactive management promotes outcome in extremely preterm infants: a population based comparison of two perinatal management strategies. Pediatrics 114:58–64

Hintz SR, Slovis T, Bulas D et al (2007) Interobserver reliability and accuracy of cranial ultrasound scanning interpretation in premature infants. J Pediatr 150:592–596

Horbar JD (1995) The Vermont-Oxford Neonatal Network: integrating research and clinical practice to improve the quality of medical care. Semin Perinatol 19:124–131

Horbar JD (1999) The Vermont Oxford Network: evidence-based quality improvement for neonatology. Pediatrics 103:350–359

Horbar JD, Badger GJ, Carpenter JH (2002) Trends in mortality and morbidity for very low birth weight infants, 1991–1999. Pediatrics 110:143–150

Horbar JD, Carpenter JH, Buzas J et al (2004) Collaborative quality improvement to promote evidence based-surfactant for preterm infants: a cluster randomised trial. BMJ 329:1004

Hoyert DL, Freedman MA, Strobino DM et al (2001) Annual summary of vital statistics: 2000. Pediatrics 108:1241–1255

Institute of Medicine (2001) Crossing the quality chasm: a new health system for the 21st century. National Academy Press, Washington DC

Institute of Medicine (IOM) (2001) Crossing the quality chasm: a new health system for the 21st century. National Academy Press, Washington, DC

Jarjour IT (2015) Neurodevelopmental outcome after extreme prematurity: a review of the literature. Pediatr Neurol 52(2):143–152

Jobe AH (2011) The new bronchopulmonary dysplasia. Curr Opin Pediatr 23(2):167–172

Jobe AH, Bancalari E (2001) Bronchopulmonary dysplasia. Am J Respir Crit Care Med 163:1723–1729

Johnson S, Marlow N (2011) Preterm birth and childhood psychiatric disorders. Pediatr Res 69:11R–18R

Johnson S, Hennessy E, Smith R et al (2009) Academic attainment and special educational needs in extremely preterm children at 11 years of age: the EPICure study. Arch Dis Child Fetal Neonatal Ed 94(4):F283–F289

Kribs A, Roll C, Göpel W (2015) Nonintubated surfactant application vs conventional therapy in extremely preterm infants: a randomized clinical trial. JAMA Pediatr 169(8):723–730

Linder N, Haskin O, Levit O et al (2003) Risk factors for intraventricular haemorrhage in very low birth weight premature infants: a retrospective case control study. Pediatrics 111:e590–e595

Mainz J (2003) Developing evidence-based clinical indicators: a state of the art methods primer. Int J Qual Health Care 15(1):i5–i11

Markestad T, Kaaresen PI, Ronnestad A et al (2005) Early death, morbidity and need of treatment among extremely premature infants. Pediatrics 115:1289–1298

Marlow N, Gill AB (2007) Establishing neonatal networks: the reality. Arch Dis Child Fetal Neonatal Ed 92: F137–F142

McIntosh N, Youle L (2008) National Neonatal Audit Project annual report. Royal College of Paediatrics and Child Health

Moore T, Hennessy EM, Myles J (2012) Neurological and developmental outcome in extremely preterm children born in England in 1995 and 2006: the EPICure studies. BMJ 345, e7961

Morley CJ, Davis PG, Doyle L et al (2008) Nasal CPAP or intubation at birth for very preterm infants. NEJM 358:700–708

Nguyen TP, Amon E, Al-Hosni M et al (2012) "Early" versus "late" 23-week infant outcomes. Am J Obstet Gynecol 207(3):226.e1–6

Peerzada JM, Schollin J, Hakansson S (2006) Delivery room decision making for extremely preterm infants in Sweden. Pediatrics 117:1988–1995

Petrou S, Johnson S, Wolke D et al (2013) The association between neurodevelopmental disability and economic outcomes during mid-childhood. Child Care Health Dev 39(3):345–347

Productive Time Delivery Board and NHS Benchmarking Club (2006) Delivering quality and value: focus on benchmarking. http://www.dh.gov.uk/en/Publicationsandstatistics/Publications/PublicationsPolicyAndGuidance/DH_4139062

Provonost P, Needham D et al (2006) An intervention to decrease catheter-related bloodstream infections in the ICU. N Engl J Med 355:2725–2732

Richardus JH, Graafmans WC, Verloove-Vanhorick SP, Mackenbach JP (2003) Differences in perinatal mortality and suboptimal care between 10 European regions: results of an international audit. BJOG 110:97–105

Roberts D, Dalziel SR (2006) Antenatal corticosteroids for accelerating fetal lung maturation for women at risk of preterm birth. Cochrane Database Syst Rev 3, CD004454

Rysavy MA, Li L, Bell EF et al (2015) Between-hospital variation in treatment and outcomes in extremely preterm infants. N Engl J Med 372(19):1801–1811

Schmidt B, Asztalos EV, Roberts RS et al (2003) Impact of bronchopulmonary dysplasia, brain injury, and severe retinopathy on the outcome of extremely low-birth-weight infants at 18 months. JAMA 289:1124–1129

Slattery M, Morrison J (2002) Preterm delivery. Lancet 360:1489–1497

Smith LK, Draper ES, Manktelow BN et al (2007) Socioeconomic inequalities in very preterm birth rates. Arch Dis Child Fetal Neonatal Ed 92:F11–F14

Stevens TP, Harrington EW, Blennow M et al (2007) Early surfactant administration with brief ventilation vs. selective surfactant and continued mechanical ventilation for preterm infants with or at risk for respiratory distress syndrome. Cochrane Database Syst Rev 4, CD003063

Stevens TP, Finer NN, Carlo WA et al (2014) Respiratory outcomes of the surfactant positive pressure and oximetry randomized trial (SUPPORT). J Pediatr 165(2):240–249

Stoelhurst GM, Rijken M, Martens SE et al (2005) Changes in neonatology: Comparison of two cohorts of very preterm infants (gestational age <32 weeks): the project on preterm and small for gestational age infants 1983 and the Leiden follow up project on prematurity 1996–1997. Pediatrics 115:396–404

Stoll BJ, Hansen NI, Bell EF et al (2010) Neonatal outcomes of extremely preterm infants from the NICHD neonatal research network. Pediatrics 126(3):443–456

Sweet DG, Carnielli V, Greisen G et al (2013) European consensus guidelines on the management of neonatal respiratory distress syndrome in preterm infants – 2013 update. Neonatology 103:353–368

Taylor HG, Klein N, Minich NM et al (2000) Middle-school-age outcomes in children with very low birthweight. Child Dev 71:1495–1511

The Victorian Infant Collaborative Study Group (1997) Outcome at 2 years of children 23–27 weeks' gestation born in Victoria in 1991–2. J Pediatr Child Health 33:161–165

Topp M, Huusom LD, Langhoff-Roos J et al (2004) Multiple birth and cerebral palsy in Europe: a multicenter study. Acta Obstet Gynecol Scand 83(6):548–553

Wolke D, Strauss VY, Johnson S et al (2015) Universal gestational age effects on cognitive and basic mathematic processing: 2 cohorts in 2 countries. Pediatrics 166(6):1410–1416

Wood NS, Costeloe K, Gibson AT et al (2005) The EPICure study: associations and antecedents of neurological and developmental disability at 30 months of age following extremely preterm birth. Arch Dis Child Fetal Neonatal Ed 90:F134–F140

Yeo KT, Lee QY, Quek WS et al (2015) Trends in morbidity and mortality of extremely preterm multiple gestation newborns. Pediatrics 136(2):263 271

Zeitlin J, Draper ES, Kollee L et al (2008) Differences in rates and short-term outcome of live births before 32 weeks of gestation in Europe in 2003: results from the MOSAIC cohort. Pediatrics 121: e936–e944

Cerebral Plasticity and Functional Reorganization in Children with Congenital Brain Lesions

17

Viviana Marchi, Andrea Guzzetta, and Giovanni Cioni

Contents

Abstract

Mechanisms of cerebral plasticity are more powerful during development. This however does not necessarily lead to better outcomes in case of early brain injuries, as opposed to later ones, due to the complex interaction of brain plasticity, vulnerability, and maturation. A deep understanding of the mechanisms underlying the reorganization of brain functions after early damage will give us the opportunity to target the intervention in terms of timing, quality, and duration so to maximize the processes of adaptive plasticity and limit the maladaptive ones. New techniques of advanced brain mapping are providing a unique opportunity to explore this matter in humans, both in the acute and post-acute phase, during the early stages of development, and in the chronic phase, when the plastic reorganization has for a large part already occurred. We will review here the current knowledge on the main mechanisms of plastic reorganization in subjects with congenital lesions, with particular reference to the language, sensorimotor, and visual systems. The main differences with the effects of later injuries will be underlined.

V. Marchi (✉) · A. Guzzetta · G. Cioni
IRCCS Stella Maris, Department of Developmental Neuroscience, Pisa, Italy

University of Pisa, Department of Clinical and Experimental Neuroscience, Pisa, Italy
e-mail: giovanni.cioni@fsm.unipi.it

G. Buonocore et al. (eds.), *Neonatology*,
https://doi.org/10.1007/978-3-319-29489-6_166

17.1 Salient Points

- Damage during brain development affects functional outcome differently from lesions of mature brains due to the complex interaction of brain plasticity, vulnerability, and maturation.
- Knowledge of the neurobiological and neurophysiological principles of plastic reorganization after early brain damage allows for a therapeutic strategy to maximize the processes of adaptive plasticity and limit the maladaptive processes by appropriate timing, nature, and duration.
- The recent application of advanced brain imaging has provided answers to questions related to the mechanism of plasticity after early brain lesions, although a full knowledge of affects on the young brain is still far from being achieved.

17.2 Introduction

The substrates of developmental neuroplasticity span across molecular alterations, cellular adaptations, cortical electrophysiological changes, and structural and functional neuronal networks assembly and are expressed vigorously during time-sensitive periods of brain development (Johnston et al. 2009). Mechanisms of cerebral plasticity are thought to be more powerful during development. For example, children are more fast-paced than adults in learning a new language (Klein et al. 2014; Li et al. 2014) or in achieving complex skills such as playing a musical instrument (Barrett et al. 2013). In a classic experiment on string players, the extent of the cortical representation of the left digits was found to be inversely correlated with the age at which the person had begun to play, indicating a larger amount of cerebral plasticity in subjects with earlier exposition to training (Elbert et al. 1995; Vaquero et al. 2016). Similarly, children lacking proper environmental inputs early in life are more prone to have an abnormal development of the functions related to those inputs (the concept of critical periods) (Lewis and Maurer 2005; Mowery et al. 2016).

The presence of more powerful mechanisms of neuronal plasticity during early phases of development should imply that recovery from brain damage is more effective for early lesions compared to similar lesions occurred later in life. This principle was first suggested by Paul Broca in 1865 (Berker 1986) and then more systematically explored by Margaret Kennard in the late 1930s (Finger 1988). Since then, most of the studies carried out in different species have not denied this general principle although describing a more complex picture, which takes into consideration several other aspects beyond the timing of the insult, including the location and extension of injury (e.g., focal versus diffuse), the clinical correlates (e.g., presence of seizures), or the genetic susceptibility of the subject (Anderson et al. 2009; Dennis et al. 2013).

One of the most important predictors of the efficacy of functional reorganization seems to be the distribution, diffuse versus focal, of the damage (Lidzba et al. 2009; Kolb and Gibb 2014; Sweatt 2016). Most strikingly, children with early unilateral left hemisphere damage can develop normal language abilities, while lesions of similar site and extent in the adult brain would produce obvious patterns of aphasia. (Bates et al. 2001) Even if an entire hemisphere is removed at an early stage of development (for instance, for the treatment of severe epilepsy), children can develop normal language and cognitive function (Liégeois et al. 2008; de Bode et al. 2015). Also, children with unilateral ischemic stroke are able to develop normal cognitive functions and maintain them over time (Ballantyne et al. 2008). In contrast, evidence suggests that sustaining an early generalized cerebral insult (e.g., global hypoxia or traumatic brain injury) is usually associated with slower recovery and poorer outcome, compared to what is observed in adults with similar lesions (Anderson 2005; Anderson et al. 2011). The mechanism most often invoked for this higher vulnerability of early damage is that, at an early stage, cognitive development is highly dependent on the integrity of diffuse neural networks, and so the transient disruption of the developing attention, memory, and learning functions undermines the efficient acquisition of new abilities (Kolb and

Gibb 2014). Conversely, at an older age, the general, already acquired, cognitive abilities can be spared, and the impairment is limited to functions directly related to the final area of damage.

The aim of the present chapter will be to outline the major discoveries of the last years concerning the mechanisms of functional reorganization typical of a young brain in different systems, in the light of future possible directions of new non-pharmacological therapeutic interventions.

17.3 How Early Is Early

The time boundaries of early brain damage have never been clearly defined. This is probably due not to the absence of effort but rather to the complexity of the task. The changes of cerebral plasticity, which influences the effects of brain damage, are gradual during development, and the sensitive periods are now known to be different for the various functional subsystems (Lewis and Maurer 2005). Also, the types of brain insult are extremely variable during development and affect the nervous system in ways that are directly dependent on the level of maturation at the moment they occur. For these and other reasons, the boundaries between early and late lesions are necessarily blurry. As here we are interested to explore how different can the young brain be in response to damage, we will focus on the lesions occurring before or around birth (also called congenital lesions), which are more frequent and have been more extensively studied, compared to later ones.

A relevant aspect of the pathophysiology of congenital brain insult is the stage of cerebral development at the moment of the insult, either prenatal or perinatal. Because of the complexity and speed of the maturational phenomena occurring during gestation, the response to a harmful event varies significantly accordingly to gestational age and leads to different pictures both from the neuropathological and the clinical point of view. For the understanding of these mechanisms, an essential contribution is provided by the noninvasive neuroimaging techniques, first with ultrasonography and more recently with computed tomography and magnetic resonance imaging. These new methodologies, increasingly applied also in children, allow to perform in vivo investigations of cerebral lesions, monitoring their evolution, and so providing further insight on the relation between lesion and function and on the different types of reorganization.

In broad terms, types of congenital brain damage can be grouped according to timing (Fig. 1). Lesions occurring during the first half of gestation (and in particular the first trimester) give rise to malformations of cortical development. These lesions are very complex in terms of their characterization as they can be extremely variable in size, location, and distribution, resulting in completely different clinical pictures. The underlying mechanisms of cerebral plasticity are likely to be similarly complex and variable. The second group of lesions is those occurring around the early third trimester of gestation (~25–34 weeks of gestation). The most typical of this group are periventricular leukomalacia and intraventricular hemorrhage. The first is an ischemic, bilateral, and diffuse lesion, while the second is a hemorrhagic lesion, usually limited inside the ventricles, but that sometimes complicates into a periventricular parenchymal infarction, usually unilateral. Finally, the third group includes lesions around term (typically lesions of the term infant at around birth). The most relevant are the hypoxic-ischemic encephalopathy and the focal cerebral stroke, of arterial origin. The first is an ischemic lesion, bilateral and diffuse, while the second is a focal lesion, similar from the neuropathological point of view to the stroke observed in adults.

As previously mentioned, the distribution of the lesion, namely, focal unilateral versus diffuse bilateral, is likely to be the single most relevant factor to influence the efficacy of plastic reorganization of brain functions. In this sense, congenital lesions provide an interesting model for studying cerebral reorganization as they naturally encompass the different combinations of distribution (focal, diffuse) and timing (early gestation, late gestation, and term) of damage.

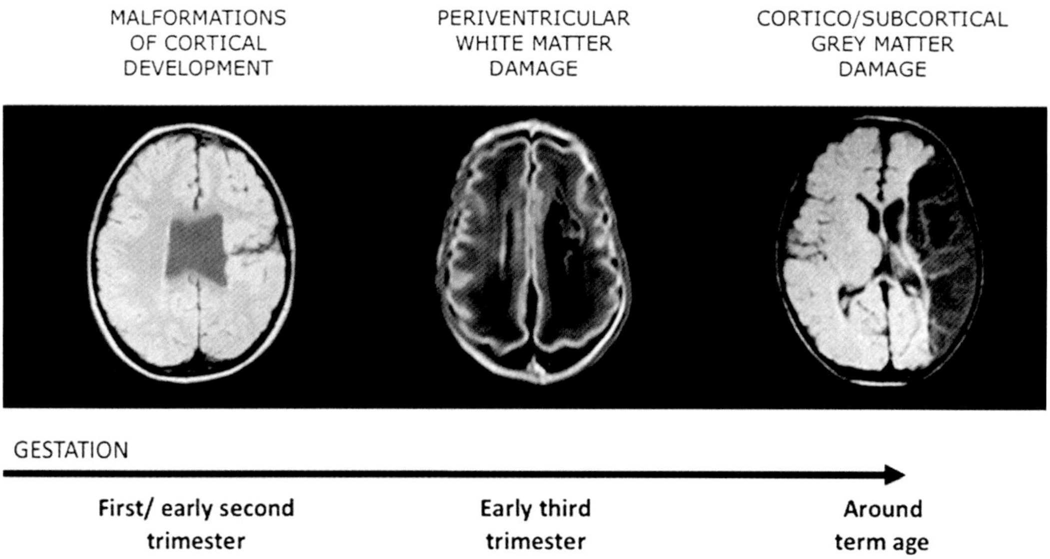

Fig. 1 Correlation between timing of insult and type of brain injury. Three examples are shown of typical congenital brain lesions on MRI, in which the correlation between timing and characteristics of the lesion is clear. In the *left* column, a case of schizencephaly, a malformation of cortical development secondary to an insult, occurred during the early phases of brain development. In the *central* column, a case of periventricular white matter damage secondary to an intraventricular hemorrhagic insult occurred at the beginning of the third trimester of gestation. In the *right* column, a case of ischemic infarction of the territory of the middle cerebral artery occurred around birth in a term-born infant

17.4 Cerebral Plasticity and the Different Systems

The effects of a cerebral lesion are clearly connected with the site of the lesion. This implies a different involvement of the various systems in different subjects, with complex and heterogeneous functional correlates. Although it is common to observe clinical pictures consisting of the impairment of multiple interconnected systems, especially in subjects with congenital cerebral damage, for the purpose of clarity, the principal systems will be considered independently, focusing in particular on the aspects of cerebral plasticity differentiating the effects of an early and a late lesion.

17.4.1 Language

With few exceptions, the left hemisphere of the brain deals with language processing. It has been estimated that this specialization interests between 95 and 98% of adults. How this special ability develops, what is its nature, and what happens when the left hemisphere is damaged by a cerebral lesion in early phases of development are still matters of debate. Indeed, more than 30 years ago, invasive techniques such as the Wada test have demonstrated that, in patients with early left-hemispheric brain lesions, the right hemisphere is able to develop a specialization for language, in the absence of significant language disabilities (Rasmussen and Milner 1977). How this happens and what are the consequences for brain function are starting to be clarified only more recently, thanks to the application of advanced functional neuroimaging techniques, such as positron emission tomography (PET) and functional magnetic resonance imaging (fMRI).

An important study of 2002 by Martin Staudt and his coworkers with an fMRI language task explored the topography of language organization following early left brain injury (namely, unilateral periventricular lesions) to discover where (and indirectly how) language function organizes in the right hemisphere. They revealed a remarkable similarity between the activation in normal controls (in the left hemisphere) and the activation in brain-injured patients (in the right hemisphere), with a perfectly specular distribution of the known cortical areas of the language circuit (Staudt 2002).

These findings indicate that reorganization of language in the right hemisphere occurs in areas that are perfectly homotopic to those normally involved in normal conditions, strongly suggesting a near equipotentiality of the two hemispheres at birth as to the ability of developing language control.

Similar findings had already been found in patients with malformations of cortical development (Hertz-Pannier et al. 1997; Müller et al. 1998). In those subjects, however, epileptic seizures, which are known to alter cerebral reorganization, were almost invariably present, thus making it hard to explore whether shifting of language could happen also in the absence of seizures and/or in case of later damage (early third trimester). Those findings were then further extended showing a similar pattern of contralateral homotopic reorganization even in patients with arterial stroke occurred at term age (Fig. 2) (Guzzetta et al. 2008). In that study, authors also showed that shifting of language function after a stroke at term is even more common than for earlier lesions, when accounting for the variable of seizures, suggesting a direct influence of timing on the pattern of reorganization suggesting, as for other systems (see below), that the hemispheric specialization of language develops as a result of a competitive process between the two hemispheres. When a left (non-epileptogenic) lesion occurs within the early third trimester of gestation, when cerebral plasticity is highly effective, the affected hemisphere is more likely to maintain its genetic advantage over the contralateral and eventually develop control over language. When a left lesion occurs at term or during early development, when the plastic potential is reducing, the non-affected hemisphere might prevail upon the affected one and take over language control. This option becomes gradually less available during development, with later lesions invariably resulting in an intra-hemispheric reorganization of function and different degrees of language disturbance (i.e., the "right-hemisphere-take-over" theory) (Szaflarski et al. 2014).

Interestingly, other studies observed subtle differences in language outcome in right versus left congenital lesions, thus getting more complex idea of language plasticity and reinforcing the idea of a specialization of the two hemispheres, in spite of their plastic potential (Guzzetta et al. 2008; Kolk et al. 2011). Convincing data support the hypothesis that a price for language function plasticity has to be paid by right-hemispheric functions, the so-called crowding effect. (Fiori

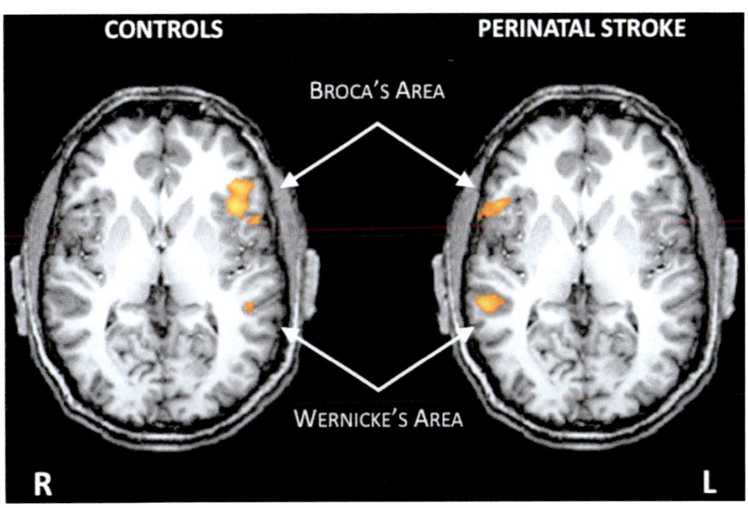

Fig. 2 Language representation in patients with left perinatal stroke and right-hemispheric reorganization of language. fMRI shows the activation of regions of the right hemisphere which are contralateral and homotopic to the regions of the language circuit activated in normal controls (group analysis performed on eight patients and ten normal controls; see (Bates et al. 2001))

and Guzzetta 2015) fMRI studies on language plasticity reveal that children with left-lesion-induced right-hemispheric language organization, despite the relatively well-preserved language functions, show deficits in visuospatial abilities, and the degree of visuospatial dysfunction is proportional to the degree of right language representation (Lidzba et al. 2006; Ilves et al. 2014).

17.4.2 The Sensorimotor System

When a cerebral lesion, either cortical or subcortical, involves the motor system, neuroplastic mechanisms should be able to drive recovery of voluntary movements, restoring an adequate cortical impulse to the spinal motor neurons and interneurons. Two major mechanisms are available to restore an efficient reconnection of the motor cortex with the spinal cord circuitry in case of a cerebral lesion. The first one involves a reorganization of the ipsilateral cortex, within the primary motor cortex or in non-primary motor areas. The second mechanism is specific for lesions occurring during the early phases of development. It is based on the existence, during the first weeks of life, of bilateral motor projections originating in the primary motor areas, which connect each hemisphere with both sides of the body. These fibers generally withdraw during development, but they can persist in case of cerebral damage, giving rise to a contralesional reorganization of motor function. This type of reorganization is specific for unilateral early brain lesions, as it requires, at the time when damage occurs, the presence of a bilateral innervation of motoneuronal pools and a developmental increase in the number of both fast-conducting ipsilateral and contralateral corticospinal axons from the intact hemisphere (Fig. 3).

The application of fMRI can provide relevant information on the type of reorganization occurring in each patient. Nevertheless it has to be integrated with techniques providing a high temporal resolution such as transcranial magnetic stimulation (TMS), in order to document the

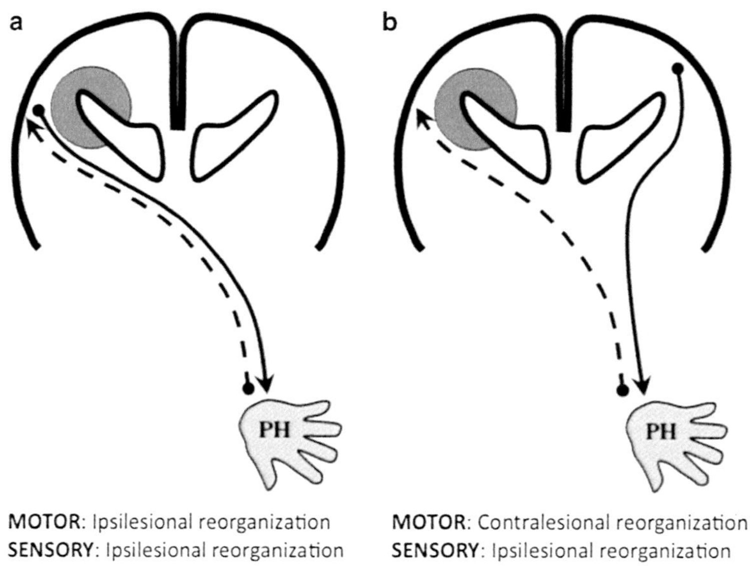

Fig. 3 Schematic representation of the main types of reorganization of sensorimotor function following early brain damage. (**a**) Ipsilesional reorganization of motor and sensory function. Both functions are reorganized in the affected hemisphere, in regions around the lesion. In this case, functional impairment is mainly related to the extent of the damage of the sensorimotor system. (**b**) Contralesional reorganization of motor function and ipsilesional reorganization of sensory function. Motor and sensory function of the affected limb is processed by different hemispheres. In this case, functional impairment is not only related to the extent of the damage of the sensorimotor system but also to the presence of the functional dissociation

existence of cortical-spinal monosynaptic connections. TMS can document that in many subjects with an early lesion of the motor cortex, a significant corticospinal bilateral innervation of spinal motoneuronal pools persists in the healthy hemisphere. In these subjects activation of the intact motor cortex elicits large responses in both the ipsi- and the contralateral muscles, with similar latencies and thresholds. (Zsoter et al. 2012)

Cerebral lesions interestingly the motor system often involve the sensory system as well and may lead to a functional deficit of different severity. These functions can be studied in vivo with techniques like somatosensory evoked potentials, magnetoencephalography, and fMRI with sensorial tasks.

In contrast to primary motor function, the intrahemispheric (ipsilesional) reorganization of primary sensory function is the principal compensatory mechanism following damage to the sensory system, even when it occurs during the very early stages of development (Zsoter et al. 2012; Staudt et al. 2004). Of critical interest is the fact that the different reorganizational potential of the sensory and the motor systems leads in many cases to an interhemispheric dissociation of these functions, with the first being reorganized in the affected hemisphere and the second being shifted contralaterally (Fig. 3b). Some evidence seems to support the hypothesis that such a dissociation could determine some functional deficits in tasks requiring a strong sensorimotor integration (such as stereognosis). This is probably due to the lack of anatomical substrates for contralesional reorganization, even in the early stages of development. However, previous studies indicated how this pattern of SM reorganization (contralesional reorganization) is already determined during the first year of life and possibly even within the first few months (Eyre et al. 2007; Guzzetta et al. 2010).

This appeared as not a mere consequence of the size and site of the lesion, but is strongly influenced by the experience following damage (action-dependent reorganization), in the sense of the complex interaction between residual motor output from the affected hemisphere and somatosensory feedback from the affected limb (hypothesis of the "amblyopia of the corticospinal system") (Eyre et al. 2007).

Should this hypothesis be confirmed, the importance of an early time window (first months of life) for therapeutic intervention would be greatly emphasized. This is especially true when considering that children with contralesional reorganization, i.e., with the unaffected hemisphere directly controlling both hands, reach lower levels of hand motor performance, making this pattern of reorganization as potentially maladaptive (Staudt et al. 2004; Guzzetta et al. 2007).

The mechanisms underlying this phenomenon are not fully understood; however two elements seem to be of special relevance. The first is the lack of an anatomical substrate for contralesional reorganization, even in the early stages of development, at variance with what happens for the motor system. The second is the possibility that thalamocortical fibers, at least for some types of early lesions, are still developing when the insult occurs and are thus able to bypass the lesion and reconnect with the sensory cortex within the damaged hemisphere (Staudt et al. 2006a; Papadelis et al. 2012). This evidence comes from the combined use of structural imaging methods, such as diffusion MRI-based tractography (Rose et al. 2011), which identify the likely trajectories of thalamocortical white matter bundles, and functional imaging methods, such as MEG, which are capable of reliably mapping the cortical location of primary sensory processing (Staudt et al. 2006b).

Moreover, diffusion studies performed during the chronic phases of the disorder, i.e., in adolescents and young adults with unilateral cerebral palsy, showed that the asymmetry of the corticospinal tract is less correlated with sensory and motor function than the asymmetry of other projections such as the thalamocortical ones. Not surprisingly, the early structural asymmetries of the corticospinal tract are not always able to predict the presence and, most of all, the severity of later hemiplegia. These data suggest an essential role of higher-order compensatory mechanisms in shaping the long-term functional outcome, and a growing body of evidence supports the hypothesis that the reorganization of motor function also heavily involves subcortical structures such as the thalamus, brainstem or spinal cord, and cerebellum (Dinomais et al. 2012). On the light of these findings, the specific target of an early therapeutic intervention should be the activation of the sensorimotor cortex of the affected hemisphere, to enhance the competitive ability of a damaged corticospinal system during development and thus mitigate the consequences of the lesion on motor outcome.

17.4.3 The Visual System

Among all the systems described, the reorganization of the visual system after early lesions in humans is maybe the less investigated. Conversely, more than any other system, visual function has been extensively studied in the animal model and especially the cat. The sparse scientific evidence in humans on the specificity of reorganizational mechanisms after early damage is summarized below (Fig. 4).

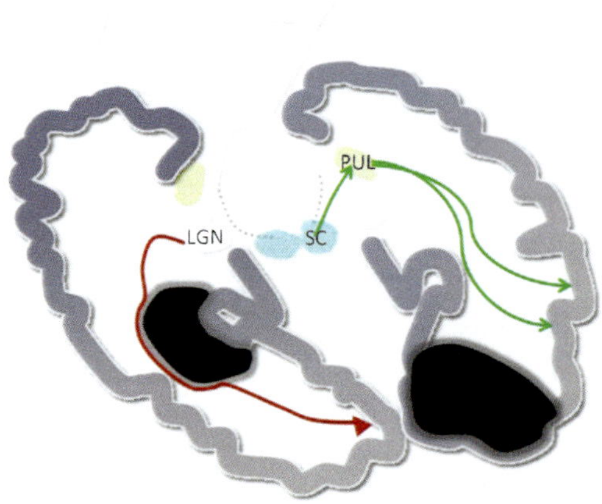

Fig. 4 Schematic representation of the main types of reorganization of visual function following early brain damage. On the *left*, a possible type of reorganization following early damage of the optic radiations. The thalamocortical connections are able to bypass the lesion and reach the final cortical target (primary visual cortex). A full recovery of conscious vision can be achieved. On the *right*, the reorganization mechanisms following early damage to the primary visual cortex. Circuits connecting the retina with extrastriatal visual structures are expanded, in particular involving the superior colliculus and the pulvinar. A full recovery of conscious vision cannot be achieved, but a high degree of functional compensation is obtained, consisting of near-normal exploratory visual behavior and navigation. *LGN* lateral geniculate nucleus, *SC* superior colliculus, *Pul* pulvinar

The correlation between damage to the optic radiations or the occipital cortex and the correspondent visual field deficit is far less strong in case of early lesion than of a lesion occurring later in life. This might be the direct expression of more powerful cerebral plasticity mechanisms in the young child that have at least in part similar neurophysiological bases to what is observed for the somatosensory system and in particular the possibility that thalamocortical fibers develop after the lesion, bypassing it (Guzzetta et al. 2013). As our knowledge, along the typical brain development, between the 22nd and 34th week of gestation, when periventricular parenchymal lesions mostly occur, afferents ascending from the thalamus make synaptic contact with the maturing neurons in the subplate region, which regulate the formation of the cortical plate. When focal periventricular brain damage occurs, geniculostriate fibers are expected to bypass the damaged tissue, reaching the visual cortex, with a full sparing of visual fields. The exact characteristics and limits of this specific type of plasticity involving thalamocortical networks are not fully understood. Some data suggest that up to term age structural modifications of the geniculostriate pathway can support functional reorganization of the visual system. Some authors recently studied longitudinally an infant with perinatal left arterial stroke, sparing the primary visual cortex but involving the optic radiations, using a combination of fMRI and diffusion tensor tractography (Seghier et al. 2004, 2005). When the infant was tested at 3 months of age with visual fMRI, cortical activation could only be observed in the unaffected side, and DTI was unable to show the presence of the optical radiations in the affected hemisphere (Seghier et al. 2004). At 20 months, the infant was tested again with the same protocol and surprisingly showed a clear fMRI activation, indirect sign of functional reorganization, further supported by clear structural modifications on diffusion tractography (Seghier et al. 2004, 2005). Unfortunately, the assessment of visual fields was not performed due to the young age of the subject. However, regardless of the possible presence of a functional impairment, the imaging data seem to support the existence of a process of reorganization at the level of the thalamocortical pathway, able to restore, at least partially, the functional connection between the lateral geniculate body and the occipital cortex.

Even when a visual field deficit is present, the subject with early damage seems to show fewer difficulties in environmental navigation and exploration. In accordance to previous studies, Tinelli and colleagues measured sensitivity to several visual tasks in a group of children with congenital unilateral brain lesions involving optic radiations compared to children with similar lesions, acquired in childhood. Children with congenital (but not with acquired) postnatal brain lesions show spared visual perception (although unconscious) in the affected hemifield clear evidence for blindsight. In children with congenital hemianopia, they also mapped the calcarine BOLD activity for visual field quadrants stimulation with fMRI. They showed that the V1 region of the intact hemisphere also responds to stimuli in the ipsilateral "blind" hemifield (Tinelli et al. 2013). Their data perfectly agree with animal model findings, which detected clearly how the ablation of the whole primary visual cortex in the newborn animal does not affect its visual orientation performances, that on the contrary are massively impaired after a similar lesion in the adult animal (Fagiolini et al. 1994). Studies on the cat model showed how this phenomenon is linked to a reorganization of the pathways connecting subcortical visual structures (lateral geniculate nucleus, superior colliculus, and pulvinar) directly to the extrastriatal ipsi- and contralateral visual centers. Some evidence shows that this could also apply to humans, at least to a certain degree, as shown, for example, by the increase in activation of extrastriatal structures on fMRI after the stimulation of the affected hemifield (Leh et al. 2006).

Previous findings have been also confirmed by a recent study of Ajina and colleagues who studied human blindsight, the phenomenon described as the ability to detect visual information within the blind region and functional brain connectivity in individuals with damage of primary visual cortex acquired during adulthood. They concluded that blindsight after the adult brain lesion is mainly mediated by persistence of an intact geniculo-extrastriate pathway, while this pathway was significantly impaired or not measurable in blindsight negative individuals (Ajina et al. 2015).

However, available data support a more effective mechanism of reorganization of visual function after early brain damage that may consist either in a reconnection with the targeted structures or in an enhanced use of compensating circuitries.

In the study of Tinelli et al. (2013), they found that congenitally lesioned subjects have strong activation of the contralesional calcarine cortex for both stimuli in the contra- and ipsilateral visual field, indicating a rewiring involving primary visual processes and not limited to compensatory circuits involving extrastriate cortices. One possibility for explaining ipsilateral activity in the spared V1 is that some of the retinal ipsilateral projections to lateral geniculate nucleus and superior colliculus, observed during early development in young animals and possibly also in human infants (Arroyo and Feller 2016), did not degenerate given the massive lesions to one hemisphere at birth.

Interestingly, in a systematic review of Guzzetta and collaborators on visual functions reorganization in preterm infants with periventricular hemorrhagic infarction, they observed that the involvement of the optic radiations was often associated with normal visual fields; conversely, the presence of basal ganglia/thalamus involvement apparently prevented such reorganization, resulting in unilateral field restriction (Guzzetta et al. 2013), These findings support the existence of effective mechanisms of plastic reorganization that allow a rewiring of geniculo-calcarine connections with restoration of full-field vision but which are hindered by the involvement of the basal ganglia and thalamus.

17.5 Conclusions

How can we summarize present knowledge on cerebral plasticity and reorganization following early brain damage? The concept that is clearly emerging, both from human and nonhuman studies, is that functional reorganization in children is neither better nor worse than in adults, but it is simply different and gives rise to a really different brain. Full knowledge of how different the young brain becomes (after damage), i.e., the specific mechanisms of cerebral plasticity in infancy, is far from being achieved. The effort is however highly meritorious as this knowledge will be essential to the definition and tuning of therapeutic programs based on solid neurobiological and neurophysiological principles. And with this is intended not only the type of treatment but also its timing, its dosage, and its means of administration. Brain mapping techniques and in particular fMRI developed over the last few years provided answers to many questions that had been at the center of scientific debate for long periods. Next implementations of these techniques, for example, the dissemination of ultrahigh-field MRI machines integrated with functional approaches, will provide a new insight to the remaining questions.

References

Ajina S, Pestilli F, Rokem A, Kennard C, Bridge H (2015) Human blindsight is mediated by an intact geniculo-extrastriate pathway. Elife 4:e08935

Anderson V (2005) Functional plasticity or vulnerability after early brain injury? Pediatrics 116:1374–1382

Anderson V et al (2009) Childhood brain insult: can age at insult help us predict outcome? Brain 132:45–56

Anderson V, Spencer-Smith M, Wood A (2011) Do children really recover better? Neurobehavioural plasticity after early brain insult. Brain 134:2197–2221

Arroyo DA, Feller MB (2016) Spatiotemporal features of retinal waves instruct the wiring of the visual circuitry. Front Neural Circuits 10:54

Ballantyne AO, Spilkin AM, Hesselink J, Trauner DA (2008) Plasticity in the developing brain: intellectual, language and academic functions in children with ischaemic perinatal stroke. Brain 131: 2975–2985

Barrett KC, Ashley R, Strait DL, Kraus N (2013) Art and science: how musical training shapes the brain. Front Psychol 4:713

Bates E et al (2001) Differential effects of unilateral lesions on language production in children and adults. Brain Lang 79:223–265

Berker EA (1986) Translation of Broca's 1865 report. Arch Neurol 43:1065

de Bode S, Smets L, Mathern GW, Dubinsky S (2015) Complex syntax in the isolated right hemisphere: receptive grammatical abilities after cerebral hemispherectomy. Epilepsy Behav 51:33–39

Dennis M et al (2013) Age, plasticity, and homeostasis in childhood brain disorders. Neurosci Biobehav Rev 37:2760–2773

Dinomais M, Groeschel S, Staudt M, Krägeloh-Mann I, Wilke M (2012) Relationship between functional connectivity and sensory impairment: red flag or red herring? Hum Brain Mapp 33:628–638

Elbert T, Pantev C, Wienbruch C, Rockstroh B, Taub E (1995) Increased cortical representation of the fingers of the left hand in string players. Science 270:305–307

Eyre JA et al (2007) Is hemiplegic cerebral palsy equivalent to amblyopia of the corticospinal system? Ann Neurol 62:493–503

Fagiolini M, Pizzorusso T, Berardi N, Domenici L, Maffei L (1994) Functional postnatal development of the rat primary visual cortex and the role of visual experience: dark rearing and monocular deprivation. Vis Res 34:709–720

Finger S (1988) The 'Kennard effect' before Kennard: the early history of age and brain lesions. Arch Neurol 45:1136

Fiori S, Guzzetta A (2015) Plasticity following early-life brain injury: insights from quantitative MRI. Semin Perinatol 39:141–146

Guzzetta A et al (2007) Reorganisation of the somatosensory system after early brain damage. Clin Neurophysiol 118:1110–1121

Guzzetta A et al (2008) Language organisation in left perinatal stroke. Neuropediatrics 39:157–163

Guzzetta A et al (2010) Hand movements at 3 months predict later hemiplegia in term infants with neonatal cerebral infarction. Dev Med Child Neurol 52:767–772

Guzzetta A, Fiori S, Scelfo D, Conti E, Bancale A (2013) Reorganization of visual fields after periventricular haemorrhagic infarction: potentials and limitations. Developmental Medicine & Child Neurology 55:23–26

Hertz-Pannier L et al (1997) Noninvasive assessment of language dominance in children and adolescents with functional MRI: a preliminary study. Neurology 48:1003–1012

Ilves P et al (2014) Different plasticity patterns of language function in children with perinatal and childhood stroke. J Child Neurol 29:756–764

Johnston MV et al (2009) Plasticity and injury in the developing brain. Brain Dev 31:1–10

Klein D, Mok K, Chen J-K, Watkins KE (2014) Age of language learning shapes brain structure: a cortical thickness study of bilingual and monolingual individuals. Brain Lang 131:20–24

Kolb B, Gibb R (2014) Searching for the principles of brain plasticity and behavior. Cortex 58:251–260

Kolk A, Ennok M, Laugesaar R, Kaldoja M-L, Talvik T (2011) Long-term cognitive outcomes after pediatric stroke. Pediatr Neurol 44:101–109

Leh SE, Johansen-Berg H, Ptito A (2006) Unconscious vision: new insights into the neuronal correlate of blindsight using diffusion tractography. Brain 129: 1822–1832

Lewis TL, Maurer D (2005) Multiple sensitive periods in human visual development: evidence from visually deprived children. Dev Psychobiol 46:163–183

Li P, Legault J, Litcofsky KA (2014) Neuroplasticity as a function of second language learning: anatomical changes in the human brain. Cortex 58:301–324

Lidzba K, Staudt M, Wilke M, Krägeloh-Mann I (2006) Visuospatial deficits in patients with early left-hemispheric lesions and functional reorganization of language: consequence of lesion or reorganization? Neuropsychologia 44:1088–1094

Lidzba K, Wilke M, Staudt M, Krägeloh-Mann I (2009) Early plasticity versus early vulnerability: the problem of heterogeneous lesion types. Brain 132:e128. author reply e129

Liégeois F, Cross JH, Polkey C, Harkness W, Vargha-Khadem F (2008) Language after hemispherectomy in childhood: contributions from memory and intelligence. Neuropsychologia 46:3101–3107

Mowery TM, Kotak VC, Sanes DH (2016) The onset of visual experience gates auditory cortex critical periods. Nat Commun 7:10416

Müller R-A et al (1998) Brain organization of language after early unilateral lesion: a PET study. Brain Lang 62:422–451

Papadelis C, Leonardelli E, Staudt M, Braun C (2012) Can magnetoencephalography track the afferent information flow along white matter thalamo-cortical fibers? NeuroImage 60:1092–1105

Rasmussen T, Milner B (1977) The role of early left-brain injury in determining lateralization of cerebral speech functions. Ann N Y Acad Sci 299:355–369

Rose S, Guzzetta A, Pannek K, Boyd R (2011) MRI structural connectivity, disruption of primary sensorimotor pathways, and hand function in cerebral palsy. Brain Connect 1:309–316

Seghier ML et al (2004) Combination of event-related fMRI and diffusion tensor imaging in an infant with perinatal stroke. NeuroImage 21:463–472

Seghier ML et al (2005) Visual recovery after perinatal stroke evidenced by functional and diffusion MRI: case report. BMC Neurol 5:17

Staudt M (2002) Right-hemispheric organization of language following early left-sided brain lesions: functional MRI topography. NeuroImage 16:954–967

Staudt M et al (2004) Reorganization in congenital hemiparesis acquired at different gestational ages. Ann Neurol 56:854–863

Staudt M et al (2006a) Extensive peri-lesional connectivity in congenital hemiparesis. Neurology 66:771

Staudt M et al (2006b) Developing somatosensory projections bypass periventricular brain lesions. Neurology 67:522–525

Sweatt JD (2016) Neural plasticity and behavior – sixty years of conceptual advances. J Neurochem 139 (Suppl 2):179–199

Szaflarski JP et al (2014) Age at stroke determines post-stroke language lateralization. Restor Neurol Neurosci 32:733–742

Tinelli F et al (2013) Blindsight in children with congenital and acquired cerebral lesions. Cortex 49:1636–1647

Vaquero L et al (2016) Structural neuroplasticity in expert pianists depends on the age of musical training onset. NeuroImage 126:106–119

Zsoter A, Pieper T, Kudernatsch M, Staudt M (2012) Predicting hand function after hemispherotomy: TMS versus fMRI in hemispheric polymicrogyria. Epilepsia 53:e98–e101

Part II

Perinatal and Neonatal Care

Organization of Perinatal Care: Training of Doctors and Nurses

18

Neil Marlow

Contents

Abstract

Medical and nursing care for the newborn is organized differently in different health systems. Whereas general support in terms of screening and routine care is provided for a large number of babies in a maternity setting, in comparison neonatal intensive care for sick and immature babies is a low throughput but high cost service. Increasing medical costs and difficulty in staffing intensive care services make it important to evaluate the organization of neonatal care, and new data on the relationship between throughput and outcome are driving centralization of care for the smallest and sickest children. In this chapter, the elements of service organization are described.

18.1 Salient Points

- Sick newborn infants need to be treated in specialist neonatal units.
- Neonatal care cannot take place in isolation from pediatric, obstetric, and fetal medicine services.
- Outcomes are improved for babies born in tertiary centers, particularly in terms of antenatal and delivery room mortality.
- Neonatal staff are responsible for the organization and training of all obstetric, midwifery, and neonatal staff in neonatal stabilization and resuscitation.

N. Marlow
Institute for Women's Health, University College London, London, UK
e-mail: n.marlow@ucl.ac.uk

G. Buonocore et al. (eds.), *Neonatology*,
https://doi.org/10.1007/978-3-319-29489-6_167

- With more enlightened views about the role of the parent in enhancing their baby's progress during the neonatal period, parents are now welcomed into the neonatal unit and encouraged to participate in their child's care.
- The provision of recommended neonatal nurse staffing levels again will vary between health systems, depending on the roles that are undertaken by nurses and the availability of other professionals, such as respiratory therapists.
- The numbers of neonatologists required to staff a neonatal service depend on the model of health care provision. Mortality was increased in areas of the USA with very low numbers of neonatologists (<4.3 doctors per 10,000 births).
- Clinical audit is key to the assessment of service quality and audit of structure and outcome can provide valuable information when bidding for increased resources and redesigning services. It also helps to confirm that we are achieving our aims in terms of outcomes and activity.
- It is important to establish an external reference for the performance of a neonatal service, and there are important resources available to support this, such as EuroNeoNet and the Vermont Oxford Network, in addition to national or local benchmarking systems.
- Target groups for follow-up programs are very preterm or very low birth weight children, children who have been encephalopathic, and any others considered to be at risk. Combined with mortality data, this information is useful in terms of monitoring outcomes and providing center-based information for parents.

18.2 Overview

Medical and nursing care for the newborn is organized differently in different health systems. Whereas general support in terms of screening and routine care is provided for a large number of babies in a maternity setting, neonatal intensive care for sick and immature babies is a low throughput high cost service. The development of neonatal intensive care has undoubtedly been one of the success stories of modern medicine. Its rapid evolution since the early 1970s has led to dramatic changes in mortality at low gestational ages and a reduction in immediate and later morbidities.

The extent to which different models of organization of neonatal services have contributed to this is hotly debated. Services evolve as the technical aspects of care change and are rarely planned on a geographic basis. However, there is a general agreement that a sick newborn infant needs to be treated in a specialist neonatal unit. Thus, a neonatal transport system must be a basic element for any regional program that aims at reducing morbidity and mortality (see ▶ Chap. 19, "Neonatal Transport Services").

Organization is very dependent on how the healthcare system is financed and managed and on the regulatory framework of a particular country. In this chapter, we describe the recent changes in organization within the United Kingdom healthcare system to illustrate the thinking and evidence base on which service changes may be planned and from which the reader may derive concepts relevant to their own local health system.

Briefly, in the UK, healthcare is organized independently in each of the four constituent countries. Within the UK, the majority of births occur in hospital (approximately 600,000 out of 680,000 annually), and healthcare is organized under the auspices of the National Health Service. The NHS is regionalized into 10 Regional Hubs that are responsible for "purchasing" health services for their population from Hospital and Primary Care Trusts (the "providers"). However, low volume services, such as neonatal intensive care, are "commissioned" (purchased or contracted) centrally.

Neonatal care is delivered in maternity hospital settings within the UK, except for highly specialist areas, for example such as cardiac surgery. Since 2000, hospitals have become increasingly focused on the areas of neonatal care they undertake based around a three tier model, where some units provide only basic noninvasive care, some more invasive care (usually including short periods of intensive care), and other hospitals provide a full neonatal intensive care service; more specialist services – surgery, extracorporeal membrane oxygenation, cardiac surgery – are provided in only a few centers around England to optimize efficiency and maximize quality outcomes.

18.3 Models of Care

Neonatal care cannot take place in isolation from other services. In particular pediatric, obstetric, and fetal medicine services are interdependent, so it makes sense that these are colocated. In many non-UK systems, however, neonatal intensive care takes place within a children's hospital setting, which has implications for family integrity and support but may provide optimal support for some of the highly technical aspects of care and management. In contrast, there are increasing moves in some countries to enhance the concept of family-centered care by colocating maternal and neonatal care for mother and child in the same area. This model does allow for some separation for the periods of necessary intensive care but optimizes the family experience and is designed to minimize parental and infant psychological morbidity. Neonatal care should be organized in a manner appropriate to the societal setting and resources available.

The issue of centralized versus dispersed services has been the subject of much debate. Apart from research carried out in the UK (Field and Draper 1999), studies in other health systems have seen advantages in terms of mortality and morbidity where services are centralized to provide care for the sickest and smallest infants in large "tertiary" units (Marlow and Gill 2007; Lasswell et al. 2010). It has been suggested that the reason that this has not been shown in England relates to under-capacity within the large neonatal services (Tucker et al. 1999; BLISS the premature baby charity 2005), as there is evidence that mortality is related to the number of nurses available each shift (Tucker et al. 2002).

To address this problem we have developed a series of "managed clinical networks" of neonatal care. A managed clinical network may be defined as linked groups of health professionals and organizations from primary, secondary, and tertiary care working in a coordinated manner to ensure equitable provision of high-quality clinically effective services, unconstrained by existing professional and Health Board boundaries. Further description of the roles and responsibilities of Managed Neonatal Networks is available (Marlow and Gill 2007), but in essence all hospitals serving a population agree to work together to deliver the whole range of care. Where possible this is carried out as close to the mother's area of residence but where specialist care (i.e., intensive care) is required then the mother and baby are transferred to the appropriate center. This way hospitals that provide different levels of care act together to make sure that the baby and family are appropriately supported. Service standards and descriptors are available (Department of Health 2009; Neonatal Critical Care Clinical Reference Group 2015).

As part of EPICure2 an analysis of variation by place of birth was undertaken which demonstrated improved outcomes for babies born in tertiary centers, particularly in terms of antenatal and delivery room mortality (Marlow et al. 2014), which was subsequently confirmed for neonatal unit admissions (Watson et al. 2014). In addition, there is the intriguing suggestion that higher throughput units have better survival at extremely low gestational ages, which does require confirmation.

18.4 Care of High-Risk Newborn Infants

Within a neonatal service a range of areas require planning and monitoring:

Antenatal counseling and support
Delivery room care and resuscitation
Screening and acute care following "normal" births
Care in the neonatal unit
Discharge care and support
Follow-up of at-risk children

18.4.1 Antenatal Counseling and Support

Central to good perinatal care is the availability of neonatal staff to discuss forthcoming deliveries with women and their partners. This is a key role for the neonatologist and the neonatal nurse. Discussions may simply include information about the process of birth for an at-risk child and a predelivery visit to the neonatal unit. In other situations, the neonatologist must be involved in discussions of prognosis where delivery is anticipated very prematurely or where fetal anomaly has been detected and on occasions must be part of the decision-making process as to where a baby is best delivered to receive optimal care. Most fetal medicine services now involve the relevant pediatric specialist, where a fetal problem has been identified to help develop a delivery plan, but of equal importance is the neonatal team who will often have a different perspective on the early management of the baby, which may alter the initial proposal.

18.4.2 Delivery Room Care and Resuscitation

Neonatal staff are usually responsible for the organization and training of all obstetric, midwifery, and neonatal staff in neonatal stabilization and resuscitation. In most countries, formalized training is available through nationally accredited neonatal life support courses, and all staff that are likely to be involved in neonatal stabilization should be properly accredited (Resuscitation Council (UK) 2015; Perlman et al. 2015a). Clear written arrangements for checking that resuscitation apparatus is always available and for calling appropriate staff when necessary should be agreed. Management plans where comfort or palliative care is anticipated need to be agreed and, given the ethical difficulties that surround, in particular, birth at extremely low gestations each neonatal unit should agree with their obstetric and midwifery colleagues a policy for communicating risk to prospective parents facing such deliveries.

18.4.3 Screening and Acute Care Following "Normal" Births

Within our health system the neonatologist is responsible for carrying out a screening examination for the newborn baby and troubleshooting where the midwife has identified potential postnatal problems. This involves identifying babies who are at high risk of particular conditions such as neonatal infection, hip dysplasia, and congenital heart disease. Screening for metabolic disease is also undertaken in most countries.

most hospitals the screening examination is delegated to trainees or to specifically trained midwifery staff, although in some settings it may be undertaken by the family pediatrician. A single neonatal examination is usually sufficient to identify major anomalies, although problems that become apparent later in the neonatal period such as duct or pressure dependent congenital heart disease and jaundice may need separate assessments (Perlman et al. 2015b). Screening with saturation monitors for heart disease may enhance the detection rate of screening examinations (Moss et al. 1991). Hospitals need to ensure that they have a range of protocols for treating babies at risk of infection (Mahle et al. 2009) and babies who develop new problems after birth (Royal College of Obstetricians and Gynaecologists 2003).

18.4.4 Care in the Neonatal Unit

18.4.4.1 Designation of Neonatal Care and Services

Neonatal units have a range of service available to them that differ from hospital to hospital. Often the quanta of care that is provided depend upon staffing levels and colocated facilities. In many countries, a three level system operates formally or informally with a fourth level designating those hospitals which provide "super-specialist" care such as cardiac surgery, neonatal surgery, etc. The detail will vary from one health system to another. The British Association of Perinatal Medicine (BAPM) grading (Royal College of Obstetricians and Gynaecologists et al. 2007) is shown in Table 1.

Table 1 Designation of neonatal services within a neonatal network

Level 1 or *Special Care Units* – provide special care but do not aim to provide any continuing high dependency or intensive care; this includes units with or without resident medical staff
Level 2 or *Local Neonatal Units* – provide high dependency care and some short-term intensive care as agreed within the network; medical staffing at middle grade and consultant level is shared with a general pediatric service
Level 3 or *Neonatal Intensive Care Units* – provide the whole range of medical neonatal care but not necessarily all specialist services such as neonatal surgery; medical staffing at all grades is dedicated to the neonatal service

Adapted from Royal College of Obstetricians and Gynaecologists et al. (2007)

Within these designations it is important that we define what activity occurs within each service. Again these definitions will vary widely between health systems. The BAPM definitions of normal, special, high dependency, and intensive care are shown in Table 2. One of the key features about the use of definitions such as these is that they reflect the level of support required by the baby and that this is independent of the setting in which the care is delivered. For example, if a baby required intensive care while awaiting transfer to a neonatal unit, the referring hospital should be able to provide the equipment and manpower immediately available to cope with the baby's needs. This may cause problems in that if the staff are needed for an emergency elsewhere in the hospital; other staff members should be available to deal with that leaving experienced staff to care for the baby who needs intensive care. Similarly, often babies who fall into the category "special care" are cared for alongside their mothers. This requires enhanced nursing support but may occur outside the confines of a neonatal unit. Sometimes, this is known as "transitional care." Neonatal units have used transitional care as a means of enhancing the care they give (promoting mother-baby contact) and also of enhancing the capacity of their neonatal unit but need extra resources to do it properly. In our system, the nursing requirements also follow the care category as indicated in Table 2. Because staff costs are the greater proportion of total unit costs this allows reimbursement to be made for care on a bed day basis.

18.4.4.2 Family-Centered Neonatal Care

Traditionally, parents were observers while medical and nursing experts assumed responsibility for care. Indeed many units were designed with viewing galleries or corridors to prevent contact. With the advent of more enlightened views of the role of the parent in enhancing the baby's progress through the neonatal period, parents are now welcomed into the neonatal unit and encouraged to participate in their child's care. The advantages of this in engendering better psychological support for parents are clear, and there is evidence that skin-to-skin contact is of great importance in promoting infant stability and well-being. Encouraging close parental involvement in their child's care demands organizational changes in the way neonatal services are run, the facilities available for parents such as sitting rooms and overnight bedrooms, and for privacy when they are with their child (The Neonatal Taskforce 2009). Some units have developed the concept of single room care to accommodate this more appropriately, but staffing, space, and cost constraints make this an expensive, if desirable, option and is not suitable for all families. Caring for a child in a single room without family present may reduce stimulation and opportunity for the baby to interact, potentially increasing parental stress (British Association of Perinatal Medicine 2001).

Within a neonatal service it is possible to draw up a range of standards for family-friendly care to ensure that a baby and his family are afforded due respect and that communication and involvement occur. An example of one such set of standards is included in Table 3. Importantly, these should be auditable so that the neonatal service should be able to demonstrate its commitment to this important area.

Further organizational issues center around the discharge of the baby home at the completion of the episode of perinatal care. The process of taking a baby home is highly stressful for parents. Units need to develop expertise and clear arrangements for preparing families for home

Table 2 Definitions of categories of neonatal care (see http://bapm.org/publications/)

Intensive care
These babies have the most complex problems. They need 1:1 care by a nurse with a neonatal qualification. The possibility of acute deterioration is such that there should be the constant availability of a competent doctor
1. Receiving any respiratory support via a tracheal tube and in the first 24 h after its withdrawal
2. Both noninvasive respiratory support and parenteral nutrition
3. The day of surgery (including laser therapy for retinopathy)
4. The day of death
5. A day during which any of the following occur: Presence of an umbilical arterial line Presence of an umbilical venous line Presence of a peripheral arterial line Insulin infusion Presence of a chest drain Exchange transfusion Therapeutic hypothermia Prostaglandin infusion Presence of replogle tube Presence of epidural catheter Presence of silo for gastroschisis Presence of external ventricular drain Dialysis (any type)
High dependency care
A nurse should not be responsible for the care of more than two babies in this category
1. Any day where a baby receives any form of noninvasive respiratory support (e.g., nasal CPAP, SIPAP, BIPAP, HHFNC)
2. Any day receiving any of the following: Parenteral nutrition Continuous infusion of drugs (except prostaglandin and/or insulin) Presence of a central venous or long line (PICC) Presence of a tracheostomy Presence of a urethral or suprapubic catheter Presence of trans-anastomotic tube following esophageal atresia repair Presence of NP airway/nasal stent Observation of seizures/CF monitoring Barrier nursing Ventricular tap
Special care
A nurse should not be responsible for the care of more than four babies receiving Special or Normal Care
Any day where a baby does not fulfill the criteria for intensive or high dependency care and requires any of the following: Oxygen by nasal cannula Feeding by nasogastric, jejunal tube, or gastrostomy Continuous physiological monitoring (excluding apnoea monitors only) Care of a stoma Presence of IV cannula Baby receiving phototherapy Special observation of physiological variables at least 4 hourly
Routine care
• Is provided for babies who themselves have no medical indication to be in hospital

and if possible supporting them in the transition. Information packs, training in resuscitation techniques, and supportive outpatient follow-up are important steps in the discharge process.

18.4.4.3 Nurse Staffing

The provision of recommended neonatal nurse staffing levels again will vary between health systems, depending on the roles that are undertaken

Table 3 Examples of family-friendly standards for NICU

1. Where admission to a neonatal unit is predicted, a prenatal opportunity to visit the neonatal unit and meet key personnel should be offered to the family
2. All parents should be introduced to facilities, routines, staff, and equipment on admission to a neonatal unit
3. Every parent should have unrestricted access to his or her baby, unless individual restrictions can be justified in the baby's best interest
4. Parents should be encouraged and supported to participate in decision-making about the care and treatment of their baby. Written and regularly updated care plans should be shared with parents. Clinical care decisions, including end-of-life decisions, should be made by experienced staff in partnership with the parents and discussions held in an appropriate setting
5. Parents are encouraged and supported to participate in their baby's care at the earliest opportunity, including: Regular skin-to-skin care Providing comforting touch, comfort holding, particularly during painful procedures Feeding Day-to-day care, such as nappy changing
6. Every baby should be treated with dignity and respect: Appropriate positioning is promoted and encouraged Clinical interventions are managed to minimize stress, avoid pain, and conserve energy Noise and light levels are managed to minimize stress Appropriate clothing is used at all times, taking into account parents' choice Privacy is respected and promoted as appropriate to the baby's condition
7. Every parent will have the opportunity to discuss their baby's diagnoses and care with a senior clinician within 24 h following admission or a significant change in condition
8. Written information should be available (in languages and formats appropriate to the local community) to all users of the service on medical and surgical treatments, to permit early and effective communication with parents covering at least: Condition/diagnosis Treatment options available Likely outcomes/benefits of treatment Possible complications/risks Possible tests and investigations Who to contact with queries or for advice Where to go for further information, including useful websites Circumstances requiring consent (written and verbal)
9. Maternity and neonatal services should encourage breastfeeding and the expression of milk through the provision of information and dedicated support, including: Whenever possible, initiation of breast feeding as soon as possible after birth When necessary, support to start expression as soon after delivery as the mother's condition allows to maximize the benefit of colostrum The availability of a comfortable, dedicated, and discrete area The facility to express discretely at the cotside The availability of breast pumps and associated equipment for every mother who requires them Supporting breastfeeding as part of the discharge process Promotion of safe and hygienic handling and storage of breast milk Possible availability of donor breast milk

Adapted from The Neonatal Taskforce (2009)

by nurses and the availability of other professionals, such as respiratory therapists. Within the UK system there have been few studies of nursing input on which to base the recommendations set out in Table 2, although recent evidence suggests that one-to-one nursing provision may be associated with lower mortality (BLISS the premature baby charity 2009). Nonetheless, it is apparent that adequacy of nurse staffing is a key issue within neonatal units in relation to mortality (Watson et al. 2016). Further research is needed to support recommendations in this area.

In systems where nurses take on more technical roles (cannulation, intubation, ventilator management), enhanced nursing support is required. With appropriate training many units have developed the role of Advanced Nurse Practitioner; such individuals form an intermediate tier between junior and senior resident doctors and assume many of the roles previously taken on by medical staff (at least in the UK) and may contribute to on call rosters (Hamilton et al. 2007). In some settings, they may act without medical staff in supporting low risk deliveries, whereas in other settings they provide intensive care activity. Both these and other roles require different and bespoke training.

18.4.4.4 Medical Staffing

Medical staffing is equally dependent upon the health service model. In the UK, medical trainees and Advanced Neonatal Nurse Practitioners support neonatal intensive care services at a technical grade (junior resident) and as experienced senior resident support. The number of staff neonatologists in this system is relatively few and they have more of an executive and managerial role. Changes to working hours (for example, the European Working Time Directive) and availability of resident staff to work in these high intensity settings mean that such systems are under threat. In many other settings, staff neonatologists (nationally qualified doctors) provide medical care.

Research into the numbers of neonatologists required to staff a neonatal service is unusual. One epidemiologic approach determined that mortality rose in areas of the USA where there was a very low supply of neonatologists (<4.3 doctors per 10,000 births) but that increasing the number did not result in further reductions (Hall and Wilkinson 2005). In the UK, the number of consultants was not related to mortality or nosocomial infection rates (Goodman et al. 2002).

18.4.4.5 Clinical Governance

Within any neonatal service a strong clinical governance framework is required in order to maximize safety and efficiency. Clinical governance comprises a range of organizational structures which we use as professionals in order to quality assure the care we provide, the most useful of which are:

The clinical audit process
The use of standards, guidelines, and perinatal audit tools
Benchmarking and the application of evidence-based care

Although all three are interwoven they merit consideration separately.

Clinical Audit

The key to the process or cycle of audit is the setting of standards, the appraisal of your service against the standard, and the revision of your standard consequent upon the audit to be followed by a reaudit to make sure it is appropriate. The areas that are amenable to audit cover the range of activities of a neonatal service and include the structure of the service (people/facilities available); the process of care (are we consistently doing what we think we are?); and the outcome of care (Is our prophylactic indomethacin effective?; Is our mortality rate appropriate for our population?).

Clinical audit is a key part of assessing the service we are giving and audit of structure and outcome can provide valuable information when bidding for resources and redesigning services. It also helps to confirm that we are achieving what we aim to achieve in terms of outcomes and activity. More information on the use of clinical audit in neonatal care is to be found elsewhere.

Standards and Guidelines

Part of the way in which we develop our service is to provide a range of policy that is based around the best evidence we have. In the USA, the Fetus and Newborn Committee of the American Academy of Pediatrics produces regular guidance based on best evidence. In the UK, guidance on aspects of clinical care is sometimes available from professional organizations and may be specified as part of the process of resourcing the service. The series of Green-top guidelines produced by the Royal College of Obstetricians and Gynaecologists, for example, contain much of relevance to neonatal care and guide practice widely in the UK. The Royal College of Paediatrics and Child Health publishes a range of documents, which although not primarily aimed at neonatal care are of great importance in neonatal practice, for example, Withholding or Withdrawing Life Sustaining Treatment in Children: A Framework for Practice (2004), which guides practice around end-of-life decisions. The British Association of Perinatal Medicine (BAPM) also produces a range of practical guidance, for example:

- Management of extremely preterm babies (2008)
- Use of Central Venous Catheters in Neonates – a Framework for Practice (2015)
- Newborn Early Warning Trigger & Track (NEWTT) – a Framework for Practice (2015)
- Practical guidance for the management of palliative care on neonatal units (2014)
- Position Statement on Therapeutic Cooling for Neonatal Encephalopathy (2010)
- Guideline for the Screening and Treatment of Retinopathy of Prematurity (2008)

Further guidance is published on an ad hoc basis, for example, the recent European Guidance on the Management of Respiratory Distress Syndrome (Tucker et al. 2002).

Most neonatal intensive care units are busy places, and it is helpful to have a range of guidance easily assessable to staff. It is also helpful to work to protocols so that audit of care is more meaningful. Key aspects of guidelines are that they should:

- Be evidence based
- Explain in principle why a treatment/process is preferred
- Be auditable to ensure they are working

Within the UK neonatal networks, guidelines are usually shared for key areas of practice: referral, transfer, and early care for very preterm babies, for example, and shared between units via their websites.

Benchmarking

Comparing the performance of one unit with another is fraught with difficulty. Population risks are different and can lead to erroneous conclusions (see ▶ Chap. 133, "Epidemiology of Adverse Cerebral Outcome of Newborns").

However, it is important to establish an external reference for the performance of a neonatal service and there are important resources available to support this – such as EuroNeoNet (https://www.euroneostat.org) and the Vermont Oxford Network (https://www.vtoxford.org), in addition to national or local benchmarking systems. Whereas the exact ranking in such datasets is not really helpful, progress against the reference population and the identification of areas where a service is an outlier are invaluable pieces of information. The most valuable benchmarking process in the UK is the MBRRACE-UK: Mothers and Babies: Reducing Risk through Audits and Confidential Enquiries across the UK (www.npeu.oc.ac.uk/mbrrace-uk), whereby there is national monitoring of perinatal and maternal mortality with focused confidential enquiries and other audit projects.

Alongside the benchmarking process, the Vermont Oxford Network offers a range of quality improvement programs, which serve to help a service deliver state-of-the-art care and minimize morbidity, in areas such as nosocomial infection, chronic lung disease, and intraventricular hemorrhage through a process of audit.

Data Collection

The key to all aspects of clinical governance is the collection of robust and accurate information about the unit and the babies it looks after. There is a range of datasets available but all require close attention to details to ensure that what is collected is accurate and useful. BAPM initially produced a UK national dataset to support the writing of annual reports that could then be compared (Sweet et al. 2013) and the international benchmarking groups require similar datasets. The UK Neonatal Collaborative has more recently codified a national dataset which is collected universally for all neonatal unit admissions (British Association of Perinatal Medicine 1997).

18.4.4.6 Follow-up After Discharge

Most neonatal services now provide follow-up for groups who are at high risk of disability. In the

Table 4 Recommended format for reporting perinatal outcomes at 2 years (BAPM 2008)

Gestational age at birth		22 w	23 w	. . .	31 w
Number of births (exclude terminations of pregnancy)[a]					
Number of live births					
Number of babies offered active care					
Number of admissions for intensive care					
Number of survivors discharged home					
No. of deaths between discharge and 2y					
No. of survivors evaluated at 2y					
No. with cerebral palsy					
No. with motor impairment GMFCS 2[b]					
No. with motor impairment GMFCS 3–5[c]					
No. with cognitive score <−2 SD[b]					
No. with cognitive score <−3 SD[c]					
No. with hearing aids but not severe hearing impairment[b]					
No. with severe hearing impairment[c]					
No. with speech and language impairment[b]					
No. with severe speech and language disability[c]					
No. with visual impairment but not severe visual impairment[b]					
No. with severe visual impairment[c]					
Total with neurodevelopmental impairment (moderate or severe)[b]					
No. with moderate disability					
No. with severe neurodevelopmental disability (SND)[c]					
Moderate impairment	% survivors evaluated				
	% admissions for NIC				
	% births[b]				
Death or moderate impairment	% admissions for NIC				
	% births[b]				
Severe impairment	% survivors evaluated				
	% admissions for NIC				
	% births[b]				
Death or severe impairment	% admissions for NIC				
	% births[b]				
No. with other disability					
Describe					

GMFCS gross motor function classification system

[a]"Births" may be total births or particular groups (e.g., gestational age) in a defined population – this could be hospital based, network based, or population based depending upon the need

[b]Components of moderate disability – a child with an impairment in any category (but none in the severe category) is classified as having moderate disability

[c]Components of severe disability – a child with any one severe disability or impairment in any category is classified as having severe impairment

UK, a recent working party has revisited the criteria for defining health status as an outcome measure for perinatal care, recommending a formal assessment and recording of data at 2 years of age (The UK National Neonatal Dataset). These are similar to those used within the The Eunice Kennedy Shriver National Institute of Child Health and Human Development (NICHD) Neonatal Network in North America. Target groups for follow-up are very preterm or very low birth weight children, children who have been encephalopathic, and any that are identified by other routes to be at risk. Combined with mortality data, this powerful information is useful in terms of monitoring outcomes and providing center-based information for parents. An example of the output from such a service is shown in Table 4.

References

BLISS the premature baby charity (2005) Special care for sick babies-choice or chance? BLISS, London

BLISS the premature baby charity (2009) The Bliss baby charter standards. BLISS, London

British Association of Perinatal Medicine (1997) The BAPM neonatal dataset for the annual reporting of data by neonatal intensive care units. BAPM, London

British Association of Perinatal Medicine (2001) Standards for hospitals providing intensive and high dependency care. BAPM, London

British Association of Perinatal Medicine (2008) Report of a BAPM/RCPCH working group: health status at two years as a perinatal outcome. BAPM, London

Department of Health (2009) Toolkit for high quality neonatal services. Department of Health, London

Field D, Draper ES (1999) Survival and place of delivery following preterm birth: 1994–96. Arch Dis Child Fetal Neonatal Ed 80:F111–F114

Goodman DC, Fisher ES, Little GA et al (2002) The relation between the availability of neonatal intensive care and neonatal mortality. N Engl J Med 346:1538–1544

Hall D, Wilkinson AR (2005) Quality of care by neonatal nurse practitioners: a review of the Ashington experiment. Arch Dis Child Fetal Neonatal Ed 90:F195–F200

Hamilton KE, Redshaw ME, Tarnow-Mordi W et al (2007) Nurse staffing in relation to risk-adjusted mortality in neonatal care. Arch Dis Child Fetal Neonatal Ed 92: F99–F103

Lasswell SM, Barfield WD, Rochat RW et al (2010) Perinatal regionalization for very low-birth-weight and very preterm infants: a meta-analysis. JAMA 304(9):992–1000

Mahle WT, Newburger JW, Matherne GP et al (2009) Role of pulse oximetry in examining newborns for congenital heart disease: a scientific statement from the American Heart Association and American Academy of Pediatrics. Circulation 120:447–458

Marlow N, Bryan Gill A (2007) Establishing neonatal networks: the reality. Arch Dis Child Fetal Neonatal Ed 92:F137–F142

Marlow N, Bennett C, Draper ES et al (2014) Perinatal outcomes for extremely preterm babies in relation to place of birth in England: the EPICure 2 study. Arch Dis Child Fetal Neonatal Ed 99(3):F181–F188

Moss GD, Cartlidge PH, Speidel BD, Chambers TL (1991) Routine examination in the neonatal period. BMJ 302:878–879

Neonatal Critical Care Clinical Reference Group (2015) Neonatal Service Specification 2015 Available from: https://www.england.nhs.uk/commissioning/spec-services/npc-crg/group-e/e08/

Perlman JM, Wyllie J et al (2015a) Part 7: Neonatal Resuscitation: 2015 International consensus on cardiopulmonary resuscitation and emergency cardiovascular care science with treatment recommendations. Circulation 132:S204–S241

Perlman JM, Wyllie J, Kattwinkel J et al (2015b) Part 7: Neonatal Resuscitation: 2015 international consensus on cardiopulmonary resuscitation and emergency cardiovascular care science with treatment recommendations. Pediatrics 136(Suppl 2):S120–S166

Resuscitation Council (UK) (2015) Resuscitation and support of transition of babies at birth. https://www.resus.org.uk/resuscitation-guidelines/resuscitation-and-support-of-transition-of-babies-at-birth

Royal College of Obstetricians and Gynaecologists (2003) Prevention of early onset neonatal Group B streptococcal disease (Greentop Guideline no. 36). RCOG, London

Royal College of Obstetricians and Gynaecologists, Royal College of Anaesthetitsts, Royal College of Paediatrics and Child Health (2007) Safer childbirth: minimal standards for the organisation, delivery of care in labour. RCOG, London

Sweet DG, Carnielli V, Greisen G et al (2013) European consensus guidelines on the management of neonatal respiratory distress syndrome in preterm infants–2013 update. Neonatology 103(4):353–368

The Neonatal Taskforce (2009) A framework for commissioning neonatal services. Department of Health, London

The UK National Neonatal Dataset. Available from: https://www1.imperial.ac.uk/neonataldataanalysis/data/data/

Tucker J, UK Neonatal Staffing Study Group (2002) Patient volume, staffing, and workload in relation to risk-adjusted outcomes in a random stratified sample of UK neonatal intensive care units: a prospective evaluation. Lancet 359:99–107

Tucker J, Tarnow-Mordi W, Gould C et al (1999) UK neonatal intensive care services in 1996. On behalf of the UK Neonatal Staffing Study Collaborative Group. Arch Dis Child Fetal Neonatal Ed 80:F233–F234

Tucker J, McCabe C, McCabe C et al (2002) Patient volume, staffing, and workload in relation to risk-adjusted outcomes in a random stratified sample of UK neonatal intensive care units: a prospective evaluation. Lancet 359:99–107

Watson SI, Arulampalam W, Petrou S et al (2014) The effects of designation and volume of neonatal care on mortality and morbidity outcomes of very preterm infants in England: retrospective population-based cohort study. BMJ Open 4(7), e004856

Watson SI, Arulampalam W, Petrou S et al (2016) The effects of a one to one nurse to patient ratio on the mortality rate in neonatal intensive care: a retrospective, longitudinal, population-based study. Arch Dis Child Fetal Neonatal Ed 101(3):F195–F200

19 Neonatal Transport Services

Rocco Agostino, Roberto Aufieri, and Maurizio Gente

Contents

R. Agostino (✉)
Ethics Committee, Pediatric Hospital Bambino Gesù, Rome, Italy
e-mail: rocco.agostino@uniroma1.it

R. Aufieri
Division of Neonatology and Neonatal Intensive Care, Casilino General Hospital, Rome, Italy

M. Gente
Department of Pediatrics and Infant Neuropsychiatry, Neonatal Emergency Transport Service, Sapienza University of Rome, Rome, Italy

G. Buonocore et al. (eds.), *Neonatology*,
https://doi.org/10.1007/978-3-319-29489-6_168

Abstract

Neonatal transfer is necessary when a newborn baby needs care that cannot be provided in the referral center. Since it represents an additional risk factor for a critically ill neonate, it should be performed, when possible, by a well-organized neonatal transport service. In a network, aimed at the regionalization of perinatal care, high-risk pregnancies should be transferred "in utero" in order to minimize risks for both mother and neonate. However, there will always be a number of neonates who need to be transferred for unpredicted or unpredictable reasons. Every maternity unit should therefore be able to provide effective neonatal resuscitation in the delivery room, be able to maintain a sick baby in a stable condition in the short term, and have access to a neonatal emergency transport service (NETS) for the provision of neonatal intensive care when appropriate. Thus, NETS provides a bridge between birth centers and neonatal intensive care units (NICUs).

Organization of NETS, quality evaluation, transport process, family-centered care, and challenging situations that can be encountered during neonatal transport are some of the topics treated in this chapter.

19.1 Salient Points

- Newborn babies requiring care that cannot be provided in the referral center should be transferred by a neonatal emergency transport service (NETS) that can guarantee a safe transport with minimization of risk.
- The organization of NETS should be appropriate to the needs and characteristics of the region covered. Each regional network should ideally have a NETS coordinating center.
- Transfer requests should be appropriately assessed and a transport plan formulated to determine level and characteristics of admitting hospital, road, vehicles, and personnel required.
- Referring centers should be able to perform basic resuscitation and stabilization before the arrival of the transport team: Insufficient performances may result in clinical deterioration during the transfer.
- Good communication between transport team, referring staff, and neonate's family is mandatory, along with audit for evaluation and improvement of the service. Efficiency and effectiveness measures should be assessed after each transport.

19.2 Introduction

Neonatal transfer is necessary when a newborn baby needs care that cannot be provided in the referral center. Since it represents an additional risk factor for a critically ill neonate (Arora et al. 2014; Lim and Ratnavel 2008), it should be performed, when possible, by a well-organized neonatal transport service.

In a network, aimed at the regionalization of perinatal care, high-risk pregnancies should be transferred "in utero" in order to minimize risks for both mother and neonate (Arora et al. 2014; Kollèe et al. 1992). However, there will always be a number of neonates who need to be transferred for unpredicted or unpredictable reasons (Finnstrom et al. 1997). Every maternity unit should therefore be able to provide effective neonatal resuscitation in the delivery room, be able to maintain a sick baby in a stable condition in the short term, and have access to a neonatal emergency transport service (NETS) for the provision of neonatal intensive care when appropriate. Thus, NETS provides a bridge between birth centers and neonatal intensive care units (NICUs).

19.3 NETS: A Mission Statement

NETS should aim to guarantee:

- Optimal care for every neonate in the most appropriate location
- Safe and quick transport with minimization of risk
- Good communication between transport team, parents, and centers involved
- Rational resource use with optimized cost-benefit ratio
- An outreach education program relating to resuscitation and pre-transport stabilization
- Guidelines for referral centers and transport personnel

The establishment of a NETS therefore requires planning and organization. There should be regular auditing to monitor its efficiency and effectiveness (see ▸ Chap. 18, "Organization of Perinatal Care: Training of Doctors and Nurses").

19.4 Organization

The organization of a NETS should be appropriate to the needs and characteristics of the region covered and resources available. Account should be taken of:

- Demography (birth rate and distribution)
- Place, number, and levels of perinatal units
- Number of transports per year and patient flow between centers
- Neonatal transport index (NTI; see below)
- Available economic resources, personnel, vehicles, and equipment
- Regular clinical audits

There are different models of perinatal networks for the provision of the most appropriate service. The choice between the two models in terms of cost-benefit ratio depends mainly on the number of transports per year and on the referral area (Agostino et al. 1998, 1999), as follows:

- *Dedicated service*: all transports carried out by a team devoted full time to this service. The optimal number of transports per year is 400–600. Fewer than 400 increase costs and more than 600 decrease efficiency.
- *On-call service*: in this organizational model, transports integrated into the overall activity of an individual NICU and carried out by "in-house" personnel. The optimal number of transports per year to minimize costs and maximize efficiency is 150–200.

The characteristics of each model are summarized in Table 1. In Europe, the most usual models for regional networks are dedicated or on-call NETS.

The NTI is an expression of the number of neonates transferred per 100 live births. This index can be used to compare the flow of newborns between facilities in each area. A low NTI

Table 1 Characteristics of the two NETS models

	Dedicated	On-call
Activation times	Usually shorter	Usually longer
Availability	Around the clock	Available on-call
Distances covered	Longer	Shorter
Area covered	Usually larger	Usually smaller
Receiving center	All NICUs (interfacility transports)	Only NICU where NETS is based
Individual-specific transport expertise	More, because mainly appointed to transport service	Less, because temporarily detached from NICU
Costs	More expensive	Less expensive

(around 1%) indicates a good distribution of perinatal facilities and well-organized maternal-neonatal transport services. Programs of regionalization of high-risk perinatal care, in the past years, have been effective in reducing NTI in most of European countries (Kempley et al. 2007; Zeitlin et al. 2004; Neto 2006).

To account for regional diversity, it is also possible to organize a network with more than one type of NETS.

19.5 NETS Coordinating Center

Each regional network should ideally have a NETS coordinating center. Its role is to:

- Triage requests for transfers.
- Monitor cot availability and find appropriate cots.
- Activate the appropriate transport team and coordinate the transfer.
- Prioritize simultaneous requests.
- Give advice to referring clinicians and to the transport team.
- Supervise staff, plan audits, and education.
- Ensure the provision of appropriate resources.

19.6 Types of Transfers

Transfers can be classified on the basis of the degree of emergency and destination:

- Acute:
  - Primary transfers: to a NICU or a higher level center, depending on the requirement for intensive or high dependency care
  - Intertertiary: between NICUs, if there is a lack of cots or the need for surgical or specialized care
- Elective:
  - Back transports: usually from a NICU to the local hospital, when a neonate is stable, to maintain the availability NICU cots and minimize costs and discomfort for families (Argus et al. 2009)
  - Return transfers: for diagnostic investigations (e.g., MRI) or procedures (laser treatment for ROP)

19.7 Transport Process

The transport process (Table 2) starts with a request for transfer by the referring center. Each transport should be coordinated by the coordinating center or by a senior neonatologist at the admitting center.

19.7.1 Triage and Cot Search

When the coordinating center (or the transport team) receives the transfer request from the referral center, severity and requirements of infant conditions should be appropriately assessed and an initial transport plan formulated. Level and characteristics of admitting hospital, road, vehicles, and personnel needed should be identified. Prioritization of simultaneous transfer requests has to be performed adopting validated scoring systems. The Mortality Index for Neonatal

Table 2 Transport process

Events	Operative approach
Request for transfer	Discussion, triage, advice and support for referring center, plan of action
Cot search	Finding the most appropriate cot and activation of the transport team
Transport team departs from base hospital	Continuing advice and support for the referring center, which is responsible for pre-transport stabilization
Transport team at the referring hospital	Assessment and further stabilization prior to transport
Transfer of the baby to admitting hospital	Monitoring, continuous assessment, specific treatment if needed
Transport team at the admitting hospital	Final assessment, hand over to admitting team
Transport team returns to base hospital	Check and replacement of used equipment and medical gases, communicate new availability

Table 3 Mortality Index for Neonatal Transportation (MINT) score. (Modified from Broughton et al. 2004)

Parameter	Value	MINT score points
pH	<6.9	10
	6.91–7.1	4
	>7.1	0
Age	0–1 h	4
	>1 h	0
Apgar score at 1 min	0	8
	1	5
	2	2
	3	2
	>3	0
Birth weight	<750 g	5
	751–1,000 g	2
	1,001–1,500 g	1
	>1,500 g	0
PaO_2	≤3 kPa (≤22,56 mmHg)	2
	>3 kPa (>22,56 mmHg)	0
Congenital abnormality	Yes	5
	No	0
Intubated at time of call	Yes	6
	No	0

Transportation (MINT) score (Table 3) is a validated, easy-to-use mortality prediction score for retrieved neonates, which can be used to determine priority of request and resource allocations (Broughton et al. 2004). All of the data used in the MINT score can be collected at the time of the telephone call requesting transfer. Particular attention should be given to the evaluation of requests of transfer for patients with unconfirmed diagnosis or need for specialized care and treatments (i.e., in the suspect of hypoxic-ischemic encephalopathy (HIE), congenital heart disease (CHD), or surgical conditions).

Systems ensuring the online monitoring of NICU and surgical cots available in the area covered can help to reduce activation times.

19.7.2 Patient Stabilization

It is important that staff at the referring hospital should be able to perform basic resuscitation and stabilization before the arrival of the transport team. It has been shown how birth and stabilization in a tertiary center can improve outcomes (Gente et al. 2015). An epidemiological analysis of 1,495 infants transported in Lazio region (Italy) showed that factors that significantly increased stabilization time were the lower gestational age, the lower level of care of the referring hospital, the medical reason for transport (compared to surgical), and the location of the referring hospital outside the main city area (Di Lallo et al. 2010).

The baby's clinical condition should be carefully evaluated to establish the initial diagnosis and a therapeutic plan. Stabilization involves basic physiological support and is defined as the treatment or correction of those processes which, if not addressed, may lead to deterioration in the baby's condition. After stabilization, preparations for transfer are started. These include ensuring that physiological parameters are satisfactory, that airway and vascular access are secure, and that appropriate monitoring is in place. Insufficient attention to resuscitation and stabilization may result in clinical deterioration during the transfer, and the environment during transport (limited space, vibration, noise, etc.) is not conducive to optimal patient care (Arora et al. 2014; Lim and Ratnavel 2008; Bouchut et al. 2011, Karlsson et al. 2012).

19.7.3 Personnel

The choice of personnel for a transport team varies widely between NETS, depending on organizational preferences, budgets, and availability of professional groups (Agostino et al. 1998; Lupton and Pendray 2004). The traditional view that a neonatologist and a nurse should constitute a neonatal transport team is no longer generally accepted. Retrieval teams with different professional backgrounds do not appear to affect the outcome of transports (Leslie and Stephenson 2003; Morrison and Cheema 2007). The nature of the professional background of transport team members is less important than training in transport practice with specific core competencies (Fenton and Leslie 2009). Poor transport experience reduces quality of NETS (Macnab 1991). Time devoted to stabilization of the neonate prior to transport increases with operator experience (James 1993). There should be regular rotation of personnel between NICU and the transport service to prevent burnout and allow for professional updating.

19.7.4 Equipment

Equipment taken on transfer needs to be suitable for a variety of babies, from the extremely low birth weight to term, and for the range of medical or surgical problems that require different therapies in transit. The transport itself requires a transport incubator system with a mechanical ventilator, infusion pumps, suction pump, and monitors (Fig. 1). A neonatal resuscitation kit, including drugs, should be carried in a separate bag.

Equipment should be dedicated exclusively for neonatal transport, to ensure its ready availability and that the battery is fully charged. Some recommendations have been provided by the European Committee for Standardization (European Committee for Standardization 2003a, b). Difficult working conditions and mechanical stresses, caused by vibrations and sudden forceful impact, mean that equipment should be checked and tested regularly. Staff should be trained in their use and should be aware of the more frequent minor causes of malfunctioning so they are able to fix them.

19.7.5 Road and Vehicles

The choice of road and vehicle should aim to guarantee the quickest, safest, and most comfortable transport for the baby, taking account of clinical conditions, regional geography, and weather, road, and traffic conditions (Sedin et al. 1999). Different scenarios should be considered and guidelines prepared to determine the choice of vehicle and appropriate response to emergency situations. Vehicles that can be used by NETS are ambulance, helicopter, and fixed wing aircraft. Ambulances are most commonly used because of lower costs, universal availability, short activation times, and the possibility of reaching hospitals directly. Dedicated vehicles guarantee shorter activation times and better compatibility between equipment. Air transport, including by helicopter, is indicated for longer

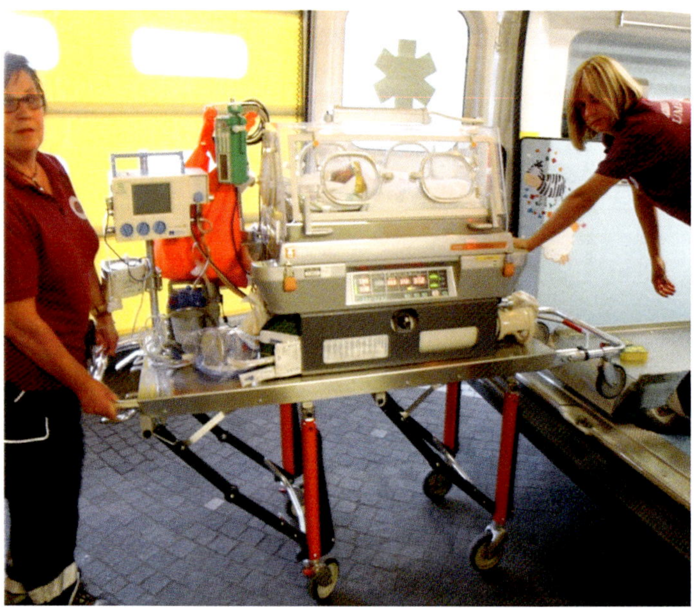

Fig. 1 Transport incubator system

distances and for regions with poor weather conditions during winter or peculiar geographic characteristics (e.g., mountain regions). Account should also be taken of the possible need for an additional ambulance journey, depending on whether there are facilities for landing at the hospital. Air transport is characterized by the presence of high noise and vibration levels and changes in gas pressures, temperatures, humidity, and gravitational forces that may affect care and possibly worsen the condition of the critically ill neonate and, for these reasons, should only be performed by specifically trained personnel (Bouchut et al. 2011; Karlsson et al. 2012; Jackson and Skeoch 2009). Global positioning systems (GPS) on vehicles allow the coordinating center to monitor and localize their positions and eventually redirect the team to a different destination in case of emergencies or change of priorities.

19.8 Challenging Situations During Neonatal Transport

Critically ill infants with special requirements that until a few years ago were to be considered as "untransportable," or should have discontinued special treatments during transport, nowadays, can be safely transported with a similar level of care provided in a NICU. A few of these situations, along with some of the most challenging scenarios to be faced by a NETS team, are depicted below.

19.8.1 Surgical Conditions

Ideally, pregnant women with antenatally diagnosed congenital surgical conditions should deliver in a tertiary level center with the availability of a pediatric surgery. However, for sometime unpredictable reasons (i.e., undiagnosed conditions, preterm labor), births of infants with surgical conditions in non-tertiary centers continue to occur.

Management of the surgical neonates requires a multidisciplinary approach with support of multiple experts. Continuous advice from the coordinating center and the pediatric surgeons of the receiving center should be guaranteed. Few basic considerations about the most common surgical conditions are summarized in Table 3 (Puri and Doodnath 2011). For further indications, please refer to the chapters in the books dedicated to the mentioned surgical condition.

19.8.2 Duct-Dependent Congenital Heart Disease (CHD)

Differential diagnosis and treatment plan in case of a suspected duct-dependent CHD represent one of the most challenging dilemmas to solve for the NETS team and the coordinating center. For infants born in centers without the availability of a pediatric cardiologist consultation, a first telephone triage should be performed, using the available tools as the Simplified Congenital heart disease-Oriented for Urgencies and emergencies Triage (SCOUT) system (Warren et al. 2001).

Transport team at the referring center has to distinguish a duct-dependent CHD from other conditions (i.e., persistent pulmonary hypertension of the newborn (PPHN), non-duct-dependent CHD, severe sepsis) and take the decision to start or not to start treatment with prostaglandin E1, relying often only on a clinical basis. Accuracy of clinical diagnosis in identifying CHD by NETS team varies from 77% to 88% depending on authors (Shivananda et al. 2010; Gupta et al. 2014). A recent study, who retrospectively analyzed 144 newborns with suspected CHD, showed how combined clinical findings, chest X-rays, SpO_2 and blood gases may assist in the diagnosis of duct-dependent CHD. Labile saturation and mean blood arterial pressure at referral <40 mmHg were the only significant predictors of non-duct-dependent CHD at the multivariate analysis; meanwhile none of the clinical factors considered were significantly associated with duct-dependent CHD on multivariate analysis. The authors conclude that in the absence of a reliable single clinical discriminator, prostaglandin E1 should be used when duct-dependent CHD is suspected (Gupta et al. 2014). For detailed information about diagnosis, stabilization, and preoperative management of infants with CHD, PGE1 indications, and adverse effects, please refer to ▶ Chaps. 67, "Cardiovascular Physiology, Pathology, and Clinical Investigation in Neonatal Medicine," and ▶ 68, "Early Diagnosis of Congenital Heart Disease: When and How to Treat" of this book.

19.8.3 Persistent Pulmonary Hypertension of the Newborn (PPHN)

Infants with clinical suspect or diagnosis of persistent pulmonary hypertension of the newborn (PPHN) can be treated and transported following current evidences and recommendations (Dhillon 2012; Steinhorn 2010). Infants should be intubated, ventilated (HFOV can be beneficial), and sedated. A central line should be positioned at the referring center. Oxygen therapy should be targeted to maintain pre-ductal $SpO_2 \geq 94\%$. If necessary, consider inotropes to maintain mean blood pressure about 55–60 mmHg and fluids to increase preload.

Inhaled nitric oxide (iNO) therapy should be started if severe hypoxia is present. The use of iNO therapy during transport has been described by several authors (Lowe and Trautwein 2007; Lutman and Petros 2008; Gaddam Bhoomaiah et al. 2014). The use of intravenous vasodilators as PGE1 has been also described during transport of infants with PPHN (Gupta et al. 2013). Transportation of infants on extracorporeal membrane oxygenation (ECMO) can be performed by specialized ECMO teams, when critical hypoxemic infants are not responsive to treatment (Broman et al. 2015; Rambaud et al. 2016). Refer to ▶ Chaps. 60, "Persistent Pulmonary Hypertension of the Newborn," ▶ 61, "Pulmonary Hypertension in Congenital Diaphragmatic Hernia," and ▶ 64, "Extracorporeal Membrane Oxygenation for Neonates" for further information about PPHN and iNO therapy.

19.8.4 Neonates with Hypoxic-Ischemic Encephalopathy (HIE) Requiring Hypothermia

Randomized controlled trials involving term and near-term infants with evidence of perinatal asphyxia showed how moderate hypothermia (33–34 °C), if started within 6 h after delivery, reduced the risk of death and disabilities at 18–24 months of age and improved neurocognitive outcome in middle childhood (Jacobs et al. 2013; Azzopardi et al. 2014).

Therefore, cooling should be initiated for neonates with GA ≥35 weeks with evidence of perinatal asphyxia and moderate or severe HIE that meet the eligibility criteria for therapeutic hypothermia (as specifically defined and adapted by each center or network) and they should be transferred to referral specialized centers for hypothermia as soon as possible (within 6 h after birth).

Referring centers, after confirming with the NETS coordinating center infant's eligibility criteria, should immediately start passive cooling, turning the warmer off, undressing, and monitoring infant's temperature, aiming at a target temperature of 35 °C, meanwhile waiting for the NETS team.

The coordinating center and NETS team should provide advice to the referring center and give priority to transports of HIE neonates, transferring them to the referral center within the shortest time possible.

NETS team at the referring center should provide further metabolic (correct acidosis and deficits), cardiocirculatory (guarantee a venous access, fluid restriction, monitor blood pressure and diuresis), and respiratory (avoid hypocapnia) stabilization, if needed. Treatment for seizures should be avoided, unless strictly necessary, for its possible interference with the EEG evaluation at the referral center. Fentanest and Midazolam can be used, if required. Eligibility criteria should be rechecked, and parental informed consent to therapeutic hypothermia should be collected.

During transport a target rectal temperature of 35 °C should be maintained, using passive or active cooling (applying cold packs in the incubator or using servo-controlled cooling systems). Continuous ECG and temperature monitoring by a rectal probe are mandatory to avoid severe hypo thermia (32–33 °C) and bradycardia (heart rate <80 bpm).

Both processes of active and passive cooling have been used and described during neonatal transport (Kendall et al. 2010; Chaudhary et al. 2013; Akula et al. 2015).

Please refer to the dedicated chapters in the book for more information about stabilization of infants with HIE and treatment with hypothermia.

19.8.5 Severe Hyperbilirubinemia

Whenever possible, it should be avoided to suspend phototherapy during neonatal transport, for neonates with severe unconjugated hyperbilirubinemia at risk of developing bilirubin encephalopathy. The adoption of a portable phototherapy unit during transport has been showed to be safe and effective and may result in a decreased requirement for exchange transfusion (Waterham et al. 2016).

19.9 Family-Centered Care

Good communication among team members and transport team, referring staff, and neonate's family is mandatory. Transferring a neonate in a center different from the birthplace means a disruption of the familiar unity and of the ongoing mother/father-baby bonding. Parents should be encouraged to see the baby before transportation and during stabilization and to visit the receiving hospital as soon as it will be possible, considering also maternal conditions.

Informed signed parental consent to transportation and emergency procedure foreseen to be performed should be requested (i.e., blood transfusion, emergency surgical procedures).

Baby's pictures in the receiving center should be taken and showed to the mother. She should be also encouraged to express her milk with breast pump to promote lactation and to include her in the caring process of the neonate.

In case of a multiple birth, especially if neonates are at risks of prolonged hospitalizations, every effort should be performed to admit all siblings in the same hospital. This would reduce parental stress, avoiding frequent trips between hospitals, in an already difficult situation. Whenever this would not be possible, siblings should be reunited in the same center as soon as their condition will be stable enough (Mosher 2013).

19.10 Quality Evaluation and Costs

Audit is essential for the evaluation and improvement of the service (Leslie and Stephenson 1997, 1994). Data collection should include demographics, staffing, pre- and intra-transport times, as well as clinical parameters (Table 4).

NETS availability and time required can be considered as indicators of efficiency (Ramnarayan 2009). Time investment includes:

1. The response time (period between call for transport and departure for referring hospital)
2. The waiting time (time between call for transport and arrival at referring hospital)
3. The stabilization time (time required to assist neonate at referring hospital)
4. "On-the-road" time (time with baby in transport between departure from referring unit to admission at receiving hospital)
5. The total transfer time (from departure, to referring hospital, to the availability of the team for another transfer)

Measures of effectiveness can be based on changes in the infant's core temperature during transfer, validated transport scores (Hermansen et al. 1998; Zupancic et al. 2007; Lee et al. 2001), and monitoring complications during transport. The Transport Risk Index of Physiologic Stability (TRIPS) score is a validated and reliable tool used to assess effectiveness of transport services, protocols, and policies (Lee et al. 2001) (Table 5).

The annual budget for running a NETS includes fixed and variable costs. Fixed costs are independent of the number of the transports and include equipment amortization, insurance cover, training and education, organization, and communication. Variable costs depend on the number of

Table 4 Stabilization and management of neonates with surgical conditions prior to and during transport to a referral center (Puri and Doodnath 2011)

Surgical condition	Stabilization and management prior to and during transport
Gastroschisis	Keep baby warm and monitor incubator's temperature (higher risk for hypothermia). Assess and treat respiratory distress. Intravenous fluids and correct deficits. To minimize heat loss and trauma, exposed viscera should be placed in clear plastic bag or silo. If not available, localize loops in the center of the abdomen and use cling film to encircle the exposed intestine and wrap film around infant. Nasogastric tube, antibiotics, vitamin K
Omphalocele	Assess and treat respiratory distress. Stabilize the sac in the middle of the abdomen, and cover it with a sterile, dry, nonadherent dressing to prevent trauma, heat loss, and vessels kinking. If the sac is a ruptured sac, treat as it for gastroschisis. Nasogastric tube, intravenous fluids, antibiotics, vitamin K
Pierre Robin syndrome	Place infant in prone position and insert an oropharyngeal airway to prevent tongue swallowing and asphyxiation
Choanal atresia	Secure in place an oral airway (appropriately sized, with the end or teeth cut off to keep the mouth open) to prevent intermittent hypoxia
Myelomeningocele	Place infant in prone position to prevent trauma and pressure on the spinal area. Place a warm, sterile, saline-soaked dressing over the lesion and cling film wrapped around the baby to prevent drying and dehiscence. If the sac is ruptured and CSF leaking, or if myelomeningocele is open, cover with Betadine-soaked gauze and start intravenous antibiotics. Prevent fecal contamination in sacral lesions. Evaluate and document neurological function, including sensorimotor level and degree of hydrocephalus
Bladder exstrophy	Remove umbilical clamp and ligate umbilical cord close to the abdominal wall to prevent mechanical damage. Cover the defect with cling film wrapped around the baby to avoid the mucosa from sticking to clothes. Wash the surface of the bladder with warm saline at each diaper change, and apply a clean cling film layer. Prophylactic antibiotics
Esophageal atresia with tracheoesophageal fistula	Intubation and ventilation if required (tip of the ET tube should be placed proximal to the carina but distal to the fistula). Handle with care and avoid crying to reduce risk of aspiration and abdominal distension. Provide oxygen if necessary. Place infant with head slightly elevated, prone, or in a right lateral position. The upper esophageal pouch should be kept empty positioning a Replogle sump catheter connected to low-intermittent or low-continuous suction (irrigate to prevent blockage by mucus). Intravenous fluids and electrolytes to compensate esophageal secretion losses. Antibiotics, vitamin K
Congenital diaphragmatic hernia	Avoid mask ventilation. Perform intubation and initiate gentle ventilation (risk of barotraumas due to hypoplastic lungs). Sedation and HFOV (if available) can help to reduce barotrauma. Prevent pulmonary hypertension (hyperventilate, low pressures, high oxygen, correct acidosis, prevent thermal and metabolic stress). Insert a nasogastric tube to prevent lung compression. Administer intravenous fluids to maintain adequate peripheral perfusion (consider inotropes, if necessary), maintain warm environment, check arterial pre-ductal blood gases, and administer antibiotics and vitamin K. Exclude pneumothorax in case of acute deterioration
Intestinal obstruction	Same principles of care, irrespective of level and cause of obstruction: decompress bowel and prevent aspiration, correct fluid losses, and prevent heath loss. Insert a nasogastric tube, and suction every 15–30 min. Correct electrolyte, acid-base, and volume deficits. Prophylactic antibiotics
Necrotizing enterocolitis	Ensure appropriate infant's stabilization. IPPV is often required. Correct shock and acidosis if present, monitor blood pressure and blood glucose, nasogastric tube, antibiotics

transports and include supplies, equipment maintenance, and ambulance expenses. Personnel salaries depend on the type of NETS: in the "dedicated" model, this is a fixed cost, whereas in the "on-call" model, it affects both fixed costs (depending on availability) and variable costs (actual hours). The total cost of the NETS and the average cost of each transport depend on the fixed and variable costs, which in turn depend on the organizational model adopted and the load of scheduled jobs (Agostino et al. 1998).

19.11 Training and Outreach Education

Continued improvement of perinatal outcomes depends on all health professionals recognizing their responsibility to keep up to date with recent advances in perinatal care, by updating their knowledge and clinical skills. Transport personnel must receive appropriate training and supervision. Core competencies include clinical, procedural, communication, and teamwork skills and the ability to work in the transport environment (Fenton and Leslie 2009). Continuing education in neonatal transport involves training and supervision of all members of the transport team. It relates not only to clinical care but also to safety and communication, as well as to administrative and other relevant topics. Extending continuing education throughout the referral region (outreach education) is also important for the health-care professionals responsible for referring and stabilizing infants for transport (Agostino et al. 1998).

19.12 Future Perspectives of NETS

Neonatal transport equipment has been massively improving over the years, and nowadays dedicated ambulances can be considered as proper mobile NICUs (Whyte et al. 2015).

The goal is a further reduction of number and rates of infants transported and promoting "in utero" transfer of high-risk pregnancies, when indicated. As already seen for certain branches, programs of outreach medical and surgical specialized care should be planned and implemented (Maka et al. 2015; Huang et al. 2008).

Personnel should be trained to face with the worst scenarios. High-fidelity simulation, even if different from the "live setting," can help to train less-experienced personnel to deal with clinical and environmental difficult situations.

Clinical computerized notes, containing images and videos of patient and exams, that can be shared, updated, and seen on smartphones or tablets "on the road" could represent the future of neonatal transport in higher-resource settings.

Table 5 Transport Risk Index of Physiologic Stability (TRIPS) score. (Modified from Lee et al. 2001)

Parameter	Value	TRIPS score points
Temperature (°C)	<36.1 or >37.6	8
	36.1–36.5 or 37.2–37.6	1
	36.6–37.1	0
Respiratory status	Severe (apnea, gasping, intubated)	14
	Moderate (RR >60/min and/or SpO_2 <85 %)	5
	None (RR <60/min and SpO_2 >85 %)	0
Systolic blood pressure (mmHg)	<20	26
	20–40	16
	>40	0
Response to painful stimuli	None, seizure, muscle relaxant	17
	Lethargic response, no cry	6
	Withdraws vigorously, cries	0

RR respiratory rate, *SpO_2* pulse oximetry

References

Agostino R, Chabernaud JL, Di Renzo GC (1998) Neonatal transport service, types, cost/benefit ratio, indicators of efficiency and effectiveness. Dev Physiopathol Clin 8:113–115

Agostino R, Fenton AC, Kollée LAA et al (1999) Organization of neonatal transport in Europe. Prenat Neonatal Med 4:20–34

Akula VP, Joe P, Thusu K et al (2015) A randomized clinical trial of therapeutic hypothermia mode during transport for neonatal encephalopathy. J Pediatr 166:856–861

Argus BM, Dawson JA, Wong C et al (2009) Financial costs for parents with a baby in a neonatal nursery. J Paediatr Child Health 45:514–517

Arora P, Bajaj M, Natarajan G et al (2014) Impact of interhospital transport on the physiologic status of very low-birth-weight infants. Am J Perinatol 31:237–244

Azzopardi D, Strohm B, Marlow N et al (2014) Effects of hypothermia for perinatal asphyxia on childhood outcomes. N Engl J Med 371:140–149

Bouchut JC, Van Lancker E, Chritin V et al (2011) Physical stressors during neonatal transport: helicopter compared with ground ambulance. Air Med J 30:134–139

Broman LM, Holzgraefe B, Palmér K et al (2015) The Stockholm experience: interhospital transports on extracorporeal membrane oxygenation. Crit Care 19:278

Broughton SJ, Berry A, Jacobe S et al (2004) The mortality index for neonatal transportation score: a new mortality prediction model for retrieved neonates. Pediatrics 114: e424–e428

Chaudhary R, Farrer K, Broster S et al (2013) Active versus passive cooling during neonatal transport. Pediatrics 132:841–846

Dhillon R (2012) The management of neonatal pulmonary hypertension. Arch Dis Child Fetal Neonatal Ed 97: F223–F228

Di Lallo D, Franco F, Farchi S et al (2010) Pre-transport stabilization time and characteristics of the referring hospital: an epidemiological study on neonatal transport in Lazio. Eur J Public Health 20:118

European Committee for Standardization (2003a) EN 13976-1:2003 rescue systems – transportation of incubators – part 1: interface conditions (harmonised standard under the Directive 93/42/EEC)

European Committee for Standardization (2003b) EN 13976-2:2003 rescue systems – transportation of incubators – part 2: system requirements (harmonised standard under the Directive 93/42/EEC)

Fenton AC, Leslie A (2009) Who should staff neonatal transport teams? Early Hum Dev 85:487–490

Finnstrom O, Otterblad Olausson P, Sedin G et al (1997) The Swedish national prospective study on extremely low birth weight (ELBW) infants. Incidence, mortality, and survival in relation to level of care. Acta Paediatr 86:503–511

Gaddam Bhoomaiah S, Chandra P, Leslie A (2014) Inhaled nitric oxide therapy during transport of neonates – experience of CenTre transport service. Arch Dis Child Fetal Neonatal Ed 99:A44

Gente M, Di Lallo D, Franco F et al (2015) Stabilization of the critically ill neonate awaiting transport. Ital J Pediatr 41(Suppl1):A15

Gupta N, Kamlin CO, Cheung M et al (2013) Prostaglandin E1 use during neonatal transfer: potential beneficial role in persistent pulmonary hypertension of the newborn. Arch Dis Child Fetal Neonatal Ed 98:F186

Gupta N, Kamlin CO, Cheung M et al (2014) Improving diagnostic accuracy in the transport of infants with suspected duct-dependent congenital heart disease. J Paediatr Child Health 50:64–70

Hermansen MC, Hasan S, Hoppin J et al (1998) A validation of a scoring system to evaluate the condition of transported very low birth weight neonates. Am J Perinatol 5:74–78

Huang T, Moon-Grady AJ, Traugott C et al (2008) The availability of telecardiology consultations and transfer patterns from a remote neonatal intensive care unit. J Telemed Telecare 14:244–248

Jackson L, Skeoch CH (2009) Setting up a neonatal transport service: air transport. Early Hum Dev 85:477–481

Jacobs SE, Berg M, Hunt R et al (2013) Cooling for newborns with hypoxic ischaemic encephalopathy. Cochrane Database Syst Rev 1:CD003311

James AG (1993) Resuscitation, stabilization, and transport in perinatology. Curr Opin Pediatr 5:150–155

Karlsson BM, Lindkvist M, Lindkvist M et al (2012) Sound and vibration: effects on infants' heart rate and heart rate variability during neonatal transport. Acta Paediatr 101:148–154

Kempley ST, Baki Y, Hayter G et al (2007) Effect of a centralized transfer service on characteristics of interhospital neonatal transfers. Arch Dis Child Fetal Neonatal Ed 92:F185–F188

Kendall GS, Kapetanakis A, Ratnavel N et al (2010) Cooling on Retrieval Study Group: passive cooling for initiation of therapeutic hypothermia in neonatal encephalopathy. Arch Dis Child Fetal Neonatal Ed 95:F408–F412

Kollèe LA, Brand R, Schreuder A et al (1992) Five-year outcome of preterm and very low birth weight infants: a comparison between maternal and neonatal transport. Obstet Gynecol 80:635–638

Lee SK, Zupancic JA, Pendray M et al (2001) Transport risk index of physiologic stability: a practical system for assessing infant transport care. J Pediatr 139:220–226

Leslie AJ, Stephenson TJ (1994) Audit of neonatal intensive care transport. Arch Dis Child 71:F61–F66

Leslie AJ, Stephenson TJ (1997) Audit of neonatal intensive care transport – closing the loop. Acta Paediatr 86:1253–1256

Leslie A, Stephenson T (2003) Neonatal transfers by advanced neonatal nurse practitioners and paediatric registrars. Arch Dis Child Fetal Neonatal Ed 88: F509–F512

Lim MT, Ratnavel N (2008) A prospective review of adverse events during interhospital transfers of neonates by a dedicated neonatal transfer service. Pediatr Crit Care Med 9:289–293
Lowe CG, Trautwein JG (2007) Inhaled nitric oxide therapy during the transport of neonates with persistent pulmonary hypertension or severe hypoxic respiratory failure. Eur J Pediatr 166:1025–1031
Lupton BA, Pendray MR (2004) Regionalized neonatal emergency transport. Semin Neonatol 9:125–133
Lutman D, Petros A (2008) Inhaled nitric oxide in neonatal and paediatric transport. Early Hum Dev 84:725–729
Macnab A (1991) Optimal escort for interhospital transport of pediatric emergencies. J Trauma 31:205–209
Maka E, Imre L, Somogyvári Z et al (2015) Laser treatment for retinopathy of prematurity in neonatal intensive care units. Premature Eye Rescue Program. Orv Hetil 156:192–196
Morrison J, Cheema I (2007) Neonatal transfers by advanced neonatal nurse practitioners: is it time to end the debate? Early Hum Dev 83:134
Mosher SL (2013) The art of supporting families faced with neonatal transport. Nurs Womens Health 17:198–209
Neto MT (2006) Perinatal care in Portugal: effects of 15 years of a regionalized system. Acta Paediatr 95:1349–1352
Puri P, Doodnath R (2011) Transport of the surgical neonate in "Newborn Surgery 3E" Prem Puri. CRC Press, Boca Raton, pp 83–90
Rambaud J, Léger PL, Larroquet M et al (2016) Transportation of children on extracorporeal membrane oxygenation: one-year experience of the first neonatal and paediatric mobile ECMO team in the north of France. Intensive Care Med 42:940–941
Ramnarayan P (2009) Measuring the performance of an inter-hospital transport service. Arch Dis Child 94:414–416
Sedin G, Agostino R, Chabernaud JL et al (1999) Technical aspects of neonatal transport in Europe. Prenat Neonatal Med 4:35–45
Shivananda S, Kirsh J, Whyte HE et al (2010) Accuracy of clinical diagnosis and decision to commence intravenous prostaglandin E1 in neonates presenting with hypoxemia in a transport setting. J Crit Care 25(174): e1–e9
Steinhorn RH (2010) Neonatal pulmonary hypertension. Pediatr Crit Care Med 11:S79–S84
Warren D, Jarvis A, Leblanc L et al (2001) Canadian paediatric triage and acuity scale: implementation guidelines for emergency departments. CJEM 3: S1–S27
Waterham M, Bhatia R, Donath S et al (2016) Phototherapy in transport for neonates with unconjugated hyperbilirubinaemia. J Paediatr Child Health 52:67–71
Whyte HEA, Jefferies AL, Canadian Paediatric Society, Fetus and Newborn Committee (2015) The interfacility transport of critically ill newborns. Paediatr Child Health 20:265–275
Zeitlin J, Papiernik E, Bréart G et al (2004) Regionalization of perinatal care in Europe. Semin Neonatol 9:99–110
Zupancic JA, Richardson DK, Horbar JD et al (2007) Revalidation of the score for neonatal acute physiology in the Vermont Oxford network. Pediatrics 119: e156–e163

Risk Management of Newborns

20

Isabelle Ligi and Sophie Tardieu

Contents

Abstract

Neonates are highly vulnerable to iatrogenesis owing to their immaturity and an important exposure to invasive therapies. Recent studies highlight the problem in terms of financial, medicolegal, and particularly human costs. The concept of clinical risk management evolved from industry to assess and reduce

I. Ligi (✉)
Division of Neonatology, La Conception Hospital, Marseille, France
e-mail: Isabelle.ligi@ap-hm.fr

S. Tardieu
Medical Evaluation Department, Public Health Department, La Conception Hospital, Marseille, France

G. Buonocore et al. (eds.), *Neonatology*,
https://doi.org/10.1007/978-3-319-29489-6_170

the risk and finally to improve patient safety. In complex and multifaceted systems like neonatal intensive care units, incident occurrence is often multifactorial and reveals system failures rather than individual error. The identification of incidents by voluntary, anonymous, and nonpunitive reporting system followed by a causation analysis is a major step to risk assessment and prevention. But risk management is first of all a behavior based on culture safety and leadership.

List of Abbreviations

CPOE	Computerized provider order entry
FMEA	Failure mode and effects analysis
IE	Iatrogenic event
ME	Medication error
NICU	Neonatal intensive care unit

20.1 Salient Points

- Neonatology is a high-risk speciality for iatrogenesis.
- Risk management is a structured process that can improve quality of health.
- Nosocomial infections and unplanned extubations are severe iatrogenic events; medication errors and cutaneous injuries are common but usually trivial.
- Many tools have been developed to assess risk.
- Incident reporting systems and causation analysis are key components of risk management.
- Leadership is critical to promote patient safety and create a safety culture.

20.2 Introduction

Rapid advances in neonatal medicine have caused a substantial reduction in neonatal mortality, especially in low birth weight babies. However, caring for newborn infants in the neonatal intensive care unit (NICU) exposes them to invasive therapies and therefore to iatrogenic damage. Moreover, NICU is a complex system with an environment of continuous and emergency care prone to error. Iatrogenesis is defined as an unintended harm or suffering arising from any aspect of health-care management (Thomas et al. 2000). The report To Err Is Human by the Institute of Medicine revealed the importance of medical errors in terms of patient harm, death, and cost in the USA (Kohn et al. 1999). Despite newborn infants constituting a high-risk population, data are still scarce. Incidence of iatrogenesis varies strongly between studies according to the methods of data collection and the definition used, but recent prospective studies have reported high incidences of 0.4–0.74 iatrogenic events (IEs) per patient (Ligi et al. 2008; Sharek et al. 2006; Kugelman et al. 2008; Frey et al. 2000). Many iatrogenic events result in permanent harm and more than a third is considered to be preventable (Ligi et al. 2008; Sharek et al. 2006; Kugelman et al. 2008). They have huge financial, human, and medicolegal costs for the patient, their families, and the staff (Kohn et al. 1999; Donn 2005).

In response to improve patient safety, the concepts and practice of risk management evolved during the last decade. Clinical risk management can be defined as organizational systems or processes that aim to improve the quality of health care and maintain safe systems of care (Scholefield 2005). It is based on a system approach, rather than an individual approach to error, taking account that human beings are fallible and that IE occurrence is a consequence of a successive lost of protective defenses, barriers, and safeguards (Reason 2000). That is why risk management is an ongoing process based on attitude (awareness of potential risk and liability), the knowledge, and understanding of hazards, skills, and commitment.

20.3 Epidemiology of Iatrogenesis in Neonatology

20.3.1 Definitions of Patient Safety Terms

Many definitions are commonly used in the patient safety literature. Using precise definitions helps interpreting the findings in the studies as there is no standardized nomenclature.

Error: a failure of a planned action to be completed as intended or use of a wrong plan to achieve an aim (Kohn et al. 1999).

Serious medical error: a medical error that could harm or injure a vulnerable patient if it reached the patient uninterrupted (Morriss 2008).

Adverse (medical) event: an injury caused by medical management rather than the underlying condition of the patient (Kohn et al. 1999).

IE: any event that compromised the safety of the patient in the presence or the absence of harm. It may or may not have been preventable and may or may not have involved an error by the health-care team (Ligi et al. 2008).

Critical incident: any event which could have reduced, or did reduce, the safety margin for the patient (Frey et al. 2000).

Severe IE: any unintended injury or complication that resulted in disability, death, or extended hospital stay and which was caused by health-care management.

Preventable IE: any avoidable iatrogenic event based on available knowledge and accepted practices (Woods et al. 2005).

Near-miss event: an event that could have resulted in an injury, fatality, or property damage if it had not been prevented.

Adverse drug event: any injury resulting from medical intervention related to a drug.

Medication error (ME): any preventable event that occurs in the process of ordering, transcribing, dispensing, administering, or monitoring a drug, irrespective of whether an injury occurred or the potential for injury was present (Kaushal et al. 2001).

20.3.2 General Epidemiology of Iatrogenesis: Frequency, Severity, Preventability, and Type

Data on epidemiology of iatrogenesis in neonatology are scarce and heterogeneous depending of definitions and methodology used. Table 1 shows data of eight studies reviewed. Undoubtedly, retrospective chart reviews underestimate broadly rates of iatrogenesis estimating that medical errors affect between 1.2% and 1.5% of admitted neonates (Brennan et al. 1991; Kanter et al. 2004). Actually, recent studies highlight the importance of iatrogenesis among neonates, as expected, in terms of frequency and severity. These studies (most of them based on a prospective, anonymous, voluntary, and nonpunitive system) reported high incidences of 0.4–1.25 events per patient (Ligi et al. 2008; Sharek et al. 2006; Kugelman et al. 2008; Frey et al. 2000; Snijders et al. 2009). Two studies reported rates of 20–25 IEs ‰ patient-days (Ligi et al. 2008; Kugelman et al. 2008). As 30–50% of the incidents were judged to be severe and harmful, the impact on patient morbidity is considerable (Ligi et al. 2008; Sharek et al. 2006; Kugelman et al. 2008; Frey et al. 2000). Preventability is often high from 35% to 83% of events (Ligi et al. 2008; Sharek et al. 2006; Kugelman et al. 2008).

Frequency of incident by category is heterogeneous, varying with local environments and patterns of problems. Nosocomial infections and respiratory events are reported to be common and often severe events. Particularly, unplanned extubations are a frequent (0.14–6.6 per 100 ventilation days), severe, but largely preventable incident (Sadowski et al. 2006; Merkel et al. 2014). MEs and cutaneous injuries (Fig. 1) occur frequently in NICU but are often minor. ME rates vary widely between studies, partly due to differences in the definitions of an error and the methodology used to their identification. Kaushal and coworkers found an incidence as high as 5.7 MEs per 100 NICU prescriptions (91 MEs per 100 admissions) but including near miss (Kaushal et al. 2001). Near miss excluded, Raju and colleagues reported a rate of 15 ME per 100 admissions (Raju et al. 1989). Dose error, occurring during the prescribing and particularly the administration stage, is reported to be the most common type of ME (Chedoe et al. 2007). Tenfold MEs are common and mainly related to errors in programming of flow rates of electric infusion pumps. Lastly, cutaneous injuries were found to be a frequent incident. Although skin necrosis was rare, scars constituted a severe and significant event with aesthetic and sometimes functional troubles.

As expected, the major risk factors of iatrogenesis are low birth weight and use of invasive

Table 1 Epidemiology of iatrogenesis in neonatal intensive care

Reference	Study design	Population	Characteristics of reporting	Definition	Results		
					Incidence/ n reports	Severe	Preventable
Frey 2000 (Frey et al. 2000) Switzerland	Prospective 1 year	467 admissions (56 % neonates)	Comprehensive, anonymous, nonpunitive	Critical incident	0.45 CI per admission	30 %	Not described
Suresh 2004 (Suresh et al. 2004) USA	Prospective Period 1: 17 months Period 2: 10 months	54 NICU	Nonpunitive, anonymous, voluntary, externally, Internet based, free text (period 1), or structured form (period 2)	Medical errors, near-miss, adverse events	1,230 reports	27 %	Not described
Kanter 2004 (Kanter et al. 2004) USA	Retrospective 1 year	66,146 premature	Discharge records	Medical error	1.2 % premature neonates	Not described	Not described
Sharek 2006 (Sharek et al. 2006) USA	Cross-sectional, retrospective	749 charts, 15 NICU	Trigger tool	Adverse event	0.74 AE per patient	40 %	56 %
Ligi 2008 (Ligi et al. 2008) France	Prospective 8 months	388 neonates	Anonymous, nonpunitive, voluntary	Iatrogenic event	25.6 IE ‰ patient-days 0.69 IE per patient	29 %	34 %
Kugelman 2008 (Kugelman et al. 2008) Israel	Prospective Period 1: 3 months Period 2: 3 months	4 NICU 697 neonates	Anonymous, daily report by a iatrogenesis advocate. Medical staff aware of the study in period 2	Iatrogenic event, medical errors, near-miss event	20.2 IE ‰ patient-days 0.4 IE per patient	48.5 %	83 %
Snijders 2008 (Snijders et al. 2008) Netherlands	Prospective 12 months	8 NICU, 1 PICU 3,859 neonates	Anonymous, voluntary, nonpunitive	Critical incident	1.25 CI per admission	1.4 %	Not described
De Franco 2014 (De Franco et al. 2014) Italy	Cross-sectional, 2 months	1 NICU, 1 subintensive 166 neonates	Anonymous, voluntary	Errors	0.43 error per patient	Not described	Not described

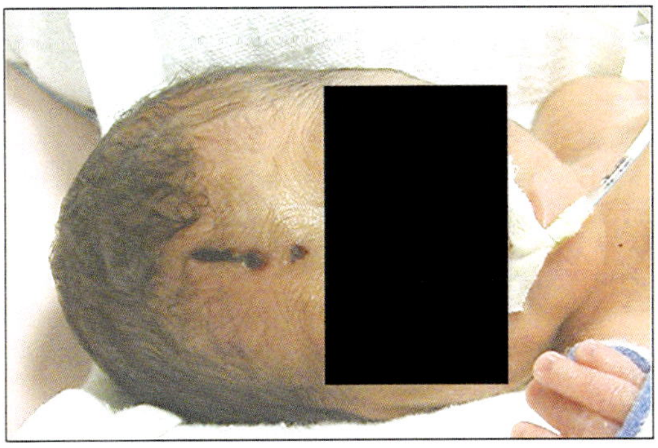

Fig. 1 Skin necrosis related to extravasation of fluids from peripheral venous catheter

procedure (central venous line and mechanical ventilation). Moreover, iatrogenesis is independently associated with an increased length of stay (Ligi et al. 2008; Sharek et al. 2006; Kugelman et al. 2008).

20.4 Learning from Iatrogenic Events

Four steps are fundamental in developing risk management policy: identification, analyze, assessment and graduation, and control of the risk.

20.4.1 Factors Contributing to Iatrogenic Event Occurrence

Multiple factors are invariably involved in the sequence of events that results in iatrogenesis occurrence. As described by James Reason in the "Swiss cheese" model of iatrogenic event occurrence, a set of circumstances coincide both in time and space to cause an event (Reason 2000). Human errors can contribute or cause an event in an active or a latent way. Active failures comprise the unintentional lapses or slips (misinterpretation, error of attention or memory, or selection) and the intentional mistakes (rule or knowledge based) or procedural violations. Active failures are immediate causes of an iatrogenic event. Latent failures are local and organizational conditions that facilitate event occurrence by providing a point of weakness. Factors include individual (training, health, awareness, fatigue) and team (communication, supervision) conditions, institutional (financial resources, safety culture) and environmental (staffing levels, equipment) factors, task conditions (workload, protocols), and patient attributes (age, language, personality, general health, social conditions).

20.4.2 Barriers Contributing to Iatrogenic Event Limitation

A safety system is composed by three different types of barriers.

20.4.2.1 Prevention Barriers

Such barriers prevent error or iatrogenic event occurrence.

20.4.2.2 Recovering Barriers

Error is made but recovered prior to generating an iatrogenic event (also called a near-miss event).

20.4.2.3 Reducing Barriers

Incident occurred but barriers limited their consequences and effects.

20.4.3 Tools to Assess Risk: Corrective Methods

20.4.3.1 Incident Reporting Systems (Ahluwalia and Marriott 2005)

Methodologies

Incident reporting systems refer to structured reporting, collation, and analysis of iatrogenic events. Reporting systems are a key strategy for learning from errors. Mandatory reporting systems, on the basis of retrospective chart reviews, focus on errors associated with serious injuries or death. But errors resulting in serious harm are only part of the problem, and iatrogenesis is certainly underestimated by these systems. However, Sharek and colleagues recently described a trigger tool chart review that retrospectively and efficiently identifies adverse events in NICU (Sharek et al. 2006). Trigger tool methodology is a rapid tool to screen for adverse events using a predetermined list of specified "word signals" that are associated with adverse events (Resar et al. 2003). By contrast, voluntary reporting systems focus on incidents that often result in slight injury, no harm, or even intercepted (so-called near miss). The intent is to identify and remedy vulnerabilities in systems to improve patient's safety. Leape and coworkers emphasize the importance of a nonpunitive, anonymous, and timely reporting system to effectively monitor adverse events. This approach has been shown to be effective in improving the report (Frey et al. 2000; Leape 2002; Suresh et al. 2004). Reporting can be facilitated by adding a trigger list of key incidents that reflect the nature of local clinical practice and areas of concern. Moreover, prospective methods of data collection demonstrate their superiority to cross-sectional or retrospective method (Michel et al. 2004). Indeed, they seem more appropriate to identify preventable events, to assess the impact of error-prevention strategies, to study organizational and human factors, and to assess the consequences of incidents. Furthermore, prospective incident report can be used as an educational process to convince clinical teams that errors contribute significantly to adverse events. WHO established guidelines for adverse event reporting and learning systems (WHO 2005).

Limitations of Incident Reporting Systems

The prospective incident reporting systems are time-consuming in reporting and investigating incidents. Moreover, voluntary reporting can be inadvertently perceived as a means to blame and can paradoxically encourage defensive clinical practices. Another bias important to bear in mind is the underestimation of incidents by underreporting or undetecting.

Our Local Experience of Iatrogenic Event Reporting

Since 2005, we use an anonymous, nonpunitive, and voluntary incident reporting system. The reporting form had been composed by a work group that consisted of neonatologists, one epidemiologist, and referent nurses on the basis of published work, professional expert devices, and a pilot study in 2003. The form consisted of three sections: administrative data (neonatal unit, patient identification, date of birth, discharge date, hospital length of stay, or death), patient characteristics (birth weight, gestational age, sex, mechanical and/or continuous positive pressure support, central venous line), and narrative sections about incidents (date, age and weight, description, causative mechanisms). At the back of the form, a trigger list of 53 potential incidents was established to help in reporting. Before the introduction of the form, several tutorial sessions and group discussions were held to familiarize nursing and medical staff with the incident report. The form was placed in the baby's chart from the time of admission until the discharge or death. Every month, two pediatricians independently reviewed the reported incident to confirm the diagnosis and to rate severity and preventability of each event. A monthly meeting is organized by the work group to discuss rates and to enact preventive measures. A monthly bulletin composed of general data (number of admissions, activity level), of a summary of IE reports and nosocomial infections, and of clinical lessons or guidelines is posted in units for feedback. Every 4 months, a staff meeting is organized with the nursing and medical team to discuss the rates and measures (Ligi et al. 2008).

20.4.3.2 Investigation and Causation Analysis of Incident

Investigations are needed for serious incidents or for recurrent ones. Root cause analysis (standardized debriefing) is a key process to understand incident genesis and to learn from the incident to improve patient safety. Debriefing process has to be confidential, nonthreatening, structured, and timely. It is a collaborative process used to dissect events. The objectives are to determine what happened, to identify why it happened (underlying causative human and system factors), and to pinpoint lessons learned to make recommendations for improvement in a blame-free way. The lessons learned need to be fed back timely to the staff via meeting and/or a monthly bulletin.

20.4.3.3 Morbidity and Mortality Committee

Mortality and morbidity clinical review meeting is a regular, structured, multidisciplinary (medical and nursing staff) process that analyzes critically the circumstances surrounding outcomes of care (death, serious morbidity, and significant aspect of regular clinical practice). Such process focuses on systems dysfunction and failures in ways to develop recommendations, change systems, and improve care.

20.4.4 Tools to Assess Risk: Preventive (Proactive) Methods

Assessment and graduation of medical risk in terms of probability of occurrence and harm potential is important for organizations in health care. Many proactive approaches have been developed: comparison with standards, analysis of processes, and of quality indicators.

20.4.4.1 Audits and Patient Safety Walk Rounds

Independent assessment of care and risk can be useful to implement preventive measures and to assess their effect during reaudit. Performance is reviewed to ensure that what should be done is being done through a systematic review of care (structure, processes, and outcomes) against explicit criteria. Patient safety walk rounds are regular rounds of seniors' leaders for the purpose of discussing safety with staff. This method has been shown to improve the safety culture of hospitals.

20.4.4.2 Failure Mode and Effects Analysis (FMEA) Tools

The reliability and potential failures of any new system, process, equipment, or service are systematically evaluated prior to exposure of patient and staff. FMEA is a systematic, proactive method for evaluating a process to identify where and how it might fail and to assess the relative impact of different failures, failures modes or "what could go wrong?", failure causes or "why would the failure happen?", and failure effects or "what would be the consequences of each failure?", in order to identify the parts of the process that are most in need of change. Even if it is time-consuming, the proactive analysis facilitates assessment of potential risk prior to its implementation.

20.4.4.3 Quality Indicators and Benchmarking

Neonatal-specific quality indicators (like breast milk nutrition, central catheter-related infections, etc.) exist and can be used to compare patient outcomes between different national and international NICU. Benchmarking is a strong tool to measure performance and improve care and neonatal outcomes.

20.5 Strategies to Reduce the Risk: Components of Risk Management

The goal of safety is not to remove all errors but is to manage errors in ways to reduce serious incidents or recurrent ones and identify and recover (near-miss incidents) errors (Fig. 2). Local safety program can be developed to improve quality of care and is based on leadership, communication, training, quality tools, and standards of care (Ligi 2010).

20.5.1 Leadership and Safety Culture

They are critical to convince that hazard and risk are not inevitable and can be managed to improve patient safety. Leaders must sensitize and encourage the entire staff in a collaborative and nonhierarchical process. The objectives are to convince that patient safety is a primary goal, that the system can be improved, and that

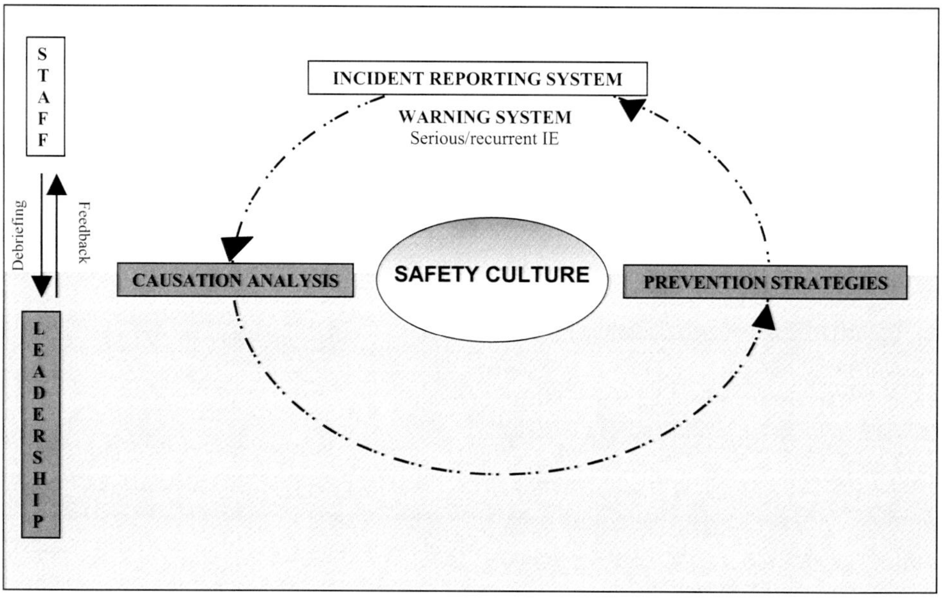

Fig. 2 Organization of risk management

the risk can be reduced. Leaders emphasize the importance of a blame-free incident monitoring as a positive mean to improve quality, empower changes, and allow development of targeted interventions. Leaders organize feedback, communication, and promotion of patient safety.

20.5.2 Communication

Communication with the parents is a major issue to limit claims and complaints. Parent consent and information are key areas. Transparency is capital in case of iatrogenic event occurrence. Communication between professionals is also essential to reduce risk and hazards.

20.5.3 Training, Induction, and Competence

As inexperience and unfamiliarity are key factors in error occurrence, continuous training is needed. Moreover, turnover is high in NICU and new staff is usual. All new staff must be aware of guidelines, policies, and procedure.

20.5.4 Guidelines, Protocols, and Checklist

Standards developed from evidence-based medicine are useful to assist professionals in decision in every steps of the care.

20.5.5 Five Steps for Implementation of a Safety Program

The Plan-Do-Act-Study method can be applied to develop safety program using quality tools to identify risk, forces, and weaknesses of local systems and processes (Table 2).

20.5.6 Prevention of MEs: An Example of Risk Management

MEs occur frequently in NICU with a real potential for harm. Prescription and administration, in particular smart pump programming, are two high-risk stages. Inexperience and intensity of workload are the major risk factors for occurrence. Even if medication management is a complex and multifaceted system,

Table 2 Risk management tools and the five steps for implementation of a safety program

Tools	Selection of situation with safety risk and safety program organization	Analysis of situation and identification of safety risk	Assessment and prioritization of risk	Risk treatment	Following and results longevity and sustainability
Trigger tools	+				
Continuous prospective incident reporting	+		+		+
Clinical audits		+			+
Safety walk rounds	+	+			
Quality indicators	+				+
Root cause analysis		+			
Mortality and morbidity review	+	+			+
FMEA		+			
Checklist				+	
Guidelines				+	
Protocols				+	

studies show that risk can be efficiently reduced and MEs prevented. First, the involvement of a NICU-based pharmacist significantly reduces dosing errors (Simpson et al. 2004). Strategies to reduce error at the prescribing stage include clinical staff education (indication documentation, formulation, and dose regimen information), improving environment conditions at the time of prescription, implementation of standardized dosing references, and perhaps use of computerized provider order entry (CPOE). CPOE could prevent 66% of MEs. However, CPOE may contribute to new types of errors and more studies are needed to assess the impact of such technology on MEs so CPOE are expensive systems (Chedoe et al. 2007). Strategies to reduce errors at the administration stage include use of standard concentrations for infusion, restriction of verbal orders to emergency situations, limitation of handwritten orders, requirement of double-checking at each step of the medication process specially for high-alert drugs (opiates, sedatives, insulin, anticoagulants, concentrated electrolyte solutions), storage of these drugs separately from ward stock, strict identification of syringes, and handoff verification check. These measures demonstrated their efficiency in reducing MEs.

References

Ahluwalia J, Marriott L (2005) Critical incident reporting systems. Semin Fetal Neonatal Med 10:31–37

Brennan TA et al (1991) Incidence of adverse events and negligence in hospitalized patients. N Engl J Med 324:370–376

Chedoe I et al (2007) Incidence and nature of medication errors in neonatal intensive care with strategies to improve safety. Drug Saf 30(6):503–513

De Franco S et al (2014) The error in neonatal intensive care: a multicenter prospective study. Minerva Pediatr 66(1):1–6

Donn S (2005) Medical liability, risk management, and the quality of health care. Semin Fetal Neonatal Med 10:3–9

Frey B et al (2000) Comprehensive critical incident monitoring in a neonatal-pediatric intensive care unit: experience with the system approach. Intensive Care Med 26:69–74

Kanter D, Turenne W, Slonim A (2004) Hospital-reported medical errors in premature neonates. Pediatr Crit Care Med 5(2):119–123

Kaushal R et al (2001) Medication errors and adverse drug events in pediatric inpatients. JAMA 285(16): 2114–2120
Kohn L, Corrigan J, Donaldson M (1999) In: I.o. Medicine (ed) To Err is human: building a safer health system. National Academy Press, Washington, DC
Kugelman A et al (2008) Iatrogenesis in neonatal intensive care units: observational and interventional, prospective, multicenter study. Pediatrics 122:550–555
Leape LL (2002) Reporting of adverse events. N Engl J Med 347(20):1633–1638
Ligi I (2010) Iatrogenic events in neonates: beneficial effects of prevention strategies and continuous monitoring. Pediatrics 126(6):1461–1468
Ligi I et al (2008) Iatrogenic events in admitted neonates: a prospective cohort study. Lancet 371:404–410
Merkel L et al (2014) Reducing unplanned extubations in the NICU. Pediatrics 133(5):1367–1372
Michel P et al (2004) Comparison of three methods for estimating rates of adverse events and rates of preventable adverse events in acute care hospitals. BMJ 328:1–5
Morriss F (2008) Adverse medical events in the NICU: epidemiology and prevention. Neoreviews 9:e8–e23
Raju T et al (1989) Medication errors in neonatal and paediatric intensive-care units. Lancet 12(2):374–376
Reason J (2000) Human error: models and management. BMJ 320(7237):768–770
Resar RK et al (2003) Methodology and rationale for the measurement of harm with trigger tools. Qual Saf Health Care 12(Suppl 2):39–45
Sadowski R et al (2006) Continuous quality improvement: reducing unplanned extubations in a pediatrics intensive care unit. Pediatrics 114(3):628–632
Scholefield H (2005) Risk management in obstetrics. Curr Obstet Gynaecol 15:237–243
Sharek PJ et al (2006) Adverse events in the neonatal intensive care unit: development, testing, and findings of an NICU-focused trigger tool to identify harm in north american NICUs. Pediatrics 118(4):1332–1340
Simpson J, Lynch R, Alroomi L (2004) Reducing medication errors in the neonatal intensive care unit. Arch Dis Child Fetal Neonatal Ed 89:F480–F482
Snijders C et al (2009) Specialty-based, voluntary incident reporting in neonatal intensive care: description of 4846 incident reports. Arch Dis Child Fetal Neonatal Ed. 94(3):F210–F215
Suresh G et al (2004) Voluntary anonymous reporting of medical errors for neonatal intensive care. Pediatrics 113(6):1609–1618
Thomas E et al (2000) A comparison of iatrogenic injury studies in Australia and the USA. I: context, methods, casemix, population, patient and hospital characteristics. Int J Qual Health Care 12:371–378
WHO (2005) Who draft guidelines for adverse event reporting and learning systems. From information to action. WHO Press, Geneva
Woods D et al (2005) Adverse events and preventable adverse events in children. Pediatrics 115:155–160

Guidelines and Protocols for Newborns

21

Rinaldo Zanini and Roberto Bellù

Contents

Abstract

The principal aim of the guidelines is to offer recommendations to assist in clinical decisions. In neonatology systematic evaluation of scientific evidence is even more important than in other fields because of variability between the methodology of clinical studies and the difficulty to perform studies in the neonatal population. Guidelines are "statements that include recommendations, intended to optimize patient care, that are informed by a systematic review of evidence and an assessment of the benefits and harms of alternative care options." In this framework they can help clinicians and healthcare providers in taking best decisions in specific conditions and setting. Methodology issues are of paramount importance in developing and evaluating guidelines. The GRADE approach is actually the standard framework to develop clinical guidelines. From an evaluation point of view, according to an approach to systematically develop guidelines, the AGREE II approach reached an elevated degree of validity and feasibility also for busy clinician and healthcare operator. Based on evidence-based guidelines, clinical pathways emerged as an important way to implement guidelines at the local level, looking at the specific processes of a given patient. Evidence-based guidelines can be effective in improving patient care; the focus is increasingly shifting toward how to encourage the use of guidelines throughout clinical practice. CP framework is one of the most promising approaches to reach this goal.

21.1 Salient Points

- Guidelines are statements that include recommendations, intended to optimize patient care, that are informed by a systematic review of

R. Zanini (✉) · R. Bellù
NICU, Ospedale Manzoni, Lecco, Italy
e-mail: r.zanini@ospedale.lecco.it

G. Buonocore et al. (eds.), *Neonatology*,
https://doi.org/10.1007/978-3-319-29489-6_171

evidence and an assessment of the benefits and harms of alternative care options.
- They can help clinicians and healthcare providers in taking optimal decisions in specific conditions and settings.
- In neonatology, systematic evaluation of scientific evidence is very important because of the variability between the methodology of clinical studies and difficulty in performing studies in the neonatal population.
- Guidelines are systematic, repeatable, shared, and transparent and may also be considered as tools for reducing the gap between current practice and alternative practices.
- Guidelines must be regularly updated.
- The GRADE approach is actually the standard framework to develop clinical guidelines.
- AGREE II approach reached an elevated degree of validity and feasibility for busy clinician and healthcare operator.
- Clinical pathways are common components of guideline implementation mainly used for specific and homogeneous group of patients sharing similar conditions.

21.2 Introduction

The principal aim of the guidelines is to offer recommendations to assist in clinical decisions, based on relevant and updated scientific evidence. In neonatology systematic evaluation of such scientific evidence, the evaluation of the quality and relevance of the information, as well as their subsequent adaptability to local circumstances to allow its implementation acquire even more importance than in other fields. The variability between the methodology of clinical studies; the difficulty to study the neonatal population, often with expert opinions; and adapting age neonatal scientific results related to later ages or even to adults underlines the urgent need for neonatal evidence-based guidelines.

The complexity of modern medical procedures, joining different branches of medicine (obstetrics and neonatology to make perinatology), increased knowledge, and available technology, has contributed to the actual good outcomes for the newborn population. However, this has also imposed new behavioral and organizational models to physicians and healthcare workers to ensure that all these opportunities result in improved and consistent clinical outcomes for patients.

Organizational processes to promote teamwork are needed to facilitate the support and management of a healthcare process that is no longer in the hands of a single physician. The costs of healthcare have increased enormously because of advancing technology, the complexity of interventions, and a continuing demand for better outcomes. These increased costs affect the healthcare systems of all industrialized countries, and there is a risk that they will stunt medical progress in the future years. Increased costs have tended to reduce the fairness of the healthcare system, making access less easy and decreasing its availability to users.

Because guidelines (GLs) are systematic, repeatable, shared, and transparent, their use can contribute to a response to both control of costs and ease of access (Kurtin and Stucky 2009).

Complexity and cost are linked by the increasingly pressing need to provide high-quality treatment with six fundamental attributes: safety, appropriateness, efficacy, efficiency, fairness, and centrality for the user and his/her family.

21.3 The Guidelines

A definition of GL has been agreed by the Institute of Medicine, USA: Guidelines are "statements that include recommendations, intended to optimize patient care, that are informed by a systematic review of evidence and an assessment of the benefits and harms of alternative care options" (Consensus Report, Institute of Medicine 2011).

Rather than being an imposition, GLs are an aid to obtaining the most appropriate healthcare results, through clearly defined criteria of scientific validity, which take into account the viewpoints of different stakeholders and which must therefore balance the interests of patients (clinical outcomes), physicians, and healthcare providers (availability of resources).

The increasing use of GL has highlighted several problems, mainly related to the non-unicity of definitions and to not observing essential methodological prerequisites. The spread of low-quality GL and GLs that give contradictory recommendations is of growing concern (Grilli et al. 2000; Shaneyfelt et al. 1999).

GLs require validity, which can be defined as the capacity to obtain an improvement in health. Validity in this sense is measurable. It is analogous to the efficacy of a drug, which can be evaluated for specific, determinable interventions, for example, by way of randomized clinical trials, or of a diagnostic procedure, which can be characterized in terms of sensitivity, specificity, predictive value, and probability ratio. The validity of the diffusion and implementation of a GL may then be evaluated in terms of the outcomes it produces (Bellù and Zanini 2001).

Systematic reviews of these studies showed that in some contexts GL can change the behavior of healthcare practitioners and in some cases they can lead to significant improvements in clinical outcomes for patients (Shaneyfelt et al. 1999; Bellù and Zanini 2001; NHS Centre for Reviews and Dissemination and Nuffield Institute for Health 1994). These systematic reviews showed how a greater chance of obtaining positive results was associated with certain characteristics of GL. These include simplicity, local adaptability, and the involvement of relevant professionals in their development.

An important problem highlighted by systematic reviews was the identification of methodological weakness of the available studies. This limited the ability to draw definitive conclusions about the validity of some treatments (NHS Centre for Reviews and Dissemination and Nuffield Institute for Health 1994).

Assessment of the validity of a set of GL should be based on the positive changes its implementation induces on a specific pathological process. Such an assessment is made difficult by numerous confusing elements and by the complexity of the studies required. The concept of the validity of a GL has therefore shifted toward evaluation of adherence of a specific GL to the reference methodology, which is considered a guarantee of achieving the desired results.

GLs may also be considered as tools for reducing the gap between current practice and alternative practices. They are therefore supporting tools to help make decisions for individual patients and for organizations by spelling out the benefits, risks, and costs of different healthcare choices.

Based on these assumptions, the following methodological criteria have been identified:

1. The development of a GL and its evaluation must be oriented toward the results of the healthcare: the start of the process of forming (or using) a GL must always start from a precise healthcare context which is seen (or, even better, evaluated) as problematic and therefore targeted for improvement.
2. The GL must be based on the best evidence available. This should also take into account the paucity of clinical studies in several clinical areas, typically diagnosis.
3. The method used to summarize the available evidence must be rigorous and follow a series of agreed steps: definition of the topic, formation of the writing group, definition of the method of bibliographical research and evaluation of the studies, dissemination, and implementation.
4. The GL must contain an explicit classification of the strength of the recommendation: this is crucial and requires the need to give a "strength" to the various recommendations, based on criteria arising directly from the quality of the studies which support the different recommendations of a GL. At this regard, recent work produced a more comprehensive way for classifying the strength of the recommendations, based not only on the quality of the evidence (type and quality of the primary studies) but also on the relevance of the clinical outcomes (Neumann et al. 2016; Mustafa et al. 2013; Atkins et al. 2004; Guyatt et al. 2008). This is known as the "GRADE approach" or framework. In this way more strength recommendations are

given for more relevant clinical outcome (such as mortality or disability).

5. The process of developing a GL must be multidisciplinary and involve users and patients. Experts in a discipline must not be the only ones to deal with a certain topic, and others, who are in some way involved with the clinical management, including the patients, must also be included.
6. A GL must be adapted to the specific local circumstances. At this regard one should consider to develop specific, local documents, such as clinical pathways, for example, based on more general guidelines.
7. A GL must take into consideration the available resources. This bridges the gap between experimental situations and the actual clinical context in which the individual practitioners work. Again, locally developed clinical pathways are tools very used to deploy general recommendations.
8. Once produced, GL must be disseminated and implemented in an appropriate manner. The simple act of publishing a set of GL in journals or congresses is not an effective way of promulgating their use in clinical practice.
9. The implementation of GL must be carefully monitored.
10. A GL must be regularly updated.

The main steps required for the formulation of GL are:

1. Formation of the work group.
2. An evaluation of the literature, aimed at establishing the best available research-based evidence for practice and researching GL already in existence.
3. Drafting the GL:
   - Systematic search of the literature.
   - Evaluation of the methodology of the studies.
   - Evaluation of the quality of the studies.
   - Production of a table of evidence, setting out the results of each study in terms of its conclusions and level of evidence. This step is the most difficult methodologically, as it assumes knowledge of epidemiology and the methodology of research. The table of evidence should state the strength of evidence on which the GL is based, using an approach such as the GRADE (Neumann et al. 2016; Mustafa et al. 2013; Atkins et al. 2004; Guyatt et al. 2008) (Table 1).
   - Formulation of recommendations. On the basis of identified studies, recommendations for best practice can be made. These are then graded, according to the GRADE criteria listed in Table 2.
4. Dissemination and implementation. These steps are an integral part of creating a set of GL. This section covers the identification of problems that may arise during the application of the GL and approaches for their resolution (e.g., incentivizing initiatives, structural and organizational changes, the use of specific tools such as reminders (paper or electronic), etc.) which can reach the site where the clinician actually makes the healthcare decisions (US Agency for Health Care Policy and Research (AHCPR) 1993). By conducting an

Table 1 Criteria for grading of evidence (according to GRADE)

1. *Type of evidence*
Randomized clinical trial = high
Observational study = low
Any other evidence = very low
2. *Decrease grade if*:
Serious (−1) or very serious (−2) limitation to study quality
Important inconsistency (−1)
Some (−1) or major (−2) uncertainty about directness
Imprecise or sparse data (−1)
High probability of reporting bias (−1)
3. *Increase grade if*:
Strong evidence of association – significant relative risk of >2 (<0.5) based on consistent evidence from at least two observational studies with no plausible confounders (+1)
Very strong evidence of association – significant risk of >5 (<0.2) based on direct evidence with no major threats to validity (+2)
Evidence of a dose-response gradient (+1)
All plausible confounders would have reduce the effect (+1)

Table 2 Strength of recommendation (according to GRADE)

Strong recommendation against a given action	Conditional (weak) recommendation against a given action	Only in research	Conditional (weak) recommendation for a given action	Strong recommendation for a given action

analysis of 431 sets of GL produced by international scientific societies between 1988 and 1998, evaluating them on the basis of essential criteria, such as their multidisciplinary applicability, completeness of the systematic review of the literature, and gradation of the evidence, Grilli et al. (2000) demonstrated that 67% did not provide information on the staff involved, 88% did not provide information on the bibliographic search strategies, and 82% did not grade the evidence. Only 5% of GL reviewed satisfied all the criteria. However, there was an improvement with time, especially in respect of the search strategy (from 2% to 18%) and grading of the evidence (from 6% to 27%). Similar studies revealed the same problems, meaning that tracking down good-quality GL cannot be taken for granted.

If it is possible to find GL with good validity, what strategies can be used to identify valid GL? It might be possible to adopt GLs that have already produced positive results in terms of health out comes. However, such experiences are relatively scarce and cannot be reproduced in different contexts. Account needs to be taken therefore of the local situation, ensuring the relevance of GL, which may lead to recommendations that are different to the originals.

An alternative strategy is to adopt stringent, validated methodological criteria to assess the available GL or to construct evaluation "grids," which can be used by clinicians and by the final users. A recent systematic review analyzed available studies on this topic. It came to the conclusion that more than one of the tools had characteristics of such validity as to be of practical use, the one developed within the context of the European project AGREE (AGREE Collaboration 2003; Brouwers et al. 2010), being one of the most widespread and useful. The AGREE II tools are accessible at www.agreetrust.org. The AGREE evaluation tool focuses attention on the methodological and formal aspects described above, structuring the analysis and the evaluation of them in a format that is easily understood and usable. In particular, the AGREE focuses on six major domains with 23 items and an overall assessment:

1. Scope and purpose (3 items)
2. Stakeholder involvement(3 items)
3. Rigor of development(8 items)
4. Clarity of presentation(3 items)
5. Applicability(4 items)
6. Editorial independence(2 items)

In this way it is possible to evaluate a set of GL, adhere to a good development process, and, therefore, by inference, achieve the desired health effect. Actually, the tool is based on theoretical assumptions and on empirical evidence, which it is now accumulating with the wide diffusion of the instrument in the last years (Brouwers et al. 2012).

21.4 Clinical Pathways (CPs)

CPs are a common component of guideline implementation. More specifically that in GL, they aim to organize and standardize care processes, thus trying to maximize patient outcomes (Rotter et al. 2010). Originating in the USA, CPs have been used since the 1980s. Their goal is to improve patient outcomes, such as mortality rate and others, while containing costs and, possibly, improving quality (Kinsman et al. 2010). They are also a means of improving systematic collection and abstraction of clinical data for audit and of promoting change in practice. Different terms, including care maps, critical pathways, local protocols, or algorithms, are used to describe the construct of CPs.

CPs are mainly used for specific and homogeneous groups of patients sharing similar conditions. The implementation of CPs may be driven by a variation in the quality of care and outcomes for patients with similar health conditions; in neonatology they have been used since many years. Usually, the aim of the implementation is to reduce a pre-identified variation in patient outcomes and costs and, more recently, to keep patients and families informed about their course of treatment or care.

Recently, an operational definition for CPs was developed, including four major criteria for developing and evaluating CPs (Lawal et al. 2016):

1. CP is a structured multidisciplinary care plan.
2. Is it used to direct the translation of guidelines or evidence into local structures.
3. CPs detail the steps of care in a plan, pathway, algorithm, guideline, protocol, or other "inventory of actions" (i.e., the intervention had time frames or criteria-based progression).
4. CPs aim to standardize care for a specific clinical problem, procedure, or episode of care in a specific population.

Given the above definition, Campbell (Campbell et al. 1998) proposed the following steps to develop CPs:

1. Select an important area of practice. Selection criteria could include common or costly clinical conditions, those where there is a high level of interest among local staff or those where variations in practice occur and affect patient outcome.
2. Gather support for the project.
3. Form a multidisciplinary group to compare current practice with established clinical guidelines.
4. Identify established guidelines.
5. Review practice, both current and past.
6. Involve local staff from all disciplines providing care for the condition.
7. Identify key areas for service development for that clinical condition and express appropriate goals for the service.
8. Develop a care pathway which specifies elements of care detailed in local protocol, the sequence of events, and expected patient progress over time.
9. Prepare documentation for the CP.
10. Educate staff in the use of the CP.
11. Pilot then implement the integrated CP.
12. Regularly analyze variances from the integrated care pathway. Investigation of the reasons why current practice is different from that recommended in the CP can be used to identify common variations from agreed best practice, alert staff to patients who are failing to progress as expected, update the CP by incorporating agreed changes, and identify research issues.
13. Discuss variations from the CP and identify avoidable and unavoidable variations; then identify and implement solutions to avoidable variations.

Integration of CP into clinical record is an essential issue, characterizing this instrument. The CP should be placed in the patient's clinical record. It records essential clinical information in way that is easy to complete and to extract data for audit; for example, checklists of all necessary activities to tick and boxes for specific results to be recorded. This can result in more legible and complete clinical records and contains a minimum essential data set for auditing and reviewing. Separate sheets should be used to record all variations from the CP so that it can be easily extracted for audit purposes. Integration of CP into electronic medical record (EMR) should improve ease of use and implementation of CP.

In conclusion, evidence-based guidelines can be effective in improving patient care; the focus is increasingly shifting toward how to encourage the use of guidelines throughout clinical practice. CP framework is one of the most promising approaches to reach this goal.

References

AGREE Collaboration (2003) Development and validation of an international appraisal instrument for assessing the quality of clinical practice guidelines: the AGREE project. Qual Safety Health Care 12:18–23

Atkins D, Best D, Briss PA, Eccles M, Falck-Ytter Y, Flottorp S, Guyatt GH, Harbour RT, Haugh MC, Henry D, Hill S, Jaeschke R, Leng G, Liberati A, Magrini N, Mason J, Middleton P, Mrukowicz J, O'Connell D, Oxman AD, Phillips B, Schünemann HJ, Edejer T, Varonen H, Vist GE, Williams JW Jr, Zaza S, GRADE Working Group (2004) Grading quality of evidence and strength of recommendations. BMJ 328:1490

Bellù R, Zanini R (2001) Sono valide le Linee Guida che utilizziamo in reparto? Riv Ital Pediatr 27:645–650

Brouwers MC, Kho ME, Browman GP, Burgers JS, Cluzeau F, Feder G, Fervers B, Graham ID, Grimshaw J, Hanna SE, Littlejohns P, Makarski J, Zitzelsberger L, AGREE Next Steps Consortium (2010) AGREE II: advancing guideline development, reporting and evaluation in health care. J Clin Epidemiol. 63:1308–1311

Brouwers MC, Kho ME, Browman GP, Burgers JS, Cluzeau F, Feder G, Fervers B, Graham ID, Grimshaw J, Hanna SE, Littlejohns P, Makarski J, Zitzelsberger L, AGREE Next Steps Consortium (2012) The Global Rating Scale complements the AGREE II in advancing the quality of practice guidelines. J Clin Epidemiol 65:526–534

Campbell H, Hotchkiss R, Bradshaw N, Porteous M (1998) Integrated care pathways. BMJ 316:133–137

Consensus Report, Institute of Medicine (2011) Clinical practice guidelines we can trust. http://nationalacademies.org/hmd/~/media/Files/Report%20Files/2011/Clinical-Practice-Guidelines-We-Can-Trust/Clinical%20Practice%20Guidelines%202011%20Report%20Brief.pdf. Accessed on 23 Oct 2016

Grilli R, Magrini N, Penna A et al (2000) Practice guidelines developed by specialty societies: the need for a critical appraisal. Lancet 355:103–106

Guyatt GH, Oxman AD, Vist GE, Kunz R, Falck-Ytter Y, Alonso-Coello P, Schünemann HJ, GRADE Working Group (2008) GRADE: an emerging consensus on rating quality of evidence and strength of recommendations. BMJ 336:924–926

Kinsman L, Rotter T, James E, Snow P, Willis J (2010) What is a clinical pathway? Development of a definition to inform the debate. BMC Med 8:31

Kurtin P, Stucky E (2009) Standardize to excellence: improving the quality and safety of care with clinical pathway. Pediatr Clin N Am 56:893–900

Lawal AK, Rotter T, Kinsman L, Machotta A, Ronellenfitsch U, Scott SD, Goodridge D, Plishka C, Groot G (2016) What is a clinical pathway? Refinement of an operational definition to identify clinical pathway studies for a Cochrane systematic review. BMC Med 14:35

Mustafa RA, Santesso N, Brozek J, Akl EA, Walter SD, Norman G, Kulasegaram M, Christensen R, Guyatt GH, Falck-Ytter Y, Chang S, Murad MH, Vist GE, Lasserson T, Gartlehner G, Shukla V, Sun X, Whittington C, Post PN, Lang E, Thaler K, Kunnamo I, Alenius H, Meerpohl JJ, Alba AC, Nevis IF, Gentles S, Ethier MC, Carrasco-Labra A, Khatib R, Nesrallah G, Kroft J, Selk A, Brignardello-Petersen R, Schünemann HJ (2013) The GRADE approach is reproducible in assessing the quality of evidence of quantitative evidence syntheses. J Clin Epidemiol 66:736–742

Neumann I, Santesso N, Akl EA, Rind DM, Vandvik PO, Alonso-Coello P, Agoritsas T, Mustafa RA, Alexander PE, Schünemann H, Guyatt GH (2016) A guide for health professionals to interpret and use recommendations in guidelines developed with the GRADE approach. J Clin Epidemiol 72:45–55

NHS Centre for Reviews and Dissemination and Nuffield Institute for Health (1994) Implementing clinical guidelines. Can guidelines be used to improve clinical practice? Effective Health Care 1:1–12

Rotter T, Kinsman L, James E, Machotta A, Gothe H, Willis J (2010) Clinicalpathways: effects on professional practice, patient outcomes, length of stayand hospital costs. Cochrane Database Syst Rev 3: CD006632

Shaneyfelt TM, Mayo-Smith MF, Rothwangl J (1999) Are guidelines following guidelines? The methodological quality of clinical practice guidelines in the peer-reviewed medical literature. JAMA 281:1900–1905

US Agency for Health Care Policy and Research (AHCPR) (1993) Program note: clinical practice guidelines development. AHCPR publication no. 93-0023. US Department of Health and Human Services

Physical Environment for Newborns: The Thermal Environment

22

Daniele Trevisanuto and Gunnar Sedin

Contents

D. Trevisanuto (✉)
Department of Women's and Children's Health, Azienda Ospedaliere di Padova, University of Padua, Padua, Italy
e-mail: daniele.trevisanuto@gmail.com

G. Sedin
Department of Women's and Children's Health, University Children's Hospital, Uppsala, Sweden

G. Buonocore et al. (eds.), *Neonatology*,
https://doi.org/10.1007/978-3-319-29489-6_172

Abstract

The exchange of heat between the infant's skin and the environment is influenced by insulation provided by the skin, the permeability of the skin, and the environmental factors such as the ambient temperature and humidity, airflow velocity, and characteristics of surfaces where the infant is positioned. High incidence of postnatal hypothermia has been reported in high- as well as low-resource countries, and it is an independent predictor of neonatal morbidity and mortality. All efforts should be put in place to prevent heat losses at birth, especially in very preterm infants. Interventions include delivery room temperature >25 °C, use of infant warmers, exothermic mattress, woolen caps, plastic wraps, and humidified and heated gases. Skin-to-skin contact has be considered, especially in low-resource settings. In addition to specific interventions, quality improvement initiatives, including the use of checklists and continuous feedbacks with the staff involved in the management of the neonate, contribute to reduce postnatal thermal losses in very preterm infants. In this chapter, we report the mechanisms of thermal homeostasis in the newborn infant and describe the clinical management of the neonates, especially very preterm infants, to prevent heat losses at birth.

22.1 Salient Points

- Physiological mechanisms involved in the maintenance of temperature include convection, radiation, conduction, and evaporation.
- The high evaporative losses of heat from the infant's skin, especially in preterm infants, will gradually decrease with increasing postnatal age.
- In very preterm infants, hypothermia at NICU admission is significantly associated with adverse neonatal outcomes such as mortality, intracranial hemorrhage, necrotizing enterocolitis, and late-onset sepsis.
- Maintaining delivery room temperature >25 °C, use of infant warmers, exothermic mattress, woolen caps, plastic wraps, and

humidified and heated gas are effective in preventing postnatal thermal losses in preterm infants.

- More than the single intervention, their sum associated to the use of checklists and continuous feedbacks to the staff is the "secret" to prevent delivery room thermal losses in preterm infants.
- Skin-to-skin contact has be considered, especially in low-resource settings.

22.2 Overview

During intrauterine life, heat production by the fetus results in a fetal temperature that is about 0.5 °C higher than the maternal temperature (Bruck 1978). After birth, the newborn infant is exposed to air and surfaces, which have a much lower temperature than that previously experienced in utero. The skin surface at birth is covered with amniotic fluid, causing heat loss through evaporation in an environment with a low vapor pressure (Hammarlund et al. 1980). As a result, the body temperature of the infant is lowered, and the rate of this reduction is influenced by the temperature of the environmental air in the delivery room and the delivery of its flow. This gives rise to thermogenic responses that increase basal heat production (Bruck 1978; Dahm and James 1972), and the skin circulation may decrease to lower the heat losses (Sjors et al. 1994).

Heat balance in the newborn infants depends on the heat transfer between the infant and the environment (Hammarlund and Sedin 1982; Hammarlund et al. 1986, 1988; Sedin 1995). This transfer is related to the temperature and the humidity of environmental air (the vapor pressure), the flow velocity of that air (which causes a sense of cooling of the skin), the temperature of the surfaces facing the infant (ceiling, walls of the room or incubator, or bedding material), and the temperature of the surfaces in direct contact with the infant (Hammarlund and Sedin 1982; Hammarlund et al. 1986; Sedin 1995, 2004).

After birth, the immediate interventions required to avoid body cooling are to carefully wipe off the amniotic fluid from the skin surface with cotton fabrics to lower the loss of heat through evaporation and to cover the infant with a warm, dry towel or blanket, or both, to lessen the exposure of the infant's skin to the environment (Hammarlund et al. 1980, 1986). This intervention is recommended for infants with gestational age higher than 32 weeks. The infant born at term or moderately preterm can be covered with a blanket and then placed on the mother's chest (Bauer et al. 1997, 1998; Whitelaw et al. 1988), but extremely preterm infants usually need other types of measures to maintain their body temperature, usually placement in an incubator or under a radiant heater (Hammarlund and Sedin 1982, 1979; Hammarlund et al. 1986; Kjartansson et al. 1995; Marks et al. 1980; Sjörs et al. 1992a) and, if necessary, mechanical ventilation with warm and humidified gas (Hammarlund et al. 1988; Riesenfeld et al. 1994, 1995; Sedin 1996a).

This chapter is divided into parts: the first part includes the mechanisms of thermal homeostasis in the newborn infant; in the second part, we will describe the clinical management of the neonates, especially very preterm infants, to prevent heat losses at birth.

22.3 Thermal Homeostasis

22.3.1 Routes of Heat Exchange

Heat exchange between the infant and its environment occurs through the skin and through the respiratory tract. About 30 years ago, the introduction of new techniques to measure the evaporation rate from the skin (Hammarlund et al. 1985, 1986; Kjartansson et al. 1995; Nilsson 1977) and from the respiratory tract (Hammarlund et al. 1988, 1985; Kjartansson et al. 1992a) has permitted to determine the heat loss through evaporation (Hammarlund et al. 1986). It is also possible to calculate the heat losses through other modes of heat exchange, such as radiation, convection (air movements), and conduction (in direct contact with a piece of material or skin), and to determine the heat loss per unit surface area and from the total body surface area (Riesenfeld et al. 1995) and also to take into consideration the proportions of the surface area of the body participating in the different modes of heat exchange (Hammarlund and Sedin 1982; Hammarlund et al. 1986). In addition, the modes of heat exchange between the infant's respiratory tract and the environment can be determined.

22.4 Water and Heat Exchange Between the Infant's Body Surface and the Environment

Heat exchange through evaporation, radiation, convection, and conduction can be calculated with knowledge of the transepidermal water loss (loss of water through the skin), the temperature of the infant's skin (T_{skin}), the temperature of the ambient air (T_{amb}), the temperature of the material on which the infant is placed (T_{bed}), and the characteristics of the material in the infant's environment (Hammarlund et al. 1980; Hammarlund and Sedin 1982).

22.4.1 Determination of Water Loss from the Skin

In the absence of forced convection (air movements), and if the effect of thermal diffusion is disregarded, the process of water exchange through a stationary water-permeable surface can be expressed in terms of the vapor pressure gradient immediately adjacent to the surface (Nilsson 1977).

The evaporation rate (ER; g/m^2 h) from the infant's skin can thus be determined by a method based on calculation of the water vapor pressure in the layer of air immediately adjacent to the vapor pressure and the distance from the evaporating surface (Nilsson 1977). In this zone, the relationship between the vapor pressure and the distance from the evaporating surface is linear (Nilsson 1977). If the gradient in this layer is known, the amount of water evaporated per unit time (transepidermal water loss, TEWL; g/m^2 h, which is a mean value of cutaneous water loss) can be calculated (Nilsson 1977) according to the following equation:

$$\mathrm{TEWL} = 0.92 \times \mathrm{ER}_{(a,b,c)} + 1,32$$

where $ER_{(a,b,c)}$ is the arithmetic mean of ER measured from the chest, an interscapular area, and a buttock (Sedin 1995, 2004; Hammarlund et al. 1985; Kjartansson et al. 1992a).

The gradient method (Evaporimeter, Servomed AB, 511 21 Varberg, Sweden) allows quick measurements of free evaporation without disturbing the infant (Nilsson 1977; Kjartansson et al. 1992a).

22.4.2 Calculation of Heat Exchange Between the Infant and the Environment

22.4.2.1 Exchange at the Surface

Heat exchange through evaporation (H_{evapor}) can be calculated if TEWL is known (Sedin 1995, 2004; Nilsson 1977; Hammarlund et al. 1985; Kjartansson et al. 1992a) according to the equation:

$$H_{evapor} = k_1 \times \mathrm{TEWL}\left(3.6 \times 10^3\right)^{-1}\left(\mathrm{W/m^2}\right)$$

where K1 is the latent heat of evaporation (2.4×10^3 J/g) and 3.6×10^3 is the correction factor for time (s).

Heat exchange through radiation (H_{rad}) can be determined if the mean temperature of the skin (T_1; K) and the mean temperature of the surrounding walls (T_2; K) are known:

$$(H_{rad}) = S_0 \times e_1 \times e_2 \times \left(T_1^{\,4} - T_2^{\,4}\right)\left(\mathrm{W/m^2}\right)$$

where S_0 is Stefan-Boltzmann's constant (5.7×10^{-8} W/m^2 K^4), e_1 is the emissivity of the skin, and e_2 is the emissivity of the surrounding walls (0.97).

Heat exchange through convection (H_{conv}) can be calculated if the mean temperature of the skin (T_1; K) and the mean temperature of the ambient air (T_3; K) are known:

$$H_{con} = K_2(T_1 - T_3)\left(W/\mathrm{m^2}\right)$$

where K_2 is the convection coefficient (2.7 W/m^2 K). The coefficient for convection given above and used in many studies referred to this chapter has usually been determined in measurements in adult human skin (Okken et al. 1982). A convection coefficient suggested as being more valid for newborns infants (Wheldon 1982) can alternatively be used, and Hconv will then be 48% higher.

Heat exchange through conduction (H_{cond}) can be determined if the temperature of the skin (T_{skin}; K) and the temperature of the bed (T_{bed}; K) are known:

$$H_{\mathrm{cond}} = K_0(T_{\mathrm{skin}} - T_{\mathrm{bed}})(W/m^2)$$

In this equation, K_0 is a conductive heat transfer coefficient. With the thermal conductivity characteristics of most regular mattresses, the heat loss through conduction is very low.

The extent of heat exchange between the body surface area and the environment thus depends on the type of heat exchange, on the position and geometry of the body (Hammarlund et al. 1986; Sedin 1995), and on the magnitude and frequency of body movements. As different modes of heat exchange are unequally influenced by changes in the body position, the relative contribution of different modes of heat exchange might vary with time. Heat exchange is often presented per area of body surface exposed to the ambient air or facing the walls of the incubator.

22.4.2.2 Heat Exchange Between the Infant's Respiratory Tract and the Environment

The expired air is usually more humid than the inspired air and has a higher water vapor pressure. This implies that evaporative loss of water and heat takes place from the respiratory tract. Convective heat transfer, usually of low degree, also occurs in the respiratory tract. In research, these two processes are considered together (Houdas and Ring 1982). In the newborn, heat can also be gained through the respiratory tract if the infant inspires very warm air with a high humidity. Because of the alternating displacement of air during the respiratory cycle, convective and evaporative heat transfer in the respiratory tract is complex. When ambient air, which is cooler than the body, passes along the mucosa of the infant during inspiration, it gains heat by convection and gains water vapor by evaporation from the mucosa. On reaching the alveoli, the air is at thermal equilibrium with the central body temperature and is saturated with water. During expiration, the expired air may become a little cooled than the body temperature before it leaves the infant (Hammarlund et al. 1985, 1988).

22.4.2.3 Determination of Water Loss from the Airway

Respiratory water loss (RWL) is usually included in measurements of total insensible water loss when these are performed with ventilated chambers, but it can be estimated separately (Hey and Katz 1969; Sulyok et al. 1973). Hey and Katz (1969) and Sulyok and colleagues (Sulyok et al. 1973) found that the respiratory water loss was higher at a low ambient humidity than at a high humidity. In other studies, data on respiratory water loss, oxygen consumption, and carbon dioxide production were provided (Hammarlund et al. 1985, 1988; Riesenfeld et al. 1994, 1995, 1987a, b, 1988, 1990; Sjörs et al. 1992b).

22.4.2.4 Calculation of Heat Exchange Between the Infant's Respiratory Tract and the Environment

The exchange of heat through convection in the respiratory tract, $H_{conv\text{-}r}$, is calculated from the air volume ventilated per unit time (V = ventilation volume) and from the temperature difference between expired and inspired air (T_e–T_I) according to the following relationship:

$$H_{\mathrm{conv-r}} = V \times r \times c\ (T_{\mathrm{e}} - T_{\mathrm{I}})\mathrm{m}^{-1}(W/\mathrm{Kg})$$

where V is ventilation volume per unit time, r is the density (1 g = 0.880 L), c is the specific heat (1 J × g^{-1} × °C^{-1}), and m is the body weight (kg) (Sedin 1995).

Because of the alternating inspiratory warming and expiratory cooling of the air, the convective heat exchange in the respiratory tract depends mainly on the temperature of the inspired air. In human infants nursed in an incubator, there is a very small difference between the temperatures of the inspired and expired air, and convective losses are small.

Evaporative heat exchange from the airway, H_{evap-r}, depends on the difference in water content between the expired and inspired air. This is the respiratory water loss (Riesenfeld et al. 1994; Sedin 1996a; Hey 1969). As the formation of water vapor in the respiratory tract requires thermal energy, the amount of heat exchange by evaporation per unit time is expressed by the following equation:

$$H_{\text{evap-r}} = K_1 \times \text{RWL}\left(3.6 \times 10^3\right)^{-1}(W/\text{Kg})$$

where k_1 is the latent heat of evaporation of water ((2.4 × 10^3 J/kg), RWL is the respiratory water loss (mg/kg min), and (3.6 × $10^3)^{-1}$ is the correction factor for time.

22.5 Heat Exchange in Incubators, Under Radiant Heaters and Heated Beds

When it was realized that a good thermal environment increases the chances of survival of the newborn infants, attempts were made to provide them with a warm environment. The ambient temperature influences the survival rate and oxygen consumption in newborn infants (Dahm and James 1972; Hey and Katz 1969; Hey 1969), and a body temperature of around 37 °C is appropriate for newborn infants at rest (Riesenfeld et al. 1990). At a high ambient temperature, full-term infants start to sweat, and if they are fed cold glucose through a gastric tube, sweating is inhibited (Stromberg et al. 1983).

22.5.1 Incubators

In a convectively heated incubator, the warm air supplied should be directed so that both the air temperature of the incubator and the incubator walls are kept warm. If the airflow velocity is lower than 0.1 m/s, the convective heat transfer will depend on the gradient between the skin and the air temperature, and the vapor pressure gradient close to the skin surface will be maintained, avoiding an increased evaporative rate due to increased airflow velocity (Sedin 1995; Okken et al. 1982; Wheldon 1982)

An evaluation of environmental and climate control in incubators has shown that the airflow velocities and capacity for humidification vary markedly between the different types of incubators. Also, the wall temperature varies considerably between different incubators (Sjörs et al. 1992b), and it is therefore necessary to determine the airflow velocities, humidity, and wall temperatures carefully before calculating heat exchange. With airflows higher than 0.2 m/s, there will be a forced convection.

22.5.2 Radiant Heaters

A radiant warmer placed over an open bed platform provides good accessibility and visibility for the care of the newborn infant and has therefore become widely used in neonatal intensive care.

Infants nursed under a radiant heater gain heat, but they may also have extensive heat losses through evaporation and convection, and also, from surfaces, through radiation (Kjartansson et al. 1992b, 1995; Marks et al. 1980; Baumgart 1982; Sjörs et al. 1997; Sosulski et al. 1983), making it difficult to estimate the relative contributions of different modes of heat exchange. Because of the free movements of air above the infant's body surface, both evaporative and convective heat loss may increase as a result of a high air velocity.

22.5.3 Heated Beds

In the 1990s, Sarman and co-workers found that infants weighting 1,000 g or more can be kept warm by placing them on a heated water-filled mattress early after birth (Sarman et al. 1989). By covering most parts of the body except the face, direct heat exchange between the infant's skin and the environment trough other modes can be almost eliminated in a large proportions of the body surface.

Preterm and term infants can maintain a normal body temperature during skin-to-skin care, if they are placed lying naked except for a diaper on the mother's or father's chest and are covered with the mother's clothing or a blanket (Bauer et al. 1997, 1998; Whitelaw et al. 1988). Only parts of the head are exposed to the environmental air and will exchange heat with the environment (Bauer et al. 1997, 1998; Whitelaw et al. 1988).

22.6 Water and Heat Exchange Between the Skin and Environment

In a series of studies, water evaporation from the skin surface of infants nursed in incubators has been determined by the use of the gradient method (the ServoMed Evaporimeter), and transepidermal water loss (TEWL) (Hammarlund and Sedin 1979; Hammarlund et al. 1983, 1985; Kjartansson et al. 1992a) and heat exchange have been calculated (Hammarlund et al. 1980, 1986; Hammarlund and Sedin 1982). In these studies, the body temperature has been maintained at 36–37 °C, except when the effect of warming has been investigated, and the ambient humidity has been kept at 50% except when the effects of different humidities have been analyzed. Evaporative heat loss is usually insensible but might become sensible when term infants are nursed in a warm environment and start to sweat (Stromberg et al. 1983). Some infants born at term and nursed in a warm environment do not begin to sweat (Stromberg et al. 1983), and if they do, the sweating is preceded by an increase in skin blood flow. In preterm infants, the sweat glands are nonfunctional (Hey and Katz 1969).

22.6.1 Heat Exchange During the First Hours After Birth

Immediately after birth, when the infant's skin is covered with amniotic fluid, there is an enormous evaporative heat loss from the skin surface. This evaporative heat loss decreases gradually during the first hours, whether the infant is nursed in the delivery room or in an incubator (Hammarlund et al. 1980; Fig. 1, top two diagrams). Heat loss through radiation is high if the infant's skin is facing the walls of the delivery room and is much lower if it is facing the inner walls of the incubator (Hammarlund et al. 1980), (Fig. 1, middle diagrams). The heat loss through convection is lower than through radiation but is much higher when the infant is nursed in room air (Fig. 1, lower left diagram) than when nursed in the incubator (Fig. 1, lower right diagram).

22.6.2 Transepidermal Water Loss During the First 4 Postnatal Weeks

The transepidermal water loss from the skin surface of the newborn infant depends primarily on the gestational age (GA) at birth (Hammarlund and Sedin 1979), but it is also influenced by the postnatal age (Hammarlund et al. 1983). The transepidermal water loss in newborn infants is also lower in small for gestational age (SGA (Hammarlund et al. 1985) than in appropriate for gestational age (AGA) (Hammarlund and Sedin 1979; Hammarlund et al. 1983, 1985) infants. There is an exponential relationship between TEWL and gestational age in AGA infants when measurements are made during the first day after birth (Hammarlund and Sedin 1979). This relationship prevails over the first 4 weeks after birth, even though the difference in TEWL between the most preterm and full-term AGA infant gradually diminishes with increasing age. The evaporation rate and TEWL both depend on the ambient relative humidity or ambient vapor pressure (Hammarlund and Sedin 1979; Hammarlund et al. 1985). This relationship seems to be valid for all gestational ages and is also valid for all postnatal ages studied (Hammarlund and Sedin 1979; Hammarlund et al. 1983, 1985; Sedin 1996b).

22.6.3 Heat Exchange During the First Day After Birth

The evaporative heat exchange is directly proportional to the amount of water that evaporates from the infant's skin and shows the same type of

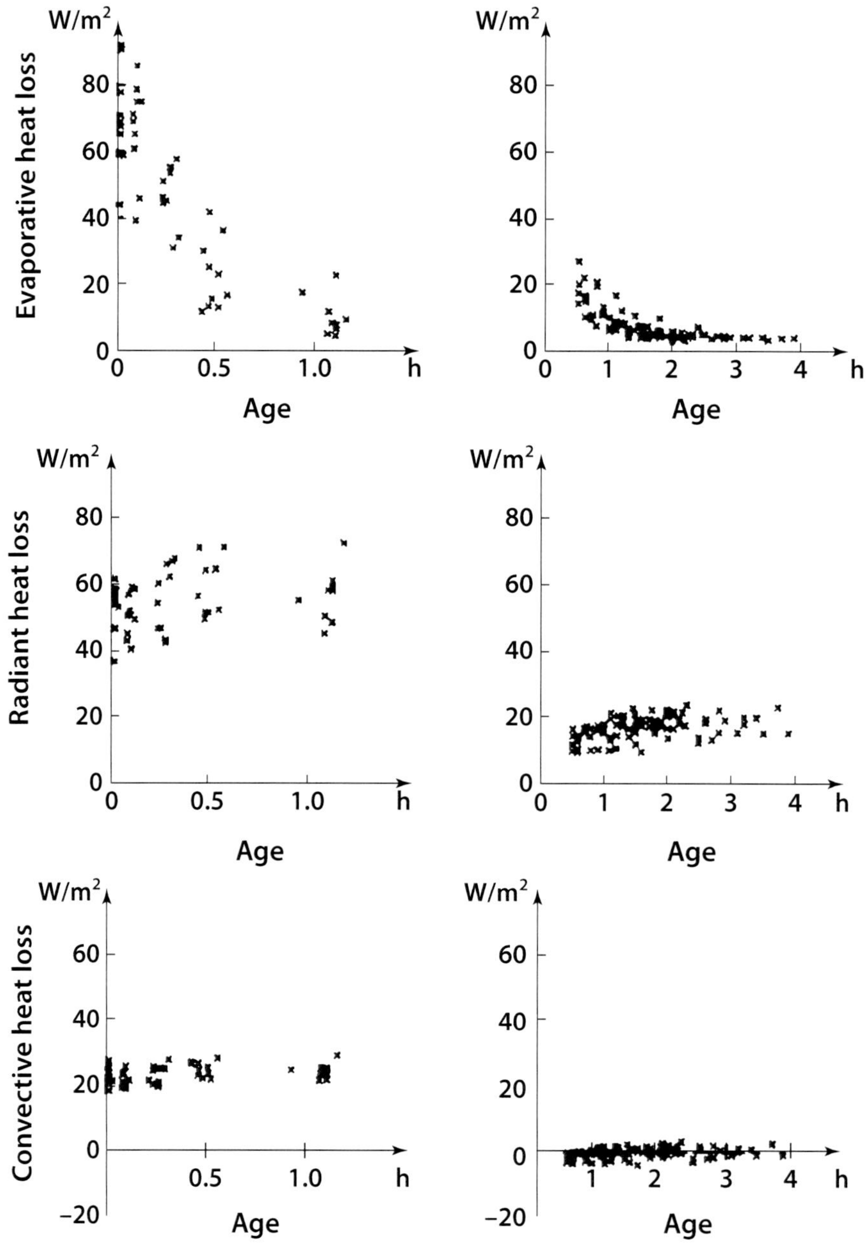

Fig. 1 Heat exchange between the skin of full-term infants and the environment immediately after birth and during the first 1–4 h postnatally. The infants were not washed or wiped. Data presented in the left-hand scatter diagrams are based on measurements in infants initially placed at the delivery bed or at the mother's chest and later in a cot. After the measurements made at 1 and 5 min after birth, the infants were covered with a towel between the measurements. Data in the right-hand diagrams are based on measurements in infants who were covered with a towel after birth and until they were placed in an incubator (Hammarlund et al. 1980)

relationship to GA as TEWL (Hammarlund and Sedin 1982; Hammarlund et al. 1985). When infants are nursed in an ambient humidity of 50%, the evaporative heat exchange may reach 50 W/m^2 of the body surface area in the most preterm infants (Hammarlund and Sedin 1982), whereas in term infants, it is close to 5 W/m^2 (Fig. 2). The high evaporative heat loss in very

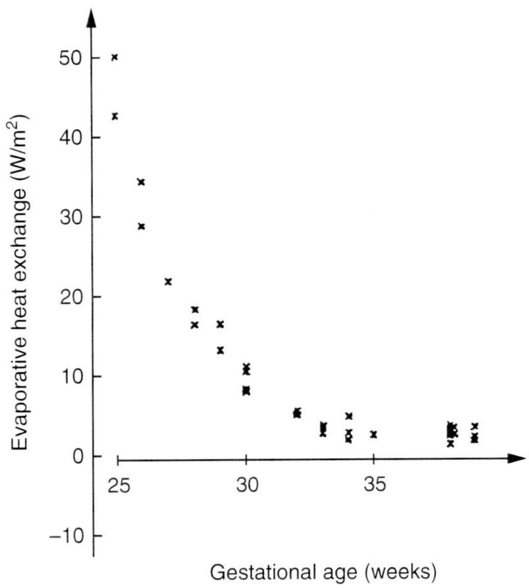

Fig. 2 Heat exchange through evaporation at ambient humidity of 50 % in relation to gestational age. Measurements were made during the first 24 h after birth in preterm infants and during the first 30 h in term infants (Hammarlund and Sedin 1982)

preterm infants makes it necessary to have a very high ambient temperature in the incubator to maintain a normal body temperature of 36.0–37.0 °C in these infants.

The servocontrol system of the incubator that controls the skin temperature regulates the temperature of the air, which also lead to changes in temperature of the incubator walls and thereby influences the heat exchange through convection and radiation.

The most preterm infants can even gain heat through these modes of heat exchange. Preterm infants were nursed in an incubator with a relative humidity of 50%, at a higher ambient vapor pressure than the more mature infants need (Hammarlund et al. 1983, 1985). This means that the heat exchange between the very preterm infants and their environment could have been ever greater, if comparisons had been made at equal ambient vapor pressures instead of at equal ambient humidities.

In studies on the effects of different ambient humidities, it was found that infants born at a GA of less than 28 weeks need a T_{amb} of around 40 °C to maintain a normal body temperature at an ambient humidity of 20%, whereas full-term infants need a T_{amb} of around 34 °C at this ambient humidity (Fig. 3). Nursing very preterm infants at a higher ambient humidity means that a lower ambient temperature can be sufficient to maintain a normal body temperature (Hammarlund and Sedin 1982).

22.6.4 Heat Exchange at Different Ambient Humidities

Evaporative heat exchange between the skin of very preterm infants and the environment is highest at a low humidity (Hammarlund and Sedin 1982) and lower at higher ambient humidity. In fact, heat exchange through evaporation in the most preterm infants is twice as high at 20% as at 60% ambient humidity. Other modes of heat exchange are all influenced by the ambient humidity (Fig. 4). The sum of the different modes of heat exchange in the different GA groups is almost the same, but the total heat loss cannot be calculated in this way, as the proportions of the body surface area exchanging heat in different ways are not known.

22.6.5 Heat Exchange During the First Weeks After Birth

The high evaporative losses of heat from the infant's skin that are seen in the most preterm

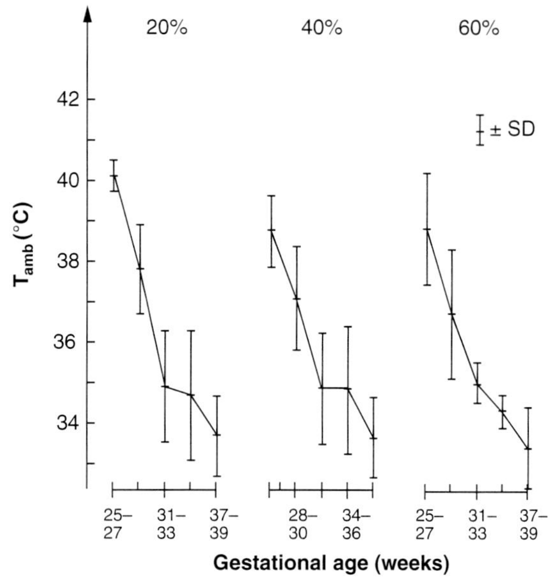

Fig. 3 The relationship between gestational age and the ambient temperature needed to maintain a normal body temperature at three different humidities of 20 %, 40 %, and 60 %. Measurements were made during the first 24 h after birth in preterm infants and during the first 30 h in term infants (Hammarlund and Sedin 1982)

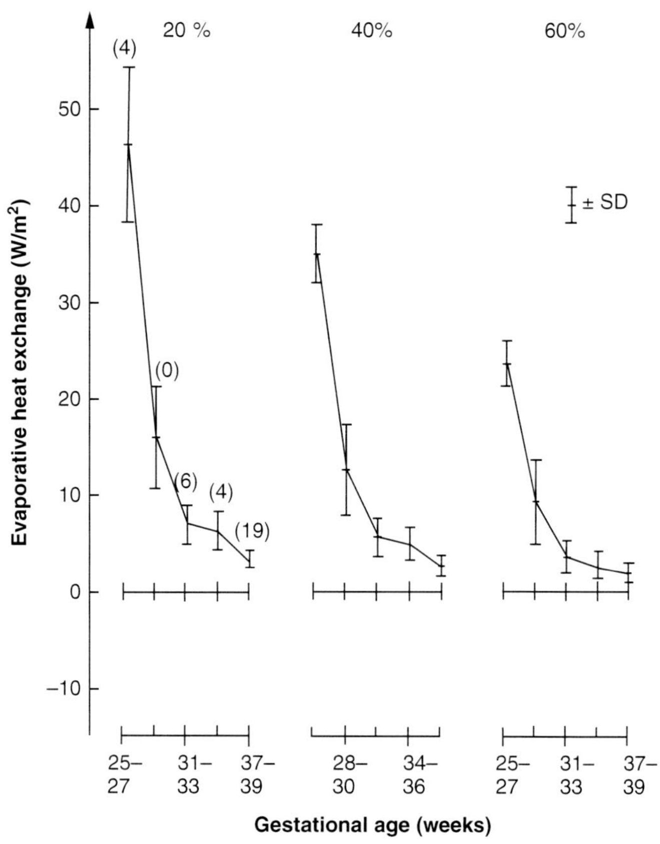

Fig. 4 Heat exchange through evaporation in relation to gestational age at relative ambient humidities of 20 %, 40 %, and 60 %. SD, standard deviation (Hammarlund and Sedin 1982)

infants during the first days after birth will gradually decrease with increasing postnatal age (Hammarlund et al. 1986). Heat loss through radiation is low early after birth in the most preterm infants born at 25–27 weeks of gestation. Heat loss from radiation will, however, be the most important mode of heat exchange after the first postnatal week. In infants born at a GA of 28 or more weeks, the radiative heat exchange is the most important mode of heat exchange from birth, and it gradually increases with age. The heat exchange through convection is low in infants nursed in incubators. Initially there is a gain of heat through convection in the most preterm infants early after birth.

During the first weeks after birth, the relative magnitude of the different modes of heat exchange markedly depends on the ambient humidity (Fig. 5). In infants born at 25–27 weeks of gestation and nursed in a dry environment, evaporative heat exchange will be the most important mode of heat exchange for more than 10 days after birth. At an ambient humidity of 60%, this mode of exchange is the highest only during the first 5 days. Thereafter, the radiative heat exchange is the most important mode of heat loss (Hammarlund et al. 1986).

The total heat exchange between the infant's skin and the environment can be calculated if the body surface area of the infant and the fractions of this area that participate in the different modes of heat exchange are known (Hammarlund et al. 1985, 1986; Hey and Katz 1969). This is very difficult with available methods, especially if estimations are to be made over a longer period of time (Hammarlund et al. 1986). The total heat exchange is basically dependent on the metabolic rate.

22.6.6 Heat Exchange Between Infant's Skin and the Environment During Care Under Radiant Heaters

Several authors have considered that a lower vapor pressure in the ambient air (Bell et al. 1980) and more convective air currents under the radiant heater (Baumgart 1982) cause an increase in evaporative water loss and heat exchange. More recent determination of the

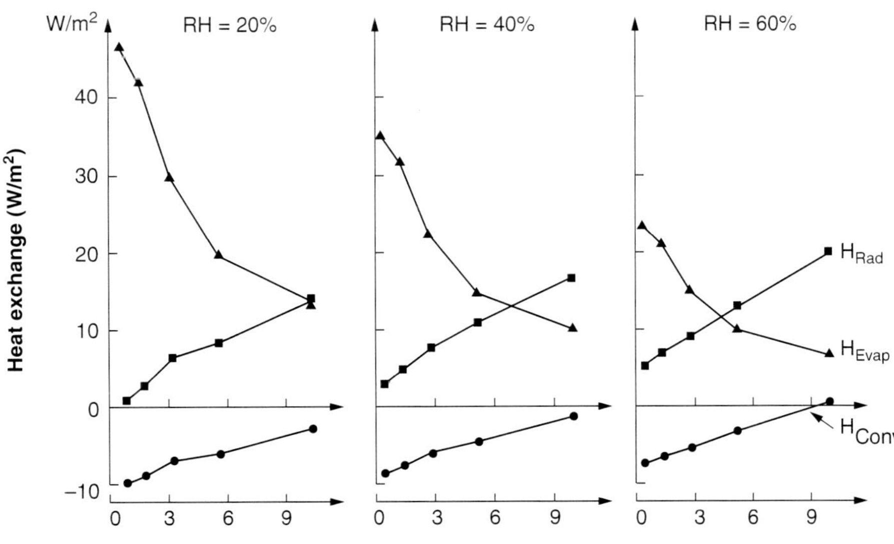

Fig. 5 Heat exchange between the infant and the environment in relation to postnatal age at relative ambient humidities (RH) of 20 %, 40 %, and 60 % in infants born at 25–27 weeks of gestation (Hammarlund et al. 1986)

evaporation rate from the skin of term, moderately preterm, and very preterm infants nursed in incubators with 50% ambient humidity and under a radiant heater has shown that the evaporation rate from the skin surface of full-term infants is significantly higher under a radiant heater than in an incubator (Kjartansson et al. 1995). In moderately preterm infants born at 30–34 weeks of gestation, the evaporation rate from the skin is significantly higher at an environmental humidity of 30% than at 50%, and in very preterm infants with GA of less than 30 weeks, the evaporation rate is higher under a radiant heater than in an incubator at an environmental humidity of 50%. A transparent heat shield positioned over the infant can lower the heat exchange (occurring through both convection and evaporation) between the infant and its environment, decrease convective air currents, increase humidification (Baumgart 1982), and diminish the water loss (Bell et al. 1980; Fanaroff et al. 1972; Flenady and Woodgate 2003). It has been suggested that a bed platform that can be used with a radiant heater or with a hood might make it easier to adapt to the mode of care that such an infant needs (Greenspan et al. 2001).

22.6.7 Ambient Humidity Influence on the Rate of Skin Barrier Maturation in Extremely Preterm Infants

In infants born at 24–25 completed weeks of gestation and nursed in incubators at 50% ambient humidity, water loss was higher than that previously found in infants born at 25–27 weeks of gestation (Agren et al. 1998).

To investigate if the level of radiant heaters (RH) in which the preterm infants are nursed might influence their postnatal skin maturation, TEWL was determined in twenty preterm infants (GA 23–27 weeks) nursed at postnatal ages (PNA) of 0, 3, 7, 14, and 28 days (Agren et al. 2006). The results indicate that the level of RH influences skin barrier development, with more rapid barrier formation in infants nursed at a lower RH. The findings have an impact for promoting skin barrier integrity in extremely preterm infants (Fig. 6; Agren et al. 2006). The individual decrease in $TEWL_{50}$ was consistently more pronounced in the RH_{50} than in the RH_{75} group. There were no differences in body temperature, skin temperature, or ambient temperatures (T_{amb} and T_{wall}) between the two study groups. The total fluid intake and serum sodium levels during the period 0–14 days of PNA are presented in Fig. 6.

Table 1 further documents that there are no significant differences between the group of infants that were nursed at an RH of 75% and those nursed at an RH of 50% (Table 1).

22.6.8 Heat Exchange Between the Infant's Skin and the Environment During Phototherapy

Phototherapy has been reported to increase insensible water loss in newborn infants (Baumgart 1982; Bell et al. 1980). This loss of water and heat might be caused by altered barrier properties in the skin or by increased respiratory water loss. However, other studies have indicated that in thermally stable term and preterm infants (Kjartansson et al. 1992b), there is no increase in the evaporation rate from the skin surface during phototherapy.

22.6.9 Heat Exchange Between the Infant's Skin and the Environment During Care on a Heated Bed

An infant on a heated bed gains heat through conduction. Some losses of water and heat from the airway will take place, depending on the vapor pressure of the room air. Sarman and colleagues showed that infants weighting $\leq$1,000 g could be kept warm when nursed on a heated water-filled mattress (Sarman et al. 1989). In a 2-week trial with infants whose birthweights were between 1,300 and 1,500 g, Gray and Flenady found that

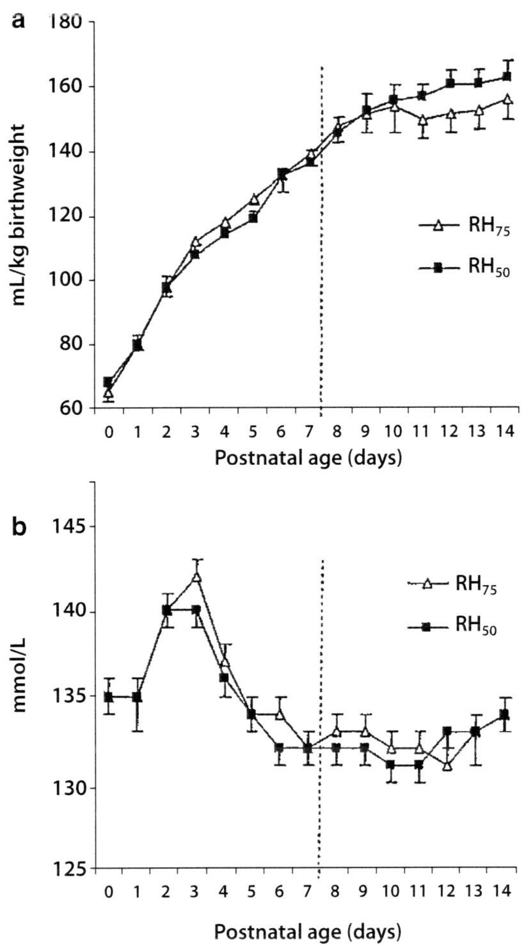

Fig. 6 Daily total fluid intake (**a**) and serum sodium levels (**b**) at postnatal ages (*PNA*) of 0–14 days in infants nursed at RH_{75} or RH_{50} from PMA 7 days (*indicated by dotted lines*). There are no statistically significant differences between study groups (Agren et al. 1998)

Table 1 Effect of activity levels on insensible water loss and oxygen consumption

Activity level	IWLS	IWLR	IWLT	VO2
0	6	6	12	8
1		8		9
2		9		10
3		10		11
4		12		12
5	7	16	23	13

Insensible water loss from the skin (IWLS) and from the respiratory tract (IWLR) and their sum (IWT) in g/kg/24 h, and oxygen consumption (VO2; L/kg/24 h), in full-term appropriate for gestational age infants at different levels of activity (From Riesenfeld et al. (1987b))

weight gain was lower and body temperature higher in those who were cot-nursed with warming than in those who were nursed in an incubator (Gray and Flenady 2003).

22.6.10 Heat Exchange Between the Infant's Skin and the Environment During Skin-to-Skin Care

After the introduction of skin-to-skin care for newborn infants (Whitelaw et al. 1988), Bauer and colleagues showed that preterm infants less than 1 week of age and with a birthweight of less than 1,500 g were not exposed to cold stress during 60-min skin-to-skin care in stable preterm infants (Bauer et al. 1997). Similarly, preterm infants born at 28–30 weeks of gestation and studied during the first and second week after birth increased their body temperature during 1 h of skin-to-skin contact with no significant change in oxygen consumption (Bauer et al. 1998). More immature infants, born at 25–27 weeks of gestation, showed no increase in oxygen consumption but a decrease in rectal temperature during the same duration of skin-to-skin contact during the first week after birth.

During the second postnatal week, the body temperature did not change in infants born at 25–27 weeks of gestation during skin-to-skin care (Bauer et al. 1998). It has been suggested that infants born at 25–27 weeks of gestation might have a very high evaporative heat loss during the first week after birth, causing cold stress (Hammarlund et al. 1986; Hammarlund and Sedin 1979).

22.6.11 Keeping the Very Preterm Infant Warm Early After Birth: The Effect of Thin Clothing

Newborn infants are at risk of losing heat soon after birth. It is therefore of great importance to wipe off amniotic fluid from the skin surface, remove wet linen, and wrap the infant in pre-warmed blankets or, alternatively, place the infant skin to skin on the mother's chest to use her body as a heat source (Whitelaw et al. 1988).

When an infant is placed in an environment where the temperature and humidity are low, the evaporative heat and water exchange will be high, and air movements in the environment may further increase the loss of heat through evaporation, conduction, convection, and radiation. It is therefore of outmost importance to keep the infant warm. In a laboratory setting, we present data on the evaporation rate from a semipermeable membrane positioned above a membrane (Hammarlund et al. 1980; Hammarlund and Sedin 1979, 1982; Adamson et al. 1965).

22.7 Water and Heat Exchange Between the Respiratory Tract and Environment

Water and heat exchange from the respiratory tract takes place with each expiration. Using indirect methods, it has been shown that respiratory water loss depends on the humidity of the inspired air, with lower losses occurring at a high humidity (Hey and Katz 1969; Sosulski et al. 1983). The respiratory water loss (mg/kg min) can be determined using a flow-through system with a mass spectrometer for measurement of gas concentrations (Hammarlund et al. 1988; Sedin 1995, 2004; Riesenfeld et al. 1987a, b, 1988, 1994, 1995; Sjörs et al. 1992b). In an environment with an ambient humidity of 50%, the evaporative heat loss from the airway will be moderate (Riesenfeld et al. 1987a), i. e., in term AGA infants, the insensible water loss from the respiratory tract (IWL_R) and that from the skin (IWL_s) will be of equal magnitude (Riesenfeld et al. 1987a). The evaporative heat loss from the respiratory tract ($H_{evap\text{-}r}$) and the evaporative heat loss ($H_{evap\text{-}s}$) from the skin will also be of equal magnitude under these conditions.

The evaporative loss of water and heat from the airways depends on the ambient humidity both in lambs (Hammarlund et al. 1988) and infants (Riesenfeld et al. 1987a), with lower losses at a high than at a low humidity. Whereas IWL_s decreased from 9 to 2 g/Kg/24 h in term infants when the ambient humidity was increased from 20% to 80%, the corresponding change in IWL_R was much smaller, i.e., from 9 to 5 g/Kg/24 h (Riesenfeld et al. 1987a). In infant placed in a calorimeter, Solyok et al. (1973) found that the respiratory heat loss was between 0.07 and 0.22 W/Kg or 3–10% of the total heat production from metabolism and about 40% of the insensible heat loss. In term infants, RW_L and $H_{evap\text{-}r}$ may increase during activity by up to 140% of the values at rest (Riesenfeld et al. 1987b).

In Table 2, data are presented on IWL_s and IWL_R. During moderate heat stress, both lambs and infants can increase their RWL and $H_{evap\text{-}r}$ without increasing their oxygen consumption and CO_2 production (Riesenfeld et al. 1988, 1994). Exposure to radiant heat can alter the respiratory water loss in a lamb while leaving the oxygen consumption and CO_2 production unchanged. RWL is directly proportional to the rate of breathing (Riesenfeld et al. 1988, 1990, 1994), which means that lambs and infants will lose more water and heat when they have a high rate of breathing (Fig. 7). The oxygen consumption will increase if

Table 2 Effect of phototherapy on respiratory value in neonates

	n	RWL (mg/kg/min)	VO_2 (mL/kg/min)	VCO_2 (mL/kg/min)	RR (breath/min)
Before	11	4.4 ± 0.7	5.9 ± 0.9	4.0 ± 0.7	48 ± 7
12 min	11	4.4 ± 0.6	5.9 ± 1.0	3.9 ± 0.6	
24 min	10	4.1 ± 0.8	5.5 ± 1.1	3.8 ± 0.7	
36 min	9	4.2 ± 1.0	5.4 ± 1.0	3.6 ± 0.6	
48 min	11	4.4 ± 0.7	5.9 ± 1.1	3.9 ± 0.7	51 ± 11
60 min	9	4.6 ± 0.9	5.9 ± 1.1	4.1 ± 0.8	
After	9	4.8 ± 0.8	6.1 ± 0.9	4.1 ± 0.4	

Respiratory water loss (*RWL*), oxygen consumption (VO_2), carbon dioxide production (VCO_2; mean ± SD), and respiratory rate (*RR*) in full-term infants before, during, and after 60 min of phototherapy (From Kjartansson et al. (1992a))

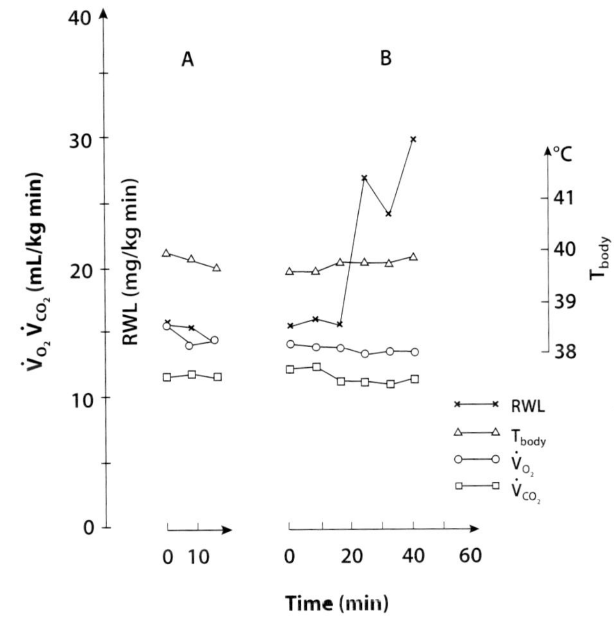

Fig. 7 Respiratory water loss (RWL), body temperature (T_{body}), oxygen consumption (VO_2), and CO_2 production (VCO_2) in 6-day-old lamb before (**a**) and during (**b**) heat stress (Riesenfeld et al. 1988)

the heat stress induces bodily movements with higher levels of activity (Riesenfeld et al. 1987b).

22.7.1 Respiratory Water and Evaporative Heat Exchange Before and After Intubation

In non-intubated lambs, exposed to a radiant heat source, RWL increased from 10.5 to 33.4 mg/kg/min, while the respiratory rate increased from 54 to 161 breaths/min, and the oxygen consumption and CO_2 production were unaltered (Hammarlund et al. 1985). During exposure to the same heat source, intubated lambs increased their respiratory water loss from 8.1 to 18.7 mg/kg/min and their rate of breathing from 46 to 125 breaths/min. In intubated lambs, both the oxygen consumption and CO_2 production increased significantly (Hammarlund et al. 1985).

22.7.2 Respiratory Water and Evaporative Heat Loss in Relation to GA

RWL was found to be highest in the most preterm infants and lower in more mature infants; they were usually asleep during the measurements (Riesenfeld et al. 1995). Studies were performed in incubators with 50% ambient relative humidity and an ambient temperature that allowed the infant to maintain a normal and stable body temperature. RWL per breath (mg/kg) was almost the same at all gestational ages, and the higher RWL values found in the most preterm infants as compared to the more mature ones were thus due to the higher rate of breathing (Agren et al. 1998).

22.7.3 Respiratory Water and Evaporative Heat Exchange During Phototherapy

When term and preterm infants were exposed to phototherapy in the absence of heat stress, there were no significant changes in RWL, oxygen consumption, CO_2 production, or rate of breathing (Kjartansson et al. 1992a; Table 2).

22.7.4 Respiratory Water and Heat Exchange During Mechanical Ventilation

In clinical neonatal care with warm and humid environment or with warm and humidified gas supplied from a respirator, heat exchange through evaporation and convection between the respiratory tract and the environment is low (Hammarlund et al. 1988; Sulyok et al. 1973; Riesenfeld et al. 1987a). Infants who inspire cold air with low water vapor pressure will have high evaporative loss from the respiratory tract and will also lose heat through convection. These losses may become clinically significant, for example, during transport in a cold climate (Sedin 1996a).

The concept of an optimum thermal environment for newborn infants evolved during the 1960s (Adamson et al. 1965). This idealized setting, called the neutral thermal environment, is characterized as the range of an environmental temperature within which the metabolic rate is at minimum and within which temperature regulation is achieved by non-evaporative physical processes alone. There is no reason to believe that normal temperature of infants is different from that of adults. An infant's internal temperature within the range of 36.5–37.5 °C (with a diurnal variation of 0.5 °C) is probably normal. Because of the balance between heat production and net heat loss, a normal body temperature should be not confused with "normal" metabolic rate (Adamson et al. 1965).

A cold-stressed infant depends primarily on mechanisms that cause chemical thermogenesis. When an infant is stimulated by cold, norepinephrine is released (Stern et al. 1965), inducing lipolysis in brown fat stores principally found in the interscapular, paraspinal, and perirenal areas. Because of the protein thermogenin, brown fat can decouple oxidative phosphorylation and break down fats to produce heat, without the inhibitory feedback loop of adenosine triphosphate (ATP) production. Triglycerides in the fat are broken down to fatty acids and glycerol. The fatty acids enter thermogenic metabolic paths that end in the common pool of metabolic acid. Brown fat is turned on in response to skin thermoreceptors prior to a decrease in core temperature, and shivering is initiated by a decrease in core temperature.

Glycolysis may also be stimulated during stress when epinephrine released from the adrenals activates glycogen stores, which may result in transient hyperglycemia (Pribylova and Znamenacek 1966). Lowered blood sugars in cold-stressed infants also have been reported (Cornblath and Schwrtz 1966), possibly caused by inhibition of glycolysis, by lipolysis, or by exhaustion of glycogen stores.

22.8 Clinical Management

22.8.1 Introduction

In very low-birth-weight infants, hypothermia (temperature <36 °C) at NICU admission is significantly associated with adverse neonatal outcomes such as mortality, intracranial hemorrhage, necrotizing enterocolitis, and late-onset sepsis (Miller et al. 2011; Laptook et al. 2007).

A recent observational study assessed the association between admission temperature and neonatal outcomes and estimated the admission temperature associated with lowest rates of adverse outcomes in 9,833 preterm infants born at fewer than 33 weeks' gestation (Lyu et al.

2015). The results show that the lowest rates of adverse outcomes were associated with admission temperatures between 36.5 °C and 37.2 °C. Furthermore, the study showed that the relationship between admission temperature and adverse neonatal outcomes was U-shaped. These data suggest that hypothermia and hyperthermia at NICU admission negatively influence neonatal outcomes.

Therefore, all efforts should be focused on preventing hypothermia and hyperthermia during the first minutes of life.

22.8.2 Thermal Delivery Room Management

The physiological mechanisms involved in the maintenance of temperature are convection, radiation, conduction, and evaporation (http://www.slideshare.net/drdilipbharodiya/nursing-care-of-elbw-and-lbw-babies-41344677) (Fig. 8).

Of these, evaporation plays the most important role in extremely preterm infants.

In relation to the pathophysiological mechanisms, clinicians have to consider four major interventions for preventing heat losses in preterm infants (Fig. 9).

22.8.2.1 Delivery Room Temperature

Increasing the delivery room temperature for an anticipated preterm delivery is recommended by the American Heart Association and European Guidelines for Neonatal Resuscitation (Wyckoff et al. 2015; Wyllie et al. 2015).

Similarly, the World Health Organization (WHO) also advocates maintaining the temperature in the delivery room at 25 °C (WHO Library Cataloguing-in-Publication Data. World Health Organization 2003). This goal, however, is rarely achieved in clinical practice. A recent study including 39 Vermont Oxford Network centers showed that 86% of the 801 infants with gestational age between 24 and 27 weeks received their initial resuscitation in a room with a temperature <25 °C (Reilly et al. 2015).

Previous observational studies with historical controls showed increasing the environmental temperature in the operating theater improved admission temperature (Kent and Williams 2008; Knobel et al. 2005). In a randomized controlled trial, admission rectal temperatures of newborns <32 weeks' gestation delivered in rooms with temperature set at 24–26 °C were compared with those of similar newborns delivered in rooms with temperature set at 20–23 °C. Premature newborns delivered in rooms with mean temperature 25.1 ± 0.6 °C (n. 43), compared with those delivered in rooms with mean temperature 22.5 ± 0.6 °C (n. 48), had a lower incidence (34.9% vs. 68.8%, $p < 0.01$) of admission rectal temperature <36 °C and higher admission rectal temperatures (36.0 ± 0.9 °C vs. 35.5 ± 0.8 °C, $p < 0.01$) (Jia et al. 2013).

22.8.2.2 Infant Warmer

Newborn infants, in particular those needing resuscitation maneuvers at birth, must be readily positioned under a radiant infant warmer (RIW)

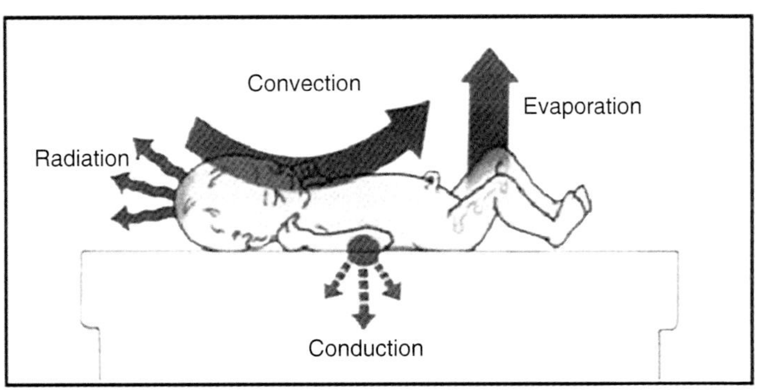

Fig. 8 Mechanisms of heat loss (http://www.slideshare.net/drdilipbharodiya/nursing-care-of-elbw-and-lbw-babies-41344677)

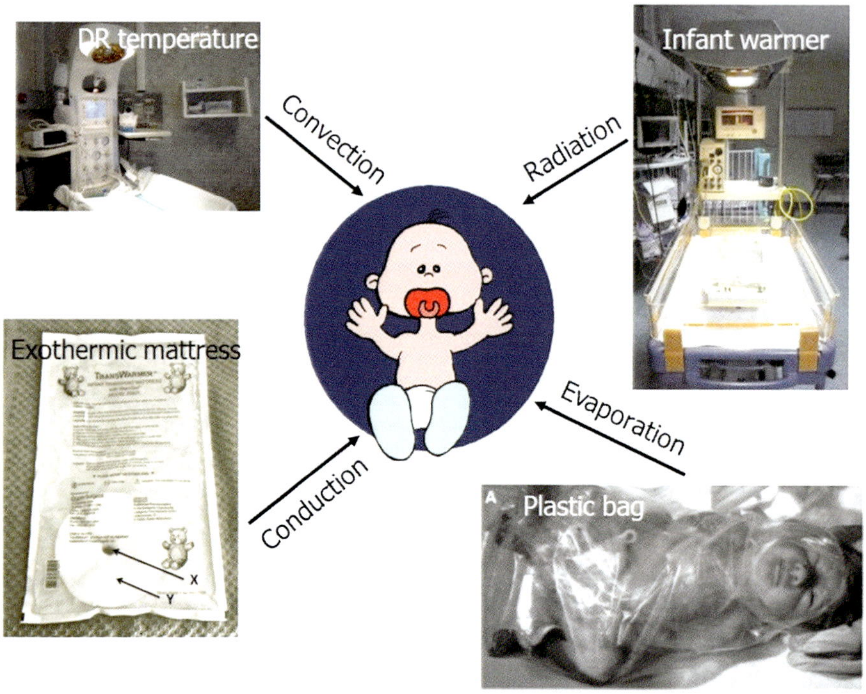

Fig. 9 Interventions to prevent heat loss in preterm infants

turned on, but further details, such as temperature of exposure and/or level of RIW power to set up, are not specified (Wyckoff et al. 2015; Wyllie et al. 2015). In a bench study, Trevisanuto et al. assessed the exposure temperature generated by three different RIWs (Trevisanuto et al. 2011). One of them did not reach the target temperature (37 °C) in all studied settings; in contrast, the other two were always above this target when set in full-power manual mode. This study shows that patient's exposure temperature under RIW (turned on preselected power outputs) significantly varies among commercially available devices, suggesting that neonates can be easily put in conditions of hypo- or hyperthermia.

22.8.2.3 Exothermic Mattress

The use of exothermic mattresses is mentioned as a thermoregulatory strategy for preterm infants in 2010 ILCOR guidelines (Kattwinkel et al. 2010). Gel-filled mattresses used in published studies reach 38–42 °C in 1–3 min; the price is about €35 [$46.50] each. Results from observational studies show that the use of the exothermic mattresses in preterm infants managed in a plastic bag/wrap under a radiant warmer from delivery room to NICU improves temperature at NICU admission (Chawla et al. 2011; Ibrahim and Yoxall 2010; McCarthy and O'Donnell 2011; Singh et al. 2010). In a RCT, McCarthy et al. randomized infants <31 weeks to treatment with or without an exothermic mattress before birth (McCarthy et al. 2013). All infants were placed in a polyethylene bag and under radiant heat immediately after birth and brought to NICU in a transport incubator. Infants randomly assigned to exothermic mattress were placed on a mattress immediately after delivery and remained on it until admission. Fewer infants in exothermic mattress group had temperatures within the target range (41% vs. 77%, $p = 0.002$) and more had temperatures >37.5 °C (46% vs. 17%, $p = 0.009$). The data safety monitoring committee recommended stopping the study for efficacy after analyzing data from half the planned sample. This study shows that placing polyethylene-wrapped very preterm infants on exothermic mattresses in the delivery room results in more infants with abnormal temperature and more hyperthermia on admission to the NICU. As hyperthermia could be harmful, a word of caution on the use of the exothermic mattress is needed.

22.8.2.4 Plastic Bag/Wrap

In very preterm infants, a diminished capacity for metabolic heat production coupled with a high surface area-to-volume ratio and an immature epidermal barrier leads to extraordinarily high evaporative heat losses. In view of this, the use of polyethylene bags to reduce evaporative heat loss while permitting radiant warming has been evaluated by several studies (Knobel et al. 2005; Cordaro et al. 2012; Vohra et al. 1999, 2004). Two systematic reviews concluded that infants wrapped immediately after birth had significantly greater admission temperatures compared with non-wrapped infants and that wrapping significantly reduced the incidence of hypothermia (McCall et al. 2010; Cramer et al. 2005). A recent RCT assessed whether the application of occlusive wrap applied immediately after birth reduced mortality in very preterm infants (Reilly et al. 2015). Eight hundred one infants were enrolled. Wrap infants had statistically significant greater baseline temperatures (36.3 °C wrap vs. 35.7 °C no wrap, $p < 0.0001$) and post-stabilization temperatures (36.6 °C vs. 36.2 °C, $p < 0.001$) than non-wrap infants. However, there were no significant differences in mortality rate (OR 1.0, 95% CI 0.7–1.5) between the two groups.

22.8.2.5 Cap/Hat

Despite the relative success of wrapping infants in food or hospital standard polythene bags, some infants still develop hypothermia. In the Heat Loss Prevention study of infants <28 weeks' gestational age, the infants wrapped in polythene bags had a mean ± SD rectal admission temperature of 36.5 ± 0.8 °C (Vohra et al. 2004). In this study, the polyethylene occlusive skin wrap covered the body up to the shoulders, but the infants' head was dried and left uncovered. The method consisting of putting the infant inside a polyethylene or polyurethane bag, with the head protruding from the bag, minimizes heat loss from the trunk, but not heat losses from the head. The brain of the newborn infant has high oxygen consumption and generates a significant amount of the total heat produced. The surface area of the head represents 20.8% of the total body surface area (Klein and Scammon 1930). Therefore, if the head were to be insulated by provision of a cap, heat loss should be reduced. Doglioni et al. evaluated whether a polyethylene total body wrapping (covering both the body and head) was more effective than conventional treatment (covering up to the shoulders) in reducing perinatal thermal losses in very preterm infants (Doglioni et al. 2014). They found that axillary temperature on NICU admission was similar in the two groups (36.5 ± 0.6 °C total body vs. 36.4 ± 0.8 °C controls; $P = 0.53$), but the rate of moderate hypothermia (temperature <36 °C) was slightly lower in the total body group (12%) than in the control group (20%).

Only a few studies have examined the effect of head insulation on neonatal heat loss after delivery (Chaput de Saintonge et al. 1979; Rowe et al. 1983; Stothers 1981; Lang et al. 2004). These studies, conducted in healthy full-term infants, show that neonatal heat loss following delivery may be reduced or prevented by the application of simple woolen hats.

22.8.2.6 Humidified and Heated Gas

The use of humidified and heated gas is the standard of care for preterm infants who need respiratory support in the NICU, but international resuscitation guidelines do not stipulate the use of this therapy during stabilization at birth (Kattwinkel et al. 2010).

One observational study with two historical cohorts (Pas et al. 2010) and one RCT (Meyer et al. 2015) from the same group assessed the impact of the use of the heated gases in preterm infants <32 weeks' gestation needing respiratory support (CPAP or intubation) at birth. The results show that the use of humidified and heated gases from birth added to the other measures to prevent hypothermia (i.e., use of a radiant heater in delivery room, suitable ambient temperature, body wrap, and head covering) may be of benefit for preterm infants <32 weeks and particularly for those <28 weeks.

22.8.2.7 Combination of Interventions

More than a single intervention, the sum of interventions is the "secret" to prevent delivery room thermal losses in preterm infants. In addition, a quality improvement intervention involving all the staff seems to be fruitful to reach this goal. For example, the introduction of checklists for preparation of material and the opportunity to give continuous feedbacks to the team were other important organizational aspects (Wyckoff et al. 2015; Wyllie et al. 2015).

A recent meta-analysis including four American studies shows that this strategy is effective to reduce hypothermia at NICU admission in preterm infants (Trevisanuto D, De Almeida MF, unpublished data) (Fig. 10).

2015 international guidelines for neonatal resuscitation recommend that the application of all these measures associated with checklists and frequent feedbacks on the team are able to optimize the thermal management of preterm infants (Wyckoff et al. 2015; Wyllie et al. 2015). Following this practice, the frequency of hypothermia in extremely low-birth-weight infants at NICU admission significantly declined over time at our institution (Rech Morassutti F et al. 2015; Fig. 11).

22.8.2.8 Skin-to-Skin Contact

Early skin-to-skin contact (SSC) begins ideally at birth and involves placing the naked baby, head covered with a dry cap and a warm blanket across the back, prone on the mother's bare chest. A recent Cochrane review assessed the effects of early SSC on breastfeeding, physiological adaptation, and behavior in healthy mother-newborn dyads (Moore et al. 2012). For the outcome "infant thermoregulation," only three studies were reported including a total of 168 dyads (mother and neonate). Two studies showed a positive effect of SSC on temperature control during the first 90 postnatal minutes (RR 0.40, 95% CI 0.19–0.61, and RR 0.50, 95% CI 0.17–0.83 respectively), whereas in one study temperatures were on average slightly higher for the control group at this time point (RR −0.10, 95% −0.24 to 0.04). A further study, conducted in a low-resource setting, assessed the impact of early SSC provided for the first 24 h on incidence of hypothermia in stable newborns weighing 1,800 g or more during the first 48 h of life (Nimbalkar et al. 2014). In the intervention group, mothers followed the SSC procedure. In the control group, after providing routine care under radiant warmer, newborns were kept clothed (including head cap) and covered with blanket with their mother (bedding in) for the first 48 h. The results showed that mean temperature in the SSC group was higher compared with the control group at all stages of reading during the first 48 h of life.

Temperature of newborns in SSC groups progressively increased after birth, whereas in the control group, there was reduction in temperature at 1 h of birth and never matched with the SSC group for the first 48 h. This study also showed that early SSC for the first 24 h can

Study or Subgroup	Intervention Events	Intervention Total	Control Events	Control Total	Weight	Odds Ratio M-H,Fixed, 95%CI
DeMauro SB, 2013	1	80	11	80	1.5%	0.08 [0.01, 0.63]
Lee HC, 2014	328	4132	633	4179	80.6%	0.48 [0.42, 0.56]
Pinheiro JMB, 2o14	20	440	56	164	10.8%	0.09 [0.05, 0.16]
Russo A, 2014	12	193	36	66	7.0%	0.06 [0.03, 0.12]
Total (95% CI)		4845		4489	100.0%	0.40 [0.35, 0.46]
Total events	361		736			

Heterogeneity: $Chi^2 = 62.53$, df = 3 ($P < 0.00001$); $I^2 = 95\%$
Test for overall effect: Z = 13.38 ($P < 0.00001$)

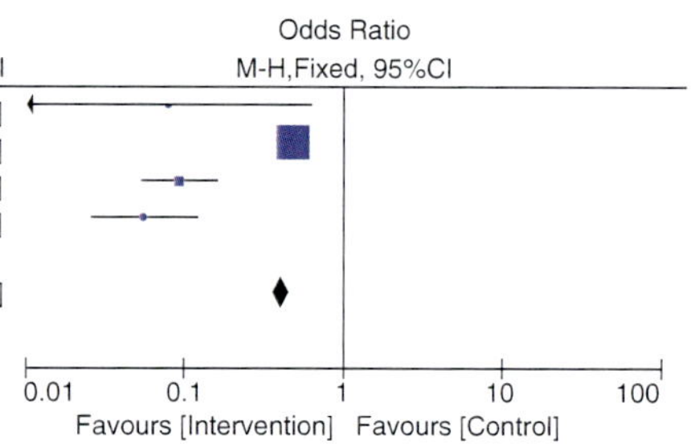

Fig. 10 Effect of an approach based on the combination of interventions associated with the use of checklists and feedback on reducing hypothermia at NICU admission in preterm infants (Trevisanuto D, De Almeida MF, unpublished data)

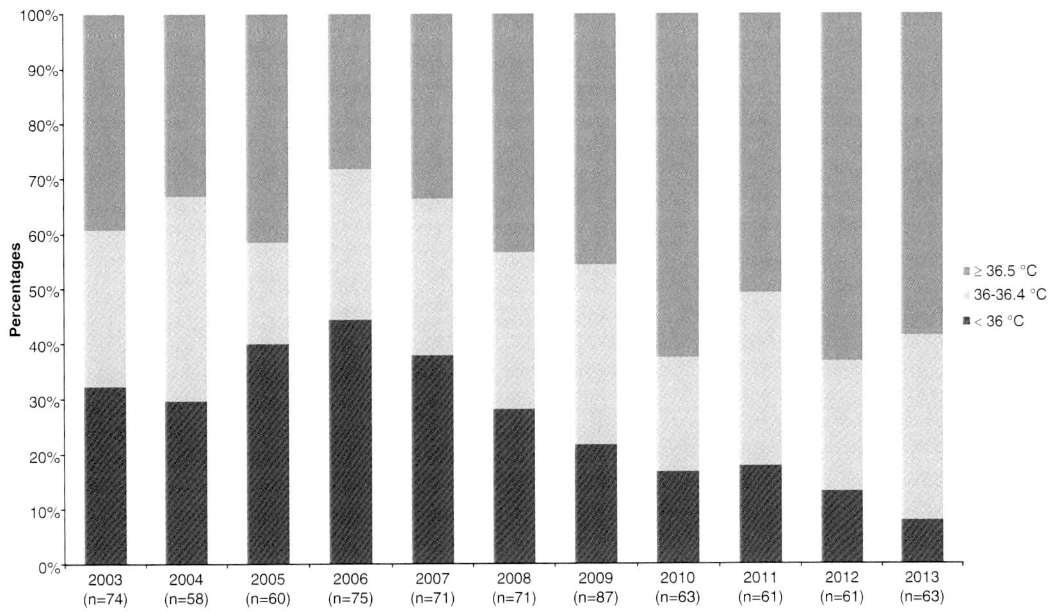

Fig. 11 Distribution of temperature at NICU admission over time at the Department of Women's and Children's Health, Azienda Ospedaliera di Padova, University of Padua (Rech Morassutti F et al. 2015)

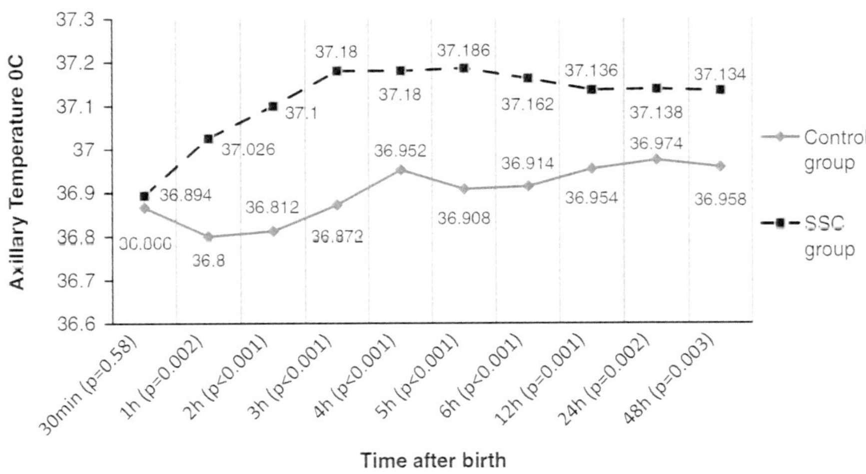

Fig. 12 Mean temperature during the first 48 postnatal hours in SSC and control group (Nimbalkar et al. 2014)

reduce the risk of hypothermia at 48 h of life (Fig. 12).

The results of these studies suggest that early SSC is effective, and it should be promoted to prevent hypothermia in term and late-preterm newborns, especially in low-resource settings.

In conclusion, hypothermia at NICU admission is a worldwide problem and is an independent predictor of neonatal morbidity and mortality. Effective interventions to prevent heat losses at birth, especially in very preterm infants, comprise increase of environmental temperature, use of infant warmers, exothermic mattress, woolen caps, plastic wraps, and humidified and heated gas. Skin-to-skin contact has been considered, especially in low-resource settings.

References

Adamson SK Jr, Gandy GM, James LS (1965) The influence of thermal factors on oxygen consumption of newborn human infants. J Pediatr 66:495–508

Agren J, Sjors G, Sedin G (1998) Transepidermal water loss in infants born at 24 and 25 weeks of gestation. Acta Paediatr 87:1185–1190

Agren J, Sjors G, Sedin G (2006) Ambient humidity influences the rate of skin barrier maturation in extremely preterm infants. J Pediatr 148:613–617

Bauer K, Uhrig C, Sperling P et al (1997) Body temperature and oxygen consumption during skin-to-skin (kangaroo) care in stable preterm infants weighting less than 1500 grams. J Pediatr 130:240–244

Bauer K, Pyper A, Sperling P et al (1998) Effects of gestational and postnatal age on body temperature, oxygen consumption, and activity during early skin-to-skin contact between preterm infants of 25–30 week gestation and their mothers. Pediatr Res 44:247–251

Baumgart S (1982) Radiant energy and insensible water loss in the premature newborn infant nursed under a radiant warmer. Clin Perinatol 9:483–503

Bell EF, Weinstein MR, Oh W (1980) Heat balance in premature infants: comparative effects of convectively heated incubator and radiant warmer, with and without plastic heat shield. J Pediatr 96:460–465

Bruck (1978) Heat production and temperature regulation. In: Stave U, Weech A (eds) Perinatal physiology. Plenum Medical Book Company, New York

Chaput de Saintonge DM, Cross KW, Hathorn MKS et al (1979) Hats for the newborn infant. BMJ 2:570–571

Chawla S, Amaram A, Gopal SP et al (2011) Safety and efficacy of Trans-warmer mattress for preterm neonates: results of a randomized controlled trial. J Perinatol 31:780–784

Cordaro T, Gibbons Phalen A et al (2012) Hypothermia and occlusive skin wrap in the low birthweight premature infant: an evidentiary review. Newborn Infant Nurs Rev 12:78–85

Cornblath M, Schwrtz R (1966) Disorders of carbohydrate metabolism in infancy. WB Saunders, Philadelphia

Cramer K, Wiebe N, Hartling L et al (2005) Heat loss prevention: a systematic review of occlusive skin wrap for premature neonates. J Perinatol 25:763–769

Dahm LS, James LS (1972) Newborn temperature and calculated heat loss in delivery room. Pediatrics 49:504–513

Doglioni N, Cavallin F, Mardegan V et al (2014) Total body polyethylene wraps for preventing hypothermia in preterm infants: a randomized trial. J Pediatr 165:261–266.e1

Fanaroff AA, Wald M, Gruber HS et al (1972) Insensible water low in low birth weight infants. Pediatrics 50:236–245

Flenady VJ, Woodgate PG (2003) Radiant warmers versus incubators for regulating body temperature in newborn infants. Cochrane Database Syst Rev 2, CD000435

Gray PH, Flenady V (2003) Cot-nursing versus incubator care in preterm infants. Cochrane Database Syst Rev 1, CD003062

Greenspan JS, Cullen AB, Touch SM et al (2001) Thermal stability and transition studies with a hybrid warming device for neonates. J Perinatol 21:167–173

Hammarlund K, Sedin G (1979) Transepidermal water loss in newborn infants. III. Relation to gestational age. Acta Paediatr Scand 68:795–801

Hammarlund K, Sedin G (1982) Transepidermal water loss in newborn infants. VI. Heat exchange with the environment in relation to gestational age. Acta Paediatr Scand 71:191–196

Hammarlund K, Nilsson GE, Oberg PA et al (1980) Transepidermal water loss in newborn infants. V. Evaporation from the skin and heat exchange during the first Hours of life. Acta Paediatr Scand 69:385–392

Hammarlund K, Sedin G, Stromberg B (1983) Transepidermal water loss in newborn infants. VIII. Relation to gestational age and post-natal age in appropriate and small for gestational age infants. Acta Paediatr Scand 72:721–728

Hammarlund K, Norsted T, Riesenfeld T et al (1985) Endotracheal intubation influences respiratory water loss during heat stress in young lambs. J Appl Physiol 79:801–804

Hammarlund K, Sromberg B, Sedin G (1986) Heat loss from the skin of preterm and fullterm newborn infants during the first weeks after birth. Biol Neonat 50:1–10

Hammarlund K, Reisenfield T, Sedin G (1988) Measurements of respiratory water loss in newborn lambs. Acta Physiol Scand 127:61–65

Hey EN (1969) The relation between environmental temperature and oxygen consumption in newborn baby. J Physiol 200:589–603

Hey EN, Katz G (1969) Evaporative water loss in newborn baby. J Physiol 200:605–619

Houdas Y, Ring EFJ (1982) Human body temperature. Its measurement and regulation. Plenum Press, New York

Ibrahim CPH, Yoxall CW (2010) Use of self-heating gel mattresses eliminates admission hypothermia in infants born below 28 weeks gestation. Eur J Pediatr 169:795–799

Jia YS, Lin ZL, Lv H et al (2013) Effect of delivery room temperature on the admission temperature of premature infants: a randomized controlled trial. J Perinatol 33:264–267

Kattwinkel J, Perlman JM, Aziz K et al (2010) Part 15: neonatal resuscitation: 2010 American Heart Association Guidelines for Cardiopulmonary Resuscitation and Emergency Cardiovascular Care. Circulation 122: S909–S919

Kent AL, Williams J (2008) Increasing ambient operating theatre temperature and wrapping in polyethylene improves admission temperature in premature infants. J Paediatr Child Health 44:325–331

Kjartansson S, Hammarlund K, Riesenfeld T et al (1992a) Respiratory water loss and oxygen consumption in newborn infants during phototherapy. Acta Paediatr 81:769–773

Kjartansson S, Hammarlund K, Sedin G (1992b) Insensible water loss from the skin during phototherapy in term and preterm infants. Acta Paediatr 81:764–768

Kjartansson S, Arsan S, Hammarlund K et al (1995) Water loss from the skin of term and preterm infants nursed under a radiant heater. Pediatr Res 37:233–238

Klein AD, Scammon RE (1930) The regional growth of the surface area of the human body in prenatal life. Proc Soc Exp Med Biol 27:463–466

Knobel RB, Wimmer JE Jr, Holbert D (2005) Heat loss prevention for preterm infants in the delivery room. J Perinatol 25:304–308

Lang N, Bromiker R, Arad I (2004) The effect of wool vs. cotton head covering and length of stay with the mother following delivery on infant temperature. Int J Nurs Stud 41:843–846

Laptook AR, Salhab W, Bhaskar B et al (2007) Neonatal Research Network. Admission temperature of low birth weight infants: predictors and associated morbidities. Pediatrics 119:e643–e649

Lyu Y, Shah PS, Ye XY et al (2015) Association between admission temperature and mortality and major morbidity in preterm infants born at fewer than 33 weeks' gestation. JAMA Pediatr 169, e150277

Marks KH, Gunther RC, Rossi JA et al (1980) Oxygen consumption and insensible water loss in premature infants under radiant heaters. Pediatrics 66:228–232

McCall EM, Alderdice F, Halliday HL et al (2010) Interventions to prevent hypothermia at birth in preterm and/or low birthweight infants. Cochrane Database Syst Rev 17(3), CD004210

McCarthy LK, O'Donnell CP (2011) Warming preterm infants in the delivery room: polyethylene bags, exothermic mattresses or both? Acta Paediatr 100:1534–1537

McCarthy LK, Molloy EJ, Twomey AR et al (2013) A randomized trial of exothermic mattresses for preterm newborns in polyethylene bags. Pediatrics 132: e135–e141

Meyer MP, Hou D, Ishrar NN et al (2015) Initial respiratory support with cold, dry gas versus heated humidified gas and admission temperature of preterm infants. J Pediatr 166:245–250

Miller SS, Lee HC, Gould JB et al (2011) Hypothermia in very low birth weight infants: distribution, risk factors and outcomes. J Perinatol 31(Suppl 1):S49–S56

Moore ER, Anderson GC, Bergman N et al (2012) Early skin-to-skin contact for mothers and their healthy newborn infants. Cochrane Database Syst Rev 16(5), CD003519

Nilsson GE (1977) Measurement of water exchange through skin. Med Biol Eng Comput 15:209–218

Nimbalkar SM, Patel VK, Patel DV et al (2014) Effect of early skin-to-skin contact following normal delivery on incidence of hypothermia in neonates more than 1800 g: randomized control trial. J Perinatol 34:364–368

Okken A, Blijham C, Franz W et al (1982) Effects of forced convection of heated air on insensible water loss and heat loss in preterm infants in incubators. J Pediatr 101:108–112

Pribylova H, Znamenacek K (1966) The effect of body temperature on the level of carbohydrate metabolites and oxygen consumption in the newborn. Pediatrics 37:743–749

Rech Morassutti F, Cavallin F, Zaramella P (2015) Association of rewarming rate on neonatal outcomes in extremely low birth weight infants with hypothermia. J Pediatr 167:557–561.e1-2

Reilly MC, Vohra S, Rac VE et al (2015) Randomized trial of occlusive wrap for heat loss prevention in preterm infants. J Pediatr 166:262–268.e2

Riesenfeld T, Hammarlund K, Sedin G (1987a) Respiratory water loss in fullterm infants on their first day after birth. Acta Paediatr Scand 76:647–653

Riesenfeld T, Hammarlund K, Sedin G (1987b) Respiratory water loss in relation to activity in fullterm infants an their first day after birth. Acta Paediatr Scand 76:889–893

Riesenfeld T, Hammarlund K, Sedin G (1988) Influence of radiant heat stress on respiratory water loss in newborn lambs. Biol Neonate 53:290–294

Riesenfeld T, Hammarlund K, Sedin G (1990) The effect of a warm environment on respiratory water loss in fullterm newborn infants on their first day after birth. Acta Paediatr Scand 79:893–898

Riesenfeld T, Hammarlund K, Norsted T et al (1994) The temperature of inspired air influences respiratory water loss in young lambs. Biol Neonate 65:326–330

Riesenfeld T, Hammarlund K, Sedin G (1995) Respiratory water loss in relation to gestational age in infants on their first day after birth. Acta Paediatr 84:1056–1059

Rowe MI, Weinberg G, Andrews W (1983) Reduction of neonatal heat loss by an insulated head cover. J Pediatr Surg 18:909–913

Sarman I, Can G, Tunell R (1989) Rewarming preterm infant on a heated, water filled mattress. Arch Dis Child 64:687–692

Sedin G (1995) Physics of neonatal heat transfer, routes of heat loss and heat gain. In: Okken A, Kock J (eds) Thermoregulation of sick and low birth weight neonates. Springer, Berlin, p 21

Sedin G (1996a) Fluid management in the extremely preterm infant. In: Hansen TN, McIntosh N (eds) Current topics in neonatology. WB Saunders Company, London, pp 50–66

Sedin G (1996b) Heat loss from the respiratory tract of newborn infants ventilated during transport. In: The proceeding of the XV European Congress on Perinatal Medicine. Glasgow, p 511

Sedin G (2004) Physics and physiology of human neonatal incubator. In: Polin R, Fox W (eds) Fetal and neonatal physiology. Saunders Company, Philadelphia, p 570

Singh A, Duckett J, Newton T et al (2010) M. Improving neonatal unit admission temperatures in preterm babies: exothermic mattresses, polythene bags or a traditional approach? J Perinatol 30:45–49

Sjörs G, Hammarlund K, Sedin G (1992a) Thermal balance in term and preterm newborn infants nursed in an incubator equipped with a radiant heat source. Pediatr Res 32:631

Sjörs G, Hammarlund K, Oberg PA et al (1992b) An evaluation of environment and climate control in seven infant incubators. Biomed Instrum Technol 26:294–301

Sjors G, Hammarlund K, Kjartasson S et al (1994) Respiratory water loss and oxygen consumption in fullterm infants exposed to cold air on the first day after birth. Acta Paediatr 83:802–807

Sjörs G, Hammarlund K, Sedin G (1997) Thermal balance in term and preterm infants nursed in an incubator with a radiant heat source. Acta Paediatr 86:403–409

Sosulski R, Polin R, Baumgart S (1983) Respiratory water loss and heat balance in intubated infants receiving humidified air. J Pediatr 103:307–310

Stern L, Lees MH, Leduc J (1965) Environmental temperature on the level of carbohydrate and catecholamine excretion in newborn infants. Pediatrics 36:367–373

Stothers JK (1981) Head insulation and heat loss in the newborn. Arch Dis Child 56:530–534

Stromberg B, Oberg PA, Sedin G (1983) Transepidermal water loss in newborn infants. X Effects of central cold-stimulation on evaporation rate and skin blood flow. Acta Paediatr Scand 71:735–739

Sulyok E, Jequier E, Prod'hom LS (1973) Respiratory contribution to the thermal balance of the newborn infant under various ambient conditions. Pediatrics 51:641–650

te Pas AB, Lopriore E, Dito I et al (2010) Humidified and heated air during stabilization at birth improves temperature in preterm infants. Pediatrics 125: e1427–e1432

Trevisanuto D, Coretti I, Doglioni N et al (2011) Effective temperature under radiant infant warmer: does the device make a difference? Resuscitation 82:720–723

Vohra S, Frent G, Campbell V et al (1999) Effect of polyethylene occlusive skin wrapping on heat loss in very low birth weight infants at delivery: a randomized trial. J Pediatr 134:547–551

Vohra S, Roberts RS, Zhang B et al (2004) Heat loss prevention (HeLP) in the delivery room: a randomized controlled trial of polyethylene occlusive skin wrapping in very preterm infants. J Pediatr 145: 750–753

Wheldon AE (1982) Energy balance in the newborn baby: use of a manikin to estimate radiant and convective heat loss. Phys Med Biol 27:285–296

Whitelaw A, Heisterkamp G, Steatlh K et al (1988) Skin to skin contact for very low birth weight infants and their mothers. Arch Dis Child 63:1377–1381

WHO Library Cataloguing-in-Publication Data. World Health Organization (2003) Managing newborn problems: a guide for doctors, nurses, and midwives. World Health Organization pp. F30–F31

Wyckoff MH, Aziz K, Escobedo MB et al (2015) Part 13: neonatal resuscitation: 2015 American Heart Association guidelines update for cardiopulmonary resuscitation and emergency cardiovascular care. Circulation 132:S543–S560

Wyllie J, Bruinenberg J, Roehr CC et al (2015) European resuscitation council guidelines for resuscitation 2015: section 7. Resuscitation and support of transition of babies at birth. Resuscitation 95:249–263

Neonatology and the Law

23

Vittorio Fineschi, Francesca Maglietta, and Emanuela Turillazzi

Contents

Abstract

Neonatology is one of the areas of medicine that in recent years has received much attention. This interest primarily concerns the constant progress in this field and the inherent ethical and medico legal problems. The extensive debate about some issues reflects both the technical and scientific progresses that have been made in the neonatological field. On the other hand, tightly argued issues such as medical malpractice litigation have reached crisis proportions in the neonatological and pediatric field. Moreover, pediatric claims are very expensive because the damages cover the life of the child and the juries tend to be very sympathetic toward children and their families. Care at the limits of viability and cerebral palsy are some of the more contentious areas of legal medicine on the neonatological field. Since recognizing "red flags" can lessen chances of malpractice claims against neonatologists, this chapter

V. Fineschi (✉)
Department of Anatomical, Histological, Forensic Medicine and Orthopaedic Sciences, "Sapienza" University of Rome, Rome, Italy
e-mail: vittorio.fineschi@uniroma1.it

F. Maglietta · E. Turillazzi
Department of Legal Medicine, University of Foggia, Foggia, Italy
e-mail: maglietta.f@gmail.com; emanuela.turillazzi@unifg.it

G. Buonocore et al. (eds.), *Neonatology*,
https://doi.org/10.1007/978-3-319-29489-6_173

focuses on some issues which have a high vulnerability to claims of medical negligence and on high-risk situations. The principles are primarily the same for any doctor working in any country under any clinical circumstances; of course, subtle differences in the law can appertain to an individual case depending on where it arose and the jurisdiction that applies.

23.1 Salient Points

- Malpractice suits in neonatology mostly arise from delivery room care, poor neurologic outcome, infusion line complications, and delay in diagnosis/treatment.
- Medical decisions regarding care at the limits of viability (between 22 and 25 weeks) should be based on the individual circumstances of each newborn rather than on inflexible guidelines, especially if these are based only on gestational age.
- Neurologic damage in newborns frequently leads to allegations of peripartum mismanagement; thus, new markers providing more accurate information about the timing of perinatal hypoxia would be of paramount importance to medical and legal professionals.
- The most prevalent cause of malpractice suits against pediatricians involves errors in diagnosis; for this reason, many physicians have resorted to defensive medicine, ordering unnecessary additional tests or diagnostic procedures.
- Malpractice claims are often caused by inadequate informed consent.Good communication, using layman's terms and avoiding medical jargon, is critical in reducing malpractice lawsuits.

23.2 Introduction

Neonatology is one of the areas of medicine that in recent years has received much attention. This interest primarily concerns the constant progress in this field and the inherent ethical and medico legal problems. The extensive debate about some issues reflects both the technical and scientific progresses that have been made in the neonatological field. On the other hand, tightly argued issues such as medical malpractice litigation have reached crisis proportions in the neonatological and pediatric field. In general, children are more vulnerable when treated in any healthcare environment, but especially in the acute care setting, thus neonatologic and pediatric care carry unique factors that increase the risk of litigation (Greve 2011). Malpractice suits in neonatology most commonly arise from delivery room care, poor neurologic outcome (cerebral palsy/hypoxic-ischemic encephalopathy), line complications (thrombus and vascular accidents related to central lines), and delay in diagnosis/treatment – acidosis, hypotension, antibiotics, developmental dysplasia of the hip, and congenital heart disease. Pediatric claims are very expensive because the damages cover the life of the child and the juries tend to be very sympathetic toward children and their families (Donn 2005). Very few data are available on neonatal malpractice claims. Italian data reported that among over 190 claims, the majority regards events in delivery room and nursery (almost 40% each) while a lower percentage in NICU (about 20%) and a minimum number of cases in the transport system (almost 1%) (Fanos et al. 2012). The NICHD workshop on patient safety in 2011 pointed out some specific issues of patient safety in neonatology. In particular, the substantial sources of errors were:

(a) Medication and total parenteral nutrition
(b) Resuscitation and respiratory care
(c) Invasive procedures
(d) Nosocomial infections
(e) Patient identification
(f) Diagnostics

Factors that could increase the injury risk are likely to be related to size, prematurity, vulnerability, and underlying disease conditions of newborn patients, but also to multidisciplinary teams involved in the care of sick newborn infants, working conditions providing fatigue, a large variety of treatment, and investigative modalities needed in the care of high-risk newborn infants (e.g., ventilator, central catheter, medications, bed-side tests) (Raju et al. 2011). In developed countries, the insurance costs due to malpractice claims in conjunction with childbirth are steadily increasing, and today, they amount to 25% of all health insurance costs, primarily due to lifelong compensation for severe disabilities caused by asphyxia (Berglund and Norman 2012).

Neonatologists' concerns about a potential complaint, inquiry, or lawsuit influence their practice of medicine in potentially positive ways such as developing audit procedures, maintaining better communication with parents and families, ensuring timely documentation of procedures, and communication of complications, but also negatively such as increased prescribing of drugs, referrals, and diagnostic testing, and avoiding treatment of certain conditions.

Since recognizing "red flags" can lessen chances of malpractice claims against neonatologists (Donn et al. 2003), this chapter focuses on some issues which have a high vulnerability to claims of medical negligence and on high-risk situations. The principles are primarily the same for any doctor working in any country under any clinical circumstances; of course, subtle differences in the law can appertain to an individual case depending on where it arose and the jurisdiction that applies (Cowan 2005).

23.3 Neonatal Resuscitation Practices

23.3.1 Presuppositions

In recent decades, a lively debate has developed concerning the decision to interrupt or not to initiate resuscitation procedures on low gestational age newborns (Chiswick 2008; Pinter 2008; Sklansky 2001). In many countries, all over the world the flourishing of rulings by multidisciplinary study groups is evidence of the importance of this debate, with neonatologists, pediatricians, obstetricians, and bioethicists working together in the attempt to support decisions regarding whether to resuscitate "at risk" newborns or not (Brunkhorst et al. 2014; Arora et al. 2016; Liu et al. 2016) mostly at the gray zone of viability. At the same time there has been an increasingly insistent request for juridical regulation of neonatal resuscitation practices as well as for clarification of the role of parents in decisions regarding this kind of assistance.

The practice approach to the resuscitation of extremely low birth weight (ELBW) infants varies greatly between the countries and, in the same country, between different centers, reflecting a paucity of evidence and consequent uncertainty among clinicians. Different and increasing possibilities to intervene in ELBW infants' care necessarily require special attention, reflecting both the need to ensure that the mother and the newborn are offered adequate assistance and spare them useless, painful, and ineffective therapies.

The central issue regards the "of uncertain vitality" infants born between 22 and 25 weeks of gestational age whose treatment at birth is one of the most challenging concerns for neonatologists (Pignotti and Donzelli 2008). Advances in medical technology enable doctors to save the lives of newborn infants who would have previously died. Some of these infants have a low chance of survival with treatment or may survive with significant morbidity and shortened life expectancy. Even with full resuscitation efforts, two of three newborns delivered at 23 weeks of gestation die, and approximately 90% of survivors have moderate to serious disability.

When we are confronting with extremely low gestational age 22 weeks' gestational age (154–160 days' intrauterine life), a quite general agreement seems to exist that decisions regarding the treatment of the mother must be based on her health conditions, cesarean section must be performed only when indicated by the mother's clinical conditions, and the newborn should be provided with comfort therapies. On the other hand, with the growth of gestational age if the newborn shows capacity to survive, the newborn's vitality must be carefully assessed at birth and resuscitation must be performed. On the basis of favorable objective clinical criteria (presence of attempts at respiration, valid cardiac frequency, recovery of skin color) which suggest proceeding with extraordinary therapies, intensive treatment of the newborn can become more advisable. It is widely believed that when gestational age is at 25 weeks, cesarean section may be performed for fetal reasons; newborns must be resuscitated and subjected to intensive, extraordinary therapies, except those cases presenting severely compromised clinical conditions suggesting the impossibility of survival.

In this scenario and after years of discussion across this troubled terrain, some crucial issues are intensely debate and still remain to be solved.

23.3.2 Some Critical Assumptions

First is the assumption that gestational age could be taken as a reference parameter for medical decisions. In fact, there is a fair margin of error in the estimation of gestational age, so that in dubious cases, clinical evaluation of the newborn is of fundamental importance. Neonatologists should take into account particularly the newborn's conditions at birth, obstetric history, and response to resuscitation procedures. A subtle decisional distinction exists in that gray zone in which even a temporal oscillation of a few days may lead to abstention from neonatal resuscitation procedures or, conversely, the initiation of resuscitation therapies. On the other hand, neonatal prognosis is conditioned by many independent predictive factors (birth weight, use of steroids before birth, multiplicity of pregnancy) (Patel 2016).

In general, the literature has established as the limit of viability the interval between 22 and 25 weeks of gestational age. Below this limit it is considered that the degree of developmental immaturity is a limiting factor to life and the benefit of treatment is not challenged (Seri and Evans 2008; Blackmon 2003). However, the chronological criterion of gestational age alone might lead to a dangerous simplification in evaluating decisional paths, giving an excessive value to one single parameter. It is well known that the prognosis for very preterm children varies with the place of birth (level III perinatal center or not), the attitude of both obstetricians and pediatricians toward care and hence the interventions they use, gestational age, postnatal age, and then later comorbidities (Patel 2016). Thus, there is a great difficult in defining the proper management for newborns in this gray zone (Haward et al. 2011; Nadroo 2011; April and Parker 2007; Savulescu and Kahane 2009).

Furthermore, no other area of medicine has been as focused upon such policies or as specific in delineating treatment limitations. Instead, in other areas, guidelines are broad and general, with much room for individual clinical judgment and professional discretion. What some authors find, in fact, is that policies for newborns appear very different from those for other patient populations (Janvier et al. 2007). In fact, even in critical situations burdened by high mortality or morbidity (e.g., adult patients with cardiac arrest after trauma; cardiac arrest in children following severe trauma; adult patients with a primary hemorrhagic stroke), the low percentages of survival or even the prevision of long term significant and disabling sequelae certainly do not lead to abstention from the resuscitation procedures laid down in rigorous protocols or guidelines (Savulescu and Kahane 2009; Janvier et al. 2007; Janvier et al. 2008).

Finally, a point of fundamental importance is the centrality of parents in the decision-making process regarding the therapies administered to their premature newborns. It being understood that resuscitation treatment requires immediate decisions and prompt and timely actions, the parents should be provided with understandable and exhaustive information about the newborns' conditions and their life expectancy, offering them understanding and all possible psychological support. In the event of a conflict between the parents' requests and the physician's decision, a shared solution should be sought, taking into consideration the safeguard of the fetus and newborn's life and health.

23.3.3 The Crux of the Matter

Not only guidelines differ but also international, national, and local variations in actual practice do exist and recent data suggest there may be a gap between policy recommendations calling for shared decision making and actual clinical practice in resuscitation decision for periviable births (Tucker Edmonds et al. 2016).

The crux of the matter is whether strict guidelines, reference standards based on the gestational age parameter, and authority rules are necessary. We personally believe that the right answer to this question is "no". In a decisional sphere burdened by such limited prognostic certainties, an individual approach is infinitely more acceptable than a statistical approach: any decision ought to be based upon the individual circumstances of each newborn rather than on reference to guidelines, especially if these are based on gestational age (Turillazzi and Fineschi 2009). Physicians do not need rigid rules based on inflexible gestational age and birthweight guidelines but guidance to address the difficult and trying issues associated with infants born at the margins of viability with a realistic assessment of the infant's clinical condition (Fanaroff 2008). We firmly think that as the principles regarding treatment of low or very low gestational age newborn should be the same of those followed for other patients, there is no need for specific policy statement. Generally, the purposes of guidelines have to improve knowledge regarding neonatal outcomes, to provide consistency in periviability counseling, and to promote informed, supportive, responsible choices. Flexible guidelines are well accepted and can be used by all neonatologists, obstetricians, and nurses who provide care to pregnant women and infants at extremely early gestational ages, but resuscitation decisions for extremely preterm infants should be approached in the same way as for other patients. They should be individualized with objective and the most accurate individual prognostication, taking into account all the relevant clinical characteristics.

23.4 Cerebral Palsy and Perinatal Hypoxia

23.4.1 Presuppositions

Despite the recognition that cerebral palsy (CP) is rarely related to medical malpractice, there are many instances where clinicians face litigation when a child is diagnosed with cerebral palsy.

Advances in science and technology have allowed researchers to gain a better understanding of the pathophysiology leading to long-term neurologic damage in newborns. Intrapartum events are now known to be an infrequent cause of adverse neurologic outcome. New insights into the origins of cerebral palsy have recently transformed the old concept that most cases of cerebral palsy begin in labor. Many factors can damage the "developing" fetal brain including prepartum, intrapartum and postpartum ischemia/hypoxemia, developmental abnormalities, genetic factors, metabolic disease, infections, autoimmune and coagulation disorders, and maternal and fetal drug use (MacLennan 1999). Clinical signs of brain damage are often considered to result from intrapartum asphyxia and a marker of perinatal obstetric and/or neonatologic mismanagement leading to medico-legal problems. Contrary to previous beliefs and assumptions, clinical epidemiological studies indicate that in most cases the events leading to cerebral palsy occur in the fetus before the onset of labor, or in the newborn after delivery. Actually it is suggested that 70–80% of cases of CP are due to prenatal factors and that birth asphyxia plays a relatively minor role. Intrapartum asphyxia is believed to account for around 10% of CP in term and near-term infants (Graham et al. 2008). Notwithstanding many advances in research into the causation of cerebral palsy, defining a causal relation between acute intrapartum events and cerebral palsy still remains very difficult.

Since the event of a brain damaged newborn frequently led to allegations of peripartum mismanagement, understanding the time of onset of the brain lesion is of paramount importance to medical and legal professionals. In Courts, in fact, much of the debate focuses on whether or not there is evidence of acute intrapartum hypoxia and if so, whether the care provided was timely and adequate (Greenwood et al. 2003; Freeman 2008).

23.4.2 The Timing of Perinatal Hypoxia

The timing of perinatal hypoxia is complex and incompletely understood. It is traditionally based on clinical, laboratory and instrumental criteria which are nonspecific markers of a difficult birth (Paneth 2001; Blair and Stanley 1997). These nonspecific intrapartum markers provide poor information on the timing and duration of an asphyxiating insult (Nielsen et al. 2008). Autopsy, placental and cord examination, laboratory tests, and genetic studies may explain both the cause of death and the time of onset of the neuropathology. Brain histological examination can provide useful information on the timing of an hypoxic-ischemic lesion; the patterns of perinatal brain injury depend on the etiology and the stage of development of the fetal nervous system, since the vulnerabilities of gray and white matter differ depending on postconceptional age and on neuroanatomic site (Folkerth 2007; Squier 2002). New insights into the mechanisms involved in neonatal hypoxic-ischemic brain injury have recently transformed the old concept that most cases are the results of an acute hypoxia during labor and delivery.

Since October 1999, the International Cerebral Palsy Task Force published a consensus statement for defining a causal relationship between acute intrapartum events and cerebral palsy in the aim to attempt "to define an objective template of evidence to better identify cases of cerebral palsy where the neuropathology began or became established around labour and birth." Three "essential criteria," which should be met before attributing cerebral palsy to an intrapartum hypoxic event and a number of "criteria that together suggest an intrapartum timing, but are non- specific" were established (Greenwood et al. 2003).

Laboratory studies, that is, acid-base disturbance assessed by means of umbilical-artery pH measurement, serum concentration of brain-specific creatine kinase isoenzyme BB (CK-BB), other serum factors (blood lactate, hypoxanthine, aspartate-aminotransferase, erythropoietin beta-endorphin), factors measured in the CSF (lactate, neuron-specific enolase, lactate dehydrogenase, hydroxybutyrate dehydrogenase, fibrinogen degradation products, ascorbic acid) may have an utility in defining the timing of an hypoxic event. Imaging studies such as head ultrasonography may be very useful for the detection of typical injuries' patterns (PVL, lesions of the basal ganglia, cerebral edema, ischemic infarcts). Cranial CT may depict ischemic or hemorrhagic lesions, generalized or focal edema, and diffuse cerebral atrophy with ex vacuo ventricular dilatation due to severe hypoxemic insult. On CT, PVL can be well visualized appearing as a region of decreased attenuation, occasionally intermixed with areas of increased attenuation due to secondary hemorrhage. However, MRI is the imaging modality of choice in the assessment of cerebral hypoxic lesion.

In cases of neonatal death, it is essential that the contribution of autoptic examination is complemented by toxicological, microbiological, and genetic investigations (Squier and Cowan 2004). The histological study of the brain with traditional histochemical techniques can provide relevant data since it is well known that depending on mechanism, severity, and timing of the insult, the distribution and the histological pattern of lesions in the brain changes dramatically. The international scientific panorama is actually rich of studies aiming to the research of histological, histochemical, and immunohistochemical markers which can provide more and more accurate information about the time of onset of hypoxic-ischemic brain damage. However, data reported by literature appear fragmentary and contradictory, often concerning experimental studies performed only on animals. Moreover, it should be underlined that most reports concern experimental studies which have used markers with late expression (>24 h) which, therefore, are scarcely reliable in cases of perinatal hypoxic-ischemic brain damage due to intrapartum asphyxia (Squier 2002). These neurobiological insights into the mechanisms of the cellular responses implicated in perinatal brain damages, and the characterization of the various mechanisms involved might open new horizons for understanding the time of onset of a brain hypoxic-ischemic lesion and for effective therapeutic strategies (Kadhim et al. 2005). By means of immunohistochemical techniques applied in studies both on animals and humans, it has been possible to identify in the brain tissue some markers of hypoxic-ischemic damage with reliable and reproducible results. The immunohistochemical picture obtained using a panel of selected antibodies (chaperonins HSPs, ORP-150, COX2) can help to identify a rather precise chronology of expression of the different markers of hypoxic-ischemic brain damage in newborns, which is correlated to the duration of the same insult and is to be ascribed, essentially, to a different stimulation of the different cellular types and also to a different response by the same cells to the ischemic insult. Some immunohistochemical markers seem to be more reliable than others in the evaluation of the timing of the neonatal hypoxic-ischemic damage (Riezzo et al. 2010). The results of histologic and immunohistochemical investigation would suggest a message to the clinicians to extend the differential diagnosis of a too large neonatal hypoxic-ischemic insult chronological category to delineate a more accurate judgment (Kadhim et al. 2005).

23.5 Informed Consent

Inadequate informed consent represents a very frequent basis alleged for medical malpractice also in the neonatological field where some issues are absolutely unique since consent is not obtained from the patient but from the family and, often, during a very emotionally stressful period. In the neonatological scenario, inadequate communication (between the obstetrician and pediatrician/neonatologist, the nurse and physician, or the healthcare team and the family) often led to malpractice claims (Donn 2005).

In the relation between physician and patient's parents and families, the problem of language and of the quality and the amount of the information becomes central: on one side there is the news, like mere description of a situation, and on the other side there is the information, as relationship with the person who receives the news. The two dimensions are not equivalent: to provide news and to provide information are not the same thing. In this regard, a fundamental issue is that of truth and of the amount of information which is to be provided to the newborns' family. How and how much is to be told about the newborn's disease, outcome, and prognosis? Which are the risks of a certain treatment that are to be explained? Which predictable sequelae are to be concealed to the newborn's parents?

The purpose of information and communication is to enable parents to make informed choices about health care of their newborns. However, in this perspective one crucial matter is the fact that we must distinguish the rights of the newborn and the capacity to make autonomous choices. A great caution is necessary when we are dealing with this issue; our attention must be focused on what is to be done with the newborn or the infant who have never had the capacity to make autonomous choices. Moreover, the dimension of informed consent has become more difficult to manage not only because technologies, widening the sphere of intervention and the possibilities of diagnosis and cure, have paradoxically sharpened the question but also because this question is more frequently transferred in judicial suits.

When we are dealing with the issue of informed consent in the neonatological and pediatric field, there are some unique challenges that differ somewhat from adult medicine.

One of the crucial questions which has major ethical importance is that of parents' role in the decision-making process. Many elements related to the newborn's parents, that is, to the recipient of the informative message are to be taken in account by the physician: their real desire of knowledge; their desire to participate to the therapeutic choices; their psychological condition; their level of knowledge. The risk is that information became only a moment of learned, specialistic, and iperspecialistic disquisitions to which parents remain completely stranger; a special burden is placed on the neonatologist to ensure that the newborn or infant's parents comprehended the explanation and information given.

Since malpractice claims are filed by parents whose newborns are died or have suffered poor outcomes, the value of the informed consent process in reducing malpractice losses may be undermined by the tendency to approach informed consent as a means to "protect" the physician rather than to communicate with the parents and to share clinical decisions, often very challenging, with them.

Open communication with parents and families should represent the gold standard of the physician- parents' patients relationship in which the physician and the parents, each with his/her background of competences and specificities, technical and scientific to those of the physician, human, of pain, perception, and quality of life to those of the parents, cooperate to the achievement of the aim health of the newborn. Parents are active participant in a dialogue that is important to the shared decision-making process; the physician has the burden to ensure that comprehension is achieved and that the parents themselves are acting in the best interests of the child.

Finally, the focus is on genomics testing in the neonatological context. Genomic testing could be used at multiple different time points, for example, preconception, preimplantation, antenatally or postnatally, and will play a role in neonatal treatment decisions. Neonatal intensive care units are especially suitable for early adoption of genetic testing because many of the 3528 monogenic diseases of known cause are present during the first 28 days of life (Online Mendelian Inheritance in Man 2012).

Genomic testing may be used for diagnosis and prognostically for critically ill infants. Aims of genetic testing may be summarized in: *treatment modification* to identify potential treatments; *anticipation or information*, providing parents with advance knowledge of potential future problems as well as the risk of recurrence in future offspring; *treatment limitation*, either because it is relevant to the best interests of the infant, to parental preferences for treatment or to resource allocation (Wilkinson et al. 2016).

Deep ethical challenges arise from these different use of genomic testing in neonatal care (Goldenberg and Sharp 2012; Stark et al. 2013). Traditional targeted diagnostic testing (such as those used for infants with a suspected not be diagnosed by conventional biochemical screening) is obviously the least problematic from an ethical point of view. When targeted prognostic testing is proposed, the balance between potential benefits and burdens of the test is substantial. Is prognostic information potentially actionable? Is the information unhelpful? Do the best interest of newborn (and future adolescent) coincide or conflict with that of parents? Facilitating parents' informed consent is substantial, but it could be not straightforward.

The complexity of what can be revealed with genetic testing and the parents' right to obtain a complete information before agreeing to genomic testing are key issues in the approach to genomic newborn testing (Cohen et al. 2013).

Genetic testing may reveal very troubling information, including potential, secondary incidental findings, so that clinicians and parents have to be prepared for the implications of the results (Lucassen 2012). As well as medical geneticists and genetic counselors, neonatologists may help families understand testing options and potential implications and can address the wide range of associated medical, psychosocial, and ethical issues that may arise before and after results are known. Given the background of uncertainty and future implications surrounding genomic testing in newborn, it is important for parents and families understanding the real meaning and scope of such a test. It is essential that parents have appropriate expectations and limitations of genetic testing for their newborn; neonatologists may play a substantial role in the decision-making process to enable parents to understand the testing being offered and make informed choices (Frati et al. 2017).

23.6 Conclusion

During the last years, a host of issues have emerged from the explosive growth of neonatological science. In fact, neonatology is one of the areas of medicine that, in recent years, has received much attention, both in the scientific literature and in the ethical and juridical debate. This interest primarily concerns the constant progress in resuscitation of extremely preterm newborns and the inherent ethical problems which is a still debated question. Prior to the new technologies, we accepted the death of extremely preterm newborns as a natural and inevitable event. The new technologies may represent wonderful means to save life of viable newborns; however, the problem emerges when it becomes evident that the strategies deployed could achieve desirable outcomes. Is it appropriate to continue therapies on an extremely preterm newborn when their only effect is to preserve life or to postpone death, irrespective of any question on the quality of life of that newborn? Are the rights and whishes of the parents to be considered when it is evident that the continuance of therapies is medically futile? Are guidelines and law regulations appropriate places for these determinations? Or, on the contrary, should these be made at the bedside by physicians and parents together?

Furthermore, we stressed on the fact that a reality of the current practice of medicine is that physicians will likely be faced with a malpractice claim at some point in their career. Neonatologists and pediatrics are not immune from this reality. Issues involved in documentation and communication are substantial also in neonatologists' practice. Consequently, neonatologists are encouraged to explore parents' lived experiences and expectations and engage in trusting empowering relationships. Finally, it calls on neonatologists to the need for thorough and accurate documentation in practice.

References

April C, Parker M (2007) End of life decision-making in neonatal care. J Med Ethics 33:126–127

Arora C, Savulescu J, Maslen H, Selgelid M, Wilkinson D (2016) The intensive care lifeboat: a survey of lay attitudes to rationing dilemmas in neonatal intensive care. BMC Med Ethics 17(1):69

Berglund S, Norman M (2012) Neonatal resuscitation assessment: documentation and early paging must be improved! Arch Dis Child Fetal Neonatal Ed 97(3): F204–F208

Blackmon LR (2003) Biologic limits of viability: implications for clinical decision-making. NeoReviews 4: e140–e146

Blair E, Stanley FJ (1997) Issues in the classification and epidemiology of cerebral palsy. Ment Retard Dev Disabil Res Rev 3:184–193

Brunkhorst J, Weiner J, Lantos J (2014) Infants of borderline viability: the ethics of delivery room care. Semin Fetal Neonatal Med 19(5):290–295

Chiswick M (2008) Infants of borderline viability: ethical and clinical considerations. Semin Fetal Neonatal Med 13:8–15

Cohen J, Hoon A, Wilms Floet AM (2013) Providing family guidance in rapidly shifting sand: informed consent for genetic testing. Dev Med Child Neurol 55(8):766–768

Cowan PJ (2005) Litigation. Semin Fetal Neonatal Med 10:11–21

Donn SM (2005) Medical liability, risk management, and the quality of health care. Semin Fetal Neonatal Med 10:3–9

Donn SM, Chiswick ML, Whittell P, Anderson S (2003) Medico-legal implications of hypoxic ischemic brain injury. In: Donn SM, Sinha SK, Chiswick ML (eds) Birth asphyxia and the brain: basic science and clinical implications. Futura Publishing, Armonk, pp 379–401

Fanaroff AA (2008) Extremely low birthweight infants – the interplay between outcomes and ethics. Acta Paediatr 97:144–145

Fanos V, Tagliabue P, Greco L, Agostiniani R, Carbone MT, D'Agostino P, Correra A (2012) Neonatal malpractice claims in Italy: how big is the problem and which are the causes? J Matern Fetal Neonatal Med 25(5):493–497

Folkerth RD (2007) The neuropathology of acquired pre- and perinatal brain injuries. Semin Diagn Pathol 24:48–57

Frati P, Fineschi V, Di Sanzo M, La Russa R, Scopetti M, Severi FM, Turillazzi E (2017) Preimplantation and prenatal diagnosis, wrongful birth and wrongful life: a global view of bioethical and legal controversies. Hum Reprod Update 23(3):338–357

Freeman RK (2008) Medical and legal implications for necessary requirements to diagnose damaging hypoxic-ischemic encephalopathy leading to later cerebral palsy. Am J Obstet Gynecol 199:585–586

Goldenberg AJ, Sharp RR (2012) The ethical hazards and programmatic challenges of genomic newborn screening. JAMA 1:307(5). https://doi.org/10.1001/jama.2012.68

Graham EM, Ruis KA, Hartman AL et al (2008) A systematic review of the role of intrapartum hypoxia – ischemia in the causation of neonatal encephalopathy. Am J Obstet Gynecol 199:587–595

Greenwood C, Newman S, Impey L et al (2003) Cerebral palsy and clinical negligence litigation: a cohort study. BJOG 110:6–11

Greve P (2011) Pediatrics: a unique and volatile risk. J Healthc Risk Manag 31(2):19–29

Haward MF, Kirshenbaum NW, Campbell DE (2011) Care at the edge of viability: medical and ethical issues. Clin Perinatol 38:471–492

Janvier A, Bauer KL, Lantos JD (2007) Are newborns morally different from older children? Theor Med Bioeth 28:413–425

Janvier A, Leblanc I, Barrington KJ (2008) The best-interest standard is not applied for neonatal resuscitation decisions. Pediatrics 121:963–969

Kadhim H, Evrard P, Kahn A et al (2005) Insights into etiopathogenic mechanisms involved in perinatal cerebral injury: implications for neuroprotection. In: Fong HD (ed) Focus on cerebral palsy research. Nova Science Publishers, Hauppauge, pp 1–26

Liu J, Chen XX, Wang XL (2016) Ethical issues in neonatal intensive care units. J Matern Fetal Neonatal Med 29(14):2322–2326

Lucassen A (2012) Ethical implications of new genetic technologies. Dev Med Child Neurol 54:196

MacLennan A (1999) A template for defining a causal relation between acute intrapartum events and cerebral palsy: international consensus statement. BMJ 319:1054–1059

Nadroo AM (2011) Ethical dilemmas in decision making at limits of neonatal viability. J IMA 43:188–192

Nielsen LF, Schendel D, Grove J et al (2008) Asphyxia-related risk factors and their timing in spastic cerebral palsy. BJOG 115:1518–1528

Online Mendelian Inheritance in Man. McKusick-Nathans Institute of Genetic Medicine, Johns Hopkins University; Baltimore. Accessed 13 July 2012. Available at www.omim.org/statistics

Paneth N (2001) Cerebral palsy in term infants–birth or before birth? J Pediatr 138:791–792

Patel RM (2016) Short- and long-term outcomes for extremely preterm infants. Am J Perinatol 33(3):318–328

Pignotti MS, Donzelli G (2008) Perinatal care at the threshold of viability: an international comparison of practical guidelines for the treatment of extremely preterm births. Pediatrics 121:e193–e198

Pinter AB (2008) End-of-life decision before and after birth: changing ethical considerations. J Pediatr Surg 43:430–436

Raju TNK, Suresh G, Higgins RD (2011) Patient safety in the context of neonatal intensive care: research and educational opportunities. Pediatr Res 70(1):109–115

Riezzo I, Neri M, De Stefano F, Fulcheri E, Ventura F, Pomara C, Turillazzi E, Fineschi V (2010) The timing of perinatal hypoxia/ischemia events in term neonates: HSPs, ORP-150 and COX2 are reliable markers to classify acute, perinatal events. Diagn Pathol 5:49. doi:10.1186/1746-1596-5-49

Savulescu J, Kahane G (2009) The moral obligation to create children with the best chance of the best life. Bioethics 23:274–290

Seri I, Evans J (2008) Limits of viability: definition of the gray zone. J Perinatol 28:S4–S8

Sklansky M (2001) Neonatal euthanasia: moral considerations and criminal liability. J Med Ethics 27:5–11

Squier W (2002) Pathology of fetal and neonatal brain damage: identifying the timing. In: Squier W (ed) Aquired damage to the developing brain, timing and causation. Arnold, London, pp 110–127

Squier W, Cowan FM (2004) The value of autopsy in determining the cause of failure to respond to resuscitation at birth. Semin Neonatol 9:331–345

Stark Z, Gillam L, Walker SP, McGillivray G (2013) Ethical controversies in prenatal microarray. Curr Opin Obstet Gynecol 25(2):133–137

Tucker Edmonds B, McKenzie F, Panoch JE, White DB, Barnato AE (2016) A pilot study of neonatologists' decision-making roles in delivery room resuscitation counseling for periviable births. AJOB Empir Bioeth 7(3):175–182

Turillazzi E, Fineschi V (2009) How old are you? Newborn gestational age discriminates neonatal resuscitation practices in the Italian debate. BMC Med Ethics 12:10–19

Wilkinson DJC, Barnett C, Savulescu J, Newson AJ (2016) Genomic intensive care: should we perform genome testing in critically ill newborns? Arch Dis Child Fetal Neonatal Ed 101(2):F94–F98

Environment and Early Developmental Care for Newborns

24

Dominique Haumont

Contents

Abstract

Preterm infants are exposed in the neonatal intensive care unit (NICU) to an environment of important and often chaotic neurosensory stimulation. There is substantial scientific evidence to support the negative effects of pain and stress, prolonged periods of intense light and noise, sleep disturbances, and difficulties of parenting. It is against this background that early developmental care (EDC) has been proposed. The important elements of early developmental care are parental physical and emotional closeness, fine-tuning of care according to appropriate assessment of the preterm infant behavior, strategies to reduce stress, and a NICU design adapted to provide this type of care.

Among the different strategies of EDC, restoring the mother-infant dyad (couplet care) and the Neonatal Individualized Developmental Care and Assessment Program (NIDCAP) are the most complex and holistic interventions.

Abbreviations

AS	Active sleep
EDC	Early developmental care
KMC	Kangaroo mother care
Nicu	Neonatal intensive care unit
NIDCAP	Neonatal individualized developmental care and assessment program
OS	Oxidative stress

D. Haumont (✉)
Department of Neonatology, Saint – Pierre University Hospital, Brussels, Belgium
e-mail: Dominique_haumont@stpierre-bru.be

G. Buonocore et al. (eds.), *Neonatology*,
https://doi.org/10.1007/978-3-319-29489-6_174

QS	Quiet sleep
REM	Rapid eye movement
VLBW	Very low birth weight

24.1 Salient Points

- EDC reduces pain and stress.
- EDC include restoring parents in their role as primary caregiver.
- NIDCAP is the most holistic teaching tool.
- Couplet care (mother-infant dyad) from birth to discharge is the aim.
- Architectural adaptations are recommended.

24.2 Introduction

The spectacular development of neonatal intensive care since the 1960s allowed a drop in neonatal mortality of very-low-birth-weight (VLBW) infants from 50% to less than 15% in the last decades (Horbar et al. 2002). In Europe, there is an important variation among countries, regions, and even units which is not completely understood (Zeitlin et al. 2015). In the gray zone of 22–24 weeks of gestation, survival increased dramatically in the recent years, but interestingly the decision to resuscitate according to birth weight or gestational age has not changed over the last 20 years (Condie et al. 2012). Despite better care, 15–25% of the VLBW infants will present neurodevelopment impairment in the following fields: motor function, vision, auditory function, cognition, behavior, attention deficit and hyperactivity disorders, visual-motor integration, and language (Marlow et al. 2007). Compared to their term pairs, there is substantial scientific evidence of altered early brain development. These differences are now well documented in brain magnetic resonance imaging, including diffusion tensor imaging, resting state functional connectivity, and magnetic resonance spectroscopy (Lubsen et al. 2011; Kwon et al. 2014). Some of these differences persist at later age (Constable et al. 2008).

Preterm infants spend weeks and sometimes months in the neonatal intensive care unit (Nicu) which is a quite different environment compared to what they would experience in utero. At this young age, brain growth and development are particularly critical and are in an extremely active process. It is well known that very low gestational age and birth weight, gender, perinatal infection and inflammation, intracranial hemorrhage, periventricular white matter disease, postnatal use of steroids, nutritional imbalances, or unfavorable socioeconomical situation impact brain development or later outcome. Which underlying mechanisms are responsible for these developmental difficulties is very complex and not totally understood. Interactions between genetic background, epigenetic effects, vulnerability to oxidative stress, and other metabolic disturbances will result in individual consequences for each baby. The existing evidence of interaction between environment and brain development has been extensively reviewed and better practices encouraged (Liu et al. 2007; White et al. 2013). Outcome will further depend on the family environment of the infants. The importance of neurodevelopmentally supportive care, the NICU environment, and parental closeness is the new challenge for changing practices (Haumont 2014).

24.3 The NICU Environment, the Early Developmental Care, and the Neonatal Individualized Developmental Care and Assessment Program

Babies in the NICU are overwhelmed by sensory inputs. They perceive noise, vestibular, olfactory, visual stimuli, pain, thermal changes, and movements. Social interactions with parents are not natural. Moving away from the traditional way of care in the NICU toward patient- and family-centered care and adapting the environment accordingly are now sustained by scientific evidence.

Noise. Against noisy open wards, the focus has evolved to very silent NICUs with single rooms. These have been shown to reduce infections and favor parental presence and breastfeeding (Domanico et al. 2011). However, in a recent study, adverse outcome was attributed to silence of single rooms (Pineda et al. 2013). It might be indeed inadequate to keep preterm infants too much in silence. But what is appropriate auditory stimulation? Another paper demonstrated that the exposure to parental talk was a significantly stronger predictor of infant vocalizations at 32 weeks and conversational turns at 32 and 36 weeks than language from other adults (Caskey et al. 2014). Single rooms should be seen as an incentive to favor parental presence which is the most important priority when implementing EDC.

Light. The development of the visual system has been fairly extensively investigated (Haumont and Hansen 2005).

During gestation, the synchronous ganglion cell waves are targeting the different neurons to allow appropriate transmission toward the visual cortex. The protection of rapid eye movement (REM) sleep is in this regard essential for normal development of ocular dominance columns (Graven 2004; Penn and Shatz 2002).

The preterm neonatal eye shows specific characteristics. The pupillary light reflex appears only after 30 weeks of gestation, and mydriasis is physiological until 32 weeks. Light acts also as a stimulus for the production of free radicals in retinal membrane lipids. It has been suggested that the immature antioxidant status of the preterm infant might play a role on their susceptibility to retinal damage. Preterm infants should be protected from direct bright light in the eyes. Input pathways entrained by light are relayed to the SCN which will express output signals. These include temperature, cortisol, melatonin, sleep-wake cycle, behavior, and cardiovascular function. In utero, the fetus has a biological clock responding to maternal entraining signals. If the baby is born preterm, he will be deprived of this circadian rhythm and submitted to an often chaotic NICU environment. Preterm infants have ultradian rhythms (period lengths much less than 24 h), which parallels the maturation of sleep pattern (Rivkees and Hao 2000). There is some clinical evidence that babies in cycled lighting grow and sleep better (Liu et al. 2007).

Pain and stress. It is well known that newborn infants in the NICU undergo many painful procedures (Carbajal et al. 2008). The fear of side effects of long-term exposure to narcotics on brain development and not recognizing pain and stress symptoms results in inappropriate pain relief in newborns. Non-pharmacological interventions like oral sucrose, nonnutritive sucking, swaddling, and facilitated tucking have been proven efficient against pain (Cignacco et al. 2007). In a study of infants born at <30 weeks gestation, the Neonatal Infant Stressor Scale scores were correlated with magnetic resonance imaging (brain metrics, diffusion, and functional magnetic resonance imaging) and neurobehavioral examinations at term equivalent postmenstrual age. Exposure to stressors in the Neonatal Intensive Care Unit was associated with regional alterations in brain structure and function. The most stressed infants showed decreased parietal and frontal cerebral width, altered diffusion measures, and functional connectivity in the temporal lobes and abnormalities in motor behavior on neurobehavioral examination (Smith et al. 2011).

Some units will claim an aggressive pain management with very liberal use of medication for medical procedures. However, the first step in medical care is "do no harm," and therefore, each procedure should be questioned. It is very likely that many routine interventions are historical and suppressible. Positioning and handling these babies matters. Even routine care like a diaper change induces significant variations in cerebral hemodynamics (Limperopoulos et al. 2008). Swaddling has been practiced for a long time and is associated with better sleep and diminished pain and stress response (van Sleuwen et al. 2007). Babies with respiratory problems do often better in prone position (Bauer 2005). The strong neck extensor muscles have to be counterbalanced to support later motor development (Amiel – Tison 1995). Healthy preterm infants have been shown to benefit from positioning in nests with flexed posture favoring more elegant movements and reducing frozen postures (Ferrari et al. 2007).

Protection of sleep. The term newborn has sleeps around 70% of the time with about half of the time in well recognizable active sleep (AS or REM sleep) and quiet sleep (QS) patterns. Before 27 weeks, it is not possible to identify a sleep pattern comprising AS and QS in the same cycle

(Dreyfus – Brisac 1968). REM sleep is considered in the ontogeny theory as a very intense cerebral activity playing an important role in brain maturation. The ultradian cycles of the preterm infant will progressively mature toward a circadian model of sleep-wake cycles. Maturation of sleep will be characterized by progressive change in the proportion of REM sleep toward a predominance of quiet sleep after term. The endogenous synaptic proliferation during REM sleep will prepare the brain for further refinement with exogenous stimulation.

There is growing evidence in animal and human research that supports the importance of sleep during early brain development. Animal studies on sleep deprivation showed structural and functional deterioration in several models. The need of endogenous synchronous waves during REM sleep has been well established for the development of synaptogenesis in the visual system (Frank and Stryker 2003). Routine unnecessary care interrupting sleep should be avoided.

Kangaroo Mother Care (*KMC*). KMC was started in 1978 in Columbia to support low-birth-weight infants in a low-cost way (Charpak et al. 2005). The proven effectiveness and safety have since enlarged this practice in countries with no limited resources. The benefits attributed to KMC are decreased morbidity, improved weight gain, breastfeeding, neurobehavioral assessment, and more mature sleep patterns. KMC is beneficial for the mother because it favors attachment and diminishes stress. Although less research about KMC in industrialized countries has been undertaken, it is now a recommended practice (Boundy et al. 2016).

Oxidative stress (*OS*). OS is one of the main causes of injury in preterm infants (Saugstad 2005). Many clinical situations will produce excessive free radical production: ischemia reperfusion injury, hypoxia and hyperoxia, inflammatory diseases, phototherapy, and intravenous nutrition with long-chain polyunsaturated fatty acids. Their immature antioxidant defenses will put them at increased risk for OS.

Any intervention in the NICU, which causes hypoxia, is potentially source of OS. Intensive care procedures like intubation, chest drainage, or intratracheal suctioning are well known to destabilize the baby. But even routine procedures like chest X-ray, changing electrodes, physiotherapy, excessive noise, weighing, or even diaper change are accompanied by an acute decrease in transcutaneous oxygen tension (Limperopoulos et al. 2008). EDC is also avoiding any hypoxic event or unnecessary care.

Early developmental care (EDC) has emerged against all potential harmful effects of the NICU environment with pain, stress, and neglected parental role. The term EDC is confusing because it ranges from very simple interventions like light and noise control, positioning, or nonnutritive sucking to the very complex Neonatal Individualized Developmental Care and Assessment Program (NIDCAP). The NIDCAP model is an early intervention program based on the observation of the preterm infant's behavior (Als et al. 1994). The theory behind developed by Als is designated as "synactive theory." The concept derives from the interdependency, differentiation, modulation, and regulation of five behavioral subsystems: autonomic, motor, state organizational (maturation of well-defined sleep and wake states), attentional/ interactional, and self-regulatory system. The assessment tool in NIDCAP is a formal and repeated observation of the infant behavior before, during, and after a care. These observations describe the reactions of the baby toward the sensory inputs and his capacity of self-regulation. The developmental goals for each infant will be defined according to his own skills and weaknesses. Individual caregiving plans and environmental adaptations will be recommended. As the NIDCAP implementation evolves in the unit, the caregivers become more and more aware of the signs shown by the baby, and handling is adjusted accordingly. The families are empowered in the caregiving and put in a central position. NIDCAP is an extensive and complex teaching program. The competence of the NIDCAP observer has to be validated by certified NIDCAP trainers. The level of developmental care in the NICU can be evaluated by the NIDCAP Nursery Certification. In this evaluation, all aspects of developmental care are analyzed: from the architecture of the unit to the behavioral assessment of the baby, the collaboration with the parents, and the skills of the staff (NIDCAP Nursery Assessment and Certification). The awareness of caregivers has dramatically increased over the last decades. In Europe, the first NIDCAP training center opened in Stockholm in 1999. Now 11 training centers are established and more are on the way. There is an important demand for teaching developmental care, and it is likely that new approaches will emerge to respond to this growing need. Parents are also increasingly involved in the care of baby. They want and deserve to fulfill their role as primary caregiver of their infant (EFCNI Rights of Parents and Newborns).

24.4 Couplet Care or Restoring the Mother-Infant Dyad: The New Challenge

Despite the fact that the importance of early mother-infant relations is well known since a long time, parental access to the unit has been very often limited (Fanaroff et al. 1972). Today the parents have theoretically permanent access, but local resistance toward this rule still exists. In northern Europe, it is less often the case (Greisen et al. 2009).

Neonatal care units and maternity wards are generally run by a different nursing and medical team. Moreover, they are geographically not always contiguous, and in most units when babies need special care after birth, it is difficult to have the mother next to her baby. Restoring the physical closeness between mothers and babies from birth to discharge is a concrete challenge for modern neonatology: introducing couplet care.

Emotional and physical closeness are linked. The mother who is separated from her newborn child will show anxiety and stress and is at risk for depression (Davis et al. 2003). It is not only a question of a humane attitude, but there is growing evidence of the importance of parent-infant closeness (Flacking et al. 2012). A group of babies born from mothers who had benefit from an early sensitivity training program showed better maturation and white matter connectivity at diffusion tension brain imaging (DTI) compared to controls (Milgrom et al. 2010). In animal studies, variations in early life maternal stimulation can alter offspring gene expression via epigenetic mechanism receptor genes (Curley et al. 2011).

Human milk is widely recommended as the best nutrient for term and preterm infants (American Academy of Pediatrics 2012). It reduces the risk of infection, necrotizing enterocolitis, and is associated with better cognitive development. The unique components of colostrum, an immune juice, are especially important in VLBW infants. Closeness of the mother and skin to skin contact are mandatory to reach successful breastfeeding.

Some places in Sweden have a long-lasting experience in caring for infants with permanent parental presence and fully restored mother-infant dyad. In those "couplet care" settings, parents and infants live together from the very first minutes after birth until discharge. This option resulted in a significant reduction of the length of stay (Örtenstrand et al. 2010).

24.5 Conclusion

Neonatal units are facing a period of important conceptual changes, a real paradigm shift. The traditional unit appeared to be inadequate, with harmful effects on brain development during this particularly vulnerable period. New strategies in caring for the baby in a holistic way and integrating his level of development and his reactions toward the different treatments have been elaborated.

Moving away from traditional units toward family-centered developmentally supportive units is the challenge of modern neonatology. The important elements of early developmental care are parental physical and emotional closeness, fine-tuning of care according to appropriate assessment of the preterm infant behavior, strategies to reduce stress, and a NICU design adapted to provide this type of care.

Keeping mothers and babies in absolute proximity from birth to discharge is the driving trend of the couplet care. In order to achieve these changes, reference strategies have to be used and the transitional period is still ongoing. At the moment, NIDCAP is the most complete tool to achieve these changes, but concepts are evolving. They will have to adapt according to further research, changes in caregiving, and local strategies. EDC is the first step to help parents in understanding their baby, a task which does not stop at discharge from the unit.

References

Als H, Lawhon G, Duffy FH et al (1994) Individualized developmental care for the very low – birth – weight preterm infant. Medical and neurofunctional effects. JAMA 272:853–858

American Academy of Pediatrics (2012) Breastfeeding and the use of human milk. Pediatrics 129:e827–e841

Amiel – Tison C (1995) Clinical assessment of the infant nervous system. In: Levene MI, Lilford RJ (eds) Fetal and neonatal neurology and neurosurgery. Churchill Livingstone, Edinburgh, pp 83–104

Bauer K (2005) Effect of positioning and handling on preterm infants in the neonatal intensive care unit. In: Sizun J, Browne JV (eds) Research on early developmental care for preterm neonates. John Libbey, Paris, pp 39–44

Boundy EO, Dastjerdi R, Spiegelman D et al (2016) Kangaroo mother care and neonatal outcome: a meta-analysis. Pediatrics 137(1):1–16

Carbajal R, Rousset A, Danan C et al (2008) Epidemiology and treatment of painful procedures in neonates in intensive care units. JAMA 300:60–70

Caskey M, Stephens B, Tucker R et al (2014) Adult talk in the NICU with preterm infants and developmental outcomes. Pediatrics 133(3):e578–e584. https://doi.org/10.1542/peds.2013-0104

Charpak N, Ruiz JG, Zupan J et al (2005) Kangaroo mother care: 25 years after. Acta Paediatr 94:514–522

Cignacco E, Hamers JP, Stoffel L et al (2007) The efficacy of non – pharmacological interventions in the management of procedural pain in preterm and term neonates. A systematic literature review. Eur J Pain 11:139–152

Condie J, Caldarelli L, Tarr L et al (2012) Have the boundaries of the "grey zone" of perinatal resuscitation changed for extremely preterm infants over 20 years? Acta Paediatr. https://doi.org/10.1111/apa.12119

Constable RT, Ment LR, Vohr BR et al (2008) Prematurely born children demonstrate white matter miscrostructural differences at 12 years of age, relative to term control subjects: an investigation of group and gender effect. Pediatrics 121:e306–e316

Curley JP, Jensen CL, Mashoodh R et al (2011) Social influences on neurobiology and behavior: epigenetic effects during development. Psychoneuroendocrinology 36(3):352–371

Davis L, Edwards H, Mohay H et al (2003) The impact of very premature birth on the psychological health of mothers. Earl Hum Dev 73(1–2):61–70

Domanico R, Davis DK, Coleman F et al (2011) Documenting the NICU design dilemma: comparative patient progress in open-ward and single family rooms units. J Perinatol 31(4):281–288

Dreyfus – Brisac C (1968) Sleep ontogenesis in early human prematurity from 24 to 27 weeks of conceptual age. Dev Psychobiol 1:162–169

EFCNI rights of parents and newborns. www.efcni.org

Fanaroff AA, Kennell JH, Klaus MH (1972) Follow – up of low birth weight infants – the predictive value of maternal visiting patterns. Pediatrics 49(2):287–290

Ferrari F, Bertoncelli N, Gallo C et al (2007) Posture and movement in healthy preterm infants in supine position in and outside the nest. Arch Dis Child Fetal Neonatal Ed 92:F386–F390

Flacking R, Lehtonen L, Thomson G et al (2012) Closeness and separation in neonatal intensive care. Acta Paediatr 101(10):1032–1037

Frank M, Stryker M (2003) The role of sleep in the development of central visual pathways. In: Maquet P, Smith C, Stickgold R (eds) Sleep and brain plasticity. Oxford University Press, New York, pp 190–206

Graven SN (2004) Early neurosensory visual development of the fetus and newborn. Clin Perinatol 31:199–216

Greisen G, Mirante N, Haumont D et al (2009) Parents, siblings and grandparents in the Neonatal Intensive Care Unit a survey of policies in eight European countries. Acta Paediatr 98:1744–1750

Haumont D (2014) NIDCAP and developmental care. J Pediatr Neonatal Individ Med 3(2):e030240

Haumont D, Hansen V (2005) Neonatal development: effects of light. In: Sizun J, Browne JV (eds) Research on early developmental care for preterm neonates. John Libbey, Paris, pp 33–37

Horbar JD, Badger GJ, Carpenter JH et al (2002) Trends in mortality and morbidity for very low birth weight infants, 1991–1999. Pediatrics 110:143–151

Kwon S, Vasung L, Ment L, Hüppi P (2014) The role of neuroimaging in predicting neurodevelopmental outcomes of preterm neonates. Clin Perinatol 41:257–283

Limperopoulos C, Gauvreau KK, O'Leary H et al (2008) Cerebral hemodynamic changes during intensive care of preterm infants. Pediatrics 122:e1006–e1013

Liu WF, Laudert S, Perkins B et al (2007) The development of potentially better practices to support the neurodevelopment of infants in the NICU. J Perinatol 27:S48–S74

Lubsen J, Vohr B, Myers E, Hampson M et al (2011) Microstructural and functional connectivity in the developing preterm brain. Semin Perinatol 35:34–43

Marlow N, Hennessy E, Bracewell M et al (2007) Motor and executive function at 6 years of age after extremely preterm birth. Pediatrics 120:793–804

Milgrom J, Newnham C, Anderson PJ et al (2010) Early sensitivity training for parents of preterm infants: impact on the developing brain. Pediatr Res 67(3):e330–e335

NIDCAP nursery assessment and certification. www.NIDCAP.org

Örtenstrand A, Westrup B, Berggren Broström E et al (2010) The Stockholm Neonatal Family Centered Care Study: effects on length of stay and infant morbidity. Pediatrics 125(2):e278–e285

Penn AA, Shatz CJ (2002) Principles of endogenous and sensory activity – dependent brain development. The visual system. In: Lagercrantz H, Hanson M, Evrard P (eds) The newborn brain: neuroscience and clinical applications. Cambridge University Press, New York, pp 204–225

Pineda RG, Neil J, Dierker D et al (2013) Alterations in brain structure and neurodevelopmental outcome in preterm infants hospitalized in different NICU environments. J Pediatr 164(1):52–60.e2

Rivkees SA, Hao H (2000) Developing circadian rhythmicity. Semin Perinatol 24:232–242

Saugstad OD (2005) Oxidative stress in the newborn-a 30 year perspective. Biol Neonate 88:228–236

Smith GC, Gutovich J, Smyser C et al (2011) Neonatal Intensive Care Unit stress is associated with brain development in preterm infants. Ann Neurol 70: e541–e549

van Sleuwen BE, Engelberts AC, Boere – Boonekamp MM et al (2007) Swaddling: a systematic review. Pediatrics 120:e1097–e1106

White R, Smith J, Shepley M et al (2013) Recommended standards for newborn ICU design. J Perinatol 33 (Suppl 1):S2–S16

Zeitlin J, Mortensen L, Cuttini M et al (2015) Declines in stillbirth and neonatal mortality rates in Europe between 2004 and 2010: results from the Euro-Peristat project. J Epidemiol Community Health. https://doi.org/10.1136/jech.207013

25 Neonatal Pain: Neurophysiology, Recognition, Prevention, and Management with Nonpharmacological Interventions

Carlo V. Bellieni, Celeste Johnston, Marsha Campbell-Yeo, Britney Benoit, and Timothy Disher

Contents

C. V. Bellieni
Neonatal Intensive Care Unit, Siena University Hospital, Siena, Italy
e-mail: cvbellieni@gmail.com

C. Johnston (✉)
School of Nursing, McGill University, Montreal, Canada
e-mail: celeste.johnston@mcgill.ca

M. Campbell-Yeo (✉)
Departments of Pediatrics, Psychology and Neuroscience, Dalhousie University School of Nursing, Halifax, Canada
e-mail: marsha.campbell-yeo@dal.ca

B. Benoit (✉)
School of Nursing, Centre for Pediatric Pain Research, Maternal-Newborn Program, Dalhousie University, IWK Health Centre , Halifax, Canada
e-mail: britney.benoit@dal.ca

T. Disher (✉)
Centre for Pediatric Pain Research, Dalhousie University School of Nursing and IWK Health Centre, Halifax, Canada
e-mail: tim.disher@dal.ca

G. Buonocore et al. (eds.), *Neonatology*,
https://doi.org/10.1007/978-3-319-29489-6_175

Abstract
Evidence indicates that the experience of pain begins in the second trimester of pregnancy, well before the third and last trimester of pregnancy human gestation: thus preterm babies can perceive pain. When babies are born preterm, they undergo painful experiences that should be avoided. These experiences can result in important short-term stress responses as well as long-term effects on development. Pharmacological agents should be used to alleviate extensive pain from surgery, but most pain is from daily procedures. Decreasing the number of procedures or clustering the procedures is the first step to overcome it. Also several non-pharmacological interventions supported by strong evidence, such as sensorial saturation, can be used by nursing staff and, more importantly, by parents.

25.1 Salient Points

- The anatomy and physiology of the fetus are sufficiently developed in the second trimester to experience nociception.
- Babies in the neonatal intensive care unit (NICU) experience painful procedures that have long-term effects.
- Decreasing the number of painful procedures is an obvious means of decreasing pain exposure.
- Multiple non-pharmacological interventions, many usable by parents, have strong supportive evidence to decrease pain response to procedures.

25.2 Anatomy

To feel pain, it is necessary for stimuli to involve neural connections between the peripheral receptors and the spinal cord and upward transmission via the spinal cord to the thalamus and from there to the outer cerebral layers. The development of the human nervous system is a progressive and ascending process, with the cerebral cortex being the last region to develop. Thus, to experience pain, an intact system of pain transmission must be available.

25.3 Development of Connections

Peripheral receptors develop from the seventh gestational week (Vanhatalo and Van Nieuwenhuizen 2000). Connections from the periphery to the spinal cord are formed early, at about 8 weeks (Okado 1981). C fibers begin to grow into the spinal cord at about 10 weeks. Early in gestation, after the tenth week of gestation, substance P and enkephalin-positive fibers appear (Yew et al. 2001). From 13 weeks' gestation, the afferent system located in the substantia gelatinosa of the dorsal horn of the spinal cord develops (Okado 1981; Bijlani et al. 1988; Yew et al. 2001). Spinothalamic connections start to develop from 14 weeks and are complete at 20 weeks' gestation, and thalamocortical connections are present from 17 weeks and completely developed at 26–30 weeks' gestation (Kostovic and Goldman-Rakic 1983). From 15 weeks, there is a subplate zone which lies beneath the cortex. This is a layer of neurons below the cortex that is specific to the fetus (see later). The thalamus plays a pivotal role in regulating the spinal-brainstem-spinal loops that mediate context-dependent descending facilitation or inhibition, coordinated through the key mechanisms underlying consciousness. In contrast to direct thalamocortical fibers, which are not visible until almost the third trimester, thalamic afferents begin to reach the somatosensory subplate at 20 weeks' gestation (Kostović and Rakic 1990) and the visual subplate at 20–22 weeks' gestation (Hevner 2000). Thalamic fibers penetrate the cortical plate from 24 to 28 weeks' gestation. From 20 weeks' gestation, peripheral receptors are present on the whole body (Valman and Pearson 1980; Bijlani et al. 1988). Recent studies have noted robust activation of the somatosensory cortex in preterm neonates exposed to tactile or painful stimuli, modulated by gestational maturity, postnatal age, sex, laterality, and sleep-wake states (Bartocci et al. 2006; Slater et al. 2006). Cortical development starts only at about 17 weeks' gestation, but continues until long after birth. Synapses appear within the cortical plate from mid-gestation.

25.4 Subplate Zone and Cortex

The role of the cerebral cortex is crucial for pain sensitivity, but we should not ignore the role of the subplate in the development of sentience and consciousness. The subplate zone is a prominent, transient laminar compartment of the cerebral wall of the human fetus. The importance of the subplate as the main synaptic zone of the human fetal cortex is based on the rich input of "waiting" afferents from the thalamus and cortex during the crucial phase of cortical target area selection. Recent neurobiological evidence shows that the subplate is an important site of spontaneous endogenous activity, building a framework for the development of cortical columnar organization (Kostović and Jovanov-Milosevic 2008). The conscious perception of pain requires peripheral pain receptors, connections to the spinal cord through an afferent system, fibers that connect the spine and the thalami, and, most importantly, connections between the thalamus and the subplate zone or cerebral cortex. It is also important to know that pain impulses may be processed in other subcortical structures, including the hypothalamic pituitary system and amygdala (important for the emotional modulation of pain) (Lowery et al. 2007). The subplate zone expands considerably between 17 and 20 weeks and recedes after 30 weeks' developmental age (Kostoví and Judaš 2002); from about 17 weeks, there is a shifting population of connections from the thalamus to this region. Neurons in the subplate zone initiate excitatory amino acid or peptide neurotransmission in the cortex, influencing the development of fetal cortical circuits (Kostović et al. 1991; Clancy et al. 2001), while the cortical plate matures into the six layers of the cerebral cortex (Mrzljak et al. 1988). Differentiation of subplate neurons at 17–25 weeks' gestation produces five cellular subtypes whose distinct dendritic and axonal patterns correspond to different functional roles in development (Kostović et al. 2002; Perkins et al. 2005). From 16 weeks' gestation, pain transmission from a peripheral receptor to the cortex is possible and is certainly completely developed from 26 weeks' gestation. Assuming that activity in the cerebral cortex or subplate zone is necessary for consciousness, then for the fetus to be conscious of an external experience, these regions need to be connected with incoming nervous activity. This starts to happen at about 16 weeks and puts an early limit on the time point at which it is likely the fetus might feel what is going on in its body or elsewhere (Van de Velde et al. 2006). Serotonin-releasing inhibitory descending pain fibers only develop after birth, and it is therefore possible that preterm babies and fetuses feel more pain than small infants.

25.5 Stress Responses

25.5.1 Hemodynamic and Neuroendocrine Responses

Neonatal responses to painful stimuli have been evaluated using a variety of measures within three classes of responses (biochemical, physiological, and behavioral). Plasma catecholamine assays may provide the most valid and reliable measures of the biochemical responses of neonates to painful stimuli (Franck and Miaskowski 1997). As early as 16 weeks' gestational age, the human fetus mounts a cerebral hemodynamic response to invasive procedures involving transgression of the fetal body, which is consistent with the "brain-sparing" effect (Teixeira et al. 1999). Increased cerebral blood flow is not necessarily indicative of pain, as this response is thought to constitute a "brain-sparing" mechanism associated with hypoxia (Woo et al. 1987) and intrauterine growth restriction (Wladimiroff et al. 1987). Nevertheless, fetal plasma concentrations of cortisol, endorphin, and noradrenaline increase after intrauterine needling of the hepatic vein to a greater degree than of the umbilical cord (Giannakoulopoulos et al. 1994, 1999).

25.5.1.1 Long-Term Consequences

The evidence for adverse consequences on future neural development due to early exposure to noxious stimuli is increasing. Ruda et al. studied an animal neonatal model of persistent hind paw peripheral inflammation. They found that, as adults, these animals exhibited spinal neuronal circuits with increased input and segmental changes in nociceptive primary afferent axons and altered responses to sensory stimulation (Ruda et al. 2016). Preterm infants who spend postconceptional weeks 28 through 32 in a NICU are less mature in their pain response to heel prick than newborn premature infants of 32 weeks' postconceptual age (PCA) (Johnston and Stevens 1996). Differences in these response patterns were strongly correlated with the number of invasive procedures experienced since birth, rather than other clinical factors (e.g., age, severity of illness, Apgar score, birth weight). These data suggest that repetitive pain and stress might alter the neurological response to pain, leading to altered neurobehavioral reactions to subsequent painful events (Van de Velde et al. 2006). According to Anand et al., repetitive pain in neonatal rat pups may lead to an altered development of the pain system associated with decreased pain thresholds during development (Anand et al. 1999). Increased plasticity of the neonatal brain may allow these and other changes in brain development to increase the vulnerability of these animals to stress disorders and anxiety-mediated adult behavior. Similar behavioral changes have been observed during the later childhood of ex-preterm neonates who were exposed to prolonged periods of neonatal intensive care: infants who are born prematurely or seriously ill are commonly exposed to multiple painful and stressful events as part of their prolonged hospitalizations and required medical procedures. There is now evidence that early events not only induce acute changes, but that permanent structural and functional changes may also result (Porter et al. 1999). Recent studies suggest that although early painful memories are not accessible to conscious recall, they might be encoded in "procedural memory" and lead to abnormal behavioral patterns or altered sensory processing in later life. Taddio et al. demonstrated that infants circumcised at birth without analgesia showed a stronger pain response to subsequent routine vaccination than uncircumcised infants or than those who underwent the procedure with analgesia (Taddio et al. 1997). It is becoming increasingly clear that neonatal painful experiences may leave a legacy of altered sensitivity to subsequent pain, perhaps for the entire life of the individual (Anand 1996, 2000; Valeri et al. 2015).

25.6 Overcoming Procedural Pain

25.6.1 Prevention

Manipulations and painful procedures must be reduced in number. Younger babies have a lower pain threshold than older babies "because of the immaturity of their pain inhibition system" (Ranger et al. 2015), and they undergo a mean number of 14 painful procedures/day when in the NICU (Simons et al. 2003). Any manipulation is potentially stressful if not painful: changes in temperature, light, and noise can disrupt their behavioral states with harmful consequences.

Reduction of stress induced by clinical trials. Clinical trials often provoke manipulations unnecessary to a baby's health. Moreover, studies of painkillers should never have placebo (Bellieni and Johnston 2015) treated babies as a reference group, because we cannot impose pain on anyone without his/her consent: parents should not be given the burden of deciding whether to enter their baby in a painful experiment, since pain must never be part of neonatal research (for a control group, a commonly recognized painkiller should be used). Unfortunately, preventing pain is not among the preeminent concerns of researchers: 75% of the studies considered in a recent review (Bellieni et al. 2008) showed that infants suffered pain during the research because placebo, no treatment, or otherwise inadequate pain management was applied.

Providing newborns with an environment tailored to their needs. Babies in incubators are exposed to very high electromagnetic fields (Bellieni et al. 2008), loud noises, disturbing lights, and stressful manipulations, and sometimes they are isolated from their family. Studies (Bellieni et al. 2003, 2004a, 2005) to overcome some of these forms of environmental pollution have been performed, and effective developmental care, centered on the single baby and his/her family, is now recommended (Als et al. 2004). It is important to treat the baby with humanity during the procedures, with special attention to non-pharmacologic analgesia and a baby-tailored environment: both can reduce the risks of neurodevelopmental compromise.

25.6.2 Recognition

Caregivers should be able to recognize the main physical signs associated with pain. Most are nonspecific: babies can cry for reasons other than pain, and pain is expressed through complex behavior. This does not mean that a crying baby should be ignored "because we are not sure" that he/she is crying for pain. On the contrary, this should alarm us as if it were pain: our duty is to exclude it and/or to treat it. Newborns show a distinct pattern of behavior to painful stimuli. This includes a wide range of expressions including screwing up the eyes, frowning, opening the mouth, extending the fingers, kicking, as well as clenching. For a thorough assessment, pain scales exist.

Chronic pain scales. It is mandatory to monitor pain in order to prevent its occurrence, mainly after surgery or in ventilated babies. For this purpose, scales exist to evaluate the level of pain and stress in intubated babies or after surgery, in order to adjust or introduce an effective analgesia.

Acute pain scales. Many scales exist in this field and are scarcely used. There are two reasons for this: first, the difficulty of applying scales where many items have to be assessed simultaneously (Bellieni et al. 2007b) and, second, the lack of any point in assessing pain after it has occurred. Acute pain scales are useful for research purposes. It is not always useful for clinical practice to assess the actual level of pain; it is more useful to be aware of whether we are actually provoking pain or rather if we might provoke it before we start. Acute pain scales are retrospective and assess pain only after it has been provoked. So it has been proposed to assess pain preventively: acute pain scales include many data, but the type of the stimulus and the region of the body (with or without nociceptors) where it is applied are decontextualized. It has been proposed (Bellieni et al. 2015) to foresee pain using a contextual model. The context of the stimulus is crucial: stimuli that might provoke pain applied to an innervated area will not be painful if applied where nociceptors are absent, and the invasiveness of a procedure often is proportional to the pain it provokes. Thus we should proceed first assessing if the site and the stimulus are adequate to provoke

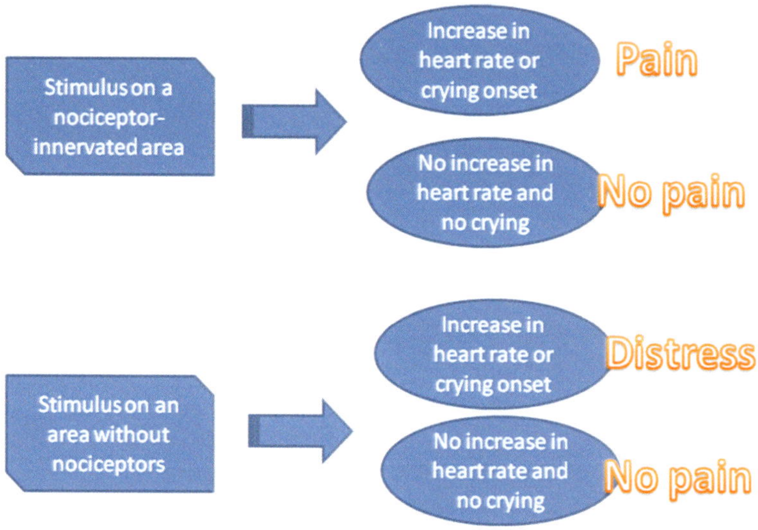

Fig. 1 Detecting pain. A congruous stimulus applied on a place full of nociceptors provokes pain, and this is pointed out by an increase of heart rate or by crying onset

pain and then assessing the reaction to this stimulus (Fig. 1) to detect if pain has been felt. When we may provoke pain-activating nociceptors, we should use easily noticeable signs such as crying or heart rate to detect pain. Crying and increased heart rate both show a high sensitivity for pain in studies made for the validation of pain scales (Codipietro et al. 2008; Mandel et al. 2012): neither crying nor heart rate is specific to pain (Barr 2000), but the sudden appearance of a reaction (crying or increase of heart rate) overcomes this limit. The first cry after a heel prick is high pitched if it is very painful. Babies cry in 1-s bursts separated by short and regular pauses when pain is high (Bellieni et al. 2004b). The ABC scale stands on this basis (Bellieni et al. 2004b, 2007c), which, unlike most other scales, can be used by the caregiver who is performing the procedure, without interrupting it to score pain, as it is uniquely based on recognizing the acoustic features of crying (Table 1).

Table 1 ABC pain scale

	Absent	Intermediate	Full
Acuteness of the first cry	0	/	2
Burst rhythmicity	0	/	2
Continuity in time of crying loudness	0	1	2

25.7 Overcoming Parents' Pain/Anxiety

In the treatment of neonatal pain, it is important to consider additional but often concealed parental pain, also because parents play an important role in the improvement of the baby. Caregivers should give adequate relationship-based care and help couples to become true parents. In the NICU this often happens through the foresight of the caregivers. Parents should be accompanied to meet their baby, gently be encouraged to call him/her by name, and dedicate all the time needed to them; in some cases, they may require the help of a psychologist (Arockiasamy et al. 2008). Parents' pain and stress will have two negative consequences: they may increase the difficulty of communication with physicians, leading to bad compliance and discussion, and will be transferred to the baby who may change his/her behavior accordingly.

25.8 Overcoming Healthcare Professionals' Pain/Anxiety

Healthcare professionals' pain/anxiety pain is often underestimated (Bellieni and Buonocore 2009), but it is useful to consider that people work in a NICU side by side with death and pain on a daily basis, sometimes in difficult conditions. These people bear all this along with their own fears and anxieties. Much should be done to help them to find ways to cope with all this pain, to avoid their beautiful and important work becoming a routine, losing much of its usefulness, and sometimes reflecting upon the type of treatment they give babies (Barr 2007). Caregivers should be trained to have a positive vision of the baby and encouraged to exploit any effort of the parents and any progress of the baby. Caregivers' anxieties can lead to unnecessary overtreatment or undertreatment (Wyatt 2007).

25.9 A Therapeutic Tripod

The therapeutic tripod represents an approach to pain relief. Neonatal pain can be relieved only by taking care of all of the legs (Fig. 2), considering not only procedural pain but also caregivers' suffering (Carbajal et al. 2003; Bellieni et al. 2007a; Bellieni and Buonocore 2008; Butler and Als 2008). Medical intervention should not be limited to drugs and technical procedures. What is required is "advocacy." Nurses and neonatologists should be advocates. They should also support parents to become active advocates; not to be frightened by their baby's apparent fragility, immaturity, and lack of reactivity; and to be able to interpret their baby's discomfort.

25.10 Procedural Pain Management with Non-pharmacological Interventions

Neonates who are born preterm spend weeks in the neonatal intensive care unit (NICU) and undergo numerous painful procedures as part of their routine care (Simons et al. 2003). In spite of evidence of negative effects and published guidelines on pain control, about one third of procedures remain unmanaged

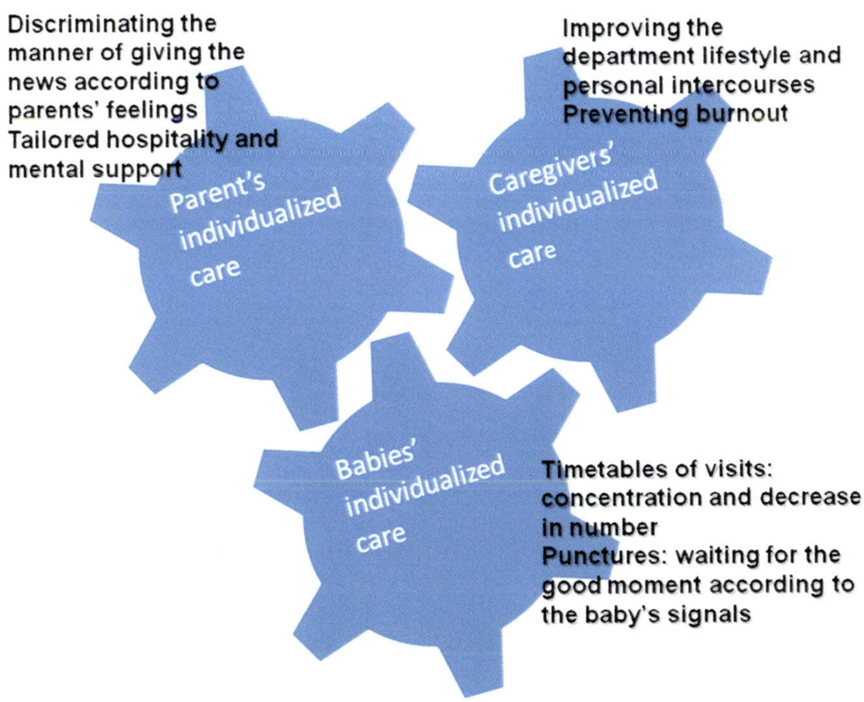

Fig. 2 Representation of neonatal pain (NP). Treating only one of the three legs of this tripod will be utterly insufficient

(Carbajal et al. 2008; Johnston et al. 2011). While pain requires management, common approaches with older populations are not appropriate for neonates, particularly preterm neonates. To date, there are several difficulties with pharmacological interventions for procedural pain. Topical anesthetics have been shown not to be effective with heel lance or venipuncture, the most common painful procedures in neonates (Stevens et al. 1999). Systemic drugs, specifically opiates, have significantly slower clearance in neonates (Zuppa et al. 2009) and are also not necessarily effective for acute procedural pain (Carbajal et al. 2005). Given the frequency of painful procedures in NICUs and the difficulties with pharmacological management, different approaches are required. Effective non-pharmacological interventions with strong supportive evidence will be reviewed.

25.11 Oral Sweet Solutions

Oral sweet solutions are currently recommended in rigorously developed clinical practice guidelines (CPGs) for the optimal management of mild to moderately painful procedures in infants (Lee et al. 2014; Committee on Newborn Pain 2016). Studies using sucrose, the most studied sweet taste, began in the late 1980s (Blass et al. 1987; Blass and Hoffmeyer 1991) and have been meta-analyzed (Stevens et al. 2013). Cumulative data from 57 randomized controlled trials including 4,730 infants with gestational ages ranging from 25 to 44 weeks concluded that sucrose is safe and effectively reduces biobehavioral response during single acute needle or lance-related procedures and the inclusion of placebo control groups are no longer considered ethical when designing sucrose trials (Stevens et al. 2013; Bellieni and Johnston 2015). Similarly, a meta-synthesis of non-sucrose sweet-tasting solutions, most notably oral glucose or dextrose, demonstrated similar pain-reducing benefits for procedural pain in infants (Bueno et al. 2013). The degree of effectiveness of sweet-tasting solutions varies across procedures; the strongest and most studied examine needle-related procedures such as venipuncture and heel lance although benefit has also been demonstrated for non-tissue breaking yet commonly performed stressful procedures such as insertion of orogastric tubes (Nimbalkar et al. 2013) while less so for echocardiogram (Lavoie et al. 2015; Potana et al. 2015). In one study pain scores measured using the Premature Infant Pain Profile (PIPP) (Stevens et al. 1996) were significantly lower for infants assigned to receive sucrose prior to undergoing echocardiogram compared to a no-treatment control arm (Potana et al. 2015), but another study found no added benefit of 25% glucose compared to the provision of nonnutritive sucking with a pacifier (Lavoie et al. 2015).

Adjuvant strategies such as nonnutritive sucking, swaddling, or facilitated tucking when combined with sweet taste have been associated with a greater benefit (Stevens et al. 2013; Pillai Riddell et al. 2015) especially for immunizations (McNair et al. 2013; Taddio et al. 2015). Minimal (da Costa et al. 2013) or no benefit (Kataria et al. 2015; Nesargi et al. 2015) has been reported when 25% glucose was provided for the reduction of the moderate to severe pain associated with eye examination for retinopathy of prematurity or treatment using laser therapy with or without concomitant topical anesthesia.

Concentrations of studied sweet-tasting solutions have varied from 5% to 50%. Although one study reports a flat dose-response function (Blass and Shah 1995), there seems to be a dose-response effect in the reduction of crying with increasing concentration of sucrose (Abad et al. 1996) with concentrations greater than 18% being considered most effective (Stevens et al. 2013). While the exact mechanism of action remains unknown, sweet-tasting solutions appear to be mediated by taste and are most efficacious when administered orally to the anterior portion of the tongue 2 min before a painful stimulus, with effects lasting up to 4 min (Johnston et al. 1999; Lefrak et al. 2006; Stevens et al. 2013).

Despite extensive and rigorous evidence, numerous questions remain related to optimal dose, sustained effect, potential for long-term adverse outcome, and concern regarding sedative versus analgesic properties related to the repeated use of sweet-tasting solutions to reduce infant pain. Currently, a 20-fold variation of recommended doses from 0.05 ml of 24% to 2.0 ml of 50% solution of sucrose exists, and the minimum effective dose (i.e., the smallest dose associated with a clinically significant reduction in pain intensity scores) has not yet been established (Stevens et al. 2013). Few studies have examined the repeated use of sucrose related to sustained efficacy or potential for associated consequences. The first study conducted by Johnston, examining outcomes associated with repeated use of sucrose, reported delayed neurobehavioral development (alertness and orientation, motor vigor) in infants who had received higher doses of sucrose over the first week of life (Johnston et al. 2002). Conversely, a study conducted over 4 weeks found no difference in neurobiological risk scores but did not measure development (Stevens et al. 2005), and another over 3 days only examined sustained efficacy and did not report on any long-lasting effects (Taddio et al. 2008). Two recent studies examining the effect of sucrose exposure in infants born preterm have been conducted with varying results. Plasma markers of ATP degradation and oxidative stress measured before and after the heel lance in 131 preterm infants were found to be significantly higher in those infants receiving a single dose of oral sucrose given just prior to heel lance when compared to those provided with nonnutritive sucking or no-treatment control (Asmerom et al. 2013). In a similar group of preterm infants, receiving 0.5 ml of 25% sucrose for every painful procedure for three consecutive days during hospitalization, there did not appear to be any adverse effect on outcomes related to feeding patterns or weight gain compared to infants in the no-treatment control group (Linhares et al. 2014). One study found that although sucrose decreased pain scores according to the Premature Infant Pain Profile (PIPP), there was still a nociceptive-specific potential measured on EEG, raising concern that additional examination of the exact analgesic properties of sucrose use is warranted (Slater et al. 2010).

25.12 Breastfeeding

Several studies have also examined the possible benefits of breastfeeding or supplemental breast milk in full-term neonates. In a systematic review of 20 clinical trials, breastfeeding (ten studies) and breast milk (ten studies) were shown to provide analgesia during routine procedural pain from heel stick and venipuncture (Shah et al. 2012). Supplemental breast milk alone does not appear to be as analgesic as sweet taste or direct breastfeeding (Shah et al. 2012). Six studies have examined breastfeeding and breast milk analgesia in preterm neonates. Supplemental breast milk was not found to be as effective as sweet taste (Skogsdal et al. 1997; Bueno et al. 2012; Simonse et al. 2012; Ou-Yang et al. 2013), and direct breastfeeding was not found to provide more analgesia than nonnutritive sucking (Holsti et al. 2011) in preterm infants undergoing heel lance. One study examining the analgesic effect of breastfeeding combined with standard care (anesthetic drops, swaddling, and nesting) for retinopathy of prematurity exams found that the addition of breastfeeding significantly reduced pain scores when compared to standard care alone (Rosali et al. 2015). On the other hand, breastfeeding has been shown to be as effective as sucrose for the relief of procedural pain (Carbajal et al. 2003). There is some evidence that breastfeeding may be superior to sucrose (Codipietro et al. 2008; Marín Gabriel et al. 2013) and glucose (Weissman et al. 2009). The benefits of glucose and breastfeeding during heel lance (Gradin et al. 2004) and EMLA and breastfeeding during immunization (Gupta et al. 2013) may be cumulative when provided simultaneously.

Maternal presence appears to play a valuable role. Healthy full-term infants cried and grimaced less by 91% and 84%, respectively, when held during breastfeeding rather than swaddled in a bassinet during heel stick (Gray et al. 2002). Breastfeeding and maternal holding with pacifier significantly reduced full-term infants' crying behavior during heel stick when compared to the group being held by an assistant with pacifier (Phillips and Chantry 2002). During heel lance, being held by a mother and breastfed was compared to being held by a mother with pacifier and to being held by a non-mother with pacifier (Phillips et al. 2005). In the first two conditions, infants cried significantly less (33% and 45%) compared to being held by a non-mother (66%, $p < 0.01$ and $p = 0.03$, respectively). However, other components of the breastfeeding intervention must play a role in efficacy beyond maternal presence, as breastfeeding has been shown to significantly reduce behavioral and biobehavioral pain scores compared to maternal holding without breastfeeding during immunization (Modarres et al. 2013) and heel lance (Leite et al. 2009; Weissman et al. 2009; Obeidat and Shuriquie 2015). There is some evidence to suggest that the analgesic efficacy of direct breastfeeding in preterm infants is dependent on sucking pattern maturity (Holsti et al. 2011).

25.13 Skin-to-Skin Care or Kangaroo Care

Interest in kangaroo care (KC), described as the mother holding the baby naked with only a diaper in a prone upright position against her bare breasts, for pain is recent. The effects of KC on infants' pain response were first studied in full-term infants (Gray et al. 2000) and were shown to reduce crying by 82% and grimacing by 65%, compared to infants who stayed in the crib during heel lance. Similar results have been reported in full-term neonates receiving intramuscular injection (Kashaninia et al. 2008). The first study in preterm infants of 32–36 weeks' gestational age was in 2003 (Johnston et al. 2003) and other studies followed. These studies consistently show that KC significantly reduced biobehavioral responses. A Cochrane systematic review (Johnson et al. 2014) for KC for pain in term and preterm neonates (19 studies, $n = 1{,}594$) found that KC was associated with improved heart rate recovery, serum, and salivary cortisol; PIPP scores at 30, 60, and 90 s; neonatal facial coding system scores; neonatal infant pain scale scores; and sleep-wake state. The addition of rocking, singing, and sucking in infants of 32–36 weeks of gestational age did not prove better than KC alone. Since this review, four studies (Marin Gabriel et al. 2013; Mosayebi et al. 2014; Gao et al. 2015; Liu et al. 2015) ($n = 320$) have evaluated the efficacy of KC to reduce pain from heel lance, one (Kostandy et al. 2013) ($n = 36$) from intramuscular injection and one (Nanavati et al. 2013) ($n = 50$) from tape removal. KC was associated with decreased NIPS scores, cry time, grimacing, heart rate, DAN score, and PIPP. The duration of KC has not been systematically compared, although studies in the review ranged from 2 min to 3 h nor has the repeated use of KC been studied. A few studies compared sweet taste or breastfeeding to KC with results showing either no difference (Okan et al. 2010), KC to be more effective (Freire et al. 2008; Chermont et al. 2009) or to have a cumulative effect (Marin Gabriel et al. 2013). No adverse effects have been reported.

25.14 Nonnutritive Sucking

Among non-pharmacological interventions, nonnutritive sucking (NNS), or pacifier use, was the first to be studied in the mid-1980s. Its use in term and preterm infants treated in neonatal intensive care and in minimal care shows that behavioral distress, namely, percent time spent in the fussing and crying state, is reduced during and after heel stick (Bellieni 2007a). In a recently updated Cochrane systematic review of non-pharmacological strategies for pain, six studies examined the effect of NNS on pain reactivity (reactions immediately after painful stimuli) and immediate pain regulation (reactions after the initial pain response period) for preterm infants (Pillai Riddell et al. 2015). For pain reactivity, NNS was not found to be effective for preterm infants (SMD −0.31, 95% CI −0.65 to 0.04, $I^2 = 72\%$), but there were statistically significant benefits for full-term neonates (SMD −1.20, 95% CI −1.54 to −0.25, $I^2 = 84$) (Pillai Riddell et al. 2015). For immediate pain regulation, there was a statistically significant effect for preterm infants (SMD −0.43, 95% CI −0.63 to −0.23, $I^2 = 0$) and neonates (SMD −0.90, 95% CI −1.54 to −0.25, I^2 = 84%) (Pillai Riddell et al. 2015).

25.15 Containment/Facilitated Tucking and Swaddling

Containment refers to restricting the premature infants' motions by holding or using an arm to place the neonate's arms and legs near the trunk to maintain a flexed in utero posture with limbs placed in body midline (Huang et al. 2004). It is also referred to as facilitated tucking (Axelin et al. 2006). The effects of facilitated tucking have been examined in preterm infants undergoing commonly performed tissue-breaking procedures in the NICU and have been shown to diminish the magnitude of physiological, behavioral, and composite biobehavioral indicators of pain response (Corff et al. 1995; Axelin et al. 2006, 2009; Cignacco et al. 2012; Liaw et al. 2012, 2013; Peyrovi et al. 2014; Pillai Riddell et al. 2015).

Similar to facilitated tucking in respect to containment and midline positioning, swaddling consists of wrapping the infant in a sheet or blanket (Aucott et al. 2002). The first study was published almost 30 years ago (Campos 1989) where it was less efficacious in reducing pain than a pacifier. In preterm infants with a postconceptual age greater than 31 weeks, swaddling improved pain response (Shu et al. 2014) and recovery (Fearon et al. 1997) after heel lance compared to no treatment, but may have less of an effect in infants with a postconceptual age less than 31 weeks (Fearon and Kisilevsky 1997) and may not be more efficacious than heel warming (Shu et al. 2014). A meta-analysis of four studies in Thailand reports that the effect size of swaddling compared to no intervention on pain scores during heel lance was greater in term infants (0.79 (95% CI = 0.53, 1.05)) than in preterm infants (0.53 (95% CI = 0.27, 0.80)) (Prasopkittikun 2003). Comparing containment to swaddling, there is little difference between their effects, and therefore these interventions can be used interchangeably (Huang et al. 2004; Pillai Riddell et al. 2015).

25.16 Rocking

Rocking, compared to pacifiers and routine care after heel lance, promoted arousal levels, while pacifiers promoted sleep and reduced heart rate (Campos 1994). Based on studies of rocking being effective in full-term neonates and on studies of simulated rocking promoting quiet sleep (Campos 1994), simulated rocking was tested for pain in 85 preterm neonates, and rocking alone was no better than control unless coupled with sucrose. In a randomized controlled trial comparing maternal holding to lying supine during immunization, holding was found to not significantly reduce Neonatal Facial Coding Scale indicators, cry duration, or visual analog scale scores in full-term born infants ranging from 2 to 6 months (Ipp et al. 2004). As such, the evidence for the analgesic efficacy of holding and rocking is limited.

25.17 Auditory Recognition/Music

The human fetus is thought to be capable of auditory perception by 29 weeks of gestational age (Hepper and Shahidullah 1994) and have the ability to remember auditory stimuli from their intrauterine environment (Fifer et al. 1995). There is a paucity of high-quality, recently conducted trials from which to draw conclusions. The most comprehensive Cochrane systematic review of non-pharmacological interventions included a single crossover trial (n = 19) assessing efficacy of a recording of the mother's voice modified to simulate the in utero environment. This was not found to be effective (SMD −0.29, 95% CI −0.94 to 0.35) (Pillai Riddell et al. 2015). In a three-arm repeated measures RCT, 35 preterm infants were randomized to one of the three conditions during heel lance: music, glucose, or control. Groups were compared based on the change from baseline PIPP score, with the music (median = +2) and glucose (median = +1) conditions showing significant improvement over the control (+3) conditions (p = 0.008). In a crossover design study with infants 30–41 weeks' gestational age, music therapy alone consisting of intrauterine maternal pulse sounds with soothing music, music therapy combined with nonnutritive sucking, nonnutritive sucking alone, and no intervention were compared when used for 5 min after heel lance (Bo and Callaghan 2000). Music therapy alone had the strongest effect on neonates' heart rate. Butt and Kisilevsky (Butt and Kisilevsky 2000), in a randomized crossover design, exposed 16 preterm neonates to vocal or instrumental music for 10 min after the end of a heel lance. Infants above 31 weeks in the music group had a significantly more rapid recovery.

Similar findings were not observed in a study examining a recorded and filtered maternal "sing-song" voice versus no voice during heel stick procedure (Johnston et al. 2007). These results may have been affected by the high volume of the recorded sound (70 db) or may indicate that familiar sound alone may not be sufficient to ameliorate the effects of a tissue-breaking procedure in younger more immature infants.

25.18 Olfactory/Aromatherapy Recognition

There is now compelling evidence that both term and preterm infants remember, recognize, and prefer smell that is associated with their intrauterine environment and their mothers and that olfactory stimuli can provide infants with comfort and modulate pain response (Goubet et al. 2003, 2007). These results were seen in both full term (Rattaz et al. 2005; Goubet et al. 2007) and preterm (average 32.3 weeks' gestational age) (Goubet et al. 2003). Pillai-Ridell et al. (2015), in a recent Cochrane systematic review, included one RCT ($n = 90$) in an analysis of the effect of familiar and unfamiliar odor on immediate pain regulation (definition). Familiar odor was determined to be effective (SMD −1.04, 95% CI −1.47 to −0.61).

25.19 Sensorial Saturation

As described by Bellieni, sensorial saturation is an intervention consisting of a combination of tactile, gustative, auditory, and visual stimuli (Bellieni et al. 2012). In a rapid review of all trials employing sensorial saturation for the reduction of pain response in neonates, eight papers ($n = 709$) were retrieved (Bellieni et al. 2012). Procedures were primarily heel lance (7/8) with a single study assessing response to endotracheal suctioning. Outcomes included validated pain scales, cry time, and intracranial pressure. Most (7/8) studies found results indicating the sensorial saturation was effective. The group that conducted this review tested the feasibility of training mothers to use sensorial saturation with the removal of baby oil to scent the hands and found that they were as effective as highly trained staff and more effective than glucose and pacifier by two points on their pain score based on crying (Bellieni et al. 2007a, c). Several trials found that sensorial saturation is more effective than any other procedure in preventing pain from heel-prick.

25.20 Conclusions

The above review provides strong evidence for the efficacy of a variety of non-pharmacological interventions. By engaging sensory modalities such as olfactory, touch, oragustatory, auditory, temperature, and vestibular, the nociceptive sensations can be dampened. The precise mechanisms, whether it is simply the competing sensations or that these sensations evoke endogenous opiates or regulatory hormones, are not known. However, given the efficacy of numerous non-pharmacological interventions (Cignacco et al. 2007) for procedural pain in neonates, and the difficulties with pharmacological agents in this population for common painful procedures such as heel lance and venipuncture, non-pharmacological interventions should be the first choice in uncompromised infants (American Academy of Pediatrics: Committee on Fetus and Newborn, Section on Surgery and Canadian Paediatric Society: Fetus and Newborn Committee 2006). They are cost-effective and easy to administer. Mothers are clearly implicated in breastfeeding and kangaroo care, but can also be included in other interventions such as sensorial saturation (Bellieni et al. 2007a;

Axelin et al. 2009). Initially, there is a requirement to train staff and parents in these methods, and it may seem easier to give a solution in an intravenous line than to coordinate care to coincide with parental visiting. Nevertheless, parents find pain the most distressing aspect of the NICU and also wish to actively participate in comforting their infant (Franck et al. 2004). These approaches are consistent with modern family-centered care in neonatal units in which the best interests of the infant and family are put ahead of staff convenience.

References

Abad F, Diaz N, Domenech E et al (1996) Oral sweet solution reduces pain-related behaviour in preterm infants. Acta Paediatr Int J Paediatr 05:54–58

Als H, Duffy FH, McAnulty GB et al (2004) Early experience alters brain function and structure. Pediatrics 113:846–857. https://doi.org/10.1542/peds.113.4.846

American Academy of Pediatrics: Committee on fetus and newborn, section on surgery and S on A and PM, Canadian paediatric society: fetus and newborn committee (2006) prevention and management of pain in the neonate : An Update. https://doi.org/10.1542/peds.2006-2277

Anand KS (1996) New perspectives on the definition of pain. Pain 67:3–6

Anand KJ (2000) Pain, plasticity, and premature birth: a prescription for permanent suffering? Nat Med 6:971–973. https://doi.org/10.1038/79658

Anand KJ, Coskun V, Thrivikraman KV et al (1999) Long-term behavioral effects of repetitive pain in neonatal rat pups. Physiol Behav 66:627–637. https://doi.org/10.1016/S0031-9384(98)00338-2

Arockiasamy V, Holsti L, Albersheim S (2008) Fathers' experiences in the neonatal intensive care unit: a search for control. Pediatrics 121:e215–e222. https://doi.org/10.1542/peds.2007-1005

Asmerom Y, Slater L, Boskovic DS et al (2013) Oral sucrose for heel lance increases adenosine triphosphate use and oxidative stress in preterm neonates. J Pediatr. https://doi.org/10.1016/j.jpeds.2012.12.088

Aucott S, Donohue PK, Atkins E, Allen MC (2002) Neurodevelopmental care in the NICU. Ment Retard Dev Disabil Res Rev 8:298–308

Axelin A, Salantera S, Lehtonen L (2006) "Facilitated tucking by parents" in pain management of preterm infants-a randomized crossover trial. Early Hum Dev 82:241–247. https://doi.org/10.1016/j.earlhumdev.2005.09.012

Axelin A, Salantera S, Kirjavainen J, Lehtonen L (2009) Oral glucose and parental holding preferable to opioid in pain management in preterm infants. Clin J Pain 25:138–145. https://doi.org/10.1097/AJP.0b013e318181ad81

Barr R (2000) Crying as a sign, a symptom, & a signal: clinical, emotional and developmental aspects of infant and toddler crying. Mac Keith Press, London

Barr P (2007) Relationship of neonatologists' end-of-life decisions to their personal fear of death. Arch Dis Child Fetal Neonatal Ed 92:F104–F107. https://doi.org/10.1136/adc.2006.094151

Bartocci M, Bergqvist LL, Lagercrantz H, Anand KJ (2006) Pain activates cortical areas in the preterm newborn brain. Pain 122:109–117. https://doi.org/10.1016/j.pain.2006.01.015

Bellieni CV, Buonocore G (2008) Neonatal pain treatment: ethical to be effective. J Perinatol 28:87–88. https://doi.org/10.1038/sj.jp.7211899

Bellieni CV, Buonocore G (2009) Flaws in the assessment of the best interests of the newborn. Acta Paediatr Int J Paediatr 98:613–617. https://doi.org/10.1111/j.1651-2227.2008.01185.x

Bellieni CV, Johnston CC (2015) Analgesia, nil or placebo to babies, in trials that test new analgesic treatments for procedural pain. Acta Paediatr Int J Paediatr. https://doi.org/10.1111/apa.13210

Bellieni CV, Buonocore G, Pinto I et al (2003) Use of sound-absorbing panel to reduce noisy incubator reverberating effects. Biol Neonate 84:293–296. https://doi.org/10.1159/000073637

Bellieni C, Pinto I, Stacchini N (2004a) Vibration risk during neonatal transport. Minerva Pediatr 56:207–212

Bellieni CV, Sisto R, Cordelli DM, Buonocore G (2004b) Cry features reflect pain intensity in term newborns: an alarm threshold. Pediatr Res 55:142–146. https://doi.org/10.1203/01.PDR.0000099793.99608.CB

Bellieni CV, Bagnoli F, Pinto I et al (2005) Reduction of exposure of newborns and caregivers to very high electromagnetic fields produced by incubators. Med Phys 32:149–152. https://doi.org/10.1118/1.1829404

Bellieni CV, Cordelli DM, Marchi S et al (2007a) Sensorial saturation for neonatal analgesia. Clin J Pain 23:219–221

Bellieni CV, Cordelli DM, Caliani C et al (2007b) Inter-observer reliability of two pain scales for newborns. Early Hum Dev 83:549–552. https://doi.org/10.1016/j.earlhumdev.2006.10.006

Bellieni CV, Maffei M, Ancora G et al (2007c) Is the ABC pain scale reliable for premature babies? Acta Paediatr Int J Paediatr. https://doi.org/10.1111/j.1651-2227.2007.00355.x

Bellieni CV, Acampa M, Maffei M et al (2008) Electromagnetic fields produced by incubators influence heart rate variability in newborns. Arch Dis Child Fetal Neonatal Ed 93:F298–F301. https://doi.org/10.1136/adc.2007.132738

Bellieni CV, Tei M, Coccina F, Buonocore G (2012) Sensorial saturation for infants' pain. J Matern Neonatal Med 25 (Suppl 1):79–81. https://doi.org/10.3109/14767058.2012.663548

Bellieni CV, Tei M, Buonocore G (2015) Should we assess pain in newborn infants using a scoring system or just a detection method? Acta Paediatr Int J Paediatr 104:221–224. https://doi.org/10.1111/apa.12882

Bijlani V, Rizvi T, Wadhwa S (1988) Development of spinal substrate for nociception in man. Pain 87:167–179

Blass EM, Hoffmeyer LB (1991) Sucrose as an analgesic for newborn infants. Pediatrics 87:215–218. https://doi.org/10.1097/00132586-199112000-00033

Blass EM, Shah A (1995) Pain-reducing properties of sucrose in human newborns. Chem Senses 20:29–35

Blass E, Fitzgerald E, Kehoe P (1987) Interactions between sucrose, pain and isolation distress. Pharmacol Biochem Behav 26:483–489

Bo L, Callaghan P (2000) Soothing pain-elicited distress in Chinese neonates

Bueno M, Stevens B, de Camargo PP et al (2012) Breast milk and glucose for pain relief in preterm infants: a noninferiority randomized controlled trial. Pediatrics 129:664–670. https://doi.org/10.1542/peds.2011-2024

Bueno M, Yamada J, Harrison D, et al (2013) A systematic review and meta-analyses of nonsucrose sweet solutions for pain relief in neonates. Pain Res Manag 18(3):153–161

Butler S, Als H (2008) Individualized developmental care improves the lives of infants born preterm. Acta Paediatr Int J Paediatr 97:1173–1175. https://doi.org/10.1111/j.1651-2227.2008.00916.x

Butt ML, Kisilevsky B (2000) Music modulates behaviour of premature infants following heel lance. Can J Nurs Res 31:17–39

Campos RG (1989) Soothing pain-elicited distress in infants with swaddling and pacifiers. Child Dev 60:781–792

Campos RG (1994) Rocking and pacifiers: two comforting interventions for heelstick pain. Res Nurs Heal 17:321–331

Carbajal R, Veerapen S, Couderc S et al (2003) Analgesic effect of breast feeding in term neonates: randomised controlled trial. BMJ 326:13

Carbajal R, Lenclen R, Jugie M et al (2005) Morphine does not provide adequate analgesia for acute procedural pain among preterm neonates. Pediatrics 115:1494–1500

Carbajal R, Rousset A, Danan C et al (2008) Epidemiology and treatment of painful procedures in neonates in intensive care units. JAMA 300:60–70. https://doi.org/10.1001/jama.300.1.60

Chermont AG, Falcão LFM, de Souza Silva EHL et al (2009) Skin-to-skin contact and/or oral 25% dextrose for procedural pain relief for term newborn infants. Pediatrics 124: e1101–e1107. https://doi.org/10.1542/peds.2009-0993

Cignacco E, Hamers JP, Stoffel L et al (2007) The efficacy of non-pharmacological interventions in the management of procedural pain in preterm and term neonates. A systematic literature review. Eur J Pain 11:139–152. https://doi.org/10.1016/j.ejpain.2006.02.010

Cignacco EL, Sellam G, Stoffel L et al (2012) Oral sucrose and “facilitated tucking” for repeated pain relief in preterms: a randomized controlled trial. Pediatrics 129:299–308. https://doi.org/10.1542/peds.2011-1879

Clancy B, Silva-Filho M, Friedlander MJ (2001) Structure and projections of white matter neurons in the postnatal rat visual cortex. J Comp Neurol 434:233–252. https://doi.org/10.1002/cne.1174

Codipietro L, Ceccarelli M, Ponzone A (2008) Breastfeeding or oral sucrose solution in term neonates receiving heel lance: a randomized, controlled trial. Pediatrics 122:e716–e721. https://doi.org/10.1542/peds.2008-0221

Committee on Newborn Pain APP (2016) Prevention and management of procedural pain in the neonate: an update. Pediatrics 137:1–13. https://doi.org/10.1542/peds.2015-4271

Corff KE, Seideman R, Venkataraman PS et al (1995) Facilitated tucking: a nonpharmacologic comfort measure for pain in preterm neonates. J Obstet Gynecol Neonatal Nurs 24:143–147. https://doi.org/10.1111/j.1552-6909.1995.tb02456.x

da Costa MC, Unchalo Eckert G, Gastal Borges Fortes B, Borges Fortes Filho J, Silveira R, Procianoy R, Coelho de Costa M (2013) Oral glucose for pain relief during exam for ROP. Clin Sci 62:199–203

Fearon I, Kisilevsky BS, Hains S, Muir DW, Tranmer J (1997) Swaddling after heel lance: age specific effects on behavioral recovery in preterm infants. J Dev Behav Pediatr 18(4):222–232

Fifer WP, Moon C LJ et al (1995) The effects of fetal experience with sound fetal development. A psychobiological perspective. In: Lawrence Erlbaum Associates. Hillsdale, pp 351–366

Franck LS, Miaskowski C (1997) Measurement of neonatal responses to painful stimuli: a research review. J Pain Symptom Manag 14:343–378. https://doi.org/10.1016/S0885-3924(97)00222-4

Franck LS, Cox S, Allen A, Winter I (2004) Parental concern and distress about infant pain. Arch Dis Child Fetal Neonatal Ed 89:F71–F75. https://doi.org/10.1136/fn.89.1.F71

Freire NB, Garcia JB, Lamy ZC (2008) Evaluation of analgesic effect of skin-to-skin contact compared to oral glucose in preterm neonates. Pain 139:28–33. https://doi.org/10.1016/j.pain.2008.02.031

Gao H, Xu G, Gao H et al (2015) Effect of repeated Kangaroo Mother Care on repeated procedural pain in preterm infants: a randomized controlled trial. Int J Nurs Stud 52:1157–1165. https://doi.org/10.1016/j.ijnurstu.2015.04.006

Giannakoulopoulos X, Sepulveda W, Kourtis P et al (1994) Fetal plasma cortisol and β-endorphin response to intrauterine needling. Lancet 344:77–81. https://doi.org/10.1016/S0140-6736(94)91279-3

Giannakoulopoulos X, Sepulveda W, Kourtis P (1999) Human fetal and maternal noradrenaline responses to invasive procedures. Pediatr Res 45:494–499

Goubet N, Rattaz C, Pierrat V et al (2003) Olfactory experience mediates response to pain in preterm newborns. Dev Psychobiol. https://doi.org/10.1002/dev.10085

Goubet N, Strasbaugh K, Chesney J (2007) Familiarity breeds content? Soothing effect of a familiar odor on full-term newborns. J Dev Behav Pediatr. https://doi.org/10.1097/dbp.0b013e31802d0b8d

Gradin M, Finnstrom O, Schollin J (2004) Feeding and oral glucose – additive effects on pain reduction in newborns. Early Hum Dev 77:57–65. https://doi.org/10.1016/j.earlhumdev.2004.01.003

Gray L, Watt L, Blass EM (2000) Skin-to-skin contact is analgesic in healthy newborns. Pediatrics 105, e14

Gray L, Miller LW, Philipp BL, Blass EM (2002) Breastfeeding is analgesic in healthy newborns. Pediatrics 109:590–593

Gupta NK, Upadhyay A, Agarwal A et al (2013) Randomized controlled trial of topical EMLA and breastfeeding for reducing pain during wDPT vaccination. Eur J Pediatr 172:1527–1533. https://doi.org/10.1007/s00431-013-2076-6

Guyatt GH, Oxman AD, Vist GE et al (2009) GRADE: an emerging consensus on rating quality of evidence and strength of recommendations. Chin J Evid-Based Med 9:8–11. https://doi.org/10.1136/bmj.39489.470347.AD

Hepper PG, Shahidullah S (1994) Development of fetal hearing. Arch Dis Child 71:8–1

Hevner RF (2000) Development of connections in the human visual system during fetal mid-gestation: a DiI-tracing study. J Neuropathol Exp Neurol 59:385–392

Holsti L, Oberlander TF, Brant R (2011) Does breastfeeding reduce acute procedural pain in preterm infants in the neonatal intensive care unit? A randomized clinical trial. Pain 152:2575–2581. https://doi.org/10.1016/j.pain.2011.07.022

Huang CM, Tung WS, Kuo LL, Ying-Ju C (2004) Comparison of pain responses of premature infants to the heelstick between containment and swaddling. J Nurs Res 12:31–40

Ipp M, Taddio A, Goldbach M et al (2004) Effects of age, gender and holding on pain response during infant immunization. Can J Clin Pharmacol J Can Pharmacol Clin 11:2–7

Johnston CC, Stevens BJ (1996) Experience in a neonatal intensive care unit affects pain response. Pediatrics 98:925–930

Johnston CC, Stremler R, Horton L et al (1999) Effect of repeated doses of sucrose during heel stick procedure in preterm neonates. Biol Neonate 75:160–166

Johnston CC, Filion F, Snider L et al (2002) Routine sucrose analgesia during the first week of life in neonates younger than 31 weeks' postconceptional age. Pediatrics 110:523–528

Johnston CC, Stevens B, Pinelli J et al (2003) Kangaroo care is effective in diminishing pain response in preterm neonates. Arch Pediatr Adolesc Med 157:1084–1088. https://doi.org/10.1001/archpedi.157.11.1084

Johnston CC, Filion F, Nuyt AM (2007) Recorded maternal voice for preterm neonates undergoing heel lance. Adv Neonatal Care 7:258–266. https://doi.org/10.1097/01.ANC.0000296634.26669.13

Johnston C, Barrington KJ, Taddio A et al (2011) Pain in Canadian NICUs have we improved over the past 12 years? Clin J Pain 27:225–232

Johnston C, Campbell-Yeo M, Fernandes A, Inglis D, Streiner D, Zee R (2014) Skin-to-skin care for procedural pain in neonates. Cochrane Database Syst Rev (1):CD008435. https://doi.org/10.1002/14651858.CD008435.pub2

Kashaninia Z, Sajedi F, Rahgozar M, Noghabi FA (2008) The effect of kangaroo care on behavioral responses to pain of an intramuscular injection in neonates. J Spec Pediatr Nurs 13:275–280. https://doi.org/10.1111/j.1744-6155.2008.00165.x

Kataria M, Narang S, Chawla D et al (2015) Oral dextrose for pain management during laser treatment of retinopathy of prematurity under topical anesthesia. Indian J Pediatr 82:694–697. https://doi.org/10.1007/s12098-015-1718-2

Kostandy RR, Anderson GC, Good M (2013) Skin-to-skin contact diminishes pain from hepatitis B vaccine injection in health full-term neonates. Neonatal Netw 32:274–280

Kostoví I, Judaš M (2002) Correlation between the sequential ingrowth of afferents and transient patterns of cortical lamination in preterm infants. Anat Rec 267:1–6. https://doi.org/10.1002/ar.10069

Kostovic I, Goldman-Rakic PS (1983) Transient cholinesterase staining in the mediodorsal nucleus of the thalamus and its connections in the developing human and monkey brain. J Comp Neurol 219:431–437

Kostović I, Jovanov-Milosevic N (2008) Subplate zone of the human brain: historical perspective and new concepts. Coll Antropol 32:3–8

Kostović I, Rakic P (1990) Developmental history of the transient subplate zone in the visual and somatosensory cortex of the macaque monkey and human brain. J Comp Neurol 297:441–470

Kostović I, Fucic A, Mrzljak L (1991) Prenatal and perinatal development of the somatostatin containing neurons in the human prefrontal cortex. Neurosci Lett 124:153–156

Kostović I, Judas M, Rados M, Hrabac P (2002) Laminar organization of the human fetal cerebrum revealed by histochemical markers and magnetic resonance imaging. Cereb Cortex 12:536–544. https://doi.org/10.1093/cercor/12.5.536

Lavoie PM, Stritzke A, Ting J et al (2015) A randomized controlled trial of the use of oral glucose with or without gentle facilitated tucking of infants during neonatal echocardiography. PLoS ONE. https://doi.org/10.1371/journal.pone.0141015

Lee GY, Yamada J, Kyololo OM et al (2014) Pediatric clinical practice guidelines for acute procedural pain: a systematic review. Pediatrics 133:500–515. https://doi.org/10.1542/peds.2013-2744

Lefrak L, Burch K, Caravantes R et al (2006) Sucrose analgesia: identifying potentially better practices. Pediatrics 118:S197–S202. https://doi.org/10.1542/peds.2006-0913R

Leite AM, Linhares MBM, Lander J et al (2009) Effects of breastfeeding on pain relief in full-term newborns. Clin J Pain 25:827–832. https://doi.org/10.1097/AJP.0b013e3181b51191

Liaw J-J, Yang L, Katherine Wang K-W et al (2012) Non-nutritive sucking and facilitated tucking relieve preterm infant pain during heel-stick procedures: a prospective, randomised controlled crossover trial. Int J Nurs Stud 49:300–309. https://doi.org/10.1016/j.ijnurstu.2011.09.017

Liaw JJ, Yang L, Lee CM et al (2013) Effects of combined use of non-nutritive sucking, oral sucrose, and facilitated tucking on infant behavioural states across heel-stick procedures: a prospective, randomised controlled trial. Int J Nurs Stud. https://doi.org/10.1016/j.ijnurstu.2012.08.021

Linhares MBM, Gaspardo CM, Souza LO et al (2014) Examining the side effects of sucrose for pain relief in preterm infants: a case-control study. Braz Med Biol Res. https://doi.org/10.1590/1414-431X20143659

Liu M, Zhao L, Li XF (2015) Effect of skin contact between mother and child in pain relief of full-term newborns during heel blood collection. Clin Exp Obstet Gynecol 42:304–308

Lowery CL, Hardman MP, Manning N et al (2007) Neurodevelopmental changes of fetal pain. Semin Perinatol 31:275–282. https://doi.org/10.1053/j.semperi.2007.07.004

Mandel R, Ali N, Chen J et al (2012) Nitrous oxide analgesia during retinopathy screening: a randomised controlled trial. Arch Dis Child Fetal Neonatal Ed 97: F83–F87. https://doi.org/10.1136/adc.2011.210740

Marin Gabriel MA, Del Rey Hurtado de Mendoza B, Jimenez Figueroa L et al (2013) Analgesia with breastfeeding in addition to skin-to-skin contact during heel prick. Arch Dis Child Fetal Neonatal Ed. https://doi.org/10.1136/archdischild-2012-302921

Marín Gabriel MÁ, del Rey Hurtado de Mendoza B, Jiménez Figueroa L et al (2013) Analgesia with breastfeeding in addition to skin-to-skin contact during heel prick. Arch Dis Child Fetal Neonatal Ed 98:F499–F503. https://doi.org/10.1136/archdischild-2012-302921

McNair C, Campbell-Yeo M, Johnston C, Taddio A (2013) Nonpharmacological management of pain during common needle puncture procedures in infants: current research evidence and practical considerations. Clin Perinatol 40:493. https://doi.org/10.1016/j.clp.2013.05.003

Modarres M, Jazayeri A, Rahnama P, Montazeri A (2013) Breastfeeding and pain relief in full-term neonates during immunization injections: a clinical randomized trial. BMC Anesthesiol 13:22. https://doi.org/10.1186/1471-2253-13-22

Mosayebi Z, Javidpour M, Rahmati M, et al (2014) The effect of kangaroo mother care on pain from heel lance in preterm newborns admitted to neonatal intensive care unit : a crossover randomized clinical trial. J Compr Ped 5(4)

Mrzljak L, Uylings HB, Kostovic I (1988) Prenatal development of neurons in the human prefrontal cortex: I. A qualitative golgi study. J Comp Neurol 271:355–386

Nanavati RN, Balan R, Kabra NS (2013) Effect of kangaroo mother care vs expressed breast milk administration on pain associated with removal of adhesive tape in very low birth weight neonates: a randomized controlled trial. Indian Pediatr 50:1011–1015

Nesargi SV, Nithyanandam S, Rao S et al (2015) Topical anesthesia or oral dextrose for the relief of pain in screening for retinopathy of prematurity: a randomized controlled double-blinded trial. J Trop Pediatr 61:20–24. https://doi.org/10.1093/tropej/fmu058

Nimbalkar S, Sinojia A, Dongara A (2013) Reduction of neonatal pain following administration of 25% lingual dextrose: a randomized control trial. J Trop Pediatr. https://doi.org/10.1093/tropej/fms072

Obeidat HM, Shuriquie MA (2015) Effect of breast-feeding and maternal holding in relieving painful responses in full-term neonates. J Perinat Neonatal Nurs 29:248–254. https://doi.org/10.1097/JPN.0000000000000121

Okado N (1981) Onset of synapse formation in the human spinal cord. J Comp Neurol 201:211–219

Okan F, Ozdil A, Bulbul A et al (2010) Analgesic effects of skin-to-skin contact and breastfeeding in procedural pain in healthy term neonates. Ann Trop Paediatr 30:119–128. https://doi.org/10.1179/146532810X12703902516121

Ou-Yang MC, Chen IL, Chen CC et al (2013) Expressed breast milk for procedural pain in preterm neonates: a randomized, double-blind, placebo-controlled trial. Acta Paediatr Int J Paediatr 102:15–21. https://doi.org/10.1111/apa.12045

Perkins L, Hughes E, Glover A (2005) Exploring subplate evolution of the fetal cortex using magnetic resonance imaging. In: Neonatal Society

Peyrovi H, Alinejad-Naeini M, Mohagheghi P, Mehran A (2014) The effect of facilitated tucking position during endotracheal suctioning on physiological responses and coping with stress in premature infants: a randomized controlled crossover study. J Matern Neonatal Med. https://doi.org/10.3109/14767058.2013.868429

Phillips RM, Chantry CJ (2002) Is breastfeeding more analgesic than pacifier? In: Pediatric Academic Societies' Annual Meeting. Baltimore

Phillips RM, Chantry CJ, Gallagher MP (2005) Analgesic effects of breast-feeding or pacifier use with maternal holding in term infants. Ambul Pediatr 5:359–364

Pillai Riddell RR, Racine NM, Turcotte K, et al (2015) Non-pharmacological management of infant and young child procedural pain. Cochrane Database Syst Rev CD006275. https://doi.org/10.1002/14651858.CD006275.pub2

Porter FL, Grunau RE, Anand KJ (1999) Long-term effects of pain in infants. J Dev Behav Pediatr 20:253–261

Potana NT, Dongara AR, Nimbalkar SM et al (2015) Oral sucrose for pain in neonates during echocardiography: a randomized controlled trial. Indian Pediatr 52:493–497

Prasopkittikun TTF (2003) Management of pain from heel stick in neonates: an analysis of research conducted in Thailand. J Perinat Neonatal Nurs 17: 304–312

Rainville P, Duncan GH, Price DD et al (1997) Pain affect encoded in human anterior cingulate but not somatosensory cortex. Science 277(5328):968–971

Rainville P, Carrier B, Hofbauer RK et al (1999) Dissociation of sensory and affective dimensions of pain using hypnotic modulation. Pain 82:159–171. https://doi.org/10.1016/S0304-3959(99)00048-2

Ranger M, Zwicker JG, Chau CMY et al (2015) Neonatal pain and infection relate to smaller cerebellum in very preterm children at school age. J Pediatr 167:292–298. https://doi.org/10.1016/j.jpeds.2015.04.055

Rattaz C, Goubet N, Bullinger A (2005) The calming effect of a familiar odor on full-term newborns. J Dev Behav Pediatr. https://doi.org/10.1097/00004703-200504000-00003

Rosali L, Nesargi S, Mathew S et al (2015) Efficacy of expressed breast milk in reducing pain during ROP screening – a randomized controlled trial. J Trop Pediatr 61:135–138. https://doi.org/10.1093/tropej/fmu073

Ruda MA, Ling Q, Hohmann AG, et al (2016) Altered nociceptive neuronal circuits after neonatal peripheral inflammation. 289:628–630

Shah PS, Herbozo C, Aliwalas LL, Shah VS (2012) Breastfeeding or breast milk for procedural pain in neonates. Cochrane Database Syst Rev 12, CD004950. https://doi.org/10.1002/14651858.CD004950.pub3

Shu SH, Lee YL, Hayter M, Wang RH (2014) Efficacy of swaddling and heel warming on pain response to heel stick in neonates: a randomised control trial. J Clin Nurs. https://doi.org/10.1111/jocn.12549

Simons SH, van Dijk M, Anand KS et al (2003) Do we still hurt newborn babies? A prospective study of procedural pain and analgesia in neonates. Arch Pediatr Adolesc Med 157:1058–1064. https://doi.org/10.1001/archpedi.157.11.1058

Simonse E, Mulder PG, van Beek RH (2012) Analgesic effect of breast milk versus sucrose for analgesia during heel lance in late preterm infants. Pediatrics 129:657–663. https://doi.org/10.1542/peds.2011-2173

Skogsdal Y, Eriksson M, Schollin J (1997) Analgesia in newborns given oral glucose. Acta Paediatr Int J Paediatr 86:217–220

Slater R, Cantarella A, Gallella S et al (2006) Cortical pain responses in human infants. J Neurosci 26:3662–3666. https://doi.org/10.1523/jneurosci.0348-06.2006

Slater R, Cornelissen L, Fabrizi L, et al (2010) Oral sucrose as an analgesic drug for procedural pain in newborn infants: a randomised controlled trial. Lancet 376 (9748):1225–1232. https://doi.org/10.1016/S0140-6736(10)61303-7

Stevens B, Johnston C, Petryshen P, Taddio A (1996) Premature infant pain profile: development and initial validation. Clin J Pain 12:13–22

Stevens B, Johnston C, Taddio A et al (1999) Management of pain from heel lance with lidocaine-prilocaine (EMLA) cream: is it safe and efficacious in preterm infants? J Dev Behav Pediatr 20:216–221

Stevens B, Yamada J, Beyene J et al (2005) Consistent management of repeated procedural pain with sucrose in preterm neonates: is it effective and safe for repeated use over time? Clin J Pain 21:543–548

Stevens B, Yamada J, Gy L et al (2013) Sucrose for analgesia in newborn infants undergoing painful procedures. Cochrane Database Syst Rev 1, CD001069. https://doi.org/10.1002/14651858.CD001069.pub4

Taddio A, Katz J, Ilersich AL, Koren G (1997) Effect of neonatal circumcision on pain response during subsequent routine vaccination. Lancet 349:599–603. https://doi.org/10.1016/S0140-6736(96)10316-0

Taddio A, Shah V, Hancock R et al (2008) Effectiveness of sucrose analgesia in newborns undergoing painful medical procedures. C Can Med Assoc J 179:37–43. https://doi.org/10.1503/cmaj.071734

Taddio A, McMurtry CM, Shah V et al (2015) Reducing pain during vaccine injections: clinical practice guideline. CMAJ 187:975–982. https://doi.org/10.1503/cmaj.150391

Teixeira JMA, Glover V, Fisk NM (1999) Acute cerebral redistribution in response to invasive procedures in the human fetus. Am J Obstet Gynecol 181:1018–1025. https://doi.org/10.1016/S0002-9378(99)70340-6

Valeri BO, Ranger M, Chau C, et al (2015) Neonatal invasive procedures predict pain intensity at school age in children born very preterm

Valman HB, Pearson JF (1980) What the fetus feels. Br Med J 280:233–234

Van de Velde M, Jani J, De Buck F, Deprest J (2006) Fetal pain perception and pain management. Semin Fetal Neonatal Med 11:232–236. https://doi.org/10.1016/j.siny.2006.02.012

Vanhatalo S, Van Nieuwenhuizen O (2000) Fetal pain? Brain Dev 22:145–150. https://doi.org/10.1016/S0387-7604(00)00089-9

Weissman A, Aranovitch M, Blazer S, Zimmer EZ (2009) Heel-lancing in newborns: behavioral and spectral analysis assessment of pain control methods. Pediatrics 124:e921–e926. https://doi.org/10.1542/peds.2009-0598

Wladimiroff JW, van den Wijngaard JA, Degani S et al (1987) Cerebral and umbilical arterial blood flow velocity waveforms in normal and growth-retarded pregnancies. Obstet Gynecol 69:705–709

Woo JS, Liang ST, Lo RL, Chan FY (1987) Middle cerebral artery doppler flow velocity waveforms. Obstet Gynecol 70:613–616

Wyatt J (2007) End-of-life decisions, quality of life and the newborn. Acta Paediatr Int J Paediatr 96:790–791. https://doi.org/10.1111/j.1651-2227.2007.00349.x

Yew DT, Luo CB, Luo JM et al (2001) Substance P and enkephalin containing fibers in the developing nucleus dorsalis of the human spinal cord. Neurosci Lett 312:87–90. https://doi.org/10.1016/S0304-3940(01)02200-5

Zuppa AF, Mondick JT, Davis L, Cohen D (2009) Population pharmacokinetics of ketorolac in neonates and young infants. Am J Ther 16:143–146

Neonatal Anesthesia

26

Nicola Disma, Leila Mameli, Rachele Bonfiglio, Clelia Zanaboni, and Pietro Tuo

Contents

Abstract

Administration of the anesthetic drugs, surgery and the underlying disease, can interfere with the developmental changes of the neonatal life. For this reason, it is mandatory for the pediatric anesthetist to know the pathophysiology of the neonatal age, in order to correctly apply the principles of the neonatal anesthesia. The perinatal period and the delivery provide us important details for the complete medical history, and the complete preoperative anesthetic evaluation should be focussed on the infants' transition from the fotal to the neonatal life. Moreover, the techniques for induction and maintenance of anesthesia may vary with the infant's size, the gestational age, medical status, and surgical procedure. Regional anesthesia is widely used for intra- and postoperative analgesia and spinal anesthesia, and it can be considered a useful

N. Disma (✉) · L. Mameli · R. Bonfiglio · C. Zanaboni · P. Tuo
Department of Anesthesia, Pediatric and Neonatal Intensive Care, Istituto Giannina Gaslini, Genoa, Italy
e-mail: nicoladisma@tin.it; NicolaDisma@Gaslini.org; leilamameli@yahoo.it; lea.bonfiglio@gmail.com; lea.bonfiglio@gmail.com; pietrotuo@gaslini.org

G. Buonocore et al. (eds.), *Neonatology*,
https://doi.org/10.1007/978-3-319-29489-6_176

alternative to general anesthesia, especially to prevent the risk of postanesthesia apnea.

Postoperative pain can be pharmacologically safely treated with opioid, paracetamol, or regional anesthesia, when handled by an experienced pediatric acute pain service.

26.1 Salient Points

- Neonates represent a fragile population, prone to perioperative complications and life-threatening events.
- Appropriate perioperative management is mandatory for improving short- and long-term outcomes.
- Isotonic fluids should be used for intra- and immediate postoperative management.
- Regional anesthesia has to be considered as part of multimodal analgesia program, whenever applicable.
- Inadequate pain treatment has detrimental effects on postoperative outcome.
- Recent studies performed in animals have raised concern that anesthetic drugs can be neurotoxic. The GAS Study is the only RCT that has demonstrated no negative effects on long-term neurological outcome in children.

26.2 Anesthesia

About 1.5 million neonates are exposed to anesthesia every year, and it is well established that this population of patients is very fragile and prone to perioperative complications and life-threatening events. This is due to several factors: the peculiar physiology of neonates, the immaturity of organs and systems, the frequent coexisting comorbidities (such as extreme prematurity, congenital malformations, congenital heart disease and others), and the incomplete understanding of the pharmacology of the routinely used anesthetics drug. Moreover, even when anesthesia is correctly delivered, there could be the risk that it interferes with the normal development of the neonatal brain. In fact, there is increased awareness of the potential neurotoxicity of anesthetic drugs administered to this vulnerable population and the consequent long-term cognitive effects. This task will be discussed in detail at the end of this chapter.

For all the above mentioned reasons, pediatric anesthesiologists should know the pathophysiology of the neonatal age, the interference of underlying diseases with anesthesia, and the correct application of basic principles for neonatal anesthesia. In addition, neonates and young infants should undergo anesthesia and surgery only in specialized centers, where a neonatal resuscitation or intensive care is available. All neonates and small infants should always receive the most appropriate, timely and safe treatment.

26.2.1 Preanesthesia Assessment

The intrauterine, the perinatal, and the delivery period are all relevant parts of the medical history and the preanesthesia assessment for those neonates undergoing anesthesia. In particular, the intrauterine environment can interfere with the growth and the ability of the neonate to adapt to extrauterine life.

Maternal exposure to some drugs (e.g., phenytoin, alcohol, steroids) or placental blood flow abnormalities may result in poor growth of the fetus or premature labor. A complicated labor and delivery may result in respiratory, cardiovascular, and metabolic instability for a variable length of time. Also the gestational age and the weight can be related to some perinatal problems.

The physical examination starts with the gestational age and the weight of the baby. Infants are classified as "term" if greater than 37 weeks gestational age and "low birth weight" if weight less than 2.5 kg. A complete examination must be performed before withholding anesthesia in an infant, with particular care to some body areas and systems, as summarized in the Table 1.

26.2.2 Intraoperative Management

Safe and effective intraoperative management of the newborn depends on a profound understanding

Table 1 Interaction between anesthesia and neonatal physiology

Organs/ systems	Pathophysiology	Anesthetic implication
Head and neck	Micrognathia CHARGE syndrome	Possible difficulties in airway management Peculiar embryology and anatomy in preterm and term infants
Respiratory	Immaturity of control mechanism More compliant chest wall 10–25% type I fibers Surfactant deficiency Oxygen toxicity	Respiratory depression in case of hypoxia Airway collapse Predisposition to respiratory fatigue RDS BPD development
Cardiovascular	Hypoxemia or acidosis	Return to fetal circulation, persistent fetal circulation (PFC), persistent pulmonary hypertension of the newborn (PPHN)
CNS	Fragile vessels Immaturity of cerebral blood flow	Increased risk of hemorrhage Hypoxia, acidosis, seizures may disrupt autoregulation
Renal	Immaturity	Lost of electrolytes
Metabolic	Active transplacentar delivery of calium and transient hypoparathyroidism Delay in normal feeding	Hypocalcemia Hypoglicemia

Table 2 Airway management in neonate

Anatomy of the newborn	Action during tracheal intubation
Prominent occiput and large head	"Sniffing position" without the additional support of a pillow under the head neck
Larynx is cephalad (C4) and anterior	Extension of the neck may impede visualizing of the vocal cords, gentle pressure with finger can facilitate larynx view
Epiglottis	Large and with "Ʊ form", difficult visualization of the vocal cords
Narrow nostril and large tongue	Obligate nasal breathing, airway obstruction, possible bleeding
Cricoids	Is the narrowest airway of the newborn, small and uncuffed tubes

of physiology and pharmacology. Moreover, technical aspects of monitoring and anesthesia equipments have to be considered.

26.2.2.1 Induction of Anesthesia and Tracheal Intubation

The techniques for induction of anesthesia vary with the infant's size, the gestational age, medical status, and surgical procedure.

A specific case is the infant with a full stomach. An "awake" or a rapid sequence intubation should be performed, but the first is associated with significant morbidity (increased intracranial pressure, bradycardia, desaturation, etc) and the second is a real challenge especially in small preterms.

Neonates with expected difficult airway management (micrognathia, macroglossia, protruding maxilla, cleft palate, masses obstructing the airway) must not be paralyzed. Tracheal intubation can be performed with a pharmacological sedation and the infant in spontaneous breathing. Topic anesthesia with lidocaine on the vocal cords can facilitate tracheal intubation.

The anatomical peculiarities of the neonate and the subsequent anesthetic implications are summarized in Table 2.

The Miller-0 straight laryngoscope blade is the most commonly recommended device for visualizing the airway for tiny neonate, preterm or of low birth weight, and the Miller-1 is used in the term neonate. Uncuffed 3.0–3.5 mm endotracheal tubes are usually the appropriate size to intubate the trachea in neonates, and the choice of cuffed tubes is an effective alternative if the pressure of the cuff is carefully monitored (<20 cmH_2O). A tightly fitting tube can damage the subglottic mucosa, causing edema and postoperative stridor or more rarely subglottic stenosis. A small leak around the tube during manual positive breath (about 20 cmH_2O pressure) ensures that the size of the endotracheal tube is adequate.

Ensuring the appropriate depth in the trachea of the newborn also requires attention. The distance from the vocal cords to the carina in the term infant is about 4 cm.

26.2.2.2 Intraoperative Fluid Therapy

It has four components:

1. *Maintenance fluid*. Fluid loses consist primarily of insensible water loss from the respiratory system, evaporation from the skin, and urinary and fecal loss. 100 ml/kg/day is the normal requirement. Isotonic fluids are mandatory during anesthesia to minimize the risk of cerebral edema.
2. *Fluid deficits*. They are caused primarily by preoperative fasting or excessive gastrointestinal losses without parenteral replacement. It is calculated by multiplying the hourly maintenance requirement by the number of hours since the last fluid intake.
3. *Third space fluid loss*. Surgical trauma can result in translocation of extracellular fluid from the intravascular space into the interstitial space (edema in bowel wall and mesentery during intraabdominal surgery). Guidelines for replacement of third space losses include the following:
   (a) Superficial surgery: 1–2 ml/kg/h
   (b) Abdominal, chest of hip surgery: 3–4 ml/kg/h
   (c) Extensive abdominal surgery: 6–10 ml/kg/h or more

   Third space loss must be replaced with an isotonic or isoosmotic solution such as normal saline solution, lactate ringer's solution, or other balanced salt solutions.
4. *Other fluid losses*. They include those from suction or removal of gastric intestinal or drainage of an ileostomy, diarrhea, or excessive sweat losses. In these cases the electrolyte content of the fluid losses should be measured to determine replacement fluids.

Urine output indicates normal hydratation (0.5–2 ml/kg/h). Serum osmolarity is also a useful monitor of electrolyte and fluid therapy.

Standard hemodynamic intraoperative monitoring contributes to assessing the adequacy of fluid therapy.

Similar to older infants, the decision to deliver blood during surgery depends on the underlying and current cardiorespiratory status, ongoing blood loss, anticipated further blood loss, and baseline hemoglobin. Transfusion of other components of blood should be guided by a combination of laboratory studies and the clinical status.

26.2.2.3 Anesthetic Drugs: Inhaled and Intravenous Agents

The aim of anesthesia is to provide insensibility to pain and immobility during surgery. Anesthesia may be provided by regional or general anesthesia or the combination of both. General anesthesia can be delivered using both inhaled and intravenous drugs for a variety of surgical procedures.

Minimum alveolar concentration (MAC) defines the anesthetic depth for inhaled agents at which 50% of patients respond to painful stimulus with movement. It has been found that MAC is considerably less in preterm than in full-term infants and that 1 MAC of inhaled drugs results in 20–30% reduction in arterial pressure. Sevoflurane, newer inhaled agent, affords a rapid induction and emergence from general anesthesia and is widely used for anesthesia in infants. Moreover, sevoflurane possesses less airway irritability than isoflurane and desflurane, and it can be used for inhaled induction and in infants with bronco pulmonary dysplasia. The traditional mask induction of anesthesia is accomplished with incremental increases in sevoflurane up to 7–8%, in a mixture of oxygen and air. Maintenance of anesthesia is performed with up to 1 MAC of sevoflurane, and

Table 3 Principal drugs used for neonatal anesthesia and their doses

	Induction	Maintenance
Sevoflurane	Incremental, up to 8%	0.5–2 MAC
Ketamine	1–2 mg/kg	Not recommended
Propofol	2–5 mg/kg	50–200 μ/kg/min
Thiopentanl	4–6 mg/kg	Not recommended
Midazolam	0.05–0.2 mg/kg	100–200 μ/kg/h
Fentanil	0.5–3 μ/kg	Up to 100 μ/kg for cardiac or major surgery
Remifentanil	0.1–1 μ/kg/min	0.1–1 μ/kg/min

it can be reduced in case of opioid administration or combination with regional anesthesia.

Intravenous drugs for anesthesia may include opioids, benzodiazepines, propofol, ketamine, barbiturates, and dexmedetomidine, which is recently introduced in clinical practice. Opioids possess analgesic and sedative properties, and they are usually combined with hypnotic drugs as propofol or benzodiazepines. Pharmacokinetic of fentanyl has been studied in infants and the elimination half-time has been found to be from 6 to 32 h, which is significantly longer than in adults. Remifentanil, a synthetic short acting opioid, is rapidly inactivated by esterases in blood and tissues and due to its short half-life is administered by continuous infusion. For this reason it is now largely used in all ages and is a suitable opioid even in small infants (Sammartino et al. 2010).

Doses of some anesthetic drugs are summarized in Table 3.

26.2.3 Anesthesia for Preterm and Ex-Premature Infants

Preterm and ex-premature infants undergoing elective surgery are more likely to encounter perioperative apnea than term infants. Factor predisposing premature infants to apnea include hypoglycemia, hypoxia, hyperoxia, sepsis, anemia, hypocalcemia, and pharmacologic effects of general anesthesia on the immature respiratory centers. As a consequence, postoperative monitoring is mandatory for the 24 h following anesthesia.

Preterm and ex-premature infants may have dramatic responses to narcotics and potent inhaled anesthetics. The benefit of providing adequate anesthesia and analgesia must be carefully balanced with the significant risk of cardiorespiratory depression in this fragile population.

26.2.4 Regional Anesthesia

Epidural analgesia in combination with light general anesthesia is a useful alternative for infants and neonates undergoing major surgery, avoiding the adverse effects related to systemic administration of opioids and other agents. Apart from providing good intraoperative and postoperative analgesia, epidural blockade has beneficial effects on the humoral, metabolic, hemodynamic responses to surgery and it may improve postoperative respiratory performance.

The complication rate of epidural analgesia performed by experienced hands is very low.

Caudal epidural anesthesia remains the most frequently performed regional anesthesia technique in infants and children. It is a popular "single shot" technique characterized by a high level of efficacy and safety.

Because the level of the plasma protein α1-acid glycoprotein, albumin, and bicarbonate reserves are lower in neonates compared with children, neonates are at gratest risk of local anesthetic toxicity, like severe cardiac dysrhythmia, hemodynamic instability, respiratory arrest, or seizures that are the most common clinical presentation. This can be avoided using bolus doses and infusion rates within recommended guidelines and by taking into account pharmacokinetics of local anesthetics in neonates.

Table 4 Dose of local anesthetics for regional block in use at Gaslini Hospital

Regional anesthesia	Local anesthetic (LA)	Bolus		Continuous infusion	
		Concentration (%)	Dose LA/adjuvant	Concentration	Infusion rate
Caudal	Naropine Levobupivacaine	0.2	1 ml/kg Clonidine 1–2 mcg/kg	–	Not frequently used
Lumbar epidural	Naropine Levobupivacaine	0.2	0.8–1 ml/kg Clonidine 1–2 mcg/kg	0.1%	0.2–0.4 ml/kg/h
Thoracic epidural	Naropine Levobupivacaine	0.2	0.6–0.8 ml/kg Clonidine 1–2 mcg/kg	0.1%	0.2–0.4 ml/kg/h
Spinal	Naropine Levobupivacaine Bupivacaine	0.5–0.75	1 mg/kg (minimum 2.5 mg) Clonidine 1 mcg/kg (selected cases)	–	–

The low intrinsic toxicity of new local anesthetics like ropivacaine and levobupivacaine make them ideal for regional anesthesia in children.

The use of **spinal anesthesia** for hernia repair in premature infants with or without RDS is reportedly a safe and satisfactory alternative to general anesthesia. Even if the review of Craven recently published in The Cochraine Database of Systematic Reviews (Craven et al. 2003) shows no reliable evidence of the effects of spinal anesthesia compared to general anesthesia on the incidence of apnea, bradycardia, or oxygen desaturation in ex-preterm infants, spinal anesthesia can be considered a safe procedure to avoid general anesthesia-related risks.

Data from the recently published GAS study provided evidence that the incidence of early apnea (from the end of anesthesia up to the first 30 min) is significantly reduced with spinal anesthesia compared with general anesthesia, but not the incidence of late apnea. In fact, the overall incidence of apnea after both regional or general anesthesia is comparable in infants undergoing inguinal hernia repair. The interpretation of this recently published data is that with modern anesthesia based on sevoflurane and caudal block the incidence of postoperative anesthesia is similar to spinal anesthesia alone, but a successful regional anesthesia significantly reduces the incidence of early apnea. The commonly used dosage of local anesthetics for spinal anesthesia is of 1 mg/kg (minimum 2.5 mg) of ropivacaine, levobupivacaine, or bupivacaine 0.5% (less frequently 0.75%) . Adjuvants like clonidine at the dose of 1 mcg/kg can be added in case of expected prolonged surgery (Davidson et al. 2015a).

Doses of local anesthetics for regional anesthesia are displayed in Table 4.

26.2.5 Anesthesia Outside the Operating Room

Sedation outside the operating room or in remote locations is increasingly called, particularly for radiologic procedures and medical interventions. Providing anesthesia in locations far from the operating room requires familiarity with the procedures as well as careful and extensive planning and resources in order to manage life-threatening situations. Some of remote locations that may require sedation include dental clinics, gastroenterology suites, cardiology sites, plastic surgery centers, radiology suites, and oncology areas. It is advisable to delegate a team of anesthetists that is committed to providing off-site anesthesia care. Each member of the anesthesia team should rotate regularly through the different off-site areas to maintain a familiarity not only with the procedures and personnel but also with the particular anesthesia demands unique to each area. A standard anesthesia cart should be at each anesthesia site, fully stocked with essential medications, necessary adjuvant equipment, a variety of oral/nasopharyngeal airways, spare Ambu bag, laryngoscope handles and blades, endotracheal tubes, alternate airway devices including laryngeal mask airways (LMAs), suction catheters, and intravenous supplies.

The most important topic to be considered before performing a sedation outside the operating room, especially in infants younger than 1 month of age, are:

- History of ongoing apnea or prematurity with postconceptual age less than 60 weeks
- Respiratory compromise and abnormal airway
- Congenital cardiac disease or unstable cardiac status
- High-risk procedure
- Inadequate qualified personnel or inadequate anesthesia and resuscitation equipment

A clear understanding of the definition of sedation is mandatory to recognize when the child has progressed to a deeper level of sedation than anticipated and is at increased risk (i.e., from moderate sedation to deep sedation or from deep sedation to general anesthesia). Recognition of this transition allows escalation of monitoring and care to avoid complications.

The following are the definitions of the American Academy of Paediatrics (AAP) and the American Society of Anaesthesiologists (ASA) (American Society of Anesthesiologists Task Force on Sedation and Analgesia by Non-Anesthesiologists 2002), strong considering that infants may quickly move from one level of sedation to another.

Minimal sedation	A drug-induced state during which patients respond normally to verbal commands.
Moderate sedation	A drug-induced depression of consciousness during which patients respond to light tactile stimulation. No interventions are required to maintain a patent airway, and spontaneous ventilation is adequate.
Deep sedation	A drug-induced depression of consciousness during which patients cannot be easily aroused but respond after pain ful stimulation. The ability to independently maintain ventilatory function may be impaired. Patients may require assistance in maintaining a patent airway, and spontaneous ventilation may be inadequate.
General anesthesia	A drug-induced loss of consciousness during which patients are not arousable, even to painful stimulation. The ability to independently maintain ventilatory function is often impaired. Patients often require assistance in maintaining a patent airway, and positive pressure ventilation may be required because of depressed spontaneous ventilation or drug-induced depression of neuromuscular function. Cardiovascular function may be impaired.

Several anesthetics drugs (Michel and Constantin 2009; Cravero 2009) can be used for sedation in infants (Table 5). Our experience at Gaslini Hospital with neonatal sedation for MRI and TC is with sevoflurane. Induction and maintenance in full-term babies without other comorbidities is performed with sevoflurane as a single anesthetic drug. Airway manipulation is minimized maintaining patients in spontaneous breathing through a face mask or LMA, and tracheal intubation is decided uniquely in case of respiratory or cardiac instability. About 1,200–1,500 pediatric sedations each year are performed at Gaslini, and the incidence of respiratory depression or airway obstruction is negligible.

26.3 Analgesia

Interest in newborn and preterm pain has greatly increased in the last three decades, including the pain associated with intensive care and surgery. In the past, pain relief in these very vulnerable

Table 5 Sedative drugs and doses for infants

Drug	Doses	Comments
Midazolam	0.5–0.75 mg/kg PO or ER 0.025–0.05 mg/kg IV 0.02–0.03 mg/kg intranasal	Possible paradoxical effects. Doses must be reduced in case of concomitant opioid administration
Dexmedetomidine	2–5 mcg/kg PO 1–2 mcg/kg IV (bolus in 10–15 min)	Possible hemodynamic effects Excellent respiratory drive
Ketamine	1–2 mg/kg IV 3–4 mg/kg IM 4–6 mg/kg PO or ER	Possible laryngospasm, apnea, agitation, hallucinations. Anticholinergic to control secretions. Frequent associated tachycardia, hypertension, and bronchodilatation. No antagonist available
Nitrous oxide	50% in 50% oxygen for "minimal sedation," up to 70% for moderate sedation	Requires specialized equipment for delivery, monitoring, and scavenging. When used alone or with local anesthesia is considered "minimal sedation." Contraindications include respiratory failure, altered mental status, otitis media, bowel obstruction, and pneumothorax
Sevoflurane	1–2 MAC inhalational	Safely used for MRI and TC. It has little toxicity and it is hemodynamic, and respiratory depressive effects are moderate and well tolerated
Naloxone	0.01–0.1 EV or IM, may be repeated every two minutes	Specifically antagonizes opioid effects. Adverse reactions: nausea, vomiting, tachycardia, hypertension. Reversal after long-term opioid use may lead to acute withdrawal
Flumazenil	0.01–0.02 EV, may be repeated every one minute	Specific benzodiazepine antagonist. Does not antagonize opioids or other sedatives. Resedation may occur in 1 h. Prolonged observation (2 h) required. Not for routine sedation reversal

subjects has been neglected, reflecting the current beliefs and the resistance to change the normal practice.

26.3.1 Effects of Pain

The fetus is able to respond to noxious stimuli increasing stress hormone levels and cerebral blood flow, whereas fentanyl dampens the stress response of preterms undergoing surgery (Lowery et al. 2007). These observations support that autonomic and metabolic reactions are triggered before the pain pathways are completed. Between 17 and 25 weeks of gestational age, several neuronal types and dendritic and axonal network differentiate from subplate neurons, assigned to guide the development of cortical and thalamic structures. Because of the nervous system plasticity, repetitive noxious stimuli reaching the subplate neurons may result in formation of permanent abnormal synapses and hyperactivity of pain responses, resulting in possible future behavior disorders.

26.3.2 Pain in the Neonatal Intensive Care Unit

Though guidelines to manage pain in the Neonatal Intensive Care Unit (NICU) have been issued (American Academy of Pediatrics et al. 2006), many newborns undergo repetitive noxious procedures without adequate pain relief. Acute pain assessment can be a difficult task, either in discriminating pain from other causes of distress or in recognizing the pain cues in the most compromised babies. Moreover, signs of ongoing pain can be missing because of limited energy reserves and exhaustion in the sickest populations. Other obstacles in pain management can be the fear of respiratory depression, routine practice, old beliefs, and lack of validated prolonged pain assessment scales (Ranger et al. 2007).

Beyond procedural, perioperative and disease-related pain relief, sedation in neonates mechanically ventilated has been advocated, aiming at promoving stress reduction, blood pressure stability, and ventilator synchrony, leading finally to a decrease of cerebral injury and death. In 2004 the NEOPAIN multicenter trial evaluated 898 ventilated preterm newborns randomized to receive morphine or placebo. The study did not demonstrate any difference in the incidence of intraventricular hemorrhage, periventricular leukomalacia, and death between the groups, while the morphine group reported hypotension, prolonged ventilation, and feeding intolerance (Anand et al. 2004).

Even if at the moment opioids cannot be recommended for routine sedation in ventilated neonates, they should be routinely administrated during surgery, invasive procedures, and inflammatory diseases, on the basis of pain evaluation and clinical judgement (Bellu et al. 2005).

26.3.3 Opioids

The most commonly used opioids in NICU are morphine and fentanyl. Morphine shows an onset time of 5 min and a peak effect at 10–30 min. The duration lasts 3–8 h, owing to the neonate drugs' half-life prolongation. Clearance reaches adult values at 6 months. The relative permeability of the newborn blood–brain barrier facilitates the penetration of morphine into the central nervous system compared to older subjects. Morphine is administrered for perioperative analgesia, while it has not proven to be so effective during procedural acute pain. Usual intravenous dosage in infants receiving ventilatory support is 50–100 μg/kg as a single dose, followed by infusion of 10–30 μg/kg/h. Lower dosages are adequate for lower gestational ages, and small incremental doses (25–50% of the usual) are advised for nonventilated infants.

Fentanyl is more lipid soluble and has a potency of 100-fold that of morphine. The peak effect is reached by 5–15 min, and the duration time is 1–2 h. Fentanyl is less sedating and has minimal cardiovascular effects, suitable for hemodynamically unstable patients. Nevertheless, disadvantages of fentanyl are rapid development of tolerance and chest wall rigidity, particularly harmful in non-intubated infants. Fentanyl is usually administered intravenously at the dosage of 1–3 μg/kg as a single dose, followed by infusion of 0.5–2 μg/kg/h.

Tolerance develops more rapidly with fentanyl (3–9 days) than with morphine and with continuous infusion than with intermittent doses. Non-pharmacological measures and switching from opioids to sedatives (when appropriate) can reduce the risk of developing tolerance. Moreover, opioid tapering protocols should be implemented in every NICU.

Codeine is a prodrug administered only by enteral route, needing CYP2D6 to be metabolized to morphine. Poor and intermediate metabolizers can udergo dose-related toxicity or therapeutic failure. On the contrary, ultrarapid metabolizers under tramadol treatment that are breast-feeding mothers can expose their babies to the risk of life-threatening respiratory depression (Madadi et al. 2008).

Tramadol is an analogue of codeine, acting both as μ-receptor agonist and monoamines reuptake inhibitor. CYP2D6 metabolizes tramadol to O-demethyl tramadol, which shows a much higher affinity for μ-receptors than the parent compound. In term neonates, CYP2D6 activity seems to be equal to adult slow metabolizers and reaches adult activity level at 44 weeks. Tramadol is administered at the dose of 1–2 mg/kg as a bolus and 5–8 mg/kg/day as a continuous infusion (Allegaert et al. 2008).

26.3.4 Paracetamol

Paracetamol is a very common analgesic in infancy, but in neonates poor pain relief is reported after its administration for painful procedures, probably depending on its inadequacy for this type of pain. Newborns are relatively protected from the paracetamol hepatotoxicity, because of lower CYP450 level and lower glucuronide/sulfate metabolism ratio (Palmer et al. 2008). Increased unconjugated hyperbilirubinemia reflects the hepatic conjugating ability and can be a marker of reduced paracetamol clearance.

The relative bioavailability of rectal versus oral formulations is higher in neonates and approaches unity, while the rate of duodenal absorption is slower, and the rate of rectal absorption is slower and more erratic in neonates, when compared with older infants. To reach the target plasma concentration of 10–20 μg/ml, a loading dose is recommended. Doses should be adjusted in relation to weight, gestational age, postnatal age, and route of administration. Term newborns should not receive more than 60 mg/kg/day of drug at dosing interval of 6 h, whereas preterms should receive lower doses (30–40 mg/kg/day) at longer intervals (8–12 h) (Bartocci and Lundberg 2007). Intravenous paracetamol can be given alone or associated with opioid as opioid sparing drug. According to Allegaert et al. neonates aged between 32 and 44 weeks should receive a loading dose of 20 mg/kg of intravenous paracetamol, followed by 10 mg/kg every 6 h. The full dosage should not be continued for more than 4 days (Allegaert et al. 2011).

26.3.5 Ketamine

Ketamine is a "dissociative" drug, providing anesthesia, analgesia and amnesia, while displaying a safe respiratory and hemodinamic profile. The new S(+) ketamine seems to be more favorable when compared with the older racemic compound. Drug action is mediated mainly by *N*-methyl-D-aspartate (NMDA) receptors antagonism. An intravenous dose of 1–2 mg/kg exhibit an onset time of 1 min, a peak effect by 5–10 min, and a duration of 30–60 min. In NICU procedural pain, ketamine reduces the discomfort associated with tracheal suctioning (Saarenma et al. 2001). Recently the Food and Drug Administration have invited the anesthesia community to address the issue of the potential neurotoxicity of anesthetic agents in neonates, on the basis of their neurodegenerative effects on the developing brain in experimental trials (Mellon et al. 2007). Indeed NMDA receptors antagonists and γ-aminobutyric acid (GABA) agonists, in doses and durations of exposure exceeding those clinically used, induce neuronal injury and death in the brain of juvenile rodents. The main part of these studies regards ketamine, as the first observations had suggested a possible role of NMDA antagonists in neuropoprotective mechanisms, contradicted by subsequent studies demonstrating its neurotoxic effects. However, the applicability of these reports to clinical situations needs further confirmations.

26.3.6 Midazolam

Benzodiazepines (BDZs) are the most popular sedative drugs used in children, often combined with opioids. They share the same GABA-ergic mechanism of action with propofol and barbiturates, resulting in hyperpolarization of the neuronal membrane and producing anxyolisis, amnesia, sedation, muscle relaxation, and anticonvulsant effects. Potential adverse effects are hypoventilation/apnea and hypotension. Midazolam is characterized by faster onset time and shorter duration than others such as diazepam and lorazepam. The immaturity of enzyme systems involved in the metabolism of the drug (CYP450 and glycuronil-tranferase), linked to gestational and postnatal age, organ dysfunction, and drug interactions, explains the marked interpatient variability in dosage requirements to produce sedation in critically ill pediatric patients (Ng et al. 2003).

In the last years the use of midazolam in NICU has been reassessed on the grounds of both clinical and experimental observations. The NEOPAIN trial showed a statistically significant higher incidence of adverse neurologic events and death in the midazolam group compared with the morphine or placebo groups (Anand et al. 1999). More recently, the potential of midazolam to induce apoptotic neurodegeneration in the brain, while failing to sedate and sensitizing cutaneous reflexes in neonatal rats, has raised concerns about the safety of midazolam in the first days of life. At the moment, the use of midazolam infusion for sedation in NICU cannot be recommended.

26.3.7 Neonatal Anesthesia and the Risk of Neurotoxicity

A great deal of concern has recently arisen regarding the safety of anesthesia in infants. The first study on the possible neurotoxic effects of anesthetics was published in 1999, when a similarity between the ethanol, antiepileptic drugs, and general anesthetic was demonstrated in puppy rats. The pathohistological changes found in animals were subsequently shown to be associated with both short- and long-term behavioral changes. These preclinical findings have raised concern that similar effects can happen in humans and that young children undergoing anesthesia for surgical or diagnostic procedures may suffer from long-term neurocognitive consequences (Sanders et al. 2008; Sun 2010; Loepke and Soriano 2008). Several epidemiological studies have also been performed to investigate if an association between anesthesia exposure in early life and long-term neurological effects exists, but results have been contradictory. Two large prospective trials are currently running in children, with the aim to show if early exposure to anesthesia may result to long-term neurological consequences: the GAS and the PANDA. The first is a trial comparing general and regional anesthesia for infants undergoing hernia repair, with administration of validated scales for neurocognitive assessment at 2 and 5 years of age as primary outcomes (https://clinicaltrials.gov/ct2/show/NCT00756600). Results from the first interim follow-up of the GAS study have recently been published in the Lancet (Davidson et al. 2016). This secondary outcome, based on a neurocognitive assessment plus the administration of the full scales of the Bayley III test, showed that a sevoflurane-based anesthesia of about one hour at the average postmenstrual age of 45 weeks do not produce significant neurocognitive changes compared with awake regional anesthesia for inguinal hernia repair. The other trial is the PANDA, which is an ambidirectional study that includes a large population of children exposed to anesthesia before the age of 3 years and prospectively followed up to the age of 8 and 15 years (https://clinicaltrials.gov/ct2/show/NCT00881764). Unfortunately, the GAS and PANDA studies can only answer some of the questions regarding pediatric anesthesia and the associated risk of neurotoxicity, and multiple different questions readily emerge that will need to be addressed, e.g., the effect of different drugs and doses, age at exposure, duration of exposure, multiple exposures, as well as the impact of surgery and underlying conditions (Davidson et al. 2015b; Disma et al. 2016).

26.4 Conclusion

Physiology and pathophysiology of the neonatal age and the pharmacology of the anesthetic and analgesic drugs are the basis for a correct anesthesia management of the newborn. Small infants, preterms and neonates with complex syndromes should be managed by experienced pediatric anesthetists only.

References

Allegaert K, van den Anker JN, de Hoon JN et al (2008) Covariates of tramadol disposition in the first months of life. Br J Anaesth 100:525–532

Allegaert K, Palmer G, Anderson B (2011) The pharmacokinetics of intravenous paracetamol in neonates: size matters most. Arch Dis Child 96:575–580

American Academy of Pediatrics, Committee on Fetus and Newborn and Section on Surgery, Canadian Paediatric Society and Fetus and Newborn Committee (2006) Prevention and management of pain in the neonate: an update. Pediatrics 118:2231–2241

American Society of Anesthesiologists Task Force on Sedation and Analgesia by Non-Anesthesiologists (2002) Practice guidelines for sedation and analgesia by non-anesthesiologists. Anesthesiology 96(4):1004–1017

Anand KJ, Barton BA, McIntosh N et al (1999) Analgesia and sedation in preterm neonates who require ventilatory support: results from the NEOPAIN trial. Neonatal Outcome and Prolonged Analgesia in Neonates. Arch Pediatr Adolesc 153:331–338

Anand KJ, Hall RW, Desai N et al (2004) Effects of morphine analgesia in ventilated preterm neonates: primary outcomes from the NEOPAIN randomized trial. Lancet 363:1673–1682

Bartocci M, Lundberg S (2007) Intravenous paracetamol: the "Stockolm protocol" for postoperative analgesia of term and preterm neonates. Pediatr Anesth 17:1111–1121

Bellu R, de Waal KA, Zanini R (2005) Opioids for neonates receiving mechanical ventilation. Cochrane Database Syst Rev 1, CD004212

Craven PD, Badawi N, Henderson-Smart DJ, O'Brian N (2003) Regional (spinal, epidural, caudal) versus general anaesthesia in preterm infants undergoing inguinal herniorrhaphy in early infancy. Cochrane Database Syst Rev (3), CD003669

Cravero JP (2009) Risk and safety of pediatric sedation/anesthesia for procedures outside the operating room. Curr Opin Anaesthesiol 22(4):509–513

Davidson AJ, Morton NS, Arnup SJ, de Graaff JC, Disma N, GAS Consortium (2015a) Apnea after awake regional and general anesthesia in infants: the general anesthesia compared to spinal anesthesia study-comparing apnea and neurodevelopmental outcomes, a randomized controlled trial. Anesthesiology 123:38–54

Davidson AJ, Becke K, de Graaff J, Giribaldi G, Habre W, Hansen T et al (2015b) Anesthesia and the developing brain: a way forward for clinical research. Paediatr Anaesth 25:447–452

Davidson AJ, Disma N, de Graaff JC, Withington DE, Dorris L, Bell G et al (2016) Neurodevelopmental outcome at 2 years of age after general anaesthesia and awake-regional anaesthesia in infancy (GAS): an international multicentre, randomised controlled trial. Lancet 387:239–250

Disma N, Mondardini MC, Terrando N, Absalom AR, Bilotta F (2016) A systematic review of methodology applied during preclinical anesthetic neurotoxicity studies: important issues and lessons relevant to the design of future clinical research. Paediatr Anaesth 26:6–36

Loepke AW, Soriano SG (2008) An assessment of the effects of general anesthetics on developing brain structure and neurocognitive function. Anesth Analg 106(6):1681–1707

Lowery CL, Hardman MP, Manning N, Whit Hall R, Anand KJS (2007) Neurodevelopmental changes of fetal pain. Semin Perinatol 31:275–282

Madadi P, Shirazi F, Walter FG, Koren G (2008) Establishing causality of cerebral nervous system depression in breastfed infants following maternal codeine use. Paediatr Drugs 10:399–404

Mellon RD, Simone AF, Rappaport BA (2007) Use of anesthetic agents in neonates and young children. Pediatr Anesth 104:509–520

Michel F, Constantin JM (2009) Sevoflurane inside and outside the operating room. Expert Opin Pharmacother 10(5):861–873

Ng E, Taddio A, Ohlsson A (2003) Intravenous midazolam infusion for sedation of infants in the neonatal intensive care unit. Cochrane Database Syst Rev (1), CD002052

Palmer GM, Atkins M, Anderson BJ et al (2008) I.V. acetaminophen pharmacokinetics in neonates after multiple doses. Br J Anaesth 101:523–530

Ranger M, Johnstone CC, Anand KJS (2007) Current controversies regarding pain assessment in neonates. Semin Perinatol 31:283–288

Saarenma E, Neuvonen PJ, Huttunen P et al (2001) Ketamine for procedural pain relief in newborn infants. Arch Dis Chil Fetal Neonatal Ed 85:F53–F56

Sammartino M, Garra R, Sbaraglia F, De Riso M, Continolo N (2010) Remifentanil in children. Paediatr Anaesth 20(3):246–255

Sanders RD, Ma D, Brooks P, Maze M (2008) Balancing paediatric anaesthesia: preclinical insights into analgesia, hypnosis, neuroprotection, and neurotoxicity. Br J Anaesth 101(5):597–609

Sun L (2010) Early childhood general anaesthesia exposure and neurocognitive development. Br J Anaesth 105(Suppl 1):i61–i68

Neonatal Care in the Delivery Room: Initial Management and Approach to Low Risk Newborns

27

Tara M. Randis and Jennifer M. Duchon

Contents

T. M. Randis
Department of Pediatrics, New York University School of Medicine, New York, NY, USA
e-mail: Tara.randis@nyumc.org

J. M. Duchon (✉)
Division of Neonatology, St. Joseph's Regional Medical Center, Paterson, NJ, USA
e-mail: jmd2116@columbia.edu

G. Buonocore et al. (eds.), *Neonatology*,
https://doi.org/10.1007/978-3-319-29489-6_177

Abstract
Successful resuscitation hinges upon preparedness. Newborn infants who do not require resuscitation can be rapidly identified upon delivery by answering the following three critical questions:

1. Term gestation?
2. Good tone?
3. Breathing or crying?

If the answer to all three questions is "yes," the newly born infant may stay with the mother for routine care. Most initial care of low risk, healthy newborns can be provided while skin-to skin contact with the mother is maintained. Breastfeeding should be initiated as soon as possible. Policies relating to routine newborn care should be continually assessed to provide the best care while minimizing unnecessary invasive interventions, as well as adhering to national and international standards as appropriate.

27.1 Salient Points

- Successful resuscitation hinges upon preparedness.
- Newly born infants who do not require resuscitation can be generally identified upon delivery by rapidly assessing the answers to the following three critical questions (Wyckoff et al. 2015):
  - Term gestation?
  - Good tone?
  - Breathing or crying?
- Skin-to-skin contact is adequate for providing thermal stability, facilitates mother-infant bonding, and should occur as soon as possible after delivery.
- Breast feeding should be initiated in the delivery room without delay.
- Practices relating to healthy newborns in the first few hours of life should be geared towards:
- The needs and practices of the surrounding community
- National and international evidence-based standards of care
- And most importantly
- The health of the newborn through maternal-infant bonding and breastfeeding

27.2 Introduction

Ancient accounts of neonatal resuscitation strategies may be found in the Old Testament, the Talmud, and early writings of Hippocrates (O'Donnell et al. 2006). Mouth-to-mouth resuscitation of newborns was described as early as 1472 in a textbook on childhood diseases written by Bagellardeus (Wiswell and Gibson 2005). While, some of these early resuscitation practices were truly revolutionary, the vast majority reflected a limited understanding of the dramatic physiologic changes that take place during birth. Techniques including swinging the infant upside down, immersion in cold water, electric shock, shaking, yelling, slapping, and even insufflation of tobacco smoke into the rectum were widely practiced as recently as the early twentieth century (O'Donnell et al. 2006; Wiswell and Gibson 2005; Raju 1999). In 1953, Virginia Apgar wrote the following regarding the resuscitation of newborn infants:

> Seldom have there been such imaginative ideas, such enthusiasm, and dislikes, and such unscientific observations and study about one clinical picture. There are outstanding exceptions to these statements, but the poor quality and lack of precise data of the majority of papers concerned with infant resuscitation are interesting. (Apgar 2015)

Over the past several decades, an improved understanding of neonatal transition to extra-uterine life accompanied by major advancements in medical technology have led to dramatic improvement in the care of the compromised newborn. Recognition of the growing need for standardization of delivery room practices has led to the development of national committees dedicated to the establishment of consensus guidelines for newborn resuscitation. A global movement towards the practice of evidence-based care in the delivery room emerged, and in 1992 the International Liaison Committee on Resuscitation (ILCOR) was established to provide a forum for liaison between resuscitation organizations in the developed world (Chamberlain and Founding Members of the International Liaison Committee on Resuscitation 2005). Importantly, this committee not only provides recommendations regarding the care of the newborn but also has acknowledged ongoing controversies and identified areas in which additional research is needed. In addition, the training of caregivers in the delivery room has become the focus of recent clinical investigations, as innovative educational strategies such as video recording of resuscitations and simulator-based teaching become an integral part of many pediatric training programs (Halamek 2008; Carbine et al. 2000). The following text is based primarily on evidence presented in the 2015 International Consensus on Cardiopulmonary Resuscitation and Emergency Cardiovascular Care Science With Treatment Recommendations (Wyckoff et al. 2015).

27.3 Delivery Room Preparation

Successful resuscitation hinges upon preparedness. Nearly 10% of newborns require some assistance to begin breathing at birth and approximately 1% will require extensive resuscitation. Personnel trained in basic resuscitation skills (including initiation of positive pressure ventilation and chest compressions) should be present at every delivery. A person trained in Advanced Life Support techniques should be readily available for low-risk deliveries and present in the delivery room for those considered high-risk. Because a newborn without apparent risk factors may unexpectedly require resuscitation, each institution should have a procedure in place for rapidly mobilizing a team with complete newborn resuscitation skills for any birth. Published recommendations regarding the necessary equipment and drugs for resuscitation of the newly born infant exist and delivery rooms should be stocked accordingly (Table 1) (American Academy of Pediatrics et al. 2016). Delivery rooms should be maintained at a temperature between 36.5 °C and 37.5 °C.

Table 1 Neonatal resuscitation supplies and equipment (Adapted from American Academy of Pediatrics et al. (2016))

Suction equipment
Suction bulb syringe
Mechanical suctioning and tubing
Suction catheters (5 F or 6 F, 8 F, 10 F, 12 F or 14 F)
8 F feeding tube and large syringe
Meconium aspirator
Positive-pressure ventilation equipment
Device for delivery of positive pressure ventilation
Face masks, newborn and premature sizes
Oxygen source
Compressed air source
Oxygen blender to mix oxygen and compressed air (flow rate set to 10 L/min) and tubing
Pulse oximeter with sensor and cover
Target oxygen saturation table
Intubation equipment
Laryngoscope with straight blade, No. 0 (preterm) and No. 1 (term)
Extra bulbs and batteries for laryngoscope
Endotracheal tubes (sizes 2.5, 3, and 3.5 mm ID)
Stylet (optional)
Scissors
Tape or other securing device for endotracheal tube
Alcohol sponges
CO_2 detector or capnograph
Laryngeal mask and 5-mL syringe
5 F or 6 F orogastric tube if insertion port present on laryngeal mask
Medications
Epinephrine: 1:10,000 concentration (0.1 mg/mL) [3 mL or 10 mL ampules]
Normal saline for volume expansion, 100 or 250 mL
Dextrose 10 %, 250 mL
Normal saline for flushes
Syringes (1-mL, 3-mL or 5-mL, 20–60-mL)
Umbilical vessel catheterization supplies
Sterile gloves
Antiseptic prep solution
Umbilical tape
Small clamp
Forceps (optional)
Scalpel
Umbilical catheters (3.5 F, 5 F)
Three-way stopcock
Syringes (3–5 mL)
Needle or puncture device for needless system
Normal saline for flushes

(continued)

Table 1 (continued)

Clear adhesive dressing to temporarily secure umbilical venous catheter to abdomen (optional)
Miscellaneous
Gloves and appropriate personal protection
Radiant warmer or other heat source
Temperature sensor with sensor cover for radiant warmer (for use during prolonged resuscitation)
Firm, padded resuscitation surface
Timer/clock with second hand
Warmed linens
Hat
Stethoscope (with neonatal head)
Tape, 1/2 or 3/4 in.
Electronic cardiac (ECG) monitor leads and ECG monitor
Interosseous needle (optional)
For very preterm babies
Size-00 laryngoscope blade (optional)
Food-grade plastic bag (1 gal size) or plastic wrap
Thermal mattress
Transport incubator to maintain baby's temperature during move to the nursery

Communication with maternal care providers is critical, as a thorough maternal history will often identify those neonates most likely to require resuscitation. In 2008, Aziz et al. (2008) published a prospective, clinical trail identifying both antepartum and intrapartum factors that were strongly associated with the need for positive pressure ventilation in the delivery room. These included multiple pregnancy, maternal infection, maternal hypertension, oligohydramnios, preterm delivery, breech presentation, meconium-stained amniotic fluid, nonreassuring heart rate patterns, and emergency C-section.

Current evidence suggests that cord clamping should be delayed for at least 30–60 s for most vigorous term and preterm newborns. If placental circulation is not intact, such as after a placental abruption, bleeding placenta previa, bleeding vasa previa, or cord avulsion, the cord should be clamped immediately after birth. There is insufficient evidence to recommend an approach to cord clamping for newborns who require resuscitation at birth.

27.4 Determining Need for Resuscitation

Newly born infants who do not require resuscitation can be generally identified upon delivery by rapidly assessing the answers to the following three critical questions (Wyckoff et al. 2015):

4. Term gestation?
5. Good tone?
6. Breathing or crying?

If the answer to all three questions is "yes," the newly born infant may stay with the mother for routine care. In this context, "routine care" means the infant is dried, placed skin to skin with the mother, and covered with dry linen to maintain a normal temperature. Note that observation of breathing, activity, and color must be ongoing. If the answer to any of these assessment questions is "no," the infant should be moved to a radiant warmer and the providers should proceed with the initial steps in stabilization which include: warming and maintaining normal temperature, positioning, clearing of secretions if necessary, drying, and providing stimulation which are discussed in more detail below. The decision to progress beyond these initial steps is determined by simultaneous assessment of two vital characteristics: respirations and heart rate. If there is apnea, labored breathing, or heart rate less than 100 beats per minute maneuvers to achieve ventilation (positive pressure ventilation, continuous positive airway pressure) should be initiated. These initial stabilization steps, subsequent reevaluation of infant, and initiation of ventilation if needed should occur within the first 60 s of life, aptly referred to as "The Golden Minute" (Wyckoff et al. 2015).

27.5 Thermal Stability in the Delivery Room

Fetal temperature in utero is tightly regulated. Fetal metabolism results in a net production of heat that is removed by placental blood flow and is ultimately dispersed through the mother. As a result, there is a slight temperature gradient, with fetal temperature approximately 0.5 °C greater than the maternal core temperature (Walker et al. 1969). Upon parturition, the neonate rapidly loses heat through a variety of mechanisms as the ambient temperature falls dramatically from 37 °C in utero to approximately 25 °C in the delivery room. Because the newborn is coated with amniotic fluid, there is substantial evaporative heat loss. Circulating air currents in the delivery room contribute to convective heat loss. Conductive heat loss occurs when the infant is placed upon cooler surfaces such as unwarmed mattresses and blankets. Finally, heat is lost through radiation to cooler surfaces surrounding the infant but not in direct contact with the infant. The newborn is capable of sensing this cold stress and immediately triggers homeothermic mechanisms to minimize further heat loss. Vasoconstriction of the dermal arterioles minimizes the flow of warm blood to the cooler surface of the skin. Non-shivering thermogenesis, in which brown fat stores undergo exothermic reactions thereby generating heat, is initiated. Despite these adaptive measures, the core temperature of the newborn will continue to fall unless interventions by caretakers occur in a timely manner. Recent guidelines state that the temperature of newly born non-asphyxiated infants be maintained between 36.5 °C and 37.5 °C after birth through admission and stabilization (Wyckoff et al. 2015). Furthermore, they recommend that admission temperature should be recorded as a predictor of outcomes as well as a quality indicator.

The low birth weight infant is exquisitely susceptible to heat loss in the immediate postnatal period as they have a larger surface area to weight ratio and limited subcutaneous fat. The preterm infant, in particular, is less able to adapt to these environmental changes secondary to an immature epidermal barrier and a paucity of brown fat stores. For these reasons, the preterm infant has often been referred to as a functional poikilotherm. It is generally accepted that the newborn should have a core body temperature at or near 37 °C. However, it is important to recognize that even a newborn with a normal core body temperature may be exerting a tremendous amount of energy to maintain this temperature and therefore is cold stressed. While it has been recognized for decades that cold stress at birth has a negative impact upon infant survival, particularly in low birth weight infants (Silverman et al. 1958), it is surprising to learn that despite dramatic advances in neonatal care, temperature management in the delivery room remains an ongoing challenge. A large, multicenter, observational study published by Laptook et al. examined the distribution of body temperatures in low birth weight infants admitted to the neonatal intensive care unit. The study included more than 5,000 very low birth weight infants and found that nearly 47% had low admission temperatures defined as less than 36 °C (Laptook et al. 2007). Furthermore, there was a significant association between the extent of reduced temperature upon admission and late-onset sepsis and in-hospital mortality. These findings were similar to those published earlier in the EPIcure study, where approximately 40% of infants less than 26 weeks gestation had admission temperatures below 35 °C, and this was correlated with decreased survival (Costeloe et al. 2000). Intraventricular hemorrhage (Gleissner et al. 2000; Van de Bor et al. 1986), hypoglycemia (Lenclen et al. 2002; Zayeri et al. 2005), and respiratory compromise (Zayeri et al. 2005, Russo et al. 2014) have also been linked to low admission temperatures. Interventions to limit heat loss in the delivery room include maintaining delivery room temperature between 36.5 °C and 37.5 °C, prewarming of blankets and mattresses, rapidly drying the newborn, and removing wet blankets from infant contact. Swaddling infants in a warmed blanket is generally sufficient for stable, term infants. Early initiation of kangaroo care, allowing for direct skin-to-skin contact with the parent, is another effective means of maintaining the newborn's temperature (Anderson et al. 2003). Overhead heaters are necessary for those infants requiring further resuscitative efforts. Occlusive wraps (polyurethane, polyethlylene, or polyvinyl) may be beneficial in minimizing heat loss in extremely preterm infants, as their use has been associated with higher admission temperatures to the intensive care unit (Cramer et al. 2005).

While it has long been recognized that neonatal hypothermia is associated with decreased survival, potential morbidities related to hyperthermia have more recently been described (Perlman 2006). Neonatal hyperthermia may occasionally be iatrogenic in nature (inappropriate use of radiant warmers, occlusive wraps). However, it most often results from an elevated maternal temperature secondary to epidural anesthesia, prolonged labor or chorioamnionitis. Shalak et al. examined a cohort of term infants with clinical chorioamnionitis and found that elevated temperature at 30 min of life was correlated with neonatal depression at birth (requiring positive pressure ventilation or Apgar score less than 5 at 5 min) and admission to the neonatal ICU (Shalak et al. 2005). Other investigators have demonstrated an association between maternal fever and neonatal encephalopathy (Impey et al. 2001). Because these studies utilize maternal fever as a surrogate for neonatal hyperthermia, it remains unclear if maternal fever alone is sufficient to cause neurologic insult or if it is simply a marker for other intrapartum risk factors.

27.6 Positioning and Clearing the Airway

Placement of the newborn on his or her back under a radiant warmer with the head in a slightly extended position will open the airway. If respiratory efforts are present but ineffective (retractions, inadequate chest wall movement or poor air entry), the airway may be obstructed. Secretions should be cleared first from the oropharynx and then the nasopharynx with either a bulb syringe or suction catheter. Care must be taken to avoid deep or vigorous suctioning as this may result on laryngeal spasm and/or vagal bradycardia.

27.7 Stimulation

Most infants cry spontaneously upon delivery and establish regular respiration by 1 min of age. If this does not occur, the majority of infants will respond to tactile stimulation such as gentle rubbing of the back, as occurs with drying of the infant, or gently flicking the bottom of the feet. Failure of the infant to respond to these measures indicates the infant may be experiencing secondary apnea and will require positive pressure ventilation. Resuscitative measures beyond these initial few steps are discussed in detail in subsequent chapters.

27.8 Assessment of Resuscitation Efforts: The Apgar Score

In 1952, Virginia Apgar created a scoring system to rapidly assess the physical condition of infants shortly after birth in order to recognize those infants in need of further interventions to establish breathing (Apgar 2015). The Apgar score, which includes evaluation of heart rate, respiratory effort, muscle tone, reflex irritability, and color, remains widely used today as a measure of the infants response to resuscitative efforts. Several investigators have attempted to expand the utility of the Apgar score beyond the scope of the delivery room, using it as a measurement of risk for later impairment. While there is some evidence to suggest that a low 5-min Apgar score may be associated with future neurologic disability, the American Academy of Pediatrics cautions against its use as a predictor of long-term outcome or as a specific marker of intrapartum asphyxia, as this was not the original intent (American Academy of Pediatrics Committee on Fetus and Newborn and American College of Obstetricians and Gynecologists Committee on Obstetric Practice 2015). Apgar score has limitations, and it is inappropriate to use it alone to establish the diagnosis of asphyxia. Numerous factors may influence the Apgar score, including maternal sedation or anesthesia, congenital malformations, gestational age, trauma, and interobserver variability (Executive Summary 2014). A low 5-min Apgar score (0–3) is a valid predictor of neonatal mortality (Casey et al. 2001). The Apgar score is affected by gestational age and therefore its significance in preterm infants remains unclear.

27.9 Postnatal Assessment

Early assessment of the low risk newborn should be geared towards identification and prevention of conditions that may require more extensive care or evaluation.

- Skin-to-skin contact is adequate for providing thermal stability, facilitates mother-infant bonding, and should occur as soon as possible after delivery.
- Breast feeding should be initiated in the delivery room without delay.
- There is no evidence for routine sampling of hematocrit or blood glucose in healthy, low risk newborns.
- Prophylaxis against neonatal ophthalmia and vitamin K deficiency should be provided, but may wait until after the first breastfeed.
- Practices relating to healthy newborns in the first few hours of life should be geared towards:
  1. The needs and practices of the surrounding community
  2. National and international evidence-based standards of care

     And most importantly
  3. The health of the newborn through maternal-infant bonding and breastfeeding

Several key aspects of continuing care of the well newborn in the delivery room and during the recovery period will be discussed. In the healthy term newborn the goal of delivery room care should be to assess the newborn for any features that may confer the need for closer monitoring and follow up, and to promote the natural bonding between mother and infant. In this regard, much of the continuing care of the newborn can be done in such as way as to be minimally invasive to the infant and not disruptive to the mother–infant dyad.

27.10 Physical Exam

Every newborn should be assessed with a brief physical examination in the delivery room. The complete physical exam of the newborn will be discussed in detail in later chapters and has a different goal. As previously stated, the purpose of the physical exam in the delivery room should be to assess the newborn for any features that may indicate the need for immediate intervention or for further investigations and follow up during the nursery stay. Important findings to identify are:

- Visually patent and normally placed anus
- Normal external genitalia
- Presence of cleft lip or palate
- Intact spine and sacral area

Most major congenital malformations are discovered during routine prenatal care, and second trimester ultrasound at 18–22 weeks gestational age remains the most common imaging modality. When performed at tertiary care or University affiliated institutions, second trimester ultrasound has been shown to have good specificity and fair sensitivity for the detection of fetal anomalies (Fadda et al. 2009). However, defects such as those listed above, especially small facial anomalies, are frequently difficult to detect with traditional two-dimensional ultrasound techniques. As more sophisticated techniques such as three-dimenstional ultrasound or fetal MRI come into wider use, the detection rate for these anomalies, especially spinal and facial defects, may improve (Lee and Simpson 2007). It is not recommended to perform a rectal probe exam, such as a rectal temperature, to document patency of the anus. Deep suctioning of the nasal and/or oral cavities is also neither necessary nor recommended to determine patency of the nares or esophagus, as this may lead to trauma or perforation of the mucosal tissues. This is supported by recommendations from The American Academy of Pediatrics (AAP) section on breastfeeding, which states that unnecessary, excessive, and over-vigorous suctioning of the oral cavity, esophagus, and airways may traumatize the infant and lead to aversive feeding behavior (Pediatrics 2005). The initial physical examination of the infant can also document normal variants such as molding or caput of the scalp, Mongolian spots or sucking blisters, whereby the pediatrician may reassure parents of the benign nature of such findings. The initial physical assessment of the baby can be performed while skin-to-skin contact with the mother is taking place.

27.11 Initiation of Breastfeeding

The full physiology and nutrition of breastfeeding and breast milk will be discussed in a dedicated section of this manual. For the purpose of the care of the infant in the delivery room, the initiation of breastfeeding may be considered one of the most important contributions to the health and well being of a newborn. Briefly, the AAP recommendations for breastfeeding and breast milk include:

- Breast milk for all infants for whom it is not medically contraindicated
- Exclusive breastfeeding for the first 6 months of life
- Continuation of breastfeeding for at least 1 year
- Peripartum practices that facilitate breastfeeding

The alert, healthy newborn infant is capable of latching on to a breast without specific assistance within the first hour after birth (Section on Breastfeeding 2012; Righard and Alade 1990). In keeping with the previous discussion on temperature regulation, the AAP recommendations to promote breastfeeding in the delivery encourage that well, full term infants be placed and remain in direct skin-to-skin contact with their mothers immediately after delivery until the first feeding is accomplished (Section on Breastfeeding 2012; Righard and Alade 1990). Weighing, measuring, bathing, and other non-urgent interventions should be delayed until after the first feed is completed. For both bonding and breastfeeding purposes, the newborn infant should remain with the mother throughout the recovery period. A Cochrane review confirms that institutional changes in maternity care practices effectively increased rates of breastfeeding initiation and duration (Dyson et al. 2005). Institutional policies surrounding routine care of healthy newborn should be developed with the goal of safety and the promotion of the mother-infant bond, as opposed to convenience of the medical and ancillary staff.

27.12 Vital Signs and Measures

27.12.1 Vital Signs

Noninvasive vital signs, such as heart rate, respiratory rate, and temperature, as well as the procedure of weighing and measuring the infant, are often performed in the delivery room. Some institutions also have protocols involving more invasive measures, such as screening for oxygen saturation, hypoglycemia, anemia, or polycythemia. A vigorous term infant who has been ascribed good Apgar scores is unlikely to have major derangements in pulse or respiratory rate. Mild tachypnea may be a physiologic part of the transition from fetal to extrauterine life. The increased pulmonary vascular resistance of the newborn as manifest by oxygen saturation takes time to normalize. Studies have demonstrated that healthy full term neonates rarely reach oxygen saturations of greater than 90% until after the first 10 min of life, and may have lower postductal saturations for an even longer period (Mariani et al. 2007; Altuncu et al. 2008).

27.12.2 Hemoglobin and Hematocrit

Healthy full term infants have, in past years, been targeted for treatment of anemia or polycythemia based on values obtained from routine screening at birth. This can be troublesome from several perspectives. The definition of both anemia and polycythemia can vary. Most practitioners define anemia as a greater than two standard deviations below the mean hemoglobin, or less than the fifth percentile. For full term neonates, this is approximately 13 g/dL from a sample of blood drawn centrally, or 14.5 g/dL drawn from capillary sampling. Symptoms of anemia in the immediate newborn period may range from pallor to tachypnea to severe respiratory distress and circulatory collapse. Polycythemia can be defined in a similar manner, but has traditionally been diagnosed as a hematocrit greater than 65% drawn centrally or 70% drawn from a capillary specimen. Risk factors include macrosomic infants, or infants who are born to mothers who have conditions that affect placental blood flow, as a compensatory mechanism from the fetus. Symptoms of polycythemia include CNS manifestations such as lethargy and tremulousness, hypoglycemia, as well as evidence of organ failure such as respiratory distress, renal failure, congestive heart failure, or intestinal symptoms. Both obstetric practices, such as method of delivery and timing of cord clamping and positioning of the infant relative to cord clamping, can affect these values, as do the timing of blood sampling relative to delivery (Hutton and Hassan 2007; Merenstein et al. 1993). The degree to which an individual infant is symptomatic at a particular hemoglobin or hematocrit is extremely variable. It is also very difficult to differentiate the clinical effects, both short and long term, of polycythemia and anemia in an asymptomatic infant from the effects of the cause of the abnormal indices. Especially for polycythemia, there is no evidence to suggest that the treatment modality, partial exchange transfusion, of an asymptomatic infant improves outcome. The most sensible approach would be to consider screening infants who are at risk for anemia from fetal or intrapartum complications, and may warrant closer follow up, or for any infant who displays symptoms of abnormal hemoglobin or hematocrit (Merenstein et al. 1993).

27.12.3 Monitoring of Glucose

There has been much discussion in recent years as to the measurement and management of glucose levels in the low risk infant.

The fetus has a complete and continuous supply of glucose from the mother from placental transfer, via carrier-mediated facilitated diffusion. After birth, when this supply is abruptly cutoff, there are several mechanisms to maintain adequate energy to the infant:

- Glycogenolysis
- Gluconeogenesis
- Lipolysis
- Fatty acid oxidation and ketogenesis
- Hormonal/endocrine regulation of these systems

Serum glucagon, catecholamines, and growth hormone rise after cord clamping and insulin levels fall, favoring glycogenolysis, lipolysis, and gluconeogenesis. Full term infants are born with adequate glycogen stores, but these are depleted within the first several hours after birth unless feeding is established. Lipolysis can occur shortly after birth and releases free fatty acids that can be used as an energy source by many tissues, although not by the brain. Fatty acid oxidation and ketogenesis take place in the liver and produce ß-hydroxybutyrate, acetoacetate, and ketones which can be used by as an energy source for the brain. Several of the major hormones required for control of these systems rise in the first few hours of life, leaving the production of usable energy from both gluconeogenesis and hepatic ketogenesis delayed. This leaves free fatty acids from lipolysis and glucose from breakdown of glycogen stores as the major energy sources immedi ately after birth (Taeusch et al. 2005; Polin et al. 2011). In infants with poor stores of adipose tissue or glycogen, such as preterm or growth-restricted infants, maintaining an adequate supply of fuel for the metabolic needs of the brain becomes of great concern. Infants who are well may also be at risk. Nonshivering thermogenesis is the major mechanism of heat production in the neonate, and cold stress in the delivery room can occur. A newborn infant left unattended in an environment at typical "room temperature" experiences energy losses of approximately 150 kcal per minute, rapidly using up energy stores (Soll 2008). Delay in enteral feeding for routine newborn care can also exacerbate hypoglycemia. This provides further evidence for care to be performed skin to skin with the mother with early initiation of breastfeeding.

Many nurseries still monitor serum glucose levels in low risk, healthy infants as part of routine care. A problem can then arise, as debate occurs what level of serum glucose should be considered abnormal and require intervention in an asymptomatic, otherwise well newborn. When it was first recognized as a pathologic state, hypoglycemia was defined as less than 20 mg/dl (1.1 mmol/l) in preterm infants and less than 30 mg/dL (1.7 mmol/l) in full term infant. Cohort studies later showed that infants with symptomatic hypoglycemia had poorer neurodevelopmental outcomes (Pildes et al. 1974). Since that time, there has been little agreement about minimum acceptable level of glucose in healthy term infants (Adamkin and Polin 2016). Some authors portend that 45 mg/dl (2.5 mmol/l) is the lower limit for all infants (Cornblath et al. 2000; Inder 2008). Others maintain that due to the key time in development, and lack of evidence for compensatory mechanisms that protect the neonatal brain from hypoglycemic injury, glucose values should be similar in newborns as in older children, greater than 60 mg/dl or 3.3 mmol/l (Taeusch et al. 2005). Symptoms from hypoglycemia include tremulousness, lethargy, seizures, hypothermia, or can mimic respiratory distress. Infants who are considered at risk for hypoglycemia are those who are small or large for gestational age, or who have maternal risk factors for abnormal glucose such as gestational diabetes or medications affecting glucose metabolism. Also at high risk for sequelae from hypoglycemia are those infants who have evidence of infection, hypothermia, polycythemia, or hypoxia-ischemia (Cornblath et al. 2000; Inder 2008). It is generally accepted that healthy term infants, either breastfed or formula fed, who do not have risk factors for compromised metabolic adaptation and who are asymptomatic need not have routine glucose monitoring (Merenstein et al. 1993; Committee on Fetus and Newborn and Adamkin 2011). Any infant who appears symptomatic from hypoglycemia, or in whom risk factors for increased altered glucose metabolism exists, should be evaluated and treated if necessary (Committee on Fetus and Newborn and Adamkin 2011).

27.13 Common Routine Treatments

27.13.1 Eye Care

Neonatal ophthalmia is defined as conjunctivitis that occurs within the first 28 days of life. It is a relatively common illness, occurring in 1–12% of newborn infants. Historically, neonatal ophthalmia referred to conjunctivitis in the newborn caused by infection with *Neisseria gonorrhoeae*, but now the term refers to any conjunctivitis in this age group, regardless of the cause (Embree 2002). Gonococcal ophthalmia was, in the past, a leading cause of blindness, but is now rare in most developed populations with access to screening and treatment during pregnancy. It is for this historical reason that delivery room prophylaxis was geared towards prevention of blindness from this pathogen. Since the diminishment of gonococcal ophthalmia, there has been debate about which agent, if any, to use as prophylaxis against conjunctivitis in the delivery room. Most cases of conjunctivitis in the neonatal period are due to either chemical conjunctivitis or nonsexually transmitted colonizing bacteria. *Chlamydia trachomatis* also comprises a portion of ophthalmia, depending on local incidence. With the exception of Gonococcal and Chlamydial conjunctivitis, the condition is mild, and usually responds well to local treatment with no long-term sequelae with appropriate therapy. For these reasons, the Canadian Paediatric Society (CPS) no longer recommends routine eye prophylaxis be given (Moore et al. 2016). However, this practice is still endorsed by the AAP and legally mandated in many states and provinces/territories in North America. If prophylaxis must be given, 0.5% erythromycin ointment is recommended. The medication should be instilled as soon as possible in the delivery room and should not be wiped off. There is no data suggesting that delaying administration until after the first breastfeed in any way affects efficacy. Erythromycin ointment has replaced other forms of prophylaxis in the United States (USA) and Canada, as data suggested that there may be protection against Chlamydial species. Later studies disproved this (Chen 1992) probably due to the fact that local treatment will not eradicate nasophargyngeal colonization of the organism. Erythromycin potentially causes less chemical conjunctivitis than silver nitrate or aminoglycosides, and the drug remains in wide usage. This is not the case in other countries, where aminoglycoside, chloramphenicol, or no prophylaxis is used (Guala et al. 2005).

27.13.2 Vitamin K

Due to limited stores at birth, neonates are prone to vitamin K deficiency if no sufficient intake is provided. The clinical syndrome associated with vitamin K deficiency has been termed hemorrhagic disease of the newborn and comprises three distinct presentations. The very early form presents within 24 h of birth and is almost exclusively seen in infants of mothers taking drugs that inhibit vitamin K. These drugs include certain anticonvulsants, some antibiotics and vitamin K antagonists, many of which are now avoided in pregnancy. Clinical presentation can be severe, with cephalohematomas and intracranial and intraabdominal hemorrhage. Classical vitamin K deficiency occurs between 24 h and 7 days of life and is associated with delayed or insufficient feeding. Clinical presentation is often mild, with bruises, gastrointestinal bleeding, or bleeding from the umbilicus and puncture sites. The late presentation of vitamin K deficiency is associated with exclusive breastfeeding. It occurs between the ages of 2 and 12 weeks and infants can be gravely ill, with a mortality rate of 20%. Intracranial hemorrhage occurs in up to 50% of those affected (Van Winckel et al. 2009). After the discovery of vitamin K in the mid twentieth century, it was shown that treatment with vitamin K could abolish hemorrhagic disease of the newborn. It then became standard practice to administer the drug soon after birth to all infants. Controversy has arisen about this practice for several reasons. Both classic and late vitamin K deficiency are relatively rare; recent reviews cite estimates of 0.01–0.44% in the general population for the classic form, and between 4.4/100,000 and 7.2/100,000 births for the late form in fully breastfed infants who did not receive vitamin K at birth (Van Winckel et al. 2009). The present dose of 1 mg represents a very large amount when compared to the daily requirement of 5–10 μg in infants. The dose of 1 mg appears to have been chosen fairly arbitrarily, with no formal studies being performed to establish what dose might be appropriate. Intramuscular form became the route of choice based primarily on the available formulation at the time (Hey 2003). In the 1990s, a study from Britain linked the administration of intramuscular vitamin K at birth to childhood cancers and leukemia (Golding et al. 1990). Later studies failed to confirm this association, but the guidelines for universal prophylactic vitamin K were revised in many countries to include enteral dosage. It is universally accepted that vitamin K is necessary to prevent all forms of clinical disease in newborns. However, the method of administration and timing remain nonuniform across guidelines. For infants at risk from maternal medications, traumatic delivery, or prematurity, the intramuscular route is preferred. For healthy term newborns at low risk, the AAP recommends that vitamin K should be given as a single intramuscular dose of 1.0 mg to all newborns within the first 6 h after birth (Pediatrics 2003). For infants whose parents refuse an intramuscular injection, an oral dose of 2.0 mg of vitamin K at the time of the first feeding with dosages repeated at 2–4 weeks and 6–8 weeks of age may be used (McMillan 1997). Some countries have investigated the use of a small daily dose of enteral vitamin K in lieu of large doses less frequently in breastfeeding infants who did not receive the injection at birth, with apparent success (Van Winckel et al. 2009). Parents choosing oral dosing should be advised of the necessity of follow-up doses and be cautioned that their infants remain at an increased risk of late vitamin K deficiency (including the potential for intracranial hemorrhage) using the oral as opposed to parenteral route (McMillan 1997).

27.14 Conclusion

A 1995 study performed across several Italian nurseries showed that despite the availability of evidence-based national and international guidelines pertaining to routine newborn care, practices were guided by long standing habit and previously developed experiences (Guala et al. 2005). This can be extrapolated to many aspects of neonatal care. However, in the low risk, well newborn, the guiding principle should be to ensure the health and well being of the baby, and facilitate practices that will encourage continued health through maternal child interaction.

References

The Task Force on Neonatal Encephalopathy: D'Alton M, Hankins G, Berkowitz R, Bienstock J, Ghidini A, Goldsmith J, Higgins R, Moore T, Natale R, Nelson K, Papile L, Peebles D, Romero RJ, Schendel D, Spong CY, Waldman R, Wu Y, American College of Obstetricians and Gynecologists' staff: Joseph G, Hawks D, Politzer A, Emig C, Thomas K. (2014) Executive summary: neonatal encephalopathy and neurologic outcome, second edition. Report of the American College of Obstetricians and Gynecologists' task force on neonatal encephalopathy. Obstet Gynecol 123:896–901. https://doi.org/10.1097/01.AOG.0000445580.65983.d2

Adamkin DH, Polin R (2016) Neonatal hypoglycemia: is 60 the new 40? The questions remain the same. J Perinatol 36:10–12. https://doi.org/10.1038/jp.2015.125

Altuncu E, Özek E, Bilgen H et al (2008) Percentiles of oxygen saturations in healthy term newborns in the first minutes of life. Eur J Pediatr 167:687–688. https://doi.org/10.1007/s00431-007-0540-x

American Academy of Pediatrics Committee on Fetus and Newborn, American College of Obstetricians and Gynecologists Committee on Obstetric Practice (2015) The Apgar score. Pediatrics 136:819–822. https://doi.org/10.1542/peds.2015-2651

American Academy of Pediatrics, American Heart Association, Weiner GM, Zaichkin J (2016) Textbook of neonatal resuscitation (NRP), 7th edn. American Academy of Pediatrics, Elk Grove Village

Anderson GC, Moore E, Hepworth J, Bergman N (2003) Early skin-to-skin contact for mothers and their healthy newborn infants. Birth 30:206–207

Apgar V (2015) A proposal for a new method of evaluation of the newborn infant. Anesth Analg 120:1056–1059. https://doi.org/10.1213/ANE.0b013e31829bdc5c. Originally published in July 1953, 32:250–259

Aziz K, Chadwick M, Baker M, Andrews W (2008) Ante- and intra-partum factors that predict increased need for neonatal resuscitation. Resuscitation 79:444–452. https://doi.org/10.1016/j.resuscitation.2008.08.004

Carbine DN, Finer NN, Knodel E, Rich W (2000) Video recording as a means of evaluating neonatal resuscitation performance. Pediatrics 106:654–658

Casey BM, McIntire DD, Leveno KJ (2001) The continuing value of the Apgar score for the assessment of newborn infants. N Engl J Med 344:467–471. https://doi.org/10.1056/NEJM200102153440701

Chamberlain D, Founding Members of the International Liaison Committee on Resuscitation (2005) The International Liaison Committee on Resuscitation (ILCOR)-past and present: compiled by the Founding Members of the International Liaison Committee on Resuscitation. Resuscitation 67:157–161. https://doi.org/10.1016/j.resuscitation.2005.05.011

Chen J-Y (1992) Prophylaxis of ophthalmia neonatorum: comparison of silver nitrate, tetracycline, erythromycin and no prophylaxis. Pediatr Infect Dis J 11:1026

Committee on Fetus and Newborn, Adamkin DH (2011) Postnatal glucose homeostasis in late-preterm and term infants. Pediatrics 127:575–579. https://doi.org/10.1542/peds.2010-3851

Cornblath M, Hawdon JM, Williams AF et al (2000) Controversies regarding definition of neonatal hypoglycemia: suggested operational thresholds. Pediatrics 105:1141–1145. https://doi.org/10.1542/peds.105.5.1141

Costeloe K, Hennessy E, Gibson AT et al (2000) The EPICure study: outcomes to discharge from hospital for infants born at the threshold of viability. Pediatrics 106:659–671

Cramer K, Wiebe N, Hartling L et al (2005) Heat loss prevention: a systematic review of occlusive skin wrap for premature neonates. J Perinatol 25:763–769. https://doi.org/10.1038/sj.jp.7211392

Dyson L, McCormick F, Renfrew MJ (2005) Interventions for promoting the initiation of breastfeeding. Cochrane Database Syst Rev CD001688. https://doi.org/10.1002/14651858.CD001688.pub2

Embree J (2002) Recommendations for the prevention of neonatal ophthalmia. Paediatr Child Health 7:480–488

Fadda GM, Capobianco G, Balata A, Litta P, et al (2009) Routine second trimester ultrasound screening for prenatal detection of fetal malformations in Sassari University Hospital, Italy: 23 years of experience in 42,256 pregnancies. Eur J Obstet Gynecol Reprod Biol; e-publication

Gleissner M, Jorch G, Avenarius S (2000) Risk factors for intraventricular hemorrhage in a birth cohort of 3721 premature infants. J Perinat Med 28:104–110. https://doi.org/10.1515/JPM.2000.013

Golding J, Paterson M, Kinlen LJ (1990) Factors associated with childhood cancer in a national cohort study. Br J Cancer 62:304–308

Guala A, Guarino R, Zaffaroni M et al (2005) The impact of national and international guidelines on newborn care in the nurseries of Piedmont and Aosta Valley, Italy. BMC Pediatr 5:1. https://doi.org/10.1186/1471-2431-5-45

Halamek LP (2008) The simulated delivery-room environment as the future modality for acquiring and maintaining skills in fetal and neonatal resuscitation. Semin Fetal Neonatal Med 13:448–453. https://doi.org/10.1016/j.siny.2008.04.015

Hey E (2003) Vitamin K—what, why, and when. Arch Dis Child Fetal Neonatal Ed 88.F80–F83. https://doi.org/10.1136/fn.88.2.F80

Hutton EK, Hassan ES (2007) Late vs early clamping of the umbilical cord in full-term neonates: systematic review and meta-analysis of controlled trials. JAMA 297:1241–1252. https://doi.org/10.1001/jama.297.11.1241

Impey L, Greenwood C, MacQuillan K et al (2001) Fever in labour and neonatal encephalopathy: a prospective cohort study. BJOG 108:594–597

Inder T (2008) How low can I go? The impact of hypoglycemia on the immature brain. Pediatrics 122:440–441. https://doi.org/10.1542/peds.2008-1417

Lee YM, Simpson LL (2007) Major fetal structural malformations: the role of new imaging modalities. Am J Med Genet C Semin Med Genet 145:33–44

Laptook AR, Salhab W, Bhaskar B, Neonatal Research Network (2007) Admission temperature of low birth weight infants: predictors and associated morbidities. Pediatrics 119:e643–e649. https://doi.org/10.1542/peds.2006-0943

Lenclen R, Mazraani M, Jugie M et al (2002) Use of a polyethylene bag: a way to improve the thermal environment of the premature newborn at the delivery room. Arch Pediatr 9:238–244

Mariani G, Dik PB, Ezquer A et al (2007) Pre-ductal and post-ductal O2 saturation in healthy term neonates after birth. J Pediatr 150:418–421. https://doi.org/10.1016/j.jpeds.2006.12.015

McMillan DD (1997) Routine administration of vitamin K to newborns. Paediatr Child Health 2:429–434

Moore ER, Bergman N, Anderson GC, Medley N (2016) Early skin-to-skin contact for mothers and their healthy newborn infants. Cochrane Database of Systematic Reviews. Issue 11. Art. No.: CD003519. https://doi.org/10.1002/14651858.CD003519.pub4.

O'Donnell CPF, Gibson AT, Davis PG (2006) Pinching, electrocution, ravens' beaks, and positive pressure ventilation: a brief history of neonatal resuscitation. Arch Dis Child Fetal Neonatal Ed 91:F369–F373. https://doi.org/10.1136/adc.2005.089029

Perlman JM (2006) Hyperthermia in the delivery: potential impact on neonatal mortality and morbidity. Clin Perinatol 33:55–63–vi. https://doi.org/10.1016/j.clp.2005.11.002

Pildes RS, Cornblath M, Warren I et al (1974) A prospective controlled study of neonatal hypoglycemia. Pediatrics 54:5–14

Policy statement: breastfeeding and the use of human milk (2005) Pediatrics 115:496–506

Raju TN (1999) History of neonatal resuscitation. Tales of heroism and desperation. Clin Perinatol

Righard L, Alade MO (1990) Effect of delivery room routines on success of first breast-feed. Lancet 336:1105–1107. https://doi.org/10.1016/0140-6736(90)92579-7

Russo A, McCready M, Torres L et al (2014) Reducing hypothermia in preterm infants following delivery. Pediatrics 133:e1055–e1062. https://doi.org/10.1542/peds.2013-2544

Section on Breastfeeding (2012) Breastfeeding and the use of human milk. Pediatrics 129:e827–e841. https://doi.org/10.1542/peds.2011-3552

Shalak LF, Perlman JM, Jackson GL, Laptook AR (2005) Depression at birth in term infants exposed to maternal chorioamnionitis: does neonatal fever play a role? J Perinatol 25:447–452. https://doi.org/10.1038/sj.jp.7211326

Silverman WA, Fertig JW, Berger AP (1958) The influence of the thermal environment upon the survival of newly born premature infants. Pediatrics 22:876–886

Soll RF (2008) Heat loss prevention in neonates. J Perinatol 28:S57–S59. https://doi.org/10.1038/jp.2008.51

Stanley C, Pallotto E (2005) Avery's diseases of the newborn. Taeusch HW, Ballard RA, Gleason CA, Avery ME, (Eds). Elsevier Health Sciences, pp 1410–1422

Van de Bor M, Van Bel F, Lineman R, Ruys JH (1986) Perinatal factors and periventricular-intraventricular hemorrhage in preterm infants. Am J Dis Child 140:1125–1130

Van Winckel M, De Bruyne R, Van De Velde S, Van Biervliet S (2009) Vitamin K, an update for the paediatrician. Eur J Pediatr 168:127–134. https://doi.org/10.1007/s00431-008-0856-1

Walker D, Walker A, Wood C (1969) Temperature of the human fetus. J Obstet Gynaecol Br Commonw 76:503–511

Wiswell TE, Gibson AT (2005) Historical evolution of neonatal resuscitation. American Academy of Pediatrics, Neonatal Resuscitation Program, Instructor Resources

Wyckoff MH, Aziz K, Escobedo MB et al (2015) Part 13: Neonatal resuscitation: 2015 American Heart Association guidelines update for cardiopulmonary resuscitation and emergency cardiovascular care. Circulation 132:S543–S560, Lippincott Williams & Wilkins

Zayeri F, Kazemnejad A, Ganjali M et al (2005) Hypothermia in Iranian newborns. Incidence, risk factors and related complications. Saudi Med J 26:1367–1371

Early Detection of Neonatal Depression and Asphyxia

28

Paolo Biban and Davide Silvagni

Contents

Abstract

Neonatal depression is a general term to describe the condition of any newborn showing a prolonged transition from intrauterine to extrauterine life, in the immediate postnatal period. The variable degree of depression is inversely related to the Apgar score, with 1 min scores of 0–3 indicating the most severe forms, which may include perinatal asphyxia.

Despite major advances in obstetric and neonatal care, perinatal asphyxia remains a serious condition which may occur in the intrapartum, immediate postpartum, and early neonatal period.

P. Biban (✉) · D. Silvagni
Azienda Ospedaliera Universitaria Integrata Verona, Verona, Italy
e-mail: paolo.biban@aovr.veneto.it

G. Buonocore et al. (eds.), *Neonatology*,
https://doi.org/10.1007/978-3-319-29489-6_178

Perinatal asphyxia can be associated either with an uneventful course or with significant mortality and long-term morbidity. Therefore, reliable diagnostic and prognostic indicators are essential for a prompt recognition and treatment of newborns at risk for subsequent negative outcome.

However, the early detection of perinatal asphyxia still constitutes a challenging target in neonatology.

Despite several biochemical markers of asphyxia are available nowadays, none of them have shown sufficient reliability in predicting long-term neurological outcome.

Electrophysiological and neuroimaging investigations, such as aEEG, diffusion weighted MRI, or magnetic resonance spectroscopy, may provide early valuable information, but may be not easily available. Further research is still needed to validate prediction models capable to identify neonates at risk of dismal outcome due to perinatal asphyxia, allowing an adequate and timely diagnosis, treatment, and counselling.

28.1 Salient Points

- Neonatal depression refers to any newborn showing a prolonged transition from intrauterine to extrauterine life, in the immediate postnatal period.
- Perinatal asphyxia remains a serious condition which may occur in the intrapartum, immediate postpartum, and early neonatal period.
- Perinatal asphyxia can be associated either with an uneventful course or with significant mortality and long-term morbidity. Accurate diagnostic and prognostic indicators are essential for a prompt recognition and treatment of newborns at high risk of injury.
- The combination of clinical, instrumental, and biochemical indicators could provide predictive models to identify neonates at risk of dismal outcome due to perinatal asphyxia, allowing timely diagnosis, treatment, and counselling.

28.2 Introduction

Perinatal asphyxia is an insult to the fetus or newborn due to hypoxia and/or ischemia, persisting long enough to cause pathological biochemical changes and a variable degree of injury to various organs, including the brain. The effects of hypoxia and ischemia are often difficult to separate clinically. Hypoxia refers to an arterial concentration of oxygen that is less than normal, while ischemia occurs when the blood flow to the cells or organs is insufficient to maintain normal function. In its more severe forms, the impaired gas exchange secondary to asphyxia is also associated with tissue lactic acidosis and hypercapnia (Aurora and Snyder 1997).

Neonatal depression is a general term to describe the condition of any newborn in the immediate postnatal period (approximately the first hour after birth) showing a prolonged transition from intrauterine to extrauterine life. The degree of depression may be described using the Apgar score: a 1 min score of 4–6 is considered as moderate depression, and a score of 0–3 indicates severe neonatal depression, which usually requires immediate resuscitative interventions. Notably, the Apgar score cannot be used to determine the need for initial resuscitation.

28.3 Incidence and Definition of Neonatal Asphyxia

Despite major advances in monitoring technology, obstetric care, and knowledge of fetal and neonatal pathologies, asphyxia remains a serious condition causing significant mortality and long-term morbidity. According to the World Health Organisation (WHO), 4–9 million cases of newborn asphyxia occur each year (World Health Organization 2005). More than a million newborns that survive asphyxia at birth develop long-term problems such as cerebral palsy, mental retardation, speaking, hearing, visual, and learning disabilities (World Health Organization 2005). Globally, it is estimated that out of four million neonatal deaths annually, nearly one fourth are attributable to asphyxia (Lawn et al. 2005). In the developing world, the incidence of asphyxia is believed to be considerably higher due to the increased prevalence of risk factors. However, the incidence of birth asphyxia may vary markedly, depending on the definition used, as well as the gestational age of the infant. Many definitions of perinatal asphyxia can be found throughout the available literature, but a universal definition is still lacking (Low 1997; The Task Force on Cerebral Palsy and Neonatal Asphyxia of the Society of Obstetricians and Gynecologists of Canada 1996; Phelan et al. 2005). One of the most utilized is that promulgated in 2003 by the American Academy of Pediatrics and the American College of Obstetrician and Gynecologists, which includes the following criteria (American College of Obstetricians and Gynecologists et al. 2003):

1. Metabolic or mixed acidosis (pH < 7.00) in an arterial cord blood sample
2. Apgar score 0–3 for more than 5 min after birth
3. Evidence of neurologic signs in the immediate neonatal period
4. Evidence of multiorgan failure in the immediate neonatal period

More recently, the following neonatal signs have been proposed as consistent with an acute peripartum or intrapartum event (American College of Obstetrics and Gynecology et al. 2014):

(a) Apgar score of less than 5, at 5 and 10 min
(b) Umbilical artery acidemia (pH less than 7.0 and/or base deicit $\geq$ 12 mmol/L)
(c) Evidence of brain injury consistent with hypoxia-ischemia, by means of brain magnetic resonance imaging or magnetic resonance spectroscopy
(d) Multisystem organ failure consistent with hypoxic-ischemic encephalopathy

Newborn infants suffering episodes of perinatal asphyxia are at high risk of dying or developing brain damage. Postasphyxial hypoxic-ischemic encephalopathy (HIE) is viewed as the hallmark and most important consequence of asphyxia, being a major cause of death and of disability in term and near-term newborn infants in developed countries (Volpe 2008).

Approximately 1–2 infants per 1000 live term births are affected by hypoxic-ischemic encephalopathy, with outcomes ranging from complete recovery to death (Levene et al. 1985). HIE is a well-recognized clinical syndrome, with a large spectrum of clinical manifestations ranging from mild to severe. The clinical staging of Sarnat and Sarnat has been widely used since the 1970s to estimate the severity of the hypoxic-ischaemic insult in infants of 36 or more weeks of gestation (Sarnat and Sarnat 1976). In most cases, the severity of the encephalopathy predicts the risk of death and long-term neurodisability (Sarnat and Sarnat 1976; Shankaran 2009). However, an hypoxic ischemic encephalopathy secondary to intrapartum asphyxia cannot reliably predict the consequent neurodevelopmental outcome (Volpe 2008; Perlman and Risser 1996). Most term newborns with perinatal asphyxia have uneventful courses and a low likelihood of subsequent neurological sequelae (Volpe 2008; Goodwin 1999). Perinatal depression, when defined as low Apgar scores in the first minutes of life, may be not only related to birth asphyxia but also to other factors carrying a much lower risk of unfavorable short- and long-term outcome, including a vagal response due to nasopharyngeal stimulation, low gestational age, depression because of maternal anaesthesia (Volpe 2008). The prognosis for any given baby remains uncertain and reliable diagnostic and prognostic indicators related to perinatal asphyxia are still needed. Accurate markers of severe asphyxia and predictors of outcome would facilitate parental counselling as well as the choice of appropriate levels of care, which may include withdrawal of intensive care or the initiation of neuroprotective strategies.

Perinatal asphyxia may be categorized as occurring in three phases: (1) intrapartum; (2) immediate postpartum; and (3) early neonatal period.

28.4 Intrapartum Asphyxial Markers

Assessment of the intrapartum condition of the fetus includes electronic fetal heart rate monitoring (EFM), the observation of meconium in the amniotic fluid, fetal scalp blood sampling for acid–base, and lactate measurements (see the comprehensive ▸ Chap. 2, "Risk Factors for Gestational Diseases" by Petraglia and coll.).

Electronic Fetal Monitoring Electronic fetal monitoring (EFM) has been used to predict fetal distress or well being. Heart rate abnormalities have been identified as a marker of asphyxia during labor, fetal bradycardia being one of the most serious (Williams and Galerneau 2003). However, EFM has been shown to be imprecise in detecting fetuses with metabolic acidosis and predicting those likely to develop an hypoxic-ischemic encephalopathy (Larma et al. 2007; Graham et al. 2008).

A recent study evaluated the accuracy of EFM in predicting neonatal encephalopathy requiring hypothermia therapy. Disappointingly, the fetal heart tracing during the last hour before delivery was poorly predictive of neonatal encephalopathy requiring whole-body cooling treatment (Graham et al. 2014). Nonetheless, another study determined that some EFM features best predicated fetal acidemia, including repetitive prolonged decelerations, baseline tachycardia, repetitive variable decelerations, and repetitive late decelerations (Cahill et al. 2012). Newer technologies, such as fetal pulse oximetry and fetal electrocardiography, have been investigated to identify fetuses at risk more accurately. In particular, fetal electrocardiogram analysis of the ST segment (STAN) monitoring has been adopted in several European countries in addition to conventional EFM. However, a recent large controlled trial performed in the USA, comparing conventional EFM versus conventional EFM with STAN, did not find any substantial difference in terms of perinatal morbidity, mortality, or operative delivery rates (Belfort et al. 2015). Other techniques, such as Doppler measurement of blood flow velocity, near infrared spectroscopy, and fetal electroencephalogram, are less suitable for a routine clinical application (Volpe 2008).

Meconium Passage in Utero Meconium passage in utero is frequently cited as a sign of fetal stress, but several studies have failed to demonstrate a correlation between meconium stained amniotic fluid and permanent neurological sequelae (Nelson and Grether 1998). Currently, meconium passage in utero is considered neither a significant nor a specific marker of fetal distress unless associated with other abnormalities (Volpe 2008; Glantz and Woods 2004).

Fetal Scalp Blood Sampling Fetal scalp blood sampling (FBS) was introduced by Bretscher and Saling in 1962 and was primarily based on pH analysis (Bretscher and Saling 1967). They defined pH cut-off values as normal (>7.25), preacidotic (7.20–7.25), and acidotic (<7.20), recommending prompt delivery for cases with acidosis. These guidelines are still regarded as the "gold standard" for diagnosing intra-partum fetal distress. Fetal acidemia due to an hypoxic-ischemic insult is usually metabolic and a consequence of anaerobic glycolysis due to prolonged intrauterine hypoxia. In a large retrospective study, Kruger et al. (1999) performed 814 lactate and/or 1221 pH scalp blood measurements when fetal distress was suspected. In terms of sensitivity and specificity, lactate performed better than pH in the prediction of severe neonatal morbidity (Kruger et al. 1999). In addition, Kruger et al. (1998) demonstrated a good correlation between lactate obtained by FBS close to delivery and from cord arterial blood immediately after delivery. The potential usefulness of fetal scalp and cord blood lactate measurements to monitor the peripartum conditions of the fetus has been recently reviewed by Nordstrom (2004). Fetal scalp blood acid–base and lactate measurements, especially when combined with fetal heart rate monitoring, seem to be of value in predicting the condition of newborns at birth. However, this invasive approach can be performed only after rupture of membranes and is not widely used. Associated complications, although rarely observed, are soft tissue damage and scalp infections (Carbonne and Nguyen 2008).

28.5 Immediate Postpartum Asphyxial Markers

Common markers of asphyxia used immediately after birth include low Apgar scores, umbilical artery acidemia, and high blood lactate concentrations.

28.5.1 Apgar Score

In a classic paper appeared in 1953 (Apgar 1953), Dr. Virginia Apgar, an obstetric anesthesiologist at Columbia University in New York, proposed a scoring system based on five signs pertaining to the condition of the infant at birth, including heart rate, respiratory efforts, color, muscle tone, and reflex irritability. Each sign was given a score of 0, 1, or 2, somewhat quantifying the degree of neonatal depression by checking the presence of bradycardia, apnea or gasping, cyanosis or pallor, hypotonia, as well as depressed reactivity. In the following years, the Apgar score was rapidly adopted by most perinatal centres worldwide, being originally used as a rapid method of assessing the need for newborn resuscitation and to define newborn asphyxia. However, the Apgar score has a number of limitations, mainly due to a considerable interobserver variability and the different physiological implications of the five factors which make up the final score. Furthermore, causes other than asphyxia may result in low Apgar scores but without a high risk of brain injury, such as resuscitation procedures, infections, congenital malformations, and maternal anesthesia (American College of Obstetricians and Gynecologists et al. 2003). Moreover, Apgar scores assigned during resuscitation are not equivalent to scores assigned to spontaneously breathing infants. In fact, many of the components which contributes to the score calculation are altered by the resuscitation manoeuvres, To this end, the adoption of an expanded Apgar score report form, accounting for resuscitative interventions, has been recently encouraged by the ACOG and the AAP (American College of Obstetrics and Gynecology et al. 2015).

Finally, the significance of low Apgar scores calculated in extremely premature babies are likely to differ from those awarded to term or near-term infants. In fact, score elements such as color, tone, and reflex irritability may markedly affect the score value in preterm infants, and even healthy preterm newborns with no signs of depression at birth may be assigned a low score because of their immaturity (Hegyi et al. 1998).

Although the Apgar score has been used to predict specific neurological outcome in the term infant, several studies have demonstrated a weak correlation between low Apgar scores and severe birth asphyxia and subsequent adverse neurological development (Goodwin 1999; Ehrenstein 2009). Nevertheless, the Apgar score is still widely used and is useful for describing the condition of newly born infants and their response to resuscitation. While it is not appropriate to use it alone to establish the diagnosis of asphyxia, when combined with other conventional markers, such as arterial umbilical cord pH and base deficits, it has some predictive value for the development of hypoxic-ischemic encephalopathy (Kruger et al. 1999; Carter et al. 1998). Conversely, according to the ACOG, if the Apgar score at 5 min is greater than or equal to 7, it is unlikely that severe hypoxic-ischemic events have occurred in the peripartum period (American College of Obstetrics and Gynecology et al. 2014).

28.5.2 Acid–Base Measurements in Umbilical Cord Blood

Because Apgar scores are poor markers of severe birth asphyxia, some investigators have suggested the use of early acid–base status as a more objective indicator and the finding of a severe metabolic acidosis in the umbilical cord arterial blood at birth are probably the most objective assessment of intrapartum hypoxic ischemia (American College of Obstetricians and Gynecologists et al. 2003). Metabolic acidosis occurs because of a prolonged tissue oxygen deficit, reflecting hypoxia or impaired blood gas exchange of significant duration to allow the accumulation of fixed acids, mainly lactic acid. Most studies assess acid–base status on the arterial cord blood as soon as possible after birth (American College of Obstetricians and Gynecologists et al. 2003). The acid–base criteria commonly used to diagnose intrapartum asphyxia are a pH <7.00 and a base deficit (BD) value >16 mmol/L in umbilical arterial blood at birth or during the first postnatal hour (The Task Force on Cerebral Palsy and Neonatal Asphyxia of the Society of Obstetricians and Gynecologists of Canada 1996; American College of Obstetricians and Gynecologists et al. 2003; MacLennan 1999). In a cohort of term infants with an umbilical arterial Ph <7.00, nearly two-thirds did not require admission in NICU and had no apparent neurological sequelae (Perlman and Risser 1993). The need for cardiopulmonary resuscitation and adrenaline administration in the delivery room identified those neonates with pH <7.00 at greatest risk for a short-term adverse outcome (Perlman and Risser 1993). In a comprehensive review, Graham et al. (2008) searched for studies reporting the incidence of umbilical arterial pH <7.00. Combining data from seven different studies, they found the mean incidence of umbilical arterial pH <7.00 at term in 3.7/1000 infants. Of 386 infants, about 17% survived with neurological morbidity, 16% developed seizures, and 6% died during the neonatal period. The combined incidence of neonatal neurological morbidity and mortality for term infants with an umbilical arterial pH <7.00 at birth was 23%, with the remaining 77% being neurologically normal at the time of neonatal discharge (Graham et al. 2008). In another study, the incidence of encephalopathy in 109 term infants with umbilical artery pH <7.00 was 31%: seizures occurred in 9% of infants with pH between 6.90 and 6.99, and in 80% of those with pH between 6.61 and 6.70 (Goodwin et al. 1992). In a smaller study, Nagel et al. (1995) reviewed 21 infants born with a pH <7.00 over a 19-month period. Two out of 21 infants died in the neonatal period, but when the survivors were evaluated at 1–3 years, they showed normal developmental scores. Therefore, even though a pH value <7.00 at delivery seems to be a good marker of severity of acidosis, it appears less well related to short- and long-term neurological outcomes. Conventionally, in the newborn, the degree of metabolic acidosis is measured also by the umbilical artery base deficit. Studies have shown that a base deficit excess greater than 16 mmol/L is predictive of neonatal encephalopathy. Low et al. (1997) observed a significant increase in moderate and severe encephalopathy with an umbilical artery base deficit >12 mmol/L, suggesting that a base deficit excess measured in arterial cord blood is a good index of prolonged asphyxia, reflecting the severity and duration of intra-partum asphyxia. Shah et al. (2003) evaluated the rate of recovery of base deficit in 244 term infants with HIE due to intrapartum asphyxia. In their series, BD values normalized by the first 4 h in the 96% of infants. Notably, infants with severe adverse outcome at 12 months had a similar BD recovery rate compared to those with a relatively good outcome. Thus, although the rate of recovery of base deficit may reflect the ability of the infant to recuperate from the oxygen debt, it is not predictive of long-term outcome (Shah et al. 2003). More recently, the ACOG and AAP confirmed an arterial cord blood gas pH less than 7.0 and/or a base deficit ≥ 12 mmol/L as neonatal signs of perinatal asphyxia (American College of Obstetrics and Gynecology et al. 2014). In a cohort study, Knutzen et al. compared arterial umbilical cord elevated base deficit to decreased pH. They hypothesized the addition of base excess would have not further increased the ability of low pH to identify term infants at-risk of neurologic sequelae (Knutzen et al. 2015). In fact, in the setting of acidemia, they did not observe any additional value in identifying term infants with neurologic morbidity when the metabolic component was included.

28.5.3 Blood Lactate at Birth

Lactate is produced as a consequence of hypoxia and poor tissue perfusion (da Silva et al. 2000). When a critical reduction in oxygen and substrate delivery occurs, aerobic metabolism through Kreb's cycle cannot be sustained and tissues use anaerobic metabolism to meet their energy requirements. This in turn leads to an increase in the production and accumulation of blood lactate (Deshpande and Ward Platt 1997). A significant association has been found between blood lactate concentrations and neurological evolution. da Silva et al. (2000) measured blood lactate at 30 min of life in 115 term infants with suspected asphyxia. Significantly higher blood lactate concentrations were observed in neonates with moderate to severe HIE (da Silva et al. 2000). In a group of 61 full-term infants with suspected asphyxia, Shah et al. (2004a) observed that blood lactate concentrations were significantly higher and took longer to normalize in neonates with moderate to severe HIE, compared to those with mild or no HIE. Furthermore, blood lactate concentrations greater than 7.5 mmol/L at 1 h of age were associated with a higher risk of neurological and systemic complications, with a sensitivity of 94% and a specificity of 67%. Of note, sensitivity and negative predictive value of lactate in the first hour of life were higher than either pH or base deficit (Shah et al. 2004a) These findings have been recently confirmed in a retrospective cohort study by Tuuli and co-workers, who found that a high umbilical arterial lactate (>3.9 mmol/L) was more specific and sensitive for neonatal morbidity if compared with low pH or elevated base excess (Tuuli et al. 2014). Interestingly, a recent study by Murray et al. (2008) found that a normalization time of blood lactate concentrations greater than 10 h was associated with a high risk of encephalopathy (Murray et al. 2008).

However, despite ongoing efforts of researchers, the value of available surrogate markers to identify infants at high risk of morbidity still remains to be elucidated. Even though umbilical arterial measures will continue to provide useful clinical information, it must be emphasized that most term infants with low pH, high base excess, and elevated lactate level will not yield obvious neurological abnormalities at short- and long-term follow-up.

28.6 Asphyxial Markers in the Early Neonatal Period

Suspected intrapartum asphyxia causing brain injury can be confirmed in the first hours after birth by various clinical, biochemical, and other measures. Some authors have attempted to develop models able to predict early and reliably the development of HIE and/or subsequent neurological sequelae in asphyxiated newborns. In a large retrospective cohort study, Shah et al. (2006) tried to validate a prognostic model for term infants with moderate to severe postasphyxial HIE. They used relatively simple clinical and laboratory observations available within the first 4 h of life and identified three significant predictors: chest compressions >1 min, onset of spontaneous breathing >30 min and a base deficit value >16 mmol/L in any blood gas analysis within the first 4 h. In this cohort of term infants with HIE, a severe adverse outcome was found in 93% of subjects in whom all three predictors were present. However, infants with none of the three predictors also had a high possibility of adverse outcome (46%) (Shah et al. 2006).

Therefore, more accurate prediction models are still needed for the early identification of those infants most likely to benefit from interventions. At present, the occurrence of abnormal neurological features after signs of intrauterine asphyxia, namely postasphyxial hypoxic-ischemic encephalopathy, remains the best indicator of a newborn infant at risk of subsequent neurological impairment (Volpe 2008). Other early markers include multiorgan dysfunction, urinary lactate/creatinine ratio, and nucleated red blood cells counts. Finally, several techniques are available to evaluate the presence and degree of neurological injury, including early electrophysiological and neuroimaging studies, such as amplitude integrated electroencephalogram (aEEG), cranial ultrasound, magnetic resonance imaging (MRI), and computed tomography (CT) (see also ▶ Chap. 132, "The Timing of Neonatal Brain Damage".

28.6.1 Postasphyxial Neonatal Encephalopathy

Neonatal encephalopathy (NE) is characterized by abnormal consciousness, tone and reflexes, and seizure activity. The main cause of NE is intrapartum hypoxic ischemia, followed by trauma, infections, metabolic diseases, and developmental abnormalities. Prognosis is related to the severity of the HIE syndrome, the onset of seizures, and the duration of the neurological abnormalities. Although several classifications are available, the most popular remains that proposed by Sarnat and Sarnat in 1976, to indicate the severity of the hypoxic ischemic insult in infants of 36 or more weeks of gestation (Sarnat and Sarnat

1976). The sequential appearance and resolution of the various transient clinical signs in the first 2 weeks suggest the extent of neurologic impairment and define different clinical categories in the early assessment of infants with HIE (Aurora and Snyder 1997). The Sarnat and Sarnat staging of HIE ranges from mild (grade I) to severe (grade III). Grade I comprises a mild encephalopathy with the infant being hyper alert, irritable, and oversensitive to stimuli, but with a normal EEG. Virtually all these patients have a normal neurological outcome. In grade II, there is a moderate encephalopathy, with the infant displaying lethargy, hypotonia and proximal weakness, low resting heart rate, and small pupils. The EEG is abnormal and 70% of the infants will have seizures. About 20% of these patients may manifest abnormal neurological outcome. In grade III, there is a severe encephalopathy with the infant stuporous, flaccid, and no reflexes. EEG is abnormal with decreased background activity and/or voltage suppression. About half of these patients die, whereas the surviving 50% suffer major neurological injury, with epilepsy and mental retardation (Aurora and Snyder 1997; Sarnat and Sarnat 1976). Recently, a revised definition by the ACOG and AAP describes neonatal encephalopathy associated with a peripartum event as a disturbance of neurologic function, which is evident in the first days after birth in an infant born at or beyond 35 weeks of gestation. NE is characterized by a subnormal level of consciousness and depressed tone and reflexes, with or without seizures, and often with impaired respiration and feeding abilities, both considered of presumed central origin (American College of Obstetrics and Gynecology et al. 2014; McAdams and Juul 2016).

28.6.2 Multiorgan Failure Consistent with Neonatal Encephalopathy

Multiple organ failure is a marker of a perinatal hypoxic ischemic insult. It can include renal, hepatic or gastrointestinal injury, hematologic abnormalities, cardiac dysfunction, metabolic derangements, or a combination of these. In 1998, the American College of Obstetrician and Gynaecologists considered multiorgan failure (MOF) as a constant feature of the neonatal postasphyxial syndrome (American College of Obstetricians and Gynecologists Committee Opinion 1998). However, this assumption has been questioned by several authors and the incidence of MOF in asphyxiated infants is variable. Such variability may partly depend on differences of selection criteria, definitions of MOF, or timing of the diagnosis of MOF.

In term newborns with arterial cord pH <7.00, Goodwin et al. (1992) observed an incidence of MOF of 30%. In a retrospective cohort study, all infants with severe HIE had evidence of MOF. However, the presence of MOF, regardless of the combination of different organs involved, did not correlate with long-term neurological outcome (Shah et al. 2004b). Thus, MOF may reinforce the suspicion of intrapartum hypoxic ischemia in newborns with HIE, but it is not a useful criterion for the early identification of infants at risk for an adverse neurological outcome. Recently, the Task Force on neonatal encephalopathy has released an updated report on neonatal encephalopathy and neurologic outcome (American College of Obstetrics and Gynecology et al. 2014). Although the presence of organ dysfunction increases the risk of hypoxic–ischemic encephalopathy in the setting of neonatal encephalopathy, the severity of brain injury seen on neuroimaging does not always correlate with the degree of injury to other organ systems.

28.6.3 Urinary Lactate/Creatinine

Huang and coworkers investigated the role of urinary lactate/creatinine ratio to differentiate normal infants (58 subjects) from infants with asphyxia (40 subjects) (Huang et al. 1999). The measurements of urinary lactate and creatinine were obtained by proton nuclear magnetic resonance spectroscopy (1H NMR) within 6 h of birth and at 48 and 72 h. Sixteen of the infants with asphyxia went on to develop an encephalopathy. Within 6 h after birth, the mean lactate/creatinine ratio in infants who subsequently developed encephalopathy was 186 times as high as the ratio in normal controls, and 88 times as high as that in infants with asphyxia not progressing to HIE. A urinary lactate/creatinine ratio of 0.64 or higher showed 94% sensitivity and 100% specificity for predicting the development of HIE.

Thus, even if measurement technique by 1H NMR is expensive and not readily available, urinary lactate/creatinine ratio could be a potentially useful marker for the early identification and treatment of infants at high risk for HIE (Huang et al. 1999). More recent papers partially confirmed the good predictive value of elevated urinary lactate to creatinine ratios for the development of neonatal encephalopathy and subsequent neurodevelopmental abnormalities. In a multicenter trial, Oh et al. reported that urinary lactate to creatinine ratios were significantly associated with death or moderate/severe neurodevelopmental disability (William et al. 2008). However, there was a large variability and considerable overlap of the data between infants with a normal outcome and those with a poor outcome, thus limiting the predictive value of this marker (William et al. 2008).

28.6.4 Nucleated Red Blood Cells

The nucleated red blood cell (NRBC) count is a marker of fetal hypoxia in term and preterm infants. In 1996, Korst et al. (1996) reported a raised NRBC in cord blood from a group of neurologically impaired term infants compared with controls. In a prospective study, Buonocore et al. (1999) observed that the NRBC count in umbilical cord blood was significantly higher in infants showing abnormal neurodevelopment at age 3 when compared to normal controls. In a more recent study a relationship between HIE staging and nucleated RBC was found: the higher the HIE staging the higher was the mean NRBC/100 WBC. In the same study NRBC count as marker for fetal asphyxia had a positive predictive value of 98%, negative predictive value of 94% with an overall accuracy of 96% (Goel et al. 2013).

28.6.5 Amplitude Integrated EEG

Continuous monitoring by amplitude integrated EEG (aEEG) can be done soon after admission to a NICU. It is helpful in the early assessment of the asphyxiated term newborn (Shalak et al. 2003). Changes in background activity and seizure activity are relatively easy to identify, allowing for prompt intervention. aEEG may provide useful information about the functional integrity of the brain, presence or onset of subclinical seizure activity, and the effect of anticonvulsant drugs. It may also aid the selection of patients suitable for neuroprotective interventions and in the early prediction of neurodevelopmental outcome (Gluckman et al. 2005; de Vries and Hellstrom-Westas 2005; Eken et al. 1995). A systematic review reported that aEEG performed within 24 h of birth has a sensitivity of 93% and specificity of 91% (Van Laerhoven et al. 2013).

28.6.6 Early Neuroimaging Investigations

Advanced neuroimaging techniques such as cranial ultrasonography (CUS), MRI, and CT can be used in the early postpartum phase. CUS is a noninvasive and widely available technique. Up to 50% of newborns with HIE may initially show a normal CUS. Furthermore, it is not difficult to visualize parasagittal cerebral lesions, cortical, or brain stem injuries. CUS is of value in the identification of focal areas of necrosis (especially if hemorrhagic) in the thalamus and basal ganglia as well as for the detection of necrotic and cystic components of periventricular white matter injury (PVL) and, although not optimal, in the evaluation of focal ischaemic injuries. CUS may also be used to study the evolution of brain lesions (Volpe 2008).

MRI is considered the gold standard for the early evaluation of the infant with hypoxic-ischemic injury. Particularly with the development of diffusion weighted imaging (DWI), MRI is considered by some to be the method of choice to assess the newborn brain even in the first few days of life, providing valuable information on the location and extent of the neurological damage in moderately to severely asphyxiated infants (Barkovich et al. 2006; Rutherford et al. 2006). DWI MRI typically shows modifications due to ischemia earlier than conventional MRI, but it may underestimate the extent of tissue injury during the first 24 h following birth. Although DWI is complementary to conventional MRI, visual analysis of DWI does not seem to significantly improve the prognostic accuracy of MRI in infants with HIE during the first week after birth (Van Laerhoven et al. 2013).

Because of radiation exposure and its poorer imaging definition compared to MRI, CT is less frequently used for infants with hypoxic-ischaemic injury. CT is, however, still occasionally useful for the identification of focal ischemic or hemorrhagic brain injuries and when MRI is not readily available (Volpe 2008).

28.6.7 Magnetic Resonance Spectroscopy

Magnetic Resonance Spectroscopy (MRS) enables in vivo quantitative analysis of cerebral metabolites (such as N-acetyl aspartate, choline-containing compounds, creatine plus phosphocreatinine, lactate, myoinositol, alanine, glutamine, and glutamate), detecting patterns of impairment of cerebral energy metabolism in infants with HIE. Impairment of cerebral metabolism occurs following a delay of several hours after resuscitation in moderately or severely encephalopathic infants. Characteristic changes in spectral peaks are observed in infants with HIE according to cerebral metabolic disturbances due to asphyxia. Elevation of lactate, which indicates tissue ischaemia and hypoxia, as well as a fall in N-acetyl aspartate, which reflects neuronal injury, is typically found in HIE. Concentration or peak area ratios are commonly described, but MRS is reported to have a low specificity (approximately 58%) during the first week after birth (Cheong et al. 2012).

28.6.8 Biochemical Markers in Early Detection of Neonatal Asphyxia

Serum, urine, and cerebrospinal fluid have been used to measure biomarkers of brain injury. Some of the biomarkers which have been evaluated include urine lactate, urine S100, cord blood interleukin (IL)-6, serum non-protein-bound iron, serum CD14, NFKB activation, creatine kinase brain band (CK-BB), S100b, serum IL-8, serum ionized calcium, cerebrospinal fluid NSE, cerebrospinal fluid or serum IL-1b, and serum IL-6 (Gazzolo et al. 2009; Merchant and Azzopardi 2015; Savman et al. 1998). Among these markers, S100b and NSE are proved to be an early index of CNS damage and correlate to the extent of brain damage due to hypoxia/asphyxia (Massaro et al. 2013). Interestingly, the evolution of serum NSE and S100b during the first 72 h following birth has been reported in neonates treated for HIE with hypothermia: NSE and S100b levels at baseline and at 72 h strongly predicted death or neurological abnormalities, or MRI-detected brain injury, at 14 days of age. Thus, early measurement of NSE and S100b levels may be useful as biomarkers of brain injury following HIE, even though information on long-term outcomes is still lacking (Massaro et al. 2013).

Since multiple organ dysfunction is commonly seen in HIE and circulating proinflammatory cytokines are involved in the final common pathway of brain injury, inflammatory cytokines (interleukins 1b, 6, and 8 and tumor necrosis factor) levels in cord, serum, and cerebrospinal fluid have been used to predict adverse outcomes following HIE. However, at present no definitive and univoque data allow the use of these markers in a clinical setting to predict neurological outcome (Chalak et al. 2013).

Novel biomarkers, possibly with better specificity for predicting brain injury, have recently been evaluated, along with the effects of therapeutic hypothermia. For instance, glial fibrillary acidic protein (GFAP), which is a cytoskeletal intermediary filament protein found in astrocytes, as well as ubiquitin carboxyl-terminal hydrolase L1 (UCHL1), which is a neuron-specific cytoplasmic enzyme present in dendrites and neuronal cytoplasm, are involved in the pathogenesis of traumatic brain injury. These biomarkers have been shown to reflect the severity of neuronal injury (Fraser et al. 2011). Furthermore, in recent studies cord GFAP and UCHL1 levels seemed to correlate with the severity of HIE and were significantly higher in infants with adverse outcomes than in those with favorable outcomes (Massaro et al. 2013; Chalak et al. 2013). Moreover, GFAP was able to correctly identify infants with abnormal outcomes at 20 months (Massaro et al. 2013; Chalak et al. 2013).

28.7 Conclusions

Early detection of perinatal asphyxia still constitutes a challenging target in neonatology. In addition, birth asphyxia can be associated either with an uneventful course or with significant mortality and long-term morbidity. Therefore, reliable diagnostic and prognostic indicators are essential for a prompt recognition and treatment of newborns at risk for subsequent negative outcome. In the last decades, many biochemical markers of asphyxia have been identified, both in cord blood and in blood samples after birth, including arterial pH, base excess, and lactate. However, such indicators have shown a limited value in predicting long-term neurological outcome. Other promising biochemical markers, e.g., urinary lactate/creatinine ratio, nucleated red blood cells, S100 B protein, NSE, GFAP, and UCHL1 still need further evaluation before their inclusion in the routine assessment of asphyxia.

Some recent electrophysiological and neuroimaging investigations, such as amplitude integrated EEG, diffusion weighted MRI, or magnetic resonance spectroscopy, may also provide early valuable information on brain damage and outcome of asphyxiated babies. However, these techniques are not always available and could be difficult to perform in critically ill neonates. Further research is still required to overcome the limitations due to the assessment of perinatal asphyxia by single parameters. The combination of clinical and biochemical indicators should aim to validate prediction models capable to identify neonates at risk of dismal outcome due to asphyxia, allowing an adequate and timely diagnosis, treatment, and counselling.

References

American College of Obstetricians and Gynecologists Committee Opinion (1998) Inappropriate uses of the terms fetal distress and birth asphyxia. Int J Gynecol Obstet 61:309–310

American College of Obstetricians and Gynecologists, Task Force on Neonatal Encephalopathy and Cerebral Palsy, American Academy of Pediatrics (2003) Neonatal encephalopathy and cerebral palsy: defining the pathogenesis and pathophysiology. American College of Obstetricians and Gynecologists, Washington, DC

American College of Obstetrics and Gynecology, Task Force on Neonatal Encephalopathy, American Academy of Pediatrics (2014) Neonatal encephalopathy and neurologic outcome, 2nd edn. American College of Obstetricians and Gynecologists, Washington, DC

American College of Obstetrics and Gynecology, Committee on Obstetric practice, American Academy of Pediatrics (2015) The Apgar score. Committee opinion N. 644. Obstet Gynecol 126:e52–e55

Apgar V (1953) A proposal for a new method of evaluation of the newborn infant. Curr Res Anesth Analg 32:260–267

Aurora S, Snyder EY (1997) Perinatal asphyxia. In: Cloherty JP, Eichenwald EC, Stark AR (eds) Manual of neonatal care, 4th edn. Lippincott Williams & Wilkins, Philadephia, pp 536–555

Barkovich AJ, Miller SP, Bartha A et al (2006) MR imaging, MR spectroscopy, and diffusion tensor imaging of sequential studies in neonates with encephalopathy. AJNR Am J Neuroradiol 27:533–547

Belfort MA, Saade GR, Thom E et al (2015) A randomized trial of intrapartum fetal ECG ST-segment analysis. N Engl J Med 373:632–641

Bretscher J, Saling E (1967) pH values in the human fetus during labor. Am J Obstet Gynecol 97:906–911

Buonocore G, Perrone S, Gioia D et al (1999) Nucleated red blood cell count at birth as an index of perinatal brain damage. Am J Obstet Gynecol 181:1500–1505

Cahill AG, Roehl KA, Odibo AO et al (2012) Association and prediction of neonatal acidemia. Am J Obstet Gynecol 207:206.e1–206.e8

Carbonne B, Nguyen A (2008) Fetal scalp blood sampling for pH and lactate measurement during labour. J Gynecol Obstet Biol Reprod 375:S65–S71

Carter BS, McNabb F, Merenstein GB (1998) Prospective validation of a scoring system for predicting neonatal morbidity after acute perinatal asphyxia. J Pediatr 132:619–623

Chalak LF, Sanchez PJ, Adams-Huet B et al (2013) Biomarkers for severity of neonatal hypoxic–ischaemic encephalopathy and outcomes in newborns receiving hypothermia therapy. J Pediatr 164:468–474

Cheong JL, Coleman L, Hunt RW et al (2012) Prognostic utility of magnetic resonance imaging in neonatal hypoxic–ischaemic encephalopathy: substudy of a randomized trial. Arch Pediatr Adolesc Med 166: 634–640

da Silva SD, Hennebert N, Denis R, Wayenberg JL (2000) Clinical value of single postnatal lactate measurement after intrapartum asphyxia. Acta Paediatr 89:320–323

de Vries LS, Hellstrom-Westas L (2005) Role of cerebral function monitoring in the newborn. Arch Dis Child Fetal Neonatal Ed 90:F201–F207

Deshpande SA, Ward Platt MP (1997) Association between blood lactate and acid base status and mortality in ventilated babies. Arch Dis Child Fetal Neonatal Ed 76:F15–F20

Ehrenstein V (2009) Association of Apgar scores with death and neurologic disability. Clin Epidemiol 1: 45–53

Eken P, Toet MC, Groenendaal F et al (1995) Predictive value of early neuroimaging, pulsed Doppler and neurophysiology in full term infants with hypoxic-ischaemic encephalopathy. Arch Dis Child Fetal Neonatal Ed 73: F75–F80

Fraser DD, Close TE, Rose KL et al (2011) Severe traumatic brain injury in children elevates glial fibrillary acidic protein in cerebrospinal fluid and serum. Pediatr Crit Care Med 12:319–324

Gazzolo D, Frigiola A, Bashir M et al (2009) Diagnostic accuracy of S100B urinary testing at birth in full-term asphyxiated newborns to predict neonatal death. PLoS One 4(2):e4298

Glantz JC, Woods JR (2004) Significance of amniotic fluid Meconium. In: Creasy RK, Resnik R, Iams JD (eds) Maternal-fetal medicine: principles and practice, 5th edn. WB Saunders, Philadelphia

Gluckman PD, Wyatt JS, Azzopardi D et al (2005) Selective head cooling with mild systemic hypothermia after neonatal encephalopathy: multicentre randomised trial. Lancet 365:663–670

Goel M, Dwivedi R, Gohiya P, Hegde D (2013) Nucleated red blood cell in cord blood as a marker of perinatal asphyxia. J Clin Neonatol 2:179–182

Goodwin TM (1999) Clinical implications of perinatal depression. Obstet Gynecol Clin North Am 26: 711–723

Goodwin TM, Belai I, Hernandez P et al (1992) Asphyxial complications in the term newborn with severe umbilical acidemia. Am J Obstet Gynecol 167:1506–1512

Graham EM, Ruis KA, Hartman AL et al (2008) A systematic review of the role of intrapartum hypoxia-ischaemia in the causation of neonatal encephalopathy. Am J Obstet Gynecol 199:587–595

Graham EM, Adami RR, McKenney SL et al (2014) Diagnostic accuracy of fetal heart rate monitoring in the identification of neonatal encephalopathy. Obstet Gynecol 124:507–513

Hegyi T, Carbone T, Anwar M et al (1998) The Apgar score and its components in the preterm infant. Pediatrics 101:77–81

Huang CC, Wang ST, Chang YC et al (1999) Measurement of the urinary lactate:creatinine ratio for the early identification of newborn infants at risk for hypoxic-ischaemic encephalopathy. N Engl J Med 341:328–335

Knutzen L, Svirko E, Impey L (2015) The significance of base deficit in acidemic term neonates. Am J Obstet Gynecol 213:373.e1–373.e7

Korst LM, Phelan JP, Ahn MO et al (1996) Nucleated red blood cells: an update on the marker for fetal asphyxia. Am J Obstet Gynecol 176:843–846

Kruger K, Kublickas M, Westgren M (1998) Lactate in scalp and cord blood from fetuses with ominous fetal heart rate patterns. Obstet Gynecol 92:918–922

Kruger K, Hallberg B, Blennow M et al (1999) Predictive value of fetal scalp blood lactate concentration and pH as marker for neurologic disability. Am J Obstet Gynecol 181:1072–1078

Larma JD, Silva AM, Holcroft CJ et al (2007) Intrapartum electronic fetal heart rate monitoring and the identification of metabolic acidosis and hypoxic- ischaemic encephalopathy. Am J Obstet Gynecol 197:301. e1–301.e8

Lawn JE, Cousens S, Zupan J (2005) 4 million neonatal deaths: when? where? Why? Lancet 365:891–900

Levene ML, Kornberg J, Williams TH (1985) The incidence and severity of post-asphyxial encephalopathy in full-term infants. Early Hum Dev 11:21–26

Low JA (1997) Intrapartum fetal asphyxia: definition, diagnosis, and classification. Am J Obstet Gynecol 176:957–959

Low JA, Lindsay BG, Derrick EJ (1997) Threshold of metabolic acidosis associated with newborn complications. Am J Obstet Gynecol 177:1391–1394

MacLennan A (1999) A template for defining a causal relation between acute intrapartum events and cerebral palsy: international consensus statement. BMJ 319: 1054–1059

Massaro AN, Jeromin A, Kadom N et al (2013) Serum biomarkers of MRI brain injury in neonatal hypoxic ischaemic encephalopathy treated with whole-body hypothermia: a pilot study. Pediatr Crit Care Med 14: 310–317

McAdams RM, Juul SE (2016) Neonatal encephalopathy: update on therapeutic hypothermia and other novel therapeutics. Clin Perinatol 43:485–500

Merchant N, Azzopardi D (2015) Early predictors of outcome in infants treated with hypothermia for hypoxic–ischaemic encephalopathy. Dev Med Child Neurol 57(Suppl 3):8–16

Murray DM, Boylan GB, Fitzgerald AP (2008) Persistent lactic acidosis in neonatal hypoxic-ischaemic encephalopathy correlates with EEG grade and electrographic seizure burden. Arch Dis Child Fetal Neonatal Ed 93: F183–F186

Nagel HT, Vandenbussche FP, Oepkes D et al (1995) Follow-up of children born with an umbilical arterial blood pH < 7. Am J Obstet Gynecol 173:1758–1764

Nelson KB, Grether JK (1998) Potentially asphyxiating conditions and spastic cerebral palsy in infants of normal birth weight. Am J Obstet Gynecol 179:507–513

Nordstrom L (2004) Fetal scalp and cord blood lactate. Best Pract Res Clin Obstet Gynaecol 18:467–476

Perlman JM, Risser R (1993) Severe fetal acidemia: neonatal neurologic features and short term outcome. Pediatr Neurol 9:277–282

Perlman JM, Risser R (1996) Can asphyxiated infants at risk for neonatal seizures be rapidly identified by current high-risk markers. Pediatrics 97:456–462

Phelan JP, Martin GI, Korst LM (2005) Birth asphyxia and cerebral palsy. Clin Perinatol 32:61–76

Rutherford M, Srinivasan L, Dyet L et al (2006) Magnetic resonance imaging in perinatal brain injury: clinical presentation, lesions and outcome. Pediatr Radiol 36: 582–592

Sarnat HB, Sarnat MS (1976) Neonatal encephalopathy following fetal distress: a clinical and electroencephalographic study. Arch Neurol 33:696–705

Savman K, Blennow M, Gustafson K et al (1998) Cytokine response in cerebrospinal fluid after birth asphyxia. Pediatr Res 43:746–751

Shah PS, Raju NV, Beyene J, Perlman M (2003) Recovery of metabolic acidosis in term infants with postasphyxial hypoxic-ischaemic encephalopathy. Acta Paediatr 92: 941–947

Shah S, Tracy M, Smyth J (2004a) Postnatal lactate as an early predictor of short-term outcome after intrapartum asphyxia. J Perinatol 24:16–20

Shah P, Riphagen S, Beyene J, Perlman M (2004b) Multiorgan dysfunction in infants with post-asphyxial hypoxic-ischaemic encephalopathy. Arch Dis Child Fetal Neonatal Ed 89:F152–F155

Shah PS, Beyene J, To T et al (2006) Postasphyxial hypoxic-ischaemic encephalopathy in neonates: outcome prediction rule within 4 hours of birth. Arch Pediatr Adolesc Med 160:729–736

Shalak LF, Laptook AR, Velaphi SC, Perlman JM (2003) Amplitude-integrated electroencephalography coupled with an early neurologic examination enhances prediction of term infants at risk for persistent encephalopathy. Pediatrics 111:351–357

Shankaran S (2009) Neonatal encephalopathy: treatment with hypothermia. J Neurotrauma 26:437–443

The Task Force on Cerebral Palsy and Neonatal Asphyxia of the Society of Obstetricians and Gynecologists of Canada (1996) Policy statement (part I). J Soc Obstet Gynecol Can 18:1267–1279

Tuuli MG, Stout MJ, Shanks A et al (2014) Umbilical cord arterial lactate compared with pH for predicting neonatal morbidity at term. Obstet Gynecol 124:756–761

Van Laerhoven H, de Haan TR, Offringa M et al (2013) Prognostic tests in term neonates with hypoxic–ischaemic encephalopathy: a systematic review. Pediatrics 131:88–98

Volpe JJ (2008) Hypoxic-ischaemic encephalopathy: clinical aspects. In: Volpe JJ (ed) Neurology of the newborn, 5th edn. WB Saunders, Philadelphia

William OHW, Perritt R, Shankaran S et al (2008) Association between urinary lactate to creatinine ratio and neurodevelopmental outcome in term infants with hypoxic-ischemic encephalopathy. J Pediatr 153:375–378

Williams KP, Galerneau F (2003) Intrapartum fetal heart rate patterns in the prediction of neonatal acidemia. Am J Obstet Gynecol 188:820–823

World Health Organization (2005) The World health report 2005. Make every mother and child count. http://www.who.int/entity/whr/2005/whr2005_en.pdf

Resuscitation of the Newborn

29

Ola D. Saugstad

Contents

Abstract

In 2015, the International Liaison Committee on Resuscitation estimated that 85% of babies born at term will initiate spontaneous respirations within 10–30 s of birth. In the USA, 5–10% of all newborn infants require basic life support in the delivery room or nursery. There are similar figures for Western Europe.

Approximately 1% of newborns require more extensive resuscitation procedures. Recent estimates indicate that worldwide 814,000 die and an equal number develops sequels after birth asphyxia. Thus, it is

O. D. Saugstad (✉)
Department of Pediatric Research, Rikshospitalet, Oslo University Hospital, University of Oslo, Oslo, Norway
e-mail: odsaugstad@rr-research.no

G. Buonocore et al. (eds.), *Neonatology*,
https://doi.org/10.1007/978-3-319-29489-6_179

important to anticipate which infants are at risk, and the antepartum and intrapartum history often can be a help in predicting which infants will need resuscitation.

29.1 Salient Points

- Always be prepared that a newborn infant might require resuscitation immediately after birth.
- 3–5% of all newborn infants receive positive pressure ventilation at birth. However, <1 per 1000 needs chest compressions and/or adrenaline. Therefore ventilation constitutes the backbone of basic newborn resuscitation.
- The "golden minute" is crucial and starts when the whole body is out.
- A satisfactory response in heart rate is the best assessment of the success of resuscitation. A 20 bpm increase the first 30 s of adequate ventilation is a satisfactory response.
- Term and near-term infants in need of positive pressure ventilation are started with air. Immature infants probably need at least 30% oxygen initially. An oxygen blender is needed in all delivery units.
- Thermal care – to avoid hypothermia – is of great importance.

29.2 Introduction

Each year 6–10 million of the approximately 130 million newborn infants born in the world need some kind of resuscitation at birth. Recently the International Liaison Committee on Resuscitation (ILCOR) estimated that 85% of babies born at term will initiate spontaneous respirations within 10–30 s of birth (Perlman et al. 2015). In the USA, 5–10% of all newborn infants require basic life support in the delivery room, or nursery, constituting at least 200,000 newborn infants in the USA alone. In Western Europe, there are similar figures. Approximately 1% of newborns require more extensive resuscitation procedures (Perlman et al. 2010; Kattwinkel et al. 2010; Richmond and Wyllie 2010). Recent estimates indicate that worldwide 814,000 die and an equal number develop sequels after birth asphyxia (Black et al. 2010).

However, data from, for instance, California indicate that birth asphyxia is decreasing from 14.8 to 1.3 per 1000 in the period of 1991–2000, and data from England show that there is a reduced need of ventilation at birth (Wu et al. 2004; Little et al. 2007). In spite of that, there is no doubt that both in industrialized and low-income countries, a large number of newborn infants are in need of resuscitation at birth. Therefore and because a vast number of deliveries throughout the world still occur at home without authorized health personnel present, it is also important to develop simple resuscitation routines.

29.3 Preparation for Resuscitation and Selection of Risk Cases

Approximately 95% of deliveries are uneventful, and the adaptation to extrauterine life occurs smoothly. Only in some infants should more vigorous resuscitation procedures be carried out. As mentioned above, as many as 5% or more need basic resuscitation including ventilation using a bag and mask. However, only a few newborn infants need advanced resuscitation. In 1:100 to 1:700, endotracheal intubation is needed, 1:1000 needs chest compression, 6:10,000 need epinephrine (adrenaline), and as few as 1:12,000 of near-term and term infants need volume therapy (Wyckoff et al. 2005; Barber and Wyckoff 2006). For preterm infants, these numbers are higher (Fig. 1).

It is important to anticipate which infants are at risk, and the antepartum and intrapartum history often can be a help in predicting which infants will need resuscitation. Fetal movement counting, non-stress testing, fetal biophysical profile, electronic fetal monitoring, and scalp pH measurement all contribute to an identification of infants at risk for low Apgar scores and need of resuscitation. Electronic fetal heart monitoring combined with scalp pH determinations improves the specificity; however, sensitivity is low. In spite of these measures, the need for resuscitation can often not be foreseen, and 20–50% of the infants requiring resuscitation have no identifiable risk factors. This

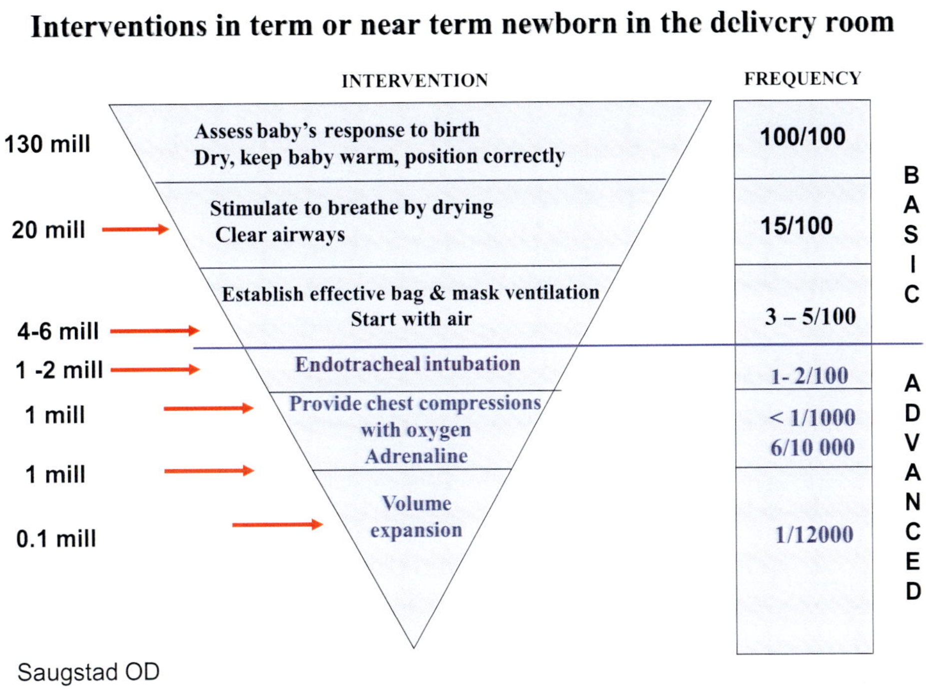

Fig. 1 Need of different interventions related to new born stabilization/resuscitation. Note the distinction between basic and advanced resuscitation (*blue horizontal line*)

implies that at every delivery, the health provider should be prepared to perform resuscitation. Equipment and facilities should be ready. Further, every health personnel attending deliveries needs to be trained in resuscitation skills. If a preterm (<37 weeks gestation) is expected, special preparation is required.

29.4 Indication for Resuscitation

The decision to resuscitate is based on clinical judgment. By observing breathing movements, tone, color, and not least heart rate, it is decided whether the infant is in need of resuscitation or not. Every time a child is delivered, the following three questions should according to the ILCOR and American Heart Association's guidelines (Perlman et al. 2010) be answered: (1) Is the baby born at term? (2) Is the baby breathing or crying? (3) Is there a good muscle tone? If the answer is "no" to any of these questions, resuscitation should be considered. In former guidelines (Kattwinkel et al. 1999; International Liaison Committee on Resuscitation 2005), a fourth and a fifth question were included: (4) Is the color pink? (5) Is amniotic fluid clear of meconium? Recent data, however, indicate that a newborn baby not necessarily needs to be pink the first few minutes of life; in fact there are strong indications this may be harmful. This question therefore was removed from the 2005/2006 ILCOR guidelines (Perlman et al. 2015; International Liaison Committee on Resuscitation 2005). In the 2010 ILCOR guidelines, no firm recommendations for suctioning of babies with meconium-stained amniotic fluid were given, and consequently this fifth question was removed (Perlman et al. 2010).

29.5 Guidelines for Resuscitation of the Newly Born

There are several sets of international guidelines for newborn resuscitation. The World Health Organization (WHO) published their revised guidelines for basic newborn resuscitation in 2012 (World Health Organization, Department of Reproductive Health and Research 1998). These are applicable for most children around the world. The ILCOR and American Heart Association's guidelines are widely used internationally; these were first published in 1992 (Emergency Cardiac Care Committee and Subcommittees of the American Heart Association 1992) and revised in 1999 (Kattwinkel et al. 1999), 2005 (International Liaison Committee on Resuscitation 2005), 2010 (Perlman et al. 2010), and 2015 (Perlman et al. 2015). American Heart Association (AHA) and American Academy of Pediatrics (AAP) and European Resuscitation Council (ERC) in close collaboration with ILCOR produced their own guidelines (Kattwinkel et al. 2010; Richmond and Wyllie 2010). A number of countries have their own national guidelines modifying the ILCOR guidelines.

29.6 Physiological and Biochemical Changes

The physiological changes during asphyxia are well described in animal experiments.

Traditionally the asphyxial process has been divided into primary and secondary apnea. During primary apnea, heart rate is still present even as high as 100 beats per minute (bpm), and there is cyanosis in mucus membranes and the skin. In secondary apnea, the baby is pale, and the heart rate is low or not present. In some guidelines, different approaches are recommended for a primary and a secondary apneic situation. However, it is probably not wise to spend time to figure out in which of these stages the infant is. Preterm infants have a more rapid drop in heart rate than term infants, and the distinction between primary and secondary apnea in the smallest infants probably is not very useful.

A metabolic and respiratory acidosis exists in newborns with birth asphyxia. Both animal and clinical studies have shown that base deficit is eliminated at a constant rate of 6–7 mmol/L/h (Saugstad et al. 2005). This elimination seems to be constant independently of the severity of birth asphyxia. Therefore, if the acid base status at birth is not known, this figure can be used to extrapolate back to the situation at birth. For instance, if base deficit is 10 mmol/L at 1 h of age, it probably was approximately 16–17 mmol/L at birth. Such calculations can be useful for assessing prognosis and for court cases.

29.7 Initial Evaluation and Stabilization

ABCD for resuscitation is the same whatever size of the patient.

A: Airways should be cleared and the infant positioned correctly.

B: Breathing should be stimulated or performed.

C: Circulation should be assessed by heart rate and skin color.

D: Drugs are rarely needed in the newborn.

29.7.1 Response to Birth

Resuscitation is a team work: optimally, two trained persons should actually perform the resuscitation, and one should assist. Each team member should identify themselves, and it should be clear who the team leader is. Each order should be stated clearly and repeated by the recipient.

As soon as the infant is delivered, that is when the whole body is out (Saugstad 2015), a clock is started, and, during the transport to the resuscitation table, the personnel should make a preliminary opinion regarding the seriousness of the situation. First and foremost, the respiratory efforts are assessed, and the heart rate is recorded. Heart rate should, after the short initial stabilization, be monitored more precisely. Bradycardia combined with no respiratory efforts or gasping is a warning of immediate intervention. Central cyanosis indicates insufficient oxygenation. Pallor may be a sign of reduced cardiac output, anemia, hypovolemia, hypothermia, or acidosis. Apgar scoring is not performed before 1 min of life, and in addition it takes some time. Apgar score therefore in itself should never be used as a criterion for resuscitation.

The golden minute, the first 60 s of life, is of importance. During the first 30 s, the infant should be positioned correctly, dried, and stimulated to breathe as needed. Infants <28 weeks of gestation should be place in polythene bags without drying.

During the last 30 s, heart rate and respiration rate should be assessed, and a pulse oximeter, if available, is connected to the right wrist. If needed positive pressure ventilation should be initiated.

29.7.2 Initial Stabilization

Start out by assessing the baby's response to birth and keep the baby warm and position it correctly; supine with the head close to the examiner, and keep airways clear.

Most infants require only to be delivered into a warm room where they can be dried immediately. The umbilical cord should be cut with sterile equipment, and the breathing pattern should be observed. The mother herself is most often the best caregiver and provider of warmth, food, and protection from infections.

The cord is usually cut after 60 s. At that time approximately 70% of the placental blood has been transfused to the baby. In an emergency cord milking might be an alternative, even in extremely low birth weight infants (Saugstad 2015).

Heat loss should be prevented, and this is one important reason why deliveries should be performed in a warm room. For preterm infants, a temperature in the room of 23–25 °C is recommended. The newborn should be quickly dried with towels, giving particular attention to the drying of the head, and swept into preferably pre-warmed towels or other linens. It is recommended that the infant be placed supine under a radiant heater on a table designed for resuscitation with the head toward the person performing resuscitation. Infants <28 weeks are put into polythene plastic bags before dried. This secures a more stable temperature until the child is put into an incubator. Hypothermia (<36 °C) as well as hyperthermia (>38 °C) should be avoided.

29.7.2.1 A: Airways

Stimulate the infant to breathe by drying. Airways are secured both by suctioning and by positioning the infant correctly in the supine position. There is, however, no justification for the practice of routine suctioning in the mouth and pharynx or gastric emptying not even after C-section, because such suctioning might even be harmful. A child who starts to breathe spontaneously within 10–15 s most probably does not need to be suctioned. In addition, it seems that the esophagus functions as a seal and a closed esophagus therefore helps in blowing air into the lungs instead of the stomach during bag and mask ventilation. Opening the esophagus with a suctioning catheter will result in more air into the stomach in case of bag and mask ventilation. However, occasionally the mouth, nose, and pharynx should be suctioned to clear airways. Remember that the mouth should be suctioned before the nose to prevent aspiration if the newborn should gasp when his or her nose is suctioned. Suctioning deep in the pharynx or the larynx, especially the first 5 min of life, may elicit bradycardia and bronchospasm. Airways are best opened with the head in the "sniffing position"; overextension should be avoided. Tactile stimulation as gentle rubbing of the back may be useful, but do not shake the baby and do not waste time by tactile stimulating an apneic child.

29.7.2.2 B: Breathing

According to a study from the UK in 2000, bag and mask ventilation was performed in 2.6% of all deliveries. This was a decrease from 3.9% in 1988 (Wyckoff et al. 2005). These figures are lower than given above from the USA and indicate that the need for bag and mask ventilation may vary throughout the world and is less than 5% in Western Europe. Still the number who would need bag and mask ventilation is high.

Clinical judgment for when to initiate ventilation should be based on heart rate, breathing efficiency, color, and tone. However, the formal indications are very simple:

Start ventilation

If the newborn is apneic or there is insufficient breathing movements and/or heart rate < 100 bpm after administration of the initial steps as drying and stimulation.

If the newborn is breathing with heart rate > 100 bpm but is persistently cyanotic.

Apneic infants with heart rate >100 bpm probably represent those with primary apnea, and they often require tactile stimulation and a few inflations with a bag and mask only. Apnea and heart rate <100 bpm may represent secondary apnea, and ventilation should be initiated. In most of these cases, the heart rate improves, and spontaneous ventilation quickly develops. Ventilation, when needed, should start within the golden minute, preferably not later than 30 s after birth.

The recommended rate of ventilation according to the AHA/AAP is 40–60 breaths per minute. An initial inflation pressure of 20 cm H_2O is often sufficient; however, even greater pressures as 30 cm H_2O or even more may occasionally be needed for term babies in order to open the lungs. For preterm infants, peak inspiratory pressure of, for instance, 20 cm H_2O is often adequate, however, depending on the size of the baby. The best way to monitor successful ventilation is to follow the heart rate which should be rapidly increasing. In addition, observe improvement in color and muscle tone and movements. Recently it has been shown that it is difficult to make an assessment of color (O'Donnell et al. 2007), and in the most recent guidelines, there is therefore less emphasis on color assessment. Observation of the chest wall movements is difficult. Recent data indicate that tidal volumes may be too high when there is a clear rise and fall of the chest during the respiratory cycle. It has also been shown that assessment of tidal volume by observing chest rise is extremely difficult (Poulton et al. 2011; Schmölzer et al. 2010a).

Heart Rate

Traditionally a cutoff for heart rate < or >100 bpm has been used. This has been based on the assumption that a heart rate <100 bpm in a newborn indicates bradycardia which in most cases is caused by asphyxia. It was demonstrated two decades ago that it takes 1–2 min to establish an efficient gas exchange in vaginally delivered babies and a few more minutes are needed after C-section (Palme-Kilander et al. 1993; Palme-Kilander and Tunell 1993). Because there is a relation between gas exchange and heart rate, it may be normal not to achieve a heart rate of 100 bpm or more even at an older age than 1 min. Supporting this are the recently published values for heart rate the first 10 min of life in normal non-asphyxiated newborns with no medical intervention (Dawson et al. 2010a). At 1 min of age, term infants have in mean a heart rate of 99 bpm with interquartile range of 66–132 bpm. For preterm infants, the values are 96 (72–122) bpm. Recent studies indicate that the heart rate is underestimated by auscultation (Kamlin et al. 2006).

New ECG devices pick up heart rate quickly, within seconds of birth. It seems that the initial drop in pulse rate found by pulse oximetry the first seconds of life to some extent represents an artifact.

In term or near-term infants, the pulse very quickly picks up during a successful resuscitation procedure, for instance, increasing from typically 90 beats per minute (bpm) at 1 min of age to 110 bpm at 90 s of life. In babies with the lowest Apgar score, heart rate is initially lower but typically increases with 20 bpm during the first 30 s of resuscitation (Saugstad et al. 1998, 2005). In infants <30 weeks of gestation, the heart rate increase is slower. It takes in median 73 s (interquartile range 24–165 seconds) to reach a heart rate of 100 bpm and 243 (191–351) s to reach 120 bpm. The heart rate in such small babies is not stable until it reaches 120 bpm (Dawson et al. 2010a). An adequate response to adequate ventilation therefore should for most term and near-term infants be approximately 20 bpm increase the first 30 s of bag and mask ventilation, however slower in preterm infants. After adequate ventilation has been established for 30 s, the heart rate should be recorded for not longer than 10 s. If the heart rate is at least 100 bpm and spontaneous respirations are established, positive pressure ventilation may be discontinued. If the heart rate is >60 bpm and improving, ventilation should continue. If the heart rate is less than 60 bpm and not improving, assisted ventilation is continued, and external heart massage is started (Perlman et al. 2015; Kamlin et al. 2006; Saugstad et al. 1998; Yam et al. 2011).

Auscultation of the heart with a stethoscope is still the gold standard for heart rate assessment, although ILCOR suggests the use of ECG. Pulse oximetry is reliable; however, the response time is slow (Saugstad 2016).

Ventilation

A self-inflating bag, a flow-inflating bag, or a T-piece resuscitator can be used. Recently a T-piece device was compared with self-inflating bags. There was no difference between the T-piece resuscitator and a self-inflating bag in achieving an HR of ≥100 bpm at 2 min in newborns ≥26 weeks gestational age resuscitated at birth. However, the use of the T-piece decreased the intubation rate and the maximum pressures applied. However, air leaks, use of drugs/chest compressions, mortality, and days on mechanical ventilation did not differ significantly between groups (Szyld et al. 2014). The use of a bag and mask requires experience, and it is possible to practice on mannequins. By inserting a resuscitation monitor which is a hot-wire anemometer placed between a ventilation device and the face mask or endotracheal tube, the operator can minimize leaks by adjusting the face mask position (Finer et al. 2009; Schmölzer et al. 2010b). In an Australian study, an average of 60% leaks were found around the face mask; however after the operators adjusted the mask position, the leak was reduced to 10% (Schmölzer et al. 2010b).

It is not easy to deliver an adequate tidal volume by bag and mask ventilation. However, it seems that starting ventilation in many instances stimulates the baby to breathe because the inflation pressure induces the baby to make inspiratory efforts (Head's paradoxical reflex) securing an adequate tidal exchange (Milner et al. 1984). The optimal tidal volume for newborn resuscitation is not known. However, a range between 4 and 8 mL/kg is often recommended. Excessive tidal volume may lead to volutrauma (Björklund et al. 1997), and a too low tidal volume leads to atelectasis and inadequate gas exchange. Both conditions may trigger cytokine release and inflammatory changes in the lung (Jobe and Ikegami 1998; Jobe et al. 2002). Recommended ventilator rate is 40–60 per minute.

PEEP or CPAP?

In order to oxygenate, the lungs must be ventilated to develop a functional residual capacity. Infants who do not breathe will need respiratory support. Positive end-expiratory pressure (PEEP) has been tested out in animal models (Jobe et al. 2002; Probyn et al. 2004). There is, however, not much evidence regarding the use of PEEP or not in the delivery room. However, one randomized controlled trial in preterm infants showed that more infants were subsequently intubated and ventilated in a group without continuous positive airway pressure (CPAP)/PEEP compared with a group ventilated with a 10 s prolonged inflation followed immediately by CPAP/PEEP (Polglase et al. 2008). It is becoming more and more common to apply PEEP during ventilation in the delivery room. CPAP in many centers is applied immediately for low birth or extremely low birth weight infants (ELBWI). More and more centers are using a T-piece device when ventilating the newborn in the delivery room. This delivers a PEEP that can be adjusted to the wanted level. Figure 2 shows recording when a mannequin is ventilated by the author with a self-inflating bag (Fig. 2a) and a T-piece device (Fig. 2b). By using a T-piece device, peak inspiratory pressure and volume are similar from breath to breath.

Studies have shown that a T-piece device delivers more exact peak inspiratory pressures than a self-inflating or a flow-inflating bag, in addition to delivering an exact PEEP.

In premature infants, especially in ELBWI, ventilation may be difficult because of airway obstruction. In such cases, airways and the mask must be repositioned (Finer et al. 2009). Figure 3 illustrates leak during bag and mask ventilation of a 27 weeks gestation newborn (Schmölzer et al. 2010a).

Sustained inflation (inspiration time >5 s) is not recommended by ILCOR. Some guidelines recommend a few opening ventilations with prolonged inspiration time; however this is not evidence based.

Endotracheal Intubation

Endotracheal intubation is necessary when bag-mask ventilation is not efficient to normalize the heart rate and establish spontaneous respiration. If chest compressions do not quickly improve, heart rate or prolonged assisted ventilation is anticipated; endotracheal intubation should also be carried out. A newborn infant without any heart beat or respiratory movement should also promptly be

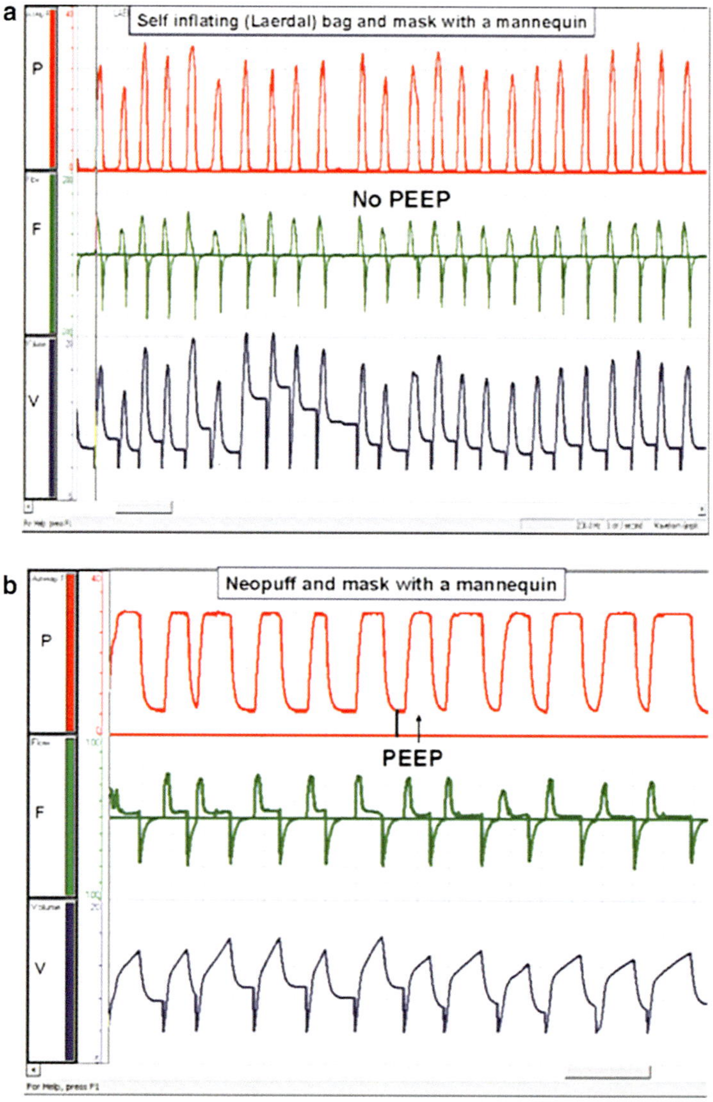

Fig. 2 (**a**) Ventilation of a mannequin with a self-inflating bag. Notice the variable peak inspiratory pressure (*P*), flow (*F*), volume (*V*), and the lack of positive end-expiratory pressure (*PEEP*). (**b**) Ventilating a mannequin with a T-piece device. Notice the identical and exact peak inspiratory pressures (*P*), the presence of PEEP, and the uniform flow and volume delivered

intubated, as bag and mask ventilation probably is not very efficient. Some infants in secondary apnea also need intubation and the most immature infants who often do not have sufficient muscle strength for their respiratory drive. The ILCOR guidelines recommend that exhaled CO_2 is monitored for confirmation of tracheal tube placement by, for instance, a colorimetric detector. Their use and limitations have been described in the literature and is reliable in most cases (Leone et al. 2006a; Schmölzer et al. 2011; Garey et al. 2008). By using a resuscitation monitor, a correct placement of the endotracheal tube can in most cases be established after the first breath by observing the gas flow in and out of the trachea (Wood et al. 2008; Schmörzel et al. 2010). By observing the leak, it is also possible to make an assessment whether the size of the tube is correct or not (see Fig. 4).

Endotracheal intubation is rarely needed in term infants. In one study from the USA, it was carried out in approximately 1 per 1000 deliveries (Wu et al. 2004). A study from the UK has shown a decrease in the need of intubation between 1993 and 1997 from 2.4% but still as high as 1.2%, of all live born (Little et al. 2007). This indicates a wide variation in intubation practice from approximately 1 per 100 to less than 1 per 1000 babies.

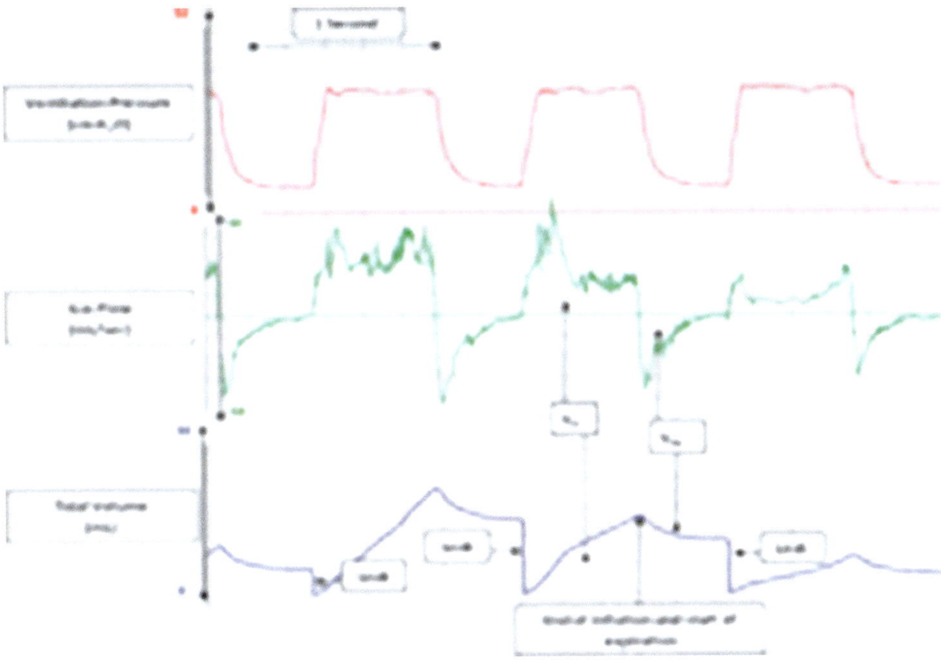

Fig. 3 Airway leak in a 27-week infant ventilated with face mask. The area underneath the inflation flow curve is greater than that under the expiratory flow curves. Leak is displayed as a straight line in the tidal volume curve. Notice the variable leaks (From Schmölzer et al. 2010a, with permission)

In another UK study, the need of endotracheal intubation for all weight groups decreased in the period 1988–2000 from 0.51% to 0.07% (Little et al. 2007). However, for infants with birth weight <1500 g, this decrease was not very evident, and their intubation need was 50-fold increased compared with babies with birth weight 3000–3500 g. If Apgar score at 5 min was 0–3, intubation rate was increased 234-fold. Even an Apgar score at 5 min of 4–5 increased the intubation rate 100-fold. Emergency C-section and breech delivery increased the need of intubation two- to threefold (Allwood et al. 2003). This dramatic reduction in intubation rates indicates both a reduction in birth asphyxia and an increase in C-section and also a more restrictive attitude regarding need of newborn intubation.

Oxygen Supplementation

High concentration of supplemental oxygen (80–100%) was used until 2010 recommended by most textbooks and guidelines dealing with newborn resuscitation. There was, however, no scientific basis for such recommendations. New studies have shown that even the most depressed term or near-term newborn infants are adequately resuscitated with room air. Several meta-analyses (Rabi et al. 2007; Saugstad et al. 2008), now including ten studies enrolled more than 2000 newly born infants in need of resuscitation (Saugstad et al. 2008), have shown that early recovery is faster if resuscitation is carried out with ambient air instead of 100% O_2; time to first breath was registered 30 s earlier, and heart rate at 90 s and 5 min Apgar score were higher (Saugstad et al. 1998). More importantly is that neonatal mortality is significantly reduced with 30–40% in room air resuscitated babies (Rabi et al. 2007; Saugstad et al. 2008). In a meta-analysis from European countries, relative risk for neonatal death was in fact reduced 69% from 3.2% to 1.1% in those resuscitated with 21% compared with 100% oxygen (Saugstad et al. 2008). For this reason, 100% oxygen should be avoided as a routine for newborn resuscitation. The 2010 ILCOR guidelines state it is for term babies

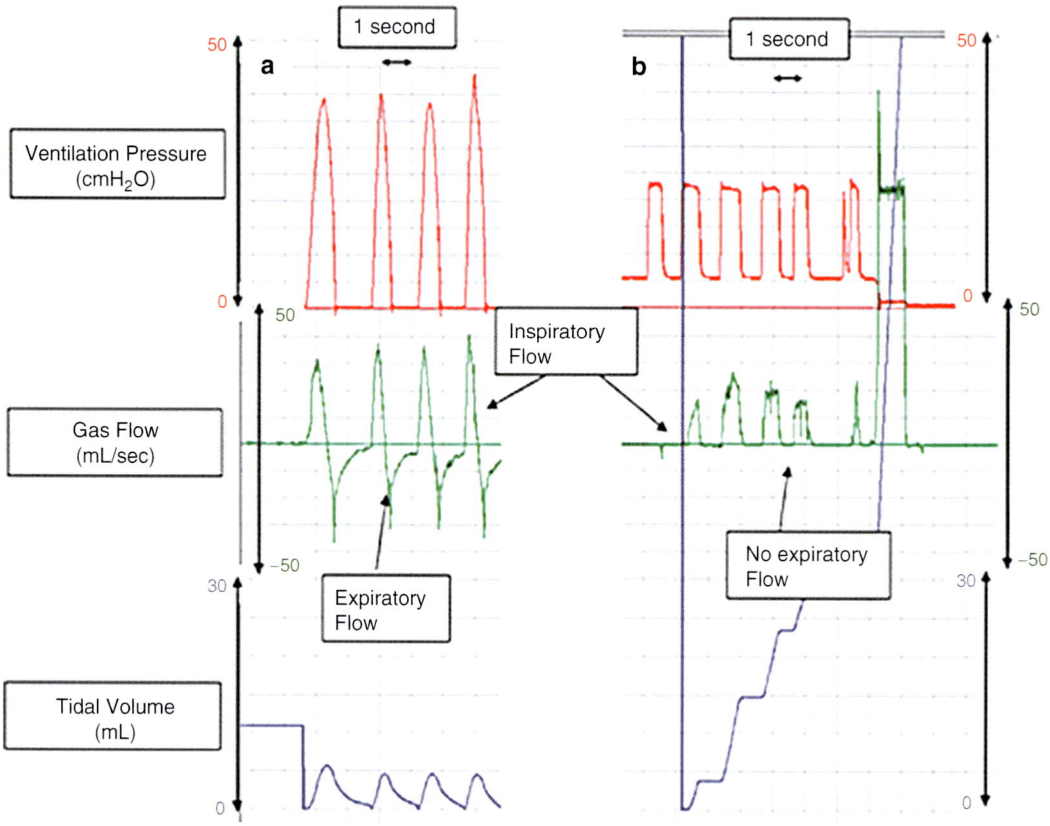

Fig. 4 (**a**) Correct endotracheal tube placement in a 26-week infant. Both inflation and expiratory flow curves return to baseline, indicating a correct placement of the endotracheal tube. (**b**) Esophageal tube placement in a piglet. The inspiratory flow curve returns to baseline indicating gas flow toward the endotracheal tube. In contrast there is no expiratory flow curve indicating endotracheal tube placement in esophagus (From (Schmölzer et al. 2010a), with permission)

"best to start resuscitation with air." For babies <32 weeks, a blender is often needed, and for babies with gestational age between 32 and 37 weeks, the optimal initial FiO_2 is not known (Perlman et al. 2010). For newborn infants <28 weeks gestation, it is recommended to start with 30% or more for stabilization/resuscitation.

Recent animal data also show that the pulmonary resistance by and large is reduced as efficiently with 21% as with 100% oxygen (Lakshminrusimha et al. 2007). In addition, it seems that the exposure of hyperoxia increases the reactivity of the pulmonary vessels subsequently increasing the risk of pulmonary hypertension (Lakshminrusimha et al. 2006).

As mentioned above, extremely low birth weight infants may need some oxygen to get started. However, some smaller studies have so far shown that 30% oxygen is at least as efficient as 90% oxygen. ELBWIs who need resuscitation therefore can be initiated with FiO_2 of 0.30 and adjust according to response in SpO_2 (Escrig et al. 2008; Wang et al. 2008; Vento et al. 2009a). However, the optimal FiO_2 for these smaller newborns is not known.

If room air resuscitation is not successful within 90 s, we still supplement with oxygen. In such case, it probably is optimal to monitor the arterial oxygen saturation by pulse oximetry. The arterial oxygen saturation at 1 min of life in non-asphyxic term or near-term babies is typically 60–70% and may be as low as 40% the first 3–4 min of life. Within 5–7 min, approximately 50% of these babies have reached a SaO2 of 90%.

After C-section, the saturation is in general 2 min behind the values found in babies born after vaginal delivery (Saugstad 2006). In high altitude, the SaO_2 is lower than at sea level; still it is recommended to start resuscitation with air also in such areas of the world.

The oxygen supply in all delivery units should have a blender, so that the oxygen concentration can be adjusted to the requirement. If justified to give supplemental oxygen, it is recommended to start with not more than 30–40% oxygen and adjust according to the clinical response, preferably following oxygen saturation measured by pulse oximetry. It is in case recommended that oxygen saturation follow the 10th to 25th percentile of recently published nomograms for normal SpO_2 values the first minutes of life of non-asphyxiated newborn babies (Dawson et al. 2010b). The aim is to reach a SpO_2 of 90% after 5–10 min in term and near-term infants and 85% in premature infants less than 32 weeks.

29.7.2.3 C: Circulation

Chest compressions are rarely needed and not included for basic newborn resuscitation. If bradycardia persists with a heart rate of less than 60 per minute and no signs of improvement after adequate ventilation, chest compressions should be started. This is needed in 0.5 to 1 per 1000 births (Wyckoff et al. 2005).

Chest compression should always be carried out simultaneously with adequate ventilation (Wyckoff and Berg 2008). Chest compressions and ventilatory rate of 3:1 should be synchronized giving 90 compressions and 30 breaths per minute. The two-thumb technique is recommended (Christman et al. 2011). An adequately performed resuscitation with chest compressions obviously requires at least two trained persons. Heart rate should be assessed after 30 s of well-coordinated chest compressions and ventilation. When the spontaneous pulse rate has reached 60 per minute, chest compressions should be discontinued, and positive pressure ventilation is continued at a rate of 40–60 breaths per minute. There are not much data, if any, supporting why a ratio of 3:1 between compressions and ventilation is chosen for newborns.

If the cardiac arrest is not of asphyxial genesis, a ratio of 15:2 may be considered (Perlman et al. 2010).

Animal studies show no advantage regarding the use of 100% oxygen for chest compressions. ILCOR still suggests it is prudent to try increasing supplementary oxygen concentrations during this procedure. If supplementary oxygen is used, it should be weaned as soon as the heart rate has recovered (Wyckoff and Wyllie 2006).

29.7.2.4 D: Drugs

When oxygenation is established through an adequate ventilation of the asphyxiated infant, it is extremely rare that drugs are needed. Epinephrine (adrenaline) was in one study indicated in 1:1200 deliveries (Barber and Wyckoff 2006) and is indicated in asystole or in sustained bradycardia (Hr <60 bpm) in spite of adequate ventilation and oxygenation and at least 30 s of coordinated chest compressions and ventilations. One study showed that even trained resuscitators are not able to give epinephrine earlier than 4–5 min of age (Barber and Wyckoff 2006). Epinephrine (1:10,000 solution) is given as a bolus as rapid as possible preferably intravenously in a dose of 0.01–0.03 mg/kg (0.1–0.3 mL/kg) which may be repeated every 3–5 min if needed. If the endotracheal route is chosen (Solevåg et al. 2010), a higher dose can be used (0.05–0.01 mg/kg). Bradycardia due to insufficient ventilation technique should be corrected by adequate ventilation before administration of epinephrine. The optimal epinephrine dose for newborn resuscitation has not been studied systematically.

Volume Therapy

Hypovolemia is rare, and volume infusion was in one study administered in 1:3000 deliveries; however hypovolemia was found in only 25% of these. Thus hypovolemia is an extremely rare event occurring in only 1:12,000 near-term or term infants (Wyckoff et al. 2005). Hypovolemic shock should be suspected if there is an obvious hemorrhage, there is pallor, there is delayed capillary refill, there are weak pulses, there is persistently low heart rate, or the circulatory status does not improve in response to the treatment steps described above. Shock may be treated with repeated transfusions of volume expanders, usually 10 mL/kg. As volume expanders, normal saline or Ringer's lactate is recommended. The volume expander may be given over 5–10 min and repeated. Albumin or other plasma substitutes are not so much recommended anymore. Blood volume expanders during acute resuscitation are only indicated when there are unmistakable signs of shock with evidence of acute blood loss, including feto-maternal hemorrhage. If there has been blood loss, O-negative blood cross-matched with the mother's blood is given. Avoid rapid boluses of volume expanders or hyperosmolar solutions to premature newborn infants. In one experimental study in hypovolemic and asphyxiated newborn piglets, the use of volume therapy seemed to be counterproductive (Wyckoff et al. 2007). Volume therapy therefore should be given on strict indications only.

Sodium bicarbonate, THAM, or naloxone has no routine place in newborn resuscitation (Perlman et al. 2010; Wyckoff and Perlman 2006).

29.8 Meconium Aspiration

If the amniotic fluid is meconium stained, there is no evidence that suctioning the oropharynx before the thorax is delivered has any beneficial effects. There are today no indications that an infant with thick meconium-stained amniotic fluid benefits from routine intubation and suctioning.

The previous practice of tracheal suctioning does not seem to have reduced the incidence of meconium aspiration syndrome or mortality (Gupta et al. 1996). It is therefore not anymore recommended that suctioning of the nose, mouth, and posterior pharynx be carried out thoroughly before delivery of the shoulder and thorax. According to previous guidelines, the trachea should be suctioned in "non-vigorous" child. If the child is vigorous, the mouth and nose should be suctioned only and resuscitation proceeded as required. "Vigorous" is defined as a newborn having strong respiratory efforts, good muscle tone, and a heart rate greater than 100 bpm. In the 2010 ILCOR guidelines, it is written that "the available evidence does not support or refute the routine endotracheal suctioning of depressed infants born through meconium-stained amniotic fluid" (Perlman et al. 2010). Thus, there has been a shift in recent years from a very active to a less active approach in these children. In 2015, this has been taken a step further when ILCOR is stating it is insufficient published human evidence to suggest routine tracheal intubation for suctioning of meconium in non-vigorous infants born through meconium-stained amniotic fluid.

29.9 Preterm Infants

There are no or very few studies on optimal resuscitation of premature infants. This means that even the extremely low gestational age newborn infants are often resuscitated according to the guidelines and principles established for term and near-term infants. Recent studies have shown that cardiorespiratory resuscitation of these in the delivery room is not futile and a more active approach seems therefore to be established (Finer et al. 1999) and this has led to a more active approach (Leone et al. 2005, 2006b; Finer and Leone 2009; Brugada 2008; Vento et al. 2009b). It is also clear that preterm infants need intervention more often than near-term or term newborn infants. In one study from the USA, 5% of babies with birth weight between 500 and 1500 g needed chest compressions and 4% received epinephrine (Finer et al. 1999).

Babies with gestational age < 28 weeks should be put into polyethylene wraps or a plastic bag up to their neck, before drying, in order to maintain the temperature (Perlman et al. 2015). They often need to be intubated given surfactant, and in some centers, they are immediately extubated, the so-called INSURE (INtubation SURfactant Extubation) approach (Victorin et al. 1990). Ventilation should be carried out using a PEEP of 5–6 cm H_2O. Today it is recommended to start these babies directly on CPAP (Morley and Davis 2008). These infants should be handled as gently as possible. Avoid rapid boluses of fluid and quick changes in body positions.

Preliminary data indicate that the extremely low birth weight infant in need of resuscitation often would need a brief exposure of oxygen, for instance, start out with 30% O_2 in order to get an adequate heart rate response (Escrig et al. 2008; Wang et al. 2008; Vento et al. 2009a). More data are needed before firmer recommendation for these tiny infants are given.

In newborn infants <32 weeks delivery room temperature should be between 23 °C and 25 °C; the babies should be covered by warm blankets and, if <28 weeks, put in plastic wrapping before drying and a cap. ILCOR recommends the use of thermal mattresses to reduce hypothermia (<36 °C); however thermal mattresses seem to increase hyperthermia (>38 °C).

29.10 Withholding and Withdrawing Resuscitation

In some cases, resuscitation should be withheld or withdrawn (Skupski et al. 2010). The ILCOR recommendations state that resuscitation could be withheld for neonates at the margins of viability or those with conditions which predict a high risk of mortality or morbidity. Many centers do not resuscitate newborn infants with gestational age of less than 23 weeks. In earlier recommendations, resuscitation was not recommended if there was anencephaly, bilateral renal agenesis, spinal muscular atrophy type I (Werdnig-Hoffmann disease) with neonatal onset, trisomy 13, or trisomy 18. However, according to the newer guidelines (Perlman et al. 2010) and I agree in that, strict indications should not be given for which newborns who should not be resuscitated. This author resuscitates and tries to stabilize infants with a gestational age of 23 weeks or more. Recent data, for instance, from the Express study from Sweden support this practice (Serenius et al. 2013).

Often, neither the exact diagnosis nor the gestational age is known at birth. A liberal policy of resuscitation is recommended whenever doubt about the care of the individual infant exists. This allows the doctor to collect more information about the clinical status and prognosis of the child. This also allows one to inform the parents so that they can become prepared and participate in the discussion and decisions about subsequent therapy. An Apgar score of 0 at 10 min is a strong predictor of mortality and morbidity. The ILCOR committee suggests that in babies with an Apgar score of 0 after 10 min of resuscitation, if the heart rate remains undetectable, it may be reasonable to stop resuscitation. However, it is underlined that the decision whether or not to redirect care should be individualized (Perlman et al. 2015).

In babies with Apgar score of 1–3 at 20 min of age and gestational age > 34 weeks, ILCOR suggests that it may be reasonable to stop assisted ventilation in babies with no spontaneous breathing despite the presence of heart rate or Apgar score of 1–3 at 20 min or more.

29.11 Post-Resuscitation Care

After a successful resuscitation, heat loss should be prevented. The child should be labeled and frequently checked with regard to breathing efforts, respiratory rate, color, heart rate, and signs of birth injury or malformations. If the resuscitation was brief and the situation was not too dramatic, the newborn could be monitored in the nursery provided an adequate respiration is established. The child could be placed so that skin-to-skin contact with the mother is obtained. However, this depends on the local conditions and the possibilities for adequate observation by a trained observer.

Even if the infant is not in need of artificial ventilation following resuscitation, the child is often brought to the intensive care unit for further close follow-up which includes monitoring of the heart rate, ventilation, determination of arterial pH and blood gases, treatment of any hypotension with volume expanders or pressors, appropriate fluid therapy, and treatment of any seizures. Any hypoglycemia or electrolyte disturbances should be corrected. Breast-feeding should be encouraged, if possible, as soon as 1 h after birth. If the resuscitation was unsuccessful and the child died, the parents need a close follow-up.

Every baby who has been resuscitated, even briefly, is at risk and should be followed up carefully both at short and long term. Blood glucose should be kept within normal ranges (McGowan and Perlman 2006).

29.11.1 Hypothermia Therapy

Moderate hypothermia as a protective treatment to term infants with hypoxic ischemic encephalopathy is recommended. Hypothermia should in case be induced in a controlled way following written protocols (Azzopardi et al. 2009). In the delivery room, it is important to avoid hyperthermia because this may augment any brain injury in severe asphyxia (Perlman 2006).

29.12 Documentation

It is useful if one attending person observes and immediately writes down the procedures performed. A thorough documentation in the medical record of all observations and actions and names of the participants is required before the resuscitation is complete. Each institution should keep records documenting the condition and procedures carried out at birth. Every institution that provides deliveries must develop its own standards for newborn resuscitation, and a plan of action should exist. The personnel should gain and maintain skills in newborn resuscitation by training using manikins, and an evaluation of the training is necessary.

29.13 Conclusions

Newborn resuscitation is not yet fully evidence based. However, recent years a rapid development has occurred, and a more evidence-based practice has been established. Still there are numerous unanswered questions.

The optimal PEEP has not been determined. Today a low oxygen approach should be chosen for newborn resuscitation starting with air in near-term and term babies. However, there are still uncertainties regarding the use of oxygen supplementation for premature infants and which oxygen saturation one should aim at in term babies not responding adequately to the initial resuscitation. How the optimal use of supplemental oxygen during chest compressions is not known. The optimal adrenaline concentration and the effect of volume therapy are uncertain. Further, the optimal procedure for chest compressions is not defined. None of the guidelines discuss the importance of pCO_2 and a moderate hypercapnia in order to restore cerebral blood flow. This should be an area of research for the coming years.

In spite of that, there is general agreement that the most important is to start ventilation as soon as this is indicated. In most cases a few blows of air is sufficient to restore the heart rate and help the baby start breathing on its own. By avoiding non-evidence-based detrimental procedures such as hyperoxygenation of the child, the results will be much improved. The new resuscitation program named Helping Babies breathe is rolled out in many parts of the world. This program was made possible when air substituted 100% oxygen for resuscitation of term and near-term newborns. "Give a breath – save a life" was the name of a large Indian campaign for newborn resuscitation launched in the 1990s. This is what it is all about, to give breaths and to save lives.

References

Allwood AC, Madar RJ, Baumer JH et al (2003) Changes in resuscitation practice at birth. Arch Dis Child Fetal Neonatal Ed 88:F375–F379

Azzopardi DV, Strohm B, Edwards AD, TOBY Study Group et al (2009) Moderate hypothermia to treat perinatal asphyxial encephalopathy. N Engl J Med 361:1349–1358. [Erratum in: N Engl J Med 2010;362:1056]

Barber CA, Wyckoff MH (2006) Use and efficacy of endotracheal versus intravenous epinephrine during neonatal cardiopulmonary resuscitation in the delivery room. Pediatrics 118:1028–1034

Björklund LJ, Ingimarsson J, Curstedt T et al (1997) Manual ventilation with a few large breaths at birth compromises the therapeutic effect of subsequent surfactant replacement in immature lambs. Pediatr Res 42:348–355

Black RE, Cousens S, Johnson HL, Child Health Epidemiology Reference Group of WHO and UNICEF et al (2010) Global, regional, and national causes of child mortality in 2008: a systematic analysis. Lancet 375:1969–1987

Brugada M (2008) Using intensive care technology in the delivery room: a new concept for the resuscitation of extremely preterm neonates. Pediatrics 122:1113–1116

Christman C, Hemway RJ, Wyckoff MH, Perlman JM (2011) The two-thumb is superior to the two-finger method for administering chest compressions in a manikin model of neonatal resuscitation. Arch Dis Child Fetal Neonatal Ed 96:F99–F101

Dawson JA, Kamlin CO, Wong C et al (2010a) Changes in heart rate in the first minutes after birth. Arch Dis Child Fetal Neonatal Ed 95:F177–F181

Dawson JA, Kamlin CO, Vento M et al (2010b) Defining the reference range for oxygen saturation for infants after birth. Pediatrics 125:e1340–e1347

Emergency Cardiac Care Committee and Subcommittees of the American Heart Association (1992) Guidelines for cardiopulmonary resuscitation and emergency cardiac care, IV: pediatric basic life support. J Am Med Assoc 268:2276–2281

Escrig R, Arruza L, Izquierdo I et al (2008) Achievement of targeted saturation values in extremely low gestational age neonates resuscitated with low or high oxygen concentrations: a prospective, randomized trial. Pediatrics 121:875–881

Finer N, Leone T (2009) Oxygen saturation monitoring for the preterm infant: the evidence basis for current practice. Pediatr Res 65:375–380

Finer NN, Horbar DH, Carpenter JH, the Vermont Oxford Network (1999) Cardiopulmonary resuscitation in the very low birth weight infant: the Vermont Oxford Experience. Pediatrics 104:428–434

Finer NN, Rich W, Wang C, Leone T (2009) Airway obstruction during mask ventilation of very low birth weight infants during neonatal resuscitation. Pediatrics 123:865–869

Garey DM, Ward R, Rich W et al (2008) Tidal volume threshold for colorimetric carbon dioxide detectors available for use in neonates. Pediatrics 121:e1524–e1527

Gupta V, Bhatia BD, Mishra OP (1996) Meconium stained amniotic fluid: antenatal, intrapartum and neonatal attributes. Indian Pediatr 33:293–297

International Liaison Committee on Resuscitation (2005) International consensus on cardiopulmonary resuscitation and emergency cardiovascular care science with treatment recommendations. Part 7: neonatal resuscitation. Resuscitation 67:293–303

Jobe AH, Ikegami M (1998) Mechanisms initiating lung injury in the preterm. Early Hum Dev 53:81–94

Jobe AH, Kramer BW, Moss TJ et al (2002) Decreased indicators of lung injury with continuous positive expiratory pressure in preterm lambs. Pediatr Res 52:387–392

Kamlin CO, O'Donnell CO, Everest NJ et al (2006) Accuracy of clinical assessment of infant heart rate in the delivery room. Resuscitation 71:319–321

Kattwinkel J, Niermeyer S, Nadkarni V et al (1999) Resuscitation of the newly born infant: an advisory statement from the pediatric working Group of the International Liaison Committee on resuscitation. Resuscitation 40:71–88

Kattwinkel J, Perlman JM, Aziz K et al (2010) Part 15: neonatal resuscitation: 2010 American Heart Association guidelines for cardiopulmonary resuscitation and emergency cardiovascular care. Circulation 122(18 Suppl 3):S909–S919

Lakshminrusimha S, Russell JA, Steinhorn RH et al (2006) Pulmonary arterial contractility in neonatal lambs increases with 100% oxygen resuscitation. Pediatr Res 59:137–141

Lakshminrusimha S, Russell JA, Steinhorn RH et al (2007) Pulmonary hemodynamics in neonatal lambs resuscitated with 21%, 50%, and 100% oxygen. Pediatr Res 62:313–318

Leone TA, Rich W, Finer NN (2005) Neonatal intubation: success of pediatric trainees. J Pediatr 146: 638–641

Leone TA, Lange A, Rich W, Finer NN (2006a) Disposable colorimetric carbon dioxide detector use as an indicator of a patent airway during noninvasive mask ventilation. Pediatrics 118:e202–e204

Leone TA, Rich W, Finer NN (2006b) A survey of delivery room resuscitation practices in the United States. Pediatrics 117:e164–e175

Little M, Järvelin M-R, Neasham DE et al (2007) Factors associated with fall in neonatal intubation rates in the United Kingdom-prospective study. Br J Obstet Gynaecol 114:156–164

McGowan JE, Perlman JM (2006) Glucose management during and after intensive delivery room resuscitation. Clin Perinatol 33:183–196

Milner AD, Vyas H, Hopkin IE (1984) Efficacy of facemask resuscitation at birth. Br Med J (Clin Res Ed) 289:1563–1565

Morley CJ, Davis PG (2008) Advances in neonatal resuscitation: supporting transition. Arch Dis Child Fetal Neonatal Ed 93:F334–F336

O'Donnell CP, Kamlin CO, Davis PG et al (2007) Clinical assessment of infant colour at delivery. Arch Dis Child Fetal Neonatal Ed 92:F465–F467

Palme-Kilander C, Tunell R (1993) Pulmonary gas exchange during facemask ventilation immediately after birth. Arch Dis Child 68:11–16

Palme-Kilander C, Tunell R, Chiwei Y (1993) Pulmonary gas exchange immediately after birth in spontaneously breathing infants. Arch Dis Child 68:6–10

Perlman JM (2006) Hyperthermia in the delivery: potential impact on neonatal mortality and morbidity. Clin Perinatol 33:55–63

Perlman JM, Wyllie J, Kattwinkel J, Neonatal Resuscitation Chapter Collaborators et al (2010) Part 11: neonatal resuscitation: 2010 International consensus on cardiopulmonary resuscitation and emergency cardiovascular care science with treatment recommendations. Circulation 122(16 Suppl 2):S516–S538

Perlman JM, Wyllie J, Kattwinkel J, Wyckoff MH et al (2015) Neonatal resuscitation chapter collaborators. Part 7: neonatal resuscitation: 2015 international consensus on cardiopulmonary resuscitation and emergency cardiovascular care science with treatment recommendations. Circulation 132(16 Suppl 1): S204–S241

Polglase GR, Hillman NH, Pillow JJ et al (2008) Positive end-expiratory pressure and tidal volume during initial ventilation of preterm lambs. Pediatr Res 64:517–522

Poulton DA, Schmölzer GM, Morley CJ, Davis PG (2011) Assessment of chest rise during mask ventilation of preterm infants in the delivery room. Resuscitation 82:175–179

Probyn ME, Hooper SB, Dargaville PA et al (2004) Positive end expiratory pressure during resuscitation of premature lambs rapidly improves blood gases without adversely affecting arterial pressure. Pediatr Res 56:198–204

Rabi Y, Rabi D, Yee W (2007) Room air resuscitation of the depressed newborn: a systematic review and meta-analysis. Resuscitation 72:353–363

Richmond S, Wyllie J (2010) European resuscitation council guidelines for resuscitation 2010 section 7. Resuscitation of babies at birth. Resuscitation 81:1389–1399

Saugstad OD (2006) Oxygen saturations immediately after birth. J Pediatr 148:569–570

Saugstad OD (2015) Delivery room management of term and preterm newly born infants. Neonatology 107(4):365–371

Saugstad OD, Soll RF (2016) Assessing heart rate at birth: auscultation is still the gold standard. Neonatology 110:238–240

Saugstad OD, Rootwelt T, Aalen O (1998) Resuscitation of asphyxiated newborn infants with room air or oxygen: an international controlled trial: the Resair 2 study. Pediatrics 102:e1

Saugstad OD, Ramji S, Rootwelt T, Vento M (2005) Response to resuscitation of the newborn: early prognostic variables. Acta Paediatr 94:890–895

Saugstad OD, Ramji S, Soll RF, Vento M (2008) Resuscitation of newborn infants with 21% or 100% oxygen: an updated systematic review and meta-analysis. Neonatology 94:176–182

Schmölzer GM, Kamlin OC, O'Donnell CP et al (2010a) Assessment of tidal volume and gas leak during mask ventilation of preterm infants in the delivery room. Arch Dis Child Fetal Neonatal Ed 95:F393–F397

Schmölzer GM, Dawson JA, Kamlin CO et al (2010b) Airway obstruction and gas leak during mask ventilation of preterm infants in the delivery room. Arch Dis Child Fetal Neonatal Ed 96(4):F254–F257

Schmölzer GM, Poulton DA, Dawson JA et al (2011) Assessment of flow waves and colorimetric CO(2) detector for endotracheal tube placement during neonatal resuscitation. Resuscitation 82:307–312

Schmörzel GM, Kamlin CO, Dawson JA et al (2010) Respiratory monitoring of neonatal resuscitation. Arch Dis Child Fetal Neonatal Ed 95:F295–F303

Serenius F, Källén K, Blennow M et al (2013) Neurodevelopmental outcome in extremely preterm infants at 2.5 years after active perinatal care in Sweden. JAMA 309:1810–1820

Skupski DW, Chervenak FA, McCullough LB et al (2010) Ethical dimensions of periviability. J Perinat Med 38:579–583

Solevåg AL, Dannevig I, Nakstad B, Saugstad OD (2010) Resuscitation of severely asphyctic newborn pigs with cardiac arrest by using 21% or 100% oxygen. Neonatology 98:64–72

Szyld E, Aguilar A, Musante GA, Vain N, Prudent L, Fabres J, Carlo WA, Delivery Room Ventilation Devices Trial Group (2014) Comparison of devices for newborn ventilation in the delivery room. J Pediatr 165:234–239

te Pas AB, Walther FJ (2007) A randomized, controlled trial of delivery-room respiratory management in very preterm infants. Pediatrics 120:322–329

Vento M, Moro M, Escrig R et al (2009a) Preterm resuscitation with low oxygen causes less oxidative stress, inflammation, and chronic lung disease. Pediatrics 124:e439–e449

Vento M, Cheung PY, Aguar M (2009b) The first golden minutes of the extremely-low-gestational-age neonate: a gentle approach. Neonatology 95:286–298

Victorin LH, Deverajan LV, Curstedt T, Robertson B (1990) Surfactant replacement in spontaneously breathing babies with hyaline membrane disease—a pilot study. Biol Neonate 58:121–126

Wang CL, Anderson C, Leone TA et al (2008) Resuscitation of preterm neonates by using room air or 100% oxygen. Pediatrics 121:1083–1089

Wood FE, Morley CJ, Dawson JA, Davis PG (2008) A respiratory function monitor improves mask ventilation. Arch Dis Child Fetal Neonatal Ed 93:F380–F381

World Health Organization, Department of Reproductive Health and Research (1998) Basic newborn resuscitation: a practical guide. WHO, Geneva. http://whqlibdoc.who.int/hq/1998/WHO_RHT_MSM_98.1.pdf

Wu YW, Backstrand KH, Zhao S et al (2004) Declining diagnosis of birth asphyxia in California: 1991–2000. Pediatrics 114:1584–1590

Wyckoff MH, Berg RA (2008) Optimizing chest compressions during delivery-room resuscitation. Semin Fetal Neonatal Med 13:410–415

Wyckoff MH, Perlman JM (2006) Use of high-dose epinephrine and sodium bicarbonate during neonatal resuscitation: is there proven benefit? Clin Perinatol 33:141–151

Wyckoff MH, Wyllie J (2006) Endotracheal delivery of medications during neonatal resuscitation. Clin Perinatol 33:153–160

Wyckoff MH, Perlman JM, Laptook AR (2005) Use of volume expansion during delivery room resuscitation in near-term and term infants. Pediatrics 115:950–955

Wyckoff M, Garcia D, Margraf L et al (2007) Randomized trial of volume infusion during resuscitation of asphyxiated neonatal piglets. Pediatr Res 61:415–420

Yam CH, Dawson JA, Schmölzer GM et al (2011) Heart rate changes during resuscitation of newly born infants <30 weeks gestation: an observational study. Arch Dis Child Fetal Neonatal Ed 96:F102–F107

Oxygen Toxicity in Newborns

30

Rodolfo Bracci, Serafina Perrone, Maximo Vento, and Giuseppe Buonocore

Contents

Abstract

The first evidence of a relationship between oxygen toxicity and neonatal diseases emerged in the early 1950s, when retinopathy was observed in premature infants breathing high concentrations of oxygen. Oxygen toxicity is due to the development of reactive oxygen species (ROS), such as the superoxide anion (O_2^-), hydrogen peroxide (H_20_2), lipid peroxide (LOOH), peroxyl radicals RO˙, electron delocalized phenoxyl radical (C_6H_50), nitric oxide (NO), and the hydroxyl radical (OH˙). OH˙ is one of the strongest oxidants in nature and may damage tissues. There is no specific

R. Bracci (✉) · G. Buonocore
University of Siena, Siena, Italy
e-mail: rodolfo.bracci@virgilio.it; giuseppe.buonocore@unisi.it

S. Perrone
Department of Molecular and Developmental Medicine, University Hospital of Siena, Siena, Italy
e-mail: saraspv@yahoo.it

M. Vento
Neonatal Research Unit, Health Research Institute Hospital La Fe, University and Polytechnic Hospital La Fe, Valencia, Spain
e-mail: maximo.vento@uv.es

G. Buonocore et al. (eds.), *Neonatology*,
https://doi.org/10.1007/978-3-319-29489-6_180

scavenger for this radical, and once released, $OH^{\cdot}$ reacts with lipoproteins, cell membranes, lipids, proteins, DNA, amino acids, and other molecules causing structural and functional damage to these structures. The main sources of ROS are NADPH oxidase reactions (principally in phagocytes after activation upon exposure to microbes, microbial products, or inflammatory mediators), mitochondrial metabolism, hypoxia-reoxygenation (hypoxanthine-xanthine oxidase reaction), hyperoxia, and paradoxically hypoxia. Abnormal percentage of ROS generation can have pathological consequences if they are lower as well as they are higher than normal. An excess of ROS, in relation to detoxification capacity, is called oxidative stress, a term which expresses the imbalance between oxidants and antioxidants that is a potential cause of damage. If oxidative stress is mild, cell defenses may increase by a mechanism which generally involves enhanced gene expression of ROS scavenging activities. Severe oxidative stress is generally followed by cell injury and plays a role in many kinds of cell death, i.e., apoptosis, necrosis, autophagy, and mitophagy. Oxidative stress has been suggested as a causative agent in pregnancy-related disorders such as recurrent pregnancy loss, preeclampsia, preterm premature rupture of membranes, intrauterine growth restriction, and fetal death. In the fetal-to-neonatal transition, both blood oxygen content and oxygen availability abruptly increase in the first few minutes after birth, eliciting the generation of a burst of ROS. Oxidative stress following hyperoxia has been recognized to be responsible for lung, retina, and red blood cell injury and possibly generalized tissue damage.

Several methods have been proposed in the attempt to detect the presence and the severity of the oxidative stress. Measurements of protein, lipid, and DNA bases oxidation and intracellular redox status are accurate methods. Prevention of ROS tissue damage involves the avoidance of conditions such as infections, asphyxia, hyperoxia, and retinal light exposure, under which excessive ROS occurs. When supplemental oxygen is needed for care, the most prudent approach would be not to tolerate possible hypoxia and not to accept SpO_2 values associated with potential hyperoxia, setting the low alarm never <85% and the high alarm never more than 95%. It is imperative to avoid a flip-flop phenomenon that leads to acute and significant changes and fluctuations in SpO_2. Preterm infants should be fed early with human expressed milk, which offers an additional protection against free radicals. Although the usefulness of antioxidant protection during pregnancy and in the neonatal period is still under investigation, the risk of tissue damage due to oxidative stress in perinatal period should not be underestimated.

30.1 Salient Points

- Oxygen is one of the most important elements in newborn resuscitation, and inappropriate oxygen administration would profoundly affect the outcomes of babies.
- Oxygen toxicity is due to the development of reactive oxygen species (ROS), such as superoxide anion (O_2^-), hydrogen peroxide (H_2O_2), lipid peroxide (LOOH), peroxyl radicals ($RO^{\cdot}$), electron delocalized phenoxyl radical (C_6H_50), nitric oxide (NO), and the hydroxyl radical ($OH^{\cdot}$).
- The main sources of ROS are NADPH oxidase reactions (principally in phagocytes after activation upon exposure microbes, microbial products, or inflammatory mediators), mitochondrial metabolism, hypoxia-reoxygenation (hypoxanthine-xanthine oxidase reaction), hyperoxia, and paradoxically hypoxia.
- ROS contribute to worsen cellular function by oxidizing and damaging numerous cellular components, in particular impairing mitochondrial function and oxygen utilization. Moreover a systemic inflammatory response that can be triggered by the ischemia-reperfusion injury can contribute to tissue injury.
- An excess of ROS, in relation to detoxification capacity, is called oxidative stress, a term which expresses the imbalance between oxidants and antioxidants that is a potential cause of damage.

- Severe oxidative stress is generally followed by cell injury and plays a role in many kinds of cell death, i.e., apoptosis, necrosis, autophagy, and mitophagy.
- In the fetal-to-neonatal transition, both blood oxygen content and oxygen availability abruptly increase in the first few minutes after birth, eliciting the generation of a burst of ROS.
- Hyperoxia has been recognized to be responsible for lung, retina, and red blood cell injury and possibly generalized tissue damage.
- Measurements of protein, lipid, and DNA base oxidation and intracellular redox status are accurate methods to detect the presence and the severity of the oxidative stress.
- Prevention of ROS tissue damage involves the avoidance of conditions such as infections, asphyxia, hyperoxia, and retinal light exposure, under which excessive ROS occurs.
- Because of the limited benefit of maintaining potentially harmful supranormal oxygen levels, oxygen supplementation and mechanical ventilation should be titrated to maintain an oxygen saturation between 85% and 95% in preterm babies.

30.2 Reactive Oxygen Species

Although the toxic effects of oxygen were already noticed at the end of the nineteenth century (Smith 1899), the first evidence of a relationship between oxygen toxicity and neonatal diseases emerged only in the early 1950s, when retinopathy was observed in premature infants breathing high concentrations of oxygen (Patz et al. 1952). At about the same time, the red blood cells of newborns were demonstrated to have increased susceptibility to oxygen damage and a fetal and neonatal deficiency of antioxidant factors became evident (Gordon et al. 1955). Great advances in our understanding of the toxic effects of oxygen were made in the years that followed when oxygen toxicity was recognized to be due to the development of reactive oxygen species (ROS). The main ROS are the superoxide anion (O_2^-), hydrogen peroxide (H_20_2), lipid peroxide (LOOH), peroxyl radicals ($RO^{\cdot}$), and the hydroxyl radical ($OH^{\cdot}$). Other important radicals are the highly reactive electron delocalized phenoxyl radical (C_6H_50) and nitric oxide (NO). The term ROS includes free radicals, which are atoms or molecules with one or more unpaired electrons. Free radicals may react with other radicals, the unpaired electrons forming a covalent bond. The resulting molecule may decompose other molecules into toxic products. Free radicals may react with non-radical molecules in free radical chain reactions, which are stopped by antioxidant molecules, enzymes, or protein reactions. Superoxide anion is the precursor of most ROS and is a mediator in oxidative chain reactions. Dismutation of O_2^- by superoxide dismutase (SOD) produces H_2O_2 that in turn may be fully reduced to water by glutathione peroxidase (GSH-Px) and catalase (Cat) or, alternatively, partially reduced to the $OH^{\cdot}$. The latter reaction is called the Fenton-Haber-Weiss reaction and is catalyzed by reduced transition metals, particularly iron, but also copper and zinc (Jankov et al. 2001; Fig. 1).

There is no specific scavenger for the hydroxyl radical, and once released, $OH^{\cdot}$ reacts with lipoproteins, cell membranes, lipids, proteins, DNA, amino acids, and other molecules causing structural and functional damage to the cell. $OH^{\cdot}$ is one of the strongest oxidants in nature and may damage tissues. Since the $OH^{\cdot}$ is formed by the Fenton reaction, which is dependent on nonprotein-bound iron (NPBI), the condition of intracellular or extracellular availability of nonprotein-bound iron is one of the most important sources of ROS-dependent tissue damage. Superoxide has low activity and poor

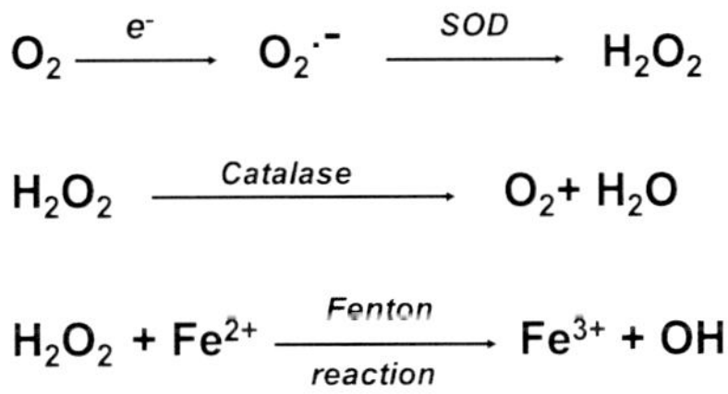

Fig. 1 **Iron-mediated oxygen radical formation.** Schematic representation of the sequence of events involved in Fenton reaction. Initially, electron donors can convert oxygen to superoxide anion. Superoxide anion is rapidly converted to hydrogen peroxide. Hydrogen peroxide can further form hydroxyl radicals ($OH^{\cdot}$) in the Fenton reaction in the presence of ferrous ions which are oxidized to form ferric ions

reactivity. However it may participate in nitric oxide-mediated reactivity generating oxidative tissue damage. Superoxide and nitric oxide readily react to form an extremely reactive substance called peroxynitrite ($ONOO^-$) (Jankov et al. 2001).

In general, the main sources of ROS are NADPH oxidase (NOX) reactions, mitochondrial metabolism, hypoxia-reoxygenation (hypoxanthine-xanthine oxidase reaction), hyperoxia, and paradoxically hypoxia (Jankov et al. 2001; Ullrich and Bachscmid 2000; Koenig and Yoder 2004; Sies 1991; Halliwell 2007). Each of these will be discussed in turn.

The NOX Enzyme has been found in virtually every tissue and modulates fundamental biological processes (Murphy 2009) While the most relevant generation of ROS by NOX occurs in **phagocytes** after activation upon exposure microbes, microbial products, or inflammatory mediators, ROS are produced via NOX in a variety of cell types in response to normal physiological signals such as insulin, angiotensin II, growth factors, and various classes of receptors such as formyl peptide receptors (FPRs) and Toll-like receptors (TLRs) (Murphy 2009; Lambeth and Neish 2014). Furthermore, NOX-dependent ROS generation has been suggested to trigger adaptive response of a variety of stressors (Lambeth and Neish 2014). However, NOX-induced ROS generation can activate the NRF2 pathway which increases antioxidant protection during inflammation (Menshicova et al. 2010). ROS released inside phagocytes during infection and cytokine production is an essential defense mechanism. It also alters the extracellular oxidative balance and harms tissues, since the cells undergo an efflux of O_2^- (Koenig and Yoder 2004). Opsonization and activation of phagocytes are also known to occur not only following infection but even as a consequence of asphyxia and particularly hypoxanthine-xanthine oxidase reaction and therefore during hypoxia-reoxygenation (Sies 1991; Halliwell 2007; Fig. 2).

The complex mechanism of ROS production has been extensively investigated in **mitochondria** where ROS generation can have physiological and pathological effect (Ullrich and Bachscmid 2000). The mitochondrial respiratory chain is a major source of ROS in eukaryotic cells (Fig. 3).

The role of mitochondria goes beyond the creation of molecular fuel. The organelle also generates ROS that are deeply involved in signaling pathways which regulate a wide variety of physiological events. ROS generation by mitochondria is mainly dependent on complexes I and III and is highly dependent on metabolic conditions and on the intramitochondrial balance between oxidative and antioxidative factors (Lismont et al. 2015; Kalogeris et al. 2014). The respiratory chain process involves a set of distinct electron carriers designed to minimize the unwanted leak of electrons from reduced cofactors onto molecular oxygen and hence ROS generation, at least under normal circumstances. Mitochondria comprise a very effective antioxidant defense which provides

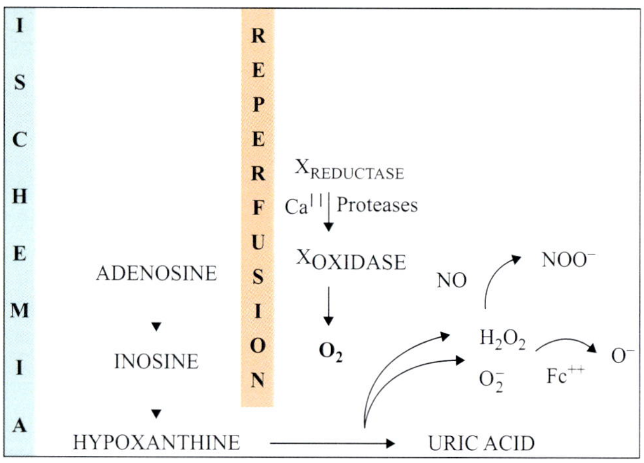

Fig. 2 Xanthine oxidoreductase system

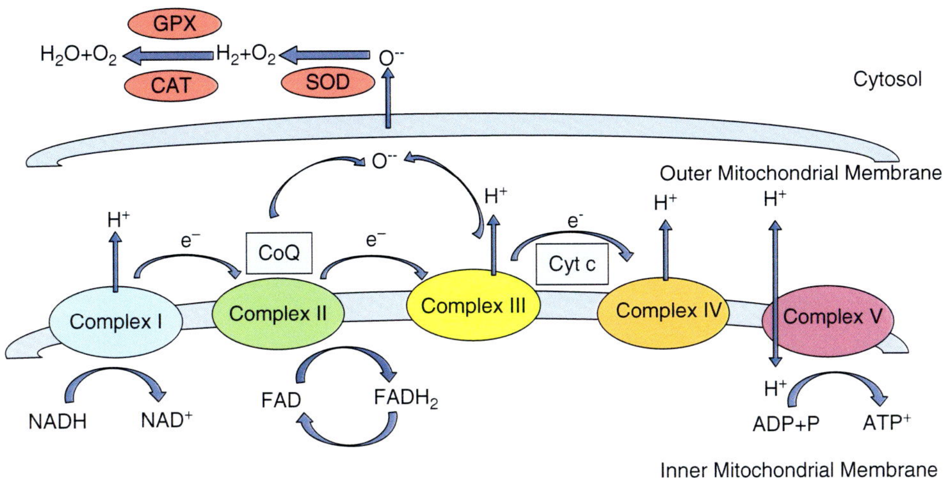

Fig. 3 Mitochondrial oxygen radical formation. Schematic representation of the sequence of events involved in oxidative phosphorylation. This process, which takes place in mitochondria, is the major source of ATP in aerobic organisms. ATP is formed as a result of the transfer of electrons from NADH to O_2 by a series of electron carriers. Initially, electron donors can convert oxygen to superoxide anion. Superoxide anion is rapidly converted to hydrogen peroxide. Hydrogen peroxide can further form hydroxyl radicals (OH$^·$) in the Fenton reaction in the presence of ferrous ions which are oxidized to form ferric ions. *SOD* superoxide dismutase, *CAT* catalase, *GPX* glutathione peroxidase, *CoQ* coenzyme Q, *Cyt c* cytochrome c.

redox status stability (Dröse and Brandt 2012). Therefore, mitochondrial function actively contributes to the redox balance through the equilibrium between pro-oxidant and antioxidant processes.

This complex variability leads to a serious difficulty in the detection and analysis of oxidative stress in adults and particularly in newborns (Fig. 4).

Under physiologic conditions, approximately 98% of O_2 undergoes a complete reduction to form H_2O_2. A 2% of electrons will leak, causing a partial reduction of the oxygen and producing ROS. The monovalent reduction of O_2 produces superoxide anion, and monovalent reduction of anion superoxide generates H_2O_2. A third monovalent reduction generates the highly reactive hydroxyl radical. The reactivity of superoxide is relatively low. However, when elevated levels of NO• are present, nitric oxide binds to mitochondrial-generated superoxide. Subsequently, ONOO- is formed with the rate constant close to that of the reaction between OH$^·$ and ascorbic acid. Then, ONOO- produces hydroxyl radicals and nitrogen dioxide and oxidizes and nitrates DNAs, lipids, and proteins. Free radicals generated from mitochondria could play a role in many kinds of cell death, i.e., apoptosis, necrosis, autophagy, and mitophagy (Vento 2014).

The release of ROS from mitochondria as well as from peroxisomes strongly depends upon physiological or pathological state of the cell. Damage of mitochondrial DNA appears to damage mitochondrial DNA-encoded proteins in electron-transporting chain, causing more superoxide to be produced. Therefore, the normal limit of 2–3% O2- release by the ETC can be greatly increased if substrates are available but energy consumption is low (Kohlhaas and Maack 2013). This theory, called "A Mitochondrial Superoxide Theory" (Indo et al. 2015), has been proposed to explain the initiation of numerous chronic diseases. Reducing excess amounts of mitochondria-generated superoxide seems important to protecting against oxidative stress-related diseases.

It is important to note that abnormally low levels of ROS can also have pathological consequences (Zorov et al. 2014). Metabolic conditions and O_2 levels modify the rate of ROS generation (Hoffman and Brookes 2009). During **hypoxia**, redox signals to and from mitochondria are activated (Collins et al. 2012). In particular, the

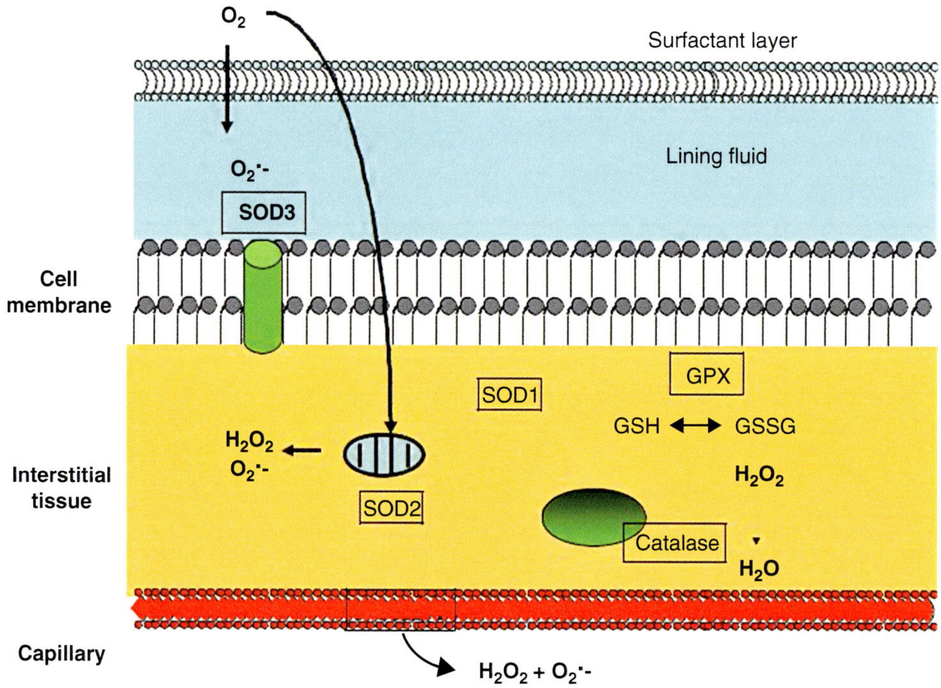

Fig. 4 Oxidative stress following hyperoxia

respiratory chain increases ROS production stimulating the signaling pathway to induce hypoxia-induced factor (HIF)-dependent gene expression. Intermittent hypoxia increases the ROS content of carotid bodies, which induces increased synthesis and stability of hypoxia-inducible factor 1a (HIF-1a) and calpain-dependent degradation of H1F-2a (Semenza and Prabhakar 2012). Thus, intermittent hypoxia will cause a disruption of the equilibrium between HIF-1α and HIF-2a, causing a loss of redox homeostasis (Semenza and Prabhakar 2012; Yuan et al. 2013). Although an increase in mitochondrial ROS is important to activate HIF, a sustained increase in ROS production can be detrimental under chronic hypoxia and can induce cell death (Kalogeris et al. 2014).

Reperfusion is the second phase of ischemia/reperfusion (I/R) injury and is characterized by the generation of ROS after reintroduction of molecular oxygen to the tissues. Xanthine oxidase- and phagocyte NADPH oxidase- derived ROS can damage biomolecules in cells and tissues. In this phase, the blood supply to ischemic tissues causes the delivery of blood-borne elements that are activated by and release ROS. ROS may also induce cell dysfunction and death by indirect mechanisms by interacting with NO, fatty acids, or free iron to form peroxynitrite, peroxyl radicals, and hydroxyl radicals. Oxygen-derived ROS also acts to enhance the inflammatory response to reperfusion via formation of oxidant-dependent pro-inflammatory mediators (Kalogeris et al. 2014; Vento 2014).

A third stage of I/R injury constitutes the reparative phase and involves ROS-dependent generation of growth factors that promote angiogenesis, vascular remodeling, and activation of matrix metalloproteinases and other factors that contribute to fibrosis, tissue remodeling, and formation of scar tissue (Kalogeris et al. 2014).

30.3 Oxidative Stress in Perinatal Period

It is important to emphasize that ROS reactions are a normal occurrence in living organisms and ROS are involved in a myriad of physiological reactions.

They have a key role in oxidation reduction, or "redox," reactions, which are an integral part of signaling pathways in various cellular processes such as energy metabolism, gene expression, protein import, and folding (Lismont et al. 2015). Hydrogen peroxide and superoxide are deeply involved in cell signaling and transcriptional regulation (Kaludercic et al. 2014). ROS are also produced in response to a variety of ligands including growth factors cytokines and G protein-coupled receptors (Lambeth 2014). The mechanism by which ROS affect these pathways may be direct or indirect, though certain cysteine-containing proteins are direct target of oxidation.

Shift in redox potential may favor beneficial or detrimental consequences according to various factors. High levels of ROS and excessive low levels of ROS can alter the balance between prooxidant and antioxidant elements which is essential for biological processes (Lismont et al. 2015). An excess of ROS, in relation to detoxification capacity, is called oxidative stress, a term which expresses the imbalance between oxidants and antioxidants that is a potential cause of damage. If oxidative stress is mild, cell defenses may increase by a mechanism which generally involves enhanced gene expression of ROS scavenging activities (Halliwell et al. 1992). Severe oxidative stress is generally followed by cell injury. ROS can be responsible for a wide range of molecular damage: lipid peroxidation, protein oxidation and nitration, protein-thiol depletion, nucleic acid hydroxylation and nitration, and DNA strand breakage (Vento 2014). ROS can damage DNA bases which can result in mutagenesis (Lambeth and Neish 2014). Lipid peroxidation can alter membrane structure disrupting membrane permeability properties and alter cellular components. At lower concentrations ROS can perturb cells and tissue functions by more subtle and often transient and reversible mechanism (Lambeth and Neish 2014). Under stressful conditions ROS may induce apoptosis and/or necrosis (Vento 2014). Excess of ROS can also induce abnormalities in cell membrane proteins with numerous functional consequences including, for instance, for recognition of cells in the immune response (Lambeth and Neish 2014).

Oxidative balance, therefore, is an intriguing problem, and much recent research has increased our knowledge of the relations between ROS and human diseases.

Oxidative stress in the fetus and newborn may result from decreased antioxidants, increased ROS, or both. The various pathways of ROS generation should be considered, and it is necessary to take into account the complexity of redox equilibrium and therefore correctly interpret the origin of oxygen toxicity in fetus and newborn. The well-known deficiency of antioxidant factors, characteristic of the neonate, is only a piece of a cohort of factors which can be involved in the fetal and neonatal oxidative stress.

Antioxidant capacity is lower in the newborn and particularly the premature infant in comparison to adults. Free radical scavenger enzyme activity and many other components of the antioxidant system increase during intrauterine life and are low in the neonate (Saugstad 2005; Chandel and Shumacker 2000).

Therefore, premature infants are almost certainly developmentally unprepared for extrauterine life in an oxygen-rich environment and exhibit a unique sensitivity to oxidant injury. Furthermore, the greater the prematurity, the higher is the associated risk of oxidant injury.

The main antioxidant enzymes include copper, zinc, and manganese containing superoxide dismutase (SOD), GSH peroxidase (GPx), catalase (Cat), thioredoxin (TRX), peroxiredoxin (PRDX), glutathione reductase (GSR), and thioredoxin reductase (TXNRD). The major nonenzymatic antioxidants are GSH, coenzyme A ubiquinol, vitamin C, and vitamin E (Lismont et al. 2015).

Of note is that the level and activity of the most relevant antioxidant enzymes such as superoxide dismutases, catalase, and glutathione peroxidase change dynamically during development and mature in the last weeks of gestation, preparing the fetus for lung respiration (Frank and Sosenko 1987; Friel et al. 2004; Tiina et al. 1998).

Nonenzymatic antioxidant factors are reported to be lower in the fetus and newborn than in adults and older babies (Rogers et al. 2000). One of the most studied antioxidant deficiencies of the fetus and newborn is tissue and erythrocyte low α-tocopherol. Other factors are important. Reduced glutathione (GSH) is the most abundant intracellular nonenzymatic antioxidant and is involved in the GSH-GPx and GSH-T enzyme activity. There are also complex interactions with environmental factors triggering oxidative stress (Njålsson and Norgren 2005). Since, in the cell, the glutathione tripeptide is assembled from cysteine and glycine and then glutamate by consecutive actions of enzymes such as y-cystathionase, y-glutamylcysteine synthetase, and glutathione synthetase, the possible problems with this mechanism may be due to recognizable inborn errors of metabolism or nutritional deficiencies (Njålsson and Norgren 2005; Yeung 2006). Several observations have shown that, depending on age, preterm infants have lower plasma concentrations of GSH and higher concentrations of glutathione disulfide (GSSO) than adults (Smith et al. 1993). This occurrence may due to low OSH and low activity of GSH synthetase in VLBW infants (Yeung 2006).

In this regard, there have been conflicting reports in the literature as to whether L-cysteine is an essential amino acid for the preterm infant as the result of the low activity of hepatic g-cystathionase. Thus, studies performed in preterm infants revealed that plasma cystathionine concentrations in ELBW infants were significantly higher than in term infants, whereas cysteine concentrations were higher in term than in preterm. Furthermore, erythrocytes from preterm infants synthesize glutathione at a much lower rate than term infants when incubated with methionine, a process dependent on the g-cystathionase pathway. These findings underscore the immaturity of the trans-sulfuration pathway and the conditional essentiality of L-cysteine in the parenteral and enteral nutrition of very preterm neonates. Moreover, it also explains the tendency toward oxidative stress (Viña et al. 1995). Iron-binding proteins have major antioxidant activity, protecting against metal-induced OH• production (Halliwell and Gutteridge 1990). Therefore, among nonenzymatic antioxidant factors, the metal transporter proteins have an important function. In particular, transferrin concentration has a key role in protecting against the nonprotein-bound iron (NPBI)-promoted oxidative stress due to OH· release (Buonocore et al. 2001; Berger et al. 1995). In this regard, low ceruloplasmin and transferrin may play an important role in neonatal susceptibility to oxidative stress and particularly to metal-induced OH• production (Lindeman et al. 2000). The finding of increased bleomycin-detectable iron in premature and some full-term infants is evidence of the real risk of the increased pro-oxidant effects of iron in neonates (Evans et al. 1992). High saturation of transferrin is therefore probably a risk factor for oxidative stress. It is generally accepted that NPBI is a pathological manifestation and in fact is extremely rare in adults (Buonocore et al. 2001). Levels of NPBI in plasma of newborns are correlated with other markers of oxidative stress and are higher in hypoxic newborns (Marzocchi et al. 2005). Interestingly, plasma-esterified F2-isoprostanes not only correlate with NPBI in the samples of cord blood of newborns, but they increased after incubation of plasma with ammonium iron sulfate (Signorini et al. 2008). This observation strongly suggests the role of NPBI in enhancing oxidative stress in the neonate. High plasma NPBI has been found in hypoxic newborns with poor outcome (Buonocore et al. 2003).

Oxidative stress has been suggested as a causative agent in pregnancy-related disorders such as recurrent pregnancy loss, preeclampsia, preterm premature rupture of membranes, intrauterine growth restriction, and fetal death. In utero stressors contribute to ROS production and resulting in tissue damage. Markers of oxidative stress, such as nonprotein-bound iron, have been measured in cord blood as an indicator of intrauterine ROS production. These markers have been associated with the development of several postnatal disease processes, suggesting that in utero oxidative stress is a significant risk factor, especially in premature neonates (Perrone et al. 2010). Pregnancy, in fact, is a state associated with enhanced oxidative stress due to the high metabolic turnover and elevated tissue oxygen requirements. During intrauterine life, many factors such as hypoxia, inflammation, and infections can induce overproduction of ROS. Whenever produced, these toxic species can induce oxidative stress and tissue injury. The placenta represents an important source of lipid peroxides, because of its high polyunsaturated fatty acid content (Marseglia et al. 2014).

The process is well balanced in healthy pregnancy by the enzymatic and nonenzymatic antioxidant redox systems. The ability of placental antioxidant defenses to reduce the effects of highly reactive and potentially damaging ROS is critical for healthy placental function and the optimal growth and development of the fetus. Occasionally, however, the developing fetus may be exposed to high levels of oxidative stress due to an overproduction of ROS and/or reduced antioxidant defense capability (Marseglia et al. 2014). Fluctuating oxygen conditions can contribute to increased ROS production, as ROS act as signaling molecules for this condition. This may be particularly pertinent to tissues which have a high-energy demand or those which contain large amounts of mitochondria, such as the placenta and fetal tissues. Another important factor which can be responsible for ROS increase in fetus and newborn is the inflammation (Pereira et al. 2015; Poggi and Dani 2014).

Individual genetic characteristics may condition the onset and the magnitude of the inflammatory and immune responses triggered by specific stimuli in the fetus and in the preterm newborn (Poggi and Dani 2014). Particularly, a recent model of the pathogenesis of the complications of prematurity suggests that a hyperresponsive phenotype activating excessive inflammatory cytokines and ROS production increases the risk of oxidative stress-related complications (Poggi and Dani 2014).

30.4 Hyperoxia

In the fetal-to-neonatal transition, both blood oxygen content and oxygen availability abruptly increase in the first few minutes after birth to their adult values, eliciting the generation of a burst of ROS (Comporti et al. 2004; House et al. 1987; Vento et al. 2002). Free radicals in the fetal-to-neonatal transition may act as signaling molecules modulating maturation of specific metabolic pathways (Forman et al. 2008; Martín et al. 2007).

Oxidative stress following hyperoxia has been extensively investigated and has been recognized to be responsible for lung injury and possibly generalized tissue damage (Saugstad 2005). The sequence of, first, the inhalation of a high level of oxygen (even for a short time), followed by membrane-bound NADPH oxidase activation, ROS production, and DNA damage with cell apoptosis has been suggested as a consequence of exposure to high oxygen concentration (Chandel and Shumacker 2000).

Hyperoxic resuscitation showed accumulation of 8-oxoG in a newborn mouse model (Sejersted et al. 2009) pointing at insufficient repair and a possible risk for genetic instability after the use of supplementary oxygen during resuscitation. Oxidative stress due to supplementary oxygen use in newborn piglets may reduce nucleotide-excision repair which could be compensated for by antioxidant supplementation (Langie Sabine et al. 2010).

Modification of neuronal nuclear membrane function leading to increased nuclear Ca^{++} influx, activation of Ca^{++}/Calmodulin-dependent protein kinase, and protein-mediated apoptotic protein expression have been reported in animals exposed to high oxygen concentration (Chang et al. 2007). An important example of the various conditions capable of modifying ROS production and creating serious oxidative stress occurs in the endothelium. It is well known that endothelium dysfunction is mainly due to oxidative stress enhanced by various factors such as cytokines, ischemia reoxygenation, glucose, LDL cholesterol, angiotensin II, shear stress, and vascular endothelial growth factor (VEGF) (Li and Shah 2004). The occurrence of endothelium oxidative stress is important in neonatology, taking into account that endothelium is deeply involved in infection-mediated alteration of the coagulation system and vascular troubles in the neonate.

Oxygen toxicity is particularly harmful for the lungs. The mechanism of damage is complex. Lung injury may be caused directly by ROS production in response to hyperoxia or indirectly by

ROS due to phagocyte activation and inflammation. The two mechanisms seem to be integrated.

In vitro and in vivo exposure to hyperoxia results in downregulation of peroxisome proliferator-activated receptor gamma (PPARy) augmenting the transdifferentiation of pulmonary lipofibroblasts (LIFs), which provide protection against oxygen free radicals, to myofibroblasts (MYFs). Transdifferentiated lipofibroblasts (Myf) are unable to maintain pulmonary epithelial cell growth and differentiation, resulting in failed alveolarization, seen characteristically in bronchopulmonary dysplasia (BPD) (Torday and Rehan 2016).

The hyperoxia-induced morphologic, molecular, and immunohistochemical changes are almost entirely prevented by pretreatment with a potent PPARc signaling pathway agonist, rosiglitazone (RGZ), suggesting the possibility of treatment of BPD based on physiological principles rather than pure pharmacology (Richter et al. 2016).

The particular toxicity of ROS in the immature lung is mainly due to the low antioxidant capacity of premature infants, as well as to the possibly high toxicity of ROS in rapidly developing tissues (Frank 1991). Increased production of ROS under certain conditions may also play a role. The main sources of ROS production in the immature lung are ischemia, reperfusion, phagocytosis, and hyperoxia (Vento et al. 2009a, b). The lung is highly susceptible to high oxygen concentrations especially when administered with positive pressure. In a prospective clinical study, extremely low gestational age (ELGA) neonates were randomly assigned to become ventilated with higher (90%) and lower (30%) oxygen concentrations as initial inspiratory fraction of oxygen. Of note is that those neonates receiving more oxygen load during fetal-to-neonatal transition had a higher oxidative stress as detected by a decreased GSH/GSSG ratio. Moreover, urinary determination of ortho-tyrosine/phenylalanine ratio and 8-oxo-dihydroguanosine/2-de-oxyguanosine ratio revealed that premature infants who received more oxygen had increased oxidation of circulating proteins and higher damage to nuclear DNA. In addition, markers of inflammation (interleukin-8 [IL8] and tumor necrosis factor-α [TNF-α]) increased at the same time. Interestingly, infants with increased markers of oxidative stress and inflammation in the first days of life developed with significantly higher incidence of BPD and stayed more days on oxygen and mechanical ventilation (Vento et al. 2009b). Effects of hyperoxia in the lung and a close relationship between oxidative stress and inflammation have been demonstrated (Denis et al. 2001; Bhandari 2008). Magnetic resonance studies have confirmed the previously reported experimental data on the consequences of hyperoxia in the lungs of premature newborn animals, namely, edema, congestion, immune cell infiltration, and decreased number of alveoli per square meter (Appleby and Towner 2001). The finding of a large number of neutrophils and high concentrations of IL-8 and leukotrienes in bronchopulmonary lavage of infants with severe chronic lung disease (CLD) demonstrates the role of inflammatory reactions and ROS production in the development of this disease (Kotecha et al. 1995).

However, in extremely premature infants, the combination of an immature antioxidant system and predisposition to altered redox potential plus a surfactant-deficient lung and the need for therapy with oxygen supplementation and mechanical ventilation together predispose the newborn to oxidative stress, lung-stretch damage, inflammation, and impairment of alveolar development, ultimately increasing the risk of chronic lung disease (Asikainen and White 2004; Halliday 2008). Generalized use of antenatal steroids has significantly reduced mortality and the incidence of severe complications in preterms younger than 34 weeks of gestational age. ELGA neonates with antenatal steroids spend less days on oxygen and on mechanical ventilation and have less severe complications such as BPD, patent ductus arteriosus (PDA), intra-periventricular hemorrhage (IPVH), or retinopathy of prematurity (ROP). Moreover, in spite of the increased antioxidant enzyme (AOE) activity and reduced oxidative stress and damage to proteins and DNA after antenatal steroid administration, the level of AOE activity was significantly lower than assessed in term infants or adults. Intriguingly, the response to antenatal steroids is conditioned both by when they are administered before birth and also by gender, with female neonates having a significantly increased response compared to male neonates (Vento et al. 2009a).

The key role of oxygen toxicity in the development of the retinopathy has been recognized for more than half a century and will be discussed in . ▶ Chap. 136, "Retinopathy of Prematurity."

Oxidative stress is involved in the increased hemolysis and anemia of the newborn and particularly of the premature infant. The red cells of newborns appear to be more susceptible to the toxic effects of oxidative stress than those of adults (Gross et al. 1967), and the free iron content of red cells, a risk factor for hemolysis, is higher in newborns in comparison with the adults (Buonocore et al. 1998). It is interesting that during aerobic and also hypoxic incubation, increased $O2^-$ production, free iron release, and senescence antigen production showed the highest significant differences between adults and neonates (Ciccoli et al. 2004).

Increased markers of oxidative stress such as hypoxanthine, total hydroperoxide, and advanced oxidation protein products have been reported in hypoxic newborns and in preterm neonates at birth and on the seventh day of life (Buonocore et al. 2000, 2002). Increased F2-isoprostanes have been also found in growth-restricted fetuses suggestive of oxidative stress and hypoxia (Longini et al. 2005). These observations demonstrate that oxidative stress follows hypoxia with a mechanism of hypoxia reoxygenation, NADP oxidase reactions, or, paradoxically, by release of ROS by hypoxic cells. Oxidative stress is also involved in tissue damage induced by infection and sepsis. Although there is general agreement that neonatal phagocytes, especially those of premature infants, have abnormalities of various functions, active neonatal secretion of pro-inflammatory cytokines suggests a very complex situation in which oxidative stress following infection may be more dangerous in newborns, especially if premature, than in adults (Bracci and Buonocore 2003). This finding suggests that hyperoxia and hypoxia may generate red cell damage via ROS and possibly have a role in the increased hemolysis in the neonate. In conclusion, experimental studies and clinical observations demonstrated high susceptibility of the fetus and newborn to oxidative stress. Increased release and decreased detoxification in the newborn appear to be negatively correlated with the gestational age.

30.5 Clinical Aspects and Prevention

30.5.1 Diagnostic Procedures

ROS have an important role in the development of retinopathy, chronic lung disease, necrotizing enterocolitis, renal failure, hemolytic anemia, septic shock, and also brain damage. The clinical care of these pathologies is treated in the corresponding chapters. Several methods have been proposed in the attempt to detect the presence and the severity of the oxidative stress. Some frequently used approaches such as the measurement of erythrocyte antioxidant defenses are not accurate since the red cell enzyme activities are age dependent and values may be an expression of an old or young red cell population (Halliwell and Whiteman 2004).

30.5.2 Lipids

The thiobarbituric acid (TBA) test should not be used to measure lipid peroxidation because most of TBA-reactive material is not related to lipid peroxidation. Measurements of malondialdehyde (MDA) by HPLC, 4-hydroxynoneal, and particularly isoprostanes are more accurate (Halliwell and Whiteman 2004). The most work has been done with F2 isoprostanes which arises from arachidonic acid non-cyclooxygenase (COX) peroxidation. Neuroprostane or F4 isoprostanes has also been measured (Halliwell and Whiteman 2004).

30.5.2.1 Isofurans

The prostanoid profile can be affected by oxygen tension. An oxygen insertion step blocks the intermediates from the IsoPs pathway to form various compounds termed isofurans (IsoFs) that contain a substituted tetrahydrofuran ring. Like the IsoPs, the IsoFs are chemically and metabolically stable and are well suited to act as in vivo biomarkers of oxidative damage. The ratio of IsoFs to IsoPs also provides information about the relative oxygen tension where the lipid peroxidation is occurring. This was clearly shown in pigs, in which exposure to high oxygen tension increased IsoFs production and reduced IsoPs levels in the brain (Solberg et al. 2012; de La Torre et al. 2014).

30.5.2.2 Neuroprostanes

The oxidation both in vivo and in vitro of docosahexaenoic acid (DHA), a major component of neuronal membranes, leads to the formation of IsoPs-like compounds termed neuroprostanes (NPs) (Arneson and Roberts 2007). The most studied series is the four-series NeuroPs, mainly F4-NeuroPs. The NPs are the only quantitative in vivo biomarker of oxidative damage selective for neurons, and thus they are specific and reliable marker of cerebral gray matter lipid oxidation.

30.5.2.3 Neurofurans

Similarly to IsoFs, in high oxygen tension conditions, an alternative pathway of oxidation of DHA leads to the formation of compounds termed neurofurans (NFs). Thus hyperoxic or hypoxic conditions can be detected through quantitative assessment of NFs and IsoFs in vivo. Given the abundance of DHA in the brain, analysis of NFs may have particular value in the quantitative assessment of lipid peroxidation in brain damage (Tataranno et al. 2015). Isofurans and neurofurans are new promising markers, and recently their potentialities are being investigated since they can be good markers of oxidative injury in conditions of high oxygen tension, but few data exists in humans, mostly due to a lack of commercially standard references (Milne et al. 2011; Song et al. 2008).

30.5.3 Proteins

Detection of oxidation of proteins can be obtained by measurement of carbonyl groups, and the use of proteomics appears to be a promising method in order to identify specifically oxidized proteins (Halliwell and Whiteman 2004). Assay of total hydroperoxides represents a measure of overall oxidative stress given that they are the intermediate oxidative products of lipids, peptides, and amino acids (Halliwell and Whiteman 2004). Allantoin and 8-hydroxydeoxyguanosine can be measured in plasma and urine, and the levels are high in conditions of oxidative stress (Mikami et al. 2000; Drury et al. 1998). Nitrosyn levels have been reported as a marker of $ONOO^-$ production from leukocyte activation (Eiserich et al. 1998). A very specific, useful, and noninvasive mean to monitor oxidative damage to circulating proteins and amino acids is the measurement of ortho-tyrosine. Oxidation of phenylalanine produces three different metabolites, ortho-, para-, and meta-tyrosine, which can be detected in urine by high-performance liquid chromatography coupled to mass spectrometry (Lubec et al. 1997). This works since only ortho-tyrosine is produced by physiologic metabolic pathways and derives from hydroxyl-derived oxidation of phenylalanine. A significant correlation between the amount of oxygen given during resuscitation and the urinary elimination of ortho-tyrosine has been detected (Solberg et al. 2007); moreover, the increased antioxidant capacity of preterm human milk has also been assessed by this methodology (Ledo et al. 2009).

30.5.4 Intracellular Redox Status

A major marker of oxidative stress is the GSH/GSSG ratio which directly reflects changes in the intracellular redox status since, when oxidative stress exceeds the reductive capacity of GSH reductase, the cell loses glutathione, exporting the excess of oxidized glutathione (Njålsson and Norgren 2005). NPBI levels appear to be a very reliable marker of oxidative stress, particularly in newborns, as previously indicated. Measurements of ethane in expired air may also be useful in detecting oxidative stress (Halliwell and Whiteman 2004).

30.5.5 DNA Damage

Determination of oxidized bases of DNA has been carried out by HPLC coupled to MS/MS (Ledo et al. 2009).

30.5.6 Prevention of ROS Tissue Damage

Avoidance of conditions such as infections, asphyxia, hyperoxia, and retinal light exposure, under which excessive free radical release occurs, is the best defense against development of imbalances in pro-oxidant and antioxidant factors in the neonate. Frequent reports of NPBI in plasma of neonates suggest that indiscriminate iron supplementation should also be avoided.

The concept of optimal oxygenation of newborns has recently been revised in order to clarify whether the optimal oxygen saturation unanimously accepted for normal infants and adults is also the best for sick neonates, especially if premature. In an attempt to avoid the risk of tissue damage caused by ROS in the first hours of life, when susceptibility to oxidative stress is particularly high, the effects of O_2 were investigated. As previously reported, hyperoxia-induced lung injury has been demonstrated. Indications on the use of oxygen were reported by Chow et al. (Chow et al. 2003) in a 5-year study in a tertiary neonatal center where oxygen therapy was adjusted to optimize neonatal care and decrease the incidence of ROP. They recommended avoidance of repeated increase and decrease in FiO_2 in response to the oxygen saturation monitor and maintenance of oxygen saturation within "acceptable" limits. They also recommended setting an alarm for oxygen saturation below 85% and above 93% for newborns under 32 weeks of age. More recently, comparison of two populations of high-risk newborns kept at O_2 saturations of 88–98% and 70–90% showed a significant reduction in ROP in the group at lower O_2 saturation but no differences in mortality or morbidity (Tin and Gupta 2007). Data from clinical outcomes seem to demonstrate that low birth weight infants cared for with liberal approaches had more cognitive disability compared with those cared for with more restrictive approaches after 10 years (Tin and Gupta 2007). Data collected from the Oxford Vermont Network in extremely low birth newborns demonstrate significant lower incidence of chronic lung disease and ROP among babies carried with target oxygen saturation of <95% compared to those kept at more than 95% (Sun 2002). Shulze et al. (1995) did not observe signs of mismatch between systemic oxygen delivery and demand in low birth weight infants kept at 93–96% O_2 and 89–92% saturation. However, Poets et al. (Poets et al. 2003) reported higher incidence of ROP in infants <30 weeks' gestation using oxygen saturation limits of 80–92% in comparison with 92–97%. Therefore, the relationship between haemoglobin oxygen saturation, risk of oxidative stress, and oxygen toxicity is still a problem. This is presumably due to the complex mechanism of oxygen toxicity which may be expressed at different percentages of O_2 saturation under different conditions. Conventional indications suggest that optimal oxygen tension should be maintained between 50 and 70 mmHg (Wolkoff and Narula 2000). However, it should be taken into account that the ability of pulse oximetry to reliably detect hyperoxia remains controversial, and it has been shown that oxygen saturation of more than 90% can be associated with an arterial oxygen tension of more than 80 mmHg (Tin and Gupta 2007). Based on all the actually available evidence, the most prudent approach would be not to tolerate possible hypoxia and not accept SpO_2 values associated with potential hyperoxia in infants breathing supplemental oxygen. For infants breathing supplemental oxygen, setting the low alarm at 1% below the lower SpO_2 chosen in the clinically intended range has been suggested, but never <85%, and setting the high alarm at 1% above the higher SpO_2 chosen, but never more than 95%. For example, if the intended range is 91–94%, the alarms would be set at 90% and 95%. Finally, the delay time should not be longer than 20 sec, to ensure that significant events are not missed (Sola et al. 2014). It is imperative to control the low limit but also to increase compliance with the upper limit and avoid a flip-flop phenomenon that leads to acute and significant changes and fluctuations in SpO_2 (Bancalari and Claure 2012; Zapata et al. 2014).Recent guidance from the American Academy of Pediatrics Committee on Fetus and Newborn advises that "recent RCTs suggest that a targeted oxygen saturation range of 90% to 95% may be safer than 85% to 89%"

(Cummings and Polin 2016). The results from the Cochrane review concur with this conclusion (Askie et al. 2017). This metaanalysis of five randomised trials found no significant difference in the primary outcome of death or major disability in extremely preterm infants when targeting a lower (SpO 85% to 89%) versus higher (SpO 91% to 95%) oxygen saturation range. Compared with a higher target range, a lower target range significantly increased the incidence of death and necrotising enterocolitis. Conversely, targeting the lower range significantly decreased the incidence of severe or treated retinopathy of prematurity.

30.5.7 Protective Effect of Human Milk in the Preterm Infant

The antioxidant properties of human milk are reported widely in the literature. In a recent study, Friel et al. (2002) confirmed that human milk of term and of preterm mothers provided better antioxidant protection. They found that human milk produced less ascorbate whether or not oxidative stress was present. Elevated concentrations of ascorbate are pro-oxidant in the extracellular milieu. Moreover, the antioxidant enzyme activity of catalase, superoxide dismutase, and glutathione peroxidase increased with time in human milk. Additional studies have shown that human milk-fed neonates had a higher plasma total antioxidant and vitamin C content. Biomarkers of oxidative status, such as total peroxide and oxidative stress index, were higher in formula-fed neonates at 3–6 months' postnatal age (Aycicek et al. 2006). Human milk of preterm mothers at 35–36 weeks' post-conceptional age also seemed to have a positive effect on the oxidant status of their infants. In a recent study, preterm infants fed with preterm human milk have significantly lower elimination of markers of hydroxyl radical aggression to protein and DNA, meaning that they produce lower amounts of free radicals. Thus, in the clinical setting even in the acute stage, preterm infants should be fed early with human expressed milk, which offers an additional protection against free radicals (Ledo et al. 2009).

30.5.8 Antioxidants

Substances inhibiting phagocyte activation or xanthine oxidase and arachidonic acid metabolism, or decompartmentalizing free iron and making it available for the Fenton reaction, have also been investigated, together with those scavenging ROS directly or repairing ROS-induced membrane injury, like calcium antagonists and beta-blockers. The subject has been reviewed by Buonocore and Groenendal (2007). On the whole, the results obtained in newborns have been uncertain. Several antioxidant substances have been used in newborn animals and humans in an attempt to improve the worst prognosis of damage, presumed to be due to ROS. Many, such as superoxide dismutase (SOD), showed the same disadvantages in newborns. Other drugs, such as allopurinol and desferrioxamine, have shown good results in animals, but no advantages in human newborns.

Among the antioxidants, melatonin has a special place since it has been reported to have several interesting effects such as enhancement of antioxidant enzyme activities and neutralization of H2O2 singlet oxygen and peroxynitrite; it appears to scavenge OH• (Tan et al. 1993). Administration of melatonin has been reported to decrease the concentrations of pro-inflammatory cytokines and markers of oxidative stress in RDS and in septic newborns (Gitto et al. 2001, 2004). In animals, a study of Carloni et al. (2008) demonstrated that melatonin has long-lasting beneficial effects in cases of brain damage following hypoxia ischemia which occurs during development. However, the effects of the melatonin may be due to a combination of effects since the melatonin, in addition to the antioxidant effects, possesses also endocrine, autocrine, and paracrine activity and appears to decrease inflammation. Vitamin E is a powerful, widely tested antioxidant. Conclusions of a recent Cochrane review are that vitamin E supplementation to preterm infants reduces the risk of intracranial hemorrhage but increases the risk of sepsis; in very low birth weight infants, it seems to reduce the risk of retinopathy and blindness (Brion et al. 2003). There is no evidence to support the use of vitamin E at high doses or the aim of keeping serum tocopherol levels above 3.5 mg/dL (Silvers et al. 2001).

It should be remembered that some formulations of vitamin E are poorly adsorbed (Italian Collaborative Group on Preterm Delivery 1991).

The efficacy of lutein as an antioxidant agent has been confirmed in experimental and clinical studies, but its routine use is not recommended in perinatal period (Perrone et al. 2014). Innovative frontiers concerning lutein supplementation are orientated toward cardiometabolic health improvement and cognitive benefits (Perrone et al. 2016). Peroxidation products in stored lipid emulsions have been shown to increase lipid peroxidation in vivo in newborns and adults. Since parenteral nutrition has been associated with increased formation of ROS, it is necessary to protect intralipids from light and add vitamins (Pitkanen et al. 2004). Finally, although hyperbilirubinemia can be regarded as a natural antioxidant factor, the risk of brain damage due to high plasma levels of this molecule, particularly in premature babies, should not be underestimated.

30.6 Conclusions

The mechanism by which the oxidative stress is deeply involved in the development of several diseases of the fetus and newborn is complex and probably not yet fully understood. However, multiple observations strongly suggest that increased free radical and ROS play a considerable role as does the deficiency of antioxidants. In particular, hyperoxia and inflammation as well as the episode of hypoxia reoxygenation appear to be a source of increased ROS release which may cause tissue injury, particularly in the preterm infant, either by direct effect or as consequences of endothelium dysfunction.

References

Appleby C, Towner RA (2001) Magnetic resonance imaging of pulmonary damage in the term and premature rat neonate exposed to hyperoxia. Pediatr Res 50:502–507

Arneson KO, Roberts LJ 2nd (2007) Measurement of products of docosahexaenoic acid peroxidation, neuroprostanes, and neurofurans. Methods Enzymol 433:127–143

Asikainen TM, White CW (2004) Pulmonary antioxidant defenses in the preterm newborn with respiratory distress and bronchopulmonary dysplasia in evolution: implications for antioxidant therapy. Antioxid Redox Signal 6:155–167

Asikainen TM, Raivio KO, Saksela M, Kinnula VL (1998) Expression and developmental profile of antioxidant enzymes in human lung and liver. Am J Respir Cell Mol Biol 19:942–949

Askie LM, Darlow BA, Davis PG, Finer N, Stenson B, Vento M, Whyte R (2017) Effects of targeting lower versus higher arterial oxygen saturations on death or disability in preterm infants. Cochrane Database Syst Rev 4:CD011190

Aycicek A, Erel O, Kocyigit A et al (2006) Breast milk provides better antioxidant power than does formula. Nutrition 22:616–619

Bancalari E, Claure N (2012) Control of oxygenation during mechanical ventilation in the premature infant. Clin Perinatol 39:563–572

Berger HM, Mumby S, Gutteridge JMC (1995) Ferrous ions detected in iron-overloaded cord blood plasma from preterm and term babies: implications for oxidative stress. Free Radic Res 22:555–559

Bhandari V (2008) Molecular mechanism of hyperoxia induced acute lung injury. Front Biosci 13: 6653–6661

Bracci R, Buonocore G (2003) Chorioamnionitis: a risk factor for fetal and neonatal morbidity. Biol Neonate 83:85–96

Brion LP, Bell EF, Raghuveer TS (2003) Vitamin E supplementation for prevention of morbidity and mortality in preterm infants. Cochrane Database Syst Rev 3: CD003665

Buonocore G, Groenendal F (2007) Antioxidant strategy. Semin Fetal Neonatal Med 12:287–295

Buonocore G, Zani S, Perrone S et al (1998) Intraerythrocyte non protein bound iron and plasma malondialdehyde in the hypoxic newborn. Free Radic Biol Med 25:766–770

Buonocore G, Perrone S, Longini M et al (2000) Total hydroperoxide and advanced oxidation protein products in preterm hypoxic babies. Pediatr Res 47:221–224

Buonocore G, Perrone S, Bracci R (2001) Free radicals and brain damage in the newborn. Biol Neonate 79:180–186

Buonocore G, Perrone S, Longini M (2002) Oxidative stress in preterm neonate at birth and on seventh day of life. Pediatr Res 52:46–49

Buonocore G, Perrone S, Longini M et al (2003) Non protein bound iron as early predictive marker of neonatal brain damage. Brain 126:1224–1230

Carloni S, Perrone S, Buonocore G (2008) Melatonin protects from the long-term consequences of a neonatal hypoxic-ischemic brain injury in rats. J Pineal Res 44:157–164

Chandel NS, Shumacker PT (2000) Cellular oxygen sensing by mitochondria: old question, new insight. J Appl Physiol 88:1880–1889

Chang E, Hornick K, Fritz KI et al (2007) Effects of hyperoxia on cortical neuronal nuclear function and programmed cell death mechanism. Neurochem Res 32:1142–1149

Chow LC, Wright KW, Sola A et al (2003) Can changes in clinical practice decrease the incidence of severe retinopathy of prematurity in very low birth weight infants? Pediatrics 111:339–345

Ciccoli L, Rossi V, Leoncini S et al (2004) Iron release, superoxide production and binding of autologous IgG to band 3 dimers in newborn and adult erythrocytes exposed to hypoxia and hypoxia-reoxygenation. Biochim Biophys Acta 1672:203–213

Collins Y, Chouchani ET, James AM et al (2012) Mitochondrial redox signaling at a glance. J Cell Sci 125:801–806

Comporti M, Signorini C, Leoncini S et al (2004) Plasma F2-isoprostanes are elevated in newborns and inversely correlated to gestational age. Free Radic Biol Med 37:724–732

Cummings JJ, Polin RA (2016) Oxygen targeting in extremely low birth weight infants. Pediatrics 138(2): e20161576–e20161576

Denis D, Fayon MJ, Berger P et al (2001) Prolonged moderate hyperoxia induced hyperresponsiveness and airway inflammation in newborn rats. Pediatr Res 50:515–519

Dröse S, Brandt U (2012) Molecular mechanism of superoxide production by the mitochondrial respiratory chain. Adv Exp Med Biol 348:145–169

Drury JA, Jeffers G, Cooke RW (1998) Urinary 8-hydroxydeoxyguanosine in infants and children. Free Radic Res 28:423–428

Eiserich JP, Hristova M, Cross CE et al (1998) Formation of nitric oxide-derived inflammatory oxidants by myeloperoxidase in neutrophils. Nature 391:393–339

Evans PJ, Evans P, Kovar IZ et al (1992) Bleomycin-detectable iron in the plasma of premature and full-term neonates. FEBS Lett 303:210–212

Forman HJ, Fukuto JM, Miller T et al (2008) The chemistry of cell signaling by reactive oxygen species and nitrogen species and 4-hydroxynonenal. Arch Biochem Biophys 477:183–195

Frank L (1991) Developmental aspects of experimental pulmonary oxygen toxicity. Free Radic Biol Med 11:463–494. 52

Frank L, Sosenko IRS (1987) Prenatal development of lung antioxidant enzymes in four species. J Pediatr 110:106–110

Friel JK, Martin SM, Langdon M et al (2002) Milk from mothers of both premature and full-term infants provides better antioxidant protection than does infant formula. Pediatr Res 51:612–618

Friel JK, Friesen RW, Harding SV, Roberts LJ (2004) Evidence of oxidative stress in full-term healthy infants. Pediatr Res 56:878–882

Gitto E, Karbownik M, Reiter RJ et al (2001) Effects of melatonin treatment in septic newborns. Pediatr Res 50:756–760

Gitto E, Reiter RJ, Cordaro SP et al (2004) Oxidative and inflammatory parameters in respiratory distress syndrome of preterm newborns: beneficial effects of melatonin. Am J Perinatol 21:209–216

Gordon HH, Nitowsky HM, Cornblath M (1955) Studies of tocopherol deficiency in infants and children. I. Hemolysis of erythrocytes in hydrogen peroxide. Am J Dis Child 90:669–681

Gross RT, Bracci R, Rudolph N et al (1967) Hydrogen peroxide toxicity and detoxification in the erythrocytes of newborn infants. Blood 29:481–493

Halliday H (2008) Surfactant, past, present and future. J Perinatol 28(Suppl 1):S47–S56

Halliwell B (2007) Biochemistry of oxidative stress. Biochem Soc Trans 35:1147–1150

Halliwell B, Gutteridge JMC (1990) The antioxidants of human extracellular fluids. Arch Biochem Biophys 280:1–8

Halliwell B, Whiteman M (2004) Measuring reactive species and oxidative damage in vivo and in cell culture: how should you do it and what do the results mean? Br J Pharmacol 142:231–253

Halliwell B, Gutteridge JMC, Cross CE (1992) Free radicals, antioxidants, and human disease: where are we now? J Lab Clin Med 1:598–620

Hoffman DL, Brookes PS (2009) Oxygen sensitivity of mitochondrial reactive oxygen species generation depends on metabolic conditions. J Biol Chem 284:16236–16245

House JT, Schultetus RR, Gravenstein N (1987) Continuous neonatal evaluation in the delivery room by pulse oximetry. J Clin Monit 3:96–100

Indo HP, Yen HC, Nakanishi I, Matsumoto K, Tamura M, Nagano Y, Matsui H, Gusev O, Cornette R, Okuda T, Minamiyama Y, Ichikawa H, Suenaga S, Oki M, Sato T, Ozawa T, Clair DK, Majima HJ (2015) A mitochondrial superoxide theory for oxidative stress diseases and aging. J Clin Biochem Nutr 56:1–7

Italian Collaborative Group on Preterm Delivery (1991) Absorption of intramuscular vitamin E in premature babies. Dev Pharmacol Ther 16:13–21

Jankov RP, Negus A, Tanswell AK (2001) Antioxidants as therapy in the newborn: some words of caution. Pediatr Res 50:681–687

Kalogeris T, Bao Y, Korthuis RJ (2014) Mitochondrial reactive oxygen species: a double edge sword in ischemia/reperfusion vs preconditioning. Redox Biol 2:702–714

Kaludercic N, Deshwal S, Dilisa F (2014) Reactive oxygen species and compartmentalization. Front Physiol 5:1–15

Koenig JM, Yoder MC (2004) Neonatal neutrophils: the good, the bad and the ugly. Clin Perinatol 31:39–51

Kohlhaas M, Maack C (2013) Calcium release microdomains and mitochondria. Cardiovasc Res 98:259–268

Kotecha S, Chan B, Azam N et al (1995) Increase in interleukin-8 and soluble intercellular adhesion molecule-1 in bronchoalveolar lavage fluid from premature infants who develop chronic lung disease. Arch Dis Child 72:F90–F96

de La Torre A, Lee YY, Oger C, Sangild PT, Durand T, Lee JC, Galano JM (2014) Synthesis, discovery, and quantitation of dihomo-isofurans: biomarkers for in vivo adrenic acid peroxidation. Angew Chem Int Ed Engl 53:6249–6252

Lambeth JD, Neish AS (2014) Nox enzymes and new thinking on reactive oxygen: a double-edged sword revised. Annu Rev Pathol 9:119–145

Langie Sabine AS, Pawel K, Barbara T et al (2010) The effect of oxidative stress on nucleotide-excision repair in colon tissue of newborn piglets. Mutat Res 695(1–2):75–80

Ledo A, Arduini A, Asensi MA et al (2009) Human milk enhances antioxidant defenses against hydroxyl radical aggression in preterm infants. Am J Clin Nutr 89:210–215

Li JM, Shah AM (2004) Endothelial cell superoxide generation: regulation and relevance for cardiovascular pathophysiology. Am J Physiol Integr Comp Phys 287:R1014–R1030

Lindeman JHN, Lentjes EG, van Zoeren-Grobben D et al (2000) Postnatal changes in plasma ceruloplasmin and transferrin antioxidant activities in preterm babies. Biol Neonate 78:73–76

Lismont C, Nordorem M, Van Veldohoven PP, Fransen M (2015) Redox interplay between mitochondria ad peroxisomes. Front Cell Dev Biol 3:1–19

Longini M, Perrone S, Kenanidis A et al (2005) Isoprostanes in amniotic fluid: a predictive marker for fetal growth restriction in pregnancy. Free Radic Biol Med 38:1537–1541

Lubec G, Widness JA, Hayde M et al (1997) Hydroxyl radical generation in oxygen-treated infants. Pediatrics 100:700–704

Marseglia L, D'Angelo G, Manti S et al (2014) Oxidative mediated aging during the fetal and perinatal period. Oxidative Med Cell Longev 2014:1–8

Martín JA, Pereda J, Martínez-López I et al (2007) Oxidative stress as a signal to up-regulate gamma-cystathionase in the fetal to neonatal transition in rats. Cell Mol Biol (Noisy-le-Grand) 53(Suppl): OL1010–OL1017

Marzocchi B, Perrone S, Paffetti P et al (2005) Non protein bound and plasma protein oxidant stress at birth. Pediatr Res 58:1–5

Menshicova F, Tkachev V, Zencov N (2010) Redox-dependent signaling system Nrf2/ARE in inflammation. Mol Biol 44(343):57

Mikami T, Kita K, Tomita S et al (2000) Is allantoin in serum and urine a useful indicator of exercise-induced oxidative stress in humans? Free Radic Res 32:235–244

Milne GL, Yin H, Hardy KD, Davies SS, Roberts LJ II (2011) Isoprostane generation and function. Chem Rev 111:5973–5996

Murphy MP (2009) How mitochondria produce reactive oxygen species. Biochem J 417:1–13

Njålsson R, Norgren S (2005) Physiological and pathological aspects of GSH metabolism. Acta Paediatr 94:132–137

Patz A, Hoeck I, de la Cruz E (1952) Studies on the effect of high oxygen administration in retrolental fibroplasia. Am J Ophthalmol 35:1248–1253

Pereira RD, De Long NE, Wang R et al (2015) Angiogenesis in the placenta: the role of reactive oxygen species signaling. Biomed Res Int 2015:814543

Perrone S, Tatarrano ML, Negro S, Longini M et al (2010) Early identification of the risk for free radical-related diseases in preterm newborns. Early Hum Dev 86:241–244

Perrone S, Tei M, Longini M, Santacroce A, Turrisi G, Proietti F, Felici C, Picardi A, Bazzini F, Vasarri P, Buonocore G (2014) Lipid and protein oxidation in newborn infants after lutein administration. Oxidative Med Cell Longev 2014:781454

Perrone S, Tei M, Longini M, Buonocore G (2016) The multiple facets of lutein: a call for further investigation in the perinatal period. Oxidative Med Cell Longev 2016:5381540

Pitkanen OM, Luukkainen P, Andersson S (2004) Attenuated lipid peroxidation in preterm infants during subsequent doses of intravenous lipids. Biol Neonate 85:184–187

Poets C, Arand J, Hummler H et al (2003) Retinopathy of prematurity: a comparison between two centers aiming for different pulse oximetry saturation levels. Biol Neonate 84:A267

Poggi C, Dani C (2014) Antioxidant strategy and respiratory disease of the preterm newborn: an update. Oxidative Med Cell Longev 2014:1–10

Richter J, Toelen J, Nagatomo T, Jimenez J, Vanoirbeek J, Deprest J (2016) Transplacental administration of rosiglitazone attenuates hyperoxic lung injury in a preterm rabbit model. Fetal Diagn Ther 39(4):297–305

Rogers S, Witz G, Anwar M et al (2000) Antioxidant capacity and oxygen radical diseases in the preterm newborn. Arch Pediatr Adolesc Med 154:544–548

Saugstad OD (2005) Oxidative stress in the newborn – a 30-year perspective. Biol Neonate 88:228–236

Schulze A, White K, Way RC et al (1995) Effect of the arterial oxygenation level on cardiac output, oxygen extraction, and oxygen consumption in low birth weight infants receiving mechanical ventilation. J Pediatr 126:777–784

Sejersted Y, Aasland AL, Bjørås M, Eide L, Saugstad OD (2009) Accumulation of 8-oxoguanine in liver DNA during hyperoxic resuscitation of newborn mice. Pediatr Res 66:533–538

Semenza GL, Prabhakar NR (2012) The role of hypoxia-inducible factors in oxygen sensing by the carotid body. Adv Exp Med Biol 758:1–5

Sies H (1991) Role of reactive oxygen species in biological processes. Klin Wochenschr 69:965–968

Signorini C, Perrone S, Sgherri C (2008) Plasma esterified F2-Isoprostanes and oxidative stress in newborns: role of non protein bound iron. Pediatr Res 63:287–291

Silvers KM, Sluis KB, Darlow BA et al (2001) Limiting light-induced lipid peroxidation and vitamin loss in infant parenteral nutrition by adding multivitamin preparations to Intralipid. Acta Pediatr 90:242–249

Smith JL (1899) The pathological effects due to increase of oxygen tension in the air breathed. J Physiol 24:19–35

Smith CV, Hansen TN, Martin NE et al (1993) Oxidant stress responses in premature infants during exposure to hyperoxia. Pediatr Res 34:360–365

Sola A, Golombek SG, Montes Bueno MT et al (2014) Safe oxygen saturation targeting and monitoring in preterm infants: can we avoid hypoxia and hyperoxia? Acta Paediatr 103:1009. ISSN 0803-5253

Solberg R, Andresen JH, Escrig R et al (2007) Resuscitation of hypoxic newborn piglets with oxygen induces a dose dependent increase in markers of oxidative stress. Pediatr Res 62:559–563

Solberg R, Longini M, Proietti F, Vezzosi P, Saugstad OD, Buonocore G (2012) Resuscitation with supplementary oxygen induces oxidative injury in the cerebral cortex. Free Radic Biol Med 53:1061–1067

Song WL, Lawson JA, Reilly D, Rokach J, Chang CT, Giasson B, GA FG (2008) Neurofurans, novel indices of oxidant stress derived from docosahexaenoic acid. J Biol Chem 283:6–16

Sun SC (2002) Relation of target SpO_2 levels and clinical outcome in ELBW infants on supplemental oxygen. Pediatr Res 51:A350

Tan DX, Chen LD, Poeggeler B et al (1993) Melatonin: a potent, endogenous hydroxyl radical scavenger. Endocr J 1:57–66

Tataranno ML, Perrone S, Buonocore G (2015) Plasma biomarkers of oxidative stress in neonatal brain injury. Clin Perinatol 42(3):529–539

Tiina MA, Kari OR, Mika S, Vuokko LK (1998) Expression and development profile of antioxidant enzymes in human lung and liver. Am J Respir Cell Mol Biol 19:942–949

Tin W, Gupta S (2007) Optimum oxygen therapy in preterm babies. Arch Dis Child Fetal Neonatal Ed 92: F143–F147

Torday JS, Rehan VK (2016) On the evolution of the pulmonary alveolar lipofibroblast. Exp Cell Res 340(2):215–219

Ullrich V, Bachscmid M (2000) Superoxide as a messenger of endothelial function. Biochem Biophys Res Commun 278:1–8

Vento M (2014) Oxygen supplementation in the neonatal period: changing the paradigm. Neonatology 105(4): 323–331

Vento M, Asensi M, Sastre J et al (2002) Hyperoxemia caused by resuscitation with pure oxygen may alter intracellular redox status by increasing oxidized glutathione in asphyxiated newly born infants. Semin Perinatol 26:406–410

Vento M, Aguar M, Escobar J et al (2009a) Antenatal steroids and antioxidant enzyme activity in preterm infants: influence of gender and timing. Antioxid Redox Signal 11:2945–2955

Vento M, Moro M, Escrig R et al (2009b) Preterm resuscitation with low oxygen causes less oxidative stress, inflammation, and chronic lung disease. Pediatrics 124:439–449

Viña J, Vento M, Garcia-Sala F et al (1995) L-cysteine and glutathione metabolism are impaired in premature infants due to a cystathionase deficiency. Am J Clin Nutr 61:1067–1069

Wolkoff LI, Narula P (2000) Issue in neonatal and pediatric oxygen therapy. Respir Care Clin N Am 6: 675–691

Yeung MY (2006) Influence of early postnatal nutritional management on oxidative stress and antioxidant defence in extreme prematurity. Acta Paediatr 95:153–163

Yuan G, Peng YJ, Reddy VD et al (2013) Mutual antagonism between hypoxia-inducible factors 1á and 2 á regulates oxygen sensing and cardiorespiratory homeostasis. Proc Natl Acad Sci 110: E1788–E1796

Zapata J, Gomez JJ, Araque Campo R, Matiz Rubio A, Sola A (2014) A randomised controlled trial of an automated oxygen delivery algorithm for preterm neonates receiving supplemental oxygen without mechanical ventilation. Acta Paediatr 103:928

Zorov DB, Juhaazova M, Sollott SJ (2014) Mitochondrial reactive oxygen species (ROS) and ROS-induced ROS release. Physiol Rev 94:909950

Physical Examination of the Newborn

31

Alessandra Coscia, Paola Di Nicola, Enrico Bertino, and Claudio Fabris

Contents

A. Coscia (✉) · P. Di Nicola · E. Bertino · C. Fabris
Neonatal Unit, University of Turin, Turin, Italy
e-mail: alessandra.coscia@unito.it;
paola_dinicola@hotmail.it; enrico.bertino@unito.it;
claudio.fabris@unito.it

G. Buonocore et al. (eds.), *Neonatology*,
https://doi.org/10.1007/978-3-319-29489-6_181

Abstract

A complete physical examination of every newborn should be performed within 24 h from birth: although there is not international standard, routine examination is regarded as a good practice in the guidelines for postnatal care.

Aims of the routine neonatal examination are to detect problems arising from maternal or familiar diseases; to confirm or not some conditions suspected during antenatal period; to detect any acute condition requiring urgent diagnosis and therapy; to diagnose congenital problems not already identified at birth; to screen some specific conditions, such as developmental dysplasia of the hip and congenital cataract; and to provide initial health and educational advice for the newborn. In any case, routine examination may be an opportunity for the healthcare provider to discuss with the parents any questions or worries about their baby, to reassure them and to give them appropriate advice.

31.1 Salient Points

- The initial examination of the newborn is an important opportunity to detect congenital anomalies and assess the infants' transition from fetal to extra-uterine life.
- Risk factors such as pre- and post-term birth, small for gestational age and large for gestational age, all have associated clinical medical challenges of which providers should be aware.
- Although a rapid check of the newborn takes place immediately after birth, every newborn should have at least one complete examination before discharge, usually within 24 h of life.
- It would be better first to perform a general "gestalt," whole inspection, and then continue with a systematic physical examination. The healthcare provider must make sure he has not omitted any item, and he must record all the findings.

A complete physical examination of every newborn should be performed within 24 h from birth: although there is not international standard, routine examination is regarded as a good practice in the guidelines for postnatal care (Royal College of Anaesthetists et al. 2007; Demott et al. 2006; Royal College of Obstetricians and Gynaecologists 2016).

On this purpose, some questions are needed to be answered.

31.2 Why Should Routine Physical Examination Be Performed?

Aims of the routine neonatal examination are:

1. To detect problems arising from maternal or familiar diseases or from complications of labour and delivery
2. To confirm or not some conditions suspected during antenatal period (e.g., congenital malformations) and to provide information about management
3. To detect any acute condition requiring urgent diagnosis and therapy
4. To diagnose congenital problems not already identified at birth (e.g., congenital heart disease, developmental dysplasia of the hip)
5. To screen some specific conditions, such as developmental dysplasia of the hip and congenital cataract
6. To provide initial health and educational advice for the newborn (e.g., breastfeeding, SIDS prevention, late HDN prevention, safe transport in cars, vaccination)

In any case, routine examination may be an opportunity for the healthcare provider to discuss with the parents any questions or worries about their baby, to reassure them and to give them appropriate advice.

31.3 Who Should Perform Physical Examination?

A complete physical examination of the newborn should be performed by a trained healthcare provider, usually by a neonatologist. However in some countries (e.g., UK), other professionals have recently begun to look after the baby's examination, such as neonatal nurse practitioners or experienced midwives, and the satisfaction level of mothers is usually very high (Wolke et al. 2002).

31.4 When Physical Examination Should Be Performed?

Although a rapid check of the newborn takes place immediately after birth, every newborn should have at least one complete examination before discharge, usually within 24 h of life.

31.5 Where to Perform Physical Examination?

The first quick examination should be performed immediately after birth, in the delivery room. This first step, mainly based on inspection, should check that the infant looks well and there are no pathological conditions requiring information to the parents (e.g., congenital malformations or any doubt about the baby's gender) or immediate management (e.g., respiratory distress).

Complete routine examination should be performed in presence of the mother or both parents, in a quiet warm room, with adequate lighting.

31.6 Full Examination

Before introducing himself to the mother, the healthcare provider must check basic information regarding maternal (e.g., maternal age, socioeconomical status, smoking, drug or alcohol abuse, any chronic disease) and family history, previous obstetric history. It is very important to inquire if there were any complications in current pregnancy and to know the results of pregnancy screening tests and diagnostic procedures (e.g., ultrasound examinations, amniocentesis). It is necessary to get information about problems during labor and delivery, as well as about baby's gender, birthweight, and gestational age. All these items should be collected in the infant's medical record.

The newborn can be properly examined only without clothes except the nappy.

31.7 In Which Order Examination Should Be Performed?

There is not any strict rule regarding the order of the examination, but some tips can be given. It would be better first to perform a general "gestalt," whole inspection, and then continue with a systematic review (e.g., from head to foot), as well as take advantage of any period of quiet or sleeping to check the anterior fontanelle, to examine the eyes, and to perform the auscultation of the heart and the lungs and the palpation of the abdomen. It is better to leave the examination of the hips at the end, because the Ortolani-Barlow test is unpleasant for the newborn.

Regardless the order of examination, the healthcare provider must make sure he has not omitted any item, and he must record all the findings. A suggested sequence is given below:

1. General observation, including posture, tone, and movements
2. Measurement of head circumference, length, and recording them, together with the weight
3. Skin (color and characteristics)
4. Head (facial appearance, fontanelle)
5. Examination and auscultation of heart and lungs
6. Femoral pulses
7. Palpation of abdomen
8. Eyes, ears, nose, and mouth
9. Neck, including the clavicles
10. Arms, hands, legs, and feet
11. Genitalia and anus
12. Evaluation of nervous system
13. Hips
14. Prone position: back and spine

31.8 What Should Be Examined?

Many conditions that can be observed during the examination are very common, and they have little clinical importance or usually resolve spontaneously. On the other hand, there are some conditions, less frequent, that require further investigation or urgent therapy.

31.8.1 General Observation and Measurements

General observation includes weight, length, and head circumference measurements. These variables must be evaluated using standardized instruments and following the techniques required for accurate measurements as described by Cameron (Cameron 2004).

Values obtained should be plotted on appropriate neonatal anthropometric charts such as the new international standards (Intergrowth-21st project) (Villar et al. 2014).

If there is any doubt regarding gestational age, it should be determined by a scoring scheme (Dubowitz and Dubowitz 1981; Ballard et al. 1991) (Fig. 1).

Simple observation allows to notice short arms and legs that can indicate the presence of skeletal dysplasia.

Healthy term babies spend most time in quiet or active sleep, but transition between behavioral states can be rapid: crying is a usual finding during the examination (Brazelton 1973). Healthy full-term infant usually lies in flexion position (flexion of the arms at the elbows and of the legs at the knees), with a relatively symmetric limb position and posturing: however, the presentation at birth can influence posture in the first days of life. Asymmetric tonic neck reflex can be noted if the head is turned to one side: in this case, there is extension of the ipsilateral arm and leg and flexion of the contralateral extremities. Infants manifest spontaneous motor activity that consists in moving their limbs in an alternating fashion (Swaiman 1999).

31.8.2 Skin

The skin of a healthy newborn should be reddish pink, but peripheral cyanosis (hands, feet, and circumoral area) is a common finding during the first 48 h, as well as traumatic cyanosis, often associated with petechiae, affecting presenting part.

Some conditions may be present:

- Central cyanosis. It is best observed on the tongue and it requires urgent investigation for pulmonary disease or congenital heart malformations. Plethoric newborns can appear cyanotic because they have more than 5 g per 100 ml of reduced hemoglobin.
- Pallor. When generalized it can be associated with anemia or shock.
- Jaundice. Jaundice appearing within the first 24 h of life most indicates hemolysis and requires further investigation and treatment.
- Capillary hemangioma (stork bites). These pink macules appear on the upper eyelids, the mid forehead, and the nape of the neck: those on the forehead and eyelids disappear or fade over the first year, whereas those on the neck are covered with hair (Fig. 2).
- Neonatal urticaria (erythema toxicum neonatorum). White papules appear on an erythematous skin, usually on the second or third day of life, and migrate to different sites.
- Milia. Retention of keratin and sebum may cause these benign white cysts distributed on the nose and cheeks.
- Mongolian blue spots. They are blue-black maculae, more frequent in African-American or Asian babies, located at the base of the spine or on the buttocks and in some cases also on the legs or in other parts. They fade slowly over the first few years of life (Fig. 3).
- Harlequin color change. This is a vasomotor instability which causes a longitudinal reddening down one half of the body and a blanching down the other side.
- Edema. It may be generalized or localized: if present, it is always pathologic in the newborn. Pedal edema may be a sign of Turner syndrome (Fig. 4).

Neuromuscular Maturity

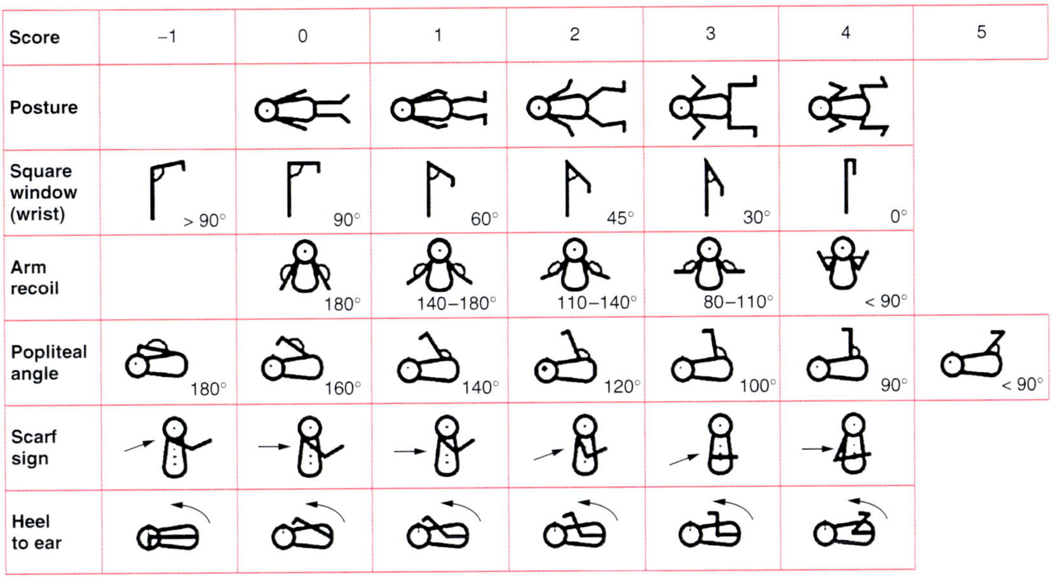

Score	−1	0	1	2	3	4	5
Posture							
Square window (wrist)	> 90°	90°	60°	45°	30°	0°	
Arm recoil		180°	140–180°	110–140°	80–110°	< 90°	
Popliteal angle	180°	160°	140°	120°	100°	90°	< 90°
Scarf sign							
Heel to ear							

Physical Maturity

	−1	0	1	2	3	4	5
Skin	Sticky, friable, transparent	Gelatinous, red, translucent	Smooth, pink; visible veins	Superficial peeling and/or rash; few veins	Cracking, pale areas; rare veins	Parchment, deep cracking; no vessels	Leathery, cracked, wrinkled
Lanugo	None	Sparse	Abundant	Thinning	Bald areas	Mostly bald	
Plantar surface	Heel-toe 40–50 mm: −1 < 40 mm: −2	> 50 mm, no crease	Faint red marks	Anterior transverse crease only	Creases anterior 2/3	Creases over entire sole	
Breast	Imperceptible	Barely perceptible	Flat areola, no bud	Stippled areola, 1–2 mm bud	Raised areola, 3–4 mm bud	Full areola, 5–10 mm bud	
Eye/Ear	Lids fused loosely: −1 tightly: −2	Lids open; pinna flat; stays folded	Slightly curved pinna; soft; slow recoil	Well curved pinna; soft but ready recoil	Formed and firm, instant recoil	Thick cartilage, ear stiff	
Genitals (male)	Scrotum flat, smooth	Scrotum empty, faint rugae	Testes in upper canal, rare rugae	Testes desoending, few rugae	Testes down, good rugae	Testes pendulous, deep rugae	
Genitals (female)	Clitoris prominent, labia flat	Clitoris prominent, small labia minora	Clitoris prominent, enlarging minora	Majora and minora equally prominent	Majora large, minora small	Majora cover citoris and minora	

Maturity Rating

Score	Weeks
−10	20
−5	22
0	24
5	26
10	28
15	30
20	32
25	34
30	36
35	38
40	40
45	42
50	44

Fig. 1 Assessment of gestational age by revised Ballard method (From Ballard et al. 1991)

– Port-wine stain (nevus flammeus). They are a vascular malformation of the capillaries in the dermis, and they are usually evident at birth, whereas strawberry nevi (cavernous hemangioma) appear only after 1 or 2 months of life. When port-wine stain affects distribution of the trigeminal nerve, it may suggest underlying intracranial vascular malformations (Sturge-Weber syndrome), whereas large lesions on the limbs may be associated with

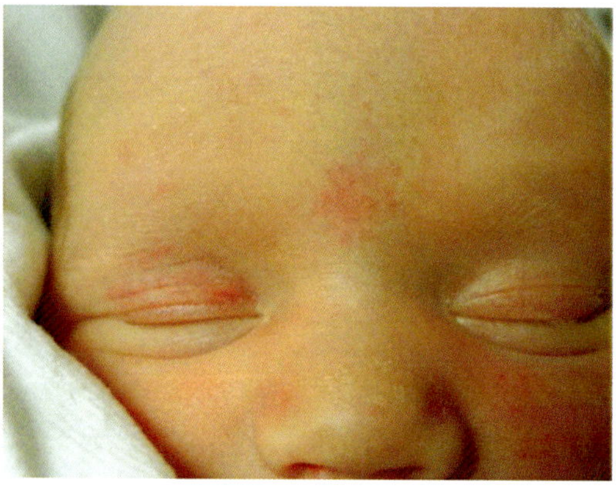

Fig. 2 Capillary haemangioma (stork bites)

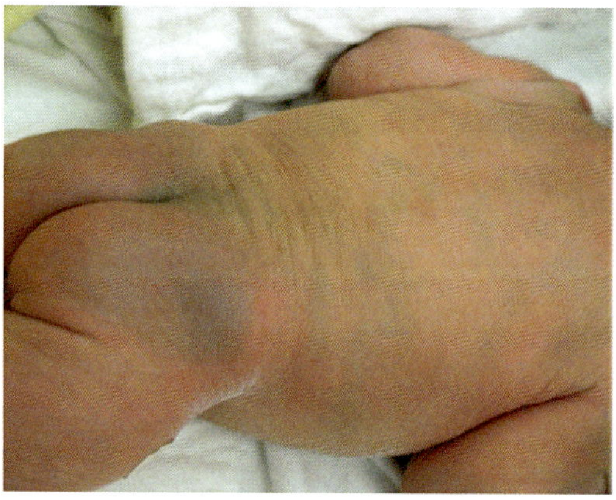

Fig. 3 Mongolian blue spots

bone hypertrophy (Klippel-Trénaunay syndrome).

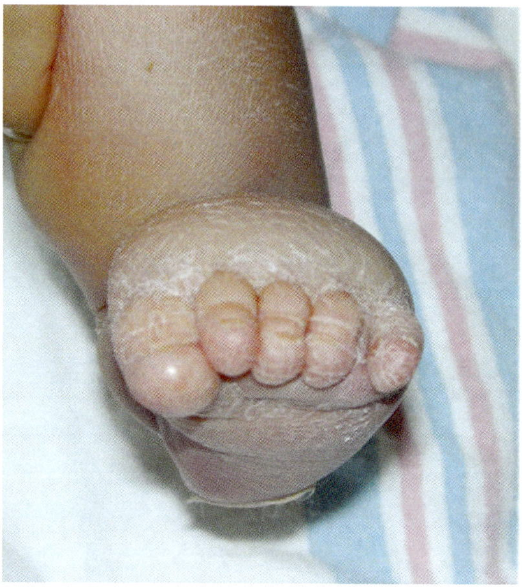

Fig. 4 Pedal oedema in Turner syndrome

31.8.3 Head and Face

Head dimensions and shape should be evaluated, and fontanelle and sutures should be palpated. The head can be considerably molded during labor and delivery. Babies in the breech presentation in utero often have the so-called breech head (prominent occipital shelf).

There may be some transient phenomena:

- **Bruising and abrasions** from the use of forceps, vacuum extractor, or scalp electrodes

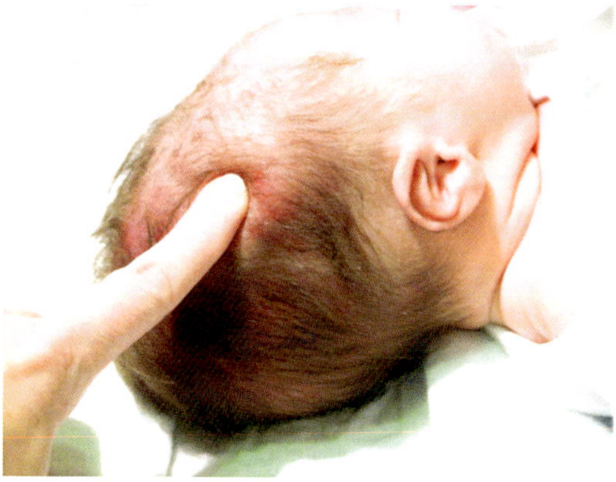

Fig. 5 Caput succedaneum

- **Caput succedaneum,** edema and bruising of the presented part, that extends beyond the sutures (Fig. 5)
- **Cephalhematoma,** collection of blood between the periosteum and the skull bone, that does not extend beyond the sutures and usually affects parietal bone

Anterior fontanelle can measure up to 3×3 cm, but its dimension can be variable: its tension (when the baby is not crying) may indicate raised intracranial pressure, from cerebral edema, intracranial hemorrhage, hydrocephalus, or meningitis.

After delivery, the coronal sutures are often overriding, but ridging at the suture lines implies premature fusion of the sutures (craniosynostosis).

Asymmetrie is a frequent finding due to pressure in utero and during labor and delivery.

Palpation of the skull bones can evidence areas of craniotabes, caused by pressure in utero from maternal pelvis, that occur in 2% of normal full-term newborns and more frequently in the preterm baby.

Cutis aplasia (small defect of the scalp) is a congenital malformation with risk of bleeding or infection of dural venous sinuses, and it may be a clue to the presence of a syndrome.

Most newborns resemble one or other parent, but when the face appears unusual, the examiner should search for other dysmorphic manifestations, to exclude a syndrome.

31.8.4 Ears

General shape, size, and position have to be evaluated. Malformations can be associated with hearing loss and require hearing check. Preauricular pits, skin tags anterior to the ear, and accessory auricles may be associated with an increased risk of renal abnormalities (Kugelman et al. 1997, 2002).

Low-set ears (when the top of the pinna falls below a line drawn from the outer canthus of the eye at right angles to the face) are a characteristic of several syndromes.

31.8.5 Nose

Newborns have to breathe through the nose, so complete nasal obstruction (i.e., from choanal atresia) causes intense respiratory distress and requires prompt investigation and treatment. If there is any doubt, a fine catheter should be passed through each nostril to ensure that both nares are patent.

Flaring of the alae nasi is always abnormal and indicates the presence of respiratory distress that requires further investigation.

31.8.6 Eyes

The eyes should be examined both by inspection and with an ophthalmoscope. If the lens is opaque from a congenital cataract or glaucoma, the red reflex cannot be elicited: any abnormality of the red reflex requires urgent evaluation by an ophthalmologist. Congenital cataract is the commonest form of preventable childhood blindness.

Swelling of the eyelids is common; a mucoid discharge ("sticky eye") is often present in the first 2 days of life and usually resolves spontaneously. A purulent discharge, accompanied by redness and swelling of the eyelids, requires microbiological investigation and treatment.

Subconjunctival hemorrhages are very common due to delivery and usually resolve within 1 to 2 weeks.

The iris is normally blue or gray in the newborn. Partial defect is called "colobomata," and it could be associated with a defect in the retina; complete absence is called "aniridia," and it is associated with an increased risk of Wilms tumor.

Size of the cornea has to be checked: if the corneal diameter is greater than 13 mm, there might be a congenital glaucoma.

31.8.7 Mouth

Direct inspection of the inside of the mouth is important, in order to exclude cleft palate, even mild defects (submucous cleft or posterior cleft palate).

Other harmless findings may be seen, including Epstein pearls (small white pearls of microkeratosis along the midline of the palate), mucus-retentioncysts of the gums (epulis) or on the floor of the mouth (ranula), and short frenulum ("tongue tie"). These conditions usually do not need treatment. Natal teeth (rare in Caucasian race) are best removed.

31.8.8 Neck

The newborn has a relatively short neck, but a very short neck may indicate abnormalities of the cervical spine (Klippel-Feil syndrome). A webbed neck is one of the characteristics of Turner syndrome, and posterior redundant skin may suggest Down's syndrome. Palpation of sternomastoid muscle can evidence "tumors," caused by bleeding or ischemia, sometimes resulting in fibrosis.

Clavicle fractures may occur during delivery with shoulder dystocia: it is possible to palpate a lump on the clavicle that results from a callus around the fracture and usually recovers without treatment.

31.8.9 Examination of Chest and Auscultation of the Heart and Lungs

A certain degree of breast enlargement is normal in newborns of either sex, and a few drops of milk ("witch's milk") may be discharged.

Neonatal routine examination detects only a half of the infants with congenital heart disease (CHD), even if the baby has significant structural heart lesion. At birth, the pressure difference between left and right side may be still low and then newborns with ventricular septal defects might not have a heart murmur.

Moreover, ductus-dependent lesions can present symptoms only a few days after birth, and femoral pulses are often palpable at first examination (Wren et al. 1999; Farrer and Rennie 2003).

Cardiorespiratory state can be deducted by simple inspection (respiratory rate and signs of respiratory distress, such as retractions or grunting). If cyanosis is present, pulse oximetry should be performed.

Normal respiratory rate is 40–60 breaths/min: if a baby has a rate persistently above 55/min, he needs to be carefully evaluated. In a full-term newborn, there should be no grunting, no retractions, and no flaring of the alae nasi: if present, they are symptoms of respiratory distress.

Palpation of the precordium may detect thrills or a pronounced ventricular heave.

Peripheral pulses, in particular femoral pulses, should be always palpated: patent ductus arteriosus produces a bounding pulse, whereas absence or difficulty to feel femoral pulses suggests coarctation. If coarctation is suspected, it can be confirmed by comparing blood pressure in the arms and legs: a difference of 20 mmHg or more suggests coarctation.

A heart murmur may be heard, but most are innocent: 60% of normal newborns have a systolic murmur at 2 h of life: the origin of an innocent murmur may be the acute angle at the pulmonary artery bifurcation, or patent ductus arteriosus, or tricuspid regurgitation (Ainsworth et al. 1999). Features that suggest a significant murmur are the following (McCrindle et al. 1996):

- Pansystolic
- $\geq 3/6$
- Harsh quality
- Best heard in the upper left sternal border
- Abnormal second heart sound
- Difficulty to feel femoral pulses

ECG or chest XR rarely changes clinical diagnosis (Smythe et al. 1990). Due to the availability of the ultrasound evaluation, this evaluation, with an expert consultation, should be performed in any infant with a suspected significant murmur.

Abnormal findings upon physical examination in the newborn nursery that are consistent with a differential diagnosis of congenital heart disease (CHD), including the presence of murmurs, tachypnea, and overt cyanosis, are not always present prior to discharge from the hospital (Mahle et al. 2009).

Physical examination alone has an approximated 50% sensitivity for CHD (Goldstein 2013).

Riede et al. (2010) found that in screening for CHD, pulse oximetry had a sensitivity and specificity of 77.78% and 99.90%, respectively. Pulse oximetry is found to be very effective in early identification of CHD in which hypoxemia is characteristic, such as hypoplastic left heart syndrome, pulmonary atresia with an intact septum, tetralogy of Fallot, total anomalous pulmonary venous return, transposition of the great arteries, tricuspid atresia, and truncus arteriosus (Mahle et al. 2009; Centers for Disease Control and Prevention (CDC) 2013c). It is not as effective in the early identification of CHD that may present without hypoxemia, such as aortic arch atresia or hypoplasia, coarctation of the aorta, interrupted aortic arch, double-outlet right ventricle, Ebstein anomaly, pulmonary stenosis, atrioventricular septal defect, and ventricular septal defect: these are considered secondary targets of pulse oximetry CHD screening in newborns (Mahle et al. 2009; Centers for Disease Control and Prevention (CDC) 2013c).

Given this, there is no consensus about the use of pulse oximetry as routine clinical practice.

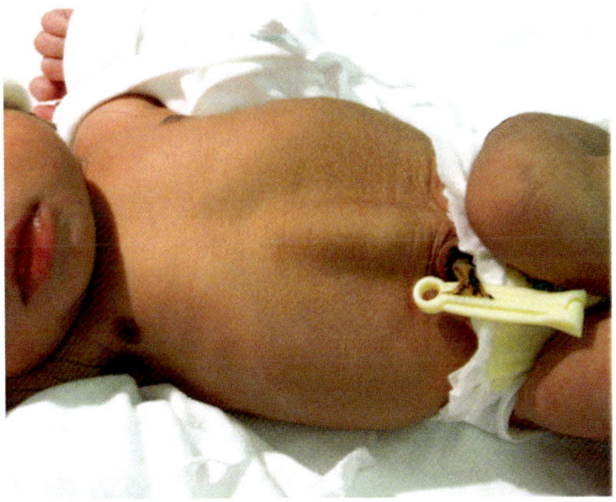

Fig. 6 Diastasis of the recti muscles

31.8.10 Abdomen

Simple observation may reveal any anomaly. Umbilicus is a common source of infection, so any discharge or redding of the skin requires attention.

A single umbilical artery occurs in 0.3% of newborns, and it is associated with an increased risk of congenital malformations, in particular renal abnormalities. Ultrasound of renal tract is probably only reserved for babies who have other problems, other than single umbilical artery (Thummala et al. 1998).

An umbilical hernia is a common finding, especially in African-American babies.

A diastasis of the recti is frequently appreciated by palpation; the liver edge is usually palpable 1 to 2 cm below the right costal margin (Fig. 6). Also the spleen tip and the kidney are palpable: it is important to detect abnormal renal mass or enlargement of the bladder that may be a sign of urinary outflow obstruction in a male infant.

31.8.11 Genitalia

31.8.11.1 Male

Hydroceles occur very frequently in neonatal period and usually resolve spontaneously. Inguinal herniae are common, in particular in preterm babies. The penis should be checked for length (usually about 3 cm) and position of urethral meatus. Sometimes penis looks short, but a normal organ is buried in sovrapubic fat. An abnormal position of urethral meatus indicates a hypospadia (glandular, coronal, mid-shaft, or perineal): ventral curvature reveals the presence of a chordee. Glandular hypospadia without chordee does not require any treatment.

In a full-term baby, testes should be palpable, but about 6% of newborns have one testis undescended at birth: if at 3 months of age the testis is still undescended, a pediatric surgeon or urologist should be consulted.

Neonatal testicular torsion usually occurs before birth: neonatologists should consult a pediatric surgeon, although the testis has usually already undergone infarction (Driver and Losty 1998).

31.8.11.2 Female

At full term, the labia majora cover the labia minora; in preterm baby the clitoris and the labia minora appear prominent. There is often a white or bloodstained discharge, due to maternal hormone withdrawal. Small hymenal skin tags, mucoid cysts, or a ring of vaginal mucosa are common.

The position and the tone of the anus must be checked, and passage of meconium should be recorded.

31.8.12 Spine

Swelling, dimple, hairy patch, or nevus along the spine or over the base of the skull might indicate underlying vertebral, spinal cord, or brain anomalies. Simple sacrococcygeal pits are common and harmless; simple dimples (less than 2.5 cm from the anus, less than 5 mm wide, without other cutaneous signs) do not indicate occult dysraphism (Gibson et al. 1995; Kriss and Desai 1998; Medina et al. 2001).

31.8.13 Limbs

Extremities are examined to inspect shape, posture, symmetry and size. About 45% of individuals with Down's syndrome have single transverse palmar creases, but the same finding may occur in 4% of the Caucasian and in 16.8% of the Chinese population. Polydactyly is often a familial trait, but it may be caused by a dysmorphic syndrome.

Digital remnants should be removed surgically.

Observation of spontaneous arm movements and testing passive movements allows to suspect a fracture or a brachial plexus lesion. Lack of active movement and pain on passive movements indicates a fracture or an infection. In a brachial plexus lesion, there is initially a lack of movement in the arm. After 48 h, in an upper root palsy (Erb's palsy: C5, C6, and sometimes C7), the arm is internally rotated, without active abduction. In a complete palsy of upper and lower roots (Klumpke's palsy: C5, C6, C7, C8, and T1), the arm is flail and there may be ptosis and Horner's syndrome; the hand may be clawed (Evans-Jones et al. 2003). Most brachial plexus lesions recover spontaneously: if recovery does not occur by 3 months of age, the baby should be referred to a specialist (Pondaag et al. 2004; Malessy and Pondaag 2009).

31.8.14 Hips

The incidence of developmental dysplasia of the hip (DDH) and instable hip is about 1–2 per 1000 births and 10 per 1000 births, respectively. The risk of DDH is increased in some conditions: female sex, breech presentation, positive family history, oligohydramnios, any abnormality of the lower limb, and any other anomaly suggesting intrauterine compression (i.e., torticollis) (Chan et al. 1997).

Clinical screening of DDH (the Ortolani's and Barlow's tests) has not reduced the number of babies requiring surgery (0.7 per 100 live births) (Godward and Dezateux 1998): moreover, most infants with abnormal neonatal examination have normal hips. Clinical examination by an unexperienced examiner is only little better than no screen (Dezateux et al. 2003).

There is another screening strategy, that is, ultrasound screening, that can also detect clinically stable but anatomically abnormal hips: unfortunately universal ultrasound screening is expensive and produces a high false-positive rate.

There is not any universal agreement concerning the best way of DDH screening. Many clinicians suggest that clinical neonatal examination is the best strategy, if performed by properly trained examiners and followed by selective ultrasound, based on risk factors (American Academy of Pediatrics 2000).

In the Ortolani-Barlow maneuvers, the baby lies supine, with the legs relaxed. For the Ortolani's test, first the examiner should straighten out the legs and then flex the hips to a right angle: after placing the middle finger over the greater trochanter of each leg and the thumbs over the internal aspects of the thighs, the examiner slowly abducts and externally rotates the hips: a definite "clunk" indicates that a previous dislocated femoral head has slipped into the acetabulum (Ortolani 1937). The next maneuver is the Barlow's test that allows to dislocate an unstable hip. Holding the hips and knees as in the Ortolani's test, with the hips at about 70° abduction, the examiner presses forward and medially each hip in turn: if the hip is dislocated, the femoral head slips into the acetabulum with a "clunk" (Barlow 1962).

31.8.15 Neurological Examination

Formal testing is only required in newborns with neuromuscular problems. The evaluation should be performed with minimal discomfort to the infant, and the main goal is to exclude any suspicious neurological signs (Ballard et al. 1991).

Neonatal neurological evaluation includes the following tests:

- General observation
- Level of consciousness and behavioral states
- Mechanical signs: head, spine, and limbs
- Motor system: muscle strength and tone and spontaneous movements
- Reflexes (deep tendon reflexes and primitive reflexes, i.e., Moro, grasp, suck, root)
- Autonomic function (heart and respiratory rate, bladder and bowel function)

Motor system function can be assessed by testing skeletal muscle posture, tone, and movements.

Full-term infants usually exhibit flexion of the limbs. Muscular tone consists in an active or passive resistance to stretch, and it results from a complex interaction between agonistic and antagonistic muscles: then any alteration in muscle tone could represent a sign of a variety of underlying neurological diseases.

The assessment of muscle tone includes the observation of posture and movement, the evaluation of resistance to passive movements, and the production of active or passive movement by specific maneuvers, such as pull-to-sit maneuver and ventral suspension. In the pull-to-sit maneuver, as the infant is pulled up from the supine position by his wrist, there should be some flexion of elbows and slight flexion of the neck, with the head coming up almost in line with the body. In the ventral suspension, as the newborn is held in the air with the examiner's hand under the chest, flexed arms and the head lie almost on a plane with the body for a few seconds.

Increased resistance to passive movement may indicate hypertonicity, often associated with an opisthotonic posture and obligate extension during ventral suspension.

Babies with reduced resistance to passive movements and unrestricted movements usually tend to drape over the examiner's hands in the horizontal plane: these findings indicate hypotonia, whereas weakness is a reduction in muscle power or strength, and it may occur together or not with hypotonia. Hypotonia combined with weakness usually indicates an involvement of peripheral nervous system, whereas hypotonia without weakness indicates an involvement of central nervous system (brain or spinal cord).

Rooting, sucking, grasp, and Moro responses are the most important primitive or developmental reflexes: they should disappear in the first months of life. When they persist, an underlying central nervous system dysfunction should be suspected.

Crossed extension, placing, and stepping reaction are other primitive reflexes.

The main aim of the neurological evaluation in the routine examination is to exclude the presence of suspicious neurological signs.

The findings that require further evaluation are the following:

- Persistent hypotonia and paucity of spontaneous movements
- Abnormal posture: frog posture, opisthotonus, excessive fisting, and fisted thumbs
- Asymmetric movements
- Failure to suck
- High-pitched cry
- Persistent and extreme irritability
- Convulsions
- Lesions over the spine

31.8.16 Assessment of Gestational Age

The most reliable guide for assigning gestational age is an early antenatal ultrasound, combined with the mother's last menstrual period: early antenatal ultrasound estimation is accurate with a margin of less than 7 days.

Several methods can be used to assess gestational age: those based on physical criteria, those based on neurological development, and those that combine physical and neurological examination.

Physical criteria progress in orderly fashion with increasing gestational age and can be assessed immediately after delivery. Neurological criteria include the assessment of posture, passive and active tone, reflexes, and righting reaction and require the infant to be in an alert rested state, not so easy to obtain until the second day of life.

The most accurate method to assess gestational age is to combine the physical criteria and the neurological assessment: Dubowitz and Dubowitz scoring system involves 11 physical criteria and 10 neurological findings (Dubowitz and Dubowitz 1981), whereas simplified Ballard system includes 6 physical and 6 neurological criteria to shorten the time taken (Fig. 1). The new Ballard score is valid for extremely premature infants (Ballard et al. 1991; Ballard and Novak 1979).

In any case, these methods are accurate only to ±2 weeks, with an overestimation in extremely premature infants.

References

Ainsworth SB, Wyllie JP, Wren C (1999) Prevalence and clinical significance of cardiac murmurs in neonates. Arch Dis Child Fetal Neonatal Ed 80:F43–F45

American Academy of Pediatrics (2000) Clinical practice guideline: early detection of developmental dysplasia of the hip. Pediatrics 105:896

Ballard JL, Novak KK, Driver MA (1979) A simplified score of fetal maturation of newly born infants. J Pediatr 95:769–774

Ballard JL, Khoury JC, Wedig K et al (1991) New Ballard score, expanded to include extremely premature infants. J Pediatr 119:417–423

Barlow TG (1962) Early diagnosis and treatment of congenital dislocation of the hip. J Bone Joint Surg Br 44: B292–B301

Brazelton TB (1973) Neonatal behavioural assessment scale. Spastics International Medical, London

Cameron N (2004) Measuring techniques and instruments. In: Nicoletti I, Benso L, Gilli G (eds) Physiological and pathological auxology. Firenze, Edizioni Centro Studi Auxologici, pp 117–159

Centers for Disease Control and Prevention (CDC) (2013c) Screening for critical congenital heart defects: morbidity and mortality weekly report (MMWR) podcasts. Retrieved 3 Mar 2013, from http://www.cdc.gov/nvbddd/pediatricgenetics/pulse.html

Chan A, McCaul KA, Cundy PJ et al (1997) Perinatal risk of factors for developmental dysplasia of the hip. Arch Dis Child Fetal Neonatal Ed 76:F94–F100

Demott K, Bick D, Norman R, et al (2006) Clinical guidelines and evidence review for post natal care: routine post natal care of recently delivered women and their babies last updated: February 2015

Dezateux C, Brown J, Arthur R et al (2003) Performance, treatment pathways, and effects of alternative policy options for screening for developmental of the hip in the United Kingdom. Arch Dis Child 88:753–759

Driver CP, Losty PD (1998) Neonatal testicular torsion. Br J Urol 82:855–858

Dubowitz L, Dubowitz V (1981) The neurological assessment of the preterm and full-term newborn infant. Clin Dev Med No 79. SIMP/Heinemann, London

Evans-Jones G, Kay SPJ, Weindling AM et al (2003) Congenital brachial palsy: incidence, causes and outcome in the UK and Republic of Ireland. Arch Dis Child Fetal Neonatal Ed 88:F185–F189

Farrer KFM, Rennie JM (2003) Neonatal murmurs: are senior house officers good enough? Arch Dis Child Fetal Neonatal Ed 88:F147–F151

Gibson P, Britton J, Hall DMB et al (1995) Lumbosacral skin markers and identification of occult spinal dysraphism in neonates. Acta Pediatr 84:208–209

Godward S, Dezateux C (1998) Surgery for congenital dislocation of the hip in the UK as a measure of outcome of screening. Lancet 351:1149–1152

Goldstein M (2013) Critical complex congenital heart disease (CCHD). Congenital Cardiology Today 11(3):1–10

Kriss VM, Desai NS (1998) Occult spinal dysraphism in neonates: assessment of high risk cutaneous stigmata on sonography. AJR Am J Roentgenol 171:1687–1693

Kugelman A, Hadab B, Ben-David J et al (1997) Preauricular tags and pits in the newborn: the role of hearing tests. Acta Paediatr 86:170–172

Kugelman A, Tubi A, Bader D et al (2002) Preauricular tags and pits in the newborn: the role of renal ultrasonography. J Pediatr 141:388–391

Mahle WT, Newburger JW, Matherne GP et al (2009) Role of pulse oximetry in examining newborns for congenital heart disease: a scientific statement from the AHA and AAP. Pediatrics 124(2):823–836

Malessy MJ, Pondaag W (2009) Obstetric brachial plexus injuries. Neurosurg Clin N Am 20(1):1–14

McCrindle BW, Shaffer KM, Kan JS et al (1996) Cardinal clinical signs in the differentiation of hearth murmurs in children. Arch Pediatr Adolesc Med 150:169–174

Medina LS, Crone K, Kuntz KM (2001) Newborns with suspected occult spinal dysraphism: a cost effectiveness analysis of diagnostic strategies. Pediatrics 108:e101

Ortolani M (1937) Un segno poco noto e sua importanza precoce di prelussazione congenita dell'anca. Pediatrica (Napoli) 45:129–136

Pondaag W, Malessy MJA, Thomeer RTWM (2004) Natural history of obstetric brachial plexus palsy: a systematic review. Dev Med Child Neurol 46:138–144

Riede FT, Worner C, Dahnert I et al (2010) Effectiveness of neonatal pulse oximetry screening for detection of critical congenital heart disease in daily clinical routine – results from a prospective multicenter study. Eur J Pediatr 169(8):975–981

Royal College of Anaesthetists, Royal College of Midwives, Royal College of Obstetricians and Gynaecologists,

Royal College of Paediatrics and Child Health (2007) Safer childbirth- minimum standards for the organisation and delivery of care in labour. RCOG Press, London
Royal College of Obstetricians and Gynaecologists (2016) Providing quality care for women a framework for maternity service standards, London
Smythe JF, Teixeira OH, Vlad P et al (1990) Initial evaluation of heart murmurs: are laboratory tests necessary? Pediatrics 86:497–500
Swaiman KF (1999) Neurologic examination of the term and preterm infant. In: Swaiman KF, Ashwal A (eds) Pediatric neurology: principles and practice, 3rd edn. Mosby, St Louis, p 69
Thummala MR, Raju TN, Langeberg P et al (1998) Isolated single umbilical artery anomaly and the risk for congenital malformations: a meta-analysis. J Pediatr Surg 33:580–585
Villar J, Cheikh Ismail L, Victora CG et al (2014) International standards for newborn weight, length, and head circumference by gestational age and sex: the newborn cross-sectional study of the INTERGROWTH-21st project. Lancet 384(9946):857–868
Wolke D, Dave S, Hayes J et al (2002) Routine examination of the newborn and maternal satisfaction: a randomised controlled trial. Arch Dis Child Fetal Neonatal Ed 86:F155–F160
Wren C, Richmond S, Donaldson L (1999) Presentation of congenital heart disease in infancy: implications for routine examination. Arch Dis Child Fetal Neonatal Ed 80:F49–F53

Primary Investigations in the Term and Preterm Newborn

32

Diego Gazzolo, Francesco Risso, and Andrea Sannia

Contents

Abstract

Admission to nursery or to neonatal intensive care unit represents one of the topic moments in newborn's early post-natal life. Moving from adequate obstetrical history documentation according to maternal-fetal risk factors and to gestational age at birth, the neonatal team have to decide which clinical, laboratory and diagnostic procedure need to be performed. Some primary investigations such as metabolic screening are generally regulated by national governments, independently from clinical conditions, whilst others depend from perinatal risk factors and by clinical evaluation at birth. This refers to the occurrence in term and preterm newborns of the main post-natal complications such as infections, glucose and bilirubinemia metabolism disturbances.

D. Gazzolo (✉)
Neonatal Intensive Care Unit, Department of Maternal, Fetal and Neonatal Medicine, S. Arrigo Children's Hospital, Alessandria, Italy
e-mail: dgazzolo@hotmail.com

F. Risso · A. Sannia
Neonatal Intensive Care Unit, Department of Emergency Medicine, G. Gaslini Children's Hospital, Genoa, Italy

G. Buonocore et al. (eds.), *Neonatology*,
https://doi.org/10.1007/978-3-319-29489-6_182

Although respiratory, cardiovascular and cerebral complications account in the majority of preterm infants, these clinical aspects have to be taken into the due consideration also in term newborns. In the present chapter on overview on new insight on neonatal laboratory technique and in non-invasive monitoring devices currently used in nursery and in intensive care is provided.

32.1 Salient Points

- Metabolic screening varies from country to country, and each nation applies its own program of neonatal screening. A multi-disciplinary report by the ACMG, HRSA, and AAP recommended a panel of 29 tests. Universal newborn screening for metabolic disorders is available in many developed countries.
- Newborns at risk of sepsis need careful physical examination and standard laboratory investigations such as WBC differential count, immature-to-total neutrophil (I:T ratio), and C reactive protein (CRP).
- Based on potential multi-organ damage due to prematurity, close monitoring in the early phases after birth is essential.
- Temperature should be monitored and recorded at 30 min intervals until thermostability is achieved.
- Monitoring of blood pressure is essential for the optimal management of premature infants.
- RDS incidence is inversely proportional to gestational age and occurs most frequently in infants of less than 1,200 g and 30 weeks' gestation.
- Transcutaneous (tc) measurements of PCO_2 and PO_2 are important monitoring parameters in the NICU allowing continuous and less invasive monitoring of blood gas levels.
- Recognition that preterm newborn are at risk for disturbances of glucose homeostasis is the most important step for the prevention of both hypoglycemia and hyperglycemia.
- Routine screening for GM-IVH is performed in infants <30 weeks or <1250 g at birth. Hemorrhage occurs mostly within the first 3 days of life.

32.2 The Term Newborn

32.2.1 Newborn Screening

Newborn screening, started in 1960, is primarily directed at disorders in which clinical complications develop during the immediate postnatal period.

32.2.1.1 Metabolic Screening

Metabolic diseases result from biochemical abnormalities that are manifest during the first days after birth (Taeusch et al. 2005). Phenylketonuria (PKU) was the first metabolic disorder known to benefit from early diagnosis and immediate dietary treatment. Infants with PKU were identified early, in large numbers, and developed normal while receiving treatment (O'Flynn 1992). The success of such screening led to further progress in the investigation of additional tests for metabolic diseases, such as galactosemia, maple syrup disease (MSUD), and homocystinuria. These tests could be applied to the same blood specimen obtained for PKU screening. In 1990, tandem mass spectrometry (MS/MS) started a new era in newborn screening (Levy 1998). The technology allows for the detection of more than 30 biochemical genetic disorders with a single assay with high specificity and with a very low of false positive rate. Currently, the disorders detected by most MS/MS newborn screening programs can be divided into three major categories: amino-acid disorders (including urea cycle defects), organic acid disorders and fatty acid oxidation defects (Levy 1998). In 1999, the American Academy of Pediatrics (AAP) Newborn Screening Task Force recommended that Human Resources and Services Administration (HRSA) developed and implemented nationally recognized newborn screening system standards and policies in collaboration with the Maternal and Child Health Bureau (MCHB) of HRSA and the American College of Medical Genetics (ACMG) (Maternal and Child Health Bureau 2006). Criteria included: (1) the current availability of an effective and rapid screening test; (2) an efficacious treatment and adequate understanding of the natural history.

Table 1 Newborn screening panel recommended by ACMG expert panel (Maternal and Child Health Bureau 2006)

MS/MS detectable disorder
Organic acids
Isovaleric acidemia
Glutaric aciduria 1
3-Hydroxy-3-methylglutaric aciduria
Multiple carboxylase deficiency
Methylmalonic acidemia due to mutase deficiency
3-Methylcrotonyl CoA carboxylase deficiency
Methylmalonic acidemia due to cobalamin A and B defects
Propionic acidemia
3-Ketothiolase
Fatty acid oxidation
Medium chain acyl-CoA dehydrogenase
Very long chain acyl-CoA dehydrogenase
Long chain 3-hydroxyacyl-CoA dehydrogenase
Trifunctional protein deficiency
Carnitine uptake defect
Amino acids/urea cycle
Phenylketonuria
Maple syrup urine disease
Homocystinuria
Citrullinemia
Argininosuccinic aciduria
Tyrosinemia type
Disorders detected by other methods
Hemoglobinoathies
Hb SS-Sickle cell anemia
Hb S/Beta-thalassemia
Hb S/C disease
Others
Congenital hypothyroidism
Biotinidase deficiency
Congenital adrenal hyperplasia
Galactosemia due to GALT deficiency
Congenital hearing loss
Cystic fibrosis

Metabolic screening varies from country to country and each nation applies its own program of neonatal screening. A multidisciplinary report by the ACMG, HRSA and AAP recommended a panel of 29 tests and there is universal newborn screening for metabolic disorders in, many developed countries (Marsden et al. 2006) (Table 1).

Conditions most commonly screened for are congenital hypothyroidism, galactosemia, adrenal hyperplasia (cah), biotinidase deficiency, sickle cell disease, cystic fibrosis are performed by immunoassays, radioimmunoassay (RIA), fluoroimmunoassay (FIA), and enzyme-linked immunosorbent assay (ELISA) techniques. The topic is considered in more detail in ▶ Chap. 111, "Inborn Errors of Metabolism and Newborns."

Today the use of MS/MS for second-tier tests and confirmatory testing has been shown to provide useful information especially in the early detection of new disorders such as some lysosomal storage disorders, ADA and PNP SCIDs, X-adrenoleucodistrophy (X-ALD), Wilson disease, guanidinoacetate methyltransferase deficiency (GAMT), and Duchenne muscular dystrophy. The new bulk of investigation will be focused to: (i) reduce the false positive rate by using second-tier tests, (ii) avoid false negative results by using new specific biomarkers, and finally (iii) introduce new treatable disorders in NBS programs (Ombrone et al. 2016).

32.2.2 Infections

A wide variety of infectious agents may affect newborn such as bacteria, viruses, fungi, protozoa, and mycoplasmas. This topic is considered in more detail in ▶ Chaps. 103, "Fetal Infections: Cytomegalovirus, Herpes Simplex, and Varicella," ▶ 104, "Fetal Infections: Rubella, HIV, HCV, HBV, and Human Parvovirus B19," ▶ 105, "Fetal Infections: Congenital Syphilis and Tuberculosis," ▶ 106, "Toxoplasmosis in the Fetus and Newborn," ▶ 107, "Neonatal Bacterial and Fungal Infections," ▶ 108, "Neonatal Septic Shock," and ▶ 109, "Neonatal Viral Infections: Enteroviruses and Respiratory Syncytial Virus."

Several laboratory tests have been evaluated for their ability to predict which at risk infants may develop symptomatic or culture-proven sepsis, but there is at present no single test that is sufficiently reliable. Investigators have proposed different combinations of laboratory tests but these various combinations were not more diagnostic than single laboratory tests although more predictive for negative cases (Kite et al. 1988).

Newborns at risk of sepsis need careful physical examination and standard laboratory investigation may be useful such as: WBC differential count, immature-to-total neutrophil (I:T ratio) and C reactive protein (CRP) (Kite et al. 1988). Although sensitivity/specificity is limited, total WBC count and differential and I:T ratio can indicate bacterial infection. Taken together: (1) an elevated WBC is not predictive of infection in newborn infants; neutropenia is more common than neutrophilia in severe neonatal sepsis, but also occurs in association with maternal diseases (PIH, IUGR); (2) thrombocytopenia is a nonspecific indicator of infection; (3) longitudinal WBC monitoring in the first 24 h from birth is more predictive of infection than a single determination (Schelonka et al. 1994; Escobar et al. 2000; Rodwell et al. 1993).

CRP is an acute-phase reactant that increases in the presence of inflammation caused by infection or tissue injury. Raised levels of CRP are found in bacterial sepsis or meningitis. After inflammation onset, CRP synthesis increases within 4–6 h, doubling every 8 h, and peaks at about 36–50 h. Levels remain elevated with ongoing inflammation, but with resolution they decline rapidly due to a short half-life of 4–7 h. CRP demonstrates high sensitivity and negative predictive value. A single normal value of CRP at birth cannot rule out infection because the sampling may have preceded the rise in CRP. Serial CRP measurements may be helpful (Benitz et al. 1998; Gabay and Kushner 1999; DuClos 2000). Although CRP is widely used in neonatal intensive care unit (NICU), several biomarkers have been recently proposed for early (2–12 h) and late (12–24 h) neonatal sepsis. The former refers to IL-6, IL-8, nCD64, and TNF-α, while the latter point regards procalcitonin (Meem et al. 2011). Anyway, on the basis of the aforementioned findings, it is reasonable to suggest that CRP combined with other biomarkers will constitute the new perspective for the early diagnosis of neonatal sepsis (Delanghe and Speeckaert 2015).

For asymptomatic term infants with positive laboratory tests, blood culture and antibiotic therapy are recommended until cultures are negative. Asymptomatic infants born before 35 weeks with risk factors for sepsis should have blood cultures before antibiotic therapy is started and before the results of laboratory tests. The duration of therapy should be guided by the baby's clinical condition and the results of the tests (Jeffrey and Gerdes 2004).

All together, future perspectives will regard molecular biology improvement with the inclusion in clinical guidelines of trustable, quick, and low-cost tests able to provide, for example, microbiological diagnosis and to identify more microorganisms than blood cultures (Suberviola et al. 2016).

32.3 The Preterm Newborn

Preterm birth affects more than 500,000 babies in the United States each year (Green et al. 2005). In Italy the incidence of preterm birth is 6.7% at <36 weeks of gestation, 5.2% between 32 and 36 weeks of gestation and 0.9% <32 weeks (Campi and Bonati 2007). Preterm birth is one of the leading causes of infant mortality and morbidity (Challis et al. 2001). It accounts for more than 70% of neonatal deaths and almost half the children with long-term neurological disabilities were born prematurely (Mathews et al. 2004). Since 1981, the US preterm birth rate has increased from approximately 9% to 12% (Green et al. 2005; Institute of Medicine, Committee on Understanding Premature Birth and Assuring Healthy Outcomes 2007). Research indicates that preterm birth is a multifactorial disease caused by genetic, social and environmental factors, which most likely interact to increase risk (Wilcox et al. 1995; Wang et al. 2002; Moore et al. 2004; Macones et al. 2004; Kogan 1995; Johnson et al. 2005; Genc et al. 2004; Crider et al. 2005). There are striking disparities in the rates and consequences of preterm birth across racial and ethnic groups in the US that are unexplained (Institute of Medicine, Committee on Understanding Premature Birth and Assuring Healthy Outcomes 2007).

32.3.1 The Problem of Preterm Labor

The factor(s) controlling the spontaneous onset of labor are not known. This is frustrating from a physiological point of view, and also a major clinical problem. The last trimester of pregnancy is necessary for the maturation of the fetal lungs and other organs in preparation for extrauterine life. If this process is interrupted by an early delivery the chances of survival of the newborn are severely decreased. The mortality rate according to different countries still remains higher and constant, at lower gestational ages, with a wide range morbidity and disability in the surviving infants (Morrison and Rennie 1997; Bibby and Stewart 2004). The factors responsible for parturition in women remain unknown and the endocrine paradigms described above do not fit primates. Therefore, more research is necessary to identify the physiological trigger for parturition and to understand why the process may be activated prematurely in some pregnancies. It is also necessary to investigate the biochemical mechanisms regulating uterine smooth muscle activity in order to develop more effective and selective therapy to control uterine contractions when this is indicated. Critical clinical findings are reported in Table 2.

Table 2 Critical assessment findings for hypo- and hyperthermia

Hypothermia
Pale, mottled skin that is cool to touch babies
Acrocyanosis
Respiratory distress
Apnea, bradycardia, central cyanosis
Irritability initially
Lethargy developing as hypothermia worsens
Hypotonia
Weak, cry and suck
Gastric residuals, abdominal distension, emesis
Shivering in more mature
Metabolic acidosis
Hypoglycemia
And temperature measurement!!
Hyperthermia
Reddened skin that is warm to touch
Tachypnea
Tachycardia
Irritability, lethargy, hypotonia, weak cry
Poor feeding
Apnea
Sweating in more mature babies
Dehydration

32.3.2 Neonatal Assessment at Birth

Based on potential multiorgan damage due to prematurity, close monitoring, in the early phases after birth, is essential. Primary investigations include vital signs recordings such as temperature determination, heart and respiratory rates, oxygen saturation monitoring in parallel with blood pH assessment.

32.3.2.1 Temperature Determination

Temperature determination is always required and might be recorded at 30 min intervals up to thermostability achievement. Furthermore, it is suggested that temperature be recorded at 1–3 h intervals by continuous monitoring with axillary determinations every 1–2 h (American Academy of Pediatrics and American College of Obstetricians and Gynecologist 2002). In this regard, recordings should include environmental temperature (i.e., air temperature in the incubator or radiant warmer settings). Measuring the skin and core temperature simultaneously may be of help differentiating between fever as a result of disease and environmental overheating. Noting that the baby's servo-controlled skin temperature is relatively stable but that the environmental temperature has dropped also may be indicative of fever as the incubator responds to the high probe reading by cooling the infant's environment.

32.3.2.2 Cardiorespiratory Monitoring

The electrical activity of an infant's heart is picked up by chest leads (usually three), placed on the infant and recorded by a cardiorespiratory monitor. The recording is displayed on a visual screen as the infant's electrocardiographic pattern. The infant's respiratory pattern also is recorded, because the chest leads electronically detect movement of the infant's chest with each respiration. The oxygen saturation monitor relies on adequate perfusion to the site and the ability to detect arterial pulsation; thus if it is placed distal to a blood pressure cuff, there will be an inaccurate reading while the cuff is inflated. Newer models of pulse oximetry reduce the artefact that results from motion and low perfusion (Goldstein et al. 1997; Sahni et al. 2003). These newer models also are indifferent to ambient light whereas older models were affected by light sources such as phototherapy.

32.3.2.3 Blood Pressure Monitoring

Monitoring of blood pressure is essential for the optimal management of premature infants. Blood pressure is one of the most important physiological parameters to evaluate clinical stability in critical care. Several medical conditions in premature infants determine changes in blood pressure (i.e., infections, drugs, dehydration, blood loss etc.). The recognition and treatment of abnormal blood pressure states has significant prognostic implications in neonatal intensive care (Nuntnarumit et al. 1999). Blood pressure in the newborn is related to weight and gestational age. Blood pressure rises with postnatal age, 1–2 mmHg/day during the first week and 1 mmHg/week during next 6 weeks in the preterm infant, just as in the full-term infant. The measurement of blood pressure can be obtained by non-invasive or invasive methods. In stable infants or when only intermittent blood pressure measurements are required, non-invasive methods are preferred. Blood pressure invasive monitoring is obtained via catheter that has been introduced into an artery. This method is indicated in very small or instable infants, especially those with severe hypotension. For more details, see ▶ Chap. 71, "Blood Pressure Disorders in the Neonate: Hypotension and Hypertension."

32.3.2.4 Transcutaneous Blood Gas Monitoring

PCO_2 and PO_2 are important monitoring parameters in NICU. Compared to conventional blood gas measurements that cause significant blood loss in preterms, transcutaneous (tc) measurements allow continuous, non-invasive monitoring of blood gas levels (Brouillette and Waxman 1997). Preterm infants are vulnerable to alterations in arterial oxygen or carbon dioxide tension.Changes in oxygen supply contribute to the subsequent development of retinopathy of prematurity or bronchopulmonary dysplasia. Hypocarbia has been associated with the subsequent development of periventricular leukomalacia and cerebral palsy, and may cause retardation of retinal vascularization (Holmes et al. 1998). Transcutaneous measurement of oxygen ($PtcO_2$) and carbon dioxide ($PtcCO_2$) tension is a non-invasive method that has recently offered some promise. Several studies have shown a good correlation between tc and arterial values (Binder et al. 1994; Geven et al. 1987).

32.4 The Preterm Baby

32.4.1 Specific Risks for the Preterm Neonate

Preterm infants usually show multiorgan failure in reverse proportion to the gestational age.

The main target-organs are:

- central nervous system (CNS): including apnea of prematurity, intracranial hemorrhage, development disability, and cerebral palsy;
- retinopathy of prematurity (ROP);
- cardiovascular complications may arise from the failure of the ductus arteriosus to close after birth: Patent ductus arteriosus (PDA) is typical in preterm babies. Other congenital cardiac malformations will further analyzed in ▶ Chap. 68, "Early Diagnosis of Congenital Heart Disease: When and How to Treat";
- respiratory problems that can range from lung malformations (pulmonary hypoplasia, see ▶ Chap. 59, "Rare Lung Diseases of Newborns") to wet lung and finally to chronic lung disease (see ▶ Chap. 57, "Bronchopulmonary Dysplasia/Chronic Lung Disease of the Newborn");
- gastrointestinal and metabolic issues can arise from glycemia and ion disorders, feeding difficulties, and finally necrotizing enterocolitis (NEC). However of particular interest are kidney diseases that are extensively described in ▶ Chaps. 114, "Pathophysiology of Fetal and

Neonatal Kidneys," and ▶ 115, "Acute and Chronic Renal Failure in the Newborn Infant";
- hematologic complications including anemia of prematurity, thrombocytopenia, and hyperbilirubinemia, and (jaundice) that can lead to Kernicterus (for review see ▶ Chap. 75, "Kernicterus, Bilirubin-Induced Neurological Dysfunction, and New Treatments for Unconjugated Hyperbilirubinemia in Neonates");
- neonatal sepsis including viral and bacterial forms that can be characterized by general (septicemia) or localized sepsis (pneumonia, urinary tract infection, meningitis etc.).

32.4.2 Patent Ductus Arteriosus (PDA)

The ductus arteriosus' function in the unborn baby is to allow blood to bypass the lungs, because oxygen for the blood comes from the mother and not from breathing air. In fullterm babies, the ductus arteriosus closes shortly after birth, but it frequently stays open in premature babies. When this happens, excess blood flows into the lungs and can cause breathing difficulties and sometimes heart failure. More details about PDA and other congenital cardiac disorders are analyzed in ▶ Chap. 69, "Patent Ductus Arteriosus."

32.4.3 Respiratory Distress Syndrome

Clinical, diagnostic and therapeutic strategies in RDS management are described in ▶ Chap. 53, "Respiratory Distress Syndrome: Predisposing Factors, Pathophysiology, and Diagnosis." One of the most common and immediate problems facing premature infants is difficulty breathing. Although there are many causes of breathing difficulties in premature infants, the most common is called respiratory distress syndrome (RDS). Its incidence is inversely proportional to gestational age and occurs most frequently in infants of less than 1200 g and 30 weeks' gestation. RDS affects male infants twice as frequently as in female infants (2:1) In RDS, the infant's immature lungs fail to produce surfactant and its administration is highly required according to RDS severity. Prophylactic and or rescue surfactant administration modalities are reported in ▶ Chap. 63, "Lung Diseases: Surfactant Replacement Therapy in Newborns."

In RDS respiratory drive recording is generally irregular in rate and depth, and is chiefly abdominal, rather than thoracic, with a rate of 30–60 breath/min. Tachypnea, a rate above 60 breaths/min after the first hour of life, is the earliest symptom of respiratory diseases. Periodic respirations are cyclic respirations of apnea (5–10 s) and ventilation (10–15 s) (Holditch-Davis et al. 2004). Apnea is a non-breathing episode lasting longer than 20 s and accompanied by physiologic alterations. Use of accessory muscle of respirations is indicative of a marked increase in the work of breathing. Retractions reflect the inward pull of the thin chest wall on inspiration. Retracting is best observed in relation to the sternum (substernal and suprasternal) and the intercostals, supracostal, and subcostal spaces. The increased negative intra-thoracic pressure necessary to ventilate the stiff, non-compliant lung causes the chest wall to retract. This further compromises the lung's expansion. The degree of retraction is directly proportional to the severity of the disease. Nasal flaring is a compensatory mechanism that attempts to take in more oxygen by increasing the size of the nostrils and thus decreasing the resistance (by as much as 40) of the narrow airways. Grunting is forced expiration through a partially closed glottis.

Because the clinical presentation of many respiratory and non-respiratory diseases is the same, a chest X-ray examination may be the only way to differentiate cause and establish the proper diagnosis. More recently, lung ultrasound pattern has been recently proposed. In detail, an ultrasound severity score has been shown to correlate with oxygenation status in both term and preterm neonates, and to be a good predictor of surfactant need in preterm babies requiring respiratory support (Brat et al. 2015).

Measurement of arterial blood gases is used to demonstrate alterations in oxygenation and acid-base balance and to differentiate between respiratory and metabolic components.

32.4.4 Hyperbilirubinemia

A common treatable condition of premature babies is hyperbilirubinemia, which affects 80% of premature infants. Although mild jaundice is fairly common in full-term babies (about 60%), it is much more common in premature babies. In premature infants, the bilirubin peak usually is on the fourth-fifth day of life and may be 10–12 mg/dL, possibly rising to greater than 15 mg/dL without any specific abnormality of bilirubin metabolism. Therefore for bilirubin screening it is enough to take sample blood on the fourth-fifth day of life. Neonatal jaundice is completely analyzed in ► Chaps. 73, "Bilirubin Metabolism, Unconjugated Hyperbilirubinemia, and Physiologic Neonatal Jaundice," and ► 74, "Pathologic Unconjugated Hyperbilirubinemia–Isoimmunization, Abnormalities of Red Blood Cells, and Infections."

32.4.5 Hypoglycemia and Hyperglycemia

Recognition that preterm newborn are at risk for disturbances in glucose homeostasis is the most important step in preventing both hypoglycemia and hyperglycemia (Table 3). Maintenance of a neutral thermal environment is especially critical to minimize energy expenditure in those infants at risk for hyperglycemia. Other conditions associated with hypoglycemia, such as asphyxia and hypothermia, may be avoided through appropriate obstetric and neonatal intervention. When hypoglycemia is suspected, the plasma or blood glucose concentration must be determined immediately. Ideally this determination should be made with one of the laboratory enzymatic methods, such as the glucose oxidase or hexokinase method, but even bedside reagent test strip glucose analyzers (i.e., glucometers) can be used if the test is performed carefully with awareness of the more limited accuracy of these devices. A number of current references use 40–45 mg/dL as the lower limit of "normal" plasma glucose concentrations in the first 72 h of life (Cornblath and Schwartz 1993).

Table 3 Indications for routine monitoring of blood glucose for prevention of neonatal hypoglycemia

Maternal conditions
Presence of diabetes or abnormal glucose tolerance test
Preeclampsia and pregnancy-induced or essential hypertension
Previous macrosomic infants
Substance abuse
Treatment with beta-agonist tocolytics
Treatment with oral hypoglycemic agents
Neonatal conditions
Prematurity
Intrauterine growth restriction
Perinatal hypoxia-ischemia
Sepsis
Hypothermia
Polycythemia-hyperviscosity
Erythroblastosis fetalis
Iatrogenic administration of insulin
Congenital cardiac malformations
Persistent hyperinsulinemia
Endocrine disorders
Inborn errors of metabolism

32.4.6 Intracranial Hemorrhage

Intracranial hemorrhage (ICH) can affect newborns of all gestational ages and often is clinically "silent". Among ICH, germinal matrix hemorrhage and intraventricular hemorrhage (GM-IVH) are the most common in the premature population (see ► Chap. 128, "Cerebral Hemorrhage in Newborns"). More recently, due to increase in extreme prematurity survival rate, cerebellar hemorrhage constitutes a common pattern affecting 2–9% of preterm infants weighting less that 750 g (de Vries et al. 2015). Routine screening for GM-IVH is performed in infants < 30 weeks or < 1250 g at birth. The timing of hemorrhage occurrence is mostly within the first three days of life. "Late" hemorrhage (i.e., after 3 days of age) may be associated with pneumothorax and its restriction of venous return to the heart.

Indications for cerebral ultrasound scan are discussed in ▶ Chap. 122, "Neuroimaging Studies."

References

American Academy of Pediatrics, American College of Obstetricians and Gynecologist (2002) Guidelines for perinatal care, 5th edn. American Academy of Pediatrics, Elk Grove Village

Benitz WE, Han MY, Madan A, Ramachandra P (1998) Serial serum C-reactive protein levels in the diagnosis of neonatal infection. Pediatrics 102:E41

Bibby E, Stewart A (2004) The epidemiology of preterm birth. Neuro Endocrinol Lett 25(Suppl 1):43–47

Binder N, Atherton H, Thorkelsson T, Hoath SB (1994) Measurement of transcutaneous carbon dioxide in low birthweight infants during the first two weeks of life. Am J Perinatol 11:237–241

Brat R, Yousef N, Klifa R, Reynaud S, Shankar Aguilera S, De Luca D (2015) Lung ultrasonography score to evaluate oxygenation and surfactant need in neonates treated with continuous positive airway pressure. JAMA Pediatr 169(8):e151797. https://doi.org/10.1001/jamapediatrics.2015.1797. Epub 2015 Aug 3

Brouillette RT, Waxman DH (1997) Evaluation of the newborn's blood gas status. Clin Chem 43:215–221

Campi R, Bonati M (2007) Italian child health statistic review: births and deaths. Ital J Pediatr 33:67–73

Challis JR, Lye SJ, Gibb W (2001) Understanding preterm labor. Ann N Y Acad Sci 943:225–234

Cornblath M, Schwartz R (1993) Hypoglycemia in the neonate. J Pediatr Endocrinol 6:113–129

Crider KS, Whitehead N, Buus RM (2005) Genetic variation associated with preterm birth: a HuGE review. Genet Med 7:593–604

de Vries LS, Benders MJ, Groenendaal F (2015) Progress in neonatal neurology with a focus on neuroimaging in the preterm infant. Neuropediatrics 46(4):234–241. https://doi.org/10.1055/s-0035-1554102. Epub 2015 Jun 29

Delanghe JR, Speeckaert MM (2015) Translational research and biomarkers in neonatal sepsis. Clin Chim Acta 451(Pt A):46–64. https://doi.org/10.1016/j.cca.2015.01.031. Epub 2015 Feb 4. Review

DuClos T (2000) Function of C-reactive protein. Ann Med 32:274–278

Escobar GJ, Dekun L, Armstrong MA et al (2000) Neonatal sepsis workups in infants 2000 grams at birth: a population-based study. Pediatrics 106:256–263

Gabay C, Kushner I (1999) Mechanisms of disease: acute-phase proteins and other systemic responses to inflammation. N Engl J Med 340:448–454

Genc MR, Onderdonk AB, Vardhana S et al (2004) Polymorphism in intron 2 of the interleukin-1 receptor antagonist gene, local midtrimester cytokine response to vaginal flora, and subsequent preterm birth. Am J Obstet Gynecol 191:1324–1330

Geven WB, Nagler E, deBoo T, Lemmens W (1987) Combined transcutaneous oxygen, carbon dioxide tensions and end-expired CO2 levels in severely ill newborns. Adv Exp Med Biol 220:115–120

Goldstein MR, Martin GI, Sindel BD et al (1997) Novel pulse oximetry technology resistant to noise artifact and low perfusion: "the neonatal model". Am J Respir Crit Care Med 155:A717

Green NS, Damus K, Simpson JL et al (2005) Research agenda for preterm birth: Recommendations from the March of Dimes. Am J Obstet Gynecol 193:626–635

Holditch-Davis D, Scher M, Schwartz T (2004) Respiratory development in preterm infants. J Perinatol 24:631–639

Holmes JM, Zhang S, Leske DA, Lanier WL (1998) Carbon dioxide-induced retinopathy in the neonatal rat. Curr Eye Res 17:608–616

Institute of Medicine, Committee on Understanding Premature Birth and Assuring Healthy Outcomes (2007) Preterm birth: causes, consequences, and prevention. National Academies Press, Washington, DC

Jeffrey S, Gerdes MD (2004) Diagnosis and management of bacterial infections in the neonate. Pediatr Clin North Am 51:939–959

Johnson WG, Scholl TO, Spychala JR et al (2005) Common di- hydrofolate reductase 19-base pair deletion allele: a novel risk factor for preterm delivery. Am J Clin Nutr 81:664–668

Kite P, Millar MR, Gorham P et al (1988) Comparison of 5 tests in diagnosis of neonatal bacteraemia. Arch Dis Child 63:639–643

Kogan MD (1995) Social causes of low birth weight. J R Soc Med 88:611–615

Levy HL (1998) Newborn screening by tandem mass spectrometry: a new era. Clin Chem 44:2401–2402

Macones GA, Parry S, Elkousy M et al (2004) A polymorphism in the promoter region of TNF and bacterial vaginosis: preliminary evidence of geneenvironment interaction in the etiology of spontaneous preterm birth. Am J Obstet Gynecol 190:1504–1508

Marsden D, Larson C, Levy HL (2006) Newborn screening for metabolic disorders. J Pediatr 148:577–584

Maternal and Child Health Bureau (2006) Newborn Screening: Toward a Uniform Screening Panel and System. http://www.mchb.hrsa.gov/screening

Mathews TJ, Menacker F, MacDorman MF (2004) Infant mortality statistics from the 2002 period: linked birth/infant death data set. Natl Vital Stat Rep 53:1–29

Meem M, Modak JK, Mortuza R, Morshed M, Islam MS, Saha SK (2011) Biomarkers for diagnosis of neonatal infections: a systematic analysis of their potential as a point-of-care diagnostics. J Glob Health 1 (2):201–209

Moore S, Ide M, Randhawa M et al (2004) An investigation into the association among preterm birth, cytokine gene polymorphisms and periodontal disease. BJOG 111:125–132

Morrison JJ, Rennie JM (1997) Clinical, scientific and ethical aspects of fetal and neonatal care at extremely preterm periods of gestation. Br J Obstet Gynaecol 104:1341

Nuntnarumit P, Yang W, Bada-Ellzey HS (1999) Blood pressure measurements in the newborn. Clin Perinatol 26:981–996

O'Flynn ME (1992) Newborn screening for phenylketonuria: thirty years of progress. Curr Probl Pediatr 22:159–165

Ombrone D, Giocaliere E, Forni G, Malvagia S, la Marca G (2016) Expanded newborn screening by mass spectrometry: new tests, future perspectives. Mass Spectrom Rev 35(1):71–84. https://doi.org/10.1002/mas.21463. Epub 2015 May 7

Rodwell RL, Taylor KM, Tudehope DI, Gray PH (1993) Hematologic scoring system in early diagnosis of sepsis in neutropenic newborns. Pediatr Infect Dis J 12:372–376

Sahni R, Gupta A, Ohira-Kist K et al (2003) Motion resistant pulse oximetry in neonates. Arch Dis Child Fetal Neonat Ed 88:F505–F508

Schelonka RL, Bradley YA, desJardins SE et al (1994) Peripheral leukocyte count and leukocyte indexes in healthy newborn term infants. J Pediatr 125:603–606

Suberviola B, Márquez-López A, Castellanos-Ortega A, Fernández-Mazarrasa C, Santibáñez M, Martínez LM (2016) Microbiological diagnosis of sepsis: polymerase chain reaction system versus blood cultures. Am J Crit Care 25(1):68–75. https://doi.org/10.4037/ajcc2016728

Taeusch HW, Ballard RA, Gleason CA (2005) Avery's disease of the newborn, 8th edn. Elsevier Saunders, Philadelphia

Wang X, Zuckerman B, Pearson C et al (2002) Maternal cigarette smoking, metabolic gene polymorphism, and infant birth weight. JAMA 287:195–202

Wilcox MA, Smith SJ, Johnson IR (1995) The effect of social deprivation on birthweight, excluding physiological and pathological effects. Br J Obstet Gynaecol 102:918–924

33 Oxygen Saturation Monitoring in Neonatal Period

Augusto Sola and Sergio Golombek

Contents

A. Sola (✉)
Ibero American Society of Neonatology (SIBEN),
Wellington, FL, USA
e-mail: augusto.sola@siben.net

S. Golombek (✉)
New York Medical College, New York, USA
e-mail: sergio.golombek@siben.net

G. Buonocore et al. (eds.), *Neonatology*,
https://doi.org/10.1007/978-3-319-29489-6_291

Abstract
Oxygen (O_2) is a potent drug that is often used inappropriately in the clinical environment. Its administration needs to be improved in neonatal care. Healthcare providers never induce hypoxemia, and the same is not true for hyperoxemia. Clinical signs (cyanosis and tongue color) are of no value to detect hypoxemia and hyperoxemia. Pulse oximetry (SpO_2) is the most important method for monitoring O_2 saturation. The hazards of hyperoxemia and hyperoxia should be avoided or minimized. Undesired effects of maternal and fetal oxidative stress and short- and long-term O_2 therapy involve every organ system and many genes. The SpO_2 in normal newborns and in those who are treated with CPAP or assisted ventilation breathing room air (FiO_2 0.21) is 95–100%. The intention to "target SpO_2" in infants breathing supplemental O_2 should not include values associated with potential hyperoxia nor possible hypoxia and also must aim to avoid recurring periods of hypoxemia-hyperoxemia-reperfusion. It is impossible to maintain newborn infants within narrow SpO_2 target ranges all the time. Choosing wider intermediate SpO_2 ranges for treatment allows for easier care and better compliance, and such ranges have been associated with a decreased rate of severe ROP, without an increased morbidity or mortality.

33.1 Salient Points

- Oxygen (O_2) is a very potent drug that is often used inappropriately in the clinical environment. Its administration needs to be improved in neonatal care.
- Healthcare providers never induce hypoxemia and all measures are implemented clinically to try to overcome it when present. The same is not true for hyperoxemia.
- Clinical signs, such as cyanosis and tongue color, are of little or no value to detect hypoxemia and hyperoxemia.
- The most widely used tool to guide its administration and dosage is noninvasive monitoring of O_2 saturation by pulse oximetry (SpO_2).
- Cellular oxygenation is complex and not easy to assess in clinical practice. Hypoxemia does not necessarily cause tissue hypoxia and there are situations where there is tissue hypoxia without hypoxemia.
- The hazards of hyperoxemia and hyperoxia are many and should be avoided or minimized. Undesired effects of maternal and fetal oxidative stress and short- and long-term O_2 therapy involve every organ system and many genes.
- The SpO_2 in normal newborns and in those who are being treated with CPAP or assisted ventilation breathing room air (FiO_2 0.21) is 95–100%.
- The intention to treat ("target SpO_2") in infants breathing supplemental O_2 should not include SpO_2 values associated with potential hyperoxia nor possible hypoxia and also must aim to avoid recurring periods of hypoxemia-hyperoxemia-reperfusion.
- It is impossible to maintain newborn infants within the desired intention to treat all the time. When tight or narrow SpO_2 target ranges are intended, there is even more time spent outside of the desired intention to treat.
- A narrow intention to treat in low ranges (i.e., SpO_2 target 85–89%) should not be used clinically. On the other hand, there is no evidence that a narrow SpO_2 target of 91–95% or 90–95% should be universally used in clinical practice for preterm infants in the initial periods of life.
- Choosing wider intermediate SpO_2 ranges for the intention to treat allows for easier care and better compliance, and such ranges have been associated with a decreased rate of severe ROP, without an increased morbidity or mortality.

33.2 Introduction

Many times clinical interventions in neonatal medicine are not based on proven benefit but on anecdotal evidence, expert opinion, and tradition. The administration of oxygen (O_2) is one of such clinical interventions. The history of the use of O_2

is fascinating and has been burdened with errors (Comroe et al. 1950; Van Den Brenk and Jamieson 1962; Phibbs 1977; Silverman 1980) but its description escapes the content of this chapter. Perinatal interest about O_2 and noninvasive monitoring of O_2 saturation by pulse oximetry (SpO_2) has increased markedly in this century (Askie et al. 2003; Chow et al. 2003; Deulofeut et al. 2006, 2007; Hagadorn et al. 2006; Saugstad 2007; Sola et al. 2007, 2008, 2014; Sola 2008; Castillo et al. 2008, 2011; Lim et al. 2014; Bizzarro et al. 2014; Rabi et al. 2007; Dawson et al. 2010, 2012; Vento et al. 2013; Saugstad et al. 2014; Sola and Zuluaga 2013; Saugstad and Aune 2014; Schmidt et al. 2013, 2014a, b; Vento 2014; Noh et al. 2014; Yalcin et al. 2013; Hamel et al. 2014; Lye et al. 2013; Klimova et al. 2013; Klingel and Patel 2013; Thomson and Paton 2014; Carlo et al. 2010; Stenson et al. 2013; Darlow et al. 2014; Kaindl et al. 2006; Wollen et al. 2014; Farrow et al. 2012; Spector et al. 2005; Wellmann et al. 2014; Hay et al. 2002; Baquero et al. 2011; Polin et al. 2014; Ahmed et al. 2010; Vagedes et al. 2013; Zhang et al. 2011; Niermeyer et al. 1995; Laman et al. 2005; de Wahl Granelli et al. 2009; Ewer et al. 2011; Zapata et al. 2014; Bancalari and Claure 2012; Claure and Bancalari 2013, 2015); only in 2015 there have been more than 16 publications on the topic (Sola 2015; Lakshminrusimha et al. 2015; Manja et al. 2015; Synnes and Miller 2015; Suwattanaphim et al. 2015; Ketko et al. 2015; van Kaam et al. 2015; Lim et al. 2015; Paul 2015; Narayen et al. 2015; Rawat et al. 2015; Clarke et al. 2015; Hassan et al. 2015; Eghbalian 2014; Samiee-Zafarghandy et al. 2015; Arawiran et al. 2015; Terrill et al. 2015).

When an infant is hypoxemic or suspected of being hypoxemic, healthcare professionals become appropriately concerned. However, the same has not been the case with hyperoxemia, which is frequent, and it is induced by excess O_2 administration. Because of the association of hyperoxemia with brain damage, gene changes, and cancer, there is a need for education about the judicious use of O_2 supplementation, SpO_2 management, and the potential damaging effects of hyperoxemia.

In this chapter we will cover several topics in relation to O_2 administration and SpO_2, including O_2 administration, assessment of O_2 in blood, arterial saturation (SaO_2) and SaO_2 monitors, physiology of tissue oxygenation, and the hazards of hyperoxia, to end with the clinical concepts of intention to treat and SpO_2 targets in neonatal care, emphasizing on the importance of avoiding abnormal amounts of O_2 in the blood (i.e., hyperoxemia or hypoxemia).

33.3 Oxygen Administration

The administration of supplemental O_2 should be considered in the same meticulous way as it is done when any drug is given to a newborn infant. Therefore, the dose or fraction of inspired O_2 (FiO_2) should be clearly indicated and the prescription should be carefully followed and monitored. Basic issues need to be taken into consideration at all times when supplemental O_2 is provided in order to avoid risks and potential damage. They are summarized in Table 1.

In clinical practice we must provide supplemental O_2 and any adjustment of FiO_2 based only on the objective assessment of O_2 in blood, which is described below.

33.4 Assessment of Oxygen in Blood

The first premise we must keep in mind is that the amount of O_2 in arterial blood does not equate with tissue oxygenation because there are many other factors that contribute to tissue oxygenation, as it will be shown later. Be this as it may, the most common method to assess O_2 in blood is the noninvasive continuous estimate of SaO_2 by SpO_2, currently being considered as the fifth vital sign.

Table 2 provides a summarized description of various methods of O_2 assessment. Clinical signs, such as cyanosis and tongue color, are of little or no value (Zhang et al. 2011; Niermeyer et al. 1995; Laman et al. 2005; de Wahl Granelli et al. 2009; Ewer et al. 2011). Intermittent invasive arterial or venous samples can be obtained to

Table 1 Guidelines in relation to administration of supplemental O_2

Do not provide $FiO_2 > 0.21$ based on previous maternal or neonatal history, gestational age, color, apnea, tachypnea, grunting, or any other clinical symptom
Provide $FiO_2 > 0.21$ only if the need is objectively demonstrated by low O_2 in blood as measured by SpO_2 monitor or others
O_2 should be blended with air and the FiO_2 clearly prescribed and measured
The gas delivered should be heated and humidified at all times
$FiO_2$1.0 (pure O_2) is very rarely truly necessary in neonatal care and less so in the delivery room
Avoid as much as possible making large increases of FiO_2 when an infant has an episode of acute decrease of SpO_2
The practice of "preoxygenation" for endotracheal tube suctioning, before or during anesthesia and before extubation, is very risky and potentially dangerous and is not supported by any (current) evidence
The use of manual ventilation with non-blended high FiO_2 and with dry and cold gas should be eradicated from clinical practice
The treatment of apnea is not to provide supplemental O_2, but to ventilate
In any case that there is cardiorespiratory arrest, resuscitative measures call for ventilation and circulation
Hyperoxygenation could be potentially dangerous due to the hypoxemia-hyperoxemia-reperfusion injury that can occur to many organs
Ventilation and cardiac massage can (and should) be provided with the same FiO_2 the infant was receiving

directly measure PaO_2 or PvO_2 and/or arterial or venous saturation (SaO_2 or SvO_2). Nevertheless, they are not ideal to closely monitor an unstable neonate as these measurements are only obtained at one point in time and therefore are not fully representative of the whole clinical picture. Additionally, the only way to measure SaO_2 is with a co-oximeter, ideally a last generation one, with multiple wavelengths. Therefore, the SaO_2 reported from a "regular" arterial blood gas determination should not be used for clinical management. The reason is that this value of Sa O_2 is not a measured SaO_2 but a calculated one. As shown in Table 2, such calculation is done using formulas or algorithms that are based on multiple factors, none truly applicable to a neonate and worse so if the infant is clinically ill. Finally, noninvasive continuous monitoring can assess the amount of O_2 in blood. Continuous transcutaneous PO_2 ($TcPO_2$) monitors had been widely used before SpO_2 became available, but they are almost never used currently. With $TcPO_2$, high PaO_2 had been more easily detected. Nonetheless, currently SpO_2 is the method used for continuous monitoring of O_2 in blood. Its advantages and disadvantages are discussed next.

33.5 Saturation and Assessment of Saturation with SpO_2 Monitors in Clinical Care

O_2 is a very insoluble molecule, and the main function of hemoglobin (Hb) is to solubilize O_2 and transport it from the lungs to the tissues. Hb is composed of four polypeptide chains, and each chain contains one heme group. Saturation is derived from the Latin word "saturare," which means to fill, and it refers to reaching a maximum capacity. The standard unit of O_2 saturation is percent; when all available hemoglobin-binding sites are completely occupied by O_2 molecules, the arterial O_2 saturation (SaO_2) is 100%. Therefore, SaO_2 can never be higher than 100%, regardless of the FiO_2 the infant breathes. One gram of hemoglobin can carry approximately 1.34 ml of O_2 when fully saturated, a concept known as the maximum oxygen-carrying capacity.

SaO_2 and Hb are the key factors that determine the arterial oxygen content (CaO_2), whereas the contribution of O_2 dissolved in plasma is minimal (0.003 ml of O_2 per millimeter of mercury of PaO_2 which is to say 0.3 ml of O_2 per deciliter of plasma when the PaO_2 is 100 mmHg). The following two examples reveal the significance of the Hb concentration in determining CaO_2:

1. With SaO_2 of 100% and Hb of 8 g/dl, CaO_2 is 10.72 ml/dl calculated by multiplying the 8 g/dl of Hb by 1.34 (and the amount of dissolved O_2 is minimal).
2. With SaO_2 of 100% and Hb of 20 g/dl, the CaO_2 is 26.8 ml/dl, using the same calculation.

Table 2 Oxygen in blood

Method	Comments
Cyanosis: a clinical sign that has been used to assess O_2 needs and to try to tailor O_2 administration	Bluish discoloration of skin and membranes Many studies have shown the poor predictive value of this clinical sign It could be due to an increased concentration of reduced (not saturated) Hb but may be due to several other factors It is unreliable because human beings perceive color with variability It depends on total Hb concentration, race, skin thickness, and illumination Unreliable because of "blind spot" for detecting cyanosis on the face of even significant Hb desaturation; such "spot" is accentuated in cases of low total Hb concentration Many infants who do not show cyanosis are hypoxemic and with a need for some evaluation and consideration of therapy Some infants who show what appears to be cyanosis do not need supplemental O_2
Tongue color (in the delivery room)	Specific but insensitive sign. When the tongue is pink, it is likely that an infant has $SpO_2 > 70$ % and may not require supplemental O_2
Measurements of PaO_2 in arterial (or venous) blood	Frequent blood samples may lead to anemia and/or hypovolemia Not fully representative, as these measurements are only at one point in time
Co-oximeters for intermittent direct measurements of SaO_2 (gold standard for measuring SaO_2)	Modern co-oximetry: spectrophotometers measuring light absorbance at 100–130 wavelengths Expensive, require blood sampling and provide only intermittent monitoring Not ideal to closely monitor an unstable neonate
Calculation of SaO_2 from an arterial blood gas by means of formulas or algorithms (based on PaO_2 measured and other factors) (should not be used for clinical management)	Is of no value in newborns Assumes a normal adult O_2 dissociation curve and O_2 affinity Assumes normal adult 2 3 DPG, hemoglobin (Hb) concentration, temperature, pH, and $PaCO_2$ and that the patient has no dyshemoglobinemia and is without fetal Hb In newborns: Hb concentration is variable and a large and variable proportion of Hb is Hb F (not A), and 2–3 DPG is low and variable in relation to transfusions In ill newborns pH, $PaCO_2$, and temperature are variable, with frequent changes It is incorrect to base clinical decisions on the reported (calculated) SaO_2 derived from the PaO_2 measured in an arterial blood gas Many places customize the output of blood gas analyzers so they do not report SaO_2 The monitor, which measures Hb-O_2 saturation, does not measure the same thing as a calculated SaO_2 from an arterial blood gas A SaO_2 value calculated from a blood gas must never be compared to continuous SpO_2
Noninvasive pulse oximetry (SpO_2) **Transcutaneous PO_2 was routinely monitored in the past, but not currently**	Please see description in text

If, in the second case, only 90% of the hemoglobin-binding sites were occupied with O_2 molecules, then CaO_2 would be 24.12 ml/dl, still much higher than in the first example with 100% SaO_2. Thus, even if all binding sites are occupied (as in the first example above), there can still be tissue hypoxia because the CaO_2 may be low because of anemia.

The hemoglobin-oxygen (Hb-O_2) dissociation curve is an italic sigmoid curve that shows a predictable relation between PaO_2 and SaO_2 when the curve is more verticalized, which happens at levels of SaO_2 of about 50–93% and SaO_2 of about 30–75 mmHg (Fig. 1). However, at higher SaO_2 levels, the Hb-O_2 is more horizontal and the predictability is lost. In addition, the curve can move to the right and to the left depending on several factors, shown in Fig. 1. As shown in the example in this figure, when the curve is shifted to the right, a PaO_2 of 52 mmHg will be associated with a SaO_2 of about 80%. With the curve shifted to the left, the SaO_2 will be about 91% with the same PaO_2. This means that with a larger amount of fetal hemoglobin (HbF), there is greater affinity for O_2 (higher SaO_2 at the same PaO_2) and that there is less O_2 release to the tissues. The reverse happens when the Hb is mostly of the adult type (HbA). As shown in Fig. 1, other conditions also affect shifts of the Hb-O_2 dissociation curve.

When a healthy neonate is breathing room air (FiO_2 0.21), the normal room air SaO_2 is 95–100%, except during the transition to extra uterine life when it is lower since, as described later, the newborn may take 15–20 min to achieve this normal SaO_2. Figure 2 shows an example of the Hb-O_2 dissociation curve in an infant receiving supplemental O_2. When the SaO_2 is about 86–93%, the corresponding PaO_2 will be about 50–68 mmHg based on the Hb-O_2 curve (Fig. 2). However, when the SaO_2 is 95–100%, the PaO_2 is unpredictable, as the relation between SaO_2 and PaO_2 is lost. In this case, if an infant is receiving 100% O_2 (FiO_2 1.0), the PaO_2 can be anywhere between 85 and up to 400 mmHg (Fig. 2), depending on the presence of lung disease and shunting and their severity. This is an important reason not to allow SaO_2 higher than about 95% when an infant is breathing $FiO_2 > 0.21$. In such cases there is a high probability of elevation of O_2 in blood or hyperoxemia, which could be associated with more dissolved free O_2 in plasma, potentially damaging tissues, cells, and genes.

A normal or even high PaO_2 and a normal SpO_2 (normoxemia or hyperoxemia) do not

Fig. 1 Hemoglobin-oxygen (Hb-O_2) dissociation curve. With HbF the curve is shifted to the left (see description in text)

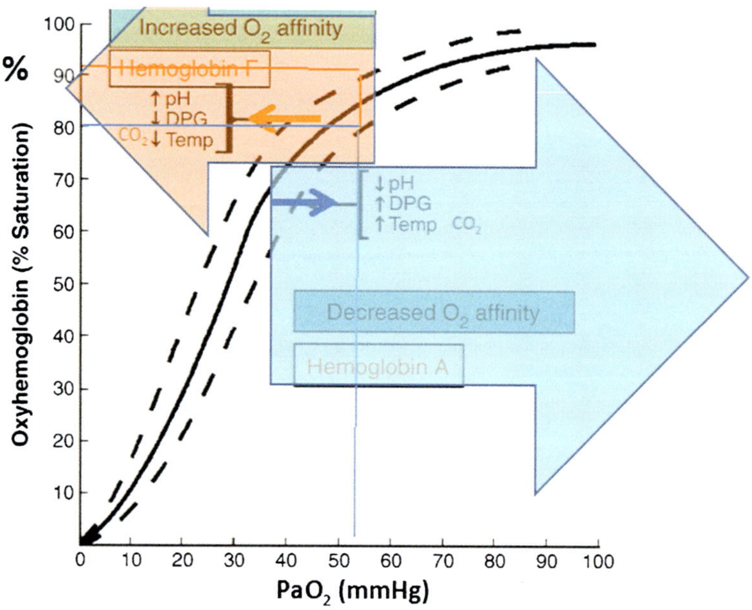

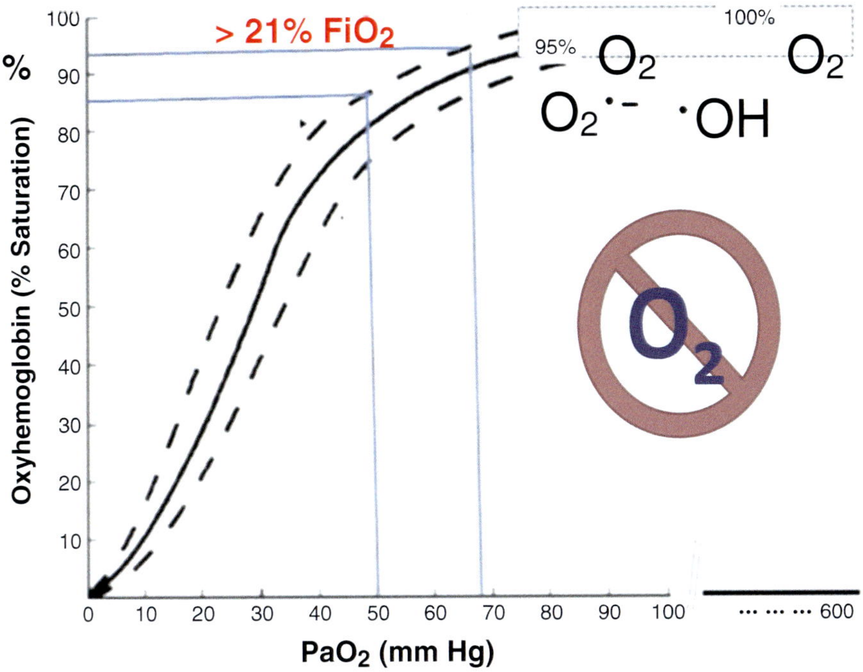

Fig. 2 **Hb-O_2 relationship when breathing supplemental O_2 (FiO_2 > 0.21)**. With SaO_2 95–100 % (measured by pulse oximetry), PaO_2 could be > 80 mmHg and free dissolved O_2 will be circulating

guarantee that the tissues are receiving enough O_2. Insufficient tissue oxygenation is called hypoxia and can exist in various circumstances on the face of normal or high PaO_2 as shown in Table 3. On the other hand, a low PaO_2 in blood (i.e., hypoxemia) is not necessarily associated with hypoxia because tissue oxygenation is a complex phenomenon, as described later. Several factors, such as an increase in cardiac output, can help to prevent hypoxia.

Table 3 Factors associated with tissue hypoxia on the face of normal or high PaO_2

1. Anemia
2. Altered affinity of Hb for binding O_2 (i.e., in cases of methemoglobinemia or when Hb-O_2 curve shifts markedly to the right)
3. Poor perfusion (altered cardiac output and vascular resistance)
4. Decreased O_2 delivery
5. Altered microcirculation and related factors

33.5.1 SpO_2 Monitors

The most common method to assess oxygenation is the noninvasive continuous measurement of arterial oxygen saturation by pulse oximetry (SpO_2), currently being considered as a fifth vital sign. However, SpO_2 does not equate with tissue oxygenation because there are many other factors that contribute to tissue oxygenation as shown in a later section.

SpO_2 monitors work by establishing the ratio between red and infrared wavelengths and display this ratio as a percentage of Hb saturated with O_2. These devices are very useful in the diagnosis of desaturation (i.e., hypoxemia) and evaluation of pulse rate, but they are of little or no value in diagnosing hyperoxemia unless some important physiological factors are entered into the assessment.

The following concepts are based on more than 200 peer-reviewed publications on the subject since the late 1990s; a few of them are listed in the bibliography (Sola et al. 2008, 2014; Castillo et al. 2011; Carlo et al. 2010; Stenson et al. 2013; Schmidt et al. 2013; Darlow et al. 2014; Hay et al. 2002; Baquero et al. 2011; Ahmed et al. 2010; Vagedes et al. 2013; Zapata et al. 2014; Sola 2015; Lakshminrusimha et al. 2015; Manja et al. 2015; Synnes and Miller 2015). Similar to most other pieces of medical equipment, all SpO_2 monitors available in the market have an inherent bias (equipment error). The bias (or SD) is not the same for monitors of different manufacturing companies and is as low as 2% or a bit lower in some and as high as 5% or higher in others. Due to equipment bias and in line with the Gaussian curve of normal distribution, the SpO_2 readout is within one standard deviation (SD) of the true arterial saturation 68% of the time. This means that when an SpO_2 with equipment bias of 1% displays a value of 90%, it does not mean that the true arterial saturation is 90%, but that 68% of the time the true arterial saturation will be either 89%, 90%, or 91%. If, on the other hand, the monitor from another company has a bias of 3%, then when the monitor reads an SpO_2 of 90%, the true arterial saturation will be between 87% and 93% for 68% of the time. Of course, based on simple statistics, the spread is more with two standard deviations. According to the Gaussian curve of normal distribution or bell-shaped curve, 95% of the time, the SpO_2 reported will be within two standard deviations of the true arterial saturation. This explains why with the same monitor in the same individual the SpO_2 readout could be different by 1–3% or more, depending on the bias of the equipment. Additionally, the true arterial saturation is not necessarily the same in two different individuals who have exactly the same SpO_2 readout. The difference could be as high as 3–4% or more. This clearly explains why it is nonsensical to emphasize differences in SpO_2 values of 1–2% in clinical care

The specificity and sensitivity to provide accurate readings also varies between SpO_2 monitors. Different monitors offer different accuracy levels and precision and they differ in the time they take to respond and in the number of false alarms, missed events, and detection of true events. False-positives and false-negatives, and therefore receiver operating curves, are also different between different SpO_2 monitors. Finally, they also differ in their ability to provide accurate measurements through motion and low perfusion. In summary, the function, strengths, limitations, and differences of oximetry monitors are well studied. The SpO_2 monitor with Signal Extraction Technology (SET®), (Masimo Corporation, Irvine, CA, USA) functions more accurately and precisely than any other SpO_2 monitor in the market. It has been proven to have better specificity and sensitivity and fewer false alarms and missed events and to function best during critical illness and is approved by the FDA to measure through motion and low perfusion states. In addition, it can use more than the classic 2 wavelengths (red and infrared) and can therefore measure hemoglobin, methemoglobin, and carboxyhemoglobin in addition to SpO_2. Based on all these concepts, the SpO_2 monitor was chosen by different investigators in the important neonatal randomized clinical trials published in the last few years (Carlo et al. 2010; Stenson et al. 2013; Schmidt et al. 2013; Darlow et al. 2014) features SET®.

33.5.1.1 Alarms in SpO_2 Monitors

There are many alarms in the NICU over the course of a day, and this has been identified as a safety issue. It is therefore important to choose monitors and other equipment that provide very few or no false alarms. This is also important for SpO_2 monitors, and as mentioned before, the amount of false alarms is different among different monitors. With SpO_2 there are also alarms that are true alarms but do not require any clinical intervention.

It cannot be overemphasized that it is clinically mandatory to choose and set alarms appropriately and to ensure the alarm system is always operative. *The low alarm limit for SpO_2 monitors should always be $\geq$85%, to avoid hypoxemia.* When the low alarm sounds, all clinicians pay attention to the potential problem of the infant. Unfortunately there is less response and much more frequent violations to high alarms in clinical care. The high alarm value to be chosen varies according to whether the infant is breathing room air or receiving any amount of supplemental O_2

($FiO_2 > 0.21$). In room air the normal SpO_2 is 95–100% and therefore the high alarm should not be on. However, in infants breathing supplemental O_2, the high alarm should be set at 95% to avoid hyperoxemia. *The high alarm should always be operative and responded to when an infant is breathing $FiO_2 > 0.21$.*

In clinical care it is not only important to detect and prevent significant periods of hypoxemia and hyperoxemia of prolonged duration (>20 s). It is also important to detect repeated shorter frequent episodes of desaturation, as they may not be inconsequential. A feature available in some monitors is the so-called alarm delay, which could be set by the clinician, just as the averaging time and sensitivity discussed below. These three variables impact when will an episode provide an audible alarm or not. If the delay is set at 10 s, the alarm will sound 10 s after the SpO_2 has been below (or above) the limits chosen. This may be necessary for some infants, as repeated and frequent brief periods of hypoxemia may have undesired long-term effects, but the alarms will sound more frequently. A delay time at 20 s means that if an infant has repeated episodes of 15 s of hypoxemia the alarms will not sound. Usually the delay should not be longer than 20 s, to ensure that significant hypoxemic events are not missed. In some babies this may need to be adjusted according to individualize care and infant's needs.

33.5.1.2 Averaging Time and Sensitivity in SpO_2 Monitors

Pulse oximeter saturation values are not really beat-to-beat and are usually obtained by averaging preceding measurements. Some SpO_2 monitors allow clinicians to modify the averaging time and sensitivity or both at the same time. This has an impact on the monitor's response and therefore on what the clinicians observe in the digital display in the same infant at the same time. With monitors that provide this function, the number of desaturations, and therefore alarms, is greater using short, 2-s averaging time. On the other hand, a long averaging time of 16 s reduces the detection of brief periodic desaturation events and of those of greater severity. It may also interpret a cluster of shorter events as a single, prolonged episode and, as a result, potentially overestimate the frequency of long events (Ahmed et al. 2010). One study recorded 339 desaturations of SpO_2 < 80% when using an average time of 16 s and 1958 when the average time was set at 3 s (Vagedes et al. 2013). Careful attention should therefore be paid to averaging time and sensitivity in the monitors used for clinical care. The performances of monitors manufactured by different companies vary, and some have default settings that cannot be modified. In the delivery room, when changes may occur rapidly during resuscitation, maximum sensitivity and an average time of 2 s are recommended. However, this is not the case for a critically ill infant in the NICU, as these settings could alarm the clinician by alerting him or her to very brief and clinically insignificant episodes. In the NICU setting, an average time of 8–12 s with intermediate sensitivity may be adequate (Sola et al. 2014; Sola 2015).

33.6 Physiology of Tissue Oxygenation

The PaO_2 depends on the amount of O_2 within alveoli (i.e., alveolar partial pressure of oxygen [PAO_2]), the ability of O_2 to enter adjacent pulmonary capillaries (i.e., O_2 diffusion), and the degree of intrapulmonary and extrapulmonary shunts. Of course the PAO_2 depends on the alveolar gas equation, which is related to the atmospheric pressure, the alveolar CO_2, and the relative humidity or water vapor pressure. At sea level the PAO_2 is about 110 mmHg in newborns and adults. The PaO_2 in healthy children and adults is approximately 100 mmHg at sea level; in neonates, however, the PaO_2 is lower (45–75 mmHg and rarely >80 mmHg) because of intrapulmonary and extrapulmonary shunting. When healthy adults are breathing 100% oxygen and the SaO_2 is 95–100%, the PaO_2 is > 600 mmHg, but it is lower, approximately 280–400 mmHg in healthy newborn infants because of the neonatal intrapulmonary and extrapulmonary shunts.

There are many factors involved in tissue oxygenation, which are summarized in Table 4. As mentioned previously, hypoxemia does not necessarily cause tissue hypoxia and there are situations where there is tissue hypoxia without hypoxemia. Some of the factors involved in tissue oxygenation mentioned in Table 4, like peripheral vascular resistance, O_2 delivery and consumption, microcirculatory changes, and the function of precapillary sphincters and post capillary venules, cannot be well evaluated in clinical care. Thus, it becomes of great significance to make an effort to avoid practices that lead to hyperoxemia that may induce unnecessary oxidative stress and oxidant injury.

33.7 Hazards of Hyperoxemia and Hyperoxia

Oxygen is a very potent drug that is often used inappropriately in the clinical environment. At high level of arterial O_2, there will be an increase in both free dissolved oxygen and reactive oxygen species (ROS). Measurements of PaO_2, when providing supplemental oxygen, help avoid unnecessary hyperoxemia and hyperoxia, but it is more important to monitor SpO_2 continuously when an infant is breathing supplemental O_2.

Excessive O_2 administration can lead to overproduction of ROS. Other chapters of this text discuss in detail the antioxidant system and the potential damage of ROS, peroxides, and free radicals to all components of the cell (proteins, lipids, and DNA). Suffice to say here that oxidative damage is less controlled in infants and therefore oxidative damage and possible cell death occur more easily with excess O_2 administration (Kaindl et al. 2006; Wollen et al. 2014; Farrow et al. 2012; Spector et al. 2005; Wellmann et al. 2014). Thus, we must change the way we administer supplemental O_2 when a newborn infant is not hypoxemic and stop using pure free-flowing O_2 in order to avoid causing conditions associated with hyperoxia, oxidative stress, and damage.

Table 4 Factors related to tissue oxygenation

PaO_2 (mmHg)	O_2 Consumption
Hb concentration (anemia) and quality (Hb F; Hb A; dyshemoglobins)	Pulmonary vascular resistance
Hb-O_2relationship (saturation in %)	Pulmonary blood flow
Oxygen content (CaO_2; in ml of O_2/dl) [(SaO_2 x Hb x 1.34) + .003 ml O_2/mmHg PaO_2]	Hematocrit (hyperviscosity)
Cardiac output (Heart rate, stroke volume, minute volume)	pH
Peripheral vascular resistance	CO_2 (local and systemic)
Systemic blood flow	Temperature
O_2 delivery	Glycemia
	Local PO_2 (4–20 mmHg)
	Distance to mitochondria
	Microcirculation

A summary of undesired effects of maternal and fetal oxidative stress and short- and long-term O_2 therapy is presented in Tables 5, 6, 7, and 8. During normal birth without supplemental O_2 administration, there is already altered lipid peroxidation levels and antioxidant capacity, which is worsened if the delivery is by cesarean section (Noh et al. 2014). Excess O_2 during labor and in cesarean deliveries induces much more damage and is potentially dangerous for the pregnant woman and the fetus, as shown in Table 5 (Yalcin et al. 2013; Hamel et al. 2014; Lye et al. 2013; Klimova et al. 2013; Klingel and Patel 2013). Therefore, the practice of providing supplemental O_2 to pregnant women should be reserved only for documented maternal hypoxemia.

Table 6 summarizes undesired effects of acute O_2 therapy and Table 7 several clinical conditions associated with hyperoxia, oxidative stress, and damage. In the neonatal and pediatric populations, excess O_2 is potentially very damaging. Our current understanding of its potentially injurious effects is summarized in Table 8, and they include increase in cancer risk, retinopathy of prematurity (ROP), bronchopulmonary dysplasia (BPD), injury to the developing brain, disruption of the circadian rhythm, and alteration of enzymes, proteins, and genes by hyperoxia (Lye et al. 2013; Klimova et al. 2013; Klingel and Patel 2013; Kaindl et al. 2006; Wollen et al. 2014; Farrow et al. 2012; Spector et al. 2005; Wellmann et al. 2014) (Table 8). O_2 excess is a concern at any time and this includes anesthesia and recovery after surgery (Table 8). Some anesthetic and

Table 5 Hyperoxemia and hyperoxia in the prenatal period

Cesarean section: higher oxidative stress and alteration of the oxidant and antioxidant system compared to vaginal deliveries (additional risk associated with planned elective cesarean sections)
Unnecessary use of O_2 during C-sections and labor and delivery
1. Increases markedly the potential damage being caused to mothers, placenta, and fetus
2. FiO_2 0.4 in elective cesarean sections under spinal anesthesia: significantly worse fetal and maternal total antioxidant capacity, total oxidant status, and oxidative stress index than with room air
3. Significant differences in healthy pregnant women who received supplemental O_2 during C-S with regional anesthesia (higher PaO_2, free O_2 radicals, and ROS in both mother and neonate)
4. Supplemental O_2 in intrauterine resuscitation: this practice should not be considered an indicated intervention for nonreassuring fetal status since it is of unproven benefit and is potentially harmful due to increase free radical activity
Effects of hyperoxia on placental functions:
1. In explants of villi of human placentas: a protein of resistance to breast cancer (ABCG2 mRNA), which also protects the fetus against maternally derived toxins, drugs, chemical substances, and pollutants (i.e., xenobiotics), increases after hours of hyperoxia. It is possible, therefore, that placental changes in O_2 tension and delivery may alter resistance to drugs and toxins during fetal life
2. Increased PaO_2 reduces the cellular pro-inflammatory response to *E. coli* and promotes an abnormal anti-inflammatory cytokine profile in the membranes. Therefore, tissue injury may occur as a result of injurious O_2 by-products secondary to hyperoxia in utero

sedative drugs have been associated with hyperoxia-induced oxidative stress and therefore should be used judiciously. Worse even is the combination of these drugs with hyperoxemia. The practice of preoxygenation must be carefully evaluated and not used routinely (Sola 2008).

Benefits of changing clinical practice to try to reduce PAO_2 and/or maintain SpO_2 values to decrease hyperoxemia have been proven (Chow et al. 2003; Deulofeut et al. 2006; Bizzarro et al. 2014; Castillo et al. 2011). Using excess O_2 for the treatment of non-hypoxemic humans is definitely a health hazard (Sola et al. 2007). More so, periods of fluctuating hypoxemia-hyperoxemia-reperfusion are potentially very damaging in newborn infants. O_2 should never be denied when necessary, but providing unnecessary O_2 should be avoided at all times during the birthing process and after birth, including in the delivery room, during resuscitation, and in the neonatal intensive care unit, as well as before,

Table 6 Undesired effects of acute O_2 therapy

Altered respiratory control and chemo- and baroreceptors responses
Raised blood pressure
Redistribution of blood in the microcirculation
Decrease blood flow in the cerebral and renal beds
Decrease cardiac index
Decrease heart rate
Decrease myocardial contractility
Decrease cardiac oxygen consumption
Lower capillary density

Table 7 Conditions associated with hyperoxia, oxidative stress, and damage

Aging	Other
DNA impact – cancer	Fragile X syndrome
Alteration of gene expression	Sickle cell disease
Central nervous system	Lichen planus
Parkinson's disease	Vitiligo
Alzheimer's disease	Infection
Neuronal degeneration	Inflammation – fibrosis
Autism	Chronic fatigue syndrome
Altered blood flow	Altered renal function
Cardiovascular	*Perinatal: specific to mother, fetus, and neonate*
Atherosclerosis	Placental defenses and genes
Heart failure	ROP
Myocardial infarction	BPD – lung injury
Decreased contractility	Developing brain
Altered chemo- and baroreceptors	Increased PVR
Endocrine	Abnormal response to iNO
Insulin	Altered clock genes
Glucagon	Altered ocular genes
Lung	Thymus (T cells)
Atelectasis	
Alveolar collapse	

ROP retinopathy of prematurity, *BPD* bronchopulmonary dysplasia, *PVR* pulmonary vascular resistance, *iNO* inhaled nitric oxide

Table 8 Undesired effects of pediatric and neonatal O_2 excess

ROP and BPD
Cell death in the developing brain
Worse long-term neurodevelopment outcomes; contributing factor to the pathogenesis of cerebral palsy (Study of 1105 preterm infants; risk of disabling cerebral palsy was double in those exposed to hyperoxia and it was eightfold in the highest quintiles of O_2 exposure)
Enzyme and gene alteration
Proteome changes induced by oxidative stress have been described
In models of persistent pulmonary hypertension (PPHN):
100 % O_2 increases ROS in the mitochondrial matrix prior to the cytosol and can produce significant changes in critical cellular signaling pathways
100 % O_2 increases PDE5 activity and decreases NO-mediated cGMP-dependent vasorelaxation
100 % O_2 decreases the response to iNO, produces oxidative stress in the lung and vessels, and alters pulmonary artery contractility
Some of these alterations are prevented with the use of antioxidants such as superoxide dismutase and catalase, confirming the role of oxidative stress in these responses
Two minutes of 100 % O_2 in children ages 8–15: abnormal activation of hippocampus, hypothalamus, and insula, areas that regulate blood pressure, heart rate, and response to stress
Risk of leukemia and cancer in childhood: threefold increase with exposure to 100 % O_2 in the delivery room for 3 min or more
Newborn eyes of experimental animals: hyperoxia at birth alters whole-genome expression (If this were to occur during induced hyperoxia after birth of preterm infants, predisposition for ROP could be markedly increased at that time)
Circadian rhythm disruption
Key circadian genes are Rev-erbα, Per, and Bmal
Rev-erbα is degraded in hyperoxia; its disruption exacerbates hyperoxic lung injury, which is associated with decreased cell proliferation and distorted alveolar architecture. Stabilizing lung Rev-erbα prevents the loss of cell proliferation
Combined effect of O_2 and phototherapy: potential cytotoxicity and disruption of circadian gene expression is concerning. This cytotoxic effect can be partly reversed in animals by stabilizing Rev-erbα and this improves mitochondrial efficiency conferring a survival advantage
Hyperoxia during anesthesia or recovery post-surgery:
Potentiation of brain damage and ROP
Negative impact of sedatives like midazolam and ketamine; both affect long-term neurodevelopmental outcome, alter NMDA receptors, and enhance human neural stem cell proliferation and neuronal apoptosis
High FiO_2 worsens compliance and lung units with low ventilation to perfusion ratios become more unstable when breathing O_2
Pure O_2 results in reabsorption atelectasis shortly after its application; rapid recurrence of the atelectasis, together with decreased FRC and alteration of ventilation homogeneity, occurs more frequently
Pure O_2 aggravates central hypoventilation and apnea, can induce mental changes, and increases the risk for postoperative atelectasis
Rev-erbα is degraded in hyperoxia; its disruption exacerbates hyperoxic lung injury, which is associated with decreased cell proliferation and distorted alveolar architecture
Diagnostic hyperoxic challenge test, nitrogen washout for pneumothorax:
Please see text. Both practices should be eradicated from clinical care
Pure O_2 (i.e., 100 % O_2, FiO_2 1.0) is almost never indicated in neonatal care. In the few cases when it is really necessary, it should be weaned as soon as possible

during, and after neonatal anesthesia and other procedures.

33.8 Intention to Treat: SpO_2 Target Ranges for Preterm Infants

The SpO_2 in normal newborns breathing room air (FiO_2 0.21) is 95–100%. The same is true for neonates who are being treated with CPAP or assisted ventilation when they are breathing room air. However, this is not the case for infants breathing supplemental O_2 in whom the most prudent approach is not to tolerate possible hypoxia and at the same time not to accept SpO_2 values associated with potential hyperoxia to avoid issues mentioned in Table 8. This is not easy to accomplish all of the time in clinical practice, and some recommendation are described below and summarized in Table 9, based on current available evidence.

First and foremost, we must take into consideration three important factors when we make decisions on the intention to treat for SpO_2 targeting. As discussed in a previous section,

Table 9 What to do with SpO_2 in clinical practice in 2016 in tiny preterm infants who are breathing supplemental oxygen?

Try to avoid $SpO_2 > 94$ % to avoid high PaO_2 values
Avoid inducing significant fluctuations in SpO_2 because a higher incidence of intermittent hypoxemic-hyperoxemic episodes is associated with severe ROP
Evaluate in detail the infant who has frequent wide swings in SpO_2 and consider modifying other aspects of care (i.e., PEEP, position, other) and not just adjustments of FiO_2, which actually could be part of the cause of the significant fluctuations
When FiO_2 is increased, return it gradually to baseline levels without leaving the infant with high SpO_2
Choose an intention to treat which is wide and not with narrow SpO_2 ranges and oximetry alarm settings, with enforcement of adherence to those alarm settings, with frequent audits and feedbacks. For example, intention to treat not less than 86 %and not more than 94 %, with low alarm at 85% and high alarm at 95%
The intention to treat for SpO_2 ranges could be, for example, between 86 % and 94 % (high alarms at 85 % and 95 %, respectively), according to the patient and the diagnosis. Of course, if somebody chooses to set alarms at 86 % and 94 % (with SpO_2 range 87–93 %), there is no supporting evidence against such practice
On the basis of evidence to date, do not use intention to treat with SpO_2 ranges as narrow as 85–89 % or 91–95 %
If the SpO_2 levels remain steadily ("stable") in the low end (85–87 %), it may also be prudent to evaluate carefully and modify settings if necessary
The intention to treat may not be the same for each NICU:
In a NICU with low rates of mortality and necrotizing enterocolitis (NEC) but high rates of severe ROP, it has been suggested that consideration is given to set the lower alarm at 85–86 % (or even lower in the tiniest of infants) and the upper alarm at 93 % or 94 %
In a NICU that has high rates of mortality and necrotizing enterocolitis but low rates of severe ROP, the lower alarm could be at 88 % and the upper alarm at 95 %
SpO_2 alarms must always be operative when a neonate is receiving supplemental O_2; the low alarm should be 1 % below the intended low SpO_2, and the high alarm at the same 1 % above the intended high SpO_2

SpO_2 monitors have a bias or error and therefore it does not make much sense to spend much time arguing if an SpO_2 of 89% is significantly worse than an SpO_2 of 91% for an individual baby at any given time. Secondly, one SpO_2 monitor is not the same as another SpO_2 monitor. All the randomized trials and descriptive studies with large sample size were performed with one SpO_2 monitor which has SET®, and therefore, it is not clear if the same planned intention to treat based on these monitors would be valid in centers using different SpO_2 monitors. Thirdly, the clinically optimal or ideal SpO_2 range for extremely preterm infants breathing supplemental O_2 is currently unknown and likely varies with advancing gestational and postnatal age and clinical condition. However, in more than a decade of many publications, prevention of severe ROP in preterm infants through changes in clinical practice and SpO_2 technology has been established (Chow et al. 2003; Deulofeut et al. 2006; Bizzarro et al. 2014; Castillo et al. 2011; Sola et al. 2014). For these preterm infants when they are receiving supplemental O_2, a prudent clinical approach is presented in Table 9, based on available publications to date.

It may be sensible to consider a lower SpO_2 limit of >85% and a higher limit of ≤95% when a preterm infant is breathing $FiO_2 > 0.21$ (Schmidt et al. 2014a, b; Sola et al. 2014; Lakshminrusimha et al. 2015; Manja et al. 2015). This is an intended range of SpO_2, which is very different to saying that an SpO_2 of 85% or 95% is normal. If one so chooses, the low and high alarm limits should be set at 85% and 95%, respectively. The alarms should be operative at all times and a clinical response would be initiated when the low or high alarm sounds.

It is a challenge to maintain infants within the intention to treat chosen. It is well known that some preterm infants breathing O_2 have more oscillation in SpO_2 than others, and it is impossible to maintain the SpO_2 within the intended target all the time. It has been shown that adherence to planned SpO_2 targets varies between shifts and centers, mainly due to the SpO_2 targets chosen, differences in education, staff commitment to this issue, workload, and accuracy and precision of monitors used. This means that actual versus intended SpO_2 levels are very variable (Dawson et al. 2010; Saugstad and Aune 2014; Schmidt et al. 2014a; Noh et al. 2014; Yalcin et al. 2013). In some places of the world, there are now equipments that provide automated control of FiO_2 for infants on noninvasive and invasive respiratory support (Zapata et al. 2014; Bancalari and Claure 2012; Claure and Bancalari 2013, 2015; van Kaam et al. 2015). Even though these methods reduce the percent time spent outside of the limits of the intention to treat, babies are still off target between 40% and 50% of the time. The percent time spent below the lower SpO_2 value chosen in the intention to treat or in hypoxemia with $SpO_2 < 80\%$ is reduced but not eliminated. The time spent above the maximum SpO_2 chosen or at extreme hypoxemia with $SpO_2 > 98\%$ is also reduced during automated FiO_2 but these episodes are not eliminated (Zapata et al. 2014; van Kaam et al. 2015). When tight or narrow SpO_2 target ranges are intended, there is more time spent outside of the desired range whether, with manual or automated control of the FiO_2 (Hagadorn et al. 2006; Deulofeut et al. 2007; Sola et al. 2007, 2008, 2014; Castillo et al. 2008; Lim et al. 2014; Bizzarro et al. 2014; Schmidt et al. 2013, 2014a, b; Carlo et al. 2010; Stenson et al. 2013; Darlow et al. 2014; Zapata et al. 2014; van Kaam et al. 2015), there are more fluctuations in SpO_2. If the narrow SpO_2 range is on the low end (SpO_2 85–89%), there are more periods of hypoxemia, which are followed by hyperoxemia by the clinical response of increasing the FiO_2. Also, the narrower the SpO_2 targeting range and alarm limits chosen, the greater will be the number of alarms. An intended narrow SpO_2 target, for example, 90–93%, is almost never the actual SpO_2 values, even when the nurse to patient ratio is one-to-one, which very rarely happens. In addition, the education programs in most nursing and medical schools emphasize the problems of hypoxia and the need to correct it, much more than what they do about the complications of hyperoxia. This is another reason why infants are outside the desired range and explains why the % time in hyperoxemia is much higher than the % time with hypoxemia. Therefore, in clinical care there are more violations and less response to high alarms with and an increased tolerance of $SpO_2 \geq 95\%$ as compared to the responses to low alarms and to $SpO_2 < 85\%$. Therefore, a narrow high target like 91–95% is not only difficult to achieve but can lead to increased tolerance of an SpO_2 level >95%. In a study of 1000 samples, we found that when SpO_2 is > 94%, hyperoxemia (PaO_2 i > 80 mmHg) occurs in 60% of the samples (Castillo et al. 2008). Therefore, with narrow SpO_2 ranges, the % time with hyperoxemia increases much more than the one spent in hypoxemia (Sola et al. 2014).

Based on these considerations, a narrow low SpO_2 target of 85–89% should not be used clinically. Even though this may not be associated with increased mortality (Schmidt et al. 2013; Darlow et al. 2014; Manja et al. 2015), it may potentially lead to more periods of hypoxemia-hyperoxemia-reperfusion damage. On the other hand, at the high end of SpO_2, there is no evidence that a narrow SpO_2 target of 91–95% or 90–95% should be universally used in clinical practice for preterm infants in the initial periods of life, since they may increase the time in hyperoxemia, which may be associated with severe ROP and other damaging effects. In one study, when the intended target SpO_2 was 91–95%, the actual SpO_2 was 85–95% 54% of the time, > 95% for 36% of the time and <85% for only 10% of the time. One study of random observations, after clinical practice was changed to aiming for SpO_2 in the 88–93% range, showed that the target was achieved 72% of the time; SpO_2 was 96–100% in 18% of the time and it was <85% for 10% of the time. Wider intermediate targets allow for easier care and better compliance and, with an SpO_2 monitor with SET ® as the one used in the large clinical studies, such ranges have been associated with a decreased rate of severe ROP, without an increased morbidity or mortality (Chow et al. 2003; Deulofeut et al. 2006, 2007; Bizzarro et al. 2014; Schmidt et al. 2014a). Therefore, in the early periods of care of small preterm infants, rather than using narrower intended targets, like 85–89%, 90–93%, or 91–95%, it may be safer to use wider intermediate SpO_2 targets such as 86%, 87%, or 88% for the lower value and 93% or 94% for the higher one. However, these intermediate target ranges may be not very different from one another, due to the inherent bias of SpO_2 monitors and the significant difference between monitors described previously.

In summary, in any infant breathing supplemental O_2, it is of clinical significance to avoid hypoxemia, hyperoxemia, and recurring episodes of hypoxemia-hyperoxemia-reperfusion. A summary of important issues for clinical care of tiny preterm babies breathing supplemental O_2 early in life and until the retina is mature is presented in Table 9. The challenges to try to keep actual SpO_2 within the intended range most of the time must be overcome to improve infant safety. For this to happen, it is necessary to ensure teamwork among all neonatal healthcare providers and to include parents in the objective of avoiding hyperoxemia in these tiny fragile infants.

33.9 Intention to Treat with SpO_2 Target Ranges in the Delivery Room and in Other Neonatal Conditions

All the measures to try to avoid both hypoxemia and hyperoxemia are just as important as in the delivery room during neonatal resuscitation, in other neonatal conditions, and during endotracheal tube suctioning, transport, anesthesia, surgery, and other procedures (Sola 2008).

Indeed, specific guidelines for targeting SpO_2 in newborns soon after birth have recently been recommended and are based on normal fetal oxygen physiology and the expected physiologic changes during transition from intrauterine to extrauterine life. A summary is presented in Table 10. During gestation, human fetuses have an extremely low SpO_2, with the highest SpO_2 in the umbilical vein (70–75%). Despite this relatively hypoxemic environment, fetal tissues are not affected in this state and are not hypoxic. Just before birth, the SpO_2 in the fetus is 60% and can decrease to 30% during labor. Healthy newborns cannot be expected to transition from fetal to neonatal life in a few seconds or minutes. In the postnatal transition period, the SpO_2 to preductal tissues (brain, right arm, coronary arteries) is higher than postductal tissues. Then the SpO_2 increases steadily but slowly in both the preductal and postductal regions (Table 10). Infants born by elective cesarean delivery take a bit longer to attain an SpO_2 above 94% (Dawson et al. 2010, 2012; Vento et al. 2013; Saugstad et al. 2014).

It is clear that in many cases there is no need to provide supplemental O_2 during neonatal resuscitation, and less so 100% O_2. A similar situation occurs in periods of apnea, when the treatment is to ventilate the alveoli (breathe) and circulate, but not to give supplemental O_2. Undeniably, many adult human beings have been successfully resuscitated by mouth-to-mouth resuscitation. In such

Table 10 SpO_2 targeting in the delivery room during neonatal resuscitation

SpO_2 increases steadily over time during the normal neonatal transition, reaching >90 % in approximately 8 min in term infants and requiring a little more time in preterm infants and after cesarean deliveries

As a general concept, if a term or preterm infant breathing room air has an SpO_2 < 90 % at or after age 10 min, detailed evaluation should be performed

In term or near-term infants:

When there is an absence of lung disease, there is no need to provide any supplemental O2

It is recommended to start resuscitation with room air

If significant lung disease is anticipated, use higher FiO2 (i.e., 0.30–0.40)

In tiny preterm infants: start with SpO_2 of 0.21–0.30

Subsequently, in both term and preterm infants, adjust FiO_2 aiming to maintain preductal SpO_2 within published nomograms, as below:

1 min of age: 10th and 90th percentiles of SpO2 are 40–85 %

2 min of age: 10th and 90th percentiles of SpO2 are 46–91 %

3 min of age: 10th and 90th percentiles of SpO2 are 55–92 %

5 min of age: 10th percentile 73 % (90th percentile is 97 %)

Age	Preductal SpO_2 in term newborns	Preductal SpO_2 in preterm newborns
3 min	55–80 %	55–80 %
5 min	75–90 %	75–85 %
10 min	90–97 %	85–90 %

If CPAP is used in tiny infants breathing room air, the increase in SpO_2 occurs more rapidly than those described above. No one knows whether this is of any benefit or whether it is actually risky because of faster exposure to potential oxidation

Always decrease FiO_2 if SpO_2 > 93–95 %

cases the FiO_2 is approximately 17% as a result of the CO_2 in exhaled gas. Similarly, studies have found that O_2 is not necessary in many cases of newborn resuscitation (Rabi et al. 2007; Dawson et al. 2010, 2012; Vento et al. 2013; Saugstad et al. 2014).

Several publications describe nomograms for what is considered normal SpO_2 during the first minutes of life or transitional period from fetal to neonatal life (Table 10). Values were obtained from preductal territory and are not the same for term and preterm infants and vary according to mode of delivery and maybe even sex (Rabi et al. 2007; Dawson et al. 2010, 2012; Vento et al. 2013; Saugstad et al. 2014). Because of study design issues and changes that have occurred in the physiology of transition by modifications in the time of cord clamping, the SpO_2 values in the nomograms may change in the near future. However, *hypoxemia should not be accepted during neonatal resuscitation, and it is as important to avoid hyperoxemia*. For this reason, in all hospital settings, including birthing centers, a heater humidifier (to provide adequately conditioned inhaled gas) and a blender (to accurately measure the dose of O_2) are mandatory. In addition, an adequate SpO_2 monitor that can rapidly measure SpO_2 despite poor perfusion and motion is necessary to more accurately adjust the amount of supplemental O_2.

Table 11 summarizes issues related to other neonatal practices and conditions in which careful attention to FiO_2 and SpO_2 also needs to be considered. Included are apnea, persistent pulmonary hypertension, BPD, and others. Currently, there is no published solid definitive research that provides concrete evidence for targeted SpO_2 in these clinical disorders. In general, in infants beyond the immediate newborn period, supplemental O_2 should be decreased when SpO_2 > 95%. Indeed, targeting a higher SpO_2 range >95% in preterm infants who were O_2 dependent with BPD conferred no significant benefit with respect to prevention of worsening ROP or improved growth and development. Worse so, it resulted in worse pulmonary outcomes, increased burden on health services, and a greater need for medications (Askie et al. 2003)

Table 11 Clinical recommendations for SpO_2 targeting in various neonatal conditions (without any published solid or definitive evidence)

Apnea
Start ventilation with the same FiO_2 the infant was receiving, even if it was room air
CPAP and room air (FiO_2 0.21)
SpO_2 of 95–100 % is normal. If SpO_2 < 94 %: evaluate and decide if more pressure or supplemental FiO_2 or both are needed
Nasal cannula (high or low flow):
As for CPAP, SpO_2 of 95–100 % is normal in room air
The FiO_2 from the wall or from a blender does not match the PiO_2 in the airways and alveoli
When an infant is in the hospital and not close to discharge, it is safer to use a blender and wean the FiO_2 all the way to room air if the SpO_2 > 95 %
If 100 % FiO_2 is used, then the only alternative is to decrease flow if SpO_2 > 95 %, but this is more unpredictable
Persistent pulmonary hypertension of the newborn and congenital diaphragmatic hernia
SpO_2 in the preductal territory (right hand) should be 91–96 %
Wean respiratory pressures and $FiO_2$when the preductal SpO_2 is >96 %
Avoid using 100 % oxygen as much as possible
Established BPD:
Persistent hypoxia must be avoided because it can lead to right ventricular hypertrophy, pulmonary vasoconstriction and hypertension, cor pulmonale, and bronchoconstriction. When breathing supplemental oxygen, it may be prudent to adjust the FiO_2 to try maintain SpO_2 at approximately 91–96 %, cautiously weaning the FiO_2 when SpO_2 > 95 %
Suction of endotracheal tube:
Do not "pre-oxygenate"
Avoid hypoxemia and hyperoxemia
If SpO_2 decreases do not increase FiO_2 abruptly or unnecessarily for recovery
Surgery and anesthesia:
Do not use preoxygenation
Avoid hypoxemia and hyperoxemia
If SpO_2 is 96–100 %, the FiO_2 should be weaned

Hyperoxemia should not be induced in any neonate before, during, and after endotracheal tube suction or invasive procedures, including surgery, and it should not be caused in periods before and after extubation. Preoxygenation is a dangerous and ineffective practice for endotracheal tube suction, before or during anesthesia and before extubation, that should be eradicated in newborns of any gestational age, and this has been summarized elsewhere (Sola 2008). Lastly, as shown in Table 8, practices that can lead to severe and prolonged hyperoxemia, like nitrogen washout without any proven benefit in important outcomes of pneumothoraces and the hyperoxic challenge test to try to differentiate heart versus lung disease, should also be eliminated from clinical practice. Some recommendations for SpO_2 targeting in various neonatal conditions are shown in Table 11.

As much as the ideal and best SpO_2 targets for tiny preterm infants breathing O_2 during the first weeks after birth is still a matter of controversy, it has been studied in much more detail than for any of the conditions mentioned in Tables 10 and 11. Therefore, we must be vigilant of future studies that may find that some of these recommendations need to be modified. Additionally, five similarly designed randomized controlled trials compared only two SpO_2 target ranges (intention to treat 85–89% versus 9–95%). The different results reported partially or completely to date, and the various publications that have analyzed such studies in detail, suggest that none of those SpO_2 ranges of intention to treat should be chosen in clinical practice. There are many more than these two possible SpO_2targets and we should not keep repeating the same mistakes of the past due to simplification and immoderation. The observed limitations in the existing evidence about optimal SpO_2 in the premature infant early in life make it essential to avoid any firm recommendation. Therefore the paragraphs in the section of "Intention to Treat: SpO_2 Target Ranges for Preterm Infant" and the concepts in Table 9 should be read and analyzed with great caution.

33.10 Summary

Cellular oxygenation is complex and not easy to assess in clinical practice. Hopefully, in the future we will be able to do this better at the bedside. In the meantime, we must do everything possible to ensure sufficient O_2 delivery to the tissues while minimizing O_2 toxicity and oxidative stress. Therefore, the intention to treat should include not only the avoidance and rapid treatment of hypoxemia but being extremely vigilant to avoid inducing or causing hyperoxemia and not allowing SpO_2 to be > 95% when supplemental O_2 is used.

Most of the available evidence derived from randomized clinical trials, physiology, and large descriptive studies have been the foundation for what is included in this chapter with the aim to provide tools for clinical practice. Based on the available evidence and on thorough review of each center's own data, infant safety and outcomes can be improved. We cannot disregard that changes in clinical practice in O_2 administration and monitoring can improve outcomes, like lower rates of severe ROP without an increase in mortality or long-term morbidity. Decreasing hyperoxemia and episodes of hypoxemia followed by hyperoxemia reperfusion from the time of birth will prevent many if not all of the problems mentioned in the various sections and tables of this chapter.

The limitations in the existing evidence (Sola and Zuluaga 2013; Saugstad and Aune 2014; Schmidt et al. 2013, 2014a, b; Sola et al. 2014; Carlo et al. 2010; Stenson et al. 2013; Darlow et al. 2014; Sola 2015; Lakshminrusimha et al. 2015; Manja et al. 2015), and the fact that the "magic" SpO_2 range for all infants at all times is not truly known, and it is likely that it will never be known, make it essential that all recommendations in regard to FiO_2 and SpO_2 are meticulously reviewed. When infants breathe supplemental O_2, we must know the dose of O_2; avoid the use of pure, dry, and cold O_2; and continuously monitor SpO_2 with the best monitors available in the market. With this and a concerted team effort to try to avoid tissue hypoxia, significant fluctuations in SpO_2, and hyperoxemia, many infants will be healthier and safer.

References

Ahmed SJ, Rich W, Finer NN (2010) The effect of averaging time on oximetry values in the premature infant. Pediatrics 125:e115–e121

Arawiran J, Curry J, Welde L, Alpan G (2015) Sojourn in excessively high oxygen saturation ranges in individual, very low-birthweight neonates. Acta Paediatr 104 (2):e51–e56

Askie LM, Henderson-Smart DJ, Irwig L, Simpson JM (2003) Oxygen-saturation targets and outcomes in extremely preterm infants. N Engl J Med 349 (10):959–967

Bancalari E, Claure N (2012) Control of oxygenation during mechanical ventilation in the premature infant. Clin Perinatol 39:563–572

Baquero H, Alviz R, Castillo A, Neira F, Sola A (2011) Avoiding hyperoxemia during neonatal resuscitation: time to response of different SpO_2 monitors. Acta Paediatr 100(4):515–518

Bizzarro MJ, Li FY, Katz K, Shabanova V, Ehrenkranz RA, Bhandari V (2014) Temporal quantification of oxygen saturation ranges: an effort to reduce hyperoxia in the neonatal intensive care unit. J Perinatol 34(1):33–38

Carlo WA, Finer NN, Walsh MC, SUPPORT Study Group of the Eunice Kennedy Shriver NICHD Neonatal Research Network et al (2010) Target ranges of oxygen saturation in extremely preterm infants. N Engl J Med 362(21):1959–1969

Castillo A, Sola A, Baquero H et al (2008) Pulse oxygen saturation levels and arterial oxygen tension values in newborns receiving oxygen therapy in the neonatal intensive care unit: is 85% to 93% an acceptable range? Pediatrics 121(5):882–889

Castillo A, Deulofeut R, Critz A, Sola A (2011) Prevention of retinopathy of prematurity in preterm infants through changes in clinical practice and SpO_2 technology. Acta Paediatr 100(2):188–192

Chow LC, Wright KW, Sola A, CSMC Oxygen Administration Study Group (2003) Can changes in clinical practice decrease the incidence of severe retinopathy of prematurity in very low birth weight infants? Pediatrics 111(2):339–345

Clarke A, Yeomans E, Elsayed K, Medhurst A, Berger P, Skuza E, Tan K (2015) A randomised crossover trial of clinical algorithm for oxygen saturation targeting in preterm infants with frequent desaturation episodes. Neonatology 107(2):130–136

Claure N, Bancalari E (2013) Role of automation in neonatal respiratory support. J Perinat Med 41(1):115–118

Claure N, Bancalari E (2015) Closed-loop control of inspired oxygen in premature infants. Semin Fetal Neonatal Med 20(3):198–204

Comroe JH Jr, Bahnson ER, Coates EO Jr (1950) Mental changes occurring in chronically anoxemic patients during oxygen therapy. J Am Med Assoc 143(12):1044–1048

Darlow BA, Marschner SL, Donoghoe M, Benefits Of Oxygen Saturation Targeting-New Zealand (BOOST-NZ) Collaborative Group et al (2014) Randomized controlled trial of oxygen saturation targets in very preterm infants: two year outcomes. J Pediatr 165 (1):30–35, e2

Dawson JA, Kamlin CO, Vento M et al (2010) Defining the reference range for oxygen saturation for infants after birth. Pediatrics 125(6):e1340–e1347

Dawson JA, Vento M, Finer NN et al (2012) Managing oxygen therapy during delivery room stabilization of preterm infants. J Pediatr 160(1):158–161

de Wahl Granelli A, Wennergren M, Sandberg K, Mellander M, Bejlum C, Ingana L et al (2009) Impact of pulse oximetry screening on the detection of duct dependent congenital heart disease: a Swedish prospective screening study in 39,821 newborns. BMJ 338: a3037

Deulofeut R, Critz A, Adams-Chapman I, Sola A (2006) Avoiding hyperoxia in infants < or 1⁄4 1250 g is associated with improved short- and long-term outcomes. J Perinatol 26(11):700–705

Deulofeut R, Dudell G, Sola A (2007) Treatment-by-gender effect when aiming to avoid hyperoxia in preterm infants in the NICU. Acta Paediatr 96(7):990–994

Eghbalian F (2014) A comparison of supine and prone positioning on improves arterial oxygenation in premature neonates. J Neonatal Perinatal Med 7 (4):273–277

Ewer AK, Middleton LJ, Furmston AT, Bhoyar A, Daniels JP, Thangaratinam S et al (2011) Pulse oximetry screening for congenital heart defects in newborn infants (PulseOx): a test accuracy study. Lancet 378:785–794

Farrow KN, Lee KJ, Perez M et al (2012) Brief hyperoxia increases mitochondrial oxidation and increases phosphodiesterase 5 activity in fetal pulmonary artery smooth muscle cells. Antioxid Redox Signal 17 (3):460–470

Hagadorn JI, Furey AM, Nghiem TH, AVIOx Study Group et al (2006) Achieved versus intended pulse oximeter saturation in infants born less than 28 weeks' gestation: the AVIOx study. Pediatrics 118(4):1574–1582

Hamel MS, Anderson BL, Rouse DJ (2014) Oxygen for intrauterine resuscitation: of unproved benefit and potentially harmful. Am J Obstet Gynecol 211 (2):124–127

Hassan MA, Mendler M, Maurer M, Waitz M, Huang L, Hummler HD (2015) Reliability of pulse oximetry during cardiopulmonary resuscitation in a piglet model of neonatal cardiac arrest. Neonatology 107 (2):113–119

Hay WW Jr, Rodden DJ, Collins SM, Melara DL, Hale KA, Fashaw LM (2002) Reliability of conventional and new pulse oximetry in neonatal patients. J Perinatol 22 (5):360–366

Kaindl AM, Sifringer M, Zabel C et al (2006) Acute and long-term proteome changes induced by oxidative stress in the developing brain. Cell Death Differ 13 (7):1097–1109

Ketko AK, Martin CM, Nemshak MA, Niedner M, Vartanian RJ (2015) Balancing the tension between hyperoxia prevention and alarm fatigue in the NICU. Pediatrics 136(2):e496–e504

Klimova NG, Hanna N, Peltier MR (2013) Effect of oxygen tension on bacteria-stimulated cytokine production by fetal membranes. J Perinat Med 41 (5):595–603

Klingel ML, Patel SV (2013) A meta-analysis of the effect of inspired oxygen concentration on the incidence of surgical site infection following cesarean section. Int J Obstet Anesth 22(2):104–112

Lakshminrusimha S, Manja V, Mathew B, Suresh GK (2015) Oxygen targeting in preterm infants: a physiological interpretation. J Perinatol 35(1):8–15

Laman M, Ripa P, Vince J, Tefuarani N (2005) Can clinical signs predict hypoxaemia in Papua New Guinean children with moderate and severe pneumonia? Ann Trop Paediatr 25:23–27

Lim K, Wheeler KI, Gale TJ et al (2014) Oxygen saturation targeting in preterm infants receiving continuous positive airway pressure. J Pediatr 164 (4):730–736.e1

Lim K, Wheeler KI, Jackson HD, Sadeghi Fathabadi O, Gale TJ, Dargaville PA (2015) Lost without trace: oximetry signal dropout in preterm infants. Arch Dis Child Fetal Neonatal Ed 100(5):F436–F438

Lye P, Bloise E, Dunk C et al (2013) Effect of oxygen on multidrug resistance in the first trimester human placenta. Placenta 34(9):817–823

Manja V, Lakshminrusimha S, Cook DJ (2015) Oxygen saturation target range for extremely preterm infants: a systematic review and meta-analysis. JAMA Pediatr 169(4):332–340

Narayen IC, Smit M, van Zwet EW, Dawson JA, Blom NA, te Pas AB (2015) Low signal quality pulse oximetry measurements in newborn infants are reliable for oxygen saturation but underestimate heart rate. Acta Paediatr 104(4):e158–e163

Niermeyer S, Yang P, Shanmina D, Zhuang J, Moore LG (1995) Arterial oxygen saturation in Tibetan and Han infants born in Lhasa, Tibet. N Engl J Med 333:1248–1252

Noh EJ, Kim YH, Cho MK et al (2014) Comparison of oxidative stress markers in umbilical cord blood after vaginal and cesarean delivery. Obstet Gynecol Sci 57 (2):109–114

Paul M (2015) Oxygen administration to preterm neonates in the delivery room: minimizing oxidative stress. Adv Neonatal Care 15(2):91–103

Phibbs RH (1977) Oxygen therapy: a continuing hazard to the premature infant. Anesthesiology 47(6):486–487

Polin RA, Bateman DA, Sahni R (2014) Pulse oximetry in very low birth weight infants. Clin Perinatol 41 (4):1017–1032

Rabi Y, Rabi D, Yee W (2007) Room air resuscitation of the depressed newborn: a systematic review and meta-analysis. Resuscitation 72(3):353–363

Rawat M, Chandrasekharan PK, Williams A, Gugino S, Koenigsknecht C, Swartz D, Ma CX, Mathew B, Nair J, Lakshminrusimha S (2015) Oxygen saturation index and severity of hypoxic respiratory failure. Neonatology 107(3):161–166

Samiee-Zafarghandy S, Saugstad OD, Fusch C (2015) Do we have an answer when it comes to providing extremely preterm infants with optimal target oxygen saturation? Acta Paediatr 104(3):e130–e133

Saugstad OD (2007) Take a breath—but do not add oxygen (if not needed). Acta Paediatr 96(6):798–800

Saugstad OD, Aune D (2014) Optimal oxygenation of extremely low birth weight infants: a meta-analysis and systematic review of the oxygen saturation target studies. Neonatology 105(1):55–63

Saugstad OD, Aune D, Aguar M, Kapadia V, Finer N, Vento M (2014) Systematic review and meta-analysis of optimal initial fraction of oxygen levels in the delivery room at <32 weeks. Acta Paediatr 103 (7):744–751

Schmidt B, Whyte RK, Asztalos EV, Canadian Oxygen Trial (COT) Group et al (2013) Effects of targeting higher vs lower arterial oxygen saturations on death or disability in extremely preterm infants: a randomized clinical trial. JAMA 309(20):2111–2120

Schmidt B, Whyte RK, Roberts RS (2014a) Trade-off between lower or higher oxygen saturations for extremely preterm infants: the first benefits of oxygen saturation targeting (BOOST) II trial reports its primary outcome. J Pediatr 165(1):6–8

Schmidt B, Roberts RS, Whyte RK, Canadian Oxygen Trial Group et al (2014b) Impact of study oximeter masking algorithm on titration of oxygen therapy in the Canadian oxygen trial. J Pediatr 165 (4):666–671, e2

Silverman WA (1980) Retrolental fibroplasia: a modern parable. Grune & Stratton, New York

Sola A (2008) Oxygen in neonatal anesthesia: friend or foe? Curr Opin Anaesthesiol 21(3):332–339

Sola A (2015) Oxygen saturation in the newborn and the importance of avoiding hyperoxia-induced damage. NeoReviews 16:e393. https://doi.org/10.1542/neo.16-7-e393

Sola A, Zuluaga C (2013) Oxygen saturation targets and retinopathy of prematurity. J AAPOS 17:650–652

Sola A, Rogido MR, Deulofeut R (2007) Oxygen as a neonatal health hazard: call for détente in clinical practice. Acta Paediatr 96(6):801–812

Sola A, Saldeño YP, Favareto V (2008) Clinical practices in neonatal oxygenation: where have we failed? what can we do? J Perinatol 28(Suppl 1):S28–S34

Sola A, Golombek SG, Montes Bueno MT et al (2014) Safe oxygen saturation targeting and monitoring in preterm infants: can we avoid hypoxia and hyperoxia? Acta Paediatr 103(10):1009–1018

Spector LG, Klebanoff MA, Feusner JH, Georgieff MK, Ross JA (2005) Childhood cancer following neonatal oxygen supplementation. J Pediatr 147(1):27–31

Stenson BJ, Tarnow-Mordi WO, Darlow BA, BOOST II United Kingdom Collaborative Group; BOOST II Australia Collaborative Group; BOOST II New Zealand Collaborative Group et al (2013) Oxygen saturation and outcomes in preterm infants. N Engl J Med 368(22):2094–2104

Suwattanaphim S, Yodavuhd S, Puangsa-art SJ (2015) Time duration of oxygen adaptation immediately after birth; monitoring by pulse oximeter in perinatal period of the infants at Charoenkrung Pracharak Hospital. J Med Assoc Thai 98(7):656–663

Synnes A, Miller SP (2015) Oxygen therapy for preterm neonates: the elusive optimal target. JAMA Pediatr 169(4):311–313

Terrill PI, Dakin C, Hughes I, Yuill M, Parsley C (2015) Nocturnal oxygen saturation profiles of healthy term infants. Arch Dis Child 100(1):18–23

Thomson L, Paton J (2014) Oxygen toxicity. Paediatr Respir Rev 15(2):120–123

Vagedes J, Poets CF, Dietz K (2013) Averaging time, desaturation level, duration and extent. Arch Dis Child Fetal Neonatal Ed 98:F265–6

Van Den Brenk HA, Jamieson D (1962) Potentiation by anaesthetics of brain damage due to breathing high-pressure oxygen in mammals. Nature 194:777–778

van Kaam AH, Hummler HD, Wilinska M, Swietlinski J, Lal MK, te Pas AB, Lista G, Gupta S et al (2015) Automated versus manual oxygen control with different saturation targets and modes of respiratory support in preterm infants. J Pediatr 167 (3):545–550.e1-2

Vento M (2014) Oxygen supplementation in the neonatal period: changing the paradigm. Neonatology 105(4):323–331

Vento M, Cubells E, Escobar JJ et al (2013) Oxygen saturation after birth in preterm infants treated with continuous positive airway pressure and air: assessment of gender differences and comparison with a published nomogram. Arch Dis Child Fetal Neonatal Ed 98(3):F228–F232

Wellmann S, Bührer C, Schmitz T (2014) Focal necrosis and disturbed myelination in the white matter of newborn infants: a tale of too much or too little oxygen. Front Pediatr 2(14):143

Wollen EJ, Kwinta P, Bik-Multanowski M, Madetko-Talowska A, Sejersted Y, Wright MS et al (2014) Hypoxia-reoxygenation affects whole-genome expression in the newborn eye. Invest Ophthalmol Vis Sci 55(3):1393–1401

Yalcin S, Aydoğan H, Kucuk A et al (2013) Supplemental oxygen in elective cesarean section under spinal anesthesia: handle the sword with care [in Spanish]. Rev Bras Anestesiol 63(5):393–397

Zapata J, Gómez JJ, Araque Campo R, Matiz Rubio A, Sola A (2014) A randomised controlled trial of an automated oxygen delivery algorithm for preterm neonates receiving supplemental oxygen without mechanical ventilation. Acta Paediatr 103(9):928–33

Zhang L, Mendoza-Sassi R, Santos JC, Lau J (2011) Accuracy of symptoms and signs in predicting hypoxaemia among young children with acute respiratory infection: a meta-analysis. Int J Tuberc Lung Dis 15:317–325

Part III

Nutrition

Physiology of the Gastrointestinal Tract in Newborns

34

Arieh Riskin, Carlo Agostoni, and Raanan Shamir

Contents

A. Riskin (✉)
Department of Neonatology, Bnai Zion Medical Center, Rappaport Faculty of Medicine, Technion, Israel Institute of Technology, Haifa, Israel
e-mail: arik.riskin@gmail.com; arik.riskin@b-zion.org.il

C. Agostoni
Pediatric Clinic, Department of Clinical Sciences and Community Health, University of Milan Fondazione, IRCCS Ca Granda, Ospedale Maggiore Policlinico, Milano, Italy
e-mail: carlo.agostoni@unimi.it

R. Shamir
Institute of Gastroenterology Nutrition and Liver Diseases, Schneider Children's Medical Center, Sackler Faculty of Medicine, Tel-Aviv University, Petach-Tikva, Israel
e-mail: shamirraanan@gmail.com

G. Buonocore et al. (eds.), *Neonatology*,
https://doi.org/10.1007/978-3-319-29489-6_183

Abstract
The chapter will discuss the different elements of the developmental physiology of the gastrointestinal tract, including organogenesis, vascularization, neural control, and host defense mechanisms. The development of gastrointestinal motility and of the digestive and absorptive functions and how they relate to feeding and nutrition of the preterm and term neonates will be outlined. Aspects of morphology, physiology, and biochemistry of the developing gastrointestinal tract as well as more recent findings at the molecular biology level will be discussed. Application of this basic knowledge on intestinal functional development should be used in order to improve nutrition for preterm infants and prevent short- and long-term morbidities that may be related to inadequate or poor feeding and nutrition:

(A) Development of the gastrointestinal tract – organogenesis and function
(B) Vascularization
(C) Neural control of motor function and gastrointestinal motility
(D) Digestion and absorption
(E) Host defense
(F) Gastrointestinal hormones and peptides (These are discussed in ▶ Chap. 35, "Hormones and Gastrointestinal Function of Newborns")

34.1 Salient Points

- The gastrointestinal tract develops from the primitive digestive tube that originates from the dorsal part of the yolk sac. By the second trimester, all anatomic structures of the gastrointestinal tract are well formed and recognizable. The process of maturation involves a rapid increase in the mucosal surface area followed by folding that forms the villi and microvilli. However, functional maturation, including the appearance of digestive enzymes in the villi and the development of swallowing and mature motility patterns, occurs much later than structural development; some functions are not fully established until 2–4 years of age.
- Mechanisms regulating intestinal vascular resistance in the neonate are nitric oxide, endothelin, and calcium-induced phosphorylation of myosin light chain kinase.
- Mesenteric blood flow is regulated by changes in the tone of the arteriole and the precapillary sphincter.
- Peristaltic activity allows intestinal contents to move along the intestine and can occur through a variety of mechanisms regulated by enteric nervous system, a subsystem of the autonomic system that includes two major nerve plexuses situated in the bowel wall.
- Gastrointestinal motility, secretion, and vascular flow are controlled by the central nervous and enteric nervous systems, comprising afferent sensory neurons, efferent motor neurons, synapses to the effector (e.g., muscle) cells, and interneurons that integrate the messages.
- Between 24 and 28 weeks' gestation, only unorganized irregular contractions are recorded with few quiescent intervals. By 28–32 weeks, periods of quiescence appear, alternating with short bursts of phasic activity called clusters. Between 32 and 36 weeks, motor patterns become more organized and the periods of quiescence and clusters lengthen. Migratory-motor complexes are first seen around 33 weeks.
- Lingual and gastric lipases are essential for the digestion of milk fat in the newborns. They are present from as early as 26 weeks' gestation and compensate for the limited action of bile acids and pancreatic lipases that are found in low amounts, especially in preterm infants.

The contribution of lingual lipase declines significantly later in life.

- Proteolysis in the stomach is affected by gastric content and motility and most importantly by gastric acidity. The pH of gastric juice is neutral or slightly acid at birth and decreases within hours. Gastric acid flow doubles during the next 2 months.
- Lactase activity appears in the differentiating brush border of the fetal small intestine along with other disaccharidases as from early as 12 weeks of gestation, although in low levels. Lactase activity exhibits relatively higher levels from 37 weeks of gestation. However, lactase activity remains decreased during the first weeks after birth, and this is reflected by the limited capacity of term and especially preterm infants to digest and absorb lactose in the small intestine.
- Prenatal exposure of the gut to bacteria may modulate postnatal adaptations inducing tolerance toward colonization of certain bacteria. Aberrant bacterial colonization immediately after birth may lead to feeding intolerance in a newborn.
- Defense factors in human milk include antimicrobial agents, anti-inflammatory factors, immunomodulators, and leukocytes. Gastric acidity and pancreato-biliary secretions decrease the load of viable microorganisms and intact dietary protein antigens.
- The use of probiotics significantly reduces the occurrence of NEC and death in VLBW premature infants.
- More randomized trials on preterm infants are needed to support the potential beneficial effects of prebiotics on feeding tolerance and the reduced incidence of NEC and hospital-acquired infections.

34.2 Development of the Gastrointestinal Tract: Organogenesis and Function

The gastrointestinal tract develops from the primitive digestive tube that originates from the dorsal part of the yolk sac. Initially the yolk sac is attached to the midgut of the digestive tube, but as early as the fourth week of gestation, the gut becomes distinct from the yolk sac. The yolk sac is connected to the digestive tube through the omphalomesenteric (vitelline) duct. The dorsal mesentery separates the digestive tube from the dorsal wall of the embryo, and at this stage there is also a ventral mesentery that separates the anterior part from the ventral embryonic wall. Continuity with the exterior environment is formed only after the rupture of the buccopharyngeal and cloacal membranes. The anatomic formation of the esophagus, stomach, intestine, pancreas, and liver is achieved by the fourth week through a series of evaginations, elongations, and dilatations. Further development through cell proliferation, growth, and morphogenesis then follows.

The pharynx, esophagus, stomach, liver, gallbladder, pancreas, and upper duodenum originate from the foregut. The distal portion of the duodenum, jejunum, ileum, cecum, appendix, and ascending colon and two-thirds of the transverse colon arise from the midgut. The hindgut differentiates into the third distal part of the transverse colon, the descending colon, the sigmoid colon, the upper two-thirds of the rectum, and the urogenital sinus (Beck 2002). Arterial supply delineates the boundaries: the celiac axis supplies the foregut, and the superior and inferior mesenteric arteries supply the midgut and hindgut, respectively.

The rapid elongation of the gut during the first trimester leads to its herniation into the umbilical cord. The gut reenters into the abdominal cavity and rotates counterclockwise around the superior mesenteric artery to reach its final position by 20 weeks of gestation (Fig. 1). Failure of this process results in malrotation.

By the second trimester, all the anatomic structures of the gastrointestinal tract are well formed and recognizable. The process of maturation involves rapid increase in the mucosal surface area followed by folding forming the villi and microvilli. However, functional maturation, including the appearance of digestive enzymes in the villi and the development of swallowing and mature motility patterns, occurs much later than structural development; some functions are not fully established until 2–4 years of age.

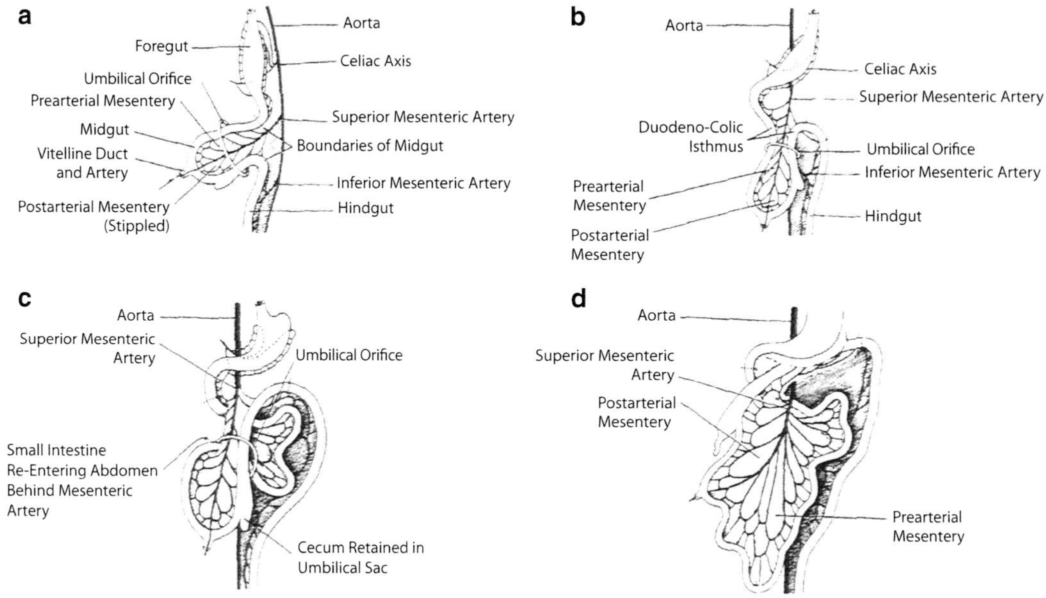

Fig. 1 Diagram showing normal rotation of alimentary tract. (**a**) Fifth week of intrauterine life (*lateral view*). The foregut, midgut, and hindgut are shown with their individual blood supply supported by the common dorsal mesentery in the sagittal plane. The midgut loop has been extruded into the umbilical cord. (**b**) Eighth week of intrauterine life (*anteroposterior view*). The first stage of rotation is being completed. Note the narrow duodenocolic isthmus from which the midgut loop depends and the right-sided position of the small intestine and left-sided position of the colon. Maintenance of this position within the abdomen after birth is termed *nonrotation*. (**c**) About the 10th week of intrauterine life, during the second stage of rotation (*anteroposterior view*). The bowel in the temporary umbilical hernia is in the process of reduction; the most proximal part of the prearterial segment entering the abdomen to the right of the superior mesenteric artery is held forward close to the cecum and ascending colon, permitting the bowel to pass under it. As the coils of small intestine collect within the abdomen, the hindgut is displaced to the left and upward. (**d**) Eleventh week of intrauterine life at the end of the second stage of rotation. From its original sagittal position, the midgut has rotated 270 degrees in a counterclockwise direction about the origin of the superior mesenteric artery. The essentials of the permanent disposition of the viscera have been attained. (Originally from Gardner and Hart (1934), Copyright American Medical Association)

Maturation tends to follow a cephalocaudal progression from the proximal to the distal part of the gastrointestinal tract (Table 1).

The regulation of timing and nature of growth and maturation of the gastrointestinal tract is complex and involves many factors. These include not only intrinsic factors like signals arising from gene expression (Montgomery et al. 1999), biologic clock or regulatory hormones, and peptide growth factors but also extrinsic environmental factors acting also at the molecular level. The gastrointestinal tract is in continuity with the environment; the fetal gut is thus exposed to the amniotic fluid content as the neonatal gut is exposed to enteral feedings, nutrients, and even microbes. This is related to the advantages of breast milk with its immunologic and trophic growth factors to the newborn (Calder et al. 2006). At the cellular level, regulation occurs by homeodomain transcription factor genes (Beck 2002) and cell to cell interactions, especially epithelial-mesenchymal interactions (de Santa et al. 2003). The pluripotent stem cell located in the crypt of the villus continuously differentiates into the four gut cell lineages: absorptive enterocytes, mucous (goblet), Paneth, and endocrine cells (Simon-Assmann et al. 2007). This process that involves continuous proliferation, migration, and loss of epithelial cells along the mucosal surface is also regulated genetically by homeodomain transcription factors (Beck 2002).

Table 1 Anatomic and functional maturation of the gastrointestinal tract (Originally Table 70.1 page 1073 from Berseth (2005), now Copyright Elsevier

Postconceptional age (weeks)					
15	20	25	30	35	40
Mouth	Salivary glands	Swallow	Lingual lipase	*Sucking*	
Esophagus	Muscle layers present	Striated epithelium present	*Poor lower esophageal sphincter tone*		
Stomach	Gastric glands present	G cells appear	Gastric secretions present	*Slow gastric emptying*	[a]
Pancreas	Exocrine and endocrine tissue differentiate	Zymogen present	*Reduced trypsin lipase*		[a]
Liver	Lobules form	Bile secreted	*Fatty acids absorbed*		[a]
Intestine	Crypt and villus form	*Glucose transport present*	*Dipeptidase, sucrase, and maltase active*	*Lactase active*	
Colon		Crypts and villi recede		*Meconium passed*	

Reproduced with permission from Berseth, CL. Developmental anatomy and physiology of the gastrointestinal tract. In: Taeusch HW, Ballard RA (eds) Avery's diseases of the newborn, 8th edn. W.B. Saunders Company. Philadelphia, Copyright W.B. Saunders
Italics indicate functional maturation
[a]Full functional maturation occurs postnatally

For detailed aspects on structural anatomic development of the different parts and organs along the gastrointestinal tract, refer to the first chapters in section on the gastrointestinal tract, where congenital malformations are discussed.

34.3 Vascularization

Vascular supply to the intestine develops concurrently with its anatomic development. The arterial supply develops as three ventral out-buddings of vessels from the aorta: The celiac trunk supplies the stomach, pancreas, and duodenum via its splenic, left gastric, and hepatic branches; the superior mesenteric artery supplies the jejunum and ileum; and the inferior mesenteric artery supplies the colon and rectum. Smaller branches of the superior mesenteric artery form arcades before entering the intestinal wall that along with anastomoses with branches of the inferior mesenteric artery provide rich collateral flow. Watershed areas of marginal blood supply however exist in the distal transverse colon and upper rectum. Since there is high metabolic activity in the intestinal mucosal layer, it has rich vascular supply, yet it is still the most sensitive layer to any derangements in blood supply.

Based on animal studies, it is assumed that intestinal basal vascular resistance decreases in the immediate postnatal period, thus doubling blood flow and oxygen delivery in the neonate to compensate for the higher metabolic activity related to nutrient absorption that was not needed in fetal life. However, later on between postnatal days 12–30 vascular resistance increases again due to maturation of the intestinal extrinsic adrenergic innervation, as well as changes in the geometry of the intestinal vasculature in response to the rapid increase in size (length and surface area) of the gut that happens concomitantly (Reber et al. 2002).

Basal vascular resistance is mediated by nitric oxide (NO) that is continuously produced by the endothelial cell NO synthase isoform (ecNOS) or is increased in response to mechanical or chemical stimuli. NO causes vasodilatation of the adjacent vascular smooth muscle via production of cGMP by activated guanylate cyclase. Rates of NO production and its relaxation effect on the mesenteric artery bed are maximal immediately after birth. Its role in determining vascular tone lessens over the first month of life. The essential role of endothelial production of NO in maintaining newborn intestinal hemodynamics may be important in the pathogenesis of necrotizing enterocolitis (NEC), because endothelial dysfunction that would limit NO production may lead to vasoconstriction and substantial intestinal ischemia (Reber et al. 2002).

Individual vascular smooth muscle cells respond to stretch stimulus by contracting via stimulation of calcium-induced phosphorylation of myosin light chain kinase (Davis and Hill 1999). This intrinsic myogenic response is the second mechanism mediating vascular response in the neonatal intestine, and it has important role in setting basal intestinal vascular resistance in the first days of life (Reber et al. 2002). It causes vasoconstriction in response to increase in intravascular pressure in some of the blood vessels.

Endothelin, the third mediator of vascular resistance, is a vasoactive peptide mainly produced by the vascular endothelium. ET-1, the intestinal form, is continuously produced by the intestinal vascular endothelium in an age-specific manner. Its production is greater in young subjects, especially in newborns, probably reflecting its essential role in angiogenesis at this time of exceptionally rapid growth of the intestine. Endothelin binding to ET_A receptors on vascular smooth muscle induces potent sustained contraction, while its binding to ET_B receptors causes NO-mediated vasodilatation. The force of ET_A-induced vasoconstriction exceeds the modest ET_B-induced NO-dependent vasodilatation; thus, the net effect of constitutive ET-1 production is vasoconstriction (Nankervis and Nowicki 2000).

The significance of these three mechanisms regulating intestinal vascular resistance in the neonate is markedly diminished after the first postnatal month of life. Thereafter, the greater degree of extrinsic adrenergic innervation causes increased basal vascular resistance with more robust responses to baro- and chemoreflexes.

Mesenteric blood flow is regulated by changes in the tone of the arteriole and the precapillary sphincter. Control of blood flow is intrinsic and extrinsic (Reber et al. 2002). Intrinsic control is achieved by local factors that react to changes in arterial pressure (pressure-flow autoregulation) and tissue oxygenation, such as functional postprandial hyperemia in response to feeding or reactive hyperemia in response to vessel occlusion. Modest arterial hypoxemia (PO2 around 50 mmHg) causes vasodilatation and increased perfusion to the gut, yet profound hypoxemia (PO2 $<$ 40 mmHg) causes vasoconstriction and gut ischemia. These different responses probably reflect NO regulation of vascular tone (Reber et al. 2002). Extrinsic regulation is mediated by sympathetic input from the splanchnic nerves. However, the vasoconstriction response to adrenergic nerve stimulation is short-lived, and gut blood flow is slowly restored to its baseline by a process termed autoregulatory escape.

Circulating endogenous and exogenous factors (e.g., hormones, histamine, and prostaglandins) can also modulate vascular tone. The presence of nutrients in the gut triggers the postprandial hyperemic response with brisk vasodilatation and increased blood flow and oxygen delivery. Postprandial hyperemia in the newborn is mediated by dilatation of the intestinal circulation in response to substance P, which is a peptide neurotransmitter in the enteric nervous system (Nowicki 1998). Both postprandial hyperemia and autoregulatory escape phenomena are present in newborns. However, unlike term infants, healthy preterm infants require compensatory systemic hemodynamic changes in response to feeding and postprandial hyperemic response because the increased mesenteric flow causes cardiac output increase and systemic blood pressure decrease (Martinussen et al. 1996). Drugs used in neonatal care such as indomethacin (Gork et al. 2008), dopamine, and caffeine (Hoecker et al. 2002) as well as other treatments (e.g., hyperalimentation and CPAP) (Havranek et al. 2006) may diminish intestinal mesenteric blood flow, thus disrupting compensatory mechanisms.

34.4 Neural Control of Motor Function and Gastrointestinal Motility

A major function of the gut is motor activity that moves the content forward along the gastrointestinal tract. This includes sucking, swallowing, gastric emptying, propagation of the food along the small intestine, and evacuation of wastes from the colon. Neural crest cells migrate into the developing gut and with muscle cells differentiate to form three layers of muscle that surround the mucosa (by 14 weeks of gestation) and a neural network that control motor activity (by 20–24 weeks of gestation). This neural network comprises the enteric nervous system (ENS). The phasic contractions of the gastrointestinal tract are regulated by a complex interplay between the myogenic, neural, and chemical control mechanisms (Sarna and Otterson 1988).

Peristaltic activity allows intestinal contents to move along the intestine and can occur through a variety of mechanisms. Phasic contractions are responsible for the mixing and propulsive movements of the gut after a meal. These are called migrating action potential complexes (MAPCs), and they are prominent postprandially (Sarna and Otterson 1988; Huizinga et al. 1998). During fasting, organized groups of contractions called cyclic motor activity and migrating motor complex (MMC) keep the upper digestive tract clean of residual food and debris (Sarna and Otterson 1988; Huizinga et al. 1998). MMC cyclic motor contractions originate from the antrum and progress to the ileum. They are characterized by periods of quiescence followed by irregular contractions and then a period of regular contractions and return to the quiescent state. In addition, the small intestine and the colon generate giant migrating contractions which are several-fold stronger than the postprandial phasic contractions and migrate uninterrupted over long distances. The giant migrating contractions are effective in rapid propulsion. The upper small intestine and the gastric antrum may also generate retrograde giant contractions that generally precede vomiting (Sarna and Otterson 1988). Movements of MMCs and MAPCs are orchestrated by the ENS.

34.4.1 Myogenic Control

Contractile activity can also propagate toward the anus in association with propagating slow-wave activity (Siegle et al. 1990), expressing myogenic control. Muscle cells generate this spontaneous electrical activity through fluctuations in resting membrane potential, and these periodic depolarizations are called slow waves, electrical control activity, basic electrical rhythm, or pacemaker activity. This myogenic pacemaker slow-wave activity originates from specialized smooth muscle cells, the interstitial cells of Cajal (ICC) (Lecoin et al. 1996), that form an electrical syncytium with the smooth muscle layers. The network of ICC is also associated with Auerbach's plexus (Huizinga et al. 1995). There is evidence that the absence of ICC network may contribute to abnormalities in intestinal transit in humans, including infantile hypertrophic pyloric stenosis and Hirschsprung's disease (Vanderwinden et al. 1996a, b). The fact that ICC are always very intimately associated with neural structures suggests a close cooperation between myogenic and neural control. Contractions occur when a slow wave under the influence of a neural or chemical stimulation exceeds the excitation threshold necessary for an action potential called electrical response activity or spike potential. Following this depolarization of the smooth muscle cell, intracellular calcium levels increase, calcium binds to the regulatory protein calmodulin, and this permits the binding of the contractile proteins actin and myosin, resulting in a contraction. It can be seen that the contraction caused by the electrical response activity occurs on the background of the electrical control activity, i.e., the slow waves of myogenic control (Sarna and Otterson 1989). This background slow-wave activity controls timing, speed, and direction of the intestinal contractions. There is probably cooperation between the neural and myogenic control of intestinal motility to ensure proper transit (Huizinga et al. 1998). Denervated gut muscle cell has thus basal contraction rate like cardiac muscle cell.

34.4.2 Enteral Nervous System (ENS)

The ENS is a subsystem of the autonomic system that includes two major nerve plexuses situated in the bowel wall. The myenteric (Auerbach) plexus lies between the external circular and longitudinal muscle layers, and the submucosal (Meissner) plexus lies between the circular muscle layer and the muscularis mucosa. The ENS also includes six minor plexuses located in the different layers of the bowel wall (Fig. 2). The ENS is integrated within the central nervous system (CNS) control of the gut, but it also provides the final regulation and is even able to regulate gut motility, secretion, and vascular flow independent of the CNS and spinal nervous control. The ENS with its large number of neurons compared to the relatively sparse central innervation of the gut is thus termed the "little brain of the gut," stressing its uniqueness compared to other peripheral nerve systems (Holle and Forth 1990).

The basic unit of the ENS is the nerve cell. Neurotransmitters are released to other neurons or directly act upon striated or smooth muscle cells. Acetylcholine is the main excitatory neurotransmitter mediating smooth muscle contractions (Vanneste et al. 2008). Glutamate is also an excitatory neurotransmitter acting on *N*-methyl-D-aspartate (NMDA)-type receptors in the myenteric plexus in conjunction with cholinergic stimuli (Wiley et al. 1991). Glutamate can be synthesized from exogenous L-glutamine in myenteric neurons and be released in response to neuronal depolarization (Wiley et al. 1991). Norepinephrine is a main inhibitory neurotransmitter. Nitric oxide (NO) mediates non-adrenergic non-cholinergic (NANC) relaxation of gastrointestinal smooth muscle (Stark et al. 1993). NO synthase (NOS) and NO-containing enteric neurons have been demonstrated in the ENS (Vanneste et al. 2008). Vasoactive intestinal peptide (VIP), another inhibitory neurotransmitter, may mediate NO effects (Grider and Murthy 2008). The absence of NO has been implicated in the pathogenesis of infantile hypertrophic pyloric stenosis (Saur et al. 2004) and Hirschsprung's disease (VanderWall et al. 1995).

Enteric neurons and glial cells of the ENS originate from the neural crest (Anderson et al. 2006). Cells from the vagal region migrate to the whole length of the gastrointestinal tract, but cells from the truncal and sacral regions populate only the foregut and the post-umbilical hindgut, respectively (Gershon et al. 1993). Like intestinal smooth muscle development, neural cells from the vagal region develop in a craniocaudal direction, as opposed to neural cells originating from the sacral region that migrate into the distal bowel in a caudocranial direction. Neural cells that migrate from the outer mesenchyme of the gut to the inner mucosa proliferate. At this stage, the cells are pluripotent and transiently express catecholamines (Baetge et al. 1990). Later in gestation, the neural cells in the gut wall mature and differentiate into enteral neurons that do not express catecholamines anymore. Differentiated neurons express serotoninergic and peptidergic (e.g., substance P and neuropeptide Y) neurotransmitters. Some of the neural crest-

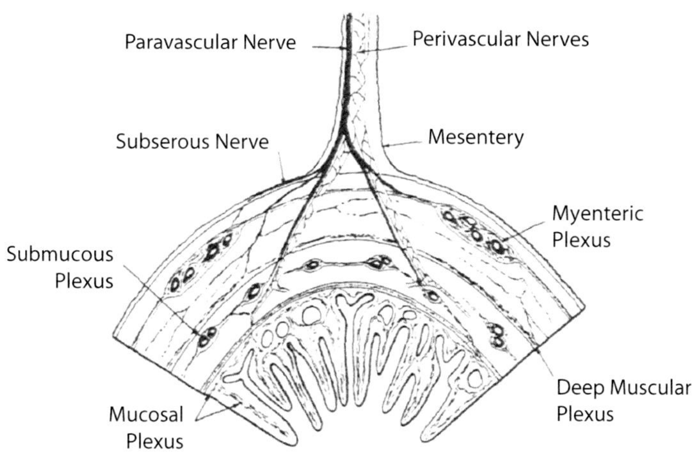

Fig. 2 Arrangement of enteric plexuses in whole mounts of intestine. In addition to the large myenteric and submucosal plexuses, several smaller plexuses are shown. (originally from Furness and Costa (1987), now Copyright Elsevier)

derived cells that colonize the fetal bowel cluster and form ganglion cells that form the two ganglionated plexuses described above (Faure et al. 2007). These ganglion cells are distributed normally by 24 weeks gestation, although their density continues to change over the first years of life (Wester et al. 1999). In the human fetus by the tenth week of gestation, the circular muscle layer is formed, followed by the appearance of a primitive myenteric plexus and the longitudinal smooth muscle layer in the 12th week of gestation. Most neurons in the myenteric ganglia at the tenth week of gestation are undifferentiated neuroblasts. The time between the 10th and 18th week of gestation is important for both morphological and functional maturation of the ENS. In the 18-week-old human fetus, most neurons in the myenteric ganglia are already differentiated and mature, and the organization of smooth muscle cells and the primary strands of the myenteric plexus provide a satisfactory basis for an integrated peristaltic movement that is already seen in the gut (Fekete et al. 1996). Neurotransmitters are evident by 24–26 weeks, although their distribution along the gut may change and reach adult pattern only close to term.

Abnormalities in migration and differentiation of neural crest cells may cause a number of gastrointestinal disorders (Newgreen and Young 2002a, b), and the main one is Hirschsprung's disease that results from the absence of enteric ganglia in the distal hindgut.

34.4.3 Central Nervous System (CNS) Control

CNS and ENS that control gastrointestinal motility, secretion, and vascular flow consist of afferent sensory neurons, efferent motor neurons, synapses to the effector (e.g., muscle) cells, and interneurons that integrate the messages. Sensory afferent fibers travel with parasympathetic preganglionic fibers in the vagus nerve and sympathetic postganglionic fibers in the splanchnic nerves. Vagal afferents conduct impulses from the mucosal and muscular layers of the whole gut, from the soft palate to the distal colon (Altschuler et al. 1989). They reach the liver, gallbladder, and pancreas too. Splanchnic afferents innervate the mucosal and muscular layers, the serosa, and the bowel mesenterium. Motor innervation is made of sympathetic and parasympathetic components of the autonomic nervous system. Preganglionic sympathetic neurons are found in segments T2-L2 of the spinal cord. Postganglionic sympathetic neurons are found in the prevertebral sympathetic trunk (celiac, superior, and inferior mesenteric ganglia). Preganglionic parasympathetic neurons are present in the medulla and in the sacral region of the spinal cord. Postganglionic parasympathetic neurons are located within the gastrointestinal tract. Most of the parasympathetic innervation of the gut comes from the vagus. Vagal efferents end up in the enteric ganglia of the ENS (Kirchgessner and Gershon 1989). Sacral nerves innervate only the distal colon from the middle of the transverse colon. Since the vagus innervates most of the gut and has both afferent and efferent fibers, it needs precise central viscerotropic organization of inputs and outputs. Afferent fibers reach the nucleus tractus solitarius and the vagal sensory nucleus. Efferent fibers originate from the motor nuclei and dorsal motor nucleus of the vagus and the nucleus ambiguous (Altschuler et al. 1989; Berthoud et al. 1990). The nucleus tractus solitarius is an important synaptic site where interneurons coordinate afferent inputs with efferent outputs delivered to the nucleus ambiguous and the dorsal motor nucleus of the vagus in order to control esophageal and gastrointestinal motility. Glutamate, an excitatory amino acid, is considered one of the neurotransmitters involved in this brain-stem synaptic transmission via NMDA receptors, specifically involved in esophageal motor activity in response to swallowing (Kessler 1993).

34.4.4 Gastrointestinal Motility

The motor activity of the gastrointestinal tract is critical for feeding, digestion, and absorption of nutrients. It is responsible for the transit of food from the esophagus, the stomach, and then throughout the intestine and promotes mixing of the nutrients with pancreatic, biliary, and intestinal secretions. Smooth muscles of the intestine are arranged in outer longitudinal and inner circular layers. They develop in a craniocaudal direction that resembles the development of the vagal neural crest-derived ENS. By the end of the first trimester, longitudinal and circular muscles are detectable in the ileum. During the rest of gestation, muscle thickness increases. By 28 weeks gestation, contraction of the gut can produce 60% of the intraluminal pressures measured at term. These pressures are sufficient for preterm infants to be able to move intestinal content forward. There is a gradual maturation of gut motility during fetal life that continues in the first years of postnatal life (Berseth 1996). The gradual maturation of gut motility is the result of muscular and neural maturation. Motor activity is immature in preterm infants. Normal propulsive motility of the gut is evident by 30 weeks gestation. The classical MMC (migrating motor complexes) are demonstrated by 33 weeks but at slower propagation rates and without being abolished by feeding as happens in older children and adults.

Sucking and swallowing involve skeletal and smooth muscles. Although sucking and swallowing reflexes appear early in gestation, their maturation is not complete until after birth. Fetuses can swallow amniotic fluid by 15–17 weeks gestation. Exposure to swallowed amniotic fluid including its growth factors such as the epidermal growth factor (EGF) is important for gastrointestinal development (Kelly et al. 1997). Close to term, the fetus swallows 450–750 ml of amniotic fluid each day. Esophageal or intestinal atresia results in polyhydramnios. Nonnutritive sucking appears between 18 and 20 weeks, but nutritive sucking that involves coordinated mechanisms of sucking, swallowing, and breathing develops only by 34–35 weeks of gestation (Lau et al. 2003), but has been described earlier (as early as 30–32 weeks) in preterm infants after early oromotor stimulation of nonnutritive sucking and use of pacifiers in preterm infants (Simpson et al. 2002). The maturation of nutritive sucking is parallel to the rapid growth in gastric size and maturation of gastric emptying, gastric antral and small intestinal motility, and stimulation of secretion of gastrointestinal enzymes and peptides that enhance weight gain as well. Early introduction of oral feeding to preterm infants accelerates maturation of nutritive sucking and the transition time from tube to full oral feeding (Simpson et al. 2002). Maturation of sucking skills correlates better with postmenstrual gestational age than with postnatal age in preterm infants (Gewolb et al. 2001). Lau et al. characterized five developmental stages of sucking in preterm infants that were found to be in correlation with postmenstrual age, feeding progress, and the number of daily oral feedings. Rhythmicity of sucking and rate of transfer of milk into the posterior pharynx were enhanced when infants reached the more mature stages of sucking, and general oral feeding performance improved as infants' sucking skills matured (Lau et al. 2000). The first stage of swallowing is an involuntary reflex in preterm and term infants induced by the presence of milk in the posterior pharynx. At term, sucking is followed in an orderly manner by swallowing, esophageal peristalsis, relaxation of the lower esophageal sphincter (LES), and relaxation of the gastric fundus.

The esophagus serves as a connecting tube between the oropharynx and the stomach, but its peristaltic activity is essential for adequate passage of nutrients and for adequate clearing of refluxed materials. Coordinated esophageal peristalsis is present by 32 weeks of gestation, and by that time upper esophageal sphincter (UES) tone is already present. Esophageal sphincters are not anatomic but rather functional. The LES is an area of increased muscular tone in the distal esophagus. Its main functions are to prevent gastric acid reflux and to propel food into the stomach. In term infants, LES tone is 20–40 mmHg. However, contraction amplitudes, propagation of pressure waves, and LES tone are lower in preterm compared to term infants. LES tone in a preterm infant less than 29 weeks gestation is lower than 5 mmHg (Newell et al. 1988). Gastroesophageal reflux (GER) that is more common in preterm infants is probably related to low LES tone and poor regulation of its relaxation (Omari et al. 1999). Using impedance pH monitoring nonacid as well as acid GER has been demonstrated (Wenzl et al. 2002) though norms for premature as well as term infants are yet to be established. The esophagus also provides aerodigestive defenses that exist in the healthy term infant and prevents aspiration of bolus feed or secretions. These mechanisms include: basal UES and LES tonic contractions, primary peristalsis of the esophagus triggered by swallowing, and secondary peristalsis with increase in UES tone in response to esophageal provocation. These defenses may not function in infants with neurodevelopmental abnormalities or maldevelopment of the foregut. Also, these defenses may not be fully mature in preterm infants, especially those with chronic lung disease (Gupta et al. 2009).

Gastric emptying of liquid feeds is regulated by the fundus and proximal third of the stomach that dilate to accommodate the milk volume and is dependent on the pressure gradient between the proximal stomach and the duodenum. Accommodation of large volumes of milk in the fundus is poor immediately after birth. During the first three postnatal days, the newborn stomach becomes more compliant and develops more receptive relaxation, associated with a larger volume capacity. This is in accordance with the small feedings that neonates ingest in the first days of life (Zangen et al. 2001). Gastric emptying of more solid contents is regulated by the distal portion of the body of the stomach, the antrum, and the pylorus where mixing is taking place. Gastric emptying requires adequate and coordinated antral and duodenal motor activities. As opposed to antral motor activity that seems to be mature as early as 24 weeks gestation (Ittmann et al. 1992), the coordination and the level of duodenal motor activity are decreased in preterm infants. In half of the preterm infants, duodenal contractions cease in response to feeding resulting in delayed gastric emptying (Al-Tawil et al. 2002). Reduced osmolality and increased volumes of feeding seem to increase gastric emptying, but gastric emptying remains strongly related to gestational age at birth even at the age of 1 month (Ramirez et al. 2006).

Maturation of gastrointestinal motility with increasing gestational age is most evident in the small intestine. This is shown by longer transit times as infants are more immature, especially before 30 weeks when ineffective gut motility may interfere with enteral feeding. The migratory motor complexes (MMCs), described above, act as "housekeepers" that propel luminal content caudally along the small intestine. Term and late preterm infants born after 36 weeks gestation present organized MMC pattern (Ittmann et al. 1992) with periods of quiescence followed by irregular contractions and then regular contractions and return to the quiescent baseline (Fig. 3). This pattern is rarely found in preterm infants. Between 24 and 28 weeks gestation, only unorganized irregular contractions

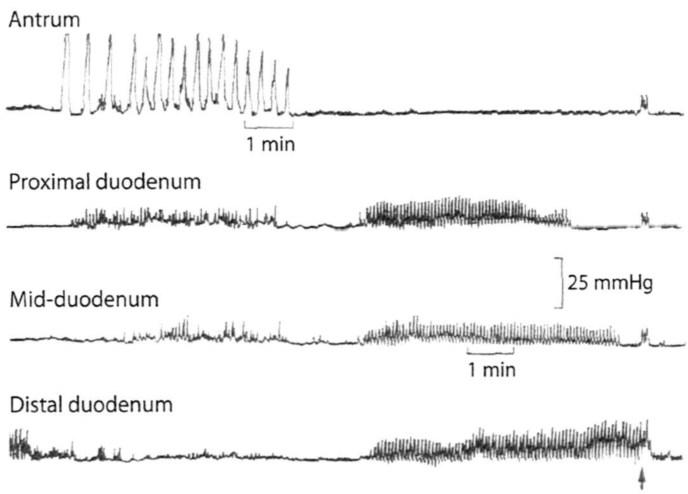

Fig. 3 Migrating motor complex in a term infant. Upper tracing: motor contractions recorded from the antrum. Lower three tracings: motor contractions recorded from the duodenum. Phasic activity present in the antrum is temporally associated with the appearance of intense phasic activity that migrates distally to the three duodenal leads. (originally from Ittmann et al. (1992), now copyright Springer)

are recorded with little quiescence intervals (Berseth 1996; Ittmann et al. 1992). By 28–32 weeks, periods of quiescence appear alternating with short bursts of phasic activity called clusters. Between 32 and 36 weeks, motor patterns become more organized and the periods of quiescence and clusters lengthen. MMCs are first seen around 33 weeks (Berseth 1996; Ittmann et al. 1992) (Fig. 4). Feeding should normally disrupt MMC pattern by creating strong contractions originating from the gastric antrum and pylorus that mix gastric content and propagate it through the pylorus and along the small intestine. These contractions are the migrating action potential complexes (MAPCs) discussed above. Berseth suggested that early feeding may accelerate the maturation of gut motility in preterm infants (Berseth 1992). Composition and caloric content of the food, but not its volume, also has an effect on the maturation and intensity of the gut motor response, suggesting that diluted formula may not provide an optimal stimulant for the preterm intestinal functional responses to feeding (Koenig et al. 1995).

Ninety-four percent of term newborn infants pass meconium within the first 24 h and close to 100% do so within the first 48 h. Passage of meconium may be delayed in preterm infants, up to 10 days and more in the very-low-birth-weight preterm infants (Wang and Huang 1994). Normal

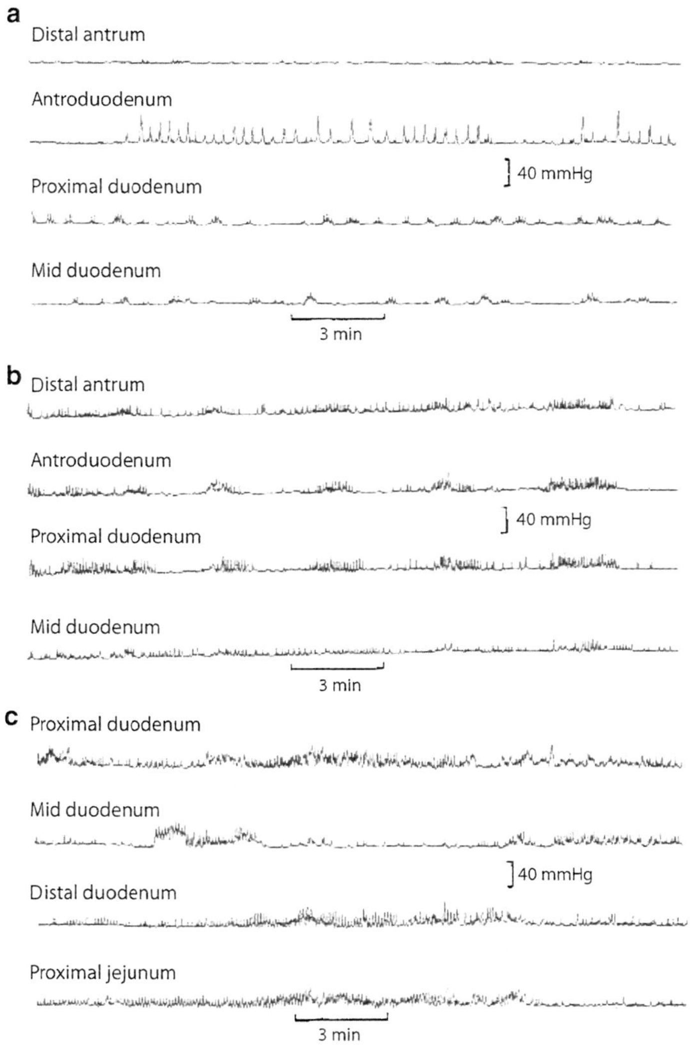

Fig. 4 Motor activity in the small intestine of preterm infants at different gestational ages. Representative serial tracings from an individual subject, at postconceptional age of (**a**) 32 weeks, (**b**) 34 and (**c**) 36 weeks, demonstrating increasing cluster duration and decreasing cluster frequency (Fig. 3 page 649 from Berseth (1989), now Copyright Elsevier)

colonic function is necessary for successful defecation. However, not many studies were done on colonic motility, especially in preterm infants. The colon transports nonabsorbable substances for excretion and facilitates exchange of water and electrolytes. Transit is slow and is achieved by mass movements that sweep the colon. Colonic motility is characterized by irregular alterations of quiescence with non-propagating and propagating contractions (Nurko 2005). Colonic propagated events are defined as low- and high-amplitude propagated contractions (LAPCs and HAPCs), and HAPCs are responsible for the mass movements. A colonic motor response to a meal is comprised of segmental contractions, increased colonic smooth muscle tone, and possibly also HAPCs. These were described in children as well, HAPCs being more frequent (Di et al. 1995). The only colonic cyclic activity is distal to the rectosigmoid junction. It is called recto motor complex and it is not synchronous with the small bowel MMCs. It keeps the rectum empty, especially at night, and thus helps maintaining continence (Rao and Welcher 1996). It seems that colonic motility in term neonates is similar to that found in older children. However, colonic motility is immature in preterm infants. This is supported by the fact that term newborns that develop hypoxemia pass meconium in utero, while preterm infants rarely do so, suggesting the production of contractions that create mass stool movements is immature in preterm babies. Hirschsprung's disease is the most common motility disorder affecting the colon. Neuronal intestinal dysplasia (NID) of the colonic submucous plexus is considered a congenital malformation of the enteric nervous system causing symptoms resembling those of Hirschsprung's disease. It is a poorly understood colonic motility disorder that is often associated with Hirschsprung's disease and is also associated with chronic intestinal pseudo-obstruction, anorectal malformations, and the multiple endocrine neoplasia (MEN) II syndrome (Koletzko et al. 1999). Anal sphincter function is mature in term infants, but may be immature in less than 30 weeks gestation premature infants. However, delayed meconium passage in preterm infants could not have been related to the absence of a recto anal inhibitory reflex (Lorijn et al. 2005).

34.5 Digestion and Absorption

Three steps can be defined in the process of nutrient absorption: digestion, which is the processing of nutrients within the intestinal lumen and at the terminal digestive sites of the brush border membrane of the mucosal epithelial cells; absorption in the epithelial absorptive surfaces, which involves the membrane transport systems of the small intestinal epithelium; and transport of nutrients into the circulation (Phillips 1997).

34.5.1 Fat Digestion and Absorption

Fat is the major source for energy (provides half of the caloric intake) (Hamosh 1995) and polyunsaturated fatty acids in newborns (Koletzko et al. 1998). It is an essential cell membrane component (Koletzko et al. 1998), and it facilitates the absorption of fat-soluble vitamins. Most of the lipids are absorbed in the proximal two-thirds of the jejunum.

Digestion and transport of fat in the lumen of the gastrointestinal tract requires solubilization of the dietary lipids, mostly triglycerides, in the aqueous medium of the gut content, i.e., emulsification. This involves mechanical actions of mastication and gastric mixing to form fat droplets, as well as coating by phospholipids (mostly phosphatidylcholine in food with the addition of bile phospholipids in the duodenum) to stabilize the emulsion. Emulsification allows exposure of large surface area to the action of the lipolytic enzymes. Hydrolysis of fat to form mono- or diglycerides and free fatty acids begins, especially in newborns, in the stomach by lingual lipase secreted from Ebner's glands near the circumvallate papillae (Kawai and Fushiki 2003) and by gastric lipase secreted by gastric glands. Lingual and gastric lipases are essential for the digestion of milk fat in the newborns because they can penetrate into the milk fat globule and initiate the digestive process, contrary to the pancreatic or milk digestive lipases (Hamosh 1990). In newborns, lingual lipase contributes significantly to lipid hydrolysis, and nonnutritive sucking stimulates its release from the posterior part of the tongue. Lingual and gastric lipases that are present as early as 26 weeks gestation compensate for the limited action of bile acids and pancreatic lipases that are found in low amounts, especially in preterm infants (Hamosh 1987). The contribution of lingual lipase significantly declines later in life.

Gastric hydrogen ions enter the duodenum and stimulate the release of secretin that enhances bicarbonate secretion from the pancreas. This process that raises the intraluminal pH to 6.5, which is more suitable for further fat digestion, is less effective in newborns. The optimum pH of lingual lipase which is 3.5–6.0 is compatible with its continued activity in the upper small intestine, especially in newborns, where the luminal pH is under 6.5 (Hamosh 1987). The initial gastric phase of lipolysis generates modest amounts of diglycerides, monoglycerides, and free fatty acids that are required with bile salts for optimal activity of the intestinal phase of lipolysis. The bile salts further enhance fat emulsification rendering it more susceptible to the action pancreatic lipase that degrades it to monoglycerides and fatty acids. The coactivity of the enzyme colipase is critical to facilitate its attachment to the triglyceride droplets and to prevent bile salts from deactivating pancreatic lipase. All pancreatic lipase levels are low after birth, especially in preterm low-birth-weight infants (Hamosh 1987), and increase to adult levels only by 6 months of age. The colipase-dependent pancreatic lipase catalyzes the intraduodenal phase of triglyceride digestion in formula-fed infants. However, in breastfed infants, this process is also mediated by the bile salt-stimulated lipase (BSSL), the main lipase in breast milk that is capable of hydrolyzing all three ester bonds of triglycerides, thus shifting the final products of triglyceride digestion to glycerol and free fatty acid that promote efficient fat absorption (Hernell and Blackberg 1994). BSSL is identical to the pancreatic bile salt-stimulated lipase that is responsible also for hydrolyzing intestinal cholesteryl esters and phospholipids (Shamir et al. 1995), and its presence in human milk may serve as a bridge until the pancreas secretes it in adequate amounts. BSSL is not destroyed and does not lose its activity in the stomach; thus, it can reach the duodenum and be activated by the concentrations of bile acids as found in the infant's duodenum. Breast milk also contains lipoprotein lipase (LPL) that has been described as related to the prolonged neonatal jaundice in breastfed infants. Lingual, gastric, and milk lipases compensate for the low pancreatic lipase activity in term and preterm newborns (Hamosh 1987), and since they all function well also in the presence of low bile acid concentrations, they can also function well in preterm infants where bile acid synthesis in the liver is decreased and their intraluminal concentration is half of the critical micellar concentration required for fat absorption (Hamosh 1987).

The source of dietary fat influences absorption (Ramirez et al. 2001), human milk being the best source for term and preterm newborns (Schanler 1995). Unsaturated fatty acids are absorbed better than saturated ones, and short- and medium-chain triglycerides are absorbed better than long-chain triglycerides (Ramirez et al. 2001). Yet, long-chain fatty acids ($\geq$16C) may have a growth-promoting effect on intestinal cells, as can be seen in short bowel syndrome (Niot et al. 2009). Intraluminal calcium concentration also influences fat absorption. High calcium intake, as found in cow's milk, can impair fat absorption in term and preterm newborns. In human milk, palmitic acid esterified at the sn-2 position of the triacylglycerol molecule is well absorbed as 2-monopalmitin (Kennedy et al. 1999). Lower digestibility of fat in bovine milk-based infant formulas compared to human milk is related to the different position of palmitic acid in both fat sources (Bracco 1994).

After the luminal phase of digestion and processing of the lipids is completed, the mixture of all lipolytic products in the lumen is mixed with bile salts to form small aggregates of mixed micelles or liposomes, which are larger aggregates that are ready for the next mucosal phase of absorption. The bile salts that have both lipid- and water-soluble domains allow the passage of micelles through the water layer at the mucosal cell surface and the lipid-rich microvillus membrane. The bile salts that are not absorbed remain in the intestinal lumen and are actively reabsorbed at the terminal ileum and into the portal system to be resecreted into the bile. This enterohepatic circulation plays an important role in the pathogenesis of neonatal hyperbilirubinemia. Monoglycerides and free fatty acids diffuse into the cells. A significant proportion of this phase of lipid absorption is not by passive diffusion, but involves active, protein-mediated transport (Thomson et al. 2001; Iqbal and Hussain 2009). The major fatty acid protein transporter so far identified is FATP4 that is mainly involved in long-chain fatty acid absorption (Stahl et al. 1999). These fatty acid transporter proteins are located on the apical side of the enterocyte (Thomson et al. 2001). Inside the absorptive cells of the villus, fatty acids are transported to the smooth endoplasmic reticulum where the triglycerides are resynthesized. The triglycerides along with cholesteryl esters, phospholipids, and apoproteins are packed together as chylomicrons that bind to the basolateral membrane and are transported via the intestinal lymphatics into the circulation (Iqbal and Hussain 2009). Fat absorption seems to be fully developed at birth to suit the high fat intake of newborn infants (Hamosh 1995). This seems to be true for preterm infants too, thus suggesting that the relative inefficiency of fat absorption in preterm infants (40–90%) is mostly attributed to immaturity of the intraluminal digestive mechanisms, as described above.

34.5.2 Protein Digestion and Absorption

Although proteins encompass 10–15% of the caloric intake, they are important for somatic growth and synthesis of intracellular structures and enzymes. Adequate protein intake is critical for the premature infant, especially for brain development (Thureen and Heird 2005). The initial step of protein digestion takes place in the stomach and includes denaturation by gastric acidity and proteolysis mostly into large polypeptides by gastric pepsins. Pepsinogens 1 and 2 are the proenzymes of pepsin that are activated in low pH. Proteolysis in the stomach is affected by gastric content and motility and most importantly by gastric acidity. The pH of gastric juice is neutral or slightly acid at birth and decreases within hours. Gastric acid flow doubles within the next 2 months (Mouterde et al. 1992). Parietal cell activity is noted in the body, antrum, and pyloric regions of the fetal stomach as early as 13 weeks (Kelly et al. 1993a). However, although the fetus has the capacity to produce gastric acid from the middle of the second trimester, gastric acid secretion is significantly reduced in preterm infants (Kelly et al. 1993b) and increases with growing postnatal and gestational age. Parietal cells disappear from the antrum of the stomach in the third trimester of pregnancy, but this process fails to occur in approximately 20% of the population (Kelly et al. 1993a). Milk entry into the infant's stomach sharply raises gastric pH followed by slower return to lower pH compared to older children (Lopez-Alonso et al. 2006). The outflow of pepsin is also diminished in the newborn infant and increases until 3 months of age (Mouterde et al. 1992). Thus, gastric proteolysis is limited in term and especially in preterm infants because of low pepsin levels combined with low gastric acidity. However, gastric proteolysis does not seem to be critical for further digestion and absorption of proteins.

In the duodenum, several proteases act together to digest proteins into amino acids and oligopeptides (di- or tripeptides). Pancreatic enzymes are secreted as inactive proenzymes that are activated by hydrolysis of a peptide bond. Bile salts in the duodenum induce enterokinase release from the microvillus membrane of the absorptive cells. Enterokinase converts trypsinogen to trypsin that in turn activates all the other pancreatic proteases and the release of more trypsinogen. The concentrations of the proteolytic enzymes (e.g., trypsin, chymotrypsin) excreted from the exocrine pancreas only modestly increase during the first hours to months after delivery, and they are fairly efficient in proteolysis from birth on. This is true for premature infants as early as 23 weeks gestation (Kolacek et al. 1990). However, feeding preterm infants with high-protein diet stimulates increased trypsin secretion into the duodenum. Lower chymotrypsin concentration are found in infants who are small for gestational age (SGA) (Kolacek et al. 1990) suggesting a deleterious effect of intrauterine growth retardation on pancreatic exocrine function, which may limit postnatal catch-up growth. Concerns regarding protease inhibitors in human milk and colostrum that may interfere with the digestion of proteins in the intestine of breastfed babies (Chowanadisai and Lonnerdal 2002) were disputed by others (Henderson et al. 2001).

Following the digestion by pancreatic proteases, amino acids and oligopeptides are passively absorbed at the brush border membrane by secondary active transport via sodium-dependent amino acid cotransporters (Stevens and Preston 1998). The low intracellular sodium concentration creates gradient for sodium entry that drives the absorption of the coupled amino acid. The energy is indirectly provided by the sodium-potassium ATPase pump. There are different classes of amino acid transporters as well as transporters for oligopeptides. There are also peptidases on the brush border membrane, as well as in the cytoplasm of the absorptive cell. In the embryonic period (4–8 weeks), the activity of proteases is mainly detected on the luminal surface of the fetal intestine. Later on, villi are formed from the duodenum up to the ileum. After 9 weeks of gestation, differentiation of Lieberkuhn crypts can be observed. The activity of proteases is high in the differentiating microvillous zone of the primitive enterocytes (Lichnovsky and Lojda 1992). Thus, the peptide transport system and the brush border and cytosolic peptidases are well developed and functional in preterm infants. In addition, preterm and term newborns have increased small intestinal permeability that allows them to absorb intact macromolecules by active pinocytosis (Walker 2002). Amniotic fluid proteins are swallowed in utero and food and other proteins are ingested during the neonatal period. These include albumin, beta-lactoglobulin, immunoglobulins (A and G) and other immunologic factors, hormones (chorionic gonadotropin and growth hormone), and even intact lactoferrin of maternal origin.

34.5.3 Carbohydrate Digestion and Absorption

Carbohydrates provide about 40% of the caloric intake of the newborn. Lactose is the major source of carbohydrates in human milk. Lactase activity appears in the differentiating brush border of the fetal small intestine along with other disaccharidases (mainly sucrase) as early as 12 weeks of gestation (Lichnovsky and Lojda 1992), although in low levels. Lactase activity exhibits relatively higher levels at 37 weeks of gestation (Villa et al. 1992). Lactase activity is still decreased during the first weeks of life, and this is reflected by the limited capacity of term and especially preterm infants to digest and absorb lactose in the small intestine (Shulman et al. 2005). Nevertheless, preterm infants fed lactose-containing milk or formulas grow well and have no diarrhea. The elevation of breath hydrogen in these infants apparently represents a successful adaptation of the colonic microflora that converts malabsorbed lactose to volatile organic acids that are subsequently absorbed (Kien et al. 1989). Glucose polymers are polysaccharides that require hydrolysis by amylase. Since pancreatic alpha-amylase levels are low in young infants and increase only later during postnatal life, glucose polymers are either hydrolyzed by salivary alpha-amylase whose activity increases earlier or by the intestinal brush border enzyme, glucoamylase. Alpha-amylase in breast milk probably also participates in digestion, because it can survive the mild acidity (Lindberg and Skude 1982) and low pepsin levels in the stomach of newborn babies.

Glucose and other monosaccharide products of hydrolysis are then absorbed from the jejunum and ileum either by active sodium-dependent D-glucose cotransport carrier system (SGLT1) or by the GLUT family of facilitative glucose transporters (Davidson et al. 1992). The sodium-dependent D-glucose cotransport carrier systems demonstrate early differentiation of a functional heterogeneity in glucose transport capacity along the human fetal small intestine (Malo and Berteloot 1991). These brush border cotransport systems develop in the jejunum and ileum of the fetus as early as 17–20 weeks gestation and can be differentiated not only by their kinetic properties but also by their differences in both substrate and inhibitor specificities (Malo 1990). The facilitative glucose transporter isoforms GLUT2 and GLUT5 are also developmentally modulated with highest levels in adult small intestine. By contrast, GLUT1 expression is higher in the fetal small intestine. In the adult small intestine, GLUT5 is localized to the luminal brush border surface of mature enterocytes. Yet, in the fetal small intestine, GLUT5 is localized along the intercellular junctions of the developing villus. Thus, both the expression and localization of GLUT 5 are developmentally regulated. In a mature absorptive epithelial cell, GLUT5 is localized to the luminal surface (Davidson et al. 1992). Postnatal glucose absorption in infants is less efficient than in adults, and the kinetics of glucose absorption is related to gestational and postnatal ages, as well as to the diet and exposure to glucocorticoids (Murray et al. 1990).

Carbohydrates that are not digested and absorbed in the small intestine reach the colon where they are degraded by colonic bacteria. The last step of this degradation is fermentation that results in the formation of short-chain fatty acids, methane, carbon dioxide, and hydrogen. These short-chain fatty acids, particularly butyrate (Wong et al. 2006), are the preferred energy source for the colonic epithelial cells. In the premature infant, colonic fermentation serves as a major important route for lactose carbon absorption (as discussed above) (Kien et al. 1989). Developmental aspects of colonic fermentative activity; effects of systemic antibiotic treatment on colonic microflora; the effects of various fermentation pathways on energy balance; the capacity for absorption of sugars, short-chain fatty acids, and electrolytes by colonic epithelia; and the effects of fermentation products on metabolism and on the mucosal cells are all important to premature infants especially in relation to colonic disease or surgical resection (Kien et al. 1989).

34.5.4 Micronutrient Absorption

The absorption of the different micronutrients matures at varying rates during infancy.

Water and electrolytes: Water is absorbed passively following the gradients of sodium and other electrolytes. Stimulation of intestinal sodium absorption by adding solutes (sugars or amino acids) that are absorbed by sodium-coupled mechanisms increase net fluid absorption (Schultz 2007).

The intestinal epithelium is more susceptible to diarrhea in young infants. Protracted diarrhea of infancy (PDI) describes infants with loose and frequent stools of sufficient severity to require nutritional support, often in the form of parenteral alimentation (Sherman et al. 2004). The most common cause for PDI is postinfectious diarrhea with failure of the injured gut to recover rapidly. The causes of PDI can be classified into two categories based on the findings of intestinal biopsy: PDI with normal villi and PDI with villus atrophy. The most common cause of protracted diarrhea with villous atrophy is microvillus inclusion disease, an autosomal recessive disorder that is present upon birth with striking secretory diarrhea. Diagnosis is based on typical electron microscopy findings including the diagnostic finding of microvilli inside involutions of the apical membrane (Bar et al. 2007). During pregnancy, ultrasound demonstrates multiple fluid-filled dilated intestinal loops and polyhydramnios. Other causes of congenital diarrhea with villus destruction include tufting enteropathy, autoimmune enteropathy, and IPEX syndrome (Sherman et al. 2004), as well as carbohydrate-deficient glycoprotein syndrome (Sparks 2006) and enterocyte heparin sulfate deficiency (Murch et al. 1996).

In the category of normal villous PDI, congenital ion transport defects cause secretory diarrhea presenting at birth. The most common congenital ion transport defect is in the chloride-bicarbonate anion exchanger that is located in the distal ileum and colon. This transmembrane protein belongs to the sulfate transporter family that has three known members in humans, all associated with a distinct genetic disease (Kere et al. 1999). Members of the gene family can transport other anions as well (chloride, sulfate, and oxalate) (Lohi et al. 2002). In these cases of congenital chloride diarrhea, $HCO3^-$ is not secreted into the gastrointestinal tract lumen, leading to alkalosis. Fecal chloride concentration exceeds the sum of fecal sodium and potassium levels, establishing the diagnosis (Kere et al. 1999). Congenital sodium diarrhea, a disorder of the intestinal H^+/Na^+ exchanger located in the small intestine and colon, is characterized by hyponatremia, alkaline diarrhea, and high concentration of stool sodium (Keller et al. 1990). In the other congenital ion transport defects (sodium cotransporters), abnormal reabsorption of sodium is involved, which usually results in hyponatremia (Sherman et al. 2004).

The colon has an important role in absorbing sodium and water from the intestinal lumen. Active absorption of sodium ion can be increased three- to fourfold by the presence of aldosterone (Harvey et al. 2008), suggesting that colonic absorption of sodium is central to maintaining salt and water homeostasis. Colonic mucosa in the fetus has well-developed villi that allows it to be involved in nutrient absorption in contrast to the adult (Menard et al. 1994). Thus, in addition to its role in salt and water homeostasis, it can also absorb essential nutrients by active (sodium-coupled) transport of glucose and amino acids that may also compensate for decreased absorption in the developing small intestine.

Minerals and trace elements: Trace elements and mineral absorption depends on the milieu in which they are presented to the intestine. The bioavailability of iron, calcium, and other minerals for absorption is better from human breast milk (Bosscher et al. 2001). Preterm infants may absorb as much as 50% of the iron in breast milk, as opposed to formulas. This is true for other minerals that are more bioavailable for preterm infants in human milk. This does not alter the need to supplement some of these nutrients (mainly calcium and phosphorus) to preterm infants to compensate for their increased demands (Schanler and Rifka 1994).

Calcium and phosphorus absorption and requirements are discussed in ▸ Chap. 41, "Calcium and Phosphorus Homeostasis: Pathophysiology."

Vitamins: Human milk is a good source for most vitamins. In healthy breastfed infants of well-nourished mothers, there is little risk for vitamin deficiencies, and the need for vitamin supplementation is rare. The exceptions to this, to avoid deficiencies, are a need for vitamin K supplementation in the immediate newborn period and the need to supplement vitamin D in breastfed infants with dark skin or inadequate sunlight exposure (Greer 2001; Mimouni and Shamir 2009). Most vitamins appear to be absorbed adequately in term and preterm infants.

Fat-soluble vitamins: Fat-soluble vitamins include vitamins A, D, E, and K. Vitamins A (retinoids) and E (tocopherols) are two potent antioxidant nutrients that also play a significant role in immune function.

Vitamin D (calciferol) plays a major role in intestinal calcium absorption and bone mineralization (Mimouni and Shamir 2009). Cholesterol-derived precursor uses UV sunlight to convert to previtamin D3, which is then converted to inactive form of vitamin D3. Vitamin D3 is then hydroxylated in the liver (25-(OH)D) and in the kidneys to make active vitamin D (1,25-$(OH)_2D$). Vitamin D crosses the placenta mainly in the form of 25-(OH)D. The transport is passive or facilitated, with lower values in the fetus, and therefore fetal 25-(OH) D concentrations correlate with those of the mother. Exogenous vitamin D_3 (from animal source) or D_2 (ergocalciferol, synthesized by plants) can also be absorbed in the duodenum and the jejunum, although vitamin D_2 appears to be absorbed to a much lesser extent than vitamin D_3 (Houghton and Vieth 2006).

Vitamin K intervenes in the synthesis of coagulation factors particularly in prothrombin synthesis. Fat-soluble vitamins are totally dependent on micelles in order to be presented to the brush border membrane. Absorption is also dependent on the presence of bile salts in the small intestine (Greer 2000). Ingested carotene and dietary retinyl esters are converted to free retinol in the proximal small intestine by pancreatic hydrolases and are the dietary sources for vitamin A. Retinol absorption into the intestinal cells is facilitated by retinol-binding protein, RBP II, which is found almost exclusively in absorptive cells. In the enterocyte, fat-soluble vitamins are re-esterified and incorporated into the developing chylomicron. Chylomicrons travel through the lymphatic system and then enter the bloodstream. Some of the vitamins use protein carrier for transport in the bloodstream (retinol-binding protein, RBP I, for carrying retinol to target tissue and D-binding protein to take hydroxylated vitamin D from the liver to the kidney for further hydroxylation). Excess is stored in liver and adipose tissue and released as needed by the body. The risk of toxicity may be relevant for high doses of vitamins D, A, and E and is less relevant for vitamin K. Disorders affecting fat absorption, such as short bowel syndrome, cholestasis, and other diseases associated with bile acid deficiency, may cause fat-soluble vitamin deficiency. Vitamin K2 (menaquinones) is synthesized by bacteria in the large intestine. Because the transfer of the vitamin K across the placenta during pregnancy is poor and the sterile gut of the infant is unable to produce menaquinones, newborn babies are routinely given supplements of vitamin K (Greer 2000).

Water-soluble vitamins: Water-soluble vitamins are required as enzyme cofactors in a wide variety of metabolic reactions. Riboflavin (vitamin B2), niacin, and vitamin C (ascorbic acid) are essential for oxidation-reduction reactions. Thiamine (vitamin B1) and biotin are involved in macronutrient metabolism. Folate, vitamin B12, pyridoxine (vitamin B6), and riboflavin play important roles in the regulation of S-adenosylmethionine production and DNA synthesis. Each of these water-soluble vitamins requires its own membrane transport process for absorption across the enterocyte. Most of the water-soluble vitamins are absorbed from the proximal small intestine (Greer 2000; Halsted 2003). Folate, biotin, and riboflavin can be transported across colonic epithelial cells as well, although the clinical significance of this is uncertain (Halsted 2003). Riboflavin is light sensitive and is rapidly photodegraded. Phototherapy is a possible cause for riboflavin deficiency in neonates (Bohles 1997). This may affect antioxidant mechanisms in preterm infants. The absorption of vitamin B12 (cobalamin) is unique in requiring multiple steps from the stomach to the ileum and the involvement of at least four different binding proteins (Halsted 2003). Its absorption is complex. In the gastric acidic environment, it is released from the food to form complexes with R-binders that are proteins found in the saliva, gastric juice, bile, and milk and have high affinity for vitamin B12. At the alkaline environment of the duodenum, pancreatic proteases degrade R-binders allowing vitamin B12 to bind to the intrinsic factor that is produced by the parietal cells of the stomach. The complex of vitamin B12 and intrinsic factor is absorbed intact in the distal ileum. Inside the ileal mucosal cells, vitamin B12 is released from the intrinsic factor and binds to a specific transport protein, transcobalamin II, to be delivered to the liver via circulation. It is excreted mainly in the bile, but has a very long half-life due to very effective enterohepatic circulation. It is actively transported across the placenta so that newborns have concentrations twice as high as mothers (Greer 2000). Hepatic stores correlate with the duration of pregnancy and are thus large in full-term newborns, but lower in preterm infants. Clinical manifestations of vitamin B12 deficiency appear only in late infancy, because of the hepatic stores and the long half-life (Greer 2000). There are several congenital defects that can affect the complex absorption of vitamin B12, but they are rare compared to dietary deficiency that is not evident in neonatal period.

34.6 Host Defense

The microbiota is a large and diverse community of microorganism that resides in the human gut. It is dominated by bacteria and is known to have a critical role in the evolution of intestinal functions and overall health of the host. The bacterial cells outnumber human cells of the host, and their total amount of genes, which is called the microbiome, estimated to be about two to four million genes, exceed the number of human genes by more than 100-fold. The microbiota is considered as an "organ within an organ," because through expression of the microbiome, these intestinal bacteria can execute numerous enzymatic reactions that mammalian host is not able to catalyze. Microbes of the intestinal tract are important in nutrient processing and absorption, may play a role in growth and is important in the development of the immune system and maintaining its integrity. The microbiota functions include modulating the expression of genes involved in strengthening mucosal barrier, angiogenesis and postnatal intestinal maturation, support of normal digestion, and consumption and storage of energy from the diet, usually by fermenting unused energy substrates to short-chain fatty acids (SCFAs) (Di Mauro et al. 2013).

Fetal gastrointestinal tract was originally thought to be sterile. However, recent studies using molecular techniques suggest that the fetal intestine may be exposed to microbes via swallowing of colonized amniotic fluid, which can be associated with preterm delivery, the so-called fetal inflammatory response syndrome (FIRS) (Park et al. 2009). Prenatal exposure of the mother to bacterial components can influence intestinal epithelial development and function in newborn, as well as sensitivity to inflammatory diseases such as NEC. Prenatal exposure of the gut to bacteria may modulate postnatal adaptations inducing tolerance toward colonization of certain bacteria. During birth the intestinal mucosa undergoes a dramatic transition to a densely colonized environment. This heavy colonization of the gastrointestinal tract of newborn infants occurs within a few days but starts immediately after birth. Initially, the type of delivery (passage through the birth canal versus cesarean section) and the type of diet (breast versus formula feeding) affect the colonization pattern (Salminen and Isolauri 2006). Other environmental factors such as developed versus developing countries and the use of antibiotics in the neonatal period may also affect the microflora composition (Guarner and Malagelada 2003). The gut interacts with intestinal bacteria to develop and mature the intestinal barrier protective mechanisms against foreign harmful molecules while maintaining appropriate responses toward commensal bacteria and nutrients by means of immune modulation and immune tolerance (Di Mauro et al. 2013) (Fig. 5). Thus, aberrant bacterial colonization may lead to feeding intolerance in a newborn (Di Mauro et al. 2013).

The immune system of preterm infants is immature. Thus, preterm infants are prone to a delayed gastrointestinal colonization, reduced microbial diversity in the bowel, acquisition of antibiotic-resistant strains, loss of strains associated with antibiotic treatment, and increased intestinal bacterial translocation (Caicedo et al. 2005). The gut of extremely low-birth-weight infants is colonized by a paucity of bacterial species (Gewolb et al. 1999). This can favor the overgrowth of microorganisms such as *Enterobacteriaceae* and *coagulase-negative staphylococci*, which are the most frequent pathogens of nosocomial infection in neonatal intensive care units (Gaynes et al. 1996). These factors also make the preterm infant more susceptible to antibiotic-resistant infections, systemic inflammatory response syndrome, and necrotizing enterocolitis (NEC) (Neu and Caicedo 2005). Breast milk and reduction of antibiotic exposure have been found to be important in increasing fecal microbial diversity in these premature infants (Gewolb et al. 1999). Microbes of the intestinal tract serve several roles, including nutrition, growth, and maintenance of function and development of the immune system (Hooper et al. 2002).

The gut is in continuity with the environment and thus exposed to bacteria and antigens. The gastrointestinal tract presents the largest surface area in the body exposed to microbes and other antigens. On the other hand, it needs to allow the entrance of nutrients and other beneficial molecules. Host defenses include nonspecific and specific components. The innate immune system responds in a nonspecific way, and the adaptive immune system responds specifically by humoral and cellular components that specifically react to particular antigens.

Defense factors in human milk include antimicrobial agents (secretory IgA, lactoferrin, lysozyme, glycoconjugates, oligosaccharides, and digestive products of milk lipids), anti-inflammatory factors (antioxidants, epithelial growth factors, cellular protective agents, and enzymes that degrade mediators of inflammation), immunomodulators (nucleotides, cytokines, and

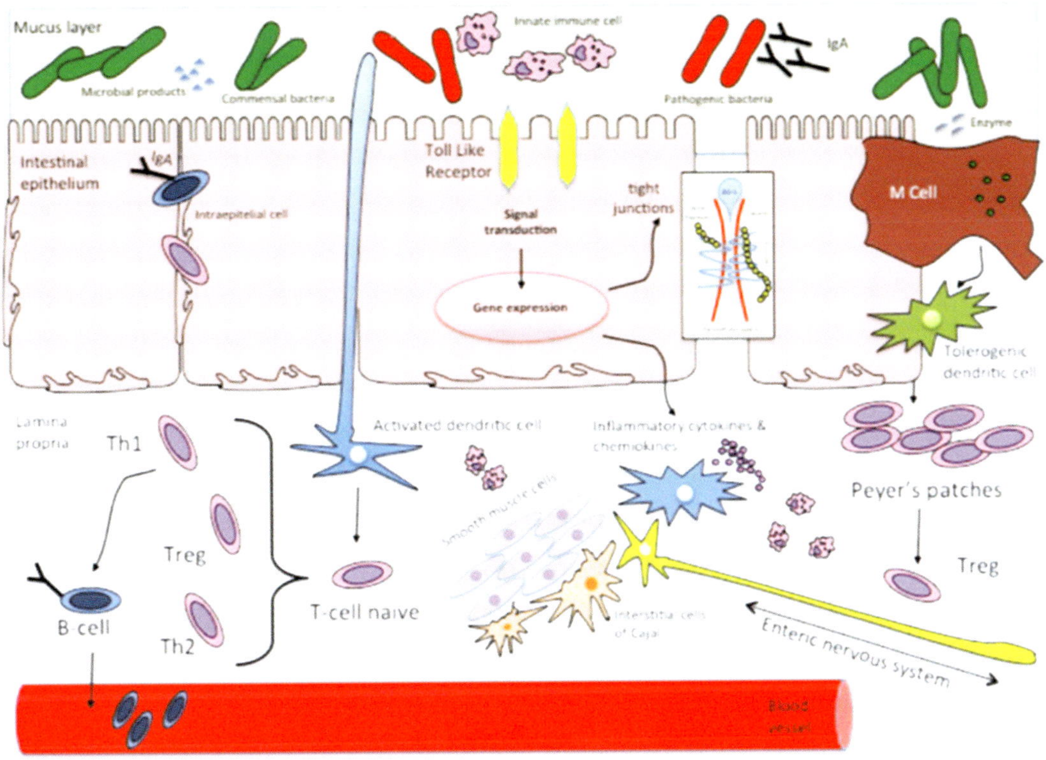

Fig. 5 Intestinal function and microbiota – cells involved in antigen sampling at the gastrointestinal barrier: Commensal bacteria inhabiting the human intestine participate in the development and maintenance of gut immunologic, sensory, and motor functions. Under normal conditions, the gastrointestinal tract provides a stable habitat for commensal bacteria that supports its structural and functional integrity. The ENS influences the gut directly with the activity related to the contraction and indirectly influencing the cells of the gut immune system. The functional bidirectional interaction act via neuroimmune peptide receptor on immune cells and on several receptors for immune mediators expressed on enteric nerves. Immune cells release mediators in response to neural stimuli – Fig. 1 page 3 from: Di Mauro et al. (2013) (http://www.ijponline.net/content/39/1/15)

anti-idiotypic antibodies), and leukocytes (neutrophils, macrophages, and lymphocytes). The presence and function of immunomodulatory and anti-inflammatory factors present in human milk help protecting the mature newborn as well as the premature infant against infections. Some of these factors present in human milk may actively modulate the synthesis and maturation of the recipient immune system. This complex interactive system of bioactive substances in human milk seems to be designed to operate in a complementary manner with other noninflammatory mechanisms in order to resist digestion of these factors in the recipient gastrointestinal tract and to supplement the infant with developmentally delayed immune factors. This is consistent with the theory of the evolution of the mammary gland from the immune system (Vorbach et al. 2006). In addition to the well-known passive protection against infections during lactation (mainly via secretory IgA antibodies and also via several other factors like bactericidal lactoferrin), breastfeeding may also actively stimulate the immune system of the infant (via anti-idiotypic antibodies, cytokines, growth factors, T and B lymphocytes, and macrophages) with other long-term positive effects (e.g., better immunological response to infections and vaccines) (Garofalo and Goldman 1999; Chirico et al. 2008).

Gastric acidity and pancreatobiliary secretions also decrease the load of viable microorganisms and intact dietary protein antigens. These defenses are all decreased in the newborn, especially the preterm infant, as described above. The use of H2-blocking agents or proton pump inhibitors that further decrease gastric acidity contributes to a decreased defense and may result in higher rates of infections (Beck-Sague et al. 1994).

Mechanical factors that appear early in gestation are also involved in host defense by creating physical barrier of mucous secretion and by gastric emptying and intestinal peristalsis that prevent stasis and bacterial overgrowth. In preterm infant gastric emptying, MMCs and peristalsis may be delayed, as discussed above. Intestinal mucus secreted into the lumen from storage vacuoles in the goblet cells, found throughout the small and large intestine, plays a significant role in intestinal defense. It contains mucins, glycoproteins, immunoglobulins, glycolipids, and albumin that form a slippery gel over the intestinal surface that enhances forward propulsion. Mucous gel can also trap large foreign antigenic molecules, thus preventing their diffusion into the gut wall. Mucin secretion changes in amount and composition during development and maturation of the newborn infant and in response to stress and hypoxia (Louis et al. 2006). Microvilli also constitute a significant barrier because of their size and negative charge that prevent large macromolecules from penetrating.

The intestinal single-cell layer of columnar epithelial cells is present by the end of the first trimester. It is the cellular site of innate immunity of the intestine separating the host from the intestinal lumen. It is arranged in crypts and villi. Stem cells at the base of the crypts proliferate and differentiate into enterocytes that migrate to the villus tip. They eventually slough into the lumen by physiologic apoptosis (anoikis), thus allowing reconstitution of the epithelium every 5 days (Pinto and Clevers 2005). This renewal mechanism serves as a defense mechanism against epithelial injury. Epithelial integrity is further protected by intracellular contacts of membrane proteins and cytoskeletal anchor proteins that form the apical junction complexes (AJCs) that are the basis for the series of tight junctions between the cells. The AJCs and their cytoskeletal connections are dynamic structures that closely regulate the flow of fluids, electrolytes ions, and even small molecules between the cells but prevent passage of larger molecules (Nusrat et al. 2000). Epithelial cells also regulate transcellular permeability to ions and small molecules through alterations in the expression of selective membrane ion channels and pores. Control of water and chloride secretion through the channels can result in secretory diarrhea that can flush away toxins and pathogens from the lumen (Hecht 1999).

In addition to mechanical barriers, and in addition to mucin secretion, the gut elaborates chemical defenses secreted by the absorptive enterocytes and Paneth cells. Paneth cells are specialized secretory enterocytes located at the base of the small intestinal crypts, where they can control microbial populations and protect neighboring stem cells. Paneth cells secrete lysozyme, phospholipase A2, and antimicrobial peptides. Antimicrobial peptides are divided into defensins (alpha and beta), which are the predominant class, and cathelicidins. These small cationic peptides are able to insert into the membranes of a broad range of microbes (including bacteria, fungi, and enveloped viruses), where they play an active role in oxygen-independent killing. It is possible that low levels of Paneth cell defensins, characteristic of normal intestinal development, may predispose preterm infants to necrotizing enterocolitis (NEC) (Salzman et al. 2007).

An important non-constitutive defense component of the gut innate immunity is the carefully programmed and regulated inflammatory response that is activated when potentially injurious stimuli cross the barrier of the intestinal epithelium. This activated inflammatory response induces recruitment of leukocytes (polymorphonuclear and macrophages) as well as complement, defensins, and cytokines to aid in defense. Multiple endogenous or exogenous signals can start the inflammatory process by inducing the local release of soluble inflammatory mediators and chemotactic agents that increase vascular permeability and attract inflammatory cells, resulting in edema and inflammation (Medzhitov 2007).

The human genome contains evolutionary ancient components of innate immunity that are transmitted in the germ cells without exposure to the microbes and encode at least ten toll-like receptors (TLRs). TLRs are transmembrane receptors that recognize pathogen-associated molecular patterns (PAMPs) or microbial associated molecular patterns (MAMPs) that are found only on microbes, like lipopolysaccharides, peptidoglycans, and lipoproteins. The binding of MAMPs to TLRs or intracytoplasmic NOD proteins results in the activation of cytoplasmic signaling circuits. These pathways include the classic nuclear factor kappa-B (NF-kappa-B), the mitogen-activated protein kinase (MAPK), and the interferon regulatory factor (IRF) pathways. During the initial events of bacterial perception by the intestinal epithelial cells, all these three pathways are activated within minutes. Modulation of these pathways involves a regulated series of phosphorylation and ubiquitination, leading to nuclear translocation of these three transcription factors and transcriptional activation of a battery of effector inflammatory molecules (Louis and Lin 2009; (Sharma and Tepas 2010) (Figs. 6 and 7). This results in induction of the expression of enzymes important for bacterial killing and wound healing, as well as antibacterial peptides, cytokines, adhesion molecules, chemotactic messengers, and antiapoptotic proteins (Neish 2009). The sterile fetal gut is naïve to MAMPs in utero. Within the first days, the neonatal gut is challenged by multiple MAMPs as the luminal flora is introduced. TLRs are expressed at the basolateral aspects of fetal intestinal crypts as early as 20 weeks of gestation (Fusunyan et al. 2001).

Membranous or microfold cells, commonly referred to as M cells, are specialized epithelial cells of the gut-associated lymphoid tissues (GALT) that play a major role in the intestinal immune system by delivering luminal antigens to the underlying immune cells. M cells in the intestine lack well-developed microvilli and allow macromolecular transport, as opposed to the absorptive enterocytes with their developed villi. M cells are present only in follicles overlying lymphoid tissue to which they can immediately present foreign antigens and microorganisms that they transport as macromolecules (Miller et al. 2007) (Fig. 5).

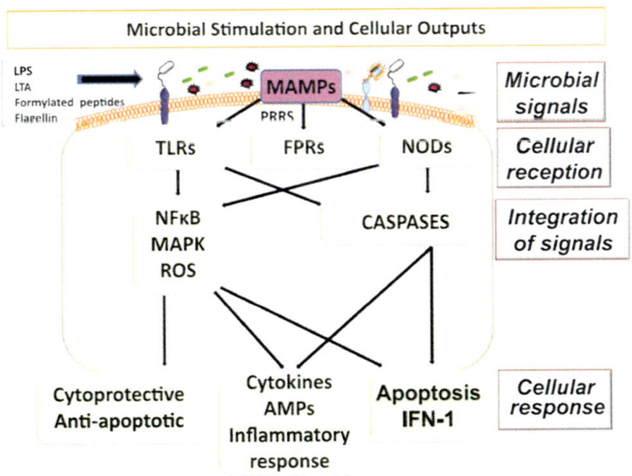

Fig. 6 Microbial associated molecular pattern (MAMP) activation and signaling in the cells of the gastrointestinal barrier: Microbial components such as lipopolysaccharides (LPS), lipoteichoic acid (LTA), formylated peptides, and flagellin serve as microbial associated molecular patterns (MAMPs) and signal pattern recognition receptors (PRRs) including toll-like receptors (TLRs), formylated peptide receptors (FPRs), or nucleotide-binding oligomerization domain-like receptors (NODs). Integration of these signals evokes cellular outputs based on the initial perception of the triggering organism. Output can be a protective response to commensal microbiota, an inflammatory response to pathogenic organism(s), or it can trigger apoptosis (Fig. 1 page 13 from: Sharma et al. (2010), copyright Springer)

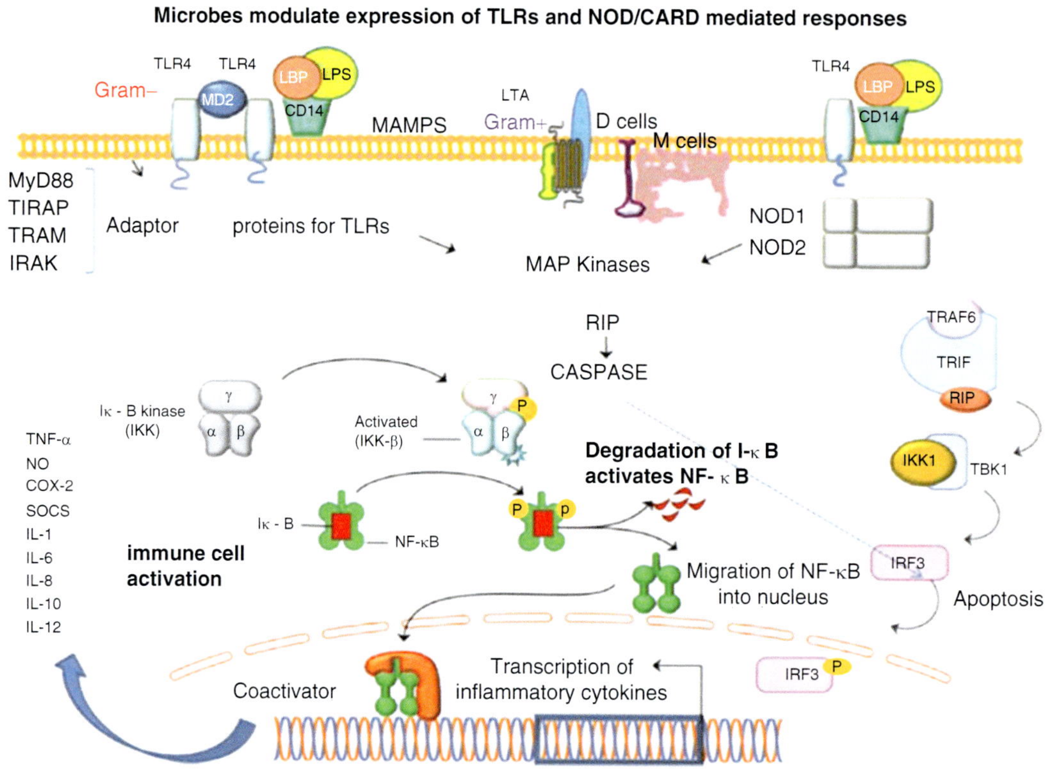

Fig. 7 Microbes modulate expression of receptors on the cells of the gastrointestinal barrier activating downstream signaling: a schematic illustration of the recognition of microbial associated molecular patterns (MAMPs), such as lipopolysaccharides (LPS), by pattern recognition receptors (PRRs) on epithelial cells and immune cell activation or apoptotic response. Transmembrane toll-like receptors (TLRs) are triggered by MAMPs and stimulate PRRs. Four adaptor proteins for TLRs are involved in propagation of signals and activation of MAP kinases that can result in transcription of pro-inflammatory cytokines or apoptotic response through activation of NF-kB (NF-kappa-B) (Fig. 2 page 14 from: Sharma et al. (2010), copyright Springer)

Subepithelial cells include follicular dendritic cells that are located in the lymphoid follicles and are important in non-phagocytic presentation of antigens to T cells as well as B cells. Peyer's patches are aggregates of lymphoid tissue that are present by 19 weeks of gestation, but become more prominent in the jejunum and ileum between 24 and 40 weeks. M cells occur in follicle-associated epithelium over areas of Peyer's patches (Miller et al. 2007) (Fig. 5). Mast cells bind immunoglobulin E and subsequently release histamine and serotonin that stimulate mucus production by adjacent goblet cells and increase enterocyte permeability, chemotaxis of granulocytes, contraction of smooth muscle cells, and lymphocyte function.

The immune system of host defense is composed of cellular and humoral components. T and B lymphocytes are produced as early as 12 weeks gestation, and are present with macrophages in the fetal intestine by 20 weeks gestation. Interspersed between the intestinal epithelial enterocytes are blood-derived intraepithelial lymphocytes (IELs) that are immune components of the host defense. They are located in the basolateral side of the epithelial layer where cells are exposed to various food and microbial antigens. They are cytotoxic and capable of producing cytokines in order to protect the host from invasion of microorganisms through the gut. Immature human enterocytes react with excessive pro-inflammatory cytokine production after inflammatory stimulation in premature infants exposed to initial colonizing bacteria, and this may lead to necrotizing enterocolitis (NEC) (Nanthakumar et al. 2000). On the other hand, antigenic stimulation of the lymphoid tissues cannot be demonstrated before 46 weeks of postmenstrual age, which poses a challenge for preterm infants whose gut can absorb macromolecules directly by pinocytosis. Secretory IgA is present by 22 weeks of gestation, although in small amounts, because the newborn intestine has few IgA-producing plasma cells. In addition preterm infants are not able to form antibodies in response to exogenous food proteins.

Enteral nutrients and food supplements may also contribute to host defense. These include amino acids (glutamine and arginine), nucleotides, long-chain fatty acids, probiotics, and prebiotics.

Glutamine contributes to maintenance of small intestinal inter-epithelial junctional integrity (Potsic et al. 2002), intestinal epithelial cell growth and proliferation (DeMarco et al. 1999), inflammatory responses, and active healing. Glutamine-deficient diet increased bacterial translocation in vitro by altering intestinal tight junctions (Potsic et al. 2002; Li and Neu 2009), and glutamine supplementation decreased the incidence of sepsis in very-low-birth-weight infants (Neu et al. 1997). Glutamine and glutamic acid together with taurine are the only free amino acids that their concentrations are increased in human milk during the first 3 months of lactation (Agostoni et al. 2000).

Arginine also plays an important role in immune function. Low plasma arginine levels in preterm infants were associated with increased risk for subsequent NEC (Becker et al. 2000), and its supplementation may prevent NEC (Shah and Shah 2007).

Exogenous nucleotides may influence cell proliferation, differentiation and apoptosis in the crypt, and villus epithelium of the fetal and neonatal small intestine (Tanaka et al. 1996). Nucleotides in infant formulas have been associated with enhanced humoral antibody responses to immunizations (Pickering et al. 1998) and with a favorable effect on the lipid profile of preterm infants (Siahanidou et al. 2004). Since endogenous nucleotides are continuously produced as the result of the cell recycling within the gut, the functional role of the contribution from exogenous nucleotide supply is still unclear.

Long-chain polyunsaturated fatty acids (LC-PUFA), arachidonic acid (AA), and docosahexaenoic acid (DHA), which are metabolites of the essential n-3 and n-6 fatty acids, are known to modulate inflammation. Supplementation of preterm infants' food with LC-PUFA may reduce the risk of NEC (Caplan and Jilling 2001; Lu et al. 2007) and also has beneficial effects on the developing visual system and cognitive development during the first year of life (Heird and Lapillonne 2005).

Although the cause of NEC is not entirely known, milk feeding and bacterial growth play a role. Probiotics are dietary supplements containing potentially beneficial bacteria or yeast, which have been used to prevent NEC (AlFaleh and Anabrees 2014a). Probiotic bacteria have been shown to reinforce the different lines of gut defense, which are immune exclusion, immune elimination, and immune regulation. They also stimulate nonspecific host resistance to microbial pathogens, thereby aiding in pathogen eradication. Documented effects include the alleviation of intestinal inflammation, normalization of gut mucosal dysfunction, and downregulation of hypersensitivity reactions. Thus, modification of gut microflora by probiotic therapy may be suitable for clinical conditions associated with gut barrier dysfunction and inflammatory response (Isolauri 2001). Consequently, probiotics are used in the treatment of acute diarrhea in children (Szajewska et al. 2007). Probiotics modify the fecal flora, can reduce the overgrowth of pathogens in the bowel of preterm infants, and thus contribute to the reduction of the incidence of nosocomial infections in neonatal intensive care units (Dani et al. 2002). *Bifidobacterium* species are the most common bacteria in human milk-fed infants. Infants consuming *Bifidobacterium breve* supplemented feedings had higher rates of fecal bifidobacteria colonization with some clinical advantages including decreased gastric aspirates and improved weight gain and feeding tolerance with no identified side effects (Kitajima et al. 1997). Significant reduction in the incidence of NEC and NEC-associated fatalities was shown by Hoyos et al. in preterm infants given daily doses of live *L. acidophilus* and *B. infantis* with no documented complications (Hoyos 1999). Dani et al. found that the incidence of NEC (Bell stage $\geq$2) was lower in preterm infants supplemented with *Lactobacillus GG* (LGG) (Dani et al. 2002). Lin et al. have shown that supplementation of human milk (Lin et al. 2005) or formula feedings (Lin et al. 2008) with a mixture of *Lactobacillus acidophilus* and *Bifidobacterium infantis* (Lin et al. 2005) or *bifidum* (Lin et al. 2008) significantly reduced the combined incidence of NEC or death in very-low-birth-weight (VLBW) infants, i.e., premature infants born weighing less than 1,500 g. There was a significant effect on NEC (Bell stage $\geq$2) itself as well. Bin-Nun et al. showed that a probiotic mixture (*Bifidobacterium infantis*, *Streptococcus thermophilus*, and *Bifidobacterium bifidum*) had a significant protective effect on NEC of any Bell stage in VLBW infants, even when Bell stage $\geq$2 NEC was only considered (Bin-Nun et al. 2005). Recent meta-analyses conclude that the use of probiotics significantly reduces the occurrence of NEC and death in VLBW premature infants (birth weight $\leq$1,500 g) born after less than 34 weeks gestation (AlFaleh and Anabrees 2014a, b; Deshpande et al. 2010). There is insufficient data with regard to the benefits and potential adverse effects in the most at risk infants weighing less than 1,000 g at birth (AlFaleh and Anabrees 2014a, b). The issue of safety (Land et al. 2005) in routine use of probiotics in young premature infants with immature defense systems (Agostoni et al. 2004a) has not yet been fully settled. Nevertheless, based on all the studies done, it seems to be very low and disproportionate when compared to the advantages of their use in VLBW premature infants, including the most premature ones weighing less than 1,000 g at birth. Practice guidelines for their routine use in neonatal intensive care units have been suggested (Deshpande et al. 2011). It must be emphasized that not all probiotics are efficacious in preventing NEC and only probiotic strains that have been shown to be efficacious should be used (Mihatsch et al. 2012). Furthermore, probiotics are usually marketed as food supplements, and as such rigorous surveillance of the products must be guaranteed before their use.

Another approach is to use prebiotic supplementation. Prebiotics are defined as nondigestible substances that, when ingested, selectively promote the growth and establishment of beneficial probiotic-like bacteria normally present in the gut (Agostoni et al. 2004b). There are few studies on the use of oligosaccharide prebiotic products in preterm infants that have been shown to increase the counts of fecal bifidobacteria, reduce stool pH, reduce stool viscosity, accelerate gastrointestinal transport, and improve mineral absorption (Moro et al. 2002; Lidestri et al. 2003; Knol et al. 2005; Mihatsch et al. 2006) with no negative impact on weight gain. More randomized trials in preterm infants are needed to support their potential beneficial effects on feeding tolerance and on the reduction of the incidence of NEC and hospital-acquired infections (Knol et al. 2005; Riskin et al. 2010; Underwood et al. 2009, 2014). In a meta-analysis including some of the above mentioned studies, it was found that prebiotic supplemented formula for premature infants increased stool colony counts of bifidobacteria and lactobacilli without adversely affecting weight gain. However, the evidence was limited, and routine oligosaccharide supplementation could not have been recommended for NEC prevention or improving gut health (Srinivasjois et al. 2009).

References

Agostoni C, Carratu B, Boniglia C, Lammardo AM, Riva E, Sanzini E (2000) Free glutamine and glutamic acid increase in human milk through a three-month lactation period. J Pediatr Gastroenterol Nutr 31 (5):508–512

Agostoni C, Axelsson I, Braegger C, Goulet O, Koletzko B, Michaelsen KF et al (2004a) Probiotic

bacteria in dietetic products for infants: a commentary by the ESPGHAN Committee on Nutrition. J Pediatr Gastroenterol Nutr 38(4):365–374
Agostoni C, Axelsson I, Goulet O, Koletzko B, Michaelsen KF, Puntis JW et al (2004b) Prebiotic oligosaccharides in dietetic products for infants: a commentary by the ESPGHAN Committee on Nutrition. J Pediatr Gastroenterol Nutr 39(5):465–473
AlFaleh K, Anabrees J (2014a) Probiotics for prevention of necrotizing enterocolitis in preterm infants. Evid Based Child Health: Cochrane Rev J 9(3):584–671
AlFaleh K, Anabrees J (2014b) Probiotics for prevention of necrotizing enterocolitis in preterm infants. Cochrane Database Syst Rev 4:CD005496
Al-Tawil Y, Klee G, Berseth CL (2002) Extrinsic neural regulation of antroduodenal motor activity in preterm infants. Dig Dis Sci 47(12):2657–2663
Altschuler SM, Bao XM, Bieger D, Hopkins DA, Miselis RR (1989) Viscerotopic representation of the upper alimentary tract in the rat: sensory ganglia and nuclei of the solitary and spinal trigeminal tracts. J Comp Neurol 283(2):248–268
Anderson RB, Newgreen DF, Young HM (2006) Neural crest and the development of the enteric nervous system. Adv Exp Med Biol 589:181–196
Baetge G, Pintar JE, Gershon MD (1990) Transiently catecholaminergic (TC) cells in the bowel of the fetal rat: precursors of noncatecholaminergic enteric neurons. Dev Biol 141(2):353–380
Bar A, Riskin A, Iancu T, Manov I, Arad A, Shaoul R (2007) A newborn infant with protracted diarrhea and metabolic acidosis. J Pediatr 150(2):198–201
Beck F (2002) Homeobox genes in gut development. Gut 51(3):450–454
Becker RM, Wu G, Galanko JA, Chen W, Maynor AR, Bose CL et al (2000) Reduced serum amino acid concentrations in infants with necrotizing enterocolitis. J Pediatr 137(6):785–793
Beck-Sague CM, Azimi P, Fonseca SN, Baltimore RS, Powell DA, Bland LA et al (1994) Bloodstream infections in neonatal intensive care unit patients: results of a multicenter study. Pediatr Infect Dis J 13 (12):1110–1116
Berseth CL (1989) Gestational evolution of small intestine motility in preterm and term infants. J Pediatr 115:646–651
Berseth CL (1992) Effect of early feeding on maturation of the preterm infant's small intestine. J Pediatr 120 (6):947–953
Berseth CL (1996) Gastrointestinal motility in the neonate. Clin Perinatol 23(2):179–190
Berseth CL (2005) Developmental anatomy and physiology of the gastrointestinal tract. In: Taeusch HW, Ballard RA (eds) Avery's diseases of the newborn, 8th edn. W.B. Saunders Company, Philadelphia
Berthoud HR, Jedrzejewska A, Powley TL (1990) Simultaneous labeling of vagal innervation of the gut and afferent projections from the visceral forebrain with dil injected into the dorsal vagal complex in the rat. J Comp Neurol 301(1):65–79
Bin-Nun A, Bromiker R, Wilschanski M, Kaplan M, Rudensky B, Caplan M et al (2005) Oral probiotics prevent necrotizing enterocolitis in very low birth weight neonates. J Pediatr 147(2):192–196
Bohles H (1997) Antioxidative vitamins in prematurely and maturely born infants. Int J Vitam Nutr Res 67 (5):321–328
Bosscher D, Van Caillie-Bertrand M, Robberecht H, Van DK, Van CR, Deelstra H (2001) In vitro availability of calcium, iron, and zinc from first-age infant formulae and human milk. J Pediatr Gastroenterol Nutr 32(1):54–58
Bracco U (1994) Effect of triglyceride structure on fat absorption. Am J Clin Nutr 60 (6 Suppl):1002S–1009S
Caicedo RA, Schanler RJ, Li N, Neu J (2005) The developing intestinal ecosystem: implications for the neonate. Pediatr Res 58(4):625–628
Calder PC, Krauss-Etschmann S, de Jong EC, Dupont C, Frick JS, Frokiaer H et al (2006) Early nutrition and immunity – progress and perspectives. Br J Nutr 96 (4):774–790
Caplan MS, Jilling T (2001) The role of polyunsaturated fatty acid supplementation in intestinal inflammation and neonatal necrotizing enterocolitis. Lipids 36 (9):1053–1057
Chirico G, Marzollo R, Cortinovis S, Fonte C, Gasparoni A (2008) Antiinfective properties of human milk. J Nutr 138(9):1801S–1806S
Chowanadisai W, Lonnerdal B (2002) Alpha(1)-antitrypsin and antichymotrypsin in human milk: origin, concentrations, and stability. Am J Clin Nutr 76 (4):828–833
Dani C, Biadaioli R, Bertini G, Martelli E, Rubaltelli FF (2002) Probiotics feeding in prevention of urinary tract infection, bacterial sepsis and necrotizing enterocolitis in preterm infants. A prospective double-blind study. Biol Neonate 82(2):103–108
Davidson NO, Hausman AM, Ifkovits CA, Buse JB, Gould GW, Burant CF et al (1992) Human intestinal glucose transporter expression and localization of GLUT5. Am J Physiol 262(3 Pt 1):C795–C800
Davis MJ, Hill MA (1999) Signaling mechanisms underlying the vascular myogenic response. Physiol Rev 79 (2):387–423
de Lorijn LF, Voskuijl WP, Omari TI, Kok JH, Taminiau JA, Benninga MA (2005) Assessment of the rectoanal inhibitory reflex in preterm infants with delayed meconium passage. J Pediatr Gastroenterol Nutr 40 (4):434–437
de Santa BP, van den Brink GR, Roberts DJ (2003) Development and differentiation of the intestinal epithelium. Cell Mol Life Sci 60(7):1322–1332
DeMarco V, Dyess K, Strauss D, West CM, Neu J (1999) Inhibition of glutamine synthetase decreases proliferation of cultured rat intestinal epithelial cells. J Nutr 129 (1):57–62
Deshpande G, Rao S, Patole S, Bulsara M (2010) Updated meta-analysis of probiotics for preventing necrotizing enterocolitis in preterm neonates. Pediatrics 125 (5):921–930

Deshpande GC, Rao SC, Keil AD, Patole SK (2011) Evidence-based guidelines for use of probiotics in preterm neonates. BMC Med 9:92

Di Mauro A, Neu J, Riezzo G, Raimondi F, Martinelli D, Francavilla R et al (2013) Gastrointestinal function development and microbiota. Ital J Pediatr 39:15

Di LC, Flores AF, Hyman PE (1995) Age-related changes in colon motility. J Pediatr 127(4):593–596

Faure C, Chalazonitis A, Rheaume C, Bouchard G, Sampathkumar SG, Yarema KJ et al (2007) Gangliogenesis in the enteric nervous system: roles of the polysialylation of the neural cell adhesion molecule and its regulation by bone morphogenetic protein-4. Dev Dyn 236(1):44–59

Fekete E, Benedeczky I, Timmermans JP, Resch BA, Scheuermann DW (1996) Sequential pattern of nerve-muscle contacts in the small intestine of developing human fetus. An ultrastructural and immunohistochemical study. Histol Histopathol 11(4):845–850

Furness JB, Costa M (1987) Arrangement of the enteric plexuses. In: Furness JB, Costa M (eds) The enteric nervous system. Churchill Livingstone, New York

Fusunyan RD, Nanthakumar NN, Baldeon ME, Walker WA (2001) Evidence for an innate immune response in the immature human intestine: toll-like receptors on fetal enterocytes. Pediatr Res 49(4):589–593

Gardner CE Jr, Hart D (1934) Arch Surg 29:942

Garofalo RP, Goldman AS (1999) Expression of functional immunomodulatory and anti-inflammatory factors in human milk. Clin Perinatol 26(2):361–377

Gaynes RP, Edwards JR, Jarvis WR, Culver DH, Tolson JS, Martone WJ (1996) Nosocomial infections among neonates in high-risk nurseries in the United States. National Nosocomial Infections Surveillance System. Pediatrics 98(3 Pt 1):357–361

Gershon MD, Chalazonitis A, Rothman TP (1993) From neural crest to bowel: development of the enteric nervous system. J Neurobiol 24(2):199–214

Gewolb IH, Schwalbe RS, Taciak VL, Harrison TS, Panigrahi P (1999) Stool microflora in extremely low birthweight infants. Arch Dis Child Fetal Neonatal Ed 80(3):F167–F173

Gewolb IH, Vice FL, Schwietzer-Kenney EL, Taciak VL, Bosma JF (2001) Developmental patterns of rhythmic suck and swallow in preterm infants. Dev Med Child Neurol 43(1):22–27

Gork AS, Ehrenkranz RA, Bracken MB (2008) Continuous infusion versus intermittent bolus doses of indomethacin for patent ductus arteriosus closure in symptomatic preterm infants. Cochrane Database Syst Rev 1:CD006071

Greer FR (2000) Vitamin metabolism and requirements in the micropremie. Clin Perinatol 27(1):95–118, vi

Greer FR (2001) Do breastfed infants need supplemental vitamins? Pediatr Clin North Am 48(2):415–423

Grider JR, Murthy KS (2008) Autoinhibition of endothelial nitric oxide synthase (eNOS) in gut smooth muscle by nitric oxide. Regul Pept 151(1–3):75–79

Guarner F, Malagelada JR (2003) Gut flora in health and disease. Lancet 361(9356):512–519

Gupta A, Gulati P, Kim W, Fernandez S, Shaker R, Jadcherla SR (2009) Effect of postnatal maturation on the mechanisms of esophageal propulsion in preterm human neonates: primary and secondary peristalsis. Am J Gastroenterol 104(2):411–419

Halsted CH (2003) Absorption of water-soluble vitamins. Curr Opin Gastroenterol 19(2):113–117

Hamosh M (1987) Lipid metabolism in premature infants. Biol Neonate 52(Suppl 1):50–64

Hamosh M (1990) Lingual and gastric lipases. Nutrition 6 (6):421–428

Hamosh M (1995) Lipid metabolism in pediatric nutrition. Pediatr Clin North Am 42(4):839–859

Harvey BJ, Alzamora R, Stubbs AK, Irnaten M, McEneaney V, Thomas W (2008) Rapid responses to aldosterone in the kidney and colon. J Steroid Biochem Mol Biol 108(3–5):310–317

Havranek T, Thompson Z, Carver JD (2006) Factors that influence mesenteric artery blood flow velocity in newborn preterm infants. J Perinatol 26(8):493–497

Hecht G (1999) Innate mechanisms of epithelial host defense: spotlight on intestine. Am J Physiol 277(3 Pt 1):C351–C358

Heird WC, Lapillonne A (2005) The role of essential fatty acids in development. Annu Rev Nutr 25:549–571

Henderson TR, Hamosh M, Armand M, Mehta NR, Hamosh P (2001) Gastric proteolysis in preterm infants fed mother's milk or formula. Adv Exp Med Biol 501:403–408

Hernell O, Blackberg L (1994) Human milk bile salt-stimulated lipase: functional and molecular aspects. J Pediatr 125(5 Pt 2):S56–S61

Hoecker C, Nelle M, Poeschl J, Beedgen B, Linderkamp O (2002) Caffeine impairs cerebral and intestinal blood flow velocity in preterm infants. Pediatrics 109 (5):784–787

Holle GE, Forth W (1990) Myoelectric activity of small intestine after chemical ablation of myenteric neurons. Am J Physiol 258(4 Pt 1):G519–G526

Hooper LV, Midtvedt T, Gordon JI (2002) How host-microbial interactions shape the nutrient environment of the mammalian intestine. Annu Rev Nutr 22:283–307

Houghton LA, Vieth R (2006) The case against ergocalciferol (vitamin D2) as a vitamin supplement. Am J Clin Nutr 84(4):694–697

Hoyos AB (1999) Reduced incidence of necrotizing enterocolitis associated with enteral administration of Lactobacillus acidophilus and Bifidobacterium infantis to neonates in an intensive care unit. Int J Infect Dis 3 (4):197–202

Huizinga JD, Thuneberg L, Kluppel M, Malysz J, Mikkelsen HB, Bernstein A (1995) W/kit gene required for interstitial cells of Cajal and for intestinal pacemaker activity. Nature 373(6512):347–349

Huizinga JD, Ambrous K, Der-Silaphet T (1998) Co-operation between neural and myogenic mechanisms in the control of distension-induced peristalsis in the mouse small intestine. J Physiol 506 (Pt 3):843–856

Iqbal J, Hussain M (2009) Intestinal lipid absorption. Am J Physiol Endocrinol Metab 296:E1183

Isolauri E (2001) Probiotics in human disease. Am J Clin Nutr 73(6):1142S–1146S

Ittmann PI, Amarnath R, Berseth CL (1992) Maturation of antroduodenal motor activity in preterm and term infants. Dig Dis Sci 37(1):14–19

Kawai T, Fushiki T (2003) Importance of lipolysis in oral cavity for orosensory detection of fat. Am J Physiol Regul Integr Comp Physiol 285(2):R447–R454

Keller KM, Wirth S, Baumann W, Sule D, Booth IW (1990) Defective jejunal brush border membrane sodium/proton exchange in association with lethal familial protracted diarrhoea. Gut 31(10):1156–1158

Kelly EJ, Lagopoulos M, Primrose JN (1993a) Immunocytochemical localisation of parietal cells and G cells in the developing human stomach. Gut 34 (8):1057–1059

Kelly EJ, Newell SJ, Brownlee KG, Primrose JN, Dear PR (1993b) Gastric acid secretion in preterm infants. Early Hum Dev 35(3):215–220

Kelly EJ, Newell SJ, Brownlee KG, Farmery SM, Cullinane C, Reid WA et al (1997) Role of epidermal growth factor and transforming growth factor alpha in the developing stomach. Arch Dis Child Fetal Neonatal Ed 76(3):F158–F162

Kennedy K, Fewtrell MS, Morley R, Abbott R, Quinlan PT, Wells JC et al (1999) Double-blind, randomized trial of a synthetic triacylglycerol in formula-fed term infants: effects on stool biochemistry, stool characteristics, and bone mineralization. Am J Clin Nutr 70 (5):920–927

Kere J, Lohi H, Hoglund P (1999) Genetic disorders of membrane transport III. Congenital chloride diarrhea. Am J Physiol 276(1 Pt 1):G7–G13

Kessler JP (1993) Involvement of excitatory amino acids in the activity of swallowing-related neurons of the ventro-lateral medulla. Brain Res 603(2):353–357

Kien CL, Heitlinger LA, Li BU, Murray RD (1989) Digestion, absorption, and fermentation of carbohydrates. Semin Perinatol 13(2):78–87

Kirchgessner AL, Gershon MD (1989) Identification of vagal efferent fibers and putative target neurons in the enteric nervous system of the rat. J Comp Neurol 285 (1):38–53

Kitajima H, Sumida Y, Tanaka R, Yuki N, Takayama H, Fujimura M (1997) Early administration of Bifidobacterium breve to preterm infants: randomised controlled trial. Arch Dis Child Fetal Neonatal Ed 76 (2):F101–F107

Knol J, Boehm G, Lidestri M, Negretti F, Jelinek J, Agosti M et al (2005) Increase of faecal bifidobacteria due to dietary oligosaccharides induces a reduction of clinically relevant pathogen germs in the faeces of formula-fed preterm infants. Acta Paediatr Suppl 94(449):31–33

Koenig WJ, Amarnath RP, Hench V, Berseth CL (1995) Manometrics for preterm and term infants: a new tool for old questions. Pediatrics 95(2):203–206

Kolacek S, Puntis JW, Lloyd DR, Brown GA, Booth IW (1990) Ontogeny of pancreatic exocrine function. Arch Dis Child 65(2):178–181

Koletzko B, Demmelmair H, Socha P (1998) Nutritional support of infants and children: supply and metabolism of lipids. Baillieres Clin Gastroenterol 12(4): 671–696

Koletzko S, Jesch I, Faus-Kebetaler T, Briner J, Meier-Ruge W, Muntefering H et al (1999) Rectal biopsy for diagnosis of intestinal neuronal dysplasia in children: a prospective multicentre study on interobserver variation and clinical outcome. Gut 44(6):853–861

Land MH, Rouster-Stevens K, Woods CR, Cannon ML, Cnota J, Shetty AK (2005) Lactobacillus sepsis associated with probiotic therapy. Pediatrics 115(1):178–181

Lau C, Alagugurusamy R, Schanler RJ, Smith EO, Shulman RJ (2000) Characterization of the developmental stages of sucking in preterm infants during bottle feeding. Acta Paediatr 89(7):846–852

Lau C, Smith EO, Schanler RJ (2003) Coordination of suck-swallow and swallow respiration in preterm infants. Acta Paediatr 92(6):721–727

Lecoin L, Gabella G, Le DN (1996) Origin of the c-kit-positive interstitial cells in the avian bowel. Development 122(3):725–733

Li N, Neu J (2009) Glutamine deprivation alters intestinal tight junctions via a PI3-K/Akt mediated pathway in Caco-2 cells. J Nutr 139(4):710–714

Lichnovsky V, Lojda Z (1992) Early prenatal development of the brush border enzymes in the embryonal intestine. Acta Univ Palacki Olomuc Fac Med 134:27–31

Lidestri M, Agosti M, Marini A, Boehm G (2003) Oligosaccharides might stimulate calcium absorption in formula-fed preterm infants. Acta Paediatr Suppl 91 (441):91–92

Lin HC, Su BH, Chen AC, Lin TW, Tsai CH, Yeh TF et al (2005) Oral probiotics reduce the incidence and severity of necrotizing enterocolitis in very low birth weight infants. Pediatrics 115(1):1–4

Lin HC, Hsu CH, Chen HL, Chung MY, Hsu JF, Lien RI et al (2008) Oral probiotics prevent necrotizing enterocolitis in very low birth weight preterm infants: a multicenter, randomized, controlled trial. Pediatrics 122 (4):693–700

Lindberg T, Skude G (1982) Amylase in human milk. Pediatrics 70(2):235–238

Lohi H, Kujala M, Makela S, Lehtonen E, Kestila M, Saarialho-Kere U et al (2002) Functional characterization of three novel tissue-specific anion exchangers SLC26A7, -A8, and -A9. J Biol Chem 277 (16):14246–14254

Lopez-Alonso M, Moya MJ, Cabo JA, Ribas J, del Carmen MM, Silny J et al (2006) Twenty-four-hour esophageal impedance-pH monitoring in healthy preterm neonates: rate and characteristics of acid, weakly acidic, and weakly alkaline gastroesophageal reflux. Pediatrics 118 (2):e299–e308

Louis NA, Lin PW (2009) The intestinal immune barrier. NeoReviews 10(4):e180–e190

Louis NA, Hamilton KE, Canny G, Shekels LL, Ho SB, Colgan SP (2006) Selective induction of mucin-3 by hypoxia in intestinal epithelia. J Cell Biochem 99 (6):1616–1627

Lu J, Jilling T, Li D, Caplan MS (2007) Polyunsaturated fatty acid supplementation alters proinflammatory gene expression and reduces the incidence of necrotizing enterocolitis in a neonatal rat model. Pediatr Res 61 (4):427–432

Malo C (1990) Separation of two distinct Na^+/D-glucose cotransport systems in the human fetal jejunum by means of their differential specificity for 3-*O*-methylglucose. Biochim Biophys Acta 1022(1):8–16

Malo C, Berteloot A (1991) Analysis of kinetic data in transport studies: new insights from kinetic studies of Na(+)-D-glucose cotransport in human intestinal brush-border membrane vesicles using a fast sampling, rapid filtration apparatus. J Membr Biol 122(2):127–141

Martinussen M, Brubakk AM, Vik T, Yao AC (1996) Mesenteric blood flow velocity and its relation to transitional circulatory adaptation in appropriate for gestational age preterm infants. Pediatr Res 39(2):275–280

Medzhitov R (2007) Recognition of microorganisms and activation of the immune response. Nature 449 (7164):819–826

Menard D, Dagenais P, Calvert R (1994) Morphological changes and cellular proliferation in mouse colon during fetal and postnatal development. Anat Rec 238 (3):349–359

Mihatsch WA, Hoegel J, Pohlandt F (2006) Prebiotic oligosaccharides reduce stool viscosity and accelerate gastrointestinal transport in preterm infants. Acta Paediatr 95(7):843–848

Mihatsch WA, Braegger CP, Decsi T, Kolacek S, Lanzinger H, Mayer B et al (2012) Critical systematic review of the level of evidence for routine use of probiotics for reduction of mortality and prevention of necrotizing enterocolitis and sepsis in preterm infants. Clin Nutr 31:6–15

Miller H, Zhang J, Kuolee R, Patel GB, Chen W (2007) Intestinal M cells: the fallible sentinels? World J Gastroenterol 13(10):1477–1486

Mimouni FB, Shamir R (2009) Vitamin D requirements in the first year of life. Curr Opin Clin Nutr Metab Care 12 (3):287–292

Montgomery RK, Mulberg AE, Grand RJ (1999) Development of the human gastrointestinal tract: twenty years of progress. Gastroenterology 116(3):702–731

Moro G, Minoli I, Mosca M, Fanaro S, Jelinek J, Stahl B et al (2002) Dosage-related bifidogenic effects of galacto- and fructooligosaccharides in formula-fed term infants. J Pediatr Gastroenterol Nutr 34 (3):291–295

Mouterde O, Dacher JN, Basuyau JP, Mallet E (1992) Gastric secretion in infants. Application to the study of sudden infant death syndrome and apparently life-threatening events. Biol Neonate 62(1):15–22

Murch SH, Winyard PJ, Koletzko S, Wehner B, Cheema HA, Risdon RA et al (1996) Congenital enterocyte heparan sulphate deficiency with massive albumin loss, secretory diarrhoea, and malnutrition. Lancet 347(9011):1299–1301

Murray RD, Boutton TW, Klein PD, Gilbert M, Paule CL, MacLean WC Jr (1990) Comparative absorption of [13C]glucose and [13C]lactose by premature infants. Am J Clin Nutr 51(1):59–66

Nankervis CA, Nowicki PT (2000) Role of endothelin-1 in regulation of the postnatal intestinal circulation. Am J Physiol Gastrointest Liver Physiol 278(3):G367–G375

Nanthakumar NN, Fusunyan RD, Sanderson I, Walker WA (2000) Inflammation in the developing human intestine: a possible pathophysiologic contribution to necrotizing enterocolitis. Proc Natl Acad Sci U S A 97 (11):6043–6048

Neish AS (2009) Microbes in gastrointestinal health and disease. Gastroenterology 136(1):65–80

Neu J, Caicedo R (2005) Probiotics: protecting the intestinal ecosystem? J Pediatr 147(2):143–146

Neu J, Roig JC, Meetze WH, Veerman M, Carter C, Millsaps M et al (1997) Enteral glutamine supplementation for very low birth weight infants decreases morbidity. J Pediatr 131(5):691–699

Newell SJ, Sarkar PK, Durbin GM, Booth IW, McNeish AS (1988) Maturation of the lower oesophageal sphincter in the preterm baby. Gut 29(2):167–172

Newgreen D, Young HM (2002a) Enteric nervous system: development and developmental disturbances – part 1. Pediatr Dev Pathol 5(3):224–247

Newgreen D, Young HM (2002b) Enteric nervous system: development and developmental disturbances – part 2. Pediatr Dev Pathol 5(4):329–349

Niot I, Poirier H, Tran TT, Besnard P (2009) Intestinal absorption of long-chain fatty acids: evidence and uncertainties. Prog Lipid Res 48(2):101–115

Nowicki PT (1998) Postnatal changes in gut hemodynamics: a possible role for substance P. Am J Physiol 274 (6 Pt 1):G1142–G1150

Nurko S (2005) What's the value of diagnostic tools in defecation disorders? J Pediatr Gastroenterol Nutr 41 (Suppl 1):S53–S55

Nusrat A, Turner JR, Madara JL (2000) Molecular physiology and pathophysiology of tight junctions. IV. Regulation of tight junctions by extracellular stimuli: nutrients, cytokines, and immune cells. Am J Physiol Gastrointest Liver Physiol 279(5):G851–G857

Omari TI, Benninga MA, Barnett CP, Haslam RR, Davidson GP, Dent J (1999) Characterization of esophageal body and lower esophageal sphincter motor function in the very premature neonate. J Pediatr 135(4): 517–521

Park CW, Moon KC, Park JS, Jun JK, Romero R, Yoon BH (2009) The involvement of human amnion in histologic chorioamnionitis is an indicator that a fetal and an intra-amniotic inflammatory response is more likely and severe: clinical implications. Placenta 30(1):56–61

Phillips SF (1997) The growth of knowledge in human digestion and absorption. Gastroenterology 112 (4):1404–1405

Pickering LK, Granoff DM, Erickson JR, Masor ML, Cordle CT, Schaller JP et al (1998) Modulation of the immune system by human milk and infant formula containing nucleotides. Pediatrics 101(2):242–249

Pinto D, Clevers H (2005) Wnt control of stem cells and differentiation in the intestinal epithelium. Exp Cell Res 306(2):357–363

Potsic B, Holliday N, Lewis P, Samuelson D, DeMarco V, Neu J (2002) Glutamine supplementation and deprivation: effect on artificially reared rat small intestinal morphology. Pediatr Res 52(3):430–436

Ramirez M, Amate L, Gil A (2001) Absorption and distribution of dietary fatty acids from different sources. Early Hum Dev 65(Suppl):S95–S101

Ramirez A, Wong WW, Shulman RJ (2006) Factors regulating gastric emptying in preterm infants. J Pediatr 149 (4):475–479

Rao SS, Welcher K (1996) Periodic rectal motor activity: the intrinsic colonic gatekeeper? Am J Gastroenterol 91 (5):890–897

Reber KM, Nankervis CA, Nowicki PT (2002) Newborn intestinal circulation. Physiology and pathophysiology. Clin Perinatol 29(1):23–39

Riskin A, Hochwald O, Bader D, Srugo I, Gabi N, Kugelman A et al (2010) The effects of lactulose supplementation to enteral feedings in premature infants: a pilot study. J Pediatr 156(2):209–214

Salminen S, Isolauri E (2006) Intestinal colonization, microbiota, and probiotics. J Pediatr 149:S115–S120

Salzman NH, Underwood MA, Bevins CL (2007) Paneth cells, defensins, and the commensal microbiota: a hypothesis on intimate interplay at the intestinal mucosa. Semin Immunol 19(2):70–83

Sarna SK, Otterson MF (1988) Gastrointestinal motility: some basic concepts. Pharmacology 36(Suppl 1):7–14

Sarna SK, Otterson MF (1989) Small intestinal physiology and pathophysiology. Gastroenterol Clin North Am 18 (2):375–404

Saur D, Vanderwinden JM, Seidler B, Schmid RM, De Laet MH, Allescher HD (2004) Single-nucleotide promoter polymorphism alters transcription of neuronal nitric oxide synthase exon 1c in infantile hypertrophic pyloric stenosis. Proc Natl Acad Sci U S A 101(6):1662–1667

Schanler RJ (1995) Suitability of human milk for the low-birthweight infant. Clin Perinatol 22(1):207–222

Schanler RJ, Rifka M (1994) Calcium, phosphorus and magnesium needs for the low-birth-weight infant. Acta Paediatr Suppl 405:111–116

Schultz SG (2007) From a pump handle to oral rehydration therapy: a model of translational research. Adv Physiol Educ 31(4):288–293

Shah P, Shah V (2007) Arginine supplementation for prevention of necrotising enterocolitis in preterm infants. Cochrane Database Syst Rev 3:CD004339

Shamir R, Johnson WJ, Zolfaghari R, Lee HS, Fisher EA (1995) Role of bile salt-dependent cholesteryl ester hydrolase in the uptake of micellar cholesterol by intestinal cells. Biochemistry 34(19):6351–6358

Sharma R, Tepas JJ 3rd (2010) Microecology, intestinal epithelial barrier and necrotizing enterocolitis. Pediatr Surg Int 26(1):11–21

Sharma et al (2010) Microecology, intestinal epithelial barrier and necrotizing enterocolitis. Pediatr Surg Int 26:11–21. https://doi.org/10.1007/s00383-009-2536-2

Sherman PM, Mitchell DJ, Cutz E (2004) Neonatal enteropathies: defining the causes of protracted diarrhea of infancy. J Pediatr Gastroenterol Nutr 38(1):16–26

Shulman RJ, Wong WW, Smith EO (2005) Influence of changes in lactase activity and small-intestinal mucosal growth on lactose digestion and absorption in preterm infants. Am J Clin Nutr 81(2):472–479

Siahanidou T, Mandyla H, Papassotiriou I, Anagnostakis D (2004) Serum lipids in preterm infants fed a formula supplemented with nucleotides. J Pediatr Gastroenterol Nutr 38(1):56–60

Siegle ML, Buhner S, Schemann M, Schmid HR, Ehrlein HJ (1990) Propagation velocities and frequencies of contractions along canine small intestine. Am J Physiol 258(5 Pt 1):G738–G744

Simon-Assmann P, Turck N, Sidhoum-Jenny M, Gradwohl G, Kedinger M (2007) In vitro models of intestinal epithelial cell differentiation. Cell Biol Toxicol 23(4):241–256

Simpson C, Schanler RJ, Lau C (2002) Early introduction of oral feeding in preterm infants. Pediatrics 110 (3):517–522

Sparks SE (2006) Inherited disorders of glycosylation. Mol Genet Metab 87(1):1–7

Srinivasjois R, Rao S, Patole S (2009) Prebiotic supplementation of formula in preterm neonates: a systematic review and meta-analysis of randomised controlled trials. Clin Nutr 28(3):237–242

Stahl A, Hirsch DJ, Gimeno RE, Punreddy S, Ge P, Watson N et al (1999) Identification of the major intestinal fatty acid transport protein. Mol Cell 4(3):299–308

Stark ME, Bauer AJ, Sarr MG, Szurszewski JH (1993) Nitric oxide mediates inhibitory nerve input in human and canine jejunum. Gastroenterology 104(2):398–409

Stevens BR, Preston RL (1998) Sodium-dependent amino acid transport is preserved in lyophilized reconstituted apical membranes from intestinal epithelium. Anal Biochem 265(1):117–122

Szajewska H, Skorka A, Ruszczynski M, Gieruszczak-Bialek D (2007) Meta-analysis: lactobacillus GG for treating acute diarrhoea in children. Aliment Pharmacol Ther 25(8):871–881

Tanaka M, Lee K, Martinez-Augustin O, He Y, Sanderson IR, Walker WA (1996) Exogenous nucleotides alter the proliferation, differentiation and apoptosis of human small intestinal epithelium. J Nutr 126 (2):424–433

Thomson AB, Keelan M, Thiesen A, Clandinin MT, Ropeleski M, Wild GE (2001) Small bowel review:

normal physiology part 1. Dig Dis Sci 46(12): 2567–2587

Thureen P, Heird WC (2005) Protein and energy requirements of the preterm/low birthweight (LBW) infant. Pediatr Res 57(5 Pt 2):95R–98R

Underwood MA, Salzman NH, Bennett SH, Barman M, Mills D, Marcobal A et al (2009) A randomized placebo-controlled comparison of two prebiotic/probiotic combinations in preterm infants: Impact on weight gain, intestinal microbiota, and fecal short chain fatty acids. J Pediatr Gastroenterol Nutr 48(2): 216–225

Underwood MA, Kalanetra KM, Bokulich NA, Mirmiran M, Barile D, Tancredi DJ et al (2014) Prebiotic oligosaccharides in premature infants. J Pediatr Gastroenterol Nutr 58(3):352–360

VanderWall KJ, Bealer JF, Adzick NS, Harrison MR (1995) Cyclic GMP relaxes the internal anal sphincter in Hirschsprung's disease. J Pediatr Surg 30(7):1013–1015

Vanderwinden JM, Liu H, De Laet MH, Vanderhaeghen JJ (1996a) Study of the interstitial cells of Cajal in infantile hypertrophic pyloric stenosis. Gastroenterology 111(2):279–288

Vanderwinden JM, Rumessen JJ, Liu H, Descamps D, De Laet MH, Vanderhaeghen JJ (1996b) Interstitial cells of Cajal in human colon and in Hirschsprung's disease. Gastroenterology 111(4):901–910

Vanneste G, Van Nassauw NL, Kalfin R, Van Colen I, Elinck E, Van Crombruggen K et al (2008) Jejunal cholinergic, nitrergic, and soluble guanylate cyclase activity in postoperative ileus. Surgery 144(3): 410–426

Villa M, Menard D, Semenza G, Mantei N (1992) The expression of lactase enzymatic activity and mRNA in human fetal jejunum. Effect of organ culture and of treatment with hydrocortisone. FEBS Lett 301 (2):202–206

Vorbach C, Capecchi MR, Penninger JM (2006) Evolution of the mammary gland from the innate immune system? Bioessays 28(6):606–616

Walker WA (2002) Development of the intestinal mucosal barrier. J Pediatr Gastroenterol Nutr 34(Suppl 1): S33–S39

Wang PA, Huang FY (1994) Time of the first defaecation and urination in very low birth weight infants. Eur J Pediatr 153(4):279–283

Wenzl TG, Moroder C, Trachterna M, Thomson M, Silny J, Heimann G et al (2002) Esophageal pH monitoring and impedance measurement: a comparison of two diagnostic tests for gastroesophageal reflux. J Pediatr Gastroenterol Nutr 34(5):519–523

Wester T, O'Briain DS, Puri P (1999) Notable postnatal alterations in the myenteric plexus of normal human bowel. Gut 44(5):666–674

Wiley JW, Lu YX, Owyang C (1991) Evidence for a glutamatergic neural pathway in the myenteric plexus. Am J Physiol 261(4 Pt 1):G693–G700

Wong JM, de Souza R, Kendall CW, Emam A, Jenkins DJ (2006) Colonic health: fermentation and short chain fatty acids. J Clin Gastroenterol 40(3):235–243

Zangen S, Di Lorenzo C, Zangen T, Mertz H, Schwankovsky L, Hyman PE (2001) Rapid maturation of gastric relaxation in newborn infants. Pediatr Res 50(5):629–632

Hormones and Gastrointestinal Function of Newborns

35

Flavia Prodam, Simonetta Bellone, Roberta Ricotti, Alice Monzani, Giulia Genoni, Enza Giglione, and Gianni Bona

Contents

Abstract

Development is a continuous process that does not stop after birth but progresses along a continuum. The intestinal absorptive process is only partially mature before 26 weeks of gestation, and gastroenteropancreatic peptides and hormones are secreted in a basal rate and can be completely stimulated or inhibited after delivery, in particular with the nutrient contact. A growing knowledge about this complex interplay among nutrients, gut peptides, and the gut under development is an important tool in the clinical care of preterm newborns. The investigation of this system in fetal and neonatal life is still ongoing. This chapter will review the data about secretion of gut peptides (GLP-1, GLP-2, oxyntomodulin, GIP, PYY, ghrelin, obestatin, motilin, and cholecystokinin) in the neonatal period with respect to full-term or preterm birth, weight status, and feeding conditions. More detailed studies on this topic could offer the physiological basis for correct nutritional supports to preterm infants as well as therapies for the necrotizing enterocolitis.

F. Prodam (✉) · S. Bellone · R. Ricotti · A. Monzani · G. Genoni · E. Giglione · G. Bona
Department of Health Sciences, Division of Pediatrics, University of Piemonte Orientale, Novara, Italy
e-mail: flavia.prodam@med.uniupo.it; simonetta.bellone@med.uniupo.it; robertaricotti@gmail.com; alice.monzani@med.uniupo.it; genonigiulia@gmail.com; enza.giglione@gmail.com; gianni.bona@maggioreosp.novara.it

G. Buonocore et al. (eds.), *Neonatology*,
https://doi.org/10.1007/978-3-319-29489-6_184

35.1 Salient Points

- Many peptides produced from the gut are involved in the development of gut functions as well as in the acute and chronic regulation of weight and energy balance.
- Glucagon-like peptide 1 (GLP-1) and Glucagone-like peptide 2 (GLP-2) are secreted from endocrine L cells of intestinal mucosa predominantly located at the ileum and colon level.
- GLP-1 shows several activities including the enhancement of insulin secretion, accumulation of fat, and suppression of glucagon secretion in the postprandial phase, thus increasing body weight.
- GLP-2 increases gut epithelial absorptive capacity and mucosal growth with a peak of secretion from 30 to 40 weeks of gestational age, acting both on endocrine pathways and enteric neurons.
- Glucose-dependent insulinotrophic polypetide has a precocious role on fat accrual and is linked to glucose metabolism.
- Peptide YY may predict postnatal growth since it negatively correlates with gestational age and anthropometric measures.
- Ghrelin plays a role in the regulation of food intake and energy expenditure but further studies are needed to clarify its exact role in neonates.
- Motilin and cholecystokinin are responsible respectively for gut and gallbladder motility and are potential therapeutic agents for the treatment of colic dysfunction and the prevention of parenteral nutrition-associated cholestasis.

35.2 Introduction

Development is a continuous process that does not stop after birth but progresses along a continuum. Nutrition, environment, and stress act on this development modulating the programming in an epigenetic manner. Prenatal and perinatal nutrition can be imprinting factors and turn on different genes that provide organisms of different phenotypes such as the thrifty phenotype (de Moura et al. 2008). Indeed, the nutritional support of gastrointestinal growth and function is an important tool in the clinical care of newborn babies, in particular preterm neonates. In fact, before birth, although amniotic fluid is not the nutritional mainstay of fetus, it contributes up to 15% of fetal nutrition requirements and plays a key role in its development and maturation (Mulvihill et al. 1985; Wagner 2002). Accordingly, by 20 weeks of gestation, the anatomy of fetal gut resembles that of a neonate. However, the intestinal absorptive process is only partially mature before 26 weeks of gestation and gastroenteropancreatic peptides are secreted in a basal rate and can be completely stimulated or inhibited after delivery, in particular with the nutrient contact (Lebenthal and Lebenthal 1999; Burrin and Stoll 2002). At the age of 2 years, the intestine reaches its full range of functions (Corpeleijn et al. 2008). Gut hormones, peptides, and growth factors clearly have a role in gut growth after birth and mediate directly and indirectly the trophic actions of the enteral nutrition in a still incompletely understood manner (Burrin and Stoll 2002). On the other hand, hormones and growth factors which are present in breast milk seem to co-exert trophic activities on gut development and immune function in a complex interplay (de Moura et al. 2008; Wagner 2002). Even less is known about the development of these regulatory systems in the human neonate, and, as a consequence, in premature infants there are still ongoing higher morbidity and mortality associated with feeding problems (Corpeleijn et al. 2008). Indeed, at present, clinical nutrition support to preterm babies consists in enteral and parenteral nutrition, but many complications are associated with both of them (Corpeleijn et al. 2008; Amin et al. 2008). Furthermore, if enteral feeding is important to gut development, several acute or chronic diseases could be due to formula fed with respect to human breast milk. In fact, formula milks contain higher amounts of proteins and lack many endogenous hormones and growth factors (Burrin and Stoll 2002; Corpeleijn et al. 2008; Agostoni 2005). An improvement in the knowledge of factors linked to gastrointestinal function, and as a consequence of energy metabolism, could improve strategies to better support nutrition of preterm newborns as well as their follow-up.

The aim of this chapter is to review the knowledge about the secretion of gut peptides in neonatal period with respect to weight status and feeding conditions. It has to be underlined that many data are still anecdotical with respect to the knowledge in childhood or adulthood and also contrasting probably due to sample size, methods of measurements, or stratification of subjects.

35.3 Etiology, Pathogenesis, and Clinical Aspects: Gut Peptides

In recent years, many peptides produced from the gut have been discovered that are strictly involved in the development of gut functions as well as in the acute and chronic regulation of weight and energy balance. They are also modulated by nutrient ingestion and could influence pancreatic secretion and beta-cell proliferation and survival. The large accumulation of data about them regards obesity and type 2 diabetes in adulthood. However, the investigation of their role in neonatal period is ongoing and could offer interesting results for the treatment of preterm babies.

35.3.1 Peptides from Proglucagon

35.3.1.1 Glucagon-Like Peptide 1 (GLP-1)

GLP-1 is a peptide of 30 amino acids expressed and secreted from endocrine L cells of intestinal mucosa predominantly located at the ileum and colon level. GLP-1 derives from the same precursor of glucagon, the proglucagon, that in L cells is processed by the prohormone convertase 1/3 (PC1/3). Proglucagon is also expressed in the brain, in particular in arcuate and paraventricular nuclei. Three hormonal products, GLP-1, GLP-2, and oxyntomodulin (OXM), derive simultaneously from its processing in neurons. In the gut, its truncated peptides (GLP-1 (7-36) amide or GLP-1 (7-37)) are the active forms, while the full-length native GLP-1 is inactive (Holst 2007). In addition, almost all secreted GLP-1 from L cells is C-terminal amidated with an improved stability. Only 10–15% of the secreted GLP-1 reaches systemic circulation in the intact form. This rapid initial whole-body clearance is due to specific tissue metabolism in the liver and also to the activity of dipeptidyl peptidase-4 (DPP-4) which is expressed in both enterocytes and endothelial cells of the lamina propria capillaries (Holst 2007).

GLP-1 shows several activities including the enhancement of insulin and suppression of glucagon secretion in the postprandial phase thus modulating the pancreatic glucose response (Neary et al. 2004; Hellstrom et al. 2004). The amplification of insulin secretion related to glucose levels has been named the incretin effect by hormones produced by the gut (Holst 2007).

GLP-1 levels have been shown to be modulated by ingested micro- and macronutrients through a direct activation of the secretion by L cells mainly via an interaction with nutrient-sensing receptors and with vagus nerve (Holst 2007). A role for neural, endocrine mediators or both in the rapid, nutrient-stimulated increase in plasma GLP-1 has been demonstrated (Spreckley and Murphy 2015). The meal size and composition seem to be key factors of GLP-1 secretion in adulthood, correlating with gastric emptying. In fact, smaller meals in particular those where nutrients are rapidly absorbed could not elicit measurable GLP-1 secretion, whereas they were able to stimulate glucose-dependent insulinotropic polypeptide (GIP) in large amounts. In contrast, larger meals containing more complex nutrients, namely, complex carbohydrates and monounsaturated lipids, were followed by high and rapid GLP-1 secretion (Holst 2007; Spreckley and Murphy 2015; Pais et al. 2016; Vilsboll et al. 2003).

GLP-1 plays a role in mediating appetite and feeding behavior. A reduction in hunger, coupled with the sensation of fullness, has been reported after its administration (Naslund et al. 1999). Consistent with animal studies, in humans, GLP-1 induces a mild but significant dose-dependent inhibition of food intake in both lean and obese subjects as well as in patients with type 2 diabetes (Verdich et al. 2001).

A role of GLP-1 in the development of gut functions was hypothesized because of its incretin action and, namely, on direct regulation by nutrients (Holst 2007).

In the context of developing of fetus and gut maturation from prenatal to postnatal life, studies on GLP-1 are limited. It has been demonstrated that it is involved in regulation of pancreatic beta-cell mass also in neonatal period (Holst 2007; Drucker 2002). Furthermore, it has been recently shown that preterm and term neonates present higher fasting GLP-1 levels than children and adults, with premature babies presenting the highest levels in both conditions, probably due to an increase in production or a decrease in metabolism secondary to immaturity of DPP-4 and/or reduced glomerular filtration rate (Amin et al. 2008; Konturek et al. 2004; Padidela et al. 2009). More recently, also GLP-1 levels during feeding have been shown to be higher in preterm neonates than in older children or adults without being linked to hypoglycemic episodes. The majority of infants of this study were fed by nasogastric tube, suggesting a direct stimulus on enteric pathways without activation of cephalic vagal tone (Amin et al. 2008). Notably, the premature neonatal gut is able to function as it typically does suggesting an ontogenic key role of GLP-1 (Amin et al. 2008). This role seems to be crucial in the first months after birth in premature newborns, with a peak 2–4 weeks after birth, more pronounced in those born before 30 weeks of gestational age, and with levels higher than the normal range in adults (Nagasaki and Ohta 2015; Kawamata et al. 2014, 2015; Shoji et al. 2016). GLP-1 levels remain persistently high at least until 38 weeks of life in both preterm and term infants (Nagasaki and Ohta 2015; Kawamata et al. 2014). This enhanced GLP-1 could also regulate enteroendocrine systems by increasing beta-cell mass and regeneration. In fact, GLP-1 production in preterm infants is related to the stimulation of insulin secretion in early postnatal period, although associated with lower insulin sensitivity (Shoji et al. 2016). However, it is not known if increased GLP-1 levels derive also from a higher gut or pancreatic production rate (Amin et al. 2008; Konturek et al. 2004). GLP-1-stimulated insulin secretion may affect fat accumulation in terms of catch-up fat in the early postnatal period, as evidenced by a higher increase in body weight associated to higher GLP-1 levels in early preterm than in late preterm neonates (Shoji et al. 2016). High GLP-1 as well as high insulin and low insulin sensitivity in the early postnatal period in very preterm infants may contribute to obesity in the future. This hypothesis seems to be also supported by the evidence that small for gestational age (SGA) neonates had fasting GLP-1 levels similar to AGA neonates when breastfed, meanwhile higher GLP-1 levels when formula fed at 4 weeks of age (Díaz et al. 2015), by considering SGA condition and the formula feeding, two of the main risk factors for later obesity and type 2 diabetes. Few preliminary studies conducted in adults born SGA with fasting and fed GLP-1 levels were similar to healthy controls (Konturek et al. 2004) without diurnal variations in the secretory profile (Brøns et al. 2016), although these studies did not evaluate nutrition contribution in the first months of life, suggesting that more investigations are needed.

35.3.1.2 Glucagon-Like Peptide 2 (GLP-2)

GLP-2 is a 33-amino acid peptide also produced by the endocrine L cells by posttranslational processing of proglucagon and is secreted in response to food intake together with GLP-1 (Holst 2007). It is also produced in the brain (Drucker and Yusta 2014). It is rapidly cleaved in inactive GLP-2 (3–33) by DPP-4 with a half-life of 7 min which is longer than that of GLP-1 (Amin et al. 2008). It binds and activates an own receptor, the GLP-2 receptor (GLP-2R), which presents homology with those of GLP-1, GIP, and glucagon and is expressed predominantly in myofibroblasts and neurons in the intestinal tract and only in a subset of epithelial cells, indicating an indirect mechanism of action (Burrin and Stoll 2002; Amin et al. 2008; Drucker and Yusta 2014). As GLP-1, it is modulated by ingested macronutrients, namely, carbohydrates and lipids (Xiao et al. 1999), short-chain fatty acids (Burrin and Stoll 2002), and fibers (Amato et al. 2016). In adulthood, after an oral feeding, GLP-2 secretion presents a biphasic increase with a first peak within 15 min and a second one more prolonged after 1 h, suggesting not only a direct stimulation by nutrients but also several factors, in particular GIP and vagus nerve (Burrin and Stoll 2002; Drucker and Yusta 2014).

In contrast to GLP-1, the role of GLP-2 in the regulation of feeding and fasting balance is more unclear. Intracerebroventricular administration of the peptide suppresses food intake in rodents in similar fashion to GLP-1 (Tang-Christensen et al. 2000). In humans, no variations in feeding behavior as well as gastric emptying have been observed after administration of GLP-2 (Schmidt et al. 2003). On the other hand, knockout mice with GLP-2R deletion selectively in hypothalamic arcuate nucleus neurons expressing pro-opiomelanocortin (POMC) display hyperphagic behavior and late-onset obesity (Guan et al. 2012).

Different from GLP-1, GLP-2 is mainly a trophic peptide of intestinal mucosa and seems to act on gastric motility with a slowing effect at least in fasting conditions (Burrin and Stoll 2002; Amin et al. 2008). Its acute administration also inhibits gastric secretion (Burrin and Stoll 2002). GLP-2 is able to increase gut epithelial absorptive capacity and mucosal growth, acting both on endocrine pathways and enteric neurons (Amin et al. 2008; Drucker and Yusta 2014; Martin et al. 2006). GLP-2 is involved in controlling the absorptive capacity of the proximal bowel. In fact, after gut resection, the residual bowel secretes higher amounts of GLP-2 after feeding in both animals and humans (Martin et al. 2006). Indeed, GLP-2 regulates the adaptative intestinal regrowth after a period of fasting or in response to enteritis caused by several agents (Drucker and Yusta 2014). The malabsorpted dietary carbohydrates which stimulate production of short-chain fatty acids are the hypothesized trigger mechanism of the increased GLP-2 secretion (Burrin and Stoll 2002; Garcia-Diaz et al. 2007). GLP-2 has been shown to also act on gut barrier functions reducing bowel permeability to macromolecules, decreasing bacteria translocation, and suppressing local expression of pro-inflammatory cytokines (Burrin and Stoll 2002; Drucker 2002; Drucker and Yusta 2014; Martin et al. 2006). GLP-2R signaling is required for prebiotic-induced increases in intestinal barrier function (Cani et al. 2009) and involves both IGF-1 and the intestinal-epithelial IGF-1 receptor (IE-IGF-1R) (Dong et al. 2014).

If GLP-2 secretion is regulated by carbohydrates and lipids, a feedback loop is present. In fact, GLP2 increases the uptake of sugars by augmenting the activity and the expression of their transporters and by enhancing the expression of several enzymes involved in digestion (Amato et al. 2016). It also plays a role in lipid physiology by facilitating their intestinal absorption of lipids and by increasing and regulating chylomicron secretion from the gut predominantly via CD36 (Amato et al. 2016; Xiao et al. 2015).

The main role of GLP-1 is to be an incretin hormone, as discussed above. Conversely, an action on glucose metabolism by GLP-2 was largely ignored. GLP-2R knockout mice do not present an impairment in glucose tolerance or in glucagon secretion (Bahrami et al. 2010), and treatments with a GLP-2R antagonist in animals or agonist in humans failed to change glucose or insulin levels (Drucker and Yusta 2014; Baldassano et al. 2015). On the contrary, GLP-2 iv administration seems to increase glucagon secretion in healthy subjects (Amato et al. 2016). GLP-2 may act as a protective factor against the deregulation of the glucose metabolism in conditions related to increased uptake of energy, such as obesity, at least in animal models (Amato et al. 2016). GLP-2 acts to improve glucose metabolism in a concentration-dependent manner in mice with high-fat diet-induced obesity (Baldassano et al. 2016). Accordingly, in obese subjects without type 2 diabetes, GLP-2 concentrations are higher than controls (Valderas et al. 2014), suggesting a protective feedback, although GLP-2 levels have been shown associated with insulin resistance in a pilot study (Geloneze et al. 2013). It has been hypothesized that GLP-2 increased secretion could be the cause of insulin resistance as GLP-2 increases absorption of nutrients, especially fatty acids, a key factor for insulin resistance or for its glucagonotrophic action in humans (Amato et al. 2016). Because of so few data, more investigations are needed to elucidate the intriguing role of GLP-2 in metabolism.

According to its trophic activity, a role in development and maturation of gastrointestinal function has been investigated. Although the specific functions of GLP-2 in controlled gut development are still largely unknown, it is active in the immature bowel, with a peak of secretion in the late weaning period (Burrin and Stoll 2002; Drucker and Yusta 2014). However, studies in mutant mice have demonstrated that it is not necessary on bowel development during fetal life (Hill et al. 1999), although its secretion mechanism has been considered established at 24 weeks of gestation in humans (Yoshikawa et al. 2006). In addition, its levels in utero would be expected lower with respect to postnatal life because of higher levels and activity of DPP-4 in the placenta (Lambeir et al. 2003).

It has been clearly demonstrated that both fasting and fed GLP-2 levels are higher in neonates when compared to older children or adults. As discussed for GLP-1, these findings could be due to either an increase in production and/or a decrease in metabolism by DPP-4 immaturity or lower glomerular filtration (Amin et al. 2008; Yoshikawa et al. 2006). Increasing GLP-2 levels in preterm babies may have an effect on the developing gut acting as a stimulus. Of note, preterm neonates with feeding intolerance showed significantly lower levels of GLP-2 and increased duration to achieve full enteral feeding and hospitalization (Ozer et al. 2009). Notably, normal infants with an age of 48 weeks have lower fed GLP-2 levels with respect to the time of their delivery at 40 weeks. These data suggest that gestational age may influence GLP-2 secretion and that its peak of secretion could correspond with the time of the most rapid growth of gut which ranges from 30 to 40 weeks of gestational age (Amin et al. 2008). However, different from previously discussed data in animals and adults, infants with intestinal dysfunction or residual small bowel with intact colon do not appear able to produce GLP-2 in response to feeding stimulation (Sigalet et al. 2004). The reason of these discordant findings remains unexplained. The lack of GLP-2 secretion could be due to resection of the L cell bearing ileum as well as an age-related inability to produce an appropriate response or ischemic components that may alter GLP-2 secretion in the remnant gut (Sigalet et al. 2004). Then, these results questioned if trying to stimulate GLP-2 secretion in infant gut dysfunction or in preterm newborns. Teduglutide, a long-acting DPP-4-resistant analog of GLP-2, has recently been approved for the treatment of adult short bowel syndrome and is in clinical trials for Crohn's disease in adults (http://www.ema.europa.eu/ema/index.jsp?curl=pages/medicines/human/orphans/2009/11/human_orphan_000210.jsp&mid=WC0b01ac058001d12b&source=homeMedSearch). GLP-2 supplementation could have a therapeutic role in neonatal conditions of gut dysfunction, and further studies which address to investigate the ontogeny of GLP-2 axis are mandatory. Although studies on the therapeutic application of GLP-2 in early life conducted on newborn pigs are encouraging (Baldassano and Amato 2014), dose, time, and route of administration are crucial and need to be investigated. As an example, it has been shown that trophic effects of enteral vs parenteral nutrition were evident on gut growth, strongly linked to increased GLP-2 secretion, and optimal when given intermittently vs continuously in neonatal pigs (Stoll et al. 2012). A recent pilot study on seven infant patients with intestinal failure has been published. Native human GLP-2 was well tolerated in children, with a pharmacokinetic profile similar to that of adults (Sigalet et al. 2015). Studies on teduglutide are still missing. Moreover, it is mandatory to verify acute and chronic side effects, in particular if GLP-2 by stimulating mucosal proliferation which also encourages the growth of malignant cells in children considering that they might need the treatment over a longer time and/or in a crucial window of development.

35.3.1.3 Oxyntomodulin (OXM)

OXM is a 37-amino acid peptide derived the from posttranslational processing of tissue-specific proglucagon molecule in intestinal cells, in particular in L cells in the distal portion of the small bowel (Konturek et al. 2004; Cohen et al. 2003). OXM co-localizes with GLP-1, GLP-2, and PYY expression and secretion (Konturek et al. 2004;

Cohen et al. 2003). Limited data are available about a possible feedback system among these peptides also in adults. OXM is also produced in the brain (Cohen et al. 2003). Like GLP-1 and GLP-2, it is inactivated in large amounts by DPP-4 (Baldassano and Amato 2014). The only known receptors for OXM are the same as for GLP-1 and glucagon (GCG-R); however, the existence of other unknown receptor subtypes has been suggested (Konturek et al. 2004; Gardiner et al. 2008; Dakin et al. 2001; Pocai 2013; Irwin and Flatt 2015).

Similar to GLP-1, OXM is released into the circulation after food ingestion in proportion to the caloric intake (Chaudhri et al. 2008). However, it possesses a lower incretin effect when compared to GLP-1 itself (Konturek et al. 2004; Gardiner et al. 2008). This is because several data demonstrated that activation of GCG-R contributes to the insulinotropic effect of OXM and, as a consequence, partially reduces its beneficial effects on glucose metabolism (Du et al. 2012). OXM also acts as an anorectic peptide (Konturek et al. 2004; Cohen et al. 2003; Gardiner et al. 2008). Its administration induces a prompt decrease in the sensation of hunger, food intake, and gastric emptying (Dakin et al. 2004). However, the mechanisms of action for OXM are not been fully investigated at present. The reduction in energy intake after OXM administration is followed by weight reduction in both animals and humans (Wynne et al. 2006). This effect was found to be not only due to the OXM anorectic action but also to an increase in energy expenditure (Gardiner et al. 2008). In vitro and in vivo rodent studies suggest OXM induces these catabolic effects that favor weight loss and subsequently improved metabolic control through both GLP-1 R and GCG-R agonisms (Pocai 2013). OXM levels also increase after gastric bypass, in a similar fashion to GLP 1 (Mechanick et al. 2008). No studies have compared activities of OXM with those of GLP-2. However, iv administrations of OXM and glucagon increase intestinal glucose uptake in rats. Because GLP-1 does not stimulate glucose absorption, GLP-2 and glucose-dependent insulinotropic peptide (GIP) and their receptors could be involved in this action (Pocai 2013).

Although the role of OXM is intriguing, no studies have been performed in neonatal time as well as in childhood. This proglucagon-derived peptide which shares both effects of GLP-1 and GLP-2 could be a good marker of nutritional status and gut development in infants (Ranganath 2008a).

35.3.2 Glucose-Dependent Insulinotropic Polypeptide (GIP)

GIP is a peptide of 42 amino acids which is synthesized by K cells located mainly in the proximal small intestine (duodenum and jejunum) (Holst 2007). GIP is frequently found to be co-localized with GLP-1 while rarely with PYY. As with other incretin hormones, GIP is cleaved and inactivated by DPP-4 with a half-life of approximately 5 min (Ranganath 2008a, b; Flatt 2007). GIP receptors (GIP-R) are expressed in several tissues, including the alpha and beta cells, stomach, adipose tissue, pituitary, heart, and brain (Ranganath 2008b; Flatt 2007).

GIP secretion rises 15 min following nutrient ingestion of mainly glucose and fats (Pais et al. 2016; Wynne et al. 2006) and is also inhibited by glucagon (Ranganath 2008b; Lu et al. 1993).

GIP can be considered as another incretin hormone (Holst 2007). However, it is clear that GIP alone cannot account for the full incretin effect normally associated with a mixed meal, with the main effect exerted by GLP-1 (Holst 2007; Jia et al. 1995). GIP, like GLP-1, is also able to promote beta-cell neogenesis, proliferation, and differentiation (Irwin and Flatt 2015; Ranganath 2008b).

The administration of GIP improves glucose tolerance and insulin sensitivity in animals (Naitoh et al. 2008; Althage et al. 2008). However, it has been demonstrated that GIP receptor KO mice subjected to a high fat diet do not gain weight and have a preserved insulin sensitivity (Gault et al. 2005). The biological effects of GIP appear to be markedly reduced in patients with type 2 diabetes when compared to normal individuals probably due to GIP-R downregulation or desensitization (Irwin and Flatt 2015; Skow et al.

2016), because its secretion is intact (Calanna et al. 2013). On the other hand, the reduced insulinotropic effect of GIP in type 2 diabetes seems an inducible and reversible pathophysiological phenomenon when glucose levels normalize. In contrast to the reduced insulinotropic effect, the glucagonotropic effect of GIP seems to be preserved in patients with diabetes (Irwin and Flatt 2015; Skow et al. 2016).

Overexpression of GIP has also been shown to be associated with reduced body weight in diet-induced obese (DIO) mice (Kim et al. 2012). The pronounced weight decrease after gastric bypass seems to be dependent by surgical ablation of GIP secretion by the duodenum (Flatt 2008), suggesting it has an obesogenic role more than an anti-obesity or incretin hormone role (Skow et al. 2016; Heptulla et al. 2000; Stock et al. 2005; Higgins et al. 2008).

Several studies on GIP were conducted in children to investigate the integrity of its response during the first phases of life.

The signals regulating the differentiation and the number of each endocrine cell type in embryonic and adult intestinal tract is quite unknown. Notably most GLP-1 cells of the ileum of e-17 embryos co-express GIP and, therefore, are LK cells that are more numerous than that in adult mouse ileum, suggesting a developmental role in glucose homeostasis (Grigoryan et al. 2012). In both term and preterm neonates, the entero-insular axis has a functional role in response to glucose with rising plasma GIP, which partially and progressively contributes to an enhanced insulin response to enterally infused glucose as well as to oral feeding (Konturek et al. 2004). However, as for GLP-1 and GLP-2, it has been shown that parenteral and enteral nutrition when given continuously decreased the secretion of GIP at least in neonatal pigs (Stoll et al. 2012). One preliminary study has shown that GIP levels are lower in both term and preterm neonates on cord blood at birth with respect to adults. Furthermore, its bloodstream concentration increases 2 h after birth (Knip et al. 1993) and is persistently high until 33 weeks of life with a following decrease (Nagasaki and Ohta 2015; Kawamata et al. 2014). However, basal GIP levels progressively increased when babies were orally fed and started to also increase after meals by the 24th day of life (Lucas et al. 1980). Fasting and post-meal GIP levels have also been shown to be similar between young subjects born SGA when compared with AGA controls (King et al. 1989).

The infants of diabetic mothers and the large for gestational age (LGA) newborn babies have a more rapid insulin response to oral glucose without differences in GIP levels when compared to AGA controls (Fallucca et al. 1985). Furthermore, amniotic fluid presents a higher GIP/insulin ratio in diabetic pregnant women who delivered overweight infants with respect to nondiabetic pregnant women or those who delivered normal-weight babies (Heijboer et al. 2006). These data suggest that the role of GIP on fat accrual is precocious and linked to glucose metabolism.

35.3.3 Peptide YY (PYY) 3–36

Peptide YY (PYY) is a 36-amino acid polypeptide hormone, a member of the PP family. There are two existing forms of PYY, differing by two amino acids, PYY1–36 and PYY3–36, the most abundant one in the bloodstream (Hellstrom et al. 2004; Konturek et al. 2004; Heijboer et al. 2006). PYY1–36 is released from distal intestinal L cells in response to luminal nutrient stimulation. In the blood, PYY1–36 is rapidly converted to PYY3–36 by the DPP-4, which cleaves the two N-terminal amino acids. PYY is able to bind to the receptor of the neuropeptide Y (NPY). Whereas PYY1–36 has similar affinities for the Y1 and Y2 receptor, PYY3–36 is a high-affinity Y2 receptor ligand (Stadlbauer et al. 2015). Plasma PYY3–36 levels increase after meal ingestion and remain elevated for several hours (Gault et al. 2005; Stadlbauer et al. 2015). Both isoforms, in addition to exerting secretory and motor activities throughout the gut, are involved in the central regulation of food intake and energy balance (Stadlbauer et al. 2015). PYY itself has been defined as an orexigenic peptide; in particular PYY3–36 shows more potent anorectic effects after either peripheral or central administration acting on Y2 receptor at the hypothalamic level via the vagal-brainstem-hypothalamic pathway

(Heijboer et al. 2006; Batterham et al. 2002). In humans, the administration of PYY3–36 is followed by a 30% reduction of ingested nutrients and is coupled with fullness sensation (Degen et al. 2005) and nausea at higher doses (Holst 2007). Signaling at the Y2 receptor has been further implicated in other behavioral and cognitive domains such as central information processing, salience learning, and working memory, throughout highly complex interactions among homeostatic, hedonic, motivational, and associative processes, being indeed involved in the pathways of rewarding (Stadlbauer et al. 2015). In mouse models, PYY is involved in regulating glucose homeostasis but differently from other gut peptides, as it directly inhibits glucose-mediated insulin secretion (Van den Hoek et al. 2004). These effects are associated with an improvement of insulin action in glucose disposal independently of those effects on food intake and weight (Adams et al. 2006). Moreover, its production by pancreatic islet cells, the presence on islets of NPY receptors, and the demonstration that Y1 activation promotes proliferation of beta cells and protects them from apoptosis suggest a role for this peptide in modulating beta-cell mass. Thus, a potential significance of PYY in fetal pancreas formation is hypothesized (Persaud and Bewick 2014). PYY also directly promotes higher fat combustion in animals (Batterham et al. 2003). According to this data, fasting plasma PYY3–36 levels are lower in obese rather than in lean subjects (Konturck et al. 2004), suggesting an involvement in the long-term control of weight. Therefore, weight loss in obese children may restore a higher postprandial level of PYY in contrast with adults whose levels remain low (Wojcicki 2012).

There are increasing data describing the role of PYY in neonates and infants (Misra et al. 2007, 2008). In newborn and infants, PYY3–36 levels seem to account for almost half of the total circulating PYY (Siahanidou et al. 2005, 2007), whose levels are higher in comparison with school-age children and adults (Wojcicki 2012). It negatively correlates with gestational age and anthropometric measures and is higher either in cord blood or in the bloodstream of preterm than full-term infants, probably to compensate the negative body weight balance (Siahanidou et al. 2007; Berseth et al. 1992; Chen et al. 2012). PYY may predict postnatal growth; thus, the negative correlation between PYY concentration and rate of weight gain in preterm infants suggests that those who have higher PYY levels at birth will exhibit a lower rate of weight gain later (Chen et al. 2012). PYY also increases after enteral feeding with formula milk in preterm babies also when affected by necrotizing enterocolitis (Chen et al. 2012; Sharman-Koendjbiharie et al. 2002), without an effective role in the inflammatory response (Siahanidou et al. 2015). An increase in postnatal age was associated with a concomitant increase in PYY (Chen et al. 2012), which remains persistently high until 10 weeks of life (Kawamata et al. 2014), and its fasting concentration decreases in 9-month-old infants (Adrian et al. 1986). Thus, it suggests that the postnatal surge is a feature of early adaptation to the extrauterine life and could have effects not only on energy homeostasis but also on the gut, including absorptive, trophic, and proliferative actions (Siahanidou et al. 2005, 2007; Adrian et al. 1986). Moreover, an early growth seems to have a role in programming appetite regulatory hormone secretion, such as PYY, in later life, considering that greater satiety responses after the meal are described among subjects who grew slowly during early life (Perala et al. 2013). Many data are needed to confirm these hypotheses.

35.3.4 Peptides from Preproghrelin

35.3.4.1 Acylated (AG) and Unacylated (UAG) Ghrelin

Ghrelin is a 28-amino acid peptide, recently isolated from the stomach, but also shown to be expressed in other tissues such as the pancreas, adrenal gland, thyroid, breast, testes, placenta, pituitary and hypothalamus, myocardium, muscle, and colon (Müller et al. 2015). Ghrelin has been identified as an endogenous ligand of the orphan GH secretagogue (GHS) receptor type 1a (Kojima and Kangawa 2005; Ghigo et al. 2001). It circulates in the blood in two forms, acylated (AG) and unacylated ghrelin (UAG) (Müller et al. 2015; Kojima and Kangawa 2005). The acyl group, which binds to ghrelin at the serine-3 residue, seems to be essential for the binding to GHSR1a and the resulting neuroendocrine functions, namely, GH secretion (Müller et al. 2015; Kojima and Kangawa 2005). UAG, which is devoid of the acyl group, represents the most abundant circulating form (Gauna et al. 2005; Wiedmer et al. 2007). UAG is biologically active, although it does not have direct neuroendocrine actions (Müller et al. 2015; Kojima and Kangawa 2005; Broglio et al. 2004) suggesting the existence of some GHS-R subtypes that are activated independently of its acylation (Müller et al. 2015; Wiedmer et al. 2007; Gil-Campos et al. 2006). The mechanism of acylation of the preproghrelin or UAG is largely unknown. Recently, the acyltransferase has been identified, which was named GOAT, that octanoylates ghrelin throughout lipids, at least in part, directly recruited from the pool of ingested dietary lipids (Müller et al. 2015; Yang et al. 2008). GOAT and ghrelin share a similar tissue expression profiles and are highly conserved across vertebrates (Müller et al. 2015).

Moreover, since its discovery, AG was identified first followed by UAG; ghrelin emerged as a player in the regulation of food intake and energy expenditure, with AG as the most potent peripheral orexigenic hormone known to date (Müller et al. 2015; Wiedmer et al. 2007; Choi et al. 2003). In animals and humans, AG, both after central and peripheral administration, has been shown to induce appetite and food intake in a diverse fashion to other described anorectic gut peptides (Wiedmer et al. 2007). Despite these clear orexigenic effects of AG, the actual physiological role of UAG in the regulation of appetite is still a matter of debate (Choi et al. 2003), but it seems able to induce a negative energy balance by decreasing food intake and delaying gastric emptying via the hypothalamus (Delhanty et al. 2012). It has also been clearly shown that both forms of ghrelin also influence energy metabolism at the peripheral level, most likely influencing fat oxidation (Wortley et al. 2004, 2005). Reduced cellular fat oxidation and promotion of adipogenesis each contributes to an increase in fat mass induced either by AG or UAG (Wiedmer et al. 2007; Thompson et al. 2004; Zhang et al. 2004). Consistent with its effects on food intake and its involvement in energy balance, circulating ghrelin levels are negatively associated with body mass index in humans (Wiedmer et al. 2007; Paik et al. 2006; Leite-Moreira and Soares 2007). Several studies indicate that ghrelin hyposecretion in essential obesity is a functional impairment in response to body weight alteration (Cummings et al. 2002). Roux-en-Y gastric bypass has been shown to be associated with alterations in glucose kinetics and glucoregulatory hormone secretion likely secondary to the anatomic rearrangement of the foregut, with increased PYY and GLP-1 concentrations and decreased ghrelin levels (Barazzoni et al. 2007; Zwirska-Korczala et al. 2007). Furthermore, the majority of the data come from studies that have analyzed exclusively the total ghrelin levels. Recent findings have also shown that UAG is decreased in obesity, while there are no concordant results for AG also in children (Gualillo et al. 2001; Cortelazzi et al. 2003; Chanoine et al. 2002; Bellone et al. 2004, 2012a; Soriano-Guillen et al. 2004). Ghrelin is also implicated in the regulation of glucose homeostasis by modulating insulin secretion and action as described previously for other gut peptides with incretin action (Yang et al. 2008; Thompson et al. 2004). In particular, UAG and AG play opposite effects on pancreatic beta-cell secretion and glucose metabolism (Müller et al. 2015; Prodam et al. 2008). In fact, if AG may contribute to the worsening of insulin sensitivity, suggesting a diabetogenic function, UAG could exert its metabolic actions counterbalancing those of AG, at least in part at the pancreatic level (Gauna et al. 2005; Wiedmer et al. 2007). In childhood, adolescence, and adulthood, it has also been demonstrated that insulin modulates ghrelin levels through inhibition (Müller et al. 2015; Wiedmer et al. 2007; Baldelli et al. 2006). Ghrelin secretion is also modulated by nutrients, namely, carbohydrates, whereas the role of fats and proteins is not completely understood due to discordant results (Müller et al. 2015; Wiedmer et al. 2007). In fact, if proteins result more effective in lowering ghrelin levels than lipids (Müller et al. 2015), in other hand, both lipids and amino acids seem to play a negligible role in the acute control of ghrelin secretion (Prodam et al. 2006). Nevertheless it is noteworthy that administration of a mixed meals in children does not inhibit total ghrelin levels unlike adults, suggesting a modulation by age and suggesting a functional profile oriented to anabolic processes of growth (Müller et al. 2015; Wiedmer et al. 2007; Nakahara et al. 2008; Prodam et al. 2014a). Particularly, its inhibition seems to start from puberty at least in lean children, except for obese children and adolescents. Conversely, total ghrelin levels decrease after OGTT at any age and weight (Prodam et al. 2014a).

Furthermore, increasing evidence indicates that the action of ghrelin affects a more complex pathway not completely known, including additional physiological functions such as learning and memory, psychological stress, mood and anxiety, depression, sleep/wake rhythm, anticonvulsant effect, thymopoiesis, and aging (Müller et al. 2015; Prodam et al. 2011).

Since pregnancy, ghrelin, both maternal and placental derived, seems to play an important role in fetal and neonatal development by increasing maternal appetite and promoting nutrient supplies to the fetus resulting in its positive energy balance (Valsamakis et al. 2014). Therefore, ghrelin regulation and secretion in fetal and neonatal period are not fully understood yet but intensively investigated in the last years. It has been demonstrated that ghrelin has been detected in human cord blood starting from 20 to 22 weeks of life; it remains relatively constant throughout the gestation and at birth and then increases peaking during the first 2 years of life (Soriano-Guillen et al. 2004; Whatmore et al. 2003; Bideci et al. 2008; Kasa-Vubu et al. 2007; Pomerants et al. 2006; Savino et al. 2012a). Even though it may also originate from the maternal compartment or may be secreted by the placenta, these ghrelin levels are directly produced by the fetus (Savino et al. 2012a; Warchoł et al. 2014). In fact, immune-reactive ghrelin cells have been shown in the fetal stomach, duodenum, pancreas, and lung from the tenth week of gestation (Mitrovic et al. 2014). Moreover, its concentration is similar between arterial and venous, and its expression is almost absent in the placenta during the third trimester (Cortelazzi et al. 2003; Bellone et al. 2006).

Higher ghrelin levels are detected in SGA newborns than in AGA or LGA neonates (Stock et al. 2005; Soriano-Guillen et al. 2004; Bunt et al. 2003) and in IUGR newborns (Chiesa et al. 2008), suggesting a role in fetal adaptation to intrauterine malnutrition. Moreover, lower cord blood ghrelin is associated with slower weight from birth to 3 and 12 months of age, at least in breastfed infants (James et al. 2004; Savino et al. 2005); this evidence, however, does not definitely rule out a role of ghrelin in the control of somatotroph secretion but clearly suggests an involvement in both short- and long-term energy balance (Bellone et al. 2006; Savino et al. 2005). Furthermore, preterm AGA newborns have higher total ghrelin levels at birth (Chen et al. 2012; Cortelazzi et al. 2003; Bellone et al. 2006; Chiesa et al. 2008; Lanyi et al. 2008). Higher ghrelin levels during the neonatal period could also influence hormone levels later in life. In fact, increased ghrelin levels in preterm born children are sustained up to prepubertal ages (Savino et al. 2012a). It is still questioned if ghrelin concentration at birth in preterm neonates was independent or not by gender, body weight, and type of delivery (Bellone et al. 2006). However, it recently found a positive correlation between ghrelin levels and gestational age, birth weight, body mass index, head circumference of babies at birth, and anthropometric values on day 15 (Kahveci et al. 2015). Moreover, in preterm infants, the positive correlations of ghrelin at birth with time to reach recommended daily intake and with weight gain rate indicate that ghrelin may predict postnatal growth. Thus, it is suggested that those babies with elevated neonatal ghrelin concentrations will be delayed in reaching recommended daily intake (Chen et al. 2012). On the other hand, what is clear is that ghrelin levels increase from birth to fourth day of life and seem to negatively correlate with weight and anthropometric parameters at that time in preterm and at birth in full-term newborns (Soriano-Guillen et al. 2004; Bellone et al. 2006).

Notably, ghrelin secretion is refractory to feeding in preterm AGA neonates in the first days of life, suggesting that it could represent an anabolic drive in newborns (Bellone et al. 2006; James et al. 2004). Accordingly, ghrelin positively correlates with the enteral nutrition intake in both preterm and full-term babies on the second day after birth (Hubler et al. 2006). However, it is modulated by feeding, progressively increasing with prolonging fasting in full-term AGA infants from the first month of life (Savino et al. 2006a). Ghrelin secretion seems to be modulated by the type of enteral nutrition, suggesting a role of this peptide in gut development and maturation. In fact, at 4 months of age, formula-fed infants have higher ghrelin and IGF-I levels without anthropometrical differences with respect to breastfed ones (Savino et al. 2005). At 6 months of age, ghrelin levels are higher in infants with a mixed nutrition of solids and milk with respect to those exclusively milk fed (Savino et al. 2005). It has been demonstrated that ghrelinemia negatively correlated with BMI at the first month in breastfed full-term infants (Cesur et al. 2012) and weight gain at 12 months of age only in breastfed but not in formula-fed infants (Savino et al. 2005, 2006a). These data suggest that a precocious derangement in ghrelin regulation could be linked to the higher risk of elevated weight gain in children who are breastfed for less than 6 months (Kalies et al. 2005). Furthermore, infant formula milks are devoid of many constituents, ghrelin among others, and this fact could influence gut maturation and fat accrual. Accordingly, mature breast milk has higher ghrelin levels than those of colostrum, with lower concentrations in preterms (Han et al. 2014). Particularly, both total ghrelin and AG progressively increase in breast milk during lactation in the first 6 months, and their concentration in milk positively correlated with those in plasma of the breastfed infants (Savino et al. 2006a; Cesur et al. 2012; Ilcol and Hizli 2007; Savino et al. 2012b). Moreover, ghrelin levels in colostrum and weight and anthropometric parameters at least at birth seem to positively correlate (Han et al. 2014). Instead, there is a positive correlation between the level of fourth month breast milk AG and early postnatal weight gain of infants (Cesur et al. 2012).

Furthermore, it is also recently hypothesized a possible role of ghrelin in the inflammatory responses in adults (Prodam and Filigheddu 2014), with the evidence of higher circulating levels in neonates with infection (Siahanidou et al. 2015).

Some preliminary studies have also analyzed AG levels in newborns. It has been demonstrated that AG is present in both fetal and neonatal circulation. AG and AG to total ghrelin ratio seem to be higher in venous cord blood suggesting that the placenta can produce AG with a small part of it transferred to the fetal circulation (Yokota et al. 2005). AG is also higher in preterm and SGA newborns when compared to full-term and AGA ones (Shimizu et al. 2007; Holst et al. 2007). Interestingly, umbilical cord AG concentration is lower than in maternal blood, and the acylation process seems to be affected by cortisol partly through a placental role (Lanyi et al. 2008). Further studies are needed to clarify the exact role of the different ghrelin forms in neonates. In fact, newborns in physiological conditions, compared with children in later life, seem to have higher UAG and lower AG levels. Moreover, their AG to UAG ratio results to be lower than in normal-weight and obese children, thus suggesting a different metabolic function for the two forms at birth (Bellone et al. 2012b).

35.3.4.2 Obestatin

In 2005, Zhang and coworkers from a conserved region of preproghrelin sequence identified a 23-amino acid peptide which was named obestatin based on previously reported activities in animal models. Obestatin is amidated like GLP-1 for bioactivity. It was initially characterized as the active ligand of the orphan receptor GPR39 (Bellone et al. 2006), but more recently, this result is discussed (Müller et al. 2015; Tang et al. 2008; Gourcerol et al. 2007). Obestatin, like ghrelin, is expressed in several tissues which include among others the stomach, duodenum, pancreas, and brain (Zhang et al. 2005). Obestatin initially appeared to be a new regulator of appetite and body weight (Holst et al. 2007), inhibiting food intake, jejunum peristalsis, and weight gain, and thus is considered an antagonist of ghrelin (Zhang et al. 2014). Following studies, however, failed to reproduce obestatin's anorectic and anti-obesity effects and questioned its existence as just a ghrelin-associated peptide (Qader et al. 2008). In contrast to other gut peptides, previous data regarding the modulation of insulin secretion are limited and controversial (Tang et al. 2008; Gourcerol et al. 2007). On the other hand, preliminary studies in vivo recently observed that obestatin is reduced in subjects with type 2 diabetes, type 1 diabetes at the onset, and obesity, while it is increased in anorexia (Müller et al. 2015; Harada et al. 2008; Prodam et al. 2014b).

In line with the abundant studies on ghrelin, the youngest gut peptide obestatin also started to be investigated in pediatric subjects (Nakahara et al. 2008; Zou et al. 2009), but with limited data in neonates. Its association with birth weight is not well characterized with conflicting results, and its role during neonatal period remains unclear. Obestatin levels seem to be high at fasting in SGA neonates with respect to those in LGA, without differences in those preterm and term (Zhang et al. 2014). No differences in cord blood obestatin levels were observed between AGA and LGA newborns in one published paper, probably due to the sample size (Boutsikou et al. 2013). Moreover, obestatin has been detected in breast milk with a positive correlation between lactating mothers and breastfed infants (Savino et al. 2012b). These data suggest that obestatin could play a role either in fetal or neonatal development and growth, also exerting effects on feeding behavior. However, further studies are required to understand the relationship between ghrelin, obestatin, and pre-/postnatal development.

35.3.5 Motilin

Motilin is a 22-amino acid peptide produced by the endocrine cells of the duodenum and jejunum. It is able to bind and activate the receptor GPR38 through which it stimulates motility of digestive organs (Poitras and Peeters 2008). In fact, it regulates gastrointestinal motility via migrating motor complex activity in its phase III of contraction (Itoh 1997). This consists of cyclical increases every 90–120 min during the interdigestive fasting periods (Poitras and Peeters 2008; Itoh 1997). The mechanism by which motilin induces gut motility is still unclear. The gut motilin-containing cells and enteric neurons are separated only by a sheet of the basal lamina of mucosal epithelium. However, the GPR38 has not been demonstrated in the vagus nerve or nodose ganglion although migrating motor complex activity is atropine sensitive and abolished by vagotomy (Itoh 1997; Nishikubo et al. 2005). Otherwise, the GPR38 is expressed in the brain, suggesting a role of motilin in feeding regulation (Savino et al. 2006a). It has to be underlined that motilin and ghrelin precursors share almost 50% similarity in their sequences, and, as a consequence, Tomasetto initially named it motilin-related peptide (Tomasetto et al. 2000). More recently, motilin has been included in the ghrelin peptide family. The GPR38 and GHS-R1a are also part of the same family of G-protein-coupled receptors with an overall sequence identity of 53% (Poitras and Peeters 2008). Furthermore, ghrelin and motilin are located in the same endocrine cells and in the same secretory granules at duodenum and jejunum level (Wierup et al. 2007).

Motilin role in gut development has been investigated in neonatal period. Motilin-secreting cells appear at 8–11 weeks of gestation in fetus with a distribution similar to that in adulthood at 12–15 weeks of gestation (Bryant et al. 1982). It has been shown that motilin is present in duodenal epithelial cells of premature infants of <32 weeks of gestation (Nishikubo et al. 2005). Its levels are higher in preterm and SGA infants after receiving enteral nutrition with respect to older children or adults (Janik et al. 1982; Mahmoud et al. 1988; Shulman and Kanarek 1993). It has been recently demonstrated that motilin secretion in preterm newborn could be modulated by prebiotics: a prebiotic-enriched formula containing dietary oligosaccharides (short-chain galacto-oligosaccharides/long-chain fructo-oligosaccharides) resulted in significant surge of motilin with consequently reduced gastric residue, compared with a common preterm formula (Dasopoulou et al. 2015). Motilin is also present in human milk, and its digestion in the stomach is retarded by milk itself, suggesting a biological role in the gut of newborns (De Clercq et al. 1998). It has also been shown a positive correlation between motilin concentration and age at 18 months of life which has not been explained yet (Savino et al. 2006a). Furthermore, colicky infants present higher motilin levels which could have a role in this gut disorders (Lothe et al. 1987; Savino et al. 2006b). Motilin-receptor antagonists could be a potential therapeutic agent for colic dysfunctions when they will become available for clinical exploration (Poitras and Peeters 2008).

35.3.6 Cholecystokinin (CCK)

CCK was the first gut hormone described as inhibitor of food intake in rodents (Gibbs et al. 1973). CCK is widely expressed both at the central and peripheral levels, in particular in I cells in the duodenum and jejunum mucosa (Moran 2000). CCK is also detectable in the bloodstream in different forms, in particular CCK-8, CCK-33 and CCK-39 (Konturek et al. 2004). Two CCK receptor subtypes have been isolated: CCK_A receptor which is expressed in the vagus nerve, enteric neurons, pancreas, and at central level and CCK_B expressed in the afferent vagus nerves, brain, and stomach (Moran 2000).

CCK possesses several activities on different tissues, among others the stimulatory effect on pancreatic enzyme excretion and the induction of gallbladder contraction (Neary et al. 2004).

CCK has been demonstrated to be a satiety signal, in particular in the short-term regulation of feeding behaviors (Konturek et al. 2004; Moran 2000; Woods 2004). It acts, synergistically with leptin, on hypothalamic region (Konturek et al. 2004; Gibbs et al. 1973). Its effect is reduced by vagotomy (Konturek et al. 2004; Moran 2000; Woods 2004).

Peripheral CCK administration is followed by a rapid but short-term lasting effect on inhibition of food intake, with an activity peak at 30 min (Shulman and Kanarek 1993). High doses of CCK determine nausea, vomiting, and taste aversion (West et al. 1987). Notably, CCK mainly inhibits fat ingestion (Covasa et al. 2001). The inhibitory effect of CCK on food intake undergoes a functional desensitization after high-dose administration as well as during continuous infusion (Moran 2000). When administered intermittently before eating, CCK maintains its anorectic effect, but a compensatory effect by increasing the daily number of meals, with only a mild result on total food intake and body weight, is observed (West et al. 1987).

According to its anorectic activity as well as the stimulation of gallbladder contraction, CCK has been investigated in neonatal life. It has been demonstrated that it increases immediately after breastfeeding, and this peak is followed by a decline 10 min later; a secondary rise occurs 30 and 60 min after it. The first increase of CCK levels may exert a stimulatory effect on digestion, while the secondary increase could, namely, have an anorectic effect (Uvnas-Moberg et al. 1993). Higher CCK levels correspond to a higher volume of ingested milk during breastfeeding (Marchini and Linden 1992). The mechanisms of CCK effect on infant satiety have been investigated in mice, and the anorectic effect of CCK seems to be mediated by the temporary expression of cholecystokinin-1 receptors on ependymal cells lining the third ventricle (Ozaki et al. 2013). CCK levels soon after birds and later on were also analyzed in mice-born IUGR by restricting the food intake of the mothers during pregnancy. Notably, gastrointestinal gene expressions and plasma levels of CCK were elevated in the male newborns, decreasing in adulthood, suggesting that, along with the altered gene expressions of other orexigenic and anorexigenic gut peptides, an early increase followed by reduction of CCK expression may provide a potential mechanism to explain hyperphagia and obesity seen in maternal undernutrition-induced IUGR offspring (Nagata et al. 2011). CCK levels are negatively correlated with age in full-term infants (Uvnas-Moberg et al. 1993). Preterm infants present an increase of CCK concentration in cord blood 1 h later after the delivery without differences in AGA and SGA babies (Tornhage et al. 1995, 1996). Notably, plasma CCK concentration increases after nasogastric tube feeding only in preterm neonates who underwent kangaroo care. These results are still under investigation (Tornhage et al. 1998). Furthermore, CCK prophylaxis in high-risk neonates seems to help in preventing parenteral nutrition-associated cholestasis (Teitelbaum et al. 1997). However, the role of CCK on gut maturation has never been explored yet. Finally, a role of CCK in visceral sensitivity could be hypothesized: it has been proven that an early-life antibiotic-induced disturbance of the gut microbiota induces visceral hypersensitivity in male rats, mediated by parallel decrease in cholecystokinin B receptor (O'Mahony et al. 2014).

35.4 Therapy and Treatments

Bioactive peptide, hormones, and factors present in human milk and produced by the gut have been shown to stimulate gut development and functions and to be modulated by nutrients themselves. The majority of findings come from studies on preterm or SGA infants. However, the knowledge about this topic is still largely incomplete with many studies performed 20 years ago and abandoned and many others linked to the new gut peptides discovered in the last years. Various compounds derived by all these hormones can be hypothesized or are in trial for the treatment of preterm newborns and colic dysfunctions. However, both the physiological and pharmaceutical researches have to better explore this field. It has to look to the future for more detailed studies to elaborate completely the functions of all these peptides and the interaction of breastfed and formula milk and solids with the gut. Nutrient sensing is a new crucial topic, and the influence of this complex process in relation to hormones in the first steps of nutrition is a challenge.

References

Adams SH, Lei C, Jodka CM et al (2006) PYY[3-36] administration decreases the respiratory quotient and reduces adiposity in diet-induced obese mice. J Nutr 136:195–201

Adrian TE, Smith HA, Calvert SA et al (1986) Elevated plasma peptide YY in human neonates and infants. Pediatr Res 20:1225–1227

Agostoni C (2005) Ghrelin, leptin and the neurometabolic axis of breastfed and formula-fed infants. Acta Paediatr 94:523–525

Althage MC, Ford EL, Wang S et al (2008) Targeted ablation of glucose-dependent insulinotropic polypeptide-producing cells in transgenic mice reduces obesity and insulin resistance induced by a high fat diet. J Biol Chem 283:18365–18376

Amato A, Baldassano S, Mulè F (2016) GLP2: an underestimated signal for improving glycaemic control and insulin sensitivity. J Endocrinol 229:R57–R66

Amin H, Holst JJ, Hartmann B et al (2008) Functional ontogeny of the proglucagon-derived peptide axis in the premature human neonate. Pediatrics 121:e180–e186

Bahrami J, Longuet C, Baggio LL et al (2010) The glucagon-like peptide-2 receptor modulates islet adaptation to metabolic stress in the ob/ob mouse. Gastroenterology 139:857–868

Baldassano S, Amato A (2014) GLP-2: what do we know? What are we going to discover? Regul Pept 194-195:6–10

Baldassano S, Rappa F, Amato A et al (2015) GLP-2 as beneficial factor in the glucose homeostasis in mice fed a high fat diet. J Cell Physiol 230:3029–3036

Baldassano S, Amato A, Caldara GF, Mulè F (2016) Glucagon-like peptide-2 treatment improves glucose dysmetabolism in mice fed a high fat diet. Endocrine 54(3):648–656

Baldelli R, Bellone S, Castellino N et al (2006) Oral glucose load inhibits circulating ghrelin levels to the same extent in normal and obese children. Clin Endocrinol 64:255–259

Barazzoni R, Zanetti M, Ferreira C et al (2007) Relationships between desacylated and acylated ghrelin and insulin sensitivity in the metabolic syndrome. J Clin Endocrinol Metab 92:3935–3940

Batterham RL, Cowley MA, Small CJ et al (2002) Gut hormone PYY(3-36) physiologically inhibits food intake. Nature 418:650–654

Batterham RL, Cohen MA, Ellis SM et al (2003) Inhibition of food intake in obese subjects by peptide YY3-36. N Engl J Med 349:941–948

Bellone S, Rapa A, Vivenza D et al (2004) Circulating ghrelin levels in the newborn are positively associated with gestational age. Clin Endocrinol 60:613–617

Bellone S, Baldelli R, Radetti G et al (2006) Ghrelin secretion in preterm neonates progressively increases and is refractory to the inhibitory effect of food intake. J Clin Endocrinol Metab 91:1929–1933

Bellone S, Prodam F, Savastio S et al (2012a) Acylated and unacylated ghrelin levels in normal weight and obese children: influence of puberty and relationship with insulin, leptin and adiponectin levels. J Endocrinol Investig 35(2):191–197

Bellone S, Prodam F, Savastio S et al (2012b) Acylated/unacylated ghrelin ratio in cord blood: correlation with anthropometric and metabolic parameters and pediatric lifespan comparison. Eur J Endocrinol 166:115–120

Berseth CL, Nordyke CK, Valdes MG et al (1992) Responses of gastrointestinal peptides and motor activity to milk and water feedings in preterm and term infants. Pediatr Res 31:587–590

Bideci A, Camurdan MO, Yesilkaya E et al (2008) Serum ghrelin, leptin and resistin levels in adolescent girls with polycystic ovary syndrome. J Obstet Gynaecol Res 34:578–584

Boutsikou T, Briana DD, Boutsikou M et al (2013) Cord blood chemerin and obestatin levels in large for

gestational age infants. J Matern Fetal Neonatal Med 26 (2):123–126
Broglio F, Gottero C, Prodam F et al (2004) Non-acylated ghrelin counteracts the metabolic but not the neuroendocrine response to acylated ghrelin in humans. J Clin Endocrinol Metab 89:3062–3065
Brøns C, Saltbæk PN, Friedrichsen M et al (2016) Endocrine and metabolic diurnal rhythms in young adult men born small vs appropriate for gestational age. Eur J Endocrinol 175:29–40
Bryant MG, Buchan AM, Gregor M et al (1982) Development of intestinal regulatory peptides in the human fetus. Gastroenterology 83:47–54
Bunt JC, Salbe AD, Tschop MH et al (2003) Cross-sectional and prospective relationships of fasting plasma ghrelin concentrations with anthropometric measures in pima Indian children. J Clin Endocrinol Metab 88:3756–3761
Burrin DG, Stoll B (2002) Key nutrients and growth factors for the neonatal gastrointestinal tract. Clin Perinatol 29:65–96
Calanna S, Christensen M, Holst JJ et al (2013) Secretion of glucose-dependent insulinotropic polypeptide in patients with type 2 diabetes: systematic review and meta-analysis of clinical studies. Diabetes Care 36:3346–3352
Cani PD, Possemiers S, Van de Wiele T et al (2009) Changes in gut microbiota control inflammation in obese mice through a mechanism involving GLP-2-driven improvement of gut permeability. Gut 58:1091–1103
Cesur G, Ozguner F, Yilmaz N, Dundar B (2012) The relationship between ghrelin and adiponectin levels in breast milk and infant serum and growth of infants during early postnatal life. J Physiol Sci 62(3):185–190
Chanoine JP, Yeung LP, Wong AC, Birmingham CL (2002) Immunoreactive ghrelin in human cord blood: relation to anthropometry, leptin, and growth hormone. J Pediatr Gastroenterol Nutr 35:282–286
Chaudhri OB, Wynne K, Bloom SR (2008) Can gut hormones control appetite and prevent obesity? Diabetes Care 31(Suppl 2):S284–S289
Chen X, Du X, Zhu J et al (2012) Correlations of circulating peptide YY and ghrelin with body weight, rate of weight gain, and time required to achieve the recommended daily intake in preterm infants. Braz J Med Biol Res 45:656–664
Chiesa C, Osborn JF, Haass C et al (2008) Ghrelin, leptin, IGF-1, IGFBP-3, and insulin concentrations at birth: is there a relationship with foetal growth and neonatal anthropometry? Clin Chem 54:550–558
Choi K, Roh SG, Hong YH et al (2003) The role of ghrelin and growth hormone secretagogues receptor on rat adipogenesis. Endocrinology 144:754–759
Cohen MA, Ellis SM, le Roux CW et al (2003) Oxyntomodulin suppresses appetite and reduces food intake in humans. J Clin Endocrinol Metab 88:4696–4701
Corpeleijn WE, van Vliet I, de Gast-Bakker DA et al (2008) Effect of enteral IGF-1 supplementation on feeding tolerance, growth, and gut permeability in enterally fed premature neonates. J Pediatr Gastroenterol Nutr 46:184–190
Cortelazzi D, Cappiello V, Morpurgo PS et al (2003) Circulating levels of ghrelin in human fetuses. Eur J Endocrinol 149:111–116
Covasa M, Marcuson JK, Ritter RC (2001) Diminished satiation in rats exposed to elevated levels of endogenous or exogenous cholecystokinin. Am J Phys Regul Integr Comp Phys 280:R331–R337
Cummings DE, Weigle DS, Frayo RS et al (2002) Plasma ghrelin levels after diet-induced weight loss or gastric bypass surgery. N Engl J Med 346:1623–1630
Dakin CL, Gunn I, Small CJ et al (2001) Oxyntomodulin inhibits food intake in the rat. Endocrinology 142:4244–4250
Dakin CL, Small CJ, Batterham RL et al (2004) Peripheral oxyntomodulin reduces food intake and body weight gain in rats. Endocrinology 145:2687–2695
Dasopoulou M, Briana DD, Boutsikou T et al (2015) Motilin and gastrin secretion and lipid profile in preterm neonates following prebiotics supplementation: a double-blind randomized controlled study. JPEN J Parenter Enteral Nutr 39(3):359–368
De Clercq P, Springer S, Depoortere I, Peeters TL (1998) Motilin in human milk: identification and stability during digestion. Life Sci 63:1993–2000
de Moura EG, Lisboa PC, Passos MC (2008) Neonatal programming of neuroimmunomodulation–role of adipocytokines and neuropeptides. Neuroimmunomodulation 15:176–188
Degen L, Oesch S, Casanova M et al (2005) Effect of peptide YY3-36 on food intake in humans. Gastroenterology 129:1430–1436
Delhanty PJ, Neggers SJ, van der Lely AJ (2012) Mechanisms in endocrinology: ghrelin: the differences between acyl- and des-acyl ghrelin. Eur J Endocrinol 167:601–608
Díaz M, Bassols J, Sebastiani G et al (2015) Circulating GLP-1 in infants born small-for-gestational-age: breast-feeding versus formula-feeding. Int J Obes 39:1501–1503
Dong CX, Zhao W, Solomon C et al (2014) The intestinal epithelial insulin-like growth factor-1 receptor links glucagon-like peptide-2 action to gut barrier function. Endocrinology 155:370–379
Drucker DJ (2002) Biological actions and therapeutic potential of the glucagon-like peptides. Gastroenterology 122:531–544
Drucker DJ, Yusta B (2014) Physiology and pharmacology of the enteroendocrine hormone glucagon-like peptide-2. Annu Rev Physiol 76:561–583
Du X, Kosinski JR, Lao J et al (2012) Differential effects of oxyntomodulin and GLP-1 on glucose metabolism. Am J Physiol Endocrinol Metab 303:E265–E271
Fallucca F, Kuhl C, Lauritsen KB et al (1985) Gastric inhibitory polypeptide (GIP) concentration in human amniotic fluid. Horm Metab Res 17:251–255
Flatt PR (2007) Effective surgical treatment of obesity may be mediated by ablation of the lipogenic gut hormone gastric inhibitory polypeptide (GIP): evidence and

clinical opportunity for development of new obesity-diabetes drugs? Diab Vasc Dis Res 4.151–153

Flatt PR (2008) Dorothy Hodgkin Lecture 2008. Gastric inhibitory polypeptide (GIP) revisited: a new therapeutic target for obesity-diabetes? Diabet Med 25:759–764

Garcia-Diaz D, Campion J, Milagro FI, Martinez JA (2007) Adiposity dependent apelin gene expression: relationships with oxidative and inflammation markers. Mol Cell Biochem 305:87–94

Gardiner JV, Jayasena CN, Bloom SR (2008) Gut hormones: a weight off your mind. J Neuroendocrinol 20:834–841

Gault VA, Irwin N, Green BD et al (2005) Chemical ablation of gastric inhibitory polypeptide receptor action by daily (Pro3)GIP administration improves glucose tolerance and ameliorates insulin resistance and abnormalities of islet structure in obesity-related diabetes. Diabetes 54:2436–2446

Gauna C, Delhanty PJ, Hofland LJ et al (2005) Ghrelin stimulates, whereas des-octanoyl ghrelin inhibits, glucose output by primary hepatocytes. J Clin Endocrinol Metab 90:1055–1060

Geloneze B, Lima MM, Pareja JC et al (2013) Association of insulin resistance and GLP-2 secretion in obesity: a pilot study. Arq Bras Endocrinol Metabol 57:632–635

Ghigo E, Arvat E, Giordano R et al (2001) Biologic activities of growth hormone secretagogues in humans. Endocrine 14:87–93

Gibbs J, Young RC, Smith GP (1973) Cholecystokinin decreases food intake in rats. J Comp Physiol Psychol 84:488–495

Gil-Campos M, Aguilera CM, Canete R, Gil A (2006) Ghrelin: a hormone regulating food intake and energy homeostasis. Br J Nutr 96:201–226

Gourcerol G, St-Pierre DH, Tache Y (2007) Lack of obestatin effects on food intake: should obestatin be renamed ghrelin-associated peptide (GAP)? Regul Pept 141:1–7

Grigoryan M, Kedees MH, Guz Y, Teitelman G (2012) Phenotype of entero-endocrine L cells becomes restricted during development. Dev Dyn 241:1986–1992

Gualillo O, Caminos J, Blanco M et al (2001) Ghrelin, a novel placental-derived hormone. Endocrinology 142:788–794

Guan X, Shi X, Li X, Chang B et al (2012) GLP-2 receptor in POMC neurons suppresses feeding behavior and gastric motility. Am J Physiol Endocrinol Metab 303: E853–E864

Han L, Li M, Yu X et al (2014) Assay of adiponectin, leptin, true insulin and ghrelin levels in preterm human milk, and its relationship with infants growth. Zhonghua Er Ke Za Zhi 52(7):510–515

Harada T, Nakahara T, Yasuhara D et al (2008) Obestatin, acyl ghrelin, and des-acyl ghrelin responses to an oral glucose tolerance test in the restricting type of anorexia nervosa. Biol Psychiatry 63:245–247

Heijboer AC, Pijl H, Van den Hoek AM et al (2006) Gut-brain axis: regulation of glucose metabolism. J Neuroendocrinol 18:883–894

Hellstrom PM, Geliebter A, Naslund E et al (2004) Peripheral and central signals in the control of eating in normal, obese and binge-eating human subjects. Br J Nutr 92(Suppl 1):S47–S57

Heptulla RA, Tamborlane WV, Cavaghan M et al (2000) Augmentation of alimentary insulin secretion despite similar gastric inhibitory peptide (GIP) responses in juvenile obesity. Pediatr Res 47:628–633

Higgins PB, Fernandez JR, Garvey WT et al (2008) Entero-insular axis and postprandial insulin differences in African American and European American children. Am J Clin Nutr 88:1277–1283

Hill ME, Asa SL, Drucker DJ (1999) Essential requirement for Pax6 in control of enteroendocrine proglucagon gene transcription. Mol Endocrinol 13: 1474–1486

Holst JJ (2007) The physiology of glucagon-like peptide 1. Physiol Rev 87:1409–1439

Holst B, Egerod KL, Schild E et al (2007) GPR39 signaling is stimulated by zinc ions but not by obestatin. Endocrinology 148:13–20

http://www.ema.europa.eu/ema/index.jsp?curl=pages/medicines/human/orphans/2009/11/human_orphan_000210.jsp&mid=WC0b01ac058001d12b

Hubler A, Rippel C, Kauf E et al (2006) Associations between ghrelin levels in serum of preterm infants and enteral nutritional state during the first 6 months after birth. Clin Endocrinol 65:611–616

Ilcol YO, Hizli B (2007) Active and total ghrelin concentrations increase in breast milk during lactation. Acta Paediatr 96:1632–1639

Irwin N, Flatt PR (2015) New perspectives on exploitation of incretin peptides for the treatment of diabetes and related disorders. World J Diabetes 6:1285–1295

Itoh Z (1997) Motilin and clinical application. Peptides 18:593–608

James RJ, Drewett RF, Cheetham TD (2004) Low cord ghrelin levels in term infants are associated with slow weight gain over the first 3 months of life. J Clin Endocrinol Metab 89:3847–3850

Janik JS, Track NS, Filler RM (1982) Motilin, human pancreatic polypeptide, gastrin, and insulin plasma concentrations in fasted children. J Pediatr 101:51–56

Jia X, Brown JC, Ma P et al (1995) Effects of glucose-dependent insulinotropic polypeptide and glucagon-like peptide-I-(7-36) on insulin secretion. Am J Phys 268:E645–E651

Kahveci H, Laloglu F, Kilic O, Ciftel M, Kara M, Laloglu E, Yildirim A, Orbak Z, Ertekin V, Cesur Y (2015) Fasting and postprandial glucose, insulin, leptin, and ghrelin values in preterm babies and their mothers: relationships among their levels, foetal growth, and neonatal anthropometry. J Matern Fetal Neonatal Med 28(8):916–921

Kalies H, Heinrich J, Borte N et al (2005) The effect of breastfeeding on weight gain in infants: results of a birth cohort study. Eur J Med Res 10:36–42

Kasa-Vubu JZ, Rosenthal A, Murdock EG, Welch KB (2007) Impact of fatness, fitness, and ethnicity on the relationship of nocturnal ghrelin to 24-hour luteinizing hormone concentrations in adolescent girls. J Clin Endocrinol Metab 92:3246–3252

Kawamata R, Suzuki Y, Yada Y et al (2014) Gut hormone profiles in preterm and term infants during the first 2 months of life. J Pediatr Endocrinol Metab 27(7–8):717–723

Kawamata R, Suzuki Y, Yada Y et al (2015) Gut hormones of preterm infants with abdominal symptoms and hypothyroxinemia. Pediatr Int 57:614–619

Kim SJ, Nian C, Karunakaran S et al (2012) GIP-overexpressing mice demonstrate reduced diet-induced obesity and steatosis, and improved glucose homeostasis. PLoS One 7:e40156

King KC, Oliven A, Kalhan SC (1989) Functional enteroinsular axis in full-term newborn infants. Pediatr Res 25:490–495

Knip M, Kaapa P, Koivisto M (1993) Hormonal enteroinsular axis in newborn infants of insulin-treated diabetic mothers. J Clin Endocrinol Metab 77:1340–1344

Kojima M, Kangawa K (2005) Ghrelin: structure and function. Physiol Rev 85:495–522

Konturek SJ, Konturek JW, Pawlik T, Brzozowski T (2004) Brain-gut axis and its role in the control of food intake. J Physiol Pharmacol 55:137–154

Lambeir AM, Durinx C, Scharpe S, De Meester I (2003) Dipeptidyl-peptidase IV from bench to bedside: an update on structural properties, functions, and clinical aspects of the enzyme DPP IV. Crit Rev Clin Lab Sci 40:209–294

Lanyi E, Varnagy A, Kovacs KA et al (2008) Ghrelin and acyl ghrelin in preterm infants and maternal blood: relationship with endocrine and anthropometric measures. Eur J Endocrinol 158:27–33

Lebenthal A, Lebenthal E (1999) The ontogeny of the small intestinal epithelium. JPEN J Parenter Enteral Nutr 23:S3–S6

Leite-Moreira AF, Soares JB (2007) Physiological, pathological and potential therapeutic roles of ghrelin. Drug Discov Today 12:276–288

Lothe L, Ivarsson SA, Lindberg T (1987) Motilin, vasoactive intestinal peptide and gastrin in infantile colic. Acta Paediatr Scand 76:316–320

Lu M, Wheeler MB, Leng XH, Boyd AE III (1993) Stimulation of insulin secretion and insulin gene expression by gastric inhibitory polypeptide. Trans Assoc Am Phys 106:42–53

Lucas A, Sarson DL, Bloom SR, Aynsley-Green A (1980) Developmental aspects of gastric inhibitory polypeptide (GIP) and its possible role in the enteroinsular axis in neonates. Acta Paediatr Scand 69:321–325

Mahmoud EL, Benirschke K, Vaucher YE, Poitras P (1988) Motilin levels in term neonates who have passed meconium prior to birth. J Pediatr Gastroenterol Nutr 7:95–99

Marchini G, Linden A (1992) Cholecystokinin, a satiety signal in newborn infants? J Dev Physiol 17:215–219

Martin GR, Beck PL, Sigalet DL (2006) Gut hormones, and short bowel syndrome: the enigmatic role of glucagon-like peptide-2 in the regulation of intestinal adaptation. World J Gastroenterol 12:4117–4129

Mechanick JI, Kushner RF, Sugerman HJ et al (2008) American Association of Clinical Endocrinologists, the obesity Society, and American Society for Metabolic & Bariatric Surgery Medical guidelines for clinical practice for the perioperative nutritional, metabolic, and nonsurgical support of the bariatric surgery patient. Endocr Pract 14(Suppl 1):1–83

Misra M, Miller KK, Cord J et al (2007) Relationships between serum adipokines, insulin levels, and bone density in girls with anorexia nervosa. J Clin Endocrinol Metab 92:2046–2052

Misra M, Prabhakaran R, Miller KK et al (2008) Prognostic indicators of changes in bone density measures in adolescent girls with anorexia nervosa-II. J Clin Endocrinol Metab 93:1292–1297

Mitrovic O, Cokic V, Dikic D et al (2014) Ghrelin receptors in human gastrointestinal tract during prenatal and early postnatal development. Peptides 57:1–11

Moran TH (2000) Cholecystokinin and satiety: current perspectives. Nutrition 16:858–865

Müller TD, Nogueiras R, Andermann ML et al (2015) Ghrelin. Mol Metab 4:437–460

Mulvihill SJ, Stone MM, Debas HT, Fonkalsrud EW (1985) The role of amniotic fluid in foetal nutrition. J Pediatr Surg 20:668–672

Nagasaki H, Ohta T (2015) Extra-uterine growth and adipocytokines in appropriate-for-gestational-age preterm infants. Pediatr Int. https://doi.org/10.1111/ped.12896

Nagata E, Nakagawa Y, Yamaguchi R et al (2011) Altered gene expressions of ghrelin, PYY, and CCK in the gastrointestinal tract of the hyperphagic intrauterine growth restriction rat offspring. Horm Metab Res 43(3):178–182

Naitoh R, Miyawaki K, Harada N et al (2008) Inhibition of GIP signaling modulates adiponectin levels under high-fat diet in mice. Biochem Biophys Res Commun 376:21–25

Nakahara T, Harada T, Yasuhara D et al (2008) Plasma obestatin concentrations are negatively correlated with body mass index, insulin resistance index, and plasma leptin concentrations in obesity and anorexia nervosa. Biol Psychiatry 64:252–255

Naslund E, Barkeling B, King N et al (1999) Energy intake and appetite are suppressed by glucagon-like peptide-1 (GLP-1) in obese men. Int J Obes Relat Metab Disord 23:304–311

Neary NM, Goldstone AP, Bloom SR (2004) Appetite regulation: from the gut to the hypothalamus. Clin Endocrinol 60:153–160

Nishikubo T, Yamakawa A, Kamitsuji H et al (2005) Identification of the motilin cells in duodenal epithelium of premature infants. Pediatr Int 47(3):248–251

O'Mahony SM, Felice VD, Nally K et al (2014) Disturbance of the gut microbiota in early-life selectively affects visceral pain in adulthood without impacting cognitive or anxiety-related behaviors in male rats. Neuroscience 277:885–901

Ozaki T, Mohammad S, Morioka E et al (2013) Infant satiety depends on transient expression of cholecysto kinin-1 receptors on ependymal cells lining the third ventricle in mice. J Physiol 591(5):1295–1312

Ozer EA, Holst JJ, Duman N et al (2009) The relationship between glucagon-like peptide 2 and feeding intolerance in preterm infants. J Trop Pediatr 55:276–277

Padidela R, Patterson M, Sharief N et al (2009) Elevated basal and post-feed glucagon-like peptide 1 (GLP-1) concentrations in the neonatal period. Eur J Endocrinol 160:53–58

Paik KH, Choe YH, Park WH et al (2006) Suppression of acylated ghrelin during oral glucose tolerance test is correlated with whole-body insulin sensitivity in children with Prader-Willi syndrome. J Clin Endocrinol Metab 91:1876–1881

Pais R, Gribble FM, Reimann F (2016) Stimulation of incretin secreting cells. Ther Adv Endocrinol Metab 7:24–42

Perala MM, Kajantie E, Valsta LM et al (2013) Early growth and postprandial appetite regulatory hormone responses. Br J Nutr 110:1591–1600

Persaud SJ, Bewick GA (2014) Peptide YY: more than just an appetite regulator. Diabetologia 57:1762–1769

Pocai A (2013) Action and therapeutic potential of oxyntomodulin. Mol Metab 3:241–251

Poitras P, Peeters TL (2008) Motilin. Curr Opin Endocrinol Diabetes Obes 15:54–57

Pomerants T, Tillmann V, Jurimae J, Jurimae T (2006) Relationship between ghrelin and anthropometrical, body composition parameters and testosterone levels in boys at different stages of puberty. J Endocrinol Investig 29:962–967

Prodam F, Filigheddu N (2014) Ghrelin gene products in acute and chronic inflammation. Arch Immunol Ther Exp (Warsz) 62(5):369–3684

Prodam F, Me E, Riganti F et al (2006) The nutritional control of ghrelin secretion in humans: the effects of enteral vs. parenteral nutrition. Eur J Nutr 45:399–405

Prodam F, Bellone S, Corneli G et al (2008) Ghrelin: a molecular target for weight regulation, glucose and lipid metabolism. Recent Patents Endocrine Metab Immune Drug Discov 2(3):1–1

Prodam F, Bellone S, Ricotti R et al (2011) Ghrelin regulation in epilepsy. Underlying mechanisms of epilepsy. InTech, Prof. Fatima Shad Kaneez (ed). ISBN:978–953–307-765-9, pp 151–180. Available from: http://www.intechopen.com/books/underlying-mechanisms-ofepilepsy/ghrelin-regulation-in-epilepsy

Prodam F, Monzani A, Ricotti R et al (2014a) Systematic review of ghrelin response to food intake in pediatric age, from neonates to adolescents. J Clin Endocrinol Metab 99(5):1556–1568

Prodam F, Cadario F, Bellone S et al (2014b) Obestatin levels are associated with C-peptide and antiinsulin antibodies at the onset, whereas unacylated and acylated ghrelin levels are not predictive of long-term metabolic control in children with type 1 diabetes. J Clin Endocrinol Metab 99(4):E599–E607

Qader SS, Hakanson R, Rehfeld JF et al (2008) Proghrelin-derived peptides influence the secretion of insulin, glucagon, pancreatic polypeptide and somatostatin: a study on isolated islets from mouse and rat pancreas. Regul Pept 146:230–237

Ranganath LR (2008a) The entero-insular axis: implications for human metabolism. Clin Chem Lab Med 46:43–56

Ranganath LR (2008b) Incretins: pathophysiological and therapeutic implications of glucose-dependent insulinotropic polypeptide and glucagon-like peptide-1. J Clin Pathol 61:401–409

Savino F, Fissore MF, Grassino EC et al (2005) Ghrelin, leptin and IGF-I levels in breast-fed and formula-fed infants in the first years of life. Acta Paediatr 94:531–537

Savino F, Grassino EC, Fissore MF et al (2006a) Ghrelin, motilin, insulin concentration in healthy infants in the first months of life: relation to fasting time and anthropometry. Clin Endocrinol 65:158–162

Savino F, Grassino EC, Guidi C et al (2006b) Ghrelin and motilin concentration in colicky infants. Acta Paediatr 95:738–741

Savino F, Lupica MM, Liguori SA et al (2012a) Ghrelin and feeding behaviour in preterm infants. Early Hum Dev 88:S51–S55

Savino F, Benetti S, Lupica MM et al (2012b) Ghrelin and obestatin in infants, lactating mothers and breast milk. Horm Res Paediatr 78(5–6):297–303

Schmidt PT, Naslund E, Gryback P et al (2003) Peripheral administration of GLP-2 to humans has no effect on gastric emptying or satiety. Regul Pept 116:21–25

Sharman-Koendjbiharie M, Hopman WP, Piena-Spoel M et al (2002) Gut hormones in preterm infants with necrotizing enterocolitis during starvation and reintroduction of enteral nutrition. J Pediatr Gastroenterol Nutr 35:674–679

Shimizu T, Kitamura T, Yoshikawa N et al (2007) Plasma levels of active ghrelin until 8 weeks after birth in preterm infants: relationship with anthropometric and biochemical measures. Arch Dis Child Fetal Neonatal Ed 92:F291–F292

Shoji H, Watanabe A, Ikeda N et al (2016) Influence of gestational age on serum incretin levels in preterm infants. J Dev Orig Health Dis 25:1–4

Shulman DI, Kanarek K (1993) Gastrin, motilin, insulin, and insulin-like growth factor-I concentrations in very-low-birth-weight infants receiving enteral or parenteral nutrition. JPEN J Parenter Enteral Nutr 17:130–133

Siahanidou T, Mandyla H, Vounatsou M et al (2005) Circulating peptide YY concentrations are higher in preterm than full-term infants and correlate negatively with body weight and positively with serum ghrelin concentrations. Clin Chem 51:2131–2137

Siahanidou T, Mandyla H, Militsi H et al (2007) Peptide YY (3-36) represents a high percentage of total PYY immunoreactivity in preterm and full-term infants and correlates independently with markers of adiposity and serum ghrelin concentrations. Pediatr Res 62:200–203

Siahanidou T, Margeli A, Tsirogianni C et al (2015) Elevated circulating ghrelin, but not peptide YY(3-36) levels, in term neonates with infection. Clin Chem Lab Med 53(11):1815–1824

Sigalet DL, Martin G, Meddings J et al (2004) GLP-2 levels in infants with intestinal dysfunction. Pediatr Res 56:371–376

Sigalet DL, Brindle M, Boctor D et al (2015) A safety and dosing study of glucagon-like peptide 2 in children with intestinal failure. JPEN J Parenter Enteral Nutr. 56(3):371–376

Skow MA, Bergmann NC, Knop FK (2016) Diabetes and obesity treatment based on dual incretin receptor activation – "twincretins". Diabetes Obes Metab 18 (9):847–854. https://doi.org/10.1111/dom.12685

Soriano-Guillen L, Barrios V, Chowen JA et al (2004) Ghrelin levels from foetal life through early adulthood: relationship with endocrine and metabolic and anthropometric measures. J Pediatr 144:30–35

Spreckley E, Murphy KG (2015) The L-Cell in nutritional sensing and the regulation of appetite. Front Nutr 2:23

Stadlbauer U, Woods SC, Langhans W, Meyer U (2015) PYY3–36: beyond food intake. Front Neuroendocrinol 38:1–11

Stock S, Leichner P, Wong AC et al (2005) Ghrelin, peptide YY, glucose-dependent insulinotropic polypeptide, and hunger responses to a mixed meal in anorexic, obese, and control female adolescents. J Clin Endocrinol Metab 90:2161–2168

Stoll B, Puiman PJ, Cui L et al (2012) Continuous parenteral and enteral nutrition induces metabolic dysfunction in neonatal pigs. JPEN J Parenter Enteral Nutr 36:538–550

Tang SQ, Jiang QY, Zhang YL et al (2008) Obestatin: its physicochemical characteristics and physiological functions. Peptides 29:639–645

Tang-Christensen M, Larsen PJ, Thulesen J et al (2000) The proglucagon-derived peptide, glucagon-like peptide-2, is a neurotransmitter involved in the regulation of food intake. Nat Med 6:802–807

Teitelbaum DH, Han-Markey T, Drongowski RA et al (1997) Use of cholecystokinin to prevent the development of parenteral nutrition-associated cholestasis. JPEN J Parenter Enteral Nutr 21:100–103

Thompson NM, Gill DA, Davies R et al (2004) Ghrelin and des-octanoyl ghrelin promote adipogenesis directly in vivo by a mechanism independent of the type 1a growth hormone secretagogue receptor. Endocrinology 145:234–242

Tomasetto C, Karam SM, Ribieras S et al (2000) Identification and characterization of a novel gastric peptide hormone: the motilin-related peptide. Gastroenterology 119:395–405

Tornhage CJ, Serenius F, Uvnas-Moberg K, Lindberg T (1995) Plasma somatostatin and cholecystokinin levels in preterm infants and their mothers at birth. Pediatr Res 37:771–776

Tornhage CJ, Serenius F, Uvnas-Moberg K, Lindberg T (1996) Plasma somatostatin and cholecystokinin levels in preterm infants during the first day of life. Biol Neonate 70:311–321

Tornhage CJ, Serenius F, Uvnas-Moberg K, Lindberg T (1998) Plasma somatostatin and cholecystokinin levels in preterm infants during kangaroo care with and without nasogastric tube-feeding. J Pediatr Endocrinol Metab 11:645–651

Uvnas-Moberg K, Marchini G, Winberg J (1993) Plasma cholecystokinin concentrations after breast feeding in healthy 4 day old infants. Arch Dis Child 68:46–48

Valderas JP, Padilla O, Solari S et al (2014) Feeding and bone turnover in gastric bypass. J Clin Endocrinol Metab 99:491–497

Valsamakis G, Papatheodorou DC, Naouma A et al (2014) Neonatal birthwaist is positively predicted by second trimester maternal active ghrelin, a pro-appetite hormone, and negatively associated with third trimester maternal leptin, a pro-satiety hormone. Early Hum Dev 90:487–492

Van den Hoek AM, Heijboer AC, Corssmit EP et al (2004) PYY3-36 reinforces insulin action on glucose disposal in mice fed a high-fat diet. Diabetes 53:1949–1952

Verdich C, Flint A, Gutzwiller JP et al (2001) A meta-analysis of the effect of glucagon-like peptide-1 (7-36) amide on ad libitum energy intake in humans. J Clin Endocrinol Metab 86:4382–4389

Vilsboll T, Krarup T, Sonne J et al (2003) Incretin secretion in relation to meal size and body weight in healthy subjects and people with type 1 and type 2 diabetes mellitus. J Clin Endocrinol Metab 88:2706–2713

Wagner CL (2002) Amniotic fluid and human milk: a continuum of effect? J Pediatr Gastroenterol Nutr 34:513–514

Warchoł M, Krauss H, Wojciechowska M et al (2014) The role of ghrelin, leptin and insulin in foetal development. Ann Agri Env Med 21(2):349–352

West DB, Greenwood MR, Marshall KA, Woods SC (1987) Lithium chloride, cholecystokinin and meal patterns: evidence that cholecystokinin suppresses meal size in rats without causing malaise. Appetite 8:221–227

Whatmore AJ, Hall CM, Jones J et al (2003) Ghrelin concentrations in healthy children and adolescents. Clin Endocrinol 59:649–654

Wiedmer P, Nogueiras R, Broglio F et al (2007) Ghrelin, obesity and diabetes. Nat Clin Pract Endocrinol Metab 3:705–712

Wierup N, Bjorkqvist M, Westrom B et al (2007) Ghrelin and motilin are cosecreted from a prominent endocrine cell population in the small intestine. J Clin Endocrinol Metab 92:3573–3581

Wojcicki JM (2012) Peptide YY in children: a review. J Pediatr Endocrinol Metab 25(3–4):227–232

Woods SC (2004) Gastrointestinal satiety signals I. An overview of gastrointestinal signals that influence food intake. Am J Physiol Gastrointest Liver Physiol 286:G7–13

Wortley KE, Anderson KD, Garcia K et al (2004) Genetic deletion of ghrelin does not decrease food intake but influences metabolic fuel preference. Proc Natl Acad Sci U S A 101:8227–8232

Wortley KE, del Rincon JP, Murray JD et al (2005) Absence of ghrelin protects against early-onset obesity. J Clin Invest 115:3573–3578

Wynne K, Park AJ, Small CJ et al (2006) Oxyntomodulin increases energy expenditure in addition to decreasing energy intake in overweight and obese humans: a randomised controlled trial. Int J Obes(Lond) 30: 1729–1736

Xiao Q, Boushey RP, Drucker DJ, Brubaker PL (1999) Secretion of the intestinotropic hormone glucagon-like peptide 2 is differentially regulated by nutrients in humans. Gastroenterology 117:99–105

Xiao C, Dash S, Morgantini C et al (2015) Gut peptides are novel regulators of intestinal lipoprotein secretion: experimental and pharmacological manipulation of lipoprotein metabolism. Diabetes 64:2310–2318

Yang J, Brown MS, Liang G et al (2008) Identification of the acyltransferase that octanoylates ghrelin, an appetite-stimulating peptide hormone. Cell 132: 387–396

Yokota I, Kitamura S, Hosoda H et al (2005) Concentration of the n-octanoylated active form of ghrelin in foetal and neonatal circulation. Endocr J 52:271–276

Yoshikawa H, Miyata I, Eto Y (2006) Serum glucagon-like peptide-2 levels in neonates: comparison between extremely low-birthweight infants and normal-term infants. Pediatr Int 48:464–469

Zhang W, Zhao L, Lin TR et al (2004) Inhibition of adipogenesis by ghrelin. Mol Biol Cell 15:2484–2491

Zhang JV, Ren PG, Avsian-Kretchmer O et al (2005) Obestatin, a peptide encoded by the ghrelin gene, opposes ghrelin's effects on food intake. Science 310:996–999

Zhang S, Zhai G, Zhang J et al (2014) Ghrelin and obestatin plasma levels and ghrelin/obestatin prepropeptide gene polymorphisms in small for gestational age infants. J Int Med Res 42(6):1232–1242

Zou CC, Liang L, Wang CL, Fu JF, Zhao ZY (2009) The change in ghrelin and obestatin levels in obese children after weight reduction. Acta Paediatr 98:159–165

Zwirska-Korczala K, Adamczyk-Sowa M, Sowa P et al (2007) Role of leptin, ghrelin, angiotensin II and orexins in 3 T3 L1 preadipocyte cells proliferation and oxidative metabolism. J Physiol Pharmacol 58 (Suppl 1):53–64

Human Milk and Formulas for Neonatal Nutrition

36

Riccardo Davanzo, Jenny Bua, and Laura Travan

Contents

R. Davanzo (✉)
Department of Mother and Child Health, Madonna delle Grazie Hospital, Matera, Italy
e-mail: riccardo.davanzo@gmail.com

J. Bua · L. Travan
Division of Neonatology, Institute for Maternal and Child Health IRCCS 'Burlo Garofolo', Trieste, Italy
e-mail: jennybua@gmail.com; lauratravan@gmail.com

G. Buonocore et al. (eds.), *Neonatology*,
https://doi.org/10.1007/978-3-319-29489-6_185

Abstract

Human milk is a unique highly individualized nutritional liquid, with multiple biological effects. Extensive research has demonstrated health benefits for both the nursed infant and her/his mother. Moreover, breastfeeding carries social, economic, and environmental benefits. Consequently, International Health Agencies and Pediatric Scientific Societies recommend early initiation of breastfeeding, exclusive breastfeeding for around 6 months, and continuing breastfeeding after the start of weaning.

Breastfeeding should be promoted among the population of healthy term infants as well as among the NICU population. Effective promotion of breastfeeding requires adequate knowledge of the physiology of lactation, of the factors facilitating and constraining the beginning and the continuation of breastfeeding, and of the true contraindications to breastfeed.

36.1 Salient Points

- Breastfeeding is proven to be beneficial for the nursed infant and the mother.
- Pediatricians should be trained to support breastfeeding.
- There are very few true contraindications to breastfeeding such as HIV infection or few drugs.
- Breastfeeding should be supported with efficient and clearly stated hospital-based strategies.
- Breast milk is the optimal form of nutrition in the preterm babies.
- Besides the other benefits, kangaroo mother care (KMC) has been demonstrated to be a galactagogue.
- When breastfeeding is not achievable or desirable, cow milk formula should be started.
- While preterm formulas are recommended for VLBW preterm babies, evidence on post-discharge formulas is still controversial.

36.2 The Uniqueness of Human milk

Human milk is a species- and individual-specific nutritional and biological liquid. Mature human milk contains 4 g/dL fat, 0.9 g/dL protein, 7 g/dL carbohydrate calculated as lactose, and 0.2 g/dL mineral constituents expressed as ash. Its energy content is around 67 kcal/dl. As 87% of human milk is water, the exclusively breastfed infant does not need extra water. Despite individual variation in maternal nutrition, the macronutrient content in human milk, as a whole, appears to be sufficient to ensure adequate infant nutrition.

About 50% of the energy in mature human milk is derived from *fat*, which is present as globules; it is essential for growth and development, particularly of the brain and the retina. The fat content (around 4 g/dL in both human and bovine milk) increases by nearly 10% during the second semester of lactation, during afternoon and evening as compared to night and morning, and during the course of each breastfeed. In fact, the last milk of a feed (hind milk) contains three times the fat concentration in the initial milk of a feed (foremilk). *Triglycerides* constitute more than 98% of human milk lipids, while the remaining 2% are composed of cholesterol and phospholipids. Each triglyceride contains three fatty acids derived from endogenous synthesis in the lactocytes of the mammary glands or from maternal plasma. Most triglycerides are structured in long-chain fatty acids plus several medium-chain fatty acids. Human milk fat has a high content of palmitic and oleic acids. The former is heavily concentrated in the 2-position of triglycerides and the latter in the 1- and 3-positions, which facilitate gut absorption.

Human milk also contains 10–15 mg/dL *cholesterol*. Though its cholesterol content is much higher than in infant formula, cholesterol intake during early infancy seems beneficial. In fact, adults who were breastfed in infancy have lower cholesterol levels than those who were bottle-fed, supporting the theory that activation of homeostatic mechanisms in early infancy downregulates cholesterogenesis.

Long-chain polyunsaturated fatty acids (*LC- PUFAs*) make up 15% (0.6 g/dL) of the fat content in human milk. Arachidonic (ARA) and docosahexaenoic (DHA) acids are the most abundant LC-PUFAs in the brain, where they constitute important components of neuronal membranes and play a role in neural development. Moreover, DHA is also a component of photoreceptors and is implicated in visual acuity. DHA is one of the most variable fatty acids in human milk, its concentration being directly influenced by the amount of DHA in the mother's diet. The lowest values are found in milk from vegan mothers and generally with little or no preformed sources of DHA (i.e., fatty fish).

Protein content is markedly higher in colostrum than in mature milk and higher in preterm than in term milk. Human milk contains two types of proteins: casein (beta and kappa) (about 40%) and whey proteins (about 60%) which protect against infection. The principal whey proteins of human milk are alpha-lactalbumin, lactoferrin, immunoglobulins (particularly IgA), lysozyme, and serum albumin. In the whey fraction, *enzymes* (particularly, bile salt-stimulated lipase, amylase, and protease) are present in sufficient quantities to aid infants in digestion and absorption. About 25% of the total nitrogen content of human milk is composed of nonprotein compounds, including urea, uric acid, creatine, creatinine, a large variety of free amino acids (predominantly glutamic acid, glutamine, alanine, and taurine), and nucleotides. Moreover, *nucleotides* and their related metabolic products (nucleosides) play an essential role in cell replication, particularly in rapidly growing infants. Nucleotides have a beneficial effect on gut microflora: they reduce the number of episodes of diarrhea, enhance immune function, increase natural killer cell activity, and stimulate antibody response to immunization with *Haemophilus influenzae* vaccine, diphtheria toxoid, and oral polio vaccine. Nucleotides can be synthesized de novo or recycled through salvage pathways; however, the capacity for nucleotide synthesis in the neonate is low. It is estimated that an infant consuming human milk as a primary nutrition source will ingest 1.4–2.1 mg of nucleotide nitrogen per day.

Carbohydrate content is lower in colostrum (5.8 g/dL) than in mature milk. The principal sugar of human milk is *lactose*, a disaccharide that promotes the gut growth of bifidobacteria and that, as compared to glucose, has a more stabilizing effect on plasma glycemia. Other significant carbohydrates are human milk *oligosaccharides* (HMOs, approximately 1 g/dL). The more than 100 *HMOs* so far identified are not digested by the infant gut and so make up part of the intestinal flora. They help to prevent infectious diseases by acting as decoy receptors at receptor sites on the intestinal, urinary, and respiratory mucosa where they block the attachment of disease-causing pathogens. HMOs may also alter immune cell responses, which may benefit the infant.

Table 1 Bioactive substances in human milk (Modified from Ballard and Morrow 2013)

Component	Function
Cells	
Macrophages	Protect against infection
Stem cells	Potential regeneration
Immunoglobulins	Inhibit pathogens; activate phagocytosis and complement
Cytokines (IL, IFN-gamma, TGF-beta, TNF-alpha) and cytokine inhibitors	Modulate inflammatory responses (pro- and anti-inflammatory)
Chemokines	
G-CSF	Granulocyte colony-stimulating factor, a trophic intestinal factor
MIF	Macrophage migratory inhibitory factor
Growth factors	
EGF	Stimulate epithelial cell proliferation
HB-EGF (heparin binding-EGF)	Protect against hypoxia and ischemia
VEGF	Vascular endothelial growth factor promoting angiogenesis
NGF	Stimulate neuron growth angiogenesis
IGF	Stimulate growth and maturation
Erythropoietin	Stimulate growth; increase formation of red blood cells and hemoglobin
Hormones	
Calcitonin	Development of enteric hormones
Somatostatin	Regulate gastric epithelial growth
Adiponectin	Reduce weight
Ghrelin	Regulate energy conversion and appetite
Leptin	Made by adipose cells that helps to regulate energy balance by inhibiting hunger
Antimicrobial factors	
Lactadherin	Antiviral
Lactoferrin	Binding and gut transport of iron ions
	Broad-spectrum antimicrobial and immunomodulatory milk glycoprotein
	Promote bifidus flora
Oligosaccharides (prebiotics)	Stimulate beneficial gut microbiome
	Block attachment of pathogens to mucosa
	Anti-inflammatory action
Mucins	Block infection by viruses and bacteria

Human milk also provides a source of various different types of micronutrients, including minerals, vitamins, and hormones.

Iron content appears to be adequate (0.3–0.5 mg/L) even in the milk produced by iron-deficient or anemic mothers, although breastfeeding may worsen maternal iron deficiency. The iron bioavailability in human milk is higher than in infant formulas (nearly 30% vs. <20%).

Similar to intracellular fluids, the *potassium* level in human milk is much higher than *sodium* (57 mEq/L vs. 7 mEq/L). In contrast, the sodium level in cow milk (22 mEq/L) is threefold that in human milk, accounting for the well-known higher risk of hypernatremic dehydration in newborns with diarrhea.

The *calcium* and *phosphorus* content of human milk is 35 mg/dL and 57 mg/dL, respectively. The Ca/P ratio (2:1) facilitates the high bioavailability of calcium from human milk.

Regardless of maternal diet, *vitamin K* is low in human milk; therefore, intramuscular injection at birth and/or repeated oral administration of vitamin K is recommended to prevent both early and late vitamin K deficiency bleeding (VKDB). The only infants who are not fully protected against late VKDB by repeated oral doses of vitamin K are those with yet unrecognized malabsorption/cholestasis (McNinch et al. 2007).

The mean level of *vitamin D* in human milk in healthy lactating women, unsupplemented or supplemented, ranges from 10 to 80 IU/L. The prevalence of serum 25(OH)D <25–37.5 nmol/L in exclusively breastfed infants is high, particularly in those born to mothers with low exposure to sunshine, hence warranting postnatal vitamin D supplementation in breastfed infants (400 IU/day) to prevent osteopenia and/or overt rickets. Actually, the cutoff values of serum 25(OH)D levels

<25–37.5 nmol/L (<10–12 μg/L) reported in most studies are very conservative, because the current recommended cutoff value for vitamin D deficiency in children is defined as serum 25(OH) D <50 nmol/L (<20 μg/L).

Human milk also contains many hundreds of *bioactive substances* (Table 1) (Ballard and Morrow 2013) with multiple nutritional, biological, and immunological roles in protecting against infection and inflammation and to promote immune maturation, organ development, and healthy microbial colonization.

The passage from nutrition with mother's milk to formula feeding has long been recognized as having short- and long-term implications for both the nursed infant and the mother. Formula-fed individuals are more prone to a wide range of diseases (infectious, immunomediated, noncommunicable, cancer) (Table 2) (Department of Health and Human Services 2011) leading to increased cost for ambulatory and hospital care of formula-fed infants (Cattaneo et al. 2006) and to slightly impaired cognitive development (von Stumm and Plomin 2015) and poorer social achievement (Sacker et al. 2013). On their part, women formula feeding their babies are at increased risk of postpartum hemorrhage, breast, and ovarian cancer (Luan et al. 2013) and will lack the same empowerment related to their successful nursing role within their family and society.

Table 2 Benefits of breastfeeding and nutrition with human milk, expressed as excess risk in different health outcomes for both the infant and the mother (Modified from US Department of Health and Human Services 2011)

Outcome	Excess risk (%)
Acute ear infection (otitis media)	100
Eczema (atopic dermatitis)	47
Diarrhea and vomiting (gastrointestinal infection)	178
Hospitalization for lower respiratory tract disease in the first year	257
Asthma, with family history	67
Asthma, no family history	35
Childhood obesity	32
Type 2 diabetes mellitus	64
Acute lymphocytic leukemia	23
Acute myelogenous leukemia	18
Sudden infant death syndrome	56
Among preterm infants	
Necrotizing enterocolitis	138
Among mothers	
Breast cancer	4
Ovarian cancer	27

36.3 Recommendations on Infant Feeding

In view of the demonstrated benefits of breastfeeding, international health agencies (World Health Organization [WHO] (http://www.who.int/mediacentre/factsheets/fs342/en/) and the United Nations Children's Fund [UNICEF]), governmental entities (Centers for Disease Control and Prevention 2013), and professional pediatric societies (Johnston et al. 2012; Davanzo et al. 2015a) strongly make the followingfeeding recommendations: (1) exclusive breastfeeding from the very beginning, (2) until about 6 months of age, (3) continuing during weaning, and (4) possibly keeping some occasional breastfeeding beyond 1–2 years of life.

36.4 From the Physiology of Lactation to Breastfeeding Management

36.4.1 Lactogenesis

Colostrum, the first breast milk, is already produced during late pregnancy under the influence of *prolactin* (*PRL*) and human placental lactogen (HPL) (stage I of lactation or *lactogenesis I*). It is normally available for the breastfeeding newborn from childbirth until the milk comes in (stage II of lactation or *lactogenesis II*), usually around 40–48 h postpartum. The decrease in maternal serum progesterone levels after delivery of the placenta triggers the shift in production from limited amounts of colostrum (the daily intake by newborn infants is usually 10–100 mL/day) to the sharply increased amounts of mature human milk over the following days and weeks. Although lactogenesis II is an automatic phenomenon, it can be anticipated nearly 12 h in pluriparous women or by the active and frequent sucking of a newborn properly latched on to the breast. Lactogenesis II may be postponed beyond

72 h after childbirth due to maternal conditions (obesity, diabetes, prolonged bed rest, acute illness at childbirth), mode of delivery (cesarean versus vaginal), and obstetric procedures (vacuum or forceps extraction for assisted vaginal delivery, induction of labor) (De Bortoli and Amir 2016).

36.4.2 From Calibration to Maintenance

The supply of breast milk subsequent to lactogenesis II follows the demand of the newborn at the breast. This cycle from stimulation to secretion is called the prolactin (PRL) reflex or the *milk secretion reflex*. The more the baby sucks at the breast, the larger the volume of milk produced. A proper, efficient suck at the breast determines PRL release and breast milk production by lactocytes in the subsequent hours. In other words, sucking at the breast is not only the way the newborn obtains breast milk immediately but is also an investment for the following feeds.

Oxytocin (*OXT*), a hormone produced by the posterior pituitary gland, is responsible for contraction of the myoepithelium around the mammary acini and ejection of the milk. Because OXT is produced in response to stimulation of the nipple by sucking, as well as by the thought, sight, or sound of the baby, it may activate breast milk ejection even before the baby gets to the breast. Furthermore, because OXT release is affected by the mother's emotions, a relaxed and confident attitude helps elicit this *milk ejection reflex*. On the other hand, psychological distress, pain (due to stitches, hemorrhoids, nipple fissures, etc.), and lack of confidence hinder milk flow. This underlines the importance of having a supportive environment and empathetic health professionals to reassure the mother and help her gain confidence so that she can successfully breastfeed. The milk intake by the nursing newborn during a single breastfeed depends not only on the ability of the baby to suck efficiently but also on the contribution of the letdown reflex in the mother. During a single breastfeed, one or more ejections of milk mediated by OXT may occur. Two subsequent ejections are separated by an interval of 2–3 min due to the refractory period of the myoepithelial cells.

The supply of breast milk progressively increases during the first weeks postpartum (*calibration phase*) and reaches an average production of around 700 mL/day at 6–8 weeks postpartum. The secretion of PRL from the anterior pituitary gland in response to sucking is not per se the only determinant of milk production. By this time, PRL secretion is merely a prerequisite for the production of breast milk, while efficient milk removal from the breast is more relevant. If breast milk is not removed, the alveolar level of a peptide hormone known as*feedback inhibitor of lactation* (*FIL*) increases, hindering the ability of PRL to act at the alveolar level, thus limiting or impeding further breast milk production. This is the basis for independent autocrine regulation of lactation in each mammary gland, which explains the differences in the rate of milk production between the two breasts.

36.5 Hospital Practices and the Baby-Friendly Hospital Model

A series of practices have been shown to promote breastfeeding in hospital settings (Table 3) (Holmes et al. 2013). As most of these practices are interdependent, the WHO and the UNICEF have developed a global program for the promotion, protection, and support of breastfeeding in maternity hospitals: the Baby-friendly Hospital Initiative (BFHI) (Cleminson et al. 2015). The BFHI program was launched to credit maternity hospitals that have implemented evidence-based practices that better enable mothers to breastfeed. Becoming baby-friendly compels facilities to examine and modify their long-standing policies and procedures. It requires training, education, and skill building of health professionals.

A maternity facility can be designated "baby-friendly" when it is compliant with the International Code of Marketing of Breast-milk Substitutes (Table 4) and when it has implemented the Ten Steps to support successful breastfeeding (Table 5) (Joint WHO/UNICEF statement 1989). Each of the ten steps has its own evidence base. Current scientific evidence demonstrates that the baby-friendly hospital practices lead to higher breastfeeding rates at hospital discharge and longer duration of breastfeeding. Moreover, a

Table 3 Hospital-based practices and breastfeeding (Holmes et al. 2013; Davanzo et al. 2015a)

Information to expectant mothers. During pregnancy, expectant mothers should be informed about the unique characteristics of breast milk and its benefits for the child and the mother, the correct breastfeeding positions, and the concept of breastfeeding on demand.
Rooming-in. Rooming-in implies that the newborn and the mother should be allowed to remain together in the same room 24 h a day. Separate care for the mother and the infant should to be limited to specific cases and after having informed the mother on the importance of rooming-in.
Breastfeeding on demand. Mothers should be encouraged to breastfeed on demand, without restricting the number and duration of feeds, and to recognize early signs of hunger in newborns other than crying (i.e., open eyes, sucking movements, sucking hands). Breastfeeding on demand helps improve lactation. Health professionals should support mothers during the first days after delivery as some newborns may be especially demanding.
Proper positioning on the breast. How the baby latches on the breast and how he/she sucks should be observed and evaluated using an appropriate scoring system (e.g., LATCH score). Many common problems (e.g., cracked nipples, breast engorgement, infant frustration while breastfeeding, slow growth) can be avoided and in some cases completely solved by improving and correcting the baby's position on the breast.
Formula supplementation. Before giving milk formula to a breastfed newborn, the health conditions of baby and mother should be carefully evaluated; mothers should be adequately informed about whether formula supplementation is absolutely necessary, as it may interfere with breastfeeding.
Pacifiers. The use of pacifiers, soothers, and dummies should be limited as much as possible since it may create nipple confusion or nipple preference, especially if begun before breastfeeding has been fully established. In breastfed babies, pacifiers may be used, given their protective role in the prevention of sudden infant death syndrome (SIDS), but only after the third to fourth week of life
Cup versus *bottle*. Bottles are often used to feed babies with expressed breast milk or formulas. However, sucking on a bottle teat is different from sucking at the breast and may contribute to nipple confusion. The use of small cups may reduce this risk.
Expressed breast milk. Whenever maternal (e.g., intolerable pain during breastfeeding, breast engorgement, return to work) or newborn problems are present (e.g., difficulty to latch on because of prematurity, congenital malformations, or other conditions), mothers should be advised and taught to express their milk.
Breastfeeding and early jaundice. Early physiological jaundice appears between 2 and 7 days of life and resolves within a few days. Jaundice can make a baby sleepy so that he or she sucks less. Early initiation of breastfeeding and frequent breastfeeding reduce the severity of early jaundice. If phototherapy is initiated, breastfeeding on demand should be encouraged, and expressed breast milk may be given to the baby at the end of the breastfeed. Glucose solution does not help; indeed, it may even worsen jaundice and make a baby suckle less at the breast. Routine formula supplementation in babies undergoing phototherapy should be avoided, and formula should be offered only when breast milk production is insufficient. In newborns with bilirubin values close to exchange transfusion, expressed breast milk may be recommended.
Breastfeeding and late jaundice. Late jaundice occurs in about 1 in 200 newborns. It starts or persists after the first week of life and usually peaks during the second or third week. It is most often due to substances in the mother's milk that interfere with the ability of the infant's liver to metabolize bilirubin (so-called breast milk jaundice). Breast milk jaundice does not cause any serious problems, whether treated or not, and it is usually not a reason to stop nursing. Nevertheless, infants still jaundiced at 2–3 weeks of age, particularly if pale stools and/or dark urine are passed or there is suspicion of enlarged liver or spleen, should be assessed and tested (total and direct bilirubin) to rule out cholestasis.
Breastfeeding and newborns at risk of hypoglycemia. Newborns at risk of hypoglycemia (e.g., small for gestational age or born to a mother with diabetes) should undergo glycemic monitoring according to local hospital protocols. If glycemia is normal, preventive formula feeding should be avoided in order not to interfere with exclusive breastfeeding.
Newborns at risk of infection. Newborns at risk of infection (e.g., born to mothers with premature rupture of membranes [PROM], fever, or a positive group B strep [GBS] vaginal/rectal swab) should undergo clinical monitoring without separating them from their mothers; this allows rooming-in and does not interfere with breastfeeding. However, routine clinical monitoring may not be sufficient in babies born to mothers with chorioamnionitis, who may need to receive antibiotics; in such cases, newborns will be admitted to a different ward from their mothers.
Discharge home. When discharging babies home, formula prescription should be given only when necessary. In exclusively breastfed babies who are not yet growing, a follow-up visit with weight check should be scheduled within 24–72 h after discharge.
Support for breastfeeding mothers. Mothers should be informed about the professional help with breastfeeding available in hospitals or healthcare centers. Many mothers stop breastfeeding before they want to because of all sorts of problems, many of which are preventable with good care and support. To help mothers reach their breastfeeding goals, extra support (face to face or by telephone) can be obtained from professionals and/or trained or untrained lay people. Reassurance, information, praise, and practical help are all part of the support that should be tailored to the particular cultural and socioeconomic setting. Health professionals should recognize the effectiveness in supporting breastfeeding provided by *peer counselors* and *lactation consultants* and should be ready to cooperate fruitfully with them.

Table 4 WHO international code of marketing of breast-milk substitutes

Breast milk substitute companies may not:
Promote their products in hospitals, shops, or to the general public
Give free samples to mothers or free/subsidized supplies to hospitals
Give gifts to health workers or mothers
Promote their products to health workers: any information provided by companies must contain only scientific and factual matters
Promote foods or drinks for babies
Give misleading information
Have direct contact with mothers
Infant formula package should:
Show labels in a language understood by the mother
Include a clear health warning
Not use baby pictures idealizing formula feeding

Table 5 The revised Ten Steps to successful breastfeeding (WHO/UNICEF 2018)

1. a) Comply fully with the International Code of Marketing of Breast-milk Substitutes and relevant World Health Assembly resolutions; b) Have a written breastfeeding policy that is routinely communicated to staff and parents; c) Establish ongoing monitoring and data-management systems.
2. Ensure that staff have sufficient knowledge, competence and skills to support breastfeeding
3. Discuss the importance and management of breastfeeding with pregnant women and their families.
4. Facilitate immediate and uninterrupted skin-to-skin contact and support mothers to initiate breastfeeding as soon as possible after birth.
5. Support mothers to initiate and maintain breastfeeding and manage common difficulties.
6. Do not provide breastfed newborns any food or fluids other than breast milk, unless medically indicated.
7. Enable mothers and their infants to remain together and to practice rooming-in 24 hours a day.
8. Support mothers to recognize and respond to their infants' cues for feeding.
9. Counsel mothers on the use and risks of feeding bottles, teats and pacifiers.
10. Coordinate discharge so that parents and their infants have timely access to ongoing support and care.

dose–effect relationship has been documented for the number of steps implemented in a maternity hospital and the success of breastfeeding among the served population of women. Eventually, even partial amelioration of hospital practices is valuable in facilities that are not candidates for a full designation of baby-friendly hospital.

In 2010, the Joint Commission International (JCI) included "exclusive breast milk feeding" in the Perinatal Care Core Measure set as a standardized performance measurement for the assessment of care in maternity hospitals, thus underscoring their responsibility as agents to facilitate the successful start of breastfeeding and recognizing the evidence connecting promotion of breastfeeding as a process of care to improved outcome (https://manual.jointcommission.org/releases/TJC2015A1/PerinatalCare.html).

36.6 Skin-to-Skin Contact and the Prevention of Neonatal Collapse

Prolonged skin-to-skin (STS) contact between the mother and her healthy newborn soon after birth (particularly in the first 2 h postpartum) and continuing in the first days of life is recommended for a variety of reasons: to improve mother–infant bonding, facilitate breastfeeding, aid in colonization of the skin and the gastrointestinal tract of the newborn infant with mother's nonpathogenic microorganisms, and facilitate metabolic, cardiorespiratory, and thermal adaptation to extrauterine life. STS is recommended by step 4 of the Ten Steps of UNICEF-BFHI.

In view of the reported association between STS contact and increased risk of sudden unexpected postnatal collapse (SUPC) (Herlenius and Kuhn 2013) of apparently healthy term infants, STS contact in the delivery room has come under criticism for health safety reasons. In many such cases, the mother is primiparous, very tired, not observed by health professionals when initiating STS contact and breastfeeding, and sometimes distracted by smartphone use.

Surveillance protocols that promote safe mother–infant bonding and early beginning of breastfeeding have recently been proposed while correcting the risk factors for SUPC. The surveillance protocol developed at the Maternal and Child Health Institute of Trieste (Italy) is especially focused on the first 2 h of life (Davanzo et al. 2015b). Interventions include antenatal and

Table 6 Protocol checklist to prevent SUPC in the delivery room. Checks by midwife and/or pediatrician are done at 10, 30, 60, 90, and 120 min of life

Infant positioned with visible and unobstructed mouth and nose
Pink color (skin and mucous membranes)
Normal breathing (no retractions nor grunting nor flaring of the nares)
Normal respiratory rate 30–60 breaths/min
Normal $SpO_2 > 90\%$ (only if deemed necessary)
Subaxillary temperature at 60 and/or 120 min after birth (normal range 36.5–37.5 °C)
Mother never left alone with her infant

early postnatal oral and written information to parents and periodic assessment (position, color, breathing) of the infant (at 10, 30, 60, 90, and 120 min of life) by midwifes and/or pediatrician in the delivery room (Table 6), ensuring that mothers are not left alone with their baby in the first hours after birth, particularly during STS contact and first breastfeeding attempts. Since there is no evidence concerning which interventions may be effective to prevent SUPC, our protocol simply represents a potential best practice.

STS may be not possible in newborns requiring resuscitation or when the mother is not well. The first baby bath can be postponed (up to 6 h of life according to the WHO) in order not to interfere with STS and breastfeeding.

36.7 The First Days of Life and Neonatal Weight Loss

Concern over sufficient milk supply is one of the main reasons why mothers wean their infants from the breast, particularly during the first days after birth when physiological weight loss occurs. On their part, health professionals may sometimes prescribe unnecessary formula supplementation to prevent hypernatremic dehydration and infant malnutrition or simply to deal with a fussy/crying baby or an unconfident mother.

Mothers should be given correct information on the feeding behavior of the healthy newborn in the first days of life. Most babies need frequent feeds, between 2 and 3 h apart or even more often and 8–15 feeds every 24 h, particularly in the period between 24 and 72 h after childbirth, until

Table 7 Clinical approach to neonatal weight loss (Davanzo et al. 2013a)

Percentage of weight loss compared to birth weight		
<8%	8–10%	≥10%
Routine care for the mother–baby couple	Newborn clinical assessment	Newborn clinical assessment
	Assess and improve breastfeeding	Assess and improve breastfeeding
	Consider expressed breast milk	Consider expressed breast milk and/or formula
	Verify mother's capability to respond to the baby's demand	Verify mother's capability to respond to the baby's demand
	Recheck weight 12 h later	Recheck weight 12 h later
		Measure serum sodium level

the breast milk comes in. In the first days postpartum during hospital stay, taking the daily weight of the newborn and recording it on a weight graph are an established method to assess breast milk intake by the newborn and breastfeeding success. Weighing a healthy term newborn before and after feeds in order to estimate the amount of breast milk ingested yields inconsistent and only partial information about the success of breastfeeding, and moreover, it can be stressful for new mothers.

Postnatal weight loss has a nadir at 48–72 h postpartum (Bertini et al. 2015) and results not only from feeding practices and milk intake during the first days postpartum but also from the physiological fall in extracellular fluid after birth and the elimination of parenteral fluids in excess given to the mother intrapartum. The average normal weight loss in the exclusively breastfed newborn is around 6–7% of birth weight, possibly less (≤5%) in formula-fed newborns. The upper limit of a safe weight loss is around 10%. Although some healthy newborns will tolerate a weight loss of up to 12%, the 10% upper safety limit virtually excludes the possible coexistence of dehydration and hypernatremia.

When interpreting early neonatal weight loss, and before prescribing the use of expressed breast milk and/or formula, we should routinely consider three other factors (Table 7)

(Davanzo et al. 2013a): (1) the infant's general condition, including hydration status; (2) the mother's general condition in relation to her capability to meet the newborn's feeding demand; and (3) the assessment of a breastfeed.

Delayed onset of lactation, defined as >72 h after delivery, is a recognized risk factor for excessive weight loss and should be considered when deciding whether to prescribe formula supplementation.

Accurate feeding assessment of infant position and latch on to the breast is essential because it allows to determine the neurobehavioral maturation of the neonate, anticipates proper breast milk intake, and provides information on maternal competence in breastfeeding, all of which need to be considered before hospital discharge after childbirth. Close attention to these factors by healthcare professionals assisting the new mother in these early days and weeks may prevent or resolve many common breastfeeding problems (breast engorgement, nipple fissures, mastitis, poor growth) that arise in the first months after childbirth.

The *LATCH charting system* (Jensen et al. 1994) is a simple, effective tool health professionals can use to assess breastfeeding in maternity wards, to record data and communicate information on breastfeeding to colleagues and to identify mother–infant pairs requiring extra help and follow-up (Tornese et al. 2012). The LATCH system assigns a numerical score (0, 1, or 2) to five key breastfeeding components designated by the letters of the acrostic L.A.T.C.H.: "L" denotes how well the infant latches on to the breast, "A" the amount of audible swallowing noted, "T" the mother's nipple type/condition, "C" the mother's level of comfort, and "H" the amount of help the mother needs to hold her infant to the breast. The total score ranges from 0 to 10, where a higher score indicates a better breastfeeding technique. A LATCH score >7 or higher at subsequent assessments predicts breastfeeding at discharge (Table 8).

In newborns with a neonatal weight loss of 8–10%, special support during breastfeeds is given to both mother and baby. Aneonatal weight loss of >8% in postterm newborns and >10% in term newborns is an indicator of possible hypernatremic dehydration. Serum sodium concentration is measured in newborn infants with a weight loss ≥10% and in those with a weight loss between 8 and 10% and either clinical signs of dehydration or "unconvincing" appearance. Such infants are given at least some expressed breast milk and/or formula, and weight is measured after 12 h.

Healthy newborns can be discharged from hospital at postnatal age ≥36 h. Newborns with a neonatal weight loss >10% are not considered ready for discharge. A postdischarge weight check can be scheduled 24–72 h after discharge depending on (1) percentage of in-hospital weight loss, (2) need for jaundice assessment, and (3) uncertainty about breastfeeding.

36.8 Low Breast Milk Supply

Sooner or later, most mothers feel that they do not have enough milk because the baby cries continuously and does not seem to be satisfied with feeds or because the baby wants to feed very often or the breasts are soft, or attempts to express breast milk are unsuccessful. These are not reliable signs of low breast milk production. If a mother is worried about her milk supply, we must try to understand whether the problem of low milk supply (hypogalactia) is true or simply perceived as such. Two reliable signs that a baby is not getting enough milk are poor weight gain and low urine output.

Weight gain. Each baby follows his/her own pattern of weight gain; accurate assessment relies on recording weight changes on a graph during the first 14 days of life. Birth weight recovery is generally expected within the first 2 weeks of life, although most healthy babies will regain weight by the end of the first week of life. If breastfeeding problems (difficulty latching on, breast engorgement, crackled nipples, etc.) persist beyond the first 2 weeks of life, the upper time limit for birth weight recovery may be extended up to 21 days of life, and if the baby is otherwise healthy, the breastfeeding techniques and patterns and mother–baby interaction are adequate.

If the infant does not gain weight properly, efforts to improve latch on to the breast and the use of expressed breast milk should be advised before suggesting formula supplementation.

Table 8 The LATCH score (Jensen et al. 1994)

	0	1	2
L Latch	Too sleepy or reluctant No latch obtained	Repeated attempts Must hold nipple in mouth Must stimulate to suck	Grasps breast Tongue down and forward Lips flanged Rhythmic suckling
A Audible swallowing	None	A few with stimulation	Spontaneous, intermittent (<24 h old) Spontaneous, frequent (>24 h old)
T Type of nipple	Inverted	Flat	Everted (after stimulation)
C Comfort (breast/nipple)	Engorged Cracked, bleeding, large blisters, or bruises Severe discomfort	Filling, small blisters, or bruises Mother complains of pinching Mild/moderate discomfort	Soft tender intact nipples (no damage)
H	Full assist (staff holds infant at breast)	Minimal assist (i.e., elevate head of bed, place pillows)	No assist from staff
Hold (positioning)		Teach one side, mother does the other	Mother able to position/hold infant
Help		Staff help, mother takes over feeding	

From the recovery of the birth weight onward, exclusively breastfed infants are expected to gain at least 150–200 g per week during the first 3 months of life. A proper reference chart is essential for accurate assessment of infant growth. Old, outdated weight charts are an inadequate reference as they were based predominantly on formula-fed infants. The growth pattern of healthy breastfed infants deviates significantly from bottle-fed infants and is characterized by more rapid growth occurring in the first 3 months of life followed by slower growth over subsequent months. This major difference in growth rate can be due to the different nutrient composition of breast milk and formula, the presence of growth factors in breast milk, and a better control of food intake by the breastfed infant.

The WHO charts (de Onis 2006) (http://www.who.int/childgrowth/standards/en/) report the growth patterns of children who were predominantly breastfed for at least 4 months and still breastfeeding at 12 months, with complementary foods introduced by 6 months of age. The current WHO standards establish growth of the breastfed infant as the norm for growth for the whole population of infants, both breastfed and bottle-fed.

Low urine output. After the breast milk comes in (>72 h postpartum), an exclusively breastfed baby who is passing urine (especially dark yellow) <5 times per day is not getting enough fluid. In infants with low milk intake, but otherwise healthy, the breastfeeding technique or pattern should be evaluated to see whether it can be improved before prescribing an infant formula. In fact, when an infant takes only part of the milk from the breast, milk production increases when the baby takes more or if the breast milk is expressed and given to the baby by bottle or an alternative means (cup or syringe). If the breastfeeding technique or pattern is adequate, other causes of low breast milk production should be considered (Table 9).

Factors affecting the rate of milk production include the frequency and completeness of milk removal and also the mass of tissue actively synthesizing milk. The mammary gland tissue may be reduced in such conditions as congenital hypoplastic breast anomalies, acquired breast hypoplasia following postinfectious scar or radiotherapy, reduction mammoplasty, or partial mastectomy and more often after preterm delivery which misses the mammary gland development of late pregnancy. Low milk production may also occur after prolonged

Table 9 Causes of low breast milk intake (Modified from UNICEF/WHO)

Breastfeeding factors	Maternal psychological factors	Maternal physical factors	Infant-related factors
Common		Uncommon	
Delayed start	Lack of confidence	Contraceptive pill, diuretics	Illness
Feeding at fixed times	Depression	Pregnancy	Prematurity
Infrequent feeds	Worry, stress	Severe malnutrition	Low birth weight
No night feeds	Dislike of breastfeeding	Alcohol use	Some specific congenital malformations
Short feeds	Rejection of baby	Smoking	
Poor attachment		Retained piece of placenta	
Bottles, pacifiers		Pituitary failure (rare)	
Other food or fruit (water, teas)		Poor breast development (very rare)	

reduced drainage (e.g., secondary to mastitis) that leads to apoptosis of lactocytes and results in decreased breast gland functioning. The role of maternal diet in low milk production has been overemphasized. The overall maternal nutrition status (except in severe malnutrition) has little influence on milk quantity and quality. In addition, neither increased nor restricted fluid intake affects the volume of milk produced; however, maternal fever and dehydration (e.g., due to diarrhea or a flu-like syndrome) may limit the fluid available for optimal breast milk production.

In brief, because new mothers are often concerned about their breast milk production, true hypogalactia should be assessed and confirmed according to reliable criteria. Nevertheless, some mothers may not be completely reassured by health professionals that hypogalactia is not true and will decide to begin formula supplementation. Ultimately, the choice of an informed mother should be accepted and supported by health professionals.

36.9 Controversies Surrounding Breastfeeding

36.9.1 Infection

Isolation of infectious agents (particularly viruses) from breast milk is important; in most cases, however, breast milk has not been shown to be a vector of transmission.

36.9.1.1 Hepatitis B Virus (HBV)

There is wide consensus that HBV-positive mothers can safely breastfeed their newborn infants provided that the infant receives active and passive prophylaxis (Chen et al. 2013).

36.9.1.2 Hepatitis C Virus (HCV)

The percentage of HCV-infected mothers that demonstrate milk positivity to HCV varies widely across studies (from 10% to 100%). Viral load is usually very low, and HCV is inactivated by gastric acidity. Moreover, transplacental antibodies are active against HCV, and lactoferrin may also play a role in inactivating the virus. Vertical mother-to-child transmission occurs in about 3–7% of mothers testing positive to HCV-RNA by PCR techniques. Because it has not been documented whether breastfeeding increases the risk of infection, breastfeeding by an HCV-positive mother is allowed (Tosone et al. 2014). No specific prophylaxis is currently recommended, although there is some concern from the Centers for Disease Control and Prevention (CDC) (http://www.cdc.gov/breastfeeding/disease/hepatitis.htm) about possible virus transmission by cracked nipples. Some authors have suggested temporary suspension of breastfeeding and expression of breast milk until bleeding fissures have healed.

36.9.1.3 Cytomegalovirus (CMV)

Between 50% and 85% of women are CMV positive, and CMV can be isolated in 14–69% of their expressed breast milk. While postnatal CMV infection is not a matter of concern in healthy term infants, postnatal CMV transmission via human milk may produce a late-onset sepsis-like syndrome in very low birth weight (BW <1,500 g) preterm infants and possibly also minor longterm neurodevelopmental abnormalities at 4 and 14 years of age (Goelz et al. 2013; Brecht et al. 2015), although these long-term consequences have not been confirmed by recent literature (Gunkel et al. 2018).

Freezing expressed breast milk has been shown to reduce CMV positivity from 40% to 10–15% (Hayashi et al. 2011), but it also lowers the benefits of expressed fresh mother's milk for high-risk preterm newborns.

Holder pasteurization (heating at 62.5 °C for 30 min) or high-temperature short pasteurization (72 °C for 5–10 s) eliminates CMV from the milk (Harmsen et al. 1995), but it also reduces the bioactive factors in human milk and possibly affects protection against necrotizing enterocolitis (NEC). Finally, in order to prevent NEC (Chowning et al. 2015; Kurath and Resch 2010), it is preferable to use fresh mother's own milk also in very low birth weight infants (VLBWIs) and/or preterms <32 weeks of gestational age, including those born to CMV-positive mothers.

36.9.1.4 Group B Streptococcus (GBS)

The incidence of the breast carriage rate of GBS in lactating mothers is 3.5%. There is inconclusive documentation on the use of breast milk of GBS-positive mothers after late-onset GBS infections (sepsis and meningitis). Although clinical protocols have been proposed (Davanzo et al. 2013b), the best strategy has yet to be developed (Filleron et al. 2014). The recommended pasteurization of maternal milk does not change the overall incidence of late-onset GBS infections in preterm infants. Some authors have suggested temporary discontinuation of breastfeeding until eradication of infection (rifampicin for 7 days for mother and infant, especially in preterms) (Gagneur et al. 2009; Soukka et al. 2010). In recurrent GBS infections and coexistent GBS-positive mother's milk, maintaining breastfeeding remains controversial, although the causative role of GBS-positive mother's milk as a vector of mother-to-infant transmission has not been definitively proven. Nevertheless, maternal compliance with professional advice to continue breastfeeding is low.

36.9.2 Environmental Contamination

The transfer of persistent organic pollutants (POPs) from mother to infant via breastfeeding is characterized by their lipophilic nature. POPs are known to accumulate in the food chain and can be detected in human milk. Nevertheless, breastfeeding seems to counteract adverse developmental effects after prenatal exposure to POPs, and breast milk remains superior to infant formula from the perspective of overall child health, after "weighing the risks against the benefits of breastfeeding" (Mead 2008).

36.9.3 New Pregnancy

In the past, mothers were advised to stop breastfeeding when they became pregnant because it was claimed that breastfeeding during pregnancy posed a higher risk for the embryo/fetus and the breastfed newborn infant. Based on current knowledge, breastfeeding can be continued during the first two trimesters of pregnancy and possibly extended into the third trimester. Caution may be warranted in women at risk of premature delivery, although no evidence exists that breastfeeding can trigger labor-inducing uterine contractions (Cetin et al. 2014).

36.9.4 Medications and Mothers' Milk

Few drugs (mainly cytostatic and some psychotropic or cardiovascular drugs) produce significant adverse effects on the breastfed infant. The risk for a nursed infant exposed to a hazardous drug is higher when he/she is exclusively breastfed or metabolism is still immature (preterm or younger than 2 months). This risk significantly decreases after 2 months of life or complementary feeding is given, that is, mixed feeding or when weaning foods are introduced. Lists of medications declared safe or hazardous during lactation are inherently limited by the fact that they are not comprehensive and often are not updated. These limitations notwithstanding, such lists serve to simply orient professional advice. In general, the assessment of potential effects a medication may have on lactation should be based on a precise methodology (Davanzo et al. 2016) and taken from authoritative sources, such as LactMed (http://toxnet.nlm.nih.gov/newtoxnet/lactmed.htm).

36.9.5 Radiological Contrast Agents

The majority of radiological contrast agents pose no additional health risk for the nursing infant of any postconceptional age (Cova et al. 2014). As a precaution, only gadolinium-based agents considered at high risk of nephrogenic systemic fibrosis (gadopentetate dimeglumine, gadodiamide, gadoversetamide) should be avoided in breastfeeding mothers. There is no need to temporarily discontinue breastfeeding or to express and discard breast milk following the administration of contrast agents declared compatible with breastfeeding.

36.9.6 Contraception

Breastfeeding is compatible with a wide range of safe and effective contraceptive methods for family planning (World Health Organization 2015). Copper intrauterine devices (IUDs) may be a first choice from the end of the first month of life onward. Progestin-only contraceptives (POC) and implants are a first choice during the whole lactation period. Combined oral contraceptives (COCs) are recommended only after 6 months postpartum. Although less effective, female condoms, male condoms, and the lactational amenorrhea method are other appropriate contraceptive options for breastfeeding women.

36.10 Human Milk Sharing

Human milk sharing, defined as cross nursing or exchange of expressed milk, is a potential source of microbial transmission, including transmission of the human immunodeficiency virus (HIV). Informal milk sharing agreements are arranged via private donor networks as well as via the Internet. Online sites that connect people interested in buying and selling human milk are growing in popularity, although recent research (Reyes-Foster et al. 2015) has shown that most mother-to-mother milk exchanges happen in person as gifts and that selling and shipping breast milk are actually rare.

Concern has been raised after the demonstrated microbial contamination of human milk purchased in the USA via the Internet (Keim et al. 2013). Another risk is purchasing milk through the Internet that is not 100% human in origin. In fact, 10% of analyzed samples ordered from popular websites were "topped off" with cow's milk. All samples contained human DNA, but 11 out of 102 also contained bovine DNA (Keim et al. 2015). In conclusion, health professionals should be aware of the increasing trend of human breast milk sharing and the potential risks due to adulteration and microbial contamination.

36.11 Nutrition with Human Milk in the Neonatal Intensive Care Unit (NICU)

36.11.1 The NICU Population and Breastfeeding Epidemiology

Human milk is the optimal form of nutrition for high-risk newborn infants admitted to the NICU, including the entire category of preterm infants (<37 weeks of gestational age [GA]), low birth weight infants (<2,500 g at birth), asphyxiated term newborns, newborns with congenital malformations, or otherwise compromised infants. Notwithstanding the variety of this case mix, the literature on the impact of early nutrition has mainly focused on very low birth weight infants (VLBWIs) and preterm infants <32 weeks GA, as these two groups represent a well-characterized subpopulation of NICU patients with very special nutritional needs. Obviously, this is not to say that the type of nutrition is irrelevant for preterm infants with higher birth weight (BW 1,500–2,499 g) or gestational age

(32–36 weeks), but simply that differences in short- and long-term outcome are less clinically remarkable and perceptible.

Breastfeeding (at the breast, expressed) is generally low for infants discharged from NICUs, regardless of their birth weight or gestational age. However, breastfeeding prevalence varies according to the specific setting. In accordance with international data from the Vermont Oxford Network Database, in 2013 only 11.3% of VLBWIs were breastfed at NICU discharge. A multicenter Italian study reported that, as compared with other birth weight categories of infants fed exclusively with human milk at NICU discharge, the breastfeeding rates are markedly lower for the two intermediate birth weight categories (25% for BW 1,500–2,000 g and 22% for BW 2,000–2,499 g vs. 31% for BW <1,500 g and 33% for BW ≥2,500 g) (Davanzo et al. 2013c).

Although intermediate birth weight newborn infants are expected to show better motor competence in the transition from parenteral nutrition to enteral tube feeding and finally to breastfeeding, the breastfeeding rate for this subpopulation is surprisingly lower. One explanation for the low rates of exclusive breastfeeding seen for the BW 1,500–2,499 g category is that NICU feeding protocols do not adequately recognize the oromotor competence of these infants and do not encourage the use of human milk. Another factor hindering the promotion of breastfeeding in the NICU is that infants in this birth weight group have a shorter length of hospital stay than those in the lower birth weight category. Recent UK data on GA categories show that late preterm infants (34–36.6 weeks GA) are less breastfed than either moderately preterm infants (32–33.6 weeks) or term infants, confirming that the intermediate GA category is the most disadvantaged (Boyle et al. 2015).

Many other factors can interfere with the use of human milk and breastfeeding in a NICU, including mother/baby separation, fragility and limited neurological competence of preterm and sick infants, anxiety and stress following the birth of a high-risk baby, maternal difficulty in milk production, and, last but not least, suboptimal knowledge about lactation and potential opposition toward breastfeeding among NICU staff.

Although interventions promoting nutrition with human milk in the NICU population have proven effective (Renfrew et al. 2010), they are often inconsistently applied. Such interventions will involve (1) providing open access to the NICU for parents, (2) improving knowledge of the science of lactation and the breastfeeding competence of the high-risk infant, (3) fostering peer support in hospital settings, (4) offering kangaroo mother care, and (5) having a clear plan in place for breast milk expression.

36.11.2 Nutrition on NICU Admission

Three subpopulations of newborn infants can be identified based on birth weight and gestational age, each of which requires a specific nutritional approach:

1. Term newborn infants, small for gestational age infants (SGA), infants 35–36 weeks GA, and, in general, neonates with a BW >2 kg can be expected to be able to take milk by mouth. If not breastfed, infants can be given donor milk or a starting formula using a cup or a bottle. Tube feeding is reserved for infants unable to feed autonomously. Intake should be 40–80 mL/kg/day. Glucose monitoring can be scheduled in the first 12 h of life, as indicated by current hypoglycemia protocols.
2. Preterm infants born at 33–34 weeks GA or newborn infants with BW 1.5–2 kg can be given mother's or donor milk or a nutrient-enriched formula via tube, initially as continuous enteral feeding of milk, then as bolus feeding. Intake should be 80 mL/kg/day. Mother's own milk will be fortified in infants showing poor growth or abnormal nutritional indexes. Fortification of human milk and nutrient-enriched formula will be continued until NICU discharge. Glucose monitoring can be scheduled in the first 12 h of life, as indicated by current hypoglycemia protocols.
3. VLBWIs need parenteral nutrition. Minimal enteral feeding is started possibly within 48–72 h, while expecting the mother's colostrum. Appropriate lab tests are selected and

scheduled according to the infant's general health conditions.

36.11.3 Oropharyngeal Colostrum

Small quantities of maternal colostrum (0.2 mL, 8–12 times/day) can be administered into the inner buccal mucosa of severe preterm infants (Rodriguez et al. 2010; Lee et al. 2015). This method is feasible, safe, and effective in increasing the blood levels of immunoactive factors and may reduce the risk of neonatal infections (Lee et al. 2015).

36.11.4 Minimal Enteral Feeding

Minimal enteral feeding (MEF) or trophic feeding (Lucas et al. 1986) involves the administration of small amounts of milk (possibly the mother's colostrum) 5–25 mL/kg/day via tube to the VLBWI. MEF is started as soon as possible within the first 72 h and is maintained for 7–10 days depending on the risk category and health conditions of the preterm infant. Unless otherwise motivated, delaying MEF carries no advantages and can reduce gut feeding tolerance with later attainment of full enteral feeding, increase the risk of neonatal infections (also because of longer duration of parenteral nutrition), and lengthen hospital stay (Flidel-Rimon et al. 2004). Colostrum-based MEF is an optimal way to prevent NEC.

36.11.5 Advancement of Enteral Feeding

Advancing enteral feed volumes at daily increments of 30–40 mL/kg (rather than 15–24 mL/kg) does not increase the risk of NEC or death in VLBW infants (Morgan et al. 2015). On the contrary, advancing the volume of enteral feeds by smaller steps delays the establishment of full enteral feeds by several days and increases the risk of invasive infection. Nevertheless, great caution is warranted when applying these findings to extremely preterm, extremely low birth weight, or growth-restricted infants. Advancement of enteral nutrition entails careful assessment for signs of gut intolerance: elevated gastric residual and abdominal distention.

The reference growth rate for the preterm infant is the same as for the fetus at the corresponding gestational age: 20 g/kg/day for VLBWIs and 15 g/kg/day for infants with a birth weight 1,500–2,200 g (Ziegler 2011). This can be assumed at least after the first 2 weeks of life, a phase of possible instability and birth weight recovery. Achieving normal growth is an essential nutritional goal for the preterm infant and is closely related to neurodevelopmental outcome (Weisglas-Kuperus et al. 2009). Nevertheless, extrauterine growth retardation is frequently due to the poor health conditions of the high-risk infant and possibly also because of suboptimal nutrition during the NICU stay.

36.11.6 Benefits of Human Milk for the Preterm Infant

Breast milk (preferably fresh; frozen only as a second choice) ranks first in the biological and nutritional hierarchy for the high-risk newborn (Davanzo and Pastore 2011) and should definitely be preferred over pasteurized donated bank milk and preterm formula (Section on Breastfeeding 2012). Nutrition of preterm infants with breast milk confers a variety of short- and long-term health benefits: better feeding tolerance, faster achievement of full enteral regimen, less risk of serious neonatal infections (e.g., sepsis, meningitis) (de Silva et al. 2004) and NEC (Meinzen-Derr et al. 2009; Maayan-Metzger et al. 2012), lower risk of retinopathy of premature (ROP) (Zhou et al. 2015), and better visual acuity, neurobehavioral, and cognitive development (Rozé et al. 2012).

36.11.7 Fat in Preterm Human Milk

Preterm milk has a higher mean fat content (4.7 g/dL) (Moltó-Puigmartí et al. 2011) and energy content (around 77–79 kcal/dL) than

Table 10 Comparison of the content of selected nutrients between preterm and breast milk (Modified from Moltó-Puigmartí et al. 2011)

	Gestational age (weeks)			
Nutrient	<28 extremely preterm	28–31 severely preterm	32–33 moderately preterm	Term
Protein (g/dL)	2.3 ± 0.5	2.1 ± 0.3	1.9 ± 0.3	1.6 ± 0.4
Carbohydrates (g/dL)	7.6 ± 0.6	7.5 ± 0.6	7.5 ± 0.5	6.2 ± 0.9
Fat (g/dL)	4.4 ± 0.9	4.4 ± 0.8	4.8 ± 1.0	4.1 ± 0.7
Energy (kcal/dL)	77.8 ± 8.4	77.6 ± 5.9	76.7 ± 6.5	67.7 ± 3.9
Sodium (mmol/L)	10.6 ± 1.9	10.6 ± 2.2	10.4 ± 1.9	11.2 ± 2.1
Calcium (mmol/L)	6.2 ± 1.4	6.5 ± 1.0	7.4 ± 1.1	5.4 ± 0.8

term milk. The fat concentration in human milk varies considerably between foremilk (32 g/dL ± 15 SD; range 11–86) and hind milk (83 g/dL ± 25 SD; range 36–149). As hind milk is remarkably energy dense (87 kcal /100 mL ± 18 SD), it may be preferentially used for the nutrition of preterm newborn infants with poor growth, even before giving medium-chain triglycerides (MCT) (Meier et al. 2013).

The fat intake by the high-risk newborn infant varies with the mode of breast milk administration. Continuous enteral feeding (CEF) of milk by nasogastric tube varies up to 25% in fat content, with recovery of much of the fat content in tubing, as nutrient losses can result from adherence to the delivery system. Practical solutions include (1) placing the syringe containing the milk vertically (exit upward), so that the floating fat is administered; (2) using a shorter set since the fat adheres to the tube's inner surface; and (3) using a bolus or infusion for 30 min instead of continuous feeds.

36.11.8 Protein in Preterm Breast Milk and Fortification

Nutritional protein requirements increase with decreasing gestational age (GA): 1.5–2 g/kg/day at >36 weeks GA, 2.3 g/kg/day at 30–36 weeks GA, and 3.6–4 g/kg/day at 24–30 weeks GA (Hay 2008). In parallel, preterm milk has a higher protein content than term milk, proportional to the degree of prematurity: 2.3 g/dL at <28 weeks GA, 2.1 g/dL at 28–31 weeks GA, and 1.9 g/dL at 32–33 weeks GA (Bauer and Gerss 2011) (Table 10). This variability is teleologically fascinating; however, because the protein concentration in preterm milk declines over the first few weeks postpartum unpredictably, it no longer meets the nutritional needs of most preterm infants. Therefore, preterm milk for VLWBIs needs to be fortified with a commercially available product containing protein, calcium, and phosphorus. The common practice is to add a fixed amount of fortifier to human milk, assuming that the milk has an average protein content.

At the recommended dosage, common products provide 1 g/dL extra protein. Fortification of human milk is usually started when the enteral feeding volume reaches 100 mL/kg per day (Klingenberg et al. 2012).

Milk fortification is expected to improve short-term growth, increase bone mineralization and prevent rickets, increase nitrogen retention, and improve neuromotor development (Arslanoglu et al. 2010). Currently, human breast milk-derived fortifiers are also available; although expensive, they seem to further reduce the risk of NEC (Assad et al. 2015; Sullivan et al. 2010).

The two proposed methods for individualized fortification are targeted fortification and adjustable fortification (Arslanoglu et al. 2010).

Targeted fortification is based on the periodic analysis of human milk with a specific instrument (milk analyzer). The amount of added fortifier is based on the protein intake with the milk. Milk analysis may be useful for deciding when to start breast milk fortification for VLBWI or how

Table 11 Nutritional assessment of the high-risk newborn infant and the need for human milk fortification

	Parameter	Abnormality cutoff values
Auxological indexes	Weight	<20 g/day
	Length	<0.5 cm/week
	Cranial circumference	<0.5 cm/week
Laboratory tests	BUN	<5 mg/dL
	Blood phosphorus	<4.5 mg/dL
	Alkaline phosphatase	>450 U/L

to adjust protein fortification, particularly when the infant does not show adequate growth. *Adjustable fortification* seems to be more practical and is calibrated to infant metabolic response, as measured by blood urea nitrogen (BUN) and, in general, by other nutritional indexes (Table 11).

While the need for milk fortification during hospital stay is unanimously recognized, its use after hospital discharge is controversial due to its possible interference with feeding directly from the breast (Zachariassen et al. 2011; Young et al. 2013).

36.11.9 Expression and Storage of Breast Milk

The hospitalized high-risk newborn infant may be unable to suck at the breast and so may be separated from its mother, possibly for extended periods of time. Mothers should start expressing their breast milk manually or with a milk pump as soon as possible (i.e., within the first 48 h postpartum). Milk should be expressed at least six times a day.

Breast milk expression alongside the incubator or cot or while looking at the baby's photograph has been shown to have a positive psychological effect and to increase breast milk production. Breast pumps for simultaneous expression of both breasts maximize stimulation and save time. During the first days postpartum, the recommended duration of expression is about 10–15 min per breast, which can later be prolonged until the final drops are expressed.

Breast pump accessories and milk containers should be washed and disinfected with physical (saturated steam) or chemical agents. Milk expressed in hospital or at home should be collected in a sterile container. After each milk collection, the container should be placed in the coldest part of the refrigerator and kept at 4 °C up to 72–96 h (Slutzah et al. 2010). If not used immediately, expressed breast milk should be frozen (−20 °C) and can be stored for up to 3 (for feeding high-risk infants) or 6 months (for healthy term newborns). Frozen milk can be thawed slowly in the refrigerator for up to 24 h or quickly in a water bath (maximum 37 °C). After thawing, the milk should be used within 24 h, if kept refrigerated. Fresh milk should not be refrozen.

36.11.10 Human Milk Bank

Human milk bank (HMB), or breast milk bank, is a service which collects, screens, processes, and dispenses by prescription human milk donated by nursing mothers, who are not biologically related to the recipient infant. The milk provided by milk banking is predominantly a pool of donated expressed term breast milks, but some milk banks may also provide preterm breast milk.

Holder pasteurization (62.5 °C for 30 min) of banked human milk is the method of choice to eliminate potential microbiological contaminants. Although indispensable, pasteurization alters the nutritional (5% loss of fat and 4% of protein) and the biological quality (loss of IgA, lactoferrin, lysozyme, IgA, lymphocytes, etc.) (Vieira et al. 2011), reducing its protective capacity against NEC. Because HMB is a kind of "mature" milk, it needs to be fortified if given to VLBWIs.

36.11.11 Kangaroo Mother Care

Kangaroo mother care (KMC) is the practice of skin-to-skin contact between the preterm low birth weight infant and his/her mother (or father). During KMC, the infant, clad in a diaper, is held in an upright prone position against the bare chest of the mother and covered with clothing and/or a blanket and a cap. KMC is effective and beneficial for thermal control, breastfeeding, maternal–infant relationship, and the health of preterm low birth weight and full-term infants. There is mounting evidence for the benefits of KMC in high-income settings (Table 12) (Davanzo et al. 2013d), and enhanced KMC practice has been strongly recommended also in high-tech settings (Nyqvist et al. 2010; Boundy et al. 2016).

The original KMC method, ideally with 24 h/day of mother–infant skin-to-skin care, termed continuous KMC, was intended as an alternative to conventional care in incubators in low-income settings. In many NICUs in affluent settings, KMC implemented as limited sessions with mother–infant skin-to-skin contact in kangaroo position for 1–2 h is termed Intermittent Kangaroo Mother Care (I-KMC) (Davanzo et al. 2013d). Each KMC session should last at least 1 h in order to facilitate the infant's state of adaptation. KMC creates an opportunity for the feeding competence of the preterm infant to emerge and spontaneously promotes breastfeeding.

The decision to practice KMC does not depend per se on either the degree of neurodevelopment or postgestational age but rather is based on infant stability and maternal information and readiness. Parents should be examined for skin infections and may need skin cleansing before contact with the infant. A recliner chaise lounge is provided to mothers for comfort, as well as a peaceful, diffusely lit environment. During I-KMC, correct infant's position should be assessed and vital parameters monitored (including temperature). Most nursing procedures can be performed during I-KMC, including oral/nasal or endotracheal suctioning, feeding tube insertion, parental nutrition administration, and i.v. injections. There is no upper time limit for the duration of an I-KMC session, and there is no evidence that slow is preferable to rapid and/or casual progression from short to longer and longer sessions, provided the mother enjoys the experience and the baby remains stable. Parents can sleep or read during sessions.

Table 12 Benefits of KMC in high-tech care settings (Modified from Davanzo et al. 2013d)

Benefits for infant
Prevents hypothermia by warmth transfer from mother to child
Improves and/or maintains stability even in very preterm infants. Heart and respiratory rates show lower variation in oxygen saturation and fewer episodes of apnea and bradycardia
Reduces stress, decreasing cortisol release during KMC
Positive effects on infant sleep patterns as a result of improved brain maturation
Improves neurobehavioral and psychomotor development
Decreases pain response in preterm infants during painful procedures
Benefits for parents
Improves parent–infant interaction
Increases psychological well-being and improves psychological adaptation and recovery after preterm delivery
Promotes recovery from postpartum depression
Salivary cortisol decreases in mothers of infants born at 25–33 weeks GA and who practice KMC
Benefits for breastfeeding
Facilitates access to breast and increases human milk production
Increases breastfeeding rate, proportion of exclusive breastfeeding at NICU discharge, and longer breastfeeding duration
Other possible benefits
Facilitates earlier hospital discharge
Could be implemented for back transport of high-risk preterm infants between hospitals

36.11.12 Feeding Competence of the Preterm Newborn and the Transition from Tube to Breast

Attainment of full oral feeds, via either bottle or breast, is considered one of the goals for preterm infants to meet prior to discharge. In many settings, "full oral feeding" is unfairly interpreted as full bottle feeding, not recognizing the fact that the experience of feeding directly at the breast during hospital stay is key to attaining successful breastfeeding at and after hospital discharge. Bottle feeding is often considered an obvious and necessary intermediate step along the pathway from tube feeding to breastfeeding, based on the assumption that it is less energetically expensive than breastfeeding. On the contrary, bottle feeding is less physiological for preterm infants, and it may disregard emerging neurodevelopmental competences and eventually divert from breastfeeding. In NICUs, unjustified delays in and restrictions on breastfeeding often occur due to persistent nonevidence-based opinions about the feeding capacity of preterm infants.

Although swallowing is first detected at 11 weeks gestation, coordinated suck–swallow is commonly, but dogmatically, believed not to be present until 32–24 weeks and even then considered to be immature. Swallowing and respiration must be coordinated since the two processes share the same channel, that is, the pharynx. In preterm infants, the difficulty in coordinating swallowing and respiration during the transition from tube to oral feeding may create a significant barrier to the establishment of full breastfeeding. In addition, weak sucking at the breast can complicate breast milk production.

In clinical practice, the decision to commence direct breastfeeds is based on various categories of long-standing guiding principles. These categories mostly refer to gestational age (GA), nonnutritive sucking of the pacifier, capability to feed at the bottle, and a repertoire of readiness cues from an infant that has been observed to be alert and active and makes sucking motions with his/her mouth. Although checklists assessing the readiness cues of preterm infants are commonly used in NICUs in the management of feeding, we must admit that there is no evidence that they can reliably predict the successful introduction of oral (breast or bottle) feeding. Moreover, as it concerns the GA category, we must observe that consistent with individual variability, infant breastfeeding competence can emerge across a wide spectrum of gestational ages rather than at any specific time. Exclusive breastfeeding in preterm infants is possible despite their immature sucking pattern, which is characterized by slow sucking, short sucking bursts with long pauses, and oxygen desaturation events during feeding. In order to obtain a satisfactory result with the breastfeed, the mother–infant couple should be offered adequate information and support, and breast milk should be expressed prior to the breastfeed, thus facilitating latch on with the technique known as "sucking at the emptied breast." Eventually, preterm infants can be frequently fed small milk volumes in combination with another adequate complementary feeding method such as tube feeding. Preterm infants should be given very small volume, frequent (12 better than 8 per day) feeds for a more physiological feeding pattern. This "preterm pattern" should be adopted in routine clinical practice whenever possible and sustainable. Preterm infants show a gradual transition, at varying postconceptual ages, to a mature sucking pattern, as observed also in healthy term infants. In other words, for preterm infants, successful breastfeeding should be defined only as the ability to consume a sufficient daily milk volume, independent of the sucking pattern, to support sustained growth. Reasonable expectations about the normal breastfeed of a preterm infant can help to promote the breastfeeding process and avoid hasty decisions by health professionals, as well as frustration in mothers.

The studies by Pineda (2011) and Nyqvist (2008) have demonstrated that the feeding competences of preterm newborns can emerge much earlier than expected, although the mean post-conceptional age (PCA) for a full breastfeed remains fixed at around 33 weeks and the mean PCA for full breastfeeding at around 36 weeks (Table 13).

Table 14 presents the relative gestational ages for the emergence and development of feeding competence. The gestational ages reported in the

Table 13 Variability of the emergence of oromotor competence in the preterm infant (Pineda 2011; Nyqvist 2008)

	Feeding competence	First attempt to the breast	First breastfeed	Full breastfeeding
	PCA[a] (weeks; range)	31; 29.6–33.6	33; 30–37	36; 33–39
Study (author and year)		Pineda (2011)	Nyqvist (2008)	

[a]*PCA* denotes postconceptional age

Table 14 Steps from tube feeding to breastfeeding (The minimal age at onset of each competence is given in the *shaded box*) (Modified from Davanzo et al. 2014)

GA (weeks)	24–25	26	27	28	29	30	31	32	33	34	35
Oropharyngeal colostrum											
Minimal enteral feeding											
Kangaroo mother care			+/–								
Nonnutritive sucking											
Initial attempts at the breast					+/–						
Syringe feeding of expressed breast milk					+/–	+/–	+/–				
First feed at the breast											
Cup feeding											
Bottle feeding								+/–			
Semi-demand feeding											
Full breastfeeding									+/–	+/–	

table do not indicate the recommended time to offer a feeding practice but rather are intended as the minimal age for the emergence of a specific competence, given the health conditions of the preterm infant and optimal facilitation by existing NICU organizational policies and protocols. Providing mothers the opportunity of having unlimited time with their babies and to engage in prolonged kangaroo mother care without unjustified restrictions is a relevant prerequisite for breastfeeding experience and success. Therefore, the table does not represent a standardized approach to testing infant skills in the breastfeeding process; instead, it depicts the flexible sequence of highly individualized development of feeding capacities in preterm infants.

36.11.13 Semi-demand Feeding

Feeding preterm infants in response to their hunger and satiation cues, rather than at scheduled intervals and with a predefined amount of milk, is referred to as semi-demand feeding. Semi-demand feeding for preterm infants during the transition from scheduled to full demand feeding in response to their hunger and satiation cues has been proposed to promote the establishment of self-regulated oral feeding, without affecting growth, risk of hypoglycemia, and length of hospital stay. The protocol can be applied for 33–36 weeks PCA preterm infants, on exclusive enteral nutrition with at least one successful breastfeeding in the previous 24 h and an adequate weight gain in the previous days (Davanzo et al. 2014). Mothers who are candidates for semi-demand feeding should have a basic breast milk production, be informed about the nutritional plan for their preterm infants, and be motivated to breastfeed their infants and to provide their extended presence in the NICU granted during the semi-demand feeding period (minimum 6 h). During each semi-demand session, mothers should test-weigh the infant and record the breast milk intake at each feed. Although the precision of this method has been criticized, test weighing is considered more accurate and reliable than clinical indicators in feeding preterm infants. During the session, the infant may be fed ad libitum. The use of pacifiers and dextrose solution is discouraged during the session as long as the mother is present. At the end of the session, the total amount of milk taken should be determined to assess whether supplementation is necessary. If the infant does not ingest the total prescribed milk volume orally over the 6-h session, supplementation should be given by gavage and divided in nightly feeds.

A predischarge 48-h period of intensive rooming-in in the NICU for the preterm infant and her/his mother may be a useful practice to establish breastfeeding and to better define the feeding plan at discharge.

Once the infant has fed the total milk volume required in a 24-h period, without any gavage, it is considered to have attained "full oral feeding." At this point, the infant may be permitted to feed ad libitum in the last few days before hospital discharge.

36.12 Infant Formula

36.12.1 General Principles

Even though the best health choice for both newborn and mother is exclusive breastfeeding, this may not always be achievable. Formula feeding should be considered particularly when (1) there are *medical contraindications against breastfeeding*, (2) *true low breast milk production is present* (*see related section*), and (3) the *fully informed* mother has *decided that bottle feeding is the better alternative*. Medical contraindication to breastfeeding may be defined as "acceptable medical reasons for the use of breast-milk substitutes." Several health conditions (WHO, UNICEF 2009) (Table 15) related to the health of the infant or the mother may justify avoidance of breastfeeding, temporarily or permanently. Whenever stopping breastfeeding is considered, the benefits of breastfeeding should be weighed against the risks posed by the specific conditions listed in the table.

When prescribing formulas, health professionals should educate parents on adequate (safe and correct) bottle preparation, particularly when powdered milk is used (FAO, WHO 2007). Summarizing, parents should check the "best before" date and the condition of the container, wash their hands before preparing the formula, dilute the powdered formula with water (heated to at least 70 °C to the volume according to the manufacturer's or the doctor's instructions), offer the bottle after the formula has cooled to a temperature appropriate for consumption, safely store unopened formula containers in a cool dry environment, and keep diluted formula in a refrigerator at 4 °C until use.

Table 15 Modified from WHO document of acceptable medical reasons for use of breast milk substitutes (WHO, UNICEF 2009)

Infant conditions
Infants who should not receive breast milk or any other milk except special formula
Classic galactosemia: special galactose-free formula
Maple syrup urine disease: special formula free of leucine, isoleucine, and valine
Phenylketonuria: a special phenylalanine-free formula (some breastfeeding under careful monitoring is possible) Infants for whom breast milk remains the best feeding option but who may need other food in addition to breast milk for a limited period
Very low birth weight ($<$1,500 g)
Infants born $<$32 weeks of gestation Newborn infants at risk of hypoglycemia because of impaired metabolic adaptation or increased glucose demand (preterms, small for gestational age, intrapartum hypoxic/ischemic stress, newborns born to diabetic mothers) if their blood sugar fails to respond to optimal breastfeeding or breast milk feeding
Maternal conditions
Maternal conditions that may justify permanent avoidance of breastfeeding
HIV infection: if replacement feeding is acceptable, feasible, affordable, sustainable, and safe
Maternal conditions that may justify temporary avoidance of breastfeeding
Severe illness that prevents a mother from caring for her infant, e.g., sepsis
Herpes simplex virus type 1 (HSV-1): direct contact between lesions on the mother's breasts and the infant's mouth should be avoided until all active lesions have resolved Maternal medications judged to be hazardous while breastfeeding
Maternal conditions during which breastfeeding can still continue, although health problems may be of concern
Breast abscess: breastfeeding should continue on the unaffected breast; feeding from the affected breast can resume once treatment has started
Hepatitis B: infants should be given im hepatitis B vaccine within the first 48 h or as soon as possible thereafter and im Hepatitis B immune globulins (HBIG)
Hepatitis C Mastitis: if breastfeeding is very painful, milk should be removed by expression to prevent progression of the condition
Tuberculosis: mother and baby should be managed according to national tuberculosis guidelines substance abuse

Since powdered infant formulas are usually not supplied sterile, they may be contaminated by bacteria. *Cronobacter* species, previously known as *Enterobacter sakazakii*, is one of the most harmful and is considered a potential causative agent of sepsis and meningitis in newborns and preterm infants during the first weeks of life. There is wide consensus that a powdered formula should be used immediately after being diluted or, if not, stored at <5 °C until use. Current knowledge suggests the use of hot water (70 °C) to dilute powdered infant formula in order to prevent *Cronobacter* contamination and growth (Silano et al. 2016). The use of liquid formula (sterilized after bottling) may be a more convenient option, especially for preterm infants and in the first month of life.

Contamination of infant formula. There have been recent reports of contamination of infant formula, including the epidemic of melamine contamination of baby formula in China associated with the development of urinary tract stones. Such episodes are not expected to occur when rigorous standards are followed and comprehensive testing regimens are implemented.

36.12.2 Nutritional Characteristics of Starting Formula

When breastfeeding is not possible, the first alternative is a cow milk-based formula adapted to human infant needs. Formulas are used for infant nutrition for several months. Starting formulas, for example, are indicated until 6 months of age, but their composition remains unchanged. In striking contrast, the nutrient composition of breast milk changes continuously during lactation and most dramatically during the early days. Except for follow-up formulas, which are marketed in Europe for the nutrition of infants 6–12 months of age, there have been no systematic attempts to graduate the change in the composition of infant formula as occurs naturally in breast milk.

Nutritional research on the novel components of human milk and new technologies applied by the food industry have led to the development of new formulas more similar to human milk. Advances in molecular biology may open the way for the large-scale production of recombinant human milk proteins, including bioactive substances and functional nutrients. Nevertheless, the need, safety, and efficacy of introducing these substances into infant formulas will need to be carefully assessed before they can be used in infant nutrition.

Currently available data are still inadequate to reach a consensus on the mandatory supplementation of infant formula with components that have been identified in human milk, are recognized to have a relevant biological and immunological effect, and are already included in many marketed products. This is the case for DHA/ARA (Sun et al. 2015), nucleotides (European Food Safety Authority (EFSA) 2014), probiotics and prebiotics (European Food Safety Authority (EFSA) 2014; Braegger et al. 2011), and taurine (European Food Safety Authority (EFSA) 2014), which do not per se provide the same health benefits to the formula-fed infant as human milk to the breastfed infant.

Given these uncertainties, the European Food Safety Authority (EFSA) Panel on Dietetic Products, Nutrition, and Allergies (DNA) has issued a document on the essential composition of infant formulas (Table 16) (European Food Safety Authority (EFSA) 2014).

Energy. The EFSA suggests an energy density of a formula between 60 and 70 kcal/100. The mean formula intake in the first month of age is around 150 mL/kg/day. The estimated energy requirement for physiological weight gain in healthy infants is 115 kcal/kg/day in the first month of life, then 100 kcal/kg/day at 3 months of age (Butte et al. 2000).

Lipids. Lipids represent 40–50% of the daily energy intake for a formula-fed infant. The recommended intake is 4.4–6.0 g/100 kcal. The endogenous synthesis of *LC- PUFAs* (chain length >18 carbons) may be insufficient, leading to low DHA content in plasma, red blood cell membranes, and cerebral cortex cells (Lauritzen et al. 2001).

Table 16 Compositional requirements of infant starting formulas for energy and selected nutrients according to the EFSA panel on NDA

Component in formula	Compositional requirement
Energy (kcal/100 ml)	60–70
Total fat (g/100 kcal)	4.4–6
Linoleic acid (LA) (mg/100 kcal)	500–1,200
Alpha-linolenic acid (ALA) (mg/100 kcal)	50–100
Docosahexaenoic acid (DHA) (mg/100 kcal)	20–50
Protein (g/100 kcal)	1.8–2.5
Total carbohydrates (g/100 kcal)	9–14
Lactose (g/100 kcal)	>4.5
Oligosaccharides (g/100 ml)	≤0.8
Calcium (mg/100 kcal)	≥50
Phosphorus (mg/100 kcal)	≥25–30
Magnesium (mg/100 kcal)	≥5
Sodium (mg/100 kcal)	≥25
Chloride (mg/100 kcal)	≥60
Potassium (mg/100 kcal)	≥80
Iron (mg/100 kcal)	≥0.3
Vitamin A (μg retinol equivalents or RE/100 kcal)	≥70
Vitamin D (μg/100 kcal)	≥2
Vitamin E (mg alpha-tocopherol (100 kcal)	≥0.6
Vitamin K (μg/100 kcal)	≥1
Inositol (mg/100 kcal)	≥4
Carnitine (mg/100 kcal)	≥1.2

Recognizing the important role LC-PUFAs play in the development and maturation of the neonatal nervous system, the European Society for Paediatric Gastroenterology, Hepatology, and Nutrition (ESPGHAN) (unlike the EFSA) recommends their addition to infant formula (European Food Safety Authority (EFSA) 2014).

Proteins. Healthy infants need no more than 12% of energy from proteins. Some studies have shown a positive association between early protein intake and later obesity: a higher body mass index ([BMI] weight in kg divided by height in m ^{2}) was observed in the high-protein as compared to the low-protein group (Michaelsen et al. 2012; Gunther et al. 2007). The EFSA recommends a minimum protein content of 1.8 g/100 kcal and a maximum no higher than 2.5 g/100 kcal. Protein sources can be cows' milk proteins (also in hydrolyzed form) and soy protein isolates. There is some evidence that bovine lactoferrin is highly homologous to human *lactoferrin*; however, few formulas marketed in Italy contain this immunomodulating protein.

Carbohydrates. These nutrients are the second source of energy intake after lipids. The minimum recommended amount is 9.0 g/100 kcal and the maximum 14 g/100 kcal. Lactose (at least 4.5 g/100 kcal) is the preferable carbohydrate in formulas, whereas sucrose and fructose should not be added as they may increase the risk of fructose intolerance and saccharase deficiency in infants. Due to the marked increase in osmolality, the addition of glucose to infant formula is also discouraged, but it is permitted for infant formulas containing hydrolyzed protein to counteract the bitter taste. Maltose and maltodextins are two other suitable carbohydrates for infant formula. Starches may be added up to 30% of total carbohydrates (2 g/100 mL). *Human milk oligosaccharides* (HMOs) constitute the third largest component after lactose and lipids in human milk and have several effects. The EFSA recommends ≤0.8 g/100 kcal. A combination of 90% galacto-oligosaccharides (GOS) and 10% fructo-oligosaccharides (FOS) is suggested to increase bifidobacteria and lactobacilli and to reduce stool pH and consistency (Ziegler et al. 2007). However, the clinical significance of this finding is still unclear (Braegger et al. 2011).

36.12.3 Special Formulas

Cow's milk formula is suitable for most full-term newborns. Moreover, special formulas are available for infants with special nutritional needs and/or specific diseases. In this section, we will focus on some selected formulas to be used during the first 6 months of life: soy formula, hydrolyzed formula, elemental formula, and nutrient-enriched formula (preterm formula and postdischarge formula). The composition of and indications for special formulas are presented in Table 17 (Amesz et al. 2010; Morgan et al. 2012).

Table 17 Composition in energy and selected nutrients and indications for the use of special formulas (Amesz et al. 2010; Morgan et al. 2012)

	Type of special formula				
	Term (starting formula)	Preterm	Post-discharge	Hydrolyzed	Hypercaloric
Indications	Healthy term and late preterm newborns	Preterm (<1,500 g) continued until 3,500 g or 40 weeks postconceptual age	Possibly for infants discharged with lower than normal weight for postconceptional age	Food allergy, malabsorption disorders	Neurologic conditions, fluid restriction
Energy (kcal/100 mL)	67–68	80–90	72–74	67	100
Proteins (g/100 mL)	1.4–1.5	2.2–2.4	1.8–1.9	1.8	2.6
Lipids (g/100 mL)	3.6	4.3	4.0	3.4	5.4
Carbohydrates (g/100 mL)	7.3	8.6	7.6	7.2	10.3
Calcium (mg/100 mL)	35–54	100–140	70–80	65.6	100
Phosphorus (mg/100 mL)	30	75	50	47.1	50

Special formulas for managing inborn errors of metabolism and formula for severe infant cholestasis are outside the scope of the present review.

Soy formula. Soy formulas contain a protein (soy) and carbohydrates (either glucose or sucrose) different from milk-based formulas. According to the American Academy of Pediatrics (Bhatia et al. 2008), the only real indications for soy formula use are for infants with congenital galactosemia, for use by families who are strict vegans, or for infants who are truly lactose intolerant. The safety of soy infant formula has been a topic of continuing debate because it contains isoflavones, naturally occurring compounds found primarily in beans and other legumes. These isoflavones are referred to as phytoestrogens because they are found in plants (phyto) and because of their ability to act like the hormone estrogen in the body. Nevertheless, no deleterious hormonal effects have been detected in growing infants fed soy formula. Although normal growth has been reported in term newborns, less weight gain and osteopenia have been documented among preterm infants fed soy formula. Consequently, soy formula should not be given to preterm infants. Finally, the possible interaction of soy-based formula with thyroxine replacement therapy should be considered in children with thyroid disorders.

Hydrolyzed formula. This is a cow's milk formula that has been processed to break down the proteins into smaller particles. There is limited evidence that as compared with cow's milk formula, the use of hydrolyzed formula reduces infant risk of allergy. Moreover, its use for supplementary feeds in maternity hospitals during the first days of life has not been demonstrated effective in preventing allergy. Conversely, infants with proven cow's milk allergy who are not breastfed should be given hydrolyzed infant formula.

Amino acid-based formula (elemental formula). This formula contains component nutrients including individual amino acids, making it easily digestable. Amino acid-based formulas are most commonly indicated in infants with multiple food intolerances and malabsorption disorders, including the short bowel syndrome.

Goat milk formula. Although popular for the treatment of allergy, it is not recommended for preventing or treating allergic disease.

Nutrient-enriched formulas. Preterm formulas and *postdischarge formula* (PDF) were developed to meet the higher requirements of energy, protein calcium, phosphorus, and magnesium in preterm infants. Their nutritional composition is an intermediate between term formula and preterm formula. Preterm infants, particularly the most immature, are often growth-restricted at hospital discharge. Feeding infants after hospital discharge with nutrient-enriched formula rather than standard term formula is expected to facilitate "catch-up" growth and improve development. Nevertheless, feeding preterm infants with PDF rather than term formula does not carry clear short- or long-term benefit (Young et al. 2012) probably because ad libitum fed infants reduce their intake relative to the calorie density of the milk. Current evidence does not support prescribing "post-discharge formula" for preterm infants following hospital discharge, whereas feeding preterm infants with "preterm formula" following hospital discharge may increase growth rates and is recommended for the most premature newborn infants (BW <1,500 g) at least until 40 weeks postconceptual age.

Hypercaloric formula. This type of formula provides over 1 kcal/mL and should be given only to infants requiring both higher energy intake and fluid restriction. Hypercaloric formula can be given to infants with severe perinatal brain damage that have higher energy and protein requirements (120% recommended average intake) in their first postnatal year in order to promote brain and corticospinal tract growth (Dabydeen et al. 2008).

References

Amesz EM, Schaafsma A, Cranendonk A, Lafeber HN (2010) Optimal growth and lower fat mass in preterm infants fed a protein-enriched postdischarge formula. J Pediatr Gastroenterol Nutr 50(2):200–207. https://doi.org/10.1097/MPG.0b013e3181a8150d

Arslanoglu S, Ziegler EE, Moro GE, World Association of Perinatal Medicine Working Group On Nutrition (2010) Donor human milk in preterm infant feeding: evidence and recommendations. J Perinat Med 38(4): 347–351. https://doi.org/10.1515/JPM.2010.064

Assad M, Elliott MJ, Abraham JH (2015) Decreased cost and improved feeding tolerance in VLBW infants fed an exclusive human milk diet. J Perinatol 36(3): 216–220. https://doi.org/10.1038/jp.2015.168

Ballard O, Morrow AL (2013) Human milk composition: nutrients and bioactive factors. Pediatr Clin North Am 60(1):49–74. https://doi.org/10.1016/j.pcl.2012.10.002

Bauer J, Gerss J (2011) Longitudinal analysis of macronutrients and minerals in human milk produced by mothers of preterm infants. Clin Nutr 30:215–220

Bertini G, Breschi R, Dani C (2015) Physiological weight loss chart helps to identify high-risk infants who need breastfeeding support. Acta Paediatr 104(10): 1024–1027

Bhatia J, Greer F, American Academy of Pediatrics Committee on Nutrition (2008) Use of soy protein-based formulas in infant feeding. Pediatrics 12(5): 1062–1068. https://doi.org/10.1542/peds.2008-0564

Boundy EO, Dastjerdi R, Spiegelman D, Fawzi WW, Missmer SA, Lieberman E, Kajeepeta S, Wall S, Chan GJ (2016) Kangaroo mother care and neonatal outcomes: a meta-analysis. Pediatrics 137(1):1–16. https://doi.org/10.1542/peds.2015-2238, Epub 2015 Dec 23. Review

Boyle EM, Johnson S, Manktelow B, Seaton SE, Draper ES, Smith LK, Dorling J, Marlow N, Petrou S, Field DJ (2015) Neonatal outcomes and delivery of care for infants born late preterm or moderately preterm: a prospective population-based study. Arch Dis Child Fetal Neonatal Ed 100(6):F479–F485. https://doi.org/10.1136/archdischild-2014-307347

Braegger C, Chmielewska A, Decsi T, Kolacek S, Mihatsch W, Moreno L, Pieścik M, Puntis J, Shamir R, Szajewska H, Turck D, van Goudoever J, ESPGHAN Committee on Nutrition (2011) Supplementation of infant formula with probiotics and/or prebiotics: a systematic review and comment by the ESPGHAN committee on nutrition. J Pediatr Gastroenterol Nutr 52(2):238–250. https://doi.org/10.1097/MPG.0b013e3181fb9e80

Brecht KF, Goelz R, Bevot A, Krägeloh-Mann I, Wilke M, Lidzba K (2015) Postnatal human cytomegalovirus infection in preterm infants has long-term neuropsychological sequelae. J Pediatr 166(4):834–839. https://doi.org/10.1016/j.jpeds2014.11.002

Butte NF, Wong WW, Hopkinson JM, Heinz CJ, Mehta NR, Smith EO (2000) Energy requirements derived from total energy expenditure and energy deposition during the first 2 y of life. Am J Clin Nutr 72(6):1558–1569

Cattaneo A, Ronfani L, Burmaz T, Quintero-Romero S, Macaluso A, Di Mario S (2006) Infant feeding and cost of health care: a cohort study. Acta Paediatr 95(5): 540–546

Centers for Disease Control and Prevention (2013) Strategies to prevent obesity and other chronic diseases: the

CDC guide to strategies to support breastfeeding mothers and babies. U.S. Department of Health and Human Services, Atlanta, http://www.cdc.gov/breastfeeding/pdf/BF-Guide-508.PDF

Cetin I, Assandro P, Massari M, Sagone A, Gennaretti R, Donzelli G, Knowles A, Monasta L, Davanzo R, Working Group On Breastfeeding, Italian Society Of Perinatal Medicine And Task Force On Breastfeeding, Ministry Of Health, Italy (2014) Breastfeeding during pregnancy: position paper of the Italian Society of Perinatal Medicine and the Task Force on Breastfeeding, Ministry of Health, Italy. J Hum Lact 30:20–22

Chen X, Chen J, Wen J, Xu C, Zhang S, Zhou YH, Hu Y (2013) Breastfeeding is not a risk factor for mother-to-child transmission of hepatitis B virus. PLoS One 8(1), e55303. https://doi.org/10.1371/journal.pone.0055303

Chowning R, Radmacher P, Lewis S, Serke L, Pettit N, Adamkin DH (2015) A retrospective analysis of the effect of human milk on prevention of necrotizing enterocolitis and postnatal growth. J Perinatol 36(3): 221–224. https://doi.org/10.1038/jp.2015.179

Cleminson J, Oddie S, Renfrew MJ, McGuire W (2015) Being baby friendly: evidence-based breastfeeding support. Arch Dis Child Fetal Neonatal Ed 100: F173–F178

Cova MA, Stacul F, Quaranta R, Guastalla P, Salvatori G, Banderali G, Fonda C, David V, Gregori M, Zuppa AA, Davanzo R (2014) Radiological contrast media in the breastfeeding woman: a position paper of the Italian Society of Radiology (SIRM), the Italian Society of Paediatrics (SIP), the Italian Society of Neonatology (SIN) and the Task Force on Breastfeeding, Ministry of Health, Italy. Eur Radiol 24(8):2012–2022

Dabydeen L, Thomas JE, Aston TJ, Hartley H, Sinha SK, Eyre JA (2008) High-energy and -protein diet increases brain and corticospinal tract growth in term and preterm infants after perinatal brain injury. Pediatrics 121: 148–156

Davanzo R, Pastore S (2011) Promoting mother's milk use in very low birth weight infants: when nutritional hierarchy deals with the professional value system. J Hum Lact 27(4):329–330. https://doi.org/10.1177/0890334411422705

Davanzo R, Cannioto Z, Ronfani L, Monasta L, Demarini S (2013a) Breastfeeding and neonatal weight loss in healthy term infants. J Hum Lact 29(1):45–53

Davanzo R, De Cunto A, Travan L, Bacolla G, Creti R, Demarini S (2013b) To feed or not to feed? Case presentation and best practice guidance for human milk feeding and group B streptococcus in developed countries. J Hum Lact 29:452–457. https://doi.org/10.1177/0890334413480427

Davanzo R, Monasta L, Ronfani L, Brovedani P, Demarini S, Breastfeeding in Neonatal Intensive Care Unit Study Group (2013c) Breastfeeding at NICU discharge: a multicenter Italian study. J Hum Lact 29(3):374–380. https://doi.org/10.1177/0890334412451055

Davanzo R, Brovedani P, Travan L, Kennedy J, Crocetta A, Sanesi C, Strajn T, De Cunto A (2013d) Intermittent kangaroo mother care: a NICU protocol. J Hum Lact 29(3):332–338

Davanzo R, Strajn T, Kennedy J, Crocetta A, De Cunto A (2014) From tube to breast: the bridging role of semi-demand breastfeeding. J Hum Lact 30(4):405–409. https://doi.org/10.1177/0890334414548697

Davanzo R, Romagnoli C, Corsello G (2015a) Position statement on breastfeeding from the Italian Pediatric Societies. Ital J Pediatr 41:80. https://doi.org/10.1186/s13052-015-0191-x

Davanzo R, De Cunto A, Paviotti G, Travan L, Inglese S, Brovedani P, Crocetta A, Calligaris C, Corubolo E, Dussich V, Verardi G, Causin E, Kennedy J, Marrazzo F, Strajn T, Sanesi C, Demarini S (2015b) Making the first days of life safer: preventing sudden unexpected postnatal collapse while promoting breastfeeding. J Hum Lact 31(1):47–52

Davanzo R, Bua J, De Cunto A, Farina ML, De Ponti F, Clavenna A, Mandrella S, Sagone A, Clementi M (2016) Advising mothers on the use of medications during breastfeeding: a need for a positive attitude. J Hum Lact 32(1):15–19. https://doi.org/10.1177/0890334415595513

De Bortoli J, Amir LH (2016) Is onset of lactation delayed in women with diabetes in pregnancy? A systematic review. Diabet Med 33(1):17–24

de Onis M, Garcia C, Onyango AW, et al (2006) WHO Child Growth Standards based on length/height, weight and age. Acta Paediatr Suppl 450:76

de Silva A, Jones PW, Spencer SA (2004) Does human milk reduce infection rates in preterm infants? A systematic review. Arch Dis Child Fetal Neonatal Ed 89(6): F509–F513

Department of Health and Human Services (2011) The surgeon general's call to action to support breastfeeding. Washington, DC. http://www.ncbi.nlm.nih.gov/books/NBK52687/

European Food Safety Authority (EFSA) (2014) EFSA Panel on Dietetic Products, Nutrition and Allergies (NDA). Scientific Opinion on the essential composition of infant and follow on formulae. EFSA J 12(7):3760

Filleron A, Lombard F, Jacquot A, Jumas-Bilak E, Rodière M, Cambonie G, Marchandin H (2014) Group B streptococci in milk and late neonatal infections: an analysis of cases in the literature. Arch Dis Child Fetal Neonatal Ed 99:F41–F47. https://doi.org/10.1136/archdischild-2013-304362

Flidel-Rimon O, Friedman S, Lev E, Juster-Reicher A, Amitay M, Shinwell ES (2004) Early enteral feeding and nosocomial sepsis in very low birthweight infants. Arch Dis Child Fetal Neonatal Ed 89(4):F289–F292

Gagneur A, Héry-Arnaud G, Croly-Labourdette S, Gremmo-Feger G, Vallet S, Sizun J, Quentin R, Tandé D (2009) Infected breast milk associated with late-onset and recurrent group B streptococcal infection in neonatal twins: a genetic analysis. Eur J Pediatr 168:1155–1158

Goelz R, Meisner C, Bevot A, Hamprecht K, Kraegeloh-Mann I, Poets CF (2013) Long-term cognitive and neurological outcome of preterm infants with postnatally acquired CMV infection through breast milk. Arch Dis Child Fetal Neonatal Ed 98:F430–F433. https://doi.org/10.1136/archdischild-2012-303384

Gunkel J, de Vries LS, Jongmans M, Koopman-Esseboom C, van Haastert IC, Eijsermans MCJ et al (2018) Outcome of preterm infants with postnatal cytomegalovirus infection. Pediatrics 141(2). pii: e20170635. https://doi.org/10.1542/peds.2017-0635

Gunther AL, Remer T, Kroke A, Buyken AE (2007) Early protein intake and later obesity risk: which protein sources at which time points throughout infancy and childhood are important for body mass index and body fat percentage at 7 y of age? Am J Clin Nutr 86:1765–1772

Harmsen MC, Swart PJ, de Béthune MP, Pauwels R, De Clercq E, The TH, Meijer DK (1995) Antiviral effects of plasma and milk proteins: lactoferrin shows potent activity against both human immunodeficiency virus and human cytomegalovirus replication in vitro. J Infect Dis 172:380–388

Hay WW Jr (2008) Strategies for feeding the preterm infant. Neonatology 94(4):245–254. https://doi.org/10.1159/000151643

Hayashi S, Kimura H, Oshiro M, Kato Y, Yasuda A, Suzuki C, Watanabe Y, Morishima T, Hayakawa M (2011) Transmission of cytomegalovirus via breast milk in extremely premature infants. J Perinatol 31(6): 440–445. https://doi.org/10.1038/jp.2010.150

Herlenius E, Kuhn P (2013) Sudden unexpected postnatal collapse of newborn infants: a review of cases, definitions, risks, and preventive measures. Transl Stroke Res 4:236–247

Holmes AV, McLeod AY, Bunik M (2013) ABM clinical protocol #5: peripartum breastfeeding management for the healthy mother and infant at term, revision 2013. Breastfeed Med 8(6):469–473. https://doi.org/10.1089/bfm.2013.9979

Jensen D, Wallace S, Kelsay P (1994) LATCH: a breastfeeding charting system and documentation tool. J Obstet Gynecol Neonatal Nurs 23(1):27–32

Johnston M, Landers S, Noble L, Szucs K, Viehmann L (2012) Breastfeeding and the use of human milk. Section on Breastfeeding. Pediatrics 129(3):e827–e841. https://doi.org/10.1542/peds.2011-3552. Epub 2012 Feb 27

Joint WHO/UNICEF statement (1989) Protecting, promoting, and supporting breastfeeding: the special role of maternity services. WHO, Geneva, http://www.who.int/nutrition/publications/infantfeeding/9241561300/en/

Keim SA, Hogan JS, McNamara KA, Gudimetla V, Dillon CE, Kwiek JJ, Geraghty SR (2013) Microbial contamination of human milk purchased via the Internet. Pediatrics 132(5):e1227–e1235. https://doi.org/10.1542/peds.2013-1687

Keim SA, Kulkarni MM, McNamara K, Geraghty SR, Billock RM, Ronau R, Hogan JS, Kwiek JJ (2015) Cow's milk contamination of human milk purchased via the internet. Pediatrics 135:e1157–e1162. https://doi.org/10.1542/peds.2014-3554

Klingenberg C, Embleton ND, Jacobs SE, O'Connell LA, Kuschel CA (2012) Enteral feeding practices in very preterm infants: an international survey. Arch Dis Child Fetal Neonatal Ed 97(1):F56–F61. https://doi.org/10.1136/adc.2010.204123

Kurath S, Resch B (2010) Cytomegalovirus and transmission via breast milk: how to support breast milk to premature infants and prevent severe infection? Pediatr Infect Dis J 29:680–681

Lauritzen L, Hansen HS, Jørgensen MH, Michaelsen KF (2001) The essentiality of long chain n-3 fatty acids in relation to development and function of the brain and retina. Prog Lipid Res 40:1–94

Lee J, Kim HS, Jung YH, Choi KY, Shin SH, Kim EK, Choi JH (2015) Oropharyngeal colostrum administration in extremely premature infants: an RCT. Pediatrics 135(2):e357–e366. https://doi.org/10.1542/peds.2014-2004

Luan NN, Wu QJ, Gong TT, Vogtmann E, Wang YL, Lin B (2013) Breastfeeding and ovarian cancer risk: a meta-analysis of epidemiologic studies. Am J Clin Nutr 98(4): 1020–1031. https://doi.org/10.3945/ajcn.113.062794

Lucas A, Bloom SR, Aynsley-Green A (1986) Gut hormones and 'minimal enteral feeding'. Acta Paediatr Scand 75(5):719–723

Maayan-Metzger A, Avivi S, Schushan-Eisen I, Kuint J (2012) Human milk versus formula feeding among preterm infants: short-term outcomes. Am J Perinatol 29(2):121–126. https://doi.org/10.1055/s-0031-1295652

McNinch A, Busfield A, Tripp J (2007) Vitamin K deficiency bleeding in Great Britain and Ireland: British Paediatric Surveillance Unit Surveys, 1993-94 and 2001-02. Arch Dis Child 92(9):759–766, Epub 2007 May 30

Mead MN (2008) Contaminants in human milk: weighing the risks against the benefits of breastfeeding. Environ Health Perspect 116:A427–A434

Meier PP, Patel AL, Bigger HR, Rossman B, Engstrom JL (2013) Supporting breastfeeding in the neonatal intensive care unit: Rush Mother's Milk Club as a case study of evidence-based care. Pediatr Clin North Am 60(1):209–226. https://doi.org/10.1016/j.pcl.2012.10.007

Meinzen-Derr J, Poindexter B, Wrage L, Morrow AL, Stoll B, Donovan EF (2009) Role of human milk in extremely low birth weight infants' risk of necrotizing enterocolitis or death. J Perinatol 29(1):57–62. https://doi.org/10.1038/jp.2008.117

Michaelsen KF, Larnkjær A, Mølgaard C (2012) Amount and quality of dietary proteins during the first two years of life in relation to NCD risk in adulthood. Nutr Metab Cardiovasc Dis 22:781–786

Moltó-Puigmartí C, Castellote AI, Carbonell-Estrany X, López-Sabater MC (2011) Differences in fat content and fatty acid proportions among colostrum, transitional, and mature milk from women delivering very preterm,

preterm, and term infants. Clin Nutr 30(1):116–123. https://doi.org/10.1016/j.clnu.2010.07.013

Morgan JA, Young L, McCormick FM, McGuire W (2012) Promoting growth for preterm infants following hospital discharge. Arch Dis Child Fetal Neonatal Ed 97(4):F295–F298. https://doi.org/10.1136/adc.2009.170910

Morgan J, Young L, McGuire W (2015) Slow advancement of enteral feed volumes to prevent necrotising enterocolitis in very low birth weight infants. Cochrane Database Syst Rev 10:CD001241. https://doi.org/10.1002/14651858.CD001241.pub6, Review

Nyqvist KH (2008) Early attainment of breastfeeding competence in very preterm infants. Acta Paediatr 97(6):776–781

Nyqvist K, Expert Group of the International Network on International Network on Kangaroo Mother Care, Anderson G, Bergman N, Cattaneo A, Charpak N, Davanzo R, Ewald U, Ludington-Hoe S, Mendoza S, Pallás-Allonso C, Peláez J, Sizun J, Widström AM (2010) State of the art and recommendations Kangaroo mother care: application in a high-tech environment. Acta Paediatr 99(6):812–819. https://doi.org/10.1111/j.1651-2227.2010.01794.x

Pineda R (2011) Direct breast-feeding in the neonatal intensive care unit: is it important? J Perinatol 31(8):540–545. https://doi.org/10.1038/jp.2010.205

Renfrew MJ, Dyson L, McCormick F, Misso K, Stenhouse E, King SE, Williams AF (2010) Breastfeeding promotion for infants in neonatal units: a systematic review. Child Care Health Dev 36(2):165–178. https://doi.org/10.1111/j.1365-2214.2009.01018.x

Reyes-Foster BM, Carter SK, Hinojosa MS (2015) Milk sharing in practice: a descriptive analysis of peer breastmilk sharing. Breastfeed Med 10(5):263–269. https://doi.org/10.1089/bfm.2015.0009

Rodriguez NA, Meier PP, Groer MW, Zeller JM, Engstrom JL, Fogg L (2010) A pilot study to determine the safety and feasibility of oropharyngeal administration of own mother's colostrum to extremely low-birth-weight infants. Adv Neonatal Care 10(4):206–212

Rozé JC, Darmaun D, Boquien CY, Flamant C, Picaud JC, Savagner C, Claris O, Lapillonne A, Mitanchez D, Branger B, Simeoni U, Kaminski M, Ancel PY (2012) The apparent breastfeeding paradox in very preterm infants: relationship between breast feeding, early weight gain and neurodevelopment based on results from two cohorts, EPIPAGE and LIFT. BMJ Open 2(2):e000834. https://doi.org/10.1136/bmjopen-2012-000834, Print 2012

Sacker A, Kelly Y, Iacovou M, Cable N, Bartley M (2013) Breast feeding and intergenerational social mobility: what are the mechanisms? Arch Dis Child 98(9):666–671

Section on Breastfeeding (2012) Breastfeeding and the use of human milk. Pediatrics 115(2):496–506

Silano M, Paganin P, Davanzo R (2016) Time for the 70°C water precautionary option in the home dilution of powdered infant formula. Ital J Pediatr 42:17. https://doi.org/10.1186/s13052-016-0228-9

Slutzah M, Codipilly CN, Potak D, Clark RM, Schanler RJ (2010) Refrigerator storage of expressed human milk in the neonatal intensive care unit. J Pediatr 156(1):26–28

Soukka H, Rantakokko-Jalava K, Vähäkuopus S, Ruuskanen O (2010) Three distinct episodes of GBS septicemia in a healthy newborn during the first month of life. Eur J Pediatr 169(10):1275–1277

Sullivan S, Schanler RJ, Kim JH, Patel AL, Trawöger R, Kiechl-Kohlendorfer U, Chan GM, Blanco CL, Abrams S, Cotten CM, Laroia N, Ehrenkranz RA, Dudell G, Cristofalo EA, Meier P, Lee ML, Rechtman DJ, Lucas A (2010) An exclusively human milk-based diet is associated with a lower rate of necrotizing enterocolitis than a diet of human milk and bovine milk-based products. J Pediatr 156(4):562–567. https://doi.org/10.1016/j.jpeds.2009.10.040, Epub 2009 Dec 29

Sun H, Como PG, Downey LC, Murphy D, Ariagno RL, Rodriguez W (2015) Infant formula and neurocognitive outcomes: impact of study end-point selection. J Perinatol 35(10):867–874. https://doi.org/10.1038/jp.2015.87, Epub 2015 Aug 6

Tornese G, Ronfani L, Pavan C, Demarini S, Monasta L, Davanzo R (2012) Does the LATCH score assessed in the first 24 hours after delivery predict non-exclusive breastfeeding at hospital discharge? Breastfeed Med 7(6):423–430

Tosone G, Maraolo AE, Mascolo S, Palmiero G, Tambaro O, Orlando R (2014) Vertical hepatitis C virus transmission: main questions and answers. World J Hepatol 6(8):538–548. https://doi.org/10.4254/wjh.v6.i8.538

Vieira AA, Soares FV, Pimenta HP, Abranches AD, Moreira ME (2011) Analysis of the influence of pasteurization, freezing/thawing, and offer processes on human milk's macronutrient concentrations. Early Hum Dev 87(8):577–580. https://doi.org/10.1016/j.earlhumdev.2011.04.016, Epub 2011 May 17

von Stumm S, Plomin R (2015) Breastfeeding and IQ growth from toddlerhood through adolescence. PLoS One 10(9):e0138676

Weisglas-Kuperus N, Hille ET, Duivenvoorden HJ, Finken MJ, Wit JM, van Buuren S, van Goudoever JB, Verloove-Vanhorick SP, Dutch POPS-19 Collaborative Study Group (2009) Intelligence of very preterm or very low birthweight infants in young adulthood. Arch Dis Child Fetal Neonatal Ed 94(3):F196–F200. https://doi.org/10.1136/adc.2007.135095, Epub 2008 Sep 19

FAO, WHO (2007) Safe preparation, storage and handling of powdered milk formula. Guidelines, Geneva

WHO, UNICEF (2009) Acceptable medical reasons for use of breast-milk substitutes. WHO, Geneva

WHO, UNICEF (2018) Implementation guidance: protecting, promoting and supporting breastfeeding in facilities providing maternity and newborn services – the revised Baby-friendly Hospital Initiative. WHO, Geneva

World Health Organization. Department of reproductive health and research. Medical eligibility criteria wheel for contraceptive use. http://www.who.int/reproductivehealth/publications/family_planning/MEC-5/en/. Published August 2015. Accessed 20 Dec 2015

Young L, Morgan J, McCormick FM, McGuire W (2012) Nutrient-enriched formula versus standard term formula for preterm infants following hospital discharge. Cochrane Database Syst Rev 3:CD004696. https://doi.org/10.1002/14651858.CD004696.pub4, Review

Young L, Embleton ND, McCormick FM, McGuire W (2013) Multinutrient fortification of human breast milk for preterm infants following hospital discharge. Cochrane Database Syst Rev 2:CD004866. https://doi.org/10.1002/14651858.CD004866.pub4

Zachariassen G, Faerk J, Grytter C, Esberg BH, Hjelmborg J, Mortensen S, Thybo Christesen H, Halken S (2011) Nutrient enrichment of mother's milk and growth of very preterm infants after hospital discharge. Pediatrics 127(4):e995–e1003. https://doi.org/10.1542/peds.2010-0723, Epub 2011 Mar 14

Zhou J, Shukla VV, John D, Chen C (2015) Human milk feeding as a protective factor for retinopathy of prematurity: a meta-analysis. Pediatrics 136(6):e1576–e1586. https://doi.org/10.1542/peds.2015-2372, Epub 2015 Nov 16. Review

Ziegler EE (2011) Meeting the nutritional needs of the low-birth-weight infant. Ann Nutr Metab 58(Suppl 1):8–18. https://doi.org/10.1159/000323381, Epub 2011 Jun 21

Ziegler E, Vanderhoof JA, Petschow B, Mitmesser SH, Stolz SI, Harris CL, Berseth CL (2007) Term infants fed formula supplemented with selected blends of prebiotics grow normally and have soft stools similar to those reported for breast-fed infants. J Pediatr Gastroenterol Nutr 44:359–364

Nutritional Recommendations for the Very-Low-Birth-Weight Newborn

37

Ekhard E. Ziegler

Contents

Abstract

To ensure uninterrupted growth and development of the prematurely born infant, all nutrients must be provided in the necessary amounts at all times. Delivery of nutrients meets with a variety of obstacles in very low birth weight (VLBW) infants, which is why VLBW infants frequently receive less than the required amounts of nutrients. As a consequence they often fail to grow like they would have in utero and, more importantly, suffer impairment of their neurocognitive development. The main obstacles to delivery of nutrients historically have been concerns regarding presumed risks attendant to the administration of nutrients. Recent years have seen a gradual dissipation of these concerns as scientific evidence of the safety of providing nutrients has accumulated. This reassessment of the risks of nutrient administration has nearly been completed in the area of parenteral nutrition but is an ongoing process in the area of enteral nutrition. The more realistic assessment of risks, together with a desire to prevent postnatal growth failure and thereby minimize the risk of impaired neurocognitive

E. E. Ziegler (✉)
Department of Pediatrics, University of Iowa, Iowa City, IA, USA
e-mail: ekhard-ziegler@uiowa.edu

G. Buonocore et al. (eds.), *Neonatology*,
https://doi.org/10.1007/978-3-319-29489-6_186

impairment, has led to more aggressive regimens of nutrient administration.

37.1 Salient Points

- Premature birth entails an interruption of the nutrient flow to the fetus/premature baby, which must be kept to a minimum if not avoided altogether.
- Nutrient needs of the VLBW baby for growth like the fetus are exceedingly high.
- Failure to meet the high protein needs leads to growth failure, which carries the risk of impaired cognitive development.
- Immaturity of the gastrointestinal tract necessitates initial delivery of nutrients via the parenteral route.
- Gut priming is needed until the gut is functionally mature enough to accept feedings.
- Human milk is the preferred feeding because of its trophic effect on the gut and its protective effect against sepsis and NEC.
- But human milk is nutritionally deficient and must be supplemented with substantial amounts of all nutrients.

37.2 Introduction

To ensure uninterrupted growth and development of the prematurely born infant, all nutrients must be provided in the necessary amounts at all times. Delivery of nutrients meets with a variety of obstacles in very low birth weight (VLBW) infants, which is why VLBW infants frequently receive less than the required amounts of nutrients. As a consequence they fail to grow like they would have in utero and, more importantly, suffer impairment of their neurocognitive development. The main obstacles to delivery of nutrients historically have been concerns regarding presumed risks attendant to the administration of nutrients. Recent years have seen a gradual dissipation of these concerns as scientific evidence of the safety of providing nutrients has accumulated. This reassessment of the risks of nutrient administration has nearly been completed in the area of parenteral nutrition but is an ongoing process in the area of enteral nutrition. The more realistic assessment of risks, together with a desire to prevent postnatal growth failure and thereby minimize the risk of impaired neurocognitive development has led to more aggressive regimens of nutrient administration.

There is principal agreement that postnatal growth of the premature infant should emulate that of the fetus in utero. Such "normal" growth would be proof of the absence of substantive nutrient deficiency and would provide assurance of unimpaired neurocognitive development. The American Academy of Pediatrics (Committee on Nutrition and American Academy of Pediatrics 1985) recommends that "postnatal growth that approximates the in utero growth of a normal fetus of the same postconception age" should be the basis for estimating nutrient requirements. It is recognized that birth engenders a permanent contraction of body water spaces, amounting to about 10–15% of extracellular fluid space. However, there are no known reasons why other body components should not be accumulating in the premature infant as they would have in the fetus. The fetal model is therefore appropriate for the estimation of nutrient intakes needed for normal growth and development.

Nutrient needs of the premature infant have been determined principally by two methods, the factorial method and the empirical method. Although both methods are ultimately based on the fetal model, they use very different approaches. In the factorial approach, fetal accretion of body components is used as the starting point. After correction for inevitable losses, inefficiency of conversion of nutrients into body components (in the case of protein), and absorptive inefficiency, the required intake for a nutrient is obtained. An important advantage of this approach is that it yields requirements for all nutrients for which fetal accumulation is known, which includes, besides protein and energy, all major minerals and most trace minerals. The factorial approach can also provide needs specifically for parenteral administration of nutrients. In the empirical approach, the intake of a nutrient is experimentally manipulated and a response, such as weight gain or, in the case of protein, nitrogen balance, is observed. This approach has been applied to protein end energy and yields energy and/or protein intakes that produce weight gain or protein accretion comparable to the fetus.

37.3 Protein Requirements Determined by the Factorial Approach

The factorial approach derives nutrient requirements as the sum of two (in the case of parenteral requirements) or three components (in the case of enteral requirements). The largest component, and the component that changes most with body size, is nutrient accretion. The other components are inevitable losses and, in the case of enteral requirements, efficiency of nutrient absorption.

Nutrient accretion is derived from body composition of the fetus. Going back to the nineteenth century, the chemical composition of a sizable number of term and preterm infants, who were stillborn or died soon after birth, has been reported by a number of investigators. Sparks (1984) and Forbes (1987, 1989) have provided comprehensive summaries of the chemical data derived from whole body chemical analyses of over 160 infants. The data permit derivation of fetal accretion rates of the various body components (Sparks 1984; Forbes 1987, 1989).

Utilizing a different approach, Ziegler et al. (1976) used select data for the construction of a "reference fetus" and derived fetal accretion rates. Accretion rates by the different approaches are similar and the fetal accretion rates in Table 1 represent a composite of the different approaches (Sparks 1984; Forbes 1987, 1989; Ziegler et al. 1976) in combination with contemporary fetal growth data (Kramer et al. 2001). Fetal accretion rates shown in Table 1 are corrected for presumed inefficiency (90%) of the conversion of dietary protein to body protein. Energy accretion values include the energy cost of growth, estimated by Micheli et al. (1992) at 10 kcal/kg/day.

Inevitable losses of protein (nitrogen) through desquamation of skin were assumed to be 27 mg/kg/day (Snyderman et al. 1969) and urinary losses in the form of urea to be 133 mg/kg/day (Saini et al. 1989; Rivera et al. 1993). Energy losses in the form of resting energy expenditure were assumed to be 45 kcal/kg/day in infants <900 g and 50 kcal/kg/day in larger infants, and other expenditures, e.g., for occasional cold exposure

Table 1 Estimated nutrient intakes needed to achieve fetal weight gain

Body weight (g)	500–700	700–900	900–1,200	1,200–1,500	1,500–1,800	1,800–2,200
Fetal weight gain (g/day)	13	16	20	24	26	29
(g/kg/day)	21	20	19	18	16	14
Protein (g/kg/day)						
Loss	1.0	1.0	1.0	1.0	1.0	1.0
Growth (accretion)	2.5	2.5	2.5	2.4	2.2	2.0
Required intake						
Parenteral	3.5	3.5	3.5	3.4	3.2	3.0
Enteral	4.0	4.0	4.0	3.9	3.6	3.4
Energy (kcal/kg/day)						
Loss	60	60	65	70	70	70
Resting expenditure	45	45	50	50	50	50
Other expenditure	15	15	15	20	20	20
Growth (accretion)	29	32	36	38	39	41
Required intake						
Parenteral	89	92	101	108	109	111
Enteral	105	108	119	127	128	131
Protein/energy (g/100 kcal)						
Parenteral	3.9	3.8	3.5	3.1	2.9	2.7
Enteral	3.8	3.7	3.4	3.1	2.8	2.6

and physical activity, were assumed to be 15 kcal/kg/day in infants <1,200 g and 20 kcal/kg/day in larger infants (DeMarie et al. 1999; Olhager and Forsum 2003). The requirements for parenterally administered protein and energy (Table 1) are calculated as the sum of accretion plus inevitable losses. Enteral requirements are derived from parenteral requirements by application of corrections for percentage absorption, assumed to be 88% for protein and 85% for energy.

Absolute fetal weight gain (g/day) increases with increasing body size, but fractional fetal weight gain (g/kg/day) decreases markedly with increasing body size. In spite of this, the rate of protein accretion remains constant up to a weight of 1,200 g. This is so because the protein content of fat-free body mass increases with increasing body size/age, offsetting the effect of the decrease in fractional growth rate. Energy accretion, on the other hand, increases with increasing body weight due to a marked increase in fetal body fat content. As the accumulation of body fat is not an absolute necessity, lesser energy intakes do not limit growth of lean body mass as long as they are greater than 100 kcal/kg/day (Micheli et al. 1992).

37.4 Protein Requirements Determined by the Empirical Approach

The empirical approach utilizes feedings (formulas or human milk) that provide precisely known intakes of energy and protein, with growth and/or nitrogen balance as outcomes. Because of the fragility of extremely immature infants, the necessary studies have been performed for the most part with infants weighing >1,200 g. As requirements are strongly influenced by body size, estimates by the empirical approach are generally applicable only to infants weighing >1,200 g. Data published before 1986 (Ziegler 1986) showed that weight gain (g/day) increased with increasing protein intake all the way to the highest intake studied (3.6 g/kg/day). Weight gain did not seem to be influenced by energy intake. The high protein intake of 3.6 g/kg/day was shown to produce a weight gain of about 30 g/day, which was more than the weight gain of the fetus and therefore represented catch-up growth. Kashyap et al. (1986, 1988, 1990) performed a series of growth and metabolic balance studies with feedings (human milk, formulas) that varied in protein and energy content. They used the data to derive equations predicting protein and energy intakes necessary to duplicate fetal weight gain. The authors estimated that protein intake necessary for infants with birth weight greater than 1,200 g to duplicate fetal weight gain was about 3.0 g/kg/day (Table 2). Using a variety of end points, including growth, body composition, and nitrogen balance, Rigo (2005) estimated the protein requirements ("advisable recommendation") of infants born at 26–30 weeks gestation (corresponding to weight of about 800–1,500 g) at 3.8–4.2 g/kg/day (3.3 g/100 kcal) and those of infants born at 30–36 weeks gestation (corresponding to weight of 1,500–2,700 g) at 3.4–3.6 g/kg/day (2.8 g/100 kcal).

Table 2 Protein requirements by the factorial method (Ziegler) and by empirical methods

	Weight <1,200 g		Weight >1,200	
	g/kg/day	g/100 kcal	g/kg/day	g/100 kcal
Ziegler (Table 1)	4.0	3.7	3.6	2.8
Kashyap and Heird (Kashyap et al. 1986; 1988; 1990)	–	–	3.0	2.5
Rigo (2005)	3.8–4.2	3.3	3.4–3.6	2.8

Table 2 provides a summary of the different estimates of requirements for infants weighing less than 1,200 g and those weighing more than 1,200 g. It is apparent that there is reasonably close agreement among the different estimates in spite of differences in methods and end points used.

37.5 Recommended Protein Intakes

Current recommendations (van Goudoever et al. 2014) are to provide initially (i.e., from birth) 2.0–2.5 g/kg/day and to gradually increase to 3.5 g/kg/day. At full enteral nutrition, infants need 3.5–4.5 g/kg/day of protein.

37.6 Requirements for Energy and Other Nutrients

Estimates of energy requirements are available by the factorial method (Table 1). However, estimates by the empirical method are considered more relevant with regard to energy. Empirical estimates (Micheli et al. 1992) indicate that energy needs are 90–100 kcal/kg/day. Energy taken in excess of this amount is used for storage in adipose tissue.

Requirements for major minerals and electrolytes derived by the factorial method are summarized in Table 3. Because there is considerable uncertainty regarding the minimal urinary losses of electrolytes and phosphorus, and because there is large variation of the efficiency of intestinal absorption of calcium, the required intakes shown in Table 2 are somewhat uncertain. Since accumulation of less than the fetal amounts of bone mineral (Ca, P) seems to be compatible with reasonable bone health, there is even uncertainty with regard to the minimum amount of Ca and P that must be accrued. Nevertheless, fetal accretion rates are considered the norm and deviations from them need to be justified. Table 4 summarizes the mineral and vitamin intakes for fully enterally fed premature infants as recommended in 2014 by Koletzko et al. (2014).

37.7 Catch-Up Growth

Growth restriction, whether occurring before birth (intrauterine) or postnatally, is associated with impaired neurocognitive development. Although postnatal growth restriction may lead to lower cardiovascular and metabolic risks later in life (Singhal et al. 2003), the overriding concern is with neurocognitive development. Therefore, in order to minimize the adverse effects of growth restriction, efforts should be made to allow infants to make up any growth deficit as soon as possible. Accelerated growth following a period of growth restriction is referred to as catch-up growth.

Most infants are capable of catch-up growth, and catch-up growth will occur if the requisite amounts of nutrients are provided. Nutrient needs for catch-up growth are above and beyond the needs for growth like the fetus. Since most premature infants will have incurred some growth deficit during the immediate postnatal period, it is advisable to provide all VLBW infants with sufficient nutrients for making up the growth deficit. Attempts to estimate nutrient needs of growth-restricted infants and needs for catch-up growth have been made (Ziegler 2005).

Table 5 presents nutrient requirements of hypothetical growth-restricted infants. The first column gives nutrient requirements of a normally grown 26-week gestation infant weighing 900 g. The next column shows requirement of a growth-restricted infant of similar weight and growing at the same rate as the normally grown infant. Because the lean body mass of this infant has a more mature composition (lower water content), the infant's metabolic rate is higher and accordingly its energy requirement is higher than that of the normally grown infant. The hypothetical infant in the far right column is also growth restricted but is assumed to undergo catch-up growth. As shown, this increases the requirements for energy and, especially for protein, by a considerable margin. If the infant is to undergo catch-up growth, these high needs have to be met.

Table 3 Requirements for major minerals and electrolytes determined by the factorial method (all values per kg/day)

	500–1,000 g		1,000–1,500 g		1,500–2,000 g	
	Accretion	Required intake	Accretion	Required intake	Accretion	Required intake
Ca (mg)	102	184	99	178	96	173
P (mg)	66	126	65	124	63	120
Mg (mg)	2.8	6.9	2.7	6.7	2.5	6.4
Na (meq)	1.54	3.3	1.37	3.0	1.06	2.6
K (meq)	0.78	2.4	0.72	2.3	0.63	2.2
Cl (meq)	2.26	2.8	0.99	2.7	0.74	2.5

Table 4 Recommended nutrient intakes of fully enterally fed preterm infants (Koletzko et al. 2014)

Amounts per 100 kcal	
Minerals	
Na (mg)	63–105
K (mg)	71–177
Cl (mg)	95–161
Ca (mg)	109–182
P (mg)	55–127
Mg (mg)	7.3–13.6
Fe (mg)	1.8–2.7
Zn (mg)	1.3–2.3
Cu (μg)	90–210
Mn (μg)	0.9–13.6
F (μg)	1.4–55
I (μg)	9–50
Se (μg)	4.5–9
Cr (ng)	27–2,045
Mo (μg)	0.27–4.5
Vitamins	
A (μg RE)	365–1,000
D (IU)	100–350
E (mg α-TE)	2–10
K (μg)	4–25
Thiamin (μg)	127–273
Riboflavin (μg)	181–364
Niacin (mg)	0.9–5
B6 (μg)	45–273
B12 (μg)	0.09–0.73
Folic acid (μg)	32–91
Pantothenic acid (μg)	300
Biotin (μg)	1.5–15
C (mg)	18–50

Table 5 Nutrient requirements of growth-restricted VLBW infants without and with catch-up growth

Gestational age	26 weeks	30 week	30 week
Weight (g)	900	900	900
Weight status	NG	GR	GR
Catch-up growth	No	No	Yes
Weight gain (g/day)	20	20	34
Required intake			
Protein (g/kg/day)	4.0	4.0	4.9
Energy (kcal/kg/day)	119	126	141
Protein/energy (g/100 kcal)	3.4	3.2	3.5

NG normally grown, *GR* growth restricted

37.8 Nutrient Delivery

Ideally, the flow of nutrients should continue without interruption and at the same level as the fetus transitions to become an infant. Although the goal of an uninterrupted flow of nutrients is difficult to attain, it should be the goal that the caretaker strives to achieve. After all, it is not known what degree of shortfall from the goal, if any, is safe in terms of neurocognitive outcome.

Nutrients are initially delivered to VLBW infants parenterally. While nutrients are provided parenterally, trophic feedings are initiated with the objective of fostering maturation of the immature intestinal tract. When maturation has advanced to the point where full feedings can be administered, parenteral nutrition can be terminated. This marks the beginning of the late feeding period, during which enteral feedings are the exclusive source of nutrients. Growth similar to the fetus, or faster than the fetus, is by consensus optimal. Yet, growth frequently proceeds at a slower rate (postnatal growth failure). The reason for growth failure is inadequate protein intake, which is caused by the low protein content of most feedings. Inadequate protein intake is thus ultimately responsible for the poor neurocognitive development with which growth failure is associated (Ehrenkranz et al. 2006). Therefore, the achievement of adequate protein intake is mandatory if neurocognitive impairment is to be minimized.

37.8.1 Parenteral Nutrition

Delivery of nutrients via the parenteral route should commence immediately at birth. Nutrients may initially be limited to amino acids, energy in the form of glucose, and certain minerals, such as calcium, phosphorus, and magnesium. Full parenteral nutrition, including intravenous lipids, should be instituted within 24 h of birth. Parenteral nutrition starting within 2 h of birth has been shown to be effective and safe (te Braake et al. 2005). Delivery of amino acids in the needed amounts (Table 1) presents no difficulty, whereas delivery of energy can usually not be achieved for some days without incurring hyperglycemia, even if lipids are provided. The best strategy is to start glucose at a rate of 4.2 mg/kg/min and to increase delivery stepwise as long as euglycemia is maintained. Lipid emulsions based on soy oil provide needed energy and deliver modest amounts of the essential long-chain polyunsaturated fatty acids, docosahexaenoic acid, and arachidonic acid. Premature reduction and/or discontinuation of parenteral nutrition before enteral nutrition has reached full levels leads to inadequate protein and energy intakes and slows growth (Miller et al. 2014). Parenteral nutrition should therefore be continued until enteral feedings provide all the nutrients that are needed.

37.8.2 Early Enteral Nutrition

While adequate amounts of nutrients are being delivered via the parenteral route, enteral feedings should be started soon after birth. The sole objective of early (trophic) feeding is to stimulate the immature intestinal tract to undergo maturation. A marker of the intestinal tract's immaturity is the frequent gastric residuals, which can therefore be used to follow the intestinal tract's maturation. The best trophic feeding is human milk because of its superior ability to mature the gut while keeping the risk of necrotizing enterocolitis to a minimum. Because it usually takes some days for the mother's milk to become available, donor milk may be used to initiate gut priming in a timely manner, i.e., on the first day of life.

Gastric residuals should be monitored and their size taken into account in advancing feedings. It is probably prudent to keep the volume of trophic feedings low (<10 mL/kg/day) until gastric residuals are substantially diminished. When they are, cautious advancement of feeds can begin. Contrary to earlier perceptions, neither the age at which trophic feedings are started nor the rate of advancement of feedings has an impact on the risk of necrotizing enterocolitis (Chauhan et al. 2008). Regardless of how feedings are advanced, it is important not to withhold feedings for more than a few hours because persistent feeding is crucial for optimal bowel maturation. Vigilance for signs of necrotizing enterocolitis must be maintained at all times. However, gastric residuals are not an early sign of necrotizing enterocolitis, and their monitoring is not of proven value in the prevention of necrotizing enterocolitis. Delays in reaching full feedings should be minimized as early achievement of full feedings offers relative protection against late-onset sepsis (Ronnestad et al. 2005).

37.8.3 Late Enteral Nutrition

It is widely appreciated that human milk does not provide the nutrients required by premature infants (Tables 1 and 3). The nutrient intake from human milk must therefore be increased by the addition of nutrient supplements (fortifiers). Infants fed unsupplemented human milk show slow growth, which carries the risk of impaired neurocognitive development. In addition, premature infants can develop deficiency states of specific nutrients, such as osteopenia (Ca, P) or zinc deficiency. Commercially available human milk fortifiers provide protein, energy, and the necessary minerals and vitamins. The amounts of minerals and vitamins are designed to meet or exceed, together with the nutrients intrinsically present in human milk, the concentrations specified in Table 4. Fortifiers provide energy in the form of carbohydrates and lipids. The protein provided by powder fortifiers (1.0–1.1 g/100 mL) is insufficient to meet the needs for protein at all times. The newer liquid fortifiers provide between 1.6 and 1.8 g of protein/100 ml milk and thereby ensure adequate protein intakes most of the time. Adequate protein intakes can be achieved if, in addition to a powder fortifier, protein is added in able form or in the form of additional fortifier. Additional protein can also be added as part of a targeted fortification regimen (Polberger et al. 1999) or in an adjustable fortification regimen (Arslanoglu et al. 2006). There is no consensus regarding which of these methods is preferred. There is, however, no question that the amount of protein provided by commercial powder fortifiers is inadequate and that additional protein must be provided in some form.

References

Arslanoglu S, Moro GE, Ziegler EE (2006) Adjustable fortification of human milk fed to preterm infants: does it make a difference? J Perinatol 26:614–621, PubMed CrossRef

Chauhan M, Henderson G, McGuire W (2008) Enteral feeding for very low birth weight infants: reducing the risk of necrotising enterocolitis. Arch Dis Child Fetal Neonatal Ed 93:F162–F166, CrossRef

Committee on Nutrition, American Academy of Pediatrics (1985) Nutritional needs of low-birth-weight infants. Pediatrics 75:976–986

DeMarie MP, Hoffenberg A, Biggerstaff SLB et al (1999) Determinants of energy expenditure in ventilated preterm infants. J Perinat Med 27:465–472

Ehrenkranz RA, Dusick AM, Vohr BR et al (2006) Growth in the neonatal intensive care unit influences neurodevelopmental and growth outcomes of extremely low birth weight infants. Pediatrics 117:1253–1261, PubMed CrossRef

Forbes GB (1987) Human body composition. Springer-Verlag, New York, pp 101–124, CrossRef

Forbes G (1989) Nutritional adequacy of human breast milk for prematurely born infants. In: Lebenthal E (ed) Textbook of gastroenterology and nutrition in infancy. Raven Press, New York, pp 27–34

Kashyap S, Forsyth M, Zucker C et al (1986) Effects of varying protein and energy intakes on growth and metabolic response in low birth weight infants. J Pediatr 108:955–963, PubMed CrossRef

Kashyap S, Schulze KF, Forsyth M et al (1988) Growth, nutrient retention, and metabolic response of low birth weight infants fed varying intakes of protein and energy. J Pediatr 113:713–721, PubMed CrossRef

Kashyap S, Schulze KF, Forsyth M et al (1990) Growth, nutrient retention, and metabolic response of low-birth-weight infants fed supplemented and unsupplemented preterm human milk. Am J Clin Nutr 52:254–262

Koletzko B, Poindexter B, Uauy R (eds) (2014) Nutritional care of preterm infants. Karger, Basel

Kramer MS, Platt RW, Wen SW et al (2001) A new and improved population-based Canadian reference for birth weight for gestational age. Pediatrics 108:1–7, CrossRef

Micheli JL, Schutz Y, Jequier E (1992) Protein metabolism of the newborn. In: Polin RA, Fox WW (eds) Fetal and neonatal physiology. Saunders, Philadelphia, pp 462–472

Miller M, Vaidya R, Rastogi D, Bhutada A, Rastogi S (2014) From parenteral to enteral nutrition: a nutrition-based approach for evaluation of postnatal growth failure in preterm infants. J Parenter Enteral Nutr 38:489–497

Olhager E, Forsum E (2003) Total energy expenditure, body composition and weight gain in moderately preterm and full-term infants at term postconceptional age. Acta Paediatr 92:1327–1334, PubMed CrossRef

Polberger S, Räihä NCR, Juvonen P et al (1999) Individualized protein fortification of human milk for preterm infants: comparison of ultrafiltrated human milk protein and a bovine whey fortifier. JPGN 29:332–338, PubMed

Rigo J (2005) Protein, amino acid and other nitrogen compounds. In: Tsang RC, Uauy R, Koletzko B, Zlotkin S (eds) Nutrition of the preterm infant, 2nd edn. Digital Educational Publishing, Cincinnati

Rivera JA, Bell EF, Bier DM (1993) Effect of intravenous amino acids on protein metabolism of preterm infants during the first three days of life. Pediatr Res 33:106–111, PubMed CrossRef

Ronnestad A, Abrahamson TG, Medbo S et al (2005) Septicemia in the first week of life in a Norwegian national cohort of extremely premature infants. Pediatrics 115: e262–e268, PubMed CrossRef

Saini J, Macmahon P, Morgan JB et al (1989) Early parenteral feeding of amino acids. Arch Dis Child 64:1362–1366, PubMed CrossRef

Singhal A, Fewtrell M, Cole TJ, Lucas A (2003) Low nutrient intake and early growth for later insulin resistance in adolescents born preterm. Lancet 361:1089–1097, PubMed CrossRef

Snyderman SE, Boyer A, Kogut MD et al (1969) The protein requirement of the premature infant. I. The effect of protein intake on the retention of nitrogen. J Pediatr 74:872–880, PubMed CrossRef

Sparks JW (1984) Human intrauterine growth and nutrient accretion. Semin Perinatol 8:74–93, PubMed

te Braake FWJ, van den Akker CHP, Wattimena DJL et al (2005) Amino acid administration to premature infants directly after birth. J Pediatr 147:457–461, CrossRef

van Goudoever JB, Vlaardingerbroek H, van den Akker C, de Groof F, van der Schoor SRD (2014) Amino acids and proteins. In: Koletzko B, Poindexter B, Uauy R (eds) Nutritional care of preterm infants. Karger, Basel, pp 49–63

Ziegler EE (1986) Protein requirements of preterm infants. In: Fomon SJ, Heird WC (eds) Energy and protein needs during in-fancy. Academic, New York, pp 69–85

Ziegler EE (2005) Nutrition of SGA/IUGR newborn infants. Minerva Pediatr 57(Suppl 1):16–18

Ziegler EE, O'Donnell AM, Nelson SE et al (1976) Body composition of the reference fetus. Growth 40:329–341, PubMed

Enteral Feeding of the Very-Low-Birth-Weight Infant

38

Johannes B. (Hans) van Goudoever

Contents

Abstract

Enteral nutrition is the natural way of feeding infants. There have been concerns that preterm infants have limited digestive capacity; however, there is evidence that digestive enzymes are present in fetal life. Minimal enteral nutrition should be started as soon as possible because enteral feeding itself may induce the maturation process of digestion and absorption, enhance tolerance to larger volumes of enteral nutrition, and avoid the complications of parenteral nutrition. Adequate oral feeding is possible from 32 weeks onwards, when an infant is capable of an adequate suck-swallow reflex. As oral feeding is not possible in VLBW infants, most frequently gastric tubes are used. The most important reason for withholding enteral feedings is the fear that enteral nutrition will enhance the development of necrotizing enterocolitis (NEC); however, there is no evidence that withholding enteral nutrition prevents NEC. Own mother's human milk is

J. B. (Hans) van Goudoever (✉)
Department of Pediatrics, Emma Children's Hospital – AMC and VU University Medical Center, Amsterdam, The Netherlands
e-mail: h.vangoudoever@amc.uva.nl

G. Buonocore et al. (eds.), *Neonatology*,
https://doi.org/10.1007/978-3-319-29489-6_187

the natural choice for infant feed, even for preterm infants. However, the concentrations of nutrients decline rapidly following birth and do not meet the requirements after approximately 2–4 weeks. Fortification is thus necessary; protein fortification has been shown to increase in-hospital weight gain and head circumference. More clinical trials are needed to improve the quality of the nutrient supply.

38.1 Salient Points

- Preterm infants have limited digestive capacity; however, digestive enzymes are present in fetal life.
- Preterm infants fed with hydrolyzed formula reach full enteral feedings approximately 2 days earlier than when fed nonhydrolyzed formula.
- Parenteral nutrition might induce complications for infants.
- Enteral nutrition downregulates the intestinal inflammatory response and promotes postnatal maturation of intestinal motor activity.
- Delaying enteral feeding does not decrease the incidence of NEC, but increases the time to reach full enteral feeding.
- There is an association of the use of human milk-based fortifier with a lower NEC incidence compared to cow milk-based fortifier and preterm formula.

38.2 Introduction

Enteral nutrition is the natural way of feeding infants. The fetus receives enteral nutrition via the amniotic fluid. The amniotic fluid is largely composed of fetal urine, but lung fluids, nasopharyngeal secretions, and intra- and transmembranous fluids contribute as well. Amniotic fluid contains protein and carbohydrates, but also bacteria important for neonatal colonization (Walker 2017). The amino acid concentrations of amniotic fluid resemble the fetal plasma amino acid concentrations.

The fetus starts to swallow considerable amount of amniotic fluid in the last trimester. By term, the fetus swallows about 700 mL/day, corresponding with 170–230 mL/kg/day (Harding et al. 1984). It is estimated that up to 10–15% of the nitrogenous requirement of the fetus can be met by swallowing amniotic fluid (Pitkin and Reynolds 1975).

There have been concerns that preterm infants have limited capacity to process carbohydrates, fats, and proteins. Peptidases, brush border enzymes, and hydrolases are present in fetal life, with an increase in enzyme activity with the glucocorticoid surge just before birth (Mooij et al. 2014; Sangild and Elnif 1996). Pancreas enzymes such as trypsin, lipase, and amylase are secreted into the duodenum by 31 weeks. From approximately 26 weeks of gestation, lingual and gastric lipases are present, which might help in digestion and absorption of lipids. Bile acids are already secreted by 22 weeks, although the synthesis is much lower in preterm compared to term infants. Adding bile salt-stimulated lipase (BSSL) to infant formula did not exert an effect on weight gain rates in preterm infants, indicating that apparently enough lipase activity is present in infants born before 32 weeks of gestation (Casper et al. 2016).

The effect of extreme premature birth (<26 weeks) and antenatal steroids on digestion and absorption is not precisely known, but may enhance these processes. Lactase activity is also lower in preterm infants, but preterm infants display normal growth when they are fed lactose-containing milk. Preterm infants fed formula pretreated with lactase showed a modest increase in initial weight gain, an effect that disappeared at the end of the study (Erasmus et al. 2002). Proteins are taken up rather efficiently in preterm infants, a process that might be facilitated by pinocytosis and also, because of the increased intestinal permeability (Corpeleijn et al. 2008), intact proteins such as lactoferrin can be absorbed (Hutchens et al. 1991).

Preterm infants fed hydrolyzed formula reach full enteral feedings approximately 2 days earlier than when fed nonhydrolyzed formula, with similar protein metabolism indices (Mihatsch et al. 2002;

Rigo et al. 1995). Enteral nutrition itself may induce the maturation process of digestion and absorption and enhance tolerance to larger volumes of enteral nutrition (Berseth 1992; Meetze et al. 1992). Altogether it follows that enteral nutrition should be installed as soon as possible also to avoid the complications of parenteral nutrient administration. This chapter will focus on feeding mode and type of enteral nutrition.

38.3 Feeding Mode

38.3.1 Minimal Enteral Feeding

The most important reason for withholding enteral feedings is the fear that enteral nutrition will enhance the development of necrotizing enterocolitis (NEC). This serious gastrointestinal problem affects approximately 5% of very-low-birth-weight (VLBW) infants, but the incidence may vary widely among centers. Mortality rates are high, ranging from 20% to 40%. The multifactorial etiology includes gut hypoxia, impaired intestinal host defense mechanisms, and alterations in microbial intestinal content (in amount, diversity and timing of colonization). Enteral nutrition is considered a risk factor as well, since in preterm infants NEC develops in the second or third week of life, after the introduction of enteral feedings (Neu and Walker 2011). However, prevention of NEC by withholding enteral nutrition has not been shown. On the contrary, withholding enteral nutrition to neonatal animals reduces intestinal cell proliferation, gut mass, and enzyme activity (Burrin et al. 2003, 2000). On the other hand, introducing large amounts of enteral feeding is a way of establishing NEC in premature piglets, despite the fact that in utero large amount of amniotic fluids are ingested (Shen et al. 2015). Large amounts of enteral feedings are frequently not tolerated by the VLBW infants. Poor motility, pathogenic microorganisms, and inflammatory processes are related to the differences observed in postnatal life compared to prenatal life. At least nine trials have examined the effects of minimal enteral feeding in VLBW infants (Morgan et al. 2013). Delaying enteral feeding does not decrease the incidence of NEC, but increases the time to reach full enteral feeding (Morgan et al. 2014). Many different definitions of minimal enteral feeding/trophic feeding exist, but in general these are considered relatively small enteral volumes of human milk or formula (<25 mL/kg/day). They can be started as early as day one of life, even in extremely low-birth-weight infants. In neonatal piglets, mucosal growth is not observed before 30% of the total amount of nutrition is administered enterally, so minimal enteral feeding is not intended to serve as a nutritional source (Burrin et al. 2000). Gut hormone levels are stimulated by minimal enteral nutrition, possibly explaining the improved motility (Lucas et al. 1986). Also less need for phototherapy and reduced rates of osteopenia and cholestasis has been reported, probably all related to a reduced time on parenteral nutrition (Berseth 1992; Meetze et al. 1992; Schanler et al. 1999). Lack of any enteral nutrition is associated with an increase in neonatal late onset infections (Sohn et al. 2001). This might be due to bacterial translocation from the intestine. In addition, the intestinal immune/inflammatory response is affected by the route of feeding, with an altered balance of cytokines, lower IL-4 and IL-10 levels in the nonenterally fed state, and subsequent lower IgA production (Fukatsu et al. 2001a, b). Enteral nutrition has been demonstrated to down-regulate the intestinal inflammatory response (van Goudoever et al. 2001). However, clinical trials have not demonstrated a beneficial effect of minimal enteral feeding on invasive infections.

Although large clinical trials on minimal enteral nutrition in VLBW infants are lacking, many studies including animal studies show beneficial effects of minimal enteral feeding in growth and feeding tolerance and provide indications of improved defense mechanisms against bacterial infections and inflammatory processes. This favors initiation of minimal enteral feeding shortly following birth as no adverse effects are reported.

38.3.2 Bolus or (Semi)Continuous Feeding

Bolus feeding results in a significant increase in blood flow to the portal-drained viscera (i.e., stomach, spleen, intestine, and pancreas). There is a surge in gastrointestinal hormones, which is however not higher in bolus fed infants than when neonates are fed continuously (van Goudoever et al. 2001). Clinical trials show that even very small preterm infants tolerate bolus feeding well. Smaller infants seem to benefit more from continuous feeding (Dsilna et al. 2005) and a small trial showed that preterm infants underwent more behavioral stress when fed intermittently (Dsilna et al. 2008). However, a large randomized controlled trial with 250 VLBW infants show that even infants less than 1000 g tolerate bolus feeding well (Rovekamp-Abels et al. 2015). However, some older trials have demonstrated less tolerance to intermittent bolus feeds than continuous milk infusion. Bolus feeding may result in apnea, deteriorating respiratory mechanics with decreased tidal volumes, and transient hypoxia (Blondheim et al. 1993; Heldt 1988). These complications might aggravate in the presence of blocking materials of the nostrils such as nasogastric tubes, or CPAP devices. In conclusion, there is still not enough evidence to recommend either bolus or (semi)continuous feeding as the preferred method.

38.3.3 Oral Feeding

Oral feeding is possible when an infant is capable of an adequate suck-swallow reflex. In the term infant, the full, complex, integrated mechanism of swallowing, with the movement of the bolus of milk into the stomach, protection of the airway, inhibition of respiration, and appropriate relaxation of the esophageal sphincter and gastric fundus is achieved within 2 days of birth (Lebenthal and Leung 1988). The swallow function is present from 16 weeks of gestational age, and gastrointestinal motor activity, in small bursts, from 24 weeks onwards. Organized motility is present from around 30 weeks of gestation and nutritive and swallowing function from 32 weeks. Enteral nutrition promotes postnatal maturation of intestinal motor activity. It follows that adequate oral feeding is possible from 32 weeks onwards. Even wireless monitoring systems are present nowadays to evaluate the feeding behavior of infants quantitatively and objectively and analyze the characteristics of these actions under oral feeding (Chen et al. 2017). Oral feeding protocols (including nonnutritive suckling) can be started however even before 30 weeks of gestation, with a positive influence on time to reach full oral feeding (Kamitsuka et al. 2017; Foster et al. 2016). The preterm infant of less than 32 weeks may be put on the breast, but the likelihood that the infant will ingest a significant volume of milk is very small. However, it may offer the mother a considerable psychological benefit and should therefore be strongly encouraged. Cup-feeding might serve as alternative, although the results are mixed (Flint et al. 2016).

38.3.4 Intragastric Feeding

As oral feeding is not possible in VLBW infants, most frequently gastric tubes are used. Either nasogastric or orogastric tubes can be installed, both checked in the right position by checking the aspirate for acidity with litmus paper or by injection a small amount of air while listening with a stethoscope placed over the stomach. The nasogastric tube has the advantage of easier fixation but has the disadvantage of (partially) blocking one nostril. With the use of some CPAP devices, a nasogastric tube is not possible. With the use of tubes and syringes, one should be aware of a potential loss of nutrients such as lipids and calcium that may not reach the infant (Greer and McCormick 1988).

38.3.5 Transpyloric Feeding

Although transpyloric feeding is frequently used in pediatric intensive care (de Lucas et al. 2000), it should not be used in neonatal intensive care. The available data do not provide evidence of any beneficial effect of transpyloric feeding for preterm infants. Some evidence of harm exists, including a higher risk of gastrointestinal disturbance and mortality, but these findings should be interpreted and applied cautiously because of methodological weaknesses in the included trials. No proven benefits in tolerance, growth, or in aspiration rates have been reported consistently (Watson and McGuire 2013).

38.4 Type of Enteral Nutrition

The aim of the nutritional support of the low-birth-weight infant is to mimic intrauterine growth rate and obtain a long-term functional development similar to the term infant. The nutrient requirements for the VLBW infant are described elsewhere (see ▶ Chap. 37, "Nutritional Recommendations for the Very-Low-Birth-Weight Newborn"), but in general nutritional support should be designed to compensate for metabolic and gastrointestinal immaturity, immunological compromise, and other problems associated with prematurity. Own mother's human milk is the preferred choice, even for preterm infants although it does not provide the required nutrients. Fortification is thus necessary, as unfortified human milk leads to in hospital suboptimal growth (Brown et al. 2016). Human milk is superior to cow's milk-based formulas because of the species specificity. This results in the availability of, for instance, functional proteins and oligosaccharides important for the host defense, which might explain the reduced rates of NEC observed in human milk fed infants (Corpeleijn et al. 2012). Bioavailability of calcium and phosphorus is higher in human milk, but preterm infants still frequently need supplementation, although evidence lacks (Harding et al. 2017). Bacterial flora in infants fed preterm formula differs markedly from those who have been fed human milk (Cong et al. 2016), although the recent improvements in preterm formula facilitate the growth of *Bifidobacterium* and *Lactobacillus* species as well (Boehm et al. 2002). Human milk is better tolerated than formula, with a faster gastric emptying (Ewer et al. 1994), while human milk might reduce intestinal permeability as well (Shulman et al. 1998). Long-term benefits of human milk as compared to formula include lower blood pressure, lower LDL to HDL ratio, and possibly a reduced risk of obesity and higher IQ, although the validity of these results have been questioned (Vohr et al. 2006; Lechner and Vohr 2017; Singhal et al. 2001; Lucas et al. 1992; Isaacs et al. 2010).

38.4.1 Preterm Human Milk

The milk from mothers, who have delivered prematurely, so-called preterm human milk, varies significantly from milk from mothers who delivered at term. Concentrations of proteins, lipids (and thus energy), hormones, vitamins, calcium, sodium, and trace elements are higher. However, the concentrations of these nutrients decline rapidly following birth and do not meet the requirements after approximately 2–4 weeks (Ballard and Morrow 2013). In addition, clinical problems such as patent ductus arteriosus and bronchopulmonary dysplasia often restrict fluid intake demand fluid restrictions with the consequent need for nutrient dense feedings. The adequacy of nutrient intake is further compromised by the variability in composition. For example, the within-feed change in lipid content is well known and can be two to threefolds different between fore- and hind milk.

38.4.2 Expressed Mother's Milk

As most low-birth-weight infants are not able to drink from the breast directly, most mothers choose to express their milk and deliver the milk to the unit themselves. As human milk is not homogenized, the fat content may separate from the remaining milk. Fresh milk is favorable, since freezing and thawing reduces the function of some beneficial components in human milk. Light exposure of breast milk reduces the riboflavin and vitamin A content substantially within a few hours. Human milk, even when fortified, can be stored at refrigerator temperature for 72 h.

38.4.3 Human Milk Banks and Donor Milk

An alternative to own mother's milk is the use of milk from a milk bank (Corpeleijn et al. 2010; Nutrition ECo et al. 2013). Setting up a milk bank may be costly and after setting up the average cost per liter is around €30/l (Meier et al. 2017). Many units around the world have such a milk bank, where mothers donate their milk to be used, most often without payment.

Although some argue that banked milk does not need to be pasteurized, almost all banks do, due to fear of pathogens. Human milk can transmit infection. Donors should be screened for hepatitis B, hepatitis C, and HIV, with counseling offered when needed. Pasteurization destroys HIV (Eglin and Wilkinson 1987). HIV is the most well-recognized viral pathogen, but transmission of cytomegalovirus is not uncommon, and raw breast milk can cause serious and even fatal illness in preterm babies (Hamprecht et al. 2001). Pasteurization, freezing, and thawing lower antimicrobial factors and denature milk lipase (Evans et al. 1978). It may reduce vitamin content as well. Therefore, benefits are not as clear as with nonpasteurized, own mother's milk. On the other hand, most of the lysozyme, IgG, and almost all IgA remain intact. Pasteurization does not affect gastric emptying (de Oliveira et al. 2017).

The benefit of donor milk may be related to the avoidance of exposing the preterm gut to cow's milk proteins, but that hypothesis was rejected based on a large multicenter trial providing either donor milk or preterm formula as add on to own mothers milk during the first 10 days of life (Corpeleijn et al. 2016). No effect was observed on the cumulative incidence of mortality, NEC, and sepsis. Exposing infants for a longer period than 10 days resulted in a significant reduction of NEC in a similarly large trial (O'Connor et al. 2016), but no effect was observed on the primary outcome: neurocognitive development at 2 years of age.

Donors have usually delivered at term or have been lactating for some time, both of which result in lower nutritional content. Nowadays, commercial instruments are available that can screen the nitrogen and energy content of milk very easy, to be informed about some quality aspects of the donor milk.

38.4.4 Fortifier

Exclusively unfortified human milk fed preterm infants show lower serum albumin, total protein, and transthyretin concentrations as a result of an inadequate protein intake. Growth rates are lower than fetal growth rates (Kashyap et al. 1990). In addition, calcium and phosphorus content are too low to meet the preterm infants requirements, resulting in decreases in serum phosphorus and increases in alkaline phosphatase (Pettifor et al. 1989) in the short term and linear growth reduction in the long term (Fewtrell et al. 2000). Hyponatremia may result in a later stage, especially when diuretics are used. The protein-related deficits that might occur using unfortified milk can be corrected with supplementation. Protein fortification has been shown to increase in-hospital weight gain (Brown et al. 2016) and increase head circumference. Both human milk protein sources as well as bovine protein supplementation has been used, with similar results (Polberger et al. 1999). Recent study show an association of the use of human milk-based fortifier with a lower NEC incidence than cow milk-based fortifier and preterm formula although severe methodological issues remain (Cristofalo et al. 2013; Sullivan et al. 2010).

The vitamin K concentration of human milk is very low and for the newborn breastfed infant, a deficiency state has been described. Vitamin K is produced by *Bacteroides* and *E. coli*, bacteria that are usually not common in breastfed infants. However, if prophylactic vitamin K is given at birth, no signs of deficiency have been described for 3 months (Greer et al. 1998), although the addition of vitamin K in fortifiers is logical and current practice.

As human milk composition changes in time, even fortified milk might not meet the requirements of the rapidly growing preterm infant. Frequent monitoring of the administered amount of nutrients remains necessary. Milk analyzers should therefore be available on all units as standard of care. The policy of waiting to change the composition of the nutrient intake until growth is faltering should be considered as suboptimal therapy, which can seriously affect long-term outcome. Human milk fortifiers have been criticized for possible side effects, such as a loss of intrinsic host defense. As described above, there is an indication that infants fed a human milk-based fortifier with human milk might be less prone to develop NEC, although the largest trial to date does not support that hypothesis (O'Connor et al. 2016). Another fear of the use of fortifiers is a reduced tolerance. A recent meta-analysis has revealed no differences between infants fed fortified or unfortified human milk (Brown et al. 2016). Also no differences were observed between infants fed preterm formula or fortified human milk.

38.4.5 Preterm Formula

Although the goal of providing nutrients to the preterm infant is to achieve a functional outcome similar to that of the breastfed term infants, it is obvious that the composition of preterm formula is different from term formula, since the requirements are much higher. Until now, the factorial approach has been used, with only moderate success. With the factorial approach, estimations of requirements are made based upon intrauterine accretion rates, while accounting for endogenous losses, incomplete digestion, and absorption. Intrauterine accretion rates are obtained from carcass analyses of fetuses, with sometimes limited information of the nutritional status of the mother or possible diseases and on intrauterine growth curves. Subsequent modifications of such formulas were made following clinical studies. As stated above, this approach has yielded only limited success. Weight gain rates are lacking behind intrauterine rates, especially in the extremely low-birth-weight infants (Hulst et al. 2004). Mainly retrospective studies have shown detrimental effects of weight gain rates that are suboptimal (Ehrenkranz et al. 2006; Latal-Hajnal et al. 2003). Recent developed guidelines from the European Society for Paediatric Gastroenterology, Hepatology and Nutrition (ESPGHAN) together with a group of experts have indicated major changes in requirements, which are discussed elsewhere (see ▶ Chap. 37, "Nutritional Recommendations for the Very-Low-Birth-Weight Newborn"). Readers are referred to these published recommendations for a detailed description.

38.5 Approach to Improve Enteral Feeding

As yet, current enteral feeding strategies fail to meet the requirements of VLBW infants. Many more clinical trials are needed to improve the quality of the nutrient supply. An alternative approach would be to determine the quantity and quality of intrauterine nutrition by measuring fetal intake and fetal metabolism. Obviously, there are many differences between life in or outside the uterus. Mimicking the uterus seems still far away, although recently a lamb model was developed (Partridge et al. 2017). Compared to the fetus, preterm infants are depending on their own metabolism, use their lungs, and are subject to more gravity forces. In addition, they are frequently ill, which might demand specific nutrients to support defense mechanisms. Medication usage may alter metabolism. Their intestines start to be colonized, and bacteria have their own nutrient requirements. However, intrauterine nutrition and metabolism might provide very valuable insight in to what the fetus is capable of with regard to metabolic activity, although the mother plays a role in the conversion to and excretion of metabolic end products. Glucose is the major oxidative substrate in utero. The ovine fetus utilizes glucose at a rate of approximately 4–7 mg/kg/min, but has the capability to metabolize double (Hay et al. 1983). Lactate is also important as energy source, especially when other sources of energy are lacking (Harding and Johnston 1995). When born at term, the human baby has a large portion of fat. Fat deposition increases exponentially with gestational age. Near term, the fat accretion is 7 g/day. In the fetal sheep, large quantities of amino acids are taken up by both the placenta and the fetus (Lemons et al. 1976). About half of the retained amount is used as fuel source and the ammonia produced in this process is converted into urea by the fetal liver. The human fetus shows a very active amino acid transport as well (Van den Akker et al. 2009). Comparison of albumin synthesis rates, using stable isotope techniques, revealed that very immature fetuses produce large quantities of albumin, rates that are not reached following birth with the present nutritional strategies (Van den Akker et al. 2008; Vlaardingerbroek et al. 2016). This information provides guidelines as to which extent anabolism can occur and to which extent postnatal nutrition should be provided (van den Akker and van Goudoever 2016).

References

Ballard O, Morrow AL (2013) Human milk composition: nutrients and bioactive factors. Pediatr Clin N Am 60 (1):49–74

Berseth CL (1992) Effect of early feeding on maturation of the preterm infant's small intestine. J Pediatr 120 (6):947–953

Blondheim O, Abbasi S, Fox WW, Bhutani VK (1993) Effect of enteral gavage feeding rate on pulmonary functions of very low birth weight infants. J Pediatr 122(5 Pt 1):751–755

Boehm G, Lidestri M, Casetta P, Jelinek J, Negretti F, Stahl B et al (2002) Supplementation of a bovine milk formula with an oligosaccharide mixture increases counts of faecal bifidobacteria in preterm infants. Arch Dis Child Fetal Neonatal Ed 86(3):F178–F181

Brown JV, Embleton ND, Harding JE, McGuire W (2016) Multi-nutrient fortification of human milk for preterm infants. Cochrane Database Syst Rev 5:CD000343

Burrin DG, Stoll B, Jiang R, Chang X, Hartmann B, Holst JJ et al (2000) Minimal enteral nutrient requirements for intestinal growth in neonatal piglets: how much is enough? Am J Clin Nutr 71(6):1603–1610

Burrin DG, Stoll B, Chang X, Van Goudoever JB, Fujii H, Hutson SM et al (2003) Parenteral nutrition results in impaired lactose digestion and hexose absorption when enteral feeding is initiated in infant pigs. Am J Clin Nutr 78(3):461–470

Casper C, Hascoet JM, Ertl T, Gadzinowski JS, Carnielli V, Rigo J et al (2016) Recombinant bile salt-stimulated lipase in preterm infant feeding: a randomized phase 3 study. PLoS One 11(5):e0156071

Chen CT, Wang LY, Wang YL, Lin BS (2017) Quantitative real-time assessment for feeding skill of preterm infants. J Med Syst 41(6):95

Cong X, Xu W, Janton S, Henderson WA, Matson A, McGrath JM et al (2016) Gut microbiome developmental patterns in early life of preterm infants: impacts of feeding and gender. PLoS One 11(4):e0152751

Corpeleijn WE, van Vliet I, de Gast-Bakker DA, van der Schoor SR, Alles MS, Hoijer M et al (2008) Effect of enteral IGF-1 supplementation on feeding tolerance, growth, and gut permeability in enterally fed premature neonates. J Pediatr Gastroenterol Nutr 46(2): 184–190

Corpeleijn WE, Vermeulen MJ, van Vliet I, Kruger C, van Goudoever JB (2010) Human milk banking-facts and issues to resolve. Forum Nutr 2(7):762–769

Corpeleijn WE, Kouwenhoven SM, Paap MC, van Vliet I, Scheerder I, Muizer Y et al (2012) Intake of own mother's milk during the first days of life is associated with decreased morbidity and mortality in very low birth weight infants during the first 60 days of life. Neonatology 102(4):276–281

Corpeleijn WE, de Waard M, Christmann V, van Goudoever JB, Jansen-van der Weide MC, Kooi EM et al (2016) Effect of donor milk on severe infections and mortality in very low-birth-weight infants: the early nutrition study randomized clinical trial. JAMA Pediatr 170(7):654–661

Cristofalo EA, Schanler RJ, Blanco CL, Sullivan S, Trawoeger R, Kiechl-Kohlendorfer U et al (2013) Randomized trial of exclusive human milk versus preterm formula diets in extremely premature infants. J Pediatr 163(6):1592–5.e1

de Lucas C, Moreno M, Lopez-Herce J, Ruiz F, Perez-Palencia M, Carrillo A (2000) Transpyloric enteral nutrition reduces the complication rate and cost in the critically ill child. J Pediatr Gastroenterol Nutr 30(2): 175–180

de Oliveira SC, Bellanger A, Menard O, Pladys P, Le Gouar Y, Dirson E et al (2017) Impact of human milk pasteurization on gastric digestion in preterm infants: a randomized controlled trial. Am J Clin Nutr 105(2): 379–390

Dsilna A, Christensson K, Alfredsson L, Lagercrantz H, Blennow M (2005) Continuous feeding promotes gastrointestinal tolerance and growth in very low birth weight infants. J Pediatr 147(1):43–49

Dsilna A, Christensson K, Gustafsson AS, Lagercrantz H, Alfredsson L (2008) Behavioral stress is affected by the mode of tube feeding in very low birth weight infants. Clin J Pain 24(5):447–455

Eglin RP, Wilkinson AR (1987) HIV infection and pasteurisation of breast milk. Lancet 1(8541):1093

Ehrenkranz RA, Dusick AM, Vohr BR, Wright LL, Wrage LA, Poole WK (2006) Growth in the neonatal intensive care unit influences neurodevelopmental and growth outcomes of extremely low birth weight infants. Pediatrics 117(4):1253–1261

Erasmus HD, Ludwig-Auser HM, Paterson PG, Sun D, Sankaran K (2002) Enhanced weight gain in preterm infants receiving lactase-treated feeds: a randomized, double-blind, controlled trial. J Pediatr 141(4):532–537

Evans TJ, Ryley HC, Neale LM, Dodge JA, Lewarne VM (1978) Effect of storage and heat on antimicrobial proteins in human milk. Arch Dis Child 53(3):239–241

Ewer AK, Durbin GM, Morgan ME, Booth IW (1994) Gastric emptying in preterm infants. Arch Dis Child Fetal Neonatal Ed 71(1):F24–F27

Fewtrell MS, Cole TJ, Bishop NJ, Lucas A (2000) Neonatal factors predicting childhood height in preterm infants: evidence for a persisting effect of early metabolic bone disease? J Pediatr 137(5):668–673

Flint A, New K, Davies MW (2016) Cup feeding versus other forms of supplemental enteral feeding for newborn infants unable to fully breastfeed. Cochrane Database Syst Rev 8:CD005092

Foster JP, Psaila K, Patterson T (2016) Non-nutritive sucking for increasing physiologic stability and nutrition in preterm infants. Cochrane Database Syst Rev 10: CD001071

Fukatsu K, Zarzaur BL, Johnson CD, Lundberg AH, Hanna MK, Wilcox HG et al (2001a) Lack of enteral feeding increases expression of E-selectin after LPS challenge. J Surg Res 97(1):41–48

Fukatsu K, Kudsk KA, Zarzaur BL, Wu Y, Hanna MK, DeWitt RC (2001b) TPN decreases IL-4 and IL-10 mRNA expression in lipopolysaccharide stimulated intestinal lamina propria cells but glutamine supplementation preserves the expression. Shock 15(4):318–322

Greer FR, McCormick A (1988) Improved bone mineralization and growth in premature infants fed fortified own mother's milk. J Pediatr 112(6):961–969

Greer FR, Marshall SP, Severson RR, Smith DA, Shearer MJ, Pace DG et al (1998) A new mixed micellar preparation for oral vitamin K prophylaxis: randomised controlled comparison with an intramuscular formulation in breast fed infants. Arch Dis Child 79 (4):300–305

Hamprecht K, Maschmann J, Vochem M, Dietz K, Speer CP, Jahn G (2001) Epidemiology of transmission of cytomegalovirus from mother to preterm infant by breastfeeding. Lancet 357(9255):513–518

Harding JE, Johnston BM (1995) Nutrition and fetal growth. Reprod Fertil Dev 7(3):539–547

Harding R, Bocking AD, Sigger JN, Wickham PJ (1984) Composition and volume of fluid swallowed by fetal sheep. Q J Exp Physiol 69(3):487–495

Harding JE, Wilson J, Brown J (2017) Calcium and phosphorus supplementation of human milk for preterm infants. Cochrane Database Syst Rev 2:CD003310

Hay WW, Jr., Myers SA, Sparks JW, Wilkening RB, Meschia G, Battaglia FC. Glucose and lactate oxidation rates in the fetal lamb. Proc Soc Exp Biol Med 1983;173(4):553-563

Heldt GP (1988) The effect of gavage feeding on the mechanics of the lung, chest wall, and diaphragm of preterm infants. Pediatr Res 24(1):55–58

Hulst J, Joosten K, Zimmermann L, Hop W, van Buuren S, Buller H et al (2004) Malnutrition in critically ill children: from admission to 6 months after discharge. Clin Nutr 23(2):223–232

Hutchens TW, Henry JF, Yip TT, Hachey DL, Schanler RJ, Motil KJ et al (1991) Origin of intact lactoferrin and its DNA-binding fragments found in the urine of human milk-fed preterm infants. Evaluation by stable isotopic enrichment. Pediatr Res 29(3):243–250

Isaacs EB, Fischl BR, Quinn BT, Chong WK, Gadian DG, Lucas A (2010) Impact of breast milk on intelligence quotient, brain size, and white matter development. Pediatr Res 67(4):357–362

Kamitsuka MD, Nervik PA, Nielsen SL, Clark RH (2017) Incidence of nasogastric and gastrostomy tube at discharge is reduced after implementing an oral feeding protocol in premature (<30 weeks) infants. Am J Perinatol 34(6):606–613

Kashyap S, Schulze KF, Forsyth M, Dell RB, Ramakrishnan R, Heird WC (1990) Growth, nutrient retention, and metabolic response of low-birth-weight infants fed supplemented and unsupplemented preterm human milk. Am J Clin Nutr 52(2):254–262

Latal-Hajnal B, von Siebenthal K, Kovari H, Bucher HU, Largo RH (2003) Postnatal growth in VLBW infants: significant association with neurodevelopmental outcome. J Pediatr 143(2):163–170

Lebenthal E, Leung YK (1988) Feeding the premature and compromised infant: gastrointestinal considerations. Pediatr Clin N Am 35(2):215–238

Lechner BE, Vohr BR (2017) Neurodevelopmental outcomes of preterm infants fed human milk: a systematic review. Clin Perinatol 44(1):69–83

Lemons JA, Adcock EW, 3rd, Jones MD, Jr., Naughton MA, Meschia G, Battaglia FC. Umbilical uptake of amino acids in the unstressed fetal lamb. J Clin Invest 1976;58(6):1428-1434

Lucas A, Bloom SR, Aynsley-Green A (1986) Gut hormones and 'minimal enteral feeding'. Acta Paediatr Scand 75(5):719–723

Lucas A, Morley R, Cole TJ, Lister G, Leeson-Payne C (1992) Breast milk and subsequent intelligence quotient in children born preterm. Lancet 339 (8788):261–264

Meetze WH, Valentine C, McGuigan JE, Conlon M, Sacks N, Neu J (1992) Gastrointestinal priming prior to full enteral nutrition in very low birth weight infants. J Pediatr Gastroenterol Nutr 15(2):163–170

Meier P, Patel A, Esquerra-Zwiers A (2017) Donor human milk update: evidence, mechanisms, and priorities for research and practice. J Pediatr 180:15–21

Mihatsch WA, Franz AR, Hogel J, Pohlandt F (2002) Hydrolyzed protein accelerates feeding advancement in very low birth weight infants. Pediatrics 110(6):1199–1203

Mooij MG, Schwarz UI, de Koning BA, Leeder JS, Gaedigk R, Samsom JN et al (2014) Ontogeny of human hepatic and intestinal transporter gene expression during childhood: age matters. Drug Metab Dispos 42(8):1268–1274

Morgan J, Bombell S, McGuire W (2013) Early trophic feeding versus enteral fasting for very preterm or very low birth weight infants. Cochrane Database Syst Rev 3:CD000504

Morgan J, Young L, McGuire W (2014) Delayed introduction of progressive enteral feeds to prevent necrotising enterocolitis in very low birth weight infants. Cochrane Database Syst Rev 12:CD001970

Neu J, Walker WA (2011) Necrotizing enterocolitis. N Engl J Med 364(3):255–264

Nutrition ECo, Arslanoglu S, Corpeleijn W, Moro G, Braegger C, Campoy C et al (2013) Donor human milk for preterm infants: current evidence and research directions. J Pediatr Gastroenterol Nutr 57(4):535–542

O'Connor DL, Gibbins S, Kiss A, Bando N, Brennan-Donnan J, Ng E et al (2016) Effect of supplemental donor human milk compared with preterm formula on neurodevelopment of very low-birth-weight infants at 18 months: a randomized clinical trial. JAMA 316 (18):1897–1905

Partridge EA, Davey MG, Hornick MA, McGovern PE, Mejaddam AY, Vrecenak JD et al (2017) An extra-uterine system to physiologically support the extreme premature lamb. Nat Commun 8:15112

Pettifor JM, Rajah R, Venter A, Moodley GP, Opperman L, Cavaleros M et al (1989) Bone mineralization and mineral homeostasis in very low-birth-weight infants fed either human milk or fortified human milk. J Pediatr Gastroenterol Nutr 8(2):217–224

Pitkin RM, Reynolds WA (1975) Fetal ingestion and metabolism of amniotic fluid protein. Am J Obstet Gynecol 123(4):356–363

Polberger S, Raiha NC, Juvonen P, Moro GE, Minoli I, Warm A (1999) Individualized protein fortification of human milk for preterm infants: comparison of ultrafiltrated human milk protein and a bovine whey fortifier. J Pediatr Gastroenterol Nutr 29(3):332–338

Rigo J, Salle BL, Picaud JC, Putet G, Senterre J (1995) Nutritional evaluation of protein hydrolysate formulas. Eur J Clin Nutr 49(Suppl 1):S26–S38

Rovekamp-Abels LW, Hogewind-Schoonenboom JE, de Wijs-Meijler DP, Maduro MD, Jansen-van der Weide MC, van Goudoever JB et al (2015) Intermittent bolus or semicontinuous feeding for preterm infants? J Pediatr Gastroenterol Nutr 61(6):659–664

Sangild PT, Elnif J (1996) Intestinal hydrolytic activity in young mink (Mustela Vison) develops slowly postnatally and exhibits late sensitivity to glucocorticoids. J Nutr 126(9):2061–2068

Schanler RJ, Shulman RJ, Lau C (1999) Feeding strategies for premature infants: beneficial outcomes of feeding fortified human milk versus preterm formula. Pediatrics 103(6 Pt 1):1150–1157

Shen RL, Thymann T, Ostergaard MV, Stoy AC, Krych L, Nielsen DS et al (2015) Early gradual feeding with bovine colostrum improves gut function and NEC resistance relative to infant formula in preterm pigs. Am J Physiol Gastrointest Liver Physiol. https://doi.org/10.1152/ajpgi.00163.2015

Shulman RJ, Schanler RJ, Lau C, Heitkemper M, Ou CN, Smith EO (1998) Early feeding, antenatal glucocorticoids, and human milk decrease intestinal permeability in preterm infants. Pediatr Res 44(4):519–523

Singhal A, Cole TJ, Lucas A (2001) Early nutrition in preterm infants and later blood pressure: two cohorts after randomised trials. Lancet 357(9254):413–419

Sohn AH, Garrett DO, Sinkowitz-Cochran RL, Grohskopf LA, Levine GL, Stover BH et al (2001) Prevalence of nosocomial infections in neonatal intensive care unit patients: results from the first national point-prevalence survey. J Pediatr 139(6):821–827

Sullivan S, Schanler RJ, Kim JH, Patel AL, Trawoger R, Kiechl-Kohlendorfer U et al (2010) An exclusively human milk-based diet is associated with a lower rate of necrotizing enterocolitis than a diet of human milk and bovine milk-based products. J Pediatr 156(4):562–7.e1

van den Akker CH, van Goudoever JB (2016) Defining protein requirements of preterm infants by using metabolic studies in fetuses and preterm infants. Nestle Nutr Inst Workshop Ser 86:139–149

Van den Akker CH, Schierbeek H, Rietveld T, Vermes A, Duvekot JJ, Steegers EA et al (2008) Human fetal albumin synthesis rates during different periods of gestation. Am J Clin Nutr 88(4):997–1003

Van den Akker CH, Schierbeek H, Dorst KY, Schoonderwaldt EM, Vermes A, Duvekot JJ et al (2009) Human fetal amino acid metabolism at term gestation. Am J Clin Nutr 89(1):153–160

van Goudoever JB, Stoll B, Hartmann B, Holst JJ, Reeds PJ, Burrin DG (2001) Secretion of trophic gut peptides is not different in bolus- and continuously fed piglets. J Nutr 131(3):729–732

Vlaardingerbroek H, Schierbeek H, Rook D, Vermeulen MJ, Dorst K, Vermes A et al (2016) Albumin synthesis in very low birth weight infants is enhanced by early parenteral lipid and high-dose amino acid administration. Clin Nutr 35(2):344–350

Vohr BR, Poindexter BB, Dusick AM, McKinley LT, Wright LL, Langer JC et al (2006) Beneficial effects of breast milk in the neonatal intensive care unit on the developmental outcome of extremely low birth weight infants at 18 months of age. Pediatrics 118(1):e115–e123

Walker WA (2017) Bacterial colonization of the newborn gut, immune development, and prevention of disease. Nestle Nutr Inst Workshop Ser 88:23–33

Watson J, McGuire W (2013) Transpyloric versus gastric tube feeding for preterm infants. Cochrane Database Syst Rev 2:CD003487

Parenteral Nutrition 39

Jacques Rigo and Thibault Senterre

Contents

Abstract

Modern perinatal medicine has resulted in a dramatic decrease of mortality in premature infants, especially in very low birth weight (VLBW, <1500 g) infants. Nutrition has become one of the most debated issues in the care of low-birth-weight infants. Nutrition of VLBW infants may be divided into two subsequent periods: the immediate adaptive or "transitional" period after birth and a stable "growing" period up to discharge from the NICU. VLBW infants need parenteral nutrition from the first days of life to promote early positive nitrogen retention and growth. Parenteral nutrition may be required or prolonged during the stable "growing" period due to feeding intolerance, gastrointestinal disorders, or surgery. Parenteral nutrition can be prescribed using tailored or standard solution; the former is formulated specifically to meet the daily nutritional requirements of the individual patient, whereas the latter is designed to provide a formulation that meets most of the nutritional needs of the stable biochemical and metabolic parameters. Very recently, it was suggested that the use of unique standard parenteral solution may contribute to a significant improvement of nutritional support for both extremely and very preterm infants.

J. Rigo (✉) · T. Senterre
Department of Neonatology, University of Liège, CHR de la Citadelle, Liège, Belgium

G. Buonocore et al. (eds.), *Neonatology*,
https://doi.org/10.1007/978-3-319-29489-6_188

39.1 Salient Points

- Nutrition of VLBW infants may be divided into a "transitional" period (after birth) and a stable "growing" period (up to discharge from the NICU).
- The aim of nutritional support during the transitional period is: to reduce protein catabolism, to provide amino acid, water, and electrolytes; to promote nitrogen retention; and to limit postnatal metabolic stress.
- The aim of the nutritional support during the stable growing period is to induce the growth of body mass; to abolish the nutritional deficit during the first weeks of life; and to reach normal anthropometric parameters.

39.2 Introduction

Modern perinatal medicine has resulted in dramatic decrease of mortality in premature infants, especially very low birth weight (VLBW, <1500 g) infants. With the major advances in life-support measures, nutrition has become one the most debated issues in the care of low-birth-weight infants. In this regard, several reports have shown the major effect of quantitative and qualitative nutrition during the first period of life on early and late outcome.

Incidence of intrauterine growth restriction (IUGR) is relatively high in VLBW infants and postnatal growth restriction (PNGR) is frequently observed during the early weeks of life resulting in a major growth deficit at the time of discharge. According to population, clinical disorders and nutritional support, growth restriction affected 60–100% of VLBW and extremely low birth weight (ELBW) infants (Ehrenkranz et al. 1999).

PNGR is mainly the result of the cumulative nutritional deficit occurring during the transitional period from birth to the time of full enteral feeding (Embleton et al. 2001; Rigo et al. 2002) but additional effects during the stable growing period have also been suggested (Curtis and Rigo 2004). Therefore, several studies evaluated the effect of more optimal (aggressive) nutrition during the early weeks of life (Wilson et al. 1997; Thureen et al. 2003; Ziegler et al. 2002; Simmer 2007) and various international scientific committees reconsidered current nutritional recommendations in preterm infants focusing on ELBW and VLBW infants (Table 1) (Tsang et al. 2005; Agostoni et al. 2010).

Due to gastrointestinal tract immaturity, cardio-respiratory adaptation, clinical status and high nutritional requirements, VLBW infants require parenteral nutrition from the first days of life to promote early positive nitrogen retention and growth. In addition, parenteral nutrition could

Table 1 Recent recommendations of daily parenteral intakes for ELBW and VLBW infants

		Tsang et al. (2005)			ESPEN-ESPGHAN (Koletzko et al. 2005)		
		Day 0	Transition	Growing	Day 0	Transition	Growing
FluIDs	mL/kg/day	90–120	90–140	120–180	80–90	100–150	140–180
Energy	kcal/kg/day	40–50	75–85	90–115	50–60	60–100	100–120
Protein	g/kg/day	2	3.5	3.5–4	1.5–2.5	2.0–3.5	3.5–4
Carbohydrate	g/kg/day	7	8–15	13–17	7–10	9–15	12–18
Fat	g/kg/day	1	1–3	3–4	0–1	1–3	2–4
Sodium	mmol/kg/day	0–1	2–5	3–7	0–3	2–3	2–7
Potassium	mmol/kg/day	0	0–2	2–3	0–2	1–2	2–5
Chloride	mmol/kg/day	0–1	2–5	3–7	0–3	2–3	2–5
Calcium	mmol/kg/day	0.5–1.5	1.5	1.3–4	NP	1–2	1.3–3.0
Phosphorus	mmol/kg/day	0–1	1.5–2	1.5–2	NP	1–2	1.0–2.5
Magnesium	mmol/kg/day	0	0–0.3	0.2–0.3	NP	NP	0.2–0.4
Zinc	μmol/kg/day	0–2	2,5	6	NP	3	4

NP not provIDed

be required or prolonged during the stable "growing" period due to feeding intolerance, gastrointestinal disorders or surgery. Provision of parenteral nutrition (PN), total or suppletive, can be ordered using individualized prescription, homemade standardized parenteral solution or ready to use industrialized prepared multichamber bags.

In this chapter we discuss the most important features regarding parenteral nutrition that have been recently reviewed (Rigo and Curtis 2004; Koletzko et al. 2005; Ben 2008; Fusch et al. 2009) (Table 1), outlining more recent practical aspects and guidelines particularly for ELBW and VLBW infants.

39.3 Nutritional Support in VLBW Infants

Nutrition of VLBW infants may be divided into two subsequent periods, firstly the immediate adaptive or "transitional" period after birth, and a stable "growing" period up to discharge from the NICU. Depending on birth weight (BW) and gestational age (GA) the transitional period may be prolonged, particularly in the more vulnerable infants with major clinical disorders. The more premature a neonate, the more challenging are the influences of immaturity and the accompanying morbidity on nutritional supply. Most of these infants receive parenterally delivered nutrients as their major source of nutrition for the first days, and sometimes weeks, of life.

Nutrition during the "stable-growing" period on PN is exceptional, used only when preterm infants are recovering from surgery and/or severe gastrointestinal problems, to prevent or limit the use of the gastrointestinal tract.

39.3.1 Parenteral Nutrition During the Transitional Period

The aim of the nutritional support in VLBW infants during the transitional period is:

1. To reduce protein catabolism providing an energy intake at least at the level of energy expenditure;
2. To provide amino acids (AA) at a level sufficient to induce a positive nitrogen retention;
3. To provide water and electrolytes to control hydration status and postnatal physiological fluid adaptation;
4. To progressively increase AA, energy and mineral intake to promote nitrogen retention and early growth and to limit a possible cumulative nutritional deficit;
5. To limit postnatal metabolic stress in this high-risk population.

Recent data suggest that provision of a more "aggressive" nutritional support from the first day of life reduces postnatal growth deficit and improves neurodevelopmental outcomes in VLBW infants (Senterre and Rigo 2011a; Martin et al. 2009).

39.3.1.1 Fluids and Electrolytes

A number of adaptive processes occurring at birth affect nutritional support. During the early weeks of life, water, electrolyte and mineral homeostasis, and glucose control are more challenging. Placental clearance and placental supply of fluids, electrolytes, minerals and nutrients are discontinued. Thermoregulation and insensible water losses influence water metabolism, especially in VLBW infants. Subsequent adaptation and compensatory regulative processes need time to stabilize.

Fluid and electrolyte administration during the transitional period should allow contraction of extracellular fluid space without compromising intravascular fluid volume and cardiovascular function, maintain normal plasma electrolyte concentrations, without impairing urinary output (<0.5–1.0 mL/kg/h) for more than 12 h.

Water balance may be very unstable, especially in ELBW infants, urinary output may be high (6–10 mL/kg/h) and insensible fluid losses can be huge, especially under a radiant warmer and/or with phototherapy.

A negative net balance for sodium is allowed and intakes should be less than 2 mmol/kg initially. Restricted sodium intake in VLBW infants has a positive influence on oxygen supply and risk of later bronchopulmonary dysplasia. However, high sodium urinary excretion (10 mmol/kg) may occur, especially in case of high fluid perfusion over 170–200 mL/kg/d compromising sodium balance.

This transitional phase may last for a variable period of several hours or days and result in initial weight loss. The end of the transitional period is usually characterized by a urine volume <2.0 mL/kg/h, urine osmolarity>serum osmolarity, fractional Na excretion diminishing from >3% to <1% and specific gravity above 1012. In preterm infants, these changes complete after 3–5 days and water and electrolytes intake will be progressively increased to replete the body losses.

During the transitional period, VLBW infants should be weighted twice daily and in/out balance, plasma sodium concentration and urinary excretion should be monitored attentively during first days of life. Fluid intake on PN should be 50–100 mL/kg/d in VLBW infants according to clinical and environmental conditions and sodium and potassium intake limited to less than 2 mmol/kg/d (Koletzko et al. 2005; Fusch et al. 2009).

39.3.1.2 Amino Acids

To reduce the temporary interruption of the transfer of nutrients, to limit the high protein catabolism up to 1.5 g/kg/d and to induce a positive nitrogen balance from the first day of life a high-protein supply (>2 g amino acids/kg per day) has recently been suggested in the so-called "aggressive" nutrition (Thureen et al. 2003; Ziegler et al. 2002; Simmer 2007).

Although, long-term benefits were not clearly demonstrated, it has been suggested that high protein intake during the first week of life induces positive nitrogen balance, increases insulin secretion, improves glucose tolerance, promotes early weight gain and improves neurodevelopmental outcome at 18 months (Stephens et al. 2009). Thus, new recommendations (Koletzko et al. 2005; Fusch et al. 2009) suggest providing 2–3 g of AA on the first day of life using a parenteral solution with a high AA:energy ratio and to progressively increase the AA intake up to 4 g/kg/d at the end of the first week of life.

39.3.1.3 Energy

Energy intake is required for both protein metabolism and deposition. Theoretically, an energy intake approximating the resting energy expenditure (i.e., 40–60 kcal/kg/day) allows the minimization of protein catabolism to about 1.5 g of protein/kg/d in ELBW infants. If amino acid intake is adequate and energy intake is in excess of resting energy expenditure, weight gain is achieved. However, because of individual differences in energy expenditure, the resting energy requirement varies considerably in this population. New recommendations (Koletzko et al. 2005; Fusch et al. 2009) suggest providing 40 kcal/kg/d on the first day of life, to increase up to 75–85 kcal/kg/d during the transitional period and to reach close to 100 kcal/kg/d at the end of the first week of life.

39.3.1.4 Carbohydrates

Glucose homeostasis is still immature during the early days of life in VLBW infants who are subject to hyper or hypoglycemia. Glucose is the main carbohydrate in fetal life and approximately 7 g/kg/d (4 mg/kg/min) of glucose crosses the placenta in the last trimester of pregnancy. Glucose production around 8 mg/kg/min (11.5 g/kg/d) in preterm infants is maximal in the postnatal period and decreases gradually with age. Gluconeogenesis may be responsible for a part of glucose production. During high rates of glucose infusion, endogenous production is not completely suppressed in VLBW infants. By contrast, maximum glucose oxidation is relatively limited, 7–8.5 mg/kg/min (10–12 g/kg/d), but could be less in critically ill VLBW infants. The imbalance between glucose infusion rate and endogenous production on one hand and the maximum oxidation rate explain the increasing incidence of hyperglycemia in VLBW infants. In addition, due to their immaturity and their underlying diseases, VLBW infants are relatively resistant to insulin during the first week of life.

During the transitional phase, fluctuations in blood sugar levels are frequently observed resulting from an insufficient glucose and energy intake associated with low substrate reserves (hypoglycemia) or from a relative excess of glucose and energy intake associated with some degree of insulin resistance (hyperglycemia). Although the definition and the long-term consequences of neonatal hypo- and hyperglycemia remain controversial, plasma glucose concentration should be monitored to remain in a normal range for VLBW infants on parenteral nutrition between 50 mg/dL (2.75 mmol/L) and 150 mg/dL (8.3 mmol/L). Hyperglycemia can be decreased by reducing insensible water loss, glucose infusion rate and by providing exogenous insulin supply. Insulin administration may help to control plasma glucose concentration, to achieve increased energy intake and to promote nitrogen retention and growth, although there is need for more data on its safety and long-term consequences as a growth-promoting agent. More recently, it has been proposed that high AA intake from the first day (2–3 g/kg/d) improves glucose tolerance in ELBW infants by stimulating growth, by enhancing insulin and insulin-like growth factors secretion (Thureen et al. 2003). This approach requires further randomized control trials.

In practice, 6 g glucose/kg per day are generally well tolerated (4–5 mg/kg/min) even on the first day of life in VLBW infants. If this intake is tolerated, it may be increased progressively to 12–16 g/kg per day at the end of the first week of life. If it is not tolerated, progression of glucose intake will be reduced and insulin perfusion will be considered according to clinical and nutritional status with an initial dose of 0.05 IU/kg/h.

39.3.1.5 Lipids

Intravenous lipid emulsions are important constituents of total PN as they provide in an isotonic solution, high energy density and essential fatty acids to VLBW infants. Intravenous lipids play two separate roles in the PN of VLBW infants. The first role is as a high-density energy substrate to be readily utilized by VLBW infants. The other role is as a source of essential fatty acids as well as long-chain PUFAs. Essential fatty acid deficiency is avoided by infusions of 0.5–1.0 g lipid per kg per day. The importance of long-chain PUFAs for the development of the brain and the retina has also been recognized. Intravenous lipid emulsions contain small amounts of these fatty acids as part of the egg phospholipid used as a stabilizer. However, clearance of lipid emulsion could be impaired in ELBW infants particularly those with IUGR requiring the monitoring of triglyceridemia.

Actually, new recommendations (Koletzko et al. 2005; Fusch et al. 2009) suggest providing 1 g/kg/d on the first day increasing stepwise fashion to 3.0 g/kg/d at the end of the first week of age.

39.3.1.6 Minerals: Ca, P and Mg

Calcium and phosphorus transfer and retention is high during the last trimester of gestation. Combined with a relative immaturity of hormonal control (Vit D, PTH), VLBW infants particularly are at risk of early neonatal hypocalcemia and hypophosphoremia (see ▶ Chap. 41, "Calcium and Phosphorus Homeostasis: Pathophysiology").

Calcium supply needs to be provided from the first day of life in combination with an adequate calcium phosphorus ratio to limit the risk of hypocalcemia and/or hypophosphoremia. Phosphorus plays a critical role in energy metabolism, and deficiency of phosphorus results in clinical disease, including muscle weakness. Early phosphorus deficiency is also potentiated by IUGR. Reference values for plasma phosphorus concentration differ in adults (>1.0 mmol/L, 3 mg/dL) and in preterm infants (>1.6 mmol/L, 5 mg/dL). Unfortunately, most neonatologists are unaware that the laboratory reports plasma phosphorus concentration of VLBW infants with regard to adult references and tolerates hypophosphatemia with the risk of hypercalciuria and osteopenia. Optimal calcium to phosphorus ratio differs in parenteral and oral nutrition due to the bypass of the gastrointestinal tract; phosphorus retention is related to bone mineralization with a weight-to-weight calcium:phosphorus ratio of 2.15:1 but also to nitrogen retention with a weight-to-weight nitrogen:phosphorus ratio of 15:1. Therefore optimal Ca to P ratio in parenteral nutrition ranges between 1.5 and 1.3.

Magnesium is rarely adjusted even in the transitional period unless the infant has persistent hypocalcemia secondary to hypomagnesemia, or has abnormally high magnesium levels due to maternal levels. Serum magnesium levels should be checked in any small infant whose mother was treated for hypertension or preeclampsia.

Actually, new recommendations (Koletzko et al. 2005; Fusch et al. 2009) suggest providing around 25–40 mg (0.6–1 mmol) of Ca/kg/d, 18–31 mg (0.6–1 mmol) of P/kg/d and 2.5–4.0 mg (0.1–0.2 mmol)/kg/d of magnesium on the first day and to progressively increase the intake according to energy and AA supplies up to 65–100 mg (1.6–2.5 mmol) of Ca/kg/d, 50–78 mg (1.6–2.5 mmol) of Phosphorus and 7–10 mg (0.3–0.4 mmol/kg/d) of magnesium.

39.3.2 Parenteral Nutrition During the Stable Growing Period

The aim of the nutritional support in VLBW infants during the stable growing period is:

1. To induce growth rate and protein accretion in the range of the fetal weight gain considering the lean body mass gain as reference;
2. To abolish the development of a cumulative nutritional deficit during the first weeks of life;
3. To reach, at the time of discharge and/or of theoretical term, an anthropometric parameter in the range of reference values for term infants.

39.3.2.1 Fluids and Electrolytes

Intravenous fluid is the carrying vehicle for parenteral nutrition. A fluid intake about 140–160 mL/kg/d in both VLBW and VLBW preterm infants allows for covering the water requirement for replacing water loss and providing enough extra water to build new tissues during the stable growing period. Fat mass is relatively free of water content. By contrast, lean body mass content is about 80%. Thus a weight gain of 20 g/kg/d containing 40% of fat results in a net storage of 13 g of water and 1–1.5 mmol of Na+/kg/d.

Sodium and potassium requirements are in the range of 3–7 mmol/kg/d for Na^+ and 2–5 mmol/kg/d for K^+ in VLBW infants respectively. A mean intake of 3 mmol/kg/day of sodium and 2 mmol/kg/day of potassium seem to be appropriate to maintain normal plasma concentration for most stable growing infants. In parenteral solution, sodium is frequently provided with phosphorus in the form of sodium glycerophosphate and limitation of sodium content also limits the phosphorus content. Chloride supply requires particular attention in parenteral nutrition. Chloride requirement is generally considered similar to sodium requirement. Chloride content in parenteral solution is related to several potential components, AA solution, sodium chloride, potassium chloride or calcium chloride and is difficult to control. However, chloride intake plays a role in the acid-base homeostasis and imbalance between $Na^+ + K^+$ and Cl^- promotes metabolic acidosis or alkalosis (Kalhoff et al. 1997). Therefore, monitoring of plasma and urinary electrolyte concentrations and appropriate correction remains recommended, during parenteral nutrition.

39.3.2.2 Amino Acids

Nitrogen requirement in parenteral nutrition is close to 95% of the enteral requirement, but corresponds in terms of g AA/kg/g to the figure in g protein/kg/d recommended in enteral nutrition, due to a relatively lower nitrogen content. Protein requirement has been recently reviewed according to fetal nitrogen accretion, lean body mass gain and the need to compensate early cumulative protein deficits during the transitional period. 3.5–4.5 g of AA /kg/d is recommended during the stable growing period in ELBW and VLBW infants (Tsang et al. 2005; Agostoni et al. 2010; Rigo 2005).

39.3.2.3 Energy

In contrast to what is generally suggested, the energy requirement in PN approximates to that of enteral nutrition. In fact, the gross energy content, measured by bomb calorimetry, of 1 g of amino acid is lower than that of 1 g of protein. Similarly, gross energy content of glucose is less than that of more complex carbohydrates. In contrast, while in parenteral nutrition the metabolizable energy of amino acid and fat solutions are identical to the gross energy, the metabolizable energy of dietary protein and fat in oral nutrition represents about 90% and 80% respectively (Curtis et al. 1986). Consequently, the recommendation for energy intake during the stable-growing period in VLBW infants on parenteral nutrition is relatively similar to that in oral nutrition and corresponds to 110–130 kcal/kg per day in VLBW infants.

39.3.2.4 Carbohydrates

Glucose contributes to most of the osmolality of PN solution (510 mOsm/L for a 10% solution) by contrast to lipid solutions. An excessive glucose intake increases CO_2 production and may be responsible for hyperglycemia, cause lipogenesis, steatosis and may contribute to liver dysfunction. The maximum glucose intake should not exceed the glucose oxidation rate in parenteral nutrition of 13–18 g/kg/d and more than 60–75% of the non-protein energy during the stable growing period.

39.3.2.5 Lipids

Intravenous lipid emulsions are important constituents of total parenteral nutrition as they provide most of the energy intake and essential fatty acids (EFA). The CO_2 production is lowered compared to PN with a high proportion of carbohydrates and the nitrogen metabolism can be improved by adding lipid emulsions to PN. Lipid oxidation depends on the overall energy intake and consumption, intake of carbohydrates and triglycerides and the carbohydrate/lipid ratio. Lipid oxidation decreases as the carbohydrate intake increases and is replaced by lipid storage.

Maximum fat oxidation occur when lipid emulsions provide 40% of the non-protein energy in newborns so it is recommended that lipid intake should provide 25–40% of non-protein energy with a maximum of 3–4 g/kg/day (Koletzko et al. 2005). An increase in the concentration of plasma triglycerides is to be expected if the infusion speed of the lipid emulsion exceeds the speed of triglyceride hydrolysis that depends on lipoprotein lipase activity. In all cases, the triglyceride infusion dose should be adjusted to maintain a serum triglyceride concentration not exceeding 200–250 mg/dL, especially in ELBW or severely ill infants who may have limited lipid tolerance.

Concerns had been raised on the potentially adverse effects of lipid infusion on hemodynamics, infections or hyperbilirubinemia. It appears prudent to avoid high lipid supplies in infants with sepsis, impaired oxygenation, or severe hyperbilirubinemia and lipid emulsion infusion should be continued at least at 0.5–1.0 g/kg/day, which is sufficient to prevent essential fatty acid deficiency.

Lipid supply may result in enhanced lipid peroxidation and the formation of free radicals. An increased lipid utilization by reducing the carbohydrate/lipid ratio results in a reduction of lipid peroxidation and free radical formation. PN should be supplemented with multi-vitamin preparations including both vitamin C and vitamin E (alpha-tocopherol), which have anti-oxidative effects. Excessive exposure of the bottle to light should be avoided.

Carnitine is necessary for the transportation of long-chain fatty acids via the mitochondrial membrane and its oxidative metabolism. Because carnitine synthesis and storage are not sufficiently developed at birth, particularly in preterm infants, and because no commercial intravenous solution has carnitine, parenterally fed infants present low plasma and tissue carnitine levels that decline with postnatal age (Borum 2009). Although a meta analysis (based on 14 randomised, controlled studies) showed there to be no effect of carnitine supplementation on the metabolism of lipids, lipogenesis or weight gain (Cairns and Stalker 2000), a carnitine supplementation of 15 μmol/100 kcal could be advisible for infants on total parenteral nutrition for more than 4 weeks.

39.3.2.6 Minerals: Ca, P and Mg

Calcium and phosphorus cannot be provided through the same parenteral solution at concentrations needed to support in utero accretion, because of solubility. With a fluid intake range of 120–150 mL/kg/day, it is advisable to supply 65–100 mg (1.6–2.5 mmol) of Ca /kg/d, 50–78 mg (1.6–2.5 mmol) of iP and 7–10 mg (0.3–0.4 mmol/kg/d) of Mg, corresponding to a Ca/P ratio of 1.3:1 by weight and 1:1 by molar ratio in the TPN solution. It must be underlined that this quantity of calcium provided by parenteral route is about 55–80% of that deposited by the fetus during the last trimester of gestation (120 mg/kg/day) but similar or higher than that obtained in enteral nutrition with the available preterm formula (see ▸ Chap. 41, "Calcium and Phosphorus Homeostasis: Pathophysiology").

39.3.2.7 Trace Elements and Vitamins

Vitamin mixtures for parenteral use have been available since the early time of parenteral nutrition and the amounts provided were (and are) determined to a large extent by the preparations available. Today, additives of all trace minerals for which a deficiency has been demonstrated are available. However, little definitive information is available concerning the parenteral requirements of either trace minerals or vitamins in VLBW infants. Research concerning the parenteral requirements of these nutrients by infants, of course, is hindered by the difficulties both of measuring plasma concentrations of the nutrients using small volumes of plasma and of interpreting the physiological significance of plasma concentrations.

39.4 Practical Aspects of Parenteral Nutrition in VLBW Infants

39.4.1 Basic Components Available for Parenteral Nutrition in Preterm Infant

39.4.1.1 AA Solutions

Considerable improvement of parenteral amino acid solutions have occurred from the late 1960s when the source of intravenous protein was casein hydrolysate. More specific pediatric amino acid solutions have been designed in the early 1990s with high essential/non-essential AA ratios and conditionally essential amino acid content for use in preterm infants. At least three different "gold standards" have been proposed for premature infants: (1) the amino acid concentrations from the umbilical cord obtained following fetal cord puncture or after birth, (2) the amino acid concentrations of rapidly growing preterm infants receiving their mother's milk or human milk supplemented with human milk proteins, (3) the amino acid concentrations of healthy breast-fed term infants. Nevertheless, despite the diverse composition of parenteral amino acid solutions used in pediatric care, nitrogen utilization does not change significantly (Fig. 1) (Rigo and Curtis 2004; Rigo 2005) (Table 2).

Therefore, optimal amino acid patterns for parenteral amino acid solutions in preterm infants still need to be determined and new solutions should be developed to potentially improve sulfur and aromatic AA imbalances and to provide additional glutamine. However, up to now, the use of cystein-HCl, acetyl-cystein, acetyl-tyrosine (Goudoever et al. 1994) and the supplementation with glutamine (Tubman et al. 2008) have not demonstrated beneficial effects. The recent data evaluating the effect of bypassing the intestine on individual AA requirements has not been translated to designing and evaluating new AA solutions.

39.4.1.2 Lipid Emulsions

Intravenous lipid emulsions consist of different oils (soybean, safflower, coconut, olive and fish oils), egg yolk phospholipids and glycerol [reviewed in 12, 14, 26, 27] (see Table 3). Intravenous lipid emulsions provide high caloric, isotonic solutions and can also be given through peripheral lines Traditionally, lipid infusions are prepared from soybean oil triglycerides emulsified with egg yolk phospholipids. Typical soybean oil contains about 45–55% linoleic acid (18:2n-6) and 6–9% linolenic acid (18:3n-3), but very little saturated or monounsaturated fat. Although clinically safe, experimental reports indicated that soybean oil based lipid emulsion could exert a negative influence on immunological functions. Those findings were related to its absolute and relative excess of ω-6 polyunsaturated fatty acids (PUFA) and the low amount of ω-3 PUFA and also to its high PUFA content with an increased peroxidation risk. The new lipid emulsion was basically designed in order to obtain balanced levels in polyunsaturated (ω-6 and ω-3), monounsaturated, and saturated fatty acids. They are differentiated by their fatty acid content, as well as fatty acid source of their origin, including soy, safflower, coconut, olive, and fish oil. Newer emulsions comprise physical mixtures of either a 20:80 mixture of soy ω-6 PUFA and ω-9 medium-chain monounsaturates (MUFA) from olive oil or

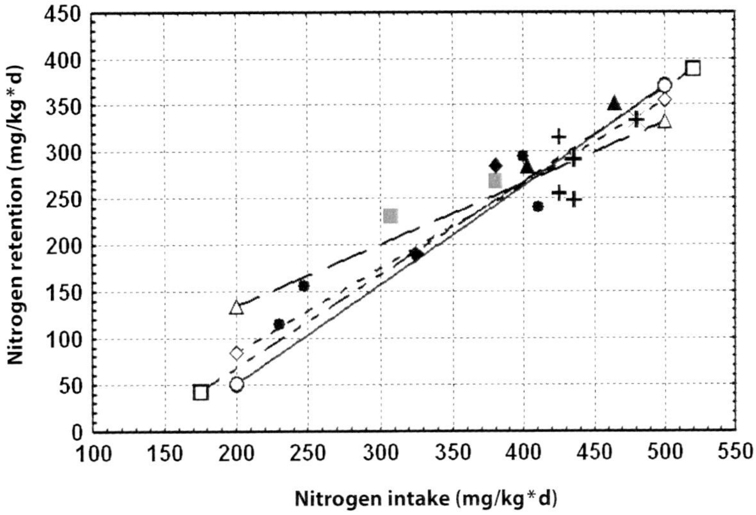

Fig. 1 Relationship between nitrogen retention and nitrogen intake in parenterally fed preterm infants computing of various studies (the different symbols represent individual studies)

Table 2 Main composition of commercial parenteral amino acID solutions for preterm infants

Product	%	Total AA (g/L)	EAA (%)	Cyst(e)ine (g/L)	Tyrosine (g/L)	Taurine (g/L)	Osmolality (mosm/L)	pH
Aminopäd	10	100	42	0.5[a]	1.1[c]	0.3	790	6.1
Aminoplasmal	10	100	42	[b]	0.4	–	864	5.7–6.3
Primene	10	100	48	1.9	0.5	0.6	780	5.5
Aminoven infant	10	100	51	0.5	4.2[c]	0.4	885	5.5–6.0
Vaminolact	6.5	65	44	1.0	0.5	0.3	510	5.2
TrophAmin	10	100	49	[b]	0.2	0.3	875	5.5

EAA Essential amino acID (n = 8)
[a]As acetyl-cystein
[b]Separately as cystein HCl
[c]As acetyl-tyrosine

Table 3 Oil content (%) in commercially manufactured intravenous lipid emulsions

Product	Soy (LCT)	Coconut (MCT)	Olive (MUFA)	Fish (ω3)
IntralipID	100	0	0	0
Lipofundin MCT/LCT	50	50	0	0
StructolipID	64	36	0	0
ClinOleic	20	0	80	0
LipoPlus	40	50	0	10
SMOFlipID	30	30	25	15
Omegaven	0	0	0	100

LCT long-chain triglycerides, *MCT* medium-chain triglycerides, *MUFA* mono unsaturated fatty acid

a 1:1 ratio of LCT with coconut oil-derived medium chain triglycerides (MCT). Structured MCT/LCT emulsions formulated from a random combination of triglycerides synthesized on the same glycerol carbon chain are cleared faster from blood in moderately catabolic patients. The newer lipid combinations with a smaller proportion of soy oil, have a much lower content of linoleic acid and linolenic acid, the potentially pro-inflammatory ω-6 PUFA, and less myristic, palmitic, and stearic acids. These long-chain SFAs are believed to have increased cardiovascular risk and can also have acute effects on cell growth and apoptosis. In MCT/LCT emulsions, MCT may be preferentially metabolized under certain clinical conditions and structured MCT may have a reduced tendency to accumulate in the reticulo-endothelial system. The olive oil-derived ω-9 MUFA appears less immunosuppressive and may inhibit release of pro-inflammatory cytokines. They are also less susceptible to peroxidation and well tolerated in critically ill neonates. Fish oil emulsions are predominantly ω-3 long-chain PUFA. Alone, they lack EFA and are formulated as a supplement to be administered with other nutritionally complete lipid products, or are manufactured as physical mixtures (10% fish: 40% soy: 50% MCT or 30% soy:30% MCT:25% olive oil:15% fish). Fish oil-derived ω-3 PUFAs appear to alleviate symptoms of cholestasis, especially in neonates. Modern lipid products, based on olive, coconut, and/or fish oils, have demonstrable formulation and clinical benefits over traditional soybean and safflower IVLE and, when combined in the new multi-chamber bags, can also offer improvements in stability and safety (Hardy and Puzovic 2009; Diamond et al. 2009; Waitzberg et al. 2006).

39.4.1.3 Mineral Sources

In parenteral nutrition, calcium may be provided in the form of calcium gluconate, calcium chloride or calcium glycerophosphate. Due to aluminium contamination calcium gluconate was progressively abandoned by industry to meet the new FDA rule of 25 μg/L of aluminium in parenteral solution but remains frequently used in home-made hospital pharmacy preparations. Calcium chloride is easy to use but its high chloride content (2 mmol Cl^-/1 mmol Ca^{++}) limits its utilization in parenteral nutrition for VLBW infants (Poole et al. 2008; Bohrer et al. 2010). Calcium glycerophosphate with a 1:1 molar ratio is an adequate source of calcium and phosphorus, but is not registered for use in parenteral nutrition and needs to be prescribed from powdered anhydrous CaGlyP.

Phosphorus may be provided in inorganic (sodium or potassium phosphate) or organic form (glucose 1 phosphate, fructose 1–6 diphosphate, sodium glycerophosphate). Potassium phosphate is frequently preferred to sodium phosphate and used as the unique source of potassium in the parenteral solution. Potassium phosphate is easy to use but its high potassium content (1 mmol P^{3-}/1 mmol K for the monobasic form, 1 mmol P^{3-}/2 mmol K for the dibasic form or 1 mmol P^{3-}/1.7 mmol K for the mixed form) limit its utilization in parenteral nutrition for VLBW infants. Organic phosphorus in the form of disodium glucose 1 phosphate (Phocytan) is widely used in parenteral solution for VLBW infants. However, as for the use of sodium glycerophosphate, 2 mmol Na^+/1 mmol P^{3-}, or fructose 1–6 diphosphate (Esafosfina) the sodium content, 3 mmol Na^+/2 mmol P^{3-}, limits its utilization in VLBW infants particularly during the first weeks of life.

Magnesium is generally provided as magnesium sulfate in parenteral solution. Magnesium chloride has also been associated with the risk of inducing anionic-cationic imbalance in the parenteral solution.

39.4.1.4 Vitamins and Trace Elements

With the daily use of hydro- and lipo-soluble vitamins combined with trace elements clinical and biochemical evidence of deficiency were no longer reported.

39.4.2 Tailored or Standard Parenteral Solutions

Parenteral solutions can be prescribed using either of two formats: tailored or standard (Poole and Kerner 1992; Lapillonne et al. 2009). Tailored solutions are formulated specifically to meet the daily nutritional requirements of the individual patient, whereas standard solutions are designed to provide a formulation that meets most of the nutritional needs of the stable biochemical and metabolic parameters. Both of these methods have advantages and disadvantages associated with their use.

Tailored solutions are based on the principle that no single parenteral regimen can be ideal for all patients, for a wide variety of pathological processes, all age groups, or for the same patient during a single disease. The main advantage of tailored solutions is flexibility. Each solution is formulated for an individual patient and can be modified when the patient's nutritional needs and metabolic, electrolyte or clinical status changes.

The disadvantage of these solutions is linked to the time involved in calculation and label preparation, which today is nevertheless diminished with the use of specific computer programs. These solutions should be prepared with strict aseptic techniques, possibly in the pharmacy, not in the ward, and stored in a refrigerator at 4 °C. The solutions thus prepared are stable for 96 h and should be allowed to reach room temperature slowly and not warmed before infusion.

Standard solutions contain fixed amounts of each component per unit volume. In some hospitals there are a few types of fixed solutions to better cover the nutritional requirements of premature infants. The advantages of these solutions are that they include all the essential nutrients in fixed amounts, which eliminates the chances of inadvertent omission or overload. The disadvantage of standard solutions is their lack of patient specificity and the need of minimal adjustment particularly during the first days of life.

Very recently, it was suggested that the use of unique standard parenteral solution contribute to a significant improvement of nutritional support in both extremely and very preterm infants (Senterre and Rigo 2011b). In addition, ready to use industrially manufactured multi-chamber bags (MCB) containing the three sterilized macro-nutrient solutions (amino acids, glucose, and lipids), in separate chambers of a single closed plastic system were evaluated in multicentric study and provides similar benefits (Rigo et al. 2011). Their guaranteed sterility and longer shelf life are major technological advances that minimize the risks of inadvertent contamination during compounding and storage.

39.4.3 Nutrient Intake

Table 4 shows the composition of a ready to use parenteral solution for VLBW infants used in our NICU and the daily nutrient intake (kg/d) given by total parenteral nutrition according to the new

Table 4 Parenteral nutrition solution and daily nutrient intake (kg/d) of very low birth weight infants (<1500 g) in total parenteral nutrition according the "aggressive approach"

Day of life	Composition	D1	D2	D3	D4	D5	D6	>D6
		/kg/d	/kg/d	/kg/d	/kg/d	/kg/d	/kg/d	/kg/d
Parenteral solution (mL)	100	50	70	100	120	140	150	150
Glucose (g)	12.5	6.3	8.8	12.5	15.0	17.5	18.8	18.8
Amino acid (g)	2.7	1.4	1.9	2.7	3.2	3.8	4.1	4.1
Calcium (mg)	72	36	50	72	86	100	108	108
Phosphorus (mg)	55	27	38	55	66	77	82	82
Magnesium (mg)	8	4.0	5.6	8.0	9.6	11.2	12.0	12.0
Natrium (mmol)	1.6	0.8	1.1	1.6	1.9	2.2	2.4	2.4
Kalium (mmol)	1.5	0.8	1.1	1.5	1.8	2.1	2.3	2.3
Chloride (mmol)	2.0	1.0	1.4	2.0	2.4	2.8	3.0	3.0
AA supplement (g)[a]		1.0	1.0	0.5	–	–	–	–
Lipid emulsion 20% (g)[a]		1.0	1.5	2.0	2.5	3.0	3.0	3.0
Total fluid (mL)		65	83	110	132	155	165	165
Total energy (kcal)[b]	57	42	69	76	91	108	113	113
Total AA g		2.4	2.9	3.2	3.2	3.8	4.1	4.1

[a]ProvIDed separately in Y route
[b]Energy (kcal) = AA × 3.75 + Glu × 3.75 + lip × 9.3

practice of "aggressive nutrition" for VLBW infants. In any case nutrient intakes are always indicative and may be modified according to each patient, his/her clinical picture, biochemical data and tolerance to nutrient intake. Thus, this standard solution could be diluted with free water according to fluid requirement and sodium intake could be adapted after a few days of life.

These nutrient intakes are a mere indication and have to be modified according to the clinical picture and biochemical data of the single patient.

The following suggestions could be useful in the management of a parenterally fed VLBW infant.

- In the first days of life fluid intake should be increased if daily weight loss is >5%, total weight loss>12–15%, serum Na >150 mmol/L, urinary osmolality >350 mOsm/L and if the infant is under phototherapy or managed in a radiant incubator. On the contrary fluid intakes should be reduced if daily weight loss <2% or there is a weight gain and serum Na <130 mmol/L.
- Glucose should be routinely administered after birth and progressively increased with the objective to increase energy intake. When a glucose infusion rate of 6 mg/kg/min or less leads to hyperglycemia, the use of insulin is advised. Insulin should be discontinued as soon as glucose tolerance is established and the energy supply necessary for growth can be delivered without hyperglycemia. If insulin is used, strict blood glucose monitoring is mandatory to avoid hypoglycemia.
- The starting dose of AA in the first day of life should be higher than what is currently advised. Intake should never be less than 1.5 g/kg/d and the starting dose should preferably be 2.0–3 g/kg/d. When energy intakes reach about 70 kcal/kg/d and there is no enteral protein intake, the dose should be increased progressively to 3.5–4.4 g/kg/d.
- Although many neonatal intensive care units start lipid infusion only after the first days, it seems logical to start parenteral lipid within the first day in order to avoid a prolonged interruption of essential fatty acids and LC-PUFA. The starting dose of 0.5–1 g/kg/d should be gradually increased to 3–3.5 g/kg/d. The lipid infusion should be adjusted to maintain a serum lipid <250 mg/dL. Using a similar approach allows to reduce the cumulative nutritional deficit and limit or abolish postnatal growth restriction in VLBW infants (Senterre and Rigo 2011a; Lapillonne et al. 2009).

References

Agostoni C, Buonocore G, Carnielli VP et al (2010) Enteral nutrient supply for preterm infants: commentary from the European Society of Paediatric Gastroenterology, Hepatology and Nutrition Committee on Nutrition. J Pediatr Gastroenterol Nutr 50:85–91

Ben XM (2008) Nutritional management of newborn infants: practical guidelines. World J Gastroenterol 28:6133–6139

Bohrer D, Oliveira SM, Garcia SC et al (2010) Aluminum loading in preterm neonates revisited. J Pediatr Gastroenterol Nutr 51:237–241

Borum PR (2009) Carnitine in parenteral nutrition. Gastroenterology 137(Suppl 5):S129–S134

Cairns PA, Stalker DJ (2000) Carnitine supplementation of parenterally fed neonates. Cochrane Database Syst Rev (4):CD000950

De Curtis M, Rigo J (2004) Extrauterine growth restriction in very-low-birthweight infants. Acta Paediatr 93:1563–1568

De Curtis M, Senterre J, Rigo J (1986) Estimated and measured energy content of infant formulas. J Pediatr Gastroenterol Nutr 5:746–749

Diamond IR, Pencharz PB, Wales PW (2009) What is the current role for parenteral lipid emulsions containing omega-3 fatty acids in infants with short bowel syndrome? Minerva Pediatr 61:263–272

Donovan R, Puppala B, Angst D, Coyle BW (2006) Outcomes of early nutrition support in extremely low-birth-weight infants. Nutr Clin Pract 21:395–400

Ehrenkranz RA, Younes N, Lemons JA et al (1999) Longitudinal growth of hospitalized very low birth weight infants. Pediatrics 104:280–289

Embleton NE, Pang N, Cooke RJ (2001) Postnatal malnutrition and growth retardation: an inevitable consequence of current recommendations in preterm infants? Pediatrics 107:270–273

Fusch C, Bauer K, Böhles HJ et al (2009) Neonatology/paediatrics. Guidelines on parenteral nutrition, Chapter 13. Ger Med Sci 7: Doc15

Hardy G, Puzovic M (2009) Formulation, stability and administration of parenteral nutrition with new lipid emulsions. Nutr Clin Pract 24:616

Kalhoff H, Diekmann L, Hettrich B et al (1997) Modified cow's milk formula with reduced renal acid load preventing incipient late metabolic acidosis in premature infants. J Pediatr Gastroenterol Nutr 25:46–50

Koletzko B, Goulet O, Hunt J et al (2005) Guidelines on Paediatric Parenteral Nutrition of the European Society Pediatric Gastroenterology, Hepatology and Nutrition (ESPGHAN) and the European Society for Clinical Nutrition and Metabolism (ESPEN), Supported by the European Society of Paediatric Research (ESPR). J Pediatr Gastroenterol Nutr 41 (Suppl 2):S1–S87

Lapillonne A, Fellous L, Mokthari M, Kermorvant-Duchemin E (2009) Parenteral nutrition objectives for very low birth weight infants: results of a national survey. J Pediatr Gastroenterol Nutr 48:618–626

Martin CR, Brown YF, Ehrenkranz RA et al (2009) Nutritional practices and growth velocity in the first month of life in extremely premature infants. Pediatrics 124:649–657

Poole RL, Kerner JA (1992) Practical steps in prescribing intravenous feeding. In: Yu VYH, MacMahon RA (eds) Intravenous feeding of the neonate. Edward Arnold, London, pp 259–264

Poole RL, Hintz SR, Mackenzie NI, Kerner JA Jr (2008) Aluminum exposure from pediatric parenteral nutrition: meeting the new FDA regulation. JPEN 32:242–246

Rigo J (2005) Protein, amino acid and other nitrogen compounds. In: Tsang RC, Uauy R, Koletzko B, Zlotkin SH (eds) Nutrition of the preterm infant: scientific basis and practice, 2nd edn. Digital educational Publishing, Cincinnati, pp 45–80

Rigo J, De Curtis M (2004) Parenteral nutrition in premature infants. In: Guandalini S (ed) Texbook of pediatric gastroenterology and nutrition. Taylor and Francis, London/New York, pp 619–638

Rigo J, De Curtis M, Pieltain C (2002) Nutritional assessment and body composition of preterm infants. Semin Neonatol 6:383–391

Rigo J, Marlowe ML, Bonnot D (2011) Practical handling, ease of use, safety, and efficacy of a new pediatric triple-chamber bag for parenteral nutrition in preterm infants. J Pediatr Gastroenterol Nutr [Epub ahead of print]

Senterre T, Rigo J (2011a) Optimizing early nutritional support based on recent recommendations in VLBW infants allows abolishing postnatal growth restriction. J Pediatr Gastroenterol Nutr [Epub ahead of print]

Senterre T, Rigo J (2011b) Reduction of postnatal cumulative nutritional deficit and improvement of growth in extremely preterm infants. Acta Paediatr [Epub ahead of print]

Simmer K (2007) Aggressive nutrition for preterm infants. Benefits and risks. Early Hum Dev 83:631–634

Stephens BE, Walden RV, Gargus RA et al (2009) First-week protein and energy intakes are associated with 18-month developmental outcomes in extremely low birth weight infants. Pediatrics 123:1337–1343

Thureen PJ, Melara D, Fennessey V et al (2003) Effect of low versus high intravenous amino acid intake on very low birth wight infants in the early neonatal period. Pediatr Res 53:24–32

Tsang RC, Uauy R, Koletzko B, Zlotkin SH (eds) (2005) Nutrition of the preterm infant: scientific basis and practice, 2nd edn. Digital educational Publishing, Cincinnati, pp 415–418

Tubman TR, Thompson SW, McGuire W (2008) Glutamine supplementation to prevent morbidity and mortality in preterm infants. Cochrane Database Syst Rev (23):CD001457

Van Goudoever JB, Sulkers EJ, Timmermans M et al (1994) Amino acid solutions for premature infants during the first week of life: The role of *N*-acetyl-L-cysteine and *N*-acetyl-L-tyrosine. JPEN 18:404–408

Waitzberg DL, Torrinhas RS, Jacintho TM (2006) New parenteral lipid emulsions for clinical use. JPEN 30:351–367

Wilson DC, Cairns P, Halliday HL et al (1997) Randomised controlled trial of an aggressive nutritional regimen in sick very low birthweight infants. Arch Dis Child 77:4F–11F

Ziegler EE, Thureen PJ, Carlson SJ (2002) Aggressive nutrition of the very low birthweight infant. Clin Perinatol 29:225–244

Postdischarge Nutrition in Preterm Infants

40

Richard J. Cooke

Contents

Abstract

Most preterm, particularly very-low-birth-weight, infants (VLBWI) are undernourished and undergrown at hospital discharge. Growth is "preprogrammed" to occur at a certain time or "critical" epoch which if missed may not be recoverable. Studies indicate that poor growth between birth-hospital discharge is associated with poorer neurodevelopmental outcome. Before hospital discharge, preterm infants fed human milk do not grow as well as infants fed nutrient-enriched formulas; also after discharge, it seems prudent to use milk fortification for all breastfed infants. The nutritional content of fortifiers differs: the level of fortification should be adjusted to ensure that growth, in terms of weight and length gain, is "tracking" in the right direction. Evidence suggests that a reduced body size is paralleled by a reduction in fat-free mass but a relative increase in fat mass, so particular attention

R. J. Cooke (✉)
Department of Pediatrics, University of Tennessee Health Science Center, Memphis, TN, USA
e-mail: richardjcooke@mac.com

G. Buonocore et al. (eds.), *Neonatology*,
https://doi.org/10.1007/978-3-319-29489-6_189

should be paid to dietary protein and energy intakes in these infants. Close communication between designated personnel in the neonatal intensive care unit and the infant's family is essential during this critical "epoch" of growth and development.

40.1 Salient Points

- Current recommendations are that the rate of weight gain parallels that of a fetus of the same gestational age once birth weight has been regained.
- Post-natal growth failure is not preventable given current recommendations and the way infants are fed.
- Close attention should be paid to the nutritional support and growth of these infants after hospital discharge. A reduced body size that is paralleled by a reduction in fat-free mass but a relative increase in fat mass suggests that particular attention should be paid to dietary protein and energy intakes in these infants.
- The extent to which "catch-up" occurs depends on many factors, including timing of the insult. Growth and development are thought to be programmed within specific time frames or critical epochs, which if missed may not be recoverable.
- Since all VLBWI accrue a significant nutrient deficit between birth and hospital discharge and mature human milk is designed for the needs of "normal" infants, it seems prudent to use milk fortification for all breastfed infants after discharge.
- The nutritional content of fortifiers differs. Further studies are needed to examine if one is better than another. In the meantime, the level of fortification should be adjusted to ensure that growth, in terms of weight and length gain, is "tracking" in the right direction.
- Irrespective of what feed is used, growth should be closely monitored and intake adjusted with the goal that birth centile, at least for weight, is reestablished between discharge and 1–2 mca.
- Continuing and close communication between designated personnel in the neonatal intensive care unit and the infant's family as well as the primary care providers is essential during this critical "epoch" of growth and development.

40.2 Introduction

The fundamental principle underlying nutritional support is that intake meets needs, thereby ensuring the best outcome, in the case of the preterm infant, optimal growth, and development. Achieving this goal is problematic and most, if not all, \very-low-birth-weight infants (VLBWI) are undernourished and undergrown when first discharged home. This has important implications for nutritional care of these high-risk infants after hospital discharge.

In this chapter the following issues will be addressed:

- Postnatal malnutrition and growth failure (PGF) between birth and hospital discharge in preterm infants
- Catch-up growth, insulin resistance, and visceral obesity in preterm infants
- Nutritional care of VLBWI after hospital discharge

40.3 Postnatal Malnutrition and Growth Failure in Preterm VLBWI

Several studies have examined postnatal growth in preterm infants during initial hospital stay and noted that most preterm, if not all very-low-birth-weight infants (VLBWI), are growth retarded at hospital discharge (Wilson et al. 1997; Carlson and Ziegler 1998; Embleton et al. 2001; Clark et al. 2003; Olsen et al. 2002; Ehrenkranz et al. 1999; Cooke et al. 2004). In studies where nutritional intake was measured, recommended dietary intakes (RDIs) took time to establish, and infants accrued a significant nutrient deficit that was directly related to the growth deficit (Wilson et al. 1997; Carlson and Ziegler 1998; Embleton et al. 2001; Clark et al. 2003; Olsen et al. 2002).

In studies where intake was not measured, poor growth was related to non-nutritional factors such as "illness" (Ehrenkranz et al. 1999; Cooke et al. 2004). In the recent study of Griffin et al. (2016), necrotizing enterocolitis was noted to have a significant negative on growth (Griffin et al. 2016). This is not surprising because intercurrent "illness" not only reduces intake but also may alter nutrient assimilation and increase requirements (Mehta et al. 2013). However, other factors underpin the development of growth failure in these infants.

Current recommendations are that the rate of weight gain parallels that of the fetus of the same gestational age once birth weight has been regained (AAPCON 1998; Klein 2002). Yet, a 24-week appropriately grown (AGA) infant weighing ~690 g at birth who regains birth weight by 2 weeks of age and grows at the recommended rate, i.e., 17 g/kg/day, will weigh 2,527 g, ~531 g less than the fetus, and be growth retarded at 37 weeks (Fig. 1). If the same infant takes 3 weeks to regain birth weight and grows at the same rate, then she/he will weigh 2,285 g, 773 g less than the fetus at 37 weeks.

Up to 40% of infants born prematurely are undergrown or small for gestational age (SGA) at birth (Larsen et al. 1990). A 24-week 550 g SGA infant who regains birth weight at 2 weeks and then gains at the recommended rate of 17 g/kg/day will weigh 1,727 g at 37 weeks, 800 g less than the 690 AGA infant at the same gestational age and ~1,300 g less than the fetus at the same gestational age (Fig. 2). Recommendations related to suboptimal weight will systematically underestimate needs and growth potential in these high-risk infants.

At the same time, current recommendations assume that nutritional requirements are consistent throughout gestation for all preterm VLBWI (AAPCON 1998; Klein 2002). However, Ziegler et al. have noted that protein and energy requirements change with advancing gestation (Ziegler et al. 2002; Table 1). In effect, a formula containing a protein-energy ratio of 3.0 g/100 kcal, as is currently fed to preterm infants, does not meet the protein needs of the infants weighing ≤1,500 g at birth, i.e., the VLBWI.

Recommended dietary intakes are based on needs for maintenance and normal growth (AAPCON 1998; Klein 2002), and no allowance is made for recovery or "catch-up" growth (Heird 2001). In the study of Embleton et al., the accrued protein deficit at hospital discharge varied from 15 to 25 g/kg (Embleton et al. 2001). An additional protein intake of 0.5–1.0 g/kg/day would have been required to recoup this deficit before

Fig. 1 Growth curve for a 24-week AGA preterm infant who regains birth weight by 7, 14, and 21 days and then grows at a rate of 17 g/kg/day

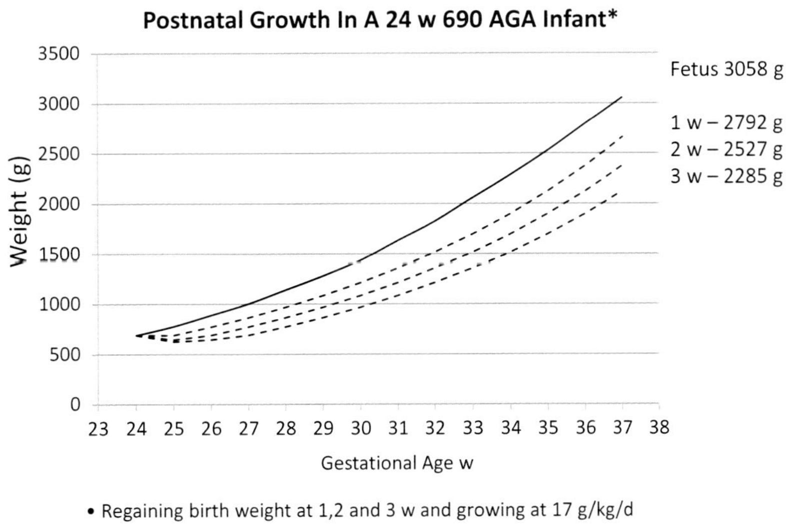

Fig. 2 Growth curve for a 24-week AGA and SGA preterm infants who regain birth weight by 14 and then grow at a rate of 17 g/kg/day

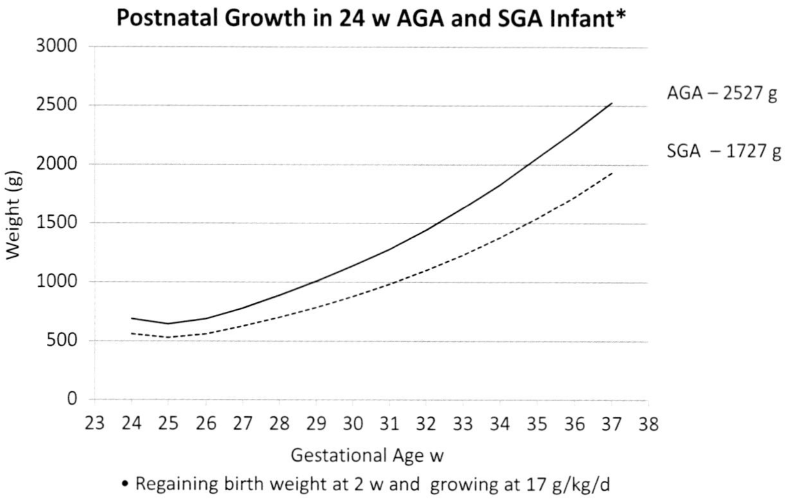

Table 1 Protein and energy needs in preterm infants

Weight g	500–700	700–900	900–1,200	1,200–1,500
Protein g/kg/day	4.0	4.0	4.0	3.9
Energy kcal/kg/day	105	108	119	127
P:E g/100 kcal	3.8	3.7	3.4	3.1

hospital discharge, further compounding the problem.

To further examine this issue, body size and body composition were measured in preterm infants ($n = 149$) at hospital discharge (Cooke and Griffin 2009). Weight, length, and head circumference were measured using standard methodology (Cooke et al. 1998). Body composition was measured using dual-emission x-ray absorptiometry (Cooke et al. 1999).

The post-menstrual age at discharge was 37 ± 1.2 weeks. However, Z-score for head circumference (−0.1 ± 0.6) was significantly greater than that for weight (−1.4 ± 0.6) which in turn was greater than for crown-heel length (−1.9 ± 0.6; $p < 0.0001$) (Cooke and Griffin 2009). Body composition results are compared to the reference infant at the same weight and same gestation in Table 2.

Table 2 Body size and composition of study infants compared to the reference infant at the same weight and same gestation (Cooke and Griffin 2009)

	Study infants[a]	Reference at 35 weeks[a]	Reference at 37 weeks[a]
Body weight g	2,369 ± 305	2,450	2,940
Fat-free mass g	2,062 ± 277[a]	2,252[a]	2,667[a]
Fat-free mass %	87 ± 3.4	91.9	90.7
Fat mass g	307 ± 130[b]	198[b]	273[b]
Fat mass %	13 ± 3.4[b]	8.1[b]	9.3[b]

[a]Study infants < reference at 35 week or 37 weeks ($p < 0.0001$)
[b]Study infants > reference at 35 week or 37 weeks ($p < 0.001$)

Global fat-free mass was less in study infants than the reference infant at the same weight (2,062 < 2,252 g; $p < 0.0001$) or gestation (2,062 < 2,667 g; $p < 0.0001$). Global fat mass was greater in study infants than the reference infant at the same weight (307 > 198 g, 13 > 8%) or gestation (307 > 273 g; 13 > 9%; $p < 0.0001$) (Cooke and Griffin 2009).

A reduced body size that is paralleled by reduced linear growth and a reduced fat-free mass indicate that dietary protein needs were not met in these infants before hospital discharge, as has been previously suggested (Ziegler et al. 2002). A reduced fat-free mass coupled with an increased global and central fat mass echoes concerns about visceral obesity and the development of insulin resistance in these high-risk infants (Uthaya et al. 2005; Yeung 2006).

Although many factors contribute to the development of PGF and the degree of which will vary, depending upon the level of maturity/size of the infant (Embleton et al. 2001), it is clear that:

1. It is not preventable given current recommendations and the way infants are fed; i.e., target growth rates related to a suboptimal body ensure that most, if not all, infants will be moderately/severely growth retarded at hospital discharge.
2. Close attention must be paid to nutritional support and growth of these infants after hospital discharge. A reduced body size that is paralleled by a reduction in fat-free mass but a relative increase in fat mass indicates that particular attention be paid to dietary protein and energy intakes in these infants.

40.4 Importance of Postnatal Malnutrition and Growth Failure

The importance of malnutrition cannot be underestimated. Nutrients play a critical role on the promotion of normal health and prevention of disease (Shils et al. 2006). It is not surprising, therefore, that it can be directly related to alterations in organ structure and function which, in turn, are paralleled by an increased morbidity and mortality in adults and children (Shils et al. 2006). However, the effects of malnutrition are greater during infancy than later in life. There are several reasons for this.

Requirements are a function of growth rate; the greater the rate, the greater the requirement and the more likely that deficiency will occur. Growth rates are greater during infancy than later in life; i.e., the term infant will double birth weight by 4–5 m, triple birth weight by 12 m, and approximately quadruple it by 24 m.

Growth is also thought to be "preprogrammed" to occur at a certain time or "critical" epoch which if missed may not be recoverable (Dobbing 1981). Thus, even short periods of nutritional deprivation may not only affect somatic but also brain growth and development (Dobbing 1981), the area of the brain that is "programmed" to grow fastest being the most affected (Bedi 1987).

In term infants, malnutrition during infancy is associated with permanent alterations in brain growth and function. Brain size is reduced (Galler et al. 1996; Stoch et al. 1982; Dobbing 1987; Winick and Rosso 1969a, b), the brain cortex is thinner (Dobbing and Sands 1971), neuronal numbers are decreased (Dobbing et al. 1971), myelination is reduced (Krigman and Hogan 1976), and dendritic morphology is altered (Benitez-Bribiesca et al. 1999; Cordero et al. 1993), all of which can be related to poorer neurodevelopmental outcome (Pryor et al. 1995; Ounsted et al. 1988; Gross et al. 1983; Hack and Breslau 1986; Hack et al. 1991; Kitchen et al. 1992a; Cooke and Foulder-Hughes 2003; Stathis et al. 1999; Peterson et al. 2006).

These concerns are greater in preterm infants. Growth rates are greater. A preterm infant is "programmed" to quadruple brain weight between 24 and 40 weeks gestation or 16 weeks (Alexander et al. 1996), almost six times faster than the term infant. Preterm infants are also more vulnerable to the effects of perinatal ischemia and inflammation, therefore the development of periventricular intraventricular hemorrhage and periventricular leukomalacia (Volpe 2008).

Compared to term, preterm infants are also more likely to be fetally and/or postnatally malnourished. Up to 40% of preterm infants are growth retarded or small for gestational age (SGA) at birth (Greisen 1992). At the same time, up to 100% of preterm VLBWI undergo significant postnatal growth failure and are SGA at hospital discharge (Ehrenkranz et al. 1999).

Poor fetal growth is paralleled by reduced organ growth as well as altered structure and function (McCance and Widdowson 1974) but not all organ systems are affected equally. This is well illustrated in the study of Myers et al. (1971). In this study, 30% reduction in body weight in SGA monkeys was associated with an 8% reduction in brain weight but ≥35% reduction in lung, liver, pancreatic, and spleen weights when compared to their AGA counterparts (Myers et al. 1971). Thus, the brain is "spared" at the expense of other organs which, e.g., through the development of chronic lung disease, sepsis, etc., may amplify undernutrition by reducing intake and/or increasing requirements.

In the late 1980s and early 1990s, studies indicated that poor growth between birth-hospital discharge was associated with poorer neurodevelopment (Morley 1999; Ehrenkranz et al. 2006) and that better growth, as achieved by feeding a nutrient-enriched formula, was associated with better developmental outcomes (Lucas et al. 1998, 1990). More recently, early parenteral nutrition coupled with the early introduction and advancement of enteral feeds has been associated with better growth but many infants continue to be SGA at hospital discharge (Evans and Thureen 2001; Dinerstein et al. 2006; Ibrahim et al. 2004; Donovan et al. 2006).

While a clear relationship exists between "catch-up" growth and development in preterm infants, the time frame within which it needs to occur is not well delineated. In most studies, infants who "catch up" or "catch back" by 6–9 m corrected age have better neurodevelopmental outcome (Morley 1999; Scott and Usher 1966; Hack et al. 1982; Hack and Fanaroff 1984; Latal-Hajnal et al. 2003). This is illustrated in the study of Latal-Hajnal et al. (2003).

In this study, infants were stratified at birth and into those who were appropriate size for gestational age (AGA weight ≥10th percentile) and SGA (weight <10th percentile). This process was repeated at 2 years of age. Four groups emerged: (a) AGA at birth and 2 years (AGA-AGA), (b) AGA at birth and SGA at 2 years (AGA-SGA), (c) SGA at birth and AGA at 2 years (SGA-AGA), and (d) SGA at birth and 2 years (SGA-SGA).

No differences were noted in development between the AGA-AGA and SGA-SGA infants. After adjusting for co-variables, infants who "caught up," i.e., SGA-AGA, had greater Bayley PDIs than those who did not (SGA-SGA). Infants who "faltered" (AGA-SGA) had lower PDIs and MDIs than those who continued to thrive (AGA-AGA). These authors concluded that the course of postnatal growth primarily determined later development.

To more closely examine this issue, Dharmaraj et al. prospectively followed growth between birth and18 months corrected age (mca) and developmental outcome at 18 mca (Dharmaraj et al. 2005). It was hypothesized that the greater the degree of early growth failure (birth to 28 days), the poorer the development at 18 mca. Infants were stratified at 28 days into those with mild (fall in weight Z-score % −1.0; MGF) and severe (fall in weight Z-score >1.0; SGF) growth failure. This process was repeated at 18 mca.

The characteristics of the study infants are presented in Table 3. No differences were noted with the exception that gestational age was less (SGR-SGR < MGR-MGR, MGR-SGR, $p < 0.05$) and the frequency of cerebral palsy tended to be greater (SGR-SGR > MGR-MGR,

Table 3 Characteristics of study infants (Dharmaraj et al. 2005)

Group (N)	MGR-MGR (50)	MGR-SGR (18)	SGR-SGR (16)	SGR-MGR (24)
Birth weight (g)	1,320 ± 339	1,348 ± 387	1,312 ± 559	1,271 ± 408
Gestation (w)	30 ± 1.6[a]	30 ± 1.8[a]	28 ± 3.0[a]	29 ± 2.3
BPD	13 (26 %)	3 (17 %)	6 (38 %)	10 (42 %)
Abnormal CUS	10 (20 %)	5 (28 %)	3 (19 %)	6 (25 %)
PVL	3 (6 %)	2 (11 %)	1 (6 %)	3 (13 %)
Cerebral palsy	4 (8 %)	3 (17 %)	5 (30 %)[b]	2 (8 %)

[a]SGR-SGR < MGR-MGR, MGR-SGR, $p < 0.05$
[b]SGR-SGR > MGR-MGR, SGR-MGR, $p < 0.10$

Fig. 3 Growth, i.e., change in weight Z-score between birth and 28 days, term and one through 18 month corrected age in infants in the study of Dharmaraj et al.

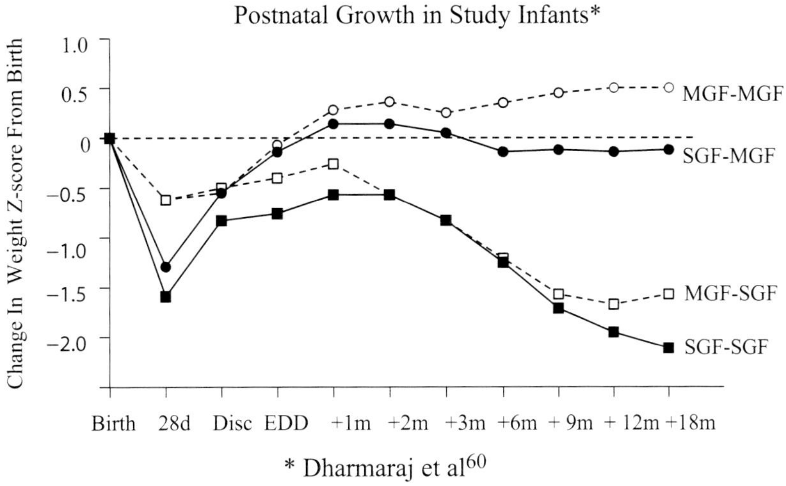

Table 4 MDI and PDI in study infants (Dharmaraj et al. 2005)

Group (N)	MGR-MGR	MGR-SGR	SGR-MGR	SGR-SGR
MDI[a]	93 ± 18	91 ± 18	95 ± 1	77 ± 19
PDI[a]	90 ± 17[a]	83 ± 19	87 ± 19[b]	77 ± 22[a]
MDI[b]	96 ± 15	93 ± 20	98 ± 16	88 ± 11
PDI[b]	94 ± 13	89 ± 15	91 ± 14	89 ± 16

MDI ~ MGR-MGR, SGR-MGR > SGR-SGR. $p < 0.05$
[a]PDI ~ MGR-MGR ($p < 0.05$), SGR-MGR ($p < 0.10$) > SGR-SGR
[b]Infants with cerebral palsy excluded. MDI ~ MGR-MGR ($p < 0.05$), SGR-MGR ($p < 0.10$) > SGR-SGR

SGR-MGR, $p < 0.10$) in infants with severe growth failure at 28 days and 18 m corrected age.

Growth of these infants is presented in Fig. 3. Between birth and 28 days, Z-scores for weight decreased and then recovered to some degree in all groups. After 28 days, growth continued to improve in infants with MGF at 28 days and 18 mca (MGF-MGF) and SGF at 28 days but mild growth failure (SGF-MGF) at 18 mca. However, growth faltered in the other groups, that is, MGF-SGF and SGF-SGF.

The developmental outcome data are presented in Table 4. MDI and PDI were less in SGF-SGF than MGF-MGF infants, supporting the primary hypothesis that poor growth between birth and 28 days is a marker for poor development. MDI and PDI were also greater in infants who recovered after 28 days (SGF-MGF) than those who did not (SGF-SGF), indicating that "catch-up" growth between 28 days and 18 mca is paralleled by markedly improved development.

Collectively, these data support the conclusions of Latal-Hajnal et al.; i.e., it is the course of postnatal growth that determines later developmental outcome in preterm infants. The data of Dharmaraj et al. also indicate that a "critical window of opportunity" exists between 28 days and 1–2 mca during which "recovery" or "catch-up" growth, to birthweight percentile, is paralleled by better neurodevelopmental outcome. If infants are to "recover," this is the time frame within which to do it.

40.5 Catch-Up Growth, Insulin Resistance, and Visceral Obesity in Preterm Infants

Despite the prevalence/severity of PGF that is paralleled by an increased morbidity/mortality before/after hospital discharge, concern has been expressed about measures taken to improve growth after hospital discharge. Concern largely relates to "catch-up" growth and the subsequent development of insulin resistance (Singhal et al. 2001, 2003) and metabolic syndrome X (Ong and Loos 2006) leading to the idea that "bigger might not be better," even in preterm VLBWI (Singhal et al. 2003).

However, a certain amount of confusion exists when the terms "rapid" and "catch-up" growth are used; i.e., they are sometimes used interchangeably (Ong and Loos 2006) but are not the same. "Rapid" growth is "an abnormal growth pattern that moves upward beyond the original growth percentile on a distance growth chart" (Hermanussen 2013a). "Catch-up" is a physiologic condition of temporary overgrowth that occurs after illness and/or starvation, and in the process, the original growth percentile is reestablished (Hermanussen 2013b).

The extent to which "catch-up" occurs depends on many factors, including timing of the insult. Growth/development is thought to be programmed within a specific time frame or critical epoch which if missed may not be recoverable (McCance and Widdowson 1974; Widdowson and McCance 1975). It also depends upon the severity and duration of the insult; the more severe and prolonged the insult, the greater the accrued nutritional deficit. Intake, therefore, must not only replace the deficit but also meet needs for maintenance and normal growth.

With acute illness, infants develop a hypermetabolic state, and there is an acute depletion of body protein to meet energy needs (Lowry and Perez 2006). With chronic protein-energy malnutrition during infancy, visceral tissue is conserved at the expense of protein and fat (Ashworth and Millward 1986). Nutritional rehabilitation in these infants with high-energy intakes largely results in increased weight gain (MacLean and Graham 1980) and body fat (MacLean and Graham 1980; Jackson 1990); i.e., the nature of the gain is dependent upon the compositional nature of intake.

At hospital discharge, all preterm VLBWI have accrued a significant protein and energy deficit (Embleton et al. 2001) and are lighter and shorter and have a reduced lean but greater fat mass than the reference infant at the same body weight or gestation (Uthaya et al. 2005). Thereafter, a diet that is relatively high in energy will promote "catch-up" that is paralleled by increased fat deposition. A diet that better meets protein needs will be paralleled by increased lean mass accretion.

Energy density is the prime determinant of volume of intake in infants (Fomon 1993a; Cooke et al. 1998). Yet at borderline low protein intakes, volume/energy intake is increased to compensate and is associated with increased fat accretion (Fomon 1993b). The energy cost of lean mass accretion is ~13.4 kcal/g and that of fat accretion is 10.6 kcal/g (Roberts and Young 1988). At equivalent energy intakes, therefore, the greater the rate of lean mass accretion, the lesser the tendency to fat accretion. A little more rather than less protein, therefore, might be considered appropriate.

The relative roles of genetic, intrauterine, and environmental factors in the pathogenesis of insulin resistance are unclear, but diet also plays a key role (Cornier et al. 2008). A high energy, i.e., glycemic or fat content, increases insulin needs, fat synthesis, storage, etc. (Bremer et al. 2012). Whether a "normal" infant diet, i.e., that appropriate for a term infant, is likely to do so in VLBWI with PGF is unclear. What is clear is that growth and nutritional need to be closely monitored during the first 1–2 m after hospital discharge, with particular attention paid to adequacy of protein intake and protein-energy status, i.e., monitoring linear growth and biochemical measures of status if needed, i.e., blood urea nitrogen, prealbumin, and albumin levels.

To more closely examine this issue, body size and composition were measured in preterm infants fed either a preterm formula (protein content = 2.7 g/100 kcal, discharge 6 m) (A), a term formula (protein content 1.8 g/100 kcal, discharge 6 m) (B), a preterm formula to term and then a term formula to 6 m (C), or unfortified breast milk (D) (Cooke et al. 1998, 1999). The results are presented in Fig. 4.

"Rapid" growth was not noted in either treatment group; i.e., Z-scores for weight did not exceed birth percentile. Between discharge and term, "catch-up" growth in weight and length occurred in the formula but not the breastfed infants. Thereafter, "catch-up" occurred in all groups and was faster and more complete in infants fed the preterm formula. Infants with the poorest growth were

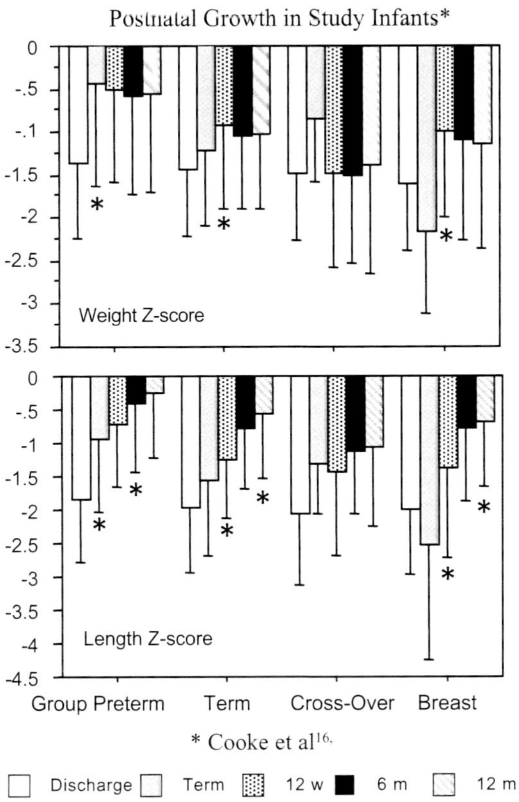

Fig. 4 Growth between discharge and 12 months in infants fed a preterm infant formula, a term formula, or a preterm formula (discharge-term)/term formula (after term, crossover) or breastfed

those fed the preterm formula between discharge and term and the term formula thereafter (Fig. 4).

More complete "catch-up" growth was paralleled by an increase in fat-free mass and total fat mass but not % fat mass (Table 5). No differences were detected in central fat mass between the groups, but leg fat mass was greater in infants fed the preterm formula (Table 6). In effect, "catch-up" growth was paralleled by an increase in linear growth, lean, and fat mass accretion, the latter reflecting increased peripheral not central fat mass accretion.

Collectively, these data:

(a) Do not support concerns about altered adiposity in preterm infants fed a nutrient-enriched formula after hospital discharge
(b) Indicate that rate and composition of growth are dependent upon the composition of the diet
(c) Do not support the recommendation that a preterm formula be fed to term and discontinued thereafter (Aggett et al. 2006)

40.6 Post-discharge Nutritional Support in Preterm Infant

40.6.1 Overview

Before hospital discharge, it is important that the method of feeding and growth patterns are well established. Nutritional status of each infant should be closely evaluated, with the information communicated to the primary care physician and arrangements for follow-up clearly defined.

Intake after discharge must not only meet needs for maintenance and normal growth but also "catch-up" growth. It is assumed that needs for normal growth are similar in preterm boys and girls. Yet, preterm boys grow faster in utero and accrete more lean mass than girls during the first 2–3 m of life (Rawlings et al. 1999). They are also more susceptible to even marginal levels of intake and benefit more when fed nutrient-enriched formulas before (Lucas et al. 1989a, 1990, 1994; Morley and Lucas 1997) and after hospital discharge (Cooke et al. 1999; Lucas et al. 2001; Carver et al. 2001; Agosti et al. 2003).

It is also assumed that needs for "recovery" are similar for all preterm infants. This is not the case. Up to 40% of infants prematurely are small for gestational age (SGA) at birth. Needs are likely to differ between the AGA and SGA infants. At the same time, the severity of PGF not only varies widely between infants discharged from a given NICU (Embleton et al. 2001); i.e., the smaller and more immature the infant, the greater the accrued nutrient deficit, but also between NICUs (Olsen et al. 2002; Cooke et al. 2004; Griffin et al. 2016; Horbar et al. 2015). In effect, needs for "recovery" are also highly variable.

Collectively, these data emphasize the importance of individualized assessment before discharge and, irrespective of what an infant is fed, close nutritional monitoring after discharge. Not surprisingly, many questions

Table 5 Body composition of preterm infants fed either preterm formula, term formula, preterm formula (to term)/term formula (after term, crossover), or breastfed (Cooke et al. 1999)

	Group	Term ($n = 148$)	12 weeks ($n = 141$)	6 months ($n = 145$)	12 months ($n = 138$)	
Fat-free mass (g)	Preterm (A)	2,745 ± 445	4,270 ± 452	5,208 ± 638	6,872 ± 806	A >
	Term (B)	2,393 ± 276	4,022 ± 411	5,139 ± 515	6,592 ± 738	B ($p < 0.05$)
	Crossover (C)	2,507 ± 244	3,948 ± 431	4,978 ± 541	6,399 ± 881	C ($p < 0.001$)
	Breastfed (D)	2,171 ± 296	3,762 ± 1,051	5,063 ± 568	6,451 ± 746	D ($p < 0.005$)
Fat mass (g)	Preterm (A)	570 ± 256	1,455 ± 461	2,033 ± 686	2,332 ± 679	A >
	Term (B)	511 ± 222	1,367 ± 419	1,940 ± 586	2,058 ± 477	B ($p < 0.05$)
	Crossover (C)	566 ± 204	1,188 ± 366	1,815 ± 632	2,077 ± 623	C ($p < 0.005$)
	Breastfed (D)	331 ± 128	1,365 ± 527	1,934 ± 658	2,153 ± 645	
Fat mass %	Preterm (A)	17 ± 5.5	25 ± 4.7	28 ± 5.9	25 ± 5.3	
	Term (B)	17 ± 6.0	25 ± 5.5	27 ± 5.1	24 ± 4.4	
	Crossover (C)	18 ± 4.7	23 ± 4.1	26 ± 5.8	24 ± 4.5	
	Breastfed (D)	13 ± 3.2	25 ± 8.2	27 ± 6.8	25 ± 4.8	

Table 6 Regional body composition of preterm infants fed either preterm formula, term formula, preterm formula (to term)/term formula (after term, crossover), or breastfed

G	Group	Term	12 weeks	6 months	12 months	
Trunk	Preterm (A)	172 ± 65	532 ± 168	651 ± 218	699 ± 249	
	Term (B)	182 ± 71	485 ± 154	635 ± 170	613 ± 160	
	Crossover (C)	186 ± 67	394 ± 136	579 ± 221	573 ± 162	
	Breastfed (D)	147 ± 54	503 ± 183	688 ± 229	657 ± 230	
Legs	Preterm (A)	159 ± 58	500 ± 155	736 ± 270	975 ± 354	A >
	Term (B)	133 ± 73	451 ± 168	652 ± 300	830 ± 271	B ($p < 0.01$)
	Crossover (C)	129 ± 75	458 ± 133	602 ± 247	822 ± 409	C ($p < 0.001$)
	Breastfed (D)	98 ± 58	454 ± 183	654 ± 289	897 ± 254	D ($p < 0.10$)

remain unanswered. How often should growth be monitored?

In the follow-up study of Dharmaraj et al. (2005), growth velocity was greatest between discharge and term, continuing to 1–2 mca, a time frame within which brain growth velocity is also greatest and likely to be functionally significant (Fig. 3). Growth monitoring during this time frame should be done at least weekly, if not more often in high-risk infants; i.e., the greater the degree of PGF, the greater the level of concern, until an acceptable growth pattern is achieved and maintained.

In the study of Cooke et al. (1998), significant growth faltering was noted:

(a) In breastfed but not formula-fed infants between discharge and term (Fig. 4)
(b) When a dietary change was made, i.e., infants fed a preterm formula between discharge and

term and then the term formula thereafter (Fig. 4)

More frequent growth monitoring would also appear prudent under these circumstances.

Which growth parameters should be monitored and evaluated? Accurate measurement of body weight and head circumference, with subsequent conversion to Z-scores, is necessary to determine whether or not an infant is "tracking" toward original birth-weight centile. Accurate measurement of body length, while difficult and time-consuming, is also important to ensure that the composition of growth is also appropriate (Singhal et al. 2003).

40.6.2 Studies

40.6.2.1 Formula Feeding

Growth

Many studies have examined post-discharge growth in preterm infants (Kitchen et al. 1992a, b; Ernst et al. 1990; Casey et al. 1990; Fitzhardinge and Inwood 1989; Fenton et al. 1990; Ross et al. 1990). Although some "catch-up" growth has been observed, preterm infants do not grow as well as their term counterparts and are smaller at 3 years (Casey et al. 1991), 8 years (Hack et al. 1993), and adulthood (Hack et al. 2003). There are several possible reasons for this.

Current in-hospital feeding practices ensure that most, if not all, VLBWI are undernourished and growth retarded at initial hospital discharge (Embleton et al. 2001; Cooke et al. 2004). A "critical epoch" of growth may, therefore, have been missed. Preterm infants also have greater morbidity than term infants during the first year of life (McCormick et al. 1980; Hack et al. 1983; Navas et al. 1992; Thomas et al. 2000; Wang et al. 1995a), and intercurrent illness will affect growth, irrespective of whether infants are admitted to hospital or not.

Until relatively recently, little attention had been paid to nutritional factors in the pathogenesis of this problem. For most early studies, infants were fed either unfortified human milk or a term infant formula after hospital discharge (Kitchen et al. 1992a, b; Ernst et al. 1990; Casey et al. 1990; Fitzhardinge and Inwood 1989; Fenton et al. 1990; Ross et al. 1990). Both feeding regimens were designed to meet nutritional needs of the term rather than the rapidly growing preterm infant. Infants, therefore, may have been partly underfed during the first 6–12 months of life.

More recently, studies have examined the effects of feeding nutrient-enriched formulas,i.e., formulas with a greater nutrient density than a term infant formula, to preterm infants after hospital discharge (Cooke et al. 1998, 1999, 2001; Lucas et al. 1992, 2001; Carver et al. 2001; Agosti et al. 2003; Bishop et al. 1993; Chan et al. 1994; Wheeler and Hall 1996; Lapillonne et al. 2004; Koo and Hockman 2006; De Curtis et al. 2002). In this respect, two meta-analyses are relevant. Reviewing the results of studies published before 2005 Henderson et al. concluded that feeding with nutrient-enriched formulas had little effect on growth (Henderson et al. 2005). As such, their conclusions on growth merit examination.

The first outcome variable evaluated was "growth during the trial period." The results of one study were used, i.e., de Curtis et al. (2002) wherein the sample size was 33 and the end point was gain in weight and crown-heel length and head circumference between 36 wca and 2 mca. Furthermore, growth velocity changes rapidly during this time frame (Fig. 5) and that which is averaged over a 12-week period may not reflect early but significant differences between the treatment groups (Cooke et al. 1998).

The second end point was "longer-term growth," i.e., weight, length, and head circumference at 6 m, 9 m, and 18 m corrected age. Data from only one study was used at 6 mca (Litmanovitz et al. 2004) and one at 9 mca (Lucas et al. 2001), again not entirely representative. The conclusions drawn by Henderson et al. on growth, therefore, must be questioned.

The more recent and more comprehensive meta-analysis of Teller et al. is very informative (Teller et al. 2016). Thirty-one eligible studies were identified which were noted to differ significantly in study design, i.e., (a) inclusion criteria,

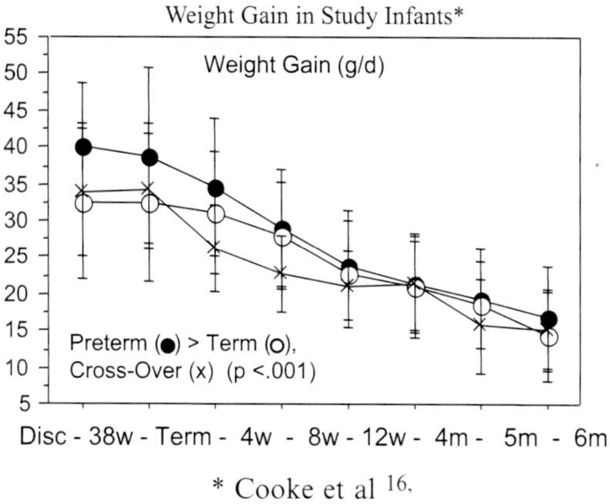

Fig. 5 Growth velocity in study infants fed either a preterm infant formula (*closed circle*), a term formula (*open circle*) or a preterm infant formula (discharge-term), or term infant formula (X)

(b) point of enrolment, (c) nutrient content of formula fed, (d) duration of intervention, and (e) outcomes evaluated.

In the main, no consistent differences were detected in body weight, length, or head circumference between treatment groups. What was noted was a consistent dose-response effect, i.e., protein-energy ratios of ≥2.5–3.0 g/100 ml were associated with increased linear growth as well as increased weight and head circumference noted at 3, 6, 9, and 12 mca (Teller et al. 2016).

Where body composition was measured using dual-emission x-ray absorptiometry (DEXA), increased linear growth was associated with increased lean mass accretion, which was paralleled by a reduced or increased fat mass but not increased adiposity (Cooke et al. 1999; Lapillonne et al. 2004; Roggero et al. 2012). An exception to these observations was the study of Koo et al. where reduced weight gain and linear growth were associated with reduced lean and fat mass accretion (Koo and Hockman 2006).

Development

In the meta-analyses of Henderson et al. (2005) and of Teller et al. (2016), no consistent effects were detected on neurodevelopment. This is not entirely surprising. In the meta-analysis of Teller et al., it was only in infants who were fed the formula with the highest protein content (≥2.5–3.0 g/100 ml) that consistent effects were noted on growth, an effect that was more pronounced in boys than girls. Yet, these studies were not "powered" to control for the confounding effect of sex on head growth and development.

In the study of Lucas et al. (1989a, 1990), sex was a confounding variable but sample size ($n = 219$) was large enough, therefore adequately "powered," to detect differences in development between treatment groups. Such was not the case for the studies of Agosti et al. (2003) ($n = 121$) and Jeon et al. (2011) ($n = 90$) and Cooke et al. (2001) ($n = 113$) where sample sizes are much smaller. In the latter study, boys fed the term formula had the poorest head growth, which in turn was paralleled by ten-point reduction in MDI when compared to girls fed the term formula, suggesting that boys are at a disadvantage when fed a term infant formula.

An additional consideration is as follows. Brain growth is rapid during the last trimester and first 2 years of life, a time when even minor insults may have significant effects (Dobbing 1981). But not all parts of the brain are developing at the same rate, therefore not equally vulnerable (Dobbing 1981). In effect global measures of function, such as Bayley's assessment, may not be sensitive enough to detect minor or focal differences in developmental outcome (Singer et al. 1994).

Dabydeen et al. prospectively randomized term and preterm infants with perinatal brain injury to either a control or high-energy and high-protein diet after perinatal brain injury during the first year of life (Dabydeen et al. 2008). Infants fed the high-energy and high-protein diet had a greater head growth and axonal diameters when compared to the control group. It was concluded that infants with significant perinatal brain injury had increased nutritional requirements and that inadequate intake, as is commonly noted in neurologically impaired infants, may compromise subsequent brain growth and development (Dabydeen et al. 2008).

Collectively, these studies (Lucas et al. 2001; Agosti et al. 2003; Cooke et al. 2001; Dabydeen et al. 2008) suggest that the feeding with a formula with a protein-energy ratio of ≥2.5–3.0 g/100 ml is associated with better head growth and trends toward better post-developmental outcome. In the case of the otherwise "normal" preterm infant, male infants are most likely to benefit. In infants with perinatal brain injury, both term and preterm infants may benefit. Further more appropriately "powered" studies are needed to address these issues.

40.6.3 Breastfeeding

Human milk has been recommended as the preferred method of feeding for preterm infants after hospital discharge (Canada 2004; AAPCON 2009; Agostoni et al. 2009; Lapillonne et al. 2013). In a nutritional sense this, at first glance, is puzzling. Before hospital discharge, preterm infants fed human milk do not grow as well as infants fed nutrient-enriched formulas (Tyson et al. 1983; Gross 1983). It is, therefore, recommended that human milk be fortified with additional nutrients (Klein 2002). Growth improves but it is still not as good as in infants fed a preterm infant formula (Carlson and Ziegler 1998). The reasons for this are not entirely clear.

Fortifiers differ in nutrient composition and it is unclear which, if any, really meets requirements. The composition of human milk varies widely (Atkinson et al. 1995), and because it is not consistently measured, there is no way of knowing what the infant is really receiving. In effect, intake less adequately meets requirements and growth is poorer. Nonetheless, because of lower rates of morbidity, e.g., sepsis and necrotizing enterocolitis (Schanler et al. 1999), and improved developmental outcome (Morley et al. 1988a), it is recommended that fortified human milk be fed whenever possible before hospital discharge (Klein 2002).

After hospital discharge, breastfed infants also grow more poorly than those fed nutrient-enriched formulas (Lucas et al. 2001; Chan et al. 1994; Wauben et al. 1998). This again is not surprising. Before discharge, intake less adequately meets requirements, the accrued nutritional deficit, and, therefore, needs for "recovery" are greater. Mature human milk is designed to meet the needs of the term infant and not the preterm infant, and there are significant differences in nutrient content between mature human milk and formulas used to feed infants before and after discharge (Table 7).

Poorer growth after discharge is paralleled by alterations in bone mineral metabolism and body composition. Bone mineral accretion is less in infants fed un-supplemented human milk after discharge (Lucas et al. 2001; Chan et al. 1994; Wauben et al. 1998; Kurl et al. 2003; Schanler et al. 1992). This, in turn, can be related to outcome on a short-term, e.g., osteopenia (Lucas et al. 1989b) and fractures (Koo et al. 1988), and long-term, e.g., poorer linear growth (Fewtrell et al. 2000), basis. Interestingly, infants fed human milk also have increased fat accretion when compared to those fed a nutrient-enriched formula (Wauben et al. 1998).

Table 7 A comparison of nutrient content of human milk with preterm, nutrient-enriched, and term infant formulas

Per liter	Human milk	Preterm	Post-discharge	Term
Energy kcal	670	810	730	67
Protein g	10	23	20	14
Fat g	35	42	40	36
Carbohydrate g	70	88	78	73
Calcium mg	260	1,400	850	530
Phosphorus mg	140	700	480	330
Sodium mmol	9	15	11	8
Chloride mmol	16	19	17	12
Zinc mg	3.2	12.1	9	6
Vitamin A mg	0.7	3	1	0.6

Thus, infants grow as they are fed. When mineral intake is inadequate, bone mineral accretion is decreased. Whether the latter in some way alters "programming" and, therefore, health in adult life is unclear. What is clear is that the assessment of bone mineral status, i.e., serum phosphorus and alkaline phosphatase, is also an important consideration during this critical time frame (Schanler 2005).

Several studies have examined the effect of nutrient fortification of human milk after hospital discharge. In a randomized controlled pilot trial, preterm infants (750–1,800 g) were fed unfortified ($n = 20$) or fortified ($n = 19$) human milk after hospital discharge-12 week (O'Connor et al. 2008). A multi-nutrient fortifier, estimated to ensure an energy and protein density of 80 kcal and 2.2 g/100 ml, was added to 50% of feeds. Weight tended to be greater (all infants), while length (all infants) and head circumference, infants $\leq$1,250 g only, were greater in the fortified group. In a follow-up of the same infants, weight, linear growth, bone mineral content, and head growth (infants <1,250 g only) but not Bayley's II developmental scores were greater in infants fed fortified human milk (Aimone et al. 2009).

In a larger more recent randomized controlled trial between hospital discharge and 4 m corrected age, Zacharisson et al. fed preterm VLBWI (24–32 weeks; 535–2,255 g) either unfortified ($n = 102$; group A) or fortified ($n = 105$; group B) human milk and compared their growth to a group of infants fed a preterm formula ($n = 113$; group C, preterm formula) (Zachariassen et al. 2011). No differences were detected in growth between groups A and B at 12 mca, and it was concluded that while fortification did not affect the durations of breastfeeding, it also did not influence growth at 1 year of age.

Yet, important and consistent differences were noted in breastfed and the formula-fed infants. Infants in C had a greater increase in weight Z-score between discharge and term and in length Z-score until 6 months CA. At 12 mca, boys in C were longer and heavier than in groups A and B, while girls in group C were longer and heavier than in group A only. Greater protein intakes in C were also related to increased serum urea nitrogen levels.

The results of this much larger scale study are puzzling in that no significant differences were detected in growth between infants fed unfortified and fortified milk. One possibility relates to the small sample size in the original study (O'Connor et al. 2008), $n \sim 20$/treatment group; i.e., the results are not generalizable. Alternatively, the level of fortification used in the latter study may have been inadequate to consistently improve growth in such a heterogeneous population. It is notable that the timing of introduction of complementary foods was later with nutrient enrichment, perhaps suggesting that energy needs were more adequately met and infants satiated longer.

The results of these studies raise more questions than answers:

(a) Should all preterm VLBWI be fortified human milk after hospital discharge? Since all VLBWI accrue a significant nutrient deficit between birth and hospital discharge and mature human milk is designed for the needs of "normal" infants, i.e., needs for maintenance and normal growth, it seems prudent to fortify in all breastfed infants after discharge.
(b) What is the best way to fortify human milk? The nutritional content of fortifiers differs. Is one better than another? Further studies are needed to examine this issue. In the meantime, the level of fortification should be adjusted to ensure that growth, in terms of weight and length gain, is "tracking" in the right direction (Arslanoglu et al. 2006; Cooke 2006).
(c) How long should fortification be continued? There are no data in this area. Data in formula-fed infants indicate that discontinuation of preterm formula and then feeding a term formula at term is paralleled by a rapid deceleration in growth that is not entirely recovered by 6 or 12 m corrected age (Fig. 4; Cooke et al. 1998). At least, 1–2 mca, therefore, seems advisable since this is also the period of greatest brain growth velocity and appears to be functionally significant (Dharmaraj et al. 2005).

40.7 Summary

Many questions remain unanswered about what to feed preterm, particularly VLBWI, infants after hospital discharge but several things are clear:

1. Nutritional status of all infants should be closely evaluated before discharge and the information relayed to the primary care physician. Infants with the greatest degree of growth failure at discharge are at greatest risk for further "growth faltering."
2. Irrespective of what is fed, growth should be closely monitored and intake adjusted with the goal that birth centile, at least for weight, is reestablished between discharge and 1–2 mca.
3. Continuing and close communication between designated personnel in the neonatal intensive care unit and the infant's family as well as the primary care providers is essential during this critical "epoch" of growth and development.

References

AAPCON (1998) Nutritional needs of preterm infants. In: Kleinman RE (ed) Pediatric nutrition handbook. American Academy of Pediatrics, Elk Grove Village, pp 55–88

AAPCON (2009) Nutritional needs of the preterm infant. In: Kleinman RE (ed) Pediatric nutrition handbook, 6th edn. American Academy of Pediatrics, Elk Grove Village, pp 79–104

Aggett PJ, Agostoni C, Axelsson I et al (2006) Feeding preterm infants after hospital discharge: a commentary by the ESPGHAN committee on nutrition. J Pediatr Gastroenterol Nutr 42:596–603

Agosti M, Vegni C, Calciolari G, Marini A (2003) Post-discharge nutrition of the very low-birthweight infant: interim results of the multicentric GAMMA study. Acta Paediatr Suppl 91:39–43

Agostoni C, Braegger C, Decsi T et al (2009) Breastfeeding: a commentary by the ESPGHAN committee on nutrition. J Pediatr Gastroenterol Nutr 49:112–125

Aimone A, Rovet J, Ward W et al (2009) Growth and body composition of human milk-fed premature infants provided with extra energy and nutrients early after hospital discharge: 1-year follow-up. J Pediatr Gastroenterol Nutr 49:456–466

Alexander GR, Himes JH, Kaufman RB, Mor J, Kogan M (1996) A United States national reference for fetal growth. Obstet Gynecol 87:163–168

Arslanoglu S, Moro GE, Ziegler EE (2006) Adjustable fortification of human milk fed to preterm infants: does it make a difference? J Perinatol 26:614–621

Ashworth A, Millward DJ (1986) Catch-up growth in children. Nutr Rev 44:157–163

Atkinson SA, Alston-Mills B, Lonnerdal B, Neville MC (1995) Major minerals and ionic constituents of human and bovine milks. In: Jensen RG (ed) Handbook of milk composition. Academic, San Diego, pp 593–622

Bedi KS (1987) Lasting neuroanatomical changes following undernutrition during early life. In: Dobbing J (ed) Early nutrition and later achievement. Academic, London, pp 1–49

Benitez-Bribiesca L, De la Rosa-Alvarez I, Mansilla-Olivares A (1999) Dendritic spine pathology in infants with severe protein-calorie malnutrition. Pediatrics 104:e21

Bishop NJ, King FJ, Lucas A (1993) Increased bone mineral content of preterm infants fed with a nutrient enriched formula after discharge from hospital. Arch Dis Child 68:573–578

Bremer AA, Mietus-Snyder M, Lustig RH (2012) Toward a unifying hypothesis of metabolic syndrome. Pediatrics 129:557–570

Carlson SJ, Ziegler EE (1998) Nutrient intakes and growth of very low birth weight infants. Perinatology 18:252–258

Carver JD, Wu PY, Hall RT et al (2001) Growth of preterm infants fed nutrient-enriched or term formula after hospital discharge. Pediatrics 107:683–689

Casey PH, Kraemer HC, Bernbaum J et al (1990) Growth patterns of low birth weight preterm infants: a longitudinal analysis of a large, varied sample. J Pediatr 117:298–307

Casey PH, Kraemer HC, Bernbaum J, Yogman MW, Sells JC (1991) Growth status and growth rates of a varied sample of low birth weight, preterm infants: a longitudinal cohort from birth to three years of age. J Pediatr 119:599–605

Chan GM, Borschel MW, Jacobs JR (1994) Effects of human milk or formula feeding on the growth, behavior, and protein status of preterm infants discharged from the newborn intensive care unit. Am J Clin Nutr 60:710–716

Clark RH, Thomas P, Peabody J (2003) Extrauterine growth restriction remains a serious problem in prematurely born neonates. Pediatrics 111:986–990

Cooke RJ (2006) Adjustable fortification of human milk fed to preterm infants. J Perinatol 26:591–592

Cooke RW, Foulder-Hughes L (2003) Growth impairment in the very preterm and cognitive and motor performance at 7 years. Arch Dis Child 88:482–487

Cooke RJ, Griffin I (2009) Altered body composition in preterm infants at hospital discharge. Acta Paediatr 98:1269–1273

Cooke RJ, Griffin IJ, McCormick K et al (1998) Feeding preterm infants after hospital discharge: effect of dietary manipulation on nutrient intake and growth. Pediatr Res 43:355–360

Cooke RJ, McCormick K, Griffin IJ et al (1999) Feeding preterm infants after hospital discharge: effect of diet on body composition. Pediatr Res 46:461–464
Cooke RJ, Embleton ND, Griffin IJ, Wells JC, McCormick KP (2001) Feeding preterm infants after hospital discharge: growth and development at 18 months of age. Pediatr Res 49:719–722
Cooke RJ, Ainsworth SB, Fenton AC (2004) Postnatal growth retardation: a universal problem in preterm infants. Arch Dis Child Fetal Neonatal Ed 89: F428–F430
Cordero ME, D'Acuna E, Benveniste S, Prado R, Nunez JA, Colombo M (1993) Dendritic development in neocortex of infants with early postnatal life undernutrition. Pediatr Neurol 9:457–464
Cornier MA, Dabelea D, Hernandez TL et al (2008) The metabolic syndrome. Endocr Rev 29:777–822
Dabydeen L, Thomas JE, Aston TJ, Hartley H, Sinha SK, Eyre JA (2008) High-energy and -protein diet increases brain and corticospinal tract growth in term and preterm infants after perinatal brain injury. Pediatrics 121:148–156
De Curtis M, Pieltain C, Rigo J (2002) Body composition in preterm infants fed standard term or enriched formula after hospital discharge. Eur J Nutr 41:177–182
Dharmaraj ST, Henderson M, Embleton ND, Fenton AC, Cooke RJ (2005) Postnatal growth retardation, catch-up growth and developmental outcome in preterm infants. Arch Dis Child 90:11A
Dinerstein A, Nieto RM, Solana CL, Perez GP, Otheguy LE, Larguia AM (2006) Early and aggressive nutritional strategy (parenteral and enteral) decreases postnatal growth failure in very low birth weight infants. J Perinatol 26:436–442
Dobbing J (1981) The later development of the brain and its vulnerability. In: Davis JA, Dobbing J (eds) Scientific foundations of pediatrics. University Park Press, Baltimore, pp 744–758
Dobbing J (1987) Early nutrition and later achievement. Academic, London
Dobbing J, Sands J (1971) Vulnerability of developing brain. IX. The effect of nutritional growth retardation on the timing of the brain growth-spurt. Biol Neonate 19:363–378
Dobbing J, Hopewell JW, Lynch A (1971) Vulnerability of developing brain. VII. Permanent deficit of neurons in cerebral and cerebellar cortex following early mild undernutrition. Exp Neurol 32:439–447
Donovan R, Puppala B, Angst D, Coyle BW (2006) Outcomes of early nutrition support in extremely low-birth-weight infants. Nutr Clin Pract 21: 395–400
Ehrenkranz RA, Younes N, Lemons JA et al (1999) Longitudinal growth of hospitalized very low birth weight infants. Pediatrics 104:280–289
Ehrenkranz RA, Dusick AM, Vohr BR, Wright LL, Wrage LA, Poole WK (2006) Growth in the neonatal intensive care unit influences neurodevelopmental and growth outcomes of extremely low birth weight infants. Pediatrics 117:1253–1261
Embleton NE, Pang N, Cooke RJ (2001) Postnatal malnutrition and growth retardation: an inevitable consequence of current recommendations in preterm infants? Pediatrics 107:270–273
Ernst JA, Bull MJ, Rickard KA, Brady MS, Lemons JA (1990) Growth outcome and feeding practices of the very low birth weight infant (less than 1500 grams) within the first year of life. J Pediatr 117: S156–S166
Evans RA, Thureen P (2001) Early feeding strategies in preterm and critically ill neonates. Neonatal Netw 20:7–18
Fenton TR, McMillan DD, Sauve RS (1990) Nutrition and growth analysis of very low birth weight infants. Pediatrics 86:378–383
Fewtrell PA, Cole TJ, Lucas A (2000) Effects of growth during infancy and childhood on bone mineralization and turnover in preterm children aged 8–12 years. Acta Paediatr 89:148–153
Fitzhardinge PM, Inwood S (1989) Long-term growth in small-for-date children. Acta Paediatr Scand – Suppl 349:27–33, discussion 4
Fomon S (1993a) Energy. In: Fomon SJ, Bell EF (eds) Nutrition of normal infants, 2nd edn. Mosby, St Louis, pp 103–120
Fomon S (1993b) Protein. In: Fomon SJ (ed) Nutrition of normal infants, 2nd edn. Mosby, St Louis, pp 121–139
Galler J, Shumsky J, Morgane PJ (1996) Malnutrition and brain development. In: Walker AW, Watkins J (eds) Paediatric nutrition. Decker, New York, pp 196–212
Greisen G (1992) Estimation of fetal weight by ultrasound. Horm Res 38:208–210
Griffin IJ, Tancredi DJ, Bertino E, Lee HC, Profit J (2016) Postnatal growth failure in very low birthweight infants born between 2005 and 2012. Arch Dis Child Fetal Neonatal Ed 101:50–55
Gross SJ (1983) Growth and biochemical response of preterm infants fed human milk or modified infant formula. N Engl J Med 308:237–241
Gross SJ, Oehler JM, Eckerman CO (1983) Head growth and developmental outcome in very low-birth-weight infants. Pediatrics 71:70–75
Hack M, Breslau N (1986) Very low birth weight infants: effects of brain growth during infancy on intelligence quotient at 3 years of age. Pediatrics 77:196–202
Hack M, Fanaroff AA (1984) The outcome of growth failure associated with preterm birth. Clin Obstet Gynecol 27:647–663
Hack M, Merkatz IR, Gordon D, Jones PK, Fanaroff AA (1982) The prognostic significance of postnatal growth in very low – birth weight infants. Am J Obstet Gynecol 143:693–699
Hack M, Caron B, Rivers A, Fanaroff AA (1983) The very low birth weight infant: the broader spectrum of morbidity during infancy and early childhood. J Dev Behav Pediatr 4:243–249
Hack M, Breslau N, Weissman B, Aram D, Klein N, Borawski E (1991) Effect of very low birth weight and subnormal head size on cognitive abilities at school age [see comments]. N Engl J Med 325:231–237

Hack M, Weissman B, Breslau N, Klein N, Borawski-Clark E, Fanaroff AA (1993) Health of very low birth weight children during their first eight years. J Pediatr 122:887–892

Hack M, Schluchter M, Cartar L, Rahman M, Cuttler L, Borawski E (2003) Growth of very low birth weight infants to age 20 years. Pediatrics 112:e30–e38

Health Canada (2004) Breast feeding duration recommendations

Heird WC (2001) Determination of nutritional requirements in preterm infants, with special reference to 'catch-up' growth. Semin Neonatol 6:365–375

Henderson G, Fahey T, McGuire W (2005) Calorie and protein-enriched formula versus standard term formula for improving growth and development in preterm or low birth weight infants following hospital discharge. Cochrane Database Syst Rev CD004696

Hermanussen M (2013a) Basics. Rapid growth. In: Hermanussen M (ed) Auxology studying human growth and development. Schweizerbart'sche, Stuttgaart, pp 18–19

Hermanussen M (2013b) Basics. In: Hermanussen M (ed) Auxology studying human growth and development. Schweizerbart'sche, Stuttgart

Horbar JD, Ehrenkranz RA, Badger GJ et al (2015) Weight growth velocity and postnatal growth failure in infants 501 to 1500 grams: 2000–2013. Pediatrics 136: e84–e92

Ibrahim HM, Jeroudi MA, Baier RJ, Dhanireddy R, Krouskop RW (2004) Aggressive early total parental nutrition in low-birth-weight infants. J Perinatol 24:482–486

Jackson AA (1990) Protein requirements for catch-up growth. Proc Nutr Soc 49:507–516

Jeon GW, Jung YJ, Koh SY et al (2011) Preterm infants fed nutrient-enriched formula until 6 months show improved growth and development. Pediatr Int. Off J Jpn Pediatr Soc 53:683–688

Kitchen WH, Doyle LW, Ford GW, Callanan C, Rickards AL, Kelly E (1992a) Very low birth weight and growth to age 8 years. II: head dimensions and intelligence. Am J Dis Child 146:46–50

Kitchen WH, Doyle LW, Ford GW, Callanan C (1992b) Very low birth weight and growth to age 8 years. I: weight and height. Am J Dis Child 146:40–45

Klein CJ (2002) Nutrient requirements for preterm infant formulas. J Nutr 132:1395S–1577S

Koo WW, Hockman EM (2006) Posthospital discharge feeding for preterm infants: effects of standard compared with enriched milk formula on growth, bone mass, and body composition. Am J Clin Nutr 84:1357–1364

Koo WW, Sherman R, Succop P et al (1988) Sequential bone mineral content in small preterm infants with and without fractures and rickets. J Bone Miner Res 3:193–197

Krigman MR, Hogan EL (1976) Undernutrition in the developing rat: effect upon myelination. Brain Res 107:239–255

Kurl S, Heinonen K, Lansimies E (2003) Pre- and post-discharge feeding of very preterm infants: impact on growth and bone mineralization. Clin Physiol Funct Imaging 23:182–189

Lapillonne A, Salle BL, Glorieux FH, Claris O (2004) Bone mineralization and growth are enhanced in preterm infants fed an isocaloric, nutrient-enriched preterm formula through term. Am J Clin Nutr 80:1595–1603

Lapillonne A, O'Connor DL, Wang D, Rigo J (2013) Nutritional recommendations for the late-preterm infant and the preterm infant after hospital discharge. J Pediatr 162:S90–S100

Larsen T, Petersen S, Greisen G, Larsen JF (1990) Normal fetal growth evaluated by longitudinal ultrasound examinations. Early Hum Dev 24:37–45

Latal-Hajnal B, von Siebenthal K, Kovari H, Bucher HU, Largo RH (2003) Postnatal growth in VLBW infants: significant association with neurodevelopmental outcome. J Pediatr 143:163–170

Litmanovitz I, Dolfin T, Arnon S et al (2004) Bone strength and growth of preterm infants fed nutrient-enriched or term formula after hospital discharge. Pediatr Res 55:274A

Lowry S, Perez JM (2006) The hypercatabolic state. In: Shils M, Shike M, Ross CA, Caballero B, Cousins R (eds) Modern nutrition in health and disease, 10th edn. Lippincott, Williams & Wilkins, Philadelphia, pp 1381–1400

Lucas A, Morley R, Cole TJ et al (1989a) Early diet in preterm babies and developmental status in infancy [see comments]. Arch Dis Child 64:1570–1578

Lucas A, Brooke OG, Baker BA, Bishop N, Morley R (1989b) High alkaline phosphatase activity and growth in preterm neonates. Arch Dis Child 64:902–909

Lucas A, Morley R, Cole TJ et al (1990) Early diet in preterm babies and developmental status at 18 months. Lancet 335:1477–1481

Lucas A, Bishop NJ, King FJ, Cole TJ (1992) Randomised trial of nutrition for preterm infants after discharge [see comments]. Arch Dis Child 67:324–327

Lucas A, Morley R, Cole TJ, Gore SM (1994) A randomised multicentre study of human milk versus formula and later development in preterm infants. Arch Dis Child Fetal Neonatal Ed 70:F141–F146

Lucas A, Morley R, Cole TJ (1998) Randomised trial of early diet in preterm babies and later intelligence quotient. BMJ 317:1481–1487

Lucas A, Fewtrell MS, Morley R et al (2001) Randomized trial of nutrient-enriched formula versus standard formula for postdischarge preterm infants. Pediatrics 108:703–711

MacLean WC Jr, Graham GG (1980) The effect of energy intake on nitrogen content of weight gained by recovering malnourished infants. Am J Clin Nutr 33:903–909

McCance RA, Widdowson EM (1974) The determinants of growth and form. Proc R Soc Lond B Biol Sci 185:1–17

McCormick MC, Shapiro S, Starfield BH (1980) Rehospitalization in the first year of life for high-risk survivors. Pediatrics 66:991–999

Mehta NM, Corkins MR, Lyman B et al (2013) Defining pediatric malnutrition: a paradigm shift toward etiology-related definitions. JPEN J Parenter Enteral Nutr 37:460–481

Morley R (1999) Early growth and later development. In: Ziegler EE, Lucas A, Moro GE (eds) Nutrition of the very low birth weight infant. Lippincott Williams and Wilkins, Philadelphia, pp 19–32

Morley R, Lucas A (1997) Nutrition and cognitive development. Br Med Bull 53:123–134

Morley R, Cole TJ, Powell R, Lucas A (1988) Mother's choice to provide breast milk and developmental outcome. Arch Dis Child 63:1382–1385

Myers RE, Hill DE, Holt AB, Scott RE, Mellits ED, Cheek DB (1971) Fetal growth retardation produced by experimental placental insufficiency in the rhesus monkey. I. Body weight, organ size. Biol Neonate 18:379–394

Navas L, Wang E, de Carvalho V, Robinson J, PICNIC (1992) Improved outcome of respiratory syncytial virus infection in a high-risk hospitalized population of Canadian children. J Pediatr 121:348–354

O'Connor DL, Khan S, Weishuhn K et al (2008) Growth and nutrient intakes of human milk-fed preterm infants provided with extra energy and nutrients after hospital discharge. Pediatrics 121:766–776

Olsen IE, Richardson DK, Schmid CH, Ausman LM, Dwyer JT (2002) Intersite differences in weight growth velocity of extremely premature infants. Pediatrics 110:1125–1132

Ong KK, Loos RJ (2006) Rapid infancy weight gain and subsequent obesity: systematic reviews and hopeful suggestions. Acta Paediatr 95:904–908

Ounsted M, Moar VA, Scott A (1988) Head circumference and developmental ability at the age of seven years. Acta Paediatr Scand 77:374–379

Peterson J, Taylor HG, Minich N, Klein N, Hack M (2006) Subnormal head circumference in very low birth weight children: neonatal correlates and school-age consequences. Early Hum Dev 82:325–334

Pryor J, Silva PA, Brooke M (1995) Growth, development and behaviour in adolescents born small-for-gestational-age. J Paediatr Child Health 31: 403–407

Rawlings DJ, Cooke RJ, McCormick K et al (1999) Body composition of preterm infants during infancy. Arch Dis Child Fetal Neonatal Ed 80:F188–F191

Roberts SB, Young VR (1988) Energy costs of fat and protein deposition in the human infant. Am J Clin Nutr 48:951–955

Roggero P, Gianni ML, Piemontese P, Amato O, Agosti M, Mosca F (2012) Effect of nutrition on growth and body composition in infants born preterm. J Matern Fetal Neonatal Med 25(Suppl 3):49–52

Ross G, Lipper EG, Auld PA (1990) Growth achievement of very low birth weight premature children at school age. J Pediatr 117:307–309

Schanler RJ (2005) Post-discharge nutrition for the preterm infant. Acta Paediatr Suppl 94:68–73

Schanler RJ, Burns PA, Abrams SA, Garza C (1992) Bone mineralization outcomes in human milk-fed preterm infants. Pediatr Res 31:583–586

Schanler RJ, Shulman RJ, Lau C (1999) Feeding strategies for premature infants: beneficial outcomes of feeding fortified human milk versus preterm formula [comment]. Pediatrics 103:1150–1157

Scott KE, Usher R (1966) Fetal malnutrition: its incidence, causes, and effects. Am J Obstet Gynecol 94:951–963

Shils ME, Shike M, Ross AC, Caballero B, Cousins RJ (2006) Modern nutrition in health and disease. Lippincott Williams and Wilkins, Philadelphia

Singer L, Arendt R, Song LY, Warshawsky E, Kliegman R (1994) Direct and indirect interactions of cocaine with childbirth outcomes. Arch Pediatr Adolesc Med 148:959–964

Singhal A, Cole TJ, Lucas A (2001) Early nutrition in preterm infants and later blood pressure: two cohorts after randomised trials. Lancet 357:413–419

Singhal A, Fewtrell M, Cole TJ, Lucas A (2003) Low nutrient intake and early growth for later insulin resistance in adolescents born preterm. Lancet 361:1089–1097

Stathis SL, O'Callaghan M, Harvey J, Rogers Y (1999) Head circumference in ELBW babies is associated with learning difficulties and cognition but not ADHD in the school-aged child. Dev Med Child Neurol 41:375–380

Stoch MB, Smythe PM, Moodie AD, Bradshaw D (1982) Psychosocial outcome and CT findings after gross undernourishment during infancy: a 20-year developmental study. Dev Med Child Neurol 24:419–436

Teller IC, Embleton ND, Griffin IJ, van Elburg RM (2016) Post-discharge formula feeding in preterm infants: a systematic review mapping evidence about the role of macronutrient enrichment. Clin Nutr 35(4):791–801

Thomas M, Bedford-Russel A, Sharland M (2000) Hospitalisation of RSV infection in ex-preterm infants – implications for RSV immune globulin. Arch Dis Child 183:122–127

Tyson JE, Lasky RE, Mize CE et al (1983) Growth, metabolic response, and development in very-low-birth-weight infants fed banked human milk or enriched formula. I. Neonatal findings. J Pediatr 103:95–104

Uthaya S, Thomas EL, Hamilton G, Dore CJ, Bell J, Modi N (2005) Altered adiposity after extremely preterm birth. Pediatr Res 57:211–215

Volpe JJ (2008) Neurology of the newborn, 5th edn. Saunders Elsevier, Philadelphia

Wang E, Law B, Stephens D, PICNIC (1995) Prospective study of risk factors and outcomes in patients hospitalised with respiratory syncytial viral lower respiratory tract infection. J Pediatr 126:212–219

Wauben IP, Atkinson SA, Shah JK, Paes B (1998) Growth and body composition of preterm infants: influence of nutrient fortification of mother's milk in hospital and breastfeeding post- hospital discharge (in process citation). Acta Paediatr 87:780–785

Wheeler RE, Hall RT (1996) Feeding of premature infant formula after hospital discharge of infants weighing less than 1800 grams at birth. J Perinatol 16:111–116

Widdowson EM, McCance RA (1975) A review: new thoughts on growth. Pediatr Res 9:154–156

Wilson DC, Cairns P, Halliday HL, Reid M, McClure G, Dodge JA (1997) Randomised controlled trial of an aggressive nutritional regimen in sick very low birthweight infants. Arch Dis Child Fetal Neonatal Ed 77:F4–F11

Winick M, Rosso P (1969a) The effect of severe early malnutrition on cellular growth of human brain. Pediatr Res 3:181–184

Winick M, Rosso P (1969b) Head circumference and cellular growth of the brain in normal and marasmic children. J Pediatr 74:774–778

Yeung MY (2006) Postnatal growth, neurodevelopment and altered adiposity after preterm birth – from a clinical nutrition perspective. Acta Paediatr 95: 909–917

Zachariassen G, Faerk J, Grytter C et al (2011) Nutrient enrichment of mother's milk and growth of very preterm infants after hospital discharge. Pediatrics 127: e995–e1003

Ziegler EE, Thureen PJ, Carlson SJ (2002) Aggressive nutrition of the very low birthweight infant. Clin Perinatol 29:225–244

Calcium and Phosphorus Homeostasis: Pathophysiology

41

Jacques Rigo, Catherine Pieltain, Renaud Viellevoye, and Franco Bagnoli

Contents

Abstract

The metabolic homeostasis of calcium, phosphorus, and magnesium and mineralization of the skeleton are complex functions that require adequate supply of nutrients, the development of the intestinal absorption process, the inter-

J. Rigo (✉) · C. Pieltain · R. Viellevoye
Department of Neonatology, University of Liège, CHR de la Citadelle, Liège, Belgium

F. Bagnoli
Department of Pediatrics, Obstetrics and Reproductive Medicine, University of Siena, Siena, Italy

G. Buonocore et al. (eds.), *Neonatology*,
https://doi.org/10.1007/978-3-319-29489-6_190

action of several hormones (such as parathyroid hormone, vitamin D, and calcitonin), and optimum renal and skeletal control. Approximately 50% of total serum calcium is in ionized form at the normal serum protein concentration and represents the biologically active component of the total serum calcium concentration. The fetus maintains higher blood calcium and phosphorus levels than the ambient maternal levels. This process is the result of the active transport of calcium across the placenta. The role of vitamin D in fetal physiology is not well understood. Calcium absorption is the main determinant of its retention in the small intestine by both active and passive processes. Acid pH in the stomach is a prerequisite for absorption. Reference values of calcium retention calculated during the last trimester of gestation (120–130 mg/kg/day) are considered the target mineral accretion rates for infants with very low birth weight. We should pay particular attention to the dosage of total and ionized serum calcium when some medications are used or when there is acidosis/alkalosis, hypomagnesemia, prematurity, infant of a diabetic mother, or birth asphyxia. In contrast to calcium, the serum phosphorus concentration varies widely depending mainly on intake and renal excretion but is also influenced by age, gender, pH, and a variety of hormones. Premature infants, particularly those born at <28 weeks' gestation, are at significant risk for reduced bone mineral content (BMC) and subsequent bone disease, variably termed metabolic bone disease (MBD), osteomalacia, osteopenia, or neonatal rickets. Several factors increase the risk for severe MBD among VLBW infants, with the most important appearing to be an inadequate supply of calcium and phosphorus associated with the use of an enteral vs. transplacental route. Early optimal parenteral and oral nutritional support, combined with biologic neonatal screening and biomarker measurements, appears to be helpful for the prevention of MBD.

41.1 Salient Points

- When calcium and phosphorus are provided together as human milk fortifiers, calcium retention and absorption rates are parallel, reaching 60 mg/kg per day.
- The ESPGHAN Committee Nutrition recommended an adequate intake of calcium 60–90 mg/kg/day (110–130 mg/100 Kcal), phosphate 65–90 mg/kg/day, Ca:P ratio 1.5–2.
- Vitamin D recommendations differ significantly between North American (400 IU/day) and European countries (800–1000 IU/day).
- Iatrogenic hypercalcemia is the most common type of hypercalcemia.
- The measurement of calcium-regulating hormones is not routinely recommended unless hypocalcemia is prolonged, refractory, or recurrent.
- When available, DEXA is more sensitive than ultrasound for quantifying osteopenia in VLBW infants.

41.2 Introduction

Ninety-eight percent of the calcium and eighty percent of the phosphorus in the body are in the skeleton; these elements are also constituents of the intracellular and extracellular spaces. The metabolic homeostasis of calcium, phosphorus, and magnesium and mineralization of the skeleton are complex functions that require the intervention of various parameters; an adequate supply of nutrients; the development of the intestinal absorption process; and the effects of several hormones, such as parathyroid hormone, vitamin D, and calcitonin, as well as optimum renal and skeletal controls (Rigo et al. 2000). Bone formation requires protein and energy for collagen matrix synthesis, and an adequate intake of calcium and phosphorus is necessary for correct mineralization. During development, nutrients are transferred mainly across the placenta. It has been calculated that during the last trimester of gestation the daily accretion per kilogram of body weight represents around 120 mg of calcium and 70 mg of phosphorus. Therefore, at birth the whole-body content of a term infant represents approximately 30 g of calcium and 16 g of phosphorus. After birth, the use of the gastrointestinal tract to provide nutrients for growth causes a reduction in calcium availability for bone accretion promoting the occurrence of relative osteopenia in preterm infants and to a lesser extent in term infants during the first weeks of life. In addition to their roles in bone formation, calcium and phosphorus play important roles in many physiologic processes, such as transport across membranes, activation and inhibition of enzymes, intracellular regulation of metabolic pathways, secretion and action of hormones, blood coagulation, muscle contractility, and nerve conduction. The 20% of phosphorus not complexed within bone is present mainly as adenosine triphosphate, nucleic acids, and cell and organelle membranes.

41.3 Calcium and Phosphorus Physiology

41.3.1 Calcium Physiology

41.3.1.1 Serum Calcium

Serum calcium is a fraction of total body calcium because only about 2% of calcium is present in extracellular fluid and soft tissues. Approximately 50% of total serum calcium is in ionized form at the normal serum protein concentration and represents the biologically active component of the total serum calcium concentration. Another 8–10% is complexed to organic and inorganic acids (e.g., citrate, lactate, bicarbonate, sulfate, and phosphate); together, the ionized and complexed calcium fractions represent the diffusible portion of circulating calcium. Approximately 40% of serum calcium is protein bound, primarily to albumin (80%) but also to globulins (20%) (Rigo et al. 2010; Hsu and Levine 2004). Ionized calcium is the only physiologically active fraction.

The protein-bound calcium is not biologically active but provides a rapidly available reserve of calcium. Under normal circumstances the serum calcium concentration is tightly regulated by parathyroid hormone (PTH) and calcitriol (1,25-dihydroxy vitamin D_3; 1,25[OH]$_2$D$_3$), which increase serum calcium (Fig. 1), and by calcitonin, which decreases serum calcium.

41.3.1.2 Placental Transport

During pregnancy there is an active calcium transfer from the mother to the fetus, reaching a peak of 120–150 mg/kg of fetal weight per day during the third trimester.

To meet the high demand for mineral requirements of the developing skeleton, the fetus maintains higher blood calcium and phosphorus levels than the ambient maternal levels. This process is the result of the active transport of calcium across the placenta by a calcium pump in the basal membrane that maintains a gradient of maternal to fetal calcium of 1:1.4. PTH has no effect on placental calcium transport.

By contrast, the main regulator of fetal ionized calcium appears to be the parathyroid hormone-related protein (PTHrP) produced by the placenta. PTHrP(1–141) or its midmolecule fragment, PTHrP(67–86), is the active form contrary to PTH (1–34) or PTHrP(1.34), suggesting that PTHrP stimulates receptor(s) distinct from the PTH/PTHrP receptor (Sato 2008).

The role of vitamin D in fetal physiology is not well understood. Cord concentrations of 25-hydroxyvitamin D and 1,25-dihydroxyvitamin D correlate significantly with those found in the maternal circulation, suggesting that the vitamin D pool of the fetus depends entirely on that of the mother. Fetomaternal relationships of 1,25-dihydroxyvitamin D concentrations are still debated.

Nevertheless, it has been demontrated that the placenta is able to synthethise and metabolize 1,25-dihydroxyvitamin D through the activity of 25-hydroxyvitamin D-1α-hydroxylase and 1,25-dihydroxyvitamin D-24 hydroxylase, two key enzymes for vitamin D metabolism (Avila et al. 2006). In addition, it has been suggested that methylation of the vitamin D-24-hydroxylase gene plays an important role in maximizing active vitamin D bioavailability at the fetomaternal interface

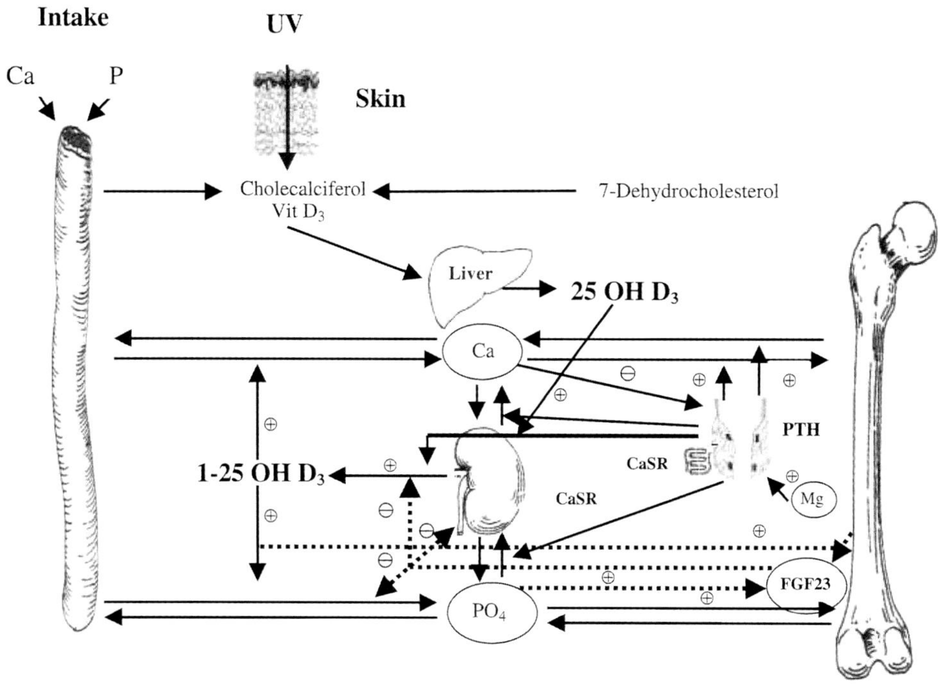

Fig. 1 Regulation of calcium and phosphate homeostasis. Parathyroid hormone (*PTH*) increases Ca release from bone, Ca resorption in the kidney, and $1{,}25(OH)_2D_3$ secretion from the kidney. PTH production is stimulated by low Ca and inhibited by low Mg and high $1{,}25(OH)_2D_3$. Vitamin D increases Ca release from bone and Ca and PO_4 absorption from the intestine. Vitamin D production is stimulated by high PTH and low PO_4. FGF23 production and release is stimulated by serum phosphate independent of PTH axis. FGF23 lowers phosphate concentration by inhibiting renal and intestinal phosphate transport as well as preventing activation of $1{,}25(OH)_2D_3$ which in turn controls levels of bone synthesis of FGF23. *CaSR* calcium-stimulating response, *UV* ultraviolet light

(Novakovic et al. 2009) and that active transplacental calcium and phosphate transfers are at least partly dependent on insulin-like growth factor-1 (IGF-1), itself a stimulating factor of fetal and placental 1,25-dihydroxyvitamin D synthesis.

Bone mass of the newborn may be related to the vitamin D status of the mother and studies of particular populations show that infants of mothers severely deficient in vitamin D may be born with rickets and can suffer fractures in the neonatal period (Salle et al. 2000; Bassir et al. 2001).

41.3.1.3 Intestinal Absorption

Calcium absorption is the main determinant of its retention; consequently, it has a significant impact on bone mineral content. Calcium absorption occurs in the small intestine by both active and passive processes. Vitamin D is essential for the active absorption of calcium, which involves carriers such as calcium-binding proteins.

After birth calcium absorption limits the rate of bone mineralization for growth although the absorption rate is higher than that during all other periods of life. The absorption of calcium occurs in the small intestine by two main routes – either through or between cells. Movement through the cell takes place by active transport dependent on vitamin D bound to a cytosolic calcium-binding protein (calbindin D_{9k}). The major role of vitamin D in transcellular calcium transport involves the biosynthesis of calcium-binding protein. Passive calcium transport is driven by chemical gradients that represent movement of calcium among the cells (paracellular transport). In addition to vitamin D status, various other factors affect calcium absorption (Rigo et al.

2010; Atkinson and Tsang 2005) Ionization of calcium compounds, which requires an acid pH, occurs in the stomach and is a prerequisite for absorption. Therefore, low availability could be the result of an insoluble fraction of calcium intake or the precipitation of calcium in the gut. Calcium chloride, citrate, and carbonate have higher solubilities than calcium phosphate, which should be avoided in formulas. By contrast, the higher solubility of organic calcium, such as that found in calcium gluconate or glycerophosphate, improves its absorption. Fat intake and LCSFA (long-chain saturated fat acids) intake may also influence calcium absorption through the formation of calcium soap. It has been showed that the free palmitate content in the gastrointestinal tract after the hydrolysis of triglyceride may impair calcium absorption. The higher bioavailability of calcium in human milk would be partly due to palmitate, which is predominantly esterified at the glycerol 2 positions (Sn-2), but also to the human milk bile salt-stimulated lipase that is not specific to the Sn-1 and Sn-3 positions. The improvement of calcium absorption with the use of medium-chain triglycerides is probably the result of the reduction of total LCSFA content in formula. At present, with the use of a well absorbed fat combination (±85% fat absorption), the influence of calcium soap formation and the B-palmitate content formula could be relatively minimal in clinical practice. A relatively low gastrointestinal pH content or the lactose and casein content of the formula may also have an additional positive effect on calcium absorption. In light of the considerable requirements of preterm infants, all of these factors probably play a significant role in the amount of calcium retained and deposited in the skeleton.

Medications also interfere with calcium absorption; for example, glucocorticoids inhibit intestinal transfer. Some anticonvulsants can also inhibit calcium absorption either directly (phenytoin) or indirectly through interference with vitamin D metabolism (phenobarbital and phenytoin). In newborn infants, a significant amount of calcium is secreted in the intestinal lumen through digestive fluid. With the use of stable isotopes, endogenous fecal calcium excretion and true calcium absorption may be evaluated. Considering that fecal calcium excretion may represent about 15 mg/kg per day in preterm infants, the true calcium absorption rate is significantly higher than the apparent rate measured by conventional metabolic balances.

Numerous metabolic balance studies have been performed in preterm infants fed human milk or a formula (Fig. 2) (Rigo et al. 2000, 2007; Rigo and Senterre 2006) to evaluate apparent calcium absorption. In preterm infants fed human milk, calcium absorption ranges from 60% to 70% depending on the calcium intake, whereas calcium retention is related to the phosphorus supply. Supplementation of human milk with phosphorus alone normalizes calciuria and allows calcium retention to reach about 35 mg/kg per day. When calcium and phosphorus are provided together or as human milk fortifiers, calcium retention and absorption rates parallel that of human milk, reaching 60 mg/kg per day. The use of new human milk fortifiers containing highly soluble calcium glycerophosphate improves calcium retention to 90 mg/kg per day (Fig. 2) (Rigo et al. 2000). In formula-fed infants, the percentage of net calcium absorption is less than that with human milk, ranging from 35% to 60%. Most of the difference probably results from the various factors affecting calcium solubility and absorption. At present, the use of a preterm formula with a high mineral content does not necessarily improve mineral retention (Rigo and Senterre 2006). Indeed, due to the poor solubility of calcium salts, especially calcium phosphate, the calcium content measured in formulas may be significantly lower than the claimed value, and an additional loss due to precipitation may occur before feeding (Rigo and Senterre 2006). In metabolic studies, the actual amount of calcium provided by feeding needs to be measured. As shown in Fig. 2, calcium retention limited to 90 mg/kg per day could presently be expected in preterm infants fed a preterm formula with a highly soluble calcium content. Nevertheless, those values are still relatively far from the reference values calculated during the last

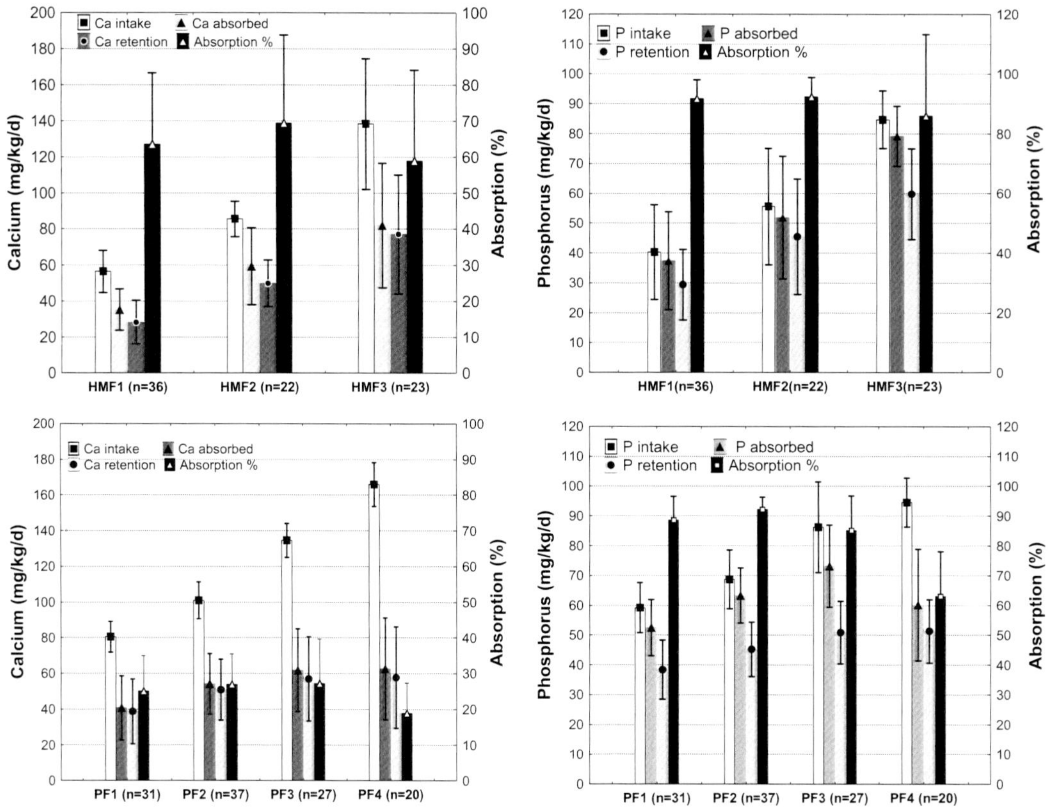

Fig. 2 Calcium and phosphorus absorption and retention in preterm infants fed human milk (without or with a human milk fortifier) and preterm formulas. In human milk groups, calcium and phosphorus absorption and retention are related to intake, in contrast to formula groups, in which a plateau is reached rapidly due to a decrease in net absorption (%). *HMF* human milk fortifier, *PF* preterm formula

trimester of gestation (120–130 mg/kg per day), which is still considered the target mineral accretion rate for infants with very low birth weight (VLBW).

41.3.1.4 Renal Excretion

Under normal circumstances, calcium status is maintained by a balance between its intestinal absorption and renal excretion. Urinary excretion is the result of glomerular filtration followed by the sum of the processes of tubular reabsorption and secretion. Approximately 70% of the filtered load of calcium is reabsorbed in the proximal tubule and 20% in the thick ascending limb of Henle's loop in association with Na^+ reabsorption. Although it is responsible for only 5–10% of Ca^{2+} reabsorption, the major regulation of Ca^{2+} reabsorption occurs in the distal convoluted tubule by a mechanism independent of Na^+ reabsorption but regulated by PTH and 1,25 $(OH)_2D_3$. Calcium reabsorption is increased by both PTH and $1,25(OH)_2D_3$. It is also regulated by ionized calcium concentration, phosphate concentration, and acid-base status and increases with Ca^{2+} depletion and alkalosis but decreases with hypercalcemia, phosphate depletion, and acidosis. The effects of diuretics on renal calcium excretion vary considerably. Furosemide markedly increases renal calcium losses and is a risk factor for neonatal nephrocalcinosis. Thiazides increase renal tubular calcium reabsorption, thereby reducing calciuria (Portal 2004).

The ability of the kidney to dispose of excess calcium represents a major homeostatic mechanism. Under normal circumstancs nearly all filtered calcium (98%) is reabsorbed in the

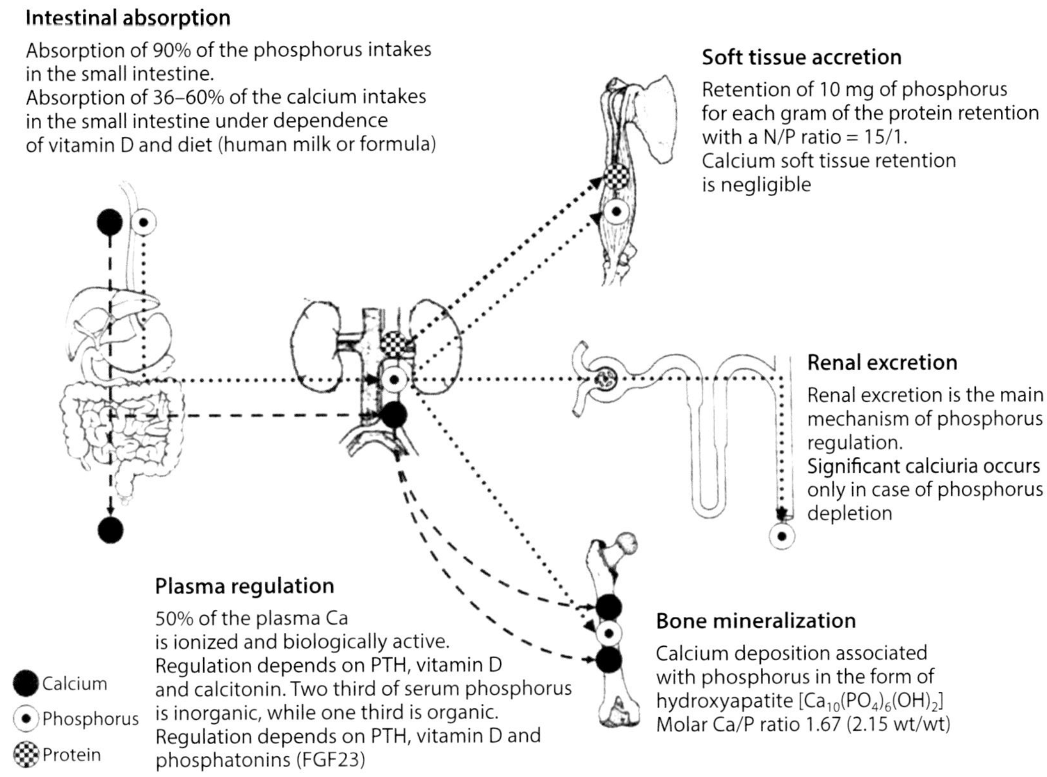

Fig. 3 Metabolism of calcium and phosphorus in term infants with feeding

renal tubule. However, preterm and term infants differ from the adult in three main aspects: (1) Renal function is far from being completely developed, (2) Mineral requirements for growth are very high and (3) Renal calcium load results solely in the difference between net absorption and net bone and soft tissue retention. Considering that calcium soft tissue retention is negligible, renal calcium load is highly dependent on bone calcium deposition associated with phosphorus in the form of hydroxyapatite $[Ca_{10}(PO_4)_6(OH)_2]$ containing a molar calcium:phosphorus ratio of 1.67 (2.15 wt/wt). Therefore, the main determinant of the urinary loss of calcium in preterm and term neonates is relative to phosphorus depletion, which has been illustrated in balance studies performed in growing preterm infants fed human milk. When human milk is provided exclusively, there is an increase in the urinary excretion of calcium associated with very low urinary phosphate excretion. In contrast, when human milk is supplemented with phosphate, significant phosphaturia appears at the same time that calciuria decreases to a minimum level. Therefore, hypercalciuria can be explained by a relative phosphate depletion that cannot meet the phosphate demand necessary for skeletal mineralization (Fig. 3).

41.3.1.5 Requirement

For preterm infants, recommendations are based on fetal accretion rates. In 1985 the American Academy of Pediatrics recommended that formulas contain 140–160 mg of calcium per 100 kcal (American Academy of Pediatric 1985). More recently, the Life Sciences Research Office recommended a calcium content of 123–185 mg/100 kcal for preterm infant formula, and an international expert panel suggested a similar value of 90–180 mg/100 kcal (Klein 2002). However, the ESPGHAN (European Society for Pediatric

Gastroenterology, Hepatology, and Nutrition) committee of nutrition considers that those calcium needs are based on data obtained in infants fed preterm formulas with low calcium bioavailability. It suggests that after birth, bone metabolism is designed to accelerate bone turnover, reducing calcium requirements and that the relative osteopenia observed in preterm infants could be considered at least partially physiologic. As a calcium retention level ranging from 60 to 90 mg/kg/day assures appropriate mineralization and decreases the risk of fracture in VLBW infants, the ESPGHAN CoN recommended the use of highly bioavailable calcium salts providing a calcium content of 110–130 mg/100 kcal (Agostoni et al. 2010).

41.3.2 Phosphorus Physiology

Unlike calcium, phosphorus remains in the soft tissues, mainly in the form of phosphate esters, and in extracellular fluid in the form of inorganic phosphate ions. It represents approximately 15% of the whole-body content. Given its widespread distribution, phosphorus plays a critical role in many biological processes, including energy metabolism, membrane composition, nucleotide structure, cellular signaling and bone mineralization. It is, therefore, not surprising that a deficiency of phosphorus results in clinical disease, including muscle weakness, impaired leukocyte function, and abnormal bone metabolization.

41.3.2.1 Serum Phosphorus

In serum about two thirds of phosphorus is organic (lipid phosphorus and phosphoric ester phosphorus) and one third inorganic. In routine clinical practice only inorganic phosphorus is measured. About 85% of the inorganic phosphorus is ionized, circulating as monohydrogen or dihydrogen phosphate; 5% is complexed with sodium, magnesium, or calcium; and 10% is protein bound (Rigo et al. 2010).

Because so many phosphorus species are present, depending on pH and other factors, the serum concentration is conventionally expressed as the mass of the elemental phosphorus (mmol/L or mg/dL). In contrast to calcium, the serum phosphorus concentration varies widely depending mainly on intake and renal excretion but is also influenced by age, gender, pH, and a variety of hormones. At birth, the mean serum phosphorus concentration is relatively low (2.6 mmol/L, or 6.2 mg/dL) but thereafter rises rapidly to reach 3.4 mmol/L, or 8.1 mg/dL, owing to both endogenous phosphorus release and low renal excretion. Serum phosphorus subsequently varies. The diet partially determines the serum phosphorus content: it is higher in formula-fed than breast-fed infants. Serum phosphorus is inversely related to serum calcium concentration. After the neonatal period, the serum phosphorus concentration progressively decreases to 2.1 mmol/L, or 5 mg/dL, at the age of 1–2 years; 1.8 mmol/L, or 4.4 mg/dL, in middle childhood; and 1.5 mmol/L, or 3.5 mg/dL, at the end of adolescence (Portal 2004).

41.3.2.2 Placental Transport

During pregnancy there is transfer of phosphorus from the mother to the fetus that reaches a peak of 60–75 mg/kg per day during the third trimester; 75% is retained for bone mineralization, and 25% is retained in other tissues. The transplacental transport of phosphorus is an active process against a concentration gradient and is sodium dependent. Both $1,25(OH)_2D_3$ and fetal PTH may be involved in the regulation of placental phosphorus transfer.

41.3.2.3 Intestinal Absorption

Intestinal phosphorus absorption takes place primarily in the duodenum, jejunum, and to a lesser extent in the ileum and colon. It occurs via two mechanisms: an active, sodium-dependent transcellular process localized to the mucosal surface and passive diffusion through the paracellular pathway. It depends on both the absolute amount of dietary phosphorus and the relative concentrations of calcium and phosphorus (an excessive amount of either can decrease the absorption of the other). Vitamin D may stimulate active phosphorus absorption, although it is largely independent of vitamin D intake. The efficiency of this absorption is high (close to 90% of intake) regardless of the type of milk given (Rigo et al. 2000, 2010). However, the use of poorly soluble phosphate salt such as calcium triphosphate in formulas is associated with a significant reduction in phosphorus absorption (Rigo et al. 2000). In contrast to calcium, only a small amount of phosphate is secreted in the intestinal lumen through digestive fluid.

41.3.2.4 Renal Excretion

The kidney contributes to a positive phosphate balance during growth by the reabsorption of a relatively high fraction of filtered inorganic phosphate (99% in newborns, 95% in infants fed human milk, and 80% in adults).

Preterm infants have an increased fractional excretion of phosphate and are at a greater risk of developing signs and symptoms of phosphate deficiency. The bulk of filtered phosphate is reabsorbed in the proximal tubule via a sodium-dependent transporter, the Na^+-phosphate cotransporter. The age-related decrease in phosphate reabsorption observed after the weaning period appears to be correlated with the smaller phosphate needs of adult and older animals than those of growing animals and is associated with a rapid downregulation of Na^+-phosphate cotransporter-2 mRNA and protein in the brush border membrane (Holtback and Aperia 2003). The kidney is the major determinant of the plasma phosphate concentration. Filtered load depends on the plasma phosphorus level and glomerular filtration rate (GFR).

Tubular reabsorption is an active and saturable process that gives rise to a maximum rate of tubular reabsorption (T_m). There is a plasma minimum threshold below which phosphorus reabsorption is almost complete and urinary excretion close to zero and a maximum threshold above which all tubular reabsorptive systems are saturated, so each additional increment in filtered load is associated with a parallel increment in excretion (Rigo et al. 2010). In preterm infants, the minimum and maximum threshold levels are 1.75 mmol/L (5.4 mg/dL) and 2.45 mmol/L (7.6 mg/dL), respectively (Fig. 4).

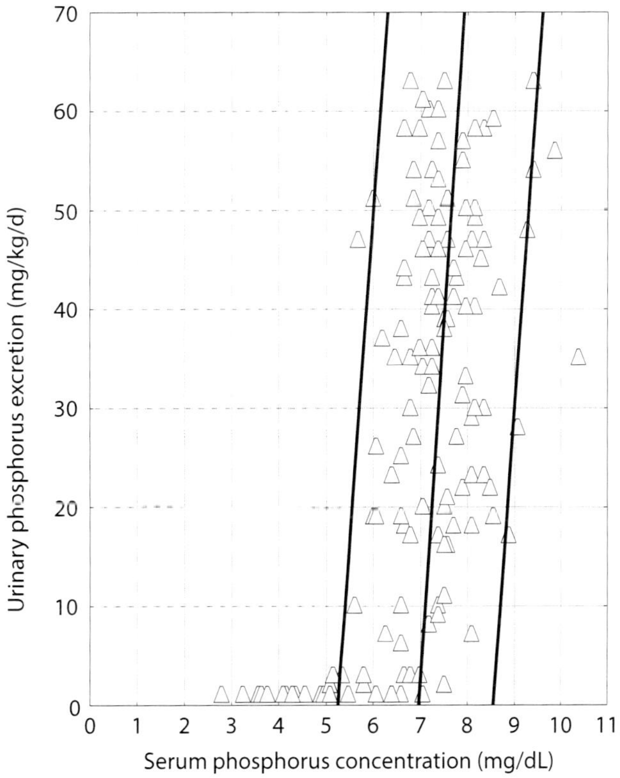

Fig. 4 Relationship between urinary excretion of phosphorus and serum phosphate level (n = 198) in preterm infants. Regression lines represent the minimum, mean, and maximum plasma phosphate concentration thresholds for tubular reabsorption of phosphate. Points to the left of the minimum threshold were considered hypophosphatemia associated with phosphorus depletion. Points to the right of the maximum threshold were considered hyperphosphatemia due to low glomerular filtration rates and relative phosphorus overload

In the intermediate zone, there is a functional relationship between GFR and T_m, known as the glomerulotubular balance, in which a change in GFR is compensated for by a change in T_m in order to regulate phosphorus excretion. The total body phosphate metabolism is tightly regulated by three hormones, namely PTH, 1,25(OH)$_2$ vitamin D and fibroblast growth factor 23 (FGF23) (Quarles 2008). The level of PTH activity in plasma is an important physiologic regulator of phosphorus excretion. PTH inhibits phosphorus reabsorption, but its activity appears to be limited to the intermediate zone between the minimum and maximum plasma threshold levels. In contrast, 1,25(OH)$_2$ vitamin D synthesis, stimulated by a decrease in plasma phosphorus concentration, has an indirect effect on phosphorus reabsorption by its effect on mineral absorption and mobilization from bone, resulting in an increase in plasma calcium concentration and the suppression of PTH release. During early postnatal life the phosphate response to PTH is blunted, whereas PTH increases tubular calcium reabsorption.

Together, these actions result in the retention of both calcium and phosphate in infants, which is favorable for growth. The role of newly discovered phosphatonin peptides such as FGF23 in the regulation of phosphorus excretion during the early life remain to be established. FGF23 principally functions as a phosphaturic factor and counter-regulatory hormone for 1,25(OH)$_2$ vitamin D production (Quarles 2008).

Absorbed phosphate enters the extracellular phosphate pool, which is in equilibrium with bone and soft tissue. In adults with neutral phosphorus balance, the amount of phosphorus excreted by the kidney is equal to the net amount absorbed by the intestine; in growing infants, it is less than the net amount absorbed due to the deposition of phosphorus in soft tissues and bone.

In growing infants, phosphorus will preferentially go to soft tissue with a weight-to-weight nitrogen:phosphorus ratio of 15:1 and to bone with a weight-to-weight calcium:phosphorus ratio of 2.15:1. The residual phosphorus constitutes the renal phosphorus load influencing plasma concentration and urinary excretion. In the face of a limited total phosphorus supply, bone mineral accretion may be limited, leading to significant calcium excretion associated with very low urinary excretion of phosphorus (Fig. 5). This particular situation is illustrated in Fig. 3, showing calcium and phosphorus metabolism in term infants.

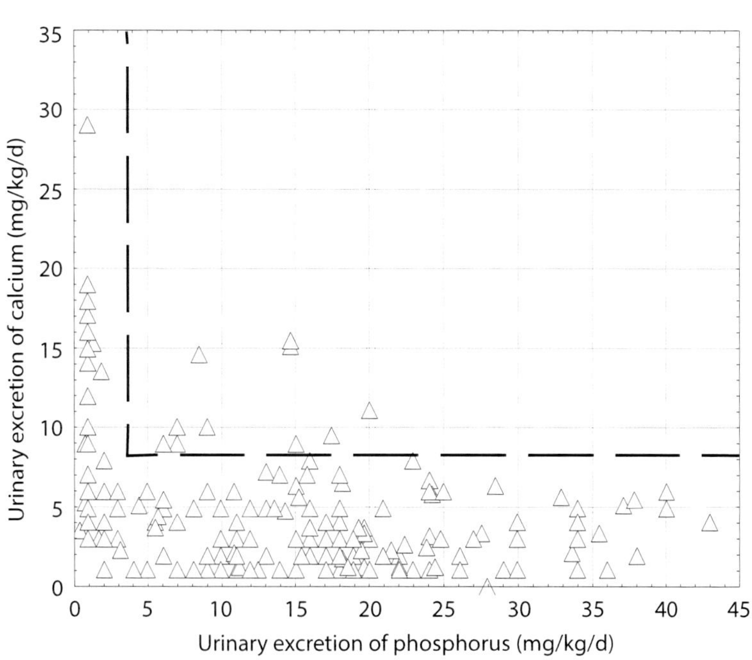

Fig. 5 Relationship between urinary excretion of calcium and urinary excretion of phosphorus in preterm infants (n = 198). Hypercalciuria (>8 mg/kg/day) is related to low phosphate excretion (<3 mg/kg/day). Conversely, urinary excretion of calcium below 8 mg/kg/day is usually observed in preterm infants with phosphorus excretion over 4 mg/kg/day

41.3.2.5 Requirement

For preterm infants the recommendations are based on fetal accretion rates. The 1985 American Academy of Pediatrics recommended 95–108 mg of phosphorus per 100 kcal for preterm formulas (American Academy of Pediatric 1985), whereas more recently, the Life Sciences Research Office and the International Expert Panel recommended similar values, with a calcium-to-phosphorus ratio maintained over 1.7:1 but less than 2.0:1 (Klein 2002). Considering a nitrogen retention ranging from 350 to 450 mg/kg/day and a calcium retention from 60 to 90 mg/kg/day. The ESPGHAN CoN recommended an adequate intake of 65–90 mg/kg/day of a highly absorbable source of phosphate (90%) with a Ca to P ratio between 1.5 and 2.0 (Agostoni et al. 2010).

41.4 Hormonal Regulation

41.4.1 Parathyroid Hormone

PTH is synthesized as a larger (115-amino acid) precursor (prepro-PTH) but is stored and secreted mainly as an 84-amino acid peptide, with the 1–34,N-terminal portion conferring bioactivity. PTH regulates large calcium fluxes across bone, kidneys, and intestine (Fig. 1). PTH increases serum calcium concentrations directly by increasing bone resorption and renal calcium reabsorption and indirectly by increasing renal synthesis of $1,25(OH)_2D_3$, thereby increasing intestinal calcium absorption. PTH also lowers serum phosphorus concentrations through its phosphaturic action on the renal proximal tubule. This action minimizes the possibly adverse effect of hyperphosphatemia related to bone resorption on calcium homeostasis.

41.4.1.1 Regulation

Serum calcium concentration regulates PTH secretion; high concentrations inhibit the secretion of PTH and low concentrations stimulate it. Low or falling serum calcium concentrations act within seconds to stimulate PTH secretion, initiated by means of a calcium-sensing receptor (CaSR) on the surfaces of parathyroid cells. Slower regulation of PTH secretion occurs over a period of hours as a result of cellular changes in PTH messenger RNA (mRNA). Vitamin D and its metabolites 25-hydroxyvitamin D and 1,25-dihydroxyvitamin D, acting through vitamin D receptors, decrease the level of PTH mRNA and hypocalcemia increase it. The slowest regulation of PTH secretion occurs over days or even months and reflects changes in the growth of the parathyroid glands. Metabolites of vitamin D directly inhibit the mass of parathyroid cells; hypocalcemia stimulates the growth of parathyroid cells independent of the contrary action of vitamin D metabolites. In the kidney, the calcium-sensing receptor (CaSR) mediates the direct inhibition of the reabsorption of divalent cations in the thick cortical ascending limb of Henle's loop (Rodriguez 2003).

41.4.1.2 Fetal Parathyroid Function

Human parathyroid glands are functionally active as early as 12 weeks of gestation. However, fetal parathyroid glands are functionally suppressed by high intrauterine calcium concentrations, and PTH levels in cord blood are frequently below the detection limit. PTH does not appear to cross the placenta in either direction, and the role of PTH in maternal-fetal calcium transport is limited. In contrast, PTHrP acts during fetal life to promote calcium transfer, high blood calcium concentration, bone development, and matrix mineralization.

Maternal hyperparathyroidism results in maternal hypercalcemia, which leads to fetal hypercalcemia and suppression of fetal and neonatal parathyroid glands. Conversely, untreated maternal hypoparathyroidism leads to maternal hypocalcemia, fetal hypocalcemia, and secondary fetal and neonatal hyperparathyroidism.

41.4.1.3 Neonatal Parathyroid Function

After birth, with the abrupt termination of the maternal calcium supply, serum calcium in the newborn decreases and serum PTH increases correspondingly. Both term and preterm infants may show a PTH response to falling serum calcium. Nevertheless, plasma PTH levels are relatively low in the neonatal period and are minimally responsive to hypocalcemia during the first 2–3 days of life leading to transient neonatal hypocalcemia. Infants with VLBW have a decreased PTH surge compared with full-term infants. Infants of diabetic mothers may have impaired PTH production during the beginning days of life. Infants with birth asphyxia may also have decreased PTH responses to hypocalcemia.

41.4.1.4 Parathyroid Hormone Reference Values

In full-term newborns, serum PTH concentrations tend to be low in cord blood but increase within the first 48 h of life in response to the decrease in serum calcium. In preterm infants the serum immunoreactive, intact PTH (1–84) concentrations increase immediately after birth, indicating that the secretion of the hormone responds physiologically to the hypocalcemic stimulus. This increase in immunoreactive PTH concentration could be blunted when premature infants receive calcium by infusion, with the calcium load buffering the postnatal depression of serum calcium. By day 10, the serum concentrations of intact PTH return to euparathyroid values (Table 1) (Salle et al. 2000). The multiplication factor for serum PTH from picograms per deciliter to picomoles per liter (pg/dL to pmol/L) is 0.11.

41.4.2 Vitamin D

41.4.2.1 Synthesis and Metabolism

Vitamin D is synthesized endogenously in the skin (cholecalciferol or vitamin D_3) after sunshine exposure or is absorbed from dietary sources as either vitamin D_3 (from animal sources) or vitamin D_2 (ergocalciferol [from vegetable sources]). Regardless of its origin, vitamin D_2 and D_3 are transported bound to the vitamin D binding protein to the liver, where it is hydroxylated at carbon 25 to form vitamin D_3 (25[OH]D_3, or calcidiol), the most abundant vitamin D metabolite. The circulating concentrations of 25[OH]D_3 provide a useful index of vitamin D status (reflecting both dietary intake and sunshine exposure). Subsequently in the kidney, 25[OH]D_3 is further hydroxylated at carbon 1 to form the final active metabolite, 1,25(OH)$_2$D$_3$, or calcitriol. This last transformation is tightly regulated and is the rate-limiting step in vitamin D metabolism. 1,25 (OH)$_2$D$_3$ can also be synthesized by various cells as well as by the placenta during pregnancy. However, this local production of 1,25(OH)$_2$D$_3$ is not associated with calcium homeostasis but could contribute to regulating cell growth.

41.4.2.2 Effects

Normal vitamin D status is necessary to maintain calcium and phosphorus homeostasis. The effects of 1,25(OH)$_2$D$_3$ (calcitriol) on target tissues are initiated by its binding to a steroid receptor (vitamin D receptor) distributed in numerous tissues, leading to the synthesis of a variety of proteins. Therefore, 1,25(OH)$_2$D$_3$ acts on the small intestine, increasing the absorption of calcium and phosphorus by the synthesis of calcium-binding (calbindin-D) proteins; on bone, mobilizing calcium and phosphorus by increasing the number of osteoclasts; and on the kidney, increasing calcium

Table 1 Evolution of intact PTH (1–84), carboxy terminal PTH, and vitamin D binding protein concentrations in 15 preterm infants

	PTH(1–84) (pmol/L)	cPTH (pmol/L)	DBP (μmol/L)
Cord Serum	11 ± 3	48 ± 8	4.43 ± 0.37
Day 1	66 ± 11[a]	125 ± 15[a]	4.40 ± 0.34
Day 2	87 ± 11[a]	168 ± 5[a]	4.96 ± 0.23
Day 5	67 ± 9[a]	152 ± 16[a]	6.21 ± 0.26[a]
Day 10	23 ± 4	69 ± 6	6.03 ± 0.30[a]
Day 30	38 ± 7	80 ± 11	5.16 ± 0.23

From (Salle et al. 2000), with permission

PTH parathyroid hormone, *cPTH* carboxy terminal PTH, *DBP* vitamin D binding protein

[a]Significantly different from cord serum, $P < 0.05$

reabsorption in the distal nephron segments by increasing the expression of the epithelial calcium influx channel. There is a natural polymorphism in the genotype of the vitamin D receptor that contributes to skeletal metabolism in early childhood and to the genetic determinant of the peak bone mass.

41.4.2.3 Regulation of Secretion

In contrast to hepatic 25-hydroxylation, renal 1-hydroxylation, which leads to the active metabolite, appears to be tightly regulated. The main factors increasing the synthesis of calcitriol via stimulation of renal $25(OH)D_3$-1α-hydroxylase are PTH, PTHrP, hypocalcemia, hypophosphatemia, and other hormonal factors, such as insulin-like growth factor-1, estrogen, prolactin, and growth hormone. The production of calcitriol is inhibited by elevated serum levels of calcium and phosphorus, but also by the newly discovered phosphatonin peptides implicated in phosphorus homeostasis. Thus, an increase in FGF23 production suppresses $1,25(OH)_2$ vitamin D via inhibition of 25-hydroxyvitamin D-1-α-hydroxylase and stimulation of 24-hydroxylase inactivating $1,25(OH)_2$ vitamin D in the proximal tubule of the kidney (Quarles 2008).

41.4.2.4 Fetal Vitamin D Function

Serum 25-hydroxyvitamin D concentration depends on vitamin D intake and production. The production of vitamin D is influenced by geographic location, season and latitude, and skin pigmentation. Vitamin D deficiency is very common during pregnancy, not only in areas with a prolonged winter season. In Belgium, vitamin D deficiency, <50 and 80 nmol/L, represent respectively 80% and 90% of the pregnant women (Pieltain et al. 2009).

Cord concentrations of the major vitamin D metabolites are consistently lower than those measured in the mother's serum. Placental vein 25-hydroxyvitamin D concentrations correlate significantly with those found in the maternal circulation, suggesting that calcidiol easily diffuses across the placental barrier and that the vitamin D pool of the fetus depends entirely on that of the mother. The fetomaternal relations of 1,25-dihydroxyvitamin D concentrations are more complex, most of the 1,25-dihydroxyvitamin D in fetal plasma is due to fetal kidney activity, as suggested by studies in fetal plasma from infants with renal agenesis. Actually, the precise role of the placental 1,25-dihydroxyvitamin D activity in the mineral homeostasis during the fetal life remains to be evaluated.

Bone mass of the newborn may be related to the vitamin D status of the mother (Pawley and Bishop 2004). Comparison of the results of dual-energy X-ray absorptiometry from different countries shows that infant whole-body bone mineral content values are lower in countries in which milk products are not supplemented with vitamin D than in those where milk products are supplemented. In contrast, vitamin D supplementation of malnourished mothers results in improved growth of the fetus and child in terms of both birth weight and subsequent linear growth during infancy.

Therefore, during pregnancy a daily vitamin D supplement of at least 400 IU/day (10 μg/day) need to be administered, whereas for at-risk populations an increased supply to 1000 IU/day [25 μg/day]) should be given at least during the last 3 months of pregnancy.

41.4.2.5 Neonatal Vitamin D: Function and Recommendations

Plasma 25(OH) D_3 concentration is a useful vitamin D biomarker reflecting vitamin D supply and usage over a period of time. Unfortunately, the cut-off used for serum 25(OH) D_3 concentrations varies among researchers, leading to various prevalence of vitamin D deficiency and/or insufficiency. Nevertheless, several surveys show a high rate of poor maternal vitamin D status throughout the world, particularly in countries without vitamin D supplementation, with poor sun exposure, extensive clothing, or with deeply pigmented skin. Thus, the rate of cord blood vitamin D severe insufficiency (<20 nmol/L; <8.3 ng/mL) may reach up to 70% in European populations (Pieltain et al. 2009; Pawley and Bishop 2004).

The concentrations of vitamin D are low in human milk (20–60 IU/L) and lower than that in regular formulas (400–600 IU/L). In breast-fed infants not receiving vitamin D supplements, vitamin D stores could be depleted within 8 weeks of delivery, suggesting the need for vitamin D supplementation (Greer 2003). A minimum daily intake of 400 IU (10 μg/day) of vitamin D is recommended by the AAP for all infants beginning soon after birth, including those who are exclusively breastfed (Wagner et al. 2008). Moreover, in breastfed full-term infants born to mothers who are vitamin D deficient, maternal supplementation with vitamin D could be required to increase the human milk vitamin D concentration and in turn improve infant vitamin D status. In addition, vitamin D is metabolized in the liver, and anticonvulsants such as phenobarbital and diphenylhydantoin increase its hepatic catabolism and requirements.

In preterm infants, as a result of the decrease in serum calcium during the first days of age, the postnatal surge in PTH induces increased synthesis of $1,25(OH)_2D_3$ during the first days day of life. Provision of 1000 IU of vitamin D_3 increases the 25-hydroxyvitamin D pool of the newborn at birth, followed by rapid renal synthesis of 1,25-dihydroxyvitamin D during the early postnatal days. In very low birth weight infants (<1500 g), immaturity of the vitamin D activation pathway, either alone or in combination with other abnormalities, particularly transient hypoparathyroidism, hypercalcitoninemia, and end-organ resistance to hormonal effects, may promote late neonatal hypocalcemia. However, after 28 weeks of gestation, activation of vitamin D is operative as early as 24 h after birth. Vitamin D supplementation just after birth improves its nutritional status, as evidenced by rises in both plasma 1,25- and 25-hydroxyvitamin D concentrations.

In countries with high vitamin D status, plasma 25-hydroxyvitamin D remained normal for 6 months while infants received around 400 IU/day (<10 μg/day). By contrast, in Europe and other countries where dairy products are not enriched with vitamin D, sunshine exposure is restricted (Salle et al. 2000), and mean cord concentrations of 25-hydroxyvitamin D are low, the administration of vitamin D (from 1000 IU/day, or 25 μg/day) results in a rapid increase in circulating concentrations of total 1,25-dihydroxyvitamin D by 5 days of age, promoting calcium absorption and mineral accretion rates during the neonatal period. Therefore, vitamin D recommendations may differ significantly between North American (400 IU/day, 10 μg/day) and European countries (800–1000 IU/day, 10–25 μg/day) (Agostoni et al. 2010).

41.4.2.6 Reference Values

New informations on the additional role of vitamin D on glucose homeostasis, immune system, cardiovascular disease, and cancer has resulted in defining vitamin D deficiency in adults as a 25-OH-D concentration < 50 nmol/L and vitamin D insufficiency as a 25-OH-D concentration of 50–80 nmol/L. At the present time, however, consensus has not been reached with regard to the concentration of 25-OH-D to define vitamin D insufficiency for infants and children (Holick 2007). Universal units of measure for 25-OH-D and $1,25\text{-}OH_2\text{-}D$ are nmol/L. Conversion to ng/mL is made by dividing the value expressed in nmol/L by 2.496. Thus, 80 nmol/L becomes 32 ng/mL.

41.4.3 Calcitonin

Calcitonin (CT) is a 32-amino acid peptide secreted by the thyroidal C cells. In addition, a group of peptide hormones, the "calcitonin family", including the calcitonin gene-related protein (CGRP), with structural similarities to calcitonin are also produced by several tissues. Although calcitonin has often been considered to be a vestigial hormone with no certain role in mammalian calcium and bone homeostasis, recent studies indicate that calcitonin has important roles in calcium and bone homeostasis that have not been previously recognized. It has been established that the major action of CT is the inhibition of bone resorption, and osteoclasts (Karsdal et al. 2008). The regulation of calcitonin is opposite to that of PTH. Mediated by the CaSR, an increase in ionized calcium stimulates calcitonin secretion, whereas a decrease in ionized calcium leads to a fall in calcitonin. Thus, the CaSR has a dual physiological response to regulate PTH and calcitonin that in the long-term will influence the maintenance of skeletal mineral content (Fudge and Kovacs 2004).

At birth, serum calcitonin concentrations are higher in cord blood than maternal blood, and they increase further in the first 24 h of life. The physiologic importance of the postnatal increase of calcitonin is unclear and it is uncertain whether calcitonin plays any specific role in calcium homeostasis and skeletal metabolism during the fetal and neonatal period (Fudge and Kovacs 2004). In contrast, CT has an important physiological role during lactation protecting the maternal skeleton against excessive resorption and attendant fragility.

41.4.4 FGF23 and Phosphatonin Peptides

"Phosphatonins" represent a number of peptides which have been recently identified as a result of the study of various diseases associated with hypophosphatemia: fibroblast growth factor 23 [FGF23], secreted frizzled-related protein 4 [sFRP-4], fibroblast growth factor 7 [FGF7] and matrix extracellular phosphoglycoprotein [MEPE] (Quarles 2008; Liu et al. 2007; Shaikh et al. 2008). FGF23 is predominantly produced by osteocytes in bone, and its principal actions are to inhibit sodium-dependent phosphate reabsorption and 1α-hydroxylase activity in the proximal tubule of the kidney, leading to phosphaturia and suppression of circulating 1,25(OH)$_2$D levels. Evidence that FGF23 is the principle phosphaturic factor comes from a variety of observations (Shaikh et al. 2008).

Fibroblast growth factor 23 regulates serum phosphate levels within a narrow range despite wide fluctuation in dietary intake via a series of classic negative endocrine feedback loops involving 1,25-dihydroxyvitamin D, parathyroid hormone, urinary phosphate excretion, and dietary phosphorus absorption. A sustained increase in dietary phosphorus intake stimulates FGF23 secretion that increases phosphaturia. At the same time, FGF23 inhibits renal synthesis of 1,25D. By contrast, a sustained reduction in phosphorus intake lowers FGF23 secretion, which enhances tubular phosphorus avidity and increases 1,25D production. A down regulation of FGF-23 could promote the relative hyperphosphatemia and the relative increase in 1,25(OH)$_2$ vitamin D promoting bone mineralization during early rapid growth in the neonatal period (Quarles 2008). The targeting of FGF23 to the kidney is mediated by a coreceptor (klotho) that enhances the binding affinity of FGF23 to the widely expressed FGF receptor 1c (Quarles 2008).

Phosphatonins have been implicated in the pathophysiology of disorders of phosphate homeostasis such as Tumor-induced osteomalacia (TIO), X-linked hypophosphatemic rickets (XLH), autosomal dominant hypophosphatemic rickets (ADHR), autosomal recessive hypophosphatemia (ARHP), tumoral calcinosis and renal failure (Shaikh et al. 2008). However, the role of newly discovered phosphatonin peptides, such as FGF 23 in the regulation of phosphorus excretion during the early life, remain to be established.

41.5 Clinical Conditions Associated with Calcium Disturbances

41.5.1 Neonatal Hypocalcemia

Serum total and ionized calcium concentrations are relatively high at birth but decrease sharply during the first hours of life to reach a nadir at 24 h and increase progressively thereafter up to the end of the first week of life (Table 2). Sudden changes

Table 2 Evolution of serum calcium concentrations (mmol/L[a]) during the first 10 days of life in term and preterm infants

	Term		Preterm	
Age	Mean	95% CI	Mean	95% CI
Birth (cord blood)	2.55	2.25–2.85	2.24	1.58–2.90
24 h	2.25	1.95–2.55	1.94	1.64–2.24
48 h	2.39	2.14–2.64	1.85	1.47–2.23
120 h	2.46	2.25–2.68	2.22	1.84–2.60
240 h	2.48	2.26–2.69	2.45	2.45–2.89

[a]Conversion to mg/dL: mmol/L × 0.2495

Table 3 Causes of neonatal calcium disorders

Hypocalcemia	Hypercalcemia
Early Hypocalcemia (1–4 days of age)	*Iatrogenic*
Prematurity	Calcium salts, vitamin A
Maternal diabetes	Hypophosphatemia (prematurity)
Perinatal stress/asphyxia	Hypervitaminosis D
Intrauterine growth restriction	Thiazide diuretics
Maternal anticonvulsants	
	Disorders of Parathyroid Function
Late Hypocalcemia (5–10 days of age)	Maternal hypocalcemia, hypoparathyroidism
Hyperphosphatemia (high phosphate load, advanced renal insufficiency)	Mutation of the parathyroid hormone-related protein receptor
Hypomagnesemia	Jansen metaphyseal chondrodysplasia
Vitamin D deficiency	Calcium-sensing receptor defects
PTH resistance (transient neonatal pseudohypoparathyroidism)	Familial hypocalciuric hypercalcemia
Hypoparathyroidism	Neonatal severe hyperparathyroidism
Primary: parathyroid agenesis, 22q11 deletion, parathyroid hormone gene mutation	
	Idiopathic Infantile Hypercalcemia
Secondary: maternal hyperparathyroidism	*Hyperprostaglandin E Syndrome*
Calcium-sensing receptor defects; autosomal dominant hypocalcemic	*Severe Infantile Hypophosphatasia*
hypercalciuria	*Other Causes*
Acquired or inherited disorders of vitamin D metabolism	Congenital carbohydrate malabsorption
Neonatal hypocalcemia associated with skeletal dysplasia	Distal renal tubular acidosis
Other causes (alkalosis, citrated blood transfusions, phototherapy, viral gastroenteritis, lipid infusions)	Tumor-related hypercalcemia
	Congenital hypothyroidism
	Williams syndrome
	Subcutaneous fat necrosis
	Blue diaper syndrome

in the distribution of calcium between ionized and bound fractions may cause symptoms of hypocalcemia even in children with functioning hormonal mechanisms for the regulation of the ionized calcium concentration (Table 3). Increases in the extracellular fluid concentration of anions such as phosphate, citrate, or bicarbonate increase the proportion of bound calcium and decrease ionized calcium. Alkalosis increases the affinity of albumin for calcium and thereby decreases the concentration of ionized calcium. In contrast, acidosis increases the ionized calcium concentration by decreasing the binding of calcium to albumin. Although it is conventional to measure the total serum calcium concentration, more physiologically relevant information is obtained by direct measurement of the ionized calcium concentration. This measurement is particularly important when evaluating patients who have abnormal circulating proteins and after blood transfusion for the correction of acidosis and hyperventilation. For example, total serum calcium decreases approximately 1 mg/dL, or 0.25 mmol/L, for each 1 g/dL of decrease in serum albumin, without any change in ionized calcium.

Neonates at the greatest risk for symptomatic or asymptomatic neonatal hypocalcemia, such as the infants of diabetic mothers or preterm or asphyxiated neonates, are frequently sick for a multitude of reasons, and the contribution of neonatal hypocalcemia to signs related to their primary illness can be easily obscured. From a clinical viewpoint, because Ca^{2+} concentrations are maintained within narrow ranges under normal circumstances, the potential risk for disturbances of physiologic function increases as the Ca^{2+} concentration decreases. A useful approach to the classification of neonatal hypocalcemia is by time of onset. The early and late forms of hypocalcemia have different causes and occur in different clinical settings.

41.5.1.1 Early Hypocalcemia: Term Infants

Early neonatal hypocalcemia occurs during the first 4 days of life and represents an exaggeration of the normal fall in serum calcium concentration that occurs during the first 24–48 h of life. At birth there is an interruption of maternal calcium supply, and the serum calcium concentration in infants is maintained by either the increased calcium flux from bone or sufficient exogenous calcium intake. Because intestinal calcium absorption is correlated with intake and dietary calcium is usually low on the first day of life, the serum calcium concentration decreases on the first day of life (Hsu and Levine 2004).

Normal serum concentrations for Ca^{2+} in full-term newborns reach a nadir at about 24 h of age (1.10–1.36 mmol/L, or 4.4–5.4 mg/dL) and rise slowly thereafter. Nenatal hypocalcemia could be reasonnably defined as a serum total calcium below 2 mmol/L or a an ionized calcium of less than 0.9–1.1 mmol/L.

Early neonatal hypocalcemia apparently results from the abrupt interruption of the placental supply and the low intake provided by oral and parenteral nutrition and also by the slow release of PTH by immature parathyroid glands or the inadequate responsiveness of the renal tubular cells to PTH.

By contrast, exaggerated rise in calcitonin secretion may not play a contributory role in premature infants. In infants with VLBW the high renal sodium excretion probably aggravates calciuric losses, and relative end-organ resistance to $1{,}25(OH)_2D_3$ may exist additionally to an 25 $(OH)D_3$ deficiency. Hypocalcemia is temporary, and the serum calcium concentration gradually reverts to normal after 1–3 days. Factors contributing to serum calcium normalization include increased calcium intake with feedings, increased renal phosphorus excretion, and improved parathyroid function. Calcium supplementation may hasten the restorative process.

41.5.1.2 Early Hypocalcemia: Preterm Infants

The frequency of hypocalcemia varies inversely with birth-weight and gestational age. In preterm infants, the postnatal decrease in the serum calcium level typically occurs more rapidly than it does in term infants, the magnitude of the depression being inversely proportional to gestation. Before routine calcium supplementation and the use of parenteral nutrition from the first day of age, many LBW infants and nearly all those with extremely low birth weight (ELBW) exhibited total calcium levels of less than 7.0 mg/dL by day 2. However, the fall in Ca^{2+} is not proportional to that in total calcium concentration, and the ratio of ionized to total calcium is higher in these infants. The reason for the maintenance of Ca^{2+} is uncertain but is probably related to low serum protein concentration and pH associated with prematurity. The sparing effect of Ca^{2+} may partially explain the frequent lack of signs in preterm infants with low total calcium levels. In preterm infants the reference values for ionized calcium are available only for large, moderately premature infants who show values very similar to those for full-term infants. These cutoff values might not apply to smaller infants, given insufficient physiologic data on ionized calcium. At present, the traditional cutoff point, a total calcium content of less than 1.75 mmol/L (7.0 mg/dL) and an ionized calcium of less than 0.9–1.1 mmol/L, remains reasonable in VLBW infants.

41.5.1.3 Perinatal Asphyxia

In asphyxiated infants, the following factors may contribute to early hypocalcemia: a decreased calcium intake due to delayed feedings and an increased endogenous phosphorus load resulting from the reduction of the glomerular filtration rate. Hyperphosphatemia may induce relative PTH resistance and a stimulation of FGF23 secretion. Theoretically, the correction of acidosis with alkali may further aggravate hypocalcemia by inducing decreased calcium flux from bone to the extracellular fluid and by lowering the ionized calcium concentration.

41.5.1.4 Maternal Conditions and Treatments

Maternal Diabetes

Infants of diabetic mothers (IDMs) demonstrate an exaggerated postnatal drop in circulating calcium levels when compared with controls of gestational age. Prematurity and birth asphyxia are frequently associated problems that independently increase the risk for hypocalcemia. In IDMs, hypocalcemia appears to be related to hypomagnesemia, the maternal form of which is caused by urinary magnesium losses with diabetes and leads to fetal magnesium deficiency and secondary functional hypoparathyroidism in the fetus and newborn. Hypocalcemia in IDMs is also correlated with the severity of maternal diabetes, which is classified by White's criteria. The natural history is usually similar to that of early neonatal hypocalcemia in preterm infants, but hypocalcemia sometimes persists for several additional days. Improved metabolic control for pregnant diabetic women has markedly diminished the occurrence and severity of early neonatal hypocalcemia in IDMs. The incidence of hypocalcemia is also increased in the infants of gestational diabetic mothers (IGDMs), and the role of hypomagnesemia has recently been demonstrated (Banerjee et al. 2003).

Maternal hyperparathyroidism with hypercalcemia, maternal chronic renal failure with secondary hyperparathyroidism, mothers with abnormal vitamin D homeostasis and mothers receiving anticonvulsants are additional factors increasing risk for neonatal hypocalcemia (Table 3).

41.5.1.5 Late Hypocalcemia

Hypocalcemia is conventionally defined as late when it occurs after the first 4 days of life. Late neonatal hypocalcemia usually develops at about 1 week of age (Table 3) and more frequently in term than preterm infants and is not correlated with maternal diabetes, birth trauma, or asphyxia. In some instances the clinical distinction between early and late hypocalcemia may not be clear.

Phosphate Loading

Hypocalcemia induced by an elevated phosphorus supply usually occurs at the end of the first week of life. Late-onset hypocalcemia is considered to be a manifestation of relative resistance of the immature kidney to PTH. In these infants the renal tubular cells are unable to respond appropriately to PTH, leading to renal retention of phosphorus and hypocalcemia. These biochemical features strongly resemble those of pseudohypoparathyroidism (Hsu and Levine 2004). The normally low neonatal glomerular filtration rate may also play a role in limiting the ability to excrete the phosphorus load.

Late hypocalcemia was frequently observed in infants fed cow's milk or evaporated milk because of their high phosphorus content. With the introduction of adapted infant formulas, late hypocalcemia, though not abolished, has become uncommon. However, even with current formulas the formula-fed infants have lower serum ionized calcium and higher serum phosphorus in the first week of life than those of breastfed infants.

These differences correlate with the absolute phosphorus amount but not with the different calcium:phosphorus ratios in formulas. The phosphate load increases calcium bone deposition, leading to hypocalcemia. The normal response to hypocalcemia is an increase in PTH secretion, inducing an increase in both the urinary excretion of phosphate and tubular resorption of calcium. The pathogenesis of this "transient hypoparathyroidism" in late neonatal hypocalcemia is poorly understood. The inadequate secretion of PTH, immaturity of PTH receptors, or transient change in the threshold of CaSR may play an important role (Stewart 2004). In these infants, serum calcium levels frequently increase when they are given human milk, lower-phosphate formulas, and calcium supplements. After several days to weeks, serum PTH usually increases and the infants are able to tolerate a higher dietary phosphate load. Some of these infants have a persistent or recurrent inability to mount an adequate PTH response to a hypocalcemic challenge and may have a form of congenital hypoparathyroidism.

Hypocalcemia Resulting from Vitamin D Disorder

Maternal vitamin D deficiency is the major risk for neonatal vitamin D deficiency presenting as hypocalcemia. Vitamin D deficiency is unusual in countries where it is common practice to supplement the diet with vitamin D dairy products and other foods. However, it occurs in women in whom both sunlight exposure and the dietary intake of vitamin D are inadequate and high incidence has been reported in most of the european countries (Pieltain et al. 2009). Therefore, if daily vitamin D supplementation during the whole pregnancy can be undertaken, the amount given should be at least 400 IU/day (10 μg/day). In countries where dairy products are not supplemented with vitamin D and sunshine exposure is low, 1000 IU/day (25 μg/day) should be given during the last 3 months of pregnancy (Salle et al. 2000).

Breastfed infants of strictly vegetarian mothers are also susceptible to vitamin D deficiency and early-onset hypocalcemic rickets.

Hypomagnesemia

Neonatal hypocalcemia usually accompanies hypomagnesemia because magnesium deficiency inhibits the secretion of PTH and reduces responsiveness to its action. Depression of the serum magnesium levels in newborns is mainly due to transient hypomagnesemia or exceptionally to primary hypomagnesemia with secondary hypocalcemia (Hsu and Levine 2004).

41.5.1.6 Other Causes of Neonatal Hypocalcemia

Bicarbonate therapy, as well as any form of metabolic or respiratory alkalosis, decreases ionized calcium levels and bone resorption of calcium. Transfusion and plasmapheresis with citrated blood can form nonionized calcium complexes, thus decreasing Ca^{2+}. Furosemide and xanthine therapy promotes calciuresis as well as nephrolithiasis. Phototherapy appears to be an additional possible cause of neonatal hypocalcemia, although the mechanism is still uncertain. Lipid infusions may increase serum free fatty acid levels, which form insoluble complexes with calcium. Most of these effects are transient, and cessation of therapy is associated with a return to normal serum calcium levels.

41.5.1.7 Clinical Manifestations of Hypocalcemia

The clinical manifestations of neonatal hypocalcemia in infants may be easily confused with other neonatal disorders (e.g., hypoglycemia, sepsis, meningitis, asphyxia, intracranial bleeding, narcotic withdrawal). The neonate with hypocalcemia may be asymptomatic; the less mature the infant, the more subtle and varied the clinical manifestations. In the neonatal period the main clinical signs of hypocalcemia are jitteriness (increased neuromuscular irritability and activity) and generalized convulsions, although focal seizures have also been reported. Infants may also be lethargic, eat poorly, vomit, and have abdominal distention. The degree of irritability does not appear to correlate with serum calcium values. Furthermore, hypocalcemia may be asymptomatic. Therefore, suspicion of hypocalcemia should be confirmed by the measurement of total serum calcium and Ca^{2+}.

The diagnostic workup for hypocalcemia includes a history, physical examination, and relevant investigations. In clinical practice, the diagnosis of hypocalcemia is based on the determination of ionized or total calcium. Serum magnesium should also be measured because hypomagnesemia may coexist and cause identical signs. The measurement of calcium-regulating hormones is not routinely recommended unless hypocalcemia is prolonged, refractory, or recurrent. Assays of calciotropic hormones and 25(OH) D may be useful in the diagnosis of uncommon causes of neonatal hypocalcemia, such as primary hypoparathyroidism, malabsorption, and disorders of vitamin D metabolism. If DiGeorge syndrome is suspected chest X-ray examination for a thymic silhouette is indicated and molecular genetic studies may be needed to confirm a microdeletion of chromosome 22q11.2.

41.5.1.8 Treatment

Early Neonatal Hypocalcemia

In asymptomatic newborns, treatment generally is indicated when the total serum calcium concentration is less than 1.5 mol/L (6 mg/dL) in the preterm infant and less than 1.75 mol/L (7 mg/dL) in the term infant. Calcium supplementation can be given either by the intravenous or oral route. Depending on the clinical status of the infant, treatment of newborns who have acute or symptomatic hypocalcemia is accomplished best by the intravenous infusion of calcium salts; 10% calcium gluconate (9.3 mg/mL of elemental calcium, maximum 2 mL/kg over 15 min followed by 75 mg/kg per day up to normal range) is used most commonly. Effective oral therapy involves adding calcium glucobionate or calcium carbonate to human milk or a low phosphate formula (calcium to phosphate ratio of 2:1).

Additional therapy depends on the cause of hypocalcemia. Infants who have hypoparathyroidism require calcitriol in addition to calcium supplementation to restore and maintain eucalcemia. Infants who have vitamin D deficiency will benefit from vitamin D supplementation. If magnesium concentrations are low, treatment with intravenous or intramuscular magnesium sulfate is essential for correction as a 50% solution of magnesium sulfate in a dose of 0.1–0.2 mL/kg.

Complications of intravenous calcium therapy include extravasation into soft tissues (with calcium deposition and sometimes cutaneous necrosis) and bradycardia. Because of the many potential risks, arterial infusions of calcium in high concentrations should be avoided. However, parenteral nutrition solutions containing standard mineral (including calcium) content can be safely infused through appropriately positioned umbilical venous or arterial catheters. The direct administration of calcium preparations with bicarbonate or phosphate solution results in precipitation and must be avoided. The duration of supplemental calcium therapy varies with the course of hypocalcemia. As few as 2 or 3 days of therapy are usually required.

Late Neonatal Hypocalcemia

There is usually little debate regarding the treatment of late hypocalcemia. Because serum calcium is not routinely measured after the first few days of life, late hypocalcemia is usually symptomatic when diagnosed and the requirement for calcium therapy may be prolonged in the case of hypocalcemia caused by malabsorption or hypoparathyroidism. In phosphorus-induced hypocalcemia, a low-phosphorus formula (or human milk) and oral calcium supplementation are indicated to decrease phosphorus absorption and increase calcium absorption. In hypomagnesemia, the magnesium deficiency usually has to be corrected before hypocalcemia can be treated successfully.

Hypoparathyroidism requires therapy with vitamin D or one of its metabolites; $1{,}25(OH)_2D_3$ (or 1 α-hydroxyvitamin D_3, a synthetic analogue that undergoes hepatic 25-hydroxylation) has the advantage f a shorter half-life, and treatment may be more easily tailored to the individual patient. Attention should be directed toward a number of concomitant treatments. Because thiazide diuretics can increase renal calcium reabsorption, the inadvertent institution or discontinuation of these drugs may increase or decrease, respectively, the plasma calcium level. In contrast, furosemide and other loop diuretics can increase the renal clearance of calcium and depress serum calcium levels. The administration of glucocorticoids antagonizes the action of vitamin D (and the analogues) and may also precipitate hypocalcemia. The development of hypomagnesemia may also interfere with the effectiveness of treatment with calcium and vitamin D (Rigo et al. 2010).

41.5.1.9 Prevention of Neonatal Hypocalcemia

The most effective prevention of neonatal hypocalcemia includes the prevention of prematurity and birth asphyxia, the judicious use of bicarbonate therapy, and mechanical ventilation to avoid secondary metabolic alkalosis. Whereas, the pharmacologic prevention of neonatal hypocalcemia, especially in VLBW infants, is based on the prophylactic use of calcium salts, phosphorus salts, and vitamin D supplementation from the first day of life, with a regular survey of serum concentrations and urinary excretion.

41.5.2 Neonatal Hypercalcemia

Hypercalcemia is defined as a pathologic elevation in plasma ionized Ca^{2+} concentration greater than 1.35 mmol/L (5.4 mg/dL) with or without a simultaneous elevation in total calcium concentration of greater than 2.75 mmol/L (11.0 mg/dL) as total calcium is more related to serum albumin concentration (Rigo et al. 2010; Rodriguez 2003). Neonatal hypercalcemia (Table 3) is relatively uncommon, but it needs to be recognized because it can result in significant morbidity or mortality. The clinical symptoms of sustained hypercalcemia are not specific. Infants with mild increases in serum calcium (2.75–3.25 mmol/L, or 11–13 mg/dL) often fail to manifest specific symptoms of hypercalcemia. Nonspecific signs and symptoms such as anorexia, vomiting, and constipation (but rarely diarrhea) may occur with moderate to severe hypercalcemia. Seizures, bradycardia, or arterial hypertension is very exceptional. On physical examination infants may appear dehydrated, lethargic, and hypotonic. Those with chronic hypercalcemia may present with failure to thrive as the principal source of physical distress. Renal function is generally impaired, and polyuria and hypercalciuria are observed. However, renal complications such as nephrocalcinosis, nephrolithiasis, and hematuria may be the earliest clinical manifestations of hypercalcemia.

41.5.2.1 Iatrogenic Hypercalcemia

Hypercalcemia may result from increased intestinal or renal calcium absorption, increased bone turnover or iatrogenic causes. Iatrogenic hypercalcemia is the most common type of hypercalcemia in the newborn and should be considered before starting extensive investigation of rare syndromes. It may result from excessive intravenous calcium administration during total parenteral nutrition or exchange transfusion but also of unbalanced calcium to phosphorus ratio in the oral or parenteral diet. Moderate hypercalcemia may also be the result of phosphorus deficiency in premature infants receiving unbalanced calcium and phosphorus regimens in oral and parenteral nutrition. In this situation, hypercalcemia is accompanied by hypophosphoremia. Infants with VLBW who are fed mineral-unsupplemented human milk may develop hypophosphatemic hypercalcemia. The low phosphorus concentration in human milk causes phosphorus deficiency, leading to an increased calcium concentration and hypercalciuria. Hypophosphatemia stimulates renal synthesis of calcitriol, which activates the intestinal absorption and skeletal resorption of calcium and phosphorus. The absorbed phosphorus is preferentially oriented for soft tissue formation, whereas the remaining phosphorus is insufficient to allow calcium deposition. Phosphorus supplementation and the use of human milk fortifiers can prevent hypophosphatemia and hypercalcemia. Similar situations have been reported in infants on parenteral nutrition, providing an unbalanced calcium:phosphorus ratio. Additionally, thiazide diuretics reduce renal calcium excretion and may represent a contributing factor. Other causes of iatrogenic hypercalcemia are the use of extracorporeal membrane oxygenation, which can cause transient hypercalcemia in up to 30% of infants, and vitamin D intoxication from the administration of excessive vitamin D supplements. Vitamin A toxicity increasing bone resorption is rare and can cause severe hypercalcemia.

41.5.3 Neonatal Hyperparathyroidism

Neonatal hyperparathyroidism frequently results in severe hypercalcemia. It may be hereditary primary hyperparathyroidism or be secondary to maternal hypocalcemia and is summarized in Table 3 with other more unusual causes of hypercalcemia.

41.5.3.1 Primary Hyperparathyroidism

Hereditary primary hyperparathyroidism manifested in neonates is associated with inactivating mutation of CaR. The serverity of hypercalcemia is related to the extent of CaR mutation, moderate with heterozygous mutation in patients with familial hypocalciuric hypercalcemia. It is an autosomal-dominant trait with a high degree of penetrance. More severe hypercalcemia occurs in neonatal hyperparathyroidism with homozygous inactivating germline mutations of the CaR gene (Toke et al. 2009).

41.5.3.2 Secondary Hyperparathyroidism

In many cases of secondary hyperparathyroidism, a thorough investigation of the infant's mother will disclose previously known but poorly treated hypoparathyroidism, pseudohypoparathyroidism, or clinically unsuspected hypocalcemia, as seen in mothers with renal tubular acidosis that had induced severe secondary hyperparathyroidism in the developing fetus during pregnancy. The clinical presentation is variable and may depend on the severity of maternal hypocalcemia. Secondary hyperparathyroidism and neonatal hypercalcemia are transient conditions with a good prognosis provided that supportive measures are instituted.

41.5.3.3 Clinical Manifestations

Most infants are asymptomatic when diagnosed. Those with mildly elevated levels of calcium often fail to manifest specific symptoms of hypercalcemia. Infants with chronic hypercalcemia may present with failure to thrive as the principal source of physical distress.

There are nonspecific signs and symptoms such as anorexia, vomiting, and constipation (but rarely diarrhea); polyuria may occur with moderate to severe hypercalcemia. In severe hypercalcemia infants are often dehydrated, lethargic, and hypotonic. Alternatively, they may present with seizures. Clinically, these infants can have bradycardia, a short QT interval, and hypertension. However, renal complications such as nephrocalcinosis, nephrolithiasis, and hematuria may be the earliest clinical manifestations of hyper- calcemia. Otherwise, the physical examination is usually normal except for the infants with subcutaneous fat necrosis, Williams syndrome, Jansen metaphyseal chondrodysplasia, and hypophosphatasia.

In clinical practice the practical approach is first to exclude the possibility of iatrogenic hypercalcemia. Secondly, a maternal history of calcium-phosphorus disease or excessive vitamin D intake during pregnancy should be investigated. Thirdly, the signs of clinical syndromes associated with hypercalcemia, such as blue diapers, fat necrosis, and elfin facies, should be sought. Finally, the initial laboratory evaluation should include serum calcium, phosphorus, alkaline phosphatase, PTH, the urinary calcium:creatinine ratio, and tubular reabsorption of phosphorus. In most cases, these tests allow the differentiation of hypercalcemia caused by parathyroid disorders from nonparathyroid conditions. In hyperparathyroidism the serum phosphorus concentration is low; renal tubular phosphorus reabsorption is decreased, usually to less than 85%; and the serum PTH concentration is elevated. Finally, additional tests may be performed: a serum $25(OH)D_3$ determination may be useful when an excess of vitamin D is suspected; long-bone X-ray films identify demineralization, osteolytic lesions, or both (hyperparathyroidism) or osteosclerotic lesions (occasionally with vitamin D excess); measurements of serum and urinary calcium in parents allow a diagnosis of familial hypocalciuric hypercalcemia; and renal sonography detects nephrocalcinosis.

41.5.3.4 Treatment

The treatment of neonatal hypercalcemia depends on the severity of the presentation. Conservative management is appropriate in the case of mild hypercalcemia in a preterm infant resulting from an inappropriate mineral supply, hypoalbuminemia, or chronic acidosis, with special emphasis on the phosphorus supply when hypercalcemia is associated with hypophosphatemia. Hypercalcemia seen in newborns exposed to maternal hypocalcemia is usually mild and transient, and treatment consists of no more than supplying the appropriate amounts of calcium and phosphorus in the milk.

Infants with moderate to severe hypercalcemia need more aggressive treatment. The initial steps are not specific: (1) Discontinue oral and intravenous calcium and vitamin D supplementation and dietary restriction; (2) increase the urinary excretion of calcium by maximizing glomerular filtration with the administration of intravenous fluids, which consist of standard saline at about twice the maintenance requirements; and (3) encourage calcium excretion with furosemide after rehydration but with particular attention to maintaining electrolyte homeostasis.

More specific therapy comprises the use of glucocorticoids, calcitonin, bisphosphonate, dialysis, and total parathyroidectomy. Glucocorticoids (2 mg/kg of prednisone) decrease intestinal calcium absorption, decrease bone resorption, and increase renal excretion. They may be useful during a short period, mainly in cases of an excess of vitamin D, but are relatively ineffective in cases of hyperparathyroidism. Calcitonin (4–6 IU/kg subcutaneously every 6 h) reduces the serum calcium concentration, but its effectiveness declines after a few days. Bisphosphonate therapy is limited in newborn infants. However, pamidronate (0.5–2.0 mg/kg) has been used in the treatment of subcutaneous fat necrosis and could be an ideal agent to stabilize cases of neonatal severe hyperparathyroidism, as recently suggested. A calcimimetic drug that reduces PTH secretion, recently approved by the FDA for chronic secondary hyperparathyroidism in dialyzed patients, could be of major interest in primary hyperparathyroidism but needs to be evaluated during infancy (Stewart 2004). Dialysis could be prescribed with a lowcalcium dialysate (1.25 mmol/L) in the face of severe and unremitting hypercalcemia. Total parathyroidectomy with partial autotransplantation could be a rescue treatment in the severe form of neonatal severe hyperparathyroidism. In the chronic phase, dietary restriction with the use of a special formula without vitamin D supplementation is the mainstay of treatment. If the dietary regimen is insufficient, corticosteroids can be used with caution. Cellulose phosphate binders have been occasionally used in children, but there is limited experience in neonates and they may contain unwanted free phosphate.

41.5.4 Nephrocalcinosis in Preterm Infants

Nephrocalcinosis is defined as ultrasound evidence of bright reflections with or without acoustic shadowing, small flecks across to completely echodense pyramids which are reproducible in both the longitudinal and transverse direction, found within the cortex or medulla. Initially, nephrocalcinosis was attributed to long-term furosemide therapy. It is now known to be multifactorial and has been associated with low gestational age and birth weight; severe respiratory disease, transient renal failure; imbalance intakes of calcium and phosphate; long duration of total parenteral nutrition; as well as pro-calciuric medications such as furosemide, corticosteroids, aminoglycosides, and xanthines. In addition, in analogy to the pathogenesis of stone formation, nephrocalcinosis is considered to result from a spontaneous or therapy-induced imbalance between promoters (e.g., calcium, oxalate, uric acid, ascorbic acid) and inhibitors (e.g., citrate, magnesium) of crystallization in urine. The prevalence of nephrocalcinosis varies between studies from 7% to 41% in recent reports (Schell-Feith et al. 2010).

The short- and long-term evolution of nephrocalcinosis has not been clearly defined. Ultrasonographic abnormalities that develop during the first months of life disappear in the majority of patients within months to years. Earlier studies had raised concerns regarding tubular function in affected patients. This has not clearly been substantiated in more recent larger studies where an unfavorable effect on renal function is seen in a small number of children (Schell-Feith et al. 2010). Nevertheless, premature children with or without nephrocalcinosis when compared with non-premature children had lower kidney size and borderline blood pressure. In addition, children with intra- or extrauterine growth retardation had an impaired GFR compared to children with appropriate pre- and postnatal growth (Bachetta et al. 2009).

In summary, nephrocalcinosis is a high incidence disease in VLBW and ELBW infants but associated with a good renal outcome and a high resolution rate. However, it has been highlighted that there could be long-term sequelae in tubular dysfunction and hypertension. This warrants close monitoring in ex-premature babies.

41.6 Disorders of Phosphate Homeostasis

41.6.1 Neonatal Hypophosphatemia

In adults, moderate hypophosphatemia is defined as a serum phosphorus concentration between 3.0 and 1 mg dL^{-1}, and is usually asymptomatic. Severe hypophosphatemia is defined as serum inorganic phosphorus concentration below 1.0 mg dL^{-1}. In children, serum phosphorus concentrations below 5 mg dL^{-1} are often considered abnormal. This level corresponds to the threshold level of tubular resorption capacity and potential increase in urinary calcium excretion (Fig. 5). Hypophosphatemia may be caused by decreased intestinal absorption of phosphate, increased urine losses of phosphate, and an endogenous shift of inorganic phosphorus from extracellular to intracellular fluid compartments. It has also been reported in various rare hereditary diseases associated or not with neonatal hyperparathyroidism (Table 4). Early hypophosphatemia was observed in IUGR. Within the 1st week of life, a significant correlation between pre eclampsia and 1st week inorganic phosphate deficiency was related in VLBW babies, whereas, the occurrence of hypercalciuria and low urinary phosphate was also observed in small-for gestational age (SGA) infants. These studies suggest that infants with extrinsic IUGR are probably insufficiently provided with phosphorus *in utero* and hence postnatally may suffer early-onset inorganic phosphate depletion from prenatal origin. This mineral imbalance has been delineated in newborns with chronic fetal hypoxia and malnutrition leading to disproportionate or type II IUGR. In those infants, hypophosphatemia as well as platelet count and high nucleated red blood cell count were closely correlated with the severity of IUGR in SGA type II.

Table 4 Causes of neonatal phosphorus disorders

Hypophosphatemia	Hyperphosphatemia
Endocrine	*Endocrine*
Hyperparathyroidism	Hypoparathyroidism
VitaminD deficiency or resistance	Hyperthyroidism
Renal losses	Growth hormone excess
Congenital tubular disorders	Vitamin D toxicity
Secondary tubular disorders	*Renal*
Diuretics	Renal failure
Volume expanders	Volume depletion
Hypercalciuria	*Increased load*
Glucosuria	Enteral, Cow milk feeding
Hypomagnesemia	Rectal enema
Gastrointestinal	Parenteral
Decrease of intake	Blood transfusion
Decrease of absorption	
Calcium salt	
Malabsorption	
Antacid	
Gene mutation	
Others	
Metabolic acidosis	
Respiratory alkalosis	
Gram-negative sepsis	
Refeeding syndrome	
Hypercalcemia	
Carbonic anhydrase inhibitors	
Dopamine	

A high incidence (i.e., 28%) of hypophosphoremia associated with a double mortality rate related to myocardial dysfunction is reported in adult intensive care patients. A short course of phosphotherapy improved the left ventricular function rapidly in inorganic phosphate depleted adults (Zazzo et al. 1995). Therefore it is tempting to speculate that early-onset inorganic phosphate depletion could be an etiologic factor in myocardial dysfunction, leading postnatally to left heart failure and ensuing pulmonary hemorrhage in the most severely growth retarded VLBW-infants.

During the first weeks of life, hypophosphatemia related to low phosphorus intake occurs in low birth weight babies who were fed soy formulas and more frequently exclusive unsupplemented human milk (Putet et al. 1987). With human milk addition of 5–10 mg/100 mL of inorganic phosphate equivalent corrects plasma concentration, reduces calcium excretion and improves calcium retention. In formula fed infants, similar hypophosphatemia is also observed in relation to an inadequate calcium phosphorus ratio resulting either from a relative phosphorus malabsorption or a relatively higher calcium absorption rate. In that situation, absorbed phosphorus is lower than that required for deposition in soft tissues and bone according to nitrogen retention and calcium absorption.

An inadequate calcium to phosphorus ratio is also observed in preterm infants with persistent metabolic acidosis or prolonged respiratory distress syndrome. In that situation, the acid-base disturbance, increased bicarbonate or hypercapnia reduced phosphorus tubular reabsorption inducing a relative hypophosphatemia and hypercalciemia associated with a concomitant urinary excretion of phosphorus and calcium increasing the risk of nephrocalcinosis.

Given its widespread distribution and critical role in vital cellular processes, it is not surprising that a deficiency of phosphorus results in various clinical symptoms including hypotension and decreased stroke volume, impaired diaphragm contractility, dyspnea and respiratory failure, paresthesia, weakness, confusion, disorientation, lethargy, areflexic paralysis, seizures and coma, leukocyte dysfunction hemolysis and thrombocytopenia, as well as rickets or osteomalacia as reported in refeeding syndrome (Fuentebella and Korner 2009).

41.6.2 Neonatal Hyperphosphatemia

Hyperphospatemia is usually due to a decrease in renal function or a PTH absence (primary or secondary hypoparathyroidism) or phosphatonin deficiency. Hyperphosphatemia is most often the result of decreased renal excretion of phosphate anions as encountered in acute or chronic renal failure, particularly when glomerular filtration rate is reduced to less than 25% of normal. Hyperphosphatemia could also be the result of increased body phosphate load from blood transfusions and hyperalimentation. Increased renal tubular reabsorption of phosphate is responsible for hyperphosphatemia seen in neonatal hypoparathyroidism and associated disorders such as infants of diabetic mothers, transient neonatal hypoparathy roidism, neonatal pseudohypoparathyroidism or in babies born to mothers with hyperparathyroidism (Table 4). Hyperphosphatemia and secondary hyperparathyroidism have been extensively investigated as inducing factors in cardiovascular calcification. Together with passive deposition of calciumphosphate in extraskeletal tissues, it has recently been demonstrated that inorganic phosphate induces arterial calcification directly through a real "ossification" of the tunica media (Caudarella et al. 2007).

41.7 Bone Mineralization

41.7.1 Factors Affecting Growth and Mineralization

During gestation, the fetus receives an ample provision of nutritional supply through the placenta. Nitrogen, energy, minerals, and vitamins allow a high velocity of body length growth, representing around 1.2 cm/week during the last trimester of gestation. The fetus maintains its hypercalcemic state in a high calcitonin and estrogen environment, promoting the modeling/remodeling ratio in favor of modeling and thus increasing endocortical bone. In addition, according to the mechanostat theory of bone development, fetal bone is also driven by the mechanical force applied to the fetal skeleton during the intrauterine resistance training provided by regular fetal kicks against the uterine wall (Rauch and Schoenau 2001, 2002). Consequently, at term the newborn skeleton has a high physical density (bone mass divided by bone volume), with elevated cortical thickness and relatively small marrow cavities.

Various factors influence the processes of growth, mineralization, and bone structure. Growth is directly related to protein and energy supplies but also to the hormonal environment comprising insulin, IGF1, and IGF2, among others. Bone formation, mineralization, and structure are related to mineral supply and hormonal factors such as PTH, PTHrP, vitamin D, and calcitonin as well as others, such as genetics and physical activity. Several factors have been found to have a significant impact on newborn bone mineral content and developing fetal bone. Reduced calcium supply, vitamin D deficiency, alcohol consumption, and smoking during pregnancy are all factors affecting fetal skeletal development in addition to low weight related to gestation and diabetes in the mother.

41.7.2 Osteopenia of Prematurity

Premature infants, particularly those born at <28 weeks' gestation, are at significant risk for reduced bone mineral content (BMC) and subsequent bone disease, variably termed metabolic bone disease (MBD), osteomalacia, osteopenia, or neonatal rickets (Rigo et al. 2007; Land and Schoenau 2008; Rigo 2008). Reduction in BMC and the development of MBD of prematurity are quite common among VLBW infants. However, due to the lack of widely adopted diagnostic criteria, the true incidence has not been determined. Fractures in premature infants typically occur several weeks after delivery and prior to the postnatal age of 6 months (Bishop et al. 2007; Harrison et al. 2008). Rib fractures, the most common type, usually occur silently and are diagnosed only if X-rays are performed. Therefore, the true incidence of fractures is difficult to determine, varying between 2.1% and 25% in 3 previous studies (Bishop et al. 2007) conducted without the use of prospective, systematic skeletal surveys.

The risk factors commonly associated with fractures include extremely low birth weight, late (> 30 days) establishment of full enteral feeds or prolonged parenteral nutrition, exclusive use of unfortified human milk, necrotizing enterocolitis, conjugated hyperbilirubinemia, chronic lung disease, use of various medications, utilization of passive respiratory physiotherapy (i.e., chest percussion), and lack of physical activity, which may be enhanced by sedatives. Recent data on fractures among VLBW infants are still lacking, but some clinical evidence suggests that the risk for fracture is greatly reduced with the use of parenteral and enteral nutrition adapted to the special nutritional needs of the premature infant.

Risk factors for MBD are commonly encountered in the preterm infant. The majority of bone mineralization, along with calcium and phosphorus accretion, occurs during the third trimester of pregnancy. Infants born before this time thus have depleted stores of these minerals (Harrison et al. 2008). Data from bone density scans (dual-energy X-ray absorptiometry [DEXA]) performed at birth in preterm and term infants suggest that bone mineral accretion during the last trimester of gestation is higher than needed, with growth in bone volume leading to a continuous increase in skeletal density. Preterm infants therefore have a large mineral deficit compared with term infants. Several factors increase the risk for severe MBD among VLBW infants, with the most important appearing to be an inadequate supply of calcium and phosphorus associated with the use of an enteral vs transplacental route. Newborn premature infants experience a diminished mineral uptake required for proper bone accretion, due, in part, to the reduced availability and to their compromised gastrointestinal (GI) absorption. Metabolic balance studies in preterm infants fed fortified human milk and formulas (Rigo et al. 2000, 2010) have reported that maximal calcium retention values may reach 60–90 mg/kg/day and maximal inorganic phosphate retention values may reach 50–75 mg/kg/day. The retention rates are relatively low compared with the fetal accretion rates. In total parenteral nutrition, similar data could be obtained with the use of organic phosphate supply and highly soluble calcium salt. In our unit, using calcium glycerophosphate, we provide up to 105 mg of calcium and 80 mg of inorganic phosphate/kg/day with a retention rate close to 95%.

Decreased bone mineralization and the development of osteopenia are the balanced result between two different factors, bone matrix growth directly related to energy balance and nitrogen retention on the one hand, and mineral accretion on the other hand (Rigo et al. 2010; Rigo and Senterre 2006). Data from DEXA scans (Rigo

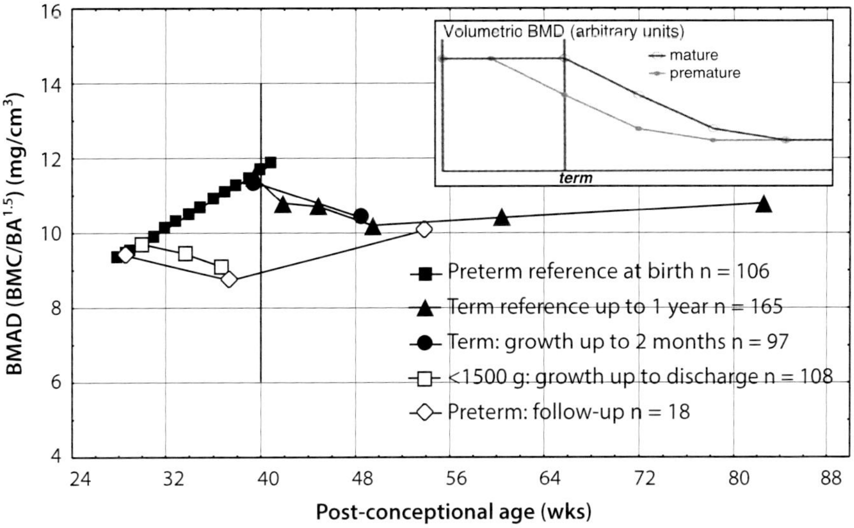

Fig. 6 Physiological evolution of DEXA apparent Bone Mineral Density during the last trimester of gestation and during the first year of life in healthy term infants (*dark symbols*) compared to that observed in premature infants (*open symbols*). Comparison to the evolution suggested by the mechanostat theory (*frame*)

et al. 2010; Rigo and Senterre 2006) performed during the first weeks after birth in both preterm and term infants suggest that bone growth, estimated by increase in bone area, is relatively higher than bone mineral accretion, leading to a continuous decrease in skeletal density (Fig. 6). Nevertheless, after a few weeks or months, with the continuous reduction in growth velocity, the balance is progressively reversed and the bone mass accrual compensates slowly for the early peak bone growth during the first few months of life. Physical activity appears to play a significant role in bone mineralization. During the neonatal period, mechanical strain on bone and joints stimulates bone formation and growth, whereas inactivity leads to bone resorption (Rauch and Schoenau 2001, 2002). This might be equally valid for preterm infants in incubators during the first weeks of life, who lack the *in utero* mechanical stimulation associated with regular kicks against the confining uterine wall (Schulzke et al. 2007). During the initial hospitalization, the movements of preterm infants usually occur without much resistance. While in the NICU, these infants are handled with little tactile stimulation in order to reduce stressful events. Moreover, the use of drugs to reduce pain aggravates the reduction in mechanical stimulation during their stay. In order to obviate the effects of reduced mechanical stimulation, systematic physical activity programs administered several times a week by nurses, therapists, and parents have been evaluated. A number of recent studies, agree that physical activity either improves bone mineralization, as determined by single-photon absorptiometry, or increases bone formation, as estimated by the measure of serum collagen C-terminal propeptide (Schulzke et al. 2007). These regimens either increased bone strength or attenuated its decrease, as evaluated by quantitative measurement of bone ultrasound transmission speed. Nevertheless, the last Cochrane review of this subject concluded that additional studies are needed before the general use of such physical activity programs can be promoted (Schulzke et al. 2007). A number of other factors may also play a significant role in bone mineralization, including genetic polymorphism, mechanical stimulation, or the use of various medications that interfere with mineral absorption or retention, such as diuretics, caffeine, and corticosteroids.

Neonatal screening for MBD in preterm infants is still controversial (Rigo 2008). Serum calcium levels are carefully regulated by hormonal secretion and are not a useful screening tool. However, a low serum phosphorus concentration < 1.8 mmol/L) that is below the renal phosphate threshold has been related to insufficient phosphorus intake and to an increased risk for osteopenia. Urinary excretion of calcium and phosphorus has been proposed as a marker of adequate postnatal mineralization when doses >1.2 mmol/L of calcium and >0.4 mmol/L of inorganic phosphorus are excreted simultaneously. However, these values are more appropriate for estimating the adequacy of the calcium to phosphate ratio than for estimating mineral accretion, especially when data on the mineral absorption rate are lacking.

In infants, 90% of alkaline phosphatase (ALP) is of bone origin and thought to reflect bone turnover. ALP concentrations usually increase during the first 2–3 weeks of life and may peak further if there are insufficient mineral supplies. Elevated levels of ALP have been reported in association with severe under mineralization based on radiologic evidence, low bone speed of sound (SOS) using quantitative ultrasound, or severe bone mineral density (BMD) deficit revealed on DEXA scans. Nevertheless, ALP is probably more sensitive for evaluating fracture risk than for assessing MBD or osteopenia.

Various radiologic investigations have been proposed for assessing bone mineralization and osteopenia among preterm infants. Plain radiography is poorly sensitive, detecting only a decrease of >20–40% of bone mineralization (Harrison et al. 2008). By contrast, DEXA technology, is sensitive, accurate, and precise, and its use has been validated in both preterm and term infants (Rigo et al. 2000, 2010; Avila-Díaz et al. 2001). Normative data on bone mineral content, projected bone area, and BMD in healthy preterm and term infants close to birth were established in order to obtain surrogate intrauterine reference values. In addition, various indices have been proposed for reducing the anthropometric dependency of the various parameters and for facilitating group or individual comparison. Thus, data obtained from various groups allow for the determination of major changes in bone mineralization during the fetal life and postnatally in preterm and term infants. These results are in agreement with the predicted time course of volumetric bone mineral density in mature newborns and premature babies, according to mechanostat theory (Land and Schoenau 2008).

The use of ultrasound has been proposed for the evaluation of bone mineralization in newborn infants (Rigo 2008). It is a simple, non-invasive, relatively inexpensive bedside procedure. Some machines have been designed to measure broadband ultrasound attenuation or SOS, commonly on the tibia. The propagation of sound waves in bone is determined by a number of factors, including mineral density, cortical thickness, elasticity, and micro-architecture, possibly providing a more complete picture of bone strength than measurements of BMD alone. In preterm and term infants at birth, there is a significant correlation among tibial SOS and gestational age, birth weight, birth length, and tibial length. However, the changes in SOS values during the last trimester of gestation are relatively small, accounting for only about 130 m/s. This value is only ±1.5 times higher than the interindividual variability (standard deviation [SD] = 95 m/s). After birth, a rapid decline in bone SOS occurs during the first days of life that cannot be completely explained by a nutritional deficit. Therefore, these data suggest that measurement of bone SOS has a lower sensitivity than DEXA for evaluating the various factors influencing bone mineralization during the neonatal period (Fig. 6).

In contrast to fetal bone metabolism, in which modeling is the main process inducing high net bone formation, with a rapid increase in trabecular thickness, neonatal bone metabolism is the result of a prevailing remodeling activity, defined as the cyclical succession of bone resorption and formation on the same bone surface (Land and Schoenau 2008; Rigo 2008). Therefore, the relative MBD of prematurity could be the result of a postnatal physiologic metabolic adaptation instead of the expression of a transitory MBD. Indeed, the relative osteopenia observed in preterm infants appears to be similar to that observed in healthy term infants during the first weeks after delivery or to that observed in early adolescence at the time of a growth spurt.

After discharge, catch-up mineralization is rapidly observed in VLBW infants (Avila-Díaz et al. 2001). At 6 months of corrected age, spine and total bone mineral density, corrected for anthropometric values, are in the range of normal term newborn infants. In fact, the catch-up mineralization observed after discharge is quite similar to that observed after the initial acceleration of growth during adolescence. Nevertheless, peak bone mass may be less during adulthood (Zamora et al. 2001). As suggested by Fewtrell and coworkers, at 8–12 years of age, formerly preterm infants were shorter, lighter, and had lower BMCs than controls. However, BMC was appropriate for the body size achieved and was not affected by early dieting or human milk feeding (Fewtrell et al. 2000).

Thus, osteopenia or rickets of prematurity seems to be a self-resolving disease, although the potential long-term consequences on the attainment of peak bone mass are not clearly known. Even if BMC improves spontaneously in most infants, this discovery does not imply that a period of demineralization is acceptable. Although the long-term consequences are unclear, the benefits of prevention and treatment include avoidance of fractures and possibly improved linear growth and peak bone mass.

In summary, after birth, the development of relative osteomalacia or osteopenia is a physiologic event resulting from a mismatch of the mineral supply and the persistent growth velocity on the one hand, and from the stimulation of bone turnover as an adaptation to extrauterine life on the other. This phenomenon is enhanced in preterm infants born with low mineral stores, an immature GI tract, and reduced physical activity, who demonstrate higher growth rates than do term infants. Several of the conditions discussed above and in the articles reviewed in this chapter might increase the severity of MBD, leading to the development of severe osteopenia and the risk for fracture. Early optimal parenteral and oral nutritional support, combined with biologic neonatal screening and measurement of serum phosphorus and ALP concentrations, as well as mineral urinary excretion, appears to be helpful for the prevention of MBD. When available, DEXA is more sensitive than ultrasound for quantifying osteopenia in VLBW infants (Rigo 2008).

References

Agostoni C, Buonocore G, Carnielli VP et al (2010) Enteral nutrient supply for preterm infants. J Pediatr Gastroenterol Nutr 50:85–91

American Academy of Pediatric (1985) Committee on nutrition: nutritional needs of low birth weight infants. Pediatrics 75:976

Atkinson SA, Tsang RC (2005) Calcium, magnesium, phosphorus, and vitamin D. In: Tsang R et al (eds) Nutrition of the preterm infant, 2nd edn. Digital Educational Publishing, Cincinnati, p 245

Avila E, Diaz L, Barrera D et al (2006) Regulation of vitamin D hydroxylaxses gene expression by 1,25-dihydroxyvitamin D3 and cyclic AMP in cultured human syncytiotrophoblasts. J Steroid Biochem Mol Biol 103:90–96

Avila-Díaz M, Flores-Huerta S, Martínez-Muñiz I, Amato D (2001) Increments in whole body bone mineral content associated with weight and length in pre-term and full-term infants during the first 6 months of life. Arch Med Res 32:288–292

Bachetta J, Harambat Jr, Dubourg L et al (2009) Both extrauerine and intrauterine growth restriction impair renal function in children born very preterm. Kidney Int 76:445–452

Banerjee S, Mimouni FB, Mehta R (2003) Lower whole blood ionized magnesium concentrations in hypocalcemic infants of gestational diabetic mothers. Magnes Res 16:127–130

Bassir M, Laborie S, Lapillonne A et al (2001) Vitamin D deficiency in Iranian mothers and their neonates: a pilot study. Acta Paediatr 90:577–579

Bishop N, Sprigg A, Dalton A (2007) Unexplained fractures in infancy: looking for fragile bones. Arch Dis Child 92:251–256

Caudarella R, Vescini F, Buffa A, Francucci CM (2007) Hyperphosphatemia: effects on bone metabolism and cardiovascular risk. J Endocrinol Investig 30(Suppl 6):29–34

Fewtrell MS et al (2000) Neonatal factors predicting childhood height in preterm infants: evidence for a persisting effect of early metabolic bone disease? J Pediatr 137:668–673

Fudge NJ, Kovacs CS (2004) Physiological studies in heterozygous calcium sensing receptor (CaSR) gene-ablated mice confirm that the CaSR regulates calcitonin release in vivo. BMC Physiol 20:5

Fuentebella J, Korner JA (2009) Refeeding syndrome. Pediatr Clin N Am 56:1201–1210

Greer FR (2003) Vitamin D deficiency-it's more than rickets. J Pediatr 143:422–423

Harrison CM, Johnson K, McKechnie E (2008) Osteopenia of prematurity: a national survey and review of practice. Acta Paediatr 97:407–413

Holick MF (2007) Vitamin deficiency. N Engl J Med 357:266–281

Holtback U, Aperia AC (2003) Molecular determinants of sodium and water balance during early human development. Semin Neonatol 8:291–299

Hsu SC, Levine MA (2004) Perinatal calcium metabolism: physiology and pathophysiology. Semin Neonatol 9:23–36

Karsdal MA, Henriksen K, Arnold M, Christiansen C (2008) Calcitonin: a drug of the past or for the future? Physiologic inhibition of bone resorption while sustaining osteoclast numbers improves bone quality. BioDrugs 22:137–144

Klein CJ (2002) Nutrient requirements for preterm infant formulas. J Nutr 132:1395S–1577S

Land C, Schoenau E (2008) Fetal and postnatal bone development: reviewing the role of mechanical stimuli and nutrition. Best Pract Res Clin Endocrinol Metab 22:107–118

Liu S, Gupta A, Quarles LD (2007) Emerging role of fibroblast growth factor 23 in a bone-kidney axis regulating systemic phosphate homeostasis and extracellular matrix mineralization. Curr Opin Nephrol Hypertens 16:329–335

Novakovic B, Sibson M, Hg HK et al (2009) Placenta-specific methylation of the vitamin D 24-hydroxylase gene: implications for feedback autoregulation of active vitamin D levels at the fetomaternal interface. J Biol Chem 284:14838–14848

Pawley N, Bishop NJ (2004) Prenatal and infant predictors of bone health the influence of vitamin D. Am J Clin Nutr 80(Suppl 6):1748S–1751S

Pieltain C, Vervoort A, Senterre T, Rigo J (2009) Intérêt de la consommation de produits laitiers et de la supplémentation en vitamine D au cours de la croissance. J Pédiatr Belge 11:24–27

Portal AA (2004) Calcium and phosphorus. In: Avner ED, Harmon WE, Niaudet P et al (eds) Pediatric nephrology, 5th edn. Lieppincott, Williams and Wilkins, Philadelphia, p 209

Putet G, Rigo J, Salle B, Senterre J (1987) Supplementation of pooled human milk with casein hydrolysate: energy and nitrogen balance and weight gain composition in very low birth weight infants. Pediatr Res 21:458–461

Quarles LD (2008) Endocrine functions of bone in mineral metabolism regulation. J Clin Invest 118:3820–3828

Rauch F, Schoenau E (2001) The developing bone: slave or master of its cells and molecules? Pediatr Res 50:309–314

Rauch F, Schoenau E (2002) Skeletal development in premature infants: a review of bone physiology beyond nutritional aspects. Arch Dis Child Fetal Neonatal Ed 86:F82–F85

Rigo J (2008) Neonatal osteopenia and bone mineralization. eNeonatal Rev 6:4

Rigo J, Senterre J (2006) Nutritional needs of premature infants: current issues. J Pediatr 149:S80–S88

Rigo J, De Curtis M, Pieltain C et al (2000) Bone mineral metabolism in the micropremie. Clin Perinatol 27:147–170

Rigo J, Pieltain C, Salle B, Senterre J (2007) Enteral calcium, phosphate and vitamin D requirements and bone mineralization in preterm infants. Acta Paediatr 96:969–974

Rigo J, Mohamed MW, De Curtis M (2010) Disorders of calcium, phosphorus, and magnesium metabolism. In: Martin R, Fanaroff A, Walsh M (eds) Neonatal-perinatal medicine, 9th edn. Elsevier Mosby, Philadelphia

Rodriguez SJ (2003) Neonatal hypercalcemia. J Nephrol 16:606–608

Salle BL, Delvin EE, Lapillonne A et al (2000) Perinatal metabolism of vitamin D. Am J Clin Nutr 71:1317S–1324S

Sato K (2008) Hypercalcemia during pregnancy, puerperium, and lactation: review and a case report of hypercalcemic crisis after delivery due to excessive production of PTH-related protein (PTHrP) without malignancy (humoral hypercalcemia of pregnancy). ocr J 55:959–966

Schell-Feith EA, Kist-van Holthe JE, van der Heijden AJ (2010) Nephrocalcinosis in preterm neonates. Pediatr Nephrol 25:221–230

Schulzke SM, Trachsel D, Patole SK (2007) Physical activity programs for promoting bone mineralization and growth in preterm infants. Cochrane Database Syst Rev (18):CD005387

Shaikh A, Berndt T, Kumar R (2008) Regulation of phosphate homeostasis by the phosphatonins and other novel mediators. Pediatr Nephrol 23:1203–1210

Stewart AF (2004) Translational implications of the parathyroid calcium receptor. N Engl J Med 351:324–326

Toke J, Patocs A, Balogh K (2009) Parathyroid hormone-dependent hypercalcemia. Wien Klin Wochenschr 121:236–245

Wagner CL, Greer FR, American Academy of Pediatrics Section on Breastfeeding, American Academy of Pediatrics Committee on Nutrition (2008) Prevention of rickets and vitamin D deficiency in infants, children, and adolescents. Pediatrics 122:1142–1152

Zamora SA, Belli DC, Rizzoli R et al (2001) Lower femoral neck bone mineral density in prepubertal former preterm girls. Bone 29:424–427

Zazzo JF, Troche G, Ruel P, Maintenant J (1995) High incidence of hypophosphatemia in surgical intensive care patients: efficacy of phosphorus therapy on myocardial function. Intensive Care Med 21:826–831

Micronutrients and Vitamins

42

Olivier Claris and Guy Putet

Contents

Abstract

Vitamins and micronutrients are essential for many cellular processes, but excessive intake may also be toxic. Iron, zinc, and copper compete for intestinal absorption. The first sign of iron deficiency is anemia, while an excessive intake may cause oxidative stress and may also impact on cardiac and liver function. Zinc deficiency may cause growth arrest, irritability, anorexia, alopecia, esophagitis, and diarrhea. Copper deficiency is associated with hypochromic anemia, hypotonia, failure to grow, diarrhea, bone abnormalities, and neutropenia. Iodine deficiency may impair growth and intellectual performance. Thiamin deficiency is known as "beriberi," while Niacin deficiency is known as pellagra. This chapter summarizes the most recent recommendations for vitamin and micronutrient intake.

O. Claris (✉)
Department of Neonatology, Hôpital Femme Mère Enfant, Bron, France

Hospices Civils de Lyon and Université Claude Bernard, Lyon, France

G. Putet
Department of Neonatology, Hopital de la Croix-Rousse, Hospices Civils de Lyon and Universite Claude Bernard, Lyon, France

42.1 Salient Points

- Iron is mainly involved in erythropoiesis, but also in neurodevelopment, cardiac, and skeletal muscle function.
- Zinc participates in carbohydrate and protein metabolism.
- Copper is involved in oxidation and reduction.
- Iodine intervenes in thyroid function.
- Thiamine is essential for carbohydrate metabolism and lipid synthesis.
- Riboflavin is implicated in energy metabolism.
- Niacin is a cofactor for electron transport and energy metabolism.
- Pyridoxine has a role in the metabolism of aminoacids, prostaglandins, carbohydrate, in the development of the immune system and neurologic function.

G. Buonocore et al. (eds.), *Neonatology*,
https://doi.org/10.1007/978-3-319-29489-6_191

- Folate is active in the biosynthesis of purines, pyrimidine, and amino acid metabolism.
- Cobalamin is involved in DNA nucleotide synthesis.
- Pantothenic acid is a precursor of Coenzyme A (energy metabolism).
- Ascorbic acid has a role in hydroxylation and as an antioxidant.
- Vitamin A is implicated in protein synthesis and epithelial cell function, growth, and immune function; it is also a strong antioxidant.
- Vitamin E is an antioxidant that prevents lipid peroxidation.
- Vitamin K is essential for hepatic synthesis of coagulation factors.
- Vitamin D plays a physiologic role in neuromuscular function and cell growth and differentiation.

42.2 Micronutrients

Table 1 summarizes the most recent recommendations (Agostini et al. 2010; Tsang et al. 2005; Koletzko et al. 2005a, b).

Iron Iron (Fe) is an important micronutrient implicated in DNA replication, cellular metabolism and oxygen delivery. It is mainly involved in erythropoesis and is the first sign of deficiency in anemia, it is also implicated in neurodevelopment, and cardiac and skeletal muscle function. On the otherhand, it is a potentially toxic nutrient and, as a powerful prooxidant, it may play a major role in the oxidative stress. Furthermore, iron overload has a direct impact on cardiac and liver function. For all these reasons, the range between requirements and toxicity is narrow.

Iron is absorbed in the duodenum as ferrous. Absorption rates depend on the iron status, the form of iron given and the age of preterm (PT) infants. Iron absorption is particularly enhanced by human milk feeding and vitamin C status, and is decreased after erythrocyte transfusion and competes with zinc and copper absorption.

Iron supplementation may be started as soon as 2 weeks of age, at a dose of 2–3 mg/kg/day (Agostini et al. 2010). Infants receiving erythropoietin treatment require higher intake, but too high an intake may cause intestinal side effects and increase retinopathy of prematurity. It is

Table 1 Micronutrients: Human milk (HM) content and intake recommendations (Agostini et al. 2010; Tsang et al. 2005; Koletzko et al. 2005a, b)

		Requirements (Tsang et al. 2005)		Requirements (Agostini et al. 2010; Koletzko et al. 2005a, b)		
	HM content FT	Enteral PT	Parenteral PT	Enteral PT	Parenteral FT	Parenteral PT
Iron	0.5–1 mg/L	2–4 mg/kg	0.25–0.67 mg/kg[a]	2–3 mg/kg	0.5–1 mg/kg	0.2 mg/kg[b]
Zinc	0.5–2.5 mg/L[c]	1–2 mg/kg	0.4 mg/kg	1.1–2 mg/kg	0.25 mg/kg	0.45–0.5 mg/kg
Copper	600–800 μg/L	120–150 μg/kg	20 μg/kg	100–132 μg/kg	20 μg/kg	
Selenium	15–20 μg/L	1.3–4.5 μg/kg	1.5–4.5 μg/kg	5–10 μg/kg	2–3 μg/kg	
Iodine	70–90 μg/L	10–80 μg/kg	1 μg/kg	11–55 μg/kg	1 μg/day	
Chromium	0.3–0.5 μg/L	0.1–2.25 μg/kg	0.05–0.3 μg/kg	0.03–1.23 μg/kg	not necessary	
Manganese	5 μg/L	0.75–75 μg/kg	1 μg/kg	<27 μg/kg	1 μg/kg	<50 μg/day
Molybdenum	2 μg/L	0.3–4 μg/kg	0.25–1 μg/kg	0.3–5 μg/kg	0.25 μg/kg	1 μg/kg
					<5 μg/day	
Fluorine				1.5–60 μg/kg		

[a]After 2 weeks of life
[b]Unnecessary before 3 weeks
[c]Decrease with postnatal days

therefore why intakes above 5 mg/kg/d are not recommended (Franz et al. 2000).

Zinc Zinc (Zn) is an ubiquitous trace metal present in numerous enzymes and participates in carbohydrate (CHO) and protein metabolism. It is required for replication, transcription and repair of DNA, and plays an important role during embryogenesis and growth. Zn is absorbed in the distal duodenum and proximal jejunum, and this is impaired by high casein intake.

Zn deficiency is characterized by growth arrest, irritability, anorexia, alopecia, esophagitis, diarrhea and functional recommendations in immunity, skin lesions of the hands and feet and poor healing. True acrodermatitis enteropathica is rarely seen in PT infants but ELBW infants on TPN without Zn, SGA, and growing PT infants fed unfortified HM are at risk of Zn deficiency (Friel et al. 1988).

Copper (Cu) It is a component of numerous enzymes (superoxide dismutase) involved in oxidation and reduction. It helps to protect cell membranes from oxidative damage. Copper competes with Zn and iron for intestinal absorption. It is absorbed in the upper part of the intestine, and this decreases by high Zn and iron intakes. Deficiency is associated with hypochromic anemia not responding to iron supplementation, hypotonia, failure to grow, diarrhea, bone abnormalities, neutropenia. In the case of hepatic cholestasis, intake has to be reduced or stopped because of potential toxicity.

Selenium (Se) It is a glutathione peroxidase component, which protects cell membranes against peroxide induced drainage. Deficiency is only seen in infants on TPN without or with too little Se, or in Keshan disease (cardiomyopathy) areas where soil is Se deficient. Addition of Se to food or TPN must be cautious as most Se compounds are toxic if given in excess (Aggett et al. 1991).

Iodine (I) It intervenes in thyroid function (T3 and T4 synthesis), and iodine deficiency (before or after birth) may impair growth and intellectual performance. Excess iodine may also create hypothyroidism. PT infants often have transitory hypothyroidism as their mechanisms to control iodine levels are immature (Rogahn et al. 2000). Based on the mean content of iodine in HM some PT infants may be on negative iodine balance. Toxicity is more often due to percutaneous intake (antiseptic solution).

Chromium (Cr) It has a role in glucose homesostasis. Hyperglycemia and insulin resistance are part of Cr deficiency, never described in infants either breast or formula fed.

Manganese (Mn) It is a component of several enzymes acting in gluconeogenesis, mitochondrial membrane maintenance and in mucopolysaccharide synthesis. Mn deficiency has not been described in human conclusively, however Mn toxicity has been seen in adults with extrapyramidal symptoms. Advisable intakes are based on what is contained in human milk.

Molybdenum (Mo) It intervenes in the function of xanthine, aldehyde and sulfite involved in purine metabolism and sulfur excretion. Deficiency is only described in adults on very long term TPN. Advisable intakes are based on what is contained in HM.

Fluorine (F) It is found in bones and teeth mainly. There are no data to make any recommendation except that it is found in human milk and crosses the placenta.

42.3 Vitamins

Table 2 summarizes the most recent recommendations for vitamin intake (Tables 3, 4, and 5).

Vitamin B1 (thiamine) Vit B1 is a coenzyme essential for CHO metabolism and lipids synthesis once transformed by the liver into thiamine pyro phosphate. It is absorbed in the proximal small intestine. Deficiency is known as "beriberi". A thiamine deficient total parenteral nutrition (TPN) may induce severe lactic acidosis and death.

Vitamin B2 (riboflavine) Vit B2 is implicated in energy metabolism (it forms flavin, adenine, dinucleotides). It is absorbed in the small intestine. Deficiency leads to stomatitis, dermatitis and anemia. Requirements are based on HM content and are related to protein intake. If protein supply is given without Vit supplementation, a deficit can occur (Lucas and Bates 1984).

Table 2 Vitamins: human milk (HM) content and intake recommendations (Agostini et al. 2010; Tsang et al. 2005)

		Requirements (Tsang et al. 2005)		Requirements (Agostini et al. 2010)	
	HM content FT	Enteral PT	Parenteral PT	Enteral PT	Equivalents
Vit A	660–1000 IU/L	750–1500 IU/kg	750–1500 IU/kg	400–1000 μg RE/kg	1 RE = 1 μg all trans retinol
					1 RE = 3.33 IU Vit A
					1 RE = 6 μg β carotene
					1 RE = 12 μg other carotenoids
Vit D	20–30 IU/L	200–1000 IU/day	60–400 IU/day	800–1000 IU/day	1 μg cholecalciferol = 40 IU Vit D
Vit E	3–4 IU/L	6–12 IU/kg	2.8–3.5 IU/kg	2.2–11 mg/kg TE	1 IU = 1 TE
					1 IU = 0.67 mg α-tocopherol
					1 IU = 1 mg dl-α-TA
Vit K	5–10 μg/L	8–10 μg/kg	10 μg/kg	4.4–28 μg/kg	

IU international units, *RE* retinol equivalent, *TE* tocopherol equivalent, *TA* tocopherol acetate

Vitamin B3 (niacin) Vit B3 can be synthesized from tryptophane (Try) in the presence of B6, once this amino acid (AA) exceeds minimal intake (60 mg of Try →1 mg of niacin expressed as Niacin Equivalent). It is also a cofactor for electron transport and energy metabolism. Absorption is effective in the small intestine. Deficiency is known as pellagra (dermatitis, diarrhea and neurological symptoms). It usually results from multiple deficiency and poor protein intake not observed in newborn infants.

Vitamin B6 (pyridoxine) Vit B6 has a role in the metabolism of AA, prostaglandins, CHO, in the development of immune system and neurologic function. Its requirement is related to protein intake (15 μg of B6 should be available per g of protein). It is absorbed in the small intestine. Deficiency leads to vomiting, irritability, dermatitis, failure to thrive, hypochromic anemia and neurological symptoms as convulsions.

Vitamin B9 (folate) Vit B9 is active in the biosynthesis of purines, pyrimidine and AA metabolism. Its activity decreases by Zn deficiency. Deficiency is associated with megaloblastic anemia, leucopenia, thrombocytopenia, growth insufficiency, and lesions in small intestine, mostly in context of malabsorption syndromes.

Table 3 Vitamins: effect of temperature and light, and toxicity

	Temperature	Light	Toxicity
Vit A	↓	Photodegraded	Intra cranial hypertension if >5000 IU/day
Vit D	Stable	Stable	Hypercalcemia, hypercalciuria, anorexia, vomiting, failure to thrive, calcifications
Vit E	Stable	Slightly affected	Large doses associated with sepsis, NEC
Vit K	Stable	↓	Not reported

Vitamin B12 (cobalamin) Vit B12 is involved in DNA nucleotides synthesis. Absorption depends on gastric pH and occurs in the small intestine. Deficiency of cobalamin is known as leading to megaloblastic anemia, glossitis and neurologic signs, but although this is not seen in FT breast fed infants, it is well established in infants of vegetarian mothers.

Vitamin B5 (pantothenic acid) It is a precursor of Coenzyme A (energy metabolism). It is absorbed

Table 4 Vitamins: daily intake recommendations (Agostini et al. 2010; Tsang et al. 2005)

		Requirements (Tsang et al. 2005)			Requirements (Agostini et al. 2010)	
	Enteral FT	Enteral PT	Parenteral FT	Parenteral PT	Enteral PT	Parenteral FT
B1	30 μg/kg	300 μg/kg	1–2 mg/day	350 μg/kg	140–300 μg/kg	350–500 μg/kg
B2	40 μg/kg	450 μg/kg	150 μg/kg	150 μg/kg	200–400 μg/kg	150–200 μg/kg
B3	0.2 mg/kg	4.5–6 mg/kg	17 mg/day	5 mg/kg	0.3–5 mg/kg	4–6.8 mg/kg
B6	14 μg/kg	180–300 μg/kg	1000 μg/day	180 μg/kg	45–300 μg/kg	150–200 μg/kg
B9	9.4 μg/kg	45–50 μg/kg	140 μg/day	56 μg/kg	35–100 μg/kg	
B12	0.05 μg/kg	0.3 μg/kg	0.75 μg/day	0.3 μg/kg	0.1–0.77 μg/kg	0.3 μg/kg
B5	1.7 mg/day	2 mg/day	5 mg/day	2 mg/kg	0.33–2.1 mg/kg	1–2 mg/kg
B8	0.7 μg/kg	4–40 μg/kg	20 μg/day	6 μg/kg	1.7–1.65 μg/kg	5–8 μg/kg
Vit C	6 mg/kg	30–40 mg/kg	80 mg/day	25 mg/kg	11–46 mg/kg	15–25 mg/kg

Table 5 Vitamins: human milk (HM) content, effects of temperature and light, and toxicity

	HM	Temperature	Light	Toxicity
B1	165–220 μg/L	↓	Photo degraded	Only in adults
B2	350–575 μg/L		↓	Not clearly defined
B3	1.8–2.5 μg/L			No side effect with nicotinamide
B6	130–310 μg/L		Inactivated	Very rare only in adults
B9	80–135 μg/L	Destroyed	Inactivated	Very rare may mask Vit B12 deficit. May depress Zn absorption
B12	0.2–1 μg/L			Not reported
B5	2.2–5 mg/L			Not reported
B8	5–9 μg/L			Not reported
Vit C	35–85 mg/L	Inactivated		Rebound scurvy in newborn only after large doses during pregnancy

in the small intestine. Deficiency has not yet been reported as diet provides sufficient amounts.

Vitamin B8 (biotin) Except in some metabolic diseases, deficiency is not seen in enterally fed infants as it is synthesized in gut, but is seen in TPN (pallor, anemia, dermatitis, lethargy, EEG abnormalities). It is also absorbed in the small intestine.

Vitamin C (ascorbic acid) Vit C has a role as a cofactor in hydroxylation reactions (proline, lysine, norepinephrin synthesis and Try) and as an antioxidant. It also has a role in folic acid conversion to folinic acid (active form) and in the oxidation of tyrosine (Tyr), and in iron absorption. 1 IU of L Ascorbic Acid corresponds to 50 μg. It is absorbed in the small intestine. Deficiency is known as scurvy. A transient elevation of plasma Tyr and Phenylalanine has been reported in VLBW infants fed high protein casein formulae.

Vitamin A This term refers to compounds (retinoids) having similar activities and structure as retinol (natural molecule derived from beta-carotene). Vit A activity is expressed as RE (retinol equivalent), 1 RE = 1 μg retinol = 3.3 IU Vit A. Vit A is mainly stored in liver and circulates in blood linked to retinol binding protein (RBP), and is implicated in protein synthesis and epithelial cell functions, growth and immune functions. It has also strong antioxidant properties. It is absorbed in the upper part of the small intestine.

No clinical deficiency is described in FT breastfed infants and precise requirements for PT infants are still unknown with recommended intakes are based mainly on biological data. Vit A supplementation may play a role as an antioxidant factor, and as a protective factor for bronchopulmonary dysplasia (BPD) (Greer 2005).

Vitamin E The term of Vit E refers to eight compounds having similar activities. The most active compound is α-tocopherol, which shows a strong antioxidant capability by protecting from lipid peroxidation. Vit E is entirely expressed as α-tocopherol equivalent (αTE), 1 mg αTE = 1 mg d-α-tocopherol = 1.49 IU, and 1 IU = 1 mg dl-α-tocopherol acetate. Vit E requirements depend on polyunsaturated fatty acid intake. It is absorbed in the small intestine. Hemolytic anemia is the main consequence of Vit E deficiency. Some controversy still persists upon the role of Vit E in BPD and retinopathy of prematurity. Large intakes of Vit E (above 50 mg/kg) have been implicated in gastro intestinal adverse effects and sepsis (Raju et al. 1997).

Vitamin K There are to two forms: Vit K1 (phyloquinone: plant form) and Vit K2 (menaquinone: synthesized by bacteria). Vit K is necessary for hepatic synthesis of coagulation factors (II, VII, IX, X, protein C and protein S). It is absorbed in the small intestine. It is needed in a very small amount and, as it is synthesized partly in the gut, synthesis is less pronounced with HM, and deficiency is seldomly seen, except in neonates and in cases of malabsorption or hepatic disease (Greer 2005).

Vitamin D Along with calcium and phosphorus homeostasis (see also ▶ Chap. 41, "Calcium and Phosphorus Homeostasis: Pathophysiology"), Vit D plays a physiologic role in neuromuscular function and cell growth and differentiation. It is absorbed in the small intestine. As Vit D deficiency in pregnant women is still frequent, recommended supply for neonates needs to be given as soon as enteral feeding is established (Salle et al. 1982).

References

Aggett PJ, Haschke F, Heine W et al (1991) Comment on the content and composition of lipids in infant formulas. ESPGAN Committee on Nutrition. Acta Paediatr Scand 80:887–896

Agostini C, Buonocore G, Carnielli VP et al (2010) Enteral supply for preterm infants. A comment of the ESPGHAN Committee on Nutrition. J Pediatr Gastroenterol Nutr 50:1–9

Franz AR, Mihatsch WA, Sander S et al (2000) Prospective randomized trial of early versus late enteral iron supplementation in infants with a birth weight of less than 1301 grams. Pediatrics 106:700–706

Friel JK, Penneys S, Reid DW, Andrews WL (1988) Zinc, copper, manganese, and iron balance of parenterally fed VLBW preterm infants receiving a trace element supplement. J Parenter Enter Nutr 12:382–386

Greer FR (2005) Vit A, E and K. In: Tsang RC, Uauy R, Koletzko B, Zlotkin SH (eds) Nutrition of the preterm infant. Scientific basis and practical application, 2nd edn. Digital Educational Publishing, Cincinnati, pp 141–172

Koletzko B, Goulet O, Hunt J et al (2005a) Iron, mineral and trace elements. J Pediatr Gastroenterol Nutr 41:S39–S46

Koletzko B, Goulet O, Hunt J et al (2005b) Vitamines. J Pediatr Gastroenterol Nutr 41:S47–S53

Lucas A, Bates C (1984) Transient riboflavin depletion in preterm infants. Arch Dis Child 59:837–841

Raju TNK, Langenberg P, Bhutani V, Quinn GE (1997) Vitamin E prophylaxis to reduce retinopathy of prematurity: a reappraisal of published trials. J Pediatr 131:844–850

Rogahn J, Ryan S, Wells J et al (2000) Randomised trial of iodine intake an thyroid status in preterm infants. Arch Dis Child Fetal Neonatal Ed 83:F86–F90

Salle B, David L, Glorieux FH et al (1982) Early oral administration of vitamin D and its metabolites in premature neonates. Effects on mineral homeostasis. Pediatr Res 16:75–78

Tsang RC, Uauy R, Koletzko B, Zlotkin SH (eds) (2005) Nutrition of the preterm infant. Scientific basis and practical application, 2nd edn. Digital Educational Publishing, Cincinnati

Part IV

Pharmacology and Infants of Smoking, Addicted, and Diabetic Mother

Safety of Medications During Pregnancy and Breastfeeding: Infants of Drug-Addicted Mothers

43

Karel Allegaert, Tim van Mieghem, and John N. van den Anker

Contents

K. Allegaert (✉)
Neonatal Intensive Care Unit, University Hospitals Leuven, Leuven, Belgium

Department of Development and Regeneration, KU Leuven, Leuven, Belgium

Intensive Care and Department of Pediatric Surgery, Erasmus MC – Sophia Children's Hospital, Rotterdam, The Netherlands
e-mail: karel.allegaert@uzleuven.be

T. van Mieghem
Department of Development and Regeneration, KU Leuven, Leuven, Belgium

Obstetrics and Gynecology, University Hospitals Leuven, Leuven, Belgium
e-mail: tim.vanmieghem@uzleuven.be

J. N. van den Anker
Division of Pediatric Clinical Pharmacology, Children's National Health System, Washington, DC, USA

Departments of Pediatrics, Integrative Systems Biology, Pharmacology and Physiology, George Washington University, School of Medicine and Health Sciences, Washington, DC, USA

Intensive Care and Department of Pediatric Surgery, Erasmus MC – Sophia Children's Hospital, Rotterdam, The Netherlands
e-mail: jvandena@childrensnational.org

G. Buonocore et al. (eds.), *Neonatology*,
https://doi.org/10.1007/978-3-319-29489-6_192

Abstract

Any decision on maternal pharmacotherapy should be balanced, comparing maternal and fetal/neonatal outcome to withholding any treatment. This is because there is a relevant body of evidence that uncontrolled maternal conditions also affect fetal outcome. The same holds true for breastfeeding.

Drugs are not thoroughly evaluated for use during pregnancy or breastfeeding. Knowledge on safety of drugs exposure during fetal and neonatal (breastfeeding) life is limited. Pregnancy category classifications for drugs are currently used, but have their limitations. Pregnancy exposure registries to build knowledge have been implemented in the recently revised version of the FDA labelling guidelines (Pregnancy and Lactation Labeling Final Rule).

Suggestive indicators of "likely safe during breastfeeding" are (i) drugs commonly administered to infants, (ii) drugs that are not absorbed following oral administration, (iii) not excreted into human milk, and finally (iv) drug considered safe during pregnancy, since fetal exposure is generally longer and more extensive. Aspects of opioids, benzodiazepines, and anti-epileptics use during fetal life or via breastfeeding have been discussed to illustrate the concepts of pregnancy-related clinical pharmacology, followed by a focused discussion on neonatal abstinence syndromes. We hereby aim to provide the practicing clinician with some guidance and sources of information.

43.1 Salient Points

- Drugs administered to the mother may have harmful effects on the fetus at any time during pregnancy. Decisions on maternal pharmacotherapy should always take account of the effects of withholding maternal treatment on maternal, fetal, and neonatal outcomes.
- The placenta should not be considered as a perfect, absolute barrier and neither is the fetus an inactive bystander following maternal and consequent fetal drug exposure.
- The same rationale holds true for breastfeeding. The goal of maternal medications during breastfeeding should fulfill two criteria: (1) provide safe and effective pharmacotherapy for maternal condition(s) and (2) assure safety or tolerance of the nursing infant from adverse events related to the maternal pharmacotherapy.
- A common misconception about drug safety is "when in doubt, do not provide breastfeeding," since breastfeeding itself provides benefits to both infant and mother.
- Suggestive indicators of "likely safe during breastfeeding" are (i) a drug commonly administered to infants (e.g., antibiotics), (ii) a drug that is not absorbed following oral administration (e.g., aminoglycosides, propofol), (iii) a drug that is not excreted into human milk (e.g., insulin, heparin), and (iv) a drug considered safe during pregnancy since fetal exposure is generally longer and more extensive.
- Breastfeeding rarely needs to be discouraged, discontinued, or interrupted when the mother needs drug therapy, but some caution should be taken with analgosedatives (opioids, benzodiazepines). Radioactive-labeled diagnostic drugs such as lithium, iodine, gold, and ergotamine alkaloids are high-risk drugs and are likely not to be compatible with breastfeeding.
- The Pregnancy and Lactation Labeling Final Rule should provide the tool to generate and collect reliable information on maternal drug use during breastfeeding.

43.2 Introduction

Drug labeling rarely includes information about dosing, efficacy, and maternal, fetal, or newborn safety and commonly states that "the drug has not been studied during pregnancy or breastfeeding." In general, drugs are not thoroughly evaluated for use during pregnancy. This is neither the case for specific pregnancy-related diseases (e.g., gestational diabetes, nausea and vomiting of pregnancy) nor for the impact of pregnancy, delivery, or the postpartum period (e.g., breastfeeding) on pharmacotherapy of nonpregnancy-related comorbidities (e.g., epilepsy, depression, pain syndromes, posttransplant, asthma, oncological diseases) (Zaijcek and Giacoia 2007; Pavek et al. 2009). A similar case can be built for early infancy and results in extensive off-label and unlicensed pharmacotherapy in both subpopulations (▶ Chap. 44, "Developmental Pharmacology and Therapeutics in Neonatal Medicine") and hence patient anxiety and prescriber liability.

Simple extrapolation from data in adults is hazardous, since pregnancy itself affects pharmacokinetics (PK, concentration-time profile) in part driven by the hormonal (e.g., estradiol) and physiological (e.g., cardiac output, renal function, plasma volume, and protein-binding capacity) changes. This results in extensive variability in drug response. In general, renal elimination capacity is increased throughout pregnancy (i.e., higher glomerular filtration rate, higher active tubular transport). Similarly, basal metabolic activity is also increased. This commonly results in higher drug metabolism (phase I and phase II processes), although these changes are in part also isoenzyme specific. This – although rare – may even result in reduced enzymatic activity during pregnancy (Ramoz and Patel-Shori 2014; Thomas and Yates 2012). Finally, changes in body weight or protein-binding capacity can affect the volume of distribution. Protein-binding capacity and the subsequent free fraction may also have an impact on the amount of drug that will be transferred from the maternal plasma to the human milk compartment (Ramoz and Patel-Shori 2014; Thomas and Yates 2012; Feghali and Mattison 2011). Despite the limited available knowledge, women during pregnancy as well as in the postpartum period need pharmacotherapy for different medical relevant conditions, either or not pregnancy related (Thomas and Yates 2012).

Drugs may have harmful effects on the fetus at any time during pregnancy. However, any decision on pharmacotherapy should always be balanced, comparing maternal and fetal/neonatal outcome to withholding maternal treatment. This is because there is also a relevant body of evidence that uncontrolled or suboptimal controlled maternal conditions in themselves also affect fetal well-being and perinatal outcome. A linear, too simplistic approach to discontinue drugs due to a perceived, association related risk, while ignoring the risks of discontinuation, is unwarranted and often dangerous (e.g., epilepsy, depression, pain syndromes, posttransplant, asthma, or oncological diseases) (Briggs et al. 2015; Gadot and Koren 2015; Amant et al. 2015).

The same rationale holds true for breastfeeding. Human milk is the obvious golden reference and the normative standard feeding for newborns and infants, but may result in breastfeeding associated drug exposure. As extensively discussed in another chapter of this textbook, drug disposition [***a***bsorption, ***d***istribution, and subsequent elimination, either through ***m***etabolic elimination or through primary renal ***e***limination (ADME) pharmacokinetics] in early infancy also differs substantially between children and adults. In general, neonates have an overall low clearance capacity with an importance between the subject explained by covariates such as organ weight and function, body composition, size, co-administration of drugs, genetic polymorphisms, growth restriction, or disease characteristics.

As a consequence, the ultimate goal of maternal medications during breastfeeding should fulfill two criteria: (1) provide safe and effective pharmacotherapy for the maternal condition(s) and (2) still assure safety or tolerance of the nursing infant from adverse events related to the maternal pharmacotherapy (Sachs and Committee on Drugs 2013). As a geneal comment before we discuss more in detail some aspects of maternal–fetal pharmacotherapy, pharmacotherapy during breastfeeding, and the neonatal abstinence syndromes, we would like to make the point that compound or class-specific information on drug use during pregnancy, postpartum, and breastfeeding is evolving and has become a field of active clinical research.

This means that updated, reliable information should be easy accessible for caregivers. Besides textbooks, LactMed is a free online database with information on drugs and lactation as one of the newest additions to the National Library of Medicine's TOXNET system. The Motherisk program has also an updated and useful website (www.motherisk.org) that can be searched and is open for advices. Another source of information with specific emphasis on teratology is the www.mothertobaby.org website. More recently (cf. infra), pregnancy exposure registries have been introduced in the FDA labeling concept, aiming to improve the available knowledge and access to knowledge on drugs and pregnancy. Also the National Center on Birth Defects and Developmental disabilities, integrated in the Centers for Disease Control (CDC), provides information on the safety of maternal drug use (www.cdc.gov/pregnancy/meds/treatingfortwo). Supported by the National Health Services (NHS) (www.rdtc.nhs.uk/services/teratology), the UK Teratology Information Service (UKTIS) website provides information, including monographs. Through the same group, the Best Use of Medicines in Pregnancy (BUMPS, www.medicinesinpregnancy.org) aims to inform and be informed by the public.

43.3 Maternal–Fetal Pharmacotherapy

Maternal pharmacotherapy may sometimes have a primary fetal indication, with maternal administration of steroids for fetal lung maturation as the best known maternal exposure, aimed for improved fetal and neonatal outcome. Transmaternal fetal therapy clearly reflects the fact that the placenta should not be considered to be a *perfect, absolute barrier* and neither is the fetus an *inactive bystander* following maternal and subsequent fetal drug exposure (Rowe et al. 2013). Consequently, effects (e.g., lung maturation, conversion of supraventricular tachycardia) but also harmful drug-related fetal side effects may occur at any time throughout pregnancy.

Structural, teratogenic effects, i.e., prenatal toxicity characterized by structural defects (e.g., mono-organ like cardiac, central nervous system, or renal, but sometimes also multi-organ) in the developing embryo or fetus, are the most commonly seen between (already) the 3rd and 11th week of pregnancy (Thomas and Yates 2012). This is of relevance when a physician considers a prescription in any female patient of childbearing age (e.g., angiotensin-converting enzyme inhibitors, coumarins, antiepileptics, isotretinoin). In contrast, drug exposure during the second and third trimester of pregnancy more generally affects either fetal growth or functional development (e.g., illicit drugs). Finally, perinatal exposure (e.g., opioids, benzodiazepines, antidepressants) may affect neonatal adaptation.

Studying the safety and the efficacy of drugs in pregnancy is obviously more limited, since it is ethically inacceptable to subject pregnant women to drugs for the sake of studying fetal and maternal safety (Briggs et al. 2015). However, capturing observations on human exposure in a structured approach may also provide relevant information despite the fact that such information may be confounded by maternal disease state. Case–control studies, observational studies and the use of prospective registration during pregnancy may provide more robust information. Such methods facilitate comparison of exposure rates to a specific compound in mothers who deliver a newborn with a specific malformation versus those who delivered a healthy baby (http://www.fda.gov/Drugs/DevelopmentApprovalProcess/DevelopmentResources/Labeling/ucm093307.html).

Largely because of these limitations, the assessment of risks and how to handle the available evidence, association, or likelihood of fetal harm related to maternal pharmacotherapy remains a difficult, balanced decision. This is also reflected by the different and evolving applied approaches: *strategies evolve, but also vary.*

Pregnancy category classifications are one approach, but classifications vary somewhat between different authorities, and these categories do not include risks related to drugs or their metabolites transferred through breast milk. The concept of pregnancy exposure registries to build knowledge has been integrated in the recently revised version of the Food and Drug Administration (FDA) labeling guidelines on medication guidelines during pregnancy and lactation. FDA defines a pregnancy exposure registry as a study that collects information from women who take prescription medicines or vaccines during pregnancy. This information includes data on the newborn and is compared with women not taken drugs during pregnancy (http://www.fda.gov/Drugs/DevelopmentApprovalProcess/DevelopmentResources/Labeling/ucm093307.html).

The FDA medication classification system initially applied a category A, B, C, D, X, and N for each compound and required a quite large amount of high-quality data to be defined as pregnancy category A (i.e., safe to the fetus). In the meanwhile, the FDA requests a more narrative description of the evidence available for use of the drug in pregnancy in three subsections, "pregnancy," "lactation," and "females and males of reproductive potentials." The "pregnancy" subsection provides information to the use of the drug in pregnant women, including dosing and potential fetal risks, and will be based on the earlier-mentioned registries. The "lactation" section will provide information about the use of the drug while breastfeeding, such as the amount of drug in human milk and potential effects on the nursing infant. This new Pregnancy and Lactation Labeling Final Rule became effective by June 30, 2015 (http://www.fda.gov/Drugs/DevelopmentApprovalProcess/DevelopmentResources/Labeling/ucm093307.html).

43.4 Breastfeeding

Lactating women are regular users of medications and are often advised to either discontinue or even stop nursing while taking drugs, despite the fact that there are only a limited number of drugs that have been identified as potentially harmful to the newborn.

A common misconception about drug safety is "when in doubt, do not provide breastfeeding," since breastfeeding itself provides relevant benefits to both the infant and the mother (Genung 2013). The earlier-described Pregnancy and Lactation Labeling Final Rule should provide the tool to generate and collect more reliable information on this topic. At present, there are still a limited number of prospective population-based studies or systematic reviews that provide some insight in the extent and the relevance of the problem (http://www.fda.gov/Drugs/DevelopmentApprovalProcess/DevelopmentResources/Labeling/ucm093307.html). Already two decades ago, Ito et al. quantified the incidence of adverse reactions (11.2%) in a cohort of 838 nursing infants with mothers on drugs (Ito et al. 1993). More importantly, all events were classified as minor and were most commonly associated with antibiotics, analgesics/narcotics, antihistamines, sedatives, antidepressants, or antiepileptics. In 2003, this overall pattern was confirmed by Anderson et al., following a systematic review of 100 published case reports. None of the cases were "definite," 47% "probable," and 53% "possible" related to breastfeeding. Central nervous system-related drugs accounted for about 50% of the events and also included three fatalities. These observations suggest that when a few simple precautions are taken in drug selection and when the infant's age is taken into account, breastfeeding rarely needs to be discontinued when the mother needs pharmacotherapy: adverse drug reactions in breastfed infants are *less than imagined* (Anderson et al. 2003).

Maternal absorption of a given dose of drug (D_m) will result in compound-specific, variable transfer of the drug into the human milk (D_i). However, concentrations in human milk usually are quite low, and the oral bioavailability following oral ingestion by the infant is also a very relevant and often forgotten covariate to estimate the subsequent exposure (RID = relative infant dose, D_m/D_i * absorption) (Fig. 1). In Fig. 1, the differences in drug concentrations in the infant (1 vs. 2) can be explained by the presence (*a*) or absence (*b*) of "*an initial concentration following fetal exposure to the drug*" since accumulation in the infant relates to dose and duration, body composition, the clearance capacity of the infant, but also the initial concentration in the newborn's compartments.

In the clinical setting, suggestive indicators of "likely safe during breastfeeding" are (*i*) a drug commonly administered to infants (e.g., antibiotics), (*ii*) a drug that is not absorbed following oral administration (e.g., aminoglycosides, propofol), (*iii*) not excreted into human milk (e.g., insulin, heparin), and finally (*iv*) a drug considered safe

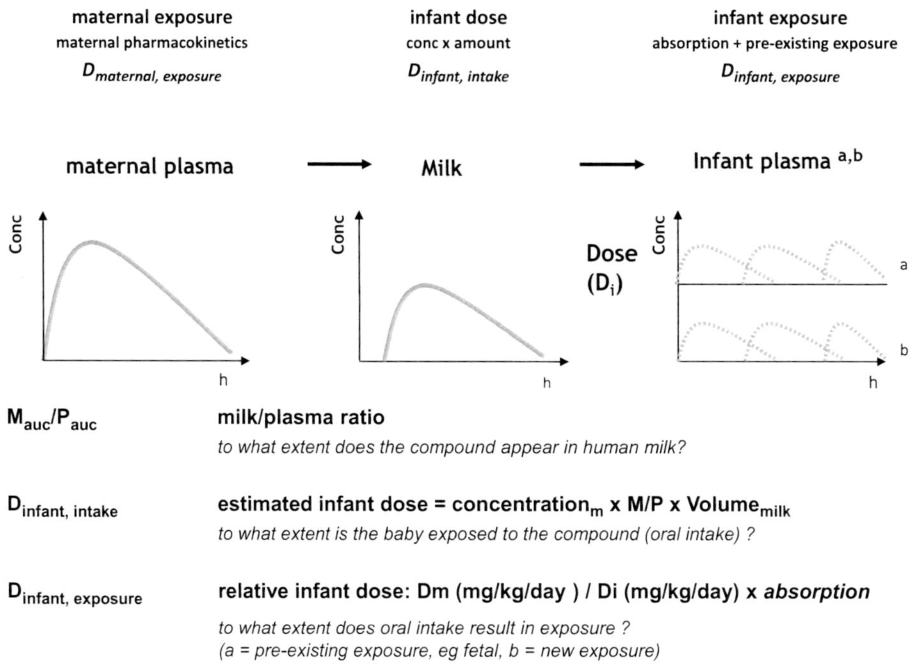

Fig. 1 Pharmacokinetics of mother–infant pairs as it relates to drug exposure through breastfeeding. Maternal absorption of a given dose of drug (D_m) will result in compound-specific, variable transfer of the drug into the human milk (D_i). However, concentrations in human milk usually are quite low, and the oral bioavailability following oral ingestion by the infant is also a very relevant and often forgotten covariate to estimate the subsequent exposure (RID = relative infant dose, D_m/D_i * absorption). The differences in drug concentrations in the infant (1 vs. 2) can be explained by the presence (*a*) or absence (*b*) of *an initial concentration following fetal exposure to the drug* since accumulation in the infant relates to dose and duration, body composition, the clearance capacity of the infant, but also the initial concentration in the newborn's compartments

during pregnancy, since fetal exposure is generally longer and more extensive. In contrast, e.g., radioactive-labeled diagnostics, lithium, iodine, gold, and ergotamine alkaloids are high-risk drugs, more likely not compatible with breastfeeding. The available data suggest that breastfeeding rarely needs to be discouraged, discontinued, or interrupted when the mother needs drug therapy, but some caution may be warranted with analgosedatives (opioids, benzodiazepines) (Van den Anker 2012; Berlin and van den Anker 2013; Hendrickson and McKeown 2012). In contrast, local anesthetics, systemic non-opioid analgesics, and intravenous or inhalational anesthetics are safe in the setting of breastfeeding (Allegaert and van den Anker 2015).

Peripartum opioid exposure became a specific focus of interest, following a case report of morphine intoxication in a breastfed neonate of a codeine-prescribed mother (Koren et al. 2006). Subsequent guidelines (lowest codeine dose possible, maternal exposure <4 days, and switch to non-opioids as soon as possible, monitor maternal and neonatal sedation) resulted in an eightfold reduction (5/238, 2.1%) in the incidence of neonatal sedation and were only associated with prolonged (>4 days) maternal codeine intake. As part of analgosedative treatment options, mothers after delivery (e.g., post-caesarean, birth-related injuries, but also preexisting pain syndromes) can be exposed to different analgosedatives that may also have impact of the breastfed infant (Van den Anker 2012; Allegaert and van den Anker 2015). This will be followed by some guidance on the use of antiepileptic drugs and breastfeeding. Aspects related to antidepressants will be covered in the section on neonatal abstinence syndrome. We hereby also cover some aspects of fetal exposure, since for some drugs, e.g., antiepileptic drugs, neonates are exposed both intrauterine and during breastfeeding.

43.4.1 Opioids

The breastfeeding rate increased steadily in the developed world (Saadeh 2012). More recently, opioid consumption in the general population – including women of childbearing age – also raised steadily (DeVane 2015). This means that the clinical experience with maternal opioids is still relatively limited with emerging data on (side) effects with codeine, oxycodone, methadone, and tramadol during breastfeeding (Rowe et al. 2013; Berlin and van den Anker 2013; Koren et al. 2006). The same phenomenon also explains the dramatic increase in the incidence of neonatal abstinence syndrome (cf infra). Referring to Fig. 1, oral absorption of opioids in neonates should be anticipated, while the extent of exposure through mother's milk will depend on maternal ingestion (dose) and metabolism. Neonatal drug elimination relates to the neonate's metabolic or renal elimination, but will be relatively limited (Allegaert et al. 2013). These circumstances have the potential to result in side effects in individual infants. A pivotal case report in 2006 of Koren et al. on codeine-related poisoning in an infant due to breastfeeding following maternal intake of codeine reinitiated the clinical interest and research on maternal–infant opioid pharmacokinetics and dynamics and its covariates (Koren et al. 2006). A pharmacogenetic link with maternal ultrafast metabolizer status for cytochrome p450 (CYP) 2D6 was documented. This genetic status results in higher and faster conversion of codeine to morphine (Koren et al. 2006). More recently, the same researchers also described that a combination of maternal genetic polymorphisms (i.c. CYP 2D6 and P-glycoprotein polymorphisms) predicted 87% of the maternal and infant central nervous system depression cases with a sensitivity of 80% and a specificity of 87% in a cohort of 111 breastfeeding mother–infant dyads (Sistonen et al. 2012). Unfortunately, this observation is not limited to codeine only.

The incidence of central nervous system depression in breastfed neonates following maternal exposure to oxycodone, codeine, or paracetamol was retrospectively compared in 533 mother–infant pairs. Lam et al. hereby clearly showed that there was a 20.1% rate of depression in infants of nursing mothers on oxycodone, as compared with 16.7% and 0.5% when treated with codeine or paracetamol, respectively (Lam et al. 2012). Finally, using a sparse sampling study design to assess transfer of tramadol and *O*-desmethyl tramadol into transitional breast milk, the relative infant dose of 2–3% remained very limited. Based on these observations, the authors concluded that short-term maternal use of tramadol is compatible with breastfeeding (Salman et al. 2011).

It remains somewhat difficult to convert the available observations in the literature to clinical guidelines for pediatricians, but we tried to provide some guidance (Van den Anker 2012; Allegaert and van den Anker 2015; DeVane 2015). Firstly – besides tramadol – it seems reasonable to anticipate that sedation may occur following maternal exposure to codeine, oxycodone, methadone, or morphine. Secondly, and clinical quite useful, there is a high concordance between maternal and neonatal somnolence. When the mother exhibits somnolence, the baby should be examined. This is likely due to the impact of genetic polymorphisms and dose on the individual maternal–infant-related effects and side effects of these drugs. Severe somnolence only emerges after 4 days of continued drug exposure and subsequent drug accumulation. When the human milk volume increases, exposure (mg/l x volume) increases and is prolonged, making subsequent accumulation in the infant more likely. As a result of the above premises, maternal opioid exposure for more than 72 h after delivery warrants specific clinical evaluation, with emphasis on signs of sedation in both the mother and the newborn (Van den Anker 2012; Salman et al. 2011; Rivers et al. 2012).

There are two additional comments to be made. Firstly (Fig. 1), this rationale does not fully apply to newborns already exposed prenatally to opioids, but these aspects will be discussed in the section on neonatal abstinence syndrome. Secondly, the route of administration of opioids obviously matters (systemic, e.g., oral, intravenous, or transcutaneous, or locoregional, e.g., spinal, epidural). Because of the much lower doses used and the lower plasma concentrations, the subsequent drug exposure through human milk will be much lower.

43.4.2 Benzodiazepines

Benzodiazepines (e.g., diazepam, lorazepam, midazolam) are commonly administered as anxiolytics. These compounds and some of their metabolites can be retrieved in human milk, but the amounts remain very low and subsequent exposure remains very limited (Cole and Hailey 1975; Nitsun et al. 2006). In 24 h of human milk collection after a single dose, only 0.005% of the maternal midazolam dose was retrieved. Taking the subsequent oral bioavailability (50–60%) into account, it is very reasonable to assume that the exposure will be very low when administered after delivery. In contrast, plasma diazepam and its active metabolite (desmethyldiazepam) could be measured up to 7–10 days of postnatal age in neonatal plasma samples after administration to the mother before or during delivery (Cole and Hailey 1975). We once again refer to Fig. 1 to explain this. Following administration during delivery, the fetus and newborn will have already a relevant concentration of benzodiazepines in the blood (Fig. 1, *level a instead of level b*), and the neonatal clearance capacity for these compounds is limited (De Wildt et al. 2002).

43.4.3 Antiepileptic Drugs

Continuation of antiepileptic treatment during pregnancy and the postpartum period is extremely important, since poor epileptic control has been associated with adverse maternal and fetal outcomes. Monitoring of maternal drug levels is often advised since pharmacokinetics may change. However, the safety of breastfeeding while taking antiepileptic drugs (AEDs) remains of some concern. This concern is also reflected in the fact that the rates of breastfeeding of women on AEDs are lower when compared to women not on AEDs living in the same region or country (Veiby et al. 2015). Moreover, women using either AED poly-therapy (75%) or lamotrigine (undergoes glucuronidation, so poorer clearance capacity in early neonatal life) had even lower breastfeeding initiation rates (70%), when compared to either the reference group (not on AEDs, 92%) or to women on AED monotherapy (80%), with a subsequent similar decline in breastfeeding rates with time (at 3 months, AED poly 67%, lamotrigine 60%, reference group 86%, AED mono 70%). Obviously, many factors affect the decision to initiate and maintain breastfeeding. Besides socioeconomic and social factors, emotional status or self-esteem but also disease-related aspects (e.g., need for day/night routine, seizure control) likely affect the individual decision of women (Veiby et al. 2015; Meador et al. 2014).

43.4.3.1 Compound-Specific Risk Assessment

Phenytoin, carbamazepine, and valproate are generally considered to be safe AEDs during breastfeeding (Veiby et al. 2015). Phenytoin and valproate have a high and carbamazepine a moderate high plasma protein binding. Consequently, the M/P ratios are quite low (phenytoin, 0.1–0.6; carbamazepine, 0.2–0.7; valproate, 0.01–0.3). Some suggest checking liver enzymes and thrombocytes in the nursing infant exposed to valproate and liver enzymes in infants exposed to carbamazepine (Veiby et al. 2015).

Lamotrigine, oxcarbazepine, levetiracetam, topiramate, gabapentin, pregabalin, vigabatrin, and tiagabine are classified as moderately safe AEDs. As mentioned earlier, lamotrigine (M/P ratio 0.4–0.67) is cleared by glucuronidation and is moderately plasma protein bound (55%). We suggest monitoring the infant for clinical signs and consider checking serum levels when the infant displays poor suckling. We hereby have to take into account that the free lamotrigine fraction in neonatal serum will be higher when compared to maternal plasma (lower binding capacity) (Veiby et al. 2015). Oxcarbazepine (M/P ratio 0.5) has the same route of metabolic elimination (glucuronidation), but clinical experience with this compound is much more limited. The M/P ratio of levetiracetam is much higher (M/P ratio 0.8–1.6), but clearance is through primary renal elimination, and there is a relevant amount of clinical experience with this compound to treat neonatal seizures (Pressler and Mangum 2013). For all the other compounds mentioned, there are only a limited number of clinical reports.

Finally, benzodiazepines, phenobarbital and primidone, ethosuximide, zonisamide, or felbamate, are classified as potential hazardous. Aspects on benzodiazepines have been discussed earlier (3.2). For phenobarbital and its prodrug primidone, accumulation may occur because of the very long elimination half-life of phenobarbital in neonates (Marsot et al. 2014). Again, clinical observation and – in the presence of symptoms – drug monitoring seem a very reasonable choice. Ethosuximide has a high M/P ratio, and the relative infant dose (32–113%) and subsequent levels in neonates are quite high (24–75%) when compared to maternal levels. Since ethosuximide is commonly part of poly-AED therapy, careful monitoring is recommended. Zonisamide also results in significant exposure (M/P ratio 0.8) and has a long elimination half-life in neonates. There are no data on felbamate, but this drug may induce hepatic failure or aplastic anemia (Veiby et al. 2015).

43.4.3.2 Impact of Prenatal and Breastfeeding-Mediated Exposure of Antiepileptic Drugs (AED) on Neurodevelopmental Outcome

Similar to the breastfeeding rates, the assessment of neurodevelopmental impact of AED exposure through breastfeeding is also hampered by several covariates (Meador et al. 2014). Firstly, postnatal exposure generally follows intrauterine exposure. Secondly, the impact of fetal exposure to AEDs during pregnancy also affects subsequent neurodevelopmental outcome (e.g., gross motor skills, fine motor skills, social skills). These neurodevelopmental observations further add to the available data on the impact of fetal exposure on the incidence of congenital malformations (Meador et al. 2014). AEDs such as valproate (9.3%, RR 5.1 to lamotrigine) and phenobarbital (4.2%, RR 2.9) are associated with a higher risk of major malformations than newer AEDs such as lamotrigine (2%) and levetiracetam, (2.4%), while topiramate (3%, RR 2.2) was associated with an increased risk of cleft lip compared with that of a reference population (Veiby et al. 2013).

As reported by the Neurodevelopmental Effects of Antiepileptic Drugs (NEAD) group, fetal valproate exposure is associated with a significantly higher risk of impaired cognitive function at 3 years (mean IQ 92, mean IQ difference of 6–9 when compared to carbamazepine, lamotrigine, or phenytoin, 258 cases of AED exposure) with a clear dose–effect relation for valproate (Meador et al. 2009). Similarly, Veiby et al. (Marsot et al. 2014) confirmed the impact of fetal AED exposure on psychomotor development. At age 6 years, infants of mothers using antiepileptic drugs ($n = 223$) had a higher risk of impaired fine motor skills compared with the reference group (11.5–4.8%, OR 2.1). The maternal treatment with multiple antiepileptic drugs was associated with adverse outcome for fine motor skills (25.0–4.8%, OR 4.3) and social skills (22.5–10.2%, OR 2.6).

Building on these background characteristics, the same study also documented that breastfeeding in infants of women using AEDs was associated with improved neurodevelopment outcome at ages 6 and 18 months, compared with those with either no breastfeeding or breastfeeding for less than 6 months (Meador et al. 2014). At 36 months, fetal AED exposure was associated with adverse development, regardless of breastfeeding. Children of women with epilepsy but without AED during pregnancy had normal development at 6 months. Based on these observations, it is fair to encourage women with epilepsy to breastfeed their infants, irrespective of antiepileptic drug treatment and taking the abovementioned suggestions on clinical monitoring into account (Meador et al. 2014).

43.5 Neonatal Withdrawal Syndromes

Neonatal withdrawal or neonatal abstinence syndrome (NAS) is a withdrawal syndrome in neonates due to acute cessation of the exposure to either illicit or prescribed drugs. Similar to tolerance or dependence, withdrawal may occur as a result of repeated or chronic administration of drugs, but also after short-term high-dose use, e.g., during neonatal stay. Consequently, NAS can appear both following discontinuation of drugs taken by the pregnant mother and following discontinuation of drugs administered intentionally to the newborn. The most commonly involved compounds are opioids, selective serotonin reuptake inhibitors (SSRIs), benzodiazepines, as well as cannabis or nicotine.

43.5.1 Opioid-Related Neonatal Abstinence Syndrome

The incidence of opioid-related neonatal abstinence syndrome (NAS) has increased significantly in the last decade, colinear with the increased medical use of prescription opioids in adults (DeVane 2015). The impact on the trends of NAS incidence throughout the Western world has been illustrated in Fig. 2 (Turner et al. 2015; Dow et al. 2012; Patrick et al. 2012, 2015; O'Donnell et al. 2009; Creanga et al. 2012). This means that NAS is no longer "restricted" to illicit drug users but also has become a frequent complication following medical prescription of opioids (DeVane 2015). The clinical picture of neonatal abstinence syndrome mimics to a large extent the syndrome of opioid withdrawal in adults ("cold turkey") and includes both neurological (e.g., agitation, crying, sleep disturbance, feeding difficulties, but also seizures) and extra-neurological symptoms (e.g., diarrhea, vomiting, perianal excoriations, sneezing, sweating, hyperthermia). The

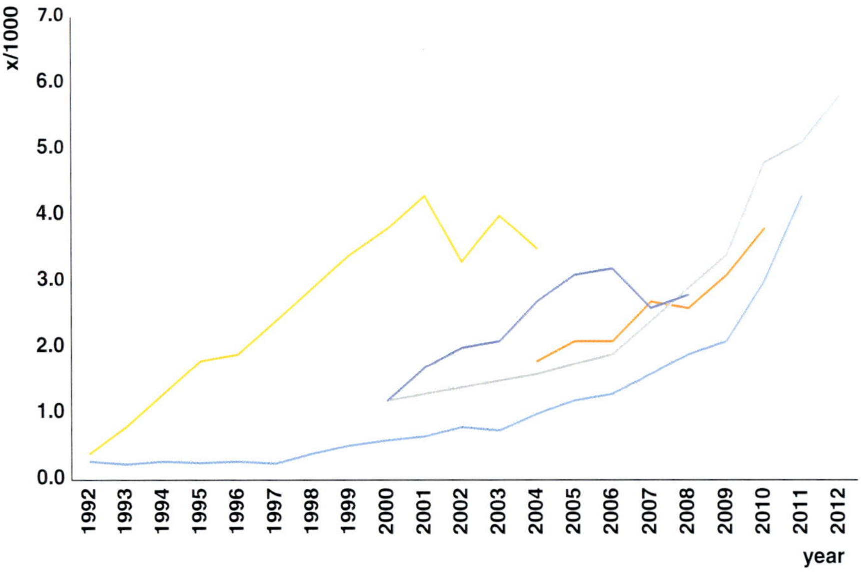

Fig. 2 The impact on the trends of NAS incidence throughout the Western world is illustrated by the trends in the annual incidence (1/1000) of neonatal abstinence syndrome in different cohorts as published between 1992 and 2012 (Turner et al. 2015; Dow et al. 2012; Patrick et al. 2012, 2015; O'Donnell et al. 2009; Creanga et al. 2012)

clinical presentation of NAS varies with the opioid (elimination half-life short or prolonged, heroin vs. methadone) used, co-drugs, maternal drug history, placental transfer, neonatal elimination capacity, but also pharmacogenetics (e.g., drug metabolism, transporters, receptor polymorphisms) (Wachman et al. 2013).

Table 1 Items and calculation of the modified Finnegan score (DeVane 2015; Hudak et al. 2012)

Central nervous system symptom-related items		
High-pitched cry	Present	2
	>2 h	3
Sleeps less than	3 h after feeding	1
	2 h after feeding	2
	1 h after feeding	3
When disturbed	Mild tremors	1
	Marked tremors	2
When undisturbed	Mild tremors	3
	Marked tremors	4
Increased muscle tone		2
Excoriation of the skin		1
Myoclonic jerks during sleep		3
Generalized convulsions		5
Autonomous/vegetative symptom-related items		
Sweating/ perspiring		1
Body temperature	37.5–38 °C	1
	>38 °C	2
Frequent yawning		1
Mottling		1
Nasal stuffiness		2
Sneezing		1
Gastrointestinal and respiratory system symptom-related items		
Frantic suckling		1
Poor feeding		2
Regurgitation		2
Projectile vomiting		3
Stools	Loose	2
	Watery	3
Tachypnea	>60/min	1
	>60/min + retractions	2

The Finnegan score (modified version, 21 items, 0–37 points, Table 1) is universally used to quantify the severity of withdrawal symptoms (Hudak et al. 2012). The score hereby reflects the central nervous system driven as well as autonomic, intestinal, and respiratory signs (Zimmermann-Baer et al. 2010). To document a threshold for suspected NAS, Zimmermann-Baer et al. documented the Finnegan score in 102 neonates (>34 weeks gestational age), up to the age of 5–6 weeks. The 95th percentile increased from 5.5 on day 1 to 7 on day 2, and at 5–6 weeks, the 95th percentile was 8 during daytime and 6 at nighttime (Zimmermann-Baer et al. 2010). Based on these observations, the authors suggest that values above 8 should raise suspicion of withdrawal. When pharmacological treatment of opiate withdrawal in neonates is deemed necessary, opiates (morphine, methadone, preferably by oral route) are the first choice, with subsequent slow weaning, although there is extensive variability in weaning and discharge practices (Hudak et al. 2012). In the event of non-opioid neonatal withdrawal, phenobarbital is the first choice. More recently, clonidine (5 μg/kg per day, divided in 8 doses) has been suggested as a novel treatment modality (Bada et al. 2015). Similarly, buprenorphine by sublingual route may also become a new treatment modality (Ng et al. 2015).

Besides pharmacological interventions, we strongly recommend to consider the impact of other interventions like swaddling, traditional supportive interventions, but also breastfeeding (MacMullen et al. 2014). Although there are no prospective randomized controlled trials, there is evidence in support of breastfeeding in women who have used methadone in pregnancy (grade C), since this reduces the incidence (NNT 5–6) and severity of NAS (grade C), without inducing clinically important sedation (grade C) (Lefevere and Allegaert 2015). Optimal NAS treatment remains undetermined and practices vary between and within hospitals. Prolonged length of stay for NAS cases may result in patient harm and impaired maternal–infant attachment, besides significant costs. The development of an educational program and a standard treatment protocol for NAS has been the most effective interventions to reduce this length of stay for NAS newborns (Asti et al. 2015). Some key messages on neonatal abstinence syndrome for the practitioner are summarized in Table 2 (DeVane 2015; Turner et al. 2015; Dow et al. 2012; Patrick et al. 2012, 2015; O'Donnell et al. 2009; Creanga et al. 2012; Wachman et al. 2013; Hudak et al. 2012; Zimmermann-Baer et al. 2010; Bada et al. 2015; Ng et al. 2015; MacMullen et al. 2014; Lefevere and Allegaert 2015; Asti et al. 2015; Siu and Robinson 2014).

Table 2 Key messages on neonatal abstinence syndrome: essentials for the practitioner (DeVane 2015; Turner et al. 2015; Dow et al. 2012; Patrick et al. 2012, 2015; O'Donnell et al. 2009; Creanga et al. 2012; Wachman et al. 2013; Hudak et al. 2012; Zimmermann-Baer et al. 2010; Bada et al. 2015; Ng et al. 2015; MacMullen et al. 2014; Lefevere and Allegaert 2015; Asti et al. 2015; Siu and Robinson 2014)

The incidence of neonatal abstinence syndrome (NAS) varies extensively (fivefold to tenfold) between units, but there is an overall relevant increase in the incidence of NAS
Besides recreational use, this increase in NAS also reflects a significant increase in the medical prescription of opioids
Fetal exposure does not necessary result in neonatal abstinence syndrome. For heroin and methadone, its incidence is about 60–80 %
The timing of appearance of NAS symptoms in part depends on the clearance characteristics of the opioid (heroin <24–48 h versus methadone 48–72 h) involved. The longer the elimination half-life, the later the symptoms appear
Treatment should be protocol driven, based on assessment (Finnegan) and followed by non-pharmacological as well as pharmacological interventions. Treatment should also cover the subsequent tapering of these drugs
Neonatal seizures are the most life-threatening complication of NAS. Furthermore, treatment aims to reduce the distress (Finnegan score, excessive crying), preserve weight gain, and improve oral feeding
Breastfeeding has a proven positive effect on the incidence and the extent of neonatal abstinence syndrome (NNT = 5–6)
Opioid withdrawal should be treated with opioids, but practices on the preferred compound (methadone, morphine) vary
Although these concepts can also be applied to withdrawal syndromes resulting from other drugs (e.g., antidepressants, sedatives), the available evidence and guidance are more limited

43.5.2 Antidepressants/SSRI-Related Withdrawal Syndromes

Selective serotonin reuptake inhibitors (SSRIs, e.g., citalopram, paroxetine, fluvoxamine) or serotonin–norepinephrine reuptake inhibitors (SNRIs, e.g., venlafaxine, duloxetine) are commonly used during pregnancy and/or breastfeeding, since depression is a highly prevalent disease in the peripartum period. This incidence is estimated to be as high as 1 in 8 women (Verreault et al. 2014). During pregnancy, antidepressants cross the placenta, but a relevant (i.e., robust and frequent) association with congenital malformations is absent and likely limited to the association between lithium and cardiopathy (RR fivefold to tenfold, but overall risk 1–5% instead of 0.5–1%), most specific for Ebstein's anomaly. Fetal exposure may result in a neonatal clinical syndrome similar to a withdrawal syndrome (poor neonatal adaptation, 30%). SSRIs have also been associated with respiratory distress, persistent pulmonary hypertension (PPHN, absolute risk <1%), and hypoglycemia. However, when evaluating the risk/benefit ratio of SSRI administration in pregnancy, the risk associated with treatment discontinuation (e.g., relapse of psychiatric problems, preterm delivery, postpartum depression) appears to outweigh the risks of therapy continuation. Moreover, maternal depression may negatively affect the child's development, emphasizing the importance of prevention by appropriate treatment during pregnancy with the least minimal effective dose (Ornoy and Koren 2014).

Recently, Reefhuis et al. applied a Bayesian analysis to combine different datasets to explore associations between birth defects and specific SSRIs. None of the earlier reported malformations associated with sertraline were confirmed, and nine previously reported associations between maternal SSRI use and birth defects were rejected (Reefhuis et al. 2015). In contrast, paroxetine (anencephaly OR 3.2; atrial septum defect OR 1.8; right ventricular outflow tract obstruction OR 2.4; gastroschisis OR 2.5; omphalocele 3.5) and fluoxetine (right ventricular outflow tract OR 2; craniosynostosis OR 1.9) have been associated with malformations (Reefhuis et al. 2015). It his hereby important to stress the fact that these are associations, not necessary reflecting causality. Secondly, the OR values observed only result in a very limited increase in the absolute risks.

43.6 Conclusions

In general, drugs are not thoroughly evaluated for use during pregnancy and/or during breastfeeding. Simple extrapolation from data in adults is hazardous, since pregnancy itself affects pharmacokinetics (PK, concentration–time profile) with a subsequent extensive interindividual variability in drug response (PD, concentration–effect profile). Despite the limited available knowledge, women need pharmacotherapy for different medical relevant conditions during pregnancy as well as in the postpartum period, either or not pregnancy related. However, any decision on pharmacotherapy should always be balanced, comparing maternal and fetal/neonatal outcome to the absence of any maternal treatment. This is because there is also a relevant body of evidence showing that uncontrolled or suboptimal controlled maternal conditions in themselves also affect fetal well-being and outcome. The same rationale holds true for breastfeeding. Compound or class-specific information on its use during pregnancy, the postpartum period, and breastfeeding is evolving. This means that updated, reliable information should be easy accessible for caregivers and suggestions on websites have been provided.

Pregnancy category classifications are one approach, but classifications vary somewhat between different authorities, and these categories do not include risks related to drugs or their metabolites via breast milk. The concept of pregnancy exposure registries to build knowledge has been integrated in the recently revised version of the FDA labeling medication guidelines during pregnancy and lactation. In the clinical setting, suggestive indicators of "likely safe during breastfeeding" are (*i*) a drug commonly administered to infants (e.g., antibiotics), (*ii*) a drug that is not absorbed following oral administration (e.g., aminoglycosides, propofol), (*iii*) not excreted into human milk (e.g., insulin, heparin), and finally (*iv*) a drug considered safe during pregnancy, since fetal exposure is generally longer and more extensive. The Pregnancy and Lactation Labeling Final Rule should also provide the tool to generate and collect more reliable information on maternal drug use during breastfeeding. Aspects of opioids, benzodiazepines, and antiepileptics used during fetal or through breastfeeding were discussed first to illustrate the concepts of pregnancy-related clinical pharmacology, followed by a focused discussion on neonatal abstinence syndrome.

43.7 Summary

Any decision on maternal pharmacotherapy should be balanced, comparing maternal and fetal/neonatal outcome to withholding any treatment. This is because there is a relevant body of evidence that uncontrolled maternal conditions also affect fetal outcome. The same holds true for breastfeeding.

Drugs are not thoroughly evaluated for use during pregnancy or breastfeeding. Knowledge on safety of drugs exposure during fetal and neonatal (breastfeeding) life is limited. Pregnancy category classifications for drugs are currently used, but have their limitations. Pregnancy exposure registries to build knowledge have been implemented in the recently revised version of the FDA labeling guidelines (Pregnancy and Lactation Labeling Final Rule).

Suggestive indicators of "likely safe during breastfeeding" are (*i*) drugs commonly administered to infants, (*ii*) drugs that are not absorbed following oral administration, (*iii*) not excreted into human milk, and finally (*iv*) drug considered safe during pregnancy, since fetal exposure is generally longer and more extensive. Aspects of opioids, benzodiazepines, and antiepileptics used during fetal life or via breastfeeding have been discussed to illustrate the concepts of pregnancy-related clinical pharmacology, followed by a focused discussion on neonatal abstinence syndromes. We hereby aim to provide the practicing clinician with some guidance and sources of information.

Acknowledgments Karel Allegaert is supported by the Fund for Scientific Research, Flanders (fundamental clinical investigatorship 1800214 N), and the research activities are further facilitated by the agency for innovation by Science and Technology in Flanders (IWT) through the SAFEPEDRUG project (IWT/SBO 130033). John van den Anker is supported by NIH (K24DA027992, R01HD048689, U54HD071601) and the European Commission (TINN [223614], TINN2 [260908]. NEUROSIS [223060]).

References

Allegaert K, van den Anker JN (2015) Maternal analgosedation and breastfeeding: guidance for the pediatrician. JPNIM 4, e04117

Allegaert K, Langhendries JP, van den Anker JN (2013) Educational paper: do we need neonatal clinical pharmacologists? Eur J Pediatr 172(4):429–435

Amant F, Han SN, Gziri MM et al (2015) Management of cancer in pregnancy. Best Pract Res Clin Obstet Gynaecol 29:741–753

Anderson PO, Pochop SL, Manoquerra AS (2003) Adverse drug reactions in breastfed infants: less than imagined. Clin Pediatr (Phila) 42:325–340

Asti L, Magers JS, Keels E et al (2015) A quality improvement project to reduce length of stay for neonatal abstinence syndrome. Pediatrics 135:e1494–e1500

Bada HS, Sithisam T, Gibson J et al (2015) Morphine versus clonidine for neonatal abstinence syndrome. Pediatrics 135:e383–e391

Berlin CM Jr, van den Anker JN (2013) Safety during breastfeeding: drugs, foods, environmental chemicals, and maternal infections. Semin Fetal Neonatal Med 18:13–18

Briggs GG, Polifka JE, Wisner KL et al (2015) Should pregnant women be included in phase IV clinical drug trials? Am J Obstet Gynecol 213:810–815

Cole AP, Hailey DM (1975) Diazepam and active metabolite in breast milk and their transfer to the neonate. Arch Dis Child 50:741–742

Creanga AA, Sabel JC, Ko JY et al (2012) Maternal drug use and its effect on neonates: a population-based study in Washington State. Obstet Gynecol 119:924–933

De Wildt SN, Kearns GL, Hop WC et al (2002) Pharmacokinetics and metabolism of oral midazolam in preterm infants. Br J Clin Pharmacol 53:390–392

DeVane CL (2015) An epidemic of opioid prescriptions. Pharmacotherapy 35:241–242

Dow K, Ordean A, Murphy-Oikonen J et al (2012) Neonatal abstinence syndrome clinical practice guidelines for Ontario. J Popul Ther Clin Pharmacol 19:e488–e506

Feghali MN, Mattison DR (2011) Clinical therapeutics in pregnancy. J Biomed Biotechnol 2011:783528

Gadot Y, Koren G (2015) The use of antidepressants in pregnancy: focus on maternal risks. J Obstet Gynaecol Can 37:56–63

Genung V (2013) Psychopharmacology column: a review of psychotropic medication lactation risks for infants during breastfeeding. J Child Adolesc Psychiatr Nurs 26:214–219

Hendrickson RG, McKeown NJ (2012) Is maternal opioid use hazardous to breast-fed infants? Clin Toxicol 50:1–14

http://www.fda.gov/Drugs/DevelopmentApprovalProcess/DevelopmentResources/Labeling/ucm093307.html. Accessed 8 July 2015

Hudak ML, Tan RC, Committee on Drugs, Committee on Fetus and Newborn, American Academy of Pediatrics (2012) Neonatal drug withdrawal. Pediatrics 129: e540–e560

Ito S, Blajchman A, Stephenson M, Eliopoloulos C, Koren G (1993) Prospective follow up of adverse reactions in breast-fed infants exposed to maternal medication. Am J Obstet Gynecol 168:1393–1399

Koren G, Cairns J, Chitayat D, Gaedigk A, Leeder SJ (2006) Pharmacogenetics of morphine poisoning in a breastfed neonate of a codeine-prescribed mother. Lancet 368:704

Lam J, Kelly L, Ciszkowski C et al (2012) Central nervous system depression of neonates breastfed by mothers receiving oxycodone for postpartum analgesia. J Pediatr 160:33.e2–37.e2

Lefevere J, Allegaert K (2015) Question: is breastfeeding useful in the management of neonatal abstinence syndrome? Arch Dis Child 100:414–415

MacMullen NJ, Dulski LA, Blobaum P (2014) Evidence-based interventions for neonatal abstinence syndrome. Pediatr Nurs 40:165–172

Marsot A, Brevaut-Malaty V, Vialet R (2014) Pharmacokinetics and absolute bioavailability of phenobarbital in neonates and young infants, a population pharmacokinetic modelling approach. Fundam Clin Pharmacol 28: 465–471

Meador KJ, Baker GA, Browning N et al (2009) Cognitive function at 3 years of age after fetal exposure to antiepileptic drugs. N Engl J Med 360:1597–1605

Meador KJ, Baker GA, Browning N et al (2014) Breastfeeding in children of women taking antiepileptic drugs. Cognitive outcomes at age 6 years. JAMA Pediatr 168:729–736

Ng CM, Dombrowsky E, Lin H et al (2015) Population pharmacokinetic model of sublingual buprenorphine in neonatal abstinence syndrome. Pharmacotherapy 35(7): 670–680

Nitsun M, Szokol JW, Saleh HJ et al (2006) Pharmacokinetics of midazolam, propofol, and fentanyl transfer to human breast milk. Clin Pharmacol Ther 79:549–557

O'Donnell M, Nassar N, Leonard H et al (2009) Increasing prevalence of neonatal withdrawal syndrome: population study of maternal factors and child protection involvement. Pediatrics 123:e614–e621

Ornoy A, Koren G (2014) Selective serotonin reuptake inhibitors in human pregnancy: on the way to resolving the controversy. Semin Fetal Neonatal Med 19:188–194

Patrick SW, Schumacher RE, Benneyworth BD et al (2012) Neonatal abstinence syndrome and associated health care expenditures: United States, 2000–2009. JAMA 307:1934–1940

Patrick SW, Davis MM, Lehman CU, Cooper WO (2015) Increasing incidence and geographic distribution of neonatal abstinence syndrome: United States 2009 to 2012. J Perinatol 35:650–655

Pavek P, Ceckova M, Staud F (2009) Variation of drug kinetics in pregnancy. Curr Drug Metab 10:520–529

Pressler RM, Mangum B (2013) Newly emerging therapies for neonatal seizures. Semin Fetal Neonatal Med 18:216–223

Ramoz LL, Patel-Shori NM (2014) Recent changes in pregnancy and lactation labeling: retirement of risk categories. Pharmacotherapy 34:389–395

Reefhuis J, Devine O, Friedman JM et al (2015) Specific SSRIs and birth defects bayesian analysis to interpret new data in the context of previous reports. BMJ 351: h3190

Rivers CM, Olsen D, Nelson LS (2012) Breastfeeding and oxycodone. J Pediatr 161:174

Rowe H, Baker T, Hale TW (2013) Maternal medication, drug use, and breastfeeding. Pediatr Clin North Am 60:275–294

Saadeh RJ (2012) The Baby-Friendly Hospital Initiative 20 years on: facts, progress, and the way forward. J Hum Lact 28:272–275

Sachs HC, Committee on Drugs (2013) The transfer of drugs and therapeutics into human breast milk: an update on selected topics. Pediatrics 132:e796–e809

Salman S, Sy SK, Ilett KF, Page-Sharp M, Paech MJ (2011) Population pharmacokinetic modeling of tramadol and its *O*-desmethyl metabolite in plasma and breast milk. Eur J Clin Pharmacol 67:899–908

Sistonen J, Madadi P, Ros CJ et al (2012) Prediction of codeine toxicity in infants and their mothers using a novel combination of maternal genetic markers. Clin Pharmacol Ther 91:692–699

Siu A, Robinson CA (2014) Neonatal abstinence syndrome: essentials for the practitioner. J Pediatr Pharmacol Ther 19:147–155

Thomas SH, Yates LM (2012) Prescribing without evidence – pregnancy. Br J Clin Pharmacol 74:691–697

Turner SD, Gomes T, Camacho X et al (2015) Neonatal opioid withdrawal and antenatal opioid prescribing. CAMJ Open 13:E55–E61

Van den Anker JN (2012) Is it safe to use opioids for obstetric pain while breastfeeding? J Pediatr 160:4–6

Veiby G, Engelsen BA, Gilhus NE (2013) Early child development and exposure to antiepileptic drugs prenatally and through breastfeeding: a prospective cohort study on children of women with epilepsy. JAMA Neurol 70:1367–1374

Veiby G, Bjork M, Engelsen BA, Gilhus NE (2015) Epilepsy and recommendations for breastfeeding. Seizure 28:57–65

Verreault N, Da Costa D, Marchand A et al (2014) Rates and risk factors associated with depressive symptoms during pregnancy and with postpartum onset. J Psychosom Obstet Gynaecol 35:84–91

Wachman EM, Hayes MJ, Brown MS et al (2013) Association of OPRM1 and COMT single-nucleotide polymorphisms with hospital length of stay and treatment of neonatal abstinence syndrome. JAMA 309: 1821–1827

Zaijcek A, Giacoia GP (2007) Obstetric clinical pharmacology: coming of age. Clin Pharmacol Ther 81:481–482

Zimmermann-Baer U, Nötzi U, Rentsch K, Bucher HU (2010) Finnegan neonatal abstinence scoring system: normal values for first 3 days and weeks 5–6 in non-addicted infants. Addiction 105:524–528

Developmental Pharmacology and Therapeutics in Neonatal Medicine

44

Karel Allegaert, Janko Samardzic, Milica Bajcetic, and John N. van den Anker

Contents

K. Allegaert (✉)
Neonatal Intensive Care Unit, University Hospitals Leuven, Leuven, Belgium

Department of Development and Regeneration, KU Leuven, Leuven, Belgium

Intensive Care and Department of Pediatric Surgery, Erasmus MC – Sophia Children's Hospital, Rotterdam, The Netherlands
e-mail: karel.allegaert@uzleuven.be; allegaertkarel@hotmail.com

J. Samardzic
Department of Paediatric Pharmacology, University Children's Hospital Basel, Basel, Switzerland

Institute of Pharmacology, Clinical Pharmacology and Toxicology, Medical Faculty, University of Belgrade, Belgrade, Serbia
e-mail: janko@med.bg.ac.rs

M. Bajcetic
Institute of Pharmacology, Clinical Pharmacology and Toxicology, Medical Faculty, University of Belgrade, Belgrade, Serbia

Clinical Pharmacology Unit, University Children's Hospital, Belgrade, Serbia
e-mail: mbajcetic@doctor.com

J. N. van den Anker
Division of Pediatric Clinical Pharmacology, Children's National Health System, Washington, DC, USA

Departments of Pediatrics, Integrative Systems Biology, Pharmacology and Physiology, George Washington University, School of Medicine and Health Sciences, Washington, DC, USA

Intensive Care and Department of Pediatric Surgery, Erasmus MC – Sophia Children's Hospital, Rotterdam, The Netherlands
e-mail: Jvandena@childrensnational.org

G. Buonocore et al. (eds.), *Neonatology*,
https://doi.org/10.1007/978-3-319-29489-6_193

Abstract

Knowledge about the safe and effective use of medicines in neonates has increased substantially but resulted in few label changes. Despite the extent of these drug exposures, newborns remain the last therapeutic orphans. Drugs, initially developed for use in adults, are reshaped and tailored to specific neonatal indications. However, neonatal pharmacotherapy not only mirrors adult pharmacotherapy but should be driven by their own specific needs. This is because both pharmacokinetics (absorption, distribution, metabolism, elimination, concentration-time) and pharmacodynamics (concentration-effect) display extensive maturation in early infancy, reflecting maturational physiology. We describe and illustrate the relevance of these maturational changes. We subsequently focus on specific aspects related to therapeutic drug monitoring, the need for population tailored neonatal formulations (*including dose flexibility and excipients*), and the difficulties related to the recognition of adverse drug reactions in neonates (*how to recognize a signal in the noise*).

44.1 Salient Points

- Critically ill newborns receive between 15 and 20 (intravenous) drugs per day, most of them either unlicensed or off-label.
- Clinical pharmacology aims to predict drug-specific (side) effects based on pharmacokinetics and pharmacodynamics.
- Pharmacokinetics (absorption, distribution, and elimination, through either metabolism or primary renal elimination) provides an estimate of the relationship between a drug concentration at a specific site and time.
- Pharmacodynamics estimates the relationship between a drug concentration and (side) effects ("what the drug does to the body").
- A specific issue in neonates is the unanticipated higher absorption of drugs administered transdermally due to proportionally higher body surface area and increased skin permeability.
- Differences in the distribution of a drug are influenced by body composition, systemic and regional blood flow, plasma protein binding, as well as the variable permeability of membranes associated with disease states.
- The primary organ for drug metabolism is the liver, but other organs (kidneys, intestines, lungs, skin, brain) can also display drug metabolizing capacity.
- Differences in neonatal physiology can also affect pharmacodynamics and may result in differences in drug potency, efficacy, or toxicity.
- Therapeutic drug monitoring may help to avoid side effects, but any measurement needs to be integrated into the clinical setting of the individual patient.
- For some drug classes, clinical monitoring (e.g., body temperature, blood pressure, analgesia, sedation) is superior to drug monitoring that is driven by a therapeutic approach.
- Neonates require tailored drug product development that utilizes both low and flexible dosing to maintain dose accuracy.
- Neonatal pharmacotherapy is a powerful tool to improve outcome, but there is an obvious and urgent need to improve our practices

through tailored adverse drug reaction prevention and management.

- Pharmacovigilance to improve adverse drug reaction prevention and management needs to be adapted to the requirements and characteristics of neonates and infants.

44.2 Introduction

44.2.1 Knowledge on Neonatal Pharmacotherapy Is Lagging Behind

Drug therapy is a very powerful tool to improve the medical outcome of neonates. Yet, caregivers still commonly prescribe drug formulations and dosing regimens that initially were developed for adults, extrapolating from indications initially validated in adult medicine and based on the pathophysiology proper to the adult patient (Fanos and Yurdakök 2010; Kearns et al. 2003; Allegaert and van den Anker 2014a).

Critically ill newborns receive between 15 and 20 (intravenous) drugs per day, most of them either unlicensed or off-label. Off-label drugs are defined as being prescribed in a different manner to label recommendations in terms of age group, dose, frequency, formulation, administration route, indication, or contraindication for use in neonates (Dessi et al. 2010; Kieran et al. 2014; Laforgia et al. 2014; Carvalho et al. 2012; Di Paolo et al. 2006; Riou et al. 2015). Figure 1 depicts the extent of the problem (at least 50% of the drugs administered, but up to >90% in extreme preterm neonates), resulting in the fact that almost

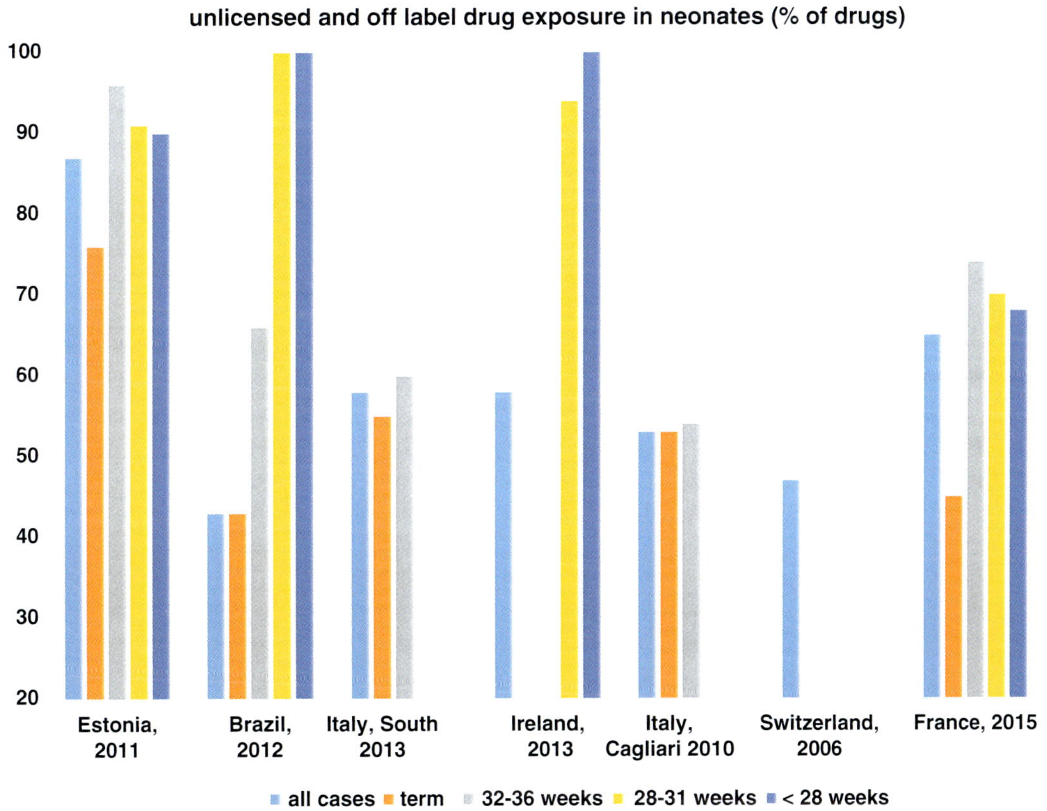

Fig. 1 Overview of recent publications on the extent of unlicensed and off-label drug exposure in neonates in different regions of Europe and beyond. This practice is even more present in the most immature neonates (Dessi et al. 2010; Kieran et al. 2014; Laforgia et al. 2014; Carvalho et al. 2012; Di Paolo et al. 2006; Riou et al. 2015; Lass et al. 2011)

all NICU patients are exposed to off-label drugs. Figure 1 hereby also shows that this is an international problem that persists (Dessi et al. 2010; Kieran et al. 2014; Laforgia et al. 2014; Carvalho et al. 2012; Di Paolo et al. 2006; Riou et al. 2015). In a survey, it was documented that the top 10 of medications most commonly prescribed in the NICU were ampicillin, gentamicin, ferrous sulfate, multivitamins, cefotaxime, caffeine citrate, furosemide, vancomycin, surfactant, and metoclopramide (Clark et al. 2006). Interestingly, drug prescription patterns differ in patient populations with raised mortality and higher disease severity (Carvalho et al. 2012; Clark et al. 2006). Over time, significant changes in drug utilization patterns occur. To illustrate this, drug utilization patterns (1997–1998 to 2001–2004) in a single NICU documented an increased utilization of antibiotics, central nervous system, endocrinology, cardiovascular, and gastrointestinal drugs. Some individual drug changes include an increased use of vancomycin, cefepime, and caffeine, whereas a decreased use of morphine was seen (Du et al. 2006).

Despite the extent of these drug exposures, newborns remain the last therapeutic orphans (Stiers and Ward 2014; Laughon et al. 2014). The federal US legislation and similar European initiatives have resulted in a relevant increase in pharmacological studies in children, with a subsequent significant increase in label changes. Unfortunately, only a few included drug label changes for neonates. To further illustrate this: there were 406 pediatric label changes (Food and Drug Administration, 1997–2010), but only 23 drugs resulted in 11 labeled indications (e.g., linezolid, rocuronium, remifentanil, sevoflurane, stavudine, nevirapine) for neonates. The absence of label change was most commonly because of unproven efficacy, despite the fact that these compounds (e.g., acetaminophen, caspofungin, valganciclovir) are relevant for neonates (Stiers and Ward 2014; Laughon et al. 2014). This may largely reflect the difficulties to proof efficacy (e.g., heterogeneity in patients, variability in outcome variables, uncertainty on biomarkers) in neonates.

44.2.2 Aiming at a Moving Target: Neonatal Physiology Affects Neonatal Pharmacotherapy

Human growth and development consists of a sequence of physiologic events that link somatic growth with maturation since weight gain coexists but is not similar to maturation. Across pediatric life, organ size and function change as does body composition, (patho)physiology, and ultimately cellular function. When we consider these physiological changes and the subsequent variability in physiological characteristics, we should be aware that maturational changes in physiology are most prominent in early infancy (Kearns et al. 2003; Allegaert and van den Anker 2014a; Smits et al. 2012a). If we focus on weight changes to further illustrate this, there is an initial decrease (6–12%) in birth weight, with a subsequent increase of 50% in the first 6 weeks of postnatal life. Moreover, weight doubles in the first 3–4 months to result in a threefold higher weight at the end of infancy. Consequently, total energy requirements change dramatically as the sum of energy expenditure and energy deposition for growth (Kearns et al. 2003; Allegaert and van den Anker 2014a; Smits et al. 2012a). These maturational physiological trends are further affected by either treatment modalities (e.g., whole body cooling, extracorporeal membrane oxygenation (ECMO), or pharmacotherapy) used or pathophysiological processes or comorbidities (e.g., perinatal asphyxia, cardiopathy, sepsis, renal failure, patent ductus arteriosus) involved. All these changes, both maturational (e.g., age, weight) and pathophysiological, result in extensive variability within the first months of postnatal life. This results in the fact that neonatal pharmacotherapy is as diverse as the neonates taken care of in our units (Kearns et al. 2003; Allegaert and van den Anker 2014a; Smits et al. 2012a).

The aim of administering a given compound is to reach effective treatment for a specific disease while avoiding disproportional side effects. Clinical pharmacology aims to predict drug-specific (side) effects based on pharmacokinetics and pharmacodynamics. Pharmacokinetics (PK,

Table 1 Examples of the developmental changes in neonatal pharmacokinetics and the clinical implications

Physiological system	Neonatal physiology compared to children and adults	Pharmacokinetic implications	Clinical implications
Gastrointestinal tract	Reduced and irregular peristalsis followed by slow gastric emptying, in part driven by the feeding regimen (breast milk vs. formula)	Slower absorption of the drug (e.g., delayed Tmax)	Possible sustained action after oral administration of the drug
	Increased gastric pH (>4) in relation to infants	Faster absorption of acid-labile and reduced absorption of weak-acid drugs	The possibility of altered bioavailability
Muscle tissue	Reduction in muscle perfusion, decreased muscle contractility	Poor perfusion limits the absorption, unpredictable pharmacokinetics	Avoid intramuscular administration of drugs
Skin	Thinner stratum corneum, increased skin perfusion, increased water content, and higher body surface area-to-weight ratio	Increased rate and extent of absorption of the drug through the skin	Increased bioavailability and potential toxicity of drugs applied topically The need for a reduced amount of the drug applied to the skin
Body composition	Lower proportion of adipose tissue (10%), decreased muscle mass, increased amount of total body water related to the body weight (80%), an increased proportion of the extracellular (45%) compared to the intracellular fluid compartment	Increased volume of distribution for water-soluble drugs and a reduced volume for drugs which are bound to muscles and adipose tissue	Consider to adjust the loading/maintenance dosing (mg/kg) to achieve therapeutic plasma concentrations of the drug
Plasma protein binding	Reduced concentrations of albumin and α-1 acid glycoprotein, with a decreased drug protein-binding affinity	Increased plasma concentration of unbound drug, with an increased volume of distribution and the possibility of occurrence of toxic effects	For drugs with high binding affinity for proteins (e.g., >70%), please consider an alternative, or maintain the plasma drug concentrations to the lower limit of the recommended therapeutic range, interaction with, e.g., indirect bilirubin
Drug metabolism	Immature isoforms of cytochrome P450 and phase II enzymes with isoenzyme-specific maturation	Isoenzyme-specific, reduced hepatic drug metabolism, with increase in half-life	To increase dosing interval of the drug and/or reduce the maintenance dose
Renal drug excretion	Decreased level of glomerular filtration rate and active tubular secretion/absorption	Accumulation of drugs and/or the active metabolites that are secreted via the kidneys with a decrease in plasma clearance	To increase dosing interval of the drug and/or reduce the maintenance dose

absorption, ***d***istribution, and elimination, through either ***m***etabolism or primary renal ***e***limination, ***ADME***) hereby estimate the relationship between a drug concentration at a specific site (e.g., plasma, cerebrospinal fluid) and time ("what the body does to the drug").

The potential impact of developmental pharmacokinetics on neonatal pharmacotherapy is illustrated in Table 1. Pharmacodynamics (PD) estimates the relationship between a drug concentration and (side) effects ("what the drug does to the body"). We will first discuss aspects of developmental pharmacokinetics and pharmacodynamics in neonates. This will provide the rationale for a focused neonatal pharmacotherapy and product development, as illustrated by the tailored use of therapeutic drug monitoring (4), specific issues on formulations (5), and pharmacovigilance (6) in neonates.

44.3 Developmental Pharmacokinetics

44.3.1 Absorption

Drug absorption is affected by age, formulation, dose, or route of administration as well as by food and other drugs that interact with the active compound (Kearns et al. 2003; Allegaert and van den Anker 2014a; Smits et al. 2012a; Choonara 1994). For example, in neonates intragastric pH is elevated (>4). This may increase the bioavailability of acid-labile compounds (penicillin G) and decrease the bioavailability of weak acids (phenobarbital) when given orally (Huang and High 1953). Additionally, gastric emptying in neonates is delayed, which means that also duodenal absorption of drugs (e.g., paracetamol) is slower in neonates. Gastric emptying in part also depends on the nutrition with a faster emptying for breast milk or extensive hydrolysate formulations (Staelens et al. 2008). There is only limited knowledge on the ontogeny of intestinal transporters and its covariates, but some data suggest that this is at least in part driven by the intestinal microflora (Mooij et al. 2012). Characteristics that affect variability in absorption, resulting in unpredictable pharmacokinetics of drugs administered intramuscularly, include decreased muscle mass, decreased contractility, and reduced overall muscular perfusion (Kearns et al. 2003). A specific issue in neonates is the unanticipated higher absorption of drugs administered transdermally due to proportionally higher body surface area and a more permeable skin. These differences are even more pronounced in premature neonates (Kearns et al. 2003; Choonara 1994).

44.3.2 Distribution

The differences in distribution of the drug are influenced by body composition, systemic and regional blood flow, plasma protein binding, as well as permeability of membranes, associated with disease states (Kearns et al. 2003; Allegaert and van den Anker 2014a; Smits et al. 2012a). The body composition in early infancy changes continuously and rapidly, resulting in an age-dependent proportion of total body water and fat. The total body water content is markedly higher in neonates (80–90% of the body weight) compared to the end of infancy (60–65%) or adults (55–60%). To further illustrate this, hydrophilic drugs like aminoglycosides have a larger volume of distribution in neonates that can be explained by a larger extracellular volume compartment (40–45% of the body weight) compared to 25–30% at the end of infancy and to 20% in adults (Kearns et al. 2003; Allegaert and van den Anker 2014a; Smits et al. 2012a). Thus, the peak plasma concentration of aminoglycosides will not only be delayed but also blunted compared to older children or adults. Protein-binding capacity is another covariate of the distribution volume. The amount and type of circulating plasma proteins does not only influence drug disposition but also drug action, since only the unbound drug can be distributed throughout the body and have a pharmacological effect (Roberts et al. 2013). Clinical implications of alterations in drug protein binding are most relevant for drugs which are highly protein bound and have a narrow therapeutic index (Roberts et al. 2013). To illustrate this, differences in protein-binding characteristics and their covariates within neonates as well as compared to other populations have recently been described for cefazolin (Smits et al. 2012b) and differences in protein binding explain the higher clearance of micafungin in neonates (Yanni et al. 2011). Specifically in neonates, unconjugated bilirubin, and free fatty acid concentrations will also display relevant competition for albumin-binding places (Kearns et al. 2003; Smits et al. 2012b).

44.3.3 Drug Elimination: Drug Metabolism and Primary Renal Clearance

To eliminate a given compound from the body through bodily fluids such a urine or bile, either drug metabolism, primary renal elimination clearance, or both are involved. Both processes display ontogeny, i.e., age-driven maturation (Hines 2013; de Wildt 2011). However, the maturation pattern of the individual hepatic or renal clearance processes differs to a large extent. This means that integration of all ontogeny-related knowledge of the different elimination routes is important to understand compound-specific, phenotypic in vivo observations in neonates (Hines 2013; de Wildt 2011; Allegaert et al. 2014).

The primary organ for drug metabolism is the liver, but also other organs (kidneys, intestines, lungs, skin, brain) can display drug metabolizing capacity. In general, drug metabolism is low in neonates and phenotypic activity of drug metabolizing enzymes is considered as a main contributor to the PK differences between neonates, children, and adults. Variation in phenotypic metabolic clearance is based on constitutional, environmental, and genetic factors (Kearns et al. 2003; Hines 2013; de Wildt 2011; Allegaert et al. 2014). In early infancy, this is mainly a reflection of the ontogeny, but other covariates may also become relevant. However, this does not exclude extensive interindividual variability within the neonatal population (Kearns et al. 2003; Allegaert and van den Anker 2014a).

Drug metabolizing enzymes are crucial in drug biotransformation and metabolic elimination. Consequently, drug metabolizing isoenzyme-specific ontogeny will affect neonatal drug clearance. Profound maturational changes in drug metabolizing enzyme activity occur during development. These changes have impact on drug clearance, drug effect, and the risk of adverse events in the neonate. The available evidence suggests that the individual hepatic drug metabolizing isoenzymes can be categorized into one of three classes based on developmental trajectories. A first group of enzymes (e.g., SULT1A3/1A4, CYP3A7) is expressed at their highest level in fetal life and subsequent decrease and disappear over the first 2 years of life. The second group contains enzymes (e.g., CYP2C19, CYP3A5, SULT1A1) that display a modest increase after birth and become more active after neonatal life or infancy. Finally, the last group (e.g., CYP2D6, CYP3A4, CYP2C9, CYP1A2) already has moderate ontogeny in the second half of pregnancy, with a subsequent more pronounced increase in phenotypic activity during early life (Kearns et al. 2003; Hines 2013; de Wildt 2011).

Most drugs or their metabolites are excreted from the body by the kidney. Again, renal elimination capacity is influenced by physiological changes depending on age, e.g., the glomerular filtration rate (GFR) in full term neonates is 35% of the adult values (Smits et al. 2012a; Schreuder et al. 2014). Term neonates have a rapid increase in GFR during the first 2 weeks of life and reach adult values by the end of the first year of life. Premature infants have similar maturational trends, but with a slower initial GFR rise because nephrogenesis is not completed before near term age, at about 34–35 weeks of gestation. Both active tubular secretion and reabsorption are also immature at birth (20–30% of adult reference values) only to reach adult values in the second part of infancy or beyond (Smits et al. 2012a; Schreuder et al. 2014).

In clinical care, a more integrated approach is needed when considering these different elimination processes: *there is no isolated neonatal liver or neonatal kidney, but only newborns in need for improved pharmacotherapy*. The maturational pattern of the individual renal or hepatic elimination processes may be different. This necessitates the integration of the ontogeny-related knowledge of the different elimination routes (metabolic vs. elimination clearance) involved to predict compound-specific, concentration-time profiles in neonates: accumulation of a given metabolite may be due to less effective (renal) elimination capacity compared to hepatic metabolic clearance (Allegaert et al. 2014).

44.4 Developmental Pharmacodynamics

Differences in neonatal physiology can also affect PD and may result in differences in drug potency, efficacy, or toxicity. However, most of the variability observed relates to differences in PK and maturational PD can only be considered once the PK aspects have been taken into account. Age-related developmental changes in the functionality and expression of receptors and differences in disease status may alter the pharmacological response to drugs (Mulla 2010; Stephenson 2005). For example, inotropic agents in neonatal myocardium act in a more limited fashion than those of the child or adult. This is due to a lower ratio of active myofilaments to noncontractile elements, greater stiffness of the ventricle, underdeveloped cardiac sympathetic nerves, and higher cardiac output per unit surface area (Bajcetic et al. 2014). Furthermore, immaturity can result in an altered risk of drug toxicity, even a decreased risk (McIntyre and Choonara 2004). To illustrate this, neonates appear to be less susceptible to renal toxicity induced by aminoglycosides compared to children and adults. A reduced intracellular accumulation of these compounds in the tubular epithelial cells of the renal cortex seems to be the underlying mechanism of this PD characteristic. More research, especially on PD in the neonatal period and the subsequent clinical implications, is needed.

44.5 Therapeutic Drug Monitoring

Therapeutic drug monitoring (TDM) aims to integrate drug measurement as an adjunct to clinical decision-making, with the aim to improve therapeutic responses and/or decrease adverse events. In essence, it is common practice to collect plasma samples at predefined time points and decrease the toxicity or efficacy by application of pharmacokinetics and pharmacodynamics (Van den Anker 2014; Young 2012).

One of the issues that really matter in the clinical decision process is the relevance of "steady state." Especially in the absence of the use of a loading dose, it takes time before the equilibrium is reached after a drug was started. This is illustrated in Fig. 2, based on the estimated concentration-time profile for a newborn, treated twice daily with 10 mg/kg vancomycin intravenously. Figure 2 nicely shows that accumulation takes time, resulting in different trough concentrations when sampled before the 3rd, 5th, or 7th administration (arrows a, b, and c) because it takes time to reach steady state.

Current observations suggest that the greatest benefit of TDM within the neonatal population

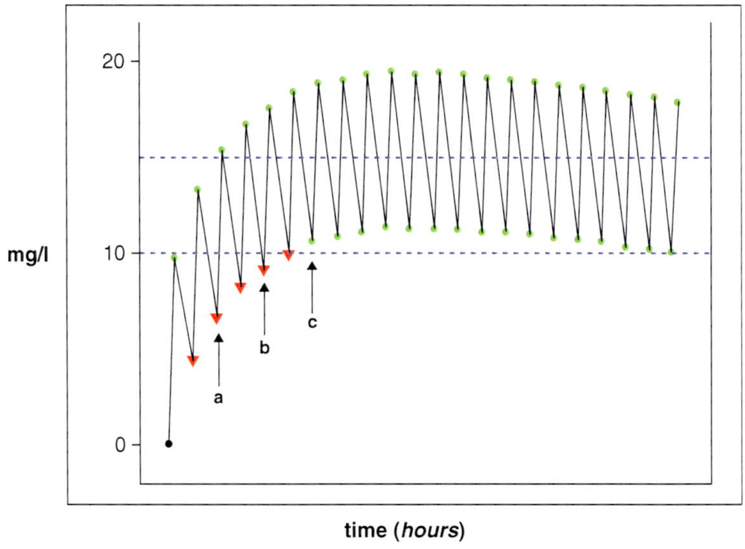

Fig. 2 The estimated concentration-time profile for a newborn, treated twice daily with 10 mg/kg vancomycin intravenously. Accumulation takes time, resulting in different trough concentrations when sampled just before the 3rd, 5th, or 7th administration (*arrows a*, *b*, and *c*)

Table 2 The general rules to assess the usefulness of therapeutic drug monitoring

It is reasonable to assume a quantitative relationship between the concentration (e.g., plasma) and a clinical (side)effect
There is only a poor correlation between the dose administered and the concentration reached (limited predictability)
The pharmacokinetics are known (a TDM result can be used to adapt the treatment)
The analytical technique is sufficiently specific, precise, and accurate in the specific population considered (e.g., neonatal plasma)
The therapeutic index of the given compound is narrow. There are significant consequences associated with either overexposure (e.g., toxicity) or underexposure (e.g., therapeutic failure)

very likely is mainly in targeted or special subpopulations: those with severely decompensated renal function, those at the extremes of age, those using immunosuppressive, specific antineoplastic, or anticonvulsant drugs, and those with anticipated drug-drug interactions. The general clinical rules before TDM is considered to be useful are provided in Table 2. We aim to discuss how these clinical rules apply to neonates, followed by some additional comments on how to integrate TDM with other clinical characteristics (Van den Anker 2014; Young 2012).

44.5.1 Limited Predictability: Is There a Poor Correlation Between Dose and Concentration?

The interindividual variability of drug disposition in neonates is – in general – pronounced: despite their small size, there is extensive variability in clearance and concentration-time profiles (Allegaert and van den Anker 2014a). To illustrate this, aminoglycosides are almost exclusively eliminated by the renal route. Birth weight, postnatal age, but also co-medication (ibuprofen, indomethacin) and peripartal asphyxia are the most relevant covariates of clearance, presumably because it predicts the time course of development of the glomerular filtration rate. However, interindividual variability in aminoglycoside clearance is high. In early life, the predictability of aminoglycoside clearance is less than 65% when these covariates are considered (De Cock et al. 2012). Taking this indicator of appropriateness into account, TDM in early neonatal life may be indicated. The same holds true for, e.g., vancomycin and for phenobarbital (Van den Anker 2014; Young 2012).

44.5.2 Is There a Quantitative Relationship Between Concentration and Effect?

For a relevant number of drug classes, clinical monitoring (e.g., body temperature, blood pressure, analgesia, sedation) is superior to any TDM-driven approach. Bedside up or down titration can be driven by the pharmacodynamic outcome variables aimed for. Obviously, the introduction of more sophisticated tools (e.g., aEEG vs. clinical seizures in neonates) may further support such clinical monitoring or may further improve the concentration (TDM)/effect relation and clinical titration (Young 2012). In contrast, it is much more difficult to evaluate the concentration-effect relation for antibiotics. Epidemiologic data on incidence of infections in neonates, the immaturity of the immune system, and the occult clinical symptoms of infection explain the frequent (over)use of antibiotics, including aminoglycosides or vancomycin in neonates (Young 2012; De Cock et al. 2012; Van den Anker 2011). Infectious diseases or septicemia are frequent causes of morbidity and mortality in preterm and term neonates.

44.5.3 Is There a Narrow Therapeutic Index: Concentration and (Side) Effects?

Besides effects, a drug may also cause side effects. Such side effects may relate to idiosyncrasy in individual cases (e.g., genetic predisposition, allergy, or pseudo-allergy). TDM may be helpful to avoid such side effects, similar to the use of the oxygen saturation monitor to avoid hyperoxia, or the measurement of thyroid function (e.g., amiodarone), liver enzymes (e.g., valproate), or renal function (e.g., ibuprofen). The extended interval dosing approach for aminoglycosides has resulted in higher peak and lower trough levels in neonates (Smits et al. 2012a; Schreuder et al. 2014; De Cock et al. 2012). This practice is supported by data on reduced nephrotoxicity in children and adults, but there is only indirect evidence for this approach in neonates (Rao et al. 2011). Raised phenobarbital levels are associated with oversedation and miosis, and raised diphantoine levels may cause arrhythmia (Young 2012; Boylan et al. 2013).

44.5.4 Significant Consequences of Therapeutic Failure Should Be Considered

Morbidity and mortality in extreme preterm neonates is extensive, relevant, and common. Consequently, in the clinical setting, it is difficult to disentangle therapeutic failure due to immaturity, comorbidity, or inappropriate choice of antibiotics (e.g., resistant pathogen), compared to "just" insufficient dosing. Similar, prolonged low concentrations of antibiotics may also induce bacterial resistance or fungal colonization (Van den Anker 2014; Young 2012). Although clinicians may feel confident to use international "reference" handbooks for drug dosing, we would like to stress that there is extensive and unexplained variability in dosing regimens between these textbooks (De Cock et al. 2012; Van den Anker 2011).

44.5.5 Therapeutic Drug Monitoring Will Not Replace Common Clinical Sense

Even if TDM is implemented, any measurement needs to be integrated in the clinical setting of the individual patient. Some relevant issues relate to, e.g., the time of sampling: is the patient already at steady state or not yet? Moreover, the specific methods used to measure either biomarkers (e.g., creatinine) or the drug itself (e.g., vancomycin measurements) may differ. Finally, we should not forget that pharmacotherapy in newborn infants remains shooting at a moving target. Using the indicators of appropriateness for TDM (Table 2), we conclude that neonates are in a rapidly evolving pharmacokinetic state. In addition to these maturational processes, most drug pharmacokinetic studies in neonates show wide interindividual variability despite similar ages. Taking this into account, and despite the relative lack of robust outcome data, TDM is a necessary tool in the neonatal intensive care unit, when combined with the clinician input of a dedicated pharmacist or pharmacologist (Van den Anker 2014; Young 2012).

44.6 Neonatal Formulations

The key characteristic of neonatal pharmacotherapy is its extensive variability, related to maturational and non-maturational covariates. This means that the neonatal community needs to have access to drug formulations tailored to the characteristics of neonates (Turner 2011). However, this does not mean that the basics of drug formulation should be neglected such as data on product stability, palatability, or compatibility (Tuleu and Breitkreutz 2013). At present, neonates are still commonly treated with drugs that have not been designed, developed, nor evaluated for use in them. As a consequence, this exposes neonates to the likely risks related to suboptimal (*too* low, *too* high, or *too* variable) dosing and side effects from potentially toxic ingredients, including excipients (Turner 2011; Tuleu and Breitkreutz 2013; Fabiano et al. 2011; Turner et al. 2014). We have illustrated the impact of dosing accuracy for two different amikacin vials (50 or 250 mg/ml) in comparing the extent of variability. The introduction of a pediatric amikacin vial resulted in a reduction in clearance variability, reflecting improved dosing precision (Allegaert et al. 2006). The issue of highly concentrated formulations is further illustrated in Table 3. This table is based on currently available vials in the Leuven NICU and reflects

Table 3 Illustrations of some highly concentrated formulations for intravenous use, compared to the doses applied in neonates. As a consequence, consecutive dilution, dosing inaccuracy, or tenfold errors are more likely to occur

Midazolam	15 mg/3 ml	0.05–0.1	mg/kg
Paracetamol/ acetaminophen	500 mg/50 ml	10	mg/kg
Propofol	200 mg/20 ml	1–3	mg/kg
Phenobarbital	200 mg/1 ml	5	mg/kg
Fentanyl	100 μgr/2 ml	1–3	μgr/kg
Insulin	300 E/3 ml	0.1–1	E/kg/h
Enoxaparin	40 mg/0.4 ml	1	mg/kg
Ranitidine	50 mg/2 ml	0.5–1	mg/kg
Dopamine	50 mg/1.25 ml	4–16	μg/kg/min
Heparin	5,000 IU/ml	10–30	IU/kg/h

the necessity of sequential dilution and subsequent reduced dosing precision (Nunn et al. 2013). In essence, neonates are in need of tailored drug product development that considers both low and flexible dosing to maintain dose accuracy.

At present, marketed formulations commonly do not meet yet the specific requirements for neonates (formulation, dose), and it is unlikely that commercially manufactured, ready-to-administer neonatal preparations will be available in the near future for all compounds prescribed. As a consequence, compounding ("extemporaneous preparation") practices will remain common practice in the near future for neonatal therapeutics (Nunn et al. 2013). Until tailored formulations will make it to the market, compounding practices for drug formulations in neonates should be evaluated to guarantee correct dosing and product stability and safety and to support pharmacists in their clinical practice. To illustrate the need to validate such compounding practices, we refer to the results of an evaluation of a pediatric oral formulation with a low amount of hydrochlorothiazide, also considered to be suited for use in neonates: only one of five hydrochlorothiazide suspensions guaranteed the correct dosing and stability after 3 weeks of storage in predefined, optimal condition (Santovena et al. 2012).

During the development of such formulations tailored for neonates, there is also a need for more guidance on excipient exposure (Fabiano et al. 2011; Turner et al. 2013). In addition to the active compounds, drug formulations also commonly contain excipients such as, e.g., cosolvents, preservatives, sweeteners, or colorants. Examples of excipients are lactose, aspartame, xylitol, propylene glycol, polyethylene glycol, benzyl alcohol, ethanol, sorbitol, or mannitol. Historical observations but also more recent case series repeatedly confronted clinicians with unanticipated, but sometimes predictable, severe side effects of neonatal drug formulations merely because of its excipients, e.g., benzyl alcohol, propylene glycol, or ethanol (Fabiano et al. 2011; Turner et al. 2013, 2014).

The use of potentially toxic excipients in medicines given to neonates is not rare, as they are present in many commonly used drug products. At least, recent observational studies confirmed the almost uniform exposure to relevant excipients (e.g., propylene glycol, ethanol, benzyl alcohol) in neonates (Fabiano et al. 2011; Turner et al. 2013, 2014). The available knowledge on the safety or toxicity of excipients is limited and difficult to retrieve, but there are initiatives (e.g., Safety and Toxicity of Excipients for Pediatrics [STEP] database initiative) to improve the present situation (Salunke et al. 2013). In addition, population-focused studies on aspects of clinical pharmacology of excipients in neonates are conducted. The propylene glycol research project and the European Study for Neonatal Excipient Exposure (ESNEE) initiative illustrate at least the feasibility to collect such information (methyl- and propyl-parabens, propylene glycol) (Salunke et al. 2013; De Cock et al. 2013; Mulla et al. 2015).

In order to improve formulations for neonates and young children, the World Health Organization has launched a global campaign: "Make medicines child size" (WHO, UNICEF). Furthermore, the European Paediatric Formulation Initiative (EuPFI) was founded with the aim of raising awareness of pediatric formulation issues (European Union Pediatric Formulations Initiative). Besides knowledge gathering on excipients (Salunke et al. 2013), novel formulations for neonates were developed, like fast-dissolving drug formulations, including orodispersible minitablets (ODMT) and oral thin (buccal wafers) and multiparticulate dosage forms that facilitate the administration of low doses (Tuleu and Breitkreutz 2013).

Specific new formulations for neonates are orodispersible minitablets (ODMTs). Such tablets disintegrate immediately upon contact with water or saliva. This permits convenient oral administration, as well as preparation of drug solutions immediately before administration. While minitablets retain some potential to stick to the esophagus, this risk is completely eliminated with ODMTs because of their rapid disintegration upon contact with water or saliva (Stoltenberg and Breitkreutz 2011). At present, an ODMT formulation of enalapril as well as hydrochlorothiazide is evaluated (Stoltenberg and Breitkreutz 2011; FP7 LENA).

44.7 Adverse Drug Reactions in Neonates: Assessment Needs a Tailored Approach

Because of the common practice to prescribe unlicensed and off-label drugs in neonates, a reasonable and relevant description for an adverse drug reaction (ADR) may be "the unintended, but harmful effect resulting from the administration of medication(s) intended for diagnostic or therapeutic reasons (irrespective of the dose)." Such a definition also covers medication errors (e.g., wrong dose, wrong route, or wrong patient) (Allegaert and van den Anker 2014b; Fabiano et al. 2012; Ligi et al. 2008). Obviously, the field of adverse drug reactions and medication errors also has a link with the growing and broader field of research on iatrogenesis, i.e., any adverse condition occurring as a result of a diagnostic procedure or treatment (Kugelman et al. 2008). History indeed repeatedly provided evidence that newborns and infants are more prone to specific adverse reactions to drugs, although some of these adverse reactions may have been anticipated based on the available knowledge on developmental pharmacology and toxicology. Table 4 provides some well-known illustrations on neonatal adverse drug reactions, including the underlying pathogenesis, since this should facilitate secondary prevention (cfr lower).

Neonatal pharmacotherapy is a powerful tool to improve outcome, but there is an obvious and urgent need to improve our practices through tailored adverse drug reaction (ADR) prevention and management. Besides the lack of labeling (e.g., eminence-based practices), inappropriate formulations (e.g., highly concentrated, excipients), (poly)pharmacy (e.g., maturational drug-drug interactions), immature organ function (how to discriminate between normal maturational function and toxicity, e.g., renal), and multiple illnesses further increase the risks for ADRs in neonates. Pharmacovigilance to improve ADR prevention and management needs to be adapted to the needs and characteristics of neonates and infants. Such a strategy should be based on *prevention* through drug prescription and administration error prevention (e.g., formulation, bedside manipulation, access) strategies, *detection* through laboratory or clinical outlier data signaling (e.g., reference laboratory values, overall high morbidity), and subsequent *assessment* (Allegaert and van den Anker 2014b; Castro-Pastrana and Carleton 2011; Lazou et al. 2013; Choonara 2013).

Assessment is of utmost importance. This is because – once a signal has been detected – differentiation of "true" ADRs from confounding events associated with immaturity, organ dysfunction, or underlying diseases remains difficult. Because of these confounding events, commonly applied ADR algorithm scoring systems do not sufficiently reliably document causality in neonates (Rieder 2012). Moreover, none of these algorithms have been validated in infants. Because of this and using a stepwise approach, a tailored algorithm was developed and subsequently validated. This new algorithm is based on 13 questions and turned out to be more reliable when compared to the classic Naranjo algorithm (Du et al. 2012). Finally, improved understanding of the developmental toxicology (Table 4) involved should further facilitate the avoidance of reoccurrence and the development of tailored guidelines (Dabliz and Levine 2012).

Table 4 Illustrative serious adverse drug reactions in neonates, with underlying pathogenesis to facilitate secondary prevention

Compound/ formulation	Clinical syndrome	Developmental pharmacology/toxicology
Sulfisoxazole	"Kernicterus"	Highly albumin-bound antibiotic, competitive with endogenous compounds, including bilirubin. This results in higher free bilirubin concentrations and subsequent kernicterus. *Similar effects can be anticipated for other high protein-bound compounds*, e.g., *ceftriaxone*
Chloramphenicol	"Gray baby syndrome"	Impaired glucuronidation, capacity, results in chloramphenicol accumulation and subsequent mitochondrial dysfunction, circulatory collapse, and death. *Similar effects can be anticipated for other glucuronidation dependent drug metabolism compounds*, e.g., *propofol*
Lopinavir/ritonavir syrup	"Alcohol accumulation"	Kaletra syrup contains both ethanol and propylene glycol. Impaired metabolic clearance results in accumulation, and subsequent hyperosmolality, lactic acidosis, renal toxicity, central nervous system impairment, cardiac arrhythmia, hemolysis, and collapse. *Explained by ethanol/propylene glycol competition for hepatic metabolic elimination*
Ceftriaxone + calcium	"Cardiovascular collapse"	Simultaneous administration of calcium-containing infusions and ceftriaxone results in intravascular precipitate, as observed during autopsy. *May be similar for other "mixtures" with calcium-containing formulations*
Topical iodide application	"Hypothyroidism"	More pronounced skin permeability and higher body surface area result in a more effective absorption of iodine with subsequent suppression of thyroid function. *Similar for other topical compounds*, e.g., *steroids or hexachlorophene*

44.8 Conclusions

Pharmacotherapy is a potential powerful tool to improve outcome in neonates, but there is still a huge lack of appropriate labeling of drugs used in the neonatal period. The knowledge on pharmacotherapy in infants is lagging behind, with often only poor and limited evidence in support of dosing regimens: "the last therapeutic orphan." Aspects to improve neonatal pharmacotherapy were discussed and these aspects interrelate with each other (Fig. 3).

Neonatal pharmacology displays extensive variability because of rapidly evolving physiology: variability is the essence of neonatal pharmacology. Related to this, the use of therapeutic drug monitoring (TDM) and the need for formulations tailored to the characteristics of newborns were discussed. Finally, pharmacovigilance also needs to be tailored to the characteristics of this population and relates to preventive strategies, signal detection, as well as assessment of causality and improved understanding. To convert the current situation into better neonatal pharmacotherapy, collaborative efforts between clinical researchers, sponsors, patient representatives, regulatory authorities, and society are needed. Clinicians should be encouraged to consult and to assess the available evidence and to contribute to more robust knowledge through collaborative networks that facilitate clinical research by covering aspects related to dosing, efficacy, safety, and formulations.

Acknowledgments Karel Allegaert is supported by the Fund for Scientific Research, Flanders (fundamental clinical investigatorship 1800214 N), and the research activities are further facilitated by the agency for innovation by Science and Technology in Flanders (IWT) through the SAFEPEDRUG project (IWT/SBO 130033). Janko Samardzic is supported by ERAWEB II scholarship for postdoctoral program at the KU Leuven, Belgium (2014–2015). Milica Bajcetic is supported by the Ministry of Education, Science and Technological Development of the Republic of Serbia (project No 173014) and the European Commission (LENA, 602295). John van den Anker is supported by NIH (K24DA027992,

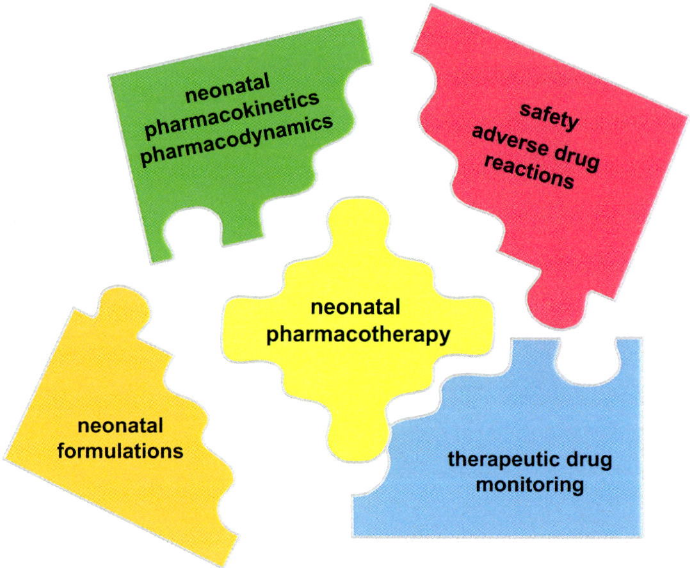

Fig. 3 Improvements in neonatal pharmacotherapy will be driven by improved knowledge on developmental pharmacokinetics and pharmacodynamics, tailored drug development, individualized therapeutic drug monitoring, and more effective recognition of adverse drug events to improve drug safety

R01HD048689, U54HD071601) and the European Commission (TINN [223614], TINN2 [260908], NEUROSIS [223060]).

References

Allegaert K, van den Anker JN (2014a) Clinical pharmacology in neonates: small size, huge variability. Neonatology 105:344–349

Allegaert K, van den Anker JN (2014b) Adverse drug reactions in neonates and infants: a population tailored approach is needed. Br J Clin Pharmacol. https://doi.org/10.1111/bcp.12430

Allegaert K, Anderson BJ, Vrancken M et al (2006) Impact of a paediatric vial on the magnitude of systematic medication errors in preterm neonates: amikacin as an example. Paediatr Perinat Drug Ther 7:59–63

Allegaert K, van de Velde M, van den Anker J (2014) Neonatal clinical pharmacology. Paediatr Anaesth 24:30–38

Bajcetic M, Uzelac TV, Jovanovic I (2014) Heart failure pharmacotherapy: differences between adult and paediatric patients. Curr Med Chem 21:3108–3120

Boylan GB, Stevenson NJ, Vanhatalo S (2013) Monitoring neonatal seizures. Semin Fetal Neonatal Med 18:202–208

Carvalho CG, Ribeiro MR, Bonilha MM et al (2012) Use of off-label and unlicensed drugs in the neonatal intensive care unit and its association with severity scores. J Pediatr (Rio J) 88:465–470

Castro-Pastrana LI, Carleton BC (2011) Improving pediatric drug safety: need for more efficient clinical translation of pharmacovigilance knowledge. J Popul Ther Clin Pharmacol 18:e76–e88

Choonara I (1994) Percutaneous drug absorption and administration. Arch Dis Child 71:F73–F74

Choonara I (2013) Educational paper: aspects of clinical pharmacology in children – pharmacovigilance and safety. Eur J Pediatr 172:577–580

Clark RH, Bloom BT, Spitzer AR, Gerstmann DR (2006) Reported medication use in the neonatal intensive care unit: data from a large national data set. Pediatrics 117:1979–1987

Dabliz R, Levine S (2012) Medication safety in neonates. Am J Perinatol 29:49–56

De Cock R, Allegaert K, Schreuder MF et al (2012) Maturation of the glomerular filtration rate in neonates, as reflected by amikacin clearance. Clin Pharmacokinet 51:105–117

De Cock RF, Knibbe CA, Kulo A et al (2013) Developmental pharmacokinetics of propylene glycol in preterm and term neonates. Br J Clin Pharmacol 75:162–171

de Wildt SN (2011) Profound changes in drug metabolism enzymes and possible effects on drug therapy in neonates and children. Expert Opin Drug Metab Toxicol 7:935–948

Dessi A, Salemi C, Fanos V, Cuzzolin L (2010) Drug treatments in a neonatal setting: focus on the off-label use in the first month of life. Pharm World Sci 32:120–124

Di Paolo ER, Stoetter H, Cotting J et al (2006) Unlicensed and off-label drug use in a Swiss paediatric university hospital. Swiss Med Wkly 136:218–222

Du W, Warrier I, Tutag Lehr V et al (2006) Changing patterns of drug utilization in a neonatal intensive care population. Am J Perinatol 23:279–285

Du W, Lehr VT, Leih-Lai M et al (2012) An algorithm to detect adverse drug reactions in the neonatal intensive care unit: a new approach. J Clin Pharmacol 53:87–95

European Union Pediatric Formulations Initiative. http://www.eupfi.org/. Accessed 19 May 2015

Fabiano V, Mameli C, Zuccotti GV (2011) Paediatric pharmacology: remember the excipients. Pharmacol Res 63:362–365

Fabiano V, Mameli C, Zuccotti GV (2012) Adverse drug reactions in newborns, infants and toddlers: pediatric pharmacovigilance between present and future. Expert Opin Drug Saf 11:95–105

Fanos V, Yurdakök M (2010) Personalized neonatal medicine. J Matern Fetal Neonatal Med 23(Suppl 3):4–6

FP7 LENA. http://www.lena-med.eu/. Accessed 19 May 2015

Hines RN (2013) Developmental expression of drug metabolizing enzymes: impact on disposition in neonates and young children. Int J Pharm 452:3–7

Huang NN, High RH (1953) Infants and children of various age groups. J Pediatr 42:657–658

Kearns GL, Abdel-Rahman SM, Alander SW et al (2003) Developmental pharmacology – drug disposition, action, and therapy in infants and children. N Engl J Med 349:1157–1167

Kieran EA, O'Callaghan N, O'Donnell CP (2014) Unlicensed and off-label drug use in an Irish neonatal intensive care unit: a prospective cohort study. Acta Paediatr 103:e139–e142

Kugelman A, Inbar-Sanado E, Shinwell ES et al (2008) Iatrogenesis in neonatal intensive care units: observational and interventional, prospective, multicenter study. Pediatrics 122:550–555

Laforgia N, Nuccio MM, Schettini F et al (2014) Off-label and unlicensed drug use among neonatal intensive care units in Southern Italy. Pediatr Int 56:57–59

Lass J, Käär R, Jõgi K et al (2011) Drug utilisation pattern and off-label use of medicines in Estonian neonatal units. Eur J Clin Pharmacol 67:1263–1271

Laughon MM, Avant D, Tripathi N et al (2014) Drug labeling and exposure in neonates. JAMA Pediatr 168:130–136

Lazou K, Farini M, Koutkias V et al (2013) Adverse drug event prevention in neonatal care: a rule-based approach. Stud Health Technol Inform 186:170–174

Ligi I, Arnaud F, Jouve E et al (2008) Iatrogenic events in admitted neonates: a prospective cohort study. Lancet 371:404–410

McIntyre J, Choonara I (2004) Drug toxicity in the neonate. Biol Neonate 86:218–221

Mooij MG, de Koning BA, Huijsman ML, de Wildt SN (2012) Ontogeny of oral absorption processes in children. Expert Opin Drug Metab Toxicol 8:1293–1303

Mulla H (2010) Understanding developmental pharmacodynamics: importance for drug development and clinical practice. Paediatr Drugs 12:223–233

Mulla H, Yakkundi S, McElnay J et al (2015) An observational study of blood concentrations and kinetics of methyl- and propyl-parabens in neonates. Pharm Res 32:1084–1093

Nunn A, Craig JV, Shah UU et al (2013) Estimating the requirement for manipulation of medicines to provide accurate doses for children. Eur J Hosp Pharm 20:3–7

Rao SC, Srinivasjois R, Hagan R, Ahmed M (2011) One dose per day compared to multiple doses per day of gentamicin for treatment of suspected or proven sepsis in neonates. Cochrane Database Syst Rev 9:CD005091

Rieder M (2012) New ways to detect adverse drug reactions in pediatrics. Pediatr Clin N Am 59:1071–1092

Riou S, Plaisant F, Maucort Boulch D et al (2015) Unlicensed and off-label drug use: a prospective study in French NICU. Acta Paediatr 104:e228–e231

Roberts JA, Pea F, Lipman J (2013) The clinical relevance of plasma protein binding changes. Clin Pharmacokinet 52:1–8

Salunke S, Brandys B, Giacoia G et al (2013) The STEP (Safety and Toxicity of Excipients for Paediatrics) database: part 2 – the pilot version. Int J Pharm 457:310–322

Santovena A, Hernandez-Paiz Z, Farina JB (2012) Design of a pediatric oral formulation with a low proportion of hydrochlorothiazide. Int J Pharm 433:360–364

Schreuder MF, Bueters RR, Allegaert K (2014) The interplay between drugs and the kidney in premature neonates. Pediatr Nephrol 29:2083–2091

Smits A, Kulo A, de Hoon JN et al (2012a) Pharmacokinetics of drugs in neonates: pattern recognition beyond compound specific observations. Curr Pharm Des 18: 3119–3146

Smits A, Kulo A, Verbesselt R et al (2012b) Cefazolin plasma protein binding and its covariates in neonates. Eur J Clin Microbiol Infect Dis 31:3359–3365

Staelens S, van den Driessche M, Barclay D et al (2008) Gastric emptying in healthy newborns fed an intact protein formula, a partially and an extensively hydrolysed formula. Clin Nutr 27:264–268

Stephenson T (2005) How children's responses to drugs differ from adults. Br J Clin Pharmacol 59:670–673

Stiers JL, Ward RM (2014) Newborns, one of the last therapeutic orphans to be adopted. JAMA Pediatr 168:106–108

Stoltenberg I, Breitkreutz J (2011) Oral disintegrating mini-tablets (ODMTs) – an novel solid oral dosage form for paediatric use. Eur J Pharm Biopharm 78:462–469

Tuleu C, Breitkreutz J (2013) Educational paper: formulation-related issues in pediatric clinical pharmacology. Eur J Pediatr 172:717–720

Turner MA (2011) Neonatal drug development. Early Hum Dev 87:763–768

Turner MA, Duncan J, Shah U et al (2013) European study of neonatal exposure to excipients: an update. Int J Pharm 457:357–358

Turner MA, Duncan JC, Shah U et al (2014) Risk assessment of neonatal excipient exposure: lessons from food safety and other areas. Adv Drug Deliv Rev 73:89–101

Van den Anker JN (2011) Getting the dose of vancomycin right in the neonate. Int J Clin Pharmacol Ther 49:247–249

Van den Anker J (2014) The impact of therapeutic drug monitoring in neonatal clinical pharmacology. Clin Biochem 47:704–705

WHO, UNICEF. Make medicines child size. http://www.who.int/childmedicines/media/backgrounder/BG2/en/index.html. Accessed 19 May 2015

Yanni SB, Smith PB, Benjamin DK Jr et al (2011) Higher clearance of micafungin in neonates compared with adults: role of age-dependent micafungin serum binding. Biopharm Drug Dispos 32:222–232

Young TE (2012) Therapeutic drug monitoring – the appropriate use of drug level measurement in the care of the neonate. Clin Perinatol 39:25–31

Infants of Smoking Mothers 45

Roberto Paludetto, Letizia Capasso, and Francesco Raimondi

Contents

Abstract

Maternal smoking during pregnancy represents a serious health hazard for the fetus and the neonate; its consequences may persist well into later life. Environmental tobacco smoke is also a threat to pre- and postnatal life. Although tobacco smoke contains thousands of compounds whose effects have not been fully studied, most of its detrimental effects are presumed to be mediated by nicotine. Cotinine, a nicotine metabolite, is used as a biomarker of tobacco exposure, and it has allowed an objective measure of smoke-related adverse events spanning from preterm birth, intrauterine growth retardation, and low birth weight to congenital malformations. Deficient cardiovascular and respiratory functions have also been linked to intrauterine and neonatal exposure to tobacco smoke such as an increased risk of metabolic syndrome in adulthood. Nicotine's complex interaction with fetal and neonatal

R. Paludetto · L. Capasso (✉) · F. Raimondi
Division of Neonatology, Department of Translational Medical Sciences, Università "Federico II" di Napoli, Naples, Italy
e-mail: paludett@unina.it; letizia.capasso@gmail.com; raimondi@unina.it

G. Buonocore et al. (eds.), *Neonatology*,
https://doi.org/10.1007/978-3-319-29489-6_194

neurotransmitters induces behavioral alterations in the newborn period and may help to explain the higher incidence of SIDS and ADHD described in offspring of smoking mothers.

45.1 Salient Points

- Smoking during pregnancy is still very common in developed countries.
- Environmental tobacco smoke is a health hazard for pregnant women and their fetuses.
- Recent studies use tobacco smoke biomarkers to document its adverse effects on the fetus and the neonate.
- In utero tobacco smoke exposure has been linked to an increased risk of some types of congenital malformations (i.e., orofacial clefts, congenital heart disease).
- Tobacco smoke exposure is associated with adverse pregnancy outcome, preterm birth, low birth weight, and intrauterine growth retardation.
- Early tobacco smoke exposure carries a higher risk of respiratory infections, poorer cardiovascular and respiratory function, and an increased risk of metabolic syndrome later in life.
- Children of smoking mothers have a higher incidence of behavioral problems, ADHD, and SIDS.

45.2 Introduction

The knowledge of adverse effects of tobacco products on adult health conditions has long been established. Scientists and clinicians are now unraveling the multifaceted relation between tobacco smoke and human development starting from the intrauterine and possibly periconceptional periods. Evidence now relates maternal smoke to deranged organogenesis, decreased organ function, poorer neurodevelopmental performance, and, recently, epigenetic changes that predispose to metabolic syndrome in adulthood. However, findings are not always unequivocal, mainly because of methodological problems. In the next paragraphs, we will critically address some of the current issues, focusing on available clinical evidence to give the reader a practical approach to the infant of the smoking mother.

45.3 Epidemiology

International authorities are monitoring the smoking habits and their consequences and consider tobacco as a "legalized health hazard" on a planetary scale. In 2007, the WHO classified 18.2% of European adult females as smokers (World Health Organization 2007). Figures vary among individual countries but have remained substantially stable since the previous report in 2002. Separate data for smoking during pregnancy are not available on this scale and have to be deduced from epidemiological surveys. Reports from Sweden and the USA, respectively, estimate a prevalence of 13% and 10.4% of women smoking during their pregnancy, but more recent work from the UK sets this figure as high as 36% (Ward et al. 2007). Whatever the data at delivery, the percentage of women who smoke around the time of conception is higher as most women who stop smoking achieve this goal very early in their gestation (Chamberlain et al. 2013). However, since many will attempt to quit smoking throughout their pregnancy, it is mandatory that they receive constant support and encouragement from healthcare professionals. This should be continued after delivery, since many women who quitted smoking during pregnancy will resume this habit shortly after giving birth. Moreover, Cnattingius et al. have demonstrated that a previous adverse pregnancy outcome has only a modest influence on smoking habits in the successive gestation (Cnattingius et al. 2006).

Besides direct smoking, a pregnant woman and her fetus can be exposed to environmental tobacco smoke (ETS). While the detrimental effects of this condition will be discussed below, it is difficult to gather good quality data on its prevalence. In 2007, Ward et al. reported in the UK that as many as 13% of infants were born to nonsmoking mothers who had had significant exposure to ETS (Ward et al. 2007). Maternal smoking during pregnancy and ETS may have additive adverse effects on infantile health.

Recently, a national study on all registered births in England between 1995 and 2011 demonstrated that national legislation in 2007 to introduce smoke-free workplaces was associated with an immediate decrease in stillbirths (7.8%), low birth weight infants (3.9%), and neonatal mortality (7.6%). The authors estimated that in the first 4 years following smoke-free legislation, 991 stillbirths, 5.470 cases of low birth weight, and 430 neonatal deaths were prevented (Been et al. 2015). Such results should encourage smoke-free legislation for all countries, especially for low- and middle-income countries where most of the burden of early life morbidity and mortality occurs.

45.4 Pharmacology of Tobacco Smoke and Its Detection in Biological Specimens

Tobacco smoke has thousands of compounds, many of which might have effects on infant's health and have not been yet investigated.

Carbon monoxide rapidly binds to both maternal and fetal hemoglobin with carboxyhemoglobin levels that eventually become higher in the fetus than in the mother because the fetus has a higher hemoglobin affinity for carbon monoxide and a longer elimination half-life than the mother. This leads to a potentially profound impairment of oxygen delivery to the tissues that can be aggravated by other smoke-derived chemicals (thiocyanates and other cyanides) also binding hemoglobin.

Nicotine is the chemical that is primarily responsible of tobacco addiction and organ toxicity. In the brain, nicotine binds to nicotinic acetylcholine receptors eliciting the release of many neurotransmitters. Nicotine can also act peripherally stimulating the release of epinephrine, ultimately increasing heart and respiratory rate and causing vasoconstriction. It also suppresses insulin release possibly affecting glucose blood levels and appetite. Nicotine passes into breast milk with concentrations that are in linear correlation with its levels in maternal serum (Pellegrini et al. 2007).

Cotinine, the major nicotine metabolite, is currently used to assess objectively an infant's exposure to tobacco smoke both before and after birth. Cotinine may be detected in plasma, urine, saliva, hair, and meconium. This sampling is expensive, may be invasive (i.e., plasma), and depends on cotinine half-life (except for hair) but often reveals a greater exposure to tobacco smoke than maternal self-reports. In the study by Puig et al., infantile exposure to ETS was significantly higher when assessed by infant urinary cotinine compared to parental self-reports (Puig et al. 2008). Similarly, 64.3% of pregnant women who claimed to be non-smokers and not exposed to ETS had plasma cotinine levels above the limit of detection (de Chazeron et al. 2007). Despite the proven value of this biomarker, much of the research published to date still relies on self -reports.

45.5 Smoke, the Pregnancy, and the Fetus

Nicotine is a powerful vasoconstrictor that significantly reduces maternal blood supply to the fetus. The latter is further impaired by placental alterations and high carboxyhemoglobin levels. These effects combined may explain why smoking during pregnancy has been associated with perinatal death, spontaneous abortion, stillbirth, abruptio placentae, placenta previa, fetal growth restriction, preterm birth, and low birth weight.

The developmental origin of health and disease is a rapidly expanding research field. Molecular mechanisms such as DNA methylation may intervene during fetal life under the influence of environmental stressors. This is an attractive model to explain the long-term effects of prenatal exposure to tobacco smoke.

From the analysis of umbilical cord blood of 418 pregnant women, prenatal exposure to cigarette smoke can cause increased methylation of the insulin-like growth factor II (*IGF2*) gene, which is associated with low birth weight, predominantly in male infants. *IGF2* plays an important role in regulating growth (Pirini et al. 2015). Also, maternal smoking during pregnancy has been linked with DNA methylation change of the AHRR gene, involved in pleiotropic responses to environmental contaminants and with the methylation of genes involved in the pathway for the detoxification of xenobiotics of tobacco smoke such as *CYP1A1*. The differential methylation of such genes persists also during adolescence; these findings support a role for epigenetics as a mediator of long-term effects of smoking exposure in utero such as increased risk of diabetes type 2, hypertension, and obesity (Novakovic et al. 2014).

In a cohort study on 7,098 pregnant women, an association with low birth weight was particularly strong for active smoking during late pregnancy, while quitting smoking early in the gestation was associated with a higher birth weight than continuing to smoke. In a cohort study on 927,424 births between 2006 and 2012, the risk for fetal growth restriction below the tenth percentile increases about 1.2-fold for cessation of smoking after the first trimester and about 1.7-fold for cessation after the second trimester; women smoking throughout pregnancy have a 2.3-fold risk for fetal growth restriction after accounting for the influence of race, low socioeconomic status, and medical comorbidities. Smoking only during the preconception period did not significantly increase fetal growth restriction risk (Blatt et al. 2015).

A slight, nonsignificant trend to a beneficial effect on birth weight has been described for reducing the number of cigarettes without quitting completely (Jaddoe et al. 2008). Each additional pack smoked during pregnancy is associated with a 2.8 g reduction in neonatal body mass composition (0.7 g decrease for fatty mass and 2.1 g for free-fatty mass) in a dose-dependent manner (Harrod et al. 2014).

Length and head circumference are also affected though probably to a lesser degree. Tobacco-related effects on fetal growth are generally reversible during the first few years of life (Kannellopoulos et al. 2007). Children with intrauterine smoke exposure show a faster increase in height and ponderal index from birth to the age of 2 years than controls, after which no difference can be documented (Harrod et al. 2012).

45.6 Neonatal Consequences of Smoke Exposure

The multifaceted damage of smoking during pregnancy on neonatal health starts with an increased rate of congenital malformations. Many questionnaire-based studies reported a greater incidence of cleft lip and palate in infants of smoking mothers (Lie et al. 2008). This piece of data has been recently confirmed by a biomarker-based study. Women with a serum cotinine above 2 ng/ml are 2.4 times more likely to deliver a child affected by an orofacial cleft (Shaw et al. 2009).

Congenital heart defects have also been associated to prenatal smoke exposure. A large questionnaire-based, case-control study conducted by Malik et al. has concluded that women who smoked around the periconceptional period were more likely to give birth to neonates with septal and right-sided obstructive defects (Malik et al. 2008). The association of congenital heart defects with prenatal smoke exposure is stronger with increasing number of daily cigarettes and among the offspring of mothers over the age of 35 years (Sullivan et al. 2015).

An impaired development of the fetal femur and/or of its vasculature has been claimed to explain the increased risk of Legg-Calvè-Perthes disease in offspring of mothers who smoked during pregnancy versus matched controls (Bahmanyar et al. 2008). More research is required to reevaluate this topic using biomarkers as an objective measure of the infant's smoke exposure.

Besides organogenesis, neonatal organ function is impaired by direct maternal smoking during pregnancy or by ETS.

Pulmonary mechanics studies in infants with prenatal exposure to tobacco smoke have shown an alteration in expiratory flow, a reduction in respiratory compliance, and an increase in airway resistance (Hanharan et al. 1992)

Prenatal smoke exposure has a long-lasting effect on expiratory flow rates as a significant reduction has been reported by Cunningham et al. in 8–12-year-old children (Cunningham et al. 1994). The respiratory function deficit was larger for black children than for white and for boys than for girls (Cunningham et al. 1995). The severity of wheezing may be further influenced by beta-2 adrenergic receptor variants in a complex gene-environment interaction (Wang et al. 2008). Offspring of nonsmoking mothers exposed to ETS during pregnancy has an increased risk of asthma in childhood too (Simons et al. 2014). In vitro and animal experiments recently showed that maternal smoking during pregnancy and lactation impairs metabolism and structural integrity of the lung in the offspring by means of epigenetic changes (Maritz and Harding 2011).

Children of mothers who smoked during pregnancy have a higher risk of respiratory tract infections both in the neonatal period and in the first year of life. The same holds true, to a milder degree, for ETS which could directly damage the respiratory epithelial lining and also suppress the innate immune system (Kum-Nji et al. 2006).

A large, questionnaire-based cohort study has evaluated the effects of maternal smoking in pregnancy on the cardiovascular function of the neonate (Geerts et al. 2007). Infants of smoking mothers had a 5.4 mmHg higher systolic pressure than offspring of nonsmoking mothers, but no significant association was found with diastolic pressure or heart rate. ETS alone (i.e., infants of nonsmoking mothers but with smoke exposure in the household) did not modify blood pressure or heart rate compared to controls.

There is concern that smoking exposure in utero may play a role in increased risk of obesity later in childhood. Children of mothers who smoked during pregnancy had higher risk of obesity at a mean age of 9 years (Oken et al. 2008; Banderali et al. 2015). Another study correlated maternal smoking with higher total fat mass at the same age (Banderali et al. 2015; Leary et al. 2006). Exposure to prenatal smoking was significantly associated with reduced neonatal fat mass and fat-free mass at birth. In contrast, at 5 months exposed offspring to prenatal smoking had greater fat-free mass and sum of skin folds. Therefore, smoking exposure in utero is significantly associated with rapid postnatal growth, which may increase the risk of metabolic diseases (Harrod et al. 2014). Nicotine-induced intrauterine starvation may directly alter the hypothalamic control on energy intake and expenditure predisposing to later obesity and to modification of brain and peripheral autonomic pathways (Oken et al. 2008; Banderali et al. 2015).

Maternal smoking during pregnancy has been associated with elevated risk of type 2 diabetes among offspring in adulthood. In an animal study, maternal nicotine exposure in utero may cause type 2 diabetes in offspring as a result of both impaired pancreatic β-cell (mass and function) and reduced peripheral insulin sensitivity (Bruin et al. 2010). Recently, newborns of smoking mothers during pregnancy have been shown to have decreased IGF1 levels and borderline low fetal β-cell function compared with newborns of nonsmoking mothers (Fang et al. 2015). Larger studies are required to confirm the hypothesis that early life metabolic alterations in fetus may predispose to metabolic syndrome in adulthood.

After birth, breastfeeding is an important source of exposure to tobacco compounds as nicotine passes into breast milk. The deleterious effect of nicotine in breast milk depends on the amount of cigarettes smoked and on the time frame between cigarette smoked and breastfeeding. Smoking mothers are less likely to breastfeed because of smoke interference with milk production and the mother's feeling of inadequate milk production; moreover, infantile colic and crying are exacerbated by tobacco smoking and increase the likelihood of the use of formula (Banderali et al. 2015).

45.7 Behavioral Aspects of the Offspring of the Smoking Mother

The profound impact of nicotine on neural cells anticipates a possible effect on neonatal behavior. Questionnaire-based research results, however, have not been entirely clear. Most studies examined tobacco in the context of other factors such as illicit substance abuse or obstetric complications (Fried and O'Connell 1987). Our group has conducted a prospective analysis of neonatal behavior, assessed by the Brazelton Neonatal Behavioral Assessment Scale, monitoring the infant's urine cotinine and administering a structured questionnaire to the parents (Mansi et al. 2002). Newborns of mothers who smoked during pregnancy had a higher urinary cotinine excretion. They were more irritable and less interactive with the environment. The same was true, although to a lesser extent, for offspring of nonsmoking mothers but smoking fathers, used as a proxy of ETS. Using a different evaluation tool, Stroud et al. came to similar conclusions (Stroud et al. 2009). Neonates of smoking mothers had an increased arousal and excitability throughout the first month of life, well past nicotine half-life. This has to be taken into account in the prevention of early disruption of maternal-infant bonding.

The adverse effects of prenatal smoke exposure on behavior extend far beyond the neonatal period. Schmitz et al. have documented an odds ratio of 3.44 for an increase of the inattentive form of attention deficit hyperactivity disorder (ADHD), and some studies show a higher rate of smokers among adolescents affected by ADHD as they self-medicated to alleviate cognitive or attentive disorders (Schmitz et al. 2006). A prospective longitudinal study by Hook et al. has linked prenatal smoke exposure to externalizing problems and aggression leading to a higher incidence of delinquent behavior both in males and females (Hook et al. 2006).

45.8 Smoke and SIDS

After the recognition that sleeping supine is associated with a decreased incidence of sudden infant death syndrome, maternal smoking has become the main preventable risk factor for SIDS. There is evidence that infants of smokers are less arousable both in REM and in non-REM phase of sleep (Chang et al. 2003) and have deficient hypoxic awakening response (Franco et al. 1999). Work in lambs exposed in utero to nicotine shows delayed arousal and reduced ventilatory and heart rate responses to hypoxia. Infants who died of SIDS had increased apoptosis in their brain stem nuclei compared to babies who had suddenly died for another diagnosis; cigarette smoke exposure was especially associated with increased apoptosis in the dorsal motor nucleus of the vagus and the arcuate nucleus (Machaalani and Waters 2008). Blanchard et al. demonstrated in preterm neonates that intrauterine smoking exposure has a negative impact on peripheral chemoreceptor tonic activity and increases the time spent in apnea (both with and without blood oxygen desaturation) and the mean duration of apneic episodes with desaturation (Blanchard et al. 2010).

These observations may provide the link between tobacco smoke, a defective cardiorespiratory control, and SIDS.

45.9 Reducing Damage from Prenatal Smoke Exposure or ETS

It is intuitive that enforcing regulations on banning smoke from public places and taxing tobacco products should reduce smoking rates and ETS. More focused programs are in place in many developed countries where smoking cessation services are available before or during the gestation offering behavioral support. The safety and efficacy of nicotine replacement therapy in pregnant women is debated (Coleman 2008; Pauly and Slotkin 2008). More recently, maternal snuff use in pregnancy (a source of nicotine containing low levels of nitrosamines and no combustion products) has been associated with the same increased risk of oral clefts as tobacco smoking (Gunnerbeck et al. 2014).

45.10 Conclusions

Perinatal health professionals need to increase their awareness about the detrimental effects of smoking during pregnancy and lactation. Further research conducted with reliable biomarkers of smoke exposure will improve the quality of our information both on direct maternal smoke and on its role as an environmental pollutant. This information is needed if measurable interventions have to be aimed toward success.

References

Bahmanyar S, Montgomery SM, Weiss RJ et al (2008) Maternal smoking during pregnancy, other prenatal and perinatal factors and the risk of Legg-Calvè-Perthes disease. Pediatrics 122:e459–e464

Banderali G, Martelli A, Landi M et al (2015) Short and long term health effects of parental tobacco smoking during pregnancy and lactation: a descriptive review. J Transl Med 13:327

Been JV, Mackay DF, Millett C et al (2015) Impact of smoke-free legislation on perinatal and infant mortality: a national quasi-experimental study. Sci Rep 5:13020

Blanchard ES, Chardon K, Leke´ A (2010) In utero exposure to smoking and peripheral chemoreceptor function in preterm neonates. Pediatrics 125(3):e592–e599

Blatt K, Moore E, Chen A et al (2015) Association of reported trimester-specific smoking cessation with fetal growth restriction. Obstet Gynecol 125(6):1452–1459

Bruin JE, Gerstein HC, Holloway AC (2010) Long-term consequences of fetal and neonatal nicotine exposure: a critical review. Toxicol Sci 116(2):364–374

Chang AB, Wilson SJ, Masters IB et al (2003) Altered arousal response in infants exposed to cigarette smoke. Arch Dis Child 88:30–33

Chamberlain C, O'Mara-Eves A, Oliver S et al (2013) Psychosocial interventions for supporting women to stop smoking in pregnancy. Cochrane Database Syst Rev 10:CD001055

Cnattingius S, Akre O, Lambe M et al (2006) Will adverse pregnancy outcome influence the risk of continued smoking in the next pregnancy? Am J Obstet Gynecol 195:1680–1686

Coleman T (2008) Reducing harm from tobacco smoke exposure during pregnancy. Birth Defects Res 84:73–79

Cunningham J, Dockery DW, Speizer FE (1994) Maternal smoking during pregnancy as a predictor of lung function in children. Am J Epidemiol 139:1139–1152

Cunningham J, Dockery DW, Speizer FE (1995) Racial differences between maternal smoking during pregnancy and lung function in children. Am J Respir Crit Care Med 152:565–569

de Chazeron I, Llorca PM, Ughetto S et al (2007) Occult exposure to environmental tobacco smoke exposure. Tob Control 16:64–65

Fang F, Luo Z-C, Dejemli A et al (2015) Maternal smoking and metabolic health biomarkers in newborns. PLoS One 10(11):e0143660

Franco P, Grosswasser J, Hassid S (1999) Prenatal exposure to cigarette smoking is associated with a decrease in arousal in infants. J Pediatr 135:34–38

Fried PA, O'Connell CM (1987) A comparison of the effects of prenatal exposure to tobacco, alcohol, cannabis and caffeine on birth size and subsequent growth. Neurotoxicol Teratol 9:79–85

Geerts CC, Grobbee DE, van der Ent CK et al (2007) Tobacco smoke exposure of pregnant mothers and blood pressure in their newborns. Hypertension 50:572–578

Gunnerbeck A, Edstedt Bonamy AK, Wikstrom AK et al (2014) Maternal snuff use and smoking and the risk of oral cleft malformations – a population-based cohort study. PLoS ONE 9(1):e84715

Hanharan JP, Tager IB, Segal MR et al (1992) The effect of maternal smoking during pregnancy on early infant lung function. Am Rev Respir Dis 145:1129–1135

Harrod CS, Reynolds RM, Chasan-Taber L et al (2012) Maternal smoking during pregnancy and offspring trajectories of height and adiposity: comparing maternal and paternal associations. Int J Epidemiol 41:722–732

Harrod CS, Reynolds RM, Chasan-Taber L et al (2014) Quantity and timing of maternal prenatal smoking on neonatal body composition: the healthy start study. J Pediatr 165:707–712

Hook B, Cederblad M, Berg R (2006) Prenatal and postnatal maternal smoking as risk factors for preschool children's mental health. Acta Paediatr 95:671–677

Jaddoe VWV, Troe EJWM, Hofman A et al (2008) Active and passive maternal smoking during pregnancy and the risks of low birthweight and preterm birth: the generation R study. Paediatr Perinat Epidemiol 22:162–171

Kannellopoulos TA, Varvarigou AA, Karatza AA et al (2007) Course of growth during the first 6 years in children exposed in utero to tobacco smoke. Eur J Pediatr 166:685–692

Kum-Nji P, Meloy L, Herrod HG (2006) Environmental tobacco smoke exposure: prevalence and mechanisms of causation of infections in children. Pediatrics 117:1745–1753

Leary SD, Smith GD, Rogers IS et al (2006) Smoking during pregnancy and offspring fat and lean mass in childhood. Obesity 14:2284–2293

Lie RT, Wilcox AJ, Taylor J et al (2008) Maternal smoking and oral clefts: the role of detoxification pathway genes. Epidemiology 19:606–615

Machaalani R, Waters KA (2008) Neuronal cell death in the sudden infant death syndrome brainstem and association with risk factors. Brain 131:218–228

Malik S, Cleves MA, Honein MA et al (2008) Maternal smoking and congenital heart defects. Pediatrics 121: e810–e815

Mansi G, Raimondi F, Pichini S et al (2002) Neonatal urinary cotinine correlates with behavioural alterations in newborns prenatally exposed to tobacco smoke. Pediatr Res 61:257–261

Maritz GS, Harding R (2011) Life-long programming implications of exposure to tobacco smoking and nicotine before and soon after birth: evidence for altered lung development. Int J Environ Res Public Health 8:875–898

Novakovic B, Ryan J, Pereira N et al (2014) Postnatal stability, tissue, and timing specific effects of AHRR methylation change in response to maternal smoking in pregnancy. Epigenetics 9(3):377–386

Oken E, Levitan EB, Gillman MW (2008) Maternal smoking during pregnancy and child overweight: systematic review and meta analysis. Int J Obes 32:201–210

Pauly JR, Slotkin TA (2008) Maternal tobacco smoking, nicotine replacement and behavioural development. Acta Paediatr 97:1331–1337

Pellegrini M, Marchei E, Rossi S et al (2007) Liquid chromatography/electrospray ionization tandem mass spectrometry assay for determination of nicotine and metabolites, caffeine and arecoline in breast milk. Rapid Commun Mass Spectrom 21:2693–2703

Pirini F, Guida E, Lawson F, Mancinelli A, Guerrero-Preston R (2015) Nuclear and mitochondrial DNA alterations in newborns with prenatal exposure to cigarette smoke. Int J Environ Res Public Health 12:1135–1155

Puig C, Garcia-Algar O, Monleon T et al (2008) A longitudinal study of environmental tobacco smoke exposure in children: parental self reports versus age dependent biomarkers. BMC Public Health 8:47–55

Schmitz M, Demarolin D, Laufer Silva T et al (2006) Smoking during pregnancy and attention-deficit/hyperactivity disorder, predominantly inattentive type: a case-control study. J Am Acad Child Adolesc Psychiatry 45:1338–1345

Shaw GM, Carmichael SM, Vollset SE et al (2009) Mid-pregnancy cotinine and risks of orofacial clefts and neural tube defects. J Pediatr 154:17–19

Simons E, To T, Moineddin R et al (2014) Maternal second-hand smoke exposure in pregnancy is associated with childhood asthma development. J Allergy Clin Immunol Pract 2(2):201–207

Stroud LR, Paster RL, Papandonatos GD et al (2009) Maternal smoking during pregnancy and newborn neurobehavior: effects at 10 to 27 days. J Pediatr 154:10–16

Sullivan PM, Dervan LA, Reiger S et al (2015) Risk of congenital heart defects in the offspring of smoking mothers: a population based study. J Pediatr 166 (4):978–984

Wang C, Salam MT, Islam T et al (2008) Effects of in utero and childhood tobacco smoke exposure and beta-2 adrenergic receptor genotype on childhood asthma and wheezing. Pediatrics 122:e107–e114

Ward C, Lewis S, Coleman T (2007) Prevalence of maternal smoking and environmental tobacco smoke exposure during pregnancy and impact on birth weight: retrospective study using Millennium Cohort. BMC Public Health 7:81

World Health Organization (2007) The tobacco atlas www.who.int/tobacco/statistics/tobacco_atlas/en/

Infants of Diabetic Mothers

46

Erin A. Osterholm, Jane E. Barthell, and Michael K. Georgieff

Contents

E. A. Osterholm · M. K. Georgieff (✉)
Division of Neonatology, Department of Pediatrics Center for Neurobehavioral Development, University of Minnesota, Minneapolis, MN, USA
e-mail: georg001@umn.edu

J. E. Barthell
Children's Hospitals and Clinics of Minnesota, Minneapolis, MN, USA

G. Buonocore et al. (eds.), *Neonatology*,
https://doi.org/10.1007/978-3-319-29489-6_195

Abstract
Ten per cent of all pregnancies are complicated by gestational diabetes mellitus or pre-conceptional diabetes and, given the increased prevalence of obesity, this percentage is expected to rise over the next few years. While advances in maternal and neonatal medical care continue to improve the outcomes for infants born to mothers with glucose intolerance during pregnancy, the risks for spontaneous abortion, stillbirth, congenital malformations, and perinatal mortality still exist. Pregnancies of mothers with diabetes are given increased surveillance, as the multifaceted metabolic changes that occur in the mother affect fetal growth, glucose and iron metabolism, cardiac anatomy and function, transition to extrauterine life, placing the infant at risk for periconceptional, fetal, neonatal, and long-term morbidities. This chapter gives a perspective on the risks of glucose intolerance during pregnancies, neonatal complications, and long-term health sequelae of infants of diabetic mothers.

46.1 Salient Points

- Appropriate periconceptional and perinatal care can improve the risks for spontaneous abortion, stillbirth, congenital malformations, and perinatal mortality and morbidity.
- Maternal hyperglycemia affects fetal growth, glucose metabolism, iron metabolism, cardiac anatomy and function, and transition to extra-uterine life.
- Maternal hyperglycemia leads to multiple issues in the neonatal period including abnormalities of neonatal body habitus, glucose, calcium and magnesium metabolism, hematologic status, cardiorespiratory function, bilirubin metabolism, and neurologic functioning.

46.2 Overview

While advances in maternal and neonatal medical care continue to improve the outcomes for infants born to mothers with glucose intolerance during pregnancy, the risks for spontaneous abortion, stillbirth, congenital malformations, and perinatal mortality and morbidity still exist. Abnormal maternal glycemic control caused by gestational diabetes mellitus or pregestational diabetes mellitus complicate up to 10% of pregnancies, and as the significantly overweight pediatric population develops into their child-bearing years, this number is likely to rise (Nold and Georgieff 2004). Pregnancies of mothers with diabetes are given increased surveillance, as the multifaceted metabolic changes that occur in the mother can place the infant at risk for periconceptional, fetal, neonatal, and long-term morbidities (Nold and Georgieff 2004; Widness 1989). Fortunately, appropriate periconceptional and prenatal care can improve the risks of perinatal complications by close monitoring of maternal glycemic control.

46.3 The Pedersen Hypothesis and Diabetic Fetopathy

In general, maternal glycemic control remains the primary factor that determines the potential complications in the conceptus and the neonate. Some sequelae, such as failure of implantation,

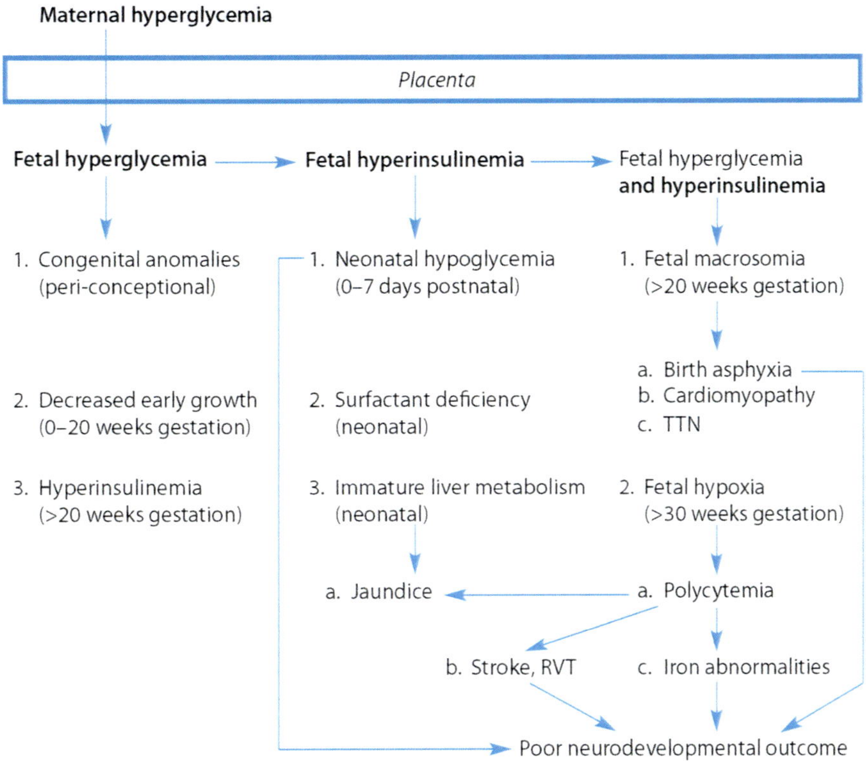

Fig. 1 The fetal and neonatal events attributable to maternal diabetes mellitus (Reproduced from (Nold and Georgieff 2004), with permission)

miscarriage, and congenital malformations, are a function of pre- and periconceptional maternal glucose control. Other sequelae, such as macrosomia, neonatal hypoglycemia, and fetal/neonatal iron deficiency, result from worsening glycemic control in the last few weeks prior to delivery (Georgieff 2006; Herranz et al. 2007). Fetal hyperglycemia, hyperinsulinemia, or the combination of the two leads to the pathologic conditions seen in the late gestation fetus and neonate (Fig. 1).

46.4 Risks of Maternal Glucose Intolerance During the Periconceptional Period

Up to 40 known congenital malformations associated with maternal diabetes have been noted (Correa et al. 2008). Indeed, a strong association between maternal glycemic control at the time of conception and early gestation and the incidence of congenital anomalies has been recognized in several epidemiological studies, with a significant decrease in congenital malformations reported in mothers with strict metabolic regulation during the periconceptional period (Fuhrmann et al. 1983; Georgieff 1995). Anomalies of the heart, musculoskeletal system, and genitourinary system have been seen at a twofold to threefold higher incidence in infants of insulin-dependent diabetic mothers compared to the normal population (Kalhan and Parimi 2006). The frequency of congenital anomalies has not been found to increase in offspring of gestationally diabetic mothers (Savona-Ventura and Gatt 2004).

The mechanisms by which these anomalies occur remain under investigation. Maternal hyperglycemia, the major teratogenic factor, may be involved in hyperglycemia-induced apoptosis that is associated with oxidative stress, lipid peroxidation, and decreased antioxidant defense capacity in the embryos (Rajdl et al. 2005; Zhao and Reece 2005). In studies of mouse embryos from diabetic mice, hyperglycemia appears to disturb cellular pathways specific for cardiac and neural tube development (Gao and Gao 2007; Kumar et al. 2007; Morgan et al. 2008). A three- to fivefold increase in major malformations in infants as well as a fivefold increase in pregnancy loss rate in mothers with HbA1c levels (>7%) early in pregnancy has been demonstrated (Galindo et al. 2006). Latest recommendations include maintaining an HbA1c less than 5% in the first trimester of pregnancy and below 6% in the third trimester in healthy pregnant women with type 1 diabetes mellitus (Radder and van Roosmalen 2005). The American College of Obstetricians and Gynecologists have recommended that all women be offered routine screening ultrasound during pregnancy most commonly between 18 and 20 weeks gestation, although the ability to identify congenital anomalies with adequate sensitivity remains controversial (Abuhamad AZ for the ACOG Practice Committee 2009). The index of suspicion when evaluating a newborn infant of a diabetic mother (IDM) should clearly be very high.

46.5 Risks of Maternal Glucose Intolerance During the Fetal Period

Maternal hyperglycemia has effects on fetal growth, glucose metabolism, oxygenation, iron metabolism, cardiac anatomy and function, and transition to extrauterine life.

46.5.1 Growth Disorders

Neonatal macrosomia is the classic presentation of an IDM and results from biochemical changes along the maternal hyperglycemia – fetal hyperinsulinemia pathway (Gomella et al. 2004; Nold and Georgieff 2004). Early in the second half of pregnancy, the pancreatic islet cells mature, and insulin production escalates in response to hyperglycemia creating an environment of hyperinsulinemia, a key anabolic hormone, coupled with hyperglycemia, a key anabolic fuel. The combination produces a large increase in fetal fat stores and some mild increase in protein content (Nold and Georgieff 2004). Hepatomegaly, splenomegaly, and cardiomegaly resulting from septal hypertrophy are often seen in the context of a macrosomic infant, while the head circumference is usually not increased. A significantly increased fetal abdominal area growth rate in the third trimester has been associated with high maternal HbA1c levels early in pregnancy (Wong et al. 2006) and has been used to effectively reduce rates of macrosomia (Schaefer-Graf and Kleinwechter 2006). The risk of shoulder dystocia, perhaps the most feared birth complication, is greater for an infant of any weight born to a mother with diabetes or gestational glucose intolerance versus a normoglycemic mother (Langer et al. 1991). Accordingly, it has been recommended that elective cesarean be strongly considered for mothers with diabetes carrying a macrosomic fetus with fetal weight estimates greater than or equal to 4,500 g (American College of Obstetricians and Gynecologists 2014).

In contrast to the pathophysiology leading to the macrosomic infant, mothers with advanced diabetic vascular disease are at risk of having fetuses with significant growth deceleration, defined as birth weight less than the fifth percentile for gestational age.

46.5.2 Disorders of Glucose Metabolism

Glucose intolerance coupled with resistance to or absence of insulin characterizes maternal diabetes during pregnancy. Although glucose crosses the placenta to the fetus, insulin that is either maternal in origin or exogenously delivered does not reach the fetus. Therefore, fetal hyperglycemia leads to pancreatic islet cell stimulation and subsequent fetal insulin production. Additionally, hypoglycemic episodes may result from sudden reductions in maternal glucose in fetuses with islet cell hyperplasia.

Both hyper- and hypoglycemia have been identified as possible mechanisms for the increased fetal mortality rate seen in pregnancies complicated by diabetes (Lucas 2001).

46.5.3 Reduced Fetal Oxygenation

Abnormalities in fetal oxygenation during diabetic pregnancies were discovered in the 1980s and account for the high rate of polycythemia in offspring of poorly controlled diabetic mothers (Nold and Georgieff 2004).

The fetal hypoxia is a consequence of an elevated fetal basal metabolic rate stimulated by chronic hyperglycemia and hyperinsulinemia. With increases in rate of substrate uptake and oxidation, the fetal environment becomes hypoxic, since the higher oxygen demand cannot be met by increased oxygen transfer by the placenta (human or ovine). Several studies have demonstrated the attempt of the fetus to increase oxygen-carrying capacity in the face of hypoxemia including elevated erythropoietin concentrations and fetal polycythemia (Bard and Prosmanne 1987; Georgieff et al. 1989, 1990; Green et al. 1992; Stonestreet et al. 1989; Widness et al. 1981). Fetal hypoxia constitutes a risk to the developing brain as does the potential for hyperviscosity and resultant fetal stroke.

46.5.4 Disorders of Fetal Iron Metabolism

Chronic fetal hypoxemia and the subsequent compensatory erythropoiesis coupled with the larger blood volume of the macrosomic fetus place a large demand on fetal iron metabolism particularly in light of limitations on maternal-fetal iron transport to support this large demand.

IDMs are at greater risk for iron deficiency of multiple organs due to the inability of the placenta to upregulate iron transport sufficiently and subsequent iron prioritization and redistribution (DeBoer et al. 2005; Deinard et al. 1986; Georgieff et al. 1997; Petry et al. 1992, 1994; Riggins et al. 2009; Schmidt et al. 2004; Siddappa et al. 2004). These deficiencies can affect neurodevelopment into infancy and beyond (DeBoer et al. 2005; Deinard et al. 1986; Riggins et al. 2009; Schmidt et al. 2004; Siddappa et al. 2004). Decreased fetal hepatic iron stores, as indexed by abnormally low cord serum ferritin concentrations, occur in 65% of live-born IDMs (Georgieff et al. 1990).

46.5.5 Acute and Subacute Nonstructural Cardiac Abnormalities

Fetal cardiac septal hypertrophy and cardiomegaly as a result of glycogen loading from chronic hyperglycemia and hyperinsulinemia are specific phenotype findings associated with pregnancies complicated by maternal diabetes. Despite good maternal metabolic control, serial evaluations of cardiac growth demonstrated cardiac hypertrophy in late gestation (34–40 weeks) in fetuses of diabetic mothers (Weber et al. 1991) making cardiomegaly a possible contribution to the increased risk of fetal death in these pregnancies (Russell et al. 2008).

46.6 Risks of Maternal Glucose Intolerance During Pregnancy on the Neonate

The abnormal metabolic milieu of hyperglycemia and hyperinsulinemia during fetal life leads to multiple issues in the neonatal period, including abnormalities of neonatal body habitus, glucose, calcium and magnesium metabolism, hematologic status, cardiorespiratory function, bilirubin metabolism, and neurologic functioning (Table 1).

46.6.1 Growth Disorders and Breastfeeding Considerations

Newborn macrosomia has been predicted by poor maternal glycemic control, particularly in the last few weeks of gestation. Occurring in 15–45% of diabetic pregnancies, macrosomia has been

Table 1 Risk, assessment and management of neonatal metabolic complications in infants of diabetic mothers

Condition	Assessment	Action value	Management
Hypoglycemia	Serum glucose	<40 mg/dL (<2.2 mmol/L) first 24 h; <50 mg/dL (<2.8 mmol/L) after 72 h	Early feedings; IV 10% dextrose solution 2 mL/kg body weight; repeat serum glucose in ½ h
Hypocalcemia	Serum ionized calcium	<3.5 mg/dL	Calcium gluconate or calcium chloride if symptomatic; treat hypomagnesemia prior to calcium treatment
Hypomagnesemia	Serum magnesium	<1.5 mg/dL	Magnesium sulfate
Polycythemia	Hemoglobin	>20–23 g/dL	Partial exchange transfusion with target hematocrit of 55%
	Hematocrit (measured centrally)	>65–70%	Partial exchange transfusion with target hematocrit of 55%
Iron deficiency	Serum ferritin	<40 mcg/L	Follow-up hemoglobin and ferritin at 6 months
Hyperbilirubinemia	Serum indirect (unconjugated) bilirubin	Dependent on age and infant size	Phototherapy, early feedings, hydration, rarely exchange transfusion

generally defined as birth weight above the 90th percentile for gestational age or greater than 4,000 g (Moore 1999).

Macrosomia at birth serves as a marker for identifying infants at risk for neonatal morbidities, including hypoglycemia, hyperbilirubinemia, and neonatal acidosis (Moore 1999). Complete anthropometric measurements, including weight, length, and head circumference, should be assessed and plotted on population-specific appropriate growth curves for each infant soon after birth.

Appropriate for gestational age IDMs have been found to have significantly greater fat mass, percent of weight that was fat, and triceps, subscapular, abdominal, flank, and thigh skinfold measurements than infants of nondiabetic women (Catalano et al. 2003). Subsequently, macrosomic IDMs generally have higher weight than length and head circumference percentiles. Fetal hyperinsulinism due to gestational diabetes mellitus (GDM) promotes the excess accretion of adipose tissue, but there are additional metabolic alterations in these infants that contribute to increased fat mass. Maternal alterations in blood leptin, retinol-binding protein 4, and adiponectin concentrations have been associated with increased overall fatty acid placental transfer resulting in higher neonatal fat mass and birth weight (Herrera and Ortega-Senovilla 2014). There also appear to be alterations in lipid metabolism with lipoproteins including long-chain polyunsaturated fatty acids essential for development being lower in the IDMs (Herrera and Desoye 2015). Infants at risk for metabolic instability in the newborn period have been better identified by body proportion measurements, such as the mid-arm-circumference-to-head-circumference ratio or body composition analysis via air displacement plethysmography (Georgieff et al. 1988).

Although there have been positive effects noted on maternal metabolism in diabetic women who breastfeed, there have been concerning reports of negative long-term effects for breastfed offspring of diabetic mothers. Hyperglycemia during pregnancy has been associated with altered breast milk immune factors with decreased glycosylation of secretory immunoglobulin A and increased glycosylation of lactoferrin suggesting that glucose dysregulation in pregnancy may have lasting consequences on the protective immune functions of breast milk (Smilowitz et al. 2013). Breast milk from obese mothers has been shown to have an increased pro-inflammatory fatty acid profile (increased omega-6 to omega-3 ratio) and decreased concentrations of fatty acids including docosahexaenoic acid, eicosapentaenoic acid, docosapentaenoic acid, and lutein that have been shown to have a critical role in neurodevelopment (Panagos et al. 2016).

GDM has been associated with delayed lactogenesis in up to one third of women, especially in those who required insulin treatment, were obese, or with suboptimal inhospital breastfeeding (Matias et al. 2014). This delay in breast milk production had a detrimental effect on both breastfeeding initiation and duration in women with GDM.

46.6.2 Neonatal Hypoglycemia

Significant hypoglycemia, defined as a blood glucose level less than 45 mg/dL (2.5 mmol/L), has been seen in up to 50% of IDMs following birth, with macrosomic or growth-restricted IDMs more likely to have hypoglycemia than IDMs of appropriate size for gestational age (Gomella et al. 2004; Nold and Georgieff 2004). The abrupt discontinuation of maternally derived glucose combined with neonatal hyperinsulinemia leads to hypoglycemia in the macrosomic infants. Normally, this interruption in glucose delivery is followed by a decrease in neonatal plasma glucose between 30 and 90 min followed by spontaneous recovery in most infants (Kalhan and Parimi 2006). Hypoglycemia seen in infants with growth restriction due to diabetic vascular disease is more likely due to decreased hepatic glycogen stores and may not appear until 6–12 h after delivery (Gomella et al. 2004). Hypoglycemia can persist and therefore requires intervention consisting of a constant intravenous dextrose infusion.

Controversy exists concerning the threshold of what constitutes hypoglycemia, as little outcome data is available for symptomatic or asymptomatic hypoglycemia. A common recommendation is that IDMs be screened at 1/2, 1, 1.5, 2, 4, 8, 12, 24, 36, and 48 h of age (Gomella et al. 2004) and be treated to maintain a glucose between 45 and 60 mg/dL (2.5 mmol/L and 3.3 mmol/L) (Schwartz 1997).

Although most infants with hypoglycemia are asymptomatic, typical symptoms can include jitteriness, sweating, tachypnea or apnea, seizures, agitation, and respiratory distress. Newborn IDMs, especially those who are macrosomic or growth restricted, should be monitored closely with regularly scheduled serum glucose measurements.

Maternal history, with attention to glycemic control, and fetal anthropometric measurements and proportion studies can help to identify infants at highest risk (Georgieff et al. 1988).

Early initiation of feedings is highly recommended, as those infants who are asymptomatic, normoglycemic, and able to tolerate feedings do not need intravenous dextrose therapy.

46.6.3 Neonatal Hypocalcemia and Hypomagnesemia

Neonatal hypocalcemia and hypomagnesemia are two frequently encountered metabolic disturbances that occur in up to 50% of IDMs during the first 3 days of life and are related to lack of maternal glycemic control (Kalhan and Parimi 2006). A physiological nadir of serum calcium has been seen in healthy term infants by 24–48 h of age during the transition from fetal to neonatal parathyroid and calcitonin regulation (Jain et al. 2008). The nadir may be exaggerated to the point of hypocalcemia, generally accepted as an ionized calcium level less than 3.5 mg/dL (Gomella et al. 2004). Ionized calcium measurements, when available, are preferable to total serum calcium measurements. Hypocalcemia in the IDM may be caused by an inadequate neonatal parathyroid response to the abrupt interruption of maternally derived calcium as well as continual high levels of calcitonin and possibly disturbances in vitamin D metabolism (Kalhan and Parimi 2006).

Recent studies correlate maternal vitamin D levels in a significant negative relationship with HbA1c, supporting a potential role for this vitamin in promoting glycemic control. Fetal cord blood vitamin D levels were directly correlated with those of the mother, with significantly lower levels seen in obese versus normal weight women (Bennett et al. 2014). Decreased bone density has been found in large for gestational age (LGA) newborns among IDMs potentially related to vitamin D status and reduced fetal movements secondary to macrosomia (Schushan-Eisen et al. 2015).

Neonatal hypomagnesemia is related to maternal hypomagnesemia and severity of maternal diabetes (Gomella et al. 2004). A serum magnesium level less than 1.5 mg/dL is considered pathologic (Gomella et al. 2004) and may complicate the treatment of hypocalcemia.

Similar to hypoglycemia, neonatal hypocalcemia and hypomagnesemia may present with symptoms such as jitteriness, sweating, tachypnea, irritability, and seizures. They present later than hypoglycemia with nadirs seen at 24–72 h following birth (Nold and Georgieff 2004). Because of this similarity of symptoms, the jittery IDMs should have serum glucose, calcium, and magnesium levels measured. Symptomatic hypocalcemic IDMs can be treated with calcium chloride or calcium gluconate preferably via a central venous catheter to reduce the chance of peripheral vein damage from the medication. Hypomagnesemia needs to be corrected in order to enable normalization of calcium homeostasis.

46.6.4 Neonatal Polycythemia

Polycythemia is present in 20–30% of IDMs, particularly if the mother's glucose control was suboptimal. The definition of polycythemia is a central venous hemoglobin concentration greater than 20 g/dL or hematocrit greater than 65% (Nold and Georgieff 2004). Blood hyperviscosity at levels higher than these leads to morbidities including vascular sludging, ischemia, and infarction of vital organ systems (Moore 1999).

The cerebral microcirculation is one area at risk for hyperviscous blood sludging, resulting in neurologic irritability, jitteriness, and a high-pitched cry. Cerebral venous sinus thrombosis must be considered in these infants, and even though neuroimaging studies may not detect pathology, symptomatic, polycythemic IDMs should be treated with partial exchange transfusion to reduce blood viscosity and the predisposition to further clot formation (Nold and Georgieff 2004).

Symptoms of vascular sludging in the renal, intestinal, and pulmonary systems may or may not be explicit. Hypertension, thrombocytopenia, hematuria, and abdominal mass are all possible signs of renal vein thrombosis. Feeding intolerance or necrotizing enterocolitis may indicate intestinal sludging. Finally, pulmonary vascular bed sludging may present as persistent pulmonary hypertension with worsening respiratory distress syndrome.

Assessment including an initial hematocrit and platelet count should be obtained soon after birth. Because of the physiologic diuresis that occurs in all newborns, an increasing hematocrit over the first 3 days of life is not uncommon. This phenomenon, however, may prolong the risk for microvascular sludging in the polycythemic IDM, emphasizing the importance of appropriate monitoring and hydration. Sludging and thrombosis of the microvasculature of any of the aforementioned organ systems may first be indicated by a declining platelet count. Asymptomatic infants with hematocrit values from 65% to 70% ought to be hydrated with intravenous fluids at a rate of at least 100 mL/kg/day, and the hematocrit should be followed daily for the first 3 days. If the infant becomes symptomatic or the hematocrit continues to increase despite appropriate therapy, a partial volume exchange transfusion should be completed. An immediate partial exchange transfusion is indicated in any IDM who is symptomatic from blood hyperviscosity or those with a central hematocrit greater than 70% (Nold and Georgieff 2004).

46.6.5 Neonatal Iron Deficiency

Abnormalities of iron metabolism, including a risk of reduced brain iron concentrations at birth, have been demonstrated in 65% of IDMs and 95% of macrosomic IDMs (Amarnath et al. 1989; Chockalingam et al. 1987; Georgieff et al. 1990). Of note, IDMs with the highest hematocrits at birth tend to also have the lowest ferritin concentrations, suggesting that the available fetal iron has been shunted into the expanded red cell mass and away from storage and non-hematologic tissue pools, including the brain. Iron deficiency presents a risk to the developing brain including effects on myelination (Connor and Menzies 1996), brain energy metabolism (de Ungria et al. 2000), and brain monoamine neurotransmitter metabolism (Beard 2003). Newborn IDMs have altered cognitive processing compared to healthy, term infants (de Regnier et al. 2000). Treatment with supplemental iron (beyond normal recommendations) in the immediate newborn period has not been assessed with respect to improving the neurodevelopmental outcome and is currently not recommended since the tissue deficiency is thought to be due to a redistribution of iron into red cells rather than a total body iron deficiency.

46.6.6 Pulmonary and Cardiac Status

Respiratory distress syndrome (RDS) and transient tachypnea of the newborn (retained fetal lung fluid) are more commonly seen in IDMs than age-matched controls (Nold and Georgieff 2004). Fetal hyperinsulinemia may inhibit the normal maturational effect of cortisol on the lung leading to a decreased production of dipalmitoyl lecithin (Moore 1999). While the infant of a nondiabetic mother reaches pulmonary maturity at a mean of 34–35 weeks gestation, the IDM is not considered to be past the risk of pulmonary immaturity until 38.5 weeks gestational age (Moore 1999). Additionally, persistent pulmonary hypertension secondary to polycythemia-associated vascular sludging may complicate RDS as both polycythemia and RDS are associated with fetal hyperinsulinemia.

Cardiopulmonary adaptation (e.g., transition) in IDMs has been shown to be significantly different than infants born to nondiabetic mothers. The classic findings of interventricular septal hypertrophy caused by glycogen loading of the septum and cardiomyopathy have been seen in up to 30% of IDMs (Moore 1999). Hypertrophic subaortic stenosis physiology has been observed with severe septal hypertrophy rendering those infants in left ventricular outflow obstructive heart failure. In such a situation, inotropes and hypovolemia worsened the condition, whereas beta-blockers and volume helped to alleviate the obstruction. Cardiomyopathy has usually been seen in conjunction with septal hypertrophy, although it may appear exclusively (Nold and Georgieff 2004).

46.6.7 Hyperbilirubinemia

Indirect hyperbilirubinemia is a common finding in IDMs as they have an increased red cell mass, ineffective erythropoiesis, and relative immaturity of hepatic bilirubin conjugation and excretion (Nold and Georgieff 2004). A 30% greater source of bilirubin is produced by the increased cell mass, and conjugation and excretion by the relatively immature glucuronosyltransferase enzyme system create elevated serum unconjugated bilirubin levels. Bilirubin levels should be assessed within the first 24 h of life and then followed until a peak has been reached. Phototherapy with appropriate hydration monitoring is the mainstay of treatment, but some infants will require exchange transfusion, using the same criteria as in hyperbilirubinemic infants born to mothers without diabetes.

46.6.8 Neuropathology

Central nervous system dysfunction can be seen immediately in the newborn period as well as manifested by neurodevelopmental and behavioral abnormalities not recognized until later infancy or childhood. The IDM is at risk for multiple morbidities that can result in neurologic injury and symptoms. Polycythemia with vascular sludging, glucose and electrolyte abnormalities, birth trauma, and perinatal asphyxia due to macrosomia all pose possible etiologies for neurologic symptoms such as seizures, jitteriness, lethargy, tone abnormalities, and movement disorders. Different neurologic symptoms typically present at specific time periods based on the etiology. Perinatal depression, birth trauma, and hypoglycemia all generally present with symptomatology within the first 24 h of life. Alternatively, symptoms due to hypocalcemia or hypomagnesemia typically present between 24 and 72 h following birth, as this is the time period at which nadir levels are expected to be reached.

Initial hypotonia followed by increased tone, jitteriness, and seizures are signs and symptoms of brain injury secondary to perinatal asphyxia. The risk for seizures due to birth asphyxia generally peaks 24 h following birth. Glucose, electrolyte, or hematologic abnormalities must be identified and corrected prior to starting anticonvulsant therapy.

Brachial plexus nerve injuries secondary to neck stretching during delivery are more commonly seen in the macrosomic IDM than appropriately grown for gestational age infants. Erb's palsy (roots C5–C7), Klumpke's paralysis (roots C–C8), diaphragmatic nerve paralysis (roots C3–C5), and recurrent laryngeal nerve damage (roots T1–T2) have all been reported.

In humans, event-related potential (ERP) studies have indicated that while healthy, term infants born to nondiabetic mothers discriminate their own mother's voice from a stranger's voice, iron-deficient IDMs do not show evidence of discrimination, suggesting abnormal cognitive processing (de Regnier et al. 2007; Siddappa et al. 2004). Research in the newborn rat has demonstrated that maternal diabetes disrupts the regulation of both insulin receptors and insulin-like growth factor-1 receptors in the developing hippocampus. These hippocampal changes may be associated with cognitive and memory impairment seen in IDMs (Hami et al. 2015).

46.7 Long-Term Health Sequelae in IDMs

Periconceptional, fetal, and neonatal events all contribute to the long-term health issues of IDMs. The future risks for development include metabolic syndrome and iron status abnormalities in conjunction with neurodevelopmental problems.

46.7.1 Metabolic Syndrome

In light of the obesity epidemic, concerns have been raised about the long-term health risks of IDMs given their fetal exposure to an abnormal metabolic milieu and macrosomic neonatal body habitus. Several studies have focused on the initial growth and ultimate likelihood of IDMs to go on to develop metabolic syndrome, characterized by increased insulin resistance often seen in the setting of obesity, hypertension, and dyslipidemia (Boney et al. 2005; Fahrenkrog et al. 2004; Plagemann 2005; Touger et al. 2005; Vohr and Boney 2008). A longitudinal study focusing on growth of Pima Indian children showed significantly different patterns of growth of offspring of diabetic mothers compared to offspring of nondiabetic mothers. Offspring of diabetic mothers showed significant "catch-down" growth during their first 1.5 years of life but by age 7 had greatly exceeded the weight of offspring of nondiabetic mothers (Touger et al. 2005). Another longitudinal study identified a trend toward a higher incidence of insulin resistance (defined as a fasting glucose/insulin ratio of <7) in 11-year-old children who were large for gestational age at birth compared to those who were appropriate despite no difference in obesity. The authors also demonstrated by multivariate logistic regression that childhood obesity and the combination of large for gestational age status and maternal gestational diabetes were associated with insulin resistance (Boney et al. 2005). A review of studies examining the consequent development of metabolic syndrome in mothers with gestational diabetes and their offspring showed that metabolic syndrome in children with increasing age is related to maternal gestational diabetes, maternal glycemia in the third trimester, maternal obesity, neonatal macrosomia, and childhood obesity (Vohr and Boney 2008). Studies evaluating lipid status in euglycemic offspring of diabetic parents have shown decreased high-density lipoprotein levels with significant association between parental diabetes status and dyslipidemia (Carlton Johnnny and Anuratha 2016).

46.7.2 Neurodevelopment

Because of the multiple morbidities for which IDMs are at increased risk, the long-term motor and cognitive developmental trajectories of these children have been studied in comparison to infants born to normoglycemic mothers. Acute perinatal events as well as abnormal intrauterine environmental affects have contributed to the long-term risks to brain development. Both newborn studies and longitudinal research have demonstrated significant neurodevelopmental differences between these groups of offspring.

For infants that experience seizures in the newborn period, the etiology of the seizures is critical for determining prognosis. Seizures caused by metabolic abnormalities such as hypoglycemia or hypocalcemia have a 10–50% risk of later developmental delays. In contrast, infants who have seizures due to hypoxic-ischemic encephalopathy carry an 80% risk for developmental problems (Volpe 2001). Transient hypoglycemia in the presence of large for gestational age infants born to normoglycemic mothers has been shown to have no harmful impact on psychomotor development at 4 years (Brand et al. 2005). Symptomatic, severe hypoglycemia (blood glucose <35 mg/dL or <2 mmol/L), however, has been shown to be associated with neurodevelopmental abnormalities and white matter injury identified on MRI (Burns et al. 2008). MRI has been recommended for routine evaluation of a newborn infant with symptomatic hypoglycemia to elucidate any cerebral injury (Inder 2008).

Specific areas of neurodevelopment of offspring born to diabetic mothers have been shown to correlate with the degree of maternal glycemic control (Nelson et al. 2003; Ornoy 2005; Riggins et al. 2009; Rizzo et al. 1997). Problems with attention span and motor functions appear to be present even in well-controlled mothers. Gross cognitive ability has appeared to be maintained unless pregnancies are associated with significant maternal nephropathy or hypertension or with neonatal iron deficiency (Riggins et al. 2009) in which case the effects negatively correlate with the level of maternal glycemic control (Ornoy 2005; Riggins et al. 2009). Another longitudinal study that followed IDMs until 11 years of age showed that poorly controlled antepartum maternal glucose and lipid metabolism correlated with poorer child performance on standard measures of neuropsychological functioning (Rizzo et al. 1997). Research in obese mothers with GDM actually demonstrated a temporary mild acceleration in cognitive development in early infancy at 6 months of age; however, by 18 months of age, there was a rapid deceleration of scores particularly in the language domain (Torres-Espinola et al. 2015). This work stressed the importance of long-term evaluation of brain development in IDMs.

46.8 Summary

Advances in medical care of pregnant women with diabetes have led to improved outcomes for mothers and their offspring. Despite this trend, the rising obesity epidemic has the potential to alter the course of progress. Metabolic syndrome characterized by insulin resistance and type II diabetes mellitus will likely continue to rise over the ensuing decade making glycemic control a more universal issue. Health-care providers who care for pregnant women ought to stress the possible implications of poor glucose control, including fetal hypoxia and iron deficiency, that can affect long-term neurodevelopmental trajectories of their infants. Women who first present with insulin resistance in pregnancy, particularly those who are overweight or obese, need to be followed for the possibility of developing type II diabetes later in life. Additionally, health-care providers of infants and children ought to be aware of the possible sequelae for offspring of diabetic mothers both in the neonatal period as well as long term. Atypical neurodevelopment and the propensity for a metabolic derangement are two arenas that warrant further research and attention as these infants are followed throughout childhood.

46.9 Disclosure

This work was sponsored in part by grants to MKG from the National Institutes of Health (HD-29421; NS-34458; HD-54490; and RR-00400-39).

References

Abuhamad AZ for the ACOG Practice Committee (2009) Ultrasonography in pregnancy. Obstet Gynecol 113:451–461, PMID: 19155920

Amarnath UM, Ophoven JJ, Mills MM (1989) The relationship between decreased iron stores, serum iron and neonatal hypoglycemia in large-for-date newborn infants. Acta Paediatr Scand 78:538–543

American College of Obstetricians and Gynecologists (2014) Safe prevention of the primary cesarean delivery. Obstet Gynecol 123:693–711

Bard H, Prosmanne J (1987) Relative rates of fetal hemoglobin and adult hemoglobin synthesis in cord blood of infants of insulin-dependent diabetic mothers. Pediatrics 75:1143–1147

Beard J (2003) Neonatal iron deficiency results in irreversible changes in dopamine function in rats. J Nutr 133:1174–1179

Bennett SE, McPeake J, McCance DR, Manderson JG, Johnston P, McGalliard R, McGinty A (2014) Maternal vitamin D status in Type 1 diabetic pregnancy: impact on neonatal vitamin D status and association with maternal glycaemic control. Pregnancy Hypertens 4:235–236, PMID: 26104623

Boney CM, Verma A, Tucker R, Vohr BR (2005) Metabolic syndrome in childhood: association with birth weight, maternal obesity, and gestational diabetes mellitus. Pediatrics 115:e290–e296

Brand PL, Molenaar NL, Kaaijk C, Wierenga WS (2005) Neurodevelopmental outcome of hypoglycaemia in healthy, large for gestational age, term newborns. Arch Dis Child 90:78–81

Burns CM, Rutherford MA, Boardman JP, Cowan FM (2008) Patterns of cerebral injury and neurodevelopmental outcomes after symptomatic neonatal hypoglycemia. Pediatrics 122:65–74

Carlton Johnnny J, Anuratha N (2016) Study of lipid status in the euglycemic offsrpin of diabetic parents with sex, age matched controls among South India population. Diabetes Metab Syndr 16 pii: S1871 – 4021. PMID: 27012159

Catalano PM, Thomas A, Huston-Presley L, Amini SB (2003) Increased fetal adiposity: a very sensitive marker of abnormal in utero development. Am J Obstet Gynecol 189:1698–1704

Chockalingam UM, Murphy E, Ophoven JC et al (1987) Cord transferrin and ferritin values in newborn infants at risk for prenatal uteroplacental insufficiency and chronic hypoxia. J Pediatr 111:283–286

Connor JR, Menzies SL (1996) Relationship of iron to oligodendrocytes and myelination. Glia 17:89–93, CrossRef

Correa A, Gilboa SM, Besser LM et al (2008) Diabetes mellitus and birth defects. Am J Obstet Gynecol 199 (237):e1–e9

de Regnier RA, Nelson CA, Thomas KM et al (2000) Neurophysiologic evaluation of auditory recognition memory in healthy newborn infants and infants of diabetic mothers. J Pediatr 137:777–784, CrossRef

de Regnier RA, Long JD, Georgieff MK, Nelson CA (2007) Using event-related potentials to study perinatal nutrition and brain development in infants of diabetic mothers. Dev Neuropsychol 31:379–396, CrossRef

de Ungria M, Rao R, Wobken JD et al (2000) Perinatal iron deficiency decreases cytochrome c oxidase (cytox) activity in selected regions of neonatal rat brain. Pediatr Res 48:169–176, CrossRef

DeBoer T, Wewerka S, Bauer PJ (2005) Explicit memory performance in infants of diabetic mothers at 1 year of age. Dev Med Child Neurol 47:525–531

Deinard AS, List A, Lindgren B et al (1986) Cognitive deficits in iron-deficient and iron-deficient anemic children. J Pediatr 108(5 Part 1):681–689

Fahrenkrog S, Harder T, Stolaczyk E et al (2004) Cross-fostering to diabetic rat dams affects early development of mediobasal hypothalamic nuclei regulating food intake, body weight, and metabolism. J Nutr 134:648–654

Fuhrmann K, Reiher H, Semmler K et al (1983) Prevention of congenital malformations in infants of insulin-dependent diabetic mothers. Diabetes Care 6:219–223

Galindo A, Burguillo AG, Azriel S, Fuente Pde L (2006) Outcome of fetuses in women with pregestational diabetes mellitus. J Perinat Med 34:323–331

Gao Q, Gao YM (2007) Hyperglycemic condition disturbs the proliferation and cell death of neural progenitors in mouse embryonic spinal cord. Int J Dev Neurosci 25:349–357

Georgieff MK (1995) Therapy of infants of diabetic mothers. In: Burg FD, Ingelfinger JR, Wald ER, Polin RA (eds) Current pediatric therapy, 15th edn. WB Saunders, Philadelphia, pp 793–803

Georgieff MK (2006) The effect of maternal diabetes during pregnancy on the neurodevelopment of offspring. Minn Med 89:44–47

Georgieff MK, Sasanow SR, Chockalingam UM, Pereira GR (1988) A comparison of the mid-arm circumference/head circumference ratio and ponderal index for the evaluation of newborn infants after abnormal intrauterine growth. Acta Paediatr Scand 77:214–219

Georgieff MK, Widness JA, Mills MM, Stonestreet BS (1989) The effect of prolonged intrauterine hyperinsulinemia on iron utilization in fetal sheep. Pediatr Res 26:467–469

Georgieff MK, Landon MB, Mills MM et al (1990) Abnormal iron distribution in infants of diabetic mothers: spectrum and maternal antecedents. J Pediatr 117:455–461

Georgieff MK, Petry CD, Mills MM (1997) Increased N-glycosylation and reduced transferrin binding capacity of transferrin receptor isolated from placentas of diabetic mothers. Placenta 18:563–568

Gomella TL, Cunningham MD, Eyal FG, Zenk KE (2004) Neonatology: management, procedures, on-call problems, diseases, and drugs, 5th edn. McGraw-Hill, New York, pp 418–433

Green DW, Khoury J, Mimouni F (1992) Neonatal hematocrit and maternal glycemic control in insulin-dependent diabetic mothers. J Pediatr 12:302–305

Hami J, Shojae F, Vafaee-Nezhad S, Lotfi N, Kheradmand H, Haghir H (2015) Some of the experimental and clinical aspects of the effects of the maternal diabetes on the developing hippocampus. World J Diabetes 15:412–422, PMID: 25897352

Herranz L, Pallardo LF, Hillman N et al (2007) Maternal third trimester hyperglycaemic excursions predict large-for-gestationalage infants in type 1 diabetic pregnancy. Diabetes Res Clin Pract 75:42–46

Herrera E, Desoye G (2015) Maternal and fetal lipid metabolism under normal and gestational diabetic conditions. Horm Mol Biol Clin Invest 23:1868–1883, PMID: 26351960

Herrera E, Ortega-Senovilla H (2014) Lipid metabolism during pregnancy and its implications for fetal growth. Curr Pharm Biotechnol 15:24–31, PMID: 247201597

Inder T (2008) How low can I go? The impact of hypoglycemia on the immature brain. Pediatrics 122:440–441

Jain A, Agarwal R, Sankar MJ (2008) Hypocalcemia in the newborn. Indian J Pediatr 75:165–169

Kalhan SC, Parimi PS (2006) Diabetes in pregnancy: the infant of a diabetic mother. In: Martin RJ, Fanaroff AA, Walsh MC (eds) Neonatal-perinatal medicine, 8th edn. Elsevier Mosby, Philadelphia, pp 1473–1478

Kumar SD, Dheen ST, Tay SS (2007) Maternal diabetes induces congenital heart defects in mice by altering the expression of genes involved in cardiovascular development. Cardiovasc Diabetol 30:34, CrossRef

Langer O, Berkus MD, Huff RW, Samueloff A (1991) Shoulder dystocia: should the fetus weighing greater than or equal to 4000 grams be delivered by cesarean section? Am J Obstet Gynecol 165(4 Pt 1):831–837

Lucas MJ (2001) Medical complications of pregnancy: diabetes complicating pregnancy. Obstet Gynecol Clin N Am 28:513–536

Matias SL, Dewey KG, Quesenberry CP, Gunderson EP (2014) Maternal prepregnancy obesity and insulin treatment during pregnancy are independently associated with delayed lactogenesis in women with recent gestational diabetes mellitus. Am J Clin Nutr 99:115–121, PMID: 24196401

Moore TR (1999) Diabetes in pregnancy. In: Creasy RK, Resnik R (eds) Maternal-fetal medicine. WB Saunders, Philadelphia, pp 964–995

Morgan SC, Relaix F, Sandell LL, Loeken MR (2008) Oxidative stress during diabetic pregnancy disrupts cardiac neural crest migration and causes outflow tract defects. Birth Defects Res A Clin Mol Teratol 82:453–463

Nelson CA, Wewerka SS, Borscheid AJ et al (2003) Electrophysiologic evidence of impaired cross-modal recognition memory in 8-month-old infants of diabetic mothers. J Pediatr 142:575–582

Nold JL, Georgieff MK (2004) Infants of diabetic mothers. Pediatr Clin N Am 51:619–637, CrossRef

Ornoy A (2005) Growth and neurodevelopmental outcome of children born to mothers with pregestational and gestational diabetes. Pediatr Endocrinol Rev 3:104–113

Panagos PG, Vishwanathan R, Penfield-Cyr A, Matthan NR, Shivappa N, Wirth MD, Herbert JR, Sen S (2016) Breastmilk from obese mothers has pro-inflamatory properties and decreased neuroprotective factors. J Perinatol 36:284–290, PMID: 26741571

Petry CD, Eaton MA, Wobken JA et al (1992) Liver, heart, and brain iron deficiency in newborn infants of diabetic mothers. J Pediatr 121:109–114

Petry CD, Wobken JD, McKay H et al (1994) Placental transferrin receptor in diabetic pregnancies with increased fetal iron demand. Am J Physiol 267: E507–E514

Plagemann A (2005) Perinatal programming and functional teratogenesis: impact on body weight regulation and obesity. Physiol Behav 86:661–668

Radder JK, van Roosmalen J (2005) HbA1c in healthy, pregnant women. Neth J Med 63:256–259

Rajdl D, Racek J, Steinerová A et al (2005) Markers of oxidative stress in diabetic mothers and their infants during delivery. Physiol Res 54:429–436

Riggins T, Miller NC, Bauer PJ et al (2009) Consequences of low neonatal iron status due to maternal diabetes mellitus on explicit memory performance in childhood. Dev Neuropsychol 34:762–779

Rizzo TA, Metzger BE, Dooley SL, Cho NH (1997) Early malnutrition and child neurobehavioral development: insights from the study of children of diabetic mothers. Child Dev 68:26–38

Russell NE, Holloway P, Quinn S et al (2008) Cardiomyopathy and cardiomegaly in stillborn infants of diabetic mothers. Pediatr Dev Pathol 11:10–14

Savona-Ventura C, Gatt M (2004) Embryonal risks in gestational diabetes mellitus. Early Hum Dev 79:59–63

Schaefer-Graf UM, Kleinwechter H (2006) Diagnosis and new approaches in the therapy of gestational diabetes mellitus. Curr Diabetes Rev 2:343–352

Schmidt AT, Waldow KJ, Salinas JA, Georgieff MK (2004) The long-term behavioral effects of fetal/neonatal iron deficiency on a hippocampally dependent learning task in the rat. Pediatr Res 55:279A

Schushan-Eisen I, Cohen M, Leibovitch L, Maayan-Metzger A, Strauss T (2015) Bone density among infants of gestational diabetic mothers and macrosomic neonates. Matern Child Health J 19:578–582, PMID: 25138627

Schwartz RP (1997) Neonatal hypoglycemia: how low is too low? J Pediatr 131:171–173

Siddappa AM, Georgieff MK, Wewerka S et al (2004) Iron deficiency alters auditory recognition memory in newborn infants of diabetic mothers. Pediatr Res 55:1034–1041

Smilowitz JT, Totten SM, Huang J, Grapov D, Durham HA, Lammi-Keefe CJ, Lebrilla C, German JB (2013) Human milk secretory immunoglobulin a and lactoferrin N-glycans are altered in women with gestational diabetes mellitus. J Nutr 143:1906–1912, PMID 24047700

Stonestreet BS, Goldenstein M, Oh W, Widness JA (1989) Effect of prolonged hyperinsulinemia on erythropoiesis in fetal sheep. Am J Physiol 257:R1199–R1204

Torres-Espinola FJ, Berglund SK, Garcia-Valdes LM, Segura MT, Jerez A, Campos D, Moreno-Torres R, Rueda R, Catena A, Perez-Garcia M, Campoy C, PREOBE Team (2015) Maternal obesity, overweight, and gestational diabetes affect the offspring neurodevelopment at 6 and 18 months of age- a follow up from the PREOBE cohort. PLoS One 10:e0133010, PMID: 26208217

Touger L, Looker HC, Krakoff J et al (2005) Early growth in offspring of diabetic mothers. Diabetes Care 28:585–589

Vohr BR, Boney CM (2008) Gestational diabetes: the forerunner for the development of maternal and childhood obesity and metabolic syndrome? J Matern Fetal Neonatal Med 21:149–157

Volpe JJ (2001) Neonatal seizures. In: Volpe JJ (ed) Neurology of the newborn, 4th edn. WB Saunders, Philadelphia, pp 178–216

Weber HS, Copel JA, Reece EA et al (1991) Cardiac growth in fetuses of diabetic mothers with good metabolic control. J Pediatr 118:103–107

Widness JA (1989) Fetal risks and neonatal complications of diabetes mellitus and metabolic and endocrine disorders. In: Brody SA, Ueland K (eds) Endocrine disorders in pregnancy. Appleton-Lang, Norwalk, pp 273–297

Widness JA, Susa JB, Garcia JF et al (1981) Increased erythropoiesis and elevated erythropoietin in infants born to diabetic mothers and in hyperinsulinemic rhesus fetuses. J Clin Invest 67:637–642

Wong SF, Lee-Tannock A, Amaraddio D et al (2006) Fetal growth patterns in fetuses of women with pregestational diabetes mellitus. Ultrasound Obstet Gynecol 28:934–938

Zhao Z, Reece EA (2005) Experimental mechanisms of diabetic embryopathy and strategies for developing therapeutic interventions. J Soc Gynecol Investig 12:549–557

9783319294872VOL01

Neonatology

Giuseppe Buonocore • Rodolfo Bracci
Michael Weindling
Editors

Neonatology

A Practical Approach to Neonatal Diseases

Second Edition

Volume 2

With 568 Figures and 386 Tables

Springer

Editors
Giuseppe Buonocore
Department of Pediatrics
Obstetrics and Reproductive Medicine
University of Siena
Siena, Italy

Rodolfo Bracci
Department of Pediatrics
Obstetrics and Reproductive Medicine
University of Siena
Siena, Italy

Michael Weindling
Liverpool Women's Hospital Neonatal Unit
Liverpool, UK

ISBN 978-3-319-29487-2 ISBN 978-3-319-29489-6 (eBook)
ISBN 978-3-319-29488-9 (print and electronic bundle)
https://doi.org/10.1007/978-3-319-29489-6

Library of Congress Control Number: 2018940273

Printed on acid-free paper

This Springer imprint is published by the registered company Springer International Publishing AG part of Springer Nature.
The registered company address is: Gewerbestrasse 11, 6330 Cham, Switzerland

Introduction

Neonatology is a science in rapid evolution. The speed of this evolution may cause some to doubt what a traditional textbook is able to achieve in bringing the most up-to-date developments to a reader's attention. Although the interested reader will use other electronic means to access current information, this is not always possible. We firmly believe that, through their own experience, experts are able to bring their own perspective and interest to a subject and act as a guide to the interested and committed reader. We therefore believe that this textbook should act as a conduit of reliable information from the expert to the clinician. We have tried to make this textbook into a genuine guide to the best and most up-to-date answers for neonatologists who are striving to give the best and highest quality care to sick babies.

All practicing clinicians work within their own culture and resources. Each has to make judgments about the best and most appropriate application of available resources to the care of their small sick patients. We hope that this textbook will support the dedicated clinician by providing the best evidence available in the various sub-specialisms of neonatology, particularly when the issue of best treatment continues to be debated. The reader who needs rapid and comprehensive information about a topic requires that the information provided should be synthetized intelligently, exhaustively, and clearly. Subjects should be updated as much as possible. We have endeavored to meet these requirements. We think that the aim of a modern textbook should be to describe the present state of the science, suggesting ways in which this might be improved, and to provide a sound understanding of pathophysiology and diagnostic and therapeutic procedures. Our overall aim is to support and optimize the care of the newborn. In this way, our approach is "practical" and aims to assist neonatologists in their daily work.

In this second edition, the text has been largely revised by experts who contributed to the previous volume. They have added new information, some of it through short- and long-term follow-up, to support the evidence that underpins good clinical practice. Some chapters are completely new.

We are grateful to all the authors for their time and contributions. We would also like to thank Andrew Spencer, Tina Shelton, Vasowati Shome, and the publication team of Springer for their great efforts in publishing this book.

We sincerely hope that this volume has built on the success of its predecessor and continues to support clinicians in a readily accessible and useful way.

Contents

Volume 1

About the Editors

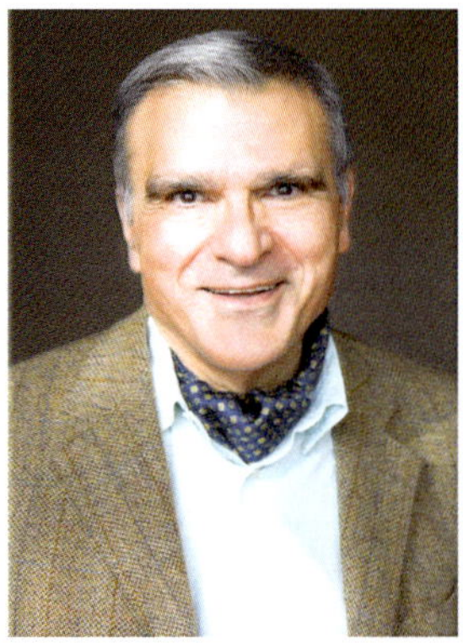

Giuseppe Buonocore is an Italian pediatrician, who is internationally recognized for his research on neonatal diseases, oxidative stress, and early identification of the newborn at high risk of brain damage. He is a full Professor of Pediatrics, Department of Molecular and Developmental Medicine, University of Siena, Italy, and Director of the Division of Pediatric-Neonatology, Azienda Ospedaliera-Universitaria of Siena, Italy. He is Chairman of Pediatrics at the School of Specialization in Pediatrics and Neonatology, University of Siena, Italy.

He is the President and Coordinator of European scientific network EURope Against Infant Brain Injury (EURAIBI). He has been a Visiting Professor at the University of Pennsylvania, the University of Florida, the University Hospitals of New York, as well as at the University of Oulu, Finland, at Taipei Medical University, and at Chang Gung Memorial Hospital at Linkou, Taiwan.

He is also the past President of ESPR and UENPS and currently President of the National College of University Full Professors of Pediatrics. He is involved in the coordination of numerous pan-European clinical trials as well as American and Australian. He has received many scientific awards: including the Seventh annual Dr. Donald V Eitzman lectures "Iron homeostasis metabolism and toxicity," University of Florida (2000), and the "Goccia d'oro 2010" for the efforts and results in the scientific research in the field of

Prenatal, Perinatal, and Neonatal Brain Damage. He also holds the patent of a scientific invention: the "Machine for automatic assessment of pain in neonates."

Dr. Buonocore has supervised more than 200 M.D./Ph.D. students (1994/2018) in Medicine and Surgery, Pediatrics, and Diagnostic Biochemistry. His current research interests are in the mechanisms of cell damage in the neonatal brain, with special reference to hypoxia, and the role of oxidant radicals in neonatal diseases and in babies with birth asphyxia. Additional research interest fields are ethics in perinatology and fetal and neonatal pain prevention. His research team is funded by several agencies including the Italian Ministry of University and Scientific Research as well as the European Community. Prof. Buonocore is author of more than 900 publications: 3 books and 27 book chapters, 300 peer-reviewed articles, and more than 617 presentations at international conferences and national meetings. He is currently Editor-in-Chief of *Current Pediatric Reviews*, Associate Editor of *Journal of Pineal Research*, and on the editorial board of several international scientific journals. He has organized more than 20 European conferences and has been the scientific coordinator or participant in several national and international clinical trials.

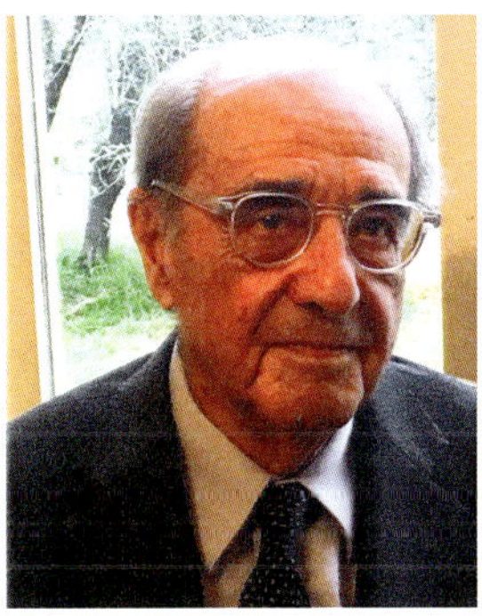

Rodolfo Bracci was born in Siena (Italy) in 1931. After graduating in Medicine and Surgery from the University of Siena Medical School in 1955, he became Assistant Professor of Pediatrics in the University of Siena. He was Post doctoral Trainee at the Albert Einstein College of Medicine, New York (1964–1965). At that time, working under the direction of Professor Ruth Gross, he made the first experiences on the antioxidant properties of the red cells of newborn. After his return to Italy, he became Assistant Professor of Pediatrics at the University of Florence and later at the University of Siena. He continued to be involved in the field of oxygen toxicity of the erythrocyte of newborn, and in 1967, he demonstrated that the red cells of newborn may have not only a low protection against reacting oxygen species but also an increased production of them.

Professor of Neonatology of the University of Siena and Director of the Neonatal Intensive Care Unit of the Siena Hospital, he was leading a staff of researchers involved in the physiopathology of the neonate, particularly in the calcium homeostasis, in the opioids metabolism, and especially in the

problems of oxygen toxicity in the red cells as well as in various organs. More than a hundred papers were published in important international journals by the doctors working under the guidance of Rodolfo Bracci. He was invited speaker in many international congresses and seminars in various cities in Europe and in America.

He has been member of the European Society of Pediatric Hematology and Immunology, the European Society for Pediatric Research, the European Society for Perinatal Medicine, the Neonatal Intensive Care Collegium, the Italian Society of Pediatrics, and the Italian Society of Neonatology.

Retired from University of Siena in 2001, he continued to publish papers, mainly together with Professor G. Buonocore.

Michael Weindling is Emeritus Professor of Perinatal Medicine at the University of Liverpool and Honorary Consultant Neonatologist at Liverpool Women's Hospital, where he was responsible for the care of newborn babies in a tertiary neonatal intensive care unit until he retired from clinical work in 2013. He is an Associate Editor of *Acta Paediatrica*. He continues with his research interest into the maintenance of appropriate brain oxygenation, cerebral hemodynamics, and the prevention of acquired damage of the developing brain.

He studied medicine at Guy's Hospital in London and qualified in 1973. His training in London included a period at the Great Ormond Street Hospital for Sick Children and then as research fellow at the University of Oxford, where he studied the cerebral hemodynamics of the developing brain. Michael Weindling was appointed a Senior Lecturer and consultant in Liverpool in 1985. During his early years as a consultant, he undertook a master's degree in medical ethics at the University of Keele with a dissertation into the changing moral status of the developing human from conceptus to neonate. He was promoted to Professor in 1996 with a personal chair entitled Professor of Perinatal Medicine, a title chosen to reflect his interest into the rapidly changing requirements of the developing brain. He has a considerable interest in medical education and for several years was Head of the School of Paediatrics in Merseyside.

Contributors

Steven H. Abman University of Colorado Denver – Anschutz Medical Campus, Denver, CO, USA

Massimo Agosti Neonatology and NICU – Maternal and Child Department, Ospedale "F del Ponte", Varese, Italy

Rocco Agostino Ethics Committee, Pediatric Hospital Bambino Gesù, Rome, Italy

Carlo Agostoni Pediatric Clinic, Department of Clinical Sciences and Community Health, University of Milan Fondazione, IRCCS Ca Granda, Ospedale Maggiore Policlinico, Milano, Italy

Munir Ahmed Division of Asthma, Allergy and Lung Biology, MRC Centre for Allergic Mechanisms of Asthma, King's College London, London, UK

Uma Sankari Ali Nephrology Division and PICU, BJ Wadia Hospital for Children, Mumbai, India

Karel Allegaert Neonatal Intensive Care Unit, University Hospitals Leuven, Leuven, Belgium

Department of Development and Regeneration, KU Leuven, Leuven, Belgium

Intensive Care and Department of Pediatric Surgery, Erasmus MC – Sophia Children's Hospital, Rotterdam, The Netherlands

Ruben E. Alvaro Department of Pediatrics, WR004 Women's Hospital, University of Manitoba, Winnipeg, MB, Canada

Gina Ancora Neonatology and Neonatal Intensive Care Unit, Ospedale Infermi, Rimini, Italy

Endla K. Anday Department of Pediatrics, Drexel University College of Medicine, St. Christopher's Hospital for Children, Neonatal-Perinatal Medicine, Philadelphia, PA, USA

Generoso Andria Department of Translational Medicine, Section of Pediatrics, Federico II University of Naples, Naples, Italy

Rajesh K. Aneja Departments of Critical Care Medicine and Pediatrics, University of Pittsburgh School of Medicine, Children's Hospital of Pittsburgh, Pittsburgh, PA, USA

Ruby V. Aneja Division of Neonatology, Temple University, West Penn Hospital, Pittsburgh, PA, USA

Molinari Angelo Claudio Thrombosis and Hemostasis Unit, Giannina Gaslini Children's Hospital, Genova, Italy

Rossella Angotti Department of Pediatrics, Obstetrics and Reproductive Medicine, Section of Pediatric Surgery, University of Siena, Siena, Italy

Carmelo Arcidiacono Department of Pediatric Cardiology, IRCCS Policlinico San Donato, San Siro, Milan, Italy

Domenico Arduini Department of Obstetrics and Gynecology, University of Rome Tor Vergata, Rome, Italy

Roberto Aufieri Division of Neonatology and Neonatal Intensive Care, Casilino General Hospital, Rome, Italy

Franco Bagnoli Department of Pediatrics, Obstetrics and Reproductive Medicine, University of Siena, Siena, Italy

Milica Bajcetic Institute of Pharmacology, Clinical Pharmacology and Toxicology, Medical Faculty, University of Belgrade, Belgrade, Serbia

Clinical Pharmacology Unit, University Children's Hospital, Belgrade, Serbia

Sarah Bajorek Department of Pediatrics, Division of Neonatology, University of Florida, College of Medicine, Gainesville, FL, USA

Antonio Balsamo Department of Medical and Surgical Sciences, Pediatric Unit, Center for Rare Endocrine Diseases (CARENDO BO), S.Orsola Malpighi University Hospital, Bologna, Italy

Jane E. Barthell Children's Hospitals and Clinics of Minnesota, Minneapolis, MN, USA

Francesco Bazzini Department of Molecular and Developmental Medicine, University of Siena, Siena, Italy

Roberto Bellù NICU, Ospedale Manzoni, Lecco, Italy

Franca Fossati-Bellani Pediatric Oncology Department, Fondazione IRCCS Istituto Nazionale dei Tumori, Milan, Italy

Carlo V. Bellieni Neonatal Intensive Care Unit, Siena University Hospital, Siena, Italy

Simonetta Bellone Department of Health Sciences, Division of Pediatrics, University of Piemonte Orientale, Novara, Italy

Elisa Belvisi Department of Molecular and Developmental Medicine, University of Siena, Siena, Italy

Britney Benoit School of Nursing, Centre for Pediatric Pain Research, Maternal-Newborn Program, Dalhousie University, IWK Health Centre, Halifax, Canada

Silvano Bertelloni Adolescent Medicine Unit, Division of Pediatrics, S. Chiara Hospital, University of Pisa, Pisa, Italy

Giovanna Bertini Neonatal Intensive Care Unit, Careggi University Hospital, Florence, Italy

Enrico Bertino Neonatal Unit, University of Turin, Turin, Italy

Natascia Bertoncelli Neonatal Intensive Care Unit, Department of Medical and Surgical Sciences of the Mother, Children and Adults, University Hospital of Modena, Modena, Italy

Giulio Bevilacqua Department of Pediatrics and Neonatology, Eastern Liguria Hospital, La Spezia, Italy

Stefania Bezzio Department of Pediatrics, University of Turin, Turin, Italy

Vineet Bhandari Neonatology/Pediatrics, St. Christopher's Hospital for Children/Drexel University College of Medicine, Philadelphia, PA, USA

Drexel University, Philadelphia, PA, USA

Paolo Biban Azienda Ospedaliera Universitaria Integrata Verona, Verona, Italy

Roberta Bilenchi Department of Medical, Surgical and Neurological Sciences, Dermatology Section, University of Siena, Siena, Italy

Caterina Bocchi Obstetrics and Gynecology, Department of Molecular and Developmental Medicine, University of Siena, Siena, Italy

Antonio Boldrini Department of Clinical and Experimental Medicine, Division of Neonatology and Neonatal Intensive Care Unit, Santa Chiara University Hospital, Pisa, Italy

Maria Elena Bolis Neonatology and NICU – Maternal and Child Department, Ospedale "F del Ponte", Varese, Italy

Gianni Bona Department of Health Sciences, Division of Pediatrics, University of Piemonte Orientale, Novara, Italy

Rachele Bonfiglio Department of Anesthesia, Pediatric and Neonatal Intensive Care, Istituto Giannina Gaslini, Genoa, Italy

Alessandro Borghesi Neonatal Intensive Care Unit, Fondazione IRCCS Policlinico 'San Matteo', Pavia, Italy

Giulio Bosco Sapienza Università di Roma, Policlinico Umberto I di Roma, Rome, Italy

Farid Boubred Division of Neonatology, La Conception Hospital, Marseille, France

Rodolfo Bracci University of Siena, Siena, Italy

Nicola Brunetti-Pierri Department of Translational Medicine, Section of Pediatrics, Federico II University of Naples, Naples, Italy

Jenny Bua Division of Neonatology, Institute for Maternal and Child Health IRCCS 'Burlo Garofolo', Trieste, Italy

Wilma Buffolano Heading Coordinating Centre for Perinatal Infection-Campania Region, Translational Medicine Department, Federico II Medical School, Naples, Italy

Giuseppe Buonocore University of Siena, Siena, Italy

Marsha Campbell-Yeo Departments of Pediatrics, Psychology and Neuroscience, Dalhousie University School of Nursing, Halifax, Canada

Letizia Capasso Division of Neonatology, Department of Translational Medical Sciences, Università "Federico II" di Napoli, Naples, Italy

Joseph A. Carcillo Departments of Critical Care Medicine and Pediatrics, University of Pittsburgh School of Medicine, Children's Hospital of Pittsburgh, Pittsburgh, PA, USA

Mario Carminati Department of Pediatric Cardiology, IRCCS Policlinico San Donato, San Siro, Milan, Italy

Virgilio P. Carnielli Division of Neonatology, Salesi Hospital, Polytechnic University of Marche, Ancona, Italy

Elisa della Casa Neonatal Intensive Care Unit, Department of Medical and Surgical Sciences of the Mother, Children and Adults, University Hospital of Modena, Modena, Italy

Alessandra Cassio Department of Medical and Surgical Sciences, Pediatric Endocrinology Unit, S. Orsola-Malpighi University Hospital, Bologna, Italy

Serena Catania Pediatric Oncology Department, Fondazione IRCCS Istituto Nazionale dei Tumori, Milan, Italy

Paolo Cavarzere Pediatric Unit, Department of Mother and Child, University Hospital of Verona, Verona, Italy

Sylvain Chemtob Departments of Pediatrics, Ophthalmology and Pharmacology, Centre Hospitalier, Universitaire Sainte-Justine, Research Center, Montréal, QC, Canada

Department of Ophthalmology, Maisonneuve-Rosemont Hospital Research Center, Montréal, QC, Canada

Stefano Chiaravalli Pediatric Oncology Department, Fondazione IRCCS Istituto Nazionale dei Tumori, Milan, Italy

Gaetano Chirico Neonatology and Intensive Neonatal Therapy Unit, Spedali Civili of Brescia, Brescia, Italy

Robert D. Christensen Divisions of Neonatology and Hematology, Department of Pediatrics, University of Utah School of Medicine, Intermountain Healthcare, Salt Lake City, UT, USA

Massimiliano Ciantelli Department of Clinical and Experimental Medicine, Division of Neonatology and Neonatal Intensive Care Unit, S. Chiara University Hospital, Pisa, Italy

Azienda Ospedaliero-Universitaria Pisana, Pisa, Italy

Elena Ciarmoli Neonatologia e Terapia Intensiva Neonatale, Fondazione MBBM, ASST-Ospedale San Gerardo-Monza, Monza, Italy

Alessandro Cicognani Department of Medical and Surgical Sciences, Pediatric Unit, Center for Rare Endocrine Diseases (CARENDO BO), S.Orsola Malpighi University Hospital, Bologna, Italy

Giovanni Cioni IRCCS Stella Maris, Department of Developmental Neuroscience, Pisa, Italy

University of Pisa, Department of Clinical and Experimental Neuroscience, Pisa, Italy

Olivier Claris Department of Neonatology, Hôpital Femme Mère Enfant, Bron, France

Hospices Civils de Lyon and Université Claude Bernard, Lyon, France

Paola E. Cogo Division of Pediatrics, Department of Medicine, S. Maria della Misericordia University Hospital, University of Udine, Udine, Italy

Richard J. Cooke Department of Pediatrics, University of Tennessee Health Science Center, Memphis, TN, USA

Giovanni Corsello Department of Sciences for Health Promotion and Mother and Child Care, University of Palermo, Palermo, Italy

Alessandra Coscia Neonatal Unit, University of Turin, Turin, Italy

Frans J. C. Cuperus Department of Gastroenterology and Hepatology, University Medical Center Groningen, Groningen, The Netherlands

Tore Curstedt Department of Molecular Medicine and Surgery, Karolinska Institutet, Karolinska University Hospital, Stockholm, Sweden

Mario De Curtis Dipartimento Materno-Infantile, Università "La Sapienza", Rome, Italy

Carlo Dani Neonatal Intensive Care Unit, Careggi University Hospital, Florence, Italy

Università degli Studi di Firenze, Florence, Italy

Riccardo Davanzo Department of Mother and Child Health, Madonna delle Grazie Hospital, Matera, Italy

Franco D'Alberton Department of Medical and Surgical Sciences, Pediatric Unit, Center for Rare Endocrine Diseases (CARENDO BO), S.Orsola Malpighi University Hospital, Bologna, Italy

Andrea De Luca Department of Medical Biotechnologies, University of Siena, Siena, Italy

UOC Malattie Infettive Universitarie, Azienda Ospedaliera Universitaria Senese, Siena, Italy

Linda S. de Vries Department of Neonatology, Wilhelmina Children's Hospital, University Medical Center, Utrecht, The Netherlands

Antonio Del Vecchio Department of Women's and Children's Health, Neonatal Intensive Care Unit, Di Venere Hospital, ASL Bari, Bari, Italy

Maria Delivoria-Papadopoulos Department of Pediatrics, Drexel University College of Medicine, St. Christopher's Hospital for Children, Neonatal-Perinatal Medicine, Philadelphia, PA, USA

Marco Della Monaca Sapienza Università di Roma, Policlinico Umberto I di Roma, Rome, Italy

Paola Di Nicola Neonatal Unit, University of Turin, Turin, Italy

Petr H. Dijk Beatrix Children's Hospital, University Medical Center Groningen, Groningen, The Netherlands

Carmelita D'Ippolito Pediatric Oncohematology and Bone Marrow Transplant, Spedali Civili Hospital, Brescia, Italy

Timothy Disher Centre for Pediatric Pain Research, Dalhousie University School of Nursing and IWK Health Centre, Halifax, Canada

Nicola Disma Department of Anesthesia, Pediatric and Neonatal Intensive Care, Istituto Giannina Gaslini, Genoa, Italy

Marcello Dòmini U.O. di Chirurgia pediatrica – Ospedale S.Orsola, Università degli Studi – Alma Mater Studiorum, di Bologna, Italy

Allison Dorfman Department of Ophthalmology/Neurology, McGill University-Montreal Children's Hospital Research Institute, Montreal, QC, Canada

Elsa Duchemin-Kermorvant INSERM UMRS1138, Centre de Recherche des Cordeliers, Paris, France

Jennifer M. Duchon Division of Neonatology, St. Joseph's Regional Medical Center, Paterson, NJ, USA

Jeroen Dudink Neonatology, Sophia Children's Hospital, Erasmus MC Rotterdam, Rotterdam, Zuid-Holland, The Netherlands

Claudio Fabris Neonatal Unit, University of Turin, Turin, Italy

Maria Teresa Fadda Sapienza Università di Roma, Policlinico Umberto I di Roma, Rome, Italy

Avroy A. Fanaroff Case Western Reserve University School of Medicine Rainbow Babies and Children's Hospital, Cleveland, OH, USA

Jonathan M. Fanaroff Case Western Reserve University School of Medicine Rainbow Babies and Children's Hospital, Cleveland, OH, USA

Vassilios Fanos Department of Surgery, Neonatal Intensive Care Unit, Neonatal Pathology and Neonatal Section, AOU and University of Cagliari, Cagliari, Italy

Maria Grazia Faticato Department of Pediatric Surgery, University of Genoa, Genoa, Italy

Giannina Gaslini Institute, Genoa, Italy

Silvia Ferranti Department of Molecular Medicine and Development, University of Siena, Siena, Italy,

Fabrizio Ferrari Neonatal Intensive Care Unit, Department of Medical and Surgical Sciences of the Mother, Children and Adults, University of Modena and Reggio Emilia, Modena, Italy

Enrico Ferrazzi Prenatal Diagnosis and Fetal Surgery Unit, Dept. of Woman, Mother and Neonate, Buzzi Children's Hospital Department of Clinical Sciences, University of Milan, Milan, Italy

Michele Fimiani Dipartimento di Medicina Clinica e Scienze Immunologiche – Sezione di Dermatologia, Università degli Studi di Siena, Policlinico "Santa Maria alle Scotte", Siena, Italy

Department of Medical, Surgical and Neurological Sciences, Dermatology Section, University of Siena, Siena, Italy

Vittorio Fineschi Department of Anatomical, Histological, Forensic Medicine and Orthopaedic Sciences, "Sapienza" University of Rome, Rome, Italy

Bobbi Fleiss UMR1141, Insem-Paris Diderot University, Hôpital Robert Debré, Paris, France

Centre for the Developing Brain, Department of Perinatal Imaging and Health, Division of Imaging Sciences and Biomedical Engineering, King's College London, King's Health Partners, St. Thomas' Hospital, London, UK

Monica Fumagalli NICU, Department of Clinical Sciences and Community Health, Fondazione IRCCS Ca' Granda Ospedale Maggiore Policlinico Milano, Università degli Studi di Milano, Milan, Italy

Clara Gabiano Department of Pediatrics, University of Turin, Turin, Italy

Silvia Garazzino Department of Pediatrics, University of Turin, Regina Margherita Childrens Hospital, AOU Città della Salute e della Scienza di Torino, Turin, Italy

Elisabetta Garetti Neonatal Intensive Care Unit, Department of Medical and Surgical Sciences of the Mother, Children and Adults, University of Modena and Reggio Emilia, Modena, Italy

Alfredo Garzi Department of Pediatrics, Obstetrics and Reproductive Medicine, Section of Pediatric Surgery, University of Siena, Siena, Italy

Università degli Studi di Salerno, Fisciano, Italy

Diego Gazzolo Neonatal Intensive Care Unit, Department of Maternal, Fetal and Neonatal Medicine, S. Arrigo Children's Hospital, Alessandria, Italy

Giulia Genoni Department of Health Sciences, Division of Pediatrics, University of Piemonte Orientale, Novara, Italy

Maurizio Gente Department of Pediatrics and Infant Neuropsychiatry, Neonatal Emergency Transport Service, Sapienza University of Rome, Rome, Italy

Michael K. Georgieff Division of Neonatology, Department of Pediatrics Center for Neurobehavioral Development, University of Minnesota, Minneapolis, MN, USA

Paolo Ghirri Department of Clinical and Experimental Medicine, Division of Neonatology and Neonatal Intensive Care Unit, Santa Chiara University Hospital, Pisa, Italy

Daniela Gianotti Department of Pediatrics and Neonatology, Eastern Liguria Hospital, La Spezia, Italy

Jason Gien University of Colorado Denver, Denver, CO, USA

Enza Giglione Department of Health Sciences, Division of Pediatrics, University of Piemonte Orientale, Novara, Italy

Mario Giuffrè Department of Sciences for Health Promotion and Mother and Child Care, University of Palermo, Palermo, Italy

Francesca Giuliani Neonatal Unit, University of Turin, Turin, Italy

Kirsten Glaser University Children's Hospital, University of Würzburg, Würzburg, Germany

Peter D. Gluckman Liggins Institute, University of Auckland, Auckland, New Zealand

Sergio Golombek New York Medical College, New York, USA

Misty Good Division of Neonatology, University of Pittsburgh School of Medicine, Children's Hospital of Pittsburgh, Pittsburgh, PA, USA

Glenn R. Gourley Department of Pediatrics, University of Minnesota, Minneapolis, USA

Paul P. Govaert Neonatology, Sophia Children's Hospital, Erasmus MC Rotterdam, Rotterdam, Zuid-Holland, The Netherlands

Anne Greenough Division of Asthma, Allergy and Lung Biology, MRC Centre for Allergic Mechanisms of Asthma, King's College London, London, UK

NIHR Biomedical Centre at Guy's and St Thomas NHS Foundation Trust and King's College London, London, UK

NICU, King's College Hospital, London, UK

Pierre Gressens UMR1141, Insem-Paris Diderot University, Hôpital Robert Debré, Paris, France

Centre for the Developing Brain, Department of Perinatal Imaging and Health, Division of Imaging Sciences and Biomedical Engineering, King's College London, King's Health Partners, St. Thomas' Hospital, London, UK

Floris Groenendaal Department of Neonatology, Wilhelmina Children's Hospital, University Medical Center Utrecht, Utrecht, The Netherlands

Salvatore Grosso Department of Molecular Medicine and Development, University of Siena, Siena, Italy,

Renzo Guerrini Pediatric Neurology and Neurogenetics Unit and Laboratories, Neuroscience Department, A. Meyer Children's Hospital – University of Florence, Florence, Italy

Isotta Guidotti Neonatal Intensive Care Unit, Department of Medical and Surgical Sciences of the Mother, Children and Adults, University Hospital of Modena, Modena, Italy

Jean-Pierre Guignard Lausanne University Medical School, Lausanne, Switzerland

Andrea Guzzetta IRCCS Stella Maris, Department of Developmental Neuroscience, Pisa, Italy

University of Pisa, Department of Clinical and Experimental Neuroscience, Pisa, Italy

Henrik Hagberg Perinatal Center, Department of Obstetrics and Gynecology, Sahlgrenska Academy, University of Gothenburg, Goteborg, Sweden

Centre for the Developing Brain, Division of Imaging Sciences and Biomedical Engineering, King's College London, King's Health Partners, St. Thomas' Hospital, London, UK

Nigel J. Hall University Surgery Unit, Faculty of Medicine, University of Southampton, Southampton, UK

Henry L. Halliday Formerly Regional Neonatal Unit, Royal Maternity Hospital, Belfast, UK

Formerly Department of Child Health, Queen's University Belfast, Belfast, UK

Mikko Hallman Department of Children and Adolescents, Oulu University Hospital, and PEDEGO Research Unit, Medical Research Center Oulu, University of Oulu, Oulu, Finland

Dominique Haumont Department of Neonatology, Saint – Pierre University Hospital, Brussels, Belgium

Axel Heep Department of Neonatology, Southmead Hospital, North Bristol NHS Trust, Bristol, UK

Lena K. Hellström-Westas Department of Women's and Children's Health, Uppsala University and University Hospital, Uppsala, Sweden

Martin J. Herman Department of Orthopaedic Surgery, Drexel University College of Medicine, St. Christopher's Hospital for Children, Philadelphia, PA, USA

Christian V. Hulzebos Beatrix Children's Hospital, University Medical Center Groningen, Groningen, The Netherlands

Petra S. Hüppi Division of Neonatology, Giannina Gaslini Children's Hospital, Genoa, Italy

Giorgio Iannetti Università degli Studi di Siena, Policlinico S. Maria alle Scotte, Siena, Italy

Sapienza Università di Roma, Policlinico Umberto I di Roma, Rome, Italy

Vincenzo Jasonni Department of Pediatric Surgery, University of Genoa, Genoa, Italy

Giannina Gaslini Institute, Genoa, Italy

Kathryn Johnson Centre for Newborn Care, Leeds Teaching Hospitals Trust, Leeds, UK

Celeste Johnston School of Nursing, McGill University, Montreal, Canada

Michael Kaplan Department of Neonatology, Shaare Zedek Medical Center, Jerusalem, Israel

The Faculty of Medicine, Hebrew University, Jerusalem, Israel,

Nandini Kataria Department of Pediatrics, University of Minnesota, Long Beach, California, USA

Tuula Kaukola Department of Children and Adolescents, Oulu University Hospital, and PEDEGO Research Center, MRC Oulu, University of Oulu, Oulu, Finland

Hirokazu Kimura Infectious Diseases Surveillance Center, National Institute of Infectious Diseases, Tokyo, Japan

John P. Kinsella University of Denver, Denver, CO, USA

Panagiotis Kratimenos Neonatologist, Children's National Medical Center, Center for Research in Neuroscience, George Washington University School of Medicine and Health Sciences, Washington, DC, USA

Edmund F. La Gamma Division of Newborn Medicine, Maria Fareri Children's Hospital, Westchester Medical Center – New York Medical College, Valhalla, NY, USA

Arianna Lamberti Department of Medical, Surgical and Neurological Sciences, Dermatology Section, University of Siena, Siena, Italy

Mariano Lanna Prenatal Diagnosis and Fetal Surgery Unit, Dept. of Woman, Mother and Neonate, Buzzi Children's Hospital Department of Clinical Sciences, University of Milan, Milan, Italy

Malcolm Levene Academic Unit of Paediatrics and Child Health, University of Leeds, Leeds, UK

Department of Neonatal Medicine, Leeds Teaching Hospitals Trust, Leeds, UK

Isabelle Ligi Division of Neonatology, La Conception Hospital, Marseille, France

Otwin Linderkamp Division of Neonatology, Department of Pediatrics, University of Heidelberg, Heidelberg, Germany

Gianluca Lista Neonatology and Neonatal Intensive Care Unit, Ospedale dei Bambini V. Buzzi, Milan, Italy

Mariangela Longini Department of Molecular and Developmental Medicine, University of Siena, Siena, Italy

Alessandra Del Longo Department of Pediatric Ophthalmology, Niguarda Ca' Granda Hospital, Milan, Italy

Vassilios Lougaris Pediatrics Clinic, Department of Clinical and Experimental Sciences, University of Brescia and Spedali Civili of Brescia, Brescia, Italy

Felicia M. Low Liggins Institute, University of Auckland, Auckland, New Zealand

Laura Lucaccioni Neonatal Intensive Care Unit, Department of Medical and Surgical Sciences of the Mother, Children and Adults, University Hospital of Modena, Modena, Italy

Licia Lugli Neonatal Intensive Care Unit, Department of Medical and Surgical Sciences of the Mother, Children and Adults, University Hospital of Modena, Modena, Italy

Giuseppe Maggiore Department of Medical Sciences-Pediatrics, University of Ferrara, University Hospital Arcispedale Sant Anna di Cona, CONA (Ferrara), Italy

Francesca Maglietta Department of Legal Medicine, University of Foggia, Foggia, Italy

Akhil Maheshwari Division of Neonatology, University of South Florida, Tampa, FL, USA

Liam Mahoney Academic Department of Paediatrics, Royal Alexandra Children's Hospital, Brighton, UK

M. Jeffrey Maisels Department of Pediatrics, Oakland University William Beaumont School of Medicine, Beaumont Children's Hospital, Royal Oak, MI, USA

Carina Mallard Department of Physiology, Institute of Neuroscience and Physiology, Sahlgrenska Academy, University of Gothenburg, Gothenburg, Sweden

Leila Mameli Department of Anesthesia, Pediatric and Neonatal Intensive Care, Istituto Giannina Gaslini, Genoa, Italy

Filomena Mandato Department of Medical, Surgical and Neurological Sciences, Dermatology Section, University of Siena, Siena, Italy

Paolo Manzoni Division of Neonatology, Department of Obstetrics and Neonatology, AOU Città della Salute e della Scienza, Turin, Italy

Viviana Marchi IRCCS Stella Maris, Department of Developmental Neuroscience, Pisa, Italy

University of Pisa, Department of Clinical and Experimental Neuroscience, Pisa, Italy

Neil Marlow Institute for Women's Health, University College London, London, UK

Richard J. Martin Rainbow Babies and Children's Hospital, Division of Neonatology, Case Western Reserve University School of Medicine, Cleveland, OH, USA

Maura Massimino Pediatric Oncology Department, Fondazione IRCCS Istituto Nazionale dei Tumori, Milan, Italy

Girolamo Mattioli Department of Pediatric Surgery, University of Genoa, Genoa, Italy

Giannina Gaslini Institute, Genoa, Italy

Liz McKechnie Centre for Newborn Care, Leeds Teaching Hospitals Trust, Leeds, UK

Stefania Mei Department of Medical, Surgical and Neurological Sciences, Dermatology Section, University of Siena, Siena, Italy

Mario Messina Department of Pediatrics, Obstetrics and Reproductive Medicine, Section of Pediatric Surgery, Policlinico "Le Scotte", University of Siena, Siena, Italy

Department of Medical, Surgical and Neurological Sciences, Section of Pediatric Surgery, University of Siena, Siena, Italy

Angelo Micheletti Department of Pediatric Cardiology, IRCCS Policlinico San Donato, San Siro, Milan, Italy

Fiorella Migliaro Division of Neonatology, Department of Translational Medical Sciences, Università "Federico II" di Napoli, Naples, Italy

Federica Mignone Department of Pediatrics, University of Turin, Regina Margherita Childrens Hospital, AOU Città della Salute e della Scienza di Torino, Turin, Italy

Francesco Molinaro Department of Pediatrics, Obstetrics and Reproductive Medicine, Section of Pediatric Surgery, Policlinico "Le Scotte", University of Siena, Siena, Italy

Department of Medical, Surgical and Neurological Sciences, Section of Pediatric Surgery, University of Siena, Siena, Italy

Davide Montin Division of Neonatology, Department of Obstetrics and Neonatology, AOU Città della Salute e della Scienza, Turin, Italy

Department of Pediatrics, University of Turin, Turin, Italy

Alice Monzani Department of Health Sciences, Division of Pediatrics, University of Piemonte Orientale, Novara, Italy

Corrado Moretti Università degli Studi di Roma "La Sapienza", Rome, Italy

Colin Morley Dept Obstetrics and Gynecology, University of Cambridge at Rosie Maternity Hospital, Cambridge, UK

Fabio A. Mosca NICU, Department of Clinical Sciences and Community Health, Fondazione IRCCS Ca' Granda Ospedale Maggiore Policlinico Milano, Università degli Studi di Milano, Milan, Italy

Michele Mussap Laboratory Medicine, Ospedale Policlinico San Martino, Genoa, Italy

Niccolò Nami Department of Medical, Surgical and Neurological Sciences, Dermatology Section, University of Siena, Siena, Italy

Diana Negura Department of Pediatric Cardiology, IRCCS Policlinico San Donato, San Siro, Milan, Italy

Josef Neu Department of Pediatrics, Division of Neonatology, University of Florida, College of Medicine, Gainesville, FL, USA

Giovanni Nigro Maternal-Infant Department, University of L'Aquila, L'Aquila, Italy

Akira Nishida Department of Neonatology, Tokyo Metropolitan Children's Medical Center, Tokyo, Japan

Giovanna Oggè Maternal-Fetal Medicine Unit, University of Turin, Turin, Italy

Robin K. Ohls Department of Pediatrics, Division of Neonatology, University of New Mexico, Albuquerque, NM, USA

Kaoru Okazaki Department of Neonatology, Tokyo Metropolitan Children's Medical Center, Tokyo, Japan

Luca Ori Neonatal Intensive Care Unit, Department of Medical and Surgical Sciences of the Mother, Children and Adults, University Hospital of Modena, Modena, Italy

Luis H. Ospina Departments of Pediatrics, Ophthalmology and Pharmacology, Centre Hospitalier, Universitaire Sainte-Justine, Research Center, Montréal, QC, Canada

Erin A. Osterholm Division of Neonatology, Department of Pediatrics Center for Neurobehavioral Development, University of Minnesota, Minneapolis, MN, USA

Roberto Paludetto Translational Medical Sciences, Università "Federico II" di Napoli, Naples, Italy

Niovi Papalexopoulou Division of Asthma, Allergy and Lung Biology, MRC Centre for Allergic Mechanisms of Asthma, King's College London, London, UK

Paola Papoff Pediatric Intensive Care Unit, Sapienza University of Rome, Rome, Italy

Giancarlo Parenti Department of Translational Medicine, Section of Pediatrics, Federico II University of Naples, Naples, Italy

Stefano Parmigiani Department of Pediatrics and Neonatology, Eastern Liguria Hospital, La Spezia, Italy

Elena Parrini Pediatric Neurology and Neurogenetics Unit and Laboratories, Neuroscience Department, A. Meyer Children's Hospital – University of Florence, Florence, Italy

Gaia Pasquali Department of Obstetrics and Gynecology, University of Rome Tor Vergata, Rome, Italy

Mary Elaine Patrinos Case Western Reserve University School of Medicine, Cleveland, OH, USA

Pierluigi Pedersini National Center for Surgical Treatment of Pediatric Hepatobiliary Malformations, Pediatric Surgery, University of Brescia, Brescia, Italy

Serafina Perrone Department of Molecular and Developmental Medicine, University Hospital of Siena, Siena, Italy

Felice Petraglia Obstetrics and Gynecology, Department of Molecular and Developmental Medicine, University of Siena, Siena, Italy

Luciane Piazza Department of Pediatric Cardiology, IRCCS Policlinico San Donato, San Siro, Milan, Italy

Catherine Pieltain Department of Neonatology, University of Liège, CHR de la Citadelle, Liège, Belgium

Agostino Pierro Division of General and Thoracic Surgery, The Hospital for Sick Children, Toronto, Canada

Alessio Pini Prato Giannina Gaslini Institute, Genoa, Italy

Elena Piozzi Department of Pediatric Ophthalmology, Niguarda Ca' Granda Hospital, Milan, Italy

Peter D. Pizzutillo Section of Orthopaedic Surgery, St. Christopher's Hospital for Children, Philadelphia, PA, USA

Tenet Healthcare, Dallas, TX, USA

Alessandro Plebani Pediatrics Clinic, Department of Clinical and Experimental Sciences, University of Brescia and Spedali Civili of Brescia, Brescia, Italy

Francesca R. Pluchinotta Department of Pediatric Cardiology, IRCCS Policlinico San Donato, San Siro, Milan, Italy

Christian F. Poets Department of Neonatology, Tübingen University Hospital, Tübingen, Germany

Simone Pratesi Neonatal Intensive Care Unit, Careggi University Hospital, Florence, Italy

Flavia Prodam Department of Health Sciences, Division of Pediatrics, University of Piemonte Orientale, Novara, Italy

Fabrizio Proietti Department of Molecular and Developmental Medicine, University of Siena, Siena, Italy

Marisa Pugliese Neonatal Intensive Care Unit, Department of Medical and Surgical Sciences of the Mother, Children and Adults, University of Modena and Reggio Emilia, Modena, Italy

Guy Putet Department of Neonatology, Hopital de la Croix-Rousse, Hospices Civils de Lyon and Universite Claude Bernard, Lyon, France

Heike Rabe Academic Department of Paediatrics, Royal Alexandra Children's Hospital, Brighton, UK

Francesco Raimondi Division of Neonatology, Department of Translational Medical Sciences, Università "Federico II" di Napoli, Naples, Italy

Luca A. Ramenghi Division of Neonatology, Giannina Gaslini Children's Hospital, Genoa, Italy

Tara M. Randis Department of Pediatrics, New York University School of Medicine, New York, NY, USA

Roberta Ricotti Department of Health Sciences, Division of Pediatrics, University of Piemonte Orientale, Novara, Italy

Henrique Rigatto Department of Pediatrics, WR004 Women's Hospital, University of Manitoba, Winnipeg, MB, Canada

Jacques Rigo Department of Neonatology, University of Liège, CHR de la Citadelle, Liège, Belgium

Arieh Riskin Department of Neonatology, Bnai Zion Medical Center, Rappaport Faculty of Medicine, Technion, Israel Institute of Technology, Haifa, Israel

Francesco Risso Neonatal Intensive Care Unit, Department of Emergency Medicine, G. Gaslini Children's Hospital, Genoa, Italy

Silvia Riva Pediatric Hepatology and Liver Transplant Unit, IRCCS-ISMETT - University of Pittsburgh Medical Center (UPMC), Palermo, Italy

José Carlos Rivera Departments of Pediatrics, Ophthalmology and Pharmacology, Centre Hospitalier, Universitaire Sainte-Justine, Research Center, Montréal, QC, Canada

Department of Ophthalmology, Maisonneuve-Rosemont Hospital Research Center, Montréal, QC, Canada

Rodney P. A. Rivers Section of Paediatrics, Department of Medicine, Imperial College, London, UK

Hector Rojas-Anaya Academic Department of Paediatrics, Royal Alexandra Children's Hospital, Brighton, UK

Maria Angela Rustico Prenatal Diagnosis and Fetal Surgery Unit, Dept. of Woman, Mother and Neonate, Buzzi Children's Hospital Department of Clinical Sciences, University of Milan, Milan, Italy

Karin Sävman Department of Pediatrics, Sahlgrenska Academy, University of Gothenburg, Gothenburg, Sweden

Timo Saarela Department of Children and Adolescents, Oulu University Hospital, Oulu, Finland

Elie Saliba Department of Neonatology and Pediatric Intensive Care, Université François Rabelais and CHRU de Tours, Tours, France

Inserm U930, France, Université François Rabelais and CHRU de Tours, Tours, France

Janko Samardzic Department of Paediatric Pharmacology, University Children's Hospital Basel, Basel, Switzerland

Institute of Pharmacology, Clinical Pharmacology and Toxicology, Medical Faculty, University of Belgrade, Belgrade, Serbia

Fabrizio Sandri Neonatology and Neonatal Intensive Care Unit, Ospedale Maggiore, Bologna, Italy

Andrea Sannia Neonatal Intensive Care Unit, Department of Emergency Medicine, G. Gaslini Children's Hospital, Genoa, Italy

Javier Fernandez Sarabia Department of Pediatric Cardiology, IRCCS Policlinico San Donato, San Siro, Milan, Italy

Paola Saracco Pediatric Hematology, Department of Pediatrics, University Hospital Città della Salute e della Scienza, Torino, Italy

Antonio Saracino Department of Pediatric Cardiology, IRCCS Policlinico San Donato, San Siro, Milan, Italy

Ola D. Saugstad Department of Pediatric Research, Rikshospitalet, Oslo University Hospital, University of Oslo, Oslo, Norway

Rosa T. Scaramuzzo Neonatology and Neonatal Intensive Care Unit, Santa Chiara University Hospital, Pisa, Italy

Kurt R. Schibler Perinatal Institute, Cincinnati Children's Hospital Medical Center, Cincinnati, OH, USA

Marco Sciveres Pediatric Hepatology and Liver Transplant Unit, IRCCS-ISMETT - University of Pittsburgh Medical Center (UPMC), Palermo, Italy

Carlo Scolfaro Department of Pediatrics, University of Turin, Regina Margherita Childrens Hospital, AOU Città della Salute e della Scienza di Torino, Turin, Italy

Gunnar Sedin Department of Women's and Children's Health, University Children's Hospital, Uppsala, Sweden

Thibault Senterre Department of Neonatology, University of Liège, CHR de la Citadelle, Liège, Belgium

Filiberto Maria Severi Obstetrics and Gynecology, Department of Molecular and Developmental Medicine, University of Siena, Siena, Italy

Raanan Shamir Institute of Gastroenterology Nutrition and Liver Diseases, Schneider Children's Medical Center, Sackler Faculty of Medicine, Tel-Aviv University, Petach-Tikva, Israel

Davide Silvagni Azienda Ospedaliera Universitaria Integrata Verona, Verona, Italy

Umberto Simeoni Division of Pediatrics, CHUV and UNIL, Lausanne, Vaud, Switzerland

Adam P. R. Smith Division of Asthma, Allergy and Lung Biology, MRC Centre for Allergic Mechanisms of Asthma, King's College London, London, UK

Augusto Sola Ibero American Society of Neonatology (SIBEN), Wellington, FL, USA

Michael Spear Department of Pediatrics, Drexel University College of Medicine, St. Christopher's Hospital for Children, Philadelphia, PA, USA

Christian P. Speer University Children's Hospital, University of Würzburg, Würzburg, Germany

David K. Stevenson Department of Pediatrics, Stanford University School of Medicine, Medical School Office Building, Stanford, CA, USA

Rosa Maria Strangi Department of Medical, Surgical and Neurological Sciences, Dermatology Section, University of Siena, Siena, Italy

Mauro Stronati Neonatal Intensive Care Unit, Fondazione IRCCS Policlinico 'San Matteo', Pavia, Italy

Veena Supramaniam Perinatal Imaging Group, Robert Steiner MR Unit, MRC Clinical Sciences Centre and Wigglesworth Perinatal Pathology Services, Hammersmith Hospital, Imperial College, London, UK

Paolo Tagliabue Neonatologia e Terapia Intensiva Neonatale, Fondazione MBBM, ASST-Ospedale San Gerardo-Monza, Monza, Italy

Sophie Tardieu Medical Evaluation Department, Public Health Department, La Conception Hospital, Marseille, France

Elena Tavella Division of Neonatology, Department of Obstetrics and Neonatology, AOU Città della Salute e della Scienza, Turin, Italy

Claire Thornton Centre for the Developing Brain, Department of Perinatal Imaging and Health, Division of Imaging Sciences and Biomedical Engineering, King's College London, King's Health Partners, St. Thomas' Hospital, London, UK

Claudio Tiribelli Liver Research Centre, University of Trieste, Trieste, Italy

Tullia Todros Maternal-Fetal Medicine Unit, University of Turin, Turin, Italy

Michela Torricelli Obstetrics and Gynecology, Department of Molecular and Developmental Medicine, University of Siena, Siena, Italy

Pier Angelo Tovo Department of Pediatrics, University of Turin, Regina Margherita Childrens Hospital, AOU Città della Salute e della Scienza di Torino, Turin, Italy

Alberto E. Tozzi Multifactorial and Complex Diseases Research Area, Bambino Gesù Children's Hospital, Rome, Italy

Laura Travan Division of Neonatology, Institute for Maternal and Child Health IRCCS 'Burlo Garofolo', Trieste, Italy

Daniele Trevisanuto Department of Women's and Children's Health, Azienda Ospedaliere di Padova, University of Padua, Padua, Italy

Pietro Tuo Department of Anesthesia, Pediatric and Neonatal Intensive Care, Istituto Giannina Gaslini, Genoa, Italy

Emanuela Turillazzi Department of Legal Medicine, University of Foggia, Foggia, Italy

Alberto G. Ugazio Institute of Child and Adolescent Health, Bambino Gesù Children's Hospital, Rome, Italy

Frank van Bel Department of Neonatology, Wilhelmina Children's Hospital, University Medical Center Utrecht, Utrecht, The Netherlands

John N. van den Anker Division of Pediatric Clinical Pharmacology, Children's National Health System, Washington, DC, USA

Departments of Pediatrics, Integrative Systems Biology, Pharmacology and Physiology, George Washington University, School of Medicine and Health Sciences, Washington, DC, USA

Intensive Care and Department of Pediatric Surgery, Erasmus MC – Sophia Children's Hospital, Rotterdam, The Netherlands

Johannes B. (Hans) van Goudoever Department of Pediatrics, Emma Children's Hospital – AMC and VU University Medical Center, Amsterdam, The Netherlands

Tim van Mieghem Department of Development and Regeneration, KU Leuven, Leuven, Belgium

Obstetrics and Gynecology, University Hospitals Leuven, Leuven, Belgium

Bart Van Overmeire Neonatology Service, Erasmus Hospital Université Libre de Bruxelles, Brussels, Belgium

Silvia Vannuccini Obstetrics and Gynecology, Department of Molecular and Developmental Medicine, University of Siena, Siena, Italy

Maximo Vento Neonatal Research Unit, Health Research Institute Hospital La Fe, University and Polytechnic Hospital La Fe, Valencia, Spain

Gennaro Vetrano U.O.C. Pediatria/Neonatologia/UTIN, Osp. "Sacro Cuore di Gesù", Benevento, Italy

Renaud Viellevoye Department of Neonatology, University of Liège, CHR de la Citadelle, Liège, Belgium

Betty R. Vohr Department of Pediatrics, The Warren Alpert Medical School of Brown University, Providence, RI, USA

Women and Infants Hospital, Providence, RI, USA

Jon F. Watchko Division of Newborn Medicine, Department of Pediatrics, University of Pittsburgh School of Medicine, Pittsburgh, PA, USA

Ronald J. Wong Department of Pediatrics, Stanford University School of Medicine, Stanford, CA, USA

Marco Zaffanello Department of Surgical Sciences, Dentistry, Gynecology and Pediatrics, University of Verona, Verona, Italy

Department of Life and Reproduction Sciences Pediatric Section, University of Verona, Verona, Italy

Department of Surgery, University of Cagliari, Cagliari, Italy

Clelia Zanaboni Department of Anesthesia, Pediatric and Neonatal Intensive Care, Istituto Giannina Gaslini, Genoa, Italy

Giacomo Zanelli Department of Medical Biotechnologies, University of Siena, Siena, Italy

Rinaldo Zanini NICU, Ospedale Manzoni, Lecco, Italy

Tianwei Ellen Zhou Departments of Pediatrics, Ophthalmology and Pharmacology, Centre Hospitalier, Universitaire Sainte-Justine, Research Center, Montréal, QC, Canada

Ekhard E. Ziegler Department of Pediatrics, University of Iowa, Iowa City, IA, USA

Luc J. I. Zimmermann Department of Pediatrics and Neonatology, School for Oncology and Developmental Biology (GROW), Maastricht University Medical Center, Maastricht, The Netherlands

Part V

Respiratory System

Neonatal Lung Development and Pulmonary Malformations

47

Corrado Moretti and Paola Papoff

Contents

C. Moretti (✉)
Università degli Studi di Roma "La Sapienza", Rome, Italy
e-mail: corrado.moretti@uniroma1.it

P. Papoff
Pediatric Intensive Care Unit, Sapienza University of Rome, Rome, Italy
e-mail: p.papoff@libero.it

G. Buonocore et al. (eds.), *Neonatology*,
https://doi.org/10.1007/978-3-319-29489-6_196

Abstract
There are five stages of lung development: embryonal, pseudoglandular, canalicular, saccular, and alveolar. Structural development of the lung may be altered by a number of prenatal conditions. The principal pulmonary malformations include intrapulmonary cystic malformations (i.e., congenital cystic adenomatoid malformation, bronchopulmonary sequestration, congenital lobar emphysema, and bronchogenic cysts), pulmonary agenesia, pulmonary hypoplasia, congenital pulmonary lymphangiectasia, and alveolar capillary dysplasia. Congenital pulmonary malformations are often diagnosed by prenatal ultrasound; however, some will present either in the neonatal period or during childhood. Symptoms vary according to the degree of lung involvement. Initial management of pulmonary malformations is supportive care, whereas surgical repair is indicated for selected cases. Prognosis is good for most pulmonary malformations except for severe pulmonary hypoplasia and alveolar capillary dysplasia.

47.1 Salient Points

- There are five stages of lung development: embryonal, pseudoglandular, canalicular, saccular, and alveolar.
- The principal pulmonary malformations include intrapulmonary cystic malformations, which encompass congenital cystic adenomatoid malformation, bronchopulmonary sequestration, congenital lobar emphysema, and bronchogenic cysts; pulmonary agenesia; pulmonary hypoplasia; congenital pulmonary lymphangiectasia; and misalignment of pulmonary veins.
- Most pulmonary malformations are often diagnosed by prenatal ultrasound.
- All patients with prenatally detected congenital cystic malformations require postnatal evaluation, preferably by CT scan.
- Symptoms vary according to the extension of lung lesion.
- Treatment is usually supportive care; surgery is reserved for selected cases.
- Maternal betamethasone is a therapeutic option for fetuses with large microcystic congenital lung lesions at risk of hydrops.

47.2 Fetal Stage of Lung Development

47.2.1 Introduction

In the early weeks of gestation, the human lung originates as a ventral endodermal pouch from the primitive foregut; it thereafter continues to grow through to adulthood until it reaches an exchange surface area of around 70–100 m^2; the air-blood barrier is some 0.2 μm thick, 1/50 of the thickness of a sheet of tissue paper.

From the structural standpoint, the lung is made up of one part that serves to convey gas extending from the trachea to the terminal bronchioles, characterized by a series of 23 branchings of the respiratory tree, and of an alveolar zone where gas is exchanged, where the acinus is the functional unit. The acinus comprises the respiratory bronchioles, often with alveoli on the walls, the alveolar ducts, and the alveoli themselves, which are characterized by a hexagonal structure (Fig. 1). The surface area of this

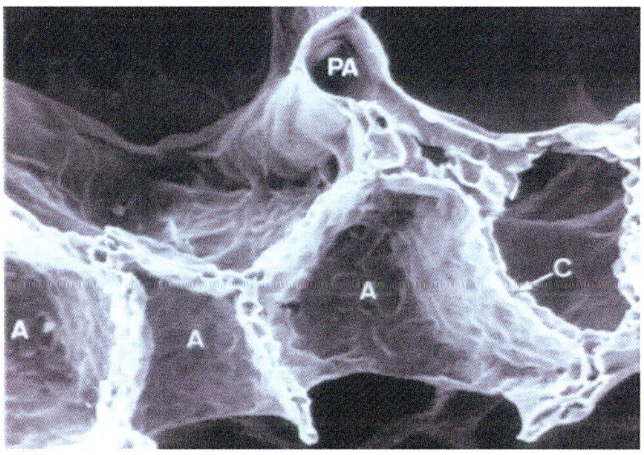

Fig. 1 The electron micrograph shows some alveoli (**A**) with a dense capillary network (**C**) between their walls. The capillaries stem from a branch of the pulmonary artery (**PA**). Reproduced from (Abrams et al. 2004), with permission

structure is vast and maintains a constant relationship with body mass during postnatal growth (about 1 m^2/kg).

The development of the human lung begins when the lung bud appears in the embryo and ends in early childhood after relatively stable and progressive growth. Even though birth is an event that implies dramatic changes in the functions of this organ, it should not be considered as a precise point of transition from one stage of development to another. Nevertheless, since this is an important event, the artifact of dividing lung development into a prenatal and postnatal stage is justified, also to emphasize that at the end of gestation, this organ has not yet reached maturity. Indeed, at the time of writing, we cannot define exactly when the lung reaches maturity (Burri 1997). Prenatal development of the respiratory system is in turn conventionally divided into five periods (Langston et al. 1984); actually, a precise watershed between these periods does not exist, but their identification can however simplify the understanding of the morphogenesis of the lung.

47.2.2 Embryonic Phase (3rd-7th Week)

The lung bud appears on the 26th day of gestation and is formed from relatively undifferentiated epithelial cells that expand into the surrounding embryonic connective tissue or mesenchyme (Fig. 2a, b). The bud begins to grow in length and to branch until, toward the fifth week, it forms five small saccular structures, two on the left and three on the right, which are the beginnings of the future secondary bronchi and of the future lobes of the mature lung (Fig. 2c, d). The developing airways will undergo further branching and are accompanied by the pulmonary arteries that derive from the sixth aortic arches.

Interactions between the epithelial cells of endodermic origin that form the respiratory tree and the mesenchymal tissue of mesodermal origin covering it are of basic importance for the branching of the airways (Alescio and Cassini 1962); this process is often referred to as "cross talk." This process is controlled through a multitude of molecular factors that include transcriptional regulators, growth factors, morphogens, and extracellular matrix molecules, all of which must be carefully controlled in both space and time to form a properly functioning lung. If some of these developmental factors do not function at the right time and/or place, then lung defects may occur.

Toward the end of the sixth week of gestation, the main airways are complete, including the segmental and subsegmental bronchi (Fig. 2e).

Developmental anomalies occurring in these first weeks of gestation may lead to many congenital malformations such as pulmonary agenesia, laryngeal or tracheal stenosis or atresia, tracheoesophageal fistula, tracheomalacia or bronchomalacia, bronchial malformations, and ectopic lobes (Table 1).

47.2.3 Pseudoglandular Phase (6th–17th Week)

During the pseudoglandular period, the airways continue to divide until they form terminal bronchioles; by the end of this period, the bronchial branching process is complete, and the airways will continue to grow in proportion with the increase in pulmonary volume. Since the newly formed epithelial tubules are surrounded by a considerable amount of mesenchyme, they make the lung look like a gland, hence the name of this phase (Fig. 3a, b). The proximal airways are covered by an epithelium that gradually becomes thinner toward the periphery, where the cells take on a cuboidal shape.

During this period the blood vessels develop in parallel to the airways so that, by the end of this phase, their hierarchical structure is already comparable to that of the adult (de Mello and Reid 1997). Also, the development of the nerves in these structures is already fairly complete.

Alterations in the development of the lung during the pseudoglandular period may give rise to many congenital malformations such as pulmonary sequestration, cystic adenomatoid

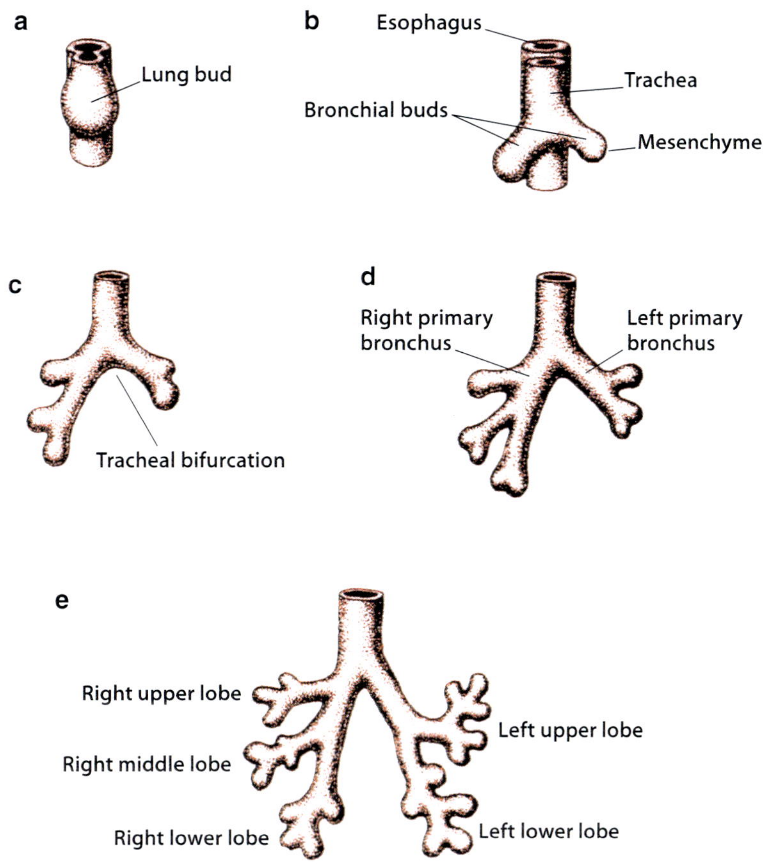

Fig. 2 Successive stages in the development of the bronchi and future lobes of the lungs: (**a**) and (**b**), four weeks; (**c**) and (**d**) five weeks; (**e**), six weeks. Modified from (Alescio and Cassini 1962)

malformation, pulmonary cysts, and congenital pulmonary lymphangiectasia (Table 1). In the early stages of this period, the pleuroperitoneal cavity starts dividing into the peritoneal and the pleural cavities due to the development of the diaphragm; when it does not divide correctly, the abdominal content in the chest becomes herniated (diaphragmatic hernia).

47.2.4 Canalicular Phase (16th–26th Week)

The canalicular period is characterized by the appearance of vascular canals (capillaries), hence the name, and by further development of the distal airways where the primitive acinar structures appear, each made up of a respiratory bronchiole, an alveolar duct, and rudimentary alveoli or saccules (Hislop 1996). The development of the terminal airways and of the capillary network determines both the progressive thinning of the mesenchyme lining and the formation of the alveolar capillary membrane (Fig. 3c, d). This phase is also characterized by the differentiation from cuboidal type-II to squamous type-I cells in the distal epithelium. Differentiation of these cell types is an important step as the type-II cells will be required to produce and secrete surfactant and the type-I

Table 1 Stage of development of congenital pulmonary malformations

Embryonic
Pulmonary agenesis
Tracheal or laryngeal agenesis or stenosis
Tracheo- or bronchomalacia
Bronchial malformations
Ectopic lobes
Pseudoglandular
Cystic adenomatoid malformation
Pulmonary sequestration
Lung cysts
Congenital pulmonary lymphangiectasia
Congenital diaphragmatic hernia
Canalicular
Pulmonary hypoplasia
Saccular/Alveolar
Pulmonary hypoplasia
Alveolar capillary dysplasia

cells will form the thin cell layer to support future gas exchange.

In this period the presence of masses inside the chest and/or changes in the physical forces, essential for lung development, produced by the presence of the pulmonary liquid and by the breathing movements of the fetus, may interfere with the development of the respiratory system and give rise to pulmonary hypoplasia.

47.2.5 Saccular Phase (25th–38th Week)

This phase is characterized by marked dilation of the terminal airways and resultant formation of saccules (Langston et al. 1984), with a considerable increase in lung volume and in the surface area for gas exchange together with a further thinning of the alveolar capillary membrane (Fig. 3e, f). In this way also, the microcirculation structure is modified because the capillary networks surrounding the saccules gradually come closer to each other and, at the end of the process, the interstitial septa, or primary septa, delimit a double network of capillaries necessary for the subsequent formation of the secondary septa (Burri 1997). The formation of the final number of alveoli, around 200–300 million, happens during the alveolar phase, which begins toward the end of gestation and ends during early infancy. The alveoli are formed through the subdivision of the saccules into subunits, thus considerably increasing the exchange surface area. It must be pointed out that, given the great difficulty in carrying out histological measurements and in standardizing findings, there is still controversy over the beginning and the end of the alveolar phase and over the final number of alveoli.

The formation of alveoli is to be considered as mainly a postnatal event since most form during the first 24–36 months after birth with a subsequent slow increase in number up to around the eighth year of life (Brody and Thurlbeck 1986).

47.3 Postnatal Lung Development

47.3.1 Alveolar Phase and Development of the Pulmonary Vasculature (36th Week of Gestation to 24 Months After Birth)

Crests, or secondary septa, grow out from the intersaccular walls, or primary septa (Fig. 4), appearing as small ridges in the epithelium (Burri 1986). Electron micrograph imaging shows the secondary septa to be formed by a thin layer of connective tissue flanked by capillaries on both sides and characterized by the presence of elastin at the tip. Elastin appears to have the function of supporting the outgrowth of the epithelium, and its presence is an essential prerequisite for the formation of the secondary septa, which takes place only after its deposition. Also, the capillary network gradually develops until maturity: in the first few weeks after birth, the interstitial layer of the septa gradually thins, drawing the two capillary networks closer until they finally merge. This transformation from a double to a single layer of the capillary network contained inside the septa is the last stage of pulmonary development (Burri 1984).

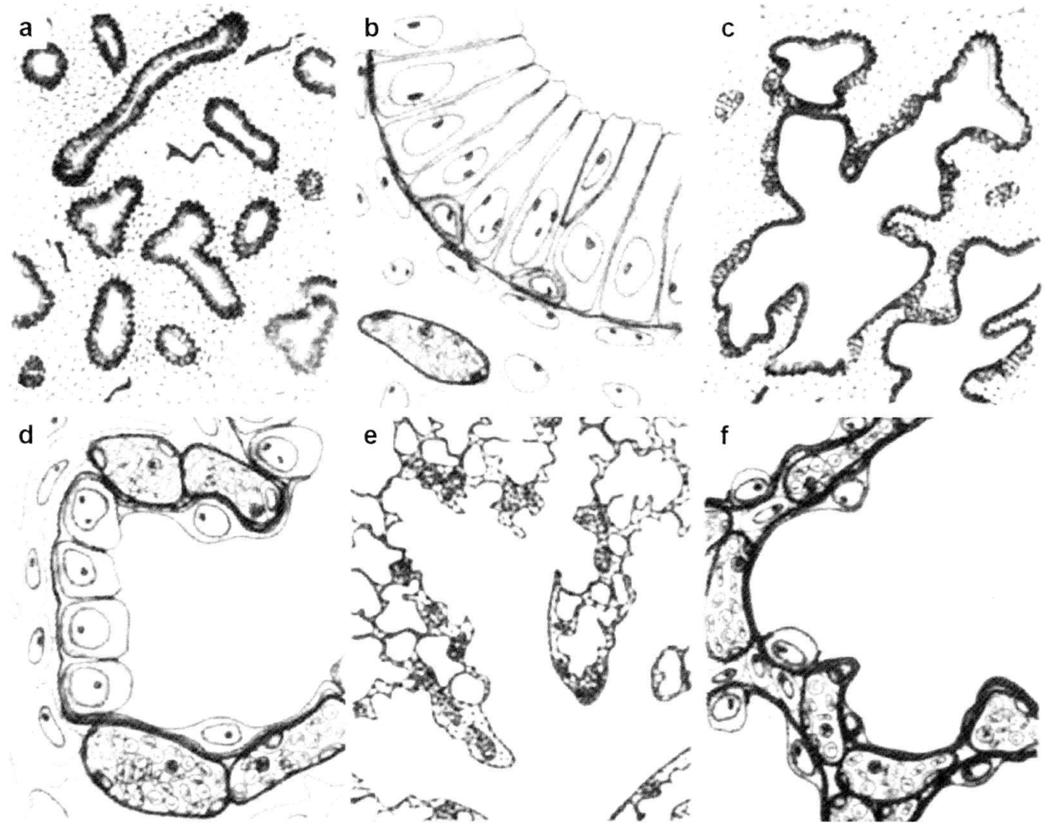

Fig. 3 Drawing that illustrates the light microscopic appearance of human lung during the glandular (**a,b**), canalicular (**c,d**) and saccular (**e,f**) stages of in utero development. Undifferentiated columnar cells of the early bronchi (**b**) rest upon a basal lamina, which has been emphasized. Mesenchymal cells and capillaries are present below the basal lamina. (**d**) shows that the epithelium overlying proliferating blood vessels thins to a squamous Type I morphology and that the most distal cells retain a cuboidal shape. At the saccular state (**f**), the septa are very thinned and the air spaces are lined by differentiated Type I and Type II cells. The low and high magnification drawings are shown at approximately the same magnification in each panel. Modified from (Asabe et al. 1994)

47.4 Physical Determinants of Lung Development

Physical forces exerted on the lung during gestation are crucial to normal development. There are two main physical factors that aid lung development: lung fluid and fetal breathing movements (FBM).

During fetal development the lung is a secretory organ that exhibits breathing-like movements without contributing to respiratory gas exchange. The lung fluid is produced by epithelial cells, especially those in the distal airways, through chloride secretion, and it flows to the upper airway where it is either swallowed or released into the amniotic space. The fluid is rich in chloride and low in bicarbonate and proteins. The rate of fluid production increases in fetal lambs from approximately 5 mL/kg at midgestation to more than 20 mL/kg near term, with hourly rates increasing from 2 to 5 mL/kg/h, respectively (Bland et al. 1982). This increase mirrors the progressive expansion of the contact surface between the alveolar epithelium and microcirculation, due to the proliferation of pulmonary capillaries and to the growth of the terminal saccules.

The production of pulmonary fluid is essential for the normal development of the respiratory apparatus since it determines the form and volume of its peripheral units; experimental evidence

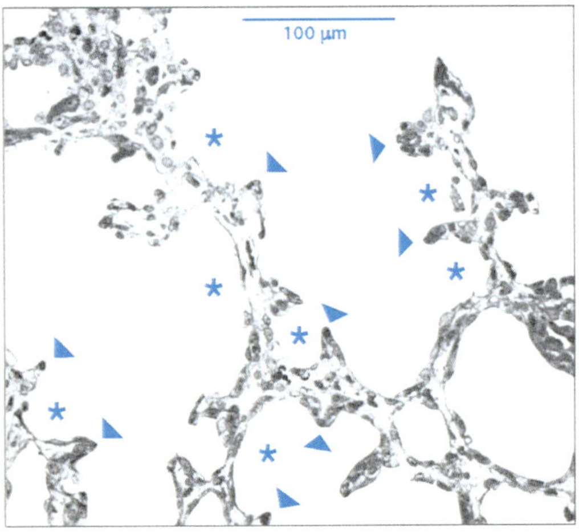

Fig. 4 Light micrograph of human lung. Air spaces are subdivided into small alveoli (*asterisks*) by secondary septa (*arrowheads*) projecting from the primary one

shows that extended drainage of tracheal fluid causes pulmonary hypoplasia (PH). The amount of pulmonary fluid that is present inside the respiratory tree depends on the balance between production at the level of the alveolar epithelium and resistance to its outflow exerted by the upper airway (Fewell and Johnson 1983); its volume at the end of gestation is around 20–30 mL/kg, a value that is comparable to that of the functional residual capacity (FRC) of a normal lung.

The other physical factor that is critical for normal lung development is FBM, periodic rhythmic contractions of the diaphragm that maintain adequate fluid volume and lung distension. During pregnancy, the fetus spends most of its time, around 30–40% during the third quarter, performing breathing movements even though ventilation is exclusively a placental function (Dawes et al. 1970). Fetal breathing appears to be related to the behavioral state of the fetus. As the fetus approaches term, the incidence of these movements is considerably greater during active periods than during periods of quiet activity (Mulder et al. 1994).

Observations of human fetuses with congenital anomalies and of experimental animals show that the breathing movements of the fetus produce distension forces that stimulate cell multiplication (Liu et al. 1992) and are necessary to ensure an adequate development of the muscular and respiratory apparatus for postnatal life. Pulmonary hypoplasia is a disorder that is frequently associated with oligohydramnios and experimentally it can be determined in the uterus through bilateral phrenectomy. These observations seem to confirm the importance of fetal respiratory activity for the development of the lung, which could undergo alterations when this activity is prevented or when there are obstacles (Porter 1999). The physiological fluctuations of PaO_2 and of $PaCO_2$ do not influence the respiratory activity of the fetus, which stops if the PaO_2 drops to a level of 16–18 mmHg. Hypoxia therefore has an inhibiting effect on breathing movements, which is not to be interpreted as a sign of neuronal immaturity but rather as a response aimed at reducing the consumption of O_2 by the fetus. In fact, intrauterine respiratory activity demands up to 15–30% of the total O_2 available. By contrast, the fetus responds to an increase in $PaCO_2$ with a corresponding increase in respiratory activity and the opposite occurs in the case of hypocapnia. These observations suggest that the central chemoreceptors are active in fetal life. Maternal ingestion of alcohol or sedatives has been shown to decrease breathing movements, but drugs such as caffeine increase them. Maternal smoking also decreases fetal breathing movements through several mechanisms including decreased uterine blood flow and hypoxia (Kotecha 2000).

The pressure inside the fetal respiratory system varies depending on the presence or absence of breathing movements. During the periods in which the fetus does not practice breathing, the pressure remains constant (Vilos and Liggins 1982): if the amniotic pressure is considered to be zero, the pressure inside the trachea is around 1–2 mmHg greater, while the intrapleural pressure is about 0.7 mmHg lower. The positive pressure inside the respiratory tree is modulated mainly by the degree of resistance of the larynx. Similarly, the negative endopleural pressure is the product of the balance between elastic return of the lungs and of the thoracic cage. The resulting force between endotracheal positive pressure and endopleural negative pressure is a transpulmonary positive pressure of around 2.5 mmHg, a force that keeps the lungs expanded hence stimulating their

growth. During the periods when the fetus performs FBM, the glottis dilates and resistance decreases at the larynx, but the rhythmic contractions of the diaphragm attenuate the outflow of fluid from the trachea and restrict the reduction of pulmonary volume (Hooper and Harding 1995).

47.5 Pulmonary Malformations

Knowledge of the various phases of pulmonary development allows us to understand the pathophysiology of the various congenital malformations of this organ, many of which, thanks to the considerable development of prenatal ultrasonography, may be diagnosed as early as between the 18th and 20th weeks of gestation.

47.5.1 Intrapulmonary Cystic Malformations

Intrapulmonary cystic malformations comprise a spectrum of congenital malformations of the lower respiratory tract that have in common the fact that cysts may represent a prominent part of the anomaly (even if not always); these include congenital cystic adenomatoid malformation (CCAM), bronchopulmonary sequestration (BPS), congenital lobar emphysemas (CLE), and bronchogenic cysts.

Intrapulmonary cystic malformations have been increasingly detected at midgestation due to improvements in ultrasound technology and the routine use of ultrasound as a screening test, but those who interpret prenatal imaging should not attempt to make a histological diagnosis, which can be definitively supported only by the direct examination of a tissue specimen. Actually, the different postnatal diagnostic entities are difficult to differentiate prenatally and there is confusion in terms of how these malformations should be described; recently a new nomenclature using the terms "congenital thoracic malformation" (CTM) and "congenital large hyperlucent lobe" have been proposed (Bush 2001). It has been suggested that many, if not all, of these defects may represent a continuum of anomalies of fetal lung development, despite some diversity in morphology. Fetal bronchial atresia or obstruction probably plays a prominent role in their pathogenesis, perhaps inducing local abnormal pulmonary growth due to the obstructed outflow of fetal lung fluid (Kunisaki et al. 2006), but it remains unknown why this mechanism may lead to different fetal chest masses.

The widespread use of antenatal ultrasound with Doppler studies has also led to a better understanding of the development of some of these anomalies and to an improvement in their management. Antenatal fast magnetic resonance imaging is also an important adjunct to prenatal ultrasound in the evaluation of CTM: it may provide further information on the nature of the lung anomaly, it may help to differentiate lung lesions from extrathoracic abnormalities such as congenital diaphragmatic hernia (CDH), and it may be useful in planning pre- or postnatal surgery.

Large congenital malformations may compress the ipsilateral lung or even the contralateral lung via mediastinal shift thus causing lung hypoplasia. Compression of the esophagus may result in polyhydramnios; the resulting uterine distension may induce premature labor. Impairment of cardiac return due to the vena cava and to cardiac compression is responsible for fetal hydrops with ascites, pleural and pericardial effusions, and skin and scalp edema.

CTM may change in size and/or appearance during pregnancy, but the growth pattern is rather unpredictable. There is a wide spectrum of clinical severity, with a relationship between the size of the malformation, concomitant lung hypoplasia, and the occurrence of pulmonary hypertension in the newborn period. Most fetuses with CTM have a good outcome, with majority of neonates being asymptomatic at birth, and also an initially large lesion does not necessarily correlate with a poor prognosis (Adzick et al. 1998; Lacy et al. 1999). Actually many lesions decrease in size over time and some of them, defined as vanishing lesions, even disappear completely on serial prenatal ultrasound scans toward the end of pregnancy (Adzick et al. 1998; MacGillivray et al. 1993; Kunisaki et al. 2015; Butterworth and Blair 2005; Calvert et al. 2006; Borsellino et al. 2006). These lesions

are often undetectable on postnatal ultrasound and chest X-ray examination, except for some extralobar lesions that may be identifiable, but in the vast majority of cases they can be detected by computed tomography (CT) scans or magnetic resonance imaging (MRI) (Blau et al. 2002; Kunisaki et al. 2015; van Leeuwen et al. 1999; Pumberger et al. 2003; Ierullo et al. 2005; Shanmugam et al. 2005). Therefore, all patients with any prenatally detected lung malformation require mandatory postnatal evaluation by CT scan, that is, the gold standard to confirm the presence or absence of a CTM. Due to the fact that many examples of hybrid lesions with features of CCAM and BPS have been described, it is also important in the postnatal period to seek an anomalous blood supply in patients who have CTM, even if prenatally color flow Doppler studies fail to identify a systemic arterial blood supply.

Most fetuses with a CTM will do well during pregnancy; however, if hydrops develops, the risk of fetal death is extremely high: up to 100% (Adzick et al. 1998; MacGillivray et al. 1993; Wilson et al. 2006a). The CCAM volume ratio (CVR), which measures the volume of the lung lesion divided by the head circumference, is a widely accepted useful prognostic tool that allows closer monitoring of fetuses at risk. Fetuses with lung lesions with a CVR > 1.6 are at increased risk of hydrops and require intervention and delivery at a high-risk center (Davenport et al. 2004; Baird et al. 2014).

In intrathoracic lesions with cystic parts, prenatal needle aspiration of the fluid has been performed but often leads to rapid re-accumulation. Therefore, fetal surgery with the implantation of shunts between the cyst and the amniotic space has successfully reduced the size of the lesion and improved hydrops fetalis; however, this intervention may cause fetal death (Calvert et al. 2006; Salomon et al. 2003).

After 32 weeks of gestation, early delivery should be considered in hydropic fetuses and, furthermore, when severe RDS is expected, the ex-utero intrapartum therapy (EXIT) procedure may be considered to allow interventions such as drainage of large pleural effusions or even resection of an affected lobe (Hedrick et al. 2005).

Recently it has been demonstrated that maternal betamethasone therapy may induce regression of CTMs and reverse fetal hydrops. Several subsequent case series have confirmed that single and multiple courses of steroid administration allow an improved survival rate and decreased CVR (Baird et al. 2014; Peranteau et al. 2015). Steroids may act at multiple levels, but the mechanism probably involves decreasing the production of lung fluid and increasing reabsorption within the CTM.

The postnatal clinical appearance of CTMs may vary from immediate respiratory distress at birth to an incidental finding on a chest X-ray at any age. In the neonatal period, a small number of patients with large lesions require surgery, which is the accepted standard of care for all symptomatic lesions. The treatment of the asymptomatic child with CCAM is controversial because most of the lesions are microcystic and do not cause mediastinal shift postnatally. Most authors would recommend resection of CTMs because of complications such as infections, hemorrhage, pneumothorax, sudden respiratory failure, and malignant transformation. The implication of operating on symptomatic patients should not be underestimated (Baird et al. 2014; Lakhoo 2009; Fitzgerald 2007; Stanton and Davenport 2006). Moreover the outcome of early surgery is generally good, most of the infants are extubated immediately after the procedure, the low complication rates are generally related to prolonged air leaks, and there is more time for compensatory lung growth, which is thought to explain the normal results of these children in pulmonary function tests (Baird et al. 2014). Furthermore, conservative management of these lesions with repeated CT scans causes significant radiation exposure. Successful expectant long-term management has been reported particularly for late-presenting asymptomatic or oligosymptomatic lobar emphysema (Ozcelik et al. 2003).

CTMs can be removed surgically between 3 and 6 months of age (Davenport et al. 2004; Calvert and Lakhoo 2007) either by open thoracotomy or, more recently, by using the minimally invasive video-assisted thoracoscopy (VATS) (Baird et al. 2014; Diamond et al. 2007; Shaw et al. 2008). But, although VATS appears safe and feasible and has clear cosmetic advantages,

this is based on its practice by experts and there is currently insufficient evidence to endorse its widespread adoption outside institutions with appropriate expertise and technical skills, which could cause excessively prolonged case durations and related complications.

47.5.2 Congenital Cystic Adenomatoid Malformation

CCAM is characterized by an adenomatoid proliferation of terminal bronchioles with the formation of solid, cystic, or mixed masses inside the pulmonary parenchyma without subsequent alveolar differentiation (Hebra et al. 2000). This lesion is usually unilateral, without a right or left prevalence, and it affects a single lobe; vascularization originates from the bronchial circulation, but in hybrid cases it may depend on an anomalous systemic vessel.

47.5.2.1 Etiology and Pathogenesis

The pathogenesis of CCAM is still unclear, but it is likely to be due to a failure of normal interaction between the mesenchymal tissue and epithelial cells during early fetal life.

47.5.2.2 Clinical Aspects

The congenital cystic adenomatoid malformation was originally classified by Stocker into three distinct histological subtypes and was subsequently expanded to five (Stocker 2002):

- Type 0: involvement of all lung lobes, incompatible with life (<2%).
- Type 1: single or multiple cysts, size >2 cm, lined by pseudostratified columnar epithelium; wall of fibromuscular and cartilaginous tissue (60–70%).
- Type 2: single or multiple cysts (<2 cm) lined by cuboidal or columnar epithelium (15–20%).
- Type 3: predominantly solid lesions, with small (<0.5 cm) cysts, lined by cuboidal epithelium (5–10%). On the whole, this constitutes a solid mass and is the form that has the worst prognosis.
- Type 4: large air-filled cysts lined by flattened epithelial cells (<10%).

This classification can obviously only be applied to resected lung specimens and it is inappropriate for describing fetal lung lesions. The emerging consensus is that imaging findings should simply describe without attempting to make a pathological diagnosis, as done by Adzick in his classification (Adzick et al. 1985) in which he simply differentiated prenatally detected cystic lesions into two types:

- Macrocystic (single or multiple echogenic cysts >5 mm)
- Microcystic (smaller echogenic cysts <5 mm)

47.5.2.3 Differential Diagnosis

The chest radiograph and clinical symptoms of CCAM may be easily confused with those of a CDH: the insertion of a nasogastric tube and instilling a few mL of barium may help locate the stomach and hence facilitate differential diagnosis (Fig. 5). Ultrasound and CT scans are also useful in determining the size of a normal lung and the position of the diaphragm.

47.5.2.4 Therapy and Treatments

The risk of infections, associated with the risk of malignant degeneration of the

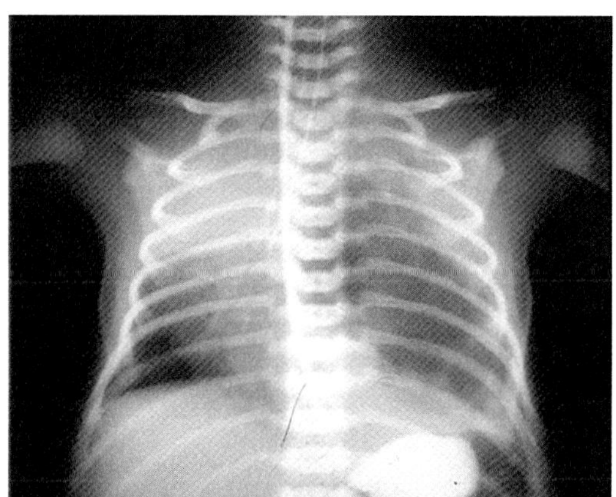

Fig. 5 Left lower lobe CCAM with mediastinal shift to the contralateral side

adenomatoid tissue into rhabdomyosarcoma or into bronchioloalveolar carcinoma or into other mesenchymal malignancies, a complication described both in children and in adults (Lakhoo 2009; Stanton and Davenport 2006), is to be considered when deciding on surgery in an asymptomatic patient. Also, in asymptomatic cases, a chest CT scan within 1 month of birth is mandatory, even if a resolution is noted on prenatal scanning (Lakhoo 2009) and bearing in mind that a true resolution of these lesions is exceptional.

When needed, assisted ventilation in these patients may determine a progressive distension of the cysts with a life-threatening mediastinal shift: one-lung ventilation may be carried out in order to achieve perioperative stabilization (Fig. 5). High-frequency oscillatory ventilation may also be successfully used in patients with pulmonary hypertension (Rossi et al. 1998).

47.5.3 Bronchopulmonary Sequestration

The term bronchopulmonary sequestration (BPS) was introduced by Pryce in 1946, who took the term from the Latin word sequestrate which means "to separate." He used it to define a portion of the pulmonary tissue that does not work and is not linked to the bronchial tree.

47.5.3.1 Etiology and Pathogenesis

The pathogenesis may be referred to an anomaly in the development of the primitive lung bud with the formation of an ancillary structure that has preserved the original arterial supply and that grows inside the pleural cavity in close contact with the normal lung (intralobular sequestration), or it may remain separate and be wrapped in its own visceral pleura (extralobular sequestration).

47.5.3.2 Clinical Aspects

Intralobular sequestration is the form most frequently found and is usually located in the paravertebral gutter in the posterior segment of the left lower lobe. Extralobular sequestration is located almost constantly on the left, may present as a subdiaphragmatic or retroperitoneal mass, and is often associated with other congenital malformations, in particular CDH. This malformation has its own vascular supply that usually originates from the lower chest or upper abdominal aorta or one of its major branches, rather than from the pulmonary artery. Usually the venous blood is normally drained into the right atrium, but occasionally the venous blood may also drain abnormally into the left atrium, the vena cava (the so-called scimitar syndrome for its characteristic chest radiograph appearance), or into the azygos system (Clements 1999). The size of abnormal arteries and veins and consequently the blood flow through the malformation is considerable and may cause heart failure and massive arteriovenous shunting (Cass et al. 1997). Recently many papers have described cystic lung lesions, defined as "hybrid lesions," with coexisting features of both CCAM (the histological features are mostly Stocker type 2 lesions) and BPS, suggesting that they may represent the two ends of a broad spectrum of disorders (Davenport et al. 2004; Rossi et al. 1998).

Only a small percentage of children with intralobular sequestration have a symptomatology characterized by respiratory distress in the neonatal period. In most cases the malformation is asymptomatic for a long time, and then it appears later in life with localized recurrent pneumonias, fever, and occasionally hemoptysis. By contrast, extralobular sequestration rarely presents respiratory symptoms and may also be found incidentally on routine chest radiography. BPSs have rarely been linked with malignancy and most likely these tumors develop in hybrid lesions (Hekelaar et al. 2000).

47.5.3.3 Differential Diagnosis

The initial detection of BPSs is currently obtained by intrauterine sonography (Fig. 6) and Doppler ultrasound is useful as it shows the characteristic vascular abnormality. Postnatally, intralobular sequestration should be suspected when the chest radiograph shows a dense lesion on the posteromedial part of the

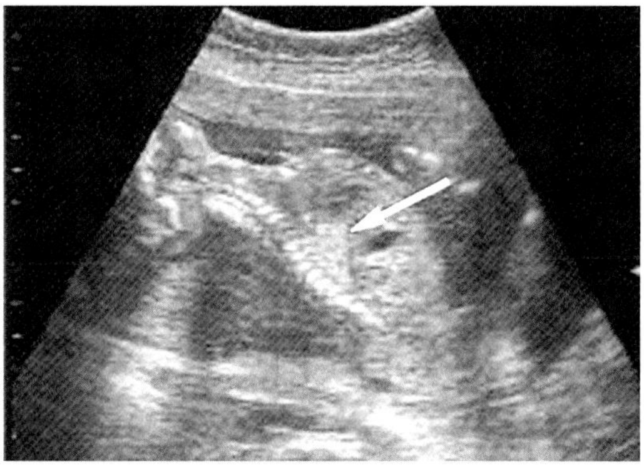

Fig. 6 Pulmonary sequestration: midtrimester fetal sonogram shows a triangular echogenic mass astride the left diaphragm

left or, less frequently, right lower zone of the lung. Multi-detector CT evaluation with intravenous contrast for CT angiogram is useful in establishing the diagnosis: this study provides the best evaluation of the vascular anatomy of the lesion, of the appearance of the lesion itself, of the diaphragm, and of the remainder of the lung (Lee et al. 2004).

47.5.3.4 Therapy and Treatments

Surgery is recommended once the infant becomes symptomatic and should be undertaken only after assessing the characteristics of the arterial supply and of the venous drainage.

47.5.4 Congenital Lung Cysts

Congenital lung cysts are divided into bronchogenic, alveolar, and combined forms. They may lie outside the normal lung structure (extrapulmonary) or within it (intrapulmonary). The cysts tend to be limited to one lung and are not associated with cystic disease elsewhere in the body. Bronchogenic cysts may vary notably in size and are rare in the newborn period.

47.5.4.1 Etiology and Pathogenesis

Congenital lung cysts result from abnormal budding of the foregut; the position within the branching pattern indicates when the cyst developed.

47.5.4.2 Clinical Aspects

Such lesions are found in the mediastinum in over two-thirds of cases. They are usually located in the right paratracheal or carinal regions, but can also be found within the parenchyma of the lung. The cysts contain a lining of respiratory epithelium and have cartilage, smooth muscle, and glands in the wall (Hebra et al. 2000). They are usually unilocular, filled with fluid or mucus, and generally do not communicate with airways. The location of the cyst is important in determining the clinical presentation: a bronchogenic cyst may cause airway compression resulting in cough, wheeze, dyspnea, or even respiratory distress, and those located in the region of the carina may determine lobar emphysema. Secondary infection of the cyst is also a very frequent complication and may cause acute distension with exacerbation of symptoms. In addition, peptic ulceration may develop in cysts containing gastric mucosa (Kirwan et al. 1973).

47.5.4.3 Differential Diagnosis

Radiographic findings are variable and range from a rounded mass to atelectasis or hyperinflation of a lobe or an entire lung (Fig. 7). The diagnosis is usually established from the chest X-ray, but the lesion must be differentiated from congenital lobar emphysema (CLE), acquired cysts complicating pulmonary interstitial emphysema (PIE), and bronchopulmonary dysplasia (BPD). Usually the latter two conditions can easily be differentiated through patient history.

47.5.4.4 Therapy and Treatments

All congenital lung cysts require surgical resection because they do not spontaneously regress, and even those that are asymptomatic may cause problems as a result of compression or infection (Stanton and Davenport 2006).

47.5.5 Congenital Lobar Emphysema

Congenital lobar emphysema (CLE), defined as a postnatal overdistension of one or more lobes of a histologically normal lung, is a rare cause of

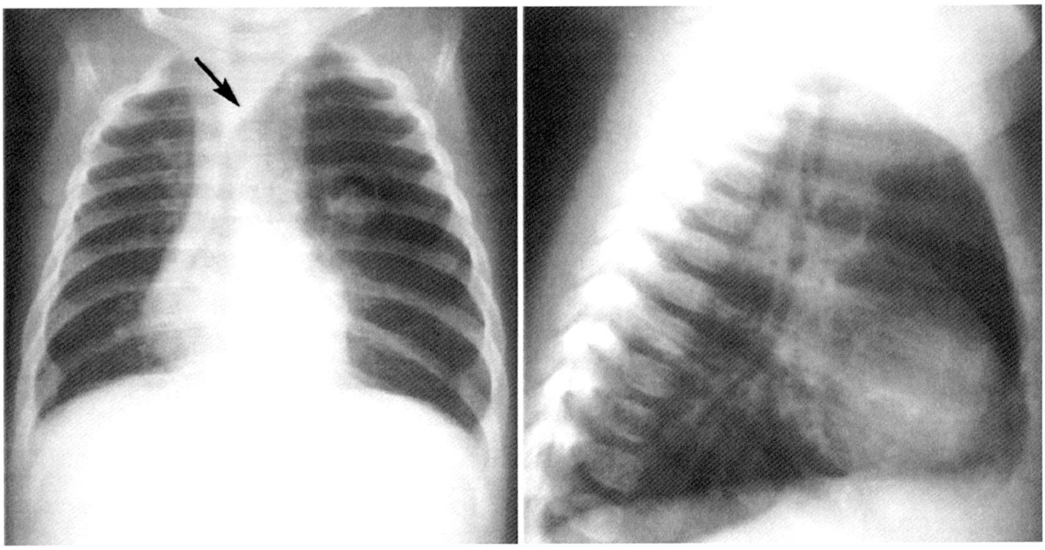

Fig. 7 Left bronchogenic cyst. The *arrow* shows upper lobe emphysema

respiratory failure in the newborn, but in most patients the diagnosis is made before 6 months of life (Berlinger et al. 1987).

47.5.5.1 Etiology and Pathogenesis

CLE may result from a malformation in the bronchial cartilage, with no or incomplete rings. It also may result from extrinsic bronchial obstruction caused by anomalous vessels or from intrathoracic masses such as bronchogenic cysts. The etiology of the intrinsic bronchial obstruction is thought to be a localized interruption of the blood supply to an already formed bronchus, resulting in bronchial infarction and luminal obstruction or developmental abnormalities of the bronchial cartilage after completion of bronchial branching (Kuhn and Kuhn 1992).

47.5.5.2 Clinical Aspects

The left upper lobe is most often involved (Fig. 8), followed by the right middle lobe; involvement of the lower lobes is very rare. Dyspnea, tachypnea, wheezing, tachycardia, and cyanosis are among the most common presenting symptoms. Chest radiograph, CT scan, ventilation scintigraphy, and bronchoscopy are usually sufficient for diagnosis. The chest radiograph will demonstrate marked hyperinflation of the affected lobe with the adjacent lobe collapsing down or up and mediastinal shift to the contralateral side.

47.5.5.3 Differential Diagnosis

CLE can easily be confused with pneumothorax, but in the latter there are no bronchovascular markings in the radiolucent area (Stanton and Davenport 2006). A CT scan is useful in the differential diagnosis of a mediastinal mass.

47.5.5.4 Therapy and Treatments

The traditional treatment for most cases of CLE with respiratory distress is lobectomy. Conservative treatment is possible in asymptomatic or mildly symptomatic cases (Thakral et al. 2001).

47.5.6 Pulmonary Agenesis

Pulmonary agenesis may be classified morphologically by the extent to which bronchopulmonary tissue is absent (Hebra et al. 2000). Pulmonary agenesis is divided into (1) bilateral complete agenesis; (2) unilateral agenesis with (a) complete absence of the lung and bronchus and no vascular supply to the affected side (agenesis), (b) rudimentary bronchus with complete absence of pulmonary parenchyma (aplasia), and

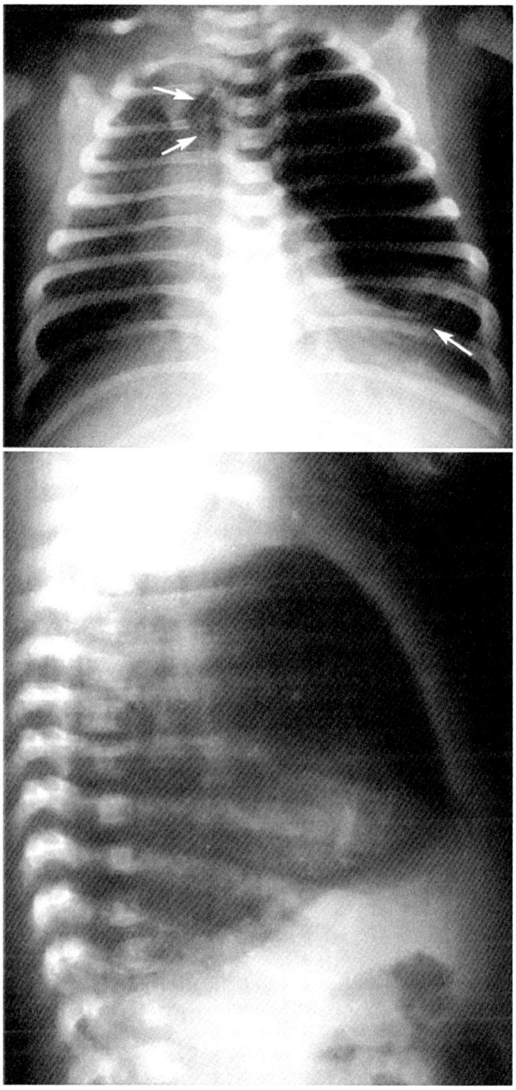

Fig. 8 Congenital left upper lobar emphysema. The *upper arrows* show retrosternal hernia. The *lower arrow* shows the collapse of the lower lobe

(c) presence of variable amounts of the bronchial tree, pulmonary parenchyma, and supporting vasculature (hypoplasia); and (3) lobar agenesis. Pulmonary agenesis is a very rare malformation and the left lung is slightly more affected than the right (Mardini and Nyhan 1985). Isolated agenesis of a lobe or lobes is more common than total unilateral lung agenesis. This abnormality occurs more often on the right than on the left, involving the upper and middle lobes.

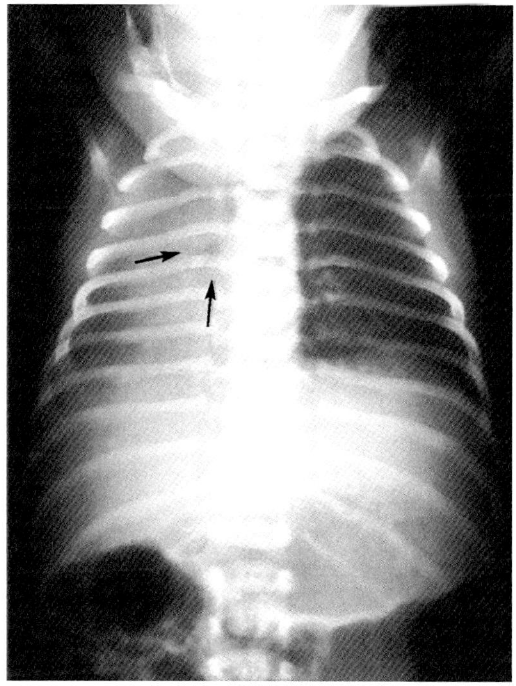

Fig. 9 Chest X-ray of a neonate with agenesis of the right lung. *Black arrows* show the right lobar bronchi ending blindly. Mediastinum shifts to the right side

47.5.6.1 Clinical Aspects

Unilateral pulmonary agenesis may present with severe respiratory distress at birth or may be asymptomatic. In this latter occurrence, recurrent respiratory symptoms secondary to respiratory tract infections may appear later in life. On auscultation, mediastinal shift and hyperresonance of the contralateral hemithorax side are usually present. Asymmetry of the chest becomes more noticeable in the adult patient (Swischuck 2004).

With postnatal compensatory growth, the remaining lung often herniates into the contralateral chest. Chest X-ray shows a mediastinal shift toward the affected side (Fig. 9), and skeletal abnormalities may be present. Absent or incomplete lung development may be associated with abnormalities of the trachea, absence of one or both kidneys, cardiac defects (patent ductus arteriosus, patent foramen ovale, ventricular defects, pulmonary veins entering the azygos vein), gastrointestinal malformations (atresia ani, esophageal atresia, short bowel), skeletal

anomalies (spina bifida, wedge-shaped vertebrae, hemivertebra, deformed ribs, absent left hand, absence of right radius, rudimentary atlas), deformed external ear, and many others. Differential diagnosis should be made with lung atelectasis, CDH, CCAM, and BPS (Gabarre et al. 2005). The difficulty of diagnosis depends on the side of the absent lung, the apparent dextrocardia induced by absence of the right lung being a striking clinical finding. Bronchoscopy has been used to establish the diagnosis of pulmonary agenesis. Typical findings include a bronchus narrowing and ending blindly.

47.5.6.2 Prognosis

About 50% of patients survive; the mortality rate is higher with agenesis of the right lung than of the left lung.

47.5.7 Pulmonary Hypoplasia

Pulmonary hypoplasia (PH) is a common and serious problem in the perinatal period with a significant mortality rate. PH is defined as a defective or incomplete development of lung tissue characterized by a reduction in the number of lung cells, airways, and alveoli, resulting in a lower organ size and weight. The pulmonary vascular bed is reduced in size with a decreased vessel count and increased pulmonary vascular muscular development (Barth and Rüschoff 1992). PH encompasses a wide spectrum of anatomic malformations ranging from total bronchial and parenchymal agenesis to mild pulmonary parenchymal hypoplasia. The lesions may be lobar, unilateral, or bilateral. Cases of isolated lobar defects have only been rarely reported. PH may be an isolated entity (primary PH) or be secondary to lesions restricting lung growth (Abrams et al. 2004). Prolonged premature rupture of membranes (PPROM) at less than 25 weeks gestation, severe oligohydramnios (amniotic fluid index <4) for more than 2 weeks, and earlier delivery are known risk factors for severe PH (de Waal and Kluckow 2015).

47.5.7.1 Etiology and Pathogenesis

Primary PH includes pulmonary agenesis (unilateral) (Abrams et al. 2004) with or without associated malformations and idiopathic PH (bilateral). The causes of primary PH have not been identified. Nakamura and colleagues (Nakamura et al. 1992) revealed five statistically significant risk factors associated with secondary PH from a large series of autopsy cases: (1) hydrops fetalis, (2) renal anomalies, (3) CDH, (4) skeletal anomalies, and (5) oligohydramnios and polyhydramnios (Table 2).

Pathologically, the hypoplastic lung shows a low ratio of lung to body weight, low DNA content, or a decreased radial alveolar count (Askenazi and Perlman 1979). Epithelial differentiation is delayed, and surfactant deficiency is associated (Asabe et al. 1994). Both pulmonary arterioles and bronchioles are decreased in size. Arterial thickness is a common finding in peripheral pulmonary blood vessels (Barth and Rüschoff 1992).

47.5.7.2 Clinical Aspects

In patients with PH, the clinical profile and the time of presentation vary depending on the extent of hypoplasia and other anomalies. Severe respiratory insufficiency resulting in a fatal outcome is the presenting symptom in a vast majority of preterm infants with severe bilateral PH. In infants with PH, the lung function is abnormal at birth with reduced tidal volume, increased respiratory rate, and reduced static lung compliance and functional residual capacity. On autopsy, the gold standard to confirm PH is a lung to body weight ratio of less than 0.015 with reduced radial alveolar count or total DNA count (Burri 1986).

The history of PH may include poor fetal movement or amniotic fluid leakage and oligohydramnios. In more mature neonates, mild to moderate hypoplasia or unilateral PH may be asymptomatic or may present with respiratory distress that requires mechanical ventilation. Newborn infants with moderate to severe PH often present with persistent pulmonary hypertension responding to inhaled nitric oxide (iNO) (Uga et al. 2004) as a result of reduced vascular bed and secondary arterial muscular hypertrophy.

Table 2 Causes of secondary pulmonary hypoplasia

Small fetal thoracic volume
CDH
Eventration of the diaphragm
Abdominal mass lesions
Exomphalos
Pleural effusions with fetal hydrops
Hydrothorax
CAM
Sequestration
Malformations of the thorax (e.g., asphyxiating thoracic dystrophy)
Achondroplasia
Thanatophoric dwarfism
Osteogenesis imperfecta
Thoracic neuroblastomas
Prolonged oligohydramnios
Fetal renal agenesis
Urinary tract obstruction
Bilateral renal dysplasia
Bilateral cystic kidneys
Prolonged rupture of membranes
Early rupture of membranes
More severe oligohydramnios (amniotic fluid index < 4)
Longer latent period before delivery
Decreased fetal breathing
CNS lesions
Lesions of the spinal cord, brain stem and phrenic nerve
Neuromuscolar disease (e.g., myotonic dystrophy, spinal muscular atrophy)
Arthrogryposis multiplex congenital
Maternal depressant drugs
Congenital heart disease with poor pulmonary blood flow
Tetralogy of Fallot
Hypoplastic right heart
Pulmonary artery hypoplasia
Scimitar syndrome causing a unilateral right-sided pulmonary hypoplasia

Pneumothorax, spontaneous or associated with mechanical ventilation, may occur (Knox and Barson 1986). Compression deformities due to prolonged oligohydramnios, contractures, and arthrogryposis may be present when PH is associated with oligohydramnios. The Potter facies (hypertelorism, epicanthus, retrognathia, depressed nasal bridge, low-set ears) suggest PH should be caused by the associated renal defects (Potter 1946a). When the etiology of the PH is a neuromuscular disease, the patient may have myopathic facies, with a V-shaped mouth, muscle weakness, and growth retardation.

A number of studies have described associated anomalies with PH including heart defects (e.g., anomalous venous return to the right atrium or the inferior vena cava or scimitar syndrome, absence of the ipsilateral pulmonary artery), skeletal and vertebral anomalies (metacarpal and radial anomalies, failure of segmentation of thoracic or other vertebrae, rib abnormalities), abdominal defects (diaphragm, abdominal wall defects), facial abnormalities, and numerous lung and tracheobronchial tree defects. There have been a number of case reports of PH and tracheoesophageal fistula and a number of reports of an association of tracheal stenosis with pulmonary agenesis. Similar to patients with a more severe degree of PH, neonates with isolated lobar hypoplasia may demonstrate other congenital malformations.

47.5.7.3 Diagnostic Methods

The diagnosis of PH can be made with certainty only at autopsy by measurement of total lung DNA content. Because of this, the incidence of PH is probably underestimated. The diagnosis should be suspected in the presence of perinatal factors suggestive of PH, unexpected respiratory distress, and specific findings at clinical examination.

Diagnosis of unilateral lobar PH requires a high index of clinical suspicion and experience with reading neonatal and infant radiographs. Characteristic findings on the chest radiograph are of a small bell-shaped chest with raised hemidiaphragms and clear lung fields, although "clear lung fields" may be masked by radiographic signs of respiratory distress in prematurely born infants. A radiographic diagnosis may be supported by clinical findings of an infant unresponsive to ventilatory support and exogenous surfactant therapy. Chest CT or MRI may be needed to better delineate the defect and to detect possible associated malformations (accessory diaphragm, BPS adjacent to a small CDH). Unilateral PH should be suspected in the presence of hyperlucency and smallness of one lung.

Hyperdistention of the contralateral lung can be seen.

The diagnosis of primary PH implies a lack of any specific pathophysiologic process that could cause fetal lung compression. For the diagnosis of secondary PH, abdominal masses, such as cystic renal diseases and an enlarged bladder, must be sought. Associated anomalies of the cardiovascular, gastrointestinal (e.g., tracheoesophageal fistula, imperforate anus, communicating bronchopulmonary foregut malformation), and genitourinary system, as well as skeletal anomalies of the vertebrae, thoracic cage, and upper limbs, may be found upon examination.

Echocardiography is fundamental to reveal possible cardiac defects. Prenatal ultrasound (Gerards et al. 2008) and, more recently, fetal MRI constitute the methods of choice to investigate the fetal lung development throughout pregnancy (Gorincour et al. 2005).

Basically, the MRI assessment of fetal lung growth and maturation consists of three diagnostic elements. First, fetal MR volumetry is used to identify restricted and insufficient lung growth. Second, the evaluation of signal intensities using different MR sequences provides information about the maturation of the fetal lung. Third, the high resolution and tissue contrast of MRI allows us to examine the structure of the fetal lung and to offer a more detailed diagnosis of fetal pulmonary pathologies (Kasprian et al. 2006).

Antenatal Prediction of Pulmonary Hypoplasia

Three-dimensional ultrasound has been used to identify PH in the high-risk fetuses. In a series of 35 fetuses (Pumberger et al. 2003), sensitivities of 85% and 92% for predicting PH were achieved when the results were adjusted for gestational age, estimated fetal weight, and two-dimensional biometric measurements. As well as reduced lung volume, these babies may also exhibit PPHN. Prediction of PPHN is difficult to assess before birth. Despite this, reduced diastolic and systolic velocities in the pulmonary arteries have been demonstrated by Doppler examination of fetuses affected by PH (Wilson et al. 2006a), but measurements can be technically difficult in the absence of amniotic fluid. A combination of clinical, biometric, and Doppler parameters may be most predictive in identifying lethal PH. Although antenatal prediction may be useful in guiding management and counseling parents, it should be noted that a lethal outcome is also dependent on the postnatal management including intention to treat and level of neonatal care offered.

47.5.7.4 Differential Diagnosis

The differential diagnosis of respiratory distress in the newborn associated with marked opacification of one side of the thorax on radiograph includes atelectasis, CDH, CCAM, BPS, chylothorax, PH, bronchogenic cyst, and a chest tumor (e.g., neuroblastoma, teratoma, fibrosarcoma). In a right-sided CDH, there may be opacification of the right hemithorax if the liver is occupying that space. A left-sided CDH will have air-filled loops of bowel in the chest except possibly in a chest radiograph taken shortly after birth or following bowel decompression. CCAM will usually appear as a cystic mass rather than a homogenous opacification. Obstruction of the bronchus with resultant opacification of the hemithorax may occur with a bronchogenic cyst or a vascular sling. Neonatal chest tumors are very rare and may present with a focal abnormality on chest X-ray.

In cases of bilateral PH with hyperlucent lungs, idiopathic PPHN should be considered in the differential diagnosis, whereas the presence of small lungs may suggest spinal thoracic dysplasia or neuromuscular diseases.

47.5.7.5 Therapy and Treatments

Treatment of PH is largely supportive, and prognosis will depend on the presence or absence of the other anomalies. iNO administered to preterm infants with PPROM, oligohydramnios, and PH improves oxygenation, survival, or other clinical outcomes (Shah and Kluckow 2011). Because of the surfactant deficiency, a significant number of infants with PH require surfactant replacement therapy and high-frequency oscillatory ventilation (HFOV) (Cacciari et al. 2001).

Conventional therapies may fail in these infants who then become candidates for ECMO

(Stevens et al. 2002). The eventual survival is limited by the underlying degree of PH.

A high level of neonatal intensive care is likely to be necessary, and delivery should take place, where possible, in a tertiary neonatal center. Initial aggressive management should be attempted even if the infant shows signs of severe respiratory failure compatible with PH. It is recognized that a subset of infants suffers from isolated PPHN, who respond well to immediate ventilatory and pulmonary vasodilator therapy with relatively few long-term complications (Alescio and Cassini 1962; Thakral et al. 2001).

The optimal ventilatory management of infants born following prolonged oligohydramnios and exhibiting signs of PH remains to be defined. There is a theoretical advantage of HFOV among infants suffering from PH, as it provides the possibility of optimal alveolar recruitment while reducing the risk of excessive barotrauma. The use of HFOV in the context of PH following PPROM has been evaluated, and a positive effect has been proposed in addition to iNO (Shah and Kluckow 2011).

Preterm infants born following midtrimester PPROM may also suffer from respiratory distress syndrome, and "conventional" surfactant therapy is indicated. Infants with severe PH, however, may fail to show a positive response to surfactant therapy alone.

Due to the high incidence of neonatal infection following prolonged oligohydramnios, appropriate investigations should be undertaken, and treatment with broad-spectrum antibiotics is mandatory if an infection with an unknown pathogen is suspected.

47.5.7.6 Prognosis

Long-term consequences of PH include: reduced exercise tolerance, even in mild cases, scoliosis in adolescent years, recurrent respiratory infections, and chronic pulmonary insufficiency. Right-sided hypoplasia has a worse prognosis than left-sided hypoplasia, probably because of the loss of the bigger right lung mass and more severe mediastinal shift and great vessel displacement (Fisher et al. 2008).

During the first 48 h of life, the best oxygenation index above 13 and the best $PaCO_2$ above 45 mmHg were predictive of poor outcome (Datin-Dorriere et al. 2008).

47.5.8 Oligohydramnios Syndrome

Bilateral PH commonly occurs in association with oligohydramnios caused by either renal disease in the fetus or chronic leakage of amniotic fluid as a consequence of PPROM. Infants subject to oligohydramnios resulting from chronic leakage of amniotic fluid over many weeks may exhibit a varying degree of PH. Oligohydramnios may act by compressing the fetal thorax or altering the dynamics of lung fluid so that full expansion of the lungs cannot be maintained. The severity of the PH is directly proportional to rupture of the membranes early in gestation, longer duration of rupture, and the presence of the oligohydramnios during the period of rupture.

For the fetal lung to develop normally, the fetal airways must be filled with fluid (Copland and Post 2004). Movement of chloride ions to the pulmonary lumen provides the main force for lung liquid secretion with a net production rate of lung fluid of about 4–5 mL/kg/h. The pressure in the fetal trachea exceeds that in the amniotic fluid by about 2 mmHg, thus amniotic fluid rarely enters the trachea. Several factors affect the volume and composition of the amniotic fluid, including amount of fetal urine and chronic leakage of amniotic fluid secondary to PPROM at 15–28 weeks' gestation.

Possible mechanisms of abnormal lung growth following oligohydramnios include: reduced lung fluid production (Blott et al. 1987) and consequent reduced production of growth factors (e.g., vascular endothelial growth factor, angiopoietins, endothelins and platelet-derived growth factor, fibroblast growth factor); reduced fetal breathing movements that are essential for lung growth; inflammation and infection which have a detrimental effect on pulmonary vascular development, such as smooth muscle hypertrophy of the distal pulmonary arterioles and decreased production of endothelial nitric oxide synthase; and other vascular growth factors.

Oligohydramnios can be associated with a spectrum of fetal positional and compression

abnormalities, such as pes equinovarus and a bell-shaped thorax.

The presence of PH in infants with bilateral renal agenesis was first recognized by Potter in 1946. It has since become apparent that a similar picture of the lethal PH is seen in conjunction with bilaterally dysplastic kidneys with or without cyst formation and in infants with congenital obstructive uropathy.

In the cases of renal agenesis, the reduction in lung volume and number of the alveoli is greater than in renal dysplasia, where these changes are more variable in their severity (Potter 1946b).

Despite attempts at in utero decompression of the urinary system, fetal surgery in this disease remains controversial and has met limited success.

47.5.8.1 Antenatal Management of Oligohydramnios

- Surveillance of infection by microbiological examination of the amniotic fluid.
- Antibiotic therapy.
- Antenatal corticosteroids should be given to women presenting with PPROM prior to 32 weeks.
- Tocolysis to delay delivery and allow for the administration of corticosteroids.
- Normalizing amniotic fluid volume with amnioinfusion.
- Promotion of fetal lung growth and development with tracheal occlusion (Keller et al. 2004).

47.5.9 Pulmonary Lymphangiectasia

Pulmonary lymphangiectasia (PL) is a rare developmental disorder involving the lung and is characterized by pulmonary subpleural, interlobar, perivascular, and peribronchial lymphatic dilatation.

Reports of occurrence in siblings suggest a genetic inheritance in some families and possibly an autosomal recessive mode of transmission (Stevenson et al. 2006); however, most cases occur sporadically (Wilson et al. 2006b). Males are more frequently affected than females (ratio 2:1). The incidence of PL is not clearly defined. Autopsy studies suggest that approximately 0.5–1% of infants who are stillborn or die in the neonatal period have congenital PL (Moerman et al. 1993).

47.5.9.1 Etiology and Pathogenesis

Noonan and colleagues classified congenital PL into three pathophysiological groups (Noonan et al. 1970):

- Type 1 – Generalized PL with thoracic and extrathoracic involvement
- Type 2 – PL secondary to pulmonary venous obstruction due to congenital heart disease
- Type 3 – Primary pulmonary developmental defect of the lung

Clinically, two forms of PL have been recognized: primary or congenital (types 1 and 3) and secondary (type 2), which occurs as a result of injury to the lymphatic vessels. The primary type has a neonatal onset and is often fatal (Esther and Barker 2004). It may be caused by a congenital defect in the primary development of the lung or may represent the localized expression of more generalized lymphatic involvement (nonimmune hydrops).

The pulmonary lymphatic system is normally well developed by the end of the 14th week of gestation. Initially, large lymph channels are present in the normal fetal lungs, which later undergo spontaneous regression. It is believed that failure of these channels to undergo the normal regression leads to congenital PL.

The secondary form results from impaired lymphatic drainage and increased lymphatic production as a consequence of increased venous and lymphatic hydrostatic pressure; it may also be due to cardiac lesions, which have been hypothesized to interfere with the normal regression of the lymphatic tissue elements after the 16th week of fetal life (Esther and Barker 2004). Hypoplastic left heart syndrome, pulmonary vein atresia, congenital mitral stenosis, cor triatriatum, and thoracic duct agenesis are the most likely causes of secondary PL.

Congenital PL may be associated with nonimmune hydrops fetalis and with congenital chylothorax (Cadichon 2008a).

47.5.9.2 Clinical Aspects

Clinical diagnosis of congenital PL can be strongly suspected in neonates who present severe respiratory distress with or without generalized or localized lymphedema and with pleural effusion (especially if chylous) either monolateral or bilateral although the disease affects both lungs.

In the postneonatal period, PL can occur any time in childhood or even adult life. During both the neonatal and postneonatal period, PL may be associated with chylothorax, chylopericardium, and chylous ascites (Dempsey et al. 2005). In older children it is frequently associated with recurrent cough, wheeze, increased respiratory effort with inspiratory crackle, and even congestive heart failure (Smeltzer et al. 1986).

Although most cases of PL are sporadic, congenital PL has been described in autosomal dominant, recessive, and X-linked syndromes. The occurrence of congenital PL in siblings and the association with a wide number of syndromes including patients with 46,XY/46,XX mosaicism, congenital ichthyosis, Noonan syndrome, Turner syndrome, Fryns syndrome, Down syndrome, and other syndromes suggest genetic predisposition (Esther and Barker 2004; Ozturk et al. 2000).

47.5.9.3 Diagnostic Methods

During the prenatal period, all causes leading to hydrops fetalis have to be taken into consideration. The diagnostic approach includes the following: complete family and obstetric history, laboratory investigations including blood type, Rhesus factor (Rh), antibody screening, TORCHES-CLAP titer (*Toxoplasma gondii*, rubella virus, *Cytomegalovirus*, herpes simplex virus, *Enterovirus*, syphilis, varicella-zoster virus, Lyme disease, AIDS (acquired immune deficiency syndrome), parvovirus B19), metabolic studies, and hemoglobin (Hb) electrophoresis (Stephenson et al. 1994). An instrumental evaluation is needed to rule out various conditions possibly related to PL and to establish whether PL is primary or secondary.

Diagnostic methods that may be useful in evaluating PL include conventional radiologic studies, echocardiography, high-resolution CT (Nobre et al. 2004) and MRI (Seed et al. 2009), lymphoscintigraphy (Sty et al. 1984), lung functionality tests (Barker et al. 2004), lung biopsy (Bellini et al. 2006), bronchoscopy, and pleural effusion examination (Bellini et al. 2006).

Chest X-rays usually show hyperinflation with interstitial markings. CT demonstrates diffuse thickening of the interstitium, both of the peribronchovascular interstitium and the septa surrounding the lobules. Coronal MRI T1 may show thickening of the interstitium, pleural fluid effusion, and atelectasia, if present. Axial MRI T2 usually shows high-signal material within the pulmonary interstitium, which is very often associated with pleural effusion. Despite the greater dose of radiation that is given during CT as compared to chest radiography, CT is preferable for the diagnosis of PL and, more generally, for the diagnosis of pediatric interstitial lung disease. Lymphoscintigraphy is a mildly invasive technique that provides valuable morpho-functional information regarding the lymphatic system (Sty et al. 1984). It highlights the accumulation of lymphatic fluid in the interstitial tissue that causes swelling, which is most evident in the limbs. In the few cases in which lung function tests were performed, they showed various patterns including restrictive, obstructive, and normal values. It is noteworthy that pulmonary function tests were stable over time in the patients who obtained multiple values. Bronchoscopic evaluation, while not specifically indicated in PL, may be useful for ruling out other pulmonary pathologies. No tracheobronchial anatomical abnormalities were reported in PL patients who were evaluated by bronchoscopy.

Lung biopsy may be useful to demonstrate the presence of dilated lymphatic spaces in the subpleural connective tissue, along the thickened interlobar septa, and around the bronchovascular axes. Great care must be taken when interpreting lung biopsies. In fact, the pathological findings in congenital PL patients may change a great deal over time, especially in case of viral infection, and, more generally, may range from initial recognition of minimal evidence of lymphatic dilatation to proof of severe lymphangiectasia. In this case, the lymphatic vessels are characterized by a thin wall, devoid of smooth muscle, and with slightly dilated lumen, lined by flattened endothelial cells.

47.5.9.4 Differential Diagnosis

During the neonatal period, transient tachypnea of the newborn and interstitial pulmonary infection are well known and are usually taken into consideration in the differential diagnosis of respiratory distress syndrome in the neonate. Rarer conditions must also be considered in the differential diagnosis of chronic interstitial lung disease in infants and include surfactant protein B deficiency, desquamative interstitial pneumonitis (familial and nonfamilial forms), pulmonary alveolar proteinosis, idiopathic pulmonary fibrosis, lymphoid interstitial pneumonitis, cellular interstitial pneumonitis, and chronic pneumonitis of infancy (Esther and Barker 2004; Bellini et al. 2008).

In older children or in adults, PL presents with a milder course. Conditions that can mimic interstitial lung disease in infants and children include neuroendocrine cell hyperplasia of infancy, acute pulmonary hemorrhage of infancy, follicular bronchiolitis, pulmonary vascular disorders (obstructive pulmonary venous disease, i.e., total and partial anomalous pulmonary venous return, pulmonary vein atresia or stenosis), hereditary hemorrhagic telangiectasia, pulmonary hemangiomatosis, various systemic diseases, and metabolic lipid storage disorders.

47.5.9.5 Therapy and Treatments

Delivery room management could be a challenge in the presence of severe respiratory distress associated with pleural effusion, and multiple procedures might be required. Tracheal intubation and assisted ventilation are usually necessary. Infants with persistent pulmonary hypertension and difficulties oxygenating should be ventilated with HFOV and could benefit from iNO administration. Sterile thoracentesis or paracentesis should be considered to reduce respiratory distress. Fluid replacement and inotropic support are often necessary. Patients with acute respiratory failure who are refractory to maximal conservative treatment might be considered candidates for ECMO. In patients with rapidly expanding pleural effusion that requires placing unilateral or bilateral chest tubes, the large amount of fluid (that is drained over days or weeks) leads to the loss of great quantities of albumin, immunoglobulin, and many other plasma factors that must be replaced. Nutrition plays a role in reducing lymphatic production. Enteral nutrition with medium-chain triglycerides and a total parenteral nutrition have been successfully employed. Octreotide has been used in PL to reduce lymph production. When the chyle leakage persists, pleurodesis by instillation of sclerosing agents or parietal pleurectomy appears to be effective.

47.5.9.6 Prognosis

Recent advances in neonatal intensive care have changed the previously nearly fatal outcome of PL at birth. However, contradictory data have been reported regarding the outcome and do not allow a consistent prognosis to be established. The outcome is more likely to be favorable if there are no associated defects. Respiratory problems can continue over the first years of life and often require home supplemental oxygen and symptomatic treatment for recurrent cough and wheeze.

47.5.10 Chylothorax

Chylothorax is an unusual entity in the neonate that commonly is associated with respiratory symptoms in the first day of life and may be expression of congenital PL. The incidence of congenital chylothorax is about 1:10,000–15,000 pregnancies, with a male-female ratio of 2:1. Chylothorax presenting at birth may be associated with cardiac anomalies, various syndromes, thoracic ductal or venous thrombosis, birth trauma or local compression of the thoracic duct, and congenital malformation of the lymphatic system (lymphangiomatosis) (Moerman et al. 1993; Mettauer et al. 2009; Ergaz et al. 2009). Chylothorax has been described as a complication of Down syndrome, in which there is presumably a significant maldevelopment of the lymphatic system. Other patients may have Turner or Noonan syndrome. Infants may have cystic hygroma malformations (Moerman et al. 1993; Rocha et al. 2006). Acquired chylothorax results from damage to the thoracic duct. It has been reported as a surgical complication in the repair of congenital diaphragmatic hernia,

tracheoesophageal fistula, and a variety of congenital heart disorder (e.g., patent ductus arteriosus ligation). Acquired chylothorax may also be the consequence of drainage of pneumothorax when the tube is inserted too far (Cadichon 2008b). In many cases, however, no underlying cause for the chylothorax is found. Chylothorax is more common on the right side: Chernick and Reed said that 53% of the cases were on the right side, 35% on the left side, and 12% were bilateral (Cadichon 2008b). Since chylothorax is typically unilateral, there may be decreased breath sounds over the side of the effusion and mediastinal shift to the contralateral side. Bilateral chylothoraces should be considered in the differential diagnosis for any infant who cannot be ventilated in the delivery room. The characteristic roentgenographic appearance is similar to that of a large pleural effusion depressing the adjacent diaphragm and displacing the mediastinum.

The evaluation of the pleural effusion is essential for the diagnosis of chylothorax. Chylothorax is usually diagnosed in the presence of "milky" pleural effusion with a triglyceride level >1.1 mmol/L and a cell count $>1{,}000$ cells/μL, with a predominance of lymphocytes (approximately 80%), according to the criteria drawn up in previous reports (Bellini et al. 2006). However, this is an unreliable diagnostic test in malnourished patients and in patients not receiving enteral nutrition, including the fetus and occasionally the neonate. Without enteral feeding, not enough chylomicron (the main triglyceride carrier) is produced to raise chyle triglyceride levels. In these patients, chylothorax may be diagnosed by detecting lymphocytes in the pleural fluid.

Treatment of chylothorax may require repeated thoracenteses or even thoracostomy tube drainage to prevent respiratory failure. The large amount of fluid that is drained over days and weeks leads to the loss of great quantities of albumin, immunoglobulin, and many other plasma factors that must be replaced, in some cases even on a daily basis. Once drainage is accomplished, these infants are placed on formulas containing medium-chain triglycerides (MCTs) to reduce thoracic duct lymph flow. Oral intake of protein and water also stimulates thoracic duct lymph flow, so in resistant cases the infant is managed with nothing by mouth, with nutritional support through a central line.

Octreotide, antiplasmin, and oral sildenafil have been used in CPL and chylothorax (Epaud et al. 2008; Malleske and Yoder 2015; Kalomenidis 2006).

A variety of approaches have been used with some success to treat the infant with persistent chylothorax, including direct attempts at repair, thoracoscopic parietal pleural clipping (Clark et al. 2015), patching with fibrin glue, or obliteration of the pleural space with sclerosing agents (Rifai et al. 2003). Congenital chylothorax also has been managed successfully using a pleuroperitoneal shunt (Podevin et al. 1999). Finally some reports suggest that ligation of the thoracic duct below the area of leakage is highly effective; this procedure is well tolerated without accumulation of fluid in the peripheral tissues or in the peritoneum (Andersen et al. 1984).

47.5.11 Misalignment of Pulmonary Veins with Alveolar Capillary Dysplasia

Alveolar capillary dysplasia (ACD) is a rare disorder typically presenting at birth with severe hypoxemia, although an unusual late onset has been reported as late as 7 months of age offering the possibility that long-term survivors with milder forms of the disease may exist (Bishop et al. 2011; Shankar et al. 2006). No gender predilection has been identified. While the cause is unknown, there have been six cases reported in siblings, indicating that in some cases this may be a familial disorder with autosomal recessive inheritance (Gutierrez et al. 2000). ACD is distinguished by immature lobular development and reduced capillary density, both of which indicate premature growth arrest.

47.5.11.1 Etiology and Pathogenesis

Pathological features include reduction of alveolar capillaries, widened alveolar septa, and increased muscularization of pulmonary arterioles (Melly et al. 2008). There is usually malpositioning

("misalignment") of pulmonary veins in the bronchovascular bundle, but this is not required for the diagnosis. As a consequence blood entering an individual lung unit can only drain via anomalous ("misaligned") veins. The obstruction that is created leads to the occlusive changes observed in the pulmonary arterial circulation. A focal distribution of disease has been described, which makes it necessary to examine multiple lung sections if ACD is suspected.

47.5.11.2 Clinical Aspects

Infants with ACD usually present with minimal or no parenchymal lung disease. Profound hypoxemia and severe metabolic acidosis consistent with severe PPHN and right ventricular failure are nearly always present. However, infants with ACD do not respond or respond only transiently to therapies that are usually effective in reversing pulmonary hypertension (iNO or ECMO) (Parker et al. 1997).

The diagnosis of ACD should be considered in infants who present with severe hypoxemia and PPHN and who do not respond appropriately after 7–10 days of standard treatment as described below. The majority of patients with ACD (approximately 75%) will have other associated anomalies of the cardiovascular, gastrointestinal, urogenital, or musculoskeletal systems. The initial chest radiograph is usually normal. The diagnosis can only be confirmed by lung biopsy or autopsy. FOXF1 mutation analysis may be useful to provide prenatal analysis for families at high risk (Bishop et al. 2011).

47.5.11.3 Differential Diagnosis

Conditions that must be considered in the differential diagnosis of ACD are idiopathic PPHN and surfactant protein B deficiency, sepsis, pneumonia, PH, CDH, or cardiac lesions (Hugosson et al. 2005).

47.5.11.4 Therapy and Treatments

Standard therapies include mechanical ventilation, high concentrations of inspired oxygen, and iNO and ECMO support. These therapies prolong life by days to weeks, but have not led to long-term survival (Tibballs and Chow 2002). Theoretically, ACD could be treated by lung transplantation. However, successful transplantation has not yet been reported. Donor availability continues to limit the utilization of lung transplantation for neonatal diseases.

References

Abrams ME, Ackerman VL, Engle WA (2004) Primary unilateral pulmonary hypoplasia: neonate through early childhood – case report, radiographic diagnosis and review of the literature. J Perinatol 24:667–670

Adzick NS, Harrison MR, Glick PL et al (1985) Fetal cystic adenomatoid malformation: prenatal diagnosis and natural history. J Pediatr Surg 20:483–488

Adzick NS, Harrison MR, Crombleholme TM et al (1998) Fetal lung lesions: management and outcome. Am J Obstet Gynecol 179:884–889

Alescio T, Cassini A (1962) Induction in vitro of tracheal buds by pulmonary mesenchyme grafted on tracheal epithelium. J Exp Zool 150:83–94

Andersen EA, Hertel J, Pedersen SA et al (1984) Congenital chylothorax: management by ligature of the thoracic duct. Scand J Thorac Cardiovasc Surg 18:193–194

Asabe K, Toki N, Hashimoto S et al (1994) An immunohistochemical study of the expression of surfactant apoprotein in the hypoplastic lung of rabbit fetuses induced by oligohydramnios. Am J Pathol 145:631–639

Askenazi SS, Perlman M (1979) Pulmonary hypoplasia: lung weight and radial alveolar count as criteria of diagnosis. Arch Dis Child 54:614–618

Baird R, Puligandla PS, Laberge JM (2014) Congenital lung malformations: informing best practice. Semin Pediatr Surg 23:270–277

Barker PM, Esther CR Jr, Fordham LA et al (2004) Primary pulmonary lymphangiectasia in infancy and childhood. Eur Respir J 24:413–419

Barth PJ, Rüschoff J (1992) Morphometric study on pulmonary arterial thickness in pulmonary hypoplasia. Pediatr Pathol 12:653–663

Bellini C, Boccardo F, Campisi C et al (2006) Congenital pulmonary lymphangiectasia. Orphanet J Rare Dis 1:43

Bellini C, Boccardo F, Campisi C et al (2008) Lymphatic dysplasias in newborns and children: the role of lymphoscintigraphy. J Pediatr 152:587–589

Berlinger NT, Porto DP, Thompson TR (1987) Infantile lobar emphysema. Ann Otol Rhinol Laryngol 96:106–111

Bishop NB, Stankiewicz P, Steinhorn RH (2011) Alveolar capillary dysplasia. Am J Respir Crit Care Med 184:172–179

Bland RD, Hansen TN, Haberkern CM et al (1982) Lung fluid balance in lambs before and after birth. J Appl Physiol 53:992–1004

Blau H, Barak A, Karmazyn B et al (2002) Postnatal management of resolving fetal lung lesions. Pediatrics 109:105–108

Blott M, Greenough A, Nicolaides KH et al (1987) Fetal breathing movements as predictor of favourable pregnancy outcome after oligohydramnios due to membrane rupture in second trimester. Lancet 2:129–131

Borsellino A, Zaccara A, Nahom A et al (2006) False–positive rate in prenatal diagnosis of surgical anomalies. J Pediatr Surg 41:826–829

Brody JS, Thurlbeck WM (1986) Development, growth and aging of the lung. In: Fishman AP (ed) Handbook of physiology, the respiratory system. American Physiological Society, Bethesda, pp 355–386

Burri PH (1984) Fetal and postnatal development of the lung. Annu Rev Physiol 46:617–628

Burri PH (1986) Development and growth of human lung. In: Fishman AP (ed) Handbook of physiology, the respiratory system. American Physiological Society, Bethesda, pp 1–46

Burri PH (1997) Postnatal development and growth. In: Crystal RG, West BG, Weibel ER, Barnes PG (eds) The lung. Lippincott- Raven, Philadelphia, pp 1013–1026

Bush A (2001) Congenital lung disease: a plea for clear thinking and clear nomenclature. Pediatr Pulmonol 32:328–337

Butterworth SA, Blair GK (2005) Postnatal spontaneous resolution of congenital cystic adenomatoid malformations. J Pediatr Surg 40:832–834

Cacciari A, Ruggeri G, Mordenti M et al (2001) High-frequency oscillatory ventilation versus conventional mechanical ventilation in congenital diaphragmatic hernia. Eur J Pediatr Surg 11:3–7

Cadichon S (2008a) Congenital pulmonary lymphangiectasia. In: Kumar P, Burton BK (eds) Congenital malformations. Mc Graw Hill Education, New York, pp 165–169

Cadichon S (2008b) Congenital hydrothorax. In: Kumar P, Burton BK (eds) Congenital malformations. Mc Graw Hill Education, New York, pp 159–164

Calvert JK, Lakhoo K (2007) Antenatally suspected congenital cystic adenomatoid malformation of the lung: postnatal investigation and timing of surgery. J Pediatr Surg 42:411–414

Calvert JK, Boyd PA, Chamberlain PC et al (2006) Outcome of antenatally suspected congenital cystic adenomatoid malformation of the lung: 10 years experience 1991–2001. Arch Dis Child Fetal Neonatal Ed 91:F26–F28

Cass DL, Crombleholme TM, Howell LJ et al (1997) Cystic lung lesions with systemic arterial blood supply: a hybrid of congenital cystic adenomatoid malformation and bronchopulmonary sequestration. J Pediatr Surg 32:986–990

Clark ME, Woo RK, Johnson SM (2015) Thoracoscopic pleural clipping for the management of congenital chylothorax. Pediatr Surg Int 31:1133–1137

Clements BS (1999) Congenital malformations of the lungs and airways. In: Taussig LM, Landau LI (eds) Pediatric respiratory medicine. Mosby, St. Louis, pp 1106–1136

Copland I, Post M (2004) Lung development and fetal lung growth. Paediatr Respir Rev 5:259–264

Datin-Dorriere V, Walter-Nicolet E, Rousseau V et al (2008) Experience in the management of eighty-two newborns with congenital diaphragmatic hernia treated with high-frequency oscillatory ventilation and delayed surgery without the use of extracorporeal membrane oxygenation. J Intensive Care Med 23:128–135

Davenport M, Warne SA, Cacciaguerra S et al (2004) Current outcome of antenatally diagnosed cystic lung disease. J Pediatr Surg 39:549–556

Dawes GS, Fox HE, Leduc BM et al (1970) Respiratory movements and paradoxical sleep in the foetal lamb. J Physiol 210:47P–48P

de Mello DE, Reid L (1997) Arteries and veins. In: Crystal RG et al (eds) The lung. Lippincott-Raven, Philadelphia, pp 1117–1127

de Waal K, Kluckow M (2015) Prolonged rupture of membranes and pulmonary hypoplasia in very preterm infants: pathophysiology and guided treatment. J Pediatr 166:1113–1120

Dempsey EM, Sant'Anna GM, Williams RL et al (2005) Congenital pulmonary lymphangiectasia presenting as nonimmune fetal hydrops and severe respiratory distress at birth: not uniformly fatal. Pediatr Pulmonol 40:270–274

Diamond IR, Herrera P, Langer JC, Kim PC (2007) Thoracoscopic versus open resection of congenital lung lesions: a case-matched study. J Pediatr Surg 42:1057–1061

Epaud R, Dubern B, Larroquet M et al (2008) Therapeutic strategies for idiopathic chylothorax. J Pediatr Surg 43:461–465

Ergaz Z, Bar-Oz B, Yatsiv I, Arad I (2009) Congenital chylothorax: clinical course and prognostic significance. Pediatr Pulmonol 44:806–811

Esther CR Jr, Barker PM (2004) Pulmonary lymphangiectasia: diagnosis and clinical course. Pediatr Pulmonol 38:308–313

Fewell JE, Johnson P (1983) Upper airway dynamics during breathing and apnoea in fetal lambs. J Physiol 339:495–504

Fisher JC, Jefferson RA, Arkovitz MS et al (2008) Redefining outcomes in right congenital diaphragmatic hernia. J Pediatr Surg 43:373–379

Fitzgerald DA (2007) Congenital cyst adenomatoid malformations: resect some and observe all? Paediatr Respir Rev 8:67–76

Gabarre JA, Izquierdo AG, Ponferrada MR et al (2005) Isolated unilateral pulmonary agenesis: early prenatal diagnosis and long-term follow-up. J Ultrasound Med 24:865–868

Gerards FA, Twisk JW, Fetter WP et al (2008) Predicting pulmonary hypoplasia with 2- or 3-dimensional ultrasonography in complicated pregnancies. Am J Obstet Gynecol 198:140–146

Gorincour G, Bouvenot J, Mourot MG et al (2005) Prenatal prognosis of congenital diaphragmatic hernia using

magnetic resonance imaging measurement of fetal lung volume. Ultrasound Obstet Gynecol 26:738–744

Gutierrez C, Rodriguez A, Palenzuela S et al (2000) Congenital misalignment of pulmonary veins with alveolar capillary dysplasia causing persistent neonatal pulmonary hypertension: report of two affected siblings. Pediatr Dev Pathol 3:271–276

Hebra A, Othersen HB Jr, Tagge EP (2000) Bronchopulmonary malformations. In: Ashcraft KW, Murphy JP, Sharp RJ et al (eds) Pediatric surgery. Saunders, Philadelphia, pp 273–286

Hedrick HL, Flake AW, Crombleholme TM et al (2005) The ex utero intrapartum therapy procedure for high-risk fetal lung lesions. J Pediatr Surg 40:1038–1043

Hekelaar N, van Uffelen R, van Vliet AC et al (2000) Primary lymphoepithelioma- like carcinoma within an intralobular pulmonary sequestration. Eur Respir J 16:1025–1027

Hislop A (1996) Fetal and postnatal anatomical development. In: Greenough A, Roberton NRC, Milner AD (eds) Neonatal respiratory disorders. Arnold, London, pp 3–12

Hooper SB, Harding R (1995) Fetal lung liquid: a major determinant of the growth and functional development of the fetal lung. Clin Exp Pharmacol Physiol 22:235–247

Hugosson CO, Salama HM, Al-Dayel F et al (2005) Primary alveolar capillary dysplasia (acinar dysplasia) and surfactant protein B deficiency: a clinical, radiological and pathological study. Pediatr Radiol 35:311–316

Ierullo AM, Ganapathy R, Crowley S et al (2005) Neonatal outcome of antenatally diagnosed congenital cystic adenomatoid malformations. Ultrasound Obstet Gynecol 26:150–153

Kalomenidis I (2006) Octreotide and chylothorax. Curr Opin Pulm Med 12:264–267

Kasprian G, Balassy C, Brugger PC et al (2006) MRI of normal and pathological fetal lung development. Eur J Radiol 57:261–270

Keller RL, Hawgood S, Neuhaus JM et al (2004) Infant pulmonary function in a randomized trial of fetal tracheal occlusion for severe congenital diaphragmatic hernia. Pediatr Res 56:818–825

Kirwan WO, Walbaum PR, McCormack MM (1973) Cystic intrathoracic derivatives of the foregut and their complications. Thorax 28:424–428

Knox WF, Barson AJ (1986) Pulmonary hypoplasia in a regional perinatal unit. Early Hum Dev 14:33–42

Kotecha S (2000) Lung growth for beginners. Paediatr Respir Rev 1:308–313

Kuhn C, Kuhn JP (1992) Coexistence of bronchial atresia and bronchogenic cyst: diagnostic criteria and embryologic considerations. Pediatr Radiol 22:568–570

Kunisaki SM, Fauza DO, Nemes LP et al (2006) Bronchial atresia: the hidden pathology within a spectrum of prenatally diagnosed lung masses. J Pediatr Surg 41:61–65

Kunisaki SM, Ehrenberg-Buchner S, Dillman JR et al (2015) Vanishing fetal lung malformations: prenatal sonographic characteristics and postnatal outcomes. J Pediatr Surg 50:978–982

Lacy DE, Shaw NJ, Pilling DW, Walkinshaw S (1999) Outcome of congenital lung abnormalities detected antenatally. Acta Paediatr 88:454–458

Lakhoo K (2009) Management of congenital cystic adenomatous malformations of the lung. Arch Dis Child Fetal Neonatal Ed 94:F73–F76

Langston C, Kida K, Reed M, Thurlbeck WM (1984) Human lung growth in late gestational and in the neonate. Am Rev Res Dis 129:607–613

Lee EY, Siegel MJ, Sierra LM, Foglia RP (2004) Evaluation of angioarchitecture of pulmonary sequestration in pediatric patients using 3D MDCT angiography. AJR 183:183–188

Liu M, Skinner SJ, Xu J et al (1992) Stimulation of fetal rat lung cell proliferation in vitro by mechanical stretch. Am J Physiol 263:L376–L383

MacGillivray TE, Harrison MR, Goldstein RB, Adzick NS (1993) Disappearing fetal lung lesions. J Pediatr Surg 28:1321–1325

Malleske DT, Yoder BA (2015) Congenital chylothorax treated with oral sildenafil: a case report and review of the literature. J Perinatol 35:384–386

Mardini MK, Nyhan WL (1985) Agenesis of the lung: report of four patients with unusual anomalies. Chest 87:522–527

Melly L, Sebire NJ, Malone M, Nicholson AG (2008) Capillary apposition and density in the diagnosis of alveolar capillary dysplasia. Histopathology 53:450–457

Mettauer N, Agrawal S, Pierce C et al (2009) Outcome of children with pulmonary lymphangiectasis. Pediatr Pulmonol 44:351–357

Moerman P, Vandenberghe K, Devlieger H et al (1993) Congenital pulmonary lymphangiectasis with chylothorax: a heterogeneous lymphatic vessel abnormality. Am J Med Genet 47:54–58

Mulder EJ, Boersma M, Meeuse M et al (1994) Patterns of breathing movements in the near-term human fetus: relationship to behavioural states. Early Hum Dev 36:127–135

Nakamura Y, Harada K, Yamamoto I et al (1992) Human pulmonary hypoplasia: statistical, morphological, morphometric, and biochemical study. Arch Pathol Lab Med 116:635–642

Nobre LF, Muller NL, de Souza Junior AS et al (2004) Congenital pulmonary lymphangiectasia: CT and pathologic findings. J Thorac Imaging 19:56–59

Noonan JA, Walters LR, Reeves JT (1970) Congenital pulmonary lymphangiectasis. Am J Dis Child 120:314–319

Ozcelik U, Gocmen A, Kiper N et al (2003) Congenital lobar emphysema: evaluation and long-term follow-up of thirty cases at a single center. Pediatr Pulmonol 35:384–391

Ozturk S, Cefle K, Palanduz S et al (2000) A case of Noonan syndrome with pulmonary and abdominal lymphangiectasia. Int J Clin Pract 54:274–276
Parker TA, Ivy DD, Kinsella JP et al (1997) Combined therapy with inhaled nitric oxide and intravenous prostacyclin in an infant with alveolar-capillary dysplasia. Am J Respir Crit Care Med 155:743–746
Peranteau WH, Boelig MM, Khalek N et al (2015) Effect of single and multiple courses of maternal betamethasone on prenatal congenital lung lesion growth and fetal survival. J Pediatr Surg 51:28–32
Podevin G, Levard G, Larroquet M et al (1999) Pleuroperitoneal shunt in the management of chylothorax caused by thoracic lymphatic dysplasia. J Pediatr Surg 34:1420–1422
Porter HJ (1999) Pulmonary hypoplasia. Arch Dis Child Fetal Neonatal Ed 81:F81–F83
Potter EL (1946a) Facial characteristics in infants with bilateral renal agenesis. Am J Obstet Gynecol 51:885
Potter EL (1946b) Bilateral renal agenesis. J Pediatr 29:68–76
Pumberger W, Hormann M, Deutinger J et al (2003) Longitudinal observation of antenatally detected congenital lung malformations (CLM): natural history, clinical outcome and long-term follow-up. Eur J Cardiothorac Surg 24:703–711
Rifai N, Sfeir R, Rakza T et al (2003) Successful management of severe chylothorax with argon plasma fulguration and fibrin glue in a premature infant. Eur J Pediatr Surg 13:324–326
Rocha G, Fernandes P, Rocha P et al (2006) Pleural effusions in the neonate. Acta Paediatr 95:791–798
Rossi R, Tjan TD, Hentschel R et al (1998) Successful perioperative management of congenital cystic adenomatoid malformation of the lung by high frequency oscillatory ventilation – report of two cases. Klin Padiatr 210:94–96
Salomon LJ, Audibert F, Dommergues M et al (2003) Fetal thoracoamniotic shunting as the only treatment for pulmonary sequestration with hydrops: favorable long-term outcome without postnatal surgery. Ultrasound Obstet Gynecol 21:299–301
Seed M, Bradley T, Bourgeois J et al (2009) Antenatal MR imaging of pulmonary lymphangiectasia secondary to hypoplastic left heart syndrome. Pediatr Radiol 39:747–749
Shah DM, Kluckow M (2011) Early functional echocardiogram and inhaled nitric oxide: usefulness in managing neonates born following extreme preterm premature rupture of membranes (PPROM). J Paediatr Child Health 47:340–345
Shankar V, Haque A, Johnson J, Pietsch J (2006) Late presentation of alveolar capillary dysplasia in an infant. Pediatr Crit Care Med 7:177–179
Shanmugam G, MacArthur K, Pollock JC (2005) Congenital lung malformations–antenatal and postnatal evaluation and management. Eur J Cardiothorac Surg 27:45–52
Shaw JP, Dembitzer FR, Wisnivesky JP et al (2008) Video-assisted thoracoscopic lobectomy: state of the art and future directions. Ann Thorac Surg 85:S705–S709
Smeltzer DM, Stickler GB, Fleming RE (1986) Primary lymphatic dysplasia in children: chylothorax, chylous ascites, and generalized lymphatic dysplasia. Eur J Pediatr 145:286–292
Stanton M, Davenport M (2006) Management of congenital lung lesions. Early Hum Dev 82:289–295
Stephenson T, Zuccollo J, Mohajer M (1994) Diagnosis and management of non-immune hydrops in the newborn. Arch Dis Child Fetal Neonatal Ed 70:151–154
Stevens TP, Chess PR, McConnochie KM et al (2002) Survival in early- and late-term infants with congenital diaphragmatic hernia treated with extracorporeal membrane oxygenation. Pediatrics 110:590–596
Stevenson DA, Pysher TJ, Ward RM et al (2006) Familial congenital non-immune hydrops, chylothorax, and pulmonary lymphangiectasia. Am J Med Genet A 140:368–372
Stocker JT (2002) Congenital pulmonary airway malformation – a new name for and an expanded classification of congenital adenomatoid malformation of the lung. Histopathology 41:424–431
Sty JR, Thomas JP Jr, Wolff MH et al (1984) Lymphoscintigraphy. Pulmonary lymphangiectasia. Clin Nucl Med 9:716
Swischuck LE (ed) (2004) Imaging of the newborn, infant, and young child. Lippincott Williams & Wilkins, Philadelphia
Thakral CL, Maji DC, Sajwani MJ (2001) Congenital lobar emphysema: experience with 21 cases. Pediatr Surg Int 17:88–91
Tibballs J, Chow CW (2002) Incidence of alveolar capillary dysplasia in severe idiopathic persistent pulmonary hypertension of the newborn. J Paediatr Child Health 38:397–400
Uga N, Ishii T, Kawase Y et al (2004) Nitric oxide inhalation therapy in very low-birthweight infants with hypoplastic lung due to oligohydramnios. Pediatr Int 46:10–14
van Leeuwen K, Teitelbaum DH, Hirschl RB et al (1999) Prenatal diagnosis of congenital cystic adenomatoid malformation and its postnatal presentation, surgical indications, and natural history. J Pediatr Surg 34:794–798
Vilos GA, Liggins GC (1982) Intrathoracic pressures in fetal sheep. J Dev Physiol 4:247–256
Wilson RD, Hedrick HL, Liechty KW et al (2006a) Cystic adenomatoid malformation of the lung: review of genetics, prenatal diagnosis, and in utero treatment. Am J Med Genet A 140:151–155
Wilson RD, Pawel B, Bebbington M et al (2006b) Congenital pulmonary lymphangiectasis sequence: a rare, heterogeneous, and lethal etiology for prenatal pleural effusion. Prenat Diagn 26:1058–1061

Neonatal Pulmonary Physiology of Term and Preterm Newborns

48

Corrado Moretti and Paola Papoff

Contents

Abstract

A knowledge of normal neonatal pulmonary development and physiology is the cornerstone for understanding the pathophysiology and optimizing the treatment of many respiratory diseases of preterm and term infants. It forms the groundwork not only for an individualized treatment but also for increasing respiratory care technology, both important factors in improving pulmonary outcomes in these vulnerable patients. Pulmonary physiology and oxygen transport in the neonate are similar to older children; however, there are critical

C. Moretti (✉)
Università degli Studi di Roma “La Sapienza”, Rome, Italy
e-mail: corrado.moretti@uniroma1.it

P. Papoff (✉)
Intensive Care Unit, Sapienza University of Rome, Rome, Italy

G. Buonocore et al. (eds.), *Neonatology*,
https://doi.org/10.1007/978-3-319-29489-6_197

differences that are important to take into consideration when treating the youngest age group, and this chapter deals with the peculiar characteristics of neonatal respiratory mechanics and the pathophysiology of the various possible causes of hypoxia.

48.1 Salient Points

- In premature infants the chest is subject to distortion owing to the poor ossification of the ribs: the inward distortion of the chest during inspiration compels the diaphragm to do more work in order to maintain tidal volume constant.
- Compliance expresses the capacity of the lung to be distended, and its reduction causes a drop in tidal volume.
- Severe neonatal respiratory diseases are characterized by a right-left shunt through fetal channels for the increase of pulmonary resistances.
- $PaCO_2$ is not usually increased in the presence of an extrapulmonary shunt because the hypoxia and hypercapnia of non-oxygenated blood cause an increase in alveolar ventilation; due to the different shape of the dissociation curve of CO_2 and O_2, hyperventilation is effective in reducing $PaCO_2$ but totally ineffective in increasing PaO_2.
- The increase in $PaCO_2$ represents a very important criterion for the diagnosis of hypoventilation because, unlike hypoxia, this is virtually the sole cause of hypercapnia.
- Alterations in diffusion never involve CO_2 given the rapidity with which it diffuses.
- Alterations in the ventilation-perfusion ratio are responsible for most of the defects in the exchange of O_2 in pulmonary diseases.

48.2 Introduction

The transfer of O_2 to the tissues and the removal of CO_2 are guaranteed by the simultaneous activity of the respiratory apparatus and of the cardiocirculatory system which ensures that O_2 reaches the tissues and that the CO_2 produced by cell metabolism is removed (Cumming et al. 1966).

The main steps in this process are:

- Pulmonary ventilation, which consists in the rhythmic introduction of fresh gases into the alveolus; tidal volume (V_T) is a term deriving from "tide" which offers an excellent representation of the flow and reflow of the gases.
- The diffusion of O_2 and CO_2 at the alveolus-capillary interface.
- Capillary perfusion, whereby O_2 and CO_2 are transported into and out of the tissues.

Unlike the respiratory apparatus, the cardiocirculatory system is a closed-loop system with a one-way flow.

48.3 Lung Mechanics

Alveolar ventilation is obtained through pulmonary expansion, which in turn occurs through dilatation of the ribcage. At rest, the lungs and ribcage are in a situation of equilibrium determined by the resultant of two contrasting forces: elastic inward recoil of the pulmonary parenchyma and outward elastic traction of the ribcage. The pulmonary volume that results from this equilibrium is defined as functional residual capacity (FRC).

The consequence of this interaction in opposite directions is the presence of a negative pressure of around −3, −5 cm H_2O in the intrapleural space, which is a virtual cavity. During normal breathing most of the V_T is ensured by the diaphragm, a muscle supplied by the phrenic nerves, whose contraction causes an increase in the vertical diameter of the ribcage; the increase in the anteroposterior diameter is due to the contraction of the internal intercostal muscles whereby the ribs rotate upwards along their axis.

Dilatation of the ribcage during inspiration causes a reduction in intrapleural pressure, and the lungs – hence the alveoli – undergo passive expansion (De Troyer 1997). The decrease in intra-alveolar pressure produces an airflow in the respiratory system; the flow stops at the end of inspiration when the alveolar pressure returns to a state of equilibrium with atmospheric pressure (Fig. 1).

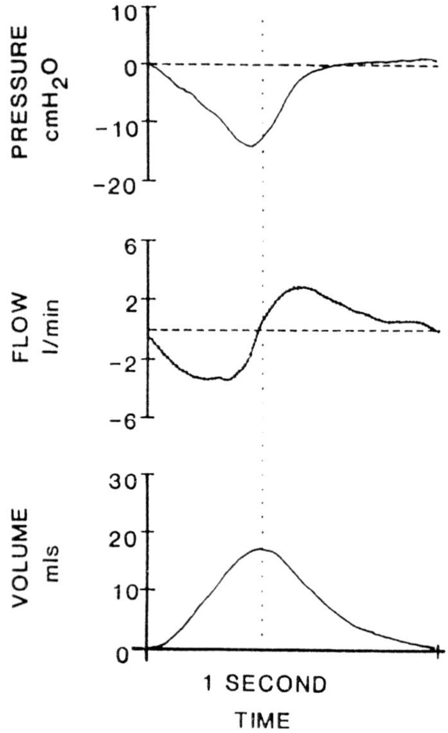

Fig. 1 Pressure, air flow, and volume signals of a respiratory cycle

In newborns, chest stability is facilitated by a relatively horizontal position of the ribs so that the intercostal muscles, which contract simultaneously with the diaphragm, can provide structural stiffness for the ribcage rather than expanding it during inspiration. Inspiration and expiration are therefore ensured above all by the activity of the diaphragm, which is less efficient in newborns compared to adults due both to its rather flat conformation that reduces its excursion and to its histological characteristics. In premature infants, in particular, the proportion of diaphragmatic slow-twitch muscle fibers that are resistant to oxidation and fatigue (Type I) is much smaller (10%) than the fast-twitch fibers which tire more easily (Type II); the proportion of Type I fibers increases progressively with age (about 25% in a term infant and 55% at eight months) (Keens et al. 1978).

Moreover, the chest of a premature infant is subject to distortion owing to the poor ossification of the ribs and sternum and because the intercostal muscles are not fully functional. The inward distortion of the chest during inspiration compels the diaphragm to do more work: indeed, in order to maintain the V_T constant, the excursion of the diaphragm must increase so as to offset the paradoxical movement of the ribcage. This phenomenon contributes to accelerating the respiratory functional exhaustion to which low birth-weight infants with respiratory distress are subject to.

The expiratory phase, by contrast, is usually a passive phenomenon determined by the forces of elastic recoil of distended tissues: the greater the expansion of the lungs during inspiration, the greater its elastic recoil. The intervention of expiration muscles, the most important ones being the muscles of the abdominal wall, occurs only in some physiological situations such as coughing and sneezing or in some pathological conditions.

48.4 Elastic Properties of the Lungs

Compliance (C) is a value that expresses the elasticity of the lung or, rather, its capacity to be distended. It is defined by correlating the pressure applied to the alveoli (P) to the ensuing volume variations (V):

$$C = V/P$$

Compliance is usually represented through pressure/volume curves: the higher its value the greater the variation of the amount of gas in the lung per unit pressure and the steeper the slope of the curve (Fig. 2). A peculiar characteristic of lung pressure/volume curves is that inflation and deflation have different pressure curves, a phenomenon that is called hysteresis.

The factors determining the degree of elasticity of the lung are the presence of elastic fibers in the parenchyma and the surface tension forces of the liquid that wets the alveoli walls (Goerke and Schurch 1997). Surface tension forces are generated by the cohesion between the molecules making up the liquid: these forces are balanced in the liquid phase but not at the air-liquid interface; the result is that the molecules on the surface exercise greater attraction towards the surrounding

molecules. The importance of the role of the surface tension forces can be demonstrated through a simple experiment: by expanding an isolated lung with saline solution, and then with air, two different pressure/volume curves are obtained. In the first case the recoil forces are entirely due to the elastic properties of the lung tissue because there is no air-liquid interface. By contrast, when the lung is expanded with gas, the surface tension forces require a greater pressure to obtain the same expansion; moreover, it must be pointed out that when the lungs are filled with saline solution the hysteresis disappears.

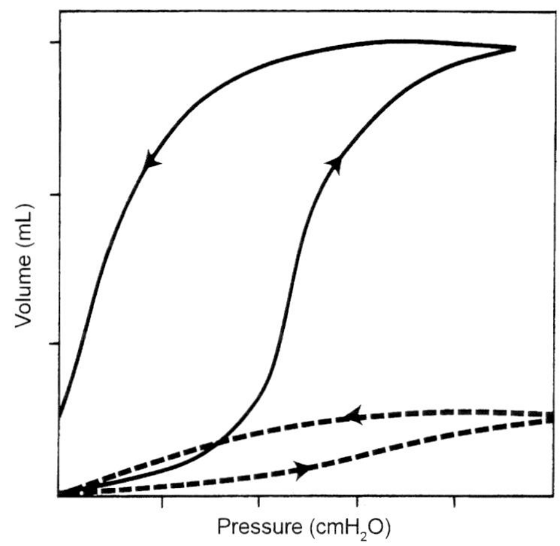

Fig. 2 Pressure/volume diagram in a neonate with RDS (dashed line) and in a normal neonate (solid line)

The presence on the surface of the alveoli of a tensioactive factor or surfactant, consisting of various phospholipids, has the function of reducing the superficial tension forces and of stabilizing the size of the alveoli.

According to Laplace's law

$$\text{Pressure} = 2 \times (\text{surface tension})/\text{radius}$$

the pressure required to maintain the alveoli expanded increases proportionally to the decrease in its radius: the consequence should be that the smaller alveoli empty out into the larger ones, but the action of the surfactant, i.e., decreasing surface tension is more effective as the alveolus decreases its size as a result of the greater concentration of surfactant molecules. The intra-alveolar pressure is thus uniformly maintained in the pulmonary parenchyma, and the size of the alveolus is kept stable.

The effects of the surfactant on lung mechanics can be easily understood from the analysis of Fig. 3, which shows two pressure/volume curves obtained by inflating a lung affected by respiratory distress syndrome (RDS), before and after treatment with surfactant.

The fundamental differences between the two curves are:

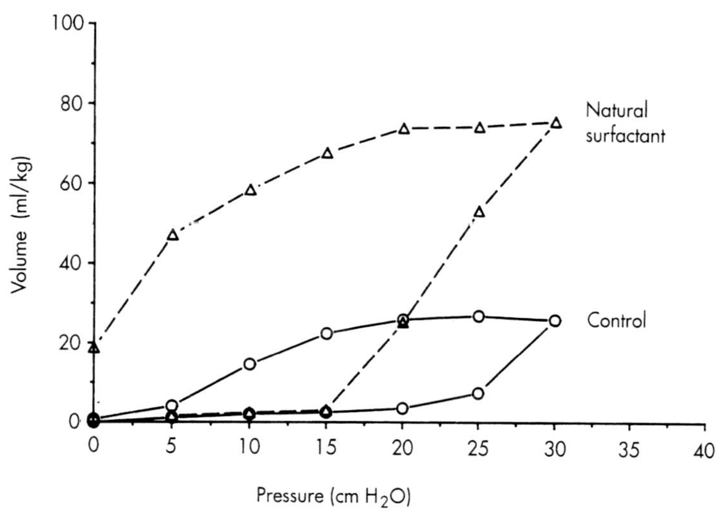

Fig. 3 Pressure-volume relationships for the inflation and deflation of surfactant-deficient and surfactant-treated preterm rabbit lungs

- The opening pressure, i.e., the pressure at which the alveoli begin to expand, is higher before being treated with surfactant.
- Lung expansion at the same peak pressure value is better after treatment with surfactant.
- Before treatment with surfactant the lung does not have stability in the expiratory phase and has a tendency to collapse and to lose FRC.

In summary, the surfactant has the following functions:

- It reduces the respiratory workload since the lung is more prone to distension.
- It increases the FRC given the lesser tendency of the lung to collapse.
- It has an anti-edema role since the increase in surface tension facilitates the attraction of liquids from the capillaries into the alveoli.
- It stabilizes the sizes of the alveoli.

A further factor that contributes to stabilizing the sizes of the alveoli is their mechanical interdependence: if an alveolus tends to collapse, the stress on the walls of the adjacent alveoli increases and this helps it remain expanded. The alveoli support each other thus contrasting any tendency towards a reduction or increase in volume of any single alveolus.

48.5 Airway Resistance

The forces that have to be overcome in order to ventilate the air inside and outside the respiratory system are not only the forces of elastic recoil of the lungs and chest but also the airway resistance.

The forces required to ensure breathing, whether the energy spent is stored and retrieved thereafter, or whether it is lost by the system in the form of heat, are defined conservative forces or dissipation forces. Conservative forces are the (volume-dependent) pressures generated by the elastic properties of the lungs and of the ribcage, forces that tend to cause these structures to return to their initial position after a deformation: the energy spent on overcoming these forces during inspiration is recovered during expiration, which is a passive phenomenon. Conversely, the dissipation forces are the (flow-dependent) energies required to overcome not only the friction of the gases against the airway walls but also the viscoelastic properties of the respiratory system determined by the molecular movements in the tissues. The dissipation forces are also defined as resistance forces: the energy required to overcome these forces is lost in the form of heat and hence can no longer be used.

In lung physiology the term airway resistance (R) is used to define the ratio between the difference in pressure between the alveoli and the mouth (ΔP) and the resulting flow ($\dot{V}$):

$$R(cmH_2O/L/s) = \Delta P(cmH_2O)/\dot{V}(L/s)$$

In the respiratory system some 30–40% of the resistance occurs at the nose, in the oropharynx and in the pharynx, while at the level of the trachea and bronchial tree the structures that resist most against the flow are the average sized bronchi and not the smaller sized airways.

The airways can indeed be schematized as a series of successive dichotomies (22 generations or bronchial branching): at each branch division the size of the segments slightly decrease in size, but since the number of elements doubles, the total cross section area increases with respect to the previous level (Fig. 4). Thanks to this architecture the resistance of the peripheral airways is very mild even if the flow runs along ducts whose size is truly very small.

The factors that determine the degree of resistance (R) of a duct include its length (l), its radius (r), and type of flow, i.e., laminar or turbulent flow

$$R = l/r^4$$

Turbulent flow, which occurs mainly at the points of branching or when the airflow is high and the radius of the duct is large, generates a larger resistance compared to laminar flow. The pressures in a laminar flow are proportional to the flow rate whereas in a turbulent flow they are proportionate to the square of the flow; in these conditions the energy needed is obviously greater. The progressive increase in total cross section area

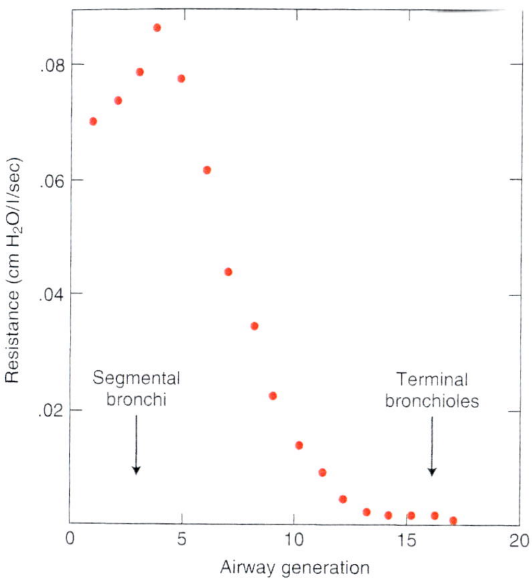

Fig. 4 Location of the main site of airway resistance. Note that the intermediate-sized bronchi contribute most of the resistance and that relatively little is located in the very small airways

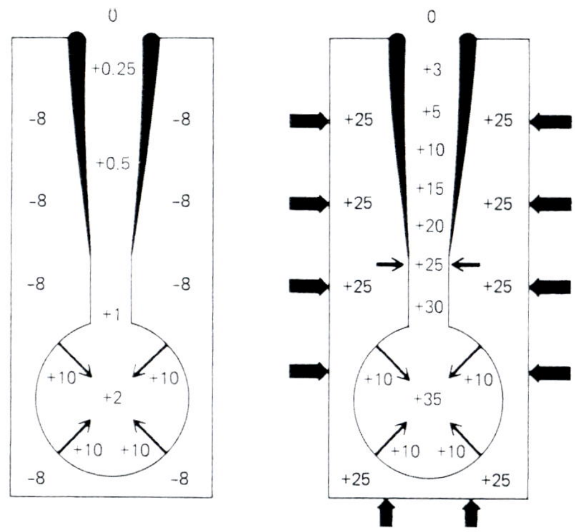

Fig. 5 Dynamic compression of airways. On the left, passive expiration: intrapleural pressure is −8 cm H_2O, pulmonary elastic recoil forces pressure is +10 cm H_2O and alveolar pressure is +2 cm H_2O. On the right, forced expiration: intrapleural pressure is +25 cm H_2O, pulmonary elastic recoil forces pressure is +10 cm H_2O and alveolar pressure is +35 cm H_2O. The arrow indicates the equal pressure point (EPP)

towards the periphery of the lung implies a progressive reduction in the linear velocity (linear velocity = airflow/cross section area) of the airflow, which is quite low and of the laminar type at the level of the smaller airways, whereas in the trachea and in the larger branches it is essentially turbulent.

Lung volume is another important factor for the resistance of the airways, above all of those with little or no cartilage structure. Indeed the small airways distend and compress very easily, and the transmural pressure gradient of the walls of the small airways is important in defining their radius: during deep inspiration the intrapleural negative pressure increases thus causing an increase in the transmural pressure gradient and hence an increase in their size. A further factor consists in increasing the elastic tension exercised by the pulmonary parenchyma on the airways during volume expansion in the inspiration phase. The resistance of the airways therefore is less during inspiration as compared to expiration; in addition, during forced expiration, as occurs in the newborn when he cries, resistance is influenced by the dynamic compression of the airways.

Making the intrapleural pressure positive determines changes in transmural pressure whose effects are clearly seen in Fig. 5, which represents the pressure values that come into play during normal expiration and forced expiration. During forced expiration the pressure inside the peripheral airways is greater than the intrapleural pressure thanks to the pulmonary elastic recoil forces; in the larger airways by contrast, the pressure comes progressively closer to atmospheric pressure and is hence lower than intrapleural pressure. The point at which the pressure inside and outside the airways is equal is defined as equal pressure point (EPP), situated in normal individuals in the central airways within the first five branchings of the bronchial tree. Downstream from this point the airways are compressed and the compression increases with greater expiration effort, which will thus not be capable of increasing the flow velocity (dynamic flow limitation).

The expiratory flow also decreases with the progressive reduction of the pulmonary volume for the attenuation of the elastic recoil forces and for the smaller size of the airways; as expiration

proceeds, the EPP moves distally towards the inside of the lung. The flow-limiting mechanism is enhanced in some pathologic conditions characterized by an increase in peripheral resistance because the pressure drop is amplified inside the airways, or in others marked by a pressure reduction of the elastic component as occurs in emphysema.

48.6 Alveolar Ventilation

The amount of fresh air ventilated into the airways in one minute, or minute volume $\dot{V}_E$ ($\dot{V}$ = volume/time unit; the minute volume is measured with the amount of expired gas and it is indicated with $\dot{V}_E$), corresponds to the V_T times the respiratory rate (RR):

$$\dot{V}_E = V_T \times RR$$

The V_T, that is to say the inspiration and expiration volume for each normal breathing cycle, measures about 6–8 mL/kg in the newborn and 4–6 mL/kg in a preterm infant; about 30% of this volume remains inside the airways without taking part in the exchange of gases with the blood (anatomic dead space) and is called the dead space volume ($\dot{V}_D$). Alveolar ventilation ($\dot{V}_A$) is the volume of fresh air that enters the respiratory zone every minute and is actually available for the exchange of gases; the $\dot{V}_A$ corresponds to:

$$\dot{V}_A = \dot{V}_E - \dot{V}_D$$

A reduction in the expansion of the lung, typical of RDS, causes a drop in V_T and hence in alveolar ventilation since the dead space remains unchanged; this compels the newborn to increase respiratory rate to keep the minute volume constant. In physiological conditions the amount of air that remains inside the lung at the end of normal expiration, or FRC, is around 20–30 mL/kg; therefore, for each breathing cycle, only a part of the air in the alveoli (around 1/5–1/6) will be replaced with new air from the atmosphere. This slow renewal of air means that the variation in gas concentration in the alveoli is only 3–4 mmHg for each breathing cycle; relative constancy in gas concentration in arterial blood therefore depends on the buffer action of the FRC.

Let us now analyze the partial gas pressures in an ideal lung, considering that barometric pressure is around 760 mmHg: 20.9% of it is generated by O_2 and 79% by nitrogen; as a consequence, the PO_2 in the air is 20.9% of 760, i.e., 159 mmHg. The air inspired is saturated with aqueous vapor in amounts proportionate to body temperature; the value of the partial pressure of aqueous vapor at 37 °C is 47 mmHg, which is to be subtracted from the relative value at total pressure of unsaturated air. The PO_2 of inspired air is hence 20.9% of 760 – 47 mmHg, therefore around 149 mmHg. The alveolar PO_2 (PAO_2) is less than that of the inspired air because the alveolar air is continuously impoverished of O_2 and enriched with CO_2 and its value is around 100 mmHg. The partial pressure values of O_2 and CO_2 at the alveoli are determined by the balance between alveolar ventilation, consumption of O_2, and production of CO_2.

Alveolar ventilation is regulated by the respiratory centers in such a way as to maintain the value of the arterial PCO_2 ($PaCO_2$) around 40 mmHg and the value of the arterial PO_2 (PaO_2) around 100 mmHg (Von Euler 1997). The value of arterial PCO_2, which is normally identical to the alveolar PCO_2 ($PACO_2$), is inversely proportionate to the degree of ventilation and is hence used as an index of alveolar ventilation; if alveolar ventilation is halved, the $PaCO_2$ doubles, if alveolar ventilation doubles, the $PaCO_2$ is halved (Fig. 6). Also the PaO_2 variations are proportionate to the degree of ventilation and inversely proportionate to the $PaCO_2$, in that the total sum of the partial pressures of the gases at the alveoli is always 760 mmHg. Actually, the partial pressure of aqueous vapor does not vary, and during ventilation the partial pressure of nitrogen varies slightly. However, the PaO_2 is not used as an index of ventilation because, unlike the $PaCO_2$, its value varies also as a function of the presence of an intra- or extrapulmonary shunt (Riley and Coumand 1951).

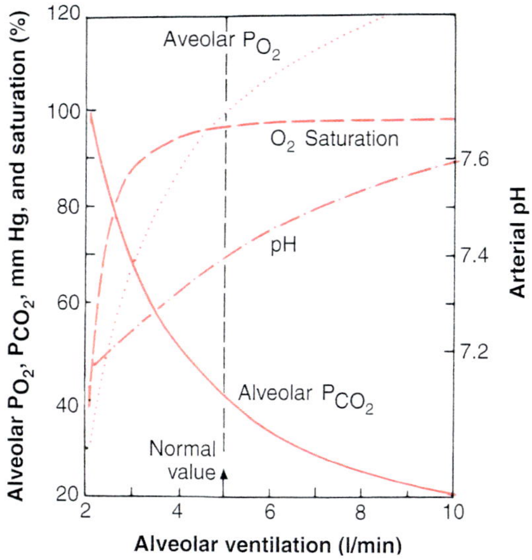

Fig. 6 Variations in analysis of blood gases related to alveolar ventilation

The amount of work that respiratory muscles must do to maintain an optimal level of $PaCO_2$ depends on the type of ventilation. Each individual, depending on the elastic and resistance characteristics of his respiratory system, has an optimal theoretical rate where a reduction in compliance implies that it increases, whereas it is reduced when resistance increases. In clinical practice most patients with a pulmonary disorder use a ventilation mode that requires less respiratory work, and respiratory rate is often close to the optimal hypothetical one. Theoretically it is therefore possible to classify pulmonary diseases as restrictive or obstructive diseases on the basis of high or reduced respiratory rate measurements, but the respiratory centers are regulated also by cortical influences and by mechanical or irritation stimuli coming from the respiratory system that may gain the upper hand over the energy advantage.

48.7 Diffusion

The next step after the cyclical renewal of alveolar air is the diffusion of O_2 from the alveoli to the blood, and of the CO_2 in the opposite direction (Scheid and Piper 1997). O_2 and CO_2 move from high partial pressure areas to others where the partial pressure is low as a result of a process of passive physical diffusion. The diffusion of the gases across the alveolar wall is described by Fick's Law:

$$\dot{V}gas = A \times K \times (P_1 - P_2)/S$$

This law states that the volume of gas that diffuses per unit of time ($\dot{V}gas$) is proportional to the surface area (A), to a diffusion constant (K) and to the partial pressure difference ($P_1 - P_2$), and it is inversely proportional to the thickness of the alveolar wall (S). The diffusion constant K is, in turn, proportional to the solubility of the gas and inversely proportional to the square root of its molecular weight. The CO_2 has a molecular weight that is not very different from that of the O_2, but it has higher solubility, and so it diffuses about 20 times more rapidly than the O_2 through the blood-gas barrier.

At the blood-gas barrier the flow pressure for the O_2 is around 60 mmHg (100 mmHg alveolar PO_2; 40 mmHg PO_2 capillary venous blood); the O_2 crosses the membrane rapidly, and the PO_2 increases just as rapidly in the blood. It must be pointed out that the blood PO_2 reaches the values corresponding to the alveolar air just before the red cells have completed half of their journey inside the lung capillaries, whose overall duration is around 0.75 s; therefore there are huge possibilities for compensation.

Moreover, thanks to the special form of the Hb dissociation curve, a high partial pressure difference persists between alveolar gas and blood also when the Hb is near total saturation. For instance, Hb is saturated at 94% with a PO_2 of 70 mmHg, when there is still a 30 mmHg gradient.

The time it takes the capillary CO_2 to equilibrate against the alveolar CO_2 is more or less the same as the time taken by the O_2 in spite of the fact that the diffusion velocity of the CO_2 is 20 times higher than that of the O_2. In this case, however, we must consider that the partial pressure gradient between capillaries and alveoli is only 5 mmHg.

48.8 Pulmonary Circulation and Ventilation/Perfusion Ratio

The fetal pulmonary arterial muscle thickness increases during the last quarter of pregnancy blocking the perfusion of the lung circulation, which is rapidly developing. Of these two phenomena, the latter is most prevalent and results in a gradual reduction in pulmonary vascular resistances. The degree of development of pulmonary circulation affects the clinical presentation of neonatal cardiorespiratory diseases where the alterations in the ventilation/perfusion ratio are determined by the capacity, or lack thereof, to increase lung vascular resistances following stimuli such as hypoxia and acidosis, with hemodynamic patterns ranging from extrapulmonary shunt to pulmonary overflow.

Let us look at the ventilation/perfusion ratio ($\dot{V}_A/\dot{Q}$) of a term newborn in physiological conditions: their cardiac index (cardiac output referred to body surface) is approximately 3.5 L/min/m^2; since body surface is around 0.25 m^2, the value of the output is 0.8–0.9 L/min. Considering a respiratory rate of around 45 breaths/min, alveolar ventilation is about 700–800 mL/min; the result is a $\dot{V}_A/\dot{Q}$ ratio of 0.8–1 as in the adult. This means that each air volume that arrives at the alveolar surface exchanges with an equal amount of capillary perfusion blood. These values are indicative, but they do give an idea of the order of magnitude of these values.

48.9 Transfer of O_2 and CO_2

In physiological conditions, O_2 is transferred to the tissues almost entirely in combination with the Hb of the red cells; only 3% is dissolved in the aqueous phase of the plasma. It must be noted that 1 g of Hb may bind to a maximum of 1.34 mL of O_2 and, since the normal concentration of Hb is about 15 g/100 mL, it may bind 20 mL of O_2 or, to use the generally accepted expression, 20 volumes of O_2 (Baumann 1987).

The amount of O_2 that binds to Hb in the erythrocytes is directly proportional to the PO_2 in the plasma and is plotted graphically as a dissociation curve of hemoglobin (Fig. 7). The italics S shape of the Hb dissociation curve is due to the functional interdependence or cooperative effect of its four hemes. As a result of this effect, while

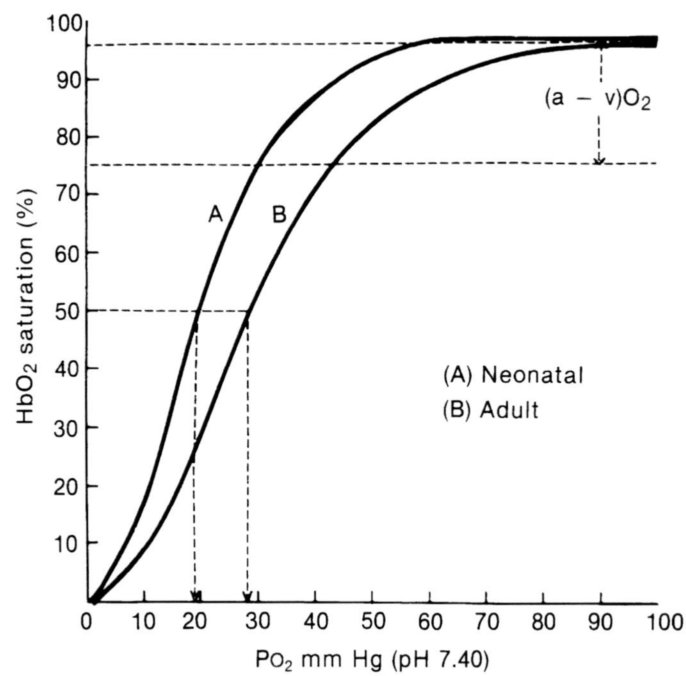

Fig. 7 Hb dissociation curve in a neonate (70% HbF) and in an adult in standard conditions (T= 37°C; pH 7.4)

the first heme combines slowly with O_2, the second, under the influence of the first that has already been assigned, will combine more rapidly, and so on. Fetal Hb has a greater affinity for O_2 compared to that of the adult; its dissociation curve is shifted to the left and has a greater saturation at the same PaO_2 (the position of the Hb curve is defined by the P_{50}, which is the PaO_2 at which the Hb is 50% saturated; the P_{50} of the HbF is 19 mmHg, that of the HbA 26 mmHg). The shift to the right of the curve, denoting a reduced affinity of the Hb for O_2, is caused by a reduction in pH; this facilitates the transfer of O_2 to the tissues (Bohr effect).

The share of Hb bounded to O_2 is expressed as percentage saturation ($SaO_2\%$); this is equal to the O_2 content in the blood (Cont. O_2) divided by the O_2 transport capacity of the Hb (Cap. O_2), times 100:

$$SaO_2\% = \text{Cont. } O_2/\text{Cap. } O_2 \times 100$$

It must be pointed out that hemoglobin saturation expresses only a percentage and not an amount or volume of O_2. The special form of the Hb dissociation curve in its upper part means that saturation decreases only slightly with considerable drops in PO_2; for the same reason, considerable increases in alveolar PO_2 do not cause a significant increase in O_2 content since maximum O_2 saturation cannot exceed 100%. The steepness of the lower part of the curve shows that the peripheral tissues receive large amounts of O_2 with small decreases in capillary PO_2. In venous blood, PO_2 is around 40 mmHg, which corresponds to a 75% saturation; this means that during tissue perfusion only 25% of the total content is used, in practice about 5 mL for every 100 mL of blood (Fig. 7).

The transport of CO_2 in the blood is not as complex as the transport of O_2 (Klocke 1997). CO_2 is found in the blood as a free gas in solution (up to 10% since it is 20 times more soluble than O_2 in the plasma) or in a chemical combination with hemoglobin and plasma protein in the form of carbamino compounds (5–10%) and above all as bicarbonate ions (70–90%). The bicarbonate is formed in the blood by the following reaction:

$$CO_2 + H_2O \rightarrow H_2CO_3 \rightarrow H^+ + HCO^-{}_3$$

CO_2 combines with water to form carbonic acid, which dissociates into hydrogen ions and bicarbonate ions; carbonic anhydrase, present in high concentrations in red cells, makes the reaction faster. Some of the released H+ ions bind to the hemoglobin according to the following reaction:

$$H^+ + HbO_2 \rightarrow H^+Hb + O_2$$

The reduced form of Hb is less acidic than the oxygenated form and it more rapidly accepts the hydrogen ions released by the dissociation reaction of carbonic acid, thus allowing a greater amount of carbon dioxide to be transported by venous blood in the form of bicarbonate ions (Haldane effect). This facilitates the uptake of CO_2 at tissue level and the inverse reaction facilitates its release into the lung capillaries where carbonic acid is converted into gas and removed from alveolar ventilation.

The acid–base status of the blood (pH) results from the ratio between bicarbonate concentration and the CO_2 in solution, and as long as this ratio is 20, the pH is stable at 7.4 (Jones 1997). (Normal arterial blood HCO_3^- concentration is 24 mmol/L, and at 37 °C about 0.03 CO_2 mmol is dissolved for every PCO_2 mmHg in 1 L of plasma; consequently the amount of CO_2 in the blood is equal to $0.03 \times PCO_2$. So in normal condition the $HCO^-{}_3/CO_2$ ratio is $24/0.03 \times 40 = 20$.)

The blood concentration of bicarbonate is determined mainly by the kidneys and the PCO_2 by the lungs. An increase in the latter reduces the pH (respiratory acidosis) and the kidneys respond by eliminating a more acid urine, secreting H^+ ions in the tubules as $H_2PO^-{}_4$ or $NH^+{}_4$, while the $HCO^-{}_3$ ions are reabsorbed. Kidney compensation, however, is hardly ever accomplished. By contrast, a reduction in PCO_2 determines an increase in pH (respiratory alkalosis), and kidney compensation occurs by eliminating a larger amount of bicarbonate. In the case of acidosis or metabolic alkalosis, respiratory compensation mechanisms step in, i.e., hyperventilation or hypoventilation, so as to maintain the $HCO^-{}_3/CO_2$ ratio, and hence the pH, within physiological limits.

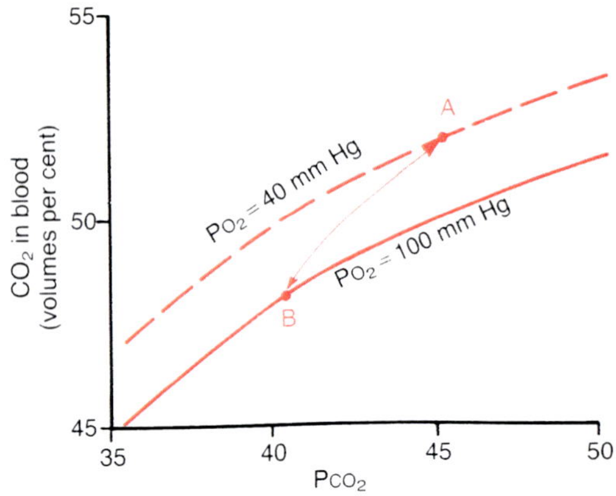

Fig. 8 Portions of carbon dioxide dissociation curves when PO_2 is 100 mmHg and 40 mmHg, respectively. Arrows represent the Haldane effect on the transport of carbon dioxide

The dissociation curve of carbon dioxide shows the relationship between PCO_2 and the total content CO_2 in the blood (Fig. 8): at physiological levels of PCO_2 the carbon dioxide content is around 50 mL or volumes per 100 mL, with an oscillation of only 4 volumes per 100 between arterial blood and venous blood (48–52 mL). In practice every 100 mL of blood that go through the lungs release 4 mL of CO_2.

In the normal range of the PCO_2 values the curve approximates a straight line without steep or flat portions; this means that an increase or slowdown in ventilation determines a proportional decrease or increase in arterial CO_2. Furthermore, the lower the PO_2, the greater the CO_2 content for a given PCO_2 (Haldane effect).

The dissociation curve of CO_2 is steeper than that of the O_2; in other words, there is greater variation in gas content for partial pressure variations. Knowing the difference between the dissociation curves of the Hb and CO_2 is essential to understand the pathophysiology of major ventilation alterations. We have seen how 100 mL of blood transport 5 mL of O_2 from the lungs to the tissues, whereas the same amount of blood transports some 4 mL of CO_2 from the tissues to the lungs. At resting conditions, therefore, for every 100 volumes of O_2 assumed by the lungs only 80 volumes of CO_2 are eliminated, where the ratio between eliminated CO_2 and O_2 uptake is defined as respiratory quotient (RQ) and is expressed by the following formula:

$$RQ = CO_2 \text{ eliminated}/O_2 \text{ uptake} = 0.8$$

48.10 Causes of Hypoxia

48.10.1 Hypoventilation

We have seen that the alveolar PO_2 and hence the arterial PO_2 is determined by the equilibrium between the speed of CO_2 removal and O_2 supply by alveolar ventilation. If the ventilation is reduced, the alveolar PO_2 drops and for the same reason the $PaCO_2$ rises, and it is the increase in $PaCO_2$ that represents a very important criterion for the diagnosis of hypoventilation because, unlike hypoxia, this is virtually the sole cause for hypercapnia. Hypoventilation is therefore characterized by an inadequate removal of CO_2 compared to its production and the relationship can be written as follows:

$$PaCO_2 = \dot{V}_{CO2}/\dot{V}_A$$

where $\dot{V}_{CO2}$ is the production of CO_2 and $\dot{V}_A$ is alveolar ventilation ($\dot{V}_E - \dot{V}_D$).

The gradual reduction in ventilation progressively brings the alveolar gas values closer to the venous blood values. Arterial PO_2 can be easily corrected by increasing the FiO_2, since the larger amount of O_2 that reaches the alveoli through each breath may offset the reduction in ventilation. Conversely, hypercapnia can be corrected only by increasing respiration frequency and/or the V_T and may require a certain amount of time because the CO_2 is stored in large amounts in the form of bicarbonates.

The causes that determine hypoventilation are mostly non-pulmonary; among the most frequent causes in newborn we may mention:

- Apnea spells in premature infants
- Depression of the CNS due to anesthetics or drugs
- Diseases of the CNS

- Diseases affecting the respiratory muscles (paralysis of the diaphragm, weak respiratory muscles in preterm infants, etc.)
- Obstruction of the upper airways (choanal atresia, Pierre-Robin syndrome, laryngomalacia, etc.)
- Obstruction or malpositioning of the tracheal tube

Hypoventilation may also be a symptom of functional exhaustion, and it may complicate pulmonary diseases when a considerable increase in work of breathing is required.

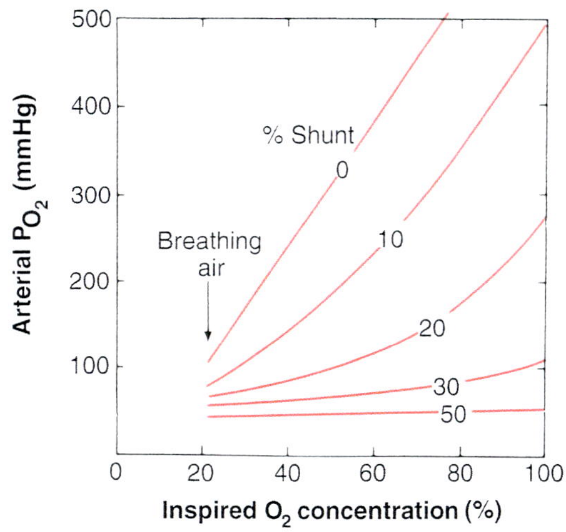

Fig. 9 Arterial PO_2 variation with different inhaled O_2 concentrations and different shunt percentage

48.10.2 Abnormal Diffusion

Normal lungs present extensive compensation possibilities to ensure O_2 diffusion. It was pointed out earlier that blood and alveolar PO_2 and PCO_2 are already in equilibrium even before the blood completes half of its journey along the pulmonary capillaries. It is, however, possible that in some pathological conditions, like pulmonary edema or interstitial fibrosis, diffusion may be slowed down to such a rate as to make the equilibrium between PO_2 of the alveolar gas and that of the capillary blood incomplete. It is not clear, as yet, what the role of diffusion is in determining hypoxia in these disorders, but it is likely that most of the pathogenic mechanism is due to alterations in the ventilation/perfusion ratio. However, hypoxia, secondary to a diffusion defect, may be rapidly redressed by administering O_2; the increase in alveolar PO_2 helps overcome the resistance to diffusion caused by changes in the membrane.

Alterations in diffusion never involve CO_2 given the rapidity with which it diffuses; in such conditions, the $PaCO_2$ is often slightly decreased because of the hyperventilation caused by hypoxia.

48.10.3 Extrapulmonary Shunt

The term extrapulmonary shunt refers to the passage of blood from the right sections to the left sections of the heart without crossing the ventilated pulmonary areas. The arterial PO_2 drops when the desaturated blood mixes with the oxygenated blood.

Figure 9 shows the effect of the increase in FiO_2 at various levels of shunting: when the latter exceeds 30%, the O_2 is no longer capable of redressing the hypoxemia, and this characteristic makes the difference between an extrapulmonary shunt and the other causes of hypoxia. The mixing of arterial blood and shunt blood causes a considerable drop in PaO_2 because the dissociation curve of the O_2 is flat in its higher portion: it is therefore possible to show up minor shunts by measuring the arterial PO_2 during 100% O_2 inhalation (hyperoxic test). By contrast, if hypoxemia is secondary to other causes (hypoventilation, limitations to diffusion, inhomogeneities in the $\dot{V}_A/\dot{Q}$ ratio), during 100% O_2 inhalation, the PaO_2 reaches levels that are virtually comparable to those observed in normal individuals, albeit over longer time intervals. A healthy individual who inhales 100% O_2 has an ideal PaO_2 of 673 mmHg (760 mmHg − 47 mmHg H_2O − 40 mmHg CO_2 = 673 mmHg).

The $PaCO_2$ is not usually increased in the presence of an extrapulmonary shunt because the hypoxia and hypercapnia of non-oxygenated blood cause an increase in alveolar ventilation; the latter is effective in reducing the $PaCO_2$, but

totally ineffective in increasing the PaO_2. As described earlier, the reason is to be found in the shape of the two dissociation curves; the CO_2 curve is virtually straight in the physiological zone, with the result that an increase in ventilation increases the elimination of CO_2. By contrast, the shape of the Hb dissociation curve, which is flat in its upper portion, does not allow the increase in ventilation to bring about an improvement in the O_2 contained in the blood.

During neonatal age, several diseases are characterized by a right-left shunt through fetal channels for the increase of pulmonary resistances; in this case oxygen therapy is a critical element in solving pulmonary vasoconstriction and in reducing the shunt.

48.10.4 Alterations in the Ventilation/Perfusion Ratio

Alterations in the ventilation-perfusion ratio ($\dot{V}_A/\dot{Q}$) are undoubtedly responsible for most of the defects in the exchange of O_2 in pulmonary diseases and rarely for CO_2 defects (West and Wagner 1997). The reason hypercapnia rarely occurs with alterations of the $\dot{V}_A/\dot{Q}$ ratio is because of the high degree of efficiency of the chemoreceptors that keeps the arterial CO_2 constant by increasing ventilation. As shown earlier, the linear shape of the CO_2 dissociation curve ensures this compensation.

Also in the healthy lung there are regional variations in the $\dot{V}_A/\dot{Q}$ ratio, but the overall effect on the total gas exchange is negligible. The distribution of ventilation in particular is regulated by tissue compliance and by the resistance of the airways; differences in these factors in the pulmonary district cause a nonuniform distribution of ventilation.

Let us now look at the consequences of the two extreme variations of the $\dot{V}_A/\dot{Q}$ ratio, bearing in mind that in practice intermediate degrees of these alterations coexist:

- $\dot{V}_A/\dot{Q} = 0$. In practice the alveoli are not ventilated but perfused (shunt effect). In this case there is no gas exchange between blood and air, but an equilibrium sets in between venous blood and the air in the nonventilated alveoli; inside the latter the partial pressures will be the same as those of venous blood (Fig. 10b). In this way an intrapulmonary shunt is caused because the blood that perfuses the nonventilated zones is not oxygenated, nor is the CO_2 removed; the consequences are identical to those caused by an extrapulmonary shunt.

  In this case an efficient compensation mechanism intervenes, hypoxic vasoconstriction, which involves the capillaries that perfuse the areas where ventilation is reduced or totally absent; the local blood flow is diverted to the ventilated alveoli, and the deleterious effects on the exchange of gases is considerably reduced. It is interesting to point out that when this occlusion of the airways persists, the alveoli end up collapsing because of the diffusion of gas in the blood, and the formation of atelectasis due to reabsorption is more rapid if the patient breathes O_2 at high concentrations. Indeed, nitrogen has a low degree of solubility, and its presence provides support for the alveoli and delays their collapse in the case of obstruction of the airways. Oxygen dependence, which is typical of children with bronchopulmonary dysplasia (BPD), is almost certainly due to the presence of multiple shunts having a low $\dot{V}_A/\dot{Q}$ ratio.
- $\dot{V}_A/\dot{Q}$ = infinite. In practice the alveoli are ventilated but not perfused (dead space effect). Also in these conditions there is no blood-air exchange; and indeed, instead of having partial pressures similar to those of venous blood, the air in the alveoli has the same partial pressures as atmospheric air. In other words, O_2 is not transferred to the blood and CO_2 is not removed. This quota of ventilation remains unused (physiological dead space) and increases the respiratory dead space thus causing a reduction in alveolar ventilation (Fig. 10c). It is not possible to describe the gas composition of the blood coming from these units because perfusion is totally absent, but clearly the PO_2 and the PCO_2 of the blood

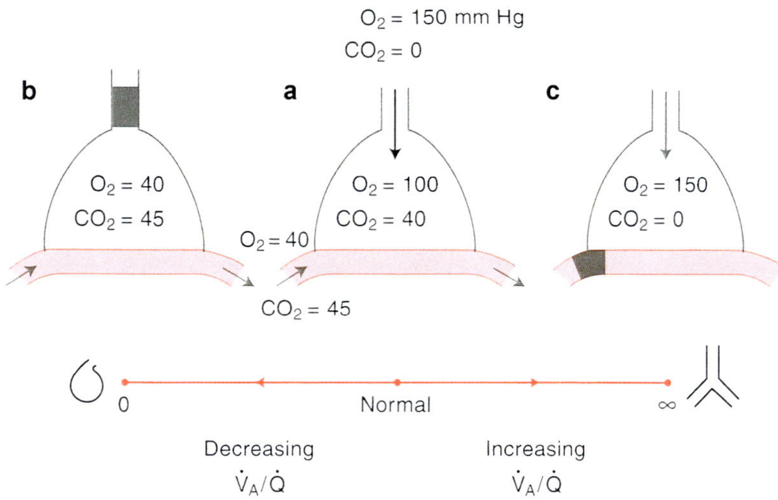

Fig. 10 Effects of altering the ventilation-perfusion ratio on the PO_2 and PCO_2 in a lung unit

will always be closer to those of inspired air as the perfusion is progressively reduced. The units with a high $\dot{V}_A/\dot{Q}$ ratio add little O_2 to the blood compared to the decrease caused by the alveoli with a low $\dot{V}_A/\dot{Q}$ ratio, and the reason is always to be sought in the shape of the Hb dissociation curve.

48.10.5 Hypoxia Due to Anemia and Hypoperfusion

It is worth remembering that to ensure an adequate O_2 supply to the tissues, a normal Hb concentration is required and also the cardiac output must be adequate. The efficacy of the latter may be determined indirectly by assessing skin color and skin temperature, peripheral pulses, gas-analysis values, diuresis and directly by means of color-Doppler echocardiography. And finally, it must be pointed out that a reduction in Hb causes a decrease in the O_2 content without any variation in the PaO_2; an anemic patient may therefore have a good PaO_2 but a low O_2 content.

48.11 Conclusions

After having schematically described the pathophysiology of the possible causes of hypoxia, it is worthwhile underlining that in practice these mechanisms often coexist and contribute to determining respiratory failure.

The most typical example in neonatology is RDS, where the lack of surfactant and an alteration in pulmonary compliance cause the formation of atelectasis and the uneven distribution of ventilation; as a consequence the $\dot{V}_A/\dot{Q}$ ratio is altered. The edema and the presence of exudates at the alveoli may have a negative impact also on the diffusion of O_2. The resulting hypoxia, combined with acidosis, further worsens the ratio due to the increase in vascular resistance with the formation of shunts in the fetal channels and hypoperfusion of the pulmonary circulation. Finally, owing to the considerable increase in respiratory work, the patient may present with hypoventilation symptoms after an initial phase characterized by tachypnea.

References

Baumann R (1987) Blood oxygen transport. In: Farhi L, Tenney SM (eds) Handbook of physiology. The respiratoty system. American Physiology Society, Bethesda, pp 147–172

Cumming G, Crank J, Horsfield K et al (1966) Gaseous diffusion in the airways of the human lung. Respir Physiol 1:58–74

De Troyer A (1997) The respiratory muscles. In: Crystal RG, West JB, Bames PJ, Weibel ER (eds) The lung: scientific foundations, 2nd edn. Lippincott-Raven Press, New York, pp 1203–1215

Goerke J, Schurch S (1997) Mechanical properties of the alveolar surface. In: Crystal RG, West JB, Bames PJ, Weibel ER (eds) The lung: scientific foundations, 2nd edn. Lippincott-Raven Press, New York, pp 1169–1176

Guyton AC (1987) Trattato di fisiologia medica. Piccin, Padova, p 572

Jones NL (1997) Acid–base physiology. In: Crystal RG, West JB, Bames PJ, Weibel ER (eds) The lung: scientific foundations, 2nd edn. Lippincott-Raven Press, New York, pp 1657–1671

Keens TG, Bryan AC, Levison H et al (1978) Developmental pattern of muscle fiber types in human ventilatory muscles. J Appl Pysiol 44:909–913

Klocke RA (1997) Carbon dioxide transport. In: Crystal RG, West JB, Bames PJ, Weibel ER (eds) The lung: scientific foundations, 2nd edn. Lippincott-Raven Press, New York, pp 1633–1642

Rider ED, Jobe AH, Ikegami M, Sun B (1992) Different ventilation strategies alter surfactant responses in preterm rabbits. J Appl Physiol 73:2089–2096

Riley RL, Coumand A (1951) Analysis of factors affecting partial pressures of oxygen and carbon dioxide in gas and blood of lungs: theory. J Appl Physiol 4:77–101

Scheid P, Piper J (1997) Diffusion. In: Crystal RG, West JB, Bames PJ, Weibel ER (eds) The lung: scientific foundations, 2nd edn. Lippincott-Raven Press, New York, pp 1592–1618

Von Euler C (1997) Neural organization and rhythm generation. In: Crystal RG, West JB, Bames PJ, Weibel ER (eds) The lung: scientific foundations, 2nd edn. Lippincott-Raven Press, New York, pp 1711–1724

West JB (1985) Ventilation/blood flow and gas exchange, 4th edn. Blackwell, Oxford

West JB (2008a) Respiratory physiology: the essentials, 8th edn. Wolters Kluwer/Lippincott Williams & Wilkins, Baltimore

West JB (2008b) Pulmonary pathophysiology. The essentials, 7th edn. Wolters Kluwer/Lippincott Williams & Wilkins, Baltimore

West JB, Wagner PD (1997) Ventilation-perfusion relationships. In: Crystal RG, West JB, Bames PJ, Weibel ER (eds) The lung: scientific foundations, 2nd edn. Lippincott-Raven Press, New York, pp 1289–1305

Control of Breathing in Newborns

49

Ruben E. Alvaro and Henrique Rigatto

Contents

Abstract

Prematurity profoundly affects breathing, making it highly irregular, with frequent pauses or apneas. This respiratory instability is secondary to the immature development of the respiratory network as well as the underdevelopment of the lungs and the resultant lung injury that occurs in this population. The increased activity of the peripheral chemoreceptors and the closeness of eupneic and threshold PCO_2 confer a great vulnerability to respiratory stability in these infants. Maintaining adequate ventilation and oxygenation during this type of breathing pattern represents a unique clinical challenge.

In this chapter, we review some of the concepts and the progress made in the area of control of breathing in the newborn. We also highlight major developments and critically analyze the scientific foundations of our knowledge in this area.

49.1 Salient Points

- In very small preterm infants, significant bradycardia and desaturation can occur with very short apneic pauses. This is likely related to their inadequate end expiratory lung volumes due to unstable chest wall secondary to the excessive chest wall compliance and to the

R. E. Alvaro (✉) · H. Rigatto
Department of Pediatrics, WR004 Women's Hospital, University of Manitoba, Winnipeg, MB, Canada
e-mail: ralvaro@exchange.hsc.mb.ca

G. Buonocore et al. (eds.), *Neonatology*,
https://doi.org/10.1007/978-3-319-29489-6_198

tonic inhibition of chest wall muscles during REM sleep.

- Most short apneas in preterm infants are central, whereas long apneas are mixed. Purely obstructive apneas are rare. Obstructive apneas are more commonly seen as part of a mixed apneic event.
- Respiratory efforts against a closed airway seem to prolong apnea and aggravate the oxygen desaturation and the decrease in heart rate that are usually associated with apneas.
- The basic reason for the respiratory instability observed in preterm infants appears to be the major contribution of the peripheral chemoreceptor drive to normal breathing and the closeness of eupneic and threshold $PACO_2$.
- Periodic breathing and apnea are more frequent in REM sleep than in quiet sleep. This is due to decreases in diaphragmatic activity, the tone of the intercostal muscles, and the tone of the adductor muscles of the upper airway producing chest distortion, impairment of the braking mechanism during expiration, pulmonary collapse, and apnea during REM sleep.
- In extremely preterm infants, periodic breathing can be associated with episodes of intermittent hypoxia. Pre- and postnatal infection together with the inflammation induced by mechanical ventilation and oxygen toxicity could alter the structure and function of the peripheral and central respiratory control system leading to chronic episodes of intermittent hypoxia.

49.2 Introduction

There are at least three important considerations regarding the study of the control of breathing during the neonatal period. First, the neonates are noncooperative subjects. This means that we must study their respiratory control without their being aware and try to compare the measurements with those of the adult under similar conditions. This is difficult to do. Second, measurements in the neonate are usually made, by necessity, in the decubitus position, whereas those in the adult subject are usually made in the sitting or standing position (Davi et al. 1979; Kalapesi et al. 1981). Third, babies are usually studied with a nosepiece because they are nose breathers; adults are usually studied using a mouthpiece. These methodological differences have made comparison of breathing in newborn with that in adult subjects difficult to interpret. There is currently a major need for studies to be done using similar methodology. Unless there is some consistency in the methodology, it is hard to define what is actually distinct or unique about the control of breathing in the neonate. In recent years, we have experienced tremendous advances in the field of respiratory control, and we are now witnessing the initial discovery of several of the genes that control the development and maturation of multiple neurally controlled respiratory functions.

In this chapter, we review some of the concepts and the progress made in the area of control of breathing in the newborn. We also highlight major developments and critically analyze the scientific foundations of our knowledge in this area.

49.3 Breathing Pattern at Rest

The neonate, and particularly the premature infant, breathes irregularly. There is significant breath-to-breath variability and long stretches of periodic breathing in which breathing and apnea alternate (Kalapesi et al. 1981; Cross and Oppé 1952; Waggener et al. 1984). Haldane's statement that "the surprising fact is not that we breathe regularly, but that we do not breathe periodically most of the time" applies more at this age than at any other (Douglas and Haldane 1908-1909). The resting breathing pattern of the neonate is not sleep state dependent, although sleep greatly modulates it (Rigatto et al. 1982a; Gabriel et al. 1976). Sleep has traditionally been divided into quiet, REM, transitional, and indeterminate states. Twenty-nine percent (29%) of sleep time in neonates is spent in quiet sleep, 33% in REM, 7% in transitional sleep, and 31% in indeterminate sleep. The proportion of quiet sleep increases with age, while the amount of REM decreases with age. The proportion of wakefulness decreases with decreasing gestational age, and in very immature infants, it

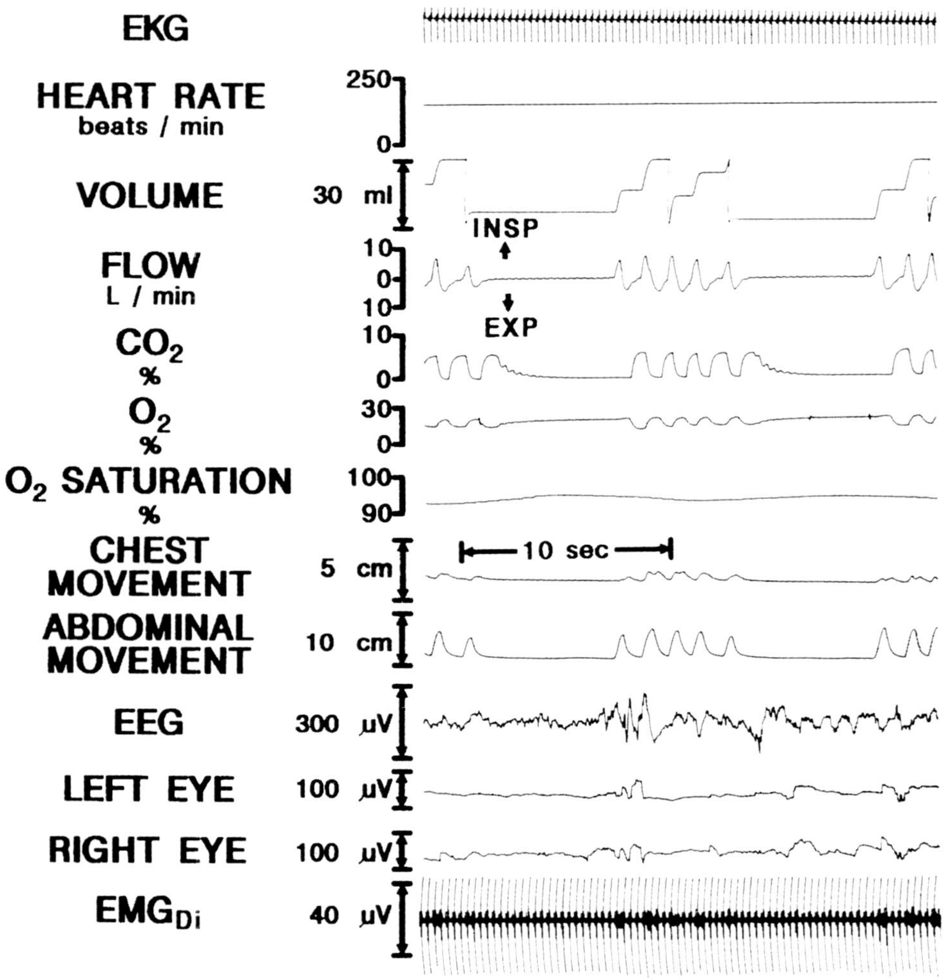

Fig. 1 Periodic breathing during quiet sleep in an 8-day-old preterm infant born at 32 weeks. Note the regular periodicity of breathing, with both apneic and breathing intervals keeping a constant length. Note also the classic trace alternant pattern on the electroencephalogram (*EEG*)

becomes difficult to define wakefulness or arousal (Curzi-Dascalova and Challamel 2000; Lehtonen and Martin 2004). We have shown that periodic breathing, a common breathing pattern in premature infants in which they alternate between breathing intervals and apneas lasting 5–10 s, occurs in the three states, wakefulness, REM, and quiet, but its prevalence is increased in REM sleep (Rigatto et al. 1982a). It is frequently stated in textbooks that in quiet sleep, in analogy with criteria used for adult subjects, breathing is regular. Prechtl and we, however, have clearly shown that periodic breathing is common in quiet sleep (Kalapesi et al. 1981; Moriette et al. 1985; Prechtl 1974). The difference is that periodic breathing in quiet sleep is regular – that is, the breathing and apneic intervals are of similar duration – and very irregular in REM sleep. The most well-defined periodic breathing observable in small babies is in quiet sleep during trace alternant (Fig. 1). Therefore, there are two major differences between neonates and adults regarding staging of sleep state. One difference relates to the patterns of breathing observed in quiet and REM sleep states and the other to the presence of the trace alternant electroencephalogram (EEG) during quiet sleep in the neonate. As this pattern subsides after 44 weeks' postconceptional age, it is not used in adults to

characterize quiet sleep. The overall minute ventilation is increased in REM sleep as compared with quiet sleep, and this is due to a primary increase in respiratory frequency with little change in tidal volume (Davi et al. 1979; Kalapesi et al. 1981; Rigatto et al. 1982a; Gaultier 1987). Increasing respiratory rate instead of tidal volume is more energy efficient to cope with higher ventilator needs (Mortola 1983). There is a well-known inverse relationship between resting respiratory rate and body size with smaller and younger infants having higher respiratory rates per unit body weight than larger, older infants (Gagliardi and Rusconi 1997). Tidal volume remains essentially unchanged from birth to adulthood (about 6 ml/kg). Minute ventilation, as expected, decreases with age as respiratory frequency and metabolic demands decrease (Polgar and Weng 1979).

49.4 Periodic Breathing and Apnea

Periodic breathing, defined as pauses in respiratory movements that last for up to 20 s alternating with breathing, is common in preterm infants. When the respiratory pause is longer than 20 s, it is called apnea (Rigatto 1988). Although the duration used to distinguish periodic breathing and apnea is arbitrary, it has proved useful and has been widely adopted. Periodic breathing is not as harmful as apnea since the respiratory pause is short and the decrease in heart rate is minor. In contrast, apnea is a more serious condition, the respiratory pause being longer and frequently associated with decreases in heart rate below 80 beats/min (Rigatto 1988, 1986). In very small preterm infants, significant bradycardia and desaturation can occur with very short apneic pauses, likely related to their higher oxygen consumption per unit weight and their relatively smaller lung volumes and oxygen stores than the term infants and adult subjects. These inadequate end expiratory lung volumes are due to excessive chest wall compliance leading to distal airway closure (Poets 2010; Poets et al. 1997) and to the tonic inhibition of chest wall muscles during REM sleep leading to unstable chest wall stability (Lopes et al. 1981a). In this instance, therefore, the length of the respiratory pause is not a very useful indicator of severity of the disruption in breathing. For this reason, many centers, including ours, have decided to rely on heart rate and oxygen saturation as the primary indicators of severity.

Apneic episodes in the neonate are classified according to the absence or presence of breathing efforts during the period of no airflow (Lee et al. 1987). Central apneas are those with no flow and no observable breathing efforts. Obstructive apneas are those with no flow despite breathing efforts. Mixed apneas begin as central and end as obstructive apnea. Breath-holding apneas are those in which flow stops at mid-expiration, and the remaining expiration occurs just before breathing starts again. A new method of classifying apneas, based on a magnified cardiac-induced pulse observed on the respiratory flow tracing, has been recently described by us. This method is able to detect the presence and timing of airway obstructions with great precision. Using this method, it is obvious that some apneas, previously classified as central because of the absence of respiratory efforts, are indeed obstructive (silent obstruction) (Fig. 2; Lemke et al. 1996; Al-Sufayan et al. 2009). We have been using this method extensively in our experimental studies, but its use in routine clinical care is not yet established.

In preterm infants with underlying disease followed longitudinally over a period of 3 months, central apneas predominated and purely obstructive apneas were rare (Fig. 3; Lee et al. 1987). Obstructive apneas are more commonly noted as part of a mixed apneic event. Most short apneas are central, whereas long apneas are mixed. The mechanism of obstruction in mixed apneas is unknown, and it is not completely clear whether the obstructed respiratory efforts prolong the apnea or whether a longer initial central pause predisposes the airway to collapse at the end of the apnea. We found that airway closure, as measured by the absence of cardiac oscillations on the respiratory flow tracing, was present in about 20% of central apneas and preceded 59% of the obstructed respiratory efforts in mixed apneas. This airway closure during central apneas did not limit the severity of oxygen desaturation or

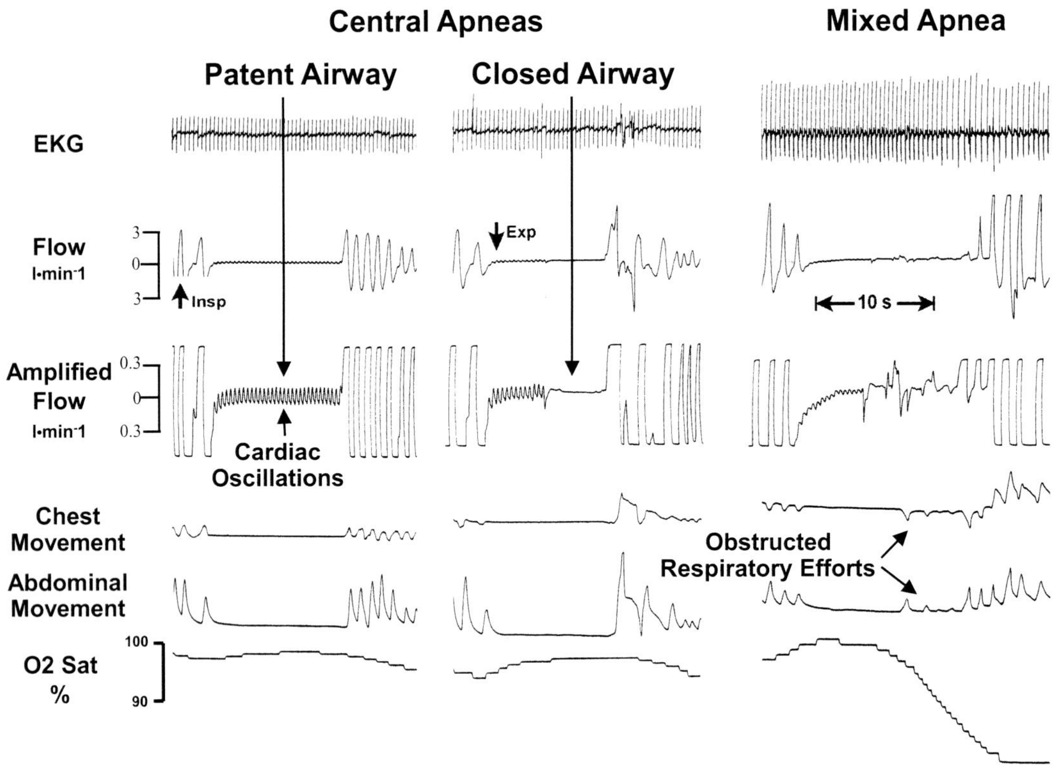

Fig. 2 Representative tracing: examples of three types of apneas diagnosed by absent (central apneas) or present obstructed respiratory efforts (mixed apnea). Central apneas are further classified using the amplified cardiac airflow oscillation into those with open airway (oscillations present) and those with closed airway (oscillations absent). Cardiac oscillations and respiratory effort signals are indicated. The flow channel shows baseline respiratory flow with minor amplification. The amplified flow represents a tenfold amplification of the flow signal by the chart recorder so that cardiac oscillation may be easily analyzed (Rigatto 1988)

the decrease in heart rate. We also found that although the length of mixed apneas was longer than central apneas, the length of the initial central component of the mixed apneas was significantly shorter than the length of central apneas, suggesting that respiratory efforts against a closed airway prolong apnea. These respiratory efforts against a closed airway also aggravated the oxygen desaturation and the decrease in heart rate that are usually associated with apneas (Al-Sufayan et al. 2009). In preterm infants recovering from respiratory support, with some degree of residual lung disease (bronchopulmonary dysplasia), the prevalence of obstructive apneas appears to be increased, comprising up to 48% of the apneas in some studies. There is no clear explanation for the obstruction, but it seems to be at the level of the larynx (Mathew et al. 1982).

Periodic breathing and apnea are clearly a consequence of a disturbance of the respiratory control system, but the precise mechanisms are unclear. Investigators in this area tend to believe that the negative feedback loop controlling respiration is affected by multiple factors related primarily to anatomic and physiologic immaturity that affect many levels of the respiratory control system including central and peripheral chemoreceptors. For example, arborization of dendrites at 30 weeks' gestation is meager, and neuroconduction and synaptic relay are impaired (Purpura 1975). Delays in traffic of neuromessages may then make the system oscillate. Unfortunately, we do not know how much immaturity is needed for a given impairment in neurophysiologic traffic. Oscillation in arterial gas tensions, changes in circulation time,

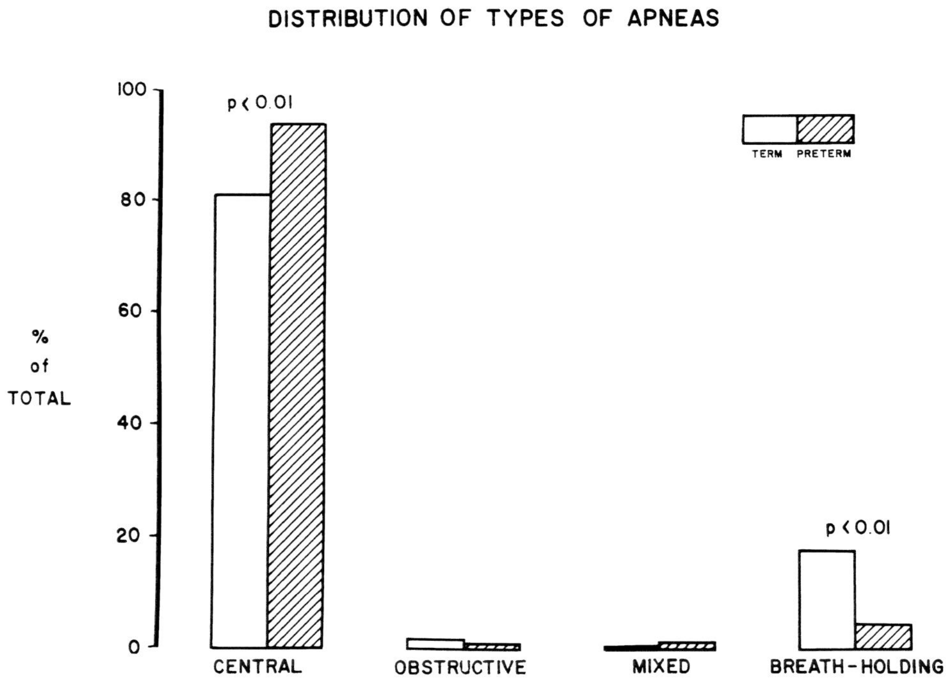

Fig. 3 Frequency distribution of the various types of apneas in healthy preterm and term infants. Central apneas are predominant. The frequency of breath-holding apneas is greater in term than in preterm infants. Obstructive and mixed types of apneas are rare (Gagliardi and Rusconi 1997)

incoordination of the respiratory pump owing to a compliant chest wall, and changes in sleep state may all contribute to this instability of the respiratory control system (Rigatto 1988). Many inhibitory neurotransmitters and neuromodulators, including adenosine, prostaglandins, endorphins, and GABA, have been also implicated in the pathogenesis of periodic breathing and apnea (Martin et al. 2004).

There has been controversy in the literature on whether periodic breathing and apnea are mechanistically different or whether long apneas are just a step further in the basic respiratory disturbance that induces the short apneas of periodic breathing. In a study carried out in our laboratory, we were able to show that (i) a prolonged apnea almost never occurred in the absence of preceding short apneas and (ii) the risk of a prolonged apnea occurring increased significantly when the preceding period contained an increased number of apneic episodes, increased duration of the longest apneic interval, or increased duration of the apneic time (Al-Saedi et al. 1997). More recently, we have shown that the periodic breathing cycles in REM but not in quiet sleep were associated with progressive decrease in minute ventilation and oxygenation likely related to the mechanical and chemoreceptor limitations known to be present in this sleep state (Ali et al. 2006). We believe that periodic breathing, especially during REM sleep, is a marker for apnea since apneas almost never occur abruptly in infants breathing regularly, but only in infants whose respiratory pattern is characterized by significant periodicity.

Compared with infants who breathe continuously, neonates breathing periodically have lower arterial PO_2 values, and their peripheral chemoreceptors are more hyperactive as reflected by the longer apneic period and more pronounced immediate decrease in ventilation in response to inhalation of high oxygen mixtures (Rigatto 1986; Rigatto and Brady 1972a; Al-Matary et al. 2004). Thus, the basic reason for background instability appears to be the major contribution of the peripheral chemoreceptor drive to normal breathing at this age. Indeed, the arterial PO_2 tension of these

infants sits on the steep portion of the minute ventilation-arterial PO_2 regression curve for human adults. This means that small changes in baseline arterial PO_2 produce large changes in baseline ventilation. Hypoxia may be a contributing factor, because inhalation of a low-oxygen mixture easily induces periodic breathing and apnea in these infants.

We found that the average CO_2 apneic threshold in preterm infants is only 1.5 Torr lower than the eupneic PCO_2, whereas in adults the average is ~3.5 Torr lower (Khan et al. 2005). The closeness of eupneic and threshold $PACO_2$ likely confers a great vulnerability to respiratory stability in these infants. It is not surprising, therefore, that brief startles, movements, or change in sleep state could allow eupneic PCO_2 to dive below the PCO_2 apneic threshold, inducing periodic breathing and apnea in these infants (Fig. 4). We believe that the key element responsible for this narrow difference is the well-known hypoxemic status of these infants. Xie et al. have recently shown in adults that the time course of the occurrence of apnea after transient hyperpnea was consistent with a peripheral chemoreceptor mechanism. In this study, hypoxia shortened the apnea latency and narrowed the eupneic-apneic $PACO_2$ threshold, while hyperoxia delayed the onset of apnea and widened the eupneic-apneic $PACO_2$ threshold (Xie et al. 2006). The same group had previously shown that the smaller difference between eupneic and apneic $PACO_2$ during hypoxia was due to a disproportionate reduction in the eupneic $PACO_2$ rather than a higher apneic threshold (Xie et al. 2001). The low arterial PO_2 in newborn infants may keep the eupneic PCO_2 relatively low, not by hyperventilation as in adult subjects but by a decrease in metabolism which parallels the decreased in arterial PO_2.

The sleep state appears also to be a contributing factor, since periodic breathing and apnea are more frequent in REM sleep than in quiet sleep. The neonate sleeps almost uninterruptedly, continuously alternating between REM sleep and quiet sleep. This pattern increases instability in the respiratory control system. Indeed, minor alterations during sleep, such as a startle or a sigh, produce apnea in these infants. The almost continuous change in baseline ventilation during sleep is what Haldane called "the hunting of the respiratory centre."

Although sleep modulates breathing, it does not cause apnea; apnea also occurs during wakefulness. The high prevalence of apnea during REM sleep may be related to muscle activity in this stage. During REM sleep, the tone of the intercostal muscles is abolished in conjunction with a decrease in diaphragmatic activity and in the tone of the adductor muscles of the upper airway – a combination of factors likely to induce chest distortion, impairment of the braking mechanism during expiration, pulmonary collapse, and

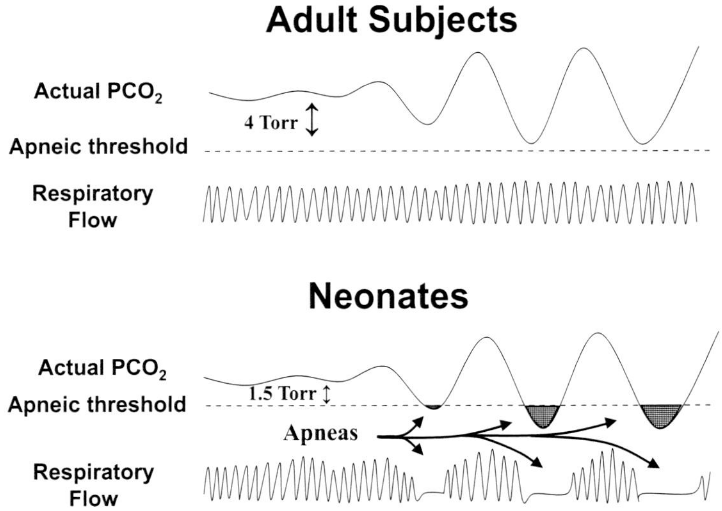

Fig. 4 Diagrammatic representation of the relationship between the CO_2 apneic threshold and the baseline or actual PCO_2 levels in neonates and adults. Because of the proximity of these two levels in neonates, PCO_2 is much more likely to dive below the apneic threshold than in the adult

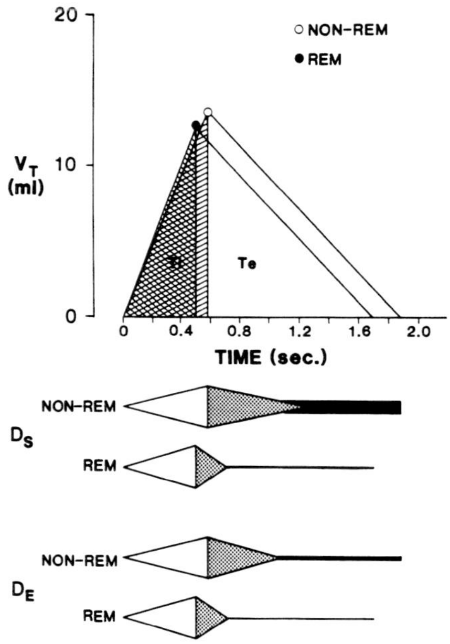

Fig. 5 Diagrammatic changes in tidal volume, timing, and diaphragmatic EMG in non-rapid eye movement (*REM*) (quiet) and REM (active) sleep. Note that total phasic activity diminishes from non-REM to REM sleep. Also, in both sleep states, it is shorter in esophageal (*DE*) than in surface EMG (*DS*). Expiratory phase activity as a proportion of total phasic activity decreases significantly from non-REM to REM sleep (Al-Saedi et al. 1997)

apnea (Rigatto 1988; Rigatto et al. 1982b; Fig. 5). When chest distortion occurs, diaphragmatic work increases by about 40%, adding to the mechanical impairment. This observation is compatible with the finding that the application of continuous negative pressure around the chest tends to abolish apnea (Thibeault et al. 1967).

In extremely preterm infants (<28 weeks), especially in those with residual lung disease, this type of breathing pattern can be associated with episodes of intermittent hypoxia. These episodes are observed in intubated and extubated patients and are a consequence of an immature respiratory control system superimposed to immature lungs (Dimaguila et al. 1997; Esquer et al. 2007; Di Fiore et al. 2013). Pre- and postnatal infection together with the inflammation induced by mechanical ventilation and oxygen toxicity not only could cause abnormal cardiopulmonary development but may also alter the structure and function of the peripheral and central respiratory control system that could lead to chronic episodes of intermittent hypoxia (Hofstetter et al. 2008; Olsson et al. 2003; Gresham et al. 2011; Balan et al. 2011). These episodes of hypoxia and reoxygenation have the potential to maintain the proinflammatory cascade and produce multisystemic morbidity (Martin et al. 2011). A recent study has shown that among extremely preterm infants who survived to 36 weeks postmenstrual age, prolonged hypoxemic episodes during the first 2–3 months after birth were associated with adverse 18-month outcomes (Poets et al. 2015).

49.5 Chemical Regulation

Inhalation of carbon dioxide increases ventilation during REM and quiet sleep in newborn infants. The response to steady-state inhalation of carbon dioxide is the same in these two sleep states, but the response during rebreathing of carbon dioxide is less in REM than in quiet sleep (Davi et al. 1979; Rigatto et al. 1982a; Moriette et al. 1985; Reed and Kellogg 1958; Fig. 6). We postulated that the differences in response with these two techniques relate to the fact that using rebreathing, it is possible to measure the response in "phasic" REM only, whereas using the steady-state technique, the response always covers both "phasic" and "tonic" REM sleep (Moriette et al. 1985). As the carbon dioxide response in "tonic" REM is the same as that during quiet sleep, the results using the steady-state method tend to resemble those in quiet sleep (Phillipson 1978; Phillipson et al. 1977).

The pattern of breathing observed with inhalation of carbon dioxide varies with the percentage of carbon dioxide inhaled. If the percentage of inhaled carbon dioxide is low (<2%) during steady-state inhalation, the response consists primarily of an increase in tidal volume (Kalapesi et al. 1981). If the percentage of inhaled carbon dioxide is high (>2%), the response in both sleep states consists of an increase in respiratory frequency and in tidal volume (Moriette et al. 1985; Rigatto and Brady 1972a). Periodic breathing is abolished with a small increase in inhaled carbon

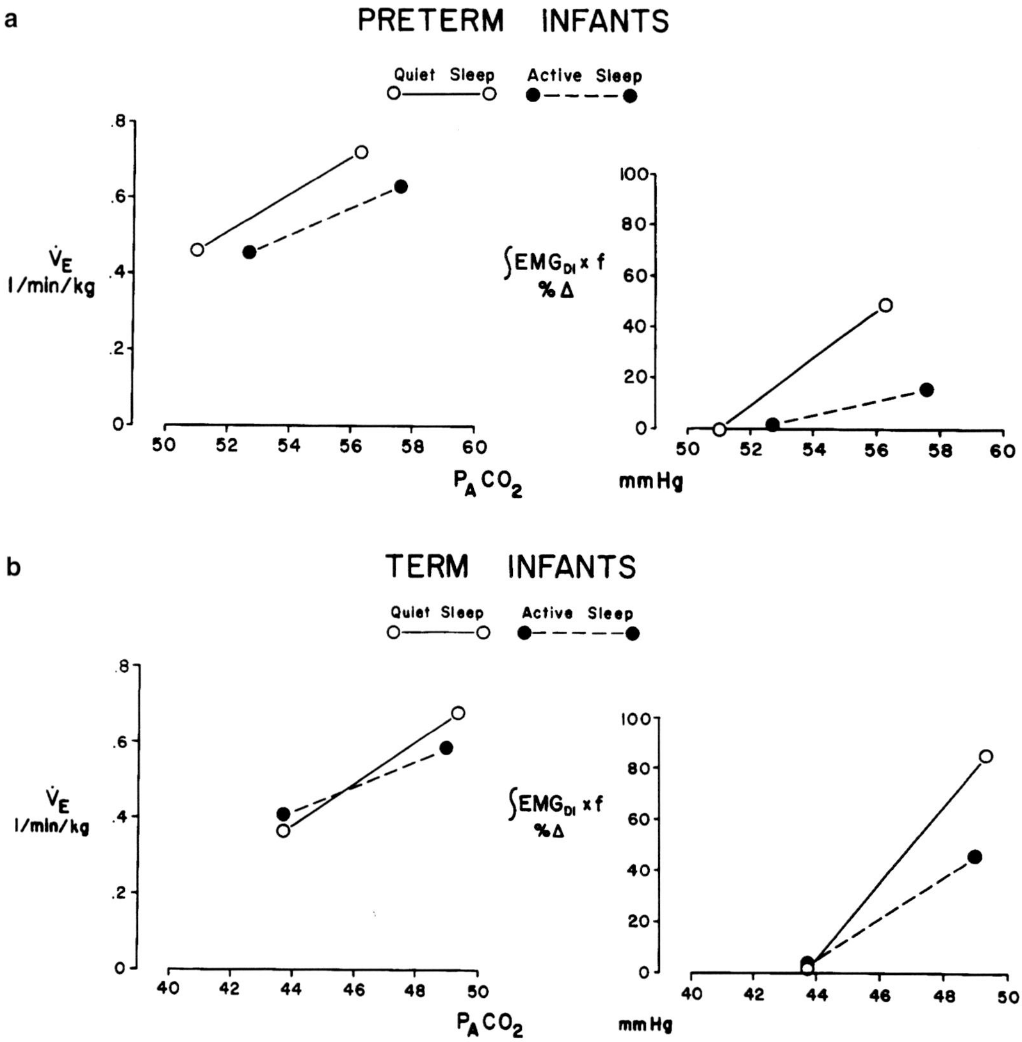

Fig. 6 The ventilatory response to CO_2 rebreathing in neonates. Note that **a** preterm and **b** term infants showed a decreased response to CO_2 in phasic rapid eye movement sleep as compared with quiet sleep (Moriette et al. 1985)

dioxide of about 1–2% (Kalapesi et al. 1981; Rigatto and Brady 1972a). This response has been attributed to the increased central drive and increased stores of carbon dioxide, with better buffering capacity for the oscillations in $PaCO_2$.

Inhalation of low oxygen produces an immediate increase in ventilation (1 min) followed by a later decrease (5 min) (Waggener et al. 1984; Rigatto and Brady 1972b; Brady and Ceruti 1966; Brady et al. 1964). The response is similar in wakefulness, REM, and quiet sleep, although hyperventilation seems slightly more sustained during late hypoxia in quiet sleep (Davi et al. 1979). The more sustained hyperventilation in these infants during quiet sleep reflects the more autonomic control during this sleep state, the system being more responsive to chemical stimuli (Phillipson 1978; Phillipson et al. 1977). The immediate increase in ventilation reflects peripheral chemoreceptor stimulation and is associated with an increase in frequency and in tidal volume. The late response is primarily manifested by a decrease in frequency (Rigatto 1986; Rigatto and Brady 1972b). The mechanism responsible for this response is still unclear and may vary according to species. In humans, it is likely related

to central release of inhibitory neuromodulators (Easton et al. 1988). This late hypoxic ventilatory depression is likely mediated through several complex mechanisms. In addition to hypoxic hypometabolism (Mortola 1999), several neuromodulators play a role in the hypoxic ventilatory depression including adenosine (Elnazir et al. 1996), γ-aminobutyric acid (GABA) (Kneussl et al. 1986), serotonin (5-HT) (Di Pasquale et al. 1992), opioids (Xia and Haddad 1991), and platelet-derived growth factor (PDGF-β) receptors (Gozal et al. 2000). However, experiments in kittens and in newborn monkeys suggest that the late decrease in ventilation may be a mechanical effect rather than a depression of the central respiratory neurons (LaFramboise et al. 1983; LaFramboise and Woodrum 1985). In these experiments, diaphragmatic activity and frequency remained elevated during hypoxia, but tidal volume decreased below control values during late hypoxia. These experiments were carried out during quiet sleep. The peculiar response of the neonate to low inhaled oxygen is of great clinical significance. Infants who are borderline hypoxic tend to breathe periodically or develop apneic spells. Hypoxia can induce periodic breathing in these infants, as shown previously (Harned and Ferreiro 1973). The relief of these apneic spells, which are frequently associated with bradycardias, can be obtained by increasing the inspired oxygen concentration (Rigatto 1986; Rigatto and Brady 1972a).

Administration of high concentrations of oxygen, on the other hand, produces an immediate decrease in ventilation followed by hyperventilation, a response that is similar during wakefulness, REM, and quiet sleep. These findings suggest a lack of major differences in the activity of the peripheral chemoreceptors during these sleep states (Rigatto 1988; Aizad et al. 1984). The immediate decrease in ventilation following the administration of 100% oxygen is related to a decrease in frequency (apnea being common in preterm infants) and a decrease in tidal volume. The late increase in ventilation with oxygen is likely related to cerebral vasoconstriction with increase H+ concentration at the chemoreceptor site (Davi et al. 1980).

49.6 Upper Airways and Pulmonary Reflexes

The laryngeal chemoreflexes (LCR) comprise a group of reflexes triggered by the contact between liquids and receptors of the laryngeal mucosa. The receptors involved appear to be unmyelinated nerve fibers located immediately beneath the laryngeal mucosal epithelium (Lucier et al. 1979). Stimulation of the laryngeal mucosa, either chemically or mechanically, causes laryngospasm, swallowing, central or mixed apnea, oxygen desaturation, and bradycardia (Thach 2001). This reflex-induced apnea is mediated through superior laryngeal nerve afferents (Martin and Abu-Shaweesh 2005). Immature LCR, characterized by exaggerated inhibitory cardiorespiratory responses, are mainly observed in preterm infants or in conditions where upper airway inflammation is present (Lindgren et al. 1992). Some authors have suggested that up to 70% of apnea of prematurity and the apneas associated with respiratory syncytial viral infection are related to LCR (Lindgren et al. 1992; Miller and DiFiore 1995; Pickens et al. 1988). With maturation, the duration and severity of apneas secondary to LCR reflexes decrease. This is in part related to decrease stimulation of the LCR due to improved coordination of upper airway muscles and to the increase in the excitatory respiratory-related neurons within the respiratory network that counterbalance the inhibitory afferent input from the LCR (Gewolb et al. 2001; Kurth et al. 1989).

The patency of the pharyngeal airway is determined by the interaction between anatomical and neural mechanisms. Impairments of either or both mechanisms result in pharyngeal airway obstruction (Isono 2008; Kuna and Remmers 2000). The anatomical forces include the mechanical properties of the pharynx and the transmural pressure. Neonates are characterized by a small maxilla and mandible compared with a relatively large cranium. This anatomical imbalance improves in the first year of life as the anatomical properties of the pharynx progressively gain stability in favor of maintaining a patent airway (Isono et al. 2000). Increase in soft tissue surrounding the tube (macroglossia, obesity, hypertrophied adenoid) and decrease in size of bony structure

(micrognathia, midfacial hypoplasia) decrease airway size. Neck extension and mandibular advancement increase the mandible enclosure size, favoring maintenance of pharyngeal airway patency. Neck flexion and bite opening narrow the pharyngeal airway. Supine position increases the gravitational force on the soft tissue and encroaches the airway within the mandibular enclosure by the tongue worsening pharyngeal airway patency (Isono 2008).

These anatomical disadvantages make the neural mechanisms important to maintain patency of the neonatal airway. These neural mechanisms regulate central drives to the pharyngeal and pump muscles and determine the size of the pharyngeal airway by the balance between two antagonistic forces: the pharyngeal muscle contraction that stiffens and maintains airway patency and the contraction of inspiratory pump muscles that narrows the pharyngeal airway by producing a negative airway pressure (Remmers et al. 1978; Brouillette and Thach 1979). This negative pharyngeal pressure sensed by upper airway receptors is known for reflexively increase pharyngeal muscle activity to stiffen airway (negative pressure reflex). Sleep depresses pharyngeal muscle activity and that suppression is greater during REM sleep (Sauerland and Harper 1976; Tangel et al. 1991). Wakefulness improves neural responses. Neonates have a strong negative pressure reflex that compensates for the relatively high collapsibility of the passive pharyngeal airway. This reflex preferentially activates the upper airway muscles without activation of the diaphragm (Cohen and Henderson-Smart 1989; Carlo et al. 1985). This negative pressure reflex diminishes later in life (Malhotra et al. 2000).

The inflation reflex of Hering-Breuer is much more active in the newborn period than in adult life (Cross et al. 1960; Olinsky et al. 1974). Small increases in lung volume cause apnea. This response is so powerful in the newborn that many have used this inflation to produce apnea and then study the mechanical properties of the respiratory system during the passive expiratory phase following apnea. The action of the stretch receptors is much influenced by sleep, being abolished during REM sleep. The irritant receptors are also poorly developed in preterm infants, and the mediated reflexes are also abolished during REM sleep (Fleming et al. 1978). Therefore, airway mechanisms responsible for clearing, such as cough, are impaired during REM sleep. The paradoxical reflex of the head is commonly observed in the neonate in the form of a sigh (Bodani et al. 1984). Many attribute the high prevalence of sighs to the greater need for lung recruitment at this age (Thach and Tauesch 1976). Sighs are more frequent in REM than in quiet sleep and are also more frequent during periodic than regular breathing. During periodic breathing, a sigh usually appears during the first or second breath after apnea. When it occurs during regular breathing, it tends to be followed by short apneas (Reed and Kellogg 1958). Efforts to discover the mechanisms triggering sighs have been fruitless. Thach and Tauesch showed that asphyxia does not seem to be a stimulus (Thach and Tauesch 1976). Alvarez and colleagues, however, have observed that airway occlusion in the presence of hypoxia predisposes to sighs (Alvarez et al. 1993).

When studying the morphology of sighs in infants and adult subjects, we have found that the sighs in infants are relatively larger than those in adults and that while post-sigh ventilation is usually increased in adults, it is decreased in infants (Qurashi et al. 2005). Since the drive to breathe early in life is dependent on the increased peripheral chemoreceptor activity, it is conceivable that the sudden increase in arterial PO_2 with sighs could produce a rapid decline in carotid body afferent discharge leading to hypoventilation and apnea. The other almost instantaneous change that occurs with a sigh includes a decrease in PCO_2. Since the CO_2 apneic threshold is much closer to the baseline CO_2 in neonates compared with adults, the decline in CO_2 below the threshold during a sigh could trigger an apnea or initiate an epoch of periodic breathing in infants with immature respiratory feedback loop (Khan et al. 2005; Bradley 2002). These findings suggest that although the ability to sigh may be an important mechanism to restore lung volume, sighs have the potential to destabilize breathing and cause hypoventilation and apnea in infants at risk for inadequate control of breathing (Henderson-Smart and Read 1979).

49.7 Respiratory Muscles

The activity of the respiratory muscles is much altered by sleep state. Tonic activity of most respiratory muscles is abolished during REM sleep (Harding et al. 1977; Dawes et al. 1982; Lopes et al. 1981b; Luz et al. 1982). The disappearance of tone in the intercostal muscles has been suggested as a major factor responsible for the increased chest distortion seen during REM sleep in infants with this condition. The lack of tone leads to chest wall collapse during inspiration, and caudal displacement of the diaphragm has to be twice as long to produce the same lung volume displacement (Henderson-Smart and Read 1979; Luz et al. 1982). Because of chest wall collapse, functional residual capacity is decreased in these infants during REM sleep (Henderson-Smart and Read 1979). We have found that distorted and nondistorted breaths produce the same instantaneous ventilation as long as they are of the same duration, although the work of the diaphragm is 40% greater when distortion is present (Luz et al. 1982).

It has been shown that in newborns, in contrast to adults, expiration is actively terminated at substantial flow rates. The role of this expiratory braking mechanism is to maintain lung volume above FRC. The newborn uses two mechanisms to actively slow expiration. The first one is the postinspiratory activity of the diaphragm (Kosch et al. 1988). This activity controls, in part, the duration of expiratory time and is also affected by sleep (Remmers and Bartlett 1977; Remmers et al. 1978). In neonates, this activity is more pronounced in the lateral than in the crural part of the diaphragm, longer in quiet than in REM sleep, and more prolonged in preterm than in term infants (Reis et al. 1994). The length and variability of this activity in preterm infants suggest that because of their highly compliant chest wall, these infants use the postinspiratory diaphragmatic activity as a braking mechanism whose role in maintaining lung volume and controlling expiratory time is much more important than in older children and adult subjects. The second mechanism that the newborn uses to slow expiration is the laryngeal narrowing during expiration (Harding et al. 1980). Sleep state profoundly affects the muscular control of upper airway resistance. Studies in fetal and neonatal lambs suggest that the abductor muscles of the larynx – the posterior cricoarytenoid and cricothyroid – have inspiratory activities in parallel with that of the diaphragm, during both quiet and REM sleep. On the other hand, the adductor muscles of the larynx – the thyroarytenoid, lateral cricoarytenoid, and intraarytenoid – have a phasic expiratory activity during quiet sleep. This activity is lost during REM sleep in the fetus and in the newborn lamb (Harding et al. 1977; Dawes et al. 1982). A reduction in adductor activity of the larynx, in conjunction with decreased intercostal and decreased postinspiratory diaphragmatic activity during REM sleep, may cause the decrease in lung volume observed during this sleep state.

A recent study using electrical activity of the diaphragm (E_{di}) measured by electrodes within a nasogastric tube positioned at the level of the diaphragm has shown that E_{di} peak was higher while the term neonates was awake than during sleep and lower in the postprandial state than preprandial and feeding states (Stein et al. 2012). The same author, using the same technique in preterm infants, has also shown that Edi peak and the tonic activity of the diaphragm do not change with postnatal maturation or with the level of noninvasive respiratory support (Stein et al. 2013)

49.8 Conclusions

In summary, although the basic mechanisms involved in the control of breathing during neonatal life are similar to those investigated more extensively in adult subjects, there are some unique aspects of this control affecting primarily in the preterm infant. First, sleep seems to have a very profound effect during this period of life. REM sleep increases the incidence of periodic breathing and apnea, decreases de ventilatory response to CO_2, enhances the late decrease in ventilation with hypoxia, increases chest distortion leading to muscle fatigue, inhibits pulmonary reflexes, and decreases upper airway tone and postinspiratory activity of the diaphragm leading

to decrease lung volume during expiration. Second, the highly compliant chest wall due to the lack of mineralization puts these newborn infants at a mechanical disadvantage which is worsened by the inhibitory effects of REM sleep. These shortcomings favor instability of the respiratory control system. Third, the low FRC of small infants means low O_2 stores with less buffering capacity and increase risk of atelectasis, leading to intrapulmonary right-to-left shunts and reduced arterial O_2 tension. This relatively hypoxic environment increases the activity of the peripheral chemoreceptors and narrows the difference between baseline PCO_2 and CO_2 apneic threshold levels favoring the establishment of periodic breathing and apneas. Thus, neonates have some unique features of their respiratory control system which may at times compromise their health. It is the understanding of these features and their intimate physiologic mechanisms by physicians and other healthcare workers that represents the best promise for a good quality of medical care at the time of birth.

References

Aizad T et al (1984) Effect of a single breath of 100% oxygen on respiration in neonates during sleep. J Appl Physiol 57:1531

Ali I, Alallah J, Kwiatkowski K, et al (2006) Morphology of Periodic Breathing (PB) in Quiet (Q) and REM sleep and its role on the control of breathing in preterm infants. Pediatr Res 59:2635.7

Al-Matary A, Kutbi I, Qurashi M et al (2004) Increased peripheral chemoreceptor activity may be critical in destabilizing breathing in neonates. Semin Perinatol 24(4):264–272

Al-Saedi SA, Lemke RP, Haider AZ et al (1997) Prolonged apnea in the preterm infant is not a random event. Am J Perinatol 14:195–200

Al-Sufayan F, Bamehrez M, Kwiatkowski K, Alvaro RE (2009) The effects of airway closure in central apneas and obstructed respiratory efforts in mixed apneas in preterm infants. Pediatr Pulmonol 44(3):253–259

Alvarez JE et al (1993) Sighs and their relationship to apnea in the newborn infant. Biol Neonate 63:139

Balan KV, Kc P, Hoxha Z, Mayer CA, Wilson CG, Martin RJ (2011) Vagal afferents modulate cytokine-mediated respiratory control at the neonatal medulla oblongata. Respir Physiol Neurobiol 178(3):458–464

Bodani J et al (1984) The effect of periodic breathing and sleep state on the incidence and "structure" of augmented breaths in neonates. Pediatr Res 18:402A

Bradley TD (2002) Crossing the threshold: implications for central sleep apnea. Am J Respir Crit Care Med 165(9):1203–1204

Brady JP, Ceruti E (1966) Chemoreceptor reflexes in the new-born infant: effects of varying degrees of hypoxia on heart rate and ventilation in a warm environment. J Physiol Lond 184:631

Brady JP et al (1964) Chemoreflexes in the newborn infant: effects of 100% oxygen on heart rate and ventilation. J Physiol Lond 17:332

Brouillette RT, Thach BT (1979) A neuromuscular mechanism maintaining extrathoracic airway patency. J Appl Physiol 46:772–779

Carlo WA, Miller MJ, Martin RJ (1985) Differential response of respiratory muscles to airway occlusion in infants. J Appl Physiol 59:847–852

Cohen G, Henderson-Smart DJ (1989) Upper airway muscle activity during nasal occlusion in newborn babies. J Appl Physiol 66:1328–1335

Cross KW, Oppé TE (1952) The effect of inhalation of high and low concentrations of oxygen on the respiration of the premature infant. J Physiol Lond 117:38

Cross KW et al (1960) The response of the new-born baby to inflation of the lungs. J Physiol 151:551

Curzi-Dascalova L, Challamel MJ (2000) Neurophysiological basis of sleep development. In: Loughlin GM, Carroll JL, Marcus CL (eds) Sleep and breathing in children. A developmental approach. Marcel Dekker, New York, pp 3–37

Davi M et al (1979) Effect of sleep state on chest distortion and on the ventilatory response to CO_2 in neonates. Pediatr Res 13:982

Davi M et al (1980) Effect of inhaling 100% O_2 on ventilation and acid-base balance in cerebrospinal fluid in neonates. Biol Neonate 38:85

Dawes GS et al (1982) Effects of hypercapnia on tracheal pressure, diaphragm and intercostal electromyograms in unanesthetized fetal lambs. J Physiol Lond 326:461

Di Fiore JM, Martin RJ, Gauda EB (2013) Apnea of prematurity – perfect storm. Respir Physiol Neurobiol 189(2):213–222

Di Pasquale E, Morin D, Monteau R, Hilaire G (1992) Serotonergic modulation of the respiratory rhythm generator at birth: an in vitro study in the rat. Neurosci Lett 143(1–2):91–95

Dimaguila MA, Di Fiore JM, Martin RJ, Miller MJ (1997) Characteristics of hypoxemic episodes in very low birth weight infants on ventilatory support. J Pediatr 130:577–583

Douglas CG, Haldane JS (1908–1909) The causes of periodic or Cheyne-Stokes breathing. J Physiol (Lond) 38:401

Easton PA, Slykerman LJ, Anthonisen NR (1988) Recovery of the ventilatory response to hypoxia in normal adults. J Appl Physiol 64:521–528

Elnazir B, Marshall JM, Kumar P (1996) Postnatal development of the pattern of respiratory and cardiovascular

response to systemic hypoxia in the piglet: the roles of adenosine. J Physiol 492(Part 2):573–585

Esquer C, Claure N, D'Ugard C, Wada Y, Bancalari E (2007) Role of abdominal muscles activity on duration and severity of hypoxemia episodes in mechanically ventilated preterm infants. Neonatology 92: 182–186

Fleming PJ et al (1978) Functional immaturity of pulmonary irritant receptors and apnea in newborn preterm infants. Pediatrics 61:515

Gabriel M et al (1976) Apneic spells and sleep states in preterm infants. Pediatrics 57:142

Gagliardi L, Rusconi F (1997) Respiratory rate and body mass in the first three years of life. The working party on respiratory rate. Arch Dis Child 76(2):151–154

Gaultier C (1987) Respiratory adaptation during sleep from the neonatal period to adolescence. In: Guilleminault C (ed) Sleep and its disorders in children. Raven, New York, pp 67–98

Gewolb IH, Vice FL, Schwietzer-Kenney EL, Taciak VL et al (2001) Developmental patterns of rhythmic suck and swallow in preterm infants. Dev Med Child Neurol 43:22–27

Gozal D, Simakajornboon N, Czapla MA, Xue YD et al (2000) Brainstem activation of platelet-derived growth factor-beta receptor modulates the late phase of the hypoxic ventilatory response. J Neurochem 74(1):310–319

Gresham K, Boyer B, Mayer C, Foglyano R, Martin R, Wilson CG (2011) Airway inflammation and central respiratory control: results from in vivo and in vitro neonatal rat. Respir Physiol Neurobiol 178:414–421

Harding R et al (1977) Laryngeal function during breathing and swallowing in foetal and newborn lambs. J Physiol Lond 272:14P

Harding R, Johnson P, McClelland ME (1980) Respiratory function of the larynx in developing sheep and the influence of sleep state. Respir Physiol 40(2):165–167

Harned HS Jr, Ferreiro J (1973) Initiation of breathing by cold stimulation: effects of change in ambient temperature on respiratory activity of the full-term fetal lamb. J Pediatr 83:663

Henderson-Smart DJ, Read DJC (1979) Reduced lung volume during behavioral active sleep in the newborn. J Appl Physiol 46:1081

Hofstetter AO, Legnevall L, Herlenius E, Katz-Salamon M (2008) Cardiorespiratory development in extremely preterm infants: vulnerability to infection and persistence of events beyond term-equivalent age. Acta Paediatr 97:285–292

Isono S (2008) Interaction between upper airway muscles and structures during sleep. In: Marcus CL, Carroll JL, Donnelly DF, Loughlin GM (eds) Sleep and breathing in children: developmental changes in breathing during sleep, 2nd edn. Informa Healthcare, New York, pp 131–156

Isono S, Tanaka A, Ishikawa T et al (2000) Developmental changes in collapsibility of the passive pharynx during infancy. Am J Respir Crit Care Med 162:832–836

Kalapesi Z et al (1981) Effect of periodic or regular respiratory pattern on the ventilatory response to low inhaled CO_2 in preterm infants during sleep. Am Rev Respir Dis 123:8

Khan A, Qurashi M, Kwiatkowski K et al (2005) Measurement of the CO_2 apneic threshold in newborn infants: possible relevance for periodic breathing and apnea. J Appl Physiol 98:1171–1176

Kneussl MP, Pappagianopoulos P, Hoop B, Kazemi H (1986) Effect of centrally administered gamma-aminobutyric acid on metabolic function. J Appl Physiol 61(2):472–476

Kosch PC, Hutchinson AA, Wozniak JA, Carlo WA et al (1988) Posterior cricoarytenoid and diaphragm activities during tidal breathing in neonates. J Appl Physiol 64(5):1968–1978

Kuna S, Remmers JE (2000) Anatomy and physiology of upper airway obstruction. In: Kryger MH, Roth T, Dement WC (eds) Principles and practice of sleep medicine, 3rd edn. WB Saunders, Philadelphia, pp 840–858

Kurth CD, Hutchison AA, Caton DC, Davenport PW (1989) Maturational and anesthetic effects on apneic thresholds in lambs. J Appl Physiol 67: 643–647

LaFramboise WA, Woodrum DE (1985) Elevated diaphragm electromyogram during neonatal hypoxic ventilatory depression. J Appl Physiol 59:1040

LaFramboise WA et al (1983) Pulmonary mechanics during the ventilatory response to hypoxemia in the newborn monkey. J Appl Physiol: Respir Environ Exerc Physiol 55:1008

Lee DSC et al (1987) A developmental study on types and frequency distribution of short apneas (3 to 15 seconds) in term and preterm infants. Pediatr Res 22:344

Lehtonen L, Martin RJ (2004) Ontogeny of sleep and awake states in relation to breathing in preterm infants. Semin Neonatol 3:229–238

Lemke RP, Al-Saedi SA, Alvaro RE et al (1996) Use of a magnified cardiac airflow oscillation to classify neonatal apnea. Am J Respir Crit Care Med 154(5):1537–1542

Lindgren C, Jing L, Graham B, Grögaard J, Sundell H (1992) Respiratory syncytial virus infection reinforces reflex apnea in young lambs. Pediatr Res 31(4 Pt 1): 381–385

Lopes J, Muller NL, Bryan MH, Bryan AC (1981a) Importance of inspiratory muscle tone in maintenance of FRC in the newborn. J Appl Physiol 51:830–834

Lopes J et al (1981b) Importance of inspiratory muscle tone in maintenance of FRC in the newborn. J Appl Physiol: Respir Environ Exerc Physiol 51:830

Lucier GE, Storey AT, Sessle BJ (1979) Effects of upper respiratory tract stimuli on neonatal respiration: reflex

and single neuron analyses in the kitten. Biol Neonate 35:82–89

Luz J et al (1982) Effect of chest and abdomen uncoupling on ventilation and work of breathing in the newborn infant during sleep. Pediatr Res 16:297A

Malhotra A, Pillar G, Fogel RB et al (2000) Genioglossal but no palatal muscle activity relates closely to pharyngeal pressure. Am J Respir Crit Care Med 162:1058–1062

Martin RJ, Abu-Shaweesh JM (2005) Control of breathing and neonatal apnea. Biol Neonate 87(4):288–295, Epub 2005 June 1

Martin RJ, Wilson CG, Abu-Shaweesh JM, Haxhiu MA (2004) Role of inhibitory neurotransmitter interactions in the pathogenesis of neonatal apnea: implications for management. Semin Perinatol 28(4): 273–278

Martin RJ, Wang K, Köroğlu O, Di Fiore J, Kc P (2011) Intermittent hypoxic episodes in preterm infants: do they matter? Neonatology 100:303–310

Mathew OP et al (1982) Pharyngeal airway obstruction in preterm infants during mixed and obstructive apnea. J Pediatr 100:964

Miller MJ, DiFiore JM (1995) A comparison of swallowing during apnea and periodic breathing in premature infants. Pediatr Res 37(6):796–799

Moriette G et al (1985) The effect of rebreathing CO_2 on ventilation and diaphragmatic electromyography in newborn infants. Respir Physiol 62:387

Mortola JP (1983) Some functional mechanical implications of the structural design of the respiratory system in newborn mammals. Am Rev Respir Dis 128: S69–S72

Mortola JP (1999) How newborn mammals cope with hypoxia. Respir Physiol 116(2–3):95–103

Olinsky A et al (1974) Influence of lung inflation on respiratory control in neonates. J Appl Physiol 36:426

Olsson A, Kayhan G, Lagercrantz H, Herlenius E (2003) IL-1 beta depresses respiration and anoxic survival via a prostaglandin-dependent pathway in neonatal rats. Pediatr Res 54:326–331

Phillipson EA (1978) Control of breathing during sleep. Am Rev Respir Dis 118:909

Phillipson EA et al (1977) Ventilatory and waking responses to CO_2 in sleeping dogs. Am Rev Respir Dis 115:251

Pickens DL, Schefft G, Thach BT (1988) Prolonged apnea associated with upper airway protective reflexes in apnea of prematurity. Am Rev Respir Dis 137(1): 113–118

Poets CF (2010) Apnea of prematurity: what can observational studies tell us about pathophysiology? Sleep Med 11:701–707

Poets CF, Rau GA, Neuber K, Gappa M, Seidenberg J (1997) Determinants of lung volume in spontaneously breathing preterm infants. Am J Respir Crit Care Med 155:649–653

Poets CF, Roberts RS, Schmidt B et al (2015) Association between intermittent hypoxemia or bradycardia and late death or disability in extremely preterm infants. JAMA 314(6):595–603

Polgar G, Weng TR (1979) The functional development of the respiratory system from the period of gestation to adulthood. Am Rev Respir Dis 120(3):625–695

Prechtl HRF (1974) The behavioural states of the newborn infant (a review). Brain Res 76:185

Purpura DP (1975) Dendritic differentiation in human cerebral cortex: normal and aberrant development patterns. In: Kreutzberg GW (ed) Advances in neurology, vol 9. Raven, New York, pp 91–116

Qurashi MJ, Khalil M, Kwiatkowski K, et al (2005) Morphology of sighs and their role on the control of breathing in preterm infants, term infants and adult subjects. Neonatology 96(1):43–49. 2009

Reed DJ, Kellogg RH (1958) Changes in respiratory response to CO_2 during natural sleep at sea level and at altitude. J Appl Physiol 13:325

Reis FJC, Cates DB, Vandriault LV et al (1994) Diaphragmatic activity and ventilation in preterm infants – the effects of sleep state. Biol Neonate 65:16–24

Remmers JE, Bartlett D Jr (1977) Reflex control of expiratory airflow and duration. J Appl Physiol: Respir Environ Exerc Physiol 42:80

Remmers JE, deGroot WJ, Sauerland EK et al (1978) Pathogenesis of upper airway occlusion during sleep. J Appl Physiol 44:931–938

Rigatto H (1986) Disorders of the control of breathing. In: US Dept. of Health and Human Services (ed) Pediatric respiratory diseases. National Institutes of Health, Bethesda, pp 20–25, Publication #86-2107

Rigatto H (1988) Control of breathing in the neonate and the sudden infant death syndrome. In: Fishman AP (ed) Pulmonary diseases and disorders, 2nd edn. McGraw-Hill, New York, pp 1363–1372

Rigatto H, Brady JP (1972a) Periodic breathing and apnea in preterm infants. I: evidence for hypoventilation possibly due to central respiratory depression. Pediatrics 50:202

Rigatto H, Brady JP (1972b) Periodic breathing and apnea in preterm infants. II: hypoxia as a primary event. Pediatrics 50:219

Rigatto H et al (1982a) Ventilatory response to 100% and 15% O_2 during wakefulness and sleep in preterm infants. Early Hum Dev 7:1

Rigatto H, Reis F, Cates D, Horvath L (1982b) Effect of sleep on phasic and "tonic" diaphragmatic EMG in preterm infants. Fed Proc 41:1103

Sauerland EK, Harper RM (1976) The human tongue during sleep: electromyographic activity of the genioglossus muscle. Exp Neurol 51:160–170

Stein HM, Wilmoth J, Burton J (2012) Electrical activity of the diaphragm in a small cohort of term neonates. Respir Care 57(9):1483–1487

Stein H, Hall R, Davis K, White DB (2013) Electrical activity of the diaphragm (Edi) values and Edi catheter

placement in non-ventilated preterm neonates. J Perinatol 33(9):707–711

Tangel DJ et al (1991) Influence of sleep on tensor palatine EMG and upper airway resistance in normal men. J Appl Physiol 70:2574–2581

Thach BT (2001) Maturation and transformation of reflexes that protect the laryngeal airway from liquid aspiration from fetal to adult life. Am J Med 111:69S–77S

Thach BT, Tauesch HW (1976) Sighing in human newborn infants: role of inflation-augmenting reflex. J Appl Physiol 41:502

Thibeault DW et al (1967) Thoracic gas volume changes in premature infants. Pediatrics 40:403

Waggener TB et al (1984) Apnea duration is related to ventilatory oscillation characteristics in newborn infants. J Appl Physiol 57:536

Xia Y, Haddad GG (1991) Ontogeny and distribution of opioid receptors in the rat brainstem. Brain Res 549(2):181–193

Xie A, Skatrud JB, Dempsey JA (2001) Effect of hypoxia on the hypopnoeic and apnoeic threshold for CO_2 in sleeping humans. J Physiol 535:269–278

Xie A, Skatrud JB, Puleo DS et al (2006) Influence of arterial O_2 on the susceptibility to posthyperventilation apnea during sleep. J Appl Physiol 100: 171–177

Meconium Aspiration Syndrome

50

Simone Pratesi and Carlo Dani

Contents

Abstract

Meconium aspiration syndrome is a disease characterized by a respiratory insufficiency of variable severity, where lung injury probably starts prenatally. The role of meconium in the pathogenesis of the disease is still partly unknown, while increasing evidence suggests that chronic in utero insults may be responsible for starting lung damage as well as triggering fetal distress and meconium passage into the amniotic fluid. Survival rate has greatly improved over the last three decades with newer and more efficient modalities of treatment. On the other hand, concern exists about the long-term neurodevelopmental and pulmonary outcome of survivors.

Abbreviations

ECMO	Extracorporeal membrane oxygenation
HFOV	High-frequency oscillatory ventilation
iNO	Inhaled nitric oxide
MAS	Meconium aspiration syndrome
MSAF	Meconium-stained amniotic fluid

50.1 Salient Points

- Approximately 13% of live-born infants are born through meconium-stained amniotic fluid (MSAF), while meconium aspiration syndrome (MAS) occurs only in 2–6% of these neonates.

S. Pratesi
Neonatal Intensive Care Unit, Careggi University Hospital, Florence, Italy
e-mail: simone.pratesi@unifi.it

C. Dani (✉)
Neonatal Intensive Care Unit, Careggi University Hospital, Florence, Italy

Università degli Studi di Firenze, Florence, Italy
e-mail: cdani@unifi.it

G. Buonocore et al. (eds.), *Neonatology*,
https://doi.org/10.1007/978-3-319-29489-6_199

- Most cases of meconium aspiration occur in utero when fetal gasping is initiated before delivery.
- Inflammation plays a major role in the pathogenesis of MAS.
- Antepartum, intrapartum, and postpartum strategies are mandatory for prevention of MAS.
- Most infants born through MSAF require no interventions; however, it is important to monitor these infants closely during the first 12 h of life.
- The percentage of newborns requiring ECMO has decreased since the introduction of treatment with inhaled nitric oxide (iNO) and high-frequency oscillatory ventilation.

50.2 Introduction

The term meconium is derived from the Greek word *mekoni*, which means poppy juice or opium due to its tarry appearance or to Aristotle's belief that it induced sleep in the fetus. Meconium constitutes the first stool of a newborn infant. The passage of meconium typically occurs within 48 h after birth; however, it can occur in utero.

The optimal care of an infant born through meconium-stained amniotic fluid (MSAF) should involve obstetrician and pediatrician together. Indeed, management of a baby at risk of meconium aspiration syndrome (MAS) starts in the delivery room or even earlier during intrauterine life. MAS is defined as respiratory distress in an infant born through MSAF whose symptoms cannot be otherwise explained; approximately 13% of live-born infants are born through MSAF, while MAS occurs only in 2–6% of these neonates (Cleary and Wiswell 1998). A retrospective review of the outcomes and treatment patterns in term neonates admitted for intensive care during a 10-year period indicates an increasing likelihood of MAS with advancing gestational age (from 1.1% at 37 weeks gestation to 24% at >42 weeks gestation), a quite constant mortality rate of about 1,2% despite changes in care during the last decade, and a higher mortality risk for infants born smaller, outborn, and delivered by C-section, who had lower Apgar scores, pulmonary hypertension, and use of cefotaxime (Singh et al. 2009).

Meconium is first noted to be present at 12 weeks gestation in human fetus. It is the by-product of fetal amniotic fluid, lanugo, skin cells, and vernix caseosa swallowing; as well it contains cells derived from the gastrointestinal tract. Meconium composition also includes four different biliary acids (cholic, chenodeoxycholic, deoxycholic, and lithocholic) and minerals of which copper, zinc, magnesium, calcium iron, and phosphorus are the most common. In addition, it contains plasmatic proteins such as α1-antitripsin and phospholipase A_2, free fatty acids, bilirubin, and enzymes. The passage of meconium from fetus into the amnion at early stage of gestation is prevented by the lack of intestinal peristalsis due to low motilin levels, tonic contraction of the anal sphincter, and a terminal cap of viscous meconium. MSAF in advanced gestation may therefore be a natural phenomenon that reflects a postterm fetus with a mature gastrointestinal tract in which motilin levels have risen. On the other hand, MSAF has been associated with perinatal conditions (such as intrauterine growth retardation, preeclampsia, eclampsia, maternal diabetes mellitus) which can compromise the uteroplacental circulation with resultant acute or chronic fetal hypoxia and acidosis, in the presence or absence of fetal distress, producing relaxation of the anal sphincter, more easily to occur in term than preterm neonates.

50.3 Pathogenesis

The traditional belief was that meconium aspiration occurs immediately after birth. Several investigators have suggested, however, that most cases of meconium aspiration occur in utero when fetal gasping is initiated before delivery. Thus, it is believed that MAS will sometimes occur despite appropriate airway management at delivery. There is currently no way to distinguish between the infant who has developed MAS by intrauterine respiration or gasping and the infant who has developed MAS by inhalation of meconium at the first breaths after delivery.

But is MAS really caused by a direct injury of meconium on the lung? It is unclear why some infants born through MSAF develop an aspiration syndrome whereas others do not. It is known that meconium presence under the vocal cords is

associated with higher risk of MAS, but its absence does not mean the infant will not develop severe respiratory failure. According to Ghidini and Spong, there are no correlations between the presence of meconium in the trachea and clinical symptoms, as two thirds of babies with meconium in the trachea do not develop any respiratory syndrome and a half of those with a respiratory syndrome did not have meconium in the lungs (Ghidini and Spong 2001). Thus, the correlation, so far considered obvious, between the presence of meconium into the airways and respiratory disease, would be not so obvious. It is suggested that other pathological events such as intrauterine asphyxia could cause the syndrome, while the presence of meconium into the amniotic fluid and the lungs only being an incidental finding or a consequence of the stress insult to the fetus. Intrauterine asphyxia would lead to a remodeling of the pulmonary vascular tree determining a thickening of the pulmonary vascular media and an abnormal vascular reactivity responsible for the persistent pulmonary hypertension associated with persistent hypoxemia frequently seen in newborn with severe MAS (Wiswell et al. 2000). Autopsy data from cases of MAS severe enough to result in neonatal demise within 48 h of birth show that muscularization of the distal pulmonary arterioles is present in close to 100% of cases. As de novo muscularization requires a minimum of 3–8 days to develop, it may actually precede the aspiration of meconium (Thureen et al. 1997). Increasing evidence suggests that a chronic in utero insult may be responsible for most cases of severe MAS as opposed to an acute peripartum event. Chronic fetal hypoxia and acidosis may lead to fetal gasping and the subsequent in utero aspiration of meconium. This is supported by autopsy findings of meconium in the alveoli of stillbirths or of infants who died shortly after birth and never developed spontaneous respirations. In contrast to these severe cases, the vigorous infant who aspirates meconium-stained fluid from the nasopharynx at birth usually develops mild to moderate disease. The pathogenic events leading to mild MAS and severe MAS seem to be different, and events antedating labor (such as chronic asphyxia or infection) are predominantly responsible for the lung disease among infants with severe MAS. This is a crucial point as it concerns the possibility to prevent severe MAS, because probably the only possible prevention could be during intrauterine life. Undoubtedly meconium in the lungs alters the pulmonary physiology, but it is not clear how much of the lung injury seen in MAS (inflammation, surfactant dysfunction, vasoconstriction, airway hyperreactivity) has to be ascribed to a direct toxicity of meconium on lung tissues or partially to other chronic or acute insults beginning before delivery or even how those injuries could be partially a consequence of the start of therapy (oxygen, ventilatory support, etc.).

Mechanisms of injury in MAS are (1) meconium mechanical obstruction of airways of variable degree, leading to zones of atelectasis with ventilation/perfusion mismatch or zones of air trapping at high risk for air leaks; (2) pneumonitis, with an inflammatory response characterized by the presence of elevated cell count and pro-inflammatory cytokines (IL8, IL6, Il1β, TNF-α), that can adversely affect tissues and cause an increase in microvascular permeability leading to hemorrhagic pulmonary edema and exudation of plasma proteins into the alveolar space leading to (3) inactivation of pulmonary surfactant through dilution and direct inhibition, besides a damage of type II alveolar pneumocytes; and (4) vasoconstriction of pulmonary vessels resulting in pulmonary hypertension and persistence of fetal circulation that in vitro studies indicate not due to the direct vasoconstrictor effect of meconium but possibly to the release of agonist humoral factors, such as thromboxane or TNF-α, by lung parenchyma capable of enhancing the pulmonary arterial constrictor potential (Tessler et al. 2008).

Inflammation plays a major role in the pathogenesis of MAS, and pulmonary function improves concomitantly with resolution of inflammation. Pro-inflammatory substances in meconium can induce lung inflammation in MAS directly via cytokines and heme present in meconium and indirectly by inducing cytokine release from epithelial cells and alveolar macrophages. IL-1b, IL-6, and IL-8 appear to be expressed at high levels in early postnatal life of infants with MAS, making it highly likely that these cytokines are already expressed in utero before birth supporting the hypothesis of perinatal timing of meconium aspiration in most cases of MAS (Cayabyab et al. 2007).

50.4 Prevention Strategies

As aforementioned, a reduction of the incidence of MAS over the past three decades has probably due to a better prenatal care, leading to a reduction of postterm pregnancies, and a better fetal surveillance before and during labor of high-risk fetuses such as those with intrauterine growth retardation. Interventions of some efficacy to further decrease the incidence of MAS could probably be done only at a prenatal or perinatal stage, removing causes of acute or above all chronic fetal asphyxia. Antepartum, peripartum, and postpartum interventions to remove meconium from the newborn's airway in order to prevent its aspiration in the presence of MSAF have been evaluated over the past three decades, including (1) amnioinfusion, (2) suctioning the infant before the first breath, and (3) intubation and tracheal suctioning of the infant immediately after delivery. Amnioinfusion has been proposed for interventions when monitoring detects variable fetal heart. Potential mechanisms through which amnioinfusion could act include mechanical cushioning of the umbilical cord, which could correct or prevent recurrent umbilical compressions, and dilution of meconium that could reduce its mechanical and inflammatory effects in the pathogenesis of MAS. It would appear that in settings where electronic fetal monitoring is routinely used, amnioinfusion confers no additional benefit in terms of prevention of MAS, while in settings without these capabilities, often in developing countries, amnioinfusion has been protective with improved neonatal outcomes, reduced MAS (4% vs. 18%), and improved maternal outcomes (Xu et al. 2007). ACOG Committee on Obstetric Practice has recently recommended that "routine prophylactic amnioinfusion for the dilution of MSAF should be done only in the setting of additional clinical trials. However, amnioinfusion remains a reasonable approach in the treatment of repetitive variable decelerations, regardless of amniotic fluid meconium status" (ACOG Committee Obstetric Practice 2006).

Intrapartum suctioning, combined with intubation after delivery of a newborn from MSAF, has been considered standard procedure for more than 25 years. The aim was to clear as much meconium as possible from the airway before the infant is able to take a breath. However, the most recent international guidelines on neonatal resuscitation suggest the suction immediately after birth only if the airway appears obstructed or if positive pressure ventilation is required to prevent the risk of induced bradycardia. Routine intervention of intubation and suction for the nonvigorous newborn with meconium-stained amniotic fluid is not recommended, while it suggests of initiating the respiratory support as indicated for each individual infant (Wyckoff et al. 2015). This is in agreement with a recent randomized controlled trial which demonstrated that endotracheal suctioning of nonvigorous infants born through MSAF does not reduce the risk and complications of MAS compared to a no-suction strategy (Chettri et al. 2015).

Also the ACOG Committee on Obstetric Practice recently recommended that "infants with MSAF should no longer receive intrapartum suctioning" (ACOG Committee on Obstetric Practice 2007). On the other hand, some have suggested an even more aggressive approach: endoscopic in utero suctioning of the fetus before delivery (Petrikovsky 2004). However, this procedure has yet to be tested and proven and therefore cannot be recommended.

Current recommended delivery room management of the meconium-stained newborn is that pressure positive ventilation should be initiated if the infant is not breathing or the heart rate is less than 100/min after the initial steps are completed (Wyckoff et al. 2015). Thus, a skilled resuscitation team should be present at all deliveries that involve MSAF to perform neonatal resuscitation as needed. Resuscitation should be initiated with air (21% oxygen at sea level), and supplementary oxygen may be administered under preductal oxygen saturation monitoring (Wyckoff et al. 2015).

50.5 Clinics and Therapy

Most infants born through MSAF require no interventions; however, it is important to monitor these infants closely for signs of respiratory distress able to develop within the first 12 h of life.

A severely compromised neonate born with MSAF should not be a priori labeled as a case of MAS until other causes of neonatal compromise have been excluded. Severe MAS should cease to be a diagnosis of inclusion (any respiratory distress in the context of MSAF with any radiologic finding), but rather become a diagnosis of exclusion. Its diagnostic criteria should be strict (i.e., the presence of meconium in the mouth or trachea at delivery, early onset of respiratory distress, and chest X-ray evidence of "patchy" areas of opacification or pulmonary air leak) and limited to cases without infection or chronic asphyxia. Infants at risk of MAS who show sign of respiratory distress (tachypnea, cyanosis, retractions, grunting, rales, and rhonchi at chest auscultation, barrel-shaped chest) must be transferred to the neonatal intensive care unit. An infant developing a severe MAS will require a wide range of intensive therapies to be rapidly available and aimed at increasing oxygenation while minimizing the barotraumas that may lead to air leak syndromes: intubation and endotracheal suction in the delivery room, mechanical ventilation (conventional or high-frequency ventilation) preferably already started in delivery room (to avoid bag ventilation at higher risk of determining air leaks), placement of a central catheter in the umbilical vein, sedation with continuous iv infusion of fentanyl and/or midazolam, administration of endotracheal surfactant as bolus or lavage, inhaled nitric oxide (iNO) if persistent pulmonary hypertension is present, inotropic drugs and/or plasma transfusion to treat hypotension, antibiotics prophylaxis (as sepsis is often in the differential diagnosis), anti-inflammatory drugs to reduce lung inflammation, strict evaluation and management of acidosis, electrolyte imbalance, and hypoglycemia. Severe case of MAS may need for extracorporeal membrane oxygenation (ECMO), even if the percentage of newborns requiring ECMO has decreased since the introduction of treatment of persistent pulmonary hypertension with iNO. A chest X-ray will be performed to evaluate if radiographic features are compatible with the diagnosis of MAS and to exclude the presence of pneumothorax, pneumomediastinum, or pulmonary interstitial emphysema, which frequently complicate MAS. Roentgenographic findings may include coarse irregular or nodular pulmonary densities, areas of diminished aeration or consolidation (atelectasis) alternating with areas of hyperinflation and generalized hyperinflation (Fig. 1). The classic findings in MAS are described as diffuse, asymmetric patchy infiltrates, but because of the diverse mechanisms that cause disease, various radiographic findings may be present. Radiographic clearing is slow over a period of days or weeks if classic radiographic findings of MAS are present. A two-dimensional echocardiogram will be performed to exclude a congenital heart defect and to assess pulmonary hypertension, myocardial contractility and cardiac output, intracardiac right to left shunts, and shunt through the ductus arteriosus. Usually in case of MAS, early blood tests are characterized by hypoxemia, metabolic acidosis, mild to severe hypercarbia, and no signs of infection (C-reactive protein negative, no leukocytosis or leukopenia). This kind of biochemical pattern prevents the physiological

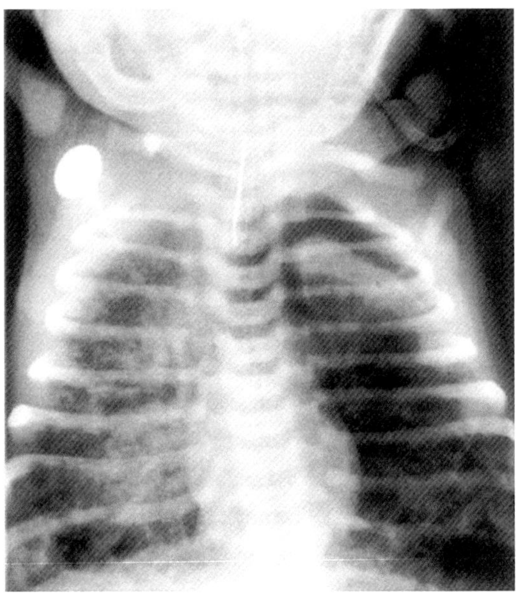

Fig. 1 Chest x ray of infant with meconium aspiration syndrome. They can be appreciated coarse irregular or nodular pulmonary densities, asymmetric areas of diminished aeration or consolidation (atelectasis) alternating with areas of hyperinflation, and left pneumothorax

drop of pulmonary arterial resistance with increase in pulmonary blood flow, resulting in right-to-left shunts at atrial and ductus arteriosus level, thus maintaining and further reducing hypoxemia into a vicious cycle. Leukopenia may present later as a consequence of the accumulation of polymorphonuclear leukocytes into the lung tissues.

Cleary and Wiswell have proposed criteria to define MAS severity: (1) mild MAS is disease that requires less than 40% oxygen for less than 48 h, (2) moderate MAS is disease that requires more than 40% oxygen for more than 48 h with no air leak, and (3) severe MAS is disease that requires assisted ventilation for more than 48 h and is often associated with persistent pulmonary hypertension (Cleary and Wiswell 1998). Pneumothorax is still a frequent complication of MAS (8–20%), and it is an important indicator of a poorer prognosis. Approximately 40% of the babies with MAS require mechanical ventilation, about 1.4% of ECMO. ECMO use is decreased during the last decade, while high-frequency oscillatory ventilation (HFOV) and iNO have been used with increasing frequency (Singh et al. 2009). However, no prospective, randomized, controlled trials have compared conventional ventilation versus HFOV in MAS. Theoretically, high-frequency ventilators should reduce air leak syndromes in MAS, but animal and clinical models have yielded conflicting results. High-frequency ventilators may slow the progression of meconium down the tracheobronchial tree and allow more time for meconium removal (Walsh and Fanaroff 2007).

Inhibition of surfactant function in the alveolar space is an important element of the pathophysiology of the disease, thus representing the rationale for administration of exogenous surfactant preparations in MAS, initially as standard bolus therapy and, more recently, in association with therapeutic lung lavage. In infants with MAS, surfactant administration may reduce the severity of respiratory illness and decrease the number of infants with progressive respiratory failure requiring support with ECMO (El Shahed et al. 2014). Bolus surfactant should be administered as early as practicable to infants who exhibit significant parenchymal disease, at a phospholipid dose of at least 100 mg/kg, rapidly instilled into the trachea. Natural surfactant or a third-generation synthetic surfactant should be used and the dosage repeated every 6 h until oxygenation has improved. Lung lavage with dilute surfactant has recently emerged as an alternative to bolus therapy in MAS, which has the advantage of removing surfactant inhibitors (hemoglobin, plasma proteins) from the alveolar space in addition to augmenting surfactant phospholipid concentration. The ideal fluid volume and technique for lavage in MAS are not yet clear; experimental data would suggest a total lavage volume of 30 mL/kg (administered as two 15 mL/kg aliquots) at a 5 mg/ml phospholipid concentration (lower concentrations make surfactant more sensitive to inactivation) as most effective in improving oxygenation and pulmonary mechanics and in attenuating lung injury. Lesser total lavage volumes or smaller aliquot volumes removed meconium less effectively, whereas a greater total lavage volume resulted in unacceptably high deposition of aqueous fluid in the lung. The advised procedure would be the following: (a) adequate stabilization of the newborn; (b) sedation and muscle relaxation to minimize bradycardia and maximize fluid recovery; (c) perform lavage in a rapid sequence, with instillation and recovery of each lavage aliquot within 60–80 s; (d) use open suction with the ventilator disconnected and manual vibratory chest squeezing to collect as much fluid as possible; and (e) ventilate with higher mean airway pressure (2–4 cm H_2O more) than the pre-lavage one for 30 min to re-recruit lung volume and clear retained lavage fluid. As large-volume lavage procedure is inevitably associated with a fall in oxygenation during and for a short time after lavage, it needs to be included in randomized controlled trial of lavage therapy in ventilated infants with severe MAS in order to assess the real benefits against the potential risk associated with the procedure (Dargaville et al. 2008). Thus, this procedure cannot be routinarily recommended, although a recent meta-analysis suggests that it may be beneficial by decreasing the risk of the composite outcome of death or use of ECMO (Hahn et al. 2013).

MAS is frequently accompanied by persistent pulmonary hypertension. iNO causes selective pulmonary vasodilation by acting directly on the vascular smooth muscle. By dilating the blood vessels in well-ventilated areas of lung, iNO decreases the ventilation perfusion ratio mismatch and improves oxygenation in infants with persistent pulmonary hypertension. Proper administration of iNO requires adequate delivery to the alveoli; thus, it may be less effective in patients with MAS, in part because of the physical "barrier" to its diffusion across the alveolar membrane produced by the meconium. Pretreatment with surfactant seems to aid the delivery of iNO to alveoli, with a resultant increase in oxygenation (Rais-Bahrami et al. 1997). Kinsella et al. showed that the combination of HFOV and iNO may be more successful than either treatment alone in patients with MAS, likely because of improved lung inflation and better delivery of the drug (Kinsella et al. 1997). iNO appears to improve outcome in hypoxemic term and near-term infants by reducing the need for ECMO, but has no apparent effect on mortality (Finer and Barrington 2006).

Since the introduction of treatment of persistent pulmonary hypertension with iNO, the need for ECMO has decreased. However, about 40% of infants with MAS treated with iNO fail to respond and require bypass. ECMO is still considered an important tool in treating the newborns with MAS and intractable respiratory failure, with the highest survival rate for any neonatal condition suitable for ECMO (on the order of 93–100%). Despite the evidence pointing to the efficacy of ECMO in severe MAS, without causing excess pulmonary or neurological morbidity (because of prolonged hypoxia), some infants are still referred late for ECMO. Recent introduction of new therapies for respiratory failure in the newborn with MAS such as iNO, surfactant, and HFOV may determine a longer pre-ECMO course in infants not responding to these therapies. A delay in ECMO initiation longer than 96 h results in a significant increase in duration of ECMO and length of post-ECMO ventilation, with also a significant increase in mortality in this group of infants. Thus, the need of ECMO in severe MAS should be predicted as early as possible to avoid ventilator-associated lung injury and to improve outcome (Kugelman et al. 2005).

Other potential therapeutic interventions for treating MAS have been indicated: synthetic surfactant, captopril, tezosentan, and pentoxifylline. Some surfactants may be more resistant to inactivation by meconium (Herting et al. 2001); however, the search for new synthetic surfactant preparations that are highly resistant to inactivation by meconium or other forms of toxic pneumonitis is ongoing.

In MAS inflammation plays an important role in the pathogenesis of lung injury. A number of anti-inflammatory agents have been investigated for their therapeutic values, such as corticosteroids, pentoxifylline, and aminophylline. A Cochrane systematic review of available clinical trials concludes that there is insufficient evidence on the use of systemic steroids in the treatment of MAS (Ward and Sinn 2003). In a recent randomized controlled study, however, both intravenous methylprednisolone and nebulized budecort were able to suppress TNF-α level in the tracheal aspirate of infants with MAS. Treated infants also had a shorter hospital stay, shorter duration of oxygen dependency, and earlier radiological clearance of the lung fields (Tripathi and Saili 2007). Local corticosteroid administration, both nebulized or intracheally administered (budesonide), could result in same benefits with lower adverse effects than systemic corticosteroid. In fact, a recent randomized controlled trial demonstrated that nebulization with budesonide of term infants with MAS improves the respiratory distress with lesser oxygen requirement and thus early discharge from NICU compared to the control group (Garg et al. 2016).

In acute lung injury following meconium aspiration, pulmonary hypertension is related to an increase of endothelin (ET)-1 levels. Recently tezosentan, an intravenous dual ETA and ETB receptor antagonist, has been shown to improve pulmonary gas exchange and hemodynamics by decreasing mean arterial pulmonary pressure and pulmonary vascular resistance in experimental meconium aspiration. Tezosentan thus seems to act predominantly in the pulmonary vasculature, the site of turnover of ET-1, and its effect to be

enhanced by the combination with an inhalational drug-like iloprost (Geiger et al. 2008).

Cell death by apoptosis in the lungs has been demonstrated in MAS. Meconium-induced apoptosis is activated by a strong vasoconstrictor, angiotensin II, which is the product of conversion of angiotensin I by angiotensin-converting enzyme (ACE) within the cell. Pretreatment with captopril, blocking the conversion of angiotensin I to the apoptotic-inducer angiotensin II, significantly inhibits meconium-induced lung apoptosis and also reduces mortality of rabbit pups from meconium. Captopril could represent another potential new therapeutic intervention for MAS (Zagariya et al. 2006).

More efficient modalities of treatment have greatly improved survival rate of MAS infants over the last three decades, but the amount of morbidity among survivors seems not changed, and growing concern exists on long-term poor neurodevelopmental and pulmonary sequelae of infants even asymptomatic at the time of discharge from the nursery.

References

ACOG Committee Obstetric Practice (2006) ACOG Committee Opinion Number 346, October 2006: amnioinfusion does not prevent meconium aspiration syndrome. Obstet Gynecol 108:1053

ACOG Committee on Obstetric Practice (2007) ACOG Committee Opinion No. 379: Management of delivery of a newborn with meconium-stained amniotic fluid. Obstet Gynecol 110(3):739

Cayabyab RG, Kwong K, Jones C et al (2007) Lung inflammation and pulmonary function in infants with meconium aspiration syndrome. Pediatr Pulmonol 42:898–905

Chettri S, Adhisivam B, Bhat BV (2015) Endotracheal suction for nonvigorous neonates born through meconium stained amniotic fluid: a randomized controlled trial. J Pediatr 166(5):1208–1213.e1

Cleary GM, Wiswell TE (1998) Meconium-stained amniotic fluid and the meconium aspiration syndrome: an update. Pediatr Clin N Am 45:511–529

Dargaville PA, Copnell B, Tingay DG et al (2008) Refining the method of therapeutic lung lavage in meconium aspiration syndrome. Neonatology 94:160–163

El Shahed AI, Dargaville P, Ohlsson A, Soll RF (2014) Surfactant for meconium aspiration syndrome in term and late preterm infants. Cochrane Database Syst Rev 12, CD002054

Finer NN, Barrington KJ (2006) Nitric oxide for respiratory failure in infants born at or near term. Cochrane Database Syst Rev 4, CD000399

Garg N, Choudhary M, Sharma D, Dabi D, Choudhary JS, Choudhary SK (2016) The role of early inhaled budesonide therapy in meconium aspiration in term newborns: a randomized control study. J Matern Fetal Neonatal Med 29(1):36–40

Geiger R, Kleinsasser A, Meier S et al (2008) Intravenous tezosentan improves gas exchange and hemodynamics in acute lung injury secondary to meconium aspiration. Intensive Care Med 34(2):368–376

Ghidini A, Spong CY (2001) Severe meconium aspiration syndrome is not caused by aspiration of meconium. Am J Obstet Gynecol 185:931–938

Hahn S, Choi HJ, Soll R, Dargaville PA (2013) Lung lavage for meconium aspiration syndrome in newborn infants. Cochrane Database Syst Rev 4, CD003486

Herting E, Rauprich P, Stichtenoth G et al (2001) Resistance of different surfactant preparations to inactivation by meconium. Pediatr Res 50:44–49

Kinsella JP, Truog WE, Walsh WF et al (1997) Randomized, multicenter trial of inhaled nitric oxide and high-frequency oscillatory ventilation in severe, persistent pulmonary hypertension of the newborn. J Pediatr 131:55–62

Kugelman A, Gangitano E, Taschuk R et al (2005) Extracorporeal membrane oxygenation in infants with meconium aspiration syndrome: a decade of experience with venovenous ECMO. J Pediatr Surg 40:1082–1089

Petrikovsky B (2004) In utero meconium suctioning may prevent meconium aspiration. Fetal Diagn Ther 19:533e5

Rais-Bahrami KRO, Seale WR, Short BL (1997) Effect of nitric oxide in meconium aspiration syndrome after treatment with surfactant. Crit Care Med 25(10):1744–1747

Singh BS, Clark RH, Powers RJ, Spitzer AR (2009) Meconium aspiration syndrome remains a significant problem in the NICU: outcomes and treatment patterns in term neonates admitted for intensive care during a ten-year period. J Perinatol 29:1–7

Tessler R, Pan J, Holmer Fiori H, Belik J (2008) Human meconium has a pulmonary vascular and airway smooth muscle relaxant effect. Pediatr Res 64(1):24–28

Thureen PJ, Hall DM, Hoffenberg A, Tyson RW (1997) Fatal meconium aspiration in spite of appropriate perinatal airway management: pulmonary and placental evidence of prenatal disease. Am J Obstet Gynecol 176:967–975

Tripathi S, Saili A (2007) The effect of steroids on the clinical course and outcome of neonates with meconium aspiration syndrome. J Trop Pediatr 53:8–12

Walsh MC, Fanaroff JM (2007) Meconium stained fluid: approach to the mother and the baby. Clin Perinatol 34:653–665

Ward M, Sinn J (2003) Steroid therapy for meconium aspiration syndrome in newborn infants. Cochrane Database Syst Rev;(4) CD003485

Wiswell TE, Gannon CM, Jacob J et al (2000) Delivery room management of apparently vigorous meconium-stained neonate: results of the multicenter, international trial. Pediatrics 105:1–7

Wyckoff MH, Aziz K, Escobedo MB, Kapadia VS et al (2015) Part 13: neonatal resuscitation: 2015 American Heart Association Guidelines update for cardiopulmonary resuscitation and emergency cardiovascular care. Pediatrics 136(Suppl 2):S196–S218

Xu H, Hofmeyr J, Roy C, Fraser WD (2007) Intrapartum amnioinfusion for meconium-stained fluid: a systematic review of randomised controlled trials. BJOG 114:383–390

Zagariya A, Bhat R, Navale S et al (2006) Inhibition of meconium-induced cytokine expression and cell apoptosis by pre-treatment with captopril. Pediatrics 117(5):1722–1727

Molecular Structure of Surfactant: Biochemical Aspects in Newborns

51

Tore Curstedt

Contents

Abstract

The surfactant-lining alveolar surface is a prerequisite for gas exchange in order to fulfill the energy needs of the living organism. Surfactant is composed of lipids, mainly phospholipids, and four surfactant-associated proteins. It facilitates alveolar increase during inspiration and prevents their collapse at end-expiration. Insufficient amounts of surfactant in premature babies can be successfully treated with surfactant preparations derived from animal lungs. Preliminary studies show that in a near future synthetic surfactants may replace or be an alternative to animal-derived preparations.

T. Curstedt (✉)
Department of Molecular Medicine and Surgery, Karolinska Institutet, Karolinska University Hospital, Stockholm, Sweden
e-mail: tore.curstedt@ki.se

51.1 Salient Points

- Surfactant forms a thin layer lining the alveolar surface.
- It facilitates alveolar increase during inspiration and prevents their collapse at the end of expiration.
- Surfactant consists of lipids, mainly phospholipids and four specific surfactant-associated proteins (SP)-A, -B, -C, and -D.
- The phospholipids, especially dipalmitoylphosphatidylcholine, reduce surface tension but need SP-B and SP-C for spreading the

G. Buonocore et al. (eds.), *Neonatology*,
https://doi.org/10.1007/978-3-319-29489-6_200

surfactant film at the alveolar air-liquid interface. The other two proteins, SP-A and SP-D, are important in host defense.
- Synthetic surfactants containing phospholipids and the two hydrophobic proteins SP-B and SP-C or their analogues seem to function very well and will probably replace or become an alternative to surfactant preparations purified from animal lungs in the near future.

51.2 Introduction

Oxygen is needed for energy production in the living organism and is a prerequisite of life. This oxygen, which is taken up from the air during breathing, has to pass from the alveoli to the blood in order to be transported to different organs where it can participate in the metabolic processes in the body. The passage from the alveoli to blood is crucial and is dependent on a barrier composed of the alveolar wall, basal laminae, and the endothelial cells. Exposure of a large alveolar surface to the air is required to facilitate an appropriate gas exchange in order to fulfill the energy needs of the living organism.

51.3 Alveolar Surface

The development of the alveoli starts in the weeks before birth and the alveolar area increases roughly linear with body weight (Fig. 1). At birth the alveolar area is 3–5 m^2 at end-expiration and about 80 m^2 in adults (Hislop et al. 1986; Parmigiani et al. 2005). Thus, the area is about 1 m^2/kg body weight. The number of alveoli increases in a curvilinear fashion with up to 150 million at birth, which is half to one third of the number in adults.

The alveoli are lined with a surface-active material, called surfactant. This material facilitates alveolar increase during inspiration and prevents alveolar collapse at end-expiration. Thus, pulmonary surfactant is essential for normal lung function and must fulfill properties such as rapid film formation through adsorption from the hypophase, low surface tension at end-expiration, and effective replenishment of the surface film during inspiration.

The surfactant lines the alveoli as a monolayer in combination with areas of multilayers (Schürch et al. 1998). The amount of surfactant needed for formation of a monolayer at end-expiration is about 3 mg/m^2, indicating that a newborn term infant needs 10 mg surfactant for the monolayer. However, during inspiration the alveolar area will increase and some of the surfactant is continuously metabolized. Thus, there must be a surplus of surfactant in the lungs and the pool in newborn full-term animals has been calculated to be about 100 mg/kg body weight (Jobe and Ikegami 1987). The alveolar subphase beneath the surfactant film has been shown in rat lungs to have an average thickness of about 0.2 µm (Bastacky et al. 1995). If humans have a similar thickness, the total

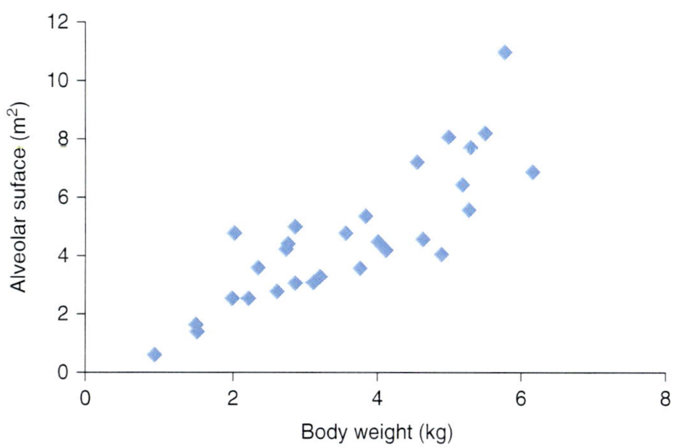

Fig. 1 Correlation between body weight and total alveolar surface area. The values are taken from Hislop et al. (1986)

aqueous alveolar phase would be about 0.2 mL/m^2 alveolar surface area. This indicates that term infants may have a mean alveolar surfactant concentration of about 500 mg/mL presuming that newborn term infants have about the same surfactant pool size as animals.

51.4 Isolation of Pulmonary Surfactant

The knowledge about the composition of pulmonary surfactant has usually been obtained from lung lavage. The lungs are lavaged using isotonic sodium chloride solution, followed by fractional centrifugation of the lavage fluid. In the first centrifugation, using 300–400 g for 10 min, cell debris is removed and the supernatant is then centrifuged at 10,000 g for 20 min. The pellets obtained contain a highly surface-active material composed of lipid-protein aggregates that are enriched in tubular myelin and lamellar bodies. Lamellar bodies are stored in type II epithelial cells and are secreted by exocytosis into the alveolar lumen and converted to tubular myelin, which is the source for the surface-active monolayer lining the alveolar surface.

51.5 Composition of Surfactant

Pulmonary surfactant lining the alveolar surface is a complex mixture of lipids and proteins. It is composed of about 80–85% phospholipids, 8–10% neutral lipids, and 8–10% proteins (Veldhuizen et al. 1998; Johansson and Curstedt 1997) (Table 1). Cholesterol is the main neutral lipid but trace amounts of triglycerides and free fatty acids are also present. Other components such as complex carbohydrates and glycolipids are also found in surfactant.

51.5.1 Phospholipid Composition

The phospholipids are mainly responsible for reducing the surface tension at the air-liquid interface. Its composition is complex and at least 50 different phospholipids may be found in surfactant (Berggren et al. 1985) and the phospholipid composition is important for surfactant activity (Calkovska et al. 2016). The most common structure is a glycerol skeleton with two ester-linked fatty acids and a phosphate group (Fig. 2). Different components, for example, choline, ethanolamine, glycerol, serine, or inositol, are usually bound to the phosphate group, thus making up the different classes of phospholipids such as phosphatidylcholine, phosphatidylethanolamine, phosphatidylglycerol, phosphatidylserine, and phosphatidylinositol. Depending on the fatty acid composition, each phospholipid class is composed of many molecular species. About 80% of the phospholipids consist of phosphatidylcholine with its surface-active disaturated species. These disaturated species, containing 40–60% of total phosphatidylcholines, are dominated by dipalmitoylphosphatidylcholine, a phosphatidylcholine containing two palmitic acids. Although phosphatidylcholines predominate among the phospholipids, phosphatidylglycerol is present in amounts up to 10% and smaller amounts of

Table 1 Composition of pulmonary surfactant

Component	%
Dipalmitoylphosphatidylcholine	30–40
Other disaturated phosphatidylcholines	3–5
Unsaturated phosphatidylcholines	35–40
Phosphatidylglycerol	5–10
Other phospholipids	5–10
Neutral lipids (mainly cholesterol)	5–10
Hydrophobic surfactant proteins (SP-B, SP-C)	1–4
Hydrophilic surfactant proteins (SP-A, SP-D)	4–8

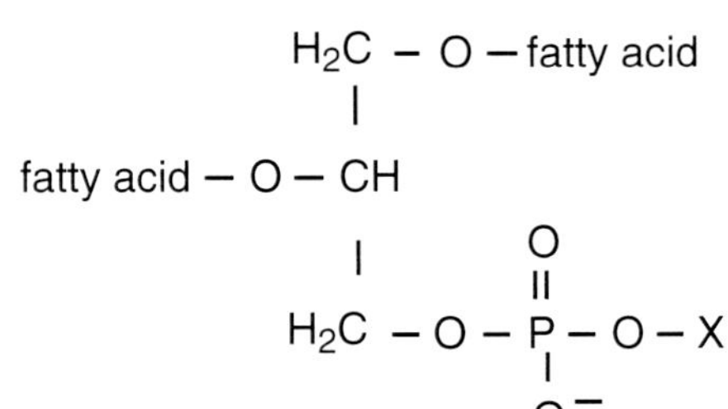

Fig. 2 General structure of phospholipids. X: e.g. choline, ethanolamine, glycerol, serine, inositol

phosphatidylethanolamine, phospatidylserine, and phosphatidylinositol are also present.

At the air-liquid interface lining the alveoli, the phospholipids are oriented in a monolayer with the hydrophilic head groups towards the aqueous phase and the hydrophobic acyl groups towards the air (Pérez-Gil 2008).

A high concentration of phospholipids, mainly dipalmitoylphosphatidylcholine, at the interface diminishes the number of water molecules exposed to the air, resulting in a lower alveolar surface tension and less force required to open up the alveoli during inspiration. This saturated phospholipid, in contrast to unsaturated species, can be packed to a very high density at the air-liquid interface and provides a large reduction of surface tension during expiration, thus preventing the alveoli from collapse at end-expiration. However, the melting point of dipalmitoylphosphatidylcholine bilayers is 41 °C, which is above the physiological temperature of the human body while that of unsaturated species is much lower. Thus, the presence of significant amounts of unsaturated phospholipids in surfactant reduces the melting temperature of the monolayers to values lower than 37 °C, which is important for the physiological properties of pulmonary surfactant. Resent results indicate that cholesterol, which constitutes 5–10% of pulmonary surfactant, may modulate the structure of surfactant membranes by decreasing the packing and increasing the mobility of phospholipids in the monolayer.

51.5.2 Surfactant-Associated Proteins

Proteins represent less than 10% of the total mass of pulmonary surfactant. Four different surfactant-associated proteins have been identified. The two hydrophobic surfactant proteins, SP-B and SP-C, increase the adsorption and spreading of the surfactant film at the alveolar air-liquid interface (Johansson and Curstedt 1997) and are crucial for obtaining a functional surfactant. The two hydrophilic surfactant proteins, SP-A and SP-D, have a primary role in host defense (Haagsman et al. 2008).

51.5.2.1 Surfactant Proteins A and D

SP-A and SP-D belong to a larger family of proteins termed collectins containing both collagenous and lectin domains. The lectin domain mediates the calcium-dependent carbohydrate binding and is also called carbohydrate recognition domain. The basic structural unit of collectins are trimers which are composed of three similar or identical polypeptides. These trimers then multimerize, resulting in differently shaped multimeric forms.

SP-A is the most abundant protein in surfactant. Each monomer with a molecular mass of about 30–36 kDa contains four structural domains with a short N-terminal segment containing interchain disulfide bonds, a collagenous region, a hydrophobic neck region, and a carbohydrate recognition domain. Three monomers form a trimer by association of the collagenous and neck regions. Six trimers form the octadecameric molecule, which is stabilized by disulfide linkages in the N-terminal regions. This octadecameric molecule forms a bouquet-like structure with an apparent molecular mass of about 650 kDa. The protein is closely associated with the phospholipids in the presence of calcium ions and together with SP-B and phospholipids tubular myelin is formed.

SP-D is composed of monomeric subunits, each with a molecular mass of about 43 kDa. Each monomer possesses similar domains as that of SP-A. SP-D usually forms a cruciform dodecamer assembled from four trimers with a molecular mass of about 520 kDa. However, SP-D can assemble into even higher-order multimers when dodecamers assemble into "fuzzy-ball" structures. SP-D binds to phosphatidylinositol and a variety of glycolipids, which are minor components of surfactant. However, only a small part of SP-D co-isolates with surfactant lipids.

SP-A and SP-D are synthesized and secreted by alveolar type II cells and by Clara cells, but SP-D especially is also expressed in other tissues such as gastric and intestinal mucosa. Both proteins interact with a variety of pathogens such as bacteria, viruses, and fungi and protect the lungs from infection by aggregation of pathogens,

stimulation of phagocytic activity, and modulation of inflammatory response. SP-A does not seem to have any effect on spreading of surfactant phospholipids, but the protein enhances the resistance to inactivation of surfactant by proteins, for example, albumin. It has also been shown that SP-A deficient mice survive and breed normally, but they lack tubular myelin and have increased susceptibility for infections.

51.5.2.2 Surfactant Proteins B and C

The hydrophobic surfactant proteins SP-B and SP-C are important for surfactant function. SP-B is expressed in alveolar type II cells and Clara cells, while SP-C is expressed only in type II cells. The proteins are structurally different, but they are both required for sustaining respiratory physiology by decreasing surface tension of the alveolar air-liquid interface and to prevent the alveoli from collapse at end-expiration. Mutations in the SP-B gene have been shown to lead to lethal respiratory failure at birth (Wert et al. 2009). However, these mutations also interact with SP-C processing by inhibiting the formation of mature SP-C from its proform. Also abnormalities in surfactant phospholipids have been observed in SP-B-deficient infants. The pathophysiology of lung disease associated with mutations in the SP-C gene is incompletely understood. These mutations are usually linked to lung disease in older children and adults. Also heterozygotes have a lack of mature SP-C leading to alveolar instability with atelectasis, inflammation, and fibrosis.

SP-B has 79 amino acid residues with three intramolecular disulfide bridges and one intermolecular disulfide bridge, thus forming a dimer. This dimer may interact with the surface of lipid bilayers by means of four or five amphipatic α-helices in each monomer. SP-B belongs to the saposin family of proteins, in which all members interact with lipids (Johansson and Curstedt 1997). However, in contrast to the other members of the saposin family, SP-B is permanently associated to the membranes, which is probably due to its high hydrophobicity. The three dimensional structure of SP-B has not been determined, but SP-B differs from the other saposins by being a covalent dimer not soluble in water. The dimeric structure of SP-B may account for its ability to cross-link juxtaposed lipid membranes, thus catalyzing the transfer of phospholipids from surfactant membranes into the interfacial surface-active film. The protein has a net positive charge, which may promote a selective interaction with anionic phospholipids, especially phosphatidylglycerol, but clear evidence about that is missing. SP-B is critical for formation of lamellar bodies and is required for formation of tubular myelin.

SP-C is a small very hydrophobic lipopeptide of 35 amino acid residues with two palmitoylated cysteines in the N-terminal part (Johansson and Curstedt 1997). It consists of a very regular and rigid α-helix covering more than 70% of the molecule and an unstructured N-terminal part. The α-helical segment adopts a transmembrane localization orientated near parallel to the phospholipid acyl groups. The length of the helix is in very good agreement with the thickness of a fluid dipalmitoylphosphatidylcholine bilayer. The primary translation product of human SP-C is a proform of 197 amino acid residues. Mutations in the C-terminal part of the molecule, not involving the mature SP-C, are seen in patients with interstitial lung diseases. These mutations may result in a conversion of the proSP-C from the native structure to b-sheets found in amyloid-like fibrils (Johansson et al. 2006). These fibrils are thought to be cell toxic and may give rise to organ malfunction and disease.

51.6 Structure of Pulmonary Surfactant

The surfactant components are synthesized in alveolar type II cells and secreted as lamellar bodies into the alveolar subphase. The lamellar bodies are transformed into tubular myelin whereupon the material adsorbs quickly to the alveolar air-liquid interface forming a surface-active film. The thin aqueous phase covering the alveolar surface contains multiple membrane structures, including lamellar bodies, tubular myelin, and the surface-active film. The

air-liquid interface is necessary for respiratory gas exchange, and the alveoli must be able to open during inspiration without collapsing during end-expiration. These criteria may be fulfilled with a complex phospholipid mixture, which can be packed to a very high density at the air-liquid interface and have a melting point below the physiological temperature of the human body. For spreading the phospholipids during breathing, the hydrophobic proteins SP-B and SP-C are necessary. The interface should also be a defense against different pathogens, and for this reason native surfactant contains the hydrophilic proteins SP-A and SP-D.

51.7 Synthetic Surfactants

Preterm babies with respiratory distress syndrome are successfully treated with exogenous surfactants purified from animal lungs (Halliday 2006). These preparations are expensive to produce and supplies are limited, and there is a need for synthetic preparations that can be produced in large amounts to a reasonable cost.

Animal experiments with synthetic surfactants based on a simple synthetic phospholipid mixture and only one peptide have shown adequate tidal volumes during inspiration, but the lungs have a tendency to collapse at end-expiration (Johansson et al. 2003). Stabilization of the lungs at end-expiration is facilitated especially if both SP-B and SP-C or their analogues are present in the surfactant preparation (Calkovska et al. 2016; Almlén et al. 2008).

Two synthetic preparations, containing phospholipids and one peptide, have been used in clinical trials. Patients with acute respiratory distress syndrome have been treated with recombinant SP-C surfactant (Venticute) (Spragg et al. 2003, 2011), but the results showed no clinical benefit (Spragg et al. 2011). Lucinactant (Surfaxin), containing a simple lipid mixture and sinapultide (KL_4), was given as prophylactic treatment to premature infants (Halliday 2006) and was approved by FDA in 2012 for prevention of respiratory distress syndrome in preterm babies.

A synthetic surfactant containing 0.2% SP-B analogue and 1.5% SP-C analogue mixed with dipalmitoylphosphatidylcholine:palmitoyloleoylphosphatidylglycerol 1:1 (w/w) has been evaluated in preterm lambs (Sato and Ikegami 2012; Seehase et al. 2012). The surfactant was as effective as Survanta under the study period of 5 h (Sato and Ikegami 2012). Treatment with the synthetic surfactant in combination with albumin gave a significantly higher survival rate after 48 h of ventilation than treatment with Cursurf and albumin (Seehase et al. 2012). The first study in humans with this synthetic surfactant has now been finished (Curstedt et al. 2015) and a phase II study has started.

Thus, synthetic surfactants containing two peptides combined with phospholipids seem to be ideal to replace natural surfactants within a near future. These preparations can be produced in large quantities to a reasonable cost for the treatment of various lung diseases with inadequate surfactant function or as carrier for different drugs.

References

Almlén A, Stichtenoth G, Linderholm B, Haegerstrand-Björkman M, Robertson B, Johansson J, Curstedt T (2008) Surfactant proteins B and C are both necessary for alveolar stability at end expiration in premature rabbits with respiratory distress syndrome. J Appl Physiol 104:1101–1108

Bastacky J, Lee CY, Goerke J et al (1995) Alveolar lining layer is thin and continuous: low-temperature scanning electron microscopy of rat lung. J Appl Physiol 79:1615–1628

Berggren P, Curstedt T, Grossmann G et al (1985) Physiological activity of pulmonary surfactant with low protein content: effect of enrichment with synthetic phospholipids. Exp Lung Res 8:29–51

Calkovska A, Linderholm B, Haegerstrand-Björkman M et al (2016) Phospholipid composition in synthetic surfactants is important for tidal volumes and alveolar stability in surfactant-treated preterm newborn rabbits. Neonatology 109:177–185

Curstedt T, Halliday HL, Speer CP (2015) A unique story in neonatal research: the development of a porcine surfactant. Neonatology 107:321–329

Haagsman HP, Hogenkamp A, van Eijk M, Veldhuizen EJA (2008) Surfactant collectins and innate immunity. Neonatology 93:288–294

Halliday HL (2006) Recent clinical trials of surfactant treatment for neonates. Biol Neonate 89:323–329

Hislop AA, Wigglesworth JS, Desai R (1986) Alveolar development in the human fetus and infant. Early Hum Dev 13:1–11

Jobe A, Ikegami M (1987) Surfactant for the treatment of respiratory distress syndrome. Am Rev Respir Dis 136:1256–1275

Johansson J, Curstedt T (1997) Molecular structures and interactions of pulmonary surfactant components. Eur J Biochem 244:675–693

Johansson J, Some M, Linderholm BM, Almlén A, Curstedt T, Robertson B (2003) A synthetic surfactant based on a poly-Leu SP-C analog and phospholipids: effects on tidal volumes and lung gas volumes in ventilated immature newborn rabbits. J Appl Physiol 95:2055–2063

Johansson H, Nordling K, Weaver TE, Johansson J (2006) The Brichos domain-containing C-terminal part of pro-surfactant protein C binds to an unfolded poly-val transmembrane segment. J Biol Chem 281: 1032–1039

Parmigiani S, Solari E, Bevilacqua G (2005) Current concepts on the pulmonary surfactant in infants. J Matern Fetal Neonatal Med 18:369–380

Pérez-Gil J (2008) Structure of pulmonary surfactant membranes and films: the role of proteins and lipid-protein interactions. Biochim Biophys Acta 1778: 1676–1695

Sato A, Ikegami M (2012) SP-B and SP-C containing new synthetic surfactant for treatment of extremely immature lamb lung. PLoS One 7(7), e39392

Schürch S, Green FHY, Bachofen H (1998) Formation and structure of surface films: captive bubble surfactometry. Biochim Biophys Acta 1408:180–202

Seehase M, Collins JJ, Kuypers E, Jellema RK, Ophelders DRMG, Ospina OL, Perez-Gil J, Bianco F, Garzia R, Razzetti R, Kramer BW (2012) New surfactant with SP-B and C analogs gives survival benefit after inactivation in preterm lambs. PLoS One 7(10), e47631

Spragg RG, Lewis JF, Wurst W, Häfner D, Baughman RP, Wewers MD, Marsh JJ (2003) Treatment of acute respiratory distress syndrome with recombinant surfactant protein C surfactant. Am J Respir Crit Care Med 167:1562–1566

Spragg RG, Taut FJH, Lewis JF, Schenk P, Ruppert C, Dean N, Krell K, Karabinis A, Günther A (2011) Recombinant surfactant protein C-based surfactant for patients with severe direct lung injury. Am J Respir Crit Care Med 183:1055–1061

Veldhuizen R, Nag K, Orgeig S, Possmayer F (1998) The role of lipids in pulmonary surfactant. Biochim Biophys Acta 1408:90–108

Wert SE, Whitsett JA, Nogee LM (2009) Genetic disorders of surfactant dysfunction. Pediatr Dev Pathol 12: 253–274

Surfactant Metabolism in Neonatal Lung Diseases

52

Virgilio P. Carnielli and Paola E. Cogo

Contents

Abstract

Surfactant treatments have been the standard of care for infants with respiratory distress syndrome (RDS) since the early 1990s. The development of surfactant is one of the great success stories in neonatal care because the therapy specifically treats surfactant deficiency and changes the pathophysiology and outcome of RDS. However, deficiency or dysfunction of pulmonary surfactant still persist in selected

V. P. Carnielli (✉)
Division of Neonatology, Salesi Hospital, Polytechnic University of Marche, Ancona, Italy
e-mail: v.carnielli@univpm.it; v.carnielli@staff.univpm.it

P. E. Cogo
Division of Pediatrics, Department of Medicine, S. Maria della Misericordia University Hospital, University of Udine, Udine, Italy

G. Buonocore et al. (eds.), *Neonatology*,
https://doi.org/10.1007/978-3-319-29489-6_201

preterm and term infants and contribute to the pathogenesis of several respiratory diseases in the newborn. After a short review of pulmonary surfactant, including the role of surfactant in selected neonatal respiratory conditions, we describe a series of studies made by applying two recently developed methods to measure surfactant kinetics. In a first set of studies which we call "endogenous studies" by using stable isotope-labelled intravenous surfactant precursors, we have shown the feasibility of measuring surfactant synthesis and kinetics in infants using several metabolic precursors including plasma glucose, plasma fatty acids, and body water. In a second set of studies, named "exogenous studies," with the use of stable isotope-labelled phosphadylcholine (PC) tracer given endotracheally, we could estimate surfactant DSPC pool size and half-life. Major finding of the surfactant kinetic studies in the newborn infant can be summarized as follow: (a) the de novo synthesis rates and turnover rates of surfactant disaturated phosphatidylcholine (DSPC) in preterm infants with respiratory distress syndrome (RDS) are very low, (b) in preterm with RDS pool size is very small and half-life much longer in comparison with animal studies, (c) patients recovering from RDS who required higher CPAP setting after extubation or reintubation had lower amount of intrapulmonary surfactant that those who did well after extubation, (d) term newborn infants with pneumonia have greatly accelerated surfactant catabolism, and (e) infants with uncomplicated congenital diaphragmatic hernia (CDH) and on conventional mechanical ventilation have normal surfactant synthesis, but those requiring ECMO do not. Information obtained from these studies in infants will help to better tailor exogenous surfactant treatment in neonatal lung diseases.

52.1 Salient Points

- The kinetics of selected surfactant components can be measured in humans and in the tiniest preterm infants with stable isotope tracers.
- The de novo synthesis rates and turnover rates of surfactant disaturated phosphatidylcholine (DSPC) in preterm infants with respiratory distress syndrome (RDS) are very low.
- Patients recovering from RDS who required higher CPAP setting after extubation or reintubation had lower amount of intrapulmonary surfactant that those who did well after extubation.
- Term newborn infants with pneumonia have greatly accelerated surfactant catabolism.
- Infants with uncomplicated congenital diaphragmatic hernia (CDH) and on conventional mechanical ventilation have normal surfactant synthesis, but those requiring ECMO do not. Information obtained from these studies in infants will help to better tailor exogenous surfactant treatment in neonatal lung diseases.

52.2 Background

Avery and Mead (1959) showed in 1959 that pulmonary surfactant deficiency is a major factor in the pathophysiology of respiratory distress syndrome (RDS). In 1980 Fujiwara et al. (1980) administered exogenous surfactant successfully to preterm infants with RDS for the first time. This was followed by numerous clinical trials, which demonstrated a marked reduction in death rates and pneumothorax, and this is nowadays a standard of care. Data, which suggest that a disturbed surfactant metabolism plays a role in several other neonatal lung diseases, such as congenital diaphragmatic hernia (CDH), meconium aspiration syndrome (MAS), pneumonia, and surfactant protein-B (SP-B) deficiency, are now accumulating. Surfactant therapy may have a therapeutic role in the management of these clinical conditions.

52.2.1 Surfactant Function and Composition

Pulmonary surfactant decreases the surface tension at the air-liquid interface in the alveoli and distal bronchioles, to promote lung expansion during inspiration and to prevent alveolar collapse

at end expiration. Surfactant also plays a pivotal role in pulmonary host defense (Phelps 2001). Pulmonary surfactant consists in complex mixture of lipids (≈90%) and proteins (≈10%), which is strikingly comparable across various species including humans (Hunt et al. 1991). Of the lipids, 80–90% are phospholipids, of which phosphatidylcholine (PC) is quantitatively the most important, accounting for 70–80% of the total. Other lipids include phosphatidylglycerol (PG), phosphatidylethanolamine, phosphatidylinositol, phosphatidylserine, sphingomyelin, cholesterol, triacylglycerols, and free fatty acids. Approximately 60% of the PC contains two saturated fatty acids (DSPC) of which dipalmitoyl (16:0/16:0; DPPC) is the most abundant. DPPC is the principal surface tension-lowering component of surfactant.

Four surfactant proteins have been identified so far (Haagsman and Diemel 2001). SP-A and -D are hydrophilic, and SP-B and -C are hydrophobic. They are either exclusively lung associated or predominately found in the lung. SP-A is the most abundant surfactant protein and is essential for the formation of tubular myelin. It functions as a regulator of phospholipid insertion into the monolayer and modulates the uptake and secretion of phospholipids by type II cells. However, mice that lack SP-A indeed have no tubular myelin but have normal lung function and surfactant metabolism even during exercise (Korfhagen et al. 1996). Furthermore, together with SP-D, SP-A has an important role in lung defense (Crouch 1998). SP-A and -D bind pathogens and facilitate their clearance (Crouch 1998). The absence of SP-D results in increased surfactant lipid pools in the airspaces and emphysema in lungs of mice (Botas et al. 1998). SP-B plays a role in formation of tubular myelin, and together with SP-C, it promotes rapid phospholipid insertion into the air-liquid interface. SP-B also influences the molecular ordering of the phospholipid layer. Infants with a genetic absence of SP-B develop lethal respiratory distress after birth, which can only be treated by lung transplantation (Nogee et al. 1993). Absence of SP-B causes a loss of lamellar bodies, tubular myelin, and an incompletely processed SP-C (deMello et al. 1994). SP-C regulates the phospholipid ordering in the monolayer, enhances the reuptake of surfactant lipids in vitro, and may have a role in surfactant catabolism. Mice that lack SP-C have normal surfactant and lung function and have no abnormalities in SP-B processing (Glasser et al. 2001). However, the stability of surfactant at low lung volumes is decreased.

Interestingly the alveolar pool of surfactant in newborn infants with RDS does not differ much from the alveolar pool of adults without respiratory disease (Rebello et al. 1996). However, without surfactant supplementation, newborns with RDS develop severe respiratory failure, possibly through a combination of mechanisms including altered surfactant composition, lung structural immaturity, and increased surfactant inactivation (Jobe and Ikegami 1994).

Limited information is available on the role of surfactant proteins in newborn infants with respiratory conditions.

52.3 Surfactant Synthesis, Secretion, and Clearance

Surfactant PC is synthesized from phospholipid precursors (e.g., fatty acids, glycerol, choline, glucose) in the Golgi apparatus (Batenburg 1992). In the fetal type II cell, intracellular glycogen stores appear to be a major source of the glycerol backbone of PC, whereas in the adult lung glucose from the circulation is a major substrate. Choline is mainly derived from the diet. The fatty acids of surfactant phospholipids are synthesized de novo in the type II cell, or taken up from the blood, or they are derived from recycling of alveolar surfactant phospholipids (Batenburg 1992).

Lamellar bodies are condensed, highly structured lipoprotein packages that serve as the intracellular storage form of surfactant. Lamellar bodies are secreted into the alveolar space by fusing of their limiting membrane with the plasma membrane. After secretion the lamellar bodies unravel to form loose membranous arrays and lattice-like structures, the tubular myelin. At alveolar surface expansion during inspiration, surfactant components insert from the hypophase

(epithelial lining fluid (ELF)) into the monolayer. At expiration the alveolar surface reduces and the monolayer is compressed, thereby squeezing out some surfactant proteins, unsaturated PC, and other lipids. By this mechanism, the monolayer comprises mainly DPPC, which is the most important surface-tension-lowering component during compression.

Alveolar surfactant can be cleared by different pathways. Surfactant components can be reutilized through uptake by the type II cell, incorporation into the lamellar bodies, and then direct re-secretion (Jacobs et al. 1983). Another way is recycling of degraded surfactant components to synthesize new surfactant lipids or proteins. Finally, surfactant can be removed from the lung, either as intact molecules or as degraded products (Wright and Dobbs 1991). The efficiency of recycling is age dependent and has been calculated to be 90% in young pigs (Martini et al. 1999), >90% in the newborn rabbit, and 50% in adult rabbits (Jacobs et al. 1985).

52.4 Surfactant Kinetics

The time required for de novo PC synthesis, secretion, and significant alveolar accumulation has been studied in animals using radioactively labelled substrates (Jobe et al. 1980). Compared to adult animals, the time to reach peak specific activity is longer in term newborns (Jobe 1988). Preterm ventilated lambs show a slow movement of surfactant PC from the synthesis sites to the alveolus similar to term ventilated lambs (Jobe et al. 1983). Recently, stable isotope techniques were used to study surfactant metabolism in human infants. Labelled precursors were infused intravenously and incorporation of label was measured by mass spectrometry in surfactant PC or DSPC isolated from tracheal aspirates. In preterm infants with RDS who received a 24-h intravenous infusion of the stable isotope [U-^{13}C]glucose, the palmitic acid of surfactant PC became labelled approximately about 17 h and was maximally labelled after ≈75 h (Bunt et al. 1998; Merchak et al. 2002). By using other precursors such as [U-^{13}C]palmitic acid, [U-^{13}C]linoleic acid, and [1-^{13}C]acetate to study surfactant kinetics, the same results were estimated (Cavicchioli et al. 2001; Bohlin et al. 2003). In term ventilated neonates without significant lung disease using infusion of [U-^{13}C]glucose, [U-^{13}C]palmitic acid or [1-^{13}C]acetate as precursor, the first appearance of label in surfactant PC was after ≈9 h from the start of the infusion and the maximal enrichment at ≈44 h (Bohlin et al. 2003; Cogo et al. 2002; Janssen 2003). As in animal studies, these results of human stable isotope studies show slower surfactant kinetics in preterm infants compared to term infants. The kind of precursor does not affect the results. The fractional synthesis rate (FSR) of surfactant after infusion of labelled glucose is a measure of the percentage of surfactant that is synthesized from glucose per day. In premature infants who received a 24-h [U-^{13C}]glucose infusion, the FSR was calculated to be ≈4%/day (Bunt et al. 1998; Merchak et al. 2002). Different values were found for different precursors: preterm infants who received labelled palmitic acid and linoleic acid had an FSR of ≈12 and ≈25%/day, respectively (Cavicchioli et al. 2001). FSR in preterm and term infants after infusion of labelled acetate was ≈2 and ≈15%/day, respectively (Merchak et al. 2002). When term infants received labelled palmitic acid, the FSR was found to be ≈17%/day (Cogo et al. 2002). After infusion with labelled glucose, term infants had a FSR of ≈8%/day (Janssen 2003). These data show a lower FSR in preterm infants compared to term infants.

The slow secretion and alveolar accumulation of surfactant are balanced in the term and preterm lungs by slow catabolism and clearance. For example, the half-life of radiolabel surfactant phospholipids given endotracheally to term lambs is about 6 days (Glatz et al. 1982). However, in premature baboons using the same method, the half-life is about 30 h (Seidner et al. 1998), which may be due to more recycling in premature animals and to species difference. Half-lives calculated in animal studies differ depending on gestational age, postnatal age, the labelled substrate used, and the surfactant pool studied.

Half-life measurements of disappearance of labelled surfactant in human infants have been performed mainly in preterm infants with RDS.

Half-lives were longer when disappearance of label in surfactant was measured after the intravenous use of labelled precursors: the half-life of ^{13}C-labeled PC-palmitate measured in tracheal aspirates of preterm infants with RDS after labelled glucose infusion was ≈96 h (Bunt et al. 1998, 2000a; Merchak et al. 2002). In preterm infants, the surfactant half-life after infusion of [U-^{13}C] palmitic acid, [U-^{13}C]linoleic acid or [1-^{13}C]acetate was ≈98, ≈47, and ≈106 h, respectively (Bohlin et al. 2003; Cogo et al. 1999). Using [U-^{13}C]palmitic acid, [U-^{13}C]glucose, or [1-^{13}C] acetate in term infants, the half-life was ≈43, ≈63, and ≈28 h, respectively (Bohlin et al. 2003; Cogo et al. 2002; Janssen 2003). Thus, surfactant half-life is different between preterm and term infants, with a lower disappearance of label in the preterm infants reflecting slower surfactant kinetics, especially in RDS.

There are in the literature two studies on critically ill term infants who were studied using different metabolic precursors for surfactant metabolism (Bohlin et al. 2003; Cogo et al. 1999). Cogo et al. after infusing labelled fatty acids in a group of critically ill infants with various diagnoses showed marked patient differences in PC kinetics (Cogo et al. 1999). Bohlin et al. reported that term infants with primary respiratory failure had a surfactant metabolism similar to that preterm infants with RDS, suggesting either delayed maturity of the surfactant system or disruption from the underlying disease (Bohlin et al. 2003).

In summary, animal studies show a slower surfactant turnover in newborns compared to adults. In human studies using stable isotopes the surfactant PC metabolism is even slower in preterm infants with RDS compared to term infants without lung disease. Moreover, term infants with respiratory failure have abnormal surfactant metabolism which resembles that of preterm infants with RDS.

52.5 Surfactant Pool Size

In most species studied, PC, and DSPC in particular, increase in the last trimester of pregnancy (Oulton et al. 1986). In amniotic fluid, surfactant concentrations increase, reflecting accumulation of alveolar surfactant. This increase is also reflected in an increasing lecithin/sphingomyelin (L/S) ratio (Gluck et al. 1974). During and shortly after birth, large amounts of surfactant are released into the alveolar space (Faridy and Thliveris 1987). Since there is no depletion of the intracellular surfactant pool, this increase in alveolar pool shortly after birth is accompanied by an increase in de novo surfactant synthesis. However, incorporation studies, as mentioned above, showed slow surfactant metabolism, which means that it takes a long time before de novo synthesized surfactant is detectable in the alveolar space. Increased lung tissue and alveolar surfactant pools can only be explained by the rapid mobilization of surfactant from other pools (lamellar bodies, small vesicles) within type II cells. The amount of lung tissue and alveolar surfactant changes with age. Surfactant pools are very high in the newborn period in all species studied to date and decrease subsequently with lung maturity. In humans total amounts of DSPC in alveolar washes at autopsy also decrease with age (Rebello et al. 1996). In preterm infants with RDS, surfactant pool sizes in the alveolus are low (2–10 mg/kg) (Jobe 1988). Total lung DSPC in the human adult, at autopsy, was ≈22 mg/kg and ≈2 mg/kg in alveolar wash (Rebello et al. 1996). In infants surfactant pool size can be estimated in vivo by measuring the dilution of a labelled surfactant component. Hallman et al. (1986) and Griese et al. (1995) showed an apparent phospholipid pool size of ≈16 mg/kg in human preterm neonates with RDS, by using PG as label to measure surfactant pool size. Pool size measurements in preterm infants with RDS using endotracheally administered stable isotope (^{13}C-DPPC) in combination with a treatment dose of surfactant (100 mg/kg) showed an endogenous surfactant PC pool size (before treatment) ranging from 1 to 15 mg/kg (Torresin et al. 2000), while term infants without RDS have three times or more that value (Cogo et al. 2003). As synthetic rates of surfactant in preterm infants are low, it is clear that pulmonary surfactant can only be rapidly increased by surfactant replacement therapy.

52.6 Effects of Surfactant Therapy on Surfactant Synthesis in Preterm Infants with RDS

Although the administration of exogenous surfactant has become the routine treatment of RDS in the preterm infant, there is very little information regarding effects of exogenous surfactant on endogenous surfactant metabolism. In healthy adult rabbits in vivo, administration of surfactant to the left lung only resulted in increased incorporation of palmitic acid from plasma into surfactant PC in the left lung but not in the right lung (Oetomo et al. 1990), suggesting stimulation of endogenous synthesis. In preterm ventilated lambs, surfactant treatment stimulated [^{3}H]palmitic acid incorporation into surfactant PC after correction for the increased surfactant pool (Ikegami et al. 1989). In 3-day-old rabbits, the administration of surfactant did not, however, influence the incorporation of labelled precursor in the total lung surfactant pool (Oguchi et al. 1985). In preterm infants with RDS, the half-life of PG was independent of the dose of exogenous surfactant (60 vs. 120 mg/kg) (Hallman et al. 1986). This indicates that the absolute turnover had doubled after two doses of surfactant compared to one dose. More recent work with stable isotopes in infants shows that the incorporation of ^{13}C from intravenous [U-^{13}C]glucose into alveolar surfactant PC palmitate increased after exogenous surfactant treatment (Bunt et al. 2000a). In summary, there is little information from animal and human studies on the effect of exogenous surfactant therapy on surfactant metabolism.

52.7 Effects of Prenatal Corticosteroids on Surfactant Synthesis in Preterm Infants with RDS

In many in vitro studies, corticosteroids increase the activity of the enzymes involved in surfactant PC synthesis (Spragg and Li 2000; Rooney et al. 1979; Ballard 1989; Pope and Rooney 1987; Post et al. 1986) and increase surfactant protein synthesis (Ballard 1989). In in vitro experiments with lung slices and isolated type II cells, corticosteroids increase the incorporation of radiolabel precursors into surfactant PC, reflecting increased PC synthesis (Rooney et al. 1979; Post et al. 1986; Gonzales et al. 1990). Prenatal corticosteroid treatment in preterm lambs rapidly increases surfactant protein mRNAs and surfactant proteins in lung tissue (Tan et al. 1999). In a study by Kessler et al. (1982) in premature baboons, a 72-h treatment with prenatal dexamethasone did not increase radioactive palmitate incorporation in lung lipids, but it increased total lung phospholipids and alveolar lavage DPPC in lung lavage fluid at birth. Bunt et al. (1999) used stable isotope labelled glucose in preterm baboons to measure the synthesis rate of surfactant PC from plasma glucose. The synthesis was doubled after a 48-h treatment with prenatal corticosteroids. In preterm infants, it was also found that two doses of prenatal corticosteroids doubled the endogenous surfactant synthesis from plasma [U-^{13}C]glucose (Bunt et al. 2000b). In summary, prenatal corticosteroids enhance surfactant PC synthesis in vivo, but de novo synthesis rates remain low, and alveolar pool sizes are not increased within 48 h. In preterm animals with RDS, prenatal corticosteroids improve pulmonary compliance within 15 h (Ikegami et al. 1996) accompanied by stimulated structural development (Beck et al. 1981; Walther et al. 1991, 1998; Ikegami et al. 1987; Ballard and Ballard 1996; Pinkerton et al. 1997). Therefore, the pathophysiology of the improved lung function after prenatal corticosteroids remains controversial.

52.8 Surfactant Status of Preterm Infants Recovering from RDS

The common belief that after surfactant replacement the exogenous surfactant is fully retained by the lung of the preterm infants suffering from RDS has been recently challenged by Verlato et al. (2008) who studied whether reduced amounts of pulmonary surfactant contribute to postextubation respiratory failure in preterm infants who had RDS, needed mechanical ventilation and

exogenous surfactant replacement for treatment of moderate/severe respiratory distress syndrome, and could not be extubated before day 3 of life. Verlato et al. studied 88 preterms by the "exogenous" tracing approach. They administered endotracheally ^{13}C-DPPC as tracer before extubation, for the estimation of surfactant DSPC pool size and half-life. Patients were retrospectively divided into three groups: that is, (a) extubation failure if, after extubation, they needed reintubation or high setting CPAP (6 or more cm H_2O of continuous positive airway pressure and a fraction of inspired oxygen greater than 0.4), (b) extubation success if they did not meet the failure criteria, and (c) not extubated if they needed ongoing ventilation. Hence, 16, 23, and 24 neonates were categorized in the extubation failure, extubation success, and not extubated groups, respectively. Mean DSPC pool size was smaller in the extubation failure group than in the extubation success group (25 vs. 43 mg/kg), and it was 37 mg/kg in the not extubated group. Mean DSPC half-life was 19, 24, and 28 h in the extubation failure, extubation success, and not extubated groups, respectively. The authors concluded that marginal surfactant deficiency may contribute to extubation failures or need for high continuous positive airway pressure settings after xtubation and perhaps more importantly they draw the attention on individual differences in exogenous surfactant handling or on individual differences in endogenous synthesis. Interestingly a recent report in abstract form showed that the administration of exogenous surfactant (Infasurf 3 ml/kg) in infants below 28 weeks of gestation and beyond 7 days of age resulted in an improvement in respiratory severity score (Merrill et al. 2006).

52.9 Neonatal Pneumonia

Pneumonia in children and newborn infants may be associated with surfactant dysfunction and severe acute respiratory distress syndrome (Herting et al. 2000, 2002; Finer 2004; Fetter et al. 1995; Rivera et al. 2004; Escande et al. 2004). There are studies involving a small number of neonates who have been treated with rescue surfactant replacement for sepsis and pneumonia. These studies demonstrated improved gas exchange compared to no surfactant treatment (Herting et al. 2000; Finer 2004; Fetter et al. 1995; Auten et al. 1991; Chinese Collaborative Study Group for Neonatal Respiratory Distress 2005; Hintz et al. 2000). Verlato et al. (2003) used the "exogenous" tracing approach with an endotracheal administration of ^{13}C labelled DPPC to study surfactant kinetics in full-terms with pneumonia, and in preterm infants with RDS. In this small study, the authors found that amount of DSPC recovered from the tracheal aspirates was not different among the study groups, whereas its half-life was significantly shorter in full-terms with pneumonia (19.3 ± 7.3 h) than in preterm infants with RDS (28.7 ± 15.9 h). Mean half-life of term control infants with normal lungs was 62 h. We recently studied a group of 28 term newborns, 13 with pneumonia, and 15 with no lung disease (Finer 2004). We measured SP-B, SP-A, disaturated-phosphatidylcholine (DSPC), and total phospholipids (PL) concentrations in tracheal aspirates at intubation and close to extubation. DSPC kinetics was also measured with stable isotope labelling. At baseline, SP-B, expressed as % of PL, was significantly different between the groups, being 3.5-fold higher in pneumonia than controls. SP-A was not different between the groups. At extubation, SP-B and SP-A concentrations had decreased significantly in newborns with pneumonia, while there was no significant change in controls. DSPC $t1/2$ was significantly shorter in the pneumonia group 11.8 versus 26.6 h confirming the early report of (Verlato et al. 2003; Herting et al. 2002). Interestingly in term newborns with pneumonia, SP-B increased relative to PL, and DSPC turned over at a significantly faster rate.

Conclusion: If it is apparent from one side that large randomized controlled studies are necessary to evaluate the effects of surfactant treatment on morbidity and mortality, it may well be that the dose and time intervals of exogenous surfactant therapy ought to be different in neonatal pneumonia from the schemes currently used for neonatal RDS.

52.10 Meconium Aspiration Syndrome (MAS)

Aspiration of meconium into the lungs directly inhibits surfactant function and induces an inflammatory response in the lung with possible detrimental effects on type II cell function and thereby surfactant metabolism. Surfactant function is inhibited by meconium in a concentration-dependent way (Moses et al. 1991; Sun et al. 1993). Meconium increases the minimum and maximum surface tensions and lowers the surface-spreading rate of surfactant (Moses et al. 1991; Sun et al. 1993; Bae et al. 1998). Studies of surfactant concentrations and composition in MAS are scarce. Cleary et al. (1997) found decreased SP-A and SP-B levels in the large aggregates of surfactant in a rat model of MAS. However, phospholipid and DPPC levels did not change significantly after meconium instillation in either lung tissue or bronchoalveolar lavage fluid (BAL). Analyses of BAL fluid from eight ventilated infants with MAS revealed no difference in phospholipid and SP-A content compared to control subjects (Dargaville et al. 2001). However, concentrations of nonsurfactant protein and albumin were more than three times those found in normal lung. In MAS infants who required ECMO, surfactant phospholipids, PC, and SP-A in tracheal aspirates increased during the ECMO treatment (Lotze et al. 1990, 1993). One study investigated the surfactant kinetics in the presence of meconium (Higgins et al. 1996). This in vitro study in type II cells of adult rats showed that meconium in low concentrations (1%) increases the PC secretion by type II cells, but had no effect on surfactant PC synthesis. Higher meconium concentrations were toxic to cultured type II cells, though the effect of these higher concentrations on surfactant synthesis is not known. Janssen et al. studied surfactant metabolism in MAS infants on ECMO with the "endogenous approach" using [U-^{13}C]glucose as a precursor for surfactant PC palmitate (Janssen 2003). The FSR in MAS infants was ≈3.3%/day (compared to controls 8%/day, $p = 0.058$) and peak enrichment was significantly lower than in controls ($p = 0.027$), suggesting lower synthesis in MAS. PC concentration in ELF in MAS was ≈4 mg/ml (significantly lower than controls: 12.8 mg/ml). The half-life of endogenous surfactant was 69 h (not different from controls). With endotracheally administered $^{2}H_{3}$-DPPC as label, surfactant pool PC size was measured to be ≈50 mg/kg in neonates with MAS requiring ECMO, which was not significantly different from controls or other ECMO infants with persistent pulmonary hypertension of the newborn (Janssen et al. 2003). Exogenous administration of surfactant in animal models of MAS improves lung function and morphology, especially when surfactant is given at a high dose (200 mg/kg) (Sun et al. 1996). Several studies showed an improvement in oxygenation after surfactant therapy, although most infants required 2 or more doses of exogenous surfactant (Halliday et al. 1996). In a randomized trial, three doses of bovine surfactant (150 mg/kg) were administered to 20 infants with MAS. Infants treated with surfactant had improved oxygenation, a reduction in severity of pulmonary morbidity, a decrease in ECMO requirement, and a decrease in hospitalization time compared to the control group ($n = 20$) (Findlay et al. 1996). Lotze et al. (1998) performed a trial in term infants with severe respiratory distress who received 4 doses of bovine surfactant (100 mg/kg/dose) at ≈30 h after birth. Half of these infants had MAS. They were unable to demonstrate a difference in oxygenation, pulmonary morbidity, or hospitalization, although the need for ECMO in the surfactant-treated group was decreased. From these studies, it seems that surfactant therapy in MAS is most effective when given in the early phase of respiratory failure, and at a high dose. Lavage with surfactant could remove meconium, inflammatory cells, edema fluid, proteins, and other debris from the lungs, leaving behind a layer of functional exogenous surfactant (Cochrane et al. 1998). Animal studies showed a beneficial effect from surfactant lavage on pulmonary function and radiographical and histological appearance. There are few reports of lavage therapy in human neonates with MAS (Moller et al. 1999). However, the patient groups were small and no control group was included. Recently, a multicenter,

randomized controlled trial comparing surfactant lavage with standard treatment of MAS has been reported (Wiswell et al. 2002). A trend towards shorter duration of ventilation and improvement in oxygenation were noted, but the differences were not statistically significant.

In conclusion, surfactant inactivation seems to play a more important role in the pathophysiology of MAS than surfactant deficiency. In the sickest MAS infants on ECMO, surfactant synthesis is disturbed. Surfactant therapy seems to be effective in MAS and should probably be given at a high dose and at an early stage in the development of the disease.

52.11 Congenital Diaphragmatic Hernia (CDH)

Although CDH lungs are immature and show morphologically some resemblance to lungs of preterm infants with RDS, it is still unclear whether a primary surfactant deficiency is present in human CDH. Several animal models have been developed to study the pathogenesis of CDH. In bronchoalveolar lavage (BAL) fluid of surgically created CDH lambs, the amounts of phospholipids, PC, SP-A, and SP-B are decreased compared to controls (Glick et al. 1992a; Wilcox et al. 1995). However, the amniotic L/S ratio is not different in CDH lambs compared to control lambs (Wilcox et al. 1995). In vitro studies in isolated type II cells of CDH lambs show a decreased incorporation of choline into PC (Glick et al. 1992a), suggesting decreased surfactant synthesis in CDH. Human studies show contradictory results; the L/S ratios in amniotic fluid have been reported to be either decreased or to be normal (Sullivan et al. 1994). SP-A and DSPC concentrations in amniotic fluid were lower in fetuses with CDH who died or required extracorporeal membrane oxygenation (ECMO) (Moya et al. 1995). Autopsy studies in CDH infants who died at birth or within the first few days of life showed decreased SP-A in lung tissue (Minowa et al. 2000). No difference in L/S ratio, PC, and PG concentrations in BAL fluid from CDH infants was found compared to age-matched controls (Ijsselstijn et al. 1998).

Cogo et al. has conducted a series of studies using the stable isotope technology to trace pulmonary surfactant in newborn infants with CDH who were treated with mechanical ventilation and did not require ECMO. In the first study using the "endogenous approach," surfactant DSPC synthesis and metabolism were compared between CDH patients and control subjects. Secretion time was 8.3 ± 5.5 and 8.5 ± 2.5 h and peak time 51.9 ± 15.2 and 51 ± 13 h in infants with CDH and in control subjects, respectively. FSR was not different for infants with CDH and control subjects ($p = 0.4$). It was concluded that surfactant DSPC synthesis and kinetics were not significantly deranged in infants with CDH compared with control subjects and speculated that other factors than surfactant deficiency, such as lower surface area or increased DSPC catabolism, may have contribute to surfactant pool alteration in CDH (Cogo et al. 2002). Cogo et al. (2003) also studied surfactant DSPC half-life, turnover and apparent pool size in CDH newborns with no ECMO by the "exogenous tracing approach." In 13 CDH infants DSPC half-life was shorter (24 vs. 53 h), turnover faster (0.6 vs. 1.5 d^{-1}), apparent pool size smaller (34 and 57 mg/kg body weight), DSPC amount from tracheal aspirates lower (2.4 and 4.6 mg/mL) Epithelial Lining Fluid (ELF) than in controls. The data from the "exogenous tracer" suggested that surfactant kinetics was grossly abnormal in mechanically ventilated CDH. This study could not ascertain whether alterations of DSPC kinetics in CDH infants were caused by a primary surfactant deficiency or were secondary to oxygen therapy and ventilator support. In the third study of this series, Cogo et al. (2004) developed a new approach to measure DSPC net synthesis and kinetics by using dual stable isotope tracer approach, i.e., combining the "endogenous" and "exogenous" techniques in the same patient. All infants received simultaneously an intratracheal (carbon-13 DPPC) and an intravenous (deuterated palmitic acid) stable isotope tracer. DSPC net synthesis from plasma palmitate was nearly identical in infants with CDH and control subjects (8.6 and 8.1 mg • kg^{-1} • d^{-1}). DSPC apparent pool size was 36.7 ± 7.5 and 58.5 ± 9.1 mg/kg, $p = 0.07$ and half-life was 26 and 50, $p = 0.03$ in infants with CDH and

control subjects, respectively. Both DSPC turnover and percentage of catabolism/recycling significantly correlated with duration of mechanical ventilation. In summary this study confirmed that synthesis was not reduced in ventilator-dependent CDH patients and that DSPC turnover was faster presumably reflecting an increased DSPC catabolism/recycling, and the authors speculate that increased catabolism may ultimately lead to a secondary surfactant deficiency.

When patients with CDH were studied on ECMO by the "exogenous" tracer (Janssen et al. 2003), surfactant PC pool size was comparable in CDH infants and in term newborn with severe respiratory failure who were not on ECMO (73 vs. 69 mg/kg, respectively). In CDH infants on ECMO, Janssen (2003) measured FSR by using [U-^{13}C]glucose as a precursor and found it to be lower than in controls (2.4 vs. 8%/day) with a similar half-life of endogenous surfactant of ≈65 h. It is unclear at present if these discrepancies in pool sizes and synthesis were due to ECMO or the severity of the patients studied. There are only a few reports of surfactant treatment in human CDH infants (Bos et al. 1991; Glick et al. 1992b; Lotze et al. 1994). Bos et al. (1991) showed an improvement of oxygenation in 3 of 5 infants with CDH after surfactant administration. When surfactant was given prophylactically to high-risk neonates with CDH, all 3 infants survived (Glick et al. 1992b). Surfactant treatment in 9 infants with CDH who required ECMO had no beneficial effect on lung function, morbidity, or survival (Lotze et al. 1994). Recent studies on surfactant supplementation in CDH (Van Meurs 2004) show no benefit associated with surfactant therapy for term infants with a prenatal diagnosis of isolated CDH and a lower survival rate in preterm infants with CDH (Lally et al. 2004).

Even today it is still not clear if there is a primary surfactant deficiency in CDH. We suggest that there is inactivation of surfactant function due to the intensive ventilation (Sakurai et al. 1999), which is often necessary in CDH infants, although a decreased surfactant synthesis due to severe hypoplasia of the lungs (especially in the more severe cases of CDH) cannot be excluded. We have recently reported that infants with CDH have a lower rate of synthesis of SP-B and less SP-B in tracheal aspirates. We speculate that in CDH infants, partial SP-B deficiency could contribute to the severity of respiratory failure and its correction might represent a therapeutic goal (Cogo et al. 2013).

52.12 Conclusions

We reviewed the role of surfactant on selected respiratory condition of the preterm and term newborn infants with emphasis on human studies and more specifically on the recent studies based on stable isotopes. These studies have produced novel information on surfactant kinetics in vivo in infants who require endotracheal intubation. This novel information is and will be proven to be very valuable to answer clinical questions concerning pulmonary surfactant in humans.

References

Auten RL, Notter RH, Kendig JW, Davis JM, Shapiro DL (1991) Surfactant treatment of full-term newborns with respiratory failure. Pediatrics 87:101–107

Avery ME, Mead J (1959) Surface properties in relation to atelectasis and hyaline membrane disease. Am J Dis Child 97:517–523

Bae CW, Takahashi A, Chida S, Sasaki M (1998) Morphology and function of pulmonary surfactant inhibited by meconium. Pediatr Res 44:187–191

Ballard PL (1989) Hormonal regulation of pulmonary surfactant. Endocr Rev 10:165–181

Ballard RA, Ballard PL (1996) Antenatal hormone therapy for improving the outcome of the preterm infant. J Perinatol 16:390–396

Batenburg JJ (1992) Surfactant phospholipids: synthesis and storage. Am J Physiol 262:L367–L385

Beck JC, Mitzner W, Johnson JW, Hutchins GM, Foidart JM, London WT, Palmer AE, Scott R (1981) Betamethasone and the rhesus fetus: effect on lung morphometry and connective tissue. Pediatr Res 15:235–240

Bohlin K, Merchak A, Spence K, Patterson BW, Hamvas A (2003) Endogenous surfactant metabolism in newborn infants with and without respiratory failure. Pediatr Res 54:185–191

Bos AP, Tibboel D, Hazebroek FW, Molenaar JC, Lachmann B, Gommers D (1991) Surfactant replacement therapy in high-risk congenital diaphragmatic hernia [letter]. Lancet 338:1279

Botas C, Poulain F, Akiyama J, Brown C, Allen L, Goerke J, Clements J, Carlson E, Gillespie AM, Epstein C, Hawgood S (1998) Altered surfactant homeostasis and alveolar type II cell morphology in mice lacking surfactant protein D. Proc Natl Acad Sci USA 95:11869–11874

Bunt JE, Zimmermann LJ, Wattimena JL, van Beek RH, Sauer PJ, Carnielli VP (1998) Endogenous surfactant turnover in preterm infants measured with stable isotopes. Am J Respir Crit Care Med 157:810–814

Bunt JH, Carnielli VP, Seidner SR, Ikegami M, Wattimena JLD, Sauer PJJ, Jobe AH, Zimmermann LJI (1999) Metabolism of endogenous surfactant in premature baboons and effect of prenatal corticosteroids. Am J Respir Crit Care Med 160:1481–1485

Bunt JE, Carnielli VP, Janssen DJ, Wattimena JLD, Hop WC, Sauer PJJ, Zimmermann LJI (2000a) Treatment with exogenous surfactant stimulates endogenous surfactant synthesis in premature infants with respiratory distress syndrome. Crit Care Med 28:3383–3388

Bunt JE, Carnielli VP, Wattimena DJL, Hop WC, Sauer PJ, Zimmermann LJ (2000b) The effect in premature infants of prenatal corticosteroids on endogenous surfactant synthesis as measured with stable isotopes. Am J Respir Crit Care Med 162:844–849

Cavicchioli P, Zimmermann LJ, Cogo PE, Badon T, Giordano G, Torresin M, Zacchello F, Carnielli VP (2001) Endogenous surfactant turnover in preterm infants with respiratory distress syndrome studied with stable isotope lipids. Am J Respir Crit Care Med 163:55–60

Chinese Collaborative Study Group for Neonatal Respiratory Distress (2005) Treatment of severe meconium aspiration syndrome with porcine surfactant: a multicentre, randomized, controlled trial. Acta Paediatr 94:896–902

Cleary GM, Antunes MJ, Ciesielka DA, Higgins ST, Spitzer AR, Chander A (1997) Exudative lung injury is associated with decreased levels of surfactant proteins in a rat model of meconium aspiration. Pediatrics 100:998–1003

Cochrane CG, Revak SD, Merritt TA, Schraufstatter IU, Hoch RC, Henderson C, Andersson S, Takamori H, Oades ZG (1998) Bronchoalveolar lavage with KL4-surfactant in models of meconium aspiration syndrome. Pediatr Res 44:705–715

Cogo PE, Carnielli VP, Bunt JEH, Badon T, Giordano G, Zacchello F, Sauer PJJ, Zimmermann LJI (1999) Endogenous surfactant metabolism in critically ill infants measured with stable isotopes labeled fatty acids. Pediatr Res 45:242–246

Cogo PE, Zimmermann LJ, Rosso F, Tormena F, Gamba P, Verlato G, Baritussio A, Carnielli VP (2002) Surfactant synthesis and kinetics in infants with congenital diaphragmatic hernia. Am J Respir Crit Care Med 166:154–158

Cogo PE, Zimmermann LJ, Meneghini L, Mainini N, Bordignon L, Suma V, Buffo M, Carnielli VP (2003) Pulmonary surfactant disaturated-phosphatidylcholine (DSPC) turnover and pool size in newborn infants with congenital diaphragmatic hernia (CDH). Pediatr Res 54:653–658

Cogo PE, Zimmermann LJ, Verlato G, Midrio P, Gucciardi A, Ori C, Carnielli VP (2004) A dual stable isotope tracer method for the measurement of surfactant disaturated-phosphatidylcholine net synthesis in infants with congenital diaphragmatic hernia. Pediatr Res 56:184–190

Cogo PE, Simonato M, Danhaive O, Verlato G, Cobellis G, Savignoni F, Peca D, Baritussio A, Carnielli VP (2013) Impaired surfactant protein B synthesis in infants with congenital diaphragmatic hernia. Eur Respir J 41:677–682

Crouch EC (1998) Collectins and pulmonary host defense. Am J Respir Cell Mol Biol 19:177–201

Dargaville PA, South M, McDougall PN (2001) Surfactant and surfactant inhibitors in meconium aspiration syndrome. J Pediatr 138:113–115

deMello DE, Heyman S, Phelps DS, Hamvas A, Nogee L, Cole S, Colten HR (1994) Ultrastructure of lung in surfactant protein b deficiency. Am J Respir Cell Mol Biol 11:230–239

Escande B, Kuhn P, Rivera S, Messer J (2004) Secondary surfactant deficiencies. Arch Pediatr 11:1351–1359

Faridy EE, Thliveris JA (1987) Rate of secretion of lung surfactant before and after birth. Respir Physiol 68:269–277

Fetter WP, Baerts W, Bos AP, van Lingen RA (1995) Surfactant replacement therapy in neonates with respiratory failure due to bacterial sepsis. Acta Paediatr 84:14–16

Findlay RD, Taeusch HW, Walther FJ (1996) Surfactant replacement therapy for meconium aspiration syndrome. Pediatrics 97:48–52

Finer NN (2004) Surfactant use for neonatal lung injury: beyond respiratory distress syndrome. Paediatr Respir Rev 5(Suppl A):S289–S297

Fujiwara T, Meata H, Chida S, Morita T, Watabe Y, Abe T (1980) Artificial surfactant therapy in hyaline membrane disease. Lancet 1:55–59

Glasser SW, Burhans MS, Korfhagen TR, Na CL, Sly PD, Ross GF, Ikegami M, Whitsett JA (2001) Altered stability of pulmonary surfactant in SP-C-deficient mice. Proc Natl Acad Sci USA 98:6366–6371

Glatz T, Ikegami M, Jobe A (1982) Metabolism of exogenously administered natural surfactant in the newborn lamb. Pediatr Res 16:711–715

Glick PL, Stannard VA, Leach CL, Rossman J, Hosada Y, Morin FC, Cooney DR, Allen JE, Holm B (1992a) Pathophysiology of congenital diaphragmatic hernia II: the fetal lamb CDH model is surfactant deficient. J Pediatr Surg 27:382–387; discussion 387–388

Glick PL, Leach CL, Besner GE, Egan EA, Morin FC, Malanowska-Kantoch A, Robinson LK, Brody A, Lele AS, McDonnell M et al (1992b) Pathophysiology of congenital diaphragmatic hernia. III: exogenous surfactant therapy for the high-risk neonate with CDH. J Pediatr Surg 27:866–869

Gluck L, Kulovich MV, Borer RC Jr, Keidel WN (1974) The interpretation and significance of the lecithin-sphingomyelin ratio in amniotic fluid. Am J Obstet Gynecol 120:142–155

Gonzales LW, Ertsey R, Ballard PL, Froh D, Goerke J, Gonzales J (1990) Glucocorticoid stimulation of fatty acid synthesis in explants of human fetal lung. Biochim Biophys Acta 1042:1–12

Griese M, Dietrich P, Reinhardt D (1995) Pharmacokinetics of bovine surfactant in neonatal respiratory distress syndrome. Am J Respir Crit Care Med 152:1050–1054

Haagsman HP, Diemel RV (2001) Surfactant-associated proteins: functions and structural variation. Comp Biochem Physiol A Mol Integr Physiol 129:91–108

Halliday HL, Speer CP, Robertson B (1996) Treatment of severe meconium aspiration syndrome with porcine surfactant. Collaborative surfactant study group. Eur J Pediatr 155:1047–1051

Hallman M, Merritt TA, Pohjavuori M, Gluck L (1986) Effect of surfactant substitution on lung effluent phospholipids in respiratory distress syndrome: evaluation of surfactant phospholipid turnover, pool size, and the relationship to severity of respiratory failure. Pediatr Res 20:1228–1235

Herting E, Gefeller O, Land M, van Sonderen L, Harms K, Robertson B (2000) Surfactant treatment of neonates with respiratory failure and group b streptococcal infection. Members of the collaborative european multicenter study group. Pediatrics 106:957–964; discussion 1135

Herting E, Moller O, Schiffmann JH, Robertson B (2002) Surfactant improves oxygenation in infants and children with pneumonia and acute respiratory distress syndrome. Acta Paediatr 91(11):1174–1178

Higgins ST, Wu AM, Sen N, Spitzer AR, Chander A (1996) Meconium increases surfactant secretion in isolated rat alveolar type II cells. Pediatr Res 39:443–447

Hintz SR, Suttner DM, Sheehan AM, Rhine WD, Van Meurs KP (2000) Decreased use of neonatal extracorporeal membrane oxygenation (ecmo): how new treatment modalities have affected ecmo utilization. Pediatrics 106:1339–1343

Hunt AN, Kelly FJ, Postle AD (1991) Developmental variation in whole human lung phosphatidylcholine molecular species: a comparison with guinea pig and rat. Early Hum Dev 25:157–171

Ijsselstijn I, Zimmermann LJ, Bunt JE, de Jongste JC, Tibboel D (1998) Prospective evaluation of surfactant composition in bronchoalveolar lavage fluid of infants with congenital diaphragmatic hernia and of age-matched controls. Crit Care Med 26:573–580

Ikegami M, Berry D, elKady T, Pettenazzo A, Seidner S, Jobe A (1987) Corticosteroids and surfactant change lung function and protein leaks in the lungs of ventilated premature rabbits. J Clin Invest 79:1371–1378

Ikegami M, Jobe A, Yamada T, Priestly A, Ruffini L, Rider E, Seidner S (1989) Surfactant metabolism in surfactant-treated preterm ventilated lambs. J Appl Physiol 67:429–437

Ikegami M, Polk D, Jobe A (1996) Minimum interval from fetal betamethasone treatment to postnatal lung responses in preterm lambs. Am J Obstet Gynecol 174:1408–1413

Jacobs H, Jobe A, Ikegami M, Conaway D (1983) The significance of reutilization of surfactant phosphatidylcholine. J Biol Chem 258:4156–4165

Jacobs HC, Ikegami M, Jobe AH, Berry DD, Jones S (1985) Reutilization of surfactant phosphatidylcholine in adult rabbits. Biochim Biophys Acta 837:77–84

Janssen DJMT (2003) Surfactant phosphatidylcholine metabolism in severe neonatal lung disease studied with studied with stable isotopes. Erasmus MC. Erasmus, Rotterdam

Janssen DJ, Tibboel D, Carnielli VP, van Emmen E, Luijendijk IH, Darcos Wattimena JL, Zimmermann LJ (2003) Surfactant phosphatidylcholine pool size in human neonates with congenital diaphragmatic hernia requiring ecmo. J Pediatr 142:247–252

Jobe A (1988) Metabolism of endogenous surfactant and exogenous surfactant for replacement therapy. Semin Perinatol 12:231–239

Jobe A, Ikegami M (1994) Movement of fluid and particles between the airspaces and pulmonary interstitium protein permeability abnormalities in the preterm. In: Effros R, Chang H (eds) Fluid and solute transport in the airspaces of the lungs (lung biology in health and disease). Marcel Dekker, New York, pp 335–355

Jobe A, Ikegami M, Sarton-Miller I, Barajas L (1980) Surfactant metabolism of newborn lamb lungs in vivo. J Appl Physiol 49:1091–1098

Jobe A, Ikegami M, Glatz T, Yoshida Y, Diakomanolis E, Padbury J (1983) Saturated phosphatidylcholine secretion and the effect of natural surfactant on premature and term lambs ventilated for 2 days. Exp Lung Res 4:259–267

Kessler DL, Truog WE, Murphy JH, Palmer S, Standaert TA, Woodrum DE, Hodson WA (1982) Experimental hyaline membrane disease in the premature monkey: effects of antenatal dexamethasone. Am Rev Respir Dis 126:62–69

Korfhagen TR, Bruno MD, Ross GF, Huelsman KM, Ikegami M, Jobe AH, Wert SE, Stripp BR, Morris RE, Glasser SW, Bachurski CJ, Iwamoto HS, Whitsett JA (1996) Altered surfactant function and structure in SP-A gene targeted mice. Proc Natl Acad Sci USA 93:9594–9599

Lally KP, Lally PA, Langham MR, Hirschl R, Moya FR, Tibboel D, Van Meurs K (2004) Surfactant does not improve survival rate in preterm infants with congenital diaphragmatic hernia. J Pediatr Surg 39:829–833

Lotze A, Whitsett JA, Kammerman LA, Ritter M, Taylor GA, Short BL (1990) Surfactant protein a concentrations in tracheal aspirate fluid from infants requiring extracorporeal membrane oxygenation. J Pediatr 116:435–440

Lotze A, Knight GR, Martin GR, Bulas DI, Hull WM, O'Donnell RM, Whitsett JA, Short BL (1993) Improved pulmonary outcome after exogenous

surfactant therapy for respiratory failure in term infants requiring extracorporeal membrane oxygenation. J Pediatr 122:261–268

Lotze A, Knight GR, Anderson KD, Hull WM, Whitsett JA, O'Donnell RM, Martin G, Bulas DI, Short BL (1994) Surfactant (beractant) therapy for infants with congenital diaphragmatic hernia on ecmo: evidence of persistent surfactant deficiency. J Pediatr Surg 29:407–412

Lotze A, Mitchell BR, Bulas DI, Zola EM, Shalwitz RA, Gunkel JH (1998) Multicenter study of surfactant (beractant) use in the treatment of term infants with severe respiratory failure. Survanta in term infants study group. J Pediatr 132:40–47

Martini WZ, Chinkes DL, Barrow RE, Murphey ED, Wolfe RR (1999) Lung surfactant kinetics in conscious pigs. Am J Physiol 277:E187–E195

Merchak A, Janssen DJ, Bohlin K, Patterson BW, Zimmermann LJ, Carnielli VP, Hamvas A (2002) Endogenous pulmonary surfactant metabolism is not affected by mode of ventilation in premature infants with respiratory distress syndrome. J Pediatr 140:693–698

Merrill J, Ballard P, Hibbs A, et al (2006) Booster surfactant therapy beyond the first week of life in ventilated extremely low gestational age infants. E-PAS2006:59:26351. Available at www.abstracts2vie w. com/pasall/index.php. Accessed 14 May 2008

Minowa H, Takahashi Y, Kawaguchi C, Sadou T, Konishi N, Nishikubo T, Yoshioka A (2000) Expression of intrapulmonary surfactant apoprotein-A in autopsied lungs: comparative study of cases with or without pulmonary hypoplasia. Pediatr Res 48:674–678

Moller JC, Kohl M, Reiss II, Diederich W, Nitsche EM, Gopel W, Gortner L (1999) Saline lavage with substitution of bovine surfactant in term neonates with meconium aspiration syndrome (MAS) transferred for extracorporeal membrane oxygenation (ECMO): a pilot study. Crit Care 3:19–22

Moses D, Holm BA, Spitale P, Liu MY, Enhorning G (1991) Inhibition of pulmonary surfactant function by meconium. Am J Obstet Gynecol 164:477–481

Moya FR, Thomas VL, Romaguera J, Mysore MR, Maberry M, Bernard A, Freund M (1995) Fetal lung maturation in congenital diaphragmatic hernia. Am J Obstet Gynecol 173:1401–1405

Nogee LM, de Mello DE, Dehner LP, Colten HR (1993) Brief report: deficiency of pulmonary surfactant protein B in congenital alveolar proteinosis. N Engl J Med 328:406–410

Oetomo SB, Lewis J, Ikegami M, Jobe AH (1990) Surfactant treatments alter endogenous surfactant metabolism in rabbit lungs. J Appl Physiol 68:1590–1596

Oguchi K, Ikegami M, Jacobs H, Jobe A (1985) Clearance of large amounts of natural surfactants and liposomes of dipalmitoylphosphatidylcholine from the lungs of rabbits. Exp Lung Res 9:221–235

Oulton M, Fraser M, Dolphin M, Yoon R, Faulkner G (1986) Quantification of surfactant pool sizes in rabbit lung during perinatal development. J Lipid Res 27:602–612

Phelps DS (2001) Surfactant regulation of host defense function in the lung: a question of balance. Pediatr Pathol Mol Med 20:269–292

Pinkerton KE, Willet KE, Peake JL, Sly PD, Jobe AH, Ikegami M (1997) Prenatal glucocorticoid and T4 effects on lung morphology in preterm lambs. Am J Respir Crit Care Med 156:624–630

Pope TS, Rooney SA (1987) Effects of glucocorticoid and thyroid hormones on regulatory enzymes of fatty acid synthesis and glycogen metabolism in developing fetal rat lung. Biochim Biophys Acta 918:141–148

Post M, Barsoumian A, Smith BT (1986) The cellular mechanism of glucocorticoid acceleration of fetal lung maturation. Fibroblast-pneumonocyte factor stimulates choline-phosphate cytidylyltransferase activity. J Biol Chem 261:2179–2184

Rebello CM, Jobe AH, Eisele JW, Ikegami M (1996) Alveolar and tissue surfactant pool sizes in humans. Am J Respir Crit Care Med 154:625–628

Rivera S, Gaugler C, Langlet C, Villega F, Astruc D, Escande B, Kuhn P, Messer J (2004) Secondary surfactant deficiencies in extremely low birth weight premature infants. Arch Pediatr 11:1346–1350

Rooney SA, Gobran LI, Marino PA, Maniscalco WM, Gross I (1979) Effects of betamethasone on phospholipid content, composition and biosynthesis in the fetal rabbit lung. Biochim Biophys Acta 572:64–76

Sakurai Y, Azarow K, Cutz E, Messineo A, Pearl R, Bohn D (1999) Pulmonary barotrauma in congenital diaphragmatic hernia: a clinicopathological correlation. J Pediatr Surg 34:1813–1817

Seidner SR, Jobe AH, Coalson JJ, Ikegami M (1998) Abnormal surfactant metabolism and function in preterm ventilated baboons. Am J Respir Crit Care Med 158:1982–1989

Spragg RG, Li J (2000) Effect of phosphocholine cytidylyltransferase overexpression on phosphatidylcholine synthesis in alveolar type II cells and related cell lines. Am J Respir Cell Mol Biol 22:116–124

Sullivan KM, Hawgood S, Flake AW, Harrison MR, Adzick NS (1994) Amniotic fluid phospholipid analysis in the fetus with congenital diaphragmatic hernia. J Pediatr Surg 29:1020–1023

Sun B, Curstedt T, Robertson B (1993) Surfactant inhibition in experimental meconium aspiration. Acta Paediatr 82:182–189

Sun B, Curstedt T, Robertson B (1996) Exogenous surfactant improves ventilation efficiency and alveolar expansion in rats with meconium aspiration. Am J Respir Crit Care Med 154:764–770

Tan RC, Ikegami M, Jobe AH, Yao LY, Possmayer F, Ballard PL (1999) Developmental and glucocorticoid regulation of surfactant protein mRNAs in preterm lambs. Am J Physiol 277:L1142–L1148

Torresin M, Zimmermann LJ, Cogo PE, Cavicchioli P, Badon T, Giordano G, Zacchello F, Sauer PJ,

Carnielli VP (2000) Exogenous surfactant kinetics in infant respiratory distress syndrome: a novel method with stable isotopes. Am J Respir Crit Care Med 161:1584–1589

Van Meurs K (2004) Is surfactant therapy beneficial in the treatment of the term newborn infant with congenital diaphragmatic hernia? J Pediatr 145:312–316

Verlato G, Cogo PE, Pesavento R, Gomirato S, Benettazzo A, Gucciardi A, Grazzini M, Carnielli VP (2003) Surfactant kinetics in newborn infants with pneumonia and Respiratory Distress Syndrome. Ital J Pediatr 29: 354–357

Verlato G, Cogo PE, Balzani M, Gucciardi A, Burattini I, De Benedictis F, Martiri G, Carnielli VP (2008) Surfactant status in preterm neonates recovering from respiratory distress syndrome. Pediatrics 122:102–108

Walther FJ, Ikegami M, Warburton D, Polk DH (1991) Corticosteroids, thyrotropin-releasing hormone, and antioxidant enzymes in preterm lamb lungs. Pediatr Res 30:518–521

Walther FJ, Jobe AH, Ikegami M (1998) Repetitive prenatal glucocorticoid therapy reduces oxidative stress in the lungs of preterm lambs. J Appl Physiol 85:273–278

Wilcox DT, Glick PL, Karamanoukian HL, Azizkhan RG, Holm BA (1995) Pathophysiology of congenital diaphragmatic hernia. XII: amniotic fluid lecithin/sphingomyelin ratio and phosphatidylglycerol concentrations do not predict surfactant status in congenital diaphragmatic hernia. J Pediatr Surg 30:410–412

Wiswell TE, Knight GR, Finer NN, Donn SM, Desai H, Walsh WF, Sekar KC, Bernstein G, Keszler M, Visser VE, Merritt TA, Mannino FL, Mastrioianni L, Marcy B, Revak SD, Tsai H, Cochrane CG (2002) A multicenter, randomized, controlled trial comparing surfaxin (lucinactant) lavage with standard care for treatment of meconium aspiration syndrome. Pediatrics 109:1081–1087

Wright JR, Dobbs LG (1991) Regulation of pulmonary surfactant secretion and clearance. Annu Rev Physiol 53:395–414

Respiratory Distress Syndrome: Predisposing Factors, Pathophysiology, and Diagnosis

53

Mikko Hallman, Timo Saarela, and Luc J. I. Zimmermann

Contents

M. Hallman (✉)
Department of Children and Adolescents, Oulu University Hospital, and PEDEGO Research Unit, Medical Research Center Oulu, University of Oulu, Oulu, Finland
e-mail: mikko.hallman@oulu.fi

T. Saarela
Department of Children and Adolescents, Oulu University Hospital, Oulu, Finland
e-mail: Timo.Saarela@ppshp.fi

L. J. I. Zimmermann
Department of Pediatrics and Neonatology, School for Oncology and Developmental Biology (GROW), Maastricht University Medical Center, Maastricht, The Netherlands
e-mail: luc.zimmermann@mumc.nl

G. Buonocore et al. (eds.), *Neonatology*,
https://doi.org/10.1007/978-3-319-29489-6_289

Abstract

Due to increased survival and new treatment strategies, new phenotypes of respiratory distress syndrome (RDS) have emerged. RDS in near-term to term infants is characterized by seemingly effortless breathing and tendency to pulmonary hypertension that can be avoided by expectant management. Common preventable cause is elective delivery before full 40 weeks of pregnancy. Sometimes these infants possess rare alleles retarding lung development. Extremely preterm infants are often affected by intrauterine inflammation, accelerating surfactant maturity. Despite new noninvasive treatment practices, initially mild RDS tends to become prolonged and develops to BPD. This is due to deficient antioxidant, anti-inflammatory, and antimicrobial capacity; predisposition to airway injury, alveolar flooding, and surfactant inactivation by multiple mechanisms are discussed. Genetic factors predisposing very preterm infants to RDS are intertwined with acquired risks: lack of labor, non-presenting twin, and adverse metabolic environment (e.g., hyperinsulinemia). Antenatal steroid, inducing structural maturity and stimulating functional maturity, is the cornerstone of prevention of RDS and the developmental diseases prior to week 34. Currently steroid supplementation in RDS is not recommended.

53.1 Salient Points

- RDS is the most common serious disease affecting the newborn.
- Advances in neonatal care have led to a decrease in mortality rates.
- Half of the infants with RDS are born between 29 and 34 weeks of gestation; symptoms of respiratory distress appear soon after birth and surfactant administration limits the progression of the disease.
- In extremely preterm infants, RDS tends to have a prolonged course and develops into BPD through many intertwined mechanisms.
- Antenatal steroid administration to the pregnant women, by inducing structural lung maturity and stimulating functional maturity, are the cornerstone of prevention of RDS.

53.2 Introduction

Respiratory distress syndrome of newborn infants (RDS), called infantile RDS or IRDS, previously idiopathic RDS or hyaline membrane disease (HMD), is the most common serious disease affecting the newborn. Since the description of hyaline membranes by Hochheim in 1903, the pathogenesis and etiology were

studied (Obladen 1992). During past 50 years, the advances in neonatal intensive have led to striking improvement in prognosis in advanced perinatal centers, changing the phenotype of RDS and allowing the decrease in RDS mortality from nearly 50% to close to 5%. In addition, infants born extremely preterm (<28 weeks) previously died at birth. Today nearly all survive long enough to develop RDS.

In 1926, Van Neergard described the hysteresis of the lung. The significance of this finding was not appreciated until surface activity was described by Clements and Pattle in the 1950s (Obladen 1992). As a consequence, Avery and Mead (1959) discovered that the airways of infants dying of HMD had high surface tension (Avery and Mead 1959). This finding was further tested several years later when dipalmitoyl phosphatidylcholine was nebulized to the airways in RDS with disappointing results (Chu et al. 1967). It took the death of President Kennedy's son Patrick on HMD in 1963 to activate the research on RDS. After defining the surfactant system and lung structures in more detail, followed by therapeutic trials using natural surfactant, an increase in the survival and an acute, dramatic decrease in the severity of RDS became evident (Robertson and Taeusch 1995). Antenatal glucocorticoid therapy (AGC) in threatened preterm birth was shown by Liggins and Howie in 1971 to decrease the risk of RDS (Liggins and Howie 1972). The acceptance of AGC in common clinical use was delayed until around the introduction of surfactant therapy in the early 1990s.

Surfactant therapy, AGC, effective ventilator treatment practices, and several supplementary treatment strategies have improved the survival and decreased the risk of RDS. Organ injuries associated with RDS and the phenotype of RDS have become remarkably less distinct ("the new RDS"). However, the risk of bronchopulmonary dysplasia (BPD) continues to be prevalent among infants born extremely preterm (ELGA, <28 weeks). Genetic and constitutional factors, most notably the length of gestation as a proxy of the degree of lung development, influence clinical management and outcome.

53.3 Risk Factors

RDS is characterized by typical features of respiratory insufficiency shortly after birth. The primary cause in most cases is lung immaturity that results in deficient gas exchange and acute lung injury. The clinical features depend on a number of interactive constitutional, genetic, and acquired factors and particularly on therapeutic practices. The risk factors have decreased as a result of improved antenatal anticipation of preterm birth, pharmacologic acceleration of fetal lung maturity, and of early treatment practices at birth.

The reported incidence of RDS among term-born infants is one in 2000 (Marttila et al. 2004). Elective delivery without labor before 40th week of pregnancy is expected to increase the risk of RDS. The incidence increases by each week of decreasing the length of gestation. At 34–36 weeks, it has ranged from 5% to 10%, at 30–33 weeks from 10% to 35%, and at 28–29 weeks from 30% to 50%, and in ELGA infants, the risk exceeds 50%. In the USA, the reported incidence is often higher. More recently the gestational age of the RDS population has decreased. This has taken place because of the successful prevention of RDS in the preterm population and increased early survival of newborn infants with very low gestation. Figure 1 shows schematically the risk and mortality of RDS and application of therapies during the past 45 years.

Increased risk of RDS is associated with elective deliveries without labor in late-preterm (34–36 weeks) and early-term (37–38 weeks) pregnancies (Gerten et al. 2005; Ramachandrappa and Jain 2008), lack of AGC before 34 weeks of pregnancy (Roberts and Dalziel 2006), and Caucasian (vs. African) ethnicity. Surfactant supplementation at preterm birth and continuous distending pressure ventilation from birth may abolish typical symptoms (Morley et al. 2008; Sandri et al. 2010). Males have a higher risk than females, the difference corresponding to a mean of 1 week of gestation (Table 1). The length of gestation interacts with other risk factors. Multiple birth increases the risk

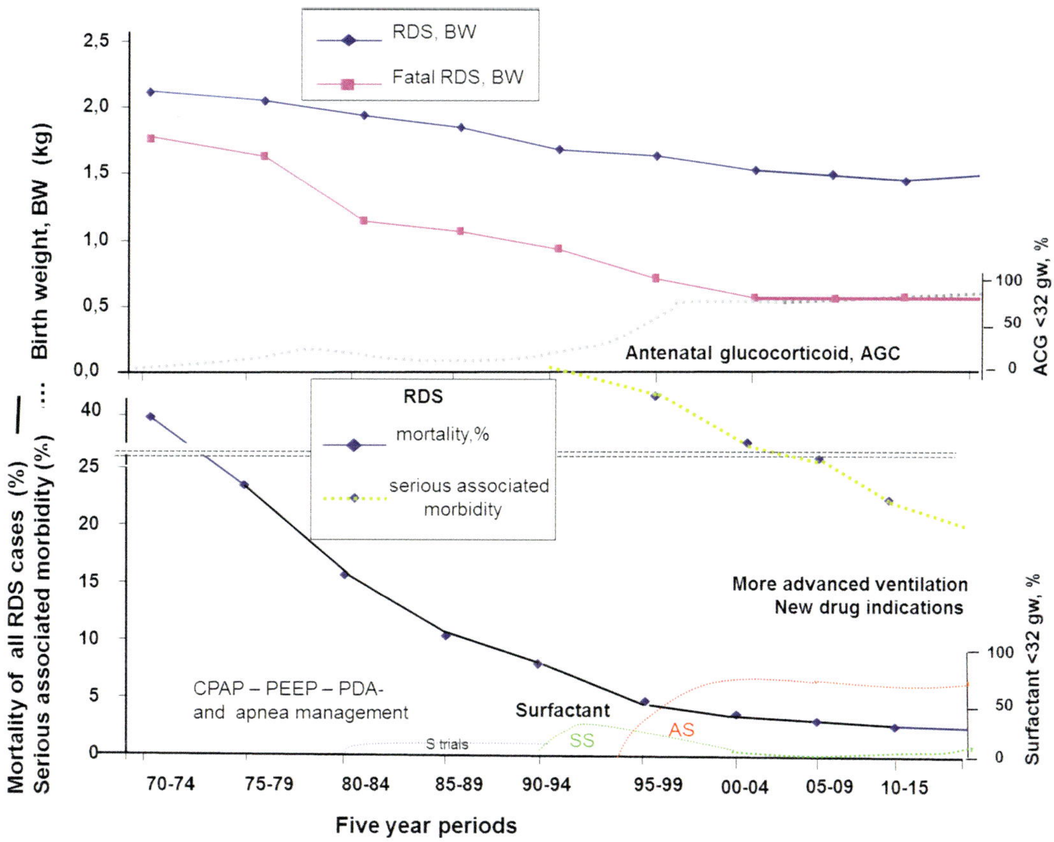

Fig. 1 Demographics of RDS during development of perinatal-neonatal treatment practices. Trends in mortality and in birth weights during 1970–2014. The figures are from Finland with prematurity rate ranging from 5.2% to 6.0% and the incidence of RDS in the range of 0.4 0.6% during the past 25 years. WHO definition of live birth was introduced in 1989. Serious associated morbidity includes bronchopulmonary dysplasia, patent ductus arteriosus, necrotizing enterocolitis, intraventricular hemorrhage gr 2–4. *S* surfactant trials, *SS* the incidence synthetic surfactant treatment of infants <32 week's gestation, *AS* animal surfactant (The figures are obtained from hospital records and from the Finnish Perinatal Register (Finnish National Institute for Health and Welfare; Dr. Mika Gissler))

of RDS in ELGA births and is a protective factor at 30 weeks or later (Marttila et al. 2004). The presenting twin has a lower risk of RDS (but higher risk of infection) than the non-presenting one. Chorioamnionitis decreases the risk of RDS in ELGA births (Watterberg et al. 1996; Kaukola et al. 2009). Maternal diabetes and fetal hydrops increase the risk of RDS. There is no consensus, whether preeclampsia or intrauterine growth restriction (IUGR) influences the risk. However, chronic retroplacental bleeding (circumvallate placenta) is associated with acceleration of lung maturity.

53.3.1 Genetic Factors Influencing Susceptibility to RDS

According to available twin studies comparing the concordance of RDS between monozygotic and dizygotic same sex preterm twins, a direct genetic contribution to the susceptibility to RDS has been small (~20%). Instead, detectable effects of individual genes are due to gene-gene or gene-environment interactions. They undermine the estimates of the genetic effects on the basis of twin studies. For instance, the presenting twin has a lower risk of RDS compared to the

Table 1 Pregnancy-related states and complications associated with altered risk of RDS as compared to gestation controls

Accelerated maturation or control	Control or delayed maturation
Vaginal birth	Elective birth with labor
Elective birth with labor	Elective low risk birth w/o labor: late preterm or early term (37–38 weeks)
Female fetus	Male fetus
Closeness to cervix in twin pregnancy (presenting)	Remote to cervix in twin pregnancy (non-presenting)
First born twin pair >28 weeks, no infection	Second born twin pair >28 weeks
Singleton <28 weeks	Twin <28 weeks
Twin 30–36 weeks	Singleton 30–36 weeks
Control <28 weeks	Preeclampsia <28 weeks
Chorioamnionitis 24–29 weeks[a]	Control 24–29 weeks
Gestation control	Poor control of maternal diabetes, fetal hydrops, severe isoimmunization

[a]Mostly histologic chorioamnionitis. Clinical chorioamnionitis, when associated with fetal infection, is associated with respiratory distress mimicking RDS

non-presenting one, and the magnitude of this difference is influenced by gene-environment interaction (Marttila et al. 2003; Hallman and Haataja 2007). RDS in late-preterm and early-term infants has likely a different genetic background compared to RDS infants with shorter gestation at birth. The rare alleles with significant adverse effect to respiratory function are more likely in RDS cases with near-term or term gestation.

Mutations that may disrupt surfactant function include *SP-B*, *ABCA3*, and *SP-C* genes. They cause fatal or severe chronic lung disease that initially resembles RDS (Wert et al. 2009). Mutations involving transcription factors TTF-1, C/EBPα, FOXA2, a glucocorticoid receptor NR3C1, and some other genes generally delay differentiation of specific functions, including the surfactant system, causing serious respiratory distress and often other symptoms (Whitsett et al. 2010). Several other proteins, including SP-A and SP-D, have important, partly redundant functions that influence the susceptibility to infections and inflammatory insults. Genes with identified roles in lung function have mutations or common allelic variants that influence surfactant function in stress or have no detectable effect. Studies thus far show that some genes expressed in type 2 cells influence the individual risk of RDS, including polymorphism of *SP-A*, *SP-B*, *SP-C*, and *ABCA3* (Hallman and Haataja 2007). According to genetic studies, mediators influencing the risk of spontaneous premature birth and the risk of RDS are partly intertwined: SP-A and SP-D influence cytokine responses mediating surfactant synthesis and preterm labor process (Karjalainen et al. 2012).

The genetic studies on the susceptibility to RDS have thus far been focused on major alleles of the likely candidate genes (i.e., surfactant proteins). For more objective data on candidate genes and alleles, very large, non-biased, population-based studies, their replicates, and meta-analyses are required. Genome-wide association analyses (GWAS) and whole-genome studies involving siblings are appropriate. Eventually research may help redefine the disease and its treatment.

53.4 Symptoms and Clinical Findings

53.4.1 Respiratory Course and Lung Function in RDS

Natural course of RDS is characterized by early rapid progression of respiratory distress leading to respiratory failure and often death in the absence of treatment within 1–48 h. The stabilization phase of respiratory distress is followed by the recovery phase, starting within 1–6 days after birth and continuing longer than progressive phase. The unifying features in RDS are the transient deficiency of surfactant in epithelial lining and the early lung injury. Cyanosis is evaluated by oxygen saturation monitoring and right-to-left circulatory shunt by measuring the arterial blood gases and calculating the alveolar-arterial O_2 tension difference. Soon after birth, the breath sounds are often diminished; later stridor may be evident.

Early RDS is characterized by low functional residual capacity, low compliance, and high venous admixture, indicating diffuse atelectasis. The early lung injury often involves peripheral airways causing obstructive small airway disease in full-blown RDS. The short inspiratory time constant early in the course of RDS increases as a sign of airway obstruction (Baldwin et al. 2006). Modest abnormalities in lung function may persist even weeks and will be evident at term after the recovery from uncomplicated RDS, and particularly when it is complicated with BPD (Hjalmarson et al. 2014). Surfactant therapy in RDS increases acutely functional residual capacity, decreases venous admixture, more gradually increases the compliance, and has little effect on airway resistance.

The post-hospitalization course of children with RDS without development of BPD reveals increased incidence of wheezing during infections and therefore higher hospitalization rates during first 2 years of life, suggesting residual lung injury or excessive immune response during infection (Koivisto et al. 2005; Jones 2009 Kotecha et al. 2013). Very premature birth (<32 weeks, VLGA), followed by treatment of RDS with modern methods and no BPD, is associated with a barely detectable impact on FEV1 and diffusion capacity in school children compared to term-born controls (Ronkainen et al. 2015).

53.4.2 Course of RDS in Preterm Infants

Half of the infants with RDS are born between 29 and 34 weeks of gestation. First symptoms are observed very soon after birth. Tachypnea, nasal flaring, subcostal and intercostal retractions, cyanosis, and expiratory grunt are characteristic, although not very specific, findings since transient tachypnea is initially nearly indistinguishable. In RDS, the symptoms continue longer than 24 h, unless specific therapies are applied.

The progression of respiratory distress is decreased or prevented by continuous distending pressures and by surfactant therapy. As a result of rather mild symptoms, the diagnosis remains suggestive, unless pre-treatment surfactant diagnostics are available or the patient has distinct favorable response to exogenous surfactant. The surfactant-induced remission is sometimes followed by relapse requiring retreatment. The response to exogenous surfactant is less predictable and generally less striking if surfactant is given later (>6 h after birth). Some develop signs of patent ductus arteriosus (PDA). Apnea, infection, and pneumothorax are rare complications.

53.4.3 Extremely Preterm Infants

Infants born before 28 weeks of gestation have simplified saccular airways, no true alveoli, and wide interstitial spaces. The highly compliant chest cage generates striking retractions despite moderate negative pleural pressures. The low surfactant pool is susceptible to abundant inhibitors. Without treatment, the infants often die before development of RDS. Providing continuous distending pressures and if necessary to gentle ventilation limits the emerging lung injury. Surfactant treatment in delivery room or within few hours after birth typically induces a sustained remission characterized by acute lowering of supplemental O_2 requirements and less acute lowering of airway pressure requirements. Relapse of respiratory failure often takes place, indicating retreatment. The course of RDS is characterized by a high incidence of cardiopulmonary complications, particularly PDA. Air leak syndrome (pneumothorax, interstitial emphysema), pulmonary hypertension, and pulmonary hemorrhage are less common. RDS particularly in this group is associated with complicating diseases: BPD, intraventricular hemorrhage (IVH), necrotizing enterocolitis (NEC), and retinopathy of prematurity (ROP). The incidence of complicating diseases varies from NICU to another.

Despite AGC, noninvasive ventilation, early surfactant, and other adjunct treatments, such as late cord clamping, caffeine, and inhaled nitric oxide or selective postnatal glucocorticoid, a significant risk of BPD and other adverse effects remain (Schmidt et al. 2008; Bassler et al. 2015).

53.4.4 Late-Preterm and Early-Term Infants

Late-preterm (35–36 gw) and early-term infants with RDS are mostly born electively without active labor. Other risk factors include acute asphyxia and poorly controlled maternal diabetes; genetic predisposition is a likely underlying cause (Ramachandrappa and Jain 2009). In RDS, the breathing is rapid but apparently effortless as the stable chest cage does not often reveal retractions and chest X-ray finding may be inconclusive. Ignoring early treatment of respiratory distress and hypoxemia escalates the later respiratory course. Persistence of pulmonary hypertension (PPHN) or pneumothorax are occasional complications. Studies reveal surfactant insufficiency despite atypical presentation.

The developmental stage explains the phenotype. The small size of newly developed true alveoli predisposes to therapy-resistant atelectasis. The stable chest cage and strong respiratory drive generates high transpulmonary pressures during inspiration, expanding alveolar ducts, improving the clearance of edema fluid. The pulmonary vasculature has a prominent smooth muscular layer that extends distally; hypoxemia-induced contractility predisposes to pulmonary hypertension.

The clinical recovery often takes place within a rather short period. Continuing severe respiratory symptoms much beyond early neonatal period raises the possibility of a rare lung disease, particularly hereditary interstitial lung disease due to multiple specific causes (▶ Chap. 59, "Rare Lung Diseases of Newborns").

53.5 Diagnostics

The diagnosis is based on a combination of characteristic symptoms, clinical findings, and the chest X-ray. Typical chest X-ray features reveal a diffuse reticulogranularity with superimposed air bronchograms (Fig. 2), indicating atelectasis and edema of respiratory units, distal to respiratory bronchioles. The prominent air bronchogram representing aerated bronchi and larger bronchioles become distinct when they are superimposed on a background of atelectatic lung parenchyma. The severity of RDS on the basis of the chest X-ray has been graded (Avery et al. 1981). The grade is likely modified several hours after exogenous surfactant. Pulmonary whiteout (grade 4) is generally a sign of a severe disease; it is also observed in mild disease very soon after birth (<1 h). Pulmonary edema and prominent heart shadow is a typical X-ray finding in RDS complicated by PDA. In near-term RDS population, reticulogranularity tends to be less distinct and the lung fields may reveal ground glass appearance. In some cases lung fields appear hyper-expanded; this entity is called type 2 RDS.

Lung ultrasound (LUS) diagnostics has been recently reported as a tool for prediction of respiratory failure (Sundell et al. 1971). LUS examined within 1 h after the admission on 59 infants with respiratory distress accurately predicted RDS ($n = 23$) with sensitivity and specificity of 95.6% and 94.4%, respectively (Vergine et al. 2014). This method is still investigational.

Analysis of surfactant component or surface activity of specimens performed on gastric or airway aspirates at birth differentiates RDS with specificity of and sensitivity of 50–75% and 80–97%, respectively (Verder et al. 2003; Hallman et al. 1986). The false-positive prediction can be due to blood contamination or to surfactant retention due to airway liquid adsorption. A simple, rapid, and accurate bedside method would be useful, if available.

53.5.1 Differential Diagnosis

Transient tachypnea (wet lung) becomes clearly distinguishable from RDS within several hours after birth. Bacterial pneumonia, mostly due to Group B *Streptococcus*, often coincides with RDS. In pulmonary infection, pleural exudate, focal infiltrates, and sepsis are common. Amniotic aspiration pneumonia, particularly meconium aspiration, is easily distinguished by the appearance of viscous, often green aspirate, typically in post-term or term infant. Congenital chylothorax is distinguished by typical milky appearance of lipid-rich

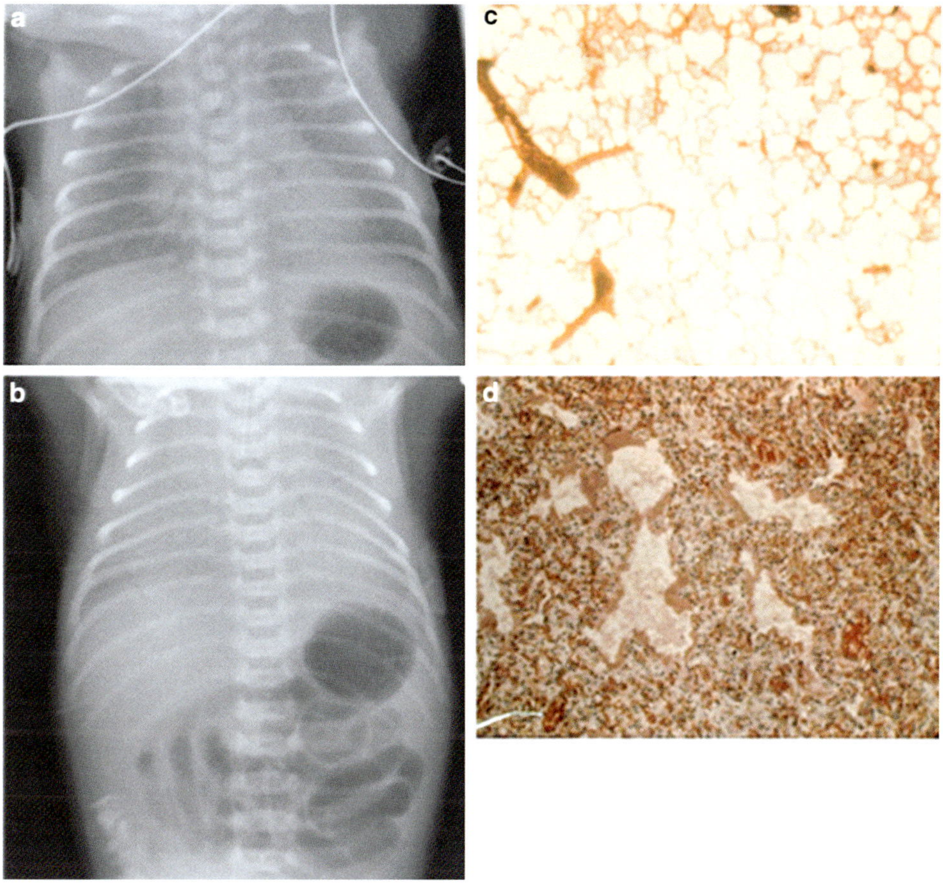

Fig. 2 Typical radiographic and pathological findings of RDS. Typical chest X-rays representing RDS of infant during surfactant (**a**) and pre-surfactant era (**b**). Autopsy findings from normal (**c**) and HMD (**d**) lungs

pleural exudate after enteral feeding. Rare cases of small preterm infants with minimal respiratory distress develop cystic interstitial emphysema soon after birth (Wilson-Mikity syndrome) (Hoepker et al. 2008), a form of obstructive inflammatory lung disease that resembles "new BPD" with minimal respiratory distress at birth.

Congenital cardiac diseases associated with respiratory distress and congestive edema, most notably anomalous pulmonary venous return with abnormal infra diaphragmatic pulmonary vein return (Scimitar syndrome), require early diagnosis and surgery. Equally critical is the prompt diagnosis and early onset of prostaglandin E2 infusion for maintenance of ductal patency and pulmonary circulation of ductus-dependent cardiac defects. Early respiratory distress due to diaphragmatic hernia, other causes of lung hypoplasia, cystic adenomatous malformation, esophagus atresia, isolated fistula, lung sequestration, tumors, and malformations require early diagnosis and specific treatment strategies.

A slow recovery from RDS may be a constitutional feature with likely genetic involvement. Failure to recover is a feature of congenital interstitial lung disease due to a mutation in genes that are essential in postnatal lung function (Wert et al. 2009). PPHN mostly develops as a consequence of primary lung disease, often RDS. Alveolar capillary dysplasia with misalignment of pulmonary vessels is suspected on the basis of persistence of acute severe defect in gas exchange; autopsy diagnosis increasingly has identified genetic background (Bishop et al. 2011).

Acute (also called acquired or adult) respiratory distress syndrome (ARDS) may develop in severe infection or asphyxia also in newborn infants. These patients often have beneficial response to a high dose of exogenous surfactant. However, surfactant therapy has not significantly improved the outcome of this severe, heterogeneous syndrome that requires proper antibiotics and comprehensive cardiopulmonary management.

53.6 Predisposing Factors

The lung has developed relatively late in evolution (~250 million years), and human evolution is recent (~5 million years). The regulation of the expression of individual genes generates much of the diversity in human genome. The regulation of the birth process and the involvement of the fetus in the transition is particularly species specific. Preterm birth is exceptionally common in human species. Spontaneous preterm birth particularly in chorioamnionitis (CA) accelerates surfactant maturity decreasing the risk of RDS. The peripheral lining of air spaces at 20–22 weeks of gestation contains epithelial cells that morphologically resemble type 2 cells, and pulmonary capillaries align with future potential airways. Later in gestation, both the number of type 2 cells and the content of lamellar bodies increase. At term, the surfactant content of the lungs reaches maximum and has a critical role in adaptation. Other pulmonary host defense systems have distinct perinatal developmental patterns as well.

53.6.1 Surfactant System

The major surfactant component, dipalmitoyl phosphatidylcholine (DPPC), concentrates at the air liquid interphase as a tightly packed lipid film (Fig. 3). Other surfactant components provide the extraordinary rapid surface adsorption of DPPC. These include phosphatidylcholine (PC) containing unsaturated fatty acids, often unsaturated phospholipids containing anionic charge [phosphatidylglycerol (PG), phosphatidylinositol (PI)] and hydrophobic surfactant proteins (SP-B and SP-C). The latter contain stretches of hydrophobic amino acids interrupted by hydrophilic amino acids with cationic charge. Natural surfactant additionally contains SP-A and SP-D: they are collagen-containing lectins that have roles in innate immunity, surfactant metabolism, and formation of tubular myelin.

The hydrophobic components are synthesized in ER, followed by serial cleavage of hydrophilic stretches of SP-B- and SP-C proproteins, and they are transported to intracellular lamellar bodies (LB) (Fig. 3). After secretion from LB into the alveolar lining, hydrophobic surfactant binds Ca^{++} and SP-A, transforming to aggregates that resemble tubular myelin and have instantaneous surface adsorption. During breathing movements, surfactant aggregates are transformed to smaller vesicles. Only a minor fraction of the surfactant complex is removed by cilia, and most of it is taken up by both alveolar macrophages (AM) and type 2 (T2) alveolar cells. Surfactant is catabolized in these cells and additionally reutilized in T2 cells.

Lowering of Surface Tension Surfactant greatly reduces surface tension thus preventing the collapse of small airspaces. Surface tension during expiration is assumed to be close to zero, and it rarely rises above 20 mN/m during normal expiration. Surfactant additionally serves as a lubricant that reduces barotrauma.

Immune Functions and Ancillary Proteins Individual surfactant components serve as immune modulators influencing together with AM and other systems in defense against microbes and other insults. Several surfactant components inhibit the signaling of the Toll-like receptors.

The coincidence of pneumonia and RDS reflects the immaturity of the innate immune system. The major defense functions of surfactant components are focused against airborne microbes, involving in their destruction without evoking excessive inflammatory response: most surfactant components are involved (PG, PI, SP-C, SP-B, SPPC, and PC). Surfactant collections, SP-A and SP-D, inhibit Toll-like receptor (TLR) signaling,

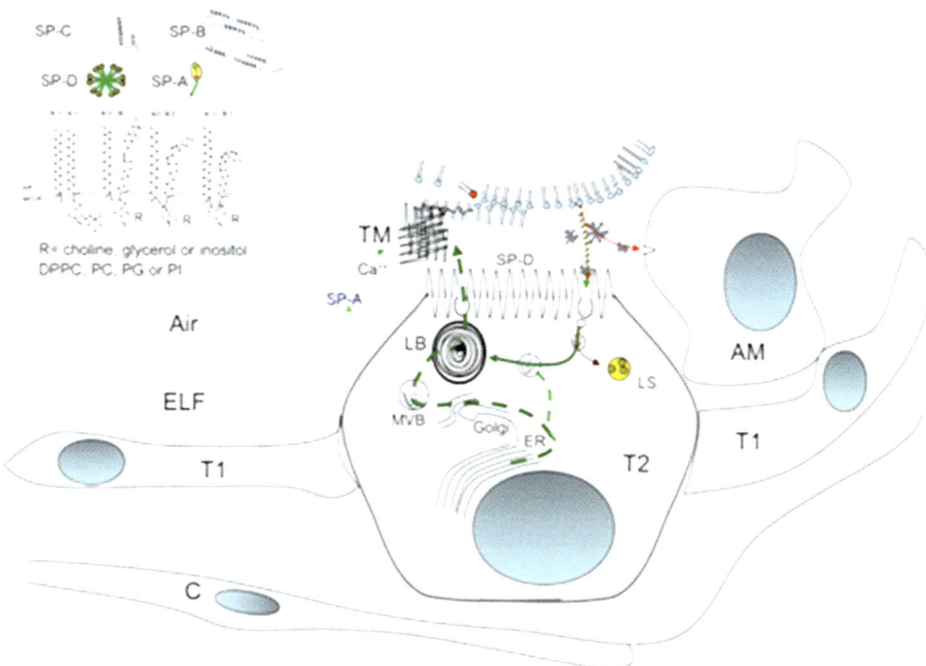

Fig. 3 Surfactant metabolism in alveolar epithelial cells and in epithelial lining fluid (*ELF*). Surfactant is synthesized endoplasmic reticulum (*ER*) of type 2 (*T2*) cells. Surfactants (DPPC, PC, PG, PI, SP-B, and SP-C) are synthesized in endoplasmic reticulum (*ER*) and processed via Golgi and multivesicular bodies (*MVB*) into lamellar bodies (*LB*). SP-A and SP-A are processed by constitutional pathway. After release of LB content into alveoli, surfactant binds SP-A and transforms to tubular myelin (*TM*) figures. In ELF, surfactant is transformed to smaller vesicles that are taken up by alveolar macrophages (*AM*) and T2 cells for either catabolism in lysosomes (*LS*) or for reprocessing into LB (recycling). In RDS, surfactant in ELF is deficient at birth, and it increases to near-control level within a few days after birth. At the same time, acquired surfactant defects appear as a result of airway and alveolar injury

aggregate viruses, and stimulate phagocytosis of bacteria. Collectins, absent in exogenous surfactants, are proposed to serve important functions in innate immunity (Wright 2005).

Regulation of Surfactant System: An Example of Antenatal Regulation of Functional Maturity - Glucocorticoid is the main hormone regulating spontaneous functional differentiation of the lung (Bird et al. 2015). The effects of glucocorticoid on the surfactant system are mediated by several pathways, one being fibroblast-derived growth factor that influences the differentiation of type 2 alveolar epithelial cells involved in surfactant synthesis and secretion. Glucocorticoid typically promotes differentiation of other functions in lung and in other organs and structural maturation of the lung. High persistent glucocorticoid activity decreases the growth. Absent glucocorticoid activity in fetus leads to lung hypercellularity, lack of functional differentiation, and respiratory failure at birth. Other hormones contributing to biochemical lung maturity include adrenergic agents, thyroid hormone, and prolactin, whereas testosterone delays lung maturity. Several other growth factors and cytokines also influence the differentiation and growth of alveolar tissue (Torday and Rehan 2015).

Besides regulation of normal differentiation, inflammatory cytokine and corticosteroid signal both the acceleration of lung maturation and spontaneous preterm labor in chorioamnionitis (Kallapur et al. 2014). IL-1 has been identified as a primary agonist upregulating the surfactant system in intrauterine inflammation (Bry et al. 1997). Lipopolysaccharide from cell wall of Gram bacteria (LPS or endotoxin) or inflammatory cytokine introduced to the amniotic fluid

accelerates differentiation of the surfactant and induces lung inflammation that extends systemically. Severe systemic infections and very high cytokine levels associate with adverse fetal consequences.

Secondary Injuries Affecting Lung and Surfactant System Pulmonary interstitium, individual lung cells, including T2 cells, and the surfactant system are exposed to multiple inflammatory and biochemical insults as part of the manifestation of lung injury in RDS: disruption of ER processing of surfactant components, inhibition, inactivation, degradation, de-aggregation, and displacement of surfactant complex have been documented (Mulugeta et al. 2015; Sáenz et al. 2010). Despite lung injury, RDS is mostly a self-healing disease, as the activation of differentiation-promoting inflammatory cytokines and of the anti-inflammatory endocrine axis promotes spontaneous maturation and healing.

In infants developing RDS, generally very low although variable quantities of surfactant are present in the airways at birth. Surfactant sufficiency is established within 2–7 days in most cases (Hallman et al. 1994; Carnielli et al. 2009). In infants at risk of BPD, the surfactant proteins and surface activity in the air spaces continue to be deficient after the first week of life. Excessive inflammation and other toxins suppress surfactant synthesis and function. The inactivated surfactant is degraded and replaced by newly synthesized surfactant. As yet unidentified step(s) in surfactant turnover is deficient in infants developing BPD.

53.6.2 Secretion of Fetal Lung Liquid and Induction of Liquid Absorption

During the second trimester, the rapidly growing fetal lung secretes Cl^- (150 mEq/L) from epithelial lining of air spaces and airways (Olver et al. 2004). This results in osmosis-driven liquid secretion of 0.2–0.5 l per 24 h of protein-poor liquid or 5–15% of total liquid intake into the amniotic cavity. At the same time, 6–9% of the cardiac output is perfusing lung tissue. A normal fetus makes periodic breathing movements with a small tidal volume (0.2–3 mL), resulting in transfer of liquid in and out from the airways. Toward the end of the second trimester, most of the amniotic fluid originates from hypotonic fetal urine, and it is cleared by fetal swallowing, with a turnover time of ~48 h.

The secretion of the lung liquid, tidal respiratory movements, and airway contractility dilate the future peripheral airways. The tidal movements of the chest wall deliver some of the amniotic fluid content to the airways. Experimental ligation of the fetal airways expands the future airways and inhibits lung maturity. Lack of fetal breathing movements leads to poor lung growth. Lack of amniotic fluid or compression of lungs (diaphragmatic hernia, intrathoracic tumor, small chest cage) causes lung hypoplasia if present from midpregnancy (Potter syndrome from fetal anuria in particular).

Chloride ion exits the epithelial cells of the airways and alveoli through apical anion-selective channels, including cystic fibrosis transmembrane regulator protein (CFTR). The driving force of the pump is linked to the Na^+,K^+-ATPase activity, generating the electrical potential difference allowing basolateral entry of Cl^- (Fig. 4).

Absorption of the Fetal Lung Liquid is Linked to Surfactant Function Toward term the secretion of lung liquid secretion decreases dramatically. The lung liquid during active term labor decreases by 40–50% as a result of active absorption of lung water and surfactant concentrates in air spaces. Lung extracellular water further decreases by another 40% during the first 6 h of life after term birth. A bulk of it exits the lung during the first breaths as the permeability of epithelium in small airways and air spaces increases acutely (Fig. 4). Both T2 and T1 epithelial cells contain amiloride-sensitive ENaC protein complex, attached in the apical plasma membrane. Besides the luminal transporters, basolateral Na^+,K^+-ATPase and voltage gated Cl^- channels transport Na^+ and Cl^- ions to lung interstitium. Aquaporins facilitate the movement of water across cell membranes. In addition, a large transepithelial leak is induced

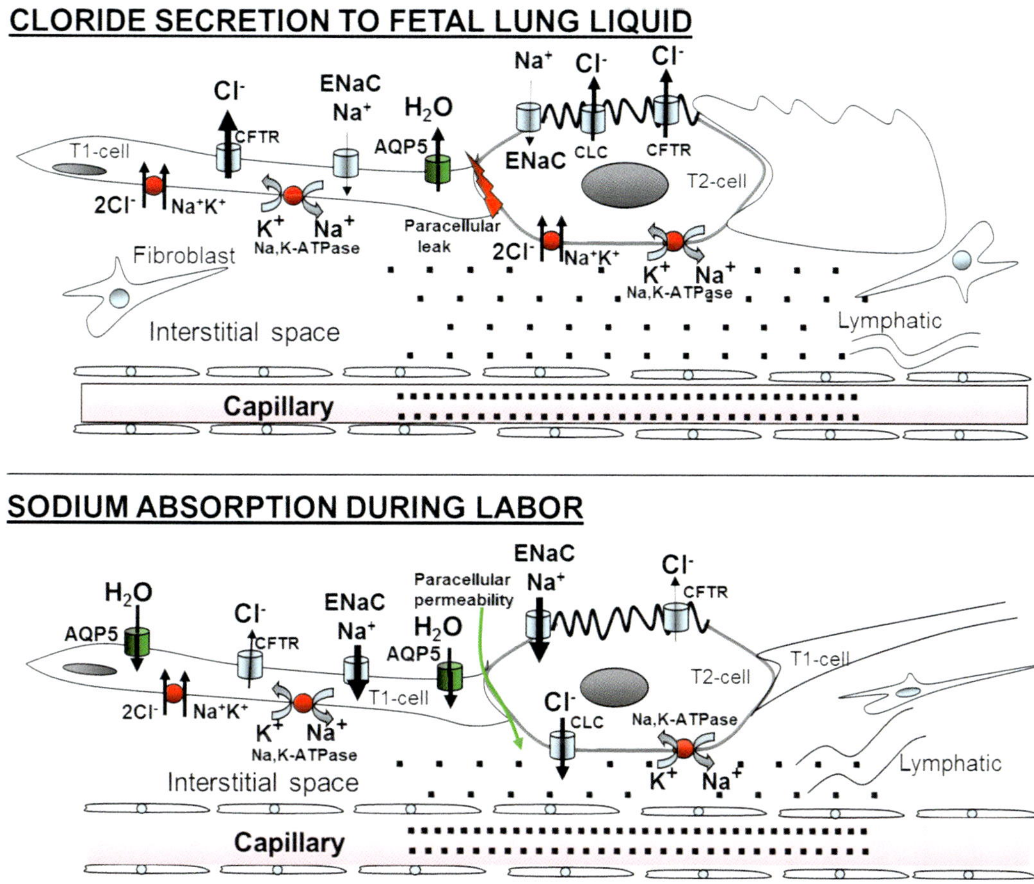

Fig. 4 Fetal lung liquid secretion (risk of RDS) and lung liquid absorption during labor (protective). Both are energy dependent driven by various transporters in the epithelial membranes. Glucocorticoid and adrenergic agents upregulate sodium channels (ENaC), promoting liquid absorption, together with aquaporins [*AQP5*] and Na^+, K^+-ATPase. Constitutional liquid secretion is driven by Na^+,K^+-Cl^- cotransporter (CLC). Cl^- exits the apical membrane through cystic fibrosis transmembrane conductance regulator (CFTR) and other channels. A paracellular leak across the epithelium is induced during first breaths after birth

at birth promoting bulk liquid from the airways (Van Driessche et al. 2007).

Adrenaline via cyclic AMP and corticosteroid induces the absorptive state of the fetal lung. Corticosteroid increases the synthesis of ENaC protein and adrenaline activates ENaC, particularly the rate-limiting ENaC-α. Cortisol increases as a result of activation of the pituitary-adrenal axis toward the term. Adrenalin increases during labor, and a further increase takes place shortly after birth.

In infants developing RDS, the ion channels responsible for clearance of the lung liquid are not active at birth. This is likely to aggravate the symptoms of RDS, and activation of ion channels involved in liquid adsorption is associated with the recovery. Wet lung syndrome is characterized by insufficient clearance of lung liquid and apparently critical deficiency of the active clearance mechanism (O'Brodovich 2005; Helve et al. 2009).

Induction of the active adsorptive state of fetal lung liquid during normal labor leads to retention and accumulation of surfactant in future air spaces and airways, providing the critical surfactant pool available at birth, thus facilitating the liquid clearance from airways and air spaces.

53.6.3 Structural Lung Development

During fetal development, there are changes in lung structure, including in the microanatomy and in the amount and composition of the extracellular matrix. These factors influence the phenotype of RDS.

During the canalicular phase between 16th and 25th weeks of gestation, the airway branching is complete and the lung transforms to organ, potentially capable of gas exchange (chapter by Moretti). This is accomplished by formation of cartilage, bronchial grands, and growth of the distal ends of the preacinar terminal bronchioles that grow and branch to two to four respiratory bronchioles. The potential gas exchange surface enlarges as a result of simultaneous vascular sprouting and acinar growth. Future airways and capillaries also approach each other, decreasing the length of gas diffusion path. The epithelium undergoes thinning from columnar to cuboidal form as type 2 cells differentiate.

During the saccular phase between 23 and 28–36 weeks, clusters of thin-walled saccules form the acinus that simultaneously expands and grows in length as the respiratory bronchioles divide into six–seven further generations by branching. Elastic fibers are deposited along the airways and capillaries. The capillaries still form a double capillary network between individual saccules.

Toward the end of gestation and particularly after birth, the elongated T1 alveolar cells expand and increasingly cover the alveolar lining, whereas surfactant-secreting T2 cells arrange around the alveolar corners. The alveolar stage involves microvascular maturation that starts preterm and continues during the first years. True alveoli grow from the walls of terminal saccules as spherical structures. They grow in size, and the inter-saccular tissue containing a double capillary network transforms into a single capillary network in close apposition to alveoli (Burri 2006).

53.7 Mechanisms of Lung Injury in RDS

Although the effect of surfactant therapy is often dramatic in reducing or even abolishing the symptoms of respiratory distress, in some cases its effect is either transient or in rare cases missing altogether. Transient effect endogenous surfactant is a sign of perturbed endogenous metabolism of surfactant and surfactant inhibitors. This emphasizes the interactive nature of factors influencing the alveolar stability, pulmonary circulation, and structural integrity, essential to the gas exchange function. These factors also include the conducting airways that are intimately involved in lung injury, pulmonary perfusion, and cardiac contractility. Ductus arteriosus increasingly remains open as the duration of pregnancy shortens, perturbing cardiopulmonary function and increasing lung edema. Regardless of length of gestation and pregnancy complications, diffuse atelectasis, lung edema, and hyaline membranes are a consequence of functional immaturity of alveolar epithelium. Infections and severe asphyxia, extreme immaturity, and other adverse events complicate and dominate the symptoms of cardiorespiratory distress. Figure 5 illustrates factors involved in pathogenesis.

53.7.1 Primary and Secondary Surfactant Deficiency

High surface tension retracts the air spaces with very small principal radii (R_1 and R_2) according to the law of Laplace: P (collapsing surface pressure) = γ (surface tension constant) × $\{1/R_1 + 1/R_2\}$.

In true alveoli or at the tip of respiratory ducts of immature lung, the two principal radii are very similar ($P = 2 \times \gamma/R$), whereas in tubular surfaces, the second radius is indefinite ($P = \gamma/R$). During inspiration, surfactant components adsorb to the lining, while during expiration, unsaturated lipids with higher surface tension are squeezed out from the lining, helping the surface tension to reach near-zero level. During tidal ventilation, surface tension increases slightly during inspiration and returns to near-zero during expiration (i.e., hysteresis) preventing atelectasis and decreasing alveolar edema. In the absence of surfactant, the tendency to atelectasis is due to the high surface pressures that increase during expiration. Surface tension in vitro is measured quantitatively using captive bubble or pulsating bubble surfactometer. These measurements have been confirmed in

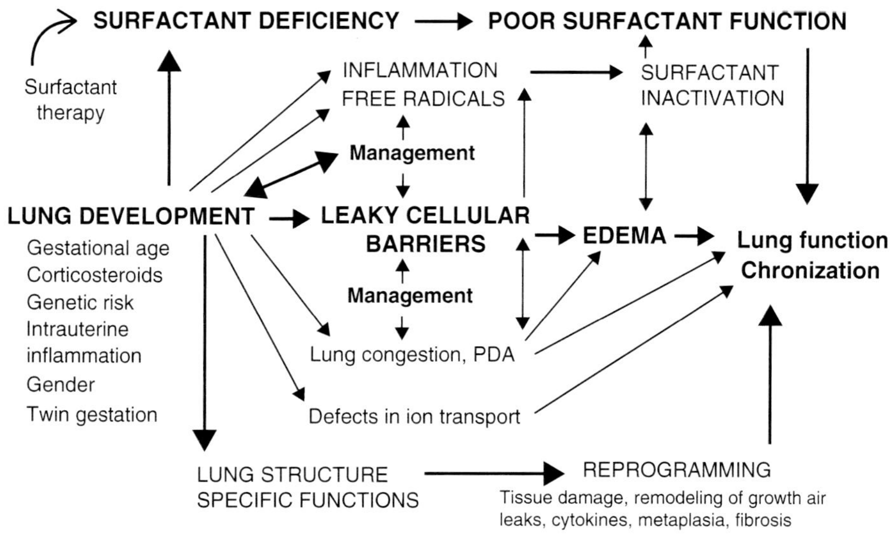

Fig. 5 Pathogenesis of RDS. Primary surfactant deficiency that is augmented by other defects in differentiation (e.g., lack of absorptive ion transport) and acquired factors (e.g., asphyxia, volutrauma). Persistence of lung injury is opposed by the lung healing, plasticity, and differentiation (e.g., induction/increase in surfactant)

situ by microscopy of the alveolar surface containing droplets of specific fluorocarbons with constant, generally low surface tension (Schürch et al. 2001).

During the first breaths, surfactant in lung liquid rapidly adsorbs and concentrates on the emerging air liquid interface. Lowering the surface tension (72 mN/m in isotonic saline) toward 0 mN/m decreases the force required for liquid clearance from narrow tubular structures and alveolar saccules; additional force required is due to viscous resistance of the small airways. Transient negative interstitial pressures generated during the first few forceful inspirations (as high as 50–70 cm H_2O) and airway pressures during forced expirations with semi-closed vocal cords, i.e., "first cry" (25–50 cm H_2O), are exceptionally high and contribute to the rapid paracellular increase in epithelial permeability and possibly injure immature airways. Low surface tension facilitates clearance of lung liquid and decreases airway injury.

Secondary surfactant defects emerge after birth. The leakage of proteinous liquid across the epithelial lining dilutes surfactant and inactivates surfactant (Hallman et al. 1991). Proteins, cationic amino acids, carbohydrates, and lipids inhibit surfactant function in vitro. Fibrin monomer is one of the most potent surfactant inhibitors described. Other mechanisms of surfactant inactivation include excess of proteolytic and phospholipase activities. Finally, oxidant injury by hydroxyl radicals and peroxynitrite and other noxious factors deteriorate surfactant function and metabolism (Sáenz et al. 2010; Hallman et al. 1994; Carnielli et al. 2009). Many of these noxious agents originate from inflammatory cells as a consequence of lung injury by barotrauma, hyperoxia, and endotoxins. ER stress and associated defect in intracellular processing and dysfunction of surfactant proteins is consistent with the observed abnormalities in surfactant composition and metabolism in infants developing BPD (Mulugeta et al. 2015).

53.7.2 Biotrauma

As a consequence of ante-, intra-, and postnatal events particularly those taking place at birth, the innate immune system is activated. The inflammatory reaction as a result of biotrauma induces both healing and tissue destruction (e.g., phagocytosis, oxidants, lytic proteins, oxidants, free radicals).

The degree of biotrauma depends on management practices, constitution, and hereditary factors. Both antenatal (e.g., antenatal steroid and antibiotics after preterm rupture of fetal membranes), delivery room (e.g., early introduction of PEEP, limitation of inspiratory pressures, noninvasive surfactant administration), and neonatal (early extubation, noninvasive ventilation, anti-inflammatory airway therapies, prevention of infections) treatment practices are primary aimed to decrease biotrauma. An experimental study by Jobe et al. illustrates an example of research on biotrauma (Hillman et al. 2007).

Besides the components of the surfactant system, other proteins, including Clara cell protein 16, SOD, eNAC, number of other anti-inflammatory peptides (e.g., defensins), signaling receptors, transcription factors, hormones, and growth factors, control the development of innate immunity.

53.7.3 Volutrauma and Barotrauma

Intubation and the associated bagging and mechanical ventilation without full control of the tidal volumes and pressures are the most important source of volutrauma and barotrauma. By increasing the airway pressure requirements, high surface tension influences volutrauma, i.e., overstretching of patent air spaces. Volutrauma predominates when large tidal volumes (>6–12 mL/kg) are delivered during mechanical ventilation shortly after birth (Hillman et al. 2007). It manifests as rupture, laceration, increase in permeability and compliance of central airways, perivascular edema, bronchiolar obstruction, and inflammatory response (biotrauma).

In RDS the minimum surface tension ranges from 20 to 50 mN/m. Distending pressures that maintain patency of alveoli with a radius of 50 μm or of alveolar ducts (very preterm) with radius of 100 μm is estimated to be 8–20 cm H_2O and 4–10 cm H_2O, respectively. High surface tension and high viscous resistance caused by airway edema and particles deteriorate lung homogeneity and predispose to volutrauma.

Volutrauma and barotrauma are decreased considerably by avoiding mechanical ventilation. Lack of lubricant property of surfactant contributes to barotrauma.

53.7.4 Delay in Clearance of Lung Liquid

Prenatal events influence the lung liquid adsorption and the amount of lung liquid at birth (Olver et al. 2004; Van Driessche et al. 2007; O'Brodovich 2005). Spontaneous labor, advanced gestation, and vaginal birth additively decrease the liquid in the airways at birth. In healthy human infants, the clearance of most airway liquid to lung interstitium takes place within seconds to minutes after the first breaths. Both active, energy-requiring, and passive pressure-driven mechanisms are stretch activated.

In normal adaptation, the clearance of liquid from lung interstitium takes place during the first day as the solute directly enters the circulation or is cleared via lymphatics. The bulk of the liquid removed from the airways accumulates in distensible perivascular spaces of large lung vessels and airways, away from the gas exchange path.

In very premature lung, low activities of developmentally regulated sodium and water transport weaken the absorptive state of premature fetal lung, delaying the accumulation of the surfactant pool before birth and the liquid clearance after birth (Van Driessche et al. 2007; Helve et al. 2009; Bland 2001). This is a major problem in elective late-preterm and early-term births: the alveolar surfactant pool at birth is small as a result of surfactant secretion into amniotic fluid and lack of adsorption of lung liquid.

Lung immaturity adversely affects lung liquid clearance as the compliant chest cage complicates generation of high negative interstitial pressures, and the activities involving ion and water transport across the epithelium toward lung interstitium are low. Diaphragmatic fatigue and particularly lack of respiratory drive due to deficient respiratory center responses contribute for alveolar edema and respiratory distress.

The passive stretch-activated bulk solute transfer takes place in both directions. It is thus responsible for either the clearance of lung fluid or the

formation of alveolar edema after very preterm birth. Edema is imminent, in case hydrostatic pressures (interstitial pressure and the airway distending pressure) fail to compensate for the high surface pressures in surfactant deficient lung.

53.7.5 High-Permeability Lung Edema

The injury of capillary endothelium and airway epithelial cells and their basement membranes is a characteristic early feature. The injury mechanisms include mechanical trauma, biotrauma, and toxins (oxygen). An important functional consequence is an increase in permeability to macromolecules soon after preterm birth. An increase in permeability exceeds the capacity of pulmonary lymphatics, resulting in interstitial edema. Small airways, bronchioles, and air spaces are susceptible to flooding and obstruction, and alveolar edema further decreases gas exchange.

Increased epithelial permeability leads to protein-rich alveolar edema and accumulation of surfactant inhibitors. Accumulation of fibrinogen into alveolar space precedes the formation of hyaline membranes. A residue of inactivated surfactant components and other residues are incorporated into the matrix of fibrin-rich hyaline membranes. They interfere with gas exchange, obstruct the air spaces, and may initiate intra-alveolar coagulation. Hyaline membranes are eventually cleared by phagocytosis and fibrinolytic activity (Idell et al. 1994).

Continuous distending pressure to the airways; avoidance of mechanical ventilation; avoidance of fluid overload, cardiac failure, and of infections; and activation of anti-inflammatory mechanisms (steroid) all contribute toward decreasing high-permeability lung edema.

53.7.6 Pulmonary Hemorrhage

Pulmonary hemorrhage complicates RDS mostly in extremely preterm infants. It may be seen as an extreme form of high-permeability lung edema that is associated with PDA, decrease in pulmonary vascular resistance, and rapidly developing left cardiac failure resulting in flooding of alveolar capillaries (e.g., in hypothermia). Hemorrhage may be precipitated by surfactant therapy as it lowers pulmonary vascular resistance increasing the left-to-right shunt through ductus arteriosus. Inadequate continuous positive airway pressure levels may further decrease pulmonary vascular resistance, allowing hydrostatic congestion and eventually rupture of capillaries and airway epithelium (▶ Chap. 55, "Pulmonary Hemorrhage, Transient Tachypnea, and Neonatal Pneumonia").

53.7.7 Abnormalities in Lung Perfusion

Acetylcholine, nitric oxide (NO), and potentially other vasoactive agents triggered dilate pulmonary arterioles during normal neonatal transition. During the early hours in RDS, the failure of alveolar capillary gas exchange may in part be due to poor perfusion of alveoli, whereas mainly in later stages of RDS, symptoms of pulmonary vascular congestion prevail. Pulmonary perfusion needs to be carefully considered throughout the respiratory course.

In extremely immature lung, the marginal size capillary bed barely provides a reservoir against hypo-hypervolemia and excessive distending pressures.

Besides lung hypoplasia, predisposition to PPHN can be the result of acute biotrauma, caused by microbes and inflammatory agents.

Prolonged rupture of fetal membranes in preterm infants is occasionally complicated by severe surfactant-nonresponsive respiratory distress, associated pulmonary hypertension, and low airway nitrite and inflammatory cytokine levels, suggesting transient immune paralysis. A dramatic, acute favorable response to inhaled NO has been demonstrated in several small studies. However, the actual improvement in the outcome has not been shown in a randomized trial (Aikio et al. 2012).

Increase in pulmonary vascular resistance in severe acute lung disease is well recognized (Steinhorn 2010). This applies also to RDS. Toward term, the muscularity of pulmonary

arteries increases. Treatment of RDS in near-term infants is often delayed, allowing progression of respiratory distress and development of PPHN that favorably responds to inhaled NO.

53.7.8 Patent Ductus Arteriosus (PDA)

Prostaglandin inhibitor-induced contraction of the fetal ductus arteriosus is detectable in the beginning in the third trimester and increases toward term. After birth, the cascade of events leading to permanent constriction followed by anatomical closure of the ductus takes place in nearly all term-born infants, whereas the degree of prematurity progressively increases the risk of hemodynamically significant PDA (Hamrick and Hansmann 2010).

PDA particularly in ELGA infants continues to be a challenge and an important factor influencing the duration of the course of RDS. A large left-to-right shunt through PDA causes pulmonary congestion at the expense of systemic perfusion. This sometimes happens within few days after birth, as a result of surfactant-induced remission of RDS that decreases pulmonary vascular resistance. Attempts to close ductus arteriosus during the first days after birth by indomethacin or ibuprofen or by ligation have been associated with serious side effects, including pulmonary hypertension and IVH. Appropriate emergency treatment of early PDA is to promote the treatment of lung edema, particularly by increasing inappropriately low continuous distending airway pressure and reducing excessive liquid intake. Adverse effects associating with PDA include pulmonary edema/IVH, NEC, ROP, and BPD. Antenatal glucocorticoid, neonatal caffeine, and inhaled budesonide decrease the risk of PDA. The potential benefit of paracetamol in early treatment of PDA is currently investigated.

53.8 Prevention of RDS

Obstetric and early neonatal management of preterm infants influence the risk and severity of RDS.

Available therapies convert RDS from lethal to manageable or preventable disease. The cost of treatment is high, and the disease may associate with complications that may be life-threatening (Gilbert 2006). In very preterm infants, RDS is a common disease that has a major influence in the risk of both acute and chronic morbidity.

53.8.1 Prevention of Premature Birth

Elimination of prematurity would be most effective in prevention. There are remarkable variation in the risk of prematurity based on the lifestyle, working conditions, risk behavior, ethnicity, socioeconomic status, and the healthcare system. In vitro fertilization practices increase the risk of premature birth.

Tocolytic agents have a limited capacity to prolong the pregnancy in threatened preterm labor. Despite side effects, they are shown to be efficacious in delaying the preterm birth for a few days required for full effect of ACG. Ca-channel antagonists delay preterm birth without causing serious adverse effects.

Supplementation of progesterone acetate from midterm pregnancies has reduced the prematurity rate only in rare cases of cervix insufficiency. Thus far, no long-term risks have been observed, and the follow-up continues (WHO 2015).

53.8.2 Pharmacological Acceleration of Fetal Lung Maturity

AGC became an accepted therapy for prevention of RDS first in the 1990s when the concerns of serious adverse long-term effects were not materialized (Liggins and Howie 1972; Roberts and Dalziel 2006). Glucocorticoid influences the development of the fetal lung, gastrointestinal tract, cardiovascular system, liver, kidney, and central nervous system. It accelerates the differentiation of the surfactant system, promotes the absorptive state of fetal lung, enhances the closure of ductus after birth, increases the generally low blood pressure of preterm infants shortly after

birth, improves the performance of the immature left ventricle, and has beneficial effects on the immune and antioxidant systems.

According to meta-analysis of randomized trials on AGC, it resulted in overall reduction of the risk of RDS (relative risk, RR 0.66, 95% CI 0.59–0.73). The most beneficial effect was observed when AGC was started 1–7 days before threatened preterm birth prior to 34 full weeks of pregnancy. According to cohort studies, AGC was efficacious of improving the postnatal survival and decreasing the risk of RDS among ELGA and preterm twin pregnancies, respectively. AGC further decreased the risks of RDS in preterm infants exposed to chorioamnionitis and rupture of fetal membranes. Although AGC decreases the risk of respiratory distress in near-term pregnancies, most fetuses are exposed only to potential adverse effects (e.g., hypoglycemia); ACG is not routinely indicated at 34 weeks or later.

AGC and exogenous surfactant supplement each other in decreasing the risk of RDS and IVH (Hallman et al. 2010). According to meta-analysis, glucocorticoid decreased neonatal mortality, IVH, and NEC and tended to decrease early neonatal infections. The cognitive and neurological problems observed in rodents following AGC have not been replicated as there is a trend toward improved neurological outcome. Exposure to AGC is associated with mild insulin resistance in young adults (Dalziel et al. 2005).

Repeating the AGC dosage in threatened preterm birth decreases the risk of RDS and of severe RDS (Peltoniemi et al. 2011). Repeating the drug weekly decreased the birth weight and head circumference dose-dependently. Although no adverse influence on growth or on neurologic or cognitive function has been detected, longer follow-up studies are required. Currently a single repeat dosage of AGC is recommended in threatened very preterm birth (<32 weeks) in case the fetus remains undelivered for more than week.

53.8.3 Diagnosis of Lung Maturity

Lung surfactant secreted into liquid-filled air spaces is carried by the lung liquid into the amniotic fluid. This amniotic surfactant pool starts emerging with imminent functional maturity of fetal lung. Surfactant increases in concentration and quality in a characteristic fashion as the pregnancy proceeds. Surfactant indices, measured in the amniotic fluid [lecithin/sphingomyelin (L/S) ratio, PG, the lung profile, saturated lecithin, LB], are used to evaluate the risk of RDS of an unborn fetus, particularly in the era when AGC or exogenous surfactant were not used (Hallman 1992). Assessment of fetal maturity in preterm and near-term pregnancies is still indicated when there is a need to balance the risk of continuing a risk pregnancy against the risk of iatrogenic RDS. The reported specificity and sensitivity of the surfactant indices in amniotic fluid have ranged from 92–100% to 30–70%, respectively. Due to surfactant retention in active labor, the sensitivity of surfactant indices in amniotic fluid or gastric aspirate at birth is likely rather low.

53.8.4 Prevention of Low-Risk Elective Births Before Term

A significant fraction of near-term (34–36 weeks) and early-term-born infants (37–38 weeks) develop RDS if delivered electively before the onset of active labor (Tita et al. 2009). In infants born at 39 weeks of pregnancy or later, RDS is very rare (<1%) regardless of the mode of delivery, whereas the risk of meconium aspiration syndrome and acute asphyxia continues to increase after term.

In elective near-term births without onset of labor, the fetus is exposed to increased risk of transient tachypnea, spontaneous pneumothorax, RDS, and persistence of fetal circulation. The induction of the adsorptive state of lung liquid allows the accumulation of surfactant in future air spaces before birth. The labor-associated hormones, cortisol, and adrenalin additionally increase the secretion of surfactant. According to available trials, AGC in elective near-term births decreases the risk of transient respiratory distress.

Before ACG treatment is accepted as a therapy in elective late-preterm and early-term births without labor, it is important to know that the mostly healthy fetuses exposed to steroid are not

adversely affected long term. In near-term births, AGC is indicated when the risk of respiratory distress is considerable. These cases include maternal diabetes with poor metabolic control, severe Rh immunization, diaphragmatic hernia, near-term RDS in the family, and documentation of immaturity of fetal lung.

References

Aikio O, Metsola J, Vuolteenaho R et al (2012) Transient defect in nitric oxide generation after rupture of fetal membranes and responsiveness to inhaled nitric oxide in very preterm infants with hypoxic respiratory failure. J Pediatr 161:397–403

Avery ME, Mead J (1959) Surface properties in relation to atelectasis and hyaline membrane disease. AMA Am J Dis Child 97(5 Part 1):517–523

Avery ME, Fletcher BD, Williams RG (1981) The lung and its disorders in the newborn infant, Major problems in clinical pediatrics, vol 1, 4th edn. Saunders, Philadelphia, pp 1–367

Baldwin DN, Pillow JJ, Stocks J, Frey U (2006) Lung-function tests in neonates and infants with chronic lung disease: tidal breathing and respiratory control. Pediatr Pulmonol 41:391–419

Bassler D, Plavka R, Shinwell ES et al (2015) Early inhaled budesonide for the prevention of bronchopulmonary dysplasia. N Engl J Med 373:1497–1506

Bird AD, McDougall AR, Seow B et al (2015) Glucocorticoid regulation of lung development: lessons learned from conditional GR knockout mice. Mol Endocrinol 29:158–171

Bishop NB, Stankiewicz P, Steinhorn RH (2011) Alveolar capillary dysplasia. Am J Respir Crit Care Med 184:172–179

Bland R (2001) Loss of liquid from the lung lumen in labor: more than a simple "squeeze". Am J Physiol Lung Cell Mol Physiol 280:L602–L605

Bry K, Lappalainen U, Hallman M (1997) Intraamniotic interleukin- 1 accelerates surfactant protein synthesis in fetal rabbits and improves lung stability after premature birth. J Clin Invest 99:2992–2999

Burri PH (2006) Structural aspects of postnatal lung development – alveolar formation and growth. Biol Neonate 89:313–322

Carnielli VP, Zimmermann LJ, Hamvas A, Cogo PE (2009) Pulmonary surfactant kinetics of the newborn infant: novel insights from studies with stable isotopes. J Perinatol 29(Suppl 2):S29–S37

Chu J, Clements JA, Cotton EK et al (1967) Neonatal pulmonary ischemia. I. Clinical and physiological studies. Pediatrics 40:709–782

Dalziel SR, Walker NK, Parag V et al (2005) Cardiovascular risk factors after antenatal exposure to betamethasone: 30-year follow-up of a randomised controlled trial. Lancet 365:1856–1862

Gerten KA, Coonrod DV, Bay RC, Chambliss LR (2005) Cesarean delivery and respiratory distress syndrome: does labor make a difference? Am J Obstet Gynecol 193:1061–1064

Gilbert WM (2006) The cost of preterm birth: the low cost versus high value of tocolysis. BJOG 113(Suppl 3):4–9

Hallman M (1992) Antenatal diagnosis of lung maturity. In: Robertson B, Van Golde LMG, Batenburg JJ (eds) Pulmonary surfactant. From molecular biology to clinical practice. Elsevier, Amsterdam, pp 425–445

Hallman M, Haataja R (2007) Genetic basis of respiratory distress syndrome. Front Biosci 12:2670–2682

Hallman M, Arjomaa P, Romu M, Tahvanainen J (1986) The lung profile in diagnosis of fetal and neonatal surfactant defects. In: Vignali M, Cosmi EV, Luerti M (eds) Diagnosis and treatment of fetal lung immaturity. Masson, Milan, pp 41–49

Hallman M, Merritt TA, Akino T, Bry K (1991) Surfactant protein A, phosphatidylcholine, and surfactant inhibitors in epithelial lining fluid. Correlation with surface activity, severity of respiratory distress syndrome, and outcome in small premature infants. Am Rev Respir Dis 144:1376–1384

Hallman M, Merritt TA, Bry K (1994) The fate of exogenous surfactant in neonates with respiratory distress syndrome. Clin Pharmacokinet 26:215–232

Hallman M, Peltoniemi O, Kari MA (2010) Enhancing functional maturity before preterm birth. Neonatology 97:373–378

Hamrick SE, Hansmann G (2010) Patent ductus arteriosus of the preterm infant. Pediatrics 125:1020–1030

Helve O, Pitkänen O, Janér C, Andersson S (2009) Pulmonary fluid balance in the human newborn infant. Neonatology 95:347–352

Hillman NH, Moss TJ, Kallapur SG et al (2007) Brief, large tidal volume ventilation initiates lung injury and a systemic response in fetal sheep. Am J Respir Crit Care Med 176:575–581

Hjalmarson O, Brynjarsson H, Nilsson S, Sandberg KL (2014) Persisting hypoxaemia is an insufficient measure of adverse lung function in very immature infants. Arch Dis Child Fetal Neonatal Ed 99:F257–F262

Hoepker A, Seear M, Petrocheilou A et al (2008) Wilson-Mikity syndrome: updated diagnostic criteria based on nine cases and a review of the literature. Pediatr Pulmonol 43:1004–1012

Idell S, Kumar A, Koenig KB, Coalson JJ (1994) Pathways of fibrin turnover in lavage of premature baboons with hyperoxic lung injury. Am J Respir Crit Care Med 149:767–775

Jones M (2009) Effect of preterm birth on airway function and lung growth. Paediatr Respir Rev 10(Suppl 1):9–11

Kallapur SG, Presicce P, Rueda CM, Jobe AH, Chougnet CA (2014) Fetal immune response to chorioamnionitis. Semin Reprod Med 32:56–67

Karjalainen MK, Huusko JM, Tuohimaa A et al (2012) A study of collecting genes in spontaneous preterm birth reveals an association with a common surfactant protein D gene polymorphism. Pediatr Res 71:93–99

Kaukola T, Tuimala J, Herva R et al (2009) Cord immunoproteins as predictors of respiratory outcome in preterm infants. Am J Obstet Gynecol 200(100):e1–e8

Koivisto M, Marttila R, Saarela T et al (2005) Wheezing illness and re-hospitalization in the first two years of life after neonatal respiratory distress syndrome. J Pediatr 147:486–492

Kotecha SJ, Edwards MO, Watkins WJ (2013) Effect of preterm birth on later FEV1: a systematic review and meta-analysis. Thorax 68:760–766

Liggins GC, Howie RN (1972) A controlled trial of antepartum glucocorticoid treatment for prevention of the respiratory distress syndrome in premature infants. Pediatrics 50:515–525

Marttila R, Haataja R, Rämet M et al (2003) Surfactant protein B polymorphism and respiratory distress syndrome in premature twins. Hum Genet 112:18–23

Marttila R, Kaprio J, Hallman M (2004) Respiratory distress syndrome in twin infants compared with singletons. Am J Obstet Gynecol 191:271–276

Morley CJ, Davis PG, Doyle LW et al (2008) Nasal CPAP or intubation at birth for very preterm infants. N Engl J Med 358:700–708

Mulugeta S, Nureki S, Beers MF (2015) Lost after translation: insights from pulmonary surfactant for understanding the role of alveolar epithelial dysfunction and cellular quality control in fibrotic lung disease. Am J Physiol Lung Cell Mol Physiol 309: L507–L525

O'Brodovich H (2005) Pulmonary edema in infants and children. Curr Opin Pediatr 17:381–384

Obladen M (1992) History of surfactant research. In: Robertson B, Van Golde LMG, Batenburg JJ (eds) Pulmonary surfactant. From molecular biology to clinical practice. Elsevier, Amsterdam, pp 1–18

Olver RE, Walters DV, Wilson SM (2004) Developmental regulation of lung liquid transport. Annu Rev Physiol 66:77–101

Peltoniemi OM, Kari MA, Hallman M (2011) Repeated antenatal corticosteroid treatment: a systematic review and meta-analysis. Acta Obstet Gynecol Scand 90:719–727

Ramachandrappa A, Jain L (2008) Elective cesarean section: its impact on neonatal respiratory outcome. Clin Perinatol 35:373–393

Ramachandrappa A, Jain L (2009) Health issues of the late preterm infant. Pediatr Clin North Am 56:565–577

Roberts D, Dalziel S (2006) Antenatal corticosteroids for accelerating fetal lung maturation for women at risk of preterm birth. Cochrane Database Syst Rev 3:CD004454

Robertson B, Taeusch HW (1995) Surfactant therapy for lung disease. In: Lefant C (ed) Lung biology in health and disease, vol 84. Marcel Dekker, New York

Ronkainen E, Dunder T, Peltoniemi O, Kaukola T, Marttila R, Hallman M (2015) New BPD predicts lung function at school age: follow-up study and meta-analysis. Pediatr Pulmonol 50:1090–1098

Sáenz A, López-Sánchez A, Mojica-Lázaro J et al (2010) Fluidizing effects of C-reactive protein on lung surfactant membranes: protective role of surfactant protein A. FASEB J 24:3662–3673

Sandri F, Plavka R, Ancora G et al (2010) Prophylactic or early selective surfactant combined with nCPAP in very preterm infants. Pediatrics 125:e1402–e1409

Schmidt B, Roberts R, Millar D, Kirpalani H (2008) Evidence based neonatal drug therapy for prevention of bronchopulmonary dysplasia in very-low-birth-weight infants. Neonatology 93:284–287

Schürch S, Bachofen H, Possmayer F (2001) Surface activity in situ, in vivo, and in the captive bubble surfactometer. Comp Biochem Physiol A Mol Integr Physiol 129:195–207

Steinhorn RH (2010) Neonatal pulmonary hypertension. Pediatr Crit Care Med 11(2 Suppl):S79–S84

Sundell H, Garrott J, Blankenship W et al (1971) Studies on infants with type II respiratory distress syndrome. J Pediatr 78:754–764

Tita AT, Landon MB, Spong CY et al (2009) Timing of elective repeat cesarean delivery at term and neonatal outcomes. N Engl J Med 360:111–120

Torday JS, Rehan VK (2015) On the evolution of the pulmonary alveolar lipofibroblast. Exp Cell Res 340:215. pii: S0014-4827(15)30174-9

Van Driessche W, Kreindler JL, Malik AB et al (2007) Interrelations/cross talk between transcellular transport function and paracellular tight junctional properties in lung epithelial and endothelial barriers. Am J Physiol Lung Cell Mol Physiol 293:L520–L524

Verder H, Ebbesen F, Linderholm B et al (2003) Prediction of respiratory distress syndrome by the microbubble stability test on gastric aspirates in newborns of less than 32 weeks' estation. Acta Paediatr 92: 728–733

Vergine M, Copetti R, Brusa G, Cattarossi L (2014) Lung ultrasound accuracy in respiratory distress syndrome and transient tachypnea of the newborn. Neonatology 106:87–93

Watterberg KL, Demers LM, Scott SM, Murphy S (1996) Chorioamnionitis and early lung inflammation in infants in whom bronchopulmonary dysplasia develops. Pediatrics 97:210–215

Wert SE, Whitsett JA, Nogee LM (2009) Genetic disorders of surfactant dysfunction. Pediatr Dev Pathol 12:253–274

Whitsett JA, Wert SE, Weaver TE (2010) Alveolar surfactant homeostasis and the pathogenesis of pulmonary disease. Annu Rev Med 61:105–119

WHO (2015) WHO recommendations on interventions to improve preterm birth outcomes. ISBN 978 924 1508988

Wright JR (2005) Immunoregulatory functions of surfactant proteins. Nat Rev Immunol 5:58–68

Treatment of Respiratory Failure in Newborn: Mechanical Ventilation

54

Colin Morley and Gianluca Lista

Contents

C. Morley (✉)
Dept Obstetrics and Gynecology, University of Cambridge at Rosie Maternity Hospital, Cambridge, UK
e-mail: colin@morleys.net

G. Lista (✉)
Neonatology and Neonatal Intensive Care Unit, Ospedale dei Bambini V. Buzzi, Milan, Italy
e-mail: gianluca.lista@icp.mi.it

G. Buonocore et al. (eds.), *Neonatology*,
https://doi.org/10.1007/978-3-319-29489-6_202

Abstract

Premature delivery is always associated with the failure of respiratory transition and a delayed achievement of an adequate functional residual capacity. For this reason preterm babies (especially the extremely low for gestational age – ELGA – infants) frequently need respiratory support. Noninvasive ventilation (NIV) is in widespread use in the management of respiratory distress even in ELGA infants without increasing neonatal mortality or neurological impairment.

The most recent meta-analysis and reviews of NIV demonstrated that NIV is a valid alternative to mechanical ventilation (MV) in the management of respiratory failure and resulted in significant reductions in the incidence of bronchopulmonary dysplasia (BPD) among surviving infants.

Nevertheless, preterm babies, mainly ELGA infants, require MV because they have unresponsive apnea, or a high and rising $PaCO_2$, and/or a high and rising FiO_2 despite treatment with continuous positive airway pressure (CPAP).

Pressure-limited ventilation continues to be the primary mode of ventilation in neonates because of its relative simplicity and ability to ventilate effectively despite large endotracheal tube (ETT) leaks.

The major disadvantage of pressure-limited ventilation is that the tidal volume (VT) varies as the baby alters its breathing pattern and with changes in lung compliance (e.g., after surfactant therapy). The consequences of such rapid improvements in compliance are inadvertent hyperventilation and lung injury from excessively large VT (volutrauma); hyperventilation may induce hypocapnia, with high risk of cerebral damage. There is strong evidence that excessive tidal volumes, rather than the ventilator pressure, are the key determinant of ventilator-induced lung injury (VILI). Inadequate (too small) VT also causes significant problems (atelectrauma): in particular inefficient gas exchange due to increased dead space to VT ratio. Therefore, in the last few years, tidal volume-targeted ventilation has

become an important standard of care in neonatal and pediatric respiratory support.

There are many volume-targeted ventilation modes used in neonatal period, but volume guarantee (VG) ventilation is the most extensively studied.

The Cochrane review on volume-targeted ventilation showed significant reductions in duration of ventilation, rates of pneumothorax (PTX), and intraventricular hemorrhage (IVH) and a borderline significant reduction in the incidence of BPD in surviving infants. Also VG ventilation plus adequate PEEP, with an open lung strategy, is an alternative to high-frequency oscillatory ventilation (HFOV) in infants ventilated for severe RDS. Nevertheless in a baby with very stiff lungs, pulmonary interstitial emphysema (PIE) or PTX, the use of HFOV still remains the best ventilator approach.

To optimize ventilatory management of infants with respiratory failure and to adjust the ventilatory settings, it is important to monitor the blood gases and perform chest X-ray. As most modern ventilators have numerical and graphical displays of ventilator parameters, these should be used to guide ventilation management and reduce the risk of lung injury.

It is important to wean babes from the ventilator and extubate them as soon as possible to reduce the risk of pulmonary infections and BPD. In many cases early caffeine administration can reduce the duration of mechanical ventilation, BPD, and the occurrence of respiratory and neurological adverse outcome. It is therefore important to have a respiratory protocol that helps the neonatologist to manage both the acute and the recovery phase of respiratory failure.

54.1 Salient Points

- Mechanical ventilation (MV) is often used to treat babies with respiratory failure initially managed with a noninvasive respiratory support.
- MV has to be tailored to optimize lung volume and improve gas exchange with less lung injury.
- Ventilation parameters may have to be modified in accordance with changes in lung mechanics of the neonates.
- When the neonatologist decides to use conventional mechanical ventilation (CMV), volume-targeted ventilation has better outcomes than pressure-limited ventilation.
- High-frequency oscillatory ventilation (HFOV) is very useful in improving oxygenation and removing carbon dioxide especially in infants with very stiff lungs.
- To reduce the occurrence of complications due to MV and to reduce the risk of BPD, it is important to wean infants from the ventilator and extubate as soon as possible.

54.2 Introduction

Respiratory diseases, with different etiologies, are one of the major problems in neonatal medicine and one of the main reasons for an infant receiving intensive respiratory support. Without respiratory support many ill newly born infants would die.

Respiratory support can be given with several different techniques. From the least intensive to the most intensive, they are: additional oxygen, high-flow nasal cannula oxygen, continuous positive airway pressure (CPAP), bi-level CPAP or nasal intermittent ventilation, untriggered mechanical ventilation, triggered mechanical ventilation, tidal volume-targeted ventilation, and high-frequency oscillatory ventilation. This chapter will only present information about mechanical ventilation.

In any discussion of mechanical ventilation, it is important to define the terminology of spontaneous breathing and mechanical ventilation because this can be confusing.

It is important to realize that patients have breaths and ventilators deliver inflations.

A breath is a spontaneous inspiration by an infant.
An inspiration is a breath taken by the baby.
An inflation is a pressure applied to the airways by a ventilator with the intention of inflating the lungs.

Spontaneous expiration is gas leaving the lung after a breath.
Ventilator exhalation is gas leaving the lung after an inflation.
Inspiratory time is the time during which a baby inspires.
Inflation time is the duration of a mechanical inflation.
Ventilator exhalation time is the exhalation time set on the ventilator.
Expiration time is the time gas leaves the lungs after an inspiration or inflation until a new inflation or inspiration occurs.

54.3 Problems with Mechanical Ventilation of Infants

Mechanical ventilation is associated with a number of problems, so it is most important not to ventilate an infant unless it is absolutely necessary.

The problems with ventilation are:

- Gas is pushed into the lungs rather than sucked in. This is unphysiological. It is much more effective for lung aeration and blood circulation through the lungs to have a negative pressure with each inspiration.
- The endotracheal tube (ETT) bypasses the larynx. This may lower the residual lung volume because the larynx is very important for maintaining lung volume during lung disease. During expiration without an ETT it may narrow or close to reduce the expiratory flow and maintain lung volume (Carlo et al. 1987).
- An ETT increases resistance to gas flow and breathing.
- Inflations can injure the airways and alveoli (Bjorklund et al. 1997). This is by several mechanisms: (1) volutrauma where the tidal volume is too high and the overdistension injures the lungs (Attar and Donn 2002); (2) repeated expansion and collapse of atelectatic areas of the lung – called atelectrauma (Donn and Sinha 2003); (3) barotrauma where repeated high ventilator pressures damage the lungs; and (4) injury from the ETT in the airway.
- Ventilation increases infection.
- Mechanical ventilation may interfere with the baby's control of breathing and blood gases.
- Unfortunately, we still do not have good evidence about when to start ventilation, how to prevent lung damage, the optimal way to wean the ventilation and extubate the infant, or when to stop ventilation.

54.4 What Are the Indications for Mechanical Ventilation?

The major reason for ventilating an infant is apnea. However, the difficult decision comes in deciding when to ventilate an infant who is very premature, or breathing with retraction of the lower chest wall, or requiring oxygen treatment, or having numerous apneic episodes.

Intubation and ventilation of very premature babies with respiratory difficulty soon after birth used to be considered mandatory. However, it is now realized that even very premature babies can often be supported with CPAP (Ammari et al. 2005) or other modes of noninvasive ventilation, particularly if treated early with caffeine.

54.4.1 Apnea

Apnea unresponsive to stimulation, nasal CPAP, caffeine, and hand ventilation for a short time is an absolute indication for mechanical ventilation.

There are few other absolute indications about when to ventilate a baby. It is often a matter of clinical judgment and local policy, consideration of the infant's gestational age, and other factors.

54.4.2 Respiratory Failure

The first question is does the infant have respiratory failure? An arterial $PaCO_2$ that has risen above 60 mmHg (~8 kPa) is a good sign of respiratory failure. However, this judgment should not be made on the first blood gas measurement, unless

the baby is obviously very ill, because many babies improve over the first hour or two with careful and gentle management, after the baby has been appropriately positioned and nasal CPAP has been used.

A capillary CO_2 is not accurate enough for making the decision to ventilate an infant because it might be spuriously high in an infant with poor peripheral circulation.

A severe uncompensated metabolic acidosis may be an indication for ventilation.

54.4.3 Oxygenation

A high and rising FiO_2, despite treatment with CPAP, is a strong pointer to the need for ventilation. There is little consensus about the FiO_2 that should be used to determine when a baby should be ventilated. To a certain extent, the FiO_2 does not matter if the PaO_2 is maintained. However, a high FiO_2 is usually a sign that there is a low lung volume if there is not a cardiac cause. Oxygen is toxic to the lungs and the higher the more likely lung injury occurs. Pragmatically, the indication for ventilation in a very premature infant being treated with CPAP is an $FiO_2 > 0.40–0.45$, especially when surfactant is still to be given, and a $pH < 7.2$ and $paCO_2 >$ 65–70 mmHg (Morley et al. 2008).

The criteria for ventilation may vary depending on the size of the baby. Babies born at <26 weeks gestation may need earlier ventilator support because of their extreme immaturity. More mature babies are stronger and ventilation should not be used unless absolutely necessary.

54.5 Investigations

54.5.1 Arterial Blood Gas Measurements

Understanding and assessing arterial blood gases is one of the most important aspects of the care of a baby with respiratory failure.

Unless the baby has mild RDS, as indicated by a low FiO_2 and minimal dyspnea, an arterial line should be inserted to enable easy and repeated measurement of arterial blood gases. A ventilated baby will require several accurate blood gases in the first days and so an arterial line is optimal for the baby and carers. Capillary blood gases can be misleading, and venous blood gases should not be used to assess the respiratory function unless the CO_2 or pH is near the normal range.

54.5.2 A Chest X-Ray

An anterior/posterior chest X-ray should be done as early as possible to confirm the respiratory diagnosis and exclude diagnoses that may need different treatment. If umbilical arterial and/or venous lines have been used, the X-ray should include the abdomen to show their position.

54.5.3 Investigate Infection

Infection must always be suspected in babies presenting with respiratory failure soon after birth because it can be present even in babies born by Cesarean section. Infection at this age usually causes septicemia and can be quickly life threatening if antibiotics are not given early. Blood cultures, gastric aspirate microscopy and culture, and blood tests for indicators of infection should be taken and then intravenous antibiotics given. Penicillin and gentamicin are safe and effective.

54.6 The Basic Principles of Mechanical Ventilation

Several aspects of ventilation need to be adjusted to optimize the blood gases, lung volume, tidal volume, and minute volume and minimize lung injury.

54.6.1 Improving Oxygenation

Oxygenation can be improved by increasing the FiO_2. However, the higher the FiO_2, the greater

the chance of lung injury because high levels are toxic to the epithelium. Therefore other techniques should be used to improve oxygenation and reduce the need for a high FiO_2.

Oxygenation is not dependent on the movement of gas in and out of the lungs. It only requires oxygen to enter the lungs and an appropriate surface area for diffusion.

Adequate oxygenation depends on ensuring the lungs are well aerated with enough surface area for gas exchange (Thome et al. 1998). Oxygenation is closely related to the PEEP or mean airway pressure (MAP) used because this is the key factor to maintain lung volume in an intubated infant with lung disease. The level of PEEP should be between 5 and 8 cm H_2O. There is no easy guide to the exact level to use in any baby at any time. PEEP can be increased when a high FiO_2 is being used or when the chest X-ray shows low lung volume.

Adjusting the PEEP depends on clinical assessment, chest X-ray appearance, and FiO_2 and the $PaCO_2$ or transcutaneous PCO_2 levels. PEEP can be increased to open the lungs if the FiO_2 is high, and the chest X-ray also shows the lungs to be underinflated. The levels of PEEP to use in different situations have not been determined.

Altering peak pressure or inflation and expiration times will alter the mean airway pressure, and have some effect on oxygenation, but adjusting these is not as effective at altering oxygenation as changing PEEP.

In a normal lung, high PEEP may cause oxygenation and $PaCO_2$ to deteriorate by overdistending the lung and reducing effective tidal volume and compressing the alveolar capillaries. Sometimes this is the first "clinical alarm", indicating too much PEEP is cardiovascular impairment by lung overinflation. However, there is no evidence this is a problem in babies ventilated for respiratory failure, because little of the inflating pressure is transmitted to the lungs unless it is increased to a very high level.

Oxygenation is dependent on the lungs being appropriately perfused. Inadequate oxygenation may be due to low blood pressure, pulmonary hypertension, or pulmonary atresia. Therefore, to ensure optimal pulmonary perfusion and oxygenation, the blood pressure must be maintained.

Primary pulmonary hypertension, with right to left shunting of venous blood past the lungs, can be recognized when a baby has a high FiO_2 to obtain a satisfactory PaO_2, yet the $PaCO_2$ is easily controlled. The chest X-ray shows lungs with a relatively normal volume and reduced vascular markings. Echocardiography is used to confirm the diagnosis.

One problem to be aware of is when the peak inflating pressure (PIP) is progressively increased to try and improve oxygenation, and the oxygenation deteriorates. This may be because the pressure is causing overdistension and interfering with pulmonary blood flow. A pointer to this is that oxygenation improves when the baby is transiently disconnected from the ventilator.

54.6.2 Controlling the Blood Level of Carbon Dioxide

CO_2 control is related to moving gas in and out of the lung. Inadequate spontaneous breathing is the primary reason for ventilation. Altering the tidal volume and ventilator rate controls the $PaCO_2$.

Careful control of the $PaCO_2$ is very important. Overventilation causing hypocarbia ($PaCO_2$ < 30 mmHg) is strongly associated with chronic lung disease and adverse neurodevelopmental outcomes (Okumura et al. 2001). Hypercarbia ($PaCO_2$ > 60 mmHg) may also be damaging because it causes acidosis and increased cerebral perfusion. The normal $PaCO_2$ range for a ventilated baby is about 35–60 mmHg.

During ventilation the tidal volume is determined by the applied pressure, i.e., PIP, PEEP, and the baby's breathing. Neonatologists think of neonatal ventilation in terms of applied pressures and the effect they have on the $PaCO_2$; however, the pressure is only a proxy for the delivered tidal volume. The higher the PIP, the greater the tidal volume delivered. Most modern neonatal ventilators measure and display tidal volume, so this can now be targeted. Large tidal volumes can damage the lungs very quickly – called volutrauma. The appropriate tidal volume for ventilated spontaneously breathing babies is around 3.5–6 ml/kg depending on the ventilator

rate. If the $PaCO_2$ is too high or too low, the tidal volume (or peak inflating pressure) is altered a little (0.5 ml/kg or 2 cm H_2O) and the $PaCO_2$ rechecked in about 30 min.

The ventilator rate should be adequate to ensure the $PaCO_2$ is in the normal range. Most babies are ventilated while breathing. They breathe between 50 and 90/min. Modern ventilators enable inflations to be triggered and synchronized with each breath to assist the baby's respiratory efforts. This is called assist/control mode of ventilation. This means that the baby triggers inflations and so controls the ventilator rate and to some extent the minute volume. With triggered ventilation, the backup rate should be set at about 30/min, well below the baby's spontaneous rate. If it is set too close to the spontaneous rate, this will reduce the proportion of triggered inflations. The product of ventilator rate and tidal volume is the minute volume. The minute volume should be ~ 200–300 ml/kg/min.

The $PaCO_2$ is related to the minute volume and so it can be increased or decreased by altering the ventilator rate. However, because ventilated babies are spontaneously breathing and triggering the ventilator, altering the set rate may have little effect on the delivered minute volume in this mode. Then the only control is adjusting the tidal volume.

54.6.3 Heating and Humidification of Ventilation Gases

Inspired gases are heated and humidified by the nose, pharynx, and upper respiratory mucosa. They are delivered to the lungs at 37 °C and with a saturation of 100%.

Medical gases are 100% dry and cold. An ETT bypasses the upper airway and so all heating and humidification of the gases must be from a heater humidifier in the circuit. Even slightly cold or dry gases quickly thicken the mucus, reduce cilial action, and damage the mucosa. It is important to ensure that all gas reaches the lungs at no less than 37 °C and carries 44 mg% H_2O (100% relative humidity) (Schulze 2007). Any condensation of water vapor in the ventilator circuit, from the inspired gas, is a loss of humidity and must be avoided by using a heated inspiratory ventilator circuit.

54.6.4 Measuring Blood Gases

During mechanical ventilation, adjusting the ventilator settings in response to frequently measured blood gases is necessary for control of $PaCO_2$ and pH. The frequency depends on the stability of ventilation. In the acute phase, when the lung function is changing, blood gases should be measured no more than 30 min after a change in ventilator settings. Transcutaneous measurements of CO_2 can be useful, give quick feedback about changes in CO_2, and reduce the number of blood gases measured but are prone to drift.

54.6.5 Monitoring Ventilator Parameters

Most modern ventilators have numerical and graphical displays of ventilator parameters. It is important these are understood and interpreted correctly. The most useful graphical display is pressure, flow, and tidal volume against time with a horizontal axis showing about 10 s worth of waveforms. See Figs. 1, 2, 3, 4, 5, and 6 for recordings during different ventilator modes and their interpretation (Schmolzer et al. 2010). Pressure volume loops are only useful when the baby is not breathing.

54.6.6 Pressure Wave

This shows the ventilator pressure wave changing with inflations. It shows the level of PEEP and how this changes with spontaneous inspirations, the onset of inflation, the rate of rise of the pressure, whether the set PIP is achieved, and whether there is any pressure plateau.

54.6.7 Flow Wave

This shows the gas flow changing as the baby breathes and the ventilator inflates. Flow

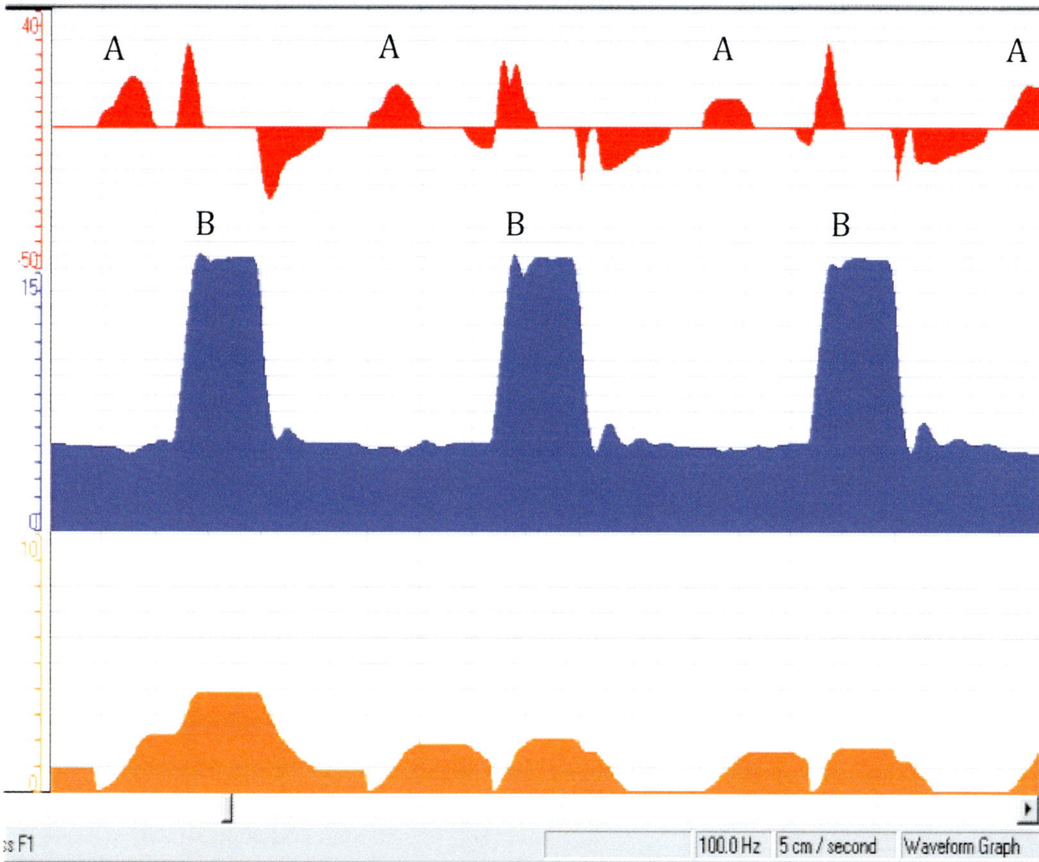

Fig. 1 This shows about 3.8 s of a recording of pressure limited fixed rate untriggered ventilation with the flow wave at the top with gas going down the ETT above the zero line and gas coming out of the ETT below the zero line. The pressure wave is in the middle showing 5 cm H_2O PEEP pressure and 16 cm H_2O peak pressure. The bottom line shows the tidal volume wave. At "A" the baby is inspiring and the ventilator pressure not rising, the PEEP falls slightly, and there is an inspiratory tidal volume. At "B" the ventilator pressure rises to a plateau for the inflation time of about 0.3 s. This result is an inflation tidal volume about the same size as the baby's inspiratory volume. It can be seen that ventilator inflations and baby's inspirations and expirations are completely out of synchrony

above the zero line is down the ETT; flow below the zero line is flow out of the tube. With spontaneous breathing triggering ventilation, it displays a small inspiratory flow immediately before inflation that triggers inflation. The display also shows any flow from spontaneous breaths not associated with inflations, the gas flow during inflations, any gas leak during inflation, any interaction between the spontaneous breaths and inflations, whether the inflation time is adequate, whether the expiratory time is appropriate for full expiration, and whether there is gas trapping, diaphragmatic braking, or any obstruction or splinting against the inflations.

54.6.8 Tidal Volume Wave

This shows the volume of gas passing down the ETT as an upstroke, the volume of gas leaving the lung as a downward curve, and any gas leak around the ETT as a vertical line at the end of each inflation.

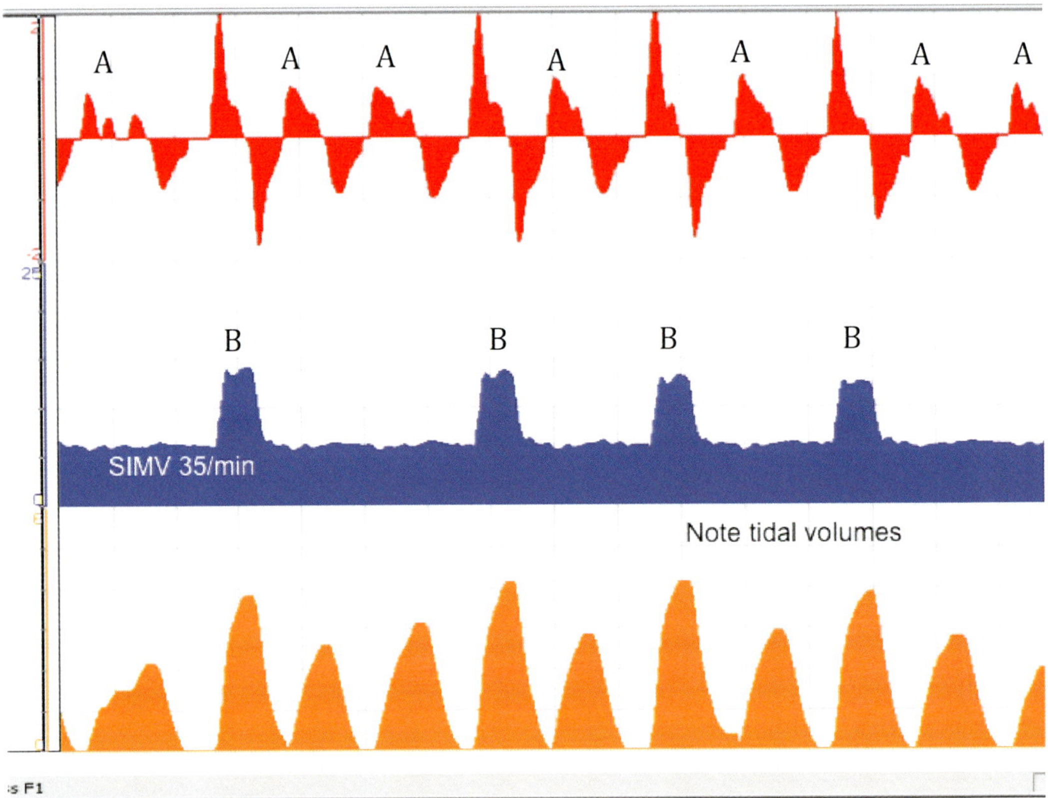

Fig. 2 This shows about 9 s of a recording of synchronised intermittent mandatory ventilation (SIMV) at a rate of 35/min with the flow wave at the top with gas going down the ETT above the zero line and gas coming out of the ETT below the zero line. The pressure wave is in the middle showing about 6 cm H_2O PEEP pressure and 14 cm H_2O peak pressure. The bottom line shows the tidal volume wave. At "A" the baby is inspiring without ventilator inflations. There is an inspiratory and expiratory tidal volume of about 2–3 ml. At "B" the ventilator pressure rises to a plateau for the inflation time of about 0.3 s. This results in an inflationary tidal volume about 20% larger than the baby's tidal volume. What cannot be seen is that these inflations were triggered by the baby's inspiratory flow, and so the tidal volumes are a combination of the baby's breathing and synchronous inflation. The baby is breathing at about 75 breaths per minute. It can be seen that the baby makes about seven inspirations without ventilator support and four with ventilator support. Out of a combined tidal volume during this time of about 34 ml, the ventilator has contributed only 4 ml. It would appear that this baby probably does not need to be ventilated

54.7 Techniques of Mechanical Ventilation

This section will be illustrated from our experience and studies using the Drager Babylog 8000+ ventilator and the Sensormedics 3100A high-frequency oscillating ventilator for many years (South and Morley 1986a, b, c, 1992; South et al. 1987, 1988; Greenough et al. 1986; Hoellering et al. 2008; Kamlin et al. 2006; McCallion et al. 2005a, b, 2008; Pellicano et al. 2009; Tingay et al. 2007; Wheeler et al. 2009a, b). Other neonatal ventilators may have slightly different modes but the general principles of use are the same.

54.7.1 Conventional Mandatory Ventilation (CMV) or Intermittent Mandatory Ventilation (IMV)

CMV and IMV are exactly the same mode and use pressure-limited, time-cycled ventilation. The ventilator is adjusted to deliver a set PIP

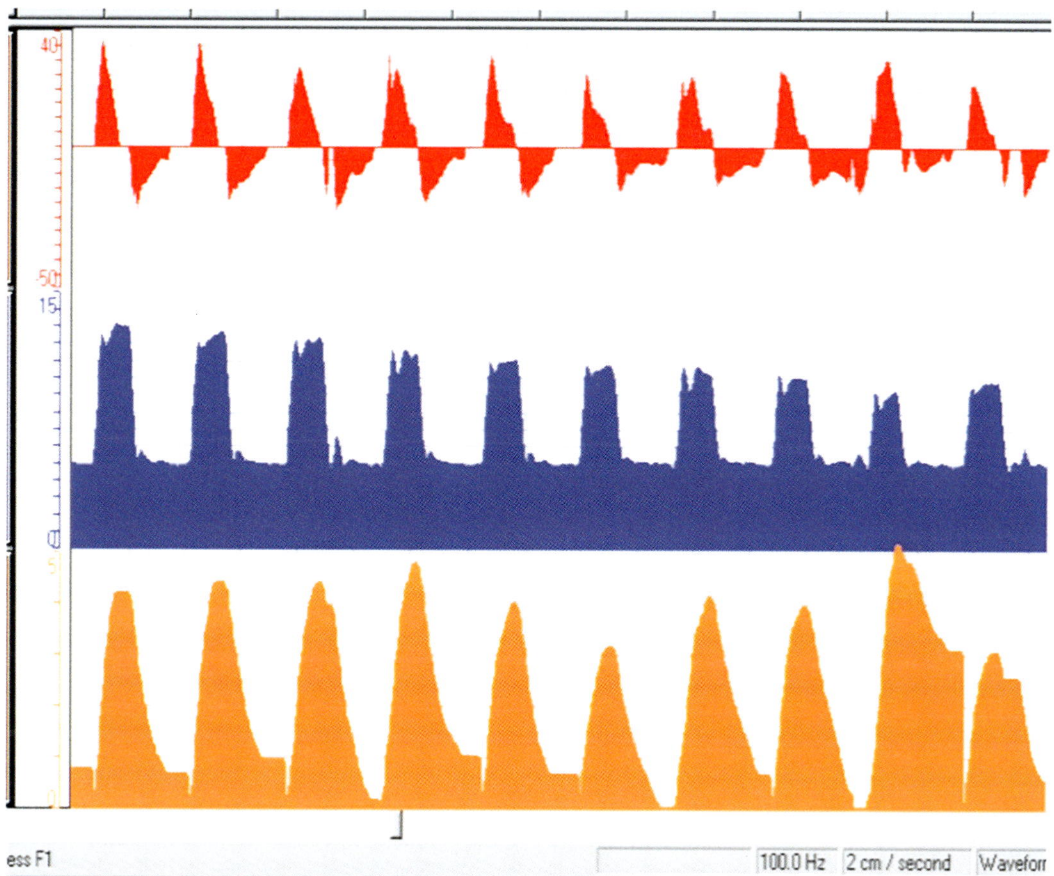

Fig. 3 This shows about 9 s of a recording of assist control ventilation A/C (SIPPV) and volume guarantee mode at a set rate of 50/min with the flow wave at the top with gas going down the ETT above the zero line and gas coming out of the ETT below the zero line. The pressure wave is in the middle showing about 6 cm H_2O PEEP pressure and the PIP changing from 13 down to 11 cm H_2O. The bottom line shows the tidal volume wave. Each of the baby's inspirations triggered an inflation and drove the ventilator at about 65/min. There is an inspiratory and expiratory tidal volume varying slightly between 4 ml and 6 ml with variable a leak. This shows how well A/C ventilation supports each of the baby's breaths and how volume guarantee changes the pressure to try and maintain the tidal volume as the baby changes its breathing

and a set PEEP with all inflations. There is no single PIP or PEEP that can be used for all babies under all circumstances. The starting PIP is chosen by experience, e.g., 20 cm H_2O and the infant's chest wall movement assessed by observation. If this is considered to be too much, the PIP is reduced. If there is none, or too little chest wall movement, the PIP is increased. When changing PIP by observing chest movement, remember in normal babies the movement with each breath is barely discernable. Subsequently, the PIP is adjusted according to the $PaCO_2$. There is no easy way to determine the appropriate PEEP for a baby and this usually starts at 5 cm H_2O.

The inflation time is usually set to 0.3 s, as this is the mean inspiratory time of a ventilated preterm infant. However, as every baby is different, it is best to adjust the inflation time by observing the flow wave. The inflation flow wave should arrive at the zero flow line when the inflation pressure finishes and then there should be little or no zero flow before expiration begins. If it is set longer, the infant may breathe out during the ventilator inflation. The expiratory time is set to provide the desired respiratory rate, ~60 per minute.

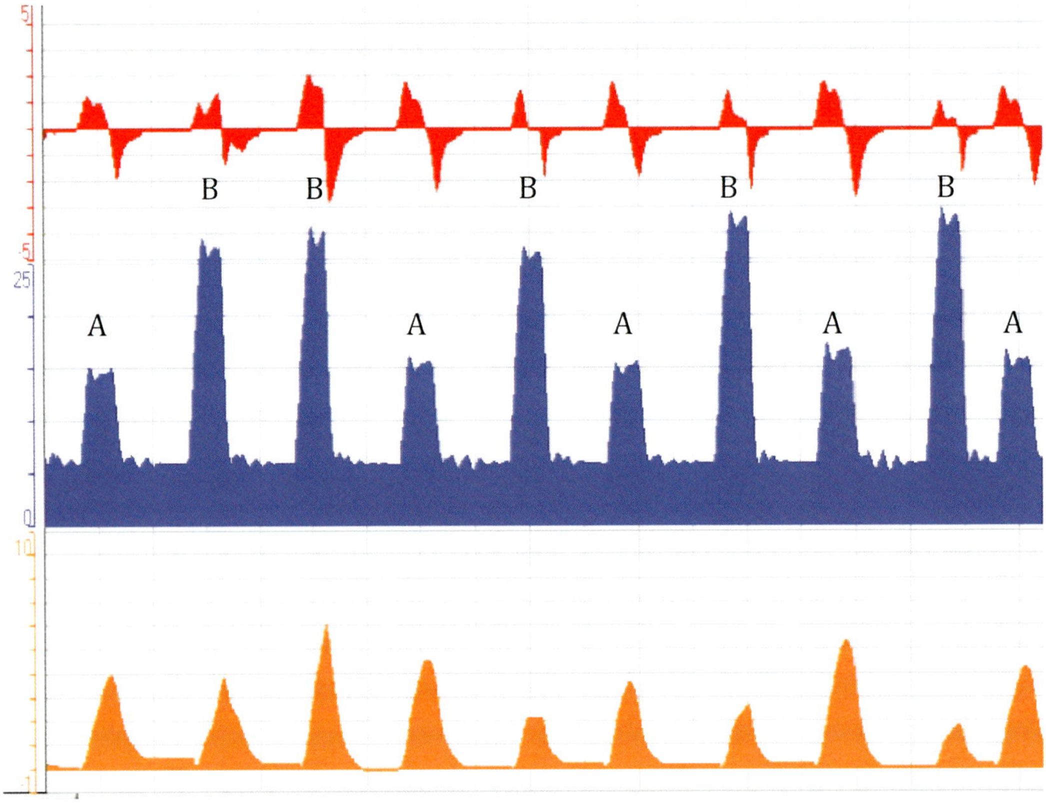

Fig. 4 This shows about 9 s of a recording of assist control ventilation A/C (SIPPV) and volume guarantee mode at a set rate of 50/min with the flow wave at the top with gas going down the ETT above the zero line and gas coming out of the ETT below the zero line. The pressure wave is in the middle showing about 6 cm H_2O PEEP pressure. The PIP changes from about 15 cm H_2O to about 30 cm H_2O. The bottom line shows the tidal volume wave. The waves marked A are triggered inflations with a lower PIP, and the waves marked B are untriggered inflations with a much higher PIP. This is happening because the volume guarantee program targets triggered and untriggered PIP separately. The pressures are changing slightly to try and produce the set tidal volume of 4.5 ml. Note that even though there is a large difference in the driving pressure, the tidal volume for triggered and untriggered inflations is similar and sometimes the untriggered inflations with the higher PIP have the smaller tidal volumes. There is an inspiratory and expiratory tidal volume varying slightly between 4 ml and 6 ml with variable a leak. This shows the problem of having the backup rate very close to the baby's spontaneous rate. The ventilator frequently changes from triggered to untriggered inflations

See Fig. 1 for a recording of ventilator, flow, and tidal volume waves during CMV showing the asynchrony between inflations and inspirations.

IMV is the only ventilator mode available on transport ventilators.

There are many problems with this mode of ventilation:

1. It is unresponsive to the infant's respiratory efforts because it is not triggered or synchronized with the infant's breathing. It may deliver an inflation when the infant is breathing out, or it may inflate on top of a large inspiration resulting in a very large tidal volume.
2. The set PIP may be too high or too low for the infant resulting in over- or underventilation. Overventilation can cause high tidal volumes and acute lung injury, and the resulting hypocarbia is associated with periventricular leukomalacia.
3. It provides little or no monitoring of the actual ventilation the baby receives.
4. The ventilator rate cannot match the infant's respiratory rate, particularly as it changes.

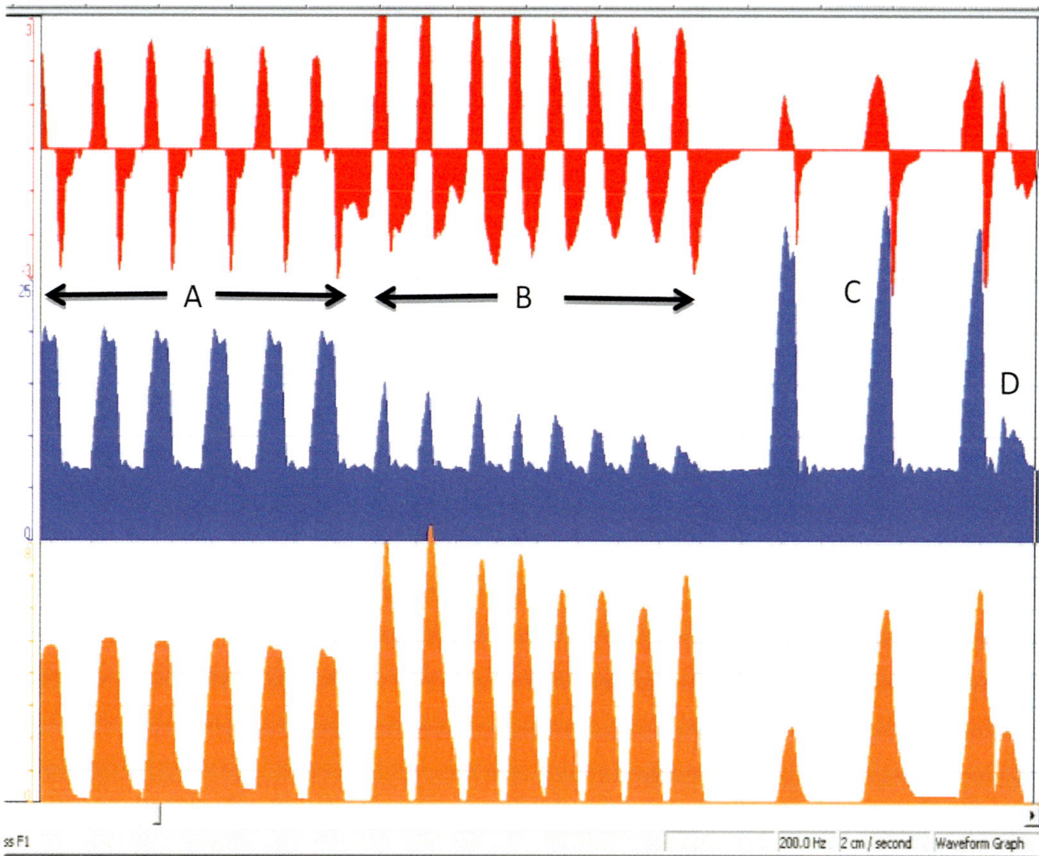

Fig. 5 This shows about 13 s of a recording of A/C (SIPPV) and volume guarantee mode at a set rate of about 50/min with the flow wave at the top with gas going down the ETT above the zero line and gas coming out of the ETT below the zero line. The pressure wave is in the middle showing about 7 cm H_2O PEEP pressure. The PIP changes to try and maintain the set tidal volume 5 ml. The bottom line shows the tidal volume wave. The group of waves marked A are all triggered inflations with a stable tidal volume. The group of waves marked B are all triggered inflations, but here the tidal volume has suddenly increased because the baby started breathing hard with inflation tidal volume of more than 130% of the set tidal volume. The volume guarantee program reacts by stopping the inflations. Note their inflation times are shorter. The PIP is lower and reducing each inflation to try and bring the tidal volumes back to the set level. At C there are three large inflations at a slower rate. These are untriggered inflations at the backup rate and have PIPs that correspond to the PIP of previous untriggered inflations. At D the baby inspires and a much smaller triggered PIP is delivered. This all shows the dynamic nature of the volume guarantee program responding to large changes in the infants' breathing pattern

54.7.2 Triggered Ventilation

The purpose of triggered ventilation is for the ventilator to inflate the infant in synchrony with the infant's inspiration and augment the inspiratory gas flow and tidal volume. With the Drager Babylog 8000+ ventilator, triggering is from a hot wire flow sensor that is placed between the wye piece of the ventilator circuit and the ETT. Two fine tungsten wires heated to 400 °C detect the gas flow by the cooling effect of the gas. It detects inspiratory gas flow, and when this has reached about 0.2 l/min, ~ 30 ms after the beginning of inspiratory flow, an inflation is started. The delay time depends on the set trigger sensitivity on a scale of 1–10 with 1 being the most sensitive. This

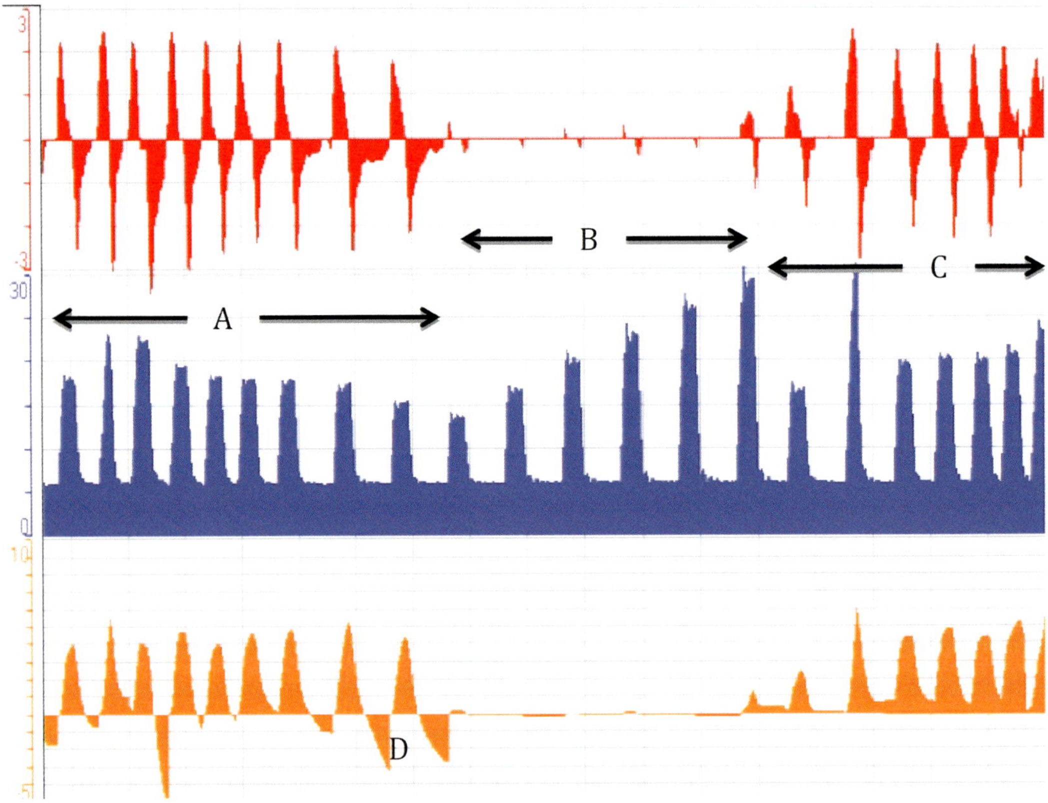

Fig. 6 This figure shows A/C volume guarantee ventilation. At A the inflations are all triggered and the PIP changes a little to maintain the tidal volume. At B the infant splints against the ventilator inflations and stops the flow and tidal volumes even though an inflation is being delivered. As the tidal volume is lower than set, the volume guarantee program uses untriggered, backup inflations and increases the PIP by 3 cm H_2O every inflation until the baby starts breathing again at C, except for one untriggered inflation. Note at D there are expiratory tidal volumes larger than the inspiratory ones. This often happens just as the baby starts splinting and blowing down the lung volume

sensitivity should always be set to 1 so that the inflation occurs as close as possible to the onset of the baby's inspiration. A higher number will mean a longer delay between the onset of inspiration and the start of inflation resulting in a nonsynchronous inflation.

A potential problem with flow triggering is that the sensor detects gas flow from condensed water bubbling in the ventilator circuit and this triggers an inflation even though the baby may not be inspiring at this time – the so-called auto-triggering. Some people reduce the sensitivity to prevent this; however, this causes an unacceptable delay between the onset of inspiration and the inflation. Ensuring the ventilator circuit is free of condensed water can prevent this.

Two other trigger mechanisms have been used:

1. A capsule stuck on the abdomen to detect abdominal movement. This may be unreliable. The effectiveness and accuracy depends on where it is placed on the abdomen.
2. Using a change in the pressure in the ventilator circuit depends on the baby making a sufficiently large inspiration to change the circuit pressure (~0.5 cm H_2O). It is inaccurate if the baby is very small or has a low inspiratory effort.

Some people worry that adding a flow sensor increases the dead space and thereby increases the infant's $PaCO_2$. For this reason, for the very preterm babies, the Vte can be increased a bit to

5–6 ml/Kg for babies <1 Kg. Increased dead space is rarely a big problem because, as an uncuffed ETT is used, there is almost always a leak around the ETT. Even with no leak, the effect on $PaCO_2$ is small and not of clinical significance compared with the clinical gain from using the sensor.

54.7.3 Synchronized Intermittent Mandatory Ventilation (SIMV)

In this mode the ventilator is pressure-limited, and time-cycled, but inflations are triggered by the baby's inspiratory gas flow in synchrony with a prior set number of inspirations. This means that not all the baby's inspirations are supported by a ventilator inflation, e.g., if the baby is breathing at 80/min and the ventilator is set to deliver 30/min, only 30 of the breaths will coincide with an inflation. For all other breaths, the inspiration is through the endotracheal tube with only PEEP for support. If the baby is apneic, the set ventilator rate is delivered.

The ventilator divides each minute by the set number of inflations, called the ventilator interval. For example, if set to 60/min because the inflation time is 0.3 s and the expiratory time 0.7 s, then the ventilator interval is 1 s. If the rate is set to 30/min, inflation time 0.3 s, and expiratory time 1.7 s, the ventilator interval is 2 s. The ventilator will deliver each inflation, triggered or untriggered, within each set ventilator interval.

See Fig. 2 for a recording of the pressure, flow, and tidal volume waves during SIMV.

The problems with SIMV ventilation are:

- Not all inspirations are supported by an inflation.
- The unsupported breaths through the ETT increase the work of breathing and can lead to exhaustion.
- The tidal volume delivered may vary considerably from the triggered inflations to the spontaneous breaths and also due to the set PIP being delivered on top of the baby's tidal volumes.

When should SIMV be used? Because of the problems with spontaneous breaths not being supported by the ventilator, it is inappropriate to use SIMV when the baby is initially ventilated or in respiratory failure. It may have a place when weaning ventilation but this can be a problem if the ventilator rate is set so low that the majority of the baby's breaths are unsupported through the endotracheal tube. It is inferior to A/C synchronized intermittent positive pressure ventilation (SIPPV).

To reduce the work of breathing of the unsupported breaths and overcome the resistance of breathing through the ETT, pressure support (PS) can be added to SIMV to partially assist the spontaneous breaths (Osorio et al. 2005). The initial preset pressure level above PEEP is generally set using the formula (PS = PIP-PEEP/2) and then reduced according to the clinical status of the baby (e.g., respiratory rate, FiO_2 to maintain the SpO_2 target, respiratory effort). The pressure used is guessed by clinical experience and not interactive with the baby's breathing. On the ventilator screen, the PS has a sinusoidal flow waveform between the SIMV inflations (Singh et al. 2007). When compared with SIMV alone, SIMV + PS reduced respiratory rate (Osorio et al. 2005), duration of mechanical ventilation, and oxygen need in preterm infants (Reyes et al. 2006; Patel et al. 2009).

54.7.4 Assist/Control (A/C) Also Called Synchronized Intermittent Positive Pressure Ventilation (SIPPV)

In this mode inflations are triggered by all the baby's inspirations. So it inflates the baby in synchrony with each spontaneous inspiration. This is the most appropriate mode to use when the baby requires full ventilatory support (Abubakar and Keszler 2005; Mrozek et al. 2000; Herrera et al. 2002).

A/C is pressure-limited, time-cycled ventilation, and the PIP, PEEP, inflation time, and expiratory time are set. However if the rate is less than the baby's breathing rate, the baby's inspiration controls the rate. It is important to realize the purpose of A/C is to support all inspirations. If the ventilator rate (the backup) is set too high, the baby does not have enough time to make a breath before the mandatory

inflation starts, the spontaneous breaths are overridden by the ventilator, and the ability to trigger inflations and assist the infant is lost, e.g., if the backup rate is 60/min, then the infant will only trigger inflations if it breathes faster than 60/min. At this backup rate, only about half the baby's breaths will trigger an inflation (McCallion et al. 2008). It is "confusing" for the baby to be trying to breathe and suddenly have inflation asynchronous with its inspiration. The main purpose of the A/C ventilation is then lost. Therefore, it is important to set the backup rate slower, about 30/min, so all the baby's breaths can trigger inflation. If the baby stops breathing, the ventilator rate will be 30/min. Spontaneously breathing ventilated babies rarely become completely apneic for very long, but obviously a rate of 30/min for several minutes after a spontaneous triggered rate of about 70/min would need careful monitoring.

See Fig. 3 for a recording of the pressure, flow, and tidal volume waves during A/C ventilation.

Some people think that with A/C mode babies are more likely to become overventilated if they trigger the ventilator too fast. In my experience this is no more of a problem than with other modes if the PIP is set to ensure reasonable average tidal and minute volumes. The clinicians need to carefully monitor the tidal volume and minute volume.

In A/C mode the baby mainly controls the ventilator rate, and so if the $PaCO_2$ is low, it is inappropriate to reduce the rate to reduce minute volume because the baby is controlling the rate. To control $PaCO_2$ PIP is the parameter to change.

54.7.5 Volume Guarantee Ventilation

One of the major complications from ventilating infants is acute lung injury leading to bronchopulmonary dysplasia. Volutrauma is one of the main causes of this. Tidal volumes of more than 8 ml/kg may cause volutrauma and so it is important to measure and control the tidal volume. This mode reduces volutrauma.

Traditionally, during neonatal ventilation altering the PIP has been used to change the $PaCO_2$. It is often forgotten, or not realized, that the PIP is a proxy for tidal volume and altering the PIP changes the tidal volume. The delivered PIP can now be changed automatically to target a specified tidal volume. This should be in the range 3.5–6.0 ml/kg depending on the baby's breathing rate and the ventilator backup rate.

The volume guarantee mode specifically targets the delivery of an expiratory tidal volume set by the clinicians (Patel et al. 2009). It works in all triggered modes: SIMV, A/C, and pressure support ventilation (PSV). The ventilator monitors expired tidal volume and determines whether it is higher, lower, or identical to the set expired tidal volume. If it is higher, the PIP is reduced for the next inflation, and if the tidal volume is lower, the PIP is increased to try and ensure the set tidal volume is achieved.

The volume guarantee mode controls the expired tidal volume very closely to the set tidal volume (Keszler and Abubakar 2004). Analyses from 6693 inflations: mean (SD) for triggered expired tidal volume =102% (29%) of set and range 0–378%; for untriggered = 97% (31%) and range 0–322% (McCallion et al. 2008). It can be seen that there can be large variations in the tidal volume. This is due to the infant's breathing. If the infant takes breaths larger than the set tidal volume, the ventilator cannot, and will not, prevent this. The ventilator response is to lower the PIP for subsequent inflations. If the inspired tidal volume is more than 130%, then the inflation is stopped. Sometimes ventilated infants "splint" or contract their abdominal muscles very hard and completely stop an inflation. The response of the ventilator will be to increase the PIP in a stepwise fashion to try and restore the tidal volume. This overcomes the splinting, and consequent hypoxia, quicker than ventilation continuing with a set PIP.

See Figs. 3, 4, 5, and 6 for recordings of assist/control with volume guarantee.

Some pressure-limited ventilators have two inflating pressures called pressure support ventilation. In this mode the PIPs are set and not related to the delivered tidal volume for many inflations. However, in volume guarantee mode, the PIP changes all the time to try and maintain the tidal volume in response to the infant's breathing.

There are several safety features with volume guarantee that ensure the tidal volume is safe and as accurate as possible:

1. If the inflating tidal volume is more than 130% of the set expired tidal volume, the current inflation is stopped.
2. The PIP does not change, up or down, by more than 3 cm H_2O from one inflation to the next. This works independently for triggered and untriggered inflations (McCallion et al. 2008).
3. There is a separate control of PIP for triggered and untriggered inflations. This is because the baby is contributing to the delivered tidal volume and the PIP required with triggered inflations will be lower than with untriggered inflations where the tidal volume has to be achieved totally by the PIP.
4. Sudden large changes in PIP can occur from one inflation to the next if the backup rate is set too close to the infant's spontaneous rate because the ventilator changes from triggered to untriggered inflations with the untriggered inflations having a larger PIP than triggered ones. However, importantly it does not result in sudden large changes in tidal volume because these are being controlled. This overrides the algorithm for the PIP not changing from one inflation to the next by more than 3 cm H_2O.
5. The expired tidal volume is used for the set tidal volume rather than inspired tidal volume because part of the inflation tidal volume is lost through leak around the ETT.
6. Volume guarantee automatically weans the PIP as the lungs heal, compliance and resistance improve, and the baby breathes more effectively. If a baby generates a tidal volume larger than the set tidal volume, the PIP may reach the PEEP level.

54.7.5.1 Setting the Maximum Inflating Pressure That Can Be Delivered in VG

In VG the maximum PIP the ventilator is allowed to deliver is called the Pmax. The Pmax should be set above the PIP being used to ventilate the baby. In VG it is important that the ventilator can pick an appropriate PIP to deliver the target Vt set. It should be set to a level the clinicians would like to be alerted about and are comfortable with. There is a debate about what pressure should be used for the Pmax. If it is set high, e.g., 30 cm H_2O, to allow the ventilator to use pressures up to that level, then it may occasionally deliver this pressure, which may concern some neonatologists. What is important is that the clinical team need to be vigilant and consider why the PIP has risen and whether there is a problem that needs correcting. Reasons may be: there is an increased leak around the ETT and so a higher pressure is needed to compensate and deliver the set Vte; the lung disease has deteriorated; and pneumothorax, PIE, atelectasis, and ETT either dislodged into the right main bronchus or nearly extubated. As the baby's condition changes, so the Pmax may need to be reset. Some experts set the Pmax about 3–5 cm H_2O above the PIP being used to maintain the set Vt. This gives a more sensitive control over the PIP delivered. If the Pmax is set too low, the ventilator may frequently alarm "low tidal volume" because it is limiting the PIP needed to deliver the set tidal volume. This can be a problem either because the frequencies of the alarms frustrate the staff or because they ignore the alarms and don't look for the cause of the alarm. It is important that the Pmax level is considered and reset if needed both if it is too high and too low. During weaning the Pmax should be reduced to avoid an inappropriately high PIP being delivered.

We consider the baby ready to be extubated from VG when the set Vt is 4–6 ml/Kg and (a) when the PIP is less than 16–14 cm H_2O), (b) the FiO_2 is <0.3, (c) there is no tachypnea or other signs of respiratory difficulty such as retraction, and (d) $pH > 7.2$ and $pCO_2 < 65$ mmHg.

When ventilating with volume guarantee, A/C mode is best so that every spontaneous breath triggers an inflation. With this combination of A/C and volume guarantee, the baby's spontaneous rate controls the ventilator rate and the volume guarantee controls the PIP. Therefore to control the $PaCO_2$, the important control is the set tidal volume. This can be increased to reduce the $PaCO_2$ or lowered to increase the $PaCO_2$, especially in chronically ventilated infants with increased pulmonary dead space and distension of the trachea.

Evidence from systematic review and meta-analysis demonstrated that preterm infants managed with tidal volume-targeted ventilation (e.g., VG ventilation) had reduced incidence of BPD,

duration of mechanical ventilation, severe IVH and PVL, pneumothorax, and risk of hypocarbia, when compared with preterm babies ventilated with pressure-limited ventilation (Wheeler et al. 2010; Peng et al. 2014). Nevertheless, the authors concluded that further multicenter RCTs are required to evaluate the impact of this ventilatory approach on long-term neurodevelopmental outcome, death, and other complications related to mechanical ventilation. We can hypothesize that a further positive effect to volume-targeted ventilation could be given by the optimization of the PEEP level. In the past PEEP has been defined as a "cheap" and effective lung protection, and the research for appropriate levels of PEEP (the so-called best PEEP) guided by SpO_2, blood gas levels, transcutaneous CO_2 monitoring, and chest X-ray (Monkman and Kirpalani 2003) is used not only in adults with ARDS but also in preterm infants with respiratory failure. It seems to be an intriguing approach to implement the protective effect of volume-targeted ventilation (Castoldi et al. 2011). A recent Cochrane review concluded, "there is insufficient evidence to guide selection of appropriate PEEP levels for RDS or CMV. There is a need for well designed clinical trials evaluating the optimal application of this important and frequently applied intervention" (Bamat et al. 2012).

54.7.6 Pressure Support Ventilation

With the Drager 8000+ ventilator, there is another triggered mode called pressure support ventilation (PSV). This is a confusing term because all the other modes are pressure supported. It is a mode that triggers ventilator exhalation and therefore automatically controls the inflation time. The ventilator tracks the inflation flow curve as it rises and falls. As the flow decreases from the peak flow to 15% of the peak flow, this triggers the ventilator to stop inflation. It automatically takes account of any leak flow. It is therefore important the inflation time is set much longer than normal ventilation to allow the ventilator to increase the expiratory time if needed. An expiratory time of 0.6 s would be appropriate even though the program will usually be choosing expiratory times nearer 0.3 s in response to the flow curve.

The shape and timing of the inflation flow curve is dependent on the gas flow in the circuit. A high gas flow will result in a shorter inflation time and a low gas flow a longer inflation time. When ventilating a baby with a low gas flow, e.g., 4 L/min, then the pressure support mode is very valuable to pick the appropriate expiratory time. The advantage of this mode is that the infant cannot exhale against inflation.

54.7.7 Neurally Adjusted Ventilator Assist (NAVA)

To reduce possible asynchrony with ventilator inflations, a new mode of mechanical ventilation has been introduced called neurally adjusted ventilator assist (NAVA) (Hummler and Schuze 2009). Using electrodes on a specially designed nasogastric tube, it detects and analyzes the diaphragmatic EMG and uses this signal to trigger ventilator inflations in proportion and in synchrony with the phasic inspiratory diaphragmatic electrical activity. Backup pressure control is provided when there is no diaphragm signal. Small preliminary studies have shown that NAVA can be successfully used in term and preterm infants (Beck et al. 2009; Stein et al. 2013). NAVA is contraindicated in some specific conditions (e.g., esophageal malformation, coagulation disorders, pace makers in use, or apnea). Large multicenter trials are needed to determine the usefulness and accuracy of NAVA and compare it with tidal volume-targeted assist/control ventilation and pressure-controlled ventilation and whether it decreases duration of ventilation and reduces BPD, rate of pneumothorax, and other major complications of prematurity.

54.7.8 High-Frequency Oscillatory Ventilation (HFOV)

This mode of ventilation is used when other modes of ventilation is unable to ensure satisfactory CO_2 exchange without using a high PIP (e.g., 30 cm H_2O or more) to deliver the tidal volume.

HFOV is done in different ways by different ventilators and so I will concentrate on the principles:

1. The lung volume is produced and maintained by a continuous high mean airway pressure ~10–20 cm H_2O, not just an end expiratory pressure of ~5 cm H_2O.
2. The tidal volume delivered is approximately equal to the infants dead space volume ~2 ml/kg
3. The ventilator rate is much higher than conventional ventilation at between 5 and 15 Hz (300 and 900/min).

Adjusting three main parameters controls the ventilation:

1. The mean airway pressure (MAP). As this controls the lung volume, and oxygenation is approximately proportional to lung volume, the MAP is increased until the FiO_2 required to produce an appropriate PaO_2 is at the lowest that can be achieved. If the MAP is increased too much, the oxygenation will deteriorate. It is best to start with a MAP slightly higher than that used on conventional ventilation and increase it until the FiO_2 is optimized. It has been recommended (Dargaville and Tingay 2012) that lung volume optimization during HFOV may be best done by stepwise increments in MAP, starting from a low MAP (e.g., 6–8 cm H_2O) and increasing the MAP to until the FiO_2 is reduced to 0.3–0.25 to obtain for the target SpO_2 and normal transcutaneous CO_2, until FiO_2 is reduced to 0.3–0.25 (De Jaegere et al. 2006). By stepwise reductions of MAP, with transcutaneous CO_2 monitoring, the minimal MAP can be found to maintain the SpO_2 targets with reduced FiO_2 and normal CO_2. Frequent chest X-rays will provide some information about the lung inflation, particularly whether the lungs are underinflated, one lung is collapsed, the lungs are seriously overinflated, or there is air leak. Changing MAP has the same effect on all HFOV ventilators.
2. The amplitude of the ventilating pressure swing (ΔP). This is the change in the pressure that is driving the change in tidal volume. This is one controller of CO_2. The higher is the ΔP, the more CO_2 is removed. The best way to judge whether the ΔP is correct is to start low and increase it until the chest is seen to be just wriggling with the ventilator. It is very easy to quickly overventilate babies with HFOV and drive the $PaCO_2$ down to dangerous levels in a few minutes. To monitor, use a transcutaneous CO_2 sensor before HFOV is started. As the $PaCO_2$ falls, ΔP is reduced accordingly. The ΔP is not very powerful with the Drager 8000+ and increasing it above 60% has little added benefit.
3. The high-frequency rate also affects the $PaCO_2$. It is important to realize this is the opposite of conventional ventilation: as the rate is reduced, the $PaCO_2$ is likely to fall, and as the rate is increased, the $PaCO_2$ rises. This is because at a lower rate, the ΔP has more time and therefore is likely to increase removing more CO_2; as the rate increases, the ΔP is reduced. It is best to start at ~8–10 Hz, adjust the MAP and ΔP to optimize the blood gases, and only adjust the frequency if the $PaCO_2$ cannot be controlled at the frequency chosen. With the Drager Babylog 8000+, changing the rate has more effect on $PaCO_2$ than changing ΔP.

The advantages of HFOV are:

1. Improvement in oxygenation by using a higher mean airway pressure than is acceptable during conventional ventilation
2. Better CO_2 removal in infants with very stiff lungs where an unacceptably high PIP would be required to produce an appropriate tidal volume

The disadvantages of HFOV are:

1. It does not synchronize with the baby's breathing.
2. It is very easy to overventilate and produce hypocarbia with HFOV.
3. The Sensormedics ventilator provides no feedback to the clinicians.
4. The Sensormedics ventilator has few alarms about the adequacy of ventilation. In fact the ETT can be clamped and no gas delivered to the baby and yet there is no alarm.

5. It is not clear how well the infant is breathing or when the infant is ready for weaning.

The Drager VN500 has a new HFOV mode of HFOV volume guarantee. More research is needed to determine if this controls and delivers the HFOV more accurately.

54.8 Weaning the Infant from Ventilation

The longer the baby is intubated and ventilated, the more likely infection will occur and neonatal chronic lung disease develops. It is therefore important to wean babies from the ventilator and extubate them as soon as possible.

The FiO_2 is reduced to maintain appropriate PaO_2 and SpO_2 and the PIP (tidal volume) is reduced to maintain the $PaCO_2$ in the normal range

When the FiO_2 and PIP have been reduced to ~ <0.40 and <16 cm H_2O, respectively, the lungs are improving, and if the baby breathes adequately, extubation may be possible. In the VG mode, the ventilator automatically weans the PIP to deliver the set Vt.

Some people advocate reducing the ventilator rate in SIMV mode so that the baby has more spontaneous and less supported breaths. One problem is the unsupported breaths are made through the ETT. This increases the work of breathing. This becomes significant if the ventilator rate is reduced below about 30/min. Lower rates are unnecessary because to maintain a normal $PaCO_2$, the baby will be breathing well.

Many babies can be extubated from A/C ventilation when the FiO_2 and PIP are low without the need for SIMV. Similarly, babies can be extubated from SIMV at 30/min.

To help decide whether a baby will breathe adequately after extubation, the ventilator can be switched to ETT CPAP for ~ 3 min, and see how well the heart rate, SpO_2, and respiratory pattern are maintained (Kamlin et al. 2006). A baby who can maintain the SpO_2 and heart rate on a few minutes of ETT CPAP has a high chance of successful extubation. A baby who becomes bradycardic or hypoxic during this time is unlikely to breathe well after extubation.

Preterm babies should be treated with caffeine (Schmidt et al. 2006, 2007) or theophylline before extubation. This increases the chance of successful extubation. They should be extubated to nasal CPAP, or NIPPV, or high-flow nasal cannula oxygen, rather than straight to unsupported breathing. These modes have been shown to reduce the incidence of reintubation (Davis et al. 1998).

54.9 Managing Complications of Ventilation

54.9.1 Endotracheal Tube Not in the Trachea

In order for a baby to be ventilated, an ETT has to be passed into the trachea. This is not a simple procedure and it has been shown that this takes two or more attempts (Lane et al. 2004; O'Donnell et al. 2006). It has also been shown that the person intubating the baby often thinks (hopes) that ETT is in the trachea, and it may take several minutes before they realize that the baby's failure to respond to the ventilation is because the ETT is not in the trachea. Some infants have been seriously compromised because the clinicians failed to appreciate they had intubated the esophagus. It is so important to ensure the ETT is in the trachea that after every intubation a CO_2 detector (Kamlin et al. 2005) or a gas flow detector is connected to the ETT so that expired CO_2 or the inspiratory and expiratory gas flow can be detected to ensure the ETT is properly placed.

54.9.2 Endotracheal Tube Inserted Too Far Down into the Right Main Bronchus

If the ETT is either inserted too far or it slips down after insertion, it will enter the right main bronchus. The left lung and right upper lobe will then not be ventilated. The diagnosis is made from a chest X-ray. The treatment is to withdraw the ETT to the appropriate level.

54.9.3 Accidental Extubation

Accidental extubation of a ventilated baby is a serious problem because the baby's condition may deteriorate quickly. Securing the ETT so it does not come loose can prevent it. Accidental extubation can be difficult to differentiate from other causes of a rapid deterioration. There are several ways to make the diagnosis. The quickest, most accurate technique is to watch the display of the ETT flow wave. If the ETT becomes dislodged, the flow pattern immediately changes so there is flow down the ETT but not back up. Placing a carbon dioxide detector on the distal end of the ETT will also rapidly show whether CO_2-containing gas is coming out of the ETT (Aziz et al. 1999). This is rapid and sensitive. Other techniques, such as auscultation of both lungs and misting of the ETT, are not so accurate. Inspection of the larynx with a laryngoscope is invasive but the only way to determine the position of the ETT if other methods are unavailable.

54.9.4 Pneumothorax

A tension pneumothorax is one cause of deterioration in a ventilated baby. This is manifest by an increased FiO_2 and/or a rising $PaCO_2$ and increased ventilatory pressures when in volume guarantee mode. Occasionally it presents with apnea.

Seeing a pneumothorax on an urgent chest X-ray confirms the diagnosis. Occasionally, the pneumothorax is not very obvious because the gas is anterior, and with the baby lying supine, the lung appears to fill the chest. One of the best radiological signs is an obvious clear demarcation around the heart, diaphragm, or mediastinum. These are normally blurred in a baby with RDS. Transillumination of the chest with a bright light in darkened surroundings usually shows the hemithorax glowing. Although this is useful in an emergency, it is not completely reliable and so a chest X-ray should always be obtained to confirm the diagnosis if possible.

The treatment is an intercostal drain, placed under strict sterile conditions, with the distal tubing underwater in a sealed bottle with suction applied to the outlet. The insertion site should be the fourth or fifth intercostal place in the anterior axillary line but away from the breast bud. The baby should be placed on his back with the affected side elevated so the body is at approximately 45° to the mattress. The drain is then inserted from the posterior lateral aspect. This ensures the drain passes anteriorly rather than posteriorly and therefore drains the air at the front of the chest. Under local anesthetic a small hole is made in the chest wall, just above a rib, and then enlarged appropriately with small artery forceps. These are used to introduce the catheter. A trocar should not be used because this increases the chance of perforating the lung.

54.9.5 Pulmonary Interstitial Emphysema (PIE)

This mostly occurs in ventilated very premature babies. It can be a serious problem and may cause death if not treated promptly and effectively. In this condition gas tracks into the interstitial tissues and compresses the airways. It commonly occurs throughout one or both lungs and probably comes from a tear in the hilum where the gas is forced into the tissues. It causes a serious deterioration in the respiratory and clinical status of the baby. The diagnosis is made from the chest X-ray.

There are two important aspects to the treatment of PIE (Swingle et al. 1984). (1) Reduce the ventilator PIP, PEEP, or set Vt, even if the $PaCO_2$ or FiO_2 rises as a consequence. However, do not compromise the baby's clinical and physiological stability to an extent where the baby may deteriorate. (2) Lay the baby with the affected side down and with the back at right angles to the mattress. The affected lung is dependent and slowly looses the PIE. This is one of the best ways of treating PIE. If both lungs are affected, lay the baby so the worst lung is dependent. This treatment may lead to complete collapse of the dependent lung. This is a transient problem and with repositioning the lung usually reinflates without PIE.

54.10 Drug Treatments During Ventilation

54.10.1 Muscle-Relaxing Drugs

In the past muscle-relaxing drugs were commonly used for ventilated babies. This has now become uncommon, as neonatologists have realized that it is better to support the spontaneous breathing of the baby rather than take overventilation completely. There is no evidence that the use of muscle-relaxing drugs improves the outcome for babies with RDS (Cools and Offringa 2005). In fact their use reduces venous return, causes edema, increases the ventilator pressure required, and prolongs ventilation. They should only be used when babies are very difficult to ventilate and oppose inflation.

54.10.2 Caffeine

Caffeine when given to ventilated very premature babies has been shown to reduce the incidence of apnea; reduce the duration of ventilation, duration of oxygen treatment, and the incidence of BPD; and reduce the incidence of neurodevelopmental problems (Schmidt et al. 2006). It appears to have few serious side effects (Schmidt et al. 2007). Caffeine should be given early to all ventilated very preterm infants, not just for treating apnea.

54.10.3 Sedation

Many people sedate ventilated infants to make them feel less stressed and more comfortable. Several different sedatives have been used. The appropriate sedative and dose has not been elucidated. There is no good evidence that they improve the outcomes for the babies, and they may adversely affect the baby's respiratory drive so that it takes longer for the baby to breathe sufficiently to be extubated (Bhandari et al. 2005; Bellu et al. 2009). The best way to keep the baby comfortable is with good nursing care and appropriate positioning.

References

Abubakar K, Keszler M (2005) Effect of volume guarantee combined with assist/control vs synchronized intermittent mandatory ventilation. J Perinatol 25 (10):638–642

Ammari A et al (2005) Variables associated with the early failure of nasal CPAP in very low birth weight infants. J Pediatr 147(3):341–347

Attar MA, Donn SM (2002) Mechanisms of ventilator-induced lung injury in premature infants. Semin Neonatol 7(5):353–360

Aziz HF et al (1999) The pediatric disposable end-tidal carbon dioxide detector role in endotracheal intubation in newborns. J Perinatol 19(2):110–113

Bamat N et al. (2012) Positive end expiratory pressure for preterm infants requiring conventional mechanical ventilation for respiratory distress syndrome or bronchopulmonary dysplasia. Cochrane Database Syst Rev CD004500.pub2

Beck J et al (2009) Patient-ventilator interaction during neurally adjusted ventilatory assist in very low birth weight infants. Pediatr Res 65(6):663–668

Bellu R et al (2009) Opioids for neonates receiving mechanical ventilation. A systematic review and meta-Analysis. Arch Dis Child Fetal Neonatal Ed 95 (4):F241–F251

Bhandari V et al (2005) Morphine administration and short-term pulmonary outcomes among ventilated preterm infants. Pediatrics 116(2):352–359

Bjorklund LJ et al (1997) Manual ventilation with a few large breaths at birth compromises the therapeutic effect of subsequent surfactant replacement in immature lambs. Pediatr Res 42(3):348–355

Carlo WA et al (1987) Control of laryngeal muscle activity in preterm infants. Pediatr Res 22(1):87–91

Castoldi F et al (2011) Lung recruitment maneuver during volume guarantee ventilation of preterm infants with acute respiratory distress syndrome. Am J Perinatol 28 (7):521–528

Cools F, Offringa M (2005) Neuromuscular paralysis for newborn infants receiving mechanical ventilation. Cochrane Database Syst Rev (2): p CD002773

Dargaville PA, Tingay DG (2012) Lung protective ventilation in extremely preterm infants. J Paediatr Child Health 48:740–746

Davis P et al (1998) Randomised controlled trial of nasal continuous positive airway pressure in the extubation of infants weighing 600 to 1250 g. Arch Dis Child Fetal Neonatal Ed 78:F1–F4

De Jaegere A et al (2006) Lung recruitment using oxygenation during open lung high-frequency ventilation in preterm infants. Am J Respir Crit Care Med 174:639–645

Donn SM, Sinha SK (2003) Can mechanical ventilation strategies reduce chronic lung disease? Semin Neonatol 8(6):441–448

Greenough A et al (1986) Fighting the ventilator–are fast rates an effective alternative to paralysis? Early Hum Dev 13(2):189–194

Herrera CM et al (2002) Effects of volume-guaranteed synchronized intermittent mandatory ventilation in preterm infants recovering from respiratory failure. Pediatrics 110(3):529–533

Hoellering AB et al (2008) Lung volume and cardiorespiratory changes during open and closed endotracheal suction in ventilated newborn infants. Arch Dis Child Fetal Neonatal Ed 93(6):F436–F441

Hummler H, Schuze A (2009) New and alternative modes of mechanical ventilation in neonates. Semin Fetal Neonatal Med 14(1):42–48

Kamlin CO et al (2005) Colorimetric end-tidal carbon dioxide detectors in the delivery room: strengths and limitations. A case report. J Pediatr 147(4):547–548

Kamlin CO et al (2006) Predicting successful extubation of very low birthweight infants. Arch Dis Child Fetal Neonatal Ed 91(3):F180–F183

Keszler M, Abubakar K (2004) Volume guarantee: stability of tidal volume and incidence of hypocarbia. Pediatr Pulmonol 38(3):240–245

Lane B et al (2004) Duration of intubation attempts during neonatal resuscitation. J Pediatr 145(1):67–70

McCallion N et al (2005) Volume-targeted versus pressure-limited ventilation in the neonate. Cochrane Database Syst Rev (3): CD003666

McCallion N et al (2005b) Volume guarantee ventilation, interrupted expiration, and expiratory braking. Arch Dis Child 90(8):865–870

McCallion N et al (2008) Neonatal volume guarantee ventilation: effects of spontaneous breathing, triggered and untriggered inflations. Arch Dis Child Fetal Neonatal Ed 93(1):F36–F39

Monkman S, Kirpalani H (2003) PEEP – a "cheap" and effective lung protection. Pediatr Resp Rev 4(1):15–20

Morley CJ et al (2008) Nasal CPAP or intubation at birth for very preterm infants. N Engl J Med 358(7):700–708

Mrozek JD et al (2000) Randomized controlled trial of volume-targeted synchronized ventilation and conventional intermittent mandatory ventilation following initial exogenous surfactant therapy. Pediatr Pulmonol 29 (1):11–18

O'Donnell CP et al (2006) Endotracheal intubation attempts during neonatal resuscitation: success rates, duration, and adverse effects. Pediatrics 117(1):e16–e21

Okumura A et al (2001) Hypocarbia in preterm infants with periventricular leukomalacia: the relation between hypocarbia and mechanical ventilation. Pediatrics 107 (3):469–475

Osorio W et al (2005) Effects of pressure support during an acute reduction of synchronized intermittent mandatory ventilation in preterm infants. J Perinatol 25 (6):412–416

Patel DS et al (2009) Work of breathing and different levels of volume-targeted ventilation. Pediatrics 123(4): e679–e684

Pellicano A et al (2009) Comparison of four methods of lung volume recruitment during high frequency oscillatory ventilation. Intensive Care Med 35(11):1990–1998

Peng WS et al (2014) Volume-targeted ventilation is more suitable than pressure-limited ventilation for preterm infants: a systematic review and meta-analysis. Arch Dis Child Fetal Neonatal Ed 99:F158–F165

Reyes ZC et al (2006) Randomized, controlled trial comparing synchronized intermittent mandatory ventilation and synchronized intermittent mandatory ventilation plus pressure support in preterm infants. Pediatrics 118(4):1409–1417

Schmidt B et al (2006) Caffeine therapy for apnea of prematurity. N Engl J Med 354(20):2112–2121

Schmidt B et al (2007) Long-term effects of caffeine therapy for apnea of prematurity. N Engl J Med 357 (19):1893–1902

Schmolzer GM et al (2010) Respiratory monitoring of neonatal resuscitation. Arch Dis Child Fetal Neonatal Ed 95(4):F295–F303

Schulze A (2007) Respiratory gas conditioning and humidification. Clin Perinatol 34(1):19–33

Singh J et al (2007) Volume-targeted ventilation of newborns. Clin Perinatol 34:9–1053

South M, Morley CJ (1986a) Synchronous mechanical ventilation of the neonate. Arch Dis Child 61 (12):1190–1195

South M, Morley CJ (1986b) Monitoring spontaneous respiration in the ventilated neonate. Arch Dis Child 61(3):291–294

South M, Morley CJ (1986c) Ventilator settings and active expiration. Arch Dis Child 61:310–311

South M, Morley CJ (1992) Respiratory timing in intubated neonates with respiratory distress syndrome. Arch Dis Child 67(4):446–448

South M et al (1987) Expiratory muscle activity in preterm babies. Arch Dis Child 62(8):825–829

South M et al (1988) A simple technique for recording the electromyogram of the external abdominal oblique muscle in the newborn. Early Hum Dev 16 (1):55–60

Stein H et al (2013) Prospective crossover comparison between NAVA and pressure control ventilation in premature neonates less than 1500 grams. J Perinatol 33 (6):452–456

Swingle HM et al (1984) New approach to management of unilateral tension pulmonary interstitial emphysema in premature infants. Pediatrics 74(3):354–357

Thome U et al (1998) The effect of positive end expiratory pressure, peak inspiratory pressure, and inspiratory time on functional residual capacity in mechanically ventilated preterm infants. Eur J Pediatr 157(10): 831–837

Tingay DG et al (2007) Effects of open endotracheal suction on lung volume in infants receiving HFOV. Intensive Care Med 33(4):689–693

Wheeler KI et al (2009a) Assist control volume guarantee ventilation during surfactant administration. Arch Dis Child Fetal Neonatal Ed 94(5):F336–F338

Wheeler KI et al (2009b) Volume-guarantee ventilation: pressure may decrease during obstructed flow. Arch Dis Child Fetal Neonatal Ed 94(2):F84–F86

Wheeler KK et al (2010) Volume-targeted or pressure-limited ventilation in the neonate. Cochrane Database Syst Rev 11:CD003666

Pulmonary Hemorrhage, Transient Tachypnea, and Neonatal Pneumonia

55

Mary Elaine Patrinos and Richard J. Martin

Contents

Abstract

The intent of this chapter is to address three other common pulmonary causes of respiratory distress in the high-risk infant. These other forms of parenchymal lung disease range in severity from mild, as seen in transient tachypnea, to severe as is often the case in pulmonary hemorrhage. It is worth noting that on occasion, one or more of these conditions may coexist in the same patient. The treatment for all conditions is largely supportive or involves the use of targeted antimicrobial therapy.

M. E. Patrinos
Case Western Reserve University School of Medicine, Cleveland, OH, USA
e-mail: maryelaine.patrinos@uhhospitals.org

R. J. Martin (✉)
Rainbow Babies and Children's Hospital, Division of Neonatology, Case Western Reserve University School of Medicine, Cleveland, OH, USA
e-mail: rxm6@case.edu

55.1 Salient Points

- Pulmonary hemorrhage occurs as a result of extreme pulmonary vascular congestion where blood-tinged secretions suctioned from the endotracheal tube may quickly evolve into frank blood. The volume of blood loss can be life-threatening, resulting in hypovolemic shock.
- The management of pulmonary hemorrhage is largely supportive with the goals of correcting hypoxic and hypercapnic respiratory failure, maintaining cardiac output, replacing blood and volume loss, and correcting abnormalities in clotting studies.
- Transient tachypnea of the newborn (TTN) is a transient early-onset respiratory distress with radiographic findings of lung hyperinflation increased pulmonary vascular markings and cardiomegaly.
- Risk factors for developing TTN include elective cesarean section without labor, prematu-

G. Buonocore et al. (eds.), *Neonatology*,
https://doi.org/10.1007/978-3-319-29489-6_203

rity, multiple gestation, male gender, maternal diabetes, macrosomia, prolonged maternal administration of hypotonic fluid, and maternal asthma.

- Neonatal pneumonia may be acquired pre- or post-natally and may be of bacterial, viral, fungal, or protozoal origin.
- The incidence of neonatal pneumonia is ten times higher for preterm infants then term infants.
- The onset of neonatal pneumonia can be congenital, early onset, and late onset. Congenital or intrauterine pneumonia is usually caused by organisms ascending from the maternal urogenital tract before or during labor or via the transplacental route. Early-onset pneumonia is usually acquired in the perinatal period. Late-onset pneumonia is diagnosed when symptoms arise after 48 h of life and the pathogens are typically acquired from the infant's environment.
- It is difficult to diagnose pneumonia, especially when it coincides with RDS. If the index of suspicion for infection is high, the accepted treatment is antibiotics for 48 h while awaiting culture results and following other clinical and laboratory parameters.

55.2 Pulmonary Hemorrhage

Pulmonary hemorrhage (PH) occurs as a result of extreme pulmonary congestion where blood-tinged secretions suctioned from the endotracheal tube may quickly evolve into frank blood. The volume of blood loss can be life-threatening, resulting in hypovolemic shock. PH usually presents in the second to fourth day of life and may be associated with lung tissue damage from respiratory distress syndrome, infection, mechanical ventilation, and oxygen-induced lung injury. Patients at highest risk for a PH include extremely preterm infants (<28 weeks' gestation) and multiples. Other predisposing factors include hypoxia, acidosis, hypervolemia, hypoproteinemia, congestive heart failure, and coagulation abnormalities. Kluckow confirmed an association between pulmonary hemorrhage and a large patent ductus arteriosus (PDA) with high pulmonary blood flow (references Kluckow and Evans 2000).

Pulmonary hemorrhage occurs when a buildup of filtrate containing plasma and whole blood produces hemorrhagic edema fluid leading to an increase in capillary pressure and subsequent rupture (Cole et al. 1973). The presence of blood in the sputum of an otherwise stable intubated infant should raise the possibility of erosion or ulceration of the carina/upper airway by an endotracheal tube or trauma from a suction catheter.

Pulmonary hemorrhage was present in the lungs of up to 68% of infants who died in the first week of life and was associated with the need for cardiopulmonary resuscitation in the neonatal intensive care unit (Kostelanetz and Dhanireddy 2004). Blood aspiration syndrome is a distinct and separate entity associated with maternal hemorrhage and early-onset respiratory distress (Gordon et al. 2003).

The clinical picture of pulmonary hemorrhage is quite dramatic and warrants immediate attention. The infant may present with signs of hypovolemic shock, cyanosis, bradycardia, and apnea. Red or pink-tinged secretions suctioned from the oropharynx or endotracheal tube may, at any time, progress to massive bleeding. The radiographic picture demonstrates patchy infiltrates, as seen in Fig. 1, or a complete white out.

The management of pulmonary hemorrhage is largely supportive with the goals of correcting hypoxic and hypercapnic respiratory failure, maintaining cardiac output, replacing blood and volume loss, and correcting abnormalities in clotting studies. The initiation of mechanical ventilation with settings adjusted to achieve high mean airway pressures may tamponade small pulmonary vessels. High-frequency oscillatory ventilation is often helpful. There is increasing evidence that closure of the patent ductus arteriosus with early medical therapy may reduce the risk of pulmonary hemorrhage. It is widely accepted that pulmonary hemorrhage in the preterm infant is secondary to a patent ductus arteriosus coupled with an acute change in pulmonary compliance and fall in pulmonary vascular resistance, resulting in pulmonary over circulation and edema. Recent data indicate

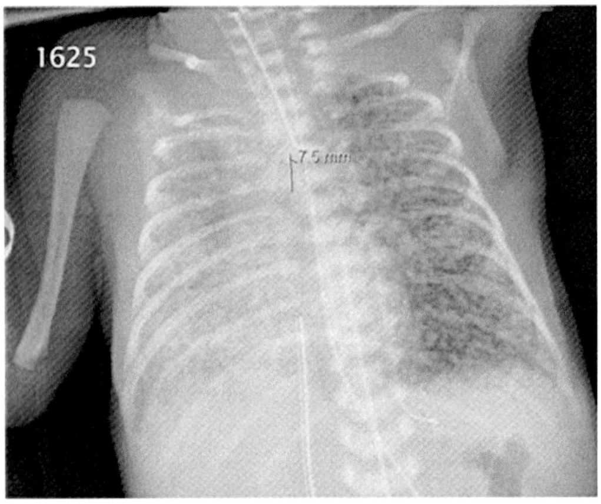

Fig. 1 Diffuse, patchy infiltrates, and right-sided atelectasis caused by pulmonary hemorrhage

that small-for-gestational-age preterm infants with a moderate to large PDA are at greatest risk (Scholl and Yanowitz 2015).

While surfactant therapy has been implicated in the pathogenesis of pulmonary hemorrhage, it also has a therapeutic role in its management (Findlay et al. 1995; Long et al. 1992; Pandit et al. 1995; Pappin et al. 1994; Raju and Langenberg 1993; Amizuka et al. 2003). This is due to the deactivation of surfactant by the hemorrhagic fluid.

In a small study, the introduction of hemocoagulase via the endotracheal tube every 4–6 h in addition to mechanical ventilation increased survival, decreased the length of pulmonary hemorrhage, and decreased the need for prolonged mechanical ventilation due to the pulmonary hemorrhage (Shi et al. 2005). The outcome of pulmonary hemorrhage depends on the severity of the infant's underlying cardiorespiratory status. Mortality rates as high as 50% occur in ELBW infants. Morbidities include periventricular leukomalacia, intraventricular hemorrhage, cerebral palsy, and cognitive delays.

55.3 Transient Tachypnea of the Newborn

Transient tachypnea of the newborn (TTN) was originally described by Avery et al. in 1966 as the clinical manifestation of delayed clearance of fetal lung fluid (Avery et al. 1966). In her work, Avery characterized early-onset respiratory distress in eight late premature infants with radiographic findings of lung hyperinflation increased pulmonary vascular markings and cardiomegaly. Symptoms were mild and transient with infants improving in a 2–5-day period. Until recently, it was believed that once TTN resolves, there are no long-term consequences for the infant (Avery et al. 1966; Martin et al. 2015; Miller et al. 1980). However, a large retrospective study of term infants suggests that TTN might be significantly associated with childhood asthma with increased propensity in males. This study also suggests that TTN is a marker of diminished pulmonary function, which may reflect an inherited susceptibility to develop asthma (Liem et al. 2007).

The incidence of TTN is approximately 1% of live births. Risks for developing TTN include elective cesarean section without labor, prematurity, multiple gestation, male gender, maternal diabetes, and macrosomia (Gross et al. 1983; Rawlings and Smith 1984). Prolonged maternal administration of hypotonic fluid and maternal asthma have also been suggested as a cause for TTN (Martin et al. 2015; Hook et al. 1997; Demissie et al. 1998) (Fig. 2).

Most of the published work related to the pathophysiology of TTN is consistent with Avery's original conclusions that TTN is the result of delayed fetal lung fluid clearance (Jain and Dudell 2006; Birnkrant et al. 2006). The lung's functional residual capacity comprises a potential air space of 20–30 mL/kg body weight. This space is filled in utero with fetal lung fluid containing high potassium and chloride and low bicarbonate and protein. Shifts between body compartments are controlled by a chloride active pump (Liem et al. 2007; Adams et al. 1963; Barker and Olver 2002; Bland 1988; Cummings et al. 1993). Two to three days prior to delivery, the fetus begins to clear lung fluid in anticipation of transition to extrauterine life. This process begins with a decrease in fetal lung fluid secretion. The major clearance takes place with the onset of labor. At this time, the lung epithelium becomes a sodium-absorbing membrane, and lung fluid flow is directed from the air space to the interstitium via the epithelial

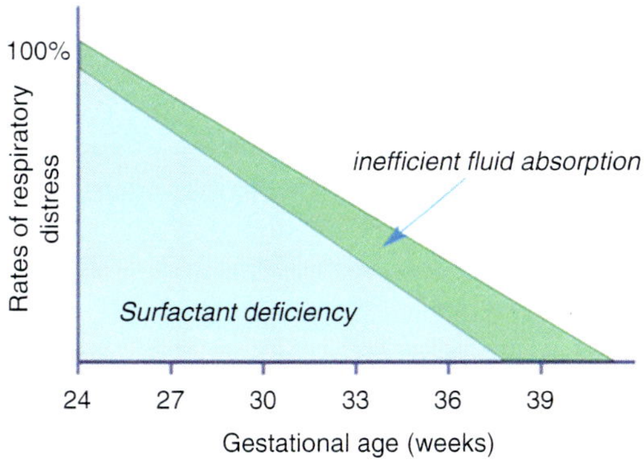

Fig. 2 Relative contribution of surfactant deficiency and insufficient fluid absorption [TTN] to neonatal respiratory distress (Adapted from Helve et al. (2009))

sodium channel (ENaC). The importance of endogenous steroids in this process is demonstrated by the relationship between low expression of serum and glucocorticoid-inducible kinase, ENaC, and poor lung liquid clearance (Janér et al. 2015). The expression of these epithelial ion transport channels is also directly related to gestational age so that TTN, like RDS, is largely a developmental condition with decreasing incidence as gestation progresses. In addition, low protein containing lung fluid exhibits low oncotic pressure, which is another driving force for lung fluid to enter the vascular system.

Mechanical compression via vaginal delivery plays a relatively minor role in lung fluid clearance. Milner et al. (1978) showed that when infants were not delivered through the vaginal canal and were not exposed to vaginal compression, they had higher interstitial and alveolar fluid volume. Furthermore, these infants also had a decrease in their lung gas volume. This hypothesis is not supported by later animal and human studies that showed no increase in functional residual capacity (FRC) in vaginally delivered infants (Jain and Dudell 2006; Hägnevik et al. 1991). Results by Birnkrant and a retrospective study by Liem et al. (2007; Birnkrant et al. 2006) found an association between TTN and the development of wheezing syndromes. These data support the hypothesis of fetal lung fluid clearance at the cell pump level and not the mechanical compression theory as the pathophysiologic basis for TTN.

TTN commonly presents soon after birth with tachypnea, grunting, nasal flaring, subcostal retractions, and possible cyanosis. An arterial blood gas is likely to show mild respiratory acidosis with hypoxemia. Chest radiographs demonstrate perihilar streaking due to periarterial lymphatic engorgement. TTN may also present in premature infants in association with respiratory distress syndrome. TTN is transient in nature with resolution of symptoms often within 8–12 h, but tachypnea may persist for up to 5 days. Infants may require oxygen support but rarely over 40% inspired oxygen. In the case of rare respiratory acidosis, CPAP may be instituted. Due to difficulty in distinguishing TTN from pneumonia, infants may receive a course of antibiotics. The radiographic findings of TTN should spontaneously resolve by 48 h (Martin et al. 2015). Lung ultrasound has been used for early diagnosis of TTN and may allow a less-invasive approach to respiratory support in infants exhibiting early signs of respiratory distress (Copetti and Cattarossi 2006; Raimondi et al. 2014).

55.4 Neonatal Pneumonia

The lungs are often a portal of entry for early onset sepsis/pneumonia in the neonatal period. Pneumonia may be acquired pre- or postnatally and be of bacterial, viral, fungal, or protozoal origin. Morbidity is high, prompting a high index of suspicion when facing an infant with signs of respiratory distress. An immature immune system and poor mechanical defense mechanisms may increase susceptibility to invasion of pathogens into the lungs. Furthermore, when an infant has comorbidities such as respiratory distress syndrome (RDS), meconium aspiration syndrome, or chronic lung disease (CLD), both vulnerability to and consequences of pneumonia may be enhanced.

The incidence of neonatal pneumonia is ten times higher for preterm infants then term infants. Barnett and Klein (Barnett and Klein 2001) reported intrauterine and early-onset pneumonia in 10–38% of stillbirths and in 20–63% of autopsies from live births that died in the first 28 days of

life. The difficulty of reporting incidence is in the inconsistency of defining pneumonia in infants less than 1 month of age. The majority of late-onset pneumonias are diagnosed in premature infants, and most were on ventilatory support at the time of diagnosis. A small single center study by Apisarnthanarak et al. (2003) showed 28% of ventilated infants developed ventilator-associated pneumonia (VAP), and, in 1986, Halliday et al. (1984) reported a 35% incidence of pneumonia in intubated patients with RDS. Despite efforts by the Center for Disease Control (CDC) and National Nosocomial Infection Surveillance System (NNIS), there is still no gold standard for diagnosing VAP in the neonatal period. For infants <1 year of age, the CDC has published clinical, radiographic, and laboratory criteria for VAP (Buonocore Chap. 55, "Pulmonary Hemorrhage, Transient Tachypnea, and Neonatal Pneumonia"). The incidence in developed countries ranges from 2.7 to 10.9 episodes per 1000 ventilator days. In developing countries, the incidence has been reported as high as 37.2 cases per 1000 ventilator days (Cernada et al. 2014). Over the last decade, VAP prevention bundles have been largely successful in reducing the incidence of hospital-acquired pneumonias.

The etiology of neonatal pneumonia can be divided into three categories: congenital, early onset, and late onset. Congenital or intrauterine pneumonia is usually caused by ascending organisms from the maternal urogenital tract before or during labor or via the transplacental route. Microorganisms such as viruses (cytomegalovirus, rubella, herpes simplex virus, adenovirus, varicella zoster virus, enteroviruses, and influenza A), bacteria (*Listeria monocytogenes*, *Mycobacterium tuberculosis*, *Treponema pallidum*), and protozoa (*Toxoplasma gondii*) are known causes of congenital pneumonia. Early-onset pneumonia is usually due to introduction of bacteria from the birth canal during the delivery process, especially in a situation of prolonged membrane rupture (Levine 1991; Airede 1992). Gasping due to asphyxia and/or meconium aspiration may introduce organisms into the respiratory system. Other factors, such as prematurity and maternal urinary tract infection, have a major role in increasing the risk of neonatal pneumonia. Group B *Streptococcus* [GBS] remains the primary cause of pneumonia in the term neonate (Apisarnthanarak et al. 2003). Overt GBS sepsis was seen in 1% of colonized infants or 1–4/1000 live births if no intrapartum antibiotic prophylaxis was given. In the USA, guidelines for intrapartum chemoprophylaxis have proven successful with a significant decrease in GBS sepsis to 0.41 per 1000 births (Stoll et al. 2011). Algorithms provide for the management of GBS-positive mothers as well as infants exposed to prophylaxis treatment. Unfortunately, other microorganisms known to cause early-onset pneumonia have increased in importance since the implementation of the GBS guidelines. The common pathogens that may influence the infant in the immediate postpartum period are *Escherichia coli [E.coli]*, *Klebsiella* spp., *Proteus mirabilis*, *H. influenzae*, group D *Streptococci*, *Listeria monocytogenes*, and pneumococci. In very low birth weight infants, rates of *E. coli* sepsis (5/1000) exceed that of GBS (2/1000). In addition, nonbacterial pneumonia may be seen in the early postnatal period such as caused by *Candida* (Gerberding et al. 1989; Aldana-Valenzuela et al. 2005), viruses (Takahashi et al. 2007; Barker et al. 1990; Faden et al. 2005), and *Chlamydia* (Numazaki et al. 2003).

Late-onset pneumonia is diagnosed when symptoms arise after 48 h of life. The pathogens are commonly acquired from the environment or nosocomial. Late-onset pneumonia is more common in premature infants or infants on prolonged ventilatory support (Yuan et al. 2007). Gram-negative bacteria (*E. coli*, *Serratia marcescens*, *Proteus* spp., *Klebsiella* spp., *Pseudomonas* spp.), coagulase-negative *Staphylococci* (Philip 1994; Chartrand and McCracken 1982), and *Staphylococcus aureus* along with GBS are among the most common bacterial organisms isolated in late-onset pneumonia. Viral organisms such as CMV (Takahashi et al. 2007; Bradshaw and Moore 2003), VZV, RSV, parainfluenza, influenzas A and B (Yusuf et al. 2007), *Rhinovirus* (Calvo et al. 2007), *Enterovirus* (Abzug 2004), and *Coronavirus* are also seen in this type of pneumonia. Recent data indicate that with increased testing, 6% of all NICU sepsis

evaluations may detect a respiratory virus via multiplex polymerase chain reaction (Ronchi et al. 2014). In addition, fungal etiologies have been implicated. Infections are acquired mainly through skin colonization and breakdown, through gastrointestinal translocation of organisms, and from the respiratory tract of family and care providers. The colonization of an infant in the intensive care unit with common or unusual flora can be due to a weak immune system, health-care provider exposure, and interventions (endotracheal tube, mechanical ventilation, and multiple courses of antibiotics) (Frakking et al. 2007; Gupta 2002; Webber et al. 1990; Garland et al. 1992).

It is difficult to diagnose pneumonia with great certainty. Isolation of bacteria or viruses from the trachea or the oropharynx does not necessarily correlate with invasive infection, but may instead, reflect colonization. Radiographic studies are difficult to interpret and cannot differentiate atelectasis or fluid from infiltrate secondary to pneumonia. The workup for suspected neonatal pneumonia includes blood and airway cultures (nasopharyngeal or tracheal if intubated). Sherman (Sherman et al. 1984) showed that tracheal secretions with a positive gram stain in relation to neonatal bacteremia had a 74% sensitivity and 47% positive predictive value and concluded that gram stain of tracheal secretions may be of practical value in the diagnosis of congenital bacteremia. Positive airway culture alone may be more suggestive of early than late-onset pneumonia; however, in neither case is it sensitive (Ruderman et al. 1994; Brook et al. 1980). Although radiographic studies are frequently nonspecific, it is more common to find pleural effusions in bacterial and fungal infections. Other nonspecific laboratory values such as C-reactive protein (CRP) and WBC counts, especially immature to mature neutrophils ratio (I/T), may aid in the diagnosis of pneumonia.

The difficulty in diagnosing pneumonia, especially when it coincides with RDS, presents the clinician with a therapeutic dilemma. Low absolute neutrophil count (ANC), high I/T ratio (>0.2), and CRP (>1) have shown to have positive predictive values of bacterial sepsis (Makhoul et al. 2006; Berger et al. 1995). Leslie et al. (1981) showed high I/T, low total neutrophil counts, and positive gram stain to be more consistent with early-onset bacterial pneumonia than RDS. However, diagnostic difficulty remains, and if the index of suspicion for sepsis is high, the accepted treatment route is antibiotics for 48 h while awaiting culture results and following the above markers trends. It is also appropriate to treat every infant who deteriorates from a respiratory standpoint, especially if the infant was asymptomatic for the first 6 h of life.

The recommended empiric choice for early-onset pneumonia is ampicillin in conjunction with an aminoglycoside (gentamicin). For late-onset pneumonia, empiric therapy may constitute nafcillin or vancomycin and an aminoglycoside. When cultures are definitive and sensitivities are known, antimicrobial therapy should be tailored for the specific organism. The prognosis of neonatal pneumonia depends on the underlying etiology and overall condition of the infant.

Acknowledgment We acknowledge the contribution of Amitai Kohn to this section in the prior addition.

References

Abzug MJ (2004) Presentation, diagnosis, and management of enterovirus infections in neonates. Paediatr Drugs 6:1–10

Adams FH, Fujiwara T, Rowshna G (1963) Surface properties and lipids from lungs of infants with hyaline membrane disease. J Pediatr 63:881–888

Airede AI (1992) Prolonged rupture of membranes and neonatal outcome in a developing country. Ann Trop Paediatr 12:283–288

Aldana-Valenzuela C, Morales-Marquec M, Castellanos-MartMart J, Deanda-Gda-G M (2005) Congenital candidiasis: a rare and unpredictable disease. J Perinatol 25:680–682

Amizuka T, Shimizu H, Niida Y, Ogawa Y (2003) Surfactant therapy in neonates with respiratory failure due to haemorrhagic pulmonary oedema. Eur J Pediatr 162: 697–702

Apisarnthanarak A, Holzmann-Pazgal G, Hamvas A et al (2003) Ventilator-associated pneumonia in extremely preterm neonates in a neonatal intensive care unit: characteristics, risk factors, and outcomes. Pediatrics 112(6 Part 1):1283–1289

Avery ME, Gatewood OB, Brumley G (1966) Transient tachypnea of newborn. Possible delayed resorption of fluid at birth. Am J Dis Child 111:380–385

Barker PM, Olver RE (2002) Invited review: clearance of lung liquid during the perinatal period. J Appl Physiol 93:1542–1548

Barker JA, McLean SD, Jordan GD et al (1990) Primary neonatal herpes simplex virus pneumonia. Pediatr Infect Dis J 9:285285J

Barnett ED, Klein JO (2001) Bacterial infections of the respiratory tract. In: Remington JS, Klein JO (eds) Infectious diseases of the fetus and newborn infant. WB Saunders, Pennsylvania, pp 1006–1018

Berger C, Uehlinger J, Ghelfi D et al (1995) Comparison of C-reactive protein and white blood cell count with differential in neonates at risk for septicaemia. Eur J Pediatr 154:138–144

Birnkrant DJ, Picone C, Markowitz W et al (2006) Association of transient tachypnea of the newborn and childhood asthma. Pediatr Pulmonol 41:978–984

Bland RD (1988) Lung liquid clearance before and after birth. Semin Perinatol 12:124

Bradshaw JH, Moore PP (2003) Perinatal cytomegalovirus infection associated with lung cysts. J Paediatr Child Health 39:563–566

Brook I, Martin WJ, Finegold SM (1980) Bacteriology of tracheal aspirates in intubated newborn. Chest 78: 875–877

Calvo C, García-García ML, Blanco C et al (2007) Role of rhinovirus in hospitalized infants with respiratory tract infections in Spain. Pediatr Infect Dis J 26:904–908

Cernada M, Brugada M, Golombek S et al (2014) Ventilator-associated pneumonia in neonatal patients: an update. Neonatology 105:98–107

Chartrand SA, McCracken GH Jr (1982) Staphylococcal pneumonia in infants and children. Pediatr Infect Dis 1:19–23

Cole VA, Normand IC, Reynolds EO, Rivers RP (1973) Pathogenesis of hemorrhagic pulmonary edema and massive pulmonary hemorrhage in the newborn. Pediatrics 51:175–187

Copetti R, Cattarossi L (2006) The 'double lung point': an ultrasound sign diagnostic of transient tachypnea of the newborn. Neonatology 91:203–209

Cummings JJ, Carlton DP, Poulain FR et al (1993) Hypoproteinemia slows lung liquid clearance in young lambs. J Appl Physiol 74:153–160

Demissie K, Marcella SW, Breckenridge MB, Rhoads GG (1998) Maternal asthma and transient tachypnea of the newborn. Pediatrics 102(1 Part 1):84–90

Faden H, Wynn RJ, Campagna L, Ryan RM (2005) Outbreak of adenovirus type 30 in a neonatal intensive care unit. J Pediatr 146:523–527

Findlay RD, Taeusch HW, David-Cu R, Walther FJ (1995) Lysis of red blood cells and alveolar epithelial toxicity by therapeutic pulmonary surfactants. Pediatr Res 37:26–30

Frakking FN, Brouwer N, van Eijkelenburg NK et al (2007) Low mannose-binding lectin (MBL) levels in neonates with pneumonia and sepsis. Clin Exp Immunol 150:255–262

Garland JS, Dunne WM Jr, Havens P et al (1992) Peripheral intravenous catheter complications in critically ill children: a prospective study. Pediatrics 89(6 Part 2):1145–1150

Gerberding KM, Eisenhut CC, Engle WA, Cohen MD (1989) Congenital candida pneumonia and sepsis: a case report and review of the literature. J Perinatol 9:159–161

Gordon E, South M, McDougall PN, Dargaville PA (2003) Blood aspiration syndrome as a cause of respiratory distress in the newborn infant. J Pediatr 142:200–202

Gross TL, Sokol RJ, Kwong MS et al (1983) Transient tachypnea of the newborn: the relationship to preterm delivery and significant neonatal morbidity. Am J Obstet Gynecol 146:236–241

Gupta A (2002) Hospital-acquired infections in the neonatal intensive care unit–*Klebsiella pneumoniae*. Semin Perinatol 26:340–345

Hägnevik K, Lagercrantz H, Sjöqvist BA (1991) Establishment of functional residual capacity in infants delivered vaginally and by elective cesarean section. Early Hum Dev 27:103–110

Halliday HL, McClure G, Reid MM et al (1984) Controlled trial of artificial surfactant to prevent respiratory distress syndrome. Lancet 1:476–478

Helve O, Pitkänen O, Janér C et al (2009) Pulmonary fluid balance in the human newborn infant. Neonatology 95:347–352

Hook B, Kiwi R, Amini SB et al (1997) Neonatal morbidity after elective repeat cesarean section and trial of labor. Pediatrics 100(3 Part 1):348–353

Jain L, Dudell GG (2006) Respiratory transition in infants delivered by cesarean section. Semin Perinatol 30:296–304

Janér C, Pitkänen OM, Süvari L et al (2015) Duration of gestation and mode of delivery affect the genes of transepithelial sodium transport in pulmonary adaptation. Neonatology 107:27–33

Kluckow M, Evans N (2000) Ductal shunting, high pulmonary blood flow, and pulmonary hemorrhage. J Pediatr 137:68–72

Kostelanetz AS, Dhanireddy R (2004) Survival of the very low birth infants after cardiopulmonary resuscitation in the neonatal intensive care unit. J Perinatol 24:279–283

Leslie GI, Scurr RD, Barr PA (1981) Early-onset bacterial pneumonia: a comparison with severe hyaline membrane disease. Aust Paediatr J 17:202–206

Levine CD (1991) Premature rupture of the membranes and sepsis in preterm neonates. Nurs Res 40:36–41

Liem JJ, Huq SI, Ekuma O et al (2007) Transient tachypnea of the newborn may be an early clinical manifestation of wheezing symptoms. J Pediatr 151:29–33

Long W, Corbet A, Allen A (1992) Retrospective search for bleeding diathesis among premature newborns with pulmonary hemorrhage after synthetic surfactant treatment. J Pediatr 120:S45–S48

Makhoul IR, Yacoub A, Smolkin T et al (2006) Values of C-reactive protein, procalcitonin, and Staphylococcus-specific PCR in neonatal late-onset sepsis. Acta Paediatr 95:1218–1223

Martin RJ, Fanaroff AA, Walsh MC (eds) (2015) Neonatal-perinatal medicine diseases of the fetus and infant, 10th edn. Mosby/Elsevier, New York

Miller LK, Calenoff L, Boehm JJ, Riedy MJ (1980) Respiratory distress in the newborn. JAMA 243: 1176–1179

Milner AD, Saunders RA, Hopkin IE (1978) Is air trapping important in the maintenance of the functional residual capacity in the hours after birth? Early Hum Dev 27: 103–110

Numazaki K, Asanuma H, Niida Y (2003) Chlamydia trachomatis infection in early neonatal period. BMC Infect Dis 3:2

Pandit PB, Dunn MS, Colucci EA (1995) Surfactant therapy in neonates with respiratory deterioration due to pulmonary hemorrhage. Pediatrics 95:32–36

Pappin A, Shenker N, Hack M, Redline RW (1994) Extensive intraalveolar pulmonary hemorrhage in infants dying after surfactant therapy. J Pediatr 124:621–626

Philip AG (1994) The changing face of neonatal infection: experience at a regional medical center. Pediatr Infect Dis J 13:1098–1102

Raimondi F, Migliaro F, Sodano A et al (2014) Use of neonatal chest ultrasound to predict noninvasive ventilation failure. Pediatrics 134:e1089–e1094

Raju TN, Langenberg P (1993) Pulmonary hemorrhage and exogenous surfactant therapy: a meta-analysis. J Pediatr 123:603–610

Rawlings JS, Smith FR (1984) Transient tachypnea of the newborn. An analysis of neonatal and obstetric risk factors. Am J Dis Child 138:869–871

Ronchi A, Michelow IC, Chapin KC et al (2014) Viral respiratory tract infections in the neonatal intensive care unit: the VIRIoN-I study. J Pediatr 165:690–696

Ruderman JW, Srugo I, Morgan MA et al (1994) Pneumonia in the neonatal intensive care unit. Diagnosis by quantitative bacterial tracheal aspirate cultures. J Perinatol 14:182–186

Scholl JE, Yanowitz TD (2015) Pulmonary hemorrhage in very low birth weight infants: a case-control analysis. J Pediatr 166:1083–1084

Sherman MP, Chance KH, Goetzman BW (1984) Gram's stains of tracheal secretions predict neonatal bacteremia. Am J Dis Child 138:848–850

Shi Y, Tang S, Li H et al (2005) New treatment of neonatal pulmonary hemorrhage with hemocoagulase in addition to mechanical ventilation. Biol Neonate 88:118–121

Stoll BJ, Hansen NI, Sánchez PJ et al (2011) Early onset neonatal sepsis: the burden of Group B Streptococcal and *E. coli* disease continues. Pediatrics 127:817–826

Takahashi R, Tagawa M, Sanjo M et al (2007) Severe postnatal cytomegalovirus infection in a very premature infant. Neonatology 92:236–236

Webber S, Wilkinson AR, Lindsell D et al (1990) Neonatal pneumonia. Arch Dis Child 65:207–211

Yuan TM, Chen LH, Yu HM (2007) Risk factors and outcomes for ventilator-associated pneumonia in neonatal intensive care unit patients. J Perinat Med 35: 334–338

Yusuf K, Soraisham AS, Fonseca K (2007) Fatal influenza B virus pneumonia in a preterm neonate: case report and review of the literature. J Perinatol 27:623–625

Pulmonary Air Leakage in Newborns 56

Paola Papoff and Corrado Moretti

Contents

P. Papoff
Pediatric Intensive Care Unit, Sapienza University of Rome, Rome, Italy
e-mail: p.papoff@libero.it

C. Moretti (✉)
Università degli Studi di Roma “La Sapienza”, Rome, Italy
e-mail: corrado.moretti@uniroma1.it

G. Buonocore et al. (eds.), *Neonatology*,
https://doi.org/10.1007/978-3-319-29489-6_204

Abstract
In neonates, the most common air leaks include pulmonary interstitial emphysema, pneumomediastinum, and pneumothorax, while pneumopericardium, pneumoperitoneum, and venous pulmonary embolism are less frequent. Air leaks are more common and severe among neonates with lung disease characterized by either poor lung compliance needing high ventilatory pressures or lung overdistention. Many affected neonates have minimal or no symptoms, while others present with signs of respiratory distress and increased oxygen requirement. Sudden collapse may occur in case of hypertensive pneumothorax or pneumopericardium. The diagnosis is suspected clinically and confirmed by chest X-ray. Treatment varies by type of air leak and severity of clinical condition.

56.1 Salient Points

- The most common neonatal air leaks include pulmonary interstitial emphysema, pneumomediastinum, and pneumothorax.
- Air leaks may occur spontaneously or develop in association with other forms of lung disease often requiring ventilatory support.
- Symptoms may vary from mild respiratory distress to severe hypoxia and hemodynamic instability.
- Diagnosis is suspected clinically and confirmed radiographically.
- Treatment varies by type and severity, ranging from watchful waiting to ventilatory pressure reduction or chest drainage.

56.2 Pulmonary Air Leaks

Pulmonary air leaks include a number of clinical conditions characterized by overdistension and rupture of the alveolar wall with air leaking from the intra-alveolar space into the surrounding tissue. The air dissects along the perivascular connective tissue sheath toward the hilum, resulting in a pneumomediastinum, or into the pleural space, producing a pneumothorax. Less commonly, air may dissect into the pericardial space, subcutaneous tissue, peritoneal space, or venous circulation causing pneumopericardium, subcutaneous emphysema, pneumoperitoneum, and venous pulmonary embolism, respectively. Air leaks are more common and more severe among neonates with pulmonary diseases that are characterized by poor lung compliance (e.g., respiratory distress syndrome) requiring high ventilatory pressures or by airway obstruction (e.g., meconium aspiration syndrome) because of alveolar overdistention.

The incidence of pulmonary air leaks is inversely related to birth weight and increase in infants who need resuscitation. Affected neonates may be asymptomatic or have various degrees of respiratory distress. Diagnosis is suspected clinically because of respiratory distress and increased oxygen requirement and confirmed by X-ray. Treatment varies by type and severity of air leak.

56.3 Structure of the Lung

Macroscopically, the lung is divided into three lobes on the right and two on the left, each of which has autonomous ventilation and blood

supply. Each lobe comprises segments, which are pyramidal in shape with the apex toward the hilum and the base toward the surface of the lung. The segments are supplied by a bronchus and by a segmentary artery and are drained by a perisegmentary venous network. Each segment comprises pulmonary lobules, each of which is supplied by a lobular bronchiole, and a branch of the pulmonary artery. The lobular bronchiole continues branching until it reaches the level of terminal bronchioles, which ventilate the alveolar sacs that comprise clusters of alveoli. There are 10–15 alveoli in each alveolar sac. These are the functional units of the lung where gas exchange occurs.

The bronchial tree and associated vessels are wrapped in a sheath of collagen and elastic tissue. The pressure on the pleural surface is transmitted through the alveolar walls to the alveoli. Each alveolar unit is interdependent with the adjacent one so that the expansion of one alveolus determines the increase in wall tension of neighboring alveoli and ensures uniform pulmonary expansion. Most of the development of the pulmonary elastic structure occurs during the fetal saccular period, which begins toward the 25th week of gestation.

The terminal bronchiole gives rise to two or more respiratory or alveolar bronchioles, which develop hemispheric evaginations called alveoli. Alveoli are more numerous in the distal portion of the respiratory bronchiolus, which ends by branching into alveolar ducts and finally the alveolar sacs, which form the terminal portion of the respiratory airways.

Each lung is enveloped by a serous membrane, the pleura.

56.4 Pulmonary Interstitial Emphysema

Pulmonary interstitial emphysema (PIE) may be defined as a collection of gas outside the airway and inside the interstitial space. It is caused by alveolar and bronchiolar rupture. The perivascular connective tissue is more abundant and less dissectible in preterm than older infants. This predisposes to air trapping in the perivascular space, resulting in pulmonary interstitial emphysema. The extent of PIE can vary. PIE may occur throughout the lungs or may be unilateral or lobar. In the former case, it may be difficult to differentiate PIE from early bronchopulmonary dysplasia (BPD).

The incidence of PIE has decreased because of treatments such as surfactant and the concept of "gentle ventilation," as well as the availability of high-frequency oscillatory ventilation (HFOV) for infants who are difficult to maintain with conventional ventilation (Helbich et al. 1998).

Risk factors for PIE are:

- Mechanical ventilation with high pressures or volumes (the most important factor)
- Low gestational age (PIE usually develops in infants younger than 32 weeks' gestation, who weigh less than 1,200 g) (Hart et al. 1983)
- Pulmonary hypoplasia
- Pulmonary diseases, e.g., severe respiratory distress syndrome (RDS), meconium aspiration syndrome (MAS), and infectious or aspiration pneumonia (Campbell 1970)
- Chorioamnionitis and funisitis (Jeffrey 2003)
- Malpositioned endotracheal tube (Greenough et al. 1984)

56.4.1 Etiology and Pathogenesis

The mechanisms involved in spontaneous, interstitial, mediastinal, and subcutaneous emphysema have been described by Macklin and Macklin (Macklin 1939). Their experimental work with various animal models led to the hypothesis that overdistended alveoli resulting from uneven ventilation rupture into the pulmonary vascular sheaths and create PIE. Predisposing factors for PIE are positive pressure ventilation (PPV) with high mean airway pressures (MAP) and reduced lung compliance.

The basic requirement for rupture is the existence of a pressure gradient between the alveolus and its surrounding structure. However, in extremely premature infants, PIE can occur at low mean airway pressures and probably

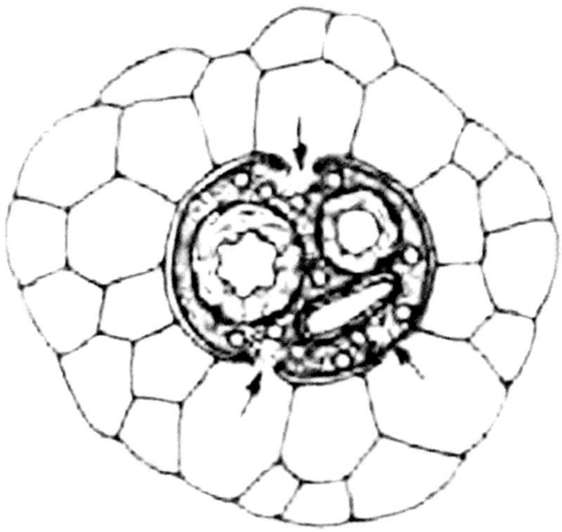

Fig. 1 Distal bronchovascular sheath surrounded by alveoli after expiratory airflow obstruction. Pressure gradient between airspace and perivascular interstitium leads to alveolar rupture (arrows) and direct introduction of air into bronchovascular sheath. Modified from (Maunder 1984)

reflects increased sensitivity to stretch by the immature lung. The pressure within adjacent alveoli is generally assumed to be similar and the interalveolar wall remains intact. As illustrated schematically in Fig. 1 (Maunder 1984), if a pressure difference develops between the alveoli, the risk of alveolar rupture is increased, causing interstitial emphysema. Since the mean pressure within the mediastinum is always rather lower than in peripheral lung parenchyma, air dissects proximally along the bronchovascular sheaths to the lung hilum and mediastinal soft tissue. Having reached the mediastinum, accumulated air may decompress into cervical and subcutaneous tissue or to the retroperitoneum, dissecting along the fascial planes. If mediastinal pressure rises abruptly or decompression via these routes is not sufficient to relieve the tension, the mediastinal parietal pleura may rupture, resulting in pneumothorax. This mechanism, rather than rupture of subpleural blebs, is thought to be responsible for spontaneous pneumothorax in a majority of cases (Caldwell et al. 1979).

The presence of air in the interstitial tissue causes reduced compliance, an increase in residual volume and dead space, and an increased ventilation perfusion (V/Q) mismatch. It also impedes pulmonary blood flow and obstructs the lymphatic drainage. These changes account for worsening oxygenation.

At an early stage of RDS, there is increased interstitial and perivascular fluid that rapidly decreases over the next few days. This fluid may obstruct the movement of gas from ruptured alveoli to the mediastinum through the bronchovascular sheaths, causing an increase of PIE. Another possible mechanism for entrapment of air in the interstitium is the increased amount of connective tissue in the immature lung. Entrapment of air in the interstitium may result in a vicious cycle that causes compression of the adjacent alveoli and a further increase in ventilation pressure with more air escaping from the overdistended alveoli into the interstitial tissues.

56.4.2 Clinical Aspects, Differential Diagnosis, and Prognosis

PIE may occur during the first 72 h of life or as a complication of prolonged positive pressure ventilation in older premature infants.

The clinical presentation of PIE varies with size and location of gas accumulation. PIE may cause compression of small airways with wheezing or diminished breath sounds because of decreased lung compliance. There may be changes in ventilator requirements, increased respiratory rate, and variations in heart rate and blood pressure. Trapped gas reduces pulmonary perfusion by compressing blood vessels, causing hypoxemia, hypercapnia, and respiratory acidosis.

The air collection along the bronchovascular sheaths is visible radiologically as small rounded, nonconfluent, microradiolucencies throughout the lungs (Fig. 2). PIE may be unilateral (Fig. 3). If there is mechanical ventilation and because of rupture of interlobular septa, PIE tends to form hypertransparent bubbles that may be quite large and look like pseudocysts. Small areas of PIE alternating with pneumatoceles have the effect of making the pulmonary parenchyma look like a honeycomb.

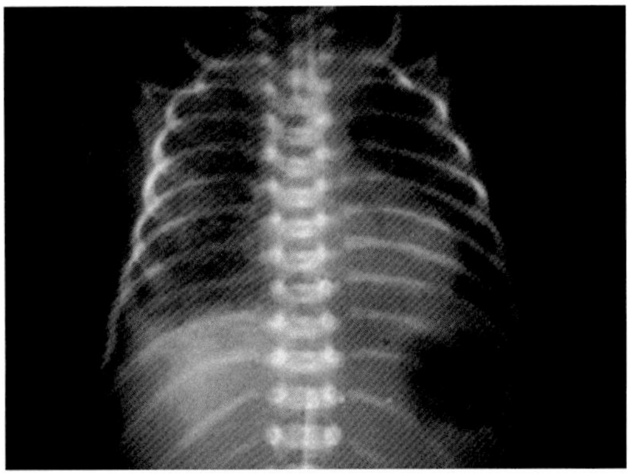

Fig. 2 Diffuse pulmonary interstitial emphysema

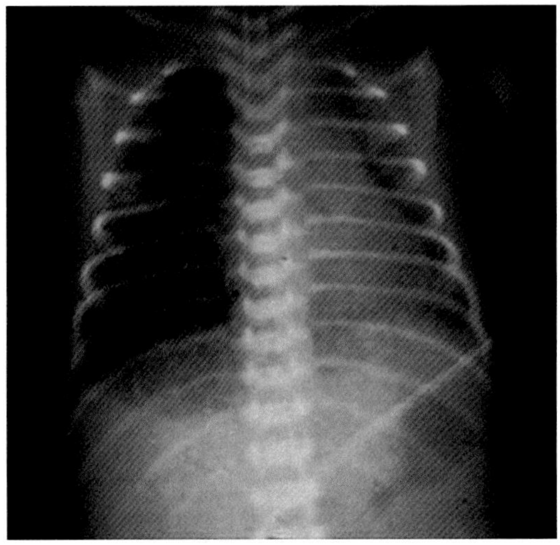

Fig. 3 Pulmonary interstitial emphysema, especially marked in the right lung

Possible complications of PIE include other air leaks, such as pneumomediastinum, pneumothorax, pneumopericardium, pneumoperitoneum, subcutaneous emphysema, and pulmonary venous embolism, intraventricular hemorrhage, possible epithelialization of the interstitial air pockets, and chronic lung disease.

PIE may be confused with severe respiratory distress syndrome (RDS), early bronchopulmonary dysplasia (BPD), cystic adenomatoid malformation, lymphangiectasia, bronchogenic cysts, congenital lobar emphysema, and pulmonary infection. PIE may take several weeks to resolve. The condition can therefore increase the length of time of mechanical ventilation and the incidence of BPD (Hart et al. 1983). Some infants may develop chronic lobar emphysema and may require surgical lobectomies.

56.4.3 Therapy and Treatments

In mechanically ventilated infants, initial treatment of PIE should be aimed at obtaining maximum patient-ventilator synchrony, securing the endotracheal tube in the appropriate position, and reducing peak inspiratory pressure (PIP) and positive end expiratory pressure (PEEP) as much as possible, consistent with blood gas values. A short inspiratory time (Ti) and a triangular pressure wave morphology should be set to avoid inflating the parenchymal cysts that have a long time constant (Meadow and Cheromcha 1985). HFOV has been found to be effective in the treatment of PIE (Helbich et al. 1998).

Treatment of the localized form includes positioning the infant with the affected side down or selectively intubating the main bronchus of the unaffected side (Brooks et al. 1977; Chan and Greenough 1992). Severely ill premature neonates may not tolerate the latter treatment because it is difficult for them to compensate for distress with one functioning lung. Physiotherapy may be useful as the presence of mucus may contribute to the formation of cysts and bubbles through a valve mechanism (Swingle et al. 1984). A short course of dexamethasone has been shown to be as an effective treatment in infants with PIE, possibly by reducing airway edema and inflammation and airway obstruction (Fitzgerald et al. 1998).

56.5 Pneumomediastinum

Pneumomediastinum is defined as a collection of gas in the mediastinal space. Free air may not be confined solely to the mediastinum but may penetrate through tissue planes, causing pneumopericardium, pneumothorax, subcutaneous emphysema, or pneumoperitoneum. Pneumomediastinum occurs in approximately 2.5 per 1,000 live births.

Risk factors for pneumomediastinum are:

- Gas trapping associated either with several lung diseases, including RDS, pneumonia, and MAS, or with mechanical ventilation
- Birth asphyxia requiring resuscitation
- Chest trauma
- Mechanical obstruction as seen with a foreign body or a tumor

56.5.1 Etiology and Pathogenesis

Pneumomediastinum is in most cases a complication of a pre-existing pulmonary disease and may be preceded by PIE. The air that leaks out of the alveoli makes its way along the bronchovascular sheaths toward the hilum and into the mediastinum. Pneumomediastinum may appear spontaneously at birth or may occur later, secondary to the formation of a valve-like mechanism and consequent rupture of the alveoli. The air moving from the mediastinum toward the neck causes the dissection of the cervical aponeurosis and the supraclavicular tissue planes, forming subcutaneous emphysema. The air in the mediastinum may also spread to the subpleural space and simulate a basal pneumothorax. Air may also leak into the peritoneal cavity through areas of lower resistance, such as the sternocostal trigone, and cause subdiaphragmatic air collections (pneumoperitoneum).

56.5.2 Clinical Aspects and Differential Diagnosis

Pneumomediastinum rarely leads to clinically significant complications. However, compression of mediastinal structures may occur when there is extensive subcutaneous and mediastinal gas. The infant with pneumomediastinum is usually asymptomatic or has mild respiratory distress. In the absence of other pulmonary disorders, it tends to regress spontaneously.

A large accumulation of trapped air may compromise ventilation and cardiac output. The first sign may be subcutaneous emphysema in the neck, face, or chest. The infant with a large pneumomediastinum may exhibit bulging in the midthoracic area, distended neck veins, and low blood pressure.

The pneumomediastinum is characterized radiologically by the presence of cardiac margins that are clearly delimited by a thin black streak. The edges of the right atrium and the left ventricle are generally well distinguished from the pulmonary parenchyma. In cases of pneumomediastinum with small quantities of air, the only sign is a radiolucent band (hyperlucency) in the retrosternal area on the lateral view (Fig. 4) (Macklin 1939; Hoffer and Ablow 1984). The main diagnostic element of pneumomediastinum is prominence of lobes of the thymus that may be more or less marked depending on the amount of air in the mediastinum (the image resembles the wings of a seagull or a spinnaker sail, Fig. 5) (Moseley 1960; Lawal et al. 2009). When there is a pneumomediastinum, the lobes of the thymus are surrounded by air, and in the lateral view, this peculiar radiographic aspect is sufficient to diagnose an anteromedial pneumothorax. The air in the mediastinum may push both thymus lobes toward the pulmonary apices, thus simulating upper lobar collapse or pneumonia. The presence of other signs suggesting pneumomediastinum allows this condition to be differentiated from pulmonary consolidation.

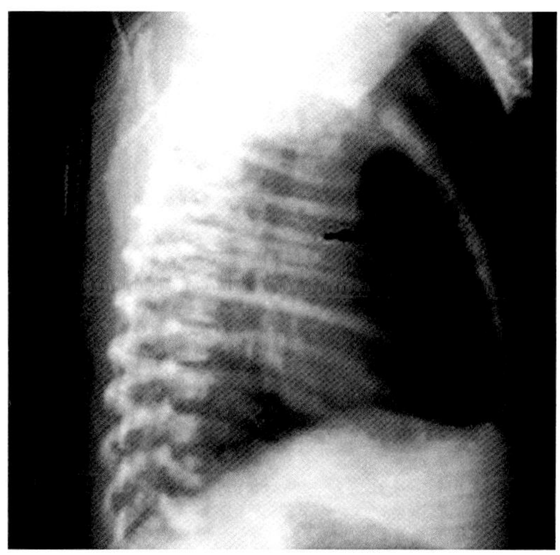

Fig. 4 Pneumomediastinum, lateral view

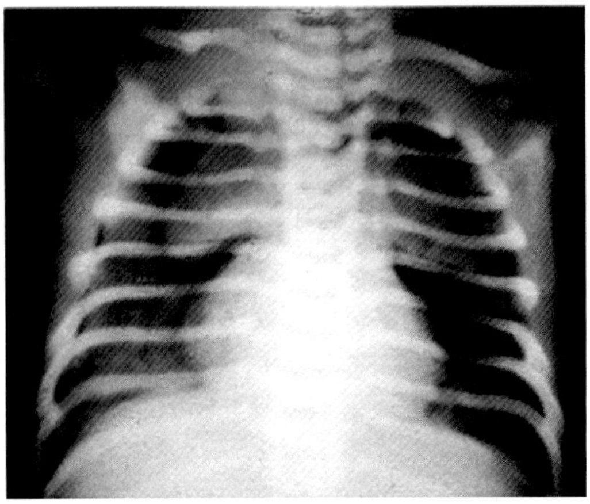

Fig. 5 Pneumomediastinum with the raised thymus lobes (spinnaker sail)

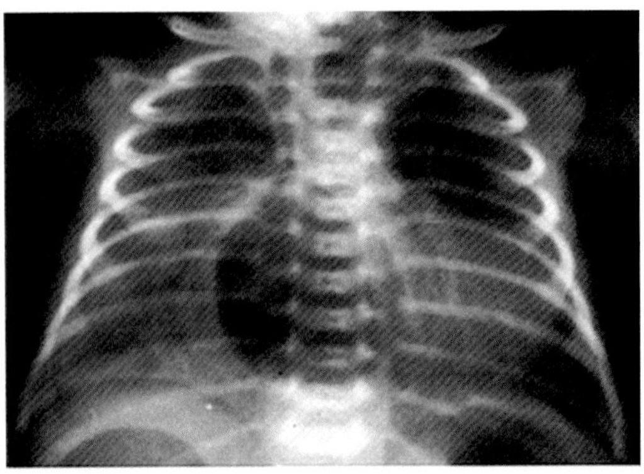

Fig. 6 Pneumomediastinum with the air collected in the triangular ligament

Air may collect in some mediastinum recesses, suchlike the triangular ligament. In such cases, the chest X-ray shows a hyperlucent paravertebral area extending from the diaphragm up to the pulmonary hilum (Fig. 6; Volberg et al. 1979).

Pneumomediastinum should be differentiated from bronchogenic cysts (Shah et al. 1999), esophageal perforation, and pneumothorax.

56.5.3 Therapy and Treatments

A conservative approach is usually adopted. Only tension pneumomediastinum with tamponade needs immediate drainage.

56.6 Pneumothorax

Pneumothorax is defined as an accumulation of air in the pleural space. Pneumothoraces have been termed small, moderate, or large if they occupy 15% or less, 15–60%, or more than 60% of the pleural space.

Spontaneous pneumothoraces develop in up to 1–1.5% of normal term infants around the time of birth owing to high transpulmonary pressure during the first breaths (only about 10% of these are symptomatic) (Steele et al. 1971). Males are more affected than females, whereas there is no difference between term and preterm infants. In the presence of lung disease, especially if mechanical ventilation is required, the incidence of pneumothorax increases dramatically (~10%). Fifteen to 20% of pneumothoraces are bilateral. Two-thirds of unilateral pneumothoraces affect the right side. There is no correlation between the incidence of pneumothorax and gestational age (Greenough et al. 1984). Reports of familial spontaneous pneumothoraces in neonates are rare (Bagchi and Nycyk 2002).

Risk factors for pneumothorax are:

- Lung diseases, such as wet lung (following cesarean section) (Benterud et al. 2009), MAS, congenital bullae, and pulmonary hypoplasia, which result in uneven lung compliance and alveolar overdistension
- PIE
- Ventilatory support. Predisposing factors during mechanical ventilation are:
  - Lack of synchronization. Asynchrony is usually secondary to trigger delay, long Ti, and an inspiratory/expiratory ratio (I/E) ≥1:1 (Primhak 1983)
  - High ventilation pressures
  - High PEEP (Klinger et al. 2008)
  - High ventilation tidal volumes (more important than increase in pressure) (McCallion et al. 2005)
  - Intubation of the right main bronchus
- Nasal CPAP (the risk is lower than during mechanical ventilation)
- Low temperature of inhaled gases (<36.5 °C). In infants weighing ≤1,500 g at birth, the

incidence of pneumothorax increases if the temperature of inhaled gases is below 36.5 °C. It is likely that lower temperatures cause a reduced content of water in the ventilation gas, which alters the mucociliary clearance (Tarnow-Mordi et al. 1989) precipitating airway obstruction

- Direct injury (suction catheter and central venous catheter positioning)

56.6.1 Etiology and Pathogenesis

In an overdistended lung, air passes from a ruptured alveolus up the bronchovascular sheath into the mediastinum and from there into the pleural cavity causing pneumothorax. The pathogenesis of pneumothorax is comparable to that of the pneumomediastinum. Rarely pneumothorax is the result of the rupture of subpleural blebs. In the neonate, the susceptibility to pulmonary rupture is further enhanced by a reduced number of alveolar connecting channels (pores of Kohn) that allow air to redistribute between ventilated and nonventilated units.

56.6.1.1 Classification

Pneumothoraces are commonly classified into three types: simple, communicating, and tension. Simple or noncommunicating pneumothorax occurs when there is no direct communication with the atmosphere. There is no mediastinal shift resulting from the accumulated air. A simple pneumothorax may occur spontaneously or as a consequence of barotrauma or volutrauma during positive pressure mechanical ventilation.

Communicating or open pneumothorax may occur in association with an open defect in the chest wall as in patent ductus arteriosus (PDA) surgery. As intrathoracic pressure is less than atmospheric pressure during spontaneous breathing, air rapidly accumulates in the pleural space. Loss of negative intrathoracic pressure results in varying degrees of lung collapse and further respiratory compromise.

Tension pneumothorax is caused by progressive accumulation of air in the pleural space. This collection of air shifts the mediastinum to the contralateral hemithorax and compresses the contralateral lung and great vessels, compromising both cardiovascular and respiratory function. Whether air enters the pleural space through a defect in the chest wall, a lacerated bronchus, or alveolus, a one-way valve effect is created so that air enters during inspiration but cannot escape during expiration. Accumulation of air continues until the intrathoracic pressure of the affected hemithorax equilibrates with atmospheric pressure. At this point, the accumulation of pressure within the thorax leads to collapse of the ipsilateral lung and displacement of the mediastinum (and associated great vessels) toward the contralateral hemithorax. While the superior vena cava is able to move to some extent, the inferior vena cava is relatively fixed within the diaphragm and will be distorted. As two-thirds of the venous return in children comes from below the diaphragm, compression of the inferior vena cava leads to a dramatic reduction in venous return to the heart and cardiovascular collapse.

56.6.2 Clinical Aspects

Diagnosis of pneumothorax is based on clinical signs, physical examination, arterial blood gases, transillumination, and imaging. Pneumothorax presents with signs of respiratory distress (grunting, increased respiratory rate, retractions), chest asymmetry, cyanosis, episodes of apnea and bradycardia, tachycardia, and hypotension. During mechanical ventilation, pneumothorax is frequently tension accompanied by compression of the mediastinal structures, which may cause impaired venous return and cardiocirculatory collapse (Ogata et al. 1976). On auscultation of the chest, breath sounds are decreased or absent in the affected side, and it may be difficult to identify the heart sounds. A pneumothorax should be suspected when there is sudden worsening of the clinical condition. However, its exact location by auscultation is not always as straightforward, especially in very low weight infants. Arterial blood gases may show a respiratory or mixed acidosis and hypoxemia.

Transillumination is an effective method for demonstrating increased transmission of light on

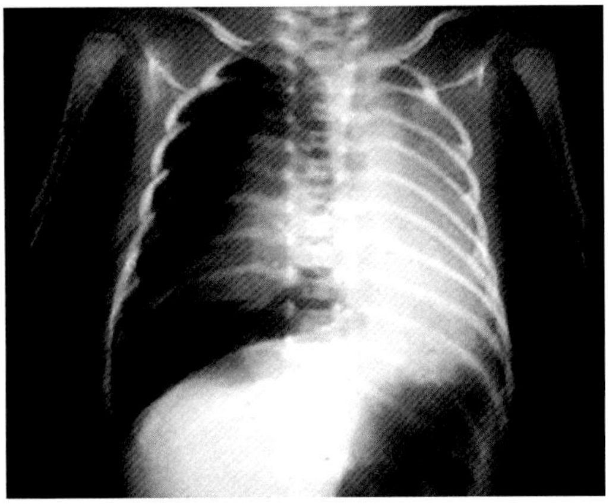

Fig. 7 Right tension pneumothorax

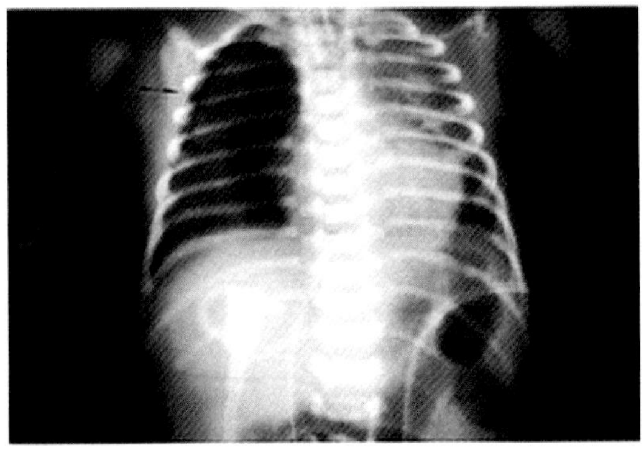

Fig. 8 Right antero-medial pneumothorax with a slight contra-lateral shift of the mediastinum

the affected side (Kuhns et al. 1975). However, chest X-ray remains the gold standard for the diagnosis of pneumothorax. Large pneumothoraces are generally easy to identify radiologically. The affected hemithorax is larger than the contralateral hemithorax, with larger intercostal spaces, and the diaphragmatic dome is lowered. The profile of the collapsed lung is sharply outlined (Fig. 7).

In tension pneumothoraces, the contralateral shift of the mediastinum is generally considerable. In the most severe cases, the diaphragm is flattened or even concave (Moseley 1960). Anterior or anteromedial collections of air inside the pleural cavity may easily be missed. The appearances are those of a lung with decreased markings and slight contralateral shift of the mediastinum (Fig. 8). In patients in whom an anteromedial pneumothorax is suspected, a lateral supine chest X-ray is useful. The thymus gland on the side of the pneumothorax may appear closely adherent to the mediastinum. A large thymus may give a false impression of a space-occupying mass in the upper mediastinum. Ultrasonography has been shown to be accurate and efficient for the early detection of clinically important pneumothoraces (Brook et al. 2009).

56.6.3 Differential Diagnosis

- Lobar emphysema
- Cystic adenomatoid malformation of the lung
- Congenital diaphragmatic hernia
- Bronchogenic cyst
- Esophageal-pleural fistula (Boerhaave syndrome)

The most common complications of pneumothorax in the neonate are respiratory or cardiac arrest, intraventricular hemorrhage, bronchopleural fistula, hemopneumothorax, and infection.

56.6.4 Therapy and Treatments

56.6.4.1 Asymptomatic Pneumothorax

The asymptomatic pneumothorax does not require any specific treatment other than close observation and may be managed conservatively. In small to moderate pneumothoraces, treatment with 100% oxygen may accelerate air reabsorption. High inspired oxygen concentrations facilitate nitrogen washout from the bloodstream (PN2 drops from 573 mmHg at room air to 0 mmHg under 100% oxygen) creating a concentration gradient between pleural gas and pleural venous circulation. This gradient favors the reabsorption of nitrogen within the pleural pockets. This technique has proved to be effective in animal models or in adult individuals with spontaneous pneumothorax (Northfield 1971), whereas in neonates 100% oxygen does not seem to offer significant advantage (Clark et al. 2014); therefore, due to the risk of oxygen toxicity, its use in neonates is controversial.

When mechanical ventilation is used, even small pneumothoraces are usually drained.

56.6.4.2 Needle Aspiration

Needle aspiration can be used to treat a symptomatic pneumothorax. It is frequently curative in infants who are not mechanically ventilated and may be a temporizing treatment in infants who are mechanically ventilated.

56.6.4.3 Thoracotomy

Chest tube drainage (thoracotomy) is usually needed for continuous drainage of pneumothoraces that develop in infants receiving positive pressure ventilation because the air leak may persist. In these cases, continuous aspiration with negative pressures of 5–10 cmH_2O may be useful.

Technique of pleural drainage:

(a) Select a chest tube of appropriate size. For small infants, 8 Fr chest tubes are adequate. For larger infants, 10 Fr chest tubes are better.
(b) Locate the fifth intercostal space in the anterior axillary line on the affected side (Brook et al. 2009).
(c) Prepare the site with antibacterial solution.
(d) Administer analgesic to the infant. Be ready for resuscitation.
(e) Inject the area with a small amount of 1% lidocaine (1 2 mg/kg).
(f) Make a small incision (approximately the size of the tube) along the intercostal space directly over the sixth rib.
(g) Insert the trocar by blunt dissection.
(h) Advance the chest tube a few centimeters and check the position radiographically.
(i) Suture the tube in place. The tube should be kept for 24–48 h from the moment the pneumothorax has stopped draining, i.e., when the intermittent air leakage stops. In the case of residual air, attach the tube to a drainage system under low continuous suction (–10 to –20 cm H_2O).

Complications of pleural drainage include:

- Infection
- Hemorrhage (laceration of intercostal vessels)
- Lung puncture
- Bronchopleural fistula, which is evidenced by persisting pneumothorax
- Chylothorax (secondary to lesions of the thoracic duct)
- Paralysis of the diaphragm (due to lesions of the phrenic nerve)
- Breast deformity (Rainer et al. 2003)

56.6.4.4 Selective Intubation

Selective intubation of the contralateral main bronchus should be reserved for cases where there is a bronchopleural fistula. In addition, a technique of single-lung ventilation using a Swan-Ganz catheter to block the main bronchus on the disease side has been successfully used on neonates unresponsive to conventional therapy (Rastogi et al. 2007).

56.6.5 Prevention

Pneumothorax may be prevented by using ventilation techniques that allow for synchronization between spontaneous and mechanical breaths so as to reduce transpulmonary pressure fluctuations. HFOV may reduce the incidence of pneumothorax in infants with severe pulmonary disease.

56.7 Pneumopericardium

Pneumopericardium is a collection of air in the pericardial space. It frequently occurs in association with pneumomediastinum. It is likely that gas enters the pericardium through a defect in the pericardial sac, probably at the pericardial reflection near the ostia of the pulmonary veins. The incidence has been estimated around 1.3% of term and preterm infants (Burt 1982). Pneumopericardium rarely occurs spontaneously (Itani and Mikati 1998).

Risk factors for pneumopericardium are:

- Prematurity
- Birth asphyxia requiring resuscitation

- Mechanical ventilation (PIP >32 cm H_2O, MAP >17 cm H_2O)
- Lung disease
- Anatomic predisposition (maldevelopment of the left pleuropericardial membrane)

56.7.1 Etiology and Pathogenesis

Pneumopericardium is frequently associated with a pneumomediastinum and/or pneumothorax since the pathogenic mechanism is the same, i.e., diffusion of air from the pulmonary interstices through the bronchovascular sheaths to the planes of pleural reflection at the level of the large vessels, where air under tension flows directly into the pericardium sac. Pericardial connective tissue is discontinuous at the reflection of parietal onto visceral pericardium near the ostia of the pulmonary veins so that there is a site of potential weakness where a microscopic dissection of air into the pericardial sac is possible. Moreover, congenital defects can be an explanation for pneumopericardium.

56.7.2 Clinical Aspects

Because of the speed at which it occurs, pneumopericardium is usually a dramatic event, causing cardiac tamponade. Symptoms appear when the pressure in the pericardium exceeds the ventricular filling pressure and cardiac output is reduced (Itani and Mikati 1998; Long 1990). Sometimes the presenting signs of pneumopericardium may be confused with those of a tension pneumothorax (sudden hypotension, bradycardia, and hypoxia). The heart sounds are muffled, but a friction rub is occasionally audible. There are low voltages on electrocardiography. The radiological appearances of pneumopericardium are of a hypertransparent image, which outlines the heart entirely, except for where the great vessels emerge (Fig. 9). Gas surrounding the heart may be confused with pneumomediastinum.

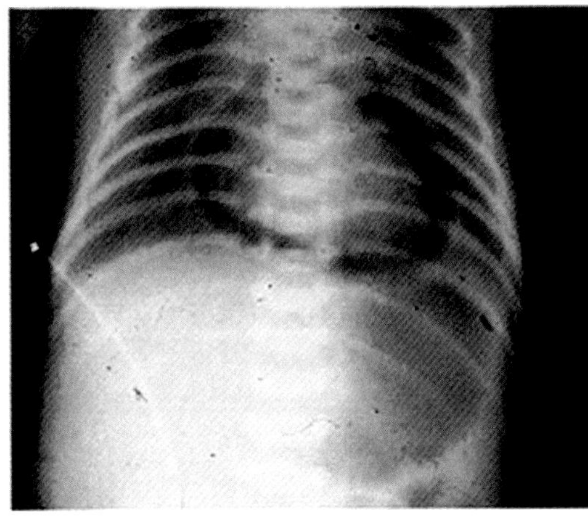

Fig. 9 Pneumopericardium: a hypertransparent image that entirely delimits the heart except for the emergence of the great vessels

56.7.3 Therapy and Treatments and Prognosis

Treatment is conservative if asymptomatic. Oxygen administration will help the reabsorption of air in cases with mild respiratory distress (Hummler et al. 1996). If cardiac tamponade occurs, drainage with a cannula needle will be performed via the subxiphoid route. Relapses are frequent and require the positioning of an indwelling drainage tube (Pfenninger et al. 1982). Mortality is high, between 70% and 90%.

56.8 Pneumoperitoneum

Pneumoperitoneum is defined as the presence of air within the peritoneal cavity.

56.8.1 Etiology and Pathogenesis

Pneumoperitoneum usually results from perforation of the gut, although in some instances it can be caused by air under pressure dissecting from the chest (pneumomediastinum, bronchopleural fistula) through the diaphragmatic apertures into the peritoneal space (Aranda et al. 1972;

Knight and Abdenour 1981). The diagnosis is made on an abdominal radiograph and usually has little clinical significance. However, it must be differentiated from intraperitoneal air due to perforated bowel.

56.8.2 Clinical Aspects, Therapy, and Treatments

Pneumoperitoneum may be an incidental finding or may present with abdominal distension or in most severe cases with cardiovascular collapse.

On the posteroanterior radiograph, pneumoperitoneum may be difficult to see if free intraperitoneal gas accumulates between intestinal loops. If gas is present on both sides of the bowel, it may outline the bowel wall, rendering it visible as a thin, linear stripe (double wall sign or Rigler's sign). If there is doubt about the diagnosis of pneumoperitoneum, consider a lateral shoot-through abdominal X-ray (with the baby lying on his back and the X-ray film at right angles to the mattress) or a lateral decubitus abdominal X-ray, both of which will demonstrate the liver clearly separates from the abdominal wall. Free abdominal air requires a surgical opinion. Either peritoneal drainage or laparotomy may be required.

56.9 Subcutaneous Emphysema

Subcutaneous emphysema occurs more commonly in the face, neck, or supraclavicular region. It typically presents as crepitus detected by palpation. Clinically, patients can develop dysphonia and dyspnea. Simple subcutaneous emphysema that does not compromise respiration can be treated with conservative management (oxygen, analgesia, antibiotic prophylaxis, reassurance, and close monitoring). More severe subcutaneous emphysema that causes respiratory obstruction is an emergency, and methods of management include infraclavicular incisions, placement of 14G fenestrated subcutaneous catheters, insertion of subcutaneous drains with or without suction, tracheostomy, or subcutaneous chest tubes (Johnson et al. 2014).

56.10 Pulmonary Gas Embolism

The presence of intravascular gas is a rare complication of positive pressure ventilation (Lee and Tanswell 1989). This condition is usually fatal and results from direct communication between airway lumen, interstitium, and small vascular channels, as demonstrated by barium studies at autopsy (Bowen et al. 1973). It can be a consequence of air leaks syndromes or lung trauma.

56.10.1 Clinical Aspects, Therapy, and Treatments

Affected infants are usually premature and have severe respiratory failure necessitating very high ventilatory pressures. Pulmonary gas embolism causes a catastrophic deterioration of the patient's condition with cardiocirculatory collapse.

The radiographs of thorax and abdomen show pulmonary interstitial emphysema and pulmonary venous air embolism (i.e., air within the heart and many vessels).

Treatment is directed to sustain cardiopulmonary function.

References

Aranda JV, Stern L, Dunbar JS (1972) Pneumothorax with pneumoperitoneum in a newborn infant. Am J Dis Child 123:163–166

Bagchi I, Nycyk J (2002) Familial spontaneous pneumothorax. Arch Dis Child Fetal Neonatal Ed 87:F70

Benterud T, Sandvik L, Lindemann R (2009) Cesarean section is associated with more frequent pneumothorax and respiratory problems in the neonate. Acta Obstet Gynecol Scand 88:359–361

Bowen FW Jr, Chandra R, Avery GB (1973) Pulmonary interstitial emphysema with gas embolism in hyaline membrane disease. Am J Dis Child 126:117–118

Brook OR, Beck-Razi N, Abadi S et al (2009) Sonographic detection of pneumothorax by radiology residents as part of extended focused assessment with sonography for trauma. J Ultrasound Med 28:749–755

Brooks JG, Bustamante SA, Koops BL et al (1977) Selective bronchial intubation for the treatment of severe localized pulmonary interstitial emphysema in newborn infants. J Pediatr 91:648–652

Burt TB (1982) Neonatal pneumopericardium. Radiology 142:81–84

Caldwell EJ, Powell RD Jr, Mullooly JP (1979) Interstitial emphysema: a study of physiologic factors involved in experimental induction of the lesion. Am Rev Resp Dis 102:516–525

Campbell RE (1970) Intrapulmonary interstitial emphysema: a complication of hyaline membrane disease. Am J Roentgenol Radium Ther Nucl Med 110:449–456

Chan V, Greenough A (1992) Severe localised pulmonary interstitial emphysema–decompression by selective bronchial intubation. J Perinat Med 20:313–316

Clark SD, Saker F, Schneeberger MT et al (2014) Administration of 100% oxygen does not hasten resolution of symptomatic spontaneous pneumothorax in neonates. J Perinatol 34:528–531

Fitzgerald D, Willis D, Usher R, Outerbridge E et al (1998) Dexamethasone for pulmonary interstitial emphysema in preterm infants. Biol Neonate 73:34–39

Greenough A, Dixon AK, Roberton NR (1984) Pulmonary interstitial emphysema. Arch Dis Child 59:1046–1051

Hart SM, McNair M, Gamsu HR, Price JF (1983) Pulmonary interstitial emphysema in very low birthweight infants. Arch Dis Child 58:612–615

Helbich TH, Popow C, Dobner MP et al (1998) Newborn infants with severe hyaline membrane disease: radiological evaluation during high frequency oscillatory versus conventional ventilation. Eur J Radiol 28:243–249

Hoffer FA, Ablow RC (1984) The cross-table lateral view in neonatal pneumothorax. AJR Am J Roentgenol 142:1283–1286

Hummler HD, Bandstra ES, Abdenour GE (1996) Neonatal fellowship.Neonatal pneumopericardium: successful treatment with nitrogen washout technique. J Perinatol 16:490–493

Itani MH, Mikati MA (1998) Early onset neonatal spontaneous pneumopericardium. J Med Liban 46:165–167

Jeffrey IJ (2003) The critical role of perinatal pathology. BJOG 110(Suppl 20):128–130

Johnson CH, Lang SA, Bilal H et al (2014) In patients with extensive subcutaneous emphysema, which technique achieves maximal clinical resolution: infraclavicular incisions, subcutaneous drain insertion or suction on in situ chest drain? Interact Cardiovasc Thorac Surg 18:825–829

Klinger G, Ish-Hurwitz S, Osovsky M et al (2008) Risk factors for pneumothorax in very low birth weight infants. Pediatr Crit Care Med 9:398–402

Knight PJ, Abdenour G (1981) Pneumoperitoneum in the ventilated neonate: respiratory or gastrointestinal origin? J Pediatr 98:972–974

Kuhns LR, Bednarek FJ, Wyman ML et al (1975) Diagnosis of pneumothorax or pneumomediastinum in the neonate by transillumination. Pediatrics 56: 355–360

Lawal TA, Glüer S, Reismann M et al (2009) Spontaneous neonatal pneumomediastinum: the "spinnaker sail" sign. Eur J Pediatr Surg 19:50–52

Lee SK, Tanswell AK (1989) Pulmonary vascular air embolism in the newborn. Arch Dis Child 64:507–510

Long WA (1990) Pneumopericardium. In: Long WA (ed) Fetal and neonatal cardiology. WB Saunders, Philadelphia, pp 377–388

Macklin CC (1939) Transport of air along sheaths of pulmonic blood vessels from alveoli to mediastinum. Arch Intern Med 64:913–926

Maunder RJ (1984) Subcutaneous and mediastinal emphysema pathophysiology, diagnosis, and management. Arch Intern Med 144:147

McCallion N, Davis PG, Morley CJ (2005) Volume-targeted versus pressure-limited ventilation in the neonate. Cochrane Database Syst Rev 3, CD003666

Meadow WL, Cheromcha D (1985) Successful therapy of unilateral pulmonary emphysema: mechanical ventilation with extremely short inspiratory time. Am J Perinatol 2:194–197

Moseley JE (1960) Loculated pneumomediastinum in the newborn. A thymic "spinnaker sail" sign. Radiology 75:788–790

Northfield TC (1971) Oxygen therapy for spontaneous pneumothorax. Br Med J 4:86–88

Ogata ES, Gregory GA, Kitterman JA et al (1976) Pneumothorax in the respiratory distress syndrome: incidence and effect on vital signs, blood gases, and pH. Pediatrics 58:177–183

Pfenninger J, Bossi E, Biesold J, Blumberg A (1982) Treatment of pneumothorax, pneumopericardium and pneumomediastinum. Helv Paediatr Acta 37:353–360

Primhak RA (1983) Factors associated with pulmonary air leak in premature infants receiving mechanical ventilation. J Pediatr 102:764–768

Rainer C, Gardetto A, Frühwirth M et al (2003) Breast deformity in adolescence as a result of pneumothorax drainage during neonatal intensive care. Pediatrics 111:80–86

Rastogi S, Gupta A, Wung JT et al (2007) Treatment of giant pulmonary interstitial emphysema by ipsilateral bronchial occlusion with a Swan- Ganz catheter. Pediatr Radiol 37:1130e4

Shah DS, Lala R, Rajegowda B, Bhatia J (1999) Bronchogenic cyst and its progress in a premature infant. J Perinatol 19:150–152

Steele RW, Metz JR, Bass JW, DuBois JJ (1971) Pneumothorax and pneumomediastinum in the newborn. Radiology 98:629–632

Swingle HM, Eggert LD, Bucciarelli RL (1984) New approach to management of unilateral tension pulmonary interstitial emphysema in premature infants. Pediatrics 74:354–357

Tarnow-Mordi WO, Reid E, Griffiths P, Wilkinson AR (1989) Low inspired gas temperature and respiratory complications in very low birthweight infants. J Pediatr 114:438–442

Volberg FM Jr, Everett CJ, Brill PW (1979) Radiologic features of inferior pulmonary ligament air collections in neonates with respiratory distress. Radiology 130: 357–360

Bronchopulmonary Dysplasia/Chronic Lung Disease of the Newborn

57

Vineet Bhandari

Contents

Abstract

Bronchopulmonary dysplasia (BPD) is a chronic lung disease associated with premature birth and characterized by early lung injury. Over the past four decades, there have been significant changes in the definition, pathology, and radiological findings of BPD. The clinical profile of infants with BPD has changed and it is uncommon in infants over 1,200 g birth weight and >30 weeks gestational age. Understanding of the basic biology of lung development and use of antenatal steroids, postnatal surfactant, new ventilatory strategies, and aggressive nutrition have resulted in major improvements in the clinical course and outcomes. Management of the early, evolving and established phases of BPD continues to improve. Despite many advances in care, however, infants with BPD have significant neurodevelopmental and pulmonary sequelae.

V. Bhandari (✉)
Neonatology/Pediatrics, St. Christopher's Hospital for Children/Drexel University College of Medicine, Philadelphia, PA, USA

Drexel University, Philadelphia, PA, USA
e-mail: vineet.bhandari@drexel.edu

G. Buonocore et al. (eds.), *Neonatology*,
https://doi.org/10.1007/978-3-319-29489-6_205

Abbreviations

α1P1	Alpha-1 proteinase inhibitor
BPD	Bronchopulmonary dysplasia
BW	Birth weight
CC10	Clara cell 10-kD protein
CCSP	Clara cell secretory protein
CMV	Conventional mechanical ventilation
CT	Computed tomography
CTGI	Continuous tracheal gas insufflation
ET-1	Endothelin-1
FGF-2	Fibroblast growth factor-2
GA	Gestational age
HFOV	High-frequency oscillatory ventilation
HGF	Hepatocyte growth factor
ICAM-1	Soluble intercellular adhesion molecule-1
ILs	Interleukins
IL-1RA	IL-1 receptor antagonist
iNO	Inhaled nitric oxide
KGF	Keratinocyte growth factor
LFA-1	Lymphocyte function-associated antigen 1
LPS	Lipopolysaccharide
MCP	Monocyte chemoattractant proteins
MIF	Macrophage migration inhibitory factor
MMPs	Matrix metalloproteinases
NAC	*N*-acetyl cysteine
NCPAP	Nasal continuous positive airway pressure
NF-kB	Nuclear factor-kappa B
NIPPV	Nasal intermittent positive pressure ventilation
PAI-1	Plasminogen activator inhibitor-1
PDA	Patent ductus arteriosus
PMA	Postmenstrual age
PTHrP	Parathyroid hormone-related protein
RCT	Randomized controlled trial
RDS	Respiratory distress syndrome
RSV	Respiratory syncytial virus
SOD	Superoxide dismutase
TA	Tracheal aspirates
TATI	Tumor-associated trypsin inhibitor
TGF-ß1	Transforming growth factor-ß1
TIMP	Tissue inhibitor of metalloproteinases
TNF	Tumor necrosis factor
TNF-α	Tumor necrosis factor-α
VEGF	Vascular endothelial growth factor

57.1 Salient Points

- BPD is the most common chronic lung disease of infancy.
- A consensus definition of BPD, with categorization of severity, has been validated with neurodevelopmental outcomes.
- While the multitude of animal studies and biomarkers associated with BPD continue to expand our scientific knowledge and understanding of the pathogenesis of BPD, there is limited data on their causal role and translational extension to the human premature neonate. Progress in this area is crucial to make an impact on BPD.
- Identification and quantification of the genetic contribution to BPD has been done.
- There is an increasing use of noninvasive ventilation techniques (SNIPPV/NCPAP) with or without less invasive modes of surfactant administration in the prevention and management of BPD.
- The efficacy and safety of caffeine in the prevention of BPD has been established.
- Pulmonary and neurodevelopmental outcome studies of the neonates surviving the "new" BPD will need to be done to assess the potential health impact of BPD in the long term.

57.2 Introduction

Bronchopulmonary dysplasia (BPD) is the commonest cause of chronic lung disease in infancy (Balany and Bhandari 2015). Recent international data report an incidence of BPD of 12–34% in very low birth weight (VLBW; <1,500 g) infants (Jensen and Schmidt 2014). Despite many advances in neonatal ventilation techniques and the widespread use of surfactant

Table 1 Diagnostic criteria for BPD

	Mild – supplemental O_2 (for 28 days) and	Moderate – supplemental O_2 (for 28 days) and	Severe – supplemental O_2 (for 28 days) and
<32 weeks GA at birth	RA at 36 weeks corrected GA or at discharge	<0.3 FiO_2 at 36 weeks corrected GA or at discharge	≥ 0.3 FiO_2
			+/– positive pressure support at 36 weeks corrected GA or at discharge
≥32 weeks GA at birth	RA by postnatal day 56 or at discharge	<0.3 FiO_2 by postnatal day 56 or at discharge	≥ 0.3 FiO_2
			+/– positive pressure support by postnatal day 56 or at discharge

BPD bronchopulmonary dysplasia, *FiO_2* fraction of inspired oxygen, *GA* gestational age, *RA* room air (From Bhandari and Bhandari (2009), with permission)

and antenatal corticosteroids, the incidence of BPD has remained the same (Smith et al. 2005) or even increased slightly (Bhandari and Bhandari 2011; Trembath and Laughon 2012). In a recent evaluation of the utility of the various definitions of BPD, the number of unclassified infants was lowest with the consensus definition (Walsh et al. 2006) (summarized in Table 1) (2.1%) and highest with the physiologic definition (Walsh et al. 2004) (16.1%) (Poindexter et al. 2015). Newer management strategies with high flow nasal cannula (up to 8 L/min) to provide positive pressure support are impacting the definition of BPD. Currently, the status of the respiratory support, with or without "physiologic" testing to ascertain the supplemental oxygen requirement, at 36 weeks postmenstrual age (PMA) is the most commonly used definition.

57.3 Pathology

Pre-surfactant era or "old" BPD lung pathology showed severe airway injury, inflammation, and parenchymal fibrosis with marked heterogeneity. Post-surfactant use, the "new" BPD lung revealed a more uniform impairment of acinar development with alveolar simplification characterized by enlargement and decreased septation of the airspaces, resulting in large-sized, thin-walled, and decreased number of alveoli. Importantly, there is absence of small and large airway epithelial metaplasia, smooth muscle hypertrophy, and fibrosis. In addition, the pulmonary microvasculature in new BPD is undoubtedly dysregulated (Coalson 2006; Baraldi and Filippone 2007). The vascular changes observed include marked angiogenesis proportionate to the growth of the air-exchanging lung parenchyma, abnormal distribution of alveolar capillaries, prominent corner vessels with variable capillary density in adjacent alveoli, or vessels that are more distant from the air surface.

57.4 Etiology and Pathogenesis

Genetic predisposition, baro- and volu-trauma from mechanical ventilation in surfactant-deficient premature lungs, pulmonary edema, pre- and postnatal infections, and reactive oxygen species from prolonged oxygen use and high oxygen concentrations have been associated with the development of BPD (Fig. 1).

1. **Genetics**: Genetic factors contribute 53–82% susceptibility (Bhandari et al. 2006a; Lavoie et al. 2008), making BPD a disease occurring secondary to "gene-environmental" factors. In the first study, it was observed that in premature twins (63 monozygotic and 189 dizygotic twin pairs), <32 weeks gestational age (GA), BPD occurred at a rate of 29% in one or more of a twin pair. After controlling for other covariates, 53% ($p = 0.004$) of BPD was explained by genetic factors alone (Bhandari et al. 2006a). These results were independently confirmed (Lavoie et al. 2008). Multiple genetic variants have been assessed in the evaluation of carrier states that predispose to the development of BPD (Bokodi et al. 2007; Bhandari and Gruen 2006; Bhandari 2012; Prosnitz et al. 2013).

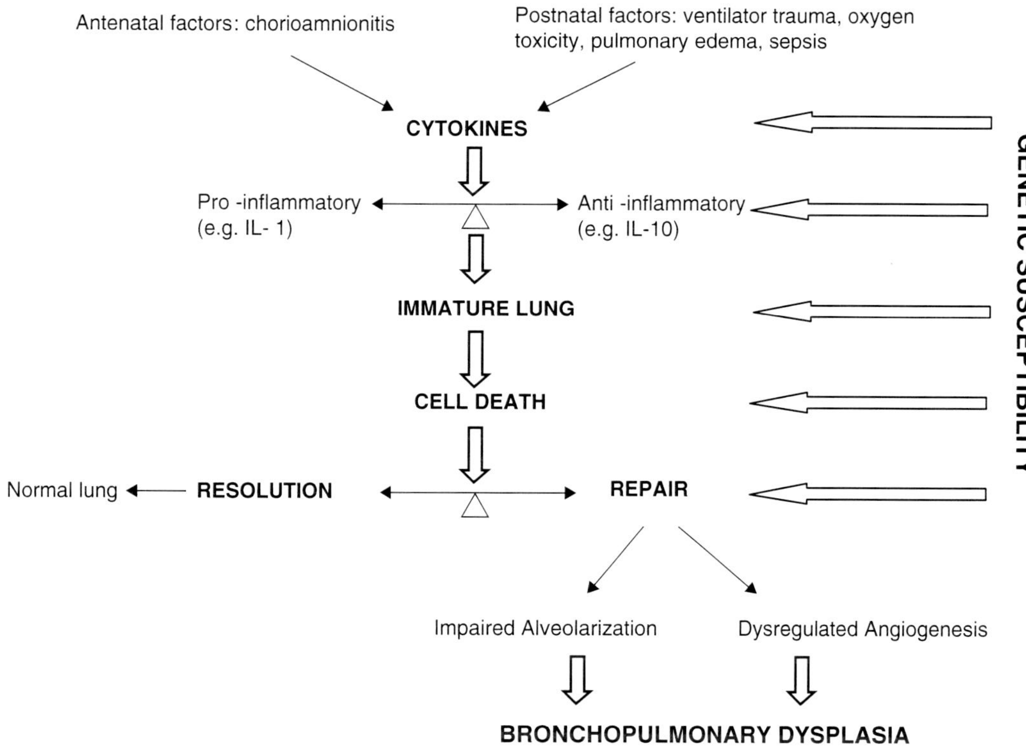

Fig. 1 Pathogenesis of "new" BPD (From Bhandari and Bhandari (2009), with permission)

2. **Prenatal infections**: Chorioamnionitis may be a risk factor for the development of BPD. Clinical observation studies suggest chorioamnionitis, and the fetal inflammatory response (FIR) syndrome increases the risk of BPD (Thomas and Speer 2014). In contrast, histological chorioamnionitis with FIR has been associated with decreased BPD (Plakkal et al. 2013).

   Given the effect of various confounding factors, the issue of antenatal infection/inflammation causing BPD in human infants remains controversial (Balany and Bhandari 2015; Ericson and Laughon 2015).
3. **Lung immaturity**: Intrinsic to the development of BPD is prematurity. Normal lung development occurs in phases which correspond to structural differences. The first phase, the embryonic phase (3–7 weeks PMA) is followed by the pseudoglandular phase (5–17 weeks). Many premature neonates are born during the late canalicular phase (16–26 weeks) of lung development. The saccular phase occurs at 24–38 weeks and accounts for the majority of infants who later develop BPD. The last phase, the alveolar phase, starts from ~32 weeks PMA till about 2–8 years after birth, with the majority of the alveolarization process occurring 5–6 months after birth. Alveolarization incorporates the processes of "elastogenesis and angiogenesis," with multiple cell to cell interactions between fibroblasts, epithelial (type I and II pneumocytes), interstitial, and endothelial cells. Premature birth, with its subsequent medical disorders and their management, alters the postnatal development of lungs, via changes in the molecular signal transduction pathways. Factors that disrupt normal angiogenesis, control of inflammation (i.e., imbalance between "pro-" and "anti-inflammatory" cytokines), and appropriate fibrin deposition or removal are at play in the pathogenesis of BPD.
4. **Hyperoxia**: Excessive oxygen induces oxidative stress with production of reactive oxygen species with increased production of

inflammatory cytokines from epithelial, endothelial, and inflammatory cells. Initial hyperoxic cellular damage induces alveolar or interstitial macrophages to express early cytokines such as IL-1 and tumor necrosis factor (TNF). Chemoattractants are then induced from multiple cell types in the lung, in turn recruiting other inflammatory cells, such as neutrophils (Bhandari and Elias 2006). An immature lung which is exposed to ante- and postnatal environmental factors contributes to the release of a variety of "pro- and anti-inflammatory" cytokines. An imbalance in these mediators leads to activation of the cellular death pathways in the lung. Thus, direct (via reactive oxygen species) or indirect (via cytokines) damage to the respiratory endothelium and epithelium occurs by inducing necrotic and/or apoptotic cell death (Bhandari and Elias 2006). This is followed by healing (resolution of injury) or repair of the lung (Bhandari and Bhandari 2003, 2007). The latter process is characterized by impaired alveolarization and dysregulated angiogenesis leading to fewer, larger simplified alveoli and a dysmorphic pulmonary vasculature (Fig. 1) – the pathologic hallmarks of BPD (Baraldi and Filippone 2007).

5. **Ventilator-induced injury (baro-, volu-, and atelecto-trauma)**: Mechanical ventilation has long been associated with the development of BPD. The initiating biophysical injury due to excessive tissue stretch leads to a cascade of inflammation-induced lung injury (Keszler and Sant'Anna 2015). Intubated neonates who ultimately develop BPD often have significantly increased levels of "pro-inflammatory" cytokines, possibly from microbial colonization and increased distention of alveolar tissue with subsequent baro-, volu-, and/or atelecto-trauma leading to increased inflammation (Speer 2006).

   The association of presence of a patent ductus arteriosus (PDA) and BPD is likely due to the increase in pulmonary circulation and subsequent pulmonary edema. This usually instigates increased ventilatory support and oxygen administration, both being important contributory factors to the development of BPD. However, a recent review concluded that a causal role for the PDA in the development of BPD could not be inferred based on data reported in controlled clinical trials (Clyman 2013). Early ductus ligation was said to be an independent risk factor for the development of BPD (Clyman 2013). In contrast, another recent study concluded that surgical ligation of PDA itself was not an independent risk factor for BPD (Schena et al. 2015).

6. **Postnatal infections**: Systemic infections predispose to the development of BPD (Van Marter et al. 2002). The inflammatory response occurring secondary to infection increases release of inflammatory and vasoactive cytokines on an already damaged pulmonary organ, increasing the need for mechanical ventilation. Airway colonization with increased neutrophilic presence and "pro-inflammatory" cytokines may also predispose to the development of BPD (Speer 2006).

7. **Role of cytokines**: The common theme of inflammation noted above is underscored by the role played by cytokines. Cytokines are chemicals produced by virtually all cell types including fibroblasts, white blood cells, and endothelial and epithelial cells. They mediate immune, inflammatory, and hematopoietic functions in response to various stimuli. In preterm infants, inciting events cause an inflammatory response, either systemically or localized to the pulmonary organ. We have only a partial understanding of how inflammation in the setting of prematurity causes BPD. Soon after birth, upon initiation of oxygen exposure and/or mechanical ventilation, there is an influx of neutrophils and macrophages into pulmonary interstitium. Neutrophils adhere to the endothelium, with interaction between these two cell types occurring via adhesion molecules (e.g., selectins and integrins). This allows for extravasation of neutrophils and macrophages toward the specific areas of injury. These inflammatory cells produce cytokines and other signaling molecules for augmentation of the inflammatory response in an attempt to mitigate the damage of the inciting insult. There is subsequent

disruption of the alveolar capillary unit and pulmonary tissue integrity. The imperfect attempt at repair, differentiation, and growth of these tissues acts in concert with the inflammation to produce the biochemical profile, signs, and symptoms we see in patients with, and those at risk, for BPD (Speer 2006; Ryan et al. 2008).

It is important to highlight the concept that the immature lung in the late canalicular/saccular phase of development is most predisposed to BPD, when exposed to the pre- and postnatal factors, as described above (Balany and Bhandari 2015). While some markers of inflammation may not be detectable within days to weeks of exposure to noxious stimuli, they have already initiated and propagated the signaling pathways of the inflammatory process/immune cascade (Bhandari 2014a). This activation and persistence of inflammation predispose to the permanent structural and functional deficits in BPD lungs (Balany and Bhandari 2015).

Many studies have been conducted to evaluate the presence of cytokines in the amniotic fluid, cord blood, plasma, and tracheal secretions of preterm neonates at risk or who have BPD in an effort to determine a biochemical profile of the condition. Many of the pulmonary biomarkers relate to the possible disruption in the above described mechanisms. A multitude of biomarkers detected in tracheal aspirates (TA), blood, and urine have been proposed for early identification of infants who subsequently develop BPD.

57.5 Biomarkers in BPD

Though there are many clinical associations indicative of an increased risk for the eventual development of BPD, currently there exists no one factor or marker that uniformly and accurately predicts its development. The inciting events that predispose to development of BPD likely occur fairly soon after birth, and we are limited by a lack of ability to distinguish very early in these neonates who will likely go on to develop this chronic disorder. A majority of the biomarkers discussed below are likely abnormal due to damage that has already occurred. Some biomarkers are capable of being perceived as either "pro-" or "anti-inflammatory" depending on their concentration in relation to their physiologic role. Given the proximity to the lung, the primary focus of most investigators has been to access pulmonary secretions to evaluate putative biomarkers for BPD.

The initial TA studies focused on the cytology of the secretions. The exfoliation of dysplastic, metaplastic bronchial cells was found to be 95% specific and 71% sensitive for the subsequent development of BPD. Categories of pulmonary biomarkers that are deranged in BPD include IL and other chemoattractant molecules, markers indicative of abnormal angiogenesis, those signifying abnormal fibrin deposition or degradation, markers of oxidative damage, and peptide growth factors. While a study has shown that TA specimens may be suitable substitutes for bronchoalveolar lavage samples in preterm infants, there has been some controversy whether measurements of the markers in the TA are valid without "normalization." While some have advocated use of total protein, secretory component of IgA, and serum urea, others have espoused that no "normalization" is required.

Table 2 summarizes the results of various TA analytes, focusing more on recent reports that would be more reflective of the "new" BPD, usually obtained in the first week of life, from babies at risk of developing BPD. More details are available from recent reviews (Thomson and Bhandari 2008; Bhandari and Bhandari 2013; Lal and Ambalavanan 2015).

Interferon-γ (IFN-γ): Increased TA levels of IFN-γ and the downstream signaling molecules interferon-γ-inducible proteins 9 and 10 (IP-9, IP-10) have been shown to be associated with increased risk of BPD and/or death (Bhandari and Bhandari 2013).

Interleukins (ILs): ILs are chemicals made by one cell type that act on other inflammatory cells. They may induce growth, differentiation, and proliferation of other leukocytes. They may also act as chemoattractants for recruitment of other cell

Table 2 Use of tracheal aspirate analytes as biomarkers for BPD

Levels associated with increased risk of BPD	Analytes
Increased	Cytokines and chemokines: IL-1β, IL-6, IL-8, IL-16, TNF-α, IFN-γ, MCP-1, MCP-2, MCP-3
	Proteases/antiproteases: MMP-8, MMP-9, trypsin-2
	Adhesion molecules: sICAM-1, L-selectin
	Oxidative injury markers: 3-chlorotyrosine, malondialdehyde, LOOH
	Peptide growth factors: TGFβ1, angiopoietin-2, endothelin-1, FGF2
	Miscellaneous: NF-kB, fibronectin, PAI-1, NGAL, pepsin
Decreased	Cytokines and chemokines: IL-10, MIF
	Proteases/antiproteases: TIMP2, cathepsin K
	Oxidative injury markers: YKL-40
	Peptide growth factors: KGF, HGF
	Miscellaneous: CCSP, PTHrP, lysozyme, PUFA, DMA
Biphasic/variable	Peptide growth factors: VEGF, sVEGFR1

For more details, see Thomson and Bhandari (2008) and Bhandari and Bhandari (2013)
IL interleukin, *TNF* tumor necrosis factor, *INF* interferon, *MCP* monocyte chemoattractant, *MMP* matrix metalloproteinase, *sICAM* soluble intracellular adhesion molecule, *LOOH* lipid hydroperoxide, *TGF* transforming growth factor, *FGF* fibroblast growth factor, *NF-kB* nuclear factor-kappa B, *PAI* plasminogen activator inhibitor, *NGAL* neutrophil gelatinase-associated lipocalin, *MIF* macrophage migration inhibition factor, *TIMP* tissue inhibitor of metalloproteinase, *YKL-40* also known as chitinase-3-like protein1, human homologue of breast regression protein 39 (BRP39), *KGF* keratinocyte growth factor, *HGF* hepatocyte growth factor, *CCSP* Clara cell secretory protein, *PTHrP* parathyroid hormone-related protein, *PUFA* polyunsaturated fatty acid, *DMA* dimethylacetals, *VEGF* vascular endothelial growth factor, *sVEGFR* soluble VEGF receptor 1

types (immune and nonimmune cells) to a site of injury and may exert "pro- or anti-inflammatory" effects. **IL-1ß**, **IL-6**, **IL-8**, and **IL-16**: IL-1ß and IL-6 are particularly active in the acute phase response to injury, while IL-8 is a potent chemotactic agent for recruitment of neutrophils. These cytokines are typically viewed as "pro-inflammatory" and have been shown to be elevated in the TA very early in the respiratory course of the preterm population that ultimately develops BPD. IL-16 acts as a chemoattractant for CD4+ T lymphocytes, monocytes, and eosinophils. Levels of IL-16 correlated significantly with neutrophil counts in the TA and subsequent development of BPD.

IL-10, **IL-4**, and **IL-13**: These cytokines usually act in an "anti-inflammatory" capacity and are responsible for the production, differentiation, and proliferation of B cells and macrophages. It has been suggested that decreased levels of "anti-inflammatory" cytokines would predispose to the development of BPD given the role that inflammation likely has in this disorder. However, there are discrepant findings regarding the levels of "anti-inflammatory" cytokines in the TA of preterm infants at risk for BPD.

IL-10: IL-10 was found to be decreased in TA samples taken in the first 7 days of life in those infants who developed BPD. Other investigators found detectable levels of IL-10 in TA of preterm ventilated infants, but could not correlate the levels with development of BPD. When lipopolysaccharide (LPS), a potent inducer of inflammation, was used to induce production of IL-10 from lung inflammatory cells (obtained from premature infants), there was a decreased ability to induce IL-10 in those infants who went on to develop BPD. A majority of preterm infants (97%) unable to constitutively express the IL-10 gene developed BPD.

IL-4 and **IL-13**: IL-4 is produced by T lymphocytes and alveolar macrophages. Levels of these potentially "anti-inflammatory" cytokines (IL-4, IL-13) could not be significantly correlated with the development of BPD.

Angiopoietin-2: Angiopoietin-2 is an angiogenic growth factor that destabilizes blood vessels, enhances vascular leak, and induces epithelial cell necrosis in hyperoxic conditions. Angiopoietin-2 concentration was observed to be increased in infants with BPD and/or death in the first week of life, when compared to those infants

with RDS who recovered (Bhandari et al. 2006b; Aghai et al. 2008). Furthermore, the levels decreased after exposure to dexamethasone (Aghai et al. 2008).

Cathepsin K: Cathepsin K is a cysteine protease, which degrades existing extracellular matrix and regulates the release of matrix proteins from fibroblasts. In one study, infants who developed BPD had declining cathepsin K levels by day 13, when compared to neonates who did not.

Chemokines: There are four families of chemokines (chemotactic cytokines); they play a role in regulating inflammation by recruiting inflammatory cells to the area of injury. The "CC" family consists of monocyte chemoattractant proteins (MCP) 1, 1α, 1β, 2, and 3. These chemokines were measured in a study to assess the role of CC chemokines in acute lung injury in the preterm, ventilated infant over the first 21 days of life. MCP-1, MCP-1α, MCP-1β, MCP-2, and MCP-3 were all increased in those infants developing BPD. However, only MCP-1, MCP-2, and MCP-3 were statistically significant, with MCP-3 being the most significant (Baier et al. 2004).

Clara cell secretory protein (CCSP): CCSP is produced by Clara cells, which are non-ciliated epithelial cells lining the respiratory and terminal bronchioles. This protein may act to modulate acute pulmonary inflammatory processes. In preterm infants with TA samples taken up to 2 weeks after birth, CCSP increased with maturity and in those neonates who had evidence of infection. In another study, the results indicated that lower levels of CCSP predisposed to development of BPD.

3-Chlorotyrosine: 3-Chlorotyrosine is a biomarker of the neutrophil oxidant, hypochlorous acid, which is utilized in the inflammatory process. Its only source is from neutrophils and monocytes which release myeloperoxidase to catalyze oxidation of chloride by hydrogen peroxide to give hypochlorous acid. In support of data that neutrophilic infiltration and subsequent oxidative injury is closely related to the development of BPD, investigators assessed levels of 3-chlorotyrosine and found that an increase in their concentration correlated with development of BPD.

Fibronectin: An extracellular matrix component, fibronectin, is important in maintaining the integrity of pulmonary tissues and microvasculature. Researchers have found a higher fibronectin level in those infants who developed BPD.

Lactoferrin and lysozyme: Lactoferrin is said to be a marker of inflammation by regulating granulocyte and macrophage proliferation, and may also have some antioxidant properties. Lysozyme is a bactericidal protein that degrades the walls of susceptible bacteria. Both are hypothesized to be released from the serous cells of the submucous glands of the respiratory tract. Both lactoferrin and lysozyme when measured in the first 3 days of life were decreased in patients with BPD as compared to those without BPD, with the decrease in lysozyme being significant.

L-selectin: Concentrations of soluble L-selectin in TA from infants are increased at 7 postnatal days of life, in infants who develop BPD (Bhandari and Bhandari 2013).

Lipid hydroperoxide (LOOH): More recently, increased LOOH levels have been noted in BPD (Fabiano et al. 2015).

Macrophage migration inhibitory factor (MIF): MIF is an upstream regulator of the innate immune response. It has been implicated in the pathogenesis of a number of inflammatory disorders including sepsis, acute RDS (in adults), asthma, and inflammatory/autoimmune diseases. MIF was quantified in TA obtained during the first 2 days of life in a cohort of neonates with RDS. There was a reduction in the concentration of MIF in the lungs of those infants who went on to develop BPD (Kevill et al. 2008).

Malondialdehyde: Malondialdehyde is a marker of oxidative damage, possibly from oxygen radicals produced under hyperoxic conditions or the respiratory burst from inflammatory cells present in the pulmonary organ. In one study of ventilated infants, its pulmonary concentrations were noted to be elevated, but weakly correlated with the development of BPD.

Matrix metalloproteinases (MMPs): MMPs are a family of endoproteinases that aid in the remodeling and degradation of extracellular matrix and basement membranes. They are secreted in inactive form and activated in

extracellular spaces and cell surfaces by oxidants and serine proteinases. They also have the capacity to activate each other. The development of BPD is partially characterized by disordered pulmonary repair after inflammation. Patients who went on to develop BPD had increased levels of tracheal MMP-8, with decreased levels of its inhibitor, "tissue inhibitor of metalloproteinases" (TIMP) (Cederqvist et al. 2001).

Neutrophil gelatinase-associated lipocalin (NGAL): TA levels of NGAL, which is part of a macromolecular complex that includes MMP9, are increased in infants with BPD (Bhandari and Bhandari 2013).

Nuclear factor-kappa B (NF-kB): NF-kB is a transcription factor activated by cellular stress, subsequently promoting expression of multiple genes including "pro-inflammatory" cytokines. TA levels of NF-kB were significantly elevated in the infants who developed BPD or died. However, this difference did not persist when GA was taken into account.

Parathyroid hormone-related protein (PTHrP): PTHrP is secreted by type II pneumocytes and plays a role in normal alveolar growth and development. Its signaling was shown to be downregulated in alveolar overdistention and under hypoxic conditions. Infants developing BPD had significantly lower levels of PTHrP in the first week of life, when compared to those who did not (Rehan and Torday 2006).

Pepsin: TA levels of pepsin (derived from gastric microaspirations) have been reported to be significantly higher in infants who had BPD and/or died in the first week and month of postnatal life (Bhandari and Bhandari 2013).

Plasminogen activator inhibitor-1 (PAI-1): PAI-1 is a regulator of fibrinolysis. It was hypothesized that inhibition of fibrinolysis may play a role in the development of BPD. Infants who developed BPD had significantly higher levels of PAI-1 than non-BPD patients.

Pulmonary trypsin-2: Trypsin-2 is a serine protease expressed in a variety of human epithelial cell types, including in the lung. It can directly attack extracellular protein matrix, basement membrane proteins, and can activate MMPs and initiate protease cascades, causing tissue destruction. It was hypothesized that when trypsin is ineffectively inhibited by its natural inhibitor tumor-associated trypsin inhibitor (TATI), it may play a role in the development of BPD. Results in TA samples from preterm infants indicated that there was significantly higher trypsin-2 to TATI ratio during first 2 weeks in those infants developing BPD.

Polyunsaturated fatty acid (PUFA) and dimethylacetals (DMA): These have been reported to be significantly decreased in infants developing BPD, but only on day 1 (Bhandari and Bhandari 2013).

Soluble intercellular adhesion molecule-1 (sICAM-1): sICAM-1 plays a role in early inflammation and is the ligand for lymphocyte function-associated antigen 1 (LFA-1). sICAM-1 is expressed by lymphocytes, eosinophils, mast, endothelial, and bronchial epithelial cells. Infants who developed BPD had significantly higher levels of soluble sICAM-1 in TA at 6–14 days of age.

Transforming growth factor-ß1 (TGF-ß1): TGF-ß1 is produced mostly by alveolar macrophages and acts on fibroblasts to increase the transcription of fibronectin and procollagen. It also inhibits synthesis of proteases and increases the synthesis of antiproteases, thus resulting in a net increase in fibrosis. Infants who developed BPD had significantly increased levels of TGF-β1 in TA.

Tumor necrosis factor-α (TNF-α): TNF-α is a pro-inflammatory cytokine that induces cell death and enhances expression of other cytokines. In a study of premature infants, TNF-α was noted to be increased early in the patients who developed BPD.

Peptide growth factors: Peptide growth factors are important for normal lung development, maturation, and repair. This group includes endothelin-1 (ET-1), fibroblast growth factor-2 (FGF-2), keratinocyte growth factor (KGF), hepatocyte growth factor (HGF), and vascular endothelial growth factor (VEGF).

ET-1: ET-1 is a potent endothelium-derived vaso- and broncho-constricting factor, produced in virtually all tissues, though its largest

concentration is in the lung. Under the influence of cytokines (IL-1β, IL-6, IL-8), production of ET can be induced in macrophages and monocytes. ET-1 has also been hypothesized to increase the production of oxygen radicals from alveolar macrophages. In preterm infants with RDS, TA concentrations of ET-1 in the first week of life were significantly elevated in infants developing BPD (Niu et al. 1998). This was, however, not confirmed by others (Ambalavanan and Novak 2003).

FGF-2: FGF plays a role in angiogenesis, by stimulating endothelial cell proliferation, degrading extracellular matrix, and appears to interact with VEGF. There was a significant elevation in the levels of FGF-2 in the TA in the BPD/death population on day 1 of life (Ambalavanan and Novak 2003).

KGF: A member of the FGF family, KGF regulates proliferation of alveolar epithelial cells and enhances synthesis of surfactant and accelerates wound closure in airway epithelium. It was noted that in premature infants who developed BPD, KGF was lower than in those who did not develop it.

Pulmonary HGF: HGF in fetal rat lungs stimulates branching of both alveolar and bronchial epithelia and contributes to growth, maturation, and maintenance of tissue homeostasis. It has been suggested that HGF also mediates repair of type II pneumocytes after acute lung injury. Infants who developed BPD had significantly lower levels of HGF in the first 2 weeks of life, when compared to non-BPD counterparts.

VEGF: VEGF promotes endothelial cell growth and remodeling. In the pulmonary system, it appears to be essential for the appropriate development of alveolar tissue; in rats its antagonism has been shown to result in dramatically impaired alveolarization (Thebaud and Abman 2007). In heavily vascularized tissues, such as the lung, VEGF exists in high concentrations. During hyperoxic episodes when damage to the microvasculature occurs, VEGF plays a role in the remodeling process, and its levels are increased, sometimes disproportionately. In preterm infants with RDS, infants developing BPD had significantly lower levels of TA VEGF closer to 1 week of life (Thomson and Bhandari 2008). Conversely, no difference in TA VEGF levels were noted between BPD and no BPD infants in another study (Ambalavanan and Novak 2003). In a recent study, a phasic pattern of VEGF concentrations was noted in infants who go on to develop BPD. These infants had an initial spike over the first 12 h of postnatal life, followed by a decrease over the next few days and then a subsequent significant increase (Bhandari et al. 2008a).

sVEGFR1: While sVEGFR1 levels were higher on day 1 in infants who developed BPD, they subsequently declined on days 3 and 7 (Bhandari and Bhandari 2013).

YKL-40: This is also known as chitinase-3-like protein 1, and low levels have been reported in infants who go on to develop BPD (Bhandari and Bhandari 2013).

Other biomarkers: Given the complexity of the pathogenesis of BPD, investigators have also attempted to use the relative concentration of TA markers to predict BPD. Infants who developed BPD had higher IL-1β concentrations and IL-1β/IL-6 ratios. Premature infants who developed BPD had higher levels of IL-1 receptor antagonist (IL-1RA) in their airways on the first day of life. IL-1β also increased significantly for BPD patients early, both compared to non-BPD patients and also within the BPD group. While the early (day 1) IL-1 antagonist/agonist molar balance offered protection, by days 5 and 7, a threshold for IL-1RA in the presence of increasing IL-1β expression favored "pro-inflammation" in the BPD group. Others have demonstrated a sustained increase of TGFβ1 levels in TA from preterm infants who developed BPD, combined with an absent or irregular secretion of IL-4, IL-10, and IL-12. Babies who developed BPD or died had lower IL-6/VEGF ratios in the TA, than those who did not have such an adverse outcome (Thomson and Bhandari 2008). In other studies, BPD infants had significantly lower TIMP-1 level with higher MMP-9/TIMP-1 ratio during the first 2 weeks of life and low TIMP-2 and MMP-2 levels during the first 3 days of life compared with no BPD infants (Ekekezie et al. 2004).

Cord blood (and TA) soluble E-selectin has been noted to be increased in infants who developed BPD. Increased serum levels of soluble

E-selectin were associated with the development of BPD. In another study, low levels of soluble L-selectin and increasing levels of soluble E-selectin were reported to be potential risk factors for BPD. The cord blood placental growth factor concentrations were noted to be increased in infants developing BPD. Serum C-IV (an antigen marker of type IV collagen, a component of basement membranes) levels were elevated in the first week of life in infants subsequently diagnosed with BPD. In another study of serial measurements of the C-terminal fragment of type I procollagen, levels at week 4 were significantly lower in infants who subsequently developed BPD. Patients with both the old and new categories of BPD had elevated serum levels of TGF-β1, though these were not statistically significant (Vento et al. 2006). Other blood markers include measures of eosinophilic activation (eosinophilic cationic protein and the cellular surface antigen CD9), which were increased in BPD. The plasma KL-6 (a circulating high molecular weight mucinous glycoprotein which is the extracellular soluble region of MUC-1 mucin possessing an undefined sialylated carbohydrate chain that is recognized by KL-6 antibody) was noted to be increased in patients with moderate/severe BPD. The plasma levels of 8-iso-prostaglandin F2alpha (a stable metabolite of F2-isoprostanes, a marker for oxidant injury) have been noted to be increased in infants who developed BPD/died. In another study, however, urinary levels of the same metabolite were not correlated with BPD.

Older infants with established BPD had higher levels of urinary leukotriene E 4 when compared to healthy infants of the same age; however, it was not found to be an early marker of BPD. Elevated urinary elevated bombesin-like peptide levels in infants at 1–4 days after birth were associated with a tenfold increased risk of developing BPD (Cullen et al. 2002). Given the importance of vascular development in the pathogenesis of BPD, investigators have postulated evaluating the vascularity of the lower gingival and vestibular oral mucosa as a marker for BPD. Infants with BPD showed a significantly lower blood vessel area as well as a higher vascular network complexity than control subjects. Increased end-tidal carbon monoxide (CO) and exhaled nitric oxide (NO) levels have been reported in infants with BPD in the first month of life (Bhandari and Bhandari 2013).

A majority of these studies comprise of a small number of babies. Appropriately so, most attempts to identify biomarkers have been to access the pulmonary compartment by collecting TA. However, TA have been collected at a variable number of time points, measurements done usually of single markers, with or without "normalization" and with variable definitions of BPD (oxygen requirement for 28 days or at 36 weeks PMA, with or without radiographic criteria). Few have been replicated in different cohorts. Those with consistent results include: elastase, IL-1β, IL-6, MCP-1, ET-1, and angiopoietin-2 (Table 2). VEGF has been replicated but showed variable results (Table 2). Most of the above comments are also true of the blood and urinary markers. Not surprisingly, none of the aforementioned markers for BPD are in general clinical use.

The majority of the above biomarkers show only an association with BPD. In order to prove a causal relationship, they need to be studied in developmentally appropriate animal models and human lungs with BPD. Some progress in this direction has been made with the following: elastin (Bland et al. 2007), cathepsin-S (Hirakawa et al. 2007), HGF (Padela et al. 2005), KGF (Frank 2003), IFN-γ (Harijith et al. 2011; Choo-Wing et al. 2013), IL-1β (Bry et al. 2007), IL-6 (Choo-Wing et al. 2007), MCP-1 (Vozzelli et al. 2004), TGF-β1 (Vicencio et al. 2004), VEGF (Thebaud et al. 2005), bombesin-like peptide (Subramaniam et al. 2007), YKL-40 (Sohn et al. 2010), and angiopoietin-2 (Bhandari et al. 2006b), but additional work is needed.

There has been an increasing focus on using "omic" techniques (genomics, epigenomics, microbiomics, transcriptomics, proteomics, and metabolomics) for detecting markers for BPD (Lal and Ambalavanan 2015; Piersigilli and Bhandari 2016). Using these approaches, biomarkers in human studies recently reported include SPOCK2, VEGF-624C > G, VEGF-460 T > C, mast cell-specific markers, miR-219

pathway, miR-152, miR-30a-3p, miR-133b, miR-206, miR-7, lactate, taurine, trimethylamine-N-oxide, gluconate, myoinositol, and alterations in surfactant lipid profile (Piersigilli and Bhandari 2016).

57.6 Clinical Aspects

Clinical diagnosis: The classical presentation is a history of a premature infant with RDS who has been intubated and mechanically ventilated and exposed to supplemental oxygen for the first week of life or longer. Usually these infants experience bouts of postnatal sepsis and have inadequate nutritional intake. Over time, these infants fulfill the diagnostic criteria for BPD, as defined earlier.

In the early phase of BPD (up to the first postnatal week of life), the clinical presentation may be indistinguishable from an infant with RDS. Such infants may require intubation and surfactant administration. Occasionally, premature infants may require minimal respiratory support with nasal continuous positive airway pressure (NCPAP) or nasal intermittent positive pressure ventilation (NIPPV), with a supplemental oxygen requirement of $<40\%$. In the evolving phase of BPD (after 1 week of life to 36 weeks PMA), such infants have not been able to be successfully extubated or have been re-intubated. These infants usually require escalation of ventilatory support and higher concentrations of supplemental oxygen. Signs and symptoms of established BPD (after 36 weeks PMA) include tachypnea, dyspnea, and chronic or intermittent crackles and wheezing. In children with subglottic stenosis secondary to prolonged intubation, there may be presence of a stridor on exam. Noisy breathing exacerbated with high airflow activities such as feeding and agitation may be heard in infants with tracheomalacia and bronchomalacia. BPD spells are episodes of tracheal obstruction associated with episodes of cyanosis and oxygen desaturations and bradycardia, usually occurring secondary to agitation, and are thought to be related to tracheomalacia and bronchomalacia. Cardiac complications of severe BPD include pulmonary hypertension and cor pulmonale. Poor growth may be related to undiagnosed hypoxia, cardiac disease, gastroesophageal reflux, and swallow dysfunction or recurrent aspiration.

Radiological findings: In the early phase of BPD, the chest X-ray shows RDS or, in some case, minimal respiratory disease. In the evolving phase, the lung fields become more hazy and dense suggesting pulmonary edema, atelectasis, or infiltrates. Recently there has been a change in the radiographic findings associated with established BPD. This change has likely been brought about by the younger GA of surviving infants, widespread use of surfactant, and less aggressive respiratory management strategies. Traditionally, in the pre-surfactant era, BPD was represented on radiographic imaging by emphysematous areas with other portions of the lung displaying volume loss. This correlated with the pathology of a pulmonary specimen that would also exhibit signs of increased inflammation, fibrosis, and small airway disease. Over the clinical course of evolving "new" BPD, the radiological signs are fairly nonspecific, and the lung fields appear hazy and dense secondary to pulmonary edema (called the leaky lung syndrome, LLS) (Hyodynmaa et al. 2012) and atelectasis (Fig. 2). Once the "new" BPD is well established, the

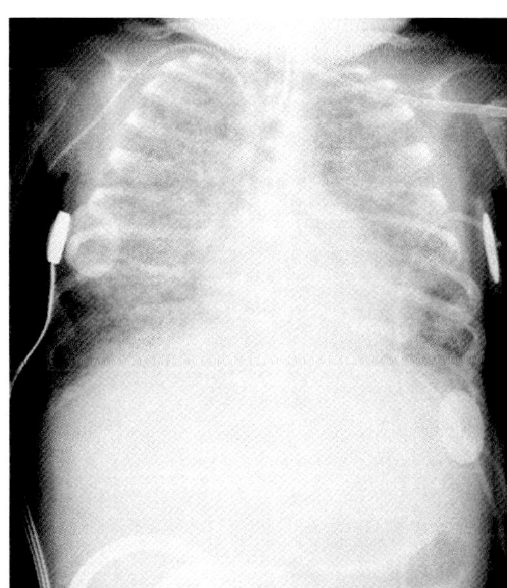

Fig. 2 Chest X-ray of an infant with established BPD

appearance of the lungs progresses to hyperinflation and cystic areas ("bubbly appearance" or cystic BPD) (Hyodynmaa et al. 2012), but without the large cysts typical of the older form of BPD (Speer 2006; Agrons et al. 2005).

57.7 Differential Diagnoses

Aspiration pneumonia: In the early phase of BPD, respiratory distress can be secondary to aspiration of amniotic fluid or maternal blood during delivery (Table 3). The radiological picture may show localized lobar infiltrates or an interstitial pattern. With supportive care that usually includes supplemental oxygen with or without mechanical ventilation, intravenous fluids, and antibiotics, such infants show significant clinical improvement within the first week of life.

Congenital heart disease: Infants with cyanotic congenital heart disease will show evidence of hypoxemia, not responsive to supplemental oxygen. In addition, there may be signs suggestive of a cardiovascular etiology (hypotension, heart murmurs, heart rhythm disturbances). Chest X-rays may be helpful in terms of the size and shape of the cardiac silhouette. Cardiac echocardiography will be diagnostic.

Infectious pneumonia: These are mostly viral or bacterial in the immediate newborn period. There may be maternal history (e.g., chorioamnionitis) that may predispose an infant to an infectious pneumonia. Chest X-rays show lobar or perihilar infiltrates. Neonates usually improve with supportive care (as mentioned above) within the first week of life.

Interstitial lung disease: In the neonatal period, genetic and developmental disorders leading to interstitial lung disease are most likely to be considered in the differential diagnoses of BPD. These include specific conditions that affect surfactant function, i.e., mutations in surfactant proteins B, C, and ABCA3. Confirmation of diagnoses may require lung biopsy and genetic testing.

Pulmonary lymphangiectasia: It is a rare developmental disorder that results in dilated and obstructed lymphatics. Confirmation of the diagnosis requires a lung biopsy. There is an association with Noonan and Turner syndromes.

Wilson-Mikity syndrome: There is significant overlap between Wilson-Mikity syndrome and the premature infants with BPD who do not have significant respiratory disease at birth (*vide supra*). Infants with Wilson-Mikity syndrome do not develop RDS. The exact etiology is unknown. Proposed predisposing factors include air trapping, fluid overload secondary to chronic PDA, recurrent aspiration, infection, rickets, and surfactant deficiency. Clinical features are characterized by features of respiratory distress. This syndrome is commonly seen between 1 and 2 months of age, and most cases slowly resolve. Chest radiographic findings are normal in the first week, but later they are similar to those of BPD, with hyperinflation, streaky infiltrates, and cystic changes. Radiographic changes persist for a few months to years after clinical findings resolve. It is perhaps a genetic variant of the "new" BPD.

Table 3 Differential diagnoses of BPD

Aspiration pneumonia
Congenital heart disease
Infectious pneumonia
Interstitial lung disease
Pulmonary lymphangiectasia
Wilson-Mikity syndrome

57.8 Prognosis

This is primarily dependent on pulmonary and neurodevelopmental outcomes.

Pulmonary outcomes (pulmonary hypertension): A major pulmonary morbidity is the development of pulmonary hypertension (PH) which is noted in ~20% of infants with birth weights <1,000 g, primarily those with moderate/severe BPD, and this persists to discharge in many infants (Ambalavanan and Mourani 2014). The gold standard for diagnosis of PH is cardiac catheterization. But given the concern that the invasive procedure would not be well tolerated in these sick BPD infants, it is usually avoided, at least, at a younger postnatal age. Echocardiography is

generally used for diagnosis. Objective measures of PH by echocardiogram include estimated right ventricular systolic pressure (RVSP) derived from the tricuspid regurgitant jet velocity (TRJV) (Mourani and Abman 2015). A threshold of RVSP greater than 35 mmHg (TRJV >3 m/s) to define PH has been used (Mourani and Abman 2015). Lack of a TRJV does not preclude the diagnosis of PH; the right ventricular myocardial performance index (MPI; also known as the Tei index) has been used as a surrogate for increased pulmonary vascular resistance in BPD (Mourani and Abman 2015). Biochemical monitoring (B-type natriuretic peptide) has been suggested to diagnose and/or monitor BPD-associated PH (Cuna et al. 2014; Montgomery et al. 2016). Management is primarily focused on maintaining oxygen saturation in the targeted range of 90–95%, in combination with inhaled nitric oxide (iNO) at 5–20 ppm (Ambalavanan and Mourani 2014). If there is a limited or no response and/or in an effort to wean off iNO, sildenafil is usually started (0.5–1 mg/kg/dose every 8 h) (Ambalavanan and Mourani 2014). Infants who do not respond to the above therapy are then usually started on a prostacyclin analog (epoprostenol, iloprost, or treprostinil) or an endothelin-receptor antagonist (bosentan or ambrisentan) (Ambalavanan and Mourani 2014). There are limited data on the use of these agents in infants with BPD and PH, and hence these need to be used with careful monitoring for efficacy and toxicity (Ambalavanan and Mourani 2014). Infants with BPD-associated PH on treatment should be closely monitored. These include assessments of oxygenation and serial echocardiograms (every 2–4 weeks initially and then 4–6 monthly), with cardiac catheterization indicated for select patients (Mourani and Abman 2015). Weaning of medications should only be done with improvement being documented by serial echocardiograms, in addition to assessment of pulmonary function and growth, over weeks (Mourani and Abman 2015).

Respiratory morbidity: Compared to non-BPD, infants with BPD have higher rates of rehospitalizations (up to 50%) in the first year and 36% in the second year of life. Reasons for rehospitalization included reactive airway disease, pneumonia, respiratory syncytial virus (RSV) infection, and worsening BPD (Bhandari and Panitch 2006). Although recurrent respiratory symptoms needing hospitalization decrease over time, this increase in respiratory symptoms persists beyond the first 2 years of life into preschool years, adolescence, and early adulthood (Bhandari and Panitch 2006). It is unclear whether it is the severity of BPD or prematurity per se that influences the persistence and severity of symptoms.

Radiological findings: In children with a history of BPD, abnormal chest x-rays with subtle radiological abnormalities have been noted later in adolescence and adulthood (Bhandari and Panitch 2006). The chest radiograph is relatively insensitive to the structural changes present in the BPD lung. In contrast, high resolution computed tomography (HRCT) is much more sensitive for visualizing radiological abnormalities in patients with BPD. Investigators have reported that there is little difference in the radiological appearance of "old" versus "new" BPD, with the absence of bronchial involvement being the only striking difference. The common findings include regions of hypoattenuation, linear opacities initiating at the pleural surface and radiating inward toward the hilum, and triangular subpleural opacities (Walkup and Woods 2015). A positive correlation between abnormal radiographic findings and pulmonary function has been reported, with severity of the clinical course being associated with extensive CT scan abnormalities (Bhandari and Panitch 2006). Chest HRCT scan scoring systems have been proposed that correlated well with clinical scores at 36 weeks PMA and duration of oxygen dependence (Walkup and Woods 2015). Magnetic resonance imaging (MRI) is also being used and has shown focal high-density areas and low-density cyst-like abnormalities in infants with BPD (Walkup and Woods 2015).

Pulmonary function: Despite many advances in neonatal care, patients with BPD continue to have significant impairment in lung function, and their lung function may continue to deteriorate into late adolescence (Doyle et al. 2006). Fortunately, this impaired lung function typically does not interfere with the patient's ability to participate in daily activities, including exercise.

Persistent airway dysfunction likely reflects severity of neonatal disease. Although there is a plethora of literature describing abnormal lung function in patients with BPD at all ages from infancy to early adulthood, there are only a few studies correlating the extent of pulmonary function impairment with various therapies used. An inverse relationship has been reported between FEV1 at school age and duration of supplemental oxygen. V'max25, a measure of flow through small airways, was reduced at school age in inverse proportion to an oxygen score that quantified neonatal supplemental oxygen exposure. Conversely, others have reported poor correlation between duration of mechanical ventilation and oxygen supplementation and forced expiratory flow in infants with BPD (Bhandari and Panitch 2006). BPD infants had low forced expiratory flow measurements at 6 and 12 months who were treated initially with either high-frequency oscillatory ventilation (HFOV) or conventional mechanical ventilation (CMV) compared with published reference values (Hofhuis et al. 2002). Infants treated initially with HFOV had significantly better lung function at 12 months than those treated with CMV (Hofhuis et al. 2002), suggesting that early HFOV in combination with surfactant treatment could lessen the neonatal lung injury that leads to BPD (Hofhuis et al. 2002). It is not known if this difference persists into adulthood. Others have found no significant difference in the degree of mild obstructive lung disease as a function of mode of ventilation at 8–9 years of age. This suggests that other factors influence long-term pulmonary outcome (Bhandari and Panitch 2006). Other studies have noted a correlation in the V'max FRC, FEV1, and FEF25–75% measured at 2 years and school age (Bhandari and Panitch 2006).

Large airways can also be affected in BPD. Prolonged endotracheal intubation and mechanical ventilation result in tracheomalacia and bronchomalacia which are associated with increased airway compliance. Other problems commonly encountered are subglottic stenosis, airway granulomas, and pseudopolyps that may require surgical intervention (Bhandari and Panitch 2006).

Most studies show no reduction in exercise capacity in children with BPD when compared to children with healthy term infants or preterm babies without lung disease (Bhandari and Panitch 2006). Decreased gas transfer and oxyhemoglobin saturations during exercise in school-aged children (6–9 years) have been reported in those with a history of BPD when compared with full-term and preterm children with no BPD. Others have shown a decrease in maximal exercise in capacity in BPD survivors aged 6–12 years when compared to healthy controls. Exercise tolerance continues be relatively unchanged in young adulthood. Higher airway obstruction and CO diffusing capacity and decreased exercise capacity but normal mean lung function in former preemies at young adulthood (mean age 19 years), when compared to controls, has been reported. This suggests that the impaired exercise tolerance in these young adults was not related to pulmonary function but perhaps poor physical fitness (Bhandari and Panitch 2006).

Many changes occur in pulmonary function with growth and development. While lung mechanics and some volumes may normalize over time, small airway dysfunction persists. While some investigators have suggested that the abnormal lung function catches up in the first year (Mello et al. 2015), others have reported no catch up during 2 years (Sanchez-Solis et al. 2016). Recent data suggest that adults with history of BPD are more likely to have airflow obstruction, bronchial hyperresponsiveness, and pulmonary gas trapping (Landry et al. 2016; Saarenpaa et al. 2015).

Neurodevelopmental outcomes: BPD children have a greater fine and gross motor skill impairment as well as cognitive function and language delay as compared to infants without BPD. Children with severe BPD had worse outcomes and required more interventions at age 8 years than did children with mild or moderate BPD (Short et al. 2007).

Most studies of BPD have been cross-sectional in nature, and the independent effect of BPD is difficult to assess, given the high likelihood of the presence of additional medical complications in these infants. While preterm infants have an

increased risk of neurodevelopmental impairment, BPD is an additional risk factor (Anderson and Doyle 2006). BPD does not appear to be associated with a specific neuropsychological but rather a global impairment (Anderson and Doyle 2006). Importantly, the spectrum of neurodevelopmental impairment appears to correlate well with the BPD disease severity (Ehrenkranz et al. 2005; Jeng et al. 2008). Recently, a single-center recent retrospective study reported that BPD (with or without chronic oxygen dependency) in children predicted abnormal neurodevelopmental outcomes at 36 months corrected age (Lodha et al. 2014). However, chronic oxygen dependency did not lead to worse neurodevelopmental outcomes in those with BPD (Lodha et al. 2014).

57.9 Therapy

The current status of the various therapeutic approaches in the three (early, evolving, and established) phases of BPD is shown in Tables 4, 5, and 6. The robustness of the evidence has been classified based on the type of clinical studies using the system developed by the US Preventive Services Task Force:

- Level I: Evidence obtained from at least one properly designed randomized controlled trial.
- Level II-1: Evidence obtained from well-designed controlled trials without randomization.
- Level II-2: Evidence obtained from well-designed cohort or case-control analytic

Table 4 Management of BPD: early phase (up to 1 postnatal week)

Therapeutic intervention	Current status	Level of evidence	Level of recommendation
Oxygen supplementation	Controversy in the acceptable oxygen saturation levels still exists across centers, but generally <95% (Samiee-Zafarghandy et al. 2015; Manja et al. 2015); usually between 87% and 93% (Lakshminrusimha et al. 2015)	I	A
Ventilatory strategy	Avoid intubation. If intubated, give "early" surfactant (Yost and Soll 2000)	I	A
	Use short inspiratory times (0.24–0.4 s), (Kamlin and Davis 2004)	I	A
	rapid rates (40–60/min)	III	B
	Low PIP (14–20 cm H_2O)	III	B
	Moderate PEEP (4–6 cm H_2O)	III	B
	Low tidal volume (3–6 mL/kg) (Ambalavanan and Carlo 2006)	III	B
	Extubate early to SNIPPV/NCPAP (Bhandari 2006)	I	A
	Blood gas targets: pH 7.25–7.35	III	B
	PaO_2 40–60 mmHg	III	B
	$PaCO_2$ 45–55 mmHg (Miller and Carlo 2007)	I	C
	High-frequency ventilation for "rescue," if conventional ventilation fails (Greenough 2007)	I	A
Methylxanthines	Improves successful extubation rate (Henderson-Smart and Davis 2003)	I	A
	Decreases BPD (Schmidt et al. 2006)	I	A
Vitamin A	If considering use, dose is 5,000 IU administered intramuscularly 3 times per week for 4 weeks. 1 additional infant survived without BPD for every 14–15 infants who received vitamin A (Tyson et al. 1999; Darlow and Graham 2007)	I	A
Fluids	Restrictive fluid intake may decrease BPD (Bhandari et al. 2005; Oh et al. 2005)	II-2	B
Nutrition	Provide increased energy intake (Lai et al. 2006)	I	B

PIP peak inspiratory pressure, *PEEP* positive end expiratory pressure, *SNIPPV* synchronized nasal intermittent positive pressure ventilation, *NCPAP* nasal continuous positive airway pressure (From Bhandari and Bhandari (2009), with permission)

Table 5 Management of BPD: evolving phase (>1 postnatal week to 36 weeks PMA)

Therapeutic intervention	Current status	Level of evidence	Level of recommendation
Oxygen supplementation	Same as in Table 4	I	A
Ventilatory strategy	Avoid endotracheal tube ventilation. Maximize noninvasive ventilation (SNIPPV/NCPAP) for respiratory support (Bhandari 2006)	I	A
	Blood gas targets: pH 7.25–7.35	III	B
	PaO_2 50–70 mmHg	III	B
	$PaCO_2$ 50–60 mmHg (Ambalavanan and Carlo 2006)	III	B
Methylxanthines	Same as in Table 4	I	A
Vitamin A	Same as in Table 4. If using, continue for 4 postnatal weeks	I	A
Steroids	Dexamethasone effective in weaning off mechanical ventilation when used "moderately early" and "delayed" (Halliday et al. 2003a, b)	I	A
	Increased incidence of neurological sequelae with early use (<96 h) (Halliday et al. 2003c)	I	D
Diuretics	Furosemide: may use daily or every other day with transient improvement in lung function (Baveja and Christou 2006)	I	B
	Spironolactone and thiazides: chronic therapy improves lung function and decreases oxygen requirements (Baveja and Christou 2006)	I	B
Nutrition	Same as in Table 4	I	B

PMA postmenstrual age, *SNIPPV* synchronized nasal intermittent positive pressure ventilation, *NCPAP* nasal continuous positive airway pressure (From Bhandari and Bhandari (2009), with permission)

Table 6 Management of BPD: established phase (>36 weeks PMA)

Therapeutic intervention	Current status	Level of evidence	Level of recommendation
Oxygen supplementation	For prevention of pulmonary hypertension and cor pulmonale. A wide variation in the acceptable oxygen saturation levels exists across centers, but generally ~95% (Greenough 2007; Khemani et al. 2007)	III	C
Ventilatory strategy	Blood gas targets: pH 7.25–7.35	III	B
	PaO_2 50–70 mmHg		
	$PaCO_2$ 50–65 mmHg (Ambalavanan and Carlo 2006)		
Steroids	Oral prednisolone may be helpful in weaning oxygen (Bhandari et al. 2008b)	II-2	C
Diuretics	Chronic therapy as in Table 5	I	B
Beta agonists	Transient relief: increased compliance and reduced pulmonary resistance (Baveja and Christou 2006)	I	C
	No significant effect on incidence or severity of BPD (Ng et al. 2001)	I	C
Anticholinergics	Used in combination with beta agonists in infants with bronchospasm. Increased compliance and decreased respiratory system resistance (Brundage et al. 1990)	II-3	C
Nutrition	Same as in Table 4	I	B
Immunization	Prophylaxis against RSV and influenza decreases incidence of rehospitalization and morbidity	I	A

PMA postmenstrual age (From Bhandari and Bhandari (2009), with permission)

studies, preferably from more than one center or research group.

- Level II-3: Evidence obtained from multiple time series with or without the intervention. Dramatic results in uncontrolled trials might also be regarded as this type of evidence.
- Level III: Opinions of respected authorities, based on clinical experience, descriptive studies, or reports of expert committees.

The recommendation for use in the clinical setting is also based on the guidelines developed by the US Preventive Services Task Force:

- Level A: Good scientific evidence suggests that the benefits substantially outweigh the potential risks.
- Level B: At least fair scientific evidence suggests that the benefits outweigh the potential risks.
- Level C: At least fair scientific evidence suggests that there are benefits provided, but the balance between benefits and risks are too close for making general recommendations.
- Level D: At least fair scientific evidence suggests that the risks outweigh potential benefits.
- Level I: Scientific evidence is lacking, of poor quality, or conflicting, such that the risk versus benefit balance cannot be assessed.

57.10 Novel Approaches/Therapies

Allopurinol: In a randomized controlled trial (RCT) of 400 preterm infants, allopurinol given for 1 week did not impact on the incidence of BPD (at 28 days).

Alpha-1 proteinase inhibitor (α1P1): Systemic treatment with α1P1 did not reveal any statistically significant differences in the rates of BPD between the treated and placebo groups of preterm infants.

Budesonide: Inhaled as well as intratracheal administration of budesonide (the latter in conjunction with surfactant) has shown to decrease BPD in 2 recent RCTs (Bassler et al. 2015; Yeh et al. 2016).

Continuous tracheal gas insufflation (CTGI): In a prospective RCT in 34 premature infants, CTGI was not found to decrease death or BPD, compared to controls.

Cromolyn: Two trials did not show any decrease in the incidence of BPD with the use of cromolyn (a mast cell stabilizer), which was confirmed in a meta-analysis.

Hydrocortisone: Low-dose hydrocortisone did not improve survival without BPD (Watterberg et al. 2004). The RCT had to be terminated early due to the hydrocortisone-treated infants receiving indomethacin having more gastrointestinal perforations (Watterberg et al. 2004).

Inositol: In a meta-analysis of RCT using inositol supplementation in premature infants, the outcome of death or BPD was reported in two trials and was found to be significantly reduced (Howlett and Ohlsson 2003).

Liquid ventilation: In an uncontrolled study of 13 premature neonates treated with partial liquid ventilation, among eight infants who survived till 36 weeks PMA, four had BPD.

Macrolide antibiotics: Erythromycin has not been shown to decrease BPD in infants when treated prophylactically or after known *Ureaplasma* colonization. Azithromycin, in a pilot study, did not reduce the incidence of BPD.

***N*-Acetylcysteine (NAC)**: In a large RCT, the use of a 6-day course of NAC did not prevent BPD or death in infants with BW $<1{,}000$ g.

Nasal continuous positive airway pressure (NCPAP): Early surfactant replacement therapy with extubation to NCPAP compared with later selective surfactant replacement and continued mechanical ventilation with extubation from low ventilator support was associated with less need for mechanical ventilation, lower incidence of BPD, and fewer air leak syndromes (Stevens et al. 2007). Use of a cutoff value of FiO_2 of 0.45 to decide on transient intubation and surfactant replacement appeared to decrease the incidence of air leaks and BPD (Stevens et al. 2007). The Cochrane review, however, did not include the results of the COIN trial which reported that in infants born at 25–28-weeks gestation, early nasal CPAP did not significantly reduce the rate of death or BPD, as compared with intubation, and the

CPAP group had a higher incidence of pneumothorace (Morley et al. 2008). In the SUPPORT study, the rates of BPD or death did not differ significantly between the CPAP group and the surfactant group (47.8% and 51.0%) after adjustment for confounding factors (Network SSGotEKSNNR et al. 2010). Follow-up studies reported improved pulmonary morbidity in the NCPAP group (Stevens et al. 2014), with no difference in neurodevelopmental outcomes (Vaucher et al. 2012).

Nasal intermittent positive pressure ventilation (NIPPV): NIPPV, both in the synchronized (SNIPPV) (Bhandari et al. 2007) and non-synchronized (Kugelman et al. 2007) modes, has been found to decrease BPD in RCT. The NIP trial did not show any difference in outcomes (Kirpalani et al. 2013), but concerns with the study design have been raised (Bhandari 2013). Combining NIPPV with a less invasive mode of surfactant administration has shown promise in a pilot RCT in decreasing the need for invasive ventilation, but no impact on BPD, after controlling for confounding factors (Oncel et al. 2015).

Nitric oxide: Inhaled nitric oxide (iNO) may or may not be beneficial in preventing BPD (Barrington and Finer 2007). Late treatment with up to five doses of surfactant in ventilated premature infants being administered iNO (TOLSURF study) did not improve survival without BPD at 36 or 40 weeks (Ballard et al. 2016). It does appear to be safe in this population, though it does not appear to impact on surfactant composition or pulmonary function. Routine use of iNO to decrease BPD in the preterm population is not recommended, pending long-term outcome data.

Patient-triggered ventilation: Studies done to date have not shown any reduction in the incidence of BPD.

Recombinant CC10: Use of an anti-inflammatory protein, recombinant human Clara cell 10-kD protein (CC10), has shown some initial promise.

Recombinant SOD: Although the antioxidant recombinant Cu-Zn superoxide dismutase (SOD) did not show any difference in outcome, infants <27 weeks of gestation that received SOD had decreased hospitalizations and emergency room visits and less frequent use of bronchodilator therapy at age 1 year, as compared to infants that did not receive it (Davis et al. 2003).

Stem cells: Intratracheal delivery of stem cells in human preterm infants is being studied to prevent BPD (Chang et al. 2014).

Synthetic surfactant: A new synthetic surfactant (lucinactant) which contains the novel peptide, sinapultide, a surfactant-associated protein B mimic, appears to be similar to animal-derived surfactant in two multicenter randomized clinical trials. A meta-analysis of the studies revealed no statistically different differences in the outcomes of death and BPD (Pfister et al. 2007).

Surfactant delivery: Use of minimally or less invasive modes of surfactant administration have shown initial promise (Dargaville et al. 2013; Kribs et al. 2015). Another attractive alternative to intubation and delivery of intratracheal surfactant would be aerosol delivery. To date, no effective aerosolized surfactant preparation is available for routine use in the clinical setting.

Thyroxine: In a RCT, postnatal supplementation of thyroxine in preterm newborns did not decrease the incidence of BPD.

Vitamin E: In a RCT, oral vitamin E supplementation did not reduce BPD in infants with BW <1,500 g.

Volume-targeted ventilation: In a meta-analysis comparing volume-targeted ventilation to pressure-limited ventilation, there was no difference in the incidence of BPD between the two groups.

More research is needed with these approaches before definite recommendations can be made.

Prevention: Among the antenatal factors, prevention of premature birth is the single most effective preventive measure for BPD. Understanding the biology of, and targeting therapies to inhibit, preterm labor safely would be an important goal. The use of progesterone in prevention of premature labor has shown promise, although the prolongation of gestation with this approach has yet to improve infant outcomes.

Antenatal steroids still remain the single most effective intervention for lung maturation and are recommended for clinical use.

The impact of antenatal steroids on BPD has been somewhat controversial with studies reporting no or some benefit; other factors may perhaps mask the benefit of antenatal steroids. Weekly courses of antenatal steroids are not recommended. Betamethasone is preferred over dexamethasone.

Considerable research has gone into understanding the role of antenatal and postnatal inflammation in the pathogenesis of BPD (Speer 2006; Ryan et al. 2008; Bhandari 2014a). Antenatal interventions to treat chorioamnionitis have not decreased BPD; postnatal interventions may be too late to be effective. In most circumstances, maintenance of target oxygen saturation ranged >85 and <95% is prudent in preterm neonates to avoid oxygen toxicity in an attempt to prevent the development of BPD, though achieving intended targets may be difficult. Restrictive fluid intake to meet physiological needs without resulting in significant dehydration showed a trend toward a lower risk for BPD (Bell and Acarregui 2008). Attempts at early extubation (Berger et al. 2014) (Jensen et al. 2015) and use of noninvasive methods of ventilation appear to show early promise in the prevention of BPD.

Given the complex nature of BPD (Fig. 1), it is unlikely that a single "magic bullet" (with the possible exception of prevention of preterm birth) will make a highly significant impact on BPD. Incremental improvements are possible by targeting multiple aspects of this condition which include early diagnosis and treatment of antenatal and postnatal sepsis, optimal maintenance of oxygenation and fluid/electrolyte status, and aggressive early parenteral/enteral nutrition, along with appropriate ventilatory strategies.

57.11 Conclusions

Focusing on aspects of basic biology (lung development, identification of biomarkers, genetics, animal models) and pharmacotherapeutic approaches (Walsh et al. 2006) has the maximum potential to make an impact on BPD. Significant improvements in the future will likely depend on our ability to identify the genetic components of BPD and to target specific and novel therapies (Bhandari 2014b).

References

Aghai ZH, Faqiri S, Saslow JG, Nakhla T, Farhath S, Kumar A et al (2008) Angiopoietin 2 concentrations in infants developing bronchopulmonary dysplasia: attenuation by dexamethasone. J Perinatol 28:149–155

Agrons A, Courtney S, Stocker J, Markowitz R (2005) From the archives of the AFIP: lung disease in premature neonates: radiologic-pathologic correlation. Radiographics 25(4):1047–1073

Ambalavanan N, Carlo WA (2006) Ventilatory strategies in the prevention and management of bronchopulmonary dysplasia. Semin Perinatol 30(4):192–199

Ambalavanan N, Mourani P (2014) Pulmonary hypertension in bronchopulmonary dysplasia. Birth Defects Res Part A Clin Mol Teratol 100(3):240–246. https://doi.org/10.1002/bdra.23241

Ambalavanan N, Novak ZE (2003) Peptide growth factors in tracheal aspirates of mechanically ventilated preterm neonates. Pediatr Res 53(2):240–244

Anderson PJ, Doyle LW (2006) Neurodevelopmental outcome of bronchopulmonary dysplasia. Semin Perinatol 30(4):227–232

Baier RJ, Majid A, Parupia H, Loggins J, Kruger TE (2004) CC chemokine concentrations increase in respiratory distress syndrome and correlate with development of bronchopulmonary dysplasia. Pediatr Pulmonol 37(2):137–148

Balany J, Bhandari V (2015) Understanding the impact of infection, inflammation, and their persistence in the pathogenesis of bronchopulmonary dysplasia. Front Med (Lausanne) 2:90. https://doi.org/10.3389/fmed.2015.00090

Ballard RA, Keller RL, Black DM, Ballard PL, Merrill JD, Eichenwald EC et al (2016) Randomized trial of late surfactant treatment in ventilated preterm infants receiving inhaled nitric oxide. J Pediatr 168:23–29. https://doi.org/10.1016/j.jpeds.2015.09.031, e4

Baraldi E, Filippone M (2007) Chronic lung disease after premature birth. N Engl J Med 357(19):1946–1955

Barrington KJ, Finer NN (2007) Inhaled nitric oxide for preterm infants: a systematic review. Pediatrics 120(5):1088–1099

Bassler D, Plavka R, Shinwell ES, Hallman M, Jarreau PH, Carnielli V et al (2015) Early inhaled budesonide for the prevention of bronchopulmonary dysplasia. N Engl J Med 373(16):1497–1506. https://doi.org/10.1056/NEJMoa1501917

Baveja R, Christou H (2006) Pharmacological strategies in the prevention and management of bronchopulmonary dysplasia. Semin Perinatol 30(4):209–218

Bell EF, Acarregui MJ (2008) Restricted versus liberal water intake for preventing morbidity and mortality in

preterm infants. Cochrane Database Syst Rev 1, CD000503

Berger J, Mehta P, Bucholz E, Dziura J, Bhandari V (2014) Impact of early extubation and reintubation on the incidence of bronchopulmonary dysplasia in neonates. Am J Perinatol 31(12):1063–1072. https://doi.org/10.1055/s-0034-1371702

Bhandari V (2006) Non-invasive ventilation of the sick neonate: evidence-based recommendations. J Neonatol 20(3):214–221

Bhandari V (2012) Genetic influences in lung development and injury. In: Bancalari E (ed) The newborn lung: questions and controversies, 2nd edn. Neonatology: questions and controversies. Saunders, Philadelphia, pp 29–55

Bhandari V (2013) The potential of non-invasive ventilation to decrease BPD. Semin Perinatol 37(2):108–114. https://doi.org/10.1053/j.semperi.2013.01.007

Bhandari V (2014a) Postnatal inflammation in the pathogenesis of bronchopulmonary dysplasia. Birth Defects Res Part A Clin Mol Teratol 100(3):189–201. https://doi.org/10.1002/bdra.23220

Bhandari V (2014b) Drug therapy trials for the prevention of bronchopulmonary dysplasia: current and future targets. Front Pediatr 2:76. https://doi.org/10.3389/fped.2014.00076

Bhandari A, Bhandari V (2003) Pathogenesis, pathology and pathophysiology of pulmonary sequelae of bronchopulmonary dysplasia in premature infants. Front Biosci 8:e370–e380

Bhandari A, Bhandari V (2007) Bronchopulmonary dysplasia: an update. Indian J Pediatr 74(1):73–77

Bhandari A, Bhandari V (2009) Pitfalls, problems and progress in bronchopulmonary dysplasia. Pediatrics 123:1562–1573

Bhandari A, Bhandari V (2011) "New" bronchopulmonary dysplasia: a clinical review. Clin Pulm Med 18(3):137–143

Bhandari A, Bhandari V (2013) Biomarkers in bronchopulmonary dysplasia. Paediatr Respir Rev 14 (3):173–179. https://doi.org/10.1016/j.prrv.2013.02.008

Bhandari V, Elias JA (2006) Cytokines in tolerance to hyperoxia-induced injury in the developing and adult lung. Free Radic Biol Med 41(1):4–18

Bhandari V, Gruen JR (2006) The genetics of bronchopulmonary dysplasia. Semin Perinatol 30(4):185–191

Bhandari A, Panitch HB (2006) Pulmonary outcomes in bronchopulmonary dysplasia. Semin Perinatol 30(4):219–226. https://doi.org/10.1053/j.semperi.2006.05.009

Bhandari V, Brodsky N, Porat R (2005) Improved outcome of extremely low birth weight infants with Tegaderm application to skin. J Perinatol 25(4):276–281

Bhandari V, Bizzarro MJ, Shetty A, Zhong X, Page GP, Zhang H et al (2006a) Familial and genetic susceptibility to major neonatal morbidities in preterm twins. Pediatrics 117(6):1901–1906

Bhandari V, Choo-Wing R, Lee CG, Zhu Z, Nedrelow JH, Chupp GL et al (2006b) Hyperoxia causes angiopoietin 2-mediated acute lung injury and necrotic cell death. Nat Med 12(11):1286–1293

Bhandari V, Gavino RG, Nedrelow JH, Pallela P, Salvador A, Ehrenkranz RA et al (2007) A randomized controlled trial of synchronized nasal intermittent positive pressure ventilation in RDS. J Perinatol 27 (11):697–703

Bhandari V, Choo-Wing R, Lee CG, Yusuf K, Nedrelow JH, Ambalavanan N et al (2008a) Developmental regulation of NO-mediated VEGF-induced effects in the lung. Am J Respir Cell Mol Biol 39(4):420–430

Bhandari A, Schramm CM, Kimble C, Pappagallo M, Hussain N (2008b) Effect of a short course of prednisolone in infants with oxygen-dependent bronchopulmonary dysplasia. Pediatrics 121(2): e344–e349

Bland RD, Xu L, Ertsey R, Rabinovitch M, Albertine KH, Wynn KA et al (2007) Dysregulation of pulmonary elastin synthesis and assembly in preterm lambs with chronic lung disease. Am J Physiol Lung Cell Mol Physiol 292(6):L1370–L1384. https://doi.org/10.1152/ajplung.00367.2006

Bokodi G, Treszl A, Kovacs L, Tulassay T, Vasarhelyi B (2007) Dysplasia: a review. Pediatr Pulmonol 42:952–961

Brundage KL, Mohsini KG, Froese AB, Fisher JT (1990) Bronchodilator response to ipratropium bromide in infants with bronchopulmonary dysplasia. Am Rev Respir Dis 142(5):1137–1142

Bry K, Whitsett JA, Lappalainen U (2007) IL-1beta disrupts postnatal lung morphogenesis in the mouse. Am J Respir Cell Mol Biol 36(1):32–42

Cederqvist K, Sorsa T, Tervahartiala T, Maisi P, Reunanen K, Lassus P et al (2001) Matrix metalloproteinases-2, -8, and -9 and TIMP-2 in tracheal aspirates from preterm infants with respiratory distress. Pediatrics 108(3):686–692

Chang YS, Ahn SY, Yoo HS, Sung SI, Choi SJ, Oh WI et al (2014) Mesenchymal stem cells for bronchopulmonary dysplasia: phase 1 dose-escalation clinical trial. J Pediatr 164(5):966–972. https://doi.org/10.1016/j.jpeds.2013.12.011, e6

Choo-Wing R, Nedrelow JH, Homer RJ, Elias JA, Bhandari V (2007) Developmental differences in the responses of IL-6 and IL-13 transgenic mice exposed to hyperoxia. Am J Physiol Lung Cell Mol Physiol 293 (1):L142–L150

Choo-Wing R, Syed MA, Harijith A, Bowen B, Pryhuber G, Janer C et al (2013) Hyperoxia and interferon-gamma-induced injury in developing lungs occur via cyclooxygenase-2 and the endoplasmic reticulum stress-dependent pathway. Am J Respir Cell Mol Biol 48(6):749–757

Clyman RI (2013) The role of patent ductus arteriosus and its treatments in the development of bronchopulmonary dysplasia. Semin Perinatol 37(2):102–107. https://doi.org/10.1053/j.semperi.2013.01.006

Coalson JJ (2006) Pathology of bronchopulmonary dysplasia. Semin Perinatol 30(4):179–184

Cullen A, Van Marter LJ, Allred EN, Moore M, Parad RB, Sunday ME (2002) Urine bombesin-like peptide elevation precedes clinical evidence of bronchopulmonary dysplasia. Am J Respir Crit Care Med 165(8):1093–1097

Cuna A, Kandasamy J, Sims B (2014) B-type natriuretic peptide and mortality in extremely low birth weight infants with pulmonary hypertension: a retrospective cohort analysis. BMC Pediatr 14:68. https://doi.org/10.1186/1471-2431-14-68

Dargaville PA, Aiyappan A, De Paoli AG, Kuschel CA, Kamlin CO, Carlin JB et al (2013) Minimally-invasive surfactant therapy in preterm infants on continuous positive airway pressure. Arch Dis Child Fetal Neonatal Ed 98(2):F122–F126. https://doi.org/10.1136/archdischild-2011-301314

Darlow BA, Graham PJ (2007) Vitamin A supplementation to prevent mortality and short and long-term morbidity in very low birthweight infants. Cochrane Database Syst Rev 4, CD000501

Davis JM, Parad RB, Michele T, Allred E, Price A, Rosenfeld W (2003) Pulmonary outcome at 1 year corrected age in premature infants treated at birth with recombinant human CuZn superoxide dismutase. Pediatrics 111(3):469–476

Doyle LW, Faber B, Callanan C, Freezer N, Ford GW, Davis NM (2006) Bronchopulmonary dysplasia in very low birth weight subjects and lung function in late adolescence. Pediatrics 118(1):108–113

Ehrenkranz RA, Walsh MC, Vohr BR, Jobe AH, Wright LL, Fanaroff AA et al (2005) Validation of the National Institutes of Health consensus definition of bronchopulmonary dysplasia. Pediatrics 116(6):1353–1360

Ekekezie II, Thibeault DW, Simon SD, Norberg M, Merrill JD, Ballard RA et al (2004) Low levels of tissue inhibitors of metalloproteinases with a high matrix metalloproteinase-9/tissue inhibitor of metalloproteinase-1 ratio are present in tracheal aspirate fluids of infants who develop chronic lung disease. Pediatrics 113(6):1709–1714

Ericson JE, Laughon MM (2015) Chorioamnionitis: implications for the neonate. Clin Perinatol 42(1):155–165. https://doi.org/10.1016/j.clp.2014.10.011, ix

Fabiano A, Gavilanes AW, Zimmermann LJ, Kramer BW, Paolillo P, Livolti G et al (2015) The development of lung biochemical monitoring can play a key role in the early prediction of bronchopulmonary dysplasia. Acta Paediatr. https://doi.org/10.1111/apa.13233

Frank L (2003) Protective effect of keratinocyte growth factor against lung abnormalities associated with hyperoxia in prematurely born rats. Biol Neonate 83(4):263–272

Greenough A (2007) How has research in the past 5 years changed my clinical practice. Arch Dis Child Fetal Neonatal Ed 92(5):F404–F407

Halliday HL, Ehrenkranz RA, Doyle LW (2003a) Delayed (>3 weeks) postnatal corticosteroids for chronic lung disease in preterm infants. Cochrane Database Syst Rev 1, CD001145

Halliday HL, Ehrenkranz RA, Doyle LW (2003b) Moderately early (7–14 days) postnatal corticosteroids for preventing chronic lung disease in preterm infants. Cochrane Database Syst Rev 1, CD001144

Halliday HL, Ehrenkranz RA, Doyle LW (2003c) Early postnatal (<96 hours) corticosteroids for preventing chronic lung disease in preterm infants. Cochrane Database Syst Rev 1, CD001146

Harijith A, Choo-Wing R, Cataltepe S, Yasumatsu R, Aghai ZH, Janer J et al (2011) A role for matrix metalloproteinase 9 in IFNgamma-mediated injury in developing lungs: relevance to bronchopulmonary dysplasia. Am J Respir Cell Mol Biol 44(5):621–630

Henderson-Smart DJ, Davis PG (2003) Prophylactic methylxanthines for extubation in preterm infants. Cochrane Database Syst Rev 1, CD000139

Hirakawa H, Pierce RA, Bingol-Karakoc G, Karaaslan C, Weng M, Shi GP et al (2007) Cathepsin S deficiency confers protection from neonatal hyperoxia-induced lung injury. Am J Respir Crit Care Med 176(8):778–785

Hofhuis W, Huysman MW, van der Wiel EC, Holland WP, Hop WC, Brinkhorst G et al (2002) Worsening of V'maxFRC in infants with chronic lung disease in the first year of life: a more favorable outcome after high-frequency oscillation ventilation. Am J Respir Crit Care Med 166(12 Pt 1):1539–1543

Howlett A, Ohlsson A (2003) Inositol for respiratory distress syndrome in preterm infants. Cochrane Database Syst Rev 4, CD000366

Hyodynmaa E, Korhonen P, Ahonen S, Luukkaala T, Tammela O (2012) Frequency and clinical correlates of radiographic patterns of bronchopulmonary dysplasia in very low birth weight infants by term age. Eur J Pediatr 171(1):95–102. https://doi.org/10.1007/s00431-011-1486-6

Jeng SF, Hsu CH, Tsao PN, Chou HC, Lee WT, Kao HA et al (2008) Bronchopulmonary dysplasia predicts adverse developmental and clinical outcomes in very-low-birthweight infants. Dev Med Child Neurol 50(1):51–57

Jensen EA, Schmidt B (2014) Epidemiology of bronchopulmonary dysplasia. Birth Defects Res Part A Clin Mol Teratol 100(3):145–157. https://doi.org/10.1002/bdra.23235

Jensen EA, DeMauro SB, Kornhauser M, Aghai ZH, Greenspan JS, Dysart KC (2015) Effects of multiple ventilation courses and duration of mechanical ventilation on respiratory outcomes in extremely low-birth-weight infants. JAMA Pediatr 169(11):1011–1017. https://doi.org/10.1001/jamapediatrics.2015.2401

Kamlin CO, Davis PG (2004) Long versus short inspiratory times in neonates receiving mechanical ventilation. Cochrane Database Syst Rev 4, CD004503

Keszler M, Sant'Anna G (2015) Mechanical ventilation and bronchopulmonary dysplasia. Clin Perinatol 42 (4):781–796. https://doi.org/10.1016/j.clp.2015.08.006

Kevill K, Bhandari V, Kettuman M, Leng L, Fan J, Mizue Y et al (2008) A role for macrophage migration

inhibitory factor in the neonatal respiratory distress syndrome. J Immunol 180(1):601–608

Khemani E, McElhinney DB, Rhein L, Andrade O, Lacro RV, Thomas KC et al (2007) Pulmonary artery hypertension in formerly premature infants with bronchopulmonary dysplasia: clinical features and outcomes in the surfactant era. Pediatrics 120(6):1260–1269

Kirpalani H, Millar D, Lemyre B, Yoder BA, Chiu A, Roberts RS et al (2013) A trial comparing noninvasive ventilation strategies in preterm infants. N Engl J Med 369(7):611–620. https://doi.org/10.1056/NEJMoa1214533

Kribs A, Roll C, Gopel W, Wieg C, Groneck P, Laux R et al (2015) Nonintubated surfactant application vs conventional therapy in extremely preterm infants: a randomized clinical trial. JAMA Pediatr 169(8):723–730. https://doi.org/10.1001/jamapediatrics.2015.0504

Kugelman A, Feferkorn I, Riskin A, Chistyakov I, Kaufman B, Bader D (2007) Nasal intermittent mandatory ventilation versus nasal continuous positive airway pressure for respiratory distress syndrome: a randomized, controlled, prospective study. J Pediatr 150(5):521–526

Lai NM, Rajadurai SV, Tan KH (2006) Increased energy intake for preterm infants with (or developing) bronchopulmonary dysplasia/chronic lung disease. Cochrane Database Syst Rev 3, CD005093

Lakshminrusimha S, Manja V, Mathew B, Suresh GK (2015) Oxygen targeting in preterm infants: a physiological interpretation. J Perinatol 35(1):8–15. https://doi.org/10.1038/jp.2014.199

Lal CV, Ambalavanan N (2015) Biomarkers, early diagnosis, and clinical predictors of bronchopulmonary dysplasia. Clin Perinatol 42(4):739–754. https://doi.org/10.1016/j.clp.2015.08.004

Landry JS, Tremblay GM, Li PZ, Wong C, Benedetti A, Taivassalo T (2016) Lung function and bronchial hyperresponsiveness in adults born prematurely. A cohort study. Ann Am Thorac Soc 13(1):17–24. https://doi.org/10.1513/AnnalsATS.201508-553OC

Lavoie PM, Pham C, Jang KL (2008) Heritability of bronchopulmonary dysplasia, defined according to the consensus statement of the national institutes of health. Pediatrics 122(3):479–485

Lodha A, Sauve R, Bhandari V, Tang S, Christianson H, Bhandari A et al (2014) Need for supplemental oxygen at discharge in infants with bronchopulmonary dysplasia is not associated with worse neurodevelopmental outcomes at 3 years corrected age. PLoS One 9(3), e90843. https://doi.org/10.1371/journal.pone.0090843

Manja V, Lakshminrusimha S, Cook DJ (2015) Oxygen saturation target range for extremely preterm infants: a systematic review and meta-analysis. JAMA Pediatr 169(4):332–340. https://doi.org/10.1001/jamapediatrics.2014.3307

Mello RR, Silva KS, Costa AM, Ramos JR (2015) Longitudinal assessment of the lung mechanics of very low birth weight preterm infants with and without bronchopulmonary dysplasia. Sao Paulo Med J 133(5):401–407. https://doi.org/10.1590/1516-3180.2014.00101812

Miller JD, Carlo WA (2007) Safety and effectiveness of permissive hypercapnia in the preterm infant. Curr Opin Pediatr 19(2):142–144

Montgomery AM, Bazzy-Asaad A, Asnes JD, Bizzarro MJ, Ehrenkranz RA, Weismann CG (2016) Biochemical screening for pulmonary hypertension in preterm infants with bronchopulmonary dysplasia. Neonatology 109(3):190–194. https://doi.org/10.1159/000442043

Morley CJ, Davis PG, Doyle LW, Brion LP, Hascoet JM, Carlin JB (2008) Nasal CPAP or intubation at birth for very preterm infants. N Engl J Med 358(7):700–708

Mourani PM, Abman SH (2015) Pulmonary hypertension and vascular abnormalities in bronchopulmonary dysplasia. Clin Perinatol 42(4):839–855. https://doi.org/10.1016/j.clp.2015.08.010

Network SSGotEKSNNR, Finer NN, Carlo WA, Walsh MC, Rich W, Gantz MG et al (2010) Early CPAP versus surfactant in extremely preterm infants. N Engl J Med 362(21):1970–1979. https://doi.org/10.1056/NEJMoa0911783

Ng GY, da S, Ohlsson A (2001) Bronchodilators for the prevention and treatment of chronic lung disease in preterm infants. Cochrane Database Syst Rev 3, CD003214

Niu JO, Munshi U, Siddiq M, Parton LA (1998) Early increase in endothelin-1 in tracheal aspirates of preterm infants: correlation with bronchopulmonary dysplasia. J Pediatr 132:965–970

Oh W, Poindexter BB, Perritt R, Lemons JA, Bauer CR, Ehrenkranz RA et al (2005) Association between fluid intake and weight loss during the first ten days of life and risk of bronchopulmonary dysplasia in extremely low birth weight infants. J Pediatr 147(6):786–790

Oncel MY, Arayici S, Uras N, Alyamac-Dizdar E, Sari FN, Karahan S et al (2015) Nasal continuous positive airway pressure versus nasal intermittent positive-pressure ventilation within the minimally invasive surfactant therapy approach in preterm infants: a randomised controlled trial. Arch Dis Child Fetal Neonatal Ed. https://doi.org/10.1136/archdischild-2015-308204

Padela S, Cabacungan J, Shek S, Belcastro R, Yi M, Jankov RP et al (2005) Hepatocyte growth factor is required for alveologenesis in the neonatal rat. Am J Respir Crit Care Med 172(7):907–914

Pfister RH, Soll RF, Wiswell T (2007) Protein containing synthetic surfactant versus animal derived surfactant extract for the prevention and treatment of respiratory distress syndrome. Cochrane Database Syst Rev 4, CD006069

Piersigilli F, Bhandari V (2016) Biomarkers in neonatology: the new "omics" of bronchopulmonary dysplasia. J Matern Fetal Neonatal Med 29:1758–1764. https://doi.org/10.3109/14767058.2015.1061495

Plakkal N, Soraisham AS, Trevenen C, Freiheit EA, Sauve R (2013) Histological chorioamnionitis and bronchopulmonary dysplasia: a retrospective cohort

study. J Perinatol 33(6):441–445. https://doi.org/10.1038/jp.2012.154

Poindexter BB, Feng R, Schmidt B, Aschner JL, Ballard RA, Hamvas A et al (2015) Comparisons and limitations of current definitions of bronchopulmonary dysplasia for the prematurity and respiratory outcomes program. Ann Am Thorac Soc 12(12):1822–1830. https://doi.org/10.1513/AnnalsATS.201504-218OC

Prosnitz A, Gruen JR, Bhandari V (2013) The genetics of disorders affecting the premature newborn. In: Rimoin DL, Connor JM, Pyeritz RE, Korf BR (eds) Emery and Rimoin's principles and practice of medical genetics, 6th edn. Elsevier, Philadelphia, pp 1–22

Rehan V, Torday J (2006) Lower parathyroid hormone related protein content of tracheal aspirates in very low birth weight infants who develop bronchopulmonary dysplasia. Pediatr Res 60(2):216–220

Ryan RM, Ahmed Q, Lakshminrusimha S (2008) Inflammatory mediators in the immunobiology of bronchopulmonary dysplasia. Clin Rev Allergy Immunol 34(2):174–190

Saarenpaa HK, Tikanmaki M, Sipola-Leppanen M, Hovi P, Wehkalampi K, Siltanen M et al (2015) Lung function in very low birth weight adults. Pediatrics 136(4):642–650. https://doi.org/10.1542/peds.2014-2651

Samiee-Zafarghandy S, Saugstad OD, Fusch C (2015) Do we have an answer when it comes to providing extremely preterm infants with optimal target oxygen saturation? Acta Paediatr 104(3):e130–e133. https://doi.org/10.1111/apa.12840

Sanchez-Solis M, Perez-Fernandez V, Bosch-Gimenez V, Quesada JJ, Garcia-Marcos L (2016) Lung function gain in preterm infants with and without bronchopulmonary dysplasia. Pediatr Pulmonol. https://doi.org/10.1002/ppul.23393

Schena F, Francescato G, Cappelleri A, Picciolli I, Mayer A, Mosca F et al (2015) Association between hemodynamically significant patent ductus arteriosus and bronchopulmonary dysplasia. J Pediatr 166(6):1488–1492. https://doi.org/10.1016/j.jpeds.2015.03.012

Schmidt B, Roberts RS, Davis P, Doyle LW, Barrington KJ, Ohlsson A et al (2006) Caffeine therapy for apnea of prematurity. N Engl J Med 354(20):2112–2121

Short EJ, Kirchner HL, Asaad GR, Fulton SE, Lewis BA, Klein N et al (2007) Developmental sequelae in preterm infants having a diagnosis of bronchopulmonary dysplasia: analysis using a severity-based classification system. Arch Pediatr Adolesc Med 161(11):1082–1087

Smith VC, Zupancic JA, McCormick MC, Croen LA, Greene J, Escobar GJ et al (2005) Trends in severe bronchopulmonary dysplasia rates between 1994 and 2002. J Pediatr 146(4):469–473. https://doi.org/10.1016/j.jpeds.2004.12.023

Sohn MH, Kang MJ, Matsuura H, Bhandari V, Chen NY, Lee CG et al (2010) The chitinase-like proteins breast regression protein-39 and YKL-40 regulate hyperoxia-induced acute lung injury. Am J Respir Crit Care Med 182(7):918–928

Speer CP (2006) Inflammation and bronchopulmonary dysplasia: a continuing story. Semin Fetal Neonatal Med 11(5):354–362

Stevens TP, Harrington EW, Blennow M, Soll RF (2007) Early surfactant administration with brief ventilation vs. selective surfactant and continued mechanical ventilation for preterm infants with or at risk for respiratory distress syndrome. Cochrane Database Syst Rev 4, CD003063

Stevens TP, Finer NN, Carlo WA, Szilagyi PG, Phelps DL, Walsh MC et al (2014) Respiratory outcomes of the surfactant positive pressure and oximetry randomized trial (SUPPORT). J Pediatr 165(2):240–249. https://doi.org/10.1016/j.jpeds.2014.02.054, e4

Subramaniam M, Bausch C, Twomey A, Andreeva S, Yoder BA, Chang L et al (2007) Bombesin-like peptides modulate alveolarization and angiogenesis in bronchopulmonary dysplasia. Am J Respir Crit Care Med 176(9):902–912. https://doi.org/10.1164/rccm.200611-1734OC

Thebaud B, Abman S (2007) Bronchopulmonary dysplasia- where have all the vessels gone? Role of angiogenic growth factors in chronic lung disease. Am J Respir Crit Care Med 175:978–985

Thebaud B, Ladha F, Michelakis ED, Sawicka M, Thurston G, Eaton F et al (2005) Vascular endothelial growth factor gene therapy increases survival, promotes lung angiogenesis, and prevents alveolar damage in hyperoxia-induced lung injury: evidence that angiogenesis participates in alveolarization. Circulation 112(16):2477–2486

Thomas W, Speer CP (2014) Chorioamnionitis is essential in the evolution of bronchopulmonary dysplasia – the case in favour. Paediatr Respir Rev 15(1):49–52. https://doi.org/10.1016/j.prrv.2013.09.004

Thomson A, Bhandari V (2008) Pulmonary biomarkers of bronchopulmonary dysplasia. Biomark Insights 3:361–373

Trembath A, Laughon MM (2012) Predictors of bronchopulmonary dysplasia. Clin Perinatol 39(3):585–601. https://doi.org/10.1016/j.clp.2012.06.014

Tyson JE, Wright LL, Oh W, Kennedy KA, Mele L, Ehrenkranz RA et al (1999) Vitamin A supplementation for extremely-low-birth-weight infants. National Institute of Child Health and Human Development Neonatal Research Network. N Engl J Med 340(25):1962–1968

Van Marter LJ, Dammann O, Allred EN, Leviton A, Pagano M, Moore M et al (2002) Chorioamnionitis, mechanical ventilation, and postnatal sepsis as modulators of chronic lung disease in preterm infants. J Pediatr 140(2):171–176

Vaucher YE, Peralta-Carcelen M, Finer NN, Carlo WA, Gantz MG, Walsh MC et al (2012) Neurodevelopmental outcomes in the early CPAP and pulse oximetry trial. N Engl J Med 367(26):2495–2504. https://doi.org/10.1056/NEJMoa1208506

Vento G, Capoluongo E, Matassa PG, Concolino P, Vendettuoli V, Vaccarella C et al (2006) Serum levels

of seven cytokines in premature, ventilated newborns, correlation with old and new forms of bronchopulmonary dysplasia. Intensive Care Med 32:723–730

Vicencio AG, Lee CG, Cho SJ, Eickelberg O, Chuu Y, Haddad GG et al (2004) Conditional overexpression of bioactive transforming growth factor-beta1 in neonatal mouse lung: a new model for bronchopulmonary dysplasia? Am J Respir Cell Mol Biol 31(6):650–656

Vozzelli MA, Mason SN, Whorton MH, Auten RL Jr (2004) Antimacrophage chemokine treatment prevents neutrophil and macrophage influx in hyperoxia-exposed newborn rat lung. Am J Physiol Lung Cell Mol Physiol 286(3):L488–L493

Walkup LL, Woods JC (2015) Newer imaging techniques for bronchopulmonary dysplasia. Clin Perinatol 42 (4):871–887. https://doi.org/10.1016/j.clp.2015.08.012

Walsh MC, Yao Q, Gettner P, Hale E, Collins M, Hensman A et al (2004) Impact of a physiologic definition on bronchopulmonary dysplasia rates. Pediatrics 114 (5):1305–1311

Walsh MC, Szefler S, Davis J, Allen M, Van Marter L, Abman S et al (2006) Summary proceedings from the bronchopulmonary dysplasia group. Pediatrics 117 (3 Pt 2):S52–S56

Watterberg KL, Gerdes JS, Cole CH, Aucott SW, Thilo EH, Mammel MC et al (2004) Prophylaxis of early adrenal insufficiency to prevent bronchopulmonary dysplasia: a multicenter trial. Pediatrics 114 (6):1649–1657

Yeh TF, Chen CM, Wu SY, Husan Z, Li TC, Hsieh WS et al (2016) Intratracheal administration of budesonide/surfactant to prevent bronchopulmonary dysplasia. Am J Respir Crit Care Med 193(1):86–95. https://doi.org/10.1164/rccm.201505-0861OC

Yost CC, Soll RF (2000) Early versus delayed selective surfactant treatment for neonatal respiratory distress syndrome. Cochrane Database Syst Rev 2, CD001456

58 Lung Ultrasound in Neonatal Diagnostic

Francesco Raimondi, Fiorella Migliaro, and Letizia Capasso

Contents

Abstract

Neonatal respiratory disease is currently diagnosed on the basis of clinical signs and chest radiographs. It has been estimated that the average extremely low birth weight infant will have 31 radiographs taken from birth to NICU discharge (Wilson-Costello et al., Pediatrics 97(3):369–374, 1996). The relevance of this radiation exposure is still debated. Moreover, the interpretation of a chest radiograph has a significant interobserver variability. Ultrasound imaging of the lung has been traditionally neglected because the high acoustic impedance of its air content prevents a clear image of the organ. The pleura is the only lung structure clearly visible with ultrasounds appearing as a homogeneous, hyperechogenic line moving synchronous with respiration.

Adult emergency physicians have shown that the interpretation at the patient bedside of these findings together with some reproducible artifacts (see below) can be very useful in critical situations where echography outperforms conventional radiology (Lichtenstein, Ann Intensive Care 4(1):1, 2014; Lichtenstein, Chest 147(6):1659–1670, 2015).

It has to be remarked that the use of artifacts (i.e., images that do not correspond to any anatomical structure) has raised a lot of concern in the scientific community. Strict methodology and close correlation with clinical data have to be used when investigating with or practicing lung ultrasound.

On this line of thought, international, evidence-based recommendations have been published with age-related comments (Volpicelli et al., Intensive Care Med 38(4):577–591, 2012). Neonatologists have learned the lesson and are now applying point-of-care lung

F. Raimondi (✉) · F. Migliaro · L. Capasso
Division of Neonatology, Department of Translational Medical Sciences, Università "Federico II" di Napoli, Naples, Italy
e-mail: raimondi@unina.it

G. Buonocore et al. (eds.), *Neonatology*,
https://doi.org/10.1007/978-3-319-29489-6_206

ultrasound to their practice (Rodríguez-Fanjul et al., Ann Pediatr (Barc), 2015; Yousef, Arch Pediatr. https://doi.org/10.1016/j.arcped.2015.12.001, 2016; Raimondi et al., Neoreviews 15(1):e2–e6, 2014). This chapter is a concise summary of their work.

58.1 Salient Points

- Ultrasound exam of the lung describes real anatomic structures (e.g., the pleura) and artifacts in the lung parenchyma.
- Artifacts and real images can be combined into profiles that accurately diagnose adult respiratory diseases.
- Neonatologists now use ultrasound mainly to diagnose lung consolidations and respiratory distress.
- Lung ultrasound is of valuable help in decision making in neonatal respiratory medicine.

58.2 From Artifacts to Clinical Correlates

A microconvex transducer is generally used to explore the adult chest. A linear, high-frequency probe is often preferred in neonates where it grants a wide view of the anterior, lateral, and possibly posterior fields both in the sagittal and transverse projections. Useful information can be gained in B-mode as well as in M-mode.

In the healthy infant (Fig. 1), a periodically moving line will be evident in B-mode below the superficial plans and between the rib images. This horizontal motion corresponds to the sliding of the pleural leaflets (the *sliding sign*). Inferiorly, the pleural image is reflected a number of times in straight and short repetitions also known as *A-lines*.

A different artifact is named *B-line*, a vertical hyperechoic image that recalls the tail of a comet (Fig. 2). B-lines can be seen as individual or multiple artifacts with a trend to coalesce into a *white lung image* of sicker patients (Fig. 3). In the adult, B-lines have been linked to the interstitial syndrome and may also be useful in evaluating the

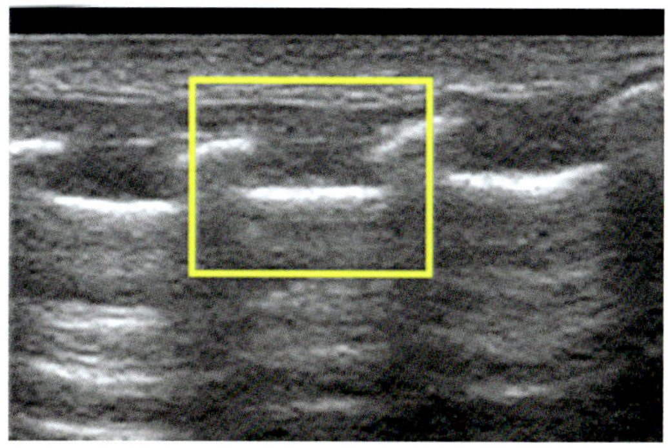

Fig. 1 Normal infant lung: the *yellow square* encircles the hyperechoic image of the pleura in between two ribs. Below the pleura, its horizontal reverberations (*white arrows*) are visible. These artifacts are known as A-lines. This image has been taken with a linear transducer

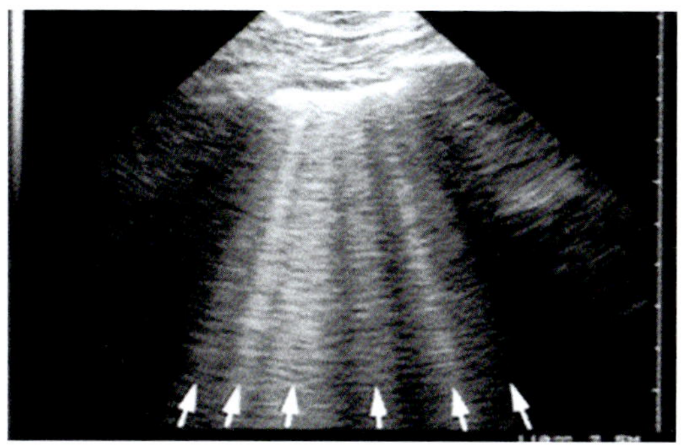

Fig. 2 B-lines: hyperechoic striae vertically departing from the pleura into the lung parenchyma (*white arrows*). This image has been taken with a microconvex transducer

patient with heart failure (Blanco and Cianciulli 2016). In the neonate, sporadic B-lines are often present after birth, especially after a C-section (Martelius et al. 2013), but a white lung image is seldom regarded as normal (see below).

Lung consolidation on ultrasonography is visualized as a subpleural echo poor or tissue-like region with blurred margins or wedge-shaped borders. Sonographic air bronchograms are hyperechoic linear elements representing air in bronchioles that appear within the hypoechoic, consolidated lung. In adults on mechanical ventilation, dynamic air bronchograms have been proven to accurately discriminate pneumonia from resorptive atelectasis (Lichtenstein et al. 2009).

The simultaneous absence of B-lines, lung sliding, and lung point is diagnostic of pneumothorax,

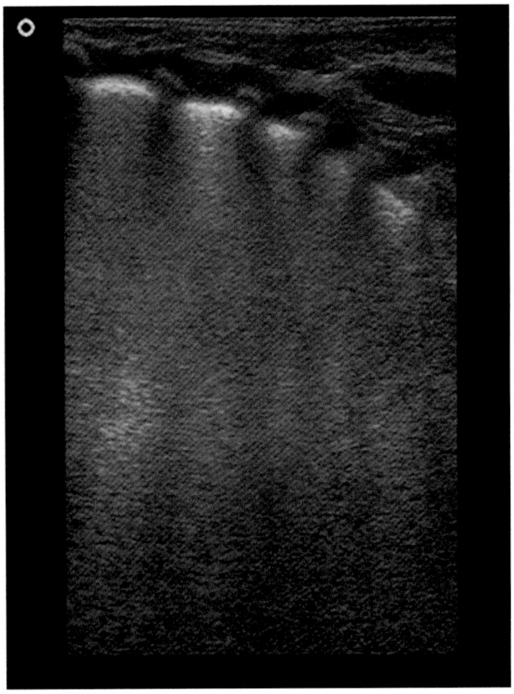

Fig. 3 White lung: thick B-lines merging in a completely *white* image with no spared areas

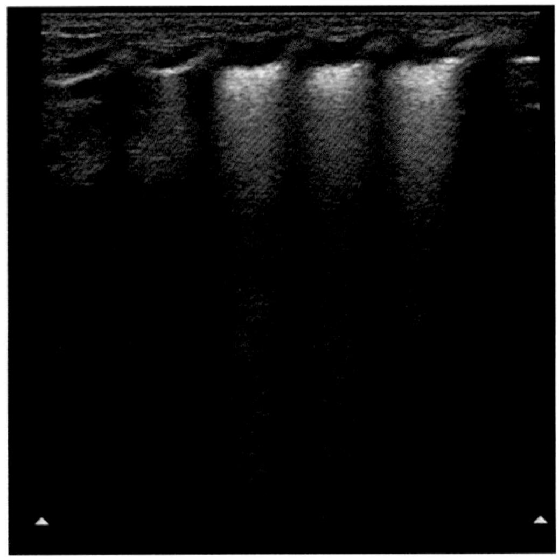

Fig. 4 The double lung point: the *white arrow* marks a sharp increase in B-lines echodensity going from the apical to the basal lung fields

even if the volume of the air leak is difficult to quantitate (Migliaro et al. 2014). Pleural effusions appear as an anechoic space between the pleural leaflets. The conventional radiograph detects as opacities images that will be differentiated as consolidations or effusion only at ultrasound scan. It is not surprising, then, that echography outperforms the radiograph in ruling in and out both pneumothorax and effusions.

58.3 "Field Validation" of Lung Ultrasound in Neonatology

Respiratory distress syndrome was initially diagnosed by Copetti et al. with the simultaneous presence of three ultrasound findings: abnormalities of the pleural line, white lung image, and absence of spared areas in all lung fields. This profile had sensitivity and specificity of 100% in their series of 55 premature infants (Copetti et al. 2008). Unfortunately, since the intratracheal administration of surfactant does not clear the picture (Cattarossi et al. 2010), chest ultrasound has limited value in the immediate follow-up of respiratory distress syndrome. The same group found that the presence of a *double lung point* (less hyperechogenic upper lung fields with thicker, brighter B-lines in dependent areas) was highly sensitive and specific of transient tachypnea of the newborn (Fig. 4) (Vergine et al. 2014).

These results have been challenged by Liu et al. in a recent unmasked, monocentric, and retrospective series of 1,358 infants; 358 neonates were classified as having RDS, while the TTN group had 228 patients (Liu et al. 2016). At ultrasound, all infants in both groups presented with an abnormal pleural line and A-line disappearance, while the double lung point had a sensitivity for TTN of only 45.6%.

These conflicting results cast a dim light on the ultrasound diagnosis of the most frequent neonatal respiratory diseases. An appropriately powered, multicenter, prospective study is warranted to settle the issue.

Irrespective of the nosologic description, lung ultrasound can be applied to neonatal medicine for important functional questions like the need of respiratory support or exogenous surfactant administration. A population of 154 unselected

term and late preterm newly born infants underwent sequential chest ultrasound scans in a well-baby nursery (Raimondi et al. 2012). The normal clearance of lung fluid was documented with progressive transition from a B-lines pattern to an A-lines one. Also, a white lung image at 2 h after birth was strictly associated with clinically significant respiratory distress and need of ventilator support. Similarly, the persistence of a white lung image after a 2 h CPAP course has been shown to be a reliable predictor of intubation and surfactant administration (Raimondi et al. 2014b). Brat et al. recently confirmed this observation building a lung hyperechogeneity score that was correlated to oxygenation status and surfactant administration (Brat et al. 2015).

58.4 Conclusions

Lung ultrasound is rapidly gaining an important role in neonatal respiratory medicine. Future research on individualized surfactant administration and other common clinical situations will make lung ultrasound a necessary tool in neonatal practice.

References

Blanco PA, Cianciulli TF (2016) Pulmonary edema assessed by ultrasound: impact in cardiology and intensive care practice. Echocardiography. https://doi.org/10.1111/echo.13182

Brat R, Yousef N, Klifa R et al (2015) Lung ultrasonography score to evaluate oxygenation and surfactant need in neonates treated with continuous positive airway pressure. JAMA Pediatr 169(8), e151797

Cattarossi L, Copetti R, Poskurica B et al (2010) Surfactant administration for neonatal respiratory distress does not improve lung interstitial fluid clearance: echographic and experimental evidence. J Perinat Med 38(5):557–563

Copetti R, Cattarossi L, Macagno F et al (2008) Lung ultrasound in respiratory distress syndrome: a useful tool for early diagnosis. Neonatology 94(1):52–59

Lichtenstein DA (2014) Lung ultrasound in the critically ill. Ann Intensive Care 4(1):1

Lichtenstein DA (2015) BLUE-protocol and FALLS-protocol: two applications of lung ultrasound in the critically ill. Chest 147(6):1659–1670

Lichtenstein D, Mezière G, Seitz J (2009) The dynamic air bronchogram. A lung ultrasound sign of alveolar consolidation ruling out atelectasis. Chest 135(6):1421–1425

Liu J, Chen XX, Li XW et al (2016) Lung ultrasonography to diagnose transient tachypnea of the newborn. Chest. https://doi.org/10.1016/j.chest.2015.12.024

Martelius L, Janér C, Süvari L et al (2013) Delayed lung liquid absorption after cesarean section at term. Neonatology 104(2):133–136

Migliaro F, Sodano A, Capasso L et al (2014) Lung ultrasound-guided emergency pneumothorax needle aspiration in a very preterm infant. BMJ Case Rep. https://doi.org/10.1136/bcr-2014-206803

Raimondi F, Migliaro F, Sodano A et al (2012) Can neonatal lung ultrasound monitor fluid clearance and predict the need of respiratory support? Crit Care 16(6):R22

Raimondi F, Cattarossi L, Copetti R (2014a) International perspectives: point-of-care chest ultrasound in the neonatal intensive care unit: an Italian perspective. NeoReviews 15(1):e2–e6

Raimondi F, Migliaro F, Sodano A et al (2014b) Use of neonatal chest ultrasound to predict noninvasive ventilation failure. Pediatrics 134(4):e1089–e1094

Rodríguez-Fanjul J, Balcells Esponera C, Moreno Hernando J et al (2015) Lung ultrasound as a tool to guide the administration of surfactant in premature neonate. Ann Pediatr (Barc). pii: S1695-4033(15) 00364-1

Vergine M, Copetti R, Brusa G et al (2014) Lung ultrasound accuracy in respiratory distress syndrome and transient tachypnea of the newborn. Neonatology 106(2):87–93

Volpicelli G, Elbarbary M, Blaivas M et al (2012) International evidence-based recommendations for point-of-care lung ultrasound. Intensive Care Med 38(4):577–591

Wilson-Costello D, Rao PS, Morrison S et al (1996) Radiation exposure from diagnostic radiographs in extremely low birth weight infants. Pediatrics 97(3):369–374

Yousef N (2016) Lung ultrasound in the newborn. Arch Pediatr. https://doi.org/10.1016/j.arcped.2015.12.001

Rare Lung Diseases of Newborns

59

Paolo Tagliabue and Elena Ciarmoli

Contents

Abstract

Rare causes of respiratory distress in the newborn, mainly in term infants, need to be considered in uncommon and atypical circumstances. Embryological, pathological, surgical, antenatal, or pediatric classifications for rare lung diseases have been reported. The following is a description of rare but not negligible pulmonary diseases causing respiratory distress with neonatal presentation.

Parenchymal diseases and cystic lung diseases are briefly dealt with in order to favor the clinical approach and the diagnostic orientation in these rare and often life-threatening conditions.

Abbreviations

ACD	Alveolar capillary dysplasia
BC	Bronchogenic cyst
BPS	Bronchopulmonary sequestration
CCAM	Congenital cystic adenomatoid malformation
CDH	Congenital diaphragmatic hernia
CLE	Congenital lobar emphysema
CPL	Congenital pulmonary lymphangiectasia

P. Tagliabue (✉) · E. Ciarmoli
Neonatologia e Terapia Intensiva Neonatale, Fondazione MBBM, ASST-Ospedale San Gerardo-Monza, Monza, Italy
e-mail: p.tagliabue@asst-monza.it; elena.ciarmoli@gmail.com

G. Buonocore et al. (eds.), *Neonatology*,
https://doi.org/10.1007/978-3-319-29489-6_207

PCD Primary ciliary dyskinesia
PPHN Persistent pulmonary hypertension of the newborn

59.1 Salient Points

- Many large lung malformations seen at the routine 20 weeks gestation scan have largely disappeared at term.
- There is even more confusion in terms of how these malformations should be described; the abnormalities are often multiple, and clinical and pathological descriptions should be kept separate.
- There are today more informations about genetic cause of these rare lung diseases.
- Advances in diagnostic imaging (including sonography, multi-detector computer tomography, magnetic resonance imaging, and angiography) have increased their detection during both antenatal and postnatal periods, and radiological characterization, which in turn influence patient counseling and management stratification.
- For some of these rare diseases, fetal surgery is possible today.

59.2 Rare Lung Disease

Rare lung diseases include a wide spectrum of conditions and are an important cause of morbidity and mortality in newborn and infants. Despite the low incidence of these lesions, neonatologists are likely to encounter these disorders through common respiratory symptoms and signs. For intensive care staff, radiologists, pathologists, and surgeons, the management and care of newborns affected by these diseases can require considerable expenditures of time and resources within a tertiary care center. Moreover, with advances in both fetal ultrasonography (US) and magnetic resonance (MR) imaging, abnormalities of the thorax are increasingly being recognized antenatally, allowing providers to (*a*) anticipate management issues at the time of delivery or later in neonatal life and (*b*) help parents comprehend the prognosis.

Numerous classifications and terminologies have been suggested for rare congenital lung malformations, attempting to incorporate a common origin and association of many of the lesions. Indeed, the most commonly encountered anomalies can be classified into three broad categories: *bronchopulmonary anomalies*, *vascular anomalies*, and *combined lung and vascular anomalies*. Moreover, chest wall deformities and solid lesions as tumor masses or thoracic manifestations of complex syndromes, including ciliopathies, must be considered (Biyyam 2010; Liechty and Flake 2008; Shanti and Klein 2008).

Although these developmental lesions usually are isolated, there are too many examples of the concurrent association of two or more in a single individual. These coexistent lesions suggest that a common pathogenetic mechanism may be involved in the development of at least some of these seemingly different lesions. According to one long-held theory, many of these lesions are due to defective foregut budding and differentiation (human lung originates as a ventral endodermal pouch from the primitive foregut (see ▶ Chap. 47, "Neonatal Lung Development and Pulmonary Malformations"). Another more recent theory of causation is that these lesions are related to airway obstruction with secondary pulmonary dysplastic changes (Langston 2003; Panicek and Heitzman 1987). It is possible that the level of airway obstruction, the completeness of the obstruction, and the timing of obstructive events may act together to produce varied patterns of malformation. Whereas there is evidence for this mechanism, the modes and timing of obstructive events and their outcomes currently are poorly understood.

For these reasons, definition and classification of these lesions are always somewhat problematic, and in reviewing the literature it is not unusual to find similar lesions called by completely different names and for the same names to be applied to very different lesions.

To address the confusing terminology used to describe many of these lesions, we have decided to classify here these heterogeneous diseases as: *Parenchymal conditions* (including bronchial ultrastructural anomalies, parenchymal molecular defects, and vascular malformations),

developmental abnormalities, and *mechanical abnormalities* (Table 1).

It is a more realistic approach as reported previously by Bush (2001). He proposed, using simple language and avoiding embryologic speculation, to describe the abnormalities actually present as well as the use of a systematic approach to search for potential multiple or associated anomalies. By reducing these lesions to their simplest components, a better understand of their etiology, natural history, associated anomalies, and treatment recommendations can be achieved.

Finally, the approach to rare lung diseases in neonates involves prenatal history, clinical features, and radiologic findings. Positive familiar history, ultrasonographic chest findings, polyhydramnios, and associated congenital anomalies are suggestive elements. The main clinical features may be: term newborn, unexpected respiratory distress, untreatable hypoxia without cyanotic heart defects, recurrent pulmonary infections, or chronic lung disease of unknown origin. The most relevant radiologic findings may present asymmetric chest imaging, dextrocardia, mediastinal shift, opacities or hypertransparencies, cystic pulmonary masses, or fluid-filled lesions (Table 2).

Table 1 Rare pulmonary causes for respiratory distress in neonates

Parenchymal conditions
Bronchial ultrastructural anomalies
Primary ciliary dyskinesia (S. Kartagener)
Parenchymal molecular defects
Congenital surfactant protein abnormalities
Surfactant protein-B gene mutations
Surfactant protein-C gene mutations
ABCA3 transporter gene mutations
Vascular malformations
Abnormalities of the arterial tree (pulmonary and systemic)
Abnormalities of the venous tree
Scimitar syndrome
Abnormalities of the connections between the pulmonary, arterial, and venous trees
Fistulae
Congenital alveolar capillary dysplasia
Abnormalities of the lymphatic tree
Congenital pulmonary lymphangiectasia
Congenital chylothorax
Developmental abnormalities
Lung underdevelopment (pulmonary agenesis/aplasia/hypoplasia)
Abnormalities of the bronchial tree (tracheal or laryngeal agenesis or stenosis)
Disorders of the bronchial walls
Congenital tracheobronchomegaly
Congenital tracheobronchomalacia
tracheo-esophageal fistula
Alveolar disorders
Congenital large hyperlucent lobe
Solid and cystic lung diseases (or congenital thoracic malformations, CTM)
Cystic adenomatoid malformation
Bronchopulmonary sequestration
Bronchogenic cyst
Other cystic lesions (Lymphatic cysts, enteric cysts, mesothelial cysts, simple parenchymal cysts, low-grade pleuropulmonary blastoma)
Abnormally placed pulmonary tissue (APPT, or "pulmonary ectopia")
Abnormal intrapleural tissue (AIPT)
Mechanical abnormalities
Rib cage anomalies
Skeletal
Muscular
Central nervous
Diaphragmatic anomalies (CDH)
Extrapleural and mediastinal masses
Isomerism

59.3 Parenchymal Conditions

59.3.1 Bronchial Ultrastructural Anomalies

59.3.1.1 Primary Ciliary Dyskinesia (PCD)

Primary ciliary dyskinesia (PCD) is a rare, autosomal recessive disorder of cilia structure, function, and biogenesis leading to chronic infections of the respiratory tract, fertility problems, and disorders of organ laterality. This genetically, functionally, and ultrastructurally heterogeneous disease affects 1:20–30,000 individuals (Noone et al. 2004). PCD was first described by Kartagener et al. in 1936. Today, *Kartagener syndrome* is a disorder characterized by a triad of bronchiectasis, dextrocardia/situs inversus, and sinusitis, with defective ciliary motility as the underlying cause but situs inversus is present in only 50% of cases of PCD (McManus

Table 2 Approach to rare lung diseases in neonates

Prenatal history
Positive familiar history
Prenatal ultrasonographic chest findings
Polyhydramnios
Associated congenital anomalies
Neonatal clinical features
Term newborn
Unexpected respiratory distress
Untreatable hypoxia without cyanotic heart defects
Recurrent pulmonary infections
Chronic lung disease of unknown origin
Radiologic findings
Asymmetric chest imaging
Dextrocardia
Mediastinal shift
Radiological opacities or hypertransparencies
Cystic pulmonary masses
Fluid-filled lesions

et al. 2003). Symptoms of PCD can occur at birth or within the first several months of life (Ferkol and Leigh 2006). Normal ciliary function is critical in the clearance of amniotic fluid from the fetal lung; more than 80% of full-term neonates with PCD have a syndrome of respiratory distress, with increased work of breathing, tachypnea, and prevalence of upper and middle lobe atelectasis on chest radiographs (Hossain et al. 2003). Most PCD patients are well immediately after birth, but develop respiratory distress at 12–24 h of life (as opposed to other causes of respiratory distress in term neonates (e.g., transient tachypnea of the newborn-TTN), which often present in the first few hours after birth). An upper and middle lobar collapse in PCD patient was reported. One possibility is that PCD is an airway disease with preferential gas trapping and hyperinflation in the lower lobes leading to atelectasis/compression in the upper lobes. An alternative explanation for collapse in the upper/middle lobes could be related to positioning. Because neonates spend the majority of their time supine, it could be that impaired mucociliary clearance leads to mucous build up and lobar collapse preferentially in the dependent lobes (Mullowney et al. 2014). A small proportion of PCD patients are discharged home on day 1 of life but are then hospitalized with respiratory distress within the first few weeks of life. Often misdiagnosed with TTN or pneumonia, PCD infants frequently require supplemental oxygen for days to weeks.

A spectrum of organ laterality defects occur with PCD, including situs inversus totalis and situs ambiguus.

The respiratory microbiology in PCD generally mirrors that of cystic fibrosis (CF); however, in PCD colonization with *Pseudomonas aeruginosa* generally occurs later, and the incidence of *Streptococcus pneumoniae* is much higher. Newborns with airway colonization with *Haemophilus influenzae*, *Staphylococcus aureus*, and *S. pneumoniae* were recently reported (Kuehni et al. 2010).

Diagnostic Tests

As PCD can result from various defects in ciliary biogenesis, structure, function, or organization, no single test captures all PCD defects.

Several older diagnostic tests are no longer recommended for PCD evaluation, including nasal saccharin testing, ciliary beat frequency calculation, and visual assessment of ciliary motion without high speed recording devices. Each of these tests has significant limitations, which can lead to frequent false positive or false negative results, especially in uncooperative newborn and children; thus, these tests are not appropriate for PCD diagnosis.

Nasal nitric oxide (NO) measurements can accurately identify patients with PCD 98.6% of the time. NO is produced by the paranasal sinus epithelium via NO–synthase and low levels are seen in PCD, CF, acute/chronic sinusitis, and nasal polyposis. In patients with PCD, however, levels of exhaled NO are extremely low (10% of normal value) when compared with other diseases.

Once the suspicion for PCD is high, the axonemal structure of the respiratory cilia may be studied using transmission electron microscopy (TEM). Thus, until recently, the identification of ultrastructural defects on TEM was the "gold standard" for the diagnosis; however, with advances in our molecular understanding in PCD, it is known that approximately 30% of patients with genetically proven PCD have normal ciliary ultrastructure.

Today, the most effective test is light microscopy analysis of transnasal brushings for ciliary beat pattern.

Transnasal brushing or nasal scrape ciliated epithelial samples can be analyzed with high-speed digital video imaging to get quantitative measurements of the ciliary beat frequency (CBF) to help differentiate between abnormally beating cilia and normal beat patterns. Normal ciliary function excludes the diagnosis of PCD. Ciliary ultrastructure may be abnormal as a primary defect or secondary to infections.

Immunofluorescent analysis using antibodies directed against the main axonemal components has been used to identify structural abnormalities of cilia; however, like many sophisticated techniques, it is restricted to a few centers that have this technology.

Finally, genetic testing for disease-causing mutations associated with PCD is recommended as part of a panel of diagnostic PCD tests. There are currently 33 known genes associated with PCD, with new genes being discovered at a rapid pace. About 80% of the mutations are loss-of-function variants (nonsense, frame shift, or defective splice mutations), while the others are conservative missense mutations or in-frame deletions. Most mutations occur in only one patient/family ("private" mutations); a few of the mutations have been seen to recur in two or more unrelated patients. At this point, with the use of next generation sequencing, approximately 66% of patients with PCD can be identified, thus facilitating early diagnosis and treatment. This is especially helpful in the cases where ciliary ultrastructural analysis is equivocal or inadequate. Specific classes of mutations are associated with specific phenotypes. Mutations in genes that lead to loss of function of the cilia also lead to low nasal NO levels (<77 nL/min). Mutations that affect the dynein arm's ultrastructure lead to situs abnormalities, while mutations that affect the central apparatus do not (Shapiro et al. 2016).

Therapies

As there are currently no therapies available that can reverse the underlying ciliary abnormalities, the goals of therapy are to prevent exacerbations and slow down the progression of the disease. Airway clearance through daily chest physiotherapy is highly recommended in PCD. Antibiotics should be given for acute respiratory exacerbations in PCD. Inhaled corticosteroids are not routinely recommend in PCD and should be reserved for PCD patients with associated asthma or airway reactivity (Lobo et al. 2015).

Finally, PCD patients should receive recommended vaccinations per local schedules.

Prognosis

The prognosis for a child with PCD is mainly good and the outcome is very different from CF, but there is a large spectrum of disease severity. These discrepancies in severity and survival may relate at least in part to the genetic and phenotypic heterogeneity of PCD as well as the usual aspects of access to care, socioeconomic backgrounds of patients, and accompanying comorbidities. Overall, the majority of patients with PCD appear to have a near-normal life expectancy when compliant with recommended therapies. A minority of patients develop progressive severe bronchiectasis, end-stage lung disease, and early death, unless they undergo lung transplant (Jain et al. 2007).

59.3.2 Parenchymal Molecular Defects

59.3.2.1 Congenital Surfactant Protein Abnormalities

Advances in physiology, biochemistry, and molecular biology have identified the chemical composition of pulmonary surfactant as well as the genes and cellular processes involved in surfactant lipid and protein homeostasis. These studies have provided molecular and genetic tools that are useful in identifying the genetic defects underlying the pathogenesis of RDS and the genetic causes of respiratory disease in newborns, infants, and children.

Pulmonary surfactant is primarily composed of phospholipids that are enriched with phosphatidylcholine (PC) and phosphatidylglycerol (PG); these phospholipids are produced in increasing amounts in late gestation by type II epithelial

cells. Four surfactant proteins (SPs), SP-A, SP-B, SP-C, and SP-D, have been identified as critical components of alveolar surfactant, each contributing to lung homeostasis via their distinct protein structures and activities. SP-D and SP-A are members of the collectin family of host defense proteins that bind pulmonary microbial pathogens and products, including viruses, fungi, and bacteria, and serve as critical innate host defense proteins with anti-inflammatory properties. SP-B and SP-C facilitate remodeling of newly secreted surfactant membranes by promoting the incorporation and spreading of lipids as the surface film expands during inhalation (For more details see ▶ Chap. 51, "Molecular Structure of Surfactant: Biochemical Aspects in Newborns").

The identification of the genes and cellular processes involved in maturation and function of the pulmonary surfactant system, as well as in alveolar development, has provided genetic tools that are useful for diagnosing rare lung diseases presenting in newborns, infants, and children.

Pathological and genetic analyses of full-term infants with refractory respiratory failure after birth have identified the role of mutations in the genes encoding SP-B (*SFTPB*), SP-C (*SFTPC*), and ABCA3 (*ABCA3*) in the pathogenesis of respiratory failure and diffuse, chronic interstitial lung disease (ILD) in newborn infants and children (Whitsett et al. 2010).

Classification of the histopathology associated with these disorders includes neonatal or congenital PAP, infantile desquamative interstitial pneumonia (DIP), chronic pneumonitis of infancy, nonspecific interstitial pneumonia (NSIP), and usual interstitial pneumonia (UIP) (in older children and adolescents) (Flidel-Rimon and Shinwell 2005). The histopathology of these disorders often overlaps and depends on the nature of the mutations, the age of the child, and the clinical therapy provided (Table 3).

Recessive mutations in the surfactant protein-B (SP-B) and the ATP-binding cassette family member A3 (ABCA3) genes present as lethal surfactant deficiency in the newborn. Usually, these mutations were found in full-term newborn infants, presenting with cyanosis, grunting, retractions, and atelectasis. Pulmonary disease associated with these mutations is unremitting despite the use of intensive care and surfactant replacement; this contrasts with RDS that is associated with premature newborns and responds to surfactant replacement.

Other recessive mutations in ABCA3 and dominant mutations in the surfactant protein-C (SP-C) gene are associated with chronic ILD in older infants, children, and adults; infants and children with chronic ILD often present with symptoms of diffuse lung disease including tachypnea, retractions, hypoxemia, and digital clubbing.

Mutations in the genes encoding receptors for GM-CSF (*CSF2RA*, *CSF2RB*) are inherited as autosomal recessive genes and are associated with progressive dyspnea and congenital PAP.

These disorders are classified as surfactant metabolism dysfunctions, pulmonary (SMDP) types 1, 2, 3, and 4 (Whitsett et al. 2015).

Deficiency of surfactant protein B (SP-B) is the most common (Fig. 1). Infants who are deficient in SP-B may have a family history of perinatal respiratory failure in siblings because the mutations are inherited as autosomal recessive alleles. *SFTPB*-related lung disease (SMDP-1) is generally fatal in the first months of life, although some infants have been supported by lung transplantation. Surfactant replacement and other ventilatory support are not effective therapies for this disorder. Histopathological diagnoses described in SP-B deficiency are associated primarily with neonatal PAP or infantile DIP (Wert et al. 2009; Nogee et al. 2000). Whereas neonatal lethality in knockout mice indicates that SP-B is indispensable for surfactant metabolism, SP-C deficiency is not lethal. The function of SP-C is less well understood, but it is likely required for optimal function of the surface film. A lack of SP-C causes progressive lung inflammation, emphysema, and remodeling as well as marked susceptibility to infection, inflammation, and fibrosis, indicating its role in innate immune responses. Acute and chronic lung diseases are associated with mutations in *SFTPC*. *SFTPC*-related disease (SMDP-2) is typically inherited as an autosomal dominant disease with variable penetrance, although sporadic mutations also have been

Table 3 Comparison of genetic disorders affecting surfactant metabolism (Downloaded from Whitsett et al. (2015))

Gene	*SFTPB*	*SFTPC*	*ABCA3*	*CSF2RA* and *CSF2RB*
Chromosome	2p11	8p21	16p13	Xp22 and 22q12
Protein	SP-B	SP-C	ABCA3	CSF2RA and CSF2RB
Phenotype	Surfactant dysfunction 1	Surfactant dysfunction 2	Surfactant dysfunction 3	Surfactant dysfunctions 4 and 5
Inheritance	Autosomal recessive	Autosomal dominant or sporadic, with variable penetrance	Autosomal recessive	Autosomal recessive
Mechanism	Loss of function	Dominant negative or toxic gain of function	Loss of function	Loss of function
Pathogenesis	Lack of SP-B	Lack of mature SP-C; misfolded protein with ER stress	Defective phospholipid transport into LBs	Defective GM-CSF signaling
Age of onset	Neonatal	Infancy to adult	Neonatal > childhood	Childhood or neonatal > childhood > adult
Clinical syndrome	RDS	ILD > RDS	RDS > ILD	Respiratory distress and/or insufficiency; dyspnea; tachypnea
Outcome	Neonatal lethal	Highly variable	Lethal if neonatal; variable severity in childhood	Variable severity
Histopathology	PAP > DIP	Depends on age and mutation Infants: CPI > PAP or DIP Children/adults: NSIP, UIP	Depends on age and mutation Infants: PAP, DIP Children/ adolescents: NSIP, UIP	PAP
LB phenotypes	Abnormal: large MVBs with no normal LBs	Variable: normal LBs and/or ↑ in large fusing LBs	Variable: small, dense LBs > normal LBs	ND[a]

[a]*ND* not determined for type II cells; large, foamy alveolar macrophages filled with surfactant material or large vacuoles containing neutral lipids, or both, were observed with electron microscopy

Abbreviations: *ABCA3* ATP-binding cassette transporter A3, *CPI* chronic pneumonitis of infancy, *CSF2R* granulocyte-macrophage colony-stimulating factor receptor, *DIP* desquamative interstitial pneumonia, *ER* endoplasmic reticulum, *ILD* interstitial lung disease, *LB* lamellar body, *MVB* multivesicular body, *NSIP* nonspecific interstitial pneumonia, *PAP* pulmonary alveolar proteinosis, *RDS* respiratory distress syndrome, *SP/SFTP* surfactant protein, *UIP* usual interstitial pneumonia

identified. Infants with *SFTPC* mutations usually exhibit features of chronic pneumonitis of infancy (Nogee 2004; Glasser et al. 2013).

Mutations in *ABCA3* on chromosome 16 are the most common cause of hereditary respiratory failure in newborns.

Mutations have been identified throughout the *ABCA3* gene that cause abnormal processing, misrouting, or impaired lipid transport as well as secondary effects on processing SP-B and SP-C. Lung histology is consistent with congenital PAP or infantile DIP. While ABCA3 is expressed in various tissues, abnormalities are found only in the lung. Pulmonary disease associated with ABCA3 deficiency is generally fatal although a number of infants have been treated by lung transplantation.

Prenatal and postnatal diagnoses are best made by identifying mutant *ABCA3* alleles. Diseases

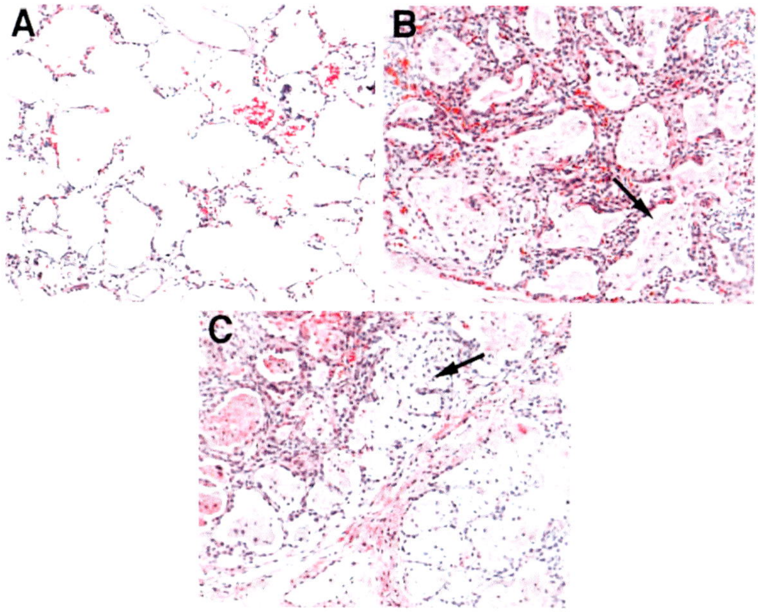

Fig. 1 Histopathology of neonatal lung. (**a**) Normal neonatal lung histology with thin alveolar septa and airspaces devoid of debris. (**b**) Histopathology of the lung from a child who had fatal SP-B deficiency demonstrates thickened alveolar septa and eosinophilic, lipoproteinaceous material intermixed with large foamy alveolar macrophages (*arrow*) filling the alveolar spaces. (**c**) Histopathology of the lung from a child who had fatal ABCA3 deficiency is similar to that for fatal SP-B deficiency, as shown in panel **b**. Original magnification is ×10 (Downloaded from Gower et al. (2008))

related to *ABCA3* and *SFTPB* are similar in onset and clinical course and are generally associated with severe respiratory failure, although several *ABCA3* mutations have been associated with chronic ILD in older infants, children, and adolescents. Histopathological findings vary depending upon the age of the patient and the mutation and often overlap with those found in deficiencies of SP-B and SP-C (Bullard et al. 2006; Shulenin et al. 2004; Doan et al. 2008).

59.3.3 Vascular Malformations

59.3.3.1 Abnormalities of the Arterial Tree (Pulmonary and Systemic)

When a lung malformation was found, it is important that also abnormal vasculature is identified or excluded.

Regarding pulmonary arterial tree, the first abnormality that is often associated with lung abnormality is the congenital origin of the left pulmonary artery from the right (pulmonary artery sling), sometimes with a cross-over arterial segment, with the right upper lobe supplied by a branch from the left pulmonary artery.

The unilateral absence of a pulmonary artery leads to the lung on that side receiving only systemic blood, either through anomalous systemic arteries or enlarged bronchial arteries.

One or both pulmonary arteries may take origin from the aorta. Bilateral origin from the aorta is part of the spectrum of common arterial trunk. Unilateral origin of a pulmonary artery from the aorta may be an isolated abnormality.

Finally, a congenitally small unilateral pulmonary artery is usually seen in association with an ipsilateral congenitally small lung (CSL). Normal pulmonary blood flow is needed for normal lung development.

Regarding systemic arterial tree, two groups of abnormalities are relevant to the lung. The first group consists of those producing a vascular ring.

The second group consists of collateral vessels which may arise from the aorta and supply all or part of one or both lungs. This last group may be seen in association with direct pulmonary arteriovenous connections (pulmonary arteriovenous malformations). Aneurysms of aortopulmonary collateral vessels were described (Chowdhury et al. 2015).

59.3.3.2 Abnormalities of the Venous Tree (Pulmonary and Systemic)

Anomalous pulmonary veins result in blood from the lungs returning to the right side of the heart.

The anomaly may be total or partial, unilateral or bilateral, and isolated or associated with other cardiopulmonary developmental defects. Anomalous pulmonary venous connections are often narrow, and this may cause relatively mild pulmonary hypertension.

Unilateral anomalous venous drainage may be part of complex lung malformations; it may also be seen in association with what appears to be a simple lung cyst.

No congenital disorders of the systemic (bronchial) venous tree have been described (Chowdhury et al. 2015).

A particular clinical problem is *Scimitar Syndrome*. Scimitar syndrome is a rare constellation, estimated to occur in two out of 100,000 births, with a 2:1 female preponderance. It consists in part of right pulmonary venous return to the inferior vena cava. In two thirds of cases, the Scimitar vein (SV) provides drainage for the entire right lung, but in one third the SV drains only the lower portion of the right lung. The developmental errors accounting for the observed anatomy in Scimitar syndrome are not understood at present. It is possible that some insult, occurring during week 11 of gestation when normally pulmonary venous drainage to the left atrium, results in the observed persistence of systemic arterial supply to the right lung from the abdominal aorta.

There are unequivocally two forms of Scimitar syndrome in terms of clinical presentation: an infantile syndrome associated with significant mortality and a child/adult presentation that is a milder form of the syndrome and in fact is frequently asymptomatic, with diagnosis being made incidentally because of radiographic abnormalities. As a rule, patients with the infantile syndrome are diagnosed in the first few months of life, the median age at presentation being 2 months. Failure to thrive, tachypnea, and heart failure are the dominant features at presentation in these severely ill patients although cyanosis may be observed if pulmonary hypertension and the anatomy at hand predispose to right-to-left shunting of blood. The elevated Qp/Qs in the infantile syndrome is often reported. Medical treatment is indicated in the infantile presentation to offset heart failure and allow growth before undertaking surgical repair. However, the presence of pulmonary hypertension or failure of response to medical therapy demands prompt surgical intervention. Mortality is quoted at 45% in infantile presentation (Gudjonsson and Brown 2006).

Abnormalities of the connections between the pulmonary, arterial, and venous trees.

59.3.3.3 Fistulae

An important group of abnormalities which potentially involves systemic and pulmonary arterial and venous trees are the various forms of pulmonary arteriovenous fistulae. They range from the diffuse and microscopic to the single or multiple large abnormalities (Chowdhury et al. 2015).

59.3.3.4 Congenital Alveolar Capillary Dysplasia (ACD)

Congenital alveolar capillary dysplasia (ACD) is a disorder of pulmonary vascular development associated with persistent pulmonary hypertension in the newborn (PPHN) and unremitting hypoxemia that is unresponsive to pulmonary vasodilators and various modes of mechanical ventilation. The incidence or prevalence of ACD is not yet known; it seems likely that some cases originally classified as idiopathic persistent pulmonary hypertension of the newborn (PPHN) may actually have been ACD. A slight male predominance (60%) has appeared in reported cases. No geographic pattern is apparent; cases have been distributed worldwide (Bishop et al. 2011).

Autosomal recessive inheritance is suspected. DNA sequencing and comparative genomic

hybridization have led to the identification of FOXF1 as one of the genes responsible for ACD and allowed for limited noninvasive diagnostic testing in some infants (Stankiewicz et al. 2009). For several reasons, these case reports almost certainly underestimate the true prevalence of ACD. The evidence is mounting to suggest that a less severe phenotype compatible with prolonged survival might exist, although definitive diagnostic criteria for this group are yet to be established.

The diagnosis of ACD is confirmed at autopsy in 90% of cases and in 10% by lung biopsy. Failure of development of alveolar capillaries leads to absence of a normal air–blood barrier. ACD is characterized by paucity of capillaries adjacent to the alveolar epithelium, anomalous distended veins, immature alveolar development, and muscularisation of the arterioles. The pathological features are diffuse in 85% and patchy in 15% of subjects (Melly et al. 2008).

The symptoms and timing of presentation are related to the distribution of capillary dysplasia and the extent of alveolar underdevelopment. More than 95% are full-term with normal transition. Respiratory distress progressing to untreatable respiratory failure is the most common presentation. The onset of symptoms is within the first hours of age in half the cases, while presentation at 2–6 weeks is reported in the 14% of cases (Boggs et al. 1994). The chest radiograph may show diffuse haziness or subtle ground-glass opacities but is often interpreted as normal. Pneumothoraces have been reported frequently in patients with fulminant disease, but it is not entirely clear whether this feature is related to abnormalities in lung architecture or surfactant function, a consequence of aggressive ventilator treatment to reverse hypoxemia, or is some combination of the two. To date, there are no reports of computed tomography or magnetic resonance lung imaging in infants with documented ACD (Cassidy et al. 2002).

There is an association with other congenital malformations in 80% of cases, the commonest being gastrointestinal (30%), cardiac (30%), and renal anomalies (23%).

The clinical approach to infants with ACD is no different than that for other neonates presenting with PPHN. However, the response to therapy is often minimal and/or not sustained, which may serve as an initial diagnostic clue. Most infants with ACD will develop progressive hypotension due to right ventricular failure and/or refractory hypoxemia. Because the hypoxemia and pulmonary hypertension cannot be effectively reversed, cardiotonic agents have only a minimal or transient effect in infants with ACD. Although transient responses to pulmonary vasodilator therapy can be observed in infants with ACD, no infant has been reported to have a sustained response to any available pulmonary vasodilator. ECMO is used at some point in the clinical course in most case series of ACD but deterioration and death followed within hours. Because none of the supportive therapies described above has changed the expected mortality due to ACD, lung transplantation is currently the only option that might prolong survival.

If here is a high index of suspicion, diagnostic lung biopsy could be considered. ACD is generally fatal (Kinugasa et al. 2002; Fliman et al. 2006).

59.3.3.5 Abnormalities of the Lymphatic Tree

Lymphatic tree disorders usually require histological confirmation. Lymphatic hypoplasia of varied distribution underlies yellow nail syndrome, in which lymphedema is accompanied by discoloration of the nails and pleural effusions.

Klippel-Trenaunay syndrome, usually characterized by varicosities of systemic veins, cutaneous hemangiomas, and soft-tissue hypertrophy, is another congenital disorder. Pleuropulmonary abnormalities are described, including pulmonary lymphatic hyperplasia, pleural effusions, pulmonary thromboembolism, and pulmonary vein varicosities (Chowdhury et al. 2015).

59.3.3.6 Congenital Pulmonary Lymphangiectasia (CPL)

A congenital malformation with presentation from fetal to early adulthood. CPL results from failure of the pulmonary interstitial connective tissue to regress, leading to dilatation of lymphatic capillaries. Radiological findings include diffuse

thickening of the peribronchovascular interstitium and the interlobular septa with pleural effusions. Supportive therapy includes albumin infusions, diuretics, thoracocentesis, and paracentesis. Nutrition plays an important role in reducing lymphatic production. Enteral nutrition with medium-chain triglycerides and total parenteral nutrition have been successfully employed. CPL often is associated with congenital and genetic diseases, including Noonan, Ullrich-Turner, Ehlers-Danlos, and Down syndromes. In rare localized disease, surgical resection is curative. When present in the newborn, the clinical course might be fatal. For the majority of patients with neonatal presentations, gradual improvement and survival are possible, particularly if there are no significant co-existing abnormalities (Bouchard et al. 2000; Pinar 2004).

59.3.3.7 Congenital Chylothorax

Congenital chylothorax may be an isolated abnormality or else associated with a congenital abnormality of the main lymphatic duct or pulmonary lymphatics. Associations with Noonan, Ullrich Turner, and Down syndrome, fetal thyrotoxicosis, H-type tracheo-esophageal fistula, and mediastinal neuroblastoma have been described; familial cases have been reported (Chowdhury et al. 2015). See also ▸ Chap. 47, "Neonatal Lung Development and Pulmonary Malformations.".

59.4 Developmental Abnormalities

Pulmonary underdevelopment has been classified into three categories: pulmonary agenesis, pulmonary aplasia, and pulmonary hypoplasia.

Pulmonary agenesis is a complete absence of the lung parenchyma, bronchus, and pulmonary vasculature.

It has been hypothesized that abnormal blood flow in the dorsal aortic arch during the 4th week of gestation (embryonic phase) is the cause. Unilateral pulmonary agenesis is difficult to diagnose with prenatal US; however, it can be suspected on the basis of mediastinal shift. More than 50% of affected fetuses have other abnormalities involving other systems.

Pulmonary aplasia is similar to agenesis, except for the presence of a short blind-ending rudimentary bronchus. Imaging findings are similar: postnatal radiography demonstrates diffuse opacification of the involved hemithorax with ipsilateral mediastinal shift (Biyyam 2010).

59.4.1 Pulmonary Hypoplasia

In this condition alveoli are reduced in number or size. Severe hypoplasia may be incompatible with extrauterine life. Lung growth before birth is dependent on blood supply, availability of space, respiratory movements, and fluid filling the airways in utero. Malformations of the rib cage, pleural effusions, thoracic masses, or intestinal loops in congenital diaphragmatic hernia (CDH) compete with the developing lung for space. Adequate amniotic fluid is essential for normal lung development and any condition that produces oligohydramnios leads to diminished lung growth. Significant and prolonged oligohydramnios can result from chronic loss of liquor after preterm premature rupture of membranes, or from inadequate production or excretion of urine because of renal and urinary tract malformations. In these conditions, airway and arterial branching is inhibited, limiting the surface for gas exchange. In the oligohydramnios sequence, the common phenotype is a flattened nose, contractures, and growth impairment of extremities, known as Potter's syndrome. The condition of prolonged preterm premature rupture of membranes is not universally lethal but depends on the degree of pulmonary hypoplasia. The following conditions increase the risk of mortality: (1) premature rupture of membranes at less than 25 weeks' gestation, (2) severe oligohydramnios (amniotic fluid index <4) for more than 2 weeks, and (3) preterm delivery earlier than 28 weeks' gestation. Serial amnioinfusions are helpful in case of oligohydramnios. Abnormalities of the thoracic cage, small, and bell shaped chest are typical radiologic findings. The lung hypoplasia is usually complicated by pulmonary hypertension therefore

high-frequency ventilation and early use of inhaled nitric oxide therapy are indicated (Biyyam 2010). See also ▶ Chap. 47, "Neonatal Lung Development and Pulmonary Malformations.".

59.4.1.1 Abnormalities of the Bronchial Tree (Tracheal or Laringeal Agenesis or Stenosis)

Absent larynx results in normal appearances from above, but intubation is impossible. The lungs are normal or hyperplastic. The commonest cause of stridor characteristically starting shortly after but not at birth is laryngomalacia, with congenital laryngeal cysts and webs entering the differential diagnosis. With total or partial absence of the trachea (*tracheal aplasia*), the main bronchi either communicates only with each other or with the esophagus. Congenital intrinsic tracheal narrowing (stenosis) may take the form of a gradual tapering or an isolated segmental narrowing or a membranous web, or it could be due to a nodule of ectopic esophageal tissue. Congenital extrinsic compression may be due to a vascular ring or pulmonary artery sling (Biyyam 2010).

59.4.1.2 Disorders of the Bronchial Walls

Bronchial wall caliber abnormalities may result in all or part of the bronchial tree being too large or too small. Congenital *tracheobronchomegaly* is associated with tracheomalacia and bronchiectasis. There are saccular bulges between cartilages. This is supported by the occasional association of Ehler-Danlos syndrome, cutis laxa, or Kenny-Caffey syndrome.

Congenital *tracheobronchomalacia* is rare, and it is caused by the presence of esophageal remnants in the wall of the trachea, which is generally seen in association with esophageal atresia and tracheo-esophageal fistula.

Congenital *bronchomalacia* may be isolated, with a generally good prognosis, and has been described in association with other congenital abnormalities, especially connective tissue disorders (Biyyam 2010).

A *tracheo-esophageal fistula* is present if the separation of those parts of the primitive foregut to become the esophagus and trachea is incomplete. Usually is associated with esophagus atresia. Histological examination of a direct connection between an otherwise normal esophagus and trachea (H-type fistula) shows that abnormalities in the wall of the trachea extend beyond the fistula; there is often widespread loss of cartilage and squamous metaplasia (For more details see ▶ Chap. 81, "Esophageal Atresia of Newborns").

59.4.1.3 Alveolar Disorders

Congenital Large Hyperlucent Lobe

Congenital large hyperlucent lobe (also know as congenital lobar overinflation (CLO) or congenital lobar emphysema (CLE)) is an example of a disorder of alveoli. CLHL is a rare anomaly of the lung development. It is defined as the postnatal overdistention of the air spaces of one or more segments or lobes of the lung that usually presents in the neonatal period with respiratory distress. This over distended portion of the lung compresses the adjacent lung lobes and compromises the ventilation. In about 50% of cases, the exact cause of CLE is not known, in the remaining 50% several mechanisms have been postulated. In some cases, it is due to partial obstruction of a lobar bronchus, leading to air-trapping. The obstruction may be caused by external compression or by intrinsic abnormalities such as mucosal taps or mucus plugs. CLHL affects the left upper lobe in about half the cases, the right middle and right upper lobes in most of the remainder, and the lower lobes in less than 10%. Curiously, the lobes almost never become infected. CLO may be associated with cardiovascular anomalies in 12 –14% of cases. Males are more frequently affected than females.

One half of the patients become symptomatic in the neonatal period, others may present months later. The presentation is with respiratory distress, which can be of varying severity. Physical examination reveals a hyper resonance in the affected area with diminished air entry on auscultation.

Chest radiography is the best diagnostic tool. Initial films may show an opaque mass on chest radiograph due to delayed clearance of lung fluid from affected lobe. The later films show a hyper

lucent overexpanded area of the lung with compression or atelectasis of the adjacent lobes of the lung, depression of the diaphragm, and mediastinal shift to the opposite side.

Most of the patients are symptomatic and require treatment. The indication for surgical treatment is life threatening, progressive, pulmonary insufficiency from compression of adjacent normal lung. Prompt resection of the involved lobe is the ideal treatment in symptomatic babies (Ankermann et al. 2004; Olutoye et al. 2000; Pariente et al. 2009).

59.4.1.4 Solid and Cystic Lung Diseases (or Congenital Thoracic Malformations, CTM)

Cystic lung lesions are the most common pulmonary lesions detected by routine antenatal ultrasound scanning. Different entities, such as congenital cystic adenomatoid malformation (CCAM), bronchopulmonary sequestrations (BPS), bronchogenic cyst (BC), and congenital lobar emphysema (CLE), may be difficult to differentiate, and antenatal MRI can provide more detail. A postnatal chest CT scan is useful in confirming the presence and extent of the lesions. Small lesions are usually asymptomatic both in utero and after birth. Large lesions may cause a mass effect resulting in esophageal compression and polyhydramnios, pulmonary hypoplasia, or vena caval obstruction with fetal hydrops. In these cases, fetal intervention may include thoracentesis or thoraco-amniotic shunting. The postnatal presentation is variable and depends on the size, location, and type of lesion. Some infants may develop PPHN and respiratory failure. If there is associated pulmonary hypoplasia or ECMO is required, the mortality rate is increased.

Congenital Cystic Adenomatoid Malformation (CCAM)

A congenital hamartomatous lesion of the lung, accounting for approximately 25% of congenital lung lesions. The incidence of CCAM is reported as between 1 in 11–35,000 live births. CCAM consists of a multicystic mass of dilated bronchiolar-like spaces that proliferate at the expense of alveoli. The cysts that enlarge following air and fluid trapping cause compression of the adjacent normal lung and mediastinum.

CCAM is categorized into four types. Type 1 is characterized by a few large cysts and is the most common (75%). In type 2, there are evenly spaced small cysts. Type 3 is very rare and appears solid on gross examination. Type 4 is characterized by acinar-type epithelium rather than the bronchiolar epithelium. Usually only one lobe is involved.

Enlarging lesions may cause progressive signs because of expansion of the cysts shortly after birth. Alternatively, abnormal signs may develop later if there are intercurrent infections. The neonatal presentation therefore ranges from respiratory failure in approximately 50% of the cases to a healthy asymptomatic infant.

Large lesions may compromise the normal development of the fetal lung, resulting in pulmonary hypoplasia or neonatal death. CCAM is a recognized cause of fetal hydrops and polyhydramnios. Infants with highly symptomatic CCAMs require surgery. Most commonly, this occurs in neonates presenting with respiratory failure of sufficient severity to require ventilatory support. When considering the timing of surgery for asymptomatic infants, some neonatologists favor operating during the neonatal period but others suggest waiting until the child is between 6 months and 2 years of age. The prognosis depends on the size of the lesion, the degree of development of the adjacent lung, and the presence of other congenital anomalies (Shanti and Klein 2008; Narendra Kumar 2008; Fitzgerald 2007; Nicolai 2009; Mendeloff 2004; Sfakianaki and Copel 2012); For more details see ► Chap. 47, "Neonatal Lung Development and Pulmonary Malformations.".

A further type of CTM is *mesenchymal cystic hamartoma* (*MCH*). The lesions may be supplied by bronchial, intercostal, or phrenic arteries. Pathological examination shows them to consist of multilocular, thin-walled cysts lined by primitive mesenchymal cells that support a ciliated cuboidal epithelium. In places, the epithelium is continuous with that lining adjacent bronchioles. The mesenchymal cells have dark oval nuclei and inconspicuous cytoplasm and show only rare mitoses. Muscular hamartomas, which are small focal proliferations of smooth muscle, are occasionally

observed incidentally in the lung, sometimes associated with similar lesions in the bowel and liver (Mark 1986).

Bronchopulmonary Sequestration (BPS)
Composed of abnormal lung tissue without connection to the normal tracheobronchial tree. There are two types of BPS based on their relationship to the pleurae, extra- and intra-lobar. Both receive an anomalous arterial supply from the systemic circulation, usually a branch of the aorta.

With extralobar BPS, the mass of pulmonary parenchyma is outside the pleurae. The lesion is found between the left lower lobe and the diaphragm in 66% of the cases. More common in males (3:1), 50% of newborns have respiratory distress because of compression of the rest of the lung parenchyma. In more than 65%, there are associated anomalies, including CDH (30%), pericardial defects, and anomalous pulmonary venous return.

Intralobar BPS is characterized by a lesion within the lobe of the lung without separate pleurae. Intralobar BPS accounts for 75% of all BPS. Usually in the lower lobe (95%), on antenatal US, BPS appears as a solid mass. The presence of hydrops or polyhydramnios is a poor prognostic factor. The majority of BPS (68%) undergo spontaneous regression before birth and survival is 95%. Early complications are usually related to the degree of associated pulmonary hypoplasia but also result from other associated anomalies. Large BPS or BPS with high systemic blood flow needs resection. Lobectomy is the treatment of choice for intralobar BPS (Liechty and Flake 2008; Shanti and Klein 2008; Mendeloff 2004). See also ► Chap. 47, "Neonatal Lung Development and Pulmonary Malformations.".

Bronchogenic Cyst (BC)
Bronchogenic cysts arise from abnormal buds from the primitive esophagus and tracheobronchial tree, which do not extend to the site were alveolar differentiation occurs.

If this separation occurs early, the system migrates into mediastinum. If it occurs late, it forms an intra pulmonary bronchogenic cyst. Bronchogenic cyst accounts for 20–30% of congenital bronchopulmonary foregut cystic malformation.

Lined with pseudostratified ciliated columnar epithelium with goblet cells and enlarged with mucous, these are considered to be infected peripheral lesions. Malignancies have been reported in these lesions. Most bronchogenic cysts are found incidentally.

Clinical presentations range from asymptomatic to recurrent nonspecific respiratory symptoms or infections to life-threatening respiratory distress. In infants, symptoms are generally caused by compression of the trachea or bronchi and esophagus, leading to wheezing, stridor, dyspnea, and dysphagia. Intraparenchymal cysts may manifest with recurrent infection. Symptomatic cysts are generally resected surgically.

Plain chest radiograph is the standard initial study. Ultrasound may show the fluid content. CT and MRI are the best confirmatory studies. Antenatal intervention is therefore rarely indicated (Shanti and Klein 2008; Mendeloff 2004).

59.4.1.5 Abnormally Placed Pulmonary Tissue (APPT, or "Pulmonary Ectopia") and Abnormal Intrapleural Tissue (AIPT)

AIPT constitutes ectopia of nonpulmonary tissues in the thorax; APPT is ectopia of lung tissue outside the thoracic cavity.

AIPT of the adrenocortical tissue, thyroid, and liver has been described in the lung, and pancreatic tissue has been noted within so-called intralobar sequestrations with gastrointestinal connections. There may be ectopic lung tissue in the neck, abdomen, or chest wall, often associated with skeletal or diaphragmatic abnormalities.

Some examples of abdominal APPT have been considered to represent extralobar sequestration.

All these are very exceptional abnormalities (Shanti and Klein 2008).

59.5 Mechanical Abnormalities

For more details about relevant abnormalities of chest wall including the diaphragm (such as CDH) see specific ► Chap. 47, "Neonatal Lung Development and Pulmonary Malformations.".

59.5.1 Isomerism

There is the usual arrangement (situs solitus) or a mirror-image arrangement (situs inversus); right isomerism; left isomerism; indeterminate; and crossover segment. Additionally, there may be absence of one lung with contralateral normal morphology. Abnormal connections may be to the esophagus, to a mediastinal cyst, or to a pulmonary parenchymal abnormality.

The term isomerism is entrenched but imprecise. Although atrial and bronchial arrangements are usually the same, they are not invariably and "Bilateral righ lung (BRL)" is a more accurate term. Nearly 80% of children with BRL (right isomerism) have associated asplenia, with a risk of overwhelming pneumococcal sepsis. A similar proportion with *bilateral left lung* (*BLL, left isomerism*) have associated polysplenia, a midline liver, malrotation of the gut, partially anomalous pulmonary venous drainage, and cardiac septal defects (Ivemark syndrome) (Chowdhury et al. 2015).

References

Ankermann T, Oppermann HC, Engler S et al (2004) Congenital masses of the lung, cystic adenomatoid malformation versus congenital lobar emphysema: prenatal diagnosis and implications for postnatal treatment. J Ultrasound Med 23:1379–84

Bishop N, Stankiewicz P, Steinhorn R (2011) Alveolar capillary dysplasia. Am J Respir Crit Care Med 184:172–179

Biyyam R (2010) Congenital lung abnormalities: embryologic features, prenatal diagnosis, and postnatal radiologic-pathologic correlation. Radiographics 30:1721–1738

Boggs S, Harris MC, Hoffman DJ, Goel R, McDonald-McGinn D, Langston C, Zackai E, Ruchelli E (1994) Misalignment of pulmonary veins with alveolar capillary dysplasia: affected siblings and variable phenotypic expression. J Pediatr 124:125–128

Bouchard S, DiLorenzo M et al (2000) Pulmonary lymphangiectasia revisited. J Pediatr Surg 35:796–800

Bullard JE, Wert SE, Nogee LM (2006) ABCA3 deficiency: neonatal respiratory failure and interstitial lung disease. Semin Perinatol 30:327–334

Bush A (2001) Congenital lung disease. A plea for clear thinking and clear nomenclature. Pediatr Pulmonol 32:328–337

Cassidy J, Smith J, Goldman A, Haynes S, Smith E, Wright C, Haworth S, Davis P, Firmin R, Kasem K et al (2002) The incidence and characteristics of neonatal irreversible lung dysplasia. J Pediatr 141:426–428

Chowdhury M et al (2015) Imaging of congenital lung malformations. Semin Pediatr Surg 24(4):168–175

Doan ML, Guillerman RP, Dishop MK, Nogee LM, Langston C et al (2008) Clinical, radiological and pathological features of ABCA3 mutations in children. Thorax 63:366–373

Ferkol T, Leigh M (2006) Primary ciliary dyskinesia and newborn respiratory distress. Semin Perinatol 30 (6):335–340

Fitzgerald DA (2007) Congenital cyst adenomatoid malformations: resect some and observe all? Paediatr Respir Rev 8:67–76

Flidel-Rimon O, Shinwell ES (2005) Respiratory distress in the term and near-term infant. NeoRevew 6:289–297

Fliman P, deRegnier R, Kinsella J, Reynolds M, Rankin L, Steinhorn RH (2006) Neonatal extracorporeal life support: impact of new therapies on survival. J Pediatr 148:595–599

Glasser SW, Senft AP, Maxfield MD, Ruetschilling TL, Baatz JE et al (2013) Genetic replacement of surfactant protein-C reduces respiratory syncytial virus induced lung injury. Respir Res 14:19

Gower WA, Wert SE, Nogee LM (2008) Inherited surfactant disorders. NeoReviews 9:e458–e467

Gudjonsson U, Brown JW (2006) Scimitar syndrome. Semin Thorac Cardiovasc Surg 9:56–62

Hossain T, Kappelman MD, Perez-Atayde AR, Young GJ, Huttner KM, Christou H (2003) Primary ciliary dyskinesia as a cause of neonatal respiratory distress: implications for the neonatologist. J Perinatol 23 (8):684–687

Jain K, Padleya SPG et al (2007) Primary ciliary dyskinesia. Clin Radiol 62:986–993

Kartagener M, Horlacher A (1936) Situs viscerum inversus and polyposisnasi in eineum Falle familiaerer Brouchiectasien. Beitr Klin Tub 87:331–333

Kinugasa H, Horigome H, Sugiura M, Saito T, Iijima T, Matsui A (2002) Intravenous prostacyclin combined with inhaled nitric oxide therapy for an infant with alveolar capillary dysplasia. Pediatr Int 44:525–527

Kuehni CE, Frischer T, Strippoli MP et al (2010) ERS Task Force on Primary Ciliary Dyskinesia in Children. Factors influencing age at diagnosis of primary ciliary dyskinesia in European children. Eur Respir J 36 (6):1248–1258

Langston C (2003) New concepts in the pathology of congenital lung malformations. Semin Pediatr Surg 12:17–37

Liechty KW, Flake AW (2008) Pulmonary vascular malformations. Semin Pediatr Surg 17:9–16

Lobo J, Zariwala M, Noone P (2015) Primary ciliary dyskinesia. Semin Respir Crit Care Med 36:169–179

Mark EJ (1986) Mesenchimal cystic hamartoma of the lung. N Engl J Med 315:1255–1259

McManus IC, Mitchison HM, Chung EM, Stubbings GF, Martin N (2003) Primary ciliary dyskinesia (Siewert's/Kartagener's syndrome): respiratory symptoms and psycho-social impact. BMC Pulm Med 3:4

Melly L, Sebire NJ et al (2008) Capillary apposition and density in the diagnosis of alveolar capillary dysplasia. Histopathology 53:450–457

Mendeloff E (2004) Sequestrations, congenital cystic adenomatoid malformations, and congenital lobar emphysema. Semin Thorac Cardiovasc Surg 16:209–214

Mullowney T et al (2014) Primary ciliary dyskinesia and neonatal respiratory distress. Pediatrics 134:1160–1166

Narendra Kumar A (2008) Perinatal management of common neonatal thoracic lesions. Indian J Pediatr 75 (9):931–937

Nicolai T (2009) Management of the upper airway and congenital cystic lung diseases in neonates. Semin Fetal Neonatal Med 14:56–60

Nogee LM (2004) Alterations in SP-B and SP-C expression in neonatal lung disease. Annu Rev Physiol 66:601–623

Nogee LM, Wert SE, Proffit SA, Hull WM, Whitsett JA (2000) Allelic heterogeneity in hereditary surfactant protein B (SP-B) deficiency. Am J Respir Crit Care Med 161:973–981

Noone PG, Leigh MW, Sannuti A et al (2004) Primary ciliary dyskinesia: diagnostic and phenotypic features. Am J Respir Crit Care Med 169(4):459–467

Olutoye OO, Coleman BG, Hubbard AM et al (2000) Prenatal diagnosis and management of congenital lobar emphysema. J Pediatr Surg 35:792–5

Panicek DM, Heitzman ER (1987) The continuum of pulmonary developmental anomalies. Radiographics 7:747–772

Pariente G, Aviram M, Landau D et al (2009) Prenatal diagnosis of congenital lobar emphysema: case report and review of the literature. J Ultrasound Med 28:1081–4

Pinar H (2004) Postmortem findings in term neonates. Semin Neonatol 9:289–302

Sfakianaki A, Copel JA (2012) Congenital cystic lesione of the lung: congenital cystic adenomatoid malformation and bronchopulmonary sequestration. Rev Obstet Gynecol 5(2):85–93

Shanti CM, Klein MD (2008) Cystic lung disease. Semin Pediatr Surg 17:2–8

Shapiro A et al (2016) Diagnosis, monitoring, and treatment of primary ciliary dyskinesia: pcd foundation consensus recommendations based on state of the art review. Pediatr Pulmonol 51:115–132

Shulenin S, Nogee LM, Annilo T, Wert SE, Whitsett JA, Dean M (2004) ABCA3 gene mutations in newborns with fatal surfactant deficiency. N Engl J Med 350:1296–1303

Stankiewicz P, Sen P, Bhatt SS, Storer M, Xia Z, Bejjani BA, Ou Z, Wiszniewska J, Driscoll DJ, Maisenbacher MK et al (2009) Genomic and genic deletions of the FOX gene cluster on 16q24.1 and inactivating mutations of FOXF1 cause alveolar capillary dysplasia and other malformations. Am J Hum Genet 84:780–791

Wert SE, Whitsett JA, Nogee LM (2009) Genetic disorders of surfactant dysfunction. Pediatr Dev Pathol 12:253–274

Whitsett JA, Wert SE, Weaver TE (2010) Alveolar surfactant homeostasis and the pathogenesis of pulmonary disease. Annu Rev Med 61:105–119

Whitsett JA et al (2015) Diseases of pulmonary surfactant homeostasis. Annu Rev Pathol 10:371–393

Persistent Pulmonary Hypertension of the Newborn

60

Jason Gien, John P. Kinsella, and Steven H. Abman

Contents

J. Gien (✉)
University of Colorado Denver, Denver, CO, USA
e-mail: Jason.Gien@ucdenver.edu

J. P. Kinsella
University of Denver, Denver, CO, USA
e-mail: john.kinsella@ucdenver.edu

S. H. Abman
University of Colorado Denver – Anschutz Medical Campus, Denver, CO, USA
e-mail: steven.abman@ucdenver.edu

G. Buonocore et al. (eds.), *Neonatology*,
https://doi.org/10.1007/978-3-319-29489-6_208

Abstract

Persistent pulmonary hypertension of the newborn (PPHN) is a clinical syndrome, characterized by failure of the pulmonary vasculature resistance to fall after birth, resulting in postnatal maintenance of a fetal circulation, which in the absence of placental gas exchange results in hypoxemia with end organ damage. Nitric oxide produced by the vascular endothelium is primarily responsible for vasodilation after birth. When delivered exogenously, inhaled nitric oxide (iNO) is the mainstay of

therapy for PPHN, with clinical studies demonstrating improved survival and decreased need for extracorporeal membrane oxygenation therapy (ECMO) with iNO treatment. However, 25–30% of cases fail to respond to iNO, most commonly in the setting of lung hypoplasia and abnormal development of the pulmonary vasculature in utero. For these infants, alternate therapies are often needed. In this chapter, we discuss the pathophysiology of PPHN, the history of PPHN therapies as they have evolved over time, mechanisms for failed responses to iNO, and the approach to PPHN that occurs in the setting of lung hypoplasia.

60.1 Salient Points

- Persistent pulmonary hypertension of the newborn (PPHN) is characterized by failure of pulmonary vasculature resistance to fall after birth, resulting in hypoxemia with end-organ damage.
- iNO is the mainstay of therapy in PPHN leading to improved survival and decreased need for extracorporeal membrane oxygenation therapy (ECMO).
- 25–30% of cases fail to respond to iNO; for these infants, alternative therapies are often needed (i.e., sildenafil, milrinone, bosentan).
- Pulmonary hypertension is a major problem in newborns with congenital diaphragmatic hernia (CDH).
- In the setting of CHD, early administration of pulmonary vasodilators plays a critical role in management of late pulmonary hypertension, with potential survival improvement.

60.2 Background

In the early 1960s, the association of respiratory distress syndrome with pulmonary hypertension and right-to-left ductal shunting was shown in the landmark studies of Rudolph et al. (1961) and the clinical observations of Stahlman (1964). Although it is now recognized that pulmonary hypertension with right-to-left veno-arterial admixture often complicates the course of newborns with diverse diseases, its recognition in term infants who were hypoxemic (but without significant lung disease) was likely first identified by Roberton et al. (1967). These authors described 13 infants born at or near-term who had marked hypoxemia but without other clinical signs of "idiopathic respiratory distress syndrome" or decreased lung compliance. They speculated that the cause of hypoxemia was right-to-left shunting, but did not specifically implicate suprasystemic levels of pulmonary vascular resistance as the cause of the hypoxemia. The first clear description of the pathophysiology of PPHN (associated with right-to-left shunting across patent fetal channels) is attributed to Gersony et al. (1969), coined the phrase "persistence of the fetal circulation" in describing two newborns with "clear lung fields" who had critical hypoxemia associated with severe pulmonary hypertension and right-to-left shunting across the oval foramen and arterial duct (Gersony et al. 1969). One infant was treated with tolazoline with only transient improvement in oxygenation. In 1970, Lees used the term "primary pulmonary hypertension" to describe this group of newborns (Lees 1970). In 1971, Siassi et al. described five infants with "persistent pulmonary vascular obstruction" associated with right-to-left shunting across the arterial duct, and in one case marked medial hypertrophy of the muscular pulmonary arteries demonstrated on autopsy (SIassi et al. 1971). This observation of a structural abnormality of the pulmonary circulation was further elucidated by Haworth and Reid in three infants who died with "persistent fetal circulation" and had extension of muscle into smaller intra-acinar arteries (Haworth and Reid 1976). The phrase "persistent pulmonary hypertension of the newborn" was first used by Levin et al. to describe a group of newborns with severe pulmonary hypertension, clear chest radiographs, and right-to-left shunting across the arterial duct demonstrated both by simultaneous temporal arterial and umbilical arterial sampling (i.e., postductal desaturation) and cardiac catheterization (Levin et al. 1976).

These initial descriptions of "PFC" focused on a discreet subset of newborns who had adequate cardiac performance without structural heart disease, absence of significant parenchymal lung disease, and suprasystemic pulmonary vascular resistance causing hypoxemia through right-to-left shunting of blood across the oval foramen and/or the arterial duct. Due to the persistence of high PVR and blood flow through these "fetal shunts," the term "persistent fetal circulation" was originally used to describe this group of patients. Although there was initial appeal to the acronym persistent fetal circulation (PFC) (Behrman 1976), this description is not quite accurate because of the absence of the placenta and onset of air breathing after delivery. It also soon became clear that "PFC" could complicate the course of other diseases of the newborn, including meconium aspiration (initially described by Stahlman (1964) and later by Fox et al. (1977), and pulmonary hypoplasia/congenital diaphragmatic hernia (Harrison and de Lorimier 1981). As a result, the term "PPHN" has been considered as a *syndrome* and over time, most authors have embraced PPHN as the proper name for this syndrome, with the classic "PFC" subtype (idiopathic PPHN) representing a relatively small percentage of the cases now commonly encountered.

Pathophysiologic mechanisms and etiologic classifications of PPHN described by Rudolph (1980) and further characterized by Geggel and Reid (1984) and Gersony (1984) provided an important framework for understanding the complex nature of this syndrome as management strategies evolved over the last two decades.

The clinical syndrome of persistent pulmonary hypertension of the newborn (PPHN) occurs in association with various neonatal diseases, including meconium aspiration syndrome, group B streptococcal sepsis, and congenital diaphragmatic hernia, as well as from undetermined causes (idiopathic). Striking differences exist between these conditions, and mechanisms that contribute to high PVR can vary between these diseases. However, these disorders are included in the syndrome of PPHN due to common pathophysiologic features, including *sustained elevation of PVR leading to hypoxemia due to right-to-left extrapulmonary shunting of blood flow across the ductus arteriosus (PDA) or foramen ovale (PFO).* In many clinical settings, hypoxemic respiratory failure in term newborns is often presumed to be associated with PPHN-type physiology; however, hypoxemic term newborns can lack echocardiographic findings of extrapulmonary shunting across the PDA or PFO. Thus, PPHN should be reserved to describe neonates in whom *extrapulmonary shunting* contributes to hypoxemia and impaired cardiopulmonary function. Recent estimates suggest an incidence for PPHN of 1.9/1000 live births, or an estimated 7400 cases/year (Walsh-Sukys et al. 2000).

Diseases associated with PPHN are often classified within one of three categories: (i) *maladaptation:* vessels are presumably of normal structural but have abnormal vasoreactivity; (ii) *excessive muscularization:* increased smooth muscle cell thickness and increased distal extension of muscle to vessels which are usually nonmuscular; and (iii) *underdevelopment:* lung hypoplasia associated with decreased pulmonary artery number. This designation is imprecise, however, and high PVR in most patients likely involves overlapping changes among these categories. For example, neonates with congenital diaphragmatic hernia (CDH) are primarily classified as having vascular "underdevelopment" due to lung hypoplasia, yet lung histology of fatal cases typically shows marked muscularization of pulmonary arteries, and clinically, these patients can respond to vasodilator therapy. Similarly, neonates with meconium aspiration often have clinical evidence of altered vasoreactivity, but excessive muscularization is often found at autopsy. As described above, autopsy studies of fatal PPHN demonstrate severe hypertensive structural remodeling even in newborns who die shortly after birth, suggesting that many cases of severe disease are associated with chronic intrauterine stress. However, the exact intrauterine events that alter pulmonary vascular reactivity and structure are poorly understood. Epidemiologic studies have demonstrated strong associations between PPHN and maternal smoking and ingestion of cold remedies that include aspirin or other nonsteroidal anti-inflammatory products

(Van Marter et al. 1996; Alano et al. 2001). Since these agents can induce partial constriction of the ductus arteriosus, it is possible that pulmonary hypertension due to antenatal ductal narrowing contributes to PPHN. Other perinatal stresses, including placenta previa and abruption, and asymmetric growth restriction, are associated with PPHN; however, most neonates who are exposed to these prenatal stresses do not develop PPHN. Circulating levels of L-arginine, the substrate for NO, are decreased in some newborns with PPHN, suggesting that impaired NO production may contribute to the pathophysiology of PPHN. It is possible that genetic factors increase susceptibility for pulmonary hypertension. A recent study reported strong links between PPHN and polymorphisms of the carbamoyl phosphate synthase gene (Pearson et al. 2001). However, the importance of this finding is uncertain, and further work is needed in this area. Studies of adults with idiopathic primary pulmonary hypertension have identified abnormalities of bone morphogenetic protein (BMP) receptor genes; whether polymorphisms of genes for the BMP or TGF-ß receptors, other critical growth factors, vasoactive substances, or other products increase the risk for some newborns to develop PPHN is unknown.

Because of the role of pulmonary hypertension in newborns with hypoxemic respiratory failure (initially severe HMD and subsequently "PFC", as described above), early approaches to management included a focus on pulmonary vasodilation using one of the few pharmacologic agents available at the time (tolazoline). Its use was first described by Cotton in 1965 in newborns with HMD (Cotton 1965) and later in infants with PPHN by Goetzman et al. (1976), Korones and Eyal (1975), and Levin et al. (1976). However, its efficacy was limited by variable responsiveness and significant complications including systemic hypotension and gastrointestinal hemorrhage (Stevenson et al. 1979).

Multiple approaches to the treatment of PPHN evolved since its first recognition as a disease marked by severe pulmonary hypertension; however, discovery of the elusive "selective pulmonary vasodilator" would markedly change our understanding and clinical management of this syndrome. Indeed, the most striking change in the management of PPHN in the last decade evolved from improved understanding of the role of endogenous NO production and exogenous NO delivery on pulmonary vasoregulation. Because the successful transition from fetal placental dependence to survival at birth requires that PVR rapidly declines and pulmonary blood flow increases, the role of NO in the transitional circulation has been intensively investigated to understand its relationship to the pathophysiology and treatment of PPHN.

NO was recognized as a potent vasodilator as early as 1979 (Furchgott and Zawadzki 1980), and in 1980, Furchgott and Zawadzki reported that acetylcholine-induced vasorelaxation was dependent on an intact endothelium through the elaboration of an endothelial-derived relaxing factor (EDRF) that diffused to the subjacent vascular smooth muscle. In 1987 investigators from two separate laboratories reported that the biologic activity of EDRF was identical to NO or an NO-containing substance. Palmer et al. (1987) induced the release of EDRF from porcine aortic endothelial cells in culture and compared the effects on superfused aortic strips with that of NO in solution. They found that the effects of EDRF were indistinguishable from those of NO. Ignarro et al. (1987) used a bioassay cascade superfusion technique with intrapulmonary arteries and veins, identified EDRF pharmacologically and chemically as NO, and found that EDRF and NO produced similar vasorelaxation and were inhibited by common antagonists. Ignarro et al. also recognized that NO was inactivated by combining with hemoproteins, and speculated that hemoglobin could trap endogenously produced NO that diffused into the vascular lumen, thus preventing any "downstream" vasorelaxation by this paracrine mediator.

The recognition that the endogenous production of this EDRF/NO mediator could be competitively blocked by modified L-arginine analogs prompted early experiments into the effects of NO in the fetal and transitional pulmonary circulation. Abman et al. (1990) performed the first experiments on the role of EDRF in the

ovine fetal circulation, demonstrating that endogenous EDRF/NO production modulates basal pulmonary vascular tone in the late-gestation fetus and that pharmacologic NO blockade inhibits endothelium-dependent pulmonary vasodilation. These investigators also showed that pharmacologic NO blockade attenuates the rise in pulmonary blood flow at delivery, thus implicating endogenous NO formation in postnatal adaptation after birth and linking this laboratory observation to the life-threatening clinical condition of PPHN. In addition, experiments using this ovine model showed that increased fetal oxygen tension augments endogenous NO release (McQueston et al. 1993; Tiktinsky and Morin 1993) and the increase in pulmonary blood flow in response to rhythmic distention of the lung and high inspired oxygen concentrations are mediated in part by endogenous NO elaboration (Tiktinsky and Morin 1993; Cornfield et al. 1992).

The observation that dilute NO gas could be therapeutically delivered by inhalation was first described by Higgenbottam et al. who reported that brief (10 min) inhalational NO treatment caused potent and selective pulmonary vasodilation in adults with severe pulmonary hypertension (Higenbottam et al. 1988; Pepke-Zaba et al. 1991). Frostell et al. demonstrated the selectivity of inhaled NO in an adult animal model of hypoxic pulmonary vasoconstriction (Frostell et al. 1991), and the first description of the potent, sustained, and selective vasodilator effect of inhaled NO in newborn lambs was reported by Kinsella et al. (1992a).

60.3 PPHN: Clinical Physiology and Evaluation

Clinically, PPHN is most often recognized in term or near term neonates, but clearly can occur in premature neonates as well. PPHN typically presents as respiratory distress and cyanosis within 6–12 h of birth. While PPHN is often associated with perinatal distress, such as asphyxia, low APGAR scores, meconium staining, and other factors, idiopathic PPHN can present without signs of acute perinatal distress. Radiographic findings are variable, depending upon the primary disease associated with PPHN. Classically, the chest x-ray in idiopathic PPHN is oligemic, normally or slightly hyperinflated, and lacks parenchymal infiltrates. In general, the degree of hypoxemia is disproportionate to the severity of radiographic evidence of lung disease.

Not all term newborns with hypoxemic respiratory failure have PPHN physiology (Abman and Kinsella 1995). Hypoxemia in the newborn can be due to *extrapulmonary shunt*, as described above, in which high pulmonary artery pressure at systemic levels leads to right-to-left shunting of blood flow across the PDA or PFO. However, in many infants *intrapulmonary shunt* or *ventilation-perfusion mismatch* is the predominant abnormality, in which hypoxemia results from the lack of mixing of blood with aerated lung regions due to parenchymal lung disease, without the shunting of blood flow across the PDA and PFO. In the latter setting, hypoxemia is related to the amount of pulmonary arterial blood that perfuses nonaerated lung regions. Although PVR is often elevated in hypoxemic newborns without PPHN, high PVR does not contribute significantly to hypoxemia in these cases.

Several factors can contribute to high pulmonary artery pressure in neonates with PPHN-type physiology. Pulmonary hypertension can be due to vasoconstriction or structural vascular lesions that directly increase PVR. Changes in lung volume in neonates with parenchymal lung disease can also be an important determinant of PVR. PVR increases at low lung volumes due to dense parenchymal infiltrate and poor lung recruitment, or with high lung volumes due to hyperinflation associated with overdistension or gas-trapping. Cardiac disease is also associated with PPHN. High pulmonary venous pressure due to left ventricular dysfunction (e.g., asphyxia or sepsis) can also elevate PAP, causing right-to-left shunting, with little vasoconstriction. In this setting, enhancing cardiac performance and systemic hemodynamics may lower PAP more effectively than promoting pulmonary vasodilation. Thus, understanding the cardiopulmonary interactions is key to improving outcome in PPHN.

PPHN is characterized by hypoxemia that is poorly responsive to supplemental oxygen. In the presence of right-to-left shunting across the PDA, "differential cyanosis" is often present, which is difficult to detect by physical exam, and is defined by a difference in PaO2 between right radial artery versus descending aorta values >10 torr, or an O2 saturation gradient >5%. However, postductal desaturation can be found in ductus-dependent cardiac diseases, including hypoplastic left heart syndrome, coarctation of the aorta, or interrupted aortic arch. The response to supplemental oxygen can help to distinguish PPHN from primary lung or cardiac disease. Although supplemental oxygen traditionally increases PaO2 more readily in lung disease than cyanotic heart disease or PPHN, this may not be obvious with more advanced parenchymal lung disease. Marked improvement in SaO2 (increase to 100%) with supplemental oxygen suggests the presence of V/Q mismatch due to lung disease or highly reactive PPHN. Most patients with PPHN have at least a transient improvement in oxygenation in response to interventions such as high levels of inspired oxygen and/or mechanical ventilation. Acute respiratory alkalosis induced by hyperventilation to achieve PaCO2 <30 torr and a pH >7.50 may increase PaO2 >50 torr in PPHN, but rarely in cyanotic heart disease.

The echocardiogram plays an important diagnostic role and is an essential tool for managing newborns with PPHN. The initial echocardiographic evaluation rules out structural heart disease causing hypoxemia or ductal shunting (e.g., coarctation of the aorta and total anomalous pulmonary venous return). Further, as stated above, not all term newborns with hypoxemia have PPHN physiology. Although high pulmonary artery pressure is commonly found in association with neonatal lung disease, the diagnosis of PPHN is uncertain without evidence of bidirectional or predominantly right-to-left shunting across the PFO or PDA. Echocardiographic signs suggestive of pulmonary hypertension (e.g., increased right ventricular systolic time intervals and septal flattening) are less helpful. In addition to demonstrating the presence of PPHN physiology, the echocardiogram is critical for the evaluation of left ventricular function and diagnosis of anatomic heart disease, including such "PPHN mimics" as coarctation of the aorta, total anomalous pulmonary venous return, hypoplastic left heart syndrome, and others. Studies should carefully assess the predominant direction of shunting at the PFO as well as the PDA. Although right-to-left shunting at the PDA and PFO is typical for PPHN, predominant right-to-left shunting at the PDA but left-to-right shunt at the PFO may help to identify the important role of *left ventricular dysfunction* to the underlying pathophysiology. In the presence of severe left ventricular dysfunction with pulmonary hypertension, pulmonary vasodilation alone may be ineffective in improving oxygenation. In this setting, efforts to reduce PVR should be accompanied by targeted therapies to increase cardiac performance and decrease left ventricular afterload. In the setting of impaired LV performance, cardiotonic therapies that increase systemic vascular resistance may further worsen LV function and increase pulmonary artery pressure. Thus, careful echocardiographic assessment provides invaluable information about the underlying pathophysiology and will help guide the course of treatment.

60.3.1 Insights into PPHN from the Laboratory

Diverse animal models have been used in order to better understand the pathogenesis and pathophysiology of PPHN. Such models have included exposure to acute or chronic hypoxia after birth, chronic hypoxia in utero, placement of meconium into the airways of neonatal animals, sepsis, and others. Each model demonstrates interesting physiologic changes that may be especially relevant to particular clinical settings, but most studies examine only brief changes in the pulmonary circulation, and mechanisms underlying altered lung vascular structure and function of PPHN remain poorly understood. Neonates with severe PPHN who die during the first days after birth already have pathologic signs of chronic pulmonary vascular disease, suggesting that intrauterine

events may play an important role in this syndrome (Geggel and Reid 1984). Adverse intrauterine stimuli during late gestation, such as abnormal hemodynamics, changes in substrate or hormone delivery to the lung, hypoxia, inflammation, or others, may potentially alter lung vascular function and structure, contributing to abnormalities of postnatal adaptation. Several investigators have examined the effects of chronic intrauterine stresses, such as hypoxia or hypertension, in animal models in order to attempt to mimic the clinical problem of PPHN. Whether chronic hypoxia alone can cause PPHN is controversial. A past report that maternal hypoxia in rats increases pulmonary vascular smooth muscle thickening in newborns, but this observation has not been reproduced in maternal rats or guinea pigs with more extensive studies (Murphy et al. 1986). Acute hypoxia alone is insufficient to account for PPHN, which is further reflected in recent clinical observations that PPHN is rare in patients with severe asphyxia who were enrolled in hypothermia studies.

Pulmonary hypertension induced by early closure of the DA in fetal lambs alters lung vascular reactivity and structure, causing the failure of postnatal adaptation at delivery and providing an experimental model of PPHN (Levin et al. 1978; Morin and Eagan 1989; Abman and Accurso 1989). Over days, pulmonary artery pressure and PVR progressively increase, but flow remains low and PaO2 is unchanged (Abman and Accurso 1989). Marked right ventricular hypertrophy and structural remodeling of small pulmonary arteries develops after 8 days of hypertension. After delivery, these lambs have persistent elevation of PVR despite mechanical ventilation with high oxygen concentrations. Studies with this model show that chronic hypertension without high flow can alter fetal lung vascular structure and function.

This model is characterized by endothelial cell dysfunction and abnormal smooth muscle cell vasoreactivity and growth, including findings of impaired NO production and activity and downregulation of lung endothelial NO synthase mRNA and protein expression (Storme et al. 1999; Villamor et al. 1997; Shaul et al. 1997; McQueston et al. 1995; Farrow et al. 2008a). Fetal pulmonary hypertension is also associated with decreased cGMP concentrations, associated with decreased soluble guanylate cyclase and upregulated cGMP-specific phosphodiesterase (PDE5) activities, suggesting further impairments in downstream signaling (Hanson et al. 1996; Steinhorn et al. 1995; Tzao et al. 2001). Thus, multiple alterations in the NO-cGMP cascade appear to play an essential role in the pathogenesis and pathophysiology of experimental PPHN, contributing to altered structure and function of the developing lung circulation and leading to failure of postnatal cardio-respiratory adaptation. Recent evidence indicates that excessive production of reactive oxygen species (ROS), such as superoxide in the pulmonary vasculature, may further contribute to the disruption in NO-cGMP signaling in this model and may contribute to poor responsiveness to inhaled NO therapy (Farrow et al. 2008a; Brennan et al. 2003; Chester et al. 2009).

Upregulation of ET-1 may also contribute to the pathophysiology of PPHN. Circulating levels of ET-1, a potent vasoconstrictor and co-mitogen for vascular smooth muscle cell hyperplasia, are increased in human newborns with severe PPHN (Rosenberg et al. 1993). In the experimental model of PPHN due to compression of the DA in fetal sheep, lung ET-1 mRNA and protein content is markedly increased, and the balance of ET receptors is altered, favoring vasoconstriction (Ivy et al. 1996, 1998;). Chronic inhibition of the ET A receptor attenuates the severity of pulmonary hypertension, decreases pulmonary artery wall thickening, and improves the fall in PVR at birth in this model (Ivy et al. 1997). Thus, experimental studies have shown the important role of the NO-cGMP cascade and the ET-1 system in the regulation of vascular tone and reactivity of the fetal and transitional pulmonary circulation.

Oxidant stress plays an important role in the pathogenesis of PPHN. Increased ROS such as superoxide ($O2^-$) and hydrogen peroxide (H2O2) have been demonstrated in pulmonary arteries in the ovine ductal ligation model of persistent pulmonary hypertension (Brennan et al. 2003; Fike et al. 2008). Mitochondrial dysfunction, increased expression and activity of NADPH oxidase, and uncoupled eNOS activity can each

generate ROS (Brennan et al. 2003; Konduri et al. 2003, 2007; Wedgwood et al. 2005). Increased ROS production promotes vasoconstriction directly and through multiple mechanisms that may include increased endothelin levels (Wedgwood and Black 2003) and oxidization of free fatty acids to create vasoconstrictor metabolites, such as isoprostanes (Lakshminrusimha et al. 2006a). $O2^-$ rapidly combines and inactivates NO and forms peroxynitrite, a potent oxidant with the potential to produce vasoconstriction and cytotoxicity. Increased ROS in the pulmonary vasculature of the ductal ligation model promotes dysfunction of NO-cGMP signaling at multiple steps in the pathway, including blunted eNOS expression, uncoupled eNOS activity (thus further promoting ROS production), and increased activity and expression of cGMP-specific phosphodiesterases, and impaired sGC activity (Farrow et al. 2008a, b; Chester et al. 2009). Superoxide dismutases (SOD) catalyze the conversion of superoxide anions to H2O2 and O2. Due to the efficiency of the reaction between NO and superoxide, the local concentration of SOD is a key determinant of the biological half-life of endogenous NO (Faraci and Didion 2004). Evidence for a critical pathologic role for ROS in PPHN includes the recent observation that administration of a single intratracheal dose of rhSOD in neonatal lambs with PPHN produced a sustained increase in oxygenation over a 24-h period, reduced production of isoprostanes and peroxynitrite, and restored normal eNOS expression and function.

In addition to vasoactive mediators, alterations of growth factors, such as VEGF and platelet-derived growth factor (PDGF), likely play key roles in PPHN. VEGF is markedly decreased in experimental PPHN, and treatment with recombinant human VEGF restores endothelial function and lowers PVR in this model (Villamor et al. 1997; Grover et al. 2003, 2005). In addition, inhibition of PDGF-B attenuates smooth muscle hyperplasia in experimental pulmonary hypertension in fetal lambs, suggesting a potential role in the pathogenesis of PPHN (Balasubramaniam et al. 2003). Additional new data suggest that maternal exposure to selective serotonin reuptake inhibitors (SSRI) during late gestation is associated with a sixfold increase in the prevalence of PPHN (Chambers et al. 2006), although it is not clear how many infants developed severe disease. Newborn rats exposed in utero to fluoxetine develop pulmonary vascular remodeling, abnormal oxygenation, and higher mortality when compared with vehicle-treated controls (Fornaro et al. 2007). However, these findings showed only mild changes in right ventricular hypertrophy and pulmonary vascular remodeling in the neonatal rat pups, with minimal changes in vasoreactivity after maternal SSRI exposure. Whether these effects were related to direct impact on the fetal lung circulation or secondary to altered maternal or umbilical-placental physiology remains unknown. As SSRIs have been reported to reduce pulmonary vascular remodeling in adult models of pulmonary hypertension, these findings also serve to highlight the unique vulnerability of fetal pulmonary vascular development.

60.3.2 Treatment of PPHN

Several pathophysiologic disturbances contribute to hypoxemia in the newborn infant, including cardiac dysfunction, airway and pulmonary parenchymal abnormalities, and pulmonary vascular disorders. In some newborns with hypoxemic respiratory failure, a single mechanism predominates (e.g., extrapulmonary right-to-left shunting without significant parenchymal lung disease seen in patients with idiopathic PPHN). These patients have systemic arterial hypoxemia despite high alveolar and pulmonary venous oxygen tensions. More commonly, the clinical manifestations of severe PPHN and hypoxemic respiratory failure are rarely attributable to a single pathophysiologic disturbance. PPHN is often associated with severe parenchymal lung disease in conditions such as meconium aspiration syndrome, bacterial pneumonia, and surfactant deficiencies or dysfunction leading to both extrapulmonary and intrapulmonary shunting. Moreover, decreased cardiac performance and reduced left ventricular output can decrease systemic blood pressure, exacerbating the right-to-left shunting of blood at the ductus arteriosus. Although severe PPHN is commonly associated with near-term and term neonates, echocardiographic studies in premature infants with

hyaline membrane disease (HMD) show that pulmonary hypertension may complicate the course of severe HMD.

The treatment of PPHN commonly focuses only on pharmacologic therapy to reduce pulmonary vascular resistance. For the relatively small subset of neonatal patients with idiopathic PPHN who have pulmonary hypertension without concomitant lung disease, selective pulmonary vasodilation alone can cause marked improvements in oxygenation. However, PPHN often occurs with more common causes of neonatal respiratory distress, including disorders characterized by moderate to severe lung disease. Moreover, sepsis neonatorum and perinatal asphyxia can severely compromise systemic vascular tone and cardiac performance, leading to systemic hypotension in addition to severe pulmonary hypertension. The pulmonary vasculature in many newborns with severe PPHN has marked structural changes, which include endothelial swelling, smooth muscle hypertrophy, and increased adventitial thickening. Moreover, functional abnormalities lead to altered responses to vasodilator and vasoconstrictor stimuli. Therefore, the therapeutic approach to PPHN requires meticulous attention to all aspects of the cardiopulmonary perturbations (pulmonary hypertension, systemic vasodilation, decreased cardiac performance, and parenchymal lung disease) that characterize this syndrome.

PPHN is a dynamic syndrome characterized by progressive changes in pulmonary vasoreactivity, cardiac performance, and parenchymal lung disease. In addition, the tendency for time-dependent changes in the relative contribution of each mechanism to hypoxemia requires continued vigilance as the disease progresses. Therefore, understanding the relative contribution of these different causes of hypoxemia becomes critically important as the inventory of therapeutic options expands. Therefore, management should be based on serial hemodynamic, echocardiographic, and radiographic assessments. Because of the diverse nature of diseases associated with PPHN, no single therapeutic approach is effective in all patients. In general, the goals of PPHN management are to optimize lung inflation and treat any underlying pulmonary parenchymal disease, to sustain cardiac performance and systemic hemodynamic stability, and to reduce pulmonary vascular resistance. In this section, management strategies for the patient with severe hypoxemic respiratory failure and PPHN are described, but it is important to recognize that many therapies advocated for the management of PPHN have not undergone rigorous evaluation with controlled clinical trials.

In general, therapy includes optimization of systemic hemodynamics with volume and cardiotonic therapy (dopamine, epinephrine, and milrinone), in order to enhance cardiac output and systemic O2 transport. Beyond these agents, another therapeutic option for stabilizing hemodynamics is arginine vasopressin. In the systemic circulation, vasopressin acts via V1a receptors of the smooth muscle, leading to vasoconstriction of both arteries and veins (Share 1988). Work in animal models has shown that despite the vasoconstrictive effect systemically, vasopressin causes dilation of the pulmonary circulation, likely mediated via nitric oxide release from the endothelium (Evora et al. 1993; Russ and Walker 1992). Outside of the neonatal period, vasopressin is used in the setting of cardiac arrest, sepsis, vasodilatory shock, and cardiac surgery with improved systemic blood pressure, a decrease in catecholamine requirements, and increased urine output (Scheurer et al. 2005; Luccini et al. 2013; Agrawal et al. 2012). In studies of patients with pulmonary hypertension, vasopressin improves systemic hemodynamics without adverse effects on the pulmonary vasculature, making it an ideal agent for treatment of infants who have pulmonary hypertension and systemic hypotension (Radicioni et al. 2012; Filippi et al. 2011). Most recently in ten infants with severe PPHN, Mohammed et al. reported improvements in oxygenation index, peak effect, a reduction in iNO dose associated with a concomitant improvement in blood pressure and urine output after initiation of vasopressin supporting the applicability of this agent in this setting (Adel Mohamed et al. 2014). A profound natriuresis is often accompanied by the increase in urine output and close monitoring of urine and serum sodium advised with vasopressin administration (Luccini et al. 2013).

Failure to respond to medical management, as evidenced by the failure to sustain improvement in oxygenation with good hemodynamic function, often leads to treatment with extracorporeal membrane oxygenation (ECMO). Although ECMO can be a life-saving therapy, it is costly and labor intensive and can have severe side effects, such as intracranial hemorrhage. Since arterio-venous ECMO usually involves ligation of the carotid artery, the potential for acute and long-term CNS injuries continues to be a major concern. Long-term follow-up of 250 neonatal ECMO survivors revealed significant abnormalities in motor performance at 12 years of age (van der Cammen-van Zijp et al. 2014) with the presence of chronic lung disease correlating with adverse motor outcomes. In this study, abnormal motor development was more subtle at 5 and 8 years of age, stressing the need for continued follow-up of neurodevelopmental outcomes in ECMO survivors (van der Cammen-van Zijp et al. 2014).

60.3.3 Nitric Oxide Therapy in PPHN

60.3.3.1 Rationale for Inhaled NO Therapy

Early laboratory studies demonstrated that inhaled nitric oxide (NO) therapy caused marked and sustained reduction in pulmonary vascular resistance (PVR) in newborn animal models (Kinsella et al. 1992a; Roberts et al. 1993), and initial pilot studies showed marked improvement in oxygenation in term newborns with PPHN (Roberts et al. 1992; Kinsella et al. 1992b). Subsequent trials confirmed the safety and efficacy of inhaled NO in this population, and it is now an integral component of PPHN therapy (Kinsella et al. 1997; Roberts et al. 1997; Wessel et al. 1997; Davidson et al. 1998a; Neonatal Inhaled Nitric Oxide Study Group 1997; Clark et al. 2000).

As described above, the physiologic rationale for inhaled NO therapy in the treatment of PPHN is based upon its ability to achieve potent and sustained pulmonary vasodilation without decreasing systemic vascular tone (Kinsella and Abman 1995). As a syndrome, PPHN is associated with diverse neonatal cardiac and pulmonary disorders that are characterized by high PVR causing extrapulmonary right-to-left shunting of blood across the arterial duct and/or oval foramen. The ability of inhaled NO therapy to selectively lower PVR and decrease extrapulmonary venoarterial admixture accounts for the acute improvement in oxygenation observed in newborns with PPHN (Kinsella et al. 1993). However, oxygenation can also improve during inhaled NO therapy in critically ill patients who do not have extrapulmonary right-to-left shunting (Abman et al. 1994; Gerlach et al. 1993). Hypoxemia in these cases is primarily due to intrapulmonary shunting caused by continued perfusion of lung units that lack ventilation (e.g., atelectasis), with variable contributions form ventilation/perfusion (V/Q) inequality. Distinct from its ability to decrease extrapulmonary right-to-left shunting by reducing PVR, low dose inhaled NO therapy can also improve oxygenation by redirecting blood from poorly aerated or diseased lung regions to better aerated distal air spaces ("microselective effect") (Rossaint et al. 1993).

Finally, the diagnostic value of inhaled NO therapy is also important, in that failure to respond to inhaled NO raises important questions about the specific mechanism of hypoxemia. Poor responses to inhaled NO should lead to further diagnostic evaluation for "unsuspected" functional/structural cardiovascular or pulmonary disease.

60.3.3.2 Inhaled NO for Treatment of PPHN

Due to its selective pulmonary vasodilator effects, inhaled NO therapy is an important adjunct to available treatments for term newborns with hypoxemic respiratory failure. Inhaled nitric oxide (iNO) therapy at low doses (5–20 ppm) improves oxygenation and decreases the need for ECMO therapy in patients with diverse causes of PPHN (Clark et al. 2000; Davidson et al. 1998; Kinsella et al. 1992b, 1997; Neonatal Inhaled Nitric Oxide Study Group 1997; Roberts et al. 1997b). Multicenter clinical trials support the use of iNO in near-term (>34 weeks gestation) and term newborns, although the use of iNO in infants less than 34 weeks gestation remains largely

investigational. Studies support the use of iNO in infants who have hypoxemic respiratory failure with evidence of PPHN, who require mechanical ventilation and high inspired oxygen concentrations. The most common criterion employed has been the oxygenation index (OI; mean airway pressure times FiO2 times 100 divided by PaO2). However, hypoxemic respiratory failure in the term newborn represents a heterogeneous group of disorders, and disease-specific responses have clearly been described. For example, patients with extapulmonary right-to-left shunting (PPHN) show acute improvement in oxygenation when PVR becomes subsystemic during NO therapy, and patients with predominantly intrapulmonary shunting (e.g., RDS) have less dramatic responses.

Clinical trials of inhaled NO in the term newborn have incorporated ECMO treatment as an endpoint. Therefore, most patients have been enrolled in the first few days of life. Although one of the pivotal studies used to support the new drug application for inhaled NO therapy included as an entry criterion a postnatal age up to 14 days, the average age at enrollment in that study was 1.7 days (Neonatal Inhaled Nitric Oxide Study Group 1997). Currently, clinical trials support the use of inhaled NO before treatment with ECMO, or usually within the first week of life. However, clinical experience suggests that inhaled NO may be of benefit as an adjuvant treatment after ECMO therapy in patients with sustained pulmonary hypertension (e.g., congenital diaphragmatic hernia). Thus, postnatal age alone should not define the duration of therapy in cases where prolonged treatment could be beneficial.

Studies support the use of inhaled NO in infants who have hypoxemic respiratory failure with evidence of PPHN, who require mechanical ventilation and high inspired oxygen concentrations. The most common criterion employed has been the oxygenation index. Although clinical trials commonly allowed for enrollment with OI levels >25, the mean OI at study entry for these studies approximated 40. Whether treatment at lower OI levels reduces ECMO use is uncertain (Konduri et al. 2004). Thus, it is unclear whether infants with less severe hypoxemia would benefit from inhaled NO therapy. However, Davidson et al. reported a controlled clinical trial in which the average OI at study entry was 24 ± 9 (Davidson et al. 1998). It is important to note that inhaled NO treatment did not reduce ECMO utilization in this study. Although entry criteria for this trial included echocardiographic evidence of pulmonary hypertension, only 9% of the patients had clinical evidence of right-to-left ductal shunting. Because of the mechanism of action of inhaled NO as a selective pulmonary vasodilator, it is likely that acute improvement in oxgyenation caused by decreased pulmonary vascular resistance and reduced extrapulmonary right-to-left shunting would be most predictive of clinical improvement. Therefore, current multicenter studies suggest that treatment with inhaled NO may include an OI >25 with echocardiographic evidence of extrapulmonary right-to-left shunting.

The first studies of inhaled NO treatment in term newborns reported initial doses that ranged from 80 ppm (Roberts et al. 1992) to 6–20 ppm (Kinsella et al. 1992b). The rationale for doses used in these clinical trials was based on concentrations which had previously been found to be effective in animal experiments by the same investigators (Geggel and Reid 1984; Levin et al. 1978). Roberts et al. reported that brief (30 min) inhalation of NO at 80 ppm improved oxygenation in patients with PPHN, but this response was sustained in only one patient after NO was discontinued (Roberts et al. 1992b). In the second report, rapid improvement in oxygenation in neonates with severe PPHN was also demonstrated, but this was achieved at lower doses (20 ppm) for 4 h (Kinsella et al. 1992b). This study also reported that decreasing the inhaled NO dose to 6 ppm for the duration of treatment provided sustained improvement in oxygenation. The relative effectiveness of low-dose inhaled NO in improving oxygenation in patients with severe PPHN was corroborated in a study by Finer et al. (1994). Acute improvement in oxygenation during treatment was not different with doses of inhaled NO ranging from 5 to 80 ppm.

These laboratory and clinical studies established the boundaries of inhaled NO dosing

protocols for subsequent randomized, clinical trials in newborns (Morin and Eagan 1989; Abman and Accurso 1989; Storme et al. 1999; Villamor et al. 1997; Shaul et al. 1997; McQueston et al. 1995). Increasing the dose to 40 ppm does not generally improve oxygenation in patients who do not respond to the lower dose of 20 ppm. The initial dose in the NINOS trial was 20 ppm, but the dose was increased to 80 ppm if the improvement in PaO2 was less than 20 torr (Neonatal Inhaled Nitric Oxide Study Group 1997). In this study, only 3 of 53 infants (6%) who had little response to 20 ppm had an increase in PaO2 >20 torr when treated with 80 ppm inhaled NO. Whether a progressive increase in PaO2 would have occurred with continued exposure to 20 ppm could not be determined with this study design. Roberts et al. initiated treatment with 80 ppm NO and subsequently weaned the inhaled NO concentration if oxygenation improved; thus, the effects of lower initial inhaled NO doses could not be evaluated and the effects on ECMO utilization were not evaluated (Roberts et al. 1992b).

These studies did not systematically evaluate individual doses in an interpretable fashion. Davidson et al. reported the results of a randomized, controlled, dose-response trial in term newborns with hypoxemic respiratory failure (Davidson et al. 1998). In this study, patients were randomized to treatment with either 0 (placebo), 5, 20, or 80 ppm NO. Each inhaled NO dose improved oxygenation compared to placebo, but there was no difference in responses between groups. However, at 80 ppm, methemoglobinemia (blood levels >7%) occurred in 13 of 37 patients (35%) and high inspired NO2 concentrations (>3 ppm) were reported in 7 of 37 patients (19%). Thus, 80 ppm inhaled NO was not more effective in improving oxygenation than 5 or 20 ppm, but was associated with adverse effects. Unfortunately, this trial was limited by early termination due to slow enrollment and the exclusion of lung recruitment approaches to optimize inhaled NO efficacy.

The available evidence, therefore, supports the use of doses of inhaled NO beginning at 20 ppm in term newborns with PPHN. Although brief exposures to higher doses (40–80 ppm) appear to be safe, sustained treatment with 80 ppm NO increases the risk of methemoglobinemia. The lowest effective *starting* dose for inhaled NO in term newborns with PPHN has not been determined. Cornfield et al. reported that initiating treatment at 2 ppm does not acutely improve oxygenation and may diminish the subsequent response to 20 ppm (Cornfield et al. 1999). However, this effect was refuted by Finer et al. who found that initial exposure to low NO doses (1–2 ppm) did not compromise subsequent responses to higher doses (10–20 ppm), and dose increases were required in 80% of the low dose group (Finer et al. 2001). Sustained improvement in oxygenation (after >4 h of treatment with 20 ppm) has been demonstrated for doses <10 ppm (Goldman et al. 1996).

Although clinical improvement during inhaled NO therapy occurs with many disorders associated with PPHN, not all neonates with acute hypoxemic respiratory failure and pulmonary hypertension respond to iNO. Several mechanisms may explain the clinical variability in responsiveness to iNO therapy (Goldman et al. 1996). A major cause of poor responsiveness to iNO is an inability to deliver NO to the pulmonary circulation due to poor lung inflation. In addition, poor NO responsiveness may be related to myocardial dysfunction or systemic hypotension, severe pulmonary vascular structural disease, and unsuspected or missed anatomic cardiovascular lesions (such as total anomalous pulmonary venous return, coarctation of the aorta, alveolar capillary dysplasia, pulmonary interstitial glycogenosis, surfactant protein deficiency, and others). Since iNO is usually delivered with high concentrations of oxygen, there is also the potential for enhanced production of reactive oxygen and reactive nitrogen metabolites, both of which may contribute to vasoconstriction and/or inadequate responses to iNO. While hyperoxic ventilation is standard therapy for PPHN, high FiO2 may be toxic to the developing lung through formation of ROS (Lakshminrusimha et al. 2006b). As noted above, iNO responsiveness may be blunted after even brief (30 min) periods of ventilation with 100% O2, and that oxidant stress alters NO responsiveness in part through increasing

expression and activity of cGMP-specific phosphodiesterases (Farrow et al. 2008b; Lakshminrusimha et al. 2007).

After improvement in oxygenation occurs with the onset of inhaled NO therapy, strategies for weaning the inhaled NO dose become important. Numerous approaches have been employed, and little differences have been noted until final discontinuation of inhaled NO treatment. In one study, inhaled NO was reduced from 20 to 6 ppm after 4 h of treatment without acute changes in oxygenation (Kinsella et al. 1992b). In another trial, inhaled NO was reduced in a stepwise fashion to as low as 1 ppm without changes in oxygenation (Davidson et al. 1998). It is important to recognize that weaning inhaled NO is a different process than discontinuation of inhaled NO therapy.

In multicenter, clinical trials of inhaled NO therapy, the typical duration of inhaled NO treatment has been less than 5 days, which parallels the clinical resolution of PPHN. However, individual exceptions occur particularly in cases of pulmonary hypoplasia (Goldman et al. 1996; Peliowski et al. 1995). If inhaled NO is required for longer than 5 days, investigations into other causes of pulmonary hypertension should be considered (e.g., alveolar capillary dysplasia), particularly if discontinuation of inhaled NO results in suprasytemic elevations of pulmonary artery pressure by echocardiography. In our practice, we discontinue inhaled NO if the FiO2 is <0.60 and the PaO2 is >60 without evidence of rebound pulmonary hypertension or an increase in FiO2 >15% after inhaled NO withdrawal.

Early clinical studies reported rapid and sometimes dramatic decreases in oxygenation and increases in PVR after abrupt withdrawal of inhaled NO during prolonged therapy. These responses are often mild and transient, and many patients with decreased oxygenation after inhaled NO withdrawal will respond to brief elevations of FiO2 and careful observation. In patients with a persistent need for treatment with higher inspired oxygen concentrations or with increased pulmonary hypertension after inhaled NO withdrawal, restarting inhaled NO treatment will generally cause rapid clinical improvement. In general, this so-called "rebound" response appears to decrease over time after more prolonged therapy. However, inhaled NO withdrawal can be associated with life-threatening elevations of pulmonary vascular resistance, profound desaturation, and systemic hypotension due to decreased cardiac output. Mechanisms that contribute to these "rebound" effects are incompletely understood, but may be related to downregulation of endogenous NO production during exogenous NO therapy. Alternatively, the rise in pulmonary vascular resistance and drop in oxygenation after inhaled NO withdrawal may simply represent the presence of more severe underlying pulmonary vascular disease with loss of treatment effect of inhaled NO. The sudden increase in pulmonary artery pressure after rapid withdrawal of vasodilator therapy is not unique to inhaled NO and has been observed in other clinical settings, such as prostacyclin withdrawal in adults with primary pulmonary hypertension and in postoperative cardiac patients.

60.3.3.3 Inhaled NO in the Premature Newborn

Early reports of iNO therapy in a premature newborn with pulmonary hypertension demonstrated marked improvement in oxygenation caused by effective treatment of severe pulmonary hypertension and resolution of extra-pulmonary right-to-left shunting (Peliowski et al. 1995), as well as other preterm infants with severe respiratory failure (Meurs et al. 1997). Subsequently, several randomized, controlled trials (RCTs) have confirmed the acute improvement in oxygenation caused by iNO treatment. However, in contrast to the direct pulmonary vasodilator effects of iNO, the focus of the most recently published studies has been on the potential beneficial effects of prolonged iNO administration on lung parenchymal and vascular development (Abman 2001).

In a small, unmasked, randomized trial of iNO (20 ppm) and dexamethasone treatment, Subhedar et al. reported no differences in survival, chronic lung disease, or ICH between iNO-treated infants and controls (Subhedar et al. 1997). In a randomized, masked, multicenter clinical trial of low dose iNO therapy (5 ppm) in severely ill premature newborns with RDS who had marked hypoxemia

despite surfactant therapy (a/A O2 ratio <0.10), iNO acutely improved PaO2, but did not reduce the incidence of mortality or BPD (Kinsella et al. 1999). Notably, there was no increase in the incidence or severity of ICH in this trial, and the incidence of the most severe ICH (grade 4) was 19% for the iNO group and 29% for the control group. The Franco-Belgium study group reported the results of an acute iNO response study (2 h oxygenation endpoint); however, the brief duration of therapy and a high rate of crossover before the 2-h trial endpoint compromised the interpretation of late outcome measures (The Franco – Belgium Collaborative NO Trial Group 1999). Hascoet et al. reported the results of an unmasked, randomized trial of iNO in 145 premature newborns with hypoxemic respiratory failure (Hascoet et al. 2005). They found no difference between the iNO and control groups in the primary outcome measure (intact survival at 28 days) and no differences in adverse events. As noted by Finer in an accompanying editorial, interpretation of the findings is limited by a relatively high rate of "open-label" iNO use and the lack of important outcomes such as death before discharge and BPD incidence at 36 weeks (Finer 2005). However, these investigators also studied the effect of low-dose iNO on serum markers of oxidative stress and found that iNO treatment apparently reduced signs of oxidative stress in these patients (Hamon et al. 2005). Field et al. described the findings of the UK INNOVO trial. In this unblinded study, 108 premature infants with severe hypoxemic respiratory failure were randomized to receive or not receive iNO (Field et al. 2005). There was no difference between the iNO and control group in the main outcome measure (death or severe disability at 1 year corrected age) and no difference in adverse events. Limitations of the study included an 8% crossover to iNO treatment and treatment with other pulmonary vasodilators in 30% of the control group. Moreover, Field et al. describe a lack of equipoise among investigators demonstrated by the observation that 75 infants eligible for enrollment were treated with iNO outside of the trial, leaving only infants with very severe lung disease enrolled in the study (Field 2005).

The largest trials of iNO therapy in premature newborns reported to date include the single center study of Schreiber et al. (2003) and the multicenter trials of Van Meurs et al. (2005), Ballard et al. (2006), and Kinsella et al. (2006) All of these studies were randomized, controlled, and masked, but have key differences in patient population, disease severity, dose and duration of therapy, and other factors.

Schreiber et al. randomized 207 infants to treatment with iNO or placebo. The main finding of the trial was a reduction in the incidence of BPD and death by 24% in the iNO group. These benefits appeared to accrue predominantly from the subset of newborns with relatively mild respiratory failure (OI <6.94). However, in addition to apparent pulmonary benefit caused by low-dose iNO, these authors also reported a 47% decrease in the incidence of severe ICH and periventricular leukomalacia (PVL). Moreover, in a subsequent report, the same group showed that the early decrease in ICH/PVL associated with iNO treatment manifested in improved neurodevelopmental outcome on follow-up examinations of this population (Mestan et al. 2005). In this follow-up study, 138 children (82% of survivors of the RCT) were evaluated for neurodevelopmental outcome at 2 years of age. In the group treated with iNO in the newborn period, 24% had abnormal outcomes (defined as cerebral palsy, blindness, hearing loss, or one score of less than 70 on the Bayley Scales of Infant Development II), in contrast to 46% in the control group.

Van Meurs et al. enrolled 420 newborns (401–1500 g birthweight) in a multicenter RCT. Although the focus of this study was on premature newborns and the major outcome measure was BPD, the design of the trial was similar to the previous NINOS trial in which term newborns were enrolled and acute changes in oxygenation determined continued treatment with study gas. That is, an acute dose-response study was performed and only patients who showed significant improvement in PaO2 were continued on study gas. In striking contrast with other studies, the average duration of iNO treatment was only 76 h. Overall, they found no difference in the incidence of death/BPD between the iNO and

control groups. However, in post hoc analyses, infants with birthweight >1000 g showed a reduction in death/BPD following treatment with iNO (50% iNO vs. 69% control). But a worrisome outcome was suggested in a post hoc analysis of newborns weighing <1000 g. This analysis showed an increased risk of ICH/PVL (43% iNO vs. 33% control). However, as noted in an editorial by Martin and Walsh (2005), baseline ultrasound examinations were not performed, and it cannot be determined whether these very severely ill infants had ICH before iNO was initiated. Indeed, the severity of illness of infants in this trial of Van Meurs et al. was also markedly different from the study of Schreiber et al. In the Van Meurs trial, the mean oxygenation index (OI) at enrollment for the iNO group was 23, compared to the median OI of 7.3 in the Schreiber study. This suggests that the degree of illness based upon the severity of respiratory failure may be related to iNO safety and efficacy in this population; however, an increased risk of ICH/PVL was not observed in a previous trial of iNO in premature newborns with severe hypoxemic respiratory failure (OI = 30) Kinsella et al. 1992a. Other differences between these two trials may offer insights into the disparate outcomes, including the duration of iNO treatment (3 days vs. 7 days), birthweight (839 g vs. 992 g), and gestational age (26 weeks vs. 27.4 weeks). Thus, Van Meurs et al. enrolled smaller, more immature infants with severe respiratory failure who were treated relatively briefly with iNO, making direct comparisons between these two trials problematic.

The results of the two largest randomized, controlled, and masked trials of iNO treatment in premature newborns were recently reported. Ballard et al. randomized 582 premature newborns with birth weights of 500–1250 g who required ventilatory support between 7 and 21 days of age (Roberts et al. 1993). Infants were treated with study gas for a minimum of 24 days and had an estimated OI of 7. They found that the incidence of survival without BPD was increased in the iNO treatment group (43.9%) compared to controls (36.8%) ($P = 0.042$). A major finding of this trial was that the benefit of BPD reduction derived almost entirely from the subset of patients enrolled between 7 and 14 days, suggesting that early treatment is important to prevent BPD. There were no differences between the iNO and control groups in adverse events, including medical or surgical treatment of PDA. There also were no differences between the groups in ICH incidence; however, infants were enrolled after the first week of life. Thus, this trial does not help inform the debate about iNO effects on brain injury in the premature newborn.

In the second trial, 793 premature newborns with birth weights of 500–1250 g and requiring mechanical ventilation in the first 48 h of life were randomized to treatment with 5 ppm iNO or placebo gas and treated for 21 days or until extubated (Kinsella et al. 1992b). Overall, there was no difference in the incidence of death or BPD between groups; however, iNO therapy reduced the incidence of BPD for infants with birth weight >1000 g by 50% ($p = 0.001$). Low-dose iNO therapy reduced the incidence of PVL ($p = 0.048$), as well as the combined endpoints of ICH, PVL, and ventriculomegaly for the entire study population ($p = 0.032$). INO therapy did not increase the incidence of adverse events, including mortality, ICH, PVL, pulmonary hemorrhage, and PDA treatment in any subgroup. In addition, this trial did not demonstrate a relationship between OI and brain injury risk, in contrast to the findings of Van Meurs et al. Despite radiographic evidence of decreased brain injury with iNO treatment, long-term follow-up of infants enrolled in these studies has failed to show improvement in neurologic outcomes with no difference in outcomes between the iNO and placebo treated groups (Mestan et al. 2005; Martin and Walsh 2005; Walsh et al. 2010).

Interestingly, while neurologic outcomes were no different between groups, long-term respiratory outcomes where significantly improved with iNO treatment decreasing the use of respiratory medications in the first year of life (Hintz et al. 2007). Subsequent studies however have failed to show any short- or long-term respiratory benefit with iNO treatment in mechanically ventilated preterm infants (Hibbs et al. 2008).

The effects of iNO in the premature newborn may be dependent on the timing, dose, and

duration of therapy, and the nature of the underlying disease. The available evidence from clinical trials suggests that routine use of iNO for the prevention and/or treatment of BPD is currently not recommended, other than for management of PPHN in preterm infants, such as in infants born preterm after prolonged rupture of membranes (Mercier et al. 2010). While a neuroprotective effect of iNO has been demonstrated in large RCTs, long-term studies have failed to show a difference in outcomes. In addition, the relationship of disease severity and ICH/PVL risk is uncertain.

60.3.4 PPHN: Ventilator Management

Perhaps the most misunderstood aspect of severe hypoxemic respiratory failure and PPHN is ventilatory management of these complex disorders. The patient with idiopathic PPHN (i.e., without significant lung disease) often requires only minimal ventilatory support. Applying inappropriately high airway pressure to the normally compliant lung can lead to air leak (e.g., pneumothorax) and adverse cardiopulmonary interactions (decreased cardiac output from reduced venous return and cardiac filling).

However, in the more common setting of severe lung disease with PPHN, lung underinflation contributes to increased PVR. Considering the important role of parenchymal lung disease in specific disorders included in the syndrome of PPHN, pharmacologic pulmonary vasodilation alone should be expected to cause sustained clinical improvement in many cases (Hibbs et al. 2008). Moreover, patients not responding to inhaled NO can show marked improvement in oxygenation with adequate lung inflation alone. High success rates in early studies were achieved by withholding inhaled NO treatment until aggressive attempts were made to optimize ventilation and lung inflation with mechanical ventilation. These early studies demonstrated that the effects of inhaled NO may be suboptimal when lung volume is decreased in association with pulmonary parenchymal disease, for several reasons (Mercier et al. 2010). First, atelectasis and air space disease (pneumonia, pulmonary edema) may decrease the effective delivery of inhaled NO to its site of action in terminal lung units. Second, in cases complicated by severe lung disease and underinflation, pulmonary hypertension may be exacerbated because of the adverse mechanical effects of underinflation on pulmonary vascular resistance. Third, attention must be given to minimize overinflation to avoid inadvertent positive end expiratory pressure and gas trapping that may elevate pulmonary vascular resistance from vascular compression. This commonly complicates the management of infants with asymmetric lung disease or airways obstruction as observed in meconium aspiration syndrome.

Treatment of the underlying lung disease is essential (and sometimes sufficient) to resolve the accompanying pulmonary hypertension. Airway pressure is poorly transmitted to the pleural space in the underinflated and poorly compliant lung, but as lung volume and compliance improve, ventilator support must be reduced to avoid injury from the adverse effects of overinflation on lung parenchyma and cardiac performance. Because of the diverse nature of diseases complicating PPHN, there is no single approach to mechanical ventilation in this syndrome. Ventilator adjustments must be made with attention to radiographic changes of the accompanying lung disease and hemodynamic status (including intravascular volume, systemic perfusion, and cardiac performance) (Gersony 1984). Mechanical ventilation in PPHN should be initiated with conventional intermittent mandatory ventilation. Alkalosis induced by mechanical hyperventilation decreases pulmonary arterial pressure and improves oxygenation in some patients with PPHN.

The goal of mechanical ventilation in PPHN is to improve oxygenation and achieve "optimal" lung volume to minimize the adverse effects of high or low lung volumes on PVR and the risk for lung injury ("volutrauma"). Mechanical ventilation using inappropriate settings can produce acute lung injury (ventilator-induced lung injury; VILI), causing pulmonary edema, decreased lung compliance, and promoting lung inflammation due to increased cytokine production and lung

neutrophil accumulation. The development of VILI is an important determinant of clinical course and eventual outcome of newborns with hypoxemic respiratory failure, and postnatal lung injury worsens the degree of pulmonary hypertension (Cole et al. 2011). On the other hand, failure to achieve adequate lung volumes (functional residual capacity) contributes to hypoxemia and high PVR in newborns with PPHN. Some newborns with parenchymal lung disease with PPHN physiology improve oxygenation and decrease right-to-left extrapulmonary shunting with aggressive lung recruitment during high frequency oscillatory ventilation (Davidson et al. 1998) or with an "open lung approach" of higher positive end-expiratory pressure with low tidal volumes, as more commonly utilized in older patients with ARDS (Kinsella and Abman 2000).

In newborns with severe lung disease, HFOV is frequently used to optimize lung inflation and minimize lung injury. The combination of HFOV with iNO often enhances the improvement in oxygenation in newborns with severe PPHN complicated by diffuse parencyhmal lung disease and underinflation (e.g., RDS, pneumonia). A randomized, multicenter trial of infants with severe PPHN demonstrated that treatment with iNO in combination with HFOV was successful in many patients who failed to respond to HFOV or iNO alone (Kinsella et al. 1997; Patterson et al. 1988). For patients with PPHN complicated by severe lung disease, response rates for HFOV+iNO were better than HFOV alone or iNO with conventional ventilation. In contrast, for patients without significant parenchymal lung disease, both iNO and HFOV+iNO were more effective than HFOV alone. This response to combined treatment with HFOV+iNO likely reflects both improvement in intrapulmonary shunting in patients with severe lung disease and PPHN (using a strategy designed to recruit and sustain lung volume, rather than to hyperventilate) and augmented NO delivery to its site of action. Although iNO may be an effective treatment for PPHN, it should be considered only as part of an overall clinical strategy that simultaneously addresses the role of parenchymal lung disease, cardiac performance, and systemic hemodynamics.

Past studies have shown that acute hyperventilation can improve PaO2 in neonates with PPHN, providing a diagnostic test and potential therapeutic strategy. However, there are many issues with the use of hypocarbic alkalosis for prolonged therapy. Depending upon the ventilator strategy and underlying lung disease, hyperventilation is likely to increase VILI, and the ability to sustain decreased PVR during prolonged hyperventilation is unproven. Experimental studies suggest that the response to alkalosis is transient and that alkalosis may paradoxically worsen pulmonary vascular tone, reactivity, and permeability edema (Acute Respiratory Distress Syndrome Network 2000; Gordon et al. 1993). In addition, prolonged hyperventilation reduces cerebral blood flow and oxygen delivery to the brain, potentially worsening neuro-developmental outcome. Overall, hyperventilation is currently not recommended for prolonged treatment of PPHN.

60.3.5 PPHN: Alternate Therapies

Additional therapies, including infusions of sodium bicarbonate, surfactant therapy and the use of intravenous vasodilators, are also highly variable between centers. Although surfactant improved oxygenation and reduced ECMO in some lung diseases, such as meconium aspiration and RDS, a multicenter trial showed benefit in infants with relatively mild disease and failed to show a reduction in ECMO utilization in the subset of newborns with idiopathic PPHN (Lakshminrusimha et al. 2006b). The use of intravenous vasodilator drug therapy, with agents such as tolazoline, magnesium sulfate, and sodium nitroprusside is also controversial due to the nonselective effects of these agents on the systemic circulation and use of these agents is no longer recommended. Systemic hypotension may worsen right-to-left shunting, impair oxygen delivery, and worsen gas exchange in patients with parenchymal lung disease.

The pulmonary vasodilator response to iNO is mediated primarily by the generation of cGMP after activation of soluble guanylate cyclase (sGC). This effect is limited by high PDE5

activity, which rapidly metabolizes cGMP, and decreases the ability of iNO or other agonists to sustain vasodilation (Walsh-Sukys et al. 2000; Laffey et al. 2000). Recently approved by the FDA for the treatment of adult chronic pulmonary hypertension, sildenafil is a potent and highly specific PDE5 inhibitor that has been used in several preclinical studies in animal models. For instance, in lambs with experimental pulmonary hypertension, both enteric and aerosolized sildenafil dilate the pulmonary vasculature and augment the pulmonary vascular response to iNO (Ziegler et al. 1998; Atz and Wessel 1999). Intravenous sildenafil was found to be a selective pulmonary vasodilator with efficacy equivalent to inhaled nitric oxide in a piglet model of meconium aspiration, although hypotension and worsening oxygenation resulted when sildenafil was used in combination with iNO (Ichinose et al. 2001; Weimann et al. 2000). In a recent open-label, dose- escalation trial in newborns with PPHN and an oxygenation index (OI) >15. Sildenafil was delivered by continuous IV infusion to evaluate the effect on OI. While the majority of infants were already receiving therapy with iNO, sildenafil use was associated with a significant decrease on OI especially in the groups receiving higher dose infusion. In a smaller subset of infants, sildenafil administration obviated the need for initiation of iNO (Shekerdemian ct al. 2002). In this study, hypotension was the most common adverse effect noted. The availability of IV sildenafil for clinical use provides an alternate option for infants with pulmonary hypertension; unresponsive to inhaled NO, however, should be administered with caution in infants with hemodynamic instability.

Prostacyclin is a potent vasodilator that causes pulmonary vasodilation through stimulation of adenylate cyclase to increase intracellular cAMP levels. Although iv prostacyclin may worsen gas exchange in PPHN patients with lung disease and systemic vasodilation, inhaled PGI2 may enhance oxygenation in infants that are poorly responsive to iNO (Shekerdemian et al. 2004). Another potential approach taking advantage of cAMP signaling is inhibition of phosphodiesterase type 3 (PDE3) that metabolizes cAMP. Milrinone, a PDE3 inhibitor, has been shown to decrease pulmonary artery pressure and resistance and to act additively with iNO in animal studies. A recent report indicates that the addition of intravenous milrinone to neonates with severe PPHN and poor iNO responsiveness was associated with improvements in oxygenation without compromising hemodynamic status (Steinhorn et al. 2007). Milrinone is of additional benefit by lowering systemic afterload in the setting of PPHN newborns with poor LV function.

Until recently, experience with bosentan, a dual endothelin-1 receptor antagonist, was limited to a few case reports in the management of PPHN. More recently a double-blind, placebo-controlled, prospective study of bosentan for the treatment of persistent pulmonary hypertension of the newborn was performed with study endpoints of oxygenation index <15, normal pulmonary artery pressure (<20 mm Hg), and no premature discontinuation of the drug because of drug-related toxicity or lack of efficacy (Kelly et al. 2002). A favorable response to bosentan was seen in 87.5% of patients as compared with 20% of those who received placebo, and no drug-related clinical or laboratory adverse events were reported. Use of bosentan is limited by its availability only in an oral formulation, as well as lack of experience with this agent; however, in severe cases of refractory pulmonary hypertension, use of this agent could be considered. Close monitoring of liver function testing is recommended when therapy is initiated with this agent (McNamara et al. 2006).

60.4 Pulmonary Hypertension in Congenital Diaphragmatic Hernia (CDH)

60.4.1 Introduction

Congenital diaphragmatic hernia (CDH) is a severe birth defect characterized by herniation of abdominal contents into the thorax caused by a defect in the diaphragm (Pierro and Thebaud 2014). Recent insight into pathophysiologic

processes responsible for CDH suggests an early role for environmental and/or genetic factors before the development of the diaphragm, leading to arrested development of both lungs. In addition, incomplete closure of the diaphragm results in a diaphragm defect, herniation of the abdominal contents into the chest, and compression of the intrathoracic structures.

Solid organ herniation exacerbates the degree of lung hypoplasia, and the most severe cases are associated with hypoplasia of the ipsilateral and contralateral lung (low lung- to-head ratio [LHR] (Lipshutz et al. 1997). Along with degree of lung hypoplasia, the severity of pulmonary hypertension (PH) and presence of left ventricular (LV) hypoplasia all contribute to the severity of the defect and adverse outcomes (Taira et al. 1998; Wynn et al. 2013). Overall survival of infants with CDH has improved in experienced centers, but mortality and morbidity remain high.

Several individual prenatal prognostic factors have been identified in CDH that can predict the clinical course after birth as well as long-term outcomes. These include liver position, severity of lung hypoplasia (as assessed by fetal lung volume on MRI: percent predicted lung volume [PPLV] and total lung volume [TLV]; LHR and observed to expected LHR by ultrasound), LV hypoplasia (right ventricle [RV]:left ventricle disproportion on fetal echocardiogram [ECHO]), and development and reactivity of the pulmonary vasculature (e.g., McGoon Index, in utero hyperoxia test). In addition, the presence of congenital heart disease or a genetic syndrome (Le et al. 2012) markedly impacts outcomes. The reliability of each individual parameter to predict survival and long-term outcome is low, and combining multiple parameters improves reliability. The CDH congenital prognostic index (CDH-CPI) is a useful tool that amalgamates ten prenatal parameters representing genetic, cardiac, hernia, and lung factors to comprehensively capture the range of severity and associated anomalies influencing prognosis (Le et al. 2012). The CDH-CPI score is correlated with survival and extracorporeal membrane oxygenation (ECMO) support, with significantly lower survival at scores below eight (Le et al. 2012).

60.4.2 Pulmonary Hypertension in CDH

The classical histological findings of CDH show pulmonary vascular remodeling superimposed on hypoplasia or pruning of the pulmonary vascular bed (Pierro and Thebaud 2014). These changes in the pulmonary vasculature are responsible for increased vascular tone and altered vasoreactivity after birth (Pierro and Thebaud 2014). Management of PH in the newborn with CDH is complicated by the structural and functional changes in the heart, pulmonary circulation, airways, and lung parenchyma. Moreover, the role and selection of pulmonary vasodilator therapies for treatment of PH change as the underlying pathophysiology evolves in the days and weeks after birth. In response, management strategies need to adjust as pulmonary vascular abnormalities progress from the acute to subacute (late) and finally chronic stages.

60.4.3 Acute Pulmonary Hypertension in CDH

After birth, infants with CDH typically present with severe hypoxemic respiratory failure (HRF) and shock. The etiology of hypoxemia is multifactorial and occurs secondary to intrapulmonary shunt as well as extrapulmonary right-to-left shunting across fetal conduits (ductus arteriosus [DA] and foramen ovale). Newborns with severe CDH often present with left-to-right shunting at the atrial septum and right-to-left shunting at the ductus arteriosus (Gien and Kinsella 2015). Differential shunting across these fetal conduits is responsible for postductal desaturation and differences in pre- and postductal arterial blood gas parameters (Gien and Kinsella 2015). The direction of atrial level shunt is determined by the relative right and left ventricular end diastolic pressures. Left-to-right shunting at the atrial septum occurs when left ventricular end diastolic pressure (LVEDP) exceeds right ventricular end diastolic pressures (RVEDP) with impaired LV filling and elevated left atrial pressure (LAP).

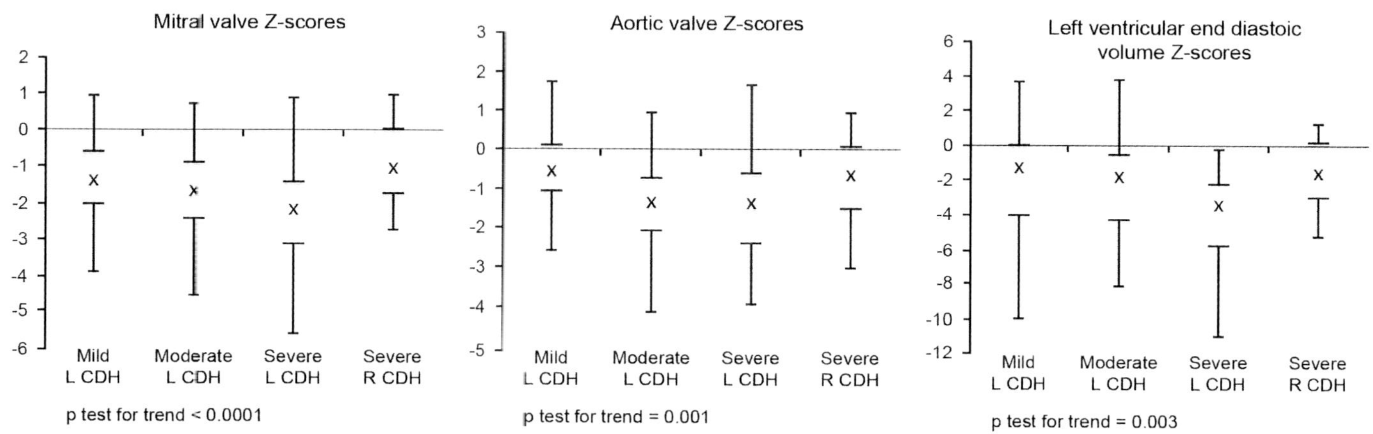

Fig. 1 Left heart hypoplasia stratified by congenital diaphragmatic hernia (CDH) side and severity at fetal assessment. Left CDH: mild (n = 42), liver down. moderate (n = 41), lung-to-head ratio (LHR) 1-1.4; severe (n = 88), LHR ≤1; Right CDH: mild (n = 2), LHR >1; severe (n = 15), LHR ≤1. For left heart measurements (mitral and aortic values, left ventricular volume) severity of hypoplasia increased with increasing severity of hernia, while the effect in the fetus with right CDH was less pronounced. Adapted with permission from Byrne et al. *Ultrasound Obstet Gynecol.*[8] CDH, congenital diaphragmatic hernia; L, left; R, right

Structural and functional LV abnormalities are responsible for impaired LV filling and contribute to the development of pulmonary venous hypertension. Baumgart et al. showed that ECMO-treated CDH infants (survivors) had significantly smaller LV mass ($P < 0.002$) than infants requiring ECMO for other diagnoses and healthy term infants (Baumgart et al. 1998). Moreover, ECMO-treated CDH neonates who died had significantly smaller LV size than other groups ($P < 0.0005$) including ECMO-treated CDH survivors (in addition to CDH and non-CDH ECMO-treated infants and well infants) (Baumgart et al. 1998). Byrne et al. reported that fetuses with severe left CDH were more likely to have smaller mitral valve ($P < 0.001$) and aortic valve sizes ($P < 0.001$), and left ventricular end diastolic volume ($P = 0.006$) Z-scores than those with mild left CDH (Fig. 1) (Byrne et al. 2015). In addition to the structural changes in the LV, their percentage LV output was also lower. Those with severe left CDH trended towards higher risk of neonatal death compared with those with mild left CDH. Although mitral and aortic valve dimensions in fetuses with right CDH were larger than in left CDH, LV outputs were similarly diminished.

The etiology of LV hypoplasia in CDH is almost certainly multifactorial reflecting mechanical compression by intra-abdominal contents as well as alteration in LV filling hemodynamics during fetal development due to changes in orientation of the inferior vena cava and venous return from the placenta. Left heart under-filling and subsequent underdevelopment may result from abnormal hemodynamics due to leftward distortion of the ductus venosus or reduced pulmonary blood flow return to the left heart (Byrne et al. 2015). In addition, after birth, compression of the LV by the RV in the presence of elevated RV pressure also impairs LV filling. The common pathway for these mechanisms is decreased filling of the left ventricle. Altered hemodynamics and compression of the heart by herniated abdominal viscera together can create strikingly abnormal left ventricular structure and function with anomalous relaxation and small chamber size, even with normal or near-normal systolic performance. Overall, altered fetal hemodynamics leading to decreased LV output can occur in both right and left CDH, but an additional compressive effect on the left heart is seen in left-sided CDH (Byrne et al. 2015).

Echocardiographic findings may be valuable in guiding the selective use of pulmonary vasodilators in management of early PH with CDH. For example, ECHO findings in the presence of severe PH may show right-to-left shunting (caused by suprasystemic pulmonary vascular resistance) at the atrial level and DA. This constellation of echocardiographic findings suggests a favorable response to pulmonary vasodilation. However, in the presence of LV dysfunction, right-to-left DA shunting is seen along with mitral insufficiency with left-to-right atrial shunting at the foramen ovale (Kinsella and Abman 2000). This constellation of findings is again consistent with suprasystemic right ventricular systolic pressure, but left-to-right atrial shunting suggests the presence of pulmonary venous hypertension and a poor response to pulmonary vasodilator therapy. Diastolic dysfunction is difficult to assess, but can be interpreted from a high LVEDP and manifests as left-to-right shunt at the atrial level. Pulmonary vasodilator therapy in the setting of left-to-right shunting at the atrial septum has the potential to exacerbate LA and pulmonary venous hypertension and contribute to pulmonary hemorrhage. In addition, as preductal saturations are maintained in this setting, pulmonary vasodilator therapy is unlikely to improve preductal saturations and may result in only a modest increase in postductal saturations. Reserving iNO therapy for infants with right-to-left atrial shunting and preductal desaturation is recommended early in the clinical course and has the potential to prevent pulmonary hemorrhage in CDH. In addition, as right-to- left shunting across the DA causes veno-arterial admixture, it is common to see significant differences in pre- and postductal arterial blood gases (ABG) measurements (Gien and Kinsella 2015). Determining the need for ECMO, degree of respiratory support and fraction of inspired oxygen (Fi02) should be based on measurement of preductal arterial gases in these infants (Gien and Kinsella 2015).

Overall, acute treatment of PH in CDH with pulmonary vasodilators is limited by the severity of LV hypoplasia, degree of impairment of LV filling, and LV systolic dysfunction. Because infants with severe CDH and acute PH are poor responders, iNO should not be routinely administered in this setting. However, careful ECHO assessment can help identify limited clinical situations that may benefit from PH therapies, including iNO, and guide the course of treatment (Kinsella and Abman 2000; Kinsella et al. 2005). In the acute management of CDH, iNO may have a selective role in stabilization for ECMO and treatment of marked preductal desaturation secondary to right-to-left atrial level shunt. Furthermore, the use of iNO for treatment of PH may be considered as LV performance improves. LV hypoplasia, and related LV output, also plays a role in the poor response to pulmonary vasodilators as diminished LV performance results in RV-dependent systemic circulation (Kinsella and Abman 2000). Initiating pulmonary vasodilator therapy in the presence of an RV-dependent systemic circulation may adversely affect systemic hemodynamics.

The Neonatal Inhaled Nitric Oxide Study (NINOS) Group conducted the largest trial of iNO in infants with CDH ($N = 53$) who were randomized to 20 ppm iNO or 100% oxygen (control) (The Neonatal Inhaled Nitric Oxide Study Group (NINOS) 1997). The oxygenation index (OI) was approximately 45 in both groups indicating more severe disease. NINOS showed no difference in the combined endpoint "death/ECMO utilization" between iNO-treated patients and controls. However, ECMO utilization was higher in the iNO-treated group (80% vs. 54% control, $P = 0.043$) pointing to an adverse effect of iNO early in the course of CDH. These results lend support to the hypothesis that LV systolic and diastolic dysfunction contribute to morbidity in severe CDH and limit the efficacy of aggressive pharmacologic pulmonary vasodilator therapy early in the course of CDH and severe PH.

Indeed, a poor response to pulmonary vasodilation is not unexpected given the structural and functional abnormalities that characterize acute CDH. Although speculative, the lack of response to pulmonary vasodilators is more likely due to left atrial/pulmonary vein hypertension than functional changes in the pulmonary arterial vasculature.

60.4.4 Subacute (Late) Pulmonary Hypertension in CDH

In addition to complicating the early course of neonates with CDH, severe PH can be protracted – persisting weeks to months after improvement in respiratory failure and cardiac performance – leading to prolonged mechanical ventilation (Kinsella and Abman 2000). In a multicenter prospective ECHO study of neonates with CDH ($N = 220$), mortality at discharge in newborns with severe PH (right ventricular systolic pressure [RVSP]/systolic blood pressure [SBP] >2/3) was 56.1% compared with 1.4% in infants with mild PH (RVSP/SBP <1/2) and 7.4% in those with moderate PH (RVSP/SBP 1/2–2/3) (Wynn et al. 2013). Recently, Lusk et al. reviewed ECHO results for 140 newborns with CDH and found that although the majority of infants had resolution of PH between 1 and 3 weeks of age, at 2 weeks the severity of PH by echocardiogram predicted mortality and need for prolonged ventilation (Lusk et al. 2015).

Treatment strategies for infants with late PH have not been carefully studied. Inhaled NO is usually the first line therapy for treatment of PH in CDH. In a subset of newborns with CDH, improvement in parenchymal lung disease may allow for the use of non invasive iNO by continuous positive airway pressure (CPAP) or nasal cannula (Kinsella et al. 2003). There is limited experience with other pharmacologic pulmonary vasodilators (e.g., prostacyclin, endothelin antagonists, and phosphodiesterase inhibitors) in infants with CDH and late PH. Olson et al. recently described two infants with CDH and severe PH at 6 weeks of age who responded favorably to treatment with trepostinil (Olson et al. 2015). Clearly, further investigation is needed to define an approach to the management of late PH in this population.

60.4.5 Chronic Pulmonary Hypertension in CDH

Chronic PH may persist in CDH over months and years, and enduring structural and functional abnormalities of pulmonary circulation in the ipsilateral and contralateral lung can complicate the course of the disease. Cardiac catheterization of seven patients with CDH who survived the neonatal period with protracted or recurrent PH revealed a range of pulmonary vascular abnormalities (Kinsella et al. 2005). These patients (age range, 3 months–12 years) had a history of severe hypoxemic respiratory failure and PH as newborns. At catheterization, therapies included supplemental oxygen ($n = 7$), iNO ($n = 2$), prostacyclin ($n = 2$), and bosentan ($n = 1$). Three of the seven patients had significant pulmonary vascular abnormalities in the lung contralateral to the initial diaphragmatic defect. Major findings at cardiac catheterization included left pulmonary artery hypoplasia or stenosis in three patients and pulmonary vein stenosis or delayed venous return in six patients. Two patients with right-sided diaphragmatic defect had striking left-sided pulmonary venous abnormalities. One patient with right-sided CDH was discharged home, but died at age 5 months with marked pulmonary vascular changes on autopsy consistent with severe PH. After a median follow-up of 12 months from catheterization, five patients were alive and discharged from hospital. The two patients with the most severe PH died from related complications at ages 8 and 19 months.

In some patients with CDH, significant PH, which may be subclinical, clearly continues beyond the neonatal period, contributing to morbidity and mortality. Understanding the pathophysiology underlying these long-term effects will require a more sophisticated view of CDH than that originating solely from in utero cardiopulmonary compression. It is possible that the injury associated with management of hypoxemic respiratory failure in newborns with CDH may cause previously unrecognized long-term effects in susceptible individuals, and/or the pulmonary circulation in patients with severe CDH may be fundamentally altered in utero, leading to abnormal responses to injury that last far beyond the newborn period (Kinsella and Abman 2000).

60.4.6 Improving Outcomes in CDH

Treatment strategies for CDH continue to evolve with increasing clinical experience and greater insight into the underlying nature of the condition. These strategies include simultaneous postductal and preductal samples to measure blood gases (adjusting ventilator support accordingly) (Table 1). Early ECHO is essential to define pulmonary artery pressure (PAP) and assess LV size

Table 1 Current approach to optimize management of CDH and related PH at Children's Hospital Colorado

Adequate access with preductal arterial line, four central venous ports
Importance of preductal ABG monitoring with R-L PDA
Postductal ABG: 7.30/56/45
Preductal ABG: 7.35/44/136
Early ECHO
Definition of PA pressure
Assessment of LV size and function
LV performance
Atrial shunt
Delayed iNO until ECHO evidence of adequate LV performance
Minimize volutrauma with low TV/PIP; early use of HFOV
LV afterload reduction with milrinone, consider maintenance of ductal patency with PGE1
Treat adrenal insufficiency
Avoid surfactant treatment
Delayed repair of defect
Achieve hemodynamic stability and decreased PVR
Consider NICU repair
Avoid interruption of ventilatory strategy
ECMO if indicated
Cardiac performance
Preductal desaturation with worsening acidemia
Nasal cannula NO postextubation for persistent PH

ABG arterial blood gas, *ECHO* echocardiogram, *ECMO* extracorporeal membrane oxygenation, *HFOV* high frequency oscillatory ventilation, *iNO* inhaled nitric oxide, *LV* left ventricle, *NICU* neonatal intensive care unit, *NO* nitric oxide, *PA* pulmonary artery, *PGE1* prostaglandin E1, *PDA* patent ductus arteriosus, *PH* pulmonary hypertension, *PVR* pulmonary vascular resistance, *TV/PIP* tidal volume/peak inspiratory pressure

and function. It is reasonable to delay the use of pulmonary vasodilator therapy until there is ECHO evidence of adequate LV performance. Reducing LV afterload pharmacologically may play an important role (e.g., milrinone), as well as maintaining ductal patency with prostaglandin E1 (PGE1) if RV-dependent systemic circulation is demonstrated by ECHO. Adrenal insufficiency also complicates the course of newborns with severe CDH and decreases catecholamine drug responsiveness (Kamath et al. 2010).

Despite refinement of postnatal interventions, limitations persist and treatment of CDH and pulmonary hypertension remain suboptimal. Consequently, new therapeutic options such as prenatal intervention or cell-based therapy are the subject of current investigation. The effects of LV dysfunction/hypoplasia on the neonatal course in severe CDH provides a compelling reason to study fetal intervention. The efficacy of prenatal intervention with percutaneous fetoscopic endoluminal tracheal occlusion (FETO) therapy in CDH has been described in case series and controlled studies (Jani et al. 2011; Ruano et al. 2012). The potential role of FETO is being investigated in CDH in a European and North American collaboration called the Tracheal Occlusion To Accelerate Lung Growth (TOTAL) Trial (Ruano et al. 2012).

Mesenchymal stem cells (MSCs) also represent an emerging therapeutic approach in CDH. Several experimental studies in animal models have shown that treatment with MSCs can reduce pulmonary injury and PH (Aslam et al. 2009; Hoffman et al. 2011). A recent study in a rat model of experimental CDH found that MSC transplantation promotes alveolar and pulmonary artery development, reducing the severity of pulmonary hypoplasia (Yuniartha et al. 2014).

60.5 Conclusion

In summary, the early course of CDH is characterized by severe PH, and cardiac, lung parenchymal, and airway abnormalities. Acute treatment of PH in CDH with pulmonary vasodilator therapy is limited by structural and functional changes of the left ventricle. In a significant subset of newborns with severe CDH, late or protracted PH occurs and may persist weeks to months following improvement in respiratory failure and cardiac performance. In contrast to early CDH, pulmonary vasodilator therapy plays a critical role in management of late PH in CDH and potentially improves survival.

Despite progress in CDH management, advances have been limited by the lack of randomized controlled trials to properly test new treatments. Major differences in clinical practice regarding the ascertainment and treatment of PH make it difficult to determine the most effective strategies to manage late PH in CDH infants. Moreover, institutional practices that lead to "improved" outcomes are slowly adopted and local changes are often guided only by experience and conviction. To overcome these barriers, centers with the best outcomes for isolated CDH should be identified from current databases and their practices disseminated to the wider community. Improving outcomes in patients with CDH will require continued vigilance, multidisciplinary collaboration, and widespread adoption of best practices.

References

Abman SH (2001) Bronchopulmonary dysplasia: a "vascular hypothesis". Am J Respir Crit Care Med 164:1755–1756

Abman SH, Accurso FJ (1989) Acute effects of partial compression of ductus arteriosus on fetal pulmonary circulation. Am J Physiol Heart Circ Physiol 26: H626–H634

Abman SH, Kinsella JP (1995) Inhaled nitric oxide for persistent pulmonary hypertension of the newborn: the physiology matters. Pediatrics 96:1153–1155

Abman SH, Chatfield BA, Hall SL, McMurtry IF (1990) Role of endothelium-derived relaxing factor activity during transition of pulmonary circulation at birth. Am J Physiol (Heart Circ Physiol 28) 259: H1921–H1927

Abman SH, Griebel JL, Parker DK et al (1994) Acute effects of inhaled nitric oxide in severe hypoxemic respiratory failure in pediatrics. J Pediatr 124:881–888

Acute Respiratory Distress Syndrome Network (2000) Ventilation with lower tidal volumes as compared

with traditional tidal volumes for acute lung injury and the ARDS. N Engl J Med 342:1301–1308
Adel Mohamed MD, Nehad Nasef MD, Vibhuti Shah MD, Patrick J, McNamara MD (2014) Vasopressin as a rescue therapy for refractory pulmonary hypertension in neonates: case series. Pediatr Crit Care Med 15:148–154
Agrawal A, Singh VK, Varma A, Sharma R (2012) Therapeutic applications of vasopressin in pediatric patients. Indian Pediatr 49:297–305
Alano MA, Ngougmna E, Ostrea EM Jr, Konduri GG (2001) Analysis of nonsteroidal antiinflammatory drugs in meconium and its relation to persistent pulmonary hypertension of the newborn. Pediatrics 107(3):519–523
Antunes MJ, Greenspan JS, Holt WJ, Vallieu DS, Spitzer AR (1994) Assessment of lung function pre-nitric oxide therapy: a predictor of response? Pediatr Res 35:212A
Aslam M, Baveja R, Liang OD, Fernandez-Gonzalez A, Lee C, Mitsialis SA et al (2009) Bone marrow stromal cells attenuate lung injury in a murine model of neonatal chronic lung disease. Am J Respir Crit Care Med 180:1122–1130
Atz AM, Wessel DL (1999) Sildenafil ameliorates effects of inhaled nitric oxide withdrawal. Anesthesiology 91:307–310
Balasubramaniam V, Le Cras TD, Ivy DD, Kinsella J, Grover TR, Abman SH (2003) Role of platelet-derived growth factor in the pathogenesis of perinatal pulmonary hypertension. Am J Phys Lung Cell Mol Phys 284:L826–L833
Ballard RA, Truog WE, Cnaan A et al (2006) Inhaled nitric oxide in preterm infants undergoing mechanical ventilation. N Engl J Med 205:343–353
Baumgart S, Paul JJ, Huhta JC, Katz AL, Paul KE, Spettell C et al (1998) Cardiac malposition, redistribution of fetal cardiac output, and left heart hypoplasia reduce survival in neonates with congenital diaphragmatic hernia requiring extracorporeal membrane oxygenation. J Pediatr 133:5762
Behrman RE (1976) Persistence of the fetal circulation. J Pediatr 89:636–637
Brennan LA, Steinhorn RH, Wedgwood S, Mata-Greenwood E, Roark EA, Russell JA, Black SM (2003) Increased superoxide generation is associated with pulmonary hypertension in fetal lambs. A role for NADPH oxidase. Circ Res 92:683–691
Byrne FA, Keller RL, Meadows J, Miniati D, Brook MM, Silverman NH et al (2015) Severe left diaphragmatic hernia limits size of fetal left heart more than right diaphragmatic hernia. Ultrasound Obstet Gynecol 46(6):688–94
Chambers CD, Hernandez-Diaz S, Van Marter LJ, Werler MM, Louik C, Jones KL, Mitchell AA (2006) Selective serotonin-reuptake inhibitors and risk of persistent pulmonary hypertension of the newborn. N Engl J Med 354(6):579–587
Chester M, Tourneux P, Seedorf G, Grover TR, Abman SH (2009) Cinaciguat, a soluble guanylate cyclase activator, causes potent and sustained pulmonary vasodilation in the ovine fetus. Am J Physiol 297:L318
Clark RH, Kueser TJ, Walker MW et al (2000) Low-dose nitric oxide therapy for persistent pulmonary hypertension of the newborn. Clinical inhaled nitric oxide research group. N Engl J Med 342:469–474
Cole FS, Alleyne C, Barks JD, Boyle RJ, Carroll JL, Dokken D, Edwards WH, Georgieff M, Gregory K, Johnston MV, Kramer M, Mitchell C, Neu J, Pursley DM, Robinson WM, Rowitch DH (2011) NIH consensus development conference statement: inhaled nitric-oxide therapy for premature infants. Pediatrics 127 (2):363–369
Cornfield DN, Chatfield BA, McQueston JA, McMurtry IF, Abman SH (1992) Effects of birth related stimuli on L-arginine-dependent vasodilation in the ovine fetus. Am J Physiol (Heart Circ Physiol 31) 262: H1474–H1481
Cornfield DN, Maynard RC, deRegnier RO, Guaing SF, Barbato JE, Milla CE (1999) Randomized, controlled trial of low-dose inhaled nitric oxide in the treatment of term and near-term infants with respiratory failure and pulmonary hypertension. Pediatrics 104:1089–1094
Cotton EK (1965) The use of priscoline in the treatment of the hypoperfusion syndrome. Pediatrics 36:149
Davidson D, Barefield ES, Kattwinkel J et al (1998) Inhaled nitric oxide for the early treatment of persistent pulmonary hypertension of the term newborn: a randomized, double-masked, placebo-controlled, dose – response, multicenter study. Pediatrics 101:325–334
Deprest J, De CP (2012) Antenatal management of isolated congenital diaphragmatic hernia today and tomorrow: ongoing collaborative research and development. Journal of pediatric surgery lecture. J Pediatr Surg 47:282–290
Evora PR, Pearson PJ, Schaff HV (1993) Arginine vasopressin induces endothelium-dependent vasodilation of the pulmonary artery. V1-receptor-mediated production of nitric oxide. Chest 103:1241–1245
Faraci F, Didion S (2004) Vascular protection: Superoxide dismutase isoforms in the vessel wall. Arterioscler Thromb Vasc Biol 24:1367–1373
Farrow KN, Lakshminrusimha S, Reda WJ, Wedgwood S, Czech L, Gugino SF, Davis JM, Russell JA, Steinhorn RH (2008a) Superoxide dismutase restores eNOS expression and function in resistance pulmonary arteries from neonatal lambs with persistent pulmonary hypertension. Am J Phys Lung Cell Mol Phys 295(6): L979–L987
Farrow KN, Groh BS, Schumacker PT, Lakshminrusimha S, Czech L, Gugino SF, Russell JA, Steinhorn RH (2008b) Hyperoxia increases phosphodiesterase 5 expression and activity in ovine fetal pulmonary artery smooth muscle cells. Circ Res 102 (2):226–233
Field DJ (2005) Nitric oxide-still no consensus. Early Hum Dev 81:1–4
Field D, Elbourne D, Truesdale A et al (2005) Neonatal ventilation with inhaled nitric oxide versus ventilatory

support without inhaled nitric oxide for preterm infants with severe respiratory failure: the INNOVO multicentre randomized controlled trial. Pediatrics 115:926–936

Fike CD, Slaughter JC, Kaplowitz MR, Zhang Y, Aschner JL (2008) Reactive oxygen species from NADPH oxidase contribute to altered pulmonary vascular responses in piglets with chronic hypoxia-induced pulmonary hypertension. Am J Phys Lung Cell Mol Phys 295(5):L881–L888

Filippi L, Gozzini E, Daniotti M, Pagliai F, Catarzi S, Fiorini P (2011) Rescue treatment with terlipressin in different scenarios of refractory hypotension in newborns and infants. Pediatr Crit Care Med 12:e237–e241

Finer NN (2005) Inhaled nitric oxide for preterm infants: A therapy in search of an indication? The search continues. J Pediatr 146:301–302

Finer NN, Etches PC, Kamstra B et al (1994) Inhaled nitric oxide in infants referred for extracorporeal membrane oxygenation: dose response. J Pediatr 124:302–308

Finer NN, Sun JW, Rich W, Knodel E, Barrington KJ (2001) Randomized, prospective study of low-dose versus high-dose inhaled nitric oxide in the neonate with hypoxic respiratory failure. Pediatrics 108:949–955

Fornaro E, Li D, Pan J, Belik J (2007) Prenatal exposure to fluoxetine induces fetal pulmonary hypertension in the rat. Am J Respir Crit Care Med 176(10):1035–1040

Fox WW, Gewitz MH, Dinwiddie R, Drummond WH, Peckham GJ (1977) Pulmonary hypertension in the perinatal aspiration syndromes. Pediatrics 59:205–211

Frostell C, Fratacci MD, Wain JC, Jones R, Zapol WM (1991) A selective pulmonary vasodilator reversing hypoxic pulmonary vasoconstriction. Circulation 83:2038–2047

Furchgott RF, Zawadzki JV (1980) The obligatory role of endothelial cells in the relaxation of arterial smooth muscle by acetylcholine. Nature 288:373–376

Geggel RL, Reid LM (1984) The structural basis of PPHN. Clin Perinatol 11:525–549

Gerlach H, Rossaint R, Pappert D, Falke KJ (1993) Time-course and dose-response of nitric oxide inhalation for systemic oxygenation and pulmonary hypertension in patients with adult respiratory distress syndrome. Eur J Clin Invest 23:499–502

Gersony WM (1984) Neonatal pulmonary hypertension: pathophysiology, classification and etiology. Clin Perinatol 11:517–524

Gersony WM, Duc GV, Sinclair JC (1969) "PFC" syndrome (persistence of the fetal circulation). Circulation 40:111

Gien J, Kinsella JP (2015) Differences in preductal and postductal arterial blood gas measurements in infants with severe congenital diaphragmatic hernia. Arch Dis Child Fetal Neonatal Ed 101:F314

Goetzman BW, Sunshine P, Johnson JD, Wennberg RP, Hackel A, Merten DF et al (1976) Neonatal hypoxia and pulmonary vasospasm: response to tolazoline. J Pediatr 89:617–621

Goldman AP, Tasker RC, Haworth SG, Sigston PE, Macrae DJ (1996) Four patterns of response to inhaled nitric oxide for persistent pulmonary hypertension of the newborn. Pediatrics 98:706–713

Gordon JB, Martinez FR, Keller PA, Tod ML, Madden JA (1993) Differing effects of actue and prolonged alkalosis on hypoxic pulmonary vasoconstriction. Am Rev Respir Dis 148:1651–1656

Grover TR, Parker TA, Zenge JP, Markham NE, Abman SH (2003) Intrauterine pulmonary hypertension decreases lung VEGF expression and VEGF inhibition causes pulmonary hypertension in the ovine fetus. Am J Phys 284:L508–L517

Grover TR, Parker TA, Hunt-Peacock C, Markham NE, Abman SH (2005) rhVEGF treatment improves pulmonary vasoreactivity and structure in an experimental model of pulmonary hypertension in fetal sheep. Am J Physiol LCMP 289:L529–L535

Hamon I, Fresson J, Nicolas MB et al (2005) Early inhaled nitric oxide improves oxidative balance in very preterm infants. Pediatr Res 57:637–643

Hanson KA, Abman SH, Clarke WR (1996) Elevation of pulmonary PDE5-specific activity in an experimental fetal ovine perinatal pulmonary hypertension model. Pediatr Res 39:334A

Harrison MR, de Lorimier AA (1981) Congenital diaphragmatic hernia. Surg Clin North Am 61:1023–1035

Hascoet JM, Fresson J, Claris O et al (2005) The safety and efficacy of nitric oxide therapy in premature infants. J Pediatr 146:318–323

Haworth SG, Reid L (1976) Persistent fetal circulation: newly recognized structural features. J Pediatr 88:614–620

Hibbs AM, Walsh MC, Martin RJ, Truog WE, Lorch SA, Alessandrini E, Cnaan A, Palermo L, Wadlinger SR, Coburn CE, Ballard PL, Ballard RA (2008) One-year respiratory outcomes of preterm infants enrolled in the nitric oxide (to prevent) chronic lung disease trial. J Pediatr 153(4):525–529

Higenbottam T, Pepke-Zaba J, Scott J, Woolman P, Coutts C, Wallwork J (1988) Inhaled "endothelium-derived relaxing factor" (EDRF) in primary hypertension (PPH). Am Rev Respir Dis 137:107S

Hintz SR, Van Meurs KP, Perritt R, Poole WK, Das A, Stevenson DK, Ehrenkranz RA, Lemons JA, Vohr BR, Heyne R, Childers DO, Peralta-Carcelen M, Dusick A, Johnson YR, Morris B, Dillard R, Vaucher Y, Steichen J, Adams-Chapman I, Konduri G, Myers GJ, de Ungria M, Tyson JE, Higgins RD, NICHD Neonatal Research Network (2007) Neurodevelopmental outcomes of premature infants with severe respiratory failure enrolled in a randomized controlled trial of inhaled nitric oxide. J Pediatr 151(1):16–22

Hoffman AM, Paxson JA, Mazan MR, Davis AM, Tyagi S, Murthy S et al (2011) Lung-derived mesenchymal stromal cell post-transplantation survival, persistence, paracrine expression, and repair of elastase-injured lung. Stem Cells Dev 20:1779–1792

Ichinose F, Erana-Garcia J, Hromi J, Raveh Y, Jones R, Krim L, Clark MWH, Winkler JD, Bloch KD, Zapol WM (2001) Nebulized sildenafil is a selective pulmonary vasodilator in lambs with acute pulmonary hypertension. Crit Care Med 29:1000–1005

Ignarro LJ, Buga GM, Wood KS, Byrns RE, Chaudhuri G (1987) Endothelium-derived relaxing factor produced and released from artery and vein is nitric oxide. Proc Natl Acad Sci U S A 84:9265–9269

Ivy DD, Ziegler JW, Dubus MF, Fox JJ, Kinsella JP, Abman SH (1996) Chronic intrauterine pulmonary hypertension alters endothelin receptor activity in the ovine fetal lung. Pediatr Res 39:435–442

Ivy DD, Parker TA, Ziegler JW, Galan HL, Kinsella JP, Tuder RM, Abman SH (1997) Prolonged endothelin A receptor blockade attenuates pulmonary hypertension in the ovine fetus. J Clin Invest 99:1179–1186

Ivy DD, Le Cras TD, Horan MP, Abman SH (1998) Increased lung preproET-1 and decreased ETB-receptor gene expression in fetal pulmonary hypertension. Am J Phys 274(4 Pt 1):L535–L541

Jani J, Valencia C, Cannie M, Vuckovic A, Sellars M, Nicolaides KH (2011) Tracheal diameter at birth in severe congenital diaphragmatic hernia treated by fetal endoscopic tracheal occlusion. Prenat Diagn 31:699–704

Kamath BD, Fashaw L, Kinsella JP (2010) Adrenal insufficiency in newborns with congenital diaphragmatic hernia. J Pediatr 156:495–497

Kelly LK, Porta NF, Goodman DM, Carroll CL, Steinhorn RH (2002) Inhaled prostacyclin for term infants with persistent pulmonary hypertension refractory to inhaled nitric oxide. J Pediatr 141:830–832

Kinsella JP, Abman SH (1995) Recent developments in the pathophysiology and treatment of persistent pulmonary hypertension of the newborn. J Pediatr 126:853–864

Kinsella JP, Abman SH (2000) Clinical approach to inhaled nitric oxide therapy in the newborn with hypoxemia. J Pediatr 136:717–726

Kinsella JP, McQueston JA, Rosenberg AA, Abman SH (1992a) Hemodynamic effects of exogenous nitric oxide in ovine transitional pulmonary circulation. Am J Phys 262:H875–H880

Kinsella JP, Neish SR, Shaffer E, Abman SH (1992b) Low-dose inhalational nitric oxide in persistent pulmonary hypertension of the newborn. Lancet 340:819–820

Kinsella JP, Neish SR, Ivy DD, Shaffer E, Abman SH (1993) Clinical responses to prolonged treatment of persistent pulmonary hypertension of the newborn with low doses of inhaled nitric oxide. J Pediatr 123:103–108

Kinsella JP, Truog WE, Walsh WF et al (1997) Randomized, multicenter trial of inhaled nitric oxide and high frequency oscillatory ventilation in severe persistent pulmonary hypertension of the newborn. J Pediatr 131:55–62

Kinsella JP, Walsh WF, Bose CL et al (1999) Inhaled nitric oxide in premature neonates with severe hypoxaemic respiratory failure: a randomised controlled trial. Lancet 354:1061–1065

Kinsella JP, Parker TA, Ivy DD, Abman SH (2003) Noninvasive delivery of inhaled nitric oxide therapy for late pulmonary hypertension in newborn infants with congenital diaphragmatic hernia. J Pediatr 142:397–401

Kinsella JP, Ivy DD, Abman SH (2005) Pulmonary vasodilator therapy in congenital diaphragmatic hernia: acute, late, and chronic pulmonary hypertension. Semin Perinatol 29:123–128

Kinsella JP, Cutter GR, Walsh WF et al (2006) Early inhaled nitric oxide therapy in premature newborns with respiratory failure. N Engl J Med 205:354–364

Konduri GG, Ou J, Shi Y, Pritchard KA Jr (2003) Decreased association of HSP90 impairs endothelial nitric oxide synthase in fetal lambs with persistent pulmonary hypertension. Am J Physiol Heart Circ Physiol 285(1):H204–H211

Konduri GG, Solimani A, Sokol GM, Singer J, Ehrenkranz RA, Singhal N, Wright LL, Van Meurs K, Stork E, Kirpalani H, Peliowski A, Group NINOS (2004) A randomized trial of early versus standard inhaled nitric oxide therapy in term and near-term newborn infants with hypoxic respiratory failure. Pediatrics 113: 559–564

Konduri GG, Bakhutashvili I, Eis A, Pritchard KA (2007) Oxidant stress from uncoupled nitric oxide synthase impairs vasodilation in fetal lambs with persistent pulmonary hypertension. Am J Physiol Heart Circ Physiol 292:H1812–H1820

Korones SB, Eyal FB (1975) Succesful treatment of "persistent fetal circulation" with tolazoline. Pediatr Res 9:367

Laffey JG, Engelberts D, Kavanaugh BP (2000) Inurious effects of hypocapnic alkalosis in the isolated lung. Am J Respir Crit Care Med 162:399–405

Lakshminrusimha S, Russell JA, Wedgwood S, Gugino SF, Kazzaz JA, Davis JM, Steinhorn RH (2006a) Superoxide dismutase improves oxygenation and reduces oxidation in neonatal pulmonary hypertension. Am J Respir Crit Care Med 174(12):1370–1377. Epub 2006 Sep 1328

Lakshminrusimha S, Russell JA, Steinhorn RH, Ryan RM, Gugino SF, Morin FC 3rd, Swartz DD, Kumar VH (2006b) Pulmonary arterial contractility in neonatal lambs increases with 100% oxygen resuscitation. Pediatr Res 59(1):137–141. Epub 2005 Dec 2002

Lakshminrusimha S, Russell JA, Steinhorn RH, Swartz DD, Ryan RM, Gugino SF, Wynn KA, Kumar VH, Mathew B, Kirmani K, Morin FC 3rd (2007) Pulmonary hemodynamics in neonatal lambs resuscitated with 21%, 50%, and 100% oxygen. Pediatr Res 62:313–318

Le LD, Keswani SG, Biesiada J, Lim FY, Kingma PS, Haberman BE et al (2012) The congenital diaphragmatic hernia composite prognostic index correlates with survival in left-sided congenital diaphragmatic hernia. J Pediatr Surg 47:57–62

Lees MH (1970) Cyanosis of the newborn. J Pediatr 77:484–498

Levin DL, Heymann MA, Kitterman JA, Gregory GA, Phibbs RH, Rudolph AM (1976) Persistent pulmonary hypertension of the newborn infant. J Pediatr 89:626–630

Levin DL, Hyman AI, Heymann MA, Rudolph AM (1978) Fetal hypertension and the development of increased pulmonary vascular smooth muscle: a possible mechanism for persistent pulmonary hypertension of the newborn infant. J Pediatr 92:265–269

Lipshutz GS, Albanese CT, Feldstein VA, Jennings RW, Housley HT, Beech R et al (1997) Prospective analysis of lung-to-head ratio predicts survival for patients with prenatally diagnosed congenital diaphragmatic hernia. J Pediatr Surg 32:1634–1636

Luccini B, Bimonetti GD, Ceschi A, Lava SA, Fare PB, Bianchetti MG (2013) Severe signs of hyponatremia secondary to desmopressin treatment for enuresis: a systematic review. J Pediatr Urol 9:1049–1053

Lusk LA, Wai KC, Moon-Grady AJ, Steurer MA, Keller RL (2015) Persistence of pulmonary hypertension by echocardiography predicts short-term outcomes in congenital diaphragmatic hernia. J Pediatr 166: 251–256

Martin RJ, Walsh MC (2005) Inhaled nitric oxide for preterm infants – who benefits? N Engl J Med 353:82–84

McNamara PJ, Laique F, Muang-In S, Whyte HE (2006) Milrinone improves oxygenation in neonates with severe persistent pulmonary hypertension of the newborn. J Crit Care 21(2):217–222

McQueston JA, Cornfield DN, McMurtry IF, Abman SH (1993) Effects of oxygen and exogenous L-arginine on EDRF activity in fetal pulmonary circulation. Am J Physiol Heart Circ Physiol 264:865–871

McQueston JA, Kinsella JP, Ivy DD, McMurtry IF, Abman SH (1995) Chronic pulmonary hypertension in utero impairs endothelium-dependent vasodilation. Am J Physiol Heart Circ Physiol 268:H288–H294

Mercier JC, Hummler H, Durrmeyer X, Sanchez-Luna M, Carnielli V, Field D, Greenough A, Van Overmeire B, Jonsson B, Hallman M, Baldassarre J, EUNO Study Group (2010) Inhaled nitric oxide for prevention of bronchopulmonary dysplasia in premature babies (EUNO): a randomised controlled trial. Lancet 376 (9738):346–354

Mestan KK, Marks JD, Hecox K et al (2005) Neurodevelopmental outcomes of premature infants treated with inhaled nitric oxide. N Engl J Med 353:23–32

Meurs KP, Rhine WD, Asselin JM, Duran DJ (1997) Response of premature infants with severe respiratory failure to inhaled nitric oxide. Preemie NO collaborative group. Pediatr Pulmonol 24:319–323

Mohamed WA, Ismail M (2012) A randomized, double-blind, placebo-controlled, prospective study of bosentan for the treatment of persistent pulmonary hypertension of the newborn. J Perinatol 32(8):608–613

Morin FC III, Eagan EA (1989) The effect of closing the ductus arteriosus on the pulmonary circulation of the fetal sheep. J Dev Physiol 11:245–250

Murphy J, Aronovitz M, Reid L (1986) Effects of chronic in utero hypoxia on the pulmonary vasculature of the newborn guinea pig. Pediatr Res 20:292–295

Neonatal Inhaled Nitric Oxide Study Group (1997) Inhaled nitric oxide in full-term and nearly full-term infants with hypoxic respiratory failure. N Engl J Med 336:597–604

Olson E, Lusk LA, Fineman JR, Robertson L, Keller RL (2015) Short-term treprostinil use in infants with congenital diaphragmatic hernia following repair. J Pediatr 167:762–764

Palmer RMJ, Ferrige AG, Moncada S (1987) Nitric oxide release accounts for the biological activity of endothelium-derived relaxing factor. Nature 327: 524–526

Parker TA, Ivy DD, Kinsella JP, Torielli F, Ruyle SZ, Thilo EH, Abman SH (1997) Combined therapy with inhaled nitric oxide and intravenous prostacyclin in an infant with alveolar-capillary dysplasia. Am J Respir Crit Care Med 155:743–746

Patterson K, Kapur SP, Chandra RS (1988) PPHN: pulmonary pathologic effects. In: Rosenberg HS, Berstein J (eds) Cardiovascular diseases, perspectives in pediatric pathology, vol 12. Karger, Basel, pp 139–154

Pearson DL, Dawling S, Walsh WF, Haines JL, Christman BW, Bazyk A, Scott N, Summar ML (2001) Neonatal pulmonary hypertension-urea-cycle intermediates, nitric oxide production, and carbamoyl-phosphate synthetase function. N Engl J Med 344(24):1832–1838

Peliowski A, Finer NN, Etches PC, Tierney AJ, Ryan CA (1995) Inhaled nitric oxide for premature infants after prolonged rupture of the membranes. J Pediatr 126:450–453

Pepke-Zaba J, Higenbottam TW, Dinh-Xuan AT, Stone D, Wallwork J (1991) Inhaled nitric oxide as a cause of selective pulmonary vasodilation in pulmonary hypertension. Lancet 338:1173–1174

Pierro M, Thebaud B (2014) Understanding and treating pulmonary hypertension in congenital diaphragmatic hernia. Semin Fetal Neonatal Med 19:357–363

Radicioni M, Troiani S, Camerini PG (2012) Effects of terlipressin on pulmonary artery pressure in a septic cooled infant: an echocardiographic assessment. J Perinatol 32:893–895

Roberton NRC, Hallidie-Smith DA, Davis JA (1967) Severe respiratory distress syndrome mimicking cyanotic heart disease in term babies. Lancet 2: 1108–1110

Roberts JD, Polaner DM, Lang P et al (1992) Inhaled nitric oxide in persistent pulmonary hypertension of the newborn. Lancet 340:818–819

Roberts JD, Chen TY, Kawai N et al (1993) Inhaled nitric oxide reverses pulmonary vasoconstriction in the hypoxic and acidotic newborn lamb. Circ Res 72:246–254

Roberts JD, Fineman JR, Morin FC et al (1997) Inhaled nitric oxide and persistent pulmonary hypertension of the newborn. N Engl J Med 336:605–610

Rosenberg AA, Kennaugh J, Koppenhafer SL, Loomis M, Chatfield BA, Abman SH (1993) Elevated

immunoreactive endothelin-1 levels in newborn infants with persistent pulmonary hypertension. J Pediatr 123:109–114

Rossaint R, Falke KJ, Lopez F et al (1993) Inhaled nitric oxide for the adult respiratory distress syndrome. NEJM 328:399–405

Ruano R, Yoshisaki CT, da Silva MM, Ceccon ME, Grasi MS, Tannuri U et al (2012) A randomized controlled trial of fetal endoscopic tracheal occlusion versus postnatal management of severe isolated congenital diaphragmatic hernia. Ultrasound Obstet Gynecol 39:20–27

Rudolph AM (1980) High pulmonary vascular resistance after birth: pathophysiologic considerations and etiologic classification. Clin Pediatr 19:585–590

Rudolph AM, Drorbraugh JE, Auld PAM, Rudolph AJ, Nadas AS, Smith CA, Hubbell JP (1961) Studies in the circulation in the neonatal period. The circulation in the respiratory distress syndrome. Pediatrics 27:551–556

Russ RD, Walker BR (1992) Role of nitric oxide in vasopressinergic pulmonary vasodilatation. Am J Phys 262:H743–H747

Scheurer MA, Scott MB, Atz AM (2005) Vasopressin to attenuate pulmonary hypertension and improve systemic blood pressure after correction of obstructed total anomalous pulmonary venous return. J Thorac Cardiovasc Surg 129:464–466

Schreiber MD, Gin-Mestan K, Marks JD et al (2003) Inhaled nitric oxide in premature infants with the respiratory distress syndrome. N Engl J Med 349:2099–2107

Share L (1988) Role of vasopressin in cardiovascular regulation. Physiol Rev 68:1248–1284

Shaul PW, Yuhanna IS, German Z, Chen Z, Steinhorn RH, Morin FC III (1997) Pulmonary endothelial NO synthase gene expression is decreased in fetal lambs with pulmonary hypertension. Am J Phys Lung Cell Mol Phys 272:L1005–L1012

Shekerdemian L, Ravn H, Penny D (2002) Intravenous sildenafil lowers pulmonary vascular resistance in a model of neonatal pulmonary hypertension. Am J Respir Crit Care Med 165:1098–2002

Shekerdemian LS, Ravn HB, Penny DJ (2004) Interaction between inhaled nitric oxide and intravenous sildenafil in a porcine model of meconium aspiration syndrome. Pediatr Res 55(3):413–418. Epub 2004 Jan 2007

SIassi B, Goldberg SJ, Emmanouilides GC, Higashimo SM, Lewis E (1971) Persistent pulmonary vascular obstruction in newborn infants. J Pediatr 78:610–615

Stahlman M (1964) Treatment of cardiovascular diseases of the newborn. Pediatr Clin N Am 11:363–400

Steinhorn RH, Russell JA, Morin FC III (1995) Disruption of cyclic GMP production in pulmonary arteries isolated from fetal lambs with pulmonary hypertension. Am J Physiol Heart Circ Physiol 268: H1483–H1489

Steinhorn RH, Kinsella JP, Butrous G, Dilleen M, Oakes M, Wessel DL (2007) Open-label, multicentre, pharmacokinetic study of IV sildenafil in the treatment of neonates with persistent pulmonary hypertension of the newborn (PPHN). Circulation 116:II–614

Stevenson DK, Kasting DS, Darnall RA et al (1979) Refractory hypoxemia associated with neonatal pulmonary disease: the use and limitations of tolazoline. J Pediatr 95:595–599

Storme L, Rairigh RL, Parker TA, Kinsella JP, Abman SH (1999) Acute intrauterine pulmonary hypertension impairs endothelium dependent vasodilation in the ovine fetus. Pediatr Res 45:575–581

Subhedar NV, Ryan SW, Shaw NJ (1997) Open randomised controlled trial of inhaled nitric oxide and early dexamethasone in high risk preterm infants. Arch Dis Child 77:F185–F190

Taira Y, Yamataka T, Miyazaki E, Puri P (1998) Comparison of the pulmonary vasculature in newborns and stillborns with congenital diaphragmatic hernia. Pediatr Surg Int 14:30–35

The Franco – Belgium Collaborative NO Trial Group (1999) Early compared with delayed inhaled nitric oxide in moderately hypoxaemic neonates with respiratory failure: a randomised controlled trial. Lancet 354:1066–1071

The Neonatal Inhaled Nitric Oxide Study Group (NINOS) (1997) Inhaled nitric oxide and hypoxic respiratory failure in infants with congenital diaphragmatic hernia. Pediatrics 99:838–845

Tiktinsky MH, Morin FC (1993) Increasing oxygen tension dilates fetal pulmonary circulation via endothelium-derived relaxing factor. Am J Phys 265:H376–H380

Tzao C, Nickerson PA, Russell JA, Gugino SF, Steinhorn RH (2001) Pulmonary hypertension alters soluble guanylate cyclase activity and expression in pulmonary arteries isolated from fetal lambs. Pediatr Pulmonol 31:97–105

van der Cammen-van Zijp MH, Janssen AJ, Raets MM, van Rosmalen J, Govaert P, Steiner K, Gischler SJ, Tibboel D, van Heijst AF (2014) IJsselstijn H; Dutch ECMO follow-up team. Motor performance after neonatal extracorporeal membrane oxygenation: a longitudinal evaluation. Pediatrics 134(2):e427–e435

Van Marter LJ, Leviton A, Allred EN (1996) PPHN and smoking and aspirin and nonsteroidal antiinflammatory drug consumption during pregnancy. Pediatrics 97:658–663

Van Meurs KP, Wright LL, Ehrenkranz RA et al (2005) Inhaled nitric oxide for premature infants with severe respiratory failure. N Engl J Med 353:13–22

Villamor E, LeCras TD, Horan MP, Halbower AC, Tuder RM, Abman SH (1997) Chronic intrauterine pulmonary hypertension impairs endothelial nitric oxide synthase in the ovine fetus. Am J Phys Lung Cell Mol Phys 272:L1013–L1020

Walsh MC, Hibbs AM, Martin CR, Cnaan A, Keller RL, Vittinghoff E, Martin RJ, Truog WE, Ballard PL, Zadell A, Wadlinger SR, Coburn CE, Ballard RA, NO CLD Study Group (2010) Two-year neurodevelopmental outcomes of ventilated preterm infants treated with inhaled nitric oxide. J Pediatr 156(4):556–61.e1. https://doi.org/10.1016/j.jpeds.2009.10.011. Epub 2010 Feb 6

Walsh-Sukys MC, Tyson JE, Wright LL, Bauer CR, Korones SB, Stevenson DK, Verter J, Stoll BJ, Lemons

JA, Papile LA, Shankaran S, Donovan EF, Oh W, Ehrenkranz RA, Fanaroff AA (2000) Persistent pulmonary hypertension of the newborn in the era before nitric oxide: practice variation and outcomes. Pediatrics 105:14–20

Wedgwood S, Black SM (2003) Role of reactive oxygen species in vascular remodeling associated with pulmonary hypertension. Antioxid Redox Signal 5(6):759–769

Wedgwood S, Steinhorn RH, Bunderson M, Wilham J, Lakshminrusimha S, Brennan LA, Black SM (2005) Increased hydrogen peroxide downregulates soluble guanylate cyclase in the lungs of lambs with persistent pulmonary hypertension of the newborn. Am J Phys Lung Cell Mol Phys 289(4):L660–L666. Epub 2005 Jun 2003

Weimann J, Ullrich R, Hromi J, Fujino Y, Clark MWH, Bloch KD, Zapol WM (2000) Sildenafil is a pulmonary vasodilator in awake lambs with acute pulmonary hypertension. Anesthesiology 92:1702–1712

Wessel DL, Adatia I, Van Marter LJ et al (1997) Improved oxygenation in a randomized trial of inhaled nitric oxice for persistent pulmonary hypertension of the newborn. Pediatrics 100:e7

Wynn J, Krishnan U, Aspelund G, Zhang Y, Duong J, Stolar CJ et al (2013) Outcomes of congenital diaphragmatic hernia in the modern era of management. J Pediatr 163:114–119

Yuniartha R, Alatas FS, Nagata K, Kuda M, Yanagi Y, Esumi G et al (2014) Therapeutic potential of mesenchymal stem cell transplantation in a nitrofen-induced congenital diaphragmatic hernia rat model. Pediatr Surg Int 30:907–914

Ziegler JW, Ivy DD, Wiggins JW, Kinsella JP, Clarke WR, Abman SH (1998) Effects of dipyridamole and inhaled nitric oxide in pediatric patients with pulmonary hypertension. Am J Respir Crit Care Med 158: 1388–1395

Pulmonary Hypertension in Congenital Diaphragmatic Hernia

61

Jason Gien, John P. Kinsella, and Steven H. Abman

Contents

Abstract

Congenital diaphragmatic hernia (CDH) is a severe congenital anomaly, where a defect in the diaphragm results in herniation of the abdominal contents into the chest and compression of the intrathoracic structures. In utero compression of the lungs results in pulmonary hypoplasia and pulmonary hypertension after birth. Along with the degree of lung hypoplasia and pulmonary hypertension, underdevelopment of the left ventricle also determines severity in CDH and contributes to adverse outcomes. After birth, CDH patients present with severe hypoxemic respiratory failure and shock, secondary to structural and functional changes in the heart, pulmonary circulation, airways, and lung parenchyma. The optimal approach to management of respiratory failure, pulmonary hypertension, and shock changes as the underlying pathophysiology evolves in the days and weeks after birth. In this chapter, we describe the approach to CDH management as shock which predominates early resolves and systemic hemodynamics stabilize and pulmonary vascular

J. Gien (✉)
University of Colorado Denver, Denver, CO, USA
e-mail: Jason.Gien@ucdenver.edu

J. P. Kinsella
University of Denver, Denver, CO, USA
e-mail: john.kinsella@ucdenver.edu

S. H. Abman
University of Colorado Denver – Anschutz Medical Campus, Denver, CO, USA
e-mail: steven.abman@ucdenver.edu

G. Buonocore et al. (eds.), *Neonatology*,
https://doi.org/10.1007/978-3-319-29489-6_292

abnormalities progress from acute to subacute (late) and finally chronic stages.

61.1 Salient Points

- Congenital diaphragmatic hernia (CDH) is a severe birth defect characterized by herniation of abdominal contents into the thorax and arrested development of both lungs.
- Presence of left ventricular hypoplasia contributes to the severity of the defect and adverse outcome.
- Pulmonary hypertension (PH) can persist months to years, and structural and functional abnormalities of pulmonary circulation can complicate the course of the disease.
- Pulmonary vasodilator therapy can be used in acute treatment; it plays a critical role in management of late PH in CDH and potentially improves survival.

61.2 Introduction

Congenital diaphragmatic hernia (CDH) is a severe birth defect characterized by herniation of abdominal contents into the thorax caused by a defect in the diaphragm (Lipshutz et al. 1997). Recent insight into pathophysiologic processes responsible for CDH suggests an early role for environmental and/or genetic factors before the development of the diaphragm, leading to arrested development of both lungs. In addition, incomplete closure of the diaphragm results in a diaphragm defect, herniation of the abdominal contents into the chest, and compression of the intrathoracic structures. Solid organ herniation exacerbates the degree of lung hypoplasia, and the most severe cases are associated with hypoplasia of the ipsilateral and contralateral lung (low lung to head ratio [LHR]) (Taira et al. 1998). Along with degree of lung hypoplasia, the severity of pulmonary hypertension (PH) and presence of left ventricular (LV) hypoplasia all contribute to the severity of the defect and adverse outcomes (Wynn et al. 2013; Le et al. 2012). Overall survival of infants with CDH has improved in experienced centers, but mortality and morbidity remain high.

Several individual prenatal prognostic factors have been identified in CDH that can predict the clinical course after birth as well as long-term outcomes. These include liver position, severity of lung hypoplasia (as assessed by fetal lung volume on MRI: percent predicted lung volume [PPLV] and total lung volume [TLV]; LHR and observed to expected LHR by ultrasound), LV hypoplasia (right ventricle [RV]:left ventricle disproportion on fetal echocardiogram [ECHO]), and development and reactivity of the pulmonary vasculature (e.g., McGoon Index, in utero hyperoxia test). In addition, the presence of congenital heart disease, or a genetic syndrome (Le et al. 2012), markedly impacts outcomes. The reliability of each individual parameter to predict survival and long-term outcome is low, and combining multiple parameters improves reliability. The CDH congenital prognostic index (CDH-CPI) is a useful tool that amalgamates 10 prenatal parameters representing genetic, cardiac, hernia, and lung factors to comprehensively capture the range of severity and associated anomalies influencing prognosis (Le et al. 2012). The CDH-CPI score is correlated with survival and extracorporeal membrane oxygenation (ECMO) support, with significantly lower survival at scores below 8 (Le et al. 2012).

61.3 Pulmonary Hypertension in CDH

The classical histological findings of CDH show pulmonary vascular remodeling superimposed on hypoplasia or pruning of the pulmonary vascular bed (Lipshutz et al. 1997). These changes in the pulmonary vasculature are responsible for increased vascular tone and altered vasoreactivity after birth (Lipshutz et al. 1997). Management of PH in the newborn with CDH is complicated by the structural and functional changes in the heart, pulmonary circulation, airways, and lung parenchyma. Moreover, the role and selection of pulmonary vasodilator therapies for treatment of PH change as the underlying pathophysiology

evolves in the days and weeks after birth. In response, management strategies need to adjust as pulmonary vascular abnormalities progress from the acute to subacute (late) and finally chronic stages.

61.4 Acute Pulmonary Hypertension in CDH

After birth, infants with CDH typically present with severe hypoxemic respiratory failure (HRF) and shock. The etiology of hypoxemia is multifactorial and occurs secondary to intrapulmonary shunt as well as extrapulmonary right-to-left shunting across fetal conduits (ductus arteriosus [DA] and foramen ovale). Newborns with severe CDH often present with left-to-right shunting at the atrial septum and right-to-left shunting at the ductus arteriosus (Baumgart et al. 1998). Differential shunting across these fetal conduits is responsible for postductal desaturation and differences in pre- and postductal arterial blood gas parameters (Baumgart et al. 1998). The direction of atrial level shunt is determined by the relative right and left ventricular end diastolic pressures. Left-to-right shunting at the atrial septum occurs when left ventricular end diastolic pressure (LVEDP) exceeds right ventricular end diastolic pressures (RVEDP) with impaired LV filling and elevated left atrial pressure (LAP).

Structural and functional LV abnormalities are responsible for impaired LV filling and contribute to the development of pulmonary venous hypertension. Baumgart et al. showed that ECMO-treated CDH infants (survivors) had significantly smaller LV mass ($P < 0.002$) than infants requiring ECMO for other diagnoses and healthy term infants (Byrne et al. 2015). Moreover, ECMO-treated CDH neonates who died had significantly smaller LV size than other groups ($P < 0.0005$) including ECMO-treated CDH survivors (in addition to CDH and non-CDH ECMO-treated infants and well infants) (Byrne et al. 2015). Byrne et al. reported that fetuses with severe left CDH were more likely to have smaller mitral valve ($P < 0.001$) and aortic valve sizes ($P < 0.001$) and left ventricular end diastolic volume ($P = 0.006$) Z-scores than those with mild left CDH (Fig. 1) (Kinsella and Abman 2000). In addition to the structural changes in the LV, their percentage LV output was also lower. Those with severe left CDH trended towards higher risk of neonatal death compared with those with mild left CDH. Although mitral and aortic valve dimensions in fetuses with right CDH were larger than in left CDH, LV outputs were similarly diminished.

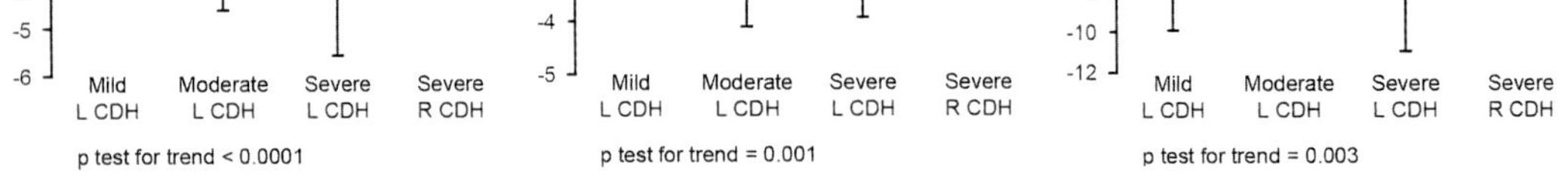

Fig. 1 Left heart hypoplasia stratified by congenital diaphragmatic hernia (CDH) side and severity at fetal assessment. Left CDH: mild (n = 42), liver down; moderate (n = 41), lung-to-head ratio (LHR) 1 to 1.4; severe (n = 88), LHR ≤1; Right CDH: mild (n = 2), LHR 41; severe (n = 15), LHR ≤1. For left heart measurements (mitral and aortic values, left ventricular volume) severity of hypoplasia increased with increasing severity of hernia, while the effect in the fetus with right CDH was less pronounced. Adapted with permission from Byrne et al. L, left; R, right

The etiology of LV hypoplasia in CDH is almost certainly multifactorial reflecting mechanical compression by intra-abdominal contents as well as alteration in LV filling hemodynamics during fetal development due to changes in orientation of the inferior vena cava and venous return from the placenta. Left heart underfilling and subsequent underdevelopment may result from abnormal hemodynamics due to leftward distortion of the ductus venosus or reduced pulmonary blood flow return to the left heart (Kinsella and Abman 2000). In addition, after birth, compression of the LV by the RV in the presence of elevated RV pressure also impairs LV filling. The common pathway for these mechanisms is decreased filling of the left ventricle. Altered hemodynamics and compression of the heart by herniated abdominal viscera together can create strikingly abnormal left ventricular structure and function with anomalous relaxation and small chamber size, even with normal or near-normal systolic performance. Overall, altered fetal hemodynamics leading to decreased LV output can occur in both right and left CDH, but an additional compressive effect on the left heart is seen in left-sided CDH (Kinsella and Abman 2000).

Echocardiographic findings may be valuable in guiding the selective use of pulmonary vasodilators in management of early PH with CDH. For example, ECHO findings in the presence of severe PH may show right-to-left shunting (caused by suprasystemic pulmonary vascular resistance) at the atrial level and DA. This constellation of echocardiographic findings suggests a favorable response to pulmonary vasodilation. However, in the presence of LV dysfunction, right-to-left DA shunting is seen along with mitral insufficiency with left-to-right atrial shunting at the foramen ovale (Kinsella and Abman 2000). This constellation of findings is again consistent with suprasystemic right ventricular systolic pressure, but left-to-right atrial shunting suggests the presence of pulmonary venous hypertension and a poor response to pulmonary vasodilator therapy. Diastolic dysfunction is difficult to assess, but can be interpreted from a high LVEDP and manifests as left-to-right shunt at the atrial level. Pulmonary vasodilator therapy in the setting of left-to-right shunting at the atrial septum has the potential to exacerbate LA and pulmonary venous hypertension and contribute to pulmonary hemorrhage. In addition, as preductal saturations are maintained in this setting, pulmonary vasodilator therapy is unlikely to improve preductal saturations and may result in only a modest increase in postductal saturations. Reserving iNO therapy for infants with right-to-left atrial shunting and preductal desaturation is recommended early in the clinical course and has the potential to prevent pulmonary hemorrhage in CDH. In addition, as right-to-left shunting across the DA causes veno-arterial admixture, it is common to see significant differences in pre- and postductal arterial blood gases (ABG) measurements (Baumgart et al. 1998). Determining the need for ECMO, degree of respiratory support, and fraction of inspired oxygen (Fi02) should be based on measurement of preductal arterial gases in these infants (Baumgart et al. 1998).

Overall, acute treatment of PH in CDH with pulmonary vasodilators is limited by the severity of LV hypoplasia, degree of impairment of LV filling, and LV systolic dysfunction. Because infants with severe CDH and acute PH are poor responders, iNO should not be routinely administered in this setting. However, careful ECHO assessment can help identify limited clinical situations that may benefit from PH therapies, including iNO, and guide the course of treatment (Kinsella et al. 2005; Pediatrics 1997). In the acute management of CDH, iNO may have a selective role in stabilization for ECMO and treatment of marked preductal desaturation secondary to right-to-left atrial level shunt. Furthermore, use of iNO for treatment of PH may be considered as LV performance improves. LV hypoplasia, and related LV output, also play a role in the poor response to pulmonary vasodilators as diminished LV performance results in RV-dependent systemic circulation (Pediatrics 1997). Initiating pulmonary vasodilator therapy in the presence of an RV-dependent systemic circulation may adversely affect systemic hemodynamics.

The Neonatal Inhaled Nitric Oxide Study (NINOS) Group conducted the largest trial of iNO in infants with CDH ($N = 53$) who were

randomized to 20 ppm iNO or 100% oxygen (control) (Lusk et al. 2015). The oxygenation index (OI) was approximately 45 in both groups, indicating more severe disease. NINOS showed no difference in the combined endpoint "death/ ECMO utilization" between iNO-treated patients and controls. However, ECMO utilization was higher in the iNO-treated group (80% vs 54% control, $P = 0.043$) pointing to an adverse effect of iNO early in the course of CDH. These results lend support to the hypothesis that LV systolic and diastolic dysfunction contribute to morbidity in severe CDH and limit the efficacy of aggressive pharmacologic pulmonary vasodilator therapy early in the course of CDH and severe PH.

Indeed, a poor response to pulmonary vasodilation is not unexpected given the structural and functional abnormalities that characterize acute CDH. Although speculative, the lack of response to pulmonary vasodilators is more likely due to left atrial/pulmonary vein hypertension than functional changes in the pulmonary arterial vasculature.

61.5 Subacute (Late) Pulmonary Hypertension in CDH

In addition to complicating the early course of neonates with CDH, severe PH can be protracted – persisting weeks to months after improvement in respiratory failure and cardiac performance –leading to prolonged mechanical ventilation (Pediatrics 1997). In a multicenter prospective ECHO study of neonates with CDH ($N = 220$), mortality at discharge in newborns with severe PH (right ventricular systolic pressure [RVSP]/systolic blood pressure [SBP] >2/3) was 56.1% compared with 1.4% in infants with mild PH (RVSP/ SBP <1/2) and 7.4% in those with moderate PH (RVSP/SBP 1/2 to 2/3) (Le et al. 2012). Recently, Lusk et al. reviewed ECHO results for 140 newborns with CDH and found that although the majority of infants had resolution of PH between 1 and 3 weeks of age, at 2 weeks the severity of PH by echocardiogram predicted mortality and need for prolonged ventilation (Kinsella et al. 2003).

Treatment strategies for infants with late PH have not been carefully studied. Inhaled NO is usually the first-line therapy for treatment of PH in CDH. In a subset of newborns with CDH, improvement in parenchymal lung disease may allow for the use of noninvasive iNO by continuous positive airway pressure (CPAP) or nasal cannula (Olson et al. 2015). There is limited experience with other pharmacologic pulmonary vasodilators (e.g., prostacyclin, endothelin antagonists, and phosphodiesterase inhibitors) in infants with CDH and late PH. Olson et al. recently described two infants with CDH and severe PH at 6 weeks of age who responded favorably to treatment with treprostinil (Kamath et al. 2010). Clearly, further investigation is needed to define an approach to the management of late PH in this population.

61.6 Chronic Pulmonary Hypertension in CDH

Chronic PH may persist in CDH over months and years, and enduring structural and functional abnormalities of pulmonary circulation in the ipsilateral and contralateral lung can complicate the course of the disease. Cardiac catheterization of seven patients with CDH who survived the neonatal period with protracted or recurrent PH revealed a range of pulmonary vascular abnormalities (Pediatrics 1997). These patients (age range, 3 months–12 years) had a history of severe hypoxemic respiratory failure and PH as newborns. At catheterization, therapies included supplemental oxygen ($n = 7$), iNO ($n = 2$), prostacyclin ($n = 2$), and bosentan ($n = 1$). Three of the seven patients had significant pulmonary vascular abnormalities in the lung contralateral to the initial diaphragmatic defect. Major findings at cardiac catheterization included left pulmonary artery hypoplasia or stenosis in three patients and pulmonary vein stenosis or delayed venous return in six patients. Two patients with right-sided diaphragmatic defect had striking left-sided pulmonary venous abnormalities. One patient with right-sided CDH was discharged home, but died at age 5 months with marked pulmonary vascular changes on autopsy consistent with severe PH. After a median follow-up of 12 months from catheterization, five

patients were alive and discharged from hospital. The two patients with the most severe PH died from related complications at ages 8 and 19 months.

In some patients with CDH, significant PH, which may be subclinical, clearly continues beyond the neonatal period, contributing to morbidity and mortality. Understanding the pathophysiology underlying these long-term effects will require a more sophisticated view of CDH than that originating solely from in utero cardiopulmonary compression. It is possible that the injury associated with management of hypoxemic respiratory failure in newborns with CDH may cause previously unrecognized long-term effects in susceptible individuals, and/or the pulmonary circulation in patients with severe CDH may be fundamentally altered in utero, leading to abnormal responses to injury that last far beyond the newborn period (Pediatrics 1997).

61.7 Improving Outcomes in CDH

Treatment strategies for CDH continue to evolve with increasing clinical experience and greater insight into the underlying nature of the condition. These strategies include simultaneous postductal and preductal samples to measure blood gases (adjusting ventilator support accordingly) (Gien and Kinsella 2015). Early ECHO is essential to define pulmonary artery pressure (PAP) and assess LV size and function. It is reasonable to delay the use of pulmonary vasodilator therapy until there is ECHO evidence of adequate LV performance. Reducing LV afterload pharmacologically may play an important role (e.g., milrinone), as well as maintaining ductal patency with prostaglandin E1 (PGE1) if RV-dependent systemic circulation is demonstrated by ECHO. Adrenal insufficiency also complicates the course of newborns with severe CDH and decreases catecholamine drug responsiveness (Jani et al. 2011).

Despite refinement of postnatal interventions, limitations persist and treatment of CDH and pulmonary hypertension remains suboptimal. Consequently, new therapeutic options such as prenatal intervention or cell-based therapy are the subject of current investigation. The effects of LV dysfunction/hypoplasia on the neonatal course in severe CDH provide a compelling reason to study fetal intervention. The efficacy of prenatal intervention with percutaneous fetoscopic endoluminal tracheal occlusion (FETO) therapy in CDH has been described in case series and controlled studies (Ruano et al. 2012; Deprest and De 2012). The potential role of FETO is being investigated in CDH in a European and North American collaboration called the Tracheal Occlusion To Accelerate Lung Growth (TOTAL) Trial (Hoffman et al. 2011).

Mesenchymal stem cells (MSCs) also represent an emerging therapeutic approach in CDH. Several experimental studies in animal models have shown that treatment with MSCs can reduce pulmonary injury and PH (Aslam et al. 2009; Yuniartha et al. 2014). A recent study in a rat model of experimental CDH found that MSC transplantation promotes alveolar and pulmonary artery development, reducing the severity of pulmonary hypoplasia (145).

61.8 Conclusion

In summary, the early course of CDH is characterized by severe PH, and cardiac, lung parenchymal and airway abnormalities. Acute treatment of PH in CDH with pulmonary vasodilator therapy is limited by structural and functional changes of the left ventricle. In a significant subset of newborns with severe CDH, late or protracted PH occurs and may persist weeks to months following improvement in respiratory failure and cardiac performance. In contrast to early CDH, pulmonary vasodilator therapy plays a critical role in management of late PH in CDH and potentially improves survival.

Despite progress in CDH management, advances have been limited by the lack of randomized controlled trials to properly test new treatments. Major differences in clinical practice regarding the ascertainment and treatment of PH

make it difficult to determine the most effective strategies to manage late PH in CDH infants. Moreover, institutional practices that lead to "improved" outcomes are slowly adopted and local changes are often guided only by experience and conviction. To overcome these barriers, centers with the best outcomes for isolated CDH should be identified from current databases and their practices disseminated to the wider community. Improving outcomes in patients with CDH will require continued vigilance, multidisciplinary collaboration, and widespread adoption of best practices.

References

Aslam M, Baveja R, Liang OD, Fernandez-Gonzalez A, Lee C, Mitsialis SA et al (2009) Bone marrow stromal cells attenuate lung injury in a murine model of neonatal chronic lung disease. Am J Respir Crit Care Med 180:1122–1130

Baumgart S, Paul JJ, Huhta JC, Katz AL, Paul KE, Spettell C et al (1998) Cardiac malposition, redistribution of fetal cardiac output, and left heart hypoplasia reduce survival in neonates with congenital diaphragmatic hernia requiring extracorporeal membrane oxygenation. J Pediatr 133:5762

Byrne FA, Keller RL, Meadows J, Miniati D, Brook MM, Silverman NH et al (2015) Severe left diaphragmatic hernia limits size of fetal left heart more than right diaphragmatic hernia. Ultrasound Obstet Gynecol 46(6):688–94

Deprest J, De CP (2012) Antenatal management of isolated congenital diaphragmatic hernia today and tomorrow: ongoing collaborative research and development. J Pediatr Surg 47:282–290

Gien J, Kinsella JP (2015) Differences in preductal and postductal arterial blood gas measurements in infants with severe congenital diaphragmatic hernia. Arch Dis Child Fetal Neonatal Ed 101(4):F314

Hoffman AM, Paxson JA, Mazan MR, Davis AM, Tyagi S, Murthy S et al (2011) Lung – derived mesenchymal stromal cell post – transplantation survival, persistence, paracrine expression, and repair of elastase – injured lung. Stem Cells Dev 20:1779–1792

Jani J, Valencia C, Cannie M, Vuckovic A, Sellars M, Nicolaides KH (2011) Tracheal diameter at birth in severe congenital diaphragmatic hernia treated by fetal endoscopic tracheal occlusion. Prenat Diagn 31:699–704

Kamath BD, Fashaw L, Kinsella JP (2010) Adrenal insufficiency in newborns with congenital diaphragmatic hernia. J Pediatr 156:495–497

Kinsella JP, Abman SH (2000) Clinical approach to inhaled nitric oxide therapy in the newborn with hypoxemia. J Pediatr 136:717–726

Kinsella JP, Parker TA, Ivy DD, Abman SH (2003) Noninvasive delivery of inhaled nitric oxide therapy for late pulmonary hypertension in newborn infants with congenital diaphragmatic hernia. J Pediatr 142:397–401

Kinsella JP, Ivy DD, Abman SH (2005) Pulmonary vasodilator therapy in congenital diaphragmatic hernia: acute, late, and chronic pulmonary hypertension. Semin Perinatol 29:123–128

Le LD, Keswani SG, Biesiada J, Lim FY, Kingma PS, Haberman BE et al (2012) The congenital diaphragmatic hernia composite prognostic index correlates with survival in left – sided congenital diaphragmatic hernia. J Pediatr Surg 47:57–62

Lipshutz GS, Albanese CT, Feldstein VA, Jennings RW, Housley HT, Beech R et al (1997) Prospective analysis of lung – to – head ratio predicts survival for patients with prenatally diagnosed congenital diaphragmatic hernia. J Pediatr Surg 32:1634–1636

Lusk LA, Wai KC, MoonGrady AJ, Steurer MA, Keller RL (2015) Persistence of pulmonary hypertension by echocardiography predicts short – term outcomes in congenital diaphragmatic hernia. J Pediatr 166:251–256

Olson E, Lusk LA, Fineman JR, Robertson L, Keller RL (2015) Short – term Treprostinil use in infants with congenital diaphragmatic hernia following repair. J Pediatr 167:762–764

Ruano R, Yoshisaki CT, da Silva MM, Ceccon ME, Grasi MS, Tannuri U et al (2012) A randomized controlled trial of fetal endoscopic tracheal occlusion versus postnatal management of severe isolated congenital diaphragmatic hernia. Ultrasound Obstet Gynecol 39: 20–27

Taira Y, Yamataka T, Miyazaki E, Puri P (1998) Comparison of the pulmonary vasculature in newborns and stillborns with congenital diaphragmatic hernia. Pediatr Surg Int 14:30–35

The Neonatal Inhaled Nitric Oxide Study Group (NINOS) (1997) Inhaled nitric oxide and hypoxic respiratory failure in infants with congenital diaphragmatic hernia. Pediatrics 99:838–845

Wynn J, Krishnan U, Aspelund G, Zhang Y, Duong J, Stolar CJ et al (2013) Outcomes of congenital diaphragmatic hernia in the modern era of management. J Pediatr 163:114–119

Yuniartha R, Alatas FS, Nagata K, Kuda M, Yanagi Y, Esumi G et al (2014) Therapeutic potential of mesenchymal stem cell transplantation in a nitrofen – induced congenital diaphragmatic hernia rat model. Pediatr Surg Int 30:907–914

Continuous Positive Airways Pressure and Other Noninvasive Respiratory Techniques in Newborns

62

Fabrizio Sandri, Gina Ancora, Gianluca Lista, and Luc J. I. Zimmermann

Contents

F. Sandri (✉)
Neonatology and Neonatal Intensive Care Unit, Ospedale Maggiore, Bologna, Italy
e-mail: f.sandri@ausl.bologna.it

G. Ancora
Neonatology and Neonatal Intensive Care Unit, Ospedale Infermi, Rimini, Italy
e-mail: gina.ancora@auslromagna.it

G. Lista
Neonatology and Neonatal Intensive Care Unit, Ospedale dei Bambini V. Buzzi, Milan, Italy
e-mail: gianluca.lista@asst-fbf-sacco.it

L. J. I. Zimmermann
Department of Pediatrics and Neonatology, School for Oncology and Developmental Biology (GROW), Maastricht University Medical Center, Maastricht, The Netherlands
e-mail: luc.zimmermann@mumc.nl

G. Buonocore et al. (eds.), *Neonatology*,
https://doi.org/10.1007/978-3-319-29489-6_209

Abstract

Continuous positive airways pressure (CPAP) is a method of assisted respiration that consists of the application of continuous positive pressure to a spontaneously breathing patient's airways throughout the entire respiratory cycle. The first use of a CPAP was in the 1930s (Poulton EP, Oxon DM, Lancet 228:981–983, 1936; Bullowa JGH, The management of the Pneumonias. Oxford University Press, New York, 1937; Barach AL, Martin J, Eckman M, Proc Am Soc Clin Invest 16:664–680, 1937), but its first notable application in the neonatal field was in 1971 when CPAP was used in the treatment of RDS (respiratory distress syndrome) in spontaneously breathing newborns undergoing tracheal intubation (Gregory GA, Kittermann JA, Phibbs RH et al. N Engl J Med 284:1333–1340, 1971). Nowadays, nasal CPAP (N-CPAP) is considered a valid approach in the management of respiratory failure of the preterm infant from birth reducing occurrence of bronchopulmonary dysplasia (BPD) and death, without increasing risk of neurological damage.

62.1 Salient Points

- CPAP is a valid approach in the management of respiratory failure of the newborn infant.
- Nasal CPAP (N-CPAP), which is CPAP delivered with nasal prongs, is the most used and effective system for the administration of CPAP in the newborn.
- N-CPAP stabilizes airways, prevents alveoli collapse, and allows spontaneously breathing patient to achieve a functional residual capacity.
- N-CPAP can be delivered by continuous or variable flow systems.
- N-CPAP is considered a valid alternative to tracheal intubation and mechanical ventilation in the acute phase of RDS by reducing occurrence of bronchopulmonary dysplasia and death.
- Surfactant replacement and caffeine prophylaxis can reduce N-CPAP failure in preterm infants with RDS.
- N-CPAP after mechanical ventilation can prevent extubation failure.
- Nasal intermittent ventilation (NIV) especially if synchronized could be a promising approach in case of N-CPAP failure before tracheal intubation.
- Nursing care is determinant to reduce N-CPAP failure.

62.2 Background

The premature lung is prone to collapse due to low presence of endogenous surfactant and reduced capacity of the preterm baby to generate an

adequate positive pressure to maintain open the alveoli. Therefore, many premature infants at birth (especially when born before 32 weeks' GA) show signs of respiratory failure and need to be managed with respiratory support and surfactant therapy.

Continuous positive airways pressure (CPAP) is a method of assisted respiration that consists of the application of continuous positive pressure to a spontaneously breathing patient's airways throughout the entire respiratory cycle. The first use of a CPAP dates back to1930s (Poulton and Oxon 1936; Bullowa 1937; Barach et al. 1937), but its first notable application in the neonatal field was in 1971 when CPAP was used in the treatment of RDS (respiratory distress syndrome) in spontaneously breathing newborns undergoing tracheal intubation (Gregory et al. 1971).

There is a distinction between CPAP and PEEP (positive end expiratory pressure). CPAP maintains a constant pressure of a level above ambient air pressure, thus providing a continuous transpulmonary pressure gradient during the various phases of the respiratory cycle. Another term for CPAP is continuous distending pressure (Morley 1999). Administered through the nose, (N-CPAP, a technique first proposed by Italian authors in the early 1970s (Agostino et al. 1973; Caliumi-Pellegrini et al. 1974)) CPAP became a cornerstone of respiratory support in the 1990s. When PEEP is used, positive pressure is applied to the airways of a patient undergoing mechanical ventilation in the phases between artificial breaths.

62.3 Physiopathology

62.3.1 Respiratory System

The main purpose of CPAP in the newborn is to reduce the work of breathing (WOB). Work is expressed as the function of force × distance and specifically, in the case of respiratory work, as pressure × volume ($P \times V$). It is necessary to create a pressure gradient between the atmosphere and the alveoli so that a volume of air comes into contact with the alveolar-capillary membrane during each inspiration. The pressure generated must be capable of overcoming the elastic properties and resistance of the respiratory system, thus

$$P_{\text{tot}} = P_{\text{el}} + P_{\text{res}} = V/C + FR$$

where P_{tot} is the total pressure, P_{el} is the pressure necessary to overcome the elastic forces, P_{res} is the pressure required to overcome the resistance, C is compliance, R is resistance, V is volume, and F is flow (equation of motion of the respiratory system).

In the neonate, increased WOB is clinically manifested by the presence of tachypnea, intercostal/diaphragmatic retractions, and paradoxical breathing.

The amount of work expended in order to expand the rib cage depends principally on:

- The elasticity of the lungs (the work is inversely proportional to the compliance of the lungs)
- The resistance to airflow imposed by the airways
- The elastic and resistive properties of the rib cage

We will examine below the physiopathological characteristics of the neonatal respiratory system, with particular attention to aspects relating to premature infants, and we will analyze the effects of CPAP application with respect to neonatal respiratory physiology.

The neonate, particularly if premature, has a double disadvantage in performing respiratory work:

- There is increased pulmonary elastic resistance
- The airways provide considerable resistance
- The compliance of the rib cage is increased

62.3.1.1 Increased Pulmonary Elastic Resistance

The lungs are elastic in nature – elasticity describes the tendency of a structure to return to its initial state after the application of a force causes it to depart from its initial conditions. Compliance (the change in volume created by change in pressure, $\Delta V/\Delta P$) is the inverse of elasticity and measures the distensibility of a structure.

Premature newborns present with reduced compliance for various reasons:

Low surfactant production with consequent increase in pulmonary surface tension and reduction in pulmonary volume at the end of expiration (functional residual capacity, FRC).

Excessive quantity of pulmonary fluid: the clearance of the pulmonary fluid is slower in the premature newborn, particularly when delivered by elective cesarean section. In fact, the premature infant is often unable to generate an adequate delta pressure to move the fluid throughout the airways until the distal space of the lung where it is reabsorbed by the interstitial venous and lymphatic vessels. In addition, fluid and sodium absorption mechanisms are immature. Furthermore, the left-to-right shunt that occurs when there is a patent ductus arteriosus (PDA), especially during the recovery phase of RDS, can contribute to an increase in pulmonary fluid.

62.3.1.2 Greater Resistance of the Airways

The premature newborn presents increased resistance above all due to the proximal airways for various reasons:

Absence of the superficial layer of adipose tissue in the neck that helps to stabilize the airways, thus keeping them patent (Wilson et al. 1980; Cohen and Henderson-Smart 1986).

Reduced mobility of the genioglossus muscle that normally stabilizes the pharynx (Gauda et al. 1987).

Reduced diameter of the airways.

Increased compliance of the airways, which creates a tendency for them to collapse during inspiration; this increased compliance also increases the ventilation of the dead space.

The premature newborn also presents increased resistance at the level of the peripheral airways. The reasons for this are:

The structural composition of the lungs is insufficient to keep the smaller airways open.

The reduction of FRC causes a reduction in diameter of the smaller airways.

62.3.1.3 Increased Compliance of the Rib Cage

Compliance of the rib cage is inversely proportional to gestational age. The compliance of the rib cage is around five times greater than that of the lungs in premature newborns (for normal values of pulmonary compliance) and around three times greater in full-term newborns. In adults the ratio is 1:1 (Gerhardt and Bancalari 1980). As such, the newborn's rib cage is much weaker and more flexible and is therefore incapable of maintaining adequate transpulmonary pressure at the end of expiration. This brings a reduction in FRC, ventilation at near-closing volumes, alveolar collapse, imbalance in the ratio of ventilation to perfusion, hypoxemia, and hypercapnia with acidosis (see ▶ Chap. 48, "Neonatal Pulmonary Physiology of Term and Preterm Newborns").

The combined effect of reduced pulmonary compliance and increased compliance of the rib cage results in a reduced FRC (Fig. 1) with a tendency toward atelectasis and a reduction in gaseous exchange.

A mechanism enacted by the newborn to maintain an adequate FRC is the partial closure of the epiglottis during expiration (grunting): the premature newborn often cannot maintain adequate laryngeal tone and so may undergo a loss of pulmonary volume. It has been shown that the suppression of grunt caused by endotracheal intubation creates a reduction in paO_2 (Harrison et al. 1968).

Aside from the cry, the newborn has two further mechanisms to increase FRC: (1) maintaining the contraction of the inspiratory muscles during the first phase of expiration and (2) commencing the inspiration before expiration has finished. This strategy, which has the effect of increasing the FRC (dynamic increase of FRC), can facilitate gaseous exchange but is disadvantageous from the point of view of the amount of energy expended (Schulze et al. 1990). Fatigue or the presence of apnea in the newborn with respiratory

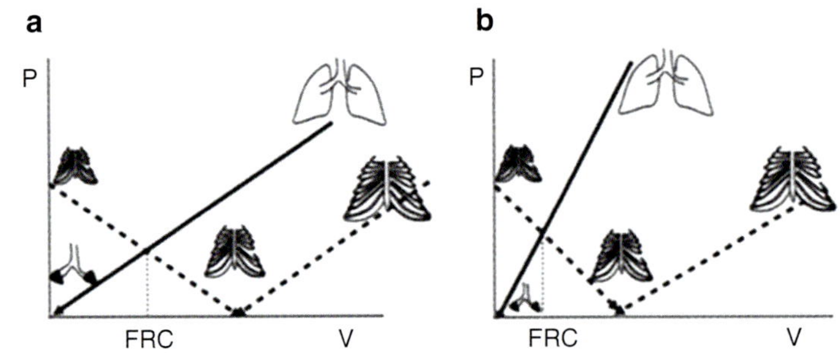

Fig. 1 Schematic representation of lung elastic (*continuous line*) and of chest wall (*discontinuous line*) forces in static conditions: the lung tends to a volume equal to zero, whereas the chest wall tends to a volume different from zero; the functional residual capacity (*FRC*) is achieved when the retraction force of the lung is equal to the expanding force of the chest wall. FRC is lower in the preterm (**b**) compared to the term newborn (**a**) due to both an higher force of lung retraction (lower lung compliance) and to a lower force of chest wall expansion. *P* pressure, *V* volume

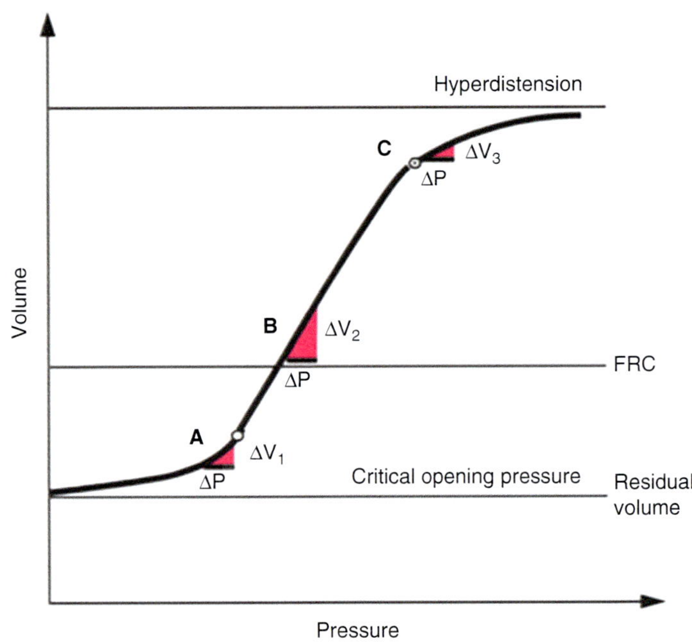

Fig. 2 Pressure/volume curve of the lung (compliance curve). ΔV, change in volume; ΔP, change in pressure; *FRC* functional residual capacity. Normal compliance in *B*; low compliance in *A* and *C*

distress syndrome can defeat the abovementioned mechanism and can encourage the development of atelectasis with consequent respiratory insufficiency (Morley 1999).

The reduction in FRC means that the newborn is working in the lower part of the compliance curve (Fig. 2, part A) and so is constrained to develop high pressures in order to gain small increases in volume. A low volume at the end of inspiration also induces closure of the small airways, followed by collapse of the alveoli. This necessitates greater pressures during inspiration in order to reopen the collapsed alveoli (critical opening pressure). Pulmonary collapse also causes epithelial damage with consequent protein exudates and surfactant consumption (see ▸ Chap. 63, "Lung Diseases: Surfactant Replacement Therapy in Newborns"). This reduction in pulmonary volume also brings a change in the ratio of ventilation to perfusion with a consequent

increase in the alveolar-arterial gradient and CO_2 concentration.

62.3.1.4 Respiratory Effects of CPAP

The application of continuous positive pressure to the airways amplifies the effect of the strategies by the spontaneously breathing newborn that are aimed at maintaining an adequate volume at the end of expiration, minimizing the energy expended to stabilize the respiratory system, and carrying out the mechanical work of respiration. This prevents collapse of the airways and improves many critical situations that bring about an increase in the respiratory workload required of the newborn. In summary, CPAP acts on the respiratory system by the following mechanisms:

1. Increasing FRC (Fig. 2, Part B), eliminating dynamic elevation of FRC reducing resistance in the airways. The reduction in airway resistance is obtained by:
   Increasing the transverse section of the pharynx (the oropharynx can account for 66% of supraglottidal resistance (Miller et al. 1990)).
   Dilating the airways and making them more rigid, stabilizing them, and preventing their collapse. In particular, an increase from 12.5% to 47% of the ratio of the width to the length of the larynx at the moment of maximum abduction of the vocal cords has been shown following CPAP application (Gaon et al. 1999).
   Increasing the FRC thus can favor caudal traction across the supraglottidal airways reducing their resistance (Van de Graaff 1988).
2. Reducing the R-L shunt, thanks to the improved oxygenation and the consequent vasodilation of the pulmonary circulation.
3. Stabilizing the thoracic wall, reducing its distortion and curbing paradoxical movement. Regularizing and slowing respiratory frequency (Kurz 1999).
4. Regularizing and slowing respiratory frequency (Kurz 1999).
5. Improving the capacity to generate a valid inspiratory force and thus to reopen collapsed alveoli following an obstructive event, probably through the elimination of the Hering-Breuer deflation reflex which is activated by a distortion in the inferior portion of the rib cage (Martin et al. 1977). In this way, it also reduces the incidence of obstructive apnea.
6. Increasing the average pressure in the airways (mean airways pressure, MAP) increasing the ventilation-perfusion ratio.
7. Preserving the surfactant on the surface of the alveoli.
8. Reducing alveolar edema.

Normalizing pulmonary volume, ventilations/minute, and the ventilation-perfusion ratio, CPAP improves oxygenation, increases the elimination of CO_2, and reduces the WOB (Poulton and Oxon 1936).

62.3.2 Cardiocirculatory System

CPAP results in a reduced preload in the right ventricle and consequently systolic output. The extent of these effects depends on how much pressure is applied by the lungs to the vascular spaces: the lower the compliance, the lower the applied pressure (Perlman and Thach 1988). In the premature newborn, in the presence of a highly compliant rib cage and often low pulmonary compliance, the pressure applied by the airways to the pleural spaces is only 5–10%, with little effect on cardiac output. In full-term newborns with normal lungs, 25% of the pressure in the airways (Paw) can be transferred to the pleural spaces, and therefore the use of high pressure in these babies can have a significant effect on cardiac output. The increased thoracic compliance of the premature newborn therefore protects the intrathoracic vascular structure from a large increase in intrapleural pressure and from a consequent reduction in central venous return (Gerhardt and Bancalari 1980). On the other hand, CPAP reduces pulmonary resistance in babies with RDS because of the vasodilatation of the pulmonary circulation resulting from improved oxygenation; this is the most important effect in newborns with respiratory pathologies treated with CPAP.

62.3.3 Renal Function

Renal function depends largely on the hemodynamic situation of the patient (Ahumada and Goldsmith 1996). In cases of low pulmonary compliance, the application of CPAP brings an improvement in oxygenation, and renal function can only be positively affected. In the presence of restricted water intake for the treatment or prevention of a PDA – a common situation in cases which require the application of CPAP – the administration of dopamine at renal doses may be useful (approx. 3 μ/kg/min).

62.3.4 Intracranial Pressure

A reduction in cerebral perfusion has been reported in the course of the application of PEEP. This is related to the level of the PEEP.

An increase in intracranial pressure was found during the application of CPAP by a box around the head, due to compression of the veins in the neck. It does not appear that CPAP applied by endotracheal or nasal tube results in an increase of intracranial pressure (Ahumada and Goldsmith 1996).

62.4 Technical Aspect

CPAP can be delivered by a variety of devices and interfaces. There are two main types of CPAP devices, categorized on the basis of the flow characteristics: continuous and variable flow systems.

An important prerequisite for success in the use of CPAP is a circuit that allows the pressure to remain at the desired level throughout the respiratory cycle. Excessive inspiratory or expiratory fluctuations directly increase WOB and offset any benefits in pulmonary mechanics produced by CPAP (Gherini et al. 1979).

Substantial differences were found in the fluctuations of Paw in different respiratory circuits hooked up to a mechanical lung model (Rasanen and Leijala 1991).

62.4.1 Continuous Flow Systems

These systems use a resistance to flow at the end of the respiratory circuit to produce pressure above that of atmospheric pressure. These CPAP systems include bubble CPAP. This device uses a fixed gas flow, and the column of water in the expiratory limb generates CPAP equal to the length of the tube that is immersed under water, which creates chest vibrations through bubbling. All these devices are also fitted with systems to humidify and heat the air. Continuous-flow mechanical ventilators can also be used to produce CPAP by the means of the PEEP valve to maintain continuous positive pressure throughout the entire respiratory cycle.

62.4.2 Variable Flow Systems

62.4.2.1 Benveniste System

The positive pressure is generated by a jet of gas directed toward an opening into a small chamber from which the mixture for the newborn comes out. Flow rates of 4–20 L/min serve to generate pressures in the chamber from 0 to 13 cmH_2O. These pressures are comparable to those measured at the oropharynx in the course of CPAP administered via one or two nasal prongs (this is indifferent, as long as the mouth is kept closed by the use of a pacifier) (Pedersen and Nielsen 1994).

62.4.2.2 Infant Flow System

A generator is connected to a circuit composed of a three-channel tube (Figs. 3 and 4): one channel (inspiratory limb) provides gas flow and is connected to the nasal cavity via nasal prongs or mask, one (expiratory limb) is open to ambient pressure, and one is used to measure the level of pressure created at the generator level. The flow provided by the infant flow driver is accelerated in the twin injector nozzles of the N-CPAP generator. When the patient makes a spontaneous inspiratory breathing effort, the generator provides assistance by converting the kinetic energy of the flow to pressure energy. When the infant makes a spontaneous expiratory effort, a pressure is applied at the nasal attachment of the N-CPAP

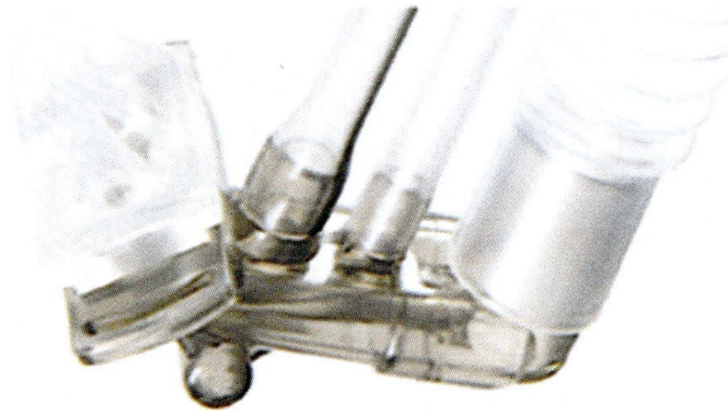

Fig. 3 Infant flow generator

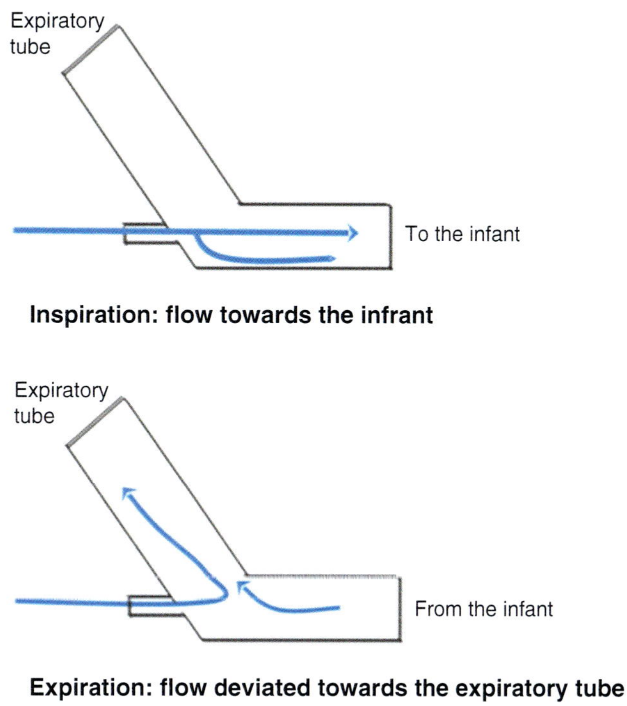

Fig. 4 Functioning of the infant flow generator

generator. This causes the flow to flip round and leave the generator via the expiratory limb. CPAP is maintained at the nasal connection throughout. When the expiratory breathing effort stops, the flow instantly flips back to the inspiratory position. The operating principle is that the high-pressure jet flows in different directions in response to the pressure generated at the level of the nasal cavities and the respiratory effort of the patient. During inspiration, the drop in pressure in the nasal cavities creates a pressure gradient that directs the flow toward the nasal cavities, thus assisting inspiration. During expiration, there is an inversion of the direction of the jet that helps the expiration (Coanda effect). The kinetic energy of this high-velocity flow is transformed into pressure in the area of the nasal cavities, thus generating CPAP. Flow rates between 5 and 11 L/min generate pressures between 2 and 10 cmH_2O. As such, the system does not require an expiratory valve. Tests on mechanical lung models have demonstrated that a CPAP circuit achieves greater stability in Paw and a reduction in WOB of around one quarter compared to traditional circuits (Moa et al. 1988; Moa and Nilsson 1993; Klausner et al. 1996). Available clinical studies have, on the

other hand, reported conflicting results. Two studies did not show any difference between this system and traditional ones in terms of improving pulmonary compliance, reducing oxygen requirements and improving respiratory frequency (Ahluwalia et al. 1998; Kavvadia et al. 2000).

A recent study comparing three circuits (infant flow system, double nasal prongs, and single nasal prong fed by mechanical ventilators) for the application of NCPAP in newborns weighing less than 1800 g with light respiratory distress or apnea demonstrated better pulmonary recruitment using the infant flow circuit (Courtney et al. 2001).

62.5 Methods of Administering CPAP

Endotracheal Tube This method entails a notable resistance (directly proportional to its length and inversely proportional to its radius) and as such involves a significant increase in WOB. At this time, it is no longer recommended as a system for the administration of CPAP. Furthermore, by bypassing the nasal and pharyngeal mucosa, it creates an alteration in the humidification and heating of the inhaled gases. Also the potential trauma applied to the vocal cords and the respiratory mucosa makes its use inadvisable for newborns who do not need mechanical ventilation.

Head-Box (Helmet CPAP) This system is of low efficacy below 1500 g bodyweight and extremely noisy and cumbersome and does not allow access to the newborn's head. Furthermore, it has been associated with an increased incidence of cerebral hemorrhage due to compression of the neck (Vert et al. 1973). Aspiration pneumonia has also been reported during feeding.

Face Mask This system too is rarely used, particularly for premature infants. The mask should cover the nose and mouth and should always be used with an orogastric feeding tube to avoid excessive abdominal distension. In the premature newborn, apart from the problem of keeping the mask in place and the consequent difficulty of generating a sufficient level of CPAP with adequate flow, there are also problems of excessive dead space that can be two or three times greater than in a full-term newborn. Cases of cerebral hemorrhaging have been reported in very low birth weight newborns undergoing this therapy due to the forces applied to the back of the head by the mask's attachments (Pape et al. 1976).

Facial Chamber The entire face protrudes into a chamber held in place by a latex ring filled with styrene particles. This system too is now not used as it does not permit access to the newborn's face for alimentation or aspiration.

Nasopharyngeal Tube (Mono-nasal CPAP) The same type of tube used for tracheal intubation is inserted through the nostril as far as the pharynx. This is a simple technique, which is widely used during the transport of the baby from the delivery room to the NICU or yet in the NICU, in case of mild forms of respiratory distress or apnea in the premature. The disadvantages lie in the fact that this tube provides elevated resistance, particularly if it is of small diameter, and that the tube also totally bypasses the humidifying-heating action provided by the nasopharyngeal mucous. In addition, it can give more nasal trauma than nasal prongs.

Nasal Prongs (Bi-nasal CPAP) Currently, this is the most used and effective system for the administration of CPAP in the newborn. The baby has to breathe through the nose; the nasal prongs also allow the air to be humidified and heated by most of the nasopharyngeal mucous. The mouth in this case acts as a pop-off pressure valve. The nasal prongs are easily applied and less invasive than the endotracheal tube; first examples of nasal prongs were put into use in the early 1970s (Agostino et al. 1973; Caliumi-Pellegrini et al. 1974; Kattwinkel et al. 1973). Particular attention has been paid to the work required of the newborn in order to overcome the resistance due to the small diameter of the nasal prongs (the so-called superimposed work of breathing). A study reported an increase of 100% in WOB during CPAP administered with nasal prongs compared to CPAP with a face mask (Goldman et al. 1979). A closer evaluation of the study, however, revealed that this increase could, in part, be put down to the increased resistance caused by the catheter placed inside the prongs to relieve pressure. Recently, these prongs have been redesigned

with a precise angle and structure in order to minimize resistance to the airflow (Klausner et al. 1996). Another problem with these prongs is related to the loss of flow (and hence of pressure) around the prongs themselves if they are not secured properly. Nowadays, the prongs are made from a soft silicon material that expands slightly in contact with the warmth and humidity of the nostrils, adapting to their dimensions and so favoring a good fit.

Nasal Masks These devices, which consist of silicone masks that completely cover the nose, are sometimes a useful alternative to nasal prongs, in particular in extremely low birth weight infants.

62.6 Clinical Applications

62.6.1 Respiratory Distress Syndrome (RDS)

The main physiopathological aspects of RDS, whose principal cause is a deficit of surfactant (Avery and Mead 1959), are reduction in pulmonary compliance, reduction in FRC, and alteration in the ratio of ventilation to perfusion. The rigidity of the rib cage is also reduced with a paradoxical distortion during inspiration which is greater the larger the reduction in pulmonary compliance, with a consequent reduction in tidal volume (Morley 1999; Greenough and Roberton 1996). These alterations lead to a profound alteration in gas exchange and increase the respiratory workload; the consequences of which are the presence of hypoxemia, hypercapnia, and acidosis.

62.6.1.1 Clinical Evidence

The first clinical experience of neonatal CPAP application came in 1971 with a case report of 20 patients affected by RDS (Morley 1999). This was followed by others (Bancalari and Sinclair 1991; Cordero et al. 1997; Tarnow-Mordi et al. 1986).

The rationale behind the use of early N-CPAP in the VLBW newborn lies in the facilitation of the acquisition and maintenance of an adequate pulmonary volume (FRC). As well as improved gas exchange, a normal air-liquid interface is maintained at the level of the terminal alveoli. This promotes the liberation of reserves of pulmonary surfactant, which in turn further stabilize the air spaces preventing the formation of hyaline membranes and the following atelectasis that is typical of surfactant deficiency. This should lead to a decrease in the requirement for mechanical ventilation with a reduction in its complications, in particular bronchopulmonary dysplasia.

The main reason for the interest in adopting N-CPAP, especially in very low birth weight newborns (VLBW, i.e., <1500 g), came from the publication of two multicenter retrospective studies. They showed that the incidence of chronic lung disease, assessed as the percentage of VLBW survivors who were oxygen dependent at 28 days from birth, was significantly lower in centers that had been early adopters of N-CPAP, despite having among the highest survival rates. The early adoption of N-CPAP at these centers was part of a low-invasiveness strategy consisting of the tolerance of relatively high pCO_2 values, up to 60 mmHg (permissive hypercapnia), before proceeding to intubation and mechanical ventilation, and the nonuse of paralyzing drugs (Avery et al. 1987; Horbar et al. 1988).

Early N-CPAP was largely used in VLBW infants with recourse to intubation and mechanical ventilation only when it was held to be essential, based on well-established criteria (Jonsson et al. 1997; Kamper and Ringsted 1990; Kamper et al. 1993; Lundstrom 1996). The common denominators of these clinical experiences are:

- Intubation in the delivery room only if considered essential for cardiopulmonary resuscitation
- Early N-CPAP, i.e., application of N-CPAP to all newborns within the first 30 min of life or at the appearance of the first signs of respiratory distress
- Intubation and, if necessary, mechanical ventilation only if one or more of the following criteria are met (criteria for failure of N-CPAP): untreatable apnea, respiratory acidosis ($pCO_2 > 65–70$ mmHg and pH <7.20), and requirement of exogenous surfactant

In Scandinavia, where the N-CPAP is widespread and long-term used, the success of

N-CPAP in treating VLBW infants avoiding mechanical ventilation, was proportional to the gestational age (76% of newborns ≤26 weeks' GA require ventilation compared to 43% of newborns >26 weeks) regardless the use of prenatal prophylaxis with steroids (Jonsson et al. 1997).

There is a general tendency to tolerate higher pCO_2 values than in the past (Avery et al. 1987; Kamper and Ringsted 1990; Kamper et al. 1993), and this has reduced the need for intubation. Even when mechanical ventilation is undertaken, it does not require the use of aggressive ventilation strategies in search of blood gas values that are obtained at the cost of high baro-volutrauma (Jonsson et al. 1997).

A study carried out on 67 newborns of <1000 g birthweight (extremely low birth weight, ELBW) who underwent early N-CPAP, if they were not intubated in the delivery room for primary resuscitation, demonstrated that it was not necessary to intubate and start mechanical ventilation in 73% of the newborns >28 weeks and in 32% of the newborns ≤28 weeks (Lindner et al. 1999). In another study, Finer et al. (Finer et al. 2004) found that all infants of 23 weeks' gestation required intubation in the delivery room, whereas only 3 of 21 (14%) infants of 27 weeks' GA required such intubation.

The reduction in the percentage of mechanically ventilated newborns did not cause an increase in mortality or negative side effects such as cerebral hemorrhage (Jonsson et al. 1997; Kamper et al. 1993; Lindner et al. 1999; Gittermann et al. 1997; Jacobsen et al. 1993; Sandri et al. 1999).

However, despite uncontrolled and cohort studies suggesting the efficacy of N-CPAP in avoiding MV and ventilatory-induced lung injury, there were few randomized clinical trials confirming the benefit of N-CPAP as the primary type of respiratory support in preterm newborns. Morley et al. published the COIN trial in 2008 (Morley et al. 2008). In this trial, N-CPAP was compared with intubation and ventilation on the hypothesis that the use of N-CPAP shortly after birth would reduce the rates of death and bronchopulmonary dysplasia. The main eligibility criteria were a gestational age at delivery between 25 and 28 weeks and an ability to breathe at 5 min after birth but needing respiratory support. Infants were ineligible if they had been intubated before randomization or if they required no respiratory support or oxygen. At 5 min after birth, the allocated treatment was started. In infants who were assigned to receive N-CPAP, this was started at a pressure of 8 cm of water with nasal prongs. They were intubated and underwent ventilation only if they had any of the following clinical signs: apnea unresponsive to stimulation and methylxanthine treatment, an arterial pH of less than 7.25 with a partial pressure of arterial carbon dioxide ($paCO_2$) of more than 60 mmHg (8.0 kPa), a metabolic acidosis not responsive to treatment, or treatment with more than a 60% concentration of oxygen. Infants receiving N-CPAP were treated with surfactant only after intubation. Surfactant treatment, ventilation settings, and extubation and reintubation criteria were not mandated in either group and followed local protocols. Half the infants in the N-CPAP group were subsequently intubated. Infants in the N-CPAP group had a better outcome at 28 days than those in the intubation group. The two groups had similar outcomes at 36 weeks' gestational age, but there was an increased incidence of pneumothorax in the N-CPAP group.

In 2010, Finer et al. published the SUPPORT trial (Finer et al. 2010).In this randomized multicenter trial, inborn infants of 24.0–27.6 weeks' GA were randomly assigned to intubation and surfactant treatment (within 1 h after birth) or to N-CPAP treatment initiated in the delivery room. The primary outcome was death or BPD at 36 weeks' postmenstrual age. A total of 1318 infants were enrolled in the study. The rates of primary outcome did not differ significantly between the two groups (47.8% and 51.0%, respectively) without any other differences in terms of adverse neonatal outcomes. The authors concluded that CPAP has to be considered as an alternative to intubation and surfactant in preterm infants.

There are studies of great interest that have demonstrated the efficacy of an approach that prescribes the use of early N-CPAP together with the administration of surfactant in the treatment of

RDS. This approach, known as the INSURE approach (intubation-surfactant-extubation), is based upon the adoption of the following procedure. In a newborn undergoing N-CPAP, whenever administration of surfactant is indicated, the patient is intubated, surfactant is administered in the usual doses, and the patient is then placed again in N-CPAP after extubation (assuming that the patient is breathing spontaneously). Mechanical ventilation is only applied when indicated by well-defined criteria of failure (Blennow et al. 1999).

A multicenter study carried out in Sweden compared the incidence of mechanical ventilation in two groups of newborns affected by moderate-to-severe RDS to whom early CPAP was applied (e.g., application at the first clinical signs of respiratory distress). The treatment group received the INSURE approach if their oxygen requirement exceeded 60%. The control group received treatment only with N-CPAP and surfactant was reserved for cases where mechanical ventilation was required. The criteria for application of mechanical ventilation (apnea and or oxygen requirement gt, 80%) were the same for both groups. Recourse to mechanical ventilation was reduced from 85% in the control group to 43% in the treatment group (Verder et al. 1994).

The same authors later carried out a multicenter study on newborns with RDS below 30 weeks' gestational age and who were undergoing early N-CPAP. They demonstrated that when the INSURE approach was adopted early in RDS, i. e., at an oxygen requirement between 40% and 60%, there was a reduction in the need for mechanical ventilation and of death in the first 7 days postpartum from 63% to 21% compared to a later approach (oxygen requirement >60%) (Verder et al. 1999).

This last work, aside from demonstrating the efficacy of the INSURE approach, permitted the establishment of a limit to the oxygen requirement in patients with RDS undergoing N-CPAP (FiO2 about 40%) above which the administration of surfactant is indicated.

A study conducted in Italy on 155 newborns of gestational age $\geq$ 28 and <32 weeks treated by the INSURE approach at oxygen requirements >40% showed no difference in requirements for surfactant and mechanical ventilation comparing two groups to which N-CPAP had been applied: in the first group, N-CPAP was applied within 30′ of birth, regardless of the clinical picture; in the second group, N-CPAP was applied only in the presence of respiratory distress with oxygen requirements >40% (Sandri et al. 2004).

A systematic review of the INSURE approach reported a reduced need for MV in the first week of life, when used early in respiratory distress syndrome (Stevens et al. 2007).

Either prophylactic surfactant or delivery room N-CPAP to maintain functional residual volume was identified as potentially beneficial practice which, if adopted in extremely preterm infants, could reduce lung injury (Burch et al. 2003).

Recently, the CURPAP study compared the administration of prophylactic surfactant followed by N-CPAP (prophylactic INSURE) with early N-CPAP followed by early selective surfactant given through a brief course of endotracheal intubation (early rescue INSURE) to preterm newborns of GA 25–28 weeks not intubated at birth (Sandri et al. 2010). In both groups, MV was started after surfactant in the absence of good respiratory drive. Infants who were extubated to N-CPAP after surfactant were eligible for MV if the following N-CPAP failure criteria occurred: $FiO_2 > 0.40$ on N-CPAP to maintain oxygen saturation of 85–92% for at least 30 min unless rapid clinical deterioration occurred, intractable apnea, respiratory acidosis defined as $pCO_2 > 65$ mmHg (8.5 kPa), and pH <7.20. This study showed that, in spontaneously breathing preterm newborns treated with N-CPAP, prophylactic surfactant given within 30 min from birth is not superior to early selective surfactant in terms of requirement of MV in the first 5 days of life.

The main implication for clinical practice of the CURPAP study is that N-CPAP should be started soon after birth in spontaneously breathing infants of 25–28 weeks' gestation, and early selective surfactant should be given once signs of respiratory distress have developed. Extubation after surfactant administration should be attempted as soon as possible. With this strategy,

more than 50% of infants will need only N-CPAP, 49% intubation and surfactant, and nearly one third also mechanical ventilation in the first 5 days of life. Overall, the respiratory approach used in this study resulted in a very good respiratory outcome: 78–79% of infants, in both arms, survived without any supplementary oxygen or respiratory support at 36 weeks' postmenstrual age. The incidences of moderate/severe BPD were 14.3 and 11.7%, respectively, in the prophylactic surfactant and N-CPAP groups, which is lower than the 30% incidence reported in other studies (Walsh et al. 2003; Payne et al. 2006).

Finally, Dunn MS et al. published the VON trial (Dunn et al. 2011). In this multicenter randomized trial, three approaches were compared for the initial respiratory management of preterm infants (26.0–28.6 weeks' GA): prophylactic surfactant (PS) and mechanical ventilation, prophylactic surfactant given as INSURE procedure (ISX) followed by N-CPAP (bubble CPAP), or N-CPAP (bubble CPAP) and selective surfactant treatment. Primary outcome was the incidence of death and BPD at 36 weeks' postmenstrual age. Six hundred forty eight infants were enrolled in 27 centers. Preterm infants initially managed with INSURE approach or N-CPAP plus selective surfactant therapy showed similar outcomes to those treated with PS and mechanical ventilation. Therefore, the authors concluded that early N-CPAP approach may be recommended as a less invasive and potentially less expensive method of management in this category of patients.

In the past, doubts have been cast on the possibility of generalizing low-invasiveness treatment strategies in VLBW infants (Roberton 1993). Currently, similar doubts may be raised for ELBW infants, in whom the application of results from studies (Finer et al. 2004; Morley et al. 2008; Sandri et al. 2010) should take into account the rate of prenatal steroid use and the type of antenatal healthcare program.

Nevertheless, two meta-analysis that analyzed the results of the most recent RCTs (e.g., CURPAP, COIN, SUPPORT, etc.) demonstrated that using a non-invasive respiratory approach in the DR and beyond can lead to a small but significant reduction in the rate of BPD in very premature infants (Schmölzer et al. 2013; Fischer and Bührer 2013). This concept is reinforced in the current neonatal resuscitation guidelines (Wylie et al. 2015).

In conclusion, the available published data suggests that:

VLBW infants, not intubated at birth for cardiopulmonary resuscitation, can be treated conservatively using NCPAP, with the administration of surfactant and mechanical ventilation only being used if precise clinical, laboratory test and instrumental criteria are met.

Prenatal steroids, higher GA, and female sex are associated with higher chances of being treated noninvasively.

A precise limit of gestational age or birth weight below which N-CPAP cannot be used with success has not yet been established.

Using NCPAP together with early selective surfactant to avoid more invasive strategies does not entail an increase in mortality rates or negative side effects.

62.6.2 Neonatal Apnea

Apnea is traditionally classified into three categories based on the presence or absence of obstruction of the upper airways: central, obstructive, and mixed (see ▶ Chap. 66, "Apnea of Prematurity and Sudden Infant Death Syndrome") (Kattwinkel 1977; Miller et al. 1985).

Because most apneic episodes have an obstructive component, CPAP appears to be one of the most effective strategies. It splints the upper airway with positive pressure and decreases the risk of pharyngeal or laryngeal obstruction. CPAP probably also improves apnea by increasing functional residual capacity (FRC) and so improving oxygenation status (Kattwinkel 1977; Miller et al. 1985). The positive effect of CPAP is also due to the stabilization of the rib cage, (Miller et al. 1990; Van de Graaff 1988; Kattwinkel 1977) that contributes to the airways opening and to the reduction of the Hering-Breuer reflex (Martin et al. 1977).

Given that N-CPAP does not have a direct effect on apnea of central origin, its use in

association with stimulants of the respiratory centers such as methylxanthine below 32 weeks of gestational age is generally accepted (AARC (American Association for Respiratory Care) 1994; Aranda and Turmen 1979; Schmidt et al. 2006).

In case of persistent and severe apnea of prematurity, before deciding to intubate the baby, it could be useful to switch the infant from N-CPAP to other form of noninvasive respiratory approach (e.g., bi-level CPAP or NIPPV), even better if synchronized with the patient effort, as suggested from a recent randomized crossover trial (Gizzi et al. 2015).

62.6.3 Weaning the Patient from Mechanical Ventilation (Post-extubation Phase)

It is well known that after a period (long or short) of intubation and mechanical ventilation, extubation can fail, leading to the re-intubation of the newborn (Fox et al. 1981). The reasons for this failure are substantially as follows:

Apnea

An increase in oxygen requirements (this can be correlated to a loss of volume from a malfunction of the glottis after intubation or to atelectasis)

Respiratory acidosis

Various contributors have demonstrated the efficacy of N-CPAP application in the post--extubation phase following mechanical ventilation. N-CPAP compared to direct extubation reduces the need of re-intubation, both in newborns weighing <1500 g (16% failure rate vs. 52%) (So et al. 1995) and in those weighing <1000 g (24% failure rate vs. 79%) (Higgins et al. 1991). The factors that necessitate re-intubation, principally apnea but also an increase in oxygen requirement due to loss of pulmonary volume and respiratory acidosis, are counteracted by N-CPAP. A meta-analysis confirmed the efficacy of N-CPAP in weaning of patients from mechanical ventilation and thus recommended its adoption as an elective method for use after extubation, if necessary in combination with a methylxanthine (Davis and Henderson-Smart 2000). To achieve successful extubation to N-CPAP, it is also important to choose the most appropriate moment in terms of parameters of mechanical ventilation. This should be at a point where the respiratory problem can be considered overcome by ventilation ($FiO_2 < 0.35$, mean airways pressure [MAP] <7 cmH_2O, ventilatory frequency ≤ 20/min) (So et al. 1995; Higgins et al. 1991; Davis and Henderson-Smart 2000). A recent study comparing a continuous flow with a variable flow CPAP device (bubble CPAP vs. infant flow system) concluded that both devices were effective in the post-extubation management of infants with RDS. However, in infants ventilated for $\leq$14 days, bubble CPAP is associated with a significantly higher rate of successful extubation and with a significantly reduced duration of CPAP support (Gupta et al. 2009). Even if previous RCTs have shown that N-CPAP is a useful method for providing respiratory support after extubation, nevertheless this approach sometimes fails and physicians use as alternative nasal intermittent positive pressure ventilation (NIPPV). A recent meta-analysis (Lemyre et al. 2017) has compared effects of management with N-CPAP versus NIPPV in preterm infants after extubation. The Cochrane review concluded that NIPPV reduces the incidence of extubation failure and the need for re-intubation within 48 h to 1 week more effectively than N-CPAP. However, nasal ventilation has no effect on BPD nor on mortality. The authors suggested that synchronization may be important in increasing the efficacy of NIPPV. Last but not least, a recent meta-analysis (Wilkinson et al. 2016) demonstrated that high-flow nasal cannulae (HFNC) have similar rates of efficacy than other forms of noninvasive respiratory support in preterm infants to prevent failure of extubation. Therefore, HFNC could be considered a valid alternative to N-CPAP in this

phase of the management of preterm infants with respiratory distress.

62.6.4 Other Clinical Applications

Transient Tachypnea of the Newborn (TTN) Some doubts have been raised regarding the safety of N-CPAP in TTN (see ▸ Chap. 55, "Pulmonary Hemorrhage, Transient Tachypnea, and Neonatal Pneumonia") due to the theoretical risk of air trapping and pneumothorax. There are, however, no relevant published data (Greenough 1996). Authoritative guidelines include TTN in indications for N-CPAP application (AARC (American Association for Respiratory Care) 1994; Jonzon 1991), and our personal experience is that the early application of N-CPAP for TTN brings about a reduction in the clinical signs of respiratory distress without a significant increase in the incidence of pneumothorax.

Meconium Aspiration Syndrome (MAS) The application of a continuous distending pressure could be beneficial, resolving the areas of atelectasis and reopening and stabilizing the airways (Ahumada and Goldsmith 1996; Fox et al. 1975). However, it should be reserved for the less severe forms of MAS (see ▸ Chap. 50, "Meconium Aspiration Syndrome"). More serious cases will require intubation (bronchoalveolar lavage with) surfactant, and mechanical ventilation (Lam 1999; Mosca et al. 1996).

Congenital Cardiopathies with Hyperafflux Pulmonary hyperafflux can lead to a reduction in pulmonary compliance and to a change in the ventilation-perfusion ratio, with consequent hypoxemia, which is potentially correctable with CPAP (Ahumada and Goldsmith 1996).

Tracheobronchomalacia CPAP resolves the collapse of the airways present in this condition, considerably relieving the respiratory distress correlated with it (AARC (American Association for Respiratory Care) 1994; Miller et al. 1986).

Atelectasis The onset of atelectasis can be due to different factors but its resolution will require the removal of the root cause in each case. However, in many situations, e.g., post-extubation atelectasis, CPAP may be used electively (AARC (American Association for Respiratory Care) 1994).

Bronchiolitis Early CPAP (predominantly nasal) can rapidly aid respiratory muscles and improve respiratory distress symptoms (retractions, tachypnea, agitation) and blood gas measurements (pO_2, pH, pCO_2). These effects have been attributed to widening of the bronchioli by positive pressure, followed by emptying of the lung and restoration of a normal FRC. This leads to a reduction in the use of mechanical ventilation (Beasley and Jones 1981; Soong et al. 1993). N-CPAP has also demonstrated its efficacy in the treatment of apnea associated with RSV infection (McNamara and Sullivan 1997).

Paralysis of the Phrenic Nerve Cases have been published in which paralysis of the phrenic nerve was successfully treated with N-CPAP application, which corrects the deficit in transmural pressure caused by paralysis of the diaphragm (Bucci et al. 1974).

Nebulization of Pharmaceuticals N-CPAP has recently been used for the respiratory administration of pharmaceuticals (beta-blockers, steroids, acetylcysteine, and adrenaline), although this does not currently seem to be of great clinical interest (Smedsaas-Lofvemberg et al. 1999).

62.7 Side Effects

System Malfunctions The obstruction of the nasal prongs or the tube by mucous (like the obstruction of the nasal passages) is common during N-CPAP, with potentially serious consequences (sudden decrease in oxygenation) due to the lack of airflow delivered to the patient (AARC (American Association for Respiratory Care) 1994).

Pulmonary Overdistention Pulmonary hyperdistension is the most serious complication that can occur during N-CPAP. This condition can occur whenever the positive pressure applied is excessive with respect to the patient's pulmonary compliance.

The presence of a hyperdistended lung leads to an increased risk of pneumothorax, a worsening

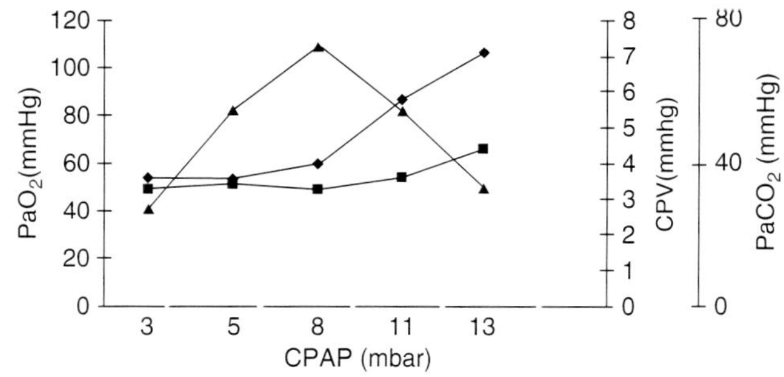

Fig. 5 Effects of different CPAP levels on the central venous pressure (CVP (■), PaO_2 (▲), and $PaCO_2$ (◆) (Modified from Gregory (1986))

of the ventilation-perfusion ratio, and an increase in CO_2 retention and WOB. It is also known that the higher the pulmonary compliance, the greater the transmission of positive pressure to the posterior mediastinum, followed by an increase in central venous pressure with a decrease in venous return and cardiac output. Figure 5 shows the effects of rising CPAP values on central venous pressure, on paO_2, and on $paCO_2$, the onset of which correlates directly with hemodynamic and respiratory interferences (Fig. 2, part C) (Gregory 1986). These hemodynamic effects can have serious consequences on gastrointestinal, renal, and cerebral perfusion and can cause an increase in intracranial pressure due to the decrease in venous drainage (Ahumada and Goldsmith 1996; AARC (American Association for Respiratory Care) 1994).

Gastric Distension It can cause reduced ventilatory excursion due to compression of the diaphragm or even gastric perforation (CPAP belly syndrome) (Ahumada and Goldsmith 1996; AARC (American Association for Respiratory Care) 1994; Leone and Krasna 2000). It can be prevented by properly affixing the nasal prongs, by positioning a permanent orogastric tube, and by periodically checking the degree of abdominal distension.

Nasal Lesions Nasal-cutaneous lesions have been described during N-CPAP with possible permanent deformities (Loftus et al. 1994; Robertson et al. 1996). These lesions can be prevented by choosing silicone nasal prongs (which permit good contact without being harmful), nasal prongs of the correct dimensions with relation to the newborn's nostrils and ensuring their correct positioning.

62.8 Suggestions for N-CPAP Use in the Clinical Practice

62.8.1 Pressure Level

There have been few data published to evaluate a method that would allow the establishment of an optimum pressure for CPAP, and its clinical applicability in practice is very limited (Tanswell et al. 1980; Elgellab et al. 2001).

It is advisable to:

Start with a level of CPAP between 5 and 7 cmH_2O.

Individualize the CPAP level on the basis of respiratory dynamics, respiratory frequency, grunting, and thoracic retraction. The level of CPAP can be increased up to 8–10 cmH_2O.

Choose higher values if there is reduced pulmonary volume.

Once an improvement in the respiratory dynamics has been reached, adjust the FiO_2 so as to maintain PaO_2 between 60 and 80 mmHg or tcO_2 saturation (measured by pulse oximetry, SpO_2) at target range (e.g., 90–95% in preterm infants as suggested by the recent European RDS guidelines) (Sweet et al. 2017).

Reduce the level of CPAP as long as lung compliance, lung volume, and oxygenation improve in order to avoid hyperdistension and transmission of positive pressure to the mediastinum.

62.8.2 Monitoring

The use of N-CPAP therapy requires accurate monitoring to both evaluate the evolution of the illness and to identify negative side effects:

Blood gas analysis from arterial or an arterialized capillary blood represents the gold standard for blood gas measurement. It should be carried out within 15–30 min of starting therapy and whenever clinically indicated (Ahumada and Goldsmith 1996).

Pulse oximetry. Despite its universally known limitations, this is the method of choice for the continuous monitoring of oxygenation level, particularly when the situation has stabilized, . It is advisable to target O_2 saturation values according to the recent guidelines (e.g., 90–95%) (Sweet et al. 2017).

Transcutaneous PO_2 and PCO_2. This type of monitoring, though potentially very useful, has in reality many limitations that require great caution in interpreting the values it obtains, which should be verified and checked frequently against the blood gas values.

ECG and systemic arterial pressure. The potential side effects of CPAP on circulation require continuous monitoring of heart rate and periodic measurement of systemic blood pressure.

Chest X-ray provides valuable information in evaluating the effect of CPAP on the evolution of the disease, such as improvement of the radiological picture or the development of complications such as hyperdistension or pneumothorax.

62.8.3 How to Try to Prevent Failure of N-CPAP?

Since the incidence of N-CPAP failure in large RCTs evaluating CPAP versus routine intubation is close to 50% (Wright et al. 2016) and CPAP failure occurs early (at about 8 h of life) above all because of increasing of oxygen requirements, it seems to be reasonable that early interventions used to establish an effective FRC may help N-CPAP a success. After delivery, the lung is fluid-filled and the reabsorption of the liquid from the lung, in the past attributed to the epithelial sodium channel, is initially related to the delta pressure generated by the first breaths that move the lung fluid in the airway until the alveoli, where the fluid is pumped into the interstitium and reabsorbed by the lymphatic and vein vessels in the hours following birth (Hooper et al. 2015). The term infant is able to generate this delta pressure with the first three to five initial prolonged inspiration to clear the lung fluid (Karlberg 1960). On the contrary, the preterm infants are often unable to do it. In animal experiment, it has been demonstrated that the use of sustained inflation (SI) (a deep and prolonged inflation), especially when followed by an adequate PEEP, is an intriguing approach to allow the preterm animal to create the FRC (Te Pas et al. 2009). Also in humans, the use of SI (e.g., a peak pressure of 20–25 cmH_20 maintained for 10–15 sec) seems to facilitate the respiratory transition at birth. In fact, a recent meta-analysis that compared SI versus positive pressure ventilation at birth in preterm infants at risk for RDS or with signs of respiratory failure concluded that SI improved short respiratory outcomes (reduced the need of mechanical ventilation in the first 72 h of life), even if death and BPD occurrence were not improved (Schmolzer et al. 2014). For this reason, the recent neonatal resuscitation guidelines suggest against the routine use of SI in the resuscitation of infants with signs of respiratory failure, but suggest the use only in individual clinical circumstances or in research settings (Wylie et al. 2015). Some authors suggest to use two ancillary therapies in the delivery room to reduce the N-CPAP failure: early surfactant administration and caffeine (Kribs and Hummler 2016). Surfactant in fact allows to achieve an early FRC by improving lung compliance (Davis et al. 1998), and caffeine is a determinant in promoting spontaneous breathing in premature infants that are at risk for apnea (Henderson-Smart and Steer 2001). Surfactant is delivered by less invasive surfactant application (LISA) by inserting a small catheter in the trachea and delivering the surfactant through this catheter without intubation (Kribs and Hummler 2016). The authors concluded that these two approaches can be considered a "bridge" between the delivery room and the NICU in order to facilitate the initial success of the N-CPAP. Future research is needed to identify which preterm infants can have benefits from this early approach yet in the delivery suite instead of in the NICU. Further studies will also

make clear whether the LISA procedure, or similar procedures, can replace INSURE (see section "Clinical Evidence") or what the place of both LISA and INSURE are in the treatment of infants with RDS on N-CPAP. Indeed, both procedures have advantages and disadvantages.

62.8.4 Weaning from N-CPAP

Once clinical improvement has been obtained as previously described, the improved situation is shown by the ability to progressively reduce FiO_2 (in 2–5% steps down to 21%) and the level of positive pressure (1 cmH_2O at a time down to 2–3 cmH_2O). Once minimal values have been reached for both parameters, the N-CPAP therapy can be stopped more or less gradually, taking into account the weight and gestational age of the baby monitoring an eventual increase of WOB (clinically manifested, e.g., by tachypnea and or intercostal and diaphragmatic retractions) and depending on the presence or lack of other indications for therapy, e.g., apnea of prematurity.

62.9 Nursing of the Neonate in N-CPAP

The importance of nursing is particularly important when CPAP is administered via nasal prongs. The following require particular attention (Sahni et al. 2016):

Correct attachment (headset and nasal prongs)
Correct positioning (circuit and infant)
Correct temperature setting on the humidifier
Correct aspiration of the airways and feeding

62.9.1 Attachment (Headset and Nasal Prongs)

The attachments for the nasal prongs always include a bonnet, which the prongs themselves are fixed to. The bonnet must be large enough to reach the level of the eyebrows and to cover the ears completely. If it is too small, it will tend to ride up, forcing the circuit toward the neonate's nose. The prongs generally come in three sizes (small, medium, and large): the size that is most compatible with the patient's nostrils must be chosen. It is wrong to assume that the smallest prongs are for the most delicate neonate. If the prongs are too small, they do not give an adequate hold, which is necessary to maintain a constant level of CPAP and to avoid an increase in airways resistance. This does not allow a reduction in WOB and may cause it to increase.

The silicone nasal prongs warm up when inserted into the nostrils, and in doing so, they become softer and expand slightly, improving their hold. The use of creams or plasters around the nose is not recommended. Once the circuit has been positioned, care must be taken that the edge of the prongs does not adhere to the nasal septum: the base of the prongs must always be visible (Fig. 6) (see also section "Positioning of the Circuit").

The prongs can increase the production of nasal secretions, and for this reason, the system for humidifying and heating the administered gas

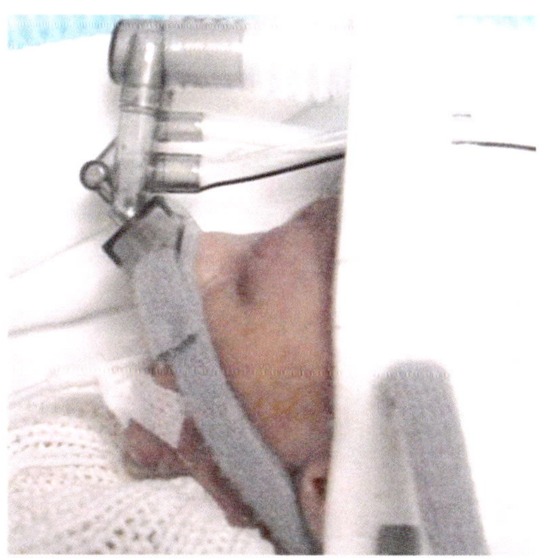

Fig. 6 Correct positioning of the nasal prongs

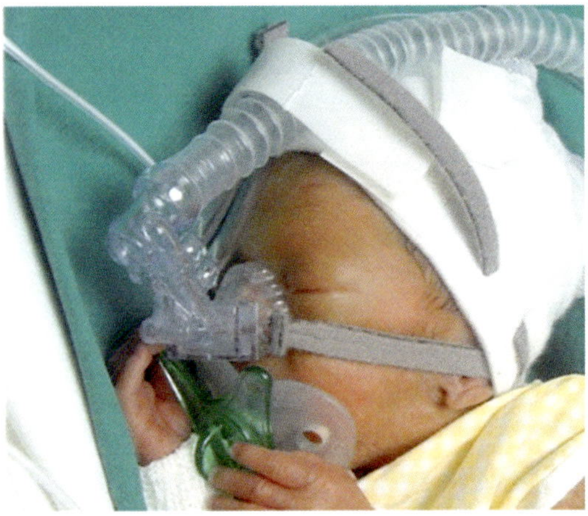

Fig. 7 Nasal mask for the application of nasal CPAP

is very important (see section "Humidification and Heating"). When the infant cries, there may be a loss of pressure: therefore, correct nursing is extremely important during the administration of CPAP (see also section "Positioning the Infant"). Silicone masks are available as an alternative to nasal prongs for very small or large infants (Fig. 7).

62.9.2 Positioning of the Circuit

The tubes should be positioned so as not to pull on the flow generator or put pressure on the neonate's nose.

The flow generator is connected to the nasal mask by ribbons, which must not be too tight. Once the ribbons have been fixed, they should be directed downward, that is, toward the base of the ears and away from the eyes in order to avoid swelling at this level. Plasters or knots between the ribbons and the nasal mask should be avoided to facilitate the rapid adjustment of the prongs. Only the gas arrival tube should be attached to the bonnet while the others should be left free.

In the case of the infant flow generator, it is important that the outlet tube be positioned outside the incubator in order to minimize noise: if necessary use the extension tube.

62.9.3 Positioning the Infant

The infant can be placed in a prone, supine (with support), or lateral position. The neck, however, must always be slightly extended. The prone position has been shown to be better for the premature neonate with respiratory distress (Sahni et al. 2016).

Kangaroo care is possible during N-CPAP. It is important to keep the infant's mouth closed. This confers at least three benefits:

It avoids loss of pressure and consequent instability of CPAP, therefore reducing WOB.

It avoids drying of the mucous and the formation of dense, whitish secretions because it favours the deglutition of saliva.

It keeps the jaw in the forward position, thus avoiding the tongue falling backward and guaranteeing the patency of the airways.

The infant can be helped to keep their mouth closed. Initially, it can be of use to place a support (e.g., roll of gauze) under the neonate's chin. The use of a pacifier favors deglutition and reduces the formation of saliva in the infant's mouth. It also helps keep the jaw in the forward position.

62.9.4 Humidification and Heating

Adequate humidification is important in order to avoid drying of the mucous and the accumulation of dense secretions, which can block the airways. The recommended gas temperature is 37 °C: this is obtained by setting the resistance temperature of the circuit at 39 °C and that of the gas at 2 °C less. It is always important to ensure that the temperature sensor is placed outside the incubator. If the neonate is positioned under an infant warmer, the sensor should be thermally isolated.

62.9.5 Airways Suction

It is not necessary to regularly suction the infant in N-CPAP and this maneuver should be performed only when necessary. To reduce the formation of oral and nasal secretions, the following measures can be used:

Set the humidifier to a suitable temperature (see previous paragraph): if the temperature is too low, it can favor the formation of dry secretions.

Keep the infant's mouth closed (see section "Positioning the Infant").

62.9.6 Feeding

The use of N-CPAP does not prevent feeding. Food intake should be encouraged (via orogastric feeding tube or bottle and also nipple feeding). Additionally, fed newborns will avoid swallowing air, thus reducing abdominal distension. An orogastric tube is not always necessary.

References

AARC (American Association for Respiratory Care) (1994) Application of continuous positive airway pressure to neonates via nasal prongs or nasopharyngeal tube. Respir Care 39:817–823

Agostino R, Orzalesi M, Nodari S et al (1973) Continuous positive airway pressure (CPAP) by nasal cannula in the respiratory distress syndrome (RDS) of the newborn. Pediatr Res 7:50

Ahluwalia JS, White DK, Morley CJ (1998) Infant flow driver or single prong nasal continuous positive airway pressure: short term physiological effects. Acta Pediatr 87:325–327

Ahumada CA, Goldsmith JP (1996) Continuous distending pressure. In: Goldsmith JP, Karotkin EH (eds) Assisted ventilation of the neonate. WB Saunders, Philadelphia, pp 151–165

Aranda JV, Turmen T (1979) Methylxanthines in apnoea of prematurity. Clin Perinatol 6:87–108

Avery ME, Mead J (1959) Surface properties in relation to atelectasis and hyaline membrane disease. Am J Dis Child 97:517–523

Avery ME, Tooley WH, Keller JB et al (1987) Is chronic lung disease in low birth weight infants preventable? A survey of eight centers. Pediatrics 79:26–30

Bancalari E, Sinclair JC (1991) Mechanical ventilation. In: Sinclair JC, Brachen MB (eds) Effective care of the newborn infant. Oxford University Press, Oxford, pp 200–220

Barach AL, Martin J, Eckman M (1937) Positive pressure respiration and its application to the treatment of acute pulmonary edema and respiratory obstruction. Proc Am Soc Clin Invest 16:664–680

Beasley JM, Jones SEF (1981) Continuous positive airway pressure in bronchiolitis. Br Med J 283:1506–1508

Blennow M, Jonsson B, Dahlstrom A et al (1999) Lung function in premature infants can be improved. Surfactant therapy and CPAP reduce the need of respiratory support. Lakartidningen 96:1571–1576

Bucci G, Marzetti G, Picece-Bucci S et al (1974) Phrenic nerve palsy treated by continuous positive pressure breathing by nasal cannula. Arch Dis Child 49:230–232

Bullowa JGH (1937) The management of the pneumonias. Oxford University Press, New York

Burch K, Rhine W, Baker R et al (2003) Implementing potentially better practices to reduce lung injury in neonates. Pediatrics 111:e432–e436

Caliumi-Pellegrini G, Agostino R, Orzalesi M et al (1974) Twin nasal cannula for administration of continuous positive airway pressure to newborn infants. Arch Dis Child 49:228–230

Cohen G, Henderson-Smart D (1986) Upper airway stability and apnoea during nasal occlusion in newborn infants. J Appl Physiol 60:1511–1517

Cordero L, Ayers LW, Davis K (1997) Neonatal airway colonization with gram-negative bacilli: association with severity of bronchopulmonary dysplasia. Pediatr Infect Dis J 16:18–23

Courtney SE, Pyon KH, Saslow JG et al (2001) Lung recruitment and breathing pattern during variable versus continuous positive airway pressure in premature infants. An evaluation of three devices. Pediatrics 197:304–308

Davis PG, Henderson-Smart DJ (2000) Nasal CPAP immediately after extubation for preventing morbidity in preterm infants. Cochrane Database Syst Rev 3: CD000143

Davis AJ, Jobe AH, Häfner D et al (1998) Lung function in premature lambs and rabbits treated with a recombinant SP-C surfactant. Am J Respir Crit Care Med 157(2): 553–559

Dunn MS, Kaempf J, de Klerk A et al (2011) Randomized trial comparing 3 approaches to the initial respiratory management of preterm neonates. Pediatrics 128(5): e1069–e1076

Elgellab A, Riou Y, Abbazine A et al (2001) Effects of nasal continuous airway positive pressure (NCPAP) on breathing pattern in spontaneously breathing premature newborn infants. Intensive Care Med 27: 1782–1787

Finer NN, Waldemar AC, Duara S et al (2004) Delivery room continuous positive airway pressure/positive end-expiratory pressure in extremely low birth weight infants: a feasibility trial. Pediatrics 114:651–657

Finer NN, Carlo WA, Walsh MC et al (2010) Early CPAP versus surfactant in extremely preterm infants. N Engl J Med 362(21):1970–1979

Fischer HS, Bührer C (2013) Avoiding endotracheal ventilation to prevent bronchopulmonary dysplasia: a meta-analysis. Pediatrics 132(5):e1351–e1360

Fox WW, Berman LS, Downes JJ Jr, Peckham GJ (1975) The therapeutic application of end-expiratory pressure in the meconium aspiration syndrome. Pediatrics 56: 214–217

Fox WW, Schwartz JG, Shaffer TH (1981) Successful extubation of neonates: clinical and physiological factors. Crit Care Med 9:823–826

Gaon P, Lee S, Hannan S et al (1999) Assessment of effect of nasal continuous positive pressure on laryngeal opening using fibre optic laryngoscopy. Arch Dis Child Fetal Neonatal Ed 80:F230–F232

Gauda EB, Miller MJ, Carlo W et al (1987) Genioglossus response to airway occlusion in apneic versus non-apneic infants. Pediatr Res 22:683–687

Gerhardt T, Bancalari E (1980) Chestwall compliance in full-term and premature infants. Acta Pediatr Scand 69:359–364

Gherini S, Peters RM, Virgilio RW (1979) Mechanical work on the lungs and work of breathing with positive end expiratory pressure and continuous positive airway pressure. Chest 76:251–256

Gittermann MK, Fusch C, Gittermann AR et al (1997) Early nasal continuous positive airway pressure treatment reduces the need for intubation in very low birth weight infants. Eur J Pediatr 156:384–388

Gizzi C, Montecchia F, Panetta V et al (2015) Is synchronised NIPPV more effective than NIPPV and NCPAP in treating apnoea of prematurity (AOP)? A randomised cross-over trial. Arch Dis Child Fetal Neonatal 100(1):F17–F23

Goldman SL, Brady JP, Bchir MB et al (1979) Increased work of breathing associated with nasal prongs. Pediatrics 64:160–164

Greenough A (1996) Transient tachypnoea of the newborn. In: Greenough A, Roberton NRC, Milner AD (eds) Neonatal respiratory disorders. Arnold, London, pp 280–285

Greenough A, Roberton NRC (1996) Respiratory distress syndrome. In: Greenough A, Roberton NRC, Milner AD (eds) Neonatal respiratory disorders. Arnold, London, pp 238–279

Gregory GA (1986) Continuous positive airways pressure. In: Thibeault DW, Gregory GA (eds) Neonatal pulmonary care, 2nd edn. Appleton & Lange, Norwalk, p 355

Gregory GA, Kittermann JA, Phibbs RH et al (1971) Treatment of the idiopathic respiratory distress syndrome with continuous positive airway pressure. N Engl J Med 284:1333–1340

Gupta S, Sinha SK, Tin W, Donn SM (2009) A randomized controlled trial of post-extubation bubble continuous positive airway pressure versus infant flow driver continuous positive airway pressure in preterm infants with respiratory distress syndrome. J Pediatr 154:645–650

Harrison VC, de Heese Hde V, Klein M (1968) The significance of grunting in hyaline membrane disease. Pediatrics 41:549–559

Henderson-Smart DJ, Steer P (2001) Methyl-xanthine treatment for apnea in preterm infants. Cochrane Database Syst Rev 3:CD000140

Higgins RD, Richter SE, Davis JM (1991) Nasal continuous positive airway pressure facilitates extubation of very low birth weight neonates. Pediatrics 88:999–1003

Hooper SB, Siew ML, Kitchen MJ (2015) Respiratory transition in the newborn: a three phase process. Arch Dis Child Fetal Neonatal Ed 101(3):F266–F271

Horbar JD, McAuliffe TL, Adler SM et al (1988) Variability in 28- day outcomes for very low birth weight infants: an analysis of 11 neonatal intensive care units. Pediatrics 82:554–559

Jacobsen T, Gronvall J, Petersen S et al (1993) "Minitouch" treatment of very low birth weight infants. Acta Pediatr 82:934–938

Jonsson B, Katz-Salamon M, Faxelius G et al (1997) Neonatal care of very low birth weight infants in special care units and neonatal intensive care units in Stockholm. Early nasal continuous positive airway pressure versus mechanical ventilation: gains and losses. Acta Pediatr Suppl 419:4–10

Jonzon A (1991) Indications for continuous positive airway pressure and respiratory therapy. Int J Technol Assess Health Care 7(Suppl 1):26–30

Kamper J, Ringsted C (1990) Early treatment of idiopathic respiratory distress syndrome using binasal continuous positive airway pressure. Acta Pediatr Scand 79: 581–586

Kamper J, Wulff K, Larsen C et al (1993) Early treatment with nasal continuous positive airway pressure in very low birth weight infants. Acta Pediatr 82:193–197

Karlberg P (1960) The adaptive changes in the immediate postnatal period, with particular reference to respiration. J Pediatr 56:585–604

Kattwinkel J (1977) Neonatal apnoea: pathogenesis and therapy. J Pediatr 90:342–347

Kattwinkel J, Fanaroff A, Cha C et al (1973) Controlled trial of continuous positive airway pressure (CPAP) in RDS and a simplified application by the nasal route. Pediatr Res 7:396

Kavvadia V, Greenough A, Dimitriou G (2000) Effect on lung function of continuous positive airway pressure administered either by infant flow driver or a single nasal prong. Eur J Pediatr 159:289–292

Klausner JF, Lee AY, Hutchinson AA (1996) Decreased imposed work with a new nasal continuous positive airway pressure device. Pediatr Pulmonol 22:188–194

Kribs A, Hummler H (2016) Ancillary therapies to enhance success of non-invasive modes of respiratory support – approaches to delivery room use of surfactant and caffeine? Semin Fetal Neonatal Med 21(3): 212–218

Kurz H (1999) Influence of nasopharyngeal CPAP on breathing pattern and incidence of apnoeas in preterm infants. Biol Neonate 76:129–133

Lam BC (1999) Surfactant lavage for the management of severe meconium aspiration syndrome. Biol Neonate 76(Suppl 1):10–14

Lemyre B, Davis PG, De Paoli AG et al (2017) Nasal intermittent positive pressure ventilation (NIPPV) versus nasal continuous positive airway pressure (NCPAP) for preterm neonates after extubation. Cochrane Database Syst Rev 2:CD003212. https://doi.org/10.1002/14651858.CD003212.pb3)

Leone RJ, Krasna IH (2000) "Spontaneous" neonatal gastric perforation: is it really spontaneous? J Pediatr Surg 35:1066–1069

Levy J, Habib RH, Liptsen E et al (2006) Prone versus supine positioning in the well preterm infant: effects on work of breathing and breathing patterns. Pediatr Pulmonol 41:754–758

Lindner W, Vossbeck S, Hummler H et al (1999) Delivery room management of extremely low birth weight infants: spontaneous breathing or intubation? Pediatrics 103:961–967

Loftus BC, Ahn J, Haddad J (1994) Neonatal nasal deformities secondary to nasal continuous positive airway pressure. Laryngoscope 104:1019–1022

Lundstrom KE (1996) Initial treatment of preterm infants–continuous positive airway pressure or ventilation? Eur J Pediatr 155(Suppl 2):S25–S29

Martin RJ, Nearman HS, Katona PG et al (1977) The effect of a low continuous positive airway pressure on the reflex control of respiration in the preterm infant. J Pediatr 90:976–981

McNamara F, Sullivan CE (1997) Nasal CPAP treatment in an infant with respiratory syncitial virus-associated apnoea. Pediatr Pulmonol 24:218–221

Miller MJ, Carlo WA, Martin RJ (1985) Continuous positive airway pressure selectively reduces obstructive apnoea in preterm infants. J Pediatr 106:91–94

Miller RW, Pollack MM, Murphy TM et al (1986) Effectiveness of continuous positive airway pressure in the treatment of bronchomalacia in infants: a bronchoscopic documentation. Crit Care Med 14:125–127

Miller MJ, DiFiore JM, Strohl KP et al (1990) Effects of nasal CPAP on supraglottic and total pulmonary resistance in preterm infants. J Appl Physiol 68:141–146

Moa G, Nilsson K (1993) Nasal continuous positive airway pressure: experiences with a new technical approach. Acta Pediatr 82:210–211

Moa G, Nilsson K, Zetterstrom H et al (1988) A new device for administration of nasal continuous positive airway pressure in the newborn: an experimental study. Crit Care Med 16:1238–1242

Morley C (1999) Continuous distending pressure. Arch Dis Child Fetal Neonatal Ed 81:F152–F156

Morley CJ, Davis PG, Doyle LW et al (2008) Nasal CPAP or intubation at birth for very preterm infants. N Engl J Med 358:700–708

Mosca F, Colnaghi M, Castoldi F (1996) Lung lavage with a saline volume similar to functional residual capacity followed by surfactant administration in newborns with severe meconium aspiration syndrome. Intensive Care Med 22:1412–1413

Pape KE, Armstrong DL, Fitzhardinge PM (1976) Central nervous system pathology associated with mask ventilation in the very low birth weight infant: a new etiology for intracerebellar hemorrhages. Pediatrics 58:473–483

Payne NR, LaCorte M, Karna P et al (2006) Reduction of bronchopulmonary dysplasia after participation in the Breathsavers Group of the Vermont Oxford Network Neonatal Intensive Care Quality Improvement Collaborative. Pediatrics 118:S73–S77

Pedersen JE, Nielsen K (1994) Oropharyngeal and esophaegeal pressure during mono-and binasal CPAP in neonates. Acta Pediatr 83:143–149

Perlman J, Thach B (1988) Respiratory origin of fluctuations in arterial blood pressure in premature infants with respiratory distress syndrome. Pediatrics 81:399–403

Poulton EP, Oxon DM (1936) Left-sided heart failure with pulmonary edema: its treatment with the "pulmonary plus pressure machine". Lancet 228:981–983

Rasanen J, Leijala M (1991) Breathing circuit respiratory work in infants recovering from respiratory failure. Crit Care Med 19:31–35

Roberton NRC (1993) Does CPAP work when it really matters? Acta Pediatr 82:206–207

Robertson NJ, McCarthy LS, Hamilton PA, Moss ALH (1996) Nasal deformities resulting from flow driver continuous positive airway pressure. Arch Dis Child Fetal Neonatal Ed 75:F209–F212

Sahni R, Schiaratura M, Polin RA (2016) Strategies for the prevention of continuous positive airway pressure failure. Semin Fetal Neonatal Med 21(3):196–203

Sandri F, Ancora G, Rinaldi M et al (1999) Incidence of intact survival in a group of ELBWI and permissive hypercapnia. Pediatr Res 45:223A

Sandri F, Ancora G, Lanzoni A et al (2004) Prophylactic nasal continuous positive airways pressure in newborns of 28–31 weeks gestation: multicentre randomised controlled clinical trial. Arch Dis Child Fetal Neonatal Ed 89:F394–F398

Sandri F, Plavka R, Ancora G et al (2010) Prophylactic or early selective surfactant combined with nCPAP in very preterm infants. Pediatrics 125:e1402–e1409

Schmidt B, Roberts RS, Davis P et al (2006) Caffeine therapy for apnea of prematurity. N Engl J Med 355:958–959

Schmölzer GM, Kumar M, Pichler G et al (2013) Non-invasive versus invasive respiratory support in preterm infants at birth: systematic review and meta-analysis. BMJ 347:f5980

Schmolzer GM, Kumar M, Aziz K et al (2014) Sustained inflation versus positive pressure ventilation at birth: a systematic review and meta-analysis. Arch Dis Child Fetal Neonatal Ed 100(4):F361–F368

Schulze A, Madler HJ, Gehrhardt B et al (1990) Titration of continuous positive airway pressure by the pattern of breathing: analysis of flow-volume-time relationships

by a non-invasive computerized system. Pediatr Pulmonol 8:96–103

Smedsaas-Lofvemberg A, Nilsson K, Moa G et al (1999) Nebulization of drugs in a nasal CPAP system. Acta Paediatr 88:89–92

So BH, Tamura M, Mishina J et al (1995) Application of nasal continuous positive airway pressure to early extubation in very low birth weight infants. Arch Dis Child Fetal Neonatal Ed 72:F191–F193

Soong WJ, Hwang B, Tang RB (1993) Continuous positive airway pressure by nasal prongs in bronchiolitis. Pediatr Pulmonol 16:163–166

Stevens TP, Blennow M, Myers EH, Soll R (2007) Early surfactant administration with brief ventilation vs. selective surfactant and continued mechanical ventilation for preterm infants with or at risk for respiratory distress syndrome. Cochrane Database Syst Rev 3: CD003063

Sweet DG, Carnielli V, Greisen G et al (2017) European consensus guidelines on the management of respiratory distress syndrome – 2016 update. Neonatology 111:107–125

Tanswell AK, Clubb RA, Smith BT et al (1980) Individualized continuous distending pressure applied within 6 hours of delivery in infants with respiratory distress syndrome. Arch Dis Child 55:33–39

Tarnow-Mordi WO, Sutton P, Wilkinson AR (1986) Inadequate humidification of respiratory gases during mechanical ventilation of the newborn. Arch Dis Child 61:698–700

Te Pas AB, Siew M, Wallace MJ et al (2009) Establishing functional residual capacity at birth: the effect of sustained inflation and positive end-expiratory pressure in a rabbit model. Pediatr Res 65(5):537–541

Van de Graaff WB (1988) Thoracic influence on upper airway patency. J Appl Physiol 65:2124–2131

Verder H, Robertson B, Greisen G et al (1994) Surfactant therapy and nasal continuous positive airway pressure for newborns with respiratory distress syndrome. N Engl J Med 331:1051–1055

Verder H, Albertsen P, Ebbesen F et al (1999) Nasal continuous positive airway pressure and early surfactant therapy for respiratory distress syndrome in newborns of less than 30 weeks' gestation. Pediatrics 103:e24

Vert P, Andre M, Silbout M (1973) Continuous positive airway pressure and hydrocephalus. Lancet 302:319

Walsh MC, Wilson-Costello D, Zadell A et al (2003) Safety, reliability, and validity of a physiologic definition of bronchopulmonary dysplasia. J Perinatol 23:451–456

Wilkinson D, Andersen C, O'Donnell CP et al (2016) High flow nasal cannula for respiratory support in preterm infants. Cochrane Database Syst Rev 2:CD006405. https://doi.org/10.1002/14651858.CD006405.pub3. Review

Wilson SL, Thach BT, Brouillette RT et al (1980) Upper airway patency in the human infant: influence of airway pressure and posture. J Appl Physiol Respir Environ Exerc Physiol 48:500–504

Wright CJ, Polin RA, Kirpalani H (2016) Continuous positive airway pressure to prevent neonatal lung injury: how did we get here, and how do we improve? J Pediatr 173:17–24.e2

Wylie J, Perlman JM, Kattwinkel J et al (2015) Part 7: neonatal resuscitation:2015 international consensus on cardiopulmonary resuscitation and emergency. Cardiovascular care science with treatment recommendations. Resuscitation 95:e171–e203

Lung Diseases: Surfactant Replacement Therapy in Newborns

63

Henry L. Halliday

Contents

Abstract

In the past three decades, introduction of prenatal steroid treatment, postnatal surfactant therapy, and assisted ventilation has contributed to better outcomes for neonates with respiratory distress syndrome (RDS). Improved survival is directly related to more effective prevention or treatment of the disease. RDS is caused by surfactant insufficiency leading to alveolar collapse and increased work of breathing with consequent hypoxia, respiratory failure, and mixed respiratory and metabolic acidosis. Following unsuccessful clinical trials in the 1960s with nebulized synthetic surfactants, comprised of phospholipids without surfactant proteins, a number of randomized controlled trials in the 1980s demonstrated benefits of surfactant instilled directly into the lungs of preterm infants. Currently, because of increased use of prenatal steroids and early

H. L. Halliday (✉)
Formerly Regional Neonatal Unit, Royal Maternity Hospital, Belfast, UK

Formerly Department of Child Health, Queen's University Belfast, Belfast, UK
e-mail: henry.halliday@doctors.org.uk

G. Buonocore et al. (eds.), *Neonatology*,
https://doi.org/10.1007/978-3-319-29489-6_210

CPAP, it is clear that early selective use of surfactant is superior to routine prophylactic treatment. However, there are still some occasions when surfactant should be administered in the delivery room including cases when intubation of very preterm infants is needed for stabilization.

63.1 Salient Points

- Respiratory distress syndrome is caused by surfactant insufficiency which leads to progressive hypoxia, respiratory failure, and mixed respiratory and metabolic acidosis as a result of alveolar collapse and increased work of breathing.
- The use of prenatal steroids and early CPAP make early selective use of surfactant superior to routine prophylactic treatment. There are still some occasions when surfactant should be administered in the delivery room including cases when intubation of very preterm infants is needed for stabilization.
- The dose of surfactant required for optimal effects is not known. It is possible that 100 mg/kg is sufficient for prophylactic treatment, but 200 mg/kg may give better outcomes for the later treatment of RDS.
- The INSURE (INtubateSURfactant Extubate to CPAP) technique minimizes the duration of ventilation and is useful for babies initially treated with CPAP who may avoid mechanical ventilation altogether.
- Less invasive surfactant administration (LISA) and nebulization are techniques that show promise and help to avoid endotracheal intubation.
- Other indications for surfactant include meconium aspiration syndrome (reducing the need for ECMO) and pneumonia, but in other cases the treatment is experimental.
- Surfactant may be used as a vehicle to deliver drugs to the lungs, and trials with budesonide show promise as a means of reducing bronchopulmonary dysplasia.

63.2 Introduction

In the past three decades, introduction of prenatal steroid treatment, postnatal surfactant therapy, and assisted ventilation has contributed to improved neonatal outcomes (Speer et al. 2013). Improved survival is directly related to more effective prevention or treatment of respiratory distress syndrome (RDS), which prior to the 1990s had a high mortality. Following unsuccessful clinical trials with nebulized synthetic surfactants, comprised of phospholipids without surfactant proteins, in the 1960s (Soll 2000a) a number of randomized controlled trials in the 1980s demonstrated benefits of surfactants instilled directly into the lungs of preterm infants (Soll 2000a, b; Seger and Soll 2009; Soll and Ozek 2010). These surfactants were of two main types: natural (derived from animal lungs or human amniotic fluid) (Soll 2000a; Seger and Soll 2009) containing surfactant proteins B and C (SP-B and SP-C) and synthetic (Soll and Ozek 2010; Soll 2000b) (containing phospholipids and other agents to facilitate spreading and adsorption). Both types of surfactant, given either prophylactically (in the delivery room within 15 min of birth) (Soll 2000a; Soll and Ozek 2010) or for treatment of RDS (Seger and Soll 2009; Soll 2000b), increased neonatal survival and reduced pulmonary air leaks such as pneumothorax and pulmonary interstitial emphysema.

More recently, further randomized clinical trials helped determine the best surfactant (Pfister et al. 2007, 2009; Ardell et al. 2015), the optimal timing for initial treatment (Singh et al. 2015; Rojas-Reyes et al. 2012; Bahadue and Soll 2012; Stevens et al. 2007), the need for redosing (Soll and Ozek 2009), and the dose of phospholipids needed for best outcomes (Speer et al. 2013). Results from these trials have provided guidelines for best practice, and these are now available in Europe (Sweet et al. 2013), the USA (Polin et al. 2014), and Canada (Davis et al. 2005). The aim of this chapter is to summarize the recommendations for surfactant treatment based on evidence from clinical trials and systematic reviews and to point out areas where controversy still exists.

63.3 Respiratory Distress Syndrome and Rationale for Surfactant Therapy

Respiratory distress syndrome (RDS) is caused by surfactant insufficiency (Avery and Mead 1959) which leads to progressive hypoxia, respiratory failure, and mixed respiratory and metabolic acidosis as a result of alveolar collapse and increased work of breathing (Halliday 2003). Surfactant deficiency is strongly associated with prematurity, and progressive acidosis further reduces surfactant production. The normal surfactant phospholipid pool size at birth is about 100 mg/kg, but in preterm infants this is often reduced to below 25 mg/kg, and if severe RDS is present, less than 5 mg/kg (Halliday 2003). Surfactant may also be inactivated by leaking of inhibitory proteins from the plasma into the alveoli. Prior to introduction of surfactant therapy, infants with RDS who survived began to produce their own endogenous surfactant after 2–3 days, and this heralded their recovery (Halliday 2003). Those infants who did not survive either developed progressive respiratory failure with irreversible hypoxic injury to the cardiovascular and central nervous systems or acute deterioration associated with pulmonary air leaks or intraventricular hemorrhage.

Surfactant therapy prevents or overcomes alveolar collapse, especially at end expiration, increases lung volumes and pulmonary compliance, and reverses respiratory failure (Halliday 2003). The result is improved survival and significant reduction in pulmonary air leaks following surfactant treatment (Soll 2000a, b; Seger and Soll 2009; Soll and Ozek 2010). There is evidence from both animal studies and clinical trials that natural surfactants, containing SP-B and SP-C, act more rapidly than synthetic preparations containing mainly phospholipids, leading to improved outcomes with regard to survival and pulmonary air leaks (Pfister et al. 2007; Ardell et al. 2015). There may also be differences when natural (animal-derived) surfactants are compared (Singh et al. 2015). Timing of surfactant therapy may also be important in determining outcome with evidence pointing to earlier therapy being superior to later treatment (Rojas-Reyes et al. 2012; Bahadue and Soll 2012). However, with increased use of prenatal steroids and early CPAP, prophylactic surfactant treatment may not be superior to delayed selective treatment (Rojas-Reyes et al. 2012). The incidence of RDS varies from about 80% at 28 weeks' gestation or below to about 50% at 30 weeks, 30% at 32 weeks, and 10% at 34 weeks (Halliday 2003).

63.4 Results from Randomized Trials and Systematic Reviews

These are discussed under the following subheadings: efficacy, timing of first dose, size of first dose, method of administration, need for redosing, type of surfactant, concomitant interventions, and other indications for surfactant therapy.

63.4.1 Efficacy

Randomized clinical trials of synthetic (protein-free) and natural (containing SP-B and SP-C) surfactants, given both prophylactically (within 10–15 min of birth in the delivery room) or as treatment for established RDS in the neonatal unit, reduce neonatal mortality and pulmonary air leaks such as pneumothorax and pulmonary interstitial emphysema (Speer et al. 2013; Soll 2000a, b; Seger and Soll 2009; Soll and Ozek 2010). Although most of these trials took place in the 1980s and 1990s, when prenatal corticosteroid treatment was less frequent than today, there is no reason to believe that surfactant treatment does not continue to have a positive impact on the outcome of preterm infants (Speer et al. 2013). Indeed prenatal corticosteroids and postnatal surfactant have synergistic effects (Jobe et al. 1993), and both should be considered when preterm birth is likely. The sizes of the effects of prophylactic surfactant administration on neonatal mortality, pneumothorax, and other selected outcomes are shown in Table 1.

Table 1 Meta-analyses of prophylactic surfactant treatment of preterm infants

	Natural surfactant				Synthetic surfactant			
Outcome	RR	95% CI	NNT	95% CI	RR	95% CI	NNT/H	95% CI
Neonatal mortality	0.60	0.44–0.83	14	9–35	0.70	0.58–0.85	15	10–31
Pneumothorax	0.35	0.26–0.49	7	5–9	0.67	0.50–0.90	20	12–67
Pulmonary interstitial emphysema	0.46	0.35–0.60	6	4–8	0.68	0.50–0.93	16	9–77
Pulmonary hemorrhage	–	–	–	–	3.28	1.50–7.16	33	20–100
Intraventricular hemorrhage	0.89	0.84–1.15	–	–	0.96	0.81–1.14	–	–
Severe IVH	1.22	0.90–1.66	–	–	1.01	0.75–1.38	–	–
Persistent ductus arteriosus	1.08	0.94–1.24	–	–	1.11	1.00–1.22	21	11–500
Retinopathy of prematurity	1.37	0.63–2.98	–	–	0.96	0.86–1.07	–	–
Severe ROP	0.58	0.27–1.24	–	–	0.89	0.58–1.36	–	–
Bronchopulmonary dysplasia	0.93	0.80–1.07	–	–	1.06	0.83–1.36	–	–

Data obtained from Cochrane Library (Soll 2000a; Soll and Ozek 2010). *RR* relative risk, *CI* confidence interval, *NNT/H* number needed to treat or harm; *IVH* intraventricular hemorrhage, *ROP* retinopathy of prematurity, *BPD* bronchopulmonary dysplasia

63.4.2 Timing of First Dose

It is clear that the earlier surfactant is given in the course of RDS, the better the outcomes with reduction in pulmonary air leaks, neonatal mortality, and CLD (Bahadue and Soll 2012). In early trials of prophylactic surfactant in infants <31 weeks' gestation, neonatal mortality and pneumothorax were reduced compared to later treatment of established RDS (Rojas-Reyes et al. 2012). However, recent large trials that reflect current practice (including greater use of prenatal steroids and early stabilization with CPAP) do not support these benefits and show reduced risk of CLD or death when using early CPAP with selective surfactant administration for infants needing intubation (Rojas-Reyes et al. 2012). Administration of surfactant generally requires endotracheal intubation, and routine prophylaxis of infants <31 weeks' gestation might lead to unnecessary treatment in up to 50% of cases (Speer et al. 2013). This will increase costs of care and could cause unwanted lung injury leading to BPD. Currently, because of increased use of prenatal steroids and early CPAP, it is clear that early selective use of surfactant is superior to routine prophylactic treatment (Rojas-Reyes et al. 2012). However, there are still some occasions when surfactant should be administered in the delivery room including cases when intubation of very preterm infants is needed for stabilization (Sweet et al. 2013).

63.4.3 Size of First Dose

Clinical trials used surfactant doses ranging from 25 to 200 mg phospholipids/kg (Morley 1991). These doses are all much larger by at least tenfold than the amount of lipids needed to form a monolayer on the alveolar surface of the lungs (Robertson and Halliday 1998). For licensed surfactant preparations, the recommended doses vary from 50 to 200 mg/kg with dose volumes of 1.2–5 mL/kg (Table 2) (Sweet et al. 2013; Polin et al. 2014; Walsh et al. 2013). Larger doses of surfactant are superior to smaller ones (Konishi et al. 1988; Gortner et al. 1994). Surfactant TA in a dose of 120 mg/kg (100 mg phospholipids/kg) improved oxygenation and reduced BPD compared to 60 mg/kg (Konishi et al. 1988). When 100 mg/kg of bovactant was compared with 50 mg/kg, the larger dose was associated with better improvement in oxygenation (Gortner et al. 1994). For poractant alfa 200 mg/kg gives a better acute response than 100 mg/kg (Halliday et al. 1993; Ramanathan et al. 2004) and probably improved survival (Ramanathan et al. 2004). The

Table 2 Some surfactant preparations in clinical use

Generic name	Trade name	Source	Phospholipids (mg/mL)	Dose (mg/kg)	Volume (mL/kg)	Manufacturer (country)
Beractant	Survanta	Bovine mince	25 (50% DPPC)	100	4	Abbott Labs (USA)
BLES	bLES	Bovine lavage	27	135	5	BLES Biochemicals (Canada)
Bovactant	Alveofact	Bovine lavage	42	50	1.2	Lyomark Pharma (Germany)
Calfactant	Infasurf	Bovine lavage	35 (74% DPPC)	105	3	ONY and Forest Labs (USA)
Poractant alfa	Curosurf	Porcine mince	80 (70% DPPC)	100–200	1.25–2.5	Chiesi Farmaceutici (Italy)
Surfactant TA	Surfacten	Bovine mince	30 (48% DPPC)	120	4	Tokyo Tanabe and Mitsubishi Pharma (Japan)

All preparations contain SP-B and SP-C in varying amounts. *BLES* bovine lipid extract surfactant

dose of surfactant required for optimal effects is not known but is probably at least 100 mg phospholipids/kg which is close to the 100–250 mg/kg estimated to form the total pulmonary surfactant pool in a full-term neonate (Robertson and Halliday 1998; Hallman 1989). It is possible that 100 mg/kg is sufficient for prophylactic treatment (Speer et al. 2013), but 200 mg/kg may give better outcomes for later treatment of RDS (Ramanathan et al. 2004).

63.4.4 Method of Administration

Surfactants usually need to be administered directly into the lungs during at least a brief period of endotracheal intubation (Speer et al. 2013). Preterm infants at high risk of developing RDS should be born in centers where personnel and equipment are readily available to allow appropriate care to begin from birth (Sweet et al. 2013). In some of the earlier clinical trials, surfactant was administered as a bolus into each main bronchus or as a single bolus into the lower trachea, whereas in other trials it was given as divided doses directed into each lung lobe by positioning the baby (Morley 1991). After instillation the baby is either manually ventilated for a short time or reconnected to the ventilator to distribute the surfactant. A sterile feeding tube is often used to deliver the surfactant through the endotracheal tube. Bolus administration has been compared with infusion over 30 min in an animal model with the former giving more uniform distribution (Ueda et al. 1994). However, a small clinical trial with beractant found no differences in outcome when three dosing procedures were compared (Zola et al. 1993), and this was supported by a study with poractant alfa, which compared a bolus dose with a 1 min infusion through a dual lumen tube (Valls-i-Soler et al. 1998). It is important to minimize duration of mechanical ventilation after surfactant administration as this is an independent risk factor for development of BPD (Vento et al. 2009). The INSURE (INtubate SURfactant Extubate to CPAP) technique minimizes duration of ventilation and is useful for babies initially treated with CPAP who may avoid mechanical ventilation altogether (Bohlin et al. 2008). Although more surfactant is used with INSURE (RR 1.62, 95%CI 1.41–1.86), the benefits of reduced air leak (RR 0.52, 95%CI 0.28–0.96), BPD (RR 0.51, 95%CI 0.26–0.99), and need for mechanical ventilation (RR 0.67, 95%CI 0.57–0.79) (Stevens et al. 2007) mean that this technique is recommended (Sweet et al. 2013). The benefits appear to be even greater when infants are treated at a lower threshold oxygen requirement of less than 45% (Stevens et al. 2007).

Other methods to forgo the need for endotracheal intubation include nebulization (Berggren et al. 2000), direct tracheal instillation at laryngoscopy using a fine feeding catheter (Kribs

et al. 2008), intrapartum pharyngeal deposition (Kattwinkel et al. 2004), and use of a laryngeal mask (Trevisanuto et al. 2005). Of these, less invasive surfactant administration (LISA) is the most widely accepted (Kribs et al. 2008, 2015), but the technique needs considerable expertise and may not prove to be widely applicable (Speer et al. 2013). Studies with nebulization of surfactant are ongoing, and this technique shows promise (Pillow and Minocchieri 2012).

63.4.5 Need for Redosing

At least two studies demonstrated that multiple doses (up to three) are superior to a single dose (Dunn et al. 1990; Speer et al. 1992), and this is confirmed in a systematic review showing reduced pneumothorax (RR 0.51, 95%CI 0.30–0.88) and a trend toward reduced mortality (RR 0.63, 95%CI 0.39–1.02) (Soll and Ozek 2009). Multiple dose treatment with poractant alfa reduced both neonatal mortality and pneumothorax in preterm infants with severe RDS (Speer et al. 1992). This study used retreatment criteria based on continued need for mechanical ventilation and oxygen supplementation at 12 and 24 h after the first dose, and about two-thirds of babies needed retreatment. Currently, babies with RDS are being treated with surfactant earlier or even prophylactically, and the need for retreatment is much less than before. Poractant alfa in an initial dose of 200 mg/kg compared to 100 mg/kg leads to reduced need for second and third doses (Halliday et al. 1993; Ramanathan et al. 2004). Although criteria for redosing in the past were fixed, it is best to adopt a more flexible approach (Speer et al. 2013; Sweet et al. 2013). Redosing of infants needing more than 30% oxygen has been compared with more than 40% in a randomized trial using calfactant (Kattwinkel et al. 2000). Babies with uncomplicated RDS did equally well with the higher threshold retreatment criterion, but about one-quarter of those enrolled had complicated RDS (associated with birth asphyxia or sepsis), and they had a lower mortality when retreated earlier (Kattwinkel et al. 2000).

Specific recommendations by surfactant manufacturers differ slightly: for beractant retreatment may be given at intervals of at least 6 h for up to four doses; for poractant alfa treatment may be repeated 12 hourly for two further doses if still intubated and after prophylaxis may be repeated 6–12 h later and after a further 12 h (Speer et al. 2013). However, the Canadian Paediatric Society recommends retreatment of infants needing more than 30% oxygen as early as 2 h after the first dose (Davis et al. 2005), and the European Association of Perinatal Medicine recommends retreatment if there is ongoing RDS indicated by need for mechanical ventilation and supplemental oxygen (Sweet et al. 2013). The latter also recommends that babies extubated to CPAP should be retreated (with the INSURE technique) when they need more than 50% oxygen or if they are likely to need mechanical ventilation (Sweet et al. 2013).

63.4.6 Type of Surfactant

Surfactant preparations studied in the 1990s were either synthetic (containing phospholipids without surfactant proteins) or natural (derived from animal lungs and containing both phospholipids and SP-B and SP-C) (Speer et al. 2013). Of these, the best known synthetic surfactants were colfosceril palmitate and pumactant, but they are no longer available for clinical use. The best known natural surfactants are beractant, calfactant, surfactant TA, and bovactant (all of bovine origin) and poractant alfa (of porcine origin) (Table 2). Recently, other surfactants have been produced in Cuba (Surfacen), Korea (Newfacten), Brazil, and India, but there is little information about them (Speer et al. 2013; Halliday 2006). Also, more recently studied are the so-called new-generation synthetic surfactant preparations (Pfister et al. 2007, 2009) which contain phospholipids and surfactant peptide analogues such as lucinactant (Moya et al. 2005; Sinha et al. 2005) and recombinant SP-C surfactant (Curstedt and Johansson 2006).

As noted earlier, studies comparing synthetic and natural surfactants provide evidence that the latter act more rapidly to improve pulmonary status, and in the longer term they show improved survival with fewer pulmonary air leaks (Ardell et al. 2015). As a result, the older synthetic surfactants, colfosceril palmitate and pumactant, are no longer available as commercial products. There have been 16 trials comparing various natural surfactant preparations (Singh et al. 2015), and the largest of these compared beractant with calfactant for both prevention and treatment of RDS (Bloom and Clark 2005). Unfortunately, the planned sample size was not reached, although more than 2,000 infants had been recruited to the two arms of the study, due to slow recruitment, but in those studied there was no trend to suggest different outcomes including survival without BPD (Bloom and Clark 2005). Studies comparing beractant and poractant alfa are smaller but show that the latter produces a more rapid onset of action in preterm infants with RDS (Ramanathan et al. 2004). This US trial of 293 preterm infants with moderately severe RDS compared two doses of poractant alfa (200 mg/kg and 100 mg/kg) with a 100 mg/kg dose of beractant and found that there was a reduced need for redosing with the higher dose of poractant alfa (Ramanathan et al. 2004). Furthermore, there was improved survival for infants of less than 32 weeks' gestation treated with the 200 mg/kg dose of poractant alfa compared with those treated with beractant. A meta-analysis of nine randomized trials comparing beractant with poractant alfa confirmed an increased mortality prior to discharge with the former (RR 1.44, 95%CI 1.04–2.00; NNH 20, 95%CI 10–100), although the benefit seemed to be limited to those infants treated with the higher dose (200 mg/kg) of poractant alfa (Singh et al. 2015). Despite the numbers of infants studied in these comparisons being modest and the American Academy of Pediatrics stating that it is still "unclear whether significant differences in clinical outcomes exist among the available animal-derived surfactant products" (Polin et al. 2014), poractant alfa is now the most widely used surfactant preparation worldwide (Curstedt et al. 2015).

63.4.7 Concomitant Interventions

Prenatal steroids, methods of respiratory support including CPAP, and caffeine treatment will be considered in this section. There have been at least 21 randomized trials of prenatal steroids involving over 4,000 infants at risk of RDS (Roberts and Dalziel 2006). Treatment with prenatal steroids is associated with an overall reduction in neonatal mortality (RR 0.69, 95%CI 0.58–0.81), RDS (RR 0.66, 95%CI 0.59–0.73), intraventricular hemorrhage (RR 0.54, 95%CI 0.43–0.69), necrotizing enterocolitis (RR 0.46, 95%CI 0.29–0.74), respiratory support and intensive care admissions (RR 0.80, 95%CI 0.65–0.99), and systemic infections in the first 48 h of life (RR 0.96, 95%CI 0.38–0.85) (Roberts and Dalziel 2006). As prenatal steroids are also effective in women with premature rupture of membranes and pregnancy-related hypertension, they should be given in most cases where preterm birth is anticipated before 35 weeks' gestation. Furthermore, there is evidence of synergistic effects of prenatal steroids and postnatal surfactant (Jobe et al. 1993), and therefore both are indicated in cases with high risk of RDS.

The combination of early surfactant treatment and CPAP was assessed in many studies (Dani et al. 2004; Sandri et al. 2010; Verder et al. 1999; Morley et al. 2008; Finer et al. 2010) with two studies comparing nasal CPAP with intubation at birth in very preterm infants (Morley et al. 2008; Finer et al. 2010). It is clear that the combination of CPAP and early surfactant administration reduces the need for mechanical ventilation particularly in infants of greater than 27 weeks' gestation (Bohlin et al. 2008; Sandri et al. 2010; Verder et al. 1999) although the reduction in BPD is rather modest (Bohlin et al. 2008). CPAP started in the delivery room without prophylactic surfactant in infants of 25–28 weeks' gestation does not significantly reduce the rate of death or BPD compared to intubation and is associated with a threefold increased risk of pneumothorax (Morley et al. 2008). However, prophylactic surfactant is not superior to CPAP and early selective surfactant in infants of

25–28 weeks' gestation (Sandri et al. 2010). To facilitate extubation after early surfactant administration by the INSURE technique, the use of respiratory stimulants such as caffeine has been recommended (Bohlin et al. 2008).

There are other reasons for recommending caffeine administration for treatment of apnea of prematurity as this has been shown to reduce risks of BPD, persistent ductus arteriosus (PDA), and need for ductus ligation (Schmidt et al. 2006). The reduced incidence of BPD in infants less than 1,250 g may be due to shortening the duration of mechanical ventilation by about 1 week, and at 18–20 months the surviving caffeine-treated infants had better neurodevelopmental outcomes with less cerebral palsy (Schmidt et al. 2007). Follow-up studies at 5 years of age suggest that these improved neurodevelopmental outcomes may be limited to a reduction in developmental coordination disorder (Doyle et al. 2014). There are clear benefits from treatment of very preterm infants with caffeine for apnea of prematurity and to facilitate extubation following surfactant therapy. There is no clear evidence that early inhaled nitric oxide will prevent BPD in these very immature babies.

Management of PDA in surfactant-treated infants is discussed below with treatment of pulmonary hemorrhage. It is good practice to monitor surfactant-treated infants for PDA and to use prostaglandin synthetase inhibitors (indomethacin or ibuprofen) early to prevent relapse of respiratory status and/or pulmonary hemorrhage.

63.4.8 Other Indications for Surfactant Therapy

Secondary surfactant dysfunction may occur in neonatal respiratory disorders other than RDS where the deficiency is primary. Surfactant inactivation and secondary dysfunction probably occur in meconium aspiration syndrome, congenital pneumonia, pulmonary hemorrhage, acute lung injury or acute respiratory distress syndrome (ARDS), and early stages of BPD (Polin et al. 2014; Robertson and Halliday 1998). There are varying degrees of evidence of effectiveness of surfactant replacement therapy in these conditions, and the evidence base is much weaker than for RDS (Speer et al. 2013; Polin et al. 2014). Four randomized trials (326 infants) of surfactant treatment in meconium aspiration syndrome are included in a systematic review that found improved oxygenation and a reduced need for extracorporeal membrane oxygenation (ECMO) in treated infants (RR 0.64, 95%CI 0.46–0.91; NNT 6, 95%CI 3–25) (El Shahed et al. 2014). However, there were no differences in risk of pneumothorax, CLD, or mortality (RR 0.98, 95%CI 0.41–2.39). These studies used a six-hourly dosing regimen with up to 150 mg/kg of bovine surfactant for up to four doses, and in general the improvement in oxygenation was not seen until after the third dose of surfactant (El Shahed et al. 2014). More recently dilute surfactant lavage has been used to try to remove meconium particles from the lungs (Dargaville et al. 2008), and studies have shown a reduced composite outcome of death or need for ECMO (RR 0.33, 95%CI 0.11–0.96; NNT 5, 95%CI 3–33), but further controlled clinical trials are needed to confirm treatment effect, refine the method of lavage, and compare this technique with standard bolus dosing (Hahn et al. 2013; Choi et al. 2012).

Surfactant inactivation is also present in neonatal pneumonia, and a subgroup of term infants with this condition showed improved oxygenation and reduced need for ECMO in a small, randomized trial of beractant (Lotze et al. 1998). A larger observational study of poractant alfa in infants with group B streptococcal pneumonia showed similar short-term improvements in oxygenation, but these were less impressive than those in preterm infants with RDS (Herting et al. 2000). Although the number of infants with pneumonia and respiratory failure treated with surfactant is relatively small, improved oxygenation warrants further study and continued use of surfactant for this indication.

Pulmonary hemorrhage is now relatively uncommon but may still occur in very preterm infants following surfactant therapy, and it has been postulated that this is due to rapidly improving pulmonary vascular resistance and large left-to-right shunt through a PDA (Halliday and Speer 1995). It is

advisable to monitor preterm infants after surfactant therapy for PDA clinically, echographically, and by blood pressure assessment and to use either indomethacin or ibuprofen at an early stage to prevent pulmonary hemorrhage. Surfactant has been used to treat massive pulmonary hemorrhage and the rationale is that blood inhibits surfactant function. There is evidence of modest improvement in oxygenation after surfactant treatment, but this comes from observational studies rather than randomized trials, which clearly would be difficult to perform (Aziz and Ohlsson 2012). A small randomized trial comparing poractant alfa and beractant to treat preterm infants with pulmonary hemorrhage showed improvements in oxygenation index with both surfactants but no differences in BPD or mortality (Bozdag et al. 2015).

In acute lung injury or ARDS, surfactant is inactivated by proteins and other substances leaking into the alveolar spaces. Pneumonia and sepsis are frequently underlying causes, and surfactant is at least partially effective in reversing signs of respiratory failure in these term infants (Robertson and Halliday 1998; Lotze et al. 1998; Herting et al. 2000). In some preterm infants born to mothers with severe preeclampsia, there may be delayed onset of respiratory distress which could be due to surfactant inactivation, a form of ARDS, and in these infants surfactant may be only partly effective with multiple doses being needed. Acute lung injury may be a prelude to the development of BPD, and surfactant has been used to treat infants with early CLD in a small observational study, which showed transient improvement in oxygenation (Pandit et al. 1995). Late booster doses of calfactant given to preterm infants still ventilated at 7–10 days transiently improved the respiratory severity score without long-term benefits (Merrill et al. 2011). In a large ($n = 511$) randomized trial, similar infants were treated with inhaled nitric oxide and either calfactant or sham instillation every 1–3 days to a maximum of five doses (Ballard et al. 2016). The primary endpoint, survival without BPD, was almost identical in both groups. Recently beractant has been used as a vehicle to deliver budesonide to the airways of preterm infants with severe RDS with a view to preventing BPD (Yeh et al. 2008). In this relatively small randomized trial, there was an unexpectedly large reduction in the combined outcome of death and BPD in infants treated with beractant plus budesonide compared to those treated with beractant alone (32% versus 61%; $p = 0.003$) (Yeh et al. 2008). Recently a larger trial ($n = 265$) of this approach to preventing BPD reported a reduction of the composite outcome, BPD or death, from 66% to 42% ($p < 0.001$; RR 0.58, 95%CI 0.44–0.77; NNT 4, 95%CI 3–8) (Yeh et al. 2016).

Congenital diaphragmatic hernia is also associated with surfactant insufficiency (Cogo et al. 2013), but surfactant treatment in a large series of infants did not improve outcomes (Polin et al. 2014). On the contrary, there were increased rates of CLD, mortality, and need for ECMO in surfactant-treated infants (Keiser and Bhandari 2016). Until more evidence is forthcoming, surfactant replacement cannot be recommended for infants with congenital diaphragmatic hernia although a recent survey found that 45% of pediatric surgeons administer surfactant (Zani et al. 2016).

63.5 Future Developments

Further research is needed to more precisely determine if there any infants who benefit more from prophylactic surfactant as opposed to early selective treatment after CPAP failure. Efforts should continue to reduce rates of BPD while maximizing survival, and this will mean limiting the duration of mechanical ventilation with judicious use of CPAP and perhaps caffeine. There will be further studies aimed to widen indications for surfactant use beyond RDS (Speer et al. 2013; Keiser and Bhandari 2016). Alternative means of administering surfactant without the need for endotracheal intubation will be pursued and tested in large randomized trials. LISA is showing promise but needs special expertise, whereas aerosolization, if perfected and shown to be efficacious, should be easier to administer (Speer et al. 2013). New-generation synthetic surfactants are likely to eventually replace natural surfactants especially if they can be produced more cheaply and in greater quantities (Speer et al. 2013; Polin et al. 2014). In

particular it is likely that surfactants will be used in the future to deliver other drugs, such as budesonide (Yeh et al. 2008, 2016) or other anti-inflammatory agents, directly to the airways to ameliorate acute lung injury and prevent BPD.

References

Ardell S, Pfister RH, Soll R (2015) Animal derived surfactant extract versus protein free synthetic surfactant for the prevention and treatment of respiratory distress syndrome. Cochrane Database Syst Rev 8:000144

Avery ME, Mead J (1959) Surface properties in relation to atelectasis and hyaline membrane disease. Am J Dis Child 97:517–523

Aziz A, Ohlsson A (2012) Surfactant for pulmonary hemorrhage in neonates. Cochrane Database Syst Rev 7, CD005254

Bahadue FL, Soll R (2012) Early versus delayed selective surfactant treatment for neonatal respiratory distress syndrome. Cochrane Database Syst Rev 11, CD001456

Ballard RA, Keller RL, Black DM et al (2016) Randomized trial of late surfactant treatment in ventilated preterm infants receiving inhaled nitric oxide. J Pediatr 168:23–29.e4

Berggren P, Liljedahl M, Winbladh B et al (2000) Pilot study of nebulized surfactant therapy for neonatal respiratory distress syndrome. Acta Paediatr 89:460–464

Bloom BT, Clark RH (2005) Comparison of Infasurf (calfactant) and Survanta (beractant) in the prevention and treatment of respiratory distress syndrome. Pediatrics 116:392–399

Bohlin K, Jonsson B, Gustafsson AS et al (2008) Continuous positive airway pressure and surfactant. Neonatology 93:309–315

Bozdag S, Dilli D, Gokmen T et al (2015) Comparison of two natural surfactants for pulmonary hemorrhage in very low-birth-weight infants: a randomized controlled trial. Am J Perinatol 32:211–218

Choi HJ, Hahn S, Lee J et al (2012) Surfactant lavage therapy for meconium aspiration syndrome: a systematic review and meta-analysis. Neonatology 101:183–191

Cogo PE, Simonato M, Danhaive O et al (2013) Impaired surfactant protein B synthesis in infants with congenital diaphragmatic hernia. Eur Respir J 41:677–682

Curstedt T, Johansson J (2006) New synthetic surfactants–how and when? Biol Neonate 89:336–339

Curstedt T, Halliday HL, Speer CP (2015) A unique story in neonatal research: the development of a porcine surfactant. Neonatology 107:321–329

Dani C, Bertini G, Pezzati M et al (2004) Early extubation and nasal continuous positive airway pressure after surfactant treatment for respiratory distress syndrome among preterm infants 30 weeks' gestation. Pediatrics 113:e560–e563

Dargaville PA, Copnell B, Tingay DG et al (2008) Refining the method of therapeutic lung lavage in meconium aspiration syndrome. Neonatology 94:160–163

Davis DJ, Barrington KJ, Fetus and Newborn Committee, Canadian Paediatric Society (2005) Recommendations for neonatal surfactant therapy. Paediatr Child Health 10:109–116 [updated Jan 2015]

Doyle LW, Schmidt B, Anderson PJ et al (2014) Reduction in developmental coordination disorder with neonatal caffeine therapy. J Pediatr 165:356–359

Dunn MS, Shennan AT, Possmayer F (1990) Single versus multiple- dose surfactant replacement therapy in neonates of 30 to 36 weeks' gestation with respiratory distress syndrome. Pediatrics 86:567–571

El Shahed AI, Dargaville P, Ohlsson A et al (2014) Surfactant for meconium aspiration syndrome in full term and late preterm infants. Cochrane Database Syst Rev 12, CD002054

Finer NN, Carlo WA, Walsh MC et al (2010) Early CPAP versus surfactant in extremely preterm infants. N Engl J Med 362:1970–1979

Gortner L, Pohlandt F, Bartmann P et al (1994) High-dose versus low-dose bovine surfactant treatment in very premature infants. Acta Paediatr 83:135–141

Hahn S, Choi HJ, Soll R et al (2013) Lung lavage for meconium aspiration in newborn infants. Cochrane Database Syst Rev 4, CD003486

Halliday HL (2003) Respiratory distress syndrome. In: Greenough A, Milner AD (eds) Neonatal respiratory disorders, 2nd edn. Arnold, London, pp 247–271

Halliday HL (2006) Recent clinical trials of surfactant treatment for neonates. Biol Neonate 89:323–329

Halliday HL, Speer CP (1995) Strategies for surfactant therapy in established neonatal respiratory distress syndrome. In: Robertson B, Taeusch HW (eds) Surfactant therapy for lung disease. Marcell Dekker, New York, pp 443–459

Halliday HL, Tarnow-Mordi WO, Corcoran JD et al (1993) Multicentre randomised trial comparing high and low dose surfactant regimens for the treatment of respiratory distress syndrome (the Curosurf 4 trial). Arch Dis Child 69:276–280

Hallman M (1989) Recycling of surfactant: a review of human amniotic fluid as a source of surfactant for treatment of respiratory distress syndrome. Rev Perinat Med 6:197–226

Herting E, Gefeller O, Land M et al (2000) Surfactant treatment of neonates with respiratory failure and group B streptococcal infection. Pediatrics 106:957–964

Jobe AH, Michell BR, Gunkel JH (1993) Beneficial effects of the combined use of prenatal corticosteroids and postnatal surfactant on preterm infants. Am J Obstet Gynecol 168:508–513

Kattwinkel J, Bloom BT, Delmore P et al (2000) High-versus low threshold surfactant retreatment for neonatal respiratory distress syndrome. Pediatrics 106:282–288

Kattwinkel J, Robinson M, Bloom BT et al (2004) Technique for intrapartum administration of surfactant

without requirement for an endotracheal tube. J Perinatol 24:360–365

Keiser A, Bhandari V (2016) Surfactant therapy in nonrespiratory distress syndrome conditions in neonates. Am J Perinatol 33:1–8

Konishi M, Fujiwara T, Naito T et al (1988) Surfactant replacement therapy in neonatal respiratory distress syndrome. A multicenter randomised clinical trial: comparison of high versus low-dose of Surfactant TA. Eur J Pediatr 147:20–25

Kribs A, Vierzig A, Hunseler C et al (2008) Early surfactant in spontaneously breathing with nCPAP in ELBW infants – a single center four year experience. Acta Paediatr 97:293–298

Kribs A, Roll C, Gopel W et al (2015) Nonintubated surfactant application vs conventional therapy in extremely preterm infants: a randomized clinical trial. JAMA Pediatr 169:723–730

Lotze A, Mitchell BR, Bulas DJ et al (1998) Multicenter study of surfactant (beractant) use in the treatment of term infants with severe respiratory failure. J Pediatr 132:40–47

Merrill JD, Ballard PL, Courtney SE et al (2011) Pilot trial of late booster doses of surfactant for ventilated premature infants. J Perinatol 31:599–606

Morley CJ (1991) Surfactant treatment of premature babies: a review of clinical trials. Arch Dis Child 66:445–450

Morley CJ, Davis PG, Doyle LW et al (2008) Nasal CPAP or intubation at birth for very preterm infants. N Engl J Med 358:700–708

Moya F, Gadzinowski J, Bancalari E et al (2005) A multicenter, randomized, masked, comparison trial of lucinactant, colfosceril palmitate, and beractant for the prevention of respiratory distress syndrome in very preterm infants. Pediatrics 115:1018–1029

Pandit PB, Dunn MS, Kelly EN et al (1995) Surfactant replacement in neonates with early chronic lung disease. Pediatrics 95:851–854

Pfister RH, Soll RF, Wiswell T (2007) Protein containing synthetic surfactant versus animal derived surfactant extract for the prevention and treatment of respiratory distress syndrome. Cochrane Database Syst Rev 4, CD006069

Pfister RH, Soll R, Wiswell TE (2009) Protein-containing synthetic surfactant versus protein-free synthetic surfactant for the prevention and treatment of respiratory distress syndrome. Cochrane Database Syst Rev 4, CD006180

Pillow JJ, Minocchieri S (2012) Innovation in surfactant therapy II: surfactant administration by aerosolization. Neonatology 101:337–344

Polin RA, Carlo WA, Committee on Fetus and Newborn (2014) Surfactant-replacement therapy for preterm and term neonates with respiratory distress. Pediatrics 133:156–163

Ramanathan R, Rasmussen MR, Gerstmann DR et al (2004) A randomized, multicenter masked comparison trial of poractant alfa (Curosurf) versus beractant (Survanta) in the treatment of respiratory distress syndrome in preterm infants. Am J Perinatol 21:109–119

Roberts D, Dalziel S (2006) Antenatal corticosteroids for accelerating fetal lung maturation for women at risk of preterm birth. Cochrane Database Syst Rev 3, CD004454

Robertson B, Halliday H (1998) Principles of surfactant replacement. Biochim Biophys Acta 1408:346–361

Rojas-Reyes MX, Morley CJ, Soll R (2012) Prophylactic versus selective use of surfactant in preventing morbidity and mortality in preterm infants. Cochrane Database Syst Rev 3, CD000510

Sandri F, Plavka R, Ancora G et al (2010) Prophylactic or early selective surfactant combined with nCPAP in very preterm infants. Pediatrics 125:e1402–e1409

Schmidt B, Roberts R, Davis P et al (2006) Caffeine therapy for apnea of prematurity. N Engl J Med 354:2112–2121

Schmidt B, Roberts RS, Davis P et al (2007) Long-term effects of caffeine therapy for apnea of prematurity. N Engl J Med 357:1893–1902

Seger N, Soll R (2009) Animal derived surfactant extract for treatment of respiratory distress syndrome. Cochrane Database Syst Rev 2, CD007836

Singh N, Halliday HL, Stevens TP et al (2015) Comparison of animal-derived surfactants for the prevention and treatment of respiratory distress syndrome in preterm infants. Cochrane Database Syst Rev 12, CD010249

Sinha S, Lacaze-Masmoneil T, Valls-i-Soler A et al (2005) A randomized, controlled trial of lucinactant versus poractant alfa in very premature infants at high risk for respiratory distress syndrome. Pediatrics 115:1030–1038

Soll RF (2000a) Prophylactic natural surfactant extract for preventing morbidity and mortality in preterm infants. Cochrane Database Syst Rev 2, CD000511

Soll RF (2000b) Synthetic surfactant for respiratory distress syndrome in preterm infants. Cochrane Database Syst Rev 2, CD001149

Soll R, Ozek E (2009) Multiple versus single doses of exogenous surfactant for the prevention or treatment of neonatal respiratory distress syndrome. Cochrane Database Syst Rev 1, CD000141

Soll R, Ozek E (2010) Prophylactic protein free synthetic surfactant for preventing morbidity and mortality in preterm infants. Cochrane Database Syst Rev 1, CD001079

Speer CP, Robertson B, Curstedt T et al (1992) Randomized European multicenter trial of surfactant replacement therapy for severe neonatal respiratory distress syndrome: single versus multiple doses of Curosurf. Pediatrics 89:13–20

Speer CP, Sweet DG, Halliday HL (2013) Surfactant therapy: past, present and future. Early Hum Devel 89 (Suppl 1):S22–S24

Stevens TP, Harrington EW, Blennow M, Soll R (2007) Early surfactant administration with brief ventilation

vs. selective surfactant and continued mechanical ventilation for preterm infants with or at risk for respiratory distress syndrome. Cochrane Database Syst Rev 4, CD003063

Sweet DG, Carnielli V, Greisen G et al (2013) European consensus guidelines on the management of neonatal respiratory distress syndrome in preterm infants – 2013 update. Neonatology 103:353–368

Trevisanuto D, Grazzina N, Ferrasse P et al (2005) Laryngeal mask airway used as a delivery conduit for the administration of surfactant to preterm infants with respiratory distress syndrome. Biol Neonate 87:217–220

Ueda T, Ikegami M, Rider ED et al (1994) Distribution of surfactant and ventilation in surfactant-treated preterm lambs. J Appl Physiol 76:45–55

Valls-i-Soler A, Fernandez-Ruanova B, Lopez-Heredia J et al (1998) A randomized comparison of surfactant dosing via a dual-lumen endotracheal tube in respiratory distress syndrome. Pediatrics 101, E4

Vento M, Cheung P-Y, Aguar M (2009) The first golden minutes of the extremely-low-gestational-age neonate: a gentle approach. Neonatology 95:286–298

Verder H, Albertsen P, Ebbesen F et al (1999) Nasal continuous positive airway pressure and early surfactant therapy for respiratory distress syndrome in newborns of less than 30 weeks' gestation. Pediatrics 103, e24

Walsh BK, Daigle B, DiBlasi RM et al (2013) AARC clinical practice guideline. Surfactant replacement therapy: 2013. Respir Care 58:367–375

Yeh TF, Lin HC, Chang CH et al (2008) Early intratracheal instillation of budesonide using surfactant as a vehicle to prevent chronic lung disease in preterm infants: a pilot study. Pediatrics 121:e1310–e1318

Yeh TF, Chen CM, Wu SY et al (2016) Intratracheal administration of budesonide/surfactant to prevent bronchopulmonary dysplasia. Am J Respir Crit Care Med 193:86–95

Zani A, Eaton S, Puri P et al (2016) International survey on the management of congenital diaphragmatic hernia. Eur J Pediatr Surg 26:38–46

Zola EM, Gunkel JH, Chan RK et al (1993) Comparison of three dosing procedures for administration of bovine surfactant to neonates with respiratory distress syndrome. J Pediatr 122:453–459

Extracorporeal Membrane Oxygenation for Neonates

64

Anne Greenough, Niovi Papalexopoulou, Munir Ahmed, and Adam P. R. Smith

Contents

Abstract

Extracorporeal membrane oxygenation (ECMO) is a modified form of cardiopulmonary bypass such that patients can be supported for a prolonged period, even up to weeks, until the patient's respiratory and/or cardiac function recovers or definitive treatment is administered. A systematic review of results of 244 infants entered into randomized trials demonstrated that ECMO was associated with a reduction in mortality (relative risk 0.44, 95% CI 0.31–0.61) and the number needed to treat was three. Survival is best in neonates with meconium aspiration syndrome and worse in those with congenital diaphragmatic hernia. Chronic respiratory, neurological, and growth problems have been reported following ECMO. Overall, follow-up of infants into the

A. Greenough (✉)
Division of Asthma, Allergy and Lung Biology, MRC Centre for Allergic Mechanisms of Asthma, King's College London, London, UK

NIHR Biomedical Centre at Guy's and St Thomas NHS Foundation Trust and King's College London, London, UK

NICU, King's College Hospital, London, UK
e-mail: anne.greenough@kcl.ac.uk

N. Papalexopoulou · M. Ahmed · A. P. R. Smith
Division of Asthma, Allergy and Lung Biology, MRC Centre for Allergic Mechanisms of Asthma, King's College London, London, UK
e-mail: niovi.papalexopoulou@nhs.net; Munir.Ahmed@worcsacute.nhs.uk; adamprsmith@gmail.com

G. Buonocore et al. (eds.), *Neonatology*,
https://doi.org/10.1007/978-3-319-29489-6_211

largest randomized trial, the UK ECMO trial, showed at 7 years of age a continuing benefit of ECMO for the primary outcome of death or severe disability (relative risk 0.64, 95% CI 0.47–0.86; $p = 0.004$). While treatment was cost-effective in most diagnostic groups, the cost ratio for infants with CDH was far poorer. Subsequent advances in other respiratory support techniques for term and near-term infants, including high-frequency oscillation and nitric oxide, and, however, have reduced the number of cases referred for ECMO and altered the profile of such patients.

64.1 Salient Points

- Extracorporeal membrane oxygenation (ECMO) is a form of cardiopulmonary bypass that supports neonates until their pulmonary and/or cardiac function recovers.
- There are two methods of ECMO: venoarterial (VA ECMO) providing support for both pulmonary and cardiac function and venovenous (VV ECMO) in which the artificial lung is in series with the patient's lung and pulmonary and systemic perfusion relies on the patient's ventricular function.
- VA ECMO has disadvantages which include possible systemic emboli and lower myocardial oxygen delivery, and the carotid artery is cannulated, and arterial reconstruction may be difficult, particularly in small infants.
- The overall survival to hospital discharge is greatest in infants with a primary diagnosis of meconium aspiration syndrome and lowest in those with a congenital diaphragmatic hernia.
- Advances in other respiratory support techniques for term and near-term infants, including high-frequency oscillation and nitric oxide, have reduced the number of cases referred for ECMO and altered the profile of such patients.
- A potential concern with the institution of newer methods of respiratory support is that it may delay ECMO treatment, which in non-randomized studies has been associated with prolongation of both ECMO and conventional treatment, as well as increased mortality.

64.2 Introduction

Extracorporeal membrane oxygenation (ECMO) is a modified form of cardiopulmonary bypass such that patients can be supported for a prolonged period, even up to weeks, until the patient's respiratory and/or cardiac function recovers or definitive treatment is administered, for example, in cardiac anomalies. Gibbon designed and used a heart-lung machine during the first successful open-heart surgery in 1953 (Gibbon 1954). In the following decades, membrane oxygenators began to be used for infants with respiratory failure and congenital cardiac defects and in 1975 Bartlett and colleagues demonstrated the potential of ECMO for neonates (Bartlett et al. 1976). Since 1989, the Extracorporeal Life Support Organization (ELSO) has maintained a registry of ECMO use in over 200 centers (Rais-Bahrami and Van Meurs 2014). Approximately 35,500 "neonatal ECMO patients" have been recorded, comprising approximately half (51.4%) of all ECMO cases. ECMO in adults was almost abandoned as initial trials failed to show better survival than that achieved by conventional respiratory support (Zapol et al. 1979; Morris et al. 1994). There has, however, been a resurgence of ECMO use in adults following the positive outcomes during the 2009 influenza A (H1N1) pandemic (Peek et al. 2009; Noah et al. 2011). Conversely, survival rates and the use of ECMO in neonates reached a peak in the early 1990s and have thereafter been declining (Frenckner and Radell 2008). In this chapter, the techniques used, the management of a neonate on ECMO, and the indications for ECMO are described. In addition, the results achieved and the impact of the advent of new respiratory support techniques and therapies on the use of ECMO are discussed.

64.3 Techniques

There are two methods of providing ECMO: venoarterial (VA) and venovenous (VV). In VA ECMO, blood is drained from the right jugular vein and returned via the right carotid artery. The

major advantage of VA ECMO is that it provides support for both lung and heart functions, as 80% cardiopulmonary bypass is achieved. VA ECMO, however, has disadvantages which include possible systemic emboli, lower myocardial oxygen delivery, and potentially worse organ perfusion from loss of pulsatile flow (Rais-Bahrami and Van Meurs 2014). In addition, the carotid artery is cannulated and arterial reconstruction may be difficult, particularly in small infants. In VV ECMO, the artificial lung is in series with the patient's lung, and pulmonary and systemic perfusion relies on the patient's ventricular function. A double lumen catheter may be sited in the right atrium via the right jugular vein: venous blood is drained from one lumen into the ECMO circuit and oxygenated blood is returned through the other lumen into the right atrium (Rais-Bahrami and Van Meurs 2014). Alternatively the blood is drained from the internal jugular vein and returned to the inferior vena cava via the femoral or, less commonly, the umbilical vein. VV ECMO obviates the need for carotid artery cannulation, but leg edema can occur following femoral vein ligation after decannulation. Advantages of VV ECMO include perfusion of myocardium with oxygenated blood, risk of pulmonary emboli rather than systemic, and maintenance of pulsatile flow. There is, however, recirculation of blood with overall lower oxygen delivery. Both techniques share similar hemorrhagic and mechanical risks.

64.3.1 ECMO Circuit

Venous blood is pumped through an oxygenator, which has blood and gas compartments separated by semipermeable membranes, through which the diffusion of oxygen and carbon dioxide occurs. The circuit contains a "bladder" – a reservoir which stops the pump from working if venous drainage becomes too low, preventing air bubbles and clots. Oxygen transfer is dependent on the surface area of the membrane, pump flow, and the degree of saturation of the venous blood. Carbon dioxide elimination is affected by the flow rate. Heat is lost, particularly due to the large surface area of the oxygenator; hence, a heat exchanger warms the blood before it is returned to the infant.

64.3.2 Management During ECMO

Prior to cannulation, infants are heparinized and remain on a heparin continuous infusion (20–50 units/kg/h) while on ECMO to maintain an activated clotting time of 180–200 s. Systemic anticoagulation is administered in the circuit to prevent thromboembolic events resulting from activation of the clotting cascade from blood coming into contact with the tubing. As a result of anticoagulation, bleeding complications do occur, most commonly during cannulation and at surgical wounds. This is exacerbated as platelets become sequestered in the oxygenator. Bleeding complications can be minimized by maintaining adequate platelet counts (>100,000 cells/mm3), a normal international normalized ratio of prothrombin time (INR), and adequate levels of fibrinogen. Additional respiratory support is required during ECMO, but it is important to use settings that minimize further lung injury while avoiding atelectasis. Typical "lung rest" settings are peak pressures less than 30 cmH_2O, PEEP levels of 8–10 cmH_2O, rates of 10–25 breaths per minute, and an inspired oxygen concentrations of 0.21–0.40. Medications and fluids can be added into the circuit; the pharmacokinetics of certain drugs during ECMO, however, are not entirely clear, with unknown dosing implications (Rehder et al. 2013). Weaning is achieved by gradually reducing the pump flow rate. Serial cranial ultrasound examinations should be undertaken during ECMO.

64.3.3 Eligibility for ECMO (ELSO 2015)

ECMO is used in term or near-term infants with reversible respiratory or cardiac failure unresponsive to maximal conventional therapy. Furthermore, the underlying pathology should have short-term reversibility.

The oxygenation index (OI) is usually used to determine the need for ECMO.

$$OI = \frac{\text{Mean airway pressure} \times FiO_2 \times 100}{\text{Postductal } PaO_2}$$

FiO_2 = fraction of the inspired oxygen

An OI > 40 has been used, as it had predicted a mortality of > 80%, but in the UK ECMO trial, an OI > 40 on conventional ventilation was only associated with a mortality of 41% (UK Collaborative ECMO Trial Group 1996).

ELSO indicates ECMO in neonatal respiratory failure in the following cases (ELSO 2015):

1. OI > 40 for >4 h
2. OI > 20 with lack of improvement despite prolonged (>24 h) maximal medical therapy or persistent episodes of decompensation
3. Severe hypoxic respiratory failure with acute decompensation (PaO_2< 40 mmHg) unresponsive to intervention
4. Progressive respiratory failure and/or pulmonary hypertension with evidence of right ventricular dysfunction or continued high inotropic requirement

Contraindications include:

- Lethal chromosomal (includes trisomy 13 and 18 but not 21) or congenital disorder
- Irreversible brain damage
- Uncontrolled bleeding
- Grade ≥ III intraventricular hemorrhage

Relative contraindications include:

1. Irreversible organ damage, unless candidate for transplantation.
2. Weight less than 2 kg and/or gestation less than 34 weeks as such infants are at increased risk of intracranial hemorrhage.
3. Mechanical ventilation greater than 10–14 days.
4. In infants with congenital diaphragmatic hernia, the absence of an initial period with a preductal saturation >85% and a $PaCO_2$ <65 mmHg is strongly associated with a worse prognosis attributable to pulmonary hypoplasia and constitutes exclusion criteria for ECMO in some centers.

ECMO has most commonly been used for meconium aspiration syndrome, persistent pulmonary hypertension, and congenital diaphragmatic hernia. Newer uses include intractable primary arrhythmias (Dyamenahalli et al. 2012) and congenital hypertrophic cardiomyopathy caused by maternal diabetes (Arzuaga and Groner 2013).

64.3.4 Mortality

There are four randomized control trials comparing neonatal ECMO with conventional therapy for respiratory failure (UK Collaborative ECMO Trial Group 1996; O'Rourke et al. 1989; Bartlett et al. 1985; Gross et al. 1994). The largest randomized neonatal ECMO trial recruited 185 neonates with severe respiratory failure from 55 neonatal intensive care units in the UK (UK Collaborative ECMO Trial Group 1996). Parental consent to entry into the trial was requested if the OI was greater than 40 or the arterial partial pressure of CO_2 was >12 kPa for 3 h. Infants were then randomized to either remain on conventional therapy at their neonatal unit or be transferred for ECMO at one of five UK centers. Overall, there was a significant reduction in mortality for the ECMO group (relative risk (RR) 0.55, 95% CI 0.39–0.77; $p = 0.0005$). There was a benefit for ECMO in all diagnoses, although the effect in CDH infants was marginal; 17 CDH infants supported conventionally died before discharge and 14 of 18 supported with ECMO died before 1 year of age (ELSO 2015). A systematic review of results of 244 infants entered into randomized trials demonstrated that ECMO was associated with a reduction in mortality (RR 0.44, 95% CI 0.31–0.61) and the number needed to treat was three (Mugford et al. 2008).

Up to July 2015, over 35,500 cases of neonatal ECMO have been reported to the ELSO registry;

the majority (28,271) received ECMO for respiratory causes. The cumulative survival to hospital discharge or transfer is currently 74%. In 2015 survival of neonatal respiratory cases was 63% compared to 81% in 1990, while the average "run" time has increased to 203 h from 144 h in 1990 (Vasavada et al. 2011). Those data (Vasavada et al. 2011) reflect the change in the nature of the population now undergoing ECMO (see later). Survival remains best in neonates with MAS (94%) and worst in those with CDH (51%). VA ECMO was used in approximately 72% of cases with a cumulative survival of 71% and VV ECMO in 28% of cases with 82% survival (Rais and Van Meurs 2014). Late mortality (>90 days post ECMO) has been reported to occur in 5.5% of patients, those with CDH being at the most risk (Ijsselstijn and van Heijst 2014).

Approximately 17% of cases reported to the ELSO Registry had a primary cardiac problem, with an overall survival of 41%. ECMO is also used during cardiopulmonary resuscitation ($n = 1,188$) with 41% survival (Organization ELS 2015). Overall survival to hospital discharge of 641 infants who received extracorporeal cardiopulmonary resuscitation was 39% (McMullan et al. 2014). Lower birth weight and pre-extracorporeal cardiopulmonary resuscitation oxygenation, as well as complications including CNS hemorrhage, increased the odds of death (McMullan et al. 2014). Analysis of data from the ELSO registry has demonstrated that neonates requiring prolonged ECMO support (>20 days) have only a 24% survival to hospital discharge; many had CDH (Prodhan et al. 2014). Complications were common with prolonged ECMO, but only receipt of inotropes was shown to be independently associated with mortality (Prodhan et al. 2014).

64.3.5 Morbidity

Chronic respiratory, neurological, and growth problems have been reported following ECMO. Review of 7,910 neonates supported by ECMO between 2005 and 2010 demonstrated that 1,412 (20%) had neurological complications (brain death, cerebral infarction, intracranial hemorrhage, or seizures) during ECMO support. Mortality was higher in patients with neurological complications (62% vs. 36%, $p < 0.001$) (Polito et al. 2013). The only long-term data on outcome following randomization to ECMO or conventional management, however, comes from the UK ECMO trial. Follow-up at 1 year revealed that ECMO was associated with a reduction in mortality without an increase in severe disability (defined as having a Griffiths quotient less than 50 or being unable to participate in quantitative developmental assessment due to severity of disability). At 4 years of age, more of the ECMO surviving infants had no disability (50% vs. 37%) (Bennett et al. 2001). Ninety of the infants (56 ECMO; 34 conventional) were seen at 7 years, and there were no significant differences in overall cognitive ability between the two groups; 76% of infants had an overall performance within the normal range (McNally et al. 2006). Overall, the study showed a continuing benefit of ECMO for the primary outcome of death or severe disability (relative risk 0.64, 95% CI 0.47–0.86; $p = 0.004$). Longitudinal assessment of motor performance at 5, 8, and/or 12 years after neonatal ECMO of a Dutch cohort of 254 survivors demonstrated that motor problems persist throughout childhood and become more obvious with time (Van der Cammen-van Zijp et al. 2014).

Beardsmore et al. showed that ECMO-supported infants from the UK RCT had better lung function at 1 year of age than those who remained on conventional ventilation (Beardsmore et al. 2000). At 7 years of age, more children from the "conventional" group had evidence of respiratory morbidity, 32% had intermittent wheeze during the 12 months prior to questioning, and 41% regularly used inhalers, compared to 11% and 25%, respectively, of the ECMO group (McNally et al. 2006). Spoel et al. undertook a prospective longitudinal study evaluating outcomes of 121 infants supported by ECMO at 5, 8, and/or 12 years. They demonstrated long-term pulmonary sequelae in the CDH patients with a tendency for lung function to deteriorate with time (Spoel et al. 2012).

64.3.6 Cost-Effectiveness of ECMO

The costs of ECMO at 1 year are dominated by the expense of initial hospital care, reflecting partly the cost of ECMO provision itself, but also that the reduced mortality results in an increased average duration of stay in conventional neonatal intensive care. Cost-effectiveness improves over time, with the 7-year follow-up analysis from the UK ECMO trial estimating that the incremental cost per life year gained was £13,385 (2002–2003 prices) (Petrou et al. 2006). While treatment of infants was cost-effective in most diagnostic groups, the cost ratio for infants with CDH was far poorer.

64.3.7 Changes in ECMO Requirements with Time

Advances in other respiratory support techniques for term and near-term infants, including high-frequency oscillation and nitric oxide, have reduced the number of cases referred for ECMO and altered the profile of such patients. Data from the ELSO registry highlight that neonatal respiratory cases fell from a peak of 1,516 in 1992 to 627 in 2015 and that the proportion of cases with MAS fell from 35% to 25%, while CDH cases rose from 18% to 28% (Qureshi et al. 2013). Conversely the number of neonatal cardiac cases has been increasing with improved survival. Infants with CDH are now the commonest patient population requiring ECMO (Rais and Van Meurs 2014). A retrospective review of 18,130 all neonates undergoing noncardiac ECMO between 1990 and 2010 demonstrated that neonates of ethnic minorities have continued to disproportionally require ECMO support compared to their birth rates (Qureshi et al. 2013). A comparison of infants with severe respiratory failure treated at a single center during two time periods showed a decrease in ECMO utilization from 42.8% to 27.7% (Hintz et al. 2000). There were concomitant increases in the use of HFOV (36.7–87.2%), surfactant (26.5–89.3%), and iNO (0–44.7%). One potential concern with the institution of newer methods of respiratory support is that it may delay ECMO treatment, which in non-randomized studies has been associated with prolongation of both ECMO and conventional treatment, as well as increased mortality (Prodhan et al. 2014; Coppola et al. 2008).

Acknowledgments We thank Dr Nicholas Barrett (Consultant in Critical Care at Guy's and St Thomas's Hospital NHS Foundation Trust) for providing data on the current mortality and Mrs Deirdre Gibbons for secretarial assistance.

The research was supported by the National Institute for Health Research (NIHR) Clinical Research Facility at Guy's and St Thomas' NHS Foundation Trust and NIHR Biomedical Research Centre based at Guy's and St Thomas' NHS Foundation Trust and King's College London. The views expressed are those of the authors and not necessarily those of the NHS, the NIHR, or the Department of Health.

References

Arzuaga BH, Groner A (2013) Utilization of extracorporeal membrane oxygenation in congenital hypertrophic cardiomyopathy caused by maternal diabetes. J Neonatal Perinatal Med 6:345–348

Bartlett RH, Gazzaniga AB, Jefferies MR et al (1976) Extracorporeal membrane oxygenation (ECMO) cardiopulmonary support in infancy. Trans Am Soc Artif Int Organs 22:80–93

Bartlett RH, Roloff DW, Cornell RG et al (1985) Extracorporeal circulation in neonatal respiratory failure: a prospective randomized study. Pediatrics 76:479–487

Beardsmore C, Dundas I, Poole K et al (2000) Respiratory function in survivors of the United Kingdom Extracorporeal Membrane Oxygenation Trial. Am J Respir Crit Care Med 161:1129–1135

Bennett CC, Johnson A, Field DJ et al (2001) UK collaborative randomised trial of neonatal extracorporeal membrane oxygenation: follow-up to age 4 years. Lancet 357:1094–1096

Coppola CP, Tyree M, Larry K et al (2008) A 22-year experience in global transport extracorporeal membrane oxygenation. J Pediatr Surg 43:46–52

Dyamenahalli U, Tuzcu V, Fontenot E et al (2012) Extracorporeal membrane oxygenation support for intractable primary arrhythmias and complete congenital heart block in newborns and infants: short- term and medium-term outcomes. Pediatr Crit Care Med 13:47–52

ELSO (2015) Guidelines for neonatal respiratory failure 2013. [Cited 18 Dec 2015]. Available from: https://www.elso.org/Portals/0/IGD/Archive/FileManager/8588d1a580cusersshyerdocumentselsoguidelinesforneonatalrespiratoryfailure13.pdf

Frenckner B, Radell P (2008) Respiratory failure and extracorporeal membrane oxygenation. Semin Pediatr Surg 17:34–41

Gibbon JH Jr (1954) Application of a mechanical heart and lung apparatus to cardiac surgery. Minn Med 37: 171–185

Gross SJ, Bifano EM, D'Euqenio DB et al (1994) 86 prospective randomized controlled trial of conventional treatment or transport for ecmo in infants with severe persistent pulmonary hypertension (PPHN): two year follow up. Pediatr Res 36:17A-A

Hintz SR, Suttner DM, Sheehan AM et al (2000) Decreased use of neonatal extracorporeal membrane oxygenation (ECMO): how new treatment modalities have affected ECMO utilization. Pediatrics 106: 1339–1343

Ijsselstijn H, van Heijst AF (2014) Long-term outcome of children treated with neonatal extracorporeal membrane oxygenation: increasing problems with increasing age. Semin Perinatol 38:114–121

McMullan DM, Thiagarajan RR, Smith KM et al (2014) Extracorporeal cardiopulmonary resuscitation outcomes in term and premature neonates. Pediatr Crit Care Med 15:e9–e16

McNally H, Bennett CC, Elbourne D et al (2006) United Kingdom collaborative randomized trial of neonatal extracorporeal membrane oxygenation: follow-up to age 7 years. Pediatrics 117:e845–e854

Morris AH, Wallace CJ, Menlove RL et al (1994) Randomized clinical trial of pressure-controlled inverse ratio ventilation and extracorporeal CO_2 removal for adult respiratory distress syndrome. Am J Respir Crit Care Med 149:295–305

Mugford M, Elbourne D, Field D (2008) Extracorporeal membrane oxygenation for severe respiratory failure in newborn infants. Cochrane Database Syst Rev 3, CD001340

Noah MA, Peek GJ, Finney SJ et al (2011) Referral to an extracorporeal membrane oxygenation center and mortality among patients with severe 2009 influenza A (H1N1). JAMA 306:1659–1668

O'Rourke PP, Crone RK, Vacanti JP et al (1989) Extracorporeal membrane oxygenation and conventional medical therapy in neonates with persistent pulmonary hypertension of the newborn: a prospective randomized study. Pediatrics 84:957–963

Organization ELS (2015) ECLS registry report – international summary 2015 July. Available from: https://www.elso.org/Registry/Statistics/InternationalSummary.aspx

Peek GJ, Mugford M, Tiruvoipati R et al (2009) Efficacy and economic assessment of conventional ventilatory support versus extracorporeal membrane oxygenation for severe adult respiratory failure (CESAR): a multicentre randomised controlled trial. Lancet 374: 1351–1363

Petrou S, Bischof M, Bennett C et al (2006) Cost-effectiveness of neonatal extracorporeal membrane oxygenation based on 7-year results from the United Kingdom Collaborative ECMO Trial. Pediatrics 117:1640–1649

Polito A, Barrett CS, Wypij D et al (2013) Neurologic complications in neonates supported with extracorporeal membrane oxygenation. An analysis of ELSO registry data. Intensive Care Med 39:1594–1601

Prodhan P, Stroud M, El-Hassan N et al (2014) Prolonged extracorporeal membrane oxygenator support among neonates with acute respiratory failure: a review of the extracorporeal life support organization registry. ASAIO J 60:63–69

Qureshi FG, Jackson HI, Brown J et al (2013) The changing population of the United States and use of extracorporeal membrane oxygenation. J Surg Res 184: 572–576

Rais BK, Van Meurs KP (2014) Venoarterial versus venovenous ECMO for neonatal respiratory failure. Semin Perinatol 38:71–77

Rais-Bahrami K, Van Meurs KP (2014) Venoarterial versus venovenous ECMO for neonatal respiratory failure. Semin Perinatol 38:71–77

Rehder KJ, Turner DA, Cheifetz IM (2013) Extracorporeal membrane oxygenation for neonatal and pediatric respiratory failure: an evidence-based review of the past decade (2002–2012). Pediatr Crit Care Med 14: 851–861

Spoel M, Laas R, Gischler SJ et al (2012) Diagnosis-related deterioration of lung function after extracorporeal membrane oxygenation. Eur Respir J 40: 1531–1537

UK Collaborative ECMO Trial Group (1996) UK collaborative randomised trial of neonatal extracorporeal membrane oxygenation. Lancet 348:75–82

Van der Cammen-van Zijp M, Janssen A, Raets M et al (2014) Motor performance after neonatal extracorporeal membrane oxygenation: a longitudinal evaluation. Pediatrics 134:e427–e435

Vasavada R, Feng Q, Undar A (2011) Current status of pediatric/neonatal extracorporeal life support: clinical outcomes, circuit evolution, and translational research. Perfusion 26:294–301

Zapol WM, Snider MT, Hill JD et al (1979) Extracorporeal membrane oxygenation in severe acute respiratory failure. A randomized prospective study. JAMA 242: 2193–2196

Lung Diseases: Problems of Steroid Treatment of Fetus and Newborn

65

Henry L. Halliday

Contents

Abstract

Corticosteroids given in the perinatal period have a multitude of biologic effects on the developing lung. Clearly, some of these will be beneficial to the immature fetus or neonate, while others will be detrimental. For the fetus at risk of preterm birth, a single course of betamethasone or dexamethasone leads to lung maturity and reduces the risk of RDS and other important complications of prematurity. Consensus seems to support repeat courses of prenatal steroids when there is a high risk of preterm birth before 29 weeks' gestation even if there are some controversies. The beneficial pulmonary effects of early postnatal dexamethasone, in the first week of life, do not seem to outweigh the adverse effects on neurodevelopment. However, late postnatal steroid therapy, after the first week of life, seems to be associated with similar beneficial pulmonary effects without significant increase in neurodevelopmental sequelae. Late steroid therapy with dexamethasone is probably still indicated for preterm infants with CLD who cannot be weaned from ventilation. Thus, administration of corticosteroids in the perinatal period must be based upon clinical judgment of the balance of benefits and risks. Further evaluation should be done considering long-term follow-up in order to confirm their safety before they can be recommended for routine use.

H. L. Halliday (✉)
Formerly Regional Neonatal Unit, Royal Maternity Hospital, Belfast, UK

Formerly Department of Child Health, Queen's University Belfast, Belfast, UK
e-mail: henry.halliday@doctors.org.uk

65.1 Salient Points

- Corticosteroids given in the perinatal period have a multitude of biological effects on the developing lung and other organs.

G. Buonocore et al. (eds.), *Neonatology*,
https://doi.org/10.1007/978-3-319-29489-6_212

- Prenatal steroids accelerate fetal lung maturity reducing neonatal mortality, respiratory distress syndrome, intraventricular hemorrhage, and necrotizing enterocolitis without affecting maternal health.
- Betamethasone and dexamethasone have been used to enhance fetal lung maturity.
- Repeat doses improve neonatal outcomes except for a reduction in some measures of weight at birth.
- Early (first week) postnatal steroids lead to earlier extubation and decreased bronchopulmonary dysplasia (BPD), patent ductus arteriosus, and retinopathy of prematurity (ROP) but increased gastrointestinal (GI) bleeding and perforation, hyperglycemia, hypertension, hypertrophic cardiomyopathy (HOCM), growth failure, and cerebral palsy (CP), although an outcome combining death and CP is not increased.
- Hydrocortisone (low dose) and dexamethasone were used in these trials, and benefits and adverse effects were limited to treatment with the latter.
- The recent PREMILOC trial of early low dose hydrocortisone suggests an increase in survival without BPD although there was increased sepsis in infants of 24–25 weeks' gestation.
- Inhaled budesonide (first 12 h) reduced BPD in one large trial, but there was a trend toward increased neonatal mortality.
- Late (after first week) postnatal steroids lead to earlier extubation and reduced neonatal mortality, BPD, death, or BPD, while there is increased GI bleeding, hyperglycemia, hypertension, HOCM, and severe ROP, but no significant increase in CP.
- It is prudent to reserve late postnatal steroids for infants who cannot be weaned from ventilation.
- Early low dose hydrocortisone improves survival without BPD (OR 1.48; 95%CI 1.02–2.16; $p = 0.04$) with higher sepsis rate in infants of 24–25 weeks' gestation.

65.2 Introduction

Corticosteroids given in the perinatal period have many biologic effects on the developing lung (Grier and Halliday 2004). These include reduced alveolarization, increased production of surfactant lipids and proteins, increased absorption of lung fluid, and increased antioxidant activity. Clearly, some of these will be beneficial to the immature fetus or neonate, while others will be detrimental. Thus administration of corticosteroids in the perinatal period must be based upon clinical judgment of the balance of benefits and risks.

The first randomized trials of corticosteroids in the perinatal period were published in 1972 in the same issue of a pediatric journal (Liggins and Howie 1972; Baden et al. 1972). They were aimed at either preventing or treating respiratory distress syndrome (RDS), a condition of predominantly preterm infants, which then had a high mortality rate. RDS is due to primary deficiency of pulmonary surfactant (Avery and Mead 1959), and Mont Liggins, an obstetrician in New Zealand, had shown that an infusion of cortisol into fetal lambs seemed to prevent RDS (Liggins 1968). He and a colleague from pediatrics, Ross Howie, performed a large randomized trial of prenatal betamethasone that showed this not only decreased the risk of RDS in neonates but also reduced mortality (Liggins and Howie 1972). Since 1972, many randomized trials have confirmed the benefits of prenatal corticosteroids (Roberts and Dalziel 2006), and long-term follow-up of the original cohort at age 31 years has been published (Dalziel et al. 2005). Detrimental effects of prenatal corticosteroids and the controversy over any additional benefit of repeat courses will be discussed in this chapter.

The trial of Baden et al. recruited only 44 infants with RDS to test the effects of hydrocortisone on blood gases, need for assisted ventilation and survival (Baden et al. 1972). Unfortunately, there were no beneficial effects of hydrocortisone, and the authors also concluded that there were no immediate detrimental effects of the therapy. However, two subsequent follow-up publications raised concerns about an excess of severe intraventricular hemorrhage (IVH) and neurosensory and electroencephalographic abnormalities (Fitzhardinge et al. 1974; Taeusch et al. 1973) in hydrocortisone-treated infants. Despite these early concerns, dexamethasone was used to treat infants with bronchopulmonary

dysplasia (BPD) and ventilator dependence less than a decade later (Mammel et al. 1983; Avery et al. 1985). The rationale for dexamethasone therapy was to reduce inflammation in the lung, an important precursor to the development of BPD. However, the doses of dexamethasone used in these trials were very large (about 0.5 mg/kg/day as a starting dose) giving pharmacologic rather than physiologic effects. It was not surprising that the acute beneficial effects on lung function (Mammel et al. 1983; Avery et al. 1985) would later be shown to have had adverse long-term effects on the developing central nervous system when dexamethasone was given in the first week of life (Yeh et al. 1998).

65.3 Results from Randomized Trials of Prenatal Corticosteroids

The most recent Cochrane Review of a single course of prenatal steroids for accelerating fetal lung maturation includes 21 studies and 4,269 infants (Roberts and Dalziel 2006). The authors conclude that prenatal steroid treatment does not increase risk of death to the mother, chorioamnionitis, or puerperal sepsis. However, treatment was associated with an overall reduction in neonatal death (RR 0.69, 95%CI 0.58–0.81), RDS (RR 0.66, 95%CI 0.59–0.73), IVH (RR 0.54, 95%CI 0.43–0.69), necrotizing enterocolitis (NEC) (RR 0.46, 95%CI 0.29–0.74), respiratory support and intensive care admissions (RR 0.80; 95%CI 0.65–0.99), and systemic infections in the first 48 h of life (RR 0.56, 95%CI 0.38–0.85). Prenatal steroid use is also effective in women with premature rupture of membranes and pregnancy-related hypertension syndromes (Roberts and Dalziel 2006). The authors concluded that a single course of prenatal steroids should be considered routinely for preterm delivery with few exceptions. Further information is needed concerning optimal dose to delivery interval, optimal steroid to use, effects in multiple pregnancies, and confirm long-term effects into adulthood (Roberts and Dalziel 2006; Wapner and Jobe 2011). A recent review assessed different steroid regimens for accelerating lung maturity and concluded that no clear advantages were found, although dexamethasone may have some benefits compared to betamethasone with less IVH and a shorter length of NICU stay (Brownfoot et al. 2013). An Australasian trial is currently underway to address this question (Crowther et al. 2013). In 2015 a systematic review concluded that a single course of prenatal steroids in women at high risk for preterm birth appears to improve most neurodevelopmental outcomes in offspring born before 34 weeks of gestation (Sotiriadis et al. 2015).

Recently, however, there has been concern about the ineffectiveness of prenatal steroids in low-income and middle-income countries (Azad and Costello 2014; Dalziel et al. 2014). This concern is based on the findings of the WHO Multicountry Survey on Maternal and Newborn Health involving more than 300,000 births in 359 hospitals in 29 countries (Vogel et al. 2014). The results have been criticized because of poor treatment coverage and underreporting of preterm birth, but it is agreed that prenatal steroids are not a panacea for preterm mortality in low-income and middle-income countries, and drugs should be included in a package of simple efficacious measures (Dalziel et al. 2014).

The most recent systematic review of repeat doses of prenatal steroids for women at risk of preterm birth for preventing RDS included ten trials and involved 4,733 women and 5,700 babies (Crowther et al. 2015). Treatment with repeat dose(s) of steroids was associated with a reduction in RDS (RR 0.83, 95%CI 0.75–0.91) and serious infant outcome (RR 0.84, 95%CI 0.75–0.94). Mean birth weight was reduced by 75.9 g (95%CI 34.0–117.6 g) with repeat doses, but after adjustment of birth weight for gestational age, these differences disappeared. The authors concluded that repeat dose(s) of prenatal steroids reduces the occurrence of RDS and serious health problems in the first few weeks of life. The short-term benefits for babies support the use of repeat dose(s) of prenatal steroids for women at risk of preterm birth. However, these benefits are associated with a reduction in some measures of weight at birth, and more research is needed on the longer-term benefits and risks (Crowther et al. 2015).

65.4 Results from Randomized Trials of Postnatal Steroids

The most recent systematic reviews of postnatal steroids for preventing (Doyle et al. 2014a) and treating chronic lung disease (CLD) (Doyle et al. 2014b) in preterm infants were published in the Cochrane Library in 2014. Twenty-nine trials enrolling 3,750 infants were included in the systematic review of postnatal steroids given in the first week of life to try to prevent CLD in preterm infants (Doyle et al. 2014a). There were significant benefits of early postnatal steroids as regards earlier extubation and decreased risks of CLD at both 28 days (RR 0.87, 95%CI 0.81–0.93) and 36 weeks' postmenstrual age (PMA) (RR 0.79, 95%CI 0.71–0.88). There were also decreases in persistent ductus arteriosus (PDA) (RR 0.79, 95% CI 0.72–0.85), retinopathy of prematurity (ROP) (RR 0.88, 95%CI 0.80–0.97), and severe ROP (RR 0.79, 95%CI 0.64–0.94). There were no significant differences in rates of mortality, infection, severe IVH, periventricular leukomalacia, NEC, or pulmonary hemorrhage. Important adverse effects included gastrointestinal (GI) bleeding (RR 1.86, 95%CI 1.35–2.55), intestinal perforation (RR 1.81, 95%CI 1.33–2.48), hyperglycemia (RR 1.33, 95% CI 1.20–1.47), hypertension (RR 1.85, 95%CI 1.54–2.22), hypertrophic cardiomyopathy (RR 4.33, 95%CI 1.40–13.4), and growth failure (RR 6.67, 95%CI 2.27–19.6). Twelve of 29 trials reported late outcomes, and several adverse effects were found including cerebral palsy (RR 1.45, 95% CI 1.06–1.98) and abnormal neurological examination (RR 1.81, 95%CI 1.33–2.47). However, the rates of the combined outcomes of death or cerebral palsy and death or major neurosensory disability were not significantly increased (Doyle et al. 2014a).

Dexamethasone was used in 20 studies and hydrocortisone in nine. In a subgroup analysis, most of the beneficial and harmful effects were attributable to dexamethasone although with hydrocortisone there was an increase in intestinal perforation (RR 2.02, 95%CI 1.13–3.59) and a borderline reduction in PDA (RR 0.85, 95%CI 0.73–0.99) (Doyle et al. 2010, 2014a). A French randomized clinical trial recently reported an increase in survival without BPD (OR 1.48; 95 %CI 1.02–2.16; p = 0.04) in preterm infants (<28 weeks' gestation) treated with low dose hydrocortisone for 10 days starting before 24 h after birth (Baud et al. 2016). In a subgroup of infants of 24–25 weeks' gestation there was an increase in sepsis (sub-hazard ratio 1.87; 95 %CI 1.09–3.21; p = 0.02). A recent follow-up study from Finland reported neurodevelopmental impairment in 61% of children at 5–7 years who had been treated with early hydrocortisone to prevent BPD compared to 39% of placebo-treated infants (Peltoniemi et al. 2016). The authors of the Cochrane Review concluded that the benefits of early postnatal steroid treatment (<8 days), particularly with dexamethasone, may not outweigh the known or potential adverse effects of this treatment. Although early steroid treatment facilitates extubation and reduces risk of CLD and PDA, it causes short-term adverse effects including GI bleeding, intestinal perforation, hyperglycemia, hypertension, hypertrophic cardiomyopathy, and growth failure. Long-term follow-up studies report increased risks of abnormal neurological examination and cerebral palsy. There is a compelling need for more long-term follow-up and reporting of late outcomes, especially neurological and developmental outcomes, among surviving infants who participated in all randomized trials of early postnatal steroids. Hydrocortisone in the doses and regimens used in these trials had few beneficial or harmful effects and cannot be recommended for prevention of CLD (Doyle et al. 2010, 2014a).

Inhaled steroids have been used to try to prevent CLD in the hope that they would have fewer adverse effects. A recent large randomized trial of high-dose inhaled budesonide reported a reduction in BPD (RR 0.74, 95%CI 0.60–0.91) in preterm infants treated within 12 h of birth (Bassler et al. 2015). Although there was also a reduction in the combined outcome of death or BPD (RR 0.86, 95%CI 0.75–1.00), the authors were concerned that the advantage of reduced BPD may have come at the expense of increased neonatal mortality (Bassler et al. 2015). Further studies of inhaled steroids with long-term follow-up are needed before this treatment can be recommended as a routine.

Twenty-one trials enrolling a total of 1,424 infants were included in the systematic review of late (>7 days) postnatal steroids for CLD in

preterm infants (Doyle et al. 2014b). Late steroid treatment was associated with a reduction in neonatal mortality (RR 0.49, 95%CI 0.28–0.85) but not at discharge (RR 0.86, 95%CI 0.66–1.13). Other beneficial effects included earlier extubation and reductions in CLD at both 28 days (RR 0.87, 95%CI 0.81–0.94) and 36 weeks' PMA (RR 0.82, 95%CI 0.70–0.96), need for late treatment with dexamethasone (RR 0.47, 95%CI 0.38–0.59), discharge on home oxygen therapy (RR 0.71, 95%CI 0.54–0.94), and death or CLD at both 28 days (RR 0.84, 95%CI 0.78–0.89) and 36 weeks' PMA (RR 0.76, 95%CI 0.68–0.85). There was a trend toward an increased risk of GI bleeding but not NEC. Short-term adverse effects included hyperglycemia (RR 1.50, 95%CI 1.25–1.80), glycosuria (RR 8.03, 95%CI 2.43–26.5), and hypertension (RR 2.12, 95%CI 1.45–3.10). There was an increase in hypertrophic cardiomyopathy (RR 2.76, 95%CI 1.33–5.74) and severe ROP (RR 1.38, 95%CI 1.07–1.79), but no significant increase in blindness. There was a trend toward reduction in severe IVH (RR 0.44, 95%CI 0.19–1.02), and trends toward an increase in cerebral palsy (RR 1.12, 95%CI 0.79–1.60) and abnormal neurological examination were partly offset by a trend in the opposite direction in death before late follow-up. The combined rate of death or cerebral palsy was not significantly different between steroid and control groups. Major neurosensory disability and the combined rate of death or major neurosensory disability were not significantly different between groups. There were no substantial differences between groups for other outcomes in later childhood, including respiratory health or function, blood pressure, or growth (Doyle et al. 2014b). The authors concluded that the benefits of late steroid therapy (>7 days) may not outweigh actual or potential adverse effects. Although there continues to be concern about an increase in adverse neurological outcomes in infants treated with early postnatal steroids, this review of late steroids suggests that this may reduce neonatal mortality without significantly increasing the risk of adverse long-term neurodevelopmental outcomes. However, the methodological quality of the studies determining long-term outcomes is limited in some cases, and no study was sufficiently powered to detect increased rates of important long-term outcomes. Given the evidence of both benefits and harms of treatment and the limitations of the evidence at present, it appears prudent to reserve the use of late postnatal steroids to infants who cannot be weaned from mechanical ventilation and to minimize the dose and duration of any course of treatment (Doyle et al. 2014b).

65.5 Conclusions

There are some problems with steroid treatment of the fetus and newborn, but on the whole if used according to accepted guidelines, the benefits outweigh the risks. For the fetus at risk of preterm birth, a single course of betamethasone or dexamethasone leads to lung maturity and reduces the risk of RDS, neonatal mortality, and other important complications of prematurity (Roberts and Dalziel 2006). The current recommendation is to give two doses of 12 mg betamethasone, 24 h apart, to women who may deliver within 7 days and are less than 35 weeks pregnant (Sweet et al. 2013). There remains some controversy about repeat courses of prenatal steroids, as they are associated with reduced fetal growth, but consensus seems to support their use when there is a high risk of preterm birth before 29 weeks' gestation (Wapner and Jobe 2011).

The beneficial pulmonary effects of early postnatal dexamethasone, in the first week of life, do not outweigh the adverse effects on neurodevelopment (Doyle et al. 2014a). However, late postnatal steroid therapy, after the first week of life, seems to be associated with similar beneficial pulmonary effects without significant increase in neurodevelopmental sequelae (Doyle et al. 2014b). Infants at higher risk of BPD have increased rates of survival free of cerebral palsy after postnatal steroid treatment (Doyle et al. 2014c). Late steroid therapy, with low-dose, short duration dexamethasone, is probably still indicated for preterm infants with CLD who remain ventilator dependent and have severe respiratory disease (Halliday 2011).

Inhaled steroids may be a promising method of reducing BPD with reduced adverse effects, but further evaluation in randomized clinical trials with long-term follow-up is needed to confirm their

safety before they can be recommended for routine use (Bassler et al. 2015; Halliday 2011).

References

Avery ME, Mead J (1959) Surface properties in relation to atelectasis and hyaline membrane disease. Am J Dis Child 97:517–523

Avery GB, Fletcher AB, Kaplan M et al (1985) Controlled trial of dexamethasone in respirator-dependent infants with bronchopulmonary dysplasia. Pediatrics 75:106–111

Azad C, Costello A (2014) Extreme caution is needed before scale-up of antenatal corticosteroids to reduce preterm deaths in low-income settings. Lancet Glob Health 2:e191–e192

Baden M, Bauer CR, Colle E et al (1972) A controlled trial of hydrocortisone therapy in infants with respiratory distress syndrome. Pediatrics 50:526–534

Bassler D, Plavka R, Shinwell ES et al (2015) Early inhaled budesonide for the prevention of bronchopulmonary dysplasia. N Engl J Med 373:1497–1506

Baud O, Maury L, Lebail F et al (2016) Effect of early low-dose hydrocortisone on survival without bronchopulmonary dysplasia in extremely preterm infants (PREMILOC): a double-blind, placebo-controlled, multicentre, randomised trial. Lancet 387: 1827–1836

Brownfoot FC, Gagliardi DI, Bain E et al (2013) Different corticosteroids and regimens for accelerating fetal lung maturation for women at risk of preterm birth. Cochrane Database Syst Rev 8, CD006764

Crowther CA, Harding JE, Middleton PF et al (2013) Australasian randomized trial to evaluate the role of maternal intramuscular dexamethasone versus betamethasone prior to preterm birth to increase survival free of childhood neurosensory disability. BMC Pregnancy Childbirth 13:104

Crowther CA, McKinlay CJ, Middleton et al (2015) Repeat doses of prenatal corticosteroids for women at risk of preterm birth for improving health outcomes. Cochrane Database Syst Rev 7, CD003935

Dalziel SR, Lim VK, Lambert A et al (2005) Antenatal exposure to betamethasone: psychological functioning and health related quality of life 31 years after inclusion in randomised controlled trial. BMJ 331:665–668

Dalziel SR, Crowther CA, Harding JE (2014) Antenatal steroids 40 years on: we can do better. Lancet 384:1829–1831

Doyle LW, Ehrenkranz RA, Halliday HL (2010) Postnatal hydrocortisone for preventing or treating bronchopulmonary dysplasia in preterm infants: a systematic review. Neonatology 98:111–117

Doyle LW, Ehrenkranz RA, Halliday HL (2014a) Early (<8 days) postnatal corticosteroids for preventing chronic lung disease in preterm infants. Cochrane Database Syst Rev 5, CD001146

Doyle LW, Ehrenkranz RA, Halliday HL (2014b) Late (>7 days) postnatal corticosteroids for chronic lung disease in preterm infants. Cochrane Database Syst Rev 5, CD001145

Doyle LW, Halliday HL, Ehrenkranz RA et al (2014c) An update on the impact of postnatal systemic corticosteroids on mortality and cerebral palsy in preterm infants: effect modification by risk of bronchopulmonary dysplasia. J Pediatr 165:1258–1260

Fitzhardinge PM, Eisen A, Lejtenyi C (1974) Sequelae of early steroid administration to the newborn infant. Pediatrics 53:877–883

Grier DG, Halliday HL (2004) Effects of glucocorticoids on fetal and neonatal lung development. Treat Respir Med 3:295–306

Halliday HL (2011) Postnatal steroids: the way forward. Arch Dis Child Fetal Neonatal Ed 96:F158–F159

Liggins GC (1968) Premature parturition after infusion of corticotrophin or cortisol into foetal lambs. J Endocrinol 42:323–329

Liggins GC, Howie RN (1972) A controlled trial of antepartum glucocorticoid treatment for prevention of the respiratory distress syndrome in preterm infants. Pediatrics 50:515–525

Mammel MC, Green TP, Johnson DE et al (1983) Controlled trial of dexamethasone therapy in infants with bronchopulmonary dysplasia. Lancet 1:1356–1358

Peltoniemi OM, Lano A, Yliherva A, Kari MA, Hallman M, Neonatal Hydrocortisone Working Group (2016) Randomised trial of early neonatal hydrocortisone demonstrates potential undesired effects on neurodevelopment at preschool age. Acta Paediatr 105:159–164

Roberts D, Dalziel S (2006) Antenatal corticosteroids for accelerating fetal lung maturation for women at risk of preterm birth. Cochrane Database Syst Rev 3, CD004454

Sotiriadis A, Tsiami A, Papatheodoros S et al (2015) Neurodevelopmental outcome after a single course of antenatal steroids in children born preterm: a systematic review and meta-analysis. Obstet Gynecol 125: 1385–1396

Sweet DG, Carnielli V, Greisen G et al (2013) European consensus guidelines on the management of neonatal respiratory distress syndrome in preterm infants – 2013 update. Neonatology 103:353–368

Taeusch HW Jr, Wang NS, Baden M et al (1973) A controlled trial of hydrocortisone therapy in infants with respiratory distress syndrome: II. Pathol Pediatr 52:850–854

Vogel JP, Souza JP, Gulmezoglu AM et al (2014) Use of antenatal corticosteroids and tocolytic drugs in preterm births in 29 countries: an analysis of the WHO Multicountry Survey on Maternal and Newborn Health. Lancet 384:1869–1877

Wapner R, Jobe AH (2011) Controversy: antenatal steroids. Clin Perinatol 38:529–545

Yeh TF, Lin YJ, Huang CC et al (1998) Early dexamethasone therapy in preterm infants: a follow-up study. Pediatrics 101, e7

Apnea of Prematurity and Sudden Infant Death Syndrome

66

Christian F. Poets

Contents

Abstract

Apnea of prematurity is a self-resolving, yet very common condition in preterm infants. Recent observational data suggest that the intermittent hypoxemia often occurring with it may be associated with an increased risk of adverse outcome, including cerebral palsy, retinopathy of prematurity, and death. Treatment should follow an incremental approach, starting with head elevated positioning, followed by caffeine administration and nasal respiratory support.

Sudden infant death syndrome has decreased markedly in incidence following primary prevention campaigns in many countries, yet continues to be a leading cause of death beyond the neonatal period. Although still incompletely understood, it seems that death is the result of an external trigger (e.g., prone sleep position) occurring in a vulnerable infant (e.g., born to a mother who smoked during pregnancy) during a critical developmental period (e.g., 2–4 months of age). Memory monitor recordings obtained during SIDS suggest that bradycardia, probably resulting from severe hypoxemia, is the primary abnormality in the sequence of events ultimately resulting in these deaths. Prevention should focus on a safe sleep environment, i.e., supine sleep position, a smoke-free environment, avoidance of overheating, use of a sleeping bag, and room but not bed sharing.

C. F. Poets (✉)
Department of Neonatology, Tübingen University Hospital, Tübingen, Germany
e-mail: Christian-f.poets@med.uni-tuebingen.de

G. Buonocore et al. (eds.), *Neonatology*,
https://doi.org/10.1007/978-3-319-29489-6_213

List of Abbreviations

AAP	American Academy of Pediatrics
ALTE	Apparent life-threatening event
AOP	Apnea of prematurity
BPD	Bronchopulmonary dysplasia
CDC	Centers for Disease Control
CI	Confidence interval
CO_2	Carbon dioxide
IH	Intermittent hypoxemia
LQTS	Long-QT-syndrome
MCAD	Medium-chain acyl-CoA dehydrogenase
N-CPAP	Nasal continuous positive airway pressure
N-IPPV	Nasal intermittent positive pressure ventilation
NNT	Number needed to treat
OR	Odds ratio
PaO_2	Partial pressure of oxygen in arterial blood
PAR	Population-attributable risk
RCT	Randomized controlled trial
ROP	Retinopathy of prematurity
RR	Relative risk
SIDS	Sudden infant death syndrome
SpO_2	Arterial oxygen saturation measured by pulse oximetry
TPN	Total parenteral nutrition
VLBW	Very low birth weight

66.1 Salient Points

- Apnea of prematurity is a self-resolving and very common condition in preterm infants.
- The intermittent hypoxemia accompanying it may be associated with an increased risk of adverse outcome (cerebral palsy, retinopathy of prematurity, and death).
- Treatment consists of head elevated positioning, followed by caffeine administration and nasal up to nasal respiratory support.
- The incidence of sudden infant death syndrome (SIDS) has markedly decreased even if it remains a leading cause of death in the postneonatal period.
- It seems that death is the result of an external trigger (position) occurring in a vulnerable infant during a critical developmental period.
- Prevention should focus on a safe sleep environment (supine positioning), a smoke-free environment, and avoidance of overheating.

66.2 Apnea of Prematurity (AOP)

66.2.1 Introduction

Apnea of prematurity (AOP) is a developmental and thus self-resolving disorder, which nonetheless may cause serious long-term sequelae through accompanying hypoxemia. Almost every infant born at less than 29 weeks gestation exhibits AOP, but little was known when it became potentially harmful. Recently, a secondary analysis of pulse oximeter saturation (SpO_2) and pulse rate data recorded for a mean duration of 68 days in 1035 participants in the Canadian Oxygen Trial (COT), who were born at 23–27 weeks GA and survived to 36 weeks postmenstrual age (PMA), showed the following (Poets et al. 2015):

- Mean percentages of recorded time with hypoxemia (pulse oximeter saturation (SpO_2) <80% for at least 10 s) for the least and most affected 10% of infants was at 0.4 and 13.5%, respectively, while bradycardia (pulse rate <80/min.) was rarer at 0.1 and 0.3%.
- Being in the highest decile for % time with intermittent hypoxemia (IH) was associated with three to fivefold increased odds of developing the primary outcome of death beyond 36 weeks or disability at 18 months, with these associations being significant only for events lasting at least 1 min.
- Odds ratios for secondary outcomes (motor impairment, cognitive, or language delay and severe retinopathy of prematurity) were similarly increased after prolonged hypoxemia.
- Bradycardia, in the absence of concomitant hypoxemia, did not significantly add to the risk of adverse outcome.
- The severity of IH, expressed as the area-under-the-curve (AUC), and the rate with

which desaturation occurred, added little prognostic value.

- Associations between hypoxemic exposure and adverse outcomes were stronger at later postnatal ages (i.e., at 8–10 week) and for infants assigned to a target range of 91–95% compared to a target range of 85–89% SpO_2.

Thus, of the three components contributing to AOP (apnea, bradycardia, hypoxemia), it seems prudent to focus on the avoidance of IH, particularly episodes lasting for 1 min, or longer, if we want to avoid adverse effects of AOP in extremely preterm infants. Up to now, however, most studies on interventions for AOP focussed on apnea.

Although not fully in line with the above data, the approach taken in the author's institution for the last 10 years has been to grade the intensity of the treatment provided for AOP based on a severity score that relies largely on the nurses' acute intervention to events (e.g. stimulation, bagging; Fig. 1). Neither the score nor any treatment threshold used with it has ever been validated. However, the low rates of retinopathy of prematurity (ROP; <2% for stage 3 or higher in infants <1500 g birth weight in 2010–2015) and high Bayley scores (Moll et al. 2011) associated with implementation of this apnea scoring paradigm suggest its potential as a protocol that warrants further study. In any case, such a severity score may only serve as an example for how apnea severity may be assessed more objectively without documentation via continuous recordings, which would be preferable but is yet impractical in most units.

66.2.2 Treatment

In the following, interventions to improve AOP will be grouped into those that have been shown to be beneficial and those where the effect is questionable and/or needs further study (Table 1).

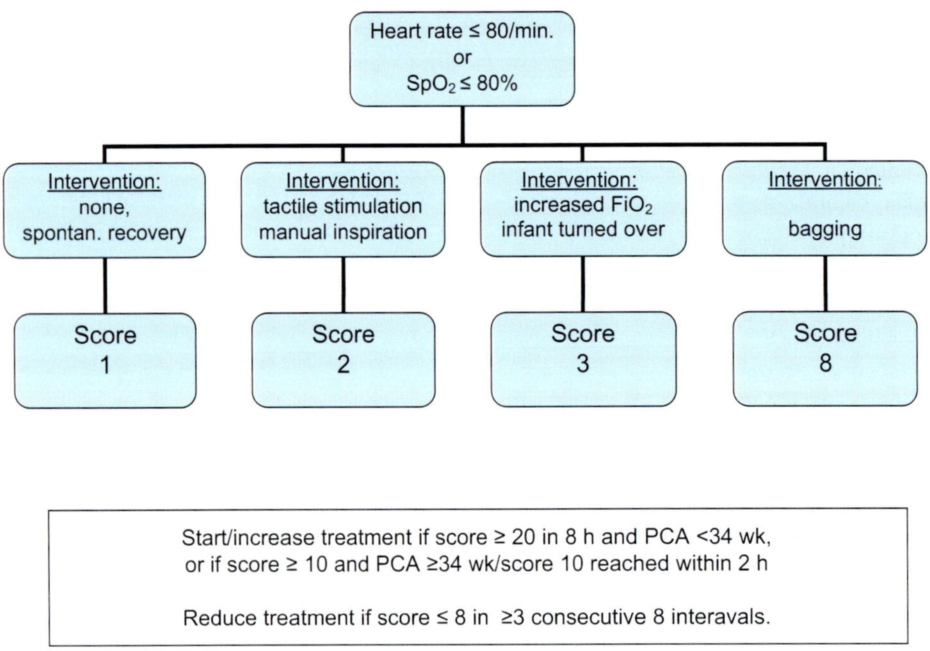

Fig. 1 A proposed apnea severity score to standardize assessment across different raters/infants. The values in the lower row of boxes indicate the respective score. The threshold for an increase in treatment severity is lower in more mature infants as these are considered more vulnerable to the detrimental effects of intermittent hypoxemia (Modified based on Poets CF (2010). Interventions for apnoea of prematurity: a personal view. Acta Paediatr 99; 2172–2177, with permission)

Table 1 Suggested incremental treatment plan for AOP

First Step: 15° head-up tilt position
Second Step: Caffeine[a]
Third Step: Variable flow CPAP or synchronized N-IPPV
Fourth Step: Intubation and mechanical ventilation[b]

[a]Consider caffeine as first-line treatment in infants <29 weeks GA

[b]High-dose caffeine or doxapram may be considered as alternatives in infants who continue to exhibit recurrent hypoxemia despite mechanical ventilation

66.2.2.1 Interventions with Proven Benefit

Head-Elevated Positioning

While a recent Cochrane analysis demonstrated *no* advantage of the prone position in reducing apnea rates in preterm infants (data on intermittent hypoxia were not reported), a head-elevated 15° tilt position was associated with a 49% reduction in desaturations to <85% in a study involving 12 preterm infants. A reinvestigation of the effectiveness of this position, however, triggered by the observation that infants appear more comfortable when only the chest and head rather than the entire body are being tilted showed only a modest (−6%) and nonsignificant reduction in hypoxemia rates in the head elevated tilt compared to the horizontal position (Reher et al. 2008), and also no significant advantage (22%) for the head-and-chest elevated position. This much less clear advantage of the head-up tilt position may be due to the fact that several infants in the earlier study had received no other treatment for AOP, whereas in the more recent one, all had received methylxanthines and/or continuous positive airway pressure (CPAP) in addition to positioning (Reher et al. 2008). Thus, a head-up tilt position may be considered a first step in an incremental treatment plan for AOP, while this intervention may be less effective in infants already receiving other treatments for AOP, such as caffeine or CPAP (see below).

Continuous Positive Airway Pressure (CPAP) and Synchronized Nasal Ventilation (S-NIPPV)

CPAP has been shown to reduce extubation failure in preterm infants and can be applied via a nasopharyngeal tube or (bi-)nasal prongs. Reintubation rates are 40% lower with the latter (relative risk (RR) 0.59 [95%-confidence interval (CI) 0.41; 0.85], number needed to treat (NNT) 5) (De Paoli et al. 2008), suggesting nasal prongs as the preferred patient interface when applying CPAP. An extension of CPAP is nasal intermittent positive pressure ventilation (N-IPPV), with better effectiveness than CPAP in preventing extubation failure if used in synchrony with the infant's own breathing efforts. Typically, an inspiratory pressure of 15–20 cm H_2O, applied at a rate of 10–20/min, is combined with a CPAP level of 5–6 cm H_2O. A recent meta-analysis investigating the effects of synchronised and nonsynchronized nasal ventilation versus CPAP on respiratory failure rates found a significant effect only for the former, making this the preferred mode of nasal ventilatory support if a trial of CPAP fails (Lemyre et al. 2014). Interestingly, gastric distension, a theoretical concern with nasal ventilation, was not an issue in the studies contributing to this meta-analysis (Lemyre et al. 2014).

An even more recent study investigated different synchronized nasal ventilation system in 19 infants at a mean PMA of 30 week and reported a decrease in bradycardia (<80/min) and desaturation (<80%) from 6.1/h with CPAP to 2.9/h with S-NIPPV. With nonsynchronized NIPPV, this rate was similar to that with CPAP (5.9 events/h) (Gizzi et al. 2014). An earlier study comparing nonsynchronized N-IPPV with nasal CPAP, delivered via a variable flow CPAP device that reduces work of breathing (InfantFlow, CareFusion, San Diego, CA), showed a decrease in bradycardia and desaturation rate by approximately 50% compared to both, nonsynchronized N-IPPV or CPAP (Pantalitschka et al. 2009). Thus, a reduced work of breathing and/or effective synchronization with the infant's own breathing efforts may be key to success for nasal respiratory support applied to ameliorate AOP.

Caffeine

Methylxanthines increase chemoreceptor sensitivity as well as respiratory drive and can also improve diaphragmatic function. Of the substances available, caffeine has a wider therapeutic range and

fewer side effects than theophylline. Its effectiveness in improving patient outcome was proven in a large placebo-controlled RCT enrolling over 2000 infants (the CAP study (Schmidt et al. 2007)). Caffeine (or placebo) was started during the first 10 postnatal days in infants of 500–1250 g birth weight at a dose of 5–10 mg/kg caffeine citrate in infants considered eligible for caffeine treatment and given until no longer considered necessary for AOP treatment. Mechanical ventilation, CPAP, and oxygen could all be discontinued approximately 1 week earlier in infants treated with caffeine. Somewhat unexpected, and not a primary outcome, was the finding of a 40% lower risk of bronchopulmonary dysplasia (BPD; 36% vs. 47%; OR 0.6; 95% CI 0.5; 0.8), a 30% lower risk of developing a symptomatic patent ductus arteriosus (OR 0.7; [0.5; 0.8]), and a 40% reduction in the risk of developing stage 4 or 5 retinopathy of prematurity (ROP) or requiring treatment for ROP in the caffeine group (OR 0.61 [0.42; 0.89]) (Schmidt et al. 2007). Most important, however, are the data on the primary outcome, showing a 23% reduction in death or disability at 18 months corrected age in addition to a reduction in cerebral palsy in infants in the caffeine group (Schmidt et al. 2007).

Results from the 5-year follow-up of this study still showed an effect of caffeine on death or disability, but this was no longer significant. Neonatal caffeine therapy, however, reduced motor impairment (OR 0.66; 0.48; 0.91) (Schmidt et al. 2012). Motor dysfunction not associated with cerebral palsy or cognitive impairments is referred to as developmental coordination disorder. At 5 years of age, this condition was found in 11% of caffeine-group infants compared to 15% of placebo-group infants. Regarding other long-term (side)effects, sleep studies, performed in 201 former CAP participants at age 5–12 years, showed no difference in sleep disorders in subjects treated with neonatal caffeine compared to placebo (Marcus et al. 2014).

In subgroup analysis, the effect of caffeine on the primary outcome was found to be restricted to those requiring ventilatory support at randomization, i.e. caffeine had no effect on death or disability in infants *not* requiring CPAP or IPPV. Interestingly, the reduced duration of the need for ventilatory support was only evident in those who were randomized within the first 3 postnatal days, and the effect on death or disability was only significant for infants receiving at least 3.5 mg/kg/day of caffeine base (7 mg/kg/day caffeine citrate). Also in secondary data analysis, a significant difference in the rate of cerebral palsy between caffeine- and placebo-group infants was only found in those receiving caffeine for at least 45 days. Thus, caffeine administration should be started within the first 3 days of age in infants <1250 g requiring respiratory support and being likely to develop AOP.

It is important also to consider when to discontinue caffeine treatment. In the CAP study, caffeine was given until a mean PMA of 34.4 weeks (Schmidt et al. 2007). However, caffeine continues to be effective in reducing intermittent hypoxia rates until 35 weeks PMA (Rhein et al. 2014). With no current standards for discontinuing caffeine therapy, the use of an apnea severity score such as that proposed in Fig. 1 may provide a treatment guideline in the clinical setting.

At what dose should caffeine be given? First, it has to be remembered that caffeine is usually available as caffeine citrate, in which the active component (caffeine) comprises only 50% of the total dose. In this chapter, all data will be on this active component. In the CAP study, a loading dose of 10 mg/kg (iv or orally) and a maintenance dose of 2.5–5 mg/kg once daily were used. Another recent randomized controlled trial compared a loading dose of 40 mg/kg caffeine (maintenance dose 10 mg/kg/day) with a "conventional" 10/2.5 mg/kg regimen in 234 infants born at a mean GA of 27 weeks. Infants in the high dose group had only half the risk of failing extubation within 48 h of caffeine loading or to require reintubation and mechanical ventilation or doxapram within 7 days of caffeine loading (15.0% vs. 29.8%, RR 0.51 [0.31; 0.85]) (Steer et al. 2004). They received mechanical ventilation for 14.4 days (SD 11.1), compared to 22.1 (17.1) days for infants in the lower dose group. This better efficacy was not at the expense of an increased risk of side effects, including no difference in Griffith's mental development scales at age 12 months. Given the

extremely sparse data on doxapram (see below), clinicians may consider starting caffeine at the standard dose of 10 mg/kg loading, 5 mg/kg/day maintenance, but to switch to a higher dose if AOP persists in an occasional infant. It has to be kept in mind, however, that the follow-up study on high dose caffeine was underpowered to detect a difference in neurodevelopmental outcome between the low- and the high-dose group that at this dose the serum level should occasionally be checked to identify those approaching toxic levels (>50 mg/l), and that a recent RCT testing the same dose as used by Steer et al. (2004) was stopped prematurely because of an unexpectedly high rate of cerebellar hemorrhages (36% vs. 10%) in infants receiving high-dose caffeine (McPherson et al. 2015). There are no indications that tachyphylaxis occurs with caffeine, but higher doses and a 12-h dosing interval may be necessary in infants approaching term-equivalent age because of a more rapid caffeine metabolism in this age group.

66.2.2.2 Interventions That Are Potentially Effective but Require Further Study

Doxapram

Doxapram stimulates peripheral chemoreceptors at low and central ones at high doses. It shows a clear dose–response curve, with a 50% reduction in apnea rate occurring in 47%, 65%, 82%, and 89% of infants at doses of 0.5, 1.5, 2.0, and 2.5 mg/kg/h, respectively. In an own longitudinal study, desaturation rates to ≤80% SpO_2 were reduced from a median of 8/h to 2/h, with this effect continuing for the follow-up period of 6 days (Poets et al. 1999a). Most studies used a continuous intravenous infusion, although some suggest that the iv solution may also be given orally at twice the dose with good effect (enteral absorption is approximately 50%) (Poets et al. 1999a). Short-term side effects become quite common at doses above 1.5 mg/kg/h and include irritability, myoclonus, elevated blood pressure, and gastric residuals. Of concern is the fact that the long-term effects of doxapram are unknown. This is particularly worrisome given that in a study on factors associated with poor development in extremely low birth weight infants, the only difference found was that infants with developmental delay (defined as a Mental Development Index <70) had received a mean cumulative doxapram dose of 2233 mg, compared to 615 mg in matched controls without delay ($p < 0.01$) (Sreenan et al. 2001). Although such a retrospective analysis cannot distinguish whether this reflects sequelae of severe AOP (for which doxapram had been given) or a direct drug effect, it clearly raises concern. In the CAP study (Schmidt et al. 2007), placebo group infants not only had been more likely to develop cerebral palsy but were also three times more likely to have received doxapram. Given these data (or lack thereof), doxapram cannot be recommended as a standard treatment for AOP, although it seems to be rather widely used in some countries.

Oxygen Administration

That oxygen stabilizes neonatal respiration was first observed in 1923 and responsible for an epidemic in ROP in the following years. Several crossover trials in infants with and without BPD have since shown that the application of low-flow oxygen results in a reduced rate of apnea and IH. Application of this therapy, however, has to be weighed against side effects potentially resulting from oxygen toxicity. The issue has resurfaced with the recent data from RCTs comparing an SpO_2 target range of 85–89% with 91–95%. As perhaps to be expected, there was a higher rate of ROP in infants randomized to the higher range, but – unexpectedly – also a lower mortality in two of these studies, which was confirmed in meta-analysis (Saugstad and Aune 2014). Interestingly, however, the study achieving the widest separation in SpO_2 between study groups was also that where no difference was found for either ROP or mortality (Schmidt et al. 2013). Infants randomized to the lower target range indeed also had more episodes of IH (SpO_2 < 80%) (Poets et al. 2015). Whether these data are sufficient to recommend keeping the SpO_2 at a

target range of 91–95% to prevent some episodes of IH is yet open to debate.

Increased Inspiratory CO_2 Concentration

One determinant of respiratory drive is CO_2. If CO_2 levels fall below the eupneic baseline value, apnea occurs. A Canadian group performed an RCT in 87 infants of 27–32 weeks GA to test whether adding 0.5 l/min. of CO_2 to the inspired air (corresponding to a CO_2 concentration of 1%) was as effective as theophylline in reducing apnea duration and rate (Alvaro et al. 2012). They found that apnea time indeed decreased with CO_2 inhalation from 183 ± 44 to 101 ± 26, 105 ± 29, and 94 ± 26 s/h during the 3 days of intervention, but this was still twice as high as the apnea time seen in infants randomized to theophylline. No data on oxygenation were provided.

Red Blood Cell Transfusions

An increase in respiratory drive resulting from an increased tissue oxygenation is also one of the proposed mechanisms for red cell transfusions potentially to ameliorate AOP, and anemia has indeed been implicated in the pathophysiology of AOP. It would thus seem only logical to hypothesize that giving a blood transfusion is an effective treatment modality in infants with AOP who are anemic. Data on the effect of blood transfusions on the frequency of these episodes, however, are conflicting. In two crossover studies from the author's group, no effect of transfusion was found on bradycardia and IH. In contrast, others found an age-dependent improvement in frequency and severity of IH after transfusion beyond the first week of life when IH events begin to increase. A meta-analysis of 4 RCTs comparing the effects of a liberal with a more restrictive transfusion policy found no statistically significant differences in the combined outcomes of death or serious morbidity at first hospital discharge (Whyte and Kirpalani 2011). While this result doesn't exclude some minor effects on apnea rate, it clearly suggests that such effects, if they exist, do not improve clinical outcomes and make it therefore difficult to justify blood transfusions as a means to treat AOP.

Oscillating Waterbed/Mechanosensory Stimulation

The theory behind this intervention is that entrainment can be achieved between an infant's own breathing rhythm and an external rhythm generator, e.g., an inflatable mattress connected to a respirator. A meta-analysis of 3 RCTs testing this intervention, involving a total of 165 infants, showed no effect on apnea or bradycardia. This may be explained by the observation that synchronization with an external rhythm generator is significantly better beyond than before 35 weeks GA, but at that age AOP is no longer a major issue. As a result, this intervention has largely been abandoned. More recently, however, it has resurfaced in the form of a stochastic mechanosensory stimulation, where actuators are embedded in a specially designed mattress (Bloch-Salisbury et al. 2009) trying to simulate the cutaneous stimulation given by maternal licking of the newborn as observed in many animal species after birth. Using such a device in a crossover design in 10 preterm infants with a mean PMA of 33 weeks and a study duration of 2×1.5 h, a 65% reduction in time with $SpO_2 < 85\%$ was found. Confirmation of the effectiveness of this approach in a larger sample and longer study duration is necessary.

In summary, treatment for AOP may follow an incremental approach, starting with infant care procedures such as prone head-up tilt positioning, followed by methylxanthines and CPAP/N-IPPV.

66.3 Sudden Infant Death Syndrome (SIDS)

Sudden deaths in infants are known since biblical times, but it was only in 1970 that Bergman et al. coined the term SIDS. More recently, it was redefined by an expert panel as "the sudden unexpected death of an infant <1 year of age, with onset of the fatal episode apparently occurring during sleep, that remains unexplained after a thorough investigation, including performance of a complete autopsy and review of the

circumstances of death and the clinical history." To facilitate research, this definition was stratified into cases with the "classic" features of SIDS present and completely documented (so-called Category 1A SIDS), those with these features present but incompletely documented (IB), and those meeting Category I criteria except for one or more of the following: age <3 weeks or >270 days, similar deaths in siblings, close relatives or infants in the custody of the same caregiver, perinatal conditions such as a history of premature birth, suspected mechanical suffocation, or marked inflammatory changes not sufficient to be assigned a cause of death (i.e., Category II) (Krous et al. 2004). According to this definition, all cases not meeting criteria for category I or II SIDS, including those for which an autopsy has not been performed, are now called "Unclassified Sudden Infant Death" (Krous et al. 2004). To also include cases of sudden unexpected death attributed to positional suffocation (previously often classified as SIDS), in 2010 the Centers for Disease Control (CDC) introduced the term "sudden unexpected infant death (SUID)," which includes SIDS, ill-defined and unknown causes of death, and accidental sleep-related suffocation (Shapiro-Mendoza et al. 2014). In an initial evaluation of this classification system, 88% of 436 SUID were classified as unexplained, with 73% occurring in an unsafe sleep environment, while 12% were assigned to suffocation, and 22% to possible suffocation with unsafe sleep factors. With the increased recognition of positional suffocation as a potential cause of death, it seems important from an epidemiological and preventive point of view not to dismiss cases that previously had been classified as SIDS, but now as suffocation (Malloy and MacDorman 2005).

66.3.1 Epidemiology

66.3.1.1 Incidence

Despite a recent decline in incidence, SIDS continues to be the leading cause of postneonatal mortality in developed countries after excluding perinatal event-related deaths (Table 2). Because of the misclassification problem mentioned above, it is important always to report changes in both SIDS and postneonatal mortality rates and to uniformly use a classification system that includes SIDS and deaths ascribed to accidental suffocation, such as that introduced by the CDC (see above).

66.3.1.2 Age and Time of Death

One of the most striking epidemiological features in SIDS is its characteristic age distribution. Some 75% of deaths occur between 2 and 4 months of age, and 95% before 9 months of age (Poets 2008). Early beliefs that SIDS is extremely rare in the neonatal period cannot be maintained: 6–7% of SIDS victims are younger than 1 month of age, and 11% of all neonatal deaths are due to SIDS (Poets 2008). There is also the recent recognition that sudden deaths or near-death events may occur in apparently healthy neonates only a few hours after delivery. Here, many risk factors otherwise largely abandoned in recent years (see below), such as prone position, overheating, or maternal fatigue, continue to be highly prevalent. Caregivers need to be alerted to the possibility of these events to occur

Table 2 SIDS and postneonatal mortality (PNM) rates in different countries, 1990 vs. 2003 (Data taken from Hauck FR, Tanabe KW: International Trends in Sudden Infant Death Syndrome: Stabilization of rates requires further action. Pediatrics 2007; 122:660–666)

Country	PNM1990	PNM2003	Change(%)	SIDS1990	SIDS2003	Change(%)
Netherlands	2.3	1.2	−48	0.56	0.10	−82
Sweden	2.4	0.96	−60	1.0	0.23	−77
Germany	3.3	1.4	−58	1.42	0.43	−70
USA	3.38	2.67	−31	1.30	0.54	−58
New Zealand	4.21	1.90	−55	2.90	0.80	−72

and infants closely monitored already in the delivery room (Poets et al. 2012).

Throughout the year, there used to be a preponderance of the cold season, but this has almost disappeared following the back-to-sleep campaigns.

66.3.1.3 Risk Factors

A large number of factors associated with an increased risk of SIDS have been identified (Poets 2008) (Table 3). Many underscore the importance of social factors in the pathogenesis of SIDS; others, such as maternal smoking or anemia during pregnancy, suggest that there must already be a disturbance during intrauterine life that poses an infant at risk. Factors that are potentially amenable to modification include maternal smoking, not breast feeding, not using a pacifier, overheating, and a nonsupine sleep position, and these are the factors targeted by most intervention campaigns. Subsequently, however, additional modifiable risk factors have been identified. These include head covering, which has a pooled adjusted OR of 16.9 (95% CI 13.6; 22.7) and a population-attributable risk (PAR) of 27% (Blair et al. 2008), and prone sleeping in preterm and low birth weight infants. Parents of the latter infants may get confused by the common use of the prone position in hospital; it is thus particularly important to place these infants on their back before hospital discharge and to explain the importance of supine sleeping to their parents. Bed-sharing is also a relatively "new" risk factor. This practice seems particularly dangerous if taking place on a sofa or with a parent who drank alcohol or who smokes and cosleeps with an infant <3 months of age (Blair et al. 2014).

Table 3 Risk factors for SIDS (Derived from Poets (2008) with permission)

Maternal factors	Infantile factors
Young age	Male gender
Multiparity	Low birth weight
Smoking during pregnancy	Low birth length
Maternal drug abuse	Premature birth
Previous fetal deaths	Blood type B
Anemia during pregnancy	Low Apgar scores
Placenta praevia	Low hematocrit at 48 h
Premature rupture of membranes	Not using a pacifier
Low social class	Prone or side sleeping position
Low family income	Bed-sharing
Short interpregnancy interval	Overheating
Unmarried mother	Not breastfed
Partner unemployed	Siblings in family
Late attendance of antenatal clinic	Sleeping in own room
Postnatal depression	Previous SIDS in family
Attendance to psychiatrist	Previous cyanotic episode
Urinary tract infection in pregnancy	

66.3.2 Pathology

66.3.2.1 Intrathoracic Petechial Hemorrhages

As implied by its definition, there is no morphological finding in SIDS that sufficiently explains death. There are, however, a number of characteristic findings in these infants, such as serosal petechiae, which are so consistent that they appear to support the concept that SIDS may indeed form a specific disease entity. Other characteristic findings in SIDS include the occurrence of (often bloody) froth around the nose and mouth. Both may result from high transpulmonary pressure swings, such as occurring during breathing against an obstructed upper airway (Poets 2008).

66.3.2.2 Abnormalities in Brainstem Serotonergic System

Serotonin is a neurotransmitter involved in regulating various processes potentially related to SIDS, e.g., sleep and arousal, control of breathing, airway reflexes, and autonomic function (Paterson et al. 2007). Endogenously released serotonin is also required for gasping. Comparative studies on the binding properties of neurotransmitter receptors found multiple brainstem abnormalities in SIDS compared to control infants, suggesting

that such abnormalities may be involved in some SIDS deaths (Paterson et al. 2007).

66.3.3 Genetic Studies in SIDS

Some infants who die suddenly and unexpectedly do so because they have an inherited disease such as the A984G mutation in the medium-chain acyl-CoA dehydrogenase (MCAD) gene or in genes encoding cardiac ion channels resulting in long-QT syndrome. These well-defined diseases, however, contribute only a few percent to all cases of SIDS (and, by definition, prohibit defining SIDS as the cause of death). More relevant to SIDS may be recent data on gene polymorphisms that may predispose infants to SIDS under certain circumstances, such as those found in the serotonin transporter gene, although there are also strong arguments to question this proposed link (Paterson et al. 2007; Weese-Mayer et al. 2007; Paterson 2013).

66.3.4 Pathophysiology

There are now a number of recordings from cardiorespiratory monitors that were obtained during SIDS. Despite some limitations, these recordings have for the first time provided us with objective data on the pathophysiological mechanisms immediately preceding SIDS. In an analysis of nine recordings of chest wall impedance and heart rate from infants who had an autopsy diagnosis of SIDS or mild BPD, gasping was the predominant pattern, being already present at the time of the monitor alarm in three infants and occurring within 3 min after it in a further four (Fig. 2) (Poets et al. 1999b). Primary trigger for the monitor alarm had been bradycardia in all but two infants, but there was no indication of heart block or ventricular tachycardia. These observations, confirmed by a similar, more recent study (Sridhar et al. 2003), suggest that prolonged apnea is unlikely to be a primary mechanism in the sequence of events leading to most cases of SIDS, while the "primary" bradycardia is most likely caused by hypoxemia. In addition, there seems to be a failure or depression of arousal and gasping. The underlying causes of both the hypoxemia and the failure of these infants to resuscitate themselves from this hypoxemia remain to be determined.

66.3.5 Prevention

66.3.5.1 Primary Prevention

Dissemination of advice on safe sleeping has been one of the most effective health interventions ever performed. Recommendations are reviewed in regular intervals to incorporate new data. The current advice given by the American Academy of Pediatrics (AAP) includes the following (abbreviated) (American Academy of Pediatrics 2011):

- Infants should be placed for sleep in a supine position for every sleep.
- Use a firm sleep surface. Pillows or sheepskins should not be placed under a sleeping infant.
- Room-sharing without bed-sharing is recommended.
- Keep soft objects and loose bedding out of the crib.
- Pregnant women should receive regular prenatal care.
- Avoid smoke exposure during pregnancy and after birth.
- Avoid alcohol and illicit drug use during pregnancy and after birth.
- Breastfeeding is recommended.
- Consider offering a pacifier at nap time and bedtime.
- Avoid overheating. Bedroom temperature should be comfortable for a lightly closed adult.
- Do not use home cardiorespiratory monitors as a strategy for reducing the risk of SIDS.
- Infants should be immunized in accordance with recommendations of the AAP and CDC.
- Avoid commercial devices marketed to reduce the risk of SIDS.
- Supervised, awake tummy time is recommended to facilitate development and to minimize development of positional plagiocephaly.

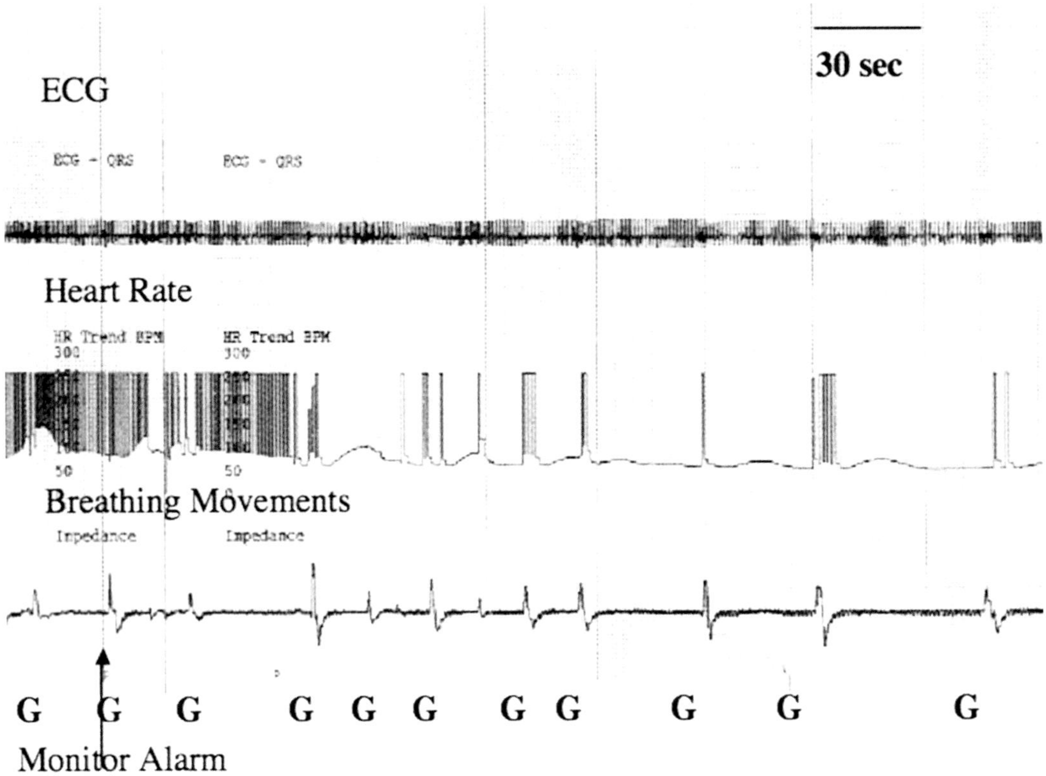

Fig. 2 Section from a memory monitor printout of a 1-month old infant born at 34 weeks gestation and with an autopsy diagnosis of SIDS. There are 11 gasps which progressively decrease in amplitude. There is an increase in heart rate from 72 to 140 bpm during the first 20 s of recording, followed by several smaller increases in heart rate that appear to occur in response to the gasps and are also decreasing in amplitude over time (From Poets et al. (1999b), with permission). G, gasp

66.3.5.2 Secondary Prevention

For many years, the use of home monitors in specific risk groups, i.e., secondary prevention, has been the only method to prevent SIDS, but its effectiveness in reducing its incidence has never been proven, and the AAP now clearly discourages its use to prevent SIDS. Nonetheless, home monitoring may be prescribed as a diagnostic tool or as an early warning of potentially dangerous pathophysiology. The first indication comprises infants after an apparent life-threatening event (ALTE) and infants from families who had two or more sudden unexpected infant deaths. Here, documented monitoring may help to reach a diagnosis. A detailed description of the diagnostic work-up of infants with ALTE would go beyond the scope of this chapter; the reader is referred to a recent Clinical Practice Guideline (Tieder et al. 2016). The second group involves technology-dependent infants (e.g., with a tracheostomy), infants with respiratory control disorders, and preterm infants with persistent AOP. AOP is not associated with an increased risk of SIDS, but monitoring may be indicated to prevent potential sequelae of IH (see above). Whatever the indication, a pulse oximeter with motion-resistant technology to reduce the frequency of false alarms is currently the preferred monitoring device. Although there are no controlled trials on this issue, there is evidence to suggest that apnea and hypoxemia may occur too late during the events leading to death always to allow for successful resuscitation. Monitoring should continue for 4 weeks after the last (true)

monitor alarm except for siblings from families with multiple deaths who should be monitored until the age of the oldest infant who died.

References

Alvaro RE, Khalil M, Qurashi M et al (2012) CO_2 inhalation as a treatment for apnea of prematurity: a randomized double-blind controlled trial. J Pediatr 60:252–257

American Academy of Pediatrics (2011) Policy Statement: SIDS and other sleep-related infant deaths: expansion of recommendations for a safe infant sleeping environment. Pediatrics 128:1030–1039

Blair PS, Mitchell EA, Heckstall-Smith EMA, Fleming PJ (2008) Head covering – a major modifiable risk factor for sudden infant death syndrome: a systematic review. Arch Dis Child 93:778–783

Blair PS, Sidebotham P, Pease A, Fleming PJ (2014). Bed-sharing in the absence of hazardous circumstances: is there a risk of sudden infant death syndrome? An analysis from two case-control studies conducted in the UK. PLoS One 9:e1077999

Bloch-Salisbury E, Indic PP, Bednarek F, Paydarfar D (2009) Stabilizing immature breathing patterns of preterm infants using stochastic mechanosensory stimulation. J Appl Physiol 107:1017–1027

De Paoli AG, Davis PG, Faber B et al (2008) Devices and pressure sources for administration of nasal continuous positive airway pressure (NCPAP) in preterm neonates. Cochrane Database Syst Rev: CD002977

Gizzi C, Montecchia F, Panetta V et al (2014) Is synchronised NIPPV more effective than NIPPV and NCPAP in treating apnoea of prematurity (AOP)? A randomised cross-over trial. Arch Dis Child Fetal Neonatal Ed 100:F17–F23

Krous HF, Beckwith JB, Byard RW et al (2004) Sudden infant death syndrome and unclassified sudden infant deaths: a definitional and diagnostic approach. Pediatrics 114:234–238

Lemyre B, Davis PG, De Paoli A, Kirpalani H (2014) Nasal intermittent positive pressure ventilation (NIPPV) versus nasal continuous pressure (NCPAP) for preterm neonates after extubation. Cochrane Database Syst Rev 9:CD003212

Malloy MH, MacDorman M (2005) Changes in the classification of sudden unexpected infant deaths: United States, 1992–2001. Pediatrics 115:1247–1253

Marcus CL, Meltzer LJ, Roberts RS, Caffeine for Apnea of Prematurity-Trial group et al (2014) Long-term effects of caffeine therapy for apnea of prematurity on sleep at school age. Am J Respir Crit Care Med 190:791–799

McPherson C, Neil JJ, Tjoeng TH, Pineda R, Inder TE (2015) A pilot randomized trial of high-dose caffeine therapy in preterm infant. Pediatr Res 78:198–204

Moll M, Schöning M, Goelz R et al (2011) 2-year follow-up examinations (Bayley II) in infants born at <32 weeks in a German perinatal center. Klin Paediatr 223:251–254

Pantalitschka T, Sievers J, Urschitz MS et al (2009) Randomised crossover trial of four nasal respiratory support systems for apnoea of prematurity in very low birthweight infants. Arch Dis Child Fetal Neonatal Ed 94:F245–F248

Paterson DS (2013) Serotonin gene variants are unlikely to play a significant role in the pathogenesis of the sudden infant death syndrome. Respir Physiol Neurobiol 189:301–314

Paterson DS, Trachgenberg FL, Thompson EG et al (2007) Multiple serotonergic brainstem abnormalities in sudden infant death syndrome. J Am Med Ass 296:2124–2132

Poets CF (2008) Apnea of prematurity, sudden infant death syndrome, and apparent life-threatening events. In: Taussig LM, Landau LI (eds) Pediatric respiratory medicine, 2nd edn. Mosby, Philadelphia, pp 413–434

Poets CF, Darraj S, Bohnhorst B (1999a) Effect of doxapram on episodes of apnoea, bradycardia and hypoxaemia in preterm infants. Biol Neonate 76:207–213

Poets CF, Meny RG, Chobanian MR et al (1999b) Gasping and other cardiorespiratory patterns during sudden infant deaths. Pediatr Res 45:350–354

Poets A, Urschitz MS, Steinfeldt R, Poets CF (2012) Risk factors for early sudden deaths and severe apparent life-threatening events. Arch Dis Child Fetal Neonatal Ed 97:F395–F397

Poets CF, Roberts RS, Schmidt B, Canadian Oxygen Trial Investigators et al (2015) Association between intermittent hypoxemia or bradycardia and late death or disability in extremely preterm infants. JAMA 314:595–603

Reher C, Kuny KD, Pantalitschka T et al (2008) Randomised crossover trial of different postural interventions on bradycardia and intermittent hypoxia in preterm infants. Arch Dis Child Fetal Neonatal Ed 2016;93(4):F289–91

Rhein LM, Dobson NR, Darnall RA, Caffeine Pilot Study Group et al (2014) Effects of caffeine on intermittent hypoxia in infants born prematurely: a randomized clinical trial. JAMA Pediatr 168:250–257

Saugstad OD, Aune D (2014) Optimal oxygenation of extremely low birth weight infants: a meta-analysis and systematic review of the oxygen saturation target studies. Neonatology 105:55–63

Schmidt B, Roberts RS, Davis P, Caffeine for Apnea of Prematurity Trial Group et al (2007) Long-term effects of caffeine therapy for apnea of prematurity. N Engl J Med 357:1893–1902

Schmidt B, Anderson PJ, Doyle LW et al (2012) Survival without disability to age 5 years after neonatal caffeine therapy for apnea of prematurity. JAMA 307:275–282

Schmidt B, Whyte RK, Asztalos EV et al (2013) Effects of targeting higher vs lower arterial oxygen saturations on death or disability in extremely preterm infants: a randomized clinical trial. JAMA 309:2111–2120

Shapiro-Mendoza CK, Camperlengo L, Ludvigsen R (2014) Classification system for the Sudden

Unexpected Infant Death Case Registry and its application. Pediatrics 134:e210–e219

Sreenan CEP, Demianczuk N, Robertson CMT (2001) Isolated mental developmental delay in very low birth weight infants: association with prolonged doxapram therapy for apnea. J Pediatr 139:832–837

Sridhar RTB, Kelly DH, Henslee JA (2003) Characterization of successful and railed autoresuscitation in human infants, including those dying of SIDS. Pediatr Pulmonol 36:113–122

Steer P, Flenady V, Shearman A et al (2004) High dose caffeine citrate for extubation of preterm infants: a randomised controlled trial. Arch Dis Child Fetal Neonatal Ed 89:F499–F503

Tieder JS, Bonkowsky JL, Etzel RA et al (2016) Brief resolved unexplained events (formerly apparent life-threatening events) and evaluation of lower-risk infants. Pediatrics 137:e20160590

Weese-Mayer DE, Ackerman MJ, Marazita ML, Berry-Kravis EM (2007) Sudden infant death syndrome: review of implicated genetic factors. Am J Med Gen 143A:771–788

Whyte R, Kirpalani H (2011) Low versus high haemoglobin concentration threshold for blood transfusion for preventing morbidity and mortality in very low birth weight infants. Cochrane Database Syst Rev: CD000512. https://doi.org/10.1002/14651858.CD000512.pub2

Part VI

Cardiovascular System

Cardiovascular Physiology, Pathology, and Clinical Investigation in Neonatal Medicine

67

Luciane Piazza, Angelo Micheletti, Javier Fernandez Sarabia, Diana Negura, Carmelo Arcidiacono, Antonio Saracino, Mario Carminati, and Francesca R. Pluchinotta

Contents

Abstract

A thorough understanding of cardiovascular physiology is essential for proper management of congenital heart disease. The clinical evaluation and treatment of neonates with a suspected congenital heart disease is challenging given the unique nature and complexity of neonatal cardiac physiology. The transition from fetal to neonatal circulation is

L. Piazza (✉) · A. Micheletti · J. F. Sarabia · D. Negura · C. Arcidiacono · A. Saracino · M. Carminati · F. R. Pluchinotta
Department of Pediatric Cardiology, IRCCS Policlinico San Donato, San Siro, Milan, Italy
e-mail: Luciane.Piazza@grupposandonato.it; mario.carminati@grupposandonato.it; mario.carminati@grupposandonato.it

G. Buonocore et al. (eds.), *Neonatology*,
https://doi.org/10.1007/978-3-319-29489-6_214

characterized by physiologic changes that start when the newborn takes its first breaths. After birth a careful clinical examination may seem normal, and the affected neonate may be discharged home undiagnosed. Signs and symptoms of severe heart disease in the newborn period include cyanosis, irritability, sweating, crying with feeding, and respiratory difficulties; these symptoms may be also present in metabolic disease and sepsis. To confirm the diagnosis, two-dimensional and color Doppler echocardiography should be used to define the anatomy, physiology, and myocardial function. Cardiac catheterization is reserved for special cases where echocardiography is not diagnostic.

67.1 Salient Points

- The transition from fetal to neonatal circulation is characterized by physiologic changes that start when the newborn takes its first breaths.
- In the fetal circulation, the right and left ventricles work in a parallel circuit.
- At birth the pulmonary circulation is established due to a rapid increase in systemic vascular resistance, removal of the very-low-resistance placenta circulation, and closure of the ductus venosus.
- Physical aeration of the lungs results in decreased pulmonary vascular resistance, fall in pulmonary pressure, and increased pulmonary blood flow.
- The most common presentation of critical CHD is the presence of a murmur, cyanosis, respiratory distress, heart failure, and shock.
- A hyperoxia test should be considered to make the differential diagnosis between oxygen desaturation due to heart disease and that due to pulmonary disease.
- Diagnosis relays on two-dimensional and color Doppler echocardiography.
- Cardiac catheterization is reserved for special cases where echocardiography is not diagnostic.

67.2 Introduction

Congenital heart defects (CHD) are a heterogeneous entity, representing the most common malformations in the fetal and neonatal period. The incidence of moderate to critical structural CHD that will require expert cardiologic care is 2.5–3 per 1,000 live births. It is the most common form of the birth defect. Specialized cardiologic care is not needed for most minor forms of CHD, such as tiny ventricular septal defect (VSD) or atrial septal defect (ASD) (Hoffman and Kaplan 2002). Most infants with congenital heart disease are identified by the end of neonatal period. Critical congenital heart disease (CCHD) has been defined as a structural malformation of the heart that is present at birth and requires intervention in the first year of life (Olney Richard et al. 2015). CCHD is responsible for 20% of deaths in the neonatal period (Lee et al. 2001). Congenital heart disease has a public health importance because the early diagnosis can help to prevent complications and decrease the mortality. For this reason, all over the world, the screening on the newborn is implemented. The pulse oximetry screening and a prenatal ultrasound detection have become a significant contributor to early identification CHD.

67.3 The Fetal and Neonatal Circulation

Fetal circulation is shown in Fig. 1.

In the fetal circulation, the right and left ventricles work in a parallel circuit. Three cardiovascular structures, unique to the fetus, are important for maintaining this circulation: ductus venosus, foramen ovale, and ductus arteriosus. The umbilical vein carries oxygenated blood (PO_2 about 30–35 mmHg) from the placenta to the inferior vena cava (IVC) through the ductus venosus, where it partially mixes with poorly oxygenated IVC blood derived from the lower part of the fetal body. When it reaches the right atrium (RA), oxygenated blood preferentially

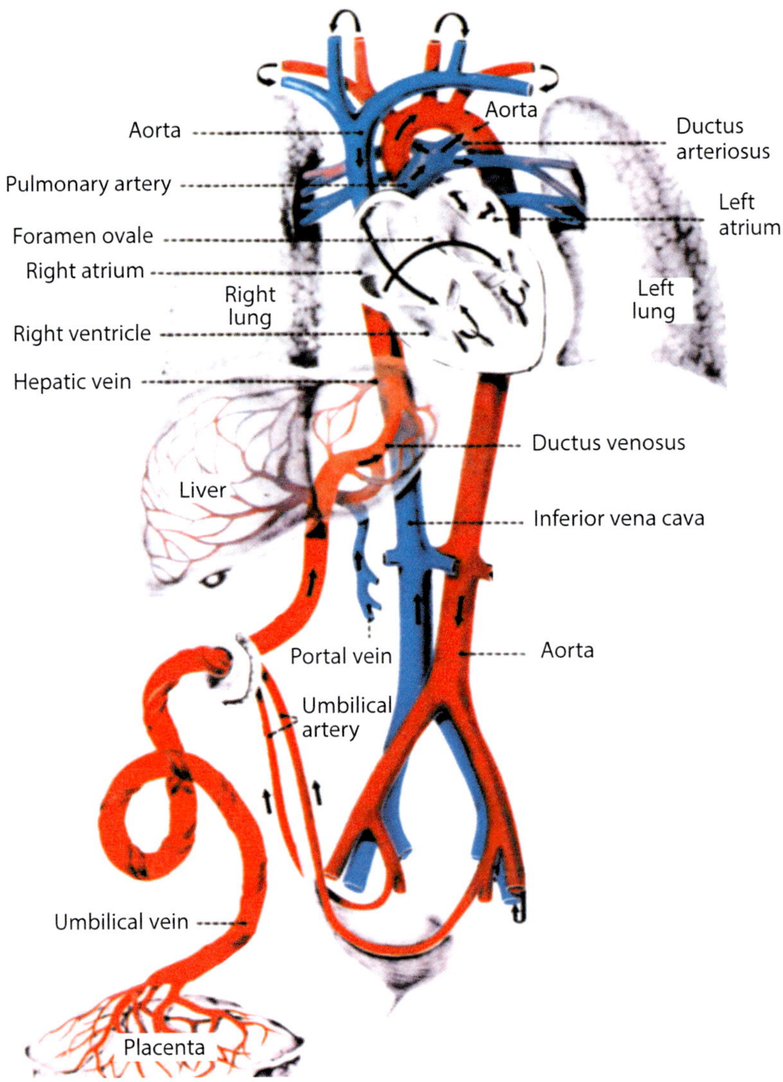

Fig. 1 Diagram of fetal circulation showing the four sites of shunt: placenta, ductus venosus, foramen ovale, and ductus arteriosus (Modified with permission from Fesslova V. Ecocardiografia fetale. Raffaello Cortina Editore, Milano 2008, p. 39)

streams across the foramen ovale (FO) and enters the left atrium (LA), where it mixes with the pulmonary venous return before entering the left ventricle (LV). From the LV, the ascending aorta supplies fully oxygenated blood (PO_2 about 28 mmHg) flows to the coronary arteries, the head, and the upper extremities. Only a small portion of the LV output flows through the aortic arch and supplies the thoracic aorta. Superior caval vein blood, which is considerably less oxygenated (PO_2 12–14 mmHg), enters the RA where it is directed to the RV. Just about 10% of RV output is ejected into the pulmonary arteries (PA) because the fetal lungs are still not expanded and ventilated, and pulmonary vascular resistances is therefore very high. Most RV output bypasses the lungs and flows through the ductus arteriosus into the descending aorta and the inferior part of the fetal body, after which it returns to the placenta via the two umbilical arteries.

A distinctive feature of fetal circulation is the role of the placenta, low-resistance vascular bed, where oxygenation and metabolite exchange occur. The placenta is not only an organ for a

gas exchange, and the fetus adapts itself producing fetal hemoglobin which has a higher affinity for oxygen, at about 70–80% of fetal hemoglobin compared to adult hemoglobin.

The dimensions of fetal cardiac chambers reflect the differences between right- and left-sided blood volume, with the RV and pulmonary artery being larger than the LV and ascending aorta, although the pressure in both circuits is equal due to the patency of the ductus arteriosus.

67.4 Pulmonary and Hemodynamic Transition

The transition from fetal to neonatal circulation is characterized by physiologic changes that start when the newborn takes the first breaths. The main circulatory and respiratory changes are as follows: first, the placental circulation disappears (clamping the umbilical cord), and the pulmonary circulation is established due to (i) a rapid increase in systemic vascular resistance (SVR) as a result of very-low-resistance placenta circulation removal and (ii) closure of the ductus venosus. Second, physical aeration of the lungs results in: (i) decreases of the pulmonary vascular resistance (PVR), fall in PA pressure, and increment of pulmonary blood flow; (ii) mechanical and passive closure of the FO due to a difference between left and right atrial pressure; pressure in the left exceeds that in the right because of increased pulmonary venous return to the LA and decreased venous return to the RA after ductus venosus closure; and (iii) closure of patent ductus arteriosus (PDA) secondary to increased arterial oxygen saturation. The ductus venosus will remain patent days after birth and mostly does not influence the cardiovascular system.

67.5 Regulation of Pulmonary Vascular Resistance and Pulmonary Blood Flow

In fetal life, the PVR is high and the oxygen concentration, at the level of smooth muscle cells in the pulmonary arteriolar walls, is low. Fetal respiratory movements are controlled by hypoxia and hypercapnia, and they are discontinuous, occurring <50% of the time. The mechanisms controlling the switch to continuous breathing after birth are currently unknown (van Vonderen et al. 2014), although the activation of chemoreceptors such as an increase in arterial, PCo2, and physical stimulants such as light, temperature, and handling are considered stimuli for large inspiratory movements.

At birth, as gas exchange occurs in the lungs, PVR promptly decreases and simultaneously pulmonary blood flow increases. Those events are associated with thinning of the medial layer of the pulmonary arterioles as well as hyperplasia of alveolar units and their own circulatory vessels. After the initial sudden decrease in PVR and pressure, there is a slow progressive decrease within 2–6 weeks. Several factors may interfere with the pulmonary flow or pulmonary vascular resistance, causing conditions such as persistent pulmonary hypertension or delay in PVR normalization process:

- Hypoxia and/or altitude
- Acidosis
- Severe hyaline membrane disease or other pulmonary diseases
- Congenital heart defects such as large VSD or PDA, which are characterized by high PA pressure, secondary to direct transmission of the systemic pressure to the PA through the large defect
- Increased pressure in the LA or pulmonary veins

67.6 Closure of the Ductus Arteriosus

During fetal life, the ductus arteriosus is fully patent and pulmonary and aortic pressures are therefore equal. The immediate consequence of the neonatal transition is the reversal of vascular shunts through the foramen ovale and ductus arteriosus. Once the ductus arteriosus closes, pulmonary artery pressure decreases as the resistance in the pulmonary vascular bed falls. The functional closure of the PDA

occurs because of constriction of medial, smooth muscle cells within 10–15 h after birth. The following factors are relevant to ductal closure:

- *Oxygen*. A postnatal increase in systemic circulatory oxygen saturation is the strongest stimulus for smooth muscle cell constriction.
- *Gestational age of the newborn*. The ductus arteriosus is more likely to remain open in preterm infants because of immaturity of the constrictor response to oxygen by ductal smooth muscle cells.
- *Prostaglandin E (PGE)*. An acute decrease in PGE levels results in constriction of the ductus arteriosus. This event is determined by placenta removal, since the placenta is a significant source of PGE. Drugs like indomethacin, a prostaglandin synthetase inhibitor, can be used to effect closure of PDA.
- *Hypoxia and acidosis* relax the ductus arteriosus but constrict pulmonary arterioles which are also constricted by sympathetic stimulation and α-adrenergic stimulation.
- *Oxygen* constricts the ductus arteriosus but relaxes pulmonary arterioles.

67.7 Measurements for Evaluating Transition

The hemodynamic and general status of the patient is determined by the interpretation of the data obtained through the monitoring of the patient and with an understanding of the fetal circulation and mechanisms of transition. Nowadays, noninvasive physiological measurements are made during extrauterine life:

- Heart rate (HR) – A cutoff value of HR of 100 beats per minute by Virginia Apgar is characterized as adequate transition. At the same time in some newborns, we can observe short moments of bradycardia followed by a rapid increase of the HR.
- Oxygen saturation (SO_2) is measured peripherally. The pink color described by the clinicians is very subjective and variable compared to the objective measurement of saturation. SO_2 should preferably be measured preductally using pulse oximetry.
- Cardiac output (CO) and stroke volume (SV) (CO = HR.SV). Echocardiography has been used to monitor CO during the neonatal transition.
- Blood pressure (BP) is considered an important value for hemodynamic monitoring of critically ill infants. It is useful to measure BP preductally (right arm) to evaluate the hemodynamic transition and assess the cardiac output. The BP is influenced by crying, gestational age, and administration of fluids.
- Gas exchange measurements, i.e., parameters such as tidal volume, respiratory rate, inspiratory time, and expiratory time.
- Tissue Perfusion:

  Two methods can be used: perfusion index and infrared spectroscopy (NIRS), which may be used to monitor the perfusion of the brain tissue

  The accurate recognition of cardiovascular instability and the perinatal complications can prevent the failure of compensatory mechanism and may potentially improve both short- and long-term outcomes.

67.8 Clinical Presentation of the Congenital Heart Disease

In spite of a wide spectrum of CHD, clinical presentation does not vary much. The first approach to the newborn with suspected CHD is crucial in improving the mortality and morbidity associated with these malformations. Prenatal diagnosis by echocardiography has also been associated with improved morbidity and mortality. However, a large number of cases are not identified in utero, and some defects can be challenging to identify using the fetal cardiac ultrasonography. After birth, a careful clinical examination may seem normal, and the affected neonate is discharged home undiagnosed. Table 7 summarizes the most common presenting CHD after discharge.

- Coarctation of the aorta
- Interruption of the aortic arch

- Aortic valve stenosis
- Total anomalous pulmonary return
- Hypoplastic left heart syndrome

Signs and symptoms of severe heart disease in the newborn period include cyanosis, irritability, sweating, crying with feeding, and respiratory difficulties. For this reason, it is very difficult to differentiate in the newborn between an error of metabolism, sepsis, and congenital heart disease. The most common presentation of critical CHD is the presence of a murmur, cyanosis, respiratory distress, heart failure, and shock. In this last scenario, the treatment of shock and clinical stabilization should precede definitive anatomic diagnosis.

67.8.1 Cyanosis

Cyanosis is a blue discoloration of the skin caused by deoxygenated blood within the capillary network. Detection of cyanosis depends on the skill and experience of the physician and environmental light (it is more evident in natural than in artificial light). Cyanosis does not always indicate hypoxemia: a neonate may be severely hypoxemic but not clinically cyanosed. Cyanosis can be detected on many parts of the body: lips, fingernails, toenails, tip of the nose, oral mucous membranes, conjunctivae, and tip of the tongue.

By definition cyanosis is determined by a deoxygenated hemoglobin (Hb) concentration exceeding 3 g/dL in arterial blood or 5 g/dL in a capillary bed.

Fetal and adult hemoglobin are different in terms of oxygen affinity, which is indicated by the P50 value. P50 is the level of partial pressure of oxygen (PaO_2) at which 50% of hemoglobin is bound to O_2. It is about 27 mmHg in adults.

The P50 of fetal hemoglobin is about 20 mmHg; the venous oxygen saturation (O_2 sat) is therefore higher in the neonate (about 80%) than in the adult (about 70% or less). As a consequence, cyanosis in neonates becomes clinically evident at a lower level of PaO_2 than in adults or children, about 38–39 mmHg and 52–54 mmHg, respectively.

The level of hemoglobin influences the appearance of cyanosis. In patients with polycythemia, cyanosis is detectable at a higher level of oxygen saturation; conversely in patients with anemia, cyanosis appears at a lower level of oxygen saturation. In the polycythemic neonate (Hb 22 g/dL), cyanosis becomes evident when O_2 saturation approaches 85–92%. In a normal neonate, the usual level of Hb is about 17 g/dL, and cyanosis becomes evident when O_2 saturation approaches 82% and PaO_2 38–39 mmHg. Often preterm babies have a reduced Hb concentration, about 12 g/dL or less, in which case cyanosis appears at an O_2 saturation level of about 75%.

Cyanosis may be either peripheral or central. Peripheral cyanosis is a bluish discoloration limited to the extremities, associated with normal arterial O_2 saturation and pink color of mucous membranes; it can be seen with acrocyanosis or exposure to cold. The blue color may reflect intermittent vasomotor changes in the skin. A pathological cause of acrocyanosis is cutaneous arterial constriction resulting from low cardiac output state with sluggish peripheral blood flow. Central cyanosis is cyanosis associated with arterial oxygen desaturation.

Unlike cyanosis secondary to lung disease, cyanosis related to CHD is generally not associated with respiratory distress. Exceptions to this rule are:

- Central cyanosis with low PaO_2 in the 20s or less associated with tachypnea.
- Cyanosis associated with low cardiac output. This is commonly seen with left heart obstructive lesions if the ductus arteriosus becomes restrictive. The pulse volume will be poor and the extremities cool.
- Cyanosis associated with obstruction of pulmonary venous drainage resulting in pulmonary edema, such as what is seen in obstructed total anomalous pulmonary venous return:
  - Differential cyanosis. This occurs when cyanosis is more evident in the lower extremities than the upper or vice versa.
- Upper limb saturation higher than the lower limb: deoxygenated blood coming from RV

shunts from pulmonary artery to distal aorta through the ductus arteriosus because of either elevated PVR or aortic obstruction proximal to the ductus, such as in critical aortic coarctation or interrupted aortic arch.

- Lower limb saturation higher than upper limb: typical of this condition is a reversed flow into the ascending aorta and the aortic arch from the pulmonary artery through a large ductus arteriosus, such as in transposition of great arteries, large PDA, and pulmonary hypertension.

Differential cyanosis is fairly uncommon and is of little practical diagnostic use.

67.8.1.1 Differential Diagnosis

Cyanosis is one of the most common clinical presentations of diverse disease processes, including cardiac, lung, and central nervous system abnormalities. Table 1 summarizes the differential diagnosis of cyanosis.

A suggested plan for investigation of the cyanotic newborn baby includes:

Table 1 Differential diagnosis of cyanosis

Newborns with CHD	
CHD with increased pulmonary vascularity	**CHD with decreased pulmonary vascularity**
D-Transposition of great arteries	Tetralogy of Fallot
Total anomalous pulmonary venous return	Double outlet right ventricle with PS
Taussig-Bing anomaly	Ebstein's anomaly
PPHN	Pulmonary atresia
Truncus arteriosus	Tricuspid atresia
Single ventricle without PS	Single ventricle with PS
TGA and VSD	TGA and PS
Pulmonary disease	
Pneumothorax or pleural effusion	
Diaphragmatic hernia	
Persistent fetal circulation syndrome	
Perinatal asphyxia	
Central nervous system	
Cyanosis with normal PaO_2	

PS pulmonary stenosis, *PPHN* persistent pulmonary hypertension of the newborn, *TGA* transposition of the great arteries, *VSD* ventricular septal defect

1. Clinical evaluation of cyanosis: central or peripheral, extension, and localization. The heart rate, arterial pulses, blood pressure, respiratory rate, and presence of respiratory distress.
2. Chest X-ray: may reveal a pulmonary or cardiac cause and the severity of the problem.
3. Arterial blood gas analysis in room air: confirms or excludes central cyanosis.
4. Hyperoxia test: helps in differentiating pulmonary or central nervous system causes from cardiac causes.
5. Umbilical arterial line: PaO_2 in a preductal artery (e.g., a radial artery) 10–15 mmHg higher than the PaO_2 in a postductal artery (e.g., from an umbilical arterial line) suggests a right-to-left ductal shunt.
6. Prostaglandin E1: to be commenced if a cyanotic defect is suspected as a result of investigations.

Table 2 summarize the differential diagnoses of CHF in the neonate.

67.8.2 Heart Failure in the Newborn

Congestive heart failure (CHF) as clinical presentation accounts for about 30% of infants and children with CHD (Olney Richard et al. 2015). CHF is a clinical syndrome in which cardiac output is insufficient to meet the metabolic demands of the tissues, including oxygen and nutrient delivery and waste removal. In the early stages, infants may be tachypneic and tachycardic with increased respiratory effort, and there may be hepatomegaly and delayed capillary refill. In worsening CHF, dyspnea with grunting and intercostal and subcostal recession may appear. Feeding difficulties, failure to thrive, and sweating may occur later. The challenge for the clinicians is an early identification of the patients with the potential rapid decompensation. An acute form with pulmonary edema and circulatory collapse may occur with "left-sided" lesions. Left obstructive lesions have the highest postdischarge mortality rate. Almost all infants (68%) with this form of CHD discovered within 3 weeks of age present in heart failure (Ashley and Lu Le 2015) .

Table 2 Causes of heart failure in newborns

1. Structural heart disease	
Anomalies of coronary circulation	At birth
Ebstein's anomaly of tricuspid valve	
Hypoplastic left heart syndrome	
Transposition of the great arteries	First week
Premature infants with large patent ductus arteriosus	
Total anomalous pulmonary venous return	
Critical aortic or pulmonary stenosis	1–4 weeks
Coarctation of the aorta	
Structural cardiac disease with left-to-right shunt at level of ventricles	
Tetralogy of Fallot or pulmonary atresia with aortopulmonary collaterals	
2. Myocardial disease	
A) Primary	
Myocarditis	
Transient myocardial ischemia (with or without birth asphyxia)	
Cardiomyopathy (as seen in infants of diabetic mothers)	
B) Secondary	
Sustained tachyarrhythmias (atrial flutter or fibrillation)	
Congenital heart block	
Birth asphyxia resulting in transient myocardial ischemia	
Severe anemia (as seen in hydrops fetalis)	
Overtransfusion or fluid overload	
Metabolic causes: hypoglycemia, hypocalcemia	
Neonatal sepsis	

67.8.3 Initial Evaluation

67.8.3.1 History

The history can provide useful information leading to the suspicion of CHD: (1) maternal disease during first trimester of gestation due to viral infections, X-ray exposure, drug intake, alcohol abuse, and diabetes and (2) problems in the perinatal period (low Apgar score and/or the need of cardiopulmonary resuscitation).

67.8.3.2 Physical Examination

Physical examination of the neonate can provide important clues to the anatomic diagnosis.

Inspection: Look for the presence of cyanosis with or without respiratory distress and respiratory pattern including the effort of breathing and use of accessory muscles, a general appearance typical of a syndrome, chromosomal abnormalities, or malformations that may be associated with CHD.

Palpation: Reduced or absent distal pulses are highly suggestive of obstruction of the aortic arch. Weak arterial pulses are characteristic of critical aortic valve stenosis, hypoplastic left heart syndrome, or cardiogenic shock. Palpation of the precordium may detect the presence of a thrill that usually indicates at least moderate outflow tract obstruction or a restrictive VSD with low right ventricular pressure. A hyperdynamic precordium suggests heart disease with high volume overload such as left-to-right shunt lesions and/or severe valvular regurgitation. A cool neonate with prolonged capillary refill time should always raise the possibility of severe CHD.

Auscultation: Rarely conclusive for CHD diagnosis. More than 50% of full-term newborn infants have an innocent murmur at some time during the first week of life. Most pathological murmurs should be audible during the first month of life. Heart murmurs audible immediately after birth are due to stenotic lesions (e.g., aortic stenosis, pulmonary stenosis, and coarctation of aorta) or left-to-right shunt lesions (e.g., a small VSD). The onset of a murmur due to a large VSD may be delayed until the first or second week of life. The continuous murmur of a PDA may not appear for 2–3 weeks. Diastolic murmurs are always indicative of cardiovascular disease. During auscultation, the physician must pay attention to the heart rate, noting its regularity and/or variability.

67.8.3.3 Four-Limb Blood Pressure

Blood pressure should be measured in the upper and lower limbs. A difference between arms and legs of more than 10 mmHg is suggestive of coarctation of the aorta, aortic arch hypoplasia, or interrupted aortic arch. Blood pressure measurements are highly specific but not sensitive

for the diagnosis. Moreover, coarctation cannot be ruled out even in the absence of significant blood pressure gradient as it may occur when a large ductus arteriosus is still patent.

67.8.3.4 Chest X-Ray

Chest X-ray can give important clues leading to the diagnosis of CHD and/or associated lung disease. The cardiothoracic ratio of normal newborn infants is > 0.5; the normal value in older children and adults is < 0.5. Therefore, the evaluation of heart size should take into consideration the degree of inspiration, judged by the level of the diaphragm. Particularly in newborns, the heart size may be difficult to determine due to an overlying thymus. In addition to the size of the heart, its position within the chest should be considered to assess visceral and cardiac situs (e.g., dextrocardia, right or left isomerism, is frequently associated with CHD).

Cardiac silhouette may be typical in some CHD as the "egg shape" in transposition of the great arteries (Fig. 2). Evaluation of pulmonary vascular markings in neonates can be difficult. It is often hard to distinguish between increased pulmonary blood flow and pulmonary venous congestion. A poorly perfused lung field suggests decreased pulmonary blood flow and indicates serious cyanotic congenital heart defects or significant left atrial hypertension.

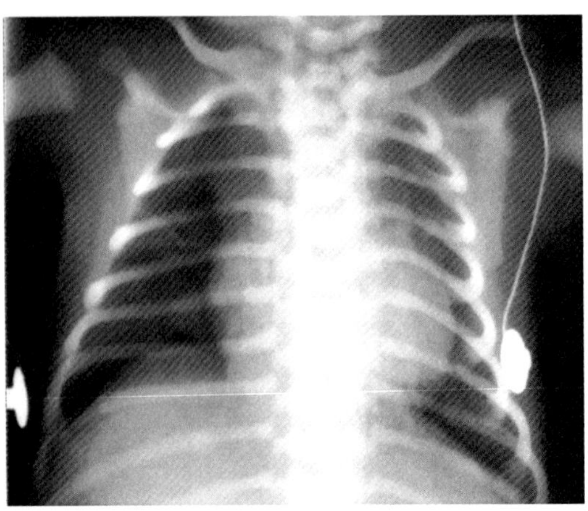

Fig. 2 Transposition of the great vessels. The heart is enlarged and has an egg-shaped configuration

In neonates with infracardiac total anomalous pulmonary venous drainage (which is almost always "obstructed"), the chest X-ray shows a small heart, upper lobe blood diversion, and fluid in the fissures (signs of pulmonary edema). Differentiating between primary pulmonary disease and respiratory distress syndrome is sometimes difficult.

67.8.3.5 Electrocardiogram (ECG)

The normal ECG of a newborn is different from that of an older child because it reflects the hemodynamic relations existing in utero. Usually it shows: (1) tachycardia with a rate as high as 160 beats/min; (2) right-sided deviation of the QRS axis with a mean of +125° and a maximum of +180°; (3) relatively small QRS complex voltages and T wave; (4) right ventricular dominance with tall R waves in V4R, V1, and V2; and (5) occasional Q waves in V1. The diagnostic value of an ECG during the newborn period is highly nonspecific and the precise diagnosis of CHD is generally obtained by other diagnostic tools, in particular echocardiography.

67.8.3.6 Hyperoxia Test

In newborns with suspected CHD, a hyperoxia test should be considered to make the differential diagnosis between oxygen desaturation due to heart disease and that due to pulmonary disease. Although this test does not give a complete diagnosis, it remains useful, especially when an echocardiogram is not easily or quickly available. The hyperoxia test is obtained by measuring the oxygen tension in room air (if tolerated), followed by repeated measurements with the patients receiving 100% inspired oxygen for 5 min. If possible, the arterial partial pressure of oxygen (PO2) should be measured directly by arterial puncture, although PO2 values obtained from a properly applied transcutaneous oxygen monitor are also acceptable. The measurements should be taken at both "preductal" and "postductal" sites.

- When a baby breathes 100% oxygen, an arterial PO2 of 250 mmHg in both upper and lower limbs virtually eliminates critical structural cyanotic heart disease (positive test).

- Patients with pulmonary disease only will show a significant increase in PO2.
- Stable intracardiac right-to-left shunting (failed or negative test). An arterial PO2 of <100 mmHg in the absence of lung disease is most likely due to intracardiac right-to-left shunting. There is only a mild increase of oxygen saturation, but it is usually below basal levels.
- Patients with large left-to-right shunting and systemic hypoxemia. In this situation, there is a high level of oxygenation, because the inspired oxygen normalizes the saturation of pulmonary venous blood, which can be low due to pulmonary edema and oxygen diffusion gradient (an example of this situation is represented by obstructed total anomalous pulmonary venous return).
- Patients with PO_2 between 100 and 250 mmHg may be affected by a structural cardiac lesion with intracardiac mixing and greatly increased pulmonary blood flow as seen when there is a single ventricle.
- Markedly higher oxygen content in the upper versus the lower part of the body. This is an important diagnostic clue to lesions that include all forms of critical aortic arch obstruction or left ventricular outflow tract obstruction.
- Reverse differential cyanosis. This occurs in neonates with transposition of the great arteries and those with abnormal pulmonary to aortic shunting due to coarctation, interruption of the aortic arch, or suprasystemic pulmonary vascular resistance (persistent fetal circulation).

Patients with a positive hyperoxia test are likely to have a duct-dependent CHD, and prostaglandin E_1 should be given, until the anatomic abnormality can be defined.

67.8.3.7 Laboratory Analysis

Initial investigations should include: complete blood count for anemia, electrolyte, methemoglobin level, lactic acid, pH, ammonia, blood culture, urine culture, uric organic acids, thyroid-stimulating hormone, and free thyroxine. Brain natriuretic peptide (BNP)/N-terminal pro-BNP (NT-pro-BNP) can be used.

67.8.3.8 Stabilization and Transport

After the initial evaluation, attention should continue to be focused on the basic neonatal life support. Airways should be stabilized, vascular access secured, volume status and inotropic support maintained, and systemic and pulmonary circulation kept in balance. The neonate may need to be transferred to a medical center with full pediatric cardiological facilities.

Each CHD has multiple anatomic variations and these anatomical details may change the physiology. On the basis of this assumption, it might be easier to consider the physiology and analyze an assessment between the systemic vascular resistance (SVR) and pulmonary vascular resistance.

For example, (i) if PVR is decreased or SRV is increased, blood will flow to the lungs and become oxygenated. (ii) If SVR is decreased or PVR in increased, blood flows to the systemic vasculature but receives inadequate oxygenation in the lungs.

The equation to guide this balance is based on Fick's principle:

$$Qp : Qs = (SaO_2 - SvO_2) : (Spvo_2 - SpaO_2)$$

- SaO_2 is the oxygen saturation.
- SvO_2 is the mixed venous oxygen saturation.
- $SpvO_2$ is the pulmonary venous desaturation.
- $SpaO_2$ is the pulmonary arterial oxygen saturation.

The PVR and SRV may be manipulated to obtain the Qp:Qs ratio 1:1.

It is crucial to define or identify those who can take advantage from prostaglandin E1 administration.

67.8.3.9 Prostaglandin E1

When systemic perfusion depends on patency of the ductus arteriosus, a continuous infusion of PGE_1 may be lifesaving. PGE is indicated for the treatment of duct-dependent lesions. Indications and treatment recommendations are shown in Tables 3 and 4.

The mechanism of action of PGE_1 action consists of the relaxation of the smooth muscle

Table 3 Indications for prostaglandin E_1

Cyanotic heart disease with severely limited or no pulmonary blood flow
Tricuspid atresia
Pulmonary atresia and critical pulmonary stenosis
Children with obstructed systemic blood flow may depend on ductal patency, e.g., in the following conditions
Aortic atresia
Critical aortic stenosis
Critical coarctation of the aorta
Interrupted aortic arch
Hypoplastic left heart syndrome

Patients with transposition of great arteries benefit from patency of the ductus arteriosus because the pulmonary and systemic circulation is in parallel

Table 4 Recommendations for treatment with prostaglandin E_1

The usual starting dose is 0,05 mcg/kg/min
When the desired effect is achieved, reduce to 0.025 mcg/kg/min
Secure vascular access

fibers forming the ductal tissue. In other tissues, PGE_1 has been shown to result in increased levels of nitric oxide and nitric oxide synthetase (Bichell et al. 2006). When ductal dilatation occurs, systemic perfusion increases (peripheral vasodilatation) and pulmonary congestion may decrease. This change is accompanied by a rise in PH and a decrease in lactate accumulation because of improved tissue perfusion.

Adverse effects include respiratory depression; PGE can cause apnea in 10–12% of the neonates and a stable airway must be maintained. Generally all neonates receiving PGE_1 infusion should be intubated for transport. Systemic hypotension and bradycardia have also been seen. Sometimes additional side effects are observed, e.g., bradycardia (7%), tachycardia (3%), and edema and cardiac arrest (1%) (Mitchell et al. 1971). PGE_1 inhibits platelet aggregation and may impair clotting. Prolonged use of PGE_1 has been associated with gastric obstruction and cortical hyperostosis of the long bones. Patients receiving PGE_1 need to be monitored for vital signs, including pulse oximetry, and arterial blood gas analysis.

Following the initial diagnosis and medical stabilization, the neonate should be transferred to a tertiary pediatric cardiac center that is fully equipped for any required additional treatment.

67.8.4 Confirming the Diagnosis

To confirm the diagnosis, two-dimensional and color Doppler echocardiography is used to define the anatomy, physiology, and myocardial function.

Echocardiography is the most commonly used noninvasive diagnostic tool. It is harmless, but some precautions have to be taken if the patient is very sick: for example, temperature stability should be maintained, and extension of the neck for suprasternal views of the arch may be problematic, particularly in a neonate with respiratory distress. Careful specialized nursing assistance is recommended.

67.8.4.1 Cardiac Catheterization

Cardiac catheterization is reserved for special cases where echocardiography is not diagnostic, as in the definition of the anatomy of peripheral pulmonary branches, aortopulmonary collaterals, some complex pulmonary venous anomalies, or in other situations where the decision making process can be hampered by an incomplete or incorrect diagnosis. Echocardiography is fully diagnostic for intracardiac anatomy, in virtually all the cases.

Interventional catheterization: nowadays, a wide range of interventional procedures can be carried out in very small babies (Table 5). These procedures include a preoperative palliation, for instance, by balloon atrial septostomy, or as an alternative to surgery, e.g., by balloon dilatation of a pulmonary or aortic stenosis. PDA stent implantation in newborn with hypoplastic left heart syndrome. Interventional catheterization can also play a role in a wide spectrum of postoperative sequelae, such as residual pulmonary branch stenosis. See the following text for further details on catheter interventional procedures.

Table 5 Indications for neonatal interventional catheterization

Atrial septostomy (Rashkind)	
Balloon valvuloplasty	Pulmonary valvular stenosis
	Aortic valvular stenosis
Balloon angioplasty of native coarctation of the aorta	
Transcatheter radiofrequency perforation and valvuloplasty → atretic pulmonary valve	
Miscellaneous	Coil embolization of abnormal vascular communications
	Stenting of a PDA
	Stenting of the right ventricle outflow

Table 6 Duct-dependent pulmonary blood flow

Critical pulmonary valve stenosis
Pulmonary atresia with intact ventricular septum
Severe tetralogy of Fallot
Complex congenital heart disease with severe pulmonary stenosis or pulmonary atresia

Table 7 Lesion specific: ductus arteriosus dependent systemic blood flow

Aortic stenosis
Coarctation of the aorta
Interrupted aortic arch
Hypoplastic left heart syndrome

Cardiac catheterization of newborns, either interventional or diagnostic, carries more risks than when performed on older patients. Basic medical stabilization, airway management, sedation and body temperature control are crucial. The baby's hemodynamic condition should be as stable as possible. Intravenous lines should be secured and intravenous infusion pumps adequately prepared. For example, a prostaglandin infusion should be given by a dedicated intravenous line.

67.8.4.2 Computed Tomography and Magnetic Resonance

Neonatal cardiovascular tomographic angiography (CTA) and magnetic resonance imaging (MRI) require the immobilization of the neonate and breath holding and contrast injection may be necessary. Neonatal MRI is technically difficult at this age because the required imaging time to complete a study is longer and the patients is less accessible for monitoring and (or) intervention than CTA. The choice of modality should be based on evaluation of the risks and benefits: radiation dose, efficacy, and image quality. During the neonatal period, echocardiography is the better imaging tool for the evaluation congenital heart disease. CTA and MRI can be used to offer additional anatomical information that could not be obtained through echocardiography, e.g., anomalous coronary arteries and anomalous pulmonary venous connection.

67.9 CHD in the Newborn

The types of CHD that may present during the newborn period differ from those recognized later in infancy. During the neonatal period, CHD can be classified according to anatomy, physiopathology, or timing of presentation. In each of the following sections, specific lesions will be discussed focusing on pathophysiology and clinical presentation.

67.9.1 Duct-Dependent Pulmonary Blood Flow

This group of CHD is characterized by obstruction of pulmonary blood flow due to severe pulmonary stenosis or pulmonary atresia. In this situation, pulmonary blood flow depends mainly on the patency of the duct (Tables 6 and 7).

67.9.1.1 Critical Pulmonary Valve Stenosis

Congenital obstruction to RV outflow can be classified as valvar, subvalvar, or involving pulmonary trunk and peripheral pulmonary artery branches. This pathology (pulmonary stenosis, PS) is relatively common; the frequency approaches 8–10% of all cardiac defects. There are many anatomical descriptions of the pulmonary valve: dome-shaped valve; dysplastic hypertrophy of the pulmonary valve leaflets; uni-commissural, bicuspid, and tricuspid valve; and hypoplastic annulus with

dysplastic valve (Gikonyo et al. 1987; Bichell et al. 2006). The main cardiac consequence of PS is an elevated RV pressure because of obstruction to right ventricular cardiac output. The rise in pressure causes RV hypertrophy that is proportional to the degree of obstruction. This hypertrophy is particularly evident in the infundibular region, producing dynamic narrowing of the outflow tract. Because the ventricular septum is intact, the systolic pressure generated in the RV may exceed the LV systolic pressure. Moreover, the higher diastolic pressure in the RV caused by muscular hypertrophy results in a noncompliant RV and increased right atrial filling pressure. When the right atrial pressure exceeds the left atrial pressure, a right-to-left shunt at the foramen ovale appears, resulting in central cyanosis or hypoxemia. There may be associated RV dysfunction and/or tricuspid regurgitation.

In critical pulmonary stenosis or pulmonary atresia, the pulmonary flow is duct dependent, as previously explained.

Newborns with critical PS present within the first week of life with cyanosis and hypoxemia and signs of CHF with peripheral vasoconstriction. Cardiac auscultation reveals a single second heart sound. The systolic murmur of PS may be soft or even absent, reflecting diminished flow across the right ventricle outflow tract. More often, a systolic regurgitant murmur due to tricuspid insufficiency is heard at the left mid-sternal border.

ECG reveals RV hypertrophy and right axis deviation. Chest X-ray reveals reduction of pulmonary blood flow.

Normal or severe cardiomegaly is present, as in case with severe tricuspid regurgitation.

Differential diagnosis during the neonatal period: TGA, pulmonary atresia with intact ventricular septum, Ebstein's anomaly. The definitive diagnosis is made by echocardiography (Figs. 3 and 4)

67.9.1.2 Pulmonary Atresia with Intact Ventricular Septum

Pulmonary atresia with intact ventricular septum (PA-IVS) is a rare lesion occurring in an estimated 8 of 1,000 live births (Bichell et al. 2006). PA-IVS is characterized by abnormalities proximal to the RV-PA junction. This pathology includes a spectrum of disease ranging from imperforate pulmonary valve with a well- developed RV to a severely hypoplastic-rudimentary RV with RV coronary fistulae and absent infundibulum. Focusing on pathophysiology, in the case of rudimentary RV, systemic venous blood, brought to the right atrium from caval veins and coronary sinus, passes mainly into the left side of the heart across the foramen ovale without passing the lungs. Anatomically, the pulmonary valve is often well formed with definable fused commissures. There is also a form when the valve is more dysmorphic with unicuspid or quadricuspid configurations, as well as complete absence of some valvular architecture with a fibrous ventriculoarterial junction (Kutsche and Van Mierop 1983). Typically, the tricuspid valve (TV) is smaller than normal. The TV is commonly dysplastic and variably regurgitant. The size of the TV correlates with the RV cavity size, and this is important in the prognosis of PA-IVS. The RV is hypertrophied with a small cavity in 90% of cases and severely hypoplastic in more than 50%. RV may be unipartite (inlet only), bipartite (inlet and outlet), or tripartite (inlet, outlet, and trabecular portions). Coronary artery abnormalities are common, including areas of stenosis or complete atresia. Retrograde blood flow from the hypertensive RV into coronary circulation through ventriculo-coronary connections (sinusoids) may be necessary for myocardial perfusion (Fig. 5). Ventriculo-coronary fistulae are not present in cases of significant tricuspid regurgitation, presumably because RV hypertension does not develop. After birth, with ductal runoff, diastolic pressure is relatively low and in competition with the suprasystemic RV pressure for coronary artery perfusion. The pulmonary arteries are usually confluent, supplied by a left-sided ductus arteriosus. Usually, because of the obligatory right-to-left shunt at the atrial level, these patients have a foramen ovale or an atrial septal defect (ASD).

Newborns with this malformation become cyanotic and hypoxemic immediately after functional closure of the PDA. When the ASD is restrictive, the cardiac output may be affected. Cyanosis is usually apparent within hours of birth, worsening progressively. In the absence of significant acidosis and reduced cardiac output, tachypnea may be evident. Cardiac examination reveals single first and second heart sounds. A soft pansystolic

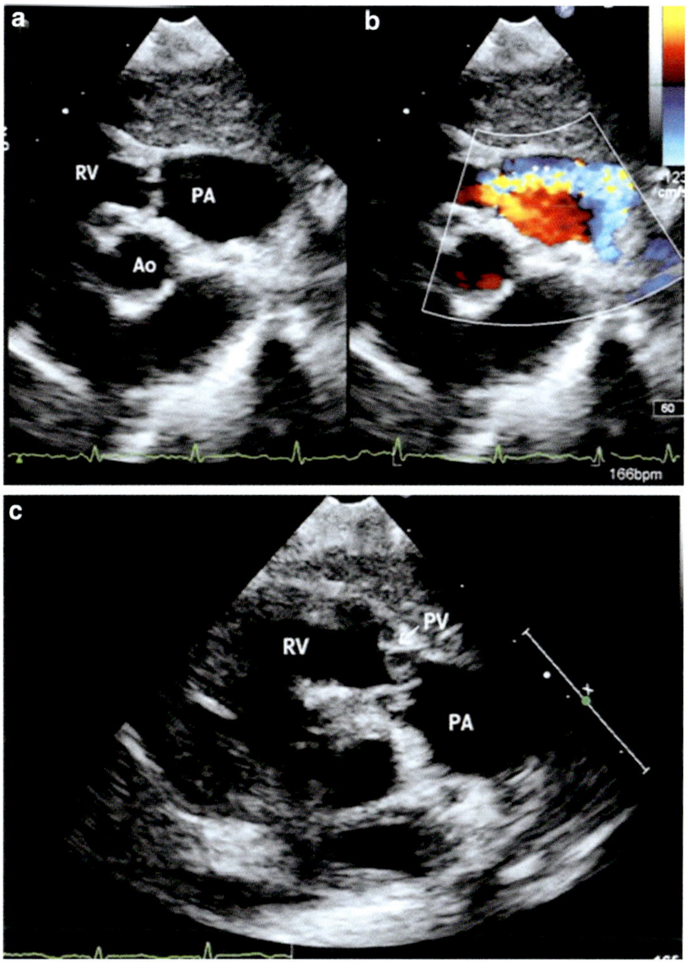

Fig. 3 Two-dimensional echocardiogram in newborn with severe pulmonary valve stenosis. (**a**) A parasternal right ventricular outflow tract view demonstrating a systolic doming of the pulmonary valve leaflets. (**b**) Two-dimensional color Doppler echocardiogram (parasternal long axis) demonstrating a central jet (*asterisks*) across the pulmonary valve. The pulmonary trunk is dilated. *Ao* aortic valve, *RV* right ventricle. (**c**) Thickened pulmonary valve cusps (*arrow*)

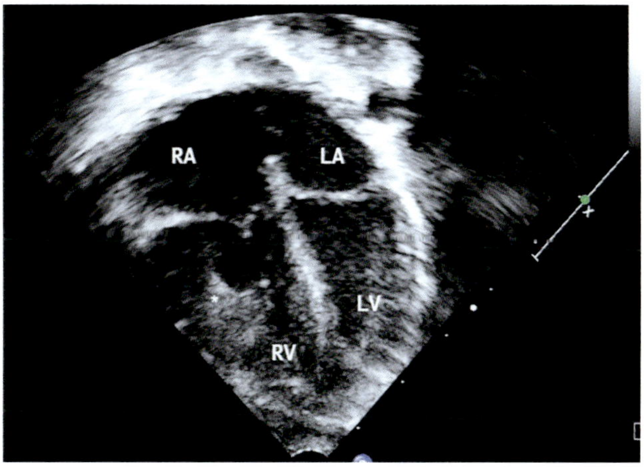

Fig. 4 Two-dimensional echocardiogram (apical four-chamber view, anatomical orientation) demonstrating a significant right ventricle hypertrophy. *RV* right ventricle, *RA* right atrium, *LA* left atrium, *LV* left ventricle

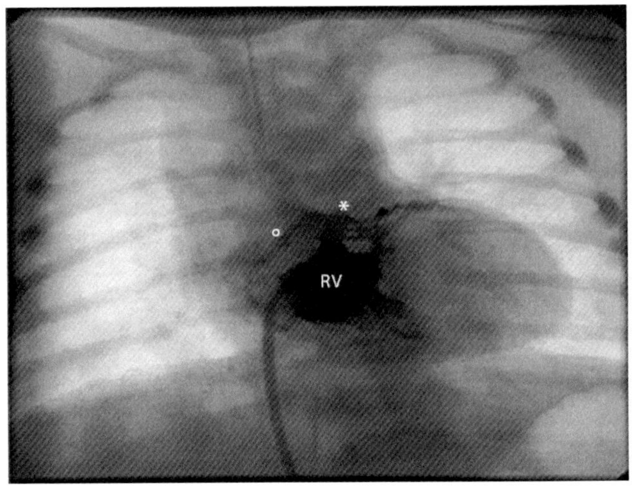

Fig. 5 Angiogram of a newborn with pulmonary atresia with intact ventricular septum. The right outflow tract (*asterisk*) ends blindly at the level of the atretic pulmonary valve (*circle*). Coronary sinusoids. *RV* right ventricle

murmur is often audible at the left lower sternal border. Sometimes the murmur of TR is prominent.

Chest X-ray reveals a variable degree of cardiomegaly. Pulmonary vascular markings are decreased.

ECG reveals LV dominance or significant LV hypertrophy. There are right atrial enlargement and ST-T abnormalities, consistent with some degree of subendocardial ischemia.

Echocardiography is effective in making the diagnosis. Catheterization is indicated for the precise assessment of the possible presence of sinusoids, RV to coronary fistulae, and stenosis of the coronary vessels when there is a severely hypoplastic RV ("RV-dependent coronary circulation"). However, when there is a tripartite RV, perforation of the atretic pulmonary valve followed by balloon dilation can be performed as an alternative to surgical valvulotomy.

67.9.1.3 Tetralogy of Fallot

Tetralogy of Fallot (TOF) occurs in 3–6 infants per 10,000 live births (Mitchell et al. 1971). The etiology is multifactorial but reported associations include untreated maternal diabetes, phenylketonuria and an increased intake of retinoic acid. Some associated chromosomal anomalies have been described: trisomies of chromosomes 21, 18, and 13; however, the most frequent association is with 22q11 chromosome microdeletion (Bailliard and Anderson 2008). This deletion, manifested by varying degrees of palatal abnormalities, dysmorphic facies, learning difficulties, immune deficiencies, and hypocalcemia, is typical of DiGeorge syndrome.

Anatomically, TOF results from anterior and cephalad deviation of the infundibular portion of the ventricular septum. This deviation causes: (1) aortic overriding over the crest of interventricular septum, (2) a malaligned subaortic ventricular septal defect, (3) obstruction of right ventricular outflow tract (RVOTO) (the level of the obstruction can be subvalvular, valvular, and supravalvular, in the pulmonary artery or its branches, and either isolated or in combination), and (4) systemic pressure in the RV with secondary hypertrophy (Fig. 6).

In case of TOF with pulmonary atresia (PAVSD), the right and left pulmonary arteries are confluent in approximately 50%, with blood to the pulmonary arteries flowing through the PDA. In the other 50%, pulmonary supply is multifocal. In these patients, the pulmonary blood supply may originate partly from the "true" pulmonary arteries and partly from aortopulmonary collateral arteries (MAPCAS). If the pulmonary arteries are discontinuous or absent, pulmonary supply is only from MAPCAS or from a combination of MAPCAS and PDA.

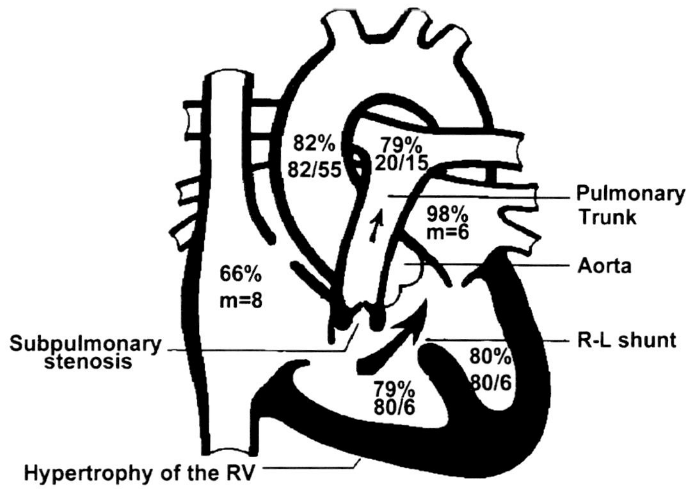

Fig. 6 Schematic diagram of oxygen saturation (%) and pressures in anatomy of Tetralogy of Fallot. The findings include: equal right and left ventricular pressures, a right-to-left (R-L) shunt at ventricular level, an anteriorly displaced infundibular septum resulting in subpulmonary stenosis

Other associated lesions include atrial septal defects, additional ventricular septal defects, and anomalous origin of coronary arteries. A right aortic arch is present in one-quarter of patients with TOF.

The initial presentation of TOF depends on the severity of obstruction of the right ventricular outflow tract.

Neonates with the most severe forms of TOF present with marked cyanosis. Pulse oximetry is equal in all limbs and demonstrates oxygen saturation of 70–80% in air. Arterial blood gas analysis demonstrates hypoxemia. Patients with less severe variants present during the neonatal period with mild-to-moderate cyanosis, but typically without respiratory distress.

The neonatal ECG usually shows right ventricular hypertrophy and right QRS axis deviation. A chest X-ray classically shows a small or absent main pulmonary artery with decreased pulmonary blood flow and, over time, a "boot-shaped" heart silhouette.

Diagnosis is confirmed by echocardiography and cardiac catheterization is not usually required.

67.9.1.4 TOF with Absent Pulmonary Valve

Approximately 2–6% of patients described as TOF also have absent pulmonary valve leaflets (Rao et al. 1971). The presence of rudimentary valvar leaflets results in free pulmonary regurgitation throughout fetal life. This chronic phenomenon produces RV overload which is transmitted to the pulmonary arteries, with concomitant dilatation of these vessels.

There may be cyanosis in a neonate when the RV pressure is relatively high and when relatively low compliance of the RV decreases the antegrade flow toward the pulmonary circulation and causes right-to-left shunting through the VSD. As the RV pressure decreases, the cyanosis becomes less evident, and more left-to-right shunt develops. Congestive heart failure signs might appear when PVR drops, causing an increased pulmonary blood flow. Some babies can present with inspiratory and expiratory stridor due to tracheobronchial tree compression by aneurysmal pulmonary arteries. In most of these cases, PDA is absent.

67.9.1.5 Severe Ebstein's Anomaly

Ebstein's anomaly (EA) is an uncommon but severe anatomic lesion when it presents in the neonatal period. Some familial cases have been reported. Overall, recognized EA is rare, accounting for less than 1% of CHD (MacLellan-Torbert and Porter 1998).

Ebstein's anomaly is characterized by abnormal attachment of the posterior and septal tricuspid leaflets in the RV cavity far from a normally positioned tricuspid valve annulus. The degrees of leaflet displacement are variable. The anterior leaflet is large, often with abnormal cordal attachments. This leaflet may obstruct the RV outlet. The inlet portion of the

RV is usually functionally integrated into the right atrium ("atrialization of the RV") and the functional RV cavity is small. Nearly all patients have a coexisting ASD or PFO. Ebstein's anomaly can be associated with accessory atrioventricular conduction pathways (Wolff-Parkinson-White syndrome).

Clinical presentation depends on the type and severity of EA. At birth, pulmonary vascular resistance is high, and the degree of cyanosis can vary with the degree of right-to-left shunting at the atrial level. In neonates with relatively mild tricuspid valve displacement and no RV outflow tract obstruction, right-to-left shunting usually decreases over the first weeks of life due to pulmonary vascular resistance decrease, with a concomitant reduction in cyanosis. If there is a significant portion of RV atrialized or if the tricuspid valve anterior leaflet obstructs the outflow tract, cyanosis persists and the severity of CHF increases. Ebstein's anomaly is one of the few disorders that may cause a thrill in a neonate.

There are several characteristic ECG appearances: right QRS axis deviation, right bundle branch block, low-voltage QRS complex in the right precordial leads, right atrial enlargement, and first degree AV block. Arrhythmias can occur in more than 50% of patients; most frequently, there are tachyarrhythmias, including paroxysmal supraventricular tachycardia, atrial fibrillation, and atrial flutter.

Cardiac size may vary from nearly normal to extreme cardiomegaly, which is rather typical of EA.

67.9.1.6 Complex CHD with Severe Pulmonary Stenosis or Pulmonary Atresia

Some patients with tricuspid atresia, single ventricle, and transposition of the great arteries may have severe pulmonary valve stenosis or pulmonary valve atresia. Postnatally, the degree of restriction to pulmonary flow will determine the clinical presentation and physical findings. Most babies present with cyanosis or murmur. In some of these neonates, restrictive ASD may be an important problem, especially in neonates with single ventricle and atrioventricular valve stenosis.

67.9.2 Duct-Dependent Systemic Blood Flow

In this group, there is a unique physiology related to left ventricular outflow obstruction (LVOTO) characterized by total or partial arterial duct-dependent systemic perfusion (Table 7). During intrauterine development, systemic perfusion is not compromised, being maintained by the ductal flow from the right ventricle to aorta. Postnatally, acute impairment of systemic perfusion follows

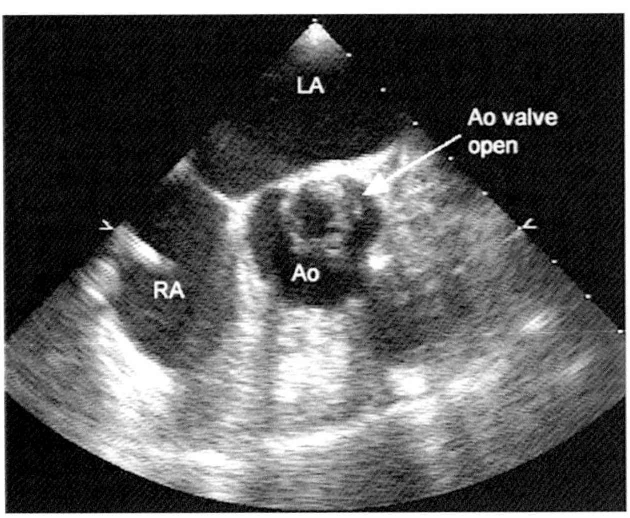

Fig. 7 Two-dimensional echocardiogram (parasternal short axis) demonstrates a unicuspid and thickened aortic valve

ductal constriction. When the PDA closes, infants present with cardiovascular collapse and symptoms of CHF.

67.9.2.1 Aortic Stenosis

The normal aortic valve has three leaflets of approximately equal size with a semilunar shape at the level of the free margins. Abnormalities of the aortic valve account for 70–80% of left ventricular outflow tract obstruction. In severe neonatal aortic stenosis (AS), the valve is often unicuspid or bicuspid (Fig. 8).

During fetal development, normal growth and development of the fetus is generally maintained in spite of valvar aortic stenosis. LVOTO exposes the left ventricle to increased afterload and results in ventricular hypertrophy and myocardial dysfunction. Moreover, chronic in utero subendocardial ischemia secondary to hypertrophy and increased intracavitary pressure can lead to coronary ischemia and development of endocardial fibroelastosis which further impairs the ventricular function. Additionally, reduced antegrade blood flow through the aortic valve predisposes to underdevelopment of the left heart structures and hypoplasia of the mitral valve, left ventricle, and aortic arch. The RV supplies an increased proportion of systemic blood flow via the PDA because LV output is reduced.

Neonates with critical aortic stenosis present dramatically soon after birth. As the ductus arteriosus begins to close, severe systemic hypoperfusion occurs resulting in decreased coronary perfusion, acute hemodynamic deterioration with cardiovascular collapse, acidosis, organ injury, and shock. Once the baby is stabilized, a complete echocardiographic evaluation is required to assess the severity and levels of the obstruction, associated cardiac abnormalities, and related hypoplasia of the aortic arch and left heart structures.

Neonates and infants with less severe obstruction may present with failure to thrive and tachypnea due to the increased work of breathing in association with pulmonary vascular congestion due to left atrial hypertension.

ECG findings vary widely in newborns and infants with AS. The right ventricular hypertrophy is the predominant pattern in neonates.

Chest X-ray shows global cardiomegaly in most cases. Pulmonary vascular markings are usually normal, but in 30–50% of cases congestion may be evident.

Following the anatomic definition by echocardiography (Figs. 7, 8 and 9), treatment strategy depends on: (i) the degree of aortic stenosis and the presence of aortic regurgitation, (ii) associated cardiac lesions, and (iii) the severity of this disease that can also affect other organs causing serious injury, for example, necrotizing enterocolitis.

67.9.2.2 Coarctation of the Aorta

Coarctation of the aorta (CoAo) occurs in 8–10% of all cases of CHD. It is a hemodynamically significant narrowing of the aorta located mostly at the insertion of the ductus arteriosus. It could be isolated or associated with other abnormalities, e.g., tubular hypoplasia of the aortic arch, left ventricular

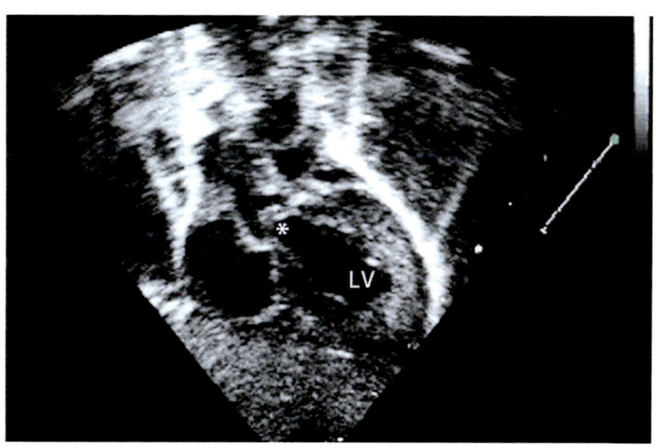

Fig. 8 Subcostal coronal view: Neonate with aortic valvar stenosis, concentric left ventricle (*LV*) hypertrophy. Aortic valve (*asterisk*)

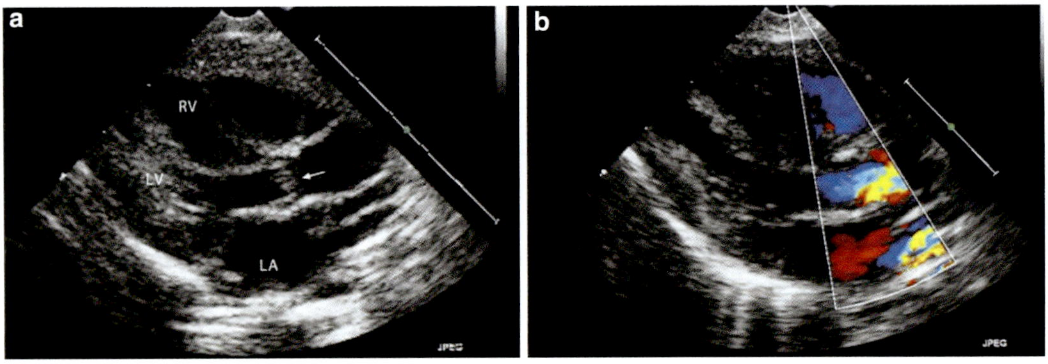

Fig. 9 Parasternal long-axis view in systole. (**a**) The valve has a domed appearance, with thickening of cusps (*arrow*). *LA* left atrium, *RV* right ventricle, *LV* left ventricle. (**b**) Color Doppler demonstrating a turbulent flow across the aortic valve

outflow obstruction, bicuspid aortic valve, VSD, and ASD. CoAo has been classified as preductal, ductal, and postductal. It is frequently seen in some chromosomal syndromes such as Turner syndrome. In newborns or young infants, the presentation is often dramatic as shock or severe congestive heart failure. A concomitant large PDA may make the diagnosis difficult. The most common signs and symptoms are tachypnea, diaphoresis at feeding, poor perfusion, hepatomegaly, and metabolic acidosis. If the duct is partially open, preductal is higher than postductal saturation; there is upper limb hypertension and weak palpable femoral pulses. If the duct is completely closed, there is no discrepancy between upper and lower limb saturation, femoral pulses are absent, and cyanosis or lower limb mottling and upper limb hypertension are present. CoAo and the absence of four-limb systolic pressure gradient can occur in the following anatomical and physiological conditions. (i) The duct is still patent, so the RV provides flow to the lower part of the body; these neonates have a differential cyanosis with lower O_2 saturation taken from lower limbs. (ii) LV dysfunction and systemic hypotension are so severe that it becomes impossible to detect a pressure gradient. (iii) Aberrant right subclavian artery arises distally to the coarctation site; therefore, right arm pressure reflects post-coarctation pressure. The key point is not to exclude diagnosis of CoAo solely through the absence of a gradient in pulse volume or systolic pressure between upper and lower limbs.

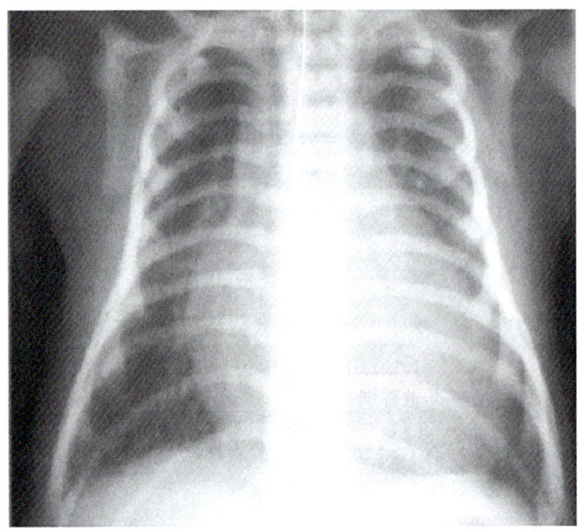

Fig. 10 Severe coarctation of the aorta. Heart is enlarged. Pulmonary arterial markings are normal, but there are distended pulmonary veins

The most common ECG pattern shows right ventricular hypertrophy initially, while biventricular hypertrophy usually appears later. Chest X-ray reveals the hallmarks of cardiomegaly and pulmonary congestion (Fig. 10). Echo color Doppler is the most sensitive and specific method for making the diagnosis (Figs. 11 and 12).

67.9.2.3 Interrupted Aortic Arch

Interrupted aortic arch (IAA) is an uncommon congenital cardiovascular malformation. The incidence is 1% of all congenital heart diseases, carrying a mortality rate higher than 90% in the neonatal period (Schumacher et al. 1986).

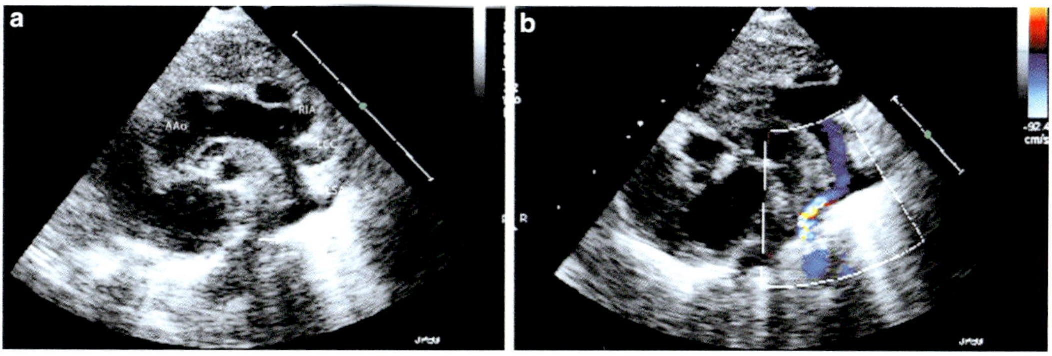

Fig. 11 Two-dimensional echocardiography of a typical coarctation viewed from the high left sagittal plane. (**a**) The aortic coarctation is visualized distal to the origin of the left subclavian artery (*LSA*). Ascending aorta (*AAo*); right innominate artery (*RIA*); left common carotid (*LCC*). (**b**) Color flow picture showing the isthmic coarctation

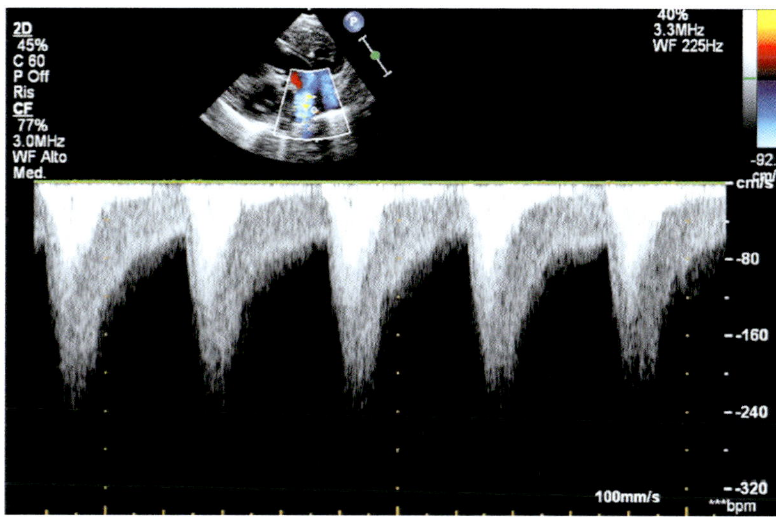

Fig. 12 Doppler sample: a continuous wave Doppler pattern at the level of the coarctation showing significant diastolic tail

IAA is defined as either a complete discontinuity or non-patent fibrous strand in the transverse arch or aortic isthmus. It is classified into three types according to the site of interruption: type A, the interruption is distal to the left subclavian artery origin; type B, between the origin of left subclavian and left common carotid artery; type C, the rarest one, between the origin of the right brachiocephalic and the left common carotid artery.

The hemodynamic condition is totally dependent on PDA patency that supplies the lower part of the body. Furthermore, most patients have only an isolated VSD but IAA can be associated with a variety of complex cardiovascular anomalies (Table 8) (Mishra 2009).

Table 8 Anomalies associated with interrupted aortic arch

VSD with posterior malalignment
Left ventricular outflow tract obstruction
Truncus arteriosus
Transposition of great arteries
Double outlet right ventricle
DiGeorge syndrome

In most cases, the pathophysiology of interrupted aortic arch is similar to critical CoAo in the newborn. Systemic blood flow is dependent on ductal patency. When the PDA closes, the baby develops poor perfusion, acidosis, shock, and renal

failure. On physical examination, tachycardia, systolic murmur, hepatomegaly, and weak femoral pulses are present. Differential cyanosis between the upper and lower limbs is usually difficult to appreciate when there is a VSD. If there is a concordant ventriculoarterial connection, pulse oximetry may show higher oxygen saturation in the preductal upper limbs compared with postductal lower limbs. If the great arteries are transposed, the oxygen saturation could be higher in the lower limbs (reversal differential cyanosis).

IAA type B is commonly associated with DiGeorge syndrome (broad nasal bridge, malar hypoplasia, narrow palpebral fissures, hypertelorism, low-set posteriorly rotated ears, retrognathia, small mouth, and submucosal palatal cleft, variable thymus, and parathyroid deficiencies). These physical features are difficult to recognize in neonates; therefore, all neonates with IAA should be genetically investigated to confirm DiGeorge syndrome. The major risk in these patients is graft-versus-host disease after blood transfusion with nonirradiated blood.

ECG and chest X-ray are not specific. Echocardiography is fundamental to make the diagnosis and to detect coexisting defects.

67.9.2.4 Hypoplastic Left Heart Syndrome

Hypoplastic left heart syndrome (HLHS) represents a group of defects characterized by varying degrees of underdevelopment of left-sided heart structures. Most of the patients have combinations of aortic and mitral valve atresia or stenosis (Garson et al. 1998). The severity is determined by the severity of outflow tract obstruction and the degree of aortic hypoplasia. This syndrome accounts for 1–3.8% of all CHD (Abbot 1936).

The LV is a rudimentary non-pumping chamber; the pulmonary venous return goes to the RA through a foramen ovale or atrial septal defect, causing complete venous blood mixing. The RV maintains the pulmonary and systemic output in a parallel fashion. The pulmonary arteries receive blood from the RV, while cerebral and cardiac perfusion are supplied retrogradely through the arterial duct into the transverse arch and ascending aorta.

During fetal life, the PVR is higher than systemic vascular resistance, and the RV maintains normal perfusion in the aorta and placenta through the patent duct. After birth, there is reversal of vascular resistance in the two circuits, with systemic pressure being higher than pulmonary, and PDA closure occurs. Additionally, an important anatomic element is the presence of an appropriately restrictive interatrial communication. With pulmonary and systemic parallel circulation, the ratio of pulmonary to systemic flow (Qp:Qs) depends on the balance between pulmonary and systemic vascular resistances. At birth, PVR is elevated but eventually decreases even in children with HLHS, resulting in increasing pulmonary blood flow and increasing RV overload, to preserve adequate systemic output. As Qp:Qs increases, more saturated blood passes from the LA to the RA across a nonrestrictive ASD; consequently, systemic oxygen saturation approaches normal values despite progressive clinical signs of CHF. This mechanism represents the most common cause of CHF in the first weeks of life (O'Donnel and McIlroy 1962). A different clinical presentation occurs when the pathophysiology is characterized by reduced pulmonary blood flow secondary to a small or restrictive interatrial communication. These babies always present critically with deep cyanosis, marked tachypnea, metabolic acidosis, hypoxemia characterized by PaO_2 values of 20 mmHg or less, and cardiovascular collapse.

All infants with HLHS should be promptly commenced on a prostaglandin infusion to maintain ductal patency and systemic perfusion. Clinical stabilization includes endotracheal intubation, vascular access placement, correction of metabolic acidosis, and oxygen delivery. After the diagnosis is made by echocardiography, prompt left atrial decompression is necessary by Rashkind maneuver and stent implantation at the fossa ovalis or surgical procedure.

Newborns with HLHS are generally full-term babies who initially appear well and healthy; only a few are affected by extracardiac anomalies, like structural brain malformations typical of chromosomal abnormalities (Natowicz et al. 1988; Gaynor et al. 2002). The magnitude and

distribution of acquired vital organ dysfunction usually relates to the circulatory impairment at the time of diagnosis. All the interventions in the preoperative period should be done in order to (i) preserve ductal patency and (ii) set or maintain Qp:Qs ratio of 1:1.

Differential diagnosis should include all the other left-sided obstructive lesions characterized by arterial duct-dependent systemic circulation (Table 7) and other nonstructural cardiac diseases with shock-like state clinical presentation such as neonatal sepsis or neonatal myocarditis; these conditions can be easily differentiated by echocardiography.

67.9.3 Parallel Circulation/ Transposition of the Great Arteries

Transposition of the great arteries (TGA) is a common form of cardiac anomaly, accounting for approximately 75–80% of all congenital heart defects (Bichell et al. 2006). TGA is defined anatomically as concordant atrioventricular (AV) connection and discordant ventriculoarterial connection. In this setting, the morphological RA is connected to the morphological RV, which gives rise to all or most of the aorta; the morphological LA is connected to the morphological LV from which the pulmonary trunk emerges (Fig. 13) (Ho et al. 1995). This condition is known as simple transposition. By contrast, complex transposition includes VSD, left ventricular outflow tract obstruction, aortic arch anomalies, and anomalous venous return.

Ventricular septal defect is present in 20% of TGA (Kirklin et al. 1986; Musumeci et al. 1988), typically in the outlet portion. Malalignment of the outlet septum deviated to the right results in variable degrees of PA overriding representing an anatomical entity called double-outlet right ventricle with subpulmonary ventricular septal defect (Taussig-Bing anomaly).

Left ventricular outflow tract obstruction can be demonstrated in over 30% of the patients with TGA (Park et al. 1983). Aortic arch obstruction is rare in TGA without VSD. Coronary anatomy may show different patterns (Ho et al. 1995). In 10% of the cases, this cardiac defect is associated with other noncardiac malformations (Kirklin et al. 1986).

67.9.3.1 Transposition Physiology

Systemic blood goes from RA to RV and then into the aorta without being oxygenated in the lungs. On the contrary, fully oxygenated pulmonary venous blood returns from the pulmonary veins into LA and LV and returns to the lungs via the pulmonary artery: in this setting, the systemic and pulmonary circulations describe parallel loops. Survival depends on the presence of one or more

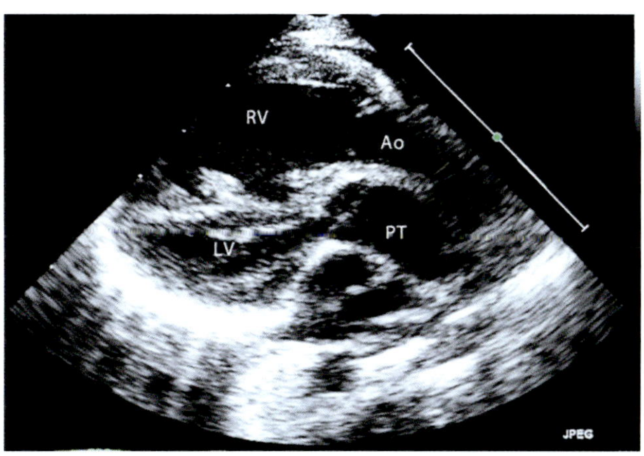

Fig. 13 Echocardiography; long-axis view demonstrating the anterior aorta arising from the right ventricle (*RV*) and the pulmonary trunk (*PT*) arising from the left ventricle (*LV*)

mixing sites between these two circulations such as an atrial septal defect, ventricular septal defect, or PDA, to achieve arterial oxygen saturation compatible with life.

Following separation of the placenta, newborns with TGA without VSD and small PFO or ASD have severe cyanosis (a very low PaO_2: 15–20 mmHg) on the first day of life, associated with high $PaCO_2$ and metabolic acidosis due to a severely decreased effective pulmonary blood flow.

67.9.3.2 Diagnosis

The hyperoxia test is suggestive of a cyanotic congenital heart condition (Martins and Castela 2008). Chest X-ray and ECG may be helpful, but findings are not specific. The definitive diagnosis relies on echocardiography.

The initial management aims at increasing FiO_2 and maximizing mixed venous oxygen saturation opening the arterial duct with prostaglandin. Resuscitation with mechanical ventilation can be necessary, and the foramen ovale should be emergently enlarged by balloon atrial septostomy. This procedure is usually performed under fluoroscopy in the cardiac catheterization laboratory. Balloon atrial septostomy, also known as the Rashkind procedure, consists of placing a balloon-tipped catheter in the LA, via the foramen ovale; the balloon is then inflated and pulled back into the RA, tearing the atrial septum. Echocardiographic guidance is mandatory. The aim of this procedure is to create an interatrial communication big enough to cause an increase in oxygen saturation due to improved blood mixing. In addition to these measures, medical support is usually necessary to optimize the clinical condition: correction of metabolic acidosis with hyperventilation and sodium bicarbonate to promote alkalosis, lower pulmonary vascular resistance, and increase pulmonary blood flow.

In case of good atrial septostomy but persisting desaturation, oxygen saturation could be improved by: (i) decreasing the whole body oxygen consumption (muscle relaxants, sedation, mechanical ventilation), (ii) increasing cardiac output with inotropic agents, and (iii) increasing oxygen-carrying capacity by treating anemia.

The arterial switch operation is the procedure of choice, and it is used to achieve complete physiological and anatomical correction.

67.9.4 Lesions with Complete Intracardiac Mixing

67.9.4.1 Total Anomalous Pulmonary Venous Return

Total anomalous pulmonary venous return (TAPVR) is a con- genital defect in which the pulmonary veins drain anomalously into the systemic venous circulation causing a complete blood mixing. TAPVR is classified in four types based on the anatomical sites of the abnormal connection: supracardiac, cardiac, infracardiac, and mixed.

1. *Supracardiac*: the veins drain into a common confluence behind the LA which drain through an anomalous vein into the systemic venous circulation, usually in the right- sided superior vena cava or the innominate vein through a persistent vertical vein.
2. *Cardiac*: the common venous confluence drains either into the coronary sinus or posterior portion of RA.
3. *Infracardiac*: the common venous confluence passes across the diaphragm through the esophageal hiatus and drains either into the portal vein or ductus venosus or hepatic vein or inferior caval vein.
4. *Mixed type*: this anatomical configuration is the result of combination of different forms of TAPVR. It is commonly associated with other major cardiac anomalies.

In addition, drainage can be obstructed or unobstructed. The majority of supracardiac TAPVR cases have some degree of obstruction which could be secondary to: (i) ascending vein compression between bronchi and pulmonary artery or aorta, (ii) vertical vein orifice stenosis, or (iii) a small and restrictive atrial communication.

Heterotaxy syndrome, especially right isomerism, is usually associated with TAPVR (Fyler

1992). TAPVR is associated with other cardiac anomalies such as single ventricle, truncus arteriosus, transposition of the great arteries, pulmonary atresia, and coarctation of the aorta (Lucas 1983).

There is an obligatory left-to-right shunt from pulmonary veins to the right heart and an obligatory right-to-left shunt from RA to the left heart to maintain the systemic output. The factors that determine blood flow distribution in these two circuits include: (i) relative size of the atrial communication and (ii) severity of any obstruction in the extracardiac pulmonary venous channel.

In the most common form of TAPVR, pathophysiology is a combination of pulmonary vein obstruction and increased pulmonary blood flow. This situation results in RV volume overload. Neonates with significant pulmonary vein obstruction present with severe cyanosis, tachypnea, and hemodynamic instability. These babies are frequently misdiagnosed as having persistent fetal circulation or sepsis or severe respiratory distress syndrome (Cobanoglu and Menashe 1993).

The clinical presentation of TAPVR varies with the degree of obstruction and pulmonary blood flow. Frequently the newborn presents with tachypnea due to RV volume overload, whereas babies with the significant pulmonary vein obstruction show frank respiratory distress, pulmonary edema, poor peripheral perfusion, hypotension, and metabolic acidosis. Identification of this pathology is crucial in critically ill neonates, and the diagnosis is usually made by echocardiography.

67.9.4.2 Truncus Arteriosus

This defect consists of a single great artery arising from the heart which gives rise to systemic arteries, pulmonary and coronary arteries. Depending on the anatomical origin of the pulmonary arteries, four types of truncus arteriosus exist (Collett and Edwads 1949):

1. Type I, pulmonary trunk arises from common arterial trunk.
2. Type II, right and left pulmonary arteries arise separately but close to one another from the left posterolateral aspect of common arterial trunk.
3. Type III, each pulmonary artery arises from the ipsilateral aspect of common arterial trunk.
4. Type IV, the main pulmonary artery is absent with the lungs receiving their blood supply through aortopulmonary collaterals.

The common arterial trunk overrides a VSD which is often large, nonrestrictive, with the superior border being formed by the truncal valve. The truncal valve may have a variable number of cusps, most commonly three; it is often anatomically abnormal showing different grade of regurgitation and/or stenosis. The pulmonary arteries are usually of normal caliber although stenosis of the origin and diffuse hypoplasia can occur. Coronary anomalies, in terms of origin and epicardial course, can coexist. Truncus arteriosus may also be associated with a right-sided aortic arch. The extracardiac anomalies are common and can contribute to the mortality; association with DiGeorge syndrome, chromosome 22q11 deletion (Bove et al. 1993), is reported in about 30% of cases (Goldmuntz et al. 1998).

In most cases, the dominant physiology is a left-to-right shunt at the level of the great arteries. The pulmonary and the systemic blood flow are determined, respectively, by pulmonary vascular resistance and systemic vascular resistance. Newborns affected by truncus arteriosus generally have an elevated pulmonary vascular resistance and are therefore asymptomatic. As pulmonary resistance gradually decreases and PBF increases, signs of CHF occur. Subsequently the volume and pulmonary pressure overload leads to pulmonary vascular disease. Furthermore, signs of CHF can be worsened by concomitant significant truncal valve regurgitation or stenosis. Echocardiography provides accurate diagnosis (Figs. 14 and 15). Definitive repair of truncus arteriosus consists of PA branches separation, RV-PA conduit implantation and VSD closure.

67.9.4.3 Complex Single Ventricle

Physiology of complex single ventricle is characterized by complete mixing of the systemic and pulmonary venous circulations. An anatomical definition describes the single ventricle as a malformation where both atrioventricular valves enter

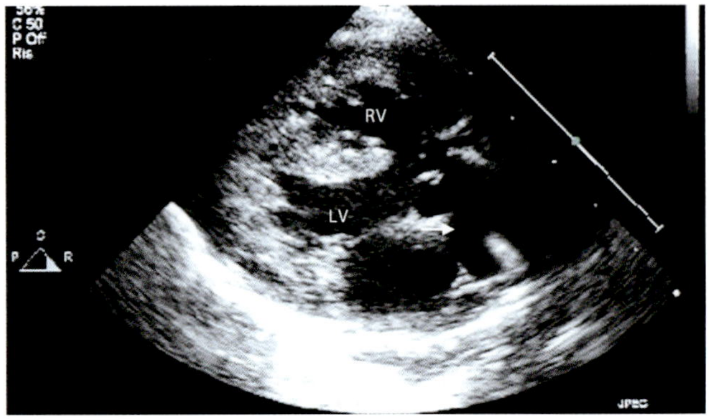

Fig. 14 Echocardiogram (long-axis parasternal view) of truncus arteriosus. Truncal vessel gives rise to the aorta and the pulmonary arteries (*arrow*). *RV* right ventricle, *LV* left ventricle

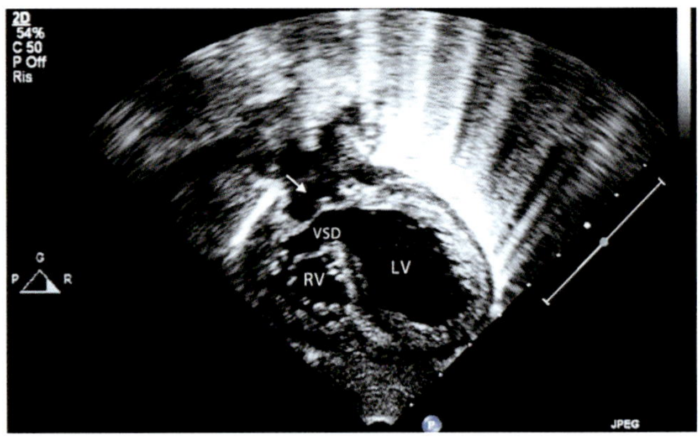

Fig. 15 Subcostal view demonstrating the ventricular septal defect (*VSD*) overriding the truncal valve. *RV* right ventricle, *LV* left ventricle

one ventricle, and there is only one identifiable ventricular sinus (Schultz and Kreutzer 2006). A large variety of anatomic lesions exist, generally associated with atresia of atrioventricular or semilunar valves. The great vessels usually arise from the heart in an abnormal fashion; frequently variable degrees of pulmonary or aortic obstruction may be present. Most complex single ventricles are associated with heterotaxy syndrome: polysplenia or asplenia, systemic venous return anomalies, anomalous pulmonary venous connection, visceral situs abnormalities, and atrioventricular septal defect.

The hemodynamic characteristics and the clinical presentation depend on the balance of anatomy and/or resistance in the systemic and pulmonary circulation. Patients without pulmonary stenosis show increased pulmonary blood flow and soon develop signs of congestive heart failure. In cases with pulmonary stenosis, cyanosis is present according to the degree of obstruction.

Patients with pulmonary or aortic atresia or severe hypoplasia of the aortic arch have a duct-dependent circulation, and they need treatment with PGE_1 as long as palliative surgery is performed.

67.9.5 Left-to-Right Shunt Lesions

In the group of left-to-right shunt lesions, the most common in neonates are PDA, ventricular septal defect, atrioventricular septal defect, and atrial septal defect. PDA will be fully described in Chap. 69, "▸ Patent Ductus Arteriosus."

67.9.5.1 Ventricular Septal Defect

Ventricular septal defect (VSD) is one of the most common isolated congenital cardiac malformations. A ventricular septal defect is a hole in the interventricular septum resulting in direct communication between the left and right ventricles. A clinical useful classification schema

divides VSD in four types, considering interventricular septum from the RV aspect:

1. Perimembranous, which partially or totally involves the membranous septum. It can extend into the inlet, trabecular, or outlet portions of the septum. This accounts for the majority of the cases.
2. Subarterial, located just beneath the pulmonary valve. This defect, also known as "doubly committed," occurs most often among Asians.
3. Inlet defect, beneath the septal cusp of the tricuspid valve.
4. Muscular defect, located anywhere in the muscular septum with all muscular margins (Fig. 16).

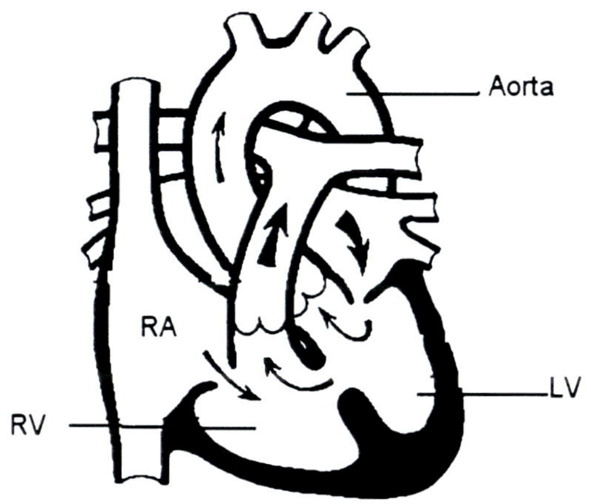

Fig. 16 Ventricular septal defect: VSD may occur anywhere in the ventricular septum. This defect is located in the muscular portion of the septum. *RV* right ventricle, *LV* left ventricle

VSD may be either isolated or form part of complex CHD as in TOF, truncus arteriosus, and double-outlet RV.

67.9.5.2 Atrioventricular Septal Defect

Atrioventricular septal defect (AVSD) is a malformation involving structures normally derived from the endocardial cushion tissue: ostium primum atrial septal defect, inlet VSD, and the common atrioventricular valve (Fig. 17). Different forms of AVSD exist but two are the most common: partial and complete. Partial AVSD indicates an atrioventricular septal defect with interatrial communication (ostium primum ASD), common AV valve but not inlet VSD; the term complete atrioventricular septal defect describes an AVSD with both ostium primum ASD and inlet VSD. There is a strong association between complete AVSD and Down syndrome, whereas partial AVSD is more seen in DiGeorge and Ellis-van Creveld syndromes.

Most neonates with left-to-right shunt defects present with signs of cardiac failure after 2 weeks of age. During fetal life, even large defects do not

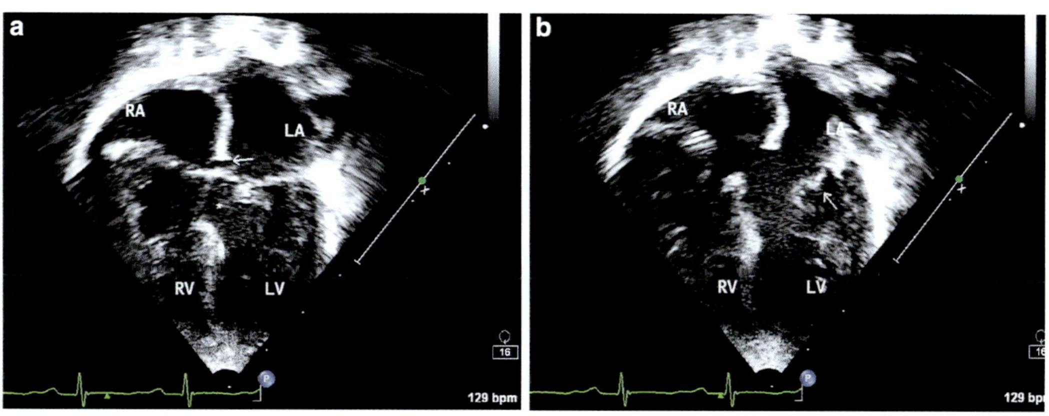

Fig. 17 (**a**) Two-dimensional echocardiogram (apical four-chamber view, anatomical orientation) demonstrating ostium primum atrial septal defect. Inlet ventricular septal defect (*asterisk*). (**b**) Two-dimensional echocardiogram (apical four-chamber view, anatomical orientation) demonstrating a complete atrioventricular septal defect. The common atrioventricular valve is indicated (*arrow*). *RA* right atrium, *LA* left atrium, *RV* right ventricle, *LV* left ventricle

have major physiological effects because of high PVR. After birth the normal decline of PVR occurs within the first 2 weeks. In the presence of a large shunt, this decline may be delayed by 1–3 months. When this phenomenon happens, pulmonary artery blood flow increases, resulting in left heart volume overload.

Babies with small left-to-right shunt defects usually come to the attention of pediatricians because of cardiac murmurs without symptoms. Children with moderate left-to-right shunt defects show varying degrees of growth retardation. Large defects cause signs and symptoms of cardiac failure, such as tachypnea, nasal flaring, rib and sternal retraction, feeding difficulties, irritability, and excessive sweating. It is extremely rare for partial AVSD to cause abnormal physical signs during neonatal period, unless there is significant AV valve regurgitation.

All the neonates with signs of cardiac failure should be investigated by echocardiography.

References

Abbot ME (1936) Atlas of congenital cardiac disease. American Heart Association, New York

Ashley SM, Lu Le N (2015) The critically Ill infant with congenital heart disease. Emerg Med Clin N Am 33:501–518

Bailliard F, Anderson RH (2008) Tetralogy of Fallot. Orphanet J Rare Dis 13:4–2

Bichell DP et al (2006) Pulmonary atresia with intact ventricular sep- tum. In: Nichols D, Ungerleider R, Spevak P (eds) Critical heart disease in infants and children. Mosby Elsevier, Philadelphia, pp 767–776

Bove EL, Lupinetti FM, Pridjian AK et al (1993) Results of a policy of primary repair of truncus arteriosus in the neonate. J Thorac Cardiovasc Surg 105:1057–1065

Cobanoglu A, Menashe VD (1993) Total anomalous pulmonary ve- nous connection in neonates and young infants: repair in the cur- rent era. Ann Thorac Surg 55:43–48

Collett RW, Edwads JE (1949) Persistent truncus arteriosus: a classification according to anatomic types. Surg Clin North Am 29:1245

Fyler DC (1992) Total anomalous pulmonary venous return. In: Fyler DC (ed) Nadas' pediatric cardiology. Hanley & Belfus, Philadelphia, pp 683–691

Garson A Jr, Bricker JT, Fisher DJ, Neish SR (1998) The science and practice of pediatric cardiology. Williams & Wilkins, Baltimore

Gaynor JW, Mahle WT, Cohen MI et al (2002) Risk factors for mortality after the Norwood procedure. Eur J Cardiothorac Surg 22:82–89

Gikonyo BM, Lucas RV, Edwards JE (1987) Anatomic features of congenital pulmonary valve stenosis. Pediatr Cardiol 8:109

Goldmuntz E, Clark B, Mitchell L et al (1998) Frequency of 22q11 deletions in patients with conotruncal defects. J Am Coll Cardiol 32:492–498

Ho SY, Baker EJ, Riggby ML, Anderson RH (1995) Color atlas of congenital heart disease – morphologic and clinical correlations. Mosby-Wolfe, London

Hoffman JIE, Kaplan S (2002) The incidence of congenital heart disease. J Am Coll Cardiol 39:1890–1900

Kirklin JW, Pacifico AD, Blackstone EH et al (1986) Current risks and protocols for operations for double-outlet right ventricle. J Thorac Cardiovasc Surg 92:913–930

Kutsche LM, Van Mierop LHS (1983) Pulmonary atresia with and without ventricular septal defect: a different etiology and pathogenesis for the atresia in the 2 types? Am J Cardiol 51:932–935

Lee K, Khoshnood B, Chen L et al (2001) Infant mortality from congenital malformation I the United States, 1970–1997. Obstet Gynecol 98:620–627

Lucas RV (1983) Anomalous venous connection, pulmonary and systemic in heart disease in infants, children and adolescents. In: Adams FH, Emmanoulides GC (eds) Heart disease in infants, chil- dren, and adolescents, 3rd edn. Williams & Wilkins, Baltimore

MacLellan-Torbert SG, Porter CJ (1998) Ebstein's anomaly of the tricuspid valve. In: Garson A, Bricker JT, Fisher DJ, Neish SR (eds) The science and practice of pediatric cardiology, 2nd edn. Williams & Wilkins, Baltimore, pp 1303–1315

Martins P, Castela E (2008) Transposition of the great arteries. Orphanet J Rare Dis 3:27

Mishra PK (2009) Management strategies for interrupted aortic arch with associated anomalies. Eur J Cardiothorac Surg 35:569–576

Mitchell SC, Korones SB, Berendes HW (1971) Congenital heart disease in 56,109 births: incidence and natural history. Circulation 43:323–332

Musumeci F, Shumway S, Lincoln C, Anderson RH (1988) Surgical treatment for double-outlet right ventricle at the Brompton Hospital, 1973 to 1986. J Thorac Cardiovasc Surg 96:278–287

Natowicz M, Chatten J, Clancy R et al (1988) Genetic disorders and major extracardiac anomalies associated with the hypoplasia left heart syndrome. Pediatrics 82:698–706

O'Donnel TV, McIlroy MB (1962) The circulatory effects of squat-ting. Am Heart J 64:347

Olney Richard S, Ailes EC, Sontag MK (2015) Detection of critical congenital heart defects: review of contributions from prenatal and newborn screening. Semin Perinatol 39:230–237

Park SC, Neches WH, Mathews RA et al (1983) Hemodynamic function after the Mustard operation for the

transposition of the great arteries. Am J Cardiol 51:1514–1519

Rao BNS, Anderson RC, Edwards JE (1971) Anatomic variations in the tetralogy of Fallot. Am Heart J 81:361

Schultz AH, Kreutzer J (2006) Cyanotic heart disease. In: Vetter VL (ed) Pediatric cardiology: the requisites in pediatrics, 1st edn. Mosby, London, pp 66–67

Schumacher G, Schreiber R, Meisner H et al (1986) Interrupted aortic arch: natural history and operative results. Pediatr Cardiol 7:89–93

van Vonderen J, Arno R, Siew ML, Walther FJ, Hooper SB, Pas AB (2014) Measuring physiological changes during the transition to life after birth. Neonatology 105:230–242

Early Diagnosis of Congenital Heart Disease: When and How to Treat

68

Francesca R. Pluchinotta, Luciane Piazza, Angelo Micheletti, Javier Fernandez Sarabia, Diana Negura, Carmelo Arcidiacono, Antonio Saracino, and Mario Carminati

Contents

Abstract

Cardiovascular malformation is the most common group of congenital malformations. The prevalence is 5.3 cases per 1,000 live births. These malformations represent a significant cause of neonatal morbidity and mortality. Advances in medical and surgical treatment of congenital heart disease (CHD) have resulted in improved outcome for conditions which previously carried high mortality. Unrecognized neonatal cardiac malformation carries a serious risk of avoidable mortality, morbidity, and handicap. Routine neonatal examination fails to detect many affected babies, because a normal physical examination does not exclude serious cardiac malformation, including hypoplastic left

F. R. Pluchinotta (✉)
Department of Pediatric Cardiology, IRCCS Policlinico San Donato, San Siro, Milan, Italy
e-mail: mario.carminati@grupposandonato.it

L. Piazza · A. Micheletti · J. F. Sarabia · D. Negura · C. Arcidiacono · A. Saracino · M. Carminati
Centro Cardiologia Pediatrica Policlinico San Donato, Milano, Italy
e-mail: Luciane.Piazza@grupposandonato.it

G. Buonocore et al. (eds.), *Neonatology*,
https://doi.org/10.1007/978-3-319-29489-6_215

heart syndrome or interruption or coarctation of the aortic arch. Babies with a cardiac murmur detected over the first few days of life should be referred for early pediatric cardiological evaluation and definitive diagnostic echocardiography. All syndromic babies such as those with Down's syndrome should be referred for early echocardiographic examination. Echocardiography is an essential tool in the evaluation of neonates and has dramatically improved the accuracy of diagnosis of congenital heart disease. The antenatal diagnosis of CHD by fetal echocardiography carries important advantages: less hypoxia and preoperative acidosis, fewer adverse neurological events and earlier surgery, opportunities for parental counseling, and the optimization of perinatal care with the selection of an optimal site for delivery.

68.1 Salient Points

- About half the babies with cardiac murmur detected over the first few days of life have structural heart disease.
- The preoperative management of patients with critical congenital heart defects has a dramatic impact on overall outcome.
- A few palliative procedures are used for specific indications: systemic-to-pulmonary artery shunt (prostaglandin and modified Blalock-Taussing shunt), pulmonary artery banding, and Norwood procedure.
- Pathologies which require correction in the neonatal period are: truncus arteriosus, transposition of the great arteries, total anomalous pulmonary venous return, Ebstein's anomaly, and tetralogy of Fallot with severe right ventricular outflow obstruction, pulmonary atresia with intact ventricular septum, and coarctation of the aorta.

68.2 Introduction

Cardiovascular malformation is the most common group of congenital malformations. The prevalence is 5.3 cases per 1,000 live births (Wren et al. 1999; Ferencz et al. 1985; Kidd et al. 1993). These malformations represent a significant cause of neonatal morbidity and mortality. Advances in medical and surgical treatment of congenital heart disease (CHD) have resulted in improved outcome in conditions which previously carried high mortality. The antenatal diagnosis of CHD, by fetal echocardiography, carries important advantages:

1. Prenatal diagnosis is associated with less hypoxia, less preoperative acidosis, fewer neurologic events, and earlier age to surgery (Tworetzky et al. 2001).
2. It provides opportunities for parental counseling.
3. It may optimize perinatal care in terms of changes in obstetric and neonatal management with multidisciplinary approach which should reduce mortality and morbidity (Berkley et al. 2009; Chew et al. 2006).

Routine neonatal examination fails to detect many affected babies, because a normal examination does not exclude serious cardiac malformation, including hypoplastic left heart syndrome or other pathologies such as interruption or coarctation of the aortic arch. Considering that about half the babies with cardiac murmur, detected over the first few days of life, have a structural heart disease (Ainsworth et al. 1999), these patients should be referred for early pediatric cardiological evaluation and definitive diagnostic echocardiography. Unrecognized neonatal cardiac malformation carries a serious risk of avoidable mortality, morbidity, and handicap (Silove 1994). Regardless of this, all syndromic babies such as Down's syndrome-affected babies who have a high prevalence of congenital heart disease should be referred for early echocardiographic examination (Wren et al. 1999). The key point is that echocardiography is an essential tool in the evaluation of neonates and has dramatically improved the accuracy of diagnosis of congenital heart disease.

68.3 When and How to Treat: Preoperative Management of Neonates with CHD

The preoperative management of patients with critical congenital heart defects has a dramatic impact on overall outcome; it requires a

Table 1 Indications for palliative procedure

1. Systemic-to-pulmonary arterial shunt
Right-sided obstructive lesion varying in severity from mild pulmonary stenosis to pulmonary atresia
Tetralogy of Fallot
Single ventricle with pulmonary stenosis
Tricuspid atresia
Atrioventricular septal defect with severe pulmonary stenosis
2. Pulmonary artery banding
Tricuspid atresia with unrestrictive VSD
Single ventricle with unrestrictive pulmonary blood flow
3. Norwood procedure
Hypoplastic left heart syndrome

coordinated, multidisciplinary approach with pediatric cardiologist, pediatric intensivist, surgeon, anesthesiologist, pediatric nurses, respiratory therapists, and family members. The major goal is to provide supportive care, clinical stabilization, and adequate cardiac output to ensure adequate tissue delivery. Advances in the surgical repair of congenital heart defects have allowed a trend toward a single-stage repair. Nevertheless, there are still two palliative procedures used for specific indications (Table 1): systemic-to-pulmonary artery shunt and pulmonary artery banding (PAB).

68.3.1 Systemic-to-Pulmonary Artery Shunt

The systemic-to-pulmonary artery shunt is a palliative procedure that is used to increase pulmonary blood flow (PBF) in cardiac defects characterized by pulmonary outflow obstruction and clinical cyanosis. In these conditions, before surgery, the ductus arteriosus is the main source of pulmonary blood flow; as the ductus closes spontaneously, severe hypoxemia, metabolic acidosis, and death can occur. That is why prostaglandin should be administrated by continuous intravenous infusion to maintain patency of the ductus arteriosus. In many cases, supporting therapy is necessary to prevent vasoconstriction and avoid hypoxia, acidosis, and hypercapnia, which may increase pulmonary vascular resistance (PVR). It is important to maintain normal blood glucose, calcium levels, and preservation of a neutral thermal environment (Nichols et al. 2006). The modified Blalock-Taussig shunt (MBTS) is the most commonly created systemic-to-pulmonary shunt in neonates (Ahamad et al. 2008). This procedure consists of a polytetrafluoroethylene (Gore-Tex) graft placement between the innominate or subclavian artery and the ipsilateral pulmonary artery (de Leval et al. 1981); it aims at increasing pulmonary blood flow (PBF) and making pulmonary arteries grow in order to achieve a favorable anatomic condition for future correction. In particular situations such as Ebstein's anomaly, pulmonary atresia with intact ventricular septum or hypoplastic left heart syndrome, transcatheter arterial duct recanalization, and stenting can be considered as an alternative technique to a surgical shunt (Santoro et al. 2008a, b; Gewilling et al. 2004). The postoperative management after Blalock-Taussig shunt insertion in neonates is generally uncomplicated. The saturation is about 75–80% in most of the cases. The extubation is deferred until pulmonary blood flow is adequate and the arterial saturation is stable. When the saturation is not adequate, the following problems should be excluded: (i) hypotension; (ii) excessive overload volume until pulmonary edema, requiring if necessary reoperation to narrow the shunt size; (iii) low diastolic pressure, leading to coronary insufficiency; and (iv) acute thrombosis. If shunt narrowing or obstruction is detected, feasible treatment could be percutaneous balloon angioplasty (Fig. 1a–c), thrombolysis, or surgery. Immediate postoperative anticoagulation with heparin is used, followed by daily aspirin therapy as long as the shunt is open.

In some centers, the transcatheter placement of a stent to maintain ductal patency has been used as an alternative method to provide a source of pulmonary blood. The stenting for PDA appears to be an acceptable alternative to the MBTS. The potential advantages compared to the shunt include a reduced procedural-related risks, avoidance of cardiopulmonary bypass, and better distribution of blood through the pulmonary arteries In some cases, after the shunt, we can observe asymmetry or pulmonary blood flow irregularity caused by distortion (sprain, twist) or localized stenosis of

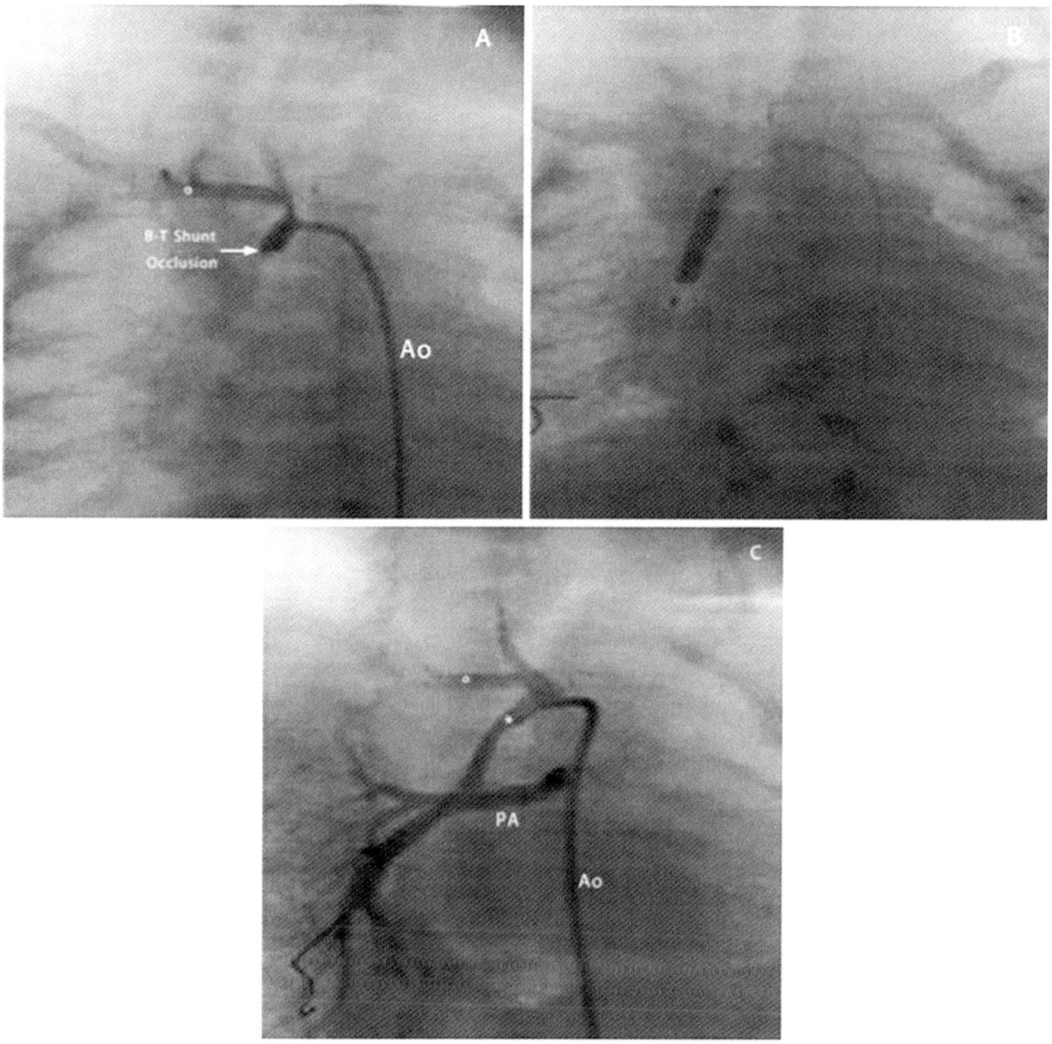

Fig. 1 (**a**) Injection in the right Blalock-Taussig shunt; the shunt is completely occluded. (**b**) Recanalization of the shunt with a balloon catheter. (**c**) Post-balloon angioplasty: injection in the right modified Blalock-Taussig shunt; complete recanalization (*asterisk*). Right subclavian artery (*circle*), *AO* aorta, *PA* pulmonary artery

pulmonary arteries, mainly at the level of the anastomosis of the shunt in the pulmonary artery.

68.3.2 Pulmonary Artery Banding

Pulmonary artery banding (PAB) is a palliative procedure performed in neonates affected by CHD associated with high pulmonary blood flow and CHF poorly controlled by medical therapy. The aim is to control the symptoms, to make the child grow properly, and to prevent the development of pulmonary vascular disease.

The banding procedure consists of surrounding the main pulmonary artery with a synthetic band in order to create a stenosis limiting the pulmonary blood flow (Fig. 2) It can be performed either through sternotomy or anterolateral thoracotomy.

PAB is an initial palliative strategy for select patients, mainly in patients suffering from single ventricle and unrestricted pulmonary blood with or without arch aortic obstruction.

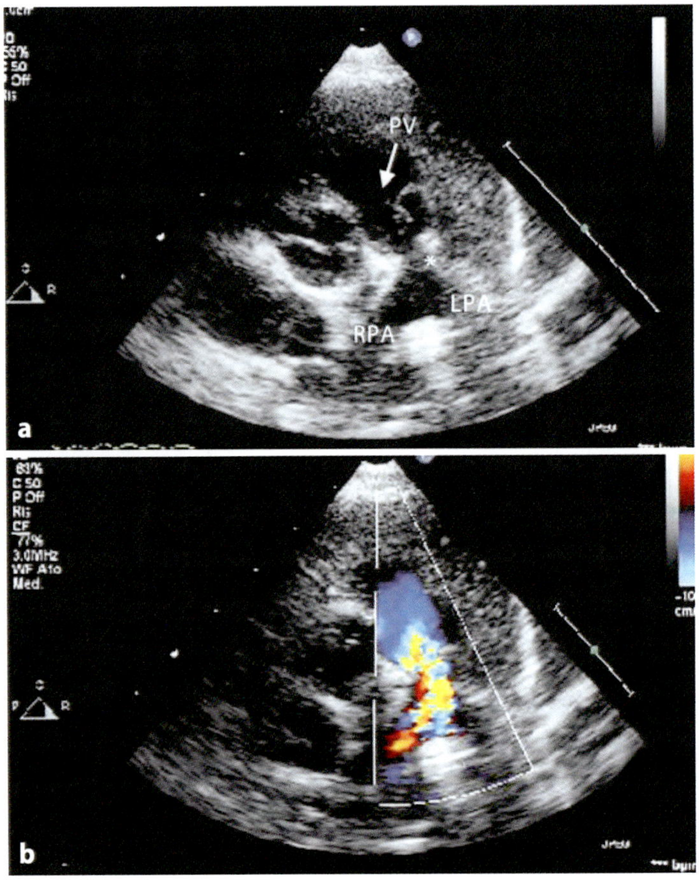

Fig. 2 Echocardiogram picture of pulmonary artery banding. (**a**) Pulmonary valve (*PV*); pulmonary banding (*asterisk*). *LPA* left pulmonary artery, *RPA* right pulmonary artery. (**b**) Color flow picture showing flow acceleration across the banding

68.3.3 Norwood Procedure

The Norwood procedure is performed to treat the conditions that result in single ventricle circulation. Since in these conditions, the most urgent problem is that the heart is unable to pump blood to the systemic circulation, the object of the Norwood procedure is to connect the single ventricle to the systemic circulation. This procedure is prescribed in the treatment of hypoplastic left heart syndrome (HLHS), an association of anatomical anomalies involving the left side of the heart. HLHS includes varying degrees of hypoplasia of the left ventricle (LV), critical stenosis, or atresia of the mitral and/or aortic valve, with some degree of hypoplasia in the aortic arch (Tworetzky et al. 2001). It is fatal without surgical interventions. The HLHS survival estimate is increate in the recent years but still accounts for 25–40% of all neonatal cardiac mortality. The prematurity, low weight, genetic syndromes, and extracardiac anomalies affect survival of these patients, although periodical and surgical management advances might neutralized the effect of anatomic factor survival.

The surgical treatment for HLHS consists of three steps:

1. Initial palliative reconstruction (Stage I – Norwood procedure)
2. Bidirectional Glenn shunt
3. Fontan operation
4. Transplantation

The first stage (Norwood procedure) is performed to provide a systemic perfusion independent from the arterial duct, to preserve function to the single ventricle by minimizing excess pressure and volume work, and to allow normal maturation of the pulmonary vasculature. An extensive aortic arch reconstruction, the pulmonary artery and aorta are used to create the “neoaorta.” A connection with

the systemic right ventricle (RV) with the systemic circulation and a modified Blalock-Taussig shunt or Sano shunt (RV to main pulmonary artery conduit) is performed. Septectomy is performed to avoid obstruction of pulmonary venous return and to allow blood flow from the left atrium (LA) to the right atrium (RA) (Kilian 2006).

The Sano shunt, compared with the BT shunt, determines in a higher elevation of the diastolic blood pressure. Because the coronary arteries are perfused in diastole, the advantage expected in the Sano strategy is supposed to be a better coronary perfusion (Bradley et al. 2001).

A new approach to the HLHS is known as "hybrid" procedure which consists of transcatheter stent implantation in the ductus arteriosus for maintenance of systemic output, as well as surgical bilateral PA branches banding to prevent pulmonary overcirculation. The stent maintains systemic perfusion, whereas the bands limit pulmonary blood flow (Lim et al. 2006; Akintuerk et al. 2002). This procedure should be performed either in a catheterization laboratory or in a theater where both angiographic and surgical capabilities and equipment should be available. The hybrid approach avoids cardiopulmonary bypass surgery and theoretically is better for the preservation of the RV function. (20) On the other hand, the complication of PA obstruction due to the banding has a negative clinical implication. This condition needs a diagnosis based on a method of image like cardiac catheterization or computed tomography The cardiac catheterization is the most used because it not only allows to put in evidence the stenosis of pulmonary branch end or band migration, but, in the same session, also stenosis with angioplasty and stent implantation could be treated.

68.4 Pathologies Which Require Correction in the Neonatal Period

68.4.1 Truncus Arteriosus

Complete mixing at the ventricular and arterial levels, with blood flow to the systemic and pulmonary circulation determined by pulmonary and systemic resistance is the consequence of truncus arteriosus. In the absence of pulmonary artery stenosis, the normal fall in pulmonary vascular resistance (PVR) results in significant left-to-right shunting, pulmonary overcirculation, and symptoms of CHF. Due to the rapid development of pulmonary overcirculation, pulmonary hypertension and subsequent vascular obstructive, disease can occur as early as 3 months of life. Therefore, the policy of many centers is to perform complete correction during the neonatal period (Grotenhuis et al. 2016). The surgical repair consists of ventricular septal defect (VSD) patch closure, pulmonary artery removal from the common arterial trunk, and RV to PA conduit implantation.

The combination of other cardiac malformations and truncus arteriosus, such as aortic arch interruption, outflow tract obstruction, and multiple VSDs, carries high mortality with high risk of reintervention in survivors (Konstantinov et al. 2006).

68.4.2 Transposition of the Great Arteries (TGA)

TGA is a ventriculoarterial discordant lesion in which the aorta arises from the RV and the pulmonary artery from the LV. (The physiology is described in ▸ Chap. 67, "Cardiovascular Physiology, Pathology, and Clinical Investigation in Neonatal Medicine") Once fetal diagnosis is made, a multidisciplinary team approach helps to improve outcomes. Most infants with TGA are diagnosed shortly after birth. This malformation requires early surgical repair during the neonatal period. Usually, the babies need a balloon atrial septostomy (Fig. 3). Additional medical support is necessary to optimize clinical conditions. A continuous infusion of prostaglandin is indicated to maintain opened the PDA and improve the mixing.

The arterial switch operation (ASO) is the procedure of choice used to achieve complete physiological and anatomic correction. Current indications for ASO in newborns and infants must be taken into account in planning operative strategy, because the optimal time depends on anatomic features such as multiple VSDs or unbalanced ventricles. The key point is the morphologically left ventricular pressure at the time of presentation. Currently, the optimal

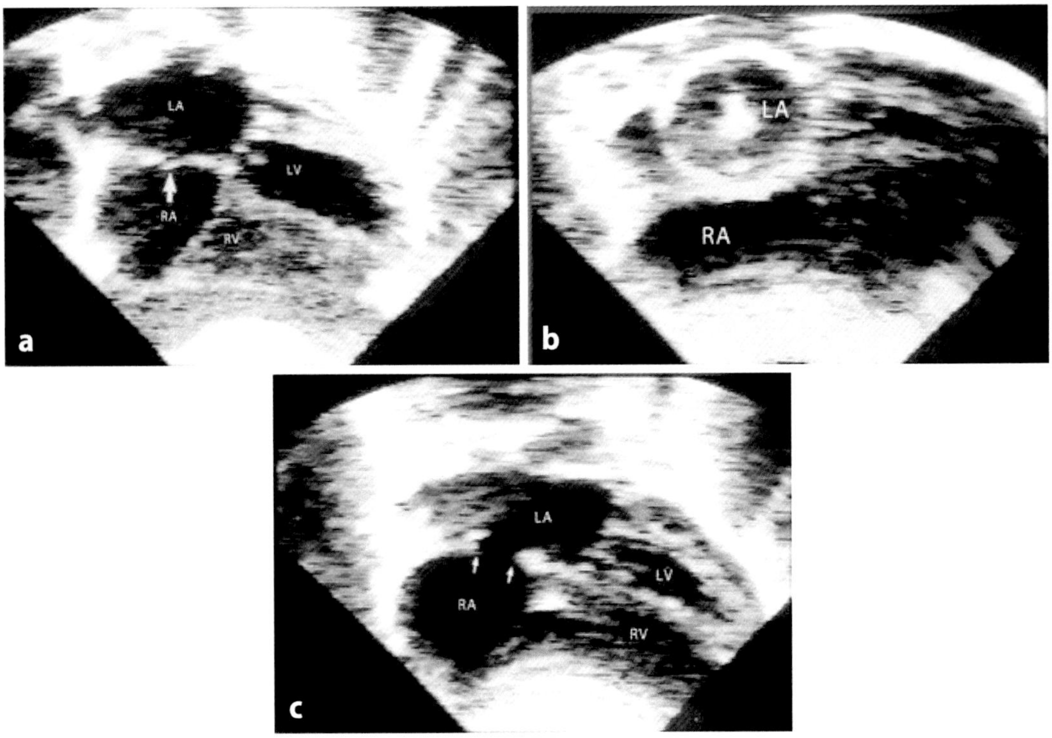

Fig. 3 Cross-sectional echocardiography from the subcostal approach demonstrating the septostomy procedure. (**a**) Short frame demonstrating the interatrial septum before the septostomy. (**b**) Catheter in the *left* atrium across the interatrial septum. (**c**) The interatrial communication (*arrows*) after balloon septostomy. *LA* left atrium, *RA* right atrium, *RV* right ventricle, *LV* left ventricle

timing of ASO for babies with TGA without VSD varies from 5 to 15 days. Occasionally, newborns with TGA do not undergo early surgery because of later presentation, later diagnosis, or both or coexisting medical problems such as septic conditions or necrotizing enterocolitis (NEC). Delaying the surgery allows the LV to pump against the lower resistance pulmonary circulation, determining myocardial deconditioning. In such cases during the postsurgery period, the LV could develop acute ventricular failure requiring cardiac pacing, extracorporeal membrane oxygenation (ECMO), and peritoneal dialysis. It results in a poor outcome. There is benefit in waiting several days after birth to perform the ASO when physiological conditions have normalized. These benefits could be (i) more complete transition from fetal to neonatal circulation, (ii) pulmonary functional improvement, and (iii) kidney and liver function improvement. (23) - However, the possible disadvantages of delaying operation may be prolonged exposure to PGE, longer duration of hypoxemia, and lower cerebral oxygen delivery, and for these reasons, the potential improvements obtained by this delay must be closely monitored. The timing of ASO may be extremely difficult for premature and low-birth-weight neonates.

In the ASO operation, the aorta and pulmonary artery are sectioned, and their distal extremities are transposed and anastomosed; (LeCompte maneuver) coronary arteries are then translocated to the neoaorta (Villafañe et al. 2014). This transfer of the coronary origins is the key to successful ASO. The next step is for the surgeon to close any intracardiac communication.

An alternative procedure is an atrial switch operation (Senning or Mustard operation) leaving the morphological right ventricle in the systemic circuit. Despite the technical difficulties associated with the arterial switch operation and the problems

related to postoperative management, early mortality is now similar to that of the atrial switch operation, whereas long-term results are better for the former procedure (Castaneda 1999; Daebritz et al. 2000; HassF et al. 1999).

68.4.3 Total Anomalous Pulmonary Venous Return (TAPVR)

TAPVR is a congenital defect in which the pulmonary veins drain anomalously into a systemic venous structure (see ▶ Chap. 67, "Cardiovascular Physiology, Pathology, and Clinical Investigation in Neonatal Medicine"). In obstructed TAPVR, correction is usually performed at the time of presentation, especially when the child is markedly cyanotic (da Cruz et al. 2007). In unobstructed TAPVR, timing of correction varies with the severity of the clinical features: generally, babies present with symptoms of CHF later in infancy; at that time correction should be carried out.

68.4.4 Ebstein's Anomaly

Hemodynamic abnormalities in this malformation are related to the severity of tricuspid regurgitation, the size of the functional RV, and the degree of right-to-left shunting across the atrial septal defect (ASD). Ebstein's anomaly may be associated with ASD and pulmonary outflow obstruction. If there is severe tricuspid regurgitation in utero, massive cardiomegaly, secondary pulmonary hypoplasia, hydrops fetalis, or a combination of these can occur (Lang et al. 1991). Ebstein's anomaly has a clinical spectrum that varies from severe cyanosis and circulatory collapse in the newborn to minimal or no symptoms in the child or adult. Once the diagnosis is made, the newborn may require support with PGE1 infusion and nitric oxide, and definitive surgical management is undertaken. For neonates, therapy is tailored to the severity of the malformation and the degree of RV outflow tract obstruction. Surgery may involve ligation of the duct, placement of a systemic-to-pulmonary shunt, creation of a functional tricuspid atresia, or tricuspid valve repair (da Cruz et al. 2007). Mortality is strongly related to severe tricuspid regurgitation and pulmonary hypoplasia.

68.4.5 Right-Sided Obstructive Lesions

68.4.5.1 Tetralogy of Fallot (TOF)

There is a wide spectrum of anatomical variability in TOF with and without pulmonary atresia (TOF/PA). As noted in the previous section, clinical presentation depends on the severity of the anatomical defects, particularly on the degree of right ventricular outflow tract obstruction, the amount of right-to-left shunt through the ventricular septal defect, and the size of pulmonary arteries. Echocardiographic examination provides all the information required to plan surgical strategy (Figs. 4 and 5). Therefore, cardiac catheterization is needed only when the diagnostic dilemma is still not sorted out like pulmonary or coronary artery anatomy and the presence of aortopulmonary collateral arteries.

All patients with TOF and TOF/PA require surgical intervention. Initial medical management depends on clinical presentation, which also depends on the severity of right ventricular outflow tract obstruction (RVOTO). When RVOTO is significant, neonates present with cyanosis, hypoxemia, and metabolic acidosis: prostaglandin infusion should be started to maintain ductal patency, and surgical palliation or repair after stabilization should be planned. Most commonly, palliation consists of a subclavian-pulmonary artery shunt such as the modified Blalock-Taussig shunt, performed without cardiopulmonary bypass. Due to advances in neonatal cardiac surgery, some centers have been performing complete repair during the neonatal period (Lang et al. 1991; da Cruz et al. 2007). Major concerns remain regarding cardiopulmonary bypass complications, associated risk of longer stay in the intensive care unit, neurobehavioral abnormalities (Bailliard and Anderson 2008; Limeropoulos et al. 1999), and anatomical issues. In this setting, percutaneous RVOT stenting could serve as an alternative treatment to a surgically constructed systemic-to-pulmonary artery shunt or ductal

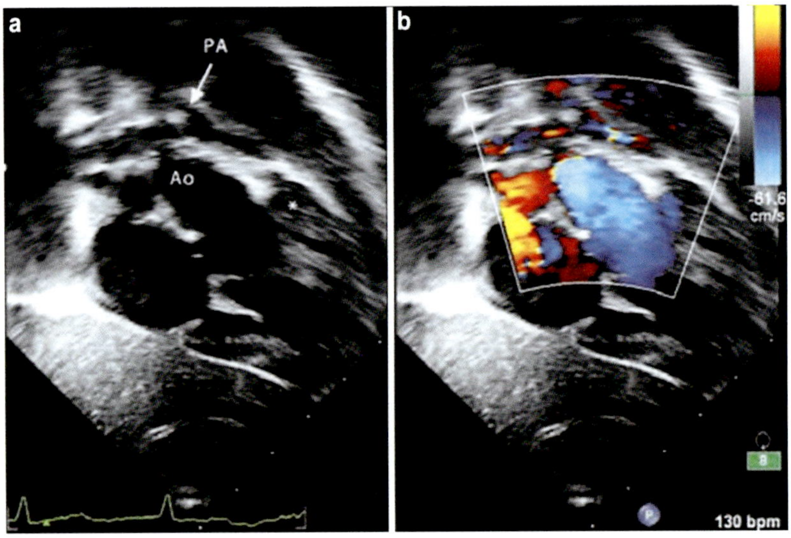

Fig. 4 (**a**) *Right* subcostal anterior oblique view in tetralogy of Fallot demonstrating the antero-cephalad deviation of the outlet septum into the right ventricular outflow tract. Infundibular pulmonary stenosis (*asterisk*). Significant hypoplasia of the pulmonary trunk and pulmonary arteries. Aorta (*AO*), pulmonary artery (*PA*). (**b**) Color Doppler imaging showing turbulence and flow acceleration in the right ventricular outflow tract. The turbulence continues into the pulmonary trunk and pulmonary arteries

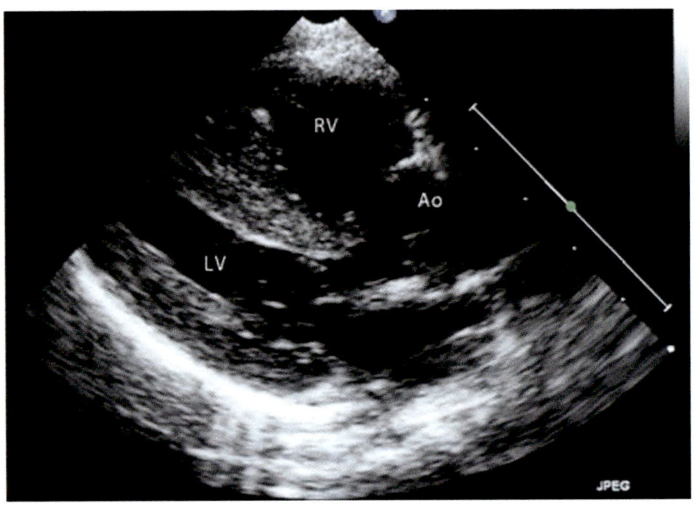

Fig. 5 Two-dimensional echocardiogram (modified parasternal long axis view) demonstrating large ventricular septal defect, aortic override, and the right ventricular hypertrophy typical of tetralogy of Fallot

stenting. This procedure is feasible and achieves increased pulmonary blood flow in a physiological direction with correct pulsating inflow resulting in an immediate increase in oxygen saturation and the patient's condition. Other concerns include VSD patch closure, subpulmonary obstruction relief, and pulmonary artery reconstruction using a transventricular approach (Hirsch et al. 2000; Stewart et al. 2005). The ideal age for complete correction is still under discussion (Tamesberger et al. 2008; Bailliard and Anderson 2008; Nicholls et al. 2006) although it is a common practice to proceed to complete correction within 4–6 months of age.

68.4.6 Pulmonary Valve Stenosis (PS)

PS is characterized by thickened, doming pulmonary valve leaflets with a hypertrophied RV and normal tricuspid valve annulus. In critical PS, transcatheter balloon dilatation is the procedure

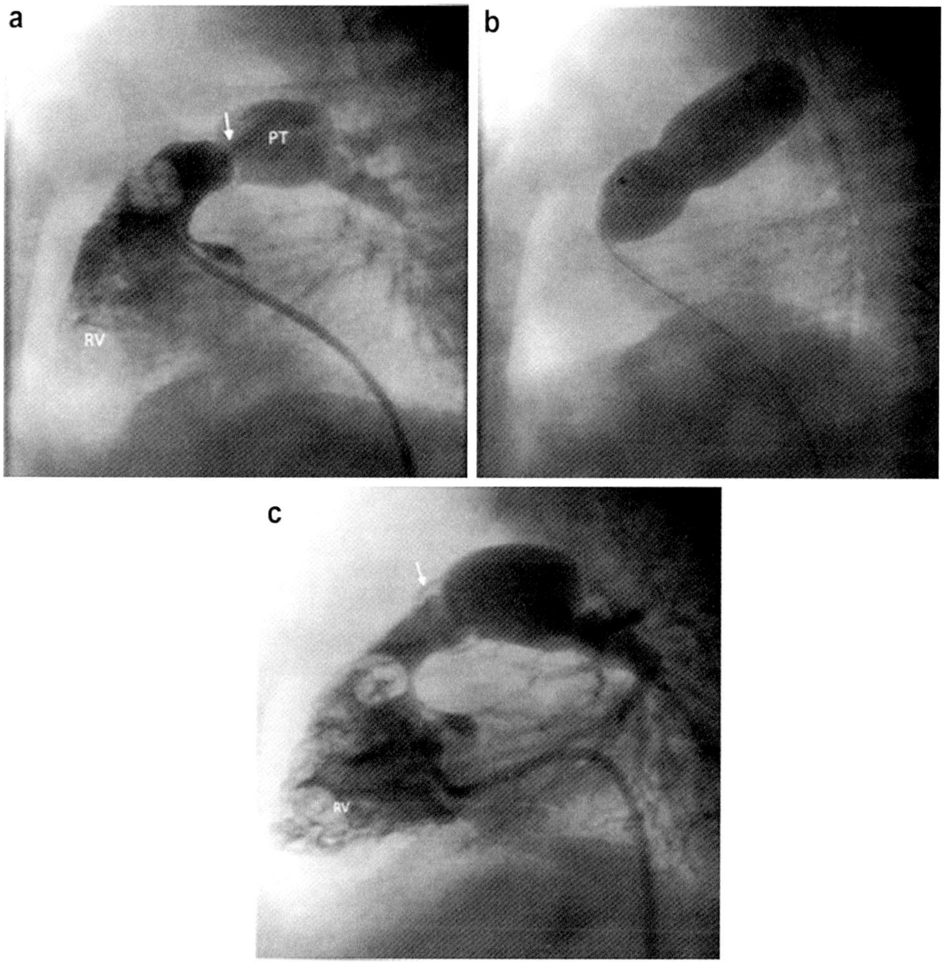

Fig. 6 A right ventriculogram in neonate with pulmonary valve stenosis. (**a**) A lateral view demonstrating systolic doming of the stenotic leaflets and narrow jet of contrast into PA (*arrow*). Right ventricle (*RV*), pulmonary artery (*PA*). (**b**) A guidewire is passing through the catheter from the right ventricle (*RV*). The balloon is inflated with diluted contrast until the balloon "waist" disappears. (**c**) A repeat right ventriculogram showing markedly improved antegrade flow through the stenotic pulmonary valve (*arrow*)

of choice. The procedure is also recommended when RV pressure exceeds half the systemic pressure. Angiography and invasive pressure measurements during cardiac catheterization confirm the echocardiographic diagnosis and allow measurement of the pulmonary valve which is fundamental to performing balloon valvuloplasty (Fig. 6). An oversized balloon, 1.2–1.4-fold the size of the annulus is used. Balloon valvuloplasty is effective and restenosis is uncommon (Stewart et al. 2005). In the presence of dysplastic valves such as in Noonan syndrome, valvuloplasty is less effective, requiring subsequent surgical valvotomy. Quite often, after critical PS balloon dilatation, cyanosis persists due to a persistent right-to-left shunt at the level of the foramen ovale as a result of significant RV hypertrophy and diastolic dysfunction; in this situation, adequate pulmonary flow may be achieved either by keeping the arterial duct open with PGE1 infusion or stent implantation or by performing an MBT shunt between the aorta and pulmonary artery.

68.4.7 Pulmonary Atresia with Intact Ventricular Septum (PA/IVS)

PA/IVS is a congenital heart defect with wide morphological heterogeneity. Morphology varies with respect to tricuspid valve size, RV hypoplasia, infundibular development, and the presence of coronary stenosis or coronary-RV cavity fistulas, called sinusoids. These connections are considered persistent communications, which do not involute during intrauterine life due to the development of RV suprasystemic pressure; they are found in up to 50% of cases (Joshi et al. 1966). Morphological aspects should be investigated by echocardiography and cardiac catheterization. Complete hemodynamic and angiographic study is essential even if a detailed diagnosis is carried out by echocardiography.

Transcatheter pulmonary valve radiofrequency perforation followed by pulmonary valve balloon dilatation is an effective procedure (Fig. 7) to decompress the right ventricular cavity and to reduce tricuspid valve regurgitation (Alwi et al. 2000). Subsequent postcatheterization management may be challenging because of arterial duct stenting, or an MBT shunt insertion may be necessary to optimize the effective pulmonary blood flow.

Another alternative approach could be surgical pulmonary valvotomy with or without MBT shunt at the same time.

Babies with sinusoidal-coronary artery-dependent circulation should not undergo right ventricular decompression as this procedure could cause myocardial infarction due to an acute reduction of RV cavity pressure and consequently in the coronary artery perfusion pressure (Santos and Azevedo 2004). Therefore a palliative surgical approach (MBT shunt and atrial septostomy in case of restrictive ASD) could be a good option for these cases.

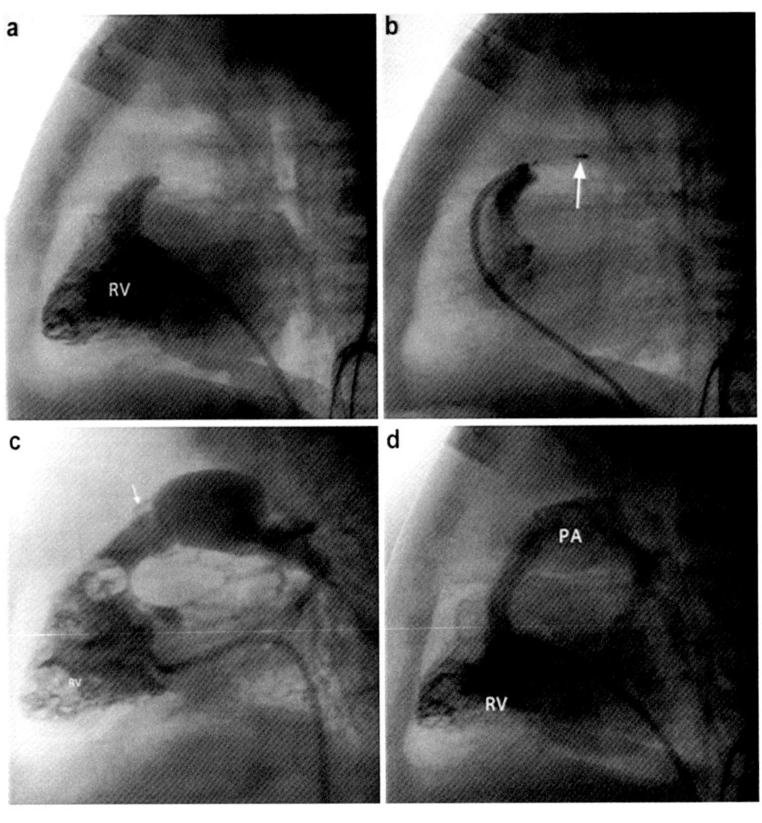

Fig. 7 Transcatheter intervention for pulmonary atresia. (**a**) Lateral view of a right ventricular (*RV*) injection in neonate with pulmonary atresia and intact ventricular septum (*asterisk*). The RV outflow tract ends blindly at the level of the atretic pulmonary valve. No contrast crosses the pulmonary valve plate. (**b**) The lateral view angiography in the infundibulum: the tip of the radiofrequency perforation wire just positioned below the atretic pulmonary valve (*arrow*). (**c**) A balloon catheter submaximally inflated across the atretic valve. (**d**) Injection in the right ventricle (*RV*) demonstrating the continuity created between the RV and the pulmonary artery (*PA*)

68.4.8 Left-Sided Obstructive Lesions

68.4.8.1 Aortic Valve Stenosis (AS)

The treatment of AS depends on the degree of obstruction and the presence of systemic hypoperfusion. Neonates presenting with collapse or congestive heart failure need emergency treatment. PGE1 infusion should be started to maintain ductal-dependent systemic flow. In many cases, inotropic support is also required. The treatment of choice for neonatal congenital aortic stenosis is transcatheter balloon valvuloplasty (Fig. 8). Vascular access is usually retrograde using the carotid artery. However, an antegrade approach using the umbilical or the femoral arteries has been described. The antegrade approach is associated with a lower morbidity compared with the retrograde approach (Maeno et al. 1997; Magee et al. 1997). Balloon valvuloplasty in neonates may be markedly effective; however, limited long-term data have shown development of significant aortic valve regurgitation in up to 25% of patients treated with this technique (Maeno et al. 1997).

68.4.8.2 Coarctation of the Aorta (CoAo)

The most common type of coarctation is located at the level of the isthmus, in the thoracic aorta, distal to the origin of the left subclavian artery. Neonates with CoAo develop symptoms once the duct closes. At that time, systemic perfusion fails, and hypotension and acidosis occur. PGE1 infusion should be given to keep ductal patency and supply systemic circulation as a palliative measure until surgical intervention is performed.

Treatment options vary from surgery to transcatheter intervention. Surgery with coarctation resection and end-to-end anastomosis or the subclavian artery flap technique is currently the first choice. However, balloon angioplasty may be performed in circumstances where the infant is a poor candidate for surgery because of cardiovascular collapse (Kilian 2006). Surgery for neonatal CoAo is associated with fewer reinterventions, improved aortic arch growth, no aortic aneurism formation, and a decreased need for antihypertensive medications when compared with neonates treated primarily with balloon angioplasty (Andrew et al. 2005).

68.4.8.3 Interrupted Aortic Arch (IAA)

IAA consists of a disconnection between the ascending and descending aorta. Clinical presentation, preoperative management, and timing of surgery are similar to critical CoAo. AVSD and patent ductus arteriosus are present in more than 90% of the cases (Fyler 1992). VSD patch closure could be approached either during the same operation or in a second stage after having performed pulmonary artery banding at the same time as IAA repair.

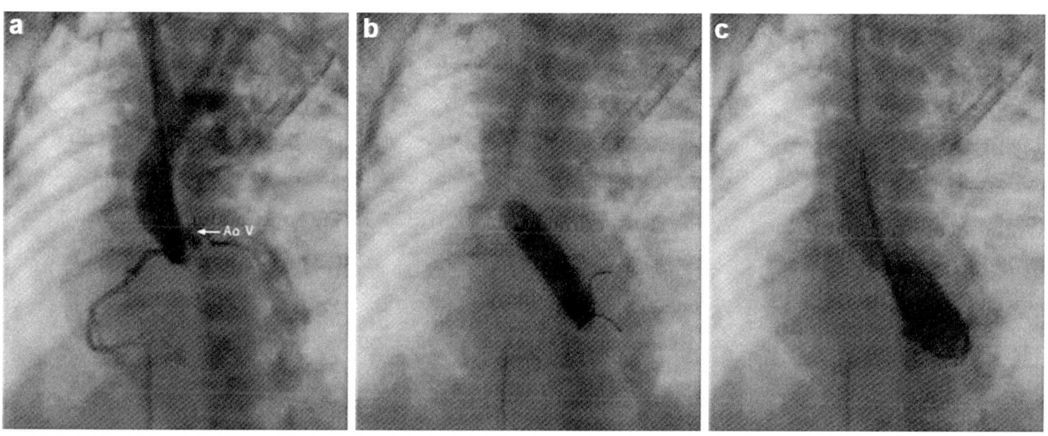

Fig. 8 (**a**) Carotid artery injection showing bicuspid aortic valve. (**b**) Balloon inflated across the aortic valve for valvuloplasty. (**c**) Injection in the left ventricle (*LV*) after valvuloplasty

References

Ahamad U, Fatimi SH, Naqvi I et al (2008) Modified blalock-taussig shunt: immediate and short-term follow-up results in neonates. Heart Lung Circ 17:54–58

Ainsworth SB, Wyllie JP, Wren C (1999) Prevalence and clinical significance of cardiac murmurs in neonates. Arch Dis Child 80:F43–F45

Akintuerk H, Miche-Behnke I, Valeske K et al (2002) Stenting of the arterial duct and banding o f the pulmonary arteries: basis for combined Norwood stage I and II repair in hypoplastic left heart syndrome. Circulation 105:1009–1103

Alwi M, Geetha K, Bilkins AA et al (2000) Pulmonary atresia with intact ventricular septum: percutaneous radiofrequency-assisted valvulotomy and balloon dilatation versus surgical valvotomy and Blalock-Taussig shunt. J Am Coll Cardiol 35:468–476

Andrew CF, Fischer LK, Schwartz T et al (2005) Comparison of angioplasty and surgery for neonatal aortic coarctation. Ann Thorac Surg 80:1659–1665

Bailliard F, Anderson RH (2008) Tetralogy of fallot. Orphanet J Rare D 4:2

Berkley EMF, Goens MB, Karr S, Rappaport V (2009) Utility of fetal echocardiography in postnatal management of infants with prenatally diagnosed congenital heart disease. Prenat Diagn 29:654–658

Bradley SM, Simsic JM, Atz AM (2001) Hemodynamic effects of inspired carbon dioxide after the norwood procedure. Ann Thorac Surg 72:2088–2094

Castaneda AR (1999) Arterial switch operation for simple and complex TGA: indication criteria and limitations relevant to surgery. Thorac Cardiovasc Surg 39:151–154

Chew C, Stone S, Donath SM, Penny DJ (2006) Impact of antenatal screening on the presentation of infants with congenital heart disease to a cardiology unit. J Pediatr Child Health 42:704–708

da Cruz E, Billieux MH, Beghetti M (2007) A neonate with isolated combined aortic and pulmonary valvar stenosis. J Cardiol 116:e13–e14

Daebritz SH, Noller G, Sachweh JS et al (2000) Anatomical risk factors for mortality and cardiac morbidity after arterial switch operation. Ann Thorac Surg 69:1880–1886

de Leval MR, Mckay R, Jones M et al (1981) Modified blalock-taussig shunt: use of subclavian artery orifice as flow regulator in prosthetic systemic pulmonary artery shunts. J Thorac Cardiovasc Surg 81:112–119

El B, Lupinetti FM, Pridjian AK et al (1993) Results of a policy of primary repair of truncus arteriosus in the neonates. J Thorac Cardiovasc Surg 105:1057–1065

Ferencz C, Rubin JD, McCarter RJ et al (1985) Congenital heart disease: prevalence at live birth. Am J Epidemiol 121:31–36

Fyler DC (ed) (1992) Nadas' pediatric cardiology. Hanley & Bel- fus, Philadelphia

Gewilling M, Boshoff DE, Dens J et al (2004) Stenting the neonatal arterial duct in duct-dependent pulmonary circulation: new techniques, better results. J Am Coll Cardiol 43:107–112

Grotenhuis HB, Ruijsink B, Chetan D et al (2016) Impact of norwood versus hybrid palliation on cardiac size and function hypoplastic left heart syndrome. Heart 0:1–9

Hass F, Wottke M, Popper H, Meisner H (1999) Long-term survival and functional follow-up in patients after arterial switch operation. AnnThorac Surg 68:1962–1967

Hirsch J, Mosca R, Bove E (2000) Complete repair of tetralogy of fallot in the neonate: results in the modern era. Ann Surg 232:508–514

Joshi VS, Brawn WJ, Mee RB (1966) Pulmonary atresia with intact ventricular septum. J Thorac Cardiovasc Surg 91:192–197

Kidd SA, Lancaster PAL, McCredie RM (1993) The incidence of congenital heart disease in the first year of life. Am Paediatric Child Health 29:3444–3449

Kilian K (2006) Left-sided obstructive congenital heart defects. Newborn Infant Nurs Rev 6:128–136

Konstantinov IE, Karamlou T, Blackstone EH et al (2006) Truncus arteriosus associated with interrupted aortic arch in 50 neonates: a congenital heart surgeons society study. Ann Thorac Surg 81:214–222

Lang D, Obenhoffer R, Cook A et al (1991) Pathologic spectrum of malformations of the tricuspid valve in prenatal and neonatal life. J Am Coll Cardiol 17:1161–1167

Lim DS, Peeler BB, Matherne GP et al (2006) Risk-stratified approach to hybrid transcatheter-surgical palliation of hypoplastic left heart syndrome. Pediatr Cardiol 27:91–95

Limeropoulos C, Majnemer A, Shevell MI et al (1999) Neurologic status of newborns with congenital heart defects before open heart surgery. Pediatrics 103:402–408

Lincoln CR, Rigby ML, Mercanti C et al (1988) Surgical risk factors in total anomalous pulmonary venous connection. Am J Cardiol 61:608–611

Maeno Y, Akagi T, Hashino K et al (1997) Carotid artery approach to balloon aortic valvuloplasty in infants with critical aortic valve stenosis. Pediatr Cardiol 18:288–291

Magee AG, Nykanen D, McCrindle BW et al (1997) Balloon dilation of severe aortic stenosis in the neonate: comparison of antegrade and retrograde catheter approaches. J Am Coll Cardiol 30:1061–1066

Martins P, Castela E (2008) Transposition of the great arteries. Orphanet J Rare D 3:27

Mckrindle BW, Kan JS (1991) Long-term results after balloon pulmonary valvuloplasty. Circulation 83:1915–1922

Nicholls DG, Ungerleider RM, Spevak PJ et al (2006) Critical heart disease in infants and children, 2nd edn. Mosby Elsevier, Philadelphia, pp 755–766

Nichols DG, Ungerleider RM, Spevak PJ et al (eds) (2006) Critical heart disease in infants and children, 2nd edn. Philadelphia, Mosby Elsevier

ParK M (2002) Pediatric cardiology for practitioners, 4th edn. CV Mosby, St. Louis

Rao S (2005) Diagnosis and management of acyanotic heart disease. Part 1: obstructive lesions. Indian J Pediatr 72:495–502

Santoro G, Palladino MT, Russo G, Calabrò R (2008a) Neonatal patent ductus arteriosus recanalization and stenting in critical Ebstein's anomaly. Pediatr Cardiol 29:176–179

Santoro G, Gaio G, Palladino MT et al (2008b) Stenting of the arterial duct in newborns with duct-dependent pulmonary circulation. Heart 94:925–929

Santos MA, Azevedo VMP (2004) Angiographic morphologic characteristics in pulmonary atresia with ventricular septum. Arq Bras Cardiol 82:5

Silove ED (1994) Assessment and management of congenital heart disease in the newborn by the district Paediatrician. Arch Dis Child 70:F71–F74

Stewart RD, Backer CL, Young L, Mavroudis C (2005) Tetralogy of fallot: results of a pulmonary valve-sparing strategy. Ann Thorac Surg 80:1431–1439

Tamesberger MI, Lechner E, Mair R et al (2008) Early primary repair of tetralogy of fallot in neonates and infants less than four months of age. Ann Thorac Surg 86:1928–1935

Tworetzky W, McElhinney DB, Reddy VM et al (2001) Improved surgical outcome after fetal diagnosis of hypoplastic left heart syndrome. Circulation 103:1269–1273

Villafañe J, Lantin-Hermoso R, Tweddell JS et al (2014) D-transposition of the great arteries. The current era of the arterial switch operation. J Am College Cardiol 64:498–511

Wren C, Richmond S, Donaldson L (1999) Presentation of congenital heart disease in infancy: implications for routine examination. Arch Dis Child Fetal Neonatal Ed 80:49–53

Patent Ductus Arteriosus

69

Bart Van Overmeire

Contents

Abstract

Patent ductus arteriosus (PDA) continues to be a frequent complication of extremely premature birth, despite the more generalized use of antenatal steroids, postnatal surfactant administration, and the improvement of noninvasive ventilatory strategies. Its incidence is inversely related to gestational age, such that it affects almost 60% of infants less than 28 weeks' gestation. Spontaneous closure of the ductus occurs in 30% of infants with very low birth weight (<1500 g). When the PDA is hampering the neonate's well-being, judicious evaluation and tailoring of the best therapeutic strategy should be performed. Ibuprofen actually seems to be the preferred drug for pharmacological treatment because of its favorable risk/benefit ratio; the therapeutic response of the most immature infants however is limited. Surgical ligation of the duct should be considered as a backup treatment due to the risks of serious complications during and after the procedure.

B. Van Overmeire (✉)
Neonatology Service, Erasmus Hospital Université Libre de Bruxelles, Brussels, Belgium

G. Buonocore et al. (eds.), *Neonatology*,
https://doi.org/10.1007/978-3-319-29489-6_219

69.1 Salient Points

- PDA continues to be a frequent complication of extremely premature birth (60% of infants less than 28 weeks' gestation), despite the more generalized use of antenatal steroids, postnatal surfactant administration, and the improvement of noninvasive ventilatory strategies.
- A large left to right shunt may cause profound hemodynamic disturbances to local organs and the brain.
- Ibuprofen actually seems to be the preferred drug for pharmacological treatment because of its favorable risk/benefit ratio; the therapeutic response of the most immature infants however is limited.
- Surgical ligation of the duct should be considered as a backup treatment due to the risks of serious complications during and after the procedure.

69.2 Epidemiology

Patent ductus arteriosus (PDA) is the most common cardiac abnormality of the preterm infant. Its incidence is inversely related to gestational age, such that it affects almost 60% of infants less than 28 weeks' gestation. Data published in 2007 demonstrated that spontaneous closure of the ductus occurs in 30% of infants with birthweights below 1500 g (very low birth weight [VLBW]) (Fanaroff et al. 2007). It is obvious that percentages are decreasing for each lower birthweight category (Table 1), but also that a markedly wide variation exists among centers. This may reflect the influence of varying factors on the closure of the ductus.

Higher closing rates, and as a consequence lower incidences of PDA, have been reported in several papers for European infants. A randomized comparative multicenter trial that compared early (day 3) versus late (day 7) indomethacin treatment for PDA in preterm infants with gestational ages between 26 and 31 weeks and suffering from respiratory distress syndrome (RDS), revealed that 281 of 380 (74%) spontaneously closed their duct by the age of 7 days (Overmeire et al. 2001a). In 210 infants who received placebo

Table 1 Closed or non-symptomatic PDA among VLBW infants surviving >12 h

501–750 g	750–1000 g	1001–1250 g	1251–1500 g
n = 4,046	n = 4,266	n = 4,557	n = 5,284
51 (17–80)	62 (40–89)	77 (52–91)	87 (67–93)

Data expressed as % (center range) from (Fanaroff et al. 2007)

Table 2 Spontaneous closure of PDA in 210 VLBW infants

Birthweight (g)	Closed ductus (%)	Gestational age (w)	Closed ductus (%)
500–750	44	24–25	54
751–1000	62	26–27	54
1001–1250	60	28–29	60
1251–1500	74	30–31	79

Data from (Overmeire et al. 2004a)

in a double blind randomized trial of ibuprofen prophylaxis, high spontaneous closing rates on the 3rd to 4th day of life were confirmed by echocardiographic assessment (Overmeire et al. 2004a). Data are displayed for five birthweight and gestational age categories (Table 2).

Data from the neonatal registry of the Belgian college of physicians, demonstrate a closed or non-symptomatic PDA in 46.7% of 2635 VLBW infants for the years 2007–2009 (College of Physicians for the Mother and Newborn, Section Neonatology). As compared to these numbers, the closure rates described by Koch et al (2006) in the United States seem lower, e.g., 34% on the third day of life in a group of 122 infants with birth weights below 1000 g. Other US data report 31% closure below 1000 g and 67% in a group of 65 VLBW infants (Nemerofsky et al. 2008). It is clear that a wide variation exists in spontaneous ductal closure in preterm infants. In addition to immaturity, which is the factor that contributes most to PDA, various cofactors affect the occurrence of PDA. For many years, the presence of severe RDS has been recognized as a delaying factor for closure (Bancalari et al. 2005), as is the association with sepsis (Gonzalez et al. 1996). Intrauterine growth restriction also affects the behavior of the ductus (Robel-Tillig et al. 2003). The group of Rakza demonstrated convincingly that hypotrophic infants had significantly larger

left to right shunts appearing earlier after birth and needing earlier treatment than eutrophic controls (Rakza et al. 2007). The authors explain that chronic hypoxia in utero may have caused a faster decrease of the pulmonary vascular resistance through the production of higher noradrenaline levels. Additionally, major anomalies of both the intima and media of the ductal vessal wall have been described (Ibara et al. 1994). It is a common belief that excessive fluid administration during the first days of life is associated with the occurrence of PDA. Unfortunately, poor evidence exists to support this view. A systematic meta-analysis on this topic was last updated in 2008. Four of the five included trials date from the era before antenatal steroids and exogenous surfactant therapy and the one from 1999 shows very weak evidence. Nevertheless, the authors conclude that the practice of restricting water intake to physiological needs in preterm infants might be expected to decrease the risk of PDA (Bell and Acarregui 2008). The role of cortisol was highlighted by the studies of Watterberg demonstrating an inverse relationship between serum cortisol levels on postnatal days 3–4 and 5–6 and the occurrence of PDA (Watterberg et al. 2000). It is known that both antenatal (Abbasi et al. 2000; Chorne et al. 2007a) and postnatal steroid administration are associated with lower incidences of PDA (Halliday et al. 2001; Doyle et al. 2010). The prenatal use of NSAIDs as tocolytics has an impact on the postnatal reactivity of the ductus. Indomethacin and ibuprofen freely cross the placenta (Hammerman et al. 1998; Norton et al. 1993). During pregnancy they have a vasoconstrictive effect on the ductus and fetal pulmonary circulation which increases with advancing gestational age. Antenatally induced changes in the fetal ductal wall lead to a decreased reactivity of the ductus to postnatal NSAID treatment with an increased rate of treatment failure (Reese et al. 2009; Soraisham et al. 2010). The use of magnesium sulfate in pregnant women has been associated with a higher risk of developing PDA in extremely low birth weight infants (Moral et al. 2007) and with a reduced responsiveness to indomethacin prophylaxis (Katayama et al. 2010). Other large studies did not confirm these observations (Rouse et al. 2008).

Many pharmacologic agents that are commonly used in the early neonatal period may influence the behavior of the ductus. Although caffeine has no direct effect on preterm sheep ductus' contractility (Clyman and Roman 2007), markedly less treatment for PDA was observed in the group of infants who received caffeine in a large multicenter clinical trial including 2,006 subjects (Schmidt et al. 2006a). In contrast to what was suggested years ago, there actually seems less evidence for a reducing effect of the postnatal administration of thyroid hormone (Osborn and Hunt 2007) and the shielding of the thorax during phototherapy (Travadi et al. 2006) on the occurrence of PDA. The administration of furosemide, by increasing circulating prostaglandin E2 levels, has been associated with an increased incidence of PDA in a study of 66 infants with RDS (Green et al. 1983). Six of seven studies that investigated the use of furosemide in preterm infants with RDS of less than 5 days of age were performed before the systematic application of prenatal steroids, surfactant or fluid restriction. However, a systematic review combining the trials indicated an increased risk of PDA and hypovolemia (Brion and Soll 2008). More recent data on the concomittant use of furosemide during NSAID treatment for PDA underscore the risk of inducing transient renal failure (Toyoshima et al. 2010) but do not confirm the clinical effect of delaying the closure of the ductus (Andriessen et al. 2009; Lee et al. 2009).

Various other frequently used drugs in the NICU may have unexpected vasodilatory actions on the ductus. To date, no clinically relevant effect on the behavior of the ductus has been described by the inhalation of nitric oxide (Schreiber et al. 2003; Askie et al. 2010; Mercier et al. 2010). Aminoglycosides, cimetidine, ranitidine and heparin are other possible candidates with dilating effects on the ductus meriting further prospective evaluation (Reese et al. 2010).

69.3 Physiology and Pathogenesis

During fetal life the patency of the ductus is essential. It allows 90% of the right ventricular output to bypass the highresistance pulmonary vascular bed.

Fetal patency of the ductus before birth and the closure after birth is the result of a balanced interaction of locally produced and circulating mediators, low oxygen tension and the unique structure of the vessel wall. Prostaglandins, converted from arachidonic acid by COX enzymes, play a major role in maintaining ductal patency in utero. There are two separate genes encoding COX proteins, COX-1 and COX-2, and a variant of COX-1 informally termed COX-3 has also been identified (Chandrasekharan et al. 2002). COX-1 is mostly constitutive whereas COX-2 is highly expressed during inflammation. COX-2 has been found to be increasingly expressed in the fetal ductus arteriosus with advancing gestation and is the main contributor to local PGE_2 generation in the ductus at term (Smith et al. 2001). Of the five major prostanoids (PGE_2, $PGF_{2\alpha}$, PGD_2, PGI_2 and TXA2), predominantly PGE2 and PGI_2 have high levels in the fetus because of high placental production and low clearance by the fetal lungs. They are the most potent ductal relaxants.

The increase in postnatal oxygen tension along with a decreased sensitivity of the ductus to PGE_2 as the fetus approaches term, initiate the closure of the ductus (Schneider and Moore 2006). In the term infant constriction begins within the first few hours after birth and functional closure is usually completed within 24–48 h of age.

After the initial functional constriction, a phase of neointimal thickening and remodeling occurs, leading to anatomical occlusion after several days (Clyman et al. 1998). Recent experiments have shown that platelets play a crucial role by promoting a thrombotic sealing and supporting luminal remodeling for the definite closure of the ductus (Echtler et al. 2010; Clyman and Chemtob 2010).

In the preterm infant the closure usually takes longer. The immature ductus has an increased sensitivity to PGE_2 and its constriction after birth is weaker. At comparable O_2 concentrations the ductus of the very immature fetus generates far lower tensions than those observed in the near-term fetus precluding definitive closure. NO synthase expression in the vasa vasorum of the vessel media is further increased and impedes the critical degree of contraction which is essential to elicit tissue hypoxia, initate remodeling and ultimately definitive closure of the ductus (Kajino et al. 2001). This carries an increased risk of reopening. A similar mechanism is believed to contribute to the failure of ductal closure of fetus previously exposed to maternal indomethacin (Clyman et al. 2001). In addition, there is evidence that the major vasorelaxant nitric oxide (NO) plays a role in the very immature ductus. Inhibition of NO synthase was found to exert a greater effect in closing the ductus of the more immature fetus whereas COX inhibition exerted a greater effect in the near-term fetus. The combined treatment with NO synthase and COX inhibitors was more effective than simply using COX inhibitors, but severe side effects precluded the introduction of this approach in clinical practice (Seidner et al. 2001).

69.4 Pathophysiology

Almost all morbidity associated with PDA in preterm infants may be explained by the persistent left to right shunt through the vessel, causing a systemic hypoperfusion and a pulmonary hyperperfusion. In most infants, the heart can cope with the increasing demands by increasing left ventricular stroke volume and heart rate.

69.4.1 Pulmonary Effects

The lungs receive an increased perfusion which may lead to decreased lung compliance, lung edema, and increased risk of pulmonary hemorrhage (Stefano et al. 1991; McCurnin et al. 2008). Symptoms and signs appear as the limits of compensatory mechanisms are reached. An association between the duration of the left to right shunt and the development of bronchopulmonary dysplasia has been demonstrated (Marshall et al. 1999), although the simultaneous presence of an infection largely increases the risk (Gonzalez et al. 1996). Unfortunately, in studies of prophylactic treatment of PDA the incidence of BPD was not reduced. This may be explained by the study design, as all infants in the control group were given a back-up

treatment only 1–3 days after the randomization. Alternatively, indomethacin may promote BPD in itself by inducing moderate renal dysfunction leading to increased lung fluid (Schmidt et al. 2006b). Experiments in baboons confirmed that a negative influence of a moderate left to right shunt increases clearly pulmonary to systemic flow ratio and exerts a negative effect on pulmonary mechanics. The most striking observation was an arrested alveolar growth and a reduced alveolar branching causing a significantly lower alveolar surface area and complexicity in the subjects that were exposed to persisted shunting (McCurnin et al. 2008).

69.4.2 Systemic Effects

Other organ systems may suffer hypoperfusion, including the gut, kidneys and the brain. A persistent patency of the ductus has been shown to be a risk factor for increased mortality. (Brooks et al. 2005; Noori et al. 2009). Disturbances in renal perfusion have been shown (Romagnoli et al. 2000). The decrease in mesenteric blood flow (Meyers et al. 1991; McCurnin and Clyman 2008) has been associated with increased risk of gut ischemia, necrotizing enterocolitis (Coombs et al. 1990), and causing a prolonged interval to full feeds (Patole et al. 2007). In infants with PDA the superior mesenteric artery flow velocities were significantly lower postprandially as compared to those with closed duct (McCurnin and Clyman 2008).

69.4.3 Cerebral Effects

Already in the early 1980s hypoperfusion of the neonatal brain as a result of ductal left to right shunt was demonstrated by Doppler flow studies (Perlman et al. 1981) and confirmed repeatedly on many occasions with other imaging techniques (Lundell et al. 1986; Shortland et al. 1990).

More recently, an impressive lowering of the regional oxygen saturation in the brain could be visualized in infants with a moderate ductal shunt by use of near infrared spectroscopy (NIRS), and a prompt amelioration after closure of the ductus (Lemmers et al. 2008). Although PDA has been clearly associated with all above-mentioned morbidities, in many situations, its causal role is not straightforward.

69.5 Pharmacological Treatment

Because left to right shunt through the ductus is associated with increased morbidity and mortality and because prostaglandins play a major role in patency of the ductus, for decades cyclooxygenase inhibitors have been used to treat PDA (Evans 2003). Successful closure of the duct has been reported to occur in 40–80% of treated infants. The risk of reopening increases to above 20% in the smallest infants. Because the process of intimal cushion formation during closure of the duct is inhibited by blockade of prostaglandins in the most immature infants, COX inhibitors are paradoxically less effective in extremely preterm neonates (Yokoyama et al. 2006; Ivey and Srivastava 2006). Until 2004, indomethacin was the only COX inhibitor approved for treatment of PDA in most countries. Since late 1990s ibuprofen has been studied as an alternative for the treatment and prophylaxis of PDA.

The decision to start with pharmacological treatment in an individual infant depends on many factors. It is obvious that if factors in favor of a spontaneous closure of the duct are present, many clinicians will postpone pharmacological treatment by a few days. The appearance of signs and symptoms in the lungs or other organ systems should motivate to the initiation of more prompt treatment.

Schematically, three approaches are possible. Firstly, a conservative management with restriction of fluids combined with optimized respiratory support including positive end expiratory pressure; secondly, the pharmacological treatment with either ibuprofen or indomethacin; and finally surgical ligation of the ductus. Benefits and risks of each approach should be balanced, taken into account the specific characteristics of the infant such as birth weight, postnatal age, antenatal exposure to corticosteroids or NSAIDs, and the presence of comorbidities or infection.

69.5.1 Hemodynamic Significance of the PDA-Shunt

Because invasive catheterization is not possible in small preterm infants, echocardiographic assessment is the method of choice to evaluate ductal patency and magnitude of PDA shunting (Kluckow et al. 2008). The technique allows monitoring the effects of intervention and has been used to guide both doses and the duration of pharmacological treatment (Sperandio et al. 2005; Carmo et al. 2009; Waal and Kluckow 2010). It is generally accepted that a left atrium-to-aortic-root diameter ratio of $\geq$1.4 in the parasternal long axis view, a ductal diameter of 1.4 mm/kg body weight, and flow reversal in diastole in the descending aorta, indicate a hemodynamically significant left to right shunt (El Hajjar et al. 2005). When the mean end diastolic flow velocity in the left pulmonary artery exceeds 0,2 m/s, there needs to be an additional high index of suspicion of significant left to right shunt (Sehgal and McNamara 2009).

Because frequent echocardiographic studies may destabilize the infant and in some NICUs it is not easy to obtain a bedside cardiac ultrasound, biomarkers such as B-type natriuretic peptide (BNP), NT-pro-BNP and cardiac troponin T (cTNT) are now more frequently used to detect "symptomatic" PDA and to guide treatment (Holmström et al. 2001; Choi et al. 2005; Sanjeev et al. 2005; Attridge et al. 2009). BNP is a vasoregulatory peptide that is released by the ventricles in response to increases in cardiac volume and pressure (El-Khuffash and Molloy 2008). BNP levels did correlate very well with the magnitude of the left to right shunt as examined by echocardiography and reflected the moment of closure. Nevertheless, the high variability in the BNP measurements preclude their use as monitoring for changes in shunt magnitude (Chen et al. 2010). The combination of measurement of biomarkers as a screening tool in those centers where echocardiography is not readily available, a high clinical suspicion and a comprehensive cardiac ultrasound and Doppler assessment, is probably an optimal approach to guide timely treatment of PDA (Chiruvolu et al. 2009).

69.5.2 Prophylaxis

A vast amount of studies have investigated the timing of pharmacological treatment of PDA. Prophylactic, early pre-symptomatic and symptomatic treatment strategies have been compared (Clyman 1996). More than 30 studies and reviews addressed prophylaxis with non-steroidal anti-inflammatory drugs (NSAIDs) in preterm infants. The last updated meta-analyses available demonstrate that both prophylactic indomethacin and ibuprofen reduce significantly the risk of developing a symptomatic PDA and the need for ductal ligation (Ohlsson and Shah 2011; Fowlie et al. 2010). Nineteen prophylactic indomethacin trials were eligible in which 2,872 infants were included. The incidence of symptomatic PDA was very significantly reduced: typical relative risk (RR) 0.44; 95% confidence interval (CI) 0.38–0.50. In the studies eligible for the ibuprofen review the ductus had closed spontaneously in 58% of the infants of the control group by the third day of life. Based on available data the prophylactic administration of ibuprofen cannot be recommended. Indomethacin offers the additional effect of reducing the occurrence of intraventricular hemorrhage (IVH) (typical RR 0.66 95% CI 0.53–0.82). No positive effect on any other outcome parameter could be demonstrated. In particular, no decrease in the rates of bronchopulmonary dysplasia, death, necrotizing enterocolitis, or white matter disease. Notwithstanding the decrease of IVH, no improved neurodevelopmental outcome has been demonstrated (Fowlie et al. 2010; Schmidt et al. 2001).

69.5.3 Treatment

Indomethacin and ibuprofen have also been extensively studied for the treatment of PDA. Ibuprofen disturbs significantly less regional circulations, which may offer less dysfunction of kidney, intestines, and brain (Overmeire et al. 1997; Patel et al. 2000; Pezzati et al. 1999). Urine production was less affected in preterm infants (n = 148) that were treated on day 2–3 of life with ibuprofen than in those receiving

indomethacin (Overmeire et al. 2000). This observation resulted in ibuprofen being introduced for clinical use in preterm infants. Necrotizing enterocolitis was diagnosed twice as often in the indomethacin group (8 versus 4; $p = 0{,}37$) (Overmeire et al. 2000). Cerebral oxygen availability has repeatedly been shown to be less affected with ibuprofen (Patel et al. 2000; Mosca et al. 1997). Systematic reviews of the trials that evaluated indomethacin or ibuprofen for early treatment of a non-symptomatic or symptomatic PDA confirmed a comparable efficacy of both drugs (Thomas et al. 2005). The most recently updated systematic meta-analysis included 20 studies (Ohlsson et al. 2010). There was no statistically significant difference between indomethacin and ibuprofen efficacy or in failure to close the ductus in 19 comparative studies including 956 infants with a typical relative risk (RR) of 0.94 (95% CI 0.76–1.17). Infants receiving ibuprofen treatment have less evidence of transient renal failure and less risk of developing necrotizing enterocolitis: 15 studies including 865 infants; typical RR 0.68 (95% CI 0.47–0.99). No other differences were noted, e.g., mortality, reopening of the ductus, need for ligation, duration of ventilatory support, duration of supplementary oxygen and development of BPD.

The conventional doses of indomethacin and ibuprofen are different, based on their respective pharmacokinetic parameters. Adapted dosing schemes have been tried to augment efficacy/side effect ratio of indomethacin, however, with variable success (Herrera et al. 2007) (see also section "NSAID Dosing Schemes").

69.5.4 Risks of Treatment

Indomethacin and ibuprofen are not devoid of adverse drug reactions. Due to their vasoconstrictive effects, both drugs affect the perfusion of various organ systems to a certain extent, e.g., the gut, kidney and brains. Although ibuprofen initially seemed to have a more favorable safety profile with less disturbance of regional circulations (Overmeire et al. 1997, 2000; Patel et al. 2000; Pezzati et al. 1999; Mosca et al. 1997), the occurrence of unexpected hypoxemia caused a lot of concern. Acute pulmonary hypertension developed in three preterm infants immediately after the infusion of ibuprofen THAM-buffered solution (Gournay et al. 2002). A clear explanation for this phenomenon is lacking. One infant of 169 treated with ibuprofen-lysine presented the same adverse effect, but no causal relationship could be found between PPHN and ibuprofen-lysine in another 229 treated infants (Overmeire et al. 2004a; Mosca et al. 2002; Aranda et al. 2009). Additional studies could not confirm a clear association between the use of ibuprofen-lysine and severe hypoxemia. Although the trial that first reported this serious adverse effect was halted by the national authorities (Gournay et al. 2004), the ibuprofen formulation under investigation became registered for clinical use in Europe in 2004. Ibuprofen-lysine was registered for treatment and prophylaxis of PDA in preterm infants in the US in 2006. Ibuprofen is insoluble in water and more than 90% bound to serum albumine (Aranda et al. 1997). An in vitro model demonstrated that at higher ibuprofen concentrations (750 μmol/L or 150 mg/L) in infant serum containing bilirubin, the fraction of unbound bilirubin increases fourfold (Ahlfors 2004). This displacement of bilirubin from albumin binding sites may be clinically relevant in jaundiced preterm infants, as high levels of free bilirubin are associated with brain damage, hearing loss and kernicterus (Ahlfors 2004; Ahlfors et al. 2006). When ibuprofen is administered in the recommended dosages of 10, 5 and 5 mg/kg at 24 hourly intervals to neonatal infants, ibuprofen serum peak levels of 20–40 mg/L are reached (Overmeire et al. 2001b). According to the in vitro model, an increase of 10% of the free fraction of bilirubin can be expected at such ibuprofen levels. Three smaller studies exploring the rise of unbound bilirubin were rather reassuring (Overmeire et al. 2004b; Amin and Miravalle 2011; Diot et al. 2010).

Additional risks of NSAID use for closing PDA in preterm infants are the occurrence of an isolated ileal perforation, particularly when there is concomitant use of steroids (Watterberg et al. 2004; Paquette et al. 2006). Although predominantly reported for indomethacin, the risk may be similar for ibuprofen as its mechanism is related to microvascular changes and not to disturbances of the

regional perfusion of the gut (Tatli et al. 2004). Increased bleeding tendency has been described after indomethacin use (Corazza et al. 1984), but except for some increased occult blood appearing in stools this does not seem to cause clinically relevant problems. Some neonatal intensive care units are reluctant to continue or introduce enteral feedings during NSAID treatment. Eighty percent of the infants that participated in the European trials of prophylactic and early therapeutic NSAID for PDA were receiving trophic feedings without any apparent untoward effect (Overmeire et al. 2000, 2001a, 2004a; Gournay et al. 2004). The most recent meta-analysis showed that necrotizing enterocolitis is less likely to occur post ibuprofen than post indomethacin treatment (Ohlsson et al. 2010).

69.5.5 NSAID Dosing Schemes

The pharmacokinetic parameters vary widely in preterm infants due to physiological changes that occur after birth. Studies have shown large prolonged half-life for indomethacin (11–36 h) and reduced clearance rate in the preterm infant, both of which reveal marked interindividual variations (Thalji et al. 1980; Shaffer et al. 2002). The volume of distribution also varies and is influenced by the patency of the ductus (Gal et al. 1991). Accordingly, optimal therapeutic dosing is difficult to establish (Guimarães et al. 2009). The most widely used doses for indomethacin are three times 0.1–0.25 mg/kg administered every 12–24 h. The lower dose with longer interval is recommended when treatment is initiated on the first day. The registered dosing scheme for ibuprofen consists of a first dose of 10 mg/kg followed by a second and third dose of 5 mg/kg at 24 hourly intervals.

In order to improve efficacy/side effect ratio of NSAID during treatment for PDA, a variety of adapted dosing schemes have been studied. As it has been observed that PGE2 production resurges within 5 days of indomethacin treatment (Seyberth 1983), a prolonged course consisting of additional indomethacin doses has been tried (Herrera et al. 2007). Unfortunately, no significant benefit for closure rates, not less reopenings or ligations, and no improvement for BPD, IVH or mortality rates has been obtained. A lower proportion of infants with diminished urine output was observed (typical RR 0.27; 95% CI 0.13–0.6) but at the expense of an increased risk of NEC (RR 1.87; 95% CI 1.07–3.27) (Herrera et al. 2007).

The continuous infusion of indomethacin has been advocated to avoid disturbances in cerebral perfusion (Christmann et al. 2002), but was reported later to be less effective in extremely low birthweight infants (Vries et al. 2005). Interestingly, by applying a stepwise increasing dosage of indomethacin based on echographic evaluation, the group of Sperandio et al (Sperandio et al. 2005) obtained ductal closing rates up to 80% without apparently increasing side effects. After an initial standard treatment, subsequent doses were given if the ductus persisted as assessed by echocardio-Doppler. Cumulative indomethacin doses were as high as 6 mg/kg (Sperandio et al. 2005). As the efficacy of ibuprofen at extremely low gestational ages is comparably reduced to indomethacin (Su et al. 2008), the administration of additional doses has been investigated. In a group of 25 VLBW infants that received a second course of three doses of ibuprofen the additional closure was 48% (Lago et al. 2002). Su et al (Su et al. 2008) obtained an additional closure rate of 50% by administrating up to six doses of ibuprofen. Similar efficacy was demonstrated after the first and second course in a study population of 160 infants with birthweight below 1000 g with a cumulative closure rate of 65% (Richards et al. 2009). In order to optimize the efficacy of ibuprofen, an adapted dosing scheme based on postnatal age has been proposed (Hirt et al. 2008). Further studies are warranted to investigate whether an individualized ibuprofen dosing scheme would result in an increased benefit/risk ratio.

69.6 Surgical Treatment

Since the introduction of indomethacin in the 1980s, surgical ligation has been reserved for those infants for whom treatment with NSAIDs fails or is contraindicated (Gersony et al. 1983). Beyond the third to fourth week of life, efficacy of

COX-inhibitors rapidly declines as the patency of the ductus is less regulated by prostaglandins. Ligation then becomes an option, however it remains nonetheless associated with a number of complications such as pneumothorax, bleeding, IVH, chylothorax as a result of thoracic duct injury, vocal cord paralysis, wound infection, hypotension, and left ventricular dysfunction in the days after the procedure (Little et al. 2003; Sørensen et al. 2010; McNamara et al. 2010; Seghaye et al. 1997; Moin et al. 2003). The morbidity rate ranges from 1 to 16% and mortality from 0% to 10%. In a large retrospective study, surgical ligation and indomethacin treatment for significant PDA were associated with a comparable risk for NEC or NEC-related gastrointestinal complications (O'Donovan et al. 2003) but mechanics of breathing significantly improved after ligation (Szymankiewicz et al. 2004). However, there are no recent controlled comparisons between pharmacological, conservative and surgical methods of PDA closure. Only one trial in 1983 enrolling 154 infants, compared initial surgical ligation versus medical treatment (Gersony et al. 1983). No statistically significant difference was found between the groups for mortality, chronic lung disease, NEC or IVH. An increase in pneumothorax (RR = 2.68; CI 1.45–4.03) and retinopathy of prematurity (RR = 3.80; CI 1.12–12.93) was observed in the ligated group. The use of prophylactic ligation cannot be recommended based on the limited current evidence (Mosalli and Alfaleh 2008). Additional data from the TIPP study indicated that ligation of the ductus was associated with a higher risk of BPD, severe retinopathy of prematurity and neurosensory impairment (Kabra et al. 2007). A retrospective analysis of 446 infants showed that ligation was significantly associated with chronic lung disease (Chorne et al. 2007b). In a group of 20 infants, a further decrease of oxygenation of the brain was observed by use of near infra red spectroscopy (Lemmers et al. 2010). No increased brain injury, however, was noted in a preterm baboon model (Loeliger et al. 2009). Because of the associated risks of ductal ligation in preterm infants in recent papers and the absence of recent comparative clinical trials, the primary surgical closure of the ductus does not seem advisable (Malviya et al. 2008).

69.7 Conclusions

PDA continues to be a frequent complication of extremely premature birth, despite the more generalized use of antenatal steroids, postnatal surfactant administration and the improvement of non-invasive ventilatory strategies. Many perinatal factors influence the development of a symptomatic PDA. A large left to right shunt may cause profound hemodynamic disturbances to local organs and the brain. From the NSAIDs studied, ibuprofen actually seems to be the preferred drug for pharmacological treatment because of its more favorable benefit/risk ratio. The therapeutic response of the most immature infants, however, is limited for all investigated COX-inhibitors. Surgical ligation of the duct should be considered as a backup treatment, because it carries the risk of serious complications and destabilization of the infant. Unfortunately, in spite of many studies, investigations and trials, there is no generally accepted and conclusive evidence to decide at which moment and to which infants the treatment of the ductus should be pursued in order to improve their long-term outcome.

References

Abbasi S, Hirsch D, Davis J et al (2000) Effect of single versus multiple courses of antenatal corticosteroids on maternal and neonatal outcome. Am J Obstet Gynecol 182:1243–1249

Ahlfors CE (2004) Effect of ibuprofen on bilirubin-albumin binding. J Pediatr 144:386–388

Ahlfors CE, Marshall GD, Wolcott DK et al (2006) Measurement of unbound bilirubin by the peroxidase test using zone fluidics. Clin Chim Acta 365:78–85

Amin SB, Miravalle N (2011) Effect of ibuprofen on bilirubin-albumin binding affinity in premature infants. J Perinat Med 39:55–58

Andriessen P, Struis NC, Niemarkt H et al (2009) Furosemide in preterm infants treated with indomethacin for patent ductus arteriosus. Acta Paediatr 98:797–803

Aranda JV, Varvarigou A, Beharry K et al (1997) Pharmacokinetics and protein binding of intravenous ibuprofen in the premature newborn infant. Acta Paediatr 86:289–293

Aranda JV, Clyman R, Cox B et al (2009) A randomized, doubleblind, placebo-controlled trial on intravenous ibuprofen l-lysine for the early closure of non-symptomatic patent ductus arteriosus within 72 hours of birth in extremely low-birth-weight infants. Am J Perinatol 26:235–245

Askie LM, Ballard RA, Cutter G et al (2010) Inhaled nitric oxide in preterm infants: a systematic review and individual patient data meta-analysis. BMC Pediatr 10:15

Attridge JT, Kaufman D, Lim DS (2009) B-type natriuretic peptide to guide therapy of patent ductus arteriosus. Arch Dis Child Fetal Neonatal Ed 94:F178–F182

Bancalari E, Claure N, Gonzalez A (2005) Patent ductus arteriosus and respiratory outcome in premature infants. Biol Neonate 88:192–201

Bell EF, Acarregui MJ (2008) Restricted versus liberal water intake for preventing morbidity and mortality in preterm infants. Cochrane Database Syst Rev (1):CD000503

Brion LP, Soll RF (2008) Diuretics for respiratory distress syndrome in preterm infants. Cochrane Database Syst Rev (1):CD001454

Brooks JM, Travadi JN, Patole SK et al (2005) Is surgical ligation of patent ductus arteriosus necessary? The Western Australian experience of conservative management. Arch Dis Child 90:F235–F239

Carmo KB, Evans N, Paradisis M (2009) Duration of indomethacin treatment of the preterm patent ductus arteriosus as directed by echocardiography. J Pediatr 155:819–822

Chandrasekharan NV, Dai H, Roos KL et al (2002) COX-3, a cyclooxygenase-1 variant inhibited by acetaminophen and other analgesic/antipyretic drugs: cloning, structure, and expression. Proc Natl Acad Sci 99:13926–13931

Chen S, Tacy T, Clyman R (2010) How useful are B-type natriuretic peptide measurements for monitoring changes in patent ductus arteriosus shunt magnitude? J Perinatol 30:780–785

Chiruvolu A, Punjwani P, Ramaciotti C (2009) Clinical and echocardiographic diagnosis of patent ductus arteriosus in premature neonates. Early Hum Dev 85:147–149

Choi BM, Lee KH, Eun BL et al (2005) Utility of rapid B-type natriuretic peptide assay for diagnosis of symptomatic patent ductus arteriosus in preterm infants. Pediatrics 115:e255–e261

Chorne N, Jegatheesan P, Lin E et al (2007a) Risk factors for persistent ductus arteriosus patency during indomethacin treatment. J Pediatr 151:629–634

Chorne N, Leonard C, Piecuch R, Clyman RI (2007b) Patent ductus arteriosus and its treatment as risk factors for neonatal and neurodevelopmental morbidity. Pediatrics 119:1165–1174

Christmann V, Liem KD, Semmekrot BA, van de Bor M (2002) Changes in cerebral, renal and mesenteric blood flow velocity during continuous and bolus infusion of indomethacin. Acta Paediatr 91:440–446

Clyman RI (1996) Recommendations for the postnatal use of indomethacin: an analysis of four separate treatment strategies. J Pediatr 128:601–607

Clyman R, Chemtob S (2010) Vessel remodeling in the newborn: platelets fill the gap. Nat Med 16:33–35

Clyman RI, Roman C (2007) The effects of caffeine on the preterm sheep ductus arteriosus. Pediatr Res 62:167–169

Clyman RI, Waleh N, Black SM et al (1998) Regulation of ductus arteriosus patency by nitric oxide in fetal lambs: the role of gestation oxygen tension and vasa vasorum. Pediatr Res 43:633–644

Clyman RI, Chen YQ, Chemtob S et al (2001) In utero remodeling of the fetal lamb ductus arteriosus: the role of antenatal indomethacin and avascular zone thickness on vasa vasorum proliferation, neointima formation, and cell death. Circulation 103:1806–1812

College of Physicians for the Mother and Newborn, Section Neonatology. Federal Public Health Services, Belgium

Coombs RC, Morgan ME, Durbin GM et al (1990) Gut blood flow velocities in the newborn: effects of patent ductus arteriosus and parenteral indomethacin. Arch Dis Child 65:1067–1071

Cooper-Peel C, Brodersen R, Robertson A (1996) Does ibuprofen affect bilirubin-albumin binding in newborn infant serum? Pharmacol Toxicol 79:297–299

Corazza MS, Davis RF, Merrit TA et al (1984) Prolonged bleeding time in preterm infants receiving indomethacin for patent ductus arteriosus. J Pediatr 105: 292–296

de Vries NK, Jagroep FK, Jaarsma AS et al (2005) Continuous indomethacin infusion may be less effective than bolus infusions for ductal closure in very low birth weight infants. Am J Perinatol 2:71–75

de Waal K, Kluckow M (2010) Functional echocardiography; from physiology to treatment. Early Hum Dev 86:149–154

del Moral T, Gonzalez-Quintero VH, Claure N et al (2007) Antenatal exposure to magnesium sulfate and the incidence of patent ductus arteriosus in extremely low birth weight infants. J Perinatol 27:154–157

Diot C, Kibleur Y, Desfrere L (2010) Effect of ibuprofen on bilirubin-albumin binding in vitro at concentrations observed during treatment of patent ductus arteriosus. Early Hum Dev 86:315–317

Doyle LW, Ehrenkranz RA, Halliday HL (2010) dexamethasone treatment in the first week of life for preventing bronchopulmonary dysplasia in preterm infants: a systematic review. Neonatology 98:217–224

Echtler K, Stark K, Lorenz M et al (2010) Platelets contribute to postnatal occlusion of the ductus arteriosus. Nat Med 16:75–82

El Hajjar M, Vaksmann G, Rakza T et al (2005) Severity of the ductal shunt: a comparison of different markers. Arch Dis Child Fetal Neonatal Ed 90:F419–F422

El-Khuffash AF, Molloy EJ (2008) Influence of a patent ductus arteriosus on cardiac troponin t levels in preterm infants. J Pediatr 153:350–353

Evans N (2003) Current controversies in the diagnosis and treatment of patent ductus arteriosus in preterm infants. Adv Neonatal Care 3:168–177

Fanaroff AA, Stoll BJ, Wright LL et al (2007) Trends in neonatal morbidity and mortality for very low birthweight infants. Am J Obstet Gynecol 196(147):e1–e8

Fowlie PW, Davis PG, McGuire W (2010) Prophylactic intravenous indomethacin for preventing mortality and morbidity in preterm infants. Cochrane Database Syst Rev (7):CD000174

Gal P, Ransom JL, Weaver RL et al (1991) Indomethacin pharmacokinetics in neonates: the value of volume of distribution as a marker of permanent patent ductus arteriosus closure. Ther Drug Monit 13:42–45

Gersony WM, Peckham GJ, Ellison RC et al (1983) Effects of indomethacin in premature infants with patent ductus arteriosus: results of a national collaborative study. J Pediatr 102:895–906

Gonzalez A, Sosenko IR, Chandar J et al (1996) Influence of infection on patent ductus arteriosus and chronic lung disease in premature infants weighing 1000 grams or less. J Pediatr 128:470–478

Gournay V, Savagner C, Thiriez G et al (2002) Pulmonary hypertension after ibuprofen prophylaxis in very preterm infants. Lancet 359:1486–1488

Gournay V, Roze JC, Kuster A et al (2004) Prophylactic ibuprofen versus placebo in very premature infants: a randomised, doubleblind, placebo-controlled trial. Lancet 364:1939–1944

Green TP, Thompson TR, Johnson DE, Lock JE (1983) Furosemide promotes patent ductus arteriosus in premature infants with the respiratory-distress syndrome. N Engl J Med 308:743–748

Guimarães H, Rocha G, Tomé T et al (2009) Non-steroid anti-inflammatory drugs in the treatment of patent ductus arteriosus in European newborns. J Matern Fetal Neonatal Med 22(Suppl 3):77–80

Halliday HL, Patterson CC, Halahakoon CW, Behalf of the European Multicenter Steroid Study Group (2001) A multicenter, randomized open study of early corticosteroid treatment (OSECT) in preterm infants with respiratory illness: comparison of early and late treatment and of dexamethasone and inhaled budesonide. Pediatrics 107:232–240

Hammerman C, Glaser J, Kaplan M et al (1998) Indomethacin tocolysis increases postnatal patent ductus arteriosus severity. Pediatrics 102:E56

Herrera C, Holberton J, Davis P (2007) Prolonged versus short course of indomethacin for the treatment of patent ductus arteriosus in preterm infants. Cochrane Database Syst Rev (2):CD003480

Hirt D, Van Overmeire B, Treluyer JM et al (2008) An optimized ibuprofen dosing scheme for preterm neonates with patent ductus arteriosus, based on a population pharmacokinetic and pharmacodynamics study. Br J Clin Pharmacol 65:629–636

Holmström H, Hall C, Thaulow E (2001) Plasma levels of natriuretic peptides and hemodynamic assessment of patent ductus arteriosus in preterm infants. Acta Paediatr 90:184–191

Ibara S, Tokunaga M, Ikenoue T et al (1994) Histologic observation of the ductus arteriosus in premature infants with intrauterine growth retardation. J Perinatol 14:411–416

Ivey KN, Srivastava D (2006) The paradoxical patent ductus arteriosus. J Clin Invest 116:2863–2865

Kabra NS, Schmidt B, Roberts RS et al (2007) Neurosensory impairment after surgical closure of patent ductus arteriosus in extremely low birth weight infants: results from the Trial of Indomethacin Prophylaxis in Preterms. J Pediatr 150:229–234

Kajino H, Chen YQ, Seidner SR et al (2001) Factors that increase the contractile tone of the ductus arteriosus also regulate its anatomic remodeling. Am J Phys Regul Integr Comp Phys 281:R291–R301

Katayama Y, Minami H, Enomoto M et al (2010) Antenatal magnesium sulfate and the postnatal response of the ductus arteriosus to indomethacin in extremely preterm neonates. J Perinatol 31:21–24

Kluckow M, Seri I, Evans N (2008) Echocardiography and the neonatologist. Pediatr Cardiol 29:1043–1047

Koch J, Hensley G, Roy L et al (2006) Prevalence of spontaneous closure of the ductus arteriosus in neonates at a birth weight of 1000 grams or less. Pediatrics 117:1113–1121

Lago P, Bettiol T, Salvadori S et al (2002) Safety and efficacy of ibuprofen versus indomethacin in preterm infants treated for patent ductus arteriosus: a randomised controlled trial. Eur J Pediatr 161:202–207

Lee BS, Byun SY, Chung ML et al (2009) Effect of furosemide on ductal closure and renal function in indomethacin-treated preterm infants during the early neonatal period. Acta Paediatr 98:797–803

Lemmers PMA, Toet MC, van Bel F (2008) Impact of patent ductus arteriosus and subsequent therapy with indomethacin on cerebral oxygenation in preterm infants. Pediatrics 121:142–147

Lemmers PM, Molenschot MC, Evens J et al (2010) Is cerebral oxygen supply compromised in preterm infants undergoing surgical closure for patent ductus arteriosus? Arch Dis Child Fetal Neonatal Ed 95: F429–F434

Little DC, Pratt TC, Blalock SE et al (2003) Patent ductus arteriosus in micropreemies and full-term infants: the relative merits of surgical ligation versus indomethacin treatment. J Pediatr Surg 38:492–496

Loeliger M, Inder TE, Dalitz PA et al (2009) Developmental and neuropathological consequences of ductal ligation in the preterm baboon. Pediatr Res 65:209–214

Lundell BP, Sonesson SE, Cotton RB (1986) Ductus closure in preterm infants. Effects on cerebral hemodynamics. Acta Paediatr Scand Suppl 329:140–147

Malviya M, Ohlsson A, Shah S (2008) Surgical versus medical treatment with cyclooxygenase inhibitors for symptomatic patent ductus arteriosus in preterm infants. Cochrane Database Syst Rev (1): CD003951

Marshall DD, Kotelchuck M, Young TE et al (1999) Risk factors for chronic lung disease in the surfactant era: a North Carolina population-based study of very low

birth weight infants. North Carolina Neonatologists Association. Pediatrics 104:1345–1350

McCurnin D, Clyman RI (2008) Effects of a patent ductus arteriosus on postprandial mesenteric perfusion in premature baboons. Pediatrics 122:e1262–e1267

McCurnin D, Seidner S, Chang LY et al (2008) Ibuprofen-induced patent ductus arteriosus closure: physiologic, histologic, and biochemical effects on the premature lung. Pediatrics 121:945–956

McNamara PJ, Stewart L, Shivananda SP et al (2010) Patent ductus arteriosus ligation is associated with impaired left ventricular systolic performance in premature infants weighing less than 1000 g. J Thorac Cardiovasc Surg 140:150–157

Mercier JC, Hummler H, Durrmeyer X et al (2010) Inhaled nitric oxide for the prevention of bronchopulmonary dysplasia in premature babies (EUNO): a randomised controlled trial. Lancet 376:346–354

Meyers RL, Alpan G, Lin E, Clyman RI (1991) Patent ductus arteriosus, indomethacin, and intestinal distension: effects on intestinal blood flow and oxygen consumption. Pediatr Res 29:569–574

Moin F, Kennedy KA, Moya FR (2003) Risk factors predicting vasopressor use after patent ductus arteriosus ligation. Am J Perinatol 20:313–320

Mosalli R, Alfaleh K (2008) Prophylactic surgical ligation of patent ductus arteriosus for prevention of mortality and morbidity in extremely low birth weight infants. Cochrane Database Syst Rev (1):CD006181

Mosca F, Bray M, Lattanzio M et al (1997) Comparative evaluation of the effects of indomethacin and ibuprofen on cerebral perfusion and oxygenation in preterm infants with patent ductus arteriosus. J Pediatr 131:549–554

Mosca F, Bray M, Stucchi I, Fumagalli M (2002) Pulmonary hypertension after ibuprofen prophylaxis in very preterm infants. Lancet 360:1023–1024

Nemerofsky SL, Parravicini E, Bateman D et al (2008) The ductus arteriosus rarely requires treatment in infants 1000 grams. Am J Perinatol 25:661–666

Noori S, McCoy M, Friedlich P et al (2009) Failure of ductus arteriosus closure is associated with increased mortality in preterm infants. Pediatrics 123:e138–e144

Norton ME, Merrill J, Cooper BA et al (1993) Neonatal complications after the administration of indomethacin for preterm labor. N Engl J Med 329:1602–1607

O'Donovan DJ, Baetiong A, Adams K et al (2003) Necrotizing enterocolitis and gastrointestinal complications after indomethacin therapy and surgical ligation in premature infants with patent ductus arteriosus. J Perinatol 23:286–290

Ohlsson A, Shah S (2011) Ibuprofen for the prevention of patent ductus arteriosus in preterm and/or low birth weight infants. Cochrane Database Syst Rev (7): CD004213

Ohlsson A, Walia R, Shah S (2010) Ibuprofen for the treatment of patent ductus arteriosus in preterm and/or low birth weight infants. Cochrane Database Syst Rev (4):CD003481

Osborn DA, Hunt RW (2007) Prophylactic postnatal thyroid hormones for prevention of morbidity and mortality in preterm infants. Cochrane Database Syst Rev (1): CD005948

Paquette L, Friedlich P, Ramanathan R, Seri I (2006) Concurrent use of indomethacin and dexamethasone increases the risk of spontaneous intestinal perforation in very low birth weight neonates. J Perinatol 26:486–492

Patel J, Roberts I, Azzopardi D et al (2000) Randomized doubleblind controlled trial comparing the effects of ibuprofen with indomethacin on cerebral hemodynamics in preterm infants with patent ductus arteriosus. Pediatr Res 47:36–42

Patole SK, Kumaran V, Travadi JN et al (2007) Does patent ductus arteriosus affect feed tolerance in preterm neonates? Arch Dis Child Fetal Neonatal Ed 92: F53–F55

Perlman JM, Hill A, Volpe JJ (1981) The effect of patent ductus arteriosus on flow velocity in the anterior cerebral arteries: ductal steal in the premature newborn infant. J Pediatr 99:767–771

Pezzati M, Vangi V, Biagiotti R et al (1999) Effects of indomethacin and ibuprofen on mesenteric and renal blood flow in preterm infants with patent ductus arteriosus. J Pediatr 135:733–738

Rakza T, Magnenant E, Klosowski S et al (2007) Early hemodynamic consequences of patent ductus arteriosus in preterm infants with intrauterine growth restriction. J Pediatr 151:624–628

Reese J, Waleh N, Poole SD et al (2009) Chronic in utero cyclooxygenase inhibition alters PGE2-regulated ductus arteriosus contractile pathways and prevents postnatal closure. Pediatr Res 66:155–161

Reese J, Veldman A, Shah L et al (2010) Inadvertent relaxation of the ductus arteriosus by pharmacologic agents that are commonly used in the neonatal period. Semin Perinatol 34:222–230

Richards J, Johnson A, Fox G, Campbell M (2009) A second course of ibuprofen is effective in the closure of a clinically significant PDA in ELBW infants. Pediatrics 124:e287–e292

Robel-Tillig E, Knüpfer M, Vogtmann C (2003) Cardiac adaptation in small for gestational age neonates after prenatal hemodynamic disturbances. Early Hum Dev 72:123–129

Romagnoli C, De Carolis MP, Papacci P et al (2000) Effects of prophylactic ibuprofen on cerebral and renal hemodynamics in very preterm neonates. Clin Pharmacol Ther 67:676–683

Rouse DJ, Hirtz DG, Thom E et al (2008) A randomized, controlled trial of magnesium sulfate for the prevention of cerebral palsy. N Engl J Med 359:895–905

Sanjeev S, Pettersen M, Lua J et al (2005) Role of plasma B-type natriuretic peptide in screening for hemodynamically significant patent ductus arteriosus in preterm neonates. J Perinatol 25:709–713

Schmidt B, Davis P, Moddemann D et al (2001) Long-term effects of indomethacin prophylaxis in extremely-low-birth-weight infants. N Engl J Med 344:1966–1972

Schmidt B, Roberts RS, Davis P et al (2006a) Caffeine therapy for apnea of prematurity. N Engl J Med 354:2112–2121

Schmidt B, Roberts RS, Fanaroff A et al (2006b) Indomethacin prophylaxis, patent ductus arteriosus, and the risk of bronchopulmonary dysplasia: further analyses from the Trial of Indomethacin Prophylaxis in Preterms (TIPP). J Pediatr 148:713–714

Schneider DJ, Moore JW (2006) Patent ductus arteriosus. Circulation 114:1873–1882

Schreiber MD, Gin-Mestan K, Marks JD et al (2003) Inhaled nitric oxide in premature infants with the respiratory distress syndrome. N Engl J Med 349:2099–2107

Seghaye MC, Grabitz R, Alzen G et al (1997) Thoracic sequelae after surgical closure of the patent ductus arteriosus in premature infants. Acta Paediatr 86:213–216

Sehgal A, McNamara PJ (2009) Does echocardiography facilitate determination of hemodynamic significance attributable to the ductus arteriosus? Eur J Pediatr 168:907–914

Seidner SR, Chen YQ, Oprysko PR et al (2001) Combined prostaglandin and nitric oxide inhibition produces anatomic remodeling and closure of the ductus arteriosus in the premature newborn baboon. Pediatr Res 50:365–373

Seyberth HW (1983) Effect of prolonged indomethacin therapy on renal function and selected vasoactive hormones in VLBW infants with symptomatic patent ductus arteriosus. J Pediatr 103:979–984

Shaffer CL, Gal P, Ransom JL et al (2002) Effect of age and birth weight on indomethacin pharmacodynamics in neonates treated for patent ductus arteriosus. Crit Care Med 30:343–348

Shortland DB, Gibson NA, Levene MI et al (1990) Patent ductus arteriosus and cerebral circulation in preterm infants. Dev Med Child Neurol 32:386–393

Smith GC, Wu WX, Nijland MJ et al (2001) Effect of gestational age, corticosteroids, and birth on expression of prostanoid EP receptor genes in lamb and baboon ductus arteriosus. J Cardiovasc Pharmacol 37:697–704

Soraisham AS, Dalgleish S, Singhal N (2010) Antenatal indomethacin tocolysis is associated with an increased need for surgical ligation of patent ductus arteriosus in preterm infants. J Obstet Gynaecol Can 32:435–442

Sørensen CM, Steensberg JN, Greisen G (2010) Surgical ligation of patent ductus arteriosus in premature infants. Dan Med Bull 57:A4160

Sperandio M, Beedgen B, Feneberg R et al (2005) Effectiveness and side effects of an escalating, stepwise approach to indomethacin treatment for symptomatic patent ductus arteriosus in premature infants below 33 weeks of gestation. Pediatrics 116:1361–1366

Stefano JL, Abbasi S, Pearlman SA et al (1991) Closure of the ductus arteriosus with indomethacin in ventilated neonates with respiratory distress syndrome; effects on pulmonary compliance and ventilation. Am Rev Respir Dis 143:236–239

Su BH, Lin HC, Chiun HY et al (2008) Comparison of ibuprofen and indomethacin for early-targeted treatment of patent ductus arteriosus in extremely premature infants: a randomized controlled trial. Arch Dis Child 93:F94–F99

Szymankiewicz M, Hodgman JE, Siassi B, Gadzinowski J (2004) Mechanics of breathing after surgical ligation of patent ductus arteriosus in newborns with respiratory distress syndrome. Biol Neonate 85:32–36

Tatli MM, Kumral A, Duman N et al (2004) Spontaneous intestinal perforation after oral ibuprofen treatment of patent ductus arteriosus in two very-low-birthweight infants. Acta Paediatr 93:999–1001

Thalji AA, Carr I, Yeh TF et al (1980) Pharmacokinetics of intravenously administered indomethacin in premature infants. J Pediatr 97:995–1000

Thomas RL, Parker GC, Van Overmeire B, Aranda JV (2005) A meta-analysis of ibuprofen versus indomethacin for closure of patent ductus arteriosus. Eur J Pediatr 164:135–140

Toyoshima K, Momma K, Nakanishi T (2010) In vivo dilatation of the ductus arteriosus induced by furosemide in the rat. Pediatr Res 67:173–176

Travadi J, Simmer K, Ramsay J et al (2006) Patent ductus arteriosus in extremely preterm infants receiving phototherapy: does shielding the chest make a difference? A randomized, controlled trial. Acta Paediatr 95: 1418–1423

Van Overmeire B, Follens I, Hartmann S et al (1997) Treatment of patent ductus arteriosus with ibuprofen. Arch Dis Child 76:F179–F184

Van Overmeire B, Smets K, Lecoutere D et al (2000) A comparison of ibuprofen and indomethacin for closure of patent ductus arteriosus. N Engl J Med 343:674–681

Van Overmeire B, Van de Broek H, Van Laer P et al (2001a) Early versus late indomethacin treatment for patent ductus arteriosus in premature infants with respiratory distress syndrome. J Pediatr 138:205–211

Van Overmeire B, Touw D, Schepens PJC et al (2001b) Ibuprofen pharmacokinetics in preterm infants with patent ductus arteriosus. Clin Pharmacol Ther 70:336–343

Van Overmeire B, Allegaert K, Casaer A et al (2004a) Prophylactic ibuprofen in premature infants: a multicentre, randomised, doubleblind, placebo-controlled trial. Lancet 364:1945–1954

Van Overmeire B, Vanhagendoren S, Schepens PJ, Ahlfors CE (2004b) The influence of ibuprofen-lysine on unbound bilirubin plasma levels in preterm neonates. Pediatr Res 55:474A

Watterberg KL, Scott SM, Backstrom C et al (2000) links between early adrenal function and respiratory outcome in preterm infants: airway inflammation and patent ductus arteriosus. Pediatrics 105:320–324

Watterberg KL, Gerdes JS, Cole CH et al (2004) Prophylaxis of early adrenal insufficiency to prevent bronchopulmonary dysplasia: a multicenter trial. Pediatrics 114:1649–1657

Yokoyama U, Minamisawa S, Quan H et al (2006) Chronic activation of the prostaglandin receptor EP4 promotes hyaluronan-mediated neointimal formation in the ductus arteriosus. J Clin Invest 116:3026–3034

Cardiac Emergencies in the Newborn 70

Liam Mahoney, Hector Rojas-Anaya, and Heike Rabe

Contents

Abstract

There are a number of different cardiac emergencies that can face the neonatologist. Many of these relate to the initial presentation of congenital cardiac lesions (incidence 6–13 per 1,000 live births). Rarer causes also include cardiac arrhythmias (1 in 25,000 for supraventricular tachycardia) and cardiomyopathies (5–9 per 100,000 infants) which can lead to hemodynamic decompensation in the neonate. Furthermore, iatrogenic injuries caused by interventions can lead to emergencies such as cardiac tamponade. These particular pathologies can present acutely and require prompt treatment by the attending physician. For the purposes of this chapter, the pathologies are split into four common presentations with the aim of providing a practical approach to cardiac emergencies in newborn: shock/circulatory failure, cyanosis, acute heart failure, and arrhythmias.

L. Mahoney · H. Rojas-Anaya · H. Rabe (✉)
Academic Department of Paediatrics, Royal Alexandra Children's Hospital, Brighton, UK
e-mail: heike.rabe@bsuh.nhs.uk

G. Buonocore et al. (eds.), *Neonatology*,
https://doi.org/10.1007/978-3-319-29489-6_216

These particular pathologies can present acutely and require prompt treatment by the attending physician. For the purposes of this chapter, the pathologies are split into four common presentations with the aim of providing a practical approach to cardiac emergencies in newborn.

- Shock/circulatory failure
- Cyanosis
- Acute heart failure
- Arrhythmias

70.1 Salient Points

- Various cardiac emergencies can face the neonatologist. Four common presentations are shock and circulatory failure, cyanosis, acute heart failure, and arrhythmias.
- Many relate to the initial presentation of congenital cardiac lesions (incidence 5–13 per 1,000 live births) but rarer causes include cardiac arrhythmias (1 in 25,000 for supraventricular tachycardia) and cardiomyopathies (5–9 per 100,000 infants), which can lead to hemodynamic decompensation in the neonate.
- Iatrogenic injuries, caused by interventions such as central venous line migration, can lead to cardiac tamponade. The most common presentation in a neonate is sudden cardiovascular collapse, and it can be readily detected on echocardiography via a simple subcostal or apical view. It carries a high mortality (50%).
- The most common cardiac arrhythmia in the newborn is supraventricular tachycardia. When such an arrhythmia has been sustained throughout the antenatal period, the infant may present as hydrops fetalis. A fetal tachycardia detected during labor by cardiotococardiography may be interpreted as fetal distress and prompt the delivery of an infant.

70.2 Shock/Circulatory Failure

Circulatory failure is defined as a state of circulatory dysfunction which leads to lack of adequate oxygen and nutrients to tissues or organs resulting in anaerobic respiration. Its etiology is split commonly into four categories (Table 1).

This chapter focuses on obstructive shock with sudden onset requiring immediate actions. Pathologies in the other categories, while in need of prompt intervention, either may present more indolently or are covered extensively by other chapters in this book.

70.2.1 Cardiac Tamponade

Cardiac tamponade is the accumulation of fluid or air in the pericardial space that causes increased pressure sufficient to impair passive filling of the heart and leading to impaired myocardial contraction and consequent cardiorespiratory decompensation (Iyer et al. 2014). The most common presentation in a neonate is of sudden

Table 1 Types of shock/circulatory failure

Type of shock	Etiology	Example pathologies
Distributive	Abnormalities in vessel tone secondary to the release of inflammatory cytokines, problems with endothelial nitric oxide production, or immature neurovascular regulatory pathways	Sepsis, PPHN
Hypovolemic	Loss of fluid from the intravascular space through blood loss or from movement of fluid to extracellular spaces (e.g., third spacing)	Twin-to-twin transfusion, IVH, DIC, sepsis, NEC
Cardiogenic	Immature or impaired contractility of the heart's myocardium leading to poor cardiac output	Perinatal asphyxia, cardiomyopathy, myositis
Obstructive	A physical obstruction to blood flow from the heart resulting in poor cardiac output	Congenital cardiac lesions, tension pneumothorax, cardiac tamponade

cardiovascular collapse. Classical features such as distended neck veins or muffled heart sounds are often hard to detect in a newborn baby. However, it can be readily detected on echocardiography via a simple subcostal or apical view (Fig. 1) (Iyer et al. 2014). The urgent need for intervention in this condition means that often emergency treatment needs to be instigated before the diagnosis is confirmed.

There are numerous causes of pericardial effusions leading to tamponade (Table 2). The most common cause that will present to neonatologist is secondary to central venous line migration. Thus, cardiac tamponade needs to be considered in any infants with a central venous catheter (CVC) that suddenly clinically deteriorates. The quoted incidence is around 1% of neonates with a central venous catheter (CVC) and carries a high mortality (50%) (Cartwright 2004; Beardsall et al. 2003; Warren et al. 2013; Abdellatif et al. 2012). This highlights the need to frequently image the position of the CVC in neonatal intensive care to ensure they are in a safe position (Warren et al. 2013).

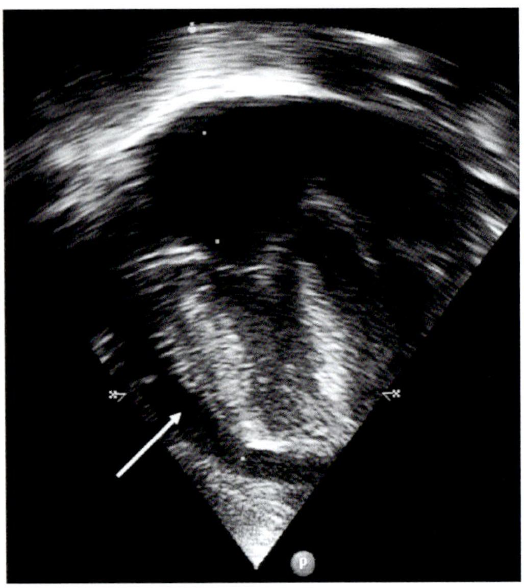

Fig. 1 Cardiac echocardiogram of a pericardial effusion (*white arrow*)

Table 2 Cause of cardiac tamponade

Classification	Underlying pathology
Iatrogenic	CVC line migration
	Chest drain misplacement
Cardiac	Hydrops fetalis
	Myocarditis
	Infectious pericarditis (viral, bacterial, and fungal)
	Pericardial tumors e.g., rhabdomyomas
Respiratory	Pneumopericardium secondary to lung pathology, e.g., PIE
Metabolic	Disorders of glycosylation
	Pompe disease

70.2.1.1 Stepwise Emergency Treatment of Cardiac Tamponade via Pericardiocentesis

- Adequate respiratory and circulatory support as per an ABC approach.
- Attach a venous cannula to a three-way tap and a 10 ml syringe (Fig. 2).
- Clean the skin below the xiphisternum with an alcohol wipe.
- Aim to enter the skin just below and to the left of the infant's xiphisternum.
- Advance the cannula though the skin at an angle of about 30° aiming toward the left shoulder (Fig. 3).

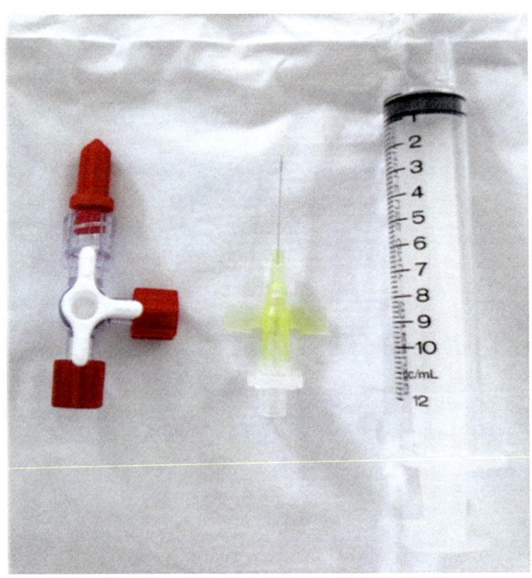

Fig. 2 Equipment needed for an emergency pericardiocentesis

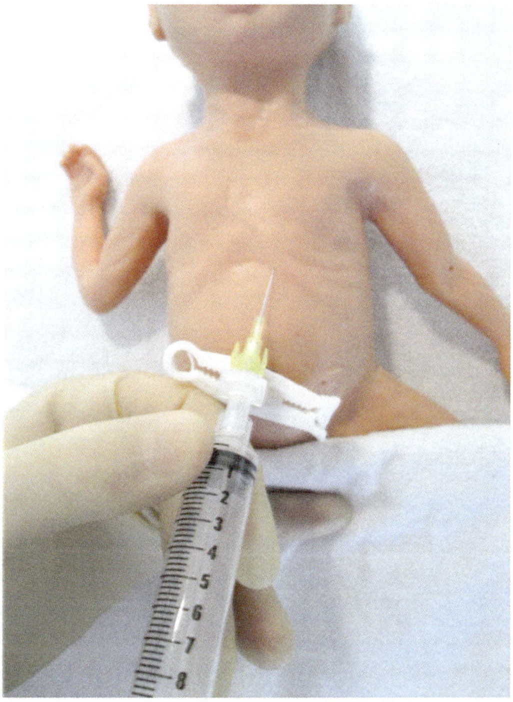

Fig. 3 Insertion point for pericardiocentesis

- Gently aspirate the syringe while advancing the cannula. Air or fluid should begin to aspirate at a depth of 1–2 cm.
- Once fluid or air is aspirated, slide the cannula over the needle so it lies in the pericardial space.
- Gently remove the needle from the cannula.
- With the syringe, aim to remove around 10 ml of fluid or air.
- Secure the cannula and the three-way tap to allow further aspiration if needed.

During this procedure, a marked improvement in clinical condition of the neonate is noted if successfully performed. There is a danger of puncturing the coronary vessels, causing cardiac arrhythmias, or a pneumothorax by pericardiocentesis. However, the baby will be in such extremis that it negates these risks.

Put the fluid gained from the procedure into sterile containers that should be sent to the laboratory to determine the cause of the effusion. Useful tests include red cell count, protein, cytology, glucose, lactate dehydrogenase, gram stain, bacterial culture, fungal culture, tuberculosis culture, and polymerase chain reaction for viral pathogens.

70.2.2 Tension Pneumothorax

A pneumothorax is the progressive increase of an air collection in the pleural space leading to the collapse of lung tissue. It is classified as exhibiting tension when the pneumothorax begins to push the contents of the mediastinum into the contralateral thoracic space. This obstructs the venous return of blood to the heart and cardiovascular collapse. It is estimated to affect up to 2% of neonates in intensive care and is much more prevalent in neonates with underlying lung pathology (e.g., respiratory distress syndrome) or those who are mechanically ventilated (Apiliogullari et al. 2011). Infants with a tension pneumothorax exhibit rapid clinical deterioration with tachypnea, pallor, and shock. An early sign of pneumothorax can be a sudden increase in oxygen requirement especially in newborns on CPAP support. The cardiac impulse is displaced to the contralateral side of the pneumothorax, and there is absent breath sounds with resonant percussion on the affected side. There can also be abdominal distension owing to diaphragmatic distortion leading to displacement of the liver. Infants will be hypotensive and tachycardic. A blood gas will also show increase partial pressures of CO_2. The affected side will transilluminate with the use of a cold light and chest x-ray will make the definitive diagnosis. However, due to the clinical condition of the infant, there is often not enough time to instigate these investigations, and urgent needle thoracocentesis is required (Fig. 4).

70.2.2.1 Stepwise Emergency Treatment of Tension Pneumothorax via Thoracocentesis

- Adequate respiratory and circulatory support as per an ABC approach.
- Prepare a butterfly needle (21–25 G) and a sterile pot filled with sterile water. Wear sterile gloves (Fig. 5).
- Clean the skin over the second intercostal space in the midclavicular line.

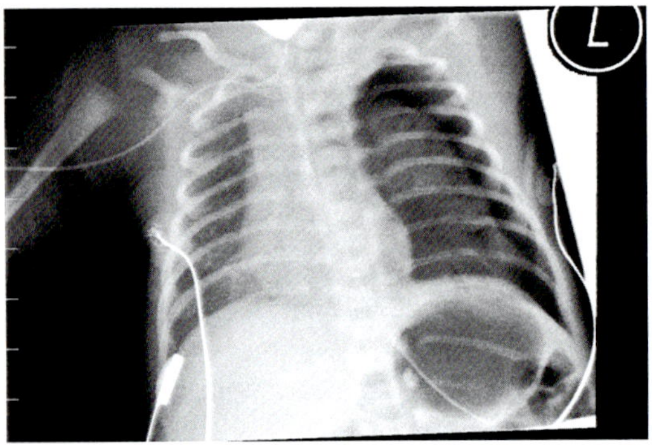

Fig. 4 Chest x-ray of a tension pneumothorax (Courtesy of Dr Neil Aiton, Brighton, UK)

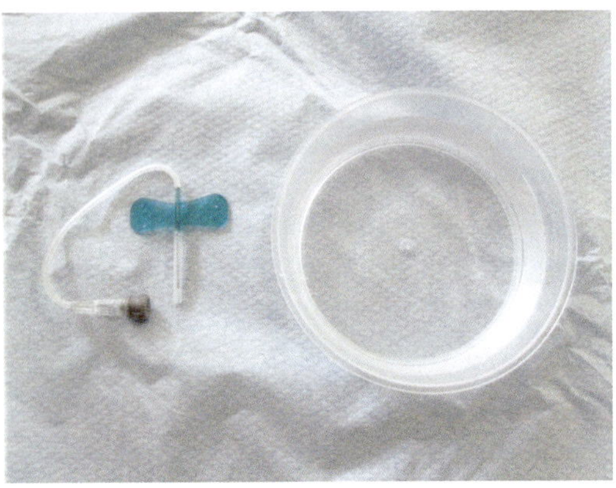

Fig. 5 Equipment needed to perform an emergency thoracocentesis

- Advance the butterfly needle through the chest wall in the second intercostal space in the midclavicular line (Fig. 6).
- The water in the sterile pot will begin to bubble confirming the diagnosis.
- Leave the needle in situ and prepare to insert a formal chest drain in the neonate.
- You will notice a marked improvement in the clinical condition of the neonate.

After treatment of the pneumothorax, it is important to check for intraventricular hemorrhages. A pneumothorax is commonly associated with a marked increase in cerebral blood flow, so when stabilized a cranial ultrasound should be performed on the affected infant looking for intracerebral bleeds (Hill et al. 1982).

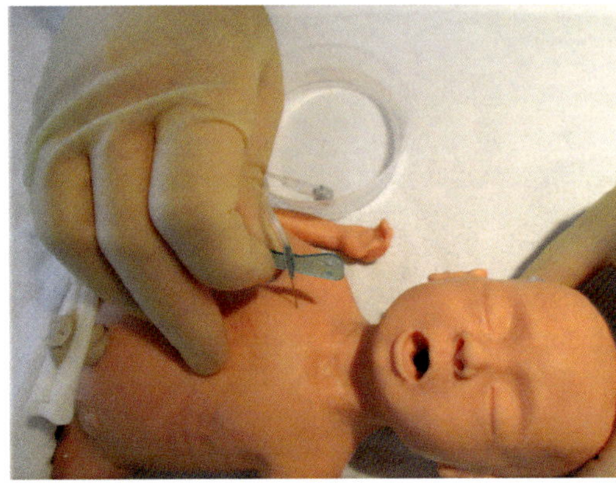

Fig. 6 Equipment pneumothorax position

70.2.3 Duct-Dependent Systemic Circulation Lesions

The incidence of congenital heart disease is about 0.8% of live births. Around 10% of these lesions, if undetected early, can present as cardiovascular collapse in the neonatal period (Hoffman and Kaplan 2002; Pradat et al. 2003; Abu-Harb et al. 1994a; Mellander and Sunnegårdh 2006; Wren 2006). Up to 9% of all infant deaths are due to cardiac causes with 30% diagnosed at postmortem (Abu-Harb et al. 1994b). Duct-dependant systemic circulation lesions are defined as congenital cardiac lesions when the systemic circulation is dependent on the ductus arteriosus being patent. The most common pathologies encountered are coarctation of the aorta (CoA), critical aortic stenosis (AS), interrupted aortic arch (IAA), and hypoplastic left heart syndrome (HLHS).

Many of these lesions can be diagnosed antenatally with fetal echocardiography. However, population studies have found that up 30% are not detected on newborn examination and are sent home with CoA being the most commonly missed condition (Ainsworth et al. 1999; Mellander 2013). Such infants may not be identified on newborn examination as only half of such infants will have a murmur at birth and the ductus arteriosus may be widely patent allowing for adequate systematic perfusion. As the duct closes, the infant will become symptomatic with poor peripheral perfusion. They will be tachypneic,

tachycardic, and irritable. It is sometimes very difficult to discriminate from neonatal sepsis or the presentation of a metabolic disorder. This is further complicated by the fact that blood gases will also show metabolic acidosis owing to a reduction in renal perfusion. But infants who present collapsed with duct-dependant systemic circulation lesions at this point will exhibit a gallop rhythm or murmur on auscultation. In the case of CoA and IAA, the femoral pulses will not be present, and the blood pressure and oxygen saturations will be lower in the legs compared to the right arm in these lesions.

Further investigations such as ECGs and chest x-rays may provide clues as the diagnosis. However, they can be normal. A definitive diagnosis is usually made on echocardiography; however, this may not be readily available and should not delay treatment of the infant. Treatment centers on reopening the duct to improve systemic circulation prior to surgical intervention (Fig. 7 and Table 3).

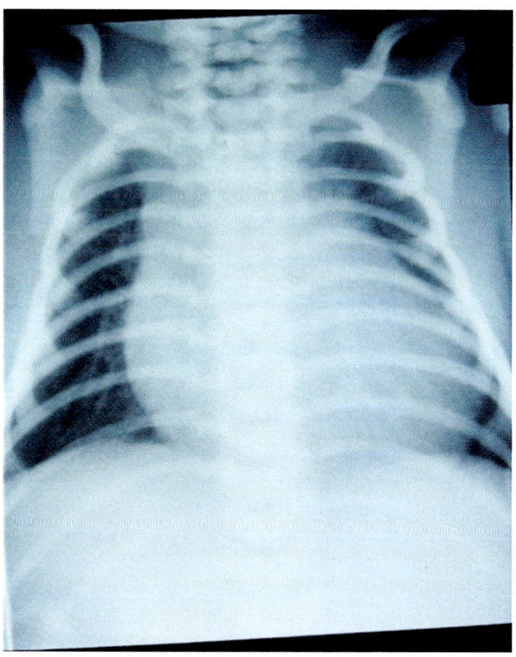

Fig. 7 Chest x-ray of a neonate with CoA exhibiting cardiomegaly and pulmonary edema (Courtesy of Dr Neil Aiton, Brighton, UK)

70.2.3.1 Stepwise Emergency Treatment of Duct-Dependant Systemic Circulation Lesion

- Airway and Breathing
  - Monitor pre- and post-ductal oxygen saturations.
  - Administer supplementary oxygen to reach a saturation range of 75–85%.
  - Intubate if necessary.
  - If echocardiography is not available, then consider using the hypoxia test.
- Circulation
  - Establish IV access (two peripheral cannulas).
  - Consider central access. In a newborn, this is easiest via an umbilical venous catheter.
  - Collect bloods for full blood count (FBC), urea and electrolyte concentrations (U&Es), c-reactive protein (CRP), liver function tests (LFTs), blood clotting studies, and blood gas.
  - Commence IV prostaglandin (5–100 ng/kg/min). Increase until improvements in oxygen saturations are noted.
  - Give 20 ml/kg 0.9% saline to support the infant's blood pressure.
  - If the infant remains clinically in shock, give a further 20 ml/kg of 0.9% saline. Give no more than this as this may exacerbate or precipitate cardiac failure.
  - If still hypotensive, commence central dopamine (5–20 mcg/kg/min).
  - If still hypotensive, consider a second-line inotrope such as noradrenaline or adrenaline.
- Further Management
  - The diagnosis could still be sepsis, so give empirical IV antibiotics such as benzylpenicillin (50 mg/kg) and gentamicin (8 mg/kg).
  - Prostaglandin causes apnea, hypoglycemia, and hypotension. Therefore, the use of this drug at doses greater than 15 ng/kg/min may require intubation. Frequent glucose monitoring is also needed.
  - Chest x-ray.
  - ECG.
  - Cardiac echocardiography if available.
  - Refer to a cardiology center for clinical advice and transfer.

Table 3 Clinical features of duct-dependant systemic circulation lesions

Condition	Clinical features	Auscultation findings	Chest x-ray findings
Aortic coarctation (CoA)	Absent femoral pulses with brachial pulses strong proximal to the lesion	Systolic murmur in the aortic region radiating to between the scapula and gallop rhythm	Normal, cardiomegaly with pulmonary edema. Rib notching can be present
Interrupted aortic arch (IAA)	Absent femoral pulses with brachial pulses strong proximal to the lesion	Systolic murmur in the aortic region, gallop rhythm	Normal, cardiomegaly with pulmonary edema
Aortic stenosis (AS)	Weak peripheral pulses, active precordium	Systolic murmur in the aortic region with an ejection click. Gallop rhythm	Normal, cardiomegaly with pulmonary edema
Hypoplastic left heart syndrome (HLHS)	Weak peripheral pulses, active precordium	Gallop rhythm	Normal, cardiomegaly with pulmonary edema

Many countries have now implemented a newborn pulse oximetry screening program to identify congenital cardiac pathology early. Discrepancies of 3% between oxygen saturations taken in the pre-ductal and post-ductal position or a saturation <95% when taken from the foot has a 99% sensitivity and 76% specificity for the detection of congenital cardiac disease (Thangaratinam et al. 2015). However, CoA, HLHS, and IAA may be missed by such screening methods, even when combined with physical examination (Mellander 2013).

70.3 Cyanosis

This is the bluish discoloration of the skin and mucous membrane due to the reduced amount of hemoglobin that is saturated with oxygen. It is evident when the arterial concentration of deoxygenated hemoglobin is greater than 3 g/dL or when the oxygen saturations are less than 80%. Its causes can broadly be distinguished as either cardiac or respiratory in nature (Table 4).

The hypoxia test can be used to assess further whether the underlying cyanosis is due to cardiac or respiratory disease. The infant is placed in 100% oxygen for over 10 min. An arterial blood gas is then taken, and if the partial pressure of O_2 rises above 20 kPa, it makes respiratory pathology more likely. If the partial pressure of O_2 rises above stays below 20 kPa, it makes cardiac pathology more likely. However, particular cardiac lesion and respiratory illnesses will not always follow the above rule (e.g., severe RDS, PPHN) (Comitis 2011; Enriques et al. 1986). Thus, the hypoxia test should be used as an adjunct for clinical decision making. In cases of cyanosis, an echocardiogram is needed urgently as it will readily diagnose congenital cardiac conditions and will also help in the management of cases of PPHN.

As sepsis and PPHN are covered elsewhere in this book, the next paragraph focuses on the treatment of duct-dependent pulmonary circulatory lesions that commonly cause sudden cardiovascular collapse.

70.3.1 Duct-Dependent Pulmonary Circulation Lesions

These congenital cardiac lesions cause cyanosis due to impeding oxygenation of blood through physically obstructing flow to the pulmonary artery or redirecting blood away from the pulmonary artery. Similar to duct-dependant systemic circulatory lesions, symptoms may not always arise until the ductus arteriosus begins to close. Once this occurs, there is reduced pulmonary blood flow and cyanosis will become more pronounced. This is exampled by the fact that infants with transposition of the great arteries (TGA) can

Table 4 Distinguishing features of respiratory and cardiac causes of cyanosis

	Respiratory	Cardiac
History	Cyanosis present from birth. Birth may have been complicated by meconium aspiration or risk factors for sepsis (e.g., group B strep) may be present	Cyanosis present in the hours to days after birth. Infant of a diabetic mother, family history of congenital cardiac pathology
Examination	Tachypnea, respiratory distress, and grunting. Crepitations and reduced air entry on auscultation	Relatively comfortable looking infant unless the PDA is closing. Auscultation reveals clear lung fields and a murmur may be present
Chest x-ray	Lungs may show focal lung pathology, e.g., consolidation congenital pneumonia. The heart shadow will appear normal	The lung fields may be normal or plethoric. The heart silhouette may be normal or enlarged or show pathognomonic changes (Fig. 8)
Blood gas	High partial pressure of CO_2	Normal or low partial pressure of CO_2

Table 5 Clinical features of duct-dependent pulmonary circulation lesions

Condition	Clinical features	Auscultation findings	Chest x-ray findings
Tetralogy of Fallot (ToF)	Normally asymptomatic at birth. If pulmonary obstruction is severe enough, it will lead to cyanosis at birth	Load harsh murmur in the pulmonary region	Upturned apex (boot-shaped heart) with reduced vascular markings
Transposition of the great arteries (TGA)	Cyanotic and severely unwell when duct closes	May be associated with a VSD or ASD	Cardiac contours show an "egg on its side" appearance
Critical pulmonary stenosis	Cyanotic and can present with sudden cardiovascular collapse	Systolic murmur in the pulmonary region	Normal heart contours with decreased pulmonary vascular markings
Tricuspid atresia with intact ventricular septum	Cyanotic and can present with sudden cardiovascular collapse	No murmur usually	Normal heart contours with increased or decreased pulmonary vascular markings
Pulmonary atresia with intact ventricular septum	Cyanotic and can present with sudden cardiovascular collapse	No murmur usually	Normal heart contours with decreased pulmonary vascular markings

be discharged home as mixing of blood at both the ductal and atrial levels can be so good that cyanosis is not visible to the naked eye (de-Wahl Granelli et al. 2009). Table 5 outlines the clinical features of common cyanotic heart lesions that where urgent intervention to reopen the duct is required (Fig. 8).

70.3.1.1 Stepwise Emergency Treatment of Duct-Dependant Pulmonary Circulation Lesion

- Airway and Breathing
  - Monitor pre- and post-ductal oxygen saturations.
  - Administer supplementary oxygen to reach a saturation range of 75–85%.
  - Intubate if necessary.
- Circulation
  - Establish IV access (two peripheral cannulas).
  - Consider central access. In a newborn, this is the easiest via an umbilical venous catheter.
  - Collect bloods for FBC, U&Es, CRP, LFTS, clotting, and a blood gas.
  - Commence IV prostaglandin (5–100 ng/kg/min). Increase until improvements in oxygen saturations are noted.
  - Give 20 ml/kg 0.9% saline to support blood pressure.
  - If the infant remains clinically in shock, give a further 20 ml/kg of 0.9% saline.

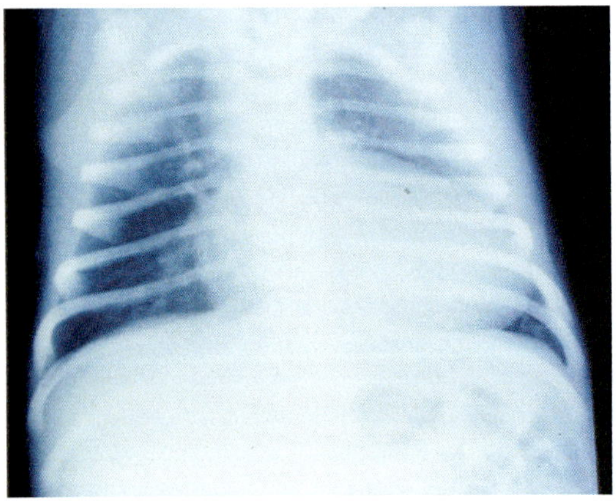

Fig. 8 Chest x-ray showing "boot-shaped" heart of ToF in a newborn (Courtesy of Dr Neil Aiton, Brighton, UK)

Give no more than this as this may exacerbate or precipitate cardiac failure.
  - If still hypotensive, commence central dopamine (5–20 mcg/kg/min).
  - If still hypotensive, consider a second-line vasopressor such as noradrenaline or adrenaline. This will support systemic circulation but may promote left to right shunting of blood across the ductus by increasing systemic vascular resistance.
- Further Management
  - The diagnosis could still be sepsis, so give empirical IV antibiotics such as benzylpenicillin (50 mg/kg) and gentamicin (8 mg/kg).
  - Prostaglandin causes apnea, hypoglycemia, and hypotension. Therefore, the use of this drug at doses greater than 15 ng/kg/min may require intubation. Frequent glucose monitoring is also needed.
  - Chest x-ray.
  - ECG.
  - Cardiac echocardiography if available.
  - Refer to a cardiology center for clinical advice and transfer.

It is important to note that PPHN and methemoglobinemia are also causes of cyanosis. The former can also coexist with congenital cardiac pathology and the latter diagnosis is rare and normally considered after cardiac pathology has been excluded.

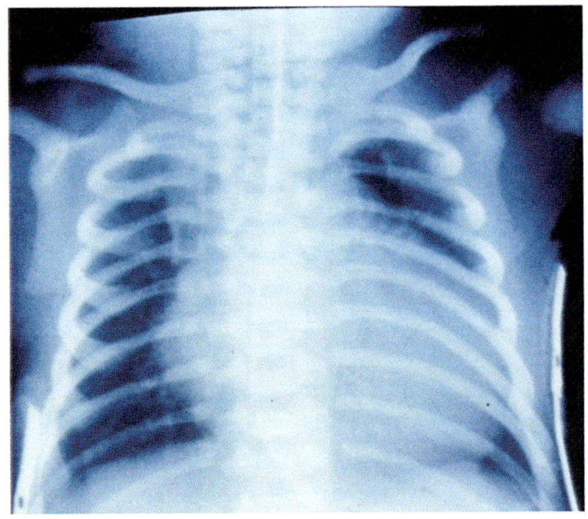

Fig. 9 A chest x-ray of an infant in cardiac failure cardiomegaly and pulmonary edema (Courtesy of Dr Neil Aiton, Brighton, UK)

70.4 Acute Heart Failure

This is defined as a complex clinical and pathophysiological state that indicates impairment of the heart's ability to contract and maintain physiological circulation. Clinical signs and symptoms are associated with tachycardia, tachypnea, bounding pulses, and hepatomegaly (Hsu and Pearson 2009). In neonates, the history may reveal excessive weight gain owing to the development of peripheral edema and an inability to feed due to breathlessness. Depending on the cause, a cardiac murmur may also be found on examination. Auscultation of the lungs may also reveal bilateral crepitations due to pulmonary edema. A chest x-ray can show cardiomegaly with pulmonary venous congestion (Fig. 9).

When looking at presentations of heart failure to tertiary cardiac centers, literature shows that over 50% are due to congenital cardiac disease, followed by cardiomyopathies, acquired heart disease, and then arrhythmias (Massin and Astadicko 2008). This reflects the fact that congenital cardiac disease is more prevalent than other types of cardiac disease (Hsu and Pearson 2009). Table 6 outlines the pathologies that may present as acute heart failure in the neonate. Some of the pathologies are also duct-dependent systemic circulation lesions, so you may need to consider the administration of

Table 6 Pathologies that may present as acute heart failure in the neonate

Classification	Underlying pathology
Congenital heart disease	Ventricular septal defect
	Atrial septal defect
	Atrioventricular septal defect
	Tetralogy of Fallot (ToF)
	CoA
	HLHS
	Patent ductus arteriosus
	Aortic stenosis
	Total anomalous pulmonary venous drainage[a]
	Truncus arteriosus
	Transposition of great arteries (TGA) with ventricular septal defect
Arrhythmia	Supraventricular tachycardia
	Atrial flutter
	Atrial fibrillation
	Third-degree heart block
	Ventricular tachycardia
Heart muscle disease	Hypertrophic cardiomyopathy
	Dilated cardiomyopathy
Acquired heart disease	Viral myositis
	Endocarditis

[a]May also present as a cyanotic infant

prostaglandin when treating a neonate in acute heart failure. The specific investigation of each type of pathology can be complex (e.g., metabolic or genetic investigations in certain cardiomyopathies) and is beyond the scope of this chapter. However, the initial treatment and stabilization of a child in cardiac failure are similar.

70.4.1 Stepwise Emergency Treatment of Duct-Dependant Systemic Circulation Lesion

- Airway and Breathing
  - Monitor pre- and post-ductal oxygen saturations.
  - Administer supplementary oxygen to reach a saturation range of >85%.
  - Intubate if necessary.
- Circulation
  - Establish IV access (two peripheral cannulas).
  - Consider central access. In a newborn, this is easiest via an umbilical venous catheter.
  - Collect bloods for FBC, U&Es, CRP, LFTS, clotting, and a blood gas.
  - Administer IV furosemide (1 mg/kg).
  - If duct-dependent systemic lesion is suspected, consider prostaglandin (see above).
  - If still hypotensive, consider central dobutamine (5–20 mcg/kg/min) administration.
  - If still hypotensive, consider a second-line inotrope such as dopamine (5–20 mcg/kg/min).
- Further Management
  - Restrict fluid intake (e.g., 90 ml/kg/day).
  - Chest x-ray.
  - ECG.
  - Cardiac echocardiography is available.
  - Refer to a cardiology center for clinical advice and transfer.

70.5 Arrhythmias

The most common cardiac arrhythmia to present in the newborn is supraventricular tachycardia (Kothari and Skinner 2006). Cardiac arrhythmias in the newborn period most often present as cardiac failure in newborns (Wren 2006). They may also present with more subtle signs like persistent tachypnea or difficulty with feeding. When such an arrhythmia has been sustained throughout the antenatal period, the infant may present as hydrops fetalis. Incidental identification of arrhythmias may present because of bradycardia (heart rate less than 90), tachycardia (heart rate greater than 180), or an irregularity of rhythm (Table 7) (Davignon et al. 1980; Moak and Hamra 1998). When detected during labor via tococardiography, this may be interpreted as fetal distress and prompt the delivery of an infant.

The relative immaturity of the conduction systems, neurological regulatory systems, and the myocardium makes arrhythmias common. Identification of the arrhythmia is key in determining its origin and appropriate emergency treatment. Once emergency treatment has been administered and the infant has been stabilized, a tertiary center should be contacted for further advice. It must also be remembered that the origin of arrhythmias may be due to abnormalities in cardiac structure, electrolyte imbalances, thyroid function, cardiomyopathy, myocarditis, intracardiac tumors, and also maternal pathology (e.g., SLE). Therefore, after cessation of the arrhythmia has taken place, appropriate further investigation needs to be pursued.

As mentioned previously when presenting as an emergency, arrhythmias often present as an infant in cardiac failure. The stepwise management of cardiac failure should therefore be instigated before definitive management of the underlying arrhythmia is administered. A caveat to this is that ideally a 12 lead ECG should be attached to the infant and a rhythm strip should be running throughout the treatment period in order to get good capture of the underlying arrhythmia and its response to treatment (Fig. 10).

70.5.1 Atrial Tachyarrhythmias

70.5.1.1 Supraventricular Tachycardia (SVT)

There are a number of mechanisms that can lead to SVT. The common factor between them is that the heart is always over 200 beats per minute and usually above 270 beats per minute (Fig. 11).

Atrioventricular reentry tachycardia (AVRT) on an ECG will show a narrow complex tachycardia with a retrograde p wave that is inscribed within the T wave. This occurs because the ventricle is depolarized by the normal conduction system, but it can take some for the electrical impulse to travel back through the ventricle and accessory pathway (orthodromic pathway). Wolff-Parkinson-White syndrome presents with similar ECG findings but also can present with a delta wave (a slurred upstroke in the QRS complex) when the tachycardia is terminated. This is because electrical signals can travel forward and backward in the accessory pathway (antidromic pathway). This forward conduction can lead to preexcitation of the ventricular and thus the manifestation of a delta wave (Fig. 12).

Atrioventricular nodal reentry tachycardia on an ECG will show a narrow complex tachycardia with no obvious p waves as they are superimposed on the QRS complex. This is due to a slow and fast conduction pathway existing in the AV node allowing simultaneous depolarization of the atria

Table 7 Normal values for heart rate and ECG intervals for a newborn

Heart rate	PR interval (seconds)	QRS interval (ms)	Cardiac axis (degrees)
90–180	0.072–0.14	0.02–0.079	+60–+190

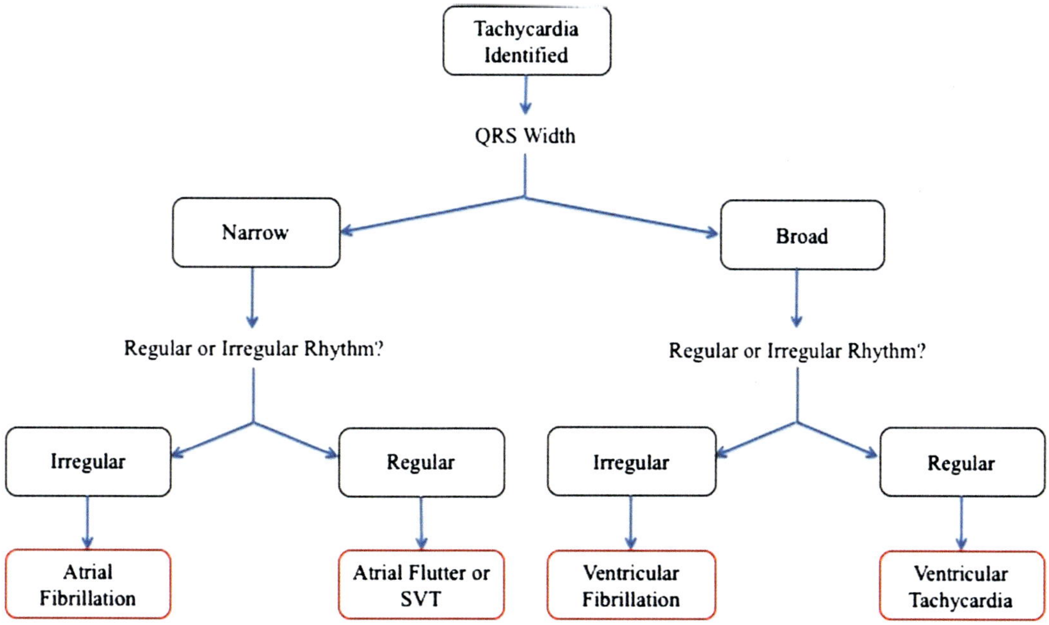

Fig. 10 Clinical algorithm for the identification of cardiac arrhythmias

Fig. 11 Rhythm strip on an ECG showing SVT

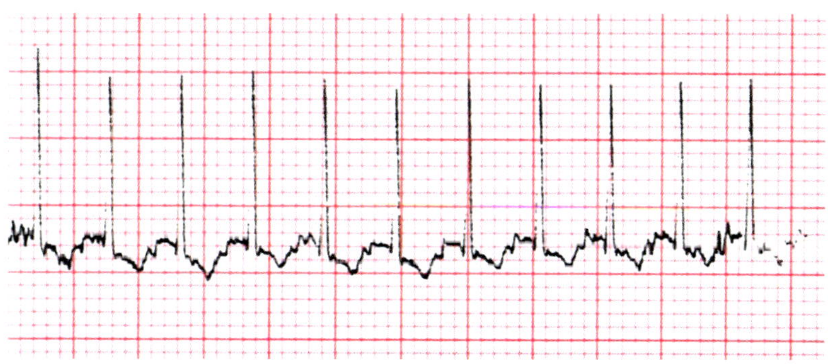

and ventricles. This is more common in older children and rare in the neonatal period.

70.5.1.2 Stepwise Emergency Treatment for SVT in an Unstable Infant

- Adequate respiratory and circulatory support as per an ABC approach.
- Vagal maneuvers: emersion of the face in ice water or application of an ice pack to the face for over 10 s (Sreeram and Wren 1990).
- Rapid IV adenosine bolus: 150 mcg/kg dose. This can be repeated and increased by 50 mcg/kg; a maximum dose of 300 mcg/kg is reached (Dixon et al. 2005).
- DC synchronized cardioversion of 1 J/kg. This can be repeated and increased by 1 J/kg up to 4 J/kg. If possible, sedate the infant.

The cessation of SVT after treatment is sudden often associated with a marked clinical improvement in the infant. SVT often can reoccur, so it is prudent to contact a tertiary center to gain advice about longer-term maintenance therapy. A variety of drugs including beta-blockers, amiodarone, digoxin, and flecainide can be used (O'Sullivan et al. 1995; Burri et al. 2003; Etheridge et al. 2001). Verapamil should never be used due to its associated cardiovascular compromise,

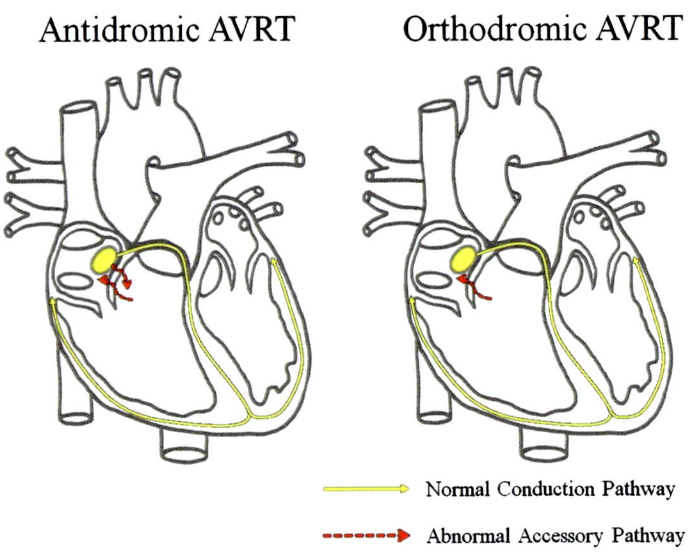

Fig. 12 Different accessory pathways that can cause SVTs in neonates SVT

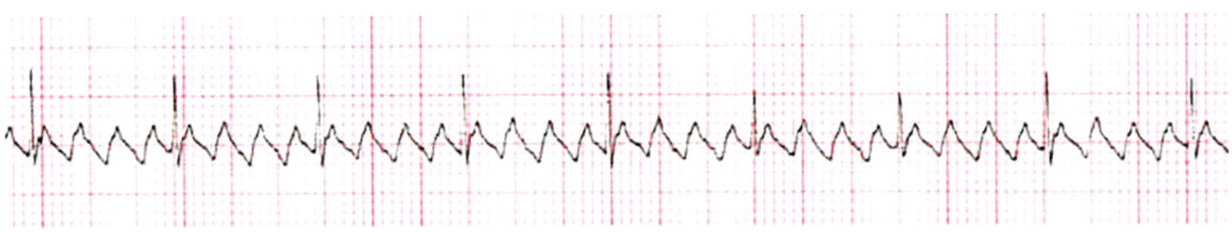

Fig. 13 An ECG showing atrial flutter in a neonate displaying 4:1 block

hypotension, and bradycardia. The majority of SVTs spontaneously resolve in the first year of life (Wren 2006).

70.5.1.3 Atrial Flutter and Atrial Fibrillation

Atrial flutter is a rare arrhythmia that does occur in neonates and is usually never encountered again until adult life. It is believed to be caused by an aberrant conduction zone between the inferior vena cavae, although the hearts are structurally normal in most cases (Kothari and Skinner 2006). It is characterized by a rapid atrial reentry with rates above 300 beats per minute. This arrhythmia is often well tolerated by neonates as the degree of AV block is often 2:1 or higher (giving its classical saw tooth pattern appearance), thus meaning the ventricular rate is 150 beats per minute and often irregular. However, if the degree of AV block changes to 1:1, an unsustainable tachycardia will ensure and lead to cardiovascular collapse (Fig. 13).

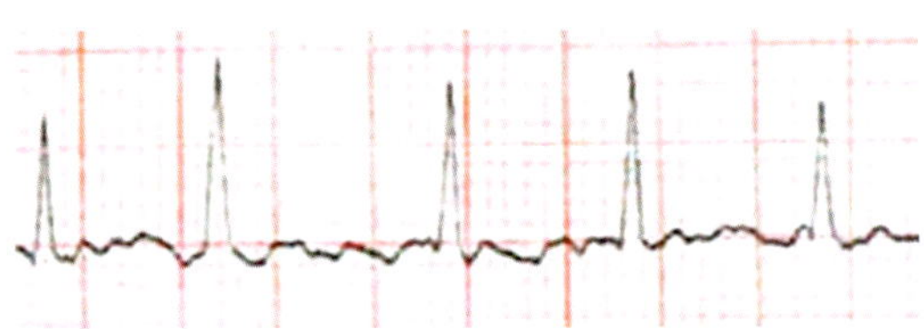

Fig. 14 A rhythm strip showing atrial fibrillation

Atrial fibrillation is virtually unknown in the neonatal period. There will be a very chaotic appearance to the P wave activity on the ECG that subsequently means the QRS complexes will also occur irregularly (Fig. 14).

70.5.1.4 Stepwise Emergency Treatment for Atrial Flutter/Fibrillation

- Adequate respiratory and circulatory support as per an ABC approach.

- DC synchronized cardioversion of 1 J/kg. This can be repeated and increased by 1 J/kg up to 4 J/kg. If possible, sedate the infant.

Often after cardioversion, atrial flutter rarely reoccurs and the outlook is excellent for these infants (Peng et al. 1998). Where it reoccurs, it is best to consult with your local tertiary cardiology center as further management may require expert input with medications such as amiodarone, digoxin, and beta-blockers and more specialist procedures such as transesophageal pacing (Kothari and Skinner 2006; Rhodes et al. 1995). Little is known about the long-term outcomes for infants with atrial fibrillation owing to its rarity.

It must be noted that atrial flutter can easily be mistaken for other types of SVT (e.g., atrioventricular nodal reentry tachycardia) when the degree of AV block is low and with a regular ventricular rate. In which case with a dose of adenosine, it will transiently block AV conduction and reveal more P waves per QRS complex. A further clue to elucidate this diagnosis is that atrial flutter will not respond to vagal maneuvers.

70.5.2 Ventricular Tachyarrhythmias

70.5.2.1 Ventricular Tachycardia

The ECG displays broad QRS complexes with a heart rate between 150 and 200 beats per minutes. There is also a disassociation from atrial activity meaning that P waves are conducted randomly (Fig. 15). In addition to the aforementioned causes of arrhythmias in the newborn, ventricular tachycardia is associated with intracardiac tumors (e.g., rhabdomyomas) and perinatal asphyxia (Perry 1997).

The most common cause of neonatal ventricular tachycardia is congenital long QT syndrome and channelopathies that can lead to "torsades de pointes" (Fig. 16). There are both autosomal dominant and recessive forms of long QT syndrome, so a family history is key when such arrhythmias are identified (Killen and Fish 2008; Skinner et al. 2005).

70.5.2.2 Stepwise Emergency Treatment for Ventricular Tachycardia

- Adequate respiratory and circulatory support as per an ABC approach.

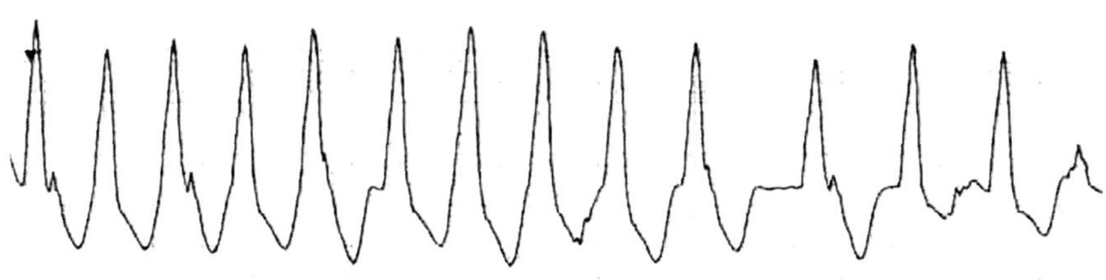

Fig. 15 Ventricular tachycardia

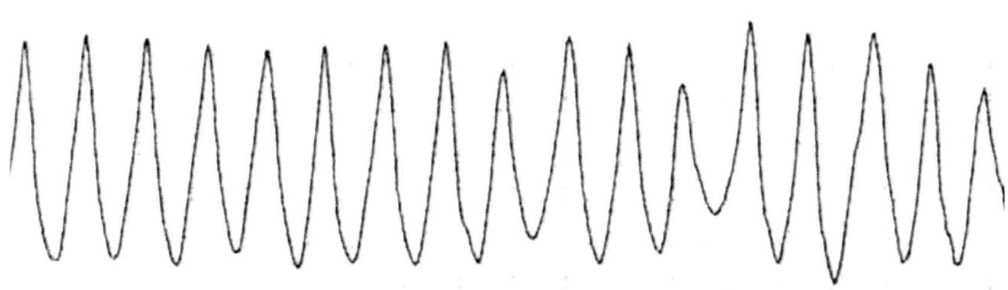

Fig. 16 Torsades de pointes

- DC synchronized cardioversion of 1 J/kg. This can be repeated and increased by 1 J/kg up to 4 J/kg. If possible, sedate the infant.

A minority of infants are well and asymptomatic and can be cardioverted chemically. Such cases need to be discussed with tertiary centers and will typically be treated with intravenous amiodarone (25 mcg/kg/min) or lidocaine (1 mg/kg). Oral preventive medication includes the use of drugs such as propranolol.

70.5.2.3 Ventricular Fibrillation

This rare arrhythmia requires full cardiopulmonary resuscitation. The uncoordinated contraction of the ventricles leads to chaotic and disorganized electrical activity that constantly changes in shape and magnitude on the ECG. If a neonate survives, then investigations for long QT syndrome are required urgently.

70.6 Bradyarrhythmias

Such arrhythmias lead to infants having heart rates less than 90 beats per minute. They are due to conduction disturbance within the sinoatrial or atrioventricular node. They can be distinguished from infants suffering from sinus bradycardia (common after perinatal asphyxia or for those undergoing cooling therapy) by the ECG morphology showing a bradycardia with either:

First-degree block: A fixed prolongation of the PR interval.

Second-degree block: Not every P wave is conducted to the ventricle leading to "dropped" QRS complexes. This includes the eponymous Wenckebach phenomenon or where the PR interval slowly increases until a P wave is not conducted leading to a "dropped" QRS complex.

Third-degree block: Complete disassociation between atrial and ventricular activity. Therefore, on an ECG, the P wave rate is usually normal because the electrical impulse from the atria is not conducted through the bundle of His. Thus the ventricles rely on their own conduction system to propagate muscular contraction. This system is slow and therefore the resulting QRS complexes are wide with a rate between 40 and 80 beats per minute (Fig. 17).

Rarely first- or second-degree heart block presents with a collapsed neonate; however, they may reflect underlying structural heart disease, especially atrial septal defects, and so require investigation. Furthermore, they may progress to third-degree heart block. This chapter focuses on the latter as this is most commonly associated with neonatal heart failure or circulatory failure.

70.6.1 Third-Degree Heart Block

This affects 1 in 22,000 live births and is frequently associated with either complex congenital heart disease such as left atrial isomerism or neonatal lupus (Kertesz et al. 1997). The latter is a result of the passive placental transmission of anti-Ro and anti-La antibodies from mothers suffering from systemic lupus or associated autoimmune disease such as Sjögren's syndrome leading to damage to the fetal conduction systems (Friedman et al. 2003). When associated with underlying cardiac pathology, the prognosis for infants is poor with mortality quoted to be as high as 85% (Kertesz et al. 1997).

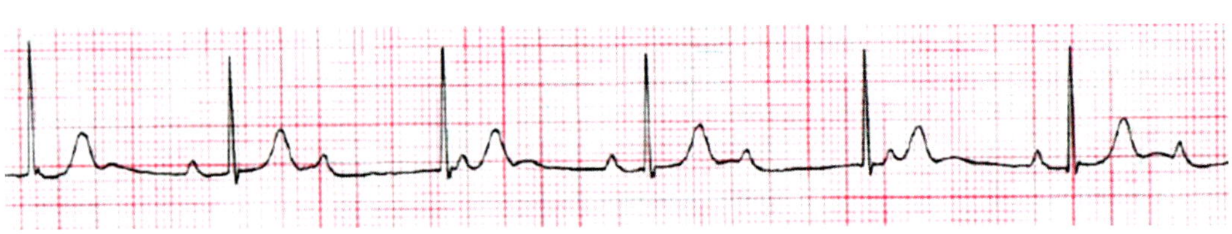

Fig. 17 An ECG rhythm strip showing third-degree heart block

70.6.1.1 Stepwise Emergency Treatment for Third-Degree Heart Block

- Adequate respiratory and circulatory support as per an ABC approach
- Infusions of positive chronotropes such as adrenaline (0.1–1.5 mcg/kg/min) or isoprenaline (0.2–10 mcg/kg/min) (Comitis 2011; Tunaoğlu et al. 2010)
- If possible transcutaneous or transesophageal pacing under sedation (Groves et al. 1995; Glatz et al. 2008)
- Transfer to a tertiary cardiac unit for permanent cardiac pacing

For mothers with systemic lupus in whom congenital heart block is detected in the fetus, antenatal corticosteroid or immunoglobulin therapy is often started to prevent damage to bundle of His. However, its efficacy is widely debated (Tunaoğlu et al. 2010).

References

Abdellatif M, Ahmed A, Alsenaidi K (2012) Cardiac tamponade due to umbilical venous catheter in the newborn. Case reports 2012:bcr–2012–6160–bcr–2012–6160. https://doi.org/10.1136/bcr-2012-6160

Abu-Harb M, Wyllie J, Hey E et al (1994a) Presentation of obstructive left heart malformations in infancy. Arch Dis Child Fetal Neonatal Ed 71:F179–F183

Abu-Harb M, Hey E, Wren C (1994b) Death in infancy from unrecognised congenital heart disease. Arch Dis Child 71:3–7

Ainsworth SB, Wyllie JP, Wren C (1999) Prevalence and clinical significance of cardiac murmurs in neonates. Arch Dis Child Fetal Neonatal Ed 80:F43–F45

Apiliogullari B, Sunam GS, Ceran S, Koc H (2011) Evaluation of neonatal pneumothorax. J Int Med Res 39:2436–2440

Beardsall K, White DK, Pinto EM, Kelsall AWR (2003) Pericardial effusion and cardiac tamponade as complications of neonatal long lines: are they really a problem? Arch Dis Child Fetal Neonatal Ed 88:F292–F295. https://doi.org/10.1136/fn.88.4.F292

Burri S, Hug MI, Bauersfeld U (2003) Efficacy and safety of intravenous amiodarone for incessant tachycardias in infants. Eur J Pediatr 162:880–884. https://doi.org/10.1007/s00431-003-1302-z

Cartwright DW (2004) Central venous lines in neonates: a study of 2186 catheters. Arch Dis Child Fetal Neonatal Ed 89:F504–F508. https://doi.org/10.1136/adc.2004.049189

Comitis GA (2011) Neonatal cardiac emergencies

Davignon A, Rautaharju P, Boisselle E, Soumis F (1980) Normal ECG standards for infants and children. Pediatric

de-Wahl Granelli A, Wennergren M, Sandberg K et al (2009) Impact of pulse oximetry screening on the detection of duct dependent congenital heart disease: a Swedish prospective screening study in 39,821 newborns. BMJ (Clin Res Ed) 338:a3037. https://doi.org/10.1136/bmj.a3037

Dixon J, Foster K, Wyllie J, Wren C (2005) Guidelines and adenosine dosing in supraventricular tachycardia. Arch Dis Child 90:1190–1191. https://doi.org/10.1136/adc.2005.077636

Dubin AM (2000) Arrhythmias in the Newborn. Neoreviews 1:e146–e151. https://doi.org/10.1542/neo.1-8-e146

Enriques AM, McKay R, Arnold RM, Wilkinson JL (1986) Misleading hyperoxia test. Arch Dis Child 61:604–606

Etheridge SP, Craig JE, Compton SJ (2001) Amiodarone is safe and highly effective therapy for supraventricular tachycardia in infants. Am Heart J 141:105–110. https://doi.org/10.1067/mhj.2001.111765

Ferencz C, Rubin JD, McCarter RJ et al (1985) Congenital heart disease: prevalence at livebirth. The Baltimore-Washington Infant Study. Am J Epidemiol 121:31–36

Friedman D, Duncanson L, Glickstein J, Buyon J (2003) A review of congenital heart block. Images Paediatr Cardiol 5:36–48

Glatz AC, Gaynor JW, Rhodes LA et al (2008) Outcome of high-risk neonates with congenital complete heart block paced in the first 24 hours after birth. J Thorac Cardiovasc Surg 136:767–773. https://doi.org/10.1016/j.jtcvs.2008.04.019

Groves AM, Allan LD, Rosenthal E (1995) Therapeutic trial of sympathomimetics in three cases of complete heart block in the fetus. Circulation 92:3394–3396. https://doi.org/10.1161/01.CIR.92.12.3394

Hill A, Perlman JM, Volpe JJ (1982) Relationship of pneumothorax to occurrence of intraventricular hemorrhage in the premature newborn. Pediatrics 69:144–149

Hoffman JIE, Kaplan S (2002) The incidence of congenital heart disease. J Am Coll Cardiol 39:1890–1900

Hsu DT, Pearson GD (2009) Heart failure in children: part I: history, etiology, and pathophysiology. Circ Heart Fail 2:63–70

Ishikawa T, Iwashima S, Ohishi A et al (2011) Prevalence of congenital heart disease assessed by echocardiography in 2067 consecutive newborns. Acta Paediatr (Oslo, Norway: 1992) 100:e55–e60. https://doi.org/10.1111/j.1651-2227.2011.02248.x

Iyer VHA, Sharma DM, Charki S, Mohanty PK (2014) Cardiac tamponade in a neonate: a dreadful condition – need for functional echo. Case reports 2014: bcr2014207040–bcr2014207040

Kertesz NJ, Fenrich AL, Friedman RA (1997) Congenital complete atrioventricular block. Tex Heart Inst J/Tex

Heart Inst St Luke's Episcopal Hosp Tex Child Hosp 24:301–307

Killen SAS, Fish FA (2008) Fetal and neonatal arrhythmias. Neoreviews 9:e242–e252. https://doi.org/10.1542/neo.9-6-e242

Kothari DS, Skinner JR (2006) Neonatal tachycardias: an update. Arch Dis Child Fetal Neonatal Ed 91: F136–F144. https://doi.org/10.1136/adc.2004.049049

Lipshultz SE, Sleeper LA, Towbin JA et al (2003) The incidence of pediatric cardiomyopathy in two regions of the United States. N Engl J Med 348:1647–1655. https://doi.org/10.1056/NEJMoa021715

Massin MM, Astadicko I, Dessy H (2008) Epidemiology of heart failure in a tertiary pediatric center. Clin Cardiol 31:388–391. https://doi.org/10.1002/clc.20262

Mellander M (2013) Diagnosis and management of life-threatening cardiac malformations in the newborn. Elsevier, pp 302–310

Mellander M, Sunnegårdh J (2006) Failure to diagnose critical heart malformations in newborns before discharge – an increasing problem? Acta Paediatr 95:407–413

Moak JP, Hamra M (1998) Cardiac electrophysiology. The science and practice of . . .

Nugent AW, Daubeney PEF, Chondros P et al (2003) The epidemiology of childhood cardiomyopathy in Australia. N Engl J Med 348:1639–1646

O'Sullivan JJ, Gardiner HM, Wren C (1995) Digoxin or flecainide for prophylaxis of supraventricular tachycardia in infants? J Am Coll Cardiol 26:991–994. https://doi.org/10.1016/0735-1097(95)00291-9

Peng CC, Chen MR, Hou CJ et al (1998) Atrial flutter in the neonate and early infancy. Jpn Heart J 39:287–295

Perry JC (1997) Ventricular tachycardia in neonates. Pacing Clin Electrophysiol 20:2061–2064. https://doi.org/10.1111/j.1540-8159.1997.tb03628.x

Pradat P, Francannet C, Harris JA, Robert E (2003) The epidemiology of cardiovascular defects, part I: a study based on data from three large registries of congenital malformations. Pediatr Cardiol 24:195–221. https://doi.org/10.1007/s00246-002-9401-6

Reller MD, Strickland MJ, Riehle-Colarusso T et al (2008) Prevalence of congenital heart defects in metropolitan Atlanta, 1998–2005. J Pediatr 153:807–813. https://doi.org/10.1016/j.jpeds.2008.05.059

Rhodes LA, Walsh EP, Saul JP (1995) Conversion of atrial flutter in pediatric patients by transesophageal atrial pacing: a safe, effective, minimally invasive procedure. Am Heart J 130:323–327. https://doi.org/10.1016/0002-8703(95)90448-4

Skinner JR, Chung S-K, Montgomery D et al (2005) Near-miss SIDS due to Brugada syndrome. Arch Dis Child 90:528–529. https://doi.org/10.1136/adc.2004.058115

Sreeram N, Wren C (1990) Supraventricular tachycardia in infants: response to initial treatment. Arch Dis Child 65:127–129. doi:https://doi.org/10.1136/adc.65.1.127

Thangaratinam S, Brown K, Zamora J et al (2015) Pulse oximetry screening for critical congenital heart defects in asymptomatic newborn babies: a systematic review and meta-analysis. Lancet 379:2459–2464. https://doi.org/10.1016/S0140-6736(12)60107-X

Tunaoğlu FS, Yildirim A, Vurali D (2010) Isolated congenital heart block. Tex Heart Inst J/Tex Heart Inst St Luke's Episcopal Hosp Tex Child Hosp 37:579–583

Warren M, Thompson KS, Popek EJ et al (2013) Pericardial effusion and cardiac tamponade in neonates: sudden unexpected death associated with total parenteral nutrition via central venous catheterization. Ann Clin Lab Sci 43:163–171

Wren C (2006) Cardiac arrhythmias in the fetus and newborn. Semin Fetal Neonatal Med 11:182–190. https://doi.org/10.1016/j.siny.2005.12.001

Blood Pressure Disorders in the Neonate: Hypotension and Hypertension

71

Jonathan M. Fanaroff and Avroy A. Fanaroff

Contents

J. M. Fanaroff (✉) · A. A. Fanaroff
Case Western Reserve University School of Medicine
Rainbow Babies and Children's Hospital, Cleveland, OH, USA
e-mail: jmf20@case.edu

Abstract

Blood pressure (BP) disorders are an extremely common problem in neonates admitted to the neonatal intensive care unit (NICU). Direct invasive measurement (via an arterial or peripheral artery catheter) is currently considered the

G. Buonocore et al. (eds.), *Neonatology*,
https://doi.org/10.1007/978-3-319-29489-6_217

optimum for measuring BP. Usually, mean blood pressure rather than systolic pressure is used. Normal blood pressure in newborns varies with gestational age, birth weight, and postnatal age, increasing by 1–2 mmHg per week for the first month. The clinical features of hypotension in the neonate include tachycardia, bradycardia, tachypnea, mottling of the skin, prolonged capillary refill time, cool extremities, and decreased urine output. Normal saline is the preferred fluid for volume expansion. Dopamine and dobutamine are the most commonly used agents to treat hypotension, although norepinephrine is preferred by some clinicians. Many hypotensive pre-term infants have low cortisol levels, and corticosteroids are being used increasingly to prevent or treat hypotension. There is an association between systemic hypotension and neonatal morbidities such as intraventricular hemorrhage and poor neurodevelopmental outcomes. Hypertension, while less common, can also lead to significant short- and long-term morbidities. It is important to determine whether any renovascular anomalies were detected prior to birth. The history may include drug abuse, perinatal asphyxia, umbilical catheter placement, or medications administered to the neonate. It is important to measure the BP in all four extremities to rule out coarctation of the aorta. Some infants may require prolonged treatment with beta-blockers, angiotensin-converting enzyme inhibitors, calcium channel blockers, and/or diuretics. Blood pressure should not be decreased too quickly in hypertensive neonates as cerebral perfusion pressure may be adversely affected.

71.1 Salient Points

- Despite many studies having looked at blood pressure ranges in neonates, there is not yet a standard definition of truly pathologic hypotension and hypertension, and blood pressure should be looked at in the context of the clinical condition.
- There is evidence that wide variations exist among NICUs in both practice styles and approaches to blood pressure disorders. The dilemma remains when to treat and how; the traditional "two standard deviations below the norm" can be applied to the term neonate, but for preterm infants "normal for age" is a challenge.
- The optimal means of restoring normal circulating blood volume, blood pressure, and cardiac output have yet to be determined; dopamine is the most widely used sympathomimetic amine in the treatment of neonatal hypotension.
- Congenital etiologies of neonatal hypertension include renal artery stenosis or hypoplasia, coarctation of the aorta, and abdominal aortic atresia.
- Beta-blockers, angiotensin-converting enzyme inhibitors, calcium channel blockers, and/or diuretics are commonly used to treat neonatal hypertension.

71.2 Introduction

Blood pressure (BP) disorders are an extremely common problem in neonates admitted to the neonatal intensive care unit (NICU). Additionally, there is an association between systemic hypotension and neonatal morbidities such as intraventricular hemorrhage and poor neurodevelopmental outcomes (Watkins et al. 1989; Batton et al. 2016). Hypertension, while less common, can also lead to significant short- and long-term morbidities. There remains, however, no standard definition of hypotension or hypertension in the neonatal period. Indeed, there is convincing evidence that wide variations exist among NICUs in both practice styles and approaches to blood pressure disorders. Barrington notes "The treatment of shock and hypotension in the preterm infant may be the area of neonatology where there is the greatest 'intervention/data imbalance'; more babies receive more treatments with less supportive evidence than in virtually any other domain" (Barrington and Janaillac 2016).

In this chapter the current status of hypotension and hypertension in the neonatal period is reviewed. First we examine the measurement of

neonatal blood pressure and then review the definitions of blood pressure disorders. Subsequently the causes, consequences, and treatment of neonatal hypotension are presented. Finally the causes, clinical features, diagnostic studies, and an approach to clinical management of neonatal hypertension are discussed.

71.3 Measurement of Neonatal Blood Pressure

The technical goal for measurement of blood pressure would be a method that is simple, reliable, noninvasive, painless, and gives a continuous measurement. Unfortunately this goal has not yet been obtained. Direct invasive measurement (via an arterial or peripheral artery catheter) is currently considered the optimum method. Usually, mean blood pressure rather than systolic pressure is used when judging the normality of data obtained from the indwelling arterial line because it is thought to be free of the artifact caused by resonance, thrombi, and air bubbles, but this may not always be true. The downside of invasive measurement relate to the risks of an indwelling catheter, such as thrombus formation, hemorrhage, or infection. Noninvasive indirect measurement includes oscillometric and automated Doppler techniques. Provided that cuff size is standardized, oscillometric measurement seems to be accurate within the normal range. However, concern has been expressed that, at the lower levels, it consistently overestimates the blood pressure providing false reassurance.

71.4 Definition of Hypotension and Hypertension

While many studies have looked at blood pressure ranges in neonates, there remains no standard definition of truly pathologic hypotension and hypertension. Figure 1 shows data obtained in a study of 608 newborns admitted to Philadelphia area NICUs during the first 99 days of life (Zubrow et al. 1995). One way to define abnormal blood pressure is based on normative values. Hence hypertension is often defined as sustained systolic (SBP) and/or diastolic (DBP) blood pressure more than two standard deviations above the mean values ($\geq$95%) (National High Blood Pressure Education Program Working Group on High Blood Pressure in Children and Adolescents 2004). However, blood pressure varies significantly, in a linear fashion, with gestational age (GA) and birth weight. Gender may also be significant on the first day of life when extremely low birth weight (ELBW) (<1,000 g) males have lower blood pressure than females (Emery et al. 1993). Blood pressure also increases daily during the week of life. Hence the definition of hypotension in the newborn has remained elusive and treatment algorithms are based upon statistically defined gestational age-dependent normative blood pressure values and clinical judgment.

The dilemma remains when to treat and how. The traditional "two standard deviations below the norm" can be applied to the term neonate, but for preterm infants "normal for age" is a challenge. Furthermore, while almost a quarter century has elapsed since Versmold published his classic paper on blood pressure in the smallest premature infants, there is a particular controversy over when to treat abnormal blood pressures in ELBW infants (Versmold et al. 1981). Whereas in adults and children, normative data for systolic, diastolic, and mean blood pressure is available, in infants most data sets have used "mean blood pressure" to define hypotension and determine when to intervene. Empirically the gestational age in weeks has been used to define the lower limits of mean blood pressure during the first day of life. But this is unreliable and the blood pressure should be looked at in the context of the clinical condition. Normal blood pressure in newborns varies with gestational age, birth weight, and postnatal age, increasing by 1–2 mmHg per week for the first month. Blood pressure rises significantly during the first 72 h of life irrespective of gestational age so that all preterm infants should have a mean pressure above 30 mmHg by this time (Fanaroff et al. 2006).

Batton et al. showed that arterial blood pressure (ABP) decreased for the first 3 h, reached a nadir at 4–5 h and then increased at an average rate of

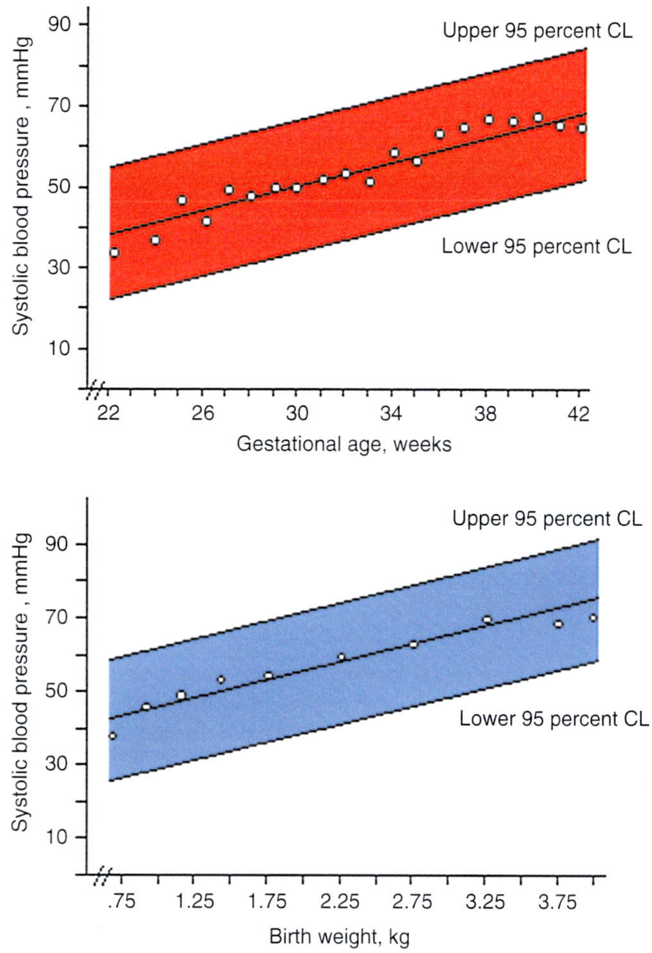

Fig. 1 Neonatal blood pressure. Linear regression of mean SBP on gestational age and birth weight in 329 infants admitted to NICU on day 1 of life. The mean SBP and 95% confidence limit (CL) for incremental gestational age and birth weight are plotted about the respective regression lines (Reproduced with permission from Zubrow et al. (1995) Copyright 1995 Nature Publishing Group)

0.2 mm Hg h^{-1}(Batton et al. 2014). The rise in ABP from hour 4 to 24 was similar for untreated infants (164) and infants given any antihypotensive therapy ($n = 203$), a fluid bolus ($n = 135$) or dopamine ($n = 92$). Gestational age-specific trends were similar. ABP tended to be lower as GA decreased, but varied widely at each GA. In a different study, Batton investigated 15 definitions of low BP: 1, 2, or ≥ 3 systolic, diastolic, or mean BP values less than or equal to the fifth percentile; 1, 2, or ≥ 3 mean arterial pressure (MAP; in mm Hg) values less than or equal to the infant's GA equivalent (in weeks); and 1, 2, or ≥ 3 MAP values ≤ 25 mm Hg (Batton et al. 2013). Low BP values were not necessarily consecutive. They concluded that factors other than BP contributed to the decision to use antihypotensive therapies. Most significantly, infant outcomes were not improved with antihypotensive therapy for any of the 15 definitions of low BP investigated.

Oxygen delivery to the tissues is influenced by cardiac output and blood flow more so than blood pressure, and, hence, values of blood pressure that are statistically abnormal are not necessarily pathologic. Shock is a complex clinical syndrome caused by acute circulatory failure. Hypotension (i.e., lower than expected blood pressure) frequently, but not always, accompanies shock. Shock is characterized (and defined) by inadequate tissue and organ perfusion, which may involve a single-organ or all-organ systems. Impaired perfusion not only results in inadequate delivery of oxygen and nutrients but also inadequate removal of metabolic waste products. Cellular function is disrupted, and eventually there is cell death. Few data are available on the relation between blood pressure and systemic flow, cardiac

output and neonatal morbidity, and mortality, but shock remains a major cause of neonatal morbidity and mortality (Barrington 2008). In most very low birth weight (VLBW) neonates, cerebral blood flow autoregulation is indeed lost when blood pressure reaches the fifth percentile (Lightburn et al. 2009). Some practices use functional echocardiography to better evaluate the circulatory status and as an indicator for interventions (Stranak et al. 2014).

The incidence of hypotension is relatively high, especially in ELBW infants. Between 16% and 98% of extremely preterm infants receive treatment for hypotension in the first few days of life. This enormous variation has arisen because of a lack of reliable information to create an evidence base for intervention (Dempsey et al. 2009; Dempsey and Barrington 2009; Efird et al. 2004). There is a significant variation among NICUs in the incidence, diagnosis, and approach to hypotension.

Al-Aweel et al. in a multicenter report found an almost threefold variation among sites in the odds of hypotension (Al-Aweel et al. 2001). Even more concerning, two of the six sites had a 5- to 30-fold higher use of vasopressors than other sites after risk adjusting for the occurrence of hypotension.

71.5 Clinical Features

In addition to low blood pressure, the clinical features of hypotension in the neonate include varying combinations of tachycardia, bradycardia, tachypnea, mottling of the skin, prolonged capillary refill time, cool extremities, and decreased urine output. A difference between the central and peripheral temperature may be indicative of hypovolemia or sepsis. Volume expansion will rapidly reduce the differential between central and peripheral temperature.

71.6 Causes of Hypotension

There are many causes of neonatal hypotension and shock syndromes. Therapy must be specifically directed at the underlying cause. Table 1 lists the various causes of hypotension. Note that there are many other causes than hypovolemia, and, indeed in ELBW infants, hypovolemia is relatively uncommon compared to other causes.

Cardiac output is the product of heart rate and stroke volume. Because of a limited ability to increase stroke volume, neonatal cardiac output is more dependent upon heart rate. Hence prolonged tachycardia or bradycardia compromises cardiac output. Stroke volume is dependent upon preload (ventricular filling), after load (systemic and pulmonary vascular resistance), and myocardial contractility. The treatment of hypotension is based upon manipulation of these parameters (Dempsey et al. 2009).

71.7 Significance of Blood Pressure Requiring Treatment in ELBW Infants

To explore the relationship between short- and long-term morbidity and neonatal blood pressure, Fanaroff et al. (2006) performed a chart review of the 156 infants with birth weight between 401 and 1,000 g who were born during the period 1998–1999 and admitted to the NICU at Rainbow Babies & Children's Hospital. Blood pressure, obtained predominantly (81%) by umbilical arterial catheter (or by oscillometer 19%), was recorded hourly for the first 24 h and then every 6 h until 72 h of life. Infants were then divided into two groups – those who received no treatment to support blood pressure ($n = 97$) and those who were treated for hypotension ($n = 59$). Infants receiving treatment weighed less at birth and were a week less mature than those who received no blood pressure support. They were also less likely to have been exposed to antenatal corticosteroids. Patients were considered to have treated hypotension if they received fluid pushes and/or pressors (dopamine and/or dobutamine) during the first 72 h of life to elevate blood pressure. The infants underwent neurologic, developmental, and formal audiologic testing. Figure 2 shows the plot of the mean blood pressure, as well as one and two standard deviations above and below the mean during the first week of life. Overall there is a spontaneous increase in mean arterial pressure (MAP) from 32 at age 1 h to 41 mmHg by the end of the first week of life. Infants

requiring blood pressure support were more likely to have severe intracranial bleeds and had a higher mortality rate. Logistic regression analyzes controlling for maternal socioeconomic status and coexisting neonatal morbidity was performed and at follow-up treated hypotension was significantly associated with delayed motor development (β–6.0, SE 3.1) and hearing loss (OR 8.9, CI 0.92–86.3) (Fanaroff et al. 2006). Batton reported that independent of early BP changes, antihypotensive therapy exposure was associated with an increased risk of death/neurodevelopmental impairment at 18–22 months' corrected age, when controlling for risk factors known to affect survival and neurodevelopment (Batton et al. 2015).

Table 1 Causes of neonatal shock

A *Hypovolemia*
a. Placental hemorrhage; abruption placenta previa
b. Feto-maternal hemorrhage
c. Twin to twin transfusion
d. Birth trauma – subaponeurotic bleed
e. Ruptured liver/spleen
f. Massive pulmonary hemorrhage
g. Disseminated intravascular coagulopathy
h. Third space losses – necrotizing enterocolitis
B *Cardiogenic shock*
a. Asphyxia
b. Arrhythmias
c. Congenital heart disease
i. Ductal dependent lesions when ductus closes
ii. Total anomalous pulmonary venous drainage
d. Cardiomyopathy
e. Myocarditis
f. Air leak syndromes
i. Pneumothorax
ii. Inadvertent positive end expiratory pressure (PEEP)
C *Sepsis and septic shock*
D *Endocrine*
a. Adrenal hemorrhage
b. Adrenogenital syndrome
E *Drug-induced hypotension*

71.8 Treatment

Successful management of neonatal hypotension and shock mandates understanding the etiology and pathophysiology of the cardiovascular compromise. The ability to establish the etiology of the condition (hypovolemia, myocardial dysfunction, or abnormal vasoregulation) at the bedside is limited. Management, despite efforts to use all the available evidence, often remains empiric. Volume replacement (fluid boluses) vasoactive medications and corticosteroids in various combinations are the foundations of therapy. It is important not to be treating a number but to consider the blood pressure in the context of the infant's total clinical condition. Frequent evaluation of vital signs, blood

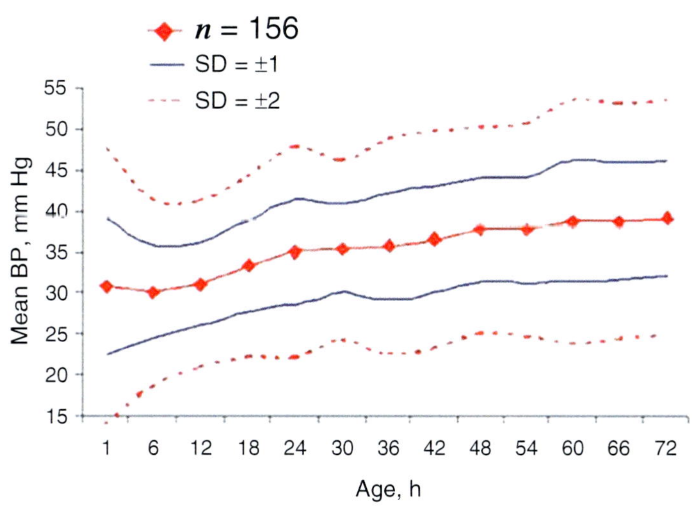

Fig. 2 Mean blood pressure of all ELBW infants in the first 72 h of life

pressure, perfusion, urine output, and neurologic status is used to guide the interventions. Although many hypotensive babies are hypovolemic, there are many other causes for hypotension and they should all be considered, including defining the hemodynamics echocardiographically, before pushing excessive volume.

The optimal means of restoring normal circulating blood volume, blood pressure, and cardiac output have yet to be determined. Whether crystalloids or colloids are preferable is also unclear in newborns. In their Cochrane review, Osborn and Evans commented: "There is no evidence from randomized trials to support the routine use of early volume expansion in very preterm infants without cardiovascular compromise. There is insufficient evidence to determine whether infants with cardiovascular compromise benefit from volume expansion. There is insufficient evidence to determine what type of volume expansion should be used in preterm infants (if at all) or for the use of early red cell transfusions" (Osborn and Evans 2004).

Normal saline has been shown to be equally effective to albumin in restoring blood pressure in hypotensive preterm infants. Because it is efficacious, safer, readily available, and inexpensive, normal saline has become the crystalloid of choice for volume expansion (Oca et al. 2003). Furthermore, in a follow-up of a randomized trial comparing crystalloid and colloid, Greenough reported that 19/131 survivors had abnormal neurodevelopmental status (Greenough et al. 2002). Although these infants differed from the normal group in birth weight, magnitude of colloid infusion received, and oxygen exposure, in addition to intraventricular hemorrhage, periventricular leukomalacia, and postnatal corticosteroid exposure, regression analysis demonstrated that only colloid infusion related significantly to abnormal neurodevelopmental outcome is independent of other variables. Thus colloid infusions should be used with caution in the perinatal period, and normal saline is the preferred fluid for volume repletion.

Although volume expansion is liberally used in newborn intensive care, little is known about its effects on hemodynamics or outcomes. Ewer et al. (2003), using data that were obtained from anonymized regional case notes of Project 27/28, a British National case-controlled study run by the Confidential Enquiry into Stillbirths and Deaths in Infancy, reported that newborns who received 30 mL/kg volume expansion in the first 48 h of life were more likely to die than those who received <30 mL/kg (OR 4.5, 95% CI 1.2, 17.2). More is not necessarily better!

Mayock and Gleason (2004), by studying the effects of volume expansion with and without hypoxia in immature lambs, provide some insight into this problem. They note that rapid volume expansion in normovolemic preterm fetal sheep did not affect blood pressure or cerebral blood flow but was associated with decreased cerebral oxygen delivery. This was further compromised when oxygen content was decreased.

We can but speculate on the long-term consequences of these findings in humans, but should be cautious about over aggressive volume correction using crystalloids or colloids which might cause hemodilution and reduce O_2 delivery to the brain.

Because systemic hypotension is associated with increased mortality as well as both short- and long-term morbidity, volume expansion, dopamine, and dobutamine have been the agents most commonly used to treat hypotension. Norepinephrine is preferred by some clinicians. Dopamine is the most widely used sympathomimetic amine in the treatment of neonatal hypotension, and a Cochrane review confirmed that it is more effective than dobutamine in raising blood pressure (Subhedar and Shaw 2003). Volume administration is less effective in the immediate postnatal period, and its extensive use is associated with significant untoward effects, especially in preterm infants. During the course of their disease, some of the sickest hypotensive newborns become unresponsive to volume and pressor administration. This phenomenon is caused by the desensitization of the cardiovascular system to catecholamines by the critical illness and relative or absolute adrenal insufficiency.

Corticosteroids have added a new wrinkle to the management of hypotension. Many hypotensive preterm infants have low cortisol levels, and corticosteroids are being used increasingly to prevent or treat hypotension in these babies. Steroids

rapidly upregulate cardiovascular adrenergic receptor expression and serve as hormone substitution in cases of adrenal insufficiency which explains their effectiveness in stabilizing the cardiovascular status and decreasing the requirement for pressor support in the critically ill newborn with volume- and pressor-resistant hypotension. Although corticosteroid therapy has resulted in improved blood pressure and circulation, many complications including unanticipated spontaneous gut perforation, hyperglycemia, and hypertension and the long-term problem of increased cerebral palsy and intellectual impairment necessitates judicious use of corticosteroids to support blood pressure in preterm infants (Yeh et al. 2004). Ibrahim's Cochrane review concluded that corticosteroids are effective in the treatment of refractory hypotension without significant adverse short-term consequences (Ibrahim et al. 2011).

However, long-term safety or benefit data is lacking. In the absence of long-term benefit or safety data, steroids cannot be recommended routinely for the treatment of hypotension in preterm infants.

Neonatal hypotension that is refractory to volume expansion, catecholamines, or corticosteroids has a mortality of about 50%. Optimization of blood pressure and tissue perfusion in refractory hypotension may be crucial to improve clinical outcomes. Vasopressin, a neuropeptide hormone, or its analog terlipressin has been used to treat refractory hypotension in neonates, but Shivanna was unable to find any reliable trials and concluded "There is insufficient evidence to recommend or refute the use of vasopressin or its analogs in the treatment of refractory hypotension in neonates" (Shivanna et al. 2013).

When the etiology of the hypotension is primary cardiac dysfunction (arrhythmia, structural heart disease, myocarditis, asphyxia), the infants may manifest the classical clinical features of congestive heart failure with edema, cardiomegaly, and hepatomegaly. Inotropic agents, with or without peripheral vasodilators, are the treatments of choice. Prostaglandin E1 to restore ductal patency is vital for infants with ductal-dependent lesions. Structural heart disease or arrhythmia often requires specific pharmacologic or surgical therapy. Fluid boluses may aggravate the condition.

71.9 Hypotension Outcomes

Batton defined low BP as $\leq$25 mmHg in the first 72 h of life (Yeh et al. 2004). He followed 67 infants with normal BP, 31 infants with untreated low BP, and 70 infants with treated low BP. Untreated infants with low BP had similar survival rates but more cerebral palsy, deafness, or any neurodevelopmental impairment when compared with infants with normal BP. Treated infants with low BP had more mortality and less survival without neurodevelopment impairment compared with infants who had normal BP (Batton et al. 2009). Kuint also reported that the early need for BP support related to intraventricular hemorrhage, periventricular leukomalacia, and major neurodevelopment impairment (Kuint et al. 2009). On the other hand, Pellicer in a prospective evaluation of the effect vasopressors/inotropes for early systemic hypotension on neurodevelopment, found no differences in the rates of abnormal neurologic status, developmental delay, or combined adverse outcome (death or cerebral palsy or severe neurodevelopmental delay between the hypotensive and normotensive groups) (Pellicer et al. 2009).

As noted above, Batton used random-intercept logistic modeling controlling for center clustering, GA, and illness severity to investigate the relationship between BP, antihypotensive therapies, and infant outcomes (Batton et al. 2016). Independent of early BP changes, antihypotensive therapy exposure was associated with an increased risk of death/neurodevelopmental impairment at 18–22 months' corrected age when controlling for risk factors known to affect survival and neurodevelopment.

Finally, despite recent advances in our understanding of the pathophysiology and management of neonatal hypotension, there are few data from well-conducted trials on the impact of the treatment on organ blood flow and tissue perfusion and on neonatal morbidity and mortality. In view of these significant problems with therapy, there is an imperative to better study this problem, define hypotension (based on hemodynamic measurements which are feasible and reproducible), and determine optimal therapy.

71.10 Hypertension

Hypertension, while not as common as hypotension, can be seen in up to 3% of NICU admissions. As noted earlier, neonatal hypertension is defined as a sustained blood pressure above the 95th percentile using available normative data. BP in newborns increases with both gestational and postconceptual age as well as with birth weight, and the data generated by Zubrow et al. (1995) provides useful parameters to define hypertension. It is important to ensure that the correct cuff size has been used, with the cuff bladder measuring two-thirds the length of the extremity. Furthermore, the diagnosis should be made based on repetitive measurements (at least three) or consistent elevation of pressure over a 2–3 day period if the infants are asymptomatic. The estimated incidence of hypertension ranges from 0.2% to 3%, and it is frequently an indicator of other renal or cardiovascular abnormalities (Adelman 1988). In Cleveland in 1983, hypertension, defined as mean blood pressure greater than 70 mmHg on three separate determinations, was noted in 2% of all neonatal admissions to the intensive and intermediate care nurseries (Skalina et al. 1986). As most infants are asymptomatic, and the onset is insidious, only by paying close attention to the vital signs, including measurement of blood pressure, will neonatal hypertension be recognized. Measures are then necessary to determine the underlying cause and institute appropriate therapy. In healthy neonates, systolic blood pressure increases rapidly during the first 6 weeks of life with the most rapid rise observed during the first 5 days. A similar pattern is observed for diastolic pressures. The observed increases in blood pressure are positively correlated with birth weight and both gestational and postnatal age (Jones and Jose 2004).

71.11 Clinical Features

In most newborns, hypertension is discovered on routine monitoring of vital signs. These infants are asymptomatic or present with the usual nonspecific features in the newborn such as hematuria, feeding difficulties, unexplained tachypnea, apnea, lethargy, irritability, or rarely seizures. Symptomatic infants are often mottled with florid features of congestive heart failure. Skalina in Cleveland reported the rapid onset of a retinopathy identical to that seen in hypertensive adults in neonates with hypertension (Skalina et al. 1983). Eleven of 21 patients with elevated blood pressure demonstrated some or all of the following abnormalities: increased ratio of venous to arterial caliber, vascular tortuosity (including arteriovenous crossing changes), superficial and deep hemorrhages, and exudates. These findings appeared to resolve after control of the hypertension.

71.12 Causes of Hypertension

There are many causes of hypertension (Table 2), but in the newborn period, hypertension is primarily is of renovascular origin, although cardiac, endocrine, and pulmonary causes must be considered as well. Neonatal hypertension may be secondary to congenital malformations or due to acquired disease states.

Congenital etiologies include: renal artery stenosis/hypoplasia, coarctation of the aorta, and abdominal aortic atresia. Renal artery stenosis has also been noted secondary to congenital rubella. Furthermore, there are a number of congenital renal parenchymal abnormalities which have been associated with hypertension in the newborn period. Both autosomal dominant or autosomal recessive polycystic kidney disease (PKD) may present in the newborn period with enlarged kidneys and hypertension. Severely affected infants with PKD are at risk of developing congestive heart failure due to severe malignant hypertension. Hypertension has also been reported in infants with unilateral multicystic dysplastic kidneys. Renal obstruction and hydronephrosis may also lead to hypertension, secondary to impingement on the renal vessels or via the renin-angiotensin system.

Acquired renal parenchymal causes of hypertension in the newborn period include severe acute tubular necrosis and cortical necrosis usually secondary to severe asphyxia. Other acquired causes of neonatal hypertension include: thromboembolic renal artery and renal

Table 2 Causes of hypertension

Renovascular conditions	Thromboembolism
	Renal artery stenosis
	Midabdominal aortic coarctation
	Renal venous thrombosis
	Compression of renal artery
	Idiopathic arterial calcification
	Congenital rubella syndrome
Renal parenchymal disease	Polycystic kidney disease
	Multicystic dysplastic kidney disease
	Ureteropelvic junction obstruction
	Acute tubular necrosis (birth asphyxia)
	Cortical necrosis
Cardiopulmonary conditions	Coarctation of thoracic aorta
	Bronchopulmonary dysplasia (BPD)
	Pneumothorax
Endocrine conditions	Congenital adrenal hyperplasia
	Hyperaldosteronism
	Hyperthyroidism
	Pseudohypoaldosteronism type II
Medications/ intoxications	Corticosteroids, e.g., dexamethasone
	Adrenergic agents
	Vitamin D intoxication
	Xanthenes – theophylline/ caffeine pancuronium
	Phenylephrine
	Maternal cocaine or heroin use
Tumors	Wilms' tumor
	Mesoblastic nephroma
	Neuroblastoma
	Pheochromocytoma
Neurologic conditions	Pain
	Intracranial hypertension
	Seizures
	Familial dysautonomia
	Subdural hematoma
Miscellaneous conditions	Closure of abdominal wall defect
	Adrenal hemorrhage
	Hypercalcemia
	Extracorporeal membrane oxygenation (ECMO)

vein complications secondary to umbilical artery catheterization or to thrombosis associated with polycythemia or hypercoagulable states. Almost 10% of the infants with indwelling umbilical arterial catheters develop hypertension (Singh et al. 1992).

Hypertension is also more common in infants with bronchopulmonary dysplasia (BPD), patent ductus arteriosus, or intraventricular hemorrhage as well as those who receive postnatal corticosteroids. Endocrinologic disorders that may produce hypertension in the newborn period include congenital adrenal hyperplasia, hyperaldosteronism, and hyperthyroidism. Salt and water overload and hypercalcemia may also be associated with hypertension in the neonate. Other factors include pain, closure of abdominal wall defects, adrenal hematoma with renal artery compression, seizures, and central nervous system disorders including those associated with inherited metabolic disorders, drug-induced hypertension, and infants of drug-dependent mothers with symptoms of withdrawal.

Medications to be aware of include aminophylline, high doses of adrenergic agents, prolonged use of pancuronium, or administration of phenylephrine ophthalmic drops. Hypertension induced by medications typically resolves when the offending agent is discontinued or its dose is reduced. Patients with certain tumors, including neuroblastoma, Wilms' tumor, and mesoblastic nephroma, may also present in the neonatal period. The hypertension results from either compression of the renal vessels or ureters by the tumor or secretion of vasoactive substances such as catecholamines associated with a pheochromocytoma or neuroblastoma.

There is also a rare disorder, known as hypertension-hyponatremia syndrome, with elevated levels of renin observed in neonates. Renal ischemia from possible microthrombi has been postulated as the precipitating cause, and with sodium supplementation and antihypertensive therapy, the condition resolves and renin levels return to normal (Daftary et al. 1999).

71.13 Diagnostic Approach

In hypertensive neonates it is important to determine whether any renovascular anomalies were detected prior to birth. The history may include

drug abuse, perinatal asphyxia, umbilical catheter placement, or medications administered to the neonate. It is important to confirm the elevated blood pressure and measure the BP in all four extremities to rule out coarctation of the aorta. The pressures are usually higher in the lower extremity and a differential pressure between the upper and lower extremity would suggest coarctation. During the physical examination, a careful search for anomalies and dysmorphic features and careful cardiac evaluation are mandatory. Tachycardia and flushing may indicate a secreting tumor such as a neuroblastoma.

Careful abdominal examination and auscultation over the renal vessels is important as well as a thorough search for features of congenital adrenal hyperplasia, such as sexual ambiguity or hyperpigmentation. Asymmetrical growth (hemihypertrophy) together with aniridia would suggest a Wilms' tumor. Remember that BPD is a common nonrenal cause of hypertension, and these infants tend to manifest the increased blood pressure late in the course of the disease unless they have been treated with corticosteroids (Alagappan and Malloy 1998). The combination of dexamethasone or aminophylline, together with repeated high doses of adrenergic agents, may all con tribute to hypertension.

The initial evaluation of neonatal hypertension includes determination of serum electrolytes, creatinine, blood urea nitrogen (BUN), and a urinalysis in order to look for renal parenchymal disease. Plasma renin levels are warranted but are normally high in neonates. Endocrinologic studies including serum and urinary measurements of cortisol, 17-hydroxyprogesterone, aldosterone and thyroxin are carried out when pertinent.

In addition to a chest radiograph, which is helpful to determine cardiomegaly and congestive heart failure, renal ultrasonography can provide important information and will identify arterial and/or venous thrombi in addition to renal anomalies. Echocardiography is also useful. Cystourethrography is performed when indicated. In selected infants aortography is used to be performed, but with magnetic resonance imaging and spiral computed tomography (CT) scans, this should no longer be necessary. In neonates, nuclear scanning has limited use to determine abnormalities of perfusion because of immature renal function.

71.14 Treatment

Therapy of neonatal hypertension should be tailored to the severity of the blood pressure elevation and to the underlying cause of hypertension as appropriate. A wide range of therapeutic agents are now available for management of neonatal hypertension in both acute and chronic settings. In most cases hypertension will resolve, but some infants may require prolonged treatment. Pharmacologic management of hypertension in the neonate includes use of beta-blockers, angiotensin-converting enzyme inhibitors, calcium channel blockers, and/or diuretics. Essential elements of therapy also include the avoidance of fluid overload (judicious diuretic therapy may be warranted or fluid restriction if renal function is impaired), relief of pain, and discontinuation of medications possibly contributing to the hypertension such as corticosteroids, aminophylline, and inotropic agents. Every effort should be made to choose the antihypertensive agent most appropriate for the clinical situation. Blood pressure must be closely monitored, and as with intravenous therapy, the BP may drop precipitously. Examples of available drugs for the treatment of hypertension are listed in Table 3. Awareness of their mechanisms of action and side effects is vital in treating these challenging patients. For example, angiotensin-converting enzyme inhibitors such as captopril are excellent antihypertensive agents but are contraindicated in the treatment of babies with coarctation of the aorta, unilateral renal artery disease, and hyperkalemia (Flynn 2000). They must also be used with care in babies with chronic hypertension because an abrupt drop in BP may adversely affect the brain and kidneys.

71.15 Follow-Up

The long-term outcomes of neonatal hypertension depend upon the underlying etiology. Although blood pressures can be controlled with

Table 3 Selected drugs for the treatment of neonatal hypertension

Drug	Dose	Comments
Chlorothiazide (diuretic)	PO: 10–20 mg/kg/dose q 12 h	Monitor electrolytes
	IV: 5–10 mg/kg/dose every 12 h	
Furosemide (diuretic)	IV: 1–2 mg/kg/dose q 12–24 h	Better for short-term use. Monitor electrolytes
	PO: 2–4 mg/kg/dose q 12–24 h	Long-term use can lead to osteopenia and renal calculi
Hydralazine (vasodilator)	IV: 0.1–0.5 mg/kg/dose q 6–8 h	May lead to tachycardia or tachyphylaxis
	PO: 0.25–1 mg/kg/dose q 6–8 h	
Captopril (ACE inhibitor)	PO: Initial: 0.25 mg/kg/dose, then 0.01–0.05 mg/kg/dose q 8–12 h	Monitor renal function and blood pressure closely; contraindicated in infants with bilateral renovascular disease
Propranolol (beta-blocker)	IV 0.01 mg/kg/dose q 6–12 h	Monitor blood pressure, heart rate, glucose
	PO: 0.25 mg/kg/dose q6 h	

antihypertensive medications, infants with parenchymal renal disease may remain hypertensive. When the hypertension is secondary to acquired renovascular disease, the blood pressure often normalizes over time and medications can be discontinued. However significant structural or functional renal abnormalities may persist. Appropriate follow-up with a pediatrician or pediatric nephrologist should be arranged.

71.16 Conclusion

Although many sick newborns are treated for hypotension and hypertension, the normal physiologic BP range ensuring appropriate organ perfusion is uncertain. Treatment decisions are based on statistically defined gestational and postnatal age-dependent normative BP values, combined with clinical intuition, because of difficulties evaluating organ perfusion and adequacy of cerebral oxygen delivery. Early-onset hypotension is usually due to the combined effects of abnormal peripheral vasoregulation, myocardial dysfunction, and hypovolemia. Volume administration is the primary initial therapy, but its use may be associated with significant untoward effects, especially in preterm infants, and should be limited to 10–20 mL/kg of isotonic saline. If the BP cannot be normalized, dopamine should be added, sometimes followed by epinephrine and corticosteroids. Hypertension, most often caused by congenital or acquired renovascular disease or volume overload, needs a thorough search for the etiology and cautious treatment so the BP does not fall too quickly or too low.

71.17 Practice Points

- Blood pressure norms are based on statistically defined gestational and postnatal age-dependent normative blood pressure values. Blood pressure increases with increasing gestational age, weight, and postnatal age.
- Treatment decisions for hypotension should be based on a combination of low blood pressure and clinical symptoms. Too much volume is associated with increased morbidity and mortality
- Care must be taken not to drop the blood pressure too quickly in hypertensive neonates as cerebral perfusion pressure will be adversely affected.

References

Adelman RD (1988) The hypertensive neonate. Clin Perinatol 15:567–585

Alagappan A, Malloy MH (1998) Systemic hypertension in very low-birth weight infants with bronchopulmonary dysplasia: incidence and risk factors. Am J Perinatol 15:3–8

Al-Aweel I, Pursley DM, Rubin LP et al (2001) Variations in prevalence of hypotension, hypertension, and vasopressor use in NICUs. Perinatology 21: 272–278

Barrington K (2008) Hypotension and shock in the preterm infant. Semin Fetal Neonatal Med 13:16–23

Barrington KJ, Janaillac M (2016) Treating hypotension in extremely preterm infants. The pressure is mounting. Arch Dis Child Fetal Neonatal Ed 101(3): F188–F189

Batton B, Zhu X, Fanaroff J et al (2009) Blood pressure, antihypotensive therapy, and neurodevelopment in extremely preterm infants. J Pediatr 154:351–357

Batton B, Li L, Newman NS, Eunice Kennedy Shriver National Institute of Child Health & Human Development Neonatal Research Network et al (2013) Use of antihypotensive therapies in extremely preterm infants. Pediatrics 131:1865–1873

Batton B, Li L, Newman NS, Eunice Kennedy Shriver National Institute of Child Health and Human Development Neonatal Research Network et al (2014) Evolving blood pressure dynamics for extremely preterm infants. J Perinatol 34:301–305

Batton B, Li L, Newman NS, et al Eunice Kennedy Shriver National Institute of Child Health & Human Development Neonatal Research Network (2015) Early blood pressure, antihypotensive therapy and outcomes at 18–22 months' corrected age in extremely preterm infants. Arch Dis Child Fetal Neonatal Ed 101(3): F201–F206

Batton B, Li L, Newman NS et al (2016) Early blood pressure, antihypotensive therapy and outcomes at 18–22 months' corrected age in extremely preterm infants. Arch Dis Child Fetal Neonatal Ed 101(3): F201–F206

Daftary AS, Patole SK, Whitehall J (1999) Hypertension-hyponatremia syndrome in neonates: case report and review of literature. Am J Perinatol 16:385–389

Dempsey EM, Barrington KJ (2009) Evaluation and treatment of hypotension in the preterm infant. Clin Perinatol 36:75–85

Dempsey EM, Al Hazzani F, Barrington KJ (2009) Permissive hypotension in the extremely low birth weight infant with signs of good perfusion. Arch Dis Child Fetal Neonatal Ed 94:F241–F424

Efird MM, Heerens AT, Gordon PV et al (2004) A Randomized-controlled trial of prophylactic hydrocortisone supplementation for the prevention of hypotension in extremely low birth weight infants. Perinatology 25:119–124

Emery EF, Greenough A, Yuksel B (1993) Effect of gender on blood pressure levels of very low birth weight infants in the first 48 hours of life. Early Hum Dev 31:209–216

Ewer AK, Tyler W, Francis A (2003) Excessive volume expansion and neonatal death in preterm infants born at 27–28 weeks gestation. Paediatr Perinat Epidemiol 17:180–186

Fanaroff JM, Wilson-Costello DE, Newman NS et al (2006) Treated hypotension is associated with neonatal morbidity and hearing loss in extremely low birth weight infants. Pediatrics 117:131–135

Flynn JT (2000) Neonatal hypertension: diagnosis and manage- ment. Pediatr Nephrol 14:332–341, Erratum in: Pediatr Nephrol 14:885

Greenough A, Cheeseman P, Kavvadia V et al (2002) Colloid infusion in the perinatal period and abnormal neurodevelopmental outcome in very low birth weight infants. Eur J Pediatr 161:319–323

Ibrahim H, Sinha IP, Subhedar NV (2011) Corticosteroids for treating hypotension in preterm infants. Cochrane Database Syst Rev 12, CD003662

Jones JE, Jose PA (2004) Neonatal blood pressure regulation. Semin Perinatol 28:141–148

Kuint J, Barak M, Morag I, Maayan-Metzger A (2009) Early treated hypotension and outcome in very low birth weight infants. Neonatology 95:311–316

Lightburn MH, Gauss CH, Williams DK, Kaiser JR (2009) Cerebral blood flow velocities in extremely low birth weight infants with hypotension and infants with normal blood pressure. J Pediatr 154:824–828

Mayock DE, Gleason CA (2004) Cerebrovascular effects of rapid volume expansion in preterm fetal sheep. Pediatr Res 55:395–399

National High Blood Pressure Education Program Working Group on High Blood Pressure in Children and Adolescents (2004) The fourth report on the diagnosis, evaluation, and treatment of high blood pressure in children and adolescents. Pediatrics 14:555–576

Oca MJ, Nelson M, Donn SM (2003) Randomized trial of normal saline versus 5% albumin for the treatment of neonatal hypotension. J Perinatol 23:473–476

Osborn DA, Evans N (2004) Early volume expansion for prevention of morbidity and mortality in very preterm infants. Cochrane Database Syst Rev 2, CD002055

Pellicer A, Bravo MC, Madero R et al (2009) Early systemic hypotension and vasopressor support in low birth weight infants: impact on neurodevelopment. Pediatrica 123:1369–1376

Shivanna B, Rios D, Rossano J, Fernandes CJ, Pammi M (2013) Vasopressin and its analogues for the treatment of refractory hypotension in neonates. Cochrane Database Syst Rev 3, CD009171

Singh HP, Hurley RM, Myers TF (1992) Neonatal hypertension. Incidence and risk factors. Am J Hypertens 5:51–55

Skalina ME, Annable WL, Kliegman RM, Fanaroff AA (1983) Hypertensive retinopathy in the newborn infant. J Pediatr 103:781–786

Skalina ME, Kliegman RM, Fanaroff AA (1986) Epidemiology and management of severe symptomatic neonatal hypertension. Am J Perinatol 3:235–239

Stranak Z, Semberova J, Barrington K, HIP consortium et al (2014) International survey on diagnosis and management of hypotension in extremely preterm babies. Eur J Pediatr 173:793–798

Subhedar NV, Shaw NJ (2003) Dopamine versus dobutamine for hypotensive preterm infants. Cochrane Database Syst Rev 3:CD001242

Versmold HT, Kitterman JA, Phibbs RH et al (1981) Aortic blood pressure during the first 12 hours of life in infants with birth weight 610 to 4,220 grams. Pediatrics 67:607–613

Watkins AM, West CR, Cooke RW (1989) Blood pressure and cerebral haemorrhage and ischaemia in very low birth weight infants. Early Hum Dev 19:103–110

Yeh TF, Lin YJ, Lin HC et al (2004) Outcomes at school age after postnatal dexamethasone therapy for lung disease of prematurity. N Engl J Med 350:1304–1313

Zubrow AB, Hulman S, Kushner H, Falkner B (1995) Determinants of blood pressure in infants admitted to neonatal intensive care units: a prospective multicenter study. J Perinatol 15:470–479

Polycythemia and Hyperviscosity in Neonates

72

Otwin Linderkamp

Contents

Abstract

Polycythemia and the resulting increase in blood viscosity are common in the neonatal period. However, neonatal blood has several favorable properties including lower plasma viscosity, RBC aggregation, and increased red blood cell deformability compared with adults. Oxygen transport to vital organs is, therefore, usually not compromised when the hematocrit (HCL) is below 0.70 L/L. Polycythemia may develop before (increased erythropoiesis, prenatal transfusion syndromes) or after birth (late cord-clamping). Nevertheless, delayed or late cord-clamping should be encouraged because of favorable circulatory effects – among other advantages. Signs of polycythemia often result from the underlying disorder (e.g., intrauterine asphyxia, maternal diabetes) rather than from the increased HCT and blood viscosity. Postnatal blood volume loss contributes to the development of polycythemia in most affected infants. Early oral feeding or, if necessary, additional i.v. fluid is therefore the first-line

O. Linderkamp (✉)
Division of Neonatology, Department of Pediatrics, University of Heidelberg, Heidelberg, Germany
e-mail: olinderkamp@yahoo.de

G. Buonocore et al. (eds.), *Neonatology*,
https://doi.org/10.1007/978-3-319-29489-6_218

treatment and prophylaxis against polycythemia. Because partial exchange transfusion (PET) did not improve the long-term neurodevelopmental outcome and even increased the risk of early complications (necrotizing enterocolitis, septicemia) in polycythemic infants, indications for PET should be restricted to symptomatic neonates with HCT ≥0.70 L/L and to asymptomatic infants with HCT ≥0.75 L/L.

Abbreviations

HCT Hematocrit
NEC Necrotizing enterocolitis
PET Partial exchange transfusion
RBC Red blood cell

72.1 Salient Points

- Neonatal polycythemia is generally defined as a central hematocrit ≥0.65 L/L, but may more appropriately be defined as hematocrit ≥0.70 L/L.
- Risk factors for polycythemia include increased fetal erythropoiesis (intrauterine hypoxia, maternal diabetes) and RBC transfusion from the placenta, the mother, or a monochorionic twin.
- Increased plasma viscosity and RBC aggregation and decreased RBC deformability may contribute to increased blood viscosity in addition to polycythemia (e.g., maternal diabetes).
- Late cord-clamping is beneficial for most infants in spite of the increased risk of polycythemia.
- Clinical signs of polycythemia and increased blood viscosity result from a decrease in blood flow to various organs. However, oxygen supply is usually not compromised up to a hematocrit of 0.70 L/L.
- Screening for polycythemia should be restricted to high-risk neonates.
- Prevention measures of polycythemia and hyperviscosity include effective control of maternal diabetes, gestosis, and smoking, and sufficient fluid administration to the newborn infant.
- Because polycythemia is aggravated or caused by hemoconcentration, additional oral and/or venous fluid administration is usually the appropriate first-line treatment.
- Partial exchange transfusion (PET) for treatment of neonatal polycythemia increased the risk of necrotizing enterocolitis and did not improve the long-term outcome in any study.
- In infants with asymptomatic polycythemia, PET may be considered if HCT ≥0.75 L/L and additional oral and i.v. fluid was insufficient.
- If additional oral and i.v. fluid failed to decrease the hematocrit sufficiently, PET may be indicated in asymptomatic infants with HCT ≥0.75 L/L and in symptomatic infants (blood glucose <40 mg/dL, platelets <100,000/μL, or respiratory distress requiring oxygen) with HCT ≥0.70 L/L.
- PET should be done with normal saline.

72.2 Introduction

Blood viscosity (V) is a measure of thickness and stickiness of the blood. With rising blood viscosity (V) the friction of blood against the vessel wall increases, thereby raising the resistance (R) to blood flow (F). R is directly proportional to V and the hindrance (Z) resulting from the vessel geometry: $R = VZ = P/F$ (Linderkamp 2007). In vessels or tubes with defined geometry (i.e., constant Z), R is directly proportional to V and the pressure (P). Thus, to provide a constant blood flow, the pressure driving the blood must increase with rising blood viscosity.

Blood viscosity is usually measured in flow devices with fixed geometry (e.g., in a rotational viscometer with a defined gap or in a tube viscometer with defined tube diameter and length). In these devices, the blood flow resistance increases linearly with the blood viscosity, and blood flow resistance is measured as pressure or force required to achieve a defined blood flow in the device ($V \approx R = P/F$). Rotational viscometers measure the force required for rotating a disk, bob, or spindle in the blood at known speed. They allow to apply various shear forces. At low shear forces RBCs aggregate, thereby increasing

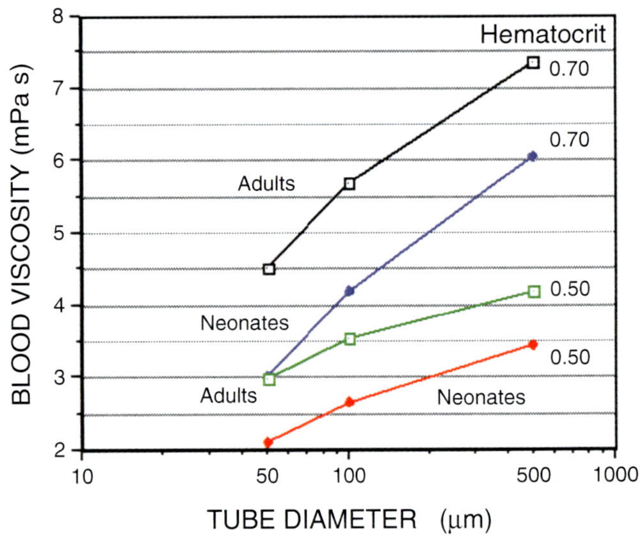

Fig. 1 Blood viscosity in adults and full-term neonates measured in tubes with diameters of 50, 100, and 500 µm. The hematocrit was adjusted to 0.50 and 0.70 L/L. Note that in 50-µm tubes the viscosity of neonatal blood with a hematocrit of 0.70 L/L was similar as the viscosity of adult blood with a hematocrit of 0.50 L/L (Adapted from Linderkamp et al. 1992a)

blood viscosity. At high shear forces blood viscosity decreases due to disaggregation and ellipsoidal deformation of RBCs. Thus, rotational viscometers provide information on RBC aggregation and RBC deformation. Tube viscometers provide better models of vessel blood flow. By using tubes with a wide range of diameters below 300 µ, the so-called Fahraeus-Lindqvist effect (decrease in blood viscosity with decreasing diameter, Fig. 1) can be determined.

72.3 Determinants of Blood Viscosity in the Neonate

Hyperviscosity is frequently used synonymously with polycythemia (i.e., high hematocrit, HCT). However, blood viscosity increases with increasing HCT, plasma viscosity, RBC aggregation, leukocyte count, and with decreasing RBC deformability. Neonatal blood has several favorable properties including lower plasma viscosity and RBC aggregation (due to lower concentrations of high molecular weight proteins) and increased RBC deformability (Linderkamp 1996, 2004, 2007; Linderkamp et al. 1986, 1992a). Plasma viscosity is about 20% lower in the neonate compared with adults, thereby decreasing blood viscosity at given HCT by 20% (Linderkamp 2004). The reduced RBC aggregation decreases blood viscosity at low shear stress and facilitates blood flow at slow flow (e.g., in veins). In preterm infants, plasma viscosity and RBC aggregation are even lower than in full-term neonates due to lower plasma protein concentrations (Linderkamp et al. 1992a).

The increased RBC deformability in neonates results from increased RBC membrane elasticity compared with adult RBCs (Linderkamp et al. 1986). RBC deformation is of great importance for effective blood flow in the microcirculation, where the 8-µm diameter RBC must negotiate 3- to 4-µm diameter vessels (Buonocore et al. 1991), but also in small arteries and arterioles, where RBC deformation is the prerequisite for the decrease in blood viscosity with decreasing vessel diameter. This Fahraeus-Lindqvist effect is more pronounced for neonatal RBCs than that of adults (Fig. 1) due to the larger volume and increased membrane elasticity of neonatal RBCs. The extent of the viscosity reduction increases with rising HCT. When going from a 500- to a 50-µm tube, the viscosity of blood with a HCT of 0.70 L/L decreases by 38% in adults and by 50% in healthy full-term neonates (Linderkamp et al. 1992a). Because of the enhanced Fåhræus-Lindqvist effect and lower plasma viscosity, blood viscosity in 50-µm tubes is similar in neonates who have a

HCT of 0.70 L/L as in adults with a HCT of 0.50 L/L. These findings may explain why circulation in neonates is less affected by a high HCT than circulation in adults.

72.4 Detection and Definition of Polycythemia and Hyperviscosity in Neonates

Definition of Polycythemia In most treatment protocols, neonatal polycythemia has been defined as venous HCT $\geq$0.65 L/L (Dempsey and Barrington 2006; Özek et al. 2010). Thus, the definition of polycythemia depends crucially on the reliability of HCT measurements.

Hematocrit Measurement HCT determined on a microcentrifuge was on average 0.057 L/L higher than the Coulter counter HCT in two studies (Villalta et al. 1989; Morag et al. 2011). Higher HCT measured by microcentrifugation may in part be the result of a small fraction of plasma remaining in the RBC column ("trapped plasma"). Trapped plasma is approximately 2–3%, thus increasing an actual HCT of 0.635–0.65 L/L. Trapped plasma can be higher (up to 8%) when the HCT is increased and the centrifugal force acting on the inner end of the blood column is <10,000 g. For this reason, only two third of the HCT tubes should be filled with blood. Villalta et al. (1989) found a closer correlation of the blood viscosity to the microhematocrit when compared to the Coulter HCT. They conclude that the microhematocrit is more reliable than the Coulter HCT. HCT in venous blood collected with excessive squeezing and prolonged tourniquet may increase. HCT measurements are similar in free flowing venous and arterial blood.

Changes in Hematocrit After Birth Cord blood HCT in healthy full-term neonates averaged 0.48–0.54 L/L in several studies (Philip and Saigal 2004). Higher values can be found in infants with increased fetal erythropoiesis, prenatal transfusion, and dehydration. The HCT increases in most newborn infants during the first 1–4 h after birth, unless neonatal blood volume is low (e.g., after early cord-clamping) (Linderkamp et al. 1992b) or the infant is born preterm (Jobling et al. 2009). In healthy full-term neonates, venous HCT increases from approximately 0.50 L/L (cord blood) to 0.54 L/L during the first 2 h after birth (Jobling et al. 2009). The dynamics of HCT changes after birth have been studied in infants with late cord-clamping. The HCT (corrected for trapped plasma) rose from 0.50 $\pm$ 0.04 L/L in cord blood to 0.63 $\pm$ 0.05 L/L at 2 h of birth and decreased to 0.59 $\pm$ 0.05 L/L at 24 h (Jobling et al. 2009). A substantial part of the HCT rise occurs within 3 min of birth (Oh et al. 1966). Shohat et al. (1984) found a HCT rise from 0.53 L/L at birth to 0.60 L/L at 2 h and a subsequent decrease to 0.52 at 12–18 h in infants with cord-clamping at 10–30 s. Other authors report little HCT changes in infants with neonatal HCT $\geq$0.65 L/L during the first days (Goldberg et al. 1982; Van der Elst et al. 1980; Bada et al. 1992), unless intravenous fluids were given (Linderkamp 2004; Morag et al. 2011; Alsafadi et al. 2014). These apparently contradictory results may be due to different feeding practices.

Cord blood is the preferred source for screening since it is routinely collected for blood gas studies and does not require vessel puncture in the infant. Shohat et al. found that the HCT at 2 h of birth can be estimated from the cord HCT multiplied by 1.13 (Shohat et al. 1984). Thus, a HCT $\geq$0.65 L/L can be expected if the cord HCT is $\geq$0.57 L/L. However, polycythemia subsequent to late cord-clamping cannot be predicted from the cord HCT, since it is in the normal range (Philip and Saigal 2004; Linderkamp et al. 1992b).

Site of Blood Sampling The skin prick ("capillary") HCT is consistently higher than the HCT measured in a simultaneously drawn venous or arterial blood sample and therefore particularly suitable for polycythemic screening. HCT measured in warmed skin prick blood is on average 0.06 L/L higher than the venous HCT over a wide range of HCT values (Rosenkrantz 2003; Linderkamp et al. 1977). This has been explained by impaired peripheral circulation and RBC

trapping in skin vessels (Linderkamp et al. 1977). Because the capillary-venous HCT differences vary widely, a venous specimen should be analyzed if the capillary HCT is $\geq$0.65 or $\geq$0.70 L/L (depending on the definition of polycythemia).

Can a Critical High Hematocrit be Defined? The definition of polycythemia as venous HCT $\geq$0.65 L/L is not based on sound scientific knowledge (Linderkamp 2004; Rosenkrantz 2003; Schimmel et al. 2004; Mimouni et al. 2011). There is some evidence that polycythemia in neonates without additional risk factors for hyperviscosity may more appropriately be defined as HCT $\geq$0.70 L/L:

- Neonatal blood demonstrates several beneficial flow properties as decreased plasma viscosity, increased RBC deformability, and a more pronounced viscosity reduction in narrow tubes when compared with adult blood (Linderkamp 1996, 2004, 2007; Linderkamp et al. 1986, 1992a).
- The red cell transport efficiency (i.e., HCT divided by blood viscosity) determined in 50-μm tubes (corresponding to small arteries) was highest over a HCT range of 0.50–0.70 L/L in the neonate (adult blood: 0.40–0.60 L/L) (Linderkamp et al. 1992a).
- Studies on circulation and oxygen supply in newborn infants with high HCT did not distinguish between infants with HCT <0.70 L/L and HCT $\geq$0.70 L/L. However, most studies including mainly infants with HCT <0.70 L/L showed normal systemic RBC transport, RBC transport in cerebral and gastrointestinal arteries, and cerebral oxygen supply (Rosenkrantz and Oh 1982; Maertzdorf et al. 1993; Mandelbaum et al. 1994; Liem et al. 1997), whereas most studies including predominantly infants with HCT $\geq$0.70 L/L showed decreased RBC transport and oxygen supply (Bada et al. 1986; Swetnam et al. 1987; Maerztdorf et al. 1989; Ergenecon et al. 2011).
- An elevated occurrence of thrombocytopenia has been noted in neonates with HCT $\geq$0.70 L/L (19%), but not in infants with HCT 0.65–0.69 L/L (5%) (Morag et al. 2011). This indicates that HCT $\geq$ 0.70 L/L increases the risk for disturbed microcirculation.
- Studies on long-term outcome did not compare infants with HCT 0.65–0.69 and $\geq$0.70 L/L. However, recent studies using a venous HCT of 0.70 L/L as critical value for intervention showed similar short-term outcome as earlier studies using a critical HCT of 0.65 L/L (Morag et al. 2011; Alsafadi et al. 2014).

Definition of Hyperviscosity Some authors propose to determine blood viscosity and not just HCT for therapeutic decisions since increased viscosity may result from increased plasma volume and RBC aggregation and decreased RBC deformability in addition to polycythemia. However, the results of blood viscosity measurements vary widely among various measuring devices and depend on the applied shear forces and (in tube viscometers) on the tube diameter (Fig. 1). Each laboratory has to establish normal values, and blood viscosity measurements are not readily available around the clock. In clinical practice, measurements of HCT or hemoglobin concentration are sufficient to detect most cases of hyperviscosity.

72.5 Causes of Polycythemia and Hyperviscosity in the Neonate

Table 1 summarizes causes of and risk factors for polycythemia and hyperviscosity in the neonate. Polycythemia is the most frequent cause of hyperviscosity. The HCT may rise as a result of an increased RBC mass, a decrease in plasma volume, or both. Late cord-clamping results in marked volume expansion by the baby's own blood from the placenta (Linderkamp 1982). Blood cells and plasma are "transfused," but approximately 20 mL/kg of plasma leave the circulation within 2 h, while the RBC mass remains constant (Oh et al. 1966). Intrauterine transfusion of blood to the fetus may occur as a result of intrauterine asphyxia, twin-twin transfusion, and maternal-fetal transfusion. In these infants, the cord HCT is usually already increased.

Table 1 Causes of polycythemia and hyperviscosity in the fetus and neonate

Cause
Increased hematocrit (≥0.65 l/l)
Red blood cell transfusion:
Placenta-to-fetus transfusion: late cord-clamping,[a] intrauterine asphyxia[a]
Twin-twin transfusion (monochorionic twins)[a]
Maternal-fetal transfusion
Transfusion of a large volume of blood or erythrocytes[a]
Increased fetal/neonatal erythropoiesis:
Chronic intrauterine hypoxia,[a] placental insufficiency,[a] maternal gestosis[a], active or passive maternal smoking[a]
Small for gestational age[a] and large for gestational age[a] infants
Hyperinsulinism (diabetic mother,[a] congenital hyperinsulinism[a])
Neonatal thyrotoxicosis,[a] adrenal hyperplasia[a]
High altitude[a]
Trisomy 13,[a] 18,[a] 21[a]
Congenital erythrocytosis
Uncontrolled treatment of the infant with erythropoietin
Dehydration
Increased plasma viscosity and RBC aggregation
Diabetic mother
Infusion of large amounts of adult plasma, immunoglobulins, fibrinogen, or plasma substitutes
Septicemia (increase in fibrinogen)
Decreased RBC deformability
Diabetic mother (glycosylated membrane proteins)
Hypoxia, acidosis
Nutritional deficiencies (vitamin E, iron, protein)
Transfusion of ATP-depleted RBC
Septicemia

[a]Discussed indications of screening for polycythemia

Increased fetal erythropoiesis is most frequently caused by intrauterine hypoxia due to maternal gestosis, maternal smoking, and placental insufficiency. In infants of diabetic mothers increased erythropoiesis has been explained by fetal hypoxemia, hyperinsulinism, hyperglycemia, and hyperketonemia (Mimouni et al. 1986). Blood volume measurements showed increased RBC mass and decreased plasma volume in polycythemic infants with intrauterine growth retardation and in macrosomic infants (including infants of diabetic mothers) (Brans et al. 1981; Maertzdorf et al. 1991). The finding of low plasma volume in polycythemic infants indicates that increased fluid administration is indicated as first intervention in neonatal polycythemia.

Increases in plasma viscosity and RBC aggregation induced by infusion of high molecular weight proteins in newborn piglets had similar negative effects on circulation as polycythemia (Goldstein et al. 1988). This explains why infusion of immunoglobulins for treatment of isoimmune thrombocytopenia and hemolytic disease or septicemia may increase the risk of thromboses (Merlob et al. 1990). Because of the higher plasma viscosity of adult plasma, fresh frozen plasma should not be used for hemodilution in polycythemic neonates (Linderkamp et al. 1984).

A marked impairment of RBC deformability is mostly found in anemic infants (e.g., iron deficiency, congenital hemolytic diseases) and in septicemia. Adult RBC are less deformable than neonatal RBC, especially in preterm infants (Linderrkamp et al. 1997). Transfusion of adult RBC should, therefore, not increase the HCT to more than 0.55 L/L. In small for gestational age infants and in infants of diabetic mothers increased plasma viscosity, increased RBC aggregation, and decreased RBC deformability may contribute to increased blood viscosity (Linderkamp 1996). Interventions to reduce the hematocrit may, therefore, be indicated in some of these infants with moderately increased HCT of 0.65–0.69 L/L.

72.6 Does Late Cord-Clamping Increase the Risk of Symptomatic Polycythemia?

Before birth, approximately 70 mL/kg of blood is contained in the fetus and another 45 mL/kg of fetal blood is in the placenta (Linderkamp 1982). If the umbilical cord is not severed immediately after birth and the infant is kept below the level of the placenta, up to 35 mL/kg of blood may flow from the placenta into the newly born infant during the following 3 min ("late cord-clamping"), thereby increasing the neonatal blood volume to 105 mL/kg. Placental transfusion occurs in a

Table 2 Effect of cord-clamping on hemorheology in full-term infants at 2 h after birth (Linderkamp et al. 1992b; Nelle et al. 1993)

	Early [a]	Leboyer [b]	Late [c]	Adults [d]	$P < 0.05$
Hematocrit [L/L]	0.47 ± 0.06	0.58 ± 0.06	0.63 ± 0.05	0.47 ± 0.05	a < b < c
Plasma viscosity [mPa s]	1.06 ± 0.09	1.06 ± 0.08	1.09 ± 0.09	1.29 ± 0.13	a = b = c < d
RBC aggregation	4.1 ± 1.0	4.2 ± 1.8	4.0 ± 1.4	10.3 ± 2.5	a = b = c < d
Blood viscosity [mPa s]	2.8 ± 0.5	3.7 ± 0.5	4.2 ± 0.4	3.5 ± 0.6	a < b < c
Red cell mass [mL/kg][a]	30 ± 0.6	39 ± 0.6	46 ± 0.6	30 ± 0.7	a < b < c
Plasma volume [mL/kg][a]	40 ± 0.6	36 ± 0.6	34 ± 0.6	40 ± 0.7	a > c
Blood volume [mL/kg][a]	70 ± 0.7	75 ± 0.11	80 ± 0.9	70 ± 0.8	a < c

[a]Calculated from residual placental blood volume and hematocrit (Nelle et al. 1993)

stepwise manner. During the first 15–20 s, about 10 mL/kg flow to the infant in relation to the uterine contractions at birth. Another 10–15 mL/kg rise of the neonatal blood volume occurs during 45–60 s and again during the third minute after birth (Yao and Lind 1982).

The blood volume expansion of up to 50% subsequent to late cord-clamping is rapidly counteracted by shifting of plasma to the extravascular space, thereby increasing the HCT and blood viscosity in relation to the amount of placental transfusion. The maximum HCT and blood viscosity are reached 2–4 h after birth (Linderkamp et al. 1992b; Yao and Lind 1982; Christensen et al. 2014). A placental transfusion of 10 mL/kg increases the HCT at 2 h of birth by about 0.04 L/L (Linderkamp et al. 1992b). Between 4 and 24 h of birth, the plasma volume expands again, thereby decreasing the HCT by approximately 0.05 L/L (Linderkamp et al. 1992b; Yao and Lind 1982). As a result of these plasma shifts, a HCT ≥0.65 L/L is found in 25% of neonates with late cord-clamping at 2–4 h of birth, but in less than 10% at 24 h (Linderkamp et al. 1992b).

Studies performed in the 1960s and 1970s demonstrated that late cord-clamping may increase the risk of circulatory overload, respiratory problems, jaundice, and polycythemia (Philip and Saigal 2004; Linderkamp 1982; Yao and Lind 1982). To avoid these risks, immediate cord-clamping (within 10 s) was recommended for infants with a high risk of polycythemia, and early cord-clamping (at 10–30 s) for low-risk infants (Yao and Lind 1982; Capasso et al. 2003). Other authors recommend to allow a medium placental transfusion of 15–20 mL/kg in full-term and preterm infants (Philip and Saigal 2004; Linderkamp 1982; Hutton and Hassan 2007; Katheria et al. 2016). A medium placental transfusion can be achieved by keeping the infant below the placenta and clamping the cord 30–60 s after birth ("delayed" cord-clamping) or by placing the infant on the mother's abdomen and clamping the cord 2–3 min after birth or when the cord stops pulsating (Leboyer birth) (Linderkamp 1982; Nelle et al. 1993).

While there is consensus that "delayed" cord-clamping is beneficial to the newborn infant, there is still concern that a maximum placental transfusion may be risky for some newborn infants However, the current state of knowledge indicates that late cord-clamping may be beneficial for most infants in spite of the marked rise of the HCT:

1. The newborn infant can rapidly compensate for a high blood volume by shifting of plasma to the extravascular space (Linderkamp 1982).
2. The resulting increase in HCT is not harmful up to a HCT of 0.70 L/L because of favorable properties of neonatal RBC and plasma (see Table 2). Moreover, the HCT decreases spontaneously after the early postnatal hours (Linderkamp et al. 1992b; Oh et al. 1966; Shohat et al. 1984).
3. Jaundice requiring phototherapy did not develop more often in late clamped neonates compared with early cord-clamping (Hutton and Hassan 2007).
4. The blood volume expansion after late cord-clamping may increase the oxygen supply of the lungs, the brain, the gut, and the kidneys (Katheria et al. 2016).

5. The increased RBC mass improves the iron supply for several months.
6. Late cord-clamping had no adverse effect on the outcome of full-term infants at 5 and 20 months of age even in children with a neonatal HCT >0.65 L/L at birth (Linderkamp et al. 2004).
7. Late cord-clamping is considered natural not only in natural cultures but also in modern societies. Psychological reasons might contribute to better neurodevelopmental outcome of children with late cord-clamping.
8. Cord blood is the baby's blood since the whole fetal blood volume circulates in the fetus and in the fetal placenta. Legally, the parents of the infant are responsible for the decision of how and when the cord is clamped and severed.
9. For infants with high risk of polycythemia, late cord-clamping combined with positioning of the baby on the mother's abdomen results in a smaller placental transfusion (approx. 15–20 mL/kg) than by keeping the infant below the placenta (approx. 35 mL/kg), and an increase of the HCT ≥0.65 L/L is unlikely (Linderkamp 1982; Yao and Lind 1982; Nelle et al. 1993).

Milking of the uncut (Christensen et al. 2014; Erickson-Owens et al. 2012) umbilical cord increased the HCT by 0.05 L/L. In prematurely born infants, delayed cord-clamping (20–60 s) and cord milking improved blood pressure and HCT, reduced blood transfusions, intraventricular hemorrhage, and late-onset sepsis in several studies (Katheria et al. 2016). Polycythemia was not observed after these relatively short periods of cord-clamping delay.

72.7 Symptoms and Complications of Polycythemia and Hyperviscosity

Frequency of Symptoms Three literature surveys on findings in neonatal polycythemia revealed considerable variation in the frequencies of symptoms and laboratory findings associated with the diagnosis of polycythemia (Rosenkrantz 2003; Schimmel et al. 2004; Pappas and Delaney-Black 2004). This may be explained by differences in the definition of polycythemia and/or hyperviscosity, the time of blood sampling, the definition of clinical signs and symptoms, and the number of infants included who had a high risk of perinatal complications independent of the occurrence of polycythemia (e.g., asphyxia, intrauterine growth retardation, diabetic mother). The knowledge of a high HCT may influence the assessment of weak clinical symptoms such as lethargy or poor feeding. Most of the clinical symptoms are unspecific and can also be observed in neonates who do not have polycythemia (Table 3). Unfortunately, most papers on clinical symptoms and signs in infants with increased HCT do not compare the results with a control group. It is particular ironic that some of the most dangerous complications such as necrotizing enterocolitis

Table 3 Clinical features ascribed to polycythemia and hyperviscosity

Central nervous system
Early effects: Hypotonia and sleepiness, irritability and jitteriness
Neurodevelopment: Long-term neurologic and developmental problems
The reported long-term sequelae are mostly caused by underlying condition as intrauterine and perinatal asphyxia or maternal diabetes
Heart and lungs
Tachycardia, tachypnea, respiratory distress
Cyanosis, plethora
Chest radiography: cardiomegaly, pulmonary plethora
Echocardiography: increased pulmonary resistance, decreased cardiac output
Gastrointestinal tract
Poor suck, vomiting
Necrotizing enterocolitis
Kidneys
Oliguria (depending on blood volume)
Metabolism
Hypoglycemia
Hypocalcemia, hypomagnesemia
Jaundice
Coagulation
Thrombocytopenia
Thrombosis

may be caused by the procedure of partial exchange transfusion (PET) rather than by the high hematocrit (Pappas and Delaney-Black 2004).

General Hemodynamics Blood flow decreases linearly with rising blood viscosity, unless increased blood viscosity is compensated for by vasodilatation or increase in blood pressure (see "Introduction"). In newborn puppies and lambs polycythemia induced by transfusion of packed RBC decreased cardiac output and blood flow to the brain, the gastrointestinal tract, the kidneys, the lungs, the limbs, and the skin (Kotagal et al. 1977; Holzman et al. 1986). However, systemic RBC flow and RBC flow to the brain and the kidneys remained stable up to a HCT of 0.70 L/L. Effects of polycythemia on blood flow dynamics in newborn infants have been studied by means of Doppler ultrasonography. Cardiac output in polycythemic newborn infants was lower than in controls, but systemic RBC transport was either similar as in controls (Mandelbaum et al. 1994) or moderately decreased (Swetnam et al. 1987). Thus, systemic RBC transport (and therefore oxygen transport) is usually maintained up to a HCT of 0.70 L/L.

Respiration Tachypnea and other signs of respiratory distress have been reported in 2–25% of infants with HCT $\geq$0.65 L/L (Van der Elst et al. 1980; Alsafadi et al. 2014; Wiswell et al. 1986; Uslu et al. 2011). Morag et al. observed respiratory distress requiring oxygen treatment in 3.8% of 53 infants with HCT 0.65–0.69 L/L and in 7.6% of infants with HCT 0.70–0.80 L/L (Morag et al. 2011). Respiratory symptoms in polycythemic neonates may develop as a result of hypervolemia, pulmonary hypertension, and right-to-left shunting through the ductus arteriosus and the open foramen ovale (Swetnam et al. 1987). Peripheral or systemic cyanosis and plethora are merely signs of a high hematocrit and blood volume, but not of compromised circulation.

Central Nervous System The focus in the care of polycythemic infants has always been on the early detection and prevention of developmental and neurological sequelae. Early neurological symptoms such as hypotonia, lethargy and sleepiness, irritability, and tremulousness are frequently seen in newborn infants with HCT $\geq$0.65 L/L (Pappas and Delaney-Black 2004). These symptoms appear to suit well to the finding of decreased cerebral blood flow in animals as in human neonates with high hematocrit. However, in newborn puppies (Kotagal et al. 1977) and in human neonates (Rosenkrantz and Oh 1982; Maertzdorf et al. 1993; Mandelbaum et al. 1994; Liem et al. 1997) RBC transport and oxygenation did not decrease up to a HCT of 0.70 L/L. Thus, decreased blood flow in neonatal polycythemia is compensated by increased oxygen content, unless a critical HCT of approximately 0.70 L/L is reached. At HCT $\geq$0.70 L/L, RBC flow to the brain and cerebral oxygenation tend to decrease (Bada et al. 1986; Swetnam et al. 1987; Maerztdorf et al. 1989; Ergenecon et al. 2011).

Nine studies on long-term neurodevelopmental outcome of children with neonatal polycythemia or hyperviscosity have been found in the literature. Four studies showed no significant differences in neurodevelopmental scores in 141 children with neonatal HCT $\geq$0.65 L/L compared with 130 control children studied at 8 months to 6 years of postnatal age (Van der Elst et al. 1980; Bada et al. 1992; Linderkamp et al. 2004; Host and Ulrich 1982). One study did not include a control group (Kumar and Ramji 2004). Four studies found signs of impaired neurodevelopment in children with neonatal polycythemia or hyperviscosity at 8 months to 7 years of age (Goldberg et al. 1982; Black et al. 1985a; Delaney-Black et al. 1989; Ratrisawada et al. 1994; Drew et al. 1997). Delaney-Black et al. (Black et al. 1985a; Delaney-Black et al. 1989) reported that neonatal polycythemia was associated with a high risk of neurologic and developmental problems at 1 and 2 years. At 7 years only small (insignificant) differences were observed between children with and without neonatal polycythemia. However, both groups included infants who had additional risks for developmental problems. PET did not improve the outcome of children with neonatal polycythemia in any study (Goldberg et al. 1982; Van der Elst et al. 1980; Bada et al. 1992; Kumar and Ramji 2004; Black et al. 1985a; Delaney-Black et al. 1989; Ratrisawada et al. 1994).

Gastrointestinal Tract In newborn dogs, increase in HCT from 0.48 to 0.70 L/L caused a decrease in gastrointestinal blood flow by 54% and of RBC transport by 32% (Kotagal et al. 1977). In polycythemic newborn infants blood flow velocity in the celiac artery was lower than in controls. However, RBC transport (blood flow velocity times HCT) was similar in both groups (Mandelbaum et al. 1994). Feeding problems have been reported in 61% of neonates with HCT ≥0.65 L/L, but also in 50% of control infants (Black et al. 1985b). Severe gastrointestinal complications are rare. Necrotizing enterocolitis (NEC) developed in 15 out of 1,122 infants (1.3%) (Morag et al. 2011; Wiswell et al. 1986). In two other studies, NEC developed in 14 out of 67 polycythemic infants after PET (30%), but in no polycythemic infant with symptomatic care (Van der Elst et al. 1980; Black et al. 1985b). Uslu et al. noted NEC grade Ia in three polycythemic infants before PET that deteriorated to grade II after PET (Uslu et al. 2011).

Renal Functions In newborns dogs and lambs polycythemia had only small effects on renal blood flow (Kotagal et al. 1977; Holzman et al. 1986). Acute renal failure, renal vein thrombosis, and renal tubular damage have been reported in individual infants with increased HCT (Rosenkrantz 2003; Pappas and Delaney-Black 2004). Oliguria (urine <1 ml/kg/h) has been noted in two out of eight neonates with HCT ≥0.70 L/L (Aperia et al. 1974), but only in one out of 101 neonates with HCT ≥0.65 L/L (Alsafadi et al. 2014). Although rare, oliguria in polycythemic infants indicates low plasma volume and should be treated immediately.

Metabolic Effects Hypoglycemia defined as serum glucose below 30–50 mg/dL was observed in 2–40% of neonates with HCT ≥0.65 L/L (Morag et al. 2011; Goldberg et al. 1982; Alsafadi et al. 2014; Wiswell et al. 1986; Uslu et al. 2011; Kumar and Ramji 2004). This wide variation can be explained by differences in hypoglycemia definitions, times and methods of blood sampling and glucose analyses, and the inclusion of different numbers of infants with a high risk for hypoglycemia (infants of diabetic mothers, intrauterine growth retardation, postmaturity). Serum glucose may be underestimated in blood with high HCT if whole blood is analyzed or the analyzed plasma has not been immediately separated from RBC and leukocytes. Rosenkrantz (Rosenkrantz 2003) suggests that decreased blood flow results in reduced glucose supply of various organs, thereby increasing the glucose extraction and decreasing especially the venous glucose concentration.

Hypocalcemia (serum calcium <2.1 mmol/L) has been reported in 0–25% (Goldberg et al. 1982; Alsafadi et al. 2014; Uslu et al. 2011; Host and Ulrich 1982; Werner 1995) and hypomagnesemia (<0.7 mmol/L) in 30% (Van der Elst et al. 1980) of infants with HCT ≥65 L/L.

Coagulation Thrombocytopenia, low antithrombin, and increased fibrin monomers have been reported in infants with polycythemia (Rivers 1975). Platelet count <100,000/μL has been found in 4.5% of infants with HCT 0.65–0.69 L/L and in 19% with HCT 0.70–0.80 L/L (Morag et al. 2011). Platelet count <50,000/μL was found mainly in infants with HCT ≥0.70 L/L, but was also independently associated with intrauterine growth restriction (Vlug et al. 2015). Thrombocytopenia in polycythemic patients may have several causes: (1) Platelets are diluted in a larger blood volume. Thus, platelet concentration may be normal in plasma but decreased in whole blood. (2) Platelet production may be decreased in infants with increased erythropoiesis. (3) Platelet consumption may be increased as a result of RBC sludging and low grade disseminated intravascular coagulation, particularly in infants with HCT ≥0.70 L/L.

Hyperbilirubinemia Jaundice has been reported in 2–46% of infants with HCT ≥0.65 (Bada et al. 1992; Alsafadi et al. 2014; Uslu et al. 2011). Phototherapy for hyperbilirubinemia was more frequently indicated in infants with HCT ≥0.70 L/L (25%) than in those with HCT 0.65–0.69 L/L (13%) (Morag et al. 2011). Increased bilirubin levels in polycythemic infants can simply be referred to the natural breakdown of the larger RBC mass. Moreover, in some infants

with increased risk of polycythemia (e.g., infants of diabetic mothers) shortened RBC life span of the less elastic RBC (Linderkamp 2004) and increased rates of ineffective erythropoiesis (Mimouni et al. 1986) my contribute to hyperbilirubinemia.

72.8 Prevention and Treatment of Polycythemia and Hyperviscosity

Prevention of Polycythemia Effective control of maternal diabetes and gestosis, cessation of active and passive smoking of the mother, and other measures for the prevention of intrauterine hypoxia may decrease the risk of neonatal polycythemia. If the risk for polycythemia is increased, delayed cord-clamping can still be recommended. However, the newly born baby should be positioned on the mother's abdomen, thereby limiting the placental transfusion to 15–20 mL/kg (Philip and Saigal 2004; Linderkamp 1982; Katheria et al. 2016; Nelle et al. 1993). Late cord-clamping in otherwise healthy neonates should not be discouraged for concern of polycythemia, since overall late cord-clamping is more beneficial for the normal neonate than early cord-clamping (Philip and Saigal 2004; Linderkamp 1982; Katheria et al. 2016).

Insufficient fluid intake may aggravate the postnatal rise in HCT observed in many infants with increased HCT at birth (Shohat et al. 1984) or late cord-clamping (Philip and Saigal 2004; Linderkamp 1982). The average milk volume of approximately 20 mL drunk on the first day may be further reduced in polycthemic infants with lethargy and poor feeding. Thus, early breastfeeding or, if necessary, early oral feeding of glucose solution may prevent symptomatic polycythemia and hypoglycemia in some high-risk infants. The efficacy of this approach has, however, not been studied.

Infusion Therapy To counterbalance the plasma volume deficiency in polycythemic infants (Linderkamp et al. 1992b; Brans et al. 1981; Maertzdorf et al. 1991), early plasma volume expansion with intravenous fluid has been recommended in several reports (Linderkamp 2004; Morag et al. 2011; Alsafadi et al. 2014; Pappas and Delaney-Black 2004; Sankar et al. 2010). However, the effect of this treatment has not been evaluated in a controlled study. Morag et al. (2011) used intravenous volume expansion (100 mL/kg/day) as first-line treatment in 110 out of 118 infants with HCT 0.70–0.75 L/L and avoided PET in 103 infants by this approach. Alsafadi et al. (2014) demonstrated that an intravenous normal saline bolus of 10–20 mL/kg was less successful (46%) than the combination of an intravenous bolus plus an increase in oral fluid intake of 10–20 mL/kg/day (67%).

Partial Exchange Transfusion (PET) Isovolemic hemodilution by a plasma substitute is the most effective method to reduce the hematocrit within a short time. However, PET did not improve the long-term outcome in six studies (Goldberg et al. 1982; Van der Elst et al. 1980; Bada et al. 1992; Black et al. 1985a; Delaney-Black et al. 1989; Ratrisawada et al. 1994; Drew et al. 1997). Moreover, severe short-term complications such as necrotizing enterocolitis (Van der Elst et al. 1980; Uslu et al. 2011; Black et al. 1985b) were more frequently seen in infants treated by PET. In one study the death rate after PET was higher than in infants with symptomatic care (23 vs. 4%) (Kumar and Ramji 2004). Two infants died of septicemia.

PET is an invasive procedure requiring a safe vascular access and the exchange of a relatively large volume of blood. Although rare, the use of umbilical vein catheterization may cause severe complications including septicemia, vasospasm, vessel perforation with hemoperitoneum or intrahepatic hematoma, air embolism, arrhythmia, thrombosis, portal hypertension, and necrotizing enterocolitis (Abiramalatha et al. 2016). The exchange transfusion itself may cause blood volume and pressure fluctuations and electrolyte abnormalities. The incidences of hypoglycemia, thrombocytopenia, and hyperbilirubinemia were not influenced by PET in published studies (Özek et al. 2010). The stress resulting from the procedure may explain that the heart rate (Rosenkrantz and Oh 1982; Swetnam et al. 1987) and energy expenditure (Dollberg et al. 2007) rose after PET.

To avoid umbilical vein catheterization, the use of a radial artery for blood withdrawal and a scalp or peripheral vein for blood replacement has been recommended (Scarcella and Gambardella 1986). To avoid large pressure fluctuations, the single exchange aliquot should not exceed 1.5 mL/kg (5 mL).

Adult plasma increases plasma viscosity and RBC aggregation and, therefore, should not be used for hemodilution (Linderkamp et al. 1984). A systematic review of the optimal fluid for PET in neonatal polycythemia showed no meaningful differences in effectiveness (decrease in hematocrit, relief of symptoms) exist between plasma, 5% albumin, and crystalloid solutions (normal saline, Ringer lactate) (De Waal et al. 2006). Plasma expanders such as hydroxyethyl starch and Hemaccel have been used for hemodilution in neonates (Supapannachart et al. 1999), but little is known about their distribution and metabolism in the neonate. Because normal saline shows the least side effects and is as effective as the other plasma substitutes, this is the optimal fluid for PET (Linderkamp et al. 1992b).

Because of the large number of infants with HCT $\geq$0.65 L/L (1–15% of all neonates), the potential side effects of PET and the limited evidence of the efficacy of PET in prevention of long-term sequelae, PET should be reserved for those polycythemic infants for whom it is unlikely that this invasive procedure is doing more harm than good. There is some evidence that a HCT $\geq$0.70 L/L increases the risk of (micro)circulatory impairment markedly. However, the study by Kumar and Ramji (2004) including only infants with HCT $\geq$0.70 L/L found no benefit of PET on the neurodevelopmental outcome during 18 months. Thus, it appears doubtful whether PET can be recommended for any infant with polycythemia.

In spite of the negative results of PET, this procedure is still recommended for two indications: (1) Persistence of HCT $\geq$0.65 L/L and serious symptoms of polycythemia in spite of intravenous fluid administration and (2) HCT $\geq$0.75 L/L in asymptomatic infants (Morag et al. 2011; Sankar et al. 2010). Morag et al. (2011) defined as serious symptoms: Blood glucose <40 mg/dl, platelet count <150.000/ µL, and respiratory distress requiring oxygen treatment.

72.9 Recommendations

Screening Routine screening of all newborn infants for polycythemia is not recommended. Screening may be done in small and large for gestational age infants, infants of diabetic mothers, and some of the rarer risk factors listed in Table 1. If risk factors or symptoms of polycythemia exist, a careful clinical examination is performed. A blood sample should be taken from a peripheral vein without prolonged tourniquet and excessive squeezing and analyzed for HCT and hemoglobin concentration, platelet and leukocyte count, glucose, and electrolytes.

Hematocrit Measurement HCT of venous or arterial blood should be measured in duplicate using the microcentrifuge technique or a Coulter counter. The microhematocrit may overestimate the actual HCT by 0.01–0.02 L/L, while the Coulter counter may underestimate the HCT by 0.05 L/L. The HCT can be estimated from the hemoglobin concentration (HCT = Hb/33).

General Care The underlying disorder is treated; hypoxia, acidosis, hypoglycemia, and electrolyte abnormalities are corrected. Body weight, cardiorespiratory, and glucose monitoring are done. Early breastfeeding or oral feeding of other fluids (e.g., 10% glucose) are indicated.

Volume Expansion If additional oral feeding is not sufficient, intravenous administration of 10 mL/kg of 10% glucose or normal saline should be given within one hour and repeated if the HCT does not decrease sufficiently. Continuous infusion of 10% glucose 100 mL/kg/day, if necessary enriched with electrolytes, has also been recommended.

Partial Exchange Transfusion (PET) PET is indicated if severe symptoms of poycythemia or a HCT $\geq$0.75 L/L in asymptomatic infants persist in spite of volume expansion. Severe symptoms are: Blood glucose <40 mg/dl, platelet count <100–150,000/μL, and respiratory distress requiring oxygen treatment. PET is performed with normal saline. A peripheral vein may be used for infusion and an umbilical artery or vein catheter or a radial artery cannula for blood withdrawal. To avoid large volume fluctuations, two persons should infuse and withdraw equal volumes simultaneously.

$$\text{Exchange volume (mL)} = \text{Blood volume} \times (\text{observed} - \text{desired HCT})/\text{observed HCT}$$

The blood volume in polycythemic infants is approximately 80–100 mL/kg, the desired HCT 0.55 L/L. Usually an exchange volume of 20–25 mL/kg is satisfactory.

In each single exchange a volume of 1–1.5 mL/kg (3–5 mL) of blood is withdrawn and the same volume simultaneously or subsequently over 2–3 min infused. PET is done in a neonatal unit and the baby is monitored for several hours after the procedure.

Informed consent of the parents must be obtained as efficacy and safety of PET for polycythemia are uncertain.

Indications for Volume Expansion and PET

- Asymptomatic HCT 0.65–0.69 L/L: early breastfeeding, extra oral fluid
- Asymptomatic HCT 0.70–0.74 L/L: extra oral fluid; if insufficient: i.v. fluid
- Asymptomatic HCT $\geq$0.75: extra oral plus i.v. fluid; if insufficient: PET
- Symptomatic HCT 0.65–0.69 L/L: oral plus i.v. fluid usually sufficient
- Symptomatic HCT $\geq$0.70: i.v. fluid; if insufficient: PET
- Symptomatic plus high risk of increased plasma volume and/or impaired RBC deformability (Table 1): consider oral plus i.v. fluid at HCT 0.65–0.69 L/L; if insufficient: PET

References

Abiramalatha T, Kumar M, Shabeer MP, Thomas N (2016) Advantages of being diligent: lessons learnt from umbilical venous cauterization in neonates. BMJ Case Rep

Alsafadi TRM, Hashmi SM, Youssef HA, Suliman AK (2014) Polycythemia in neonatal intensive care unit, risk factors, symptoms, pattern, and management controversy. J Clin Neonatol 3:93–98

Aperia A, Bergqvist G, Bomberger O et al (1974) Renal function in newborn infants with high hematocrit values before and after isovolemic hemodilution. Acta Paediatr 63:878–884

Bada HS, Korones SB, Kolni HW et al (1986) Partial plasma exchange transfusion improves cerebral hemodynamics in symptomatic neonatal polycythemia. Am J Med Sci 291:157–163

Bada HS, Korones SB, Pourcyrous M et al (1992) Asymptomatic syndrome of polycythemic hyperviscosity: effect of partial plasma exchange transfusion. J Pediatr 120:579–85

Black VD, Lubchenco LO, Koops BL et al (1985a) Neonatal hyperviscosity: randomized study of effect of partial plasma exchange transfusion on long-term outcome. Pediatrics 75:1048–1053

Black VD, Rumack CM, Lubchenko LO, Koops BL (1985b) Gastrointestinal injury in polycythemic term infants. Pediatrics 76:225–231

Brans YW, Shannon DL, Ramamurthy RS (1981) Neonatal polycythemia. II. Plasma, blood, and red cell volume estimates in relation to hematocrit levels and quantity of intrauterine growth. Pediatrics 68:175–181

Buonocore G, Bernie S, Gioia D et al (1991) Whole blood filterability in the neonate. Clin Hemorheol 11:41–48

Capasso L, Raimondi F, Capasso A et al (2003) Early cord clamping protects at-risk neonates from polycythemia. Biol Neonate 83:197–200

Christensen RD, Baer VL, Gerday E et al (2014) Whole blood viscosity in the neonate: effects of gestational age, hematocrit, mean corpuscular volume and umbilical cord milking. J Perinatol 34:16–21

De Waal KA, Baerts W, Offringa M (2006) Systematic review of the optimal fluid for dilutional exchange transfusionin in neonatal poycythaemia. Arch Dis Child Fetal Neonatal Ed 91:F7–F10

Delaney-Black V, Camp BW, Lubchenco LO et al (1989) Neonatal hyperviscosity association with lower achievement and IQ scores at school age. Pediatrics 83:662–667

Dempsey EM, Barrington K (2006) Short and long term outcomes following partial exchange transfusion in the polycythaemic newborn: a systematic review. Arch Dis Child Fetal Neonatal Ed 91:F2–F6

Dollberg S, Marom R, Mimouni FB, Littner Y (2007) Increased energy expenditure after dilutional exchange transfusion for neonatal polycythemia. J Am Coll Nutr 26:412–415

Drew JH, Guaran RL, Cichello M, Hobbs JB (1997) Neonatal whole blood hyperviscosity: the important factor influencing later neurologic function is the viscosity and not the polycythemia. Clin Hemorheol Microcirc 17:67–72

Ergenecon E, Hirfanoglu IM, Turan O et al (2011) Partial exchange transfusion results in increased cerebral oxygenation and faster peripheral microcirculation in newborns with polycythemia. Acta Paediatr 100:1432–1436

Erickson-Owens DA, Mercer JS, Oh W (2012) Umbilical cord-milking in term infants delivered by cesarean section: a randomized controlled trial. J Perinatol 32:580–584

Goldberg K, Wirth FH, Hathaway WE et al (1982) Neonatal hyperviscosity II. Effect of partial plasma exchange transfusion. Pediatrics 69:419–425

Goldstein M, Stonestreet B, Brann BS, Oh W (1988) Cerebral cortical blood flow and oxygen metabolism in normocythemic hyperviscous newborn piglets. Pediatr Res 24:486–489

Holzman IR, Tabata B, Edelstone DI (1986) Blood flow and oxygen delivery to the organs of the neonatal lamb as a function of hematocrit. Pediatr Res 20:1274–1279

Host A, Ulrich M (1982) Late prognosis in untreated neonatal polycythemia with minor or no symptoms. Acta Paediatr Scand 71:629–633

Hutton EK, Hassan ES (2007) Late vs early clamping of the umbilical cord in full-term neonates. Systematic review and meta-analysis of controlled trials. JAMA 297:1241–1252

Jobling J, Henry E, Wiedmeier SE, Christensen RD (2009) Reference ranges for hematocrit and blood hemoglobin concentration during the neonatal period: data from a multihospital health care system. Pediatrics 123: e333–e337

Katheria AC, Lakshminrusimha S, Rabe H et al (2016) Placental transfusion: a review. J Perinatol (Epub ahead of print)

Kotagal UR, Keenan WJ, Reuter JH et al (1977) Regional blood flow in polycythemia and hypervolemia. Pediatr Res 11:394A

Kumar A, Ramji S (2004) Effect of partial exchange transfusion in asymptomatic polycythemic LBW infants. Indian Pediatr 41:366–372

Liem KD, Hopman JC, Oeseburg B et al (1997) The effect of blood transfusion and haemodilution on cerebral oxygenation and in newborn infants investigated by near infrared spectrophotometry. Eur J Pediatr 156:305–310

Linderkamp O (1982) Placental transfusion: determinants and effects. Clin Perinatol 9:559–592

Linderkamp O (1996) Pathological flow properties of blood in the fetus and neonate. Clin Hemorheol 16:105–116

Linderkamp O (2004) Blood viscosity of the neonate. NeoReviews 5:e406–e416

Linderkamp O (2007) Hemorheology of the fetus and neonate. In: Baskurt OK, Hardeman MR, Rampling MW, Meiselman HJ (eds) Handbook of hemorheology and hemodynamics, vol 69, Biomedical and health research. IOS Press, Amsterdam

Linderkamp O, Versmold HT, Strohhacker I et al (1977) Capillary-venous hematocrit differences in newborn infants. I. Relationship to blood volume, peripheral blood flow, and acid–base parameters. Eur J Pediatr 127:9–14

Linderkamp O, Versmold HT, Riegel KP, Betke K (1984) Contributions of red cells and plasma to blood viscosity in preterm and full-term infants and adults. Pediatrics 74:45–51

Linderkamp O, Nash GB, Wu PYK, Meiselman HJ (1986) Deformability and intrinsic material properties of neonatal red blood cells. Blood 67:1244–1250

Linderkamp O, Stadler AA, Zilow EP (1992a) Blood viscosity and optimal hematocrit in preterm and full-term neonates in 50- to 500-μm tubes. Pediatr Res 32:97–102

Linderkamp O, Nelle M, Kraus M, Zilow EP (1992b) The effect of early and late cord-clamping on blood viscosity and other hemorheological parameters in full-term neonates. Acta Paediatr 81:745–750

Linderkamp O, Bauer J, Noecker-Ribaupierre M, Riegel KP (2004) Neonatal polycythemia resulting from late cord-clamping does not cause developmental or neurologic sequelae. Pediatr Res 56:490

Linderrkamp O, Kiau U, Ruef P (1997) Cellular and membrane deformability of red blood cells in preterm infants with and without growth retardation. Clin Hemorheol Microcirc 17:279–283

Maertzdorf WJ, Aldenhuyzen-Dorland W, Slaaf DW et al (1991) Circulating blood volume in appropriate and small for gestational age full term and preterm polycythaemic infants. Acta Paediatr Scand 80:620–627

Maertzdorf WJ, Tangelder GJ, Slaaf DW, Blanco CE (1993) Effects of partial plasma exchange transfusion on blood flow velocity in large arteries of arm and leg, and in cerebral arteries in polycythaemic newborn infants. Acta Paediatr 82:12–18

Maerztdorf WJ, Tangelder GJ, Slaaf DW, Blanco CE (1989) Effects of partial plasma exchange transfusion on cerebral blood flow velocity in polycythaemic preterm, term and small for date newborn infants. Eur J Pediatr 148:774–778

Mandelbaum VH, Guajardo CD, Nelle M, Linderkamp O (1994) Effects of polycythaemia and haemodilution on circulation of neonates. Arch Dis Child Fetal Neonatal Ed 71:F53–F54

Merlob P, Litmanovitch I, Mor N et al (1990) Necrotizing enterocolitis after intravenous immunoglobulin treatment for neonatal isoimmune thrombocytopenia. Eur J Pediatr 149:432–433

Mimouni F, Miodovnik M, Siddiqi TA et al (1986) Neonatal polycythemia in infants of insulin-dependent diabetic mothers. Obstet Gynecol 68:370–372

Mimouni FB, Merlob P, Dollberg S, Mandel D (2011) Neonatal polycythemia: critical review and a consensus statement of the Israeli Neonatology Association. Acta Paediatr 100:1290–1296

Morag I, Strauss T, Lubin D et al (2011) Restrictive management of neonatal polycythemia. Am J Perinatol 28:677–682

Nelle M, Zilow EP, Kraus M et al (1993) The effect of Leboyer delivery on blood viscosity and other hemorheological parameters in term neonates. Am J Obstet Gynecol 169:189–193

Oh W, Blankenship W, Lind J (1966) Further study of neonatal blood volume in relation to placental transfusion. Ann Paediatr 207:147–159

Özek E, Soll R, Schimmel MS (2010) Partial exchange transfusion to prevent neurodeveplopmental disability in infants with polycythemia. Cochrane Database Syst Rev 2010:CD005089

Pappas A, Delaney-Black V (2004) Differential diagnosis and management of polycythemia. Pediatr Clin North Am 51:1063–1086

Philip AGS, Saigal S (2004) When should we clamp the umbilical cord? NeoReviews 5:e142–e154

Ratrisawada V, Plubrukarn R, Trachulchang K et al (1994) Developmental outcome of infants with neonatal polycythemia. J Med Assoc Thai 77:76–80

Rivers RPA (1975) Coagulation changes associated with high hematocrit in the newborn infant. Acta Pediatr 64:449–456

Rosenkrantz TS (2003) Polycythemia and hyperviscosity in the newborn. Semin Thromb Hemost 29:515–527

Rosenkrantz TS, Oh W (1982) Cerebral blood flow velocity in infants with polycythemia and hyperviscosity: effects of partial exchange transfusion with Plasmanate. J Pediatr 101:9498

Sankar MJ, Agarwal R, Deorari A, Paul VK (2010) Management of polycythemia in neonates. Indian J Pediatr 77:1117–1121

Scarcella A, Gambardella P (1986) Partial exchange transfusion using peripheral vessels in polycythaemic newborn infants. Eur J Pediatr 144:545–546

Schimmel MS, Bromiker R, Soll RF (2004) Neonatal polycythemia: is partial exchange transfusion justified? Clin Perinatol 31:545–553

Shohat M, Merlob P, Reisner SH (1984) Neonatal polycythemia: I. Early diagnosis and evidence relating to time of sampling. Pediatrics 73:7–10

Supapannachart S, Siripoonya P, Boonwattanasoontorn W, Kanjanavanit S (1999) Neonatal polycythemia: effects of partial exchange transfusion using fresh frozen plasma, Haemaccel and normal saline. J Med Assoc Thai 82(Suppl 1):S82–S86

Swetnam SM, Yabek SM, Alverson DC (1987) Hemodynamic consequences of neonatal polycythemia. J Pediatr 110:443–447

Uslu S, Ozdemir H, Bulbul A et al (2011) The evaluation of polycythemic newborns: efficacy of partial exchange transfusion. J Matern Fetal Neonatal Med 24: 1492–1497

Van der Elst CW, Molteno CD, Malan AF, Heese H (1980) The management of polycythaemia in the newborn infant. Early Hum Dev 4:393–403

Villalta IA, Pramanik AK, Diaz-Blanco J, Herbst JJ (1989) Diagnostic errors in neonatal polycythemia based on method of hematocrit determination. J Pediatr 115:460–462

Vlug RD, Lopriore E, Janssen M et al (2015) Thrombocytopenia in neonates with polycythemia: incidence, risk factors and clinical outcome. Expert Rev Hematol 8:99–102

Werner EJ (1995) Neonatal polycythemia and hyperviscosity. Clin Perinatol 22:693–710

Wiswell TE, Cornish JD, Northam RS (1986) Neonatal polycythemia: frequency of clinical manifestations and other associated findings. Pediatrics 78:26–30

Yao AC, Lind J (1982) Placental transfusion. A clinical and physiological study. Thomas Publisher, Springfield

Part VII

Hyperbilirubinemia and Liver Diseases

Bilirubin Metabolism, Unconjugated Hyperbilirubinemia, and Physiologic Neonatal Jaundice

73

Giovanna Bertini and Carlo Dani

Contents

Abstract

Neonatal jaundice is a frequent problem in neonatology, but with the advent of phototherapy which has simplified its treatment, it no longer represents a major concern, but early hospital discharge of neonates has now resulted in a re-emergence of the risk of kernicterus. Neonatal jaundice is principally the result of an increased synthesis of bilirubin, of a transient deficiency of bilirubin conjugation, of a partial deficiency of hepatic bilirubin uptake and intracellular transport, and of an increased enterohepatic circulation of the pigment that limit bilirubin elimination. The fact that bilirubin production in the neonate is two or more times greater than in the adult per kilogram of body weight represents the mainstay of this condition. Prevention of kernicterus in full-term infants is based on the detection of neonates at risk for developing hyperbilirubinemia. The daily evaluation of transcutaneous bilirubin measurement gives additional information on the rise of serum bilirubin level and can help to distinguish physiological from nonphysiological hyperbilirubinemia. A significant hyperbilirubinemia is more frequent in infants born before term and in

G. Bertini
Neonatal Intensive Care Unit, Careggi University Hospital, Florence, Italy
e-mail: giovanna.bertini@unifi.it

C. Dani (✉)
Neonatal Intensive Care Unit, Careggi University Hospital, Florence, Italy

Università degli Studi di Firenze, Florence, Italy
e-mail: cdani@unifi.it; carlo.dani@unifi.it

G. Buonocore et al. (eds.), *Neonatology*,
https://doi.org/10.1007/978-3-319-29489-6_220

neonates who do not feed well and lose more than 10% of body weight. Each jaundiced newborn should receive a bilirubin measurement. Transcutaneous bilirubin (TcB) can be used as first step in order to reduce the number of invasive and painful blood sampling, but TSB measurement is always necessary when the level of bilirubin is high and for therapeutic decisions.

Abbreviations

C-N	Crigler-Najjar syndrome
CO	Carbon monoxide
COHbc	Carboxyhemoglobin corrected for inspired CO
TcB	Transcutaneous bilirubin
TSB	Total serum bilirubin
UGT	Uridin 5′-diphospho-glucuronosyltransferase

73.1 Salient Points

- Bilirubin is mainly produced from the catabolism of hemoglobin, and partially from non-erythroid hemeproteins, myoglobin, and ineffective erythropoiesis.
- Bilirubin production in a normal neonate is two or more times greater than the adult per kg body weight.
- Jaundice appears in newborns at a concentration of bilirubin >5 mg/ml with a typical cephalocaudal progression; the bilirubin is 99% unconjugated.
- Physiological jaundice usually appears after 24 h of life and reaches its maximum intensity by third to fifth day in term and seventh day in preterm infants.
- High levels of bilirubin (>95th percentile), especially in premature infants, can lead to bilirubin encephalopathy and subsequently to kernicterus.
- Genetic mutations in enzymes involved in bilirubin metabolism may lead to higher blood levels of bilirubin and higher risk of encephalopathy.
- Daily evaluation of transcutaneous bilirubin measurement gives information on the rise of serum bilirubin level and can help to distinguish physiological from nonphysiological hyperbilirubinemia.

73.2 Introduction

Jaundice is the most frequent condition identified in a newborn and appears at a concentration of bilirubin >5 mg/ml with a typical cephalocaudal progression. The majority of textbooks of pediatrics reported that about 60% of full-term newborns are jaundiced. However, more recent data show that about 25% of neonates have visible jaundice during their hospitalization and 5.1% have a serum total bilirubin (STB) concentration >12.9 mg/dL (Bertini et al. 2001).

73.3 Bilirubin Metabolism

The presence of jaundice implies the determination of STB concentration, and only after this determination, neonatal jaundice could be classified as an exaggerated jaundice (>20 mg/dL). In the past, jaundice was frequently classified as physiological, pathological, critical or severe, etc. Nowadays, we prefer to describe the level of STB in relation to time. But why the STB is frequently high in the first days of life? When we determine an STB, we obtain a number in mg/dL or μmol/L, but at least in the first few hours we do not know if a high STB concentration is due to excessive production of bilirubin or reduced hepatic clearance or excessive intestinal reabsorption (Fig. 1).

Bilirubin is mainly produced from the catabolism of hemoglobin, and partially from non-erythroid hemeproteins, myoglobin, and ineffective erythropoiesis (Fig. 2). The site of conversion of heme to bilirubin is the reticuloendothelial system, and together with bilirubin, a molecule of carbon monoxide (CO) and an atom of iron are products of the catabolism (Fig. 2). The determination of CO in the expired air or the measurement of CO-hemoglobin are able to quantify the production of bilirubin in newborns (Stevenson et al. 1980). To answer to the question "why the STB is frequently high in the first days of life?", it must be considered

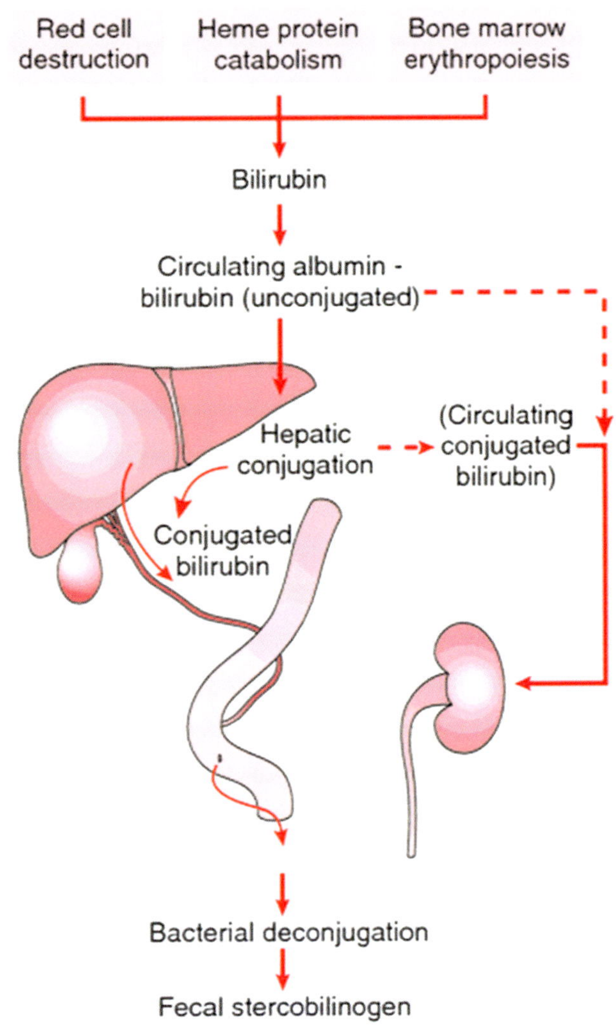

Fig. 1 Production, hepatic clearance, and intestinal absorption of bilirubin contribute to SBC

that bilirubin production in a normal neonate is two or more times greater than the adult per kg body weight. In addition, a transient deficiency of bilirubin conjugation is present at birth (during fetal life bilirubin is cleared by the mother through the placenta), a partial deficiency of hepatic bilirubin uptake and intracellular transport could exist, and in some cases an increased enterohepatic circulation of the pigment has been demonstrated (Rubaltelli 1993).

Bilirubin is insoluble in water without the alkalinization with NaOH but, in the blood, is transported bound to albumin to two binding sites (one at very high affinity) in equilibrium with a very low concentration of unbound or free bilirubin (Jori et al. 1988). About 8 mg of bilirubin is bound to each gram of albumin.

Bilirubin is conjugated to monoconjugated and diconjugated bilirubin by the enzyme system UDP-glucuronosyltransferase (UGT) 1A1 codified by UGT 1A1 gene complex (Fig. 3). When bilirubin load in newborns is high, bilirubin is mainly conjugated with only one molecule of glucuronic acid. In the intestines, monoconjugated bilirubin is more easily deconjugated by β-glucuronidase and reverted to native bilirubin which can be reabsorbed by the gut. In fact, the intestinum of neonates is almost sterile, and bilirubin is not yet degraded to sterco- and urobilinogen.

73.4 Unconjugated Hyperbilirubinemia

Neonatal jaundice is by definition a hyperbilirubinemia where the bilirubin is 99% unconjugated. In routine laboratory determinations, unconjugated bilirubin is reported as indirect-reacting bilirubin even if this equation is not right. The only utility of performing a determination of total, direct-reacting, and indirect-reacting bilirubin is the suspect of cholestatic jaundice like biliary atresia. By the way, the so-called physiologic jaundice could become a severe jaundice in a number of clinical situations. Why are the neonatologists afraid that STB reaches high levels especially in premature infants? Elevated STB can lead to bilirubin encephalopathy and subsequently to kernicterus with risk of death or permanent severe neurodevelopmental disabilities. Jaundice in absence of a hemolytic disease is frequently considered a physiologic or developmental event with very low risk, but this is not true. The right emphasis given to breastfeeding has convinced many sanitary personnel that it is important to say to mothers "feed the baby on demand, forget the balance and weight gain, and remember that any mother produces the right amount of milk for his baby." This personnel does not take into account the role of heme oxygenase and the effect of starvation on increasing the activity of this enzyme which has a key role in bilirubin production. Thus, in recent time, many infants are admitted to hospital after their discharge with a severe dehydration, hypernatremia, and hyperbilirubinemia as consequence of insufficient feeding. Two important papers reported exclusively breastfed infants at high risk of kernicterus due to very high hyperbilirubinemia consequent to insufficient nutrition (Maisels and Newman 1995; Hansen 1997). In the paper by Maisels et al. (Maisels and Newman 1995), the six studied infants had a SBC ranging from 39.0 to 49.7 mg/dL, four had a gestational age of 37 weeks, one of 38, and another of 39 weeks. All had a direct Coombs test negative. They were treated with blood exchange transfusion, but unfortunately, all

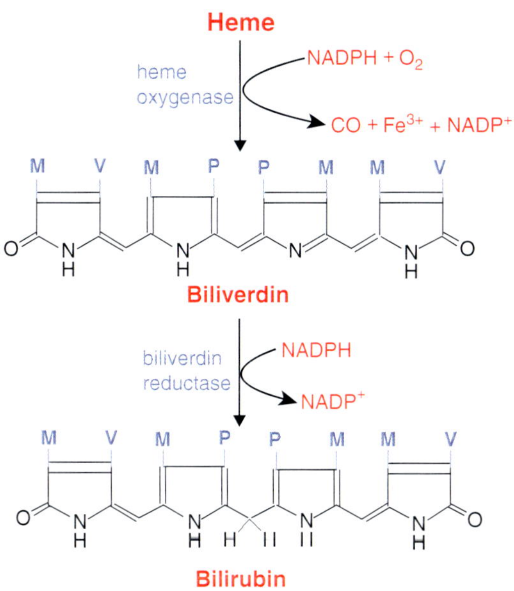

Fig. 2 The conversion of heme produces a molecule of carbon monoxide, a molecule of bilirubin, and an atom of iron

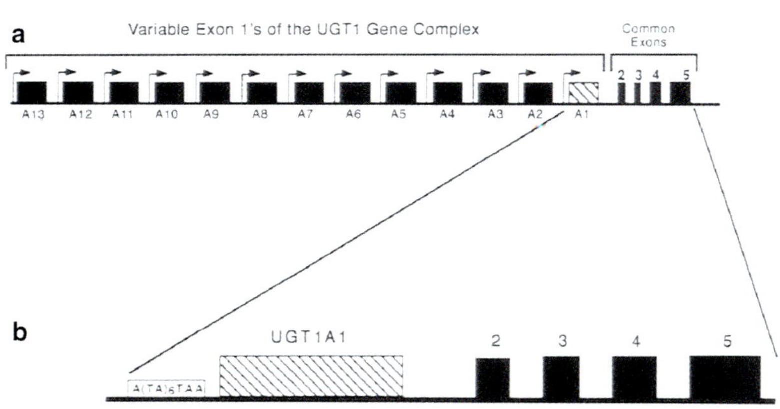

Fig. 3 Schematic representation of the genomic structure of the UGT 1 gene complex

were affected by kernicterus. Three of the four neonates reported by Hansen (1997) had a gestational age of 36 weeks, while the fourth was born at 40 weeks, but their SBC ranged from 32.1 to 36.3. Three of them were treated only with intensive phototherapy and formula feeding "ad libitum," while the fourth received an exchange transfusion when SBC was already decreased to approximately 23 mg/dL. All the infants had a normal follow-up.

73.5 Bilirubin Conjugation Genetics

Recently, new light has clarified the clinical observation that some healthy infants have more severe jaundice without evident signs of hemolysis and others have a prolonged neonatal jaundice, the so-called breast milk jaundice. An important study of Kaplan et al. (2002) has shown that white neonates with a polymorphism of the gene encoding UGT (Fig. 3), in which an additional TA base pair is inserted in the TATAA box of the gene promoter (Gilbert's syndrome), could develop a relevant hyperbilirubinemia. Affected individuals who are homozygous for the variant promoter and have seven TA repeats – $(TA)_7TAA$ (7/7) instead of the more usual six repeats $(TA)_6TAA$ (6/6) – have a higher serum total bilirubin (STB) concentration, an increased blood carboxyhemoglobin corrected for inspired CO (COHbc) which is an index of heme catabolism and bilirubin production, a decreased total conjugated bilirubin (TCB) which suggest a decrease efficacy of enzyme system UDP-glucuronosyltransferase 1A1, and an increased production/conjugation rate (COHbc)/(TCB/STB[%]). In synthesis, newborns with Gilbert's syndrome not only have a diminished enzyme activity which results from decreased expression of normally structured UGT but also an increased hemolysis which exacerbates neonatal hyperbilirubinemia. This condition is important also because white population is frequently associated with prolonged hyperbilirubinemia associated with breastfeeding; after cessation of breastfeeding, the infant's bilirubin level becomes normal (Kaplan et al. 2002). In the oriental population, a mutation of the UGT 1A1 is responsible of Gilbert's syndrome and prolonged unconjugated hyperbilirubinemia associated with breast milk. The most frequent missense mutation is G → A transition at nucleotide 211. Arginine replaces glycine at position 71 of corresponding protein product (G714) (Maruo et al. 2000).

Identification of genetic mutations of bilirubin conjugation may be investigated not only with full genetic consultation and laboratory analysis but also asking to the parents about ethnic background, risk factors, previous infants with hyperbilirubinemia, and if they were jaundiced as neonates or in later life. This is particularly important on the light of recent studies showing that Gilbert's syndrome is a determining factor for the development of neonatal hyperbilirubinemia due to ABO incompatibility (Kaplan et al. 2000) and G-6-PD deficiency (Mediterranean mutation) (Kaplan et al. 1997). Moreover, Maruo et al., studying Japanese hyperbilirubinemic infants with no obvious cause for their jaundice, determined the allele frequency of a mutated UGT 1A1 (G71R) to be more than double than that of controls (Maruo et al. 2000). Both hetero- and homozygosity for the G71R mutation were associated with hyperbilirubinemia (Maruo et al. 2000). It is possible that the high incidence of hyperbilirubinemia in Japanese newborns may be a function of the frequency of the G71R mutation in that population. In addition, a case of kernicterus in a breastfed infant with hereditary spherocytosis and Gilbert's syndrome has been recently reported (Berardi et al. 2006).

Crigler-Najjar (C-N) syndromes are very rare. However, while type 1 C-N is rarely undetected by neonatologists, C-N type 2 is more insidious. In fact, jaundice is very often confused with nonhemolytic jaundice, and infants with C-N type 2 could be discharged after phototherapy without any short-term follow-up. Infants often return to the hospital with intense jaundice and signs of bilirubin encephalopathy. C-N type 1 presents with very high hyperbilirubinemia during the first few days of life, and generally phototherapy reduces TSB below 20 mg/dL only transiently (Rubaltelli et al. 1994). The treatment with Sn-proto- or mesoporphyrin, heme oxygenase inhibitors, has been attempted (Rubaltelli et al. 1989, 1995), but it is only capable to reduce

the time spent under the lamps; the drug remains an experimental therapy. However, this treatment might be useful during diseases or starvation when SBC increases over 20–25 mg/dL. By now, the only treatment which could give to these infants a normal life is liver transplant.

73.6 The So-Called Physiological Neonatal Jaundice

Physiological neonatal jaundice occurs due to *physiologic* factors that are seen as "normal" in the newborn and differs by pathological jaundice that is due to *pathologic* factors that alter the usual process in bilirubin metabolism. Physiological jaundice usually appears after 24 h of life, reaches its maximum intensity by third to fifth day in term and seventh day in preterm infants, commonly presents a TSB <12 mg/dL which is higher in Asian infants, is not clinically detectable after 14 days, and often disappears without any treatment.

As we said before, the "physiologic jaundice" represents an old denomination because the majority of neonatologists prefer to describe the level of TSB in relation to time and to treat infants according to "risk zone" putting the TSB against the hour of life. Risk zones for late preterm (35–37 weeks of gestational age) and term (38–42 weeks of gestational age) newborns were prepared according to the percentile tracks based on the hour-specific serum bilirubin values (American Academy of Pediatrics Subcommittee on Hyperbilirubinemia 2004). On the age-specific nomogram, the zone >95th percentile was labeled as high risk and that <5th percentile was labeled as low risk. Serum total bilirubin values between the 5th and 30th, 30th and 60th, and 60th and 95th percentiles were designated as being in the low-intermediate, intermediate, and high-intermediate risk zones, respectively. The 5th and 95th percentiles on the nomogram had the highest sensitivity (100%) and specificity (98.2%), respectively, in predicting the subsequent development of hyperbilirubinemia in term newborns. In fact, as aforementioned, infants born at 35–37 weeks' gestation had significantly higher STB levels on days 5 and 7 and were 2.4 times more likely to develop significant hyperbilirubinemia than those of infants born at 38–42 weeks' gestation (American Academy of Pediatrics Subcommittee on Hyperbilirubinemia 2004). This occurs because late preterm infants have an immature hepatic system leading to decreased excretion of bilirubin, a delayed enteral feedings that leads to reabsorption of bilirubin, and a decrease in serum albumin levels that can increase the serum level of free or unbound bilirubin.

73.7 Management of Physiological Neonatal Jaundice

All jaundiced infants should be routinely monitored because the ability of physicians and other health care providers to recognize clinically significant jaundice and predict bilirubin levels is limited (Romagnoli et al. 2014).

Therefore each jaundiced newborn should receive a bilirubin measurement. Transcutaneous bilirubin (TcB) can be used as first step in order to reduce the number of invasive and painful blood sampling, but TSB measurement is always necessary when the level of bilirubin is high and for therapeutic decisions.

The evaluation of jaundice is now facilitated by the availability of different nomograms for both TcB and TSB. However, a nomogram could not perform well in one specific setting if the racial, genetic, and environmental background of that setting is too different from that of the reference population. Furthermore, predictive tools should be developed in one sample and validated in another one. This is the reason why many nomograms have been developed in different population (American Academy of Pediatrics Subcommittee on Hyperbilirubinemia 2004; Romagnoli et al. 2014) which permits to plan the need of bilirubin monitoring and/or the need of treatment (see ▶ Chap. 76, "Treatment of Hyperbilirubinemia in Newborns"). When a physiological jaundice disappears spontaneously or after phototherapy, it is not necessary to carry out

particular biochemical tests, but when jaundice is more severe and has the characteristics of pathologic hyperbilirubinemia, a careful diagnostic and therapeutic approach is needed (see ▶ Chap. 74, "Pathologic Unconjugated Hyperbilirubinemia–Isoimmunization, Abnormalities of Red Blood Cells, and Infections").

References

American Academy of Pediatrics Subcommittee on Hyperbilirubinemia (2004) Management of hyperbilirubinemia in the newborn infant 35 or more weeks of gestation. Pediatrics 114:297–316

Berardi A, Lugli L, Ferrari F et al (2006) Kernicterus associated with hereditary spherocytosis and UGT1A1 promoter polymorphism. Biol Neonate 90(4):243–246

Bertini G, Dani C, Tronchin M, Rubaltelli FF (2001) Is breastfeeding really favoring early neonatal jaundice? Pediatrics 107(3), E41

Hansen TW (1997) Acute management of extreme neonatal jaundice – the potential benefits of intensified phototherapy and interruption of enterohepatic circulation. Acta Paediatr 86:843–846

Jori G, Reddi E, Rubaltelli FF (1988) Structural and functional differences between fetal and adult serum albumin. Int J Pept Protein Res 31:17–21

Kaplan M, Renbaum P, Levi-Lahad A et al (1997) Gilbert syndrome and glucose-6-phosphate dehydrogenase deficiency: a dose-dependent genetic interaction crucial to neonatal hyperbilirubinemia. Proc Natl Acad Sci U S A 94:12128–12132

Kaplan M, Hammerman C, Renbaum P et al (2000) Gilbert's syndrome and hyperbilirubinemia in ABO-incompatible neonates. Lancet 356:652–653

Kaplan M, Hammerman C, Rubaltelli FF et al (2002) Hemolysis and bilirubin conjugation in association with UDP-glucuronosyltransferase 1A1 promoter polymorphism. Hepatology 35:905–911

Maisels MJ, Newman TB (1995) Kernicterus in otherwise healthy, breast-fed term newborns. Pediatrics 96:730–733

Maruo Y, Nishizawa K, Sato H et al (2000) Prolonged unconjugated hyperbilirubinemia associated with breast milk and mutations of the bilirubin uridine diphosphate-glucuronosyltransferase gene. Pediatrics 106:e59

Romagnoli C, Barone G, Pratesi S, Raimondi F, Capasso L, Zecca E, Dani C (2014) Task force for hyperbilirubinaemia of the Italian society of neonatology. Italian guidelines for management and treatment of hyperbilir ubinaemia of newborn infants $\geq$ 35 weeks' gestational age. Ital J Pediatr 40:11

Rubaltelli FF (1993) Bilirubin metabolism in the newborn. Biol Neonate 63:133–138

Rubaltelli FF, Guerrini P, Reddi E, Jori G (1989) Tin-protoporphyrin in the management of children with Crigler-Najjar disease. Pediatrics 84:728–731

Rubaltelli FF, Novello A, Vilei MT, Muraca M (1994) Serum and bile bilirubin pigments in the differential diagnosis of Crigler-Najjar disease. Pediatrics 94:553–556

Rubaltelli FF, Dario C, Zancan L (1995) Congenital nonobstructive, nonhemolytic jaundice: effect of tin-mesoporphyrin. Pediatrics 95:942–2

Stevenson DK, Bartoletti AL, Ostrander CR, Johnson JD (1980) Pulmonary excretion of carbon monoxide in the human infants as an index of bilirubin production: IV: effects of breast-feeding and caloric intake in the first postnatal week. Pediatrics 65:1170–1172

Pathologic Unconjugated Hyperbilirubinemia–Isoimmunization, Abnormalities of Red Blood Cells, and Infections

74

Michael Kaplan, Ronald J. Wong, and David K. Stevenson

Contents

M. Kaplan (✉)
Department of Neonatology, Shaare Zedek Medical Center, Jerusalem, Israel

The Faculty of Medicine, Hebrew University, Jerusalem, Israel,
e-mail: mkaplan@mail.huji.ac.il

R. J. Wong
Department of Pediatrics, Stanford University School of Medicine, Stanford, CA, USA
e-mail: rjwong@stanford.edu

D. K. Stevenson
Department of Pediatrics, Stanford University School of Medicine, Medical School Office Building, Stanford, CA, USA
e-mail: dstevenson@stanford.edu

G. Buonocore et al. (eds.), *Neonatology*,
https://doi.org/10.1007/978-3-319-29489-6_221

Abstract
Although pathologic unconjugated hyperbilirubinemia can be best understood in terms of primary problems with bilirubin uptake and conjugation, most pathologic unconjugated hyperbilirubinemia occurring after birth and requiring treatment is often associated with increased bilirubin production and further exacerbated by environmental or acquired factors, such as isoimmunization, abnormalities of red blood cells, and infection. This chapter will describe the etiology and pathogenesis of unconjugated hyperbilirubinemia, its genetic predisposition, as well as current screening tools and treatment strategies.

74.1 Salient Points

- Despite all efforts to prevent extreme hyperbilirubinemia, which can result in bilirubin neurotoxicity, it continues to occur even in countries with advanced medical systems.
- The major contributing factors to the development of severe hyperbilirubinemia are increased bilirubin production and diminished bilirubin conjugation and elimination – an imbalance between these processes results in hyperbilirubinemia.
- Some degree of decreased bilirubin conjugation is universal and transient in neonates; therefore, the major modulator of severe hyperbilirubinemia is increased bilirubin production due to hemolysis.
- Hemolysis is associated with increased risk of bilirubin neurotoxicity compared to neonates with similar total bilirubin concentrations, but without overt hemolysis.
- Hemolytic conditions include immune hemolysis of which Rh isoimmunization is the most severe, but preventable, while ABO heterospecificity is today the most common cause.
- Of the nonimmune causes, glucose-6-phosphate dehydrogenase (G6PD) deficiency is the most widespread and frequently associated with bilirubin encephalopathy and kernicterus.

74.2 Introduction

Unconjugated hyperbilirubinemia in the newborn is a normal phenomenon, transitional in nature, and usually harmless, if not protective, for the human neonate exposed to increased levels of oxygen and light in the environment outside the womb before antioxidant enzymatic defenses are fully upregulated. The phenomenon is called "physiologic neonatal jaundice," and the contributing biochemistry has been described in the preceding chapter.

74.3 Etiology and Pathogenesis

74.3.1 Imbalance Between Bilirubin Production and Elimination

Physiologic neonatal jaundice implies benignity, but also a causation that is developmental in nature. That is, newborn infants have normally increased bilirubin production (two to three times that of the adult on a body weight basis) (Vreman et al. 1989; Stevenson et al. 1994) because of their relatively increased red blood cell (RBC) mass responsive to their fetal state and shortened RBC lifespan, combined with transitionally impaired uptake, conjugation, and excretion of bilirubin. As long as the bilirubin production and elimination processes remain in

equilibrium, the serum/plasma bilirubin concentrations will not rise to dangerous levels. Imbalance, however, between these forces is the major determinant of transitional hyperbilirubinemia after birth. Although pathologic unconjugated hyperbilirubinemia could be defined as an exacerbation of increased bilirubin production or impairment of conjugation, the diagnosis would not even be considered if the pattern of transitional hyperbilirubinemia did not deviate from the normal one. For example, an infant might have markedly increased bilirubin production but better than usual elimination and therefore not deviate from the usual course of hyperbilirubinemia. Conceivably, it would also be possible to have greater impairment of uptake or conjugation that is counterbalanced by a lower bilirubin production rate, for example, because of anemia, so that the trajectory of bilirubin levels would not deviate from the expected course. Thus, pathologic unconjugated hyperbilirubinemia is probably best defined epidemiologically, using the Bhutani nomogram (Bhutani et al. 1999), which defines the normal trajectory of hour-specific bilirubin levels, even defining risk zones that reflect the likelihood that a particular infant tracking in that zone might deviate enough from the general population to warrant further diagnostic workup or treatment. Given that immaturity of the uridine 5′-phosphoglucuronosyltransferase 1A1 (UGT1A1) bilirubin-conjugating enzyme leading to temporarily impaired bilirubin elimination is universal, in most cases, increased bilirubin production is a major contributing cause of all kinds of neonatal jaundice. Disorders of hepatic uptake, conjugation, and intrahepatic circulation contribute to the pathologic exacerbation of transitional neonatal jaundice and are not discussed in this chapter. Treatment of pathologic jaundice is also not discussed because it depends less on the cause (although there may be some consideration of risk in this regard) and more on the extent to which an individual infant has deviated from the normal transitional pattern of hyperbilirubinemia and is at more risk for injury because of the absolute level, binding capacity, and clinical circumstances that might alter binding affinity of albumin for bilirubin.

Thus, pathologic unconjugated hyperbilirubinemia is defined as an hour-specific bilirubin value exceeding the 95th percentile for a population-based hour-specific bilirubin nomogram, appropriate for the particular ethnic and cultural circumstances (Bhutani et al. 1999). Because all neonates have relatively impaired elimination of the pigment after birth, one of the most common causes of pathologic unconjugated hyperbilirubinemia is increased bilirubin production from any cause. Such causes are the focus of this chapter and include hemolysis resulting from isoimmunization, abnormalities of red cells, and infections, but also many other conditions. Some of these other conditions are quite common, such as closed-space bleeding, most often encountered by the pediatrician in the form a cephalohematoma or bruising. Depending upon the volume of extravascular blood, bilirubin production can be increased to a rate comparable to that observed in hemolytic conditions. Thus, such infants may have a transitional trajectory of bilirubin levels in one of the higher risk zones on the Bhutani nomogram or even cross zones depending upon their conjugating capacity and the magnitude of the increase in bilirubin production. Premature infants also have increased production relative to the full-term infant, perhaps because of even shorter RBC life spans. The latter is mitigated by less of an increase in the RBC mass among infants born at earlier gestation. The situation is compounded in premature infants by a degree of UGT1A1 activity, which is even more immature than the already diminished function in the term infant. Nonetheless, the more mature and larger of the premature infants are likely to deviate from the full-term hour-specific nomogram because of an exaggerated imbalance between increased bilirubin production and impaired elimination (Kaplan et al. 2002). Finally, the infant of a diabetic mother has increased bilirubin production as a major contributing cause to their propensity for pathologic unconjugated hyperbilirubinemia (Stevenson et al. 1979, 1981). This increased bilirubin production may be the result of polycythemia, but often reflects ineffective erythropoiesis in the presence of a normal hemoglobin or hematocrit level. The likelihood of a pathologic trajectory

of bilirubin levels in the transitional period after birth is further exacerbated by impaired elimination in these infants. This latter compounding factor was revealed by higher bilirubin levels in infants of diabetic mothers compared to infants of normal mothers while controlling for bilirubin production on a body weight basis.

The most important phenomenon contributing to pathologic unconjugated hyperbilirubinemia is hemolysis from any cause. The rapid destruction of RBCs in the circulation with the consequent degradation of heme is the predominant source of bilirubin in most pathologic unconjugated hyperbilirubinemia requiring diagnostic workup and treatment. Hemolysis can occur from a variety of specific causes, including isoimmunization (Rh disease, ABO heterospecificity, and other immune globulin-mediated hemolytic conditions), red cell enzyme deficiencies (glucose-6-phosphate dehydrogenase [G6PD] deficiency, hexokinase deficiency, and other less common enzymatic deficiencies), and RBC membrane defects (hereditary spherocytosis, elliptocytosis, and other less common RBC membrane defects) (Wong et al. 2006).

Finally, there are now recognized polymorphisms of the heme oxygenase-1 (HO-1) gene promoter involving GT expansions (Shibahara et al. 2002). An increased number of GT expansions in the promoter can alter the expression of HO-1 and lead to clinically important decreases in bilirubin production and vice versa (Hua et al. 2005; Berardi et al. 2006). The effect of short GT promoter sequences on the modulation of neonatal hyperbilirubinemia is not consistent and may be influenced by ethnicity (Kaplan et al. 2014a; Katayama et al. 2015). HO-1 may have other biological consequences, including risk for vascular disease, and among pregnant women, idiopathic recurrent miscarriages, intrauterine growth restriction, and preeclampsia (Shibahara et al. 2002; Denschlag et al. 2004). What is important to understand in the context of pathologic unconjugated hyperbilirubinemia is the fact that there may be native variation in bilirubin production rates which in the context of impaired elimination in the transitional period after birth or in conditions which further limit uptake or conjugation might contribute to pathologic unconjugated hyperbilirubinemia without other apparent environmental or acquired exigencies (Beutler et al. 1998; Bosma et al. 1995; Kaplan et al. 2003; Watchko et al. 2002).

74.4 Clinical Aspects and Therapy and Treatments

74.4.1 Hemolytic Conditions

74.4.1.1 Increased Risk Associated with Hemolysis

Neonates with hemolytic disease appear to be at a higher risk of developing bilirubin-induced brain damage at lower concentrations of total serum/plasma bilirubin (TSB) compared with those without hemolysis. Indeed, the first link to be established between increasing bilirubin levels and the risk of kernicterus was in newborns with hemolytic disease due to Rh isoimmunization (Hsia et al. 1952). Subsequent reports suggested that the incidence of kernicterus in hyperbilirubinemic newborns with hemolytic disease may be higher than that in counterparts without evidence of hemolytic disease, as reviewed by Newman and Maisels (1990). In a survey of the literature up to 1983, Watchko and Oski (1983) reinforced the concept that hyperbilirubinemia among neonates without hemolytic disease was less dangerous with regard to the development of kernicterus than in cases where hemolysis was present. A similar stand was taken by Newman and Maisels (1992) several years later. However, there is little data on which to base this view. A study shedding some light on this question was performed by Ozmert et al. (1996). In 102 children aged 8–13 years, who had been treated for indirect hyperbilirubinemia ranging from 17 to 48 mg/dL (291–821 μmol/L), a positive direct Coombs test (also known as a direct antiglobulin test [DAT]), presumed to reflect ongoing hemolysis, was associated with lower IQ scores and a higher incidence of neurologic abnormalities. They also found, in these same children, that the incidence of detected

neurologic abnormalities increased proportionately to the time of exposure to high bilirubin levels. Similarly, Nilsen et al. (1984) found that, of 55 Norwegian males born in the early 1960s and had neonatal hyperbilirubinemia, those who had a positive Coombs test and hyperbilirubinemia for greater than 5 days had significantly lower IQ scores than average. The 5-year outcomes of 140 Californian children who had TSB levels >25 mg/dL (428 μmol/L) in the neonatal period were similar to controls, and there were no cases of kernicterus. However, the subgroup of nine children, who had a positive DAT and were therefore presumed hemolytic, had significantly lower IQ values than those hyperbilirubinemic children, where DAT was negative (Newman et al. 2006). In a reanalysis of data from the Collaborative Perinatal Project, Kuzniewicz and Newman found no relationship between maximum TSB and IQ scores (Kuzniewicz and Newman 2009), but the presence of a positive DAT in those with a TSB ≥25 mg/dL (428 μmol/L) was associated with a 6.7-point decrease in IQ scores.

Of 249 newborns admitted to a children's hospital in Cairo, Egypt, with TSB values ≥25 mg/dL (428 μmol/L), there was poor correlation between the admission TSB levels and the development of acute bilirubin encephalopathy or ABE (Gamaleldin et al. 2011). However, those with risk factors for hemolysis including Rh incompatibility or sepsis were at greater risk for developing ABE than those without these factors. The effect of hemolysis in exacerbating bilirubin neurotoxicity has recently been extensively reviewed (Kaplan et al. 2014b).

Although there is to date no evidence demonstrating higher levels of unbound bilirubin in hemolyzing neonates, it is still generally accepted that hemolysis is a potential factor increasing the risk for bilirubin-related brain damage. While a TSB concentration of 20–24 mg/dL (342–410 μmol/L) may be associated with kernicterus in a neonate with Rh isoimmunization, a healthy, term non-hemolyzing infant will rarely be endangered by TSB concentrations in this range. Hemolysis due to direct Coombs positive Rh and ABO immunization, other isoimmunizations, and G6PD deficiency may therefore pose an increased threat to an otherwise healthy newborn. The Subcommittee on Hyperbilirubinemia of the American Academy of Pediatrics (AAP) includes jaundice developing within the first 24 h, blood group incompatibility with a positive DAT, other known hemolytic disease including G6PD deficiency, all associated with increased hemolysis, as major risk factors for the development of severe hyperbilirubinemia (American Academy of Pediatrics 2004). The AAP recommends initiating phototherapy or performing exchange transfusions at lower levels of TSB in neonates with hemolytic conditions than in non-hemolyzing counterparts. However, one should not be lulled into a sense of false security that a hyperbilirubinemic newborn without a clearly hemolytic condition will not develop kernicterus. Cases of kernicterus have been reported in which there was no clinical evidence of hemolysis (Maisels and Newman 1995). Crigler-Najjar syndrome, a condition not associated with increased hemolysis, is frequently complicated by bilirubin-induced neurologic dysfunction (BIND).

Hemolysis may not be easily identified in the newborn. Clearly hemolytic conditions such as G6PD deficiency, immune isoimmunization, and hereditary spherocytosis will obviously suggest the presence of hemolysis. RBC indices, useful as indicators of hemolysis in older children or adults, are not reliable for this purpose in newborns (Blanchette et al. 2005). Hemolysis, while ongoing, may not be readily determinable. For example, in a multinational, multicenter study of 1,370 newborns, the level of corrected end-tidal carbon monoxide (ETCOc), an index of heme catabolism, in 92 of 120 (76%) neonates who were hyperbilirubinemic was greater than the mean value for the cohort (Stevenson et al. 2001). In a male cohort of G6PD-normal, otherwise healthy African-American neonates born to nonsmoking mothers, ETCOc values were significantly higher among hyperbilirubinemic neonates than among those who did not develop hyperbilirubinemia (Kaplan et al. 2006). Also using ETCOc, Maisels and Kring (2006) demonstrated that, before hospital discharge, most infants with TSB levels >75th percentile on the Bhutani nomogram

(Bhutani et al. 1999) produced significantly more bilirubin than those with lower TSB levels. Because bedside ETCOc testing has not been available for several years and blood typing, DAT determination, and G6PD screening are not universally performed, it is possible that an infant not actually classified as having a hemolytic condition may, in fact, be actively hemolyzing and the potentially increased risk for hyperbilirubinemia and kernicterus may therefore go unrecognized. Recent availability of a new ETCOc device should facilitate the identification of hemolysis in hyperbilirubinemic newborns without a clear hemolytic etiology (Christensen et al. 2015a; Castillo Cuadrado et al. 2015) and add to the body of ETCOc-related data already available (Tidmarsh et al. 2014).

Hemolytic conditions in the newborn are generally divided into two major etiologic groups: immune and nonimmune. The former group includes Rh isoimmunization, although nowadays Rh disease is largely preventable by antenatal and postnatal Rh_oD globulin (of which the best known commercial preparation is RhoGAM) administration. Rh disease will, nevertheless, be discussed in some detail, because much of our knowledge of the pathophysiology of kernicterus derives from studies of babies with this condition. With the virtual elimination of Rh isoimmunization in Western countries with sophisticated health systems, ABO immune disease (mother blood group O, baby group A or B) has become the most common immune hemolytic condition currently encountered. Of the nonimmune causes, G6PD deficiency is by far the most important and is highly associated with the development of extreme hyperbilirubinemia and kernicterus.

74.5 Immune Hemolytic Disease

74.5.1 Rh Isoimmune Hemolytic Disease

Rh disease in pregnancy is highly associated with both intrauterine hemolysis and severe hemolytic disease following delivery. Untreated, the condition can lead to intrauterine anemia and severe *hydrops fetalis*, with rapid postnatal evolvement of hyperbilirubinemia with the potential of kernicterus.

74.5.1.1 Background: The Immunization Process

The Rh group of antigens comprises the C, D, and E pairs of antigens. While each of these antigens may result in isoimmunization, anti-D isoimmunization is the most common and has the greatest degree of clinical significance. There is some effect of racial distribution of Rh negativity. In Caucasian populations, about 13–15% of individuals are Rh negative. About half of that number is encountered in African Americans, while Rh negativity is very rare in individuals of Asian background. The incidence of Rh isoimmunization is infrequent and is reported to be 6.8 cases per 1,000 live births (Martin et al. 2003).

The immunization process may begin if an Rh-negative woman, usually D-negative, is exposed to a D antigen. This may occur by antepartum or intrapartum transplacental fetomaternal transfusion of fetal RBCs containing a D antigen. Similar transfusion of Rh-positive RBCs may occur during abortion, blood administration, or procedures including amniocentesis, chorionic villus sampling, or fetal blood sampling. The mother's immune system may respond by forming anti-D IgG antibodies. These then cross the placenta and adhere to the fetal RBCs containing the D antigen. The antigen-antibody response leads to hemolysis and anemia. Because the mother's immune system becomes primed, the immune response may become more severe and more rapid with progressive pregnancies. In cases of prolonged and severe anemia, bone marrow stimulation may result in increased numbers of circulating immature RBCs (erythroblastosis) and even extramedullary hematopoiesis with hepatosplenomegaly. Fetal hydrops, including generalized tissue edema and pleural, pericardial, and peritoneal effusions, may result from hypoproteinemia, tissue hypoxia, and capillary leak, combined with congestive cardiac failure due to anemia and venous congestions due to poor myocardial function with diminished cardiac output (Moise 2008).

74.5.1.2 Management of the Pregnancy

Hydrops fetalis is associated with a very high mortality rate, and major efforts should be made to prevent this occurrence. The mainstay of the management of a pregnancy complicated by Rh isoimmunization includes active surveillance of the fetus to detect fetal anemia. Once the fetus does become anemic, the decision to perform an intrauterine transfusion or to deliver the infant will depend on the gestational age: the potential complications of delivering a premature infant will have to be weighed against those involved in performing an intrauterine transfusion. In the recent past, amniocentesis was the primary method of fetal monitoring (Liley 1961). The degree of hemolysis was assessed by determinations of the amount of bilirubin in the amniotic fluid readings in the high zone being indicative of severe hemolysis with a high likelihood of fetal death. This regimen has been largely replaced by a combination of advancing ultrasonographic techniques and developing genetic technologies. Because this condition is nowadays rare, and therapeutic technologies are advancing at a rapid rate, Rh-immunized women and their fetuses should be managed in a tertiary center capable of adequately managing the fetus. As the neonatologist not actively involved in this field may be unfamiliar with many of these recent advances, an outline of current management of affected pregnancies follows.

A general principle is that all pregnant women should have an antibody screen performed early in pregnancy. If a woman is RhD-negative and there is no evidence of anti-D alloimmunization, rhesus immune globulin should be administered at 28 weeks gestation (Moise 2008). By doing so, the incidence of antenatal immunization will be reduced to 0.1% (Bowman 1988). The globulin should also be administered following spontaneous or elective abortion, amniocentesis, chorionic villus sampling, or fetal blood sampling. Within 72 h of delivery, another dose should be administered, should the woman have delivered an RhD-positive infant.

The RhD gene has been localized to the short arm of chromosome 1 (Chërif-Zahar et al. 1991). Approximately 55% of individuals will be heterozygous at the RhD locus, in which case only 50% of their fetuses will be RhD-positive. Because an RhD-negative fetus requires no further testing, it is important to assess the chance of an at-risk fetus having a D antigen. Gene frequency tables, combined with the history of RhD-positive or RhD-negative infants fathered by any individual, have been used to estimate the likelihood of the father being heterozygous. Recent advances in DNA technology, however, allow for accurate determination of whether the father is heterozygous or homozygous for the RhD gene (Lo et al. 1998). Should the father be heterozygous, steps should be taken to determine the Rh type of the fetus. This can be done accurately by retrieving fetal DNA via amniocentesis (Van den Veyver and Moise 1996), but this technology is being replaced by cell-free fetal DNA techniques, which allow the presence of fetal RhD in the maternal plasma to be detected by PCR techniques (Lo et al. 1998; de Haas et al. 2015). Further advances in this field may enable fetal Rh typing to be performed noninvasively in the future.

Determination of the maternal anti-D titer is an important step in the monitoring of an RhD-sensitized woman. A critical titer is that associated with an increased risk for severe hemolytic disease of the newborn and with a high risk of severe hydrops and suggests the need for referral to a tertiary center for continued management. The critical titer varies from center to center, but a titer ranging from 8 to 32 is usually used (Moise 2008).

Doppler assessment of the blood flow velocity in the fetus' middle cerebral artery (MCA) is replacing amniocentesis as a means of detecting fetal anemia. In an anemic fetus, the blood velocity may increase due to decreased viscosity and increased cardiac output. In one study, a value of more than 1.5 multiples of the median identified all cases of moderate to severe anemia (Mari et al. 2000). In a recent study comparing diagnostic amniocentesis with MCA flow, Doppler measurements improved on optical density determinations by 9% (Oepkes et al. 2006). Should fetal anemia be detected by either Doppler or amniocentesis, fetal blood sampling may be obtained (cordocentesis) to determine hematocrit,

direct antibody titer, fetal blood type, reticulocyte count, and TSB values. Intravascular intrauterine transfusion may be considered if the hematocrit value is less than 30%; however, should the pregnancy have reached 35 weeks gestation or more, the advantages of induction of delivery may outweigh the dangers of intrauterine transfusions. Repeated intrauterine transfusion may cause fetal bone marrow suppression, and in a repeatedly transfused fetus, the RBC mass at the time of delivery may be comprised almost entirely of donor cells. In this situation, exchange transfusion may be unnecessary, although "top-up" transfusions for anemia may be required (De Boer et al. 2008). In capable hands, the outcome of intrauterine transfusion should be good. In the Netherlands, the survival rate in 254 treated fetuses was 89% (Van Kamp et al. 2005).

74.5.1.3 Postnatal Management of the Newborn

Management of a hydropic, severely anemic neonate, especially if complicated by respiratory and other problems of prematurity, is a major neonatal challenge, requiring a degree of expertise available only at a tertiary center. The infant may be generally swollen because of soft tissue edema and in addition may have large collections of fluid in the pleural, pericardial, and peritoneal spaces. Intubation may be difficult because of the soft tissue swelling. Ventilation may be difficult, and the need for emergency drainage of the fluid collections, sometimes in the delivery or operating room, may add to the challenge. Anoxic myocardial damage may necessitate use of inotropes, and respiratory ventilatory support may have to be complemented by surfactant and nitric oxide (NO) administration. High-frequency ventilation may be necessary. Metabolic acidosis should be corrected (Smits-Wintjens et al. 2008).

Because the circulatory system may be overloaded, and myocardial function poor, it may be preferable to correct the anemia by performing a partial exchange transfusion, rather than by simple blood transfusion. Following insertion of an umbilical venous or arterial catheter, small amounts of anemic blood should be removed and replaced with equivalent amounts of donor packed RBCs. This procedure may be repeated to "titrate" until the desired hematocrit value is obtained.

In the fetus, most bilirubin formed from increased heme catabolism will be eliminated via the placenta. Severe intrauterine hyperbilirubinemia is therefore not usually a problem. Once delivered, however, the placenta no longer participates in the bilirubin elimination process, and continued hemolysis combined with immature conjugation and excretion may precipitate, causing a rapid rise in TSB values with the potential, if untreated, of causing extreme hyperbilirubinemia. Once the baby has been stabilized, attention should be paid to preventing this from occurring, and rectifying this situation should it occur. This is achieved by instituting intense phototherapy as soon as possible, closely monitoring TSB levels, and performing an exchange transfusion in cases where the TSB continues (>0.2 mg/dL [3.4 μmol/L] per hour) to increase despite intensive phototherapy. In general, the principles of the 2004 AAP guideline should be adopted to guide the management of the hyperbilirubinemia. The reader is referred to a subsequent chapter in this volume for further details on the treatment of hyperbilirubinemic newborns.

Some early studies demonstrated that intravenous immune globulin (IVIG) administration may be effective in preventing or limiting the number of exchange transfusions in Rh disease (Rübo et al. 1992). Indeed, the AAP guideline recommends the use of IVIG in order to prevent exchange transfusion in cases of failing phototherapy (American Academy of Pediatrics 2004). A recent Cochrane report, however, suggested that more information, based on well-designed studies, is needed before IVIG can be routinely recommended for isoimmune hemolysis (Alcock and Liley 2002), while a Dutch study demonstrated that prophylactic IVIG use did not reduce the number of exchange transfusions necessary in cases of Rh isoimmunization or alter the long-term neurodevelopmental outcome (Smits-Wintjens et al. 2011; van Klink et al. 2016).

Very few studies have related to the long-term neurodevelopmental outcome of fetuses treated

with intrauterine transfusion. Overall, the results to date are encouraging, although future long-term follow-up studies will be necessary to fully evaluate the current therapeutic modalities offered to the fetuses and newborn infants of Rh-immunized pregnancies (Smits-Wintjens et al. 2008). Fetal exposure to moderately increased bilirubin levels for prolonged periods of time may result in sensorineural hearing loss because of the effect of bilirubin on the developing auditory neural system (Hudon et al. 1998).

74.5.2 ABO Immune Disease

74.5.2.1 Background: Blood Group Incompatibility and Direct Antibody Titer (DAT) Positivity

Now that the occurrence of Rh isoimmunization has been reduced by anti-D immune prophylaxis, ABO incompatibility has become the single most frequent cause of immune hemolytic disease, causing jaundice in the neonate. Despite its increased frequency, the clinical picture, though, is usually milder than that of Rh disease. Nevertheless, in a series of children with kernicterus, ABO incompatibility is high on the list of identifiable causes.

ABO blood group heterospecificity refers to the situation in which the mother has O blood and the baby has blood group A or B. This setup is present in approximately 12% of pregnancies. In some instances, women with blood group O have a high titer of naturally occurring anti-A or anti-B antibodies. In contrast to Rh isoimmunization, in which immune sensitization occurs progressively with subsequent pregnancies, high titers of anti-A or anti-B antibodies can sometimes be found in blood group O women before their first pregnancy or even in girls (Grundbacher 1980). Unlike blood group A or B individuals, in whom their respective anti-B or anti-A antibodies are IgM molecules, and therefore unable to cross the placenta in significant quantities, the respective antibodies of blood group O persons are predominantly IgG molecules. Being smaller than IgM, IgG molecules may cross the placenta and attach to the corresponding fetal RBCs, provided that these cells have the A or B antigen. This immune process may cause hemolysis commencing in utero. Extravascular hemolysis of the IgG-coated RBCs is probably mediated by Fc-receptor-bearing cells within the reticuloendothelial system. Prior to delivery, there is little danger of severe hyperbilirubinemia, and the immune process is usually not sufficiently severe enough to cause hydrops. Babies may sometimes be born moderately anemic, and there is a potential danger of hyperbilirubinemia in the first days following delivery.

The hallmark of isoimmunization is a positive DAT. The test is termed “direct” if the antiglobulin is detected on the RBCs. An “indirect” test refers to the antibody being detected in the serum. About one-third of blood group A or B neonates born to a blood group O mother will have a positive DAT (Ozolek et al. 1994). Measurements of endogenous formation of CO, reflective of heme catabolism, have demonstrated, overall, an increased rate of heme catabolism in hyperbilirubinemic DAT-positive, ABO-incompatible neonates compared with controls (Stevenson et al. 1994; Fallstrom and Bjure 1968; Uetani et al. 1989). In a multicenter, international study of bilirubin production using ETCOc determinations, DAT positive babies (not necessarily hyperbilirubinemic) had significantly higher ETCOc values than the total population studied (Stevenson et al. 2001). While hyperbilirubinemic, DAT positive babies had even higher ETCOc values than the general DAT positive population, these were not significantly higher than hyperbilirubinemic babies of other categories. In a recent study >50% of DAT-positive, ABO-incompatible newborns developed a TSB >95th percentile (designated hyperbilirubinemia), and carboxyhemoglobin, corrected for ambient CO (COHbc) values were globally higher than previously published newborn values. Furthermore, babies in whom hyperbilirubinemia developed had higher even COHbc values than the already high values of the babies who did not develop hyperbilirubinemia (Kaplan et al. 2010).

Not all DAT-positive neonates will develop severe hyperbilirubinemia. In one study, although a positive DAT was predictive of an elevated TSB value, only 20% of DAT-positive neonates

actually developed TSB values ≥12.8 mg/dL (218 μmol/L), and even fewer had severe jaundice (Ozolek et al. 1994). In another study, only 19.6% of DAT positive, ABO-incompatible infants required phototherapy (Meberg and Johansen 1998). Despite this apparent clinical mildness, the authors occasionally encounter newborns with severe hyperbilirubinemia of early onset, occasionally unresponsive to phototherapy or IVIG therapy and warranting exchange transfusion. As already mentioned and to complete this clinical spectrum, kernicterus has been described in association with ABO hemolytic disease (Bhutani et al. 2004; Sgro et al. 2006).

The reasons for the absence of clinical disease in the majority of DAT-positive newborns may include the paucity of A and B antigenic sites on neonatal RBCs compared with adult RBCs or weak expression of these antigens in neonates. Non-RBC A or B antigenic sites may exist and bind with transplacentally acquired antibody without affecting the RBC. ABO blood group incompatibility with a negative DAT, not usually predictive of hemolysis or hyperbilirubinemia, may sometimes cause early and rapidly progressing jaundice, reminiscent of DAT-positive, hemolytic disease.

ABO heterospecificity with a positive DAT does not necessarily indicate ABO *hemolytic disease* as many ABO-incompatible, DAT positive neonates have no clinical evidence of ongoing hemolysis and do not develop early jaundice or hyperbilirubinemia. In order to support the diagnosis of ABO hemolytic disease, some or all of the following criteria are necessary:

1. Indirect hyperbilirubinemia, especially during the first 24 h of life.
2. Mother with blood group O, baby with blood group A or B.
3. Spherocytosis on blood smear.
4. Increased reticulocyte count.
5. Availability of a clinical tool for assessing ETCOc may ease the determination of ongoing hemolysis, thereby facilitating the diagnosis of ABO hemolytic disease.

An interaction between DAT-negative ABO incompatibility and polymorphism for the $(TA)_7$ sequence in the promoter of the *UGT1A1* gene, which encodes the corresponding bilirubin-conjugating enzyme, has been described. Neonates who were both ABO incompatible and homozygous for the variant gene promoter had a significantly higher incidence of TSB ≥15.0 mg/dL (257 μmol/L) than counterparts not bearing this combination (Kaplan et al. 2000a).

74.5.2.2 Clinical Manifestations of ABO Hemolytic Disease

Most blood group A or B neonates born to blood group O mothers will not develop any signs of hemolytic disease. It is essential to closely observe any newborn born to a blood group O mother for the development of hyperbilirubinemia. Routine blood group and DAT determination on umbilical cord blood is an option, but not mandatory, but may enable those at especially high risk for hyperbilirubinemia to be assiduously followed. A transcutaneous bilirubin (TcB) or TSB measurement should be performed at the first sign of visible jaundice. Phototherapy and exchange transfusions are indicated according to the 2004 AAP guideline (American Academy of Pediatrics 2004), using the lower level of TSB on the graph intended for newborns with risk factors. IVIG may be helpful in modifying the rate of rise of bilirubin and may be particularly useful in situations in which the TSB is approaching the indications for exchange transfusion, despite a trial of intense phototherapy. It is thought that IVIG blocks the Fc receptors in the reticuloendothelial system, thereby inhibiting hemolysis and limiting bilirubin formation.

74.5.3 Isoimmunization Due to Antibodies Other Than RhD

More than 50 RBC antigens may cause hemolytic disease of the newborn (Moise 2005). The most important of these with regard to prenatal hemolysis and the need for intrauterine infection include anti-c, anti-Kell, and anti-E (Hackney et al. 2004; Joy et al. 2005; McKenna et al. 1999) although

others may also, infrequently, be problematic. Alloimmunization due to these autobodies can sometimes cause severe hemolytic disease of the fetus requiring prenatal intervention. Fetal surveillance protocols and clinical strategies developed for RhD alloimmunization are useful in monitoring all alloimmunized pregnancies. Similarly, the postnatal management should be based on the principles outlined in the management of the RhD-immunized newborn. Anti-Kell isoimmunization warrants special mention as fetal anemia often predominates the clinical picture. This may be due to erythropoietic suppression in addition to a hemolytic process (Vaughan et al. 1994).

74.6 Nonimmune Hemolytic Disease

74.6.1 Glucose-6-Phosphate Dehydrogenase (G6PD) Deficiency

G6PD deficiency is one of the most common enzyme deficiencies known and is estimated to affect hundreds of millions of people worldwide (Beutler 1994; WHO Working Group 1989). Immigration patterns have transformed this condition from one limited to its indigenous distribution, including areas in Southern Europe, Africa, the Middle East, and Asia, to one that may now be encountered virtually in any corner of the globe. G6PD deficiency is a major factor in the pathogenesis of hyperbilirubinemia and is highly associated with extreme hyperbilirubinemia and kernicterus (Kaplan and Hammerman 2004; Valaes 1994). The condition is overrepresented in recent series of neonates with extreme hyperbilirubinemia and bilirubin encephalopathy, relative to the overall frequency of this condition in the United States, Canada, and United Kingdom and Ireland, respectively (Bhutani et al. 2004; Sgro et al. 2006; Manning et al. 2007). For example, in the United States-based Pilot Kernicterus Registry (Bhutani et al. 2004), over 20% of reported neonates had G6PD deficiency, whereas the overall frequency of G6PD deficiency in that country is estimated at less than 3% (WHO Working Group 1989). Because G6PD deficiency has major public health implications as far as the neonate is concerned, it will be discussed below in some detail.

74.6.1.1 Function of G6PD

G6PD plays a major part in stabilization of the RBC membrane. The enzyme catalyzes the first step in the hexose monophosphate pathway, oxidizing glucose-6-phosphate to 6-phosphogluconolactone, thereby reducing NAPD to NADPH. NADPH is essential for the regeneration of reduced glutathione from oxidized glutathione, a substance that plays an integral part in the body's antioxidative mechanisms. The pathway is also instrumental in stimulating catalase, another important antioxidant. In the absence of G6PD, NADPH will not become available, reduced glutathione will not be regenerated, and cells may be rendered susceptible to oxidative stress. The RBC is especially vulnerable to the G6PD deficiency state, as, unlike other body cells, no alternative source of NADPH is available in that cell. Oxidative membrane damage incurred may manifest as hemolysis (WHO Working Group 1989).

74.6.1.2 Genetics of G6PD Deficiency

G6PD deficiency is an X-linked condition. Males may therefore be normal hemizygotes or deficient hemizygotes. Females may be either normal or deficient homozygotes or heterozygotes. The most common mutations are G6PD A^-, found in Africa and southern Europe and in African Americans. G6PD Mediterranean, regarded as a more severe type than G6PD A^-, is encountered in Mediterranean countries, the Middle East, and India. Another variant encountered primarily in Asia is G6PD Canton. Many other mutations have been documented (Beutler 1994).

74.6.1.3 G6PD Deficiency and Hemolysis

Most G6PD-deficient individuals will lead perfectly normal lives and for the most part be unaware of their inherited condition. However, G6PD deficiency is notoriously associated, in children and adults, with severe hemolytic episodes associated with jaundice and anemia, which may occur following exposure to a

hemolytic trigger. Classically, these episodes often occur following ingestion of or contact with the fava bean (favism). Beutler (1994) has emphasized the role of infections in the pathogenesis of acute hemolysis.

The most extreme form of G6PD deficiency-associated hemolytic jaundice in neonates is typified by acute and unpredictable onset of jaundice. Some identifiable substances which may trigger hemolysis include naphthalene used to store clothes, herbal medicines, henna applications, or menthol-containing umbilical potions. Frequently, however, no identifiable trigger can be found. Extreme jaundice may develop suddenly and with no prior warning, and the TSB concentration may increase exponentially to dangerous levels. G6PD deficiency may therefore be the one reason that kernicterus may not be completely preventable. The hemolysis may be severe and exchange transfusion may be the only recourse.

Frequently, changes in hematologic indices typical of hemolysis in older children and adults, including falling hemoglobin and hematocrit values and increasing reticulocyte count, may be absent, despite a clinical picture of hemolysis. However, studies of endogenous CO formation, reflective of the rate of heme catabolism, have demonstrated an important role of increased hemolysis in association with this condition (Necheles et al. 1976; Slusher et al. 1995). Slusher et al. (1995), for example, demonstrated significantly higher levels of COHb in Nigerian G6PD-deficient neonates who developed kernicterus, compared with neonates who were hyperbilirubinemic, but did not develop signs of kernicterus.

More frequently and less life-threatening, G6PD-deficient neonates may have a more moderate form of hyperbilirubinemia. The incidence of this form of jaundice occurs at a rate several-fold that of controls. The hyperbilirubinemia usually responds to phototherapy, although exchange transfusion may also be necessary. These infants have a low-grade hemolysis, which cannot be implicated as the primary icterogenic factor (Kaplan et al. 1996a, 2004). Diminished bilirubin conjugation has been shown to be of major importance in the pathogenesis of the hyperbilirubinemia (Kaplan et al. 1996b). An intriguing interaction has been noted between G6PD deficiency and noncoding area $(TA)_7$ promoter polymorphism in the *UGT1A1* gene (Kaplan et al. 1997). This polymorphism, also known as *UGT1A1*28*, is associated with Gilbert syndrome. The incidence of hyperbilirubinemia, defined as a TSB $\geq$15.0 mg/dL (257 μmol/L), increased in a stepwise, dose-dependent fashion, in G6PD-deficient neonates who were either heterozygous or homozygous for the polymorphism. This effect was not seen in the G6PD-normal control group. Furthermore, G6PD deficiency alone, in the absence of the promoter polymorphism, did not increase the incidence of hyperbilirubinemia over and above that of G6PD-normal counterparts. In contrast, in Asians, in whom the $(TA)_7$ polymorphism is rare, a similar interaction was noticed between G6PD deficiency and coding area mutations of the UGT1A1 gene (Huang et al. 2002).

Unlike the acute hemolytic form of jaundice, this milder form of jaundice can be predicted by predischarge TSB testing. Neonates who had a predischarge TSB concentration below the 50^{th}percentile on the Bhutani nomogram (Bhutani et al. 1999) had a very small likelihood of subsequent hyperbilirubinemia. As the predischarge TSB increased above the 50th percentile, however, the chance of subsequent hyperbilirubinemia increased significantly (Kaplan et al. 2000b).

74.6.1.4 Testing for G6PD Deficiency

Many qualitative or quantitative screening tests are available which should accurately determine the hemizygous state in males or the homozygous state in females. However, being an X-linked condition, a large section of the female population may be heterozygotes. Because of X-inactivation, heterozygotes have two RBC populations: G6PD-deficient and G6PD-normal. Nonrandom X-inactivation may result in unequal ratios of normal and enzyme-deficient RBCs. Phenotype, determined on a sample of pooled RBCs, may, as a result, have either a normal, intermediate, or deficient phenotype, rendering the heterozygote state difficult to determine using standard biochemical tests (Fairbanks and Fernandez 1969). It was previously thought that heterozygotes had sufficient enzyme activity to protect them from the

dangers of G6PD deficiency (WHO Working Group 1989). However, more recent reports suggest that heterozygotes may not be without risk (Herschel et al. 2002; Kaplan et al. 1999, 2001). Females of high risk groups should be closely followed up according to the development of jaundice, a normal reading screen notwithstanding. Also, biochemical tests may give a falsely normal result if performed during an acute hemolytic episode, as older RBCs may be destroyed, leaving younger cells, with higher enzyme activity, intact (Herschel and Beutler 2001). In such cases, G6PD testing should be performed several weeks after the acute hemolysis has subsided. An alternate method is to analyze DNA for the specific suspected mutation.

Some countries have introduced neonatal screening for G6PD deficiency combined with parental education. There is some data demonstrating the effect of screening in combination with parental education in reducing the incidence of G6PD-associated kernicterus (Kaplan et al. 2015). Parents of screened newborns and their medical attendants should be made more aware of the condition by the screening process. Parental education should lead to avoidance of potentially offending substances, and knowledge that an infant is G6PD-deficient should speed the process of approach to a medical center, evaluation, and treatment of a jaundiced neonate.

The treatment of neonatal hyperbilirubinemia associated with G6PD deficiency should follow the recommendations of the AAP (American Academy of Pediatrics 2004) for neonates with hemolytic risk factors. In the event an infant presents with neurological signs commensurate with bilirubin encephalopathy, exchange transfusion should be immediately performed.

74.6.2 Pyruvate Kinase Deficiency

Pyruvate kinase catalyzes the conversion of phosphoenolpyruvate to pyruvate and the formation of adenosine triphosphate (ATP) from adenosine diphosphate in the Embden-Meyerhof pathway. Pyruvate kinase deficiency, a condition inherited in an autosomal recessive manner (Mentzer 1998), results in a lack of ATP, an important source of energy for RBC metabolism (Zanella et al. 2007a). Lack of ATP shortens RBC longevity. As a result, in the newborn period, hemolysis with anemia, reticulocytosis, and severe jaundice may ensue (Grace et al. 2015). Exchange transfusion may be required. This RBC enzyme defect is much less frequently encountered than G6PD deficiency. Four isozymes are encoded by 2 genes, among which 180 mutations have been described (Zanella et al. 2007b). The condition should be considered in any newborn with severe hyperbilirubinemia of unknown etiology. Diagnosis is determined by enzyme assay, while molecular studies using "next-generation techniques" may be instrumental in aiding diagnosis (Christensen et al. 2014).

74.6.3 Hereditary Spherocytosis

Of the hereditary RBC membrane defects which may lead to acute hemolysis and hyperbilirubinemia in the newborn, hereditary spherocytosis is probably the most common (Iolascon et al. 1998; Steiner and Gallagher 2007). Hereditary spherocytosis is also one of the few causes of hyperbilirubinemia which does not resolve in the neonatal period. This condition may be inherited both in an autosomal dominant and recessive fashion, and frequently there may be a history of acute hyperbilirubinemia in a sibling or a parent. It is thought that protein deficiencies in the RBC membrane, including ankyrin, band 3, -α-spectrin, β-spectrin, and protein 4.2, leave microscopic patches of the lipid bilayer inner surface bare of proteins, at which points microvesiculation occur. These osmotically fragile RBCs are trapped in the spleen, the microvesicles aspirated by macrophages, and the cell destroyed. Hemolysis may result in hyperbilirubinemia, anemia, and splenomegaly. The diagnosis can be made microscopically by demonstrating spherocytes in the peripheral blood smear, with confirmation by the osmotic fragility test. The latter test may be especially important in differentiating babies with hereditary spherocytosis from those with direct Coombs-positive ABO isoimmunization, a condition that also results in microspherocytosis. Mutations of at least five genes encoding the abovementioned proteins have

been recognized. The condition can be suspected by examination of RBC indices on the complete blood count. A high mean corpuscular hemoglobin concentration (MCHC) and low mean corpuscular volume (MCV) are typical and even more specific if the MCHC is divided by the MCV. Values for this ratio >0.36 are highly indicative of hereditary spherocytosis (Christensen et al. 2015b).

The clinical spectrum of hereditary spherocytosis during the perinatal period is wide and ranges from severe fetal anemia with hydrops fetalis to the asymptomatic neonate (Christensen et al. 2015b). The condition is frequently associated with neonatal hyperbilirubinemia. Of 178 affected, Italian term, predominantly breastfed, newborns, 112 (63%) developed neonatal hyperbilirubinemia requiring phototherapy. The incidence of hyperbilirubinemia was even higher in those who also had a genetic variation in the promoter of the bilirubin UGT1A1 gene, similar to that described in G6PD deficiency (Iolascon et al. 1998). Kernicterus has been described (Berardi et al. 2006). Treatment comprises intense phototherapy with resort to exchange transfusion in cases unresponsive to light therapy. Splenectomy may become necessary later during childhood in order to control the anemia resulting from ongoing hemolysis.

74.6.4 Hereditary Elliptocytosis, Hereditary Pyropoikilocytosis, Hereditary Ovalocytosis, and Hereditary Stomatocytosis

These are rare conditions affecting the RBC membrane. The diagnosis may be made by microscopic morphological examination of the peripheral blood smear (Christensen et al. 2014). Hemolysis may occur in the neonatal period and result in anemia and hyperbilirubinemia.

74.6.5 Infection

Infection is often associated with pathologic unconjugated hyperbilirubinemia. The presence of infection also creates increased risk for injury caused by bilirubin, probably related to alterations in binding of bilirubin to albumin but also through other mechanisms that may not be well defined related to the inflammatory process (Fernandes et al. 2004). The likelihood of neurotoxic injury caused by bilirubin is increased for a given level of bilirubin in the presence of infection. Moreover, an infant is more likely to deviate from the normal trajectory of bilirubin levels because of increased bilirubin production in the presence of infection. The cause of this increased production may be hemolysis but also upregulation of HO-1 (also known as heat shock protein 32), which may respond to oxidative stress associated with the infected state.

74.7 Summary

In summary, pathologic unconjugated hyperbilirubinemia is best defined epidemiologically. Although some pathologic unconjugated hyperbilirubinemia can be understood in terms of primary problems with uptake and conjugation, most pathologic unconjugated hyperbilirubinemia encountered by the pediatrician after birth and requiring treatment is associated with increased bilirubin production, often further exacerbated by environmental or acquired factors. Thus, a treatment strategy designed to modulate bilirubin production remains rational and potentially important, if a drug with the appropriate safety profile and efficacy is approved. Meanwhile, phototherapy is the mainstay of treatment and is reviewed in a following chapter.

References

Alcock GS, Liley H (2002) Immunoglobulin infusion for isoimmune haemolytic jaundice in neonates. Cochrane Database Syst Rev:CD003313

American Academy of Pediatrics (2004) Management of hyperbilirubinemia in the newborn infant 35 or more weeks of gestation. Pediatrics 114:297–316

Berardi A, Lugli L, Ferrari F et al (2006) Kernicterus associated with hereditary spherocytosis and UGT1A1 promoter polymorphism. Biol Neonate 90:243–246

Beutler E (1994) G6PD deficiency. Blood 84:3613–3636

Beutler E, Gelbart T, Demina A (1998) Racial variability in the UDP-glucuronosyltransferase 1 (UGT1A1) promoter: a balanced polymorphism for regulation of bilirubin metabolism? Proc Natl Acad Sci USA 95:8170–8174

Bhutani VK, Johnson L, Sivieri EM (1999) Predictive ability of a predischarge hour-specific serum bilirubin for subsequent significant hyperbilirubinemia in healthy term and near-term newborns. Pediatrics 103:6–14

Bhutani VK, Johnson LH, Jeffrey Maisels M et al (2004) Kernicterus: epidemiological strategies for its prevention through systems-based approaches. J Perinatol 24:650–662

Blanchette V, Dror Y, Chan A (2005) Hematology. In: MacDonald MG, Mullett MD, Seschia MMK (eds) Avery's neonatology: pathophysiology and management of the newborn. Lippincott, Williams and Wilkins, Philadelphia, pp 1169–1234

Bosma PJ, Chowdhury JR, Bakker C et al (1995) The genetic basis of the reduced expression of bilirubin UDP-glucuronosyltransferase 1 in Gilbert's syndrome. N Engl J Med 333:1171–1175

Bowman JM (1988) The prevention of Rh immunization. Transfus Med Rev 2:129–150

Castillo Cuadrado ME, Bhutani VK, Aby JL et al (2015) Evaluation of a new end-tidal carbon monoxide monitor from the bench to the bedside. Acta Paediatr 104:e279–e282

Chërif-Zahar B, Mattéi MG, Le Van Kim C et al (1991) Localization of the human Rh blood group gene structure to chromosome region 1p34.3-1p36.1 by *in situ* hybridization. Hum Genet 86:398–400

Christensen RD, Henry E (2010) Hereditary spherocytosis in neonates with hyperbilirubinemia. Pediatrics 125:120–125

Christensen RD, Yaish HM, Lemons RS (2014) Neonatal hemolytic jaundice: morphologic features of erythrocytes that will help you diagnose the underlying condition. Neonatology 105:243–249

Christensen RD, Lambert DK, Henry E et al (2015a) End-tidal carbon monoxide as an indicator of the hemolytic rate. Blood Cells Mol Dis 54:292–296

Christensen RD, Yaish HM, Gallagher PG (2015b) A pediatrician's practical guide to diagnosing and treating hereditary spherocytosis in neonates. Pediatrics 135:1107–1114

De Boer IP, Zeestraten EC, Lopriore E et al (2008) Pediatric outcome in Rhesus hemolytic disease treated with and without intrauterine transfusion. Am J Obstet Gynecol 198(54):e51–e54

de Haas M, Thurik FF, Koelewijn JM et al (2015) Haemolytic disease of the fetus and newborn. Vox Sang 109:99–113

Denschlag D, Marculescu R, Unfried G et al (2004) The size of a microsatellite polymorphism of the haem oxygenase 1 gene is associated with idiopathic recurrent miscarriage. Mol Hum Reprod 10:211–214

Fairbanks VF, Fernandez MN (1969) The identification of metabolic errors associated with hemolytic anemia. JAMA 208:316–320

Fallstrom SP, Bjure J (1968) Endogenous formation of carbon monoxide in newborn infants. 3. ABO incompatibility. Acta Paediatr Scand 57:137–144

Fernandes A, Silva RF, Falcao AS et al (2004) Cytokine production, glutamate release and cell death in rat cultured astrocytes treated with unconjugated bilirubin and LPS. J Neuroimmunol 153:64–75

Gamaleldin R, Iskander I, Seoud I et al (2011) Risk factors for neurotoxicity in newborns with severe neonatal hyperbilirubinemia. Pediatrics 128:e925–e931

Grace RF, Zanella A, Neufeld EJ et al (2015) Erythrocyte pyruvate kinase deficiency: 2015 status report. Am J Hematol 90:825–830

Group WW (1989) Glucose-6-phosphate dehydrogenase deficiency. WHO Working Group. Bull World Health Organ 67:601–611

Grundbacher FJ (1980) The etiology of ABO hemolytic disease of the newborn. Transfusion 20:563–568

Hackney DN, Knudtson EJ, Rossi KQ et al (2004) Management of pregnancies complicated by anti-c isoimmunization. Obstet Gynecol 103:24–30

Herschel M, Beutler E (2001) Low glucose-6-phosphate dehydrogenase enzyme activity level at the time of hemolysis in a male neonate with the African type of deficiency. Blood Cells Mol Dis 27:918–923

Herschel M, Ryan M, Gelbart T et al (2002) Hemolysis and hyperbilirubinemia in an African American neonate heterozygous for glucose-6-phosphate dehydrogenase deficiency. J Perinatol 22:577–579

Hsia DY, Allen FH Jr, Gellis SS et al (1952) Erythroblastosis fetalis. VIII. Studies of serum bilirubin in relation to Kernicterus. N Engl J Med 247:668–671

Hua L, Shi D, Bishop PR et al (2005) The role of UGT1A1*28 mutation in jaundiced infants with hypertrophic pyloric stenosis. Pediatr Res 58:881–884

Huang CS, Chang PF, Huang MJ et al (2002) Glucose-6-phosphate dehydrogenase deficiency, the UDP-glucuronosyltransferase 1A1 gene, and neonatal hyperbilirubinemia. Gastroenterology 123:127–133

Hudon L, Moise KJ Jr, Hegemier SE et al (1998) Long-term neurodevelopmental outcome after intrauterine transfusion for the treatment of fetal hemolytic disease. Am J Obstet Gynecol 179:858–863

Iolascon A, Miraglia del Giudice E, Perrotta S et al (1998) Hereditary spherocytosis: from clinical to molecular defects. Haematologica 83:240–257

Joy SD, Rossi KQ, Krugh D et al (2005) Management of pregnancies complicated by anti-E alloimmunization. Obstet Gynecol 105:24–28

Kaplan M, Hammerman C (2004) Glucose-6-phosphate dehydrogenase deficiency: a hidden risk for kernicterus. Semin Perinatol 28:356–364

Kaplan M, Vreman HJ, Hammerman C et al (1996a) Contribution of haemolysis to jaundice in Sephardic Jewish glucose-6-phosphate dehydrogenase deficient neonates. Br J Haematol 93:822–827

Kaplan M, Rubaltelli FF, Hammerman C et al (1996b) Conjugated bilirubin in neonates with glucose-6-phosphate dehydrogenase deficiency. J Pediatr 128:695–697

Kaplan M, Renbaum P, Levy-Lahad E et al (1997) Gilbert syndrome and glucose-6-phosphate dehydrogenase deficiency: a dose-dependent genetic interaction crucial to neonatal hyperbilirubinemia. Proc Natl Acad Sci U S A 94:12128–12132

Kaplan M, Beutler E, Vreman HJ et al (1999) Neonatal hyperbilirubinemia in glucose-6-phosphate dehydrogenase-deficient heterozygotes. Pediatrics 104:68–74

Kaplan M, Hammerman C, Renbaum P et al (2000a) Gilbert's syndrome and hyperbilirubinaemia in ABO-incompatible neonates. Lancet 356:652–653

Kaplan M, Hammerman C, Feldman R et al (2000b) Predischarge bilirubin screening in glucose-6-phosphate dehydrogenase-deficient neonates. Pediatrics 105:533–537

Kaplan M, Hammerman C, Vreman HJ et al (2001) Acute hemolysis and severe neonatal hyperbilirubinemia in glucose-6-phosphate dehydrogenase-deficient heterozygotes. J Pediatr 139:137–140

Kaplan M, Muraca M, Hammerman C et al (2002) Imbalance between production and conjugation of bilirubin: a fundamental concept in the mechanism of neonatal jaundice. Pediatrics 110, e47

Kaplan M, Hammerman C, Maisels MJ (2003) Bilirubin genetics for the nongeneticist: hereditary defects of neonatal bilirubin conjugation. Pediatrics 111:886–893

Kaplan M, Herschel M, Hammerman C et al (2004) Hyperbilirubinemia among African American, glucose-6-phosphate dehydrogenase-deficient neonates. Pediatrics 114:e213–e219

Kaplan M, Herschel M, Hammerman C et al (2006) Studies in hemolysis in glucose-6-phosphate dehydrogenase-deficient African American neonates. Clin Chim Acta 365:177–182

Kaplan M, Hammerman C, Vreman HJ et al (2010) Hemolysis and hyperbilirubinemia in antiglobulin positive, direct ABO blood group heterospecific neonates. J Pediatr 157:772–777

Kaplan M, Renbaum P, Hammerman C et al (2014a) Heme oxygenase-1 promoter polymorphisms and neonatal jaundice. Neonatology 106:323–329

Kaplan M, Bromiker R, Hammerman C (2014b) Hyperbilirubinemia, hemolysis, and increased bilirubin neurotoxicity. Semin Perinatol 38:429–437

Kaplan M, Hammerman C, Bhutani VK (2015) Parental education and the WHO neonatal G-6-PD screening program: a quarter century later. J Perinatol 35:779–784

Katayama Y, Yokota T, Zhao H et al (2015) Association of HMOX1 gene promoter polymorphisms with hyperbilirubinemia in the early neonatal period. Pediatr Int 57:645–649

Kuzniewicz M, Newman TB (2009) Interaction of hemolysis and hyperbilirubinemia on neurodevelopmental outcomes in the collaborative perinatal project. Pediatrics 123:1045–1050

Liley AW (1961) Liquor amnil analysis in the management of the pregnancy complicated by resus sensitization. Am J Obstet Gynecol 82:1359–1370

Lo YM, Hjelm NM, Fidler C et al (1998) Prenatal diagnosis of fetal RhD status by molecular analysis of maternal plasma. N Engl J Med 339:1734–1738

Maisels MJ, Kring E (2006) The contribution of hemolysis to early jaundice in normal newborns. Pediatrics 118:276–279

Maisels MJ, Newman TB (1995) Kernicterus in otherwise healthy, breast-fed term newborns. Pediatrics 96:730–733

Manning D, Todd P, Maxwell M et al (2007) Prospective surveillance study of severe hyperbilirubinaemia in the newborn in the UK and Ireland. Arch Dis Child Fetal Neonatal Ed 92:F342–F346

Mari G, Deter RL, Carpenter RL et al (2000) Noninvasive diagnosis by Doppler ultrasonography of fetal anemia due to maternal red-cell alloimmunization. Collaborative Group for Doppler Assessment of the Blood Velocity in Anemic Fetuses. N Engl J Med 342:9–14

Martin JA, Hamilton BE, Sutton PD et al (2003) Births: final data for 2002. Natl Vital Stat Rep 52:1–113

McKenna DS, Nagaraja HN, O'Shaughnessy R (1999) Management of pregnancies complicated by anti-Kell isoimmunization. Obstet Gynecol 93:667–673

Meberg A, Johansen KB (1998) Screening for neonatal hyperbilirubinaemia and ABO alloimmunization at the time of testing for phenylketonuria and congenital hypothyreosis. Acta Paediatr 87:1269–1274

Mentzer WC (1998) Pyruvate kinase deficiency and disorders of glycolysis. In: Nathan DG, Orkin SH (eds) Nathan and Oski's hematology of infancy and childhood. WB Saunders Company, Philadelphia, pp 665–703

Moise KJ (2005) Red blood cell alloimmunization in pregnancy. Semin Hematol 42:169–178

Moise KJ Jr (2008) Management of rhesus alloimmunization in pregnancy. Obstet Gynecol 112:164–176

Necheles TF, Rai US, Valaes T (1976) The role of haemolysis in neonatal hyperbilirubinaemia as reflected in carboxyhaemoglobin levels. Acta Paediatr Scand 65:361–367

Newman TB, Maisels MJ (1990) Does hyperbilirubinemia damage the brain of healthy full-term infants? Clin Perinatol 17:331–358

Newman TB, Maisels MJ (1992) Response to commentaries re: evaluation and treatment of jaundice in the term newborn: a kinder, gentler approach. Pediatrics 89:831–833

Newman TB, Liljestrand P, Jeremy RJ et al (2006) Outcomes among newborns with total serum bilirubin levels of 25 mg per deciliter or more. N Engl J Med 354:1889–1900

Nilsen ST, Finne PH, Bergsjo P et al (1984) Males with neonatal hyperbilirubinemia examined at 18 years of age. Acta Paediatr Scand 73:176–180

Oepkes D, Seaward PG, Vandenbussche FP et al (2006) Doppler ultrasonography versus amniocentesis to predict fetal anemia. N Engl J Med 355:156–164
Ozmert E, Erdem G, Topcu M et al (1996) Long-term follow-up of indirect hyperbilirubinemia in full-term Turkish infants. Acta Paediatr 85:1440–1444
Ozolek JA, Watchko JF, Mimouni F (1994) Prevalence and lack of clinical significance of blood group incompatibility in mothers with blood type A or B. J Pediatr 125:87–91
Rübo J, Albrecht K, Lasch P et al (1992) High-dose intravenous immune globulin therapy for hyperbilirubinemia caused by Rh hemolytic disease. J Pediatr 121:93–97
Sgro M, Campbell D, Shah V (2006) Incidence and causes of severe neonatal hyperbilirubinemia in Canada. CMAJ 175:587–590
Shibahara S, Kitamuro T, Takahashi K (2002) Heme degradation and human disease: diversity is the soul of life. Antioxid Redox Signal 4:593–602
Slusher TM, Vreman HJ, McLaren DW et al (1995) Glucose-6-phosphate dehydrogenase deficiency and carboxyhemoglobin concentrations associated with bilirubin-related morbidity and death in Nigerian infants. J Pediatr 126:102–108
Smits-Wintjens VE, Walther FJ, Lopriore E (2008) Rhesus haemolytic disease of the newborn: postnatal management, associated morbidity and long-term outcome. Semin Fetal Neonatal Med 13:265–271
Smits-Wintjens VE, Walther FJ, Rath ME et al (2011) Intravenous immunoglobulin in neonates with rhesus hemolytic disease: a randomized controlled trial. Pediatrics 127:680–686
Steiner LA, Gallagher PG (2007) Erythrocyte disorders in the perinatal period. Semin Perinatol 31:254–261
Stevenson DK, Bartoletti AL, Ostrander CR et al (1979) Pulmonary excretion of carbon monoxide in the human infant as an index of bilirubin production. II. Infants of diabetic mothers. J Pediatr 94:956–958
Stevenson DK, Ostrander CR, Hopper AO et al (1981) Pulmonary excretion of carbon monoxide as an index of bilirubin production. IIa. Evidence for possible delayed clearance of bilirubin in infants of diabetic mothers. J Pediatr 98:822–824
Stevenson DK, Vreman HJ, Oh W et al (1994) Bilirubin production in healthy term infants as measured by carbon monoxide in breath. Clin Chem 40:1934–1939
Stevenson DK, Fanaroff AA, Maisels MJ et al (2001) Prediction of hyperbilirubinemia in near-term and term infants. Pediatrics 108:31–39
Tidmarsh GF, Wong RJ, Stevenson DK (2014) End-tidal carbon monoxide and hemolysis. J Perinatol 34:577–581
Uetani Y, Nakamura H, Okamoto O et al (1989) Carboxyhemoglobin measurements in the diagnosis of ABO hemolytic disease. Acta Paediatr Jpn 31:171–176
Valaes T (1994) Severe neonatal jaundice associated with glucose-6-phosphate dehydrogenase deficiency: pathogenesis and global epidemiology. Acta Paediatr Suppl 394:58–76
Van den Veyver IB, Moise KJ Jr (1996) Fetal RhD typing by polymerase chain reaction in pregnancies complicated by rhesus alloimmunization. Obstet Gynecol 88:1061–1067
Van Kamp IL, Klumper FJ, Oepkes D et al (2005) Complications of intrauterine intravascular transfusion for fetal anemia due to maternal red-cell alloimmunization. Am J Obstet Gynecol 192:171–177
van Klink JM, van Veen SJ, Smits-Wintjens VE et al (2016) Immunoglobulins in neonates with rhesus hemolytic disease of the fetus and newborn: long-term outcome in a randomized trial. Fetal Diagn Ther 39:209–213
Vaughan JI, Warwick R, Letsky E et al (1994) Erythropoietic suppression in fetal anemia because of Kell alloimmunization. Am J Obstet Gynecol 171:247–252
Vreman HJ, Rodgers PA, Gale R et al (1989) Carbon monoxide excretion as an index of bilirubin production in rhesus monkeys. J Med Primatol 18:449–460
Watchko JF, Oski FA (1983) Bilirubin 20 mg/dL = vigintiphobia. Pediatrics 71:660–663
Watchko JF, Daood MJ, Biniwale M (2002) Understanding neonatal hyperbilirubinaemia in the era of genomics. Semin Neonatol 7:143–152
Wong RJ, DeSandre GH, Sibley E et al (2006) Neonatal jaundice and liver disease. In: Fanaroff AA, Martin RJ, Walsh MC (eds) Neonatal-perinatal medicine: diseases of the fetus and infant. Mosby, Philadelphia, pp 1419–1465
Zanella A, Bianchi P, Fermo E (2007a) Pyruvate kinase deficiency. Haematologica 92:721–723
Zanella A, Fermo E, Bianchi P et al (2007b) Pyruvate kinase deficiency: the genotype-phenotype association. Blood Rev 21:217–231

75 Kernicterus, Bilirubin-Induced Neurological Dysfunction, and New Treatments for Unconjugated Hyperbilirubinemia in Neonates

Christian V. Hulzebos, Claudio Tiribelli, Frans J. C. Cuperus, and Petr H. Dijk

Contents

Abstract

Severe hyperbilirubinemia occurs worldwide and threatens neurodevelopmental outcome of many infants. Acute kernicterus is an unambiguous clinical disorder in severely jaundiced newborn infants but may also occur in preterm infants at bilirubin levels below current treatment thresholds. Bilirubin-induced neurological dysfunction (BIND) consists of more subtle, but permanent, bilirubin encephalopathy and may present with auditory dysfunction and/or mild neurologic abnormalities such as mild impairment in neurologic and/or

C. V. Hulzebos (✉) · P. H. Dijk
Beatrix Children's Hospital, University Medical Center Groningen, Groningen, The Netherlands
e-mail: c.v.hulzebos@umcg.nl

C. Tiribelli
Liver Research Centre, University of Trieste, Trieste, Italy

F. J. C. Cuperus
Department of Gastroenterology and Hepatology, University Medical Center Groningen, Groningen, The Netherlands

G. Buonocore et al. (eds.), *Neonatology*,
https://doi.org/10.1007/978-3-319-29489-6_222

cognitive performance. Early prevention of severe hyperbilirubinemia is key to reduction of neurological sequelae and implies knowledge of maternal, perinatal, and neonatal risk factors. Subsequent recognition of neonates with perceived bilirubin neurotoxicity risk factors, of which hemolysis and sepsis are the most important, will enable categorization of neonates into high-, moderate-, or low-risk groups, with individualized screening and appropriate treatment. Phototherapy is the cornerstone of current treatment, and – if unsuccessful – exchange transfusion can be performed. Phototherapy does not always prevent bilirubin accumulation, and concerns exist about aggressive use in ELBW infants. Exchange transfusions are invasive procedures and associated with significant morbidity. It is highly conceivable that new treatments which either decrease bilirubin production, increase hepatic clearance, or decrease enterohepatic circulation will find their way in patients suffering severe hyperbilirubinemia and imminent BIND despite conventional treatment in the foreseeable future.

75.1 Salient Points

- Severe hyperbilirubinemia occurs worldwide, and bilirubin neurotoxicity threatens neurodevelopmental outcome of many infants.
- Early recognition of hyperbilirubinemia-associated risk factors, timely diagnosis, and appropriate treatment are key in the management of neonatal hyperbilirubinemia.
- Conventional treatment consists of LED phototherapy and exchange transfusion.
- Novel treatment modalities aim to decrease bilirubin production, increase hepatic clearance, and/or decrease enterohepatic circulation.

75.2 Introduction

In the nineteenth century, it was already known that unconjugated hyperbilirubinemia could potentially harm the central nervous system of jaundiced newborn infants. Yellow staining of deep brain nuclei in jaundiced infants was first reported in 1847. The term kernicterus (kern (German) = nucleus, ikteros. (Greek) = yellow) was first denoted in 1903 to describe the pathological findings of this specific yellow staining pattern (Hansen 2000). Nowadays, kernicterus is not only used to describe the pathological findings but merely to describe the clinical findings of acute and/or chronic bilirubin encephalopathy in jaundiced infants. Although acute kernicterus is an unambiguous clinical disorder in severely jaundiced newborn infants with the possibility of permanent sequelae, subtle forms of bilirubin encephalopathy referred to as bilirubin-induced neurological dysfunction, also known as BIND, have evolved more recently (Shapiro 2010; Lunsing 2014). This chapter aims to describe the pathophysiology of bilirubin neurotoxicity, its clinical spectrum, and diagnostic tools. Novel treatment modalities to prevent infants from developing severe unconjugated hyperbilirubinemia and bilirubin neurotoxicity will be highlighted.

75.3 Pathophysiology: Risk Factors

The risk of kernicterus and BIND may be in part determined by the concentration of total serum bilirubin (TSB), which consists in neonates almost exclusively of unconjugated bilirubin (UCB), but is primarily determined by the concentration of non-albumin-bound free bilirubin (Bf) (Watchko and Tiribelli 2013). Bf can easily pass the blood-brain barrier and may better reflect the bilirubin load distributed in the brain (Ostrow et al. 2003a). Several cellular mechanisms of the brain protect the brain against bilirubin accumulation. One of these protective regulating mechanisms is UCB export from the brain to the blood by multidrug resistance p-glycoprotein 1 (MDR1) and most importantly by the multidrug resistance-associated protein 1 (MRP1) (Ostrow et al. 2003a; Wennberg et al. 2006). Data from in vitro and in vivo experiments have suggested that Bf, and not TSB, is the principal determinant of bilirubin neurotoxicity (Ahlfors and Shapiro 2001a; Ostrow et al. 2003b; Calligaris et al. 2007). A number of pathophysiological factors are related to the variable clinical

spectrum of bilirubin neurotoxicity. First, several mechanisms including necrosis and apoptosis are involved in bilirubin-induced neuronal damage, resulting in specific types of cellular damage and function (Ostrow et al. 2004). Second, neuronal susceptibility to bilirubin neurotoxicity is not comparable in all cell types of the brain, neurons being more susceptible than glia cells of which the exact mechanisms remain speculative (Ostrow et al. 2004). Third, the amount of UCB that enters the brain is dependent not only on the Bf concentration but also on intactness of the blood-brain barrier. The Bf concentration in plasma is determined by the concentration of unconjugated bilirubin bound to albumin at a specific plasma pH in relation to the affinity of bilirubin to bind albumin. Conditions associated with low albumin concentrations or with displacement of bilirubin from albumin (e.g., by sulfonamides or free fatty acids) increase Bf concentrations. Conditions that decrease intactness of the blood-brain barrier (e.g., hyperosmolality, hypercapnia, asphyxia, prematurity, infection, and sepsis) can result in a net increase of UCB uptake in the brain. Multiple other factors (i.e., cerebral blood flow, vascular permeability, cellular efflux pumps, and cellular recovery capacity) may affect the development of neurotoxicity at any given Bf concentration (Wennberg et al. 2006). Some of these factors are incorporated as risk factors in management guidelines of jaundiced infants. Clinical evidence of most of these risk factors is limited. Most factors are based on anecdotal clinical evidence or theoretical and experimental animal data. Although imperfect, these factors are used by many clinicians to determine TSB thresholds before starting treatment (Lucey 1972; Pearlman et al. 1980; Kim et al. 1980; Turkel 1990; Watchko and Maisels 2003; Maisels and Watchko 2003; Management of Hyperbilirubinemia in the Newborn Infant 35 or More Weeks of Gestation 2004). The risk factors that increase the susceptibility for bilirubin neurotoxicity, which sometimes also predispose to develop hyperbilirubinemia, are shown in Table 1. Risk assessment of bilirubin neurotoxicity for each individual newborn infant involves more than measurement of the TSB concentration and appears to be a dynamic process affected by continuously changing individual conditions. Unfortunately, Bf cannot be routinely measured so that concentration of TSB and the currently used risk factors are the principal parameters which determine treatment thresholds.

Table 1 Risk factors used in addition to TSB to assess the risk of bilirubin neurotoxicity in the management of jaundiced infants

Risk factors
Acidosis
Asphyxia
Hemolysis
Hypothermia
Hypoalbuminemia or less albumin available to bind bilirubin
Intracranial hemorrhage
Low birth weight
Meningitis
Prematurity
Sepsis

75.4 Clinical Symptoms

The clinical spectrum of signs of bilirubin neurotoxicity relates to the bilirubin-induced damage to specific brain areas. Specific brain stem nuclei (auditory, vestibular, and oculomotor), cerebellar Purkinje cells, basal ganglia (i.e., globus pallidus and subthalamus), and the hippocampus are particularly vulnerable for bilirubin neurotoxicity. Acute bilirubin encephalopathy in the initial phase is characterized by lethargy, hypotonia, and poor sucking. In the second or intermediate phase, most commonly within 2–3 days after the initial phase, hypertonia (retrocollis, opisthotonus), discomfort, and irritability dominate. The infant may develop fever, a typical high-pitched cry, and seizures, which may alternate with drowsiness and hypotonia. Exchange transfusion at this stage might reverse in some cases the central nervous system damage. When left untreated, this second phase progresses into a more advanced stage characterized by pronounced retrocollis-opisthotonus, shrill cry, apnea, fever, sometimes seizures, deep stupor to coma, and even death (Management of Hyperbilirubinemia in the Newborn Infant 35 or More Weeks of Gestation 2004; Shapiro 2003).

Choreoathetosis, vertical gaze paralysis, "kernicteric facies," auditory dysfunction, and dental dysplasia (Perlstein's tetrad) and motor delay are the most commonly described permanent neurologic sequelae in infants who survive the acute phase of kernicterus (Slusher et al. 2011). Intelligence is usually normal in these infants (Shapiro 2003). Less severe hyperbilirubinemia can result in subtle bilirubin encephalopathy referred to as "bilirubin-induced neurological dysfunction" (BIND) or as "bilirubin-associated neurological dysfunction" (BAND). Subtle permanent bilirubin encephalopathy can present with auditory dysfunction and/or mild neurologic abnormalities such as mild impairment in neurologic and/or cognitive performance (Oh et al. 2003; Shapiro 2005). Involvement of the auditory nervous system dysfunction may result in sensorineuronal hearing loss or deafness. Alternatively, auditory dysfunction referred to as auditory neuropathy (AN) or auditory dys-synchrony (AD) may occur. AN/AD is defined as normal neurophysiological tests of the inner ear, i.e., normal cochlear microphonic responses and otoacoustic emissions, but an abnormal or absent auditory brain stem response (ABR) resulting in abnormal sound processing. AN/AD is clinically characterized by problems in sound localization and speech discrimination. Hearing loss is not per se present and a normal audiogram is often seen.

A prospective study evaluated effects of moderate degrees of hyperbilirubinemia (TSB levels ranging from 233 to 444 μmol/L) in term infants with respect to the development of minor neurologic dysfunction up to 12 months after birth. A significant increase in minor neurologic dysfunction, i.e., mild abnormalities in muscle tone regulation in combination with significant postural and reflex dysfunction throughout the first year of life, was found in hyperbilirubinemic infants compared to control infants (Soorani-Lunsing et al. 2001).

Isolated movement disorders such as athetosis or dystonia are sometimes seen, and in a retrospective analysis of extremely low-birth-weight infants, a significant association between peak concentrations of TSB during the first 2 weeks of life and neurodevelopmental impairment was found (Shapiro 2003, 2005; Oh et al. 2003; Newman and Klebanoff 1993). Alternatively, classical kernicterus with typical MRI findings is sometimes observed in sick, very low-birth-weight preterm neonates at relatively low bilirubin concentrations, which are even under commonly applied treatment thresholds. Innate vulnerability or bilirubin neurotoxicity potentiating comorbidities (i.e., CNS damage, low albumin levels) may thus predispose for development of low bilirubin kernicterus (Watchko and Maisels 2014).

75.5 Epidemiology

In the past century, kernicterus was almost exclusively seen in the context of high concentrations of TSB related to Rh hemolytic disease. When Rh disease became rare in high-income countries due to the introduction of Rh-immune globulin, and phototherapy appeared an effective treatment for unconjugated hyperbilirubinemia, the incidence of kernicterus decreased. Subsequently, treatment criteria were liberalized. As a combined result of the more liberal treatment criteria, a trend toward earlier hospital discharge (before the maximal TSB concentration is reached), and higher survival rate of preterm infants, kernicterus never disappeared. Though largely needed, the exact incidence of kernicterus and BIND is unknown. This is at least, in part, related to differences in the definition of severe hyperbilirubinemia and in methods of assessing neurodevelopmental outcome among studies. Epidemiological data on severe hyperbilirubinemia and bilirubin encephalopathy from several developed countries show incidences of TSB concentrations ≥510 μmol/L between 2 and 13 per 100.000 live births and of bilirubin encephalopathy to be ~1 case per 100.000 live births (Manning et al. 2007; Gotink et al. 2013). It is estimated that 1–3 per 100.000 live births are at risk of developing kernicterus when untreated and that 5–10% of infants surviving severe hyperbilirubinemia suffer permanent sequelae in high-income countries (Wennberg et al. 2006; Ip et al. 2004). Low- and middle-income countries (LMICs) contribute largely to the estimated incidence of severe hyperbilirubinemia of ~0.5 million neonates per year, i.e.,

0.4% of all live births worldwide (Bhutani et al. 2013). In line with this are disproportionately higher rates of bilirubin-related morbidity and mortality data in LMICs when compared to high-income countries (Olusanya et al. 2014, 2015). Early prevention of severe hyperbilirubinemia is key to reduction of neurological sequelae but implies knowledge of risk factors for severe hyperbilirubinemia. The majority of these maternal (e.g., Asian mother, primiparity), perinatal (e.g., place of delivery), and neonatal (e.g., low gestational age) risk factors are similar in LMICs and HICs (Olusanya et al. 2015; D'Silva et al. 2014; Norman et al. 2015). Subsequent recognition of neonates with perceived bilirubin neurotoxicity risk factors, of which – for reasons not completely understood – increased bilirubin production rates due to hemolysis (blood group incompatibility, G6PD deficiency, genetic polymorphisms) and sepsis are the most important, will enable categorization of neonates into high-, moderate-, or low-risk groups, with individualized screening and appropriate follow-up for SH (Kaplan et al. 2014; Wong and Stevenson 2015). Interestingly, home deliveries do not necessarily increase the incidence of SH, provided that the perinatal care in the home setting is well organized (Gotink et al. 2013).

75.6 Diagnosis

Current management guidelines for jaundiced infants are actually based on the total serum bilirubin (TSB) concentrations. Because exact neurotoxic TSB concentrations are unknown and risk factors for imminent bilirubin neurotoxicity are not evidence based, other diagnostic tools, in addition to TSB, may be valuable to detect imminent BIND in jaundiced newborn infants (Table 2).

Though easily available in clinical settings in developed countries, the measurement of TSB in less-developed countries is much less easy. This not only prevents the assessment of TSB but also delays treatment when necessary, thus increasing the risk of acute bilirubin encephalopathy. Transcutaneous measuring of bilirubin (TcB) is available and works well up to a bilirubin concentration of 15 mg/dL. The cost of the apparatus renders TcB measurements not ideal for a widespread use. Recently, the Bilistick system has been suggested as a valuable alternative (Coda Zabetta et al. 2013). Bilistick is a point-of-care (POC) diagnostic instrument for TSB in newborns' blood, providing TSB results within 2 min. The short time allows doctors and nurses to triage neonates with hyperbilirubinemia and install appropriate prompt treatment before irreversible brain damage has occurred. This system has been tested extensively in studies in four different countries (Nigeria, Egypt, Indonesia, and Vietnam) in recent years with promising results.

Table 2 Diagnostic tools to evaluate the severity of hyperbilirubinemia and/or risk on bilirubin neurotoxicity

Diagnostic tool
Anamnestic
History of hyperbilirubinemic period
Treatment
Gestational age
Risk factors present in hyperbilirubinemic period
Symptoms of kernicterus during hyperbilirubinemic period
Abnormal physical examination
BIND (–M) score
Total serum bilirubin concentration
Free bilirubin concentration
Bilirubin/albumin ratio
Auditory brain stem response
Magnetic resonance imaging

To evaluate the risk of BIND, the history of the infant is important. Information about the gestational age, physical examination, and the presence of risk factors for severe hyperbilirubinemia and bilirubin neurotoxicity as well as the duration of the hyperbilirubinemic period, the presence of acute symptoms, and whether the child is treated or not is crucial data to diagnose BIND at a later age (Shapiro 2010).

Although preliminary clinical series and in vitro data point to a correlation between Bf and BIND, the possibility to clinically measure Bf prevented so far its introduction in clinical practice. Alternatively, the bilirubin/albumin ratio (B/A ratio) could be used as a surrogate parameter to indicate Bf concentrations (Ahlfors and Wennberg 2004;

Ahlfors and Parker 2005). However, due to the presence of bilirubin displacers, i.e., drugs that interfere with the bilirubin-albumin binding, Bf may reach values much higher than suggested by the calculated B/A ratio. In addition the individual variability in the binding affinity of the albumin for bilirubin should also be taken into account. Alternatively, other plasma constituents such as apolipoproteins may bind UCB and decrease Bf. Consequently, the B/A ratio seems an imperfect surrogate to estimate Bf. It needs to be outlined, however, that also Bf may be an imperfect predictor of bilirubin neurotoxicity, since many factors affect the development of bilirubin neurotoxicity at any given Bf level as pointed out in the pathophysiology paragraph.

The theoretical considerations and clinical evidence for the concept that additional use, i.e., next to TSB, of the B/A ratio in jaundiced premature infants might improve the prediction of BIND have been reviewed. From these data, it has been suggested that the additional use of the B/A ratio may be valuable in evaluating jaundiced premature infants (Ritter et al. 1982; Scheidt et al. 1991; Amin et al. 2001; Govaert et al. 2003; Hulzebos et al. 2008). Recently, a randomized controlled trial in 615 preterm infants of 32 weeks' gestation or less investigated the additional use of the B/A ratio in the treatment of hyperbilirubinemia in preterm infants (ISRCTN74465643) (Hulzebos et al. 2014; Iskander et al. 2014). Preterm infants were randomly assigned to treatment based on either B/A ratio and TSB thresholds, whichever threshold was crossed first, or on the TSB thresholds only. There was no difference between the groups in neurodevelopmental outcome at 18–24 months' corrected age. In another trial, in 193 near-term and term neonates with TSB levels ranging from ~290 to ~1,045 μmol/L, both TSB and the B/A ratio showed to be strong predictors for neurotoxicity, but the B/A ratio did not improve prediction of acute bilirubin encephalopathy over TSB alone (Iskander et al. 2014).

The possibility that biochemical markers, i.e., use of Tau and S100B protein concentrations, are useful in the diagnosis of bilirubin-induced neurotoxicity has been studied in hyperbilirubinemic newborn infants (Okumus et al. 2008). Tau protein is a microtubule-associated structural protein of central nervous system neurons. S100B protein, a neurotrophic factor, is synthesized in astroglial cells in the central nervous system and Schwann cells. Previous data showed increased Tau and S100B protein concentration in plasma and/or cerebrospinal fluid in patients with cerebral injury (e.g., hypoxia and trauma). In a prospective study of 92 hyperbilirubinemic non-asphyxiated infants, Tau and S100B protein concentration was positively correlated with TSB concentration. Tau and S100B concentration increased at TSB concentration above 327 μmol/L, observed in 46 infants. At lower TSB concentrations, protein concentrations remained rather unchanged. Above a TSB concentration of 327 μmol/L, clinical symptoms of bilirubin encephalopathy (i.e., auditory neuropathy, minor neurologic dysfunction, and electroencephalographic abnormalities) were present in 22 of 46 of the infants. Compared to TSB concentrations, measurement of Tau and S100B protein concentration did not improve sensitivity or specificity for any of the described clinical symptoms. The use of Tau and S100B protein concentration in the assessment of BIND is not recommended.

The neural auditory pathway is very susceptible to bilirubin toxicity putatively resulting in sensorineuronal hearing loss or auditory neuropathy also known as auditory dys-synchrony. A frequently used, noninvasive, and very sensitive tool to determine bilirubin neurotoxicity is the auditory brain stem response (ABR), which allows for determination of electrophysiological activity of the neural auditory pathway. The ABR consists of a sequence of positive waves (numbered I–V) representing the auditory pathway from the inner ear to brain stem. Waves I and II represent the peripheral auditory nerve; waves III–V represent the activity in the auditory centers at brain stem level of the pathway (cochlear nucleus and lateral lemniscus, resp.) (Amin et al. 1999). Bilirubin-induced ABR changes involve mainly waves III and V and may progress from reversible increased interwave latencies to the loss of wave amplitude. ABR changes can be transient but may also progress into permanent wave changes or even loss of any recognizable wave (Amin et al. 2001; Shapiro and Nakamura 2001;

Ahlfors and Shapiro 2001b). A bedside method to evaluate the intactness of the auditory pathway is the automated auditory brain stem response (AABR) with an ALGO hearing screening system (Natus Medical, San Carlos, CA, USA). AABR measurements are simplified ABR measurements and able to identify infants with abnormal cochlear or auditory function. A pass or refer result is shown on the ALGO machine for each ear of the infant. In an observational study of 191 patients of variable birth weight (ranging from 406 to 4,727 g) and variable gestational age (from 24 to 42 weeks), an abnormal ALGO result (bi-or unilateral refer) was associated with increased BF concentrations and BF/TSB ratio, but not with TSB concentrations alone, whereas others report that TSB as well as the B/A ratio predicted bilateral refer AABR at hospital admission and at 3 months follow-up (Iskander et al. 2014; Ahlfors et al. 2009).

Recent data, using visual-evoked potentials (VEPs) in children with moderately elevated TSB levels, suggest that BIND may also affect visuocortical function resulting in delayed visual maturation (Good and Hou 2015). Another tool to identify acute and chronic bilirubin neurotoxicity in jaundiced infants is magnetic resonance imaging (MRI) (Volpe 2009). MRI changes include bilateral hyperintensity of globus pallidus on T1-weighted scans in the early phase (first 3 weeks of life) and most commonly subtle but persistent pallidal hyperintensity, suggestive of permanent gliosis, on late T2-weighted scans (with disappearance of hyperintensity on T1-weighted scans). The subthalamic nucleus and hippocampus are affected less frequently (approximately 40% and 5% of reported cases, respectively). Bilateral damage of the globus pallidus and the subthalamic nucleus is a specific sign of bilirubin neurotoxicity, which sometimes can also be visualized with ultrasonography, and is a key in the differentiation between hypoxic-ischemic encephalopathy or metabolic disorders, which predominantly affect the thalamus (Govaert et al. 2003). The additional value of MR spectroscopy to MRI is not completely clear, but acute changes in cerebral metabolism have been shown in bilirubin encephalopathy (Groenendaal et al. 2004).

In 1999, a clinical scoring system was developed to evaluate the neurotoxicity risk of exposure to unconjugated hyperbilirubinemia. Clinical signs of bilirubin-induced neurological dysfunction (BIND) include altered mental status, muscle tone, and cry of the infant. Dependent on the level of abnormality, 0–3 points are obtained for each clinical sign, resulting in an overall BIND score between 0 and 9, representing no toxicity or advanced toxicity – associated with kernicterus or death, respectively (Johnson et al. 1999). TSB and B/A ratios appear to be positively related to this BIND score in (near-) term infants (Iskander et al. 2014). A modified BIND score (BIND-M) has been found reliable for prediction signs of acute bilirubin neurotoxicity (Radmacher et al. 2015).

75.7 Treatment

To identify newborns at risk for severe hyperbilirubinemia and to prevent bilirubin neurotoxicity, guidelines have been developed for the management of jaundiced infants. The American Academy of Pediatrics' Subcommittee on Hyperbilirubinemia has published a guideline for hyperbilirubinemic infants of 35 or more weeks of gestation in 2004 (Management of Hyperbilirubinemia in the Newborn Infant 35 or More Weeks of Gestation 2004). This "AAP" guideline, which will be adapted soon, has been adopted by many countries worldwide for the management of jaundiced "near-term" newborn infants. International guidelines for preterm infants are less common, and rather local or national guidelines or approaches for preterm infants are used (National Institute for Health and Clinical Excellence 2010; van Imhoff et al. 2011; Maisels et al. 2012; Wallenstein and Bhutani 2013). Few prospective studies have analyzed effects of different TSB thresholds on long-term outcome (Table 3). In a group of 95 low-birth-weight infants, hyperbilirubinemia was treated either with prophylactic phototherapy (starting 12 h after birth, $n = 46$) or conservative phototherapy (starting at a fixed TSB threshold of 150 μmol/L, $n = 49$) (Jangaard et al. 2007). The maximum TSB concentrations were comparable in both groups, but in a subgroup of extreme low-birth-weight infants

Table 3 Long-term outcome of randomized controlled trials on TSB thresholds

Author/year	Population	Prophylactic conservative treatment TSB threshold		Long-term outcome
Morris (2008) (Amin et al. 2001)	ELBW infants (BW <1,000 g) $n = 1974$	Direct postnatally	137 μmol/L (BW 501–750 g) or 171 μmol/L (BW 751–1,000 g)	No significant difference for the combination of death or neurological impairment. Prophylactic phototherapy reduced the risk of neurodevelopmental impairment (RR = 0.86 (95 % CI: 0.74–0.99))
				Nonsignificant higher mortality among infants with a BW of 501–750 g (RR = 1.13 (95 % CI: 0.96–1.34))
Jangaard (2007) (Scheidt et al. 1991)	LBW infants (<1,500 g) $n = 95$	12 h postnatally	150 μmol/L	Nonsignificant increase in cerebral palsy and death in a subgroup of infants (with a BW <1,000 g) in the conservative group

ELBW extreme low birth weight, i.e., birth weight less than 1,000 g; *LBW* low birth weight, i.e., birth weight less than 1,500 g; *RR* relative risk; *CI* confidence intervals

(ELBW; BW <1,000 g), the maximum TSB concentrations were significantly higher in the conservative group (171 μmol/L vs. 139 μmol/L, conservative vs. prophylactic treatment) with a concomitant higher incidence of cerebral palsy. However, since the study was not originally powered for this outcome, it failed to demonstrate significant differences in long-term neurodevelopmental outcome. Another randomized controlled trial assigned 1974 ELBW preterm infants to a prophylactic phototherapy group (started immediately postnatal) or a conservative phototherapy group (based on predefined TSB thresholds: 137 μmol/L for infants weighing 501–750 g and 171 μmol/L for infants weighing 751–1,000 g) (Morris et al. 2008). The primary outcome of this study was a combination of neurodevelopmental impairment (defined as blindness, severe hearing loss, moderate or severe cerebral palsy, or a score below 70 on the mental or psychomotor developmental index of the Bayley Scales of Infant Development II) or death. In this study, maximum TSB concentrations were significantly higher in the conservative (168 μmol/L) versus the prophylactic group (120 μmol/L). Prophylactic phototherapy significantly did not affect the combined primary outcome but did reduce the risk of neurodevelopmental impairment (relative risk (95% confidence intervals): 0.86 (0.74–0.99)). This benefit of prophylactic phototherapy seems questionable for infants with a birth weight of 501–750 because in this group a nonsignificant trend toward increased mortality was found. A recent systematic review concludes that prophylactic phototherapy results in lower TSB concentrations, and possibly in fewer exchange transfusions, and decreases the risk of neurodevelopmental impairment. Yet, the efficacy and safety of prophylactic phototherapy on long-term neurodevelopmental outcomes is not established (Okwundu et al. 2012). It has been advocated that intravenous human serum albumin (HSA) should be considered as acute treatment for jaundiced infants with hypoalbuminemia, but this recommendation lacks firm evidence of RCTs. Theoretically, HSA could reduce the risk of bilirubin neurotoxicity by binding BF in the blood compartment, thereby preventing its translocation to the brain (Fig. 1). In agreement with this, two (retrospective) cohort studies show reduced BF concentrations in jaundiced neonates after adjunct HSA treatment (Caldera et al. 1993; Hosono et al. 2001). Moreover, recent animal data show that intravenous albumin administration provided a synergistic effect to phototherapy and prevented bilirubin accumulation in the brains of hyperbilirubinemic Gunn rats (Cuperus et al. 2013). Scant data are available on the effects of albumin on neurotoxicity: a small Japanese cohort study showed beneficial effects on bilirubin neurotoxicity, as measured by auditory brain stem responses

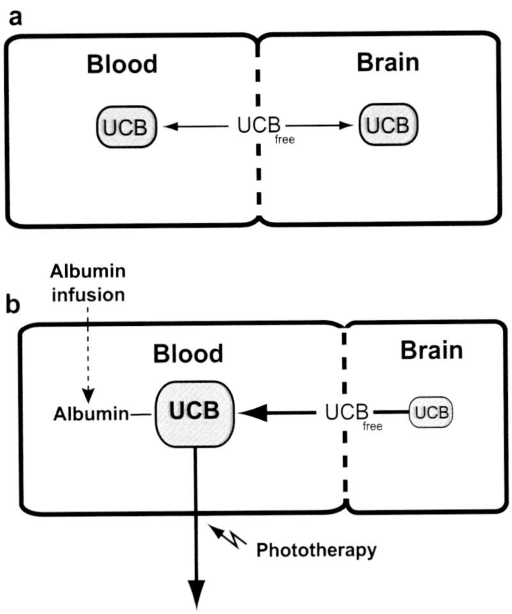

Fig. 1 Proposed mechanism of albumin infusion. (**a**) Unconjugated free bilirubin (UCB_{free}), but not unconjugated bilirubin (UCB) is able to cross the blood-brain barrier. (**b**) Albumin infusion could reduce the risk of bilirubin neurotoxicity by binding UCB_{free} in the blood compartment, thereby preventing its translocation to the brain. Simultaneously applied phototherapy will reduce UCB concentrations.

(Hosono et al. 2002). Despite the lack of firm evidence, albumin infusion is incorporated in management guidelines of jaundiced newborns, especially when exchange transfusion thresholds are reached.

75.8 New Treatments for Unconjugated Hyperbilirubinemia

Conventional treatment for severe unconjugated hyperbilirubinemia consists of phototherapy and exchange transfusion. Recently, the use of filtered sunlight for the purpose of phototherapy has been analyzed and was considered safe and noninferior to conventional phototherapy, which merits further research, especially in resource constraint settings (Slusher et al. 2015). Although conventional phototherapy is considered effective and safe, concerns exist about aggressive use in ELBW infants, and phototherapy does not always prevent toxic accumulation of bilirubin in neonates. Long-term phototherapy, as required by Crigler-Najjar patients, may take up to 16 h per day and becomes less effective with age. In spite of this intensive treatment regimen, approximately one-third of the patients with Crigler-Najjar disease type I develop mild to severe brain damage. In addition, patients still die resulting from complications related to the disease (Van Der Veere et al. 1996). Exchange transfusion should be considered if phototherapy fails to decrease plasma bilirubin below toxic levels. This "rescue treatment," however, is associated with a significant morbidity in sick newborns, and even mortality has been reported (Dennery et al. 2001). These considerations have prompted investigators to develop alternative treatments for unconjugated hyperbilirubinemia. Most of these treatments are still in an experimental phase. Nevertheless, it is highly conceivable that some of them will find their way into clinical practice in the foreseeable future.

75.8.1 Treatments that Decrease the Production of Bilirubin

Treatments that decrease the production of bilirubin could actually prevent unconjugated hyperbilirubinemia, which would be a more rational strategy compared with removing bilirubin that is already accumulated in the body. Bilirubin is produced in the macrophages of the reticuloendothelial system. These macrophages contain two essential enzymes: heme oxygenase (HO) and biliverdin reductase. Heme oxygenase converts heme, the source of bilirubin, into blue-green biliverdin. Biliverdin reductase then converts biliverdin into bilirubin. Consequently, bilirubin production can be decreased by agents that inhibit HO and/or biliverdin reductase (Fig. 1). Several agents have been developed to inhibit these enzymes such as the metalloporphyrins (Suresh et al. 2003; Cuperus et al. 2009a). Metalloporphyrins compete with heme for HO binding sites resulting in a competitive inhibition of HO and in a decreased conversion of heme into biliverdin. Currently,

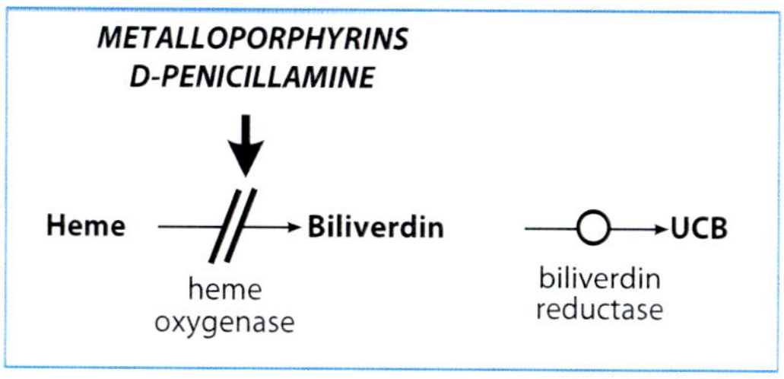

Fig. 2 Inhibitors of heme oxygenase effectively decrease the conversion of heme into biliverdin, the first essential step in bilirubin production (Reproduced from Cuperus et al. (2009a), with permission)

tin-mesoporphyrin is the most evaluated metalloporphyrin in humans. In clinical trials so far conducted, it was demonstrated that this agent mitigates unconjugated hyperbilirubinemia. Also, the use of tin-mesoporphyrin replaced the need for phototherapy in glucose-6-phosphate dehydrogenase-deficient newborns. Tin-mesoporphyrin thus seems a highly promising new treatment strategy for unconjugated hyperbilirubinemia. Currently, however, metalloporphyrins cannot be recommended for routine treatment of unconjugated hyperbilirubinemia due to insufficient evidence regarding the long-term safety of these agents (Schulz et al. 2012). D-penicillamine, a chelating agent that is used in the treatment of Wilson's disease, is another HO inhibitor (Fig. 2) (Cuperus et al. 2009a). The use of this agent decreased the number of exchange transfusions in infants with ABO hemolytic disease, but its efficacy has only been evaluated in a single clinical trial. Curiously, inhibitors of biliverdin reductase have never been explored, most likely because the accumulation of biliverdin in the blood would produce green babies.

75.8.2 Treatments that Increase the Hepatic Clearance of Bilirubin

Almost all bilirubin is excreted via the bile, and many therapies aim to enhance this excretory pathway by targeting the hepatic clearance of the bilirubin. In the hepatocyte, bilirubin is firstly bound to cytosolic ligandin, which prevents its diffusion back into the blood. The enzyme UDP-glucuronosyltransferase, which resides in the endoplasmatic reticulum of the hepatocytes, subsequently conjugates bilirubin with one or two glucuronic acid groups. This step increases the water solubility of the molecule and allows the now conjugated bilirubin to be excreted into the bile via the canalicular transporter MRP2. Several therapies target these three steps in bilirubin catabolism (Fig. 3). Clofibrate, a lipid-lowering drug, increases UGT1A1 activity (Fig. 3). This drug mitigated neonatal unconjugated hyperbilirubinemia in several clinical trials and decreased the need of phototherapy if applied as add-on treatment. Long-term clofibrate use, however, is associated with an overall increase in non-cardiovascular mortality. Although short-term clofibrate treatment has not been shown to have serious adverse effects, its safety issues must be addressed before it could be considered for clinical use. Various herbal extracts that are used in the treatment of neonatal jaundice throughout Asia, such as Yin Zhi Huang, also increase the hepatic clearance of UCB by inducing the expression of ligandin, UGT1A1, and MRP2 (Cuperus et al. 2009a). Clinical use of traditional herbal medicine during neonatal jaundice is not recommended, however, due to the danger of contamination, potential side effects, and reduced reproducibility associated with the use of an herbal mixture, rather than treatment with a well-described individual molecule. The most well-known agent that enhances hepatic bilirubin clearance, however, is phenobarbital. This antiepileptic agent enhances ligandin, UGT1A1, and MRP2 activity (Fig. 3). Since the 1960s, phenobarbital has been used extensively in the treatment of neonatal jaundice. Numerous clinical trials have shown that administering phenobarbital to pregnant women or to newborns mitigates neonatal hyperbilirubinemia and decreases the number of exchange transfusions. Nevertheless, phenobarbital is currently not used as routine treatment of neonatal jaundice. This is mainly because phototherapy is more effective, because decline of TSB concentrations in infants treated with

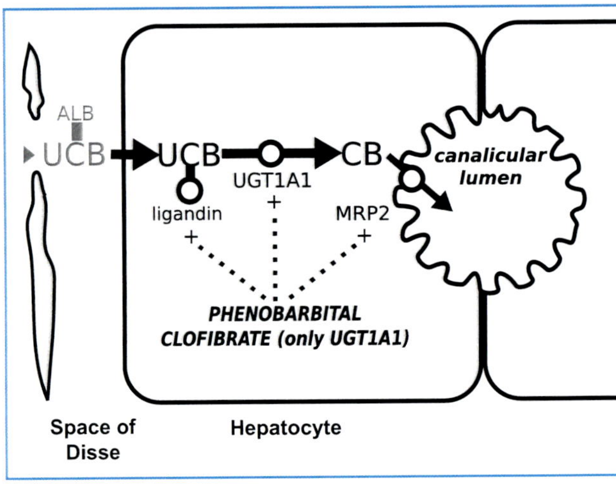

Fig. 3 Phenobarbital and clofibrate increase the hepatic clearance of bilirubin. *Alb* albumin, *UCB* unconjugated bilirubin, *UGT1A1* UDP-glucuronosyltransferase1A1 (Reproduced from Cuperus et al. (2009a), with permission)

phenobarbital and phototherapy is not faster when compared to phototherapy alone, and because its therapeutic effect is not evident until a few days after administration, in contrast to some of the adverse effects (i.e., sedation) (Cuperus et al. 2009a). Phenobarbital is still applied in Crigler-Najjar type II patients, who have a 95% decrease in UDP-glucuronosyltransferase activity. In these patients, phenobarbital is able to increase the residual enzyme activity, which effectively counteracts the development of severe unconjugated hyperbilirubinemia. Phenobarbital is not effective in the treatment of Crigler-Najjar type I, however, because these patients lack residual (e.g., inducible) UDP-glucuronosyltransferase activity. The most effective treatment for Crigler-Najjar disease type I would be repair or replace the defective UGT1A1 in the liver. Currently, this can only be achieved by a liver transplantation. In 1986 the first successful orthotopic liver transplantation (OLT) in a Crigler-Najjar patient was reported, and several other patients have undergone transplantation since. Two types of transplantation have been used: OLT in which the patients' own liver is replaced by a donor liver and auxiliary liver transplantation in which part of the own liver is left in situ and is supported by a donor graft. If successful, a liver transplant completely corrects the underlying metabolic defect, which dramatically improves the quality of life. Liver transplantation, however, remains a high-risk procedure, with a 1-year survival between 85% and 90%. Infusion of hepatocytes with an unimpaired UGT1A1 activity into the liver of Crigler-Najjar patients would be an attractive alternative to a liver transplant. This procedure, which is known as hepatocyte transplantation, could partially restore enzyme activity without the many complications that are associated with a liver transplant. So far, eight Crigler-Najjar type I patients received this treatment, often with multiple infusions of hepatocytes (e.g., via the portal vein). Hepatocyte infusion, however, decreased plasma bilirubin levels only for a limited period of 5–6 months and did not eliminate the need for a liver transplant in these patients (Forbes et al. 2015). Ultimately, gene therapy would be the most elegant method to repair or replace defective UGT1A1 within the hepatocytes of Crigler-Najjar type I patients. The results of gene therapy seem promising in animal models (van Dijk et al. 2015). Currently, however, the results of clinical trials must be awaited before gene therapy can be applied in Crigler-Najjar patients.

75.8.3 Treatments that Decrease the Enterohepatic Circulation of Bilirubin

After conjugation bilirubin enters the intestinal lumen via the bile. The intestinal conjugated

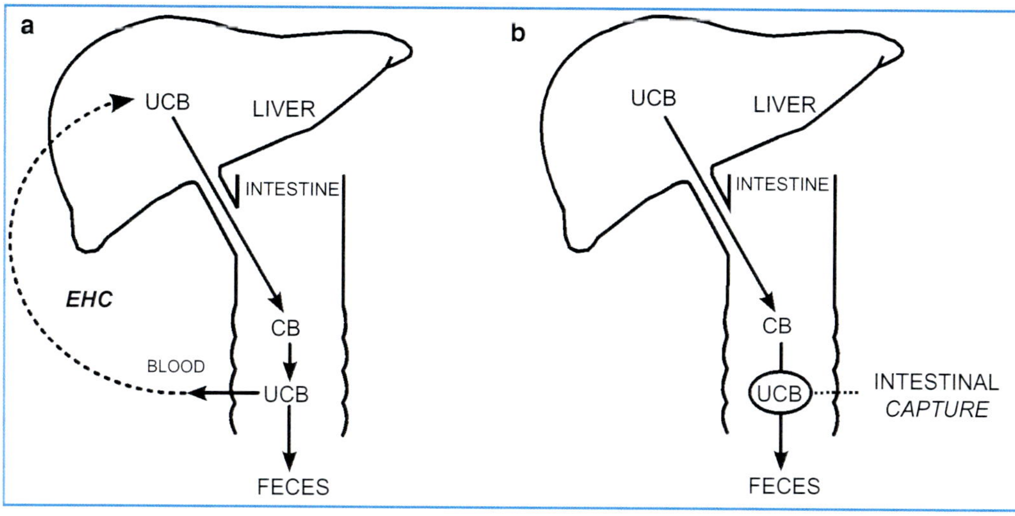

Fig. 4 (**a**) Normally, and especially in conditions that delay the intestinal transit, there is an enterohepatic circulation of unconjugated bilirubin which increases plasma bilirubin levels. (**b**) Binding unconjugated bilirubin to capture agents in the intestinal lumen may prevent this enterohepatic circulation and thus decrease plasma bilirubin levels. *UCB* unconjugated bilirubin *CB* conjugated bilirubin, *EHC* enterohepatic circulation (Reproduced from Cuperus et al. (2009a), with permission)

bilirubin is mostly hydrolyzed to UCB which can be reabsorbed into the enterohepatic circulation (Fig. 4a). The majority of this reabsorbed UCB, however, spills over into the systemic circulation due to the poor first pass extraction by the liver. Conditions that enhance this enterohepatic circulation contribute to the pathogenesis of unconjugated hyperbilirubinemia. For example, poor feeding in neonates is associated with increased plasma bilirubin levels most likely caused by a delayed gastrointestinal transit, which increases the amount of intestinal UCB available for reabsorption. Indeed, conditions that accelerate the gastrointestinal transit, such as early and frequent feedings, seem to lower plasma bilirubin levels in newborn infants (Wennberg et al. 1966). In line with this observation are data on enteral administration of the laxative polyethylene glycol (PEG) in hyperbilirubinemic Gunn rats (Cuperus et al. 2010). PEG administration accelerated gastrointestinal transit by almost 50% and concomitantly decreased UCB concentrations by ~25% after 36 h. This effect was more pronounced after 2 weeks (UCB −40%) and even more if combined with phototherapy (UCB −60%). Fecal UCB disposal in Gunn rats can also be increased by enteral bile salt administration, which results in lower UCB concentrations (Cuperus et al. 2009b). Bilirubin reabsorption could also be prevented by agents that bind and capture the pigment within the intestinal lumen (Fig. 4b). Several capturing strategies have so far been tested. Cholestyramine, a known binder of bile salts, and agar, a gelatinous substance derived from seaweed, decreased plasma bilirubin levels in hyperbilirubinemic rats but were less effective in neonates. Treatment of neonates with activated charcoal effectively decreased plasma bilirubin levels but only if it was administered within the first day of life. Charcoal, however, might also capture essential nutrients, which limits its clinical applicability. Oral amorphous calcium phosphate did lower plasma bilirubin levels, but only in Crigler-Najjar type I patients. Calcium phosphate is currently used in a number of Dutch Crigler-Najjar type I patients as an adjunct to phototherapy if plasma unconjugated bilirubin levels become dangerously elevated. Orlistat, a lipase inhibitor, increases the intestinal fat

content, which is hypothesized to capture the lipophilic unconjugated bilirubin. Orlistat has been shown to lower plasma bilirubin levels in a trial with Crigler-Najjar patients, but the decrease was considered clinically relevant (i.e., >10%) only in 7 of 16 patients. Zinc salts are also well-known binders of unconjugated bilirubin and moderately decreased plasma bilirubin levels in patients with Gilbert's syndrome (Cuperus et al. 2009a). This inherited condition is characterized by a chronic, mild unconjugated hyperbilirubinemia related to diminished hepatic UGT1A1 expression. Administration of zinc salts, however, may lead to increased zinc levels in plasma, which may limit their clinical use. In addition, a recent meta-analysis failed to demonstrate that oral zinc supplementation given to infants up to 1 week old reduces the incidence of hyperbilirubinemia or need for phototherapy (Mishra et al. 2015). Recently, effects on neonatal jaundice of oral probiotics in a rather small number of term infants have been analyzed. Preliminary data of small case-control studies suggest a bilirubin-lowering effect of specific prebiotic strains via unrevealed mechanisms, in which reduced activity of intestinal bacterial β-glucuronidase seems possible (Liu et al. 2015). Possible and documented side effects, unknown long-term effects, and inconsistent results of these aforementioned agents limit their widespread application in patients suffering severe hyperbilirubinemia and imminent BIND.

75.9 Future Prospective

The molecular events leading to BIND are still partially unsettled as the criteria are not fully defined to describe BIND when the damage may be successfully treatable. It is therefore needed to approach this increasingly present damage in a more translational way linking in vitro with in vivo models. This will hopefully provide hints on an effective prevention of the neurological damage in addition to a highly effective treatment, i.e., phototherapy. To this end, we need to understand better how unconjugated, free bilirubin may enter the cell and how the cells are handling this potentially toxic substance. We know that MRP1 may extrude UCB from cells, but data obtained in vitro suggest that the activity of this ABC transporter is not the only player in reducing UCB cytotoxicity. Intracellular oxidation of UCB may be an additional mechanism which needs to be assessed as pharmacological inducers of oxidizing pathways are available. Also still unknown is why UCB accumulates and damages specific regions of the brain. Understanding this still unexplained uneven distribution will unravel the background for regional sensitivity. Collectively these data will hopefully allow to define more effective treatment not only for the newborns but also for the patients with Crigler-Najjar type I.

References

Ahlfors CE, Parker AE (2005) Evaluation of a model for brain bilirubin uptake in jaundiced newborns. Pediatr Res 58(6):1175–1179

Ahlfors CE, Shapiro SM (2001) Auditory brainstem response and unbound bilirubin in jaundiced (jj) Gunn rat pups. Biol Neonate 80(2):158–162

Ahlfors CE, Wennberg RP (2004) Bilirubin-albumin binding and neonatal jaundice. Semin Perinatol 28(5):334–339

Ahlfors CE, Amin SB, Parker AE (2009) Unbound bilirubin predicts abnormal automated auditory brainstem response in a diverse newborn population. J Perinatol 29(4):305–309

American Academy of Pediatrics Subcommittee on Hyperbilirubinemia (2004) Management of hyperbilirubinemia in the newborn infant 35 or more weeks of gestation. Pediatrics 114(1098–4275; 1):297–316

Amin SB, Orlando MS, Dalzell LE, Merle KS, Guillet R (1999) Morphological changes in serial auditory brain stem responses in 24 to 32 weeks' gestational age infants during the first week of life. Ear Hear 20(5): 410–418

Amin SB, Ahlfors C, Orlando MS, Dalzell LE, Merle KS, Guillet R (2001) Bilirubin and serial auditory brainstem responses in premature infants. Pediatrics 107(4):664–670

Bhutani VK, Zipursky A, Blencowe H, Khanna R, Sgro M, Ebbesen F et al (2013) Neonatal hyperbilirubinemia and Rhesus disease of the newborn: incidence and impairment estimates for 2010 at regional and global levels. Pediatr Res 74(Suppl 1):86–100

Caldera R, Maynier M, Sender A, Brossard Y, Tortrat D, Galiay JC et al (1993) The effect of human albumin in association with intensive phototherapy in the

management of neonatal jaundice. Arch Fr Pediatr 50(5):399–402

Calligaris SD, Bellarosa C, Giraudi P, Wennberg RP, Ostrow JD, Tiribelli C (2007) Cytotoxicity is predicted by unbound and not total bilirubin concentration. Pediatr Res 62(5):576–580

Coda Zabetta CD, Iskander IF, Greco C, Bellarosa C, Demarini S, Tiribelli C et al (2013) Bilistick: a low-cost point-of-care system to measure total plasma bilirubin. Neonatology 103(3):177–181

Cuperus FJ, Hafkamp AM, Hulzebos CV, Verkade HJ (2009a) Pharmacological therapies for unconjugated hyperbilirubinemia. Curr Pharm Des 15(25):2927–2938

Cuperus FJ, Hafkamp AM, Havinga R, Vitek L, Zelenka J, Tiribelli C et al (2009b) Effective treatment of unconjugated hyperbilirubinemia with oral bile salts in Gunn rats. Gastroenterology 136(2):673–82.e1

Cuperus FJ, Iemhoff AA, van der Wulp M, Havinga R, Verkade HJ (2010) Acceleration of the gastrointestinal transit by polyethylene glycol effectively treats unconjugated hyperbilirubinaemia in Gunn rats. Gut 59(3):373–380

Cuperus FJ, Schreuder AB, van Imhoff DE, Vitek L, Vanikova J, Konickova R et al (2013) Beyond plasma bilirubin: the effects of phototherapy and albumin on brain bilirubin levels in Gunn rats. J Hepatol 58(1):134–140

Dennery PA, Seidman DS, Stevenson DK (2001) Neonatal hyperbilirubinemia. N Engl J Med 344(8):581–590

D'Silva S, Colah RB, Ghosh K, Mukherjee MB (2014) Combined effects of the UGT1A1 and OATP2 gene polymorphisms as major risk factor for unconjugated hyperbilirubinemia in Indian neonates. Gene 547(1):18–22

Forbes SJ, Gupta S, Dhawan A (2015) Cell therapy for liver disease: from liver transplantation to cell factory. J Hepatol 62(1 Suppl):S157–S169

Good WV, Hou C (2015) Visuocortical bilirubin-induced neurological dysfunction. Semin Fetal Neonatal Med 20(1):37–41

Gotink MJ, Benders MJ, Lavrijsen SW, Rodrigues Pereira R, Hulzebos CV, Dijk PH (2013) Severe neonatal hyperbilirubinemia in the Netherlands. Neonatology 104(2):137–142

Govaert P, Lequin M, Swarte R, Robben S, De Coo R, Weisglas-Kuperus N et al (2003) Changes in globus pallidus with (pre)term kernicterus. Pediatrics 112(6):1256–1263, 1098–4275

Groenendaal F, van der Grond J, de Vries LS (2004) Cerebral metabolism in severe neonatal hyperbilirubinemia. Pediatrics 114(1):291–294

Hansen TW (2000) Pioneers in the scientific study of neonatal jaundice and kernicterus. Pediatrics 106(2):E15

Hosono S, Ohno T, Kimoto H, Nagoshi R, Shimizu M, Nozawa M (2001) Effects of albumin infusion therapy on total and unbound bilirubin values in term infants with intensive phototherapy. Pediatr Int 43(1):8–11

Hosono S, Ohno T, Kimoto H, Nagoshi R, Shimizu M, Nozawa M et al (2002) Follow-up study of auditory brainstem responses in infants with high unbound bilirubin levels treated with albumin infusion therapy. Pediatr Int 44(5):488–492

Hulzebos CV, van Imhoff DE, Bos AF, Ahlfors CE, Verkade HJ, Dijk PH (2008) Usefulness of the bilirubin/albumin ratio for predicting bilirubin-induced neurotoxicity in premature infants. Arch Dis Child Fetal Neonatal Ed 93(5):F384–F388

Hulzebos CV, Dijk PH, van Imhoff DE, Bos AF, Lopriore E, Offringa M et al (2014) The bilirubin albumin ratio in the management of hyperbilirubinemia in preterm infants to improve neurodevelopmental outcome: a randomized controlled trial – BARTrial. PLoS One 9(6):e99466

Ip S, Chung M, Kulig J, O'Brien R, Sege R, Glicken S et al (2004) An evidence-based review of important issues concerning neonatal hyperbilirubinemia. Pediatrics 114(1):e130–e153

Iskander I, Gamaleldin R, El Houchi S, El Shenawy A, Seoud I, El Gharbawi N et al (2014) Serum bilirubin and bilirubin/albumin ratio as predictors of bilirubin encephalopathy. Pediatrics 134(5):e1330–e1339

Jangaard KA, Vincer MJ, Allen AC (2007) A randomized trial of aggressive versus conservative phototherapy for hyperbilirubinemia in infants weighing less than 1500 g: short- and long-term outcomes. Paediatr Child Health 12(10):853–858

Johnson L, Brown AK, Bhutani VK (1999) BIND – A clinical score for bilirubin-induced neurological dysfunction in newborns. Pediatrics 104:746

Kaplan M, Bromiker R, Hammerman C (2014) Hyperbilirubinemia, hemolysis, and increased bilirubin neurotoxicity. Semin Perinatol 38(7):429–437

Kim MH, Yoon JJ, Sher J, Brown AK (1980) Lack of predictive indices in kernicterus: a comparison of clinical and pathologic factors in infants with or without kernicterus. Pediatrics 66(6):852–858

Liu W, Liu H, Wang T, Tang X (2015) Therapeutic effects of probiotics on neonatal jaundice. Pak J Med Sci 31(5):1172–1175

Lucey JF (1972) Neonatal jaundice and phototherapy. Pediatr Clin North Am 19(4):827–839

Lunsing RJ (2014) Subtle bilirubin-induced neurodevelopmental dysfunction (BIND) in the term and late preterm infant: does it exist? Semin Perinatol 38(7):465–471

Maisels MJ, Watchko JF (2003) Treatment of jaundice in low birthweight infants. Arch Dis Child Fetal Neonatal Ed 88(6):F459–F463

Maisels MJ, Watchko JF, Bhutani VK, Stevenson DK (2012) An approach to the management of hyperbilirubinemia in the preterm infant less than 35 weeks of gestation. J Perinatol 32:660–664

Manning D, Todd P, Maxwell M, Platt MJ (2007) Prospective surveillance study of severe hyperbilirubinaemia in

the newborn in the UK and Ireland. Arch Dis Child Fetal Neonatal Ed 92(5):F342–F346

Mishra S, Cheema A, Agarwal R, Deorari A, Paul V (2015) Oral zinc for the prevention of hyperbilirubinaemia in neonates. Cochrane Database Syst Rev 7:CD008432

Morris BH, Oh W, Tyson JE, Stevenson DK, Phelps DL, O'Shea TM et al (2008) Aggressive vs. conservative phototherapy for infants with extremely low birth weight. N Engl J Med 359(18):1885–1896

National Institute for Health and Clinical Excellence (2010) Available at: http://www.nice.org.uk/CG98

Newman TB, Klebanoff MA (1993) Neonatal hyperbilirubinemia and long-term outcome: another look at the Collaborative Perinatal Project. Pediatrics 92(5):651–657

Norman M, Aberg K, Holmsten K, Weibel V, Ekeus C (2015) Predicting nonhemolytic neonatal hyperbilirubinemia. Pediatrics 136(6):1087–1094

Oh W, Tyson JE, Fanaroff AA, Vohr BR, Perritt R, Stoll BJ et al (2003) Association between peak serum bilirubin and neurodevelopmental outcomes in extremely low birth weight infants. Pediatrics 112(4):773–779

Okumus N, Turkyilmaz C, Onal EE, Atalay Y, Serdaroglu A, Elbeg S et al (2008) Tau and S100B proteins as biochemical markers of bilirubin-induced neurotoxicity in term neonates. Pediatr Neurol 39(4):245–252

Okwundu CI, Okoromah CA, Shah PS (2012) Prophylactic phototherapy for preventing jaundice in preterm or low birth weight infants. Cochrane Database Syst Rev 1: CD007966

Olusanya BO, Ogunlesi TA, Slusher TM (2014) Why is kernicterus still a major cause of death and disability in low-income and middle-income countries? Arch Dis Child 99(12):1117–1121

Olusanya BO, Osibanjo FB, Slusher TM (2015) Risk factors for severe neonatal hyperbilirubinemia in low and middle-income countries: a systematic review and meta-analysis. PLoS One 10(2):e0117229

Ostrow JD, Pascolo L, Shapiro SM, Tiribelli C (2003a) New concepts in bilirubin encephalopathy. Eur J Clin Invest 11(11):988–997, 0014-2972

Ostrow JD, Pascolo L, Tiribelli C (2003b) Reassessment of the unbound concentrations of unconjugated bilirubin in relation to neurotoxicity in vitro. Pediatr Res 54 (1):98–104, 0031-3998

Ostrow JD, Pascolo L, Brites D, Tiribelli C (2004) Molecular basis of bilirubin-induced neurotoxicity. Trends Mol Med 10(2):65–70, 1471–4914

Pearlman MA, Gartner LM, Lee K, Eidelman AI, Morecki R, Horoupian DS (1980) The association of kernicterus with bacterial infection in the newborn. Pediatrics 65(1):26–29

Radmacher PG, Groves FD, Owa JA, Ofovwe GE, Amuabunos EA, Olusanya BO et al (2015) A modified Bilirubin-induced neurologic dysfunction (BIND-M) algorithm is useful in evaluating severity of jaundice in a resource-limited setting. BMC Pediatr 15, 015-0355-2

Ritter DA, Kenny JD, Norton HJ, Rudolph AJ (1982) A prospective study of free bilirubin and other risk factors in the development of kernicterus in premature infants. Pediatrics 69(3):260–266

Scheidt PC, Graubard BI, Nelson KB, Hirtz DG, Hoffman HJ, Gartner LM et al (1991) Intelligence at six years in relation to neonatal bilirubin levels: follow-up of the National Institute of Child Health and Human Development Clinical Trial of Phototherapy. Pediatrics 87(6):797–805

Schulz S, Wong RJ, Vreman HJ, Stevenson DK (2012) Metalloporphyrins – an update. Front Pharmacol 3:68

Shapiro SM (2003) Bilirubin toxicity in the developing nervous system. Pediatr Neurol 29(5):410–421, 0887-8994

Shapiro SM (2005) Definition of the clinical spectrum of kernicterus and bilirubin-induced neurologic dysfunction (BIND). J Perinatol 25(1):54–59, 0743-8346

Shapiro SM (2010) Chronic bilirubin encephalopathy: diagnosis and outcome. Semin Fetal Neonatal Med 15(3):157–163

Shapiro SM, Nakamura H (2001) Bilirubin and the auditory system. J Perinatol 21(Suppl 1):S52–S55, discussion S59–62

Slusher TM, Owa JA, Painter MJ, Shapiro SM (2011) The kernicteric facies: facial features of acute bilirubin encephalopathy. Pediatr Neurol 44(2): 153–154

Slusher TM, Olusanya BO, Vreman HJ, Brearley AM, Vaucher YE, Lund TC et al (2015) A randomized trial of phototherapy with filtered sunlight in African neonates. N Engl J Med 373(12):1115–1124

Soorani-Lunsing I, Woltil HA, Hadders-Algra M (2001) Are moderate degrees of hyperbilirubinemia in healthy term neonates really safe for the brain? Pediatr Res 12;50(6):701–705

Suresh GK, Martin CL, Soll RF (2003) Metalloporphyrins for treatment of unconjugated hyperbilirubinemia in neonates. Cochrane Database Syst Rev 2:1469–493 CD004207

Turkel SB (1990) Autopsy findings associated with neonatal hyperbilirubinemia. Clin Perinatol 17(2): 381–396

Van Der Veere CN, Sinaasappel M, McDonagh AF, Rosenthal P, Labrune P, Odievre M et al (1996) Current therapy for Crigler-Najjar syndrome type 1: report of a world registry. Hepatology 24(2):311–315, 0270-9139

van Dijk R, Beuers U, Bosma PJ (2015) Gene replacement therapy for genetic hepatocellular jaundice. Clin Rev Allergy Immunol 48(2 –3):243–253

van Imhoff DE, Dijk PH, Hulzebos CV, BARTrial study group, Netherlands Neonatal Research Network (2011) Uniform treatment thresholds for hyperbilirubinemia in preterm infants: background and synopsis of a national guideline. Early Hum Dev 87(8):521–525

Volpe JJ (2009) Bilirubin and brain damage. Neurology of the newborn, 5th edn. Saunders Elsevier, Philadelphia, pp 619–651

Wallenstein MB, Bhutani VK (2013) Jaundice and kernicterus in the moderately preterm infant. Clin Perinatol 40(4):679–688

Watchko JF, Maisels MJ (2003) Jaundice in low birthweight infants: pathobiology and outcome. Arch Dis Child Fetal Neonatal Ed 88(6):F455–F458

Watchko JF, Maisels MJ (2014) The enigma of low bilirubin kernicterus in premature infants: why does it still occur, and is it preventable? Semin Perinatol 38(7):397–406

Watchko JF, Tiribelli C (2013) Bilirubin-induced neurologic damage – mechanisms and management approaches. N Engl J Med 369(21):2021–2030

Wennberg RP, Schwartz R, Sweet AY (1966) Early versus delayed feeding of low birth weight infants: effects on physiologic jaundice. J Pediatr 68(6):860–866

Wennberg RP, Ahlfors CE, Bhutani VK, Johnson LH, Shapiro SM (2006) Toward understanding kernicterus: a challenge to improve the management of jaundiced newborns. Pediatrics 117(2):474–485

Wong RJ, Stevenson DK (2015) Neonatal hemolysis and risk of bilirubin-induced neurologic dysfunction. Semin Fetal Neonatal Med 20(1):26–30

Treatment of Hyperbilirubinemia in Newborns

76

Jon F. Watchko and M. Jeffrey Maisels

Contents

J. F. Watchko (✉)
Division of Newborn Medicine, Department of Pediatrics, University of Pittsburgh School of Medicine, Pittsburgh, PA, USA
e-mail: watcjf@mail.magee.edu

M. J. Maisels
Department of Pediatrics, Oakland University William Beaumont School of Medicine, Beaumont Children's Hospital, Royal Oak, MI, USA

G. Buonocore et al. (eds.), *Neonatology*,
https://doi.org/10.1007/978-3-319-29489-6_223

Abstract

The main aim of treating hyperbilirubinemia is to prevent kernicterus and/or neurodevelopmental impairment. Recommendations for treatment are based primarily on the total serum bilirubin (TSB) levels but also as a function of gestational age, birth weight, bilirubin/albumin ratios, and risk factors that increase the risk of bilirubin neurotoxicity. Setting thresholds for intervention in the premature neonate is more challenging than in term babies. Phototherapy is effective in lowering the circulating bilirubin or preventing it from rising further; its primary purpose is to prevent the need for an exchange transfusion. Phototherapy uses visible light energy to change the shape and structure of bilirubin, converting it to molecules that can be excreted even when normal conjugation is deficient. Exchange transfusion remains an important if infrequently required intervention. It is recommended in any infant who is jaundiced and manifests signs of intermediate to advanced stages of acute bilirubin encephalopathy even if the TSB is falling. Pharmacologic agents used in the management of hyperbilirubinemia can accelerate the normal metabolic pathways for bilirubin clearance, inhibit the enterohepatic circulation of bilirubin, and interfere with bilirubin formation by blocking the degradation of heme or inhibiting hemolysis. Currently, the only drug in clinical use is intravenous immunoglobulin.

76.1 Salient Points

- Phototherapy and exchange transfusion treatment guidelines are based primarily on the TSB but importantly modulated by maturity and other factors that increase the risk of bilirubin neurotoxicity.
- Phototherapy effectiveness is dependent on the irradiance delivered by the light source and the surface area of the infant exposed to the light. The irradiance is determined by the wavelength spectrum of the light and the distance between the neonate and the light source.
- Aggressive phototherapy may increase mortality risk in extremely low birth weight (ELBW) infants.
- A double volume exchange transfusion (DVET) is indicated in infants with signs of intermediate to advanced acute bilirubin encephalopathy (ABE) (hypertonia, arching, retrocolis, opisthotonos, fever, high-pitched cry) even if the TSB is falling.
- The efficacy of a DVET is determined by the mass of albumin exchanged; therefore the target hematocrit of the blood for DVET should be 35–40%.
- Low bilirubin kernicterus is a rare but refractory cause of bilirubin-induced neurotoxicity in preterm neonates. Although low bilirubin kernicterus is multifactorial in pathogenesis, marked hypoalbuminemia is often a prominent clinical feature.

76.2 Introduction

The indications for the treatment of hyperbilirubinemia and the methods used for treatment vary according to the individual circumstances. Thus, treatment of hyperbilirubinemia can be prophylactic, when the purpose is to prevent further increase in the total serum bilirubin (TSB) level, or therapeutic, where the objective is to rapidly decrease a TSB level that is a threat to the infant. The TSB

level can be lowered (or prevented from increasing further) in one of three ways: (a) phototherapy, which converts bilirubin to products that can bypass the liver's conjugating system and be excreted in the bile or the urine without further metabolism, (b) exchange transfusion, which removes bilirubin mechanically, and (c) pharmacologic agents that interfere with heme degradation and bilirubin production, accelerate the normal metabolic pathways for bilirubin clearance, or inhibit the enterohepatic circulation of bilirubin.

76.3 Using Phototherapy and Exchange Transfusion to Prevent Kernicterus and/or Neurodevelopmental Impairment

A selection of recommendations and guidelines for the use of phototherapy and exchange transfusion in term, late preterm, and preterm infants are provided in Figs. 1 and 2 and Tables 1 and 2 (American Academy of Pediatrics, Subcommittee

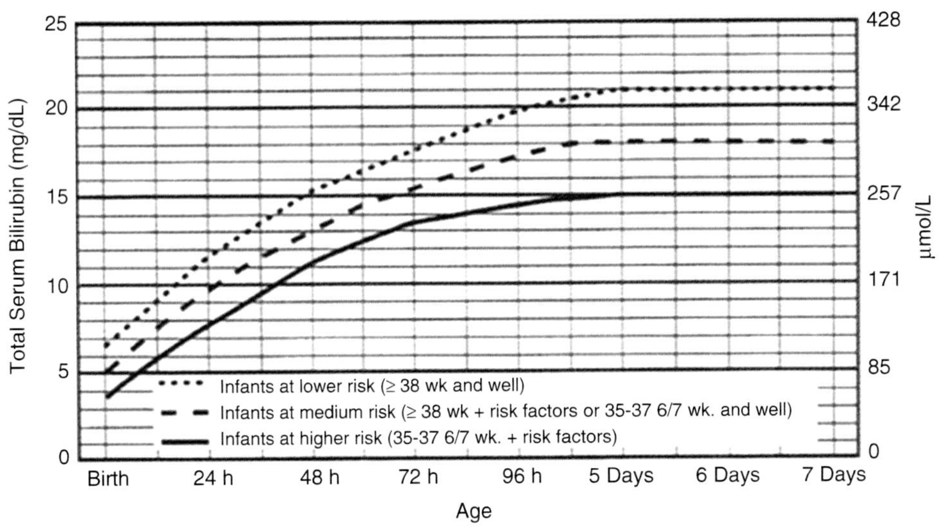

Fig. 1 Guidelines for phototherapy in hospitalized infants of 35 or more weeks' gestation

Use total bilirubin. Do not subtract direct reading or conjugated bilirubin

The lines for lower, medium, and higher risk refer to risk for neurotoxicity

Risk factors for neurotoxicity – isoimmune hemolytic disease, G6PD deficiency, asphyxia, significant lethargy, temperature instability, sepsis, acidosis, or albumin < 3.0 g/dL (if measured)

For well infants 35–37 6/7 weeks can adjust TSB levels for intervention around the medium risk line. It is an option to intervene at lower TSB levels for infants closer to 35 weeks and at higher TSB levels for those closer to 37 6/7 weeks

It is an option to provide conventional phototherapy in hospital or at home at TSB levels 2–3 mg/dL (35–50 mmol/L) below those shown, but home phototherapy should not be used in any infant with risk factors

These guidelines refer to the use of intensive phototherapy, which should be used when the TSB exceeds the line indicated for each category. Infants are designated as "higher risk" because of the potential negative effects of the conditions listed on albumin binding of bilirubin (Cashore 1980; Cashore et al. 1983a; Ebbesen and Brodersen 1982a), the blood–brain barrier (American Association of Blood Banks Technical Manual Committee 2002), and the susceptibility of the brain cells to damage by bilirubin (American Association of Blood Banks Technical Manual Committee 2002)

Intensive phototherapy implies irradiance in the blue-green spectrum (wavelengths of ~430–490 nm) of at least 30 μW/cm ^{2} per nm (measured at the infant's skin directly below the center of the phototherapy unit) and delivered to as much of the infant's surface area as possible. Note that irradiance measured below the light source center is much greater than that measured at the periphery. Measurements should be made with a spectroradiometer specified by the manufacturer of the phototherapy system

If the total serum bilirubin does not decrease or continues to rise in an infant who is receiving intensive phototherapy, this strongly suggests the presence of hemolysis (From American Academy of Pediatrics, Subcommittee on Hyperbilirubinemia (2004) with permission)

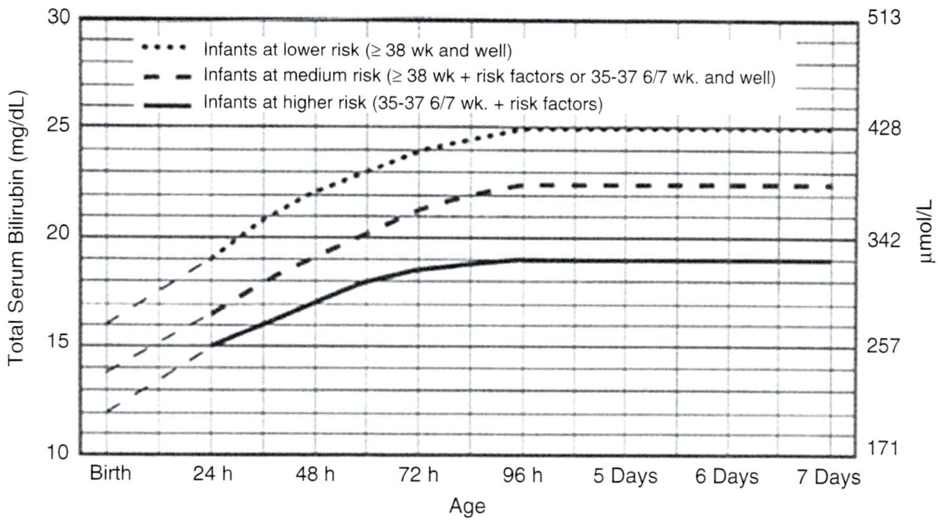

Fig. 2 **Guidelines for exchange transfusion in infants 35 or more weeks' gestation**

Immediate exchange transfusion is recommended if infant shows signs of acute bilirubin encephalopathy (hypertonia, arching, retrocollis, opisthotonos, fever, high-pitched cry) or if TSB is ≥ 5 mg/dL (85 µmol/L) above these lines

The lines for lower, medium, and higher risk refer to risk for neurotoxicity

Risk factors for neurotoxicity – isoimmune hemolytic disease, G6PD deficiency, asphyxia, significant lethargy, temperature instability, sepsis, or acidosis

Measure serum albumin and calculate bilirubin/albumin (B/A) ratio (see legend below)

Use total bilirubin. Do not subtract direct reacting or conjugated bilirubin

During birth hospitalization, exchange transfusion is recommended if the TSB rises to these levels despite intensive phototherapy. For readmitted infants, if the TSB level is above the exchange level, repeat TSB measurement every 2–3 h and consider exchange if the TSB remains above the levels indicated after intensive phototherapy for 6 h

The following B/A ratios can be used together with but not in lieu of the TSB level as an additional factor in determining the need for exchange transfusion

Risk Category	Ratio of bilirubin to albumin (B/A) **B/A ratio at which exchange transfusion should be considered**	
	TSB mg/dL/Alb, g/dL	**TSB µmol/L/Alb, µmol/L**
Infants ≥ 38 0/7 wk	8.0	0.94
Infants 35 0/7–36 6/7 wk and well or ≥ 38 0/7 wk if higher risk or isoimmune hemolytic disease or G6PD deficiency	7.2	0.84
Infants 35 0/7–37 6/7 wk if higher risk or isoimmune hemolytic disease or G6PD deficiency	6.8	0.80

If the TSB is at or approaching the exchange level, send blood for immediate type and crossmatch. Blood for exchange transfusion is modified whole blood (red cells and plasma) cross-matched against the mother and compatible with the infant (American Association of Blood Banks Technical Manual Committee 2002) (From American Academy of Pediatrics, Subcommittee on Hyperbilirubinemia (2004) with permission)

on Hyperbilirubinemia 2004; Maisels et al. 2012; Hulzebos et al. 2014). Several additional guidelines have been published for the treatment of the jaundiced newborn (National Institute for Health and Clinical Excellence 2010; Bratlid et al. 2011). These recommendations are based primarily on the TSB levels but also as a function of gestational age, birth weight, bilirubin/albumin ratios, and risk factors that increase the risk of bilirubin neurotoxicity (American Academy of Pediatrics,

Table 1 Suggested use of phototherapy and exchange transfusion in preterm infants <35 weeks gestational age (From Maisels et al. (2012) with permission (footnotes modified))

Phototherapy		Exchange transfusion
Gestational age (wk)	Initiate phototherapy total serum bilirubin (mg/dL)	Total serum bilirubin (mg/dL)
<28 0/7	5–6	11–14
28 0/7 – 29 6/7	6–8	12–14
30 0/7 – 31 6/7	8–10	13–16
32 0/7 – 33 6/7	10–12	15–18
34 0/7 – 34 6/7	12–14	17–19

This table reflects the authors' recommendations for operational or therapeutic TSB thresholds – bilirubin levels at, or above which, treatment is likely to do more good than harm. These TSB levels are not based on good evidence and are lower than those suggested in recent UK (National Institute for Health and Clinical Excellence 2010) and Norwegian (Bratlid et al. 2011) guidelines

The wider ranges and overlapping of values in the exchange transfusion column reflect the degree of uncertainty in making these recommendations

Use the lower range of the listed TSB levels for infants at greater risk for bilirubin toxicity, e.g., (1) lower gestational age, (2) serum albumin levels < 2.5 g/dL, (3) rapidly rising TSB levels, suggesting hemolytic disease, and (4) those who are clinically unstable. When a decision is being made about the initiation of phototherapy or exchange transfusion, infants are considered to be clinically unstable if they have one or more of the following conditions: (a) blood pH < 7.15; (b) blood culture positive sepsis in the prior 24 h; (c) apnea and bradycardia requiring cardio-respiratory resuscitation (bagging and or intubation) during the previous 24 h; (d) hypotension requiring pressor treatment during the previous 24 h; and (e) mechanical ventilation at the time of blood sampling (Oh et al. 2010)

Recommendations for exchange transfusion apply to infants who are receiving intensive phototherapy to the maximal surface area but whose TSB levels continue to increase to the levels listed

For all infants, an exchange transfusion is recommended if the infant shows signs of acute bilirubin encephalopathy (hypertonia, arching, retrocollis, opisthotonos, high-pitched cry) although it is recognized that these signs rarely occur in VLBW infants

Use total bilirubin. Do not subtract direct reacting or conjugated bilirubin from the total

For infants ≤ 26 weeks gestation, it is an option to use phototherapy prophylactically starting soon after birth

Use postmenstrual age for phototherapy, e.g., when a 29 0/7 week infant is 7 days old, use the TSB level for 30 0/7 weeks

Discontinue phototherapy when TSB is 1–2 mg/dL below the initiation level for the infant's postmenstrual age

Discontinue TSB measurements when TSB is declining and phototherapy is no longer required

Measure the serum albumin level in all infants

Measure irradiance at regular intervals with an appropriate spectroradiometer

The increased mortality observed in $\leq$1,000 g infants who are receiving phototherapy suggests that it might be prudent to use less intensive levels of irradiance in these infants. In such infants, phototherapy is almost always prophylactic – it is used to prevent a further increase in the TSB and intensive phototherapy with high irradiance levels usually is not needed. In infants $\leq$ 1,000 g it is reasonable to start phototherapy at lower irradiance levels. If the TSB continues to rise, additional phototherapy should be provided by increasing the surface area exposed (phototherapy above and below the infant, reflecting material around the incubator). If the TSB, nevertheless, continues to rise, the irradiance should be increased by switching to a higher intensity setting on the device or by bringing the overhead light closer to the infant. Fluorescent and LED light sources can be brought closer to the infant, but this cannot be done with halogen or tungsten lamps because of the danger of a burn

On the other hand, in the first NICHHD trial (Lipsitz et al. 1985), irradiance levels were quite low, yet there was a 19% increase in mortality in infants <1,000 g who received phototherapy ($p = 0.112$). One alternative to using lower irradiance is to decrease the length of exposure by using intensive phototherapy for a short period. Another option is to consider intermittent (cyclical) phototherapy (Lau and Fung 1984; Vogl et al. 1978). In one recent preliminary study, infants <1,000 g who received phototherapy for 15 min in the hour had mean peak bilirubin levels (6.5 $\pm$ 1.6 mg/dL) that were virtually identical to those receiving continuous phototherapy (6.3 $\pm$ 1.3 mg/dL) (Arnold et al. 2015)

Subcommittee on Hyperbilirubinemia 2004; Maisels et al. 2012; Hulzebos et al. 2014). Thus intervention at lower TSB levels is recommended in more premature infants and for those in whom risk factors for bilirubin-induced brain damage are present. It would be ideal if these guidelines were the product of evidence-based estimates of when the benefit of these interventions exceeded their risks and costs. Such estimates should come from randomized trials or high-quality, systematic observational studies, but these studies are rare (Ip et al. 2003, 2004). Treatment guidelines must,

Table 2 Bilirubin albumin ratio trial phototherapy and exchange transfusion criteria[a]

BW (g)	Phototherapy				Exchange transfusion			
	Standard risk		High risk		Standard risk		High risk	
	TSB	B/A*	TSB	B/A*	TSB	B/A*	TSB	B/A*
<1,000	5.8	2.3	5.8	2.3	9.9	3.9	9.9	3.9
1,000–1,250	8.7	3.5	5.8	2.3	12.8	5.1	9.9	3.9
1,250–1,500	11.1	3.7	8.7	2.9	15.2	6.1	12.8	5.1
1,500–2,000	12.8	4.2	11.1	3.7	16.9	6.8	15.2	6.1
2,000–2,500	14.0	4.6	12.8	4.2	18.1	7.2	16.9	6.8

[a]At 48 h of postnatal age and older
High risk: asphyxia, hypoxemia, acidosis, hemolysis, neurologic deterioration (sepsis, meningitis, intracranial hemorrhage > grade 2)
TSB is expressed in mg/dl and B/A* ratio is expressed as mg/g
From Hulzebos et al. (2014) with permission

therefore, rely on relatively uncertain estimates of risks and benefits as well as the recognition that using a single TSB to predict long-term behavioral and developmental outcomes is not reliable and will lead to conflicting results (Ip et al. 2003, 2004).

Although kernicterus has been reported in term and late preterm infants at levels below 25 mg/dL (Ip et al. 2004), such outcomes are rare, and if TSB levels meeting or exceeding the American Academy of Pediatrics (AAP) exchange transfusion criteria (Fig. 2) are treated promptly, the outcomes are generally favorable (Newman et al. 2006; Newman and Maisels 1990). Setting thresholds for intervention in the premature neonate is more challenging (Tables 1 and 2) and has been a capricious exercise at best, and one for which no claim of an "evidence-base" can be made (Maisels and Watchko 2003). Guidelines for preterm neonates are provided by different experts, none of whom would make any claim for the greater validity of one approach versus another (Maisels and Watchko 2003). A report from the United Kingdom showing a remarkably wide range of treatment thresholds for phototherapy and exchange transfusions in premature neonates, further underscores this uncertainty (Rennie et al. 2009).

Phototherapy is effective in lowering the circulating bilirubin or preventing it from rising further. Its main demonstrated value is that it reduces the need for exchange transfusion, although recent evidence suggests that it might also have a role in reducing neurodevelopmental impairment in infants of extremely low birth weight (ELBW, ≤1,000 g) (Morris et al. 2008).

76.4 Assessing the Risk of Kernicterus and Neurodevelopmental Impairment in Preterm Infants

Chronic bilirubin encephalopathy, including kernicterus at postmortem, is currently a rare event in premature neonates. In past decades, however, autopsy proven kernicterus was often reported in sick, very low birth weight infants who had only modestly elevated total serum bilirubin (TSB) levels, a condition termed low bilirubin kernicterus. Improvements in neonatal intensive care and the discontinuation of benzyl alcohol as a bacteriostatic agent in intravenous fluids and medications have been implicated in this marked reduction. Recent case series of preterm neonates, however, demonstrate that low bilirubin kernicterus has not completely disappeared, its occurrence enigmatic and unpredictable (Watchko and Maisels 2014; Watchko 2016). In a study from the Netherlands, five sick preterm infants (25–29 weeks gestation) with peak TSB levels ranging from 8.7 to 11.9 mg/dL (148–204 μmol/L) developed the classical magnetic resonance imaging (MRI) findings of kernicterus (Govaert et al. 2003). Serum albumin levels in these infants were strikingly low, ranging from 1.4 to 2.1 g/dL (Govaert et al. 2003). Two other extremely low birth weight (ELBW) neonates with complicated neonatal courses, comorbid CNS injury, and peak TSB levels of 7.5 mg/dl (128 μmol/L) and 9.9 mg/dl

(168 μmol/L) developed neurologic sequelae and MRI findings consistent with chronic bilirubin encephalopathy (Moll et al. 2011). Choreoathetosis and the classical MRI findings of kernicterus at follow-up were documented in two additional preterm infants of 31 and 34 weeks gestation (Sugama et al. 2001). The mother of one showed clinical signs of chorioamnionitis but neither infant was acutely ill in the newborn period, and their peak TSB levels were 13.1 mg/dL (224 μmol/L) and 14.7 mg/dL (251 μmol/L), respectively (Sugama et al. 2001). These reports renew concerns about low bilirubin kernicterus in the premature infant (Watchko and Maisels 2014; Watchko 2016) as does a follow-up study of 2,575 ELBW infants which showed an association between peak serum bilirubin and (a) death or neurodevelopmental impairment (odds ratio [OR] 1.068: 95% CI 1.03–1.11), (b) psychomotor developmental index (PDI) < 70 (OR 1.057: 95% CI 1.00–1.12), and (c) hearing impairment (OR 1.138: 95% CI 1.00–1.30) (Oh et al. 2003). A review of recent low bilirubin kernicterus cases, however, suggests that if phototherapy were used in each at the levels recommended in the guidelines outlined in Tables 1 or 2, it is likely that kernicterus could have been prevented in many of these preterm neonates (Watchko and Maisels 2014; Watchko 2016).

76.4.1 Unbound or Free Bilirubin and the Bilirubin/Albumin Ratio

Recognition that a peak TSB level, by itself, is a rather poor predictor of the likelihood of poor neurodevelopmental outcome or kernicterus, raises the question of whether we should be using measurements of unbound or "free" bilirubin (B_f) or the ratio of bilirubin to albumin (B/A) to predict hyperbilirubinemia risk (McDonagh and Maisels 2006; Wennberg et al. 2006). Most bilirubin in the circulation is bound to albumin, and a relatively small fraction remains unbound. Circulating B_f is in dynamic equilibrium with the extravascular tissues including the CNS and provides a measure of the relative force with which bilirubin will exit the vascular space at a given TSB, albumin concentration, and albumin-bilirubin binding constant(s). Although B_f is the vehicle of bilirubin's biologic effects in the brain, it does not by itself dictate the development of bilirubin encephalopathy as bilirubin-induced neurotoxicity depends on a complex interaction between the level and duration of CNS B_f exposure and the innate cellular characteristics of the developing CNS that may predispose or protect against bilirubin-induced neuronal injury (Watchko and Tiribelli 2013).

Elevations of B_f have been associated with kernicterus in sick preterm infants (Cashore and Oh 1982; Nakamura et al. 1992). In addition, elevated B_f concentrations are more closely associated than TSB with transient abnormalities in the brainstem auditory evoked potential (BAEP) in both term (Funato et al. 1994) and preterm (Amin et al. 2001) infants. Although in one study a B_f level of > 1.0 μg/dL predicted the presence or absence of neurotoxicity in preterm neonates with high sensitivity and specificity (Nakamura et al. 1992), there is no agreement about what constitutes the neurotoxic B_f threshold (Daood et al. 2009), i.e., the threshold at which B_f produces changes in cellular function culminating in permanent cell injury and cell death. Notably for practitioners, clinical laboratory measurement of B_f is not generally available.

The ratio of bilirubin (mg/dL) to albumin (g/dL) (B/A) does correlate with measured B_f in neonates (Ahlfors 1994) and has been used as an approximate surrogate for the measurement of B_f (Ahlfors 1994), and the AAP has endorsed this approach (American Academy of Pediatrics, Subcommittee on Hyperbilirubinemia 2004). A recent prospective, randomized controlled trial in the Netherlands (the Bilirubin/Albumin Ratio Trial or BARTrial) compared treatment of preterm neonates based on the B/A ratio or TSB (whichever was exceeded first) versus TSB only (control group) and evaluated neurodevelopmental outcome at 18–24 months corrected age (Hulzebos et al. 2014). The study failed to demonstrate an improved neurodevelopmental outcome in preterm neonates managed using the B/A ratio but may have been underpowered. Only 30% of infants in the experimental group were treated on

the basis of B/A ratio as opposed to TSB. Moreover, it is not clear how many infants had marked degrees of hypoalbuminemia that might pose a risk. The B/A ratio becomes increasingly relevant when serum albumin levels decline below 2.5 g/dl in preterm neonates and less than 3 g/dl in term neonates and may trump TSB levels as an indication when marked hypoalbuminemia is present (Watchko and Maisels 2014; Watchko 2016; Ahlfors 1994). The BARTrial treatment thresholds are outlined in Table 2 (Hulzebos et al. 2014).

It must also be recognized that albumin binding capacity can vary significantly between newborns (Ahlfors 1994; Cashore 1980), is impaired in sick infants (Cashore et al. 1983; Ebbesen and Brodersen 1982; Esbjorner 1991), and increases with increasing gestational age (Cashore et al. 1983; Ebbesen and Nyboe 1983) and postnatal age (Ebbesen and Brodersen 1982; Esbjorner 1991). A recent study of VLBW infants from one National Institute of Child Health and Human Development (NICHD) Neonatal Network institution confirmed that bilirubin-binding capacity was lower and B_f higher in unstable versus stable neonates but did not report on longer term neurodevelopmental outcomes (Bender et al. 2007). Follow-up in the phototherapy trial of 224 infants born in 1974–1976 with birth weights < 2,000 g and evaluated at age 6 years showed no relation between measures of bilirubin-albumin binding and IQ scores (Scheidt et al. 1991). It will be instructive to see how measures of B_f correlate with short- and long-term outcomes in the NICHD Neonatal Network ELBW cohort.

Crucially important in the measurement of B_f is the bilirubin-albumin binding constant k, a term whose numeric value may actually vary considerably depending on conditions including among other factors, sample dilution, albumin concentration, and the presence of competing compounds (McDonagh and Maisels 2006; Wennberg et al. 2006; Daood et al. 2009). Moreover, the risk of bilirubin encephalopathy is likely not simply a function of the B_f concentration alone or TSB level but a combination of both, i. e., the total amount of bilirubin available (the miscible pool of bilirubin) as well as the tendency of bilirubin to enter the tissue (the B_f concentration) (Ahlfors 1994). Nevertheless, markedly reduced serum albumin levels with resultant elevated B/A ratios should be considered when making decisions on when to initiate treatment (Hulzebos et al. 2014; Watchko and Maisels 2014; Watchko 2016; Ahlfors 1994). Clarifying and defining clinically germane B_f concentrations, bilirubin to albumin ratios, exposure conditions, and exposure durations, as well as improving, standardizing, and validating B_f measurements are important lines of clinical and translational research.

76.4.2 Phototherapy in Infants with Birth Weights ≤ 1,000 g

The NICHD Neonatal Research Network conducted a randomized controlled trial of "aggressive vs. conservative" phototherapy in a large cohort of infants who were followed to age 18–20 months of corrected age (Morris et al. 2008). The protocol for this study is shown in Table 3. Compared with conservative phototherapy, aggressive phototherapy did not reduce the primary outcome of death or neurodevelopmental impairment but, in surviving infants,

Table 3 Criteria for initiating phototherapy and exchange transfusions in the NICHD Neonatal Research Network Trial

	Aggressive management			Conservative management			
		Exchange transfusion		Phototherapy begins		Exchange transfusion	
Birth weight	Phototherapy begins	mg/dL	μmol/L	mg/dL	μmol/L	mg/dL	μmol/L
501–750 g	ASAP after enrollment[a]	≥13.0	≥222	≥8.0	≥137	≥13.0	≥257
751–1,000 g	ASAP after enrollment[a]	≥15.0	≥257	≥10.0	≥171	≥15.0	≥257

[a]Enrollment was expected within 12–36 h after birth, preferably between 12 and 24 h

did reduce the rates of (a) neurodevelopmental impairment (relative risk [RR] 0.86: 95% CI 0.74–0.99), (b) hearing loss (RR 0.32: 95% CI 0.15–0.68), (c) mental development index score <70 (RR 0.83: 95% CI 0.71–0.98), and (d) athetosis (RR 0.20: 95% CI 0.04–0.90) (Morris et al. 2008). The reduction in neurodevelopmental impairment was attributable almost entirely to a decrease in infants with profound impairment in the aggressive phototherapy group (RR 0.68: 95% CI 0.52–0.89) (Morris et al. 2008). A subsequent comparison of infants from the same study who never received phototherapy to those who received any phototherapy showed a similar significant decrease in the rate of profound delay in the phototherapy group (Hintz et al. 2011).

It was noteworthy, however, that there was a 5% increase in mortality in infants with birth weights of 501–750 g who received aggressive phototherapy. This was not statistically significant, but a post hoc Bayesian analysis estimated a 99% probability that aggressive phototherapy increased the rate of death in this subgroup (Tyson et al. 2012). A similar but nonsignificant increase in mortality was also observed in neonates <1,000 g in the NICHD Collaborative Phototherapy trial conducted in 1974–1976 (Lipsitz et al. 1985), in spite of low phototherapy irradiance estimated to be ~ 8uW/cm^2/nm. It is unclear why phototherapy might increase mortality in these tiny infants, but it is likely that light penetrates more deeply through the thin, gelatinous skin, reaching the subcutaneous tissues and possibly producing oxidative injury to cell membranes (Hintz et al. 2011).

What should neonatologists do with this information? Notably, infants in the aggressive phototherapy group of the Network study received 88 h of phototherapy compared with 35 h in the conventional group (Morris et al. 2008). One approach is not to use early prophylactic phototherapy. In many units, phototherapy is initiated in ELBW neonates when their TSB reaches 5 mg/dL (86 μmol/L). As the TSB at the start of phototherapy in the aggressive group was 4.8 mg/dL (82 μmol/L), instituting phototherapy at a TSB of 5 mg/dL (86 μmol/L) will likely have a similar effect on TSB levels as does prophylactic phototherapy initiated in every infant soon after birth. Another possible approach designed to reduce phototherapy exposure duration is to provide intermittent or cycled phototherapy that past studies has been shown to be as effective as continuous phototherapy (Lau and Fung 1984; Vogl et al. 1978). Preliminary data from a recent study of cycled phototherapy in infants <1,000 g found that the mean peak bilirubin levels were no different in infants who received phototherapy delivered for 15 min per hour versus infants receiving continuous phototherapy (Arnold et al. 2015). Others suggest it is reasonable to start phototherapy at lower irradiance levels and only if the TSB continues to rise, providing additional phototherapy by increasing the surface area exposed (phototherapy above and below the infant) or increasing the irradiance by switching to a higher intensity setting on the device (Maisels et al. 2012).

76.5 Phototherapy

Phototherapy uses visible light energy to change the shape and structure of bilirubin, converting it to molecules that can be excreted even when normal conjugation is deficient. Light provides an infusion of discrete photons of energy that correspond to the individual molecules of a drug in a conventional medication. Absorption of these photons by bilirubin molecules in the skin leads to a therapeutic effect in much the same way as binding of drug molecules to a receptor has a desired effect. Figure 3 provides a detailed description of how phototherapy works.

The relative contributions of the various reactions to the overall elimination of bilirubin are unknown, although in vitro and in vivo studies suggest that photoisomerization is more important than photodegradation (Lightner and McDonagh 1984). Bilirubin elimination depends on the rates of formation as well as the rates of clearance of the

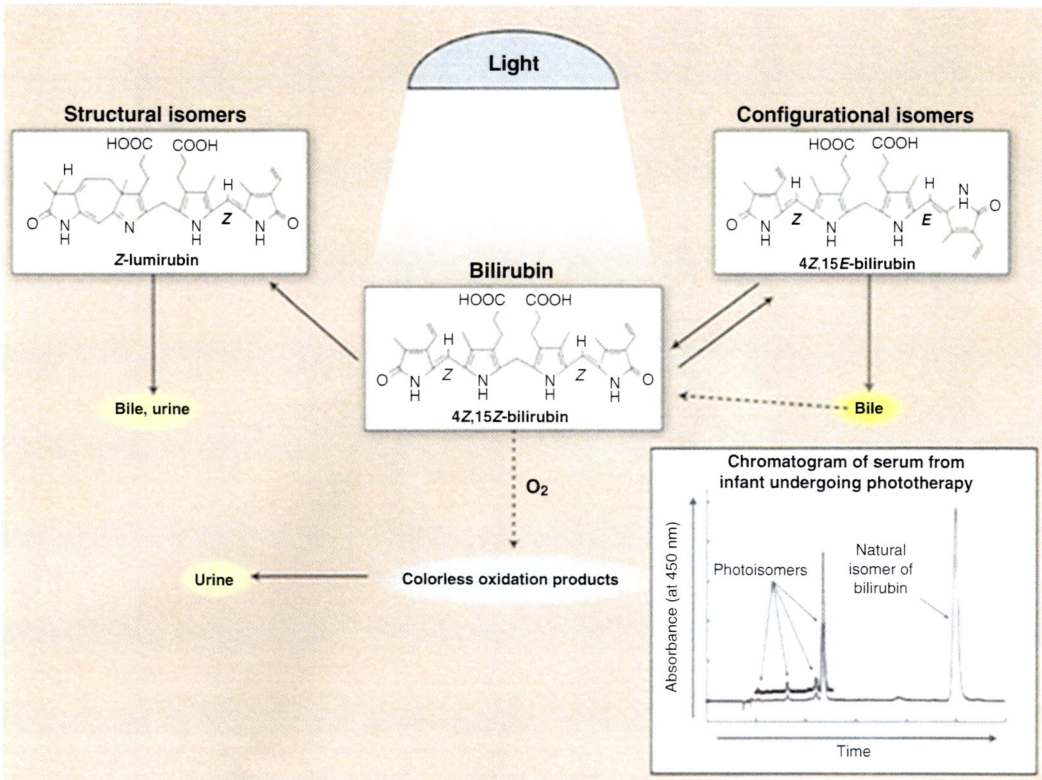

Fig. 3 Mechanism of phototherapy. The absorption of light by the normal form of bilirubin (4Z,15Z-bilirubin) generates fleeting transient excited-state bilirubin molecules. These fleeting intermediates can react with oxygen to produce colorless products of lower molecular weight, or they can undergo rearrangement to become structural isomers (lumirubins) or configurational isomers in which the configuration of at least one of the two Z-configuration double bonds has changed to an E-configuration. (Z and E, from the German zusammen (together) and entgegen (opposite), respectively, are prefixes used for designating the stereochemistry around a double bond. The prefixes 4 and 15 designate double bond positions). Only the two principal photoisomers formed in humans are shown. The photoisomers are less lipophilic than the 4Z,15Z form of bilirubin and can be excreted unchanged in bile without undergoing glucuronidation. Lumirubin isomers can also be excreted in urine. Photooxidation products are excreted mainly in urine. Once in bile, configurational isomers revert spontaneously to the 4Z,15Z form of bilirubin. Configurational isomerization is reversible and much faster than structural isomerization, but the clearance of the 4Z,15E isomer is slow. Structural isomerization is irreversible and lumirubin is cleared more rapidly and makes the major contribution to overall bilirubin elimination. Both configurational and structural isomerizations occur much more quickly than photooxidation. The graph, a high-performance liquid chromatogram of serum from an infant undergoing phototherapy, shows the presence of several photoisomers in addition to the 4Z,15Z isomer. Photoisomers are also detectable in the blood of healthy adults after sunbathing (From reference Maisels and McDonagh (2008) with permission)

photo products. Photoisomerization occurs rapidly during phototherapy, and isomers appear in the blood long before the level of plasma bilirubin begins to decline. The radiometric quantities used and the important factors that influence the dose and efficacy of phototherapy are listed in Tables 4 and 5 and illustrated in Fig. 4. A common misconception is that ultraviolet (UV) light (<400 nm) is used for phototherapy. Phototherapy lights in current use do not emit significant erythemal UV radiation. In addition, the fluorescent tube glass, the lamp plastic cover, and in the case of preterm infants, the incubator itself will filter out UV light.

Table 4 Radiometric quantities used in phototherapy

Quantity	Dimensions	Usual units of measure
Irradiance (radiant power incident on a surface per unit area of the surface)	W/m^2	W/cm^2
Spectral irradiance (irradiance in a certain wavelength band)	W/m^2 per nm (or W/m^2)	$\mu W/cm^2$ per nm

From reference (Maisels 1996) with permission

Table 5 Factors that affect the dose and efficacy of phototherapy

Factor	Technical terminology	Rationale	Clinical application
Type of light source	Spectrum of light (nm)	Blue-green spectrum is most effective at lowering total serum bilirubin (TSB); light at this wavelength penetrates skin well and is absorbed strongly by bilirubin	Use special blue fluorescent tubes or light-emitting diodes (LED) or another light source with output in blue-green spectrum for intensive phototherapy (PT)
Distance of light	Spectral irradiance source from patient (a function of both distance and light source) delivered to surface of infant	↑ Irradiance leads to ↑ rate of decline in TSB. Standard PT units deliver 8–10 $\mu W/cm^2/nm$; intensive PT delivers ≥ 30 $\mu W/cm^2/nm$	If special blue fluorescent tubes are used, bring tubes as close as possible to infant to increase irradiance. (Do not do this with halogen lamps because of danger of burn.) Positioning special blue tubes 10–15 cm above infant will produce an irradiance of at least 35 $\mu W/cm^2/nm$
Surface area exposed	Spectral power (a function of spectral irradiance and surface area)	↑ Surface area exposed leads to ↑ rate of decline in TSB	For intensive PT, expose maximum surface area of infant to PT. Place lights above and below[a] or around[b] the infant. For maximum exposure, line sides of bassinet, warmer bed, or incubator with aluminum foil
Cause of jaundice	2	Phototherapy (PT) is likely to be less effective if jaundice is caused by hemolysis or if cholestasis is present (direct bilirubin is increased)	When hemolysis is present, start PT at a lower TSB level and use intensive PT. Failure of PT suggests hemolysis is cause of the jaundice. When direct bilirubin is elevated, watch for bronze baby syndrome or blistering
TSB level at start of PT		The higher the TSB, the more rapid the decline in TSB with PT	Use intensive PT for higher TSB levels. Anticipate a more rapid decrease in TSB when TSB > 20 mg/dL

[a]Commercially available sources for light below include special blue fluorescent tubes available in the Olypmpic Bili-Bassinet (Natus Medical, San Carlos, CA), the BiliSoft Fiberoptic /LED mattress (GE Healthcare, Wauwatosa, WI), and neoBlue blanket LED (Natus Medical Inc., San Carlos, CA)
[b]The Mediprema Cradle 360 (Mediprema, Tours Cedex, France) provides 360° exposure to special blue fluorescent light

76.5.1 Clinical Use and Efficacy of Phototherapy

The factors that influence the dose and efficacy of phototherapy are listed in Table 5 and illustrated in Fig. 4. There is a clear dose–response relationship between the irradiance (energy output of the phototherapy device) delivered to the infant and the rate of decline in the TSB (Tan 1982; Vandborg et al. 2012). Although earlier studies suggested that there was a saturation point beyond which an increase in irradiance produced no

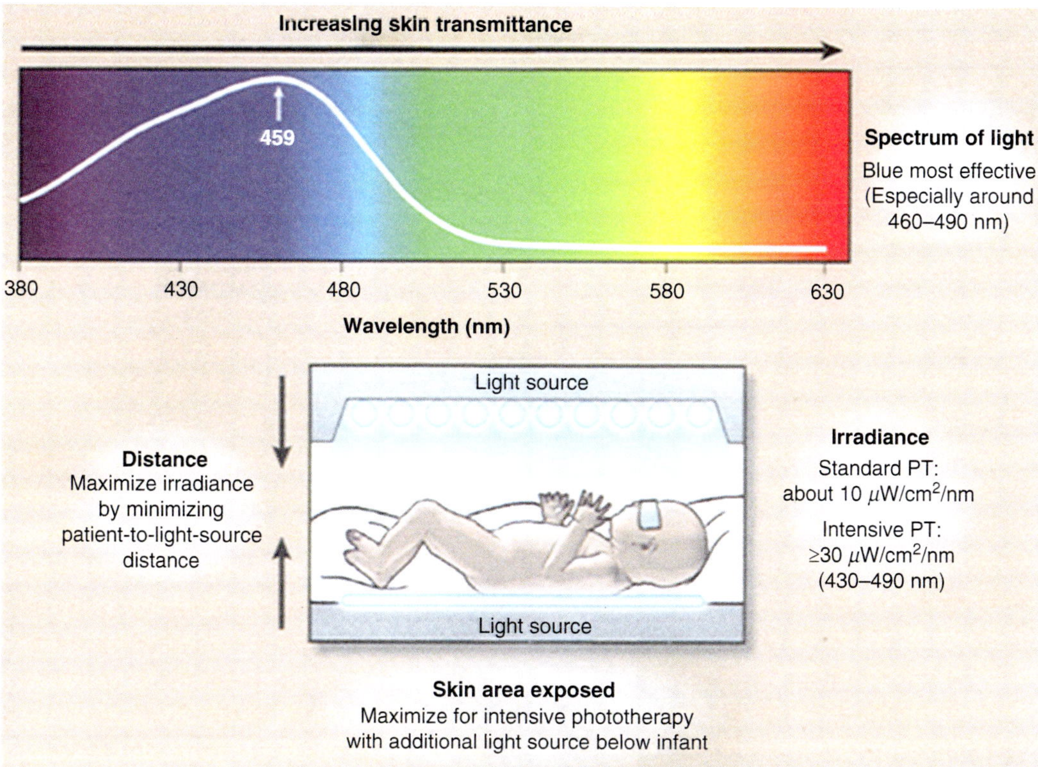

Fig. 4 Important factors in the efficacy of phototherapy. The absorbance spectrum of bilirubin bound to human serum albumin (*white line*) is shown superimposed on the spectrum of visible light. Clearly, blue light is most effective for phototherapy, but because the transmittance of skin increases with increasing wavelength, the best wavelengths to use are probably in the range 460–490 nm. Term and near-term infants should be treated in a bassinet, not an incubator, to allow the light source to be brought to within 10–15 cm of the infant (except when halogen or tungsten lights are used), increasing irradiance and efficacy. For intensive phototherapy, an auxiliary light source (fiber-optic pad, light-emitting diode [LED] mattress or pad, or special blue fluorescent tubes) can be placed below the infant or bassinet. Special blue fluorescent tubes can also be placed in a 360° configuration around the infant (see Table 5 for a list of some commercially available units) (From reference Maisels and McDonagh (2008) with permission)

added efficacy of phototherapy (Tan 1982), more recent studies show that the dose–response relationship of phototherapy for hyperbilirubinemia demonstrates no evidence of a saturation point (Vandborg et al. 2012). Although the rate of TSB decline is linearly related to the irradiance, there is a remarkably wide range of decrease in the TSB at each irradiance illustrating that there are many other factors involved in the response to phototherapy. These include among others the rate of bilirubin production of which hemolysis is key contributor, the rates of photoisomer elimination, the rates of migration of bilirubin and individual photoisomers into and out of the blood, and the rate of reabsorption of bilirubin from the intestine into the blood.

It is, therefore, important to perform regular measurements of the irradiance with a radiometer or spectroradiometer. Special blue fluorescent lamps or light-emitting diode (LED) lights have been found to be effective in clinical studies (Maisels et al. 2007; Seidman et al. 2003) and will deliver 30–45 μW/cm ^{2}/nm in the 430–490 nm band. Most recently, however, it is been shown that the rate and level of photoisomerization (the formation of ZE isomers) was not affected by increasing the irradiance or using double versus single phototherapy lights (Mreihil et al. 2015).

As only the Z,E photoisomers were measured and there was no measurement of lumirubin, it is difficult to interpret these data, but they tend to confirm previous observations suggesting that it is the formation of lumirubin and not ZE-bilirubin that is primarily responsible for the decrease in serum bilirubin levels in infants receiving phototherapy.

Commonly used phototherapy units include those that contain daylight, white, or blue fluorescent tubes, halogen lamps, and light emitting diodes (LED). When the TSB exceeds the levels indicated in Fig. 1, intensive phototherapy is recommended (American Academy of Pediatrics, Subcommittee on Hyperbilirubinemia 2004). The AAP defines intensive phototherapy as the use of high levels of irradiance in the 430–490 nm band (usually 30 $\mu W/cm^2$ per nm or higher) delivered to as much of the infant's surface area as possible (American Academy of Pediatrics, Subcommittee on Hyperbilirubinemia 2004). Thus, it is particularly important to use lamps that have an emission within the 430–490 nm bands. Increasing the surface area of the infant exposed to light significantly increases the efficacy of phototherapy and can be achieved by placing additional sources of light below or around the infant. A simple method of increasing the area exposed is to place some reflecting material such as a white sheet or aluminum foil within or around the bassinette or incubator (Djokomuljanto et al. 2006).

76.5.1.1 Where Does Phototherapy Work?

Phototherapy can act on bilirubin in the vascular (capillaries) and extra vascular (skin and subcutaneous tissue) compartments. The effect of phototherapy in the latter site produces the well-known blanching effect on the infant's skin, an effect that has been confirmed with transcutaneous bilirubin measurements (Hegyi et al. 1986). As a result, it has become a common practice to turn the infant at intervals from supine to prone and back. Several randomized studies, however, show that turning infants every few hours does not improve the efficacy of phototherapy (Shinwell et al. 2002; Yamauchi et al. 1989; Donneborg et al. 2010). If blanching of the skin is not accompanied by a decrease in the TSB, it follows that the primary site of action for the serum bilirubin lowering effect of phototherapy is the blood in the superficial capillaries. Additional evidence to support this conclusion is the documentation of the formation of bilirubin photoisomers within 15 min of initiating phototherapy (Mreihil et al. 2015; Mreihil et al. 2010).

76.5.2 Phototherapy to Prevent an Exchange Transfusion

As the primary purpose of phototherapy is to prevent the need for an exchange transfusion, it is useful to know how many infants need to be treated with phototherapy in order to prevent one exchange transfusion. Previous randomized trials of phototherapy (Brown et al. 1985; Maurer et al. 1985; Martinez et al. 1993) found that, among infants without hemolysis, 6–10 infants needed to be treated with phototherapy to prevent one from developing a TSB level $\geq$20 mg/dL (343 μmol/L) (Ip et al. 2004). These data, however, are not applicable to the current use of phototherapy because these studies included infants with lower TSB levels than those currently recommended for instituting phototherapy (American Academy of Pediatrics, Subcommittee on Hyperbilirubinemia 2004) and had as their end points lower TSB levels than those at which the AAP recommends exchange transfusions (American Academy of Pediatrics, Subcommittee on Hyperbilirubinemia 2004). A recent analysis of infants $\geq$ 35 weeks of gestation evaluated the numbers needed to treat (NNT) with phototherapy in order to prevent one infant from reaching the exchange transfusion level according to the current AAP guidelines (American Academy of Pediatrics, Subcommittee on Hyperbilirubinemia 2004). The NNT ranged from 10 (95% CI: 6–19) for < 24 h old, 36 week gestation boys to 3,041 (95% CI: 888–11,096) for $\geq$ 3 day old, 41 week girls (Newman et al. 2009). If we need to treat 3,000 infants with phototherapy to prevent one exchange transfusion, it is reasonable to ask whether, in many of these infants, phototherapy might have been avoided. In these infants, other interventions including lactation support, formula

substitution or supplementation (Martinez et al. 1993), or the use of home phototherapy should also be considered.

Nevertheless, it is relevant to note the dramatic impact that the use of phototherapy has had on reducing the number of exchange transfusions performed in term and preterm infants (Maisels 2001). Before phototherapy was introduced some 36% of infants with birth weight <1,500 g required an exchange transfusion (Keenan et al. 1985). In the recent Neonatal Research Network study only 5/1974 (0.25%) infants with birth weights ≤ 1,000 g required an exchange transfusion (Morris et al. 2008).

76.5.3 Short-Term Adverse Effects

Since phototherapy was introduced, perhaps more than 100 million infants, worldwide, have been exposed to this treatment. Reports of *clinically significant toxicity* from phototherapy are rare. There is no evidence, to date, that the products of photodecomposition have any neurotoxic effects (Haddock and Nadler 1970; Silberberg et al. 1970). Nevertheless, there are some well-documented, short-term, potentially negative effects in the human newborn receiving phototherapy. These include DNA damage (Tatli et al. 2008), decreased cytokine levels (Procianoy et al. 2010), oxidative stress (Aycicek and Erel 2007), decreased cardiac output, increased cerebral blood flow, and decreased renal blood flow (Benders et al. 1999).

Mortality in infants <1,000 g birth weight. The possible increase in mortality in infants <1,000 g has been discussed in section Phototherapy in Infants with Birth Weights ≤ 1000 g (p. 5) (Morris et al. 2008; Hintz et al. 2011; Tyson et al. 2012).

Bronze Baby Syndrome. In infants with cholestasis (direct hyperbilirubinemia), phototherapy can produce the bronze baby syndrome, in which the skin, serum, and urine develop a dark grayish-brown discoloration (Kopelman et al. 1972; Rubaltelli et al. 1983). The pathogenesis of this condition, which occurs only in infants with cholestasis, is not fully understood. When phototherapy is stopped and cholestasis resolves, the coloration disappears. Bronzing is not a contraindication for phototherapy.

Skin. Rare purpuric and bullous eruptions have been reported in infants with severe cholestatic jaundice who are receiving phototherapy (Mallon et al. 1995; Paller et al. 1997), probably as a result of sensitization by accumulating porphyrins. An erythematous rash has been reported in infants treated with tin-mesoporphyrin, who are subsequently exposed to sunlight or daylight fluorescent bulbs (Valaes et al. 1994). Congenital porphyria, a family history of porphyria, and concomitant use of photosensitizing drugs are absolute contraindications to phototherapy. Severe blistering and agitation during phototherapy could be a sign of congenital porphyria (Tonz et al. 1975).

Insensible water loss and temperature control. Conventional phototherapy can produce an acute change in the infant's thermal environment, leading to an increase in peripheral blood flow and insensible water loss (Dollberg et al. 1995; Maayan-Metzger et al. 2001). This question has not been studied with LED lights but, because of their relatively low heat output, they should be much less likely to cause insensible water loss. In term infants who are nursing or feeding adequately, additional intravenous fluids are usually not required.

Eye damage. Because light can be toxic to the retina, the eyes of infants receiving phototherapy should be protected with appropriate eye patches (Messner et al. 1978).

Other effects. Intensive phototherapy does not cause hemolysis (Maisels and Kring 2006a). Because bilirubin is a powerful antioxidant (McDonagh 1990; Sedlak and Snyder 2004), lowering the TSB, particularly in ELBW infants could have undesirable consequences (Vreman et al. 2004) but none have yet been clearly identified although, as noted above, aggressive phototherapy was associated with an increase in mortality in infants with birth weight 501–750 g (Morris et al. 2008; Hintz et al. 2011; Tyson et al. 2012).

76.5.4 Long-Term Adverse Effects

There has been little systematic research into the potential long-term adverse effects of phototherapy and the potential long-term consequences of phototherapy exposure in the newborn remain largely unknown. One study has suggested that intensive phototherapy might increase the number of atypical melanocytic nevi identified at school age (Csoma et al. 2007), but a recent systematic review and meta-analysis of five studies with a total of 2,921 subjects of whom 642 underwent phototherapy concluded that there was no evidence that phototherapy exposure significantly increased the number of melanocytic nevi (Lai and Yew 2015). Epidemiologic studies linking disease registries with perinatal databases have suggested the possible relationship between an increased risk of childhood leukemia and phototherapy (Cnattingius et al. 1995), but others have not found this (Roman et al. 1997). A Swedish study found a strong association between phototherapy and juvenile-onset diabetes (Dahlquist and Kallen 2003), but a subsequent, large, Scottish, case-control study did not (Robertson and Harrild 2010). On the other hand, the complete absence of any abnormal neurodevelopmental outcomes, including visual and auditory function, school performance, and social interactions in children with the Crigler-Najjar syndrome who have received daily phototherapy for up to 21 years, is certainly reassuring (Strauss et al. 2006).

76.5.5 Expected Rate of Decline in Serum Bilirubin

The effectiveness of phototherapy depends not only on the dose of light but also on the cause and severity of the hyperbilirubinemia. During active hemolysis, the TSB may not decline or not decline as rapidly as it would in an infant without hemolysis. On the other hand, because it is most likely that phototherapy works on bilirubin present in the capillaries in the skin and superficial subcutaneous tissue, the more bilirubin present at those sites (i.e., the higher the TSB level) the more effective phototherapy will be (Jährig et al. 1982). In some infants with a TSB > 30 mg/dL (513 μmol/L), intensive phototherapy can result in a decline of as much as 10 mg/dL (171 μmol/L) within a few hours (Hansen 1997). Hemolysis is more likely to be the cause of hyperbilirubinemia in infants who require phototherapy during the birth hospitalization than in those readmitted for such treatment (Maisels and Kring 2002; Maisels and Kring 2006b; Kaplan et al. 2006), and phototherapy in infants treated during the birth hospitalization is almost always initiated at a lower serum bilirubin level. For both of these reasons, the level of TSB tends to fall relatively slowly in such infants.

76.5.6 Discontinuing Phototherapy

Although there are no firm standards for discontinuing treatment, phototherapy can be safely stopped in infants treated during the birth hospitalization if two consecutive TSB values fall below the level at which phototherapy was initiated. In infants readmitted for phototherapy, hemolysis is less often the cause for their hyperbilirubinemia (Maisels and Kring 2002; Kaplan et al. 2006) and treatment is begun at higher initial TSB levels. In these patients, intensive phototherapy can result in a TSB decrement of 30–40% in the first 24 h (Maisels and Kring 2002) with the most pronounced decline occurring in the first 4–6 h. Phototherapy can be discontinued when the total serum bilirubin level has fallen below 13–14 mg/dL (222–239 μmol/L) (American Academy of Pediatrics, Subcommittee on Hyperbilirubinemia 2004).

76.5.7 Rebound After Phototherapy

A rebound in the TSB level of 1–2 mg/dL (17–34 μmol/L) (Maisels and Kring 2002) and occasionally more (Kaplan et al. 2006) can occur after phototherapy is discontinued. Infants at increased risk of a clinically significant rebound are those born at < 37 weeks' gestation, those with hemolytic disease, and those treated with

phototherapy during the birth hospitalization (Maisels and Kring 2002; Kaplan et al. 2006). It is usually unnecessary to keep an infant in the hospital to check for rebound (Maisels and Kring 2002; Yetman et al. 1998), but for infants who require phototherapy during their birth hospitalization and for those with well-defined hemolytic disease, a follow-up bilirubin level should be obtained 24 h after discharge.

76.5.8 Sunlight Exposure

Sunlight will lower the serum bilirubin level (Cremer et al. 1958), but the practical difficulties involved in safely exposing a naked newborn to the sun either inside or outside (and avoiding sunburn) preclude the use of sunlight as a reliable therapeutic tool in developed countries. Progress has been made, however, in adapting filtered sunlight using special filters for effective and safe phototherapy in low- and middle income countries where access to standard phototherapy equipment and a consistent source of electricity are lacking (Slusher et al. 2014, 2015).

76.5.9 Home Phototherapy

The economic and social pressures for early discharge of infants from hospital after delivery have led to the widespread use of home phototherapy in the USA. When used appropriately and with adequate monitoring of the TSB, home phototherapy poses no obvious hazards to the infant and is certainly much cheaper than hospital treatment (Slater and Brewer 1984; Rogerson et al. 1986). The development of new LED mattresses and blankets has made it easier and more effective to administer phototherapy at home.

76.6 Exchange Transfusion

Exchange transfusion remains an important if infrequently required intervention to prevent or reduce the risk for kernicterus (Watchko 2000). The prevention of Rh hemolytic disease with Rh immune globulin and the effective use of phototherapy have led to a dramatic decline in the number of exchange transfusions performed (Maisels 1996). Of 1974 ELBW infants treated with phototherapy in the NICHD Neonatal Research Network study (Morris et al. 2008), only five required an exchange transfusion (0.25%). It is now possible for a pediatric resident to complete a 3-year training program without ever having performed or even witnessed an exchange transfusion. The indications for exchange transfusions in term and in preterm infants are provided in Tables 1, 2, and 3 and in Fig. 2.

It is important to note that the efficacy of a double volume exchange transfusion is a function of the mass of albumin exchanged given that bilirubin is bound with high affinity to albumin in the vascular compartment (Valaes 1963; Sproul and Smith 1964; Watchko 2014). It follows that donor blood of high plasma volume, i.e., lower hematocrit, approximating 35–40%, should be used to enhance the amount of bilirubin-free albumin introduced into the infant's circulation during the exchange (Valaes 1963; Sproul and Smith 1964; Watchko 2014). This is a *fundamental* aspect of performing an exchange transfusion and necessary to optimize the effectiveness of this intervention.

Exchange transfusion is indictated when signs of intermediate to advanced stages of acute bilirubin encephalopathy are present. More specifically, the 2004 AAP statement on hyperbilirubinemia specifies that "immediate exchange transfusion is recommended in any infant who is jaundiced and manifests signs of intermediate to advanced stages of acute bilirubin encephalopathy (hypertonia, arching, retrocolis, opisthotonos, fever, high-pitched cry) even if the TSB is falling" (American Academy of Pediatrics, Subcommittee on Hyperbilirubinemia 2004). This recommendation is consistent with reports (Harris et al. 2001; Hansen et al. 2009) that at least some infants so treated may escape unscathed without chronic bilirubin encephalopathy (kernicterus). On the other hand, as previously observed, a spontaneous decline in TSB coincident with the clinical onset of intermediate to advanced signs of ABE

can also occur. This suggests enhanced influx of bilirubin from the serum into the brain and is often a prognostic sign for poor outcome as opposed to a sign of clinical improvement (Ackerman et al. 1971).

Given the urgency of an exchange transfusion in an infant with intermediate to advanced stages of ABE, it has been suggested that emergency release uncross-matched blood be used to provide timely treatment (Sims 2011). Although this will acutely lower the serum bilirubin level (Sisson et al. 1958) there are a number of reasons why this result might be falsely reassuring and not entirely therapeutic. First, emergency release blood is in the form of packed red blood cells (PRBC) in an additive solution of preservatives but with a limited quantity of plasma albumin; the albumin concentration in a unit of PRBC approximates only 0.3–0.5 g/dl. Given that the efficacy of a double volume exchange transfusion is determined by the mass of albumin exchanged (Valaes 1963; Sproul and Smith 1964; Watchko 2014), there is likely much less bilirubin removed using PRBC. In addition, as the PRBC concentration of albumin is very low, the infant's serum albumin level will fall along with the serum bilirubin during each successive aliquot exchanged and marked hypoalbuminemia result – an undesirable effect. Indeed, on balance it is unclear whether sufficient bilirubin will be removed using PRBC alone to prevent ongoing neurotoxicity in light of the resultant marked hypoalbuminemia. The hematocrit of PRBC range from ~55% to 70% so exchange transfusion using PRBC will also raise the hematocrit and thereby diminish the neonates plasma volume, further compromising the available intravascular albumin pool for bilirubin binding. Polycythemia and potential hyperviscosity are also concerns in a neonate receiving a large volume of PRBC. On the other hand, RBC binds bilirubin albeit at one-hundredth the affinity of albumin (Lamola et al. 1979). Nevertheless, the mass of RBC available to bind bilirubin is appreciable in a double volume exchange transfusion so some bilirubin clearance by RBC will occur. In addition, as a double volume exchange transfusion removes 87% of the infant's blood volume, the use of PRBC (that contain very little bilirubin) should provide a dilutional effect while at the same time removing blood that contains the serum with an elevated bilirubin level. Although sedimented erythrocytes have been used in the past to perform exchange transfusions (Sisson et al. 1958), data to address the above concerns are lacking.

The ideal replacement fluid for an exchange transfusion is reconstituted whole blood; PRBCs are mixed with plasma in order to achieve the desired hematocrit (typically 35–40% to optimize the amount of bilirubin-free albumin introduced into the infant's circulation during the exchange). The time required to thaw the plasma and reconstitute the PRBC is approximately 2–3 h; however, to ensure a safe transfusion, the blood bank also has to determine if there are any maternal RBC antibodies present and if so, compatible PRBC units need to be located. Determining if antibodies are present can take about an hour, and if present, determining their identity can take several more hours. Blood for double volume exchange will also need to be irradiated albeit this can be accomplished in about 5 min with an irradiator on site. Thus it usually takes the blood bank a minimum of 4 h to find compatible PRBCs and prepare whole blood for double volume exchange. It is notable that in Hansen's report on the reversibility of acute intermediate phase bilirubin encephalopathy (Hansen et al. 2009), the time interval between hospital admission and initiation of double volume exchange transfusion was between 3.5 and 9 h with a mean of 6.5 h (Watchko 2014).

76.6.1 Exchange Transfusion Risks

The potential complications of exchange transfusions are listed in Table 6 (Watchko 2000) and were recently reviewed (Ip et al. 2004). The morbidity and mortality associated with exchange transfusions are significantly dependent on the clinical state of the infant before the exchange, being much higher in sick preterm infants and quite low in term and near-term infants who are relatively well (Jackson 1997; Patra et al. 2004). It is interesting that when exchange transfusions were performed using

Table 6 Potential complications of exchange transfusion

Cardiovascular	Arrhythmias
	Cardiac arrest
	Volume overload
	Embolization with air or clots
	Thrombosis
	Vasospasm
Hematologic	Sickling (donor blood)
	Thrombocytopenia
	Bleeding (overheparinization of donor blood)
	Graft versus host disease
	Mechanical or thermal injury to donor cells
Gastrointestinal	Necrotizing enterocolitis
Biochemical	Hyperkalemia
	Hypernatremia
	Hypocalcemia
	Hypomagnesemia
	Acidosis
	Hypoglycemia
Infectious	Bacteremia
	Virus infection (hepatitis, CMV)
	Malaria
Miscellaneous	Hypothermia
	Perforation of umbilical vein
	Drug loss
	Apnea

From reference Watchko (2000) with permission

both umbilical venous (UVC) and arterial (UAC) catheters, they were significantly more likely to be associated with adverse events (Patra et al. 2004). Although this may relate to the conditions that led to the use of the UAC independent of the need for exchange transfusion, when controlling for preexisting neonatal morbidity, infants who underwent an exchange transfusion through both the UAC and UVC still had a fivefold increased risk of an adverse event compared with those exchanged through other routes (Patra et al. 2004).

76.7 Pharmacologic Treatment

Pharmacologic agents used in the management of hyperbilirubinemia can accelerate the normal metabolic pathways for bilirubin clearance, inhibit the enterohepatic circulation of bilirubin, and interfere with bilirubin formation by blocking the degradation of heme or inhibiting hemolysis.

76.7.1 Decreasing Bilirubin Production

Currently the only drug in clinical use is intravenous immunoglobulin (IVIG). IVIG inhibits hemolysis in immune-mediated hemolytic disease (Hammerman et al. 1996a) possibly by blocking Fc receptors (Hammerman et al. 1996a). Earlier controlled trials and a systematic review suggested that the administration of IVIG to infants with Rh or ABO hemolytic disease would significantly reduce the need for exchange transfusion (Rübo et al. 1992; Dagoglu et al. 1995; Voto et al. 1995; Gottstein and Cooke 2003; Hammerman et al. 1996b). In contrast, more recent randomized, controlled trials showed no benefit from the administration of IVIG to newborns with Rh hemolytic disease (Smits-Wintjens et al. 2011; Santos et al. 2013). In addition a recent systematic review and meta-analysis concluded that the efficacy of IVIG was not conclusive in Rh hemolytic disease of the newborn when such studies had a low risk of bias, while in studies with a high risk of bias there was a possible benefit (Louis et al. 2014). The authors also concluded that the role of IVIG in ABO disease was not clear because the studies that showed a benefit had a high risk of bias (Louis et al. 2014). Another concern has arisen because of anecdotal reports of an association of necrotizing enterocolitis with the administration of IVIG (Figueras-Aloy et al. 2010; Kara et al. 2013; Navarro et al. 2009; Krishnan and Pathare 2011), although this may be product specific (Krishnan and Pathare 2011; Krishnan and Pathare 2012). The doses of IVIG used have ranged from 500 mg/kg given over 2 h soon after birth to 800 mg/kg given daily for 3 days. Given the above conflicting information it is difficult to provide a firm recommendation with regard to the use of IVIG in isoimmune hemolytic disease. We would currently consider its use if the TSB is rising despite intensive phototherapy and the TSB level is within 2–3 mg/dL (34–51 μmol/L) of the exchange level (American Academy of

Pediatrics, Subcommittee on Hyperbilirubinemia 2004) (Fig. 2).

The microsomal enzyme heme oxygenase is necessary for the conversion of heme to biliverdin, the rate limiting step in bilirubin formation. Tin-mesoporphyrin (SnMP) is a potent inhibitor of heme oxygenase and is effective in reducing TSB levels and the requirements for phototherapy in term and preterm infants (Kappas 2004). SnMP has also produced a temporary reduction in TSB levels (Rubaltelli et al. 1989) in patients with the Crigler-Najjar syndrome and has prevented the need for exchange transfusion in Jehovah's Witness' newborns with Rh hemolytic disease (Kappas et al. 2001). To date, more than 1,000 newborns have received SnMP in controlled clinical trials, but the drug is still awaiting FDA approval in the USA and currently is the subject of a randomized controlled trial. Other metalloporphyrins hold clinical promise as well and are the subject of ongoing research (Schulz et al. 2012).

References

Ackerman BD, Dyer GY, Taylor PM (1971) Decline in serum bilirubin concentration coincident with clinical onset of kernicterus. Pediatrics 48:647–650

Ahlfors CE (1994) Criteria for exchange transfusion in jaundiced newborns. Pediatrics 93:488–494

American Academy of Pediatrics, Subcommittee on Hyperbilirubinemia (2004) Clinical practice guideline: management of hyperbilirubinemia in the newborn infant 35 or more weeks of gestation. Pediatrics 114:297–316

American Association of Blood Banks Technical Manual Committee (2002) Perinatal issues in transfusion practice. In: Brecher M (ed) Technical manual. American Association of Blood Banks, Bethesda, pp 497–515

Amin SB, Ahlfors CE, Orlando MS et al (2001) Bilirubin and serial auditory brainstem responses in premature infants. Pediatrics 107:664–670

Arnold C, Tyson JE, Cuadrado ME et al (2015) Cycled phototherapy: a safer effective treatment for small premature infants. EPAS 1582.605

Aycicek A, Erel O (2007) Total oxidant/antioxidant status in jaundiced newborns before and after phototherapy. J Pediatr (Rio J) 83:319–322

Bender GJ, Cashore WJ, Oh W (2007) Ontogeny of bilirubin-binding capacity and the effect of clinical status in premature infants born at less than 1300 grams. Pediatrics 120:1067–1073

Benders MJNL, van Bel F, van de Bor M (1999) Haemodynamic consequences of phototherapy in term infants. Eur J Pediatr 158:323–328

Bratlid D, Nakstad B, Hansen TW (2011) National guidelines for treatment of jaundice in the newborn. Acta Paediatr 100:499–505

Brown AK, Kim MH, Wu PYK et al (1985) Efficacy of phototherapy in prevention and management of neonatal hyperbilirubinemia. Pediatrics 75:393–400

Cashore WJ (1980) Free bilirubin concentrations and bilirubin-binding affinity in term and preterm infants. J Pediatr 96:521–527

Cashore WJ, Oh W (1982) Unbound bilirubin and kernicterus in low birthweight infants. Pediatrics 69:481–485

Cashore WJ, Oh W, Brodersen R (1983) Reserve albumin and bilirubin toxicity index in infant serum. Acta Paediatr Scand 72:415–419

Cnattingius S, Zack MM, Ekbom A et al (1995) Prenatal and neonatal risk factors for childhood lymphatic leukemia. J Natl Cancer Inst 87:908–914

Cremer RJ, Perryman PW, Richards DH (1958) Influence of light on the hyperbilirubinemia of infants. Lancet 1:1094–1097

Csoma Z, Hencz P, Orvos H et al (2007) Neonatal blue-light phototherapy could increase the risk of dysplastic nevus development. Pediatrics 119:1036–1037

Dagoglu T, Ovali F, Samanci N et al (1995) High-dose intravenous immunoglobulin therapy for haemolytic disease. J Internat Med Res 23:264–271

Dahlquist G, Kallen B (2003) Indications that phototherapy is a risk factor for insulin-dependent diabetes. Diabetes Care 26:247–248

Daood MJ, McDonagh AF, Watchko JF (2009) Calculated free bilirubin levels and neurotoxicity. J Perinatol 29: S14–S19

Djokomuljanto S, Quah BS, Surini Y et al (2006) Efficacy of phototherapy for neonatal jaundice is increased by the use of low-cost white reflecting curtains. Arch Dis Child Fetal Neonatal Ed 91:F439–F442

Dollberg S, Atherton HD, Hoath SB (1995) Effect of different phototherapy lights on incubator characteristics and dynamics under three modes of servocontrol. Am J Perinatol 12:55–60

Donneborg ML, Knudsen KB, Ebbesen F (2010) Effect of infants' position on serum bilirubin level during conventional phototherapy. Acta Paediatr 99: 1131–1134

Ebbesen F, Brodersen R (1982) Risk of bilirubin acid precipitation in preterm infants with respiratory distress syndrome: Considerations of blood/brain bilirubin transfer equilibrium. Early Hum Dev 6:341–355

Ebbesen F, Nyboe J (1983) Postnatal changes in the ability of plasma albumin to bind bilirubin. Acta Paediatr Scand 72:665–670

Esbjorner E (1991) Albumin binding properties in relation to bilirubin and albumin concentrations during the first week of life. Acta Paediatr Scand 80: 400–405

Figueras-Aloy J, Rodriguez-Miguelcz JM, Iriondo-Sanz M et al (2010) Intravenous immunoglobulin and necrotizing enterocolitis in newborns with hemolytic disease. Pediatrics 125:139–144

Funato M, Tamai H, Shimada S, Nakamura H (1994) Vigintiphobia, unbound bilirubin, and auditory brainstem responses. Pediatrics 93:50–53

Gottstein R, Cooke R (2003) Systematic review of intravenous immunoglobulin in haemolytic disease of the newborn. Arch Dis Child Fetal Neonatol Ed 88:F6–F10

Govaert P, Lequin M, Swarte R et al (2003) Changes in globus pallidus with (pre) term kernicterus. Pediatrics 112:1256–1263

Haddock JH, Nadler HL (1970) Bilirubin toxicity in human cultivated fibroblasts and its modification by light treatment. Proc Soc Exp Biol Med 134:45–48

Hammerman C, Vreman HJ, Kaplan M et al (1996a) Intravenous immune globulin in neonatal immune hemolytic disease: does it reduce hemolysis? Acat Paediatr 85:1351–1353

Hammerman C, Kaplan M, Vreman HJ et al (1996b) Intravenous immune globulin in neonatal ABO isoimmunization: Factors associated with clinical efficacy. Biol Neonate 170:69–74

Hansen TWR (1997) Acute management of extreme neonatal jaundice – the potential benefits of intensified phototherapy and interruption of enterohepatic bilirubin circulation. Acta Paediatr 86:843–846

Hansen TWR, Nietsch L, Norman E et al (2009) Reversibility of acute intermediate phase bilirubin encephalopathy. Acta Paediatr 98:1689–1694

Harris MC, Bernbaum JC, Polin JR et al (2001) Developmental follow-up of breastfed term and near-term infants with marked hyperbilirubinemia. Pediatrics 107:1075–1080

Hegyi T, Graff M, Zapanta V et al (1986) Transcutaneous bilirubinometry III Dermal bilirubin kinetics under green and blue light phototherapy. Am J Dis Child 140:994–997

Hintz SR, Stevenson DK, Wong R et al (2011) Is phototherapy exposure associated with better or worse outcomes in 501- to 1000-g-birth-weight infants? Acta Paediatr 100:960–965

Hulzebos CV, Dijk PH, van Imhoff DE et al (2014) The bilirubin albumin ratio in the management of hyperbilirubinemia in preterm infants to improve neurodevelopmental outcome: a randomized controlled trial – the BARTrial. PLoS One 9, e99466

Ip S, Glicken S, Kulig J et al (2003) Management of neonatal hyperbilirubinemia. AHRQ Publication, Rockville

Ip S, Chung M, Kulig J et al (2004) An evidence-based review of important issues concerning neonatal hyperbilirubinemia. Pediatrics 114:e130–e153

Jackson JC (1997) Adverse events associated with exchange transfusion in healthy and ill newborns. Pediatrics 99, e7

Jährig K, Jährig D, Meisel P (1982) Dependence of the efficiency of phototherapy on plasma bilirubin concentration. Acta Paediatr Scand 71:293–299

Kaplan M, Kaplan E, Hammerman C et al (2006) Post-phototherapy neonatal bilirubin rebound: a potential cause of significant hyperbilirubinaemia. Arch Dis Child 91:31–34

Kappas A (2004) A method for interdicting the development of severe jaundice in newborns by inhibiting the production of bilirubin. Pediatrics 113:119–123

Kappas A, Drummond GS, Munson DP, Marshall JR (2001) Sn-mesoporphyrin interdiction of severe hyperbilirubinemia in Jehovah's Witness newborns as an alternative to exchange transfusion. Pediatrics 108:1374–1377

Kara S, Ulu-ozkan H, Yilmaz Y et al (2013) Necrotizing enterocolitis in a newborn following intravenous immunoglobulin treatment for haemolytic disease. J Coll Physicians Surg Pak 23:598–600

Keenan WJ, Novak KK, Sutherland JM et al (1985) Morbidity and mortality associated with exchange transfusion. Pediatrics (Suppl) 75:417–421

Kopelman AE, Brown RS, Odell GB (1972) The "bronze" baby syndrome: A complication of phototherapy. J Pediatr 81:466–472

Krishnan L, Pathare A (2011) Necrotizing enterocolitis in a term neonate following intravenous immunoglobin therapy. Indian J Pediatr 78:743–744

Krishnan L, Pathare A (2012) Author's Reply. Correspondence in regard to necrotizing enterocolitis in a term neonate following intravenous immunoglobulin therapy. Indian J Pediatr 79:1677

Lai YC, Yew YW 2015 Neonatal blue light phototherapy and melanocytic nevus count in children: a systemic review and meta-analysis of observational studies. Ped Dermatology https://doi.org/10.1111/pde.12730. [Epub ahead of print]

Lamola AA, Eisinger J, Blumberg WE et al (1979) Fluorometric study of the partition of bilirubin among blood components: basis for rapidmicorassays of bilirubin and bilirubin binding capacity in whole blood. Anal Biochem 100:25–42

Lau SP, Fung KP (1984) Serum bilirubin kinetics in intermittent phototherapy of physiological jaundice. Arch Dis Child 59:892–894

Lightner DA, McDonagh AF (1984) Molecular mechanisms of phototherapy for neonatal jaundice. Acc Chem Res 17:417–424

Lipsitz PJ, Gartner LM, Bryla DA (1985) Neonatal and infant mortality in relationship to phototherapy. Pediatrics 75(Suppl):422–441

Louis D, More K, Oberoi S et al (2014) Intravenous immunoglobulin in isoimmune haemolytic disease of newborn: an updated systematic review and meta-analysis. Arch Dis Child Fetal Neonatal 99:F1–F7

Maayan-Metzger A, Yosipovitch G, Hadad E et al (2001) Transepidermal water loss and skin hydration in preterm infants during phototherapy. Am J Perinatol 18:393–396

Maisels MJ (1996) Why use homeopathic doses of phototherapy? Pediatrics 98:283–287

Maisels MJ (2001) Phototherapy – traditional and nontraditional. J Perinatol 21:S93–S97

Maisels MJ, Kring E (2002) Rebound in serum bilirubin level following intensive phototherapy. Arch Pediatr Adolesc Med 156:669–672

Maisels MJ, Kring EA (2006a) Does intensive phototherapy produce hemolysis in newborns of 35 or more weeks gestation? J Perinatol 26:498–500

Maisels MJ, Kring E (2006b) The contribution of hemolysis to early jaundice in normal newborns. Pediatrics 118:276–279

Maisels MJ, McDonagh AF (2008) Phototherapy for neonatal jaundice. N Engl J Med 358:920–928

Maisels MJ, Watchko JF (2003) Treatment of jaundice in low birthweight infants. Arch Dis Child Fetal Neonatol Ed 88:F459–F463

Maisels MJ, Kring EA, DeRidder J (2007) Randomized controlled trial of light-emitting diode phototherapy. J Perinatol 27:565–567

Maisels MJ, Watchko JF, Bhutani VK, Stevenson DK (2012) An approach to the management of hyperbilirubinemiain the preterm infant less than 35 weeks of gestation. J Perinatol 32:660–664

Mallon E, Wojnarowska F, Hope P, Elder G (1995) Neonatal bullous eruption as a result of transient porphyrinemia in a premature infant with hemolytic disease of the newborn. J Am Acad Dermatol 33:333–336

Martinez JC, Maisels MJ, Otheguy L et al (1993) Hyperbilirubinemia in the breastfed newborn: a controlled trial of four interventions. Pediatrics 91:470–473

Maurer HM, Kirkpatrick BV, McWilliams NB et al (1985) Phototherapy for hyperbilirubinemia of hemolytic disease of the newborn. Pediatrics (Suppl) 75:407–412

McDonagh AF (1990) Is bilirubin good for you? Clin Perinatol 17:359–369

McDonagh AF, Maisels MJ (2006) Bilirubin unbound: deja vu all over again? Pediatrics 117:523–525

Messner KH, Maisels MJ, Leure-DuPree AE (1978) Phototoxicity to the newborn primate retina. Invest Ophthalmol Vis Sci 17:178182

Moll M, Goelz R, Naegele T, Wilke M, Poets CF (2011) Are recommended phototherapy thresholds safe enough for extremely low birth weight (ELBW) infants? A report on 2 ELBW infants with kernicterus despite only moderate hyperbilirubinemia. Neonatology 99:90–94

Morris BH, Oh W, Tyson JE et al (2008) Aggressive vs. conservative phototherapy for infants with extremely low birth weight. New Engl J Med 359:1885–1896

Mreihil K, McDonagh AF, Nakstad B et al (2010) Early isomerization of bilirubin in phototherapy of neonatal jaundice. Pediatr Res 67:656–659

Mreihil K, Madsen P, Nakstad B et al (2015) Early formation of bilirubin isomers during phototherapy for neonatal jaundice: effects of single vs. double flourescent lamps vs. photodiodes. Pediatr Res 78:56–62

Nakamura H, Yonetani M, Uetani Y et al (1992) Determination of serum unbound bilirubin for prediction of kernicterus in low birth weight infants. Acta Paediatr Jpn 54:642–647

National Institute for Health and Clinical Excellence (2010) Neonatal jaundice. www.nice.org.uk/CG98

Navarro M, Negre S, Matoses ML et al (2009) Necrotizing enterocolitis following the use of intravenous immunoglobulin for haemolytic disease of the newborn. Acta Paediatr 98:1214–1217

Newman TB, Maisels MJ (1990) Does hyperbilirubinemia damage the brain of healthy full-term infants? Clin Perinatol 17:331–358

Newman TB, Liljestrand P, Jeremy RJ et al (2006) Outcomes among newborns with total serum bilirubin levels of 25 mg per deciliter or more. N Engl J Med 354:1889–1900

Newman TB, Kuzniewicz MW, Liljestrand P et al (2009) Numbers needed to treat with phototherapy according to American academy of pediatrics guidelines. Pediatrics 123:1352–1359

Oh W, Tyson JE, Fanaroff AA et al (2003) Association between peak serum bilirubin and neurodevelopmental outcomes in extremely low birth weight infants. Pediatrics 112:773–779

Oh W, Stevenson DK, Tyson JE et al (2010) Influence of clinical status on the association between plasma total and unbound bilirubin and death or adverse neurodevelopmental outcomes in extremely low birth weight infants. Acta Paediatr 99:673–678

Paller AS, Eramo LR, Farrell EE et al (1997) Purpuric phototherapy-induced eruption in transfused neonates: relation to transient porphyrinemia. Pediatrics 100: 360–364

Patra K, Storfer-Isser A, Siner B (2004) Adverse events associated with neonatal exchange transfusion in the 1990s. J Pediatr 144:626–631

Procianoy RS, Silveira RC, Fonseca LT et al (2010) The influence of phototherapy on serum cytokine concentrations in newborn infants. Am J Perinatol 27: 375–379

Rennie JM, Sehgal A, De A et al (2009) Range of UK practice regarding thresholds for phototherapy and exchange transfusion in neonatal hyperbilirubinaemia. Arch Dis Child Fetal Neonatol Ed 94:F323–F327

Robertson L, Harrild K (2010) Maternal and neonatal risk factors for childhood type 1 diabetes: a matched case–control study. BMC Public Health 10:281

Rogerson AG, Grossman ER, Gruber HS et al (1986) 14 years of experience with home phototherapy. Clin Pediatr 25:296–299

Roman E, Ansell P, Bull D (1997) Leukaemia and non-Hodgkin's lymphoma in children and young adults: are prenatal and neonatal factors important determinants of disease? Brit J Cancer 76:406–415

Rubaltelli FF, Jori G, Reddi E (1983) Bronze baby syndrome: A new porphyrin-related disorder. Pediatr Res 17:327–330

Rubaltelli FF, Guerrini P, Reddi E, Jori G (1989) Tin-protoporphyrin in the management of children with Crigler-Najjar disease. Pediatrics 84:728–731

Rübo J, Albrecht K, Lasch P et al (1992) High-dose intravenous immune globulin therapy for hyperbilirubinemia caused by Rh hemolytic disease. J Pediatr 121:93–97

Santos MC, Sa CA, Gomes SC, Camacho LA et al (2013) High-dose intravenous immunoglobulin therapy for hyperbilirubinemia due to Rh hemolytic disease: a randomized clinical trial. Transfusion 53:777–782

Scheidt PC, Graubard BI, Nelson KB et al (1991) Intelligence at six years in relation to neonatal bilirubin level: follow-up of the National Institute of Child Health and Human Development Clinical Trial of Phototherapy. Pediatrics 87:797–805

Schulz S, Wong RJ, Vreman HJ et al (2012) Metalloporphyrins – an update. Front Pharmacol 3:68

Sedlak TW, Snyder SH (2004) Bilirubin benefits: cellular protection by a biliverdin reductase antioxidant cycle. Pediatrics 113:17761782

Seidman DS, Moise J, Ergaz Z et al (2003) A prospective randomized controlled study of phototherapy using blue and blue-green light-emitting devices, and conventional halogen-quartz phototherapy. J Perinatol 23:123–127

Shinwell ES, Sciaky Y, Karplus M (2002) Effect of position changing on bilirubin levels during phototherapy. J Perinatol 22:226–229

Silberberg DH, Johnson L, Schutta H et al (1970) Effects of photodegradation products of bilirubin on myelinating cerebellum cultures. J Pediatr 77:613–618

Sims ME (2011) Legal briefs: Kernicterus still preventable. NeoReviews 12:e727–e730

Sisson TR, Whalen LE, Telel A (1958) A comparison of effects of whole blood and sedimented erythrocytes in exchange transfusion. Pediatrics 21:81–89

Slater L, Brewer MF (1984) Home versus hospital phototherapy for term infants with hyperbilirubinemia: a comparative study. Pediatrics 73:515–519

Slusher TM, Vreman HJ, Olusanya BO et al (2014) Safety and efficacy of filtered sunlight in treatment of jaundice in African neonates. Pediatrics 133:e1568–e1574

Slusher TM, Olusanya BO, Vreman HJ et al (2015) A randomized trial of phototherapy with filtered sunlight in African neonates. New Engl J Med 373:1115–1124

Smits-Wintjens VEHJ, Walther FJ et al (2011) Intravenous immunoglobulin in neonates with rhesus hemolytic disease: a randomized controlled trial. Pediatrics 127: 680–686

Sproul A, Smith L (1964) Bilirubin equilibration during exchange transfusion in hemolytic disease of the newborn. J Pediatr 65:12–26

Strauss KA, Robinson DL, Vreman HJ et al (2006) Management of hyperbilirubinemia and prevention of kernicterus in 20 patients with Crigler-Najjar disease. Eur J Pediatr 165:306–319

Sugama S, Soeda A, Eto Y (2001) Magnetic resonance imaging in three children with kernicterus. Pediatr Neurol 25:328–331

Tan KL (1982) The pattern of bilirubin response to phototherapy for neonatal hyperbilirubinemia. Pediatr Res 16:670–674

Tatli MM, Minnet C, Kocyigit A et al (2008) Phototherapy increases DNA damage in lymphocytes of hyperbilirubinemic neonates. Mutat Res 654:93–95

Tonz O, Vogt J, Filippini L et al (1975) Severe light dermatosis following phototherapy in a newborn infant with congenital erythropoietic uroporphyria. Helv Paediatr Acta 30:47–56

Tyson JE, Pedroza C, Langer J et al (2012) Does aggressive phototherapy increase mortality while decreasing profound impairment among the smallest and sickest newborns? J Perinatol 32:677–684

Valaes T (1963) Bilirubin distribution and dynamics of bilirubin removal by exchange transfusion. Acta Paediatr 52(suppl 149):1–115

Valaes T, Petmezaki S, Henschke C et al (1994) Control of jaundice in preterm newborns by an inhibitor of bilirubin production: studies with tin-mesoporphyrin. Pediatrics 93:1–11

Vandborg PK, Hansen BM, Greisen G et al (2012) Dose–response relationship of phototherapy for hyperbilirubinemia. Pediatrics 130:e352–e357

Vogl TP, Hegyi T, Hiatt IM et al (1978) Intermittent phototherapy in the treatment of jaundice in the premature infant. J Pediatr 92:627–630

Voto LS, Sexer H, Ferreiro G et al (1995) Neonatal adminstration of high-dose intravenous immunoglobulin and rhesus hemolytic disease. J Perinat Med 23:443–451

Vreman HJ, Wong RJ, Stevenson DK (2004) Phototherapy: current methods and future directions. Semin Perinatol 28:326–333

Watchko JF (2000) Exchange transfusion in the management of neonatal hyperbilirubinemia. In: Maisels MJ, Watchko JF (eds) Neonatal Jaundice. Harwood Academic Publishers, London, pp 169–176

Watchko JF (2014) Recent advances in the management of neonatal jaundice. Res Rep Neonatol 4:183–193

Watchko JF (2016) Bilirubin-induced neurotoxicity in the preterm neonate. Clin Perinatol 43:297–311

Watchko JF, Maisels MJ (2014) The enigma of low bilirubin kernicterus in premature infants:why does it still occur, and is it preventable? Semin Perinatol 38:397–406

Watchko JF, Tiribelli C (2013) Bilirubin-induced neurologic damage – mechanisms and management approaches. N Engl J Med 369:2021–2030

Wennberg RP, Ahlfors CE, Bhutani V et al (2006) Toward understanding kernicterus: a challenge to improve the management of jaundiced newborns. Pediatrics 117:474–485

Yamauchi Y, Casa N, Yamanouchi I (1989) Is it necessary to change the babies' position during phototherapy? Early Hum Dev 20:221–227

Yetman RJ, Parks DK, Huseby V et al (1998) Rebound bilirubin levels in infants receiving phototherapy. J Pediatr 133:705–707

Pathology and Treatment of Liver Diseases in Newborns

77

Giuseppe Maggiore, Silvia Riva, and Marco Sciveres

Contents

G. Maggiore (✉)
Department of Medical Sciences-Pediatrics, University of Ferrara, University Hospital Arcispedale Sant Anna di Cona, CONA (Ferrara), Italy
e-mail: giuseppe.maggiore@unife.it

S. Riva · M. Sciveres
Pediatric Hepatology and Liver Transplant Unit, IRCCS-ISMETT - University of Pittsburgh Medical Center (UPMC), Palermo, Italy
e-mail: sriva@ismett.edu; msciveres@ismett.edu

G. Buonocore et al. (eds.), *Neonatology*,
https://doi.org/10.1007/978-3-319-29489-6_224

Abstract

Liver disease in the newborn usually presents with two main distinct clinical syndromes: neonatal cholestasis and neonatal liver failure; in both cases, an urgent diagnosis is required. Cholestasis usually presents with *prolonged jaundice* or, less frequently, with a *hemorrhagic syndrome* related to late onset vitamin K deficiency. Cholestatic jaundice is associated with discolored stools and dark urines due to hyperbilirubinuria. Cholestasis affects approximately 1 in every 2,500 infants and its etiological spectrum is particularly wide, including conditions with severe prognosis. Diagnostic approach to a prolonged jaundice belongs to primary care pediatrician and includes diagnosing *of* its eventual cholestatic nature by evaluating abnormal stool or urine color and by measuring total and direct serum bilirubin; preventing *of* the hemorrhagic complications related to vitamin K deficiency by administrating a single intramuscular dose of vitamin K1; early suspecting biliary atresia in case of suggestive clinical picture, since the favorable outcome of surgery also relies on its precocity; and *early referring* the infant to a center experienced in the treatment of hepatobiliary disorders in childhood. Neonatal acute liver failure (NALF) is a rare and challenging condition. NALF is a multietiologic syndrome which is difficult to recognize initially. As important as the recognition of causes that may indicate specific diet and medical therapy is the selection of infants suitable for liver transplantation since mortality is high and only 25% of infants survive with their native liver. Management of *NALF* requires supporting the neonate until liver regeneration or liver transplantation takes place.

Abbreviations

AAT	Alpha-1-antitrypsin
AATD	Alpha-1-antitrypsin deficiency
AGS	Alagille syndrome
ALF	Acute liver failure
BA	Biliary atresia
EFA	Essential fatty acids
FHLH	Familial hemophagocytic lymphohistiocytosis
GALD	Gestational alloimmune liver disease
HFI	Hereditary fructose intolerance
HT1	Hereditary tyrosinemia type 1
MAS	Macrophage activation syndrome
NALF	Neonatal acute liver failure
NBAS	Neuroblastoma-amplified sequence
NH	Neonatal hemochromatosis
PFIC	Progressive familial intrahepatic cholestasis
PI	Protease inhibitor
SGA	Small for gestational age
VKDB	Vitamin K deficiency bleeding
γGT	Gamma-glutamyl transpeptidase

77.1 Salient Points

- Liver disease in the newborn usually presents with two main distinct clinical syndromes: cholestasis or neonatal liver failure; in both cases, urgent diagnosis is required.
- Cholestasis is secondary to infections, inborn errors of metabolism, genetic disorders, or biliary atresia.
- Cholestasis usually presents with prolonged jaundice or, less frequently, with a hemorrhagic syndrome related to vitamin K deficiency.
- Prolonged jaundice (more than 2 weeks) should be always considered pathological and requires a precise diagnosis by clinical features laboratory tests and ultrasonography.

- The management of neonatal cholestasis is based on early diagnosis of biliary atresia; administration of a single intramuscular dose of vitamin K to prevent hemorrhagic complications; and early referral to a center with appropriate expertise.
- Treatment of cholestasis relies on surgery for biliary atresia (Kasai procedure), specific medical therapy of the cause whenever possible, ursodeoxycholic acid, and supportive care such as nutritional therapy.
- Neonatal acute liver failure (NALF) is rare multietiologic syndrome defined by the presence of severe coagulopathy, with or without hepatic encephalopathy, appearing in a newborn with no history of known liver disease.
- NALF may have a fetal onset, with decompensation at birth, or a perinatal onset, with symptoms developing in the first 4 weeks of life.
- The most common etiologies of NALF are liver-based metabolic disorders and perinatally acquired infections.
- Management of NALF requires intensive life support and referral to a pediatric liver unit for early assessment for liver transplantation.

77.2 Neonatal Cholestasis

Cholestasis is identified by a reduction of biliary flow, with accumulation in the liver and extrahepatic tissues of substances normally excreted in the bile, such as bilirubin, cholesterol, and bile acids. In the newborn, bile acids are physiologically elevated in the serum due to a delayed maturation of biliary secretion. Cholestasis is a pathological condition secondary to a wide range of possible causes such as infections, inborn errors of metabolism, or genetic disorders of biliary transport.

Different to the more common, so-called physiologic neonatal jaundice due to increased concentration of serum indirect (unconjugated) bilirubin, cholestatic jaundice is characterized by conjugated hyperbilirubinemia. A concentration of direct bilirubin >1 mg/dl is considered abnormal for a total serum bilirubin up to 5 mg/dl. For values greater than 5 mg/dl, a direct bilirubin fraction of more than 20% of the total bilirubin is an abnormal value. It must be taken into account that the method commonly used for measuring bilirubin, the diazo or the Van den Bergh reaction, does not measure specifically conjugated bilirubin but direct bilirubin which comprises conjugated bilirubin together with the δ-bilirubin fraction.

Discolored stools and dark urines due to conjugated hyperbilirubinuria clinically identify cholestatic jaundice.

In the neonate, cholestasis usually presents with *prolonged jaundice* or, less frequently, with a *hemorrhagic syndrome* related to late onset of vitamin K deficiency. More rarely, cholestasis can present with hypocalcemic seizures due to vitamin D deficiency related to malabsorption. Hepatomegaly is a constant feature and spleen enlargement can be observed in about 50% of cases. *Pruritus* is absent in the neonatal period, but can occur from the age of 4 months on. Every newborn with a jaundice that prolongs for more than 2 weeks should be considered a pathological case and one that needs a precise diagnosis.

Cholestasis affects approximately 1 in every 2,500 infants, and its etiological spectrum is particularly wide, also including conditions with severe prognoses, such as biliary atresia, which is the single most frequent pathologic entity. Table 1 lists most of the recognized causes of neonatal cholestasis.

The diagnostic approach to a prolonged jaundice belongs to the primary care pediatrician who has the obligation to:

- *Diagnose* its eventual cholestatic nature by evaluating abnormal stool or urine color and by measuring total and direct serum bilirubin in a venous blood sample;
- *Prevent* the hemorrhagic complications secondary to vitamin K deficiency by administrating a single intramuscular dose of vitamin K1;
- *Early suspect* biliary atresia in the case of a suggestive clinical picture, given that the favorable outcome of surgery also relies on the precocity of the disease;
- *Early referral* the infant to a center experienced in the treatment of hepatobiliary disorders in childhood.

Table 1 Neonatal cholestasis: the spectrum of etiology

Site of the lesion	Disease
Whole biliary tree	Biliary atresia
	Sclerosing cholangitis with neonatal onset
	Sclerosing cholangitis and ichthyosis due to claudin I defect
Intrahepatic biliary tree	**Infections**
	Prenatal: CMV, toxoplasmosis, syphilis, rubeola
	Perinatal: disseminated bacterial infections
	Post-natal: *E. coli* pyelonephritis
	Genetic cholestasis
	Progressive familial intrahepatic cholestasis (PFIC)
	Benign recurrent intrahepatic cholestasis (BRIC)
	TJP2 cholestatic liver disease
	Alfa-1-antitrypsin deficiency
	Cystic fibrosis
	Familial cholestasis of Native Americans (Quebec)
	Niemann-Pick type II disease
	Gaucher disease
	Wolman disease
	Mucopolisaccaridosis type VI and VII
	Mucolipidosis II
	Peroxisomal disorders (Refsum disease, Zellweger disease)
	Hepatocyte nuclear factor 1β (HNF1β) deficiency
	Mitochondrial respiratory chain disorders
	Citrin deficiency
	Complex III assembly defect (GRACILE syndrome)
	Inborn error of primary bile acid synthesis
	Microvillous inclusion disease (MVID)
	Syndromic cholestasis
	Alagille syndrome
	Aagenaes syndrome
	Williams syndrome
	Kabuki syndrome
	Hardikar syndrome
	McCune-Albright syndrome
	ARC (arthrogryposis, renal dysfunction, and cholestasis) syndrome
	Donohue syndrome (Leprechaunism)
	Benign intrahepatic cholestasis
	Parenteral nutrition-induced cholestasis
	Other forms of intrahepatic cholestasis
	Cholestasis secondary to Pituitary Stalk Interruption Syndrome
	Cholestasis secondary to congenital hypothyroidism
	Cholestasis secondary to congenital hyperthyroidism or maternal Graves' disease
	Cholestasis secondary to hepatic hemangiomatosis
	Cholestasis secondary to placental chorioangioma
	Cholestasis secondary to congenital portosystemic shunt
	Cholestasis secondary to pyruvate kinase deficiency
	Post-hemolytic cholestasis
	Drug-induced cholestasis
	Cryptogenic intrahepatic cholestasis
	Cholestasis secondary to neonatal lupus
Extrahepatic biliary tree	Choledocholithiasis
	Spontaneous perforation of bile ducts
	Congenital choledochal stenosis
	Congenital choledochal dilatation (choledochal cyst)

77.3 Principal Causes of Cholestasis in the Newborn

77.3.1 Biliary Atresia

Biliary atresia (BA) is an obliterative cholangiopathy of unknown origin involving intra- and extrahepatic biliary structures. Its prevalence in Europe and the USA varies from 1:14,000 to 1:20,000 live-born. BA spontaneously progresses to cirrhosis and liver failure in the first years of life. Its treatment is principally surgical and is based on two sequential

procedures: the *Kasai procedure* or hepatoportoenterostomy corresponding to a bilio-digestive anastomosis between the porta hepatis and an intestinal Roux loop and, in case of failure of this procedure, liver transplantation (Chardot 2006). BA does not seem to be a single entity, but a pathological phenotype caused by different etiologies, including a perinatal insult that triggers an immune-mediated obliteration of the extrahepatic bile duct lumen or an embryonic or fetal defect in the normal morphogenesis of the biliary tree (Petersen and Davenport 2013). The success of the *hepatoportoenterostomy* depends on the precocity of the diagnosis and surgery (Serinet et al. 2009). Unfortunately in the early phase of the disease, the newborn with BA appears healthy, meconium is rarely discolored, stools are only moderately discolored, and jaundice is mild. In regions with high prevalence of BA, such as Taiwan (1: 2,700), a strategy based on a universal screening using a stool color card has been successfully developed (Hsiao et al. 2008). The outcome of the Kasai procedure depends on early surgery performed before the age of 6 weeks and on the caseload of the center performing the primary surgery. Long-term results of the Kasai procedure show a survival rate with the native liver at ten years in about 30% of patients and at twenty years of about 25%. At present, sequential treatment for biliary atresia results in long-term survival, with a good quality of life in more than 90% of treated patients.

77.3.2 Transitory (Benign) Neonatal Cholestasis

Transitory (benign) neonatal cholestasis is a multifactorial condition in which anoxic-ischemic factors due to perinatal disease and immaturity of bile secretions play a predominant role (Jacquemin et al. 1998). Risk factors include prematurity, perinatal asphyxia, low birth weight for gestational age, surgery, and parenteral nutrition that act synergically; SGA newborns with a perinatal hypoxic event have an incidence of cholestasis up to 33% (Champion et al. 2012).

Cholestasis develops in the first month of life. The clinical picture and course is benign and similar to that of what was formerly called *idiopathic neonatal hepatitis*. Clinical signs and abnormal liver function tests normalize within the first year of life in all patients. Liver biopsy usually shows specific findings as giant cell hepatitis, portal fibrosis and infiltration, ductular proliferation, and even steatosis.

77.3.3 Genetic Cholestasis

Genetic cholestasis includes a heterogeneous group of rare disorders of hepatobiliary transport sometimes restricted to specific geographic areas, such as the case of *Aagenaes syndrome* (also known as Norwegian cholestasis), in which recurrent cholestasis with neonatal onset is associated with lymphedema, or of *Native North American Indian childhood cirrhosis*, a familial intrahepatic cholestasis described in Ojibway-Cree children from Quebec, typically presenting with transient neonatal jaundice in an otherwise healthy infant but progressing to biliary cirrhosis. This disorder is associated with mutation of the FLJ14728 gene coding for a protein, known as cirhin, preferentially expressed in the embryonic liver, and of still unknown function.

Canalicular secretion of bile salts is the driving force behind bile flow and enterohepatic cycling of bile salts. Most of the secreted bile salts are absorbed in the terminal ileum, actively re-uptaken by the hepatocytes and finally secreted again in the bile. Most genetic diseases are caused by defects in proteins involved in this process.

Progressive familial intrahepatic cholestasis (PFIC) results from mutations in, at least, three distinct genes that encode hepatobiliary transport proteins (Davit-Spraul et al. 2009). Mutations in the FIC1 gene (also known as ATP8B1) cause a variety of different diseases according to location, severity, and zygosity of mutations. The most known is PFIC type 1, a severe, early onset form of cholestasis, described as Byler's disease, characterized by frequent progression to biliary cirrhosis. The relapsing variant of cholestasis is

called benign recurrent intrahepatic cholestasis (BRIC) type 1, while other phenotypes caused by mutations of FIC1 are *intrahepatic cholestasis of pregnancy* (*ICP*) *type 1* and *Greenland familial cholestasis*, initially described among indigenous *Inuit* families in *Greenland* and thereafter reconducted among the spectrum of the FIC1-related diseases.

Similarly, mutations in the bile salt export pump (BSEP) gene (also known as ABCB11) cause *PFIC type 2* or *BRIC type 2* as well as *ICP type 2* and even chronic gallstone disease. Serum *gamma-glutamyltransferase* (*γGT*) activity is low to normal in PFIC types 1 and 2.

PFIC type 3 is caused by mutations in the MDR3 gene (also known as ABCB4) coding for a phospholipid translocator in the canalicular membrane. Because of their inability to secrete phospholipids, patients with *PFIC type 3* produce free bile acid-rich bile that damages the cholangiocytes of intrahepatic bile ducts. Serum γGT activity is elevated in these patients.

Ursodeoxycholic acid therapy is useful for patients with a partial defect. Liver transplantation is a more definitive therapy for patients with severe defects.

A new promising tool for the treatment of monogenic defects of bile secretion is the use of chaperone drugs, which, in some instances, might be capable of enhance canalicular localizations of otherwise functional transporters. In some PFIC2 patients with missense mutations, BSEP is not detected at the canaliculus level owing to mistrafficking of BSEP mutants. In these patients, 4-phenylbutyrate (4-PB), a well-known chaperone drug, has been shown to partially correct mistrafficking both in vitro and in vivo leading to a significative improvement of the clinical picture (Gonzales et al. 2015).

Another cause of progressive cholestasis with neonatal onset is related to mutations of *TJP2*, a cytosolic component of several classes of cell-cell junctions, essential for hepatobiliary integrity. A single, incompletely penetrant, homozygous missense mutation of TJP2 has been identified in Amish individuals with familial hypercholanemia, a disorder manifesting with pruritus, fat malabsorption, and transient neonatal cholestasis but without the features of a progressive liver disease.

In contrast, more severe mutations, which probably abolish the translation of the protein, are responsible of a progressive liver disease, very similar to PFIC 1-2 (Sambrotta et al. 2014). Serum γGT may be normal or moderately elevated in these patients.

Another cholestatic disease akin to PFIC-2 may occur in children with defects of *MYO5B* gene, responsible for *microvillous inclusion disease* (MVID), a congenital disorder of the enterocyte leading to intractable diarrhea often necessitating intestinal transplantation and in children with mutations in VPS33B or in VIPAR genes in the *arthrogryposis-renal dysfunction-cholestasis* (*ARC*) *syndrome*.

In both cases the BSEP protein, although correctly expressed, could not reach the canalicular membrane because of a defect of intracellular trafficking mechanisms.

Inborn errors of bile acid synthesis are rare genetic disorders that can present as neonatal cholestasis. These disorders are characterized by a failure to synthesize normal bile acids, with an accumulation of unusual bile acids and/or bile acid intermediaries. Cholesterol is converted to cholic and chenodeoxycholic acid through a series of reactions involving modifications of the steroid nucleus and oxidation of the side chain. Inborn errors have been shown for single enzymes involved both in modifications of the sterol nucleus and in steps in modification of the side chain. Unusual bile acids or bile alcohols, once synthesized, can be identified for diagnostic purposes, using gas chromatography-mass spectrometry and fast atom bombardment mass spectrometry techniques.

Individuals with inborn errors of bile acid synthesis generally present with cholestasis, low/normal serum bile acid concentrations, normal γGT serum activity, and the absence of pruritus. Failure to diagnose any of these conditions can result in liver failure or early progressive chronic liver damage. If recognized early, most of patients have a remarkable clinical response to oral bile acid therapy.

Two main defects that influence the modifications of the steroid nucleus have been well characterized: the 3β-hydroxy-Δ5-C^{27}-steroid dehydrogenase deficiency, the most frequent, and the 3-oxo-Δ4-steroid 5β-reductase deficiency. Diagnosis of the latter can be problematic because a similar pattern of metabolite excretion can occur as a result of unspecific liver damage caused by viruses or inborn errors of pathways unrelated to bile acid synthesis. The 3β-hydroxy-Δ5-C^{27}-steroid dehydrogenase catalyzes an early step in the synthesis of bile acids from cholesterol. Patients with autosomal recessive mutations in the encoding gene, HSD3B7, fail to synthesize bile acids and develop cholestatic jaundice and malabsorption of lipids (Jacquemin et al. 1994). Pathological findings may include intralobular cholestasis with giant cell transformation and hepatic injury confined to the portal limiting plate where the smallest bile ductules may be injured and where fibrosis typically develops. Interlobular bile ducts are usually spared. Ultrastructure of the liver reveals nonspecific changes. Liver disease improves dramatically on treatment with cholic acid, which produces beneficial feedback inhibition of abnormal bile acid production and enhances choleresis.

Defective side chain oxidation in patients with cerebrotendinous xanthomatosis (CTX) leads to synthesis of bile alcohols, but patients with CTX usually do not show a cholestatic liver disease. Their major problems (neurological damage, atherosclerosis, and xanthomata) are caused by an accumulation of cholestanol and cholesterol in the tissues, while bile acid precursors are probably diverted into synthesis of cholestanol. Chenodeoxycholic acid suppresses the production of abnormal metabolites from cholesterol (by inhibition of cholesterol 7 α-hydroxylase) and leads to improvement of the neurological disease. Defective side chain oxidation also occurs in peroxisomal disorders, leading to accumulation of C^{27} bile acids such as trihydroxycoprostanic acid (THCA).

Alagille syndrome (AGS) is an autosomal-dominant disorder with variable penetrance and a prevalence of approximately 1 in 70,000 live births (Alagille et al. 1987). AGS may present in the neonatal period with cholestasis that may be severe enough to suggest biliary atresia. AGS is characterized by five principal features: chronic cholestasis resulting from paucity of interlobular bile ducts, peripheral pulmonary artery stenosis, butterfly-like vertebral arch defect, posterior embryotoxon, and peculiar *facies* (Fig. 1). In the complete form of the syndrome, all five features are observed, though incomplete or partial forms exist. Other, less frequent features include growth retardation, renal and bone abnormalities, and ocular abnormalities – such as optic disc drusen, angulated retinal vessels, pigmentary retinopathy, and vascular intracranial abnormalities.

Jagged 1 gene (JAG1) has been identified as the responsible for coding for a cell surface protein that functions in an embryologically important signaling pathway, known as the Notch signaling pathway. Defects of the Notch pathway can affect angiogenesis. Mutations in JAG1 can be identified in at least 70% of AGS, though they are inherited in only 30% of cases. These JAG1 mutations include total gene deletions, as well as mutations (frameshift, missense, and nonsense) in almost all regions of the gene.

Therapy consists in nutritional supplementation of medium-chain triglycerides, essential fatty acids, and fat-soluble vitamins. Liver transplantation has been used successfully to treat patients with liver failure, portal hypertension, or severe pruritus and xanthomatosis (Fig. 2).

Alpha-1-antitrypsin deficiency (AATD) is a genetic disorder that can manifest as neonatal cholestasis or chronic liver disease in infancy and

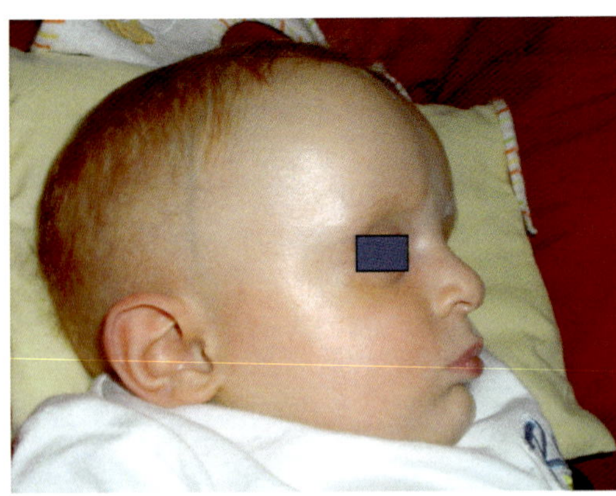

Fig. 1 Alagille syndrome: typical facies

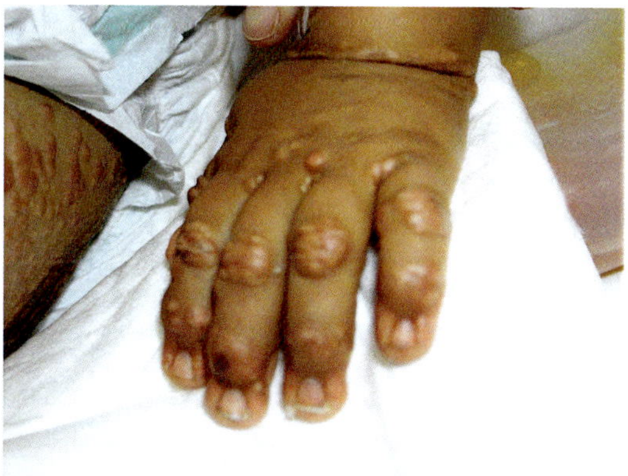

Fig. 2 Alagille syndrome: diffuse xanthomata

childhood, pulmonary emphysema in adulthood, and, more rarely, skin panniculitis or membranoproliferative glomerulonephritis (Primhak and Tanner 2001). AATD is caused by mutations in the SERPINA1 gene encoding alpha-1-antitrypsin (AAT) and is inherited as an autosomal recessive trait. AATD is characterized by low serum levels of AAT, that is, the main human protease inhibitor (PI). The prevalence of AATD in Western Europe and in the USA is estimated at approximately 1 in 2,500/5,000 newborns and is dependent on Scandinavian descent in the population. The most common deficiency alleles in Northern Europe are PI Z and PI S, and the majority of individuals with severe AATD are PIZZ. The mutant Z protein product is synthesized in hepatocytes but then accumulates intracellularly rather than being appropriately secreted, thus causing hepatocellular injury. Ten percent of PI-ZZ AATD infants present with cholestatic jaundice, with an incidence of 1:10,000/20,000 newborns, but only 5% of them will develop a severe progressive cholestatic liver disease that would need an early liver transplant. In the majority of cases, clinical jaundice disappears, but clinical and biochemical features of chronic liver disease may persist and progress to biliary cirrhosis later in the pediatric age. The variable clinical presentations suggest an important contribution of genetic and environmental disease modifiers. In PIZZ homozygotes, specific globules, due to accumulation of AAT, are seen in hepatocytes.

Ursodeoxycholic acid therapy may significantly improve clinical status and liver laboratory test results in children with liver disease associated with AATD. No beneficial effect of UDCA has been shown in children in case of a most severe liver involvement: these patients are candidates for liver transplantation.

77.4 Management of a Cholestatic Newborn

The main goal of management of an infant with cholestasis is to detect or at least to exclude biliary atresia within 45–60 days of age. History and physical examination, together with simple laboratory tests and a liver ultrasound, will allow clinicians to reach this objective in the majority of cases. Decolorized stools associated with a hard palpable liver will strongly suggest BA. Unfortunately, there is no single laboratory test that is able to confirm or exclude BA; however, biochemical evaluation will allow clinicians to (Bernard 1998):

- *Confirm* the cholestatic nature of the jaundice by measuring in a venous blood sample, the direct bilirubin, that should be greater than 1 mg/dl. Cholestasis will be confirmed by measuring the total serum bile acid levels. A non-cholestatic increase of direct bilirubin characterizes two autosomal recessive inherited inborn errors of bilirubin transport: *Dubin-Johnson syndrome*, which is due to mutations of the MRP2 gene, and *Rotor syndrome* which is due to biallelic inactivating mutations in the closely linked genes *SLCO1B1* and *SLCO1B3* that result in complete functional deficiencies of both protein products OATP1B1 and OATP1B3, respectively.
- *Distinguish* a cholestatic jaundice from a jaundice related to liver failure where a non-vitamin K-dependent coagulopathy exists.
- *Exclude* other causes of cholestasis, such as α-1-antitrypsin deficiency, by examining the protein electrophoretic pattern (the absence of α1 globulin peak) or cystic fibrosis by a normal sweat test. A normal eye examination and a column x-ray showing the absence of butterfly vertebrae will be against a diagnosis of *Alagille syndrome*.

In biliary atresia, the total bilirubin serum levels do not generally exceed 6–8 mg/dl, aminotransferase activity is generally increased with an aspecific pattern, and alkaline phosphatase activity measurement is not helpful due to the high activity physiologically present in the newborn infant.

Gamma-glutamyl transpeptidase activity has been used, in the past, to distinguish biliary atresia from intrahepatic cholestasis, but wide variability in serum activity makes interpretation of test results difficult. The degree of elevation of γGT is not useful in discriminating the etiology of the cholestasis, even if a normal γGT level suggests genetic and metabolic causes of intracellular cholestasis (Maggiore et al. 1991). Serum bile acids are, by definition, elevated in cholestasis: normal values or only slight increase in cholestatic infants with low to normal γGT level suggests an inborn error of bile acid synthesis. Urinanalysis and culture are diagnostic in case of cholestasis secondary to *E. coli* urinary infection.

Ultrasonography is recommended for the diagnostic evaluation of the infant with cholestasis. Ultrasound imaging is the most operator dependent and thus may be most appropriately performed at the referral center by experienced personnel.

Although biliary atresia could not be positively identified, there are a number of indirect signs that may synergically suggest diagnosis of AVB. The most important are the so-called triangular cord sign, an area of hyperechogenicity between the bifurcation of main portal branches and a small or absent gallbladder. Anatomic abnormalities such as poly/asplenia, pre-duodenal portal vein, complete situs inversus, or cystic dilatation at porta hepatis are commonly associated with BA. More recently, vascular findings at color-Doppler examination such us diameter and flux of portal vein, diameter and resistance index of hepatic artery, and the presence of subcapsular flow have been identified as good markers of suspicion of BA especially if combined with the other signs (Lee et al. 2009).

Hepatobiliary scintigraphy is time consuming and expensive and generally adds little to the routine evaluation of the cholestatic infant due to the low specificity (significant number of false-positive and false-negative results of the test).

Percutaneous liver biopsy can be performed safely in young infants and can provide disease-specific findings. Examples include PAS-positive granules in alpha-1 antitrypsin deficiency, ductal paucity in Alagille syndrome, necroinflammatory duct lesions in sclerosing cholangitis, and other findings that are relatively specific for metabolic and storage diseases. Liver biopsy has a very high sensitivity and specificity for the diagnosis of BA. However, because of the dynamic and progressive nature of extrahepatic biliary atresia, even this test can be misleading. Biopsy interpretation is, nonetheless, pathologist dependent and requires expertise in pediatric liver disease (Moyer et al. 2004).

77.5 Treatment of a Cholestatic Newborn Infant

Specific medical treatment of neonatal cholestasis is directed at the cause, as in the case of cholestasis, which is associated with urinary tract infection, hypothyroidism, hypopituitarism, congenital toxoplasmosis, or syphilis.

Ursodeoxycholic acid, at high dose (25 mg/kg/day), is effective and safe in some cholestatic conditions of infancy, such as parenteral nutrition-associated cholestasis, progressive intrahepatic cholestasis of infancy (particularly in PFIC 3), α-1-antitripsin deficiency, cystic fibrosis, biliary atresia after successful Kasai procedure, and post-hemolytic cholestasis. In case of severe itching, rifampicin (10 mg/kg/day) can be administered.

If there is no specific therapy, treatment is supportive and consists primarily of nutritional therapy, including supplements of vitamins A, D, E, and K.

In infants with chronic cholestasis, oral replacement therapy of the fat-soluble vitamins may prove extremely difficult because of low concentrations of intraluminal bile acids. Water-soluble forms of vitamin E, d-alpha-tocopheryl polyethylene glycol-1000 succinate, have enabled correction of vitamin E deficiency states in these patients. Exclusively, breastfed infants, in general, are at risk of hypovitaminosis D and at even greater risk in the absence of adequate exposure to sunlight or when the maternal diet is not

sufficient to provide for vitamin D requirements. Vitamin K prophylaxis at birth by intramuscular administration of 1 mg of vitamin K1 effectively prevents vitamin K deficiency bleeding. Breastfed infants with cholestasis are not fully protected against late onset vitamin K deficiency and should be given oral supplements of vitamin K.

For formula-fed infants, a formula that is high in medium-chain triglycerides should be used because it is better absorbed in the presence of bile salt deficiency. Adequate calories and protein intake are required: infants may need more than 130 cal/kg day and 2–3 g of protein/day.

Infants with persistent cholestasis are at a high risk for essential fatty acid (EFA) deficiency, particularly of the omega-6 fatty acids and linoleic and arachidonic acids. EFA deficiency appears to be related to fat malabsorption, hepatic EFA metabolism, enhanced lipid peroxidation, and dietary intake.

77.6 Neonatal Acute Liver Failure

Neonatal acute liver failure (NALF) is a rare and challenging condition. NALF is a multietiologic syndrome that has a difficult early detection. In addition to recognizing the causes that represent an indication to specific diet or medical therapy, it is also important to early select infants eligible for liver transplantation, since only 25% of infants with NALF will survive with their native liver. NALF management requires supporting the neonate until liver regeneration or liver transplantation occurs.

77.7 Definition

The definition of NALF is controversial. In adults, acute liver failure (ALF) is defined by the onset of hepatic encephalopathy within 8 weeks from the first symptoms (generally jaundice) in the absence of pre-existing liver disease. This definition is unsatisfactory in infancy because encephalopathy is a late event in the disease. Furthermore, illness duration can be difficult to assess, particularly in infants presenting ALF in the first few weeks of life secondary to a condition that may be caused by unrecognized metabolic diseases. For all these reasons, the pediatric acute liver failure study group has reached a consensus defining ALF in infancy as a "coagulopathy due to liver dysfunction, not corrected by vitamin K administration, in a patient with no history of known liver disease, with an INR >1.5, if the patient has encephalopathy, or >2.0, if the patient does not have encephalopathy" (Bucuvalas et al. 2006). Moreover, NALF can be also defined only by the presence of severe coagulopathy (prothrombin time >17 s and/or factor V <50%) appearing in the first 4 weeks of life, regardless of the presence of hepatic encephalopathy (Dhawan and Mieli Vergani 2005; Durand et al. 2001).

77.8 Etiology

NALF can be classified according to the timing of liver damage onset. In case of onset during fetal life, a chronic liver damage will develop "in utero" with decompensation at birth. In case of onset in the perinatal period, acute liver damage will develop early after birth with no underlying liver disease. Table 2 lists most of the recognized causes of NALF. The most common etiologies are liver-based metabolic disorders and perinatally acquired infections (Table 3) (McClean and Davison 2003).

77.8.1 Neonatal Hemochromatosis

Neonatal hemochromatosis (NH) is a rare clinical condition in which severe liver disease develops in the fetus and in the newborn, accompanied by massive intrahepatic and extrahepatic (pancreas, heart, thyroid, salivary glands) tissue iron storage (siderosis) sparing the reticuloendothelial system.

Liver injury has been identified as early as 28 weeks of gestation. The etiology of this condition is not fully clear and probably represents an endpoint of previous insults (viral, immunological) to the fetal liver. Previous miscarriages are generally recorded and oligohydramnios or

Table 2 Causes of neonatal acute liver failure

Causes
Fetal onset
Neonatal hemochromatosis
Hemophagocytic lymphohistiocytosis
Mitochondrial respiratory chain disorders
Mitochondrial hepatopathy
Complex I deficiency
Complex IV deficiency (SCO1 mutations)
Complex III deficiency (*BCS1L* mutations)
Multiple complex deficiencies
Mitochondria-specific tRNA-modifying enzyme, tRNA 5-methylaminomethyl-2-thiouridylate methyltransferase (*TRMU* gene)
Mitochondrial DNA depletion syndrome
Deoxyguanosine kinase (dGK) deficiency
DGUOK, MPV17, POLG gene mutations
Complex III/IV (cytochrome oxidase) assembly defect
Inborn disorders of bile acid synthesis
Oxysterol 7α-hydroxylase deficiency
Di-/trihydroxycholestanoic acidemia
Δ4-3-Oxosteroid 5β reductase deficiency
Neonatal lupus
Neonatal veno-occlusive disease
Neonatal leukemia
Perinatal onset
Viral infections
Enterovirus
Echovirus 11
Echovirus 6 and 9, *Coxsackie*
Herpes virus
Herpes simplex virus 1 and 2
HHV6
Parvovirus B19, *Adenovirus*, *Paramyxovirus*
Inborn metabolic disorders
Galactosemia
Hereditary tyrosinemia type 1
Hereditary fructose intolerance
Urea cycle disorders
Bacterial infections
Drug (paracetamol)
Ischemic (shock liver syndrome)
Undetermined

polyhydramnios can complicate the pregnancy. Due to a recurrence rate in sibships higher than the one predicted for simple Mendelian autosomal recessive inheritance, thus suggesting a possible role of maternal transmission, it has been

Table 3 Etiology and diagnostic screening in case of neonatal liver failure

Etiology	Diagnostic screening
Infections	
Enterovirus	Viral culture and detection in blood, urine, and stools
HSV 1 and 2	CSF by nuclear acid testing
HHV6	Viral serology in mother and infant
Adenovirus	
Parvovirus B19	
Bacterial	Blood culture
Metabolic	
Galactosemia	Reduced red blood cell galactose-1-phosphate uridyl transferase activity
HFI	Mutations of HFI gene
HT1	Elevated urinary excretion of succinylacetone; elevated excessive amounts of δ-aminolevulinic acid; in urine elevated serum αfetoprotein
IE bile acid synthesis	Total serum bile acids; FAB-MS and GC-MS urine analysis
Urea cycle disorders	Plasma amino acids; urinary orotic acid
CDGS	Transferrin iso-electrofocusing
NH	Serum ferritin levels, saturation of transferrin; MRI
Mitochondrial disorders	Fasting and postprandial lactate; plasma lactate/pyruvate ratio >20; genetics
Infiltrative/storage	
HLH	Bone marrow examination
Leukemia	
Niemann-Pick type II	
Others	
Neonatal lupus	Maternal autoantibodies of the Ro/La family
Drug	
Hypoxic/ischemia	

HSV herpes simplex virus, *HHV6* human herpes virus 6, *HFI* hereditary fructose intolerance, *HT1* hereditary tyrosinemia type 1, *MRCD* mitochondrial respiratory chain disorders, *IE bile salts* inborn errors of bile salt synthesis, *CDGS* congenital disorders of glycosylation syndrome, *NH* neonatal hemochromatosis, *HLH* hemophagocytic lymphohistiocytosis, *GALT* galactose-1-phosphate uridyl transferase, *FAB-MS* fast atom bombardment ionization-mass spectrometry, *GC-MS* gas chromatography-mass spectrometry, *MRI* magnetic resonance imaging, *CSF* cerebrospinal fluid

suggested that maternal alloimmunity may play a part in this recurrence. In fact, evidence suggests that most cases are due to a gestational disease with transplacental transfer of maternal IgG antibodies targeting the fetal liver resulting in immune injury.

Gestational alloimmune liver disease (GALD) is defined by a complement-mediated hepatocyte injury as a primary disease mechanism. The alloimmune target is believed to be a fetal hepatocyte cell surface antigen, with subsequent complement activation (C5b-9 complex) resulting in severe loss of hepatocytes and fetal iron overload. This cascade of events leads to ALF and neonatal death. Moreover, immunomodulation during at-risk pregnancy appears to reduce the severity of disease in most of cases.

Clinical manifestations can occur in utero or immediately after birth. Neonates affected are often premature and/or small for date. The usual presentation is an end-stage liver disease in the first few days of life with hypoglycemia, coagulopathy, hyperammonemia, jaundice, irritability and/or drowsiness, and ascites.

The diagnosis of NH should be considered in any neonate with coagulopathy; liver enzyme activity is usually normal or only slightly elevated. Diagnosis is based on the exclusion of other causes of liver disease, such as neonatal lupus or hemophagocytic lymphohistiocytosis, by evidence of an iron overload by MRI in the liver, pancreas, and/or heart. When feasible liver biopsy usually shows grade 3–4 siderosis in the hepatocyte. Biopsy of minor salivary gland is easier to document extrahepatic siderosis. An increased serum ferritin level in the neonate has been considered as a biomarker of NH; however, hyperferritinemia is nonspecific and is most likely a hallmark of hepatocellular injury regardless of etiology. In fact, hyperferritinemia may result from massive hepatic necrosis, systemic inflammation, or decreased hepatic ferritin clearance (Jimenez-Rivera et al. 2014).

For many years the only treatment for NH was liver transplantation with survival rates of 50%. Treatment with antioxidants and chelation therapy may improve symptoms but is usually associated with side effects (Table 4). In recent years the understanding that NH is probably an alloimmune disease has led to a new treatment approach utilizing exchange transfusion (ET) and intravenous immunoglobulins (IVIG) (Heissat et al. 2015).

Table 4 Antioxidant cocktail used in the management of neonatal hemochromatosis

1. *N*-Acetylcysteine (140 mg/kg orally, then 70 mg/kg over/every 4 h for 19 doses) 100 mg/kg/day
2. Selenium (3 μg/kg/day) intravenously
3. Prostaglandin E1 (0.5 μg/kg/h) intravenously
4. Desferrioxamine 30 mg/kg/day intravenously over 8 h until ferritin <500 μg/L
5. Alpha-tocopheryl polyethylene glycol succinate (20–30 IU/kg/day)

77.8.2 Hemophagocytic Lymphohistiocytosis

Hemophagocytic lymphohistiocytosis (*HLH*) comprises a group of life-threatening diseases classified in primary and secondary.

The former is caused by mutations in genes involved in granule-mediated cytotoxicity, and the latter occurs in a context of infections, malignancies, or autoimmune/autoinflammatory disorders. Both are characterized by systemic inflammation, severe cytokine storms, and immune-mediated organ damage.

Primary hemophagocytic lymphohistiocytosis, better known as *familial hemophagocytic lymphohistiocytosis* (*FHLH*), is a rare heritable disorder of immune regulation that is typically characterized by sudden onset of severe systemic illness. A functional impairment or the absence of proteins participating in lymphocyte cytotoxicity underlies the disease. The disorder, with an autosomal recessive transmission, is caused by loss-of-function mutations in genes involved in the cytotoxic function of natural killer (NK) cells and $CD8^+$ T cells.

Main clinical features include fever, marked liver and spleen enlargement, and neurological abnormalities. Laboratory investigations show pancytopenia, hypertriglyceridemia, severe coagulopathy with hypofibrinogenemia, abnormal liver enzymes, and cerebrospinal fluid pleocytosis (50% of cases). The diagnosis is difficult because hemophagocytosis can

be absent in bone marrow aspirate in the early phases of the disease.

Initial management includes chemotherapy with dexamethasone, etoposide, and cyclosporine, but the prognosis is poor, with a 5-year survival rate of 21%. Long-term survival requires a bone marrow transplant with a matched sibling, a treatment with a 5-year survival rate of 68%. Liver transplantation is contraindicated in this condition due to recurrence of the disease in the graft.

Secondary HLH is defined by a similar clinical syndrome but is assumed to lack a known genetic basis. This form of HLH is thought to occur in the context of an underlying immunological condition such as malignancy or an autoimmune or autoinflammatory disorder. Secondary HLH associated with the latter two conditions is also referred to as macrophage activation syndrome (MAS). Decreased perforin expression and reduced cytotoxicity of NK cells or $CD8^+$ T cells have been found in a few patients with MAS, as well as heterozygous mutations in genes involved in granule-mediated cytotoxicity (Filipovich and Chandrakasan 2015).

77.8.3 Mitochondrial Respiratory Chain Disorders

Structural and functional alterations of mitochondria are responsible for a number of disorders, affecting the central and peripheral nervous system, skeletal and cardiac muscles, the liver, the bone marrow, the pancreas, the kidneys, and the intestines.

Mitochondrial disorders, in the neonatal period, usually present as a multi-organ disease with severe liver failure. However, liver disease in association with a respiratory chain deficiency may be overlooked, since liver dysfunction is common in severely sick newborn infants.

A clinical picture with abnormal fetal growth, hypoglycemia with lactacidosis, coagulopathy, neurological symptoms, or renal tubulopathy should alert toward a mitochondrial disorder. A normal lactate level does not exclude respiratory chain defects.

Remarkable advances have been made recently in our understanding of mitochondrial hepatopathies, including the identification of specific mutations in nuclear genes, e.g., mitochondrial depletion syndrome caused by DGUOK, MPV17, SUCLG1, and POLG1, or in nuclear translation factor genes (TRMU, EFG1, and EFTu) of the respiratory chain enzyme complexes (Fellman and Kotarsky 2011).

Most infants show an early onset with nonspecific symptoms (lethargy, hypotonia, poor feeding) and/or extrahepatic features (neurological symptoms, myopathy, proximal renal tubular dysfunction, hypertrophic cardiomyopathy, hematological and gastrointestinal disorders), although few patients with respiratory chain defects limited to the liver have been described. A thorough investigation is necessary to exclude significant extrahepatic involvement before OLT can be proposed. Liver dysfunction may in fact precede neurologic involvement for weeks, months, or years. Laboratory tests that support diagnosis are elevated serum lactate level (>2.5 mmol/L), increased lactate/pyruvate molar ratio (>25 mol/mol), hypoglycemia, prolonged prothrombin time, hyperammonemia, and variably elevated aminotransferase and bilirubin concentrations (Lee and Sokol 2013).

77.8.4 Viral Infections

Neonatal *herpes simplex virus* (*HSV*) type 1 and 2 infection can be transmitted at delivery due to exposure to infected maternal genital secretions or lesions, although intrauterine or postnatal infection can also occur. Risk of transmission is highest in the case of primary infection in the mother, which is asymptomatic in most cases. Incidence is 1: 3,500 to 1: 20,000 live newborns, with a higher (70%) prevalence of HSV2. Delivery by cesarean section significantly reduces the risk of neonatal infection. Symptoms typically develop after day 5. ALF may occur within a disseminated disease involving the skin, eyes, mucous membranes, brain, lung, adrenals, and liver or as the only manifestation. Despite acyclovir therapy the prognosis is poor with high mortality (50–70%) and morbidity (neurologic sequelae). Successful liver transplantation has been reported. *Human herpes virus 6* infection has been reported occasionally.

Other viruses such as *Adenovirus*, *Parvovirus B19, and Paramyxovirus* have also been associated with NLF; among *Enteroviruses*, *Echovirus*, particularly serotype 11, is the most frequently identified virus. Severe infection with multi-organ involvement, including the liver, occurs almost exclusively in newborns, typically between day 4 and 7. Mortality is high, but antiviral treatment with an antiviral agent pleconaril (15 mg/kg/day) may improve the outcome.

Hepatitis B virus is vertically transmitted during delivery from a viremic mother. Infants at risk of developing ALF are those born to an HBsAg-positive, HBeAg-negative, anti-HBe-positive mother. ALF usually develops after the strict neonatal period and within 12 weeks of life. Universal screening of HBsAg-positive mothers and passive active immunizations by three to four doses of HBV vaccine in infancy associated with anti-hepatitis B immunoglobulins within 24 h of birth is the most effective way to prevent HBV infection of the newborn babies independently of the HBe antigen status of the mother. In areas with a low prevalence of HBV infection or limited resources, three doses of HBV vaccine universally in infancy, in lieu of maternal screening, can also produce good protective efficacy.

77.8.5 Inherited Metabolic Disorders

Classic galactosemia is an autosomal recessive disorder caused by a deficiency of the galactose-1-phosphate uridyl transferase enzyme. The onset usually occurs early in the neonatal period and complete elimination of dietary lactose/galactose results in resolution of liver failure. A galactose-free diet should be always started in NLF until the result of quantitative assay of erythrocyte galactose-1-phosphate uridyl transferase enzyme activity is available.

Hereditary fructose intolerance (*HFI*) is an autosomal recessive disorder caused by a deficiency of the enzyme fructose-1-phosphate aldolase. Symptoms develop only once fructose/sucrose is introduced into the diet; thus, symptoms do not usually occur in neonates fed fructose- and sucrose-free milk formulas, except for those given medications or rehydration formulas containing fructose, sucrose, or sorbitol. Complete elimination of fructose/sucrose/sorbitol results in a dramatic improvement.

Hereditary tyrosinemia type 1 (*HT1*) is an autosomal recessive disorder caused by a deficiency of *fumarylacetoacetate hydrolase*, which results in an accumulation of toxic metabolites responsible for liver and proximal renal tubular dysfunctions and porphyria-like crises. Infants most often present with coagulopathy soon after birth. Clinical signs of liver failure become apparent usually between 1 and 6 months of age and include ascites and edema secondary to hypoalbuminemia and bleeding diathesis. Jaundice is usually mild and the plasma aminotransferases may be only slightly or moderately elevated. Hypoglycemia may be caused by liver failure and hyperinsulinism.

Diagnosis is based on the finding of *succinylacetone* in the plasma or urine; this test is highly specific and sensitive, by enzyme analysis of skin fibroblast and by molecular genetic studies.

Management includes nitisinone (NTBC, Orfadin®) in a starting dose of 1 mg/kg/day once a day, as soon as the diagnosis is confirmed or even suspected. Nitisinone can only be given orally (or by nasogastric tube). The patient should also be started on a tyrosine- and phenylalanine-restricted diet, which has been proven curative in 90% of cases. Infants not responding to NTBC or with a suspicion of hepatocellular carcinoma are considered for liver transplant (Lee and Sokol 2013; Clayton 2002).

77.8.6 Inborn Error in Bile Acid Synthesis

The Δ4-3-oxosteroid 5-reductase deficiency is an autosomal recessive condition that causes defective bile acid steroid nucleus synthesis. Early diagnosis is important because oral administration of chenodeoxycholic acid and/or cholic acid can be curative. The typical presentation is neonatal cholestasis. However, without treatment liver failure rapidly ensues. There is therefore a 50% mortality rate in infants for whom diagnosis is delayed (de Laet et al. 2013).

77.8.7 Ischemic Damage

Transient acute liver dysfunction in newborns secondary to hemodynamic failure or shock liver syndrome is a well-recognized complication of reduced hepatic blood flow in low cardiac output states. The particular pattern of liver blood flow in neonates, characterized by a large intrahepatic shunt through the ductus venous and by a low arterial blood supply, produces a symmetric response to ischemia, with a significant reduction of blood flow in the right lobe compared to the left liver, which is supplied by the umbilical venous blood (Bergounioux et al. 2004).

77.8.8 ALF Related to Mutations in the Neuroblastoma-Amplified Sequence (NBAS) Gene

Biallelic mutations in the neuroblastoma-amplified sequence (NBAS) gene have been identified in patients presenting recurrent acute liver failure (RALF) in early infancy. The phenotypic spectrum of NBAS gene defect varies from isolated RALF to a multisystem disorder including short stature, skeletal dysplasia with neonatal spontaneous fractures, generalized hirsutism, gum hypertrophy, optic atrophy, and cardiomyopathy. Liver crises are triggered by febrile infections. These become less frequent with age but are not limited to childhood. Full recovery is typical, but ALF episodes can be fatal. For this reason, it is recommended to perform NBAS analysis in individuals with fever associated with acute and/or recurrent liver failure: identifying NBAS deficit allows optimizing therapy and preventing further episodes (Haack et al. 2015; Capo-Chichi et al. 2015).

77.9 Management

Management of NALF requires intensive life support and referral to a pediatric liver unit for early assessment for liver transplantation. Enteral feeding should always be preferred, and in the event that exclusive parenteral nutrition is required, enteral feeding should be restarted as soon as possible.

Fructose and galactose should be excluded from the diet until the diagnosis of galactosemia and fructosemia has been excluded. Normoglycemia should be maintained with high glucose concentrations infused through a central line. Coagulopathy, if severe, may be controlled with infusions of fresh frozen plasma. Anyway, as INR is used as a criterion for listing patients for liver transplantation, coagulopathy should not be corrected except in the event of active bleeding or if an invasive procedure is required. Fluids should be restricted to 75% of maintenance to prevent cerebral edema. Ascites may respond to infusion of serum albumin associated with diuretic therapy. Gastrointestinal bleeding should be prevented with ranitidine or proton pump inhibitors.

Ventilatory support should be considered early in cases of neurological and respiratory deterioration. Hepatic encephalopathy and cerebral edema may be treated by protein intake restriction, probiotic administration, and diuretic therapy (mannitol).

\Wide spectrum antibiotics and fluconazole target on positive cultural findings should be administered even in the absence of evidence of sepsis. Intravenous acyclovir should be continued until herpes virus infection has been excluded.

The main causes of NALF that contraindicate orthotopic liver transplantation are familial hemophagocytic lymphohistiocytosis, neonatal leukemia, mitochondrial disorders with extrahepatic involvement, multi-organ failure, and uncontrolled sepsis. Neonatal hemochromatosis and viral ALF are currently the most common indications to liver transplantation in NALF. Despite the introduction of surgical techniques such as the split liver that allow surgeons to use portions of the donor's liver, the death rate of patients on the waiting list remains high.

References

Alagille D, Estrada A, Hadchouel M et al (1987) Syndromic paucity of interlobular bile ducts (Alagille syndrome or arteriohepatic dysplasia): review of 80 cases. J Pediatr 110:195–200

Bergounioux J, Franchi-Abella S, Monneret S et al (2004) Neonatal ischemic liver failure: potential role of the ductus venosus. J Pediatr Gastroenterol Nutr 38:542–544
Bernard O (1998) Early diagnosis of neonatal cholestatic jaundice. Arch Pediatr 5:1031–1035
Bucuvalas J, Yazigi N, Squires RH Jr (2006) Acute liver failure in children. Clin Liver Dis 10:149–168
Capo-Chichi JM, Mehawej C, Delague V et al (2015) Neuroblastoma Amplified Sequence (NBAS) mutation in recurrent acute liver failure: confirmatory report in a sibship with very early onset, osteoporosis and developmental delay. Eur J Med Genet 58:637–641
Champion V, Carbajal R, Lozar J et al (2012) Risk factors for developing transient neonatal cholestasis. J Pediatr Gastroenterol Nutr 55:592–598
Chardot C (2006) Biliary atresia. Orphanet J Rare Dis 26:1–28
Clayton PT (2002) Inborn errors presenting with liver dysfunction. Semin Neonatol 7:49–63
Davit-Spraul A, Gonzales E, Baussan C, Jacquemin E (2009) Progressive familial intrahepatic cholestasis. Orphanet J Rare Dis 4:1
de Laet C, Dionisi-Vici C, Leonard JV et al (2013) Recommendations for the management of tyrosinaemia type 1. Orphanet J Rare Dis 8:8
Dhawan A, Mieli Vergani G (2005) Acute liver failure in neonates. Early Hum Dev 81:1005–1010
Durand P, Debray D, Mandel R et al (2001) Acute liver failure in infancy: a 14-year experience of a pediatric liver transplantation center. J Pediatr 139:871–876
Fellman V, Kotarsky H (2011) Mitochondrial hepatopathies in the newborn period. Semin Fetal Neonatal Med 16:222–228
Filipovich AH, Chandrakasan S (2015) Pathogenesis of hemophagocytic lymphohistiocytosis. Hematol Oncol Clin North Am 29:895–902
Gonzales E, Grosse B, Schuller B et al (2015) Targeted pharmacotherapy in progressive familial intrahepatic cholestasis type 2: evidence for improvement of cholestasis with 4-phenylbutyrate. Hepatology 62: 558–566
Haack TB, Staufner C, Ko MG et al (2015) Biallelic mutations in NBAS cause recurrent acute liver failure with onset in infancy. Am J Hum Genet 97:163–169
Heissat S, Collardeau-Frachon S, Baruteau J et al (2015) Neonatal hemochromatosis: diagnostic work-up based on a series of 56 cases of fetal death and neonatal liver failure. J Pediatr 166:66–73
Hsiao CH, Chang MH, Chen HL et al (2008) Universal screening for biliary atresia using an infant stool color card in Taiwan. Hepatology 47:1233–1240
Jacquemin E, Setchell KD, O'Connell NC et al (1994) A new cause of progressive intrahepatic cholestasis: 3 beta-hydroxy-C27-steroid dehydrogenase/isomerase deficiency. J Pediatr 125:379–384
Jacquemin E, Lykavieris P, Chaoui N et al (1998) Transient neonatal cholestasis: origin and outcome. J Pediatr 133:563–567
Jimenez-Rivera C, Gupta A, Feberova J et al (2014) Successful treatment of neonatal hemochromatosis as gestational alloimmune liver disease with intravenous immunoglobulin. J Neonatal-Perinatal Med 7:301–304
Lee WS, Sokol RJ (2013) Mitochondrial hepatopathies: advances in genetics, therapeutic approaches, and outcomes. J Pediatr 163:942–948
Lee MS, Kim MJ, Lee MJ et al (2009) Biliary atresia: color doppler US findings in neonates and infants. Radiology 252:282–289
Maggiore G, Bernard O, Hadchouel M et al (1991) Diagnostic value of serum gamma-glutamyl transpeptidase activity in liver diseases in children. J Pediatr Gastroenterol Nutr 12:21–26
McClean P, Davison S (2003) Neonatal liver failure. Semin Neonatol 8:393–401
Moyer V, Freese DK, Whitington PF et al (2004) Guideline for the evaluation of cholestatic jaundice in infants: recommendations of the North American Society for Pediatric Gastroenterology, Hepatology and Nutrition. J Pediatr Gastroenterol Nutr 39:115–128
Petersen C, Davenport M (2013) Aetiology of biliary atresia: what is actually known? Orphanet J Rare Dis 8:128
Primhak RA, Tanner MS (2001) Alpha-1-antitrypsin deficiency. Arch Dis Child 85:2–5
Sambrotta M, Strautnieks S, Papouli E et al (2014) Mutations in TJP2 cause progressive cholestatic liver disease. Nat Genet 46:326–328
Serinet MO, Wildhaber BE, Broué P et al (2009) Impact of age at Kasai operation on its results in late childhood and adolescence: a rational basis for biliary atresia screening. Pediatrics 123:1280–1286

Neonatal Cholestasis: Conjugated Hyperbilirubinemia

78

Nandini Kataria and Glenn R. Gourley

Contents

A chapter prepared for Dr. Giuseppe Buonocore's *Neonatology* textbook.

N. Kataria (✉)
Department of Pediatrics, University of Minnesota, Long Beach, California, USA
e-mail: nandini.kataria@gmail.com

G. R. Gourley
Department of Pediatrics, University of Minnesota, Minneapolis, USA

G. Buonocore et al. (eds.), *Neonatology*,
https://doi.org/10.1007/978-3-319-29489-6_225

Abstract
Jaundice during the first few weeks of life is a common finding. Frequently, such jaundice is due to elevation of the unconjugated, or indirect, bilirubin and is often the result of a benign process. More concerning is jaundice due to elevation of the conjugated bilirubin fraction. Neonatal cholestasis is defined as an accumulation of biliary substances, such as bilirubin and bile acids because of impaired canalicular bile flow. Neonatal cholestasis manifests with a conjugated hyperbilirubinemia and must be differentiated from unconjugated hyperbilirubinemia, as it is more often associated with a specific disease process. The incidence of neonatal cholestasis has been estimated at 1 in 2,500 live births.

78.1 Salient Points

- Neonatal cholestasis is defined as accumulation of biliary substances, such as bilirubin and bile acids, as a result of impaired canalicular bile flow.
- In neonates, there is structural, as well as functional, immaturity of the biliary system.
- Etiologically, the causes of cholestasis can be categorized as infectious, metabolic, toxic, chromosomal, vascular disorders, and bile duct anomalies.
- The spectrum of clinical presentation can vary from the progressively poor feeding and failure to thrive to lethargy, irritability, and coagulopathy.
- Neonatal cholestasis must be urgently evaluated in any infant who is jaundiced after 2 weeks of life, and fractionation of the total bilirubin level is crucial.
- Investigation should proceed in a logical, stepwise manner to ensure conditions requiring immediate intervention, such as biliary atresia, galactosemia, sepsis, and hypothyroidism, are not overlooked and treated in a timely manner.
- Liver biopsy is the most definitive test in the evaluation of neonatal cholestasis.
- Medical management of cholestasis is largely supportive because the underlying disease is often untreatable.
- Cholestatic infants are particularly susceptible to fat-soluble vitamin deficiency as a consequence of malabsorption.

78.2 Introduction

Jaundice during the first few weeks of life is a common finding. Frequently, such jaundice is due to elevation of the unconjugated, or indirect, bilirubin and is often the result of a benign process. Neonatal cholestasis is defined as prolonged conjugated hyperbilirubinemia in the newborn period. This can be a result of impaired canalicular bile flow which can be associated with many specific disease processes. Excretion of bile flow can be impaired due to problems with intrahepatic production of bile, transmembrane transport of bile, or mechanical obstruction in the extrahepatic transport of bile. Cholestasis results from the accumulation of bile components, i.e., bilirubin and bile acids. Conjugated hyperbilirubinemia in the neonate is defined as a conjugated bilirubin concentration >1 mg/dl when the total serum bilirubin is <5 mg/dl or greater than 20% of the total serum bilirubin when total serum bilirubin is >5 mg/dl. The incidence of neonatal cholestasis has been estimated at 1 in 2,500 live births (Walker et al. 2004).

78.3 Pathophysiology

Bile is a unique vital aqueous secretion of the liver formed by the hepatocyte and modified downstream by absorptive and secretory properties of the bile duct epithelium. Approximately 5% of bile consists of organic and inorganic solutes. The bile-secretory unit consists of a canalicular network formed by the apical membrane of adjacent hepatocytes and sealed by tight junctions. The bile canaliculi (~1 μm in diameter) conduct the flow of bile countercurrent to the direction of portal blood flow and connect with the canal of Hering and bile ducts which progressively increase in diameter prior to the entry of bile into the gallbladder, common bile duct, and intestine. Canalicular bile secretion is determined by both bile salt-dependent and bile salt-independent transport systems localized at the apical membrane of the hepatocyte and largely consists of a series of adenosine triphosphate-binding cassette transport proteins that function as export pumps for bile salts and other organic solutes. These transporters create osmotic gradients within the bile canalicular lumen that provide the driving force for movement of fluid into the lumen via aquaporins. Canalicular flow and cholangiocyte secretion is highly regulated by hormones, second messengers, and signal transduction pathways. Most determinants of bile secretion are now characterized at the molecular level in man (Boyer 2013; Soroka and Boyer 2014). The process of bile generation in the liver involves two key processes. The first process involves the uptake of bile acids from the blood into the hepatocyte. Uptake across the sinusoidal membrane of the hepatocyte is an active process and involves two receptors: the Na taurocholate cotransporting polypeptide (NTCP) and the organic anion transporting proteins (OATPs). Besides transport of bile acids, these receptors also transport other anions, such as toxins and drugs, across the sinusoidal membrane. The secretion of bile acids across the biliary canalicular membrane involves the bile salt export pump (BSEP) and the multidrug-resistant proteins (MRP2 and MDR3).

In neonates, there is structural, as well as functional, immaturity of the biliary system. Such immaturity increases susceptibility to cholestasis. The uptake of bile acids across the sinusoidal membrane can be affected by a number of ways, as with downregulation of NTCP and OATP receptors, secondary to sepsis and hepatitis, resulting in cholestasis secondary to decreased bile production. Alteration in the canalicular membrane receptors can similarly result in cholestasis, such as that seen with mutation in the BSEP or MDR3 in the progressive familial intrahepatic cholestasis (PFIC) syndromes.

78.3.1 Classification of Neonatal Cholestasis

The differential diagnosis of neonatal cholestasis is extensive (Table 1). Neonatal cholestasis can be classified according to anatomy or etiology. Anatomically, causes of cholestasis can be classified as extrahepatic or intrahepatic. Examples of extrahepatic causes of cholestasis are choledochal cysts and biliary atresia, whereas idiopathic neonatal hepatitis, congenital infections, and α_1-antitrypsin deficiency are examples of intrahepatic causes. Etiologically, the causes of cholestasis can be categorized as infectious, metabolic, toxic, chromosomal, vascular disorders, and bile duct anomalies.

78.4 Clinical Presentation

Infants with cholestasis usually present with the classic triad of prolonged jaundice, pale stools, and dark urine. Acholic stools warrant expedient evaluation. There is a wide variation in clinical presentation. Progressive failure to thrive and hypoglycemia may be seen with metabolic disease, whereas lethargy and irritability may be the only presenting symptoms with cholestasis secondary to bacterial sepsis. Bleeding may be present due to vitamin K deficiency secondary to malabsorption of fat-soluble vitamins or from deficiency of clotting factors.

On physical examination, cholestatic infants will exhibit jaundice. Hepatomegaly is common and splenomegaly can be a sign of advanced liver

Table 1 Differential diagnosis of neonatal cholestasis

Bile duct anomalies
1. Biliary atresia
2. Choledochal cyst
3. Non-syndromic bile duct paucity
4. Inspissated bile syndrome
5. Choledocholithiasis
6. Neonatal sclerosing cholangitis
7. Spontaneous perforation of bile ducts
Infections
1. Viral
HIV
CMV
HHV6
Herpes simplex
Adenovirus
Rubella
Reovirus 3
Coxsackie virus
Varicella zoster
Parvovirus B19
Hepatitis B and C
Echovirus
2. Bacterial
UTI
Sepsis
Listeriosis
Tuberculosis
Syphilis
3. Parasitic
Toxoplasmosis
Malaria
Metabolic and genetic conditions
1. Disorders of carbohydrate metabolism
Galactosemia
Fructosemia
Glycogen storage disease type 4
2. Disorders of amino acid metabolism
Tyrosinemia
Arginase deficiency
3. Disorders of lipid metabolism
Wolman syndrome
Niemann-Pick disease
Gaucher's disease
4. Disorders of bile acid synthesis
Zellweger's syndrome
5. Genetic condition
Alagille syndrome
Caroli disease
Progressive familial intrahepatic cholestasis types 1, 2, 3
Citrin deficiency
Alpha-1 antitrypsin deficiency
Dubin-Johnson syndrome
Rotor syndrome
X-linked adrenoleukodystrophy
Endocrinopathies
1. Hypothyroidism
2. Septo-optic dysplasia
Chromosomal disorders
1. Turner syndrome
2. Trisomies 13, 18, 21
3. Cat eye syndrome
4. Donohue syndrome
Toxic
1. Drugs
2. Alcohol (fetal alcohol syndrome)
3. Parenteral nutrition
Neoplastic
1. Leukemia
2. Histiocytosis X
3. Neuroblastoma
4. Hepatoblastoma
5. Hemophagocytic lymphohistiocytosis
Miscellaneous
1. Cystic fibrosis
2. Gestational alloimmune liver disease (neonatal hemochromatosis)
3. Idiopathic neonatal hepatitis
4. Aagenaes syndrome
5. North American Indian familial cholestasis
6. Neonatal lupus erythematosus
7. Le foie vide (infantile hepatic non-regenerative disorder)
8. Mitochondrial disorders
9. Intestinal obstruction
10. Congestive heart failure
11. Budd-Chiari syndrome
12. Neonatal asphyxia

disease. There can be other specific clues to the underlying illness as well. Choledochal cysts can sometimes present with a right upper quadrant mass. Alagille syndrome can present with characteristic facies and there may be other associated anatomic anomalies and a heart murmur. Growth retardation can be seen with congenital infections, such as rubella and cytomegalovirus.

78.5 Evaluation

Neonatal cholestasis should be urgently evaluated in any infant who is jaundiced after 2 weeks of life (Moyer et al. 2004). Evaluation should commence with a detailed patient history, including family, pregnancy, antenatal, and postnatal histories, and physical exam. Important clues regarding cholestatic etiology may be missed without a thorough history and exam. Fractionation of the total bilirubin level is crucial in the initial investigation of cholestasis.

Once cholestasis is established with an elevated conjugated bilirubin, further investigation should proceed in a logical, stepwise manner to ensure conditions requiring immediate intervention, such as galactosemia, sepsis, and hypothyroidism, are not overlooked and treated in a timely manner. Next, evaluation for biliary atresia is crucial as the successful surgical treatment of biliary atresia is dependent on timely diagnosis (Abdel-Kader and Balistreri 1994). After biliary atresia has been excluded, evaluation should be done to establish the cause of intrahepatic cholestasis. A suggested approach to the evaluation of infants with cholestatic jaundice is summarized in Fig. 1.

78.5.1 Laboratory Evaluations

The first step in diagnosing neonatal cholestasis is the fractionation of the total serum bilirubin. Conjugated hyperbilirubinemia is defined as a conjugated bilirubin greater than 1 mg/dl or more than 20% of the total bilirubin level. Serum alanine aminotransferase (ALT) and aspartate aminotransferase (AST) are sensitive indicators of hepatocellular injury but lack specificity or prognostic value. Elevation of alkaline phosphatase (ALP) can be seen in biliary obstruction, but also lacks specificity, as it is also found in bone and kidney. Thus, with ALP elevations, diseases in other organs, such as bone, must be excluded. The enzyme gamma-glutamyl transpeptidase (GGT) is located in the biliary epithelium, and elevations are highly sensitive for cholestatic disorders, such as biliary atresia, α_1-antitrypsin (α_1-AT) deficiency, and idiopathic neonatal hepatitis. One exception is seen in progressive familial intrahepatic cholestasis types 1 and 2 in which normal or low levels of GGT can be seen. GGT values should be evaluated in the context of the infant's age. GGT values can normally be high in neonates (six to seven times the upper limit of the adult reference range, declining to adult levels by age 5–7 months (Cabrera-Abreu and Green 2002; Hirfanoglu et al. 2014)). Values should always be interpreted with age-specific reference ranges.

78.5.2 Radiographic Investigations

There are several different modalities available to investigate neonatal cholestasis. Yang et al. compared some of these methods in 2009 (Gourley et al. 2009).

78.5.3 Abdominal Ultrasound

Abdominal ultrasonography is a simple, noninvasive procedure that is often used as the first step in the work-up of cholestatic infants. Ultrasound can provide useful information regarding size and appearance of the liver and gallbladder, visualization of gallstones and sludging of bile, and diagnosis of choledochal cysts (Bates et al. 1998). The triangular cord sign, which represents a fibrous cone of tissue at the porta hepatis, has been reported to be highly specific and sensitive for biliary atresia, with a specificity of 100% and sensitivity ranging from 85% to 100% (Kotb et al. 2001; Park et al. 1997). Abdominal ultrasound can also be used as a screen for anomalies associated with biliary atresia, such as polysplenia and interruption of the inferior vena cava (Bates et al. 1998).

78.5.4 Hepatobiliary Scintigraphy

Hepatobiliary scintigraphy using technetium-labeled iminodiacetic acid derivatives represents the only available method of imaging that can evaluate hepatobiliary physiology (Abramson et al. 1982) and can help to distinguish between

biliary atresia and other forms of neonatal cholestasis. As the test can determine the patency of the biliary tract, it is highly sensitive for biliary atresia, but lacks specificity, estimated at 83–100% and 35–50%, respectively (Park et al. 1997; Dehghani et al. 2006). Excretion of the isotope can also be delayed in forms of intrahepatic cholestasis. In biliary atresia, the uptake of the isotope occurs in a normal manner, but excretion into the biliary system and the intestines, is delayed or absent. In forms of intrahepatic cholestasis, such as in idiopathic neonatal hepatitis, the uptake of the isotope is delayed, but the isotope may ultimately be excreted into the intestines. Pretreatment with phenobarbital, 5 mg/kg/day for 5 days, can improve the sensitivity for biliary atresia by stimulating bile acid-independent flow (Walker et al. 2004); however, this may cause an unnecessary delay and may not eliminate the need for liver biopsy.

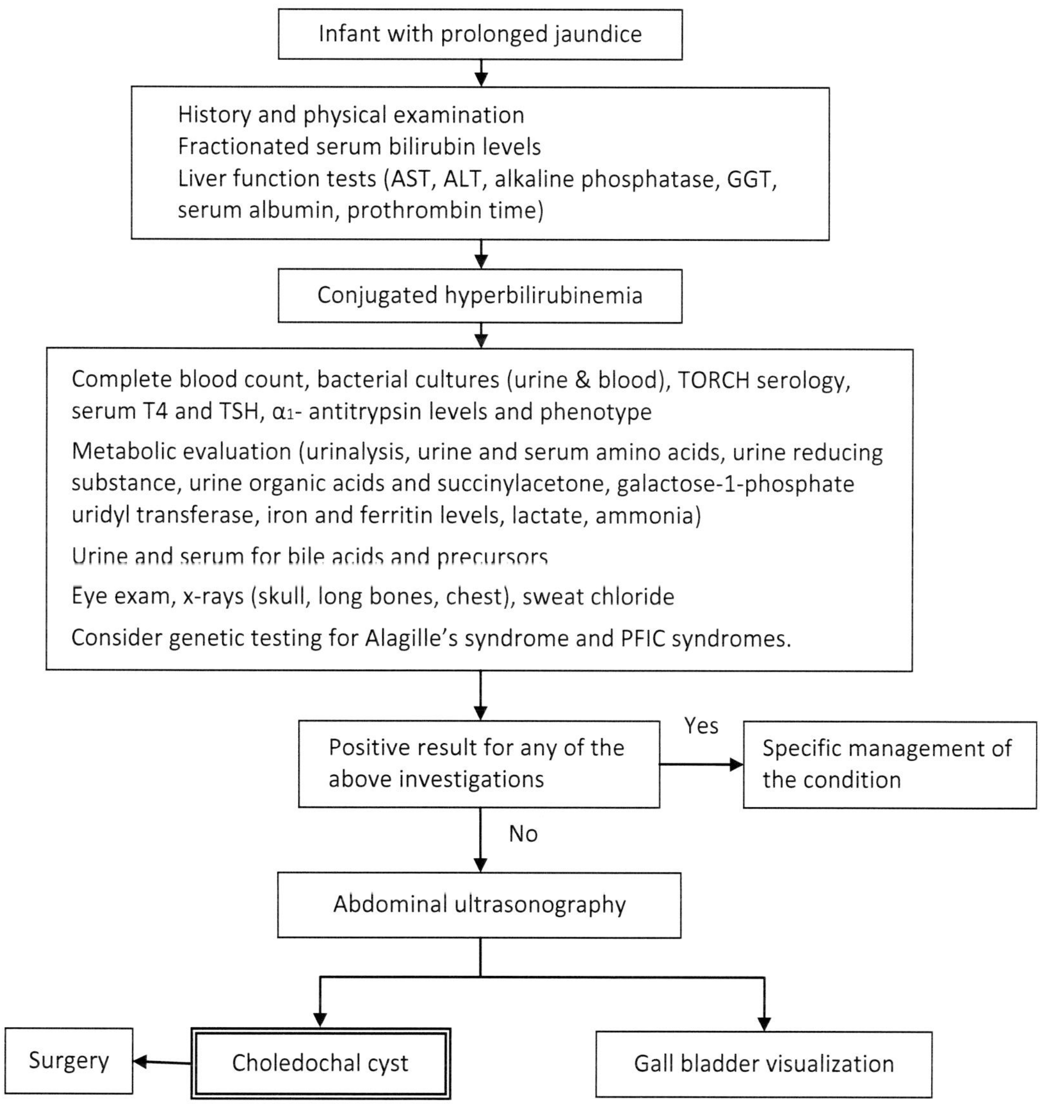

Fig. 1 (continued)

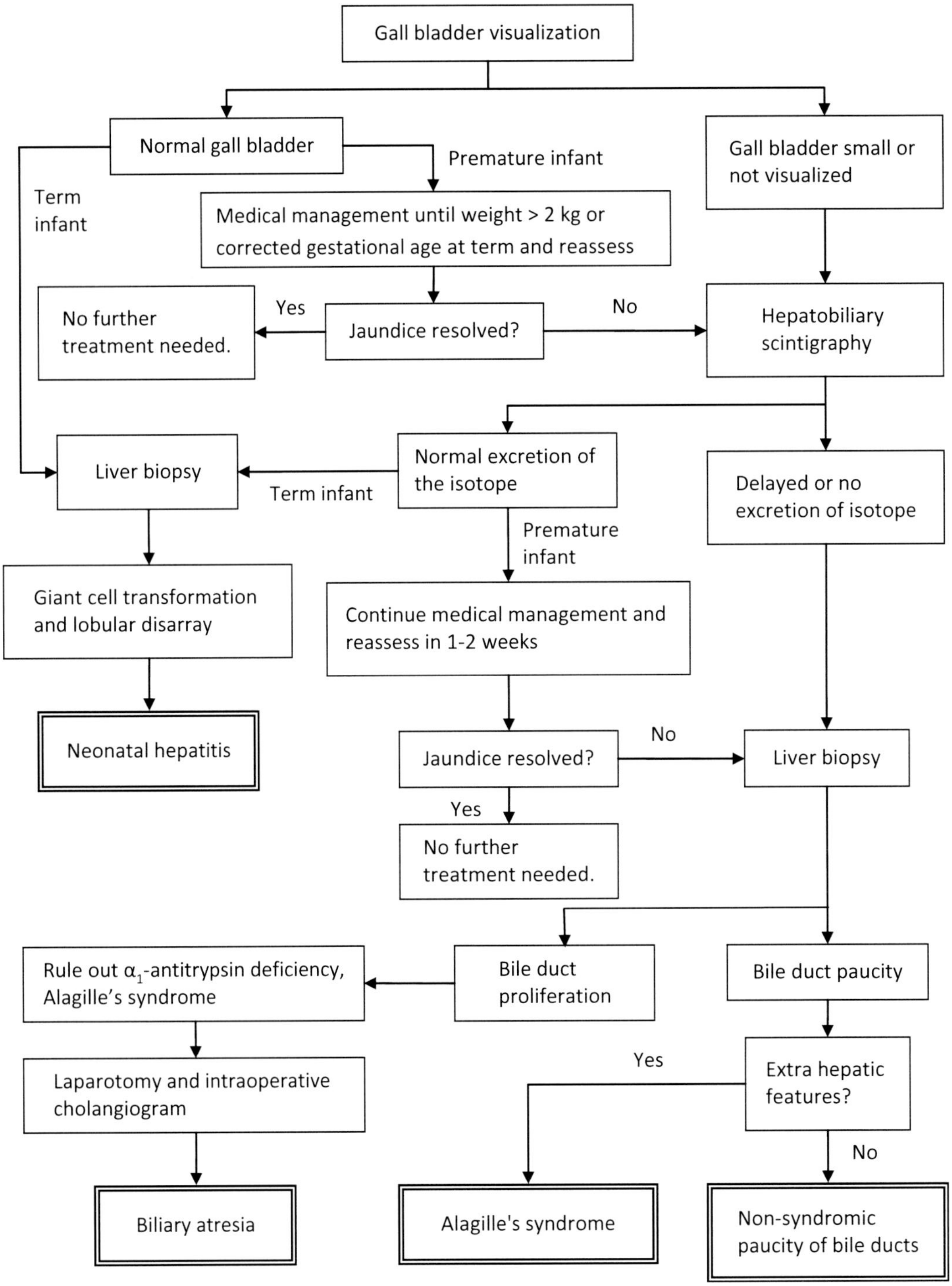

Fig. 1 An approach to a full-term or premature infant with cholestasis (Venigalla and Gourley 2004)

78.5.5 Endoscopic Retrograde Cholangiopancreatography (ERCP)

ERCP in adults or older children has both diagnostic and therapeutic indications in managing biliary tract but there are limited data in neonates. This technique uses an endoscopic approach to access the biliary and pancreatic ducts through the ampulla of Vater. Contrast material is then injected to visualize the ductal system. With good technique, nonvisualization of the common bile duct is highly suggestive of biliary atresia. For biliary disease such as choledocolithiasis, bile plug syndrome, strictures, and primary sclerosing cholangitis, therapeutic ERCP can be particularly helpful. Sphincterotomy, sphincteroplasty, stone extractions, stricture dilation, and stent placement can all be performed using ERCP. The utility of ERCP in neonates can be limited by the availability of appropriately small-sized endoscopes and will require general anesthesia. However, in inconclusive cases, ERCP may serve as an additional diagnostic tool which may prevent more invasive procedures (Shteyer et al. 2012).

78.5.6 Magnetic Resonance Cholangiography (MRCP)

MRCP is being increasingly used to assess the biliary and pancreatic ducts. Nonvisualization of the common bile duct or any portion of the extrahepatic biliary tree is thought to be diagnostic of biliary atresia. Previously, sensitivity and specificity for detecting biliary atresia by MRCP were estimated at 95% and 88%, respectively. More recent data suggests that biliary defects such as biliary stenosis and breast milk jaundice can also result in nonvisualization of the extrahepatic biliary tree resulting in false-positive results using MRCP. The sensitivity and specificity for MRCP are now suggested between 85 and 99% and 36 and 57% (Liu et al. 2014). If any portion of the biliary tracts is nonvisualized with MRCP, then the results must be interpreted in conjunction with other studies. Furthermore, neonates require general anesthesia in order to perform this study, and these risks must be considered prior to performing this study.

78.5.7 Duodenal Aspirate Analysis

Duodenal fluid can be obtained by either placement of a naso- or oroduodenal tube or using a string in the duodenum. Bilirubin concentration in the aspirate can then be assessed, and a duodenal aspirate bilirubin concentration less than that in the serum is suggestive of biliary obstruction (Larrosa-Haro et al. 2001). Although sensitivity of duodenal aspirate analysis approaches that for scintigraphy, the test is more invasive.

78.5.8 Liver Biopsy

Percutaneous liver biopsy is the most definitive test in the evaluation of neonatal cholestasis and should be performed in most infants with undiagnosed cholestasis (Moyer et al. 2004; Yang et al. 2009). Biopsy is recommended prior to a surgical procedure for biliary atresia. If biopsy results are equivocal and the infant is less than 6 weeks of age, biopsy may need to be repeated. Histologic findings in biliary atresia include bile duct proliferation and bile plugs. These findings must be differentiated from idiopathic neonatal hepatitis, in which there is giant cell transformation and focal hepatocellular necrosis. Liver biopsy can also be useful to diagnose congenital viral infection; viral inclusion bodies suggest cytomegalovirus or herpes infection. Lack of intrahepatic bile ducts in infants less than 1 year of age has been found to be an adverse prognostic factor independent of neonatal liver disease etiology (Sergi et al. 2008).

78.6 Management of Cholestasis

The medical management of cholestasis is largely supportive because the underlying disease is often untreatable. Management consists of drug therapy (Table 2) and nutritional support (Table 3) which

Table 2 Medical management of cholestasis

Class of medication	Medication	Dose	Side effects
Bile acid analogs	Ursodeoxycholic acid (UDCA)	15–20 mg/kg/day	Diarrhea, hepatotoxicity
	Cholestyramine	0.25–0.5 g/kg/day	Constipation, steatorrhea, hyperchloremic metabolic acidosis, hypoproteinemic hemorrhage
Enzyme inducers	Phenobarbital	3.5–10 mg/kg/day	Sedative effects, behavioral changes
	Rifampin	10 mg/kg/day, in two divided doses	Hepatotoxicity, drug interactions
Opioid antagonists	Naloxone	0.2 μg/kg/min	Opioid withdrawal-like phenomenon including abdominal pain, tachycardia, high blood pressure, nightmares
	Nalmefene	2–20 mg/day (titrate to effect)	
	Naltrexone	5 mg/kg/day	

Table 3 Nutritional support in cholestasis

Class	Supplement	Dose	Side effects
Vitamin A	Aquasol A	5,000–25,000 IU/day	Hepatotoxicity, hypercalcemia
			Pseudotumor cerebri
Vitamin D	Cholecalciferol	2,500–5,000 IU/day	Hypercalcemia
	25 – OH cholecalciferol	3–5 mcg/kg/day	Nephrocalcinosis
Vitamin E	Aquasol E	50–400 IU/day	Potentiation of vitamin K deficiency coagulopathy, diarrhea
	TPGS (d-alpha-tocopheryl polyethylene glycol-1000 succinate)	15–25 IU/kg/day	Potentiation of vitamin K deficiency coagulopathy, hyperosmolality, and diarrhea
Vitamin K	Phytonadione	2.5–5 mg every other day	
Water-soluble vitamins		Twice daily recommended allowance	

address complications of chronic cholestasis rather than the underlying cause (Table 1). These complications include pruritus, malabsorption, and nutritional deficiencies.

78.6.1 Pruritus

Pruritus is a common symptom of cholestatic disease though the exact cause of pruritus is unknown. Pruritus can often be excruciating and can be associated with significant morbidity. It is most commonly seen with primary sclerosing cholangitis, primary biliary sclerosis, cholangiocarcinoma, and viral hepatitis and is not generally a problem in the care of the newborn. A few theories have been suggested for the mechanism of pruritus: the first is that bile salts act as pruritogens by inducing mast cell degranulation and the second is that plasma levels of endogenous opioids such as enkephalins are increased either due to increased synthesis or due to reduced clearance. Both of these theories do not have strong supporting evidence in the literature; however, both bile acid analogs and opioid receptor antagonists have demonstrated beneficial effects on pruritus in clinical studies.

Ursodeoxycholic acid (UDCA) is a nontoxic hydrophilic bile acid and epimer of chenodeoxycholic acid. UDCA acts by altering the bile acid pool by replacing potentially toxic hydrophobic bile acids and increasing the rate of

transport of intracellular bile acids across the canalicular membrane (Venigalla and Gourley 2004). UDCA is, thus, a choleretic, often used as a first-line therapy for cholestasis and has been shown to decrease pruritus (Cies and Giamalis 2007). UDCA is generally safe although diarrhea is commonly seen in the pediatric population. The dosage of UDCA is 15–20 mg/kg/day in divided doses (Cies and Giamalis 2007).

Cholestyramine is a nonspecific anion exchange resin that binds bile acids, decreasing enterohepatic circulation by preventing their reabsorption in the terminal ileum (Walker et al. 2004). Cholestyramine also acts as a choleretic agent by promoting the conversion of cholesterol to bile acids that promote choleresis and has been shown to reduce pruritus (Cies and Giamalis 2007). Dosing is recommended at 0.25–0.5 g/kg/day and side effects of cholestyramine use, although mild, are common and include increased fat malabsorption and abdominal discomfort (Cies and Giamalis 2007). Hypoproteinemic hemorrhage and hyperchloremic metabolic acidosis after cholestyramine has also been described in case reports (Shojania and Grewar 1986; Eaves and Korman 1984). Cholestyramine also interferes with the absorption of several drugs, including UDCA and thyroxin, and no other medications should be taken within 4 h of cholestyramine ingestion when feasible (Cies and Giamalis 2007; Hegade et al. 2015).

Phenobarbital is a microsomal enzyme inducer that can stimulate bile acid-independent flow, enhance bile acid synthesis, and decrease bile acid pool size. The therapeutic dose of phenobarbital is 5–10 mg/kg/day, although its sedating side effect can limit its use (Cies and Giamalis 2007). Rifampin, another microsomal enzyme inducer, has also been reported to act as a glucocorticoid receptor ligand, which could potentiate its antipruritic affect as glucocorticoids have proven beneficial in adults with cholestatic pruritus (Calleja et al. 1998; Mitchison et al. 1989). Recommended rifampin dosage is 4–10 mg/kg/day in two divided doses (Cies and Giamalis 2007; Hegade et al. 2015). Side effects including hepatotoxicity, urine and tear discoloration, and multiple drug interactions have been reported.

Opioid antagonists have been shown to be effective as a second-line therapy in relieving cholestatic pruritus in some patients. Although most studies have failed to demonstrate a direct correlation between levels of enkephalins and itch, beneficial therapeutic effect has been demonstrated in clinical trials. The interaction between pain and itch is widely accepted, and the beneficial effect of opioid antagonists may simply be by reducing pain signaling (Oude Elferink et al. 2011). Medications that have been studied include naloxone and nalmefene, and both were relatively well tolerated, with headache and anorexia being the most common. Nalmefene has the benefit of a longer plasma half-life and greater bioavailability after oral administration, compared to naloxone. Importantly, this class of medications can induce an opioid withdrawal-like phenomenon in patients with excessive endogenous opioids (Maxwell et al. 2005; Bergasa 2008; Chang and Golkar 2008). Research of these medications is limited in the pediatric population.

Perception of pruritus is mediated in part by serotonin neurotransmission. Ondansetron, a 5-hydroxytryptamine receptor type 3 antagonist, has been shown to be effective in improving cholestatic pruritus resistant to first-line therapies (Maxwell et al. 2005; Chang and Golkar 2008; Bergasa et al. 1992). There are case reports that suggest the efficacy of ondansetron in treating intractable pruritus in the pediatric population but none in neonates so far (Frigon and Desparmet 2006; Dillon and Tobias 2013).

Antidepressants have been discovered to be associated with relief of cholestatic pruritus in adult patients. The improvement in pruritus has been found to be independent from any improvement in depression (Browning et al. 2003; Zylicz et al. 2003). Selective serotonin reuptake inhibitors have also been reported to decrease pruritus associated with polycythemia vera and the multifactorial pruritus associated with malignancy (Diehn and Tefferi 2001; Zylicz et al. 1998). Findings suggest that, in addition to the serotonin system, other neurotransmitters including noradrenalin may contribute to the pruritus of cholestasis (Bergasa and Jones 1995).

Ultraviolet B (UVB) radiation has proven to be an effective treatment of generalized pruritus, as well as pruritus in adults with primary biliary

cirrhosis (Seckin et al. 2007; Frederick Suchy 2007). UVB radiation is also the treatment of choice for pruritus in uremic patients (Seckin et al. 2007). A small pilot study in eight adult patients with pruritus and chronic liver disease treated with bright light therapy (full spectrum) showed a small, but statistically insignificant, improvement (Bergasa et al. 2001). The use of UVB phototherapy in children with cholestatic pruritus has not been investigated.

Plasmapheresis has been shown to be effective in patients with cholestatic pruritus not responsive to traditional medications (Pusl et al. 2006; Rifai et al. 2006). The pruritogenic compound removed is unknown. Relief is temporary, as pruritus often returns within several weeks after plasmapheresis. Experience is limited to plasmapheresis in adult patients.

Additional medications have been tried mainly in adults with primary biliary cirrhosis. The antiepileptic medication carbamazepine has been suggested to relieve pruritus secondary to its beneficial effect on other painful conditions. Other medications include terfenadine, androgenic steroids, azathioprine, ondansetron, and propofol (Frederick Suchy 2007).

Transient therapeutic biliary drainage has been shown to efficiently resolve pruritus, but results in the depletion of compounds including bile salts from the enterohepatic circulation. This invasive technique is particularly useful in the management of pruritus in progressive familial intrahepatic cholestasis (PFIC) and benign recurrent intrahepatic cholestasis (BRIC) (Fischler et al. 2001).

A few recent studies have shown an increase in the plasma level of autotaxin (ATX) and lysophosphatidic acid (LPA). LPA appears to potentiate itch signaling through the thin unmyelinated C-fibers which may be pruriceptive. No therapies have yet been targeted toward this pathway but have potential for targeted therapies in the future (Oude Elferink et al. 2011; Kremer et al. 2015).

78.6.2 Nutritional Management

Nutritional management should start at the initial visit and growth parameters including height and weight for age and weight for height measurements closely followed. Decreased bile acid delivery to the intestines is the end result of cholestasis regardless of etiology, resulting in fat and fat-soluble vitamin malabsorption. Malabsorption occurs when the intraluminal bile acid concentration falls below the critical micellar concentration, resulting in decreased long-chain triglyceride lipolysis. Essential fatty acid (EFA) deficiency may occur secondary to malabsorption of long-chain triglycerides and inadequate intake. Manifestations of EFA deficiency include growth impairment, dry scaly rash, thrombocytopenia, and impaired immune function (Frederick Suchy 2007).

Medium-chain triglycerides (MCTs) are more readily absorbed and are a better source of fat calories. Cholestatic infants should be started on an MCT-containing formula like Enfaport, Pregestimil, or Alimentum, which contain 84%, 55%, and 33% of fat calories as MCT oil, respectively. As a result of steatorrhea and increased energy expenditure, cholestatic infants should receive approximately 125% of recommended dietary allowance based on ideal body weight (Dani et al. 2015). Some infants may need additional calories for catch-up growth if significant malnutrition is present, and use of nocturnal enteral feeds may be required if oral intake is not adequate.

The fat-soluble vitamins A, D, E, and K require solubilization by bile acids into micelles to be absorbed across the intestines. Cholestatic infants are particularly susceptible to fat-soluble vitamin deficiency as a consequence of malabsorption. Doses of at least two to four times the recommended daily allowance are given (Dani et al. 2015). Vitamin supplementation should continue at least 3 months after resolution of jaundice. Fat-soluble vitamin levels should be followed during treatment (Table 3).

78.7 Specific Diseases

78.7.1 Biliary Atresia

Biliary atresia is a rare but life-threatening condition that presents in infancy and the etiology remains unknown. The incidence is thought to

be 1 in 10–20,000 live births. Biliary atresia is a progressive inflammatory cholangiopathy resulting in the obliteration of the intra- and extrahepatic biliary tree which eventually leads to biliary cirrhosis. It is the most common cause of neonatal cholestasis and remains the most frequent indication for pediatric liver transplantation (Haber and Russo 2003).

The etiology and pathogenesis of biliary atresia remains unclear, but many mechanisms and theories have been proposed including a defect in embryologic development of the biliary tree; a defect in the fetal/prenatal circulation; environmental toxin exposure; viral infection, i.e., rotavirus, CMV, etc.; and immune dysregulation. There are recent data that suggest a virally induced upregulation of Th1-mediated immune response that may lead to inflammation and bile duct injury (Bezerra 2005; Feldman and Mack 2012).

There are two recognized clinical forms of biliary atresia: the acquired/perinatal form and the embryonic/congenital form. The perinatal form is the most common, accounting for 80–90% of cases. These infants are usually born at term and are clinically normal. They usually present with jaundice in the first few weeks of life, followed by hepatomegaly and acholic stools. Failure to thrive, pruritus, coagulopathy, and splenomegaly develop with disease progression eventually leading to cirrhosis. In the embryonic form of biliary atresia, infants present with early onset of disease, with jaundice at or shortly after birth and have associated anomalies that can include vascular anomalies of the splenic or portal veins, hepatic artery, or inferior vena cava. Situs inversus, annular lung disease, and congenital heart disease are additional associated anomalies (Venigalla and Gourley 2004).

78.7.2 Evaluation

Thorough history taking and physical exam coupled with a systematic approach will help ensure a timely diagnosis of biliary atresia. Lab evaluation will reveal a conjugated hyperbilirubinemia, elevated transaminases, and gamma-glutamyl transferase levels. Since biliary atresia can result in the malabsorption of fat-soluble vitamins, coagulopathy can be present due to vitamin K deficiency and will result in an elevated prothrombin time.

Abdominal ultrasound often shows a small or absent gallbladder. Care must be taken during interpretation of ultrasound findings because presence or absence of a gallbladder does not confirm or exclude biliary atresia. Observation of the triangular cord sign, by an experienced ultrasonographer, is highly sensitive and specific for biliary atresia (Lee et al. 2009). Splenic and vascular anomalies associated with the embryonic form of biliary atresia may also be seen. If findings on ultrasound are inconclusive for biliary atresia, hepatobiliary scintigraphy should be used to determine the extrahepatic biliary patency. Excretion of isotope into the intestines excludes biliary atresia although lack of excretion into the intestines is not specific for the disease and further evaluation is essential. If the scan is performed when the infant is young, it may need to be repeated as the disease can progress in the first few weeks of life.

Liver biopsy can provide the diagnosis in up to 97% of cases when radiologic studies are inconclusive. In biliary atresia, classic histologic findings include bile duct proliferation, bile plugging, and portal tract edema with periportal fibrosis. As bile ductular inflammation and obliteration in biliary atresia are progressive, if liver biopsy is done early in the disease process, repeat biopsy may be necessary if results are initially equivocal (Moyer et al. 2004; Azar et al. 2002).

In the event that diagnosis is not possible after liver biopsy and radiologic evaluation, operative exploration and cholangiography are then recommended. α_1-Antitrypsin deficiency, as well as other causes of intrahepatic cholestasis, presents similarly to biliary atresia and should be excluded prior to laparotomy, as these conditions can be worsened with portoenterostomy (Lai et al. 1994).

78.7.3 Management

Prompt recognition and appropriate surgical intervention before 60 days of life significantly

improve outcomes. After confirmation of biliary atresia with an intraoperative cholangiogram, the treatment of choice is the Kasai hepatoportoenterostomy. The surgery involves removal of the fibrous tissue at the porta hepatis and formation of a roux-en-Y anastomosis between the duodenum and the hilum of the liver. The two most important prognostic factors determining success of the Kasai procedure are age at operation and experience of the surgeon (Davenport et al. 1997; McClement et al. 1985). The relationship of survival to age is not linear or stepwise and the rate of survival with native liver has been estimated at 90% for those with surgery by 100 days of age compared to 60% if the surgery is performed after 100 days of life (Davenport et al. 1997). Presence of cirrhosis prior to the procedure also accounts for poor success of the procedure and may be an indication for early transplantation (Bittmann 2005). If surgical correction or palliation is not possible, biliary atresia is uniformly fatal. It is possible for patients to live longer than 20 with their native liver following the Kasai procedure; however, 60.5% of long-term survivors have long-term liver-related complications (Bijl et al. 2013).

Complications of the Kasai procedure include ascending cholangitis and portal hypertension. Ascending cholangitis is a common and frequently recurrent postoperative complication with affected patients presenting with fever, worsening jaundice, and elevated ESR. Cholangitis can worsen the prognosis in those who have had restoration of bile flow after portoenterostomy. Recurrence of cholangitis is the single most significant variable pertaining to long-term prognosis (Houwen et al. 1989). After initial treatment with intravenous antibiotics, those with recurrent ascending cholangitis may benefit from prophylactic antibiotics, such as oral trimethoprim-sulfamethoxazole or neomycin (Bu et al. 2003).

Treatment with steroids after the Kasai procedure is controversial. One study showed lower postoperative bilirubin levels, but there was no improvement in terms of cholangitis attacks and early liver transplantation (Chung et al. 2008). Another study concluded that high-dose steroids following surgery did not result in a statistically significant treatment difference in bile drainage at 6 months and may be associated with earlier onset of adverse events in children with biliary atresia (Bezerra et al. 2014). A 2015 study was the first to show tangible longer-term benefit from high-dose steroids but emphasized the importance of early surgery (<45 days of age) (Tyraskis and Davenport 2015). A 2015 meta-analysis concluded that moderate high-dose steroid therapy (prednisolone 4–5 mg/kg/day) improves jaundice clearance particularly in infants undergoing surgery by 70 days of age (Chen et al. 2015). Portal hypertension may develop in 40–80% of patients within 5 years after the Kasai procedure (Venigalla and Gourley 2004). These patients have splenomegaly that may be complicated by ascites and variceal bleeding. Twenty percent of the patients that have portal hypertension may be noted to have portal vein thrombosis, likely secondary to ongoing portal tract inflammation. Therapeutic endoscopy with either ligation or sclerotherapy can be used to treat acute variceal bleeding. In addition to the surgical management, patients should also receive supportive care for cholestasis, including supplementation of fat-soluble vitamins and a high calorie diet.

78.7.4 α_1-Antitrypsin (α_1-AT) Deficiency

α_1-AT deficiency is the most common inherited cause of neonatal cholestasis and one of the most important indications for pediatric liver transplant. It is caused by mutations in the SERPINA 1 gene found on chromosome 14 and is inherited in an autosomal codominant fashion (Monajemzadeh et al. 2013). α_1-AT is a glycoprotein with inhibitory activity against elastase, trypsin, and other proteolytic enzymes. The primary function of this enzyme is to prevent lung and other tissue damage from these circulating proteases. Intracellular accumulation of abnormal α_1-AT is the cause of liver disease, cirrhosis, and hepatic carcinoma (Teckman 2013). More than 100 different variants of α_1-AT mutants have been found, but only a few are clinically relevant,

with M being normal and Z being the most deficient. Patients with PiZZ phenotype have greatly reduced amounts of α_1-AT, around 10–15% of normal, with an incidence of 1 in 2,000–5,000 live births in European and North American populations (Coakley et al. 2001). The PiZZ phenotype is associated with neonatal liver disease and adult emphysema. Approximately 15% of PiZZ neonates develop clinical disease within 20 years, and accumulation of the defective α_1-AT molecule in the liver is the cause of hepatic injury (Lomas et al. 1992). These infants have intrauterine growth retardation and are more likely to develop coagulopathy compounding the cholestasis. On biopsy, periodic acid-Schiff-positive diastase-resistant inclusions within hepatocytes represent the abnormal alpha-1-antitrypsin protein. Documenting low plasma α_1-AT levels and determining α_1-AT phenotype confirm the diagnosis.

As with idiopathic neonatal hepatitis, management of α_1-AT deficiency is mostly supportive and includes nutritional supplementation. Prognosis is related to the severity of the liver disease. In children with progressive liver disease, liver transplantation has shown good survival rates of 90% at 1 year and 80% at 5 years (Francavilla et al. 2000).

78.7.5 Idiopathic Neonatal Hepatitis

Idiopathic neonatal hepatitis accounts for approximately 30% of neonatal cholestasis cases. A diagnosis of exclusion, idiopathic neonatal hepatitis is diagnosed by documentation of classic histologic findings on liver biopsy. Although occasional familial cases suggest a genetic association, most cases are sporadic.

Infants with idiopathic neonatal hepatitis have often low birth weight. Jaundice is present within the first few weeks of life but not immediately after birth. The liver may be enlarged on physical examination and serum bilirubin and hepatic transaminases mildly elevated. Low or normal GGT levels may signify more severe disease and a worse prognosis, especially if GGT levels do not increase over the course of the disease (Wang et al. 2006). Imaging of the biliary tree is often normal (Torbenson et al. 2010). On liver biopsy, findings include lobular disarray with hepatocyte swelling, giant cell transformation, necrosis, and increased extramedullary hematopoiesis. In contrast to biliary atresia, management of idiopathic neonatal hepatitis is largely supportive. Prognosis is excellent with 90% resolution by 1 year of age in sporadic cases but worse in familial cases.

78.7.6 Progressive Familial Intrahepatic Cholestasis

Progressive familial intrahepatic cholestasis (PFIC) is a group of genetic disorders, with autosomal recessive inheritance, associated with progressive intrahepatic cholestasis. There are three distinct forms of PFIC which vary in presentation and diagnosis (Table 4).

Table 4 Clinical features of different forms of progressive familial intrahepatic cholestasis

	PFIC-1	PFIC-2	PFIC-3
Mutation	ATP8B1 gene, chromosome 18	ABCB11 gene, chromosome 2	ABCB4
Extrahepatic tissue involved	Pancreas, small bowel, stomach, bladder, heart, and kidney	None	None
Serum bile salt concentration	Elevated	Elevated	Elevated
GGT level	Normal	Normal	Elevated
Liver histology	Bile duct paucity, mild lobular fibrosis	Giant cell hepatitis, hepatocellular necrosis	Bile ductular proliferation
Cirrhosis	First decade of life	Early infancy	First or second decade of life

PFIC-1, the original Byler disease described in an Amish family, is caused by a mutation in the ATP8B1 gene on chromosome 18, which encodes for the FIC1 protein (Srivastava 2014; Hori et al. 2010). Normally, the activity of the FIC1 protein helps to maintain the integrity of the canalicular membrane of hepatocytes by protecting it from the high bile salt concentration in the canalicular lumen. While the exact mechanism of cholestasis and the other symptoms of PFIC-1 are not completely understood, it appears to be related to the overload of bile acids in the hepatocyte due to the loss of the protective effect of the FIC1 protein. This results in episodic cholestasis in the first month of life. With time, the jaundice resolves but the pruritus continues and end-stage liver disease ensues. The ATP8B1 FIC1 gene has a wide tissue distribution and, besides the canalicular membrane, is also expressed in the pancreas, small bowel, stomach, bladder, heart, and kidney. This might explain the extrahepatic manifestation of PFIC-1 such as diarrhea and pancreatic insufficiency with fat-soluble vitamin deficiency seen in affected patients. Importantly, serum GGT and transaminase levels are normal, with markedly elevated serum bile salts.

PFIC type 1 typically presents in infancy and can progress to cirrhosis within the first decade of life. Liver histology at biopsy shows bile duct paucity and mild lobular fibrosis. Liver transplantation for hepatic decompression may become necessary by the second decade.

PFIC-2 is caused by a mutation in the ABCB11 gene encoding the bile salt export protein (BSEP) on chromosome 2. This protein helps in the export of bile acids from the hepatocyte to the canaliculi against a concentration gradient. Loss of protein function results in decreased bile flow, accumulation of bile salts in the hepatocytes, and hepatocellular damage. PFIC-2 typically presents in the neonatal period and is more severe than PFIC-1. Clinical presentation is similar to PFIC-1, with the exception of lack of the extraintestinal manifestations, as the protein is specific to the hepatocytes. Liver biopsy usually shows more inflammation, giant cell hepatitis, hepatocellular necrosis, and portal fibrosis. Prognosis is worse for those requiring liver transplantation in the first decade of life.

PFIC-3 is caused by defect in the adenosine triphosphate-binding cassette (ABCB4) gene encoding the multidrug-resistant class III (MDR3) protein. The MDR3 protein is a phospholipid flippase present on the canalicular membrane of the hepatocyte responsible for biliary secretion. Mutations result in a loss of the detergent neutralizing properties of phospholipids resulting in injury to the biliary epithelium and ultimately cholestasis. This also results in higher concentrations of unmicellized bile salts and promotes cholesterol crystallization resulting in obstruction of bile ducts. Clinical presentation is similar to PFIC-1 and is often delayed until early adulthood but can present in late infancy. There is often a history of cholestasis of pregnancy in the mother. In contrast to PFIC-1 and PFIC-2, GGT is markedly elevated, and bile analysis shows a high bile acid to phospholipid ratio. PFIC-3 can sometimes present with GI bleeding and portal hypertension. Liver biopsy may appear consistent with biliary atresia as it shows portal fibrosis and true bile ductular proliferation with an inflammatory infiltrate, but the biliary tract will be patent on scintigraphy or cholangiography. Prognosis is variable (Srivastava 2014).

78.7.7 PFIC Management

Management of PFIC is largely supportive and the first step usually consists of medical therapies. This includes relief from pruritus, optimizing nutritional status, including correcting vitamin deficiencies and controlling symptoms of advance liver disease like variceal bleeding and coagulopathy, if present.

Biliary diversion procedures are seen to be particularly helpful in the management of PFIC as they decrease the enterohepatic circulation of toxic bile salts. There are two main types of biliary diversion procedures: external partial biliary diversion which consists of surgically creating a permanent stoma that diverts the bile from the gall bladder to the outside or internal partial biliary diversion which consists of creating a conduit from the gall bladder to the colon so no external fistula is needed. These procedures can be very

helpful in patients who are not responding to medical therapy and are not yet candidates for liver transplant (Srivastava 2014).

78.7.8 Benign Recurrent Intrahepatic Cholestasis (BRIC)

BRIC is an autosomal recessive disorder, with incomplete penetrance characterized by repeated episodes of severe pruritus and jaundice at any age, but more commonly before the second decade of life (Ermis et al. 2010; Strubbe et al. 2012). Mutation of the ATP8B1 gene on chromosome 18, encoding the FIC1 gene, is thought to be the cause. This is the same gene responsible for PFIC-1. BRIC is differentiated from PFIC based on the phenotypic presentation, mainly with episodic bouts of cholestasis. Pruritus is the most common presenting symptoms followed by jaundice. Elevation in alkaline phosphatase and conjugated bilirubin are common, while GGT, AST, and ALT are usually normal. Treatment should focus on symptomatic relief until the resolution of each episode. Prognosis is more favorable than PFIC-1 and typically does not progress to fibrosis (Nguyen et al. 2014).

78.7.9 Cholestasis in Premature Infants

Cholestasis is common in very low birth weight infants, with a multifactorial etiology. The biliary system is immature in these infants resulting in an exaggerated physiologic cholestasis. Other factors can contribute to cholestasis in premature infants, including perinatal hypoxia, sepsis, parenteral nutrition (PN), and enteral feeding difficulties (Steinbach et al. 2008; Herzog et al. 2003; Hsieh et al. 2009). Cholestasis is a frequent complication of PN. Although the exact etiology is unknown, immaturity of the enterohepatic circulation likely plays a role. Risk factors include early initiation and prolonged PN, lack of enteral feeds, sepsis, and prematurity. Conjugated hyperbilirubinemia with elevated transaminases is usually seen within 2 weeks of commencing PN. Management includes decreasing or cessation of PN and increasing enteral feeds. In those infants who cannot tolerate full enteral feeds, trophic feeds should be instituted to decrease enterohepatic circulation (Dani et al. 2015). In such infants, modifications in PN formulation should include limiting glucose intake to 15 g/kg/day, limiting intralipid, cycling of PN to 12 h daily, and reducing or eliminating manganese and copper, as these trace nutrients are primarily secreted via bile. Ursodeoxycholic acid can aid in stimulating bile acid excretion via mechanisms previously discussed.

Biliary atresia is rare in premature infants and liver biopsy and hepatobiliary scintigraphy should be delayed in these infants until corrected gestational age (CGA) is term and weight is greater than 2 kg. Liver biopsy should be performed if cholestasis persists past 2 months CGA, presence of acholic stools, and those without excretion on hepatobiliary scan.

78.7.10 Alagille Syndrome

Alagille syndrome is an autosomal dominant condition with variable penetrance that affects the heart, liver, skeletal muscle, face, and eyes. Facial features are characterized by a broad forehead, deep-set eyes, and a pointed chin giving the face a triangular appearance. Butterfly vertebra, curved phalanges, and a short ulna are common skeletal anomalies. Peripheral pulmonic stenosis, tetralogy of Fallot, pulmonary atresia, and VSD are cardiac anomalies that may be seen. Posterior embryotoxon and optic nerve drusen constitute eye findings. Supernumerary digital flexion creases are seen in one third of cases (Kamath et al. 2002). Cutaneous xanthomas secondary to hyperlipidemia can also be seen.

The incidence of Alagille syndrome is estimated at 1 in 100,000 live births. About 94–97% of cases have mutations in the JAG1 gene, while the remainder are due to mutations in the NOTCH2 gene. Both genes are part of the Notch pathway involved in intracellular signaling (Nguyen et al. 2014; McDaniell et al. 2006).

Initially, infants with Alagille syndrome present with neonatal cholestasis, as seen in biliary

atresia. Differentiation of the two disorders can be difficult because initial liver biopsies may show bile duct proliferation consistent with BA. Bile ducts are initially structurally normal and are then progressively lost. The paucity of bile ducts seen on live biopsy is characteristic of Alagille syndrome. Characteristic facies may not be evident until 2 years of age.

Management is largely supportive, with nutritional support including fat-soluble vitamin supplementation. Pruritus can be recalcitrant and require multimodal therapies. A cardiologist may be an integral part of the medical team for managing hemodynamically significant cardiac disease. These patients should also be screened for vascular anomalies such as aortic aneurysms, which can be associated with defects in the Notch signaling pathway (Kamath et al. 2004). Of those who present with cholestasis in the newborn period, over 50% will require liver transplantation by 10 years of age secondary to cirrhosis. Caution must be used in evaluation of family members as matched living donors, as there may be subclinical disease in such donors. The 5-year survival rate is 80% and can significantly improve growth in up to 90% of cases (Turnpenny and Ellard 2012).

References

Abdel-Kader HH, Balistreri WF (1994) Neonatal hepatobiliary disease. Semin Gastrointest Dis 5 (2):65–77

Abramson SJ, Treves S, Teele RL (1982) The infant with possible biliary atresia: evaluation by ultrasound and nuclear medicine. Pediatr Radiol 12(1):1–5

Azar G, Beneck D, Lane B, Markowitz J, Daum F, Kahn E (2002) Atypical morphologic presentation of biliary atresia and value of serial liver biopsies. J Pediatr Gastroenterol Nutr 34(2):212–215

Bates MD, Bucuvalas JC, Alonso MH, Ryckman FC (1998) Biliary atresia: pathogenesis and treatment. Semin Liver Dis 18(3):281–293

Bergasa NV (2008) Update on the treatment of the pruritus of cholestasis. Clin Liver Dis 12(1):219–234, x

Bergasa NV, Jones EA (1995) The pruritus of cholestasis: potential pathogenic and therapeutic implications of opioids. Gastroenterology 108(5):1582–1588

Bergasa NV, Talbot TL, Alling DW et al (1992) A controlled trial of naloxone infusions for the pruritus of chronic cholestasis. Gastroenterology 102(2):544–549

Bergasa NV, Link MJ, Keogh M, Yaroslavsky G, Rosenthal RN, McGee M (2001) Pilot study of bright-light therapy reflected toward the eyes for the pruritus of chronic liver disease. Am J Gastroenterol 96 (5):1563–1570

Bezerra JA (2005) Potential etiologies of biliary atresia. Pediatr Transplant 9(5):646–651

Bezerra JA, Spino C, Magee JC et al (2014) Use of corticosteroids after hepatoportoenterostomy for bile drainage in infants with biliary atresia: the START randomized clinical trial. JAMA 311(17):1750–1759

Bijl EJ, Bharwani KD, Houwen RH, de Man RA (2013) The long-term outcome of the Kasai operation in patients with biliary atresia: a systematic review. Neth J Med 71(4):170–173

Bittmann S (2005) Surgical experience in children with biliary atresia treated with portoenterostomy. Curr Surg 62(4):439–443

Boyer JL (2013) Bile formation and secretion. Compr Physiol 3(3):1035–1078

Browning J, Combes B, Mayo MJ (2003) Long-term efficacy of sertraline as a treatment for cholestatic pruritus in patients with primary biliary cirrhosis. Am J Gastroenterol 98(12):2736–2741

Bu LN, Chen HL, Chang CJ et al (2003) Prophylactic oral antibiotics in prevention of recurrent cholangitis after the Kasai portoenterostomy. J Pediatr Surg 38 (4):590–593

Cabrera-Abreu JC, Green A (2002) Gamma-glutamyltransferase: value of its measurement in paediatrics. Ann Clin Biochem 39(Pt 1):22–25

Calleja C, Pascussi JM, Mani JC, Maurel P, Vilarem MJ (1998) The antibiotic rifampicin is a nonsteroidal ligand and activator of the human glucocorticoid receptor. Nat Med 4(1):92–96

Chang Y, Golkar L (2008) The use of naltrexone in the management of severe generalized pruritus in biliary atresia: report of a case. Pediatr Dermatol 25(3):403–404

Chen Y, Nah SA, Chiang L, Krishnaswamy G, Low Y (2015) Postoperative steroid therapy for biliary atresia: systematic review and meta-analysis. J Pediatr Surg 50 (9):1590–1594

Chung HY, Kak Yuen Wong K, Cheun Leung Lan L, Kwong Hang Tam P (2008) Evaluation of a standardized protocol in the use of steroids after Kasai operation. Pediatr Surg Int. 2008 Sep;24(9):1001–1004.

Cies JJ, Giamalis JN (2007) Treatment of cholestatic pruritus in children. Am J Health-Syst Pharm 64 (11):1157–1162

Coakley RJ, Taggart C, O'Neill S, McElvaney NG (2001) Alpha1-antitrypsin deficiency: biological answers to clinical questions. Am J Med Sci 321(1):33–41

Dani C, Pratesi S, Raimondi F, Romagnoli C, Task Force for Hyperbilirubinemia of the Italian Society of Neonatology (2015) Italian guidelines for the management and treatment of neonatal cholestasis. Ital J Pediatr 41:69

Davenport M, Kerkar N, Mieli-Vergani G, Mowat AP, Howard ER (1997) Biliary atresia: the King's College

Hospital experience (1974–1995). J Pediatr Surg 32 (3):479–485

Dehghani SM, Haghighat M, Imanieh MH, Geramizadeh B (2006) Comparison of different diagnostic methods in infants with cholestasis. World J Gastroenterol 12 (36):5893–5896

Diehn F, Tefferi A (2001) Pruritus in polycythaemia vera: prevalence, laboratory correlates and management. Br J Haematol 115(3):619–621

Dillon S, Tobias JD (2013) Ondansetron to treat pruritus due to cholestatic jaundice. J Pediatr Pharmacol Ther 18(3):241–246

Eaves ER, Korman MG (1984) Cholestyramine induced hyperchloremic metabolic acidosis. Aust N Z J Med 14 (5):670–672

Ermis F, Oncu K, Ozel M et al (2010) Benign recurrent intrahepatic cholestasis: late initial diagnosis in adulthood. Ann Hepatol 9(2):207–210

Feldman AG, Mack CL (2012) Biliary atresia: cellular dynamics and immune dysregulation. Semin Pediatr Surg 21(3):192–200

Fischler B, Papadogiannakis N, Nemeth A (2001) Clinical aspects on neonatal cholestasis based on observations at a Swedish tertiary referral centre. Acta Paediatr 90 (2):171–178

Francavilla R, Castellaneta SP, Hadzic N et al (2000) Prognosis of alpha-1-antitrypsin deficiency-related liver disease in the era of paediatric liver transplantation. J Hepatol 32(6):986–992

Frederick Suchy RS (2007) Liver disease in children, 3rd edn. Cambridge University Press, New York

Frigon C, Desparmet J (2006) Ondansetron treatment in a child presenting with chronic intractable pruritus. Pain Res Manag: J Can Pain Soc 11(4):245–247

Gourley GR, Yang L, Higgins L, Riviere MA, David LL (2009) Proteomic analysis of biopsied human colonic mucosa. J Pediatr Gastroenterol Nutr 2010 Jul;51 (1):46–54

Haber BA, Russo P (2003) Biliary atresia. Gastroenterol Clin North Am 32(3):891–911

Hegade VS, Kendrick SF, Jones DE (2015) Drug treatment of pruritus in liver diseases. Clin Med 15(4):351–357

Herzog D, Chessex P, Martin S, Alvarez F (2003) Transient cholestasis in newborn infants with perinatal asphyxia. Can J Gastroenterol 17(3):179–182

Hirfanoglu IM, Unal S, Onal EE et al (2014) Analysis of serum gamma-glutamyl transferase levels in neonatal intensive care unit patients. J Pediatr Gastroenterol Nutr 58(1):99–101

Hori T, Nguyen JH, Uemoto S (2010) Progressive familial intrahepatic cholestasis. Hepatobiliary Pancreat Dis Int 9(6):570–578

Houwen RH, Zwierstra RP, Severijnen RS et al (1989) Prognosis of extrahepatic biliary atresia. Arch Dis Child 64(2):214–218

Hsieh MH, Pai W, Tseng HI, Yang SN, Lu CC, Chen HL (2009) Parenteral nutrition-associated cholestasis in premature babies: risk factors and predictors. Pediatr Neonatol 50(5):202–207

Kamath BM, Loomes KM, Oakey RJ, Krantz ID (2002) Supernumerary digital flexion creases: an additional clinical manifestation of Alagille syndrome. Am J Med Genet 112(2):171–175

Kamath BM, Spinner NB, Emerick KM et al (2004) Vascular anomalies in Alagille syndrome: a significant cause of morbidity and mortality. Circulation 109 (11):1354–1358

Kotb MA, Kotb A, Sheba MF et al (2001) Evaluation of the triangular cord sign in the diagnosis of biliary atresia. Pediatrics 108(2):416–420

Kremer AE, Gonzales E, Schaap FG, Elferink RP, Jacquemin E, Beuers U (2015) Serum autotaxin activity correlates with pruritus in pediatric cholestatic disorders. J Pediatr Gastroenterol Nutr 2016 Apr;62 (4):530–535

Lai MW, Chang MH, Hsu SC et al (1994) Differential diagnosis of extrahepatic biliary atresia from neonatal hepatitis: a prospective study. J Pediatr Gastroenterol Nutr 18(2):121–127

Larrosa-Haro A, Caro-Lopez AM, Coello-Ramirez P, Zavala-Ocampo J, Vazquez-Camacho G (2001) Duodenal tube test in the diagnosis of biliary atresia. J Pediatr Gastroenterol Nutr 32(3):311–315

Lee MS, Kim MJ, Lee MJ et al (2009) Biliary atresia: color Doppler US findings in neonates and infants. Radiology 252(1):282–289

Liu B, Cai J, Xu Y et al (2014) Three-dimensional magnetic resonance cholangiopancreatography for the diagnosis of biliary atresia in infants and neonates. PLoS One 9(2):e88268

Lomas DA, Evans DL, Finch JT, Carrell RW (1992) The mechanism of Z alpha 1-antitrypsin accumulation in the liver. Nature 357(6379):605–607

Maxwell LG, Kaufmann SC, Bitzer S et al (2005) The effects of a small-dose naloxone infusion on opioid-induced side effects and analgesia in children and adolescents treated with intravenous patient-controlled analgesia: a double-blind, prospective, randomized, controlled study. Anesth Analg 100(4):953–958

McClement JW, Howard ER, Mowat AP (1985) Results of surgical treatment for extrahepatic biliary atresia in United Kingdom 1980–2. Survey conducted on behalf of the British Paediatric Association Gastroenterology Group and the British Association of Paediatric Surgeons. Br Med J (Clin Res Ed) 290(6465):345–347

McDaniell R, Warthen DM, Sanchez-Lara PA et al (2006) NOTCH2 mutations cause Alagille syndrome, a heterogeneous disorder of the notch signaling pathway. Am J Hum Genet 79(1):169–173

Mitchison HC, Bassendine MF, Malcolm AJ, Watson AJ, Record CO, James OF (1989) A pilot, double-blind, controlled 1-year trial of prednisolone treatment in primary biliary cirrhosis: hepatic improvement but greater bone loss. Hepatology (Baltimore, Md) 10 (4):420–429

Monajemzadeh M, Shahsiah R, Vasei M et al (2013) Alpha 1 antitrypsin deficiency in infants with neonatal cholestasis. Iran J Pediatr 23(5):501–507

Moyer V, Freese DK, Whitington PF et al (2004) Guideline for the evaluation of cholestatic jaundice in infants: recommendations of the North American Society for Pediatric Gastroenterology, Hepatology and Nutrition. J Pediatr Gastroenterol Nutr 39(2):115–128

Nguyen KD, Sundaram V, Ayoub WS (2014) Atypical causes of cholestasis. World J Gastroenterol 20 (28):9418–9426

Oude Elferink RP, Kremer AE, Beuers U (2011) Mediators of pruritus during cholestasis. Curr Opin Gastroenterol 27(3):289–293

Park WH, Choi SO, Lee HJ, Kim SP, Zeon SK, Lee SL (1997) A new diagnostic approach to biliary atresia with emphasis on the ultrasonographic triangular cord sign: comparison of ultrasonography, hepatobiliary scintigraphy, and liver needle biopsy in the evaluation of infantile cholestasis. J Pediatr Surg 32 (11):1555–1559

Pusl T, Denk GU, Parhofer KG, Beuers U (2006) Plasma separation and anion adsorption transiently relieve intractable pruritus in primary biliary cirrhosis. J Hepatol 45(6):887–891

Rifai K, Hafer C, Rosenau J et al (2006) Treatment of severe refractory pruritus with fractionated plasma separation and adsorption (Prometheus). Scand J Gastroenterol 41(10):1212–1217

Seckin D, Demircay Z, Akin O (2007) Generalized pruritus treated with narrowband UVB. Int J Dermatol 46 (4):367–370

Sergi C, Benstz J, Feist D, Nutzenadel W, Otto HF, Hofmann WJ (2008) Bile duct to portal space ratio and ductal plate remnants in liver disease of infants aged less than 1 year. Pathology 40(3):260–267

Shojania AM, Grewar D (1986) Hypoprothrombinemic hemorrhage due to cholestyramine therapy. CMAJ 134(6):609–610

Shteyer E, Wengrower D, Benuri-Silbiger I, Gozal D, Wilschanski M, Goldin E (2012) Endoscopic retrograde cholangiopancreatography in neonatal cholestasis. J Pediatr Gastroenterol Nutr 55(2):142–145

Soroka CJ, Boyer JL (2014) Biosynthesis and trafficking of the bile salt export pump, BSEP: therapeutic implications of BSEP mutations. Mol Aspects Med 37:3–14

Srivastava A (2014) Progressive familial intrahepatic cholestasis. J Clin Exp Hepatol 4(1):25–36

Steinbach M, Clark RH, Kelleher AS et al (2008) Demographic and nutritional factors associated with prolonged cholestatic jaundice in the premature infant. J Perinatol: Off J Calif Perinat Assoc 28(2):129–135

Strubbe B, Geerts A, Van Vlierberghe H, Colle I (2012) Progressive familial intrahepatic cholestasis and benign recurrent intrahepatic cholestasis: a review. Acta Gastro-Enterologica Belgica 75(4):405–410

Teckman JH (2013) Liver disease in alpha-1 antitrypsin deficiency: current understanding and future therapy. COPD 10(Suppl 1):35–43

Torbenson M, Hart J, Westerhoff M et al (2010) Neonatal giant cell hepatitis: histological and etiological findings. Am J Surg Pathol 34(10):1498–1503

Turnpenny PD, Ellard S (2012) Alagille syndrome: pathogenesis, diagnosis and management. Eur J Hum Genet: EJHG 20(3):251–257

Tyraskis A, Davenport M (2015) Steroids after the Kasai procedure for biliary atresia: the effect of age at Kasai portoenterostomy. Pediatr Surg Int. 2016 Mar;32 (3):193–200.

Venigalla S, Gourley GR (2004) Neonatal cholestasis. Semin Perinatol 28(5):348–355

Walker WA, Kleinman R et al (2004) Pediatric gastrointestinal disease: pathophysiology, diagnosis, management, 3rd edn. B.C. Decker, Hamilton

Wang JS, Tan N, Dhawan A (2006) Significance of low or normal serum gamma glutamyl transferase level in infants with idiopathic neonatal hepatitis. Eur J Pediatr 165(11):795–801

Yang JG, Ma DQ, Peng Y, Song L, Li CL (2009) Comparison of different diagnostic methods for differentiating biliary atresia from idiopathic neonatal hepatitis. Clin Imaging 33(6):439–446

Zylicz Z, Smits C, Krajnik M (1998) Paroxetine for pruritus in advanced cancer. J Pain Symptom Manage 16 (2):121–124

Zylicz Z, Krajnik M, Sorge AA, Costantini M (2003) Paroxetine in the treatment of severe non-dermatological pruritus: a randomized, controlled trial. J Pain Symptom Manage 26(6):1105–1112

Surgical Treatment of Biliary Tract Malformations in Newborns

79

Pierluigi Pedersini

Contents

Abstract

The most common biliary malformations in newborn requiring early surgical treatment are represented by biliary atresia (BA), congenital bile duct dilatation (CBDD), and solitary liver cysts (SLCs). **Biliary atresia** (BA) is the first

P. Pedersini (✉)
National Center for Surgical Treatment of Pediatric Hepatobiliary Malformations, Pediatric Surgery, University of Brescia, Brescia, Italy
e-mail: pierluigi.pedersini@gmail.com

G. Buonocore et al. (eds.), *Neonatology*,
https://doi.org/10.1007/978-3-319-29489-6_226

cause of neonatal cholestatic jaundice. The origin of BA still remains unclear; if untreated, it usually leads to exitus within the first 2 years of life; therefore, early diagnosis is mandatory to plan a timely surgery, preferably earlier than 70 days. The Kasai operation can achieve good results in about a half of cases, but even children successfully treated suffered from liver failure, so the majority of these patients need liver transplantation later in life. Actually, the sequential use of Kasai operation and liver transplantation has dramatically increased the survival rate of patients with BA. **Congenital bile duct dilatation** is a relatively rare malformation of the pancreatobiliary system; the etiology remains essentially unclear. The cyst usually occurs with asymptomatic jaundice that may be mild and intermittent or progressive due to complete biliary obstruction. The surgical procedure of choice is total excision. **Solitary liver cyst** is a benign lesion with unknown etiology. They are often asymptomatic and identified incidentally or antenatally in the third trimester. Intervention is required among children who are symptomatic for a mass effect. On the basis of recent studies and fortieth experience of our Center, we summarize the current status of diagnosis and therapy of these biliary tract malformations.

79.1 Salient Points

- Biliary atresia (BA) is a progressive necroinflammatory obliterative cholangiopathy involving the intra- and extrahepatic bile ducts.
- Ultrasound plays a critical role in the diagnosis of BA; atretic gallbladder, "triangular cord" thickness (>3.4 mm), and hepatic subcapsular flow appear to be the most significant predictors of BA.
- The current surgical management of BA provides Kasai portoenterostomy (KPE) in neonatal period, which aims to restore bile flow, and later liver transplantation, when the KPE has failed.
- Congenital bile duct dilatation (CBDD) rarely occurs in the first months of life and is primarily a disease of older infants; it presents with jaundice, abdominal pain, and a right hypochondrial mass.
- Solitary liver cyst is a benign lesion; total excision or enucleation depends on the anatomical type of lesion.

79.2 Biliary Atresia

79.2.1 Introduction

Biliary atresia (BA) is a progressive necroinflammatory obliterative cholangiopathy involving the intra- and extrahepatic bile ducts. The disease arises during the first days of life and usually evolves into obliteration of extrahepatic bile ducts with interruption of bile flow, resulting in cholestasis and progressive liver damage. If untreated, BA leads to cirrhosis, hepatic failure, and exitus within the first 2 years of life. Early diagnosis is mandatory to plan a timely surgery, preferably within 70 days of life.

Although the surgical treatment can achieve a good relief of cholestasis in about a half of cases, even children successfully treated show the consequences of liver deterioration, namely, hepatic fibrosis or cirrhosis with portal hypertension, so the majority of BA patients need liver replacement later in life (Caccia et al. 2004). Actually, BA is still the most common indication for pediatric liver transplantation worldwide, with dramatic increase of the survival rate of BA patients during the last few decades (Lee et al. 2013).

BA is the most common cause of cholestatic jaundice in newborn, and its prevalence is about 1:10.000–15.000 live births, meaning approximately 700 newborns affected every year in Europe, with a small female preponderance. Incidence of BA is highest in Asian and Pacific populations and familial cases have been reported (Chardot 2006).

Obliteration of bile ducts can involve the extrahepatic biliary tree, partially or completely, and the types of BA are classified according to the most proximal level of obstruction: **type I** involves just the common bile duct; **type II** also involves the cystic and the hepatic ducts; and **type**

III, present in more than 95% of cases, involves all extrahepatic biliary ducts and represent the most severe form of BA.

Two forms of BA have been identified, which can be defined clinically: (**1**) **isolated BA** (~**90**%), representing the largest but not homogeneous group, because of variation in time presentation, degree of cholangiopathy, and obliteration of biliary tree, and (**2**) **syndromic BA and associated malformations** (~**10**%), with female predominance. This may be further divided into a *BA splenic malformation* (*BASM*) *syndrome*, with congenital anomalies such as polysplenia, asplenia, cardiac or intra-abdominal defects (situs inversus, preduodenal portal vein, absence of retrohepatic inferior vena cava, intestinal malrotation), and *BA with random malformations*, as esophageal or jejunal atresia (Davenport 2012).

79.2.2 Etiology and Pathogenesis

The etiology of BA still remains largely unknown. Some cases seem to be related to abnormal morphogenesis of bile ducts occurring early in pregnancy with cholestasis from birth (*embryonic or fetal BA*, 35% of cases), while many cases appear to arise from later damage to normally developing bile ducts, with onset of symptoms at the age of about 4 weeks (*perinatal or acquired BA*, 65% of cases) (Baumann and Ure 2012).

Several epidemiologic studies have pointed toward a potential association between viral infection and BA. An association with some virus infections (CMV, RSV, EBV, and HPV) has been reported, while no association with hepatitis A, B, and C viruses has been found (Chardot 2006). The viruses most commonly implicated are *Reoviridae* and *Rotaviridae*. In human neonates, the association of reovirus type III and BA has been suggested, but not confirmed otherwise. The role of rotavirus type C in the etiology of BA in humans remains still controversial, because of the few published studies and their incomplete accuracy. Thus, currently there are no studies that can definitively prove a viral etiology of BA (Saito et al. 2015).

The role of immune-mediate mechanism in the pathogenesis of BA has been based by the assumption that the initial damage of biliary epithelium is followed by the activation of immune cells and the release of proinflammatory cytokines that perpetuate the injury up to biliary destruction, which is followed by collagen deposition to produce biliary fibrosis (Besso and Bezerra 2011; Srivastava 2011; Sira et al. 2015).

The progressive liver damage, the presence of lymphocytes in the liver of patients with BA, and the association with HLA-B12 have suggested an autoimmune persistent injury against the biliary epithelium (Alvarez 2013).

Defect in fetal circulation and exposure to environmental toxins has also been proposed. Recently, the role of gene ADP ribosylation factor-6 (ARF6) in defective bile duct formation, leading to BA, has been postulated (Ningappa et al. 2015).

Therefore, BA does not seem to be a single disease, but a phenotype, resulting from a number of different and separate etiologies.

79.2.3 Clinical Aspects

The clinical signs are jaundice persisting beyond 14 days of age, alcoholic stools, dark urine, and hepatomegaly. The liver gradually increases in size and consistency along with aging. Splenomegaly also follows hepatomegaly, suggesting portal hypertension. The general condition of the newborn is usually good with adequate weight growth; mild jaundice is often missed and the diagnosis is established later. When the patients are untreated, the majority of them will die of hepatic failure, esophageal variceal bleeding, and infections (Caccia et al. 2004).

79.2.4 Diagnosis

Antenatal diagnosis of BA remains exceptional. Since early diagnosis appears essential for successful surgical treatment, neonatal jaundice lasting more than 14 days should be investigated for BA. There are many causes of pathological jaundice in the neonatal period, and the most likely to be confused with BA are neonatal hepatitis syndrome and interlobular biliary hypoplasia. When

newborn shows jaundice, alcoholic stools, dark urine, and hepatomegaly with hardening in consistence, BA should be strongly suspected (Caccia et al. 2004).

Biochemical liver function tests show increased total bilirubin (TB) with predominance of direct bilirubin (DB) more than 50% and high levels of γGT, ALT, and AST (more than two to three times of normal values). BA is very strongly suspected with the presence of TB greater than 4.5 mg/dL, DB more than 80% of TB, and γGT greater than 500 UI/L (Caccia et al. 2004).

Ultrasound (US) plays a critical role in the diagnosis of BA. Some US findings have been described as useful indicators of BA, as abnormal gallbladder morphology, "triangular cord" sign, visualization of the extrahepatic bile duct, diameter of the hepatic artery, and presence of hepatic subcapsular flow. Between these, atretic gallbladder, "triangular cord" thickness (>3.4 mm), and, more recently, hepatic subcapsular flow appear to be the most significant predictors of BA (Lee et al. 2015; El-Guindi et al. 2013). US also is helpful in the assessment of splenomegaly or associated anomalies, such as polysplenia.

Hepatobiliary scintigraphy (e.g., Tc-99m DISIDA) shows a failure of excrection of the radioisotope into the intestine, but has relatively poor discrimination with severe neonatal cholestasis from whatever cause. Endoscopic retrograde cholangiopancreatography (ERCP) (Shanmugam et al. 2009) and MR cholangiography play a limited role in the diagnosis of BA because they may be performed in selected skilled centers only.

The definitive diagnosis is based on detection of fibrosing obstruction of the extrahepatic bile ducts during exploratory laparotomy, cholangiography, and liver biopsy (Caccia et al. 2004). The main histological features suggestive of BA are ductular proliferation, portal fibrosis, and absence of sinusoidal fibrosis (Russo et al. 2011). Overall, the predictive value of liver biopsy for BA was 91%. Recently, some countries have adopted a simple population screening program for BA. In Taiwan, it has allowed to shorten the time to surgery, with the median age at intervention being <50 days, representing the best result achieved anywhere (Hsiao et al. 2008).

79.2.5 Therapy and Treatment

The current surgical management of BA provides Kasai portoenterostomy (KPE) in neonatal period, which aims to restore bile flow, and later liver transplantation, when the KPE has failed (Chardot 2006).

The KPE provides a careful dissection to locate patent bile duct remnants in the porta hepatis with the restoration of biliary flow by a 45 cm Roux-en-Y loop anastomosis to the hepatic hilum. Alternative laparoscopic approach was reported since 2002 (Estevez et al. 2002), but results are certainly not better and rarely comparable to standard open approach nowadays (Ure et al. 2011).

The best surgical results after KPE are obtained in children operated within 60 days of life, with early satisfactory biliary drainage in at least 70% of cases (Nio et al. 2010), resulting in increased pigmentation of stools and progressive resolution of jaundice. The outcome of surgery may be improved by early postoperative adjuvant high-dose steroid therapy (oral prednisolone, IV methylprednisolone, or hydrocortisone), which does have a significant benefit in reduction of postoperative bilirubin and clearance of jaundice (Tyraskis and Davenport 2015). However, the effect of steroids may be limited or inhibited by an increasing fibrosis and onset of cirrhosis, due to delayed diagnosis and surgery.

Thus, the age at treatment is one of the most important factors determining surgical outcome that can be influenced by reduced effectiveness of adjuvant therapy and postoperative complications.

The most common complications following the KPE are cholangitis and portal hypertension. Rare complications include hepatopulmonary syndrome, pulmonary hypertension, intrahepatic biliary cavities, and malignancy (Chardot 2006).

Cholangitis occurs particularly in the first weeks or months after operation in 33–60% of cases and clinically is characterized by fever, vomiting, jaundice, choluria, and alcoholic stools; treatment requires IV antibiotics and corticosteroids. Portal hypertension occurs in at least two-thirds of children after KPE, with the appearance of varices in the esophagus, stomach, and Roux loop. Treatment requires variceal sclerotherapy or band ligation. Factors shown to predict

outcome after KPE include age at operation, experience of the surgeon, anatomical type of BA, and relapse of cholangitis (Caccia et al. 2004; Lee et al. 2013; Chardot 2006; Davenport 2012).

79.2.6 Prognosis

Overall, KPE results in clearance of jaundice from 38% to 62% of patients in various series (Davenport 2012), with a mean native liver survival rate of 53% at 5 years (Shinkai et al. 2009), while the other patients develop progressive hepatic failure that leads to liver transplantation (Caccia et al. 2004; Lee et al. 2013).

The choice of sequential treatment by KPE and late liver transplantation is supported by the following reasons: firstly, performing liver transplantation in all children with BA would deprive some of these of the possibility to live with their own liver, while the long-term results of liver transplantation and prolonged immunosuppression are not entirely known; secondly, performing transplantation on all children with BA will dramatically increase the need of pediatric liver grafts at this time when the shortage of organs is as yet an unsolved problem; and lastly, liver transplantation at older age reduces the period of immunosuppressive therapy (Caccia et al. 2004).

The overall prognosis of BA has improved since the early days of pediatric liver transplantation. Currently, about 90% of children with BA, treated sequentially by KPE and liver transplantation, have an acceptable quality of life (Lee et al. 2013).

79.3 Congenital Bile Duct Dilatation

79.3.1 Introduction

Congenital bile duct dilatation (CBDD) is a relatively rare malformation of the pancreatobiliary system with an incidence of 1:100,000–200,000 and a female predominance (3:1 to 4:1). For unknown reasons, it is most common in Asian countries, especially in Japan.

A maternally inherited condition, such as an X-linked dominant trait, has been suggested recently. Several cases of familial recurrence have been reported (Iwasaki et al. 2008).

In 1977, Todani classifies CBDD in five types: **type I**, cystic dilatation of the common bile duct (80% of cases); **type II**, *diverticulum* of the common bile duct (10%); **type III**, choledochocele (4%); **type IV** (11%), (**a**) intra-extrahepatic bile duct dilatation and (**b**) plurisegmental common bile duct dilatation; and **type V**, isolated intrahepatic bile duct dilatation (<1%).

79.3.2 Etiology and Pathogenesis

The etiology of CBDD remains speculative. In majority of patients, an anomalous pancreatobiliary duct junction with a long common channel involving the common bile duct and the main pancreatic duct is present and may be a responsible factor for CBDD, allowing reflux of activated pancreatic proenzymes into the biliary system and leading to duct wall destruction and dilatation. Distal common bile duct stenosis or obstruction may add to ductal dilatation. An autonomic dysfunction by diminished ganglion cells in the distal common bile duct causing partial obstruction and proximal dilatation has been suggested.

79.3.3 Pathology

Two histopathological types of CBDD that may be present concurrently or separately have been described: the "glandular" type, in which there are microscopic cavities in the mucosal layer with chronic inflammatory infiltrate, and the "fibrotic" type, in which the wall is composed mainly of fibrous tissue with interrupted elastic fibers, well-developed collagen fibers, and lower inflammation.

79.3.4 Clinical Aspects

Rarely, it occurs in the first months of life, and in fact it is primarily a disease of older infants and young children, because more than half percent of cases presents in the first decade of life. The

classic presentation of CBDD with jaundice, abdominal pain, and a right hypochondrial mass is seen only in one-third of children. Infants usually present with asymptomatic jaundice that may be mild and intermittent or progressive due to complete biliary obstruction. Late complications in cases with delayed or escaped diagnosis are represented by cholelithiasis, cirrhosis, portal hypertension, liver abscess, spontaneous rupture, and cholangiocarcinoma (Benjamin 2003).

79.3.5 Diagnosis

There are no specific laboratory tests, and the initial diagnosis is made by US. The findings of a dilated common bile duct with US are helpful for early diagnosis of CBDD. TC may show the cystic dilatation better than US; it does not however demonstrate ductal anatomy (Takaya et al. 2003). Because preoperative biliary duct imaging is essential, the diagnosis must be confirmed by the MRC, especially when dealing with the fusiform type (Fitoz et al. 2007). ERCP requires an experienced endoscopist and must be done in older infants or young children with caution, in order to avoid infection of the cyst or precipitate pancreatitis. In most cases, CBDD have been demonstrated antenatally by US.

79.3.6 Therapy and Treatment

In the past, internal drainage by cystoenterostomy or partial cyst excision was considered the preferred surgical treatment. Nevertheless, this procedure led to significant morbidity due to recurrent cholangitis, cholelitiasis, pancreatitis, and even cholangiocarcinoma.

Today, total excision of the CBDD with a Roux-en-Y hepaticojejunostomy and cholecystectomy is widely considered the treatment of choice. Before intervention, a cholangiography through the gallbladder is performed to demonstrate accurately the anatomy of the cyst and the pancreatobiliary ductal system.

When the ductal dilatation extends into the main hepatic ducts, after excision of involved ductal structures, polyductal Roux-en-Y jejunostomy must be performed. In case of choledococele which is located inaccessibly within the distal common bile duct, complete surgical excision is precluded. The approach should be transduodenally, and the presenting wall of choledococele is excised with marsupialization of choledococele into the duodenum.

The laparoscopic excision of CBDD is an alternative surgical approach whose first large pediatric series was published in 2004 (Li et al. 2004). This is technically feasible, safe, and effective with a comparable outcome to open procedure. Additional benefits are less postoperative pain with less pulmonary complications, a shortened period of ileus, and less adhesion formation (Aspelung et al. 2007). For these reasons, this procedure should be considered as a good alternative to standard surgical approaches; nevertheless, it is technically demanding and requires advanced skills (Liem et al. 2009).

More recently, it has been proposed to use the robotic surgery for surgical treatment of CBDD, considering that the three-dimensional vision, the high motion stability, and the scaling wound effect would be a greater benefit for the hepaticojejunostomy (Naitoh et al. 2015). However, the small series reported cannot show a definitive advantage of this technique at present.

79.3.7 Prognosis

Although the surgical management of CBDD is successful in 90% of cases, early complications can occur in 2.5–25% of patients and include biliary or pancreatic fistula, biloma, and cholangitis (Takeshita et al. 2011). Late complications occur in 25% of patients and are represented by cholangitis, delayed anastomotic stricture, intrahepatic calculi, and liver failure (Ohtsuka et al. 2015). Cholangiocarcinoma was rarely observed in patients with cysts removed in infancy, but the risk of carcinogenesis increases with age (Xiao-dong et al. 2014).

79.4 Congenital Solitary Liver Cyst

79.4.1 Introduction

Solitary liver cyst (SLC) is a benign lesion more common in females (2:1), and it can be classified as simple solitary liver cyst and solitary intrahepatic biliary cyst (Macedo 2013; Berg et al. 2002). Early report suggested that their incidence was 0.17% based on autopsy findings. The spectrum of potential pathologies causing congenital solitary liver cysts in children is wide (Rogers et al. 2007).

79.4.2 Etiology and Pathogenesis

The etiology of simple congenital cysts is unknown. They are generally thought to develop from aberrant bile ducts, which are obstructed from the main biliary system or as result of a vascular disruption during the fetal period (Berg et al. 2002).

79.4.3 Pathology

Simple cysts are typically unilocular, lined by a single layer of cuboidal or columnar epithelial cells, resembling biliary cells. The cystic layer can secrete fluid similar to serum and may be clear, brown, or, occasionally, bilious (Howard 2002). They rarely communicate with the biliary tree and are not considered premalignant. They may be completely intrahepatic, partially extrahepatic, or pedunculated. The presence of septa is usually regarded as a pointer to other pathologies and the need for further investigations (Rogers et al. 2007).

79.4.4 Clinical Aspects

Most solitary liver cysts are asymptomatic and identified incidentally or antenatally in the third trimester (Berg et al. 2002; Charlesworth et al. 2007). Simple cysts rarely cause symptoms unless become enlarged. Symptoms are usually vague, and in such cases pain, hepatomegaly, abdominal distension, feeding difficulties, respiratory distress, and duodenal obstruction have been reported (Shankar et al. 2000). Infection, hemorrhage, and spontaneous rupture are other rare complications.

79.4.5 Diagnosis

US is widely used for the diagnosis of SLC (Liang et al. 2005). US should demonstrate the cyst location, loculation, wall contour and characteristics, content, and associated pathology. In the differential diagnosis, TC and MRI should be able to show a mesenchymal hamartoma and rarely embryonal sarcoma as well as cystic teratoma (Charlesworth et al. 2007; Celebi et al. 2014). In selected cases, functional hepatic scintigraphy may be useful in distinguishing simple from choledochal cyst by the different radioisotope uptake (Rogers et al. 2007).

The differential diagnosis of upper quadrant abdominal cysts and masses includes hepatobiliary lesions such as liver cysts, parasitic cysts, benign tumors (mesenchymal hamartoma, cystadenoma), malignant tumors (sarcoma), choledochal cysts, and type I BA, other intra-abdominal cysts (ovarian, omental, mesenteric, adrenal, or renal cysts), and different conditions such as dilated bowel loops and duodenum and gallbladder duplications (Soyer et al. 2007).

79.4.6 Therapy and Treatment

Because of the scarcity of case series, the optimal management of simple hepatic cyst remains controversial. Most unilocular cysts do not require intervention postnatally, and conservative management of cysts smaller than 10 mm has been suggested. Intervention is required among children who are symptomatic for a mass effect or complications such as infection, hemorrhage, or rupture with peritonitis

(Charlesworth et al. 2007; Shankar et al. 2000; Liang et al. 2005; Celebi et al. 2014). Various treatment options, including percutaneous aspiration, percutaneous injection sclerotherapy, laparoscopic excision, or fenestration, have been reported as a possible alternative to open surgery (Celebi et al. 2014).

The total excision or enucleation seems to be the treatment of choice, but will depend on the anatomical type of lesion. If this is not possible, partial excision with deroofing of the cyst wall is recommended (Berg et al. 2002; Shankar et al. 2000; Celebi et al. 2014). During surgery, communication with the extrahepatic and intrahepatic biliary system has to be ruled out by cholangiography (Berg et al. 2002). In case of a biliary cyst, a Roux-en-Y cystoenterostomy or hepaticojejunostomy as described for CBDD is recommended (Howard 2002).

79.4.7 Prognosis

The postoperative course can be complicated by bile leakage, cholangitis, septicemia, and recurrence of the cyst (Berg et al. 2002; Rogers et al. 2007). Children who undergo incomplete excision must be followed up closely for recurrence (Celebi et al. 2014).

References

Alvarez F (2013) Is biliary atresia an immune mediated disease? J Hepatol 59:648–650

Aspelung G, Ling SC, Ng V et al (2007) A role for laparoscopic approach in the treatment of biliary atresia and choledochal cysts. J Pediatr Surg 42:869–872

Baumann U, Ure B (2012) Biliary atresia. Clin Res Hepatol Gastroenterol 36:257–259

Benjamin IS (2003) Biliary cystic disease: the risk of cancer. J Hepatobil Pancreatol Surg 10:335–339

Berg C, Baschat AA, Geipel A et al (2002) First-trimester diagnosis of fetal hepatic cyst. Ultrasound Obstet Gynecol 19:287–289

Besso K, Bezerra JA (2011) Biliary atresia: will blocking inflammation tame the disease? Annu Rev Med 62:171–185

Caccia G, Ekema G, Falchetti D, Pedersini P (2004) Atresia delle vie biliari: attualità e prospettive. Prosp Pediatr 34:39–43

Celebi S, Kuthluk G, Besik Bestas C et al (2014) Current diagnosis and management of simple hepatic cysts detected antenatally and postnatally. Pediatr Surg Int 30:599–604

Chardot C (2006) Biliary atresia. Orph J Rare Dis 1:28

Charlesworth P, Ade-Ajayi N, Davenport M (2007) Natural history and long term follow-up of antenatally detected liver cysts. J Pediatr Surg 42:494–499

Davenport M (2012) Biliary atresia: clinical aspects. Semin Pediatr Surg 21:175–184

El-Guindi MA, Sira MM, Konsowa HA et al (2013) Value of hepatic subcapsular flow by color Doppler ultrasonography in the diagnosis of biliary atresia. J Gastroenterol Hepatol 28:867–872

Estevez E, Neto EC, Neto MO et al (2002) Laparoscopic Kasai portoenterostomy for biliary atresia. Pediatr Surg Int 28:737–740

Fitoz S, Erden A, Boruban S (2007) Magnetic resonance cholangiopancreatography of biliary system abnormalities in children. Clin Imaging Mar-Apr 31 (2):93–101

Howard ER (2002) Cysts. In: Surgery of the liver, bile ducts and pancreas in children, 2nd edn. Arnold Publisher, London, p 239

Hsiao CH, Chang MH, Chen HL et al (2008) Universal screening for biliary atresia using an infant stool color card in Taiwan. Hepatology 47:1233–1240

Iwasaki J, Yoshifumi O, Shunichi N et al (2008) Familial recurrence of congenital bile duct dilatation. World J Gastroenterol 14:941–943

Lee S, Park H, Moon SB et al (2013) Long-term results of biliary atresia in the era of liver transplantation. Pediatr Surg Int 29:1297–1301

Lee MS, Cheon JE, Choi YH et al (2015) Ultrasonographic diagnosis of biliary atresia based on a decision-making tree model. KJR 16:1364–1372

Li L, Feng W, Jing-Bo F et al (2004) Laparoscopic-assisted total cyst excision of choledochal cyst and Roux-en-Y hepatoenterostomy. J Pediatr Surg 39:1663–1666

Liang P, Cao B, Wang Y et al (2005) Differential diagnosis of hepatic cystic lesions with gray-scale and color Doppler sonography. J Clin Ultrasound 33: 100–105

Liem NT, Dung A, Son TN (2009) Laparoscopic complete cyst excision and hepaticoduodenostomy for cholecochal cyst: early results in 74 cases. J Laparoendosc Adv Surg Tech 19:S87–S90

Macedo FI (2013) Current management of noninfectious hepatic cystic lesions: a review of literature. World J Hepatol 5:462–469

Naitoh T, Morikawa T, Tanaka N et al (2015) Early experience of robotic surgery for type I congenital dilatation of the bile duct. J Robot Surg 9:143–148

Ningappa M, So J, Glessner J et al (2015) The role of ARF6 in biliary atresia. PloS ONE. https://doi.org/10.1371/journal.pone0138381

Nio M, Sasaki H, Wada M et al (2010) Impact of age at Kasai operation on short- and long-term outcomes of type III biliary atresia at a single institution. J Pediatr Surg 45:2361–2363

Ohtsuka H, Fukase K, Yoshida H et al (2015) Long-term outcomes after extrahepatic excision of congenital choladocal cysts: 30 years of experience at a single center. Hepatogastroenterology 62:1–5

Rogers TN, Woodley H, Ramsden W et al (2007) Solitary liver cysts in children: not always so simple. J Pediatr Surg 42:333–339

Russo P, Magee JC, Boitnott J et al (2011) Design and validation of the Biliary Atresia Research Consortium histological assessment system for cholestasis in infancy. Clin Gastroenterol Hepatol 9:357–362

Saito T, Terui K, Mitsunaga T et al (2015) Evidence of viral infection as a causative factor of human biliary atresia. J Pediatr Surg 50:1398–1404

Shankar SR, Parelkar SV, Das SA et al (2000) An antenatally diagnosed solitary, nonparasitic hepatic cyst with duodenal obstruction. Pediatr Surg Int 16:214–215

Shanmugam NP, Harrison PM, Devlin J et al (2009) Selective use of endoscopic retrograde cholangiopancreatography in the diagnosis of biliary atresia in infants younger than 100 days. J Pediatr Gastroenterol Nutr 49:435–441

Shinkai M, Ohhama Y, Take H et al (2009) Long-term outcome of children with biliary atresia who were not transplanted after Kasai operation: >20 year experience at Children's Hospital. Pediatr Gastroenterol Nutr 48:443–450

Sira MM, Sira AM, Ehsan NA et al (2015) P-selectin (CD62P) expression in the liver tissue of biliary atresia: a new perspective in etiopathogenesis. JPGN 61: 561–567

Soyer T, Karnak I, Senokar ME (2007) Congenital solitary intrahepatic biliary cist in a newborn: report of a case. Surg Today 37:521–524

Srivastava A (2011) Biliary atresia and inflammation: from pathogenesis to prognosis. Trop Gastroenterol 32:1–3

Takaya J, Muneyuki M, Tokuhara D et al (2003) Congenital dilatation of the bile duct: changes in diagnostic tools over the past 19 years. Pediatr Int 45:383–387

Takeshita N, Ota T, Yamamoto M (2011) Forty-year experience with flow diversion surgery for patients with congenital choledochal cysts with pancreaticobiliary maljunction at a single institution. Ann Surg 254:1050–1053

Tyraskis A, Davenport M (2015) Steroids after the Kasai procedure for biliary atresia: the effect of age at Kasai portoenterostomy. Pediatr Surg Int. https://doi.org/10.1007/s0038301538363

Ure BM, Kuebler JF, Schukfeh N et al (2011) Survival with native liver after laparoscopic versus conventional Kasai portoenterostomy in infants with biliary atresia. A prospective trial. Ann Surg 253:826–830

Xiao-dong H, Lei W, Wei L et al (2014) The risk of carcinogenesis in congenital choledochal cyst patients: an analysis of 214 cases. Ann Hepatol 13:819–826

Part VIII

Orofacial and Gastrointestinal Malformations and Diseases

Orofacial Malformations

80

Giorgio Iannetti, Maria Teresa Fadda,
Marco Della Monaca, and Giulio Bosco

Contents

Abstract

Orofacial malformations encompass several different syndromes. Congenital anomalies can occur in up to 15% of newborn, and many of these involve the oral, craniofacial, and dental region. Finding of a single craniofacial anomaly at birth may alert to the presence of a complex syndrome. The majority of these syndromes present a frequency ranging from between one in 5600 and one in 100,000. Many attempts of systematic classification

G. Iannetti (✉)
Università degli Studi di Siena, Policlinico S. Maria alle Scotte, Siena, Italy

Sapienza Università di Roma, Policlinico Umberto I di Roma, Rome, Italy
e-mail: iannetti.giorgio@gmail.com

M. T. Fadda · M. Della Monaca · G. Bosco
Sapienza Università di Roma, Policlinico Umberto I di Roma, Rome, Italy

G. Buonocore et al. (eds.), *Neonatology*,
https://doi.org/10.1007/978-3-319-29489-6_227

were suggested, but none is still universally accepted. The comprehensive management of orofacial syndromes required a staged multidisciplinary approach in dedicated centers with dedicated resources, high patient volume, and strong interest in improving the lives of these complex and challenging patients.

80.1 Salient Points

- The finding of a single cranio-facial anomaly at birth may alert to the presence of a complex syndrome.
- Craniostenosis is characterized by the precocious fusion of one or more sutures of the skull; the clinical pictures depend on the sutures concerned.
- Cleft lip-cleft palate can be complete or incomplete and mono- or bilateral; it can affect the lip, hard palate, and soft palate. The cleft of the soft palate may also be present in syndromic forms (Apert syndrome or Robin sequence).
- Congenital mandibular malformations provoking breathing difficulties usually need treatment soon after birth.
- The most relevant tongue malformations are divided into ankyloglossia, lingual fissures, macroglossia, microglossia, and aglossia.
- Craniofacial malformations need to be managed with a multidisciplinary approach in dedicated centers.

80.2 Etiology and Classification

Skull and facial deformations are mostly the result of a developmental abnormality that occurs during the embryonic stage, which becomes all the more serious with the early occurrence of the pathogenetic noxa.

Currently, a genetic cause has been recognized in 25% of congenital malformation, while 10% are due to external factors (chemical, physical, biological) that can act directly on the embryo–fetal development. Alcohol, cocaine, cytomegalovirus, toxoplasmosis, diabetes, methotrexate, hydantoin, radiation, retinoids (vitamin A), and rubella appear to be factors related to craniofacial malformations (Cohen 2002).

It is also known that the pathogenetic mechanisms may occur for developmental abnormalities of the central nervous system, muscles, and other soft tissues and directly involve the cartilage or bone (Johnston and Bronsky 1995).

Based on chronological pathomorphogenetic criteria, Van der Meulen proposed a classification in 1983 (Van der Meulen et al. 1983) using the term "dysplasia" to recognize three main pathogenetic mechanisms involving the bone in which most facial bone malformations converge:

- Cleft: failure to merge the embryonic process
- Dysostosis: bone growth alteration
- Synostosis premature closure of sutures (Fig. 1)

In 2001 (Cohen 2002), Cohen proposed a classification of all the craniofacial malformation considering the pathogenetic mechanisms together with current knowledge on genetics. Based on this classification, the craniofacial malformations can be divided as follows:

(a) Chromosomal abnormalities: the genetic error is due to the numerical abnormality of a chromosome (e.g., Down–Turner).
(b) Metabolic abnormalities: the genetic abnormality causes an enzyme deficiency (e.g., mucopolysaccharidosis).
(c) Soft tissue development abnormality.

This last group is rather wide and includes malformations of different origin:

- Malformations involving the skin and mucosa, such as laxa skin, ectodermal dysplasia, and epidermolysis bullosa.
- Malformations involving the vascular system and peripheral nervous system, such as the Sturge–Weber syndrome and neurofibromatosis types 1 or 2.
- Deformities involving the muscular system, Moebius syndrome.

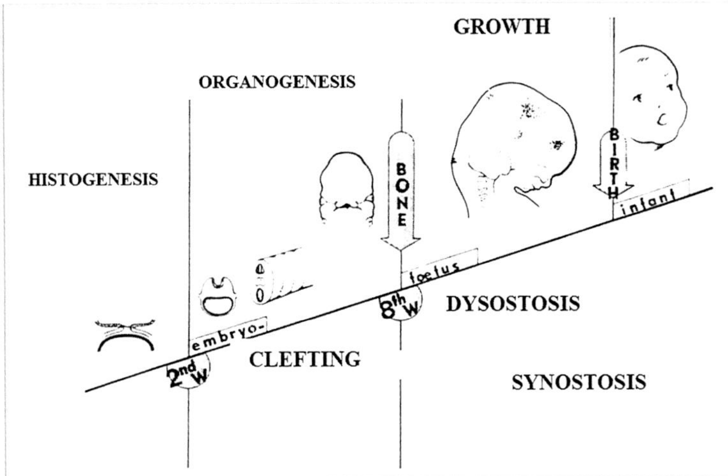

Fig. 1 From Stricker M, Van Der Meulen JC. Craniofacial Malformations. Churchill and Livingstone, London 1990

- Malformations involving the SNC, like lissencephaly, anencephaly, encephalocele, or holoprosencephaly (Figs. 2 and 3).
- Hard tissue abnormality: malformations involving cartilage or bone tissue. Among those from the cartilage, achondroplasia malformation involves a lack of formation, growth, and ossification of cartilage in the entire skeletal system and thus also of all the structures of craniofacial cartilage origin. Concerning the bone, anomalies may occur in ossification such as in osteopetrosis and in fibrous dysplasia (monostotic or polyostotic).

Due to the complexity of this classification, it is better to focus on the clinical pictures that maxillofacial surgeons have to face, illustrating all available treatment options:

- Isolated craniostenosis
- Craniostenosis syndromes
- Syndromes of branchial arches I and II
- Facial clefts and LPS
- Pierre Robin

80.3 Isolated Craniostenosis

Craniostenosis is characterized by the precocious fusion of one or more sutures of the skull. There are different clinical pictures that depend on the sutures concerned. Often, in isolated forms, the issue is limited to the alteration of the harmonious development of the skull. Syndromes with craniosynostosis may present important alterations, such as intracranial hypertension, visual disturbances, and changes in the brain, with varying frequency depending on the severity of the case.

Scaphocephaly – This condition is the most common isolated craniosynostosis. It is characterized by precocious closure of the sagittal suture and subsequent expansion of the coronal, lambdoid, and metopic sutures. The resulting morphological damage is increased growth of the skull in the sagittal direction and the reduction in the transverse direction (Fig. 4).

Frontal Plagiocephaly – This condition is divided into unilateral true and positional forms. The true form is due to the early fusion of the coronal suture of one side. Often, this alteration coexists with precocious closure of some of the sutures of the cranial base (sphenotemporal, sphenoethmoid, and sphenozygomatic). The result is the asymmetry of the skull with flattening of the frontal area and upper orbital margin on the pathological side and compensatory expansion on the opposite side. There may also be an asymmetry of the skull base that is radiographically detectable. In fact, the lines that bound the middle and posterior cranial fossa are no longer parallel but

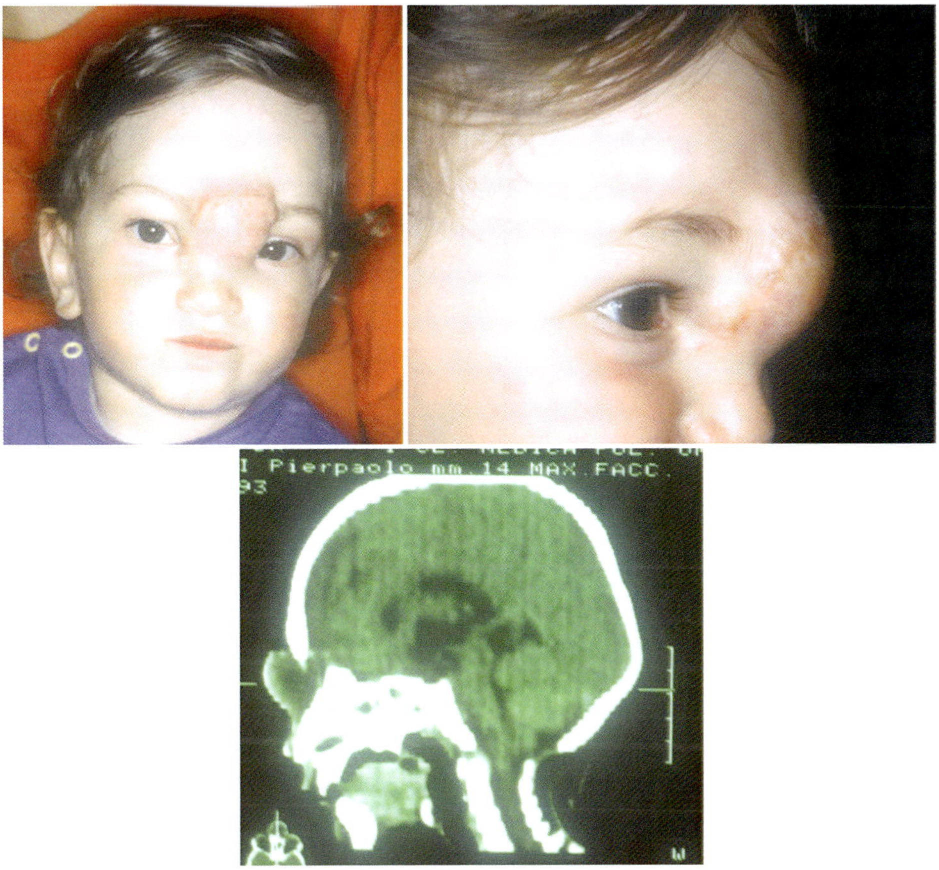

Fig. 2 Frontonasal encephalocele

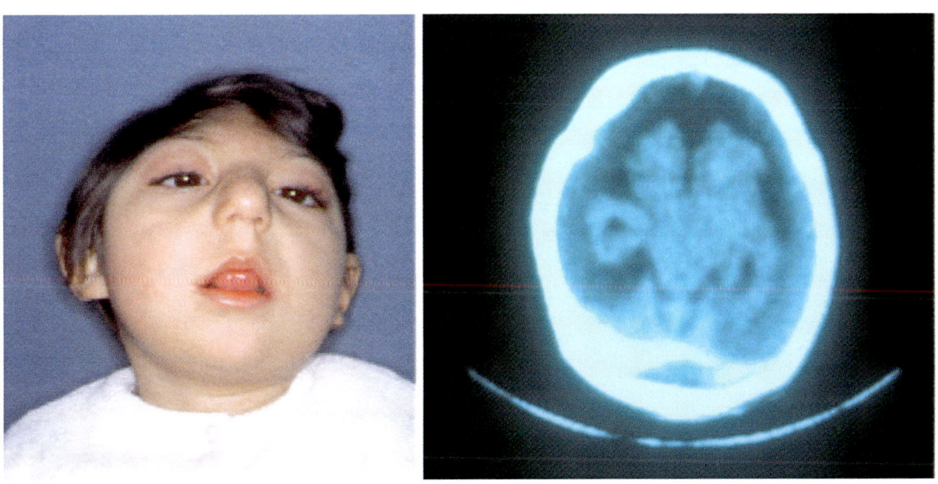

Fig. 3 Microcephaly

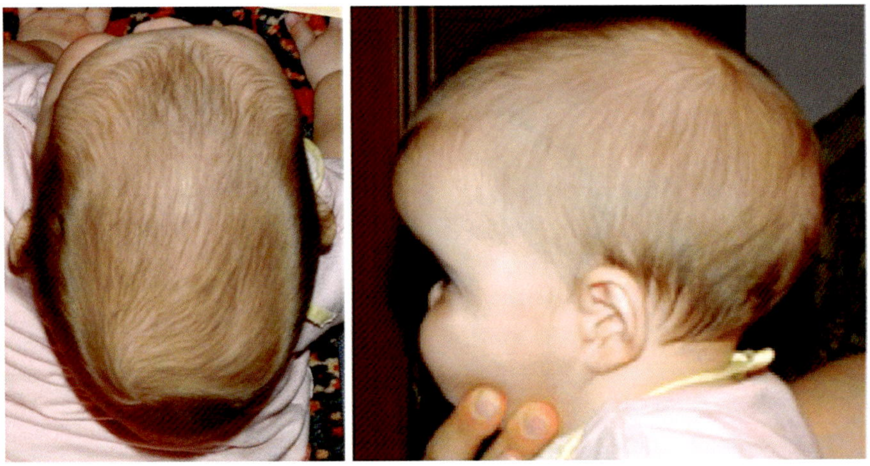

Fig. 4 Scaphocephaly

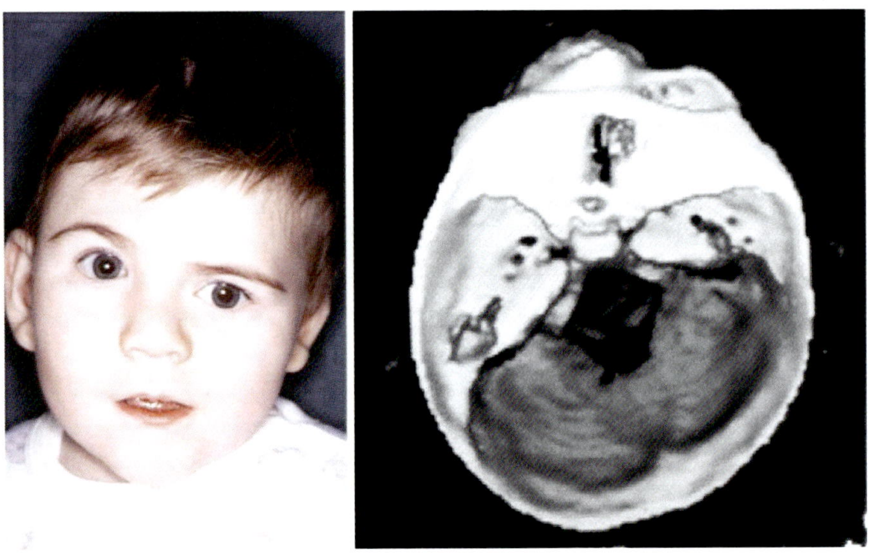

Fig. 5 Anterior plagiocephaly

form an angle of about 9° on the pathological side (Figs. 5, 6, and 7).

The positional form is only due to an abnormal position during intrauterine life. No alterations of the sutures are present, and it requires a functional nonsurgical treatment. The differential diagnosis between the true and positional form is based on the development and morphological features. From the development point of view, the positional form tends to improve, whereas the true form worsens. Based on the morphological features, the two forms are distinguished by differences in the superior orbital rim orientation, position of the ear, root of the nose, and chin deviation as suggested by Mulliken (Fig. 8 and Table 1).

Brachycephaly – This results from early closure of the coronal sutures bilaterally that causes an increased transverse and/or vertical growth of the skull and reduction in its sagittal dimension (Fig. 9).

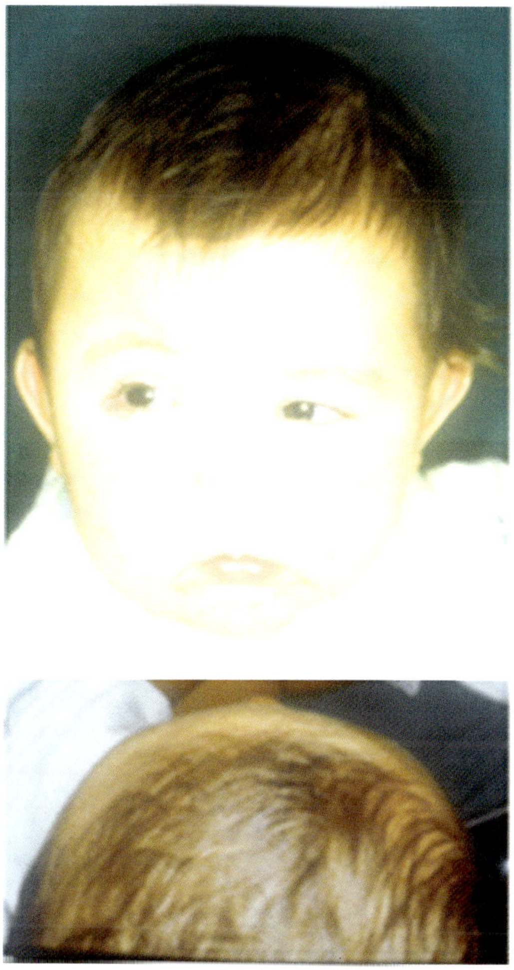

Fig. 6 Mild plagiocephaly

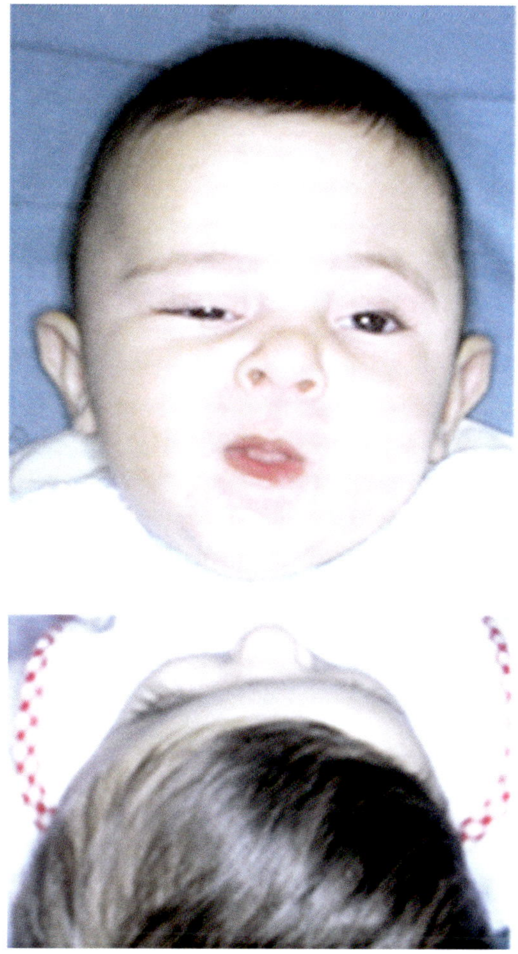

Fig. 7 Severe Plagiocephaly

Trigonocephaly – This results from the early closure of the metopic sutures. The skull shows an anterior triangular shape in the axial view, and a reduction of the anterior skull diameter is present (Fig. 10).

80.4 Treatment of Craniostenosis

Classically, the surgical treatment of skull-isolated synostosis usually takes place within the first 6 months of life. It is based on the removal of specific sutures and possibly associated with the remodeling of the cranial vault. Other suggested methods include the use of bone distractors to guide the expansion of the cranial vault or the application of springs to exert a continuous force that is more similar to that in physiological growth. Recently, less invasive treatments have been favored, such as there has been directed in favor of a less invasive treatment represented by endoscopic suturectomy with very limited cutaneous access and the possible application of helmets to encourage proper skull development (Cohen and Maclean 2000) (Figs. 11 and 12).

80.5 Craniostenosis Syndromes

Craniostenosis syndromes are caused by genetic defects that have been well identified in some cases. In particular, the most frequent forms,

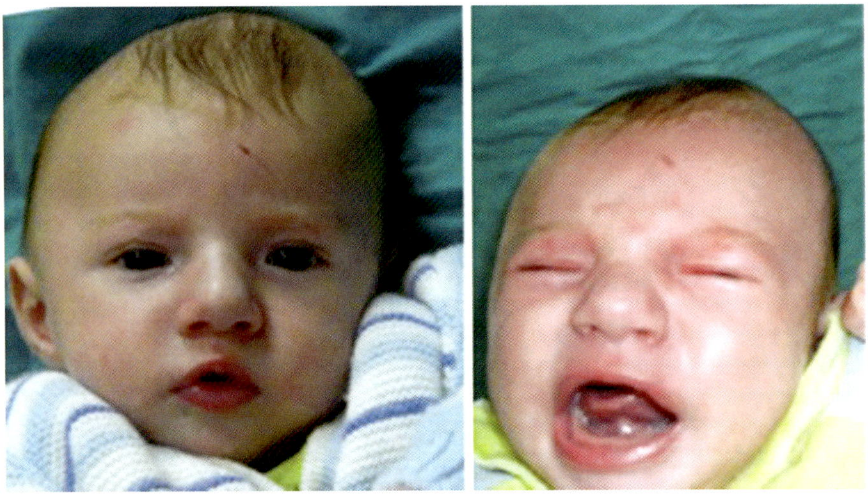

Fig. 8 Positional plagiocephaly

Table 1 From Hansen and Mulliken 1994

Features	Synostotic	Deformational
Ipsilateral superior orbital rim	Up	Down
Ipsilateral Ear	Anterior, high	Posterior, low
Nasal root	Ipsilateral	Midline
Ipsilateral malar eminence	Forward	Backward
Chin deviation	Contralateral	Ipsilateral
Ipsilateral Palpebral fissure	Wide, low	Narrow, high
Anterior fontanelle deviation	Contralateral	None

Crouzon and Apert syndromes, are caused by point mutation located on the short arm of chromosome 10 in the gene that codes for a growth factor for fibroblasts (cells of the body assigned for the production of collagen, elastin, and reticular fibers in the loose connective tissue) (Tessier 1974, 1976).

The most common syndromes are:

- *Crouzon syndrome* – This syndrome is autosomal dominant and occurs with a frequency of 1 in every 25,000 births. It owes its name to those who first described the most obvious symptoms: (1) the false exorbitism or exophthalmos due to reduced growth in posterior–anterior direction of the orbits and (2) the orbitofrontal zygomatic maxillary skeletal retrusion that determines third-class occlusion according to term of growth. The syndrome is associated with craniosynostosis that can involve at least one suture of the cranial vault to different degrees (most commonly the coronal or sagittal). It is associated with reduced growth in the posterior–anterior direction of the maxillofacial complex. The reduction of the nasal airway patency determines the prevalence of breathing orally. Hypertelorism, defined as an increase in the orbital bony distance to different degrees, is often observed and depends on the severity of craniosynostosis (Fig. 13).
- *Apert syndrome* – Apert syndrome has an incidence of 1 in 100,000 live births (Forrest and Hopper 2013). Its transmission is autosomal dominant with complete penetrance, but in most cases its development is due to a de novo mutation. The clinical picture of the syndrome is complex and it can express with other additional symptoms and different degrees of severity. The phenotype of Apert children is quite variable and does not correlate with the type of genetic mutation. The syndrome is therefore not predictable.

One of the main clinical features with which the syndrome occurs is the craniosynostosis of the coronal suture. This involves abnormal development of the cranial vault and consequently of the brain in early life period, when the baby's skull is expanding

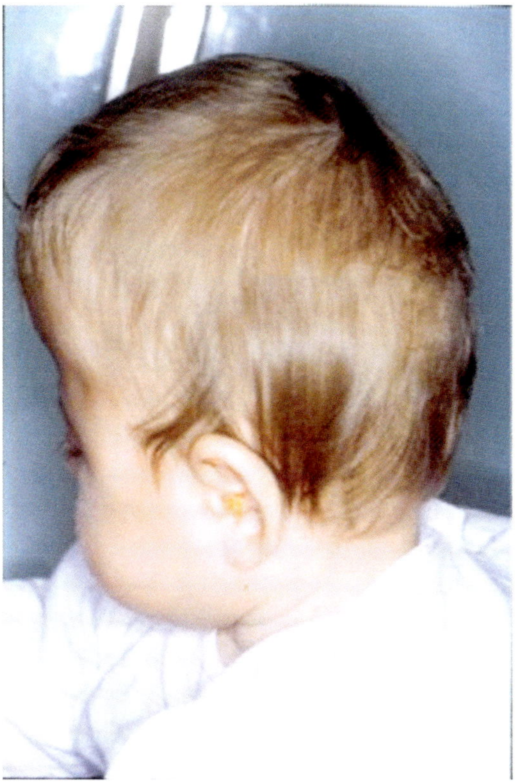

Fig. 9 Brachycephaly

rapidly under the thrust of the brain in development. The early closure of the coronal suture may also be associated with that of other sutures. This greatly exacerbates the clinical picture and can reveal a risk of hydrocephalus (increase intracranial pressure), herniation of the brain through the foramen magnum, and cardiorespiratory arrest. Other cranioencephalic deformities are agenesis of the corpus callosum (24%), abnormalities of the septum pellucidum, ventriculomegaly (45%), and fusion of the cervical vertebrae.

Hypertelorism is obvious at the orbits in association with proptosis, strabismus, antimongoloid eyelids, retrusion of the upper and lower orbital margin, and cleft eyebrow.

In these patients, the facial deformities are characterized by an underdeveloped jaw bone, narrow palate, soft palate cleft, cross bite, anterior open bite, bulbous nasal tip, depression of the glabellar region, and reduction of nose–throat space.

Teeth abnormalities are late eruption, dental inclusion, ectopy of some dental elements, dental crowding, and lack of space in the arch.

The syndactyly/fusion of the fingers and toes is always bilateral but hardly symmetrical. It can

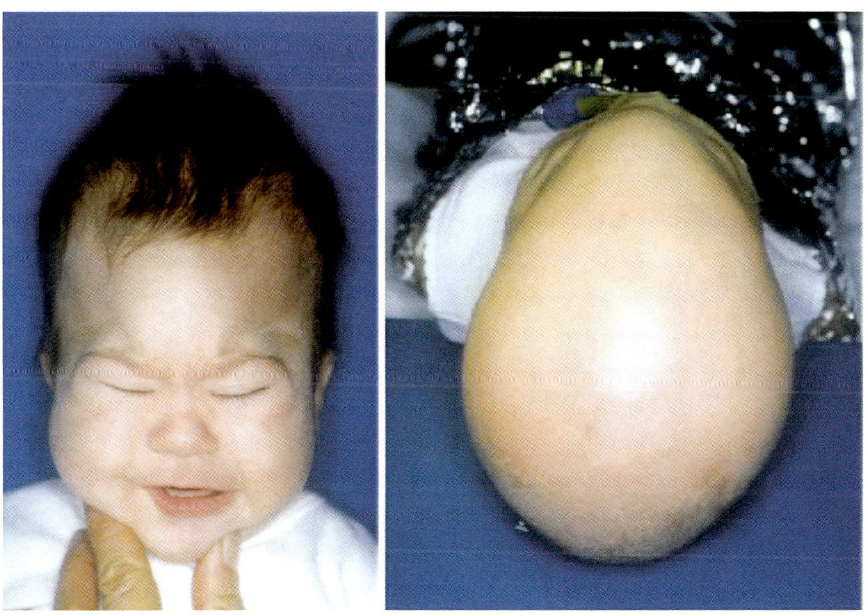

Fig. 10 Trigonocephaly

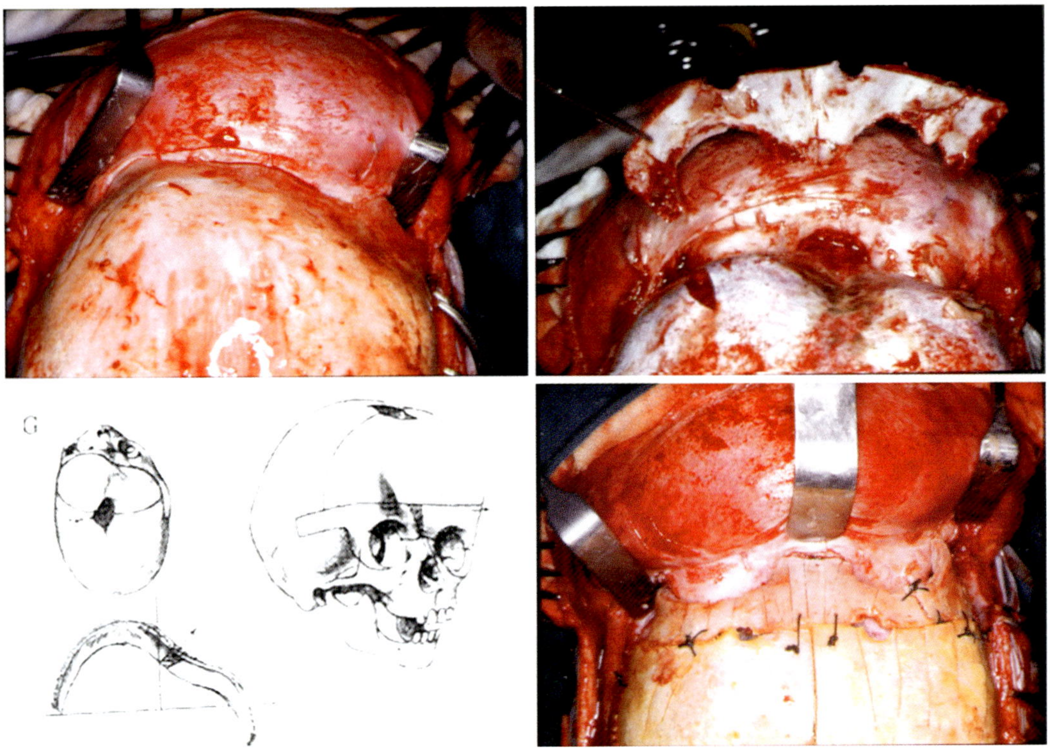

Fig. 11 Anterior plagiocephaly: open surgery

affect only the soft tissue or can involve the bone sketches too. It can manifest itself more seriously at the upper limbs and can completely prevent movements of prehension.

With varying impacts, Apert syndrome may also be associated with malformations of the urogenital system, acne, and heart and lung abnormalities.

The IQ of these children is variable, with some authors arguing that it tends to be lower than average and others that it is up to the average. The literature suggests that if there is a deficit, it is usually mild and independent of the brain abnormalities (Chiari syndrome, corpus callosum agenesis, septal abnormality). Apert syndrome can be related to cerebral or respiratory hypertension, which would involve a reduction of oxygen in the brain (Fig. 14).

Smith–Lemli–Opitz syndrome – Smith–Lemli–Opitz syndrome is a multiple congenital anomalies and mental retardation syndrome caused by a defect in cholesterol synthesis. Smith–Lemli–Opitz syndrome is an autosomal recessive genetic condition caused by deficiency of the enzyme 3 beta-hydroxysterol-delta 7-reductase, the final enzyme in the sterol synthetic pathway that converts 7-dehydrocholesterol (7DHC) to cholesterol. Prevalence of Smith–Lemli–Opitz syndrome has been estimated to be 1 in 20,000–60,000 births among whites (Forrest and Hopper 2013). Smith–Lemli–Opitz syndrome is also not uncommon in Hispanics. Its specific prevalence in different populations has not been precisely determined. The higher-than-expected prevalence of Smith–Lemli–Opitz syndrome suggests a heterozygote advantage. Severely affected individuals have multiple congenital malformations and are often miscarried or stillborn or die in the first weeks of life. Dysmorphic facial features, microcephaly, second-toe and third-toe syndactyly, other malformations, and mental retardation are typical. Mildly affected individuals may have only subtle dysmorphic features and learning and behavioral disabilities (Forrest and Hopper 2013).

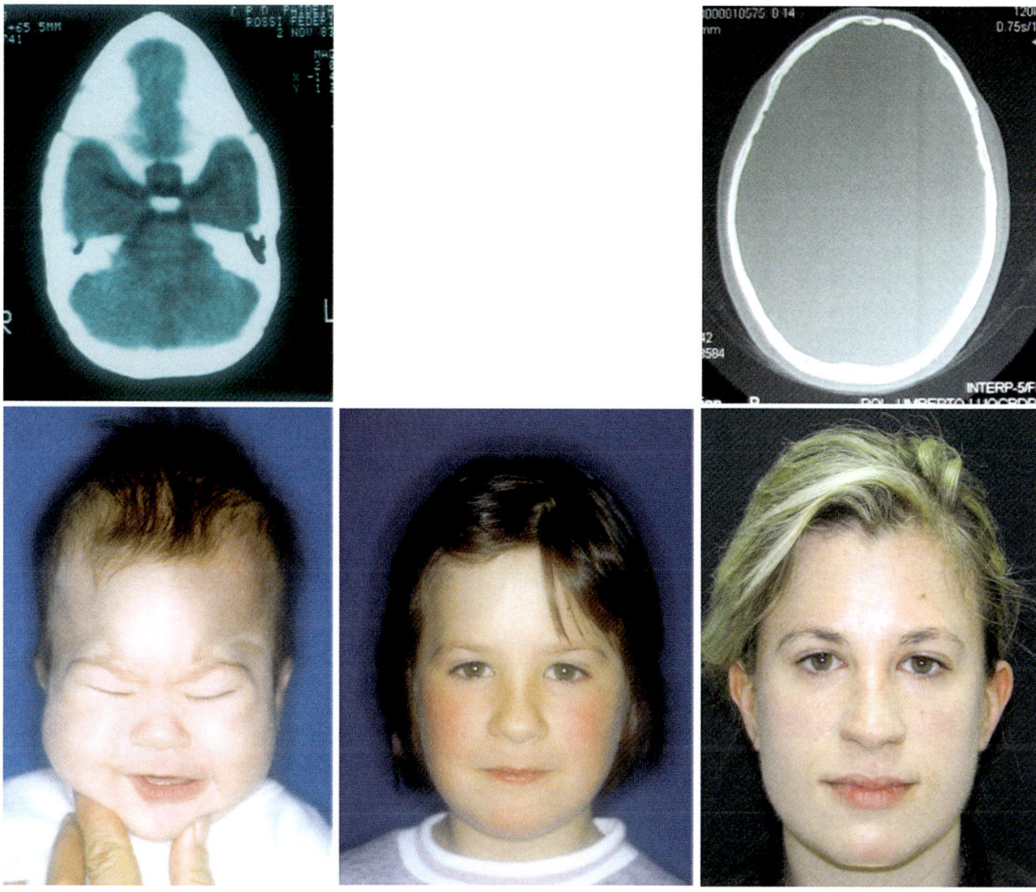

Fig. 12 Trigonocephaly: pre-, post-, and long-term view

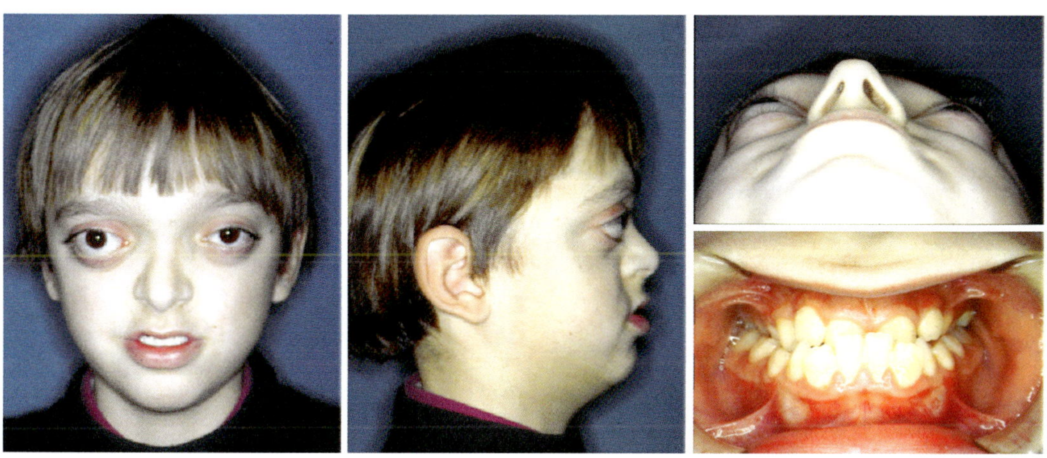

Fig. 13 Crouzon syndrome

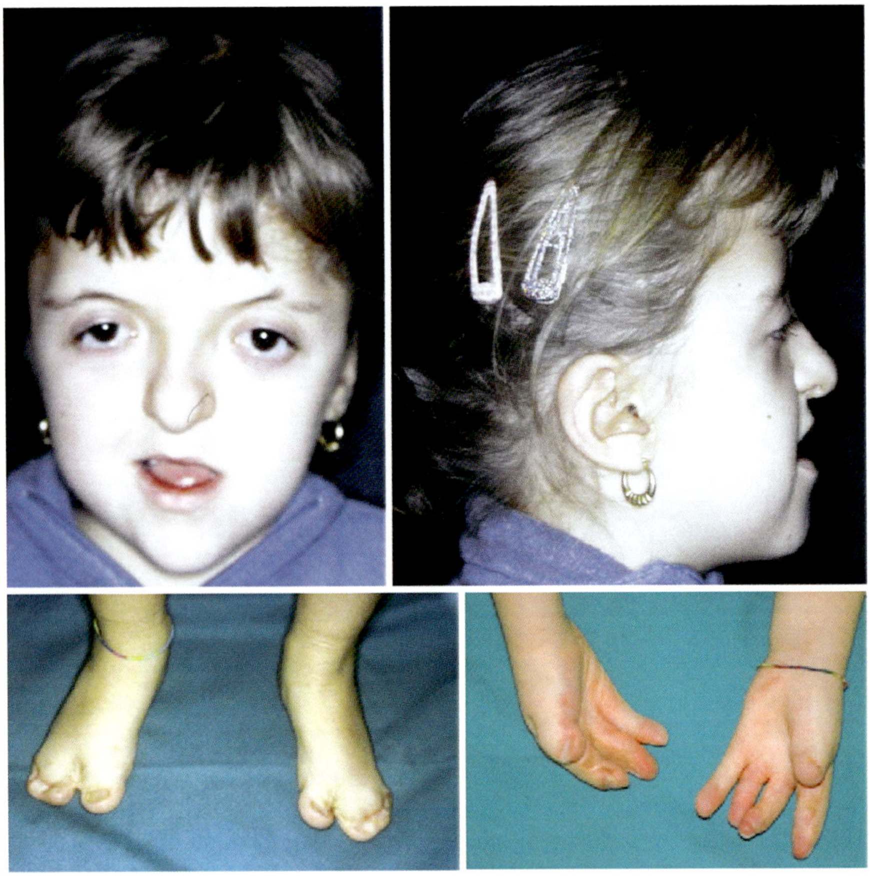

Fig. 14 Apert syndrome

Treatments of syndromic forms aim to solve the craniosynostosis, to ensure the normal patency of the upper airway, and to gain the advancement of the facial skeleton freed from the blockage from a pathological facial suture. Craniosynostosis is resolved using methods for isolated forms, while the other aims are achieved by the posterior–-anterior distraction of the facial bones after performing a Le Fort III osteotomy (Tessier 1971; Tulasne and Tessier 1986). An internal distractor can be used for advancements up to 1 cm, while an external distractor is preferred for advancements over 1 cm. The timing of this osteotomy depends on the severity of respiratory and ocular signs (Figs. 15 and 16).

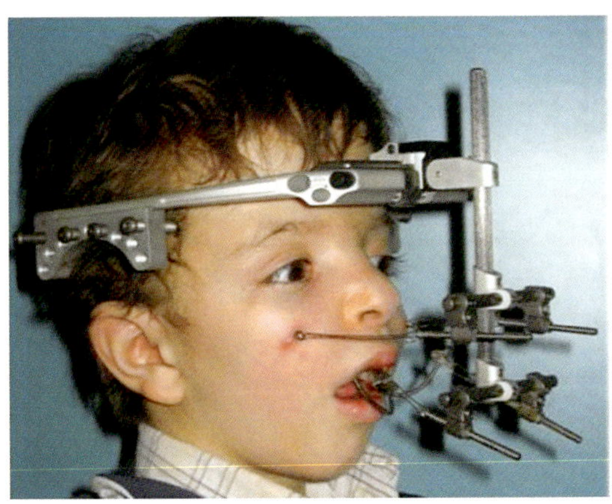

Fig. 15 External distractor device

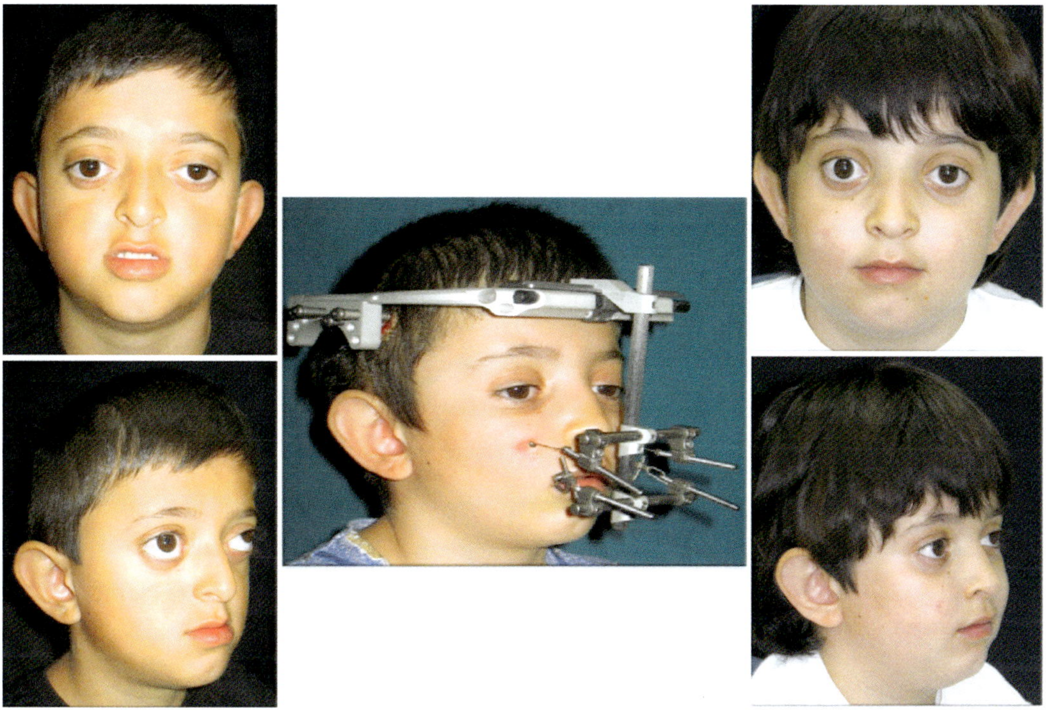

Fig. 16 Crouzon syndrome; presurgery, with external distractor device, and postsurgery views

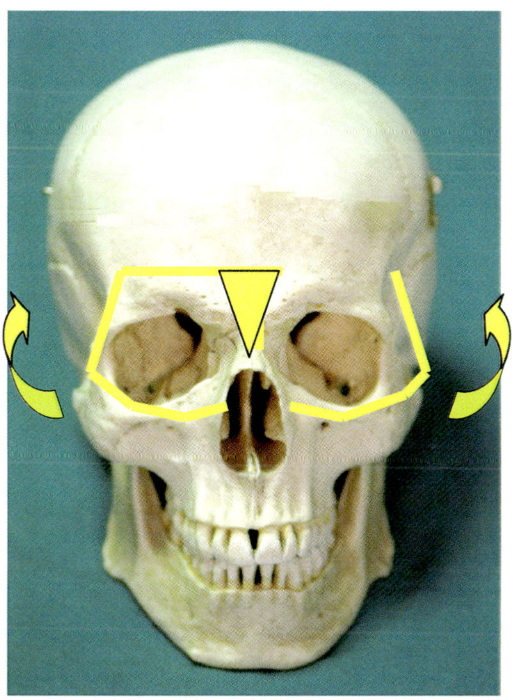

Fig. 17 Surgical scheme of orbit mobilization

In these syndromic forms, hypertelorism is corrected through surgery mobilization of the orbits. It is performed when the upper canines have at least started to descend in the arch to ensure that they will not to be damaged during the osteotomy (Figs. 17 and 18).

In the craniofacial clefts, the normalization of the infraorbital distance is corrected through the facial bipartition technique. In this technique two hemifaces are mobilized and rotated on the midline after the execution of an ethmoid–nasal osteotomy (triangle with apex at the bottom (Figs. 19 and 20a, b).

80.6 Facial Clefts and LPS

Facial clefts are caused by the nasal and maxillary embryonic lack of fusion. They may involve the middle third of the face and thus increase the symmetrical or asymmetrical infraorbital distance, with variable severity of cleft skin (Figs. 21 and 22).

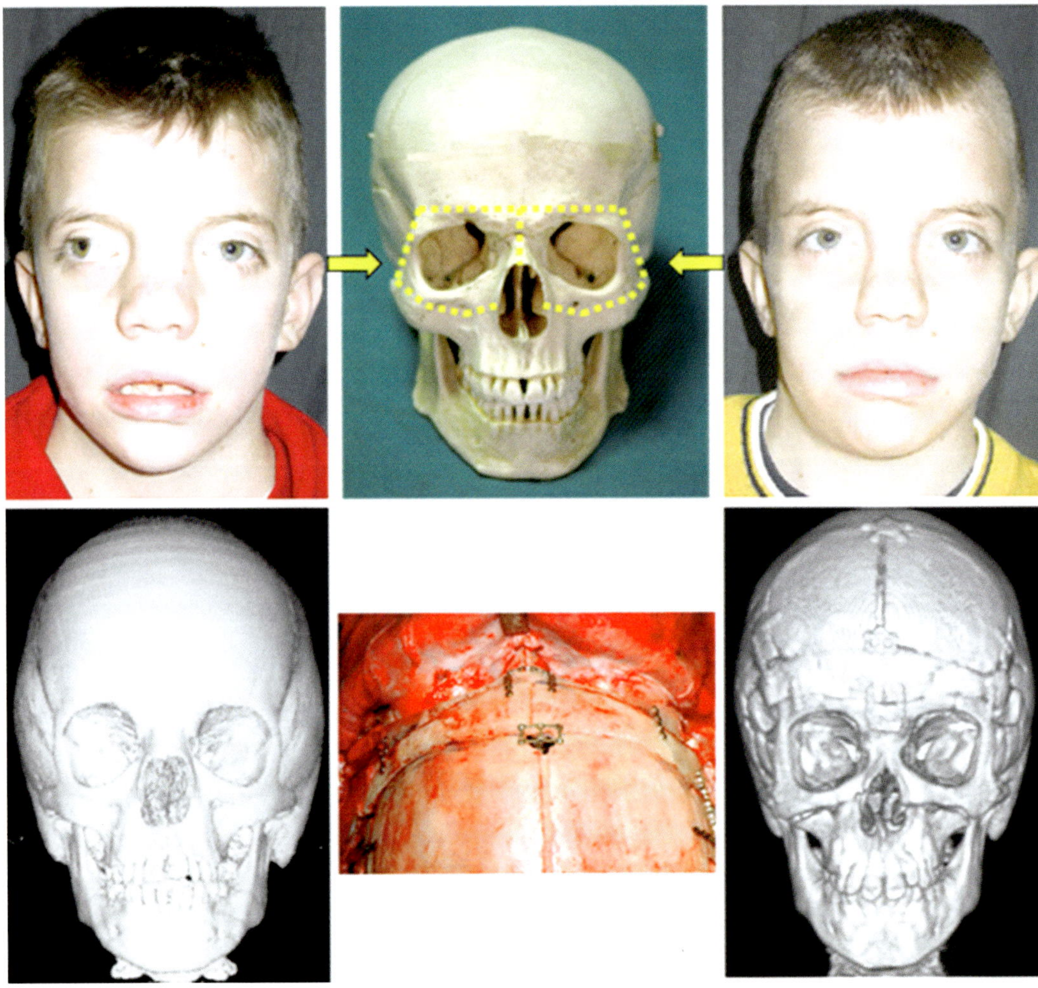

Fig. 18 Opitz syndrome; pre- and postsurgery views

80.7 Cleft Lip–Cleft Palate (Clcp)

LPS is a malformation that occurs with varying frequency depending on race. The incidence appears high among Asians (0.82–4.04 per 1000 live births), intermediate in Caucasians (0.9–2.69 per 1000 live births), and low in Africans (0.18–1.67 per 1000 live births). Males are affected twice as often as females. The data, however, are influenced by the correct registration of new cases (Neligan et al. 2013).

It is well known that genetic and external factors may facilitate the occurrence of a CLCP. Family history, parents older than 30 years old, the use of medicines, alcohol, and smoking are all factors that increase the risk of CLCP.

Several classifications have been proposed based on morphology, embryology, and clinical–therapeutic practices. The most reliable classifications are those by Veau (1938), Stark (1958), Stricker (1970), Tessier (1976), Millard (1977), and Ortiz–Posadas (2005) and that of the most recent classification by the American Cleft Palate Association and Iowa System.

Without going into surgical details, we should remember that LPS can be complete or incomplete and mono- or bilateral. It can affect the lip, hard palate (including the alveolar process), and the soft palate. Obviously, the less severe forms

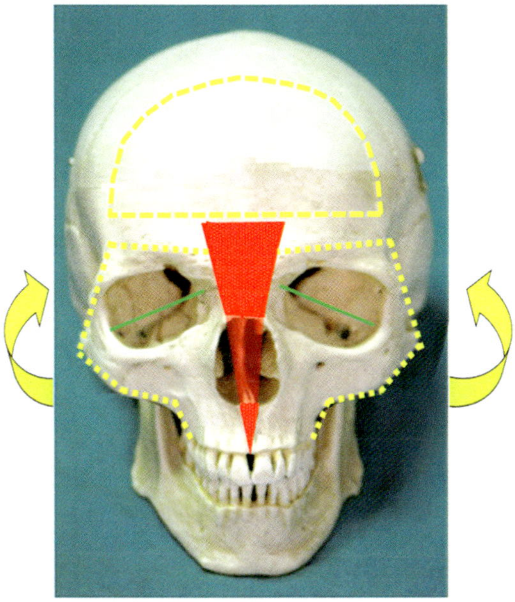

Fig. 19 Surgical scheme of facial bipartition technique

are those involving the lip or the soft palate only, while the more complex forms affect the lip and palate structures (Figs. 23 and 24).

The cleft of the soft palate may also be present in syndromic forms as in the Apert syndrome or Robin sequence. During pregnancy, the two emimaxilla cannot meet in the midline due to tongue not migrating downward.

A child born with a cleft lip and/or palate usually does not have serious difficulties in feeding, but he may benefit from the use of baby bottles with modified teats, depending on the malformation, such as nipple with one-way or a wider one to avoid liquid reflux from the oral cavity to the nose. The choice of one of these devices, which can be purchased easily, depends on the malformations and babies' attitudes.

The observation of a cleft lip and/or palate should be made as early as the fifth month of

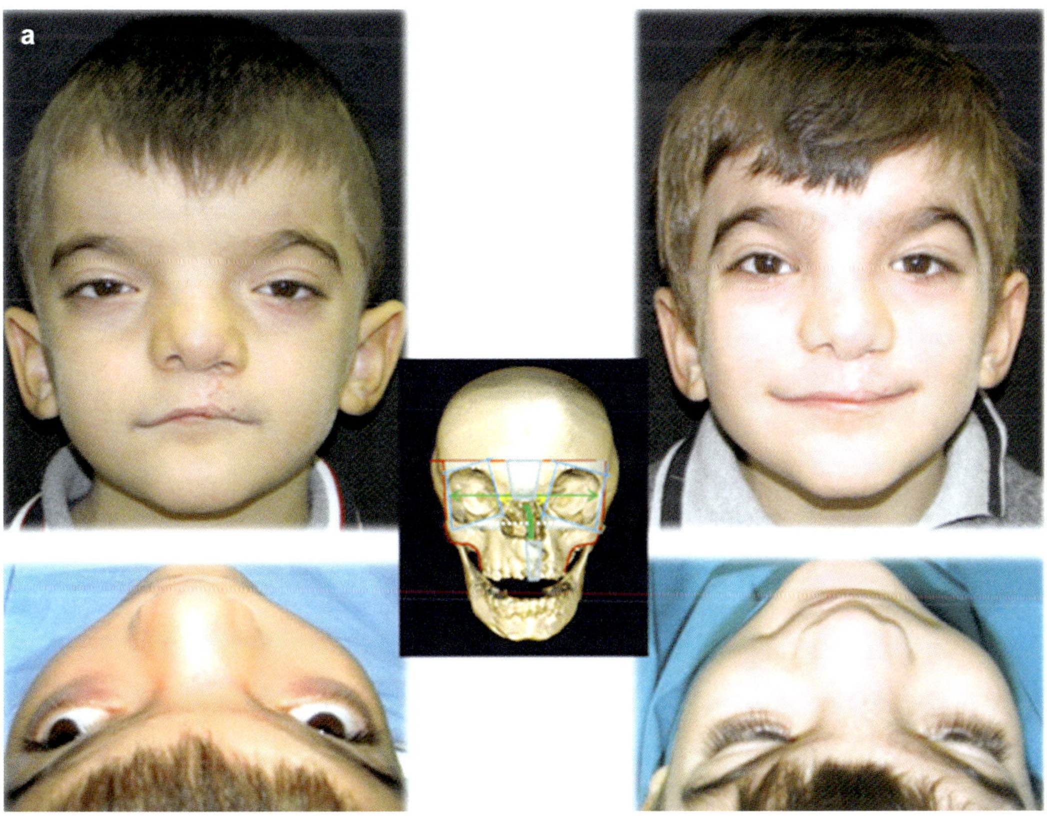

Fig. 20 (continued)

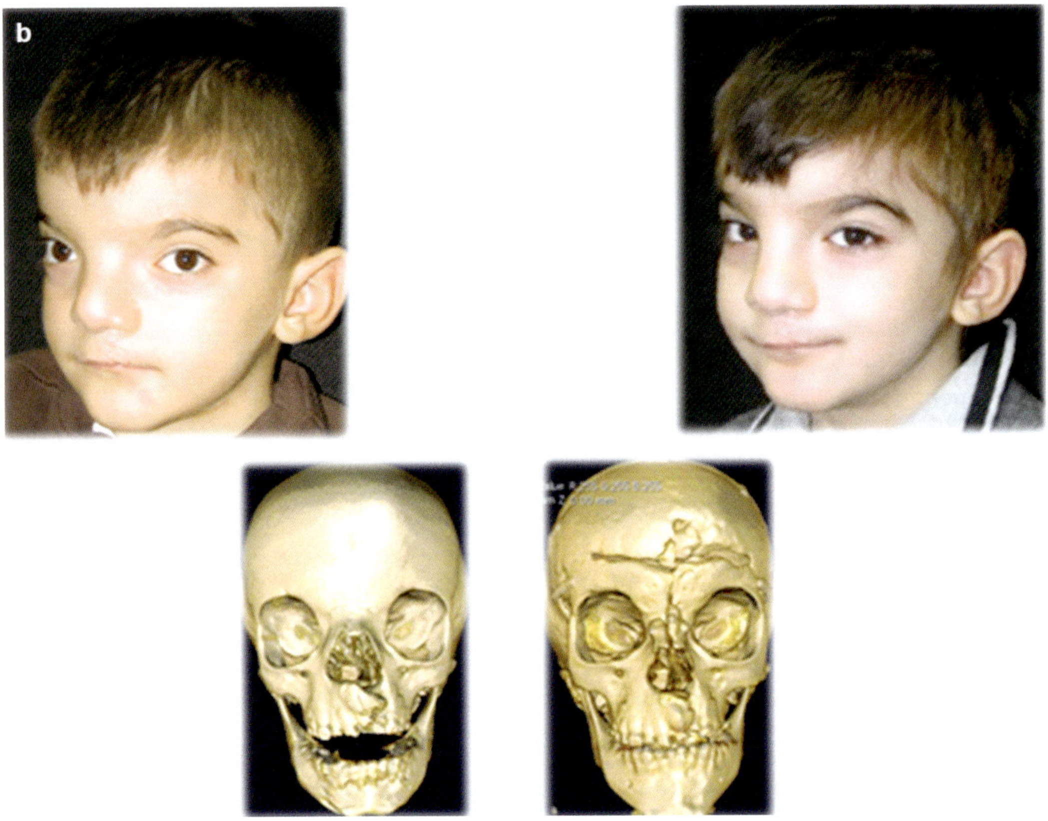

Fig. 20 (**a** and **b**) Facial median cleft; pre- and postoperative views

pregnancy through a morphological ultrasound and possibly a fetal MRI to prepare the parents. Possibly with the support of a psychologist, the situation they will face at the birth of the child should be explained along with how to provide a suitable environment.

The therapeutic treatment of a child with CLCP has often changed over the past decades, and there is still no universally accepted therapeutic strategy.

The first step of cleft care consists of preoperative molding treatment.

The nasoalveolar molding (NAM) technique utilizes wire and acrylic nasal stents attached to an intraoral plate. This appliance is used to reduce the severity of the oronasal deformity prior to surgery. It molds the nasal cartilages, columella, alveolar ridges, and premaxilla into a more physiologically symmetrical form and position during the neonatal period (1 week to 6 months). This technique takes advantage of the malleability of immature nasal cartilage and its ability to maintain a permanent correction of its form.

The reconstruction of the lip and nose and the closing of the soft palate are done under general anesthesia between 6 and 12 months to prevent language alterations.

The closing of the hard palate, gengivoperiosteoplasty, and bone graft are performed between 6 and 8 years old. The delay in the procedure helps to prevent growth alteration such as class III

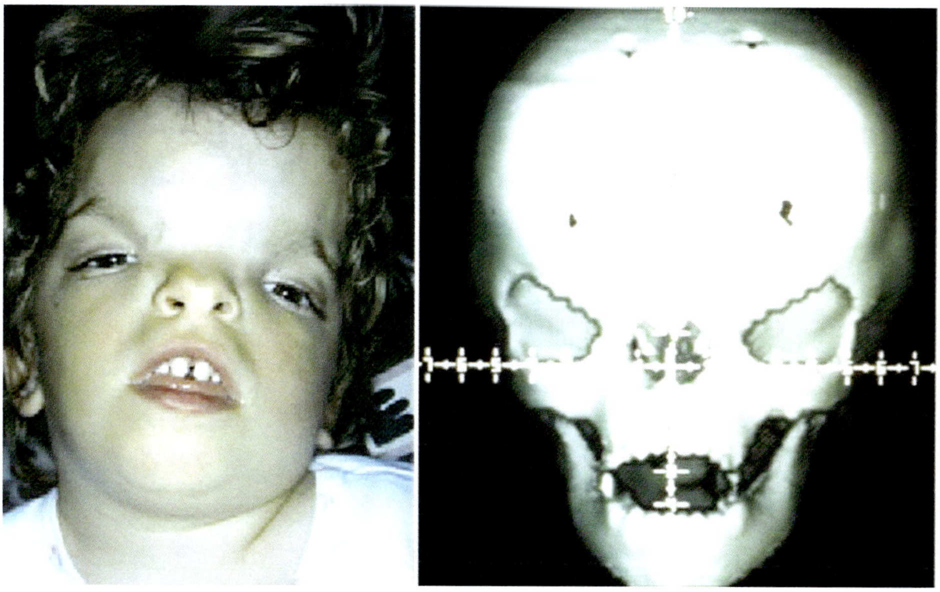

Fig. 21 Craniofacial median cleft

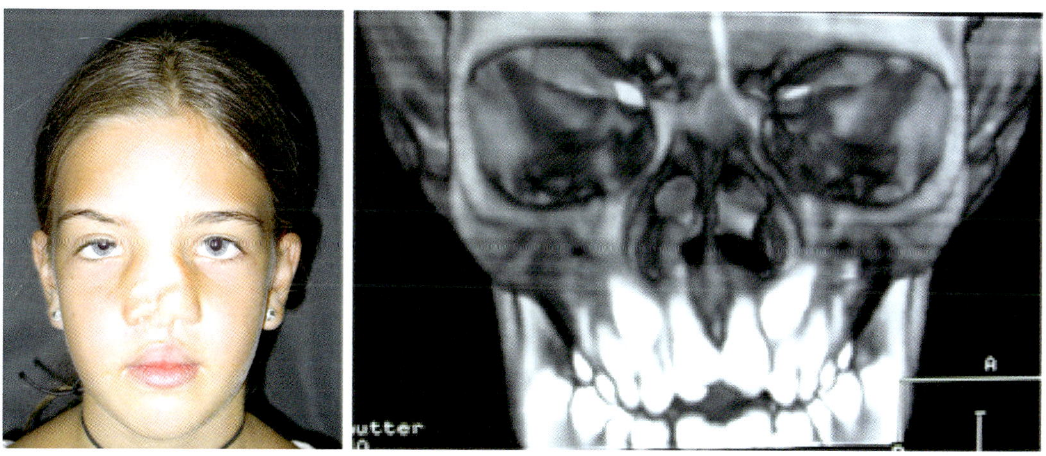

Fig. 22 Maxillary–ethmoid median cleft

occlusion deformity and to help tooth eruption (Fig. 25).

In every case, the CLCP patients will need a multidisciplinary follow-up until the end of the growth with a maxillofacial surgeon, ENT, orthodontist, speech therapist, and psychologist (Figs. 26, 27, 28, and 29).

80.8 Congenital Mandibular Diseases

The most important congenital mandibular malformations for the neonatologist are those provoking breathing difficulties. The Pierre Robin

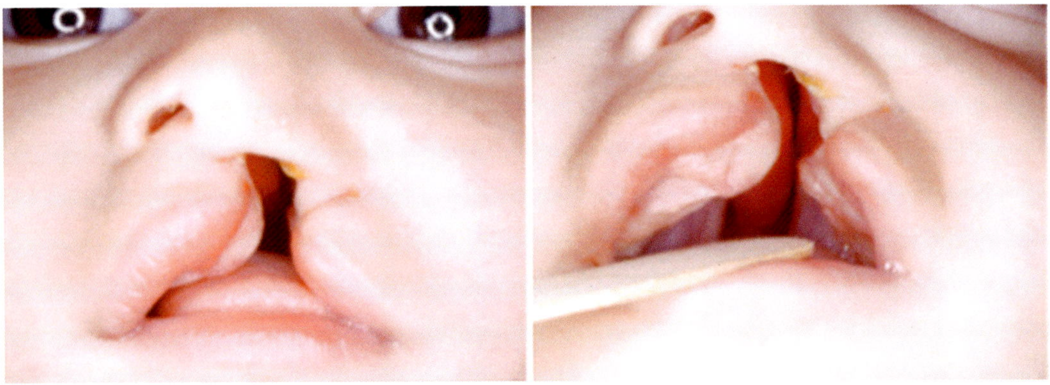

Fig. 23 Monolateral left cleft lip and plate

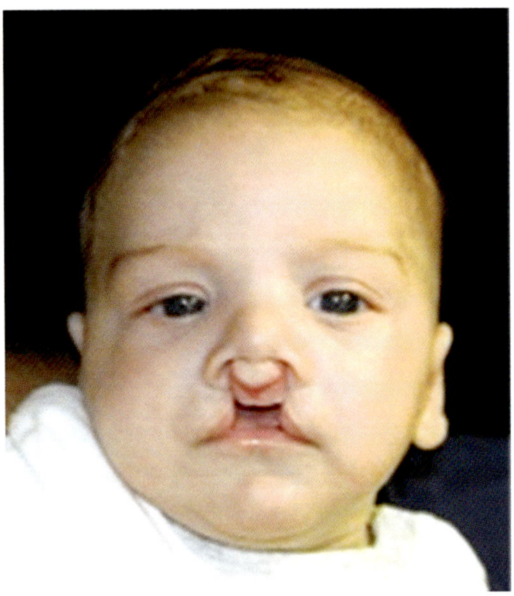

Fig. 24 Bilateral cleft lip and palate

sequence, syndromes of the first and second branchial arch, and the morphofunctional of the temporomandibular joint may require immediate treatment after birth.

80.9 Pierre Robin Sequence

The Pierre Robin sequence occurs with a frequency of 1 in 10 to 20 thousand births with a clinical picture of varying severity (Neligan et al. 2013; Breugem and Mink van der Molen 2009). The most accredited pathogenetic mechanism consists of the failure to rotate the head upward, which normally occurs in the fourth week of pregnancy. The tongue remains in the space between the palatine processes in growth so as to prevent the fusion in the midline. This would provoke a back cleft of the secondary palate, usually in the shape of an inverse "U" or "V." The altered position of the tongue (glossoptosis) results in the failure to push the tongue on the jaw, which appears smaller at birth, causing the reduction of the respiratory rhinopharyngeal space. The tongue itself has normal volume and morphology and becomes an obstacle to breathing by occupying the respiratory–nasal–pharyngeal space and causes the phenomenon of glossoptosis (Breugem and Mink van der Molen 2009).

Depending on the severity of the obstruction of the upper airways, in 1994 a classification into three groups (Caouette–Laberge) was proposed (Caoutte-Laberge et al. 1994):

1. Sufficient breathing with the child in the prone position and normal diet
2. Sufficient breathing with the child in the prone position but difficulties in feeding with the need to apply a nasal cannula
3. Difficult breathing even in the prone position and feeding difficulties

In the less severe cases, it may be enough to keep the child in a prone position or lateral

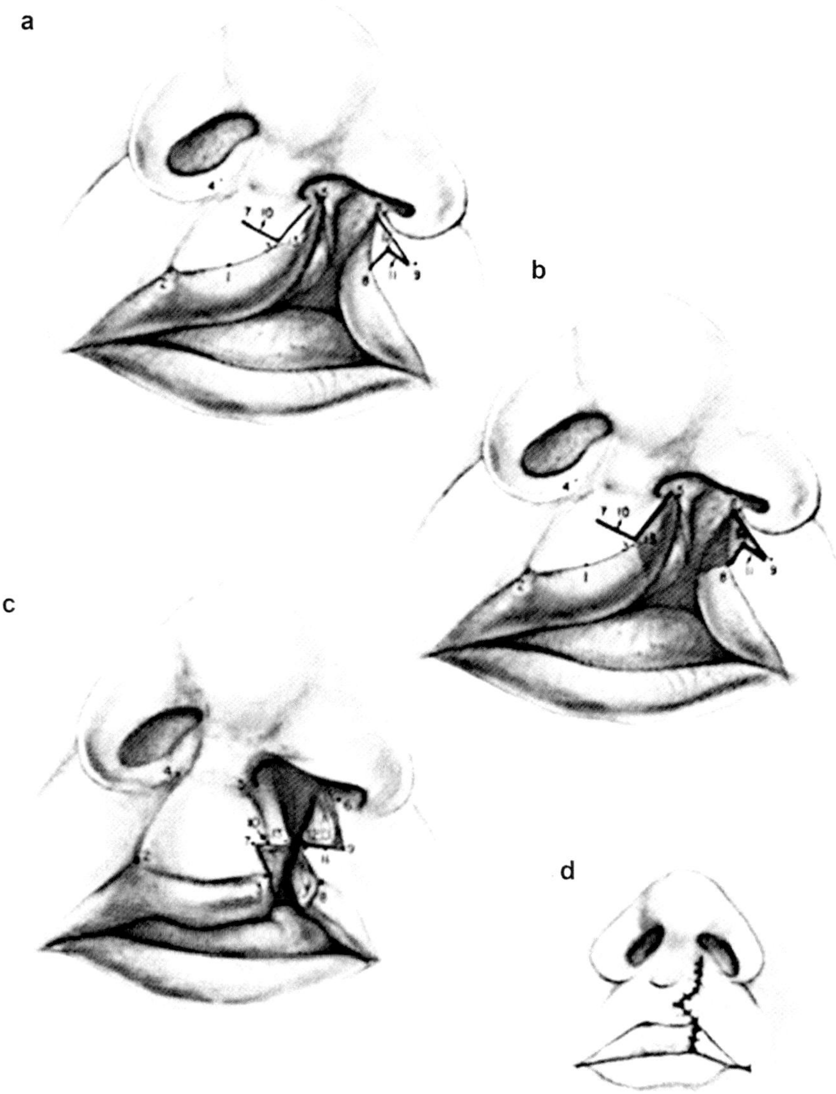

Fig. 25 Surgical scheme for monolateral cleft lip: Tennison–Randall technique

decubitus or to apply a palatal plate that prevents the tongue from occupying the nasal cavity. Alternatively, a nasal cannula can be required for a few days (before the neuromuscular recovery of the tongue). In severe cases, a mandibular lengthening osteodistraction is indicated, so to avoid a tracheotomy. It can also be performed from the first days of the child's life (Fig. 30).

80.10 First and Second Gill Arch Syndrome

Syndromes of the first and second brachial arch are also called spectrum oculoauriculovertebral, which are a group of congenital anomalies characterized by unilateral or bilateral mandibular hypoplasia.

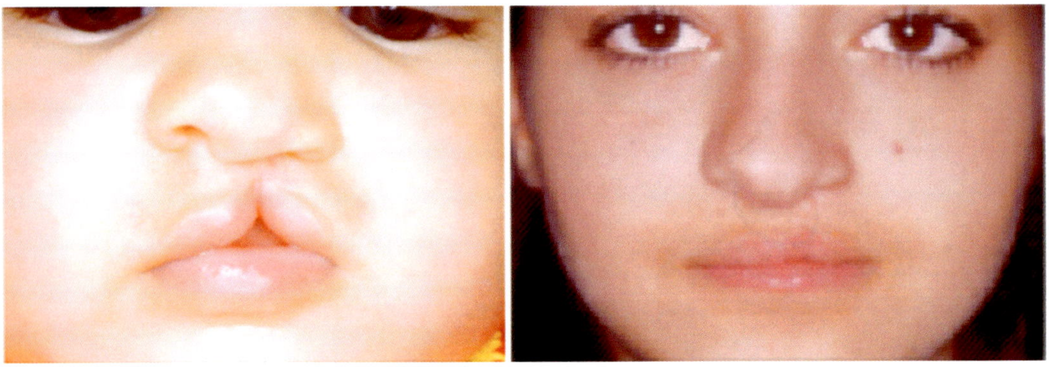

Fig. 26 Monolateral incomplete cleft lip and palate: pre- and postoperative view

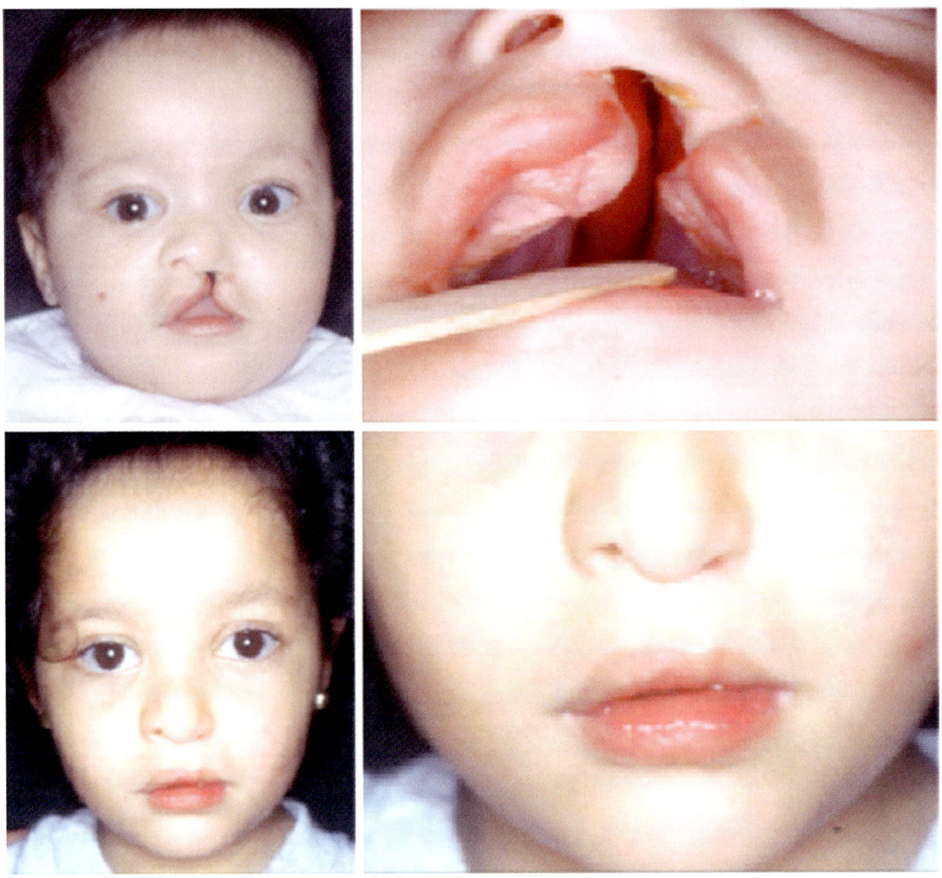

Fig. 27 Complete monolateral cleft lip and palate: pre- and postoperative views

The three-dimensional organization of the human face structures involving the mesial movements of the eyeball and the differentiations of the pharyngeal arches occurs between the fourth and the eighth week of intaruterine life.

The maxillary process is formed from the first arch and it is positioned above the stomodaeum and the mandibular process. It mainly gives rise mainly to the Meckel cartilages (which will be the guide for the formation

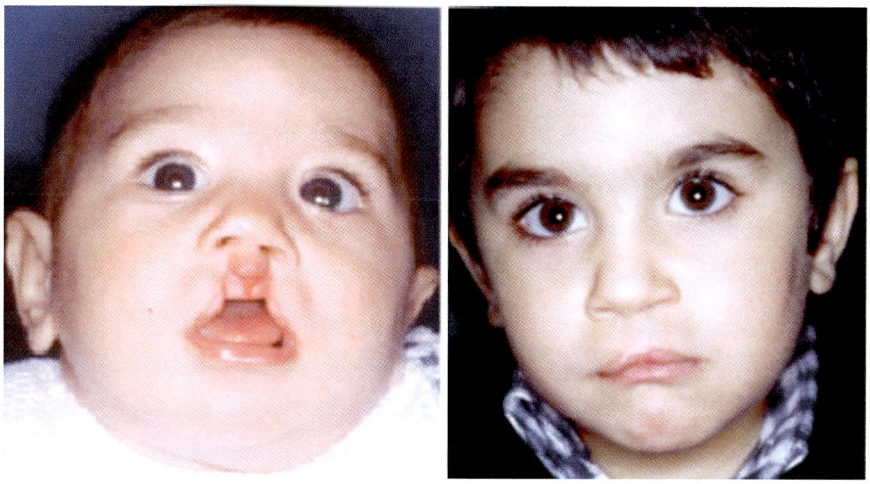

Fig. 28 Bilateral incomplete cleft lip and palate: pre- and postoperative view

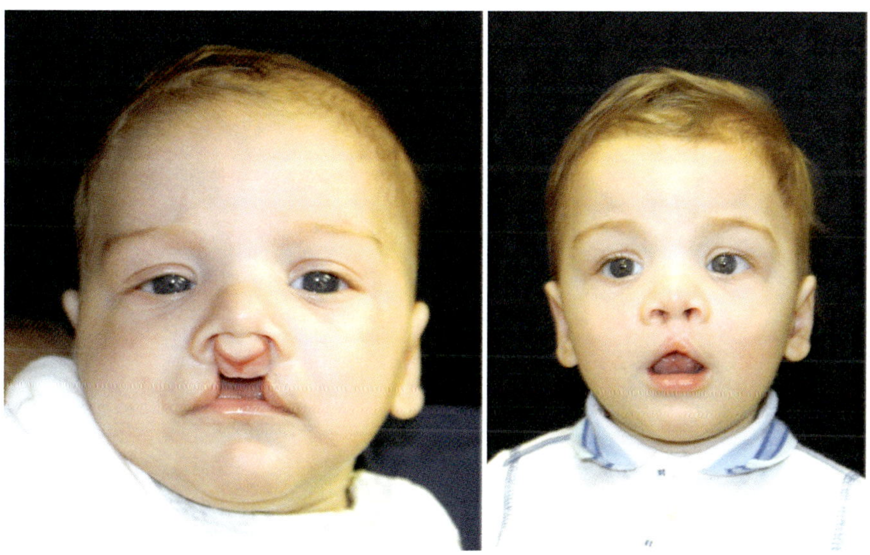

Fig. 29 Bilateral complete cleft lip and palate: pre- and postoperative view

of the mandible), as well as the anvil, the hammer, the masticatory muscles, and parts of the auricle. The bracket, much of the hyoid bone, the mimic muscles, and some other portions of the auricle differentiate from the second arch (Granstrom and Jacobsson 1999; Jacobson and Granstrom 1997).

Therefore, it is understandable that these syndromes also involve abnormalities of the ear, face muscles, and the outer and middle ear structures.

The deformity can have different degrees of severity according to the structures involved and how early pathogenic noxa occurs (Fig. 31).

Furthermore, the presence of fusion anomalies charged to the cervical vertebrae are very frequent in these syndromes. Among the asymmetrical shapes, the one mainly observed is HFM.

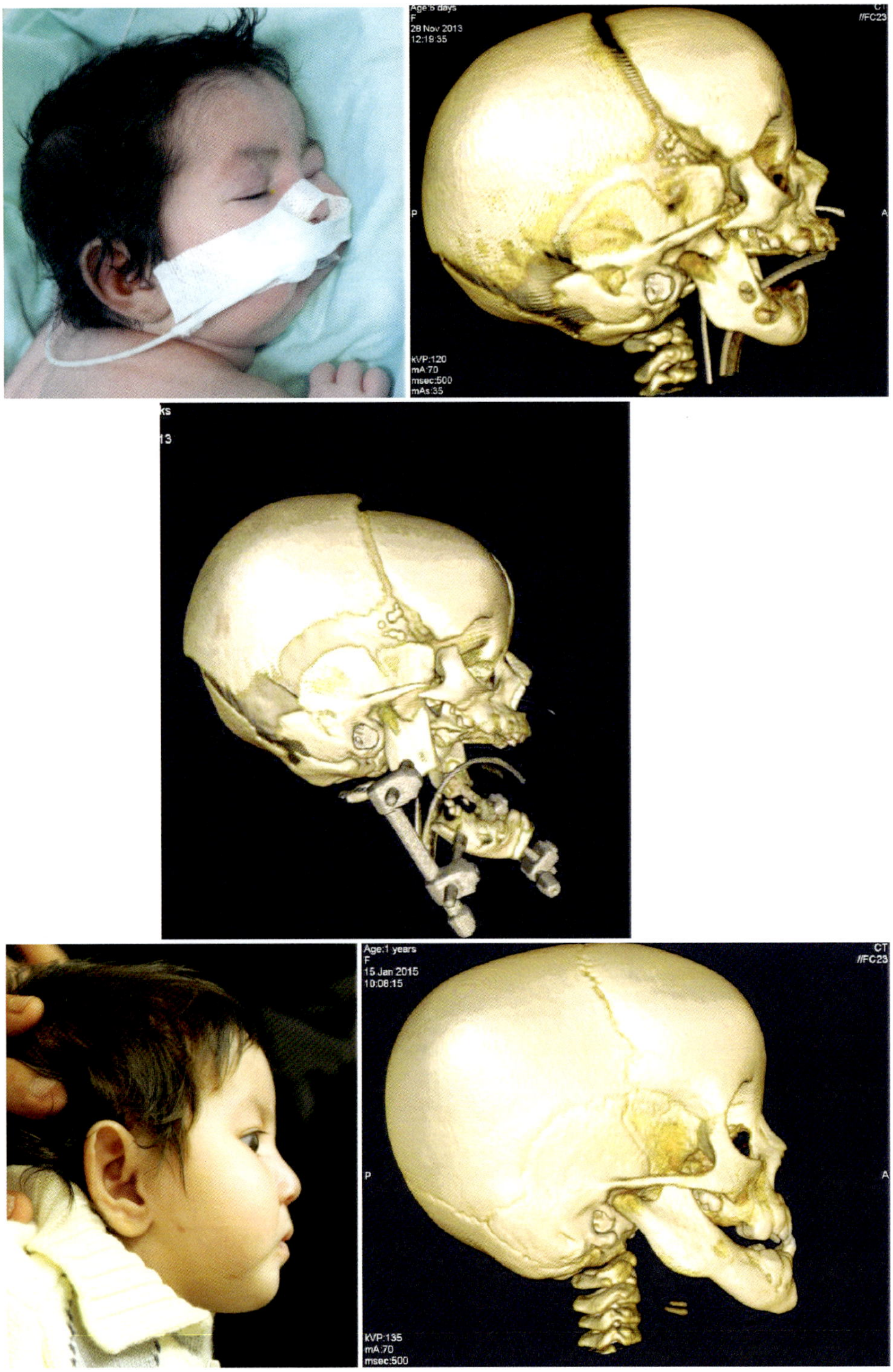

Fig. 30 Pierre Robin sequence: pre- and postoperative views

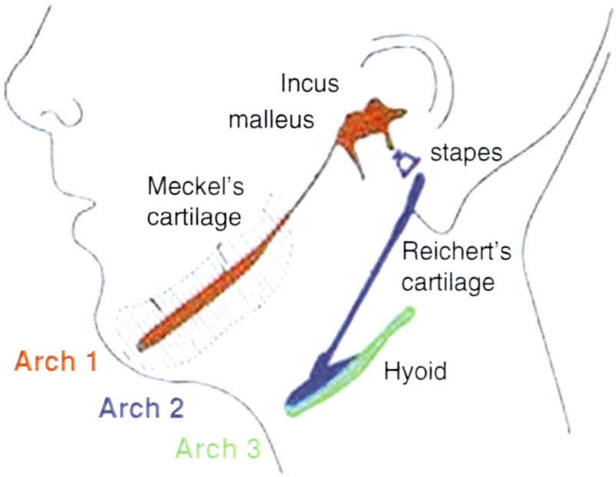

Fig. 31 Pharyngeal arch structures

Among the bilateral forms, Franceschetti or Treacher Collins syndrome deserves to be noted. It is characterized by mandibular hypoplasia with short leg, maxillary hypoplasia, and antimongoloid eyelid zygomatic inclination, a frequent abnormality with a typical down plant of the ear (Fig. 32).

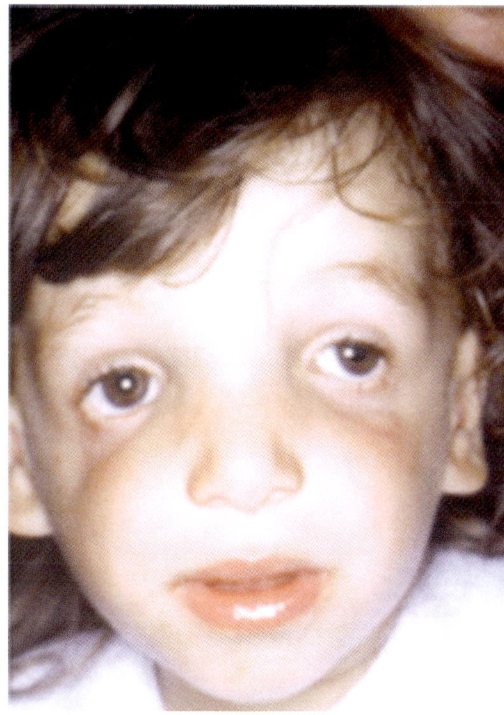

Fig. 32 Treacher Collins syndrome

80.11 Hemifacial Microsomia

Hemifacial microsomia is an asymmetrical craniofacial dysostosis with unknown pathogenesis. The etiopathogenetic mechanism of this syndrome is not yet fully understood. It occurs mostly on one side only and it can have different forms with varying severity. For this reason, various classifications have been proposed.

Currently, the most followed classification is the one proposed by Vento, who formulated the acronym OMENS (orbit, mandible, ear, nerve, and soft tissue) to assess the degree of involvement of the relevant structures. Physical examination may show auricles, absence or malformation of the ear, mandibular asymmetry due to the lack of all or a part of the branch and/or of the condyle, orbital dystopia, and, in severe cases, abnormal facial injury of the seventh cranial nerve (Kearns et al. 2000).

It has a frequency of 1:4000, but it is more frequent in females with a ratio of 3:1 (Forrest and Hopper 2013; Lowe et al. 2000; Nuckolls et al. 1999; Slavkin 1984; Slavkin and Melnick 1982; Sperber 1992; Gorlin et al. 2001; Cohen and Maclean 2000; Vig et al. 1984; Cohen 1981; Tessier 1971, 1974, 1976; Tulasne and Tessier 1986; McCarthy 1990; Neligan et al. 2013).

This malformation usually does not cause changes in breathing or swallowing at birth, but depending on the severity of the case, it may be necessary to implement a functional therapy or surgical treatment to prevent or reduce morphological and functional damages (Silvestri et al. 1996).

Goldenhar syndrome or oculoauriculovertebral sequence is a variant of hemifacial microsomia, constituting approximately 10% of patients. It is differentiated by the presence of ocular abnormalities (lipoma, lipodermoid, epibulbar dermoid, or coloboma) and cervical spine anomalies (Neligan et al. 2013) (Figs. 33, 34, and 35).

80.12 Tongue Malformations

The most relevant tongue malformations are divided into ankyloglossia, lingual fissures, macroglossia, microglossia, and aglossia.

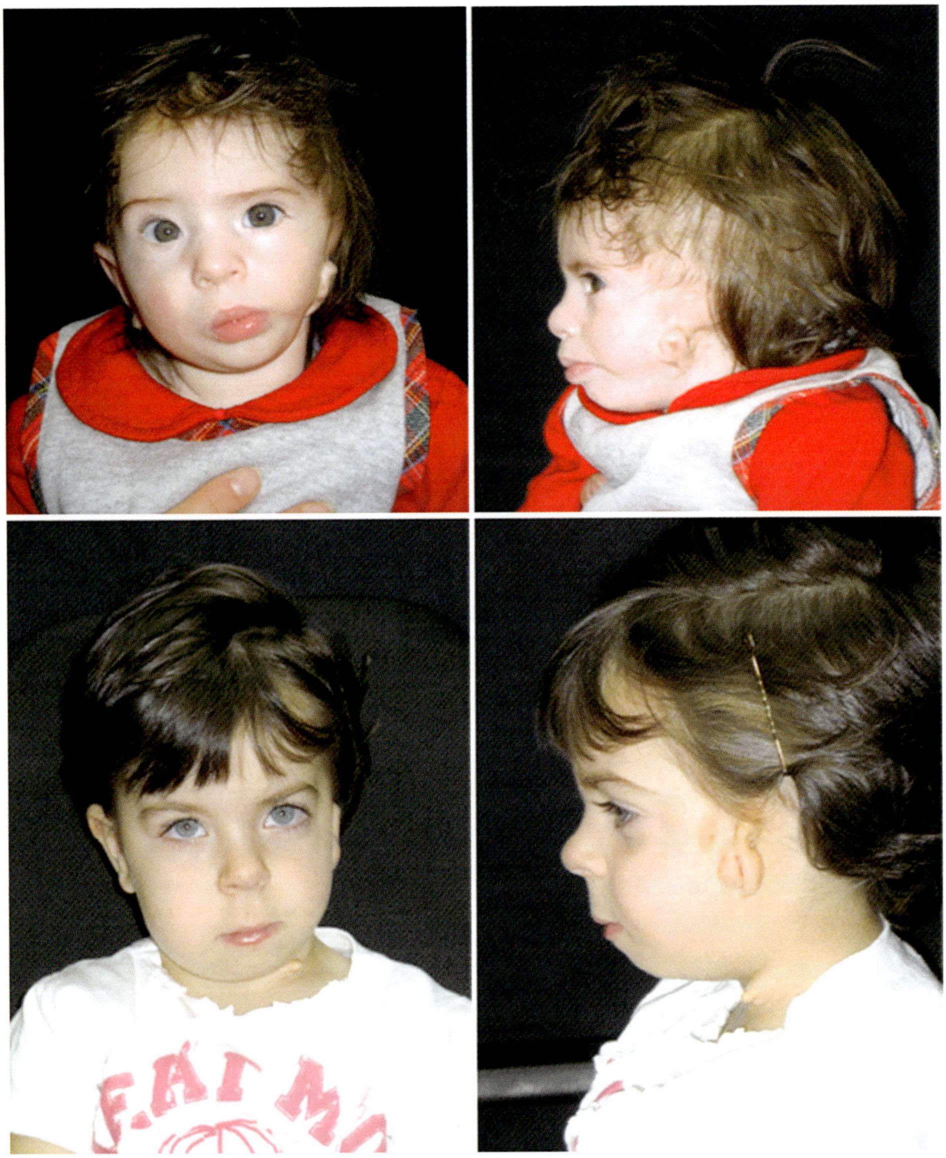

Fig. 33 HFM clinical cases

Ankyloglossia (*Tongue Tie*) – Ankyloglossia, or tongue-tie, is a congenital anomaly in which a short lingual frenulum or a highly attached genioglossus muscle restricts tongue movement (Mueller and Callanan 2007). The definition of ankyloglossia is not standardized, and there are wide variations of opinion regarding its clinical significance and optimal management.

Depending upon the study population and criteria used to define ankyloglossia, the reported prevalence varies from < 1 to 10.7% (Hall and Renfrew 2005).

The diagnosis is based on clinical signs by assessing the impossibility of reaching the palate with the tongue or protruding the tip beyond the lower teeth.

Surgery is the treatment of choice. The procedure consists of frenulum removing, including in some cases the upper bundle of genioglossus muscle.

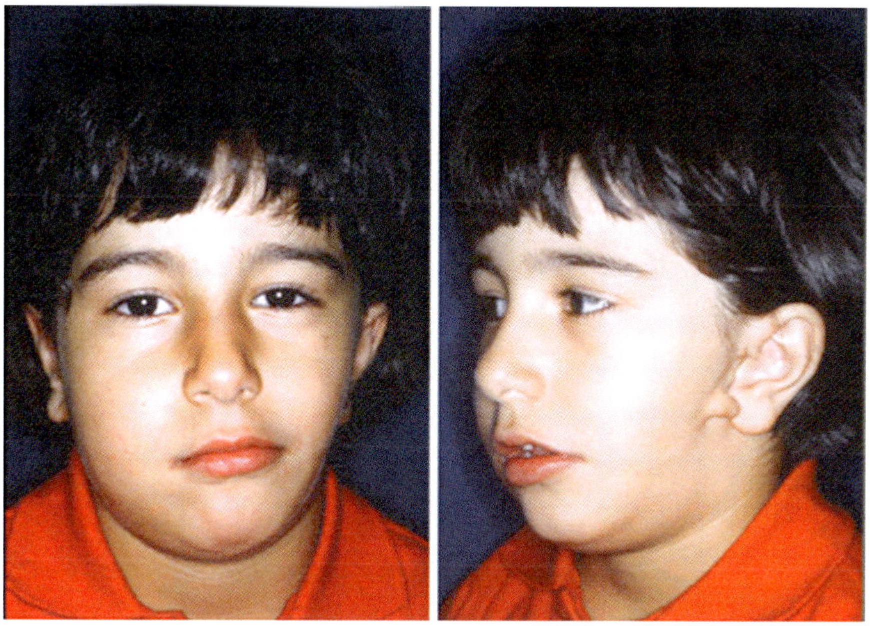

Fig. 34 HFM clinical cases

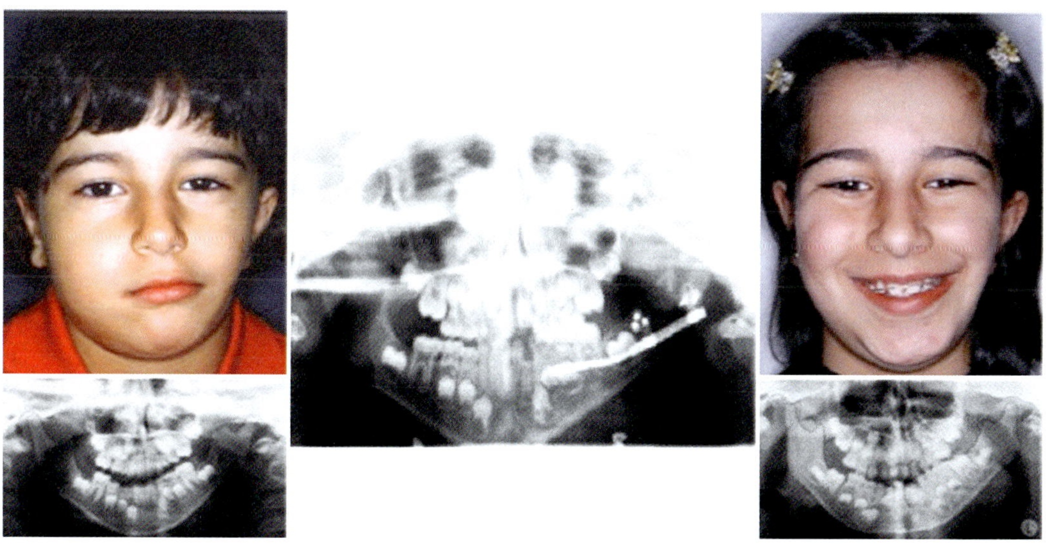

Fig. 35 Left HFM: pre- and postoperative views

Macroglossia – Although the exact incidence of macroglossia in the general population is unknown, the condition is found in some congenital syndromes, such as Down syndrome (1 per 700 live births) and Beckwith–Wiedemann syndrome (0.07 per 1000 live births). In Beckwith–Wiedemann syndrome, 97.5% of patients have macroglossia. True isolated congenital macroglossia is a rare condition with a wide range of clinical signs ranging from dental malposition to excessive mandibular growth and open bite. In very severe cases respiratory disorders may be experienced. Surgical intervention in macroglossia is reserved for severe cases that

cause functional and airway impairment. A partial glossectomy may be required as a first step in surgical care. In some cases, an elective tracheostomy is performed prior to surgical correction.

Tongue fissure – Tongue fissure is a condition frequently seen in general population that is characterized by grooves that vary in depth and are noted along the dorsal and lateral aspects of the tongue. Patients are usually asymptomatic, and the condition is initially noted on routine intraoral examination as an incidental finding. Fissured tongue is also seen in Melkersson–Rosenthal syndrome and Down syndrome and in frequent association with benign migratory glossitis (Alioglu et al. 2000)

Microglossia and aglossia – Aglossia is an extremely rare congenital defect characterizing complete absence of the tongue. This condition is usually associated with other serious developmental defects in the body, such as Hanart syndrome. Microglossia is another rare congenital anomaly in which only a tiny or rudimentary tongue has developed from the cupola. Although microglassias may develop as isolated cases, in most of the cases, they occur in association with other anomalies like oromandibular limb hypogenesis syndrome or hypoglassia–hypodactylia syndrome.

References

Alioglu Z, Caylan R, Adanir M, Ozmenoglu M (2000) Melkersson-Rosenthal syndrome: report of three cases. Neurol Sci 21(1):57–60

Breugem CC, Mink van der Molen AB (2009) What is "Pierre – Robin sequence"? J Plast Reconstr Aesthet Surg 62:1555–1558

Caoutte-Laberge L, Bayet B, Larocque Y (1994) The Pierre Robin sequence: review of 125 cases and evolution of treatment modalities. Plast Reconstr Surg 93:934e–942e

Cohen MM Jr (1981) The patient multiple anomalies. Raven, New York

Cohen MM Jr (2002) Malformations of the craniofacial region: evolutionary, embryonic, genetic, and clininical perspectives. Am J Med Gen 115(4):245–268

Cohen MM Jr, Maclean JE (2000) Craniosyn- ostosis: diagnosis, evaluation and management, 2nd edn. Oxford University Press, New York

Forrest CR, Hopper RA (2013) Craniofacial syndromes and surgery. Plast Reconstr Surg 131:86e–109e

Gorlin R, Cohen MM Jr, Hennekam RCM (2001) Syndromes of the head and neck. Oxford University Press, New York

Granstrom G, Jacobsson C (1999) First and second branchial arch syndrome: aspects on the embryogenesis, elucidations, and rehabilitation using the osseointegration concept. Clin Implant Dent Relat Res 1(2):59–69

Hall DM, Renfrew MJ (2005) Tongue tie. Arch Dis Child 115:1211

Jacobson C, Granstrom G (1997) Clinical appearance of spontaneous and induced first and second branchial arch syndromes. Scand J Plast Reconstr Surg Hand Surg 31(2):125–136

Johnston MC, Bronsky PT (1995) Prenatal craniofacial development: new insight on normal and abnormal mechanisms. Crit Rev Oral Biol Med 6(4):368–422

Kearns GJ, Padwa BL, Mulliken JB et al (2000) Progression of facial asymmetry in hemifacial microsomia. Plast Reconstr Surg 105(2):492–498

Lowe LH, Booth TN, Joglar JM et al (2000) Midface anomalies in children. Radiographics 20(4):907–922

McCarthy JG (1990) Plastic surgery. Cleft lip and palate and craniofacial anomalies, vol 4. Saunders, Philadelphia

Mueller DT, Callanan VP (2007) Congenital malformations of the oral cavity. Otolaryngol Clin North Am 40:401

Neligan PJ, Rodriguez ED, Losee JE (2013) Plastic surgery. Craniofacial, head and neck surgery, pediatric surgery, vol 3, 3rd edn. Elsevier Saunders, Philadelphia

Nuckolls GH, Shum L, Slavkin HC (1999) Progress toward understanding craniofacial malformations. Cleft Palate Craniofac J 36(1):12–26

Silvestri A, Natali G, Iannetti G (1996) Functional therapy in hemifacial microsomia: therapeutic protocol for growing children. J Oral Maxillofac Surg 54 (3):271–278

Slavkin HC (1984) Congenital craniofacial malformations: issues and perspectives. J Prosthet Dent 51(1):109–118

Slavkin HC, Melnick M (1982) Maternal influences on congenital craniofacial malformations. Am J Orthod 81(4):261–268

Sperber GH (1992) The aetiopathogenesis of craniofacial anomalies. Ann Acad Med Singapore 21(5):708–714

Tessier P (1971) Total osteotomy of the middle third of the face for fasciostenosis or for sequelae of Le Fort III fractures. Plast Reconstr Surg 48(6):533–541

Tessier P (1974) Experience in the treatment of orbital hypertelorism. Plast Reconstr Surg 53(1):1–18

Tessier P (1976) Exopthalmous in Crouzon's disease and in Apert's disease. Bull Mem Soc Fr Ophtalmol 88:357–361

Tulasne JF, Tessier PL (1986) Long – term stability results of Le Fort III advancement in Crouzon's syndrome. Cleft Palate J 23(Suppl 1):102–109

Van der Meulen JC, Mazzola R, Vermey-Keers C et al (1983) A morphogenetic classification of craniofacial malformations. Plast Reconstr Surg 71: 560–572

Vig KW, Millicovsky G, Johnston MC (1984) Craniofacial development: the possible mechanism for some malformations. Br J Orthod 11(3):114–118

Esophageal Atresia of Newborns

81

Mario Messina, Francesco Molinaro,
Alfredo Garzi, and Rossella Angotti

Contents

M. Messina (✉) · F. Molinaro
Department of Pediatrics, Obstetrics and Reproductive Medicine, Section of Pediatric Surgery, Policlinico "Le Scotte", University of Siena, Siena, Italy

Department of Medical, Surgical and Neurological Sciences, Section of Pediatric Surgery, University of Siena, Siena, Italy
e-mail: mario.messina@unisi.it

A. Garzi
Department of Medical, Surgical and Neurological Sciences, Section of Pediatric Surgery, University of Siena, Siena, Italy

Università degli Studi di Salerno, Fisciano, Italy

R. Angotti
Department of Pediatrics, Obstetrics and Reproductive Medicine, Section of Pediatric Surgery, University of Siena, Siena, Italy

G. Buonocore et al. (eds.), *Neonatology*,
https://doi.org/10.1007/978-3-319-29489-6_228

Abstract

Esophageal atresia includes a group of congenital anomalies characterized as interruption of the continuity of the esophagus combined with or without a persistent communication with the trachea. These congenital malformations occur in 1:2,500–3,000 live births.

Over the last 40 years, there has been a steady improvement in the overall survival rate due to early diagnosis and prompt referral, improvements in preoperative care and diagnosis and treatment of associated anomalies, advances in anesthetic techniques, and sophisticated neonatal intensive care.

There is increasing experience with the thoracoscopic approach to repair esophageal atresia (Brandigi et al., J Siena Acad Sci 5, 2013; Bax and van Der Zee, J Pediatr Surg 37: 192–196, 2002; Rothenberg, J Pediatr Surg 37: 869–872, 2002; Nguyen et al., J Laparoendosc Adv Surg Tech A 16: 174–178, 2006; Krosnar and Baxter, Paediatr Anaesth 15: 541–546, 2005; Rothenberg, Semin Pediatr Surg 14: 2–7, 2005a; Rothenberg, Esophageal atresia and tracheoesophageal fistula. In: Najmaldin et al. (eds) Operative endoscopy and endoscopic surgery in infants and children. Hodder Arnold, London, pp 89–97, 2005b), but this requires advanced skills in minimal invasive surgery.

81.1 Salient Points

- Prenatal diagnosis is an important step to plan an early management of patients with esophageal atresia.
- Bronchoscopy is a preoperative obliged step.
- The thoracoscopic approach is a good option for patients with esophageal atresia (Type III).

81.2 Background

Esophageal atresia includes a group of congenital anomalies characterized as interruption of the continuity of the esophagus combined with or without a persistent communication with the trachea (Chittmittrapap et al. 1980). These congenital malformations occur in 1:2,500–3,000 live births. The overwhelming majority of cases of esophageal atresia are sporadic/non-syndromic, although a small number within this nonfamilial group are associated with chromosomal abnormalities (Chittmittrapap et al. 1980). Familial/syndromic cases of esophageal atresia are extremely rare, representing less than 1% of the total. Esophageal atresia is two to three times more common in twins (Merci et al. 1998). The etiology of esophageal atresia is likely multifactorial and remains unknown (Crisera et al. 1999; Zhou et al. 1999).

81.3 Embryology

The mechanism that causes tracheoesophageal malformations is still unclear; however, the development of reproducible animal models of these anomalies has allowed detailed analysis of the various stages of faulty organogenesis (Zhou et al. 1999). By contrasting these stages with normal development, it has been possible to identify key developmental processes that may be disturbed during embryogenesis (Roessler et al. 1996). It is generally accepted that the respiratory primordium appears as a ventral evagination on the floor of the postpharyngeal foregut at the beginning of the fourth week of gestation and that the primitive lung buds are located at the caudal end of this evagination. During a period of rapid growth, the ventrally placed trachea becomes separated from the dorsally placed

esophagus (Roessler et al. 1996; Digilio et al. 1999). The presence of associated malformations could provide clues as to the possible etiology of esophageal atresia (Chittmittrapap et al. 1980; Zhou et al. 1999; Marsh et al. 2000). Such malformations are present in 50% of cases and can occur in distinct patterns. These are nonrandom associations rather than syndromes because the presence of anomalies in one system makes it more likely that defects exist in another. One of the best-described associations is the VACTERL association, which comprises vertebral, anorectal, cardiac, tracheoesophageal, renal, and limb abnormalities. The pattern of these associations is likely to be dictated by the timing of a possible insult that affects multiple morphogenetic events (Chittmittrapap et al. 1980; Marsh et al. 2000; Mee et al. 1992).

81.3.1 Classification

In 1976 Kluth (1976) published an extensive *Atlas of Esophageal Atresia* which comprised ten major types, each with numerous subtypes which is based on the original Vogt classification. It would appear to be more valuable to describe the anatomical anomaly rather than assign a label, which may not be widely recognizable (Fig. 1) (Driver et al. 2001; Poenaru et al. 1993).

81.3.1.1 Esophageal Atresia with Distal Tracheoesophageal Fistula (86%, Vogt IIIb, Gross C)

This is the most common variety in which the proximal esophagus, which is dilated, and the muscular wall thickened ends blindly in the superior mediastinum at about the level of the third or fourth thoracic vertebra. The distal esophagus, which is thinner and narrower, enters the posterior wall of the trachea at the carina or more commonly 1–2 cm more proximally in the trachea. The distance between the blind proximal esophagus and the distal tracheoesophageal fistula varies from overlapping segments to a wide gap. Very rarely the distal fistula may be occluded or obliterated leading to the misdiagnosis preoperatively of an isolated atresia (Driver et al. 2001; Poenaru et al. 1993).

81.3.1.2 Isolated Esophageal Atresia Without Fistula (7%, Vogt II, Gross A)

The proximal and distal esophagus ends blindly without any connection to the trachea. The proximal esophageal segment is dilated and thick-walled and usually ends higher in the posterior mediastinum at around the second thoracic vertebra. The distal esophagus is short and ends a variable distance above the diaphragm. The distance between the two ends will determine whether a primary repair is feasible (rarely) or whether a delayed primary anastomosis or an esophageal replacement should be performed. It is important to exclude a proximal tracheoesophageal fistula in these cases (Driver et al. 2001; Poenaru et al. 1993).

81.3.1.3 Tracheoesophageal Fistula Without Atresia (4%, Gross E)

There is a fistulous connection between an anatomically intact esophagus and trachea. The

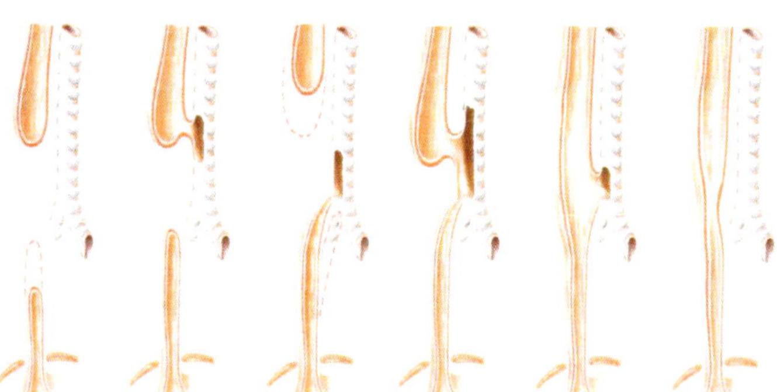

Fig. 1 Anatomical types of esophageal atresia

fistulous tract may be very narrow or 3–5 mm in diameter and is commonly located in the lower cervical region. They are usually single, but two and even three fistulas have been described (Driver et al. 2001; Poenaru et al. 1993).

81.3.1.4 Esophageal Atresia with Proximal Tracheoesophageal Fistula (2%, Vogt III, Gross B)

This rare anomaly needs to be distinguished from the isolated variety. The fistula is not at the distal end of the upper pouch but is sited 1–2 cm above the end on the anterior wall of the esophagus (Driver et al. 2001; Poenaru et al. 1993).

81.3.1.5 Esophageal Atresia with Proximal and Distal Tracheoesophageal Fistula (<1%, Vogt IIIa, Gross D)

In many of these infants, the anomaly was misdiagnosed managed as proximal atresia and distal fistula as a result of recurrent respiratory infections; investigations carried out revealed a tracheoesophageal fistula, previously mistaken for a recurrent fistula. With the increasing use of preoperative endoscopy (bronchoscopy and/or esophagoscopy), early recognition of the double fistula is made and total repair performed at the initial procedure. If the proximal fistula is not identified preoperatively, the diagnosis should be suspected by a large gas leak emanating from the upper pouch during the fashioning of the anastomosis (Driver et al. 2001; Poenaru et al. 1993).

81.4 Pathophysiology

The motility of the esophagus is always affected in esophageal atresia. The disordered peristalsis more commonly involves the distal esophageal segment. Whether the motility disorder is primarily due to abnormal innervation as evidenced by an abnormality in neuropeptide distribution or secondary to vagal nerve damage occurring during the surgical repair remains uncertain. The resting pressure in the whole esophagus is significantly higher than in normal patients, and the closing pressure of the lower esophageal sphincter is reduced. The trachea is also abnormal in esophageal atresia. The abnormality consists of an absolute deficiency of tracheal cartilage and an increase in the length of the transverse muscle in the posterior tracheal wall. When severe, these abnormalities result in tracheomalacia with collapse of the trachea over a 1–2-cm segment in the vicinity of the fistula (Spitz et al. 1994; Lopez et al. 2006).

81.5 Associated Anomalies

Over 50% of infants with esophageal atresia have one or more additional anomalies. The systems affected are as follows:

- Cardiovascular 29%
- Anorectal anomalies 14%
- Genitourinary 14%
- Gastrointestinal 13%
- Vertebral/skeletal 10%
- Respiratory 6%
- Genetic 4%
- Other 11%

There is an increased incidence of associated anomalies in pure atresia (65%) and a lower incidence in H-type fistula (10%). The VATER association first described by Quan and Smith in 1973 (Quan and Smith 1972) consists of a combination of anomalies including vertebral, anorectal, tracheoesophageal, and renal or radial abnormalities. This association was later expanded as the VACTERL association to include cardiac and limb defects (Chittmittrapap et al. 1980; Merci et al. 1998; Crisera et al. 1999; Zhou et al. 1999; Roessler et al. 1996; Digilio et al. 1999; Marsh et al. 2000). Other associations, which may include esophageal atresia, are the CHARGE association (coloboma, heart defects, choanal atresia, retarded growth and development, genital hypoplasia, and ear deformities), Potter's

syndrome (renal agenesis, pulmonary hypoplasia, typical dysmorphic facies), and Schisis association (omphalocele, cleft lip and/or palate, genital hypoplasia). Genetic defects associated with esophageal atresia include trisomies 21 and 18 and 13q deletion. Of the cardiac anomalies, the most common are ventricular septal defect and tetralogy of Fallot. Major cardiac malformations are one of the main causes of mortality in infants with esophageal atresia (Chittmittrapap et al. 1980; Marsh et al. 2000; Babu et al. 2000). The vertebral anomalies in esophageal atresia are mainly confined to the thoracic region and are responsible for later development of scoliosis. The claim that the presence of 13 ribs is associated with long-gap atresia has not been substantiated. Of the gastrointestinal anomalies, the most frequently encountered are duodenal atresia and malrotation, while there is an increased incidence of pyloric stenosis. Miscellaneous anomalies include cleft lip and palate, omphalocele, lung abnormalities, choanal atresia, and hypospadias (Babu et al. 2000; Filston et al. 1982a).

81.6 Genetic Counseling

The majority of cases of esophageal atresia are sporadic/non-syndromic, although a small number within this non-familiar group are associated with chromosomal abnormalities. Familial/ syndromic cases of esophageal atresia are extremely rare. Esophageal atresia is two to three times more common in twins. The overall risk of esophageal atresia recurrence in a sibling of an affected child is about 1 % (Digilio et al. 1999; Marsh et al. 2000).

81.7 Clinical Description and Diagnosis

The diagnosis of esophageal atresia may be suspected prenatally by the finding of a small or absent fetal stomach bubble on ultrasound scan performed after the 18th week of gestation. Overall the sensitivity of ultrasonography is 42%, but in combination with polyhydramnios, the positive predictive value is 56% (Stringer et al. 1995; Shulman et al. 2002). Available methods of improving the prenatal diagnostic rate include ultrasound examination of the fetal neck to view the blind-ending upper pouch and to observe fetal swallowing and magnetic resonance imaging (Langer et al. 2001; Litingtung et al. 1998; Cloud 1968). The newborn infant of a mother with polyhydramnios should always have a nasogastric tube passed soon after delivery to exclude esophageal atresia. Infants with esophageal atresia are unable to swallow saliva and are noted to have excessive salivation requiring repeated suctioning. A plain X-ray of the chest and abdomen will show the tip of the catheter arrested in the superior mediastinum (T2–T4), while gas in the stomach and intestine signifies the presence of a distal tracheoesophageal fistula (Fig. 2). The absence of gastrointestinal gas is indicative of an isolated atresia. A fine bore catheter may curl up in the upper pouch giving the false impression of an intact esophagus, or rarely it may pass through the trachea and proceed distally into the esophagus through the fistula (Stringer et al. 1995; Langer et al. 2001).

81.8 Management

81.8.1 Preoperative

Once the diagnosis of esophageal atresia has been established, the infant will need to be transferred to a pediatric surgical center. A suction catheter, preferably of the double lumen type, is placed in the upper esophageal pouch to suction secretions and prevent aspiration. The infant is placed on its side in the portable incubator while monitoring the usual vital signs. Vascular access should be provided as a precautionary measure, but intravenous fluid administration is not usually necessary (Filston et al. 1982a). The preterm infant with respiratory distress requires special attention. Clearly there is a need for endotracheal intubation and mechanical ventilation. In

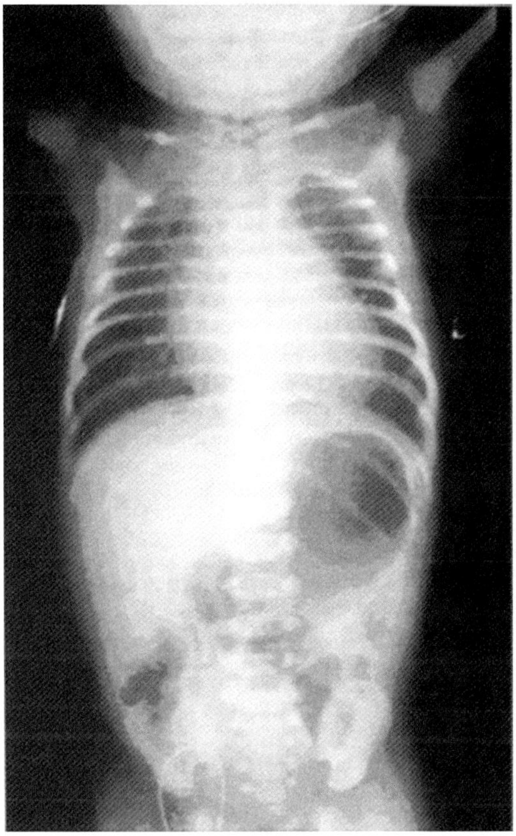

Fig. 2 Plain X-ray (chest and abdomen) showing the radiopaque tube in the blind upper esophageal pouch. Air in the stomach indicates the presence of a distal tracheoesophageal fistula

addition there is the added risk of gastric over distention and rupture of the stomach due to escape of respiratory gases down through the distal fistula into the stomach due to the increased pulmonary resistance. This sequence of events can be minimized by positioning the end of the endotracheal tube distal to entry of the tracheoesophageal fistula and by applying gentle low pressure ventilation (Lopez et al. 2006; Filston et al. 1982a; Stringer et al. 1995). All infants with esophageal atresia should have an echocardiogram prior to surgery. The ECHO and/or MR will define any structural anomaly of the heart or great blood vessels and occasionally may indicate a right-sided aortic arch, which occurs in 2.5% of cases. These diagnostic tests determine the side of approach for the operative repair (Babu et al. 2000).

81.8.2 Risk Categorization and Prognosis (Outcome)

In 1962, Waterston proposed a classification of infants born with esophageal atresia into three groups "with different chances of survival." The classification based on birth weight, associated anomalies, and pneumonia comprised:

- **Group A**: Over 5 1/2 lb (2,500 g) birth weight and well
- **Group B**:
  1. Birth weight 4–5 1/2 lb (1,800–2,500 g) and well
  2. Higher birth weight, moderate pneumonia, and congenital anomaly
- **Group C**
  1. Birth weight under 4 lb (1,800 g)
  2. Higher birth weight and severe pneumonia and severe congenital anomaly

Over the last 40 years, there has been a steady improvement in the overall survival rate due to early diagnosis and prompt referral, improvements in preoperative care and diagnosis and treatment of associated anomalies, advances in anesthetic techniques, and sophisticated neonatal intensive care (Chittmittrapap et al. 1980). The Spitz classification for survival in esophageal atresia comprises:

- Group I: Birth weight over 1,500 g with no major cardiac anomaly
- Group II: Birth weight less than 1,500 g or major cardiac anomaly
- Group III: Birth weight less than 1,500 g plus major cardiac anomaly

Major cardiac anomaly was defined as either cyanotic congenital heart disease that required palliative or corrective surgery or non-cyanotic heart anomaly that required medical or surgical treatment for cardiac failure (Spitz et al. 1994).

81.8.3 Selection for Nontreatment

Infants with Potter's disease (bilateral renal agenesis) syndrome and trisomy 18 which is fatal in

the first year of life in over 90% of affected infants should be offered by opinion of no active treatment. Similarly, infants with totally uncorrectable major cardiac defects or with grade IV intraventricular hemorrhage should be considered for nonoperative management.

81.8.4 Emergency Ligation of the Distal Tracheoesophageal Fistula

Generally, the operative correction of an esophageal atresia is not regarded as an emergency procedure. The one exception is the preterm infant with severe respiratory distress syndrome requiring ventilatory support. Ventilatory gases escaping down the distal fistula result in gastric distension, which further impedes respiratory function. With progressively increasing gastric distension, the stomach may eventually rupture causing a tension pneumoperitoneum, which renders ventilatory support even more difficult (Spitz et al. 1994; Filston et al. 1982a; Stringer et al. 1995). Many maneuvers have been advocated to alleviate the problem including positioning of the endotracheal tube distal to the fistula. However, if the fistula is sited at the level of the carina, this maneuver is impossible to achieve. Others have advocated blocking of the fistula by a Fogarty catheter passed at bronchoscopy. The affected infants are usually preterm and in critical respiratory status. The smallest-caliber bronchoscope will not permit ventilation, while maneuvering a Fogarty catheter into the distal esophagus in a cyanotic infant will aggravate the condition and further exacerbate the hypoxia (Cloud 1968; Holmes et al. 1987).

81.8.5 Operative Approach

The operation is performed under general endotracheal anesthesia with dependable vascular access and employing gentle ventilatory pressure so as not to produce gastric distension (Holmes et al. 1987; Hagberg et al. 1986).

Intraoperative endoscopy: Preliminary bronchoscopy may be carried out to define the site of entry of the distal tracheoesophageal fistula and to assess the presence of tracheomalacia. An alternative is to carry out an esophagoscopy to dame the length of the upper esophagus and to exclude an upper pouch fistula, which is more common with isolated esophageal atresia (Spitz et al. 1993; Spitz 1973; Yeung et al. 1992).

Position: The infant is placed on the left side with the right arm across the front of the chest for a right posterolateral thoracotomy.

Incision: A "conventional" incision centered 1 cm below the inferior angle of the scapula approximately 5–6 cm long is made. The muscle of the chest wall may either be split or divided with electrocautery taking care to preserve the long thoracic nerve to serratus anterior. The thorax is opened through the fourth or fifth intercostal space by dividing the intercostal muscles or by entry through the bed of the unresected rib.

An alternative incision is an axillary incision. This incision has been proposed by Bianchi and has been used for most thoracic operations over the years. The skin incision can be vertical or horizontal although a horizontal incision is cosmetically more pleasing. The subcutaneous tissue and fascia are divided to expose the serratus anterior. Tissue planes are developed between the superficial fascia and the muscle layers. Care should be taken to avoid the intercostobrachial and long thoracic nerves. Latissimus dorsi is retracted posteriorly, and the serratus anterior muscle is elevated to expose the desired rib space for thoracotomy (Bianchi et al. 1998).

Extrapleural approach: It has the advantage of conferring protection of the pleural space in the event of an anastomotic leak. Commencing posteriorly, the pleura is gently freed off the chest wall using blunt dissection. The dissection proceeds into the mediastinum to provide good access to the esophagus. The extrapleural approach is slightly more time-consuming and has theoretically advantages over the transpleural approach still used by many surgeons (Cloud 1968; Agrawal et al. 1999).

Exposure of the esophageal segments: The azygos vein is the first structure encountered on

entering the mediastinum. The azygos vein is gently mobilized and divided between ligatures to expose the esophagus. The distal esophagus usually lies directly deep to the azygos vein and is identified by the vagus nerve coursing over its anterior aspect (Duranceau et al. 1977; Filler et al. 1992; Corbally et al. 1993).

Repair of the defect: The distal esophagus is mobilized. A marking seromuscular suture is placed in the lateral wall of the distal esophagus to assist with orientation. The distal esophagus is dissected to the level of the fistula, and the upper and lower extent of the fistula is marked with fine nonabsorbable sutures before dividing the esophagus just distal to the fistula. The tracheal side of the fistula is closed with interrupted 5/0 sutures to achieve an airtight closure. The tracheal closure may be tested by instilling warm saline over the suture line while the anesthesiologist expands the lungs. An end-to-end anastomosis between the proximal and distal esophagus is fashioned using interrupted full-thickness fine sutures (Fig. 3).

If there is a wide gap, the distal esophagus can be mobilized safely well down toward the diaphragm. Just prior to the final suture being tied, a transanastomotic fine-caliber nasogastric tube may be passed. This allows gastric decompression in the early postoperative course and provides a mute for early enteral feeding (Holmes et al. 1987; Spitz et al. 1993; Spitz 1996).

In our experience a very tense anastomosis can be achieved in most cases, and if the infant is subsequently electively paralyzed and mechanically ventilated for approximately 5 days postoperatively, the anastomosis will heal without leakage.

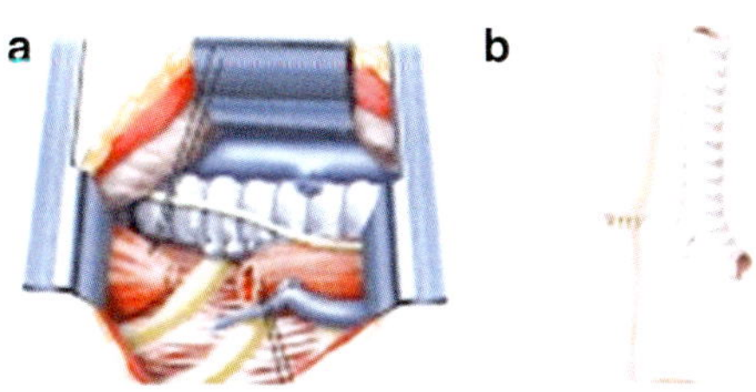

Fig. 3 The operative repair of an esophageal atresia and distal tracheoesophageal fistula. (**a**) Ligature of the fistula. (**b**) Anastomosis

However, many methods have been proposed to overcome a wide gap:

- Intracorporeal bougienage
- Extracorporeal stretching (Focker's technique)
- Circular myotomy (by Livatidis) or spiral myotomy (Kimura's technique)

Others authors have proposed tubularization of the upper pouch after creating a flap (Fig. 4).

Others, finally, prefer abandoning any attempt at initial primary anastomosis awaiting delayed primary anastomosis 6–12 weeks later (Filston et al. 1982b; Livitidis 1973). The thoracotomy incision is now closed with or preferably without intercostal drainage especially if the procedure has been totally extrapleural, and a technically satisfactory anastomosis has been performed.

81.8.6 Thoracoscopic Approach

There is increasing experience with the thoracoscopic approach to repair esophageal atresia (Brandigi et al. 2013; Bax and van Der Zee 2002; Rothenberg 2002, 2005a, b; Nguyen et al. 2006; Krosnar and Baxter 2005), but this requires advanced skills in minimal invasive surgery (Hagberg et al. 1986; Livitidis 1973; Puri et al. 1981). It is clear that there are many potential advantages of the thoracoscopic approach, as a good cosmetic appearance (minimal scarring), a magnification and excellent visualization, a less postoperative pain, and a uniform collapse of the lung that eliminates retraction trauma. However, there are also many disadvantages that must be considered by the surgeon. The main disadvantages are the small operative space and the need of good lung compliance that thoracoscopic approach always requires. Also, most surgeons use a transpleural approach although an extrapleural approach has also been described (Rothenberg 2005a), and an anastomotic leak occurs. Finally, single-lung ventilation is not always achievable in neonates. For all these reasons, not all infants are suitable for thoracoscopic repair. It is contraindicated in unstable infant or

Fig. 4 The operative repair of an esophageal atresia by flap

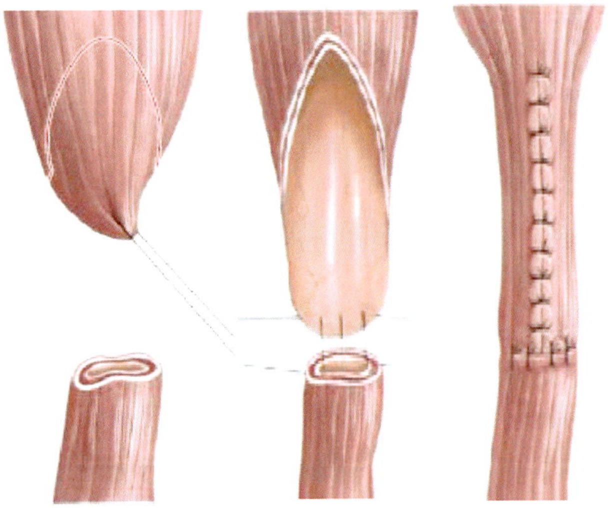

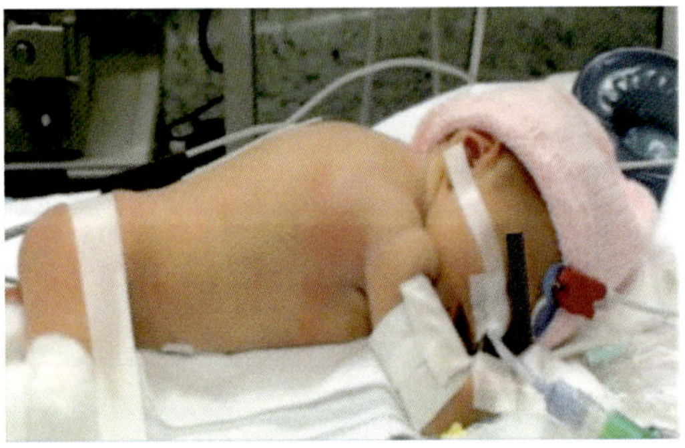

Fig. 5 Patient's position during thoracoscopic approach

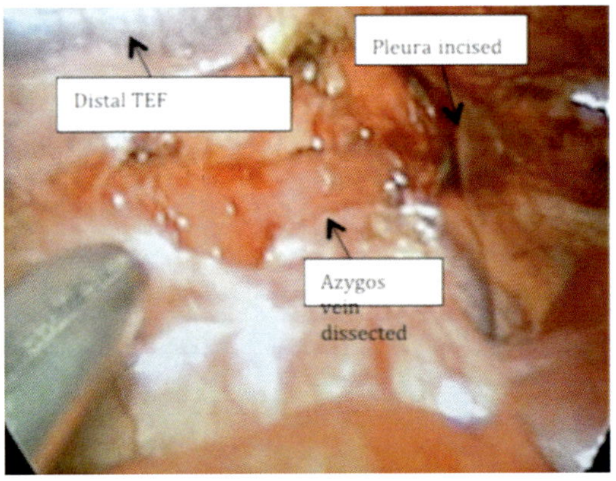

Fig. 6 TEF riveled after azygos vein dissection

extremely small. Congenital heart disease and hyaline membrane disease when the infant is able to tolerate only short periods of single-lung ventilation during ligation of the fistula should be considered relative contraindications (Rothenberg 2005b).

The patient is placed in the left lateral decubitus position, slightly prone, with the right side elevated (Fig. 5). Three 5-mm trocars are placed. A 5-mm port is placed in the fifth intercostal space in the posterior axillary, and the pneumothorax is created (0.5 l/min, 6 mmhg). A 30° scope is introduced. Two working ports are placed in the third and sixth intercostal spaces in the midaxillary line. Sometimes a fourth port is required to help retract the lung.

81.8.6.1 Closure of the Tracheoesophageal Fistula

The chest is insufflated and the lung collapsed. The pleura overlying the posterosuperior mediastinum is incised (transpleural approach), exposing the azygos vein. The azygos vein is divided by a 5-mm LigaSure. The lower esophageal pouch is identified and traced in a proximal direction to where it enters the back wall of the trachea. The fistula can be ligated using a 4-0 Vicryl suture on the tracheal side, and subsequently it is divided with scissors (Fig. 6).

81.8.6.2 Mobilization of the Upper Pouch

Downward pressure applied on the orogastric tube by the anesthetist helps identify the upper pouch. The pleura overlying the pouch is incised and the pouch mobilized toward the neck with a combination of blunt and sharp dissection. Mobilization can be continued into the thoracic inlet, to gain additional esophageal length, depending on the gap that has to be overcome to achieve an esophageal anastomosis. The most dependent part of the upper esophageal pouch is opened.

81.8.6.3 Esophageal Anastomosis

The anastomosis is performed using interrupted all-layer sutures (5/0 absorbable) tied. The knot can be tied extracorporeally using a knot pusher or intracorporeally (Fig. 7). Once the posterior wall of the anastomosis has been completed, a catheter (6-Ch nasogastric tube) is introduced through the mouth and advanced into the distal esophagus. This facilitates completion of anterior wall of anastomosis.

81.8.7 Postoperative Management

In all other instances, regular pharyngeal suction is necessary for the first few postoperative days. The suction catheter should be clearly marked to prevent the tube being passed to the site of the anastomosis and causing damage. Transanastomotic nasogastric feeds may be commenced on the second or third postoperative day, and when the infant is swallowing saliva, oral feeds may be started. A follow-up contrast study is not regularly performed, but if there is any doubt as to the integrity of the anastomosis, a water-soluble contrast study is carried out (Holmes et al. 1987). A chest tube is usually left (on the sixth intercostal space in the posterior axillary line).

81.8.8 Complications and Outcomes

81.8.8.1 Anastomotic Leaks

These occur in 15–20% of patients, but in only one-third or less is there a major disruption (Fig. 8). Major leaks occur in the early postoperative period (<48 h) and present with life-threatening tension pneumothorax. Minor leaks may be detected on the routine contrast study usually performed on the fifth to seventh day postoperatively (Spitz et al. 1994; Cloud 1968).

81.8.8.2 Anastomotic Strictures

Anastomotic stenoses develop in 30–40% of cases, most of which will respond to one or two dilatations (Fig. 9). Risk factors that have been implicated in stricture formation include anastomotic tension, anastomotic leakage, and gastroesophageal reflux. Endoscopic dilatation of the

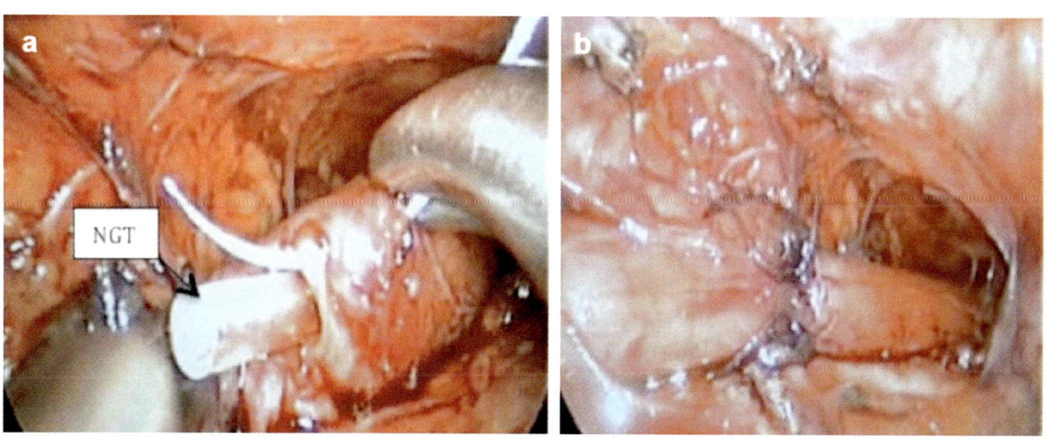

Fig. 7 (**a**) Nasogastric tube placed after performing anastomosis of the posterior wall; (**b**) completed anastomosis

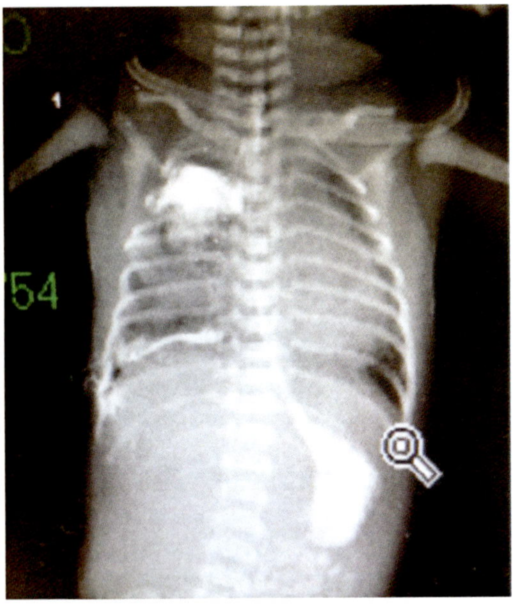

Fig. 8 Anastomotic leak in patient in tenth postoperative day

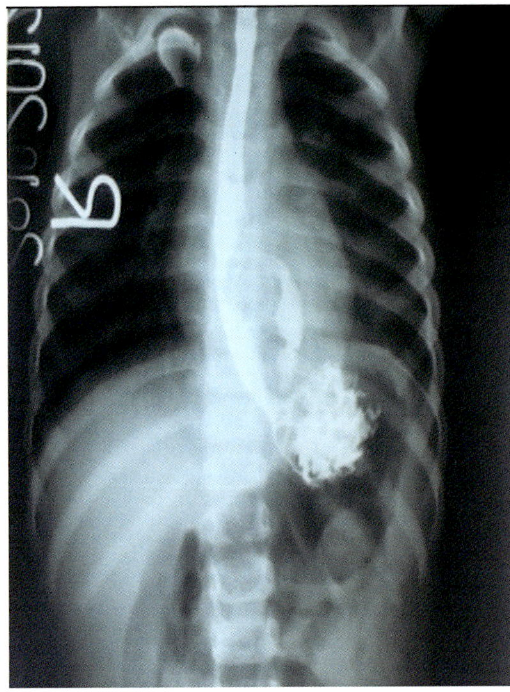

Fig. 10 Perforation of esophagus during endoscopic dilatation, in patient with originally EA type III long gap, who had underwent primary anastomosis under tension

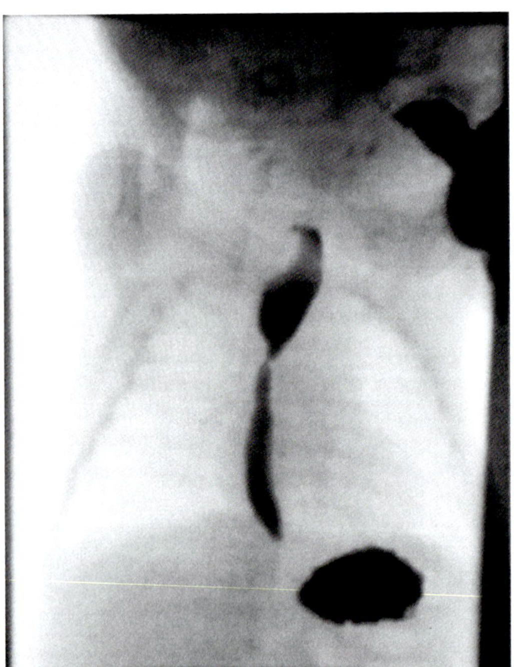

Fig. 9 Anastomotic stricture in patient in 1 month after surgery (primary end-to-end anastomosis)

stricture can be carried out either at rigid esophagoscopy using semirigid bougies (Savary-Gilliard) of progressively larger caliber or by balloon dilatation introduced either at fluoroscopy or during flexible endoscopy. Even if dilatations can be considered a simple mini-invasive surgery, it is no free from risks. The main complication is the perforation of esophagus that it is anelastic and rigid (Fig. 10). For this reason, some surgeons, at the end of the procedure, introduce contrast into the esophagus to ensure that there has been no perforation and to establish the effectiveness of the dilatation (Lividitis 1973). Only rarely is it necessary to resort to resection of an intractable anastomotic stricture.

81.8.8.3 Recurrent Tracheoesophageal Fistula

The incidence of recurrent tracheoesophageal fistula is between 5% and 14%.

A recurrent fistula should be suspected if the infant manifests respiratory symptoms (coughing

during feeds, apneic or cyanotic episodes) or has recurrent respiratory infections after "successful" repair of the esophageal atresia (Spitz et al. 1994; Stringer et al. 1995; Filston et al. 1982b). The diagnosis may be suspected on the plain chest radiograph, which shows an air esophagogram. Bronchoscopic examination will reveal the recurrent fistula at the site of the original tracheoesophageal fistula. It is essential to pass a fine ureteric catheter across the fistula into the esophagus and to view the catheter in the esophagus at endoscopy (Holmes et al. 1987).

81.8.8.4 Gastroesophageal Reflux (GOR)

GOR is common in all infants following repair of esophageal atresia – significant reflux occurs in around 40% of cases, about half of whom will require surgical management. GOR is more common following anastomosis under tension and after delayed primary repair (Parker et al. 1979). Incompetence of the lower esophageal sphincter mechanism may be due to a primary neurogenic disturbance inherent in the development of the esophageal atresia or to technical factors involved in the repair or it may be due to shortening of the intra-abdominal esophagus and/or abolishment of the gastroesophageal angle of His (Bax and van Der Zee 2002; Rothenberg 2002; Nguyen et al. 2006).

Symptoms of GOR are similar to those of recurrent fistula with acute or chronic respiratory problems but also include recurrent vomiting and stricture formation. The diagnosis can be established on contrast swallow, pH monitoring, and endoscopy and biopsy of the distal esophagus. Anti-reflux medication including gastric acid suppression is only successful in about half the cases. Surgical treatment is problematic given the inherent dysmotility present in the distal esophagus. A fundoplication may in itself produce a functional obstruction at the gastroesophageal junction. The failure rate of fundoplication carried out in the first 3 months of life is excessively high. With regard to the nature of the wrap, there are advocates for partial (Thal) as well as for a short, floppy wrap (Toupet or Nissen type) (Brandigi et al. 2013; Bax and van Der Zee 2002).

81.8.8.5 Tracheomalacia

Tracheomalacia may be defined as a structural and function weakness of the trachea resulting in partial and occasionally complete respiratory obstruction. The structural abnormality comprises a deficiency in the cartilage in the tracheal rings and an increase in the length of the transverse muscle. The result is that the airway collapses during expiration causing expiratory stridor, which varies in severity from a hoarse barking cough to recurrent respiratory infection to acute life-threatening episodes of cyanosis or apnea. The incidence of tracheomalacia is around 10%, and about half will require surgical correction (Duranceau et al. 1977). The definitive treatment consists of aortopexy in which the ascending and arch of the aorta are elevated anteriorly toward the sternum. The result is usually dramatic with immediate resolution of the obstruction to the air passages.

81.8.8.6 Dysmotility

This affects the distal esophagus particularly in relation to abnormal coordination of contractions, which in fact can be seen on contrast studies of the esophagus. The dysmotility is a major factor in the long-term swallowing problems encountered in these children (Agrawal et al. 1999).

81.8.8.7 Respiratory Function

During infancy and for the first 3 years of life, patients with esophageal atresia suffer increased frequency of respiratory infections. The tendency to respiratory infections has variously been attributed to esophageal dysmotility and/or gastroesophageal reflux with recurrent aspiration or to a primary respiratory abnormality (Filston et al. 1982a; Stringer et al. 1995).

81.9 Esophageal Replacement

The need to replace the esophagus in esophageal atresia is extremely rare and should only be considered in very long-gap situations or where repeated attempts at retaining the host esophagus have failed and the infant's survival is at risk (Spitz et al. 2004; Bax and van der Zee 2007).

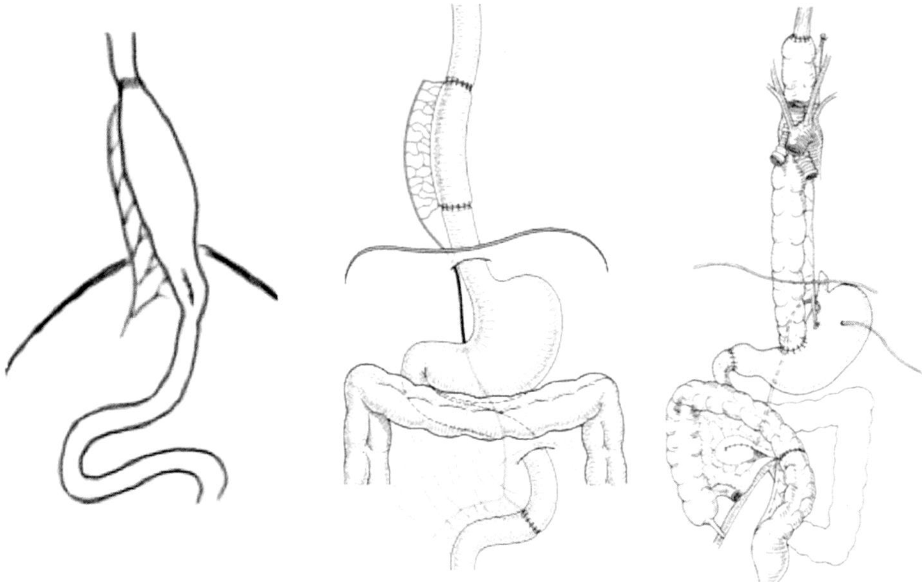

Fig. 11 Esophageal replacement. (**a**) Stomach, (**b**) jejunum, (**c**) colon

There are basically three methods of esophageal replacement currently being practiced in children – gastric transposition, colonic interposition, and jejunal interposition (Fig. 11).

References

Agrawal L, Beardsmore CS, MacFadyen UM (1999) Respiratory function in childhood following repair of oesophageal atresia and tracheoesophageal fistula. Arch Dis Child 81:404–408

Babu R, Pierro A, Spitz L et al (2000) The management of esophageal atresia in neonates with right-sided aortic arch. J Pediatr Surg 35:56–58

Bax KM, van Der Zee DC (2002) Feasibility of thoracoscopic repair of esophageal atresia with distal fistula. J Pediatr Surg 37:192–196

Bax NM, van der Zee DC (2007) Jejunal pedicle grafts for reconstruction of the esophagus in children. J Pediatr Surg 42:363–369

Bianchi A, Sowande O, Alizai NK, Rampersad B (1998) Aesthetics and lateral thoracotomy in the neonate. J Pediatr Surg 33:1798–1800

Brandigi E, Molinaro F et al (2013) Thoracoscopic repair of esophageal atresia with distal fistula in a new born: a technical case report. J Siena Acad Sci 5. Published Since 1761:85–88

Chittmittrapap S, Spitz L, Kiely EM, Brereton RJ (1980) Esophageal atresia and associated anomalies. Arch Dis Child 64:364–368

Cloud DT (1968) Anastomotic technique in esophageal atresia. J Pediatr Surg 3:561–564

Corbally MT, Spitz L, Kiely E et al (1993) Aortopexy for tracheomalacia in oesophageal anomalies. Eur J Pediatr Surg 3:264–266

Crisera CA, Connelly PR, Marmureanu AR et al (1999) Esophageal atresia with tracheoesophageal fistula: suggested mechanism in faulty organogenesis. J Pediatr Surg 34:204–208

Digilio MC, Marino B, Bagolan P et al (1999) Microdeletion 22q11 and esophageal atresia. J Med Genet 36:137–139

Driver CP, Shankar KR, Jones MO et al (2001) Phenotypic presentation and outcome of esophageal atresia in the era of the Spitz classification. J Pediatr Surg 36:1419–1421

Duranceau A, Fisher SR, Flye M (1977) Motor function of the esophagus after repair of esophageal atresia and tracheoesophageal fistula. Surgery 82:116–123

Filler RM, Messineo A, Vinograd L (1992) Severe tracheomalacia associated with esophageal atresia: results of surgical treatment. J Pediatr Surg 27: 1136–1140

Filston HC, Chitwood WR Jr, Schkolne B, Blackmon LR (1982a) The Fogarty balloon catheter as an aid to management of the infant with esophageal atresia and tracheoesophageal fistula complicated by severe RDS or pneumonia. J Pediatr Surg 17:149–151

Filston HC, Rankin JS, Kirks DR (1982b) The diagnosis of primary and recurrent tracheoesophageal fistulas: value of selective catheterization. J Pediatr Surg 17:144–148

Hagberg S, Rubenson A, Sillen U, Werkmaster K (1986) Management of long-gap esophagus: experience with end-to-end anastomosis under maximal tension. Prog Pediatr Surg 19:88–92

Holmes SJK, Kiely EM, Spitz L (1987) Tracheoesophageal fistula and the respiratory distress syndrome. Pediatr Surg Int 2:16–18

Kluth D (1976) Atlas of esophageal atresia. J Pediatr Surg 11:901–919

Krosnar S, Baxter A (2005) Thoracoscopic repair of esophageal atresia with tracheoesophageal fistula: anesthetic and intensive care management of a series of eight neonates. Paediatr Anaesth 15:541–546

Langer JC, Hussain H, Khan A et al (2001) prenatal diagnosis of esophageal atresia using sonography and magnetic resonance imaging. J Pediatr Surg 36:804–807

Litingtung Y, Lei L, Westphal H, Chiang C (1998) Sonic hedgehog is essential to foregut development. Nat Genet 20:58–61

Livitidis A (1973) Esophageal atresia: a method of overbrindging large segment gaps. Z Kinderchir 13:298–306

Lopez PJ, Keys C, Pierro A et al (2006) Oesophageal atresia: improved outcome in high-risk groups? J Pediatr Surg 41:331–334

Marsh AJ, Wellesley D, Burge D et al (2000) Interstitial deletion of chromosome 17 (del(17)(q22q23.3)) confirms a link with oesophageal atresia. J Med Genet 37:701–704

Mee RBB, Beasley SW, Auldist AW, Myers NA (1992) Influence of congenital heart disease on management of oesophageal atresia. Pediatr Surg Int 7:90–93

Merci J, Hasthorpe S, Farmer P, Hutson JM (1998) relationship between esophageal atresia with tracheoesophageal fistula and vertebral anomalies in mammalian embryos. J Pediatr Surg 33:58–63

Nguyen T, Zainabadi K, Bui T et al (2006) Thoracoscopic repair of esophageal atresia and tracheoesophageal fistula: lessons learned. J Laparoendosc Adv Surg Tech A 16:174–178

Parker AF, Christie DL, Cahill JL (1979) Incidence and significance of gastroesophageal reflux following repair of esophageal atresia and tracheoesophageal fistula and the need for anti-reflux procedures. J Pediatr Surg 14:5–8

Poenaru D, Laberge JM, Neilson JR, Guttman FM (1993) A new prognostic classification for esophageal atresia. Surgery 113:426–432

Puri P, Blake N, O'Donnell B, Guiney EJ (1981) Delayed primary anastomosis following spontaneous growth of esophageal segments in esophageal atresia. J Pediatr Surg 16:180–183

Quan L, Smith DW (1972) The VATER association: vertebral defects, anal atresia, tracheoesophageal fistula with esophageal atresia, radial dysplasia. Birth Defects 8:75–78

Roessler E, Belloni E, Gaudenz K et al (1996) Mutations in the human sonic hedgehog gene cause holoprosencephaly. Nat Genet 14:357–360

Rothenberg SS (2002) Thoracoscopic repair of tracheoesophageal fistula in newborns. J Pediatr Surg 37:869–872

Rothenberg SS (2005a) Thoracoscopic repair of esophageal atresia and tracheoesophageal fistula. Semin Pediatr Surg 14:2–7

Rothenberg SS (2005b) Esophageal atresia and tracheoesophageal fistula. In: Najmaldin A, Rothenberg S, Crabbe D, Beasley S (eds) Operative endoscopy and endoscopic surgery in infants and children. Hodder Arnold, London, pp 89–97

Shulman A, Mazkereth R, Zalel Y et al (2002) Prenatal identification of esophageal atresia: the role of ultrasonography for evaluation of functional anatomy. Prenat Diagn 22:669–674

Spitz L (1973) Congenital esophageal stenosis distal to associated esophageal atresia. J Pediatr Surg 8:973–974

Spitz L (1996) Esophageal atresia: past, present, and future. J Pediatr Surg 31:19–25

Spitz L, Kiely E, Brereton RJ, Drake D (1993) Management of esophageal atresia. World J Surg 17:296–300

Spitz L, Kiely EM, Morecrofl JA, Drake DP (1994) Oesophageal atresia: at-risk groups for the 1990s. J Pediatr Surg 29:723–725

Spitz L, Kiely E, Pierro A (2004) Gastric transposition in children a 21-year experience. J Pediatr Surg 39:276–281

Stringer MD, McKenna KM, Goldstein RB et al (1995) Prenatal diagnosis of esophageal atresia. J Pediatr Surg 30:1258–11263

Yeung CK, Spitz L, Brereton RJ (1992) Congenital esophageal stenosis due to tracheobronchial remnants: a rare but important association with esophageal atresia. J Pediatr Surg 27:852–855

Zhou B, Hutson JM, Farmer PJ et al (1999) Apoptosis in tracheoesophageal embryogenesis in rat embryos with or without adriamycin treatment. J Pediatr Surg 34:872–875

82 Gastrointestinal Malformations of Newborns

Marcello Dòmini

Contents

M. Dòmini (✉)
U.O. di Chirurgia pediatrica – Ospedale S.Orsola,
Università degli Studi – Alma Mater Studiorum,
di Bologna, Italy
e-mail: marcello.domini@unibo.it

G. Buonocore et al. (eds.), *Neonatology*,
https://doi.org/10.1007/978-3-319-29489-6_229

Abstract

The gastrointestinal tract may be subject to a variety of congenital abnormalities that arise during embryological development. The most important malformations can mainly be due to «underdevelopment» of the midgut (atresias or stenosis), to «overdevelopment» (intestinal duplications), to defects of the abdominal wall (Omphalocele and Gastroschisis), to anomalies of intestinal rotation and fixation, to persistence of embryonic structures (Meckel's diverticulum) or to abnormal formation of cellular components (e.g. nerves in Hirschsprung's disease). These disorders primarily result in symptoms of intestinal obstruction. Prenatal diagnosis is very important and to detect them the correct examination of the fetal gastrointestinal tract includes the visualization of the stomach, the small and large bowel, the abdominal wall and the insertion of the umbilical cord. The ability to diagnose these malformations prenatally is influenced by the site of obstruction, the presence of associated anomalies, and the gestational age at the time of imaging. In this chapter, we discuss and illustrate a wide spectrum of congenital anomalies affecting the gastrointestinal tract, their clinical symptoms, diagnosis and surgical therapies.

82.1 Salient Points

- Abdominal wall defects allow visceral organs to protrude outside the abdominal cavity; when possible, surgery is performed shortly after birth.
- Nonbilious projectile vomiting in a newborn should always raise the suspect of hypertrophic pyloric stenosis requiring investigation by ultrasound for the need for surgery and the prevention of alkalosis and dehydration.
- Bilious vomiting in a newborn should raise the suspect of duodenal atresia suggesting the need to perform abdomen X-ray and check for "double bubble sign."
- Intestinal obstruction usually involves the upper tract of the gut and is manifest by slow progressive abdominal distension. An abdominal X-ray should be done to check for an air-fluid interface.
- Meckel's diverticulum is a diverticulum of the terminal ileum often containing heterotrophic tissue, especially gastric, and potentially causing intestinal bleeding.

82.2 Defects of the Abdominal Wall

The stomach and intestines begin development outside the baby's abdomen and only later does the abdominal wall enclose them. Abdominal Wall defects are congenital defects that allow the stomach, the intestines, or other organs to protrude through an unusual opening that forms on the abdomen. They could have a wide spectrum of presentation that at one extreme can extend till to reach the thorax (Ectopia cordis) and in the other can manifest as an infraumbilical defect (exstrophy of the bladder). Anyway most of times these defects are limited to the umbilical region, and their two most frequent manifestations are the Omphalocele and the Gastroschisis. While infants with gastroschisis rarely have defects other than those affecting the intestines, a very large rate of children with omphalocele, have associated congenital anomalies or chromosomal abnormalities.

82.2.1 Omphalocele

It is a central defect of the abdominal wall in the umbilical region, through which can herniate hollow and parenchymatous viscera. The defect is covered with a sac that outside is formed by the amniotic membrane and inside from the peritoneal membrane. The umbilical cord always extends from the top of the sac.

The size of the defect can vary from 4 to 8–10 cm. When the defect is wide, the liver is almost always herniated together with small and large intestine and sometimes stomach, bladder, and internal genitalia (uterus ovaries and adnexa in females; intra-abdominal testes in males). The more the defect is large, the more the abdominal cavity is small and poorly developed, and the herniated viscera usually have lost their natural right to reside there.

The overall incidence is nearby 1/5,000 live births with a slight male preponderance.

82.2.1.1 Embryology

During the embryologic development of the abdominal cavity, at about 5 weeks of gestation, the gut develop within the umbilical coelom, outside the abdominal wall, and return to the peritoneal cavity nearby at 10 weeks of gestation before starting the rotation and fixation process. A failure in this course of action will bring to a defect of the abdominal wall (Klein 2006). Since the gut is physiologically outside the peritoneal cavity till the 10th week of gestational age, the prenatal diagnosis of omphalocele is not feasible until the 12th week.

82.2.1.2 Associated Anomalies

Associated anomalies are present in almost 50 % of patients with omphalocele. Most of them are cardiac anomalies (Tetralogy of Fallot, ventricular and atrial defects, ectopia cordis, and coarctation of the aorta). Chromosomal anomalies such as Down syndrome are more frequent in patients without herniation of the liver and have been reported in 15–20% of cases. The most frequent is the Beckwith-Wiedemann (BW) syndrome (7 %) that manifests as macroglossia, gigantism, visceromegaly, and hypoglycemia and often it brings to tumor development, such as Wilms tumor, hepatoblastoma, rhabdomyosarcoma, neuroblastoma. Rarely the BW can be familiar.

It is always present an intestinal malrotation due to the incomplete phase of intestinal rotation and fixation, and it could raise the incidence of an intestinal volvulus.

82.2.1.3 Diagnosis

Prenatal diagnosis is feasible following the 12th week of gestation, when the bowel return to the peritoneal cavity. The ultrasound visualization of viscera outside the abdomen covered with an amniotic sac and the umbilical cord ending at the top of the sac permits the differential diagnosis with Gastroschisis. When the surgeon informs the parents about the malformation of the incoming baby (so-called counseling) to give them every notion in order to decide whether keep the baby or interrupt the pregnancy, he must refer to two forms of omphalocele: the "intracorporeal" liver and the "extracorporeal" liver. In the second one, the defect is obviously larger and most of times it is recommended a caesarian section delivery, even if the more recent obstetric literature finds no benefit of caesarean section (How et al. 2000).

82.2.1.4 Therapy

Usually when a prenatal diagnosis is present, the delivery is programmed in a third level Centre. After birth the baby's abdominal wall is covered with tepid and wet gauzes and wrapped in a plastic bag to avoid dehydration. A nasogastric tube (it could also reveal an esophageal atresia) to deflate the stomach and a rectal probe to facilitate the meconium emission are inserted. Then it is possible to complete the preoperative clinical cardiopulmonary assessment.

82.2.1.5 Surgical Treatment

First of all is mandatory to insert a central venous line.

The aim of the operation is to put into the abdominal cavity the herniated viscera and to

close the defect, possibly in one single time (primary closure).

For small omphaloceles, the primary closure is almost ever feasible. The sac is excised and the bowel reinserted in abdomen. Most of times in order to close the defect without increasing the intra-abdominal pressure that could prejudice the cardiopulmonary system by reducing the venous return it is required to perform the so-called stretching of the abdominal muscular wall to augment the compliance (Weber 1995).

In case of very large omphaloceles in which the first attempt of primary closure would fail, a staged reduction of the intestinal content with silastic prosthesis according to the Schuster's technique will be performed (Schuster 1986). The viscera inside the silo will be gradually reduced in the following days till to reach the complete closure of the abdominal wall in a couple of week (Figs. 1–2).

Sometimes the closure of the abdominal wall can be a surgical challenge. Infants with giant omphalocele have such a large underdevelopment of the abdominal cavity that can preclude reduction of the abdominal contents and primary repair in many of these cases. It can happens that neither silo nor skin flap could be able to successfully treat those patients. The VAC device (KCI, San Antonio, Tex) is a new alternative approach that consists of a sponge applied directly to the bowel and liver, covered with impermeable transparent dressing, and attached to a low negative pressure system that gradually reduces the viscera into the abdominal cavity. The sponge is changed every 3–5 days under local sedation. The obliteration of dead space and continuous evacuation of exudate promote development of a healthy granulation bed and prevent bacterial colonization (Kilbride et al. 2006).

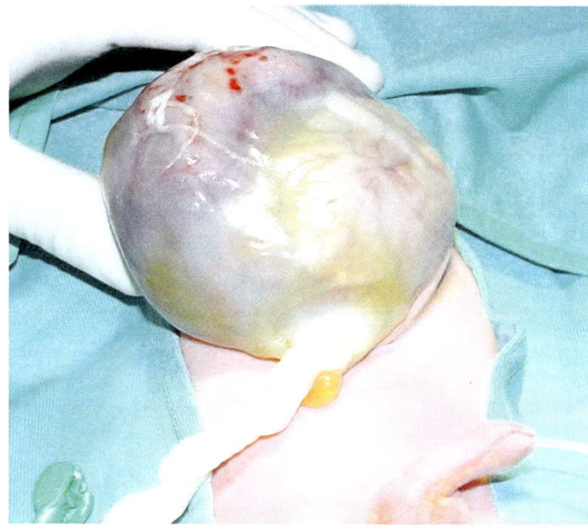

Fig. 1 Giant omphalocele. The translucent sac permits to see the liver and the intestinal loops inside. Please note the cord insertion

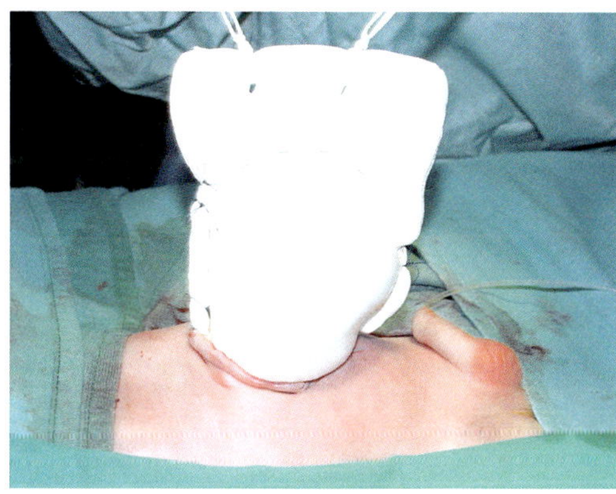

Fig. 2 Giant omphalocele. A silastic prosthesis has been sutured to the abdominal wall according to the Schuster's technique. It will be progressively reduced in the following days

82.2.1.6 Prognosis

Most of all it depends on the associated conditions, in particular the cardiac malformations, then on the abdominal complications due to the intervention and to the use of the prosthesis (infections, intestinal adhesions, occlusive conditions…).

Survival rate is nearby 75–80%.

82.2.2 Gastroschisis

It is a small defect of the abdominal wall (2 max 4 cm of size) at the right of the abdominal insertion of the umbilical cord, through which herniate intestinal loops not covered by any sac or membrane. The liver is always inside the abdomen. Often the bowel is thickened and

edematous because of the chemical action of the amniotic fluid and of eventual kinking of the mesenteric vessels ("antenatal" form). Other times it is almost normal without any sign of inflammation ("perinatal" form).

The overall incidence is nearby 1/10,000 live births with a slight male preponderance. The incidence is higher in North Europe (Klein 2006).

82.2.2.1 Embryology

It seems to be the consequence of the in utero regression of the right umbilical vein that determines the development of a locus of minoris resistentiae through which the bowel can protrude before its complete fixation.

82.2.2.2 Associated Anomalies

Since it is a tardy development, the incidence of associated anomalies is very low. Intestinal malrotation is almost always present. In 10–15% of cases, intestinal atresia or stenosis are present, probably due to an ischemic injury of the bowel. Cardiac anomalies are present in 1 % of cases.

Chromosomal anomalies are very rare.

These are very often small for date babies due to the excessive protein loss in the amniotic fluid.

82.2.2.3 Diagnosis

Prenatal diagnosis is feasible following the 12th week of gestation, with the ultrasound visualization of intestinal loops outside the abdomen, not covered with an amniotic sac, with an umbilical cord normally inserted. Polyhydramnios is quite often present.

82.2.2.4 Way of Delivery

Mode of delivery for gastroschisis is a major controversy in obstetric management. Proponents of cesarean delivery have suggested that it may improve outcomes by decreasing risk for bowel contamination and injury. On the contrary, earlier reports demonstrated no benefit for cesarean delivery. In a recent paper considering 5,985 pregnancies with gastroschisis in the USA, 63.5% attempted vaginal delivery and 36.5% underwent a planned cesarean delivery. The rate of attempted vaginal delivery increased from 59.7% in 2005 to 68.8% in 2013. The paper concludes that given the increased maternal morbidity with cesarean delivery, and lack of neonatal benefit, planned cesarean delivery specifically for gastroschisis is not recommended (Friedman et al. 2016).

In Italy, almost all cases of gastroschisis are planned for caesarian section.

82.2.2.5 Therapy

The herniated bowel is covered with tepid and wet sterile gauzes and wrapped in a plastic bag to avoid dehydration. A nasogastric tube to detend the stomach and a rectal probe to facilitate the meconium emission are inserted. Then it is possible to complete the preoperative clinical cardiopulmonary assessment.

82.2.2.6 Surgical Treatment

The first attempt of closure must be done with the Bianchi's "minimal invasive management" (Bianchi and Dickson 1998). It does not require a traditional surgical operation but only the patient, slow manual reduction of the herniated intestinal loops through the original hole. This maneuver is done with the baby asleep in his crib without general anesthesia and can be completed in 3–4 h, leaving the bowel able to adapt in the peritoneal cavity (Figs. 3–4). This approach avoids the injuries of surgical operations and has high chances to be resolutive. Anyway the bowel movements could be absent for a long time after the reduction; therefore, a parenteral nutrition must be started.

Unfortunately sometimes the reduction with this technique is impossible due to the severe thickening of the bowel and it is mandatory to perform the traditional surgical operation enlarging cranially and caudally the defect for few cm and reducing the gut in abdomen, even with the "stretching" maneuver (Schwartz 1995).

When primary abdominal wall closure is not convenient, then it will get by the staged Schuster's technique (Schuster 1986). Recently has been proposed a new device to cover unreduced viscera of a

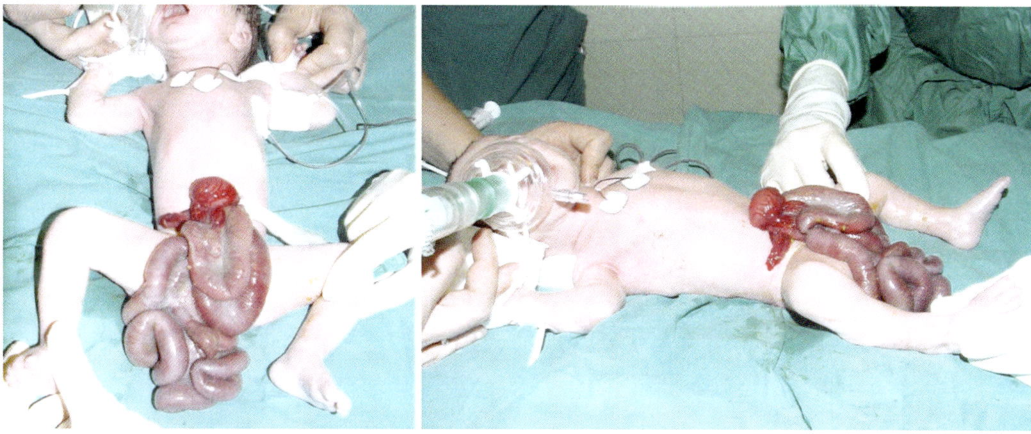

Fig. 3 Gastroschisis. The defect of the abdominal wall is on the right of the umbilical cord insertion

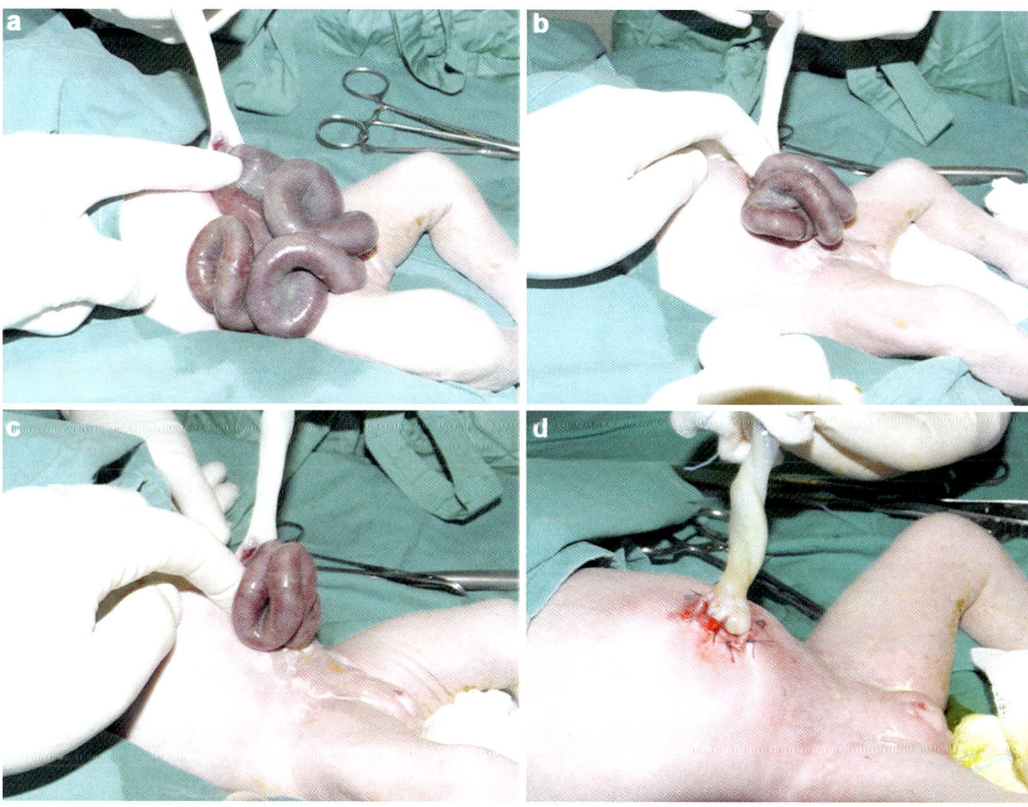

Fig. 4 (**a**–**d**) Gastroschisis: Bianchi's "minimal invasive management"

gastroschisis for staged gastroschisis closures. The Alexis wound retractor (AWR) device consists of two rings: an elastic white one that must be placed into the patient's abdomen and a rigid green one, external that is gently lifted, avoiding any leakage of peritoneal fluid out of the abdominal cavity. A plastic cylinder covers the eviscerated bowel like a silo and its upper limit is closed with a simple tie.

The cylinder is reduced with repeated tying until complete bowel reduction was obtained. AWR seems permit continuous stretching of the abdominal wall, enhancing the equalizing of the viscero-abdominal disproportion observed in gastroschisis (Ferreira et al. 2014).

82.2.2.7 Prognosis

Survival rate is high, nearby 85–90%. Mortality is principally due to the low birth weight and to the associated intestinal conditions (atresia, stenosis, bowel perforation. . .).

82.3 Pylorus

82.3.1 Pyloric Atresia, Aplasia, Web

These malformations are very rare (1/100,000 births) without sex prevalence. Less than 200 cases are described in literature. Often, they are babies with more than one malformation (i.e., esophageal atresia, multiple other gastrointestinal tract atresias, cardiac malformations) (Klein 2006). Carmi syndrome is a condition with coexistence of epidermolysis bullosa and pyloric atresia (PA–EB) that occurs that varies from approximately 18 % to 40 % of the cases of pyloric atresia (Al-Salem et al. 2014; Short et al. 2014).

The diagnosis can be obtained by prenatal echography since 3rd–4th month of gestational age observing a single gastric bubble and polyhydramnios. If a prenatal diagnosis is missing, the neonate presents a gastric vomiting (not bilious) and epigastric distension. If an incomplete pyloric web is present, the obstructive symptomatology raise later and it can be confused with the hypertrophic pyloric stenosis symptoms (Scherer 2006). In this case, the diagnosis will be achieved with ultrasound and contrast medium radiography of the stomach. Except for those cases of membranous pyloric web that could be treated by endoscopic resection only, the surgical resection of the obstruction is mandatory. In the last decade, the trans-umbilical skin incision with or without laparoscopic assistance has become the surgical approach of choice for many procedures in neonates and therefore also for the pyloric pathologies.

82.3.2 Hypertrophic Pyloric Stenosis (HPS)

82.3.2.1 Incidence

It is the most frequent cause of gastrointestinal obstruction in pediatric age. In our Country, the incidence is nearby 0.2% and male:female rate is 5:1.

82.3.2.2 Pathogenesis

Up to now, despite considerable investigations no sure causative factors have been identified. Both genetic (variability among races, male preponderance and positive family history with first-born infant prevalence) and environmental (breast-feeding babies, seasonal variability with spring/autumn prevalence) factors seem to play a role in the etiology. From the histological point of view, there is a marked muscle hypertrophy of the circular layer with complete reduction of the pyloric lumen. The pylorus appears as an enlarged and elongated pale firm mass (pyloric "olive") measuring 2–2.5 cm in length and 1–1.5 cm in diameter.

82.3.2.3 Symptoms

The onset of symptoms is at 2–8 weeks of age and consists in nonbilious projectile vomiting (sometimes with blood), progressively ingravescent, that provokes a hypochloremic hypokaliemic alkalosis (Schwartz 2006). A delay in the diagnosis leads to severe dehydration.

82.3.2.4 Diagnosis

In the past, the diagnosis was made by the clinical picture and the palpation of the pyloric "olive" in the right side of the abdomen. Nowadays, ultrasound procedure permits most of times to achieve a sure diagnosis (pyloric muscle thickness more than 3.5 mm; pyloric channel length more than 16 mm) (Schwartz 2006). In doubt cases, an upper gastric contrast examination is definitively diagnostic.

In daily practice, laboratory tests are needed to check the alkalosis and to exclude peripheral eosinophilia. In effect, symptoms of eosinophilic gastroenteritis (EGE) nonbilous, projectile vomiting, can be easily confused with HPS. Further laboratory tests, imaging, and biopsy can be needed to diagnose EGE (Choi et al. 2014).

82.3.2.5 Therapy

Preoperative preparation includes positioning of a naso-gastric tube and intravenous line for fluid resuscitation (whose length depends on the severity of the dehydration and electrolyte alterations). Oral feeding is obviously discontinued.

Surgical treatment of choice is the Fredet-Ramstedt pyloromyotomy. Traditionally it is obtained through a small right upper quadrant transverse incision, but in recent years more and more surgeons prefer the supraumbilical skin incision (Bianchi's technique) with the upper division of the midline fascia (Fig. 5) (Tan and Bianchi 1986).

Once the pyloric mass is exteriorized from the peritoneal cavity and hold by the surgeon's finger at the duodenal side, a longitudinal sero-muscular incision of the pylorus is made. The muscle is split and divaricated till the mucosa is bulging out through the incision.

Feeding starts 6 h after with initial glucose solution and afterwards with increasing volumes of milk till to reach the full regimen after 15–20 h. Discharge is in 3rd postoperative day.

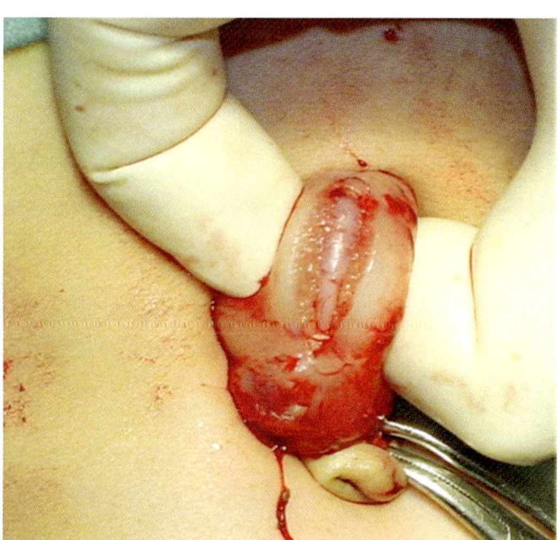

Fig. 5 Transumbilical pyloromyotomy. The muscle has been divided and split and it is possible to observe the bulging of the mucosa

In some centre, this procedure is performed by laparoscopic way (MacKinlay and Barnhart 2008), but even if we are laparoscopic surgeons in our opinion there are no real benefits on doing it. Three ports of access are needed (one transumbilical of 5 mm and two of 3 mm in left and right upper quadrants) versus the single supraumbilical incision of the Bianchi's approach and the time needed to reach the full feeding and the postoperative discharge is more or less similar, whereas the laparoscopic procedure has a greater complication rate (mucosal perforation or incomplete myotomy). Nevertheless, in the largest series of pyloromyotomy ever reported, although laparoscopy is associated with a statistically significant increase in the risk of incomplete pyloromyotomy, both open and laparoscopic pyloromiotomy are associated with low rates of mucosal perforation and incomplete pyloromyotomy in specialist centers (Hall et al. 2014).

82.3.2.6 Prognosis

Prognosis is excellent. Recurrences are exceptional.

82.4 Duodenal Obstructions

Duodenal obstruction can be "intrinsic" or "extrinsic."

The intrinsic obstructions are more frequent and consist of, with decreasing incidence:

- duodenal atresia
- duodenal web
- endoluminal diverticulum

The extrinsic forms are quite rare and include, always with decreasing incidence:

- annular pancreas
- congenital Ladd's bands (in intestinal malrotation)
- duodenal duplication
- preduodenal port vein

The clinical feature is overlapping either in intrinsic or in extrinsic forms.

82.4.1 Classification

1. Duodenal Atresia

   We can recognize three different types (Applebaum et al. 2006):

   1st type: Complete duodenal web, with mucosal and submucosal layer.

   2nd type: The two blind pouches are joined by a thin and short fibrous cord with an intact mesentery.

   3rd type: The two duodenal pouches are separated and there is a mesenteric "V-shaped" defect.
2. Partial intrinsic obstruction
   (A) *Incomplete mucous web*: It is a diaphragm with a central hole that can be primary (created together with the web) or secondary (consequent to a perforation of the web due to the increased pressure).
   (B) *Endoluminal Diverticulum*: It is a membranous fold that extends inside the lumen as a "windsock." It can be only partially obstructive and becoming progressively obstructive as time goes by either for the duodenal lumen or the biliary tree. If it goes beyond the Vater Papilla, it can provoke biliary stagnation and litiasic concretions.
3. Partial extrinsic obstruction
   (A) *Annular Pancreas*: Partially or totally obstructive. It is an embryologic consequence of the persistence of the primitive ventral pancreas that normally should rotate around the duodenum to form the head of the pancreas (Fig. 6) (Kimura et al. 1990).
   (B) *Ladd's Bands*: They are found in patients with intestinal malrotation in which the cecum is in epigastric region. These bands connect the cecum and the right abdominal wall compressing the descending part of duodenum
   (C) *Preduodenal Port Vein*: It is really exceptional and it is due to the anomalous persistence of the anterior residual of vitelline veins.

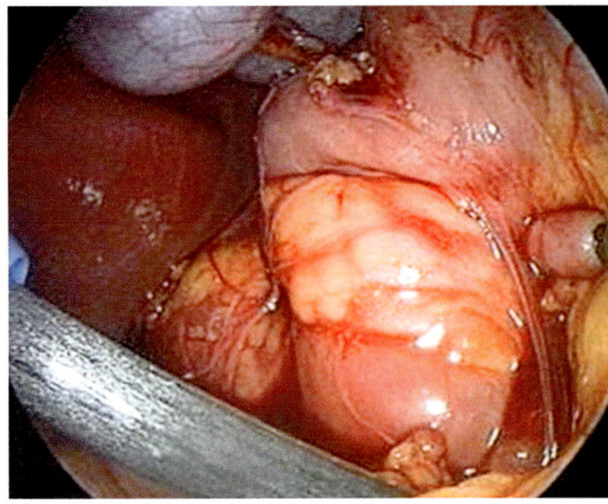

Fig. 6 Laparoscopic view of an annular pancreas

82.4.2 Duodenal Atresia

In 90 % of cases, it is located in the first or second duodenal portion near the Vater papilla, usually (75–85%) beyond the outflow of Oddi's sphincter.

82.4.2.1 Incidence

In different countries, it varies from 1 every 3,000 or 1 every 5,000 births.

82.4.2.2 Embryogenesis

It is thought to depend on a defect in the vacuolization process of the primitive gut between the eighth and the tenth week of gestational age.

82.4.2.3 Associated Anomalies

It is frequently associated to other congenital anomalies: The most frequent are the skeletal (ribs, vertebrae, sacrum, radius...) (36 %) and the intestinal (26 %) (esophageal atresia, ano-rectal malformations, Hirschsprung disease, malrotations...). In 20 % of cases, a cardiopathy can be discovered. Urinary anomalies are present in 8 % of cases.

Down syndrome is particularly frequent in subjects with duodenal atresia (30 %). When the gynecologist observes a duodenal atresia in prenatal ultrasound, he would strongly suggest to perform a fetal karyotyping.

82.4.2.4 Prenatal Diagnosis

It is possible to get a prenatal diagnosis since the 20th week of g.a. The echographic observation of polyhydramnios together with the "double bubble" sign is diagnostic (except in the extremely rare case of a coexisting I type oesophageal atresia).

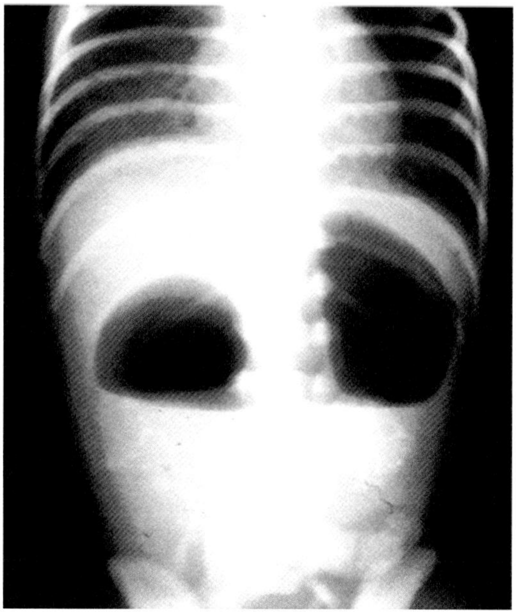

Fig. 7 Radiographic appearance of the "double bubble" sign. No air below the duodenum

82.4.2.5 Symptoms and Diagnosis

In case of lack of a prenatal diagnosis, the main symptom is vomiting that in 80 % of cases is biliary (due to the subvaterian atresia).

The direct radiography of the abdomen shows the diagnostic "double bubble" sign. If a doubt persists, a contrast medium can be given to the child to reveal the atresia or a partial duodenal obstruction (Fig. 7).

82.4.2.6 Therapy

It is not a surgical emergency. The operation can be performed after 24–72 h so that the patient can be prepared to the operation studying the cardiac functioning and performing all the preoperative assessments.

A naso gastric tube is inserted and total parenteral nutrition (TPN) substitutes the oral feeding.

In this way, in case of very low birth weight patients the surgical correction can be delayed also for many days or weeks.

The operation differs in case of web or atresia.

- If a web is present, a duodenotomy is done and the duodenal web is excised (paying attention to the Vater papilla).
- If the web is incomplete, a Fogarty catheter can be inserted in the hole and after inflating the balloon, pulled gently up in order to expose the web. In this way, the excision of the web will result easier (Fig. 8a, b)
- In case of atresia, a duodeno-duodenotomy is performed. The anastomosis is done according to the Kimura technique: a "diamond-shaped" suture with horizontal incision on the upper pouch and sagittal incision on the lower pouch (Fig. 9a, b) (Kimura et al. 1990). If the upper duodenum is particularly dilated, a "tapering" can be performed.

No gastrostomy is required.

The oral feeding can start when the biliary stagnation stops and bowel movements are noted. It can happens also after 10 days or more.

The same operation is performed also in case of Annular pancreas (paying attention to the choledocal and pancreatic ducts).

In the last few years, the surgical correction of a duodenal atresia or stenosis has been performed also by laparoscopic approach with good results (Van der Zee and Bax 2008; Parmentier et al. 2015). Since this is a very difficult operation, also due to the small space of work given by the newborn abdominal cavity, a video-assisted approach permits to identify the two duodenal pouches exteriorizing them through the umbilical incision and completing the operation by traditional surgery.

82.4.2.7 Prognosis

It is good quoad vitam and function. Nevertheless there is a 5 % of mortality due to the associated malformations (overall the cardiac ones). Obviously it is mandatory that the newborn must be operated in a Centre of III level, with a neonatal ICU.

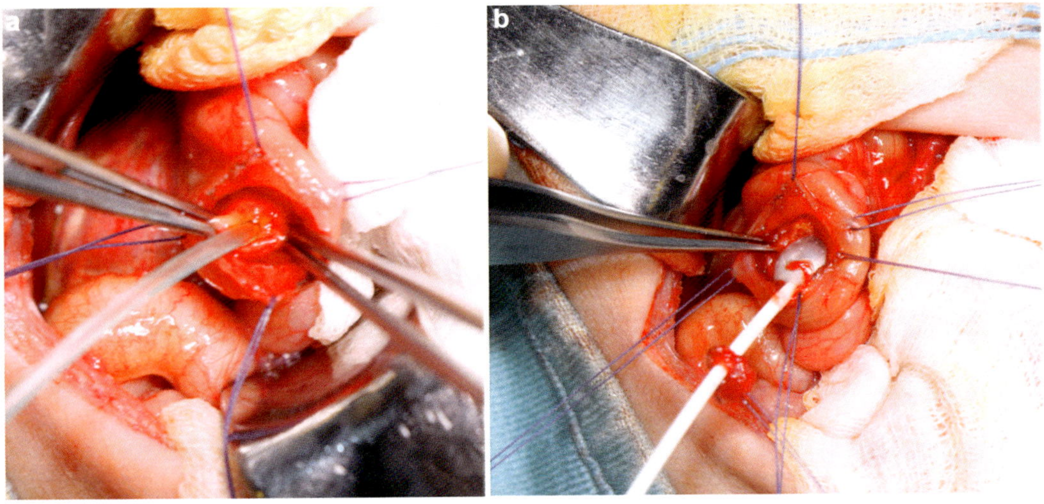

Fig. 8 (**a**) Uncomplete duodenal web with Fogarty catheter inside. (**b**) Excision of the web showing the inflated balloon in the distal side of duodenum

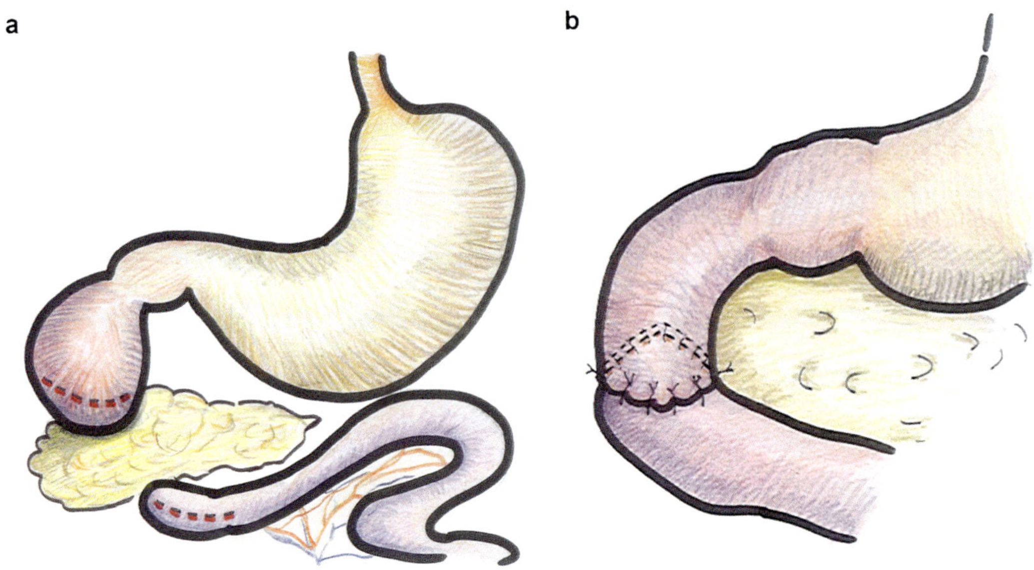

Fig. 9 (**a**, **b**) The "diamond-shaped" Kimura's anastomosis

82.5 Intestinal Obstructions

The intestinal congenital obstructions are constituted by atresias and functional disorders of the gut:

- jejunal atresia
- ileal atresia
- colic atresia
- meconium ileus

The morbidity and mortality of neonatal intestinal obstruction has improved over last few years mainly due to antenatal detection, early intervention, and meticulous resuscitation before surgery along with good NICU care.

82.5.1 Jejunal and Ileal Atresia

They represent 95 % of congenital intestinal intrinsic obstructions. The remaining 5 % is due to the intestinal stenosis.

The most represented sites are:

- Proximal jejunum (31 %)
- Distal Jejunum (20 %)
- Proximal Ileum (13 %)
- Distal Ileum (36 %)

82.5.1.1 Classification

We can distinguish five different types (Grosfeld 2006):

- *Type I*: There is not an apparent external interruption in the bowel at the level of the atresic loop; nevertheless there is a dilatation above the endoluminal mucous web.
- *Type II*: The atresic bowel is joined to the subsequent segment by a by a thin fibrous cord, with intact mesentery.
- *Type IIIa*: The atresic segments are completely separated with a "V"-shaped defect of the mesenterium.
- *Type IIIb*: There is an "apple peel" (sometimes defined also as "Christmas Tree") defect of the mesenterium (Fig. 10).
- *Type IV*: Multiple atresias.

The most frequent is the type IIIa. The most severe types are IIIb and IV.

82.5.1.2 Incidence

In literature, it varies from 1 every 1,500 or 1 every 2,000 births and therefore is more frequent than the duodenal atresia, even if in our casuistry (more than 30 years) the proportion between intestinal atresia and duodenal atresia is 2:3.

Usually these babies are low weight at birth.

82.5.1.3 Embryogenesis

Differently from other digestive atresias (oesophageal, duodenal, rectal) that derive from precocious genesis (in fact they are embryopathies), the jejunal and ileal atresias have a late genesis (they are fetopathies). For this reason, they are rarely associated to other anomalies and usually they cannot be discovered before fifth month of gestational age.

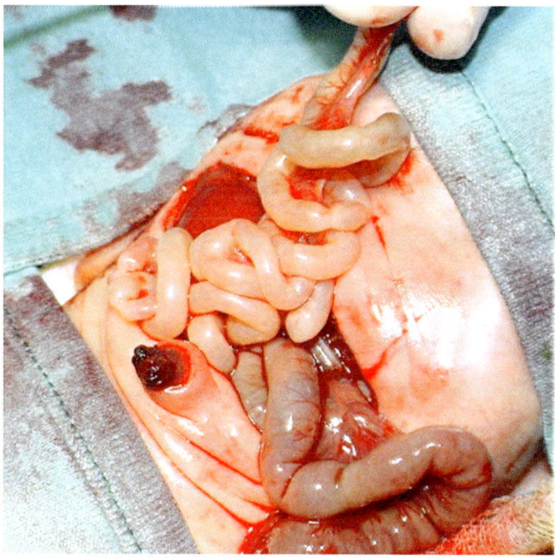

Fig. 10 "Apple peel" ileal atresia

There are two major theories that try to explain the genesis of this malformation:

- *Louw-Barnard theory (1955)*: They thought that atresias are consequent to an ischemic damage of the bowel that could be due to different causes (volvulus, internal hernia, vascular catastrophy…); it brings to the necrosis of the intestinal segment with consequent reabsorption and creation of the atresic pouch, resulting in atresia of different types. This theory seems to be more reliable than the following theory.
- *Tandler theory (1902)*: He retained that an error during the phase of recanalization that follows the solid phase of the intestinal development was responsible of the atresic condition. It seems to be a plausible theory to explain the embryogenesis of the intestinal webs.

82.5.1.4 Associated Anomalies

Intestinal atresias are usually isolated anomalies. Sometimes they can be found associated to other malformative conditions (Gastroschisis, Omphalocele, Meconium peritonitis…), but it is probably secondary to ischemic damages of the bowel consequent to these conditions.

There is a familial pattern of multiple atresias affecting the stomach, duodenum, small bowel,

and colon occurring in individuals of French-Canadian background that probably represents a rare autosomal recessive gene inheritance.

82.5.1.5 Prenatal Diagnosis

It is possible to get a prenatal diagnosis since the 20th week of gestational age. Often a polyhydramnios is found. Usually it is larger when the atresia is higher in the intestinal tube. Sonographic prenatal features of small intestinal obstruction are not unique. The prenatal ultrasound will show also multiple "bubbles" that are the expression of the intestinal loops full of amniotic fluid and secretions. In any case, antenatal dilatation of intestinal loop (more than 15 mm in length and 7 mm in diameter) suggests fetal bowel obstruction.

The observation of these findings is not pathognomonic of intestinal atresia since they can be found also in a lot of different conditions, such as Meconium Ileus, Total colonic atresia, Hirschsprung's disease, Small left colon syndrome, meconium Plug syndrome, and other more.

In a recent paper, they speculate that echogenicity of bowel content increases proportionally to the level of bowel atresia. Preliminary results indicate that the most distal the atresia is, the greater is the echogenicity of intestinal content.

High echogenicity of intestinal dilated bowel fluid content could be a new factor to consider in the study of fetal intestinal atresia. It could become a specific marker to differentiate upper intestinal obstructions from colonic atresia (Goruppi et al. 2016).

These studies are surely interesting but, from the surgical point of view, they do not change the management of these babies: Intestinal atresias must be operated independently from the level of obstruction.

82.5.1.6 Symptoms and Diagnosis

If a prenatal diagnosis has not been made, the newborn slowly will manifest an abdominal distension and later on biliary vomit.

The direct abdominal x-ray will show multiple air-fluid levels and no further gas beyond that point (Fig. 11). The more distal the atresia, the more apparent the clinical abdominal distension and the greater the number of distended intestinal loops and air-fluid levels observed. But this finding is not sufficient for the correct diagnosis. The abdominal radiography must be accurately observed to look for some calcification that is pathognomonic of meconium peritonitis.

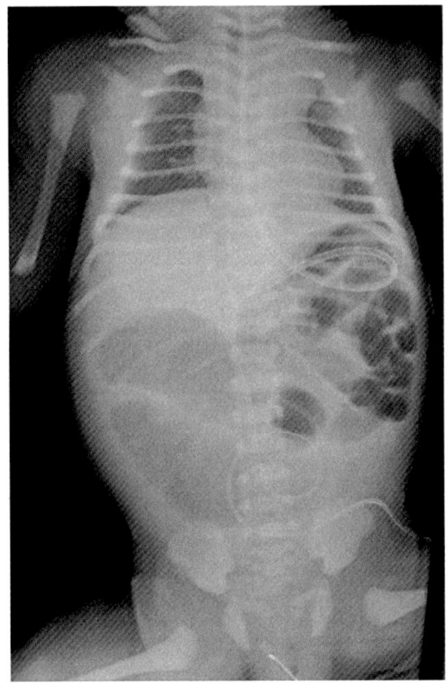

Fig. 11 Abdominal X-ray showing the ileal distension and no gas in the large bowel

A contrast enema with gastrographin let to recognize a colic atresia, will raise the suspect of Hirschsprung's disease, and could be resolutive in case of Meconium ileus or meconium plug syndrome (Fig. 12).

A care clinical evaluation of these newborns may avoid unnecessary surgery because at least 50 % of patients with uncomplicated meconium ileus may respond to nonoperative therapy.

Meconium ileus and 10 % of ileal atresias could be consequent to cystic fibrosis; therefore, these infants should undergo sweat chloride determination before hospital discharge.

82.5.1.7 Therapy

It is not a surgical emergency and the operation can be delayed till the 2nd or 3rd day of life, after positioning a naso-gastric tube and total parenteral nutrition.

The standard technique is performed through a transverse supraumbilical laparotomy, but nowadays the best technique is the video-assisted

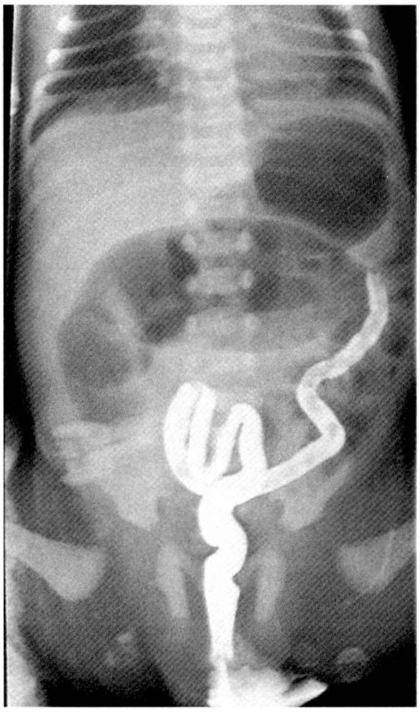

Fig. 12 Contrast enema showing the microcolon and the "soap bubbles" image typical of meconium ileus

approach in which a laparoscopy with trans-umbilical approach let to grasp and exteriorize the atresic loop through the umbilical incision (that can be enlarged laterally for 1–2 cm).

- In types I, II, and IIIa, a primary end-to-end anastomosis is performed. In case of large disproportion between the proximal and the distal ends of the atresic bowel, a tapering of the dilated proximal loop can be performed in order to consent the primary anastomosis (Fig. 13a–c)
- In type IIIb, usually a primary anastomosis is performed. Sometimes one can make a temporary ileostomy, delaying the anastomosis after some month.
- In type IV more primary anastomoses are needed (Fig. 14a, b)

Total parenteral nutrition continues till bowel movements are noted and the gastric stagnation reduces.

82.5.1.8 Prognosis

It is good quoad vitam and function. Healing is waited in 90–95% of babies if other malformations are absent. Type IIIb has a lower rate of recovery due to the worst blood supply of the gut.

Furthermore, in case of type IIIb or IV in which it is necessary to remove a large part of bowel, a fearful consequence can be the "short bowel syndrome." Anyway there are some techniques that try to elongate the residual bowel in order to augment the absorptive surface of bowel (particularly, the Bianchi's technique), and a good survival rate is get with babies with 25–30 cm of functioning small intestine when the ileo-ciecal valve is preserved (Bianchi 1999).

82.5.2 Colic Atresia

It is extremely rare. In more than 50 % of cases is above the splenic flexure. When it is beyond it is at the sigmoid level and can be confused with the rectal atresia.

82.5.2.1 Incidence

It varies from 1 every 10,000 to 1/20,000 births (Oldham and Arca 2006). In our casuistry, we observed only 8 cases in 32 years. Only the pyloric atresia is rarer than the colic one.

82.5.2.2 Classification

It is similar to the classification used for the small bowel atresias:

- *Type I*: Endoluminal mucous web (complete or partial).
- *Type II*: A thin fibrous cord, with intact mesenterium joining the two segments.
- *Type III*: The atresic segments are completely separated with a "V"-shaped defect of the mesenterium

82.5.2.3 Embryogenesis

There are the same two theories employed in the small bowel atresias.

82.5.2.4 Associated Anomalies

Skeletal malformations (syndactylism, polydactylism, radial agenesis) are quite frequent, such as the cardiac and ocular anomalies.

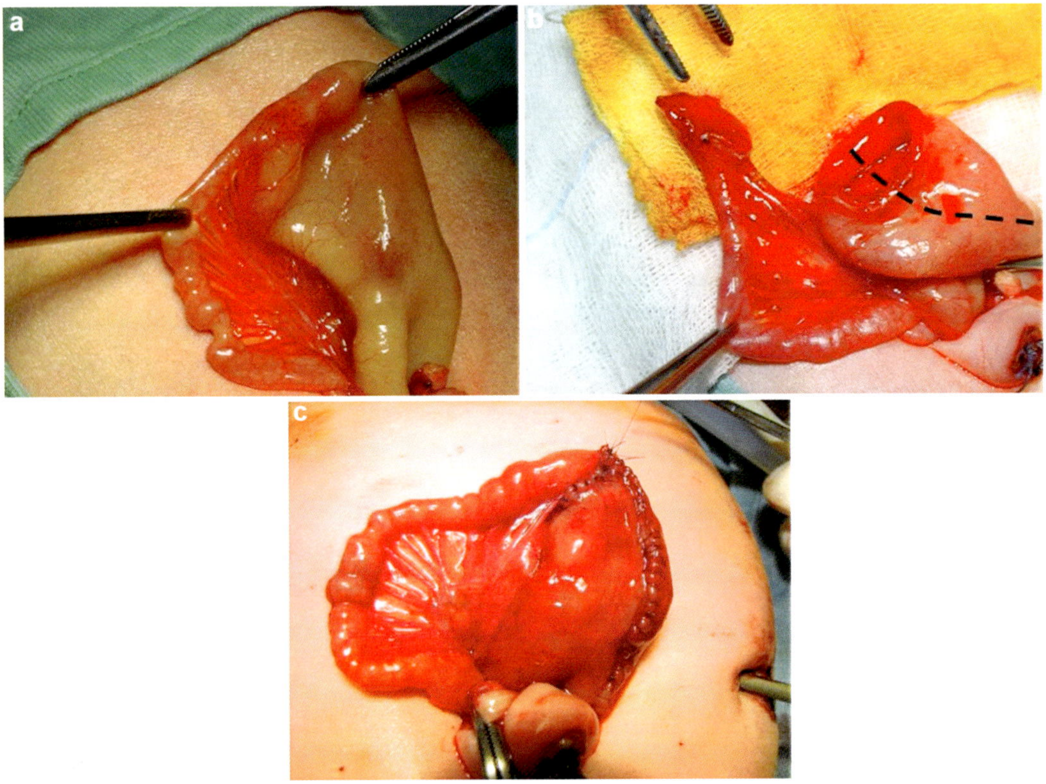

Fig. 13 (**a**) Disproportion between proximal and distal ends. (**b**) Section of the bowel. The intermittent *line* indicates the limit of the tapering of the proximal end. The distal loop has been spatulated to enlarge the diameter for the anastomosis. (**c**) The proximal bowel has been reduced and the anastomosis completed

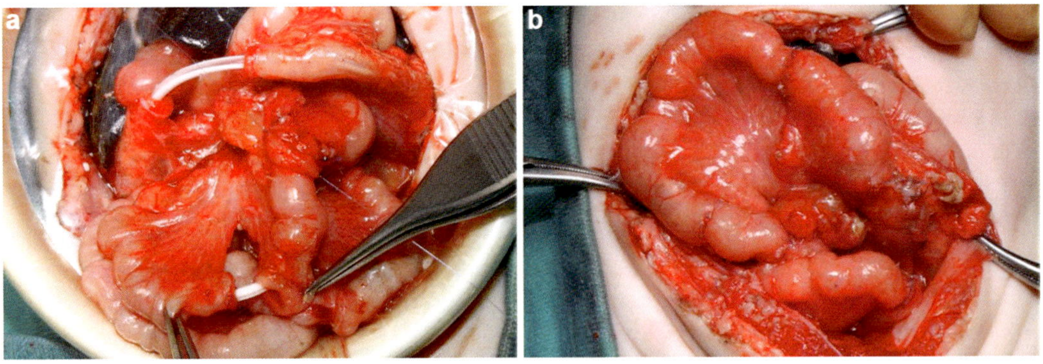

Fig. 14 (**a**) Multiple atresias. A naso-jejunal tube has been inserted through the bowel to check the patency of the bowel after the excision of the atretic segments. (**b**) Multiple atresias. Multiple anastomosis

Sometimes it is observed in patients with Omphalocele or Gastroschisis, and it is probably a consequence of an ischemic damage due to the pathology itself.

82.5.2.5 Prenatal Diagnosis

It is very difficult to recognize with prenatal ultrasound. There are no reports about the effectiveness of prenatal US in predicting colonic atresia,

probably because of the rarity of this condition and a later diagnosis in colonic atresia than in small bowel atresias is often observed. Some reports describe a sensitivity of 7.7% in prenatal detection of colonic obstructions. Most of times the amount of amniotic fluid is normal and the presence of some dilated bowel loop is not pathognomonic. These findings could be caused by the different timing and quantity of water reabsorption in small intestine and colon (Goruppi et al. 2016).

82.5.2.6 Symptoms and Diagnosis

If a prenatal diagnosis has not been made, the newborn progressively will manifest an abdominal distension with no meconium emission. Later on biliary vomit will appear.

The direct abdominal x-ray will show multiple air-fluid levels either in small or large intestine and no further gas beyond that point.

A contrast enema with gastrographin will show a microcolon and let to recognize a colic atresia, or it will raise the suspect of Hirschsprung's disease and could be resolutive in case of Meconium ileus or meconium plug syndrome (Fig. 12).

82.5.2.7 Therapy

It is not a surgical emergency as for the small bowel atresias. The video-assisted approach let to exteriorize from the umbilical incision the dilated colon and permits the primary colo-colic anastomosis. In case of a very huge proximal colon, it could be prudent to make a temporary colostomy to delay the definitive colo-colic anastomosis after some week or month. Colic biopsies must be taken for histological diagnosis of the presence of neuronal cells.

82.5.2.8 Prognosis

It is good quoad vitam and function. Healing exceeds in 90 % of babies if other malformations are absent.

82.5.3 Meconium Ileus

It is a congenital neonatal intestinal obstruction due to thickened and tenacious meconium that cannot proceed along the intestinal lumen and accumulate within it.

It is due to an autosomal recessive disease, the cystic fibrosis (CF), which is characterized by a lot of clinical manifestations of which the meconium ileus (MI) is the early and more severe one.

82.5.3.1 Incidence

It varies from 1 every 1,500 to 1/2,000 births among white population; on the contrary it is rare in blacks (1/17,000) and almost unheard in Asians and Africans (1/100,000) (Schuster 1986). A Family history of CF is present in 10–33% of patients with MI.

82.5.3.2 Embryogenesis

The defect of CF is an esocrin-eccrin gland dysfunction particularly of the mucus secreting and sweat glands. Two pathologic events in meconium ileus bring to intraluminal accumulation of tenacious meconium: the development of pancreatic exocrine enzyme deficiency and the secretion of hyperviscous mucus by pathologically abnormal intestinal glands.

82.5.3.3 Prenatal Diagnosis

Family history, amniocentesis, and prenatal ultrasound permit to predict of which infants are at risk of developing a MI (nearby 20 % of CF population) (Ziegler 2006).

82.5.3.4 Differential Diagnosis

The major differential diagnosis is with all the causes of neonatal intestinal obstruction, in particular:

- Ileal Atresia
- Meconium plug syndrome
- Neonatal small left colon
- Hirschsprung's disease

82.5.3.5 Symptoms and Diagnosis

MI manifests in newborn in two forms:

- Uncomplicated or simple MI
- Complicated MI (meconium peritonitis)

Uncomplicated MI presents at birth and abdominal distension is the main symptom. As time goes by bilious vomiting and failure to stool compare. The clinical picture is overlapping that of intestinal atresia.

Complicated MI is often recognized in utero with the observation of an intra-abdominal calcification due to intestinal perforation consequent to the intestinal obstruction. Sometimes at birth a cystic mass is palpable.

The radiological picture shows the absence of air-fluid levels since the gas cannot layer above the inspissated meconium and granular "soap bubbles" appearance due to air bubbles intermixed within the sticky meconium. In case of complicated MI, abdominal calcifications can be observed.

A contrast enema shows the microcolon.

Definitive diagnosis is obtained with the sweat test that measures the amount of sodium and chloride in the sweat. If sweat chloride exceeds 60 mEq/L, it is diagnostic of CF (Klein 2006).

The ultimate diagnostic step is the genetic test.

MI may occur also in the absence of CF in term or preterm infants with pancreatic insufficiency due to several causes.

82.5.3.6 Therapy

Nonoperative treatment consists of trying to dissolute the inspissated intraluminal meconium with solubilizing agents either taken by mouth or by enema (Noblett technique) (Friedman et al. 2016). Gastrografin enema is the standard of nonoperative treatment. It is a hyperosmolar, water-soluble, radiopaque solution that should draw fluids into the intestinal lumen helping in the release of intestinal meconium.

Nevertheless, the mainstay of MI treatment remains an operative procedure. The initial procedure is a laparotomic enterotomy with irrigation and ileal emptying from meconium (Fig. 15). An alternative procedure is the confectioning of a temporary ileostomy to relief the obstruction.

Complicated MI require almost ever a surgical operation to assess residual intestinal length and for eventual conservative resection.

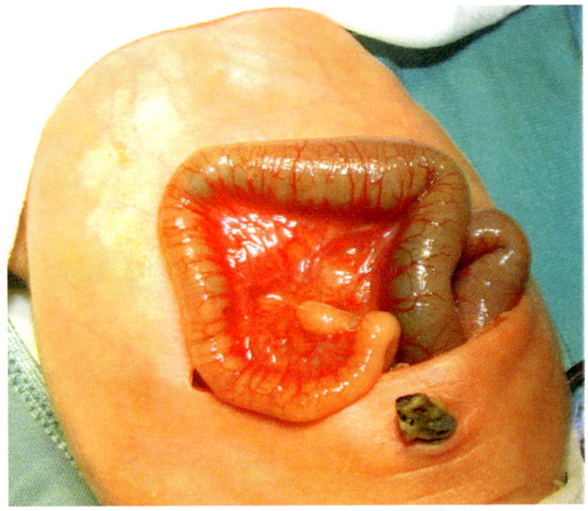

Fig. 15 Typical surgical findings of meconium ileus. The distal ileum if filled by thickened meconium that cannot proceed

82.5.3.7 Prognosis

Survival rate is now 100 % either with nonoperative or with operative treatment, whereas in 1960s it was 33 % in the first 6 months.

Longtime prognosis depends on CF course and its complications.

82.6 Persistence of the Omphalo-(mes)-enteric Duct

The pathology of the omphalo-enteric duct (improperly called "omphalo-mesenteric") consists of a wide range of congenital anomalies all due to a missed or a partial involution.

82.6.1 Classification

Five different presentations can be recognized, herein listed in decreasing order (Snyder 2006).

1. Meckel Diverticulum
2. Omphalo-enteric fistula (there is an open communication between ileum and umbilicus)
3. Fibrous cord (obliterated omphalo-mesenteric duct, from ileum to umbilicus)
4. Umbilical sinus or polyp (remnant of intestinal mucosa at the umbilicus)

5. Cyst of the vitelline duct (in the context of a fibrous cord)

The *Meckel Diverticulum* (*MD*) is the most frequent presentation with an incidence that is about 82–96% according to the different casuistics; fibrous cord is nearby 10 % and the omphalo-enteric fistula between 2 % and 6 %.

82.6.2 Meckel Diverticulum

His name is due to J.F. Meckel, German anatomic, who described it in 1809 and defined its embryological origin from the vitelline duct (Snyder 2006).

The MD is a "true" ileal diverticulum (its wall contains all the three layer of the intestinal wall), in communication with the ileal lumen and placed at 20–60 cm from the ileocecal valve. It is in the antimesenteric border of terminal ileum, and in 75 % of cases it is not connected with the internal abdominal wall; in the remaining 25 % its tip is joined to the umbilicus. Usually it has an own vascular pedicle deriving from the vitelline arteries. In 25 % of cases, it is lined with heterotopic tissues. Gastric mucosa is the most common heterotopic tissue found in MD (>50%) followed by ectopic pancreatic tissue (5 %). MD with heterotopic tissues is three time more symptomatic than the other forms of MD.

82.6.2.1 Embryopathogenesis

MD is the embryonal remnant of the omphalomesenteric duct (or vitelline duct) that connects the primitive gut with the yolk sac. As defined above, the MD anomalies are a consequence of its persistence due to an incomplete obliteration (5th–7th week of gestational age) (Skandalakis et al. 1994).

82.6.2.2 Incidence

In a wide postmortem study, MD has been found in 2 % of persons. The male/female ratio is 3:1 in symptomatic cases, whereas it is 1:1 for autoptic verifications. Eighty percent of complicated MD is less than 10 years old, and 60 % of them is younger than 2 years old.

82.6.2.3 Associated Anomalies

MD is frequently associated with other digestive malformations: omphalocele (24 %), ano-rectal malformations (11.4%), duodenal or jejunal atresia (12.7%), and oesophageal atresia (5 %). Therefore, in case of abdominal surgical exploration (laparoscopy or laparotomy), the MD must be systematically checked (Snyder 2006).

82.6.2.4 Symptoms

Only 4–6% of people who has a MD will develop some complication and become "symptomatic": The incidence of clinical manifestation is inversely proportional to age and it is prevalent in males. Complications in pediatric and adolescent age can be subdivided into five groups:

- Digestive bleeding (31–35%)
- Intestinal occlusion (27–30%)
- Diverticulitis (22–25%)
- Enteric fistula or omphalitis (4–10%)
- Other (1–10%)

Usually symptoms manifest during infancy, within 2 years of life. In neonate or toddler, intestinal occlusions or digestive bleeding are prevalent. In older ages, bleeding or diverticulitis are main manifestations.

Intestinal occlusion can be due to intussusception of the MD or volvulus. Intussusception provokes recurrent abdominal pain, emesis, rectal bleeding, palpable abdominal mass in lower quadrants and in advanced state lethargy. Volvulus can occur for twisting of intestinal loops around the fibrous remnant of the vitelline duct joined with the abdominal wall, and it can bring to intestinal ischemia and necrosis.

Bleeding is consequence of the peptic ulcer due to the hydrochloric acid (HCl) secreted by the isle of heterotopic gastric mucosa that lines the inner mucosa of the MD. The peak of incidence is within the first 2–3 years of life, but it can be observed also in scholar or adolescent boys or girls. Usually the blood is red and not dark; rarely there is a stillicidium that brings to a severe anemia. In these cases, occult blood test must be done.

Diverticulitis has a clinical picture that overlaps those of acute appendicitis. Most of times it depends on HCl produced by the heterotopic gastric mucosa, but sometimes it can be consequent to fecal impaction inside the MD. It can bring to perforation, peritonitis, or localized abscess.

In adulthood have been described other complications such as parasitic infections, fecalith, carcinoid, and other tumors.

82.6.2.5 Diagnosis

When a digestive bleeding is observed, the MD should always be suspected. The instrumental exam to confirm the presence of heterotopic gastric mucosa is the abdominal scintiscan with Tc-99 pertecnectatum (Fig. 16) (Pinar et al. 2009). It was introduced by Jewett in 1970 and it is based on the tropism of the radioisotope for the gastric mucosa, either the orthotopic or the heterotopic one. It should be better to perform the exam after 6 h of fasting. The sensibility can be improved giving the patient pentagastrin or cimetidine orally. If these parameters are respected, the sensibility is nearby 80 %.

Differential diagnosis includes all the other cases of intestinal bleeding (i.e., intestinal duplications, heterotopic gastric mucosa, blue rubber bleb naevus stndrome. . .) (Davis et al. 2015).

In cases with negative prior investigation, when the bleeding stops the cause of intestinal hemorrhage can be detected timely by applying the wireless capsule endoscopy (WCE) that can show the orifice of MD (Sokol et al. 2009; Xiniasa et al. 2012). WCE is a useful tool to investigate obscure GI bleeding in children.

For those cases in which the diagnosis remain uncertain, the minimally invasive approach given by videolaparoscopy permits to reach the diagnosis and gives the best therapeutic option: resection of the MD after taking it out from the umbilicus as we are used to do in case of acute appendicitis (TULAA technique "Trans-Umbilical-Laparoscopically-Assisted-Approach").

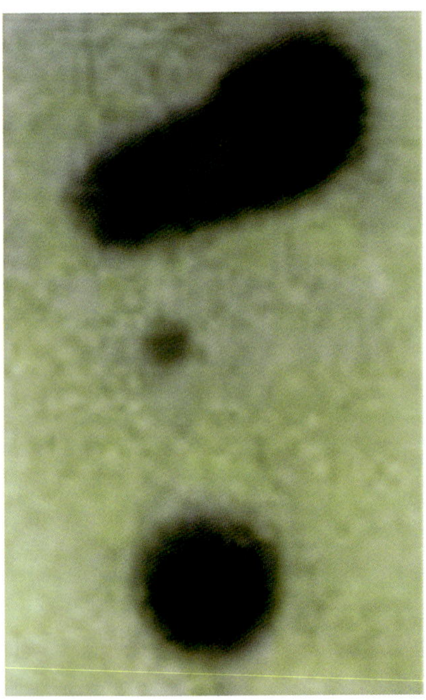

Fig. 16 Scintiscan with Tc99. At the *top* you see the gastric accumulation of radionuclide; at the *bottom* there is the bladder filled with radioactive urine and among them there is a little accumulation in correspondence of an isle of gastric mucosa inside the MD

82.6.2.6 Therapy

It is surgical and consists in the simple resection of the MD (Fig. 17) or in the resection of the intestinal loop that contains the MD and subsequent ileal anastomosis (Fig. 18a, b). Today the removal of MD should be done by laparoscopic or, better, videoassited approach. Extracorporeal diverticulectomy is preferable than intracorporeal

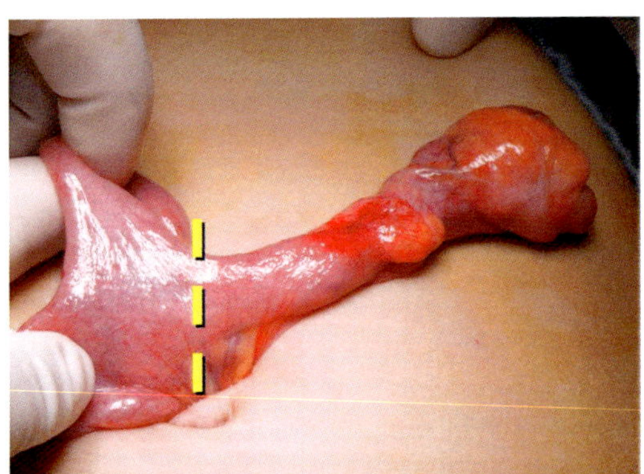

Fig. 17 Meckel diverticulum. The intermittent *line* shows the margin of antimesenteric resection

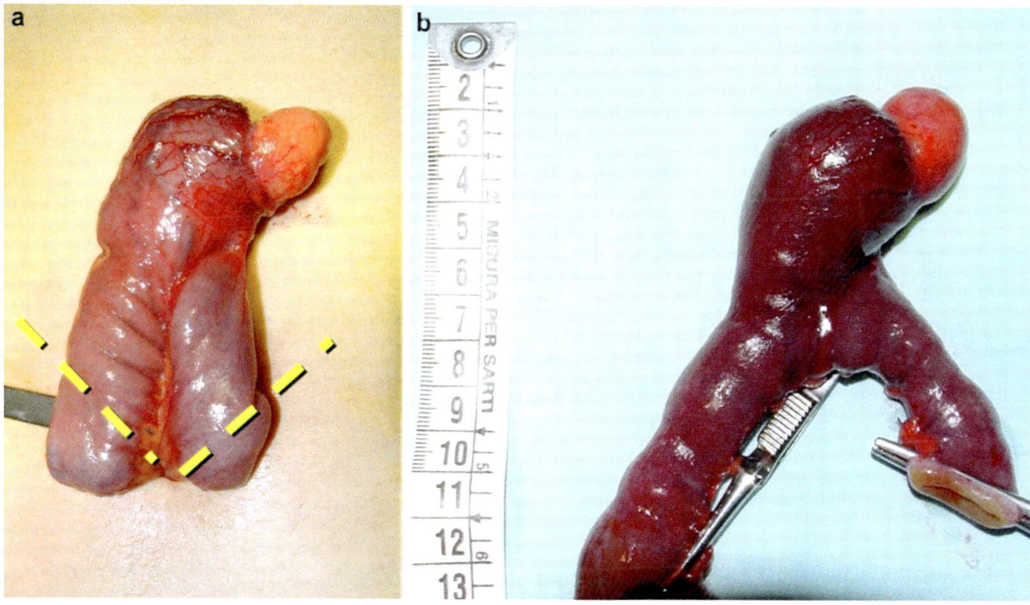

Fig. 18 (**a**) Meckel diverticulum. The intermittent *line* shows the margin of bowel resection. (**b**) Meckel diverticulum. The resected loop containing the diverticulum

diverticulectomy because it avoids the use of expensive laparoscopic staplers (Schier 2008; Chan et al. 2014), leaving the traditional laparotomic approach only for particular or complicated cases.

When a MD is casually found during a laparotomy or laparoscopy for other causes, the surgeon should ask the parents the permission for the prophylactic ablation.

82.6.2.7 Prognosis

Despite the possible complications that it can provoke, MD is a benign pathology and when promptly removed it brings to a complete resolution in every patient.

82.7 Duplications of the Alimentary Tract

Intestinal duplications are spherical or tubular ubiquitary structures (they can be found anywhere from esophagus to anus) that can be joined and sometimes communicating (the tubular ones) with the normal bowel.

82.7.1 Incidence

The incidence is low, since they represent only 0.1–0.3% of all the congenital malformations of the alimentary canal. Intraabdominal duplications account for 78 % of all duplications, and within those, 65 % are jejunoileal, 20.5% are colonic, 8 % are gastric, and 6.5% duodenal There is no sex prevalence if considered as a unique entity, whereas it has been found that in females there is prevalence of gastric duplications and in males of thoracic duplications.

82.7.2 Embryopathogenesis

Enteric duplications are believed to occur between the fourth and eighth weeks of embryonal development.

Since they are quite different from the morphologic point of view, it is difficult to set them in a unique embryological origin (Lund 2006). Therefore, three different theories have been proposed.

1. *Diverticular theory*
   Kaible in 1905 observed that in 4–8 weeks human embryo it is possible to find micro-diverticular structures inside the enteric tract. He supposed that the persistence and growing of these diverticular structures that normally should disappear is the foundation of the duplications development. As a matter of fact, it could explain the origin of spherical duplications but not that of tubular duplications.
2. *Theory of the difficult enteric recanalization*
   Bremer in 1944 believed that abnormal recanalization of the intestinal lumen after the solid stage of development of the primitive gut in the 6th–7th week of gestation could result in duplications. Unfortunately it has been demonstrated that the solid stage of development in human embryos does not usually extend beyond the duodenum.
3. *Notochord split syndrome*
   The most satisfactory of several theories of the origin of gastrointestinal duplications is that relating to the development of the neuroenteric canal. Saunders in 1943 and successively Bentley-Smith (1960) worked out the "split notochord theory," hypotizing that in these malformations everything depends on a wrong separation of the notochordal plate during the presomitic stage. According to these Authors if the notochordal plate fails to migrate as a result of adhesions to the endodermal lining, the spinal canal cannot close ventrally and a tract resembling a diverticulum is established with the primitive gut. This tract may remain open leaving a fistula between the gut and the spinal canal; however, in the majority of cases it disappears completely leaving only the duplication on the gastrointestinal tract. This theory explains well the thoracic and caudal duplications, but is weak to explain the other alimentary duplications, confirming it is impossible to create a unifying model of origin.

82.7.2.1 Pathology

Duplications are hollow structures with a muscle and a mucosal layer that could contain a small area of heterotopic lining (usually gastric mucosa but sometimes also pancreatic or respiratory). They tend to share a common muscular wall and blood supply with the adjacent normal bowel and could communicate with its lumen (rare, the tubular ones, usually on the antimesenteric border) or more frequently they do not communicate with it (the cystic form that are generally on the mesenteric edge).

1. *Cystic duplications*
   They represent nearby 90 % of cases. Most of times they are located in the small bowel (60 %) and do not communicate with the normal intestinal lumen. They must be differentiated from other cystic masses of the abdominal cavity that lack of intestinal mucosal lining.
2. *Tubular duplications*
   They are 10 % of cases, are long structures adherent to the normal lumen with whom they communicate at their terminal side, and are usually located on the antimesenteric border and their length could vary from few cm to one meter or more. In some cases, it could extend to the whole small bowel or the entire colon. Sometimes abdominal forms could go up in the thorax giving origin to the rare thoraco-abdominal duplications (usually gastro-oesophageal duplications).

82.7.2.2 Associated Anomalies

Infrequently, they principally consist of:

- Digestive malformations (oesophageal atresia, intestinal atresia...)
- Vertebral malformations
- Lumbar Myelomeningocele or complex genito-urinary malformations in case of rectal or colonic duplications

82.7.2.3 Diagnosis

When the prenatal ultrasound shows an intra-abdominal cystic formation, a cystic duplication must be considered. The tubular duplications are more difficult to be diagnosed on prenatal ultrasound even if current ultrasound technology allows detecting enteric duplications with a low false-positive rate as early as 12 weeks of gestation. There are two sonographic signs highly suggestive of enteric duplication: the "double-wall" sign due to an inner hyperechoic rim correlating to the mucosa-submucosa and an

outer surrounding hypoechoic layer reflecting muscularis propria, and the presence of peristalsis (Laje et al. 2010).

Instrumental postnatal diagnosis consists of abdominal ultrasound, contrast medium radiography of the abdomen, MR or CT and scintiscan with 99Tc pertecnectatum to look for the tubular forms with gastric mucosa in case of bleeding (Fig. 19).

82.7.2.4 Symptoms

In 70 % of cases, they manifest within first 6 months of life. The remaining 30 % manifest within 2 years of life. Clinical manifestation in older age is exceptional.

Duplications may be incidentally encountered during surgery for other medical conditions. Their clinical presentations vary according to the site of duplication. The ileum is the most common region involved. The clinical picture depends on the level of the duplication in the alimentary tract, on the morphology (cystic or tubular), and on the mucosal lining.

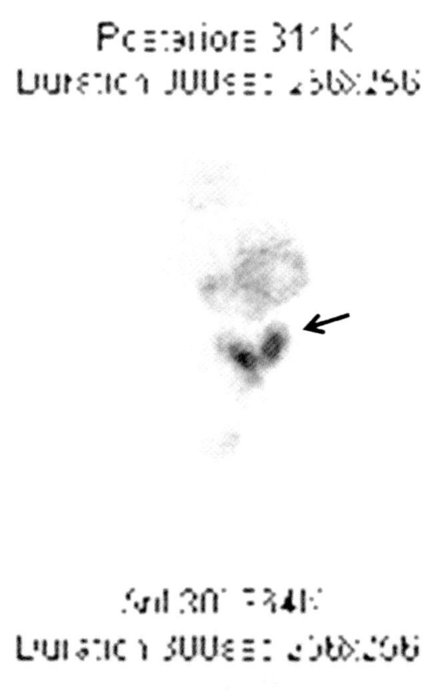

Fig. 19 Scintiscan with 99Tc pertecnectatum showing the large amount of tubular gastric mucosa

Usually the cystic forms bring to an occlusive state due to the "mass effect" consequent to the increasing volume of the internal secretions. Sometimes it could bring to volvulus or intussusception with occlusive state.

The tubular forms that frequently are lined with gastric mucosa usually manifest with a digestive bleeding or perforation.

Symptoms are different according to the involved enteric tract:

- Oesophagus: Dysfagia, respiratory distress, cardiac disturbs
- Gastrointestinal tract: Mass effect, vomiting, occlusion, digestive bleeding
- Colorectal tract: Mass effect, constipation, bleeding.

In the last years, the diagnosis with the video-capsule has become a valid tool to recognize the inner orifice of a tubular duplication of the small bowel (Sokol et al. 2009). Colonoscopy remains the gold-standard for colonic duplications.

82.7.2.5 Therapy

Cystic duplications must be removed in any case, even if not symptomatic because of the risk of malignant degeneration. For cystic duplications, usually the intestinal resection with end-to-end anastomosis is performed. In case of tubular duplication, an elegant solution is the stripping of the mucosal layer (Fig. 20a, b), as in case of oesophageal ones. Sometimes for colonic duplications, it could be sufficient to create a distal communication between normal colon and duplicated one (Klein 2006). The rectal forms should be approached by posterior sagittal way according to the Pena's operation. A subordinate approach is combined perineal and abdominal. Temporary colostomy is optional but strongly recommended in these cases.

A recent report from a large French multicentric study shows that mini-invasive surgery for abdominal duplications is feasible and safe with a low rate of adverse events (Guerin et al. 2012).

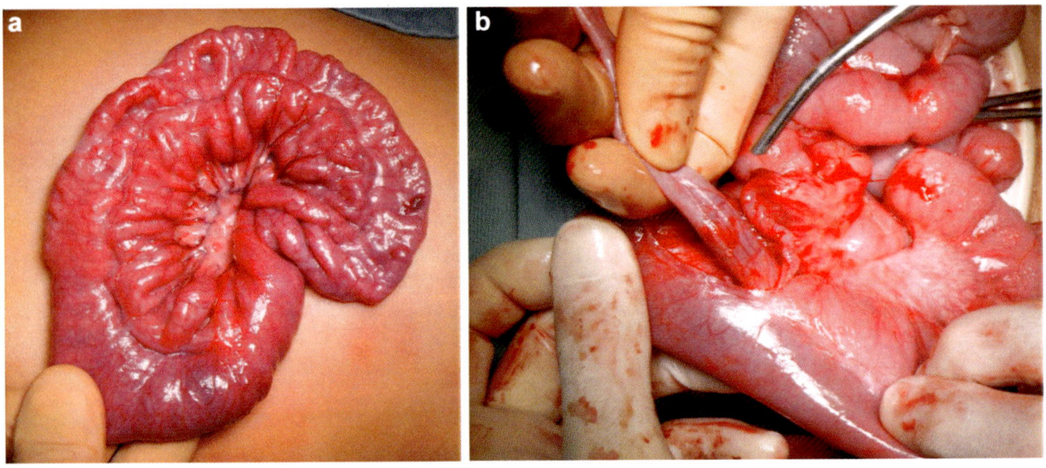

Fig. 20 (**a**) Ileal tubular duplication. The inner layer is the duplicated one. (**b**) Ileal tubular duplication. Stripping of the internal mucosa

82.7.2.6 Prognosis

It depends on the form and level of the duplication. Usually it is a good prognosis.

82.8 Intestinal Malrotation

Malrotation is a congenital anomaly resulting from the embryologic failure of normal rotation and fixation of the gut. The ascending colon instead of being in its usual position on the right flank is located under the stomach; therefore, the peritoneum that covers the colon fixing it to the posterior abdominal wall has to pass in front of the duodenum creating an external compression on it that can be occlusive.

Furthermore, the large intestine is mobile and there is a higher risk of intestinal volvulus than in normal population. Midgut volvulus can lead to irreversible intestinal necrosis, which is potentially fatal.

82.8.1 Classification

The rotation-fixation process is well defined but complex, so a stop during any stage of the development brings to a different form of malrotation (Table 1).

Table 1 Different types of intestinal malrotations and their possible consequences

Type	Anatomy	Clinical aspects
IA	No rotation	Volvulus of the midgut
IIA	No duodenal rotation; normal colic rotation	Duodenal obstruction; Ladd's bands
IIB	Inverse duodenal rotation; normal colic rotation	Intestinal occlusion
IIIA	Normal duodenal rotation; absent colic rotation	Duodenal obstruction; Ladd's bands; intestinal volvulus
IIIB	Incomplete rotation and fixation	Duodenal obstruction; Ladd's bands
IIIC	Incomplete fixation of the cecum	Volvulus of the cecum
IIID	Internal hernias	Occlusion or subocclusion

The most frequent and clinically interesting forms are (Lelli Chiesa 1993):

- *Type IA*: Lack of rotation also called "mesenterium commune": the small bowel lays in the right hemi-abdomen, while the colon is in the left.
- *Type IIIA*: The rotation is incomplete: the small bowel stays in the right hemi-abdomen; cecum and ascending colon are in the epigastrium. In

this form, there are some parietal adhesions (Ladd's band) between abdominal wall and colon that can bring to extrinsic occlusive compression of the 3rd duodenal portion.

The "volvulus neonatorum" happens most frequently in types IA and III.

82.8.1.1 Incidence

In literature, it is nearby 1 every 10,000 births, but it refers only to the symptomatic cases. Large series of postmortem examination reveal that the incidence is 1/200 or 1/300 patients. This demonstrates how this anomaly can be well tolerated and that it brings to complications only 1 every 500 patients.

There is a male prevalence 2:1.

82.8.1.2 Embryogenesis

There are no descriptions of genetic or familial causes for this pathology. The primitive gut completes the anticlockwise rotation between the 4th and the 10th week of gestation and fixates to the posterior abdominal wall when it reaches its definitive position (on the right the ascending colon, on the left the descending). When it does not happen, we have an intestinal malrotation (Filston and Kirks 1981).

82.8.1.3 Associated Anomalies

An intestinal malrotation is always present in case of Bochdalek's diaphragmatic hernia, Omphalocele, or Gastroschisis. Often is present in heterotaxy syndrome. Also in case of intestinal atresias, an intestinal malrotation can be found.

82.8.1.4 Prenatal Diagnosis

The prenatal ultrasound is not helpful in the diagnosis of an intestinal malrotation.

82.8.1.5 Symptoms and Diagnosis

Symptomatology of intestinal malrotation can be nonspecific. In a retrospective study evaluating presentations of intestinal malrotation in children, anorexia or nausea was noted in 36 %, intermittent apnoea in 24 %, and failure to thrive in 41 %. Sometimes is noted variation of stooling pattern and diarrhea.

When an acute onset happens, symptomatology is the same of an intestinal occlusion. It can manifest as a duodenal obstruction, a volvulus, or an internal hernia. Half of patients become symptomatic in the first weeks of life. The remaining 50 % usually show some sign of malrotation within 6th month of life. In the successive ages, the presentation is less frequent and atypical (Smith 2006). In a recent large series, 37.7% of patients were diagnosed less than one month of age, 34.2% were 1–11 months of age, and 28.1% of patients were 12 months or older (Kulaylat et al. 2015).

- *Duodenal Obstruction*
  In neonates and toddlers, it is an acute presentation due to the "Ladd's bands" that obstruct the third portion of duodenum provoking biliary vomit. In infants and prescholar age, pain, irritability, and other nonspecific symptoms are more common. The key for suspicion and referral in the older patients is recurrent episodes of unexplained abdominal pain, irritability, vomiting, or failure to thrive (Shalaby et al. 2013).
- *Intestinal Volvulus*
  Usually it happens clockwise and represents a true diagnostic and surgical emergency. In half of patients, it manifests in first 2 weeks of life ("volvulus neonatorum"). Most of times the lack of early signs can be falsely reassuring, with abdominal examination remaining unremarkable until intestinal ischemia is advanced. When biliary vomit and progressive painful abdominal distension appear, the surgical intervention must be considered. Later on bloody stools emission could be observed.

  The clinical conditions rapidly worsen and become critical. The baby gets a pale and suffering aspect and in very short time he precipitates in a shock state that in absence of a prompt therapeutic treatment could bring to death in few hours.

  In infancy or adolescence, symptoms are often subtle and variegated and usually consist in cramp form pain and gastric or biliary vomit.

In malrotated patients, it could be difficult to diagnose an acute appendicitis since the cecum is not in its right position but in could be in the left

iliac fossa or in hypogastrium or elsewhere in the abdomen. Therefore, the patient will go to the operative room with a generic diagnosis of acute abdomen and only at the surgical operation the acute appendicitis will be diagnosed. For this reason, the laparoscopic approach has been an improvement also in the diagnostic approach permitting to explore the whole abdominal cavity.

Sometimes these patients could manifest some degree of malabsorption due to the fact that the intestinal loops present an intermittent torsion and the twisting of lymphatic vessels bring to a stasis with consequent mesenteric lymphoadenomegaly.

82.8.1.6 Diagnosis

It is very difficult. The sooner is the diagnosis the better will be the treatment.

When a "volvulus neonatorum" happens first of all, a direct abdominal x-ray must be taken (Smith 2006). Unfortunately most of times it does not show anything that could be evocative, since generally air-fluid levels are absent. When an absence of intestinal air is noted together with a massive abdominal opacity due to a peritoneal transudate, the volvulus should be immediately suspected. If there is enough time, a contrast enema should be done and it will show the left disposition of the colon. If the clinical conditions permits to do it, also a contrast medium radiography of the abdomen must be taken. A prompt diagnosis will bring to the best treatment possible and it could let to preserve the intestine avoiding the terrible complication of the short bowel syndrome (SBS) due to the necessity of removing a large part of the necrotic bowel leaving only few cm of health gut.

Contrast enema and Upper Gastrointestinal Series (UGIS) (Smith 2006; Marine and Karmazyn 2014) are the mainstay of the diagnosis for malrotation also for older patients.

When the duodenal loop shape and position of the duodeno-jejunal junction (DJJ) is evaluated, the sensitivity of UGIS for diagnosis of malrotation ranges from 93 % to 100 % (Marine and Karmazyn 2014).

The role of ultrasonography (US) in the evaluation of malrotation is disputed. However, the use of US has been increasingly described (Hennessey et al. 2014). In a recent paper is described the US examination for malrotation after that the duodenum is distended with water by filling the stomach with water via a nasogastric tube. In this large series, 114 of the 139 children (82 %) had a normal US examination. No child with a normal US examination required an exploratory laparotomy/laparoscopy. Therefore, no false-negative results were detected.

82.8.1.7 Therapy

It is always surgical for every type of malrotation.

For types II and III, the operation consists in:

(a) Resection of the Ladd's bands
(b) Identification and resolution of eventual volvulus or internal hernia
(c) Repositioning of the whole bowel according to the anomalous (but well tolerated) anatomic condition of the "mesenterium commune," with the small bowel to the right and the large bowel to the left of the patient (Fig. 21a, b). A prophylactic appendectomy should always be performed (Spitz 1995)

In case of "volvulus neonatorum," the surgical operation must be performed as soon as possible, even if the laboratoristic analyses show a dramatic condition of the patient, without waiting for the resuscitatory therapy. A delay of few hours could bring to the necessity to remove a large part of intestinal loops with a very low prognosis.

The skin incision is supraumbilical and the volvulus must be reduced always with an anticlockwise rotation of the cyanotic bowel. It is useful to wait for some 10 min to observe the reprise of the gut. Therefore, Ladd's bands must be carefully resected and the bowel repositioned in the abdomen as described above.

If the intestinal loops appear to be necrotic (Fig. 22) and do not seem to recover after detorsion, it is suggested to perform the intestinal resection. Whereas if the loops seem to be ischemic, it is preferable to suture the abdomen leaving inside the gut and to postpone the decision if resect or not, after a new surgical laparotomy 24 h later (so called "second look"). Sometimes

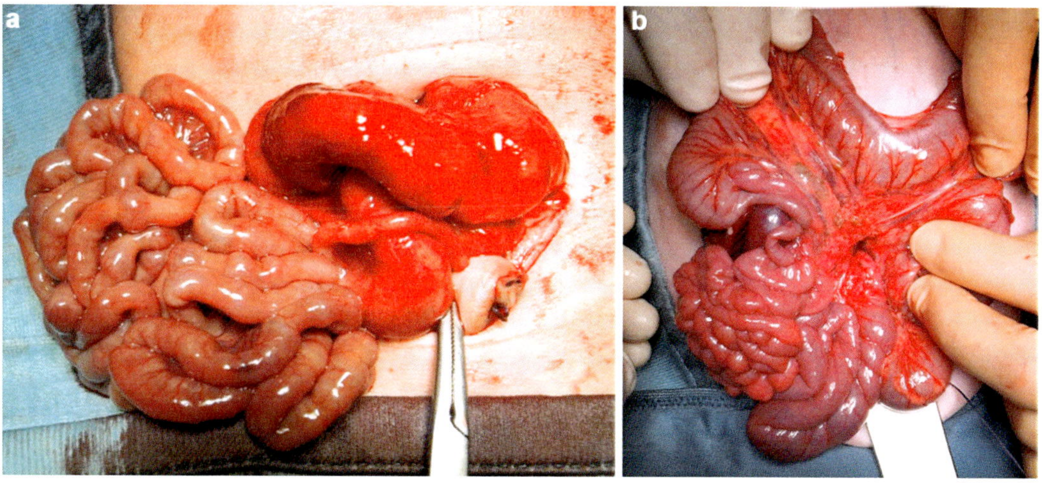

Fig. 21 (**a**) Intestinal malrotation. The colon is on the left of the patient and the small gut is on the right. (**b**) Intestinal malrotation. The mesenterium commune has been freed

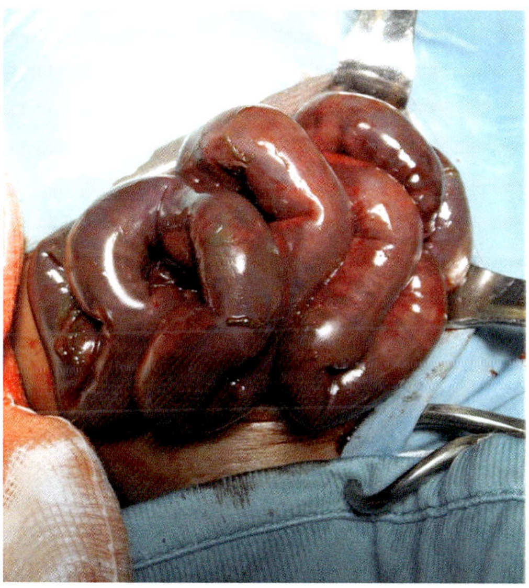

Fig. 22 Intestinal volvulus. The intestinal loops appear ischemic and necrotic

this conservative behavior let to observe that the necrosis is circumscribed and permits to perform a shorter resection.

In other cases, it could be a good attitude to perform an ileostomy in the healthy bowel with differed recanalization.

A recurrence of the volvulus is possible, but it is extremely rare.

In the last decade, the laparoscopic approach has been extended also to treat symptomatic intestinal malrotation or to separate patients with doubtful intestinal malrotation on imaging into a group that is prone to volvulus (and therefore requires treatment) and into a group that is not (Bax and Van der Zee 2008).

The whole same procedure done in traditional surgery can be performed laparoscopically. Nevertheless, a recent paper comparing open surgery with laparoscopic surgery for malrotation concludes that lap-surgery may not be indicated for the treatment of all cases of malrotation, and its role in the treatment of malrotation in neonates needs further assessment (Go Miyano et al. 2015).

82.8.1.8 Prognosis

Intestinal malrotation not complicated by a volvulus has a very good prognosis.

On the contrary, the "volvulus neonatorum" has a very poor prognosis (death, SBS) in 10–30% of patients.

Patients who suffer from SBS can survive with a lifelong total parenteral nutrition (TPN). Unfortunately TPN brings to a lot of complications (infections, sepsis, and liver failure).

In patients with only 20–30 cm of small bowel but with preserved ileo-ciecal valve, it is

possible to reach a good quality of life and the TPN is integrated with some degree of enteral nutrition.

The extrema ratio is given by the combined transplantation of liver and intestine which prognosis actually is not encouraging.

82.9 Ano-Rectal Malformations

Ano-rectal malformations (ARM) is a generic term that comprehends a large group of congenital anomalies of the anus and the rectum that go from the simple "anal stenosis" to the very complex "cloacal persistence syndrome" passing through a wide spectrum of presentations in which the ano-rectal agenesis is the most frequent.

82.9.1 Incidence

ARM are observed 1 every 4,000 births, with male prevalence for "high" and "intermediate" forms (ano-rectal agenesis) with an M:F rate = 3:1; on the contrary for "low" forms the rate is M:F = 1:3 (see classification) (Rossi 1993; Godse et al. 2015).

ARM are very challenging malformations from the diagnostic and surgical point of view and are very difficult also from the clinical and prognostic judgment even when promptly and correctly treated with a high chance of remaining problems for the duration of life (incontinence, constipation. . .) that could bring to a lot of psychological and social troubles.

82.9.2 Embryogenesis

The anus and the connected sphincter muscle complex originate from an ectodermal introflexion that successively joins the ano-rectal canal (the end of the primitive gut) that, on the contrary, origins from the endoderm. A damage occurring during these developmental phases brings to an ARM formation. ARM are due to an incomplete embryologic evolution of the primitive "cloaca." At the 4th week of gestational age, the cloaca is divided from the cloacal membrane into two parts: the "external cloaca" and the "internal cloaca."

In the *external cloaca* flow together the urethra and rectum.

In the *internal cloaca* goes the allantois, the primitive gut, and mesonephric ducts; later on it will be divided from the uro-rectal septum into the anterior "uro-genital sinus" and the posterior "ano-rectal sinus" (Rossi 1993).

From the "cloacal membrane" will develop the ventral genital tubercle, the lateral genital folds, and the posterior anal tubercles.

Due to not completely known causes, the normal evoluting process can stop giving rise to a lot of different forms of ano-rectal anomalies that go from the simple "imperforate anus," to the multiple forms of the "ano-rectal agenesis," in which the rectum ends as a fistula in the neighboring organs (bladder or urethra in the male, vagina in the female), till the extremely rare "rectal atresia," in which the anal orifice is apparently normal, but the anal canal is blind-ending after few cm, and the rectum is atresic.

The "rectal" group of the ARM depends from defects of the internal cloaca, whereas the "anal" group is due to defects of the external cloaca (perineum, genital folds, and proctodeum).

A recent paper debates about the use of the term "persistent cloaca" for severe form of female ARM. Studying a group of mice, they noted that the abnormal cloacas found are not part of the normal spectrum of cloacal development observed in normal rat embryos. They concluded that the cloaca of a normal embryo will never result in ARM and, therefore, that the term "persistent cloaca" for the human anomaly should be considered a misnomer (Kluth 2010).

82.9.3 Classification

A large discussion is still present in the international community of pediatric surgeons about the better way to classify patients with ARMs.

The most diffused and accepted classification of the different forms of ARM has been for a long

time the Melbourne Classification of the 1970, successively enlarged and completed by the Wingspread classification (1984): they are based on the radiological assessment of the height of the ARM: A direct radiography of the abdomen is taken 24 h after the birth to permit the intestinal gas to reach the rectal pouch; a radiopaque spot is painted in the perineal area where should be the anal orifice (Holschneider et al. 2005). The radiography must be taken in perfect lateral projection, then on the radiological image a line between the middle of the pubic bone and the sacrococcygeal joint at the level of the "ischiatic point" is drawn ("pubo-coccygeal line"), and the classification is based on the level of the rectal pouch with respect to this line.

- *"High ARM"*: when the intestinal air of the rectal pouch stops over the pubo-coccygeal line.
- *"Intermediate ARM"*: when the intestinal air stops between the p-c line and the ischiatic point.
- *"Low ARM"*: when the intestinal air stops under the p-c line and the ischiatic point, very near to the perineal skin.

In the Wingspread classification, the cloaca is considered as a separate form ("the clover syndrome") in its turn subdivided into three forms: high, intermediate, and low, according to the length of the common canal in which outflow rectum, urethra, and vagina.

Because of these anatomic relations, the Wingspread classification had a significant impact on the choice of surgical approach. However, some details of the Wingspread classification remained questionable. In 1995, Pena (Holschneider et al. 2005) proposed a new classification system purely descriptive with therapeutic and diagnostic implications for males and females without considering the ARM as "high," "intermediate," or "low," but only for the clinical features and presence of the fistula. He distinguished between perineal, vestibular, bulbar, prostatic, and bladder neck fistulas; imperforate anus without fistula; vaginal fistulas; cloacal fistulas; and rectal atresia or stenosis. By using both the antero-posterior and the lateral view in plain spinal radiographs, he measured the sacrum and compared it to fixed hip-girdle. He called the value obtained, the sacral ratio (SR), and thought that it could be used to predict which patients would be more likely to develop incontinence, even if undergoing technically adequate surgery. Patients who had less space on a radiological view of the sacrum would be those most likely to have a neurological disorder capable of irremediably compromising the operational capacity of the sphincter system. The mean "normal" SR was calculated as 0.74 for the anteroposterior view and 0.77 for the lateral view.

Bianchi (Khalil et al. 2010) too proposed an intuitive classification that consider the perineum ("well formed," "moderately formed," "poorly formed"), the rectal fistula according to site ("perineal," "fourchette and vestibular," "urethral," "vesical," or "absent fistula"), the urinary flow ("strong and intermittent" or "weak and dribbling"), the bladder ("normal" or "neurogenic") and the sacrum ("complete", "deform," or "hypoplastic"), considering the sacral ratio as defined by Peña.

Nevertheless, comparison of outcome data has been hindered because of confusion related to classification and assessment systems. So in 2005 the participants to the Krickenbeck Conference on ARM developed standards for an International Classification of ARM based on a modification of fistula type and adding rare and regional variants and design a system for comparable follow-up studies. This new international classification enables the different operative procedures to be more comparable to each other than with the Wingspread classification.

In the past in fact it was believed that "low" ARMs enjoyed good prognosis, but there are other factors, beyond the level of the rectum, which may influence the prognosis of these patients: the anatomy of the sacrum and the perineal muscle. So, the more recent distinction in forms with good and poor prognosis is more useful in terms of outcome compared to the old classification (Arnoldi et al. 2014).

The European consensus meeting of ARM-Net members found the Krickenbeck classification as the most appropriate in describing ARM for clinical use (van der Steeg et al. 2015).

82.9.4 Associated Anomalies

There is a high frequency of associated anomalies probably due to the gestational period in which the cloacal subdivision occurs: between the 4th and the 6th week, when begins the organogenesis. The incidence is nearby 50–60%, but it varies according to the form of ARM. In the "rectal" forms (high and intermediate ARM), the incidence and the severity of the associated malformations is almost twice than in the "anal" forms (low ARM). In decreasing order, they are interested in the uro-genital, skeletal, digestive, cardiac, nervous, and pulmonary apparatuses.

It seems to be there is no significant association between the prevalence of anorectal anomalies and maternal age (Godse et al. 2015).

- *Chromosomal anomalies*
  They are nearby 7 %. Down syndrome is present in 3.5% of patients with ARM. Genetic syndromes consist of 2.3%.
- *Uro-genital apparatus*
  They are the most frequent anomalies (20–30% in the low ARM, 50–70% in the high/intermediate ARM). The vesico-ureteral reflux (VUR) is the most frequent anomaly, overall in the female; obstructive uropathies and neurological bladder are extremely common in case of sacral agenesis.
- *Skeletal apparatus*
  Vertebral anomalies have a great incidence (40 % in the "rectal" forms, 17 % in the "anal" forms). The major part is localized in the sacrum or coccyx (sacral agenesis or hemisacrum).
  These anomalies are present in almost half of high forms; therefore, it is very important to study these forms with direct radiography, CT, and MR to evaluate the presence of a "tethered cord," which is a caudal traction on the medullar cone that can bring to nervous problems to the limbs or to a neurological bladder. If a tethered cord is present, the patient must be submitted to the neurosurgeon to get it away.
- *Digestive system*
  The incidence is nearby 10 % (15 % for "rectal" forms, 7 % in the "anal" forms). Oesophageal atresia affects 10 % of cases, duodenal atresia 2 %, and Hirschsprung's disease 3–5%)
- *Cardiovascular apparatus*
  Cardiovascular anomalies are present in 9 % of cases, independently from the form of ARM.
- *Other*
  It can be sporadically present other kind of anomalies (cleft lip, hydrocephalus, rachischisis)
- *VATER Association*
  It is an association of anomalies due to: (V) vertebral anomalies, (A) Anorectal agenesis, (TE) Tracheo-esophageal fistula with or without esophageal atresia, and (R) Renal dysplasia. This association can be also more complex (VACTER, VACTERL) if is present also a cardiac defect (C) and hypoplasia of the limbs (L). It is found in 7.7% of patients with ARM. Equal proportions of male and female cases occurred with VATER associations (Godse et al. 2015).

82.9.5 Symptoms

ARM are usually discovered immediately after birth just observing the perineal area (Fig. 23); therefore, further assessments are done before that symptoms manifest. If the objective examination is done superficially and the diagnosis is missing, the symptoms are those of an occlusive state (abdominal distension, missed meconium

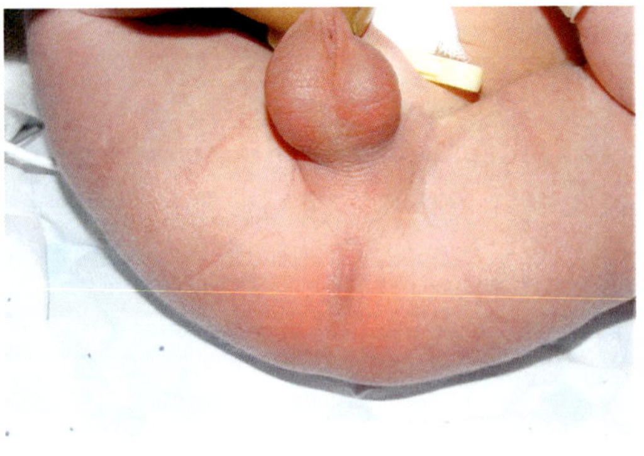

Fig. 23 ARM. Absence of the anus

evacuation, biliary vomit). In case of perineal fistula, a normal emission of meconium can be observed and sometimes the baby can grow normally with a progressive impairing constipation that can bring to a subocclusive state during infancy.

82.9.6 Diagnosis

Prenatal diagnosis of ARM is still challenging. In a recent paper of a multicentric registry considering a large series of 97 patients, only 7.2% of isolated cases were prenatally diagnosed. No cases were prenatally diagnosed from 1985 to 1990 and only two (10.5%) cases from 2006 to 2010 (Godse et al. 2015).

Images that can be seen prenatally and should raise suspicious for an anorectal malformation include: dilated and or calcified bowel, lack of meconium at the expected rectal level, hydronephrosis, absent kidney, neural tube defects, tethered cord, hydrocolpos, and vertebral anomalies (Bischoff et al. 2013).

Sometimes it is possible to observe a colonic dilatation without a polyhydramnios. The suspect can rise when a skeletal defect is discovered (radial or sacral aplasia), furthermore in presence of a concomitant uropathy or cardiopathy.

The simple examination of the perineal area after birth is usually sufficient for diagnosis. In low forms, sometimes a perineal outflow of meconium through a cutaneous fistula is present. In males this orifice can be observed ventrally in every place from anus to the tip of the penis along the raphe line. Sometimes scrotal pearls of meconium can be seen on the raphe of the scrotum and are considered to be a sign of low presentation of an anorectal malformation. In females, the orifice can be in anterior perineal region or in vestibular or vulvar site.

In high or intermediate forms, the rectal fistula is internal (recto-urethral fistula in males; recto-vaginal fistula in females) and meconium can be observed to come out from urethra or vagina.

In patients with persistence of the cloaca, meconium, and urine come out from a unique orifice, the common channel.

As told before the assessment of the level of the ano-rectal atresia is made by direct radiography of the abdomen after 24 h of life. The old "invertography" is no longer necessary since the intestinal air reaches the rectal pouch anyway, so a simple direct radiography after 24 h of life is sufficient for the diagnosis.

Furthers exams must be investigate the other apparatuses: sacral radiography, cardiac ultrasound, urinary ultrasound, CT or MR to evaluate the presence of a "tethered cord," VCU to exclude a vesico-ureteral reflux, and urodynamics for neurologic bladder. Sometimes a vaginoscopy can be useful to distinguish a "duplex vagina" from a "septa vagina" and to identify the fistula outflow in one of the two vaginas (usually is in the right one).

The study of the common channel in cloacal forms with an endoscopy is mandatory to measure its length.

When a temporary colostomy has been performed, a distal colography is useful to determine the height of the fistula.

82.9.7 Therapy

Surgical therapy changes from low forms to high or intermediate ones.

In *low ARM* the complete surgical correction is usually done at birth (within first 24–48 h of life). In these cases, the rectum is normally positioned in the "pubo-rectal sling"; therefore, it is sufficient to create an adequate new anal orifice in its natural anatomic site identifying the middle of the external sphincter by the use of an electro-muscle stimulator (Fig. 24). The patient can be placed either in prone or lithotomy position, according to the preference of the surgeon and the technique. In my personal opinion, the transanal anorectoplasty (TAP) (Khalil et al. 2010) proposed by Bianchi through the 1980s is the best technique to treat these forms. The child is placed in the lithotomy position with the gluteal region at the edge of the table and the surgeon sits between the child's legs. With the Peña muscle stimulator, the center point of the external sphincter complex is identified and marked. The rectal fistula is dissected

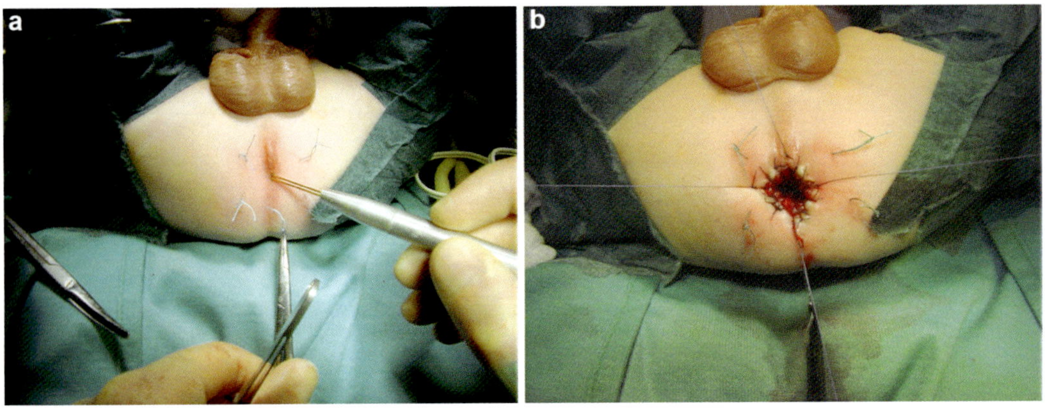

Fig. 24 (**a**, **b**) Low ARM. The electrostimulator permits to identify the correct point in which create the new anus. The rectum has been found few mm over the perineal skin

circumferentially and freed until the rectum is sufficiently mobilized to allow it to be rerouted through the anal canal decrossing it from the perineal muscles. Then it is anastomosed to the perianal skin at the anus (Fig. 25a–e)

In *high or intermediate forms*, a temporary colostomy is performed at birth till the definitive surgical correction. The most diffused surgical technique is the "Posterior Sagittal Ano-Recto-Plasty" according to Peña-De Vries (1982) (Peña and Levitt 2006; De Vries and Peña 1982). The baby is put in prone position and a sagittal posterior skin incision is done through the intergluteal line opening "as a book" the muscle structures till to reach the rectal pouch. When the fistula is found, it is sutured and sectioned. The rectal pouch is opened and separated from urethra (in males) or vagina (in females), then it is correctly positioned in its own anatomic site inside the "muscle complex," which is well identified by the use of the electro-stimulator.

The same technique is used to correct the cloacal malformation, lowering the three separated orifices to the perineal skin.

The Peña's technique has been demonstrated to be superior to every surgical technique previously described that privileged the laparotomic abdomino-perineal approach (Stephens 1953; Rehbein 1965; Swenson 1967; Kiesewetter 1967). Results are definitively better since from the functional (fecal continence) than from the aesthetical point of view. The advantages of the Pena's technique can be summarized as follows: (1) precise identification of every perineal muscle; (2) optimal surgical view; (3) homogeneous treatment of every different form of ARM (included the "persistence of the cloaca") that can be corrected in a single surgical time; (4) optimal positioning of the neo-anus (and other orifices in cloacal forms); and (5) good functional result for urinary and fecal continence. In November 2012, the patient number 3000 in Peña's database have been operated with his technique (van der Steeg et al. 2015).

The TAP Bianchi's technique (Khalil et al. 2010) can be performed also to correct high and intermediate forms of ARM in males combining a laparotomic with a minimal perineal approach. The rectourethral fistula is reached through a low Pfannenstiel incision and is divided close to the urethra. The perineal time is completed in the same way described before. This technique gained interest since it let to correct the malformation without splitting the muscle complex as in the Peña's approach.

In 2000, Georgeson introduced the "Laparoscopic Assisted Ano-Recto-Plasty" (LAARP) a new mini-invasive technique that reprises the concepts of the Bianchi's technique substituting the laparotomic time with a laparoscopic one (Georgeson et al. 2000). The fistula is identified, sutured, and sectioned using a three-trocar laparoscopic approach. In our Centre, it is considered the

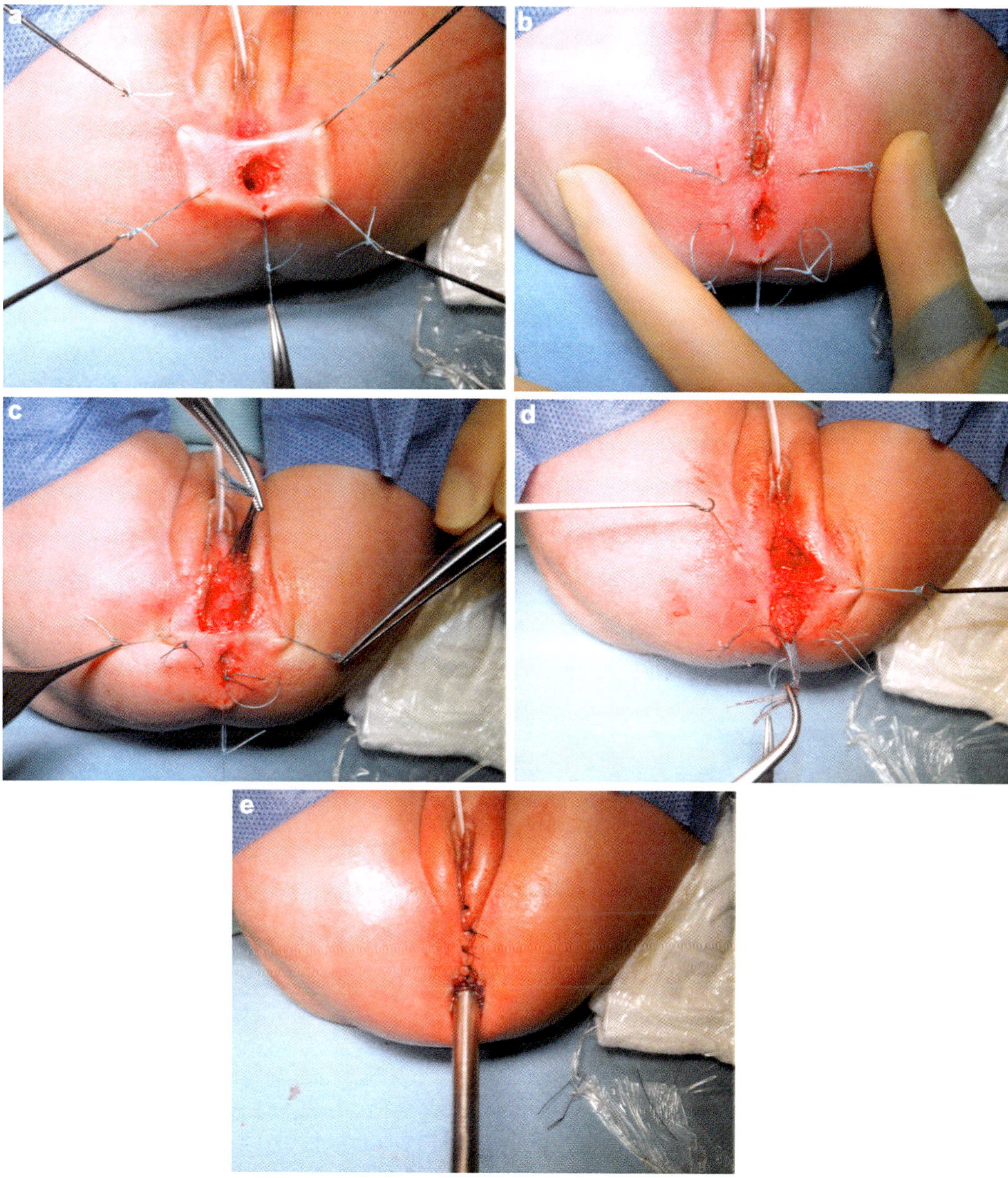

Fig. 25 (**a**) Bianchi technique. The anal canal has been prepared in the center point of the external sphincter complex. (**b**) Bianchi technique. The perineal fistula has been dissected circumferentially. (**c**) Bianchi technique. The rectum is mobilized. (**d**) Bianchi technique. The rectum is rerouted through the anal canal and decrossed from the perineal muscles. (**e**) Bianchi technique. At the end of the operation, the new-anus is calibrated with the Hegar dilator

treatment of choice in high forms of ARM, even if a specific laparoscopic skill is needed.

A video-assisted surgical technique especially fit for ARM in females has been proposed by Marcela Bailez (2008).

In 2015, Peña (Bischoff et al. 2015) published a paper about the use of laparoscopy in ARMs. He attests that the ideal indication for laparoscopy is for cases in which laparotomy is needed to repair the malformation. He

concluded that only 10 % of male patients require an abdominal approach to treat a recto-bladder neck fistula and only they represent an ideal indication for laparoscopy. In cases of rectourethral prostatic fistulas, the malformation can be repaired either way: laparoscopically or posterior sagitally. In females, only those with complex cloacae with a common channel length greater than 3 cm require a laparotomy; they represent about 30 % of the cloacae. Nevertheless, since to repair this type of cloacae sophisticated and technically demanding maneuvers that have never been done laparoscopically are required, Peña does not think laparoscopy could be indicated. In all other malformations, recto-perineal fistula, recto-urethral bulbar fistula, anorectal malformation without fistula, rectal atresia, recto-vestibular fistula, he does not find justification for laparoscopy.

82.9.8 Postoperative Treatment

It is very important the postoperative care of these children. Every child must undergo to a long cycle of postoperative anal dilatations (minimum 3–6 months), with the aim to progressively calibrate the muscle complex to gain an "elastic" anal canal. It should be better to leave in place the colostomy at least for 3 months before closing it. The patient must be carefully followed in the first 2–3 years in his "toilette training" even with the use of enemas or medical therapy till the intestinal movements regularize. The clinical evaluation of the result regarding the continence relies on four basic points based on the level of cleaning: (1) clean, (2) stained, (3) sporadic fecal soiling, and (4) constant fecal soiling.

In a recent paper, considering a large sample the authors found that the differences in SR confirm Peña's data, but there were significantly many incontinent patients with a normal SR. They concluded that the SR cannot be considered as a marker and it should be interpreted cautiously and a close follow-up of all patients with ARM maintained (Macedo et al. 2004).

82.10 Results

There is no mortality in patients with ARM except for those with severe associated life-threatening anomalies.

High and intermediate forms are loaded by 30–40% of consequent handicaps (fecal incontinence, neurologic bladder…). In 2010, Bianchi published the results of 245 patients (175 male, 70 female) underwent TAP over 21 years. Of the 212 eligible patients, 182 with good prognostic factors (well-formed/moderately formed perineum and SR <0.7) resulted to be continent but have experienced constipation. Thirty patients with poor perineal neurology (poorly formed perineum, poor sacrum, and poor stimulation response) are incontinent and require significant bowel management to avoid soiling (Khalil et al. 2010).

In 2013, Peña published a very interesting update on the current management of patients with anorectal malformation (Bischoff et al. 2013).

References

Al-Salem AH, Abdulla MR, Kothari MR, Naga MI (2014) Congenital pyloric atresia, presentation, management, and outcome: a report of 20 cases. J Pediatr Surg 49:1078–1082

Applebaum H, Lee SL, Puapong DP (2006) Duodenal atresia and stenosis – annular pancreas. In: Grosfeld JL, O'Neill JA, Fonkalsrud EW, Coran AG (eds) Pediatric surgery, 6th edn. Mosby Elsevier, Philadelphia, pp 1260–1268

Arnoldi R, Macchini F, Gentilino V, Farris G, Morandi A, Brisighelli G, Leva E (2014) Anorectal malformations with good prognosis: variables affecting the functional outcome. J Pediatr Surg 49:1232–1236

Bailez MM (2008) Laparoscopy in the treatment of female infants with ano-rectal malformations. In: Bax KMA, Georgeson KE, Rothenberg SS, Valla JS, Yeung CK (eds) Endoscopic surgery in infants and children, 2nd edn. Springer Verlag, Berlin/Heidelberg, pp 399–408

Bax KMA, Van der Zee DC (2008) Intestinal malrotation. In: Bax KMA, Georgeson KE, Rothenberg SS, Valla JS, Yeung CK (eds) Endoscopic surgery in infants and children, 2nd edn. Springer Verlag, Berlin/Heidelberg, pp 299–308

Bianchi A (1999) Experience with intestinal lengthening and tailoring. Eur J Pediatr Surg 9:256–259

Bianchi A, Dickson AP (1998) Elective delayed reduction and no anesthesia: "minimal intervention management" for gastroschisis. J Pediatr Surg 33:1338

Bischoff A, Levitt MA, Pena A (2013) Update on the management of anorectal malformations. Pediatr Surg Int 29:899–904

Bischoff A, Martinez-Leo B, Pena A (2015) Laparoscopic approach in the management of anorectal malformations. Pediatr Surg Int 31:431–437

Chan KWE, Lee KH, Wong HYV, Tsui SYB, Wong YS, Pang KYK, Mou JWC, Tam YH (2014) Laparoscopic excision of Meckel's diverticulum in children: what is the current evidence? World J Gastroenterol 20 (41):15158–15162

Choi S-J, Jang Y-J, Choe B-H, Cho SH, Ryeom H, Hong SJ, Lee D (2014) Eosinophilic gastritis with gastric outlet obstruction mimicking infantile hypertrophic pyloric stenosis. J Pediatr Gastroenterol Nutr 59(1): e9–e11

Davis JS, Hirzel AC, Rodriguez MM, Neville HL, Sola JE (2015) Heterotopic gastric mucosa mimicking a Meckel's diverticulum in a young girl. J Pediatr Surg 50:879–881

De Vries PA, Peña A (1982) Posterior sagittal ano-rectoplasty. J Pediatr Surg 17:638–643

Ferreira CG, Lacreuse I, Geslin D, Schmitt F, Schneider A, Podevin G, Becmeur F (2014) Staged gastroschisis closure using Alexis wound retractor: first experiences. Pediatr Surg Int 30:305–311

Filston HC, Kirks DR (1981) Malrotation – the ubiquitous anomaly. J Pediatr Surg 16:614

Friedman AM, Ananth CV, Siddiq Z, D'Alton ME, Wright JD (2016) Gastroschisis: epidemiology and mode of delivery, 2005–2013. Am J Obstet Gynecol (in press)

Georgeson KE, Inge TH, Albanese CT (2000) Laparoscopically assisted ano-rectal pull-through for high imperforate anus: a new technique. J Pediatr Surg 35:927–930

Go Miyano MD, Hiroaki Fukuzawa MD, Keiichi Morita MD, Masakatsu Kaneshiro MD, Hiromu Miyake MD, Hiroshi Nouso MD, Masaya Yamoto MD, Koji Fukumoto MD, Naoto Urushihara MD (2015) Laparoscopic repair of malrotation: what are the indications in neonates and children? J Laparoendosc Adv Surg Tech 25(2):155–158

Godse AS, Best KE, Lawson A, Rosby L, Rankin J (2015) Register based study of anorectal anomalies over 26 years: associated anomalies, prevalence, and trends. Birth Defects Res Part A 103:597–602

Goruppi I, Arévalo S, Gander R, Molino J-A, Oria M, Carreras E, Peiro J-L (2016) Role of intraluminal bowel echogenicity on prenatal ultrasounds to determine the anatomical level of intestinal atresia. J Matern Fetal Neonatal Med. https://doi.org/10.3109/14767058.2016.1163677

Grosfeld JL (2006) Jejunal atresia and stenosis. In: Grosfeld JL, O'Neill JA, Fonkalsrud EW, Coran AG (eds) Pediatric surgery, 6th edn. Mosby Elsevier, Philadelphia, pp 1269–1287

Guerin F, Podevin G, Petit T, Lopez M, de Lagausie P, Lardy H, Bonnard A, Becmeur F, Philippe P, Larroquet M, Sapin E, Kurzenne JY, le Mandat A, Francois-Fiquet C, Gaudin J, Valioulis I, Morisson-Lacombe G, Montupet P, Demarche M (2012) Outcome of alimentary tract duplications operated on by minimally invasive surgery: a retrospective multicenter study by the GECI (Groupe d'Etude en Coeliochirurgie Infantile). Surg Endosc 26:2848–2855

Hall NJ, Eaton S, Seims A, Leys CM, Densmore JC, Calkins CM, Ostlie DJ, St Peter SD, Azizkhan RG, von Allmen D, Langer JC, Lapidus-Krol E, Bouchard S, Piché N, Bruch S, Drongowski R, MacKinlay GA, Clark C, Pierro A (2014) Risk of incomplete pyloromyotomy and mucosal perforation in open and laparoscopic pyloromyotomy. J Pediatr Surg 49:1083–1086

Hennessey I, John R, Gent R, Goh DW (2014) Utility of sonographic assessment of the position of the third part of the duodenum using water instillation in intestinal malrotation: a single-center retrospective audit. Pediatr Radiol 44:387–391

Holschneider A, Hutson J, Pena A, Bekhit E, Chatterjee S, Coran A, Davies M, Georgeson K, Grosfeld J, Gupta D, Iwai N, Kluth D, Martucciello G, Moore S, Risto R, Durham Smith E, Sripathi DV, Stephens D, Sen S, Ure B, Grasshoff S, Boemers T, Murphy F, Soylet Y, Dubbers M, Kunst M (2005) Preliminary report on the international conference for the development of standards for the treatment of anorectal malformations. J Pediatr Surg 40:1521–1526

How HYA, Harris BJ, Pietrantoni M et al (2000) Is vaginal delivery preferable to elective caesarean delivery in fetuses with a known ventral wall defect? Am J Obstet Gynecol 182:1527

Khalil BA, Morabito A, Bianchi A (2010) Trans-anoproctoplasty: a 21-year review. J Pediatr Surg 45:1915–1919

Kilbride KE, Cooney DR, Custer MD (2006) Vacuum-assisted closure: a new method for treating patients with giant omphalocele. J Pediatr Surg 41:212–215

Kimura K, Mukohara N, Nishijima E (1990) Diamond-shaped anastomosis for duodenal atresia: an ecperience with 44 patients over 15 years. J Pediatr Surg 25:977

Klein MD (2006) Congenital defects of the abdominal wall. In: Grosfeld JL, O'Neill JA, Fonkalsrud EW, Coran AG (eds) Pediatric surgery, 6th edn. Mosby Elsevier, Philadelphia, pp 1157–1171

Kluth D (2010) Embryology of anorectal malformations. Semin Pediatr Surg 19:201–208

Kulaylat AN, Hollenbeak CS, Engbrecht BW, Dillon PW, Safford SD (2015) The impact of children's hospital designation on outcomes in children with malrotation. J Pediatr Surg 50:417–422

Laje P, Flake AW, Scott Adzick N (2010) Prenatal diagnosis and postnatal resection of intraabdominal enteric duplications. J Pediatr Surg 45:1554–1558

Lelli Chiesa PL (1993) Malrotazioni intestinali. In: Lima M, Dòmini R (eds) Chirurgia delle Malformazioni digestive. Piccin, Padova, pp 279–288

Lund DP (2006) Alimentary tract duplications. In: Grosfeld JL, O'Neill JA, Fonkalsrud EW, Coran AG (eds) Pediatric surgery, 6th edn. Mosby Elsevier, Philadelphia, pp 1389–1395

Macedo M, Martins JL, Freitas Filho LG (2004) Sacral ratio and fecal continence in children with anorectal malformations. BJU Int 94:893–894

MacKinlay GA, Barnhart DC (2008) Laparoscopic pyloromyotomy. In: Bax KMA, Georgeson KE, Rothenberg SS, Valla JS, Yeung CK (eds) Endoscopic surgery in infants and children, 2nd edn. Springer Verlag, Berlin/Heidelberg, pp 281–288

Marine MB, Karmazyn B (2014) Imaging of malrotation in the neonate. Semin Ultrasound CT MRI 35:555–570

Noblett HR (1969) Treatment of uncomplicated meconium ileus by gastrographin enema: a preliminary report. J Pediatr Surg 4:190–197

Oldham KT, Arca MJ (2006) Atresia, stenosis and other obstructions of the colon. In: Grosfeld JL, O'Neill JA, Fonkalsrud EW, Coran AG (eds) Pediatric surgery, 6th edn. Mosby Elsevier, Philadelphia, pp 1493–1497

Parmentier B, Peycelon M, Muller C-O, El Ghoneimi A, Bonnard A (2015) Laparoscopic management of congenital duodenal atresia or stenosis: a single-center early experience. J Pediatr Surg 50:1833–1836

Peña A, Levitt MA (2006) Anorectal malformations. In: Grosfeld JL, O'Neill JA, Fonkalsrud EW, Coran AG (eds) Pediatric surgery, 6th edn. Mosby Elsevier, Philadelphia, pp 1566–1590

Pinar OK, Aksoy T, Bozkurt MF, Orhan D (2009) Detection of ectopic gastric mucosa using 99mTc perthecnetate: review of the literature. Ann Nucl Med 23:97–105

Rossi F (1993) Malformazioni ano-rettali. In: Dòmini R, Lima M (eds) Chirurgia delle Malformazioni digestive. Piccin, Padova, pp 367–404

Scherer LR III (2006) Peptic ulcer and other conditions of the stomach. In: Grosfeld JL, O'Neill JA, Fonkalsrud EW, Coran AG (eds) Pediatric surgery, 6th edn. Mosby Elsevier, Philadelphia, pp 1225–1241

Schier F (2008) Laparoscopic treatment of Meckel's diverticulum. In: Bax KMA, Georgeson KE, Rothenberg SS, Valla JS, Yeung CK (eds) Endoscopic surgery in infants and children, 2nd edn. Springer Verlag, Berlin/Heidelberg, pp 281–288

Schuster SR (1986) Omphaloceles and gastroschisis. In: Welch KJ, Randolph JG, Ravitch MM, O'Neill JA, Rowe MI (eds) Rob & Smith's pediatric surgery, 4th edn. Year Book Medical Publishers, Chicago, pp 740–763

Schwartz MZ (1995) Gastroschisis. In: Spitz L, Coran AG (eds) Rob & Smith's pediatric surgery, 5th edn. Chapman & Hall Medical, London/Glasgow/Weinheim/New York/Tokyo/Melbourne/Madras, pp 249–255

Schwartz MZ (2006) Hypertrophic pyloric stenosis. In: Grosfeld JL, O'Neill JA, Fonkalsrud EW, Coran AG (eds) Pediatric surgery, 6th edn. Mosby Elsevier, Philadelphia, pp 1215–1224

Shalaby MS, Kuti K, Walker G (2013) Intestinal malrotation and volvulus in infants and children. BMJ 347:f6949. https://doi.org/10.1136/bmj.f6949 (Published 26 Nov 2013)

Short SS, Grant CN, Merianos D, Haydel D, Ford HR (2014) A case of congenital pyloric atresia with dystrophic epidermolysis bullosa. Pediatr Surg Int 30:681–684

Skandalakis JE et al (1994) The small intestines. In: Skandalakis JA, Gray SW (eds) Embryology for surgeons, 2nd edn. Williams & Wilkins, Baltimore, p 184

Smith S (2006) Disorders of intestinal rotation and fixation. In: Grosfeld JL, O'Neill JA, Fonkalsrud EW, Coran AG (eds) Pediatric surgery, 6th edn. Mosby Elsevier, Philadelphia, pp 1342–1357

Snyder CL (2006) Meckel's diverticulum. In: Grosfeld JL, O'Neill JA, Fonkalsrud EW, Coran AG (eds) Pediatric surgery, 6th edn. Mosby Elsevier, Philadelphia, pp 1304–1312

Sokol H, Seksik P, Wendum D, Bellanger J, Parc Y, Cosnes J, Beaugerie L (2009) Gastrointestinal bleeding diagnosed using video capsule endoscopy. Meckel's diverticulum. Gut 58(9):1206, 1290

Spitz L (1995) Malrotation. In: Spitz L, Coran AG (eds) Rob & Smith's operative surgery – pediatric surgery, 2nd edn. Chapman & Hall, London/New York, pp 341–347

Tan KC, Bianchi A (1986) Circumumbilical incision for pyloromyotomy. Br J Surg 73(5):399

van der Steeg HJJ, Schmiedeke E, Bagolan P, Broens P, Demirogullari B, Garcia-Vazquez A, Grasshoff-Derr S, Lacher M, Leva E, Makedonsky I, Sloots CEJ, Schwarzer N, Aminoff D, Schipper M, Jenetzky E, van Rooij IALM, Giuliani S, Crétolle C, Holland Cunz S, Midrio P, de Blaauw I (2015) European consensus meeting of ARM-Net members concerning diagnosis and early management of newborns with anorectal malformations. Tech Coloproctol 19:181–185

Van der Zee DC, Bax KMA (2008) Laparoscopic treatment of duodenal and jejunal atresia and stenosis. In: Bax KMA, Georgeson KE, Rothenberg SS, Valla JS, Yeung CK (eds) Endoscopic surgery in infants and children, 2nd edn. Springer Verlag, Berlin/Heidelberg, pp 293–297

Weber TR (1995) Omphalocele/exomphalos. In: Spitz L, Coran AG (eds) Rob & Smith's pediatric surgery, 5th edn. Chapman & Hall Medical, London/Glasgow/Weinheim/New York/Tokyo/Melbourne/Madras, pp 239–248

Xiniasa I, Mavroudia A, Fotoulakib M, Tsikopoulosa G, Kalampakasb A, Imvriosa G (2012) Wireless capsule endoscopy detects Meckel's diverticulum in a child with unexplained intestinal blood loss. Case Rep Gastroenterol 6:650–659

Ziegler MM (2006) Meconium ileus. In: Grosfeld JL, O'Neill JA, Fonkalsrud EW, Coran AG (eds) Pediatric surgery, 6th edn. Mosby Elsevier, Philadelphia, pp 1289–1303

Rare Surgical Emergencies of Newborns

83

Mario Messina, Francesco Molinaro, and Rossella Angotti

Contents

Abstract

Over the past decade, multiple factors have changed the pattern of neonatal surgical emergencies. An increase in prenatal screenings and the development of neonatal tertiary care centers have changed the clinical approach to this kind of emergencies. In fact, most conditions, leading to gastrointestinal (GI) emergencies, are uncommon, and treatment in specialist centers enables concentration of appropriate resources and expertise. Comorbidity is common, particularly in the preterm or low-birth-weight infant.

In the literature, nobody specifies the cutoff that enables to define when rare emergencies could be considered as common or uncommon.

We propose our series, compared with others in the literature, in order to specify which

M. Messina (✉) · F. Molinaro
Department of Pediatrics, Obstetrics and Reproductive Medicine, Section of Pediatric Surgery, Policlinico "Le Scotte", University of Siena, Siena, Italy

Department of Medical, Surgical and Neurological Sciences, Section of Pediatric Surgery, University of Siena, Siena, Italy
e-mail: mario.messina@unisi.it

R. Angotti
Department of Pediatrics, Obstetrics and Reproductive Medicine, Section of Pediatric Surgery, University of Siena, Siena, Italy

G. Buonocore et al. (eds.), *Neonatology*,
https://doi.org/10.1007/978-3-319-29489-6_230

emergencies, although rare, could be considered common or uncommon in neonates.

83.1 Salient Points

- Neonatal gastric perforation is associated with high mortality, particularly in premature and low-birth-weight infants.
- Excessive gastric aspirate, abdominal distention, bilious vomiting, and failure to pass meconium are typical clinical findings that suggest intestinal obstruction in the neonate.
- Abdominal radiographs can be used to confirm the diagnosis of intestinal occlusion or perforation.
- Placement of a nasogastric tube to decompress the stomach, fluid and electrolyte replacement, and surgical therapy are options for the treatment of intestinal emergency in newborns.

83.2 Background

Over the past decade, multiple factors have changed the pattern of neonatal surgical emergencies. An increase in prenatal screenings and the development of neonatal tertiary care centers have changed the clinical approach to this kind of emergencies. In fact, most conditions, leading to a gastrointestinal (GI) emergencies, are uncommon, and treatment in specialist centers enables concentration of appropriate resources and expertise. Comorbidity is common, particularly in the preterm or low-birth-weight infant (Filston 1998).

Symptoms of GI emergencies may be subtle, including irritability or feeding intolerance, or they may be more apparent, with vomiting (bilious or nonbilious), abdominal distention, and shock. Vomiting in the neonatal period should always prompt the consideration of a pathologic process. It may be difficult to differentiate a life-threatening cause from a mild viral gastroenteritis or even severe gastroesophageal reflux. The initial symptoms may be nonspecific and the history may not be helpful in a neonate who has not developed a normal pattern. Early diagnosis, availability of diagnostic service, and prompt surgical intervention with optimal pre- and postoperative care are necessary to increase survival of newborns with such problems (Filston 1998). In this chapter, we only explain the pathologies caused GI emergencies in newborn age with a rare prevalence. The problem is to define "rare disease." A disease or disorder is defined as rare in Europe when it affects fewer than 1 in 2000.

A disease or disorder is defined as rare in the USA when it affects fewer than 200,000 Americans at any given time.

One rare disease may affect only a handful of patients in the EU (European Union), and another touch as many as 245,000. In the EU, as many as 30 million people alone may be affected by one of over 6000 rare diseases existing.

- Eighty percent of rare diseases have identified genetic origins, while others are the result of infections (bacterial or viral), allergies, and environmental causes or are degenerative and proliferative.
- Fifty percent of rare diseases touch children.

If we extend this term in neonatal surgery, we find that the most part of malformation could be defined as rare disease, because the incidence is more elevated than 1–2000 neonates. For this reason, it is important to define, in the group of rare surgical emergencies in neonates, what are common and uncommon, in order to focus the discussion only in the group of uncommon diseases. In the literature, nobody specifies the cutoff that enables to define when rare emergencies could be considered as common or uncommon.

We propose our series, compared with others in the literature, in order to specify which emergencies, although rare, could be considered common or uncommon in neonates.

83.3 Incidence, Etiology, and Pathophysiology

Table 1 shows the principal causes of neonatal surgical emergencies of GI tract. We divided the list into common and uncommon ones, and we specified if they caused occlusive clinical pattern or perforative ones, derived from a review of the literature (Raffensperger et al. 1970; Lim et al. 1994). We divided our data based on the two

Table 1 Neonatal surgical emergencies of the GI tract. The table shows the principal causes of neonatal emergencies, specifying the common and uncommon ones

Common	Uncommon
Occlusion	
Malrotation (duodenal obstruction, volvulus, internal hernia)	Gastric duplications and acute stomach volvulus
Duodenal atresia, stenosis, or annular pancreas	Congenital pyloric atresia or web
Jejunal atresia or stenosis	Duodenal duplication
Ileal atresia or stenosis	Preduodenal portal vein
Simple meconium ileus	Cystic duplication of the bowel with volvulus
Meconium ileus with perforation	Colon atresia
Meconium plug syndrome	Colon duplication with volvulus
Hirschsprung's disease	Functional intestinal obstruction
Drug-induced ileus	Intestinal psuedo-obstruction
Hypertrophic pyloric stenosis	Neuronal intestinal dysplasia
Meckel's diverticulum	
Perforation	
Necrotizing enterocolitis	Spontaneous intestinal perforation
Meckel's diverticulum	
Miscellaneous	
Hemangiomas, lymphangiomas, and vascular malformations of GI	Neonatal appendicitis
	Littre's hernia

principles of clinical manifestation in neonatal age: occlusion and perforation.

83.3.1 Obstruction

Intestinal obstruction is the most common surgical emergency of the newborn. The incidence of neonatal intestinal obstruction is approximately 1 case per every 500–1000 live births. Approximately 50% of these neonates will have intestinal atresia or stenosis. Duodenal atresia and jejunal atresia occur in approximately equal numbers, although some authors report that jejunoileal atresia is the more common (De la Hunt 2006). Congenital pyloric atresia (CPA) is a very rare condition that was first described by Calder in 1749. Commonly, CPA occurs as an isolated lesion, which has an excellent prognosis, but it can also be seen in association with other malformations, which can have a negative impact on the final outcome (Messina et al. 2002). Colon atresia is an extremely rare condition (Puri 2003).

Intestinal duplications are rare congenital malformations that could cause intestinal obstruction as mass effect or causing volvulus. Duplications of the alimentary tract occur in 1 of 4500 births. Gastric duplications constitute 8% of these or roughly 17 of every 1,000,000 births. A bowel volvulus caused by the presence of a cystic intestinal duplication can lead to an intestinal perforation. The different locations and sizes of these duplications require a specific diagnostic and surgical approach. Early diagnosis and treatment of uncomplicated intestinal duplications by means of prenatal sonographic screening and laparoscopic-assisted resection, respectively, are desirable in this congenital malformation, in order to prevent the risk of occlusion/perforation (Messina et al. 2003).

Pathophysiology. Proximal intestinal obstruction as in cases of duodenal or pyloric atresia leads to fluid loss that has a high concentration of hydrogen, potassium, and chloride ions. Hypochloremic alkalosis can develop if fluid losses are not replaced. Distal intestinal obstructions lead to fluid and electrolyte loss from both emesis as well as from fluid sequestered into the lumen of dilated bowel loops. Fluid shifts and intravascular volume depletion may lead to severe dehydration, oliguria, metabolic acidosis, and inadequate peripheral perfusion. Prolonged intestinal obstruction leads to alterations in intestinal motility, accumulation of gas and fluid, and bacterial overgrowth. Severe abdominal distention in the neonate can easily impair diaphragmatic function causing respiratory acidosis. As plasma volume loss increases, alterations in blood flow may result in bowel ischemia and necrosis (De la Hunt 2006).

83.3.2 Perforation

Gastrointestinal perforation is a catastrophic condition in neonates, especially in premature neonates.

Spontaneous perforations of the gastrointestinal tract occur in the stomach, duodenum, small intestine, or colon. The problem is encountered only infrequently; so, the exact incidence is unknown. Male infants are affected more often than females (approx. 4:1). Although neonatal gastric perforation is a well-recognized entity, other spontaneous GI perforations are much rarer and often incorrectly attributed to other disease processes (i.e., necrotizing enterocolitis) (Grosfeld et al. 1996).

Gastric perforation among neonates is a rare but frequently fatal condition of uncertain etiology.

Neonatal gastric perforation is associated with high mortality, particularly in premature infants. There is also a trend toward higher mortality in lower-birth-weight infants (Touloukian 1973).

Pathophysiology. Almost all spontaneous perforations of the GI tract are considered to be the result of ischemic necrosis. The perforation is the end result of "selective circulatory ischemia," a defense mechanism of the neonate to hypoxia, physiologic stress, and shock. Microembolic phenomena may also play a role. In response to physiologic stress (hypoxia, hypovolemia, etc.), blood is selectively shunted away from mesenteric vessels to the more vital heart and brain. Local mesenteric ischemia can progress to microvascular thrombosis and subsequent gastrointestinal wall necrosis and perforation. Although ischemia is likely the underlying problem, other factors including bacterial colonization, hyperosmolar feeds, and an immature neonatal immune system may also contribute. Indomethacin may also play a causal role in spontaneous GI perforations particularly in preterm infants as it does in the etiology of necrotizing enterocolitis. Risk factors for neonatal gastrointestinal perforation include all causes of severe fetal distress (abruption, emergent c-section, etc.) (Grosfeld et al. 1996).

Specifically, in the gastric tract, gastric wall ischemia, hypothalamic mechanisms, excessive gastric acid-pepsin ulceration, and congenital muscular wall defects could account for spontaneous gastric perforation, even if many authors believe that this spontaneous rupture is due to an acute rise in the intragastric pressure at the time of parturition (Touloukian 1973).

83.3.3 Miscellaneous

Acute neonatal appendicitis is a rare condition associated with significant morbidity and mortality. The severity of this disease is caused by its tendency to occur more frequently in premature infants, an increased perforation rate with rapid progression to peritonitis, and delay in diagnosis and intervention. Although appendicitis in the perinatal period may occur as an isolated event, in many cases it occurs in association with other pathologic states, including prematurity, inguinal hernia, and others. The presentation of neonatal appendicitis can be identical to necrotizing enterocolitis, leading to misdiagnosis (Van Veenendaal et al. 2004).

Littre's hernia was originally defined by Rinke in 1841 as "the presence of a Meckel's diverticulum in any hernial sac." It is generally difficult to differentiate from other types of hernia, until complications arise. It is a rare and accidental finding at any age, but absolutely exceptional in neonates. The potential surgical risk is linked to the presence of a Meckel' diverticulum (Messina et al. 2005).

83.4 Clinical Findings

83.4.1 Occlusion

Prenatal ultrasonography can readily identify proximal obstructing lesions that can produce proximal bowel dilation with hyperperistalsis and the classic "double bubble" appearance of duodenal atresia. Distal intestinal obstructions are less likely to cause polyhydramnios but on occasion dilated loops of bowel may be identified as anechoic masses.

Over the maternal polyhydramnios, four clinical findings suggest intestinal obstruction in the neonate: excessive gastric aspirate, abdominal distention, bilious vomiting, and failure to pass meconium. The presence or absence of each of these clinical findings depends largely upon the level of gastrointestinal obstruction. Early recognition of intestinal obstruction is imperative if the complications of respiratory compromise and sepsis are to be avoided (Raffensperger et al. 1970; Lim et al. 1994).

Excessive gastric output: Passage of a nasogastric or orogastric tube is often performed in premature infants and infants with a maternal history of polyhydramnios. If the initial volume of gastric aspirate is large (>50 cc) or is bilious, then gastrointestinal obstruction should be considered.

Abdominal distention: Abdominal distension may not be apparent at birth but develops over time as ingested air accumulates proximal to an obstruction. The time of onset, degree, and characteristic appearance of the distention may suggest the level of obstruction. Gastric distention within a few hours may cause the epigastrium to protrude indicating an obstruction of the stomach or duodenum. Gradual overall abdominal distension occurring over a 12–24 h period suggests a distal gastrointestinal tract obstruction.

Bilious emesis: It is usual for healthy newborns to spit up postprandially, but bilious emesis in a term newborn is distinctly abnormal. Premature infants (<35 weeks) occasionally have bilious emesis secondary to an immature or poorly functioning pyloric sphincter but proximal gastrointestinal obstruction must still be considered. Sepsis with an associated paralytic ileus may also result in bilious emesis. Vomiting begins soon after delivery if the lesion is proximal or complete, but may be delayed in cases of distal or incomplete obstruction.

Failure to pass meconium: A normal newborn is expected to pass a large amount of thick, dark green, shiny meconium usually within the first 12 h of life and almost always by 24 h. Failed or delayed passage of meconium suggests obstruction, but neonates with proximal obstructing lesions may pass a normal amount of meconium. Because neonates with ileal atresia or distal small bowel obstruction may pass several meconium stools on the first day of life, passage of meconium does not exclude the possibility of obstruction. Preterm infants commonly have delayed passage of meconium. Approximately 20% will not pass stool during the first 48 h following birth.

Additional physical findings that suggest obstruction are the presence of intestinal patterning and peristalsis that is visible through the intestinal wall. Distended loops of bowel may be palpable as ill-defined tubular masses. The rectum may feel tight on exam if small and unused as in cases of distal bowel obstruction. Lethargy and hypotonia are late signs of intestinal obstruction and the resultant sepsis. Abdominal wall discoloration and ecchymosis suggest perforation and/or necrosis (De la Hunt 2006).

83.4.2 Perforation

Most infants can immediately present signs of perforation. In fact, in case of spontaneous gastrointestinal perforation, infants present within the first week of life (usually 4–5 days) with an abrupt onset of abdominal distention and associated tachycardia, hypovolemia, and poor systemic perfusion. With severe pneumoperitoneum, respiratory function is compromised requiring urgent intubation. Typically, the abdomen is markedly distended and tympanitic to percussion. Pneumoperitoneum is usually present in these infants. The clinical course of neonates with spontaneous gastrointestinal perforation may mimic those of NEC or other diseases associated with perforation (Grosfeld et al. 1996).

83.5 Diagnosis

In case of rare disease causing emergencies, the diagnosis can be difficult, but it is possible to research clinical grounds of intestinal obstruction or perforation.

In case of occlusion, flat and upright abdominal radiographs are obtained to confirm the diagnosis. Swallowed air serves as the contrast media to help delineate the level of obstruction. A normal neonate swallows air from birth and has air within the proximal small bowel within 30 min. Air usually reaches the colon by 3–4 h and can be identified in the rectum by 6–8 h. There should be no air-fluid levels in an upright film of a normal newborn (Steves and Ricketts 1987).

When a complete obstruction exists, the air pattern may stop abruptly leaving the remainder of the bowel airless. Bowel loops proximal to complete obstruction are dilated. Multiple dilated loops of the bowel with “stepladder” air-fluid levels on

the upright film are the pattern most often seen with distal intestinal obstruction. However, air-fluid levels are not characteristic of the distal intestinal obstruction due to meconium ileus. Partial obstructions as in stenosis may allow small amounts of air to pass beyond the level of obstruction, but the paucity of bowel gas in the bowel distal to dilated bowel segments can easily be identified as abnormal. The abdominal films should always be inspected for peritoneal and/or scrotal calcifications which may signify an intrauterine perforation with meconium peritonitis.

Barium or gastrografin contrast enema examination may be useful to distinguish between causes of distal bowel obstruction (ileal atresia, meconium ileus, Hirschsprung's disease, meconium plug, etc.) and in cases of meconium ileus or plug may also be therapeutic. Upper gastrointestinal barium studies are generally not as useful unless one is seeking patterns of abnormal bowel rotation. UGI contrast studies are reserved for cases of partial obstruction that cannot be confirmed by plain radiographs (Rosser et al. 1982). Under the suspicion of perforation, the contrast study is strictly unrecommended, and the diagnosis is confirmed by plain abdominal x-rays (flat and decubitus views) that demonstrate free intraperitoneal air. Serial abdominal films are to be obtained if perforation cannot be demonstrated initially but remains highly suspected (Grosfeld et al. 1996).

Additional laboratory evaluation includes blood cultures, blood leukocyte and platelet counts, arterial blood gases, and serum pH, especially in case of appendicitis.

83.6 Treatment

The specific management strategies and surgical considerations for the various conditions causing intestinal obstruction in the neonate are not described in this chapter. However, the initial treatment of any suspected neonatal obstruction includes placement of a nasogastric tube to decompress the stomach and to prevent vomiting/aspiration. Fluid and electrolyte replacement should be quickly undertaken to resuscitate the infant and restore circulating blood volume in anticipation of the potential need for surgical intervention. Most obstructive lesions in neonates will require surgical therapy and surgery should not be delayed once volume resuscitation is adequate. If an intestinal anastamosis is anticipated, perioperative antibiotics are indicated (De la Hunt 2006).

In the presence of clinical and radiological signs of perforation, treatment commences as soon as possible, simultaneous to the diagnostic workup. Rapid deterioration is anticipated and prevented with aggressive fluid resuscitation, intravenous antibiotics, correction of acid-base disturbances, and nasogastric decompression. Intubation and ventilatory support is required in infants with respiratory distress. Aspiration of the massively distended pneumoperitoneum can be helpful in infants with severe life-threatening respiratory compromise. Surgical exploration is indicated. The site of perforation is identified although in up to 10% of cases, the perforation site has sealed spontaneously and cannot be identified. Surgical treatment is dictated by the infant physiologic condition and the findings at laparotomy (i.e., site of perforation, tissue condition, soilage, etc.) and includes primary repair, resection with external diversion, resection with anastamosis, drainage, etc. Obstruction distal to the site of perforation is excluded whenever possible (Weinberg et al. 1989). It's not already clear the role of minivasive surgery (MIS) in case of neonatal occlusion or perforation. Without any critical sign of occlusion or perforation, MIS could be an alternative treatment in case of rare abdominal malformation.

83.7 Outcomes

A multidisciplinary team of surgeons, anesthetists, neonatologists, radiologists, cardiologists, obstetricians, nurses, physiotherapists, and other health professionals experienced in dealing with extremely small infants will provide the best outcome.

The outcomes from neonatal intestinal obstruction or perforation vary with the etiology of the disease. Overall survival is generally good but often is influenced by the associated anomalies of each condition (Raffensperger et al. 1970; Lim et al. 1994).

The prognosis is adversely affected by prematurity, the presence of other anomalies, and a delay in diagnosis (Weinberg et al. 1989; Angotti et al. 2014).

References

Angotti R, Bulotta AL, Ferrara F, Molinaro F, Cerchia E, Meucci D, Messina M (2014) Uncommon surgical emergencies in neonatology. Pediatr Med Chir 36(5–6):99

De la Hunt MN (2006) The acute abdomen in the newborn. Semin Fetal Neonatal Med 11:191–197

Filston HC (1998) Other causes of intestinal obstruction. In: O'Neill JA Jr et al (eds) Pediatric surgery, 5th edn. Mosby, St. Louis, pp 1215–1221

Grosfeld JL et al (1996) Gastrointestinal perforation and peritonitis in infants and children: experience with 179 cases over ten years. Surgery 120:650

Lim CT, Yip CH, Chang KW (1994) Meconium ileus – a rare cause of neonatal intestinal obstruction in Malaysia. Singapore Med J 35(1):74–76

Messina M, Ferruci D, Meucci D, Buonocore G, Di Maggio G (2002) Neonatal intestinal occlusion due to duodenal duplication in association with malformed gallbladder sludge. Biol Neonate 81:210–212

Messina M, Ferrucci E, Garzi A, Meucci D, Buonocore G (2003) A rare case of neonatal ileo-cecal valve stenosis due to covered iliac perforation. Biol Neonate 83:69–72

Messina M, Ferrucci E, Meucci D, Di Maggio G, Molinaro F, Buonocore G (2005) Littre's hernia in newborn infants: report of two cases. Pediatr Surg Int 21:485–487

Puri P (2003) Duplications of the alimentary tract. In: Puri P (ed) Newborn surgery. Arnold, London, pp 479–488

Raffensperger JG, Seeler RA, Moncada R (1970) Intestinal obstruction in the newborn. In: Raffensperger JG et al (eds) The acute abdomen in infancy and childhood. JB Lippincott Company, Philadelphia, pp 1–19

Rosser SB, Clark CH, Elechi EN (1982) Spontaneous neonatal gastric perforation. J Pediatr Surg 17:390–394

Steves M, Ricketts RR (1987) Pneumoperitoneum in the newborn infant. Am Surg 53(4):226–230

Touloukian RJ (1973) Gastric ischemia: the primary factor in neonatal perforation. Clin Pediatr 12:219

Van Veenendaal M, Plötz FB, Nikkels PG, Bax NM (2004) Further evidence for an ischemic origin of perforation of the appendix in the neonatal period. J Pediatr Surg 39(8):e11–e12

Weinberg G, Kleinhaus S, Boley SJ (1989) Idiopathic intestinal perforations in the newborn: an increasingly common entity. J Pediatr Surg 24:1007–1008

Meconium Plug Syndrome

84

Mario Messina, Rossella Angotti, and Francesco Molinaro

Contents

Abstract

Meconium plug syndrome is a relatively common cause of transient functional colon obstruction in newborn, characterized by delayed passage (>24–48 h) of meconium and intestinal dilatation with an obstruction of the colon with thickened plugs of mucus. The incidence is of 1 in 1,000 births. The clinical presentation is the same as that for a distal intestinal obstruction. Most infants present within their first 24–36 h of life. Clinical and radiological signs of meconium plug syndrome can overlap with other disorders. For these reasons, the diagnosis can be difficult.

M. Messina (✉) · F. Molinaro
Department of Pediatrics, Obstetrics and Reproductive Medicine, Section of Pediatric Surgery, Policlinico "Le Scotte", University of Siena, Siena, Italy

Department of Medical, Surgical and Neurological Sciences, Section of Pediatric Surgery, University of Siena, Siena, Italy
e-mail: mario.messina@unisi.it

R. Angotti
Department of Pediatrics, Obstetrics and Reproductive Medicine, Section of Pediatric Surgery, University of Siena, Siena, Italy

G. Buonocore et al. (eds.), *Neonatology*,
https://doi.org/10.1007/978-3-319-29489-6_231

The treatment of the meconium plug is conservative and consists of stimulation of the rectum or colon in some manner. In many cases, simple finger examination of the rectum or insertion of a rectal thermometer produces enough stimulation to induce peristalsis and promote evacuation of the meconium. In other cases, water-soluble contrast enema examination may induce meconium passage.

84.1 Salient Points

- Meconium plug syndrome is a relatively common cause of transient functional colon obstruction in newborn.
- Meconium plug syndrome must be considered as possible diagnosis in newborn with delayed passage (>24–48 h) of meconium and intestinal dilatation with an obstruction.
- The treatment of the meconium plug syndrome is conservative.

84.2 Definition

The term meconium plug syndrome was first reported by Clatworthy in 1956 to describe the colonic obstruction because of the inspissated meconium (Clatworthy et al. 1956). It is a relatively common cause of transient functional colon obstruction in newborn (Burge and Drewett 2004), characterized by delayed passage (>24–48 h) of meconium and intestinal dilatation. In meconium plug syndrome, a newborn has obstruction of the colon with thickened plugs of mucus (Fig. 1). The incidence of meconium plug syndrome is of 1 in 1,000 births (Al-Salem et al. 2014).

84.3 Etiology/Pathogenesis

The exact etiology of meconium plug syndrome is not known, and pathogenesis it is unproved. Several theories have been proposed. However, the main hypothesis, about pathophysiological mechanism, is that it is a transient functional immaturity of the colon. It has been suggested that the immature myenteric nervous system causes ineffective peristalsis and excessive water absorption, producing meconium plugs that obstruct the colon (Coppola 2014).

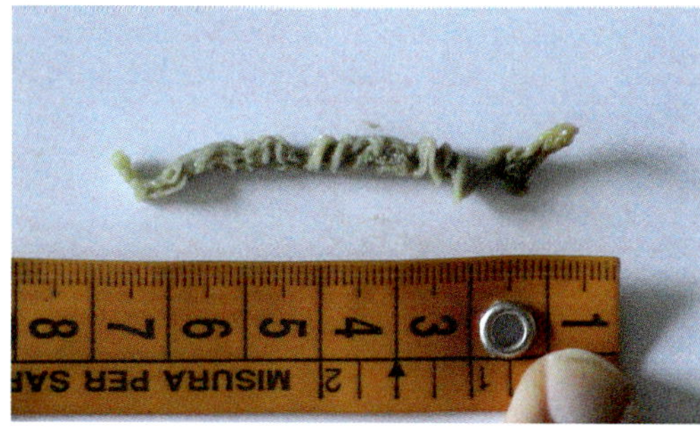

Fig. 1 Female, 4 days old with meconium plug syndrome

84.4 Associated Conditions

Meconium plug syndrome is an isolated disease up to 80% of cases. Generally it is observed in premature newborns that are otherwise normal; however, occasionally it can be associated with an underlying diagnosis. The following disorders may be encountered in order of decreasing frequency (Al-Salem et al. 2014; Coppola 2014):

- *Hirschsprung's disease and cystic fibrosis* in approximately 40% of cases.
- *Hypoglycemia/maternal gestational diabetes* in 40–50% of cases. Maternal gestational diabetes mellitus induces neonatal hypoglycemia which affects intestinal motility via activation of the autonomic nervous system and glucagon release. Glucagon release is known to decrease motility in the left colon. Neonatal hypoglycemia also stimulates the sympathetic and parasympathetic autonomic nervous system. Parasympathetic stimulation results in increased motility in its area of distribution, which ends at the splenic flexure, whereas sympathetic stimulation results in diminished motility.
- *Hypermagnesemia/eclamptic mothers*: infants born to eclamptic mothers treated with magnesium sulfate have a hypermagnesemia that can cause intestinal hypomotility.

- *Maternal drugs (psychotropic)*: maternal drugs used during the third trimester, as psychotropic drugs with known anticholinergic effects, can cross the placenta and affect the fetus, causing an intestinal hypomotility.
- *Sepsis*: it can lead to bowel immotility, and as such, it can mimic meconium plug syndrome.

84.5 Clinical Presentation

The clinical presentation is the same as that for a distal intestinal obstruction. Most infants present within their first 24–36 h of life.

Findings include:

- No passage of meconium (delayed for >48). The term of 48 h, however, should be elongated in premature infant meconium, because in these neonates evacuation may be delayed for days to weeks. The meconium plug syndrome can be considered as differential diagnosis if it is associated with obstructive signs such as distention and vomiting.
- Abdominal distension
- Bilious vomiting
- Difficulty feeding

84.6 Differential Diagnosis

Clinical and radiological signs of meconium plug syndrome can overlap with other disorders. For these reasons, the diagnosis can be difficult. The main disorders that must be considered as differential diagnosis are reportedplug syndrome below:

- Meconium ileus: this is a common cause of delayed or no meconium pass. In this case, thickened meconium blocks the small bowel, rather than the colon, and results in a small diameter colon called microcolon. So, the site of stop of meconium is at two separate locations: ileal obstruction with proximal small bowel dilatation and microcolon in meconium ileus, colon in meconium plug syndrome. Also, it should be considered that meconium ileus can result in perforation, small bowel volvulus, intestinal atresia, and peritonitis (Lim et al. 1994).
- Small left colon syndrome: this is a transient disorder of colon that, in the past, was considered a synonym of meconium plug syndrome. To date, it is known that they are two different disorders of functional obstructions of the colon. Neonatal small left colon syndrome is characterized by an abrupt colonic caliber transition at or near the splenic flexure. Most patients with neonatal small left colon syndrome are born at or near term and are of normal birth weight. However, both disorders have spontaneous resolution within several days or more frequently within 1 month or more (small left colon syndrome) (Mees et al. 1986).

  Hirschsprung's disease/ganglia: it is known that in these cases the main problem is absence of ganglion cells, even if it can be an underlying condition in patients with meconium plug syndrome.
- Imperforate anus/anorectal malformations: these can be diagnosed clinically.
- Ileal atresia: even if clinical picture can be the same and it must be involved in differential diagnosis, abdomen X-ray usually clarifies the situation.

84.7 Diagnosis

- Physical examination: neonate with softly distended abdomen, sometimes with palpable loops of intestine (Keckler et al. 2008). Nasogastric tube aspirate is bilious.
- Abdominal X-ray: the anteroposterior radiograph which includes supine and horizontal beam views (left lateral decubitus or cross-table lateral) shows multiple distended segments of bowel, and often it is impossible to distinguish if distension involves small bowel or colon (Fig. 2). Erect abdominal radiographs, albeit seldom necessary in the newborn, show a paucity of air-fluid levels, and in most cases, no gas is seen in the colon. If air is introduced into the rectum from below (e.g., on rectal examination), rectal gas may be visualized.

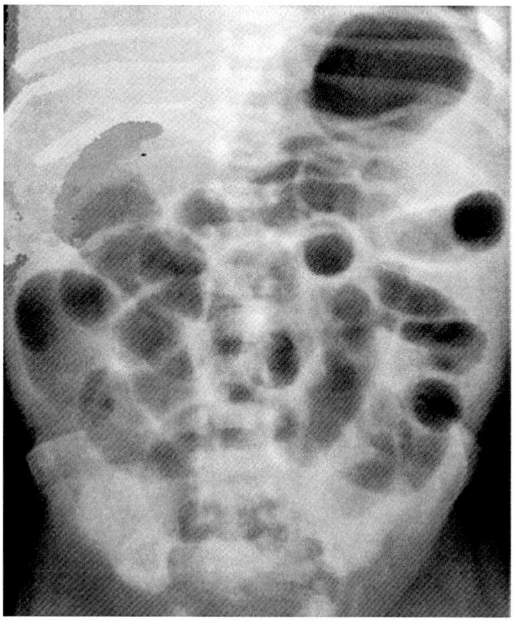

Fig. 2 Male, 1 day old with no meconium passage. Plain X-ray showing distended loops of bowel

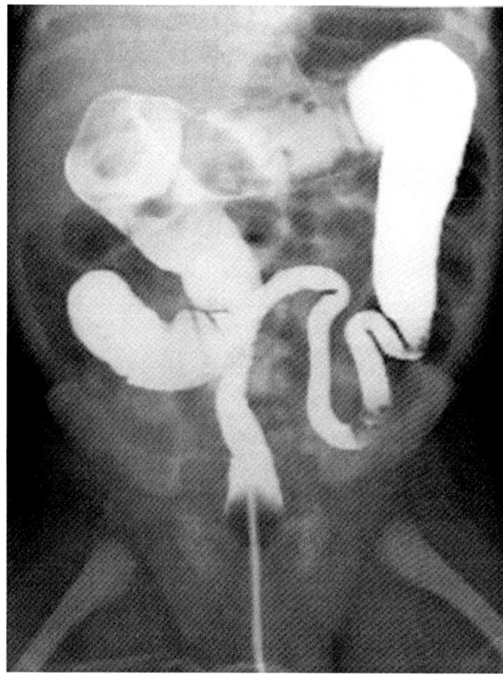

Fig. 3 Male, 1 day old, contrast enema showing microcolon (*left*) and dilated proximal bowel loops. It is evident in the transition zone* between the dilated and the normal-to-decreased caliber distal colon

In this setting, meconium in the rectum can erroneously suggest a small presacral mass. However, if air entirely surrounds the meconium mass, it will outline the contour of the mass and suggests the correct diagnosis. If peristalsis forces gas in from the small bowel into the colon and mixes with the meconium, a granular or bubbly appearance mimicking the findings of pneumatosis cystoides intestinalis and necrotizing enterocolitis (NEC) results. If a bubbly pattern is seen within the first 12 h of life, meconium plug syndrome should be considered, but if it arises after 12–18 h, NEC is more likely. NEC typically occurs in preterm infants (Pilling and Steiner 1981).

- Contrast enema: this study can be both diagnostic and therapeutic. Water-soluble contrast should be used because the risk of perforation and leak is high so the extravasation of barium will cause peritonitis. Also, barium will thicken in the lumen of the colon and can contribute to the obstruction. Contrast enema shows thick plugs and ropes of material occluding the colon and distal bowel (Fig. 3). Irrigation of the colon with the water-soluble contrast can help wash these plugs free and out of the body, and it can be sometimes therapeutic (Burge and Drewett 2004; Swischuk 1968).
- Chloride sweat testing: this test must be done to exclude or confirm the presence of cystic fibrosis that can be associated with meconium plug syndrome. However, the main limit of this test is weight of neonate that must be a minimum of 3 kg (Burge and Drewett 2004; Swischuk 1968).
- Suction rectal biopsy: also this exam could be necessary because some patients with meconium plug syndrome have Hirschsprung's disease which is diagnosed by absence of ganglion cells on a rectal biopsy (Burge and Drewett 2004; Swischuk 1968).

84.8 Management

- The treatment of the meconium plug is conservative and consists of stimulation of the rectum or colon in some manner. In many cases, simple finger examination of the rectum or insertion of a rectal thermometer produces enough

stimulation to induce peristalsis and promote evacuation of the meconium. In other cases, water-soluble contrast enema examination may induce meconium passage. Examinations with contrast materials such as these require care regarding the patient's fluid and electrolyte balance (Burke et al. 2002; Swischuk 1997; Rescorla and Grosfeld 1993). With conservative treatment, complete decompression usually occurs within hours. However, in some infants, the first contrast enema is no therapeutic, and they can be treated with serial rectal irrigations with or without acetylcysteine that can lose the thickened secretions. If it is not useful, contrast enema may take up to 2–3 days. Rarely, these children need surgical approach.

84.9 Contrast Enema Technique

- Perform the enema with attention to the delicate temperature stability of the newborn infant. Use blankets and lamps and warm the contrast to body temperature.
- Advance a small-caliber soft, rubber catheter (10–14 F) into the rectum using minimal lubricant. Hold the catheter in place primarily by taping the patient's buttocks tightly together.
- Some radiologists deploy a small Foley balloon (5 mL) to aid contrast retention. However, do not inflate the balloon until a preliminary injection of a small amount of contrast under fluoroscopy demonstrates adequate caliber of the rectum. Initial injection without an inflated balloon also assesses for a possible low-transition zone in patients with Hirschsprung disease.
- Because the internal volume of the colon may be low, at the author's institution, contrast is injected by hand using a syringe under careful and almost continuous fluoroscopic monitoring. Others use a low-capacity reservoir, such as an intravenous bag, and infuse via gravity drip.
- Opacity the entire colon both to maximize the therapeutic effect of the enema and to identify the position of the cecum.
- Carefully attempt to reflux contrast into the distal ileum in patients who may have meconium ileus.
- After the colon has been filled and the appropriate films obtained, remove the catheter without attempting to drain the colon. Allowing the patient to expel the contrast may help dislodge the meconium plug.

Response to the enema often is dramatic, with immediate passage of meconium and resolution of intestinal dilatation. In some patients, clinical findings persist, and a second enema is performed for therapy.

84.10 Surgical Procedures

Rarely meconium plug requires a surgical procedure. However, in this case, the main aim of surgery is a temporary decompression of dilated bowel that means a temporary ileostomy. The most simple form is a double-barreled ileostomy according to Mikulicz, with the two loops brought out side-to-side. This solution is quick and avoids an intra-abdominal anastomosis. Similar type of temporary ileostomy is with a skin bridge (Fig. 4) that is simpler to perform, and it ensures a better aesthetical result.

More technical alternatives have been described thereafter: a distal ileostomy with end-to-side ileal anastomosis (Bishop-Koop) has been called "distal chimney enterostomy." This procedure consists of a Roux-en-Y anastomosis between the end of the proximal segment and the side of the distal segment, at least 3–5 cm from the open end. The open limb of the distal segment is used as an ileostomy. A variation of this technique has been described, using an angulating proximal segment, which is obliquely anastomosed with the distal stump. Proximal chimney enterostomy, the so-called Santulli procedure, consists of a proximal ileostomy with end-to-side ileal anastomosis. The end of the distal limb is anastomosed to the side of the proximal limb, the end of which is used as the enterostomy. This technique should facilitate irrigation as well as decompression of the proximal small bowel. The enterostomies can be closed by an end-to-end anastomosis when uninhibited passage of intestinal contents is established, mostly between 7 and 12 days after.

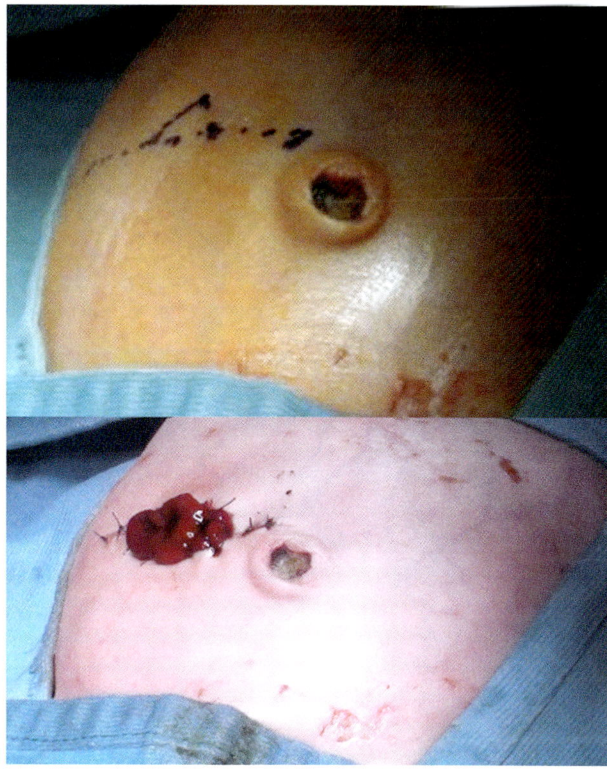

Fig. 4 Male, 1 day old, who underwent surgery. Temporary ileostomy with a skin bridge (intraoperative findings)

84.11 Prognosis

Prognosis is excellent, if no underlying disease is present (Fuchs and Langer 1998)

Main points of meconium plug syndrome
It is a transient functional disorder of the colon
It is frequent in premature patients
It is different disorder from small left colon syndrome
Clinical and radiological signs can overlap with other disorders of distal obstruction
The treatment of the meconium plug is conservative

References

Al-Salem H (2014) Meconium plug syndrome. In: An illustrated guide to pediatric surgery. Springer International Publishing, Switzerland, pp 195–197

Burge D, Drewett M (2004) Meconium plug obstruction. Pediatr Surg Int 20:108–110

Burke MS, Ragi JM, Karamanoukian HL, Kotter M, Brisseau GF, Borowitz DS, Ryan ME, Irish MS, Glick PL (2002) New strategies in nonoperative management of meconium ileus. J Pediatr Surg 37:760–764

Clatworthy HW Jr, Howard WH, Lloyd J (1956) The meconium plug syndrome. Surgery 39(1):131–142

Coppola CP (2014) Meconium plug syndrome and meconium ileus. In: Pediatric surgery. Springer International Publishing, Switzerland, pp 183–185

Fuchs JR, Langer JC (1998) Long-term outcome after neonatal meconium obstruction. Pediatrics 101:4–7

Keckler SJ, St Peter SD, Spilde TL, Tsao K, Ostlie DJ, Holcomb GW 3rd, Snyder CL (2008) Current significance of meconium plug syndrome. J Pediatr Surg 43(5):896–898

Lim CT, Yip CH, Chang KW (1994) Meconium ileus-a rare cause of neonatal intestinal obstruction in Malaysia. Singap Med J 35(1):74–76

Mees WJ, Kramer PP, Bax NM (1986) The small left colon in newborn infants. Tijdschr Kindergeneeskd 54(5):143–147

Pilling DW, Steiner GM (1981) The radiology of meconium ileus equivalent. Br J Radiol 54(643):562–565

Rescorla FJ, Grosfeld JL (1993) Contemporary management of meconium ileus. World J Surg 17(3):318–325

Swischuk LE (1968) Meconium plug syndrome: a cause of neonatal intestinal obstruction. Am J Roentgenol Radium Ther Nucl Med 103(2):339–346

Swischuk LE (1997) Imaging of the newborn, infant, and young child, 4th edn. Lippincott, Williams & Wilkins, Philadelphia

Hirschsprung's Disease in Newborns 85

Girolamo Mattioli, Maria Grazia Faticato, Alessio Pini Prato, and Vincenzo Jasonni

Contents

Abstract

Hirschsprung's disease, first described by Harald Hirschsprung in 1886, is one of the most common causes of intestinal obstruction in the newborn.

The disease occurs in roughly 1 in 5000 live births with a strong male preponderance and results as a consequence of abnormal migration of neural crest-derived neuroblasts that determines congenital absence of intestinal intramural ganglia within the enteric nervous system (ENS) with variable distal bowel involvement.

Symptoms range from neonatal intestinal obstruction to chronic progressive constipation in older children; a common severe complication presenting in many patients is enterocolitis.

The gold standard for the diagnosis of Hirschsprung is rectal suction biopsy.

The treatment is surgical and involves removing the aganglionic bowel and reconstructing the intestinal tract by bringing the normally innervated bowel down to the anus.

G. Mattioli (✉) · M. G. Faticato · V. Jasonni
Department of Pediatric Surgery, University of Genoa, Genoa, Italy

Giannina Gaslini Institute, Genoa, Italy
e-mail: girolamomattioli@ospedale-gaslini.ge.it; girolamomattioli@gaslini.org; mgfaticato@gmail.com; vincenzojasonni@ospedale-gaslini.ge.it

A. Pini Prato
Giannina Gaslini Institute, Genoa, Italy
e-mail: a.piniprato@gmail.com

85.1 Salient Points

- Hirschsprung's disease (HSCR) is one of the most common causes of intestinal obstruction in the newborn.

G. Buonocore et al. (eds.), *Neonatology*,
https://doi.org/10.1007/978-3-319-29489-6_232

- Mutations affecting the RET proto-oncogene on chromosome 10q11.2 were identified in HSCR patients.
- Hirschsprung-associated enterocolitis (HAEC) represents the most severe complication of the disease.
- The gold standard for the diagnosis of HSCR is rectal suction biopsy.
- Laparoscopic-assisted endorectal pull-through (Soave-Georgeson technique) is the procedure of choice both in newborns and infants with HSCR.

85.2 Introduction

Although sporadic reports of patients with suggestive clinical features are dated back to the seventeenth century, the first telling and concise description of the disease is that of Sir Harald Hirschsprung, a Danish pediatrician who reported the details of his series of two patients at the Society of Pediatrics in Berlin in 1886.

Hirschsprung's disease (HSCR) is one of the most common causes of intestinal obstruction in the newborn. The disease occurs as a consequence of abnormal migration/differentiation of the neural crest-derived neuroblasts into the developing gut; this determines absence of intestinal intramural ganglia. Synonyms of HSCR are congenital megacolon and intestinal aganglionosis that indicate severe bowel loops distension and absence of intramural ganglia, respectively. Most patients present in infancy, and early diagnosis is important to avoid complications. Overall prognosis is good. In fact, with proper treatment most patients live normal adult lives (Holschneider and Puri 2000).

85.3 Etiology and Pathogenesis

The disease is caused by the failure of the neural crest-derived neuroblasts to migrate cranio-caudally during weeks 5–12 of gestation. This abnormal migration determines congenital absence of intestinal intramural ganglia within the enteric nervous system (ENS) (myenteric and submucosal plexuses) with variable distal bowel involvement. This intrinsic innervation is named "gut mini brain" or enteric nervous system and coordinates movements, immune functions, and secretion of the gut. Subsequently, its abnormality determines functional bowel obstruction and facilitates the onset of severe infections known as Hirschsprung-associated enterocolitis (HAEC), which represents the most severe complication of the disease.

The pathogenesis is still unclear, but recent studies suggest that the intestinal microbiota contributes to the etiology of enterocolitis and may play an important role in the development of the disease (Frykman et al. 2015).

The diseased bowel begins at the pectinate line (anal canal shows physiologic aganglionosis) and extends proximally with variable distal bowel involvement. Aganglionosis extending up to the splenic flexure of the colon is named classic or rectosigmoid HSCR (most frequent, accounts for up to 80% of cases); the one extending beyond (confined within the large bowel) is named long HSCR (10%); whereas the one involving the whole large bowel (usually extending to at least 5–7 cm of terminal ileum) is defined total colonic aganglionosis (TCSA) or ultralong HSCR (10%). Total intestinal aganglionosis (TIA) is extremely rare and is nearly incompatible with life, even though the advent of parenteral nutrition, innovative surgical techniques, and small bowel transplantation have improved survival (Holschneider and Puri 2000; Coran and Teitelbaum 2000; Loening-Baucke and Kimura 1999; Ruttenstock and Puri 2009).

This is a complex genetic disease as suggested by the high proportion of sporadic cases, variable expressivity, incomplete sex-dependent penetrance, and variable risk of sibling recurrence. In 1994, mutations affecting the RET proto-oncogene on chromosome 10q11.2 were identified in HSCR patients, the same being also involved in different diseases such as multiple endocrine neoplasia type 2A and 2B and sporadic and familial medullary thyroid carcinoma. Since then, loss-of-function of RET tyrosine-kinase has been demonstrated in approximately 50% of familial and 10–15% of sporadic HSCR cases (Parisi and Kapur 2000; Stewart and von Allmen 2003; Eng 1996; Romeo et al. 1994). Eight other HSCR susceptibility genes

have been identified to date namely GDNF, EDN3, EDNRB, NRTN, ECE1, PHOX2B, SOX10, and ZFHX1B. Amongst these, GDNF belongs to the Ret signaling pathway.

Strong genetic background is also confirmed by the frequent presence of associated anomalies that can basically involve all systems and organs. Association can be either syndromic or not. Down syndrome (trisomy 21) is the most common chromosomal abnormality associated with the disease, accounting for approximately 10% of patients. Other syndromic associations are those with congenital central hypoventilation (Ondine's course), Waardenburg-Shah, Bardet-Biedl, Mowat-Wilson, Goldberg-Shprintzen, and others. Non-syndromic associations are those involving neurologic, cardiovascular, urogenital, gastrointestinal, and skeletal systems, metabolism, or pigmentation. Anomalies that have been encountered in HSCR patients include congenital deafness, refractive anomalies or visual impairment, hydrocephalus, bladder diverticulum, Meckel's diverticulum, imperforate anus, ventricular septal defect, renal agenesis, cryptorchidism, and neuroblastomas. Recent evidence suggested that the incidence of associated anomalies is somehow underestimated with true isolated HSCR being relatively rare (Amiel et al. 2008; Tomita et al. 2003; Pini Prato et al. 2009, 2013).

85.4 Clinical Aspects

HSCR is a congenital disease, which can be familial or sporadic. It occurs in roughly 1 in 5000 live births, but its incidence varies significantly among ethnic groups (1.5, 2.1, and 2.8 per 10,000 live births in Caucasians, African-Americans, and Asians, respectively). There is a strong male preponderance, with a male to female ratio of roughly 4:1. Familial cases are not infrequent. Approximately 3–5% of male siblings and 1% of female siblings of children with classic HSCR also have the disease. However, the risk is substantially higher (12.4–33%) in siblings of children with TCSA.

Symptoms range from neonatal intestinal obstruction to chronic progressive constipation in older children (Table 1). Although meconium delay has long been considered a characteristic feature of HSCR patients, in a review of more than one hundred patients, we demonstrated that "only" 64% percent of infants with Hirschsprung's disease fail to pass meconium in the first 24 h of life (Pini Prato et al. 2008a). More than 90% of HSCR patients had symptom onset before 1 year of age with difficult bowel movements, poor feeding, and progressive abdominal distention. Explosive bowel movements caused by functional colonic obstruction and hyperperistalsis are common in infants with Hirschsprung's disease. In fact, rectal examination may demonstrate a tight anal sphincter and explosive discharge of stool and gas. A small percentage of patients may not have symptoms until later in life. Common symptoms in older children include chronic progressive constipation, recurrent fecal impaction, failure to thrive, and malnutrition. One third of patients with Hirschsprung's disease present with the Hirschsprung associated enterocolitis rather than constipation. This severe and frightening complication is characterized by explosive smelly diarrhea, abdominal distension, and signs of impending septic or hypovolemic shock. HAEC still carries a significant morbidity (need for enterostomy) and mortality range between 5% and 50% (Khan et al. 2003; Hackam et al. 1998; Pini Prato et al. 2008b, 2011).

Table 1 Clinical features of patients with Hirschsprung's disease and incidence of symptoms

Symptoms of Hirschsprung's disease (series of 112 patients) (Pini Prato et al. 2008b)	Incidence (%)
Newborns and infants	
Abdominal distension	94
Difficult bowel movements	92
Failure to pass meconium	63
Intestinal obstruction	61
Failure to thrive	42
Enterocolitis	35
Older children	
Absence of soiling or overflow incontinence (Hackam et al. 1998)	96
Chronic constipation with onset before 1 year of age	96
Progressive abdominal distension	85
Fecal impaction	49
Failure to thrive	27

Though clinical features do not strictly correlate to length of aganglionosis, long HSCR and TCSA tend to have worse clinical features and outcome. Total bowel aganglionosis is extremely rare and is nearly incompatible with life (Pini Prato et al. 2008b, 2011; Menezes et al. 2008).

Based on typical clinical findings, HSCR can be suspected if the child is younger than 12 months at onset, complains of meconium delay, fails to thrive, does not experience overflow incontinence or soiling, and has a tight anal sphincter with empty rectum at physical examination. Symptoms may recur after previously resolving with enemas, laxatives, or feeding changes. Conditions that can mimic HSCR in the neonatal period include cystic fibrosis, meconium plug syndrome, small left colon syndrome, hindgut atresia, anorectal malformations, ENS immaturity of the preterm, hypothyroidism, intestinal neuronal dysplasia, and chronic intestinal pseudo-obstruction (Khan et al. 2003; Martucciello et al. 2005).

85.5 Diagnosis

The gold standard for the diagnosis of HSCR is rectal suction biopsy (RSB) (Pini-Prato et al. 2007). This is a safe and painless procedure that can be accomplished in an outpatient setting. The harvested specimens must be taken 1, 3 and 5 cm above the pectinate line and should contain enough submucosa to properly assess the ENS. It should be processed with histochemical and enzyme histochemical staining techniques including acetylcholinesterase, alpha-naftylesterase, NADPH-diaphorase, succinic and lactic dehydrogenases, and nitric oxide synthase for innervative assessment, and toluidine blue or hematoxylin and eosin for gross histology. The diagnostic features include absence of ganglia and thick parasympathetic nerve trunks in the submucosa and increased achetycholinesterase activity in the lamina propria (Bruder and Meier-Ruge 2010).

The diagnostic accuracy of RSB is close to 100% after 1 month of age but must be taken with care in the newborn or preterm who can only partially express all diagnostic features. In order to improve the diagnosis of HSCR, we implemented an innovative instrument to perform safe RSB at the bedside of both newborn and adult patients, which was named Solo-RBT. We reported a series of 389 biopsies performed with the instrument Solo-RBT with an incidence of complications (bleeding, perforation) lower than 1% (Martucciello et al. 2001; Pini Prato et al. 2001, 2006). Imaging can help diagnose Hirschsprung's disease. A plain abdominal radiograph may show a dilated small bowel or proximal colon. Contrast enema radiographs of the colon are commonly normal for the first few months of life and indefinitely in patients with total colonic disease. After the dilation process begins, the diseased portion of the colon will appear normal and the more proximal colon will be dilated. A "transition zone" (passage from aganglionic to normoganglionic bowel) may be visible on a contrast enema radiograph. However, the aganglionic colon will extend beyond this point in about 10% of patients (Proctor et al. 2003). Fig. 1 shows contrast enema radiographs of an infant with Hirschsprung's disease. Anal manometry (balloon distention of the rectum) demonstrates the absence of internal anal sphincter relaxation upon rectal distention. Contrast enema and anal manometry are similar in sensitivity and specificity and can only be used as adjunctive diagnostic tools with the diagnosis only being confirmed by histochemistry with a RSB (Fig. 2). The usefulness of barium enema relies in the possibility of predicting the length of aganglionosis and therefore plan surgical treatment accordingly.

85.6 Treatment

After HSCR is diagnosed, surgery is mandatory. Serial rectal irrigation helps decompress the bowel and prevent enterocolitis in the preoperative period. This treatment is essentially a temporary noninvasive colostomy to decompress the dilated colon. In otherwise healthy newborns with undistended colons and classic HSCR, radical surgery can be attempted primarily. If the child has HAEC, TCSA, or a significantly dilated colon, a decompressive enterostomy (either a colostomy or an ileostomy) can be placed for several months while the child

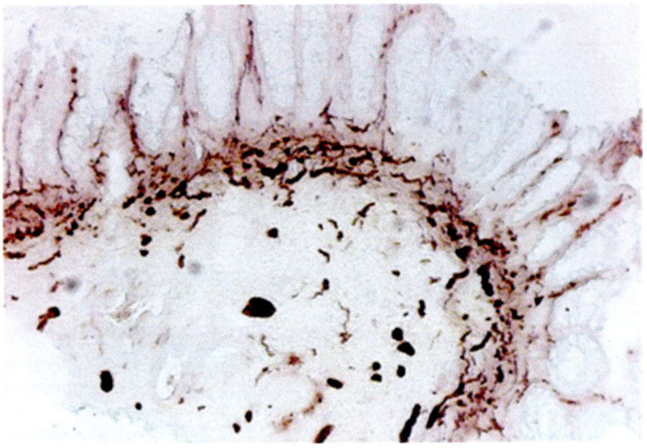

Fig. 1 Rectal suction biopsy of a neonatal Hirschsprung's disease. Acetylcholinesterase staining showing absence of ganglia, thick nerve trunks in the submucosal and increased acetylhcolinesterase activity in the lamina propria

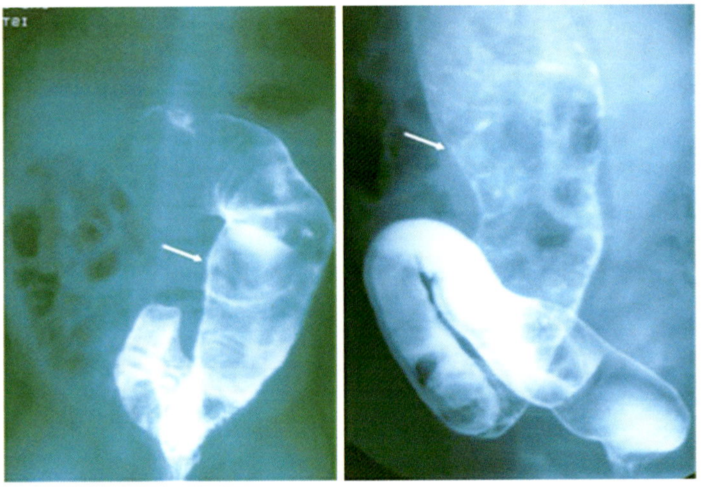

Fig. 2 Barium enema of a 2-month-old baby showing dilated descending colon (*white arrows*). These slides do not clarify the site extent of aganglionosis and the site of normoganglionic colon

recovers. There are several alternative surgical procedures to treat HSCR. All work well provided certain considerations are taken into account: (1) aganglionic bowel must be removed radically, including the rectum down to the sphincters, (2) the normoganglionic bowel must be identified with intraoperative seromuscular biopsies stained with histochemistry avoiding gross anatomical considerations and blind pull-through, (3) an experienced pathologist is required for intraoperative assessment in order to correctly identify the correct site of anastomosis as well as the possible presence of associated hypoganglionosis or intestinal neuronal dysplasia, and (4) surgeons must be well experienced to achieve better results and reduce the incidence of complications. The radical resection of the aganglionic bowel can be performed either with an endorectal, retrorectal, or perirectal approach (Soave, Duhamel, or Swenson procedure, respectively) depending on the surgeon's attitude. We have operated many patients since 1991, and we adopted either endorectal, retrorectal, or perirectal approaches with similar results (Pini Prato et al. 2008a). The advent of laparoscopy has modified the surgical approach and HSCR treatment changed accordingly (Mattioli et al. 2008; Langer et al. 2003; Ekema et al. 2003). The most frequently employed technique is, currently, the Soave-Georgeson technique, which embraces the advantages of the endorectal pull-through and those of the minimally invasive surgery (Figs. 3, 4, and 5) (Ekema et al. 2003).

We reviewed the results of a series of patients who underwent the Soave-Georgeson procedure

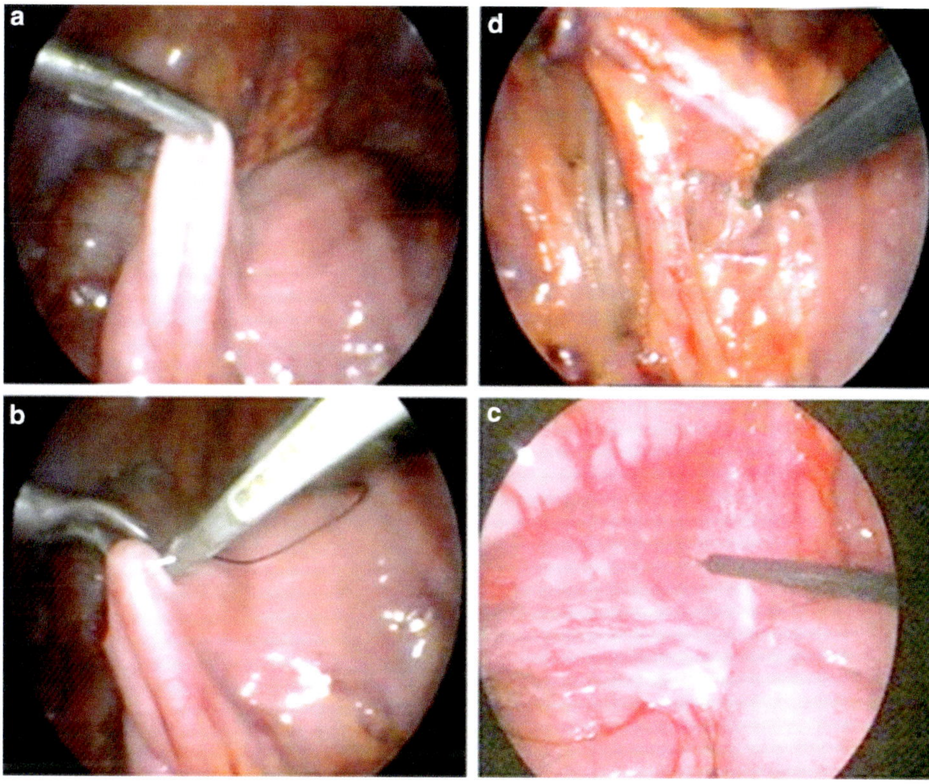

Fig. 3 Laparoscopic pictures of the intracorporeal steps of Soave-Georgeson technique. Anticlockwise: (**a**) Identification of the distended and hypertrophic colon, site of the seromuscular biopsy, (**b**) seromuscular biopsy to identify normoganglionic bowel, (**c**) commencing the preparation of the aganglionic rectum (newborn patients with virtually transparent mesentery), (**d**) nearly completed preparation of the mesentery before the perianal step of the procedure

Fig. 4 Soave-Georgeson technique: transanorectal pull-through of the aganglionic bowel previously prepared during the laparoscopic step

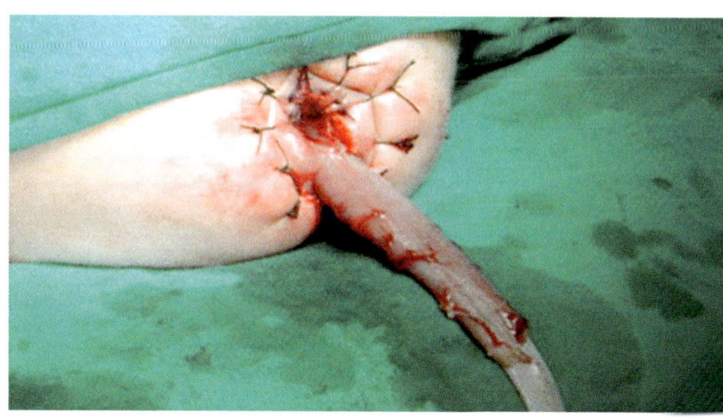

and compared them with those of a matched series of patients who underwent a Soave-Boley procedure (conventional laparotomic procedure). We observed similar results (complications, functional outcome, fecal continence, etc.) but shorter hospitalization and better cosmetic scores.

Recently the robotic approach was introduced in the pediatric surgery but our results in HSCR treatment suggest that robot-assisted procedure may play a role only for older patients affected by the disease (Mattioli et al. 2017).

Basing on these considerations, we concluded that laparoscopic-assisted endorectal pull-through (Soave-Georgeson technique) is the procedure of choice both in newborns and infants with HSCR.

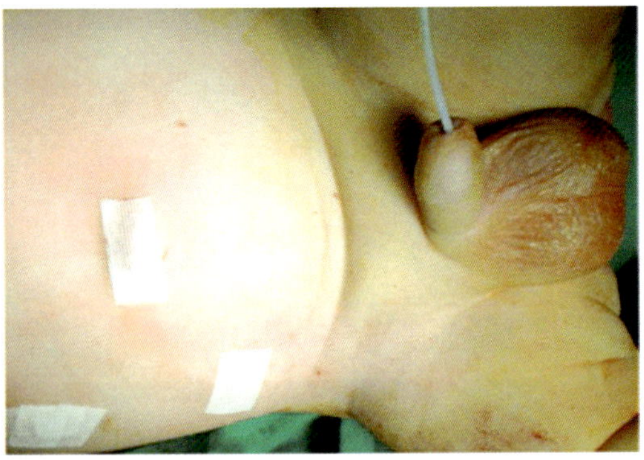

Fig. 5 Soave-Georgeson technique: final cosmetic appearance of the baby's belly

85.7 Prognosis

Mortality rate for HSCR is relatively low, being more frequent in the preoperative period as a result of severe HAEC occurrences (Pini Prato et al. 2011). Although mortality involves mainly newborns or young children, some reports described adult deaths due to septic complications secondary to severe enterocolitis. Postoperative results of the surgical treatment of HSCR appear to be satisfactory. However, despite good overall outcome, some authors showed a higher than expected incidence of problems in the long-term follow-up. Enterocolitis, constipation, failure to thrive, fecal soiling, and incontinence are the most frequent complaints regardless of the surgical technique adopted (Pini Prato et al. 2008a, b; Mattioli et al. 2008). In particular, various reports demonstrated that soiling and incontinence have an important impact on psychosocial functioning and parental criticism, and therefore on quality of life (Pini Prato et al. 2008a, b; Menezes et al. 2008).

There are many strategies for the treatment of these conditions (conservative management, pharmacological therapy, neuromodulation techniques, surgical intervention such as posterior sphincter myotomy or myectomy of the internal anal sphincter) (Ng et al. 2015). An alternative proposed management plan is the use of botulinum toxin (which is inoculated at the level of the internal anal sphincter), aiming for inducing a reversible relaxation of the internal anal sphincter (Han-Geurts et al. 2014).

Outcome of classic (rectosigmoid) HSCR can be hardly compared to that of ultralong HSCR (total colonic aganglionosis) as it is well known that the latter implies a significantly worse prognosis. Nonetheless, various reports demonstrated that overall outcome of HSCR improves with time and that this occurs during the whole childhood up to adolescence or adulthood.

In a series of 112 patients with HSCR, we observed a 15% incidence of complications (residual achalasia, stricture, adhesions, leakage, postoperative constipation, and enterocolitis) in the classic HSCR group and roughly 60% in the TCSA group. This confirmed that outcome is significantly interfered by extent of aganglionosis. With regard to long-term outcome, we observed overall good functional results. In particular, we observed 85% of excellent to good continence in the classic HSCR group of patients and 69% in the TCSA group. Psychological self-acceptance scored good to fair in 80% of classic HSCR and 55% of TCSA. Patients' perspectives were excellent to good in 98% and 100% of patients, respectively. Cosmetic results were excellent to good in 75% of classic HSCR and 18% of TCSA patients. Overall good expectations are reasonable but a number of patients with persistent issues can occur (Pini Prato et al. 2008a).

In the case of a redo operation, we can expect similar long-term results and outcome provided experienced surgeons and pathologists cooperate in the radical treatment. In our series, patients who underwent a redo pull-through for various reasons experienced results that do not significantly differ from those of a single pull-through. This allows optimistic expectations but suggests centralization of care in order to achieve the best for patients.

References

Amiel J, Sproat-Emison E, Garcia-Barcelo M, Lantieri F, Burzynski G, Borrego S, Pelet A, Arnold S, Miao X, Griseri P, Brooks AS, Antinolo G, de Pontual L, Clement-Ziza M, Munnich A, Kashuk C, West K, Wong KK, Lyonnet S, Chakravarti A, Tam PK, Ceccherini I (2008) Hirschsprung disease, associated syndromes and genetics: a review. J Med Genet 45(1):1. https://doi.org/10.1136/jmg.2007.053959

Bruder E, Meier-Ruge WA (2010) Twenty years diagnostic competence center for Hirschsprung's disease in Basel. Chirurg 81(6):572. https://doi.org/10.1007/s00104-010-1924-4

Coran AG, Teitelbaum DH (2000) Recent advances in the management of Hirschsprung's disease. Am J Surg 180(5):382. https://doi.org/10.1016/S0002-9610(00)00487-6

Ekema G, Falchetti D, Torri F, Merulla VE, Manciana A, Caccia G (2003) Further evidence on totally transanal one-stage pull-through procedure for Hirschsprung's disease. J Pediatr Surg 38(10):14577064

Eng C (1996) Seminars in medicine of the Beth Israel hospital, Boston. The RET proto-oncogene in multiple endocrine neoplasia type 2 and Hirschsprung's disease. N Engl J Med 335(13):943. https://doi.org/10.1056/NEJM199609263351307

Frykman PK, Nordenskjöld A, Kawaguchi A, Hui TT, Granström AL, Cheng J, Tang J, Underhill DM, Iliev I, Funari VA, Wester T, HAEC Collaborative Research Group (HCRG). Characterization of bacterial and fungal microbiome in children with Hirschsprung disease with and without a history of enterocolitis: a multicenter study. Worcester: Reeta Prusty Rao, Worcester Polytechnic Institute, 2015, 10(4). https://doi.org/10.1371/journal.pone.0124172

Hackam DJ, Filler RM, Pearl RH (1998) Enterocolitis after the surgical treatment of Hirschsprung's disease: risk factors and financial impact. J Pediatr Surg 33(6):9660207

Han-Geurts IJ, Hendrix VC, de Blaauw I, Wijnen MH, van Heurn EL (2014) Outcome after anal intrasphincteric Botox injection in children with surgically treated Hirschsprung disease. J Pediatr Gastroenterol Nutr 59(5):604. https://doi.org/10.1097/MPG.0000000000000483

Holschneider AM, Puri P (2000) Hirschsprung's disease and allied disorders, 2nd edn. Harwood Academic Publishers, Amsterdam

Khan AR, Vujanic GM, Huddart S (2003) The constipated child: how likely is Hirschsprung's disease? Pediatr Surg Int 19(6):439. https://doi.org/10.1007/s00383-002-0934-9

Langer JC, Durrant AC, de la Torre L, Teitelbaum DH, Minkes RK, Caty MG, Wildhaber BE, Ortega SJ, Hirose S, Albanese CT (2003) One-stage transanal soave pullthrough for Hirschsprung disease: a multicenter experience with 141 children. Ann Surg 238(4):569. https://doi.org/10.1097/01.sla.0000089854.00436.cd

Loening-Baucke V, Kimura K (1999) Failure to pass meconium: diagnosing neonatal intestinal obstruction. Am Fam Physician 60(7):10569507

Martucciello G, Favre A, Torre M, Pini Prato A, Jasonni V (2001) A new rapid acetylcholinesterase histochemical method for the intraoperative diagnosis of Hirschsprung's disease and intestinal neuronal dysplasia. Eur J Pediatr Surg 11(5):300. https://doi.org/10.1055/s-2001-18557

Martucciello G, Pini Prato A, Puri P, Holschneider AM, Meier-Ruge W, Jasonni V, Tovar JA, Grosfeld JL (2005) Controversies concerning diagnostic guidelines for anomalies of the enteric nervous system: a report from the fourth international symposium on Hirschsprung's disease and related neurocristopathies. J Pediatr Surg 40(10):1527. https://doi.org/10.1016/j.jpedsurg.2005.07.053

Mattioli G, Pini Prato A, Giunta C, Avanzini S, Della Rocca M, Montobbio G, Parodi S, Rapuzzi G, Georgeson K, Jasonni V (2008) Outcome of primary endorectal pull-through for the treatment of classic Hirschsprung disease. J Laparoendosc Adv Surg Tech A 18(6):869. https://doi.org/10.1089/lap.2007.0223

Mattioli G, Pio L, Leonelli L, Razore B, Disma N, Montobbio G, Jasonni V, Petralia P, Pini PA (2017) A provisional experience with robot-assisted soave procedure for older children with Hirschsprung disease: back to the future? J Laparoendosc Adv Surg Tech A 25:546. https://doi.org/10.1089/lap.2016.0337

Menezes M, Pini Prato A, Jasonni V, Puri P (2008) Long-term clinical outcome in patients with total colonic aganglionosis: a 31-year review. J Pediatr Surg 43(9):1696. https://doi.org/10.1016/j.jpedsurg.2008.01.072

Ng J, Ford K, Dalton S, McDowell S, Charlesworth P, Cleeve S (2015) Transanal irrigation for intractable faecal incontinence and constipation: outcomes, quality of life and predicting non-adopters. Pediatr Surg Int 31(8):729. https://doi.org/10.1007/s00383-015-3735-7

Parisi MA, Kapur RP (2000) Genetics of Hirschsprung disease. Curr Opin Pediatr 12(6):11106284

Pini Prato A, Martucciello G, Jasonni V (2001) Solo-RBT: a new instrument for rectal suction biopsies in the diagnosis of Hirschsprung's disease. J Pediatr Surg 36(9):11528606

Pini-Prato A, Martucciello G, Jasonni V (2006) Rectal suction biopsy in the diagnosis of intestinal dysganglionoses: 5-year experience with Solo-RBT in 389 patients. J Pediatr Surg 41(6):1043. https://doi.org/10.1016/j.jpedsurg.2006.01.070

Pini-Prato A, Avanzini S, Gentilino V, Martucciello G, Mattioli G, Coccia C, Parodi S, Bisio GM, Jasonni V (2007) Rectal suction biopsy in the workup of childhood chronic constipation: indications and diagnostic value. Pediatr Surg Int 23(2):117. https://doi.org/10.1007/s00383-006-1845-y

Pini Prato A, Gentilino V, Giunta C, Avanzini S, Parodi S, Mattioli G, Martucciello G, Jasonni V (2008a) Hirschsprung's disease: 13 years' experience in 112 patients from a single institution. Pediatr Surg Int 24(2):175. https://doi.org/10.1007/s00383-007-2089-1

Pini Prato A, Gentilino V, Giunta C, Avanzini S, Mattioli G, Parodi S, Martucciello G, Jasonni V (2008b) Hirschsprung disease: do risk factors of poor surgical outcome exist? J Pediatr Surg 43(4):612. https://doi.org/10.1016/j.jpedsurg.2007.10.007

Pini Prato A, Musso M, Ceccherini I, Mattioli G, Giunta C, Ghiggeri GM, Jasonni V (2009) Hirschsprung disease

and congenital anomalies of the kidney and urinary tract (CAKUT): a novel syndromic association. Medicine (Baltimore) 88(2):83. https://doi.org/10.1097/MD.0b013e31819cf5da

Pini Prato A, Rossi V, Avanzini S, Mattioli G, Disma N, Jasonni V (2011) Hirschsprung's disease: what about mortality? Pediatr Surg Int 27(5):473. https://doi.org/10.1007/s00383-010-2848-2

Pini Prato A, Rossi V, Mosconi M, Holm C, Lantieri F, Griseri P, Ceccherini I, Mavilio D, Jasonni V, Tuo G, Derchi M, Marasini M, Magnano G, Granata C, Ghiggeri G, Priolo E, Sposetti L, Porcu A, Buffa P, Mattioli G (2013) A prospective observational study of associated anomalies in Hirschsprung's disease. Orphanet J Rare Dis 8:184. https://doi.org/10.1186/1750-1172-8-184

Proctor ML, Traubici J, Langer JC, Gibbs DL, Ein SH, Daneman A, Kim PC (2003) Correlation between radiographic transition zone and level of aganglionosis in Hirschsprung's disease: implications for surgical approach. J Pediatr Surg 38(5):775. https://doi.org/10.1016/jpsu.2003.50165

Romeo G, Ronchetto P, Luo Y, Barone V, Seri M, Ceccherini I, Pasini B, Bocciardi R, Lerone M, Kääriäinen H, Martucciello G (1994) Point mutations affecting the tyrosine kinase domain of the RET proto-oncogene in Hirschsprung's disease. Nature 367(6461):377. https://doi.org/10.1038/367377a0

Ruttenstock E, Puri P (2009) A meta-analysis of clinical outcome in patients with total intestinal aganglionosis. Pediatr Surg Int 25(10):833. https://doi.org/10.1007/s00383-009-2439-2

Stewart DR, von Allmen D (2003) The genetics of Hirschsprung disease. Gastroenterol Clin N Am 32(3):14562576

Tomita R, Ikeda T, Fujisaki S, Shibata M, Tanjih K (2003) Upper gut motility of Hirschsprung's disease and its allied disorders in adults. Hepato-Gastroenterology 50(54):14696442

Gastroenteritis and Intractable Diarrhea in Newborns

86

Andrea De Luca and Giacomo Zanelli

Contents

A. De Luca (✉)
Department of Medical Biotechnologies, University of Siena, Siena, Italy

UOC Malattie Infettive Universitarie, Azienda Ospedaliera Universitaria Senese, Siena, Italy
e-mail: deluca.andrea2308@icloud.com

G. Zanelli
Department of Medical Biotechnologies, University of Siena, Siena, Italy
e-mail: giacomo.zanelli@unisi.it

G. Buonocore et al. (eds.), *Neonatology*,
https://doi.org/10.1007/978-3-319-29489-6_233

Abstract

Gastroenteritis (GE) still represents a major cause of morbidity and mortality in children worldwide. Although the implementation of effective measures resulted in a significant decrease of global mortality, much remains to be done. The burden of GE in the neonatal age

is generally reduced in relation to some protective factors (breastfeeding, minimal exposure to water and contaminated food, passive maternal immunity). In newborns, the contribution of the various causative agents could differ from that of the other pediatric age groups, nevertheless *Rotavirus* and pathogenic strains of *E. coli* remain the main etiologies. The acquisition of the pathogen generally occurs through the contaminated birth canal or by the use of contaminated tools, objects, or hands of the caregivers. The clinical presentation may vary widely from an acute, self-limiting disease to life-threatening complicated infections. The assessment of the dehydration and its rapid correction represent the cornerstones of the management of any GE. Antibiotic therapy should be reserved to cases with systemic symptoms, severe dehydration, or in the presence of bloody diarrhea. While the occurrence of diarrhea in the neonatal age is mainly caused by acute gastrointestinal infections, differential diagnosis with several other diseases including forms of severe congenital disorders should be considered.

86.1 Salient Points

- Gastroenteritis represents a major global public health challenge due to their significant impact in infants' morbidity and mortality.
- The burden of gastrointestinal infections in newborns is generally reduced in relation to some protective factors such as exclusive breastfeeding.
- *Rotavirus* and pathogenic strains of *E. coli* represent the main etiological agents of childhood gastroenteritis, probably also in newborns.
- Oral or intravenous rehydration therapy is the mainstay of the management of any gastrointestinal infection.
- Consensus exists about the importance of improving safe water supply, adequate sanitation, and proper hygiene for the prevention of diarrheal diseases.

86.2 Introduction

Gastroenteritides (GE) are infections that involve the gastrointestinal tract and are associated with diarrhea with or without vomiting. Usually acute and self-limited, they represent a major cause of morbidity and mortality in less than 5-year-old children worldwide. They may also present a persistent course (lasting more than 14 days), thus contributing to forms of malabsorption and disability. In this chapter, we describe the epidemiology, etiopathogenesis, clinical aspects, and prevention of GE in newborns.

86.3 Epidemiology

It is estimated that about 700,000 children die from infectious diarrhea worldwide each year, and that this number is particularly concentrated in the age group <2 years (Fischer Walker et al. 2013; Bhutta et al. 2013; WHO 2015). While the incidence of diarrhea in children is similar throughout the world (2.7 episodes/child/year), mortality is mainly concentrated in low-middle income countries (Southeast Asia and Africa) in relation to known risk factors (poverty, malnutrition, poor access to health facilities, vitamin deficits) (Fischer Walker et al. 2013). Although the implementation of effective measures resulted in a significant reduction of global mortality in the past two decades, the number of deaths attributable to diarrhea, most of which preventable, is still unacceptable and much remains to be done (Bhutta et al. 2013). The most urgent challenges are represented by the implementation of and access to effective strategies in poorest areas and the impact of mass population dislocation (for conflicts or disasters) as well as of climate change on the spread of infections (Bhutta et al. 2013; Hershey et al. 2011; Carlton et al. 2015). The burden of GE in the neonatal age is generally reduced in relation to some protective factors (breastfeeding, minimal exposure to water and contaminated food, passive maternal immunity); nevertheless, it is estimated that approximately 17,000 newborns die each

year for GE (WHO 2015; O'Ryan et al. 2011). The low birth weight, prematurity, and reduced gastric acidity are well-recognized risk factors for more severe gastrointestinal infections in this age group (O'Ryan et al. 2011).

86.4 Etiology

Numerous microorganisms are responsible for GE. Their prevalence may vary according to the geographic areas (Fig. 1) (Kotloff et al. 2013). The pathogenic mechanism can be summarized in "noninflammatory" and "inflammatory-invasive" diarrhea defining two clinical syndromes also known as "watery diarrhea" and "bloody diarrhea" (Table 1) (Steiner and Guerrant 2010). In newborns, the contribution of the various etiologies could differ from that of the other pediatric age groups. The main etiologies are described in the following paragraphs.

86.4.1 *Rotavirus*

Worldwide, up to 40% of hospitalizations in children aged less than 5 years with diarrhea are due to *Rotavirus* infection (Ciccarelli et al. 2013). This microorganism is considered as the most frequent cause of GE and one of the main causes of death by dehydration (O'Ryan et al. 2011; Kotloff et al. 2013). It is an RNA virus with at least three human serotypes (A, B, and C), the most frequent of which is A. *Rotavirus* probably infect

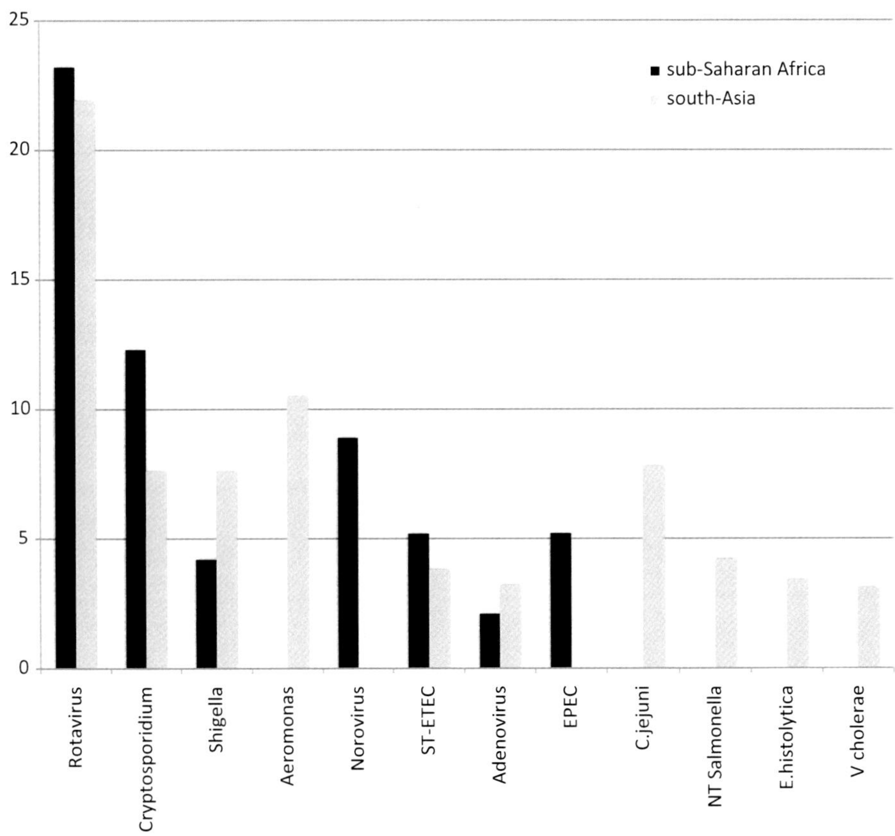

Fig. 1 Adjusted attributable fraction (expressed as weighted percent of total episodes) of pathogens significantly associated with moderate to severe diarrhea in infants aged 0–1 months in different areas (Freely adapted from Kotloff et al. 2013). *ST* heat-stable enterotoxin, *ETEC* enterotoxigenic *Escherichia coli*, *EPEC* enteropathogenic *Escherichia coli*, *NT Salmonella* nontyphoidal *Salmonella*

Table 1 Correlation between etiopathogenesis and diarrheal syndrome

Type of diarrheal syndrome	
Noninflammatory	Inflammatory
Watery – diarrhea	Bloody – diarrhea (dysentery)
Vibrio cholerae	*Shigella* spp
E. coli (ETEC, EPEC, EAEC)	*E. coli* (EIEC, EHEC)
Viruses (*Rotavirus* et al.)	NT *Salmonella*[a, b]
Giardia lamblia	*Campylobacter jejuni*[a]
Cryptosporidium parvum	*Clostridium difficile*[a]
	Yersinia spp
	Entamoeba hystolitica

[a]The attribution of specific enteric infections to a single type of diarrheal syndrome is by no means absolute. Some pathogens could determine both kinds of diarrhea (watery or bloody)

[b]*NT Salmonella* nontyphoidal *Salmonella*

newborns more commonly than previously recognized and with most infections being asymptomatic. The incubation period is short (1–3 days), and it can be responsible of outbreaks in nurseries. The pathogenetic mechanism is based on the infection of mature enterocytes located in the middle and upper villus epithelium, probably following cell entry using lactase as receptor. The alterations of the mucosal surface lead to a watery diarrhea. The reduced amount of lactase in the premature (<32 weeks) justifies the lower frequency of infection in these patients. The child may acquire the infection from the birth canal, but the most common mode of transmission is between infants through the hands of healthcare workers. The possibility of airborne transmission is still debated. Cases of meningitis-encephalitis, Reye syndrome, neonatal enterocolitis, and Kawasaki disease related to *Rotavirus* infection have also been described (O'Ryan et al. 2011).

86.4.2 Other Viruses

Nosocomial outbreaks caused by *Norovirus* or *Adenovirus* have been described in neonatal units (O'Ryan et al. 2011; Tzialla et al. 2011; Civardi et al. 2013). The clinical manifestations, which include watery diarrhea, are similar to those in other age groups. Other types of viruses (*Enterovirus*, bocavirus, astrovirus, calicivirus, coronavirus) can be involved in GE in the neonatal age although their role and frequency are not well understood (O'Ryan et al. 2011; Steiner and Guerrant 2010).

86.4.3 *Escherichia coli*

E. coli rapidly colonizes the intestinal tract of healthy newborns during the first days of life and constitutes the predominant intestinal aerobic flora throughout life. However, some pathogenic strains can cause diarrhea by different mechanisms. Enteropathogenic *E. coli* (EPEC) is considered a worldwide problem since it represents one of the main bacterial causes of childhood diarrhea in developing countries and is significantly associated with death in children 0–11 months of age (O'Ryan et al. 2011; Kotloff et al. 2013). Although its incidence is higher after 6 months of age, neonatal outbreaks have been described (O'Ryan et al. 2011). Transmission occurs through the contaminated birth canal or horizontally from other adult carriers. The disease is mediated by several genetic virulence factors, can vary widely, but usually appears as a non-bloody diarrhea (O'Ryan et al. 2011). Enterotoxigenic *E. coli* (ETEC) produces two types of toxin (LT heat-labile and ST heat-stable enterotoxin) determining a secretory response of the intestinal mucosa similar to that induced by the cholera toxin. It is considered a significant pathogen and a common cause of moderate to severe diarrhea in developing countries; neonatal outbreaks have been observed (O'Ryan et al. 2011; Kotloff et al. 2013). Enteroaggregative *E. coli* (EAEC) serotypes exhibit a characteristic aggregative pattern of adherence and produce persistent diarrhea in infants and children in resource-limited nations (Ciccarelli et al. 2013). Its frequency seems to be higher than previously recognized, and several nursery outbreaks have been described (O'Ryan et al. 2011). Enteroinvasive *E. coli* (EIEC) causes diarrhea by means of a *Shigella*-like intestinal epithelial invasion producing a dysentery-like syndrome, although the

clinical manifestations may be milder than those of shigellosis. Little is known about the epidemiology in newborns (O'Ryan et al. 2011). Shiga toxin-producing *E. coli* (STEC) has been recognized as an emerging gastrointestinal pathogens in most of the industrialized world. A particular subset of STEC, enterohemorrhagic (EHEC), produces a clinical syndrome characterized by bloody diarrhea. Its exact incidence in the neonatal age is unclear, although it has been described in children (O'Ryan et al. 2011). The most virulent EHEC belongs to serotype O157: H7, it has an animal reservoir, and is transmitted by contaminated food. Its dangerousness is related to the association with the emergence of hemolytic-uremic syndrome (HUS) (O'Ryan et al. 2011).

86.4.4 *Shigella* spp

Shigella are divided into four species and represent one of the most frequent causes of GE in childhood in developing countries (Kotloff et al. 2013). The production of a plasmid-encoded invasive toxin determines a typical dysenteric syndrome. The peak incidence is in the first 4 years of life, and neonatal cases are rare. Mothers of infected newborns are sometimes carriers, and more than half of neonatal cases occur within the first 3 days of life, consistent with a fecal-oral transmission during delivery (O'Ryan et al. 2011). Although neonatal disease is milder, complications may still occur (O'Ryan et al. 2011).

86.4.5 *Salmonella* spp

Numerous species of nontyphoidal *Salmonella* (NT *Salmonella*) can cause GE. Many animals are carriers, and human infections are due to consumption of meat and contaminated milk or to contact with colonized pets. The pathogenesis is related to the invasive capacity of the microorganism that can cause dysentery, similar to *Shigella* and other pathogens. Although the peak incidence is between 6 months and 4 years of age, neonatal infection is relatively frequent. In newborns, the route of transmission is represented by the mother during labor; items for the nursery can be contaminated, and the caregivers can be sources of infection, facilitating epidemics. Extra-intestinal complications are frequent (O'Ryan et al. 2011).

86.4.6 *Campylobacter* spp

Infection with *Campylobacter* species occurs after ingestion of contaminated food, including unpasteurized milk, poultry, and contaminated water. Many farm animals and pets are sources. *C. jejuni* causes either watery diarrhea or dysentery-like illness; usually, older infants and children are involved, but infected neonates have been reported. *C. fetus* can cause bacteremia and meningitis after perinatal infection in newborns (O'Ryan et al. 2011).

86.4.7 *Aeromonas hydrophila*

Aeromonas hydrophila is widely distributed both in animals and in the environment. Its role as a cause of diarrhea has long been debated. Several evidences seem to confirm its contribution as a pathogen even in newborns (O'Ryan et al. 2011; Kotloff et al. 2013). It typically determines a watery diarrhea mediated by toxin production.

86.4.8 Other Bacteria

Several other bacterial pathogens can cause GE (*Vibrio cholerae*, *Clostridium difficile*, *Yersinia species*), but they are infrequently observed during the neonatal period (O'Ryan et al. 2011).

86.4.9 Parasites

Certain parasites such as *Giardia intestinalis*, *Entamoeba histolytica*, and especially *Cryptosporidium parvum* are relatively frequent causes of diarrhea in children (O'Ryan et al. 2011; Kotloff et al. 2013). However, the clinical manifestations are generally observed in older children and are related to the acquisition of the germ in highly

endemic areas where neonatal care or personal and environmental hygiene are reduced (O'Ryan et al. 2011).

86.5 Transmission

Gastroenteritis is determined by the transmission of pathogens through the fecal-oral route. In most cases, the diarrheic feces of the patients represent the primary source of infection with the possibility of person-to-person transmission either directly or by water and environment contamination. Other microorganisms (NT *Salmonella*, *Campylobacter*) colonize the gut of different animal species with a risk of infection mainly related to the consumption of contaminated food. In resource-limited settings, these transmission patterns frequently overlap, and spread of gastrointestinal infections is amplified by factors such as overcrowding, poor hygiene, scarce availability of safe water, lack of efficient waste disposal, and insufficient health education (Bhutta et al. 2013; O'Ryan et al. 2011). In neonatal infection, the acquisition of the pathogen may occur by different ways: through the contaminated birth canal during the first days of life, or, especially in the nosocomial setting, through the use of contaminated tools, objects, or milk, and through the hands of the caregivers (O'Ryan et al. 2011; Ciccarelli et al. 2013). The high infectivity of *Rotavirus* infection has led to hypothesize the possibility that its transmission may also occur through the respiratory route by aerosol droplets (O'Ryan et al. 2011).

86.6 Clinical Aspects

Acute gastroenteritis is characterized by the onset of diarrhea with or without vomiting. According to the WHO, diarrhea is defined as the passage of three or more loose or liquid stools per day, or more frequently than what is considered normal for a given individual (WHO 2014). In the neonatal period, it may be difficult to define a diarrhea, since the feces of infants (especially when breastfed) may be relatively frequent, soft-liquid, and with large variability between subjects (Ciccarelli et al. 2013). In the diagnosis of GE, the previous bowel habits and the general condition of the newborn should therefore be taken into account. Typically, the GE of the neonatal period are acute, self-limiting diseases and are mild to moderate in severity. The presence of a pathogen in the intestinal tract can also result in colonization in the absence of disease. The virulence of the microorganism, the amount of the inoculum and several individual factors (e.g., prematurity, low birth weight, malnutrition, etc.) affect both the risk and severity of the disease. The clinical presentation may vary widely and some accompanying symptoms may be fever, vomiting, food refusal, dehydration, abdominal distension, and lethargy. In the management of GE, it is essential to assess the degree of dehydration and the type of diarrhea (watery or bloody), which is a relevant correlate of the presence of invasive pathogens. The risk of dehydration in children is very high and can rapidly lead to hypovolemic shock and death, regardless of the etiology. For certain bacterial infections, intestinal and extraintestinal complications are also possible (Table 2) (Bhutta et al. 2013; O'Ryan et al. 2011; Ciccarelli et al. 2013). It should be noted that while the occurrence of diarrhea in the neonatal age is generally caused by acute gastrointestinal infections, differential diagnosis with several other diseases should be considered (Table 3). In particular, it should be emphasized that diarrhea may be one of the several clinical signs of severe systemic bacterial or viral infections. The occurrence of more episodes of diarrhea in highly endemic areas, or

Table 2 Main extraintestinal complications during bacterial gastroenteritis

Complications
Sepsis and septic shock
Focal bacteremic infection
Meningitis
Osteomyelitis
Pneumonia
Convulsions
Hemolytic-uremic syndrome
Disseminated intravascular coagulation
Urinary tract infection

Table 3 Differential diagnosis of diarrhea in the newborn and causes of intractable diarrhea (Freely adapted from Ciccarelli et al. 2013)

Metabolic or anatomic disorders	Inflammatory and immune disorders
Postinfectious disaccharidase deficiency	Intolerance to cow's milk protein
Congenital disaccharidase defect	Intolerance to soy protein
Cystic fibrosis	Regional enteritis
Congenital glucose-galactose malabsorption	Ulcerative colitis
Congenital chloridorrhea	Hirschsprung's disease
Congenital defect of the Na+/H+ exchanger	Intestinal lymphangiectasia
Congenital bile acid malabsorption	Congenital microvillus atrophy
Congenital defect of enterokinases	Autoimmune enteropathy
Shwachman syndrome	Wiskott-Aldrich syndrome
Physiological pancreatic amylase deficiency	Thymic dysplasia
Enteropathic acrodermatitis	HIV hypoparathyroidism
Wolman's disease	Hyperparathyroidism
Abetalipoproteinemia	**Various**
Adrenal insufficiency	Intestinal epithelial dysplasia
Intestinal hormone hypersecretion	Systemic infection of viral or bacterial origin
Transcobalamin II deficiency	Phototherapy for hyperbilirubinemia
Hereditary tyrosinemia	Familial dysautonomia
Methionine malabsorption	Familial enteropathy
	Diarrhea from medications
	Necrotizing enterocolitis

during malnutrition, may lead to chronic diarrhea that impacts the growth and development of the child. Stunting may in turn lead to subsequent disability. Moreover, after an acute episode of GE, it is not uncommon to observe persistent diarrhea due to secondary deficiency of disaccharidases (O'Ryan et al. 2011; Ciccarelli et al. 2013).

86.7 Diagnosis

In the case of newborns with acute diarrhea, the probability of a gastrointestinal infectious cause is very high. For this reason, it is important to evaluate the history of contact with other subjects presenting similar symptoms and, if not exclusively breastfed, the possible exposure to contaminated water. The assessment of the degree of dehydration, the severity of the clinical picture, and differential diagnostic possibilities are the cornerstone of the management of every acute diarrhea (O'Ryan et al. 2011; Ciccarelli et al. 2013). The etiological diagnosis is based on the demonstration of the microorganism (or its toxins) in stools, although in many cases of mild GE it is not essential, since the disease is usually self-limited. In more severe cases, it is relevant to identify etiologies that may benefit from antibiotic therapy in addition to rehydration. In this regard, especially in countries with limited economic and diagnostic resources, clinical criteria differentiating watery versus bloody diarrhea are relevant in order to initiate empiric antibiotic treatment of invasive pathogens (Table 1). For this purpose, the microscopic search for mucous or leukocytes in the stool may be useful. In relation to the diagnosis performed by the microbiology laboratory, it is important to underline that standard stool cultures do not allow to identify pathogenic strains of *E. coli*, for which more complex diagnostic methods are required, available in reference centers only. For some pathogens (e.g., *Yersinia*, *Aeromonas*), the laboratory must be informed for the need to use specific culture media or assays which are not included in the routine workflows. In case of bloody diarrhea or *Salmonella* infection, blood cultures are required and, when clinically indicated, cerebrospinal fluid culture, in order to

exclude the possibility of disseminated infection. The main viruses causing GE (*Rotavirus* and *Adenovirus*) are detected in stool by rapid Latex or immunoenzymatic assays (ELISA). The diagnosis of toxigenic *Clostridium difficile* infection is based on the combined search for a common fecal antigen (ELISA) and the toxin gene (generally by polymerase chain reaction, PCR). The use of PCR or other nucleic acid amplification techniques may also aid the diagnosis for other viral etiologies (*Norovirus, Enterovirus, Coronavirus*, etc.) and for typing strains of bacterial pathogens (e.g., *E. coli*). In case of suspected intestinal parasitosis, it is appropriate to complete the diagnosis by repeated parasitological fecal examination especially in highly endemic areas (O'Ryan et al. 2011; Ciccarelli et al. 2013).

86.8 Therapeutic Approach

Dehydration is probably the main complication of gastroenteritis in childhood. For this reason, the assessment of the degree of dehydration is the cornerstone in the management of any diarrhea. According to current WHO recommendations, oral rehydration therapy (ORT) is considered the treatment of choice to replace fluid and electrolyte losses caused by diarrhea in children with mild to moderate dehydration (Ciccarelli et al. 2013; WHO 2014). Despite its proven efficacy, ORT remains underused (Piescik-Lech et al. 2013). Different oral rehydration solutions (ORS) are available generally with low osmolarity (210–250 mOsm/L) and variable concentration of sodium, sugar, and other electrolytes (Ciccarelli et al. 2013). Efforts to improve the palatability and the efficacy of ORS are still continuing (Piescik-Lech et al. 2013). In case of patients unable to drink or persistently vomiting, the introduction of ORT via a nasogastric tube can be considered. Intravenous rehydration is the treatment of choice in cases of failure of ORT, as well as for patients with severe dehydration (see ▶ Chap. 87, "Rehydration After Diarrhea in Newborns"). The hospitalization of an infant with diarrhea is recommended in cases of moderate to severe dehydration or in the presence of bloody diarrhea or systemic symptoms. Continuation of breastfeeding is strongly recommended, and formulated milk interruption is controversial, since enteral nutrition seems to favor the recovery of intestinal functions (WHO 2014; Piescik-Lech et al. 2013). Diarrhea is associated with significant zinc loss, and the use of zinc supplementation can reduce the duration and severity of diarrhea in children. In areas where the prevalence of zinc deficiency or the prevalence of moderate malnutrition is high, zinc supplementation may be of benefit in children aged 6 months or older. For this reason, WHO recommends zinc supplementation in children with GE (WHO 2014). Nevertheless, current evidence does not support the use of zinc in children under 6 months of age (Ciccarelli et al. 2013). Although the use of probiotics (*Lactobacillus* GG and *S. boulardii*), antisecretory drugs (racecadotril), and of antiemetics (ondansetron) have all shown efficacy in the treatment of GE in childhood, there are insufficient data to recommend them in neonatal age (Bhutta et al. 2013; Ciccarelli et al. 2013; Piescik-Lech et al. 2013; Freedman et al. 2013). Usually, neonatal GE are mild and self-limiting and do not require antibiotic therapy. The use of empiric antibiotic therapy should be reserved to cases of newborns with systemic symptoms and severe dehydration or in the presence of bloody diarrhea. The use of antibiotics is still debated for some etiologies (EPEC, ETEC, etc.), contraindicated in other (EHEC) or recommended in the presence of some enteroinvasive pathogens (*Salmonella* NT, *Campylobacter*, *Shigella*), or other microorganisms (*Vibrio cholerae*, *C. difficile*). Due to the widespread diffusion of antibiotic resistance among many enteropathogens, the evaluation of antibiotic susceptibility is always recommended (O'Ryan et al. 2011).

86.9 Preventive Measures and Control

Considering the transmission modalities of most GE, the infection control of each diarrhea episode is based on patient isolation and strengthening of hygiene measures. Consensus exists

about the importance of improving safe water supply, of adequate sanitation, and of proper hygiene for the prevention of infectious diseases, especially diarrheal diseases (Bhutta et al. 2013). It is well known that exclusive breastfeeding is protective against intestinal infections and prevents exposure to environmental contamination (O'Ryan et al. 2011; Ciccarelli et al. 2013). The protective effects of breastfeeding against GE infections have been demonstrated in several studies. Antibacterial substances, such as lactoferrin, lysozyme, phagocytes, and specific immunoglobulins, are responsible for the protective role of breast milk. Breastfeeding also promotes the formation of a competitive intestinal flora against pathogens (O'Ryan et al. 2011; Ciccarelli et al. 2013). Some of the infections causing GE are vaccine-preventable diseases. Although vaccines against *Rotavirus* and cholera have demonstrated clearly positive results in terms of safety and efficacy, these are administered after the neonatal period (Bhutta et al. 2013; Ciccarelli et al. 2013). Recent studies based on mathematical models have suggested that the implementation of all the effective strategies for the control of diarrhea (hygiene and sanitation, breastfeeding, zinc supplementation, vaccines, and adequate and prompt therapy) could reduce global deaths from GE in pediatric age from 54% to 95% by 2025 (Bhutta et al. 2013).

86.10 Intractable Diarrhea

Intractable diarrhea (ID) is a severe protracted diarrhea starting from birth that requires parenteral nutrition. Excluding forms of recurrent infections or a disaccharidase deficit consequent to an acute GE, ID is now considered a complex and heterogeneous syndrome that includes several genetic disorders associated with villous atrophy and functional or immunological bowel alterations (Table 3). Histopathological analysis and molecular analysis are mandatory to confirm the diagnosis. These cases must be managed in specialized centers (Terrin et al. 2012).

References

Bhutta ZA, Das J, Walker N et al (2013) Interventions to address deaths from childhood pneumonia and diarrhoea equitably: what works and at what cost? Lancet 381:1417–1429

Carlton EJ, Woster AP, DeWitt P et al (2015) A systemic review and meta-analysis of ambient temperature and diarrhoeal diseases. Int J Epidemiol 2016 Feb; 45(1):117–30. https://doi.org/10.1093/ije/dyv296. Epub 2015 Nov 13

Ciccarelli S, Stolfi I, Caramia G (2013) Management strategies in the treatment of neonatal and pediatric gastroenteritis. Infect Drug Resist 6:133–161

Civardi E, Tzialla C, Baldanti F et al (2013) Viral outbreaks in neonatal intensive care units: what we do not know. Am J Infect Control 41:854–856

Fischer Walker CL, Rudan I, Liu L et al (2013) Global burden of childhood pneumonia and diarrhoea. Lancet 381:1405–1416

Freedman S, Ali S, Oleszczuk M et al (2013) Treatment of acute gastroenteritis in children: an overview of systematic reviews of interventions commonly used in developed countries. Evid Based Child Health 8:1123–1137

Hershey CL, Doocy S, Anderson J et al (2011) Incidence and risk factors for malaria, pneumonia and diarrhea in children under 5 in UNHCR refugee camps: a retrospective study. Confl Heal 5:24

Kotloff K, Nataro JP, Blackwelder WC et al (2013) Burden and etiology of diarrhoeal disease in infants and young children in developing countries (the Global Enteric Multicenter Study, GEMS): a prospective, case-control study. Lancet 382:209–222

O'Ryan M, Nataro JP, Cleary TG (2011) Microorganism responsible for neonatal diarrhea. In: Klein R (ed) Infections of the fetus and newborn infants, 7th edn. Elsevier Saunders, Philadelphia, pp 359–418

Piescik-Lech M, Shamir R, Guarino A et al (2013) Review article: the management of acute gastroenteritis in children. Aliment Pharmacol Ther 3:289–303

Steiner TS, Guerrant RL (2010) Principles and syndromes of enteric infections. In: Mandell Douglas and Bennett's principles and practices of infectious diseases, 7 edn. Elsevier Churchill Livingston, Philadelphia, pp 1335–1351

Terrin G, Tomaiulo R, Passariello A (2012) Congenital diarrheal disorders: un update diagnostic approach. Int J Mol Sci 13:4168–4185

Tzialla C, Civardi E, Borghesi A et al (2011) Emerging viral infections in neonatal intensive care unit. J Matern Fetal Neonatal Med 24:156–158

WHO (2014) Integrated management of childhood illness. Chart Booklet. www.who.int. Accessed 29 Feb 2016

WHO (2015) Global Health Observatory (GHO). Child Health. www.who.int. Accessed 29 Feb 2016

87 Rehydration After Diarrhea in Newborns

Carlo V. Bellieni

Contents

Abstract

Diarrhea can threaten babies' health and life. Water alone is useless for oral rehydration. With appropriate oral solutions, most dehydrated children can be rehydrated successfully without resorting to parenteral intravenous therapy. A rapid diagnosis should be done to assess whether fluid replacement should be started and the appropriate route of administration. This chapter illustrates an easy way to recognize the grade of dehydration and the appropriate rehydration (intravenous or oral). Other options, such as ondansetron and probiotics, are discussed in the text.

C. V. Bellieni (✉)
Neonatal Intensive Care Unit, Siena University Hospital, Siena, Italy
e-mail: cvbellieni@gmail.com

87.1 Salient Points

- Sodium absorption is the main step for water absorption in oral rehydration treatment; several types of cotransporters of sodium have been proposed, although glucose is used most often.
- Babies with gastroenteritis might experience sudden severe fluid loss at the onset of gastroenteritis sufficient to cause hypovolemic shock, needing intravenous therapy: red flag signs reported in the text are useful indicators of this risk.
- Ondansetron, a serotonin receptor antagonist, is increasingly used in the treatment of diarrhea, but little is known about its impact on outcomes.

G. Buonocore et al. (eds.), *Neonatology*,
https://doi.org/10.1007/978-3-319-29489-6_234

87.2 Introduction

Babies with diarrhea undergo huge fluid loss; the main problems a physician faces are choosing the fluids for rehydration and deciding on the best way to administer them. Fluids should be rapidly absorbed from the intestinal lumen: this effect is maximized with a composition of salts and other components. The combined use of an oral rehydrating solution (ORS) and an appropriate regimen of refeeding is called oral rehydrating treatment (ORT). Fluid absorption can be promoted by the enteral administration of properly designed fluids, even in the presence of ongoing losses. Water passively follows the osmotic gradient generated by the transcellular transport of electrolytes and nutrients. This is why water alone cannot be usefully employed for oral rehydration. Nevertheless, with appropriate ORS, most dehydrated children can be rehydrated successfully without resorting to parenteral intravenous (or intraosseous, when necessary) therapy; here we will see when and how and in which cases intravenous (iv) rehydration is suggested. Oral rehydration solution, zinc treatment, continued feeding, and antibiotic treatment for certain strains of diarrhea (cholera, Shigella, and cryptosporidiosis) are effective strategies for treatment of diarrhea (Das et al. 2014). Probiotics exert positive effect in reducing the duration of acute rotavirus diarrhea compared with control (Ahmadi et al. 2015). Prebiotics are not recommended in acute diarrhea (Guarino et al. 2014).

87.3 Mechanism of Enteral Rehydration

The main mechanism by which ORS is effective is the coupled transport of sodium and glucose molecules at the intestinal brush border. This process is known as cotransport: the absorption of a molecule of an organic substrate promotes the absorption of an ion of sodium from the small intestine which, in turn, provokes the rapid absorption of a molecule of water. Cotransport across the luminal membrane is facilitated by the protein sodium glucose cotransporter 1 (SGLT1); once in the enterocyte, the transport of glucose into the blood is facilitated by glucose transporter type 2 (GLUT2) in the basolateral membrane, through the gradient promoted by the Na+/K+ ATPase (Curran 1960). This mechanism remains intact, even in patients with severe diarrhea (Pierce et al. 1968). That is why an ORS should basically contain water, sodium, and glucose or another cotransporter, in well-determined proportions.

87.4 Types of Enteral Rehydration Solutions

Glucose is the most used cotransporter, though different types of cotransporters of sodium (e.g., amino acids or cereals) have been proposed (Bhan et al. 1994; Fontaine et al. 2000). The composition of some ORS is detailed in Table 1. A high concentration of cotransporters increases the osmolarity of the solutions and may decrease rather than improve sodium and water transport into the bloodstream (McInerny et al. 2009). Solutions of lower osmolarity, but that maintain the 1:1 or 2:1 glucose to sodium ratio (Fleisher et al. 2006), perform optimally as oral solutions for diarrhea management. ORS often contain 20 mEq/L of potassium and 10–30 mEq/L of base in the form of citrate or bicarbonate (Table 1; Centers for Disease Control and Prevention 2003). In May 2004, the WHO and the United Nations Children's Fund (UNICEF) released a joint statement to decrease diarrhea deaths among the world's most vulnerable children (**Clinical management of acute diarrhoea** 2004). This statement recommended two simple and inexpensive changes from previous formulations for ORS: the switch to a new lower osmolarity formulation that reduces the need for intravenous fluids and shortens the duration of the episode (UNICEF 2001) and the introduction of zinc supplementation for 10–14 days, to decrease the duration and severity of the episode and the likelihood of subsequent infections in the 2–3 months following treatment (**Zinc Investigators' Collaborative Group** 2000; Baqui et al. 2002). It is estimated that more than three quarters of all diarrhea deaths could be prevented with full coverage and

Table 1 Compositions of WHO ORS solution and of some ORS solution products (Liberato et al. 2015; World Health Organization 2002; Koletzko and Osterrieder 2009; Munos et al. 2010)

Solution	Osmolarity Osm/L	Glucose mmol/L	Sodium mmol/L	Chloride mmol/L	Potassium mmol/L	Base mmol/L
WHO (1975)	311	111	90	80	20	30 (bicarbonate)
ESPGHAN guidelines (1977)	200–250	74–111	60	60	20	10 (citrate)
WHO (2002)	245	75	75	65	20	10 (citrate)
Dicodral (Dicofarm)	205	104	30	41	20	10 (bicarbonate)
Dicodral 60 (Dicofarm)	221	90	60	37	20	14 (citrate)
Dioralyte (Sanofi-Aventis)	240	90	60	60	20	10 (citrate)
Electrolade (Thomson & Ross)	251	111	50	40	20	30 (bicarbonate)
Pedialyte (Abbott)	250	139	45	35	20	10 (citrate)
Rapolyte (KoGEN)	250	110	60	50	20	10 (citrate)

utilization of zinc and ORS (Jones et al. 2003; Fischer Walker et al. 2009). Despite the evidence of benefit (Liberato et al. 2015), there has been little progress on the widespread introduction of low osmolarity ORS and zinc for diarrhea treatment (Fischer Walker et al. 2009).

The WHO originally developed an ORS solution composed of glucose 111, sodium 90, potassium 20, chloride 80, and bicarbonate 30, all in mmol/L (Centers for Disease Control and Prevention 2003). However, as in developed countries, viral gastroenteritis is the usual cause of diarrhea and is associated with less severe salt losses, so the sodium content of the original WHO ORS solution was considered excessive, because higher osmolarity decreased rather than increased intestinal sodium and water absorption, and hypernatremia was reported with its use (Duggan et al. 2004). In 2002, the WHO proposed a new ORS solution, composed of glucose 75, sodium 75, potassium 20, chloride 65, and citrate 10, all in mmol/L (World Health Organization 2002); this preserves the 1:1 molar ratio of sodium/glucose that is critical for efficient cotransport of sodium. It has a reduced osmolarity (245 mOsm/L) compared with the previous formulation (311 mOsm/L).

ORS with complex carbohydrates (derived from rice or carrots) should be given to infants only when they have already been eating solid food and therefore should not be given to infants who are less than 4 months old (Koletzko and Osterrieder 2009).

As countries launched diarrheal disease control programs to roll out ORS, they faced difficulties in ensuring access and achieving high coverage levels, in part due to inadequate manufacturing capacity. In an effort to improve provision of fluids in early diarrhea episodes to prevent the development of dehydration, diarrheal disease control programs promoted the use of additional fluids and homemade solutions such as rice water and sugar salt solution [collectively referred to as recommended home fluids (RHFs)]; however, there is insufficient evidence to estimate the effectiveness of RHFs against diarrhea mortality (Munos et al. 2010).

87.5 Assessing Dehydration to Decide the Type of Fluid Therapy

One of the main concerns when dealing with infantile diarrhea is the mode of fluid administration. To this aim, dehydration was formerly divided into mild, moderate, and severe, according to the amount of fluid loss calculated through a series of clinical signs; iv fluids were

Table 2 National Collaborating Centre for Women's and Children's Health (2009) assessment of dehydrated patients

Increasing severity of dehydration →			
	No clinically detectable dehydration	Clinical dehydration	Clinical shock
Symptoms (remote and face-to-face assessments)	Appears well	Appears to be unwell or deteriorating	–
	Alert and responsive	Altered responsiveness (e.g., irritable, lethargic)	Decreased level of consciousness
	Normal urine output	Decreased urine output	–
	Skin color unchanged	Skin color unchanged	Pale or mottled skin
	Warm extremities	Warm extremities	Cold extremities
Signs (face-to-face assessments)	Alert and responsive	Altered responsiveness (e.g., irritable, lethargic)	Decreased level of consciousness
	Skin color unchanged	Skin color unchanged	Pale or mottled skin
	Warm extremities	Warm extremities	Cold extremities
	Eyes not sunken	Sunken eyes	–
	Moist mucous membranes (except after a drink)	Dry mucous membranes (except for "mouth breather")	–
	Normal heart rate	Tachycardia	Tachycardia
	Normal breathing pattern	Tachypnea	Tachypnea
	Normal peripheral pulses	Normal peripheral pulses	Weak peripheral pulses
	Normal capillary refill time	Normal capillary refill time	Prolonged capillary refill time
	Normal skin turgor	Reduced skin turgor	–
	Normal blood pressure	Normal blood pressure	Hypotension (decompensated shock)

reserved for the last category (dehydration >10%). As the boundaries between the three degrees were difficult to assess, more recently only two degrees of dehydration (some dehydration and severe dehydration) have been proposed (National Collaborating Centre for Women's and Children's Health 2009).

The British Guideline Development Group (GDG) proposed a new and easy clinical assessment scheme (Table 2) that divides patients into no clinically detectable dehydration, clinical dehydration, and clinical shock (National Collaborating Centre for Women's and Children's Health 2009; Khanna et al. 2009), the last group requiring specific emergency management with administration of iv fluid boluses. When the patient has been assigned to one of the three groups, an easy flowchart helps to decide the type of rehydration needed. The GDG classification is useful because a small infant with gastroenteritis might experience sudden severe fluid loss at the onset of gastroenteritis sufficient to cause hypovolemic shock, needing iv therapy, before any signs of dehydration (e.g., dry mucous membranes or reduced skin turgor) were present. Nevertheless, some signs can be common to different classes of dehydration: both dehydration and shock might be associated with a change in conscious state, though to

different extents. The GDG concluded that when there was uncertainty, the safe approach would be to treat as though shock were present (National Collaborating Centre for Women's and Children's Health 2009). Red flag signs (altered responsiveness, sunken eyes, tachycardia, tachypnea, reduced skin turgor) should alert the clinician to a risk of progression to shock (Table 2). Children with such red flag signs require especially careful consideration and close monitoring. For instance, tachycardia (a red flag sign) would be of even greater concern if it worsened over time, pointing to a serious risk of clinical deterioration and shock.

Babies with dehydration will usually be treated with oral fluid rehydration, and those with red flag symptoms and/or evidence of deterioration will require careful management, probably in a hospital setting, while those with suspected or definite shock will require emergency iv treatment in hospital (Table 3). The GDG considered that recognition of the symptoms and signs of dehydration and shock needs considerable expertise. Clinicians therefore require training and experience in order to ensure competence in assessing children with gastroenteritis.

87.6 Modes of Alimentation

Newborns who cannot drink can be offered ORS through a nasogastric tube. If babies vomit ORS persistently, continuous infusion through a nasogastric tube may improve tolerance. The GDG (National Collaborating Centre for Women's and Children's Health 2009) counsels treating suspected or confirmed shock with a rapid intravenous infusion of 20 mL/kg of 0.9% sodium chloride solution. A second rapid intravenous infusion of 20 mL/kg of 0.9% sodium chloride solution should be administered if a child remains shocked after the first infusion, and possible causes of shock other than dehydration must be considered. If the rapid intravenous infusions resolve the symptoms/signs of shock, rehydration with intravenous fluid therapy should be started. For fluid deficit replacement and maintenance (if the baby is not hypernatremic at presentation), an isotonic solution such as 0.9% sodium chloride or 0.9% sodium chloride with 5% glucose should be used. For those who require initial rapid intravenous fluid boluses for suspected or confirmed shock, 100 mL/kg for fluid deficit replacement should be added to maintenance fluid requirements, and the clinical response should be monitored; for those who are not shocked at presentation, 50 mL/kg for fluid deficit replacement should be added to maintenance fluid requirements, and the clinical response monitored; plasma sodium, potassium, urea, creatinine, and glucose at the outset should be measured, and fluid composition and rate of administration should be monitored regularly and altered. If necessary, provision of intravenous potassium supplementation should be considered once the plasma potassium level is known. If intravenous fluid therapy is required in a newborn presenting with hypernatremic dehydration:

- Use an isotonic solution such as 0.9% sodium chloride, or 0.9% sodium chloride with 5% glucose, for fluid deficit replacement and maintenance.
- Replace the fluid deficit slowly, typically over 48 h.
- Monitor the plasma sodium frequently, aiming to reduce it at a rate of less than 0.5 mmol/L per hour (National Collaborating Centre for Women's and Children's Health 2009).

The 2014 ESPGHAN guidelines on management of acute gastroenteritis (Guarino et al. 2014) largely complement the National Institute for Health and Care Excellence (NICE) guideline published in 2009 (National Collaborating Centre for Women's and Children's Health 2009); differences are highlighted in Table 4 (Whyte et al. 2015).

87.7 Further Treatments

Diarrhea is one of the major causes of death in children under 5 years of age, disproportionately affecting children in low- and middle-income countries. Treatment of diarrhea with oral rehydration solution addresses dehydration and reduces diarrhea-related deaths. The World Health

Table 3 Fluid management (National Collaborating Centre for Women's and Children's Health 2009)

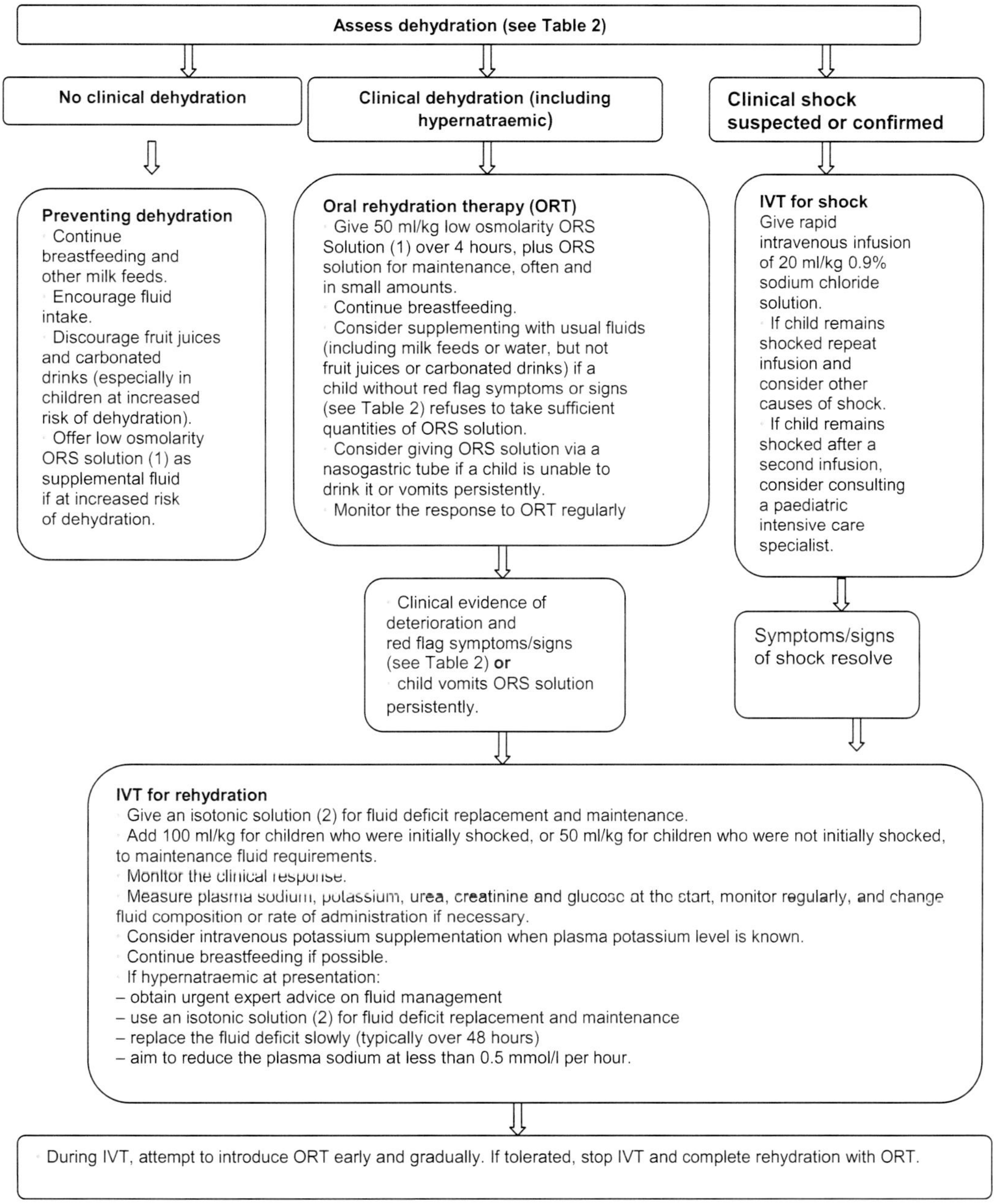

[1]240–250 mOsm/l (see Table 1)

[2]Such as 0.9 % sodium chloride or 0.9 % sodium chloride with 5 % glucose

Organization Program for the Control of Diarrheal Disease began in 1978, and while global ORS access rates have improved substantially over the past 40 years, rates of ORS use have stagnated (Lenters et al. 2013). In developing countries ondansetron hydrochloride use in children with gastroenteritis is increasing rapidly; however, little is known about its impact on outcomes (Freedman

Table 4 Comparison of ESPGHAN 2014 and NICE 2009 guidelines on acute gastroenteritis rehydration in children (Whyte et al. 2015)

	ESPGHAN 2014	NICE 2009
First-line rehydration therapy	Standard hypoosmolar ORS. Rapid rehydration with 20 mL/kg/h_ for 2–4 h followed by oral rehydration or continuous infusion of dextrose solution is adequate for initial rehydration of most patients requiring hospital assistance	Standard hypoosmolar ORS aiming at 50 mL/kg over first 4 h to treat fluid deficit plus maintenance
Management of shock	0.9 % NaCl or Ringer's lactate 20 mL/kg bolus, repeat twice if necessary (total 60 mL/kg) then maintenance fluid	0.9 % NaCl or 0.9 % NaCl + 5 % glucose bolus of 20 mL/kg then add 100 mL/kg to maintenance fluid

et al. 2014); it should be used carefully because in patients it may provoke epatopathy or increase the QT length (Freedman et al. 2014). Ondansetron and probiotics may improve patient outcomes in pediatric age. Appropriate strategies are needed to optimally integrate oral ondansetron into clinical practice to maximize its potential benefits (Schnadower et al. 2015). Although probiotics remain a promising option, there are challenges in generalizing the data available to patients presenting for outpatient care (Schnadower et al. 2015).

References

Ahmadi E, Alizadeh-Navaei R, Rezai MS (2015) Efficacy of probiotic use in acute rotavirus diarrhea in children: a systematic review and meta-analysis. Caspian J Int Med 6(4):187–195

Baqui AH, Black RE, El Arifeen S, Yunus M, Chakraborty J, Ahmed S et al (2002) Effect of zinc supplementation started during diarrhoea on morbidity and mortality in Bangladeshi children: community randomised trial. BMJ 325:1059. https://doi.org/10.1136/bmj.325.7372.1059

Bhan MK, Mahalanabis D, Fontaine O, Pierce NF (1994) Clinical trials of improved oral rehydration salt formulations: a review. Bull World Health Organ 72:945–955

Centers for Disease Control and Prevention (2003) Managing acute gastroenteritis among children: oral rehydration, maintenance, and nutritional therapy. MMWR 52 (No. RR-16)

Clinical management of acute diarrhoea (WHO/FCH/CAH/04.07) (2004) Geneva & New York: World Health Organization & United Nations Children's Fund. Available online at the following URL: http://www.emro.who.int/cah/pdf/who_unicef_statement.pdf

Curran PF (1960) Na, Cl, and water transport by rat ileum in vitro. J Gen Physiol 43:1137–1148

Das JK, Salam RA, Bhutta ZA (2014) Global burden of childhood diarrhea and interventions. Curr Opin Infect Dis 27(5):451–458

Duggan C, Fontaine O, Pierce NF et al (2004) Scientific rationale for a change in the composition of oral rehydration solution. JAMA 291:2628–2631

Fischer Walker CL, Fontaine O, Young MW, Black RE (2009) Zinc and low osmolarity oral rehydration salts for diarrhoea: a renewed call to action. Bull World Health Organ 87(10):780–786

Fleisher GR, Ludwig S, Henretig FM (2006) Textbook of pediatric emergency medicine. Lippincott Williams and Wilkins, Philadelphia, p 238, available at the following URL: http://books.google.it/books?id=oA7qSOvYZxUC&dq=Gary+Robert+Fleisher,+Stephen+Ludwig,+Fred&printsec=frontcover&source=bl&ots=Pcac8KFq8z&sig=HO6MVj8pHT0o6St0SDvBlRpTs8k&hl=it&ei=nmwuS5C6AYn7_AaurMiMCQ&sa=X&oi=book_result&ct=result&resnum=1&ved=0CAoQ6AEwAA#v=snippet&q=rehydration&f=false

Fontaine O, Gore SM, Pierce NF (2000) Rice-based oral rehydration solution for treating diarrhoea. Cochrane Database Syst Rev 2:CD001264

Freedman SB, Hall M, Shah SS, Kharbanda AB, Aronson PL, Florin TA, Mistry RD, Macias CG, Neuman MI (2014) Impact of increasing ondansetron use on clinical outcomes in children with gastroenteritis. JAMA Pediatr 168(4):321–329

Guarino A, Ashkenazi S, Gendrel D, Lo Vecchio A, Shamir R, Szajewska H, European Society for Pediatric Gastroenterology, Hepatology, and Nutrition, European Society for Pediatric Infectious Diseases (2014) European Society for Pediatric Gastroenterology, Hepatology, and Nutrition/European Society for Pediatric Infectious Diseases evidence-based guidelines for the management of acute gastroenteritis in children in Europe: update 2014. J Pediatr Gastroenterol Nutr 59(1):132–152

Jones G, Steketee RW, Black RE, Bhutta ZA, Morris SS (2003) How many child deaths can we prevent this year? Lancet 362:65–71. https://doi.org/10.1016/S0140-6736(03)13811-1

Khanna R et al (2009) Diarrhoea and vomiting caused by gastroenteritis in children under 5 years: summary of NICE guidance. BMJ 338:b1350

Koletzko S, Osterrieder S (2009) Acute infectious diarrhea in children. Dtsch Arztebl Int 106(33):539–548, Available at the following URL: http://www.ncbi.nlm.nih.gov/pmc/articles/PMC2737434/pdf/Dtsch_Arztebl_Int-106-0539.pdf

Lenters LM, Das JK, Bhutta ZA (2013) Systematic review of strategies to increase use of oral rehydration solution at the household level. BMC Public Health 13(Suppl 3):S28

Liberato SC, Singh G, Mulholland K (2015) Zinc supplementation in young children: a review of the literature focusing on diarrhoea prevention and treatment. Clin Nutr 34(2):181–188

McInerny TK et al (2009) Textbook of pediatric care. American Academy of Pediatrics, Elk Grove Village, p 2657

Munos MK, Walker CL, Black RE (2010) The effect of oral rehydration solution and recommended home fluids on diarrhoea mortality. Int J Epidemiol 39(Suppl 1):i75–i87

National Collaborating Centre for Women's and Children's Health (2009) Diarrhoea and vomiting caused by gastroenteritis. Diagnosis, assessment and management in children younger than 5 years. Available at the following URL: www.nice.org.uk/nicemedia/pdf/CG84FullGuideline.pdf

Pierce NF, Banwell JG, Rupak DM et al (1968) Effect of intragastric glucose-electrolyte infusion upon water and electrolyte balance in Asiatic cholera. Gastroenterology 55:333–343

Schnadower D, Finkelstein Y, Freedman SB (2015) Ondansetron and probiotics in the management of pediatric acute gastroenteritis in developed countries. Curr Opin Gastroenterol 31(1):1–6

UNICEF (2001) Reduced osmolarity oral rehydration salts (ORS) formulation. In: Report from a meeting of experts jointly organized by the World Health Organization and United Nations Children's Fund. New York

Whyte LA, Al-Araji RA, McLoughlin LM (2015) Guidelines for the management of acute gastroenteritis in children in Europe. Arch Dis Child Educ Pract Ed 100(6):308–312

World Health Organization (2002) Oral rehydration salts (ORS): a new reduced osmolarity formulation. World Health Organization, Geneva

Zinc Investigators' Collaborative Group (2000) Therapeutic effects of oral zinc in acute and persistent diarrhea in children in developing countries: pooled analysis of randomized controlled trials. Am J Clin Nutr 72: 1516–1522

Necrotizing Enterocolitis of Newborns 88

Sarah Bajorek and Josef Neu

Contents

Abstract

The disease necrotizing enterocolitis ("NEC") was first described over 150 years ago, however a major emphasis on understanding its pathogenesis and treatment has only burgeoned within the past 40 years (Obladen Neonatology 2009;96(4):203–210). NEC is a devastating process often progressing to death or severe morbidity within 24 hours of exhibiting initial symptoms. Currently, no clear definition of NEC exists. NEC has been a catchall term encompassing multiple pathophysiologic pathways leading to intestinal necrosis commonly seen in preterm infants. This heterogeneity and lack of a clear definition has contributed to confusion in our understanding of the pathogenesis of the most common forms of this disease. Understanding the most common form, "classical" NEC and the ability to separate that disease from other causes of intestinal damage that are termed "NEC" is important for diagnosis, prevention, and treatment. It is imperative to focus research efforts on the pathogenesis of classical NEC. We also need to find biomarkers that can

S. Bajorek (✉) · J. Neu
Department of Pediatrics, Division of Neonatology, University of Florida, College of Medicine, Gainesville, FL, USA
e-mail: sbajorek@ufl.edu; neuj@peds.ufl.edu

G. Buonocore et al. (eds.), *Neonatology*,
https://doi.org/10.1007/978-3-319-29489-6_235

be obtained noninvasively that are highly sensitive and specific and predict severity, in order to identify NEC early if we are to prevent its occurrence or be able to treat it before it progresses. This chapter will provide an overview of current concepts of NEC, including diagnosis, pathogenesis, prevention, and treatment options. Also highlighted are potential areas of future research.

88.1 Salient Points

- Despite much research, necrotizing enterocolitis (NEC) is still a major cause of morbidity and mortality in premature, low-birth weight infants.
- While the pathogenesis is still unknown, there are several factors thought to play a part in causing NEC in preterm infants, including an underdeveloped intestinal barrier, immature immune function, and aberrant bacterial colonization.
- There are many predisposing factors that increase the odds of development of necrotizing enterocolitis including antibiotics and H2 blockers. Genetic links have been found, but their clear association with NEC remains to be established.
- Classical necrotizing enterocolitis can present in several different manners; from an insidious onset with feeding intolerance and abdominal distention to a more rapid progression leading to multisystem organ failure and death within several hours.
- The measure shown to be most protective of development of NEC is feeding infants their own mother's milk.
- Further research into more representative animal and stem cell models and development of biologic markers to both diagnose and monitor development of NEC are needed.

88.2 Impact/Importance

NEC is the most common cause of gastrointestinal-related morbidity and mortality among NICU patients, disproportionately affecting premature, low-birth weight infants (Guthrie et al. 2003). The prevalence of NEC in the United States is about 7% of very low-birth weight infants based on large databases (Holman et al. 2006). A review of data from 511 centers showed that NEC carries a mortality between 16% and 42% based on birth weight (Fitzgibbons et al. 2009). These data show that the absolute risk and mortality of NEC decrease with increasing birth weight (Fitzgibbons et al. 2009). Of the patients who survive NEC, many have long-term complications including poor neurodevelopmental outcomes as well as short gut syndrome (Hintz 2005a). It is estimated that NEC accounts for nearly 20% of neonatal medical expenditure and costs over $5 billion per year in the United States (Bisquera et al. 2002).

Despite much research and advances in neonatal care, the incidence, morbidity, and mortality of NEC have not changed. Some believe this is due to saving smaller and sicker neonates. Some countries such as Sweden were previously thought to have extremely low prevalence of NEC; however, recent studies have shown an increase associated with increased survival of the smallest neonates (Ahle et al. 2013). Another likely reason for a lack of improvement in the prevalence of NEC is that the pathogenesis remains poorly understood; hence targets for prevention and treatment are sparse. Diagnosis of NEC can be difficult as well, with often subtle signs being the harbinger before full-blown disease develops. Hence, the diagnosis may be overenthusiastically made before definitive signs or at an advanced stage of the disease.

88.2.1 Historical Perspective

The commonly used Bell staging criteria for NEC and management plans were first described in 1978 and then modified in an attempt to eliminate patients with feeding intolerance or septic ileus (Bell et al. 1978; Walsh and Kliegman 1986). These staging criteria have a number of limitations, including not being able to differentiate between NEC and spontaneous intestinal perforation. Spontaneous intestinal perforation (SIP) can mimic NEC in that it presents as pneumoperitoneum without pneumatosis and

thus would be classified as stage III B per the abovementioned staging criteria. However, SIP has been shown to be a different disease, with onset typically within the first week of life, with distinctly different histologic findings, and with less associated morbidity and mortality (Chan et al. 2012, 2014; Torrazza et al. 2014).

Because current diagnostic "definitions" of NEC can easily confuse septic ileus, SIP, and NEC seen in term infants, it has been suggested that new classification systems be developed and used (Guthrie et al. 2003; Gordon 2009; Gordon et al. 2012; Neu and Walker 2011). Clinical datasets have started to differentiate SIP from NEC, which has improved their utility in delineating the disease and making the clinical data more useful for research. Other classifications seek to further delineate classical NEC from other disease states. One proposed classification separates medical from surgical NEC to obtain clean NEC data (Guthrie et al. 2003; Neu and Walker 2011). However, this method lumps babies with intestinal damage that is caused by congenital intestinal anomalies, heart disease, polycythemia, and severe perinatal asphyxia most often seen in term infants (Ostlie et al. 2003; Maayan-Metzger et al. 2004) with the more classical form of NEC seen in very low-birth weight preterm infants. It is critical to understand that what is termed "NEC" is not all the same disease. Treatment and prevention for these entities are likely to differ.

88.2.2 Pathogenesis/Causes of Classic NEC

88.2.2.1 Animal Models

Animal models have been developed to study the pathogenesis of NEC. One early rat NEC model, developed by Drs. Pitt and Barlow, prescribed formula feeding, hypoxia, and hypothermia (Barlow et al. 1974). This model has been widely used to study the pathogenesis of NEC. Other rat models include reoxygenation after hypoxia and hypothermia to enhance intestinal injury (Le Mandat Schultz et al. 2007).

This model has also been adapted for use in mice (Jilling et al. 2006). Another rat model utilizes clamping the superior mesenteric artery with subsequent reperfusion (Hammerman et al. 2002). Another model involves chemical ablation of Paneth cells in rodent modes (McElroy et al. 2013). Piglets have also been used for NEC research because they share considerable similarities to human intestinal physiology (Sangild et al. 2013). However, piglets are usually not viable until 90% of gestation is complete, and there remain significant differences in piglet and human transfer of immunoglobulins and gut closure at the time of birth (Sangild et al. 2000). Therefore, piglets remain a suboptimal animal model to aid in the understanding of NEC. Much of what is currently believed about the pathogenesis of NEC was discovered through these models. Thus, there is concern that these animal models are not representative of the pathophysiology of classical human "preterm" NEC. Although they may have the same endpoint, i.e., gut necrosis, they may lend to possible misconceptions about the actual pathophysiology of NEC. This is underlined by the fact that most preterm infants do not develop NEC shortly after birth, and classic NEC is not associated with proximal antecedent asphyxia or other major known stressors. The search for good models of human preterm NEC still needs to be determined, and this is difficult because most animals' mucosal immune systems differ from that of the preterm human. The recent development of techniques for the growth of intestinal tissue from stem cells in humans, despite several shortcomings, is one excellent step for better understanding and modeling NEC development and potential treatment strategies (Afrazi et al. 2014).

88.2.2.2 Prematurity

Prematurity is the most consistent risk factor associated with neonatal "classical" NEC, with the most premature infants being the most commonly affected (Lin and Stoll 2006). Because NEC rarely occurs in utero, it is thought that postnatal factors including feeding, hemodynamic changes, medications, and altered intestinal microbiota contribute to its pathogenesis (Huda et al. 2014). Motility of the gut, a key mechanism in the prevention of bacterial overgrowth, is dysfunctional in the

preterm neonate. Lack of motility increases the exposure time of potentially pathogenic bacteria to the immature intestinal surface that encompasses poor secretory immunoglobulin (IgA) response, decreased neutrophil function, poor macrophage activation, unbalanced cytokine production and function, and underactivity of intestinal defensins (Huda et al. 2014).

88.2.2.3 Underdeveloped Intestinal Barrier

Studies suggest that approximately 30% of neonates with NEC develop septicemia, with positive blood cultures, which is thought to be due to translocation of gut bacteria into the systemic circulation (Kazez et al. 1997). Some commonly found organisms in the blood of neonates who developed NEC include *Escherichia coli*, *Enterobacter*, and *Klebsiella* species and, occasionally, coagulase-negative *Staphylococcus* (Potoka et al. 2002). These infections are likely the result of translocation through an already injured and underdeveloped intestinal epithelium. Free radical production has been postulated to cause damage to this already fragile tissue.

The intestinal epithelium contains the most rapidly proliferating cells in the body and acts both to provide a barrier between the gut lumen and the highly immunoreactive subepithelium. It is presumed that the preterm infant has an underdeveloped intestinal barrier, caused by relatively loose tight junctions, which allows bacteria to pass into the lamina propria. Along with bacterial translocation, the toxins associated with the bacteria frequently also enter the circulation (Gatt et al. 2006). This translocation likely is enhanced through the production of nitric oxide associated with inflammation, which alters the tight junctions. The intercellular tight junction proteins are also affected by various other factors which can lead to increased permeability (Anand et al. 2007). Interaction of these microbes and toxins with subepithelial macrophages, dendritic cells, and undifferentiated lymphocytes leads to a hyperimmune response associated with high systemic levels of proinflammatory cytokines and chemokines that affect many other organs including the lung, liver, and brain.

88.2.2.4 Immature Immune Function

The neonate's GI tract is critical for various aspects of innate as well as adaptive immunity. Innate immune function of the GI tract includes tight junctions, intraluminal secretions, digestive enzymes, mucous proteins, and defensing. Paneth cells, located in the crypts of Lieberkuhn, play an important role in innate immunity by detecting the presence of bacteria (Elphick 2005). Once detected, the Paneth cells secrete antimicrobial peptides, including lysozyme and enteric alpha-defensins, which cause cell lysis (Kazez et al. 1997). Recent studies have investigated the role of Paneth cells in NEC and have found increased levels of enteric defensins (secreted by Paneth cells) in preterm infants with NEC (Salzman et al. 1998, 2007).

Gastrointestinal-associated lymphoid tissue (GALT) is found primarily in the distal small intestine (MacDonald 2003; Sedda et al. 2014). Activation of this lymphoid tissue is triggered by inflammatory mediators acting through epithelial and other cell receptors. Lipopolysaccharide (LPS), an endotoxin released by gram-negative bacteria, is a ligand for Toll-like receptor 4 (Jilling et al. 2006; Leaphart et al. 2007). Toll-like receptors on the intestinal epithelial cells signal the release of cytokines and chemokines (interferon gamma, IL-6, IL-8, IL-12, IL-18, TNF-α) to initiate the inflammatory cascade in the intestinal tract (Otte et al. 2004). The activation of TLR4 is thought to be a major contributor to NEC pathogenesis because its surface density increases during the second half of gestation until just before term, when adaptive immunity matures, and TLR4 is downregulated and actively removed from the mucosal cell surface (Otte et al. 2004).

LPS signaling is via activation of the transcription of nuclear factor-kB (NF-kB), which induces transcription of many cytokines including interleukin -1 (IL-2), interleukin-6 (IL-6), chemokines, tumor necrosis factor (TNF), and platelet-activating factor (PAF), which all have been shown to stimulate inflammation (Hawiger 2001). Immature intestinal cells have higher activation of NF-kB and release of cytokines in response to TNF-α in comparison to mature epithelial cells (Kilpinen et al. 1996). PAF, a mediator

of leukocyte functions, including platelet aggregation, has also been reported to upregulate TLR4 expression (Soliman et al. 2010). Increased circulating and luminal levels of platelet-activating factor have been associated with NEC (Soliman et al. 2010). PAF has been found to be decreased in preterm neonates initially and then increased in the stool after initiation of enteral feeding (Soliman et al. 2010). The increased action and interplay between TLR4, NF-kB, TNF, and PAF is thought to contribute to the hyperimmune response associated with NEC.

88.2.2.5 Bacterial Colonization

Four decades ago the link of bacteria NEC was first described in the literature (Santulli et al. 1975). Since that time much research has been done to better understand the link between bacterial colonization and NEC. While numerous bacteria have been implicated in causing NEC, one specific pathogen that fulfills Koch's postulates for the etiology of NEC has not been found (Falkow 2004). Rather, it appears that NEC is preceded by a "dysbiosis" or pathogenic alteration of the ecology of the intestinal microbiota (Claud and Walker 2001).

There is a long held belief that the fetus grows in a sterile uterine environment and only becomes colonized with bacteria after birth. Recent research has shown that the intrauterine environment is indeed not sterile (Ben-Amor et al. 2005; DiGiulio et al. 2008). Meconium, the infant's first stool, is formed from sloughed intestinal cells while the infant is still in utero. A recent study has shown that meconium is also not sterile and compared meconium microbiota to other sites and found that it was most similar to amniotic fluid (Ardissone et al. 2014). Currently, the role of the prenatal microbiome and perturbations in a healthy microbiome along with its interaction with the immature host intestinal mucosal immune system is being investigated – specifically the role prenatal microbiota may have on prematurity and other disease states including NEC.

After delivery and with the start of enteral feeding, the microbiota of the gut rapidly expands both in species and in number. An infant's gut microbial pattern is different than that of an older child, in that they have fewer bacterial species; however, the variability between infants in this age group is significantly higher than that between adults (Yatsunenko et al. 2012). Also, preterm infants in the NICU setting have been found to have different microbiota than healthy term infants (Björkström et al. 2009). Preterm neonates have altered microbiota as they mature over time, and there is difference in the development of microbiota in babies housed in different NICUs (Taft et al. 2014).

Neonates fed human milk have shown to harbor different bacterial taxa in their stools compared to formula-fed neonates (Wang et al. 2015). Breastfed infants had a higher percentage of *Bacteroidetes*, *Proteobacteria*, and lower *Firmicutes* compared with formula-fed infants (Donovan et al. 2012). Formula-fed neonates tend to colonize their intestines with *Actinobacteria* and *Firmicutes*, including *Clostridia* and *Staphylococcus*: organisms known to commonly cause pathogenesis (Donovan et al. 2012). The exact relationship of these differences in taxonomy as they relate to disease remains poorly understood.

A loss of microbial diversity and lack of enterococcal species in the stool have been seen before NEC develops (Stewart 2015). Also a correlation of pneumatosis intestinalis and the presence of *Clostridium* have been found (Smith et al. 2011). One study found that dysbiosis and bloom of bacteria belonging to the phylum *Proteobacteria* and a decrease in *Firmicutes* were found in patients with NEC between 1 week prior and <72 h of NEC development (Mai et al. 2011). Support for this was demonstrated in studies by Claud et al. (2013). This suggests that NEC is not caused by a single organism but more likely from a perturbation in the microbiome that either activates TLR4 or has metabolites that start the inflammation cascade.

88.2.2.6 Effects of Antibiotics on Intestinal Microbiota

Administration of antibiotics to preterm infants is a common practice in NICUs due to the concern for sepsis. Several decades ago, Goldmann's

studies suggested that neonates had bacterial overgrowth of pathogenic bacteria after 3 days of antimicrobial exposure in the NICU (Goldmann et al. 1978). More recently, it has been shown that the odds of developing NEC and mortality associated with NEC correlates with length of antibiotic exposure (Cotten et al. 2009; Alexander et al. 2011). However, in these studies it is unclear whether the initial degree of illness led to increased antibiotic usage or whether increased antibiotic usage led to increased degree of illness. The effects of antibiotic exposure on the microbial diversity of the intestine have been shown to last months after treatment is discontinued and has been shown to have long-lasting effects (Fouhy et al. 2012). Therefore, it is critical that the routine use of antibiotics in the preterm be reconsidered.

88.2.2.7 Effects of H2 Blockers

Premature infants have limited gastric acid secretion, which can be reduced even further with the use of H2 blockers that have been linked to NEC in preterm neonates (Hyman et al. 1985; Athalye-Jape et al. 2013). H2 antagonists have been used in the preterm population historically for treatment of apnea and bradycardia putatively due to gastroesophageal reflux as well as in TPN while a patient is nil per os. Several studies have shown an association between the use of H2 antagonists and an increased incidence of NEC as well as septicemia (Cucchiara et al. 1993; Orenstein et al. 2003, 2005). It is thought that H2 antagonists raise the gastric pH and reduce the bactericidal action in the stomach, which increases the total number of bacteria promoting an overgrowth of potentially pathogenic bacteria (Gupta et al. 2013). These are among the most widely misused drugs in the NICU, and their routine use has been discouraged (Ho et al. 2015).

88.2.2.8 Ischemia

The terminal ileum and proximal colon are common sites involved in NEC, and they are also watershed areas of perfusion. The intestinal mucosal surface is susceptible to fluctuations in perfusion and hypoxic-ischemic injury (Colgan and Taylor 2010). Most term neonates who develop intestinal necrosis have conditions that predispose them to ischemia, e.g., polycythemia, birth asphyxia, exchange transfusion, and congenital heart disease (Colgan and Taylor 2010). Preterm infants with a large patent ductus arteriosus have decreased gut perfusion and an increased risk for NEC (Bor et al. 1988). These findings have given way to the idea that inadequate intestinal blood flow and subsequent reperfusion injury may contribute to the pathophysiology of NEC in this class of infants.

88.2.2.9 Red Blood Cell Transfusion

Some researchers suggest that red blood cell transfusion might increase an infant's risk of NEC (Singh et al. 2011; Mally et al. 2006). However, other studies do not support transfusions as a cause of NEC (Josephson et al. 2010; Agwu 2005). It is thought that the relationship may be that an infant with a predisposition to NEC may require more RBC transfusions and the effect of transfusion may not be causal. The causal relationship between NEC and RBC transfusion needs to be further evaluated.

88.2.2.10 Genetic

Twin gestation research has supported that NEC risk may have a genetic component (Bhandari 2006). However not one single gene has been found to be a cause for NEC. Some studies have looked at the TLR4 gene and its products, with no association to NEC. However, variants of NFKB1, downstream from TLR4 have been associated with NEC (Sampath et al. 2011). It is thought that multiple genetic mutations may make an infant more likely to be susceptible to NEC.

88.2.3 Presentation/Clinical Diagnosis

Classical NEC is associated with prematurity and has a peak presentation between 29 and 31 weeks postmenstrual age (Gordon et al. 2014). Thus, a baby born at a very low gestational age (e. g., 24 weeks) would be more likely to develop NEC at a later postnatal age than a baby born at a later gestational age (e.g., 28 weeks). NEC may

start as a slowly progressing process that initially manifests with feeding intolerance and abdominal distention, followed by emesis, bloody stools, temperature instability, lethargy, apnea, and bradycardia. All too often, however, it progresses rapidly, leading to multisystem organ failure or death within a few hours of the overt onset of illness. The fulminance of disease progression is one of the most compelling reasons why predictive diagnostic tests and prevention rather than treatment strategies will be the keys to improving outcomes.

NEC is commonly found in a specific portion of the bowel, usually the terminal ileum or proximal colon. It is thought that the terminal ileum and proximal colon are commonly involved because they are watershed areas of perfusion, prone to ischemia. These are also regions that are most closely associated with GALT, and hence are highly prone to inflammatory injury. NEC can also involve noncontiguous portions of the intestine, or the entire gut referred to as "NEC totalis." NEC totalis is generally referred to widespread disease with less than 25% of viable bowel remaining (Huda et al. 2014).

88.2.4 Laboratory Findings

Laboratory findings associated with NEC can be varied, and most do not differentiate between NEC, feeding intolerance, and sepsis. However, there are several laboratory findings that have been shown to aid the clinician in assessing severity of NEC, including metabolic acidosis, neutropenia, left shift of segmented neutrophils, thrombocytopenia, hyperglycemia, and hyponatremia. Thrombocytopenia is associated with a poor prognosis (Kafetzis et al. 2003). A drop in absolute monocyte count in an infant with feeding intolerance may also be associated with NEC (Remon et al. 2014). These initial findings need to be reproducible in larger studies. A combination of some of these laboratory findings have been used in scoring systems used to predict the timing and type of surgical intervention in NEC (Hutter et al. 1976; Sola et al. 2000). However, the utility of these systems is still in question.

88.2.5 Biomarkers

Biomarkers are molecular or biologic measures that can objectively assess the state of disease or response to intervention. Many studies have been done looking for biomarkers that can distinguish NEC from other mimicking diseases. Criteria for a good biomarker include that it is both sensitive and specific, can monitor disease, and predict outcome. There are a number of biomarkers that are not specific to the GI tract, including CRP, procalcitonin, cytokines, TGF- β, inter-alpha inhibitor protein, and serum amyloid that have been investigated for their utility in diagnosing NEC (Table 1).

CRP, which is frequently used clinically, is sensitive, but not specific for NEC and has a late response to inflammation (Ng et al. 1997; Pourcyrous 2005). Procalcitonin cannot distinguish between NEC and healthy patients (Turner et al. 2007). Recently, transforming growth factor-β was found to be decreased from birth in premature infants who developed NEC (Maheshwari et al. 2014). A low level (as defined as less than 1,380 pg/mL) on the first postnatal day was associated with the development of NEC with 64% accuracy (Stoll et al. 2013).

Cytokines, cell-signaling molecules, have also been investigated as early biomarkers of disease to better understand pathophysiology and to predict outcome. Increased serum IL-1 β, IL-1 receptor antagonist, IL-6, IL-10, CXCL5, IL-8/CXCL8, CCL2, CCL3, and neurotrophin-4 have been detected in premature infants with NEC (Edelson et al. 1999; Harris et al. 2005; Ng et al. 2010; Torrazza et al. 2013). Plasma IL-8/CXCL8, epithelial-derived neutrophil chemoattractant-78/CXCL5, and IL-10 levels were higher in infants with NEC than in those with sepsis syndrome (Ng et al. 2010). IL-8/CXCL8 levels correlate with the extent of NEC, need for surgical bowel resection, and 60-day mortality in infants with NEC (Edelson et al. 1999; Ng et al. 2010).

Several biomarkers including intestinal fatty acid-binding protein, pro-apolipoprotein CII, and serum amyloid A have been shown to distinguish between feeding intolerance and NEC (Maury 1985; He 2002; Badolato 1994; Arnon et al. 2005). Lower levels of inter-alpha inhibitor protein

Table 1 Conventional biomarkers

Conventional biomarkers	Description	Usage and limitations	References
1. Non-specific biomarkers			
CRP	Bacterial infection acute phase reactant and "late phase" biomarker	CRP is widely used in the detection of NEC; elevated levels are frequently found in other inflammatory conditions. Sensitive but non-specific. Also, levels do not rise until 12–18 h after insult and so is a delay	(Ng et al. 1997; Pourcyrous 2005)
Procalcitonin	Bacterial infection acute phase reactant	PCT blood levels are lower than those with sepsis, and there is no difference between NEC and healthy infants	(Turner et al. 2007)
Cytokines and chemokines (IL-1RA, 6, IL-8, IL-10, IL-12, IL-18, IP-10, TNF- α)	Early phase inflammatory mediators	Increase in proinflammatory profile associated with development to NEC, poor prognosis, and increased mortality. However, can be triggered by various inflammatory causes and thus loss of specificity. Further study needs to be done	(Maheshwari et al. 2014; Benkoe et al. 2014; Stoll et al. 2013; Edelson et al. 1999; Harris et al. 2005; Ng et al. 2010; Torrazza et al. 2013)
Transforming growth factor-β	Protein that performs many cellular functions including cell growth, proliferation, cell death, and apoptosis	Recently found that a low level on the first postnatal day was associated with developing NEC with 64% accuracy	(Maheshwari et al. 2014)
Serum amyloid A (SAA)	An acute phase reactant induced by proinflammatory cytokines, which can be stimulated by LPS. Made by the liver	Lower levels of SAA are found in infants with NEC than in those with sepsis. Better biomarker than CRP or IL-6 because it shows an early, sensitive, sustainable response to systemic inflammation	(Maury 1985; He 2002; Badolato 1994; Arnon et al. 2005)

distinguish NEC from feeding intolerance (Ng et al. 2010). However, levels also were decreased in sepsis and so may not be able to distinguish between NEC and sepsis. Lower levels of SAA are found in infants with NEC than in those with sepsis (Arnon et al. 2005). SAA is a better biomarker than CRP or IL-6 because it shows an early, sensitive, and sustainable response to systemic inflammation (Maury 1985; He 2002; Badolato 1994; Arnon et al. 2005).

88.2.6 Bowel-Specific Biomarkers

In addition to the above non-specific biomarkers, there are a number of GI tract-specific biomarkers currently being investigated to aid in the diagnosis of NEC (Tables 2 and 3). Elevated plasma levels of claudin-3, liver fatty acid-binding protein (L-FABP), and intestinal fatty acid-binding protein (I-FABP) have been observed in infants with NEC (Thuijls et al. 2010; Aydemir et al. 2011; Derikx 2010; Lieberman et al. 1997; Ng et al. 2013; Pelsers et al. 2005; Voganatsi et al. 2001; Konikoff and Denson 2006; Zoppelli et al. 2012; Yoon et al. 2014; Bin-Nun et al. 2014; Däbritz et al. 2012; Tepas et al. 2006). L-FABP is expressed mainly in liver hepatocytes but also in enterocytes of intestinal mucosa, whereas I-FABP is predominantly expressed in mature enterocytes of the small and large intestine. Increased plasma and urinary concentrations of L-FABP and I-FABP have been found in patients having intestinal mucosal injury, including intestinal ischemia and NEC (Aydemir et al. 2011; Derikx 2010; Lieberman et al. 1997). Claudin-3 is an intestinal tight junction protein. Elevated urinary and serum claudin-3 has been reported in infants with NEC.

Table 2 Gut-specific biomarkers

Conventional biomarkers	Description	Usage and limitations	References
2. Gastrointestinal-specific biomarkers			
Intestinal fatty acid-binding protein (I-FABP)	An intracellular protein that is specifically expressed in mature enterocytes of the small and large intestine	Elevated urinary and plasma concentrations of I-FABP have been reported in infants with NEC, and it may predict disease severity. Larger trials need to be performed	(Lieberman et al. 1997; Ng et al. 2013; Pelsers et al. 2005)
Liver fatty acid-binding protein (L-FABP)	A protein expressed mainly in liver hepatocytes but also in mature enterocytes of intestinal mucosa	Elevated urinary and plasma concentrations of I-FABP have been reported in infants with NEC, and it may predict disease severity. Larger trials need to be performed	(Ng et al. 2013; Pelsers et al. 2005)
Fecal calprotectin (S100A9)	Heterodimeric complex of antimicrobial proteins released from activated leukocytes	Fecal calprotectin seems to be increased in premature infants with NEC. Does not predict severity of disease. Does not require serum. POC tests are being investigated. Also has wide intra- and inter-patient variations	(Voganatsi et al. 2001; Konikoff and Denson 2006; Zoppelli et al. 2012; Yoon et al. 2014; Bin-Nun et al. 2014)
Fecal calgranulin C (phagocyte-specific S100A12)	Protein involved in calcium-dependent signal transduction and has regulatory effects on neutrophil activities	Biochemical properties similar to fecal calprotectin and serve as marker of GI inflammation. May be helpful marker in predicting disease severity. However, much interindividual and intraindividual variability	(Däbritz et al. 2012)

However, it is less sensitive and specific than I-FABP (Ng et al. 2013; Pelsers et al. 2005). Fecal calprotectin (S100A9) is a cytosolic protein complex of human neutrophils and has been used as an inflammatory biomarker (Voganatsi et al. 2001). Its fecal concentrations are increased in various infections and inflammatory processes and have been used to differentiate inflammatory bowel disease from irritable bowel syndrome (Konikoff and Denson 2006). It has been investigated for diagnosis of NEC in preterm infants; however, it has wide intra- and interindividual variability (Zoppelli et al. 2012; Yoon et al. 2014; Bin-Nun et al. 2014). Fecal calgranulin (S100A12) is a protein involved in calcium-dependent signal transduction and has regulatory effects on neutrophil activities. It may be a helpful marker in predicting disease severity. This too has much interindividual and intraindividual variability (Däbritz et al. 2012). Despite an increasing understanding of the role of inflammation and intestinal mucosal injury in the pathophysiology of NEC, a clinically useful sensitive and specific biomarker for early diagnosis has not yet been found.

88.2.7 Radiographic Findings

Currently, the diagnosis of NEC is most commonly made using clinical criteria and abdominal plain films. Pneumatosis intestinalis, or air in the wall of the bowel (Image 1), has historically been the diagnostic finding associated with NEC, but without other signs such as pneumoperitoneum associated with perforation or deteriorating clinical status, it does not indicate the need for surgical intervention. If the air is located within the submucosa, it can take on a bubbly appearance; if in the subserosa, it will take on a linear appearance.

Table 3 Diagnostic modalities

Method	Advantages	Limitations	References
Radiography	Current method for detection of NEC. Widely understood/accepted	Late findings, imaging takes time. High interobserver differences in diagnosis of NEC	(Faingold et al. 2005)
Ultrasonography, Doppler U/S	Can better demonstrate portal venous gas. Doppler U/S can measure velocity of blood flow. Progression of initial hyperemia, followed by ischemia and bowel wall thinning has been confirmed by Doppler U/S	Artifact from air in bowel may occlude images. User variability	(Oh et al. 2010; Błaż 2014)
NIR spectroscopy	Continuous monitoring of oxygen status in splanchnic or mesenteric tissue. Noninvasive. Low cost	Optimal placement may be difficult on preterm infant. Has been evaluated in term infants with NEC associated with cardiac surgery. A trial of NEC in preterm infants has yet to be performed	(DeWitt et al. 2014)
Breath hydrogen monitoring	Measurement is related to abnormal growth of intestinal bacteria and malabsorption. Increase in breath hydrogen has been found in infants who later were found to have NEC. May provide a method for early detection of NEC	Technical difficulty in obtaining quality samples, variability based on several patient and feeding factors and calibration. Other causes of bacterial overgrowth may confound data. Low positive predictive value	(Ian et al. 1987; Cheu 1990)
Computerized auscultation	Monitoring of gastric emptying and bowel peristalsis. Has been investigated for other populations of infants	Complexity of bowel sound signal. No published data on use for NEC in preterm infants. Current sensors are not small enough for preterm infants	(Tomomasa et al. 1999)
Electronic nose (eNose)	Analyzes fecal volatile organic compounds (VOCs). Has been able to predict NEC 2–3 days prior to onset of symptoms. Noninvasive and does not use serum	Larger multicenter validation studies need to be done. Findings of ethnicity, race, and sex need to be investigated	(De Meij et al. 2015)

Plain films may also reveal portal venous gas (Image 3) or fixed dilated air-filled loops. Pneumoperitoneum (Image 4), which may present as "football sign" (Images 1 and 2) on abdominal plain film, represents bowel perforation, and a radiologic finding that usually mandates prompt surgical intervention (Tepas et al. 2006).

Radiographic imaging has several limitations. Pneumoperitoneum may be absent on plain film in a significant portion (50–60%) of infants with bowel perforation (Faingold et al. 2005). Also, there are interobserver differences in diagnosis of NEC on plain film (Rehan et al. 1999). The presence of one sign on plain film does not reliably correlate with severity of NEC (Tam et al. 2002). However, a scoring system, the Duke abdominal assessment scale (DAAS), that combines radiographic findings has been developed (Coursey et al. 2008). It is a 10-point scale with 0 representing a normal gas pattern to 10 representing pneumoperitoneum. It has shown that increasing DAAS score is associated with increasing disease severity (Coursey et al. 2008). This has several practical limitations and can be difficult to use in clinical practice.

88.2.8 Other Diagnostic Modalities

Abdominal ultrasound is being studied as a modality to diagnose and monitor NEC. Some benefits of ultrasound include that it is readily available, can be performed at the bedside, and is noninvasive (Oh et al. 2010; Błaż 2014). Institutions with experienced sonographers and radiologists have demonstrated improved sensitivity and specificity for the detection of necrotic bowel in NEC as confirmed by intraoperative findings and histologic specimens (Błaż 2014). However, there are limitations of ultrasound,

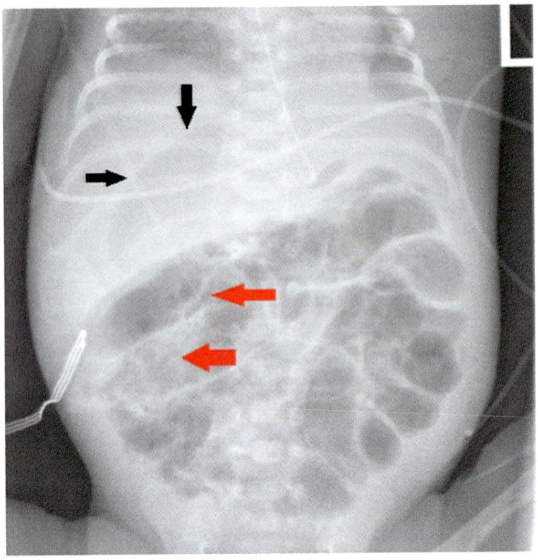

Image 1 *Black arrows* indicate pneumoperitoneum. "Football sign" depicting free air in the abdomen outlining the falciform ligament. *Red arrows* indicate pneumatosis intestinalis (intramural air) (Used with permission by Dr. Catalina Bazacliu, MD)

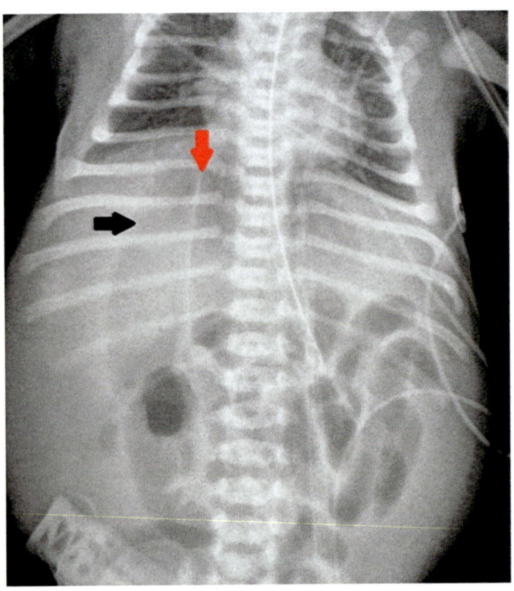

Image 2 *Black arrow* points to the "football sign" with the *Red arrow* outlining the falciform ligament (Used with permission by Dr. Jonathan Williams, MD)

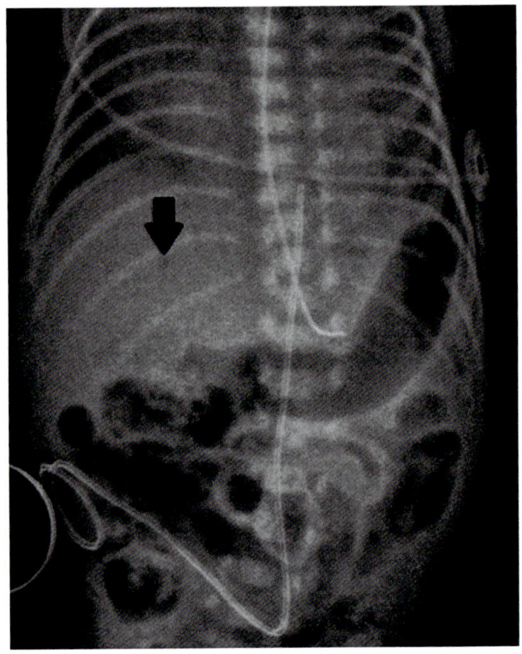

Image 3 *Black arrows* indicate portal venous gas (air within the hepatobiliary tree) (Used with permission by Dr. Jonathan Williams, MD)

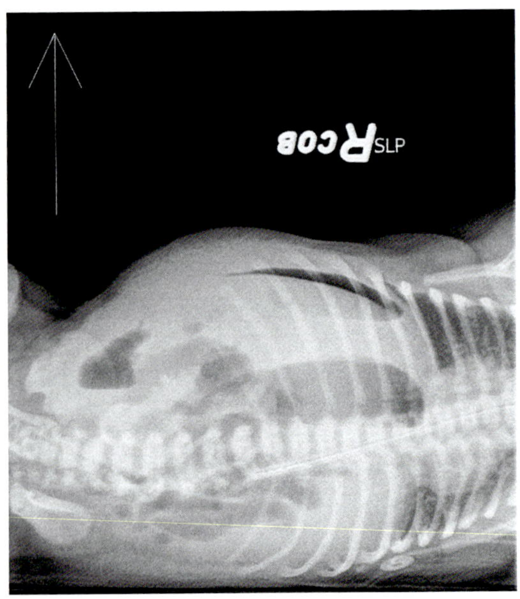

Image 4 Free air under the diaphragm (Used with permission by Dr. Jonathan Williams, MD)

including user variability, bowel gas obscuring the image, and the fact that ultrasound should not be performed in neonates who are clinically unstable or who have abdominal tenderness.

Near-infrared spectroscopy (NIRS) is a technology that uses near-infrared light between 650 and 950 nm to noninvasively probe the concentration and oxygenation of hemoglobin. It is being used to measure oxygenation of hemoglobin in the brain, muscle, and other tissues and to detect changes induced by injury or disease. A recent study has shown in a subset of infants with single ventricle congenital heart disease that it may be a useful tool in assessing risk of developing NEC (DeWitt et al. 2014). However, whether these findings would be seen in the subset of NEC that develops in preterm neonates is yet to be established. Some of the conceived advantages of NIRS are that it is noninvasive and the relatively low cost. However, there are limitations, including finding the optimal placement for monitoring and technical limitations including probe malfunction.

Other noninvasive technologies being investigated for potential early detection and monitoring of NEC include gastric tonometry/intramucosal pH, breath hydrogen monitoring, computerized auscultation, and analysis of fecal volatile compounds (Ian et al. 1987; Cheu 1990; Tomomasa et al. 1999; De Meij et al. 2015). Breath hydrogen monitoring can detect abnormal growth of intestinal bacteria and malabsorption (Ian et al. 1987). Increase in breath hydrogen has been found in infants who later were found to have NEC (Cheu 1990). However, other causes of malabsorption and different enteral food intake may lead to error. Computerized auscultation can provide monitoring of gastric emptying and motility (Tomomasa et al. 1999). Continuous monitoring would be needed, and there is much complexity to the bowel sound signal. An interesting new technology called electronic nose (eNose), which analyzes fecal volatile organic compounds (VOCs), has been shown to be able to detect a patient developing NEC prior to onset of symptoms (De Meij et al. 2015). This technology was able to identify infants 2–3 days prior to the diagnosis of NEC and was able to distinguish NEC from sepsis. Studies are underway to evaluate this modality in greater depth.

88.2.9 Management

88.2.9.1 Medical Treatment

There is lack of evidence that any specific treatment approach influences the outcome of NEC, and thus treatment remains largely supportive. Current medical treatment includes stopping feedings, providing gastric decompression (with a large bore Replogle tube), fluid resuscitation, correction of acidosis, anemia, and thrombocytopenia, and starting broad spectrum antibiotics to cover potential pathogens, including gram-positive, gram-negative, and anaerobic organisms. Optimal antimicrobial therapy for NEC is not known. One RCT assigned 42 infants with NEC receiving ampicillin and gentamicin to clindamycin or no therapy. Clindamycin did not affect mortality or intestinal perforation and increased intestinal strictures (Faix et al. 1988). A large retrospective cohort study showed that infants with medical NEC alone had no survival benefit associated with anaerobic antimicrobial therapy (Autmizguine et al. 2014). However, infants with surgical NEC treated with anaerobic antimicrobial therapy had lower mortality (Autmizguine et al. 2014). Close monitoring of patient condition is warranted and includes serial blood gases, blood counts, and abdominal radiographs. The usual treatment of nil per os (NPO) and antibiotics typically is given for 7–10 days for medical NEC; however, the length of treatment has not been carefully studied.

88.2.9.2 Surgical Treatment

Surgery is required in 30–50% of reported cases of NEC in low-birth weight infants (Blakely et al. 2005). When gangrenous or perforated bowel is suspected, surgical intervention is necessary. Surgical intervention should be considered if the patient is clinically deteriorating despite maximal medical management, in some patients with peritonitis, and those with persistent thrombocytopenia (Blakely et al. 2005). When pneumoperitoneum is found, surgeons should be involved early to

minimize the time to surgery. The two options for surgical intervention include exploratory laparotomy and primary peritoneal drainage. A meta-analysis performed in 2001 and again in 2011 demonstrated that a difference in outcome could not be assessed (Basani et al. 1996; Moss et al. 2001). Also, the timing of surgery for these complex patients has not been adequately studied.

88.2.10 Complications

The most common delayed complication after recovering from acute NEC is the formation of intestinal strictures. The incidence of intestinal stricture may be as high as 36% (Horwitz et al. 1995). As mentioned previously, recent RCTs have shown an association with antibiotics aimed at anaerobic organisms (clindamycin) and intestinal strictures (Faix et al. 1988). If intestinal strictures form, patients will present with abdominal distention, feeding intolerance, and a partial bowel obstruction. Strictures usually can be identified using retrograde contrast studies.

Approximately 8% of infants who develop NEC and undergo bowel resection were left with short bowel syndrome (SBS), which has an associated mortality of 38% (Cole et al. 2008). The total 5-year cost for just one child with short bowel syndrome has been estimated to be nearly 1.5 million US dollars (Spencer et al. 2008). Short bowel is defined as a shortened small bowel length that leads to intestinal failure (inadequate absorption of nutrients, water, or electrolytes). These patients have poor absorption of nutrients and thus poor nutrition and growth. Depending on the length of bowel left, they may need to be on very prolonged parenteral nutrition to aid in nutrition and growth. One of the common complications associated with long-term TPN use is TPN cholestasis. Recurrent NEC is relatively uncommon with the incidence being about 6% (Stringer et al. 1993).

For those children with SBS, a few treatments have been developed to help preserve and improve the function of the remaining intestine. These include autologous gastrointestinal reconstruction procedures, including the lengthening and tailoring (LILT) and serial transverse enteroplasty (STEP) procedures (Jones et al. 2010; Sudan et al. 2007). The main predictor of the ability to achieve full enteral feeds is the final length of the remaining small intestine (Goulet et al. 2005). If the final length is <40 cm, the likelihood of PN dependency is high. These recent advances in surgical care provide hope for patients with SBS.

Intestinal transplantation can be considered in patients with short bowel syndrome from NEC who develop cholestasis and other complications related to dependence on parenteral nutrition (Vennarecci et al. 2000). Long-term survival after intestinal transplantation for NEC-induced short gut syndrome has been reported. For patients undergoing intestinal transplant in 2007, a 1- and 5-year graft survival was 69.2 and 53.8% for patients less than 18 years old (Smith et al. 2014).

88.2.10.1 Long-Term Outcomes

Long-term clinical outcomes depend on severity of NEC. In general it is reported that surgical NEC survivors were more mature, larger, and older at the time of surgery. In infants with NEC requiring surgery born less than or equal to 30 weeks gestation mortality of 53% has been observed (Ladd et al. 1998).

Inflammation from NEC has effects on other organ systems such as the developing brain. Sonntag et al. reported significant neurodevelopmental delay at 12 and 20 months in a group of VLBW survivors of NEC (Sonntag et al. 2000). A large retrospective cohort study showed that those with surgical NEC had more cystic periventricular leukomalacia, bronchopulmonary dysplasia, and stunted growth in comparison to those who were medically managed (Hintz 2005b).

88.2.11 Prevention

88.2.11.1 Breast Milk

The most protective, preventative measure against the development NEC is to feed very low-birth weight infants their own mother's milk (Meier and Bode 2013). Mother's own breast milk clearly shows a beneficial role in reducing the incidence

of NEC compared with formula (Sullivan et al. 2010; Lucas and Cole 1990). Mother's own milk has been shown to contain a variety of microbes, and there is a possibility that that the microbial pattern for each mother's milk may be personalized to her infant. There have been two meta-analyses that have demonstrated a risk reduction in NEC using donor milk (Boyd et al. 2007; Quigley and McGuire 2014). However, these meta-analyses included studies of variable quality, and it is questionable whether strict criteria for NEC were used in some of the earlier studies.

There are many bioactive components in human milk including antigen-specific antibodies (IgA, IgM, AND IgG), leukocytes, enzymes, lactoferrin, growth factors, hormones, oligosaccharides, polyunsaturated fatty acids, nucleotides, stem cells, and specific glycoproteins. All of these, as well as the effect on inhibiting hyperimmune responses by inhibiting NF-kB, are thought to reduce the risk of NEC (Minekawa et al. 2004; Hanson et al. 2003). Human milk feeding does not, however, prevent all NEC. Scandinavian countries routinely feed neonates breast milk, and recent reports show an increase in the incidence of NEC (likely due to increased interventions of neonates born between 22 and 25 weeks gestation). The incidence of NEC for these extremely preterm neonates was approximately 13% (Ahle et al. 2013). Further research needs to be conducted to elucidate the factors of breast milk that protect against NEC, and whether donor milk prevents NEC.

88.2.11.2 Other Preventative Measures Currently Being Investigated

Feeding Strategies

The fear of NEC has been a major factor delaying enteral feeds in very low-birth weight infants. The optimal timing for initiating enteral feedings and its association with NEC is unknown. One meta-analysis compared early versus delayed enteral feedings (>4 days) and did not find a reduction in NEC. However, delayed enteral feedings were associated with a longer time to full feedings (Morgan and Young 2014). Later initiation of enteral feedings has been shown to be associated with increased morbidities, likely related to higher gut inflammation in those infants not fed early (Konnikova et al. 2015).

Probiotics

Probiotics, which are live microorganisms, have been suggested to be associated with reduced NEC incidence in preterm infants (Hunter et al. 2012). *Lactobacillus reuteri* strain DSM 17938 showed a decrease in feeding intolerance and duration of hospitalization in premature infants weighing less than 1,500 g (Rojas et al. 2012). Several meta-analyses of prospective randomized controlled trials (RCTs) evaluating probiotics use in preventing NEC in very low-birth weight (VLBW; <1,500 g) infants suggest that probiotics can reduce the incidence of NEC (Wang et al. 2012). None of the studies thus far shown a reduced incidence of NEC in babies less than 1,000 g birth weight. In addition, a review of the rigor of the RCTs included in these meta-analyses found that there is not sufficient data to recommend probiotics. Only two of the included studies were classified as high level of evidence and neither showed a benefit of probiotics over placebo (Mihatsch et al. 2012; Rouge et al. 2009). Since then a multicenter double-blind placebo controlled trial (ProPrem) from Australia and New Zealand not powered from NEC on secondary analysis showed a significant reduction of NEC (from 4.4% to 2%) in VLBW (<1,500 g) infants, but no effect on mortality (4.9–5.1%) (Jacobs et al. 2013). However, upon closer inspection, there was no effect on NEC in the ELBW (<1,000 g) infants. The PIPs trial in England set out to evaluate the efficacy and safety of *Bifidobacterium breve* BBG-001 in preterm infants to prevent late-onset sepsis, necrotizing enterocolitis, and death (Costeloe n.d.). There were 1,315 infants between 23 and 31 weeks gestation at 24 hospitals enrolled in this RCT. The early results show there was no significant decrease in NEC, late-onset sepsis, or death (Costeloe n.d.).

There are a few concerns with the studies on probiotics (Abrahamsson et al. 2014). One concern is that many of the studies used different strains of probiotics at different concentrations.

Another concern about the widespread use of probiotics is the side effects of probiotics, specifically sepsis, which has been described in infants (Jenke et al. 2011; Salminen et al. 2004; De Groote et al. 2005; Lin et al. 2008). Sepsis has been seen in patients receiving probiotics containing *Bifidobacterium* and *Lactobacillus* (Jenke et al. 2011; Salminen et al. 2004; De Groote et al. 2005; Lin et al. 2008). One RCT showed the incidence of sepsis was higher in the probiotic group in infants weighing less than 750 g (Lin et al. 2008). Also, recently a product called ABC Dophilus Powder, a probiotic containing *Bifidobacterium lactis*, *Streptococcus thermophilus*, and *Lactobacillus rhamnosus*, was recalled by the US Centers for Disease Control (CDC) after a fatal case of NEC caused by mucormycosis in a premature infant (CDC n.d.). The jury is still out on the routine use of probiotics to prevent NEC, and, therefore, at this time they are currently not recommended for routine use by AAP (Thomas and Greer 2010).

88.2.12 Nutritional Supplements

88.2.12.1 Lactoferrin

Lactoferrin is one of several nutritional supplements that have been studied to evaluate whether their prophylactic use could prevent NEC. A meta-analysis reported a lower risk of NEC (Bell stage II or greater) for preterm infants randomly assigned to oral as compared to placebo (Mohan and Abrams 2015). However, the studies included in this meta-analysis were of low quality. A multicenter randomized clinical trial (Elfin) is currently in process to further investigate whether lactoferrin could be a preventative supplement (Lactoferrin immunoprophylaxis for very preterm infants 2012).

88.2.12.2 Arginine

Arginine is a precursor for nitric oxide (NO) synthesis, and NO plays a significant role in normal GI functioning and mucosal integrity (Konturek and Konturek 1995). Studies have shown that reduced levels of plasma arginine were found in infants with NEC, which suggests that arginine supplementation could reduce intestinal injury and could be a potential preventative treatment (Amin et al. 2002; Shah 2004). A large multicenter RCT providing routine administration of arginine has not been performed.

88.2.13 Future

A consensus on the classification of NEC into subtypes with distinctly different pathophysiology needs to be agreed upon and applied into clinical practice so that research can be performed on each subtype of NEC. More representative animal models, the use of human stem cell derived tissue as well as evaluation of the microbiota prior to the development of NEC along with the host response will help elucidate the pathogenesis and pathophysiology of classical NEC. Diagnostic markers that can be used clinically will need to be developed that can both diagnose and monitor NEC. Treatment options are currently being explored and will be better targeted with improved understanding of the pathophysiology of classical (preterm) NEC. There is still much research to be done to better understand, treat, and prevent the different diseases we call "NEC."

References

Abrahamsson T, Rautava S, Moore A, Neu J, Sherman P (2014) The time for a confirmative necrotizing enterocolitis probiotics prevention trial in the extremely low birth weight infant in North America is now! J Pediatr 2:(165). https://doi.org/10.1016/j.jpeds.2014.05.012

Afrazi A, Branca MF, Sodhi CP et al (2014) Toll-like receptor 4-mediated endoplasmic reticulum stress in intestinal crypts induces necrotizing enterocolitis. J Biol Chem 289(14):9584–9599. https://doi.org/10.1074/jbc.m113.526517

Agwu JC (2005) In a preterm infant, does blood transfusion increase the risk of necrotizing enterocolitis? Arch Dis Child 90(1):102–103. https://doi.org/10.1136/adc.2004.051532

Ahle M, Drott P, Andersson RE (2013) Epidemiology and trends of necrotizing enterocolitis in Sweden: 1987–2009. Pediatrics 132(2):e443–e451. https://doi.org/10.1542/peds.2012-3847

Alexander VN, Northrup V, Bizzarro MJ (2011) Antibiotic exposure in the newborn intensive care unit and the risk of necrotizing enterocolitis. J Pediatr 159(3):392–397. https://doi.org/10.1016/j.jpeds.2011.02.035

Amin HJ, Zamora SA, McMillan DD et al (2002) Arginine supplementation prevents necrotizing enterocolitis in the premature infant. J Pediatr 140(4):425–431. https://doi.org/10.1067/mpd.2002.123289

Anand RJ, Leaphart CL, Mollen KP, Hackam DJ (2007) The role of the intestinal barrier in the pathogenesis of necrotizing enterocolitis. Shock 27(2):124–133. https://doi.org/10.1097/01.shk.0000239774.02904.65

Ardissone A, De La Cruz D, Davis-Richardson A et al (2014) Meconium microbiome analysis identifies bacteria correlated with premature birth. Plos One 9(3): e90784

Arnon S, Litmanovitz I, Regev R et al (2005) Serum amyloid A protein is a useful inflammatory marker during late-onset sepsis in preterm infants. Biol Neonate 87 (2):105–110. https://doi.org/10.1159/000081979

Athalye-Jape G, Rao S, Patole S, More K (2013) Association of inhibitors of gastric acid secretion and higher incidence of necrotizing enterocolitis in preterm very Low-birth-weight infants. Am J Perinatol 30(10):849–856. https://doi.org/10.1055/s-0033-1333671

Autmizguine J, Hornik CP, Benjamin DK et al (2014) Anaerobic antimicrobial therapy after necrotizing enterocolitis in VLBW infants. Pediatrics 135(1): e117–e125. https://doi.org/10.1542/peds.2014-2141

Aydemir C, Dilli D, Oguz SS et al (2011) Serum intestinal fatty acid binding protein level for early diagnosis and prediction of severity of necrotizing enterocolitis. Early Hum Dev 87(10):659–661. https://doi.org/10.1016/j.earlhumdev.2011.05.004

Badolato R (1994) Serum amyloid A is a chemoattractant: induction of migration, adhesion, and tissue infiltration of monocytes and polymorphonuclear leukocytes. J Exp Med 180(1):203–209. https://doi.org/10.1084/jem.180.1.203

Barlow B, Santulli T, Heird W, Pitt J, Blanc W, Schullinger J (1974) An experimental study of acute neonatal enterocolitis – the importance of breast milk. J Pediatr Surg. 5(9):587–595

Basani L, Simmer K, Samnakay N, Deshpande G (1996) Peritoneal drainage versus laparotomy as initial surgical treatment for perforated necrotizing enterocolitis or spontaneous intestinal perforation in preterm low birth weight infants. Cochrane Database Syst Rev. https://doi.org/10.1002/14651858.cd006182.pub2, Rao SC

Bell MJ, Ternberg JL, Feigin RD et al (1978) Neonatal necrotizing enterocolitis. Ann Surg 187(1):1–7. https://doi.org/10.1097/00000658-197801000-00001

Ben-Amor K, Heilig H, Smidt H, Vaughan EE, Abee T, de Vos WM (2005) Genetic diversity of viable, injured, and dead fecal bacteria assessed by fluorescence-activated cell sorting and 16S rRNA gene analysis. Appl Environ Microbiol 71(8):4679–4689. https://doi.org/10.1128/aem.71.8.4679-4689.2005

Benkoe T, Reck C, Pones M et al (2014) Interleukin-8 predicts 60-day mortality in premature infants with necrotizing enterocolitis. J Pediatr Surg 49(3):385–389. https://doi.org/10.1016/j.jpedsurg.2013.05.068

Bhandari V (2006) Familial and genetic susceptibility to major neonatal morbidities in preterm twins. Pediatrics 117(6):1901–1906. https://doi.org/10.1542/peds.2005-1414

Bin-Nun A, Booms C, Sabag N, Mevorach R, Algur N, Hammerman C (2014) Rapid fecal calprotectin (FC) analysis: point of care testing for diagnosing early necrotizing enterocolitis. Am J Perinatol 32 (04):337–342. https://doi.org/10.1055/s-0034-1384640

Bisquera JA, Cooper TR, Berseth CL (2002) Impact of necrotizing enterocolitis on length of stay and hospital charges in very low birth weight infants. Pediatrics 109 (3):423–428. https://doi.org/10.1542/peds.109.3.423

Björkström MV, Hall L, Söderlund S, Håkansson EG, Håkansson S, Domellöf M (2009) Intestinal flora in very low-birth weight infants. Acta Paediatr 98(11):1762–1767. https://doi.org/10.1111/j.1651-2227.2009.01471.x

Blakely M, Lally K, McDonald S, et al (2005) Postoperative outcomes of extremely low birth-weight infants with necrotizing enterocolitis or isolated intestinal perforation: a prospective cohort study by the NICHD Neonatal Research Network. Ann Surg 6(241). http://www.ncbi.nlm.nih.gov/pubmed/?term=blakely+ml+postoperative+outcomes+of+extremely+low+birth-weight+infants+with+necrotizing. Accessed 28 Sept 2015.

Błaż W (2014) Usefulness of ultrasound examinations in the diagnostics of necrotizing enterocolitis. Pol J Radiol 79:1–9. https://doi.org/10.12659/pjr.890539

Bor M, Verloove-Vanhorick SP, Brand R, Ruys JH (1988) Patent ductus arteriosus in a cohort of 1338 preterm infants: a collaborative study a. Paediatr Perinat Epidemiol 2(4).328–336. https://doi.org/10.1111/j.1365-3016.1988.tb00227.x

Boyd CA, Quigley MA, Brocklehurst P (2007) Donor breast milk versus infant formula for preterm infants: systematic review and meta-analysis. Arch Dis Child Fetal Neonatal Ed 92(3):F169–F175. https://doi.org/10.1136/adc.2005.089490

CDC. 128- moved: fatal gastrointestinal mucormycosis in an infant|fungal disease. http://www.cdc.gov/fungal/rhizopus-investigation.html. Accessed 19 Sept 2015.

Chan KYY, Leung FWL, Lam HS et al (2012) Immunoregulatory protein profiles of necrotizing enterocolitis versus spontaneous intestinal perforation in preterm infants. PLoS One 7(5):e36977. https://doi.org/10.1371/journal.pone.0036977, Neu J, ed

Chan KYY, Leung KT, Tam YH et al (2014) Genome-wide expression profiles of necrotizing enterocolitis versus spontaneous intestinal perforation in human intestinal tissues. Ann Surg 260(6):1128–1137. https://doi.org/10.1097/sla.0000000000000374

Cheu HW (1990) Breath hydrogen excretion in the premature neonate. Arch Pediatr Adolesc Med 144(2):197. https://doi.org/10.1001/archpedi.1990.02150260077032

Claud EC, Walker WA (2001) Hypothesis: inappropriate colonization of the premature intestine can cause neonatal necrotizing enterocolitis. FASEB J 15:1398–1403

Claud EC, Keegan KP, Brulc JM et al (2013) Bacterial community structure and functional contributions to emergence of health or necrotizing enterocolitis in preterm infants. Microbiome 1:20

Cole CR, Hansen NI, Higgins RD, Ziegler TR, Stoll BJ (2008) Very low birth weight preterm infants with surgical short bowel syndrome: incidence, morbidity and mortality, and growth outcomes at 18 to 22 months. Pediatrics 122(3):e573–e582. https://doi.org/10.1542/peds.2007-3449

Colgan SP, Taylor CT (2010) Hypoxia: an alarm signal during intestinal inflammation. Nat Rev Gastroenterol Hepatol 7 (5):281–287. https://doi.org/10.1038/nrgastro.2010.39

Costeloe K (2016) Probiotics in preterm infants: the PiPS trial. In: Hot topics in neonatology

Cotten CM, Taylor S, Stoll B et al (2009) Prolonged duration of initial empirical antibiotic treatment is associated with increased rates of necrotizing enterocolitis and death for extremely low birth weight infants. Pediatrics 123(1):58–66. https://doi.org/10.1542/peds.2007-3423

Coursey CA, Hollingsworth CL, Gaca AM, Maxfield C, DeLong D, Bisset G (2008) Radiologists' agreement when using a 10-point scale to report abdominal radiographic findings of necrotizing enterocolitis in neonates and infants. Am J Roentgenol 191(1):190–197. https://doi.org/10.2214/ajr.07.3558

Cucchiara S, Minella R, Iervolino C et al (1993) Omeprazole and high dose ranitidine in the treatment of refractory reflux oesophagitis. Arch Dis Child 69(6): 655–659. https://doi.org/10.1136/adc.69.6.655

Däbritz J, Jenke A, Wirth S, Foell D (2012) Fecal phagocyte-specific S100A12 for diagnosing necrotizing enterocolitis. J Pediatr 161(6):1059–1064. https://doi.org/10.1016/j.jpeds.2012.06.003

De Groote MA, Frank DN, Dowell E, Glode MP, Pace NR (2005) Lactobacillus rhamnosus GG bacteremia associated with probiotic use in a child with short gut syndrome. Pediatr Infect Dis J 24(3):278–280. https://doi.org/10.1097/01.inf.0000154588.79356.e6

De Meij TGJ, van der Schee MPC, Berkhout DJC et al (2015) Early detection of necrotizing enterocolitis by fecal volatile organic compounds analysis. J Pediatr 167(3):562–567. https://doi.org/10.1016/j.jpeds.2015.05.044, e1

Derikx JP (2010) Non-invasive markers of gut wall integrity in health and disease. World J Gastroenterol 16(42): 5272. https://doi.org/10.3748/wjg.v16.i42.5272

DeWitt AG, Charpie JR, Donohue JE, Yu S, Owens GE (2014) Splanchnic near-infrared spectroscopy and risk of necrotizing enterocolitis after neonatal heart surgery. Pediatr Cardiol 35(7):1286–1294. https://doi.org/10.1007/s00246-014-0931-5

DiGiulio DB, Romero R, Amogan HP et al (2008) Microbial prevalence, diversity and abundance in amniotic fluid during preterm labor: a molecular and culture-based investigation. PLoS One 3(8):e3056. https://doi.org/10.1371/journal.pone.0003056, Fisk NM

Donovan SM, Wang M, Li M, Friedberg I, Schwartz SL, Chapkin RS (2012) Host-microbe interactions in the neonatal intestine: role of human milk oligosaccharides. Adv Nutr (Bethesda, Md) 3:450S–455S

Edelson MB, Bagwell CE, Rozycki HJ (1999) Circulating Pro- and counterinflammatory cytokine levels and severity in necrotizing enterocolitis. Pediatrics 103(4): 766–771. https://doi.org/10.1542/peds.103.4.766

Elphick DA (2005) Paneth cells: their role in innate immunity and inflammatory disease. Gut 54(12):1802–1809. https://doi.org/10.1136/gut.2005.068601

Faingold R, Daneman A, Tomlinson G et al (2005) Necrotizing enterocolitis: assessment of bowel viability with color doppler US1. Radiology 235(2):587–594. https://doi.org/10.1148/radiol.2352031718

Faix RG, Polley TZ, Grasela TH (1988) A randomized, controlled trial of parenteral clindamycin in neonatal necrotizing enterocolitis. J Pediatr 112 (2):271–277. https://doi.org/10.1016/s0022-3476(88)80069-6

Falkow S (2004) Opinion: Molecular Koch's postulates applied to bacterial pathogenicity – a personal recollection 15 years later. Nat Rev Microbiol 2(1):67–72. https://doi.org/10.1038/nrmicro799

Fitzgibbons SC, Ching Y, Yu D et al (2009) Mortality of necrotizing enterocolitis expressed by birth weight categories. J Pediatr Surg 44(6):1072–1076. https://doi.org/10.1016/j.jpedsurg.2009.02.013

Fouhy F, Guinane CM, Hussey S et al (2012) High-throughput sequencing reveals the incomplete, short-term recovery of infant gut microbiota following parenteral antibiotic treatment with ampicillin and gentamicin. Antimicrob Agents Chemother 56(11): 5811–5820. https://doi.org/10.1128/aac.00789-12

Gatt M, Reddy BS, Macfie J (2006) Review article: bacterial translocation in the critically ill – evidence and methods of prevention. Aliment Pharmacol Ther 25(7): 741–757. https://doi.org/10.1111/j.1365-2036.2006.03174.x

Goldmann DA, Leclair J, Macone A (1978) Bacterial colonization of neonates admitted to an intensive care environment. J Pediatr 93(2):288. https://doi.org/10.1016/S0022-3476(78)80523-X

Gordon PV (2009) Understanding intestinal vulnerability to perforation in the extremely low birth weight infant. Pediatr Res 65(2):138–144. https://doi.org/10.1203/pdr.0b013e31818c7920

Gordon P, Christensen R, Weitkamp J-H, Maheshwari A (2012) Mapping the new world of necrotizing enterocolitis (NEC): review and opinion. E-J Neonatol Res 4: 145–172

Gordon PV, Clark R, Swanson JR, Spitzer A (2014) Can a national dataset generate a nomogram for necrotizing enterocolitis onset? J Perinatol 34(10):732–735. https://doi.org/10.1038/jp.2014.137

Goulet O, Baglin-Gobet S, Talbotec C et al (2005) Outcome and long-term growth after extensive small bowel resection in the neonatal period: a survey of 87 children.

Eur J Pediatr Surg 15(2):95–101. https://doi.org/10.1055/s-2004-821214

Gupta RW, Tran L, Norori J et al (2013) Histamine-2 receptor blockers alter the fecal microbiota in premature infants. J Pediatr Gastroenterol Nutr 56: 397–400

Guthrie SO, Gordon PV, Thomas V, Thorp JA, Peabody J, Clark RH (2003) Necrotizing enterocolitis among neonates in the United States. J Perinatol 23(4):278–285. https://doi.org/10.1038/sj.jp.7210892

Hammerman C, Goldschmidt D, Caplan MS et al (2002) Protective effect of bilirubin in ischemia-reperfusion injury in the rat intestine. J Pediatr Gastroenterol Nutr 35(3):344–349. https://doi.org/10.1097/00005176-200209000-00020

Hanson LÅ, Korotkova M, Telemo E (2003) Breastfeeding, infant formulas, and the immune system. Ann Allergy Asthma Immunol 90(6):59–63. https://doi.org/10.1016/s1081-1206(10)61662-6

Harris MC, D'Angio CT, Gallagher PR, Kaufman D, Evans J, Kilpatrick L (2005) Cytokine elaboration in critically ill infants with bacterial sepsis, necrotizing entercolitis, or sepsis syndrome: correlation with clinical parameters of inflammation and mortality. J Pediatr 147(4):462–468. https://doi.org/10.1016/j.jpeds.2005.04.037

Hawiger J (2001) Innate immunity and inflammation: a transcriptional paradigm. Immunol Res 23 (2-3):099–110. https://doi.org/10.1385/IR:23:2-3:099

He R (2002) Serum amyloid A induces IL-8 secretion through a G protein-coupled receptor, FPRL1/LXA4R. Blood 101(4):1572–1581. https://doi.org/10.1182/blood-2002-05-1431

Hintz SR (2005) Neurodevelopmental and growth outcomes of extremely low birth weight infants after necrotizing enterocolitis. Pediatrics 115(3):696–703. https://doi.org/10.1542/peds.2004-0569

Ho T, Dukhovny D, Zupancic JA, Goldmann DA, Horbar JD, Pursley DM (2015) Choosing wisely in newborn medicine: five opportunities to increase value. Pediatrics 136:e482–e489

Holman RC, Stoll BJ, Curns AT, Yorita KL, Steiner CA, Schonberger LB (2006) Necrotising enterocolitis hospitalisations among neonates in the United States. Paediatr Perinat Epidemiol 20(6):498–506. https://doi.org/10.1111/j.1365-3016.2006.00756.x

Horwitz JR, Lally KP, Cheu HW, David Vazquez W, Grosfeld JL, Ziegler MM (1995) Complications after surgical intervention for necrotizing enterocolitis: a multicenter review. J Pediatr Surg 30(7):994–999. https://doi.org/10.1016/0022-3468(95)90328-3

Huda S, Chaudhery S, Ibrahim H, Pramanik A (2014) Neonatal necrotizing enterocolitis: clinical challenges, pathophysiology and management. Pathophysiology 21(1):3–12. https://doi.org/10.1016/j.pathophys.2013.11.009

Hunter C, Dimaguila MAV, Gal P et al (2012) Effect of routine probiotic, lactobacillus reuteri DSM 17938, use on rates of necrotizing enterocolitis in neonates with birthweight < 1000 grams: a sequential analysis. BMC Pediatr 12(1):142. https://doi.org/10.1186/1471-2431-12-142

Hutter JJ, Hathaway WE, Wayne ER (1976) Hematologic abnormalities in severe neonatal necrotizing enterocolitis. J Pediatr 88(6):1026–1031. https://doi.org/10.1016/s0022-3476(76)81069-4

Hyman PE, Clarke DD, Everett SL et al (1985) Gastric acid secretory function in preterm infants. J Pediatr 106(3): 467–471. https://doi.org/10.1016/s0022-3476(85)80682-x

Ian W, Garstin H, Boston VE (1987) Sequential assay of expired breath hydrogen as a means of predicting necrotizing enterocolitis in susceptible infants. J Pediatr Surg 22(3):208–210. https://doi.org/10.1016/s0022-3468(87)80329-9

Jacobs S, Tobin J, Opie G (2013) Probiotic effects on late-onset sepsis in very preterm infants: a randomized controlled trial. Pediatrics 132(6):X9–X9. https://doi.org/10.1542/peds.2013-1339d

Jenke A, Ruf E-M, Hoppe T, Heldmann M, Wirth S (2011) Bifidobacterium septicaemia in an extremely low-birthweight infant under probiotic therapy. Arch Dis Childhood Fetal Neonatal Ed 97(3):F217–F218. https://doi.org/10.1136/archdischild-2011-300838

Jilling T, Simon D, Lu J et al (2006) The roles of bacteria and TLR4 in rat and murine models of necrotizing enterocolitis. J Immunol 177(5):3273–3282. https://doi.org/10.4049/jimmunol.177.5.3273

Jones BA, Hull MA, Kim HB (2010) Autologous intestinal reconstruction surgery for intestinal failure management. Curr Opin Organ Transplant 15(3):341–345. https://doi.org/10.1097/mot.0b013e328338c2c0

Josephson CD, Wesolowski A, Bao G et al (2010) Do red cell transfusions increase the risk of necrotizing enterocolitis in premature infants? J Pediatr 157(6):972–978. https://doi.org/10.1016/j.jpeds.2010.05.054, e3

Kafetzis DA, Skevaki C, Costalos C (2003) Neonatal necrotizing enterocolitis: an overview. Curr Opin Infect Dis 16(4):349–355. https://doi.org/10.1097/00001432-200308000-00007

Kazez A, Küçükaydin N, Küçükaydin M, Kontaş O, Okur H, Doğan P (1997) A model of hypoxia-induced necrotizing enterocolitis: the role of distension. J Pediatr Surg 32(10):1466–1469. https://doi.org/10.1016/s0022-3468(97)90564-9

Kilpinen S, Henttinen T, Lahdenpohja N, Hulkkonen J, Hurme M (1996) Signals leading to the activation of NF-kappaB transcription factor are stronger in neonatal than adult T lymphocytes. Scand J Immunol 44(1):85–88. https://doi.org/10.1046/j.1365-3083.1996.d01-277.x

Konikoff MR, Denson LA (2006) Role of fecal calprotectin as a biomarker of intestinal inflammation in inflammatory bowel disease. Inflamm Bowel Dis 12(6):524–534. https://doi.org/10.1097/00054725-200606000-00013

Konnikova Y, Zaman MM, Makda M, D'Onofrio D, Freedman SD, Martin CR (2015) Late enteral feedings are associated with intestinal inflammation and

adverse neonatal outcomes. PLoS One 10: e0132924

Konturek SK, Konturek PC (1995) Role of nitric oxide in the digestive system. Digestion 56(1):1–13. https://doi.org/10.1159/000201214

(2012) Lactoferrin immunoprophylaxis for very preterm infants. Arch Dis Childhood Fetal Neonatal Ed. 98(1): F2–F4. https://doi.org/10.1136/archdischild-2011-301273

Ladd AP, Rescorla FJ, West KW, Scherer L, Engum SA, Grosfeld JL (1998) Long-term follow-up after bowel resection for necrotizing enterocolitis: factors affecting outcome. J Pediatr Surg 33(7):967–972. https://doi.org/10.1016/s0022-3468(98)90516-4

Le Mandat Schultz A, Bonnard A, Berrebi D et al (2007) Expression of TLR-2, TLR-4, NOD2 and pNF-kB in a neonatal rat model of necrotizing enterocolitis. PLoS One 2(10):e1102. https://doi.org/10.1371/journal.pone.0001102, Gold J, ed

Leaphart CL, Cavallo J, Gribar SC et al (2007) A critical role for TLR4 in the pathogenesis of necrotizing enterocolitis by modulating intestinal injury and repair. J Immunol 179(7):4808–4820. https://doi.org/10.4049/jimmunol.179.7.4808

Lieberman JM, Sacchettini J, Marks C, Marks WH (1997) Human intestinal fatty acid binding protein: report of an assay with studies in normal volunteers and intestinal ischemia. Surgery 121(3):335–342. https://doi.org/10.1016/s0039-6060(97)90363-9

Lin PW, Stoll BJ (2006) Necrotising enterocolitis. Lancet 368(9543):1271–1283. https://doi.org/10.1016/s0140-6736(06)69525-1

Lin H, Hsu C, Chen H, et al (2008) Oral probiotics prevent necrotizing enterocolitis in very low birth weight preterm infants: a multicenter, randomized, controlled trial. Pediatrics 4(122). https://doi.org/10.1542/peds.2007-3007

Lucas A, Cole TJ (1990) Breast milk and neonatal necrotising enterocolitis. Lancet 336(8730-8731):1519–1523. https://doi.org/10.1016/0140-6736(90)93304-8

Maayan-Metzger A, Itzchak A, Mazkereth R, Kuint J (2004) Necrotizing enterocolitis in full-term infants: case–control study and review of the literature. J Perinatol 24(8):494–499. https://doi.org/10.1038/sj.jp.7211135

MacDonald TT (2003) The mucosal immune system. Parasite Immunol 25(5):235–246. https://doi.org/10.1046/j.1365-3024.2003.00632.x

Maheshwari A, Schelonka RL, Dimmitt RA et al (2014) Cytokines associated with necrotizing enterocolitis in extremely-low-birth-weight infants. Pediatr Res 76(1): 100–108. https://doi.org/10.1038/pr.2014.48

Mai V, Young CM, Ukhanova M et al (2011) Fecal microbiota in premature infants prior to necrotizing enterocolitis. PLoS One 6(6):e20647. https://doi.org/10.1371/journal.pone.0020647, Chakravortty D

Mally P, Golombek SG, Mishra R et al (2006) Association of necrotizing enterocolitis with elective packed red blood cell transfusions in stable, growing, premature neonates. Am J Perinatol 23(08):451. https://doi.org/10.1055/s-2006-951300

Maury CPJ (1985) Comparative study of serum amyloid a protein and C-reactive protein in disease. Clin Sci 68(2):233–238. https://doi.org/10.1042/cs0680233

McElroy SJ, Underwood MA, Sherman MP (2013) Paneth cells and necrotizing enterocolitis: a novel hypothesis for disease pathogenesis. Neonatology 103:10–20

Meier PP, Bode L (2013) Health, nutrition, and cost outcomes of human milk feedings for very low birthweight infants. Adv Nutr: Int Rev J 4(6):670–671. https://doi.org/10.3945/an.113.004457

Mihatsch WA, Braegger CP, Decsi T et al (2012) Critical systematic review of the level of evidence for routine use of probiotics for reduction of mortality and prevention of necrotizing enterocolitis and sepsis in preterm infants. Clin Nutr 31(1):6–15. https://doi.org/10.1016/j.clnu.2011.09.004

Minekawa R, Takeda T, Sakata M, Hayashi M (2004) Human breast milk suppresses the transcriptional regulation of IL-1 -induced NF- B signaling in human intestinal cells. AJP: Cell Physiol 287(5):C1404–C1411. https://doi.org/10.1152/ajpcell.00471.2003

Mohan P, Abrams SA (2015) Oral lactoferrin for the prevention of sepsis and necrotizing enterocolitis in premature infants. Cochrane Database Syst Rev. https://doi.org/10.1002/14651858.CD007137

Morgan J, Young L (2014) Delayed introduction of progressive enteral feeds to prevent necrotising enterocolitis in very low birth weight infants. Cochrane Database Syst Rev. https://doi.org/10.1002/14651858.cd001970.pub5, McGuire W

Moss LR, Dimmitt RA, Henry MCW, Geraghty N, Efron B (2001) A meta-analysis of peritoneal drainage versus laparotomy for perforated necrotizing enterocolitis. J Pediatr Surg 36(8):1210. https://doi.org/10.1053/jpsu.2001.25764

Neu J, Walker WA (2011) Necrotizing enterocolitis. N Engl J Med 364(3):255–264. https://doi.org/10.1056/nejmra1005408

Ng PC, Cheng SH, Chui KM et al (1997) Diagnosis of late onset neonatal sepsis with cytokines, adhesion molecule, and C-reactive protein in preterm very low birthweight infants. Arch Dis Childhood Fetal Neonatal Ed 77(3):F221–F227. https://doi.org/10.1136/fn.77.3.f221

Ng PC, Ang IL, Chiu RWK et al (2010) Host-response biomarkers for diagnosis of late-onset septicemia and necrotizing enterocolitis in preterm infants. J Clin Investig 120(8):2989–3000. https://doi.org/10.1172/jci40196

Ng EWY, Poon TCW, Lam HS et al (2013) Gut-associated biomarkers L-FABP, I-FABP, and TFF3 and LIT score for diagnosis of surgical necrotizing enterocolitis in preterm infants. Ann Surg 258(6):1111–1118. https://doi.org/10.1097/sla.0b013e318288ea96

Oh S, Young C, Gravenstein N, Islam S, Neu J (2010) Monitoring technologies in the neonatal intensive care unit: implications for the detection of necrotizing

enterocolitis. J Perinatol 30(11):701–708. https://doi.org/10.1038/jp.2010.9
Orenstein SR, Shalaby TM, Devandry SN et al (2003) Famotidine for infant gastro-oesophageal reflux: a multi-centre, randomized, placebo-controlled, withdrawal trial. Aliment Pharmacol Ther 17(9):1097–1107. https://doi.org/10.1046/j.1365-2036.2003.01559
Orenstein S, Gremse D, Pantaleon C, Kling D, Rotenberg K (2005) Nizatidine for the treatment of pediatric gastroesophageal reflux symptoms: an open-label, multiple-dose, randomized, multicenter clinical trial in 210 children. Clin Ther 27(4):472–483. https://doi.org/10.1016/j.clinthera.2005.04.008
Ostlie DJ, Spilde TL, St Peter SD et al (2003) Necrotizing enterocolitis in full-term infants. J Pediatr Surg 38(7):1039–1042. https://doi.org/10.1016/s0022-3468(03)00187-8
Otte J-M, Cario E, Podolsky DK (2004) Mechanisms of cross hyporesponsiveness to toll-like receptor bacterial ligands in intestinal epithelial cells☆. Gastroenterology 126(4):1054–1070. https://doi.org/10.1053/j.gastro.2004.01.007
Pelsers MMAL, Hermens WT, Glatz JFC (2005) Fatty acid-binding proteins as plasma markers of tissue injury. Clin Chim Acta 352(s 1–2):15–35. https://doi.org/10.1016/j.cccn.2004.09.001
Potoka DA, Upperman JS, Nadler EP et al (2002) NF-kB inhibition enhances peroxynitrite-induced enterocyte apoptosis. J Surg Res 106(1):7–14. https://doi.org/10.1006/jsre.2002.6423
Pourcyrous M (2005) C-reactive protein in the diagnosis, management, and prognosis of neonatal necrotizing enterocolitis. Pediatrics 116(5):1064–1069. https://doi.org/10.1542/peds.2004-1806
Quigley M, McGuire W (2014) Formula versus donor breast milk for feeding preterm or low birth weight infants. https://doi.org/10.1002/14651858.CD002971.pub3
Rehan VK, Seshia MMK, Johnston B, Reed M, Wilmot D, Cook V (1999) Observer variability in interpretation of abdominal radiographs of infants with suspected necrotizing enterocolitis. Clin Pediatr 38(11):637–643. https://doi.org/10.1177/000992289903801102
Remon J, Kampanatkosol R, Kaul RR, Muraskas JK, Christensen RD, Maheshwari A (2014) Acute drop in blood monocyte count differentiates NEC from other causes of feeding intolerance. J Perinatol 34(7):549–554. https://doi.org/10.1038/jp.2014.52
Rojas MA, Lozano JM, Rodriguez VA et al (2012) Prophylactic probiotics to prevent death and nosocomial infection in preterm infants. Pediatrics 130(5):e1113–e1120. https://doi.org/10.1542/peds.2011-3584
Rouge C, Piloquet H, Butel M-J et al (2009) Oral supplementation with probiotics in very-low-birth-weight preterm infants: a randomized, double-blind, placebo-controlled trial. Am J Clin Nutr 89(6):1828–1835. https://doi.org/10.3945/ajcn.2008.26919
Salminen MK, Rautelin H, Tynkkynen S et al (2004) Lactobacillus bacteremia, clinical significance, and patient outcome, with special focus on probiotic L. rhamnosus GG. Clin Infect Dis 38(1):62. https://doi.org/10.1086/380455
Salzman NH, Polin RA, Harris MC et al (1998) Enteric defensin expression in necrotizing enterocolitis. Pediatr Res 44(1):20–26. https://doi.org/10.1203/00006450-199807000-00003
Salzman NH, Underwood MA, Bevins CL (2007) Paneth cells, defensins, and the commensal microbiota: a hypothesis on intimate interplay at the intestinal mucosa. Semin Immunol 19(2):70–83. https://doi.org/10.1016/j.smim.2007.04.002
Sampath V, Le M, Lane L et al (2011) The NFKB1 (g.-24519delATTG) variant is associated with necrotizing enterocolitis (NEC) in premature infants. J Surg Res 169(1):e51–e57. https://doi.org/10.1016/j.jss.2011.03.017
Sangild PT, Petersen YM, Elnif J, Schmidt MH, Buddington RK, Burrin DG (2000) Premature and term newborn pigs differ in their intestinal responses to parenteral and enteral nutrition. Gastroenterology 118(4):A76. https://doi.org/10.1016/s0016-5085(00)82381-1
Sangild PT, Thymann T, Schmidt M, Stoll B, Burrin DG, Buddington RK (2013) Invited review: the preterm pig as a model in pediatric gastroenterology. J Anim Sci 91:4713–4729
Santulli T, Schullinger J, Heird W, Gongaware R, Wigger J (1975) Acute necrotizing enterocolitis in infancy: a review of 64 cases. Pediatrics 55(3):376–387
Sedda S, Marafini I, Figliuzzi MM, Pallone F, Monteleone G (2014) An overview of the role of innate lymphoid cells in gut infections and inflammation. Mediators Inflamm 2014:1–7. https://doi.org/10.1155/2014/235460
Shah P (2004) Arginine supplementation for prevention of necrotising enterocolitis in preterm infants. Cochrane Database Syst Rev. https://doi.org/10.1002/14651858.CD004339.pub2
Singh R, Visintainer PF, Frantz ID et al (2011) Association of necrotizing enterocolitis with anemia and packed red blood cell transfusions in preterm infants. J Perinatol 31(3):176–182. https://doi.org/10.1038/jp.2010.145
Smith B, Bodé S, Petersen BL et al (2011) Community analysis of bacteria colonizing intestinal tissue of neonates with necrotizing enterocolitis. BMC Microbiol 11(1):73. https://doi.org/10.1186/1471-2180-11-73
Smith JM, Skeans MA, Horslen SP et al (2014) OPTN/SRTR 2012 annual data report: intestine. Am J Transplant 14(S1):97–111. https://doi.org/10.1111/ajt.12582
Sola MC, Del Vecchio A, Rimsza LM (2000) Evaluation and treatment of thrombocytopenia in the neonatal intensive care unit. Clin Perinatol 27(3):655–679. https://doi.org/10.1016/s0095-5108(05)70044-0
Soliman A, Michelsen KS, Karahashi H et al (2010) Platelet-activating factor induces TLR4 expression in intestinal epithelial cells: implication for the pathogenesis of necrotizing enterocolitis. PLoS One 5(10):e15044. https://doi.org/10.1371/journal.pone.0015044, Unutmaz D, ed

Sonntag J, Grimmer I, Scholz T, Metze B, Wit J, Obladen M (2000) Growth and neurodevelopmental outcome of very low birthweight infants with necrotizing enterocolitis. Acta Paediatr (Oslo, Norway : 1992) 5(89):528–532

Spencer AU, Kovacevich D, McKinney-Barnett M et al (2008) Pediatric short-bowel syndrome: the cost of comprehensive care. Am J Clin Nutr 88(6):1552–1559. https://doi.org/10.3945/ajcn.2008.26007

Stewart C (2015) Early gut microbiome and polymicrobial infection. Encycl Metagenomics pp. 143–150. https://doi.org/10.1007/978-1-4899-7475-4_798

Stoll B, Cismowski M, Hamrick S, Bhatia A (2013) Cytokine levels in the preterm infant with neonatal intestinal injury. Am J Perinatol 31(06):489–496. https://doi.org/10.1055/s-0033-1353437

Stringer MD, Brereton RJ, Drake DP, Kiely EM, Capps SNJ, Spitz L (1993) Recurrent necrotizing enterocolitis. J Pediatr Surg 28(8):979–981. https://doi.org/10.1016/0022-3468(93)90496-8

Sudan D, Thompson J, Botha J et al (2007) Comparison of intestinal lengthening procedures for patients with short bowel syndrome. Ann Surg 246(4):593–604. https://doi.org/10.1097/sla.0b013e318155aa0c

Sullivan S, Schanler RJ, Kim JH et al (2010) An exclusively human milk-based diet is associated with a lower rate of necrotizing enterocolitis than a diet of human milk and bovine milk-based products. J Pediatr 156(4):562–567. https://doi.org/10.1016/j.jpeds.2009.10.040

Taft DH, Ambalavanan N, Schibler KR et al (2014) Intestinal microbiota of preterm infants differ over time and between hospitals. Microbiome 2(1):36. https://doi.org/10.1186/2049-2618-2-36

Tam AL, Camberos A, Applebaum H (2002) Surgical decision making in necrotizing enterocolitis and focal intestinal perforation: predictive value of radiologic findings. J Pediatr Surg 37(12):1688–1691. https://doi.org/10.1053/jpsu.2002.36696

Tepas JJ, Sharma R, Hudak ML, Garrison RD, Pieper P (2006) Coming full circle: an evidence-based definition of the timing and type of surgical management of very low-birth-weight (<1000 g) infants with signs of acute intestinal perforation. J Pediatr Surg 41(2):418–422. https://doi.org/10.1016/j.jpedsurg.2005.11.041

Thomas DW, Greer FR (2010) Probiotics and prebiotics in pediatrics. Pediatrics 126:1217–1231

Thuijls G, Derikx JPM, van Wijck K et al (2010) Non-invasive markers for early diagnosis and determination of the severity of necrotizing enterocolitis. Ann Surg 251(6):1174–1180. https://doi.org/10.1097/sla.0b013e3181d778c4

Tomomasa T, Takahashi A, Nako Y et al (1999) Analysis of gastrointestinal sounds in infants with pyloric stenosis before and after pyloromyotomy. Pediatrics 104(5): e60–e60. https://doi.org/10.1542/peds.104.5.e60

Torrazza M, Li N, Young C et al (2013) Pilot study using proteomics to identify predictive biomarkers of necrotizing enterocolitis from buccal swabs in very low birth weight infants. Neonatology 104(3):234. https://doi.org/10.1159/000353721

Torrazza RM, Li N, Neu J (2014) Decoding the enigma of necrotizing enterocolitis in premature infants. Pathophysiology 21(1):21–27. https://doi.org/10.1016/j.pathophys.2013.11.011

Turner D, Hammerman C, Rudensky B et al (2007) Low levels of procalcitonin during episodes of necrotizing enterocolitis. Dig Dis Sci 52(11):2972–2976. https://doi.org/10.1007/s10620-007-9763-y

Vennarecci G, Kato T, Misiakos E, et al (2000) Intestinal transplantation for short gut syndrome attributable to necrotizing enterocolitis. Pediatrics 2(105):587–595

Voganatsi A et al (2001) Mechanism of extracellular release of human neutrophil calprotectin complex. J Leukoc Biol 70(1):130–134

Walsh M, Kliegman R (1986) Necrotizing enterocolitis: treatment based on staging criteria. Pediatr Clin North Am 33(1):179–210

Wang Q, Dong J, Zhu Y (2012) Probiotic supplement reduces risk of necrotizing enterocolitis and mortality in preterm very low-birth-weight infants: an updated meta-analysis of 20 randomized, controlled trials. J Pediatr Surg 47(1):241–248. https://doi.org/10.1016/j.jpedsurg.2011.09.064

Wang M, Li M, Wu S, Lebrilla C, Chapkin R, Ivanov I, Donovan S (2015) Fecal microbiota composition of breast-fed infants is correlated with human milk oligosaccharides consumed. J Pediatr Gastroenterol Nutr 60(6):825. https://doi.org/10.1097/MPG.0000000000000752

Yatsunenko T, Rey F, Manary M, et al (2012) Human gut microbiome viewed across age and geography. Nature 7402(486). http://www.ncbi.nlm.nih.gov/pubmed/22699611. Accessed 28 Sept 2015

Yoon JM, Min J, Yi J et al (2014) Fecal calprotectin concentration in neonatal necrotizing enterocolitis. Korean J Pediatr 57(8):351. https://doi.org/10.3345/kjp.2014.57.8.351

Zoppelli L, Güttel C, Bittrich H-J, Andrée C, Wirth S, Jenke A (2012) Fecal calprotectin concentrations in premature infants have a lower limit and show postnatal and gestational age dependence. Neonatology 102(1):68–74. https://doi.org/10.1159/000337841

Surgical Treatment in Newborns of Necrotizing Enterocolitis

89

Nigel J. Hall and Agostino Pierro

Contents

Abstract

Great controversy surrounds the indications for surgery in infants with NEC. While many respond to intensive medical treatment, in up to 50% more severe NEC develops, requiring surgical intervention. As with the lack of consensus regarding indications for surgical intervention, there is a lack of consensus concerning the ideal surgical management of infants with NEC. Surgical options depend primarily on the extent of intestinal disease and the clinical stability of the infant. In addition to surgery in the acute phase, a number of infants develop late complications of NEC, either following medical or previous surgical treatment, and these complications may require surgical intervention. Clear knowledge of these outcomes is important in counseling parents and in assessing the effectiveness of treatments.

N. J. Hall (✉)
University Surgery Unit, Faculty of Medicine, University of Southampton, Southampton, UK
e-mail: n.j.hall@soton.ac.uk

A. Pierro
Division of General and Thoracic Surgery, The Hospital for Sick Children, Toronto, Canada
e-mail: agostino.pierro@sickkids.ca

G. Buonocore et al. (eds.), *Neonatology*,
https://doi.org/10.1007/978-3-319-29489-6_236

89.1 Salient Points

- Many infants with NEC respond to intensive medical treatment, while up to 50% develop more severe NEC requiring surgical intervention.
- There is little consensus as to the most appropriate timing and nature of surgery to be performed.
- Surgical options depend primarily on the extent of intestinal disease and the clinical stability of the infant.
- Mortality from NEC is related to the severity of disease, degree of prematurity, and associated anomalies.
- A number of infants develop late complications of NEC, either following medical treatment or previous surgeries; these complications require surgical intervention.

89.2 Introduction

While many infants with NEC respond to intensive medical treatment, up to 50% develop more severe NEC requiring surgical intervention (Kosloske 1985). This group of infants represents a major challenge for pediatric surgeons, and there is little consensus as to the most appropriate timing and nature of surgery. In addition to surgery in the acute phase, a number of infants develop late complications of NEC, either following medical or previous surgical treatment, and these complications require surgical intervention.

There is great controversy surrounding the indications for surgery in infants with NEC. Table 1 summarizes the indications reported in the literature. In a survey of pediatric surgeons from the United Kingdom, the indications for operation in neonates with NEC included pneumoperitoneum in 45%, clinical deterioration in 37%, and intestinal obstruction in 18% (Rees et al. 2005). The most widely accepted indication for surgery is the presence of pneumoperitoneum but this is not always demonstrable even in neonates with intestinal perforation. Other absolute indications for surgery in acute NEC include the continued deterioration of an infant that is refractory to maximal medical treatment, persisting inotrope requirement and an abdominal mass or abscess secondary to intestinal perforation. Recently abdominal ultrasound has been used to detect necrotic intestine. Although this technique is operator dependent, the information obtained can be useful in deciding whether infants not responding to medical treatment require a laparotomy (Yikilmaz et al. 2014).

Table 1 Indications for surgery in infants with NEC

Absolute indications
Pneumoperitoneum
Clinical deterioration despite maximal medical treatment
Abdominal mass with persistent intestinal obstruction or sepsis
Intestinal stricture
Relative indications
Abdominal mass
Increased abdominal tenderness, distension, and/or discoloration
Intestinal perforation associated with persistent signs of intestinal obstruction and/or sepsis
Portal venous gas

In similarity to the lack of consensus regarding indications for surgical intervention, there is a lack of consensus concerning the ideal surgical management of infants with NEC. While a number of factors may be considered in determining the type of surgical intervention including the weight and clinical status of the infant, even very low birth weight infants appear to tolerate surgery well (Anveden-Hertzberg and Gauderer 2000). Surgical options for the infant with NEC include primary peritoneal drainage (PPD) or laparotomy. At laparotomy, the principal surgical objectives are to control sepsis, remove gangrenous bowel, and preserve as much bowel length as possible (Fasoli et al. 1999; Pierro 1997; Albanese and Rowe 1998). Within these objectives, a number of surgical options exist (Table 2) depending primarily on the extent of intestinal disease and the clinical stability of the infant. At laparotomy, the extent of the disease can be classified as focal when it is limited to a single intestinal segment and multifocal if it includes two or more intestinal segments with more than 50% of the small intestine viable and panintestinal when the majority of the small and

large bowel are involved with less than 25% viable bowel remaining (Fasoli et al. 1999).

89.3 Primary Peritoneal Drainage

The use of peritoneal drainage before laparotomy, as a method of stabilizing and improving the systemic status of extremely low birth weight premature infants with intestinal perforation secondary to NEC, was first proposed by Marshall and Ein in the 1970s (Ein et al. 1977; Marshall 1975). Initially, it was hoped that the drainage of air and stools from an infant too unstable for a laparotomy would relieve symptoms of abdominal compartment syndrome and infection and subsequently improve tolerance of a laparotomy. Subsequent reports, predominantly of infants weighing <1500 g, have proposed that peritoneal drainage may be used as a definitive treatment without the need for subsequent laparotomy. In fact some reports have claimed that this method of treatment may in fact be superior to laparotomy. Subsequently, two randomized controlled trials (RCTs) have addressed the issue of whether primary peritoneal drainage (PPD) or laparotomy is superior in the smallest infants with NEC (Moss et al. 2006; Rees et al. 2008). These are summarized in Table 3.

Table 2 Surgical options for advanced NEC

Surgical options
Primary peritoneal drainage
Laparotomy
Resection with enterostomy
Resection with primary anastomosis
Proximal diverting jejunostomy
"Clip and drop" technique

Interestingly neither trial found a significant difference in primary outcome measures between infants treated with PPD or laparotomy. However, the authors of one of the trials advocate the use of a primary laparotomy as a definitive treatment on the basis of no significant difference in outcome between the groups and a need for delayed/rescue laparotomy in 74% in infants who initially had PPD (Rees et al. 2008).

89.4 Resection of Affected Bowel and Enterostomy Formation

Resection of necrotic bowel in neonates with NEC has the theoretical advantage of reducing bacterial translocation, correcting the septic state of the patient and removing the driving force behind the systemic inflammatory response. Following intestinal resection, the conventional view is that it is safer to exteriorize the bowel ends as the presence of peritonitis, inflammation of the bowel wall, and reduced intestinal blood supply in patients with NEC are unfavorable factors for the healing of an anastomosis (Andreasyan et al. 2007). Furthermore, the stoma allows adequate healing and rests the distal bowel prior to subsequent reanastomosis (Fasoli et al. 1999). There are, however, a number of potential disadvantages to this approach. It is often difficult to reestablish sufficient enteral feeding for adequate weight gain (Bethell et al. 2016). High-output stomas, in particular, carry a risk of dehydration and electrolyte imbalance, and

Table 3 RCTs comparing laparotomy with primary peritoneal drainage in infants with perforated necrotizing enterocolitis

Study	Included infants	Number	Main outcomes	Authors conclusion
Moss et al. 2006 (2006)	<1500 g	PPD 55 Lap 62	No difference in mortality or dependence on PN at 90 days or length of hospital admission	No effect of procedure on outcome
Rees et al. 2008 (2008)	<1000 g	PPD 35 Lap 34	No difference in survival, ventilator or PN dependence at 1 or 6 months or length of hospital admission 74% of infants undergoing PPD required delayed rescue laparotomy	Recommend early laparotomy

PPD primary peritoneal drain, *Lap* laparotomy, *PN* parenteral nutrition

the importance of early closure to avoid chronic salt and water loss has been highlighted. Enterostomies have also been associated with significant morbidity while present, including stenosis, prolapse, and excoriation of the surrounding skin. Stoma closure involves a second anesthesia and is usually performed once the infant is thriving and fully recovered from the acute stage of the illness. Metabolic or physical problems, however, may demand earlier surgery. In one series, the incidence of complications in infants with enterostomies for NEC was 68% (O'Connor and Sawin 1998). This high rate has prompted the search for alternative strategies that may avoid the need for repetitive surgery and complications associated with stomas, while ensuring that the underlying surgical principles of treating NEC by means of laparotomy are adhered to. Thus in many centers, a primary anastomosis is preferred following intestinal resection whenever deemed safe to do so.

89.5 Resection and Primary Anastomosis

The attractiveness of primary anastomosis following intestinal resection is that a second surgical procedure can be avoided. However, consideration must be given to the potential complications of intestinal anastomoses, particularly leakage and, in the longer term, stricture formation. Once considered a hazardous surgical option because of the risk of anastomotic leakage due to poor intraperitoneal healing in the presence of peritonitis, inflammation of the bowel wall, and compromised intestinal blood supply, this approach has gained popularity. A number of centers have published retrospective reviews of infants treated with intestinal resection and primary anastomosis with results comparable with or in some cases favorable to those obtained with stoma formation. Furthermore, while resection and primary anastomosis were initially described in selected patients with focal disease and in good general condition, it is also now gaining acceptance as a valid treatment option for severe NEC, in very low birth weight infants (Hall et al. 2005) and even for multifocal disease (Pierro 1997).

Despite a number of reports, there remains no good-quality evidence to suggest whether stoma formation or primary anastomosis confers an advantage over the other approach following intestinal resection for NEC. On ongoing trial comparing primary anastomosis with stoma formation in infants undergoing intestinal resection for NEC will hopefully help delineate the optimal surgical strategy (STAT Trial 2012).

89.6 Operations for Panintestinal Disease

The techniques described thus far are of particular use for the infant with one or more short segments of NEC. Multiple resections and primary anastomoses may be appropriate for some infants with more widespread disease, provided careful attention is paid to the viability of resection margins. Infants with NEC affecting a large proportion of the gastrointestinal tract pose a particularly difficult problem, and treatment of this group remains particularly controversial. The surgical principles in these children are difficult if not impossible to fulfill. Due to the length of bowel involved, it is often not possible to fully remove all gangrenous intestines while salvaging adequate length for sustainable life. It is for these reasons that in the infant with panintestinal NEC who is unstable and critically ill, some surgeons would forego further treatment. However, when there is doubt, a number of techniques have recently been reported with the aim of allowing time for stabilization of the infants' general condition and the possibility of some healing of the gastrointestinal tract to occur. Due to the severity of the disease, the mortality with these strategies remains high.

89.6.1 Proximal Jejunostomy

Initially proposed by Martin and Neblett (1981), surgical creation of a high jejunostomy in the presence of panintestinal disease has been reported in several small series (Thyoka et al. 2011; Sugarman and Kiely 2001). This technique allows decompression and defunctioning of the

diseased intestine but does not remove gangrenous segments and may permit continued bacterial translocation. A second laparotomy with intestinal reconstructive surgery is performed once the infant has recovered from the acute stage of the illness with the aim of preserving as much bowel length as possible. Typically, this is performed sooner (4–6 weeks) than elective stoma closure since the infant is unlikely to thrive until some form of intestinal continuity is achieved. This procedure may be useful in neonates with NEC affecting the majority of the intestine, but the high morbidity and mortality rate should be carefully considered.

89.6.2 "Clip and Drop" Technique

This method complies with surgical principles and also avoids stoma formation. For the infant with extensive bowel necrosis, Vaughan et al. (1996) advocated the resection of all segments of grossly nonviable or perforated bowel, irrigation, and aspiration of peritoneal contamination, clipping the ends of remaining bowel and returning them to the abdomen. This is followed by a second-look laparotomy with delayed anastomosis 48–72 h later. In their small series, all three infants with NEC survived (Vaughan et al. 1996), and in a subsequent report of four infants in whom this technique was employed, one died, and the remaining three required stoma formation at the second look (Molik et al. 2001). Ron et al. reported a series of 13 infants undergoing this surgical technique of whom just six were long-term survivors, all of whom had fairly extensive surgical morbidity. However, all achieved full enteral feeds (Ron et al. 2009).

89.7 Authors' Preferred Surgical Strategy

The author's preferred approach to the operative management of infants with NEC is illustrated in Fig. 1. In infants with focal disease involving a small length of small or large bowel, a resection and primary anastomosis are usually performed, with the exception of patients unstable during the operation or with unhealthy distal intestine who are managed with a stoma at the level of the affected bowel.

In infants with multifocal disease (>50% of the bowel assumed to be viable), various surgical options are available. Resection and one or more intestinal anastomoses (preferably not more than two) are performed when it is possible to ascertain the viability of the bowel distal to NEC without causing significant bleeding. Stoma (with or without intestinal resection), proximal enterostomy or clip, and drop technique are performed when (a) it is not possible to ascertain the status of the bowel distal to the NEC, (b) the distal bowel is of dubious viability, (c) attempts to dissect the distal bowel cause significant bleeding, and (d) the patient is unstable perioperatively. In these

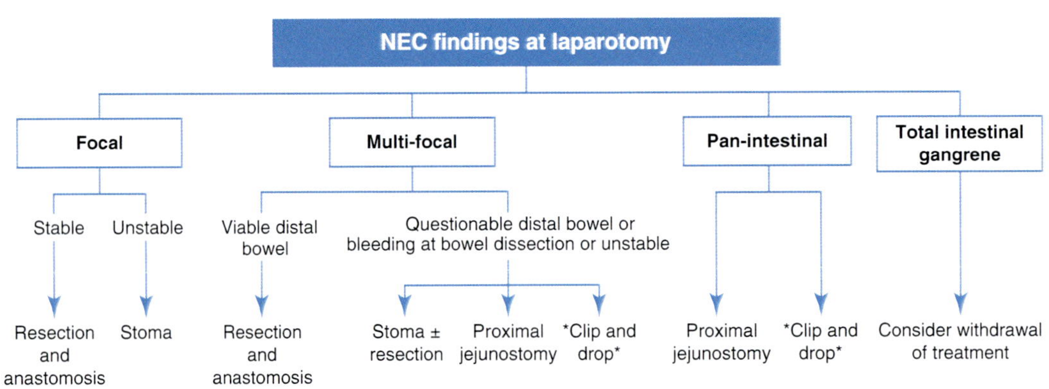

Fig. 1 Authors' preferred operative management of NEC (Adapted from Pierro and Hall (2003))

circumstances, a stoma with or without intestinal resection(s) is the preferred surgical option. However, if this would lead to massive intestinal resection, the "clip and drop" technique described earlier will be adopted in an attempt to salvage as much intestinal length as possible. If the mobilization of the bowel loops affected by NEC causes significant bleeding, a high diverting jejunostomy is preferred.

In patients with panintestinal disease (>75% of small and large bowel involved), two options are considered: (a) proximal diverting jejunostomy when the intestinal resection would cause significant bleeding or loss of the majority of the small bowel and (b) "clip and drop" technique in the attempt to salvage some of the affected bowel and avoid a short bowel syndrome. In neonates with total intestinal gangrene, closure of the abdomen and treatment withdrawal are considered.

89.8 Outcome of Surgical Intervention

Central to the decision to operate on an infant with NEC and in determining the most appropriate operation to perform is the effect of any surgical intervention on outcome. Mortality from NEC is related to severity of disease, degree of prematurity, and associated anomalies. In a study of 83 neonates who required a laparotomy for advanced NEC (Fasoli et al. 1999), the overall mortality rate was 30%. Causes of death included multisystem organ failure ($n = 10$), sepsis ($n = 14$), and congenital cardiac abnormality ($n = 1$). The mortality rate was higher (67%) in infants with panintestinal involvement compared with infants with focal (12%) or multifocal disease (30%). While mortality is clearly the most important outcome to be considered, morbidity in survivors of NEC is often significant.

Up to 30% of infants develop an intestinal stricture after NEC (Phad et al. 2014). These are commonly located in the colon, can affect multiple intestinal segments, can promote a second episode of NEC, and can occur distal to the diverting stoma. Post-NEC strictures should ideally be resected with an end-to-end anastomosis.

In addition to the "surgical" complications related to intestinal anastomoses and stomas, other medium- and long-term complications include short bowel syndrome (affecting up to 23% of survivors of NEC) (Cikrit et al. 1986), hepatic cholestasis related to long-term parenteral nutrition dependency, and malabsorption. Importantly it is now accepted that infants who develop NEC are at increased risk of adverse neurodevelopmental outcome compared with preterm infants who do not develop NEC. Infants with NEC who require surgery appear to be more severely affected than those who respond to medical treatment alone (Hintz et al. 2005; Rees et al. 2007).

Clearly knowledge of these outcomes is important in counseling parents and in assessing effectiveness of treatments. As we now progress to critically determine whether a particular surgical approach is more effective than another in the setting of randomized controlled trials, it is imperative that we consider these morbidities and in particular neurodevelopmental outcome in addition to mortality as part of our evaluations.

References

Albanese CT, Rowe MI (1998) Necrotizing Enterocolitis. In: O'Neill JA Jr, Rowe MI, Grosfeld JL, Fonkalsrud EW, Coran AG (eds) Pediatric Surgery, vol 2, 5th edn. Mosby, St Louis, pp 1297–1332

Andreasyan K, Ponsonby AL, Dwyer T, Dear K, Cochrane J (2007) Infant feeding and childhood atopy: does early introduction of non-milk fluids matter? Pediatr Allergy Immunol 18(3):250–257. https://doi.org/10.1111/j.1399-3038.2006.00509.x

Anveden-Hertzberg L, Gauderer MW (2000) Surgery is safe in very low birthweight infants with necrotizing enterocolitis. Acta Paediatr 89(2):242–245

Bethell G, Kenny S, Corbett H (2016) Enterostomy-related complications and growth following reversal in infants. Arch Dis Child Fetal Neonatal Ed. https://doi.org/10.1136/archdischild-2016-311126

Cikrit D, West KW, Schreiner R, Grosfeld JL (1986) Long-term follow-up after surgical management of necrotizing enterocolitis: sixty-three cases. J Pediatr Surg 21(6):533–535

Ein SH, Marshall DG, Girvan D (1977) Peritoneal drainage under local anesthesia for perforations from necrotizing enterocolitis. J Pediatr Surg 12(6):963–967

Fasoli L, Turi RA, Spitz L, Kiely EM, Drake D, Pierro A (1999) Necrotizing enterocolitis: extent

of disease and surgical treatment. J Pediatr Surg 34(7):1096–1099

Hall NJ, Curry J, Drake DP, Spitz L, Kiely EM, Pierro A (2005) Resection and primary anastomosis is a valid surgical option for infants with necrotizing enterocolitis who weigh less than 1000 g. Arch Surg 140(12):1149–1151

Hintz SR, Kendrick DE, Stoll BJ, Vohr BR, Fanaroff AA, Donovan EF, Poole WK, Blakely ML, Wright L, Higgins R (2005) Neurodevelopmental and growth outcomes of extremely low birth weight infants after necrotizing enterocolitis. Pediatrics 115(3):696–703

Kosloske AM (1985) Surgery of necrotizing enterocolitis. World J Surg 9(2):277–284

Marshall DG (1975) Peritoneal drainage under local anesthesia for necrotizing enterocolitis perforation. In: January 1975. Winnipeg, Manitoba

Martin LW, Neblett WW (1981) Early operation with intestinal diversion for necrotizing enterocolitis. J Pediatr Surg 16(3):252–255

Molik KA, West KW, Rescorla FJ, Scherer LR, Engum SA, Grosfeld JL (2001) Portal venous air: the poor prognosis persists. J Pediatr Surg 36(8):1143–1145

Moss RL, Dimmitt RA, Barnhart DC, Sylvester KG, Brown RL, Powell DM, Islam S, Langer JC, Sato TT, Brandt ML, Lee H, Blakely ML, Lazar EL, Hirschl RB, Kenney BD, Hackam DJ, Zelterman D, Silverman BL (2006) Laparotomy versus peritoneal drainage for necrotizing enterocolitis and perforation. N Engl J Med 354(21):2225–2234

O'Connor A, Sawin RS (1998) High morbidity of enterostomy and its closure in premature infants with necrotizing enterocolitis. Arch Surg 133(8):875–880

Phad N, Trivedi A, Todd D, Lakkundi A (2014) Intestinal strictures post-necrotising enterocolitis: clinical profile and risk factors. J Neonatal Surg 3(4):44

Pierro A (1997) Necrotizing enterocolitis: pathogenesis and treatment. Br J Hosp Med 58(4):126–128

Pierro A, Hall N (2003) Surgical treatment of infants with necrotizing enterocolitis. Semin Neonatol 8(3): 223–232

Rees CM, Hall NJ, Eaton S, Pierro A (2005) Surgical strategies for necrotising enterocolitis: a survey of practice in the United Kingdom. Arch Dis Child Fetal Neonatal Ed 90(2):F152–F155. https://doi.org/10.1136/adc.2004.051862

Rees CM, Pierro A, Eaton S (2007) Neurodevelopmental outcomes of neonates with medically and surgically treated necrotizing enterocolitis. Arch Dis Child Fetal Neonatal Ed 92(3):F193–F198

Rees CM, Eaton S, Kiely EM, Wade AM, McHugh K, Pierro A (2008) Peritoneal drainage or laparotomy for neonatal bowel perforation? A randomized controlled trial. Ann Surg 248(1):44–51

Ron O, Davenport M, Patel S, Kiely E, Pierro A, Hall NJ, Ade-Ajayi N (2009) Outcomes of the "clip and drop" technique for multifocal necrotizing enterocolitis. J Pediatr Surg 44 (4):749–754. doi:S0022–3468(08)00825–7 [pii]; https://doi.org/10.1016/j.jpedsurg.2008.09.031

STAT Trial (2012) http://www.isrctn.com/ISRCTN01700960

Sugarman ID, Kiely EM (2001) Is there a role for high jejunostomy in the management of severe necrotising enterocolitis? Pediatr Surg Int 17(2–3):122–124

Thyoka M, Eaton S, Kiely EM, Curry JI, Drake DP, Cross KM, Hall NJ, Khoo AK, De Coppi P, Pierro A (2011) Outcomes of diverting jejunostomy for severe necrotizing enterocolitis. J Pediatr Surg 46(6):1041–1044. https://doi.org/10.1016/j.jpedsurg.2011.03.024

Vaughan WG, Grosfeld JL, West K, Scherer LR III, Villamizar E, Rescorla FJ (1996) Avoidance of stomas and delayed anastomosis for bowel necrosis: the 'clip and drop-back' technique. J Pediatr Surg 31(4):542–545

Yikilmaz A, Hall NJ, Daneman A, Gerstle JT, Navarro OM, Moineddin R, Pleasants H, Pierro A (2014) Prospective evaluation of the impact of sonography on the management and surgical intervention of neonates with necrotizing enterocolitis. Pediatr Surg Int 30(12):1231–1240. https://doi.org/10.1007/s00383-014-3613-8

Part IX

Hematology, Immunology, and Malignancies

Hematology and Immunology of Newborns: Overview

90

Robert D. Christensen

Contents

R. D. Christensen (✉)
Divisions of Neonatology and Hematology, Department of Pediatrics, University of Utah School of Medicine, Intermountain Healthcare, Salt Lake City, UT, USA
e-mail: Robert.Christensen@hsc.utah.edu

G. Buonocore et al. (eds.), *Neonatology*,
https://doi.org/10.1007/978-3-319-29489-6_237

Abstract
Normal ranges for hematologic values in adult medicine are established by drawing blood from large numbers of healthy adult volunteers. These are not available for newborns; therefore, neonatal hematology utilizes the concept of "reference intervals" which consist of 5th to 95th percentile values compiled from laboratory tests performed on selected neonates from whom a complete blood count (CBC) was drawn for a clinical purpose. The various blood cell counts of neonates must be interpreted in accordance with reference intervals based on gestational and postnatal age. Making a judgment about whether a hematological value is normal or abnormal requires cognizance of other factors such as any specific illnesses involved, the level of intensive care support given, and the anatomical site of the blood sampling (venous, arterial, capillary). Reference intervals for hemoglobin, hematocrit, erythrocyte indices, reticulocyte count, neutrophil and eosinophil concentrations, platelet count, and mean platelet volume are reported in this chapter. Reference values are not available for bone marrow aspirate or biopsy, since they are usually performed on not strictly normal subjects.

90.1 Salient Points

- "Normal ranges" for hematologic values of neonates are generally not available. Instead neonatal hematology utilizes "reference intervals."
- The "reference intervals" concern erythrocytes, leukocytes, and platelets.
- A bone marrow aspirate or biopsy is useful in providing information not otherwise available.

90.2 The Reference Interval Concept

"Normal ranges" for hematologic values of neonates are generally not available. This is because blood is not drawn on healthy normal neonates to establish such ranges, as is done with the consent of healthy adult volunteers. Instead, neonatal hematology utilizes "reference intervals." These consist of 5th–95th percentile values compiled from laboratory tests that were performed on neonates thought to have minimal pathology relevant to that laboratory test or with pathology unlikely to significantly affect the test results. The premise on which the reference interval concept is based is that these values approximate normal ranges, although they were admittedly obtained for a clinical reason and not from healthy volunteers.

Defining reference intervals in neonatal hematology is complicated by the fact that ranges obtained from term infants generally do not apply to preterm infants and ranges obtained from low-birth-weight preterm infants can be very different from ranges obtained from extremely low-birth-weight preterm infants. As an example, a venous hematocrit of 38% would be within the reference range for a 2-h-old neonate born at 24 weeks gestation, but would be low for a 2-h-old term infant.

Another problem encountered in defining reference intervals in neonatal hematology is that unstable sick neonates might have values within the reference interval, yet those values might not be optimal for patient care. As an example, for a neonate born at 24 weeks gestation, now 4 weeks old, a venous hematocrit of 24% would be normal, in that it is above the lower 5th % reference interval limit. However, if such a patient develops a nosocomial infection, becomes hypoxemic and tachycardic, and is placed on a ventilator, the hematocrit of 24% might be too low for optimal patient care. A higher hematocrit might facilitate better tissue oxygenation, diminish the heart rate, and permit better caloric utilization for growth. Therefore, just because a value falls within the reference interval does not assure that it is optimal for the clinical circumstances.

Making a determination about whether a specific hematologic value is normal or abnormal often requires cognizance of the gestational age of the neonate, the age (hours after delivery) when the sample was obtained, any specific illnesses involved, the level of intensive care support

given, and the anatomical site of the blood sampling (venous, arterial, capillary). Sometimes knowledge of other factors is pertinent, such as whether delayed cord clamping occurred or "stripping or milking" of the umbilical cord was performed after delivery. This chapter describes the reference intervals that have been assembled for use in neonatal hematology and immunology and provides information needed to avoid pitfalls in interpreting these limits.

90.3 Erythrocytes

90.3.1 Hemoglobin Concentration

The concentration of hemoglobin in the blood and the hematocrit are among the most commonly performed of all clinical laboratory tests. The hemoglobin can be quantified by manual or automated techniques. The standard assay for hemoglobin determination, approved by the World Health Organization, is simple but highly reproducible (International Committee for Standardization in Haematology 1978). It involves the conversion of the several forms of hemoglobin in the blood, including oxyhemoglobin, carboxyhemoglobin, and the minor quantities of other hemoglobin species present, to a single compound, hemoglobincyanide, which is then determined spectrophotometrically. The hemoglobin concentration and the hematocrit are, for the most part, different measurements of the same biologic variable. However, because the hemoglobin concentration is a direct measurement but the hematocrit is usually calculated, as explained later, the hemoglobin concentration has sometimes been a slightly preferred method.

Reference intervals for hemoglobin values on the day of birth of newborn infants 22–42 weeks gestation (Jopling et al. 2009) are shown in Fig. 1. In keeping with the reference interval concept, values were not included in the figure if the mother had a diagnosis of placenta previa, abruptio placenta, or any antenatal hemorrhage or if the patient had a diagnosis of hemorrhage at birth. No differences occur on the basis of gender. Postmature infants do not have higher hemoglobin concentrations than those delivered at term, unless chronic hypoxemia has occurred.

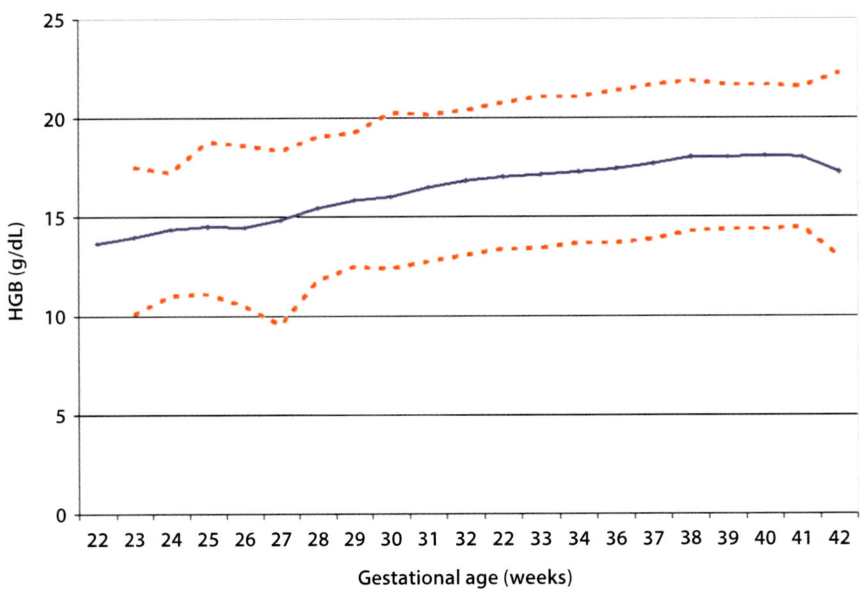

Fig. 1 Reference intervals for blood hemoglobin concentration on the day of birth ($n = 24{,}416$ patients) at 22–42 weeks gestation. The *solid line* shows the mean value, and the *dashed lines* show the 5% and 95% reference intervals (Reproduced from Jopling et al. (2009), with permission)

Reference intervals for hemoglobin over the first 28 days after birth are shown in Fig. 2 for patients 35–42 weeks gestation at birth and in Fig. 3 for patients 29–34 weeks gestation. Hemoglobin values for patients <29 weeks were not included in the report because virtually all had repeated phlebotomy and erythrocyte transfusions, thus confounding the slope of the hemoglobin reference range.

90.3.2 Hematocrit

In 1929, Dr. Maxwell M. Wintrobe described a clinical laboratory test that he called the *volume of packed red blood cells* (VPRC) (Wintrobe 1929). The test was performed by centrifuging blood in a specifically designed glass tube called a *hematocrit*. Originally, "hematocrit" was the name of the tube used in the measurement, not the measurement itself. However, usage subsequently changed, and the term hematocrit now typically indicates the measurement, and the term VPRC is rarely used.

The hematocrit is the proportion of the blood sample occupied by erythrocytes. The units for hematocrit are usually given as either a percentage or a decimal fraction (liters of red blood cells/liter of blood). Because neonates and young children do not have a liter of blood in their entire circulation, children's hospital laboratories sometimes choose to express the hematocrit as a percentage not as liters per liter.

Originally, the result of the hematocrit test was read directly from the tube, after a standardized centrifugation, as the proportion of the height of the total column of blood occupied by red cells. Although an extremely simple concept, this test constituted a significant advance in clinical medicine. It was highly successful and became widely used, probably because the results were very reproducible and useful in patient care and because the test could be performed without complicated or expensive instrumentation. Subsequent modifications of the hematocrit test to permit using small blood samples led to its applicability to neonates. Ten years after it was described for testing adults, Waugh and

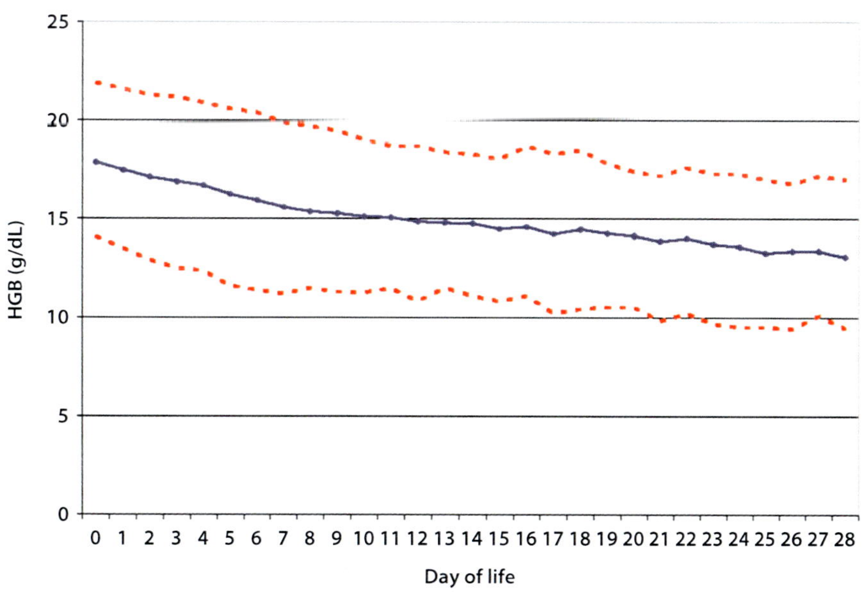

Fig. 2 Reference intervals for blood hemoglobin concentration during the 28 days after birth for neonates 35–42 weeks gestation. The *solid line* shows the mean value, and the *dashed lines* show the 5% and 95% reference intervals (Reproduced from Jopling et al. (2009), with permission)

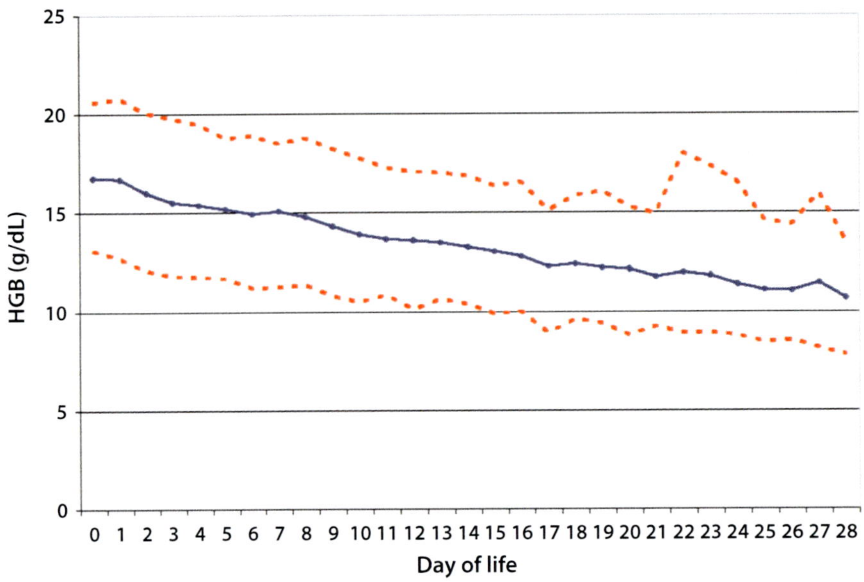

Fig. 3 Reference intervals for blood hemoglobin concentration during the 28 days after birth for neonates 29–34 weeks gestation. The *solid line* shows the mean value, and the *dashed lines* show the 5% and 95% reference intervals (Reproduced from Jopling et al. (2009), with permission)

colleagues reported that the hematocrit of normal infants, averaging 51.3%, was higher than that of normal adults (Waugh et al. 1939).

Most hospital laboratories no longer use centrifugation methods for hematocrit determinations; instead, aperture-impedance instruments calculate the hematocrit. This is done by electronically measuring the mean red blood cell volume and multiplying this number by the erythrocyte concentration, also measured electronically. The mean volume of the erythrocytes multiplied by their number per microliter yields the volume of red blood cells per microliter or the hematocrit. Other types of cell counters calculate the hematocrit using laser optics, correlating the magnitude of a light pulse generated by passing a red blood cell through a laser with the cell's volume.

Many neonatologists have noticed that when manual and electronic methods for hematocrit determination are used on an individual neonate, a consistent difference occurs between the two, a difference usually not seen in testing older children and adults. Neonates tend to have a slightly higher spun hematocrit than automated hematocrit. The reason for this involves the phenomenon of trapped plasma in the spun hematocrit. When blood is centrifuged, a small amount of plasma is always "trapped" between the erythrocytes, slightly elevating the spun hematocrit value. The amount of trapped plasma is insignificant in most cases, usually in the range of 1–3% of the plasma volume, as determined by radioiodinated serum albumin labeling experiments (Smock and Perkins 2014). However, in samples with a very high hematocrit, more plasma becomes trapped when the cells are centrifuged. Because term neonates have higher hematocrits than adults, this additional plasma trapping tends to make the spun hematocrit a higher value than the automated, calculated value (which is not subject to the plasma trapping pitfall). Few spun hematocrits are used in modern neonatology, but in any NICUs doing so, this difference between spun and automated hematocrit values should be recognized.

Hematocrit reference intervals for newborn infants on the day of birth at 22–42 weeks gestation (Jopling et al. 2009) are shown in Fig. 4. As with hemoglobin, no differences occur on the basis of gender. Reference ranges for hematocrit

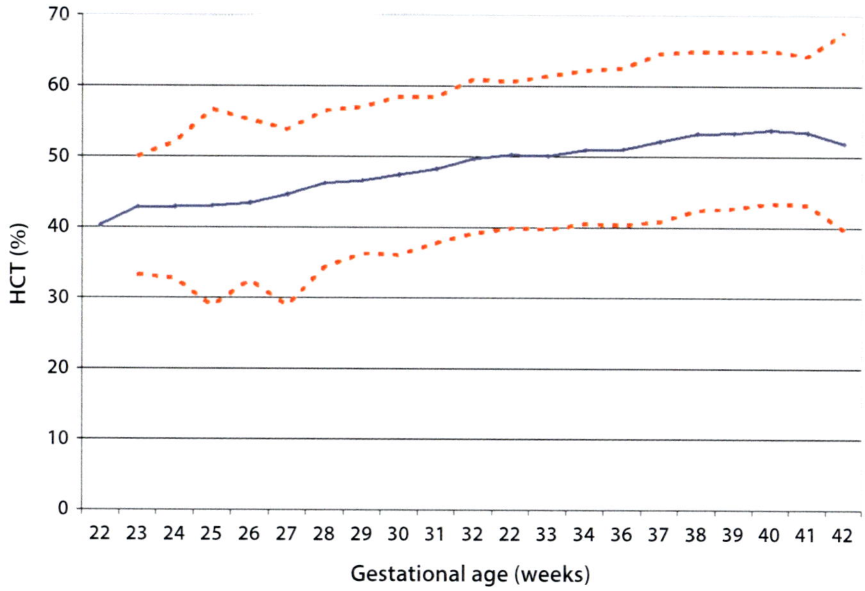

Fig. 4 Reference intervals for hematocrit on the day of birth ($n = 25{,}464$ patients) at 22–42 weeks gestation. The *solid line* shows the mean value, and the *dashed lines* show the 5% and 95% reference intervals (Reproduced from Jopling et al. (2009), with permission)

over the first 28 days after birth are shown in Fig. 5 for patients 35–42 weeks gestation at birth and in Fig. 6 for patients 29–34 weeks.

The hematocrit, like the hemoglobin and the erythrocyte count, normally increases during the first 4 h after birth. The increase, as shown in Fig. 7, might not occur in preterm infants. Gairdner et al. first reported this consistent postnatal increase in hematocrit during the hours following birth and speculated that it was the result of intravascular concentration of blood received by placental transfusion (Gairdner et al. 1952). Its absence in preterm infants might be due to early phlebotomy losses for laboratory studies or lack of a placental transfusion (because of the desire to rapidly hand the patient to the neonatology team).

90.3.3 Erythrocyte Count

The erythrocyte count is the number of erythrocytes in a volume of blood, usually expressed as cells per microliter or cells per liter. Older methods for determining the erythrocytecount used a counting chamber viewed from a microscope, but modern methods use an electronic particle counter, sampling many logs more cells than the previous methods.

90.3.4 Erythrocyte Indices

In addition to devising the hematocrit, Dr. Wintrobe introduced the concept of *erythrocyte indices* and described methods for their calculation. Virtually every CBC includes a report of these indices. The original manual methods for making the measurements with which the erythrocyte indices were calculated have been replaced by automated instruments, which provide measurements that are more precise and reproducible. These indices can provide the neonatologist with valuable information not otherwise available.

The *mean corpuscular volume* (MCV) is a measure of the average size of circulating erythrocytes, expressed in femtoliters (fL, 10^{-15} L).

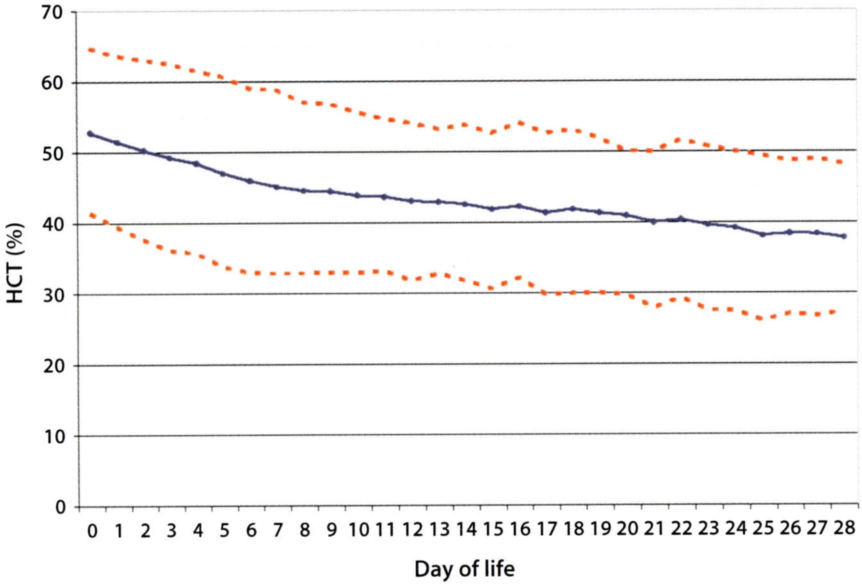

Fig. 5 Reference intervals for hematocrit during the 28 days after birth for neonates 35–42 weeks gestation. The *solid line* shows the mean value, and the *dashed lines* show the 5% and 95% reference intervals (Reproduced from Jopling et al. (2009), with permission)

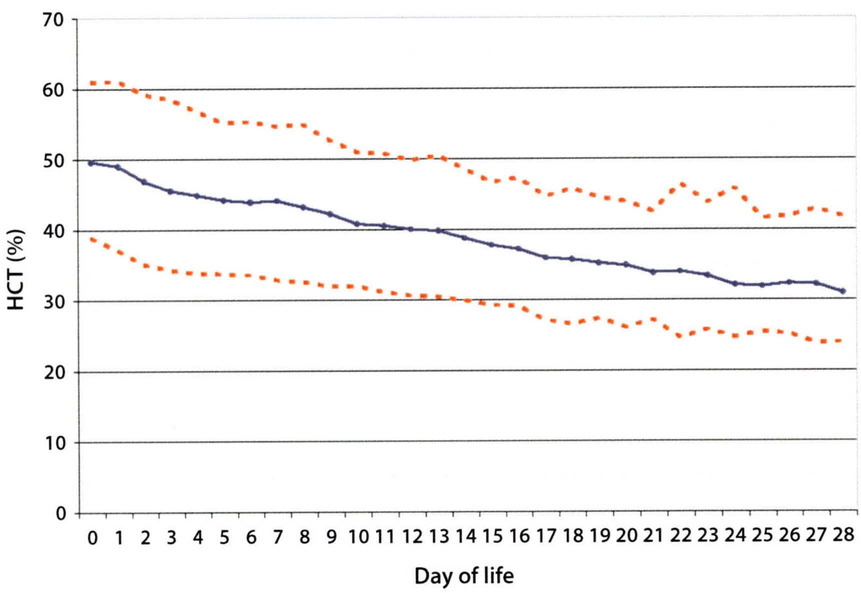

Fig. 6 Reference intervals for hematocrit during the 28 days after birth for neonates 29–34 weeks gestation. The *solid line* shows the mean value, and the *dashed lines* show the 5% and 95% reference intervals (Reproduced from Jopling et al. (2009), with permission)

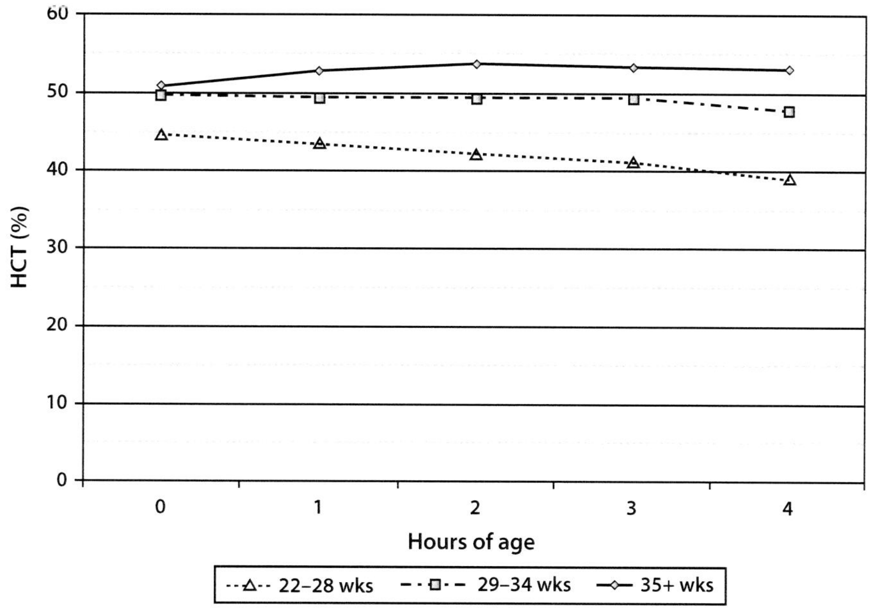

Fig. 7 Reference intervals for hematocrit over the 4-h period following birth (n = 23,534 patients). Three groups are shown based on gestational age (Reproduced from Jopling et al. (2009), with permission)

Most modern automated cell counters, using laser optics or aperture-impedance, measure the MCV of erythrocytes directly. However, as originally described, the MCV was calculated after measuring the hematocrit and the erythrocyte count by the formula:

$$\mathrm{MCV(fL)} = \frac{\mathrm{Hematocrit(L/L)} \times 1000}{\mathrm{Erythrocyte\ count}\left(\times 10^{12}/\mathrm{L}\right)}$$

The *mean corpuscular hemoglobin* (MCH) is a measure of the amount of hemoglobin in an average circulating erythrocyte. It is expressed in picograms of hemoglobin (pg, 10^{-12} g) and is given by the formula:

$$\mathrm{MCH(pg)} = \frac{\mathrm{Hemoglobin(g/L)}}{\mathrm{Erythrocyte\ count}\left(\times 10^{12}/\mathrm{L}\right)}$$

The *mean corpuscular hemoglobin concentration* (MCHC) is a measure of the concentration of hemoglobin in an average circulating erythrocyte and is expressed as units of grams of hemoglobin per deciliter of packed red blood cells (*g/dL*):

$$\mathrm{MCHC(g/dL)} = \frac{\mathrm{Hemoglobin(g/dL)}}{\mathrm{Hematocnt(L/L)}}$$

Reference ranges for MCV and MCH (Christensen et al. 2008) from 22 to 42 weeks gestation are shown in Fig. 8. A fetus at 22–24 weeks gestation, and similarly an extremely preterm neonate at 22–24 weeks gestation, has erythrocytes that are exceeding large, by comparison to those of adults. The MCV and MCH fall immediately when a preterm neonate receives an erythrocyte transfusion, because the MCV and MCH of the blood donor will be much lower. By 3–4 months after birth, the MCV and MCH have diminished to the level of a normal adult (88 ± 8 fL). Thereafter, the MCV continues to decline, reaching nadir levels during the fourth to sixth months and then slowly increasing to adult values after the first year. When a newborn infant has an MCV of less than 94 fL, alpha-thalassemia trait or iron deficiency should be considered. Erythrocyte indices of Central African neonates do not differ from those of neonates from other parts of the world, although the hematocrits of these neonates are somewhat lower (Scott-Emuakpor et al. 1985).

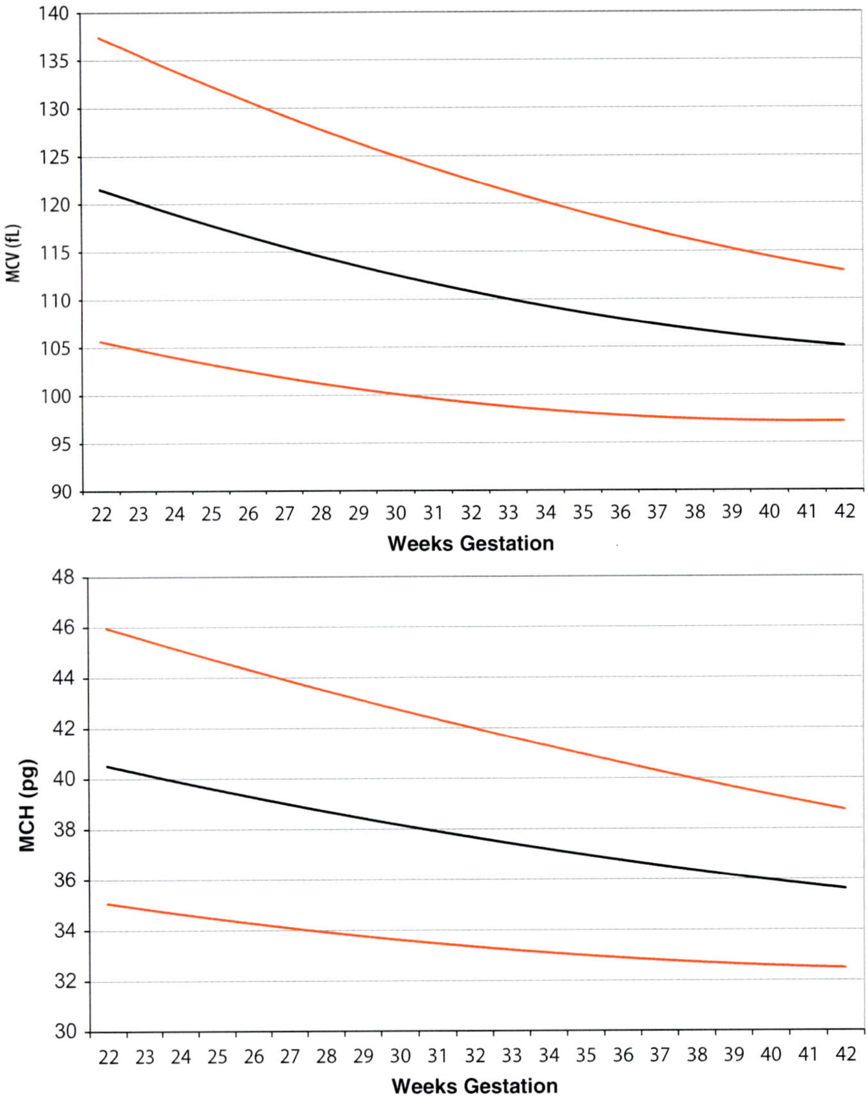

Fig. 8 Reference intervals for mean corpuscular volume (*MCV*) and mean corpuscular hemoglobin (*MCH*) for neonates on the first day after birth for neonates 22–42 weeks gestation. The *lower line* shows the 5th percentile values, the *middle line* shows the mean values, and the *upper lines* show the 95th percentile values (Reproduced from Christensen et al. (2008), with permission)

Unlike the MCV and MCH, the MCHC does not change during gestation or after delivery (Christensen et al. 2015). A reference range for MCHC of 34 ± 1 g/dL is appropriate to all ages (Christensen et al. 2008). An elevated MCHC can be useful screen for hereditary spherocytosis. Michaels and associates compared automated MCHC measurements from 112 children with hereditary spherocytosis who had not undergone splenectomy with 112 matched healthy children (Michaels et al. 1997) and observed that the MCHC of the group with hereditary spherocytosis was 35.9 gldL, significantly higher than the controls (34.3 gldL, $P < 0.001$). Similarly, newborn infants with hereditary spherocytosis have a higher MCHC (Table 1).

Table 1 An elevated mean corpuscular hemoglobin concentration (MCHC) in a neonate can suggest the possibility of hereditary spherocytosis. Values are shown as mean and 95% confidence intervals or mean ± SD (when too few values were present to calculate confidence intervals)

	N	MCHC (g/dL)
Non-transfused neonates <12 h since birth	17,624	34.0 (33.0–35.1)
Neonates with Coombs (–) jaundice	1592	34.4 (33.2–35.5)
Neonates with Coombs (+) jaundice	363	34.7 (33.3–36.0)
Neonates with hereditary spherocytosis	15	36.9 ± 0.7
P (Coombs (+) vs. Coombs (–) neonates		<0.001
P (hereditary spherocytosis vs. Coombs (–) neonates		<0.001
P (hereditary spherocytosis vs. Coombs (+) neonates		<0.001

In addition to the erythrocyte indices, the RDW and the hemoglobin distribution width (HDW) are commonly reported on automated CBCs. The RDW is a measure of the homogeneity of red blood cell size, and the HDW is a measure of the homogeneity of red blood cell hemoglobin. The RDW is expressed as a percentage, meaning the percent of erythrocytes that fall outside (smaller or larger) the standard gated population of erythrocytes. An elevated RDW value reflects an abnormal divergence of erythrocyte size. The RDW begins to increase in cases of iron deficiency before any other change in erythrocyte indices or concentrations. The HDW is expressed in grams per deciliter (*g/dL*) and provides an index of divergence of hemoglobin concentration within erythrocytes. The RDW provides a numeric assessment of anisocytosis, and the HDW provides a numeric assessment of anisochromasia.

90.3.5 Reticulocyte Count

As the erythroid precursor cells clonally mature within the bone marrow, their nucleus becomes pyknotic and is extruded (usually at the orthochromatic normoblast stage), after which the red blood cells are released into the blood. Cytoplasmic organelles, such as ribosomes, mitochondria, and the Golgi complex, generally persist for some time after the erythrocytes have reached the circulation. Supravital stains such as new methylene blue and brilliant cresyl blue stain the nucleic acid within these organelles (new methylene blue is a distinct chemical stain; regular methylene blue stains reticulocytes poorly). The circulating erythrocytes that contain organelles and thus have a reticulum of blue stain are termed reticulocytes (Smock and Perkins 2014). Reticulocytes generally circulate for 24 h or less and thereafter lose tile organelles and fail to stain as reticulocytes. The quantity of reticulum (i.e., nucleic acid) in an erythrocyte diminishes as it matures; thus, in the youngest reticulocytes, the reticulum is densely packed, while in the oldest ones only a few scattered threads are found. Reticulocytes are on average about 20% larger than mature erythrocytes (Killman 1964). Scanning electron microscopy has shown that reticulocytes are not generally bilaterally indented disks like mature erythrocytes.

A neonatologist usually orders a reticulocyte count to assess the level of erythrocyte production, because high reticulocyte counts signify increased erythropoiesis and counts of 0 signify a low level of effective erythropoiesis. Reticulocytes can be reported in at least three different ways, which can sometimes be confusing: (1) as a percentage, (2) as an absolute number, or (3) as a corrected value. The immature reticulocyte fraction (IRF) is gaining popularity among neonatologists (Christensen et al. 2016).

A reticulocyte percentage is the percentage of erythrocytes that stain as reticulocytes. An obvious limitation of this method is that it fails to account for differences in the absolute number of erythrocytes. For example, each of two neonates may have a reticulocyte count of 5%. The neonatologist may be tempted to conclude that the two

have similar levels of erythrocyte production. However, the first is anemic, with an erythrocyte count of 2 × 10^6/μL, and the other is not anemic, with an erythrocyte count of 4 × 10^6/μL. The anemic infant actually has only one-half the number of reticulocytes (5% of 2 × 10^6 or 100,000 reticulocytes/μL of blood) as does the normal infant (5% of 4 × 10^6 or 200,000 reticulocytes/μL). Failure to recognize this pitfall can give the neonatologist a false impression that the anemic patient is mounting an appropriate increase in erythrocyte production. Reporting the reticulocyte count as an *absolute number* is gaining popularity because it gives a clearer comparison of effective erythropoiesis between groups, despite differences in hematocrit (see Fig. 9).

A third method of reporting reticulocytes is by using one or two corrections. One type of correction is for hematocrit. The reticulocyte percentage is adjusted to a standard hematocrit, usually 45% (0.45 L/L), and the correction is applied as follows:

$$\text{Corrected reticulocyte count} = \frac{\text{Patient's reticulocyte count}(\%) \times \text{Patient's hematocrit}(\mathrm{L/L})}{0.45(\mathrm{L/L})}$$

This correction is appropriate for neonatal patients and provides a better framework for assessing the level of effective erythropoiesis, because it normalizes all values to a standard hematocrit. Another type of correction is sometimes made for *shift reticulocytes*. This correction accounts for the observation that whereas reticulocytes generally survive in the circulation for 1 day,

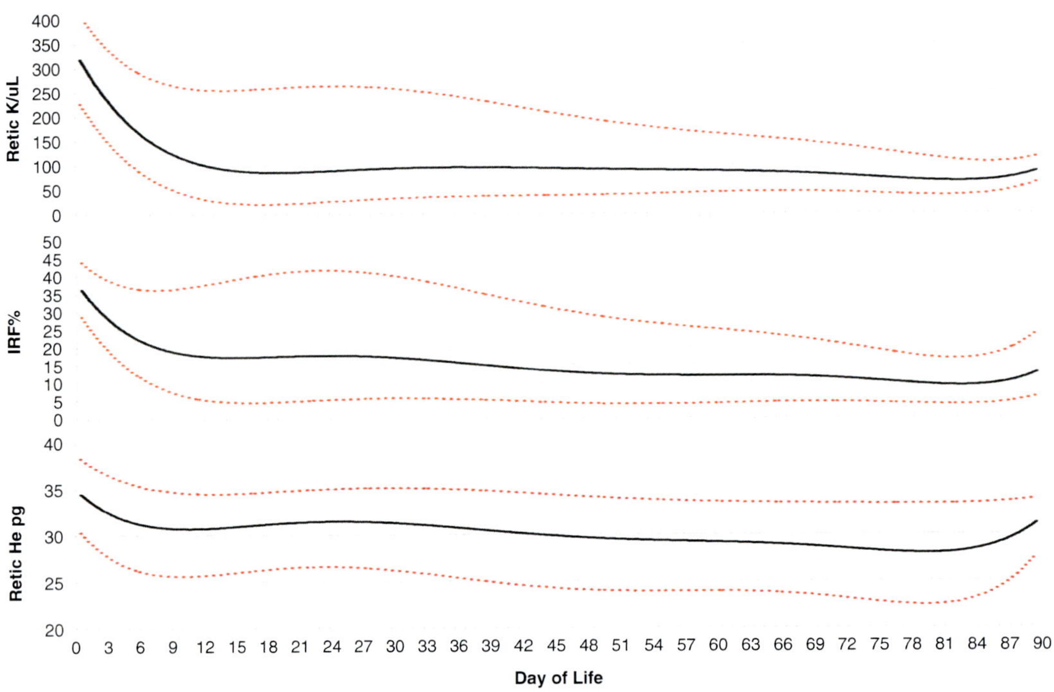

Fig. 9 Reference intervals for absolute reticulocytes/uL blood (*upper panel*), immature reticulocyte fraction (*middle panel*), and reticulocyte hemoglobin concentration (*lower panel*). In all three, the upper (95th %) and lower (5th%) reference intervals are given by *dashed lines*, and the median is shown by the *solid line*

during increased erythropoiesis, even younger reticulocytes can be released from the marrow to the blood. These shift reticulocytes, prematurely released from the marrow into the blood, survive longer than 1 day in the blood before losing their organelles, giving the false impression that the reticulocyte count is high. When reticulocytes survive in the circulation for 2 days, rather than 1 day, the correction for shift reticulocytes is made by reducing the percentage reported in half. To apply this correction, the degree of shift is assumed to be related to the intensity of stimulation of the marrow by erythropoietin. The examiner assumes that the maturation time of reticulocytes in the blood is 1 day when the hematocrit is normal, 1.5 days when it is reduced moderately, and 2.0 days when tile hematocrit is reduced markedly. With a hematocrit of 20%, the physician assumes a marked erythropoietic effort, causing a shift in premature reticulocytes that survive 2 days:

$$\text{Corrected reticulocyte count} = \frac{\text{Patient's reticulocyte count}(\%)}{2.0}$$

The shift reticulocyte count correction is rarely used by neonatologists. The correction for shift reticulocytes is only appropriate when the anemia is the result of hemorrhage or hemolysis, because it assumes that erythrocyte production has increased in response to the anemia. If the anemia is the result of hypoproduction of erythrocytes, the reticulocyte count correction for shift reticulocytes would not be valid. Because relative hypoproduction of erythrocytes is thought to be a common component of anemia in preterm infants, the use of this correction might be misleading.

The immature reticulocyte fraction (IRF) is a measure of the proportion of reticulocytes with intense reticulum staining (Christensen et al. 2016). A threshold is set and the fraction of reticulocytes staining above that threshold reflects the "young" reticulocytes. Thus, a high IRF is used as a parameter of brisk erythropoiesis. Thus, after erythropoietin treatment, the IRF might increase; contrariwise after an erythrocyte transfusion, the IRF might fall.

On the day of birth, normal term infants have reticulocyte values of 4–7% and absolute reticulocyte counts of 200,000–400,000/μL (Christensen et al. 2016). Infants delivered prematurely have somewhat higher reticulocyte counts; values of 6–10% and absolute counts of 400,000–550,000/μL are common. In healthy neonates, reticulocyte levels fall markedly over the first few days of life. By the fourth day, the reticulocytes can be 0–1%. Figure 9 shows reference intervals for absolute reticulocyte count, immature reticulocyte fraction, and reticulocyte hemoglobin content (Christensen et al. 2016). The latter is becoming popular as a measure of iron sufficiency.

90.3.6 Erythrocyte Morphology

Using erythrocytes suspended in wet preparations, Zipursky enumerated the various morphologic forms of erythrocytes in term and preterm infants and in adults (Zipursky et al. 1983). He observed considerable heterogeneity among erythrocytes of infants, particularly preterm infants. Whereas 78% of erythrocytes from adults were discocytes, only about 40% of the erythrocytes of neonates had this characteristic shape. Morphologic abnormalities of erythrocytes of neonates have also been reported using other methods. For instance, interference-contrast microscopy shows pits or craters on the surface of about 2.6% of erythrocytes of healthy adults. In contrast, about 25% of the erythrocytes of term infants and about one-half of the erythrocytes of preterm infants have pits (Pearson et al. 1978). It is believed that these pits are cytoplasmic vacuoles and represent hypofunction of the spleen or reticuloendothelial system.

90.3.7 Site of Sampling

The hematocrit, hemoglobin concentration, and erythrocyte concentration of newborn infants vary, somewhat predictably, according to the vascular source from which the sample is obtained (Table 2) (Oettinger and Mills 1949; Mollision 1951; Oh and Lind 1966; Moe 1967; Linderkamp

Table 2 The effect of site of blood sampling on hematocrit or blood hemoglobin concentrations of neonates

Author	Year	Anatomic sites of comparison	Average difference
Valquist	1941	Capillary vs. femoral vein	Capillary 10% higher
Oettinger and Mills	1949	Great toe vs. internal jugular	Capillary 21% higher
Mollision	1951	Capillary vs. venous	Capillary 5% higher
Oh and Lind	1966	Heel vs. scalp or femoral vein	Capillary 15% higher[a]
Moe	1967	Patients with erythroblastosis fetalis; heel vs. umbilical vessel	Capillary 25% higher
Linderkamp	1977	Capillary vs. umbilical vessel	Capillary 10–21% higher
Rivera and Rudolph	1982	Heel vs. antecubital vein	Capillary 12–20% higher
Thurlbeck and McIntosh[b]	1987	Heel vs. UAC	Capillary 15% higher

UAC umbilical artery catheter
[a]The capillary hematocrit was only 5% higher when the heel was warmed
[b]Preterm infants, 24–32 weeks gestation, with respiratory distress

et al. 1977). In general, erythrocyte values are higher (i.e., more concentrated) when samples are obtained by lancing capillary beds than when drawn from an artery or a vein or obtained from an indwelling arterial or venous catheter. The specific anatomic site of the vein, artery, or capillary bed sampled appears not to affect the results. For instance, values obtained from a femoral vein are equivalent to those obtained from a scalp vein (Linderkamp et al. 1977), and values from an umbilical artery are equivalent to those from a radial artery. Similarly, values from a capillary bed, such as from a heel, toe, or finger, are also equal if perfusion of those sites is similar (Linderkamp et al. 1977).

As a general rule, capillary blood obtained from a neonate's poorly perfused extremity is a poor source on which to base clinical decisions. The erythrocyte values from such a source are about 15% (range of 5–25%) above those of simultaneously obtained venous or arterial blood. The amount that a capillary hematocrit is elevated above a venous or arterial hematocrit cannot be accurately predicted in individual cases, but in general, it appears to vary with perfusion of the extremity.

When a CBC is obtained from a sick neonate with poor skin perfusion, the neonatologist interpreting the value should realize that a capillary hematocrit is less informative and less reproducible than a venous or an arterial hematocrit. Oh (Oh and Lind 1966) and Lindercamp and colleagues (1977) found that infants of the shortest gestation generally have the largest difference in capillary and venous hematocrits (Table 2). Warming the extremity before lancing the capillary bed can result in a better correlation between capillary and venous hematocrits (Oh and Lind 1966; Moe 1967; Linderkamp et al. 1977). However, when a neonatologist feels it is important to detect changes in serial hematocrit samples, it should likewise be important to keep a uniform site of sampling (i.e., all venous or all arterial). When comparing serial hematocrits of an ill neonate, it is useful to have the sample site documented.

90.3.8 Blood Sampling Relative to Delivery

About 100 mL of blood usually can be withdrawn from the placental vessels at term by using the technique of catheterizing the vessels and washing out the blood (Turner et al. 1992). Direct venipuncture of the placental end of the umbilical vein after cord clamping generally yields somewhat less blood (50–60 mL). The blood within the umbilical cord and placenta constitute about one third of the entire circulating blood volume of the fetus. Normally, after a term fetus is delivered, a placental transfusion occurs,

and the umbilical arteries constrict in response to the increasing PO_2, retarding the flow of blood from the neonate back into the placenta (Vain et al. 2014).

90.4 Leukocytes

The 1972 edition of *Holt's Pediatrics* stated, "the blood count is of relatively little help in the diagnosis of sepsis neonatorum" (Barnett and Einhorn 1972). This was a prevalent teaching of the time, and when the first cases of group B streptococcal infection were reported, no mention was made of blood leukocyte counts or differential cells counts in these neonates. The notion that the CBC was not a useful test for neonatal patients was likely based on the extreme variability of neutrophil counts in neonates and the apparent lack of correlation between neutrophil findings and the presence of infection.

Attitudes about the utility of CBCs of neonates began to change after publications of Xanthou (1970), Zipursky and colleagues (1976), Akenzua and associates (1974), and Manroe and coworkers (1979). Those reports showed differences in blood neutrophil concentrations in infected compared with noninfected neonates, and they pointed out that neutropenia, accompanied by a high ratio of immature neutrophils (bands and metamyelocytes) to total neutrophils (segmented neutrophils and band neutrophils and metamyelocytes), was particularly common in neonates with sepsis.

90.4.1 Site of Sampling

Neutrophil concentrations are lower in blood drawn from an umbilical artery catheter (or other arterial line) than in blood simultaneously drawn by venipuncture or capillary stick (Christensen and Rothstein 1979). Arterial neutrophil counts are about 75% of venous or capillary values. After moderate crying, the leukocyte counts increase to about 115% of baseline, but this is not accompanied by a change in the differential count. Lower neutrophil concentrations in arterial blood are also observed in experimental animals (Chervenick et al. 1968). The explanation appears to be related to the differences in blood flow of arterial compared with capillary or venous blood. The pulsatile flow of arterial blood appears to "push" the larger cells toward the periphery of the vessel, whereas the leukocytes and erythrocytes are more uniformly mixed in the capillary and venous circulations.

90.4.2 Leukocyte Counts in Term Infants

In 1979, Manroe and associates published reference values for blood neutrophil concentrations in neonates and for the proportion of circulating neutrophils that were immature (non-segmented) (Figs. 10 and 11). They reported values for neonates of 26–44 weeks' gestation and with birth weights of 660–5000 g (Manroe et al. 1979). The data were obtained from 1974 to 1976, when the survival of very-low-birth-weight (VLBW) infants was 42% (compared with 79% a decade later). This publication constituted a landmark; for the first time, neonatologists could determine with some confidence whether their patient had a blood neutrophil count that was low, normal, or high (Manroe et al. 1979).

Neonates at high altitude, such as those in the NICUs of Colorado (Maynard et al. 1993), Utah (Schmutz et al. 2008), and New Mexico (Carballo et al. 1991), have a higher range of neutrophil counts than do those reported from near sea level (Dallas) (Manroe et al. 1979; Mouzinho et al. 1994). Figure 12 shows reference intervals of blood neutrophils among neonates at high altitude, and Fig. 13 shows the high altitude and sea level ranges superimposed to directly compare the differences.

90.4.3 Leukocyte Counts in Preterm Infants

Several studies suggested that the normal values reported by Manroe might not be applicable to VLBW infants. One of the first of these was a report by Coulombel and coworkers of

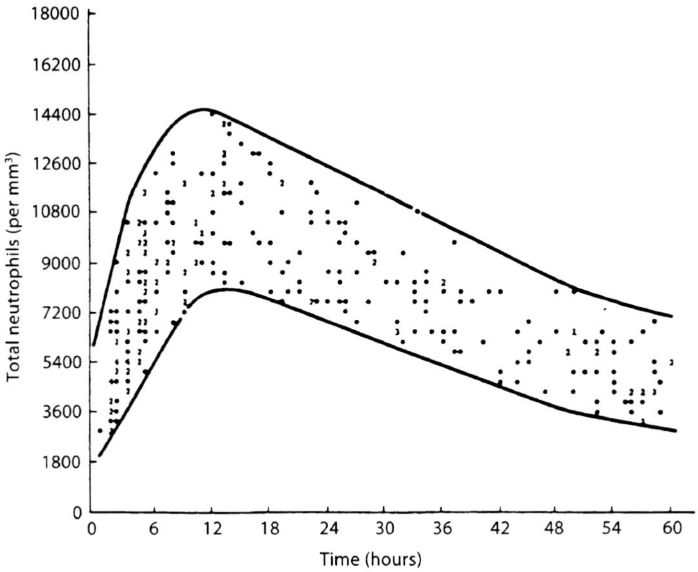

Fig. 10 Manroe chart. Reference intervals for blood neutrophil concentration of normal newborn infants in Dallas, Texas, during the first 60 h after birth. *Dots* represent single values and numbers represent the number of values at that same point (Reproduced from Manroe et al. (1979), with permission)

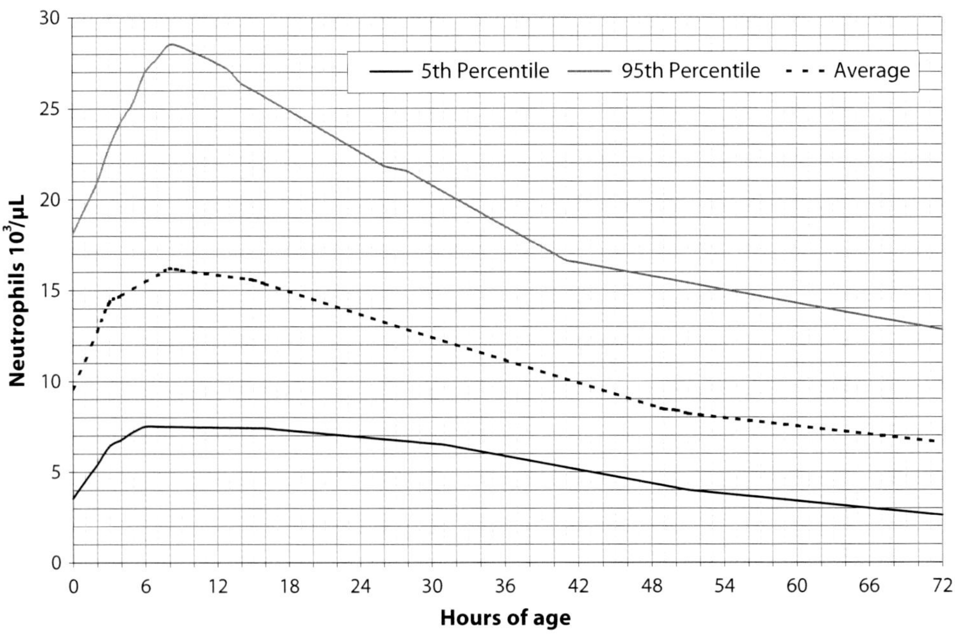

Fig. 11 Reference intervals for blood neutrophil concentrations during the first 72 h after birth of term and near term (>36 week gestation) neonates. A total of 12,149 values were used in this analysis. The 5th percentile, mean, and 95th percentile values are shown (Reproduced from Schmutz et al. (2008), with permission)

132 neonates with CBCs obtained during their first 12 h of life (Coulombel et al. 1979). Blood was sometimes obtained from capillary samples and other times from umbilical venous or arterial catheters. All 132 infants had a clinical reason for obtaining a CBC, although this report excluded those with culture-positive evidence of bacterial infection. The researchers observed an inverse relationship between gestational age and blood neutrophil concentration.

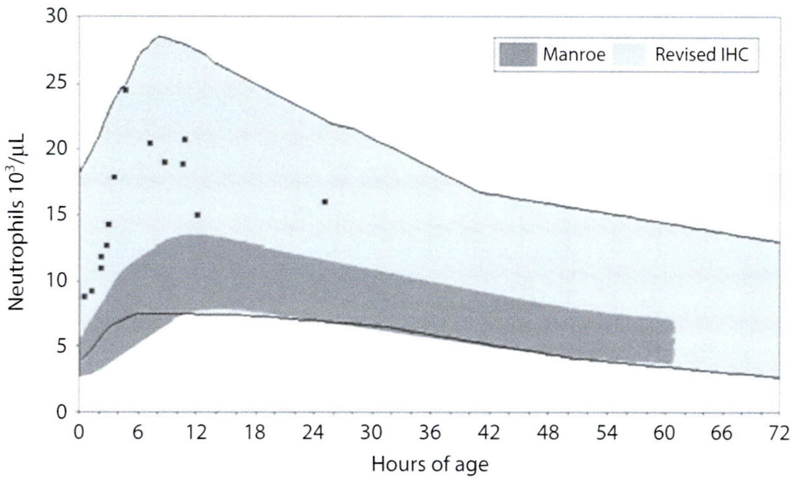

Fig. 12 Reference intervals for blood neutrophil concentrations, superimposed Manroe and Schmutz curves (revised IHC, Intermountain Healthcare)

In 1982, Lloyd and Oto reported serial leukocyte counts from 24 preterm infants, all less than 33 weeks' gestation (Lloyd and Oto 1982). They observed blood neutrophil concentration ranges that were lower than those reported by Manroe. In 1994, Mouzinho and colleagues reported the results of 1799 blood leukocyte and differential counts obtained from 193 VLBW infants (Mouzinho et al. 1994). After excluding counts from neonates with perinatal and/or neonatal complications, values from normal VLBW neonates were displayed and compared with the Manroe reference ranges (Fig. 14). Infants of younger gestations had reference ranges for blood neutrophils that differed significantly from those of larger older neonates. The VLBW infants had the same upper limit boundary for absolute neutrophil count of the larger older infants, but their lower limit boundary was significantly less than the boundary of the older infants. Reference ranges for neonates 28–6 weeks gestation are shown in Fig. 15 and for neonates <28 weeks gestation in Fig. 16.

90.4.4 Eosinophils

Eosinophilia is not a rare finding in the neonatal intensive care unit. In growing preterm infants, a nonspecific low-grade eosinophilia is so common as to warrant the label "eosinophilia of prematurity" (Calhoun et al. 2000; Sullivan and Calhoun 2007). Despite its relatively frequent occurrence, the causes and significance of this condition are uncertain.

The concentration of eosinophils in the blood can increase to very high concentrations without a concomitant increase in the concentration of other leukocytes. This attests to a unique controlling mechanism. The mechanism regulation eosinophil concentrations in blood are reviewed in ▶ Chap. 96, "Physiology and Abnormalities of Leukocytes in Newborns," and the material given here relates only to reference ranges for eosinophils.

Defining the normal range of eosinophils in the blood of neonates has been attempted in relatively few studies. Medoff and Barbero (1950) reported that during the first 12 h of life, absolute blood eosinophil concentrations range from 20 to 850/μL. On the basis of this report, eosinophilia on the first day of life would be defined as an absolute blood eosinophil count of more than 850/μL. Xanthou reported that by the fifth day, eosinophil concentrations had a much greater range than on the first day, with values of 100–2500/μL (Xanthou 1972). By day 5, eosinophilia would be diagnosed if the count was more than 2500/μL. Our group complied reference intervals for neonates using electronic CBC records of over 80,000 neonates in

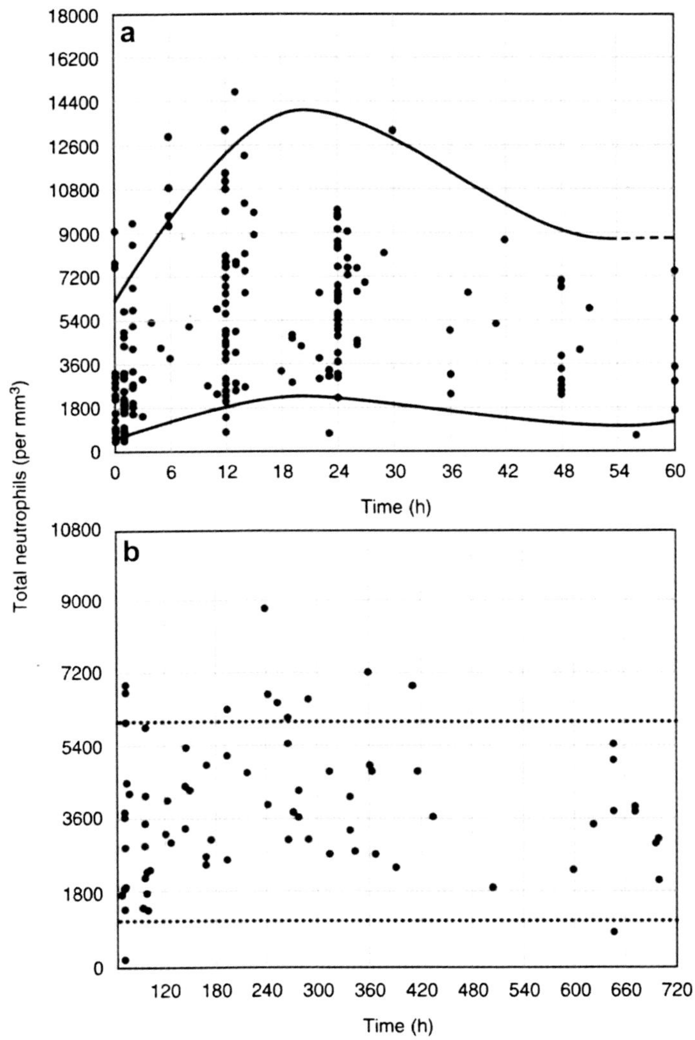

Fig. 13 Reference intervals for absolute blood neutrophil concentration of very low-birth-weight infants. Dots represent single values (Reproduced from Mouzinho et al. (1994), with permission)

a multihospital healthcare system (Christensen et al. 2010). As shown in Fig. 17, the blood concentration of eosinophils gradually increases over the interval of 22–42 weeks gestation. As shown in Fig. 18, the reference range over the first month following birth increases slightly, with the 95% value at birth being about 1200/μL and at 1 month being 1500/μL.

According to the reports of Medoff and Xanthou, absolute eosinophil counts of less than 20/μL on the first day of life and less than 100/μL after the first 5 days define eosinopenia. However, the diagnosis of eosinopenia in the neonatal intensive care unit is made rarely, because so many apparently normal infants have no eosinophils identified. In contrast to this statement, Burell suggested that a complete lack of eosinophils in neonates should be considered an abnormality (Burell 1952). Our findings (Christensen et al. 2010) are consistent with that conclusion. He found that a complete absence of eosinophils was common in infants who fared poorly and subsequently died. He reported that on the day of death there was generally a complete absence of blood eosinophils. Bass reported that blood eosinophil concentrations declined rapidly in the presence of bacterial infection (Bass 1975).

By defining eosinophilia as blood concentration of more than 700/μL (a definition of eosinophilia sometimes used in adult medicine), Gibson

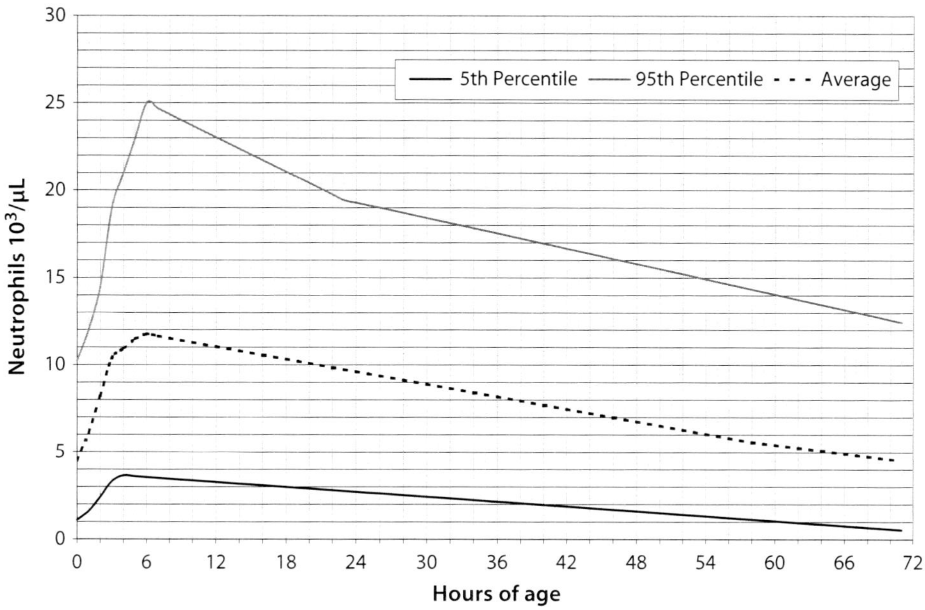

Fig. 14 Reference intervals for blood neutrophil count during the first 72 h after birth of neonates <28–36 weeks gestation. A total of 8896 values were used in this analysis. The 5th percentile, mean, and 95th percentile values are shown (Reproduced from Schmutz et al. (2008), with permission)

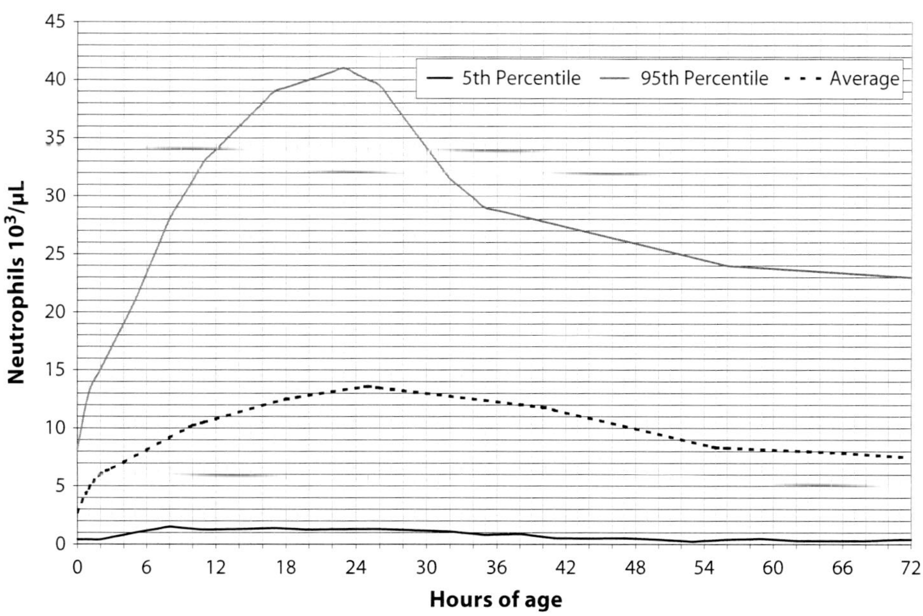

Fig. 15 Reference intervals for blood neutrophil count during the first 72 h after birth of neonates <28 weeks gestation. A total of 8896 values were used in this analysis. The 5th percentile, mean, and 95th percentile values are shown (Reproduced from Schmutz et al. (2008), with permission)

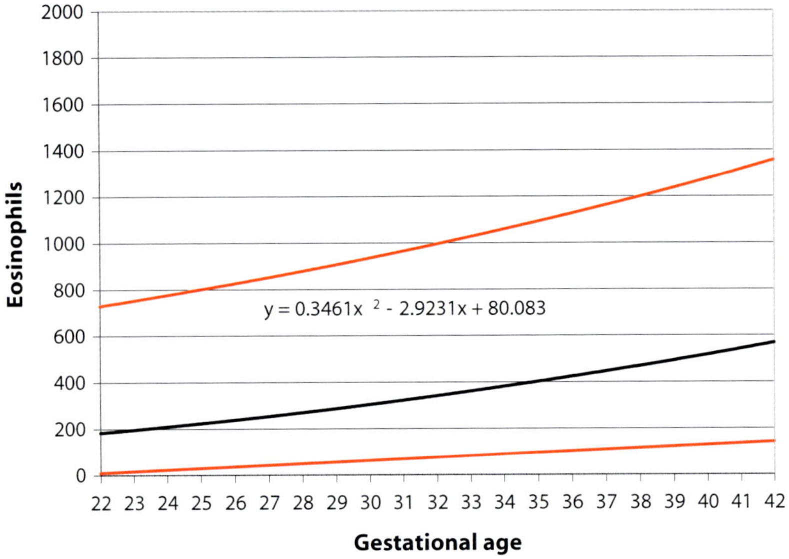

Fig. 16 Reference intervals for blood concentration of eosinophils on the day of birth from 22 to 42 weeks gestation. The 5th percentile, mean, and 95th percentile values are shown (Reproduced from Christensen et al. (2010), with permission)

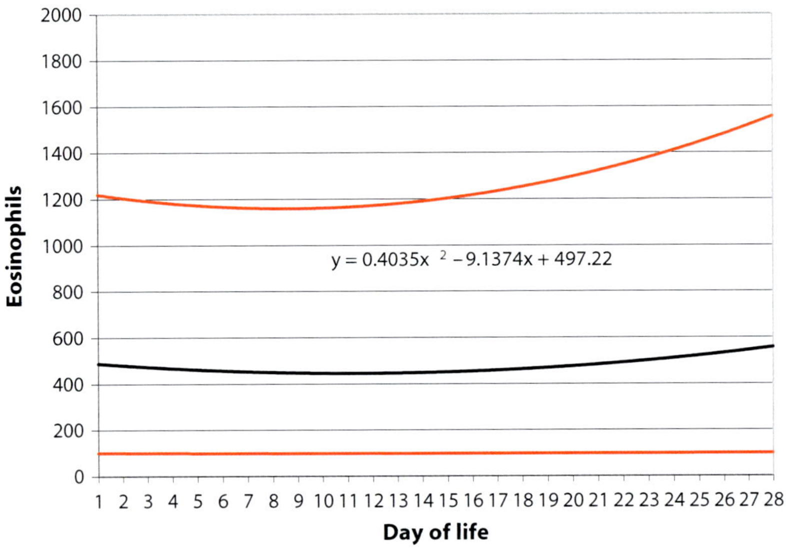

Fig. 17 Reference intervals for blood concentration of eosinophils during the first 28 days following birth. The 5th percentile, mean, and 95th percentile values are shown (Reproduced from Christensen et al. (2010), with permission)

and coworkers (1979) found that about 75% of preterm infants develop eosinophilia. This may be because 700/μL is a value well within the reference range for neonates. They reported that eosinophilia in preterm infants generally occurs during a period in which an anabolic state is established. This anabolic state and the accompanying eosinophilia usually are seen *in* the second or third week of life, and the eosinophilia persists for many days and sometimes for weeks. Portuguez-Molavasi reported that at least one episode of eosinophilia (defined as an absolute eosinophil count >1000/μL) occurred in 35% of all infants admitted to an intensive care nursery (Portuguez-Molavasi et al. 1980). Craver reported that eosinophils can be seen *in* the cerebrospinal fluid weeks after intraventricular hemorrhage (Craver 1996), but the significance of this finding is not clear, and this finding did not correlate with blood eosinophil counts.

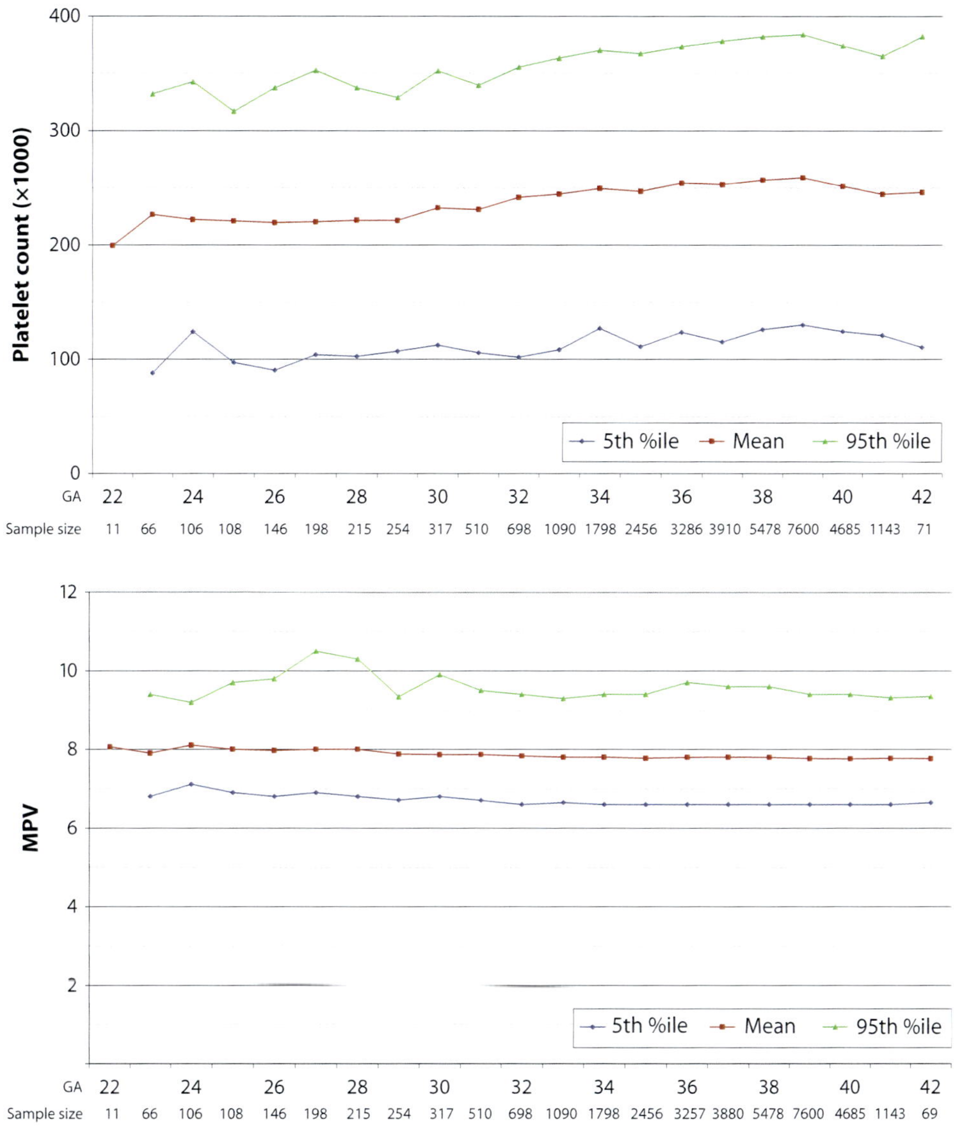

Fig. 18 Reference intervals for blood concentration of eosinophils during the first 28 days following birth. The 5th percentile, mean, and 95th percentile values are shown (Reproduced from Christensen et al. (2010), with permission)

90.5 Platelets

90.5.1 Site of Sampling

Thurlbeck and McIntosh (1987) reported no difference in the platelet counts drawn from umbilical arterial lines, venipunctures, or heel stick. Therefore, unlike the case for neutrophils and erythrocytes, it does not appear to matter what vascular source is used for drawing a platelet count. On that basis, it is common practice to obtain platelet counts of neonates from the most convenient sampling site.

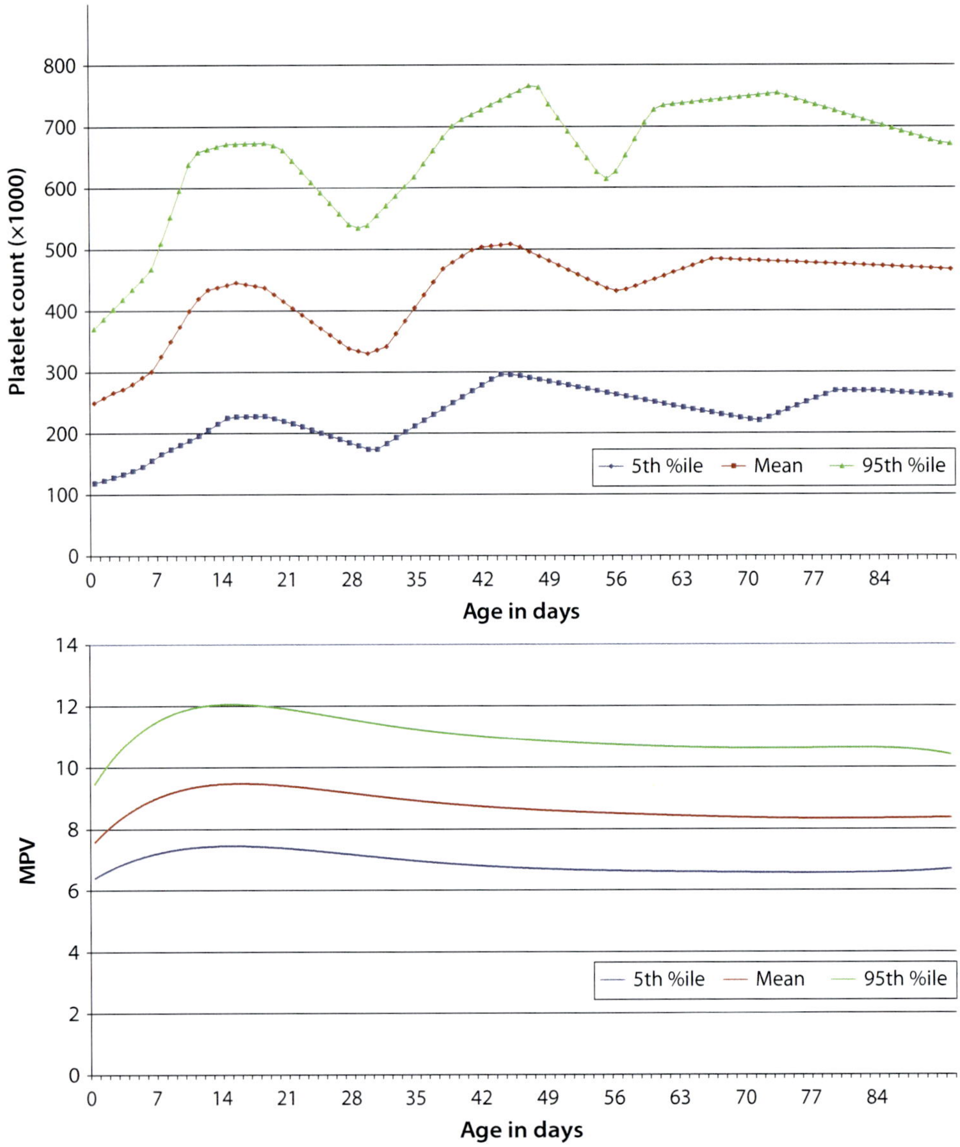

Fig. 19 Reference intervals for platelet count (*upper panel*) and mean platelet volume (*lower panel*) on the day of birth, for neonates delivered at 22–42 weeks gestation. Values are shown for the 5th percentile, mean, and 95th percentile (Reproduced from Wiedmeier et al. (2009), with permission)

90.5.2 Reference Intervals for Platelet Counts and Mean Platelet Volume on the Day of Birth

In adults, the reference interval for platelet count is 150,000–450,000/μL. This same range has been used to define thrombocytopenia and thrombocytosis in neonates (Wiedmeier et al. 2009). However, the data suggest a more complex situation. The reference range for platelet count at birth, between 22 and 42 weeks gestation, is shown in Fig. 19. Platelet counts as low as 100,000/μL can be normal for neonates >29 weeks gestation, and counts above 350,000/

μL are high for neonates >29 weeks. While the blood concentration of platelets increases gradually between 22 and 42 weeks, the mean platelet volume (MPV) does not. The MPV averages 8 fL, with a range of about 7–9.5 fL (Wiedmeier et al. 2009).

Following birth, the platelet count gradually increases. As shown in the upper panel of Fig. 20, the reference range over the first 90 days after birth has the appearance of a sign wave. We speculate that the first wave is the result of thrombopoietin (and perhaps other megakaryopoietic stimulators) surging after birth. Accompanying the increase in platelet count after birth is an increase in MPV (shown in the lower panel of Fig. 20). At 2 weeks after birth, the reference range for platelet count it is about 7.5–12 fL, but platelet size gradually falls to that at birth at a month or 2. Like the erythrocyte distribution width, is a measure of the distribution of various sized platelets in the circulation.

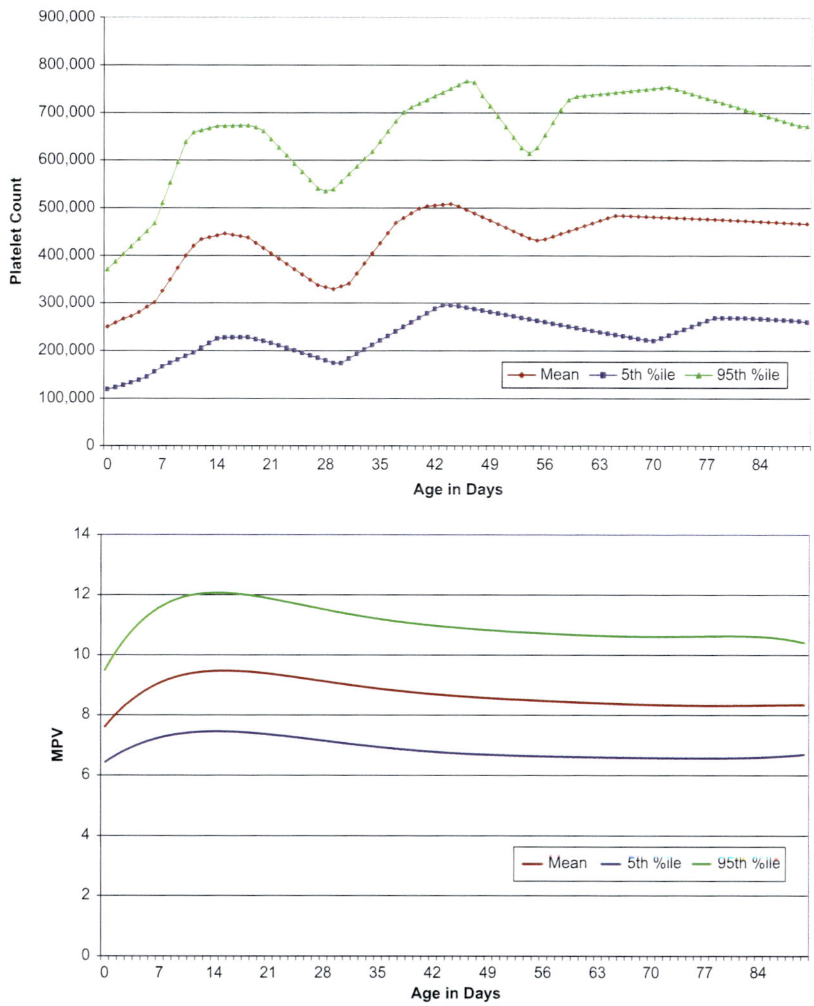

Fig. 20 Reference intervals for platelet count (*upper panel*) and mean platelet volume (*lower panel*) during the first 90 days following birth. Values are shown for the 5th percentile, mean, and 95th percentile (Reproduced from Wiedmeier et al. (2009), with permission)

90.5.3 Reticulated Platelets, Platelet Distribution Width, Plateletcrit, and Immature Platelet Fraction

Additional information on platelet characteristics can sometimes be useful in managing a thrombocytopenic neonate. Relatively new tests include the reticulated platelet count, which requires flow cytometric capability, and the platelet distribution width and plateletcrit, which can be performed on routine hematology analyzers (Beckman-Coulter), and the immature platelet fraction, which can be performed on other hematology analyzers (Sysmex Inc.).

Newly synthesized platelets generally have a higher content of ribonucleic acid than platelets that have been circulating for several days. These newly produced platelets can be recognized by flow cytometric analysis after RNA staining with thiazole orange. Such platelets have been called *reticulated platelets* to reflect their similarity to reticulocytes (Peterec et al. 1996). Between 3% and 5% of the circulating platelets of healthy term neonates and LBW infants are recognized as reticulated platelets (Table 3). Peterec and colleagues (1996) reported that infants of less than 30 weeks gestation had reticulated platelet percentages about twice those of term infants, although with a very large variation (8.8% ± 5.1%). Joseph and associates (1966) observed that adults ($n = 18$) had a slightly but significantly higher percentage of reticulated platelets than did healthy term neonates ($n = 42$). They observed no difference in reticulated platelet count between infants depending on mode of delivery.

The immature platelet fraction (IPF) is a measure somewhat analogous to the reticulocyte count. In adults the IPF ranges from 0.5% (lower reference limit) to 3% (upper reference limit) (Jung et al. 2010). Neonates typically have a broader IPF reference interval, which increases slightly over the first week following birth (Cremer et al. 2010). At birth the low reference interval is about 4% and the upper reference interval is about 11%. At day 7, these values are 5.5% (lower) and 13.5% (upper). This corresponds with an increasing MPV during the first week (Wiedmeier et al. 2009) and might be explained by a postnatal increase in platelet production. Neonates with infections tend to have lower platelet counts but do not necessarily have an increase in immature platelet fraction. This has prompted the supposition of an inadequate megakaryocytopoietic response during neonatal infection (Cremer et al. 2013).

Table 3 Differential cell counts of nucleated cells aspirated from the bone marrow of normal infants at term and from healthy adult men

Cell types	Term neonates (% [mean ± SD])	Health adults (% [mean, 95% CI])
Nucleated erythroid		
Proerythroblast	0.1 ± 0.1	0.6; 0.1–1.1
Basophilic erythroblast	0.2 ± 0.2	1.4; 0.4–2.4
Polychromatic erythroblast	13.1 ± 6.8	21.6; 13.1–30.1
Orthochromic erythroblast	0.7 ± 0.7	2.0; 0.3–3.7
Neutrophil		
Promyelocytes	0.8 ± 0.9	3.3; 1.9–4.7
Myelocytes	3.9 ± 2.9	12.7; 8.5–16.9
Metamyelocytes	19.4 ± 4.8	15.9; 7.1–24.7
Band neutrophils	28.9 ± 7.6	12.4; 9.4–15.4
Segmented neutrophils	7.4 ± 4.6	7.4; 3.8–11.0
Myeloid/erythroid ratio	4.3:1	3.1:1; 1.1–5.2:1
Eosinophils	2.7 ± 1.3	3.1; 1.1–5.2
Basophils	0.1 ± 0.2	0.1
Monocytes	0.9 ± 0.9	0.3; 0.0–0.6
Lymphocytes	14.4 ± 5.5	16.2; 8.6–23.8
Megakaryocytes	0.1 ± 0.1	0.1
Plasma cells	0.0 ± 0.1	1.3; 0.0–3.5
Undifferentiated blasts	0.3 ± 0.3	0.9:0.1–1.7
Unknown of damaged cells	6.0 ± 3.2	

Data for term neonates from Rosse et al. (1977) and from Shapiro and Bassen (1941)

90.6 Bone Marrow

A bone marrow aspirate or biopsy occasionally is useful in providing information not otherwise available. In cases of a persistent cytopenia, a neonatologist might want information relating to the state of production. For example, a persistent thrombocytopenia could be the result of decreased platelet production or of increased platelet destruction or use. A marrow examination can sometimes help differentiate these conditions because in cases of decreased platelet production, the marrow contains few megakaryocytes, but in cases of increased platelet use, the proportion of megakaryocytes should be increased.

Bone marrow aspirates of neonates are often diluted with peripheral blood, which can lead to misinterpretations about the state of production. This limitation can be minimized by taking care to withdraw the smallest possible marrow sample, thereby not over-diluting the specimen with blood, and by using a biopsy technique (Sola et al. 1999).

Marrow is accessible from essentially any bone in the neonate. We have found that the flat part of the proximal tibia is a simple and reliable site from which to obtain a marrow sample, because this site is easy to stabilize, the landmarks are obvious, and the amount of tissue between the skin and the bone is small. The (right-handed) operator holds the tibia firmly in a gloved left hand, while the right hand is used to prepare and sterilely drape the area and then to inject 1% lidocaine as a local anesthetic. Lidocaine (typically 0.1 mL without epinephrine) is injected subcutaneously, holding the needle in place for several seconds, after the needle is advanced to the bone and another 0.1 mL is injected into the periosteum. A few minutes later, the operator holds the 19-gauge, 1/2-in. needle (Osgood marrow needle fitted with a trocar) in the right hand and twists it carefully through the anesthetized periosteum with the mid-tibia clearly marked directly between the left thumb and forefinger. The needle is directed toward the middle of the tibial shaft to enter the middle of the marrow cavity. The needle is correctly positioned when it is solidly in place and when, on aspiration, marrow enters the aspirating syringe.

If only a microscopic analysis of the bone marrow cells is to be accomplished, only a few drops of marrow should be aspirated. If flow cytometry, a karyotype analysis, or a hematopoietic progenitor cell culture is needed, more cells are needed, and up to 0.25 mL of marrow can sometimes be aspirated. Volumes exceeding this amount from very small preterm infants essentially always draw significant amounts of peripheral blood through the marrow and result in a dilute specimen, which may be difficult to interpret.

Little information is available on bone marrow biopsies in neonates. Although the issue of cellularity is much more accurately assessed with a biopsy specimen than with an aspirate, we have found success in obtaining marrow needle biopsies, even in the smallest preterm infants in our neonatal intensive care unit, by using a modification of the aspiration method (Sola et al. 1999). After the operator feels the Osgood needle penetrating the cortex of the tibia, the stylet (trocar) is withdrawn. The hollow needle is then advanced into the marrow space an additional 3–5 mm. Advancing the needle without a stylet cores a small segment of marrow into the needle. A syringe is then attached to the needle hub, and minimal suction is applied for about 1 s. This process helps secure the small-core marrow biopsy specimen within the needle. The syringe and the attached needle are then withdrawn, and the core of marrow is pushed out of the needle by reintroducing the stylet. The core can be placed into fixative and subsequently sectioned and stained, or it can be smeared on cover slips.

Anticipated results of bone marrow differential counts are shown *in* Table 2. Studies in 1941 and 1952 used marrow aspirates obtained from normal neonates, but this practice is no longer permitted. The normal values for marrow nucleated cell concentrations in neonates are available, but normal values for laboratory tests that were devised since 1952 (e.g., concentrations of hematopoietic progenitor cells) are not available (Rosse et al. 1977; Shapiro and Bassen 1941). In modern practice, bone marrow aspirates are only performed on neonates if a clinical reason exists to do so or the patient is enrolled in a study that requires a bone

marrow study. These subjects therefore are not strictly normal subjects, and the results should not be considered normal values.

References

Akenzua GI, Hui IT, Milner R et al (1974) Neutrophil and band counts in the diagnosis of neonatal infection. Pediatrics 54:38–42

Barnett HL, Einhorn AH (1972) Pediatrics, 15th edn. Appleton-Century-Crofts, New York, p 597

Bass DA (1975) Behavior of eosinophil leukocytes in acute inflammation. II Eosinophil dynamics during acute inflammation. J Clin Invest 56:870–879

Burell JM (1952) A comparative study of the circulating eosinophil levels in babies. Arch Dis Child 27:337

Calhoun DA, Sullivan SE, Lunøe M et al (2000) Granulocyte-macrophage colony-stimulating factor and interleukin-5 concentrations in premature neonates with eosinophilia. J Perinatol 20:166–171

Carballo C, Foucar K, Swanson P et al (1991) Effect of high altitude on neutrophil counts in newborn infants. J Pediatr 119:464–646

Chervenick PA, Boggs DR, Marsh JC et al (1968) Quantitative studies of blood and bone marrow neutrophils in normal mice. Am J Physiol 215:353–360

Christensen RD, Rothstein G (1979) Pitfalls in the interpretation of leukocytes counts of newborn infants. Am J Clin Pathol 72:608–611

Christensen RD, Jopling J, Henry E et al (2008) The erythrocyte indices of neonates, defined using data from over 12,000 patients in a multihospital healthcare system. J Perinatol 28:24–28

Christensen RD, Jensen J, Maheshwari A et al (2010) Reference ranges for blood concentrations of eosinophils and monocytes during the neonatal period, defined using data from over 80,000 records in a multihospital healthcare system. J Perinatol 30:540–545

Christensen RD, Yaish HM, Gallagher PG (2015) A pediatrician's practical guide to diagnosing and treating hereditary spherocytosis in neonates. Pediatrics 135:1107–1114

Christensen RD, Henry E, Bennett ST et al (2016) Reference intervals for reticulocyte parameters of infants during their first 90 days after birth. J Perinatol 36:61–66

Coulombel L, Dehan M, Tehernia G et al (1979) The number of polymorphonuclear leukocytes in relation to gestational age in the newborn. Acta Paediatr Scand 68:709–711

Craver RD (1996) The cytology of cerebrospinal fluid associated with neonatal intraventricular hemorrhage. Pediatr Pathol Lab Med 16:713–719

Cremer M, Weimann A, Schmalisch G et al (2010) Immature platelet values indicate impaired megakaryopoietic activity in neonatal early-onset thrombocytopenia. Thromb Haemost 103:1016–1021

Cremer M, Weimann A, Szekessy D et al (2013) Low immature platelet fraction suggests decreased megakaryopoiesis in neonates with sepsis or necrotizing enterocolitis. J Perinatol 33:622–626

Gairdner D, Marks J, Bosco JD (1952) Blood formation in infancy: the normal bone marrow. Arch Dis Child 27:128–133

Gibson JG Jr, Vaucher Y, Corrigan JJ (1979) Eosinophilia in premature infants: relationship to weight gain. J Pediatr 95:99–101

International Committee for Standardization in Haematology (1978) Recommendations for reference method for haemoglobinometry in human blood. J Clin Pathol 31:139–143

Jopling J, Henry E, Wiedmeier SE, Christensen RD (2009) Reference ranges for hematocrit and blood hemoglobin concentration during the neonatal period: data from a multihospital healthcare system. Pediatrics 123: e333–e377

Joseph MA, Adams D, Maragos J et al (1966) Flow cytometry of neonatal platelet RNA. J Pediatr Hematol Oncol 18:277–281

Jung H, Jeon HK, Kim HJ, Kim SH (2010) Immature platelet fraction: establishment of a reference interval and diagnostic measure for thrombocytopenia. Korean J Lab Med 30:451–459

Killman SA (1964) On the size of normal human reticulocytes. Acta Med Scand 176:529–533

Linderkamp O, Versmold HT, Strohhacker I et al (1977) Capillary-venous hematocrit differences in newborn infants. 1. Relationship to blood volume, peripheral blood flow and acid-base parameters. Eur J Pediatr 127:9–14

Lloyd BW, Oto A (1982) Normal values for mature and immature neutrophils in very preterm babies. Arch Dis Child 57:233–235

Manroe BL, Weinberg AG, Rosenfeld CR et al (1979) The neonatal blood count in health and disease. 1. Reference values for neutrophilic cells. J Pediatr 95:89–98

Maynard EC, Reed C, Kircher T (1993) Neutrophil counts in newborn infants at high altitude. J Pediatr 122:990–991

Medoff HS, Barbero GJ (1950) Total blood eosinophil counts in the newborn period. Pediatrics 6:737–760

Michaels LA, Cohen AR, Zhao H et al (1997) Screening for hereditary spherocytosis by use of automated erythrocyte indexes. J Pediatr 130:957–960

Moe PJ (1967) Umbilical cord blood and capillary blood in the evaluation of anemia in erythroblastosis fetalis. Acta Paediatr Scand 56:391–394

Mollision PL (1951) Blood transfusion in clinical medicine, 3rd edn. Blackwell, Oxford

Mouzinho A, Rosenfeld CR, Sanchez PJ et al (1994) Revised reference ranges for circulating neutrophils in very-low-birth-weight neonates. Pediatrics 94: 76–82

Oettinger L Jr, Mills WE (1949) Simultaneous capillary and venous hemoglobin determinations in the newborn infant. J Pediatr 35:362–365

Oh W, Lind J (1966) Venous and capillary hematocrit in newborn infants and placental transfusion. Acta Paediatr Scand 55:38–48

Pearson HA, McIntosh S, Ritchey AK et al (1978) Developmental aspects of splenic function in sickle cell diseases. Blood 53:358–365

Peterec SM, Brennan SA, Tinder EM et al (1996) Reticulated platelet values in normal and thrombocytopenic neonates. J Pediatr 12(9):269–274

Portuguez-Molavasi A, Cote-Boileau T, Aranda JV (1980) Eosinophilia in the newborn, possible role in adverse drug reactions. Pediatr Res 14:537

Rosse C, Kraemer MJ, Dillon TL et al (1977) Bone marrow cell populations of normal infants: the predominance of lymphocytes. J Lab Clin Med 89:1228–1240

Schmutz N, Henry E, Jopling J, Christensen RD (2008) Expected ranges for blood neutrophil concentrations of neonates: the Manroe and Mouzinho charts revisited. J Perinatol 28:275–281

Scott-Emuakpor AB, Okolo M, Omene JA et al (1985) Normal hematological values of the African neonate. Blut 51:11–18

Shapiro LM, Bassen FA (1941) Sternal marrow changes during first week of life. Am J Med Sci 202:341–350

Smock LJ, Perkins SL (2014) Examination of the blood and bone marrow. In: Greer JP, Arber DA, Glader B, List AF, Means RT Jr, Paraskevas F, Rodgers GM (eds) Wintrobe's clinical hematology. Lippincott, Williams & Wilkins, Philadelphia, pp 3–5

Sola MC, Rimsza LM, Christensen RD (1999) A bone marrow biopsy technique suitable for use in neonates. Br J Haematol 107:458–460

Sullivan SE, Calhoun DA (2007) Eosinophilia in the neonatal intensive care unit. Clin Perinatol 27:603–622

Thurlbeck SM, McIntosh N (1987) Preterm blood counts vary with sampling site. Arch Dis Child 62:74–75

Turner CW, Luzins J, Hutcheson C (1992) A modified harvest technique for cord blood hematopoietic stem cells. Bone Marrow Transplant 10:89–91

Vain NE, Satragno DS, Gorenstein AN et al (2014) Effect of gravity on volume of placental transfusion: a multicenter, randomized, non-inferiority trial. Lancet 384:235–240

Waugh TF, Merchant FT, Maugham GB (1939) Blood studies on newborn; determination of hemoglobin, volume of packed red cells, reticulocytes and fragility of erythrocytes over 9 day period. Am J Med Sci 198:646–652

Wiedmeier SE, Henry E, Sola-Visner MC et al (2009) Platelet reference ranges for neonates, defined using data from over 47,000 patients in a multihospital healthcare system. J Perinatol 29:130–136

Wintrobe MM (1929) A simple and accurate hematocrit. J Lab Clin Med 15:287

Xanthou M (1970) Leukocyte blood picture in healthy full term and premature babies during the neonatal period. Arch Dis Child 45:242–249

Xanthou M (1972) Leucocyte blood picture in ill newborn babies. Arch Dis Child 47:741–746

Zipursky A, Palko J, Milner R et al (1976) The hematology of bacterial infections in premature infants. Pediatrics 57:839–853

Zipursky A, Brown E, Palko J et al (1983) The erythrocyte differential count in newborn infants. Am J Pediatr Hematol Oncol 5:45–51

Pathophysiology of Coagulation and Deficiencies of Coagulation Factors in Newborn

91

Paola Saracco and Rodney P. A. Rivers

Contents

P. Saracco (✉)
Pediatric Hematology, Department of Pediatrics, University Hospital Città della Salute e della Scienza, Torino, Italy
e-mail: paola.saracco@unito.it

R. P. A. Rivers
Section of Paediatrics, Department of Medicine, Imperial College, London, UK

G. Buonocore et al. (eds.), *Neonatology*,
https://doi.org/10.1007/978-3-319-29489-6_238

Abstract

The hemostatic system of the neonate is dynamically evolving and different from older children and very different from the adult. The main points of difference between neonatal and adult hemostasis are as follows:

Platelets show significant differences in function.

Bleeding times are shorter through increased activity of von Willebrand factor (VWF).

Many procoagulant and inhibitor levels are gestationally dependent.

Reduced procoagulant and inhibitor reserve.

Relatively impaired fibrinolysis.

This neonatal coagulopathy impacts both the diagnosis and management of hemorrhagic or thrombotic events in neonates. Diagnostic laboratories should use age-analyzer and reagent-appropriate references ranges.

91.1 Salient Points

- The hemostatic system of the neonate is dynamically evolving, and main differences compared to adults are reduced procoagulant and inhibitor reserve, altered platelet functions, and impaired fibrinolysis. This neonatal coagulopathy impacts both the diagnosis and management of hemorrhagic or thrombotic events in neonates.
- Bleeding disorders may be life-threatening, and a rapid evaluation is essential. Diagnostic laboratories should use age-analyzer and reagent-appropriate references ranges.
- Not all components of hemostasis are evaluated by routine screening tests that exhibit a nonoptimal sensitivity and specificity to predict bleeding in this high-risk population. Thromboelastography and thromboelastometry are functional assays providing a comprehensive assessment of the coagulation system and may better evaluate bleeding and bleeding risk in neonates.
- Standardized bleeding assessment tools should also be developed in order to record clinical bleeding and describe prospectively patterns of bleeding for clinical hemostatic outcomes in transfusion trials.
- The role of currently available hemostatic agents in therapy and prevention of acquired bleeding conditions should be explored.

91.2 Introduction

The hemostatic system of the neonate is dynamically evolving and different from older children and very different from the adult. Main differences are reduced procoagulant and inhibitor reserve, altered platelet functions, and impaired fibrinolysis. However, this coagulation system is protective against both hemorrhage and thrombosis in healthy newborns. Thrombin generation is equivalent to adult. In both, normal screening test results do not equate with normal hemostasis.

Hemostasis is classified into **primary** (adhesion, activation, and aggregation of platelets at a site of vessel injury), **secondary** (activation of coagulation factors resulting in the formation of covalently cross-linked fibrin that stabilizes the platelet plug), and **tertiary or fibrinolysis** (activation of fibrinolytic pathway triggering clot breakdown to maintain or restore blood flow). The principal function of the components making up the hemostatic system is to limit hemorrhage at sites of vascular injury. Subendothelial fibroblasts demonstrate strong TF protein staining and TF mRNA hybridization, as do pericytes surrounding capillaries. These sources of TF act as a "hemostatic envelope," triggering coagulation when exposed to blood.

A typical routine coagulation profile assesses a component of these pathways and consists of activated partial thromboplastin time (aPTT), prothrombin time (PT), fibrinogen, and platelet count. aPTT, PT, and fibrinogen levels are measures of the intrinsic, the extrinsic, and the final common clotting pathway, respectively.

Phases of hemostasis including inhibitors pathway and fibrinolysis have been summarized in Chap. 99 of previous edition (in Practical Approach to Neonatal Diseases, 2012) (see Figs. 1, 2, 3, 4, 5, and 6).

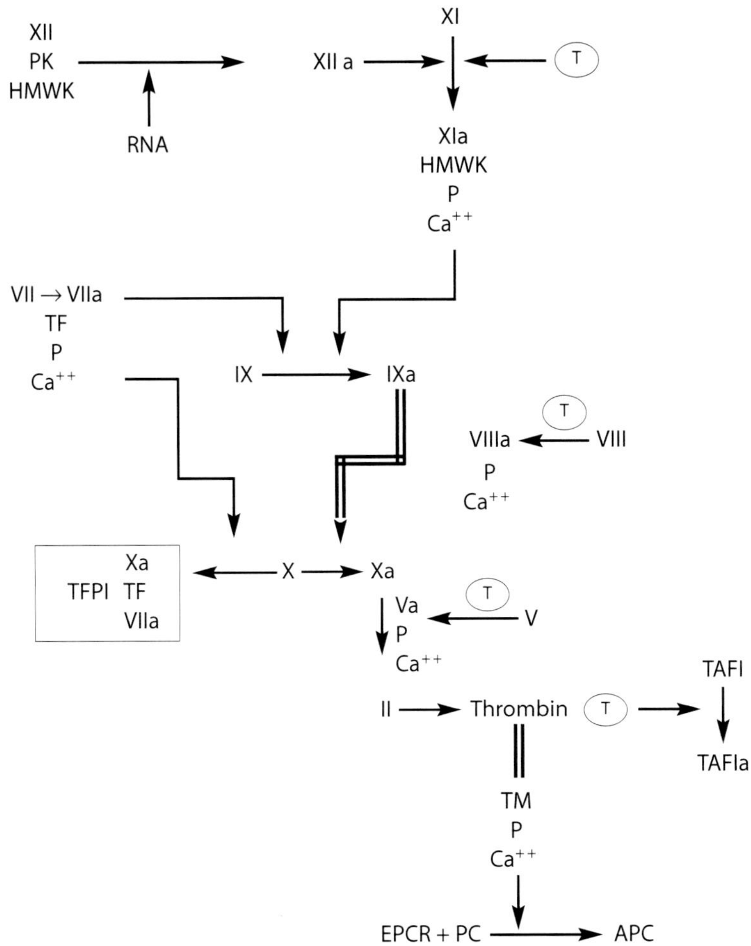

Fig. 1 Pathways of coagulation activation illustrating the importance of the intrinsic pathway of FX activation once the TF pathway of initial activation is shut down by TFPI complex formation. *PK* plasma kallikrein, *HMWK* high molecular weight kininogen. *P* phospholipid, *TF* tissue factor, *TFPI* tissue factor pathway inhibitor, *TAFI* thrombin-activatable fibrinolysis inhibitor, *TAFIa* activated thrombin-activatable fibrinolysis inhibitor, *TM* thrombomodulin, *EPCR* endothelial protein C receptor, *PC* protein C, *APC* activated protein C

91.3 Developmental Hemostasis and Hemostasis Investigation in the Neonate

91.3.1 Developmental Hemostasis

The evolution of hemostasis development has been discernable from studies on fetal (Holmberg et al. 1974) and newborn plasmas at differing gestational and postnatal ages (Barnard et al. 1979; Jensen et al. 1973; Salonvaara et al. 2004). Most coagulation proteins are measurable by 10 weeks' gestation; some display functional changes relating to differences in molecular composition. The changes associated with advancing gestation were initially reported in the 1970s and have become known as **developmental hemostasis**, a term coined by Andrew et al. (1987). The maturation of the hemostatic system in utero is reflected in hemostatic differences between preterm and term neonates (Table 1).

91.3.2 Coagulation Factors

FV, FVIII, fibrinogen, and platelet count are present at close to adult values by 24 weeks' gestation, whereas contact factors (FXI, FXII, high molecular weight kininogen, and prekallikrein) and the VK-dependent factors (II, VII, IX, and X) are reduced, with values approximate to 20% of adult levels by 28 weeks' gestation rising to around 50% at term. The physiological causes for

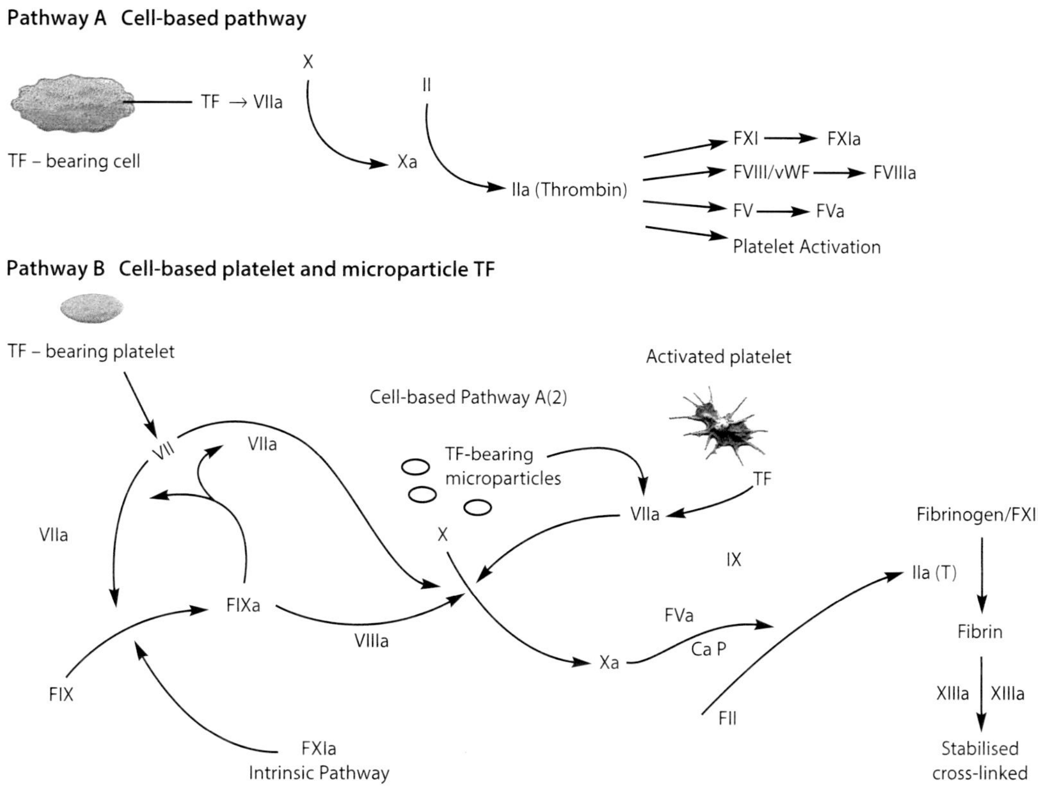

Fig. 2 Pathways of coagulation activation. Initiation membrane-linked activation pathway A and subsequent amplification intrinsic pathway B with involvement of platelet and microparticle tissue factor (*TF*) and membranes

these developmental changes are probably driven by the function of coagulation proteins in other physiological systems such as angiogenesis, inflammation, and wound repair (Ignjatovic et al. 2011).

Factor XIII shows no clear gestational dependence, remaining at 50–75% of adult from 30 weeks' gestation to term but reaching adult values by 3 weeks' postnatal age. At birth, FVIII levels are skewed toward the higher levels. Fibrinogen levels continue to rise afterward. The prolonged thrombin time (TT) obtained, even when measures to prevent in vitro fibrinogenolysis are taken, results from the "fetal" form of fibrinogen.

Levels of VWF are increased at birth; the VWF is present in larger-sized multimers than normal and displays increased activity in promoting platelet adhesion. The raised level persists for the first 3 months of life. Limited studies on ADAMTS-13 in the newborn have given discrepant results with both adult equivalent and reduced levels being reported.

91.3.3 Anticoagulant Proteins

Levels of anticoagulants are reduced at birth compared to adults. Antithrombin is 30% of adult at under 30 weeks of gestation rising to 50% at term. Protein C is present in a fetal form, but function does not appear to be affected; it is present at around 50% of the adult value, increasing slowly after birth but not achieving adult values until the early teens.

Protein S level is reduced at birth, but available PS is free and active because of the absence of C4b-binding protein. Its interaction with protein C may be affected by the level of α_2-M (Cvirn et al. 2002). The free TFPI level is also reduced to some 50–65% of adult values.

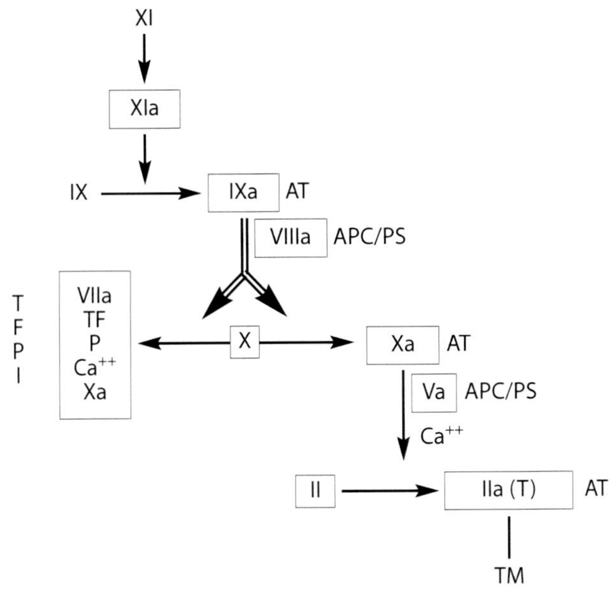

Fig. 3 Regulation of coagulation pathways: effectors of procoagulant inhibition. Sites of inhibition of thrombin generation and termination of thrombin activity on binding to thrombomodulin. The physiologic inhibitor of the TF-VIIa complex is TFPI. Once this pathway of FX activation is blocked, the FIXa-VIIIa complex or intrinsic pathway becomes the principal pathway of FX activation. In the termination phase, free thrombin loses its procoagulant and platelet-activating activity on binding to TM and to the abundant AT. *AT* antithrombin, *APC* activated protein C, *PS* protein S, *TFPI* tissue factor pathway inhibitor, *TM* thrombomodulin

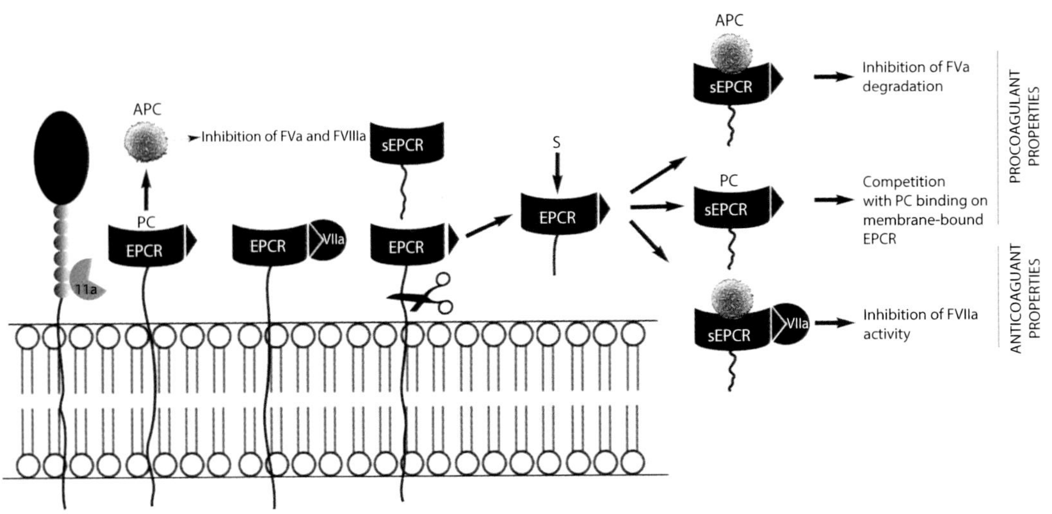

Fig. 4 EPCR and TM in coagulation/endothelium. Roles of thrombomodulin, of endothelially bound protein C receptor and of released plasma EPCR in downregulation of thrombin generation. *TM* thrombomodulin, *APC* activated protein C, *EPCR* endothelial protein C receptor, *sEPCR* soluble endothelial protein C receptor, *PC* protein C

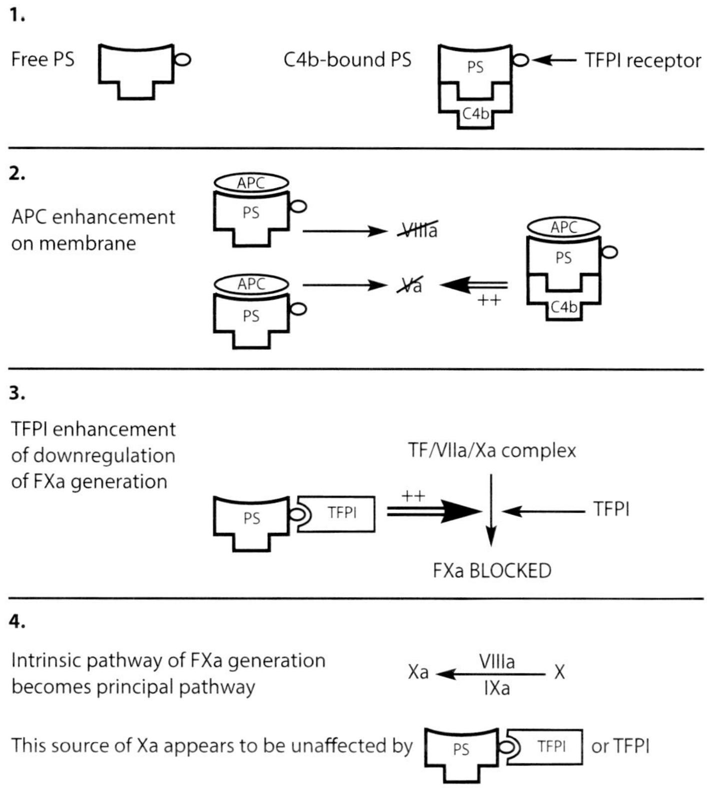

Fig. 5 Mechanisms of protein S enhancement of thrombin generation inhibition. Protease digestion of FVa and FVIIIa by protein C is enhanced by protein S. PS is active whether free or bound to C4b-binding. Enhancement of TFPI inhibition of the TF/VIIa/Xa complex is independent of protein C, but FXa generated by the intrinsic pathway is not inhibited. *PS* protein S, *TFPI* tissue factor pathway inhibitor, *APC* activated protein C

91.3.4 Fibrinolytic Proteins

Plasminogen levels are also lower than in adults, demonstrating reduced fibrinolysis. In the neonate, all major fibrinolytic proteins demonstrate age-dependent concentration variations (Andrew et al. 1992). Marked changes in the components occur following birth. TPA and PAI-1 are below adult levels in cord blood, whereas in both term and preterm neonates, tPA, uPA, and PAI-1 are transiently increased above the adult value on day 1. Plasminogen levels are some 20% of adult at 28 weeks and 50% at term, rising to the normal adult range by 6 months with α_2-AP levels being at 80% of adult at term. Fetal plasminogen exists in two major glycoforms with increased mannose and sialic acid content displaying slower activation kinetics than adult forms. Functionally they bind less well to cellular receptors, and the plasmin formed from it has less enzymatic activity. Mean α_2-AP levels are around 80% of adult at term. The inhibition of the two fetal plasmin isoforms by α_2-AP (plasmin-antiplasmin [PAP] complexes) is slower than that of the adult plasmin variants. The other principal plasmin inhibitors are α_2-M and α_1-antitrypsin. Although elevated levels of PAP complexes in healthy newborns derive from increased production of plasminogen activators at birth, inhibition of fibrinolysis predominates in the plasma of the newborn beyond day 1.

91.3.5 Neonatal Platelets

Platelets appear in human fetus at 5 weeks post-conception, increasing during fetal life to reach a mean of 150/nl by end of first trimester. Below 30 weeks' gestation, the fifth centile is 104,200/μ L, and in the late preterm and term population, it is 123,100/μL. The mean platelet volume is quite similar to that in adults (7–9 fl) with a mean of 8 fl (range 7–9.5 fl) (Wiedmeier et al. 2009). Increased numbers of circulating megakaryocyte

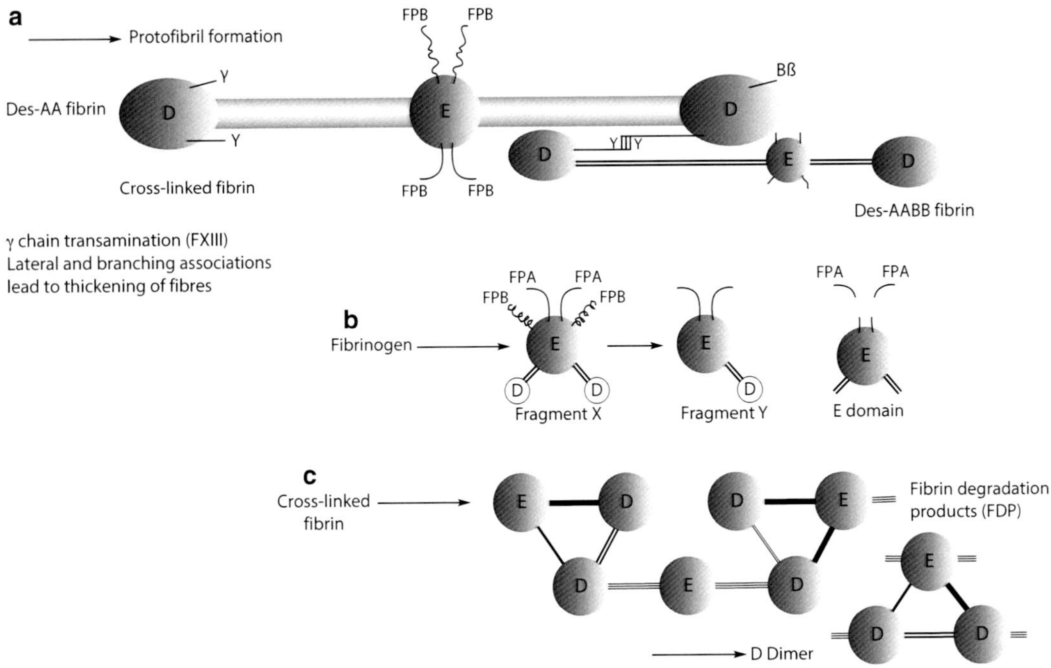

Fig. 6 Cartoon of the formation of soluble fibrins and protofibrils following removal of fibrinopeptide A by thrombin. Products of plasmin degradation of fibrinogen and fibrin. (**a**) Lengthening as fibrin monomers (soluble). (**b**) Fibrinogen degradation by plasmin. (**c**) Fibrin degradation by plasmin. *FPB* fibrinopeptide B, *FPA* fibrinopeptide A

progenitors and of mature megakaryocytes are found. Circulating precursors are proportional both to the numbers in marrow and to the blood platelet count. Newly synthesized platelets have an increased RNA content and can be identified by flow cytometry. In non-thrombocytopenic neonates, the proportion is similar to that in adults.

Thrombopoietin is detectable in the plasma of newborns of all gestations. Levels are similar to baseline adult levels in term infants (140 pg/mL), with a wide range. In the preterm, levels have been reported to be higher.

Platelets from neonates have reduced activation response; aspects of neonatal platelet function have been repeatedly reviewed (Israels et al. 2003; Saxonhouse and Manco-Johnson 2009). Platelet receptors for adhesive proteins, GP1a/GPII (collagen), GP1b/GPIX/GPV (VWF), and GPIIb/GPIIIa (fibrinogen, fibronectin, VWF), are present on fetal and cord blood platelets with receptor concentrations being similar to those on adult-derived platelets. The number of α_2-adrenergic receptors is approximately half that on adult platelets, and this is not due to receptor occupancy by catecholamines in cord blood. By 2 months of age, levels are similar to those on adult platelets. The diminished response to thromboxane analogues is not a consequence of a reduction in receptors but is due to attenuated downstream signaling.

91.3.6 Laboratory Evaluation of Hemostasis

Bleeding disorders may be life-threatening, and rapid evaluation is essential. Investigations can thus be tailored to allow rapid diagnosis and treatment.

91.3.7 PT and aPTT

Not all components of hemostasis are evaluated by routine screening tests, and so "normal" test

Table 1 Neonatal hemostasis versus older children/adults. *APCR* activated protein C resistance, *TFPI* tissue factor pathway inhibitor

	Preterm neonates vs term neonate	Neonates vs older children/adults
Primary hemostasis		
Platelet count		Same
Platelet function	Decreased	Decreased
VWF level	Decreased	Higher
VWF large multimers		Higher
Coagulation factors		
FII, FVII, FIX, FX	Lower	Lower
FV	Lower	Same or lower
FVIII	Higher	Same or higher
FXI	Lower	Lower
FXII	Lower	Lower
Fibrinogen level	Same	Same
Fibrinogen function		Decreased
Regulation of coagulation		
Antithrombin	Lower	Lower
Protein C	Lower	Lower
Protein S total	Lower	Lower
Protein S free		Higher
APCR generation		Reduced
Free TFPI		Lower
Fibrinolysis		
Plasminogen level	Lower	Lower
Plasminogen function	NA	Decreased
tPA	Same	
α_2-antiplasmin	Lower	Higher
α_2-M	same	Lower
PAI	Same	Higher

results for gestation and postnatal age do not equate with the presence of normal hemostasis.

Conventional tests utilizing the strong activators as in the PT and APTT tests only reveal deficiencies in the procoagulant pathways; they provide no information on how the balance between procoagulant and inhibitor concentrations might affect TG in the neonate.

In the early studies of TG using strong activation, TG in neonatal plasma had been found to be some 30–50% of the peak value generated in adult, the poor response being attributed to the low levels of FII encountered in the newborn. By manipulating the levels of inhibitors including TFPI, AT, and PC and by activating the PC with soluble thrombomodulin, the effects on TG using low concentrations of lipidated TF for activation have been studied. TG in cord-derived plasma was found to start earlier due to faster FX activation and to be comparable with that generated in adult plasma, the free thrombin generated being approximately 90% of the adult value. APC was found to have a greater effect on prolonging the clotting time than did increases to AT (Cvirn et al. 2002; Cvirn et al. 1999).

91.3.8 Thromboelastography/Thromboelastometry

Thromboelastography (TEG) and rotating thromboelastometry (ROTEM) are functional assays of whole blood coagulation which provide a comprehensive assessment of the coagulation system reflecting the complex interplay between coagulation factors, cellular components, enzymes, and feedback mechanisms that maintain equilibrium between clot formation and lysis. This functional test enables rapid assessment of kinetic changes, rate of clot formation, clot strength, and clot stability in a small sample (0.3 ml) of whole blood. This test is comparable if not better than standard coagulation test for evaluating bleeding and bleeding risk in neonates (Radicioni et al. 2012). Test variables are R, clotting time (time to initial fibrin formation); K, clot kinetics (time until specific clot strength of 20 mm obtained); α, α angle (rate of clot formation due to fibrin accumulation and cross linking); MA, maximum amplitude (final strength of the clot); fibrinolysis or rate of clot breakdown (amplitude 30 min after MA achieved); and CI, coagulation index (derived linear calculation of R, K, α, and MA). In general R and K values are lower, while lysis and CI values are higher in neonates compared to older children and adults.

91.3.9 Platelet Function Tests

Platelet Function Analyzer 100 (PFA): closure times are shorter for newborn than adult blood.

Aggregometry: generally, aggregation to a variety of agonists is decreased. The differences are magnified in platelets from preterm neonates. The relevance of such findings to in vivo hemostasis has been thrown into question by a report claiming to use a more physiological set of stimuli in a whole blood experiment. Using a combination of collagen and endogenous thrombin as stimulants, maximal aggregation and lag time to the start of aggregation were similar in neonatal and adult samples (Cvirn et al. 2009). This result was attributed to the faster generation of thrombin in neonatal blood and possibly offers an explanation for the "abnormally" short bleeding time of neonates. An increased response to ristocetin reflects the increased level and enhanced function of neonatal VWF.

Flow cytometry: platelets from both term and <30 weeks' gestational age preterm infants have reduced levels of activation markers following stimulation. P-selectin expression following stimulation is further reduced in preterm newborns in proportion to their gestation. Agonist-induced secretion of granule components is reduced in both term and preterm platelets due to reduced function of receptor-mediated transduction pathways (Baker-Groberg et al. 2016). Electron microscopy (EM): using whole mount EM to count calcium-rich platelet dense granules, significantly fewer dense granules were observed in fetal and neonatal platelets. This finding highlights the importance of taking developmental factors into consideration when diagnosing dense granule deficiencies in neonates (Urban et al. 2017).

91.3.10 What are Reference Ranges in Neonates

Over the years very different techniques have been utilized to record the end point of clot formation, and published reference data may not be applicable to reported results from a neonate under investigation now (Hathaway and Corrigan 1991). Moreover, reference ranges for coagulation assays in neonates vary with laboratory analyzer and reagent system, and this must be taken into consideration when comparing results from different laboratories. The Perinatal and Pediatric Haemostasis Subcommittee (SCC) of the International Society on Thrombosis and Hemostasis (ISTH) published consensus recommendations for laboratories reporting pediatric samples for hemostasis tests (Ignjatovic et al. 2012).

It is hoped that reference ranges will be produced from large centers so that other centers using similar apparatus and reagents may be able to consult them when faced with abnormal results. Factor assays and screening tests need to be interpreted using gestational age and postnatal age-adjusted ranges.

Currently age reference ranges have been established for platelet count, coagulation screening tests, coagulation, and anticoagulation proteins in preterm and term neonates (Neary et al. 2015; Attard et al. 2013) (Tables 2 and 3), and recently validated TEG reference ranges parameters have been developed in term neonates (Sewell et al. 2017).

91.4 Neonatal Bleeding Disorders

Bleeding disorders may be life-threatening, and rapid evaluation is essential. Investigations can thus be tailored to allow rapid diagnosis and treatment. Acquisition of a detailed family history is imperative. When there is a positive family history, the potential risk should the neonate have acquired the defect along with knowledge as to whether the diagnosis can be made in the neonate have to be taken into account when planning investigations and in determining whether follow-up investigations beyond 6 months of age may be required. This may be especially needed for the detection of milder congenital defects. Babies born to mothers on warfarin, anticonvulsants, or antituberculous drugs should be screened because of inhibitory effects on VK. The clinical setting is extremely important, often indicating the likely cause.

Table 2 Infants <28 weeks gestational age (<28/40 GA; n = 62) compared with those >28 weeks GA (>28/40 GA; n = 44)

Median (range)	GA < 28/40	GA > 28/40	p value
PT (s)	18.1 (12.9–28.5)	16.9 (12.3–25.5)	0.02
aPTT (s)	87.2 (53.7–139.3)	72.6 (43.6–101.1)	0.0001
Fibrinogen (g/l)	1.4 (0.7–3.8)	1.3 (0.8–4.0)	0.88

Table 3 Approximate coagulation reference ranges, coagulation, and anticoagulant proteins in preterm infants 30–36 gestational age and term infants

Test or level	Preterm infant 30–36 GA, at day 1	Preterm infant 30–36 GA, at day 30	Term infant at day 1
PT (s)	10.6–16.2	10.0–13.6	14.4–16.4
aPTT (s)	27.5–79.4	26.9–62.5	34.3–44.8
Fibrinogen (g/l)	1.5–3.25	1.50–4.14	1.92–3.74
PFA-100 collagen/ADP closure time (s)			40–92
VWF (U/ml)	0.78–2.10	0.66–2.16	0.50–2.87
Factor II (UI/ml)	0.20–0.77	0.36–0.95	0.41–0.69
Factor V (UI/ml)	0.41–1.44	0.48–1.56	0.64–1.03
Factor VII (UI/ml)	0.21–1.13	0.21–1.45	0.52–0.88
Factor VIII (UI/ml)	0.50–2.13	0.50–1.99	1.05–3.29
Factor IX (UI/ml)	0.19–0.65	0.13–0.80	0.35–0.56
Factor X (UI/ml)	0.11–0.71	0.20–0.92	0.46–0.67
Factor XI (UI/ml)			0.07–0.41
Factor XII (UI/ml)			0.43–0.8
AT (UI/ml)	0.39–0.87	0.48–1.08	0.58–0.9
α_2-macroglobulin (UI/ml)	0.95–1.83	1.06–1.94	0.95–1.83
Protein C clotting (UI/ml)	0.17–0.53	0.21–0.65	0.24–0.40
Protein S (clotting; UI/ml)	0.12–0.60	0.33–0.93	0.28–0.47

Awareness of conditions associated with disseminated intravascular coagulation (DIC) is important.

Sites of bleeding suggesting a primary coagulation disorder in neonates include puncture sites (heel prick, screen, or immunization), gastrointestinal tract, umbilical stump, extracranial hemorrhage, intraventricular hemorrhage (IVH), and pulmonary hemorrhage.

91.4.1 Bleeding Assessment Tool

Particularly in preterm and in term neonates admitted to intensive care units (ICU), standardized bleeding assessment tools should be developed in order to record clinical bleeding with secondary aim of assessing incidence of bleeding and describe prospectively patterns of bleeding for clinical hemostatic outcomes in transfusion trials. A modified WHO bleeding score has been developed for neonatal ICU setting, including recording of site, severity and duration of all clinical bleeding events, and allowing to categorize bleeding into none, mild, moderate, major, and severe hemorrhage (neonatal bleeding assessment tool, NeoBAT) (Venkatesh et al. 2013).

91.4.2 Laboratory Investigations

Screening tests should include a prothrombin time, an activated partial thromboplastin and mixture time, a thrombin-calcium time, and a fibrinogen level, and full blood count and platelet count should also be performed.

If PT prolonged and APTT normal	Acquired causes: vitamin K deficiency; Inherited causes: FVII deficiency
If PT prolonged and APTT prolonged	Acquired causes: vitamin K deficiency, DIC, liver disease; Inherited conditions: combined factor deficiency, deficiency of FII, FV, FX or fibrinogen
If PT normal and APTT prolonged	Acquired causes: heparin, lupus anticoagulants; Inherited causes (rare): deficiency of FVIII, FIX, FXI, or FXII
If PT and APTT normal	Acquired causes: thrombocytopenia; Inherited causes: FXIII deficiency

The Reptilase time with calcium is abnormal in some dysfibrinogenemias.

A D-dimer assay or fibrin degradation product measurement may be useful if DIC is suspected. Measurements of individual components of the systems involved may be required, but antigen levels do not necessarily equate with biological function.

Platelet function can be assessed by the platelet function analyzer closure time. Platelet glycoprotein (GP) expression is fully developed in term and preterm neonates; by using flow cytometry, deficiency states in receptor expression can be identified. Investigation of the parents' platelet function may be helpful.

In the disordered proteolysis of DIC, routine tests if done sequentially would be expected to reveal falls in FV and FVIII, whereas in metabolic liver disease or VK deficiency, they are conserved, unless DIC has been triggered by blood loss and shock.

Deficiencies of ADAMTS-13, FXIII, and of α_2-antiplasmin are not detected in the routine investigations. FXIII should be evaluated by measurement of the transglutaminase activity following thrombin/calcium activation (Karimi et al. 2009).

91.4.3 Inherited Coagulation Disorders

Birth is the first hemostatic challenge for a hemophiliac, but usually bleeding is rare; however, serious cerebral bleeding may occur, more likely if the birth involved assisted delivery with forceps or vacuum extraction. Exposure to surgery poses a considerable threat to an infant when a hemorrhagic diathesis has not been previously suspected. The risks entail complicating or life-threatening hemorrhage and transfusion-transmitted infections from infused plasma-derived products. Immune stimulation leading to inhibitor formation is particularly to be feared. A recent review on approved indications for factor products in the neonate has been recently published (Punzalan and Gottschall 2016).

91.4.3.1 The Hemophilias

A well term neonate with signs of bleeding and an isolated borderline or prolonged APTT may have a form of hemophilia. Along with von Willebrand disease, the hemophilias account for over 95% of all inherited bleeding disorders. Hemophilia, as it involves the neonate, has been reviewed by Chalmers et al. (2011) and Kulkarni and Soucie (2011).

There are three types arising from separate factor deficiencies: hemophilia A (FVIII deficiency), B (FIX deficiency), and C (FXI deficiency). Hemophilia A and B are indistinguishable clinically, both giving rise to bleeding of variable severity.

Prenatal carrier testing can be performed utilizing polymerase chain reaction techniques; the molecular genetic testing for hemophilia A has been reviewed by Goodeve (2008).

The genes for FVIII and FIX are present on the X chromosome, and that of FXI is on chromosome 4. A male infant with abnormal bleeding and normal screening tests except for a prolonged APTT should be screened for FVIII and FIX deficiencies. Both have been described in phenotypic girls.

FXI deficiency gives rise to less severe bleeding but should be considered in all well neonates with bleeding and an abnormal APTT; it is an autosomal recessive disorder.

Even in FVIII or FIX severe deficiency (FVIII <1%) bleeding in the first week of life is uncommon.

Raised TF availability along with the lower levels of TFPI and AT, combined with the PS

inhibition by α_2-M, may explain why bleeding in neonates with hemophilia is rare.

In one retrospective review, puncture bleeding (16%) and bleeding post circumcision (30%) were the most common; hemorrhagic shock from liver hematomata in two neonates has been reported.

Intracranial hemorrhage (ICH) is rare, and elective cesarean section is not recommended for its prevention. The subject has been reviewed by Ljung (2008). Vacuum extraction was found to be particularly associated with extracranial hemorrhages in the Swedish studies with 69% of 16 cranial hemorrhages occurring in relation to this procedure. Some 50% of those born with hemophilia are not suspected antenatally. Extracranial hemorrhage (ECH) in the form of cephalohematomas and subgaleal hemorrhages can involve massive blood loss and can be accompanied by an ICH which may be clinically unsuspected.

Prophylactic treatment of identified cases of hemophilia is not generally advocated. Screening for ICH is recommended. If an ICH is identified, treatment should continue for 2–3 weeks aiming at 100% concentration over the first 7 days and 50% over the latter part of the course.

As cesarean section does not eliminate the risk of cranial bleeding, normal vaginal delivery for known carriers is generally recommended. The management of carriers and of babies has been reviewed by Street et al. (2008).

In cases of known or suspected carriers where the fetal diagnosis is unknown, a cord blood sample should be obtained for diagnosis, and intramuscular administration of vitamin K should be withheld. Oral vitamin K prophylaxis should be commenced and continued if the diagnosis is confirmed and a cranial ultrasound performed before discharge. Circumcision should be avoided.

Because of the association of a low FVIII level in type III von Willebrand disease (VWD), VWF antigen should be measured in all infants with FVIII activity below 10%.

The FIX level may be as low as 15 IU/dL in normal neonates. Severe and moderately severe deficiency states may be discernible, but mild cases cannot be differentiated from those who are not affected and require further evaluation when the child is older unless a genetic diagnosis is possible.

Management of Bleeding

First-line treatment of bleeding and prophylaxis for patients with hemophilia A is recombinant FVIII (rFVIII) and for hemophilia B rFIX. Management of bleeding has been reviewed by Kulkarni and Lusher (2001) and by Ljung (2008). Alternatively, a monoclonally purified, viral inactivated plasma-derived product may be used. Plasma should only be used when concentrates are unavailable. There are recently approved extended half-life products studied in patients 1–18 years, but not in neonates (Powell 2015).

Limited pharmacokinetic data in the newborn indicate a shortened half-life for FVIII. In adults the half-life of rFVIII is 11–17 h, but in the neonate, it may be as short as 6 h. The volume of distribution in adults is limited to the plasma volume so that each 1 IU/kg infused raises the plasma concentration by 2%. The volume of distribution in the newborn is increased. On this basis, it has been calculated that an initial infusion of 50–60 IU/kg followed by 8–12 hourly infusions of 25–30 IU/kg should raise the FVIII to adult levels.

Proposals for the use of prophylaxis in order to reduce any bleeding consequences of birth trauma are controversial, and there is a lack of evidence-based guidelines. Prophylaxes in preterm infants, two with FVIII deficiency and one with FIX deficiency, have been reported. The FVIII was given at 50 IU/kg daily increasing to twice daily with septic episodes.

In the neonate receiving rFIX, the half-life was estimated to be 5.8 h. Because of a reported very large volume of distribution and this rapid elimination, up to 30 IU/kg each hour may be required to maintain 100% FIX activity. Experience with recombinant FIX in the USA has led to a dose recommendation of a 120 IU/kg bolus followed by 60 IU/kg 12 hourly as the maintenance dose.

Antibody (inhibitor) formation in neonates is rare. The genetic and nongenetic risk factors involved have been reviewed (Peyvandi and

Makris 2017). Although the risk of inhibitor development has been a concern, some evidence points to a reduced risk of inhibitor development with early prophylactic treatment.

91.4.3.2 Von Willebrand Disease

This bleeding disorder affects males and females and is caused by a quantitative or qualitative deficiency of VWF. It is the commonest inherited bleeding disorder with an estimated prevalence of 0.8–1.3%; in most instances, it is inherited in an autosomally dominant fashion. Evidence-based guidelines for diagnosis and management have recently been published under the aegis of the National Heart, Lung, and Blood Institute Expert Panel (USA) (Nichols et al. 2008).

There are three major types of VWD: type I, in which there is a partial quantitative deficiency, is the most common. In type II, there is a qualitative VWF defect, and in type III, there is virtually a complete lack of VWF. The bleeding tendency is usually mild, and since levels in the neonate are elevated with the high molecular weight multimers (HMWM) forms, bleeding in the neonatal period is unusual. Type III disease may however present with superficial mucosal bleeding; ICH in this form of VWD is described. Where VWD is associated with thrombocytopenia as in the type IIb subgroup or in the more severe form of type III disease, bleeding is more likely to occur.

Diagnosis of type III VWD is made by finding low levels of both FVIII and VWF antigen and of ristocetin cofactor activity. VWF multimers will also be missing. In the presence of thrombocytopenia, type IIb should be excluded. Because of the normally raised levels in the neonate, other forms of VWD can only be diagnosed by molecular techniques (Laffan et al. 2014).

Management

First-line treatment in the neonate is viricidally treated VWF/FVIII concentrate. A recombinant VWF has undergone phase 3 trial in adults. The recommended loading dose is 30–60 U/kg with maintenance doses of 20–40 U/kg every 12–48 h. A trough level of >50 IU/dL should be maintained for 3–5 days according to perceived risks of rebleeding.

Desmopressin is contraindicated in the neonate because of the danger of inducing hyponatremia. Platelet replacement may be required in bleeding associated with type IIb disease.

91.4.3.3 Rare Inherited Bleeding Disorders

These disorders have been the subject of a recent review, and guidelines on diagnosis and management have been produced (Peyvandi et al. 2009, 2012; Peyvandi and Menegatti 2016).

They are generally inherited as autosomal recessive traits, and severe bleeding is encountered in individuals with either homozygous or compound heterozygous mutations.

91.4.3.4 Disorders of Fibrinogen

Quantitative and qualitative defects including afibrinogenemia and hypofibrinogenemia (autosomal recessive) and the dysfibrinogenemias (autosomal dominant) have been reviewed (de Moerloose and Neerman-Arbez 2009) and may be identified in the neonatal age group. Afibrinogenemia and the more severe forms of hypofibrinogenemia present most often as bleeding from the umbilical cord; however mucosal bleeding is encountered, and ICH in afibrinogenemia has been reported. Significant bleeding would not be anticipated with levels above 0.5 g/L.

The dysfibrinogenemias may be detected following investigation of an abnormal coagulation test result or when screening is carried out against a background of a family history. They are associated both with bleeding and thrombotic disorders but are unlikely to present in the neonate.

Fibrinogen levels are within the normal adult range at birth. In afibrinogenemia, the PT, APTT, and TCaT are all markedly prolonged, and fibrinogen levels in functional and antigenic assays are undetectable. In hypofibrinogenemia, the level of fibrinogen ranges from 0.20 to 0.80 g/L and determines the degree of prolongation of the above tests. The TCaT and Reptilase time are the tests most likely to reveal a dysfibrinogenemia, the antigenic levels being higher than levels suggested in functional assays.

Management

Virally inactivated fibrinogen concentrates are the treatment of choice in bleeding from afibrinogenemia or hypofibrinogenemia. A minimum level of 0.5 g/L is considered necessary for hemostasis although raising the level to 1 g/L is recommended in a bleeding neonate (Kulkarni and Lusher 2001). The half-life of 3–5 days permits infrequent dosing, and prophylaxis from an early age given every 7–14 days has been used to maintain a level above 0.5 g/L. In the absence of concentrate, cryoprecipitate or fresh frozen plasma (FFP) can provide fibrinogen, but the risks of viral transmission and of volume overload are greater. Use of fibrin glue and antifibrinolytic agents may need to be considered. Primary prophylaxis is not generally recommended in afibrinogenemia. Following a severe bleed such as an ICH, secondary prophylaxis aimed at keeping a level of above 0.5 g/L is considered reasonable (Bolton-Maggs et al. 2004).

91.4.3.5 FII, FV, FVII, FX, FXI, FXII, and Combined FV/FVIII Deficiencies

Each of these deficiencies leads to a life-long bleeding disorder; the congenital disorders of the VK-dependent factors have been the subject of a review (Girolami et al. 2008). All the above are associated with a neonatal hemorrhagic diathesis. In a large Iranian series, ICH was most commonly associated with FVII and FX deficiencies. The deficiencies of factor II (Lancellotti and De Cristofaro 2009), FV (Asselta and Peyvandi 2009), FVII (Mariani and Bernardi 2009), FX (Menegatti and Peyvandi 2009), FXI (Duga and Salomon 2009), and FXIII (Karimi et al. 2009) have each been the subjects of recent reviews (Peyvandi and Menegatti 2016; Peyvandi et al. 2016).

As presented above, the levels of FII, FVII, FX, and FXI are reduced compared with adult values both at term and in a gestationally determined manner. Although severe deficiency states are diagnosable in the newborn, those infants with higher levels may need follow-up retesting to establish a heterozygote diagnosis. Undetectable FII is not compatible with life and has never been reported in a live-born baby.

In FV deficiency, the severity of the bleeding tendency is variable and has been attributed to the coexistent finding of a reduced level of TFPI. As FV is at normal adult values at birth, both homozygous and heterozygous deficiency states are usually diagnosable in the neonatal period.

FXI severe deficiency is associated with a spectrum of bleeding severity with some homozygous states being almost asymptomatic.

FXII deficiency, although causing a prolonged APTT, does not give rise to clinical bleeding.

It should be noted that a normal APTT for gestation and age does not necessarily rule out an intrinsic factor deficiency since the high FVIII level can normalize the APTT in the presence of other deficiencies.

Management

As recommended above, specific factor concentrates (e.g., FVII, FXI) should be used when available; alternatively, prothrombin complex concentrate (e.g., FII and FX) may be considered.

FVII deficiency can be rectified using plasma-derived FVII concentrate at 10–30 IU/kg twice weekly or by rFVIIa in doses of 15–25 μg/kg every 3–6 h.

FV replacement requires the use of virally inactivated FFP raising the level to 15 IU/dL with 15–20 mL/kg followed by 5 mL/kg 12 hourly. The level should be maintained at 25% after a severe bleed.

FX deficiency is treated with FFP or prothrombin complex concentrates containing FX, although the high levels of FII, FVII, and FIX in these concentrates pose a thromboembolic risk; a freeze-dried concentrate of human FIX and FX (FX P Behring, Germany) has become available which may prove useful in managing this disorder.

91.4.3.6 FXIII Deficiency

Severe deficiency most commonly present in the newborn period with umbilical stump bleeding, hematoma, and ICH (Naderi et al. 2014). Making the diagnosis is therefore particularly important because monthly infusions of FXIII concentrate or of cryoprecipitate can prevent this complication (see below), the half-life of FXIII being around 30 days.

FXIII is not involved in any of the screening coagulation tests and must be analyzed specifically utilizing a functional assay.

Neonates diagnosed with FXIII levels below 3 IU/dL should be commenced on a prophylactic replacement regimen of viricidally treated, plasma-derived FXIII concentrate. FXIII distribution is limited to the plasma volume. Each 1 IU/kg infused raises the plasma concentration by 2%. The aim is to keep the pretreatment trough at >3 IU/dL. This requires 10 IU/kg every 4 weeks initially with subsequent monitoring. FXIII is also present in cryoprecipitate and in FFP.

91.4.3.7 Hereditary Combined VK Deficiency Factor Disease

This is a very rare autosomal recessive condition arising from mutations affecting either the γ-glutamyl carboxylase enzyme or the VK epoxide enzyme complex. In the severely compromised, bleeding may occur in the neonate with umbilical and intracranial hemorrhages reported. However phenotype may be very heterogenous, and multiple disorders including bone and heart development may be expected in affected patients (Watzka et al. 2014).

The PT and APTT are variably prolonged depending on the degree of functional deficit. The condition may be difficult to distinguish from VK deficiency since some response may follow VK administration. Molecular studies may be required. VK should be administered, and ongoing prophylaxis with VK may be required. In those unresponsive to VK, both FFP and factor concentrates have been used.

91.4.3.8 Fibrinolytic Deficiency States

Inherited deficiencies of PAI-1 and of α_2-AP (autosomal recessive) are very rare; they can give rise to serious bleeding. They can be screened for using the euglobulin clot lysis time.

91.4.3.9 PAI-1 Deficiency

The uncontrollable fibrinolysis associated with PAI-1 deficiency can give rise to ICH. Infants have a very short euglobulin clot lysis time in the face of normal screening tests. Relative insensitivity of available assays to activity measurements and in antigen detection makes diagnosis of deficiency difficult. Replacement is by using FFP in combination with e-aminocaproic acid (EACA) as a fibrinolytic inhibitor. Doses of EACA of 50–100 mg/kg every 6 h orally can maintain clot stability after replacement therapy.

Alpha-1-AT deficiency can only be replaced with FFP, and EACA may be of use in controlling excessive lysis.

91.4.4 Acquired Coagulation Disorders

The most common causes of bleeding (as well as thrombosis) in neonates are acquired conditions, and particularly the sick preterm infant is much more likely to have an acquired coagulopathy such as DIC, a disorder triggered by many conditions as hypoxia or bacterial infection, and resulting in the activation and consumption of coagulation proteins and platelets and the breakdown of fibrin. The primary management of DIC is to treat the underlying cause and provide appropriate component support.

91.4.4.1 Liver Dysfunction and Liver Failure

Acute neonatal liver failure is an uncommon condition associated with coagulopathy, direct hyperbilirubinemia, and hypoalbuminemia. Causes include five main entities: intrauterine insult, sepsis, hematological disorders, inborn errors of metabolism, and primary liver disease. Liver disease can affect the synthesis of a number of coagulation proteins. Levels of procoagulants and anticoagulants can become reduced resulting both in hemorrhagic and prothrombotic tendencies. Comparisons between FV and FVIII levels are helpful in evaluating the liver dysfunction because both should be present at adult levels and FV is the only one dependent on liver synthesis. Abnormal activation can reduce FVIII. Brief responses to platelet and fibrinogen infusions are indicative of consumption. Unless the cause of the liver failure can be reversed, the associated hemorrhagic diathesis is likely to be fatal.

91.4.4.2 Vitamin K Deficiency Bleeding (VKDB)

Vitamin K-Dependent Proteins

During carboxylation of their precursor molecules in hepatocytes, vitamin K (VK) is oxidized to epoxide and is recycled via an oxidation-reduction pathway for reuse in its reduced, hydroquinone form, in the g-carboxylation reaction (Fig. 7). In hemostasis, two classes of VK-dependent proteins are identifiable, one of procoagulants, factors II, VII, IX, and X, and one of inhibitors: protein C (PC), protein S (PS), and protein Z (PZ). The serine protease domain of factors II, VII, IX, and X and of PC becomes functional after cleavage of specific peptide bonds. Neither PS nor PZ are serine proteases. All depend on g-carboxylation of glutamic acid residues for their biologic activity. Reduced carboxylation in the absence of sufficient VK is associated with reduced activity. Precursor molecules in liver microsomes serve as immediately available substrates for the g-carboxylase enzyme once VK becomes available. Precursors are released into the circulation as proteins induced by vitamin K absence (PIVKAs). With a 70 h half-life for PIVKA II, its measurement can be used to diagnose previous VK deficiency even after VK has been administered.

In the first published series of 50 cases of what he named hemorrhagic disease of the newborn, Townsend identified four key features distinguishing affected babies from cases of hemophilia: early onset, usually on day 2–3 of life, a self-limited time course, a lack of a family history, and the importance of adequate feeds in reversing the condition. The name change recommended in 1999 by the ISTH Pediatric/Perinatal Subcommittee to VKDB indicates the specific etiology and widens the inclusion to babies beyond the 4 week neonatal period (Sutor et al. 1999). Recognition of the particular dangers from the late-onset form has resulted in the widespread introduction of various prophylactic regimens. In VK deficiency, the glutamate residues of factors II, VII, IX, and X are variably, incompletely γ-carboxylated.

Their measurement has been used to detect degrees of VK deficiency. Cord blood levels of PIVKA II vary through gestation, increasing near term and in pregnancies complicated by preeclampsia.

The differences between the adult and neonatal liver contents per gram of liver are striking (McCarthy et al. 1986). No VK_2 menaquinones were detectable in the neonatal autopsy material until approximately 14 days postnatal age; in the adult, they make up 75–97% of the total liver VK.

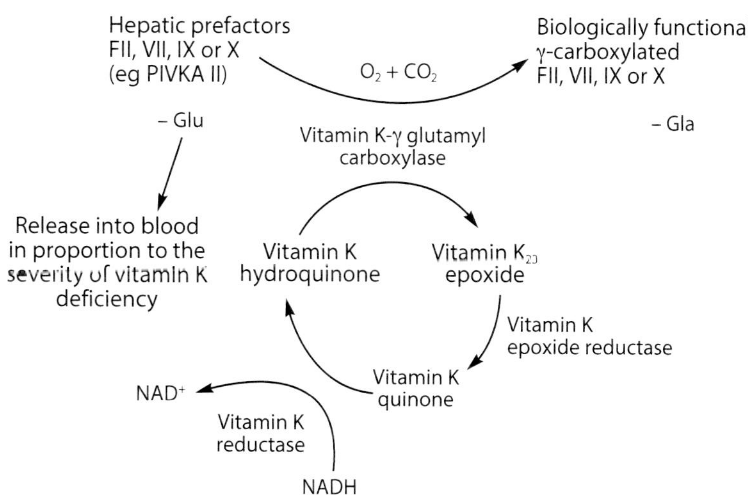

Fig. 7 Vitamin K – metabolism and dependent factors. *PIVKA* protein induced by vitamin K absence or inhibition

Table 4 Newborn and adult liver vitamin K_1 and K_2 values. Vitamin K concentrations and total values in livers from newborns and adults. Values in parentheses are median (Data from (McCarthy et al. 1986))

	Vit K_1 (ng/g)	Total Vit K_1 (μg)	Total Vit K_1 and K_2 (μg)
Adult	1.1–21.3 (5.4)	1.7–38.3 (7.8)	33–330
Term newborn	0.1–8.8 (0.1)	0.02–0.91 (0.09)	0.02–0.91
Preterm newborn	0.3–6.0 (1.4)	0.02–0.91 (0.09)	0.02–0.91

The newborn seems totally dependent on VK1 for sufficiency. Fortification of cow's milk formulae was recommended by the American Academy of Pediatrics in 1971 and continues at around 55–60 μg/L. In breast milk, the principal form of VK is phylloquinone (PhQ) with menaquinone-4 being the next highest. The average concentration of PhQ in colostrum is about 2 μg/L and in mature human milk, about 1 μg/L. Even if taking 200 mL/kg a day, it has been estimated that a baby would receive less than 1 μg VK a day. In one report, ceasing to supplement breastfed babies with formula feeds in the first days of life resulted in an incidence VKDB of 1 in 1200 live births (Table 4).

The effect of the differences in VK intake between breast- and formula-fed infants on PIVKA II detection is shown in Table 5. PIVKA II was only present in the breastfed groups. MK-4 appears to be synthesized in the mother from phylloquinone. The neonatal protective effects of 20 mg VK given daily for 14 days to mothers on anticonvulsants, where early neonatal bleeding had previously been a feature, were clear. Intramuscular VK_1 (0.5–1.0 mg) given at birth raises hepatic concentrations 1000–5000-fold at 24–48 h and at 6 days was 1.4 μg/g; by 28 days, levels remained some 200-fold above the levels encountered at birth. There is no evidence that neonatal VK1 provision enhances dependent factor protein synthesis, so in the preterm infant with gestationally determined low levels of the VK-dependent factors, postnatal VK administration will only prevent an emergence of inactive forms. Factor replacement is the only way to achieve improved hemostasis.

VKDB, delineated into three types as described by Lane and Hathaway in 1985 and accepted by the Pediatric/Perinatal Subcommittee of the International Society on Thrombosis and Haemostasis in 1999, includes the division into idiopathic and secondary forms (Sutor et al. 1999). Among the secondary causes are the frequently undiagnosed causes of fat malabsorption such as cholestasis, biliary atresia, a1-antitrypsin deficiency, and cystic fibrosis and a failure to be aware of the effects of drugs given to the mother or infant (warfarin, anticonvulsants, and antituberculous agents).

Table 5 PIVKA II measurements in breast- and formula-fed infants. Immunoassay on plasma samples from two groups of infants

		Age (months)		
		1	2	3
Breastfed	Number	62	44	32
Vit K: 2.1 μg/mL	PIVKA II + ve	3	4	2
Formula fed	Number	43	48	45
Vit K: 50 μg/mL	PIVKA II + ve	0	0	0

PIVKA protein induced by vit K absence or inhibition (Data from (Widdershoven et al. 1986))

Early VKDB is defined as bleeding due to VK deficiency in the first 24 h of life; it is usually caused by drugs administered to the mother that interfere with VK metabolism but can arise from conditions causing maternal fat malabsorption.

Classical VKDB occurs between days 2 and 7 and is regarded as idiopathic but often has its origins in the failure to establish adequate early breastfeeding (von Kries et al. 1987).

Late-onset VKDB extends the period of bleeding from day 8 to 6 months (Sutor et al. 1999). The peak incidence is between 3 and 8 weeks. It is almost always in exclusively breastfed infants. An impaired secretion of bile salts with mild abnormalities in liver function tests leading to VK malabsorption is often implicated. Although warning bleeds can be a feature, many cases present with intracranial bleeds. In one series, severe ICH was noted in 63% of cases. Of those followed up, some

40% had long-term neurological consequences. Factors contributing to the VKDB are the relatively low VK content of breast milk, the lack of gut microflora that synthesize vitamin K2, and, in preterm infants, inadequately functional VK epoxide cycles. Various chemicals in the breast milk of mothers living in industrialized countries may be acting as enzyme inducers, interfering with quinone metabolism.

Diagnostic criteria of VKDB are a prothrombin time $\geq$ four times the control value plus at least one of:

(a) A normal or raised platelet count, normal fibrinogen, and absent FDP
(b) PT returning to normal after vitamin K
(c) PIVKA (usually of FII) level above normal control values

A probable case: PT and APTT prolonged for age plus one of the above.

Use of PIVKA measurements may be helpful in differentiating VKDB from cases of non-accidental injury since retinal bleeds, often considered as pathognomonic of NAI, have been described in VKDB.

Treatment of VKDB

A slow intravenous dose of 1–2 mg Konakion will fully correct deficiency in those less than 6 months of age. The subcutaneous route can be utilized in the absence of venous access. Higher doses may be indicated for the reversal of warfarin antagonists. Increases in factor levels are detectable within 20 min of the intravenous dose, values rising to close to normal for age by 2 h. Severe bleeding may require factor replacement as well as the VK until the diagnosis can be confirmed. FFP in a dose of 15 mL/kg or prothrombin complex concentrate, where the dose extrapolated from adult data is 50 units/kg body weight, may be used but these take time to arrive and VK administration should not be delayed. rFVIIa can also be effective in life-threatening hemorrhage at 90 μg/kg.

Prevention of VKDB

Surveys on the incidence of both classical and late-onset VKDB have been evaluated in a Cochrane review (Puckett and Offringa 2000) and have been reviewed by Shearer (2009). A UK survey documented that almost all late-onset cases were breastfed babies who had received either no VK or just one oral dose. The authors commented that parental refusal of prophylaxis had become more problematic.

Efficacy of Vitamin K Prophylaxis

The single intramuscular injection of 0.5–1.0 mg of phylloquinone offers better protection than the single or most multiple oral dose regimens. A depot effect is not achieved by intravenous or oral delivery. The move toward oral regimens was triggered by Golding et al. (1990) and Golding et al. (1992) linking childhood cancer to receipt of intramuscular VK with a possible doubling of the risk of leukemia. Subsequently reviews of data from many surveys have concluded that there is no convincing evidence that vitamin K provided by any route influences cancer risk in children, but an influence cannot be totally ruled out (Parker et al. 1998; Passmore et al. 1998).

Many oral regimens were found not to prevent all cases of late-onset VKDB. However, a Danish regimen used when the Konakion Cremophor preparation was available, of a 2 mg dose at birth followed by a 1 mg dose given weekly for 3 months, resulted in no cases being reported over a 7.5 year survey period. In a randomized study in the USA with 67 infants in two groups, 2 mg Konakion MM given orally at birth, at 7 days and at 30 days, was at least as effective as a single dose of 1 mg intramuscularly at birth. Konakion MM given orally is not predictably absorbed in infants with cholestasis. Concerns remain over bioavailability and over compliance with oral dosing regimens. In the USA, a single intramuscular injection of 0.5–1.0 mg PQ remains the recommended prophylaxis. Low-dose oral regimens should be continued for 3 months.

In preterm infants, the reduced activity of the VK epoxide reductase is associated with evidence of hepatic overload at previously prescribed parenteral VK dosages. In a recent trial in which differing dosage regimens in babies <32 weeks' gestational age were compared, 0.2 mg intravenously or 0.5 mg intramuscularly led to VK_1

2,3-epoxide accumulation, whereas 0.2 mg intramuscularly did not. The protection lasted almost 3 weeks following which additional supplementation was needed (Clarke et al. 2006).

A prolonged PT in a preterm infant in the first month of life who has received intramuscular VK at birth is unlikely to be due to VK deficiency. All infants with late-onset bleeding require testing for associated disorders.

The importance of VKDB is reflected in the number of continuing reviews of the subject (Pichler and Pichler 2008; Van Winckel et al. 2009; Sankar et al. 2016) and alert reports (Schulte et al. 2014).

A recent position paper (Mihatsch et al. 2016) on prevention of VKDB by ESPGHAN Committee on Nutrition states the following recommendations:

1. All newborns infants should receive vitamin K prophylaxis.
2. Vitamin K prophylaxis and mode of administration should be documented.
3. Parental refusal after adequate information should be documented.
4. Intramuscular application is the preferred route for efficiency and reliability of administration.
5. Healthy newborns should either receive 1 mg of vitamin K1 by IM injection at birth, or 3 × 2 mg orally at birth, at 4–6 days and at 4–6 weeks or 2 mg orally at birth and a weekly dose of 1 mg orally for 6 months.
6. In case of oral policy if the infant vomits or regurgitate the formulation within 1 h, repeating the oral dose may be appropriate.
7. The oral route is not appropriate for preterm infants and for newborns, who are unwell, have cholestasis or impaired intestinal absorption, or are unable to take oral vitamin K, or those whose mothers have taken medications that interfere with vitamin K metabolism.

Future research topics are (a) robust national surveillance data of VKDB, which require accurate documentation of policies and procedures, (b) efficacy and quality control of individual vitamin K products used for supplementation, and (c) future studies to compare efficacy and safety of multiple oral doses with IM vitamin K and also evaluate the optimal dose in preterm neonates.

Intraventricular Hemorrhage (IVH)

The contribution of the immature hemostatic system to the occurrence of IVH in very low birth weight (VLBW) neonates is unclear. Preterm and VLBW neonates are at high risk of IVH especially in the first week of life as a result of immaturity of the cerebral vascular system. The higher bleeding tendency in preterm and VLBW neonates may also contribute to increase the risk. High-grade IVH was shown to coincide with severe derangement of coagulation in ELBW infants (Piotrowski et al. 2010).

The role of therapies targeting the hemostasis system (vitamin K, plasma, recombinant FVIIa, prothrombin complex concentrates) for the prevention or treatment of IVH is currently being debated (Kuperman AA IVH in preterm infants coagulation perspective Semin thromb Hemostas 2011, p. 37). Studies published in the past decades provided no definite answers to the question of whether prophylaxis with hemostatic agents can decrease the incidence of IVH and IVH-related mortality. Heterogeneity of agents, doses, and timing of the intervention, as well as the fact that no imaging modalities were used in the earlier reports, preclude any firm conclusions. It is time to reevaluate the relationship between premature coagulation and IVH and to cautiously and thoroughly study the role of currently available hemostatic agents in potential IVH therapy and prevention.

Hypoxic-Ischemic Encephalopathy (HIE) and Hypoxic-Ischemic Encephalopathy Treated with Therapeutic Hypothermia (TH)

HIE is a significant cause of neonatal morbidity and mortality, and multiorgan dysfunction is common. Disruption of hemostasis can occur from ischemic injury, systemic oxygen deprivation, acute blood loss, or DIC. Initial hemostatic dysfunction is highly prevalent among neonates with moderate to severe HIE and is associated with a high transfusion burden and increased risk of bleeding (up to 69%) (Pakvasa et al. 2017).

Additionally, therapeutic hypothermia (TH) slows enzymatic activity of the coagulation

cascade leading to constitutive prolongation of routinely assessed coagulation studies (Forman et al. 2014).

Thus, establishing evidence-based guidelines for managing coagulopathy during TH can optimize medical care and contribute to better outcomes. Routinely used coagulation tests exhibit a nonoptimal sensitivity and specificity to predict bleeding in this high-risk population; thromboelastography, a functional assay of global hemostatic status that can be performed under temperature-regulated conditions, may improve the approach to assessment and treatment of bleeding risk in these neonates. Further studies are also needed to evaluate transfusion practices as comparison between cryoprecipitate transfusion and fresh frozen plasma transfusion on bleeding risk and other outcomes among neonates with moderate to severe HIE.

91.5 Indications for Use of Plasma and Coagulant Factor Concentrates

91.5.1 Plasma

In neonatal practice, plasma is predominantly given to reduce perceived bleeding risk (prophylaxis) in non-bleeding patients; other usages include as a volume expander, bleeding with abnormal coagulation test results, intraoperative bleeding, and sepsis-related coagulopathy. It is currently not known which neonates deemed at high risk of bleeding or even actively bleeding might benefit from plasma transfusion, and so far, the overall quality of studies and numbers of included infants are very limited. A recent review (Keir and Stanworth 2016) has provided following recommendations:

1. There is no current evidence to support the prophylactic use of plasma in association with abnormalities of coagulation tests, which have limited predictive use for clinically significant bleeding.
2. There is no supporting evidence to recommend plasma for simple volume replacement or routinely for prevention of IVH in neonates.
3. We support the therapeutic use of plasma when active bleeding is present or before invasive procedures in those with a risk of significant bleeding and who have abnormal coagulation profile defined as a PT or an aPTT significantly above the normal gestational and postnatal age related reference range.

91.5.2 Recombinant Factor VIIa

Recombinant factor VIIa is thought to induce thrombin generation at sites of endothelial injury. In newborns rFVIIa is most commonly used for off-label indications, specifically treatment or prevention of intractable or life-threatening bleeding. However there is no evidence from most studies (including those on prevention of ICH or of bleeding during cardiopulmonary bypass CPB) of the efficacy of rFVIIa for bleeding in neonates, and there may be a higher rate of thrombosis (Witmer et al. 2011).

Thus, rFVIIa use should be limited to rescue therapy for intractable bleeding, mostly during CPB.

91.5.3 Prothrombin Complex Concentrate

PCC contain the vitamin K-dependent coagulant factors and are pooled from human plasma. Three-factor (II, IX, X) and four-factor (II, VII, IX, X) PCC are available.

PCC are indicated in newborns with bleeding and congenital deficiency or inhibition of vitamin K-dependent factors. The role of PCC in prevention and treatment of neonatal IVH remains to be explored.

91.5.4 Fibrinogen Concentrate

Fibrinogen concentrate is approved for use in bleeding in patients with congenital fibrinogen deficiency. There are no studies on the use of fibrinogen concentrate specifically in neonates. Prevention and management of bleeding in neonates on CPB with acquired hypofibrinogenemia needs further investigation.

References

Andrew M, Paes B, Milner R et al (1987) Development of the human coagulation system in the full-term infant. Blood 70(1):165–172

Andrew BM, Vegh P, Johnston M, Bowker J, Ofosu F, Mitchell L (1992) Maturation of the hemostatic system during childhood. Blood 80(8):1998–2005

Asselta R, Peyvandi F (2009) Factor V deficiency. Semin Thromb Hemost 35(4):382–389. https://doi.org/10.1055/s-0029-1225760

Attard C, van der Straaten T, Karlaftis V, Monagle P, Ignjatovic V (2013) Developmental haemostasis: age-specific differences in the quantity of haemostatic proteins. J Thromb Haemost 11(10). https://doi.org/10.1111/jth.12372

Baker-Groberg SM, Lattimore S, Recht M, McCarty OJT, Haley KM (2016) Assessment of neonatal platelet adhesion, activation, and aggregation. J Thromb Haemost 14(4):815–827. https://doi.org/10.1111/jth.13270

Barnard DR, Simmons MA, Hathaway WE (1979) Coagulation studies in extremely premature infants. Pediatr Res 13(12):1330–1335

Bolton-Maggs PHB, Perry DJ, Chalmers EA et al (2004) The rare coagulation disorders – review with guidelines for management from the United Kingdom Haemophilia Centre Doctors' Organisation. Haemophilia 10(5): 593–628. https://doi.org/10.1111/j.1365-2516.2004.00944.x

Chalmers EA, Williams M, Brennand J, Liesner R, Collins P, Richards M (2011) Guideline on the management of haemophilia in the fetus and neonate. Br J Haematol 154(2):208–215. https://doi.org/10.1111/j.1365-2141.2010.08545.x

Clarke P, Mitchell SJ, Wynn R et al (2006) Vitamin K prophylaxis for preterm infants: a randomized, controlled trial of 3 regimens. Pediatrics 118(6): e1657–e1666. https://doi.org/10.1542/peds.2005-2742

Cvirn G, Gallistl S, Muntean W (1999) Effects of antithrombin and protein C on thrombin generation in newborn and adult plasma. Thromb Res 93(4):183–190

Cvirn G, Gallistl S, Koestenberger M, Kutschera J, Leschnik B, Muntean W (2002) Alpha 2-macroglobulin enhances prothrombin activation and thrombin potential by inhibiting the anticoagulant protein C/protein S system in cord and adult plasma. Thromb Res 105(5):433–439

Cvirn G, Kutschera J, Wagner T et al (2009) Collagen/endogenous thrombin-induced platelet aggregation in cord versus adult whole blood. Neonatology 95(2): 187–192. https://doi.org/10.1159/000155613

Duga S, Salomon O (2009) Factor XI deficiency. Semin Thromb Hemost 35(04):416–425. https://doi.org/10.1055/s-0029-1225764

Forman KR, Diab Y, Wong ECC, Baumgart S, Luban NLC, Massaro AN (2014) Coagulopathy in newborns with hypoxic ischemic encephalopathy (HIE) treated with therapeutic hypothermia: a retrospective case-control study. BMC Pediatr 14(1):277. https://doi.org/10.1186/1471-2431-14-277

Girolami A, Scandellari R, Scapin M, Vettore S (2008) Congenital bleeding disorders of the vitamin K-dependent clotting factors. Vitam Horm 78:281–374. https://doi.org/10.1016/S0083-6729(07)00014-3

Golding J, Paterson M, Kinlen LJ (1990) Factors associated with childhood cancer in a national cohort study. Br J Cancer 62(2):304–308

Golding J, Greenwood R, Birmingham K, Mott M (1992) Childhood cancer, intramuscular vitamin K, and pethidine given during labour. BMJ 305(6849):341–346

Goodeve A (2008) Molecular genetic testing of hemophilia A. Semin Thromb Hemost 34(6):491–501. https://doi.org/10.1055/s-0028-1103360

Hathaway W, Corrigan J (1991) Report of scientific and standardization subcommittee on neonatal hemostasis. Normal coagulation data for fetuses and newborn infants. Thromb Haemost 65(3):323–325

Holmberg L, Henriksson P, Ekelund H, Astedt B (1974) Coagulation in the human fetus. Comparison with term newborn infants. J Pediatr 85(6):860–864

Ignjatovic V, Mertyn E, Monagle P (2011) The coagulation system in children: developmental and pathophysiological considerations. Semin Thromb Hemost 37(7): 723–729. https://doi.org/10.1055/s-0031-1297162

Ignjatovic V, Kenet G, Monagle P (2012) Developmental hemostasis: recommendations for laboratories reporting pediatric samples. J Thromb Haemost 10(2):298–300. https://doi.org/10.1111/j.1538-7836.2011.04584.x

Israels SJ, Rand ML, Michelson AD (2003) Neonatal platelet function. Semin Thromb Hemost 29 (4):363–372. https://doi.org/10.1055/s-2003-42587

Jensen AH, Josso F, Zamet P, Monset-Couchard M, Minkowski A (1973) Evolution of blood clotting factor leves in premature infants during the first 10 days of life: a study of 96 cases with comparison between clinical status and blood clotting factor levels. Pediatr Res 7(7):638–644. https://doi.org/10.1203/00006450-197307000-00007

Karimi M, Bereczky Z, Cohan N, Muszbek L (2009) Factor XIII deficiency. Semin Thromb Hemost 35(4): 426–438. https://doi.org/10.1055/s-0029-1225765

Keir AK, Stanworth SJ (2016) Neonatal plasma transfusion: an evidence-based review. Transfus Med Rev 30(4): 174–182. https://doi.org/10.1016/j.tmrv.2016.07.001

Kulkarni R, Lusher J (2001) Perinatal management of newborns with haemophilia. Br J Haematol 112(2):264–274. https://doi.org/10.1046/j.1365-2141.2001.02362.x

Kulkarni R, Soucie JM (2011) Pediatric hemophilia: a review. Semin Thromb Hemost 37(07):737–744. https://doi.org/10.1055/s-0031-1297164

Laffan M, Lester W, O'Donnell J et al (2014) The diagnosis and management of von Willebrand disease: a United Kingdom Haemophilia Centre Doctors Organization guideline approved by the British Committee for Standards in Haematology. Br J Haematol 167(4):453–465. https://doi.org/10.1016/j.virol.2008.08.028.Macropinocytosis

Lancellotti S, De Cristofaro R (2009) Congenital prothrombin deficiency. Semin Thromb Hemost 35(04): 367–381. https://doi.org/10.1055/s-0029-1225759

Ljung RCR (2008) Intracranial haemorrhage in haemophilia A and B. Br J Haematol 140(4):378–384. https://doi.org/10.1111/j.1365-2141.2007.06949.x

Mariani G, Bernardi F (2009) Factor VII deficiency. Semin Thromb Hemost 35(4):400–406. https://doi.org/10.1055/s-0029-1225762

McCarthy PT, Shearer MJ, Crampton O (1986) Vitamin K content of human liver at different ages. Rec Adv New Dev Hemostaseol Haemost 16:84. https://doi.org/10.1002/j.1552-4604.1988.tb03106.x

Menegatti M, Peyvandi F (2009) Factor X deficiency. Semin Thromb Hemost 35(4):407–415. https://doi.org/10.1055/s-0029-1225763

Mihatsch WA, Braegger C, Bronsky J et al (2016) Prevention of vitamin K deficiency bleeding in newborn infants: a position paper by the ESPGHAN committee on nutrition. J Pediatr Gastroenterol Nutr 63(1):123–129. https://doi.org/10.1097/MPG.0000000000001232

de Moerloose P, Neerman-Arbez M (2009) Congenital fibrinogen disorders. Semin Thromb Hemost 35(04): 356–366. https://doi.org/10.1055/s-0029-1225758

Naderi M, Dorgalaleh A, Alizadeh S et al (2014) Clinical manifestations and management of life-threatening bleeding in the largest group of patients with severe factor XIII deficiency. Int J Hematol 100(5):443–449. https://doi.org/10.1007/s12185-014-1664-1

Neary E, McCallion N, Kevane B et al (2015) Coagulation indices in very preterm infants from cord blood and postnatal samples. J Thromb Haemost 13(11): 2021–2030. https://doi.org/10.1111/jth.13130

Nichols WL, Hultin MB, James AH et al (2008) Von Willebrand disease (VWD): evidence-based diagnosis and management guidelines, the National Heart, Lung, and Blood Institute (NHLBI) expert panel report (USA). Haemophilia 14(2):171–232. https://doi.org/10.1111/j.1365-2516.2007.01643.x

Pakvasa MA, Winkler AM, Hamrick SE, Josephson CD, Patel RM (2017) Observational study of haemostatic dysfunction and bleeding in neonates with hypoxic-ischaemic encephalopathy. BMJ Open 7(2):e013787. https://doi.org/10.1136/bmjopen-2016-013787

Parker L, Cole M, Craft AW, Hey EN (1998) Neonatal vitamin K administration and childhood cancer in the north of England: retrospective case-control study. BMJ 316(7126):189–193

Passmore SJ, Draper G, Brownbill P, Kroll M (1998) Case-control studies of relation between childhood cancer and neonatal vitamin K administration. BMJ 316 (7126):178–184

Peyvandi F, Makris M (2017) Inhibitor development in haemophilia. Haemophilia 23:3–3. https://doi.org/10.1111/hae.13145

Peyvandi F, Menegatti M (2016) Treatment of rare factor deficiencies in 2016. Hematology 2016(1):663–669. https://doi.org/10.1182/asheducation-2016.1.663

Peyvandi F, Palla R, Menegatti M, Mannucci PM (2009) Introduction: rare bleeding disorders: general aspects of clinical features, diagnosis, and management. Semin Thromb Hemost 35(4):349–355. https://doi.org/10.1055/s-0029-1225757

Peyvandi F, Bolton-Maggs PH, Batorova A, De Moerloose P (2012) Rare bleeding disorders. Haemophilia 18 (Suppl. 4):148–153. https://doi.org/10.1111/j.1365-2516.2012.02841.x

Peyvandi F, Garagiola I, Biguzzi E (2016) Advances in the treatment of bleeding disorders. J Thromb Haemost 14(11):2095–2106. https://doi.org/10.1111/jth.13491

Pichler E, Pichler L (2008) The neonatal coagulation system and the vitamin K deficiency bleeding – a mini review. Wien Med Wochenschr 158(13–14):385–395. https://doi.org/10.1007/s10354-008-0538-7

Piotrowski A, Dabrowska-Wojciak I, Mikinka M et al (2010) Coagulation abnormalities and severe intraventricular hemorrhage in extremely low birth weight infants. J Matern Fetal Neonatal Med 23(7):601–606. https://doi.org/10.1080/14767050903229614

Powell JS (2015) Longer-acting clotting factor concentrates for hemophilia. J Thromb Haemost 13(Suppl 1): S167–S175. https://doi.org/10.1111/jth.12912

Puckett RM, Offringa M (2000) Prophylactic vitamin K for vitamin K deficiency bleeding in neonates. Offringa M, ed. Cochrane Database Syst Rev (4):CD002776. https://doi.org/10.1002/14651858.CD002776

Punzalan RC, Gottschall JL (2016) Use and future investigations of recombinant and plasma-derived coagulation and anticoagulant products in the neonate. Transfus Med Rev 30(4):189–196. https://doi.org/10.1016/j.tmrv.2016.07.002

Radicioni M, Mezzetti D, Del Vecchio A, Motta M (2012) Thromboelastography: might work in neonatology too? J Matern Fetal Neonatal Med 25(Suppl 4):18–21. https://doi.org/10.3109/14767058.2012.714996

Salonvaara M, Riikonen P, Vahtera E, Mahlamäki E, Heinonen K, Kekomäki R (2004) Development of selected coagulation factors and anticoagulants in preterm infants by the age of six months. Thromb Haemost 92(4):688–696. https://doi.org/10.1160/TH03-12-0769

Sankar MJ, Chandrasekaran A, Kumar P, Thukral A, Agarwal R, Paul VK (2016) Vitamin K prophylaxis for prevention of vitamin K deficiency bleeding: a systematic review. J Perinatol 36(Suppl 1):S29–S35. https://doi.org/10.1038/jp.2016.30

Saxonhouse MA, Manco-Johnson MJ (2009) The evaluation and management of neonatal coagulation disorders. Semin Perinatol 33(1):52–65. https://doi.org/10.1053/j.semperi.2008.10.007

Schulte R, Jordan LC, Morad A, Naftel RP, Wellons JC, Sidonio R (2014) Rise in late onset vitamin K deficiency bleeding in young infants because of omission or refusal of prophylaxis at birth. Pediatr Neurol 50(6): 564–568. https://doi.org/10.1016/j.pediatrneurol.2014.02.013

Sewell EK, Forman KR, Wong ECC, Gallagher M, Luban NLC, Massaro AN (2017) Thromboelastography in term neonates: an alternative approach to evaluating coagulopathy. Arch Dis Child Fetal Neonatal Ed 102(1):F79–F84. https://doi.org/10.1136/archdischild-2016-310545

Shearer MJ (2009) Vitamin K deficiency bleeding (VKDB) in early infancy. Blood Rev 23(2):49–59. https://doi.org/10.1016/j.blre.2008.06.001

Street AM, Ljung R, Lavery SA (2008) Management of carriers and babies with haemophilia. Haemophilia 14(Suppl. 3):181–187. https://doi.org/10.1111/j.1365-2516.2008.01721.x

Sutor AH, von Kries R, Cornelissen EA, McNinch AW, Andrew M, Vitamin K (1999) Deficiency bleeding (VKDB) in infancy. ISTH pediatric/perinatal subcommittee. International society on thrombosis and haemostasis. Thromb Haemost 81(3):456–461

Urban D, Pluthero FG, Christensen H et al (2017) Decreased numbers of dense granules in fetal and neonatal platelets. Haematologica 102(2):e36–e38. https://doi.org/10.3324/haematol.2016.152421

von Kries R, Becker A, Göbel U (1987) Vitamin K in the newborn: influence of nutritional factors on acarboxyprothrombin detectability and factor II and VII clotting activity. Eur J Pediatr 146(2):123–127

Van Winckel M, De Bruyne R, Van De Velde S, Van Biervliet S (2009) Vitamin K, an update for the paediatrician. Eur J Pediatr 168(2):127–134. https://doi.org/10.1007/s00431-008-0856-1

Venkatesh V, Curley A, Khan R et al (2013) A novel approach to standardised recording of bleeding in a high risk neonatal population. Arch Dis Child Fetal Neonatal Ed 98(3):F260–F263. https://doi.org/10.1136/archdischild-2012-302443

Watzka M, Geisen C, Scheer M et al (2014) Bleeding and non-bleeding phenotypes in patients with GGCX gene mutations. Thromb Res 134(4):856–865. https://doi.org/10.1016/j.thromres.2014.07.004

Widdershoven J, Motohara K, Endo F, Matsuda I, Monnens L (1986) Influence of the type of feeding on the presence of PIVKA-II in infants. Helv Paediatr Acta 41(1–2):25–29

Wiedmeier SE, Henry E, Sola-Visner MC, Christensen RD (2009) Platelet reference ranges for neonates, defined using data from over 47,000 patients in a multihospital healthcare system. J Perinatol 29(2):130–136. https://doi.org/10.1038/jp.2008.141

Witmer CM, Huang Y-S, Lynch K, Raffini LJ, Shah SS (2011) Off-label recombinant factor VIIa use and thrombosis in children: a multi-center cohort study. J Pediatr 158(5):820–825.e1. https://doi.org/10.1016/j.jpeds.2010.10.038

The Thrombotic Risk of the Newborn 92

Molinari Angelo Claudio and Paola Saracco

Contents

Abstract

The first weeks of life have the highest rate of thrombotic complications in the pediatric age, and thromboembolism mainly affects sick newborns. It is well known that despite low levels of procoagulant factors in the first months of life, newborns show a perfect hemostasis; this is probably due to the balancing effect of the low levels of physiological inhibitors (protein C, protein S, and antithrombin).

Some other pathophysiological insights are available to favor the knowledge of the process that pathological situations may lead newborns to experience thromboembolic complications. In the recent years, genetic prothrombotic conditions have been widely studied but their role in determining thrombosis in the neonates is

M. Angelo Claudio (✉)
Thrombosis and Hemostasis Unit, Giannina Gaslini Children's Hospital, Genova, Italy
e-mail: aclaudiomolinari@gaslini.org

P. Saracco
Pediatric Hematology, Department of Pediatrics, University Hospital Città della Salute e della Scienza, Torino, Italy
e-mail: paola.saracco@unito.it

G. Buonocore et al. (eds.), *Neonatology*,
https://doi.org/10.1007/978-3-319-29489-6_239

still under debate. Moreover, in the sick newborn, especially preterm, several acquired perinatal and iatrogenic conditions might result in a disturbance between coagulation and fibrinolysis, leading to thrombus formation. The use of central lines, cardiac diseases and polycythemia, renal diseases such as congenital nephrotic syndrome and neonatal hemolytic uremic syndrome, peripartum asphyxia, infants of diabetic mothers, dehydration, septicemia, necrotizing enterocolitis, acute respiratory distress syndrome, and extracorporeal membrane oxygenation lead to elevated thrombin generation and subsequent thrombus formation.

Abbreviations

ACA	Anticardiolipin antibodies
AIS	Arterial ischemic stroke
APA	Antiphospholipid antibodies
APLS	Antiphospholipid syndrome
ArT	Arterial thrombosis
AT	Antithrombin (natural anticoagulant)
CNS	Central nervous system
CSVT	Cerebral sinovenous thrombosis
CVL	Central venous line
ETP	Endogenous thrombin potential
FI	Fibrinogen
FII	Coagulation factor II
FV	Coagulation factor V
FVII	Coagulation factor VII
FVIII	Coagulation factor VIII
FVL	Factor V Leiden (prothrombotic polymorphism of FV)
FX	Coagulation factor X
FXIII	Coagulation factor XIII
LA	Lupus anticoagulant
MTHFR	Methylenetetrahydrofolate reductase
PAP	Plasmin-alpha2-antiplasmin complex
PC	Protein C (natural anticoagulant)
PE	Pulmonary embolism
PLG	Plasminogen
PRT G20210A	Prothrombotic mutation of factor II G20210A
PS	Protein S (natural anticoagulant cofactor of PC)
PVT	Portal vein thrombosis
RVT	Renal vein thrombosis
TAT	Thrombin–antithrombin complex
TE	Thromboembolic events
TF	Tissue factor
TFPI	TF pathway inhibitor
TM	Thrombomodulin
UAC	Umbilical artery catheter
UVC	Umbilical vein catheter
VWF	Von Willebrand factor

92.1 Salient Points

- Newborns comprise the largest group of children developing TE due to the peculiarities of their developmental hemostatic system.
- Given the significant differences between the plasma factor concentrations in different age groups, a detailed knowledge on the development of hemostasis is critical for the neonatologist in order to adapt pharmacological approaches and interpret results from laboratory tests in the neonate with TE.
- Coagulation laboratories should develop neonatal age-related reference ranges specific to their own testing systems. Without this, accurate diagnosis and management of neonates and children with suspected bleeding or clotting disorders is not possible.
- Neonatal symptomatic thrombosis (excluding stroke) is reported to occur in 2.4/1,000 admissions to neonatal intensive care units according to an international registry from Canada, the USA, and Europe; 64 among 97 (66%) registered events are venous thrombosis. In a German prospective nationwide 2-year registry, the incidence of clinically apparent neonatal TEs (including cerebral events) is 5.1/100,000 live births; 76% are venous events.
- Arterial thromboses (ArT) represent almost 50% of all neonatal TEs and are mainly iatrogenic complications, associated with catheterization of the femoral artery as well as peripheral arteries and the umbilical artery.
- Registry data and case studies have demonstrated that the majority of symptomatic neonatal TEs, especially spontaneous events (i.e.,

not catheter related), are associated with multiple hemostatic prothrombotic defects or with the combination of prothrombotic defects and environmental or clinical conditions.

- Numerous clinical and environmental conditions such as the use of central lines, cardiac diseases and polycythemia, renal diseases such as congenital nephrotic syndrome and neonatal hemolytic uremic syndrome, peripartum asphyxia, infants of diabetic mothers, dehydration, septicemia, necrotizing enterocolitis, acute respiratory distress syndrome, and extracorporeal membrane oxygenation lead to elevated thrombin generation and subsequent thrombus formation.
- Endothelial, coagulation, and fibrinolytic systems are activated in newborns; it might occur during birth due to the mechanical stress, the adaptation of circulation, and the short-term hypoxic state.
- The presence of an indwelling line has been identified as the most important acquired risk factor for the development of both arterial and venous systemic events, spontaneous non-catheter-related events being relatively uncommon.
- The Subcommittee for Perinatal/Pediatric Hemostasis of the International Society on Thrombosis and Hemostasis has recommended that pediatric patients with thrombosis (regardless of risk factors) should be tested for a full panel of genetic prothrombotic traits.

92.2 Introduction

The hemostatic system of the healthy neonate, although immature, is generally in balance; on the other hand, in the sick newborn, especially preterm, numerous acquired perinatal and iatrogenic conditions might result in a disturbance between coagulation and fibrinolysis, leading to thrombus formation. Nevertheless, the contribution of acquired prothrombotic disorders in the pathogenesis of thromboembolic disease in newborns remains poorly defined. Few data are currently available regarding the influence of maternal or fetal genes on thrombotic risk in the fetus and neonate.

Due to the unique peculiarities of their developmental coagulation system, newborns are at highest risk of developing TEs among pediatric patients (Andrew 1995; Stein et al. 2004; Chalmers 2006).

Recently, several studies based on national and international registries (Andrew et al. 1994; Nowak-Gottl et al. 1997a; Schmidt and Andrew 1995; van Ommen et al. 2001) have evaluated the role of risk factors for thrombosis both in children and newborns, emphasizing the differences between different pediatric age and adult age.

Nevertheless, the contribution of both inherited and acquired prothrombotic disorders in the pathogenesis of thromboembolic disease in newborns remains poorly defined and at present there is no definitive consensus about recommendations on screening for thrombophilia in newborns with TEs.

The aim of the present chapter is to provide an overview of the current knowledge on the development of the hemostatic system and the role of inherited, acquired perinatal and maternal prothrombotic risk factors as well as clinical and laboratory investigations in neonatal systemic arterial and venous thrombosis and in neonatal central nervous system (CNS) thrombotic events like cerebral sinovenous thrombosis (CSVT) and arterial ischemic stroke.

92.3 Physiological Thrombotic Risk of the Newborn

92.3.1 The Evolution of the Neonatal Hemostatic System

The hemostatic system is a dynamic evolving system which develops from the first month of gestation (Manco-Johnson 2005) and during infancy and early childhood profoundly differs from adults.

92.3.1.1 Synthesis of Coagulation Proteins

In normal neonates, the levels of coagulation factor II (FII), factor VII (FVII), factor IX, factor X (X), factor XI, prekallikrein, high-molecular-weight kininogen, heparin cofactor II, and plasminogen

(PLG) are all approximately 50% of adult levels, while the levels of factor V (FV), factor VIII (FVIII), von Willebrand factor (VWF), factor XIII, and fibrinogen (FI) are closer to adult values and sometimes higher. Adult plasma concentrations are not achieved before the sixth month of life. However, the vitamin-K-dependent inhibitors of coagulation protein C (PC) and protein S (PS) as well as antithrombin (AT) are also reduced in the neonatal period, counterbalancing the reduced clotting potential of neonatal plasma. In fact, both AT and PC concentrations are decreased to approximately 30% of adult values in term and even lower in preterm newborns (Andrew et al. 1987, 1988, 1990; Albisetti 2003; Monagle et al. 2006).

92.3.1.2 Factor VIII, Von Willebrand Factor, and ADAMTS-13

The mean level of VWF and FVIII is normal or slightly increased, and presence of qualitative abnormalities of the VWF molecule with ultra large VWF multimers is a common finding (Fukui et al. 1979; Tsai et al. 2002; Hellstrom-Westas et al. 2005).

Upon endothelial cell activation, the VWF stored in the Weibel–Palade bodies is released as ultra large multimers which are hyperactive to favor platelet function and thrombus formation. VWF multimers' size is regulated by a specific protease from the ADAMTS family (a disintegrin and metalloprotease with thrombospondin motifs) which has been named ADAMTS-13 (Perutelli and Molinari 2007).

Mean ADAMTS-13 levels were found significantly lower in newborns than in healthy children. In a further study, the mean ADAMTS-13 level in preterm infants was lower than in the term infants, with a positive correlation between ADAMTS-13 and both gestational age and birth weight (Kavakli et al. 2002).

92.3.1.3 Endothelium and Platelets

The endothelium and platelets generally appear to be less reactive in neonates than in adults though high levels of the von Willebrand factor are usually present resulting in overall normal platelet function.

Platelets are less reactive in newborns compared to adults, and hypo-aggregation induced by collagen ADP and epinephrine has been reported. However, due to the high level of high-molecular-weight multimers of VWF, enhanced ristocetin-induced agglutination has been demonstrated (Israels et al. 1990; Michelson 1998; Andrew et al. 2000). Moreover, a higher rate of activate platelets was found in neonates (Schmugge et al. 2003) and even more in newborns with central venous lines (Schmugge et al. 2007).

The concentrations of activation markers like thrombomodulin (TM), thrombin–AT complex (TAT), D-dimer, and plasmin-alpha2-antiplasmin complex (PAP) are significantly higher in newborns. During the first 12 days of life, TM, TAT, and PAP show a continuous decline, whereas the concentrations of endothelin, VWF, and D-dimers do not change (Knofler et al. 1998).

92.3.1.4 Fibrinolysis

Despite increased tissue plasminogen activator (t-PA), newborns have lower plasma levels and activity of PLG and increased concentration of PLG activator inhibitor (PAI) (Andrew et al. 1987, 1988, 1990; Albisetti 2003; Monagle et al. 2006); in addition, dysfunctional PLG with low activation by streptokinase and urokinase had been found in full-term newborns (Benavent et al. 1984).

92.3.1.5 Thrombin Activation and Generation

In neonates, thrombin generation in a capillary wound starts fast and is at least as strong as in adults, therefore supporting the data obtained with small amounts of TF for clotting activation in vitro (Muntean et al. 2004). Activation with small amounts of lipidated TF results in shorter clotting times and faster activated factor X and thrombin generation in neonates compared with adults due to the concomitant action of low TF pathway inhibitor and AT (Cvirn et al. 2003); besides, since the concentrations of both tissue

factor pathway inhibitor and AT in cord plasma are approximately 50% of the respective adult values, thrombin generation is faster in neonates than in adults (Fritsch et al. 2006). In a recent study, the endogenous thrombin potential (ETP) measured without TM was greater than the lower limit of the adult reference interval in 30% of 109 full-term and 49% of 55 preterm neonates, a finding consistent with the reduced levels of procoagulants in this setting. When the test was modified adding TM, ETP reverted into the adult reference interval in 97% and 100% full-term and preterm neonates (Tripodi et al. 2008); besides, the inhibition of thrombin was found impaired in plasma from sick neonates of GA 30–38 weeks compared with plasma from healthy neonates of GA 30–38 weeks (Shah et al. 1992).

92.3.1.6 Relevance for Laboratory Investigation of Coagulation in Newborns

Given the significant differences between the plasma factor concentrations in different age groups, a detailed knowledge on the development of hemostasis is critical for the neonatologist/intensives in order to adapt pharmacological approaches and interpret results from laboratory tests in the neonate with TE (Monagle et al. 2006). Recently, in the first large-scale study since, Andrew et al. (1987, 1988, 1990, determining the age-associated numerical changes in coagulation proteins, results clearly demonstrated that the absolute values of reference ranges for coagulation assays in neonates and children vary with analyzer and reagent systems. In this study, the authors also present for the first time age-related ranges for tissue factor (TF) pathway inhibitor (TFPI), D-dimer, and ETP (Monagle et al. 2006).

Thus, coagulation laboratories should develop age-related reference ranges specific to their own testing systems. Without this, accurate diagnosis and management of neonates and children with suspected bleeding or clotting disorders is not possible.

Additional risk factors, e.g., congenital thrombophilia or critical illness, have to be considered separately from the immaturity of neonatal hemostasis.

92.4 Additional Risk Factors for Neonatal Thromboembolism

92.4.1 Maternal Thrombophilia and Gestational Risk Factors

Few data are currently available regarding the influence of maternal thrombophilia (prothrombotic polymorphisms, dyslipidemia, antiphospholipid antibodies) and prenatal gestational risks (gestational diabetes, pregnancy-induced hypertension–preeclampsia, intrauterine growth restriction) on thrombotic risk in the fetus and neonate.

During gestation, the maternal and fetal circulation systems coexist and interact with the placenta. Association between thrombosis and infarction in the placenta and peri- and neonatal infarction, the most commonly presumed mechanism being embolization to the fetus, has been reported in literature (Adams-Chapman et al. 2002; Burke and Tannenberg 1995; Redline et al. 1998).

Pregnancy itself is a prothrombotic state as a shift toward prothrombotic reactions is seen in women as gestation progresses through the second and third trimesters and just after gestation (increased levels of vitamin-K-dependent FII, FVII, and FX; increased levels of TAT; increased endothelial activation with elevated levels of circulating VWF, FVIII, and soluble TM; increased triglyceride and Lp(a) levels; reduced levels of free and total PS; and reduced activated PC sensitivity ratio) (Clark 2003). However, maternal thrombosis during and just after pregnancy often occurs in the presence of additional risk factors (i.e., advanced maternal age, cesarean section, hypertension, gestational diabetes, infections, preeclampsia/eclampsia, antiphospholipid syndrome, and inherited thrombophilia). Some of these maternal factors may also predispose to placental infarction with subsequent cerebral infarction in the fetus.

Preeclampsia may lead to endothelial activation of coagulation. Gestational diabetes leads to maternal vascular damage which can predispose

to placental thrombosis and infarction. In case of chorioamnionitis, inflamed vessels of the placenta lead to localized thrombosis, vasospasm, and infarction, and maternal sepsis during gestation may lead to disseminated intravascular coagulation (DIC) resulting in placental thrombosis and infarction, too. Maternal smoking may lead to vasospasm and/or endothelial activation with resulting placental injury and growth retardation, and maternal cocaine use may predispose to vasoconstriction with resulting placental infarction. Moreover, thrombocytosis has been observed in neonates of mothers with history of polydrug use. At the time of delivery, placental–fetal transfusion may lead to polycythemia (Golomb 2003). Antiphospholipid syndrome (APLS) in pregnancy is characterized by the presence of autoantibodies in association with recurrent fetal loss and severe complications such as preeclampsia, fetal growth retardation, or placental insufficiency (Heilmann et al. 2003).

In a review of the literature till 2007 about infants born to mothers with antiphospholipid antibodies (APL), 16 infants with perinatal thrombosis were reported. Thromboses were arterial (13/16), mostly strokes (8/16). Hydrops fetalis with left renal vein thrombosis was associated to a lupus anticoagulant (LA) present only in the child. Additional risk factors to APL, either prenatal (preeclampsia and/or intrauterine growth retardation) or perinatal (asphyxia, sepsis, arterial or venous catheter, and congenital thrombophilia), were present (one to four of them) in nine out of the 14 evaluable babies. APL were the only risk factor found in five full-term babies who suffered from stroke in four cases and from renal thrombosis in another. Eleven of these infants with APL in their serum presented a neonatal APS with the same antibody (LA or aCL IgG) found in neonates and their mothers, while the other infants had thrombosis with APL only in their mother's blood.

92.4.1.1 Environmental and Iatrogenic Modifications

Endothelial, coagulation, and fibrinolytic systems are activated in newborns; it might occur during birth due to the mechanical stress, the adaptation of circulation, and the short-term hypoxic state (Knofler et al. 1998).

Generation and inhibition of thrombin was compared with healthy neonates. Fifty neonates with respiratory failure requiring mechanical ventilation and 40 healthy neonates were studied on the first day of life. Eight plasma pools from 40 healthy neonates of GA 30–38 weeks were compared with six plasma pools from 30 sick neonates of GA 30–38 weeks. Additional four plasma pools prepared from 20 sick neonates of GA less than 30 weeks were studied. Thrombin generation was similar for both healthy and sick neonates of GA 30–38 weeks. However, the inhibition of thrombin was impaired in plasma from sick neonates of GA 30–38 weeks compared with plasma from healthy neonates of GA 30–38 weeks (4.37 ± 0.22 versus 5.21 ± 0.21 nmol; p less than 0.05) (Shah et al. 1992).

A combined hemostatic defect consisting of a reduction in certain procoagulants, anticoagulants (AT, PC), and components of the fibrinolytic system (PLG) was demonstrated in very-low-birth-weight infants (VLBW <1,500 g) with gestational age 26–32 weeks. Sixteen of them were healthy; 28 were suffering from RDS and 24 from septicemia. The hemostatic defect was more profound in the RDS group; nevertheless, increased TAT and/or PAP values were a more frequent finding in the septicemic group of infants (91.8 vs. 17.9%). Increased D-dimers were demonstrated in 34.8% and 28.6% of the infants, respectively (Aronis et al. 1998).

The modality of delivery (spontaneous vaginal delivery vs. elective cesarean section) has been demonstrated to be able to modify the levels of PS, PC, and AT; plasma collected from the cord blood of 41 consecutive healthy newborns, 18 delivered vaginally (mean gestational age 39.7 ± 0.8) and 23 by elective cesarean section (mean gestational age 38.5 ± 0.7), were tested for AT activity, PC antigen and activity, total and free PS antigen, F1 concentration, and PLG activity. Among factors studied in the cord blood of infants born after vaginal delivery, PC antigen levels and AT activity were statistically higher (41.3 ± 9.4 vs. 33.9 ± 7.2 and 58.5 ± 10.0 vs. 48.4 ± 12.7, respectively; $P < .01$), while free PS was significantly lower (36.8 ± 11.6 vs. 46.4 ± 12.5; $P < .05$) than in newborns delivered by cesarean

section. Cord blood PLG and F1 were elevated in vaginally delivered neonates in comparison to those delivered by cesarean section, but the difference was not statistically significant (Franzoi et al. 2002). In a small group of newborns with CVL, increased platelet activation and VWF binding to platelets have been significantly recorded (Schmugge et al. 2007).

92.5 Neonatal Non-CNS Thrombotic Events

92.5.1 Epidemiology and Thrombus Location

Neonatal symptomatic thrombosis (excluding stroke) is reported to occur in 2.4/1,000 admissions to neonatal intensive care units according to an international registry from Canada, the USA, and Europe; 64 among 97 (66%) registered events are venous thrombosis (Schmidt and Andrew 1995). In a German prospective nationwide 2-year registry, the incidence of clinically apparent neonatal TEs (including cerebral events) is 5.1/100,000 live births; 76% are venous events (Nowak-Gottl et al. 1997a).

Both arterial and venous non-CNS thrombosis in the newborn may be located in several anatomic sites (i.e., venous events: deep vein thrombosis of the limbs, intrathoracic vessels, pulmonary embolism, renal veins, hepatic veins, superior and inferior caval veins, portal vein, right intracardiac thrombosis, mesenteric veins, and retinal vein; arterial events: aorta, left intracardiac thrombosis, renal artery, mesenteric artery, and limb artery).

92.5.1.1 Venous Systemic Thrombosis

Neonatal renal vein thrombosis (RVT) is the most common non-catheter-related thrombosis in infancy. It has been reported to occur in 0.5/1,000 admissions in neonatal intensive care units; according to the German registry, the incidence is of 2.2/100,000 live births (Bokenkamp et al. 2000). It usually presents within 3 days after birth in neonates born at term; in 7% of neonates, it presents in the uterus and a male predominance has been reported (Kuhle et al. 2004; Lau et al. 2007).

Central venous line (CVL)-related venous thromboses (VT) are commonly associated with indwelling central venous catheters. Compared to adults, newborns present a higher incidence of thrombosis of the superior limbs due to the strong association with CVL placement in the upper venous system (Ross et al. 1989).

Portal vein thrombosis (PVT) is described in the neonate secondary to umbilical venous catheter insertion. A retrospective analysis reported 133 infants (all but five of whom were neonates) with portal vein thrombosis, with an incidence of 3.6/1,000 admissions; an umbilical vein catheter had been inserted in 73% of the infants and was in an inappropriate position in half of them (Morag et al. 2006).

The frequency of pulmonary embolism (PE) during the newborn period is unknown but likely underestimated because the clinical features are often subtle or masked by the presence of underlying lung disease. In a retrospective autopsy series, an incidence of 14% has been reported (Sanerkin et al. 1966).

92.5.1.2 Arterial Systemic Thrombosis

Arterial thromboses (ArT) represent almost 50% of all neonatal TEs and are mainly iatrogenic complications, associated with catheterization of the femoral artery as well as peripheral arteries and the umbilical artery.

The reported incidence of umbilical artery catheter-related TE is considerably influenced by the diagnostic test chosen. Studies considering only symptomatic TEs report an incidence of 1–3%, while studies using ultrasound and angiography report an incidence of 14–35% and 64%, respectively. In autopsy series an incidence of 9–28% has been reported (Andrew 2000). Spontaneous, non-catheter-related ArT are uncommon in the newborn period and most frequently involve the aorta. Mortality rate has been reported in around 33% (Monagle et al. 2000).

92.5.1.3 Intracardiac Thrombosis

Venous intracardiac thrombosis involving the right atrium frequently occurs in newborns with central venous lines (CVL), but no incidence data are reported in literature. Thrombosis involving the

right ventriculum is uncommon. Left intracardiac thrombi (atrium and ventriculum) are rare events usually occurring in children with underlying risk factors as congenital heart disease, cardiovascular surgery, or arrhythmia (Berman et al. 1991; John et al. 2007; Marsh et al. 1988).

92.5.1.4 Specific Additional Risk Factors for Systemic Thrombosis

Inherited Thrombophilia

At present, the role of thrombophilic conditions in both arterial and venous systemic thrombotic events in the neonate remains poorly defined; on the other hand, the presence of an indwelling line is clearly identified as the most important risk factor.

Manco-Johnson et al. did not find any association between thrombophilia and catheter-related events in newborns (Manco-Johnson et al. 1999) in contrast with previously published data by Nowak-Gottl et al. who detected a high incidence of inherited prothrombotic factors in a cohort of infants and children, ranging from neonates to 18 years, with catheter-related events (Nowak-Gottl et al. 1997c).

A german group of researchers reported lipoprotein(a) as a risk factor for thrombosis in neonates and children (Nowak-Gottl et al. (1997b, 1999) but that finding was not confirmed in other cohorts. In the registry from the Netherlands, a higher incidence of thrombophilia in older children (21%, 95% CI 8–34%) than in neonates (6%, 95% CI 0–16%) was detected (van Ommen et al. 2001), while in the study by Revel-Vilk et al., the overall frequency of inherited prothrombotic proteins was similar in newborns and older children (13%) (Revel-Vilk et al. 2003).

Kosch et al. investigated the prevalence of prothrombotic risk factors in renal vein thrombosis: the study evidenced a significant association between genetic risks, especially FVL and Lp (a) (Kosch et al. 2004).

Registry data and case studies have demonstrated that the majority of symptomatic neonatal TEs, especially spontaneous events (i.e., not catheter related), are associated with multiple hemostatic prothrombotic defects or with the combination of prothrombotic defects and environmental or clinical conditions. As a result, the Subcommittee on Perinatal and Pediatric Haemostasis of the International Society on Thrombosis and Haemostasis has recommended that pediatric patients with thrombosis (regardless of risk factors) should be tested for a full panel of genetic prothrombotic traits (Manco-Johnson et al. 2002).

92.5.2 Acquired Risk Factors

The presence of an indwelling line has been identified as the most important acquired risk factor for the development of both arterial and venous systemic events, spontaneous non-catheter-related events being relatively uncommon. Neonates in the neonatal intensive care unit may have umbilical artery (UAC) and vein (UVC) catheters as well as additional intravenous lines. These can cause damage of the endothelium wall and activation of the coagulation cascade. In a large prospective study, 148 neonates with both umbilical arterial and venous catheters were serially screened for thrombosis in the abdominal aorta and inferior vena cava by 2-D ultrasonography. Abdominal aortic thrombi were detected in 32.3% of infants with UAC and small thrombi were detected in the inferior vena cava of 4.1% of infants with UVC. The only significant risk factors associated with abdominal aortic thrombosis were the presence of UAC compared with UVC and longer duration of UAC in situ (Boo et al. 1999). Excluding renal vein thrombosis, catheter-related events accounted for 89% and 94% of TEs in the Canadian and Netherland registries, respectively (Schmidt and Andrew 1995; van Ommen et al. 2001).

Central line placement is a recognized risk factor also for thrombosis involving the right atrium. Other identified risks for intracardiac events are congenital heart diseases (i.e., aortic coarctation), cardiac surgery, and ECMO (John et al. 2007; Marsh et al. 1988; Cohen et al. 1995).

Perinatal asphyxia, prematurity, dehydration, and maternal diabetes are established risk factors for renal vein thrombosis. However, in a recent

review by Lau et al. (2007) pertaining to all the available literature about venal rein thrombosis, among 271 patients (less than one-third) had a history of perinatal asphyxia, and dehydration and maternal diabetes were even less common. One-third (28%) of patients were before 36 weeks of gestation.

Numerous clinical and environmental conditions such as the use of central lines, cardiac diseases and polycythemia, renal diseases such as congenital nephrotic syndrome and neonatal hemolytic uremic syndrome, peripartum asphyxia, infants of diabetic mothers, dehydration, septicemia, necrotizing enterocolitis, acute respiratory distress syndrome, and extracorporeal membrane oxygenation lead to elevated thrombin generation and subsequent thrombus formation (Nowak-Gottl et al. 2003).

92.5.3 Clinical Investigation

The clinical picture of vascular incidents in neonates is extremely variable and largely dependent on the location and the size of the thrombus or embolus. Presentation may vary from discrete symptoms or asymptomatic events to life- or limb-threatening acute events; as several right-to-left (i.e., venoarterial) shunts remain patent for a considerable time in the neonate, a paradoxical embolus cannot be ruled out even in the absence of congenital heart disease.

92.5.3.1 Arterial Thrombosis

Arterial vascular events are almost always directly related to arterial vascular catheterization of central or peripheral arteries. This underscores the need for meticulous clinical observation in children with arterial access in place. Obvious signs include ischemia of limbs or trunk, pale or cold extremities distal to the catheterization site, weak or absent palpability of the pulse (pulse oximeters will also show this), and decreased or immeasurable blood pressure. Signs of necrotizing enterocolitis such as feed intolerance, bilious gastric aspirates, blood-stained stools, and bowel wall pneumatosis in an infant with an umbilical arterial catheter should raise the suspicion of mesenteric infarction. Diagnostic work-up for renal failure in children with UAC should include a Doppler flow study of the renal arteries to avoid missing out on the diagnosis of renal artery thrombosis. Elevated blood pressure might also hint at decreased renal perfusion.

There are some reports of aortic thrombosis in the neonate mimicking coarctation of the aorta with significant blood pressure differences in upper and lower body blood pressure readings; thus, the investigation of upper and lower body blood pressure measurements should be performed in any infant with hypertension diagnosed by measurements obtained from the upper body (Kenny and Tsai-Goodman 2007).

92.5.3.2 Venous Thrombosis

Limb swelling, pain, and cyanotic or hyperemic color should raise the suspicion of venous thrombosis.

Renal Vein Thrombosis

RVT may present with an abdominal mass and hematuria or proteinuria; hence, these symptoms should ring a bell especially in neonates with risk factors such as prematurity, asphyxia, critical illness, femoral CVL, and male sex (Kuhle et al. 2004) (Bokenkamp et al. 2000).

Portal Vein Thrombosis

Signs of impaired liver function, hepatomegaly, and splenomegaly should raise the suspicion of PVT; however, only about 10% of children with PVT develop acute clinical symptoms (Morag et al. 2006). Thrombosis of the inferior vena cava can present with signs resembling obstruction of the renal vein (hematuria, retroperitoneal mass); however, these will occur bilaterally when the inferior vena cava is affected. In addition, the lower limbs may be edematous and, if blood flow is substantially impaired, the child may be in respiratory distress and may have high blood pressure.

Pulmonary Embolism

PE is a rare event in the neonatal period. Clinical signs of massive ventilation/perfusion mismatch, difficult oxygenation, and signs of right heart

failure should raise the suspicion of PE, especially in babies with congenital heart disease. In the few cases reported in the literature, diagnosis of PE was confirmed by lung perfusion scans or angiography (Moreno-Cabral and Breitweser 1983; Gamillscheg et al. 1997; Feldman et al. 2005).

92.6 Neonatal Central Nervous System Thrombotic Events

92.6.1 Epidemiology and Thrombus Location

92.6.1.1 Neonatal Arterial Ischemic Stroke

Ischemic perinatal stroke (IPS) has been recently redefined as "a group of heterogeneous conditions in which there is focal disruption of cerebral blood flow secondary to arterial or cerebral venous thrombosis or embolization, between 20 weeks of fetal life through the 28th postnatal day, confirmed by neuroimaging or neuropathology studies"; moreover, three subcategories based on gestational age (fetal ischemic stroke) or postnatal age (neonatal ischemic stroke and presumed perinatal ischemic stroke) at diagnosis, have been further suggested (Raju et al. 2007).

IPS is surely underdiagnosed in newborns and often diagnosed in retrospect following delayed presentation at a few months of age. The Canadian Pediatric Ischemic Stroke Registry reports an incidence of 93/100,000 live births, only 25% occurring in children born at term (de Veber and the Canadian Pediatric Ischemic Stroke Study Group 2000). In other studies, incidence has been estimated at between 24–35/10,000 live births and 1/3,000–1/4000 live births (Chalmers 2005; Estan and Hope 1997).

The typical distribution is the middle cerebral artery, more commonly left than right, and small artery involvement can occur, too.

92.6.1.2 Cerebral Sinovenous Thrombosis

Similar to arterial ischemic stroke, the incidence of CSVT is underestimated in newborns. In the Canadian Paediatric Ischemic Stroke Registry, neonates accounted for 45% of registered CSVT, with an incidence of 41/100,000 live births per year. Premature and term neonates are affected with a slight prevalence of males. Among term neonates with intraventricular hemorrhage (IVH), underlying CSVT is documented in 31% and is more likely when thalamic hemorrhage is present (Monagle et al. 2000). The most susceptible vascular structures are superior sagittal sinus and lateral sinuses (DeVeber et al. 2001).

92.6.1.3 Specific Additional Risk Factors for Cerebral Thrombosis

Inherited Thrombophilia

Although there has been considerable interest in the potential role of thrombophilia in the etiology of childhood ischemic stroke, there are very few studies focused specifically on newborns. Kurnik et al. (2003) reported the largest cohorts in literature of children who presented with symptomatic arterial ischemic stroke during the neonatal period: an inherited prothrombotic state was detected in 59% neonates. Gunther et al. (2000) in behalf of the German childhood stroke study group investigated the prevalence of high levels of Lp(a), FVL mutation, PRTG20210A variant, MTHFR T677T genotype, deficiency of natural anticoagulants, and anticardiolipin antibodies (ACA) in 91 neonatal stroke patients and 182 age- and sex-matched healthy controls finding that 62/91 stroke patients (68.1%) had at least one prothrombotic risk factor compared with 44 control subjects (24.2%) (odds ratio 6.70).

In a cohort study from the UK, among 24 infants with perinatal cerebral infarction confirmed by neonatal MRI, ten (42%) had at least one prothrombotic risk factor (Mercuri et al. 2001). The presence of prothrombotic risk factors and, in particular, of FVL was significantly associated with poor outcome after perinatal cerebral infarction. Golomb et al. (2001) on behalf of the Canadian childhood stroke study detected prothrombotic abnormalities in 14/22 (64%) perinatal arterial ischemic stroke, the most common abnormality being the presence of ACA; in this series, most of prothrombotic defects were transient.

Little data from large studies are available on the incidence of prothrombotic abnormalities in neonatal CSVT. There are no published case–control studies. In the Canadian registry, prothrombotic disorders were identified in 20% of patients with neonatal CSVT (DeVeber et al. 2001).

Curry and coworkers investigated the prevalence of prothrombotic risk factors in 60 mother–child pairs with perinatal arterial stroke; the study supported the multifactorial etiology of perinatal arterial stroke and emphasized the role of maternal as well as infant thrombophilia. Prothrombotic risk factors were found in 28 of 51 mothers (55%) and 30 of 60 children (50%). Forty-one pairs (68%) had at least one abnormality in the mother, child, or both (Curry et al. 2007).

92.6.2 Acquired Risk Factors

The real incidence of acquired risk factors in perinatal ischemic stroke is poorly understood as most studies lack an appropriate control group. Only two case–control studies have been published so far. In the study from Wu (Wu et al. 2004), prepartum risk factors significantly associated with arterial ischemic stroke in neonates born at ≥36 weeks' gestation were preeclampsia (OR: 3.6; 95% CI: 1.1–11.4) and intrauterine growth restriction (OR: 5.3; 95% CI: 1.5–18.6). Newborns with stroke were also at higher risk of delivery complications, such as emergency cesarean section (OR: 6.8; 95% CI: 2.7–16.6), 5-min Apgar <7 (OR: 23.6; 95% CI: 4.1–237), and resuscitation at birth (OR: 4.5; 95% CI: 1.6–12.3). Estan (Estan and Hope 1997) reported that cases (12 neonates with unilateral infarction born at 32 weeks and above) were more likely than controls to require assisted ventilation for resuscitation at birth (OR 7.0, 95% CI 1.04–53.5), but Apgar scores at 5 min were no different. In 2004, a small study demonstrated a significant reduction in physiological anticoagulants in hypoxic neonates (El et al. 2004).

There is only one hospital-based case–control study investigating prenatal and perinatal risk factors in preterm infants (27–36 weeks) with ischemic stroke.

Twin-to-twin transfusion syndrome, fetal heart rate abnormality, and hypoglycemia have been reported as independent risk factors for stroke beside no identified maternal risk factor. Involvement of the different branches of the middle cerebral artery changed with increasing gestational age (Benders et al. 2007).

Prenatal gestational risks (infections, diabetes, hypertension), peripartum complications, asphyxia, dehydration, sepsis, infections, and heart disease have all been reported as single or associated risks for cerebral sinovenous thrombosis. However, a higher incidence of idiopathic events than in older children was reported (DeVeber et al. 2001; Fitzgerald et al. 2006).

92.6.2.1 Clinical Investigation

In contrast to the clinical picture in adults, neonatal stroke does not usually present with hemiplegia. The leading clinical symptoms in central nervous system TE in neonates are seizures and lethargy. The diagnosis of ischemic stroke as well as of sinus vein thrombosis can initially be confirmed by cerebral ultrasound through the open fontanel followed by cranial magnetic resonance imaging (MRI) (Saracco et al. 2009).

92.7 Laboratory Investigation in Newborns with Thrombosis

Initial laboratory work-up in a neonate in whom thrombosis is suspected should include a full blood count as well as a coagulation screening with determination of prothrombin time, thrombin time, and activated partial thromboplastin time.

D-dimers: D-dimers, which are elevated as an acute phase reaction in all patients with infection or systemic inflammatory response syndrome, are a positive finding in almost all critically ill neonates. Conversely, negative D-dimers might be relatively accurate in ruling out thrombosis in most patients, including neonates. Nevertheless, this needs confirmation in large clinical trials.

Platelets: In almost all neonates, platelet number decreases after birth. However, a sudden and severe drop in platelet counts should alert the intensivist. Although the differential diagnosis

for thrombocytopenia in the neonate is broad, including auto- and alloantibodies as well as effects of medications and consumption, thrombocytopenia remains one of the most sensitive indicators for micro- (in the setting of sepsis) or macro-circulatory thrombosis.

Thrombophilia testing: Current evidence does not resolve the issue of thrombophilia testing, but a stepwise thrombophilia investigation in any neonate with a significant TE event is reasonable. A limitation to this approach is the amount of blood required. This is especially important in the premature or anemic infant for whom excessive blood loss is not tolerable. Therefore, the evaluation should always take place at an experienced tertiary care center that has either a reference laboratory or a reliable referral center. The physiological reduction of some coagulation factors and anticoagulant proteins may lead to a difficult interpretation of laboratory investigations and therefore deficiencies need to be confirmed by repeat testing later in infancy (i.e., beyond 6 months or afterward in premature infants) (Williams et al. 2002). As screening all newborns with TEs for a wide range of prothrombotic disorders may be prohibitively expensive, targeted screening may be more effective.

In case of a clinically significant spontaneous TE or ischemic skin lesions, it is mandatory to look for homozygous deficiency of PC and PS, as a specific treatment option for PC defect is available. In remaining cases a stepwise approach starting with most common risk factors may be reasonable. Testing of natural anticoagulants for detecting a heterozygous defect should be performed after 6 months of age. The protein-based assays are affected by the TE event and must be repeated at 3–6 months of life before a definitive diagnosis can be made. If anticoagulation is being administered, then the protein-based assays should be obtained 14–30 days after discontinuing the anticoagulant. DNA-based assays are neither influenced by the acute thrombotic event nor by the treatment; Lp(a) concentrations tend to increase during the first year of life and should be repeated at 8–12 months if the original values are low, especially in white individuals.

In case of a positive result for genetic thrombophilia in the newborn, testing of both parents (FVL and PRT G20210A mutations, Lp(a), natural anticoagulants) may be offered; in case of negative screening, testing of the mother has been suggested for the newborn with perinatal stroke (Roach et al. 2008). All these tests should be performed in the non-acute setting as they are not useful to support management decisions but only for counseling about possible risks of parents themselves and of other or future children. However, in those countries where the health system is mainly managed by insurance companies, family members should be carefully informed about the possible consequences of this screening (i.e., potential insurance issues) without potential specific benefit to the individual being screened.

92.7.1 Thrombophilia Testing

Initial laboratory testing
Antiphospholipid antibody panel
Anticardiolipin antibodies and lupus
Anticoagulant (IgG, IgM)
Fibrinogen protein C activity and protein S activity
Antithrombin activity assay
Factor V Leiden prothrombin G20210A
Homocysteine lipoprotein(a)
Additional laboratory testing
Factor VIII activity and factor IX activity
Factor XI activity
Plasminogen activity
Heparin cofactor II activity

References

Adams-Chapman I, Vaucher YE, Bejar RF et al (2002) Maternal floor infarction of the placenta: association with central nervous system injury and adverse neurodevelopmental outcome. J Perinatol 22 (3):236–241, Ref Type: Pamphlet

Albisetti M (2003) The fibrinolytic system in children. Semin Thromb Hemost 29:339–348

Andrew M (1995) Developmental hemostasis: relevance to hemostatic problems during childhood. Semin Thromb Hemost 21:341–356

Andrew M (2000) Arterial thromboembolic complication in pediatric patients. In: Andrew M, Monagle PT, Brooker LA (eds) Thromboembolic complications during infancy and childhood. B.C. Decker, Hamilton, pp 165–199

Andrew M, Paes B, Milner R et al (1987) Development of the human coagulation system in the full-term infant. Blood 70:165–172

Andrew M, Paes B, Milner R et al (1988) Development of the human coagulation system in the healthy premature infant. Blood 72:1651–1657

Andrew M, Paes B, Johnston M (1990) Development of the hemostatic system in the neonate and young infant. Am J Pediatr Hematol Oncol 12:95–104

Andrew M, David M, Adams M et al (1994) Venous thromboembolic complications (VTE) in children: first analyses of the Canadian Registry of VTE. Blood 83:1251–1257

Andrew M, Monagle PT, Brooker LA (2000) Developmental hemostasis: relevance to thromboembolic complications in pediatric patients. In: Andrew M, Monagle PT, Brooker LA (eds) Thromboembolic complications during infancy and childhood. B.C. Decker, Hamilton/Lewiston

Aronis S, Platokouki H, Photopoulos S et al (1998) Indications of coagulation and/or fibrinolytic system activation in healthy and sick very-low-birth-weight neonates. Biol Neonate 74:337–344

Benavent A, Estelles A, Aznar J et al (1984) Dysfunctional plasminogen in full term newborn – study of active site of plasmin. Thromb Haemost 51:67–70

Benders MJ, Groenendaal F, Uiterwaal CS et al (2007) Maternal and infant characteristics associated with perinatal arterial stroke in the preterm infant. Stroke 38:1759–1765

Berman W Jr, Fripp RR, Yabek SM et al (1991) Great vein and right atrial thrombosis in critically ill infants and children with central venous lines. Chest 99: 963–967

Bokenkamp A, von KR, Nowak-Gottl U et al (2000) Neonatal renal venous thrombosis in Germany between 1992 and 1994: epidemiology, treatment and outcome. Eur J Pediatr 159:44–48

Boo NY, Wong NC, Zulkifli SS, Lye MS (1999) Risk factors associated with umbilical vascular catheter-associated thrombosis in newborn infants. J Paediatr Child Health 35:460–465

Burke CJ, Tannenberg AE (1995) Prenatal brain damage and placental infarction – an autopsy study. Dev Med Child Neurol 37:555–562

Chalmers EA (2005) Perinatal stroke – risk factors and management. Br J Haematol 130:333–343

Chalmers EA (2006) Epidemiology of venous thromboembolism in neonates and children. Thromb Res 118:3–12

Clark P (2003) Changes of hemostasis variables during pregnancy. Semin Vasc Med 3:13–24

Cohen RS, Ramachandran P, Kim EH, Glasscock GF (1995) Retrospective analysis of risks associated with an umbilical artery catheter system for continuous monitoring of arterial oxygen tension. J Perinatol 15:195–198

Curry CJ, Bhullar S, Holmes J et al (2007) Risk factors for perinatal arterial stroke: a study of 60 mother-child pairs. Pediatr Neurol 37:99–107

Cvirn G, Gallistl S, Leschnik B, Muntean W (2003) Low tissue factor pathway inhibitor (TFPI) together with low antithrombin allows sufficient thrombin generation in neonates. J Thromb Haemost 1:263–268

de Veber GA, the Canadian Pediatric Ischemic Stroke Study Group (2000) Canadian pediatric ischemic registry: analysis of children with arterial ischemic stroke. (abstract). Ann Neurol 48:514

DeVeber G, Andrew M, Adams C et al (2001) Cerebral sinovenous thrombosis in children. NEngl J Med 345:417–423

El BA, Hussein HA, bou-Elew HH, bdel Kader MS (2004) Study of protein C, protein S, and antithrombin III in hypoxic newborns. Pediatr Crit Care Med 5:163–166

Estan J, Hope P (1997) Unilateral neonatal cerebral infarction in full term infants. Arch Dis Child Fetal Neonatal Ed 76:F88–F93

Feldman JP, Feinstein JA, Lamberti JJ, Perry SB (2005) Angiojet catheter-based thrombectomy in a neonate with postoperative pulmonary embolism. Catheter Cardiovasc Interv 66:442–445

Fitzgerald KC, Williams LS, Garg BP et al (2006) Cerebral sinovenous thrombosis in the neonate. Arch Neurol 63:405–409

Franzoi M, Simioni P, Luni S et al (2002) Effect of delivery modalities on the physiologic inhibition system of coagulation of the neonate. Thromb Res 105:15–18

Fritsch P, Cvirn G, Cimenti C et al (2006) Thrombin generation in factor VIII-depleted neonatal plasma: nearly normal because of physiologically low antithrombin and tissue factor pathway inhibitor. J Thromb Haemost 4:1071–1077

Fukui H, Takase T, Ikari H et al (1979) Factor VIII procoagulant activity, factor VIII related antigen and von Willebrand factor in newborn cord blood. Br J Haematol 42:637–646

Gamillscheg A, Nurnberg JH, exi-Meskishvili V et al (1997) Surgical emergency embolectomy for the treatment of fulminant pulmonary embolism in a preterm infant. J Pediatr Surg 32:1516–1518

Golomb MR (2003) The contribution of prothrombotic disorders to peri- and neonatal ischemic stroke. Semin Thromb Hemost 29:415–424

Golomb MR, MacGregor DL, Domi T et al (2001) Presumed pre- or perinatal arterial ischemic stroke: risk factors and outcomes. Ann Neurol 50:163–168

Gunther G, Junker R, Strater R et al (2000) Symptomatic ischemic stroke in full-term neonates : role of acquired and genetic prothrombotic risk factors. Stroke 31: 2437–2441

Heilmann L, von Tempelhoff GF, Pollow K (2003) Antiphospholipid syndrome in obstetrics. Clin Appl Thromb Hemost 9:143–150

Hellstrom-Westas L, Ley D, Berg AC et al (2005) VWF-cleaving protease (ADAMTS13) in premature infants. Acta Paediatr 94:205–210

Israels SJ, Daniels M, McMillan EM (1990) Deficient collagen-induced activation in the newborn platelet. Pediatr Res 27:337–343

John JB, Cron SG, Kung GC, Mott AR (2007) Intracardiac thrombi in pediatric patients: presentation profiles and clinical outcomes. Pediatr Cardiol 28:213–220

Kavakli K, Canciani MT, Mannucci PM (2002) Plasma levels of the von Willebrand factor-cleaving protease in physiological and pathological conditions in children. Pediatr Hematol Oncol 19:467–473

Kenny D, Tsai-Goodman B (2007) Neonatal arterial thrombus mimicking congenital heart disease. Arch Dis Child Fetal Neonatal Ed 92:F59–F61

Knofler R, Hofmann S, Weissbach G et al (1998) Molecular markers of the endothelium, the coagulation and the fibrinolytic systems in healthy newborns. Semin Thromb Hemost 24:453–461

Kosch A, Kuwertz-Broking E, Heller C et al (2004) Renal venous thrombosis in neonates: prothrombotic risk factors and long-term follow-up. Blood 104:1356–1360

Kuhle S, Massicotte P, Chan A, Mitchell L (2004) A case series of 72 neonates with renal vein thrombosis. Data from the 1-800-NO-CLOTS Registry. Thromb Haemost 92:729–733

Kurnik K, Kosch A, Strater R et al (2003) Recurrent thromboembolism in infants and children suffering from symptomatic neonatal arterial stroke: a prospective follow-up study. Stroke 34:2887–2892

Lau KK, Stoffman JM, Williams S et al (2007) Neonatal renal vein thrombosis: review of the English-language literature between 1992 and 2006. Pediatrics 120: e1278–e1284

Manco-Johnson MJ (2005) Development of hemostasis in the fetus. Thromb Res 115(Suppl 1):55–63

Manco-Johnson MJ, Sifontes M, Nuss R (1999) Coagulation abnormalities in neonatal catheter related thrombosis. (Abstract). Thromb Haemost 82(suppl):384

Manco-Johnson MJ, Grabowski EF, Hellgreen M et al (2002) Laboratory testing for thrombophilia in pediatric patients. On behalf of the Subcommittee for Perinatal and Pediatric Thrombosis of the Scientific and Standardization Committee of the International Society of Thrombosis and Haemostasis (ISTH). Thromb Haemost 88:155–156

Marsh D, Wilkerson SA, Cook LN, Pietsch JB (1988) Right atrial thrombus formation screening using two dimensional echocardiograms in neonates with central venous catheters. Pediatrics 81:284–286

Mercuri E, Cowan F, Gupte G et al (2001) Prothrombotic disorders and abnormal neurodevelopmental outcome in infants with neonatal cerebral infarction. Pediatrics 107:1400–1404

Michelson AD (1998) Platelet function in the newborn. Semin Thromb Hemost 24:507–512

Monagle P, Adams M, Mahoney M et al (2000) Outcome of pediatric thromboembolic disease: a report from the Canadian Childhood Thrombophilia Registry. Pediatr Res 47:763–766

Monagle P, Barnes C, Ignjatovic V et al (2006) Developmental haemostasis. Impact for clinical haemostasis laboratories. Thromb Haemost 95:362–372

Morag I, Epelman M, Daneman A et al (2006) Portal vein thrombosis in the neonate: risk factors, course, and outcome. J Pediatr 148:735–739

Moreno-Cabral RJ, Breitweser JA (1983) Pulmonary embolectomy in the neonate. Chest 84:502–504

Muntean W, Leschnik B, Baier K et al (2004) In vivo thrombin generation in neonates. J Thromb Haemost 2:2071–2072

Nowak-Gottl U, von KR, Gobel U (1997a) Neonatal symptomatic thromboembolism in Germany: two year survey. Arch Dis Child Fetal Neonatal Ed 76:F163–F167

Nowak-Gottl U, Debus O, Findeisen M et al (1997b) Lipoprotein (a): its role in childhood thromboembolism. Pediatrics 99:E11

Nowak-Gottl U, Dubbers A, Kececioglu D et al (1997c) Factor V Leiden, protein C, and lipoprotein (a) in catheter-related thrombosis in childhood: a prospective study. J Pediatr 131:608–612

Nowak-Gottl U, Junker R, Hartmeier M et al (1999) Increased lipoprotein(a) is an important risk factor for venous thromboembolism in childhood. Circulation 100:743–748

Nowak-Gottl U, Kosch A, Schlegel N (2003) Neonatal thromboembolism. Semin Thromb Hemost 29:227–234

Perutelli P, Molinari AC (2007) von Willebrand factor, von Willebrand factor-cleaving protease, and shear stress. Cardiovasc Hematol Agents Med Chem 5:305–310

Raju TN, Nelson KB, Ferriero D, Lynch JK (2007) Ischemic perinatal stroke: summary of a workshop sponsored by the National Institute of Child Health and Human Development and the National Institute of Neurological Disorders and Stroke. Pediatrics 120:609–616

Redline RW, Wilson-Costello D, Borawski E et al (1998) Placental lesions associated with neurologic impairment and cerebral palsy in very low-birth-weight infants. Arch Pathol Lab Med 122:1091–1098

Revel-Vilk S, Chan A, Bauman M, Massicotte P (2003) Prothrombotic conditions in an unselected cohort of children with venous thromboembolic disease. J Thromb Haemost 1:915–921

Roach ES, Golomb MR, Adams R et al (2008) Management of stroke in infants and children: a scientific statement from a Special Writing Group of the American Heart Association Stroke Council and the Council on Cardiovascular Disease in the Young. Stroke 39:2644–2691

Ross P Jr, Ehrenkranz R, Kleinman CS, Seashore JH (1989) Thrombus associated with central venous catheters in infants and children. J Pediatr Surg 24:253–256

Sanerkin NG, Edwards P, Jacobs J (1966) Pulmonary thrombo-embolic phenomena in the newborn. J Pathol Bacteriol 91:569–574

Saracco P, Parodi E, Fabris C et al (2009) Management and investigation of neonatal thromboembolic events: genetic and acquired risk factors. Thromb Res 123: 805–809

Schmidt B, Andrew M (1995) Neonatal thrombosis: report of a prospective Canadian and international registry. Pediatrics 96:939–943

Schmugge M, Rand ML, Bang KW et al (2003) The relationship of von Willebrand factor binding to activated platelets from healthy neonates and adults. Pediatr Res 54:474–479

Schmugge M, Bang KW, Blanchette VS et al (2007) Platelet activation and von Willebrand factor binding to platelets in newborn infants with central venous lines. Acta Haematol 117:145–148

Shah JK, Mitchell LG, Paes B et al (1992) Thrombin inhibition is impaired in plasma of sick neonates. Pediatr Res 31:391–395

Stein PD, Kayali F, Olson RE (2004) Incidence of venous thromboembolism in infants and children: data from the National Hospital Discharge Survey. J Pediatr 145:563–565

Tripodi A, Ramenghi LA, Chantarangkul V et al (2008) Normal thrombin generation in neonates in spite of prolonged conventional coagulation tests. Haematologica 93(8):1256–1259

Tsai HM, Sarode R, Downes KA (2002) Ultralarge von Willebrand factor multimers and normal ADAMTS13 activity in the umbilical cord blood. Thromb Res 108:121–125

van Ommen CH, Heijboer H, Buller HR et al (2001) Venous thromboembolism in childhood: a prospective two-year registry in The Netherlands. J Pediatr 139:676–681

Williams MD, Chalmers EA, Gibson BE (2002) The investigation and management of neonatal haemostasis and thrombosis. Br J Haematol 119:295–309

Wu YW, March WM, Croen LA et al (2004) Perinatal stroke in children with motor impairment: a population-based study. Pediatrics 114:612–619

Coagulation Disorders: Clinical Aspects of Platelet Disorders

93

Antonio Del Vecchio

Contents

Abstract
Platelets contribute to primary hemostasis, and their function is affected by their number and condition. A moderately elevated platelet count in the range of 450,000–600,000/μL is not an uncommon finding in the neonatal population; even thrombocytopenia is common, especially in very sick newborns. An infant with clinical signs of thrombocytopenia but without coagulation abnormalities should prompt examination for hepatosplenomegaly, congenital anomalies, and/or signs of sepsis. Thrombocytopenia can be the result of increased platelet destruction. Common causes include systemic neonatal infection even in the absence of disseminated intravascular coagulation, a localized thrombus in the renal vein or

A. Del Vecchio (✉)
Department of Women's and Children's Health, Neonatal Intensive Care Unit, Di Venere Hospital, ASL Bari, Bari, Italy
e-mail: delveccant@libero.it

G. Buonocore et al. (eds.), *Neonatology*,
https://doi.org/10.1007/978-3-319-29489-6_240

attached to an indwelling catheter or in an ECMO circuit, and placental insufficiency and perinatal hypoxia, especially in preterm babies. In immune thrombocytopenias, autoantibodies, alloantibodies, or drug-dependent antibodies may combine with platelet membranes and produce impairment of platelet function. These mechanisms are responsible for various clinical syndromes, including neonatal alloimmune thrombocytopenia, post-transfusion purpura, and autoimmune thrombocytopenia, which occur in neonates born to mothers with idiopathic thrombocytopenic purpura, systemic lupus erythematosus, lymphoproliferative disorders, or hyperthyroidism. Most cases of decreased platelet production are the consequence of reduced megakaryocytes or impaired platelet production by megakaryocytes, such as congenital amegakaryocytic thrombocytopenia, thrombocytopenia with absent radii syndrome, and chromosomal anomalies. Qualitative disorders of platelets function can be acquired (occurring as a result of medications given to the mother or neonate, NO therapy, or ECMO) or hereditary, which do not cause problems during the neonatal period. Laboratory tests are mandatory for the diagnosis of platelet disorders. Treatment consists of platelet transfusions.

93.1 Salient Points

- The regulation of platelets production and their function significantly contribute to primary hemostasis, but hyporesponsiveness of neonatal platelets correlates with gestational age
- In addition to their classic role in hemostasis and thrombosis, platelets have a central role in inflammation and immune response. Developmental changes in platelet production and function in neonate influences their immune responses, especially in preterm infants.
- The use of Thromboelastography (TEG) provides a global measure of coagulation in neonates and correlates with gestational age. TEG parameters might be predictive of clinical bleeding in preterm neonates

93.2 Introduction

Platelets contribute to primary hemostasis, and their function is affected by their number and condition. Platelets arise from the fragmentation of megakaryocytes in the bone marrow and circulate in the blood as disk-shaped non-nucleated particles, with a life span of 7–10 days. Their average diameter is about 1.5 μm, 20% of the diameter of erythrocytes. Once released from the bone marrow, young platelets enter the circulation, where a large proportion pool in the spleen. It has been suggested that this splenic sequestration of young platelets is the result of a longer transit time of large platelets through the splenic cords. The spleen serves as a reservoir for platelets, containing about one-third, which are then able to enter the circulation after exercise or epinephrine administration. In addition to the spleen, the lungs also contain a small pool of platelets, perhaps 10–15% of the total number, and these are also able to enter the circulation after exercise or epinephrine administration (Sola and Christensen 2000).

Blood platelets adhere to sites of vascular injury, generate biological mediators, secrete their granule contents, form multicellular aggregates, and serve as a nucleus for plasma coagulation reactions. When endothelial continuity is disrupted, platelets adhere to the exposed basement membrane collagen and change their shape from smooth disks to spiny spheres, interacting with subendothelium-bound von Willebrand factor (vWf) via the membrane glycoprotein Ib (GPIb) complex (platelet adhesion). Subsequently, they secrete and release proaggregatory substances, such as adenosine 5′-diphosphate (ADP) and they synthesize thromboxane A2 from arachidonic acid. Additional platelets are recruited and form aggregates on those platelets that are adherent to the vessel wall to consolidate the initial hemostatic plug. A platelet glycoprotein IIb/IIIa (GPIIb–IIIa) complex mediates platelet-to-platelet interactions (platelet aggregation), a primary hemostatic plug is formed, and bleeding is stopped (primary hemostasis).

Platelets also provide an extensive phospholipid surface for the interaction and activation of

clotting factors in the coagulation cascade. Enzymes and cofactors of the coagulation system and a fibrin mesh further stabilize the initial hemostatic plug (secondary hemostasis). Collectively, they help to maintain the integrity of the vascular system (Handin 2003).

In addition to their classic role in hemostasis and thrombosis, recent studies reveal an important role in inflammation and the immune response (Li et al. 2012). Platelets produce various proinflammatory cytokines such as IL-1ß, P-selectin, CD40L, transforming growth factor-ß, and thrombospondin-1 supporting leukocyte/platelet interaction. Furthermore, in connection with various functional Toll-like receptors on their surface, platelets likely act as sentinels, recognizing invading microorganisms and activating the cross talk between innate immunity and hemostasis (Semple and Freedman 2010). In addition, activated platelets influence B-cell differentiation and proliferation, determining germinal center formation and antibody production (Elzey et al. 2005). Furthermore, platelets may play an important role in host defense stimulating also the adaptive immunity. Platelets can actively bind circulating Gram-positive bacteria and deliver them to splenic CD8 $\alpha +$ dendritic cells, supporting antibacterial CD8+ T-cell expansion (Verschoor et al. 2011). Thus, defects of platelet function not only affect hemostasis but theoretically could adversely affect innate and adaptive immune responses.

93.3 Platelet Function in Neonates

The hemostatic system of neonates matures during the early weeks and months of life. It has been well characterized with regard to plasma coagulation factors. However, because of the difficulty of obtaining adequate volumes of blood for aggregation tests, few data are available about the function of neonatal platelets. Most research on neonatal platelet function has been accomplished from the blood of term neonates, and most of those studies utilized umbilical cord blood samples, which cannot be an accurate model for neonatal platelet function over the subsequent hours and days (Haley et al. 2014).

GPIb appears on platelets early during fetal life and is present in fetuses of 18–26 weeks' gestation in greater amounts than those found in adults. The plasma of neonates contains higher concentrations of vWf than adult plasma, with an increased proportion of functional high-molecular-weight forms, which result in enhanced platelet adhesion. In the immediate newborn period, this enhanced platelet adhesion may compensate for the decreased intrinsic platelet activation in healthy neonates but may leave sick neonates at increased risk of bleeding.

Platelets also express GPIIb-IIIa early in gestation, and at 27 weeks' gestation, fibrinogen is found in concentrations similar to those in adults with normal binding to newborn platelets. Studies of platelet adhesion and platelet aggregation evaluating the responses to agonists are not easily performed in newborn infants and frequently generate conflicting results. There is diminished platelet function in neonates, as measured by aggregation in response to a number of physiological agonists (Sola and Christensen 2000; Kühne and Imbach 1998). Recent studies, using flow cytometry of cord blood and peripheral blood of neonates, demonstrated that platelets from term and preterm neonates display generalized hyporeactivity to thrombin, collagen, ADP, and U46619 (a stable thromboxane A2 analog) during the first few days of life. Platelet responses reach normal adult levels between the fifth and the ninth days of life. Persistence of platelet hyporeactivity in neonates after the tenth day of life may therefore suggest a platelet disorder.

The mechanism for the decreased reactivity of neonatal platelets has not been adequately explained. Platelet hyporeactivity was formerly considered to be the result of platelet activation and degranulation during labor and delivery, but more recent studies of platelet activation markers have not supported this theory (Blanchette and Rand 1997). Decreased activation is due to relative deficiencies of phospholipid metabolism and thromboxane production, different regulation of GPIIb/IIIa activation, impaired mobilization of calcium and intracellular signaling, granule secretion, and aggregation (Rajasekhar et al. 1997; Hezard et al. 2002). Although the

hyporesponsiveness of neonatal platelets depends on gestational age, and is indicative of the maturation of the hemostatic system, this transient dysfunction may be a developmental phenomenon to protect the neonate from the possible harmful effects of birth stress on the coagulation system (Sola and Christensen 2000).

Certain maternal diseases might influence neonatal platelet function. Neonates born to mothers with pregnancy-induced hypertension (PIH) can have thrombocytopenia and impaired platelet function. PIH can also activate maternal platelets. Altered metabolism of calcium, alteration of platelet membrane glycoproteins, increased release of plasma β-thromboglobulin, and altered NO bioavailability (El Haouari and Rosado 2009) have been considered to explain the effects of PIH on platelets. Neonates born to mothers with PIH can have decreased platelet surface expression of P-selectin and CD63, GPIIb-IIIa, and CD9 (Kuhne et al. 1996; Strauss et al. 2010a).

In gestational diabetes, maternal hyperglycemia can be accompanied by fetal hyperinsulinemia which in animal studies has been associated with impaired platelet function. The inhibition of platelet-activating factor biosynthesis, the reduction of the levels of platelet-activating factor, and the impairment of thromboxane synthesis have been proposed as potential mechanisms (Strauss et al. 2010a; Del Vecchio et al. 2015).

93.4 Clinical Aspects

Compared with adults or older children, the hemostatic system of neonates is naturally immature with a low functional reserve capacity. In spite of this, neonatal hemostasis is generally in equilibrium, and there is a relatively low incidence of inappropriate bleeding in term infants (Sola and Christensen 2000; Kühne and Imbach 1998). However, in the presence of additional risk factors such as prematurity, asphyxia, or infection, the neonatal hemostatic system is easily overwhelmed, and bleeding can be rapid and dramatic.

Abnormalities of platelet function or of platelet–vessel wall interactions should be considered, particularly in infants who have platelet-type bleeding (e.g., petechiae, purpura, mucous membrane bleeding) with a normal platelet count (Sola and Christensen 2000). A precise understanding of the type of platelet dysfunction and identification of the individual disorder allows for appropriate therapy.

93.5 Quantitative Disorders of Platelets

93.5.1 Thrombocytosis

A moderately elevated platelet count in the range of 450,000–600,000/μL is not an uncommon finding in the neonatal population, although a platelet count peak above 600,000/μL is rare. No adverse outcomes related to thrombocytosis have been described. In many preterm infants, a moderately increased platelet count has been observed at around 4–6 weeks of age, at the same time as the nadir of anemia of prematurity (Sutor 1995; Dame and Sutor 2005).

Initial studies on the administration of recombinant erythropoietin (rEPO) to preterm infants reported an increase in hematocrit and reticulocyte numbers, followed by a period of iron deficiency. This iron deficiency and decreased ferritin levels was accompanied by a significant thrombocytosis. Iron deficiency is known to cause thrombocytosis in older children (Halperin et al. 1990), but this relationship was not noticed in NICU patients before the introduction of rEPO treatment.

A secondary reactive thrombocytosis has been described in very young infants, particularly during infection. Antimicrobial therapy can also cause thrombocytosis in neonates treated with ceftriaxone, aztreonam, imipenem–cilastatin, ceftizoxime, and ceftazidime for suspected infection. No morbidity is generally associated with the elevated platelet count, and no treatment is necessary (Dame and Sutor 2005).

Early elevation of serum thrombopoietin levels is also related to subsequent thrombocytosis in low-birth-weight preterm infants (Matsubara et al. 2001). Infants with Down syndrome occasionally have a slightly raised platelet count between 6 weeks and around 1 year of age, and

thrombocytosis may occur in infants with congenital adrenal hyperplasia (CAH) (Kivivouri et al. 1996). The latter may have a normal hemoglobin, hematocrit, and red blood cell counts, while having significantly elevated white blood cell and platelet counts, possibly due to a stress-related response by marrow precursors as may occur in the course of sepsis. Usually, thrombocytosis resolves with the successful treatment of CAH (Gasparini et al. 1996). Thrombocytosis is also seen occasionally in neonates with gastroesophageal reflux disease and following maternal use of methadone, but the causes and significance of these varieties of thrombocytosis are unclear.

93.5.2 Thrombocytopenia

Thrombocytopenia is one of the commonest hematological problems in neonates, affecting 22–35% of infants admitted to the neonatal intensive care unit and almost 50% of all sick preterm neonates. The incidence of neonatal thrombocytopenia varies greatly, depending on the patient population and on the definition of thrombocytopenia. The platelet count in healthy neonates is similar to the range observed in older children and adults (150,000–450,000/μL), even though various centers, mostly in Europe, consider 100,000/μ L as the lowest limit. Premature infants may have slightly lower values than term infants, since fetal platelet counts increase linearly with gestation. Recent data suggest to define thrombocytopenia as a platelet count less than the fifth percentile reference range for gestational age and postnatal age. The fifth percentile is 104,000/μL for premature infants $<$32 weeks' gestation and 120,000/μL for late preterm and term neonates (Wiedmeier et al. 2009). Thrombocytopenia is also defined as mild when platelet count is between 100,000/μL and 150,000/μL, moderate between 50,000/μL and 100,000/μL, and severe $<$50,000/μL.

One classification of thrombocytopenia is based on the timing of onset: early ($\leq$72 h of life) vs late ($>$72 h). Early thrombocytopenia is commonly associated with fetomaternal conditions, reduced platelet production being secondary to placental insufficiency and fetal hypoxia, intrauterine growth restriction, or maternal hypertension. The resulting neonatal thrombocytopenia is usually mild to moderate, resolves spontaneously, and does not generally warrant treatment. The most frequent causes of thrombocytopenia occurring after the first 72 h of life, both in preterm and term infants, are sepsis and necrotizing enterocolitis, and the associated thrombocytopenia can be severe and protracted, often requiring therapy (Sola-Visner et al. 2009).

Variation from this pattern of thrombocytopenia suggests an immune thrombocytopenia with an increased risk of hemorrhage, since in this case the thrombocytopenia is usually severe (platelets $<$50,000/μL). Thrombocytopenia in the neonate can be asymptomatic or can present with a variety of symptoms, including petechiae, melena, hematuria, blood-stained endotracheal secretions, and bleeding from previous puncture sites. Other clinical signs of thrombocytopenia are intraventricular hemorrhage (IVH) or pulmonary hemorrhage (Murray 2002).

An infant with clinical signs of thrombocytopenia but without coagulation abnormalities should prompt examination for hepatosplenomegaly, congenital anomalies, and/or signs of sepsis.

In the mother, the platelet count, appearance of the blood smear, drug history, and evidence of transmissible infection should be investigated. Parental consanguinity and/or hematologic disease in family members should also be excluded (Bussel and Corrigan 1995). Neonatal thrombocytopenia is broadly due to the following mechanisms: decreased platelet production, increased platelet destruction, or platelet sequestration (Sola and Rimsza 2002).

93.5.2.1 Thrombocytopenia Due to Decrease Platelet Production

Overlap exists between the varieties of thrombocytopenia among neonates with intrauterine growth restriction (IUGR) and those with pregnancy-induced hypertension (PIH). Placental insufficiency and/or fetal hypoxia are likely involved in the reduced production of platelets (Watts et al. 1999). Plasma concentrations of thrombopoietin are generally elevated in these

patients, who have low to normal platelet counts (150,000–200,000/μL) or mild thrombocytopenia (100,000–150,000/μL) in the first day after delivery. Thereafter, the platelet count usually falls, with a nadir on days 4–5, generally recovering to above 150,000/μL by days 7–10. If not complicated, the nadir is rarely below 50,000/μL, and the risk of hemorrhage is not significant. These patients usually do not need platelet transfusions or other treatments for thrombocytopenia (Murray 2002).

Most cases of decreased platelet production are the consequence of reduced megakaryocytes or impaired platelet production by megakaryocytes. Congenital amegakaryocytic thrombocytopenia (CAMT) is a rare disorder with absence or near absence of megakaryocytes in the bone marrow and a risk of developing aplastic anemia. Compound heterozygosity for two-chain termination point mutations in the Mpl gene (thrombopoietin receptor) has been identified. Consequently, plasma thrombopoietin levels in these patients are significantly elevated. Both X-linked and autosomal recessive patterns of inheritance have been reported. Bone marrow transplant is currently the only treatment (Geddis 2009; MacMillan et al. 1998).

Thrombocytopenia with absent radii syndrome (TAR) is an autosomal recessive disorder with hypomegakaryocytic thrombocytopenia and bilateral absence of the radii, with the presence of functional thumbs. Bone marrow samples show decreased, absent, or immature megakaryocytes. No thrombopoietin gene mutations have been found. TAR may be associated with congenital heart disease, renal problems, defects of the lower limbs, and other hematological abnormalities, including aleukemoid reaction, eosinophilia, and anemia. There is symptomatic thrombocytopenia within the first 4 months of life in 90% of patients, often resulting in gastrointestinal or intracranial bleeding. The elevated level of thrombopoietin despite normal Mpl suggests that the imperfect thrombocytopoiesis in TAR is probably due to a lack of response to thrombopoietin in the signal transduction pathway (Geddis 2009).

Fanconi anemia is an autosomal recessive disorder associated with skeletal and genitourinary abnormalities. These patients can become pancytopenic. It is important to note that 25% of affected patients are structurally normal, and the diagnosis should be considered in the presence of thrombocytopenia, anemia, and leukopenia and in the absence of dysmorphic features.

Thrombocytopenia associated with a myeloproliferative disorder or with a wide variety of hemostatic abnormalities has been reported in Noonan syndrome, a rare autosomal dominant disorder with facial anomalies, congenital heart disease, skeletal abnormalities, and genital malformations (Bader-Meunier et al. 1997). Alport's syndrome, a genetic disorder associated with nephritis and nerve deafness, may present with thrombocytopenia and macrothrombocytes. Wiskott–Aldrich syndrome is a rare, sex-linked recessive disorder with thrombocytopenia, eczema, a tendency to severe bleeding, and an increased incidence of recurrent infections because of an impairment of cellular and humoral immunity. There is also an increased incidence of malignancy, such as lymphoma. The platelets are small, with one-half normal volume and decreased platelet mass, and their aggregation and life span also are diminished. The general prognosis is poor, and marrow transplantation is considered the treatment of choice (Bussel and Corrigan 1995).

Thrombocytopenia is also present in other chromosomal abnormalities. For instance, thrombocytopenia is found in 87% of infants with trisomy 18, in 54% of those with trisomy 13, in 31% of those with Turner's syndrome, and in 28% of those with trisomy 21 (Sola and Christensen 2000).

93.5.2.2 Thrombocytopenia Resulting from Increased Platelet Destruction

Immune Thrombocytopenias

Autoantibodies, alloantibodies, or drug-dependent antibodies may combine with platelet membranes and produce platelet impairment, resulting in platelet removal by phagocytes of the reticuloendothelial system. Immune destruction of platelets may be prompted by antibodies against a platelet membrane antigen or antibodies as part of an immune complex that binds Fc receptors on platelets. These immunologic mechanisms are

responsible for various clinical syndromes, including neonatal alloimmune thrombocytopenia (NAIT), autoimmune thrombocytopenia, and posttransfusion purpura.

NAIT is the platelet counterpart of hemolytic disease of the neonate, even though contrary to what happens in the hemolytic disease, it commonly occurs in primiparous women and is not screened during pregnancy. NAIT is secondary to placental transfer of maternal alloantibodies directed against paternally inherited antigens present on the fetal platelets but absent on maternal platelets. When this type of incompatibility between parental platelet exists, the mother may develop an immune response to antigens expressed on the fetal platelets inherited from the father. Homozygosity of the father for a specific platelet antigen results in the expression of that antigen on the fetal platelets; however, heterozygosity of the father for that antigen results in approximately 50% incidence of neonatal alloimmune thrombocytopenia (Bussel and Sola-Visner 2009; Williamson et al. 1998; Curtis 2015; Zdravic et al. 2016).

Antigens appear on fetal platelets early in the gestation, and maternal antibodies are able to cross the placenta early in the second trimester, thereby reacting with antigens on fetal platelets and inducing severe fetal thrombocytopenia. Mothers do not generally have a history of abnormal bleeding and have a normal platelet count. Neonatal alloimmune thrombocytopenia is usually a consequence of antibodies against the antigen HPA-1a, but there are also other antigens (Williamson et al. 1998).

The severity of thrombocytopenia is unpredictable. Nevertheless, certain clinical features are characteristic of neonatal alloimmune thrombocytopenia, such as severe thrombocytopenia (20,000–50,000/μL) at birth with a platelet count that continues to fall over the first days of life and then increases over the next 1–4 weeks. Intracranial hemorrhage occurs in approximately 10–15% of cases; at least one-half of these occur in utero, with death occurring in 10% of affected infants and neurological sequelae in 20%. Although controversial, prenatal treatment with percutaneous umbilical cord blood sampling and administration of IVIG to the mother may influence the natural history of the disease. Neonatal alloimmune thrombocytopenia causes more intracranial hemorrhage than any other hemostatic disorder in the newborn period. The usual presentation of an infant born to healthy mother is with purpura and/or petechiae within a few hours of birth and severe thrombocytopenia without other signs of disseminated intravascular coagulopathy (DIC) or sepsis. The full blood count is usually normal in the affected neonates apart from the severe thrombocytopenia (Bussel and Sola-Visner 2009).

In addition to a low platelet count, usually due to platelet consumption and rarely associated with reduced production, an infant's platelets may also have defective function (Roberts et al. 2008). The treatment of choice for rapidly raising the platelet count in neonates with severe neonatal alloimmune thrombocytopenia is transfusion with maternal or HPA-matched platelets because random donor platelet transfusions usually do not improve, or only briefly improve, the platelet count. Maternal platelets are usually washed to remove plasma, which may contain antiplatelet antibodies. IVIG can be used in the neonate to augment the platelet count, even though first improvement in platelet count may not be evident for 24–72 h (Bussel and Sola-Visner 2009).

Autoimmune thrombocytopenia occurs in neonates born to mothers with idiopathic thrombocytopenic purpura (ITP), systemic lupus erythematosus (SLE), lymphoproliferative disorders, or hyperthyroidism. Maternal autoantibodies bind to the maternal and the fetal platelets and result in platelet destruction (Roberts et al. 2008). Thrombocytopenia occurs in approximately 10% of cases in which the mother has ITP or SLE, and intracranial hemorrhage occurs in approximately 1% of these. The mother is usually healthy without a history of ITP or other autoimmune disorder, but with a slightly decreased platelet count that resolves after delivery. Autoimmune thrombocytopenic purpura in pregnant women can induce moderate or severe thrombocytopenia in the fetus or the newborn, but the severity of the maternal disease and maternal platelet count usually predicts the neonatal platelet count (Velat et al. 1998).

The neonate born to a mother with autoimmune disease should have platelet counts

monitored for at least the first week. The usual clinical picture includes mild to moderate thrombocytopenia, petechiae, or bruising in an otherwise healthy neonate. Intracranial hemorrhage is very rare. Thrombocytopenia usually persists 1–2 months in the infant, with spontaneous resolution.

The severity of thrombocytopenia in the first infant delivered to a woman with active ITP usually predicts the degree of thrombocytopenia of the next sibling. Monitoring the course of thrombocytopenia in breastfed neonates of mothers with ITP is recommended, since IgG antibodies are transferred via breast milk, and Bussel has reported one neonate in whom severe neonatal thrombocytopenia resolved only after stopping breastfeeding (Bussel and Sola-Visner 2009; Bussel 1997).

Treatment of infants affected by maternal ITP may include intravenous immunoglobulin (IVIG) or steroids or a combination of IVIG and steroids, platelet transfusion, or exchange transfusion (Sola and Christensen 2000).

Infections

Thrombocytopenia frequently accompanies systemic neonatal infection, even in the absence of disseminated intravascular coagulation (DIC). The reported incidence of thrombocytopenia associated with sepsis in neonates is extremely variable, depending on the definition of thrombocytopenia; 80% of neonates if thrombocytopenia is diagnosed as a platelet count of less than 150,000/μL, 55–65% if thrombocytopenia is diagnosed as a platelet count of less than 100,000/μL.

The usual mechanism responsible for thrombocytopenia in infected neonates is accelerated platelet destruction, which may be caused directly by the organism or its products, immune-mediated destruction, and adhesion of the platelets to the subendothelial layer of injured blood vessels (Sola-Visner et al. 2008).

Twenty-five percent of neonates with a bacterial infection are thrombocytopenic at the time sepsis is diagnosed. Thrombocytopenia may develop after 36–48 h, but bleeding is rare because this variety of thrombocytopenia is usually moderate. However, monitoring the platelet count is recommended, since these patients may require platelet transfusions. Recovery occurs over 5–7 days as the sepsis improves (Zipursky and Jaber 1978).

The involvement of platelets in the activity of the innate and adaptive immune system has been demonstrated in recent studies conducted in adults: the lethal effects of platelets on *P. falciparum* parasites require platelet activation (McMorran et al. 2009), and thrombocytopenic patients with primary chronic autoimmune thrombocytopenia have a significantly higher long-term risk of infection (Nørgaard et al. 2011).

It is possible to speculate that developmental changes in platelet production and function in neonate influence their immune responses, especially in preterm infants (Saxonhouse and Sola 2004; Bednarek et al. 2009) and that thrombocytopenia and disorders of platelet function may be responsible for increased susceptibility to infections.

Fungal sepsis, which is a particularly common problem among extremely low-birth-weight neonates, is frequently associated with thrombocytopenia. In contrast to the thrombocytopenia that may complicate bacterial infection, it is generally severe with platelet counts falling below 50,000/μL. Antifungal treatment is recommended while awaiting culture results in a clinically septic extremely low-birth-weight infant with thrombocytopenia (Manzoni et al. 2006).

Thrombocytopenia is common with congenital viral infections. All the viruses that cause TORCH infections, coxsackievirus B, Epstein–Barr virus, adenovirus, and echovirus can cause thrombocytopenia. The mechanism is most likely a combination of accelerated destruction, diminished production, and accelerated removal of platelets from the circulation because of the reticuloendothelial hyperactivity and splenomegaly that often accompany congenital viral infections. Vacuolization of megakaryocytes has also been reported (Sola et al. 2000; Manzoni 2015).

Disseminated Intravascular Coagulation

Disseminated intravascular coagulation (DIC) is a disorder of hemostasis, with an inappropriate systemic activation of normal clotting mechanisms

after endothelial injury, which is secondary to the underlying disease, which may include serious bacterial and viral infection, hypothermia, shock, anoxia, renal vein thrombosis, necrotizing enterocolitis, and meconium or fluid aspiration. All these disease processes are complicated by endothelial disruption and result in release of tissue factors and cytokines, and excessive activation of coagulation and fibrinolysis, and, ultimately, a consumptive coagulopathy (Edstrom et al. 2000).

Infants with DIC have low platelet counts and fibrinogen levels, prolonged prothrombin time (PT) and partial thromboplastin time (PTT), and elevated fibrin degradation products. They often present with gastrointestinal bleeding, hematuria, bleeding from venipuncture or sites of invasive procedures, pulmonary hemorrhage, and less frequently intracranial hemorrhage. Successful treatment of neonatal DIC depends on a correct diagnosis, treatment of the underlying disorders, and maintaining platelet counts greater than 50,000/μL, fibrinogen concentrations greater than 1 g/L, and PT values within the physiological range.

Necrotizing Enterocolitis

Thrombocytopenia is common in neonates with necrotizing enterocolitis (NEC). Platelet counts frequently fall to the range of 30,000–60,000/μL, and platelet transfusions do not usually maintain a normal blood platelet concentration for more than 1 or 2 days, suggesting a platelet consumptive process (Sola and Christensen 2000).

Asphyxia

Placental insufficiency can be associated with early-onset thrombocytopenia in preterm neonates, and perinatal hypoxia has been associated with severe and prolonged thrombocytopenia. Some of these infants have a decreased platelet count without DIC or persisting beyond the resolution of DIC. The decreased platelet count is probably due to the direct harmful effects of hypoxia on the megakaryocyte progenitors (Saxonhouse et al. 2006; Christensen et al. 2015).

Total body cooling, performed to improve the neurodevelopmental outcome of neonates with severe perinatal asphyxia, can be responsible for the activation of platelet and significant changes in surface antigen composition which lead to their rapid removal from the circulation (Oncel et al. 2013).

Thrombosis

Thrombocytopenia sometimes occurs in neonates who have a localized thrombus in the renal vein, or attached to an indwelling catheter, or in the ECMO circuit. It is unclear whether the thrombocytopenia is caused by platelet adhesion and aggregation to a developing thrombus or by platelet consumption at the vascular surfaces where the thrombus has begun.

Some sick neonates develop thrombocytopenia without any other coagulation defect, associated with platelet thrombi on the cardiac valves. In some neonates, platelets which have aggregated in the pulmonary capillaries release substances causing vasoconstriction with consequent pulmonary hypertension (Edstrom et al. 2000).

Kasabach–Merritt Syndrome

Consumption of platelets in giant hemangiomata can cause thrombocytopenia. These vascular tumors are usually solitary and may involve internal organs, head or neck, the trunk, or the extremities. Platelets are trapped by abnormal endothelium within the hemangioma, and the platelet counts often fall to less than 50,000/μL. In some patients, there is laboratory evidence of DIC, but thrombocytopenia may also occur in the absence of DIC. Proposed treatments have included steroids, alpha interferon, total or partial surgical excision of the hemangioma, or embolization or irradiation of the hemangioma (Clapp et al. 2001).

Drugs Producing Thrombocytopenia in Mother and Fetus

Thrombocytopenia as a result of maternal–fetal drug interaction is thought to be caused by immune reactions in which antibody is formed against a drug–haptene complex that cross-reacts with a platelet antigen. This has been reported with the maternal use of quinine, carbamazepine, phenytoin, and valproic acid (Bussel and Corrigan 1995). Thrombocytopenia induced by the maternal use of thiazide diuretics has also been reported

and may be due to impaired fetal platelet production with reduced megakaryocytes in the marrow but without inducing thrombocytopenia in the mother. In vitro studies have described thrombocytopenia with the maternal use of ampicillin and furosemide (Sola and Christensen 2000).

93.6 Qualitative Disorders of Platelets

Qualitative disorders of platelets form a large group of rare diseases in which the infant has a normal platelet count but excessive mucocutaneous bleeding. The qualitative platelet disorders are classified as either hereditary or acquired.

93.6.1 Hereditary Disorders

Most hereditary disorders of platelet function do not cause problems during the neonatal period but present later in life. Inherited functional platelet disorders are rare, but, because of diagnostic difficulties, frequency is probably underestimated. Major adhesion, aggregation, and secretion platelet defects are reported in Table 1.

Glanzmann's thrombasthenia is one type of hereditary platelet dysfunction that may present during the neonatal period. A deficiency of the glycoprotein IIb/IIIa complex, which is inherited in an autosomal recessive pattern, results in platelets that do not aggregate in response to normal stimuli, except to ristocetin. The microscopic appearance of the platelets and the platelet count are normal (Nair et al. 2002). Although platelet transfusions are effective, they should be used only for serious hemorrhage or if there is a need for surgery because these patients often develop alloantibodies. Recombinant factor VIIa may provide a therapeutic alternative to platelet transfusion for some patients (Poon 2007).

Bernard–Soulier syndrome is an autosomal recessive disorder resulting from a deficiency of

Table 1 Hereditary qualitative disorders of platelets

Adhesion defects	Aggregation defects	Secretion defects
Bernard–Soulier syndrome Absence or decreased expression of the glycoprotein complex GP Ib-IX-V on the surface of the platelets	Glanzmann thrombasthenia Abnormalities of platelet GPIIb-IIIa (fibrinogen receptor) → platelets less able to adhere to each other and to the underlying tissue of damaged blood vessels	Abnormalities of platelet granules (α, δ, α + δ) α: Gray platelet syndrome, Quebec platelet disorder (FV Quebec), Jacobsen–Paris–Trousseau syndrome δ: Storage pool disease, Hermansky–Pudlak syndrome, Chediak–Higashi syndrome, Wiskott–Aldrich syndrome α and δ combined deficiency
"Platelet-type" von Willebrand disease (pseudo von Willebrand disease) Defect of platelet GPIba → increased avidity for normal vWF → binding of the largest vWF multimers to resting platelets and clearance from the circulation → thrombocytopenia and adhesion defect	Afibrinogenemia Abnormal platelets and clotting (combined bleeding disorder)	Abnormalities of the signal transduction and secretion Impaired liberation of Arachidonic acid from membrane phospholipids Cyclooxygenase deficiency ("aspirin like disease") Thromboxane synthetase deficiency Thromboxane A2 receptor abnormalities
Collagen receptor deficiency Abnormalities of platelet GPVI and GPIa-IIa (receptors for collagen) → adhesion and collagen-induced platelet aggregation defects		

platelet glycoprotein protein Ib, which mediates the initial interaction of platelets with subendothelial components via the von Willebrand protein. This syndrome can result in a severe bleeding disorder. Platelets do not aggregate in response to ristocetin. The platelet count is low, but the platelets are usually large, often the size of red blood cells. As in Glanzmann's thrombasthenia, platelet transfusions may cause antibody formation to the absent glycoprotein, and the administration of recombinant factor VIIa for acute bleeding episodes should be considered as an alternative treatment.

May–Hegglin anomaly is a benign condition characterized by giant platelets. Giant platelets are also found in variants of Alport's syndrome. Platelet function disorders relating to platelet secretion cause mild to moderate bleeding. Included in this subset of disorders are gray platelet syndrome, dense granule deficiency, Chediak–Higashi syndrome, and Hermansky–Pudlak syndrome (Sola and Christensen 2000).

93.6.2 Acquired Disorders

Acquired disorders of platelet function are common. A primary hemostatic defect can occur as a result of medications given to the mother or neonate. Aspirin, given to the mother, crosses the placenta and may produce irreversible inhibition of the cyclooxygenase enzyme, increasing the bleeding time for the life of affected platelets. Gastrointestinal bleeding, melena, or cephalohematoma may affect neonates whose mothers received aspirin during pregnancy within 5 days of delivery (Sola and Christensen 2000).

Indomethacin and ibuprofen, commonly used for the closure of patent ductus arteriosus, can interfere with cyclooxygenase function. The influence of these drugs on platelet function is transitory, generally lasting about 24 h. Ibuprofen, administered to neonates with a PDA, has little adverse effect on platelet plug formation and prolongs the bleeding time less than indomethacin (Sheffield et al. 2009; Del Vecchio et al. 2002). Nitric oxide (NO) also has the potential to reduce platelet function, probably because of increased cGMP. In premature infants, inhaled NO may prolong bleeding time, decrease platelet aggregation, and inhibit platelet adhesion to endothelial cells, increasing the risk of intraventricular hemorrhage (Cheung et al. 1997).

Extracorporeal membrane oxygenation (ECMO) is used in neonates for the treatment of persistent pulmonary hypertension, meconium aspiration, and congenital diaphragmatic hernia. Impaired platelet function and thrombocytopenia have been described in patients on ECMO. During ECMO, platelet dysfunction persists despite platelet transfusions, and platelet function returns to normal 8 h after the discontinuation of ECMO (Sola and Christensen 2000).

Other circumstances where platelet dysfunction has been described include hyperbilirubinemia and phototherapy, although bleeding has not been reported in otherwise healthy infants in these situations (Sola and Christensen 2000).

Uremia and/or renal failure can also cause neonatal platelet dysfunction. Gastrointestinal tract bleeding is the most frequent symptom, and bleeding time is often very prolonged in these patients. Excessive production of nitric oxide by endothelial cells inhibits platelet function and may be responsible for bleeding in uremic patients. Because the prolonged bleeding time and the hemostatic abnormalities may be partly corrected by red blood cell transfusion or erythropoietin therapy, the failure of hemoglobin to turn off excess nitric oxide synthesis has been suggested as a cause of the platelet dysfunction. Another suggestion is that platelets arrive on exposed vascular subendothelium, being propelled there mainly by erythrocytes, which release ADP to activate the platelets following vessel injury. Consequently, a low hematocrit may result in a prolonged bleeding time (Sola et al. 2001).

93.7 Evaluating Platelet Function in a Neonate

The main goal of platelet function testing is to determine the cause of abnormal bleeding. However, a thorough assessment of platelet function in the neonate is difficult because of difficulties in

obtaining sufficient blood for these types of studies (Watts et al. 1999). This is particularly true for aggregometry and flow cytometric evaluation of platelet activation, but various other studies, such as those listed below, can be helpful.

93.7.1 Laboratory Studies

93.7.1.1 Peripheral Smear

Examination of the peripheral smear is useful for evaluating platelet clumping or platelets adhering to neutrophils (platelet satellitism), large platelet size (Bernard–Soulier syndrome), or platelet granularity (gray platelet syndrome).

93.7.1.2 Platelet Aggregometry

Platelet aggregometry measures the transmission of light through a platelet suspension before and after platelet response to agonists like ADP, epinephrine, collagen, and thrombin ristocetin. Aggregometry can help in the diagnosis of von Willebrand disease, Glanzmann thrombasthenia, or storage pool disorders. Using these methods, platelets of neonates do not have the high level of aggregation characteristic of adult platelets (Israels et al. 1990; Louden et al. 1994). These differences are more marked in platelets of preterm infants (Israels et al. 1997). Clinical application to neonates is significantly reduced because of the lack of appropriate neonatal reference intervals and limited availability of the technology (Halimeh et al. 2010).

93.7.1.3 Flow Cytometry

Flow cytometry is an accurate way to measure neonatal platelet activation. The need for little amount of blood (5–100 μL) and the minimal sample manipulation prior to analysis have solved many of the problems encountered in neonatal aggregometry studies. Flow cytometry detects glycoproteins on platelet surface, using monoclonal antibodies directed at platelet activation markers like as p-selectin and the fibrinogen-binding site exposed on the glycoprotein IIb/IIIa complex. Flow cytometric studies from cord blood or from neonates have confirmed the early neonatal platelet hyporesponsiveness during the first days of life (Rajasekhar et al. 1997). High costs of equipment and reagents, need for qualified laboratory staff, length of time needed for testing, and lack of neonatal reference intervals appropriate for gestational and postnatal age do not recommend the routine use of this method.

93.7.1.4 Platelet-Associated Immunoglobulin G

Assays have been developed to assess the presence of IgG on platelets. In the thrombocytopenic neonate, this may indicate platelet destruction and reduced platelet survival. The detection of increased platelet-associated immunoglobulin is observed in a variety of conditions associated with thrombocytopenia, which limits the value of this test for the diagnosis of specific disorders, such as ITP.

93.7.1.5 Bleeding Time

The bleeding time measures the time required for a platelet plug, which occurs through the interaction of platelets with the subendothelial structures of a damaged vessel, to arrest bleeding from a standardized superficial skin incision (Del Vecchio and Sola 2000; Del Vecchio 2002). It is a useful clinical tool to identify quantitative or qualitative platelet disorders or microvascular defectiveness. Its diagnostic value in neonates is controversial, due to limited experience in executing the test and highly operator dependency. A prolonged bleeding time with a normal platelet count indicates a qualitative platelet disorder. In thrombocytopenic neonates with platelet counts below about 75,000–100,000/μL, the bleeding time is prolonged proportionally to the severity of thrombocytopenia (Del Vecchio 2002).

93.7.1.6 Platelet Function Analyzer 100

The platelet function analyzer 100 (PFA-100) is an in vitro method for the assessment of primary hemostasis under shear stress, where primary hemostasis is simulated by an in vitro quantitative measurement of platelet adhesion, activation, and aggregation in whole blood. The PFA-100 uses a disposable test cartridge that contains a membrane coated with collagen and

either ADP (Col/ADP membrane) or epinephrine (Col/Epi membrane), thus mimicking exposed subendothelium. A blood sample of 0.8 mL of citrated blood is placed in a cup and is aspirated through the aperture. The shear stress and the agonists in the membrane activate platelets lead to platelet aggregation. The end point, expressed as closure time, is when blood flow stops because of occlusion of the aperture by platelet aggregates, giving a measure of platelet dependent hemostasis (Saxonhouse and Sola 2004). The closure times, similar to bleeding times, are significantly shorter in neonates than in adults and healthy children. The advantages of this instrument include simplicity and reproducibility.

93.7.1.7 Thromboelastogram (TEG) and Rotating Thromboelastogram (ROTEM)

Thromboelastography (TEG) is a point-of-care device that evaluates the process of clot formation and degradation utilizing a small whole blood volume sample. TEG analyzes the initiation of clot formation, actual clot firmness, and fibrinolysis, reflecting the complex clotting process that involves coagulation factors, cellular components, and enzymes.

Actually TEG provides a global measure of coagulation in a single test.

The use of TEG and ROTEM to evaluate clot formation in neonates has recently been reported (Chan et al. 2007; Radicioni et al. 2012; Strauss et al. 2010b), and clot formation parameters of term and preterm infants correlate with gestational age. Reference values for ROTEM clot formation parameters were established in cord blood of term and preterm neonates (Edwards et al. 2008).

Furthermore, it has been recently reported that several TEG parameters are predictive of clinical bleeding in newborns undergoing hypothermia.

93.7.1.8 Mean Platelet Volume

The mean platelet volume (MPV) is a measure of the average size of circulating platelets. Since the average platelet size is larger when the marrow produces increased numbers of platelets, high MPV in thrombocytopenic neonates can be an indirect measure of increased platelet production in bone marrow.

93.7.1.9 Reticulated Platelet Count

Reticulated platelets, similar to reticulated erythrocytes, lose their RNA content in the process of aging and senescence. Because reticulated platelets are detectable in the circulation for only 24 h, they are an excellent measure of platelet production and turnover. These new platelets can be recognized by flow cytometry, and in term neonates they represent 3–5% of circulating platelets. Increased production of platelets is expected to increase the percentage of reticulated platelet (Saxonhouse et al. 2004).

93.7.1.10 Bone Marrow Biopsy

In most cases of platelet disorders, bone marrow biopsy is not necessary. It provides important information about the state of platelet production that is not otherwise available. It is particularly useful in evaluating neonates with thrombocytopenia when an estimate of the marrow megakaryocyte mass is needed. Unlike a direct aspiration of cells from a neonate's bone marrow, which can result in a sample that is so diluted with peripheral blood that interpretation is limited, the marrow biopsy preserves the basic architecture of the marrow. Bone marrow biopsy uses a 19-gauge, half-inch Osgood needle to obtain bone marrow clots from the tibia of a baby, enabling the assessment of marrow cellularity and architecture (Sola et al. 1999).

93.8 Treatments

93.8.1 Platelet Transfusion

Platelet transfusions represent the only specific therapy currently available for most thrombocytopenic neonates. There is great variability worldwide in neonatal platelet transfusion practice, due to the lack of concrete evidence to guide transfusion decisions (Christensen 2002; Del Vecchio et al. 2001). In approximately 75% of neonates with thrombocytopenia, the condition is mild and transient and

needs no treatment. However, in 20–25% of cases, one or more platelet transfusions are given in an attempt to treat or decrease the risk of hemorrhage. Among critically ill patients, most platelet transfusions are given to prevent, rather than to treat, bleeding, with a transfusion trigger of 40,000–50,000/μL. It is not clear how many platelet transfusions in the NICU are actually unnecessary or provide more risk than benefit (Christensen 2002; Del Vecchio et al. 2008).

Baer and coworkers reported that the number of platelet transfusions administered in the NICU predicts the mortality rate, suggesting that multiple platelet transfusions may be harmful. Since platelet transfusions carry risks, eliminating unnecessary platelet transfusions would be useful (Baer et al. 2007). Improving transfusion practice requires the definition of a safe lower limit for platelet counts in stable neonates, platelet transfusion strategies for critically ill neonates, and improved treatments for conditions that are associated with severe thrombocytopenia. To avoid unnecessary transfusions, Christensen et al. proposed transfusion guidelines based on platelet mass (platelet count times mean platelet volume). In a pilot study, the use of these guidelines was associated with fewer platelet transfusions without any increase in problems due to hemorrhage (Gerday et al. 2009; Christensen et al. 2008).

Although platelet count and/or platelet mass can indicate the platelet transfusion, the evidence strongly suggests that factors other than the degree of thrombocytopenia determine the bleeding risk (Sparger et al. 2015).

While there is no scientific evidence to guide platelet transfusion practices in neonates, individual NICUs should adopt guidelines appropriate to their practice and adhere to them closely (Josephson et al. 2009; Christensen et al. 2008). As a general rule, platelets should be given to non-bleeding thrombocytopenic neonates as prophylactic transfusions to maintain platelet count >20,000/μL for clinically stable neonates and >50,000/μL for clinically unstable neonates. Platelet counts should be maintained >50,000–100,000/μL when there is significant bleeding and >50,000/μL for invasive procedures (Murray et al. 2002; Strauss 2008).

93.8.2 Thrombopoietic Factors

Inadequate megakaryocytopoiesis and platelet production are major contributors to most episodes of neonatal thrombocytopenia. As alternatives to platelet transfusion, the administration of thrombopoietic growth factors, such as recombinant thrombopoietin (rTPO) and interleukin-11 (IL-11), may be useful. The opportunity of decreasing platelet transfusions with the use of novel thrombopoiesis-stimulating agents, such as romiplostim and eltrombopag, could be also considered in thrombocytopenic neonates even though the response of neonates to these thrombopoietic factors and their non-hematopoietic effects have not been well established (Sallmon et al. 2010). Actually, thrombopoietic factors are promising agents for older patients but have potential toxicities that are likely to preclude their use for sick preterm infants.

93.8.3 Other Therapies

Recombinant activated factor VII has been used successfully off-label in controlling life-threatening bleeding during infancy, but the clinical situations in which benefits are likely, and potential toxicities, particularly thrombosis, remain unknown. The administration of intravenous immunoglobulin (IVIG) is useful for the treatment of immune thrombocytopenia. Corticosteroids were classically used for alloimmune and autoimmune neonatal thrombocytopenia, often in combination with IVIG, but are now unusual. Dosing schedules for IVIG include 400 mg/kg/d for 3–5 consecutive days or a single dose of 1000 mg/kg on day 1.

References

Bader-Meunier B, Tchernia G, Mielot F (1997) Occurrence of myeloproliferative disorders with Noon syndrome. J Pediatr 130:885–889

Baer VL, Lambert DK, Henry E et al (2007) Do platelet transfusions in the NICU adversely affect survival? Analysis of 1600 thrombocytopenic neonates in a multihospital healthcare system. J Perinatol 27:790–796

Bednarek FJ, Bean S, Barnard MR, Frelinger AL, Michelson AD (2009) The platelet hyporeactivity of extremely

low birth weight neonates is age-dependent. Thromb Res 124:42–45
Blanchette VS, Rand ML (1997) Platelet disorders in newborn infants: diagnosis and management. Semin Perinatol 21:53–62
Bussel JB (1997) Immune thrombocytopenia in pregnancy: autoimmune and alloimmune. J Reprod Immunol 37:35–61
Bussel JB, Corrigan JJ (1995) Platelet and vascular disorders. In: Miller DR, Baehner RL (eds) Blood diseases of infancy and childhood. Mosby, St. Louis, pp 866–923
Bussel JB, Sola-Visner M (2009) Current approaches to the evaluation and management of the fetus and neonate with immune thrombocytopenia. Semin Perinatol 33:35–42
Chan KL, Summerhayes RG, Ignjatovic V, Horton SB, Monagle PT (2007) Reference values for kaolin-activated thromboelastography in healthy children. Anesth Analg 105:1610–1613
Cheung PY, Salas E, Schulz R (1997) Nitric oxide and platelet function: implications for neonatology. Semin Perinatol 21:409–417
Christensen RD (2002) Advances and controversies in neonatal ICU platelet transfusion practice. Adv Pediatr Infect Dis 55:255–269
Christensen RD, Paul DA, Sola-Visner MC, Baer VL (2008) Improving platelet transfusion practices in the neonatal intensive care unit. Transfusion 48: 2281–2284
Christensen RD, Baer VL, Yaish HM (2015) Thrombocytopenia in late preterm and term neonates after perinatal asphyxia. Transfusion 55:187–196
Clapp DW, Shannon KM, Phibbs RH (2001) Hematologic problems. In: Klaus MH, Fanaroff AA (eds) Care of the high risk neonate. Saunders, Philadelphia, pp 447–479
Curtis BR (2015) Recent progress in understanding the pathogenesis of fetal and neonatal alloimmune thrombocytopenia. Br J Haematol 171:671–682
Dame C, Sutor AH (2005) Primary and secondary thrombocytosis in childhood. Br J Haematol 29:165–177
Del Vecchio A (2002) Use of the bleeding time in the neonatal intensive care unit. Acta Paediatr Suppl 91:82–86
Del Vecchio A, Sola MC (2000) Performing and interpreting the bleeding time in the neonatal intensive care unit. Clin Perinatol 27:643–654
Del Vecchio A, Sola MC, Theriaque DW et al (2001) Platelet transfusions in the neonatal intensive care unit: factors predicting which patients will require multiple transfusions. Transfusion 41:803–808
Del Vecchio A, Sullivan SE, Christensen RD et al (2002) Indomethacin prolongs the bleeding time in neonates significantly more than ibuprofen. Pediatr Res 51:466A
Del Vecchio A, Latini G, Henry E, Christensen RD (2008) Template bleeding times of 240 neonates born at 24 to 41 weeks gestation. J Perinatol 28:427–431
Del Vecchio A, Motta M, Romagnoli C (2015) Neonatal platelet function. Clin Perinatol 42:625–638
Edstrom CS, Christensen RD, Andrew M (2000) Developmental aspects of blood hemostasis and disorders of coagulation and fibrinolysis in the neonatal period. In: Christensen RD (ed) Hematologic problems of the neonate. Saunders, Philadelphia, pp 239–271
Edwards RM, Naik-Mathuria BJ, Gay AN, Olutoye OO, Teruya J (2008) Parameters of thromboelastography in healthy newborns. Am J Clin Pathol 130:99–102
El Haouari M, Rosado JA (2009) Platelet function in hypertension. Blood Cells Mol Dis 42:38–43
Elzey BD, Grant JF, Sinn HW, Nieswandt B, Waldschmidt TJ, Ratliff TL (2005) Cooperation between platelet-derived CD154 and CD4+ T cells for enhanced germinal center formation. J Leukoc Biol 78:80–84
Gasparini N, Franzese A, Argenziano A (1996) Thrombocytosis in congenital adrenal hyperplasia at diagnosis. Clin Pediatr 35:267–269
Geddis AE (2009) Congenital amegakaryocytic thrombocytopenia and thrombocytopenia with absent radii. Hematol Oncol Clin North Am 23:321–331
Gerday E, Baer VL, Lambert DK et al (2009) Testing platelet mass versus platelet count to guide platelet transfusions in the neonatal intensive care unit. Transfusion 49:2034–2039
Haley KM, Recht M, McCarty OJ (2014) Neonatal platelets: mediators of primary hemostasis in the developing hemostatic system. Pediatr Res 76:230–237
Halimeh S, Gd A, Sander A, Edelbusch C, Rott H, Thedieck S et al (2010) Multiplate whole blood impedance point of care aggregometry: preliminary reference values in healthy infants, children and adolescents. Klin Padiatr 222:158–163
Halperin DS, Washer P, Lacourt G (1990) Effects of recombinant human erythropoietin in infants with the anemia of prematurity: a pilot study. J Pediatr 116:779–786
Handin RI (2003) Blood platelets and the vessel wall. In: Nathan DG (ed) Hematology of infancy and childhood. Saunders, Philadelphia, pp 1457–1474
Hezard N, Amory C, Leroux B, Schlegel N, Potron G, Nguyen P (2002) Platelet hyporeactivity in healthy children remains beyond the neonatal period. Blood 100:69a
Israels SJ, Daniels M, McMillan EM (1990) Deficient collagen-induced activation in the newborn platelet. Pediatr Res 27:337–343
Israels SJ, Odaibo FS, Robertson C, McMillan EM, McNicol A (1997) Deficient thromboxane synthesis and response in platelets from premature infants. Pediatr Res 41:218–223
Josephson CD, Su LL, Christensen RD et al (2009) Platelet transfusion practices among neonatologists in the United States and Canada: results of a survey. Pediatrics 123:278–285
Kivivouri SM, Rajantie J, Siimes MA (1996) Peripheral blood cell counts in infants with Down's syndrome. Clin Genet 49:15–19
Kühne T, Imbach P (1998) Neonatal platelet physiology and pathophysiology. Eur J Pediatr 157:87–94
Kuhne T, Ryan G, Blanchette V, Semple JW, Hornstein A, Mody M (1996) Platelet-surface glycoproteins in healthy and preeclamptic mothers and their newborn infants. Pediatr Res 40:876–880

Li C, Li J, Li Y, Lang S, Yougbare I, Zhu G et al (2012) Crosstalk between platelets and the immune system: old systems with new discoveries. Adv Hematol 2012:384685

Louden KA, Broughton Pipkin F, Heptinstall S, Fox SC, Tuohy P, O'Callaghan C et al (1994) Neonatal platelet reactivity and serum thromboxane B2 production in whole blood: the effect of maternal low-dose aspirin. Br J Obstet Gynaecol 101:203–208

MacMillan ML, Davies SM, Wagner JE (1998) Engraftment of unrelated donor stem cells in children with familial amegakaryocytic thrombocytopenia. Bone Marrow Transplant 21:735–737

Manzoni P (2015) Hematologic aspects of early and late-onset sepsis in preterm infants. Clin Perinatol 42:587–595

Manzoni P, Arisio R, Mostert M et al (2006) Prophylactic fluconazole is effective in preventing fungal colonization and fungal systemic infections in preterm neonates: a single-center, 6-year, retrospective cohort study. Pediatrics 117:22–32

Matsubara K, Baba K, Nigami H (2001) Early elevation of serum thrombopoietin levels and subsequent thrombocytosis in healthy preterm infants. Br J Haematol 115:963–968

McMorran BJ, Marshall VM, de Graaf C, Drysdale KE, Shabbar M, Smyth GK et al (2009) Platelets kill intraerythrocytic malarial parasites and mediate survival to infection. Science 323:797–800

Murray NA (2002) Evaluation and treatment of thrombocytopenia in the neonatal intensive care unit. Acta Paediatr Suppl 438:74–81

Murray NA, Howarth LJ, McCloy MP et al (2002) Platelet transfusion in the management of severe thrombocytopenia in neonatal intensive care unit patients. Transfus Med 12:35–41

Nair S, Ghosh K, Kulkarni B et al (2002) Glanzmann's thrombasthenia: updated. Platelets 13:387–393

Nørgaard M, Jensen AØ, Engebjerg MC, Farkas DK, Thomsen RW, Cha S et al (2011) Long-term clinical outcomes of patients with primary chronic immune thrombocytopenia: a Danish population-based cohort study. Blood 117:3514–3520

Oncel MY, Erdeve O, Calisici E, Oguz SS, Canpolat FE, Uras N, Dilmen U (2013) The effect of whole-body cooling on hematological and coagulation parameters in asphyxic newborns. Pediatr Hematol Oncol 30:246–252

Poon MC (2007) The evidence for the use of recombinant human activated factor VII in the treatment of bleeding patients with quantitative and qualitative platelet disorders. Transfus Med Rev 21:223–236

Radicioni M, Mezzetti D, Del Vecchio A, Motta M (2012) Thromboelastography: might work in neonatology too? J Matern Fetal Neonatal Med 25(Suppl 4):18–21

Rajasekhar D, Barnard MR, Bednarek FJ, Michelson AD (1997) Platelet hyporeactivity in very-low-birth-weight neonates. Thromb Haemost 77:1002–1007

Roberts I, Stanworth S, Murray NA (2008) Thrombocytopenia in the neonate. Blood Rev 22:173–186

Sallmon H, Gutti RK, Ferrer-Marin F, Liu ZJ, Sola-Visner MC (2010) Increasing platelets without transfusion: is it time to introduce novel thrombopoietic agents in neonatal care? J Perinatol 30:765–769

Saxonhouse MA, Sola MC (2004) Platelet function in term and preterm neonates. Clin Perinatol 31:15–28

Saxonhouse MA, Sola MC, Pastos KM et al (2004) Reticulated platelet percentages in term and preterm neonates. J Pediatr Hematol Oncol 26:797–802

Saxonhouse MA, Rimsza LM, Stevens G et al (2006) Effects of hypoxia on megakaryocyte progenitors obtained from the umbilical cord blood of term and preterm neonates. Biol Neonate 89:104–108

Semple JW, Freedman J (2010) Platelets and innate immunity. Cell Mol Life Sci 67:499–511

Sheffield MJ, Schmutz N, Lambert DK et al (2009) Ibuprofen lysine administration to neonates with a patent ductus arteriosus: effect on platelet plug formation assessed by in vivo and in vitro measurements. J Perinatol 29:39–43

Sola MC, Christensen RD (2000) Developmental aspects of platelets and disorders of platelets in the neonatal period. In: Christensen RD (ed) Hematologic problems of the neonate. Saunders, Philadelphia, pp 273–309

Sola MC, Rimsza LM (2002) Mechanisms underlying thrombocytopenia in the neonatal intensive care unit. Acta Paediatr Suppl 438:66–73

Sola MC, Rimsza LM, Christensen RD (1999) A bone marrow biopsy technique suitable for use in neonates. Br J Haematol 107:458–460

Sola MC, Del Vecchio A, Rimsza LM (2000) Evaluation and treatment of thrombocytopenia in the neonatal intensive care unit. Clin Perinatol 27:655–679

Sola MC, Del Vecchio A, Edwards TJ et al (2001) The relationship between hematocrit and bleeding time in very low birth weight infants during the first week of life. J Perinatol 21:368–371

Sola-Visner M, Saxonhouse MA, Brown RE (2008) Neonatal thrombocytopenia: what we do and don't know. Early Hum Dev 84:499–506

Sola-Visner M, Sallmon H, Brown R (2009) New insights into the mechanisms of nonimmune thrombocytopenia in neonates. Semin Perinatol 33:43–51

Sparger K, Deschmann E, Sola-Visner M (2015) Platelet transfusion in the neonatal intensive care unit. Clin Perinatol 42:613–623

Strauss RG (2008) How I transfuse red blood cells and platelets to infants with the anemia and thrombocytopenia of prematurity. Transfusion 48:209–217

Strauss T, Maayan-Metzger A, Simchen MJ, Morag I, Shenkmean B, Kuint J, Kenet G (2010a) Impaired platelet function in neonates born to mothers with diabetes or hypertension during pregnancy. Klin Padiatr 222:154–157

Strauss T, Levy-Shraga Y, Ravid B, Schushan-Eisen I, Maayan-Metzger A, Kuint J, Kenet G (2010b) Clot formation of neonates tested by thromboelastography

correlates with gestational age. Thromb Haemost 103:344–350

Sutor AH (1995) Thrombocytosis in childhood. Semin Thromb Hemost 21:330–339

Velat AS, Caulier MT, Devos P (1998) Relationships between severe neonatal thrombocytopenia and maternal characteristics in pregnancies associated with autoimmune thrombocytopenia. Br J Haematol 103:397–401

Verschoor A, Neuenhahn M, Navarini AA, Graef P, Plaumann A, Seidlmeier A et al (2011) A platelet-mediated system for shuttling blood-borne bacteria to CD8α+ dendritic cells depends on glycoprotein GPIb and complement C3. Nat Immunol 12: 1194–1201

Watts TL, Murray NA, Roberts IAG (1999) Thrombopoietin has a primary role in the regulation of platelet production in preterm babies. Pediatr Res 46:28–32

Wiedmeier SE, Henry E, Sola-Visner MC, Christensen RD (2009) Platelet reference ranges for neonates, defined using data from over 47,000 patients in a multihospital healthcare system. J Perinatol 29:130–136

Williamson L, Hackett G, Rennie J (1998) The natural history of fetomaternal alloimmunization to the platelet specific antigen HPA-1A as determined by antenatal screening. Blood 92:2280–2287

Zdravic D, Yougbare I, Vadasz B, Li C, Marshall AH, Chen P, Kjeldsen-Kragh J, Ni H (2016) Fetal and neonatal alloimmune thrombocytopenia. Semin Fetal Neonatal Med 21:19–27

Zipursky A, Jaber HM (1978) The haematology of bacterial infection in newborn infants. Clin Haematol 7:175–193

Anemia in the Neonatal Period

94

Robert D. Christensen and Robin K. Ohls

Contents

Abstract

Anemia is a pathological reduction in the hematocrit, blood hemoglobin concentration, and circulating erythrocyte count. Neonatal reference intervals for hematocrit and hemoglobin are characteristic of this age. Neonatal red cell survival is shorter than in children and adults and the lower end of the normal range for infants of this age is approximately 9 g/dl. This nadir is called physiologic anemia. Neonates have red cells with erythrocyte membranes and distinctive metabolic characteristics that differ slightly from those of adults and so does the antigen expression. Isoimmunization caused by maternal-fetal blood group incompatibility is the most common cause of newborn hemolytic jaundice. Alloimmunization can present with unique neonatal findings, with a low reticulocyte count along with a low hemoglobin and elevated bilirubin. Causes of hemorrhage resulting in fetal or neonatal anemia are divided into prenatal, perinatal, and postnatal

R. D. Christensen (✉)
Divisions of Neonatology and Hematology, Department of Pediatrics, University of Utah School of Medicine, Intermountain Healthcare, Salt Lake City, UT, USA
e-mail: robert.christensen@hsc.utah.edu

R. K. Ohls
Department of Pediatrics, Division of Neonatology, University of New Mexico, Albuquerque, NM, USA

G. Buonocore et al. (eds.), *Neonatology*,
https://doi.org/10.1007/978-3-319-29489-6_241

varieties. The use of "early" and the use of "late" erythropoietin administration to prevent and treat the anemia of prematurity has decreased transfusion requirements in preterm infants and beneficial neurodevelopmental effects have been reported. This chapter reviews the various pathologies that give rise to anemia during the fetal and neonatal periods and provides practical approaches for dealing with these clinical issues.

94.1 Salient Points

- Various pathologies cause anemia during the fetal and neonatal periods.
- During early fetal and neonatal development, erythropoietin has biological roles in addition to that of an erythropoietic growth factor.
- "Reference intervals" are used in neonatology in place of the "normal ranges" commonly used in adult medicine.
- Neonates have erythrocyte membranes that differ slightly from those of adults. Red blood cells of neonates also have distinctive metabolic characteristics.
- Fetal and neonatal anemia can be due to abnormalities in erythrocyte membrane or cellular metabolism, immune-mediated hemolytic diseases, hemorrhage, congenital infection, and hypoproliferative disorders.
- The indications for erythrocyte transfusion deserve careful consideration.

94.2 Introduction

Anemia is a pathological reduction in the hematocrit, blood hemoglobin concentration, and circulating erythrocyte count (Kling 2013). These three laboratory measures are somewhat similar to one another, in that each quantifies the same biological variable involving the capacity of blood to deliver oxygen to tissues. However, none of the three measurements actually assesses whether oxygen demands of tissues are being adequately met. In fact, limitations in delivery of oxygen to a neonate's tissues are frequently not the result of anemia at all, but instead are due to abnormalities in oxygen intake as a result of pulmonary pathology. This chapter reviews the various pathologies that give rise to anemia during the fetal and neonatal periods and provides practical approaches for dealing with these clinical issues.

94.3 Erythropoietin in the Fetus and Neonate

During early fetal and neonatal development, erythropoietin (Epo) has biological roles in addition to that of an erythropoietic growth factor (Lundby and Olsen 2011). Epo is a constituent of amniotic fluid, typically in concentrations of 25–40 mU/mL. A normal human fetus swallows 200–300 mL of amniotic fluid/kg/day and thus swallows 10–15 U of Epo/kg/day (Juul 2000; Juul et al. 2001). In humans, Epo does not cross the placenta, and the source of the Epo in amniotic fluid is not the maternal circulation. In the second and third trimesters, amniotic fluid is largely derived from fetal urine, with minor constituents from fetal tracheal effluent and the placenta and fetal membranes. However, Epo in amniotic fluid does not come from fetal urine (Brace et al. 2006). The fetal kidney makes little Epo before delivery, and the first-voided urine of neonates generally has no detectable Epo (Juul 2000). Studies using in situ hybridization and immunohistochemistry indicate that the source of Epo in amniotic fluid is largely maternal: from mesenchymal and endothelial cells in the deciduae and from the amnion (Juul et al. 2001).

Epo is also present in colostrum and human milk in concentrations of 10–20 mU/mL, and Epo levels in milk do not correlate with Epo levels in the mother's blood (Juul 2000; Brace et al. 2006; Li et al. 2013). In fact, over the first weeks of lactation, mother's serum Epo concentrations fall, while her milk Epo concentrations increase, reaching the highest concentrations in women breastfeeding for a year or more. The source of Epo in breast milk is mammary gland epithelium (Juul 2000; Juul et al. 2000; Kling 2002).

Epo in human amniotic fluid, colostrum, and breast milk is relatively protected from proteolytic digestion in the fetal and neonatal gastrointestinal tract. However, rather than being absorbed from the gastrointestinal track into the blood, the Epo swallowed by the fetus and neonate binds to Epo receptors on the luminal surface of villous enterocytes, where it serves as an intestinal growth and development factor. Experimental animals artificially fed formulas devoid of Epo have retarded villous development, a condition that can be remedied by enteral recombinant Epo and blocked by anti-Epo antibody (Juul et al. 2001). Preliminary studies suggest that feeding recombinant Epo may protect preterm neonates from feeding intolerance and necrotizing enterocolitis (El-Ganzoury et al. 2014),

Epo is produced by cells in the developing central nervous system and is present in relatively high concentrations in fetal cerebrospinal fluid (CSF) (McPherson and Juul 2008; Dame et al. 2001; Fauchère et al. 2008; Juul et al. 1997, 1999). The highest concentrations of Epo in the CSF are in the most premature neonates, and by several years of age CSF Epo concentrations are typically <1 mU/mL (Juul et al. 1997). Epo receptors are expressed on human fetal neurons (Li et al. 1996; Juul et al. 1998a, b, 2004), and at least small quantities of recombinant Epo administered intravenously cross the blood-brain barrier and appear in the CSF (Juul et al. 2004; Nguyen et al. 2014). Epo is a neuroprotectant (Nguyen et al. 2014; Beirer et al. 2006; Fauchère et al. 2015). Its production increases rapidly in the brain during hypoxia, and when Epo binds to receptors on neurons, antiapoptotic activity is induced. The clinical utility of recombinant Epo as a neuroprotectant is a topic of current studies.

The liver is the primary site of fetal Epo production. The kidney produces only about 5% of the total Epo during midgestation. The mechanisms regulating the switch in Epo production from the liver to the kidney are not completely known but may involve developmental expression of transcription activators such as hypoxia-inducible factor and hepatic nuclear factor 4 (Ohls 2002a; Zhao et al. 2006) or developmental methylation of promoter and enhancer regions. Alternatively, the switch might involve the GATA transcription factors, particularly GATA-2 and GATA-3, which are negative regulators of Epo gene transcription.

94.4 Neonatal Reference Intervals for Erythrocytes

"Reference intervals" are used in neonatology in place of the "normal ranges" commonly used in adult medicine. The difference is reference intervals are constructed from selected clinically obtained laboratory tests, not from tests performed on healthy volunteers. In order to more closely approximate a normal range, the laboratory tests included in a neonatal reference interval include only patients with minimal pathology or with pathology not known to be related to the test under consideration. For instance, reference intervals for the hematocrit of neonates exclude data from neonates with clinical issues known to affect the hematocrit, such as recipients of red blood cell transfusions, those with a diagnosis of hemolytic disease, or those who have a diagnosis of anemia or polycythemia (Henry and Christensen 2015; Jopling et al. 2009; Christensen et al. 2009). Reference intervals for hematocrit and hemoglobin on the day of birth are shown in Fig. 1.

Fetal erythrocytes have features similar to "stress erythropoiesis" in adults. These include marked anisocytosis, poikilocytosis, macrocytosis, and the presence of nucleated erythrocytes. Marrow cellularity in the fetus is relatively high. Erythroid precursors account for 30–65% and myeloid cells 45–75% of nucleated marrow cells at birth (Christensen 2013). The myeloid to erythroid ratio at birth is approximately 1.5:1. Marrow cellularity decreases after birth, attaining a density that is normal for adults by 1–3 months. Initially, this decrease in cellularity results from a rapid decline in red cell production. At 1 week of age, erythroid elements account for only 8–12% of nucleated cells, and the myeloid to erythroid ratio exceeds 6:1. The normal adult proportion of myeloid to erythroid precursors is not established until the third month. Both the percentage and

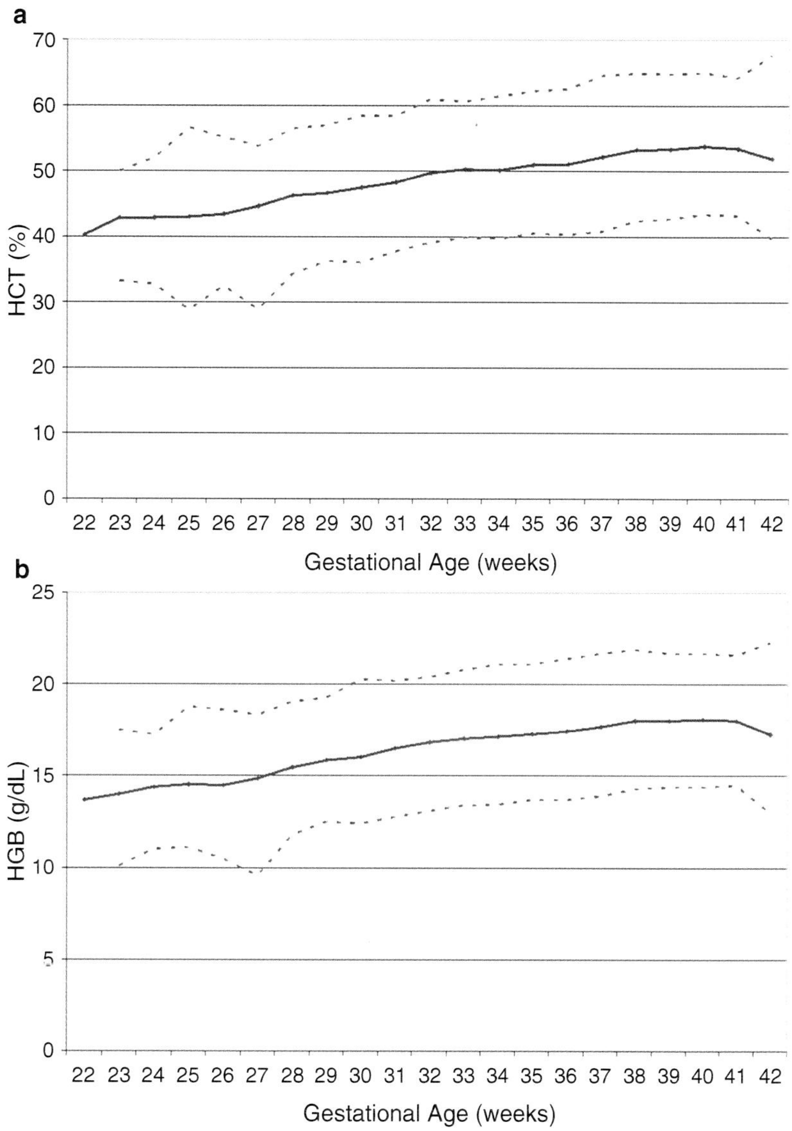

Fig. 1 Reference ranges for hematocrit (Panel **a**) and blood hemoglobin concentration (Panel **b**) on the day of birth. Values are given as a function of gestational age (From Jopling et al. 2009, with permission.) **Panel a** Hematocrit (HCT %) **Panel b** Hemoglobin (HGB g/dL)

absolute number of lymphocytes increase during the first 2 months, so that by 3 months of age they constitute nearly 50% of marrow nucleated cells. Differential counts of bone marrow aspirates from preterm infants are similar to those of term infants (Christensen 2013).

In newborn infants, the hemoglobin (Hb) concentration and hematocrit of capillary blood are 5–10% higher than those of venous blood (Christensen 2013). The difference between capillary and venous values is greatest at birth but largely disappears by 3 months of age. The discrepancy is greatest in preterm infants and in those with hypotension, hypovolemia, and acidosis (Oettinger and Mills 1949; Linderkamp 1977).

Reticulocytes at birth are approximately 5% of erythrocytes, with a range of 4–7% (Christensen 2013). Absolute reticulocyte counts during the first 90 days after birth, the immature reticulocyte fraction and the reticulocyte hemoglobin content during this period, are shown in Fig. 2.

Nucleated red blood cells (NRBC) are seen regularly on blood smears during the first day of

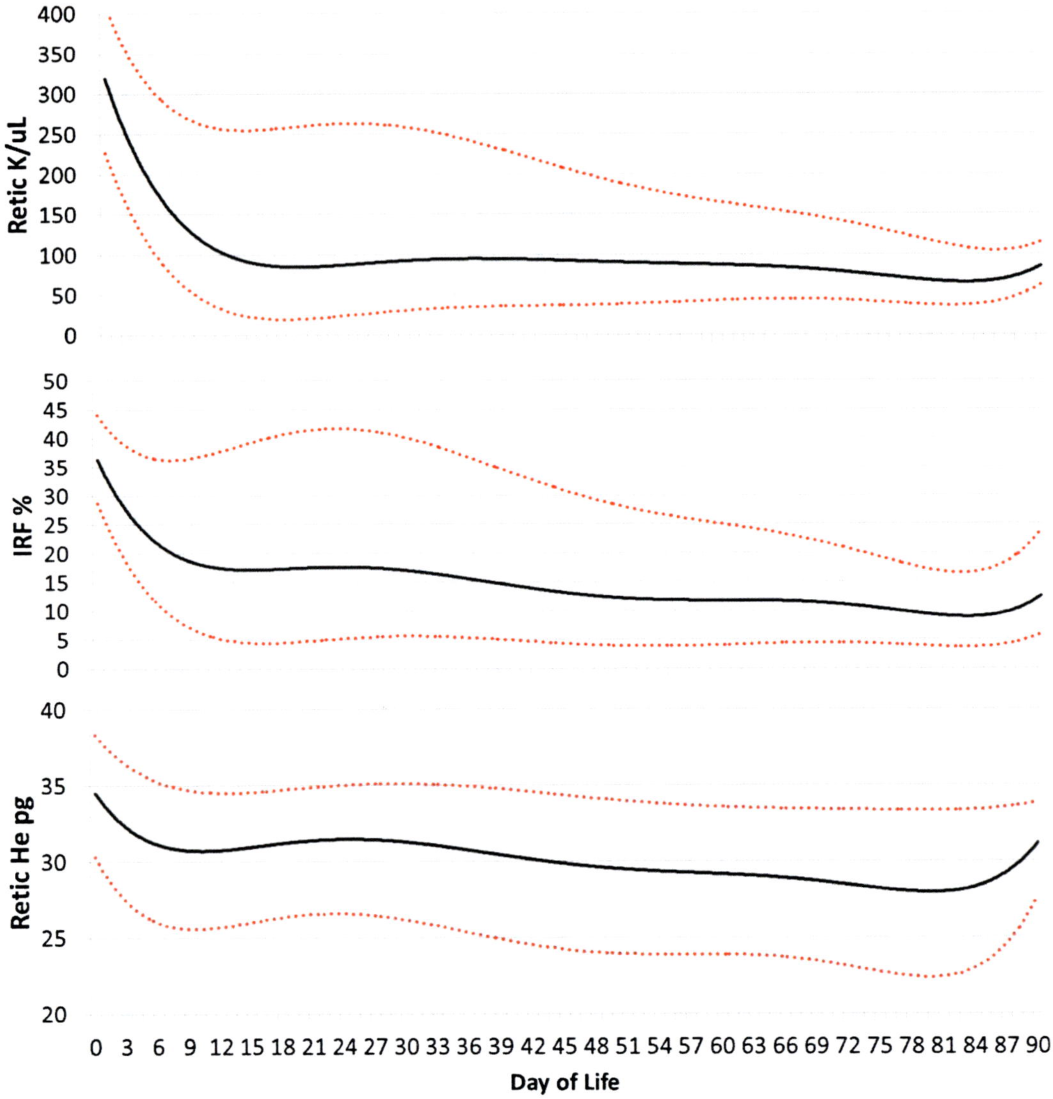

Fig. 2 Reference intervals for absolute reticulocyte count, immature reticulocyte fraction, and reticulocyte hemoglobin content during the first 90 days after birth

life, constituting about 0.1% of the red cell population (500 normoblasts/mm^3) (Christensen 2013; Buonocore et al. 1999; Perrone et al. 2005; Christensen et al. 2011), but are not common in the circulation after the first 3 days unless intermittent or chronic hypoxemia is present. Reference intervals for NRBC/μL blood, on the day of birth, according to gestational age, are shown in Fig. 3.

Red cell morphology is characterized by macrocytosis and poikilocytosis. Target cells and stomatocytes can be prominent. Similarly a high proportion of siderocytes (3.2% vs. normal adult mean of 0.1%) are seen (Zipursky 1983; Christensen et al. 2014a).

Measuring the circulating red blood cell volume in a fetus or neonate is challenging. Mock et al. used a nonradioactive method based on in vivo dilution of biotinylated RBC enumerated by flow cytometry to estimate the correlation between hematocrit and circulating RBC volume

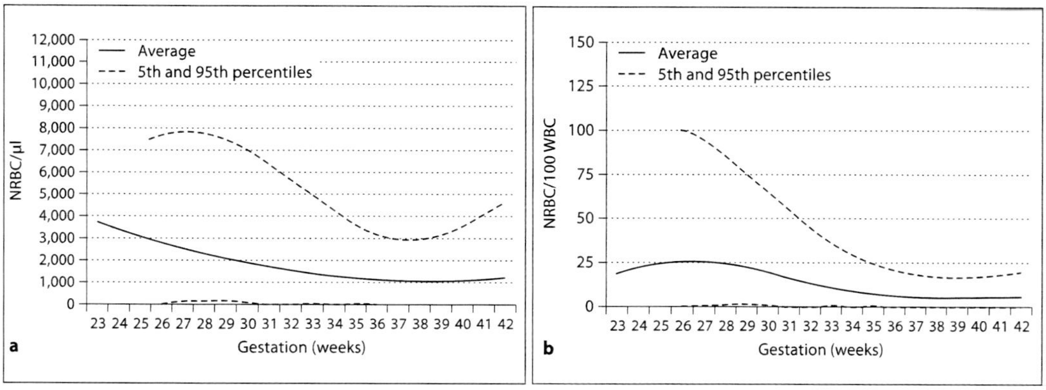

Fig. 3 Reference intervals for blood concentrations of nucleated red blood cells (*NRBC*) on the day of birth are displayed according to gestational age. In each panel, the *lower* and *upper lines* represent the 5th and 95th percentile limits and the *middle line* shows the median value. The *left* panel shows the data expressed as NRBC/μL blood and the *right* panel shows the data expressed as NRBC/100WBC (From Christensen et al. Neonatal reference ranges for blood concentrations of nucleated red blood cells. Neonatology 2010)

in infants below 1300 g. They found that venous hematocrit values correlated highly with the circulating erythrocyte volume ($r = 0.907; p < 0.0001$) (Mock et al. 2001; Strauss et al. 2003).

Neonates have a shorter red cell survival than do children and adults. The life span of red cells from term infants is estimated to be 60–80 days, using the ^{51}Cr method (Pearson and Vertrees 1961), and 45–70 days using methods involving ^{59}Fe (Pearson 1967). Fetal studies using [14C] cyanate-labeled red cells in sheep revealed an average red cell life span of 64 ± 6 days (Brace et al. 2000). The mean red cell life span increased linearly from 35 to 107 days as the fetal age increased from 97 days (midgestation) to 136 days (term). In a similar fashion, neonatal red cells transfused into adults have a short survival (Pearson 1967), indicating that factors intrinsic to the newborn red cell are responsible. This conclusion gains further support by the demonstration that adult red cells survive normally in newborn recipients (Brace et al. 2000). The life span frequency function is not parametrically distributed, in that most cells are destroyed before the mean survival is reached. Shortened red cell survival corresponds with erythropoietic rates at birth that are three to five times greater than those of normal adults.

The abrupt transition from the relative hypoxia of the uterus to an oxygen-rich environment triggers responses that have profound effects on erythropoiesis (Fig. 4). During the first 2 months of life, the infant has both the highest and the lowest Hb concentrations occurring at any time in development. Epo levels at birth are usually well above the normal adult range and fall in the immediate postnatal period (Ruth et al. 1990). By 24 h, the Epo value is below the normal adult range where it remains throughout the first month of life. The decrease in Epo is followed by a decline in the number of bone marrow precursors (Kling et al. 1996) and a fall in the reticulocyte count.

The fall in hemoglobin and hematocrit during the first days after birth occurs too rapidly to be explained by reduced red blood cell production alone and suggests an element of active, transient, mild hemolysis. The theory of a normal, physiological hemolysis during the first days after birth is supported by elevated exhaled carbon monoxide (CO) concentrations during the first week after birth. CO is released when heme is metabolized to bilirubin, and thus the higher exhaled CO levels initially suggest more rapid heme degradation during the first days to week (Maisels and Kring 2006; Christensen et al. 2015a).

The combination of initial physiological hemolysis, a shortened cell survival, decreased red blood cell production, and somatic growth with expansion of the blood volume is responsible for a progressive fall of the Hb concentration to a mean

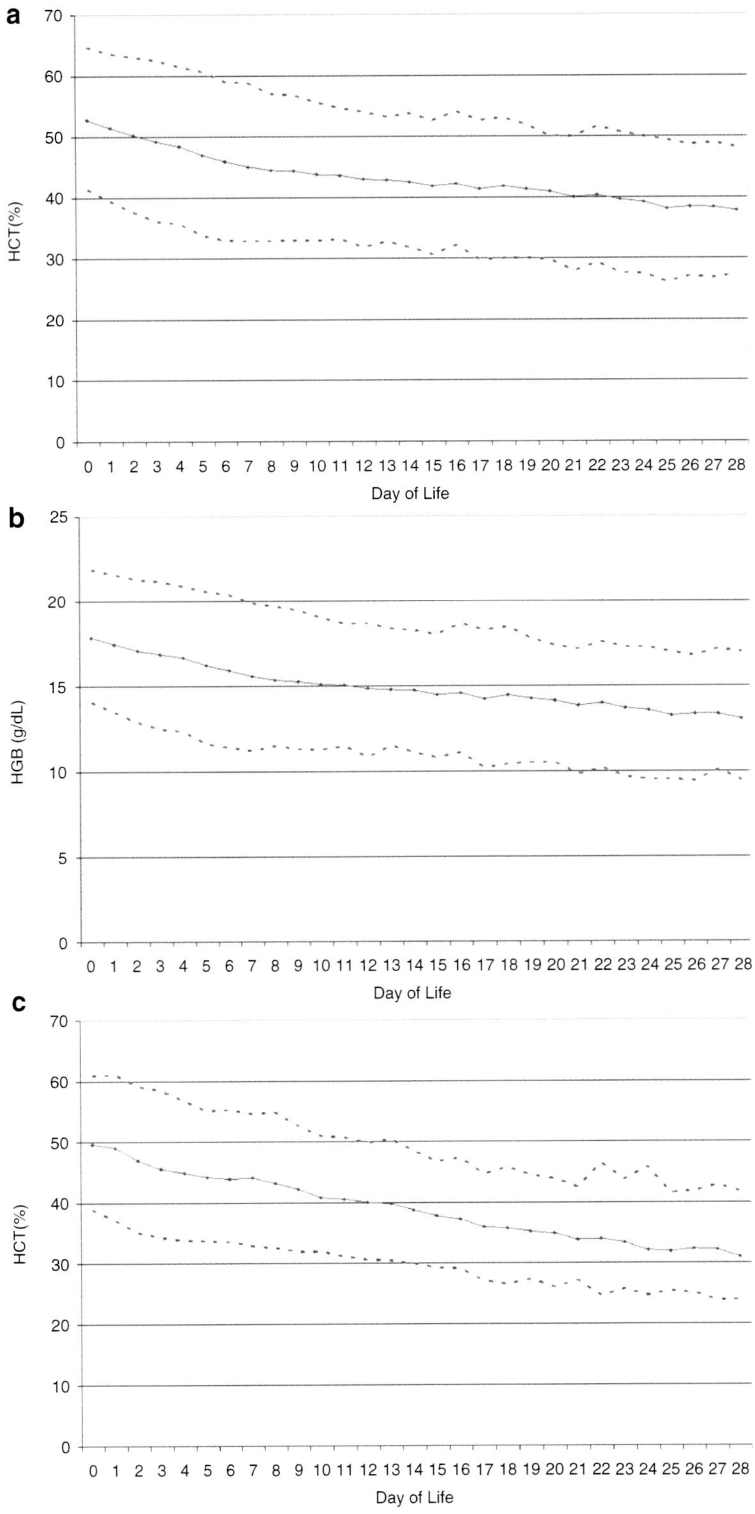

Fig. 4 (continued)

d

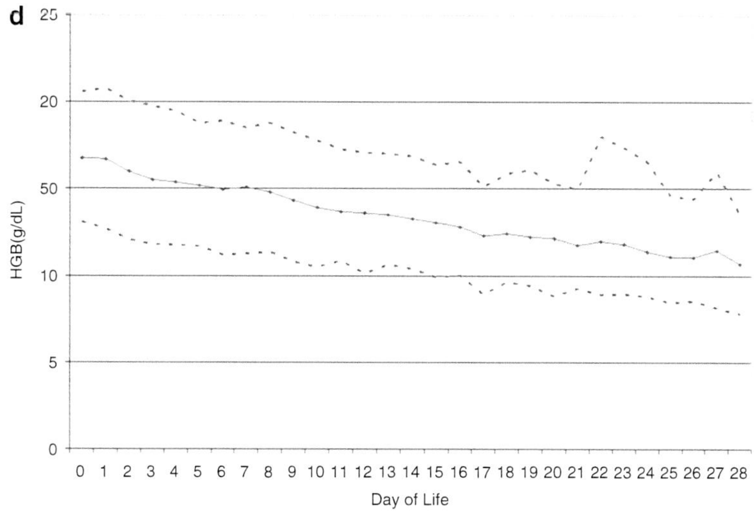

Fig. 4 Reference ranges for hematocrit and blood hemoglobin concentration during the first month after birth. Panel (**a**) shows hematocrit from late preterm and term neonates. Panel (**b**) shows hemoglobin from late preterm and term neonates. Panel (**c**) shows hematocrit from preterm neonates and Panel (**d**) shows hemoglobin from preterm infants (From Jopling et al. 2009, with permission). **Panel** (**a**) Hematocrit (HCT %) from late preterm and term neonates. **Panel** (**b**) Hemoglobin (HGB g/dL) from late preterm and term neonates. **Panel** (**c**) Hematocrit (HCT %) from preterm neonates. **Panel** (**d**) Hemoglobin (HGB g/dL) from preterm neonates

of approximately 11 g/dL at 2 months of age (Christensen 2013). The lower range of normal for infants of this age is approximately 9 g/dl. This nadir is called *physiologic anemia*, in that it is not associated with apparent distress and is not prevented with nutritional supplements. Stabilization of the Hb concentration is heralded by an increase in reticulocytes at 4–8 weeks. Thereafter, the Hb concentration rises to a mean level of 12.5 g/dL, where it remains throughout infancy and early childhood (Christensen 2013).

At term, the placenta and umbilical cord contain 75–125 mL of blood (30–40 mL/kg), or approximately one-fourth to one-third of the fetal blood volume. Umbilical arteries constrict shortly after birth, but the umbilical vein remains dilated, and blood flows in the direction of gravity. Infants held below the level of the placenta can receive half of the placental blood volume (30–50 mL, or 10–15 mL/kg) in 1 min. Some studies show that infants held above the placenta can lose 20–30 ml of blood back into the placenta per minute (Linderkamp 1978, 1992) but a more recent study from Argentina refutes this, reporting no effect of position on the volume of placental transfusion (Vain et al. 2014). The blood volume of infants with early cord clamping averages 72 ml/kg, whereas the volume of infants with delayed cord clamping averages 93 ml/kg.

Linderkamp et al. compared postnatal alterations in blood viscosity, hematocrit, plasma viscosity, red cell aggregation, and red cell deformability in the first 5 days of postnatal life in full-term neonates with early (less than 10 s) and late (3 min) cord clamping (Linderkamp 1978, 1992). The residual placental blood volume decreased from 52 ± 8 ml/kg of neonatal body weight after early cord clamping to 15 ± 4 ml/kg after clamping. The neonatal blood volume was 50% higher in the late cord-clamped infants.

Placental transfer of blood to preterm infants can occur by delayed clamping of the umbilical cord. Transfer of about 10 mL/k body weight can be expected by delaying clamping for 30–60 s and has been claimed to reduce intraventricular hemorrhage and late-onset sepsis (Aladangady et al. 2006; Mercer et al. 2006; Strauss et al. 2008). For very low birth weight (VLBW <1500 g) deliveries, delayed cord clamping or the somewhat more rapid alternative of umbilical cord milking can result in a higher 24 h hemoglobin and hematocrit and lower the risk of hypotension, early RBC

transfusion, and intraventricular hemorrhage (Baer et al. 2011a, b). Moreover, drawing all initial blood studies of VLBW neonates, on admission to the NICU, from otherwise discarded blood in the umbilical cord, after placental delivery, can result in a higher 24 h hemoglobin and hematocrit and lower the risk of initial hypotension (Christensen et al. 2014b; Baer et al. 2013).

94.4.1 Fetal and Neonatal Anemia Due to Abnormalities in the Erythrocyte Membrane or Cellular Metabolism

Neonates have erythrocyte membranes that differ slightly from those of adults (Ruef and Linderkamp 1999). The percentage of spectrin dimers are the same as in adult cells but neonatal cells have more immunoreactive myosin (Matovcik 1986). The quantity and distribution of lipids in neonatal red cells differ in several respects from adult red cells. Total lipids, phospholipid, and cholesterol are increased out of proportion to the surface area of newborn red cells (Linderkamp 1986).

Antigen expression in neonatal cells differs from that of adult cells. The A, B, S, and Lutheran antigens are present in lower amounts, membrane receptors for digoxin are 2.5 times that in adult red cells, and an increase in insulin receptors is also seen, possibly explainable by their larger surface area (Linderkamp 1986). Red cell deformability and viscoelastic properties are normal (Linderkamp 1986; Bautista et al. 2003), but the passage of newborn red cells through small pore filters is impaired as a result of larger size. Osmotic fragility of erythrocytes from preterm neonates is similar to or less than erythrocytes of term neonates.

Red cells of neonates have distinctive metabolic characteristics (Oski and Komazawa 1975; Oski and Smith 1968; Barretto et al. 1995). To some extent, these differences are explained by the young age and increased size of the red cells. The increase in activity of many of the glycolytic enzymes is comparable in magnitude to that observed in high-reticulocyte adult blood. Increased glycolytic enzyme activity is responsible for increased consumption of glucose and galactose and increased levels of adenosine triphosphate (ATP).

The concentration of 2,3-DPG falls rapidly during short periods of incubation (Soubasi et al. 2000), apparently because of accelerated breakdown. Preterm infants have lower 2,3-DPG concentrations than term infants. These concentrations gradually increase with gestation. Concentrations can be increased with the use of Epo, thereby shifting the oxygen dissociation curve to the right (van Zoeren-Grobben et al. 1997).

The activities of two key enzymes of the pentose phosphate pathway, glucose-6-phosphate dehydrogenase and 6-phosphogluconate dehydrogenase, are increased due to the young mean red cell age. The response of the pentose phosphate pathway to oxidant stimuli is normal, and the level of reduced glutathione is equal to or greater than that found in adults (van Zoeren-Grobben et al. 1997). However newborn cells have glutathione instability, increased Heinz body formation, and a propensity to increased methemoglobin generation, all indicative of greater susceptibility to oxidant-induced injury. Although red cells of the newborn infant have low levels of activities of both glutathione peroxidase and glutathione synthetase, no apparent relationship exists between these deficiencies and oxidant vulnerability.

Although elevated at birth, the red cell ATP level falls rapidly during short periods of incubation. The uptake of labeled orthophosphate by cord blood cells is slower than that by adult cells, resulting in delayed incorporation of phosphate into ATP and 2,3-DPG (Barretto et al. 1995; Soubasi et al. 2000).

Cord blood contains three types of Hb: HbF (α_2, γ_2), HbA (α_2, β_2), and HbA2 (α_2, δ_2). HbF constitutes the major fraction (50–85%). Because of this, hemoglobinopathies involving β-chain synthesis, such as sickle cell disease and β-thalassemia, are not problematic during the neonatal period. The G-γ to A-γ ratio at birth is approximately 3:1, in contrast to a ratio of 2:3 in adults (Bard 2000; Bard et al. 2001). HbA accounts for 15–40% of the Hb at birth. HbA2 is present in only trace amounts (mean, 0.3%) at birth, but it increases slowly after birth, reaching the normal adult level (2–3%) by 5 months of age.

Relative to values in adults, free erythrocyte protoporphyrin is high at birth and remains elevated through the first 6 months.

The level of HbF at birth is influenced by a number of variables, the most significant of which is gestational age. Premature infants have more HbF and postmature infants less (van Zoeren-Grobben et al. 1997). Neonates who have survived chronic intrauterine hypoxia have higher levels of HbF. Hemolytic disease is associated with lower levels of HbF. This association does not result from a difference in the synthetic ratios of β- and δ-globin chains, but rather relates to a younger population of red cells produced late in fetal life. The switch from γ-chain synthesis to β-chain synthesis is insensitive to environmental variables and appears to be developmentally programmed. Neither intrauterine transfusion nor neonatal exchange transfusion affects the synthetic rates of β- and δ-chains. Studies quantifying the specific globin mRNAs report that (G)gamma globin mRNA to total gamma globin mRNAs remains around 66% until the 44 week of postconceptual age, when a change in the (G) gamma and (A)gamma globin mRNA proportions occurred. Immature red cells of adults have a range of (G)gamma globin mRNA to total gamma globin mRNAs varying from 20% to 74%.

HbF has a higher affinity for oxygen than does HbA (Bard 2000). The oxygen tension at which the Hb of cord blood is 50% saturated is 19–21% mmHg, 6–8% mmHg lower than that of normal adult blood. This shift to the left of the Hb-oxygen dissociation curve results from poor binding of 2,3-DPG by HbF. The position of the oxygen dissociation curve is determined by both the percentage of HbA and the red cell content of 2,3-DPG. As the relative proportion of HbA increases, the oxygen dissociation curve shifts by approximately 4–6 months of age to the adult position. The increased oxygen affinity of HbF confers a physiologic advantage to the fetus in facilitating the transfer of oxygen from mother to fetus.

HbF is resistant to acid elution. Unlike HbA, HbF is not eluted from fixed blood smears immersed in an acid buffer (van Zoeren-Grobben et al. 1997). This property permits the differential staining of HbF and HbA, a technique used widely to study the distribution of HbF in red cells and to detect fetal cells in the maternal circulation, termed a Kleihauer-Betke stain.

When a neonate has Coombs negative hemolytic jaundice, considerations include an inherited disorder of erythrocyte membrane structure or erythrocyte metabolism. In neonates of Northern European ancestry with hemolytic jaundice in the first days of life and a negative Coombs test, hereditary spherocytosis (HS) or hereditary elliptocytosis (HE) should be considered (Christensen and Henry 2010; Christensen et al. 2014c, 2015b, c). HS has a prevalence estimate of about 1 case per 2000 births and HE about 1 case per 3000 births. Neonates with HS tend to have a large MCHC, as shown in Fig. 5 (Christensen et al. 2015b). When a neonate born to parents from Southeastern Asia has Coombs negative jaundice, a variety of HE called Southeastern Asian ovalocytosis should be considered. These disorders can be suspected by peripheral smear, noting the distinctive abnormalities of erythrocyte shape, and are confirmed by more specific testing, including EMF flow cytometry (Christensen et al. 2015c) or next-generation sequencing using a panel of potentially affected genes (Christensen et al. 2014c). See Table 1 and Fig. 6.

Programs to mass-screen neonates for hemoglobinopathies appear to be successful (Christensen et al. 2014d). For instance, during a 10-year evaluation in Brussels, over 100,000 neonates underwent screening for hemoglobinopathies. Sickle cell was identified in 64, 6 had beta-thalassaemia major, 4 had Hb C disease, and 3 had Hb H (Gulbis et al. 2006).

94.4.2 Fetal and Neonatal Anemia Due to Immune-Mediated Hemolytic Disease

Various causes of fetal and neonatal hemolytic disease are noted in Table 2. Fetal bilirubin is cleared by the placenta and metabolized by the maternal liver (Stevenson et al. 2004). As a result, fetal hemolytic disease does not typically present as severe jaundice at birth. However, after birth, the products of heme catabolism must be processed by the

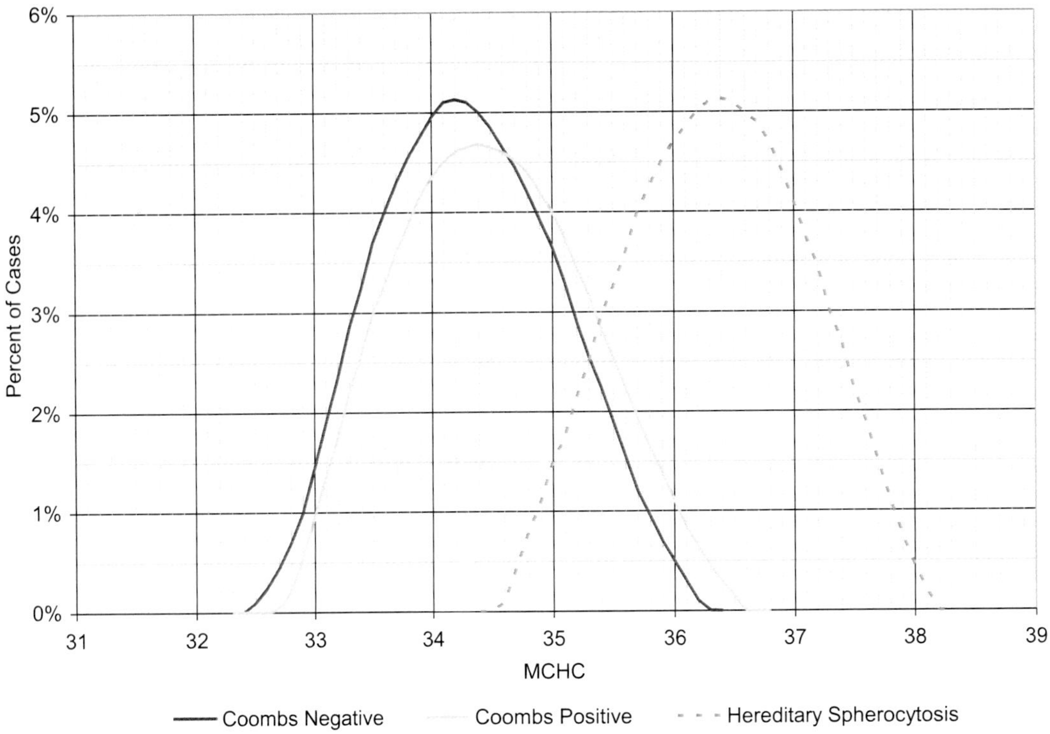

Fig. 5 Elevated mean corpuscular hemoglobin concentration in neonates with hereditary spherocytosis. The distribution of MCHC measurements is shown for three groups of neonates with hemolytic jaundice (**a**). Coombs negative jaundice, (**b**) Coombs positive jaundice, and (**c**) hereditary spherocytosis (From Christensen and Henry 2010, with permission)

Table 1 The more common varieties of Coombs negative neonatal hemolytic disease with abnormal erythrocyte shapes

Defect	*Disorder*	*Proportion with this variety*	*Inheritance*	*Severity*
Ankyrin	Spherocytosis	40–65%	Dominant	Mild to moderate
Band 3	Spherocytosis	20–35%	Dominant	Mild to moderate
	Southeast Asian ovalocytosis			
β-Spectrin	Spherocytosis	15–30%	Dominant	Mild to moderate
ά-Spectrin	Spherocytosis	<5%	Recessive	Severe
Protein 4.2	Spherocytosis	<5% (Japan)	Recessive	Mild to moderate
Protein 4.1	Elliptocytosis		Dominant	Mild to moderate

neonate's liver, which is limited in its ability to metabolize bilirubin efficiently. This limitation is due in part to a deficiency of the cytoplasmic acceptor protein ligandin and in part because of decreased activity of uridine diphosphoglucuronyl transferase (Stevenson et al. 2004; Bhutani et al. 2005).

Worldwide, isoimmunization caused by maternal-fetal blood group incompatibility is the most common cause of newborn hemolytic jaundice. Antigens in the Rh, ABO, MN, Kell, Duffy, and Vel systems are well developed on fetal red cells during early intrauterine life (Geifman-Holtzman et al. 1997). They are present in the fifth to seventh gestational week and remain through the remainder of intrauterine development. Other antigens, such as the Lutheran and XgA systems, develop more slowly but are present at birth, unlike Lewis antigens, which develop after birth. By

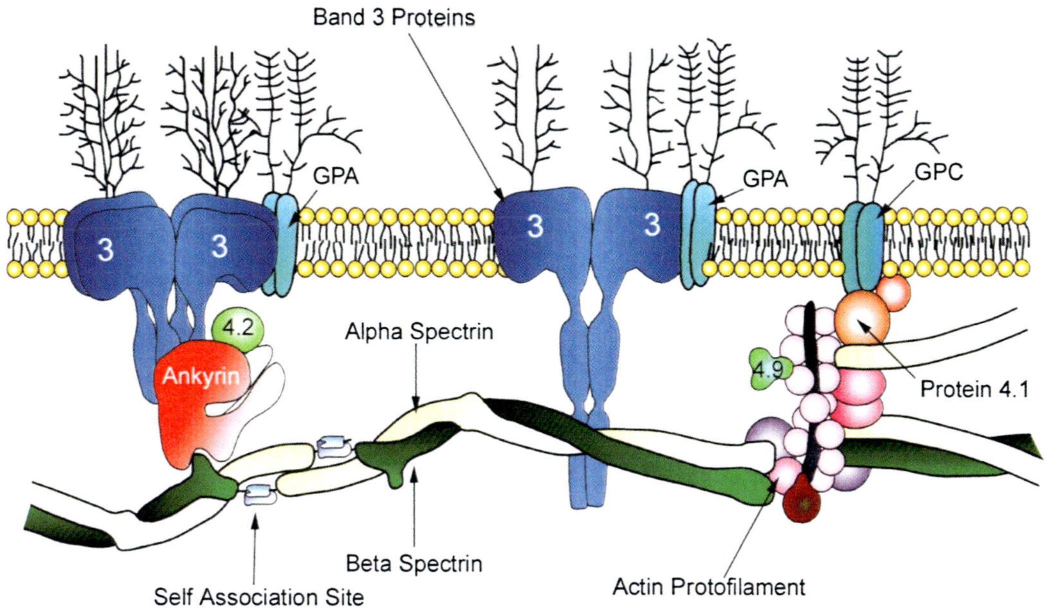

Fig. 6 A schematic drawing of the red cell membrane, noting the subunits described to have genetic defects as the basis for congenital abnormalities in erythrocyte shape, and predisposing to neonatal hemolytic jaundice (From Gallagher, PG. Disorders of erythrocyte metabolism and shape. In Hematologic Problems of the Neonate. Christensen RD editor, WB Saunders Co, 2000, with permission)

2 years of age, the red cell antigens have developed a pattern that is seen throughout the remainder of life (Geifman-Holtzman et al. 1997). Although A and B antigens are present early in utero, A and B isoagglutinin production occurs later during the second and third trimester (Lipitz et al. 1998). By 30–34 weeks' gestation, about one-half of all fetuses have measurable anti-A or anti-B antibodies.

Alloimmunization to Kell can present with unique neonatal findings. A low reticulocyte count can be seen along with a low Hb and elevated bilirubin (Weiner and Widness 1996). This is because anti-Kell antibodies can bind to erythroid progenitors and reduce red cell production (Vaughan et al. 1998).

Extremely high titers of anti-C antibody have been associated with neonatal hemolytic disease (Kozlowski et al. 1995). However, routine screening of anti-C titers during pregnancy is not warranted because antibody titers do not accurately reflect the severity of hemolytic disease (van Dijk et al. 1995; May-Wewers et al. 2006).

94.4.3 Fetal and Neonatal Anemia Due to Hemorrhage

Causes of hemorrhage resulting in fetal or neonatal anemia are noted in Table 3 and are divided into prenatal, perinatal, and postnatal varieties.

Prenatal Hemorrhage. Approximately 1 pregnancy in 400 is associated with fetal to maternal hemorrhage (FMH) of 30 ml or more, and 1 pregnancy in 2000 is associated with FMH of 100 ml or more (Kosasa et al. 1993). FMH consisting of small volumes of blood is very common. Perhaps as many as 75% of pregnancies can be shown to have 0.01–0.1 mL of fetal blood transferred into the maternal circulation. Transfer of fetal blood cells into the mother occurs during abortions as well. This has been reported in approximately 2% of spontaneous abortions and in 4–5% of induced abortions (Giacoia 1997).

The Kleihauer-Betke stain of maternal blood evaluates the acid elution of Hb from red cells (Huissoud et al. 2009). HbF resists acid elution to a greater degree than adult Hb. Therefore maternal cells appear clear (termed *ghost cells*), whereas any

Table 2 Causes of neonatal hemolytic disease

A. Immune mediated
1. Rh (anti-D) incompatibility
2. ABO incompatibility
3. Other blood group incompatibility – Duffy, Kell, Jka, MNS, Vw
4. Maternal autoimmune hemolytic anemia
B. Erythrocytes enzyme mutations
1. G6PD deficiency
2. Pyruvate kinase deficiency
3. Hexose kinase deficiency
4. Glucose phosphate isomerase deficiency
5. Pyrimidine 5′ nucleotidase deficiency
C. Erythrocyte membrane mutations
1. Hereditary spherocytosis
2. Hereditary elliptocytosis/ovalocytosis (Southeast Asian ovalocytosis)
3. Other membrane disorders
D. Infections
E. Hemoglobin defects
1. α-Thalassemia
2. γ-Thalassemia
F. Angiopathic hemolysis
1. Arterovenous malformations
2. Cavernous hemangiomas
3. Disseminated intravascular coagulation
4. Large vessel thrombosis
5. Severe valvar stenosis
G. Miscellaneous causes
1. Galactosemia
2. Hypothyroidism
3. Lysosomal storage diseases

Table 3 Causes of hemorrhage in the fetus and neonate

A. Prenatal
1. Twin-twin transfusion
2. Fetal maternal hemorrhage
3. Trauma with bleeding into cord, placenta, amniotic fluid
B. Perinatal
1. Placenta previa
2. Placental abruption
3. Vasa previa
4. Velamentous insertion of the umbilical cord
5. Nuchal cord
6. Trauma or incision of the cord or placenta during cesarean section
7. Rupture of the umbilical cord at delivery
C. Postnatal
1. Subgaleal hemorrhage
2. Cephalohematoma
3. Organ trauma after birth
4. Pulmonary hemorrhage
5. Intracranial hemorrhage
6. Iatrogenic blood loss

erythrocytes of fetal origin will appear pink. False-positive results occur when mothers have an increase in HbF (i.e., sickle cell disease, thalassemia, and hereditary persistence of HbF). Diagnosing FMH can also be difficult to detect when the mother is blood group O and the infant is A, B, or AB, because fetal cells are rapidly cleared from the maternal circulation by maternal anti-A or anti-B antibodies, and therefore they do not appear on the Kleihauer-Betke stain.

Severe FMH can be suspected before delivery by decreased fetal movements and a fetal sinusoidal heart rate pattern (Huissoud et al. 2009; Lopriore et al. 1995). Giacoia reviewed these variables to determine if they correlated with the severity of FMH (Giacoia 1997). Fetal movements for a period ranging between 24 h and 7 days were absent in 17 of 134 cases evaluated. In this group, six infants survived, five were stillborn, and five died in the neonatal period. A sinusoidal heart rate pattern was reported in 21 cases and was associated with decreased fetal movement in 40% of the cases. No significant difference was found between the cases with a hemorrhage of less than 200 ml and those less than 200 ml. Significant FMH has been described following maternal trauma (Huissoud et al. 2009). In a larger study from Intermountain Healthcare, we found an incidence of FMH of 1 case per 9160 live births, with 67% of affected neonates having an initial hemoglobin <7 g/dL (Christensen et al. 2012). Outcomes were poorer in those with the lowest initial Hgb, with death or major morbidities in 100% of those with an initial Hgb <5 g/dL, and in all who were born <35 weeks gestation (Christensen et al. 2012).

Neonates delivered after a significant FMH can be very pale, tachycardic, and tachypnec, but they generally do not have marked respiratory distress or a requirement for supplemental oxygen. Their Hb concentration can be as low as 4–6 g/dl and a

significant metabolic acidosis is often present in association with poor perfusion. Other causes of pallor can be ruled out once the infant is stable. Infants with asphyxia or chronic anemia due to hemolysis can also present with pallor. These diagnoses can be distinguished from acute hemorrhage based on differences in clinical signs and symptoms. With chronic blood loss, the signs of shock are usually absent. Asphyxiated infants are pale and floppy and may have poor peripheral circulation. The Hb will be stable, but may decrease if disseminated intravascular coagulation (DIC) and internal bleeding occur. Table 4 lists potential ways to improve the outcome after FMH.

Twin-twin transfusion is a complication of monochorionic twin gestations, occurring in 5–30% of these pregnancies (Dennis and Winkler 1997; Dommergues et al. 1995). It involves placental anastomoses that permit transfer of blood from one twin to the other. The perinatal mortality rate can be 70% or more. About 70% of monozygous twin pregnancies have monochorionic placentas. Although vascular anastomoses are present in almost all such, not all develop twin-twin transfusion.

Acute twin-twin transfusion generally results in twins of similar size but with Hb concentrations that vary by more than 5 g/dl (Dennis and Winkler 1997; Dommergues et al. 1995). In chronic twin-twin transfusion, the donor twin becomes progressively anemic and growth retarded, whereas the recipient twin becomes polycythemic, macrosomic, and sometimes hypertensive. Both can develop hydrops fetalis; the donor twin becomes hydropic from profound anemia, and the recipient twin from congestive heart failure and hypervolemia. The donor twin often has low amniotic fluid volumes, whereas the recipient twin has increased amniotic fluid, due to significant differences in blood volume, renal blood flow, and urine output.

Chronic twin-twin transfusion can be diagnosed by serial prenatal ultrasound measuring cardiomegaly, discordant amniotic fluid production, and fetal growth discrepancy of >20%. Percutaneous umbilical blood sampling can determine if Hb concentration differences of greater than 5 g/dl exist. After birth, the donor twin may require transfusions and can have neutropenia, hydrops from severe anemia, growth retardation, congestive heart failure, and hypoglycemia. The recipient twin is often the sicker of the two, with problems including hypertrophic cardiomyopathy, congestive heart failure, polycythemia, hyperviscosity, respiratory difficulties, hypocalcemia, and hypoglycemia. Neurologic evaluation and imaging are imperative because the risk of antenatally acquired neurologic cerebral lesions is 20–30% in both twins. The incidence of neurologic morbidity following the intrauterine death of one of the fetuses averages 20–25%. Morbidities include multiple cerebral infarctions, hypoperfusion syndromes from hypotension, and periventricular leukomalacia. Long-term neurologic follow-up is indicated for all survivors of twin-

Table 4 Recommendations for improving outcomes of neonates with anemia after fetomaternal hemorrhage (FMH)

Area of improvement	Potential means of improvement
Heightened suspicion of FMH by the obstetrical staff	When mother reports lack of fetal movements, consider FMH and perform nonstress test or biophysical profile. Consider FMH in such patients when non-reassuring fetal heart rate pattern is found
Availability of maternal blood testing for FMH using the Kleihauer-Betke or flow cytometric quantification of fetal erythrocytes in maternal blood	Provide FMH testing in all hospitals with a delivery service. Rapid reporting of positive results from laboratory directly to NICU attending
Rapid and clear communication by the obstetrical staff to the neonatal staff that FMH is being considered as a possible diagnosis	Prepare the neonatal staff for a possible case of FMH by communicating that this diagnosis is being considered by the obstetrical staff
Rapid involvement of the blood bank if emergency transfusion is likely	When a neonate has an initial hgb <10 g/dL and FMH is a consideration as the most likely cause, notify the blood bank immediately that emergency blood may be needed

twin transfusion (Dennis and Winkler 1997; Dommergues et al. 1995).

Prenatal treatment for twin-twin transfusion consists of close monitoring and reduction amniocenteses to decrease uterine stretch and prolong the pregnancy. Selective feticide of the hydropic twin has been advocated by some and has resulted in the survival of the healthier twin in some studies (De Lia et al. 1995). Treatment in utero has occurred during some pregnancies using laser ablation of bridging vessels, resulting in improved survival rates up to around 50%, with approximately 70% of the pregnancies having at least one survivor (Ville et al. 1995; van Heteren et al. 1998). However, the survival rate without morbidity in the surviving twin is approximately 50%. Supski et al. performed a meta-analysis of 140 cases to correlate types of treatment with outcome (Supski et al. 2002). They found no differences in outcome between amnioreduction, fetoscopy, septostomy, and close observation.

Perinatal Hemorrhage. Perinatal blood loss to the fetus can occur with various obstetric complications, such as placenta previa, placental abruption, incision or tearing of the placenta during cesarean section, and cord avulsion. When a fetus undergoes significant blood loss back into the placenta, the term *fetoplacental hemorrhage* is used. Placental anomalies such as a multilobed placenta and placental chorioangiomas can be a source of perinatal bleeding (Kramer et al. 1997).

Placental abruption occurs in 3–6 per 1000 live births. Risk factors of placental abruption include prolonged rupture of membranes, severe fetal growth restriction, chorioamnionitis, hypertension, maternal diabetes, cigarette smoking, and advanced maternal age (Kramer et al. 1997). The incidence of abruption increases with lower gestational age. Neonatal mortality rates from abruption range from 0.8 to 2.0 per thousand births, or 15–20% of the deliveries in which significant abruption occurs.

Women with a history of a previous cesarean birth and increased parity are at increased risk of placenta previa (McMahon et al. 1997), a condition where part or all of the placenta overlies the cervical os. Cigarette smoking is associated with a 2.6 to 4.4-fold increased risk of placenta previa (Chelmow et al. 1996). Prenatal diagnosis of vasa previa (anomalous vessels overlying the internal os of the cervix) can be made with transvaginal color Doppler and should be suspected in cases of antepartum or intrapartum hemorrhage. Although uncommon (1 in 3000 deliveries), the perinatal death rate is high, ranging from 33% to 100% when this condition is undetected before delivery (Chen and Konchak 1998).

Neonates delivered after placental abruption or after placenta previa can be anemic but they can also have signs of hypoxia and ischemia. The majority of blood lost in an abruption or previa is maternal blood, but the neonate can have some degree of anemia as well. Therefore, when perinatal blood loss is recognized or suspected, the neonate's Hb should be measured at birth and again 12 h or so later. A Kleihauer-Betke stain can be performed on maternal blood to determine if fetal hemorrhage can be documented. Monitoring bleeding mothers with ultrasound might detect placental abnormalities.

Cord rupture due to traction on a shortened or abnormal umbilical cord usually occurs on the fetal side. Cord aneurysms, varices, and cysts can all lead to a weakened cord. Cord infections (funisitis) can also weaken the cord and increase the risk of rupture. Infants born precipitously may be at increased risk for hemorrhage due to a ruptured cord.

Cord hematomas occur infrequently (1 per 5000–6000 deliveries) and can be a cause of fetal blood loss and perinatal mortality. Intrauterine death can occur due to compression of the umbilical vessels by a cord hematoma. Cord hematomas can result from trauma from percutaneous umbilical blood sampling. Hematomas of the cord can be diagnosed in utero by ultrasound (Chen and Konchak 1998; Deans and Jauniaux 1998).

Subamniotic hematomas can occur when chorionic vessels rupture near the cord insertion. Most subamniotic hematomas are the result of traction on a normal or shortened umbilical cord and are not noted until after delivery.

Velamentous insertion of the umbilical cord occurs when the umbilical cord enters the membranes distant from the placenta. This is present in 0.5–2.0% of pregnancies (Benirschke 1994).

Blood vessels left unprotected by Wharton jelly are more likely to tear. Rupture of anomalous vessels in the absence of traction or trauma can occur even if the cord itself attaches centrally or paracentrally. The fetal mortality remains very high in this condition, often because detection by routine ultrasound is rare (Eddleman et al. 1992).

Postnatal Hemorrhage. Loss of fetal blood into the placenta can occur during delivery. In fact, a net shift of blood from the fetus into the placenta is a rather common cause of low-grade neonatal anemia. At term, the fetal-placental-umbilical cord unit contains about 120 ml of blood per kg body weight. After delivery, but before the umbilical cord is severed, blood in this unit can flow predominantly toward or away from the neonate. A fetoplacental hemorrhage can probably occur when the neonate is held significantly higher than the placenta after birth. Also, neonates can lose up to 20% of their blood volume when born with a tight nuchal cord, which allows blood to be pumped through umbilical arteries toward the placenta, while constricting flow back from the placenta to the baby, through the umbilical vein, which is more easily constricted due to its thin wall.

As shown in Fig. 7, blood loss can occur into the subgaleal space before or after birth. This is seen most commonly with difficult deliveries requiring vacuum or forceps assistance. Subgaleal hemorrhages are potentially life-threatening and must be recognized as early as possible to prevent significant morbidity or mortality. The hemorrhage occurs when bridging veins are torn, allowing blood to accumulate in the large potential space between the galea aponeurotica and the periosteum of the skull. The subgaleal space extends from the orbital ridge to the base of the skull and can accommodate a volume equivalent to a neonate's entire blood volume (Kilani and Wetmore 2006; Uchil and Arulkumaran 2003).

Subgaleal hematomas can form because of risk factors such as coagulopathy or asphyxia, but vacuum extraction itself is a risk factor for their development. The diagnosis should be considered in the presence of a ballotable fluid collection in dependent regions of the infant's head, coupled with signs of hypovolemia (Teng and Sayre 1997). Treatment requires restoration of blood volume and control of bleeding. Exsanguination due to subgaleal hemorrhage has been reported. A suggested way to estimate the volume of blood lost is by following head circumference; 40 ml of blood has been lost for every 1 cm increase in head circumference that occurs (Chadwick et al. 1996). The duration of vacuum application is thought to be the best predictor of scalp injury, followed by duration of second stage of labor and paramedian cup placement. Of those with reported subgaleal hemorrhages, 80–90% had some history of

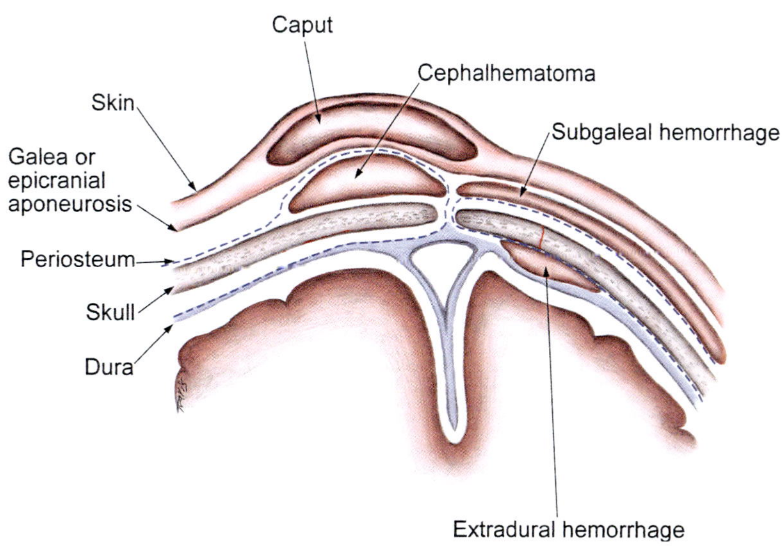

Fig. 7 A schematic drawing of the scalp and skull of a newborn infant, illustrating four distinct anatomic spaces where fluid or blood might collect during or after delivery: (1) caput, (2) cephalhematoma, (3) subgaleal hemorrhage, and (4) subdural hemorrhage (From E-Medicine, WebMD, Microsoft Corporation)

vacuum or instrument-assisted delivery (Teng and Sayre 1997; Chadwick et al. 1996). Limiting the frequency and duration of vacuum assistance in high-risk infants might decrease the incidence of subgaleal hematomas.

Anemia appearing after the first 24 h of life in a nonjaundiced infant can be a sign of hemorrhage. Hemorrhages can be visible, such as a cephalohematoma, or occult. Breech deliveries can be associated with renal, adrenal, or splenic hemorrhage into the retroperitoneal space. Delivery of macrosomic infants, such as infants born to diabetic mothers, can result in hemorrhage. Infants with overwhelming sepsis can bleed into soft tissue and organs.

In addition to causing anemia, adrenal hemorrhage can result in circulatory collapse due to the loss of organ function. The incidence of adrenal hemorrhage is 1.7 per 1000 births (Felc 1995). Adrenal hemorrhage can also affect surrounding organs. Intestinal obstruction and kidney dysfunction have been reported in infants with adrenal hemorrhage (Pinto and Guignard 1995). The diagnosis can be made using ultrasonography, during which calcifications or cystic masses are noted. Adrenal hemorrhage can be distinguished from renal vein thrombosis (RVT) by ultrasound, in that RVT generally results in a solid mass. Occasionally, both entities coexist in the same patient.

The liver of a neonate is prone to iatrogenic rupture, resulting in high morbidity and mortality (Davies 1997). Neonates with this problem can appear asymptomatic until the liver ruptures and hemoperitoneum occurs. This problem can occur in both term and preterm infants (Emma et al. 1992) and has been associated with chest compressions during cardiopulmonary resuscitation. Surgical intervention has been reported to save some infants but the mortality is very high (Emma et al. 1992).

Splenic rupture can result from birth trauma or as a result of distention caused by extramedullary hematopoiesis, such as that seen in erythroblastosis fetalis. Abdominal distension and discoloration, scrotal swelling, and pallor are clinical signs of splenic rupture; these can also be seen with adrenal or hepatic hemorrhage (Davies 1997; Emma et al. 1992; Miele et al. 1997).

More rare causes of hemorrhage in the newborn period include hemangiomas of the gastrointestinal tract (Nagaya et al. 1998), vascular malformations of the skin, and hemorrhage into soft tumors, such as giant sacrococcygeal teratomas. Occult intra-abdominal hemorrhage can occur with fetal ovarian cysts, which are usually benign and resolve spontaneously. One case of fetal anemia was diagnosed by a spontaneous hemorrhage into a fetal ovarian cyst and was managed by intrauterine blood transfusions (Abolmakarem et al. 2001).

94.4.4 Fetal and Neonatal Anemia Due to Congenital Infection

Neonatal bacterial sepsis can cause anemia on the basis of hemolysis, DIC, and hemorrhage. Some microorganisms responsible for neonatal sepsis produce hemolytic toxins that result in erythrocyte lysis, often associated with a microangiopathic process (Berkowitz et al. 1990).

Congenital viral infections can also cause hemolytic anemia. Congenital syphilis can present with hemolytic anemia. Initial maternal screening for syphilis can be negative despite overwhelming infection, a condition termed the *prozone effect* (Berkowitz et al. 1990), which occurs when a higher than optimal amount of antibody in the tested sera prevents the flocculation reaction seen in positive reagin test. In cases of nonimmune hydrops, nontreponemal testing should be repeated using serum dilutions to prevent a missed diagnosis of syphilis in women with negative syphilis serologic results.

Fetal and neonatal infection with parvovirus B19 can cause severe anemia, hydrops, and fetal demise (de Jong et al. 2006). This is generally a hypoplastic anemia, but hemolysis can occur as well. The virus replicates in erythroid progenitor cells and results in red cell aplasia. In utero transfusions for hydropic fetuses can be successful. Intrauterine fetal infusion of B19 IgG-rich high titer gamma globulin has been reported to be successful (Matsuda et al. 2005).

Other fetal infections associated with neonatal anemia include malaria and HIV. Congenital

malaria is seen rarely in the USA, generally in large cities where imported cases of malaria are increasing. In certain African countries, congenital malaria has been reported in up to 20% of neonates (Runsewe-Abiodun et al. 2006). Congenital HIV infection in a neonate is generally asymptomatic. However infants born to mothers on zidovudine can have a hypoplastic anemia due to suppressive effects of the drug on fetal erythropoiesis (Shah et al. 1996).

94.4.5 Anemia of Prematurity and Other Hypoproliferative Disorders

Impaired erythrocyte production can occur in a fetus or neonate for a variety of reasons. Lack of an appropriate or sufficient marrow environment (as seen in osteopetrosis), lack of specific substrates or their carriers (e.g., iron, folate, vitamin B_{12}, or transcobalamin II deficiency), and lack of specific growth factors (e.g., decreased Epo production or abnormalities in Epo receptors) can be causative.

Anemia of Prematurity. Infants delivered before 32 completed weeks of gestation typically develop a transient and unique anemia knows as the Anemia of Prematurity. During the first week or 2 after birth, while in an intensive care unit, anemia secondary to phlebotomy loss is common. However after this period has passed, a second anemia is sometimes seen, characterized as a normocytic, normochromic, hyporegenerative anemia, with serum Epo concentrations significantly below those found in adults with similar degrees of anemia (Brown et al. 1984). This anemia is not responsive to the administration of iron, folate, or vitamin E. Some infants with the anemia of prematurity are asymptomatic, whereas others have clear signs of anemia that are alleviated by erythrocyte transfusion. These signs include tachycardia, rapid tiring with nipple feedings, poor weight gain, increased requirements for supplemental oxygen, episodes of apnea and bradycardia, and elevated serum lactate concentrations.

The reason preterm infants do not significantly increase serum Epo concentration during this anemia is not known. Indeed, it is unclear whether production of Epo does in fact increase, yet the serum concentration does not. Certainly their erythroid progenitors are sensitive to Epo (Shannon et al. 1987; Rhondeau et al. 1988), and concentrations of other erythropoietic growth factors appear to be normal (Ohls et al. 1990).

The molecular and cellular mechanisms responsible for the anemia of prematurity remain undefined. Some explanations include the transition from fetal to adult Hb, shortened erythrocyte survival, and hemodilution associated with a rapidly increasing body mass (Donato 2005). It is unknown whether preterm infants rely on Epo produced by the liver (the source of Epo in utero), or that produced by the kidney, or a combination of the two. Regardless of the mechanism responsible for the anemia of prematurity, exogenous Epo administered to preterm infants accelerates effective erythropoiesis (Ohls 2002b). A meta-analysis of studies evaluating the use of “early” and the use of “late” Epo administration to prevent and treat the anemia of prematurity reveals a positive effect on decreasing transfusion requirements in preterm infants (Aher and Ohlsson 2014a, b). In addition, beneficial neurodevelopmental effects of recombinant Epo administration have been reported in preterm infants (Bierer et al. 2006; Ohls et al. 2004, 2014a, b, 2015; Juul 2004).

Pharmacokinetic studies of darbepoetin, the long-acting erythropoietic stimulator, have been conducted among neonates with the anemia of prematurity, with the speculation that less frequent dosing and cost savings might render darbepoetin a more attractive alternative than recombinant Epo for treating the anemia of prematurity (Warwood et al. 2005, 2006a, b; Patel and Ohls 2015). Following subcutaneous and intravenous dosing, darbepoetin has a considerably shorter terminal half-life in neonates than in adults (Table 5). Intravenous dosing appears to be as effective as subcutaneous dosing.

Other Hypoproliferative Anemias. During the neonatal period, hypoproliferative anemias are rare, with the exception of the anemia of prematurity, which is common (Table 6). Diamond-Blackfan syndrome can be diagnosed at

birth but usually is not recognized until after 2–3 months of age. At least 10–25% of infants with Diamond-Blackfan syndrome have anemia at birth (Gazda and Sieff 2006; Lipton and Ellis 2009), and severe anemia with hydrops has been reported. Aase syndrome, another congenital hypoplastic anemia syndrome involving skeletal anomalies (Aase and Smith 1969), is sometimes classified as a variant of Diamond-Blackfan syndrome. Congenital dyserythropoietic anemia is a rare disorder marked by ineffective erythropoiesis, megaloblastic anemia, and characteristic abnormalities of the nuclear membrane and cytoplasm seen on electron microscopy. Fanconi anemia is almost never manifest during the neonatal period. This autosomal-recessive disorder is characterized by marrow failure and congenital anomalies, including abnormalities in skin pigmentation, gastrointestinal anomalies, renal anomalies, and upper limb anomalies (Landmann et al. 2004).

Table 5 Terminal half-life of darbepoetin among adults, children, and neonates after subcutaneous or intravenous dosing

	After subcutaneous dosing	After intravenous dosing
Adults	49 h	25 h
Children	43 h	22 h
Neonates	22 h	10 h

Table 6 Syndromes associated with congenital anemia

Syndrome	Phenotypic features	Genotypic gestures
Adenosine deaminase deficiency	Autoimmune hemolytic anemia, reduced erythrocyte adenosine deaminase activity	AR, 20q13.11
Congenital dyserythropoietic anemias	Type I (rare), megaloblastoid erythroid hyperplasia and nuclear chromatin bridges between nuclei; type II (most common), hereditary erythroblastic multinuclearity, positive acidified serum (HEMPAS) test, increased lysis to anti-i; type III, erythroblastic multinuclearity ("gigantoblasts"), macrocytosis	Type I: 15q15.1-q15.3; type II: 20q11.2; type III: 15q21
Diamond-Blackfan syndrome	Steroid-responsive hypoplastic anemia, often macrocytic after 5 months of age	AR; sporadic mutations and AD inheritance described; 19q13.2, 8p23.3–p22
Dyskeratosis congenita	Hypoproliferative anemia usually presenting between 5 and 15 years of age	X-linked recessive, locus on Xq28; some cases with AD inheritance
Fanconi pancytopenia	Steroid-responsive hypoplastic anemia, reticulocytopenia, some macrocytic RBCs, shortened RBC life span. Cells are hypersensitive to DNA cross-linking agents	AR, multiple genes, complementation; group A: 16q24.3; B:; C: 9q22.3; D2: 3p25.3; E: 6p22-p21; F: 11p15; G: 9p13
Osler hemorrhagic telangiectasia syndrome	Hemorrhagic anemia	AD, 9q34.1
Osteopetrosis	Hypoplastic anemia from marrow compression; extramedullary erythropoiesis	AR, 16p13, 11q13.4-q13.5; AD: 1p21; lethal, reduced osteoclasts
Pearson syndrome	Hypoplastic sideroblastic anemia, marrow cell vacuolization	Pleioplasmatic rearrangement of mitochondrial DNA; X-linked or AR
Peutz-Jeghers syndrome	Iron deficiency anemia from chronic blood loss	AD, 19p13.3
X-linked α-thalassemia/mental retardation (ATR-X and ATR-16) syndromes	ATR-X, hypochromic, microcytic anemia; mild form of hemoglobin H disease ATR-16, more significant hemoglobin H disease and anemia are present	ATR-X, X-linked recessive, Xq13.3; ATR-16, 16p13.3, deletions of α-globin locus

AD autosomal dominant, *AR* autosomal recessive, *RBC* red blood cell

Osteopetrosis involves osteoclast dysfunction, resulting in a decreased marrow space (Charles and Key 1998; Fasth 2009). Developmental delay, ocular involvement, and neurodegenerative findings occur in these patients in association with hypoplastic anemia. Patients are generally treated with stem cell transplantation, but they are particularly susceptible to posttransplantation complications after myeloablation, and reduced-intensity conditioning programs may be helpful.

Pearson syndrome is a congenital hyporegenerative anemia that can progress to pancytopenia and additionally affects the exocrine pancreas, liver, and kidneys (Pearson et al. 1979). These patients can present during the neonatal period, but typically do so later in infancy. Features include failure to thrive and cytopenia. The marrow examination shows characteristic vacuoles within erythroid and myeloid precursors, hemosiderosis, and ringed sideroblasts. The syndrome is caused by a loss of large segments of mitochondrial DNA (van den Ouweland et al. 2000; Manea et al. 2009).

94.5 Considerations for Erythrocyte Transfusion

The best practices in neonatal transfusion medicine are only beginning to be defined (Widness et al. 2005). Methods of preventing early anemia in very low birth weight (VLBW) neonates have been tested, such as delayed clamping of the umbilical cord or umbilical cord milking (stripping) and drawing the initial laboratory blood studies of VLBW infants using otherwise discarded blood in the umbilical cord, not directly from the neonate (Bell et al. 2005). Guidelines to reduce phlebotomy losses of VLBW neonates, and the selected use of erythropoiesis-stimulating agents, have also been favorably tested as complementary anemia prevention approaches. Each of these strategies will be reviewed briefly below.

One very basic issue that remains unsettled is at what level to keep the Hb concentration during the NICU stay. It is not clear whether to keep a NICU patient's Hb as high as it would be in utero (often requiring multiple transfusions to do so) or whether to permit it to fall to considerably lower values, attempting to avoid or minimize transfusions. Attempts have been made to define the best Hb range for NICU patients, but study findings are discordant. In a single-centered study, Bell et al. randomized 100 neonates with birth weights <1300 g (average birth weight 956 g) to maintain a hematocrit in a "higher range" versus in a "lower range." Those kept in the lower range received fewer transfusions (average of 2/additional transfusions per patient), but were more likely to have intraparenchymal brain hemorrhage or periventricular leukomalacia (Kirpalani et al. 2006). In contrast, the Premature Infants in Need of Transfusion study (PINT), a larger multicentered study involving 451 extremely low birth weight neonates (average birth weight 770 g), concluded that neonates randomized to the lower hematocrit range had fewer transfusions but similar neurodevelopmental outcomes (Whyte et al. 2009). Longer-term follow-up of the Iowa cohort indicated that the restricted transfusion strategy resulted in better neurodevelopmental outcomes (Nopoulos et al. 2011; McCoy et al. 2011).

Various neonatal transfusion guidelines have been used over the last two decades, and research is ongoing to determine the optimal strategy for administering red cell transfusions to preterm and term neonates. The strategy developed by the University of Utah and Intermountain Healthcare is shown in Table 7. When considering a transfusion in a preterm infant with a low hematocrit, it should be determined if the infant needs an immediate increase in oxygen delivery to tissues. If so, then treatment consists of a transfusion of packed red cells. If there is no evidence that an immediate increase in oxygen delivery is necessary, then treatment with erythropoiesis-stimulating agents might be considered. As the process of stimulating erythropoiesis requires at least a week to significantly impact the reticulocyte count, and may not appreciably increase the hemoglobin concentration during that time, the infant should continue to be observed for signs consistent with anemia.

A method of reducing erythrocyte transfusions, among a subset of preterm neonatal patients, is to begin the administration of recombinant Epo or Darbepoetin to those with low hematocrits after

Table 7 Intermountain healthcare/university of Utah guidelines for red blood cell transfusions for newborn infants

Condition	Indication	Treatment
ECMO, cyanotic heart disease, PPHN	Hgb <12 g/dL or Hct <36%	15–20 mL/kg over 2–4 h
Ventilator or CPAP	Hgb <10 g/dL or Hct <30%	
Supplemental O2	Hgb <8 g/dL or Hct <24%	
Stable in room air	Hgb <7 g/dL or Hct <21%	

These guidelines provide an "indication" where transfusions are generally thought to have benefits outweighing risks. The guidelines do not mandate that a transfusion *must* be ordered for all neonates with this "indication"; rather, the guidelines are intended as reminders to *consider* a transfusion under those circumstances. Any order for blood products should always be accompanied by a note in the medical record stating the clinical reason for the transfusion

the first 3 weeks of life (Ohls et al. 2009, 2013, 2014a, b; Patel and Ohls 2015). Recombinant Epo certainly stimulates erythropoiesis in such patients, although its combination with additional folate, iron, vitamin E, and vitamin B_{12} may be superior to recombinant Epo alone. Haiden and colleagues achieved significantly greater success in preterm infants <800 g (38% of infants not transfused) when vitamin B_{12} at a dose of 21 mg/kg/week SC was added to a regimen of Epo, iron, vitamin E, and folate (Haiden et al. 2006). When combined with limited phlebotomy losses, this therapy shows great promise in ELBW infants.

Another method of reducing erythrocyte transfusions to ill neonates is to delay clamping the umbilical cord. Even a delay of 30 s can result in improved iron status, fewer transfusions, and perhaps superior neurodevelopmental outcomes (Christensen et al. 2014d, e; Rabe et al. 2004, 2009). Yet another method of reducing or postponing early erythrocyte transfusions among extremely low birth weight neonates is to draw the blood for the initial laboratory tests from the placenta not from the neonate (Baer et al. 2013). The initial phlebotomy of an extremely low birth weight neonate, on admission to the NICU, can include a blood culture, CBC, type and cross-match, metabolic screen, blood gas, electrolytes, and glucose. Sometimes other studies such as coagulation tests are also drawn at or shortly following NICU admission. The total blood volume needed for these baseline NICU laboratory studies can be 4–5 mL or more. In a 400–500 g neonate, this can exceed 10% of the total blood volume.

Early transfusions in the NICU can be reduced by careful attention to phlebotomy volumes during the first days following delivery. Transfusions given during the first week or 2 are principally to replace phlebotomy losses for laboratory tests. Employing laboratory methods that minimize blood loss will reduce early transfusions. Such methods include point of care monitors, point of care analyzers, and a concerted effort to use the smallest amount of blood possible for the needed laboratory studies (Christensen et al. 2014d; Widness et al. 2005; Henry et al. 2015).

References

Aase JM, Smith DW (1969) Congenital anemia and triphalangeal thumbs: a new syndrome. J Pediatr 74:471–474

Abolmakarem H, Tharmaratnum S, Thilaganathan B (2001) Fetal anemia as a consequence of hemorrhage into an ovarian cyst. Ultrasound Obstet Gynecol 17:527–528

Aher SM, Ohlsson A (2014a) Early versus late erythropoietin for preventing red blood cell transfusion in preterm and/or low birth weight infants. Cochrane Database Syst Rev 4:CD004863

Aher SM, Ohlsson A (2014b) Late erythropoietin for preventing red blood cell transfusion in preterm and/or low birth weight infants. Cochrane Database Syst Rev 9:CD004868

Aladangady N, McHugh S, Aitchison TC et al (2006) Infant's blood volume in a controlled trial of placental transfusion at preterm delivery. Pediatrics 117:93–98

Baer VL, Lambert DK, Henry E, Snow GL, Butler A, Christensen RD (2011a) Among very-low-birth-weight neonates is red blood cell transfusion an independent risk factor for subsequently developing a severe intraventricular hemorrhage? Transfusion 51:1170–1178

Baer VL, Lambert DK, Henry E, Snow GL, Christensen RD (2011b) Red blood cell transfusion of preterm neonates with a Grade 1 intraventricular hemorrhage is associated with extension to a Grade 3 or 4 hemorrhage. Transfusion 51:1933–1939

Baer VL, Lambert DK, Carroll PD, Gerday E, Christensen RD (2013) Using umbilical cord blood for the initial

blood tests of VLBW neonates results in higher hemoglobin and fewer RBC transfusions. J Perinatol 33: 363–365

Bard H (2000) Fetal and neonatal hemoglobin structure and function. In: Christensen RD (ed) Hematologic problems of the neonate. WB Saunders, Philadelphia

Bard H, Peri KG, Gagnon C (2001) Changes in the G gamma- and A gamma-globin mRNA components of fetal hemoglobin during human development. Biol Neonate 80:26–29

Barretto OC, Nonoyama K, Deutsch AD, Ramos J (1995) Physiological red cell, 2,3-diphosphoglycerate increase by the sixth hour after birth. J Perinat Med 23:365–369

Bautista ML, Altaf W, Lall R, Wapnir RA (2003) Cord blood red cell osmotic fragility: a comparison between preterm and full-term newborn infants. Early Hum Dev 72:37–46

Beirer R, Peceny MC, Hartenberger CH, Ohls RK (2006) Erythropoietin concentrations and neurodevelopmental outcome in preterm infants. Pediatrics 118:635–640

Bell EF, Strauss RG, Widness JA et al (2005) Randomized trial of liberal versus restrictive guidelines for red blood cell transfusion in preterm infants. Pediatrics 115: 1685–1691

Benirschke K (1994) Obstetrically important lesions of the umbilical cord. J Reprod Med 39:262–272

Berkowitz K, Baxi L, Fox HE (1990) False-negative syphilis screening: the prozone phenomenon, nonimmune hydrops, and diagnosis of syphilis during pregnancy. Am J Obstet Gynecol 163:975–977

Bhutani VK, Donn SM, Johnson LH (2005) Risk management of severe neonatal hyperbilirubinemia to prevent kernicterus. Clin Perinatol 32:125–139

Bierer R, Peceny MC, Hartenberger CH, Ohls RK (2006) Erythropoietin concentrations and neurodevelopmental outcome in preterm infants. Pediatrics 118:e635–e640

Brace RA, Langendorfer C, Song TB, Mock DM (2000) Red blood cell life span in the ovine fetus. Am J Physiol Regul Integr Comp Physiol 279:R1196–R1204

Brace RA, Cheung CY, Davis LE, Gagnon R, Harding R, Widness JA (2006) Sources of amniotic fluid erythropoietin during normoxia and hypoxia in fetal sheep. Am J Obstet Gynecol 195:246–254

Brown MS, Garcia JF, Phibbs RH et al (1984) Decreased response of plasma immunoreactive erythropoietin to "available oxygen" in anemia of prematurity. J Pediatr 105:793–798

Buonocore G, Perrone S, Gioia D et al (1999) Nucleated red blood cell count at birth as an index of perinatal brain damage. Am J Obstet Gynecol 181:1500–1505

Chadwick LM, Pemberton PJ, Kurinczuk JJ (1996) Neonatal subgaleal haematoma: associated risk factors, complications and outcome. J Paediatr Child Health 32:228–232

Charles JM, Key LL (1998) Developmental spectrum of children with congenital osteopetrosis. J Pediatr 132: 371–374

Chelmow D, Andrew DE, Baker ER (1996) Maternal cigarette smoking and placenta previa. Obstet Gynecol 87(5 Pt 1):703–706

Chen KH, Konchak P (1998) Use of transvaginal color Doppler ultrasound to diagnose vasa previa. J Am Osteopath Assoc 98:116–117

Christensen RD (2013) Reference ranges in neonatal hematology. In: deAlarcon PA, Werner EJ, Christensen RD (eds) Neonatal hematology, 2nd edn. Cambridge, UK: Cambridge University Press, pp 404–406

Christensen RD, Henry E (2010) Hereditary spherocytosis in neonates with hyperbilirubinemia. Pediatrics 125: 120–125

Christensen RD, Henry E, Jopling J, Wiedmeier SE (2009) The CBC: reference ranges for neonates. Semin Perinatol 33:3–11

Christensen RD, Henry E, Andres RL, Bennett ST (2011) Reference ranges for blood concentrations of nucleated red blood cells in neonates. Neonatology 99:289–294

Christensen RD, Lambert DK, Baer VL, Richards DS, Bennett ST, Ilstrup SJ, Henry E (2012) Severe neonatal anemia from fetomaternal hemorrhage: report from a multihospital health-care system. J Perinatol 33:429–434

Christensen RD, Yaish HM, Lemons RS (2014a) Neonatal hemolytic jaundice: morphologic features of erythrocytes that will help you diagnose the underlying condition. Neonatology 105:243–924

Christensen RD, Baer VL, Lambert DK, Ilstrup SJ, Eggert LD, Henry E (2014b) Association, among very-low-birthweight neonates, between red blood cell transfusions in the week after birth and severe intraventricular hemorrhage. Transfusion 54:104–108

Christensen RD, Nussenzveig RH, Yaish HM, Henry E, Eggert LD, Agarwal AM (2014c) Causes of hemolysis in neonates with extreme hyperbilirubinemia. J Perinatol 34:616–619

Christensen RD, Carroll PD, Josephson CD (2014d) Evidence-based advances in transfusion practice in neonatal intensive care units. Neonatology 106. 245–253

Christensen RD, Baer VL, Gerday E, Sheffield MJ, Richards DS, Shepherd JG, Snow GL, Bennett ST, Frank EL, Oh W (2014e) Whole-blood viscosity in the neonate: effects of gestational age, hematocrit, mean corpuscular volume and umbilical cord milking. J Perinatol 34:16–21

Christensen RD, Lambert DK, Henry E, Yaish HM, Prchal JT (2015a) End-tidal carbon monoxide as an indicator of the hemolytic rate. Blood Cells Mol Dis 54:292–296

Christensen RD, Yaish HM, Gallagher PG (2015b) A pediatrician's practical guide to diagnosing and treating hereditary spherocytosis in neonates. Pediatrics 135: 1107–1114

Christensen RD, Agarwal AM, Nussenzveig RH, Heikal N, Liew MA, Yaish HM (2015c) Evaluating eosin-5-maleimide binding as a diagnostic test for hereditary spherocytosis in newborn infants. J Perinatol 35:357–361

Dame C, Juul SE, Christensen RD (2001) The biology of erythropoietin in the central nervous system and its

neurotrophic and neuroprotective potential. Biol Neonate 79:228–235
Davies MR (1997) Iatrogenic hepatic rupture in the newborn and its management by pack tamponade. J Pediatr Surg 32:1414–1419
de Jong EP, de Haan TR, Kroes AC (2006) Parvovirus B19 infection in pregnancy. J Clin Virol 36:1–7
De Lia JE, Kuhlmann RS, Harstad TW et al (1995) Fetoscopic laser ablation of placental vessels in severe previable twin-twin transfusion syndrome. Am J Obstet Gynecol 172(4 Pt 1):1202–1208
Deans A, Jauniaux E (1998) Prenatal diagnosis and outcome of subamniotic hematomas. Ultrasound Obstet Gynecol 11:319–323
Dennis LG, Winkler CL (1997) Twin-to-twin transfusion syndrome: aggressive therapeutic amniocentesis. Am J Obstet Gynecol 177:342–347
Dommergues M, Mandelbrot L, Delezoide AL et al (1995) Twin-to-twin transfusion syndrome: selective feticide by embolization of the hydropic fetus. Fetal Diagn Ther 10:26–31
Donato H (2005) Erythropoietin: an update on the therapeutic use in newborn infants and children. Expert Opin Pharmacother 6:723–734
Eddleman KA, Lockwood CJ, Berkowitz GS et al (1992) Clinical significance and sonographic diagnosis of velamentous umbilical cord insertion. Am J Perinatol 9:123–126
El-Ganzoury MM, Awad HA, El-Farrash RA, El-Gammasy TM, Ismail EA, Mohamed HE, Suliman SM (2014) Enteral granulocyte-colony stimulating factor and erythropoietin early in life improves feeding tolerance in preterm infants: a randomized controlled trial. J Pediatr 165:1140–1145
Emma F, Smith J, Moerman PH (1992) Subcapsular hemorrhage of the liver and hemoperitoneum in premature infants: report of 4 cases. Eur J Obstet Gynecol Reprod Biol 44:161–164
Fasth A (2009) Osteopetrosis – more than only a disease of the bone. Am J Hematol 84:469–470
Fauchère JC, Dame C, Vonthein R et al (2008) An approach to using recombinant erythropoietin for neuroprotection in very preterm infants. Pediatrics 122:375–382
Fauchère JC, Koller BM, Tschopp A, Dame C, Ruegger C, Bucher HU, Swiss Erythropoietin Neuroprotection Trial Group (2015) Safety of early high-dose recombinant erythropoietin for neuroprotection in very preterm infants. J Pediatr. https://doi.org/10.1016/j.jpeds.2015.02.052
Felc Z (1995) Ultrasound in screening for neonatal adrenal hemorrhage. Am J Perinatol 12:363–366
Gazda HE, Sieff CA (2006) Recent insights into the pathogenesis of Diamond-Blackfan anaemia. Br J Haematol 135:149–157
Geifman-Holtzman O, Wojtowycz M, Kosmos E et al (1997) Female alloimmunization with antibodies known to cause hemolytic disease. Obstet Gynecol 89:272–275
Giacoia GP (1997) Severe fetomaternal hemorrhage: a review. Obstet Gynecol Surv 52:372–380
Gulbis B, Ferster A, Cotton F (2006) Neonatal haemoglobinopathy screening: review of a 10-year programme in Brussels. J Med Screen 13:76–78
Haiden N, Klebermass K, Cardona F (2006) A randomized, controlled trial of the effects of adding vitamin B12 and folate to erythropoietin for the treatment of anemia of prematurity. Pediatrics 118:180–188
Henry E, Christensen RD (2015) Reference intervals for CBC parameters of neonates. Clin Perinatol 42:3
Henry E, Christensen RD, Sheffield MJ, Eggert LD, Carroll PD, Minton SD, Lambert DK, Ilstrup SJ (2015) Why do four NICUs using identical RBC transfusion guidelines have different gestational age-adjusted RBC transfusion rates? J Perinatol 35:132–136
Huissoud C, Divry V, Dupont C et al (2009) Large fetomaternal hemorrhage: prenatal predictive factors for perinatal outcome. Am J Perinatol 26:227–233
Jopling J, Henry E, Wiedmeier SE, Christensen RD (2009) Reference ranges for hematocrit and blood hemoglobin concentration during the neonatal period: data from a multihospital health care system. Pediatrics 123: e333–e337
Juul SE (2000) Nonerythropoietic roles of erythropoietin in the fetus and neonate. Clin Perinatol 27:527–541
Juul SE (2004) Recombinant erythropoietin as a neuroprotective treatment: in vitro and in vivo models. Clin Perinatol 31:129–142
Juul SJ, Li Y, Christensen RD (1997) Erythropoietin is present in the cerebrospinal fluid of neonates. J Pediatr 130:428–433
Juul SJ, Li Y, Anderson DK, Christensen RD (1998a) Erythropoietin and erythropoietin receptor in the developing human central nervous system. Pediatr Res 43:40–47
Juul SE, Yachnis AT, Christensen RD (1998b) Tissue distribution of erythropoietin and erythropoietin receptor in the developing human fetus. Early Hum Dev 52:235–239
Juul SE, Stallings SA, Christensen RD (1999) Erythropoietin in the cerebrospinal fluid of neonates who sustained CNS injury. Pediatr Res 46:543–548
Juul SE, Zhao Y, Dame JB et al (2000) Origin and fate of erythropoietin in human milk. Pediatr Res 48: 600–607
Juul SE, Ledbetter DJ, Joyce AE et al (2001) Erythropoietin acts as a trophic factor in neonatal rat intestine. Gut 49:182–189
Juul SE, McPherson RJ, Farrell F et al (2004) Erythropoietin concentrations in cerebrospinal fluid of nonhuman primates and fetal sheep following high-dose recombinant erythropoietin. Biol Neonate 85:138–144
Kilani RA, Wetmore J (2006) Neonatal subgaleal hematoma: presentation and outcome – radiological findings and factors associated with mortality. Am J Perinatol 23:41–48
Kirpalani H, Whyte RK, Andersen C et al (2006) The Premature Infants in Need of Transfusion (PINT) study: a randomized, controlled trial of a restrictive (low) versus liberal (high) transfusion threshold for

extremely low birth weight infants. J Pediatr 149:301–307

Kling PJ (2002) Roles of erythropoietin in human milk. Acta Paediatr Suppl 91:31–35

Kling PJ (2013) Anemia of prematurity and erythropoietin therapy. In: de Alarcon PA, Werner EJ, Christensen RD (eds) Neonatal hematology, 2nd edn. Cambridge, UK: Cambridge University Press, pp 37–46

Kling PJ, Schmidt RL, Roberts RA et al (1996) Serum erythropoietin levels during infancy: associations with erythropoiesis. J Pediatr 128:791–796

Kosasa TS, Ebesugawa I, Nakayama RT et al (1993) Massive fetomaternal hemorrhage preceded by decreased fetal movement and a nonreactive fetal heart rate pattern. Obstet Gynecol 82:711–714

Kozlowski CL, Lee D, Shwe KH et al (1995) Quantification of anti-c in haemolytic disease of the newborn. Transfus Med 5:37–42

Kramer MS, Usher RH, Pollack R et al (1997) Etiologic determinants of abruptio placentae. Obstet Gynecol 89:221–226

Landmann E, Bluetters-Sawatzki R, Schindler D, Gortner L (2004) Fanconi anemia in a neonate with pancytopenia. J Pediatr 145:125–127

Li Y, Juul SE, Morris-Winman JA et al (1996) Erythropoietin receptors are expressed in the central nervous system of mid-trimester human fetuses. Pediatr Res 40:376–381

Li Y, Xiao Z, Yan J, Li X, Wang Q, Zhu H, Pan J, Zhu X, Wang J, Feng X (2013) Urine erythropoietin level is associated with kidney and brain injury in critically ill neonates. Neonatology 104:87–94

Linderkamp O (1977) Capillary-venous hematocrit differences in newborn infants. Eur J Pediatr 127:9–15

Linderkamp O (1978) The effect of intra-partum and intrauterine asphyxia on placental transfusions in premature and full-term infants. Eur J Pediatr 127:91–99

Linderkamp O (1986) Deformability and intrinsic material properties of neonatal red blood cells. Blood 67:1244

Linderkamp O, Nelle M, Kraus M, Zilow EP (1992) The effect of early and late cord-clamping on blood viscosity and other hemorheological parameters in full-term neonates. Acta Paediatr 81:745–750

Lipitz S, Many A, Mitrani-Rosenbaum S et al (1998) Obstetric outcome after RhD and Kell testing. Hum Reprod 13:1472–1475

Lipton JM, Ellis SR (2009) Diamond-Blackfan anemia: diagnosis, treatment, and molecular pathogenesis. Hematol Oncol Clin North Am 23:261–282

Lopriore E, Vandenbussche FP, Tiersma ES et al (1995) Twin-to-twin transfusion syndrome: new perspectives. J Pediatr 127:675–680

Lundby C, Olsen NV (2011) Effects of recombinant human erythropoietin in normal humans. J Physiol 589: 1265–1271

Maisels MJ, Kring E (2006) The contribution of hemolysis to early jaundice in normal newborns. Pediatrics 118:276–279

Manea EM, Leverger G, Bellmann F (2009) Pearson syndrome in the neonatal period: two case reports and review of the literature. Pediatr Hematol Oncol 31:947

Matovcik LM (1986) Myosin in adult and neonatal human erythrocyte membranes. Blood 67:1668

Matsuda H, Sakaguchi K, Shibasaki T et al (2005) Intrauterine therapy for parvovirus B19 infected symptomatic fetus using B19 IgG-rich high titer gammaglobulin. J Perinat Med 33:561–563

May-Wewers J, Kaiser JR, Moore EK et al (2006) Severe neonatal hemolysis due to a maternal antibody to the low-frequency Rh antigen C(w). Am J Perinatol 23:213–217

McCoy TE, Conrad AL, Richman LC, Lindgren SD, Nopoulos PC, Bell EF (2011) Neurocognitive profiles of preterm infants randomly assigned to lower or higher hematocrit thresholds for transfusion. Child Neuropsychol 17:347–367

McMahon MJ, Li R, Schenck AP et al (1997) Previous cesarean birth. A risk factor for placenta previa? J Reprod Med 42:409–412

McPherson RJ, Juul SE (2008) Recent trends in erythropoietin-mediated neuroprotection. Int J Dev Neurosci 26:103–111

Mercer JS, Vohr BR, McGrath MM et al (2006) Delayed cord clamping in very preterm infants reduces the incidence of intraventricular hemorrhage and late-onset sepsis: a randomized, controlled trial. Pediatrics 117:1235–1242

Miele V, Galluzzo M, Patti G et al (1997) Scrotal hematoma due to neonatal adrenal hemorrhage: the value of ultrasonography in avoiding unnecessary surgery. Pediatr Radiol 27:672–674

Mock DM, Bell EF, Lankford GL, Widness JA (2001) Hematocrit correlates well with circulating red blood cell volume in very low birth weight infants. Pediatr Res 50:525–531

Nagaya M, Kato J, Niimi N et al (1998) Isolated cavernous hemangioma of the stomach in a neonate. J Pediatr Surg 33:653–654

Nguyen AQ, Cherry BH, Scott GF, Ryou MG, Mallet RT (2014) Erythropoietin: powerful protection of ischemic and post-ischemic brain. Exp Biol Med (Maywood) 239:1461–1475

Nopoulos PC, Conrad AL, Bell EF, Strauss RG, Widness JA, Magnotta VA, Zimmerman MB, Georgieff MK, Lindgren SD, Richman LC (2011) Long-term outcome of brain structure in premature infants: effects of liberal vs restricted red blood cell transfusions. Arch Pediatr Adolesc Med 165:443–450

Oettinger L, Mills WB (1949) Simultaneous capillary and venous hemoglobin determinations in newborn infant. J Pediatr 35:362–369

Ohls RK (2002a) Erythropoietin and hypoxia inducible factor-1 expression in the mid-trimester human fetus. Acta Pediatr 91(Suppl A 38):27–32

Ohls RK (2002b) Erythropoietin treatment in extremely low birth weight infants: blood in versus blood out. J Pediatr 140:3–6

Ohls RK (2009) Why, when and how should we provide red cell transfusions to neonates? In: Ohls RK, Yoder MC (eds) Hematology, immunology and infections disease. Saunders Elsevier, Philadelphia, pp 44–57

Ohls RK (2013) Why study erythropoietin in preterm infants? Acta Paediatr 102:567–568

Ohls RK, Liechty KW, Turner MC et al (1990) Erythroid "burst promoting activity" in the serum of patients with the anemia of prematurity. J Pediatr 116:786–789

Ohls RK, Ehrenkranz RA, Das A (2004) Neurodevelopmental outcome and growth at 18 to 22 months' corrected age in extremely low birth weight infants treated with early erythropoietin and iron. Pediatrics 114:1287–1291

Ohls RK, Christensen RD, Kamath-Rayne BD, Rosenberg A, Wiedmeier SE, Roohi M, Lacy CB, Lambert DK, Burnett JJ, Pruckler B, Schrader R, Lowe JR (2014a) A randomized, masked, placebo-controlled study of darbepoetin alfa in preterm infants. Pediatrics 132:e119–e127

Ohls RK, Kamath-Rayne BD, Christensen RD, Wiedmeier SE, Rosenberg A, Fuller J, Lacy CB, Roohi M, Lambert DK, Burnett JJ, Pruckler B, Peceny H, Cannon DC, Lowe JR (2014b) Cognitive outcomes of preterm infants randomized to darbepoetin, erythropoietin, or placebo. Pediatrics 133:1023–1030

Ohls RK, Christensen RD, Widness JA, Juul SE (2015) Erythropoiesis stimulating agents demonstrate safety and show promise as neuroprotective agents in neonates. J Pediatr. https://doi.org/10.1016/j.jpeds.2015.03.054

Oski FA, Komazawa M (1975) Metabolism of the erythrocytes of the newborn infant. Semin Hematol 12:49

Oski FA, Smith C (1968) Red cell metabolism in the premature infant. III. Apparent inappropriate glucose consumption for cell age. Pediatrics 41:473

Patel S, Ohls RK (2015) Darbepoetin administration in term and preterm neonates. Clin Perinatol. https://doi.org/10.1016/j.clp.2015.04.016

Pearson HA (1967) Life-span of the fetal red blood cell. J Pediatr 70:166–171

Pearson HA, Vertrees KM (1961) Site of binding to chromium-51 by hemoglobin. Nature 189:1019–1021

Pearson HA, Lobel JS, Kocoshis SA et al (1979) A new syndrome of refractory sideroblastic anemia with vacuolization of marrow precursors and exocrine pancreatic dysfunction. J Pediatr 95:976–984

Perrone S, Vezzosi P, Longini M et al (2005) Nucleated red blood cell count in term and preterm newborns: reference values at birth. Arch Dis Child Fetal Neon Ed 90: F174–F175

Pinto E, Guignard JP (1995) Renal masses in the neonate. Biol Neonate 68:175–184

Rabe H, Reynolds G, Diaz-Rossello J (2004) Early versus delayed umbilical cord clamping in preterm infants. Cochrane Database Syst Rev CD003248

Rabe H, Alvarez JR, Lawn C (2009) A management guideline to reduce the frequency of blood transfusion in very-low-birth-weight infants. Am J Perinatol 26:179–183

Rhondeau SM, Christensen RD, Ross MP et al (1988) Responsiveness to recombinant human erythropoietin of marrow erythroid progenitors from infants with the "anemia of prematurity". J Pediatr 112:935–940

Ruef P, Linderkamp O (1999) Deformability and geometry of neonatal erythrocytes with irregular shapes. Pediatr Res 45(1):114–119

Runsewe-Abiodun IT, Ogunfowora OB, Fetuga BM (2006) Neonatal malaria in Nigeria – a 2 year review. BMC Pediatr 6:19

Ruth V, Widness JA, Clemons G, Raivio JO (1990) Postnatal changes in serum immunoreactive erythropoietin in relation to hypoxia before and after birth. J Pediatr 116:950–954

Shah M, Li Y, Christensen RD (1996) Effects of perinatal zidovudine on hematopoiesis: a comparison of effects on progenitors from human fetuses versus mothers. AIDS 10:1239–1247

Shannon KM, Naylor GS, Torkildson JC et al (1987) Circulating erythroid progenitors in the anemia of prematurity. N Engl J Med 31:728–733

Soubasi V, Kremenopoulos G, Tsantali C et al (2000) Use of erythropoietin and its effects on blood lactate and 2, 3-diphosphoglycerate in premature neonates. Biol Neonate 78:281–287

Stevenson DK, Wong RJ, DeSandre GH, Vreman HJ (2004) A primer on neonatal jaundice. Adv Pediatr 51:263–288

Strauss RG, Mock DM, Johnson K et al (2003) Circulating RBC volume, measured with biotinylated RBCs, is superior to the Hct to document the hematologic effects of delayed versus immediate umbilical cord clamping in preterm neonates. Transfusion 43:1168–1172

Strauss RG, Mock DM, Johnson KJ et al (2008) A randomized clinical trial comparing immediate versus delayed clamping of the umbilical cord in preterm infants: short-term clinical and laboratory endpoints. Transfusion 48:658–665

Supski DW, Gurushanthaiah K, Chasen S (2002) The effect of treatment of twin-twin transfusion syndrome on the diagnosis-to-delivery interval. Twin Res 5:1–4

Teng FY, Sayre JW (1997) Vacuum extraction: does duration predict scalp injury? Obstet Gynecol 89:281–285

Uchil D, Arulkumaran S (2003) Neonatal subgaleal hemorrhage and its relationship to delivery by vacuum extraction. Obstet Gynecol Surv 58:687–693

Vain NE, Satragno DS, Gorenstein AN, Gordillo JE, Berazategui JP, Alda MG, Prudent LM (2014) Effect of gravity on volume of placental transfusion: a multicentre, randomised, non-inferiority trial. Lancet 384(9939):235–240

van den Ouweland JM, de Klerk JB, van de Corput MP et al (2000) Characterization of a novel mitochondrial DNA deletion in a patient with a variant of the Pearson marrow-pancreas syndrome. Eur J Hum Genet 8:195–203

van Dijk BA, Dooren MC, Overbeeke MA (1995) Red cell antibodies in pregnancy: there is no "critical titre". Transfus Med 5:199–202

van Heteren CF, Nijhuis JG, Semmekrot BA et al (1998) Risk for surviving twin after fetal death of co-twin in twin-twin transfusion syndrome. Obstet Gynecol 92:215–219

van Zoeren-Grobben D, Lindeman JH, Houdkamp E et al (1997) Markers of oxidative stress and antioxidant activity in plasma and erythrocytes in neonatal respiratory distress syndrome. Acta Paediatr 86: 1356–1362

Vaughan JI, Manning M, Warwick RM et al (1998) Inhibition of erythroid progenitor cells by anti-Kell antibodies in fetal alloimmune anemia. N Engl J Med 338:798–803

Ville Y, Hyett J, Hecher K et al (1995) Preliminary experience with endoscopic laser surgery for severe twin-twin transfusion syndrome. N Engl J Med 332:224–227

Warwood TL, Ohls RD, Wiedmeier SE et al (2005) Single-dose darbepoetin administration to anemic preterm neonates. J Perinatol 25:725–730

Warwood TL, Ohls RK, Lambert DK et al (2006a) Intravenous administration of darbepoetin to NICU patients. J Perinatol 26:296–300

Warwood TL, Ohls RK, Lambert DK et al (2006b) Urinary excretion of darbepoetin after intravenous vs. subcutaneous administration to preterm neonates. J Perinatol 26:636–639

Weiner CP, Widness JA (1996) Decreased fetal erythropoiesis and hemolysis in Kell hemolytic anemia. Am J Obstet Gynecol 174:547–551

Whyte RK, Kirpalani H, Asztalos EV, Andersen C, Blajchman M, Heddle N, LaCorte M, Robertson CM, Clarke MC, Vincer MJ, Doyle LW, Roberts RS, PINTOS Study Group (2009) Neurodevelopmental outcome of extremely low birth weight infants randomly assigned to restrictive or liberal hemoglobin thresholds for blood transfusion. Pediatrics 123:207–213

Widness JA, Madan A, Grindeanu LA (2005) Reduction in red blood cell transfusions among preterm infants: results of a randomized trial with an in-line blood gas and chemistry monitor. Pediatrics 115:1299–1306

Zhao W, Kitidis C, Fleming MD, Lodish HF, Ghaffari S (2006) Erythropoietin stimulates phosphorylation and activation of GATA-1 via the PI3-kinase/AKT signaling pathway. Blood 107:907–915

Zipursky A (1983) The erythrocyte differential count in newborn infants. Am J Pediatr Hematol Oncol 5:45–52

Fetal and Neonatal Hydrops

95

Gennaro Vetrano and Mario De Curtis

Contents

Abstract
Hydrops fetalis (i.e., fetal hydrops) (HF) is a serious condition defined as abnormal accumulation of fluid in two or more fetal compartments. It presents as ascites, pleural effusion, pericardial effusion, and skin edema. In some patients, it may also be associated with polyhydramnios and placental edema. Potter was the first to distinguish nonimmune hydrops fetalis (NIHF) from immune hydrops. These days approximately 90% of cases of hydrops fetalis are due to nonimmune diseases. The basic mechanism for the formation of HF is an imbalance between interstitial fluid production and lymphatic return. The antenatal diagnosis of HF is made by the ultrasound finding of fluid accumulation in the fetus or placenta. The management of hydrops fetalis is a great challenge for fetal medicine specialists and neonatologists and the mortality rate still remains high.

G. Vetrano (✉)
U.O.C. Pediatria/Neonatologia/UTIN, Osp. "Sacro Cuore di Gesù", Benevento, Italy
e-mail: gennvet@hotmail.com

M. De Curtis
Dipartimento Materno-Infantile, Università "La Sapienza", Rome, Italy

95.1 Salient Points

- Hydrops fetalis is a serious condition defined as abnormal accumulation of fluid in two or more fetal compartments.

G. Buonocore et al. (eds.), *Neonatology*,
https://doi.org/10.1007/978-3-319-29489-6_242

- Approximately 90% of cases of hydrops fetalis are due to nonimmune diseases.
- The basic mechanism for the formation of hydrops fetalis is an imbalance between interstitial fluid production and lymphatic return.
- Main causes of hydrops fetalis are: hematological disorders, cardiovascular and infectious conditions, genetic abnormalities, tumors, and idiopathic origins.
- The management of hydrops fetalis is still a great challenge for fetal medicine specialists and neonatologists and the mortality caused by this pathology varies widely.
- The hydropic fetus is usually in a precarious state and even minimal delay in the diagnosis may hamper access to life-saving procedures.

95.2 Introduction

Hydrops fetalis (i.e., fetal hydrops) (HF) is a serious condition defined as abnormal accumulation of fluid in two or more fetal compartments. It presents as ascites, pleural effusion, pericardial effusion, and skin edema (Fig. 1). In some patients, it may also be associated with polyhydramnios and placental edema. Potter was the first to distinguish nonimmune hydrops fetalis (NIHF) from immune hydrops (Potter 1943).

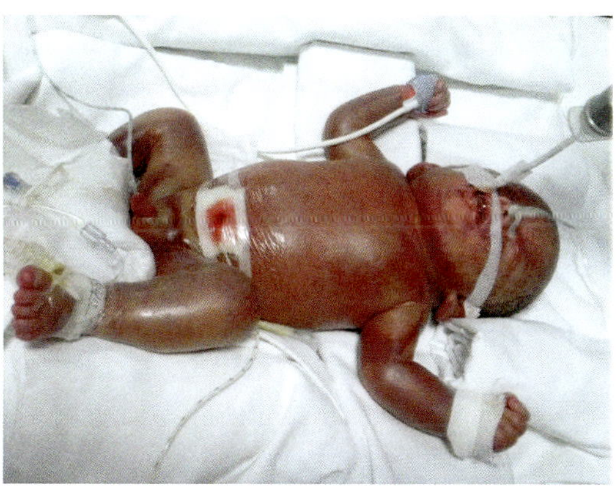

Fig. 1 Preterm newborn with NIHF

95.3 Epidemiology

In the past, hemolytic disease due to Rh incompatibility used to be the main cause of both fetal and neonatal immune hydrops. These days approximately 90% of cases of hydrops fetalis are due to nonimmune diseases, with the number of affected live born ranging from 1:1500 to 1:3800 (Santolaya et al. 1992; Warsof 1986). Hydrops fetalis is much more common in Southeast Asia; in Thailand the expected frequency of nonimmune hydrops fetalis due to homozygous alpha-thalassemia or Bart hydrops ranges from one every 500 to one every 1500 pregnancies (Suwanrath-Kengpol et al. 2005; Abrams et al. 2007). Although the availability of ultrasound technology has greatly improved antenatal diagnosis of HF, perinatal mortality (PNM) remains high.

95.4 Pathogenesis

The basic mechanism for the formation of HF is an imbalance between interstitial fluid production and lymphatic return. Fluid accumulation in the fetus can be due to (a) heart failure, (b) anemia, (c) obstructed lymphatic flow, or (d) decreased plasma osmotic pressure. The fetus is particularly susceptible to interstitial fluid accumulation because of its greater capillary permeability, compliant interstitial compartments, and predisposition to increased venous pressure because of impaired lymphatic return (Abrams et al. 2007; Apkon 1995). Clinical and animal studies have shown that high central venous pressure (CVP) has a pivotal role in the development of fetal hydrops (Shinbane et al. 1997). Increased CVP causes edema and effusions by increasing capillary hydrostatic pressure and decreasing lymphatic return (Moise et al. 1992). Albumin is the main oncotically active plasma protein and when its hepatic synthesis is impaired transcapillary fluid movement increases (Abrams et al. 2007; Apkon 1995). Hypoproteinemia and hypoalbuminemia are common in human hydrops; however, studies in humans and animals have shown that hypoalbuminemia is unlikely to trigger this condition (Pasman et al. 2006).

95.5 Etiology

Regardless of the known causes of immune hydrops, extensive pre- and postnatal investigations have improved our knowledge of the etiology of nonimmune hydrops fetalis (NIHF). Indeed, larger series and a systematic review report that a cause can be found in nearly 60% of cases prenatally (Santo et al. 2011) and in 85% when postnatal detection is included (Bellini et al. 2009). HF is an end-stage process and a nonspecific finding associated with a range of abnormalities. Its causes can be divided into six broad categories: hematological disorders, cardiovascular and infectious conditions, genetic abnormalities, tumors, and idiopathic origins. Table 1 summarizes the causes of fetal hydrops.

95.6 Diagnosis

A pregnant woman with polydramnios, severe anemia, toxemia, or isoimmune disease should undergo further investigation. The antenatal diagnosis of HF is made by the ultrasound finding of fluid accumulation in the fetus or placenta. Specifically, excess serous fluid should be identified in at least one space (ascites, pleural effusion, or pericardial effusion), accompanied by skin edema (>5 mm thick), or fluid in two potential spaces without edema (Mahony et al. 1984; Romero et al. 1988). Ascites can be detected when a minimum of 50 mL is present in the fetal abdomen (Holzgreve et al. 1984). Polyhydramnios and placental thickening (typically defined as a placental thickness ≥4 cm in the second trimester or >6 cm in the third trimester (Lee et al. 2012; Hoddick et al. 1985)) may be present, but oligohydramnios is a particularly ominous finding when it develops in nonimmune hydrops fetalis (Fleischer et al. 1981). It is important to perform middle cerebral artery Doppler studies to assess the presence of fetal anemia. The fetus with NIHF due to severe anemia will have increased velocity through the middle cerebral artery (Mari et al. 2000).

Women with NIHF may develop the mirror syndrome, also referred to as Ballantyne's syndrome. In this uncommon complication the mother presents with an edema that "mirrors" that of her hydropic fetus. The mirror syndrome may represent a form of preeclampsia and is characterized by edema in approximately 90% of cases, hypertension in 60%, and proteinuria in 40% (Braun et al. 2010).

The subsequent workup of the hydropic fetus should focus on detecting the underlying cause. In general, the first step is to collect detailed information on the mother's medical history, specifically in relation to hereditary or metabolic diseases, diabetes, anemia, exposure to infectious agents, and use of medication. The second step includes a detailed ultrasound examination of the fetus and an accurate workup of the mother. The third step, after obtaining the results on the mother's conditions, is a systematic approach to the fetus, including invasive testing, such as villocentesis, amniocentesis, cordocentesis, and sampling of any effusions. Invasive investigations of the fetus are necessary when maternal blood and ultrasound examination fail to provide a definitive cause of HF. The recommended workup of a fetus with HF is shown in Table 2.

If the etiology of HF is not identified before birth, postnatal investigations should be carried out. Blood samples for laboratory analysis are similar to those taken antenatally: blood group including Rh status, direct Coombs antibody screen, full blood cell count, karyotype, metabolic and chemistry studies, hemoglobin electrophoresis, if indicated. Structural defects should be evaluated using skeletal radiographs and ultrasound. A genetic consultation may also be helpful, particularly to determine the risk of recurrence. In case of intrauterine or neonatal death, an autopsy is mandatory.

95.7 Treatment

The management of hydrops fetalis is a great challenge for fetal medicine specialists and neonatologists. The hydropic fetus is usually in a precarious state, and even minimal delays could hamper access to life-saving procedures (Désilets et al. 2013).

Table 1 Causes of hydrops fetalis

Hematological	Genetic
Isoimmunization (immune hydrops) (hemolytic disease of the newborn, erythroblastosis)	Inborn errors of metabolism
Rh (most commonly D; also C, c, E, e)	Glycogen-storage disease, type IV
Kell	Lysosomal storage diseases
ABO	Hypothyroidism and hyperthyroidism
Others	Others
Other hemolytic disorders	Genetic syndromes
Glucose phosphate isomerase deficiency	Chromosomal syndromes
Pyruvate kinase deficiency	Beckwith-Wiedemann syndrome (trisomy 11p15)
G-6-PD deficiency	Cri-du-chat syndrome (chromosomes 4 and 5)
Disorders of red cell production	Trisomy 10, mosaic
Diamond-Blackfan syndrome	Trisomy 13
Leukemia (usually associated with Down or Noonan syndrome)	Trisomy 15
Alpha-thalassemia (Bart hemoglobinopathy)	Trisomy 18
Parvovirus B19	Trisomy 21 (Down syndrome)
Others	Turner syndrome (45, X)
Fetal hemorrhage	Others
Placental subchorial tumors	
Fetomaternal hemorrhage	
Twin-to-twin transfusion	
Isoimmune fetal thrombocytopenia	
Others	
Cardiovascular	**Tumors and others**
Structural anomalies	Intrathoracic tumors or masses
Abnormalities of left ventricular outflow	Abdominal tumors or masses
Abnormalities of right ventricular outflow	Other conditions
Other vascular malformations	Placental choriocarcinoma
Nonstructural anomalies	Placental chorangioma
Obstruction of venous return	Cystic hygroma
Supraventricular tachycardia	Intussusception
Congenital heart block	Meconium peritonitis
Prenatal closure of the foramen ovale or ductus arteriosus	Intracranial teratoma
Myocarditis	Sacrococcygeal teratoma
Idiopathic arterial calcification or hypercalcemia	
Infectious	**Idiopathic**
Parvovirus B19	
Cytomegalovirus (CMV)	
Syphilis	
Herpes simplex	
Toxoplasmosis	
Hepatitis B	
Adenovirus	
Ureaplasma urealyticum	
Coxsackievirus type B	
Listeria monocytogenes	

A woman with a hydropic fetus should be hospitalized in a level-3 perinatal centre if antenatal nonstress testing (NST) (American Pregnancy Association 2006) and biophysical profile (BPP) (Manning 1999) are not reassuring (Table 3). At the same time, efforts should be continued to determine the underlying etiology of HF. Delivery is indicated after 34 weeks' gestation, or earlier if there is evidence of a mature fetal lung profile at amniocentesis or if the fetal condition deteriorates. Delivery is also necessary in the presence of obstetric indications or compromised maternal conditions due to the mirror syndrome (maternal hydrops) (Van Selm et al. 1991; Norton et al. 2015).

Table 2 Antenatal evaluation of hydrops fetalis

Maternal history
Age, parity, gestation
Hereditary or metabolic diseases, anemia
Recent infections or contacts
Medication use
Maternal laboratory evaluation
Complete blood cell count
Blood type, Rh, indirect Coombs antibody screen
Kleihauer-Betke stain
Syphilis, TORCH, and parvovirus B19 titres
Culture for group B streptococcus, Listeria
Maternal triple screen
Oral glucose tolerance test
Optional, as indicated:
Metabolic studies
Hemoglobin electrophoresis
G6PD, pyruvate kinase
Autoimmune screen (SLE, anti-Ro and -La)
Ultrasonography
Identify anatomic abnormalities
Evaluate extent of edema and effusions
Rule out twin gestation
Doppler blood flow assessment
Fetal echocardiography
Evaluate for cardiac malformation, arrhythmia
Amniocentesis
Karyotype
Culture or PCR for TORCH, parvovirus
Amniotic fluid a-fetoprotein
Restriction endonucleases (thalassemias)
Lecithin-sphingomyelin ratio, phosphatidyl glycerol to evaluate lung maturity
Fetal blood sampling
Karyotype
Complete blood cell count
Blood type; hemoglobin electrophoresis
Blood chemistries, albumin, gases
Culture or PCR for TORCH, parvovirus
Metabolic testing (Tay-Sacks, Gaucher, GM_1 gangliosidosis)
Fetal effusion sampling
Culture or PCR for TORCH, parvovirus
Protein content
Cell count and cytology

G6PD glucose-6-phosphate dehydrogenase, *PCR* polymerase chain reaction, *SLE* systemic lupus erythematosus, *TORCH* toxoplasmosis, other agents, rubella, cytomegalovirus, herpes simplex
Modified from Swain et al.: Prenatal diagnosis and management of nonimmune hydrops fetalis. Aust N Z J Obstet Gynaecol 39:285, 1999

Table 3 Conservative management in hospital

Hospitalize the patient in case of
Fetal skin thickening
Pericardial effusion
Nonreactive NST
Biophysical profile (BPP) ≤ 6
Subjective decreased fetal movement
Gestational age below 32–34 weeks
Treat underlying cause, if possible
Administer antenatal corticosteroids
Monitor serial growth and effusion volumes
NST and BPP every 2 or 3 days

NST nonstress test

The appropriate treatment of the fetus with hydrops, which carries a high mortality risk, can only be undertaken after a precise and detailed diagnosis. Full parental involvement is essential, because the associated abnormalities may be severely debilitating or even lethal. In addition, invasive fetal treatment and elective preterm delivery remain controversial. Therefore, obstetricians, fetal medicine specialists, and neonatologists should consult themselves on the optimal timing of delivery, also involving pediatric surgeons, cardiologists, and cardiothoracic surgeons. Various anecdotal approaches are found in the literature, but no properly designed clinical trials have been performed to provide the clinician with evidence-based management. Furthermore, the hydropic process may resolve spontaneously. Thus, the available management schemes aim to correct the underlying pathophysiology, including fetal transfusion to correct anemia (regardless of the cause), drug treatments for cardiac arrhythmias, correction or reduction of space-occupying lesions that impede cardiac venous or lymphatic return, and procedures intended to stop fetal blood loss (regardless of the cause) (Watson and Campbell 1986; Muller-Hansen et al. 1998; Jones 1995).

Fetal transfusion with packed red blood cells (RBCs) given intraperitoneally has become accepted as standard care for fetuses with severe anemia. It carries low risk, despite the lack of definitive evidence from randomized clinical trials. This approach has been used successfully in

the treatment of severely anemic fetuses of isoimmunized pregnancies and to correct anemia due to various other causes – unless the pregnancy is at an advanced gestational age and the risks associated with delivery are considered to be less than those associated with the procedure (Norton et al. 2015). Alternative routes (percutaneous umbilical vein, intrahepatic umbilical vein, umbilical artery, intracardiac transfusions) for the administration of blood products to the fetus have been reported. Other approaches are aimed at the mother, fetus, and newborn baby. Maternal plasmapheresis, promethazine, or corticosteroids have been used for the mother. Fetal therapies available include partial packed-cell exchange transfusion, fetal intravenous IgG, platelet transfusion, and the administration of human granulocyte-stimulating factor. Neonatal stem cell transplantation has been used for α-thalassemia (Carr et al. 1995). However, these newer therapeutic techniques carry greater risk for the fetus than the intraperitoneal route and should therefore be used cautiously.

Highly vascularized tumor masses and acute, massive twin-to-twin hemorrhages are life-threatening diseases that may justify life-threatening treatment. Techniques such as tumor debulking surgery, surgery for active bleeding, photocoagulation, and radiofrequency thermal ablation may all be helpful in the treatment of fetal conditions such as sacrococcygcal tumors, highly vascularized fetal intraabdominal, thoracic, or placental masses, and when there is massive arteriovenous shunting (Bullard and Harrison 1995; Rubod et al. 2006).

The management of the twin-to-twin transfusion syndrome is currently an unresolved problem: treating an anemic fetus with transfusions has shown no evidence of benefit; volume reduction for the transfusion recipient or a combination of transfusion and fetal reduction has rarely been used or may not correct the ongoing pathophysiology. Furthermore, feticide of the affected twin is often followed by the development of hydrops in the previously normal surviving twin (Mahone et al. 1993).

Treatments of fetal arrhythmias include taking no action, pharmacological treatment, and immediate delivery. Maternal treatment with antiarrhythmic medications for NIHF secondary to fetal tachyarrhythmia is recommended, unless the gestational age is close to term or there is a maternal or obstetrical contraindication. On the other hand, in-utero therapy for fetal bradyarrhythmia resulting in hydrops is considered investigational and is not generally recommended outside of a research setting (Norton et al. 2015).

In the presence of fetal maturity, the simplest and most direct approach is delivery of the affected fetus and treatment of the arrhythmia directly after birth. Possible treatment options include digitalis, furosemide, flecainide, verapamil, amiodarone, propanolol, procainamide, quinidine, adenosine, sotalol, terbutaline, corticosteroids, and immunoglobulins. Various drug combinations are also used. However, the choice of the drug remains empirical and arbitrary, until definitive evidence from clinical trials becomes available (Strasburger et al. 1986; Simpson and Sharland 1998).

The management of space-occupying masses varies depending on the type of lesion and from center to center. If immediate delivery is not practicable, the mass is either reduced or removed. Pleural and pericardial effusions and ascites may be treated with single or serial drainage. Fetal surgery with definitive correction of the underlying anomaly has also been used. Successes and failures have been reported with all methods; there is no evidence suggesting that one approach is better than another (Wesolowski and Piazza 2008).

Postnatal management of HF poses a unique set of problems for the neonatologist. Treatment of the infant after delivery is facilitated by the knowledge of the underlying cause. In addition to appropriate equipment and supplies for resuscitation, a skilled team of health care professionals (neonatologists, nurses, respiratory therapists, and radiology and ultrasonography technicians) should be present in the delivery room (McMahan and Donovan 1995; American Heart Association 2006). Fluid in the pleural, pericardial, and abdominal cavities may require aspiration in the delivery room to allow adequate ventilation and circulation. Umbilical arterial and venous catheters are sited to monitor and treat arterial pressure, blood gases, venous pressure, hematocrit, and the metabolic

state of the infant. Packed red cells or whole blood cross matched with the mother should be available for the correction of severe anemia by partial exchange transfusion, even if this is due to non-immune causes. Surfactant therapy and mechanical ventilation are used to manage surfactant deficiency and pulmonary hypoplasia, which may be associated with hydrops. Fluid intake is based on an estimate of the infant's "dry weight" (e.g., 50th percentile for gestational age) and kept to a minimum (e.g., 40–60 mL/kg/day) until the edema is resolved. Inotropic support (e.g., dopamine) may be required to improve cardiac output (Mascaretti et al. 2003; Teixeira et al. 2008).

In case of death, it is mandatory to continue the investigation postmortem of the fetus or newborn with NIHF. Genetic counseling, clinical photography, and fetal X-rays should be obtained to evaluate possible dysmorphic syndrome or skeletal dysplasia. Autopsy is strongly recommended. Additional procedures include storage of fetal blood, tissue, DNA, and amniotic fluid supernatant. Placental examination (microscopy, histopathology) focusing on tumors, fetal anemia, infection, and metabolic disorder is indicated (Désilets et al. 2013).

95.8 Prognosis

Estimates of mortality vary widely. The condition has a mortality rate of virtually 100% when structural defects are present or the cause of HF is unknown. Most case series report 60–90% mortality, although notable improvements have been described (Abrams et al. 2007). The prognosis of NIHF due to cardiac structural abnormalities is poor, with combined fetal and infant mortality reported as 92%, largely due to the severity of the heart defects causing in utero congestive heart failure (Randenberg 2010). Treatable causes of hydrops, such as fetal arrhythmia or infection with parvovirus B19, have a better prognosis (Bonvicini et al. 2011). However, when the congenital infection (parvovirus) occurs in the early second trimester (<20 weeks of gestation) the risk of a poor outcome for the fetus is greatest (Lamont et al. 2011).

In cases of tachyarrhythmias, the prognosis has been improved by antenatal antiarrhythmic treatment. Cases presenting before 24 weeks' gestation have a worse prognosis, whereas those that present later may benefit from delivery and intensive neonatal care (McCoy et al. 1995).

Although idiopathic NIHF has a low recurrence risk, the risk for some cases of NIHF may be as high as 25%, making genetic counseling an integral part of the management of any patient with NIHF (Norton et al. 2015).

Czernik et al. reported that, among liveborn infants, neonatal mortality with NIHF is as high as 60%. Temporal trends suggest that the associated mortality has not improved over the past two decades. In addition to the small sample size, an explanation for the lack of improvement in survival over time may be that the more severe cases are now more frequently diagnosed prenatally and referred to tertiary centers (Czernik et al. 2011).

References

Abrams ME, Meredith KS, Kinnard P, Clark RH (2007) Hydrops fetalis: a retrospective review of cases reported to a large national database and identification of risk factors associated with death. Pediatrics 120(1):84–89

American Heart Association (2006) 2005 American Heart Association (AHA) guidelines for cardiopulmonary resuscitation (CPR) and emergency cardiovascular care (ECC) of pediatric and neonatal patients: pediatric basic life support. Pediatrics 117(5):e989–e1004

American Pregnancy Association (2006) Fetal Non-Stress Test (NST). http://www.americanpregnancy.org/prenataltesting/non-stresstest.html

Apkon M (1995) Pathophysiology of hydrops fetalis. Semin Perinatol 19:437

Bellini C, Hennekam RC, Fulcheri E et al (2009) Etiology of nonimmune hydrops fetalis: a systematic review. Am J Med Genet A 149A:844–851

Bonvicini F, Puccetti C, Salfi NC et al (2011) Gestational and fetal outcomes in B19 maternal infection: a problem of diagnosis. J Clin Microbiol 49:3514–3518

Braun T, Brauer M, Fuchs I, Czernik C, Dudenhausen JW, Henrich W, Sarioglu N (2010) Mirror syndrome: a systematic review of fetal associated conditions, maternal presentation and perinatal outcome. Fetal Diagn Ther 27:191–203

Bullard KM, Harrison MR (1995) Before the horse is out of the barn: fetal surgery for hydrops. Semin Perinatol 19 (6):462–473. Review

Carr S et al (1995) Intrauterine therapy for homozygous alpha-thalassemia. Obstet Gynecol 85:876

Czernik C, Proquitté H, Metze B, Bührer C (2011) Hydrops fetalis: has there been a change in diagnostic spectrum and mortality? J Matern Fetal Neonatal Med 24:258–263

Désilets V, Audibert F et al (2013) Investigation and management of non-immune fetal hydrops. J Obstet Gynaecol Can 35(10):923–936

Fleischer AC et al (1981) Hydrops fetalis: sonographic evaluation and clinical implications. Radiology 141:163

Hoddick WK, Mahony BS, Callen PW, Filly RA (1985) Placental thickness. J Ultrasound Med 4:479–482

Holzgreve W, Curry CJ, Golbus MS, Callen PW, Filly RA, Smith JC (1984) Investigation of nonimmune hydrops fetalis. Am J Obstet Gynecol 150:805

Jones DC (1995) Nonimmune fetal hydrops: diagnosis and obstetrical management. Semin Perinatol 19(6): 447–461

Lamont RF, Sobel JD, Vaisbuch E et al (2011) Parvovirus B19 infection in human pregnancy. BJOG 118: 175–186

Lee AJ, Bethune M, Hiscock RJ (2012) Placental thickness in the second trimester: a pilot study to determine the normal range. J Ultrasound Med 31:213–218

Mahone PR, Sherer DM, Abramowicz JS, Woods JR Jr (1993) Twin-twin transfusion syndrome: rapid development of severe hydrops of the donor following selective feticide of the hydropic recipient. Am J Obstet Gynecol 169(1):166–168

Mahony BS, Filly RA, Callen PW, Chinn DH, Golbus MS (1984) Severe nonimmune hydrops fetalis: graphic evaluation. Radiology 151:757

Manning F (1999) Fetal biophysical profile. Obstet Gynecol Clin North Am 26(4):557–577

Mari G, Deter RL, Carpenter RL et al (2000) Noninvasive diagnosis by Doppler ultrasonography of fetal anemia due to maternal red-cell alloimmunization. Collaborative Group for Doppler Assessment of the Blood Velocity in Anemic Fetuses. N Engl J Med 342:9–14

Mascaretti RS, Falcão MC, Silva AM, Vaz FA, Leone CR (2003) Characterization of newborns with nonimmune hydrops fetalis admitted to a neonatal intensive care unit. Rev Hosp Clin Fac Med Sao Paulo 58(3): 125–132. Epub 2003 Jul 22

McCoy MC, Katz VL, Gould N, Kuller JA (1995) Non-immune hydrops after 20 weeks' gestation: review of 10 years' experience with suggestions for management. Obstet Gynecol 85(4):578–582

McMahan MJ, Donovan EF (1995) The delivery room resuscitation of the hydropic neonate. Semin Perinatol 19(6):474–482

Moise KJ Jr, Carpenter RJ Jr, Hesketh DE (1992) Do abnormal Starling forces cause fetal hydrops in red blood cell alloimmunization? Am J Obstet Gynecol 167(4 Pt 1):907–912

Muller-Hansen I, Hackeloer BJ, Kattner E (1998) Pre- and postnatal diagnosis and treatment of hydrops fetalis-an interdisciplinary problem. Z Geburtshilfe Neonatol 202(1):2–9

Norton ME, Chauhan SP, Dashe JS (2015) Society for maternal-fetal medicine (SMFM) clinical guideline #7: nonimmune hydrops fetalis. Am J Obstet Gynecol 212(2):127–139. https://doi.org/10.1016/j.ajog.2014.12.018. Epub 2014 Dec 31. Review

Pasman SA, Meerman RH, Vandenbussche FP, Oepkes D (2006) Hypoalbuminemia: a cause of fetal hydrops? Am J Obstet Gynecol 194(4):972–975

Potter EL (1943) Universal edema of the fetus unassociated with erythroblastosis. Am J Obstet Gynecol 46:130

Randenberg AL (2010) Nonimmune hydrops fetalis part II: does etiology influence mortality? Neonatal Netw 29:367–380

Romero R et al (1988) Nonimmune hydrops fetalis. In: Romero R et al (eds) Prenatal diagnosis of congenital anomalies. Appleton & Lange, Norwalk, p 414

Rubod C, Houfflin V, Belot F, Ardiet E, Dufour P, Subtil D, Deruelle P (2006) Successful in utero treatment of chronic and massive fetomaternal hemorrhage with fetal hydrops. Fetal Diagn Ther 21(5):410–413

Santo S, Mansour S, Thilaganathan B et al (2011) Prenatal diagnosis of non-immune hydrops fetalis: what do we tell the parents? Prenat Diagn 31:186–195

Santolaya J, Alley D, Jaffe R, Warsof SL (1992) Antenatal classification of hydrops fetalis. Obstet Gynecol 79:256

Shinbane JS, Wood MA, Jensen DN et al (1997) Tachycardia-induced cardiomyopathy: a review of animal models and clinical studies. J Am Coll Cardiol 29 (4):709–715

Simpson JM, Sharland GK (1998) Fetal tachycardias: management and outcome of 127 consecutive cases. Heart 79(6):576–581

Strasburger JF, Huhta JC, Carpenter RJ Jr et al (1986) Doppler echocardiography in the diagnosis and management of persistent fetal arrhythmias. J Am Coll Cardiol 7(6):1386–1391

Suwanrath-Kengpol C, Kor-anantakul O, Suntharasaj T, Leetanaporn R (2005) Etiology and outcome of non-immune hydrops fetalis in southern Thailand. Gynecol Obstet Invest 59:134–137

Teixeira A, Rocha G, Guedes MB, Guimarães H (2008) Newborn with nonimmune hydrops fetalis – the experience of a tertiary center. Acta Med Port 21 (4):345–350. Epub 2008 Oct 24

Van Selm M et al (1991) Maternal hydrops syndrome: a review. Obstet Gynecol Surv 46:785

Warsof S, Nicolaides K, Rodecket CL (1986) Immune and non-immune hydrops. Obstet Gynecol 29:533

Watson J, Campbell S (1986) Antenatal evaluation and management in nonimmune hydrops fetalis. Obstet Gynecol 67(4):589–593

Wesolowski A, Piazza A (2008) A case of mediastinal teratoma as a cause of nonimmune hydrops fetalis, and literature review. Am J Perinatol 25(8):507–512

Physiology and Abnormalities of Leukocytes in Newborns

96

Kurt R. Schibler

Contents

Abstract

Leukocytes have a major role in host defence against invading microorganisms. During the fetal and neonatal periods, leukocyte physiology is peculiar and neutrophil counts vary considerably early in the neonatal period. Neonates, especially preterm children, have an immaturity of neutrophil function and production, with limited abilities to recall mature neutrophils in peripheral blood. Infections may therefore be more challenging at this age. The most common disorders of leukocytes present in newborns are quantitative abnormalities such as neutropenia, neutrophilia, and leukemoid reaction. Quantitative defects in phagocytic leukocytes may also occur in conjunction with qualitative changes. Classification of leukocyte abnormalities according to underlying kinetic mechanisms can provide useful indicators for the diagnosis and management of affected infants. When evaluating a neonate with leukocyte abnormalities, it is helpful to recall that some varieties of these abnormalities are common and others are exceedingly rare. If neutropenia persists for more than 5 days, further evaluation is indicated, particularly if the neutrophil count is less than 500 cells per microliter. Because of the immaturity of the immune system in newborns, early treatment should be initiated to prevent severe consequences. The etiology of leukocyte abnormalities and the seriousness of clinical features determine treatment (antibiotics,

K. R. Schibler (✉)
Perinatal Institute, Cincinnati Children's Hospital Medical Center, Cincinnati, OH, USA
e-mail: kurt.schibler@cchmc.org

G. Buonocore et al. (eds.), *Neonatology*,
https://doi.org/10.1007/978-3-319-29489-6_243

granulocytes transfusions, intravenous immunoglobulins, or granulocytes – colony stimulating factor administration). This chapter will focus on the features of newborns' immune system and higlight the most common causes of leukocyte abnormalities and key therapeutic options.

96.1 Salient Points

- Leukocyte physiology is peculiar in the fetus and newborn infant.
- A number of leukocyte abnormalities can present during the newborn period. They have different etiologies, pathogenesis, and clinical features. Differential diagnosis is necessary.
- Therapy and treatment include antibiotics, granulocyte transfusion, IVIG, G-CSF, and GM-CSF.

96.2 Physiology of Leukocytes in the Fetus and Neonate

96.2.1 Introduction

96.2.1.1 Kinetics

The circulating pool of neutrophils reflect a dynamic equilibrium between pools of neutrophil precursors and mature neutrophils in the bone marrow, circulating neutrophils, and activated neutrophils that have emigrated into the tissues. The bone marrow is the predominant hematopoietic organ after birth. Within the bone marrow, pluripotential hematopoietic stem and progenitor cells give rise to lineage committed neutrophil precursors. These precursors mature under the influence of growth factors such as granulocyte colony-stimulating factor (G-CSF) and granulocyte-macrophage colony-stimulating factor (GM-CSF). The bone marrow thus contains pools of immature neutrophils and of stored mature neutrophils. After emigration from the bone marrow, neutrophils enter the circulation for a brief period of hours then translocate into the tissues.

The peripheral blood neutrophil pool is estimated to contain approximately 5% of the total neutrophil pool. Neutrophil distribution studies in adults estimate approximately 1 billion neutrophils per kilogram body weight, of which 20% are in the bone marrow precursor pool, 75% are in the marrow storage pool, 3% are in the marginated vascular pool, and 2% are in the circulating blood (Luchtman-Jones and Schwartz 2002). Approximately 1.5 billion neutrophils per kilogram body weight are produced daily. The neuxtrophil life span consists of about 9 days in the bone marrow, 3–6 h in the blood, and 1–4 days in the tissues.

Myeloblasts, promyelocytes, and myelocytes are collectively referred to as the neutrophil proliferative pool (NPP) because these cells retain the capacity for cell division. As committed neutrophil precursors mature, their capacity to undergo cell division is lost. This population of postmitotic cells that includes metamyelocytes, band neutrophils, and mature segmented neutrophils is called the neutrophil storage pool (NSP). Neutrophils are released from the NSP to maintain circulating and marginated neutrophil pools in equilibrium. About 0.3×10^9 neutrophils per kilogram body weight are present in the circulating pool of healthy adults (Luchtman-Jones and Schwartz 2002).

Adults have a large NSP and can increase circulating neutrophils rapidly in response to infection (Maheshwari and Christensen 2004). To the contrary, newborn infants have a relatively small NSP (Maheshwari and Christensen 2004). These differences in the available pool of postmitotic neutrophils limit the ability of newborn infants to respond to infectious challenges. The circulating neutrophil concentration in humans is relatively low during gestation, but progressively rises until term. Postnatally, the circulating neutrophil count is much higher. Manroe and colleagues described neutrophil ranges in normal term infants during the first 28 days of life (Manroe et al. 1979). They delineated a rise in neutrophil count with a peak between 12 and 24 h with the range of neutrophil concentrations at that time between 7800 and 14,500 cells per microliter. The neutrophil count subsequently decreased and stabilized after 72 h with a lower value of 1750 cells per microliter. Mouzihno and coworkers later established a reference range for blood neutrophil concentrations in the very low

birth weight infant population (Mouzinho et al. 1994). The upper range for normal neutrophil concentration was similar to that of term infant. The lower levels defining neutropenia were about 2000 cells per microliter at 12 h and stabilized at 1000 cells per microliter by 48 h of life.

The normal circulating monocyte count in the healthy human adult is estimated to be between 300 and 450 monocytes/mm^3. Peripheral blood monocyte counts have been observed to vary in a cyclic fashion over a 3- to 6-day period (Douglas and Yoder 1996; Trubowitz and Davies 1982).

The production and kinetics of circulating human adult mononuclear phagocytes have been studied by in vivo pulse labeling of mononuclear phagocytes with tritiated thymidine followed by autotransfusion of radiolabeled leukocytes. The number of promonocytes present in bone marrow has been estimated to be between 3% and 5%, with approximately 40% of the promonocytes actively proliferating (Meuret et al. 1975). The promonocyte cell cycle rate varies between 30 and 48 h. These rapidly dividing cells achieve a production rate between 7×10^5 and 7×10^6 monocytes/kg of body weight per hour. After 60 h of maturation in the bone marrow, mature monocytes move into the intravascular space, where they circulate for approximately 3 days (Meuret et al. 1975). Van Furth and coworkers (van Furth et al. 1979) calculated that 1.66×10^{10} circulating monocytes leave the intravascular space/h. Therefore, these investigators estimated the turnover of monocytes to be 0.4×10^9 cells/day. Whitelaw (Whitelaw 1972) has suggested that the total intravascular monocyte pool is composed of a marginated pool and a circulating pool. He calculated that the marginated pool was 3.3 times greater than the circulating pool. Other investigators have failed to confirm a marginated pool of monocytes in human subjects (van Furth et al. 1979); however, experiments in mice and rats provide evidence for marginated monocyte pools (Meuret and Hoffmann 1973; van Furth and Sluiter 1986).

Analysis of tissue macrophage kinetics is difficult, given that the ultimate fate of tissue macrophages is not precisely known. Alveolar macrophages purportedly move from the respiratory tract to the alimentary tract, where they are eventually cleared (van Furth 1992). The fate of other tissue macrophages has not been determined.

Tissue macrophages are derived from bone marrow precursors. The first evidence for the bone marrow origin of macrophages was obtained in mouse chimeras (Haller et al. 1979) and rat parabiosis experiments (Parwaresch and Wacker 1984; Volkman 1966). Studies in human subjects have confirmed the data observed in animal experiments. In several patients undergoing bone marrow transplantation, isolation and characterization of lung (Thomas et al. 1976) and liver macrophages (Gale et al. 1978) provided evidence that these cells contained the karyotype of the bone marrow donor. Thus, terminally differentiated macrophages must have been derived from transplanted bone marrow. Furthermore, by following the disappearance of the Y body–containing macrophages from male patients who have received female donor marrow, the half-life of the alveolar macrophage was estimated to be 81 days.

The size of the tissue macrophage compartment is considerable. By some estimates, the number of tissue macrophages is 500–1000 times greater than the bone marrow compartment. Some organs, such as the lung and liver, may have particularly large macrophage populations that may account for between 20% and 30% of the total cell number. These cells are long lived and in a number of tissues have been estimated to survive for several months (van Furth 1992; Thomas et al. 1976; Gale et al. 1978).

96.2.1.2 Function

Leukocytes are the major effector cell for host defense against invading microorganisms. Neutrophils are present in the circulation until they encounter chemotactic factors that initiate rolling and adhesion to the vascular endothelium. Ultimately they migrate through the endothelium and move in response to a chemotactic stimulus to sites of microbial invasion. Mononuclear phagocytes (monocytes, macrophages, and dendritic cells) function primarily as cells resident within tissues where they engage in both innate and acquired immune functions. Innate functions of both neutrophils and mononuclear phagocytes include phagocytosis of opsonized microbes or targets exhibiting patterns recognition

molecules resembling components of microbes The ingested targets are degraded within intracellular vacuoles via the release of hydrolytic enzymes and reactive oxygen intermediates. Mononuclear phagocytes also process ingested materials and present them to lymphocytes generating local immune responses and initiating acquired immune functions.

96.2.1.3 Leukocyte Functional Differences Associated with Prematurity

After neutrophils have emigrated from the circulation, cell movement may occur either by random movement or by directed movement toward a chemoattractant. Random movement not related to a stimulus occurs in any direction with equal probability. The ability to undergo directed migration depends upon sensory mechanisms capable of detecting differences in concentration of chemotactic molecules and linking this information to the locomotory apparatus in the cell.

Random movement by neonatal neutrophils is normal compared to that observed in adult cells (Pahwa et al. 1977). However, a number of studies indicate that directed movement of neutrophils from preterm and term neonates to defined chemotactic stimuli is impaired (Luchtman-Jones and Schwartz 2002). Recent studies indicate that preterm neonatal neutrophil chemotaxis also may be reduced by cesarean section delivery and exposure to general or epidural anesthetic agents (Birle et al. 2015). Neutrophil recruitment in preterm neonates appears to be reduced due to diminished adherence to endothelial cells (Nussbaum et al. 2013). These adhesion-related abilities may correlate with markedly reduced expression of PSGL-1 and Mac-1 on neutrophils in preterm infants. In addition, human umbilical vein endothelial cells from extremely premature infants exhibit a severely diminished capability to recruit adult neutrophils perhaps secondary to diminished upregulation of E-selectin and ICAM-1. Neutrophil recruitment and endothelial cell adhesion-related functions are ontogenetically regulated in the fetus and preterm neonate.

Mononuclear phagocytes exhibit both random and directed movement (Miller 1978). Random or nondirected movement occurs in the absence of attracting substances. Directed movement along a concentration gradient of chemical attractants is essential for the effective localization of mononuclear phagocytes to sites of infection and inflammation. Chemoattractant molecules that bind to receptors on the cell surface govern this directional movement, called chemotaxis. Chemotactic substances are produced through activation of the complement, fibrinolytic, and kinin systems or are directly produced by microorganisms. These chemoattractants may also accentuate random migration of mononuclear phagocytes in the absence of a concentration gradient. An entire family of proinflammatory molecules called *chemokines* has been identified and many of its members have been characterized (Broxmeyer and Kim 1999). Several members of this family serve as potent chemoattractants for mononuclear phagocytes. Monocyte chemotactic protein 1, macrophage inflammatory protein 1, and regulation upon activation, normal T-cell expressed and secreted (RANTES) are key regulators of monocyte migration. Monocyte-derived dendritic cells migrate to lymphoid organs in response to secondary lymphoid chemokine (Sozzani et al. 1999; Chan et al. 1999).

Mononuclear phagocyte migration has been examined in cord blood and neonatal peripheral blood and has been compared with adult peripheral blood monocytes. In most reports, random movement by cord blood monocytes appears to be equivalent to that of adult peripheral blood monocytes (Marodi et al. 1980; Weston et al. 1977; Klein et al. 1977). To the contrary, several investigators have reported diminished directed movement by cord blood and neonatal peripheral blood compared with that of adult peripheral blood monocytes. Yegin (1983) reported that monocyte chemotaxis increased gradually during childhood and was equivalent to adult chemotactic activity after 5–6 years of age. These results are consistent with those of other investigators who reported similar chemotactic activity by cord blood and adult peripheral blood monocytes, but dramatically decreased chemotaxis by neonatal peripheral blood monocytes in the first few days of life (Raghunathan et al. 1982). Monocyte chemotaxis gradually increased but remained lower than adult peripheral blood monocyte activity over the first 6 months of life. Other groups of

investigators report a slightly increased chemotaxis of cord blood monocytes in response to endotoxin-activated adult serum or activated adult lymphocytes (Pahwa et al. 1977; Hawes et al. 1980). Differences in methods of measurements applied, patient populations examined, and monocyte isolation used likely account for the contradictory results reported by these investigators.

Neutrophils establish contact with microorgnisms through opsonins, including complement and IgG antibody. The phagocyte completely encircles the microorganisms with circumferential interactions between opsonins and receptors. Once the newly formed vacuole is internalized, the products of intracellular granules are discharged into the vacuole (Baehner 1975; Bainton 1981). Mobilization of granules appears to be normal in newborns compared to adults (Kjeldsen et al. 1996). Neutrophilic granules from newborn infants possess equivalent content of myeloperoxidase and lysozyme, but diminished quantities of lactoferrin and gelatinase (Kjeldsen et al. 1996; Ambruso et al. 1984).

In several experiments, neutrophils from healthy term infants provided opsonins from adult serum exhibited normal phagocytosis of a variety of microorganisms including *Escherichia coli*, group B *Streptococci*, *Pseudomonas aeruginosa*, *Serratia marcessans*, *Staphylococcus aureus*, and *Candida albicans* (McCracken and Eichenwald 1971; Harris et al. 1983; Forman and Stiehm 1969; Xanthou et al. 1975). Phagocytosis by neutrophils from preterm infants, while less well-studied, appears to have competent phagocytic functions for bacteria and foreign particles (McCracken and Eichenwald 1971; Forman and Stiehm 1969). Ingestion of Candida albicans by neutrophils of preterm infants was reported to be normal in one study, but diminished in others (Xanthou et al. 1975; Bektas et al. 1990; Al-Hadithy et al. 1981).

The kinetics of phagocytosis by monocytes from cord blood and adult peripheral blood have been studied by Schuit and Powell (Schuit and Powell 1980). These investigators found that monocytes isolated from adult peripheral blood ingested all polystyrene particles within 50 min. In comparison only 38% of cord blood monocytes had initiated phagocytosis in the same time period. The cord blood monocytes were able to ingest the particles by 100 min. These studies were not influenced by the presence of serum or heat-inactivated serum. Other investigators have reported that opsonized (IgG) sheep erythrocytes, *Staphylococcus aureus*, *Escherichia coli*, *Streptococcus pyogenes*, *Toxoplasma gondii*, and type II herpes simplex are ingested by cord blood monocytes as effectively as monocytes derived from adult peripheral blood (Speer and Johnston 1984). Defective phagocytosis of *Streptococcus agalactiae* by cord blood monocytes has been reported by Marodi and colleagues (Marodi et al. 1984). Monocytes derived from term cord blood ingested fewer group B *Streptococci* than monocytes isolated from adult blood. Other studies suggested that the phagocytic defect of group B *Streptococcus* by cord blood monocytes could be overcome by inclusion of adhesive glycoprotein fibronectin in the culture (Jacobs et al. 1985). Although fibronectin alone did not enhance phagocytosis, preopsonizing group B *Streptococcus* with IgG preparation in combination with fibronectin enhanced phagocytosis by cord blood monocytes.

The phagocytic activity of cord blood monocyte–derived macrophages has been compared with that of macrophages derived from adult blood monocytes. After a 10-day culture period, Speer and co-workers (Speer et al. 1988) determined that cord blood–derived macrophages ingested complement opsonized *Staphylococcus aureus* to the same extent as macrophages derived from adult blood. Other investigations compared the phagocytic activity of alveolar macrophages from intubated newborns with alveolar macrophages from bronchoalveolar lavage of adult subjects. Phagocytosis of *Candida albicans* by newborn and adult alveolar macrophages was determined to be equivalent with respect to rate and number of organisms ingested (D'Ambola et al. 1988).

96.3 Leukocyte Abnormalities

96.3.1 Etiology and Pathogenesis

The chief disorders of leukocytes observed in the newborn period include quantitative abnormalities such as neutropenia, neutrophilia, and

leukemoid reaction. Quantitative defects in phagocytic leukocytes also occur in conjunction with qualitative abnormalities and with rare hematopoietic disorders. Leukocyte disorders that occur in the neonatal period are categorized based on the frequency of the condition in Table 1.

96.3.1.1 Common Leukocyte Abnormalities

Infection

Animal studies comparing the hematopoietic response to infection between neonates and adults demonstrate the kinetic differences in the supply and release of neutrophil pools form the bone marrow (Erdman et al. 1982). These developmental differences increased susceptibility of newborn animals to exhaustion of bone marrow reserves when subjected to experimental infection and ultimately limit their capability to survive these infections (Christensen and Rothstein 1980; Christensen 1989). Septic neonates who are neutropenic have a higher mortality than nonneutropenic neonates (AlMulla and Christensen 1995; Rodwell et al. 1993). Neonates also have an immaturity of neutrophil function and production. Immaturity of granulopoiesis in preterm neonates is manifest by a low neutrophil cell mass, a reduced capacity for increasing progenitor cell proliferation, and frequent occurrence of neutropenia in response to sepsis (Carr 2000). There may be reduced ability of neonatal neutrophils in signal transduction, cell surface receptor upregulation, mobility, cytoskeletal rigidity, microfilament contraction, oxygen metabolism, and intracellular oxidant mechanisms (Hill 1987). In recent investigations, the in vitro response of cord blood neutrophils to peptidoglycan (Gram-positive bacterial components) and LPS (Gram-negative components) increased CD11b, chemotaxis, TNF-alpha, and IL-8 in neutrophils stimulated by peptidoglycan or LPS (Fong et al. 2014). Peptidoglycan, but not LPS, increased reactive oxygen species production. Moreover, neonatal neutrophils are capable of vigorous molecular and functional responses to bacterial components.

Associated with Maternal Hypertension

A high proportion of newborn infants delivered to women with hypertension have reduced circulating neutrophil concentrations (Manroe et al. 1979; Mouzinho et al. 1994). The neutrophil kinetic abnormality is decreased neutrophil production (Koenig and Christensen 1989a). This is supported by studies delineating a decrease in neutrophil progenitor cells and decreased cycling of these cells, a relatively normal NSP, and the absence of immature neutrophils in the circulation, termed a "left shift." This variety of neutropenia is particularly common in severe maternal hypertension accompanied by fetal growth restriction. The cause of reduced neutrophil production is uncertain, but does not appear to be related to maternal medications (Koenig and Christensen 1989a; Doron et al. 1994).

The significance of neutropenia associated with maternal hypertension is that nonspecific innate host defenses may be impaired. Several investigators have documented a higher incidence of

Table 1 Frequency of leukocyte abnormalities

Common	Moderately common	Rare
Bacterial and fungal infection	Twin-twin transfusion	Severe congenital neutropenia (Kostmann's syndrome)
Maternal hypertension	Isoimmune	Cyclic neutropenia
	Rh hemolytic disease	Shwachman-Diamond syndrome
	Drug induced	Reticular dysgenesis
	Viral infection (rubella, cytomegalovirus)	Autoimmune neutropenia
	Leukemoid reaction	Chediak-Higashi syndrome
		Dyskeratosis Congenita
		Chronic Granulomatous Disease
		Leukocyte adhesion deficiency types I and II

nosocomial infection among infants delivered to hypertensive mothers neutropenic infants compared to nonneutropenic infants (Koenig and Christensen 1989a; Doron et al. 1994; Cadnapaphornchai and Faix 1992).

96.3.1.2 Moderately Common Leukocyte Abnormalities

Associated with Rh Hemolytic Disease

A well-documented complication of severe Rh erythroblastosis fetalis is a reduction in the concentration of neutrophils and platelets (Koenig and Christensen 1989b; Zipursky 1993). In one series of 20 infants with Rh sensitization, 11 infants had severe disease requiring multiple exchange transfusions (Koenig and Christensen 1989b). Before exchange transfusion all infants with severe disease had neutropenia. The neutrophil kinetic defect persisted between 3 and 5 days in these infants, whereas none of the infants with mild disease exhibited neutrophil depletion.

Associated with Therapeutic Hypothermia for Hypoxic Ischemic Encephalopathy

Therapeutic hypothermia has become standard of care for term newborn infants diagnosed with hypoxic ischemic encephalopathy in the first few hours after birth (Shankaran et al. 2008; Azzopardi et al. 2009; Jacobs et al. 2011; Simbruner et al. 2010). In a randomized, controlled, multicenter trial of systemic hypothermia in neonatal hypoxic ischemic encephalopathy, total and leukocyte subsets and serum chemokine levels were measured over time in both hypothermia and normothermia groups as primary outcomes for safety (Jenkins et al. 2013). The hypothermia group had significantly lower median circulating total WBC and leukocyte subclasses than the normothermia group before rewarming. While the absolute neutrophil count rebounded after rewarming in the hypothermia group, chemokines were negatively correlated with their target leukocytes in the hypothermia group, suggesting active chemokine and leukocyte modulation by hypothermia. Relative leukopenia at 60–72 h correlated with more severe central nervous system injury in the hypothermia group.

Isoimmune Neonatal Neutropenia

Isoimmune neonatal neutropenia results from maternal production of IgG directed against antigens on fetal neutrophils (Maheshwari and Christensen 2004). This is analogous to Rh hemolytic disease in that maternal sensitization to fetal neutrophil antigens results in transplacentally acquired IgG antibody destroy the infant's neutrophils (Boxer et al. 1972). Maternal sensitization may occur during gestation and may occur even in the fetus of a primigravida (Lalezari and Radel 1974). The incidence of isoimmune neonatal neutropenia is estimated to be 0.5–2 per 1000 live births (Levine and Madyastha 1986).

Affected infants frequently develop a fever in the first days of life and are particularly susceptible to cutaneous infections caused by *Staphylococcus aureus*. *β-Hemolytic Streptococcus* and *Escherichia coli* have also been linked to infections among susceptible infants with this disorder. The onset of infection is usually concurrent with severe neutropenia. In the circulation, the concentrations of other myeloid lineages particularly monocytes and eosinophils are typically increased. Characteristic findings on bone marrow evaluation are myeloid hyperplasia with a paucity of mature neutrophils and normal erythropoietic and megakaryocytic elements.

Neutrophil antibodies are detected in the sera of mother and infant. The antibodies react against neutrophils of the patient and of the father, but they do not react against neutrophils from the mother. Several neutrophil-specific antibodies have been implicated including most commonly human neutrophil alloantigens (HNA)-1, HNA-2, and HNA-3. Other antigenic targets include NC1, SH, SAR, LAN, LEA, CN1, and certain HLA antigens. HNA-1 and NC1 have been identified as isotypes of the FcγIII receptor (Maheshwari and Christensen 2004). HNA-2 is an antigen on glycoprotein (GP)50 and HNA-3 corresponds to an antigen on GP75-90. The infant's neutrophil counts typically normalize over the first 1 to 5 weeks of life as might be expected with the half-life of maternal antibodies.

Treatment for affected infants is supportive. Therapy also includes appropriate antibiotic administration for infections and close follow-

up. The use of prophylactic antibiotics has been shown to be ineffective. Intravenous immunoglobulin (IVIG) administration and steroid therapy have not been shown to consistently improve circulating neutrophil counts. For infants with persistence of extremely low neutrophil counts, less than 500 cells per microliter, G-CSF administration might be undertaken. This therapy usually results in a prompt clinical response in circulating neutrophil concentrations.

Neonatal Autoimmune Neutropenia

Neonatal autoimmune neutropenia results from transplacental passage of maternal IgG autoantibodies directed against neutrophil antigens. Mothers of these infants can be asymptomatic or have autoimmune neutropenia from systemic lupus erythematosis or idiopathic thrombocytopenic purpura (Conway et al. 1987; Lalezari et al. 1986).

Drug-Induced Neutropenia

A significant number of medications have been implicated as causes of the development of neutropenia (Table 2). The mechanisms may involve bone marrow suppression or immune-mediated destruction. Several classes of medications including anti-inflammatory drugs, antibiotics, anticonvulsants, cardiovascular drugs, diuretics, and sedatives are commonly used on the maternity floor and in the newborn nursery. Marrow recovery generally begins several days after discontinuing the causative agent.

Leukemoid Reaction

Newborn infants may mount an exaggerated response to infection. As the neutrophil count increases and a left shift occurs, a significant increase in neutrophil precursors in the peripheral blood as well as an increase in the WBC count exceeding 50,000 cells per microliter is considered a leukemoid reaction. A leukemoid reaction in response to a severe infection in the newborn is frequently accompanied by cytoplasmic vacuoles within the neutrophils and by the appearance of toxic granulations. Infants with Down syndrome may have a type of leukemoid reaction unrelated to infection.

Table 2 Examples of drugs associated with neutropenia

Anti-inflammatory agents • Indomethacin • Pentazocine • Para-aminophenol derivatives o Acetomenophen • Pyrozolone derivatives o Aminopyrine o Dipyrone o Oxyphenbutazone o Phenylbutazone	**Antithyroid** • Carbimazole • Methimazole • Propylthiouracil
Antibiotics • Cephalosporins • Clindamycin • Gentamicin • Isoniazid • Penicillins and semisynthetic penicillins • Rifampin • Streptomycin • Trimethoprim-sulfamethoxazole • Vancomycin	**Cardiovascular** • Captopril • Dispopyramide • Hydralizine • Methyldopa • Procainamide • Propranolol • Quinidine
Anticonvulsants • Carbamazepine • Phenytoin • Valproate	**Diuretics** • Acetazolamide • Chlorthiadone • Chlorothiazide • Ethicrynic acid • Hydroclorothiazide
Antidepressants • Amitriptyline • Amoxapine • Doxepin • Imipramine	**Hypoglycemic agents** • Chlorpropamide • Tolbutamide
Antihistamines (H-2 Inhibitors) • Cimetidine • Ranitidine	**Sedatives** • Benzodiezapines • Meprobamate
Antimalarials • Amodiaquine • Chloroquine • Dapsone • Pyrimethamine • Quinine	**Phenothiazines** • Chlorpromazine • Phenothiazines

96.3.1.3 Rare Leukocyte Abnormalities

Severe Congenital Neutropenia and Cyclic Neutropenia

Severe congenital neutropenia (SCN) and cyclic neutropenia (CyN) are rare disorders of myelopoiesis usually caused by heterogeneous mutations in *ELANE*, the gene that encodes neutrophil elastase (Makaryan et al. 2015;

Horwitz et al. 1999; Dale et al. 2000). Mutations in *CSF3R*, *RAS*, and *RUNX1* are associated with evolution to MDS and AML, but the biological basis for the substantial difference in risk of leukemic evolution for CyN versus SCN is not known (Beekman and Touw 2010; Link et al. 2007; Skokowa et al. 2014).

Patients with SCN usually have ANC less than 500 cells per milliliter without regular cyclic fluctuations and a bone marrow showing maturational arrest of the myeloid lineage. CyN is characterized neutrophil fluctuations from near 2,000 cells per microliter to less than 200 cells per microliter at approximately 21-day intervals (Kostmann 1956). The duration of the neutropenic episodes ranges from 3 to 10 days. Other formed elements in the blood with short circulation times such as monocytes, platelets, and reticulocytes also cycle. Bone marrow aspirates during periods of neutropenia are noteworthy for cellular hypoplasia or maturational arrest (Bonilla et al. 1989). Individual with cyclic neutropenia have medical histories of repetitive infections occurring in tandem with cyclic episodes of depressed circulating neutrophil concentrations. The severity of infections tends to correlate with the degree of neutropenia. Although cyclic neutropenia is usually benign, death from sepsis occurs in as many as 10% of affected individuals. The disease persists throughout the patients' lifetimes (Dale et al. 1993).

A recent review of data from the Severe Chronic Neutropenia International Registry (SCNIR) including 307 patients with ELANE mutations was conducted to assess the relationships of mutations and risk for severe outcomes and MDS/AML (Makaryan et al. 2015). The diagnosis was made based on clinical data, and the *ELANE* mutations were identified later in all cases. The SCNIR population included 40 families with two or more affected members (CyN 20 families; SCN 20 families). The family members with neutropenia had *ELANE* mutations, and all members with *ELANE* mutations had neutropenia. Of the 307 patients only 10 were not exposed to G-CSF. For the SCN patients, there were 15 deaths attributable to MDS/AML and three transplant-related deaths in patients who failed to respond to G-CSF, and four others of unknown cause. For the CyN patients, there were eight deaths, none due to MDS/AML. Three deaths were attributable to sepsis; two of these patients were known not to be taking G-CSF as recommended, and one other patient was never treated with G-CSF. One death followed hematopoietic transplantation (not for MDS/ AML). The causes of the other four deaths were cancer (one), heart failure (one), stroke (one), and unknown (one).

Infections were common in these patients before G-CSF, including mouth ulcers (80%), pneumonia (49%), abscesses (19%), sepsis (17%), cellulitis (12%), and peritonitis (3%). Sixty-one of 97 patients (63%) with mutations unique to SCN reported pneumonia, compared to 31 of 73 patients (42%) with overlapping mutations and five of 26 patients (19%) with mutations only seen in CyN ($P = 3 \times 10^{-4}$). Abscesses occurred in all patient groups: overlapping mutations (four of 73, 5%), CyN (four of 26, 15%), or SCN (19 of 97, 20%).

With longitudinal follow-up, severe events (MDS/AML, stem cell transplant, or death) were far greater in SCN versus CyN patients (eight of 120 CyN vs. 62 of 187 SCN, $P < 10^{-4}$). The striking excess of severe events over time in SCN versus CyN and for mutation unique to SCN versus the overlapping mutations in patients on G-CSF was also highly statistically significant ($P < 10^{-4}$).

The investigators grouped mutations in five principal categories: missense, frameshift, termination, intronic, and deletion or insertion. The missense mutations were most common, and 94% were predicted to have a probable or possible damaging effect on the protein structure by Polyphen 2 analysis. The most striking finding was the association of frameshift mutations in congenital patients with a high risk of abscesses (8/17 evaluable patients, 47%) and evolution to MDS/AML (6/19 patients, 32%). It appears also that a higher proportion of termination mutations are associated with leukemic transformation, but the number of these patients is relatively small. Two mutations C151Y (3/4 patients) and G214R (3/9 patients) appear to confer a high risk of leukemia. The apparent high risk associated with these mutations may be attributable to major

changes in protein structure due to size and charge/polarity differences of exchanged amino acids. Overall, the study demonstrated that clinically important genotype–phenotype correlations of clinical outcomes and the results of sequencing of *ELANE* for patients with cyclic and congenital neutropenia. Some mutations appear to be linked to a relatively good prognosis, notably P139L, IVS4 + 5 G > A, and S126L, whereas other mutations, specifically C151Y and G214R, are associated with a notably poor prognosis. This analysis provides useful information to guide clinical care and to focus research on the cellular and molecular mechanisms for neutropenia and leukemogenesis in these patients.

Shwachman-Diamond Syndrome

Shwachman-Diamond syndrome is an autosomal recessive disorder, with an incidence estimated at 1 in 50,000 births, characterized by ineffective hematopoiesis, exocrine pancreatic dysfunction, and metaphyseal dysostosis, and an increased risk of leukemia (Shwachman et al. 1964). Typically, patients with Shwachman-Diamond syndrome present in the first year of life with diarrhea and failure to thrive. In addition to pancreatic insufficiency, these patients uniformly develop neutropenia. About 60% of patients are malnourished and short in stature and many also exhibit ichthyotic skin rashes. Shwachman-Diamond syndrome is also associated with other clinical findings including microcephaly, hypertelorism, retinitis pigmentosa, syndactyly, cleft palate, dental dysplasia, skin pigment defects, and myocardial fibrosis (Burroughs et al. 2009). Leukemic transformation has been known to occur. Patients are predisposed to skin infections and pneumonia as a result of the neutropenia. Supportive measures for patients with SDS include pancreatic enzymes, antibiotics, transfusions, and granulocyte colony-stimulating factor. The only definitive therapy is bone marrow transplantation.

Boocock and colleagues reported a causal mutation in the SBDS gene, named after Schwachman-Bodian-Diamond (Boocock et al. 2003). Approximately 90% of SDS patients have biallelic mutations in the SBDS gene. The structure and function of the SBDS gene has not been determined, but accumulating evidence suggests that the gene plays a role in ribosome biosynthesis and RNA processing (Ganapathi et al. 2007). SDS cells exhibit abnormal expression of multiple genes involved in ribosome biogenesis and rRNA and mRNA processing and to have decreased expression of several ribosomal protein genes involved in cell growth and survival (Rujkijyanont et al. 2009). Additionally, SBDS has been shown to co-sediment with the 60S ribosomal precursor subunit in sucrose gradients and to associate with the 28S rRNA that is a component of the 60S subunit (Ganapathi et al. 2007). Although these findings provide evidence for a role of SBDS in ribosome biogenesis, SBDS is a multifunctional protein and may contribute to nonribosomal activities that play a role in the clinical phenotype. SBDS genotyping may be used to confirm the definitive diagnosis.

Reticular Dysgenesis

Reticular dysgenesis, also called congenital aleukocytosis, is characterized by severe neutropenia associated with leukopenia, presence of rudimentary thymic lymphoid and splenic tissue, and agammaglobulinemia (Roper et al. 1985). Histological examination of the bone marrow, spleen, and lymphoid tissue reveals normal reticular structure with normal erythroid and megakaryocyte elements, but with absent or sparse myeloid cells. The mechanism of the disorder is unknown, but a defect in telomere function is suspected (Savage and Alter 2009). Bacterial and viral infections occur early in life and are severe. Aggressive antibiotic therapy and supportive care are necessary for survival. Treatment with G-CSF and GM-CSF has been ineffective. Bone marrow transplantation remains the only long-term treatment option available for infants with this disorder (Roper et al. 1985; Bertrand et al. 2002).

Dyskeratosis Congenita

Dyskeratosis congenita (DKC) is an inherited bone marrow failure syndrome caused by germline defects in telomere biology and diagnosed by the classical triad of abnormal nails,

reticular skin pigmentation, and oral leukoplakia (Savage and Alter 2009). Clinical diagnosis of DKC can be challenging due to phenotypic heterogeneity, variable age of onset of the mucocutaneous triad, and presence of several clinical variants of DKC. The presence of very short telomeres, resulting of germline mutations in key telomere biology genes, is the unifying feature of DKC and its clinical variants. Telomere length less than the first percentile for age in leukocyte subsets measured by flow cytometry with in situ hybridization (flow FISH) is highly sensitive and specific for DKC. Patients with DC are at high risk of developing trilineage bone marrow failure, pulmonary fibrosis, liver disease (cirrhosis and fibrosis), and malignancy (myelodysplastic syndrome, acute myelogenous leukemia, and squamous cell carcinoma of the head and neck and anogenital region).

DKC can be inherited in one of three forms, X-linked, autosomal dominant, or autosomal recessive (Kirwan and Dokal 2008). De novo germline mutations are also relatively frequent in DC and to date, 70% of DC patients have an identifiable germline mutation. These mutations occur in genes responsible for functioning and maintenance of telomeres. Currently, there are nine known DC-associated genes (DKC1, TERT, TERC, TINF2, WRAP53, NOP10, NHP2, CTC1, and RTEL1). X-linked DKC, which has a more severe phenotype compared with the autosomal dominant form of DKC, is caused by a mutation in *DKC1*, which encodes dyskerin (Heiss et al. 1998). Patients with the autosomal dominant form of DKC have been found to have mutations in *TERC*, and two families with the autosomal recessive form of DKC have been found to have mutation in *TERT*, suggesting that disruption of the telomerase complex alone could result in defective hematopoiesis (Marrone et al. 2007). Although it is clear that telomeres play a significant role in the pathogenesis of DKC, there may be a distinct contribution from ribosomal defects. Ongoing work examining genotype/phenotype correlations and basic mechanisms will hopefully elucidate the true contributions of telomerase activity and impaired ribosomal biogenesis to the pathophysiology of DKC.

Bone marrow failure (BMF) develops in up to 90% patients with DKC and can be life-threatening. Hematopoietic stem cell transplant (HSCT) is the only current modality for cure of BMF associated with DKC (Savage and Alter 2009). Treatment with androgen therapy is often considered for BMF in individuals who cannot or do not wish to undergo HSCT. Between 50% and 70% of DC patients treated with androgens respond and no longer be dependent on red blood cell and platelet transfusions.

Leukocyte Adhesion Deficiency Type I, Type II, and Type III

Leukocyte adhesion deficiency (LAD) encompasses a rare group of autosomal recessive disorders (Etzioni 2009). LAD-1 is associated with defects in neutrophil adhesion and chemotaxis, resulting in impaired clearance of complement-opsonized microorganisms. Infants present with delayed separation of the umbilical cord and recurrent infections despite a normal or increased neutrophil count. LAD should be suspected in any infant with unusually severe bacterial infections accompanied by normal or increased circulating neutrophils and a striking absence of purulent material at the site of infections.

The clinical presentation varies depending on the relative deficiency of CD18. CD18 is the β_2-subunit of the cell surface leukocyte integrin. These molecules are involved in adherence, chemotaxis, C3bi-mediated ingestion, degranulation, and neutrophil respiratory burst. Diagnosis of LAD-1 is made by demonstration of a severe deficiency of the β_2-subunit of neutrophil integrins. Carriers can be identified as having about 50% of the normal β_2-subunit levels in circulating neutrophils, whereas affected individuals express 0–10% levels. α/β-Integrins are common on the surface of all neutrophils and make up three distinct cell surface proteins: LFA-1 ($\alpha_1\beta_2$), MAC-1 ($\alpha_m\beta_2$), and P150,95 ($\alpha_x\beta_2$). Each of these integrins is affected because they require a common β_2-subunit that is diminished in quantity or functionally defective. Several mutations have been identified in the gene coding for the β_2-subunit. These mutations fall into several categories in which there are absent, low, or normal level of

CD18 mRNA and in which the β_2-subunit protein precursor is absent, low in abundance, or abnormal in size. There is a close genotype–phenotype correlation between the molecular defect and the clinical severity of disease.

Leukocyte trafficking from bloodstream to tissue is important for the continuous surveillance for foreign antigens as well as for rapid leukocyte accumulation at sites of inflammatory response or tissue injury. Leukocyte interaction with vascular endothelial cells is a pivotal event in the inflammatory response and is mediated by several families of adhesion molecules. The crucial role of the beta(2)-integrin subfamily in leukocyte emigration was established after leukocyte adhesion deficiency (LAD) type I was discovered.

LAD type II is a rare autosomal recessive clinical syndrome involving recurrent bacterial infections, short stature, severe mental retardation, and the hh (Bombay) RBC phenotype. Neutrophils from patients affected with this disorder exhibit markedly diminished chemotaxis in vitro, although the neutrophils display normal levels of CD18 and are able to ingest serum-opsonized particles. The molecular defect in these patients is a defect in the fucosyltransferase gene responsible for the carbohydrate linkages associated with the AB blood groups, specifically the sialyl-Lewis X structure. Neutrophil function is defective in these individuals because sialyl-Lewis X is the neutrophil cell surface ligand recognized by endothelial cell surface E-selectin and P-selectin receptors (Phillips et al. 1995).

The LAD type II disorder clarifies the role of the selectin receptors and their fucosylated ligands. Clinically, patients with LAD type II suffer not only from a less severe form of infectious episodes resembling the moderate phenotype of LAD type I, but also from severe psychomotor and growth retardation. LAD type III emphasizes the importance of the integrin-activation phase in the adhesion cascade. All hematopoietic integrin activation processes are defective, which lead to severe infection as observed in LAD type I and to marked increase tendency for bleeding problems (defective activation of beta(1), beta(2), and beta (3) integrins) (Fagerholm et al. 2014). Mutations in FERMT3 (KINDLIN3) have now been shown to be the basis for LAD-III (Rognoni et al. 2016). Mutations in FERMT3 (KINDLIN3) disrupt KINDLIN3, a cytoskeletal protein that interacts with the cytoplasmic tails of beta(1)-, beta(2)-, and beta(3)-integrins and is required for transmembrane signaling of these heterodimers. Patients with these disorders suffer from life-threatening bacterial infections, and in its severe form, death usually occurs in early childhood unless bone marrow transplantation is performed.

Chediak-Higashi Syndrome

Chediak-Higashi syndrome is a rare, autosomal recessive disorder characterized by the presence of giant cytoplasmic granules in multiple cells throughout the body. The syndrome affects neutrophil and lymphocyte function (Introne et al. 1999). Mutations in lysosomal trafficking regulator (LYST) cause Chediak-Higashi syndrome (Gil-Krzewska et al. 2016). Our understanding of how LYST regulates lytic granule exocytosis is very limited. Neutrophils display abnormal adherence and chemotaxis, delayed degranulation, and impaired ingestion and killing of microorganisms. Patients with this syndrome are highly susceptible to bacterial infections. Most patients with Chediak-Higashi syndrome exhibit lymphohistiocytic infiltration of multiple organs that appears to result from a lack of natural killer cell function (Ji et al. 2016). Death often occurs in the first decade of life from infection, bleeding, or lymphohistiocytic infiltration. With early and accurate diagnosis, bone marrow transplantation can be effective in treatment of the hematopoietic complications of Chediak-Higashi syndrome (Sanchez-Guiu et al. 2014).

Chronic Granulomatous Disease

Chronic granulomatous disease (CGD) is an inherited immunodeficiency syndrome in which generation of superoxide by the respiratory burst oxidase of phagocytic leukocytes is markedly diminished or absent (Roos 2016). The disorder, which has an incidence of approximately one per 250,000 individuals, results from mutations in any one of four essential subunits of the respiratory burst complex. Superoxide generated during the

respiratory burst is the precursor for a number of potent oxidants that are important in elimination of many microbial pathogens. Approximately two thirds of CGD cases are caused by defects in the X-linked gene encoding gp91-phox, the large subunit of the flavocytochrome b_{588}, a plasma membrane heterodimer that is the redox center of the phagocyte oxidase (Ghosh et al. 2015). A rare autosomal recessive form of CGD is caused by mutations in gene encoding the small subunit of the p22-phox flavocytochrome b_{588}. Other cases of autosomal recessive CGD are caused by gene defects in two soluble proteins that interact with flavocytochrome b588, p47-phox, or p67-phox.

The clinical manifestations of CGD are apparent during infancy or early childhood (Roos 2016 p. 103). Patients with CGD experience recurrent purulent bacterial and fungal infections that are difficult to treat and often may be life-threatening. Common sites of infection are skin, lymph nodes, lungs, bones, liver, and the gastrointestinal tract. Individuals with CGD are particularly susceptible to infections with *Staphylococcus aureus*, a variety of Gram-negative bacilli including *Pseudomonas*, *Salmonella*, and *Serratia* species and fungus such as *Aspergillus* species. Many of these microorganisms express catalase, which prevents phagocytes of CGD patients from scavenging microbe-generated hydrogen peroxide to promote microbial killing within the phagosome. The hallmark of CGD is the propensity to develop chronic inflammatory granulomas with wide spread tissue distribution.

The prognosis for individuals with CGD has improved significantly since the disorder was first described in the 1950s. Current management includes aggressive treatment of acute infections in combination of antimicrobial medications and with the use of prophylactic antibiotics during infection-free periods. Also prevention of infections through immunizations is recommended (Roos 2016). Use of prophylactic interferon-γ (IFN-γ) induces a reduction in the risk for serious infections (The International Chronic Granulomatous Disease Cooperative Study Group 1991). Suppression of inflammation with TNFα blocking agents has been successful in treating patients with severe colitis, but this therapy has been associated with significant infectious complications (Uzel et al. 2010).

Rapid diagnosis of severe forms of CGD is essential since hematopoietic stem cell transplantation (HSCT) may be curative in over 90% of patients (Roos 2016; Ghosh et al. 2015). HSCT is highly successful early in the course of the disease, but the outcomes rapidly decline with co-existing morbidity, increasing age and less well-matched donors.

Because the genetic defect of CGD affects primarily cells of the hematopoietic system, this disorder is prime candidate for gene therapy targeted at hematopoietic stem cells. Insertion of a functional copy of the involved gene into hematopoietic stem cells should reconstitute the respiratory burst oxidase activity in circulating and tissue phagocytes and thus could provide a life-long cure of the disease. Clinical trials for chronic granulomatous disease have demonstrated that gene transfer into hematopoietic stem cells and autologous transplant can result in clinical improvement and is curative for many patients. Unfortunately, early clinical trials were complicated by vector-related insertional mutagenic events for CGD and other immunodeficiency diseases (Kuo and Kohn 2016). Clinical trials for CGD using alternative retro- or lenti-viral vector constructs that are self-inactivating, and they have shown clinical efficacy without leukemic events thus far. The field of gene therapy continues to progress, with improvements in viral vector profiles, stem cell culturing techniques, and site-specific genome editing platforms (Roos 2016; Ghosh et al. 2015; Kuo and Kohn 2016).

Autoimmune Neonatal Neutropenia

Autoimmune neutropenia (AIN) is a disorder caused by increased destruction of neutrophils as a result of autoantibodies to the patient's own neutrophils (Veldhuisen et al. 2014). The incidence is approximately one per 100,000 live births (Boxer et al. 1975). Primary AIN is not associated with other autoimmune disorders such as systemic lupus erythematosis. Reports of associations with parvovirus B19 and β-lactam antibiotics suggest mechanisms such as development of cross-reacting antibodies resulting from

molecular mimicry, changes in endogenous antigens, enhanced HLA expression, or loss of suppression of self-reacting lymphocyte clones. HNA-1a (NA-1) autoimmunization has been linked to HLA-DR2, a finding implicating immune response genes (Lyall et al. 1992). Patients with this immune-mediated neutropenia are identified in the first 3 years of life with a variety of infections. In approximately 80% of patients the infections are mild, consisting of abscesses, conjunctivitis, gastroenteritis, otitis media, pyoderma, and upper respiratory infections. In the remaining cases, AIN predisposes to serious infections such as meningitis, pneumonia, and sepsis (Bux et al. 1998). Diagnosis of AIN is made by detection of neutrophil-specific antibodies (Farruggia 2016). Generally, patients with AIN do not require specific treatment for the neutropenia; however, to increase neutrophil counts in cases of severe infection or before elective surgery, some patients have been treated with corticosteroids, IVIG or G-CSF. Corticosteroids and IVIG increased neutrophil counts in about 50% of individuals, whereas GCSF increased neutrophil counts in all patients treated (Farruggia 2016). Infections are treated symptomatically with antibiotics. Infants with recurrent infections are often treated with prophylactic antibiotics.

96.3.2 Clinical Aspects

Classification of leukocyte abnormalities according to the underlying kinetic mechanism in can provide useful clues for diagnosis and management of affected infants. The complete blood count and differential white count provides an estimate of the responsible kinetic mechanism by determining the degree of left shift, or the ratio of immature to total neutrophils in the blood. Neutropenia accompanied by a large left shift is likely to be on the kinetic basis of accelerated neutrophil destruction or usage. A large left shift is defined as a ratio of immature (band neutrophils or metamyelocytes) to total neutrophils of greater than 0.3. On the contrary, neutropenias in which only mature neutrophils are observed in the blood are more likely to be on the kinetic basis of diminished neutrophil production or excessive margination (Koenig and Christensen 1991).

The variety of leukocyte abnormality is often suggested by associated findings (Table 3). For instance, neutropenia in an infant with intrauterine growth restriction delivered to a mother with hypertension is likely to have neutropenia based on diminished neutrophil production as is commonly seen in that condition (Koenig and Christensen 1991). The presence of neutropenia in the mother whose infant presented with neutropenia would prompt evaluation for maternal autoimmune antibodies causing immune-mediated neutrophil destruction. The presence of steatorrhea in a neutropenic neonate should prompt consideration of Shwachman-Diamond syndrome since this is present in the majority of infants with this condition (Shwachman et al. 1964). Severe and prolonged neutropenia, with counts typically less than 200 cells per microliter associated with monocytosis and eosinophilia on peripheral blood smear, is seen in Kostmann's syndrome (Kostmann 1956). The bone marrow examination in these infants is characterized by arrested neutrophil development at the promyelocyte or myelocyte stage. Neutrophilia with immature circulating myeloid elements

Table 3 Associated findings in newborn patients with leukocyte abnormalities that can suggest a specific disorder

Associated finding	Variety of leukocyte abnormality
Albinism	Chediak-Higashi syndrome
Anemia and multiple gestation	Donor in twin-twin transfusion
Blueberry muffin rash	Congenital cytomegalovirus
Down syndrome	Leukemoid reaction
Hydrops	Rh hemolytic disease
Monocytosis and eosinophilia	Kostmann's syndrome
Mother with hypertension	Neutropenia of PIH
Mother with neutropenia	Maternal autoimmune neutropenia
Pancytopenia	Reticular dysgenesis
Shock	Endotoxemia or sepsis
Steatorrhea	Shwachman-Diamond syndrome

observed association with a stable infant with Down syndrome would prompt a period of clinical observation. In most cases, the neutrophilia is generally transient; however, these infants require long-term follow-up as up to 30% of these infants may develop leukemia later in childhood (Homans et al. 1993). Neutrophilia or neutropenia with a left shift in conjunction with clinical signs of shock will prompt early and aggressive antibiotic treatment and supportive care in addition to and an evaluation to identify the causative microbial agent. Association of neutrophilia and the presence of a "blueberry muffin rash" often indicative of extramedullary hematopoiesis might prompt evaluation for congenital viral infections such as cytomegalovirus (CMV).

96.3.3 Differential Diagnosis

When evaluating a neonate with leukocyte abnormalities, it can be helpful to maintain the perspective that some varieties of these abnormalities are common and others are exceedingly rare. The most common causes of leukocyte abnormalities among infants have an underlying cause that is obvious. One variety of neutropenia in conjunction with a large left shift or an immature to total neutrophil ratio exceeding 0.3–0.5 accompanies overwhelming sepsis, whereas another variety of neutropenia (generally with no left shift or an immature to total neutrophil ratio of less than 0.2) occurs in an infant with intrauterine growth restriction born to a woman with pregnancy-induced hypertension. In general these common varieties of neutropenia do not require additional diagnostic evaluation. Neutropenia accompanying sepsis resolves quickly if the patient survives. However, if neutropenia in the infant with sepsis persists for several days additional evaluation should be considered. Similarly, in most cases of neutropenia accompanying pregnancy-induced hypertension, neutropenia resolves within 5 days. If neutropenia persists for more than 5 days, additional evaluation may be considered particularly if the neutrophil count is less than 500 cells per microliter.

Laboratory tests to be considered are those that provide a specific diagnosis such as alloimmune or autoimmune neutropenia. These tests, while not diagnostic, are required to complete evaluations of some rare forms of neutropenia such as congenital and cyclic neutropenia. Obtaining a complete blood count on the infant, including microscopic examination of neutrophil morphology, can be useful in identifying features such as left shift, monocytosis, eosinophilia, and the presence of cytoplasmic inclusions formed by fused lysosomes. Monocytosis and eosinophilia are commonly observed in patients with congenital neutropenia and cytoplasmic inclusions are characteristic of Chediak-Higashi syndrome (Introne et al. 1999). Also, a complete blood count on the mother to establish her neutrophil concentration can be useful to detect cases of autoimmune neutropenia in which mother has immune-mediated neutropenia, which is passively acquired by the fetus. Maternal and infant neutrophil antigen typing and antineutrophil antibody determination should identify most cases of immune-mediated neutropenia.

To evaluate neonatal immune mediated neutropenia, antibody testing is performed on both maternal and infant blood samples including two screening tests: (1) a neutrophil agglutination assay and (2) a granulocyte immunofluorescence assay. If either assay is positive, an HLA screen is performed because HLA antibodies can react with neutrophil assays and it cannot be determined whether the antibody is neutrophil specific or HLA related. When this occurs an additional test with antigen capture assay is use. In this assay monoclonal antibody immobilization of neutrophil antigens is done to differentiate between neutrophil antigen-specific antibodies from HLA antibodies (Farruggia 2016; Bux 2001). This assay can detect more than one neutrophil antigen-specific antibody.

Bone marrow study may be useful in patients with severe and prolonged neutropenia in whom isoimmune and maternal autoimmune neutropenia have been excluded. Bone marrow aspirate or biopsy can be helpful by suggesting the kinetic mechanism underlying the neutropenia by estimation of proliferative myeloid cells compared to

postmitotic myeloid cells. For example, when neutropenia is caused by diminished neutrophil production, the proliferative compartment is decreased. In accelerated neutrophil usage or destruction, the proliferative compartment responds by expanding production. In addition, mature neutrophils are rapidly released into the peripheral blood, simulating a maturational arrest or decreased postmitotic pool. Despite its utility in narrowing the differential diagnosis, bone marrow study almost never provides a precise diagnosis. For instance, no pathognomonic feature of bone marrow biopsy discriminates completely between hyporegenerative neutropenias in the neonatal period such as between neutropenia associated with maternal hypertension or Shwachman-Diamond syndrome. In a few instances, there are useful morphological clues in the bone marrow. For example, congenital neutropenia syndrome is suggested by enlargement and binucleation of promyelocytes and other myeloid precursors (Gorlin 1993). In autoimmune neutropenia, the bone marrow may contain macrophages with ingested antibody-coated neutrophils.

Neutrophil counts vary considerably early in the neonatal period with a mean about 11,000 cells per microliter and a range between 6,000 and 26, 000 cells per microliter (Manroe et al. 1979; Schelonka et al. 1994). After the first 12 h of life, neutrophil counts fall reaching a mean of 5000 cells per microliter (range 1000 to 10,000 cells per microliter). Neutrophilia, defined as an elevation of the circulating absolute neutrophil count more than two standard deviations above the mean, may occur in response to both bacterial and viral infections, stress (postoperative or after seizures), or in conjunction with hemolytic anemia or immune thrombocytopenia. Occasionally, newborn infants exhibit an exaggerated response to infection with a significant increase in total WBC count (50,000 cells per microliter) and increased early myeloid precursors in the peripheral blood, termed a leukemoid reaction. The leukemoid reaction observed with a severe infection is often accompanied by cytoplasmic vacuoles within neutrophils and by the appearance of toxic granulations. The duration of the reactions range from days to weeks. Approximately 10% of infants with Down syndrome may have a transient leukemoid reaction that resembles congenital leukemia (Homans et al. 1993). It is characterized by the presence of megakaryoblasts in the peripheral blood, hepatosplenomegaly, variable thrombocytopenia, infrequently hydrops fetalis, and severe hepatic fibrosis. Abnormalities in all three hematopoietic lineages have been described. In most cases, the leukemoid reaction is transient;, however, in up to 30% of infants with Down syndrome infants who experience a neonatal leukemoid reaction acute megaloblastic leukemia it occurs later in childhood. Leukemoid reactions have also been reported in phenotypically normal infants who have trisomy 21 mosaicism associated with a clonal trisomy 21 in bone marrow cells (Brodeur et al. 1980).

96.3.4 Prognosis

96.3.4.1 Infection

Infection remains a major cause of illness and death in the neonatal period (Gladstone et al. 1990). Newborn babies have an immature immune system and therefore may not elicit all signs of infection, and delay in treatment may lead to severe illness or death (Maheshwari and Christensen 2004). Early treatment with antibiotics has been shown to reduce mortality due to sepsis in the neonatal period (Siegel and McCracken 1981). Early treatment depends on knowledge of risk factors and picking up early signs of infection and laboratory screening for markers of infection in this age group (Philip and Hewitt 1980). However, the signs of infection tend to be nonspecific. Suspected sepsis is therefore often defined as any clinical concern for infection to warrant the starting of intravenous antibiotic therapy before laboratory or microbiological evidence of infection.

Although advances in neonatal intensive care have led to improved survival of very low birth weight (VLBW) and extremely premature infants, late onset sepsis (systemic infection after 72 h of age) continues to be a significant cause of morbidity and mortality. The incidence of late onset sepsis increases with both decreasing birthweight and gestational age and has been reported as

occurring in approximately 27% of VLBW infants (Stoll et al. 2015). Infants with the lowest birth weights are also more likely to have multiple episodes of sepsis. In developing countries, infection is estimated to cause 30–40% of neonatal deaths (Seale et al. 2015). The spectrum of organisms responsible for early onset (vertically transmitted) sepsis differs from that associated with late onset (nosocomial) sepsis (Shane and Stoll 2014). Nosocomial infections are frequently associated with clinical deterioration including increased apnea or ventilatory requirement, temperature instability, abdominal distension, acidosis, lethargy, septic shock, necrotizing enterocolitis, meningitis, and death. The complications of necrotizing enterocolitis and meningitis predispose an infant to an increased risk of future neurological impairment (Shah et al. 2012; Tsai et al. 2016) and the mortality from late onset sepsis remains high, about 7–10% (Stoll et al. 2015). This risk is secondary to immature immune responses, poorly developed skin and mucosal barriers to infection, numerous entry portals for organisms via cannulae, catheters and endotracheal tubes, and continuing exposure to opportunistic organisms during often a prolonged hospital stay.

96.3.5 Therapy and Treatment

96.3.5.1 Antibiotics

Early neonatal sepsis is mainly acquired from the mother. Vertical transmission of infection from mother to infant may take place before birth, during labor, or at the time of delivery. Most infants with peripartum acquired sepsis will develop clinical symptoms of sepsis within two days of life. After this period, nosocomial and community-acquired infections start to play a bigger role. The bacteria most commonly implicated in early neonatal sepsis are Group B *Streptococcus* and Gram-negative bacilli, particularly Escherichia coi (Stoll et al. 2011). Neonatal intensive care units or special care baby units tend to choose empirical first line antibiotic therapy that will cover both Gram-negative and Gram-positive bacteria. A combination of an aminoglycoside such as gentamicin and a beta-lactam such as ampicillin or penicillin has been the treatment of choice for early neonatal sepsis.

The range of organisms causing late onset sepsis includes Gram-positive and Gram-negative bacteria as well as fungi. Since bacterial infections predominate, empiric antibiotic regimens focus on cover for both Gram-positive and negative bacterial infection. These antibiotics can be either narrow or broad spectrum in the range of organisms that they target. The epidemiology of late onset infection differs between developing and developed countries in the incidence of infection, the organisms responsible, and the subsequent mortality rates. Historical reviews have also demonstrated that the predominant organisms responsible for neonatal sepsis have changed with time (Lamba et al. 2016; Mularoni et al. 2014; Greenhow et al. 2012).

In developing countries, the most common organisms isolated from neonatal blood cultures taken from babies in the first week of life are *Klebsiella species*, *Escherichia coli*, *and Staphylococcus aureus* (Zaidi et al. 2009). After the first week of life, *S. aureus*, group B *Streptococcus*, *Streptococcus pneumoniae*, and nontyphoidal *Salmonella species* were most frequent. *S. pneumoniae* was most common in the post-neonatal period. Gram-negatives predominated among home-delivered babies. The World Health Organization recommends that initial treatment of suspected neonatal sepsis should be with penicillin and gentamicin (The WHO Young Infants Study Group 1999). This regimen covers most of the likely organisms, but significant resistance, in particular to cotrimoxazole among all pathogens, and to gentamicin and third-generation cephalosporins among Klebsiella and emerging resistance in E. coli is a cause for concern. Recent studies support the use of simplified antibiotic regiments including oral amoxicillin rather than injectable penicillin and gentamicin when hospitalization is not possible (African Neonatal Sepsis Trial (AFRINEST) group et al. 2015a; African Neonatal Sepsis Trial (AFRINEST) group et al. 2015b).

In developed countries, staphylococcus aureus was previously responsible for the majority of late onset infections in many neonatal units with other commonly being isolated organisms coagulase

negative *Staphylococci*, *Escherichia coli*, group B *Streptococcus*, *Klebsiella pneumoniae*, *Enterococcus*, *Candida*, and *Pseudomonas*. Coagulase negative *Staphylococci* have now emerged as the leading cause of late onset sepsis in almost all developed countries and account for greater than 50% of positive blood cultures (Marchant et al. 2013). As skin commensals, these organisms are also common blood culture contaminants, and there is a lack of consensus as to how to interpret coagulase negative *Staphylococci* positive results. In the intensive care setting, the vast majority of coagulase negative *Staphylococci* are resistant to methicillin and thus infants with suspected late onset infection are typically treated with empiric broad spectrum antibiotics that include vancomycin (Rubin et al. 2002). There are concerns regarding unrestricted vancomycin use as a risk factor for the development of resistant organisms, particularly enterococci. Practice guidelines are recommended to restrict the use of vancomycin (Rubin et al. 2002). Its routine use as prophylaxis against nosocomial infection is not recommended (Craft et al. 2000).

In general prophylactic antibiotics are recommended for children with chemotherapy-induced neutropenia and children with chronic neutropenic conditions whose neutrophil count is less than 500 cells per microliter until recombinant G-CSF administration raises the neutrophil count to greater than 1000 cells per microliter (Feng et al. 2014; Ozkaynak et al. 2005). Broad use of prophylactic antibiotics for neutropenic neonates is not recommended. In most cases, neutropenia is of limited duration and general use of antibiotics may contribute to emergence of bacteria with high antibiotic resistance. Individualization of care to include prophylactic antibiotics might be considered for an infant with severe neutropenia (500 cells per microliter) continuing for several days and requiring treatment with G-CSF to increase the neutrophil count above 1000 cells per microliter. Prophylactic antibiotics might also be considered for an infant with severe prolonged neutropenia who is unresponsive to G-CSF treatment. The precise antibiotics used in such cases should be selected based on the local nursery bacterial epidemiology.

96.3.5.2 Granulocyte Transfusions

The availability of new generations of effective antibiotics, recombinant hematopoietic growth factors to counter neutropenia, the risk of transmission of infection, and the necessity for appropriate technology are some of the factors that have diminished the enthusiasm for the use of granulocyte transfusions in neonates. A recent systematic review evaluated the role of granulocyte transfusions as an adjunct to antibiotics in the treatment of neutropenic septic newborns (Pammi and Brocklehurst 2011). Authors of this systematic review found that no recent studies of granulocyte transfusion have been conducted in newborn infants. They found no significant difference in mortality of all causes during hospitalization in infants with sepsis and neutropenia who received granulocyte transfusions when compared with placebo or no granulocyte transfusion.

96.3.5.3 IVIG

Intravenous Immunoglobulin for Preventing Infection in Preterm and/or Low Birth Weight Infants

Nosocomial infections continue to be a significant cause of morbidity and mortality among preterm and/or low birth weight infants. Maternal transport of immunoglobulins to the fetus mainly occurs after 32 weeks' gestation and endogenous synthesis does not begin until several months after birth. Administration of intravenous immunoglobulin provides IgG that can bind to cell surface receptors, provide opsonic activity, activate complement, and promote antibody dependent cytotoxicity. Intravenous immunoglobulin thus has the potential of preventing or altering the course of nosocomial infections.

Ohlsson and Lacy conducted a systematic review to assess the effectiveness and safety of intravenous immunoglobulin (IVIG) administration compared to placebo or no intervention to preterm and/or low birth weight (LBW, less than 2500 g birth weight) infants in preventing nosocomial infections (Ohlsson and Lacy 2004). Nineteen studies conducted in many countries were included in this review. The most recent trial was reported in 2000. This included approximately 5,000 preterm

and/or LBW infants. Among qualifying studies the quantity of IVIG per dose varied widely from 120 mg/kg to 1 g/kg. Also, the number of doses varied from a single dose to seven doses. Several different IVIG preparations were used including Gammagard, Sandoglobulin, Gamimmune, Intraglobin; IgVena, Biotransfusion, an unnamed product, Venogamma, and Gammumine-N. When all studies were combined, the meta-analysis indicated that IVIG administration resulted in a 3% reduction in sepsis and a 4% reduction in any serious infection, one or more episodes, but was not associated with reductions in other important outcomes: sepsis, necrotizing enterocolitis, intraventricular hemorrhage, or length of hospital stay. Most importantly, IVIG administration did not have any significant effect on mortality from any cause or from infections. Prophylactic use of IVIG was not associated with any short-term serious side effects. From a clinical perspective, the small reduction in nosocomial infections without a reduction in mortality or other important clinical outcomes is felt to be of marginal importance.

Antistaphylococcal Immunoglobulins to Prevent Staphylococcal Infection in Very low Birth Weight Infants

Nosocomial infection continues to be a major problem affecting the immediate health and long-term outcome of preterm and very low birth weight neonates. More than half of these infections are caused by *Staphylococci*. Various type-specific antibodies targeted at different antigenic markers of *Staphylococcus* have been developed and have shown promise in animal studies.

Shah and Kaufman conducted a systematic review to evaluate the efficacy and safety of antistaphylococcal immunoglobulins in the prevention of *Staphylococcal* infection in very low birth weight infants (Shah and Kaufman 2009). Three eligible studies were included testing two different antistaphylococcal immunoglobulin products. Two studies used pooled generic antistaphylococcal immunoglobulin (INH-A21) and the third study used antibody against type 5 and type 8 capsular polysaccharide antigen (Altastaph). These studies enrolled a total of 2,701 neonates. No significant differences were noted in the risk of Staphylococcal infection or the risk of any infection between INH-A21 and placebo or Altastaph versus placebo. Furthermore, no significant differences were observed in the incidence of chronic lung disease, patent ductus arteriosus, necrotizing enterocolitis, intraventricular hemorrhage, retinopathy of prematurity, or duration of antibiotic and vancomycin use. At the present time, antistaphylococcal immunoglobulins (INH A-21 and Altastaph) are not recommended for prevention of *staphylococcal* infections in preterm or VLBW neonates. Further research to investigate the efficacy of other antistaphylococcal products such as Pagibaximab under development may be forthcoming in the future.

Intravenous Immunoglobulin for Treatment of Infections in Neonates

Ohlsson and Lacy conducted a systematic review to assess the effectiveness of intravenous immunoglobulin (IVIG) to reduce mortality and morbidity caused by suspected and proven infection in newborn infants (Ohlsson and Lacy 2015). A total of nine studies evaluating 3,973 infants were included in this review. The undisputable results of the largest trial included in this systematic review, INIS trial, which enrolled 3,493 infants, and our meta-analyses (n = 3973) showed no reduction in mortality during hospital stay, or death or major disability at two years of age in infants with suspected or proven infection (Inis Collaborative Group et al. 2011). Although based on a small sample size (n = 266), this update provides additional evidence that IgM-enriched IVIG does not significantly reduce mortality during hospital stay in infants with suspected infection. Routine administration of IVIG or IgM-enriched IVIG to prevent mortality in infants with suspected or proven neonatal infection is not recommended. No further research is recommended.

96.3.5.4 G-CSF and GM-CSF

In the United States, the Food and Drug Administration approve G-CSF to use in patients with severe chronic neutropenia, cancer patients receiving myelo-suppresive chemotherapy, cancer patients receiving bone marrow transplantation,

and patients undergoing peripheral blood hematopoietic stem cell collection. Patients with severe chronic neutropenia generally derive considerable benefit from G-CSF administration. Varieties of neutropenia in neonates for which G-CSF treatment is effective are Kostmann's syndrome, Shwachman-Diamond syndrome, cyclic neutropenia, and alloimmune neutropenia. Almost all patients respond to doses of 5–10 micrograms per kg administered at intervals ranging from every day to once per week to achieve neutrophil concentrations above 500–1000 cells per microliter (Corey et al. 1996).

G-CSF and GM-CSF for Treating or Preventing Neonatal Infections

Several reports in neonatal animals and in humans suggest that G-CSF or GM-CSF might benefit neonates who have neutropenia of bacterial sepsis (Cairo et al. 1990, 1991; Kocherlakota and La Gamma 1997). Carr and colleagues reported a systematic review to determine the efficacy and safety of the hematopoietic colony-stimulating factors (G-CSF or GM-CSF) in newborn infants, when used for treatment of suspected or proven systemic infection to reduce mortality, or prophylaxis, to prevent systemic infection in infants at high risk of nosocomial infection (Carr et al. 2003). This meta-analysis found no evidence from the seven published studies that treatment with G-CSF or GM-CSF in preterm infants with suspected systemic infection reduced early mortality of all causes early in the hospital course. No recent trials of G–CSF or GM-CSF for treatment of early onset sepsis have been conducted.

The decision regarding whether to administer G-CSF to a given neutropenic infant must be individualized considering risks and benefits. Animal studies suggesting benefit to colony-stimulating factor therapy for bacterial sepsis generally administered the hematopoieitic growth factor concurrently or within hours of innoculation with the bacterial agent. Under the best of circumstances, treatment of clinical sepsis with G-CSF or GM-CSF within hours of bacterial invasion may not be feasible. In the face of overwhelming sepsis, bone marrow neutrophil storage pools may already be depleted limiting the capability for response to G-CSF or GM-CSF treatment. Additionally, septic and neutropenic infants exhibit elevated circulating G-CSF concentrations, suggesting that their G-CSF receptors are saturated with endogenous G-CSF (Schibler et al. 1998). This being the case the administration of exogenous G-CSF would not be expected to be beneficial.

GM-CSF for Prophylaxis of Sepsis

Three prophylaxis studies using GM-CSF have been published. Although all three used GM-CSF, they adopted very differing treatment regimens and do not use comparable criteria for identifying episodes of systemic infection. Results of a systematic review of these studies concluded that GM-CSF prophylaxis did not lead to a significant reduction in mortality (Carr et al. 2003). A subsequent trial was conducted to examine whether GM-CSF administered as prophylaxis to preterm neonates at high risk of neutropenia would reduce sepsis, mortality, and morbidity. This was a single-blind, multicenter, randomized controlled trial conducted in 26 centers enrolling 280 preterm small for gestational age neonates less than or equal to 31 weeks' gestation (Carr et al. 2009) and below the 10th centile for birthweight. Infants were randomized within 72 h of birth to receive GM-CSF 10 microgram/kg per day subcutaneously for 5 days or standard management. The primary outcome was sepsis-free survival to 14 days from trial entry. Analysis was by intention to treat. Neutrophil counts after trial entry rose significantly more rapidly in infants treated with GM-CSF than in control infants during the first 11 days; however, there was no significant difference in sepsis-free survival for all infants. The authors concluded that early postnatal prophylactic GM-CSF corrects neutropenia but does not reduce sepsis or improve survival and short-term outcomes in extremely preterm neonates. Two- and five-year follow-up studies of this cohort found that administration of GM-CSF to very preterm SGA babies was not associated with improved or more adverse neurodevelopmental, general health, or educational outcomes at 5 years (Marlow et al. 2013, 2015).

In summary, in vitro and in vivo studies suggest that newborn infants are particularly vulnerable to infections because of qualitative and quantitative neutrophil in leukocyte-mediated immunity. The myeloid growth factors, G-CSF and GM-CSF, have been reported to increase neutrophil numbers and to enhance phagocyte function. There is currently insufficient evidence to support use of G-CSF or GM-CSF either as treatment of established systemic infection to reduce mortality or as prophylaxis to prevent systemic infection in high-risk neonates. No toxicity has been reported in association with use of either G-CSF or GM-CSF in neonates. Among infants with severe congenital neutropenia or cyclic neutropenia, it is generally accepted that G-CSF therapy is beneficial.

References

A controlled trial of interferon gamma to prevent infection in chronic granulomatous disease. The International Chronic Granulomatous Disease Cooperative Study Group. (1991) N Engl J Med 324(8): 509–516

African Neonatal Sepsis Trial (AFRINEST) group et al (2015a) Oral amoxicillin compared with injectable procaine benzylpenicillin plus gentamicin for treatment of neonates and young infants with fast breathing when referral is not possible: a randomised, open-label, equivalence trial. Lancet 385(9979): 1758–1766

African Neonatal Sepsis Trial (AFRINEST) group et al (2015b) Simplified antibiotic regimens compared with injectable procaine benzylpenicillin plus gentamicin for treatment of neonates and young infants with clinical signs of possible serious bacterial infection when referral is not possible: a randomised, open-label, equivalence trial. Lancet 385(9979):1767–1776

Al-Hadithy H et al (1981) Defective neutrophil function in low-birth-weight, premature infants. J Clin Pathol 34 (4):366–370

AlMulla ZS, Christensen RD (1995) Neutropenia in the neonate. Clin Perinatol 22(3):711–739

Ambruso DR et al (1984) Oxidative metabolism of cord blood neutrophils: relationship to content and degranulation of cytoplasmic granules. Pediatr Res 18(11): 1148–1153

Azzopardi DV et al (2009) Moderate hypothermia to treat perinatal asphyxial encephalopathy. N Engl J Med 361(14):1349–1358

Bacterial etiology of serious infections in young infants in developing countries: results of a multicenter study. The WHO Young Infants Study Group. (1999) Pediatr Infect Dis J 18(10 Suppl): S17–S22

Baehner RL (1975) Microbe ingestion and killing by neutrophils: normal mechanisms and abnormalities. Clin Haematol 4(3):609–633

Bainton DF (1981) Selective abnormalities of azurophil and specific granules of human neutrophilic leukocytes. Fed Proc 40(5):1443–1450

Beekman R, Touw IP (2010) G-CSF and its receptor in myeloid malignancy. Blood 115(25):5131–5136

Bektas S, Goetze B, Speer CP (1990) Decreased adherence, chemotaxis and phagocytic activities of neutrophils from preterm neonates. Acta Paediatr Scand 79(11):1031–1038

Bertrand Y et al (2002) Reticular dysgenesis: HLA non-identical bone marrow transplants in a series of 10 patients. Bone Marrow Transplant 29(9):759–762

Birle A et al (2015) Neutrophil chemotaxis in cord blood of term and preterm neonates is reduced in preterm neonates and influenced by the mode of delivery and anaesthesia. PLoS One 10(4):e0120341

Bonilla MA et al (1989) Effects of recombinant human granulocyte colony-stimulating factor on neutropenia in patients with congenital agranulocytosis. N Engl J Med 320(24):1574–1580

Boocock GR et al (2003) Mutations in SBDS are associated with Shwachman-Diamond syndrome. Nat Genet 33(1):97–101

Boxer LA, Yokoyama M, Lalezari P (1972) Isoimmune neonatal neutropenia. J Pediatr 80(5):783–787

Boxer LA et al (1975) Autoimmune neutropenia. N Engl J Med 293(15):748–753

Brodeur GM et al (1980) Transient leukemoid reaction and trisomy 21 mosaicism in a phenotypically normal newborn. Blood 55(4):691–693

Broxmeyer HE, Kim CH (1999) Regulation of hematopoiesis in a sea of chemokine family members with a plethora of redundant activities. Exp Hematol 27(7): 1113–1123

Burroughs L, Woolfrey A, Shimamura A (2009) Shwachman-Diamond syndrome: a review of the clinical presentation, molecular pathogenesis, diagnosis, and treatment. Hematol Oncol Clin North Am 23 (2):233–248

Bux J (2001) Molecular nature of granulocyte antigens. Transfus Clin Biol 8(3):242–247

Bux J et al (1998) Diagnosis and clinical course of autoimmune neutropenia in infancy: analysis of 240 cases. Blood 91(1):181–186

Cadnapaphornchai M, Faix RG (1992) Increased nosocomial infection in neutropenic low birth weight (2000 grams or less) infants of hypertensive mothers. J Pediatr 121(6):956–961

Cairo MS et al (1990) Seven-day administration of recombinant human granulocyte colony-stimulating factor to newborn rats: modulation of neonatal neutrophilia, myelopoiesis, and group B Streptococcus sepsis. Blood 76(9):1788–1794

Cairo MS et al (1991) Modulation of neonatal rat myeloid kinetics resulting in peripheral neutrophilia by single pulse administration of Rh granulocyte-macrophage

colony-stimulating factor and Rh granulocyte colony-stimulating factor. Biol Neonate 59(1):13 21
Carr R (2000) Neutrophil production and function in newborn infants. Br J Haematol 110(1):18–28
Carr R, Modi N, Dore C (2003) G-CSF and GM-CSF for treating or preventing neonatal infections. Cochrane Database Syst Rev (3): CD003066
Carr R et al (2009) Granulocyte-macrophage colony stimulating factor administered as prophylaxis for reduction of sepsis in extremely preterm, small for gestational age neonates (the PROGRAMS trial): a single-blind, multicentre, randomised controlled trial. Lancet 373(9659): 226–233
Chan VW et al (1999) Secondary lymphoid-tissue chemokine (SLC) is chemotactic for mature dendritic cells. Blood 93(11):3610–3616
Christensen RD (1989) Neutrophil kinetics in the fetus and neonate. Am J Pediatr Hematol Oncol 11(2):215–223
Christensen RD, Rothstein G (1980) Exhaustion of mature marrow neutrophils in neonates with sepsis. J Pediatr 96(2):316–318
Conway LT et al (1987) Natural history of primary autoimmune neutropenia in infancy. Pediatrics 79(5):728–733
Corey SJ, Wollman MR, Deshpande RV (1996) Granulocyte colony-stimulating factor and congenital neutropenia–risk of leukemia? J Pediatr 129(1):187–188
Craft AP, Finer NN, Barrington KJ (2000) Vancomycin for prophylaxis against sepsis in preterm neonates. Cochrane Database Syst Rev (2): CD001971
Dale DC, Bolyard AA, Hammond WP (1993) Cyclic neutropenia: natural history and effects of long-term treatment with recombinant human granulocyte colony-stimulating factor. Cancer Invest 11(2):219–223
Dale DC et al (2000) Mutations in the gene encoding neutrophil elastase in congenital and cyclic neutropenia. Blood 96(7):2317–2322
D'Ambola JB et al (1988) Human and rabbit newborn lung macrophages have reduced anti-Candida activity. Pediatr Res 24(3):285–290
Doron MW et al (1994) Increased incidence of sepsis at birth in neutropenic infants of mothers with preeclampsia. J Pediatr 125(3):452–458
Douglas SD, Yoder MC (1996) The mononuclear phagocyte and dendritic cell systems. In: Stiehm ER (ed) Immunological disorders in infants and children. W.B. Saunders, Philadelphia, pp 113–132
Erdman SH et al (1982) Supply and release of storage neutrophils. A developmental study. Biol Neonate 41 (3–4):132–137
Etzioni A (2009) Genetic etiologies of leukocyte adhesion defects. Curr Opin Immunol 21(5):481–486
Fagerholm SC, Lek HS, Morrison VL (2014) Kindlin-3 in the immune system. Am J Clin Exp Immunol 3(1):37–42
Farruggia P (2016) Immune neutropenias of infancy and childhood. World J Pediatr 12(2):142–148
Feng X et al (2014) Prophylactic first-line antibiotics reduce infectious fever and shorten hospital stay during chemotherapy-induced agranulocytosis in childhood acute myeloid leukemia. Acta Haematol 132(1):112–117
Fong ON et al (2014) Expression profile of cord blood neutrophils and dysregulation of HSPA1A and OLR1 upon challenge by bacterial peptidoglycan. J Leukoc Biol 95(1):169–178
Forman ML, Stiehm ER (1969) Impaired opsonic activity but normal phagocytosis in low-birth-weight infants. N Engl J Med 281(17):926–931
Gale RP, Sparkes RS, Golde DW (1978) Bone marrow origin of hepatic macrophages (Kupffer cells) in humans. Science 201(4359):937–938
Ganapathi KA et al (2007) The human Shwachman-Diamond syndrome protein, SBDS, associates with ribosomal RNA. Blood 110(5):1458–1465
Ghosh S, Thrasher AJ, Gaspar HB (2015) Gene therapy for monogenic disorders of the bone marrow. Br J Haematol 171:155–170
Gil-Krzewska A et al (2016) Chediak-Higashi syndrome: lysosomal trafficking regulator domains regulate exocytosis of lytic granules but not cytokine secretion by natural killer cells. J Allergy Clin Immunol 137(4):1165–1177
Gladstone IM et al (1990) A ten-year review of neonatal sepsis and comparison with the previous fifty-year experience. Pediatr Infect Dis J 9(11):819–825
Gorlin JB (1993) The phagocyte system: structure and function. In: Natan D (ed) Haematology of infancy and childhood. W.B. Saunders, Philadelphia, p 882
Greenhow TL, Hung YY, Herz AM (2012) Changing epidemiology of bacteremia in infants aged 1 week to 3 months. Pediatrics 129(3):e590–e596
Haller O, Arnheiter H, Lindenmann J (1979) Natural, genetically determined resistance toward influenza virus in hemopoietic mouse chimeras. Role of mononuclear phagocytes. J Exp Med 150(1):117–126
Harris MC et al (1983) Phagocytosis of group B streptococcus by neutrophils from newborn infants. Pediatr Res 17(5):358–361
Hawes CS, Kemp AS, Jones WR (1980) In vitro parameters of cell-mediated immunity in the human neonate. Clin Immunol Immunopathol 17(4):530–536
Heiss NS et al (1998) X-linked dyskeratosis congenita is caused by mutations in a highly conserved gene with putative nucleolar functions. Nat Genet 19(1):32–38
Hill HR (1987) Biochemical, structural, and functional abnormalities of polymorphonuclear leukocytes in the neonate. Pediatr Res 22(4):375–382
Homans AC, Verissimo AM, Vlacha V (1993) Transient abnormal myelopoiesis of infancy associated with trisomy 21. Am J Pediatr Hematol Oncol 15(4):392–399
Horwitz M et al (1999) Mutations in ELA2, encoding neutrophil elastase, define a 21-day biological clock in cyclic haematopoiesis. Nat Genet 23(4):433–436
Inis Collaborative Group et al (2011) Treatment of neonatal sepsis with intravenous immune globulin. N Engl J Med 365(13):1201–1211
Introne W, Boissy RE, Gahl WA (1999) Clinical, molecular, and cell biological aspects of Chediak-Higashi syndrome. Mol Genet Metab 68(2):283–303
Jacobs RF et al (1985) Phagocytosis of type III group B streptococci by neonatal monocytes: enhancement by

fibronectin and gammaglobulin. J Infect Dis 152 (4):695–700

Jacobs SE et al (2011) Whole-body hypothermia for term and near-term newborns with hypoxic-ischemic encephalopathy: a randomized controlled trial. Arch Pediatr Adolesc Med 165(8):692–700

Jenkins DD et al (2013) Altered circulating leukocytes and their chemokines in a clinical trial of therapeutic hypothermia for neonatal hypoxic ischemic encephalopathy. Pediatr Crit Care Med 14(8):786–795

Ji X et al (2016) Lysosomal trafficking regulator (LYST). Adv Exp Med Biol 854:745–750

Kirwan M, Dokal I (2008) Dyskeratosis congenita: a genetic disorder of many faces. Clin Genet 73(2):103–112

Kjeldsen L et al (1996) Granules and secretory vesicles in human neonatal neutrophils. Pediatr Res 40(1):120–129

Klein RB et al (1977) Decreased mononuclear and polymorphonuclear chemotaxis in human newborns, infants, and young children. Pediatrics 60(4):467–472

Kocherlakota P, La Gamma EF (1997) Human granulocyte colony-stimulating factor may improve outcome attributable to neonatal sepsis complicated by neutropenia. Pediatrics 100(1), E6

Koenig JM, Christensen RD (1989a) Incidence, neutrophil kinetics, and natural history of neonatal neutropenia associated with maternal hypertension. N Engl J Med 321(9):557–562

Koenig JM, Christensen RD (1989b) Neutropenia and thrombocytopenia in infants with Rh hemolytic disease. J Pediatr 114(4 Pt 1):625–631

Koenig JM, Christensen RD (1991) The mechanism responsible for diminished neutrophil production in neonates delivered of women with pregnancy-induced hypertension. Am J Obstet Gynecol 165(2):467–473

Kostmann R (1956) Infantile genetic agranulocytosis: agranulocytosis infantilis hereditaria. Acta Paediatr Suppl 45(Suppl 105):1–78

Kuo CY, Kohn DB (2016) Gene therapy for the treatment of primary immune deficiencies. Curr Allergy Asthma Rep 16(5):39

Lalezari P, Radel E (1974) Neutrophil-specific antigens: immunology and clinical significance. Semin Hematol 11(3):281–290

Lalezari P, Khorshidi M, Petrosova M (1986) Autoimmune neutropenia of infancy. J Pediatr 109(5):764–769

Lamba M et al (2016) Bacteriological spectrum and antimicrobial susceptibility pattern of neonatal septicaemia in a tertiary care hospital of North India. J Matern Fetal Neonatal Med 29(24):3993–3998

Levine DH, Madyastha PR (1986) Isoimmune neonatal neutropenia. Am J Perinatol 3(3):231–233

Link DC et al (2007) Distinct patterns of mutations occurring in de novo AML versus AML arising in the setting of severe congenital neutropenia. Blood 110(5): 1648–1655

Luchtman-Jones L, Schwartz AL (2002) Hematologic problems in the fetus and neonate. In: Fanaroff AA, Martin RJ (eds) Neonatal-perinatal medicine: diseases of the fetus and infant. Mosby, St. Louis, pp 1205–1206

Lyall EG, Lucas GF, Eden OB (1992) Autoimmune neutropenia of infancy. J Clin Pathol 45(5):431–434

Maheshwari A, Christensen RD (2004) Developmental granulopoiesis. In: Polin RA, Fox WW, Abman SH (eds) Fetal and neonatal physiology. Saunders, Philadelphia, pp 1388–1396

Makaryan V et al (2015) The diversity of mutations and clinical outcomes for ELANE-associated neutropenia. Curr Opin Hematol 22(1):3–11

Manroe BL et al (1979) The neonatal blood count in health and disease. I. Reference values for neutrophilic cells. J Pediatr 95(1):89–98

Marchant EA et al (2013) Neonatal sepsis due to coagulase-negative staphylococci. Clin Dev Immunol 2013:586076

Marlow N et al (2013) A randomised trial of granulocyte-macrophage colony-stimulating factor for neonatal sepsis: outcomes at 2 years. Arch Dis Child Fetal Neonatal Ed 98(1):F46–F53

Marlow N et al (2015) A randomised trial of granulocyte-macrophage colony-stimulating factor for neonatal sepsis: childhood outcomes at 5 years. Arch Dis Child Fetal Neonatal Ed 100(4):F320–F326

Marodi L, Csorba S, Nagy B (1980) Chemotactic and random movement of human newborn monocytes. Eur J Pediatr 135(1):73–75

Marodi L, Leijh PC, van Furth R (1984) Characteristics and functional capacities of human cord blood granulocytes and monocytes. Pediatr Res 18(11): 1127–1131

Marrone A et al (2007) Telomerase reverse-transcriptase homozygous mutations in autosomal recessive dyskeratosis congenita and Hoyeraal-Hreidarsson syndrome. Blood 110(13):4198–4205

McCracken GH Jr, Eichenwald HF (1971) Leukocyte function and the development of opsonic and complement activity in the neonate. Am J Dis Child 121(2):120–126

Meuret G, Hoffmann G (1973) Monocyte kinetic studies in normal and disease states. Br J Haematol 24(3): 275–285

Meuret G, Batara E, Furste HO (1975) Monocytopoiesis in normal man: pool size, proliferation activity and DNA synthesis time of promonocytes. Acta Haematol 54 (5):261–270

Miller ME (1978) Phagocytic cells. In: Miller ME (ed) Host defense in the human neonate. Grune & Stratton, New York, pp 59–71

Mouzinho A et al (1994) Revised reference ranges for circulating neutrophils in very-low-birth-weight neonates. Pediatrics 94(1):76–82

Mularoni A et al (2014) The role of coagulase-negative staphylococci in early onset sepsis in a large European cohort of very low birth weight infants. Pediatr Infect Dis J 33(5):e121–e125

Nussbaum C et al (2013) Neutrophil and endothelial adhesive function during human fetal ontogeny. J Leukoc Biol 93(2):175–184

Ohlsson A, Lacy JB (2004) Intravenous immunoglobulin for preventing infection in preterm and/or low-birth-

weight infants. Cochrane Database Syst Rev (1): CD000361

Ohlsson A, Lacy JB (2015) Intravenous immunoglobulin for suspected or proven infection in neonates. Cochrane Database Syst Rev (3): CD001239

Ozkaynak MF et al (2005) Randomized comparison of antibiotics with and without granulocyte colony-stimulating factor in children with chemotherapy-induced febrile neutropenia: a report from the Children's Oncology Group. Pediatr Blood Cancer 45(3):274–280

Pahwa SG et al (1977) Cellular and humoral components of monocyte and neutrophil chemotaxis in cord blood. Pediatr Res 11(5):677–680

Pammi M, Brocklehurst P (2011) Granulocyte transfusions for neonates with confirmed or suspected sepsis and neutropenia. Cochrane Database Syst Rev (10): CD003956

Parwaresch MR, Wacker HH (1984) Origin and kinetics of resident tissue macrophages. Parabiosis studies with radiolabelled leucocytes. Cell Tissue Kinet 17(1): 25–39

Philip AG, Hewitt JR (1980) Early diagnosis of neonatal sepsis. Pediatrics 65(5):1036–1041

Phillips ML et al (1995) Neutrophil adhesion in leukocyte adhesion deficiency syndrome type 2. J Clin Invest 96(6):2898–2906

Raghunathan R et al (1982) Phagocyte chemotaxis in the perinatal period. J Clin Immunol 2(3):242–245

Rodwell RL et al (1993) Hematologic scoring system in early diagnosis of sepsis in neutropenic newborns. Pediatr Infect Dis J 12(5):372–376

Rognoni E, Ruppert R, Fassler R (2016) The kindlin family: functions, signaling properties and implications for human disease. J Cell Sci 129(1):17–27

Roos D (2016) Chronic granulomatous disease. Br Med Bull 118(1):50–63

Roper M et al (1985) Severe congenital leukopenia (reticular dysgenesis). Immunologic and morphologic characterizations of leukocytes. Am J Dis Child 139(8): 832–835

Rubin LG et al (2002) Evaluation and treatment of neonates with suspected late-onset sepsis: a survey of neonatologists' practices. Pediatrics 110(4), e42

Rujkijyanont P et al (2009) Bone marrow cells from patients with Shwachman-Diamond syndrome abnormally express genes involved in ribosome biogenesis and RNA processing. Br J Haematol 145(6):806–815

Sanchez-Guiu I et al (2014) Chediak-Higashi syndrome: description of two novel homozygous missense mutations causing divergent clinical phenotype. Eur J Haematol 92(1):49–58

Savage SA, Alter BP (2009) Dyskeratosis congenita. Hematol Oncol Clin North Am 23(2):215–231

Schelonka RL et al (1994) Peripheral leukocyte count and leukocyte indexes in healthy newborn term infants. J Pediatr 125(4):603–606

Schibler KR et al (1998) A randomized, placebo-controlled trial of granulocyte colony-stimulating factor administration to newborn infants with neutropenia and clinical signs of early-onset sepsis. Pediatrics 102 (1 Pt 1):6–13

Schuit KE, Powell DA (1980) Phagocytic dysfunction in monocytes of normal newborn infants. Pediatrics 65(3):501–504

Seale AC, Obiero CW, Berkley JA (2015) Rational development of guidelines for management of neonatal sepsis in developing countries. Curr Opin Infect Dis 28 (3):225–230

Shah PS, Kaufman DA (2009) Antistaphylococcal immunoglobulins to prevent staphylococcal infection in very low birth weight infants. Cochrane Database Syst Rev (2): CD006449

Shah TA et al (2012) Hospital and neurodevelopmental outcomes of extremely low-birth-weight infants with necrotizing enterocolitis and spontaneous intestinal perforation. J Perinatol 32(7):552–558

Shane AL, Stoll BJ (2014) Neonatal sepsis: progress towards improved outcomes. J Infect 68(Suppl 1): S24–S32

Shankaran S et al (2008) Outcomes of safety and effectiveness in a multicenter randomized, controlled trial of whole-body hypothermia for neonatal hypoxic-ischemic encephalopathy. Pediatrics 122(4):e791–e798

Shwachman H et al (1964) The syndrome of pancreatic insufficiency and bone marrow dysfunction. J Pediatr 65:645–663

Siegel JD, McCracken GH Jr (1981) Sepsis neonatorum. N Engl J Med 304(11):642–647

Simbruner G et al (2010) Systemic hypothermia after neonatal encephalopathy: outcomes of neo.nEURO.network RCT. Pediatrics 126(4):e771–e778

Skokowa J et al (2014) Cooperativity of RUNX1 and CSF3R mutations in severe congenital neutropenia: a unique pathway in myeloid leukemogenesis. Blood 123(14):2229–2237

Sozzani S et al (1999) The role of chemokines in the regulation of dendritic cell trafficking. J Leukoc Biol 66(1):1–9

Speer CP, Johnston RB Jr (1984) Phagocyte function. In: Ogra PL (ed) Neonatal infections: nutritional and immunologic interactions. Grune & Stratton, Orlando, pp 21–36

Speer CP et al (1988) Phagocytosis-associated functions in neonatal monocyte-derived macrophages. Pediatr Res 24(2):213–216

Stoll BJ et al (2011) Early onset neonatal sepsis: the burden of group B Streptococcal and E. coli disease continues. Pediatrics 127(5):817–826

Stoll BJ et al (2015) Trends in care practices, morbidity, and mortality of extremely preterm neonates, 1993–2012. JAMA 314(10):1039–1051

Thomas ED et al (1976) Direct evidence for a bone marrow origin of the alveolar macrophage in man. Science 192 (4243):1016–1018

Trubowitz S, Davies S (1982) Pathophysiology of the monocyte-macrophage system. In: Trubowitz S (ed) The

human bone marrow: anatomy, physiology, and pathophysiology. CRC Press, Boco Raton, pp 95–126

Tsai MH et al (2016) Infectious complications and morbidities after neonatal bloodstream infections: an observational cohort study. Medicine (Baltimore) 95(11):e3078

Uzel G et al (2010) Complications of tumor necrosis factor-alpha blockade in chronic granulomatous disease-related colitis. Clin Infect Dis 51(12):1429–1434

van Furth R (1992) Development and distribution of mononuclear phagocytes. In: Gallin JI (ed) Inflammation: basic principles and clinical correlates. Raven, New York, pp 325–340

van Furth R, Sluiter W (1986) Distribution of blood monocytes between a marginating and a circulating pool. J Exp Med 163(2):474–479

van Furth R, Raeburn JA, van Zwet TL (1979) Characteristics of human mononuclear phagocytes. Blood 54(2): 485–500

Veldhuisen B et al (2014) Molecular typing of human platelet and neutrophil antigens (HPA and HNA). Transfus Apher Sci 50(2):189–199

Volkman A (1966) The origin and turnover of mononuclear cells in peritoneal exudates in rats. J Exp Med 124(2): 241–254

Weston WL et al (1977) Monocyte-macrophage function in the newborn. Am J Dis Child 131(11): 1241–1242

Whitelaw DM (1972) Observations on human monocyte kinetics after pulse labeling. Cell Tissue Kinet 5(4): 311–317

Xanthou M et al (1975) Phagocytosis and killing ability of Candida albicans by blood leucocytes of healthy term and preterm babies. Arch Dis Child 50 (1):72–75

Yegin O (1983) Chemotaxis in childhood. Pediatr Res 17(3):183–187

Zaidi AK et al (2009) Pathogens associated with sepsis in newborns and young infants in developing countries. Pediatr Infect Dis J 28(1 Suppl):S10–S18

Zipursky A (1993) Isoimmune hemolytic disease. In: Nathan DG (ed) Hematology of infancy and childhood. WB Saunders, Philadelphia, p 65

Neonatal Hereditary Neutropenia

97

Gaetano Chirico and Carmelita D'Ippolito

Contents

Abstract

Hereditary neutropenia includes many disorders of distinct origin and variable prognosis, characterized by a reduction of the absolute neutrophil count (ANC) below 0.5×10^9/l, that predisposes patients to bacterial infections of variable severity, in particular pyogenic infections, such as cutaneous cellulitis, deep

G. Chirico (✉)
Neonatology and Intensive Neonatal Therapy Unit, Spedali Civili of Brescia, Brescia, Italy
e-mail: gaechirico@alice.it

C. D'Ippolito
Pediatric Oncohematology and Bone Marrow Transplant, Spedali Civili Hospital, Brescia, Italy

G. Buonocore et al. (eds.), *Neonatology*,
https://doi.org/10.1007/978-3-319-29489-6_244

abscesses, pneumonia, and sepsis. The diagnosis of severe congenital neutropenia (SCN) is usually made on the basis of patient history and physical examination, and of a severe neutropenia with normal or near normal hemoglobin level and platelet count, while bone marrow examination reveals in most cases the typical defect of neutrophils, with myeloid cell differentiation arrest at the promyelocyte stage, and very few myelocytes and metamyelocytes.

The most common monogenic congenital neutropenia are usually classified according to the presence or absence of association with innate or adaptive immunodeficiency, or with extrahematopoietic manifestations, like involvement of the pancreas, central nervous system, heart, muscle, and skin.

Most of the forms of congenital neutropenia are extremely rare, about six cases per one million; some genes have been only found in a few families. The inheritance is monogenic, which may be autosomal (dominant or recessive), or X-linked. During the last few years, several genetic causes of neutropenia have been elucidated.

97.1 Salient Points

- Hereditary neutropenia is characterized by a reduction of the absolute neutrophil count (ANC) below $0.5 \times 10^9/l$.
- Neutropenia can lead to bacterial infections of variable severity, in particular pyogenic infections, such as cutaneous cellulitis, deep abscesses, pneumonia, and sepsis.
- The diagnosis of severe congenital neutropenia (SCN) is usually made on the basis of patient history and physical examination, and of a severe neutropenia with normal or near normal hemoglobin level and platelet count.
- Bone marrow examination reveals in most cases the typical defect of neutrophils with myeloid cell differentiation arrest at the promyelocyte stage, and very few myelocytes and metamyelocytes.
- The most common monogenic congenital neutropenia are usually classified according to the presence or absence of association with innate or adaptive immunodeficiency, or with extrahematopoietic manifestations, like involvement of the pancreas, central nervous system, heart, muscle, and skin.
- Most of the forms of congenital neutropenia are extremely rare, the estimated frequency is about six per one million; some genes have been only found in a few families.
- The inheritance is monogenic, which may be autosomal (dominant or recessive) or X-linked. During the last few years, several genetic causes of neutropenia have been elucidated.

97.2 Introduction

Hereditary neutropenia includes many disorders of distinct origin and variable prognosis, characterized by a reduction of the absolute neutrophil count (ANC) below $0.5 \times 10^9/l$, that predisposes patients to bacterial infections, in particular pyogenic infections, such as cutaneous cellulitis, deep abscesses, pneumonia, and sepsis (Welte et al. 2006). Susceptibility to bacterial infections, even in patients with severe neutropenia, can be quite variable, depending on the underlying etiology (Boztug et al. 2008). The diagnosis of severe congenital neutropenia (SCN) is usually made on the basis of the observation at birth, or in the following months of life, of a severe reduction of ANC ($<0.5 \times 10^9/l$) with normal or near normal levels of hemoglobin and platelets, while bone marrow examination reveals in most cases the typical defect of neutrophils with myeloid cell differentiation arrest at the promyelocyte stage and very few myelocytes and metamyelocytes (Badolato et al. 2004). Congenital neutropenia may be associated with innate or adaptive immunodeficiency or with extrahematopoietic manifestations, like involvement of the pancreas, central nervous system, heart, muscle, and skin.

All the forms of congenital neutropenia are extremely rare, except for ethnic neutropenia, which is a frequent mild congenital form, with probably polygenic inheritance. The minimal prevalence of congenital neutropenia is six cases per million inhabitants (Dale et al. 2003); the

inheritance is monogenic which may be autosomal (dominant or recessive) or X- linked.

During the last few years, several genetic causes of neutropenia have been elucidated. In this respect, scientific research is continuously evolving; some genes are extremely rare and have been only found in a few families. The classification of the most common causes of monogenic congenital neutropenia is presented below (Table 1).

97.3 Congenital Neutropenia Without Extrahematopoietic Manifestations and with Normal Adaptive Immunity

97.3.1 Severe Congenital Neutropenia (OMIM Code 202700)

Severe congenital neutropenia (SCN) is a rare disease characterized by a chronic neutropenia due to a genetic defect. The absolute neutrophil count (ANC) is short of 200 cells/mm^3 from birth. This predisposes to severe life-threatening infections (Zeidler et al. 2003; Lekstrom-Himes and Gallin 2000).

The incidence is estimated to be approximately two cases per million of the population (Xia et al. 2009). Affected patients regularly have episodes of fever, skin infections, stomatitis, pneumonia, and perirectal abscesses that usually begin in the first months of life and lead to death during infancy and childhood. Eosinophylia, monocytosis, and splenomegaly may be present. The disorder remains a paradigm in the field of congenital neutropenia. The bone marrow examination reveals the typical arrest of the myeloid cell differentiation at the promyelocytic stage with a marked depletion of mature neutrophils (Xia et al. 2009; Dale et al. 2000). Recent studies on the genetic basis of SCN have detected mutation in the neutrophil elastase gene, *ELA2 (ELANE)*; this gene defect is inherited as an autosomal dominant trait in about 60–80% of patients (Horwitz et al. 2007). More than 50 separate ELANE mutations have been hitherto found in SCN patients (Germeshausen et al. 2013).

ELA2 encodes a serine protease synthesized during the promyelocyte/myelocyte stage, which is stored in the primary granules (Horwitz et al. 2007). Correct localization of the neutrophil elastase (NE) in the primary granules requires interaction of NE with the adaptor protein complex AP3 that shuttles transmembrane cargo proteins from the Golgi network to the lysosomes. Most mutations in *ELA2* remove the tyrosine-based recognition sequence for the AP3μ subunit, thereby favoring the misallocation of the enzyme to the membrane instead of inside the granules. It was proposed that mislocalized NE must drastically reduce the production of neutrophils from the myeloid progenitor cells in favor of monocytes.

The introduction of hematopoietic growth factors has greatly improved both life span and quality of life (Freedman et al. 2000). However, patients with SCN have a heterogeneous response to G-CSF therapy and often require a gradual increase of the dosage that generally ranges from 11 to 13 μg/kg/die. In addition, 3–5% of SCN patients are refractory to G-CSF treatment.

Finally, a significant number of children who are receiving G-CSF therapy are developing myelodysplastic syndrome (MDS) or acute myeloid leukemia (AML). The exact relationship between G-CSF treatment and the risk of leukemic transformation is still unclear (Rosenberg et al. 2010). A subset of SCN patients, namely those with more severe disease, are more prone to develop MDS, AML, or both, probably because of exposure to other leukemogenic factors such as monosomy of chromosome 7, alterations of chromosome 21, activating mutations of the oncogene *ras*, and mutation in the G-CSF receptor (*CSF3R*) (Donadieu et al. 2005). At risk are patients with mutations in ELANE, HAX1, or WAS (Rosenberg et al. 2008, 2010; Devriendt et al. 2001) (see below).

The cumulative incidence of malignant transformations in SCN after 10 years of treatment with G-CSF amounts to 21% (Rosenberg et al. 2006) according to the Severe Chronic Neutropenia International Registry data. It does not appear to be a direct consequence of the treatment; indeed, cases of malignant transformation were reported in SCN patients who were not treated

Table 1 Monogenic congenital neutropenia

Subgroup of neutropenia	Disease name	OMIM code	Hematological manifestations	Extrahematological manifestations	Inheritance	Gene	Normal function of the gene
Congenital neutropenia without extrahematopoietic manifestations	Severe congenital neutropenia-cyclic neutropenia	202700-162800	Severe and permanent maturation arrest-intermittent-cyclic arrest	No	Dominant	ELANE	Protease activity antagonism with alpha 1 antitrypsin
Congenital neutropenia with extrahematopoietic manifestations	Kostmann disease	610738	Maturation arrest	SNC mental retardation, seizure	Recessive	HAX1	Control of apoptosis
	Shwachman-Diamond	260400	Mild neutropenia, dysgranulopoiesis, mild dysmegacariocytopoiesis	Exocrine pancreas deficiency chondrodysplasia mental retardation, cardiomyopathy	Recessive	SDB5	Ribosomal protein regulator of RNA expression
	Severe congenital neutropenia	612541	Maturation arrest	Increased visibility of superficial veins, cardiac and urogenital defects	Recessive	G6PC3	Glucose 6 -phosphatase complex: catalytic unit
	Barth disease	302060	No maturation arrest	Hypertrophy Cardiomyopathy Growth retardation	X linked	TAZ	Tafazzin: phospholipid membrane homeostasis
	Hermansky-Pudlak syndrome type 2	608233	No maturation arrest	Albinism	Recessive	AP3B1	Cargo protein:/ ER trafficking with ELANE interaction

	Poikilodermia type Clericuzio	604173	No maturation arrest, minor dysgranulopoetic features	Skin poikilodermia	Recessive	C160RF57	Not known
	Glycogen storage type Ib	232220	No maturation arrest	Hypoglicemia, fasting lactic acidosis, hyperlipidemia, glycogen overload of the liver	Recessive	SLC37A4	Glucose 6-phosphate complex: trans ER transporter
Congenital neutropenia without extrahematopoietic manifestations and with innate or adaptive deficiency	Severe congenital neutropenia	202700	Permanent, severe, or mild sometimes maturation arrest	Lymphopenia	Dominant	GFI1	Transcription factor encoding a regulator of *ELA2*
	Severe congenital neutropenia	300299	Severe permanent maturation arrest	Monocytopenia	X linked	WAS	Regulator of actin cytoskeleton
	WHIM	193670	Severe permanent no maturation arrest myelokathexis	Warts, hypo-gammaglobulinemia, infections and myelokathexis syndrome	Dominant	CXCR4	Chemokine receptor (CXCL12)

with G-CSF, while patients with CyN or idiopathic neutropenia showed no signs of malignant conversion after prolonged use of recombinant G-CSF (Rosenberg et al. 2006; Germeshausen et al. 2005).

Patients with SCN showed mutations in an area of the CSF3R gene that codes for the intracytoplasmic domain of the G-CSFR which were initially thought to be the cause of SCN (Dong et al. 1995). Later, those mutations turned out to be acquired somatic mutations which are associated with the transformation of leukemia in SCN (Germeshausen et al. 2001).

In the light of this finding, G-CSF treatment seams a safe option for the vast majority of patients with neutropenia, while patients at risk for leukemic transformation would benefit from hematopoietic stem cell transplantation (Fioredda et al. 2015).

97.3.2 Cyclic Neutropenia (OMIM Code 162800)

Cyclic neutropenia is an autosomal dominant or sporadic condition, characterized by periodic episodes of severe neutropenia with a nadir of less than 0.2×10^9 cells/L that occur usually every 21 days (Dale and Hammond 1988).

The neutropenic periods persist for 3–5 days and are accompanied by malaise, fever, gingivitis, oral ulcers, and lymphoadenopathy. There are also regular oscillations of the other leukocyte subsets, reticulocytes, and platelets. Symptoms begin during the first year of life, are often milder after puberty, and are usually less severe than in SCN (Horwitz et al. 2007; Germeshausen et al. 2013; Freedman et al. 2000; Rosenberg et al. 2006, 2008, 2010; Donadieu et al. 2005; Devriendt et al. 2001; Germeshausen et al. 2005; Dong et al. 1995; Germeshausen et al. 2001; Fioredda et al. 2015; Dale and Hammond 1988), even though fatal *Clostridium* bacteremia has been reported in untreated patients (Dale et al. 2003). A variety of studies suggest that cyclic neutropenia occurs because of a periodic disruption in cell production in the bone marrow (Dale et al. 2003). It has been shown that a heterozygous mutation of *ELA2* is the genetic cause of the disease. The mutations reported in cyclic neutropenia are located in the same gene associated with SCN, but in different exons resulting in preferential accumulation of NE in granules.

In the management of these patients the use of prophylactic G-CSF treatment is recommended; it has been very effective in improving peripheral blood neutrophil counts and avoiding symptoms and infections (Freedman et al. 2000). The required dose of G-CSF is usually lower than in SNC: 2–3 μg/kg/day or on alternate days; the occurrence of MDS or leukemia has not been reported in patients with cyclic neutropenia (Freedman et al. 2000).

97.4 Congenital Neutropenia with Innate and Adaptive Deficiency but Without Extrahematopoietic Manifestations

The same genetic mutations that lead to myeloid cell defects may also be associated with aberrations in cells involved in innate and adaptive immunity.

To identify the affected babies, a complete white blood cell (WBC) count and differential, with lymphocyte subpopulations and immunoglobulin levels, should be obtained.

97.4.1 Neutropenia Associated with GFI1 Mutations (OMIM Code 202700)

This cause of congenital neutropenia is extremely rare, having hitherto been found in just four patients (Karsunky et al. 2002; Person et al. 2003). The clinical phenotype is not particularly homogeneous: severe neutropenia – and marked monocytosis – was diagnosed in one patient at 4 months of age, while the father, who showed the same mutation, had a moderate form of neutropenia. On the other hand, another patient, who was diagnosed at 56 years of age with idiopathic neutropenia, was not clearly liable to infections. All those patients

had moderate lymphopenia (CD3 cells were 1–1.4 G/l), normal memory cells, and humoral immunity. Heterozygous GFI1 mutations – i.e., dominant ones – cause an increased expression of ELANE, just as ELANE mutations do.

GFI1, a transcriptional repressor and splicing control factor, plays an outstanding role in the control of the normal differentiation of hematopoietic cells (van der Meer et al. 2010). In some patients, monoallelic mutations have been observed which may lead to SCN (Armistead et al. 2010; Zhuang et al. 2006). Furthermore, GFI1 mutations are linked to aberrations in lymphoid and myeloid cells. Unsurprisingly, a defect in a significant transcriptional master switch factor provokes the impaired regulation of a number of pathways that may contribute to atypically differentiated neutrophil granulocytes.

97.4.2 Myelocathexis and WHIM Syndrome (OMIM Code193670)

Myelocathexis is a rare autosomal dominant disorder characterized by moderate to severe chronic neutropenia resulting from the retention of mature neutrophils in the bone marrow. Myelocathexis is often associated with hypogammaglobulinemia, leucopenia, and warts, a clinical picture recognized as WHIM syndrome (warts, hypogammaglobulinemia, infections, myelokathexis) (Aprikyan et al. 2000), an autosomal dominant disease. In WHIM syndrome ANCs are usually $<0.5 \times 10^9$/L, but during infectious episodes their number rises suddenly, allowing a more benign course with recurrent mild respiratory infections. Early death related to infections has not been reported. WHIM syndrome is caused by heterozygous mutations in the gene coding for the chemokine receptor CXCR4. Cells expressing the mutated CXCR4 have an increased responsiveness to chemokines and thus are not released from the bone marrow to the circulating blood pool (Aprikyan et al. 2000). The neutropenia associated with myelocathexis and WHIM is only partially corrected by administration of G-CSF (Gorlin et al. 2000).

97.4.3 SNC Due to WAS Mutation (OMIM code 300299)

Pernicious mutations in WASp are the usual causes of the Wiskott–Aldrich syndrome, which is an X-linked syndrome showing immunodeficiency, eczema, and hemorrhage (Notarangelo et al. 2008). The Wiskott–Aldrich syndrome protein (WASp) is an adaptor protein steering the polymerization of actin filaments (Thrasher and Burns 2010). Cells lacking WASp show flawed locomotion and delocalization of receptors. Unlike WASp deficiency, rare WAS mutations cause a constitutive activation of WASp, thus leading to increased actin polymers and, as a result, to abnormal cell divisions (Moulding et al. 2007; Westerberg et al. 2010). Those patients fail to show the classical signs of the Wiskott–Aldrich syndrome, but rather present congenital neutropenia (Devriendt et al. 2001; Beel et al. 2009), with myelodysplasia (Devriendt et al. 2001; Beel et al. 2009; Ancliff et al. 2006), increased myeloid cell apoptosis (Devriendt et al. 2001; Moulding et al. 2007; Westerberg et al. 2010; Beel et al. 2009; Ancliff et al. 2006) and abnormalities in lymphoid cells (Devriendt et al. 2001; Westerberg et al. 2010).

97.5 Congenital Neutropenia with Extrahematopoietic Manifestations

97.5.1 Kostmann Syndrome (OMIM code 610738)

Rolf Kostmann described, in 1956, an autosomal recessive hematological disease characterized by a chronic neutropenia with an absolute neutrophil count (ANC) below of 500 cells/mm^3 and an early eruption of severe bacterial infections in a large Swedish family with frequent intermarriages (Kostmann 1956), which was later referred to as the "Kostmann syndrome." The underlying genetic defect in this syndrome was found to be a mutation of the *HAX1* gene (Klein et al. 2007; Germeshausen et al. 2008; Kostman 1975). Its precise frequency is not known, but, apparently,

it is much lower than ELANE neutropenia, except in some areas, such as Sweden and Kurdistan. A following study published by Kostmann in 1975, which focused on the same pedigree in northern Sweden, described an improvement in survival rates linked to the use of antibiotics. On the other hand, neurological disorders began to be observed in the second decade, in particular neuropsychological deficits and epilepsy (Carlsson and Fasth 2001). The syndrome is described more accurately in a recent study of the same pedigree, where five out of six patients presented with neurological issues (Germeshausen et al. 2008; Kostman 1975; Carlsson and Fasth 2001). A HAX1gene mutation with pleiotropic functions has been found in this syndrome, while the detailed working of the HAX1 deficiency are not fully understood. HAX1 regulates the potential of the inner mitochondrial membrane (Klein et al. 2007; Han et al. 2010), while also being a cytoplasmic protein with numerous interaction partners. For instance, HAX1 binds to multiple virus proteins. Patients showing mutations only affecting isoform A have SCN without any further neuron impairments, while mutations of both isoforms (A and B) are found to be linked to neurological abnormalities, such as development delays and seizures (Germeshausen et al. 2008). Sometimes, neutropenia with ELANE mutations is improperly referred as Kostmann syndrome.

97.5.2 Hermansky-Pudlak Syndrome2 (OMIM Code 608233)

This autosomal recessive disease is characterized by neutropenia, oculocutaneous albinism, and moderate bleeding disorders (Dell'Angelica et al. 1999). It is caused by mutations of the gene encoding for the beta3 component of the AP3 complex, again preventing the transport of NE (and other proteins) from the Golgi network to the lysosomes in hematopoietic cells and in melanocytes (Dell'Angelica et al. 1999).

The severe neutropenia is responsive to G-CSF treatment.

97.5.3 Shwachman-Diamond Syndrome (OMIM Code 260400)

The Shwachman-Diamond syndrome (SDS) is a rare multiorgan disease inherited as an autosomal recessive trait that combines neutropenia, exocrine pancreatic insufficiency, skeletal abnormalities, and short stature (Dror and Freedman 2002).

The symptoms begin early in infancy with bacterial infections (pneumonia, otitis media, osteomyelitis, skin infections, sepsis) and failure to thrive because of intestinal malabsorption.

Chronic neutropenia is constantly observed in all patients and two thirds of them have a neutrophil count less than 1×10^9 cells/L; so while the neutropenia can be intermittent, it is never cyclic. Mild anemia and thrombocytopenia are described commonly (Dror and Freedman 2002).

Cytopenia reflects hematopoietic dysplasia, which, in association with cytogenetic abnormalities, may increase the risk of transformation in MDS/AML mainly in older children. For this reason, annual bone marrow aspirates are recommended in patients with SDS. Indeed, follow-up studies of SDS patients demonstrate that some cytogenetic changes my spontaneously regress.

The causative gene of the disease has been identified and was named *SDBS*. It is expressed in both hematopoietic and non-hematopoietic tissues. Treatment of patients suffering from SDS includes pancreatic enzyme replacement and administration of G-CSF, which increases ANC to normal levels and should be started in case of severe infections (Paley et al. 1991).

97.5.4 Neutropenia Associated with Glucose-6-Phosphatase Complex Disorders

Patients with glycogen-storage disease of type Ib, which is caused by mutations in the gene coding for the glucose-6-phosphate-transporter (G6PT) protein (Gerin et al. 1997), have long been known to suffer not only from hypoglycemia

and glycogen storage symptoms but also from congenital neutropenia. Glucose 6 phosphatase is a complex of three proteins bound to the endoplasmic reticulum responsible for glycogenolysis. Two of these three proteins are associated with congenital neutropenia: the translocase (SLC37A4), and G6PC3 that is a catalytic protein. Neutrophil granulocytes are particularly vulnerable to defects in glucose metabolism. The association between these molecular changes and neutropenia is not clear, because the glycogenolysis pathway is not the source of energy normally used by neutrophils, which mainly use the pentose pathway; this raises the hypothesis that the involved proteins perform a different function in neutrophils.

97.5.4.1 Glycogen Storage Disease Type Ib

It is a metabolic disorder characterized by hepatic glycogen accumulation, intolerance of fasting, hypoglycemic events, and hyperlactacidemia, as well as susceptibility to infections (Ambruso et al. 2003) and colitis resembling Crohn's. This susceptibility to infections is due to neutropenia and, sometimes, to neutrophil dysfunction (defective chemotactism). The origin of the neutropenia and neutrophil dysfunction is unknown.

97.5.4.2 G6PC3 Mutations (OMIM Code 612541)

Patients with G6PC3 mutations, which are prevalent in Turkey, are affected by a variant of congenital neutropenia disease with neutropenia from severe to moderate, typical arrested myeloid maturation, and several other congenital abnormalities. Apart from heart and urogenital deficiencies, face dysmorphic disorders, increasingly visible superficial veins, hearing loss from inner ear dysfunction, aberrant endocrine function, or myopathy may be observed (Notarangelo et al. 2014).

G6PC3 deficiency's molecular physiopathology includes an activation of the unfolded protein response and an increased stress of the endoplasmic reticulum, in addition to abnormal intracellular glucose homeostasis.

Mutations of the G6PC3 gene are generally homozygous, but a double heterozygote has been described (Boztug et al. 2009).

97.5.5 Neutropenia Associated with Poikilodermia, Clericuzio Type (OMIM Code 604173)

Clericuzio type is a neutropenia with genodermatosis that onset in the first year of life. Recurrent infections occur, especially pneumonia. The neutropenia is often severe. The poikilodermia includes skin atrophy and popular erythematous rash. Composite mutations of the C16ORF57 gene are responsible of pathology (Volpi et al. 2010). The Clericuzio type was first described among Navajos.

97.5.6 Barth's Disease (OMIM Code 302060)

This X-linked disease causes dilated cardiomyopathy as well as endomyocardial fibrosis (resulting in an early death in a few cases), myopathy, and moderate or severe neutropenia, which occasionally cause serious infections. An acidopathy involving a number of organic acids, including the 3-methylglutaconic acid, may also be observed. This syndrome is linked to G4-5 gene mutations coding for the tafazzin protein, which contributes to the phospholipid membrane homeostasis (Donadieu et al. 2011).

References

Ambruso DR, McCabe ER, Anderson DC et al (2003) Infectious and bleeding complications in patients with glycogen Ib. Am J Dis Child 139:691–697

Ancliff PJ, Blundell MP, Cory GO et al (2006) Two novel activating mutations in the Wiskott-Aldrich syndrome protein result in congenital neutropenia. Blood 108:2182–2189

Aprikyan A, Liles W, Park J et al (2000) Myelocatexis, a congenital disorder of severe neutropenia characterized by accelerated apoptosis and defective expression of bcl-x in neutrophil precursors. Blood 95: 320–327

Armistead PM, Wieder E, Akande O et al (2010) Cyclic neutropenia associated with T cell immunity to granulocyte proteases and a double de novo mutation in GFI1, a transcriptional regulator of ELANE. Br J Haematol 150:716–719

Badolato R, Fontana S, Notarangelo LD, Savoldi G (2004) Congenital neutropenia: advances in diagnosis and treatment. Curr Opin Allergy Clin Immunol 4:513–521

Beel K, Cotter MM, Blatny J et al (2009) A large kindred with X-linked neutropenia with an I294T mutation of the Wiskott-Aldrich syndrome gene. Br J Haematol 144:120–126

Boztug K, Welte K, Zeidler C, Klein C (2008) Congenital neutropenia syndromes. Immunol Allergy Clin North Am 28:259–275

Boztug K, Appaswamy G, Ashikov A et al (2009) A syndrome with congenital neutropenia and mutations in G6PC3. N Engl J Med 360:32–43

Carlsson G, Fasth A (2001) Infantile genetic agranulocytosis, morbus Kostmann: presentation of six cases from the original "Kostmann family" and a review. Acta Paediatr 90:757–764

Dale DC, Hammond WP (1988) Cyclic neutropenia: a clinical review. Blood Rev 2:178–185

Dale DC, Person RE, Bolyard AA et al (2000) Mutation in the gene encoding neutrophil elastase in congenital and cyclic neutropenia. Blood 96:2317–2322

Dale DC, Cottle TE, Fier CJ, Bolyard AA, Bonilla MA, Boxer LA, Cham B, Freedman MH, Kannourakis G, Kinsey SE et al (2003) Severe chronic neutropenia: treatment and follow-up of patients in the Severe Chronic Neutropenia International Registry. Am J Hematol 72:82–93

Dell'Angelica EC, Shotelersuk V, Aguilar RC et al (1999) Altered trafficking of lysosomal proteins in Hermansky-Pudlak syndrome due to mutations in the beta 3A subunit of the AP-3 adaptor. Mol Cell 3:11–21

Devriendt K, Kim AS, Mathijs G et al (2001) Constitutively activating mutation in WASP causes X-linked severe congenital neutropenia. Nat Genet 27:313–317

Donadieu J, Leblanc T, Bader Meunier B, French Severe Chronic Neutropenia Study Group et al (2005) Analysis of risk factors for myelodysplasias, leukemias and death from infection among patients with congenital neutropenia. Experience of the French Severe Chronic Neutropenia Study Group. Haematologica 90:45–53

Donadieu J, Fenneteau O, Beaupain B, Mahlaoui N, Chantelot CB (2011) Congenital neutropenia: diagnosis, molecular bases and patient management. Orphanet J Rare Dis 6:26

Dong F, Brynes RK, Tidow N, Welte K, Lowenberg B, Touw IP (1995) Mutations in the gene for the granulocyte colony-stimulating-factor receptor in patients with acute myeloid leukemia preceded by severe congenital neutropenia. N Engl J Med 333:487–493

Dror Y, Freedman MH (2002) Shwachman-Diamond syndrome. Br J Haematol 118:701–713

Fioredda F, Iacobelli S, van Biezen A, Gaspar B, Ancliff P, Donadieu J et al (2015) Stem cell transplantation in severe congenital neutropenia: an analysis from the European Society for Blood and Marrow Transplantation. Blood 126:1885–1892

Freedman MH, Bonilla MA, Fier C et al (2000) Myelodisplasia syndrome and acute myeloid leukemia in patients with congenital neutropenia receiving G-CSF therapy. Blood 96:429–436

Gerin I, Veiga-da-Cunha M, Achouri Y et al (1997) Sequence of a putative glucose 6- phosphate translocase, mutated in glycogen storage disease type Ib. FEBS Lett 419:235–238

Germeshausen M, Ballmaier M, Welte K (2001) Implications of mutations in hematopoietic growth factor receptor genes in congenital cytopenias. Ann N Y Acad Sci 938:305–320

Germeshausen M, Schulze H, Kratz C et al (2005) An acquired G-CSF receptor mutation results in increased proliferation of CMML cells from a patient with severe congenital neutropenia. Leukemia 19:611–617

Germeshausen M, Grudzien M, Zeidler C, Abdollahpour H, Yetgin S, Rezaei N et al (2008) Novel HAX1 mutations in patients with severe congenital neutropenia reveal isoform-dependent genotype-phenotype associations. Blood 111:4954–4957

Germeshausen M, Deerberg S, Peter Y, Reimer C, Kratz CP, Ballmaier M (2013) The spectrum of ELANE mutations and their implications in severe congenital and cyclic neutropenia. Hum Mutat 34:905–914

Gorlin RJ, Gelb B, Diaz GA et al (2000) WHIM syndrome, an autosomal dominant disorder: clinical, hematological, and molecular studies. Am J Med Genet 91:368–376

Han J, Goldstein LA, Hou W et al (2010) Deregulation of mitochondrial membrane potential by mitochondrial insertion of granzyme B and direct Hax-1 cleavage. J Biol Chem 285:22461–22472

Horwitz MS, Duan Z, Korkmaz B et al (2007) Neutrophil elastase in cyclic and severe congenital neutropenia. Blood 109:1817–1824

Karsunky H, Zeng H, Schmidt T, Zevnik B, Kluge R, Schmid KW, Dührsen U, Möröy T (2002) Inflammatory reactions and severe neutropenia in mice lacking the transcriptional repressor Gfi1. Nat Genet 30:295–300

Klein C, Grudzien M, Appaswamy G, Germeshausen M, Sandrock I, Schäffer AA et al (2007) HAX1 deficiency causes autosomal recessive severe congenital neutropenia (Kostmann disease). Nat Genet 39:86–92

Kostman R (1975) Infantile genetic agranulocytosis. A review with presentation of ten new cases. Acta Paediatr Scand 64:362–368

Kostmann R (1956) Infantile genetic agranulocytosis (agranulocytosis infantilis hereditaria): a new recessive lethal disease in man. Almqvist and Wiksells Boktryckeri, Uppsala

Lekstrom-Himes JA, Gallin JI (2000) Immunodeficiency diseases caused by defects in phagocytes. N Engl J Med 343:1703–1714

Moulding DA, Blundell MP, Spiller DG et al (2007) Unregulated actin polymerization by WASp causes defects of mitosis and cytokinesis in X-linked neutropenia. J Exp Med 204:2213–2224

Notarangelo LD, Miao CH, Ochs HD (2008) Wiskott-Aldrich syndrome. Curr Opin Hematol 15:30–36

Notarangelo LD, Savoldi G, Cavagnini S, Bennato V, Vasile S, Pilotta A, Plebani A, Porta F (2014) Severe congenital neutropenia due to G6PC3 deficiency: early and delayed phenotype in two patients with two novel mutations. Ital J Pediatr 40:80

Paley C, Murphy S, Karayalcin G et al (1991) Treatmemt of neutropenia in Shwachman-Diamond syndrome (SDS) with recombinant human granulocyte colony-stimulating factor (RH-GCSF). Blood 78:3a

Person RE, Li FQ, Duan Z, Benson KF, Wechsler J, Papadaki HA, Eliopoulos G, Kaufman C, Bertolone SJ, Nakamoto B et al (2003) Mutations in proto-oncogene GFI1 cause human neutropenia and target ELA2. Nat Genet 34:308–312

Rosenberg PS, Alter BP, Bolyard AA et al (2006) The incidence of leukemia and mortality from sepsis in patients with severe congenital neutropenia receiving long-term G-CSF therapy. Blood 107: 4628–4635

Rosenberg PS, Alter BP, Link DC et al (2008) Neutrophil elastase mutations and risk of leukaemia in severe congenital neutropenia. Br J Haematol 140:210–213

Rosenberg PS, Zeidler C, Bolyard AA et al (2010) Stable long-term risk of leukaemia in patients with severe congenital neutropenia maintained on G-CSF therapy. Br J Haematol 150:196–199

Thrasher AJ, Burns SO (2010) WASP: a key immunological multitasker. Nat Rev Immunol 10:182–192

van der Meer LT, Jansen JH, van der Reijden BA (2010) Gfi1 and Gfi1b: key regulators of hematopoiesis. Leukemia 24:1834–1843

Volpi L, Roversi G, Colombo EA et al (2010) Targeted next-generation sequencing appoints c16orf57 as clericuziotype poikiloderma with neutropenia gene. Am J Hum Genet 86:72–76

Welte K, Zeidler C, Dale DC (2006) Severe congenital neutropenia. Semin Hematol 43:189–195

Westerberg LS, Meelu P, Baptista M et al (2010) Activating WASP mutations associated with X-linked neutropenia result in enhanced actin polymerization, altered cytoskeletal responses, and genomic instability in lymphocytes. J Exp Med 207:1145–1152

Xia J, Bolyard AA, Rodger E et al (2009) Prevalence of mutations in ELANE, GFI1, HAX1, SBDS, WAS and G6PC3 in patients with severe congenital neutropenia. Br J Haematol 147:535–542

Zeidler C, Schwinzer B, Welte K (2003) Congenital neutropenias. Rev Clin Exp Hematol 7:72–83

Zhuang D, Qiu Y, Kogan SC, Dong F (2006) Increased CCAAT enhancer-binding protein epsilon (C/EBPepsilon) expression and premature apoptosis in myeloid cells expressing Gfi-1 N382S mutant associated with severe congenital neutropenia. J Biol Chem 281:10745–10751

Recombinant G-CSF Treatment of Severe Chronic Neutropenia in Neonates and Infants

98

Robert D. Christensen

Contents

Abstract

Neutropenia is a condition characterized by a diminution in the number of circulating neutrophils and increases susceptibility to local and systemic infections. Neutropenia can be a transient and benign condition, in which there is no need of specific therapy, except for intercurrent situations, such as antibiotic therapy in infections. Alternatively, it can be part of a more complex and severe situation, associated with other organ dysfunctions or malformations. Severe chronic neutropenia is a group of diagnoses characterized by hyporegenerative neutropenia, generally present from birth; these newborns and children often need the administration of recombinant granulocyte colony-stimulating factor (rG-CSF). The advent of rG-CSF dramatically improved the lives of these patients, elevating their circulating neutrophil concentrations, markedly reducing infectious illnesses, and extending life expectancy. When a transient variety of neonatal neutropenia is diagnosed, distinct from severe chronic neutropenia (SCN), the benefit of rG-CSF treatment is unproven and of dubious value.

R. D. Christensen (✉)
Divisions of Neonatology and Hematology, Department of Pediatrics, University of Utah School of Medicine, Intermountain Healthcare, Salt Lake City, UT, USA
e-mail: robert.christensen@hsc.utah.edu

G. Buonocore et al. (eds.), *Neonatology*,
https://doi.org/10.1007/978-3-319-29489-6_245

98.1 Salient Points

- Neutrophils are pivotal to the process of antibacterial defense, and patients lacking neutrophils can experience repeated local and systemic infections.
- Neutropenia in newborn is defined if the ANC (Absolute Neutrophil Count) is less than 1,000/μL or when ANC falls below the 5th% reference interval for age; severe neutropenia is defined if the ANC is less than <500/μL.
- Severe chronic neutropenia (SCN) is a group of diagnosis characterized by hyporegenerative and severe neutropenia, present at birth, which benefits from the use of recombinant granulocyte colony-stimulating factor (rG-CSF).
- rG-CSF stimulates proliferation and differentiation of neutrophil precursors and shortens their transit time through the marrow.
- The US FDA-approved algorthim rG-CSF for making the decision regarding rG-CSF use for SCN in the NICU is: initiate treatement if SCN is certain or, if SCN is uncertain, only if (1) ANC < 500/μL for 2 days or more, or (2) ANC is <1000/μL for 5 days or more.

98.2 Diagnosing Neutropenia in a Neonate

Finding a low blood neutrophil concentration can generate questions: Is the count below the reference interval? If it is, what conditions should be considered in the differential diagnosis? Is the neutropenia in this particular patient likely to be a significant clinical problem or will it be trivial and transient? Should rG-CSF be administered? This chapter will focus on these issues, reviewing the studies and the reasoning involved in answering these questions.

First, what is the definition of neonatal neutropenia? It is important to consider the number of neutrophils per microliter of blood, also known as the ANC (absolute neutrophil count) and not just the WBC (white blood cells or leukocytes per microliter). By a strict definition, if the ANC is less than 1000/μL, the neonate has neutropenia, and if the ANC is less than <500/μL, the neonate has *severe* neutropenia (Christensen et al. 2006, 2015; Schmutz et al. 2008). Counts above 1000/μL can technically be neutropenic if they fall below the 5th % reference interval for age. For instance, as shown in Fig. 1, an ANC of 3000/μL 12 h after term birth is indeed an abnormally low ANC (Christensen et al. 2006, 2015; Schmutz et al. 2008; Manroe et al. 1979; Mouzinho et al. 1992; Henry and Christensen 2015). The fact that the ANC is below the lower reference interval indicates an abnormality. However, it is doubtful that an ANC as high as 3000/μL constitutes a significant host-defense deficiency or renders the patient at high risk for acquiring an infection. Therefore, we recommend using the diagnosis "neutropenia" only if the ANC is less than 1000/μL.

98.3 The Importance of Neutrophils in Neonatal Host Defense

Neutrophils are pivotal to the process of antibacterial defense, and patients lacking neutrophils can experience repeated local and systemic infections (Maheshwari 2014). Severe chronic neutropenia (SCN) is a group of diagnoses bearing the common feature of hyporegenerative neutropenia, generally severe neutropenia, present from birth (Makaryan et al. 2015). The advent of recombinant granulocyte colony-stimulating factor (rG-CSF) dramatically improved the lives of patients with SCN, elevating their circulating neutrophil concentrations, markedly reducing infectious illnesses, and extending life expectancy (Makaryan et al. 2015).

SCN can be diagnosed in a neonate (Calhoun and Christensen 1997; Fujiu et al. 2002; Saito-Benz et al. 2015). However, the majority of patients with SCN are not diagnosed until they are several months old, following many infectious episodes that prompt evaluations into immunological deficiencies. When a transient variety of neonatal neutropenia is diagnosed,

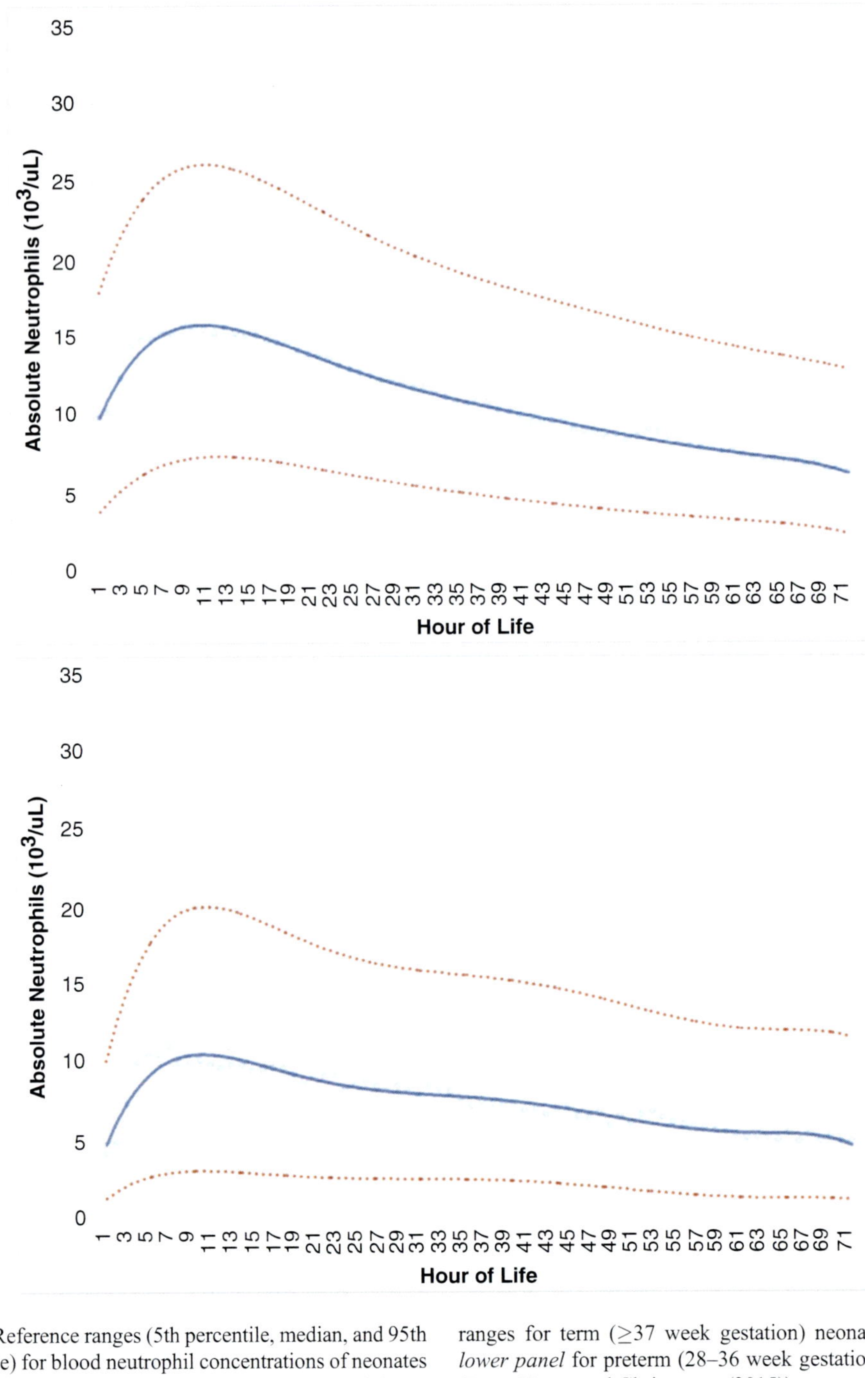

Fig. 1 Reference ranges (5th percentile, median, and 95th percentile) for blood neutrophil concentrations of neonates during their first 3 days after birth. The *upper panel* shows ranges for term (≥37 week gestation) neonates and the *lower panel* for preterm (28–36 week gestation) neonates (From Henry and Christensen (2015))

distinct from SCN, the benefit of rG-CSF treatment is unproven and of dubious value (Christensen et al. 2006; Maheshwari 2014; Christensen and Calhoun 2004). This chapter will review the biological plausibility, the animal studies, and the clinical trials aimed at testing rG-CSF and rGM-CSF treatment for neonates with neutropenia.

98.4 Severe Chronic Neonatal Neutropenia

Kostmann syndrome. Table 1 lists varieties of neutropenia that are generally considered as part of the SCN syndrome. The prototype for SCN is Kostmann syndrome, initially described in 1956 within a kindred in northern Sweden (Kostmann 1956; Carlsson and Fasth 2001; Aprikyan et al. 2004; Horwitz et al. 2013). Patients with this condition generally have circulating neutrophil concentrations <200/μL and a marrow aspirate or biopsy showing a "maturation arrest" where few neutrophilic cells are seen beyond the promyelocyte stage. The original family had what appeared to be an autosomal recessive disorder, but most kindreds subsequently reported seem to have autosomal dominant inheritance. The condition is the result of mutations in the ELA2 (neutrophil elastase) gene (Horwitz et al. 2013). Although rG-CSF treatment is effective in increasing blood neutrophils and reducing febrile illnesses, it does not generally correct the gingivitis that is a prominent feature of this condition in some families. This is probably because rG-CSF does not increase the natural antimicrobial peptide (LL-37) deficiency in Kostmann syndrome patients (Tirali et al. 2013) (Table 2).

Table 1 Varieties of neutropenia among neonates and infants that are generally considered "severe chronic neutropenia"

Kostmann syndrome
Shwachman-Diamond syndrome
Barth syndrome
Cartilage-hair hypoplasia
Cyclic neutropenia
Glycogen storage disease type 1b
Severe neonatal immune-mediated neutropenias

Table 2 Varieties of neutropenia among neonates and infants that are *not* classified as "severe chronic neutropenia"

Pregnancy-induced hypertension
Severe intrauterine growth restriction
The twin-twin transfusion syndrome
Rh hemolytic disease
Bacterial infection
Necrotizing enterocolitis
Chronic idiopathic neutropenia of prematurity

Shwachman-Diamond syndrome. This variety of SCN is generally diagnosed after manifestations of exocrine pancreatic insufficiency, with diarrhea and failure to thrive. It is generally an autosomal recessive condition where multiple organ systems are affected including the pancreas, liver, skeletal, and central nervous systems. Mutations in the Shwachman-Bodian-Diamond syndrome (SBDS) gene are present in most patients. The SBDS gene is involved in the process of ribosomal genesis. Some children with this syndrome respond favorably to rG-CSF; others progress to bone marrow failure and require marrow transplantation (Saito-Benz et al. 2015; Myers et al. 2013).

Barth syndrome. These infants are males (X-linked) with dilated cardiomyopathy, organic aciduria, growth failure, muscle weakness, and neutropenia (Bellanne-Chantelot et al. 2004; Clarke et al. 2013). The diagnosis is suggested by typical clinical findings, a marked increase in urinary 3-methylglutaconic acid, and moderately increased urinary 3-methylglutaric acid and 2-ethylhydracrylic acid. The diagnosis is established by detecting a *TAZ* pathogenic variant on molecular genetic testing (Clarke et al. 2013). rG-CSF can be helpful in these patients as an adjunct to treating infections, or as a measure to prevent infections if neutropenia is severe.

Cartilage-hair hypoplasia. This is a form of short-limbed dwarfism associated with sparse hair and frequent infections. These patients have short pudgy hands, redundant skin, and hyperextensible joints in the hands and feet but typically have flexor contractions at the elbow. The condition is the result of mutation in RMRP (the RNA component of the RNase MRP ribonuclease mitochondrial RNA processing complex). Approximately 100 different RMRP mutations have been reported in the promoter and the transcribed regions. Neutropenia occurs in some patients with cartilage-hair hypoplasia, and these can benefit from rG-CSF administration (Crahes et al. 2013; Rogler et al. 2014).

Cyclic neutropenia. This is a rare inherited autosomal dominant disorder resulting from mutations in the gene for neutrophil elastase (ELA-2 or ELANE). Infants with this condition typically have regular oscillation in their blood neutrophil count with periods of severe neutropenia occurring every 21 days. During these periods, they often have painful mouth ulcers, fevers, and bacterial infections. Some of the severe consequences are gangrene, bacteremia, and septic shock (Dale and Welte 2011). Because it generally takes several cycles before the diagnosis is considered, most infants with this condition are not diagnosed in the immediate newborn period. rG-CSF administration is useful in preventing the very low nadir counts and thereby preventing infectious complications (Dale and Welte 2011).

Glycogen storage disease type 1b. von Gierke disease is an autosomal recessive disorder caused by a deficiency of the enzyme glucose-6-phosphate translocase, which transports glucose-6-phosphate into the endoplasmic reticulum for further metabolism. In GSD-1b, glucose-6-phosphate accumulates intracellularly. Affected neonates present with hypoglycemia, hepatomegaly, growth failure, and neutropenia. Patients with GSD-1b have recurrent bacterial infections, oral ulcers, and inflammatory bowel disease. Neutropenia in infants with GSD-1b does not appear to be caused by impaired maturation of neutrophil progenitors, but involves increased levels of apoptosis and excessive egress of neutrophils from the blood to inflamed tissues, particularly the intestine (Visser et al. 2012). Vitamin E has also been reported to improve the neutrophil counts of these infants (Melis et al. 2009). The gene causing GSD-1b is located on chromosome 11q23 (Chow 2001). rG-CSF can help these patients avoid the recurrent bacterial infections that are otherwise a problematic part of the condition.

Severe immune-mediated neonatal neutropenia. The great majority of cases of severe immune-mediated neonatal neutropenia are alloimmune (van den Tooren-de Groot et al. 2014; Águeda et al. 2012; Wiedl and Walter 2010) but some are autoimmune resulting from maternal autoimmune disease (Curtis et al. 2005; Davoren et al. 2004). Rarely autoimmune neutropenia of infancy is responsible, a primary isolated autoimmune phenomenon (Lekjowski et al. 2003; Conway et al. 1987).

Alloimmune neonatal neutropenia is a relatively common condition where the mother develops antibodies to antigens present on paternal and fetal neutrophils. Antineutrophil antibodies have been found in the serum of as many as 20% of randomly surveyed pregnant and postpartum women (Bux et al. 1998). Most such antibodies cause little problem to the fetus and neonate, but up to 2% of consecutively sampled neonates have neutropenia on this basis. This variety of neutropenia can be severe and prolonged, with a median duration of neutropenia of about 7 weeks, but a range up to 6 months. Repeated infections can occur in these patients until their severe neutropenia remits. Delayed separation of the umbilical cord and skin infections are the most common infectious complications, but serious and life-threatening infections can occur. The mortality rate in this condition, due to overwhelming infection, is reported to be 5%. Severe cases have been successfully treated with rG-CSF. Unlike patients with other varieties of SCN, the neutropenia in this condition will remit spontaneously, and the rG-CSF treatment can be stopped.

Neonatal autoimmune neutropenia occurs when mothers have autoimmune diseases, and their antineutrophil antibodies cross the placenta and bind to fetal neutrophils. Clinical features are generally milder than in alloimmune neonatal neutropenia, and it is rare that a neonate with this variety of neutropenia needs rG-CSF treatment (Curtis et al. 2005; Davoren et al. 2004).

Autoimmune neutropenia of infancy is an unusual disorder where the fetus, and subsequently the neonate, has a primary isolated autoimmune phenomenon (Lekjowski et al. 2003; Conway et al. 1987). Neutrophil-specific antibodies are found in the neonate's serum, reactive against his/her own neutrophils, but no antibodies are found in the mother's serum. Most cases occur in children between 3 and 30 months of age, with a reported incidence of 1:100,000 children. Affected children most often present with minor

infections. Bux reported 240 cases and reported that 12% presented with severe infections, including pneumonia, sepsis, or meningitis (Bux et al. 1998). The neutropenia in this condition generally persists much longer than in cases of alloimmune neutropenia, with a median duration of about 30 months and a range from 6 to 60 months. This variety of neutropenia can be severe, with blood neutrophil concentrations often <500/μL. rG-CSF administration can increase the neutrophil count and reduce infection complications.

Pharmacological agents. Medications administered to women during pregnancy or to neonates rarely result in severe chronic neutropenia. A transient, typically dose-dependent, reduction in neutrophil concentration has been reported with several medications. More severe and chronic neonatal neutropenia is reported with methimazole for treatment of hyperthyroidism (Angelis et al. 2015), with valganciclovir for congenital CMV infection (Kimberlin et al. 2015), and with for treatment with monoclonal anti-TNF antibody for chronic inflammatory bowel disease in pregnant women (Guiddir et al. 2014).

98.5 Neonatal Neutropenia Not Categorized as SCN

Small for gestational age-/pregnancy-induced hypertension. This is the most common variety of neutropenia seen in the NICU (Mouzinho et al. 1992; Koenig and Christensen 1989a, 1991; Sharma et al. 2009; Procianoy et al. 2010). Perhaps one third of neonates born weighing <10th percentile for gestational age have this variety of neutropenia. The ANC can be very low, frequently <500/μL, but the count generally rises spontaneously within the first days and is almost always >1000/μL by day 3. Typically no leukocyte "left shift" is seen, and no toxic granulation, Dohle bodies, and vacuolization are present in the neutrophils. Usually the condition is so transient that such a predisposition is unlikely. The condition is probably caused by an inhibitor of neutrophil production of placental origin that might function mechanistically by depressing natural G-CSF production (Christensen et al. 2006; Tsao et al. 1999). Administering rG-CSF to neonates with this common and transient variety of neonatal neutropenia will elevate their blood neutrophil concentration to normal more rapidly, but there is no evidence that this will reduce morbidities, shorten the hospitalization, or reduce the risk of death.

The twin-twin transfusion syndrome. The donor in a twin-twin transfusion is generally neutropenic, but the recipient can also have neutropenia, although usually not as severe (Koenig et al. 1991). As with the varieties of neutropenia accompanying PIH and SGA, there is generally no leukocyte "left shift" nor are there neutrophil morphological abnormalities. This condition is also transient, with the ANC generally spontaneously rising to >1000/μL by 2 or 3 days, and thus no rG-CSF administration is warranted.

Rh hemolytic disease. Neonates with anemia from Rh hemolytic disease are almost always neutropenic on the first day of life (Koenig and Christensen 1989b). This variety of neutropenia is similar to that of PIH/SGA and donors in a twin-twin transfusion and is likely due to reduced neutrophil production. The neutropenia is transient, generally resolving in a day or 2, and thus no specific treatment is generally required for the neutropenia.

Bacterial infection. Two strategies have been proposed for rG-CSF usage during neonatal infections. Since neutropenia commonly accompanies overwhelming septic shock in neonates, perhaps rG-CSF might be a reasonable adjunct to antibiotics and intensive care treatment. Second, since neutrophil function, particularly chemotaxis, is immature among neonates, perhaps rG-CSF administration might be a reasonable way to prevent nosocomial infections among high-risk neonatal patients. Animal models for both potential uses of rG-CSF were established and supported these hypotheses. In a Cochrane review, Carr et al. examined both potential uses (Carr et al. 2003). They located seven studies where infected neonates were treated with rG-CSF

versus placebo (Carr et al. 2003; Ahmad et al. 2002; Bedford-Russell et al. 2001; Bilgin et al. 2001; Drossou-Agakidou et al. 1998; Miura et al. 2001; Schibler et al. 1998) and three studies where rG-CSF versus placebo was used as prophylaxis against infections (Gillan et al. 1994; Cairo et al. 1995, 1999). They found no evidence that the addition of rG-CSF or rGM-CSF to antibiotic therapy in preterm infants with suspected systemic infection reduces immediate all-cause mortality. No significant survival advantage was seen at 14 days from the start of therapy [typical RR 0.71 (95% CI 0.38,1.33). They conducted a subgroup analysis of 97 infants from three of the studies who, in addition to systemic infection, had a low neutrophil count (<1700/μL) at trial entry. This subgroup did show a significant reduction in mortality by day 14 [RR 0.34 (95% CI 0.12, 0.92); RD −0.18 (95% CI −0.33, −0.03); NNT 6 (95% CI 3–33)].

The three prophylaxis studies (Cairo et al. 1999; Carr et al. 1999; Rosenthal et al. 1996) did not show a significant reduction in mortality in neonates receiving rGM-CSF [RR 0.59 (95% CI 0.24,1.44); RD −0.03 (95% CI −0.08,0.02)]. The identification of sepsis as the primary outcome of prophylaxis studies has been hampered by inadequately stringent definitions of systemic infection. However, data from one study suggest that prophylactic rGM-CSF might provide protection against infection when given to preterm infants who are neutropenic (Rosenthal et al. 1996). Carr et al. concluded that there is currently insufficient evidence to support the introduction of either rG-CSF or rGM-CSF into neonatal practice, either as treatment of established systemic infection to reduce resulting mortality or as prophylaxis to prevent systemic infection in high-risk neonates. This conclusion is consistent with other meta-analyses and reviews (Carr et al. 1999; Rosenthal et al. 1996; Bernstein et al. 2001; Carr and Modi 1997, 2004; Carr 2000; Carr and Huizinga 2000; Bracho et al. 1998; Parravicini et al. 2002; Modi and Carr 2000).

Necrotizing enterocolitis. Neutropenia is relatively common among severe cases of NEC (Hutter et al. 1976; Kling and Hutter 2003; Song et al. 2012). In some cases the neutropenia is transient and resembles the neutropenia following endotoxin. One potential mechanism is influx of neutrophils into the inflamed area of bowel (Song et al. 2012). No studies have focused on using rG-CSF among neutropenic neonates with NEC.

Chronic idiopathic neutropenia of prematurity. Certain preterm neonates develop neutropenia when 4–10 weeks old. This variety of neutropenia is often associated with a patient's spontaneous recovery from the anemia of prematurity. Neutrophil counts are generally <1000/μL but rarely <500/μL (Juul et al. 1998; Juul and Christensen 2003; Mhaskar et al. 2014). The condition is transient, lasting a few weeks to perhaps a month or more. It appears to be a hyporegenerative neutropenia, because it is not accompanied by a leukocyte "left shift" nor morphological abnormalities of the neutrophils. Patients with this condition have a "rG-CSF-mobilizable neutrophil reserve," meaning that if rG-CSF is given, their neutrophil count increases within hours. This has been taken as evidence that these patients do not have a significant host-defense deficiency and they can supply neutrophils to tissues when needed. Thus, although these patients can be neutropenic for several weeks, this condition is likely benign and needs no treatment.

98.6 Leukocyte Growth Factors

G-CSF and GM-CSF are naturally occurring proteins involved in proliferation and differentiation of myeloid precursors into mature neutrophils (Mhaskar et al. 2014; Shaw et al. 2015). The genes for both have been cloned and the purified recombinant factors are commercially available in pharmacological quantities (Mhaskar et al. 2014). These factors have been widely used in adult and pediatric medicine primarily to treat neutropenia. They can shorten the duration of neutropenia after

chemotherapy for leukemia and solid tumors and after bone marrow transplantation.

Target cells for these factors differ. G-CSF is lineage specific for the committed progenitors of neutrophils. It stimulates proliferation and differentiation, expanding the available pool of neutrophil precursors and shortening their transit time through the marrow. GM-CSF acts on multilineage progenitors and on those of monocyte and neutrophil lineage and enhances bactericidal activities of mature phagocytes.

Patients with SCN generally derive considerable benefit from rG-CSF administration. Almost all respond to doses of 5–10 μg per kg administered at intervals ranging from every day to once per week in order to achieve neutrophil concentrations above 500–1000/μL (Zeidler et al. 2009; Shu et al. 2015).

Reports in neonatal animals and humans provided a rational basis to examine rG-CSF or rGM-CSF administration to neonates who have neutropenia with clinical sepsis. Carr and colleagues published a systematic review investigating the efficacy and safety of G-CSF or GM-CSF administration to newborns for treatment of suspected or proven systemic infection to reduce mortality or for prophylaxis of systemic infection in infants at high risk of nosocomial infection (Carr et al. 2003). They identified no substantial evidence that treatment with rG-CSF or rGM-CSF in preterm infants with suspected systemic infection reduces mortality.

Table 3 shows five recent studies where NICUs with a very high death rate among neonates with neutropenia and clinical sepsis showed potential benefit of rG-CSF administration (Kuhn et al. 2009; Chaudhuri et al. 2012; Khan et al. 2012; Gathwala et al. 2012; Borjianyazdi et al. 2013). As additional pertinent investigative work is published, these guidelines will be modified accordingly.

rGM-CSF administration to neonates was studied using slightly different strategies than the rG-CSF trials. It seems clear that the prophylactic use of rGM-CSF does not reduce sepsis or reduce the all-cause mortality rate or reduce morbidity among preterm infants, using follow-up studies up to 5 years (Carr et al. 2009; Marlow et al. 2013, 2015).

98.7 A Consistent Approach to the Use of RG-CSF and RGM-CSF in the Nicu

An algorithm for making the decision regarding rG-CSF administration in the NICU is given in Fig. 2. This is intended as a guideline to serve until better data accumulate to warrant a change in approach. The algorithm is in keeping with FDA-approved approaches and avoids off-label uses.

The principal question in the algorithm is whether the neutropenic neonate has a variety of severe congenital neutropenia, a question to which there are three possible answers: (1) yes, (2) no, and (3) uncertain. We propose that if the answer is "yes," the patient should be afforded the benefit of rG-CSF treatment, and if the answer is "no," rG-CSF should not be given. Cases where the answer is "uncertain" might receive rG-CSF if the neutropenia is severe (ANC <500/μL for 2 days of more) or prolonged (<1000/μL for 5 days or more), while the question of SCN is being investigated. An International Registry for SCN cases can be accessed at the website http://depts.washington.edu/registry/, using the entry criteria and exclusion criteria given in Table 4. We propose beginning rG-CSF treatment with a dose of 10 μg/kg subcutaneously, once per day for three consecutive days. Thereafter, doses are given as needed to titrate the ANC to around 1000/μL. We did not include criteria for administering rGM-CSF, as we found insufficient evidence for its use in NICU patients. If one follows this schema (Fig. 2), it will result in little use of rG-CSF in the NICU. Any rG-CSF usage in Neonatology should be focused on patients with the most to gain and least to lose by its application.

Severe chronic neutropenia includes Kostmann syndrome, Shwachman-Diamond syndrome, cyclic neutropenia, Bart syndrome, autoimmune or alloimmune neonatal neutropenia, or any syndrome or condition where severe and chronic neutropenia is a consistent finding.

G-CSF administration is not recommended for neonates with neutropenia of a non-severe or a non-chronic nature, such as the neutropenia associated with PIH, sepsis, or chronic idiopathic (mild) neutropenia.

Table 3 Randomized clinical trials testing rG-CSF treatment for neonates with clinical sepsis and neutropenia

Year	First author (reference)	Country	Eligibility	rG-CSF dose	Control	Death rate in rG-CSF-treated group	Death rate in control group	Length of stay (days) treated versus control
2009	Kuhn (Kuhn et al. 2009)	France	ANC <1500/μL × 2 days and ≤32 weeks gestation	10 μg/k/day I.V. × 3 days	5% dextrose	At 2 weeks 16% (16/102)	At 2 weeks 29% (28/98)	Not reported
						At 4 weeks 27%	(p = 0.03)	
						(28/102)	At 4 weeks 30% (29/98)	
							(p = 0.40)	
2012	Chaudhuri (Chaudhuri et al. 2012)	India	ANC <1500/μL and clinical sepsis	10 μg/k/day I.V. × 3 days	5% dextrose	10% (4/39)	35% (14/39)	Regression (accounting for deaths) $p < 0.01$
							($p < 0.05$)	
2012	Khan (Khan et al. 2012)	Bangladesh	ANC <5000/μL and clinical sepsis	10 μg/k/day S.Q. × up to 5 days	Sham	20% (3/15)	33% (5/15)	Not reported
							(p = 0.68)	
2012	Gathwala (Gathwala et al. 2012)	India	ANC <5000/μL and clinical sepsis	10 μg/k/day I.V. × 5 days	Sham	15% (3/20)	35% (7/20)	Not reported
							(p = 0.27)	
2014	Borjianyazdi (Borjianyazdi et al. 2013)	Iran	ANC <500/μL and clinical sepsis	10 μg/k/day S.Q. × up to 5 days	Saline	4% (1/23)	0% (0/23)	25 ± 6 versus 30 ± 7 $p = 0.04$
							(p = 1.00)	
Summary statistics						20% (39/199)	22% (55/195)	Unable to calculate
							(p = 0.05 chi^2 with Yates correction)	

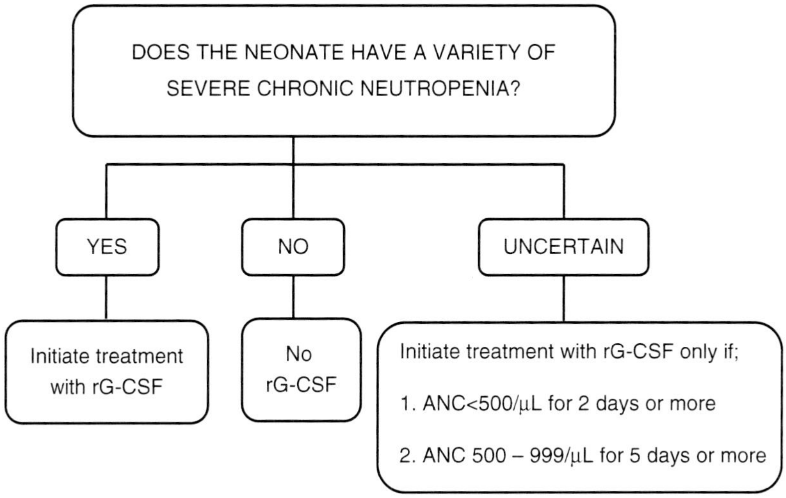

Fig. 2 The US FDA-approved rG-CSF for use in children with severe chronic neutropenia and for children receiving myelosuppressive chemotherapy of marrow transplantation. The rG-CSF used in the USA is produced by Amgen (Thousand Oaks, CA) and has a molecular weight slightly lower than natural G-CSF, because it is produced in *Escherichia coli* and is not glycosylated. It has an amino acid sequence identical to that of natural G-CSF except for the addition of an N-terminal methionine, which is necessary for its expression in *E. coli*

Table 4 Screening for severe chronic neutropenia

Inclusion questions
1. Has a blood neutrophil count of <500/μL been documented on at least three occasions in the past 3 months?
2. Is there a history of recurrent infections?
3. Is the bone marrow evaluation consistent with severe chronic neutropenia?
4. Has a cytogenetic evaluation been completed?
5. Is the patient now receiving Neupogen (rG-CSF)?
Exclusion criteria
1. The neutropenia is known to be drug induced
2. Thrombocytopenia is present (<50,000/μL) except in the case of Shwachman-Diamond syndrome or glycogen storage disease type 1b
3. Anemia is present (hgb <8 g/dL) except in the case of Shwachman-Diamond syndrome or glycogen storage disease type 1b
4. The infant has a myelodysplastic syndrome and aplastic anemia, is HIV positive, has some other hematological disease, has rheumatoid arthritis, or has had previous chemotherapy for cancer

References

Águeda S, Rocha G, Ferreira F et al (2012) Neonatal alloimmune neutropenia: still a diagnostic and therapeutical challenge. J Pediatr Hematol Oncol 34:497–499

Ahmad A, Laborada G, Bussel J, Nesin M (2002) Comparison of recombinant G-CSF, recombinant human GM-CSF and placebo for treatment of septic preterm infants. Pediatr Infect Dis J 21:1061–1065

Angelis D, Kubicky RA, Zubrow AB (2015) Methimazole associated neutropenia in a preterm neonate treated for hyperthyroidism. Case Rep Endocrinol 2015:680191

Aprikyan AA, Carlsson G, Stein S et al (2004) Neutrophil elastase mutations in severe congenital neutropenia patients of the original Kostmann family. Blood 103:389

Bedford-Russell AR, Emmerson AJB, Wilkinson N et al (2001) A trial of recombinant human granulocyte colony stimulating factor for the treatment of very low birthweight infants with presumed sepsis and neutropenia. Arch Dis Child Fetal Neonatal Ed 84: F172–F176

Bellanne-Chantelot C, Clauin S, Leblanc T et al (2004) Mutations in the ELA2 gene correlate with more severe expression of neutropenia: a study of 81 patients from the French Neutropenia Register. Blood 103:4119–4125

Bernstein HM, Pollock BH, Calhoun DA, Christensen RD (2001) Administration of recombinant G-CSF to neonates with septicemia: a meta-analysis. Pediatrics 138:917–920

Bilgin K, Yaramis A, Haspolat K et al (2001) A randomized trial of granulocyte-macrophage colony-stimulating factor in neonates with sepsis and neutropenia. Pediatrics 107:36–41

Borjianyazdi L, Froomandi M, Noori Shadkam M et al (2013) The effect of granulocyte colony stimulating factor administration on preterm infant with neutropenia and clinical sepsis: a randomized clinical trial. Iran J Pediatr Hematol Oncol 3:64–68

Bracho F, Goldman S, Cairo MS (1998) Potential use of granulocyte colony-stimulating factor and granulocyte-macrophage colony-stimulating factor in neonates. Curr Opin Hematol 5:215–220

Bux J, Behrens G, Jaeger G, Welte K (1998) Diagnosis and clinical course of autoimmune neutropenia in infancy; analysis of 240 cases. Blood 91:181–186

Cairo MS, Christensen RD, Sender LS et al (1995) Results of a phase I/II trial of recombinant human granulocyte-macrophage colony-stimulating factor in very low birthweight neonates: significant induction of circulatory neutrophils, monocytes, platelets, and bone marrow neutrophils. Blood 86:2509–2515

Cairo MS, Agosti J, Ellis R et al (1999) A randomised double-blind placebo-controlled trial of prophylactic recombinant human GM-CSF to reduce nosocomial infection in very low birthweight neonates. J Pediatr 134:64–70

Calhoun DA, Christensen RD (1997) The occurrence of Kostmann syndrome in preterm neonates. Pediatrics 99:259–261

Carlsson G, Fasth A (2001) Infantile genetic agranulocytosis, morbus Kostmann: presentation of six cases from the original "Kostmann family" and a review. Acta Paediatr 90:757–764

Carr R (2000) Neutrophil production and function in newborn infants. Br J Haematol 110:18–28

Carr R, Huizinga TWJ (2000) Low sFcRIII demonstrates reduced neutrophil reserves in preterm neonates. Arch Dis Child Fetal Neonatal Ed 83:F160

Carr R, Modi N (1997) Haemopoietic colony stimulating factors for preterm neonates. Arch Dis Child 76: F128–F133

Carr R, Modi N (2004) Haemopoietic growth factors for neonates: assessing risks and benefits. Acta Paediatr Suppl 93:15–19

Carr R, Modi N, Doré CJ et al (1999) A randomised controlled trial of prophylactic GM-CSF in human newborns less than 32 weeks gestation. Pediatrics 103:796–802

Carr R, Modi N, Dore C (2003) G-CSF and GM-CSF for treating or preventing neonatal infections. Cochrane Database Syst Rev CD003066

Carr R, Brocklehurst P, Doré CJ, Modi N (2009) Granulocyte-macrophage colony stimulating factor administered as prophylaxis for reduction of sepsis in extremely preterm, small for gestational age neonates (the PROGRAMS trial): a single-blind, multicentre, randomised controlled trial. Lancet 373:226–233

Chaudhuri J, Mitra S, Mukhopadhyay D et al (2012) Granulocyte colony-stimulating factor for preterms with sepsis and neutropenia: a randomized controlled trial. J Clin Neonatol 1:202–206

Chow JY (2001) The molecular basis of type I glycogen storage diseases. Curr Mol Med 1:25–44

Christensen RD, Calhoun DA (2004) Congenital neutropenia. Clin Perinatol 31:29–38

Christensen RD, Henry E, Wiedmeier SE et al (2006) Neutropenia among extremely low birth-weight neonates: data from a multihospital healthcare system. J Perinatol 26:682–687

Christensen RD, Yoder BA, Baer VL et al (2015) Early-onset neutropenia in small for gestational age infants. Pediatrics 136:e1259–1267

Clarke SL, Bowron A, Gonzalez IL et al (2013) Barth syndrome. Orphanet J Rare Dis 12(8):23

Conway LT, Clay ME, Kline WE et al (1987) Natural history of primary autoimmune neutropenia in infancy. Pediatrics 79:728–733

Crahes M, Saugier-Veber P, Patrier S et al (2013) Foetal presentation of cartilage hair hypoplasia with extensive granulomatous inflammation. Eur J Med Genet 56:365–370

Curtis BR, Reon C, Aster RH (2005) Neonatal alloimmune neutropenia attributed to maternal immunoglobulin G antibodies against the neutrophil alloantigen HNA1c (SH): a report of five cases. Transfusion 45:1308–1313

Dale DC, Welte K (2011) Cyclic and chronic neutropenia. Cancer Treat Res 157:97–108

Davoren A, Saving K, McFarland JG et al (2004) Neonatal neutropenia and bacterial sepsis associated with placental transfer of maternal neutrophil-specific autoantibodies. Transfusion 44:1041–1046

Drossou-Agakidou V, Kanakoudi-Tsakalidou F, Taparkou A et al (1998) Administration of recombinant human granulocyte-colony stimulating factor to septic neonates induces neutrophilia and enhances the neutrophil respiratory burst and beta2 integrin expression. Results of a randomized controlled trial. Eur J Pediatr 157: 583–588

Fujiu T, Maruyama K, Koizumi T (2002) Early-onset group B streptococcal sepsis in a preterm infant with Kostmann syndrome. Acta Paediatr 91:1397–1399

Gathwala G, Walia M, Bala H, Singh S (2012) Recombinant human granulocyte colony-stimulating factor in preterm neonates with sepsis and relative neutropenia: a randomized, single-blind, non-placebo-controlled trial. J Trop Pediatr 58:12–18

Gillan ER, Christensen RD, Suen Y et al (1994) A randomized, placebo-controlled trial of recombinant human granulocyte colony-stimulating factor administration in newborn infants with presumed sepsis: significant

induction of peripheral and bone marrow neutrophilia. Blood 84:1427–1433

Guiddir T, Frémond ML, Triki TB et al (2014) Anti-TNF-α therapy may cause neonatal neutropenia. Pediatrics 134:e1189–e1193

Henry E, Christensen RD (2015) Reference intervals in neonatal hematology. Clin Perinatol. doi:10.1016/j.cip.2015/04/005

Horwitz MS, Corey SJ, Grimes HL, Tidwell T (2013) ELANE mutations in cyclic and severe congenital neutropenia: genetics and pathophysiology. Hematol Oncol Clin North Am 27:19–41

Hutter JJ Jr, Hathaway WE, Wayne ER (1976) Hematologic abnormalities in severe neonatal necrotizing enterocolitis. J Pediatr 88:1026–1031

Juul SE, Christensen RD (2003) Effect of recombinant granulocyte colony-stimulating factor on blood neutrophil concentrations among patients with "idiopathic neonatal neutropenia": a randomized, placebo-controlled trial. J Perinatol 23:493–497

Juul SE, Calhoun DA, Christensen RD (1998) "Idiopathic neutropenia" in very low birthweight infants. Acta Paediatr 87:963–968

Khan TH, Shahidullah M, Mannan MA, Nahar N (2012) Effect of recombinant human granulocyte colony stimulating factor (rhG-CSF) for the treatment of neonates in presumed sepsis with neutropenia. Mymensingh Med J 21:469–474

Kimberlin DW, Jester PM, Sánchez PJ et al (2015) Valganciclovir for symptomatic congenital cytomegalovirus disease. N Engl J Med 372:933–943

Kling PJ, Hutter JJ (2003) Hematologic abnormalities in severe neonatal necrotizing enterocolitis: 25 years later. J Perinatol 23:523–530

Koenig JM, Christensen RD (1989a) Incidence, neutrophil kinetics, and natural history of neonatal neutropenia associated with maternal hypertension. N Engl J Med 321:557–562

Koenig JM, Christensen RD (1989b) Neutropenia and thrombocytopenia in infants with Rh hemolytic disease. J Pediatr 114:625–631

Koenig JM, Christensen RD (1991) The mechanism responsible for diminished neutrophil production in neonates delivered of women with pregnancy-induced hypertension. Am J Obstet Gynecol 165:467–473

Koenig JM, Hunter DD, Christensen RD (1991) Neutropenia in donor (anemic) twins involved in the twin-twin transfusion syndrome. J Perinatol 11:355–358

Kostmann R (1956) Infantile genetic agranulocytosis; agranulocytosis infantilis hereditaria. Acta Paediatr 45 (Suppl 105):1–78

Kuhn P, Messer J, Paupe A et al (2009) A multicenter, randomized, placebo-controlled trial of prophylactic recombinant granulocyte-colony stimulating factor in preterm neonates with neutropenia. J Pediatr 155:324–330.e1

Lekjowski M, Maheshwari A, Calhoun DA et al (2003) Persistent perianal abcess in early infancy as a presentation of autoimmune neutropenia. J Perinatol 23:428–430

Maheshwari A (2014) Neutropenia in the newborn. Curr Opin Hematol 21:43–49

Makaryan V, Zeidler C, Bolyard AA et al (2015) The diversity of mutations and clinical outcomes for ELANE-associated neutropenia. Curr Opin Hematol 22:3–11

Manroe BL, Weinberg AG, Rosenfeld CR, Browne R (1979) The neonatal blood count in health and disease. I. Reference values for neutrophilic cells. J Pediatr 95:89–98

Marlow N, Morris T, Brocklehurst P et al (2013) A randomised trial of granulocyte-macrophage colony-stimulating factor for neonatal sepsis: outcomes at 2 years. Arch Dis Child Fetal Neonatal Ed 98:F46–F53

Marlow N, Morris T, Brocklehurst P (2015) A randomised trial of granulocyte-macrophage colony-stimulating factor for neonatal sepsis: childhood outcomes at 5 years. Arch Dis Child Fetal Neonatal Ed 100:F320–F326

Melis D, Della Casa R, Parini R et al (2009) Vitamin E supplementation improves neutropenia and reduces the frequency of infections in patients with glycogen storage disease type 1b. Eur J Pediatr 168:1069–1074

Mhaskar R, Clark OA, Lyman G et al (2014) Colony-stimulating factors for chemotherapy-induced febrile neutropenia. Cochrane Database Syst Rev 10: CD003039

Miura E, Procianoy RS, Bittar C et al (2001) A randomized double-masked, placebo controlled trial of recombinant granulocyte colony-stimulating factor administration to preterm infants with the clinical diagnosis of early-onset sepsis. Pediatrics 107:30–35

Modi N, Carr R (2000) Promising stratagems for reducing the burden of neonatal sepsis. Arch Dis Child Fetal Neonatal Ed 83:F150–F153

Mouzinho A, Rosenfeld CR, Sanchez PJ, Risser R (1992) Effect of maternal hypertension on neonatal neutropenia and risk of nosocomial infection. Pediatrics 90:430–435

Myers KC, Davies SM, Shimamura A (2013) Clinical and molecular pathophysiology of Shwachman-Diamond syndrome: an update. Hematol Oncol Clin North Am 27:117–128

Parravicini E, van de Ven C, Anderson L, Cairo MS (2002) Myeloid hematopoietic growth factors and their role in prevention and/or treatment of neonatal sepsis. Transfus Med Rev 16:11–24

Procianoy RS, Silveira RC, Mussi-Pinhata MM et al (2010) Sepsis and neutropenia in very low birth weight infants delivered of mothers with preeclampsia. J Pediatr 157:434–438, 438.e1

Rogler LE, Kosmyna B, Moskowitz D et al (2014) Small RNAs derived from lncRNA RNase MRP have gene-silencing activity relevant to human cartilage-hair hypoplasia. Hum Mol Genet 23:368–382

Rosenthal J, Healey T, Ellis R et al (1996) A two year follow-up of neonates with presumed sepsis treated

with recombinant human G-CSF during the first week of life. J Pediatr 128:135–137

Saito-Benz M, Miller HE, Berry MJ (2015) Shwachman-Diamond syndrome in a preterm neonate. J Paediatr Child Health. doi:10.1111/jpc.12941

Schibler KR, Osborne KA, Leung LY et al (1998) A randomized placebo-controlled trial of granulocyte colony-stimulating factor administration to newborn infants with neutropenia and clinical signs of early-onset sepsis. Pediatrics 102:6–13

Schmutz N, Henry E, Jopling J, Christensen RD (2008) Expected ranges for blood neutrophil concentrations of neonates: the Manroe and Mouzinho charts revisited. J Perinatol 28:275–281

Sharma G, Nesin M, Feuerstein M, Bussel JB (2009) Maternal and neonatal characteristics associated with neonatal neutropenia in hypertensive pregnancies. Am J Perinatol 26:683–689

Shaw BE, Confer DL, Hwang W, Pulsipher MA (2015) A review of the genetic and long-term effects of G-CSF injections in healthy donors: a reassuring lack of evidence for the development of haematological malignancies. Bone Marrow Transplant 50(3): 334–340

Shu Z, Li XH, Bai XM et al (2015) Clinical characteristics of severe congenital neutropenia caused by novel ELANE gene mutations. Pediatr Infect Dis J 34: 203–207

Song R, Subbarao GC, Maheshwari A (2012) Haematological abnormalities in neonatal necrotizing enterocolitis. J Matern Fetal Neonatal Med 25(Suppl 4):22–25

Tirali RE, Yalçınkaya Erdemci Z, Çehreli SB (2013) Oral findings and clinical implications of patients with congenital neutropenia: a literature review. Turk J Pediatr 55:241–245

Tsao PN, Teng RJ, Tang JR, Yau KI (1999) Granulocyte colony-stimulating factor in the cord blood of premature neonates born to mothers with pregnancy-induced hypertension. J Pediatr 135:56–59

van den Tooren-de Groot R, Ottink M, Huiskes E, van Rossum A et al (2014) Management and outcome of 35 cases with foetal/neonatal alloimmune neutropenia. Acta Paediatr. doi:10.1111/apa.12741

Visser G, de Jager W, Verhagen LP et al (2012) Survival, but not maturation, is affected in neutrophil progenitors from GSD-1b patients. J Inherit Metab Dis 35:287–300

Wiedl C, Walter AW (2010) Granulocyte colony stimulating factor in neonatal alloimmune neutropenia: a possible association with induced thrombocytopenia. Pediatr Blood Cancer 54:1014–1016

Zeidler C, Germeshausen M, Klein C, Welte K (2009) Clinical implications of ELA2-, HAX1-, and G-CSF-receptor (CSD3R) mutations in severe congenital neutropenia. Br J Haematol 144:459–466

Fundamentals of Feto-Neonatal Immunology

99

Akhil Maheshwari and Edmund F. La Gamma

Contents

Abstract

The immune system in the newborn infant is in a unique state of maturational flux that is distinct from all other periods of postnatal life. Faced with a continuous barrage of novel environmental antigens, the neonatal immune system must simultaneously protect the host from potentially harmful pathogens and, at the same time, learn to tolerate commensal microbes and dietary macromolecules and allow absorption and utilization of nutrients. While some components of the immune system perform at par with adults, the immaturity of the other branches results in a physiological, developmentally regulated immunodeficient state. The teleological significance of some of these alterations is still being elucidated. This chapter highlights the most prominent quantitative and qualitative differences in the innate and adaptive arms of the neonatal and adult immune systems and provides a brief overview of the developing mucosal immune system.

A. Maheshwari (✉)
Division of Neonatology, University of South Florida, Tampa, FL, USA
e-mail: akhilm@health.usf.edu

E. F. La Gamma
Division of Newborn Medicine, Maria Fareri Children's Hospital, Westchester Medical Center – New York Medical College, Valhalla, NY, USA
e-mail: edmund_lagamma@nymc.edu

G. Buonocore et al. (eds.), *Neonatology*,
https://doi.org/10.1007/978-3-319-29489-6_246

99.1 Salient Points

- The fetal-neonatal immune system must balance its role in host defense and elimination of invading pathogens, with the need to tolerate self-antigens, nutrients, and commensals.
- Neonatal neutrophils are developmentally deficient in most host defense functions such as migration, phagocytosis, and microbial killing.
- With limited antigenic experience, the innate immune system forms the mainstay of neonatal immunity. The monocyte-macrophage lineage, natural killer cells, and the noncytotoxic innate lymphoid cells play critical roles.
- The adaptive immune system in the fetus and neonate also displays innate-like properties to compensate for limitations in antigen-specific immune responses. The presence of B-1 lymphocytes and polyspecific antibodies are two examples for such adaptive mechanisms.
- The mucosal immune system undergoes rapid development after birth, following the massive exposure to microbial and food antigens.

The transition from fetal to neonatal life at birth forms an important functional watershed in the developing immune system. In utero, the fetus is exposed to a steady stream of "foreign" antigens that are derived mainly from the mother, and must downregulate its immune response to survive. After birth, however, the neonatal immune system is exposed to a new, more diverse set of antigens and must evolve dichotomous responses to "contain" the microorganisms on various cutaneous and mucosal surfaces and, at the same time, develop tolerance to other commensal microbes and dietary macromolecules. During this remarkable transition, while some components of the immune system perform at par with adults, immaturity of the other arms results in a developmentally regulated state of immunodeficiency. This chapter highlights major quantitative and qualitative differences in the innate and adaptive arms of the neonatal and adult immune systems and provides a brief review of the developing mucosal immune system.

99.2 Innate Immune System

This section will review the developmental issues relevant to the collection of defense mechanisms human neonate is born with prior to exposure to environmental antigens and acquisition of adaptive immunity. Cell lineages, their maturation, and functional capacities or limitations will be defined.

99.2.1 Neutrophils

99.2.1.1 Development

The two major hematopoietic progenitors committed to the neutrophil lineage are the colony-forming units-mix, which give rise to a mixture of various leukocyte populations, and the CFU-GEMM, which produce granulocytes, erythrocytes, megakaryocytes, and macrophages. The mechanisms underlying this process of lineage commitment are now beginning to be understood (Starnes et al. 2009). The effect of biomechanical forces as critical regulators of hematopoiesis is a new field of investigation (Adamo et al. 2009), as is the prevention of apoptosis as a mechanism for hematopoietic progenitor cell growth and development (Boxer 2006). In the bone marrow, the neutrophil cell lineage includes the early precursors with a capacity for 4–5 cell divisions and the later, post-mitotic stages that are in process of differentiation. In adults, the neutrophil proliferating pool (NPP) contains about 2×10^9 cells/kg body weight and the neutrophil storage pool (NSP) contains about 6×10^9 cells/kg body weight (Maheshwari and Christensen 2004). The NPP and NSP together contain nearly 90% of all neutrophils in the body. The remaining 10% (0.6×10^9/kg) are equally distributed free in the circulation or attached to the microvascular endothelium.

Although umbilical cord blood and fetal blood have a 10- to 50-fold higher concentration of CFU-GM than does the blood of adults (Williams et al. 2006), the fetus has an overall much smaller pool of neutrophil progenitors (Christensen et al. 1986; Christensen 1987). In the midgestation

fetus and preterm infant, the NSP is very small in size and can be readily exhausted during sepsis (Maheshwari and Christensen 2004). Studies in experimental animals show that the NSP is considerably smaller in animals delivered prematurely (1.0–1.3 × 10^9 cells/kg) than at full-term (1.3–2.5 × 10^9 cells/kg) and in adulthood (4.5–7.5 × 10^9/kg). The NPP is also smaller, about one tenth the size (per kg body weight) of adults (Engle et al. 1983). Indirect evidence for a small granulocytopoietic pool in the human fetus comes from studies of soluble CD16, which is derived from apoptotic neutrophils, and its low concentrations in plasma of preterm neonates may reflect a low total body neutrophil mass. The low sCD16 levels of premature infants reach adult values only by the fourth postnatal week (Carr and Huizinga 2000).

During acute inflammation, neutrophils are released first from the NSP, and once these stores are exhausted, progressively immature cells are mobilized (the "left" shift of sepsis). Circulating neutrophils persist in the bloodstream for 6–8 h and then for a few hours to several days in tissues. In the fetus, as in the adult, mature neutrophils are stored within the bone marrow and also in the liver and spleen. These maturational relationships and short half-life frequently result in the presenting clinical sign of neutropenia rather than neutrophilia in newborns with bacterial sepsis.

99.2.1.2 Function

Transendothelial Migration

Circulating neutrophils leave the intravascular compartment to enter the tissues in three major steps: *margination and rolling* on vascular endothelium, *attachment* to the endothelial cells, and *transendothelial* migration (Fig. 1) (McIntyre et al. 2003; Panes and Granger 1994). Leukocyte traffic is preferentially directed to inflamed areas through regional changes in vascular flow and along concentration gradients of humoral chemoattractants such as chemokines, bacterial products (such as formyl-met-leu-phe or f-MLP), complement fragments (C5a), and leukotrienes (LTB_4). Among chemokines, members of the CXC subfamily with a glutamate-leucine-arginine (ELR) tripeptide sequence (such as interleukin-8 (IL-8/CXCL8)) have a neutrophil-specific chemotactic activity (Bagorda et al. 2006; Shaik et al. 2009).

In inflamed tissues, transient interruptions in the laminar flow of marginating neutrophils cause these cells to tumble and roll on vascular endothelial surface. This process is mediated through a process of repetitive binding and release of selectins (L-selectin on neutrophils, E- and P-selectin on endothelium) from their sialomucin receptors called addressins. The term *selectin* is derived from a key lectin domain that interacts selectively with oligosaccharide receptors bearing

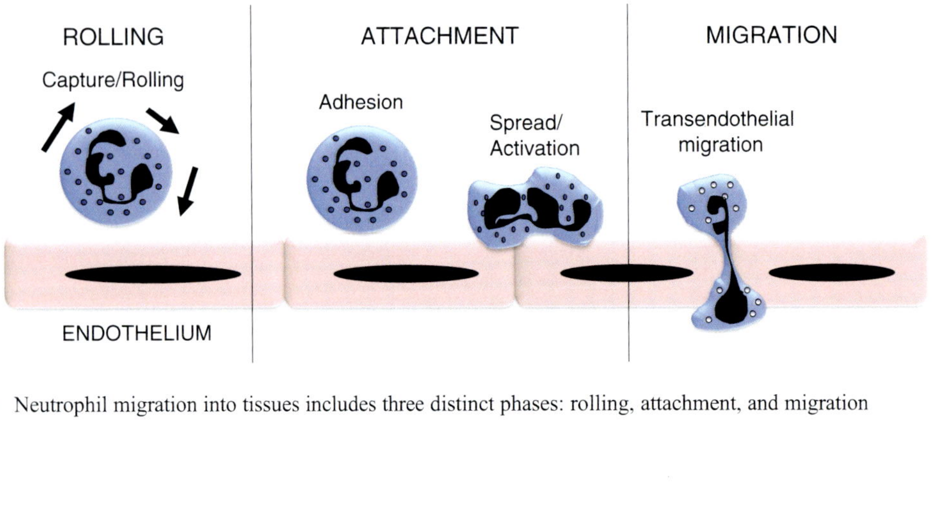

Fig. 1 Neutrophil migration into tissues includes three distinct phases: rolling, attachment, and migration

sialylated carbohydrate moieties. L-selectin is constitutively expressed on neutrophils and is shed after cellular activation (Rosen 2004). Rolling neutrophils slow down and attach to endothelium through the binding of β_2-integrins to cognate receptors on endothelial cells (Edwards 1995). The β_2-integrins expressed on neutrophils include the leukocyte function-associated antigen-1 (LFA-1, $\alpha_L\beta_2$, CD11a/CD18), Mac-1 ($\alpha_M\beta_2$, CD11b/CD18), and the p150, 95 ($\alpha_X\beta_2$, CD11c/CD18), which bind endothelial receptors such as the intercellular adhesion molecule-1 (ICAM-1) and ICAM-2. LFA-1 binds to both ICAM-1 and ICAM-2, whereas Mac-1 and p150, 95 bind exclusively to ICAM-1. These neutrophils undergo activation on the endothelial surface and migrate through the capillary/venular wall, a process that involves the platelet-endothelial cell adhesion molecule (PECAM1, CD31), the integrin-associated protein (CD47), and a series of other junctional molecules (Wagner and Roth 2000).

Compared to neutrophils from adults, neutrophils from both term and preterm infants adhere poorly to the endothelium. Neonatal neutrophils have lower selectin expression than adults at birth (Kim et al. 2003), which might be further reduced by perinatal stress such as in birth asphyxia (Hashimoto et al. 2002). In addition, neonatal neutrophils display defective shedding of L-selectin (Kim et al. 2003). This combination of decreased expression and impaired shedding of L-selectin impairs the ability of neutrophils to roll on the endothelial surface, thereby limiting the recruitment of circulating neutrophils into the tissues. Neutrophil-endothelial adherence and neutrophil transmigration is further limited in neonates due to a developmental deficiency of mac-1 (CD18/CD11b), one of the β_2 integrins (Reddy et al. 1998). The transendothelial migration of neutrophils is also limited, at least in immature cells released from the NSP during sepsis, by reduced deformability of the neutrophil membrane and cytoplasm (Linderkamp et al. 1998). For these reasons, it is generally belived that the propensity of neonates to bacteremia is more typical than a proper localization and abscess formation.

Chemotaxis

Once outside the blood vessel, neutrophils migrate along concentration gradients of various chemoattractants such as IL-8 (and other ELR$^+$ CXC chemokines), f-MLP, and C5a (Bagorda et al. 2006). These chemotactic stimuli bind to high-affinity G-protein-coupled receptors on the leukocyte surface, and minute spatial gradients in chemoattractant concentrations can cause the receptors to be distributed asymmetrically toward the migrating neutrophil pseudopodium. Cellular movement involves a number of intracellular signaling pathways and cytoskeletal proteins. A chemoattractant hierarchy has been reported, wherein bacterial products are preferred over host chemokines (Heit et al. 2002).

Neutrophils from both term and preterm neonates have an impaired chemotactic response, migrating at only about half the speed traveled by adult cells (Carr et al. 1992; Bektas et al. 1990; Fox et al. 2005). While neutrophils from term infants achieve normal chemotactic function by 2 weeks after birth, such postnatal neutrophil maturation begins 2–3 weeks after birth in immature preterm infants and proceeds very slowly (Sacchi et al. 1982). Neutrophils from preterm infants born at 34–36 weeks gestation achieve normal chemotaxis by 40–42 weeks of post-conceptional age. In more immature preterm infants (<34 weeks), neutrophil chemotaxis improves with time but remains impaired in comparison to adults even at 42 weeks PCA (Eisenfeld et al. 1990). Although minor infections may enhance chemotaxis in neonates, the migratory responses of neonatal neutrophils may become further depressed during systemic Gram-negative sepsis (Turkmen et al. 2000; Laurenti et al. 1980).

Neonatal neutrophils bind various chemoattractants normally. However, chemoattractant-induced membrane depolarization, calcium transport, and sugar uptake are relatively less efficient. The chemotactic defect in neonatal neutrophils may be multifactorial, affected by factors such as a larger, poorly motile neutrophil subpopulation, impaired calcium mobilization, and aberrations in intracellular signaling pathways such as NF-κB activation (Weinberger et al. 2001; Krause et al. 1989). Lower Mac-1 expression can also impede

chemotaxis due to impaired neutrophil interaction with the extracellular matrix (Weinberger et al. 2001; Jones et al. 1990). Inability to effectively direct neutrophils to the bacterial source contributes to the neonatal vulnerability to septicemia.

Phagocytosis

Phagocytosis is a specialized form of endocytosis directed at engulfing solid particles into an internal phagosome. This internalized phagosome "matures" through interactions with the endosomal compartment and eventually fuses with a lysosome for killing of internalized microorganisms and terminal degradation of the cargo (Segal 2005). Phagocytosis is more efficient when the target is opsonized by specific immunoglobulin G (IgG) or complement factors, which may act by neutralizing inhibitors of phagocytosis such as the capsular polysaccharide or by rendering the microbial surface more hydrophobic. Neutrophils express receptors for IgG ($F_c\gamma$ receptors I-III, or CD16, CD32, CD64), C3b (CR1), and iC3b (CR3). In some instances, microorganisms may be ingested without opsonization through lectin-carbohydrate (lectins on bacterial fimbriae interact with neutrophil glycoproteins), protein-protein (proteins such as filamentous hemagglutinin that express the arg-gly-asp or RGD amino acid sequence bind to integrins), and hydrophobic-protein (bacterial glycolipids and neutrophil integrins) interactions (Segal 2005; Ofek et al. 1995).

The interaction of IgG or complement receptors on the neutrophil surface with the opsonized particle triggers cytoskeletal rearrangements to enclose the opsonized particle within a phagosome. Phagocytosis is most efficient when organisms are coated with both IgG and C_3, which allows cooperative interaction of cognate receptors for both the opsonins. As mentioned above, neutrophils express integrin receptors for matrix proteins with the RGD tripeptide motif (such as fibronectin, laminin, and collagen), and ingest C_3-coated particles more efficiently when adherent to surfaces coated with these RGD-bearing proteins (Segal 2005; Carreno et al. 1993; Ruoslahti 1988).

Preterm neutrophils have impaired phagocytosis, which corrects only in the late third trimester to become comparable to adults (Bektas et al. 1990). Preterm neutrophils ingest particles more slowly and ingest fewer bacteria (such as *E. coli*). The lack of opsonic activity is an important consideration, as preterm infants often have lower concentration of specific antibodies (Etzioni et al. 1990). Compared to term neonates and adults, preterm neutrophils also have decreased expression of CD16 ($F_c\gamma$RIII) and CD32 ($F_c\gamma$RII), the two most abundant neutrophil IgG receptors (Payne and Fleit 1996). Whereas CD16 expression normally increases to adult levels over the first 3 weeks of life, CD32 deficiency may or may not correct with time (Payne et al. 1993).

Intracellular Killing

The phagolysosome provides an enclosed space in which an ingested microbe is exposed to high concentrations of toxic substances, while limiting the exposure of the phagocyte and other cells to these potentially injurious agents (Segal 2005). The major killing mechanism in neutrophils involves the generation of reactive oxygen species (ROS) in a "respiratory burst." An NADPH-dependent oxidase localized on the cell membrane (and therefore, the phagosome membrane) reduces molecular oxygen (O_2) to superoxide anion ($O\bullet_2^-$); (Quinn and Gauss 2004) subsequent generation of peroxide (H_2O_2) and the hydroxyl radical (OH•, formed in the presence of iron) also contributes to the microbicidal capacity of neutrophils (Clark 1999). These oxygen-dependent bactericidal mechanisms can be broadly divided into myeloperoxidase (MPO)-independent (such as hydrogen peroxide) and MPO-dependent (MPO catalyzes reactions between H_2O_2 and halides to form highly reactive products) (Klebanoff 2005). H_2O_2 is a weak bactericidal agent per se, but the MPO-H_2O_2-halide system increases its efficacy by nearly 50-fold. The bactericidal effects of free oxygen radicals are due to oxidizing effects on various components of the bacterial cell wall (Clark 1999).

Neutrophils also have elaborate nonoxidative killing mechanisms such as low pH (as low as 6.0), defensins, bactericidal/permeability-increasing protein (BPI), lactoferrin, lysozyme, and a variety of cationic proteins. Defensins are

broad-spectrum antimicrobial peptides with activity against gram-positive and gram-negative bacteria, fungi, and enveloped viruses and are also released in the gut by Paneth cells (Lehrer 2007). BPI binds lipopolysaccharide (LPS) and blocks its effects, can damage the outer membrane of gram-negative bacteria, and has some opsonic activity (Elsbach and Weiss 1998). Lactoferrin, an iron chelator, is bacteriostatic as it deprives bacteria of the iron required for growth. Lactoferrin is also involved in neutrophil degranulation, in oxygen radical production, and in granulocytopoiesis. Lysozyme hydrolyzes a glycoside bond in the bacterial cell wall peptidoglycan. Primary granules also contain other cationic antibacterial proteins such as azuricidin, indolicin, and cathelicidins (Segal 2005; Moraes et al. 2006).

The respiratory burst is depressed in preterm neutrophils, which explains the observed developmental defects in intracellular killing of bacterial pathogens such as *Staphylococcus aureus* or *Escherichia coli* (Gahr et al. 1985). The killing capacity cannot be fully explained on the basis of low opsonic activity in preterm plasma and improves only as a function of gestational age (Bektas et al. 1990; Drossou et al. 1997; Komatsu et al. 2001; Bjorkqvist et al. 2004). The neutrophil respiratory burst in infants born at 24–28 weeks is clearly less robust than in those born at 29–35 weeks and takes about 2 months to correct. However, neutrophils from preterm infants continue to have an overall weaker oxidative burst than adults and may not show any improvement in critically ill preterm infants (Strunk et al. 2004). Neonatal neutrophils are also less effective in killing group B streptococci, although the data on Candidacidal activity are conflicting. The antiviral activity of neonatal neutrophils is also diminished compared with that of adults. Indeed, the most commonly recovered bacteria in extremely low birth weight/extremely low gestational age neonates (ELBW/ELGAN) is a commensal organism called *Staphylococcal epidermidis*.

Degranulation

Neutrophils contain two major types of granules (Fig. 2): (1) the "azurophilic" granules (stain positive with the azure A dye) and (2) "specific" granules (do not stain with azure A). Azurophilic granules contain myeloperoxidase (MPO); proteolytic enzymes such as cathepsins, proteinase-3, and elastase; and antimicrobial proteins such as defensins and the bactericidal permeability-increasing protein (BPI). These granules release their contents into the phagolysosomes and are involved in intracellular killing. The specific

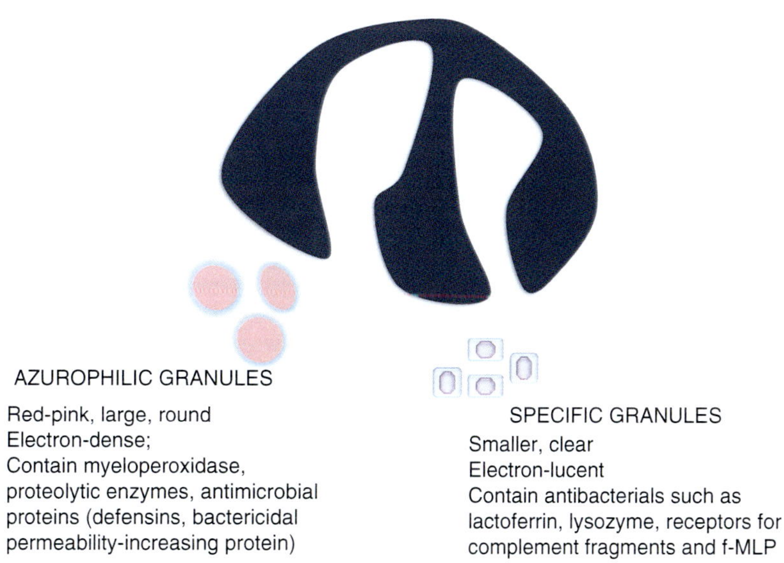

Fig. 2 Neutrophils contain two major types of granules: (1) the "azurophilic" granules (stain positive with the azure A dye) and (2) "specific" granules (do not stain with azure A)

granules contain antibacterial agents such as lactoferrin and lysozyme, receptors for complement components, and bacterial products such as f-MLP. Specific granules fuse with the cell membrane to release their contents by exocytosis and also bring functionally important membrane proteins such as integrins, cytochrome-b_{558}, and receptors for chemotactic agents and opsonins to the cell surface. Specific granules play an important role in extracellular killing (Borregaard and Cowland 1997).

Neutrophils from term neonates have granule contents and degranulation responses similar to adults (Ambruso et al. 1984). However, neutrophils from preterm infants have a lower capacity to release BPI, elastase, and lactoferrin than in adults and term infants (Bektas et al. 1990; Nupponen et al. 2002). Collectively, developmental deficiencies in neutrophil function accounts for a substantial component of neonatal susceptibility to invasive bacterial infections.

99.2.2 Monocytes and Macrophages

99.2.2.1 Development

Embryonic macrophages are first seen in the yolk sac at 3–4 weeks of gestation (Takashina 1987). Unlike macrophages in the fetus and the adult which are derived from circulating monocytes, these large-sized histiocytic cells develop in the early embryonic period from yolk sac progenitors prior to the first appearance of monocytes (Smythies et al. 2006a; Shepard and Zon 2000; Maheshwari et al. 2009). At 5 weeks of gestation, two distinct cell lineages with a dendritic/macrophage structure can be identified in the yolk sac, mesenchyme, and the fetal liver. The larger subgroup is MHC II-negative, and there is only a minor population that expresses these antigens. MHC II-negative cells also appear in the thymic cortex, in the marginal zones of lymph nodes, in the splenic red pulp, and in the bone marrow (Janossy et al. 1986). A few MHC II-positive cells are seen in the liver at 7–8 weeks of gestation, the lymph nodes at 11–13 weeks of gestation, and the T-cell areas of the developing thymic medulla by 16 weeks of gestation. Subsequently, the numbers increase gradually, and MHC class II-positive cells are also seen in the skin and gastrointestinal tract (Janossy et al. 1986; MacDonald et al. 1988).

During the second month of gestation, as hematopoiesis becomes established in the fetal liver, monocytes are seen in high proportions and constitute nearly 70% of all hematopoietic cells (Kelemen and Janossa 1980). Over the next 6 weeks, as the erythroid cells predominate, this proportion falls to 1–2% (Kelemen and Janossa 1980). The first monocytes in circulation are not seen until about the fifth month of gestation (Kelemen and Janossa 1980) and remain uncommon until the bone marrow becomes the predominant site of hematopoiesis (Porcellini et al. 1983). At 30 weeks, monocytes comprise 3–7% of hematopoietic cells (Linch et al. 1982). Term cord blood studies show a relative monocytosis, which persists during the neonatal period. The absolute monocyte counts tend to decline gradually from 1340–2200/μL in the first week to about 700 in the third week (Xanthou 1970; Weinberg et al. 1985). We are currently analyzing data from a large cohort of neonates with more than 100,000 blood counts to define the normal ranges of absolute monocyte counts.

Information on tissue macrophage kinetics in the neonatal period is mainly from autopsy studies. The size of the macrophage pool varies in different organ systems. In the gastrointestinal tract, macrophages appear in the *lamina propria* as early as 10 weeks of gestation and a sizable macrophage population can be seen during midgestation (Maheshwari et al. 2009). In contrast, the alveolar macrophage population remains small in the fetus and expands rapidly during the early neonatal period (Alenghat and Esterly 1984; Jacobs et al. 1985; Kurland et al. 1988). This increase may result both from an influx of monocytes from the circulation as well as from clonal expansion in situ.

Monocytes and macrophages can be identified using immunocytochemistry for the macrophage marker HAM56, cellular constituents such as nonspecific esterase and peroxidase, innate immune receptors such as CD11b, and the MHC complex

(Johnston 1988; Yoder et al. 1988; Santiago-Schwarz and Fleit 1988; Stiehm et al. 1984; Morris et al. 1975; Bhoopat et al. 1986; Bulmer et al. 1988; Glover et al. 1987). A lower proportion of cord blood macrophages stains for esterase, although there are no discernible differences in peroxidase activity (Yoder et al. 1988; Santiago-Schwarz and Fleit 1988; Morris et al. 1975; Stiehm et al. 1983). Neonatal monocytes have lower expression levels of the aforementioned surface markers, except for CD14 (Bhoopat et al. 1986). In certain tissues, such as in the gastrointestinal tract, resident macrophages are characteristically downregulated for the expression of innate immune receptors such as CD14 (Smith et al. 2001).

99.2.2.2 Monocyte Subsets

Increasing evidence indicates that peripheral blood monocytes are a heterogeneous population comprised of at least two subpopulations: (1) "classical" $CD14^{+}$ $CD16^{-}$ monocytes, which express CCR2, CD64, CD62L, and represent nearly 80–90% of all blood monocytes and (2) "nonclassical" $CD14^{low}$ $CD16^{+}$ monocytes that lack CCR2 (Geissmann et al. 2003). $CD14^{+}$ monocytes express the Fc γ receptors CD64 and CD32, have phagocytic activity, and produce TNF and IL-1β in response to LPS. In contrast, the nonclassical $CD14^{low}CD16^{+}$ monocytes are poorly phagocytic and do not produce TNF or IL-1β (Grage-Griebenow et al. 2001). These monocytes patrol the blood vessels in the steady state to remove senescent endothelial cells and extravasate during tissue healing (Geissmann et al. 2003).

99.2.2.3 Function

Transendothelial Migration, Chemotaxis, Phagocytosis, and Respiratory Burst

Unlike neutrophils, the major host defense functions of monocytes in cord blood of term infants are largely intact. Cord blood monocytes show adherence, random migration, chemotaxis, bactericidal activity, phagocytosis-associated chemiluminescence, production of superoxide anion (O-2), and generation of hydrogen peroxide at levels comparable to those of cells from healthy adult volunteers (Speer et al. 1985, 1986; Weston et al. 1977). The ability of fetal and neonatal monocytes to kill a variety of pathogens including *S. aureus*, *S. epidermidis*, *E. coli*, and *C. albicans* appears to be equivalent to that of adults (Speer et al. 1985; D'Ambola et al. 1988).

Cytokine production: Resident macrophages are often the first phagocytic cells of the innate immune system to encounter invading pathogens breaching the various epithelial surfaces of the skin, gut, and lung. These cells serve important host defense functions through phagocytosis and also as sentinel cells that regulate local inflammatory responses by producing various cytokines and chemokines (Denning et al. 2007; Smythies et al. 2005). Most studies on monocyte/macrophage cell function have been done on cord blood, and fetal cells have not been studied to the same extent so far. Term cord-blood monocytes produce IL-1, IFN-α, and TNF in concentrations that are comparable to adults, but the levels of IFN-γ, IL-8, IL-10, and GM-CSF are lower. These cells also produce lower concentrations of extracellular proteins like fibronectin and bioreactive lipids like leukotriene B_4 (Bryson et al. 1980; Weatherstone and Rich 1989; Wilson 1986; Bessler et al. 1987). Impaired monocyte secretory functions in neonates may be partially responsible for poorer cytokine responses of neonatal T cells (Kesson and Bryson 1991).

Emerging evidence indicates that macrophages are dynamic and heterogeneous cells, which are polarized into the classically activated M1 macrophages that express various inflammatory signals and the more-recently described M2 macrophages that function with an anti-inflammatory profile (Benoit et al. 2008). Although the effect of development on macrophage polarization is not known, the relative inability of cord blood monocytes (vs. monocytes from adults) to mount a robust inflammatory cytokine response is intriguing (Schibler et al. 1992, 1993).

99.3 Adaptive Immune System

99.3.1 Dendritic Cells

99.3.1.1 Development

Dendritic cells (DCs) are a discrete leukocyte population with a highly developed antigen-presenting function. DC populations have been grown from separated hematopoietic precursors, suggesting that there is a common granulocyte-monocyte-dendritic cell progenitor (Jaffe 1993). Cells with a dendritic/macrophage structure are present in the yolk sac, mesenchyme, and the liver at 4–6 weeks of age. DCs are detectable in skin by 6–7 weeks of gestation (Foster et al. 1986).

DCs initially derived their name from their distinctive morphology, with numerous fine dendritic cytoplasmic processes commonly found penetrating epithelial bound organ surfaces. However, phenotype alone is not sufficient to define these cells in view of functional differences between the subpopulations. A working definition requires DCs to be able to stimulate T-cells, home to T-cell dependent lymph node areas, be able to pinocytose, and have characteristic cell surface antigens.

Human peripheral blood DCs include mainly two subgroups (Grouard et al. 1997; O'Doherty et al. 1994): (1) myeloid DCs (or mDCs) are $CD11c^{+}$ cells that express myeloid markers such as CD13, CD33, and CD11b; and (2) plasmacytoid DCs (or pDCs) are $CD11c^{-}$ and have a plasmacytoid morphology with well-developed rough endoplasmic reticulum and Golgi apparatus.

99.3.1.2 Function

Cord blood DCs represent about 0.3% of all mononuclear cells. Most studies show an increased number and proportion of pDCs in cord blood compared to adult peripheral blood, with pDC:mDC ratios of 1–3:1 that contrast with the usual 1:2 ratio in adults (Velilla et al. 2006).

Due to the low frequency of DCs in peripheral blood, most studies of neonatal DCs have been carried out using in vitro monocyte-derived dendritic cells (MDDCs). Compared to pDCs from adults, cord blood DCs exhibit low or no basal expression of co-stimulatory molecules CD40, CD80, or CD86, show an impaired maturational response following stimulation with agonists for various toll-like receptors (measured as increase in the expression of co-stimulatory molecules and production of IFN-alpha, TNF-alpha, IL-1, IL-6, and IL-12), and perform poorly at accessory function (Petty and Hunt 1998; Bondada et al. 2000). Cord blood dendritic cells have lower expression levels of ICAM-1 and MHC antigens than in adults. These cells are also poor stimulators of mixed lymphocyte reactions, regardless of whether cord or adult mononuclear or T cells were used as the responders (Petty and Hunt 1998). How precisely these cells contribute to the susceptibility of neonates to maturation of adaptive immunity, prevention of invasive illness and barrier dysfunction is an area in need of further exploration.

99.3.2 T-Lymphocytes

99.3.2.1 Development

The thymus arises at about 6 weeks of gestation from the third branchial arch, with the cortex arising from its ectodermal layer and the medulla from the endoderm. Lymphoid cells migrate over the next 2–3 weeks, initially from the yolk sac and fetal liver, and then from the bone marrow to colonize the fetal thymus (Stites and Pavia 1979; Strominger 1989; Cahill et al. 1999; Wilson et al. 1991, 1992; Siegel and Gleicher 1981; Wilson 1991). These prothymocytes interact with the stroma, proliferate actively, and are triggered to differentiate with expression of the first T cell-specific surface molecules (e.g., CD2, and later CD4 and CD8) (Wilson et al. 1991; Haynes et al. 1988; Anderson et al. 1996). A clear delineation of the thymic cortical and medullary regions occurs at 12 weeks of gestation; Hassall's corpuscles appear shortly thereafter (Haynes 1984; Bodey and Kaiser 1997). The most immature thymocytes are found in the subcapsular cortical

region, and cells move into the deeper layers as they mature (Haynes 1984).

The early prothymocytes do not express CD3, the T-cell receptor (TCR), CD4, or CD8 and are often referred to as "triple-negative thymocytes" (Mathieson and Fowlkes 1984). The progeny continues to divide and rearrange their TCR genes, and since these cells express both CD4 and CD8, they are now called "double-positive" (Haynes 1984; Mathieson and Fowlkes 1984). They undergo *positive selection* by self-major histocompatability complex (MHC) restriction, and more than 95% (about 50 million) cells die each day during this stage (Mathieson and Fowlkes 1984). *Negative selection* occurs next and is mediated by the bone marrow-derived antigen-presenting cells (APC) (e.g., dendritic cells and macrophages), which eliminate autoreactive cells either by *clonal deletion* or *clonal anergy* (Chidgey and Boyd 2001; Viret et al. 1999). As these thymocytes mature and reach the medulla, they express only one of the CD4 or CD8 antigens. These single-positive T cells migrate from the thymus to the peripheral lymphoid organs at about 14 weeks of gestation (Haynes 1984). By 15 weeks, human thymocytes express a complete set of TCRs (Haynes 1984; George and Schroeder 1992).

During fetal life, thymus is the largest lymphoid tissue in terms of body proportions. It is about two thirds its mature weight at birth and reaches its peak mass at around 10 years of age. Subsequently, it continues to involute and is replaced by adipose tissue (Cooper and Buckley 1982).

99.3.2.2 T-Cell Receptor (TCR) Repertoire

The TCR is composed of two distinct functional subunits, each specialized for a different function (Teyton et al. 2000). The first, highly polymorphic, is structured unique for each T cell for antigen recognition; it is composed of two polypeptide chains, α and β (except in a specific T-cell subset where it consists of γ and δ chains) (Teyton et al. 2000; Garcia et al. 1999). The second, also known as CD3, is a trimolecular complex, involved in signal transduction and cellular activation. The extracellular region of the TCR resembles an immunoglobulin (Ig) Fab fragment and derives its structural diversity from recombinatorial permutations involving a set each of variable (V), diversity (D), and joining (J) gene segments (Hazenberg et al. 2001; Oltz 2001). The variable domain is situated in the N-terminal end of the α/β (or γ/δ) chains, whereas the C terminal is the constant region (Teyton et al. 2000). The variable domains consist of V, D, and J elements in the β chain, and V and J in the α chain (Davis and Bjorkman 1988). The antigen-binding sites are formed by three "complementarity-determining regions" (CDRs). CDR3, the most extensive of these segments, serves as a key site for antigen recognition (Schelonka et al. 1998).

By mid-gestation, all the TCR Vβ families (V here refers to the variable domain of the β chain, and should be recognized as different from the V gene segments mentioned above) are expressed, but they have shorter CDR3 regions. This is primarily due to limited expression of the enzyme terminal deoxynucleotidyl transferase (Tdt), which induces N-terminal diversity and, consequently, CDR3 heterogeneity (Bonati et al. 1992). In term infants, the T-cell Vβ repertoire is similar to that seen in adults (Schelonka et al. 1998; Garderet et al. 1998). Cord blood T cells from term infants are also able to expand the TCR β repertoire on stimulation with bacterial toxins (Garderet et al. 1998). It is the central position of T-cell function in the maturing immune system that places the capacity to adapt to a changing environment central to successful maturation of immune defenses. This is primarily a time and antigen experience-dependent process influenced by the maternal inoculation with flora during a normal birth as well as the subsequent clinical and home environments as influenced by clinicians and their use of antibiotics or other teleologically relevant experiences.

99.3.2.3 Circulating T Cells

T-cell subpopulations gradually increase in number beyond 19 weeks' gestation and continue to rise after birth to peak at about 6–9 months. The numbers decline subsequently, and adult levels are finally reached at 6–7 years of age (Erkeller-

Yuksel et al. 1992; Panaro et al. 1991). In term neonates, CD4+ cells constitute a higher proportion of T cells than adults. CD8+ cells, on the other hand, are fewer both in terms of their absolute number and as a percentage of total T cells. The CD4/CD8 ratio, consequently, is as high as 4.9:1 during the perinatal period and declines to adult values of approximately 2:1 only by 4 years of age (Erkeller-Yuksel et al. 1992; Panaro et al. 1991). Preterms have significantly higher numbers of CD4+ T cells, but the number of CD8+ T cells does not seem to change with gestational age (Thilaganathan et al. 1992; Series et al. 1991). These numbers decrease with perinatal distress but normalize by 3 weeks of age except in some very-low-birth-weight infants (Series et al. 1991).

Peripheral T cells in the fetus and neonate may be in a relatively immature transitional state; in cord blood, nearly 85% T cells express CD38 (compared with less than 5% of adult cells) but lack other markers of activation (Wilson et al. 1985). Cord blood T cells differ also in being predominantly naïve (80–90% express the CD45RA phenotype, compared with only 40–60% of the adult cells) (Pirenne et al. 1992; Hassan and Reen 1993). The percentage of memory T cells (CD45RO) increases in healthy infants during the first few years of life but reaches adult levels only by the second decade (Pirenne et al. 1992). Neonatal T cells also have lower expression of CDw29 and CD11b, providing further evidence to a lack of previous stimulation (Pirenne et al. 1992; Hoshino et al. 1993). The ratios and relationships of T-cell subtypes and the clinical relevance to invasive disease is an area of perinatal immunology that is in need of further clarification.

99.3.2.4 Function

Proliferation Cord blood T cells from premature infants have a limited capacity for mitogen-induced proliferation but these defects are corrected by full-term (Pirenne et al. 1992; Leino et al. 1981; Clerici et al. 1993). Similarly, proliferative responses to monoclonal antibodies against T-cell markers (e.g., CD3, CD2) are dramatically less than adult lymphocytes and resemble adult naïve T cells (Splawski et al. 1991; Gerli et al. 1989). These responses improve as the numbers of peripheral blood memory T cells increase. When tested with allogeneic cells (mixed lymphocyte reaction), however, cord blood lymphocytes respond better, though still somewhat less than cells from adult subjects (Pirenne et al. 1992; Clerici et al. 1993; Roncarolo et al. 1994; Reen 1998; Risdon et al. 1994).

Cytokine Production Neonatal concentrations of pro-inflammatory cytokines like IL-1, IL-6, TNF-α, IFN-α, and IFN-β are comparable to adults and also increase similarly during sepsis (Liechty et al. 1991, 2000; Muller et al. 1996; Sautois et al. 1997; Yachie et al. 1990). Premature infants, however, are known to produce lower amounts of TNF-α and IFN-α as compared to those born at term (de Bont et al. 1993; Seghaye et al. 1998; Chheda et al. 1996). Among the cytokines involved in adaptive immunity, only IL-2 concentrations are comparable; others like IL-4, IL-5, IL-10, IL-15, and IFN-γ are known to be significantly lower than adults (Seghaye et al. 1998; Chheda et al. 1996; Qian et al. 1997; Elsasser-Beile et al. 1995; Kibler et al. 1986; Lilic et al. 1997). Transforming growth factor (TGF)-β_1 and macrophage inflammatory protein-1alpha (MIP)-1α, both of which play a negative role in hematopoiesis, are also present in much lower concentrations (Chang et al. 1994).

The concentrations of hematopoietic colony stimulating factors including IL-3, granulocyte macrophage-colony stimulating factor (GM-CSF), granulocyte-CSF, and monocyte-CSF are slightly lower to comparable to adults, but even full-term infants are known to be unable to mount adequate responses during stress (Pirenne-Ansart et al. 1995; Cairo et al. 1991). Chemokines, which have emerged as important regulators of leukocyte trafficking, are currently an important area of study. The concentrations of some of these are known to be comparable to adults, including IL-8/CXCL8, epithelial neutrophil attractant (ENA)-78/CXCL5, growth-related oncoprotein (GRO)-α/CXCL1, eotaxin/CCL11, and RANTES (regulated upon activation, normal T cell expressed and secreted)/CCL5 (Sullivan et al. 2002).

Most of these deficiencies are caused by altered regulation of posttranscriptional mRNA processing (Chang et al. 1994). It is believed that lower concentrations of some of these cytokines are caused by a relative paucity of memory or primed T cells. However, genetic and other individual traits such as atopy are also likely to be important determinants of the cytokine response (Piccinni et al. 1996; Hagendorens et al. 2000; Williams et al. 2000).

During development, naïve T cells differentiate into distinct effector T-helper (Th) subsets, a process in which cytokines play a critical role. These differentiated T cells were originally categorically designated Th1 and Th2 cells based on distinct functional properties and the cytokines that drive their development (Mosmann et al. 1986). Th1 type cytokines, such as IFN-γ and IL-2, play a key role in initiating early resistance to pathogens and induction of cell-mediated immunity. Th2 cytokines drive the system toward immune tolerance rather than toward defense from microbial infections. Accumulating evidence suggests that Th1 responses in newborns are compromised at several steps including deficient production of Th1 type cytokines by neonatal CD4+ T cells and hyporesponsiveness of neonatal macrophages to stimulation by IFN-γ. These deficiencies contribute to the apparently weak cellular immunity in newborns biased toward a Th2 type response (Adkins 2003).

Since the original Th1 and Th2 description, a differentiated T-cell population, Th17 cells, has been shown to have a pathogenic role in allergic, autoimmune, and other chronic inflammatory diseases (Weaver et al. 2006; Ivanov et al. 2007). Th17 cells have also been shown to play a protective role in immunity to infection, where they take on Th1-like effector functions to promote pathogen clearance by enhancing neutrophil recruitment to sites of infection and activating macrophages (Weaver et al. 2006; Ivanov et al. 2007; Wilson et al. 2007). While the role of Th17 cells early in life remains unclear, cord blood mononuclear cells have a limited capacity to produce IL-17 (Schaub et al. 2008). In very premature infants with a history of serious bloodstream infections (BSI), we found lower serum IL-17 levels than their counterparts who never developed BSI.

The fetus occupies a unique immunologic position where the Th2 phenotype predominates in utero and transitions to a more Th1 functionality following birth. It is generally considered to be core process of evolutionary significance where both mother and fetus maintain a high level of immunologic suppression to enable continuation of pregnancy.

Antigen-Specific Responses The response of T cells to specific antigens can also be assessed in terms of proliferation or cytokine production. These responses usually require previous exposure to the corresponding antigen and are generally not detected at birth or from cord blood unless there was an intrauterine exposure. Neonatal T cells do, however, respond well to certain antigens such as tetanus/diphtheria toxoids, influenza, and mycobacterial antigens (Clerici et al. 1993). In response to superantigens, cord blood T cells produce lesser amounts of IL-2 (Takahashi et al. 1995). However, after stimulation, the percentage of Vβ_2+ T cells (which determine potential reactivity to superantigens) and the number of memory T cells increase significantly just like adults (Takahashi et al. 1995; Toubert et al. 1998). But unlike adult T cells, cord blood T cells are unable to respond if restimulated with the superantigen. This tolerance induction in cord blood T cells may again be due to the underlying immunologic naïvete (Takahashi et al. 1995; Macardle et al. 1999).

99.3.2.5 Other Subgroups

Cytotoxic T-Lymphocytes (CTLs) CTLs are important in host defense against intracellular infections, in allograft rejection, and tumor cell surveillance (Gromo et al. 1987; Liu et al. 1996). CTLs utilize two well-established mechanisms for cell lysis, one involving release of extracellular mediators (such as the pore-forming perforin/granzyme system), and a second fas/fas ligand dependent pathway that leads to target cell apoptosis (Kagi et al. 1996; Smyth et al. 2001).

CTL cytotoxicity is evident by 18 weeks of gestation but is far less efficient than adult cells even at term (<20% of adult CTL activity) (Toivanen et al. 1981). Perforin expression in

neonatal CTLs is about 30% of adult levels. CD28, which is a T-cell activation marker, is also expressed to significantly lower levels (Risdon et al. 1994). Similar results are also observed in other assays; neonatal cells showed only 33% of lectin/mitogen-dependent cytotoxicity of adult cells (Lubens et al. 1982). Circulating inhibitors such as α-fetoprotein and prostaglandins may also lead to lower CTL activity in neonates (Lubens et al. 1982).

γδT Cells The γδ T cells represent a distinct functional subset, with a majority lacking surface expression of both CD4 and CD8 (Kang and Raulet 1997; Steele et al. 2000; McVay and Carding 1999). These cells are detectable in the fetal thymus and liver at 6–8 weeks of gestation and comprise nearly 10% of the peripheral blood T cells at 16 weeks (McVay and Carding 1996; Holtmeier et al. 2001). Subsequently, the numbers decline gradually to reach about 3% at term (Peakman et al. 1992).

These cells are present mainly on skin and mucosal surfaces (McVay and Carding 1999). Although the exact functions of these T cells are not well understood, they can lyse target cells with the perforin/granzyme system like the cytotoxic T cells and can secrete cytokines like interferon (IFN)-γ and tumor necrosis factor (TNF)-α upon activation. The cytotoxicity of neonatal γδ T cells is significantly less than adults (Morita et al. 1994).

Fetal γδ T cells have a more diverse repertoire but a more limited junctional diversity than adults. This diversity is retained throughout the first year of life, and then decreases gradually over the first decade of life (Morita et al. 1994). Overall, however, γδ T cells have a relatively restricted repertoire in comparison to the αβ T- or B cells (Sloan-Lancaster and Allen 1996).

T-Regulatory Cells T-regulatory cells (Tregs) downregulate T-cell responses to both foreign and self antigens, thereby playing an important role in balancing Th1/Th2 effector lineages (Groux et al. 1997; Barrat et al. 2002). Treg cells, including both natural $CD4^{+}$ $CD25^{+}$ Tregs and the IL-10-producing Tregs, express the forkhead/winged-helix family transcriptional repressor-p3 (Foxp3) (Darrasse-Jeze et al. 2005), a commonly used but not entirely specific marker for Tregs (Hori et al. 2003). Although Tregs have been detected in cord blood, current knowledge about Treg function early in life is limited and thus their relevance to immune defense of the newborn is uncertain.

99.3.3 B-Lymphocytes

99.3.3.1 Development

B-cell progenitors, pro-B cells, are derived from pluripotent hematopoietic cells in the bone marrow (Klein 1983). The first recognizable B-cell progenitor, the large pre-B cell, is characterized by the presence of cytoplasmic μ heavy chains (Klein 1983). Immature B cells undergo a selection process analogous to T cells to eliminate self-identifying clones (*clonal selection, clonal deletion*), although there may also be other mechanisms to maintain self-tolerance (Nossal 1986; Buhl et al. 2000). Once B cells begin to express surface IgM (sIgM), they are ready to leave the bone marrow to enter the peripheral circulation (Rudin and Thompson 1998).

Pre-B cells can be identified in the fetal liver as early as 7 weeks of gestation, and in the marrow by 12 weeks. sIgM+ B cells are found in the fetal liver by 9 weeks and in the bone marrow, peripheral blood, and spleen by 12 weeks. B cells with sIgA, sIgG, and sIgD isotypes appear between 10 and 12 weeks (Gathings et al. 1977). There is also increased traffic to the lymphoid tissues, and by 22 weeks, the proportion of B cells in the spleen, peripheral blood, and bone marrow is similar to that in adults (Gathings et al. 1977; Bofill et al. 1985). By 30 weeks, there are no detectable pre-B cells in the fetal liver, and bone marrow becomes the exclusive site for B-cell maturation. Plasma cells are not generally found until 20 weeks' gestation. IgM/IgD+ B cells populate the lymph nodes by 16–17 weeks' gestation and the spleen by 16–21 weeks. In fetal lymph nodes, primary nodules develop around the follicular dendritic cells by 17 weeks' gestation (Bofill et al. 1985; Holt and Jones 2000). Considering the extreme degree of premature birth and survival in this era even

below 24 weeks, it is perhaps no surprise that effective production of antibody for opsonization and enhanced cytotoxicity is limited.

99.3.3.2 Immunoglobulin Repertoire

Receptor diversity in the antigen binding site originates from DNA recombination involving various V, D, or J gene segments giving rise to a large number of V(D)J permutations (Oltz 2001). Additional receptor diversity is generated by imprecise gene segment joins, additional nucleotides added to the splice junction of the VDJ joins by the enzyme terminal deoxynucleotidyl transferase (TdT), and somatic mutations (for B cells only, not T cells). Thereafter, these VDJ or VJ (light chains) units join to their respective constant region gene segments (Kelsoe 1999; Neuberger et al. 2005).

In the fetus and neonate, the Ig repertoire is relatively restricted. During early and mid-gestation, certain heavy chain V gene segments are preferentially expressed (Foster et al. 1986). Early in fetal life, the most J_H proximal V_H gene segments are utilized preferentially, and consequently, the CDR3 region of the rearranged VDJ gene segment is shorter than that in adults. This leads to relatively limited junctional diversity, but this altered architecture of the antigen-binding site may also allow greater polyspecificity of antigen binding (at a cost of lower antibody affinity) (Casali and Schettino 1996; Schroeder et al. 1987). The utilization of V_H gene families spreads out more evenly with increasing gestation. However, even at term, cord blood B cells have a higher usage of V_H genes of the V_H 1 and V_H 5 family with decreased V_H 3 use compared with adult B cells (Choi et al. 1995). In general, the antibody response in neonates is of low affinity and restricted to the IgM isotype. The somatic mutation of the heavy and light Ig variable region genes and the selection of higher affinity antibody-producing B cells is limited at birth but increases very slowly after 10 days of age (Ridings et al. 1997). It is significant that the maturation of antigen presenting cells and functional limitations of B cells reduces the capacity of effective defense mechanisms during the period of novel exposure to nutrient derived antigens and gut flora yet eventually acquires the ability to accurately discern self from diet.

99.3.3.3 Circulating B Cells

At birth, the proportion of B cells is similar to that of adults, but the absolute number of B cells is significantly higher (Paloczi 1999). The number peaks at about 3–4 months of age, and then declines to adult levels by 6–7 years of age (Ugazio et al. 1974). Preterm infants have comparable B cell numbers to the term infants (Thomas and Linch 1983). However, the number is smaller in growth-retarded infants (Strominger 1989). Unlike adults, most of B cells in cord blood express activation markers (CD25, CD23, transferrin receptor) (Durandy et al. 1990).

99.3.3.4 Function

Immunoglobulin Production The fetus and the neonate are capable, although at a lower intensity than adults, of mounting antigen-specific antibody responses. The presence of allergen-specific IgEs in cord blood, anti-tetanus IgM in cord sera of newborns whose mothers were vaccinated during pregnancy, and reactivity to *Ascaris* antigens in the event of maternal infestation are some examples (Johnson et al. 1996; King et al. 1998; Weil et al. 1983; Gill et al. 1983; Sanjeevi et al. 1991)

However, this response remains immature (Holt and Jones 2000). They may be unable to respond to all the antigens in a vaccine and often have delayed isotype switch (D'Angio et al. 1995). It appears that the *interval* from birth is a more important determinant of antibody response than the gestational age. Both preterm and term infants immunized with diphtheria toxoid at 0–10 days of age had poorer responses than similarly immunized adults, but the response was better when vaccination was deferred until 1–2 months of age (D'Angio et al. 1995). With certain antigens like hepatitis B, however, premature infants may show a relatively poorer early response than their term counterparts, although these deficiencies correct during later infancy (Golebiowska et al. 1999). Collectively, these observations suggest

that many of the maturational signals needed to achieve a full capacity of host defenses arise from evolutionary appropriate cues received from the neonatal environment forcing the irrevocable expansion of a wide diversity of immune capacities. Thus, the newborn is effectively, not solely limited by its ontological immaturity of cellular and humoral capacities.

Serum Immunoglobulin Levels Serum Ig levels remain very low until 18–20 weeks' gestation. Most of the newborn's serum immunoglobulins are derived from active transplacental transfer of maternal IgG (particularly IgG1 and IgG3) during the third trimester (McNabb et al. 1976; Kohler and Farr 1966; Palfi et al. 1998). In the full-term neonate, serum IgG levels are equal or even higher than maternal serum IgG levels, but in the preterm, who missed these maternal antibodies, the levels are lower (Kohler and Farr 1966). Hobbs and Davis found that nearly all infants born before 32 weeks' gestation had serum IgG levels less than 400 mg/dL at birth (compared with term infants who had serum levels around 1000 mg/dL) (Hobbs and Davis 1967). The levels fall after birth (through normal catabolism) to a nadir of 300–500 mg/dL between 3 and 5 months of age, when the infant starts producing increasing amounts of his/her own. Because of starting at a lower level, this nadir may be much lower, and earlier, in preterm infants (Ballow et al. 1986). Cord blood Ig levels also tend to be lower in growth retarded neonates (Yeung and Hobbs 1968).

The serum levels of IgA, IgM, and IgE are very low even in term infants, since these do not cross the placenta. However, when faced with an intrauterine infection, the fetus is definitely capable of producing appreciable amounts of IgM (Deorari et al. 2000). For many years, it was believed that augmenting the neonatal repertoire with exogenous pooled IgG could augment immune functions. Unfortunately, data proving efficacy of this approach for prevention or intervention for bacterial infections has not proven compelling; nevertheless, use of high titer Ig for mitigating perinatal transmission of hepatitis B is well established. Taken together, it is clear that an improved understanding of these IgG relationships may some day be exploited to enhance bacterial opsonization.

99.3.4 Other Subgroups

99.3.4.1 CD5 Expressing B Cells

B cells with surface expression of CD5, which is a T-cell antigen, may represent a functionally and ontogenically distinct subset. Some believe that CD5 positivity defines a so-called "B-1" subset of cells, distinct from the conventional adult "B2" population by virtue of their earlier appearance in ontogeny, capacity for bone marrow-independent self-renewal, and constitutively expressing signal transducer and activator of transcription-3 (STAT3) (Hardy and Hayakawa 1994; Karras et al. 1997). B-1 cells express the B-cell-lineage antigens CD19 and CD45R, although CD45R is present at lower levels on B-1 cells than on B-2 cells (Dorshkind and Montecino-Rodriguez 2007; Hardy 2006; Montecino-Rodriguez and Dorshkind 2006). B-1 cells in the peritoneal and pleural cavities can be identified by their unusual CD11b + $sIgM^{hi}$ $sIgD^{low}$ phenotype and can be further subdivided on the basis of differential expression of the cell-surface antigen CD5, into CD5+ CD11b + $sIgM^{hi}$ $sIgD^{low}$ B-1a cells and CD5- CD11b + $sIgM^{hi}$ $sIgD^{low}$ B-1b cells (Kantor and Herzenberg 1993).

These cells are the predominant B-cell type during fetal life and have a distinctive anatomic localization in the fetal spleen and the peritoneal cavity. They appear in the spleen at 15 weeks and are seen in the lymph node primary follicles at about 17 weeks of gestation (Bhat et al. 1992; Antin et al. 1986). In adults, CD5 expression can be found on about 25–35% of total B cells and 1–7% of all the peripheral blood mononuclear cells. In contrast, CD5+ B cells represent approximately 90% of the total cord blood B cells. This number decreases to 75–80% during infancy and reaches adult levels only by late adolescence (Bhat et al. 1992; Antin et al. 1986).

The exact function of B-1 cells in the fetus is still unclear. The functional characteristics of B-1

cells such as the unique localization, broad polyspecific specificities, and a restricted Ig repertoire have been considered to indicate a role of these cells in the innate, rather than in adaptive, immunity (Hardy and Hayakawa 1991). Unlike follicular B-2 cells that respond to protein antigens, and with T-cell help, undergo immunoglobulin heavy chain class-switching and affinity maturation, B-1 cells respond mainly to T-cell-independent immunogens that include carbohydrate antigens (Dorshkind and Montecino-Rodriguez 2007; Hardy 2006; Montecino-Rodriguez and Dorshkind 2006). Recent observations indicate that the two types of B-1 cell, B-1a and B-1b, show functional differences during the immune response. B-1a cells spontaneously secrete IgM, which provides a first line of defense against certain encapsulated bacteria, such as *Streptococcus pneumoniae*, whereas antibody production by B-1b cells is induced and has a role in the ultimate clearance of the pathogen and in providing long-term protection (Kantor and Herzenberg 1993; Alugupalli et al. 2004; Haas et al. 2005).

99.3.5 T- and B-Cell Interaction

T-cell signals are crucial for the proliferation, differentiation, and survival of B cells and include both antigen presentation and humoral signals (cytokines like IL-2, IL-4, IL-5, IL-6, IL-10, IL-13, and IFN-γ) (Bishop and Hostager 2001). Several pairs of other receptor-ligand molecules are also involved, including the CD40-CD40 ligand (CD40L) in B-cell immunoglobulin isotype switching, and others like B7/CD28, CD11a (LFA-1)/CD54 (ICAM-1), and CD58 (LFA-3)/CD2 in T- and B-cell activation (Bishop and Hostager 2001). Only about 30% of naïve neonatal T cells express CD40L, compared to 80% of the naïve T cells from adults (Nonoyama et al. 1998). However, once primed with mitogen (s) and IL-2, which converts naïve T-cells to the memory phenotype, neonatal T-cell CD40L expression is upregulated to adult levels (Merrill et al. 1996). The capacity of neonatal B cells to differentiate into plasma cells and undergo isotype switching can be variable (vide infra), but, in general, neonatal T cells are less efficient at providing humoral and CD40-dependent activation signals (Gerli et al. 1993; Splawski et al. 1996; Lucivero et al. 1983; Andersson 1985).

99.3.6 Natural Killer Cells

99.3.6.1 Development

NK cells share some T-cell markers but are not affected in many natural/experimental disruptions of the T-cell system (Spits et al. 1995; Puel et al. 1998; Volpe 1996). It is conceivable that the two lineages are derived from a common progenitor (Phillips et al. 1992; Sato et al. 1999). Morphologically, NK cells are large granular lymphocytes and have characteristic surface markers including the CD56/neural cell adhesion molecule and CD16/Fcγ receptor IIIa (FcγRIIIa), a low affinity IgG receptor. They also express CD2, LFA-1, and cytokine receptors such as IL-2$R_{\beta\gamma c}$, IL-12R, IFN-γR, and IL-15R_{α} (Spits et al. 1998).

NK cells can be detected as early as 6 weeks of gestation, and the number then increases progressively until birth. In cord blood, 10–15% of all lymphocytes are NK cells, which is comparable to adult peripheral blood (Phillips et al. 1992). The phenotype of fetal NK cells, however, is different from that of adult cells. Fifty to 80% of fetal NK cells express CD3γ, ε, λ, and σ proteins, unlike a much smaller number in term infants, or in adults where only CD3σ is expressed (Phillips et al. 1992; Gerli et al. 1989). On the other hand, only 30–50% of the fetal NK cells express CD16 (compared with more than 90% of neonatal and adult NK cells). Similarly, CD56 and CD57 are expressed poorly on fetal or neonatal NK cells, compared to nearly 50% positivity in adult NK cells (Phillips et al. 1992; Gaddy et al. 1995).

99.3.6.2 Function

NK cells recognize viral-infected and tumor cells by the absence or decreased expression of MHC class I molecules on the cell surface (Herberman et al. 1979; Trinchieri 1989; Leibson 1997). Their MHC-unrestricted killing is mediated by perforin/granzyme apoptotic pathways (Ortaldo et al. 1992). The other mechanism of cytolysis is

antibody-dependent cell-mediated cytotoxicity (ADCC), where target cell-bound IgG1 or IgG3 triggers the FcγRIIIa receptor on the NK cell (Leibson 1997; Trinchieri and Valiante 1993). NK cells are also believed to play a key role in maintaining immunological tolerance at the maternal-fetal interface (Gaunt and Ramin 2001).

Fetal NK cells have a significantly lower cytolytic activity (including ADCC) against tumor cell target cell lines than adults, but it increases with gestational age parallel to increasing expression of CD56 and CD16 (Merrill et al. 1996; Phillips et al. 1992). However, even at term, the cytolytic activity is only 50–80% of adult levels (Sato et al. 1999).

NK cells should not be confused with the natural killer T cells, a heterogeneous group of T cells which express an alpha beta T-cell receptor besides some of the NK cell markers. Many of these cells recognize the nonpolymorphic CD1d molecule, an antigen-presenting molecule that binds self- and foreign lipids and glycolipids. NK T cells constitute only 0.2% of all peripheral blood T cells. These cells play an important role in mucosal immunity and in the pathogenesis of inflammatory/allergic conditions; the role during fetal life remains unclear (Middendorp and Nieuwenhuis 2009). Imbalances in this system produced by chronic inflammation may be involved in the presentation of the acquired forms of hemophagocytic lymphohistiocytosis in the neonatal period.

99.3.7 Noncytotoxic Innate Immune Cells

99.3.7.1 Development

The noncytotoxic ILCs are characterized by a classic lymphoid cell morphology, but, unlike the adaptive T and B cells, do not show antigen specificity and function as a part of the innate immune system (Artis and Spits 2015). The ILCs are derived from the common lymphoid progenitor (Klose et al. 2014) and are classified into the group 1 ILCs (ILC1), group 2 ILCs (ILC2), and the group 3 ILCs (ILC3); these subsets are defined on the basis of differential requirements for transcription factors during development, cytokine expression, and other distinct effector functions (Edwards 1995). The three ILC subsets exhibit remarkable functional similarity in cytokine expression and function with the T-helper cells of the Th1, Th2, and Th17 subsets, respectively (Artis and Spits 2015). ILC1s express the T-bet transcription factor and produce Th1-associated cytokines such as interferon-γ and TNF to protect against intracellular bacteria and parasites. ILC2s express the GATA-binding protein 3 transcription factor and produce Th2-associated cytokines (including IL-4, IL-5, IL-9, and IL-13) and/or the epidermal growth factor receptor ligand amphiregulin. These cells are active during tissue repair, allergic disorders, and antihelminth immunity. ILC3s express the RAR-related orphan receptor-γT transcription factor and produce IL-17A, IL-17F, IL-22, GM-CSF, and TNF to promote antibacterial immunity, chronic inflammation, or tissue repair.

99.3.7.2 Function

There is limited information on ILCs in the fetus and neonate. ILC2 cells are detectable in cord blood and may be present in higher proportions in male than in female neonates (Forsberg et al. 2014). In a murine model of gastroschisis, organs exposed to amniotic fluid were shown to contain high numbers of ILC2 and ILC3, and eosinophilia, which was reversed by the administration of anti-IL5 antibody (Frascoli et al. 2016). In another study, ILC3s were implicated as a source of increased IL-17 levels seen in patients with preeclampsia, and gestational/chronic diabetes were associated with ILC3s (Barnie et al. 2015).

99.3.8 The Mucosal Immune System

99.3.8.1 Peyer's Patches and Other Organized Lymphoid Tissue

Peyer's patch anlagen become identifiable in fetal ileum at 11 weeks as aggregates of HLA-DR^+, $CD4^+$ lymphoid cells (Finke et al. 2002; Spencer et al. 1985). At birth, the organized lymphoid compartment is naïve but structurally complete, and the predominant activity involves

proliferative expansion (rather than primary lymphopoiesis) (MacDonald and Spencer 1994; Husband and Gleeson 1996). The number of PP increases from about 60 at birth to over 200 by 12–14 years (Cornes 1965).

In the vermiform appendix, the development of lymphoid structures lags behind the Peyer's patches (Bhide et al. 2001). Appendiceal lymphoid follicles enlarge rapidly after birth following bacterial colonization and translocation (Gebbers and Laissue 2004). The first IgA^+ plasma cells appear at 2 weeks after birth and then increase to adult levels at 4–5 months. To what extent full and appropriate capacity of this system contributes to the susceptibility of the preterm neonate to the development of necrotizing enterocolitis remains to be ascertained.

99.3.8.2 Lymphocytes in the *Lamina Propria* and Intraepithelial Compartments

Scattered B cells are first observed in the lamina propria at 14-weeks gestation (Spencer et al. 1985). The fetal intestinal B-cell population consists of two distinct cell types. The first population of large, dividing, mature B cells shares morphologic and phenotypic ($CD20^+IgM^+IgD^+$light chain$^+$) features with the thymic B cells. These are large-sized cells with extensive cytoplasmic processes, which are in contact with adjacent T cells. A second population of smaller pre-B cells (IgM^+ light chain$^-CD20^-$) has also been identified, suggesting the presence of local B-cell development (Golby et al. 2002). As extrathymic T-cell development occurs in human fetal intestine (vide infra), it has been hypothesized that as in the thymus, the B cells may play a role in the development and selection of the T cells.

The B-cell population in the fetal intestine comprises IgM^+ and IgG^+ cells (Rognum et al. 1992). The fetal intestinal B-cell repertoire is similar to B cells in circulation or other organs but differs significantly from plasma cells in postnatal intestine (Golby et al. 2002). After birth, the IgM^+ plasma cell population expands faster than IgG^+ cells, and at the same time microbial stimulation induces B cells to undergo IgA class switch in both lamina propria and organized lymphoid tissue (Fagarasan et al. 2001). IgA^+ plasma cells are first seen in the lamina propria during the second postnatal week (Crabbe et al. 1970a, b; Shroff et al. 1995). The number of IgA^+ cells in the mucosa reaches adult levels at 2 years, although serum IgA concentrations reach adult levels only during the second decade (MacDonald and Spencer 1994).

Intestinal T cells can be identified from 12 to 14 weeks of gestation (Spencer et al. 1986). Outside the organized lymphoid tissue, intestinal T cells are distributed as intraepithelial (IELs) and lamina propria lymphocytes (LPLs). The fetal gut has a small number of IELs (3–5 $CD3^+$ IEL/100 IECs compared to 6–27 cells/100 IECs in older children), which expand rapidly after birth (a tenfold expansion of the $\alpha\beta$ T cells and a two- to threefold increase in the $\gamma\delta$ cells, vide infra) (MacDonald and Spencer 1994; Cerf-Bensussan and Guy-Grand 1991). In contrast, LPLs continue to expand during fetal period and have a density similar to the postnatal intestine by 19–27 weeks gestation (Spencer et al. 1986).

Several early lineage T-cell populations can be seen in the fetal intestine, suggesting that T cells may develop locally in an extrathymic pathway (Spencer et al. 1985, 1986, 1989; Husband and Gleeson 1996; Howie et al. 1998; Gunther et al. 2005; Fichtelius 1968; Latthe et al. 1994; Koningsberger et al. 1997). These immature T-cell lineages have been shown in Fig. 3. Whereas most immature LPLs differentiate rapidly after birth, the differentiation of IELs is slower and continues through infancy (Williams et al. 2004). In addition to phenotypic changes, intestinal T cells also continue to undergo functional maturation during infancy and childhood. The TCR β-chain repertoire is polyclonal during fetal period and infancy and only gradually becomes restricted to the oligoclonal pattern characteristic of adults. This restriction is likely due to expansion of a few dominant clones which are specific for the commensal bacterial flora (Williams et al. 2004).

In the fetal intestine, about 10–30% IELs express the $\gamma\delta$ T-cell receptor (Spencer et al. 1985). Rodent studies suggest that $\gamma\delta$ cells may regulate IEC function, display cytotoxic activity,

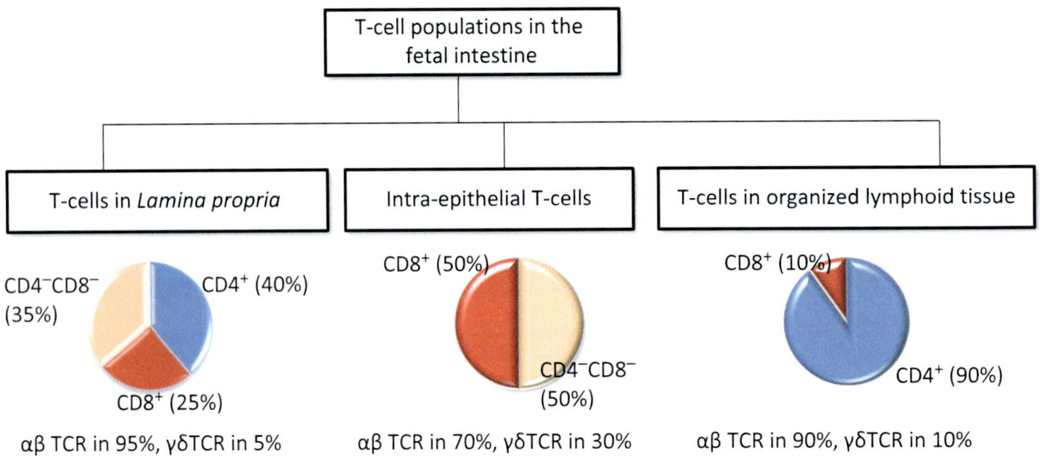

Fig. 3 T-cell lineages seen in the fetal intestine

and may promote antimicrobial immunity (Komano et al. 1995; Boismenu and Havran 1994; Kagnoff 1998). Similar to αβ T cells, the fetal/neonatal γδ repertoire is also polyclonal (Holtmeier et al. 1997).

ILC3s are abundant at the gut mucosal interface. Emerging evidence indicates that these cells may be induced in response to microbial colonization and may promote B-cell IgA production (Magri et al. 2014). IL22 production by ILCs may play an important role in shaping the composition of the intestinal microbiota (Sonnenberg et al. 2011).

99.3.8.3 Secretory Immunoglobulins

Secretory immunoglobulins, IgA and IgM, play an important role in mucosal defense. Secretory IgA (sIgA) can be detected in mucosal secretions as early as 1–8 weeks after birth (Haworth and Dilling 1966; Brandtzaeg et al. 1991; Gleeson et al. 1982; Mellander et al. 1984). sIgM, on the other hand, appears transiently during early infancy (Gleeson et al. 1982).

sIgA levels rise during neonatal period to reach an initial peak (as measured in saliva) at 4–6 weeks. In premature infants, sIgA appears in secretions at a similar chronological age as in full-term infants, although sIgA concentrations may be lower. If chronological age is corrected for prematurity, sIgA concentrations then become similar to matched full-term infants (Hayes et al. 1999; Wan et al. 2003). Salivary IgA levels continue to rise up to 18 months of age (Wan et al. 2003). A transient nadir in sIgA has been inconsistently (Mellander et al. 1984; Fitzsimmons et al. 1994) recorded at 3–6 months (Gleeson et al. 1982; Burgio et al. 1980).

Secreted immunoglobulins also change qualitatively during the first year. There is a switch from monomeric IgA to polymeric sIgA sometime during the first year, indicating maturation of the secretory immune system (Cripps et al. 1991) or, alternatively, increasing exposure to exogenous antigens (Weemaes et al. 2003). The relative amounts of IgA subclasses in mucosal secretions also change during infancy. At birth, sIgA1 is the dominant subclass, but sIgA2 increases rapidly by 6 months of age (Fitzsimmons et al. 1994).

Specific sIgA responses appear to be related more to the timing and quantum of the antigenic stimulus than to developmental factors during infancy. sIgA antibodies to *E. coli* somatic antigens appear in neonates within a few weeks after timed exposure and colonization (Lodinova et al. 1973). The strength of the stimulus also has an effect: earlier, and stronger, specific sIgA responses are seen in neonates born in areas endemic for a pathogen as compared to infants in the developed world (Cripps et al. 1991; Onyemelukwe et al. 1985).

During the neonatal period, colostrum provides an important alternative source of sIgA

(Ogra et al. 1983). Milk antibodies, amounting to about 0.5–1 g/day throughout lactation (comparable to the 2.5 g/day being produced by a 65 kg adult), are directed against antigens present in the environment shared by the mother-infant dyad (Hanson and Korotkova 2002). The presence of "enteromammary" and "bronchomammary" pathways allows immune cells stimulated by antigens in the maternal intestine and bronchial mucosa to migrate to the mammary gland (Ogra et al. 1983; Hanson et al. 1984; Takahashi et al. 2002; Goldman et al. 1998). Interestingly, sIgA levels have been reported to be higher in colostrum and milk of mothers of preterm neonates (Araujo et al. 2005).

Premature infants lack the intrinsic protective mechanisms of the adult intestinal mucosa that prevent sensitization against luminal constituents: a strong physical barrier, luminal enzymes that can alter ingested antigens, presence of regulatory T cells, and the production of sIgA (Mayer 2005). The risk of sensitization is further increased due to several developmental deficiencies within primary immune cells: (1) specific antibody responses in premature infants are abnormal due to reduced antigen affinity, increased polyreactivity, and autoreactivity (Bhat et al. 1992; Chen et al. 1998) and (2) the lengths of immunoglobulin heavy chain third complementarity determining regions (CDR3) are almost three amino acids shorter in the fetus/premature infant than adults (Bauer et al. 2002). This reduces the potential antibody diversity available to the fetus/preterm neonate by about 20^3 (= 8000) fold (Bauer et al. 2002). Moreover, antigen-binding sites with short CDR3 regions, due to their tertiary structure, are more likely to bind to peptides such as allergens (Collis et al. 2003) and (3) the short CDR3 regions of fetal CD5$^+$ B1 cells share characteristics with variable regions of IgE heavy chains (Zemlin et al. 2001; Collins et al. 2003). These observations have led to the hypothesis that B1 cells may contribute to the repertoire of allergen specific IgE$^+$ plasma cells and that premature exposure of the immature intestinal B-cell repertoire to allergens may influence the risk of sensitization (Collins et al. 2003).

99.3.8.4 Intestinal Macrophages and Dendritic Cells

Macrophages first appear in the developing intestine at 11–12 weeks of gestation, increase rapidly during the 12–22 week period, and then continue to expand at a slower pace through early childhood (Rognum et al. 1992; Maheshwari and Zemlin 2006; MacDonald and Spencer 1990; Braegger et al. 1992; Harvey et al. 1990; Spencer et al. 1987). These cells play a critical host defense role in being the first phagocytic cells of the innate immune system to encounter luminal bacteria that breach the epithelium and gain access to the lamina propria (Smythies et al. 2005, 2006b). Intestinal macrophages display avid phagocytic and bacteriocidal activity but are markedly attenuated in their inflammatory responses (Smythies et al. 2005), a unique adaptive mechanism that prevents unnecessary inflammation in the gut mucosa despite the proximity to luminal bacteria. In sick and preterm neonates who are predisposed to bacterial translocation due to an abnormally permeable gut epithelial barrier, immaturity of the local adaptive immune system, and low secretory IgA production (Gebbers and Laissue 2004; van Elburg et al. 2003; Albanese et al. 1994), intestinal macrophages assume even greater importance as a host defense system because of their ability to eliminate "previously unknown" bacteria through phagocytosis and intracellular killing. A breach of the gut mucosal barrier defense is met by tissue macrophages in the liver (Kupffer cells).

Intestinal macrophages are derived from circulating monocytes, which are recruited to the mucosa under the influence of various epithelial and mesenchymal cell-derived chemoattractants (Smythies et al. 2005, 2006b; Kelsall 2008). Because neither intestinal macrophages nor their precursor monocytes have the ability to undergo clonal expansion (Smythies et al. 2006b), the only mechanism available for the development and maintenance of the gut macrophage pool is through the continuous recruitment and differentiation of blood monocytes. In adults, interleukin-8/CXC ligand 8 (IL-8/CXCL8) and transforming

growth factor-beta (TGF-β) recruit macrophage precursors to the intestinal mucosa (Smythies et al. 2006b). However, several lines of evidence indicate that IL-8 and TGF-β may not be important as macrophage chemoattractants in the fetal intestine. In the fetus, IL-8 is comprised mainly of a longer, less-potent 77-amino acid isoform (unlike the shorter 72-amino acid isomer in the adult) (Maheshwari et al. 2008a). Similarly, TGF-β bioactivity is low in the early-/mid-gestation fetal intestine (Maheshwari et al. 2008b). Finally, macrophages appear in the fetal intestine at least a few weeks before lymphocytes or neutrophils (Maheshwari and Zemlin 2006; MacDonald and Spencer 1990; Braegger et al. 1992), suggesting that macrophage precursors are likely to be recruited to the early fetal intestine by chemoattractant(s) more specific for macrophage precursors than IL-8/CXCL8, which recruits both neutrophils and macrophage precursors (Fox et al. 2005; Smythies et al. 2006b), or TGF-β, which mobilizes macrophage precursors as well as T lymphocytes (Smythies et al. 2006b; Adams et al. 1991). We have shown recently that epithelial cells in the fetal intestine produce chemerin (previously known as tazarotene-induced gene-2/TIG2 or retinoic acid receptor responder-2/RARRES2) to recruit macrophage precursors.

We have shown recently that unlike in the adult, intestinal macrophages in the midgestation fetus/premature infant are responsive to bacterial products and produce inflammatory cytokines. This inflammatory downregulation of fetal intestinal macrophages occurs under the influence of TGF-β, particularly the TGF-β_2 isoform. Further investigations are currently in progress to determine whether the incompletely developed macrophage tolerance to bacterial products in the preterm intestine could predispose these infants to necrotizing enterocolitis.

There is very limited data on fetal/neonatal intestinal DCs (MacDonald 1996). HLA-DR$^+$ DC-like cells can be detected in both *lamina propria* as well as the Peyer's patches after 14 weeks, but these cells may have some overlap with *lamina propria* macrophages (Spencer et al. 1987). In rats and nonhuman primates, DCs have been noted in the fetal lamina propria as well in Peyer's patches (Wilders et al. 1983; Makori et al. 2003). The functional importance of these DCs is not clear.

References

Adamo L, Naveiras O, Wenzel PL, McKinney-Freeman S, Mack PJ, Gracia-Sancho J, Suchy-Dicey A, Yoshimoto M, Lensch MW, Yoder MC, Garcia-Cardena G, Daley GQ (2009) Biomechanical forces promote embryonic haematopoiesis. Nature 459:1131–1135

Adams DH, Hathaway M, Shaw J, Burnett D, Elias E, Strain AJ (1991) Transforming growth factor-beta induces human T lymphocyte migration in vitro. J Immunol 147:609–612

Adkins B (2003) Peripheral CD4+ lymphocytes derived from fetal versus adult thymic precursors differ phenotypically and functionally. J Immunol 171:5157–5164

Albanese CT, Smith SD, Watkins S, Kurkchubasche A, Simmons RL, Rowe MI (1994) Effect of secretory IgA on transepithelial passage of bacteria across the intact ileum in vitro. J Am Coll Surg 179:679–688

Alenghat E, Esterly JR (1984) Alveolar macrophages in perinatal infants. Pediatrics 74:221–223

Alugupalli KR, Leong JM, Woodland RT, Muramatsu M, Honjo T, Gerstein RM (2004) B1b lymphocytes confer T cell-independent long-lasting immunity. Immunity 21:379–390

Ambruso DR, Bentwood B, Henson PM, Johnston RB Jr (1984) Oxidative metabolism of cord blood neutrophils: relationship to content and degranulation of cytoplasmic granules. Pediatr Res 18:1148–1153

Anderson G, Moore NC, Owen JJ, Jenkinson EJ (1996) Cellular interactions in thymocyte development. Annu Rev Immunol 14:73–99

Andersson U (1985) Development of B lymphocyte function in childhood. Acta Paediatr Scand 74:568–573

Antin JH, Emerson SG, Martin P, Gadol N, Ault KA (1986) Leu-1+ (CD5+) B cells. A major lymphoid subpopulation in human fetal spleen: phenotypic and functional studies. J Immunol 136:505–510

Araujo ED, Goncalves AK, Cornetta Mda C, Cunha H, Cardoso ML, Morais SS, Giraldo PC (2005) Evaluation of the secretory immunoglobulin A levels in the colostrum and milk of mothers of term and pre-term newborns. Braz J Infect Dis 9:357–362

Artis D, Spits H (2015) The biology of innate lymphoid cells. Nature 517:293–301

Bagorda A, Mihaylov VA, Parent CA (2006) Chemotaxis: moving forward and holding on to the past. Thromb Haemost 95:12–21

Ballow M, Cates KL, Rowe JC, Goetz C, Desbonnet C (1986) Development of the immune system in very low birth weight (less than 1500 g) premature infants: concentrations of plasma immunoglobulins and patterns of infections. Pediatr Res 20:899–904

Barrat FJ, Cua DJ, Boonstra A, Richards DF, Crain C, Savelkoul HF, de Waal-Malefyt R, Coffman RL, Hawrylowicz CM, O'Garra A (2002) In vitro generation of interleukin 10-producing regulatory CD4(+) T cells is induced by immunosuppressive drugs and inhibited by T helper type 1 (Th1)- and Th2-inducing cytokines. J Exp Med 195:603–616

Barnie PA, Lin X, Liu Y, Xu H, Su Z (2015) IL-17 producing innate lymphoid cells 3 (ILC3) but not Th17 cells might be the potential danger factor for preeclampsia and other pregnancy associated diseases. Int J Clin Exp Pathol 8:11100–11107

Bauer K, Zemlin M, Hummel M, Pfeiffer S, Karstaedt J, Steinhauser G, Xiao X, Versmold H, Berek C (2002) Diversification of Ig heavy chain genes in human preterm neonates prematurely exposed to environmental antigens. J Immunol 169:1349–1356

Bektas S, Goetze B, Speer CP (1990) Decreased adherence, chemotaxis and phagocytic activities of neutrophils from preterm neonates. Acta Paediatr Scand 79:1031–1038

Benoit M, Desnues B, Mege JL (2008) Macrophage polarization in bacterial infections. J Immunol 181:3733–3739

Bessler H, Sirota L, Dulitzky F, Djaldetti M (1987) Production of interleukin-1 by mononuclear cells of newborns and their mothers. Clin Exp Immunol 68:655–661

Bhat NM, Kantor AB, Bieber MM, Stall AM, Herzenberg LA, Teng NN (1992) The ontogeny and functional characteristics of human B-1 (CD5+ B) cells. Int Immunol 4:243–252

Bhide SA, Wadekar KV, Koushik SA (2001) Peyer's patches are precocious to the appendix in human development. Dev Immunol 8:159–166

Bhoopat L, Taylor CR, Hofman FM (1986) The differentiation antigens of macrophages in human fetal liver. Clin Immunol Immunopathol 41:184–192

Bishop GA, Hostager BS (2001) B lymphocyte activation by contact-mediated interactions with T lymphocytes. Curr Opin Immunol 13:278–285

Bjorkqvist M, Jurstrand M, Bodin L, Fredlund H, Schollin J (2004) Defective neutrophil oxidative burst in preterm newborns on exposure to coagulase-negative staphylococci. Pediatr Res 55:966–971

Bodey B, Kaiser HE (1997) Development of Hassall's bodies of the thymus in humans and other vertebrates (especially mammals) under physiological and pathological conditions: immunocytochemical, electronmicroscopic and in vitro observations. In Vivo 11:61–85

Bofill M, Janossy G, Janossa M, Burford GD, Seymour GJ, Wernet P, Kelemen E (1985) Human B cell development. II. Subpopulations in the human fetus. J Immunol 134:1531–1538

Boismenu R, Havran WL (1994) Modulation of epithelial cell growth by intraepithelial gamma delta T cells. Science 266:1253–1255

Bonati A, Zanelli P, Ferrari S, Plebani A, Starcich B, Savi M, Neri TM (1992) T-cell receptor beta-chain gene rearrangement and expression during human thymic ontogenesis. Blood 79:1472–1483

Bondada S, Wu H, Robertson DA, Chelvarajan RL (2000) Accessory cell defect in unresponsiveness of neonates and aged to polysaccharide vaccines. Vaccine 19:557–565

Borregaard N, Cowland JB (1997) Granules of the human neutrophilic polymorphonuclear leukocyte. Blood 89:3503–3521

Boxer LA (2006) Severe congenital neutropenia: genetics and pathogenesis. Trans Am Clin Climatol Assoc 117:13–31; discussion-2

Braegger CP, Spencer J, MacDonald TT (1992) Ontogenetic aspects of the intestinal immune system in man. Int J Clin Lab Res 22:1–4

Brandtzaeg P, Nilssen DE, Rognum TO, Thrane PS (1991) Ontogeny of the mucosal immune system and IgA deficiency. Gastroenterol Clin North Am 20:397–439

Bryson YJ, Winter HS, Gard SE, Fischer TJ, Stiehm ER (1980) Deficiency of immune interferon production by leukocytes of normal newborns. Cell Immunol 55:191–200

Buhl AM, Nemazee D, Cambier JC, Rickert R, Hertz M (2000) B-cell antigen receptor competence regulates B-lymphocyte selection and survival. Immunol Rev 176:141–153

Bulmer JN, Morrison L, Smith JC (1988) Expression of class II MHC gene products by macrophages in human uteroplacental tissue. Immunology 63:707–714

Burgio GR, Lanzavecchia A, Plebani A, Jayakar S, Ugazio AG (1980) Ontogeny of secretory immunity: levels of secretory IgA and natural antibodies in saliva. Pediatr Res 14:1111–1114

Cahill RN, Kimpton WG, Washington EA, Holder JE, Cunningham CP (1999) The ontogeny of T cell recirculation during foetal life. Semin Immunol 11:105–114

Cairo MS, Suen Y, Knoppel E, van de Ven C, Nguyen A, Sender L (1991) Decreased stimulated GM-CSF production and GM-CSF gene expression but normal numbers of GM-CSF receptors in human term newborns compared with adults. Pediatr Res 30:362–367

Carr R, Huizinga TW (2000) Low soluble FcRIII receptor demonstrates reduced neutrophil reserves in preterm neonates. Arch Dis Child Fetal Neonatal Ed 83:F160

Carr R, Pumford D, Davies JM (1992) Neutrophil chemotaxis and adhesion in preterm babies. Arch Dis Child 67:813–817

Carreno MP, Gresham HD, Brown EJ (1993) Isolation of leukocyte response integrin: a novel RGD-binding protein involved in regulation of phagocytic function. Clin Immunol Immunopathol 69:43–51

Casali P, Schettino EW (1996) Structure and function of natural antibodies. Curr Top Microbiol Immunol 210:167–179

Cerf-Bensussan N, Guy-Grand D (1991) Intestinal intraepithelial lymphocytes. Gastroenterol Clin North Am 20:549–576

Chang M, Suen Y, Lee SM, Baly D, Buzby JS, Knoppel E, Wolpe S, Cairo MS (1994) Transforming growth factor-beta 1, macrophage inflammatory protein-1 alpha, and interleukin-8 gene expression is lower in stimulated human neonatal compared with adult mononuclear cells. Blood 84:118–124

Chen ZJ, Wheeler CJ, Shi W, Wu AJ, Yarboro CH, Gallagher M, Notkins AL (1998) Polyreactive antigen-binding B cells are the predominant cell type in the newborn B cell repertoire. Eur J Immunol 28:989–994

Chheda S, Palkowetz KH, Garofalo R, Rassin DK, Goldman AS (1996) Decreased interleukin-10 production by neonatal monocytes and T cells: relationship to decreased production and expression of tumor necrosis factor-alpha and its receptors. Pediatr Res 40:475–483

Chidgey AP, Boyd RL (2001) Thymic stromal cells and positive selection. APMIS 109:481–492

Choi Y, Rickert MH, Ballow M, Greenberg SJ (1995) Human IgH-V gene repertoire in neonatal cord blood, adult peripheral blood, and EBV-transformed cells. Ann N Y Acad Sci 764:261–264

Christensen RD (1987) Circulating pluripotent hematopoietic progenitor cells in neonates. J Pediatr 110:623–625

Christensen RD, Harper TE, Rothstein G (1986) Granulocyte-macrophage progenitor cells in term and preterm neonates. J Pediatr 109:1047–1051

Clark RA (1999) Activation of the neutrophil respiratory burst oxidase. J Infect Dis 179(Suppl 2):S309–S317

Clerici M, DePalma L, Roilides E, Baker R, Shearer GM (1993) Analysis of T helper and antigen-presenting cell functions in cord blood and peripheral blood leukocytes from healthy children of different ages. J Clin Invest 91:2829–2836

Collins AM, Sewell WA, Edwards MR (2003) Immunoglobulin gene rearrangement, repertoire diversity, and the allergic response. Pharmacol Ther 100:157–170

Collis AV, Brouwer AP, Martin AC (2003) Analysis of the antigen combining site: correlations between length and sequence composition of the hypervariable loops and the nature of the antigen. J Mol Biol 325:337–354

Cooper MD, Buckley RH (1982) Developmental immunology and the immunodeficiency diseases. JAMA 248:2658–2669

Cornes JS (1965) Peyer's patches in the human gut. Proc R Soc Med 58:716

Crabbe PA, Nash DR, Bazin H, Eyssen H, Heremans JF (1970a) Immunohistochemical observations on lymphoid tissues from conventional and germ-free mice. Lab Invest 22:448–457

Crabbe PA, Nash DR, Bazin H, Eyssen H, Heremans JF (1970b) Studies on the immunoglobulins of the mouse intestinal secretions. Prog Immunobiol Stand 4:308–311

Cripps AW, Gleeson M, Clancy RL (1991) Ontogeny of the mucosal immune response in children. Adv Exp Med Biol 310:87–92

D'Ambola JB, Sherman MP, Tashkin DP, Gong H Jr (1988) Human and rabbit newborn lung macrophages have reduced anti-Candida activity. Pediatr Res 24:285–290

D'Angio CT, Maniscalco WM, Pichichero ME (1995) Immunologic response of extremely premature infants to tetanus, *Haemophilus influenzae*, and polio immunizations. Pediatrics 96:18–22

Darrasse-Jeze G, Marodon G, Salomon BL, Catala M, Klatzmann D (2005) Ontogeny of CD4+CD25+ regulatory/suppressor T cells in human fetuses. Blood 105:4715–4721

Davis MM, Bjorkman PJ (1988) T-cell antigen receptor genes and T-cell recognition. Nature 334:395–402

de Bont ES, Martens A, van Raan J, Samson G, Fetter WP, Okken A, de Leij LH (1993) Tumor necrosis factor-alpha, interleukin-1 beta, and interleukin-6 plasma levels in neonatal sepsis. Pediatr Res 33:380–383

Denning TL, Wang YC, Patel SR, Williams IR, Pulendran B (2007) Lamina propria macrophages and dendritic cells differentially induce regulatory and interleukin 17-producing T cell responses. Nat Immunol 8:1086–1094

Deorari AK, Broor S, Maitreyi RS, Agarwal D, Kumar H, Paul VK, Singh M (2000) Incidence, clinical spectrum, and outcome of intrauterine infections in neonates. J Trop Pediatr 46:155–159

Dorshkind K, Montecino-Rodriguez E (2007) Fetal B-cell lymphopoiesis and the emergence of B-1-cell potential. Nat Rev Immunol 7:213–219

Drossou V, Kanakoudi F, Tzimouli V, Sarafidis K, Taparkou A, Bougiouklis D, Petropoulou T, Kremenopoulos G (1997) Impact of prematurity, stress and sepsis on the neutrophil respiratory burst activity of neonates. Biol Neonate 72:201–209

Durandy A, Thuillier L, Forveille M, Fischer A (1990) Phenotypic and functional characteristics of human newborns' B lymphocytes. J Immunol 144:60–65

Edwards SW (1995) Cell signalling by integrins and immunoglobulin receptors in primed neutrophils. Trends Biochem Sci 20:362–367

Eisenfeld L, Krause PJ, Herson V, Savidakis J, Bannon P, Maderazo E, Woronick C, Giuliano C, Banco L (1990) Longitudinal study of neutrophil adherence and motility. J Pediatr 117:926–929

Elsasser-Beile U, Dursunoglu B, Gallati H, Monting JS, von Kleist S (1995) Comparison of cytokine production in blood cell cultures of healthy children and adults. Pediatr Allergy Immunol 6:170–174

Elsbach P, Weiss J (1998) Role of the bactericidal/permeability-increasing protein in host defence. Curr Opin Immunol 10:45–49

Engle WA, Schreiner RL, Baehner RL (1983) Neonatal white blood cell disorders. Semin Perinatol 7:184–200

Erkeller-Yuksel FM, Deneys V, Yuksel B, Hannet I, Hulstaert F, Hamilton C, Mackinnon H, Stokes LT, Munhyeshuli V, Vanlangendonck F et al (1992) Age-related changes in human blood lymphocyte subpopulations. J Pediatr 120:216–222

Etzioni A, Obedeanu N, Blazer S, Benderly A, Merzbach D (1990) Effect of an intravenous gammaglobulin

preparation on the opsonophagocytic activity of preterm serum against coagulase-negative staphylococci. Acta Paediatr Scand 79:156–161

Fagarasan S, Kinoshita K, Muramatsu M, Ikuta K, Honjo T (2001) In situ class switching and differentiation to IgA-producing cells in the gut lamina propria. Nature 413:639–643

Fichtelius KE (1968) The gut epithelium – a first level lymphoid organ? Exp Cell Res 49:87–104

Finke D, Acha-Orbea H, Mattis A, Lipp M, Kraehenbuhl J (2002) CD4+CD3- cells induce Peyer's patch development: role of alpha4beta1 integrin activation by CXCR5. Immunity 17:363–373

Fitzsimmons SP, Evans MK, Pearce CL, Sheridan MJ, Wientzen R, Cole MF (1994) Immunoglobulin A subclasses in infants' saliva and in saliva and milk from their mothers. J Pediatr 124:566–573

Forsberg A, Bengtsson M, Eringfalt A, Ernerudh J, Mjosberg J, Jenmalm MC (2014) GATA binding protein 3(+) group 2 innate lymphoid cells are present in cord blood and in higher proportions in male than in female neonates. J Allergy Clin Immunol 134:228–230

Foster CA, Holbrook KA, Farr AG (1986) Ontogeny of Langerhans cells in human embryonic and fetal skin: expression of HLA-DR and OKT-6 determinants. J Invest Dermatol 86:240–243

Fox SE, Lu W, Maheshwari A, Christensen RD, Calhoun DA (2005) The effects and comparative differences of neutrophil specific chemokines on neutrophil chemotaxis of the neonate. Cytokine 29:135–140

Frascoli M, Jeanty C, Fleck S, Moradi PW, Keating S, Mattis AN, Tang Q, MacKenzie TC (2016) Heightened Immune activation in fetuses with gastroschisis may be blocked by targeting IL-5. J Immunol 196:4957–4966

Gaddy J, Risdon G, Broxmeyer HE (1995) Cord blood natural killer cells are functionally and phenotypically immature but readily respond to interleukin-2 and interleukin-12. J Interferon Cytokine Res 15:527–536

Gahr M, Blanke R, Speer CP (1985) Polymorphonuclear leukocyte function in term and preterm newborn infants. Biol Neonate 48:15–20

Garcia KC, Degano M, Speir JA, Wilson IA (1999) Emerging principles for T cell receptor recognition of antigen in cellular immunity. Rev Immunogenet 1:75–90

Garderet L, Dulphy N, Douay C, Chalumeau N, Schaeffer V, Zilber MT, Lim A, Even J, Mooney N, Gelin C, Gluckman E, Charron D, Toubert A (1998) The umbilical cord blood alphabeta T-cell repertoire: characteristics of a polyclonal and naive but completely formed repertoire. Blood 91:340–346

Gathings WE, Lawton AR, Cooper MD (1977) Immunofluorescent studies of the development of pre-B cells, B lymphocytes and immunoglobulin isotype diversity in humans. Eur J Immunol 7:804–810

Gaunt G, Ramin K (2001) Immunological tolerance of the human fetus. Am J Perinatol 18:299–312

Gebbers JO, Laissue JA (2004) Bacterial translocation in the normal human appendix parallels the development of the local immune system. Ann N Y Acad Sci 1029:337–343

Geissmann F, Jung S, Littman DR (2003) Blood monocytes consist of two principal subsets with distinct migratory properties. Immunity 19:71–82

George JF Jr, Schroeder HW Jr (1992) Developmental regulation of D beta reading frame and junctional diversity in T cell receptor-beta transcripts from human thymus. J Immunol 148:1230–1239

Gerli R, Bertotto A, Crupi S, Arcangeli C, Marinelli I, Spinozzi F, Cernetti C, Angelella P, Rambotti P (1989) Activation of cord T lymphocytes. I. Evidence for a defective T cell mitogenesis induced through the CD2 molecule. J Immunol 142:2583–2589

Gerli R, Agea E, Muscat C, Tognellini R, Fiorucci G, Spinozzi F, Cernetti C, Bertotto A (1993) Activation of cord T lymphocytes. III. Role of LFA-1/ICAM-1 and CD2/LFA-3 adhesion molecules in CD3-induced proliferative response. Cell Immunol 148:32–47

Gill TJ 3rd, Repetti CF, Metlay LA, Rabin BS, Taylor FH, Thompson DS, Cortese AL (1983) Transplacental immunization of the human fetus to tetanus by immunization of the mother. J Clin Invest 72:987–996

Gleeson M, Cripps AW, Clancy RL, Husband AJ, Hensley MJ, Leeder SR (1982) Ontogeny of the secretory immune system in man. Aust N Z J Med 12:255–258

Glover DM, Brownstein D, Burchett S, Larsen A, Wilson CB (1987) Expression of HLA class II antigens and secretion of interleukin-1 by monocytes and macrophages from adults and neonates. Immunology 61:195–201

Golby S, Hackett M, Boursier L, Dunn-Walters D, Thiagamoorthy S, Spencer J (2002) B cell development and proliferation of mature B cells in human fetal intestine. J Leukoc Biol 72:279–284

Goldman AS, Chheda S, Garofalo R (1998) Evolution of immunologic functions of the mammary gland and the postnatal development of immunity. Pediatr Res 43:155–162

Golebiowska M, Kardas-Sobantka D, Chlebna-Sokol D, Sabanty W (1999) Hepatitis B vaccination in preterm infants. Eur J Pediatr 158:293–297

Grage-Griebenow E, Flad HD, Ernst M (2001) Heterogeneity of human peripheral blood monocyte subsets. J Leukoc Biol 69:11–20

Gromo G, Geller RL, Inverardi L, Bach FH (1987) Signal requirements in the step-wise functional maturation of cytotoxic T lymphocytes. Nature 327:424–426

Grouard G, Rissoan MC, Filgueira L, Durand I, Banchereau J, Liu YJ (1997) The enigmatic plasmacytoid T cells develop into dendritic cells with interleukin (IL)-3 and CD40-ligand. J Exp Med 185:1101–1111

Groux H, O'Garra A, Bigler M, Rouleau M, Antonenko S, de Vries JE, Roncarolo MG (1997) A CD4+ T-cell subset inhibits antigen-specific T-cell responses and prevents colitis. Nature 389:737–742

Gunther U, Holloway JA, Gordon JN, Knight A, Chance V, Hanley NA, Wilson DI, French R, Spencer J, Steer H,

Anderson G, MacDonald TT (2005) Phenotypic characterization of CD3-7+ cells in developing human intestine and an analysis of their ability to differentiate into T cells. J Immunol 174:5414–5422

Haas KM, Poe JC, Steeber DA, Tedder TF (2005) B-1a and B-1b cells exhibit distinct developmental requirements and have unique functional roles in innate and adaptive immunity to *S. pneumoniae*. Immunity 23:7–18

Hagendorens MM, Van Bever HP, Schuerwegh AJ, De Clerck LS, Bridts CH, Stevens WJ (2000) Determination of T-cell subpopulations and intracellular cytokine production (interleukin-2, interleukin-4, and interferon-gamma) by cord blood T-lymphocytes of neonates from atopic and non-atopic parents. Pediatr Allergy Immunol 11:12–19

Hanson LA, Korotkova M (2002) The role of breastfeeding in prevention of neonatal infection. Semin Neonatol 7:275–281

Hanson LA, Ahlstedt S, Andersson B, Cruz JR, Dahlgren U, Fallstrom SP, Porras O, Svanborg Eden C, Soderstrom T, Wettergren B (1984) The immune response of the mammary gland and its significance for the neonate. Ann Allergy 53:576–582

Hardy RR (2006) B-1 B cell development. J Immunol 177:2749–2754

Hardy RR, Hayakawa K (1991) A developmental switch in B lymphopoiesis. Proc Natl Acad Sci U S A 88:11550–11554

Hardy RR, Hayakawa K (1994) CD5 B cells, a fetal B cell lineage. Adv Immunol 55:297–339

Harvey J, Jones DB, Wright DH (1990) Differential expression of MHC- and macrophage-associated antigens in human fetal and postnatal small intestine. Immunology 69:409–415

Hashimoto M, Nishida A, Minakami H, Takashima Y, Kato M, Okada Y, Ogawa Y, Itoh S, Kimura H (2002) Decreased expression of L-selectin on peripheral blood polymorphonuclear leukocytes in neonates with severe asphyxia. Biol Neonate 81:95–98

Hassan J, Reen DJ (1993) Neonatal CD4+ CD45RA+ T cells: precursors of adult CD4+ CD45RA+ T cells? Res Immunol 144:87–92

Haworth JC, Dilling L (1966) Concentration of gamma-A-globulin in serum, saliva, and nasopharyngeal secretions of infants and children. J Lab Clin Med 67:922–933

Hayes JA, Adamson-Macedo EN, Perera S, Anderson J (1999) Detection of secretory immunoglobulin A (SIgA) in saliva of ventilated and non-ventilated preterm neonates. Neuroendocrinol Lett 20:109–113

Haynes BF (1984) The human thymic microenvironment. Adv Immunol 36:87–142

Haynes BF, Martin ME, Kay HH, Kurtzberg J (1988) Early events in human T cell ontogeny. Phenotypic characterization and immunohistologic localization of T cell precursors in early human fetal tissues. J Exp Med 168:1061–1080

Hazenberg MD, Verschuren MC, Hamann D, Miedema F, van Dongen JJ (2001) T cell receptor excision circles as markers for recent thymic emigrants: basic aspects, technical approach, and guidelines for interpretation. J Mol Med 79:631–640

Heit B, Tavener S, Raharjo E, Kubes P (2002) An intracellular signaling hierarchy determines direction of migration in opposing chemotactic gradients. J Cell Biol 159:91–102

Herberman RB, Djeu J, Kay HD, Ortaldo JR, Riccardi C, Bonnard GD, Holden HT, Fagnani R, Santoni A, Puccetti P (1979) Natural killer cells: characteristics and regulation of activity. Immunol Rev 44:43–70

Hobbs JR, Davis JA (1967) Serum gamma-G-globulin levels and gestational age in premature babies. Lancet 1:757–759

Holt PG, Jones CA (2000) The development of the immune system during pregnancy and early life. Allergy 55:688–697

Holtmeier W, Witthoft T, Hennemann A, Winter HS, Kagnoff MF (1997) The TCR-delta repertoire in human intestine undergoes characteristic changes during fetal to adult development. J Immunol 158:5632–5641

Holtmeier W, Pfander M, Hennemann A, Zollner TM, Kaufmann R, Caspary WF (2001) The TCR-delta repertoire in normal human skin is restricted and distinct from the TCR-delta repertoire in the peripheral blood. J Invest Dermatol 116:275–280

Hori S, Nomura T, Sakaguchi S (2003) Control of regulatory T cell development by the transcription factor Foxp3. Science 299:1057–1061

Hoshino T, Yamada A, Honda J, Imai Y, Nakao M, Inoue M, Sagawa K, Yokoyama MM, Oizumi K, Itoh K (1993) Tissue-specific distribution and age-dependent increase of human CD11b+ T cells. J Immunol 151:2237–2246

Howie D, Spencer J, DeLord D, Pitzalis C, Wathen NC, Dogan A, Akbar A, MacDonald TT (1998) Extrathymic T cell differentiation in the human intestine early in life. J Immunol 161:5862–5872

Husband AJ, Gleeson M (1996) Ontogeny of mucosal immunity – environmental and behavioral influences. Brain Behav Immun 10:188–204

Ivanov S, Bozinovski S, Bossios A, Valadi H, Vlahos R, Malmhall C, Sjostrand M, Kolls JK, Anderson GP, Linden A (2007) Functional relevance of the IL-23-IL-17 axis in lungs in vivo. Am J Respir Cell Mol Biol 36:442–451

Jacobs RF, Wilson CB, Palmer S, Springmeyer SC, Henderson WR, Glover DM, Kessler DL Jr, Murphy JH, Hughes JP, van Belle G et al (1985) Factors related to the appearance of alveolar macrophages in the developing lung. Am Rev Respir Dis 131:548–553

Jaffe R (1993) Review of human dendritic cells: isolation and culture from precursors. Pediatr Pathol 13:821–837

Janossy G, Bofill M, Poulter LW, Rawlings E, Burford GD, Navarrete C, Ziegler A, Kelemen E (1986) Separate ontogeny of two macrophage-like accessory cell populations in the human fetus. J Immunol 136:4354–4361

Johnson CC, Ownby DR, Peterson EL (1996) Parental history of atopic disease and concentration of cord blood IgE. Clin Exp Allergy 26:624–629
Johnston RB Jr (1988) Current concepts: immunology. Monocytes and macrophages. N Engl J Med 318:747–752
Jones DH, Schmalstieg FC, Dempsey K, Krater SS, Nannen DD, Smith CW, Anderson DC (1990) Subcellular distribution and mobilization of MAC-1 (CD11b/CD18) in neonatal neutrophils. Blood 75:488–498
Kagi D, Ledermann B, Burki K, Zinkernagel RM, Hengartner H (1996) Molecular mechanisms of lymphocyte-mediated cytotoxicity and their role in immunological protection and pathogenesis in vivo. Annu Rev Immunol 14:207–232
Kagnoff MF (1998) Current concepts in mucosal immunity. III. Ontogeny and function of gamma delta T cells in the intestine. Am J Physiol 274:G455–G458
Kang J, Raulet DH (1997) Events that regulate differentiation of alpha beta TCR+ and gamma delta TCR+ T cells from a common precursor. Semin Immunol 9:171–179
Kantor AB, Herzenberg LA (1993) Origin of murine B cell lineages. Annu Rev Immunol 11:501–538
Karras JG, Wang Z, Huo L, Howard RG, Frank DA, Rothstein TL (1997) Signal transducer and activator of transcription-3 (STAT3) is constitutively activated in normal, self-renewing B-1 cells but only inducibly expressed in conventional B lymphocytes. J Exp Med 185:1035–1042
Kelemen E, Janossa M (1980) Macrophages are the first differentiated blood cells formed in human embryonic liver. Exp Hematol 8:996–1000
Kelsall B (2008) Recent progress in understanding the phenotype and function of intestinal dendritic cells and macrophages. Mucosal Immunol 1:460–469
Kelsoe G (1999) V(D)J hypermutation and receptor revision: coloring outside the lines. Curr Opin Immunol 11:70–75
Kesson AM, Bryson YJ (1991) Induction of interferon-gamma by cord blood mononuclear cells is calcium dependent. Cell Immunol 133:138–146
Kibler R, Hicks MJ, Wright AL, Taussig LM (1986) A comparative analysis of cord blood and adult lymphocytes: interleukin-2 and interferon production, natural killer cell activity, and lymphocyte populations. Diagn Immunol 4:201–208
Kim SK, Keeney SE, Alpard SK, Schmalstieg FC (2003) Comparison of L-selectin and CD11b on neutrophils of adults and neonates during the first month of life. Pediatr Res 53:132–136
King CL, Malhotra I, Mungai P, Wamachi A, Kioko J, Ouma JH, Kazura JW (1998) B cell sensitization to helminthic infection develops in utero in humans. J Immunol 160:3578–3584
Klebanoff SJ (2005) Myeloperoxidase: friend and foe. J Leukoc Biol 77:598–625
Klein M (1983) Immunological markers of human mononuclear cells. Clin Biochem 16:128–133
Klose CS, Flach M, Mohle L, Rogell L, Hoyler T, Ebert K, Fabiunke C, Pfeifer D, Sexl V, Fonseca-Pereira D, Domingues RG, Veiga-Fernandes H, Arnold SJ, Busslinger M, Dunay IR, Tanriver Y, Diefenbach A (2014) Differentiation of type 1 ILCs from a common progenitor to all helper-like innate lymphoid cell lineages. Cell 157:340–356
Kohler PF, Farr RS (1966) Elevation of cord over maternal IgG immunoglobulin: evidence for an active placental IgG transport. Nature 210:1070–1071
Komano H, Fujiura Y, Kawaguchi M, Matsumoto S, Hashimoto Y, Obana S, Mombaerts P, Tonegawa S, Yamamoto H, Itohara S et al (1995) Homeostatic regulation of intestinal epithelia by intraepithelial gamma delta T cells. Proc Natl Acad Sci U S A 92:6147–6151
Komatsu H, Tsukimori K, Hata K, Satoh S, Nakano H (2001) The characterization of superoxide production of human neonatal neutrophil. Early Hum Dev 65:11–19
Koningsberger JC, Chott A, Logtenberg T, Wiegman LJ, Blumberg RS, van Berge Henegouwen GP, Balk SP (1997) TCR expression in human fetal intestine and identification of an early T cell receptor beta-chain transcript. J Immunol 159:1775–1782
Krause PJ, Kreutzer DL, Eisenfeld L, Herson VC, Weisman S, Bannon P, Greca N (1989) Characterization of nonmotile neutrophil subpopulations in neonates and adults. Pediatr Res 25:519–524
Kurland G, Cheung AT, Miller ME, Ayin SA, Cho MM, Ford EW (1988) The ontogeny of pulmonary defenses: alveolar macrophage function in neonatal and juvenile rhesus monkeys. Pediatr Res 23:293–297
Latthe M, Terry L, MacDonald TT (1994) High frequency of CD8 alpha alpha homodimer-bearing T cells in human fetal intestine. Eur J Immunol 24:1703–1705
Laurenti F, Ferro R, Marzetti G, Rossini M, Bucci G (1980) Neutrophil chemotaxis in preterm infants with infections. J Pediatr 96:468–470
Lehrer RI (2007) Multispecific myeloid defensins. Curr Opin Hematol 14:16–21
Leibson PJ (1997) Signal transduction during natural killer cell activation: inside the mind of a killer. Immunity 6:655–661
Leino A, Ruuskanen O, Kero P, Eskola J, Toivanen P (1981) Depressed phytohemagglutinin and concanavalin A responses in premature infants. Clin Immunol Immunopathol 19:260–267
Liechty KW, Koenig JM, Mitchell MD, Romero R, Christensen RD (1991) Production of interleukin-6 by fetal and maternal cells in vivo during intraamniotic infection and in vitro after stimulation with interleukin-1. Pediatr Res 29:1–4
Liechty KW, Adzick NS, Crombleholme TM (2000) Diminished interleukin 6 (IL-6) production during scarless human fetal wound repair. Cytokine 12:671–676
Lilic D, Cant AJ, Abinun M, Calvert JE, Spickett GP (1997) Cytokine production differs in children and adults. Pediatr Res 42:237–240

Linch DC, Knott LJ, Rodeck CH, Huehns ER (1982) Studies of circulating hemopoietic progenitor cells in human fetal blood. Blood 59:976–979

Linderkamp O, Ruef P, Brenner B, Gulbins E, Lang F (1998) Passive deformability of mature, immature, and active neutrophils in healthy and septicemic neonates. Pediatr Res 44:946–950

Liu CC, Young LH, Young JD (1996) Lymphocyte-mediated cytolysis and disease. N Engl J Med 335:1651–1659

Lodinova R, Jouja V, Wagner V (1973) Serum immunoglobulins and coproantibody formation in infants after artificial intestinal colonization with *Escherichia coli* 083 and oral lysozyme administration. Pediatr Res 7:659–669

Lubens RG, Gard SE, Soderberg-Warner M, Stiehm ER (1982) Lectin-dependent T-lymphocyte and natural killer cytotoxic deficiencies in human newborns. Cell Immunol 74:40–53

Lucivero G, Dell'Osso A, Iannone A, Selvaggi L, Antonaci S, Bettocchi S, Bonomo L (1983) Phenotypic immaturity of T and B lymphocytes in cord blood of full-term normal neonates. Analysis of cell surface markers by using conventional techniques and monoclonal antibodies. Biol Neonate 44:303–308

Macardle PJ, Wheatland L, Zola H (1999) Analysis of the cord blood T lymphocyte response to superantigen. Hum Immunol 60:127–139

MacDonald TT (1996) Accessory cells in the human gastrointestinal tract. Histopathology 29:89–92

MacDonald TT, Spencer J (1990) Ontogeny of the mucosal immune response. Springer Semin Immunopathol 12:129–137

MacDonald TT, Spencer J (1994) Ontogeny of the gut-associated lymphoid system in man. Acta Paediatr Suppl 83:3–5

MacDonald TT, Weinel A, Spencer J (1988) HLA-DR expression in human fetal intestinal epithelium. Gut 29:1342–1348

Magri G, Miyajima M, Bascones S, Mortha A, Puga I, Cassis L, Barra CM, Comerma L, Chudnovskiy A, Gentile M, Llige D, Cols M, Serrano S, Arostegui JI, Juan M, Yague J, Merad M, Fagarasan S, Cerutti A (2014) Innate lymphoid cells integrate stromal and immunological signals to enhance antibody production by splenic marginal zone B cells. Nat Immunol 15:354–364

Maheshwari A, Christensen RD (2004) Developmental granulocytopoiesis. In: Polin RA, Fox WW, Abman SH (eds) Fetal and neonatal physiology, 3rd edn. WB Saunders, Philadelphia, pp 1388–1395

Maheshwari A, Zemlin M (2006) Ontogeny of the intestinal immune system. Haematol Rep 10:18–26

Maheshwari A, Voitenok NN, Akalovich S, Shaik SS, Randolph DA, Sims B, Patel RP, Killingsworth CR, Fallon MB, Ohls RK (2009) Developmental changes in circulating IL-8/CXCL8 isoforms in neonates. Cytokine 46:12–16

Maheshwari A, Kelly DR, Nicola T, Ambalavanan N, Jain SK, Murphy-Ullrich J, Athar M, Shimamura M, Bhandari V, Aprahamian C, Dimmitt RA, Serra R, Ohls RK (2011) TGF-β2 suppresses macrophage cytokine production and mucosal inflammatory responses in the developing intestine. Gastroenterology 140:242–53

Maheshwari A, Kurundkar AR, Shaik SS, Kelly DR, Hartman Y, Zhang W, Dimmitt R, Saeed S, Randolph DA, Aprahamian C, Datta G, Ohls RK (2009) Epithelial cells in fetal intestine produce chemerin to recruit macrophages. Am J Physiol Gastrointest Liver Physiol 297:G1–G10

Makori N, Tarantal AF, Lu FX, Rourke T, Marthas ML, McChesney MB, Hendrickx AG, Miller CJ (2003) Functional and morphological development of lymphoid tissues and immune regulatory and effector function in rhesus monkeys: cytokine-secreting cells, immunoglobulin-secreting cells, and CD5(+) B-1 cells appear early in fetal development. Clin Diagn Lab Immunol 10:140–153

Mathieson BJ, Fowlkes BJ (1984) Cell surface antigen expression on thymocytes: development and phenotypic differentiation of intrathymic subsets. Immunol Rev 82:141–173

Mayer L (2005) Mucosal immunity. Immunol Rev 206:5

McIntyre TM, Prescott SM, Weyrich AS, Zimmerman GA (2003) Cell-cell interactions: leukocyte-endothelial interactions. Curr Opin Hematol 10:150–158

McNabb T, Koh TY, Dorrington KJ, Painter RH (1976) Structure and function of immunoglobulin domains. V. Binding, University of immunoglobulin G and fragments to placental membrane preparations. J Immunol 117:882–888

McVay LD, Carding SR (1996) Extrathymic origin of human gamma delta T cells during fetal development. J Immunol 157:2873–2882

McVay LD, Carding SR (1999) Generation of human gammadelta T-cell repertoires. Crit Rev Immunol 19:431–460

Mellander L, Carlsson B, Hanson LA (1984) Appearance of secretory IgM and IgA antibodies to *Escherichia coli* in saliva during early infancy and childhood. J Pediatr 104:564–568

Merrill JD, Sigaroudinia M, Kohl S (1996) Characterization of natural killer and antibody-dependent cellular cytotoxicity of preterm infants against human immunodeficiency virus-infected cells. Pediatr Res 40:498–503

Middendorp S, Nieuwenhuis EE (2009) NKT cells in mucosal immunity. Mucosal Immunol 2:393

Montecino-Rodriguez E, Dorshkind K (2006) New perspectives in B-1 B cell development and function. Trends Immunol 27:428–433

Moraes TJ, Zurawska JH, Downey GP (2006) Neutrophil granule contents in the pathogenesis of lung injury. Curr Opin Hematol 13:21–27

Morita CT, Parker CM, Brenner MB, Band H (1994) TCR usage and functional capabilities of human gamma delta T cells at birth. J Immunol 153:3979–3988

Morris RB, Nichols BA, Bainton DF (1975) Ultrastructure and peroxidase cytochemistry of normal human leukocytes at birth. Dev Biol 44:223–238

Mosmann TR, Cherwinski H, Bond MW, Giedlin MA, Coffman RL (1986) Two types of murine helper T cell clone. I. Definition according to profiles of lymphokine activities and secreted proteins. J Immunol 136:2348–2357

Muller K, Zak M, Nielsen S, Pedersen FK, de Nully P, Bendtzen K (1996) In vitro cytokine production and phenotype expression by blood mononuclear cells from umbilical cords, children and adults. Pediatr Allergy Immunol 7:117–124

Neuberger MS, Di Noia JM, Beale RC, Williams GT, Yang Z, Rada C (2005) Somatic hypermutation at A.T pairs: polymerase error versus dUTP incorporation. Nat Rev Immunol 5:171–178

Nonoyama S, Etzioni A, Toru H, Ruggerie DP, Lewis D, Pollack S, Aruffo A, Yata JI, Ochs HD (1998) Diminished expression of CD40 ligand may contribute to the defective humoral immunity in patients with MHC class II deficiency. Eur J Immunol 28:589–598

Nossal GJ (1986) The Florey lecture, 1986. The regulatory biology of antibody formation. Proc R Soc Lond B Biol Sci 228:225–240

Nupponen I, Turunen R, Nevalainen T, Peuravuori H, Pohjavuori M, Repo H, Andersson S (2002) Extracellular release of bactericidal/permeability-increasing protein in newborn infants. Pediatr Res 51:670–674

O'Doherty U, Peng M, Gezelter S, Swiggard WJ, Betjes M, Bhardwaj N, Steinman RM (1994) Human blood contains two subsets of dendritic cells, one immunologically mature and the other immature. Immunology 82:487–493

Ofek I, Goldhar J, Keisari Y, Sharon N (1995) Nonopsonic phagocytosis of microorganisms. Annu Rev Microbiol 49:239–276

Ogra PL, Losonsky GA, Fishaut M (1983) Colostrum-derived immunity and maternal-neonatal interaction. Ann N Y Acad Sci 409:82–95

Oltz EM (2001) Regulation of antigen receptor gene assembly in lymphocytes. Immunol Res 23:121–133

Onyemelukwe GC, Leinoen M, Makela H, Greenwood BM (1985) Response to pneumococcal vaccination in normal and post-infected Nigerians. J Infect 11:139–144

Ortaldo JR, Winkler-Pickett RT, Nagashima K, Yagita H, Okumura K (1992) Direct evidence for release of pore-forming protein during NK cellular lysis. J Leukoc Biol 52:483–488

Palfi M, Hilden JO, Gottvall T, Selbing A (1998) Placental transport of maternal immunoglobulin G in pregnancies at risk of Rh (D) hemolytic disease of the newborn. Am J Reprod Immunol 39:323–328

Paloczi K (1999) Immunophenotypic and functional characterization of human umbilical cord blood mononuclear cells. Leukemia 13(Suppl 1):S87–S89

Panaro A, Amati A, di Loreto M, Felle R, Ferrante M, Papadia AM, Porfido N, Gambatesa V, Dell'Osso A, Lucivero G (1991) Lymphocyte subpopulations in pediatric age. Definition of reference values by flow cytometry. Allergol Immunopathol (Madr) 19:109–112

Panes J, Granger DN (1994) Leukocyte-endothelial cell interactions: implications for the pathogenesis and treatment of gastrointestinal disease. Dig Dis 12:232–241

Payne NR, Fleit HB (1996) Extremely low birth weight infants have lower Fc gamma RIII (CD 16) plasma levels and their PMN produce less Fc gamma RIII compared to adults. Biol Neonate 69:235–242

Payne NR, Frestedt J, Hunkeler N, Gehrz R (1993) Cell-surface expression of immunoglobulin G receptors on the polymorphonuclear leukocytes and monocytes of extremely premature infants. Pediatr Res 33:452–457

Peakman M, Buggins AG, Nicolaides KH, Layton DM, Vergani D (1992) Analysis of lymphocyte phenotypes in cord blood from early gestation fetuses. Clin Exp Immunol 90:345–350

Petty RE, Hunt DW (1998) Neonatal dendritic cells. Vaccine 16:1378–1382

Phillips JH, Hori T, Nagler A, Bhat N, Spits H, Lanier LL (1992) Ontogeny of human natural killer (NK) cells: fetal NK cells mediate cytolytic function and express cytoplasmic CD3 epsilon,delta proteins. J Exp Med 175:1055–1066

Piccinni MP, Beloni L, Giannarini L, Livi C, Scarselli G, Romagnani S, Maggi E (1996) Abnormal production of T helper 2 cytokines interleukin-4 and interleukin-5 by T cells from newborns with atopic parents. Eur J Immunol 26:2293–2298

Pirenne H, Aujard Y, Eljaafari A, Bourillon A, Oury JF, Le Gac S, Blot P, Sterkers G (1992) Comparison of T cell functional changes during childhood with the ontogeny of CDw29 and CD45RA expression on CD4+ T cells. Pediatr Res 32:81–86

Pirenne-Ansart H, Paillard F, De Groote D, Eljaafari A, Le Gac S, Blot P, Franchimont P, Vaquero C, Sterkers G (1995) Defective cytokine expression but adult-type T-cell receptor, CD8, and p56lck modulation in CD3- or CD2-activated T cells from neonates. Pediatr Res 37:64–69

Porcellini A, Manna A, Manna M, Talevi N, Delfini C, Moretti L, Rizzoli V (1983) Ontogeny of granulocyte-macrophage progenitor cells in the human fetus. Int J Cell Cloning 1:92–104

Puel A, Ziegler SF, Buckley RH, Leonard WJ (1998) Defective IL7R expression in T(−)B(+)NK(+) severe combined immunodeficiency. Nat Genet 20:394–397

Qian JX, Lee SM, Suen Y, Knoppel E, van de Ven C, Cairo MS (1997) Decreased interleukin-15 from activated cord versus adult peripheral blood mononuclear cells and the effect of interleukin-15 in upregulating anti-tumor immune activity and cytokine production in cord blood. Blood 90:3106–3117

Quinn MT, Gauss KA (2004) Structure and regulation of the neutrophil respiratory burst oxidase: comparison with nonphagocyte oxidases. J Leukoc Biol 76:760–781

Reddy RK, Xia Y, Hanikyrova M, Ross GD (1998) A mixed population of immature and mature leucocytes in umbilical cord blood results in a reduced expression

and function of CR3 (CD11b/CD18). Clin Exp Immunol 114:462–467

Reen DJ, Early E (1998) Cord blood 'naive' T cells demonstrate distinct immunological properties compared with their adult counterparts. Bone Marrow Transplant 22(Suppl 1):S35

Ridings J, Nicholson IC, Goldsworthy W, Haslam R, Roberton DM, Zola H (1997) Somatic hypermutation of immunoglobulin genes in human neonates. Clin Exp Immunol 108:366–374

Risdon G, Gaddy J, Stehman FB, Broxmeyer HE (1994) Proliferative and cytotoxic responses of human cord blood T lymphocytes following allogeneic stimulation. Cell Immunol 154:14–24

Rognum TO, Thrane S, Stoltenberg L, Vege A, Brandtzaeg P (1992) Development of intestinal mucosal immunity in fetal life and the first postnatal months. Pediatr Res 32:145–149

Roncarolo MG, Bigler M, Ciuti E, Martino S, Tovo PA (1994) Immune responses by cord blood cells. Blood Cells 20:573–585; discussion 85-6

Rosen SD (2004) Ligands for L-selectin: homing, inflammation, and beyond. Annu Rev Immunol 22:129–156

Rudin CM, Thompson CB (1998) B-cell development and maturation. Semin Oncol 25:435–446

Ruoslahti E (1988) Fibronectin and its receptors. Annu Rev Biochem 57:375–413

Sacchi F, Rondini G, Mingrat G, Stronati M, Gancia GP, Marseglia GL, Siccardi AG (1982) Different maturation of neutrophil chemotaxis in term and preterm newborn infants. J Pediatr 101:273–274

Sanjeevi CB, Vivekanandan S, Narayanan PR (1991) Fetal response to maternal ascariasis as evidenced by anti *Ascaris lumbricoides* IgM antibodies in the cord blood. Acta Paediatr Scand 80:1134–1138

Santiago-Schwarz F, Fleit HB (1988) Identification of nonadherent mononuclear cells in human cord blood that differentiate into macrophages. J Leukoc Biol 43:51–59

Sato T, Laver JH, Aiba Y, Ogawa M (1999) NK cell colony formation from human fetal thymocytes. Exp Hematol 27:726–733

Sautois B, Fillet G, Beguin Y (1997) Comparative cytokine production by in vitro stimulated mononucleated cells from cord blood and adult blood. Exp Hematol 25:103–108

Schaub B, Liu J, Schleich I, Hoppler S, Sattler C, von Mutius E (2008) Impairment of T helper and T regulatory cell responses at birth. Allergy 63:1438–1447

Schelonka RL, Raaphorst FM, Infante D, Kraig E, Teale JM, Infante AJ (1998) T cell receptor repertoire diversity and clonal expansion in human neonates. Pediatr Res 43:396–402

Schibler KR, Liechty KW, White WL, Rothstein G, Christensen RD (1992) Defective production of interleukin-6 by monocytes: a possible mechanism underlying several host defense deficiencies of neonates. Pediatr Res 31:18–21

Schibler KR, Trautman MS, Liechty KW, White WL, Rothstein G, Christensen RD (1993) Diminished transcription of interleukin-8 by monocytes from preterm neonates. J Leukoc Biol 53:399–403

Schroeder HW Jr, Hillson JL, Perlmutter RM (1987) Early restriction of the human antibody repertoire. Science 238:791–793

Segal AW (2005) How neutrophils kill microbes. Annu Rev Immunol:197–223

Seghaye MC, Heyl W, Grabitz RG, Schumacher K, von Bernuth G, Rath W, Duchateau J (1998) The production of pro- and anti-inflammatory cytokines in neonates assessed by stimulated whole cord blood culture and by plasma levels at birth. Biol Neonate 73:220–227

Series IM, Pichette J, Carrier C, Masson M, Bedard PM, Beaudoin J, Hebert J (1991) Quantitative analysis of T and B cell subsets in healthy and sick premature infants. Early Hum Dev 26:143–154

Shaik SS, Soltau TD, Chaturvedi G, Totapally B, Hagood JS, Andrews WW, Athar M, Voitenok NN, Killingsworth CR, Patel RP, Fallon MB, Maheshwari A (2009) Low intensity shear stress increases endothelial ELR+ CXC chemokine production via a focal adhesion kinase-p38{beta} MAPK-NF-{kappa}B pathway. J Biol Chem 284:5945–5955

Shepard JL, Zon LI (2000) Developmental derivation of embryonic and adult macrophages. Curr Opin Hematol 7:3–8

Shroff KE, Meslin K, Cebra JJ (1995) Commensal enteric bacteria engender a self-limiting humoral mucosal immune response while permanently colonizing the gut. Infect Immun 63:3904–3913

Siegel I, Gleicher N (1981) Development of the fetal immune system. Prog Clin Biol Res 70:31–40

Sloan-Lancaster J, Allen PM (1996) Altered peptide ligand-induced partial T cell activation: molecular mechanisms and role in T cell biology. Annu Rev Immunol 14:1–27

Smith PD, Smythies LE, Mosteller-Barnum M, Sibley DA, Russell MW, Merger M, Sellers MT, Orenstein JM, Shimada T, Graham MF, Kubagawa H (2001) Intestinal macrophages lack CD14 and CD89 and consequently are down-regulated for LPS- and IgA-mediated activities. J Immunol 167:2651–2656

Smyth MJ, Kelly JM, Sutton VR, Davis JE, Browne KA, Sayers TJ, Trapani JA (2001) Unlocking the secrets of cytotoxic granule proteins. J Leukoc Biol 70:18–29

Smythies LE, Sellers M, Clements RH, Mosteller-Barnum-M, Meng G, Benjamin WH, Orenstein JM, Smith PD (2005) Human intestinal macrophages display profound inflammatory anergy despite avid phagocytic and bacteriocidal activity. J Clin Invest 115:66–75

Smythies LE, Maheshwari A, Clements R, Eckhoff D, Novak L, Vu HL, Mosteller-Barnum LM, Sellers M, Smith PD (2006a) Mucosal IL-8 and TGF-{beta} recruit blood monocytes: evidence for cross-talk between the lamina propria stroma and myeloid cells. J Leukoc Biol 80:492

Smythies LE, Maheshwari A, Clements R, Eckhoff D, Novak L, Vu HL, Mosteller-Barnum LM, Sellers M, Smith PD (2006b) Mucosal IL-8 and TGF-beta recruit

blood monocytes: evidence for cross-talk between the lamina propria stroma and myeloid cells. J Leukoc Biol 80:492–499

Sonnenberg GF, Fouser LA, Artis D (2011) Border patrol: regulation of immunity, inflammation and tissue homeostasis at barrier surfaces by IL-22. Nat Immunol 12:383–390

Speer CP, Ambruso DR, Grimsley J, Johnston RB Jr (1985) Oxidative metabolism in cord blood monocytes and monocyte-derived macrophages. Infect Immun 50:919–921

Speer CP, Wieland M, Ulbrich R, Gahr M (1986) Phagocytic activities in neonatal monocytes. Eur J Pediatr 145:418–421

Spencer J, Finn T, Isaacson PG (1985) Gut associated lymphoid tissue: a morphological and immunocytochemical study of the human appendix. Gut 26:672–679

Spencer J, MacDonald TT, Finn T, Isaacson PG (1986) The development of gut associated lymphoid tissue in the terminal ileum of fetal human intestine. Clin Exp Immunol 64:536–543

Spencer J, MacDonald TT, Isaacson PG (1987) Heterogeneity of non-lymphoid cells expressing HLA-D region antigens in human fetal gut. Clin Exp Immunol 67:415–424

Spencer J, Isaacson PG, Walker-Smith JA, MacDonald TT (1989) Heterogeneity in intraepithelial lymphocyte subpopulations in fetal and postnatal human small intestine. J Pediatr Gastroenterol Nutr 9:173–177

Spits H, Lanier LL, Phillips JH (1995) Development of human T and natural killer cells. Blood 85:2654–2670

Spits H, Blom B, Jaleco AC, Weijer K, Verschuren MC, van Dongen JJ, Heemskerk MH, Res PC (1998) Early stages in the development of human T, natural killer and thymic dendritic cells. Immunol Rev 165:75–86

Splawski JB, Jelinek DF, Lipsky PE (1991) Delineation of the functional capacity of human neonatal lymphocytes. J Clin Invest 87:545–553

Splawski JB, Nishioka J, Nishioka Y, Lipsky PE (1996) CD40 ligand is expressed and functional on activated neonatal T cells. J Immunol 156:119–127

Starnes LM, Sorrentino A, Pelosi E, Ballarino M, Morsilli O, Biffoni M, Santoro S, Felli N, Castelli G, De Marchis ML, Mastroberardino G, Gabbianelli M, Fatica A, Bozzoni I, Nervi C, Peschle C (2009) NFI-A directs the fate of hematopoietic progenitors to the erythroid or granulocytic lineage and controls {beta}-globin and G-CSF receptor expression. Blood 114:1753

Steele CR, Oppenheim DE, Hayday AC (2000) Gamma (delta) T cells: non-classical ligands for non-classical cells. Curr Biol 10:R282–R285

Stiehm ER, Mann D, Newland C, Sztein MB, Steeg PS, Oppenheim JJ, Blaese RM (1983) Deficient DR antigen expression on human neonatal monocytes: reversal with lymphokines. Birth Defects Orig Artic Ser 19:295–298

Stiehm ER, Sztein MB, Steeg PS, Mann D, Newland C, Blaese M, Oppenheim JJ (1984) Deficient DR antigen expression on human cord blood monocytes: reversal with lymphokines. Clin Immunol Immunopathol 30:430–436

Stites DP, Pavia CS (1979) Ontogeny of human T cells. Pediatrics 64:795–802

Strominger JL (1989) Developmental biology of T cell receptors. Science 244:943–950

Strunk T, Temming P, Gembruch U, Reiss I, Bucsky P, Schultz C (2004) Differential maturation of the innate immune response in human fetuses. Pediatr Res 56:219–226

Sullivan SE, Staba SL, Gersting JA, Hutson AD, Theriaque D, Christensen RD, Calhoun DA (2002) Circulating concentrations of chemokines in cord blood, neonates, and adults. Pediatr Res 51:653–657

Takahashi N, Imanishi K, Nishida H, Uchiyama T (1995) Evidence for immunologic immaturity of cord blood T cells. Cord blood T cells are susceptible to tolerance induction to in vitro stimulation with a superantigen. J Immunol 155:5213–5219

Takahashi T, Yoshida Y, Hatano S, Sugita-Konishi Y, Igimi S, Yajima M, Kojima T, Kanno T, Yonekubo A, Yajima T, Kuwata T (2002) Reactivity of secretory IgA antibodies in breast milk from 107 Japanese mothers to 20 environmental antigens. Biol Neonate 82:238–242

Takashina T (1987) Haemopoiesis in the human yolk sac. J Anat 151:125–135

Teyton L, Apostolopoulos V, Cantu C 3rd, Celia H, Mallet-Designe V, Stefanko R, Stramann T, Wallace M (2000) Function and dysfunction of T cell receptor: structural studies. Immunol Res 21:325–330

Thilaganathan B, Mansur CA, Morgan G, Nicolaides KH (1992) Fetal T-lymphocyte subpopulations in normal pregnancies. Fetal Diagn Ther 7:53–61

Thomas RM, Linch DC (1983) Identification of lymphocyte subsets in the newborn using a variety of monoclonal antibodies. Arch Dis Child 58:34–38

Toivanen P, Uksila J, Leino A, Lassila O, Hirvonen T, Ruuskanen O (1981) Development of mitogen responding T cells and natural killer cells in the human fetus. Immunol Rev 57:89–105

Toubert A, Douay C, Chalumeau N, Garderet L, Dulphy N, Zilber MT, Gelin C, Mooney N, Charron D (1998) Effects of superantigenic stimulation on the cord blood alphabeta T cell repertoire. Bone Marrow Transplant 22(Suppl 1):S36–S38

Trinchieri G (1989) Biology of natural killer cells. Adv Immunol 47:187–376

Trinchieri G, Valiante N (1993) Receptors for the Fc fragment of IgG on natural killer cells. Nat Immun 12:218–234

Turkmen M, Satar M, Atici A (2000) Neutrophil chemotaxis and random migration in preterm and term infants with sepsis. Am J Perinatol 17:107–112

Ugazio AG, Marcioni AF, Astaldi A Jr, Burgio GR (1974) Peripheral blood B lymphocytes in infancy and childhood. Acta Paediatr Scand 63:205–208

van Elburg RM, Fetter WP, Bunkers CM, Heymans HS (2003) Intestinal permeability in relation to birth weight

and gestational and postnatal age. Arch Dis Child Fetal Neonatal Ed 88:F52–F55
Velilla PA, Rugeles MT, Chougnet CA (2006) Defective antigen-presenting cell function in human neonates. Clin Immunol 121:251–259
Viret C, Janeway CA Jr (1999) MHC and T cell development. Rev Immunogenet 1:91–104
Volpe R (1996) Graves' disease/model of SCID mouse. Exp Clin Endocrinol Diabetes 104(Suppl 3):37–40
Wagner JG, Roth RA (2000) Neutrophil migration mechanisms, with an emphasis on the pulmonary vasculature. Pharmacol Rev 52:349–374
Wan AK, Seow WK, Purdie DM, Bird PS, Walsh LJ, Tudehope DI (2003) Immunoglobulins in saliva of preterm and full-term infants. Oral Microbiol Immunol 18:72–78
Weatherstone KB, Rich EA (1989) Tumor necrosis factor/cachectin and interleukin-1 secretion by cord blood monocytes from premature and term neonates. Pediatr Res 25:342–346
Weaver CT, Harrington LE, Mangan PR, Gavrieli M, Murphy KM (2006) Th17: an effector CD4 T cell lineage with regulatory T cell ties. Immunity 24:677–688
Weemaes C, Klasen I, Goertz J, Beldhuis-Valkis M, Olafsson O, Haraldsson A (2003) Development of immunoglobulin A in infancy and childhood. Scand J Immunol 58:642–648
Weil GJ, Hussain R, Kumaraswami V, Tripathy SP, Phillips KS, Ottesen EA (1983) Prenatal allergic sensitization to helminth antigens in offspring of parasite-infected mothers. J Clin Invest 71:1124–1129
Weinberg AG, Rosenfeld CR, Manroe BL, Browne R (1985) Neonatal blood cell count in health and disease. II. Values for lymphocytes, monocytes, and eosinophils. J Pediatr 106:462–466
Weinberger B, Laskin DL, Mariano TM, Sunil VR, DeCoste CJ, Heck DE, Gardner CR, Laskin JD (2001) Mechanisms underlying reduced responsiveness of neonatal neutrophils to distinct chemoattractants. J Leukoc Biol 70:969–976
Weston WL, Carson BS, Barkin RM, Slater GD, Dustin RD, Hecht SK (1977) Monocyte-macrophage function in the newborn. Am J Dis Child 131:1241–1242
Wilders MM, Sminia T, Janse EM (1983) Ontogeny of non-lymphoid and lymphoid cells in the rat gut with special reference to large mononuclear Ia-positive dendritic cells. Immunology 50:303–314
Williams TJ, Jones CA, Miles EA, Warner JO, Warner JA (2000) Fetal and neonatal IL-13 production during pregnancy and at birth and subsequent development of atopic symptoms. J Allergy Clin Immunol 105:951–959
Williams AM, Bland PW, Phillips AC, Turner S, Brooklyn T, Shaya G, Spicer RD, Probert CS (2004) Intestinal alpha beta T cells differentiate and rearrange antigen receptor genes in situ in the human infant. J Immunol 173:7190–7199
Williams DA, Xu H, Cancelas JA (2006) Children are not little adults: just ask their hematopoietic stem cells. J Clin Invest 116:2593–2596
Wilson CB (1986) Immunologic basis for increased susceptibility of the neonate to infection. J Pediatr 108:1–12
Wilson CB (1991) The ontogeny of T lymphocyte maturation and function. J Pediatr 118:S4–S9
Wilson M, Rosen FS, Schlossman SF, Reinherz EL (1985) Ontogeny of human T and B lymphocytes during stressed and normal gestation: phenotypic analysis of umbilical cord lymphocytes from term and preterm infants. Clin Immunol Immunopathol 37:1–12
Wilson CB, Lewis DB, English BK (1991) T cell development in the fetus and neonate. Adv Exp Med Biol 310:17–27
Wilson CB, Penix L, Weaver WM, Melvin A, Lewis DB (1992) Ontogeny of T lymphocyte function in the neonate. Am J Reprod Immunol 28:132–135
Wilson NJ, Boniface K, Chan JR, McKenzie BS, Blumenschein WM, Mattson JD, Basham B, Smith K, Chen T, Morel F, Lecron JC, Kastelein RA, Cua DJ, McClanahan TK, Bowman EP, de Waal Malefyt R (2007) Development, cytokine profile and function of human interleukin 17-producing helper T cells. Nat Immunol 8:950–957
Xanthou M (1970) Leucocyte blood picture in healthy full-term and premature babies during neonatal period. Arch Dis Child 45:242–249
Yachie A, Takano N, Yokoi T, Kato K, Kasahara Y, Miyawaki T, Taniguchi N (1990) The capability of neonatal leukocytes to produce IL-6 on stimulation assessed by whole blood culture. Pediatr Res 27:227–233
Yeung CY, Hobbs JR (1968) Serum-gamma-G-globulin levels in normal premature, post-mature, and "small-for-dates" newborn babies. Lancet 1:1167–1170
Yoder MC, Lanker TA, Engle WA (1988) Culture medium oxygen tension affects fibronectin production in human adult and cord blood macrophages. Immunol Lett 19:1–6
Zemlin M, Bauer K, Hummel M, Pfeiffer S, Devers S, Zemlin C, Stein H, Versmold HT (2001) The diversity of rearranged immunoglobulin heavy chain variable region genes in peripheral blood B cells of preterm infants is restricted by short third complementarity-determining regions but not by limited gene segment usage. Blood 97:1511–1513

Congenital Immunodeficiencies in Newborns

100

Alessandro Plebani, Gaetano Chirico, and Vassilios Lougaris

Contents

A. Plebani (✉) · V. Lougaris
Pediatrics Clinic, Department of Clinical and Experimental Sciences, University of Brescia and Spedali Civili of Brescia, Brescia, Italy
e-mail: alessandro.plebani@unibs.it

G. Chirico
Neonatology and Intensive Neonatal Therapy Unit, Spedali Civili of Brescia, Brescia, Italy

G. Buonocore et al. (eds.), *Neonatology*,
https://doi.org/10.1007/978-3-319-29489-6_247

Abstract

Congenital immunodeficiency diseases are a group of primarily single-gene disorders of the immune system. To date, more than 300 genetic defects have been identified as responsible for congenital immunodeficiencies. Although diverse, these diseases share the common features of susceptibility to infections and result in substantial morbidity and shortened life spans. The severity of congenital immunodeficiencies largely depends on the arm of the immune system affected, and being congenital many of these disorders have their clinical symptoms early in infancy. In syndromic immunodeficiencies, the defects of the immune system may not represent the major clinical problem. Most important, prompt diagnosis and treatment can lead in marked improvement in the quality and length of life and better outcome. The possibility to apply the neonatal screening test for severe combined immunodeficiency will further ameliorate patients' outcome.

100.1 Salient Points

- Congenital immunodeficiencies may present in newborns.
- Severity of infections depends largely from the underlined defect.
- Failure to thrive and/or chronic diarrhea in infancy should lead to suspect a primary immunodeficiency.
- Admission to ICU for respiratory distress or invasive infection should alert physicians for congenital immunodeficiency.
- Persistent candidiasis and neonatal skin rush (maternal engraftment) should be carefully evaluated.
- Lymphopenia and/or hypogammaglobulinemia are strongly suggestive for congenital defects of the immune system.
- Immune defects may be associated to different syndromic conditions.

The primary immunodeficiency diseases (PIDs) are a heterogeneous group of inherited disorders with defects in one or more components of the immune system, leading to an increased susceptibility to infections. Classically, primary immunodeficiency diseases are classified into T lymphocyte, B lymphocyte, phagocytic cell, and complement deficiencies. This classification is simple and practical because clinical symptoms, mainly susceptibility to infections, are distinct according to the arm of the immune system affected.

With advances in diagnostic and therapeutics these disorders have been better understood and more successfully treated, yet their prognosis depends on early recognition of the disorder and initiation of the appropriate management.

Evaluation of immune function should be considered for children with clinical symptoms suggestive of a distinct immune disorder or with unusual, chronic, or recurrent infections such as: one or more systemic bacterial infections (sepsis, meningitis); two or more serious bacterial infections (cellulitis, suppurative otitis media, pneumonia, lymphoadenitis) within 1 year; serious infections occurring at unusual sites (liver, brain abscess); infections with opportunistic pathogens (*Aspergillus, Serratia marcescens, Pneumocisti jierovecii, Cryptosporidium, Nocardia*); and infections with common childhood pathogen but with unusual severity.

Severe or recurrent infections caused by encapsulated bacteria suggest a primary B cell or complement defect, and they occur after the first 6–12 months of age, in parallel with the decrease of the maternally acquired IgG. On the contrary severe viral (adenovirus, cytomegalovirus, respiratory syncytial virus), fungal, or opportunistic infections, occurring during the first few months of life, are more indicative of a primary T cell defect. A history of consanguineity or a positive family history for congenital immunodeficiencies are helpful for an early diagnosis, as well as the presence of typical signs, such as the absence of lymphoid tissue or the presence of syndromic features.

A complete blood count, with differential count, and assessement of immunoglobulin serum levels are the most cost-effective diagnostic screening tests. Normal neutrophil counts and

normal platelet size or counts allow to roule out neutropenia and Wiskott-Aldrich syndrome, respectively. If the absolute lymphocyte count is normal, the patient is not likely to have a severe T cell defect, because T cells normally represent 70% of circulating lymphocytes, and their absence results in severe lymphopenia. This is not the case for T^-B^+ severe combined immunodeficiencies, in which absolute lymphocyte count is normal, because of the presence of circulating B cells. In this case, cytofluorimetric analysis of B and T cell subsets will reveal that virtually all lymbcocytes belong to the B cell lineage. Functional defects of T cell lineage may account for combined immunodeficiencies with mild T cell lymphopenia. Low immunoglobulin serum levels with normal T cell counts points to a diagnosis of a primary B cell defect. Knowledge of the normal values for absolute lymphocyte counts and for immunoglobulin serum levels, at various ages in infancy and childhood, is crucial for the diagnosis of PIDs. Normal neutrophils and T and B cell counts should point to a functional defect of phagocytes. The genes for many PIDs are known, which may lead to a successful neonatal screening program. In this chapter we will focus on T and B cell defects, as defects of phagocytes and complement will be discussed elsewhere.

100.2 Defects of the B Cell Compartement

100.2.1 Agammaglobulinemia Either X-Linked (XLA or Bruton's Agammaglobulinemia) or Autosomal Recessive Agammaglobulinemia (ARA)

XLA and ARA represent the prototype of the disorders of the B cell compartment. Both disorders are characterized by absent/low immunoglobulin serum levels, defective antibody response to antigens, and absence of circulating B cells in the presence of normal T cell counts and function. Both disorders result from an early block of B cell development, caused, in XLA, by mutations in the gene encoding Bruton's tyrosine kinase (Btk), which has a crucial role in early B cell differentiation. XLA accounts for 70–90% of agammaglobulinemic patients. Six distinct autosomal recessive genetic defects have been found to cause ARA, including mutations in the genes encoding: the μ heavy chain gene; the Igα and Igβ signalling molecules; B cell linker adaptor protein (BLNK); the surrogate light chain, λ5/14.1; and the p85α subunit of PI3K (Table 1). Recently an autosomal dominant form of agammaglobulinemia due to mutation in the gene encoding for TCF3 has been reported (Boisson et al. 2013) (Table 1). Translocation involving the gene encoding for the leucine-rich repeat-containing 8 (LRRC8) has been reported to cause agammaglobulinemia in a syndromic patient. With the exception of BLNK, p85α, TCF3, and LRRC8, the other genes encode for proteins entering the B cell receptor complex which is crucial for transducing the signals leading to early B cell development (Conley et al. 2009; Mohiuddin et al. 2013). Onset of symptoms in agammaglobulinemia occurs early in infancy, usually between the ages of 6–12 months, in parallel with the decrease of the maternally acquired IgG. However, in extremely preterm infants an earlier onset of infections may be observed. A positive family history for primary immunodeficiencies is an indication for an immunological investigation even in the absence of clinical symptoms. Bacterial infections are the most common clinical manifestations of agammaglobulinemia, usually substaind by *Streptococcus pneumoniae*, *Haemophylus influenzae*, *Staphylococcus aureus*, and *pseudomonas* species. Infections include otitis media, sinusitis, pneumonia, sepsis, and meningitis. Other bacterial species, such as *Salmonella* and *Campylobacter*, have also been described and account for gastrointestinal infections. Viral infections are usually handled normally with the exception of hepatitis viruses and enteroviruses (Conley et al. 2009). Live attenuated vaccines should not be administered. On physical examination, lymphoid hypoplasia, with minimal or no tonsillar tissue and no palpable lymph nodes, is frequently observed. Patients found to have low/absent immunoglobulin serum levels should have their B cells enumerated by flow cytometry using

Table 1 Agammaglobulinemia: clinical and genetic heterogeneity

Disease	Inheritance	Gene defect	Clinical phenotype	Prevalence in agammaglobulinemia
BTK deficiency	XL	*BTK*	Early and late onset, bacterial infections	85%
μ heavy chain deficiency	AR	*IGHM*	Early and late onset, bacterial infections	15%
λ5 chain deficiency	AR	*IGLL1*	Early and late onset, bacterial infections	
Igα chain deficiency	AR	*CD79A*	Early and late onset, bacterial infections	
Igβ chain deficiecny	AR	*CD79B*	Early and late onset, bacterial infections	
BLNK deficiency	AR	*BLNK*	Early and late onset viral and bacterial infections	
p85α deficiency	AR	*PIK3R1*	Early and late onset bacterial infections	
TCF3 deficiency	AD	*E47*	Early and late onset bacterial infections	

XL X-linked, *AR* autosomal recessive, *AD* autosomal dominant

monoclonal antibodies against CD19 or CD20. Normally, approximately 10% of circulating lymphocytes are B cells. B cells are absent (<1%) in both XLA and ARA; on the contrary hypogammaglobulinemia in the presence of normal B cell counts is suggestive of a diagnosis of common variable immunodeficiency (CVID). This distinction is important, because children with hypogammaglobulinemia due to XLA/ARA or CVID can have different clinical problems, and the two conditions clearly have different inheritance patterns. Although CVID is considered a disorder of the adults, it may occur in infancy as well. However, because of the transient hypogammaglobulinemia of infancy, a definite diagnosis of CVID cannot be made early in life unless a defective antibody response to antigens is documented. Gene sequence analysis of the genes recently identified to cause CVID (*ICOS*, inducible costimulator; *TACI*, transmembrane activator, calcium modulator, and cyclophilin ligand interactor; *BAFF-R*, B cell activating factor of the TNF family receptor, *CD19*, *CD20*, *CD21*, *CD81*, *LRBA*, *NFKB1*, *NFKB2*), is a useful tool for providing a definite early diagnosis. However, mutations of these genes account only for 10–15% of CVID patients (Conley et al. 2009; Park et al. 2009; Lougaris et al. 2014).

Immunoglobulin replacement therapy is the treatment of choice in agammaglobulinemic patients. Current protocols are based on intravenous immunoglobulins (IVIG) or subcutaneous immunoglobulins (SCIG). It is widely accepted, based on different international studies, that maintaining preinfusion IgG levels >500 mg/dl assures a notable reduction in the number of infections. This protective IgG level is usually achieved by administration of 400/mg/kg every 3–4 weeks for the endovenous route or administration of 100 mg/kg/dose every week for the subcutaneous one.

100.2.2 The Hyper IgM Syndrome (HIGM)

HIGM is a heterogeneous group of genetic disorders characterized by normal/elevated IgM, associated with low IgG and IgA serum levels, as a result of a defect in the immunoglobulin class switch recombination process, and normal T and B cell counts. X-linked and autosomal recessive

forms of the disorder have been identified (Geha et al. 2007; Durandy et al. 2007) (Table 2). Recently, monoallelic dominant mutations in *PIK3R1* were described in patients with an HIGM-like syndrome (Deau et al. 2014). The X-linked forms are caused by mutations of the *CD40LG* (CD40 ligand deficiency) or *IKBKG* (NEMO deficiency) genes. The autosomal recessive forms are due to mutations of the *AICDA* (AID deficiency), *UNG* (UNG deficiency), or of the *TNFRFS5* (CD40 deficiency) genes. Distinct clinical features are associated to different genetic defects. Namely, CD40 ligand deficiency and CD40 deficiency are the most severe forms and their clinical presentation is similar to that observed in immunodeficiencies characterized by functional T cell defects. In fact, CD40L is expressed on activated CD4 T cells and CD40 on B and dendritic cells, thus a defective expression of these molecules ultimately lead to a defect of T cell priming. Most patients present in infancy with bacterial infections of the upper and lower respiratory tract and have a unique predisposition to *Pneumocystis jierovici* pneumonia (PCP). These patients are also susceptible to infection with opportunistic pathogens, such as *cytomegalovirus*, *Histoplasma capsulatum*, *Cryptococcus*, and *Cryptosporidium parvum*; the latter is associated with chronic diarrhea. Infection of the biliary tree with *Cryptosporidium parvum* may predispose patients to sclerosing colangitis and to tumor of the liver, pancreas, or biliary tree. Neutropenia is a common finding of the CD40 ligand deficiency. NEMO deficiency is easily recognizable because of the presence of anhydrotic ectodermal dysplasia with sparse scalp hear, conical teeth, and absent sweat glands.

Table 2 Immunodeficiency with Hyper IgM: clinical and genetic heterogeneity

Disease	Inheritance	Gene defect	Clinical feature
CD40 ligand (CD40L) deficiency	XL	*CD40LG*	Bacterial and opportunistic infections, neutropenia, liver disease
AID deficiency	AR	*AICDA*	Bacterial infections, enlarged lymph nodes and tonsils
CD40 deficiency	AR	*TNFRSF5*	Bacterial and opportunistic infection, liver disease
NEMO deficiency	XL	*IKBKG*	Bacterial and opportunistic infections, ectodermal dysplasia
UNG deficiency	AR	*UNG*	Bacterial infections, enlarged lymph nodes and tonsils
PI3KR1 loss of function	AD	*PIK3R1*	Viral and bacterial infections, enlarged lymph nodes and tonsils, short stature, increased risk for lymphoma development

XL X-linked, *AR* autosomal recessive, *AD* autosomal dominant

The HIGM syndromes due to mutations of AID and UNG are considered primary B cell defects. These patients have an increased susceptibility to bacterial infections, similar to that observed in agammaglobulinemic patients; lymphoid hyperplasia is typical of these disorders.

In the case of low/absent levels of serum IgG and IgA, with normal/elevated IgM, the diagnosis of CD40 ligand deficiency or CD40 deficiency is usually accomplished by demonstrating the inability of activated patients' CD4+ T cells to express functional CD40L or of patients' B cells to express the CD40 molecule, respectively. Diagnosis of HIGM caused by mutations in the remaining genes requires gene sequence analysis.

The HIGM-like syndrome associated with *PIK3R1* monoallelic mutations has been described in a small number of patients and is characterized by a B cell maturational defect leading to the classical immunological HIGM phenotype, enlarged lymph nodes, splenomegaly, short stature, viral infections, and mild T cell functional defects.

Except for CD40 ligand deficiency and CD40 deficiency, for which stem cell transplantation is

recommended (Geha et al. 2007), appropriate use of antibiotics to treat documented infections and regular administration of intravenous immunoglobulins are the only effective treatments for these disorders. In addition, patients with CD40 ligand deficiency and CD40 deficiency should receive co-trimoxasole as *Pneumocystis carinii* pneumonia prophylaxis; they should drink boiled water, and azithromycin prophylaxis may lessen the risk of *Cryptosporidium parvum* infections.

100.3 Defects of T Cell Compartment

100.3.1 Severe Combined Immunodeficiencies (SCIDs)

SCIDs are a heterogeneous group of congenital disorders characterized by block of T cell differentiation, variably associated with abnormal development of other lymphocyte lineages, such as B or natural killer (NK) cells (Fischer and Notarangelo 2004). The overall frequency of these disorders is estimated to be 1: 50,000–1:100,000 live births. SCIDs results from a large number of disorders with X-linked or AR-inheritance, most of which are now molecularly defined. The clinical presentation is quite uniform, among the various SCIDs. Affected patients present within the first few months of life with infections, mainly of the respiratory and gastrointestinal tract. Oral candidiasis, persistent diarrhea with growth impairement, and/or interstitial pneumonitis are the most frequent manifestations leading to diagnosis. These patients present increased susceptibility to infections substained by opportunistic organisms including *Candida albicans*, *Pneumocystis jiroveci*, and *Aspergillus* species or by viruses (adenovirus, cytomegalovirus, respiratory syncytial virus). Live attenuated vaccines are another cause of severe clinical manifestations. BCG vaccination may lead to disseminated and often lethal infection; progressive central nervous system poliovirus infection can occur secondary to oral polio vaccination or exposure to a recently vaccinated individual; and severe gastroenteritis with vaccine viral shedding may follow rotavirus vaccination.

Noninfectious clinical manifestations consist mainly of graft-versus-host disease (GVHD), presenting with a severe skin rash, caused by maternal engraftment or following transfusion with nonirradiated blood derivatives.

A diagnosis is possible at birth, with most affected infants having lymphopenia (less than 2000 lymphocytes/mm^3). Lymphocyte phenotyping shows severely depleted T lymphocytes number; B lymphocytes and NK cells may be present or absent depending on the type of SCID. If a high T cell count argues against a diagnosis of SCID, but the clinical symptoms are typical enough, a systematic search for the maternal origin of the circulating T cells should be performed. Serum immunoglobulin concentrations are diminished or absent, and no antibody response can be elicited after immunization. Four lymphocyte phenotypes are possible on the basis of the effect of the defective gene on T-cell, B-cell, and NK cell development. The $T^-B^+NK^+$ immunophenotype is due to CD3δ-, CD3γ, CD3e-, CD3ζ, or interleukin-7 receptor α-chain deficiency; a similar immunological phenotype with variable B cell counts is observed in PNP (Purine Nucleoside Phosphorylase) deficiency; the $T^-B^+NK^-$ form includes the X-linked SCID which is due to γc deficiency, and the autosomal recessive forms due to JAK3 (Janus kinase 3), or CD45 deficiency; the $T^-B^-NK^+$ form is caused by RAG1, RAG2 (recombination-activating gene), or Artemis deficiency; the $T^-B^-NK^-$ form is caused by ADA (adenosine-deaminase) deficiency. The presence of autoreactive autologous T lymphocytes in the absence of B cells is typical of Omenn syndrome. A total lack of both lymphocytes and granulocytes is suggestive of reticular dysgenesis which is due to mutations of AK2 (adenilate kinase 2) (Table 3).

The natural course of SCIDs is severe, with most patients dying within the first years of life, unless properly treated. Supportive therapy, which may at best prolong survival, consists in the use of intraveneous immunoglobulins, aggressive treatment of infectious episodes, prophylactic co-trimoxasole (to prevent *Pneumocystis jiroveci* pneumonia), and use of irradiated blood products. Hematopoietic stem cell transplantation (HSCT) often results in

Table 3 Clinical and immunological features of most frequent forms of primary immunodeficiencies with prevalent T cell defects

Disease	T lymphocytes	B lymphocytes	NK cells	Ig serum levels	Inheritance	Peculiar clinical features	Gene defects
SCID T−B−							
– RAG1/ 2 deficiecny	↓↓	↓↓	N	↓	AR	/	RAG1, RAG2
– Artemis deficiency	↓↓	↓↓	N	↓	AR	Radiation sensitivity,	Artemis
– Reticular dysgenesis	↓↓	No ↓	↓	↓	AR	Neutropenia, thrombocytopenia, deafness	AK2
– Adenosine deaminase (ADA) deficiency	↓↓	↓↓	↓	↓	AR	Liver disease, neurological symptoms, costochondral junction flaring	ADA
SCID T−B+							
– X-linked	↓↓	No ↑	↓↓	↓	XL		Common γc (IL-2,4,7,15,21)
– JAK3 deficiency	↓↓	No ↑	↓↓	↓	AR		JAK3
– IL-7Rα deficiency	↓↓	No ↑	N	↓	AR		IL-7 receptor α chain
– CD45 deficiency	↓↓	N	↓	↓	AR		CD45
– CD3 γ/δ/ε/ζ deficiency	↓↓	N	N	↓	AR		CD3 γ/δ/ε/ζ
Purine nucleoside phosphorylase (PNP) deficiency	↓↓	No ↓	N	↓	AR	Autoimmune hemolytic anemia, neurological impairment	PNP
Omenn syndrome	Present in variable number	↓↓	N	↓ (IgE↑)	AR	Erytroderma, adenopathies, hepatosplenomegaly, eosinophilia	RAG1, RAG2, Artemis, RMRP
Nijmegen breakage syndrome (NBS)	↓	↓	N	↓	AR	Microcephaly, developmental defects, radiation sensitivity	NBS1
Ligase IV deficiency	↓	↓	N	↓	AR	Microcephaly, developmental defects, radiation sensitivity	LIG4
Cernunnos/XLF deficiency	↓	↓	N	↓	AR	Microcephaly, developmental defects, radiation sensitivity	Cernunnos/XLP
MHC class II deficiency	CD4↓	N	N	No ↓	AR		CIITA, RFX5, RFXAP, RFXANK
Wiskott-Aldrich syndrome	↓	N	N	IgG and IgM↓, IgA and IgE ↑	XL	Thrombocytopenia with small platelets, eczema, bacterial and viral infections	WAS

N normal, *AR* autosomal recessive, *XL* X-linked

permanent cure, with a survival rate of 90% if an HLA-identical family donor is available. Excellent results (80% survival) have been obtained with HLA-matched unrelated donor and with aploidentical donor (75% survival). ADA-deficient SCID and X-linked SCID have been treated with somatic gene therapy; however, serious adverse events occurred in the case of X-SCID. ADA-deficient SCID is also managed with regular injections of polyethylene glycol conjugate to the bovine-derived adenosine deaminase (PEG-ADA).

100.3.2 Combined Immunodeficiencies (CIDs)

CID is distinguished from SCID by the presence of low but not absent T cell function. Similar to SCID, CID is a syndrome of various genetic defects. Clinical presentation overlaps that of SCID patients, although sometimes infections develop slightly later. Two representative forms of CID are hereby reported.

100.4 MHC Class II Antigen Deficiency

MHC class II antigen deficiency is an autosomal recessive primary immunodeficiency caused by the absence of MHC class II expression on cells normally expressing HLA class II molecules (Rieth et al. 2007). This disorder is caused by mutations in several different genes which code for a complex of regulatory factors controlling transcription of MHC II genes (Table 3).

MHC class II-deficient patients have a very low number of CD4 T cells but normal or elevated numbers of CD8 T cells. Lymphopenia is only moderate. Patients are hypogammaglobulinemic due to impaired antigen-specific responses caused by the absence of antigen-presenting molecules. These patients present, from early infancy, with an increased susceptibility to viral, bacterial, fungal, and protozoan infections, primarily of the respiratory and gastrointestinal tract. Curative treatment is BMT, although it has limited success in comparison with other types of SCID.

100.5 Wiskott-Aldrich Syndrome

The Wiskott-Aldrich syndrome (WAS) is an X-linked recessive disorder characterized by microplatelet thrombocytopenia, eczema, recurrent infections, and increased risk of autoimmunity and lymphoreticular neoplasia (Ochs and Thrasher 2006). Thrombocytopenia and small platelet volume in a male should raise suspicion of the diagnosis. This disorder is caused by mutation of the *WAS* (WASP protein) gene (Table 3). WASP is expressed in all hematopoietic cells, including CD34+ stem cells. Mutation of this gene not only cause WAS but also X-linked thrombocytopenia (XLT), a milder form of the disease characterized by microplatelet thrombocytopenia, but without the clinical findings associated with the classic WAS phenotype. The classic clinical symptoms (bleeding, infections, and eczema) are usually not apparent simultaneously. The earliest manifestation, often present at birth, consists of petechiae and bruises. Additional early manifestations of thrombocytopenia include bloody diarrhea and hemorrage following circumcision. Eczema and recurrent bacterial infections usually develop during the first year of life; later, infections with microorganisms such as *Pneumocystis jiroveci* and the herpesviruses become more frequent. The severity of the immune deficiency can vary depending largely on the mutation and its effect on protein expression. Both T- and B- lymphocyte functions are affected. During infancy the number of circulating lymphocytes might be normal or moderately decreased. By 6 years of age, lymphopenia, caused by a progressive T cell derangement, is a common finding in classic WAS. Consistent findings are low isohemagglutinins titers and marked decreased response to polysaccharide antigens.

Intravenous immunoglobulin, appropriate treatment and control (use of killed vaccines) of infections and eczema, and platelet transfusion for serious bleeding episodes are part of a good supportive therapy. Bone marrow transplantation is the treatment of choice and may be curative. Recently, gene therapy has been applied in a limited number of affected patients with promising results (Worth and Thrasher 2015).

100.6 Immunodeficiencies as Part of Complex Diseases

100.6.1 DiGeorge Syndrome (DGS)

DGS is one of the most common chromosomal disorder known (estimated prevalence of 1/4000–1/6000 persons) and is caused by developmental defects in the third pharyngeal pouch and fourth pharyngeal arch (Goldmuntz 2005). As a result, defects are found in the thymus, heart, and parathyroid glands. Approximately 90% of patients with DGS are hemizygous for 22q11; in rare instances, patients are hemizygous for 10p13. Although classically recognized by the triad of congenital heart defects, immunodeficiency secondary to thymic hypoplasia, and hypocalcemia secondary to parathyroid gland hypoplasia, it is now well recognized that the phenotypic features seen in patients with DGS are much more variable and extensive than previously recognized: DGS shows phenotypic overlap with other disorders including velocadiofacial syndrome (VCFS) and conotruncal anomaly face syndrome (CTAFS), both of which are frequently associated with 22q deletions. Dysmorphic facial features are present in DGS and include hypertelorism; low-set, prominent ears; micrognathia; high arched palate; and short phyltrum of the upper lip. Cardiac defects, dysmorphic facial features, and the occurrence of hypocalcemic seizures occurring during the neonatal period should raise the suspicion of DGS. All children suspected of having DGS should have an immunological work up. Most infants with DGS have a mild and transient immunodeficiency. Immunoglobulin serum levels are usually normal, T cell production is usually moderately impaired, and T cell mitogen responses are often normal or near normal. These patients usually develop normal or near-normal immunologic function over time. Total thymus aplasia is present in less than 1% of cases and accounts for complete DGS which resembles patients with SCID in their immunological phenotype and susceptibility to infections.

Bone marrow and thymus transplantations have been efficaciously performed in complete DGS.

100.6.2 Cartilage Hair Hypoplasia (CHH)

CHH is a rare autosomal recessive chondrodysplasia with growth failure, hypoplastic hair, defective immunity, and eritrogenesis. CHH is caused by mutations in the *RMRP* (ribonuclease mitochondrial RNA-processing) (Hermanns et al. 2006). The disease is prevalent among the Old Order Amish in the United States and in the Finnish population. The growth failure has its onset prenatally and is usually due to the shortness of limbs. All segments of the limbs are affected. The major radiological abnormalities are confined to the metaphyseal parts of the tubular bones, which are flared, scalloped, and irregularly sclerotic. The majority of the patients have sparse, fine, and silky hair. Hirschprung disease and predisposition to malignancies have been reported.

The defective cellular immunity is characterized by mild to moderate lymphopenia and impaired in vitro lymphocyte response to mitogens. Humoral immunity is usually intact. In a few patients a more severe immunological phenotype, similar to combined immunodeficiey (CID), has been reported. Deficient erythrocyte production presents usually as mild macrocytic anemia in early childhood, with spontaneous recovery before adulthood. Occasionally, the patients have severe congenital hypoplastic anemia. Hematopoietic cell transplantation has resulted in successful immunereconstitution in CHH patients who present with CID, but will not affect the morphologic features or dwarfism.

100.6.3 Nijmegen Breakage Syndrome (NBS)

NBS is an autosomal recessive genetic disease belonging to a group of disorders often called chromosome instability syndromes, characterized by microcephaly, particular "bird-like face", growth retardation, immunodeficiency, and predisposition to cancer (The International Nijmegen Breakage Syndrome Study Group 2000). NBS is caused by mutation of *NBS* gene which encodes

for a protein involved in the repair of DNA double-strand breaks. Intrauterine growth delay, in the presence of microcephaly and some facial features (sloping forehead, receding mandible, prominent midface, upward slant of the palpebral fissures), could raise the suspicion of NBS. Chromosomal rearrangements typically involving chromosomes 7 and 14 and chromosomal hypersensitivity to X-irradiation are a useful laboratory test to support the clinical suspicion. A definite diagnosis is achieved by gene sequence analysis; the 657del(5) mutation is present in approximately 90% of cases, simplifying the task of genetic confirmation in many cases. Hypogammaglobulinemia is common. Mild to moderate lymphopenia is present with impaired in vitro lymphocyte proliferative response to mitogens. Many patients suffer from recurrent upper and lower respiratory tract infections, and chronic lung disease is the second leading cause of death; the first cause of death is cancer, with a median of age of cancer-related death of only 10 years. Differential diagnosis should include ligase IV deficiency, Cernunnos deficiency which show overlapping clinical and laboratory findings with NBS (Table 3). Ataxia telangiectasia overlaps NBS in a number of characteristics, including chromosomal instability, radiosensitivity, and cancer predisposition; in contrast AT patients do not display the characteristic "bird-like" facial appearance, microcephaly, and growth retardation of the NBS patients.

100.6.4 Immunodysregulation, Polyendocrinopathy, Enteropathy, X-linked (IPEX)

IPEX is a rare genetic disorder of immune regulation caused by mutations in the *FOXP3* gene located in the centromeric region of the X chromosome (Moraes-Vasconcelos et al. 2008). The product of this gene is required for the development of CD4+ CD25+ T regulatory cells. In the absence of T regulatory cells, activated CD4+ T cells produce multiorgan damage resulting in autoimmune manifestations such as type I diabetes mellitus, severe enteropathy, hypothyroidism, and autoimmune skin disease resembling eczema, psoriasis, or atopic dermatitis. These clinical manifestations, often fatal, usually occur in early infancy and often appear sequentially, rather than simultaneously. Immunologic investigation reveals little beyond variably increased IgE levels, eosinophilia, mild increase in CD4:CD8 ratio, and an increase in T cell activation markers. Autoantibodies are often absent early but develop gradually or acutely. Immunosuppressive drugs have been used with some success. Unfortunately, these drugs do not maintain long-term remission of symptoms, may be toxic, and facilitate opportunistic infections. Hematopoietic stem cell transplantation can be taken into consideration at least for the most severe forms.

100.6.5 Autoimmune Polyendocrinopathy-Candidiasis Ectodermal Dystrophy Syndrome (APECED)

APECED, also known as APS-1 (autoimmune polyglandular syndrome type 1), is an autosomal recessive disorder due to mutation of the *AIRE* (autoimmune regulator) gene (Moraes-Vasconcelos et al. 2008). The product of this gene is crucial for the induction of central tolerance, through the regulation of self-antigen gene expression in the antigen-presenting cells of the thymic medulla. Thus, defects of *AIRE* lead to a defective selection of organ-specific T cells which are responsible for autoimmune manifestations. APECED is characterized by a set of three abnormal features: chronic mucocutaneous candidiasis, hypothyroidisms, and adrenal insufficiency. At least two of these major components need to be present for diagnosis. Usually the first sign of the syndrome is mucocutaneous candidiasis which may occur soon after birth, whereas the other symptoms appear in childhood or later. A characteristic finding relevant to the endocrinopathies of APECED is the existence of high-serum antibody titers reacting specifically with components of the affected endocrine organs. At present management of these patients is based on supportive therapy.

100.6.6 SCID Neonatal Screening Test

The purpose of newborn screening is early detection of inborn conditions for which prompt treatments mitigate mortality or irreversible damage. The first heritable immune disorders to which newborn screening has been applied are those that together comprise severe combined immunodeficiencies (SCID). SCID are caused by defects in any of a diverse group of genes encoding for proteins crucial for the development of adaptive immunity. A feature of all SCID is defective production of T cells. Most SCID are also defective in B cells, but even when B cells are present, they cannot produce antibodies without T cell help. SCID is the most severe primary immunodeficiency and constitutes a pediatric emergency. Affected children are higly susceptible to bacterial, viral, fungal, and opportunistic infections, ultimately leading to death in all cases by the age of 2 years. Hematopoietic stem cell transplantation (HSCT) is extremely effective and the only curative treatment for SCID, allowing the majority of affected children to live normal and fully functional lives. However, the success of HSCT is greatly influenced by age at diagnosis and clinical presentation. A worse outcome is observed for patients who have already experienced recurrent or opportunistic infections before HSCT. SCID neonatal screening test will allow for an even earlier diagnosis of infectious free patients, thus ameliorating patients' outcome. The test developed for population-based SCID newborn screening is quantification (which can be performed on dried blood spot) of an extrachromosomal nonreplicating DNA circle that indicates the presence of recently generated autologous T cells, the T cell receptor excision circle (TREC). Specific TREC sequences are detectable by polymerase chain reaction (PCR), and the number of TREC copies can be counted by quantitative PCR. Low or absent quantities of TRECs is suggestive of SCID. A definite diagnosis has to be confirmed by appropriate immunological investigation. Newborn screening for SCID has been applied in 11 States in the USA and has revealed an incidence of SCID of 1:58,000, which is lower than the one previously considered (Kwan et al. 2014). Identified affected patients underwent early HSCT with positive outcome. TRECs analysis identifies not only patients affected with SCID but also patients affected with complete Di George syndrome and idiopathic T cell lymphopenias. Tandem mass spectrometry can be applied for newborn screening for adenosine deaminase (ADA) deficiency (Azzari et al. 2011). In conclusion, and although in other countries ouside of the USA, the newborn screening program for SCIDs has only been applied in terms of pilot studies, it is likely that in the near future a wider implementation of this test may change the natural history of SCID.

References

Azzari C, la Marca G, Resti M (2011) Neonatal screening for severe combined immunodeficiency caused by an adenosine deaminase defect: a reliable and inexpensive method using tandem mass spectrometry. J Allergy Clin Immunol 127(6):1394–1399

Boisson B, Wang YD, Bosompem A, Ma CS, Lim A, Kochetkov T, Tangye SG, Casanova JL, Conley ME (2013) A recurrent dominant negative E47 mutation causes agammaglobulinemia and BCR-B cells. J Clin Invest 123:4781–4785

Conley ME, Dobbs AK, Farmer DM et al (2009) Primary B cell immunodeficiencies: comparisons and contrasts. Ann Rev Immunol 27:199–227

Deau MC, Heurtier L, Frange P et al (2014) A human immunodeficiency caused by mutations in the PIK3R1 gene. J Clin Invest 124(9):3923–3928

Durandy A, Revy P, Fischer A (2007) Autosoma hyper-IgM syndromes caused by an intrinsic B cell defect. In: Ochs HD, Smith CIE, Puck JM (eds) Primary immunodeficiencies diseases. A molecular and genetic approach. Oxford University Press, New York, pp 269–278

Fischer A, Notarangelo LD (2004) Combined immunodeficiencies. In: Stiehm ER, Ochs HD, Winkelstein JA (eds) Immunologic disorders in infants and children. Elsevier, Philadelphia, pp 447–479

Geha RS, Plebani A, Notarangelo LD (2007) CD40, CD40 ligand, and the hyper IgM syndrome. In: Ochs HD, Smith CIE, Puck JM (eds) Primary immunodeficiencies diseases. A molecular and genetic approach. Oxford University Press, New York, pp 251–268

Goldmuntz E (2005) DiGeorge sindrome: new insights. Clin Perinatol 32:963–978

Hermanns P, Tran A, Munivez E et al (2006) RMRP mutations in cartilage hair hypoplasia. Am J Med Genet 140:2121–2130

Kwan A, Abraham RS, Currier R et al (2014) Newborn screening for severe combined immunodeficiency in 11 screening programs in the United States. JAMA 312(7):729–738

Lougaris V, Tampella G, Baronio M et al (2014) The genetic heterogeneity of Common Variable Immunodeficiency (CVID): an update. J Vaccines Vaccin 5:223. https://doi.org/10.4172/2157-7560.1000223

Mohiuddin MS, Abbott JK, Hubbard N et al (2013) Diagnosis and evaluation of primary panhypogammaglobulinemia: a molecular and genetic challenge. J Allergy Clin Immunol 131(6): 1717–1718

Moraes-Vasconcelos D, Costa-Carvalho BT, Torgerson TR et al (2008) Primary immune deficiency disorders presenting as autoimmune diseases IPEX and APECED. J Clin Immunol 28:S11–S19

Ochs HD, Thrasher AJ (2006) The Wiskott-Aldrich sindrome. J Allergy Clin Immunol 117:725–738

Park MA, Li JT, Hagan JB et al (2009) Common variable immunodeficiency: a new look at an old disease. Lancet 372:489–502

Rieth W, Lisowska-Grospierre B, Fischer A (2007) Molecular basis of major histocompatibility complex class II deficiency. In: Ochs HD, Smith CIE, Puck JM (eds) Primary immunodeficiencies diseases. A molecular and genetic approach. Oxford University Press, New York, pp 227–241

The International Nijmegen Breakage Syndrome Study Group (2000) Nijmegen breakage sindrome. Arch Dis Child 82:400–406

Worth AJ, Thrasher AJ (2015) Current and emerging treatment options for Wiscott-Aldrich syndrome. Expert Rev Clin Immunol 11(9):1015–1032

Inflammatory Mediators in Neonatal Asphyxia and Infection

101

Kaoru Okazaki, Akira Nishida, and Hirokazu Kimura

Contents

K. Okazaki (✉) · A. Nishida
Department of Neonatology, Tokyo Metropolitan Children's Medical Center, Tokyo, Japan
e-mail: kaoru_okazaki@tmhp.jp; ahachioji@gmail.com; chacha.nishida0901@gmail.com

H. Kimura
Infectious Diseases Surveillance Center, National Institute of Infectious Diseases, Tokyo, Japan
e-mail: kimhiro@nih.go.jp

G. Buonocore et al. (eds.), *Neonatology*,
https://doi.org/10.1007/978-3-319-29489-6_248

Abstract

Inflammatory mediators, such as inflammatory cytokines, are closely associated with neonatal diseases, including neonatal asphyxia (NA) and infection. The pathophysiology of NA may be mainly responsible for ischemia-reperfusion injuries, leading to the damage of tissue and organs via the production of aberrant inflammatory mediators, including cytokines. Excessive cytokine production may be associated with the activation of innate immunity, leading to further exacerbation of NA. In addition, pathogenic organisms can induce an acute/excessive inflammatory response through phagocyte activation with cytokine storm. Thus, these unbalanced immunological responses may induce inflammation and tissue damage in NA and infection. Furthermore, to compensate for cytokine imbalance, anti-inflammatory cytokines may be induced. Possible causes include the fact that preterm and term neonates are susceptible to NA and infection due to their lack of an adequate immune system. Therefore, given such a milieu, proper balanced cytokine production may influence the outcome of patients with NA and infection. From these aspects, we describe the relationships between inflammatory mediators in NA and infection in this chapter.

Abbreviations

APCs	Antigen-presenting cells
APPs	Antimicrobial proteins and peptides
BBB	Blood-brain barrier
BPIs	Bactericidal/permeability-increasing proteins
CAM	Chorioamnionitis
CARS	Compensatory anti-inflammatory response syndrome
CNS	Central nervous system
CRP	C-reactive protein
DAMPs	Damage-associated with molecular patterns
Epo	Erythropoietin
FIRS	Fetus inflammatory response syndrome
G-CSF	Granulocyte-colony-stimulating factor
GM-CSF	Granulocyte-macrophage colony-stimulating factor

HMGB1 protein	High-mobility group box 1 protein
IFN	Interferon
IgG	Immunoglobulin G
IL	Interleukin
MARS	Mixed anti-inflammatory response syndrome
MCP-1	Monocyte chemoattractant protein-1
MIP	Macrophage inflammatory protein
MMPs	Matrix metalloproteinases
NA	Neonatal asphyxia
NF-κB	Nuclear factor kappa-B
NO	Nitric oxide
PG	Prostaglandins
PRRs	Pattern recognition receptors
RANTES	Regulated on activation, normal T cell expressed and secreted
ROS	Reactive oxygen species
SIRS	Systemic inflammatory response syndrome
TGF	Transforming growth factor
TLRs	Toll-like receptors
TNF	Tumor necrosis factor
TREM-1	Triggering receptor expressed on myeloid cells-1
VEGF	Vascular endothelial growth factor

101.1 Salient Points

- Inflammatory mediators, particularly cytokines, are closely associated with neonatal diseases including neonatal asphyxia.
- A relationship between the pathophysiology of neonatal asphyxia, initial production of inflammatory mediators, and inflammatory cascade has been found.
- A relationship between innate immunity, cytokine production, and reactive oxygen species in neonatal asphyxia has been also demonstrated.
- Knowledge of infection and inflammatory mediators, systemic inflammatory responses, and the pathophysiology of systemic inflammatory responses to neonatal infection is necessary to establish preventative measures and treatment.

101.2 Basic Aspects of NA and Inflammatory Mediators

101.2.1 Relationships Between the Pathophysiology of NA, Initial Production of Inflammatory Mediators, and Inflammatory Cascades

NA is caused by cardiac and respiratory failure, which induces the abrupt cessation of blood flow and oxygen delivery in the antenatal or intrapartum period and may put fetuses and neonates in a hazardous situation. Severe NA may lead to hypoxic-ischemic encephalopathy, which is a very serious neonatal disease due to the presence of a hypoxic-ischemic injury and may sometimes result in a poor outcome, such as cerebral palsy and neonatal death.

When we logically discuss the title, it is essential to understand the timescale of inflammatory mediator production and the subsequent host defense mechanisms against NA. It is suggested that hypoxia in various cells/tissues may transduce an SOS signal (Castellheim et al. 2009), for example, damage-associated with molecular patterns (DAMPs) (later mentioned in another part of the chapter), which are a group of well-known ligands that include heat shock proteins and high-mobility group box 1 (HMGB1) protein (Bianchi 2007). The recognition of DAMPs may lead to the initial overproduction of inflammatory mediators (Castellheim et al. 2009). Thus, it can be thought that the essential pathophysiology of NA is associated with inflammatory cascades that are involved with various inflammatory mediators and other host defense mechanisms. A schematic illustration of the relationships between inflammatory mediators, inflammatory cascades, and NA is shown in Fig. 1.

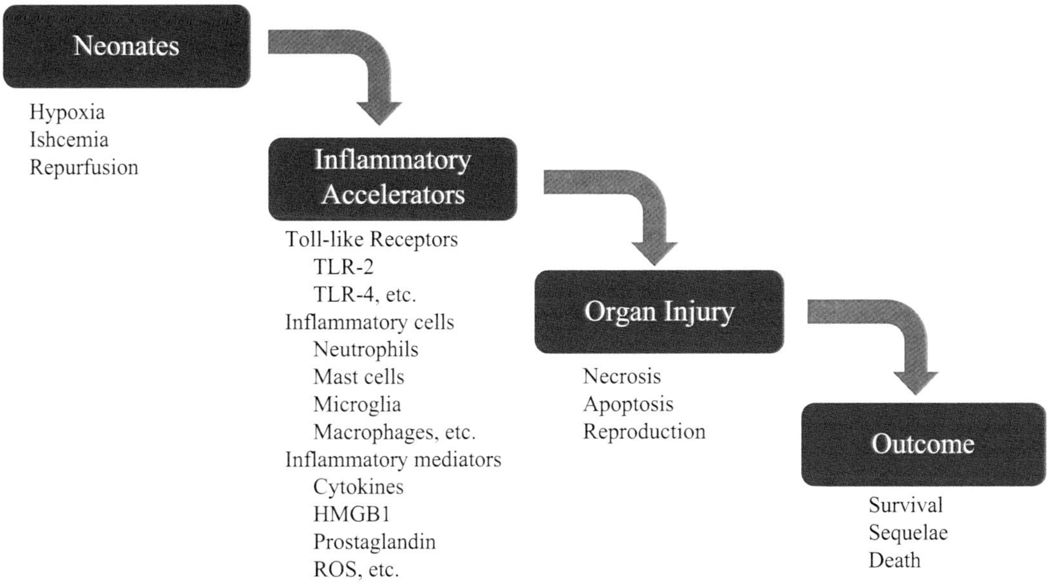

Fig. 1 Inflammatory cascades in neonatal asphyxia

101.2.2 Cytokines Are the Most Important and Representative Inflammatory Mediators in NA

Hypoxia-ischemia certainly leads to the excessive production of inflammatory mediators in NA; therefore, the main inflammatory mediator components in NA may be cytokines (Volpe 2001). Some well known inflammatory cytokines or chemokines are associated with the pathophysiology of NA, and Table 1 shows the detailed functions of these cytokines. Of them, interleukin (IL)-1β, IL-6, IL-8, tumor necrosis factor (TNF)-α, granulocyte-colony-stimulating factor (G-CSF), and vascular endothelial growth factor (VEGF) may be mainly involved in the pathophysiology of NA (Tables 2 and 3). Indeed, the serum and cerebrospinal fluid levels of various inflammatory cytokines, such as IL-1β, IL-6, and IL-8, were drastically increased in NA patients compared with healthy neonates (Okazaki et al. 2006). These elevated cytokines may activate various inflammatory cells, for example, neutrophils, microglia (brain macrophages), and T cells. Moreover, IL-6 can lead to the excess production of inflammatory proteins in NA, such as C-reactive protein (CRP). However, to prevent such an inflammatory reaction, regulation of anti-inflammatory proteins is needed. Therefore, to understand the pathophysiology of NA better, ischemia-reperfusion associated-cytokine production and other inflammatory responses need to be taken into account.

101.2.3 Relationships Among Innate Immunity, Cytokine Production, and Reactive Oxygen Species (ROS) in NA

The pathophysiology of NA may also be linked to the innate immune system, which is initialized through the recognition of various cellular ligands, for example, Toll-like receptors (TLRs). The innate immune system represents the first line of the host defense mechanism, which contains many inflammatory cells, including neutrophils, macrophages, eosinophils, and natural killer cells (Cuenca et al. 2013). However, neonatal immune cells cannot produce multiple cytokines due to their immature status (Kollmann et al. 2009).

Furthermore, hypoxia-ischemia may firstly activate neutrophils. Activated neutrophils infiltrate the central nervous system (CNS) mainly via

Table 1 Summarized cytokine functions of blood and CSF in neonatal asphyxia

Cytokine	Main functions	References
Inflammation-related cytokines		
IL-1β IL-6 IL-18 G-CSF IFN-γ TNF-α	Synthesis and release of cytokines (e.g., IL-1β, IL-8, MCP-1) Increase of inflammatory mediators (e.g., COX-2, PG, free radicals) Increased expression of adhesion molecules Increase of vascular permeability Enhancing the toxicity of excitatory amino acids Disruption or stabilization of the blood–brain barrier Aggravation of brain tissue damage Neutrophil adhesion to human cerebral endothelial cells Induction of apoptosis in nerve cells Promotion of astrocyte differentiation Protection of the central nervous system Amelioration of neuronal apoptosis Reduction of neuro-inflammation	Fisher et al. (1996); Dinarello (1998); Savman et al. (1998); Marodi (2001); Hedtjärn et al. (2002, 2004); Chiesa et al. (2003); Felderhoff-Mueser et al. (2005); Okazaki et al. (2006); Pober and Sessa (2007); Kollmann et al. (2009); Schlager et al. (2011); Okazaki et al. (2012); Roka et al. (2013); Lv et al. (2015); Li et al. (2015)
Anti-inflammation-related cytokines		
IL-10	Inhibition of leukocyte aggregation and chemokine production Neuroprotection against neonatal excitotoxic lesions Inhibition of IL-1β, IL-8, and TNF-α Reduction of inflammatory responses in the brain Reduction of the hypoxic stress response	Savman et al. (1998); Mesples et al. (2003); Kollmann et al. (2009); Roka et al. (2013); Lv et al. (2015)
Chemokines		
IL-8 MCP-1	Attraction of neutrophils, monocytes, and lymphocytes Enhancement of IL-1β and TNF-α neurotoxicity Activation of glial cells Improvement of brain injury by anti-IL-8 antibody or anti-MCP1 antibody	Baggiolini (1998); Savman et al. (1998); Fotopoulos et al. (2005); Okazaki et al. (2006); Lv et al. (2015)
Others		
HMGB1	Upregulation of adhesion molecules in endothelial cells Activation of dendritic cells and phagocytes such as granulocytes and macrophages/monocytes Induced production of pro-inflammatory cytokines from inflammatory cells	Okazaki et al. (2008b); Zhang et al. (2011); Chirico et al. (2014)
HIF-1α	Both neuroprotective and neurotoxic effects Increase of pro-apoptotic genes within 24 h after ischemia Cell survival effects in mild hypoxia Cell death effects in severe hypoxia Cell survival effects, such as erythropoiesis and angiogenesis Cell death effects, such as apoptosis and necrosis	Baranova et al. (2007); Fan et al. (2009)

(*continued*)

Table 1 (continued)

Cytokine	Main functions	References
VEGF	Angiogenesis Protective effects on neurons and glial cells Promotion of the proliferation and angiogenesis of vascular endothelial cells Promotion of neuron precursor cell proliferation Survival, repair, and regeneration of neurons in the cerebral cortex Disruption of the blood–brain barrier	Ergenekon et al. (2004); Feng et al. (2008); Aly et al. (2009); Okazaki et al. (2012)

HIF hypoxia-inducible factor

Table 2 Cytokine profile in serum and CSF levels in asphyxia within 72 h after birth

Serum		
Okazaki et al. (2006, Japan)	Cytokines	IL-1β, IL-2, IL-4, IL-6, IL-8, IL-10, TNF-α, and IFN-γ
	Subjects	Normal neonates (n = 10), asphyxiated neonates (n = 17)
	Summary	Increased: IL-6, IL-8, and IL-10 Dcreased: IFN-γ No significance: IL-1β, IL-2, IL-4, and TNF-α
CSF		
Savman et al. (1998, Sweden)	Cytokines	IL-1α, IL-1β, IL-2, IL-3, IL-4, IL-5, IL-6, IL-8, GM-CSF, TNF-α, and IFN-γ
	Subjects	Normal (n = 7), HIE: mild (n = 4), moderate (n = 8), severe (n = 8)
	Summary	Increased: IL-6 and IL-8 No significance: IL-1α, IL-1β, IL-2, IL-3, IL-4, IL-5, GM-CSF, TNF-α, and IFN-γ
Serum (plasma) and CSF		
Aly et al. (2006, USA)	Cytokines	IL-1β, IL-6, and TNF-α
	Subjects	No HIE (n = 13), HIE: mild (n = 5), moderate (n = 7), severe (n = 12)
	Summary	Increased: IL-1β, IL-6, and TNF-α

the choroid plexus, which is a possible access route to the CNS due to impermeability of the blood-brain barrier (BBB), and aggressively release many cytotoxic substances, such as ROS, toxic granules (e.g., myeloperoxidase), arachidonic acid metabolites, and cytokines, such as IL-1β, IL-6, IL-8, and monocyte chemoattractant protein-1 (MCP-1). Indeed, activated neutrophils produce pro-inflammatory cytokines, including TNF-α and IL-1β. These pro-inflammatory cytokines activate immune cells, for example, microglia, astrocytes, and endothelial cells, which produce and release many pro-inflammatory cytokines in the brain. Moreover, neutrophils are also a major source of these cytokines. However, neutrophils may not affect the initial inflammatory response in the brain because infiltration occurs within 2 h after the onset of hypoxia, and they are thus not involved in the initial response. The BBB prevents the easy infiltration of the brain by neutrophils. The initial sources of inflammatory cytokines before neutrophil recruitment may be innate immune cells in the brain, such as microglia, astrocytes, and endothelial cells.

Microglia are resident macrophages in the brain and may be associated with both hypoxia-ischemia and neonatal stroke injuries in the developing brain (Derugin et al. 2000). Microglia in the neonatal brain may induce the rapid and sustained increase of pro- and anti-inflammatory cytokines compared with those in adult brain. Activated microglia are also the main source of IL-18, which exaggerates brain tissue damage after hypoxia-ischemia in neonatal rats (Hedtjarn et al. 2002). IL-18 is a crucial pro-inflammatory factor that stimulates the expression of IL-1β and IL-8. Deletion of IL-18 protects from brain damage. In addition, activated microglia in neonatal

Table 3 Temporal alteration of cytokine levels in neonatal asphyxia with or without hypothermia

Authors	Characteristics	Contents
Okazaki et al. (2012, Japan)	Cytokines	G-CSF, VEGF
	Subjects	Non-asphyxia (n = 4), mild asphyxia (n = 5), severe asphyxia with head cooling (n = 5)
	Sampling time	0, 6, 12, 18, and 24 h
	Summary	Increased: G-CSF (head cooling) Dcreased: VEGF (head cooling)
Chalak et al. (2014, USA)	Cytokines	IL-1, IL-6, IL-8, VEGF, TNF-α, IFN-γ, RANTES, UCH-L1, and GFAP
	Subjects	Mild (n = 7) without hypothermia, moderate (n = 17) and severe (n = 3) with hypothermia
	Sampling time	0, 6–24, 48–72, 78–96 h
	Results	Increased: IL-6, IL-8, IL-1, IL-6, IL-8, TNF-α, IFN-γ, VEGF, GFAP, and UCH-L1 (hypothermia)
Jenkins et al. (2012, USA)	Cytokines	IL-1β, IL-2, IL-6, IL-8, IL-10, IL-12, IL-13, TNF-α, MCP-1, MIP-1α, IFN-γ, and IP-10
	Subjects	Systemic hypothermia of 33.0 °C for 48 h in HIE (n = 28), normothermia (n = 22)
	Sampling time	0, 12, 24, 36, 48, 60, and 72 h
	Summary	Increased: IL-6, IL-8, IL-10, and MCP-1(hypothermia) Dcreased: MIP-1α (at 60–70 h) IL-6, IL-8, and MCP-1 (a biphasic pattern in the hypothermia group)
Róka et al. (2013, Hungary)	Cytokines	IL-1α, IL-1β, IL-2, IL-4, IL-6, IL-8, IL-10, MCP-1, EGF, VEGF, IFN-γ, and TNF-α
	Subjects	TOBY trial HIE with hypothermia [33–34 °C] (n = 10), normothermia (n = 8)
	Sampling time	6, 12, 24 h
	Summary	Increased: VEGF (hypothermia) Dcreased: IL-6, IL-4 (hypothermia), and IL-10 (hypothermia and normothermia)

RANTES regulated on activation, normal T cell expressed and secreted, *UCH* ubiquitin carboxy-terminal hydrolase, *GFAP* glial fibrillary acidic protein

brains with a hypoxic-ischemic injury may secrete IL-23 by promoting the full maturation of Th17 cells as effector cells. IL-17 also shows some effects, including upregulating the expression of pro-inflammatory cytokines and attracting neutrophils to mediate defenses against different pathogens (Akdis et al. 2011). Thus, microglia may be the initial sources of pro- and anti-inflammatory cytokines in the neonatal brain with hypoxia-ischemia.

Vascular endothelial cells are also a source of cytokine production in the brain. Hypoxia induces the production of pro-inflammatory cytokines, including IL-1 and IL-6, by endothelial cells in vitro (Ala et al. 1992). In general, endothelial cells play pivotal roles in blood flow maintenance, such as inhibition of blood coagulation and control of vessel permeability. During inflammation, activated inflammatory cells may target endothelial cells for further augmentation of inflammation via the aberrant production of pro-inflammatory cytokines.

Activated inflammatory cells, such as neutrophils and mast cells, produce excessive amount of ROS including superoxide radicals and hydroxyl radicals under high oxygen conditions, resulting in tissue and organ damage (Fellman and Raivio 1997). Resuscitation with a high concentration of oxygen induces not only the synthesis of ROS but also the production of inflammatory mediators, such as cytokines. Many experimental studies have shown the

relationship between high oxygen conditions and the cytokine responses.

101.2.4 Relationships Among Signaling Pathways, HMGB1, and Cytokine Production

Cytokine production is regulated by various intercellular signaling pathways (Rossol et al. 2011). Among them, nuclear factor kappa-B (NF-κB) plays crucial roles in the production of various inflammatory cytokine mediators such as IL-1β, TNF-α, IL-6, and HMGB1 (Bonizzi and Karin 2004). The inflammatory mediator HMGB1 was discovered initially as a protein that maintained the double-stranded structure of DNA. Leukocytes produce and actively release HMGB1. Recently, HMGB1 was shown to play a critical role in several inflammatory diseases, including septic shock, rheumatoid arthritis, and acute lung inflammation. Tissue injury and microbial invasion induce the extracellular release of HMGB1 (Abraham et al. 2000). Moreover, the addition of anti-inflammatory drugs, such as corticosteroids, may effectively suppress the phosphorylation of NF-κB, resulting in the suppression of inflammatory cytokines. Thus, to prevent excessive inflammatory responses in NA, it is essential to control the activity of NF-κB.

101.2.5 Roles of IL-6, HMGB1, and IL-10 in NA

IL-6 is the most important cytokine in the inflammatory responses of the CNS and plays a central role in neuronal inflammatory responses to hypoxic-ischemic damage (Fig. 1). In the acute phase of NA, IL-6 may be produced by many inflammatory cells, such as neutrophils and macrophages. Increased levels of IL-6 in serum and cerebrospinal fluid may be associated with the severity of NA. Recently, it was reported that IL-6 shows dual roles in neuronal inflammation (Dubovy et al. 2013). Several stimuli, such as infection and hypoxia, may drastically induce IL-6 production in the brain and serum. High levels of IL-6 may cause an excessive inflammatory response, and the activation of many inflammatory cells induces tissue or organ damage. Conversely, low concentrations of IL-6 may protect neuronal cells in the brain. This neuroprotective effect of IL-6 may be due to the blockade of N-acetyl factor N-methyl-D-aspartate-induced excitotoxicity via gp130. Thus, IL-6 is also involved in both the promotion of neuronal survival and protection against neuronal damage. In addition, immediately after hypothermia, the serum concentration of IL-6 significantly increased in the hypothermia therapy group compared with the normothermia therapy group (Roka et al. 2013). The elevation of IL-6 and CRP appears to be a neuroprotective effect that protects against neural apoptosis. Hypothermia may induce the neurotrophic effect of IL-6. Thus, IL-6 may have distinct effects on neurons.

HMGB1 may induce endothelial cell activation by the upregulation of adhesion molecules and the secretion of pro-inflammatory cytokines and chemokines (Fiuza et al. 2003). Extracellular HMGB1 is a representative alarmin molecule. Binding between HMGB1 and TLRs (TLR2 and TLR4) may induce the production of many pro-inflammatory cytokines; in particular, HMGB1-TLR4 signaling may enhance neural-glutamate sensitivity (Maroso et al. 2011). In the brain of NA patients, glutamate concentration is high and excited neurons may release HMGB1. Thus, HMGB1 is an important factor in the inflammatory responses in NA.

IL-10 is a representative anti-inflammatory cytokine. In general, IL-10 acts to protect healthy fetuses and neonates against harmful inflammation. Indeed, the anti-inflammatory response may be dominant in the immunity of fetuses and neonates (Sharma et al. 2012). Innate immune cells, for example, macrophages and dendritic cells, produce IL-10 via TLR2. Released IL-10 plays a central role in both limiting the immune response and preventing host damage from inflammation (Saraiva and O'garra 2010). Thus, IL-10 is essential for the control of the increased levels of pro-inflammatory cytokines during the early phase of inflammation.

101.2.6 Relationships Between the BBB and Inflammatory Responses

Needless to say, the BBB is very important for the maintenance of intracerebral homeostasis and the separation of the peripheral circulation from direct contact with the CNS. The BBB has molecular selectivity; therefore, cytokines, including those with a large molecular size, are unable to pass through the barrier. However, robust pro-inflammatory cytokines in the brain lead to an increase of proteases, that is, matrix metalloproteinases (MMPs), which is a family of enzymes that can degrade the components of the extracellular matrix, such as collagen, proteoglycan, gelatin, laminin, and elastin. MMPs in the brain also degrade tight junctions and extracellular matrix components in the endothelial basement membrane (Rosenberg 2009). MMPs cause an increase of BBB permeability, leading to brain edema, hemorrhage, and infiltrations (Rosenberg 2009). Thus, MMPs may play pivotal roles in the destruction of the BBB. Collectively, degradation of the BBB may lead to the easy infiltration of the brain by circulating leukocytes and exacerbates inflammation and brain damage (Liu and Mccullough 2013).

Amoeboid microglia in the immature brain respond vigorously to hypoxia, accumulate in injured tissues, and produce excessive amounts of pro-inflammatory cytokines, for example, TNF-α and IL-1β, along with glutamate, nitric oxide (NO), and ROS production, resulting in oligodendrocyte death, axonal degeneration, and disruption of the immature BBB (Bona et al. 1999). Astrocytes are neural cells that play important roles in the maintenance of capillary blood cells. Astrocyte foot processes form a network that covers more than 90 % of brain capillaries, produce tight junctions, and enhance the barrier function of brain capillary endothelial cells. Within minutes of a hypoxic insult, astrocytes may be activated by inflammatory mediators and produce ROS. These activated astrocytes produce pro-inflammatory cytokines, such as TNF-α, IL-1β, and IL-6. Astrocytes also feed neurons. Thus, the failure of astrocyte functions may lead to ischemic injury and destruction of the BBB.

101.3 Clinical Aspects of NA and Inflammatory Mediators

101.3.1 Effectiveness and Theory of Hypothermia Therapy in NA

At present, hypothermia therapy may be the only evidenced-based effective therapy for NA. The main purpose of hypothermia is to protect against excessive neuronal death by apoptosis (programmed cell death). The abrupt cessation of both blood and oxygen supply may lead to primary energy failure, a reperfusion period, and a latent phase resulting in secondary energy failure. Primary energy failure is caused by rapid adenosine triphosphate deletion due to the lack of glucose supply, leading to cell death via necrosis (Sahni and Sanocka 2008). In the latent phase, pro- or anti-apoptotic proteins initiate a cascade of delayed cell death via apoptosis. At 1–6 h after birth, secondary energy failure may induce neuronal death via apoptosis and cause severe brain damage, such as seizures and cytotoxic edema. Second energy failure is also associated with an inflammatory response. The latent phase prior to second energy failure is the best period in which to initiate appropriate therapy for NA. Appropriate anti-inflammatory therapies in the latent phase (within 6 h of birth) may prevent the evolution of secondary energy failure or the initiation of anti-apoptotic pathways.

Brain protection in NA may be achieved by hypothermia, which induces the reduction of cerebral metabolism, leading to the prevention of BBB disruption and reduction of brain edema. Neuroprotective mechanisms of hypothermia therapy may be involved in the attenuation of microglia adverse reactions (e.g., activation, migration, and proliferation), inhibition of neurotoxic mediators (e.g., NO and ROS), and inhibition of apoptosis (Seo et al. 2012; Si et al. 1997). Thus, hypothermia therapies may be correlated with inflammatory responses. Hypothermia may also partially block subsequent inflammatory responses: (i) production of inflammatory mediators by activated microglia (e.g., IL-10, TNF-α, and NO), (ii) activation of NF-κB, (iii) mRNA

expression of pro-inflammatory cytokines (e.g., INF-γ, TNF-α, IL-2, IL-1β, and macrophage inflammatory protein [MIP]-2) and anti-inflammatory cytokines (e.g., IL-10) in the brain, and (iv) induction of pro-inflammatory cytokines in human peripheral blood mononuclear cells (Okazaki et al. 2015). In a rat model with ischemia-reperfusion injury, HMGB1 levels in the brain and plasma were also attenuated by hypothermia (Matsui et al. 2014). Thus, hypothermia may suppress excessive inflammatory responses in hypoxic-ischemic injury. The effects of hypothermia therapy on serum cytokine levels associated with NA are shown in Tables 1 and 3.

101.3.2 Other Therapeutic Approaches

101.3.2.1 Erythropoietin (Epo)

Epo shows not only hematopoietic effects but also anti-apoptotic, antioxidant, and anti-inflammatory effects (Rangarajan and Juul 2014; Mizuno et al. 2008). In the brain, Epo inhibits the activation of microglia and astrogliosis, leading to the activation of neurogenesis, oligodendrogenesis, and angiogenesis (Rangarajan and Juul 2014). In addition, brain immune cells, for example, astrocytes, neurons, and immature oligodendrocytes, may produce endogenous Epo to prevent neural cell apoptosis after ischemia-reperfusion damage. In contrast, various inflammatory mediators, such as ROS, NO, and inflammatory cytokines (e.g., IL-1β, TNF, and interferon [IFN]-γ), may inhibit the production of Epo, thereby aggravating brain injury. However, exogenous Epo may be able to pass to through a BBB disrupted by a hypoxic-ischemic injury and provide anti-apoptotic effects. Some clinical trials of Epo in NA are currently in progress (Fauchère et al. 2015).

101.3.3 G-CSF

G-CSF also shows non-hematopoietic effects. G-CSF production may be induced by inflammatory stimuli, and increased G-CSF levels may stimulate the proliferation of neutrophils in the bone marrow, resulting in the elevation of circulating neutrophils. However, many studies suggested that G-CSF shows neuroprotective effects against inflammation, including anti-apoptotic, anti-inflammatory, excitoprotective, and neurotrophic responses. G-CSF also leads to the increased production of anti-inflammatory cytokine (e.g., IL-10), while pro-inflammatory cytokines (e.g., NF-κB, IL-1β, TNF-α, and IL-12) and vascular adhesion molecules (e.g., vascular cell adhesion molecule-1, intercellular adhesion molecule-1) may be eliminated (Li et al. 2015; Komine-Kobayashi et al. 2006). However, systemic G-CSF administration did not improve long-term outcome, and it also adversely affected neurologic disabilities with brain injury in the hippocampus (Schlager et al. 2011). The passage of exogenous G-CSF to the brain may be limited by the BBB; therefore, intranasal G-CSF administration may cause an effective increase of G-CSF in the brain. Further clinical trials are needed.

101.3.4 Glucocorticoids

Glucocorticoids, such as dexamethasone and hydrocortisone, are representative anti-inflammatory drugs that inhibit NF-κB activation, resulting in inflammatory responses. Previous studies showed that pretreatment of neonatal neutrophils with hydrocortisone or dexamethasone could reduce the production of IL-8 and MIP-1α (Irakam et al. 2002). However, there is only little evidence showing the effects of glucocorticoid therapy in NA. In addition, dexamethasone has two incompatible effects regarding its neuroprotective and neurotoxic actions (Murphy et al. 2001; Feng et al. 2009). Hydrocortisone induced pulmonary hypertension in asphyxiated newborn piglets (Chapados et al. 2011).

101.3.5 Antioxidative Agents for NA

ROS are produced by various physiological events in vivo (Kondo et al. 2000). In addition, ROS can elicit adjacent cell injury in endothelial and glomerular mesangial cells. Superoxide dismutase is a representative antioxidant

enzyme that can pass easily through the BBB and inhibit the action of oxygen free radicals. However, superoxide dismutase only exerts neuroprotective effects when it is administered prior to a hypoxic-ischemic insult. Allopurinol, an antioxidant medication, is not only a xanthine oxidase inhibitor but also an antioxidative agent that may act as a hydroxyl radical scavenger, leading to the suppression of ROS production (Kelen and Robertson 2010). Moreover, allopurinol therapy significantly decreased the mRNA expression of pro-inflammatory cytokines in the brain. Allopurinol might suppress ROS-mediated NF-κB activation, which is a core element of inflammatory responses (Yamaguchi et al. 2015). Indeed, in moderate NA, allopurinol administration showed a better long-term outcome at 5 years of age (Kaandorp et al. 2012). Thus, the early administration of allopurinol therapy may be more effective for ischemia-reperfusion injury. Combination therapy with allopurinol and hypothermia may have the potential to improve outcome in moderately and severely asphyxiated neonates.

101.3.6 Disodium Cromoglycate (Cromolyn)

Interestingly, it may be possible to use disodium cromoglycate (cromolyn), an antiallergic drug, as a neuroprotective agent. In neonatal rats with hypoxia-ischemia, mast cells are primarily activated in the brain and initiate strong inflammatory responses in microglia, astrocytes, and neutrophils. Activated mast cells are recruited to the site of inflammation immediately after a hypoxic-ischemic insult and release pro-inflammatory cytokines, such as TNF-α. Disodium cromoglycate may suppress these immunological responses and attenuate brain injury in NA.

101.3.7 Anticonvulsants

Due to the below threshold levels of regional cerebral blood flow, changes of spontaneous electrical activity in neurons of newborns may easily lead to neonatal seizures (Nakamura et al. 2014). First-line therapeutics in neonatal seizures may be used as various anticonvulsant drugs, for example, phenobarbital, midazolam, phenytoin, and lorazepam. These anticonvulsants may affect immunity. For example, high-dose phenobarbital therapy may lead to the suppressed production of IL-2 in vitro (Yang et al. 1992). Midazolam inhibits IL-1β-induced IL-6 release in vitro. Valproic acid also increases the levels of some cytokines, such as IL-1α, IL-1β, IL-2, IL-6, and MCP-1 (Verrotti et al. 2001). Thus, many anticonvulsants may affect cytokine profiles. However, anticonvulsant therapy can lead to changes in inflammatory responses; the effects of this therapy should be monitored closely because it may aggravate the occurrence of seizures.

101.3.8 Sedation Drugs

Morphine and fentanyl are used frequently in NA for pain control and sedation. Some studies suggested that morphine suppressed the production of many cytokines, such as IL-1β, IL-6, IL-10, IL-12p70, and TNF-α (Chavez-Valdez et al. 2013). In addition, morphine may reduce chemotaxis of neonatal neutrophils due to the decreased expression of IL-8 receptors on the surface of these cells (Yossuck et al. 2008). These effects may partially contribute to the improvement of NA.

101.4 Basic Aspects of Infection and Inflammatory Mediators

101.4.1 Concept of Systemic Inflammatory Response States

Serial immunological responses in infection may occur in vivo. Conceptually, systemic inflammatory response states may be categorized as follows: fetal inflammatory response syndrome (FIRS), systemic inflammatory response syndrome (SIRS), mixed anti-inflammatory response syndrome (MARS), and compensatory anti-inflammatory response syndrome (CARS)

(Gomez et al. 1998; Hotchkiss et al. 2013a). Particularly, these concepts in sepsis may be important for understanding not only pathophysiology but also therapeutics. Both FIRS and SIRS are characterized by IL-6-centered robust pro-inflammatory cytokinemia. This excessive production of pro-inflammatory cytokines may enhance the clinical findings of sepsis, such as fever, tachycardia, dyspnea, and leukocytosis (Levy et al. 2003). Unmanaged rigorous inflammation may induce the uncontrolled overproduction of pro-inflammatory cytokines and cause death and nonreversible damage, such as white matter injury and pulmonary inflammation (Hotchkiss et al. 2013a). Against this rigorous overproduction of inflammatory mediators, a compensatory increase of anti-inflammatory cytokines occurs. MARS is classified as intermediate homeostasis in which equivalent amounts of pro- and anti-inflammatory cytokines are present, and its represents a form of temporary homeostasis between diminishing SIRS and ascending CARS. CARS is the final stage where low levels of pro-inflammatory cytokines and excessive amounts of anti-inflammatory cytokines are present, and it is the consequence of counter-regulatory mechanisms that are initiated to limit excessive inflammatory processes. Indeed, CARS play a more important role in the pathophysiology of septic shock and multiple organ failure in children than in adults (Osuchowski et al. 2012; Hotchkiss et al. 2013b; Wynn et al. 2010; Adib-Conquy and Cavaillon 2009). Tables 4 and 5 show the detailed changes of cytokine profiles during systemic inflammatory responses.

101.4.2 Pathophysiology of SIRS in Neonatal Infection

Neonatal sepsis, a representative systemic infection, may be life-threatening and can cause SIRS. Furthermore, common viral infections, such as influenza, also cause SIRS. The pathophysiology of SIRS may essentially involve the excessive production of inflammatory mediators. Obviously, the initial cause of SIRS is the invasion of various pathogens, including bacteria and viruses. Pathogen-induced inflammatory responses may be caused initially by innate immunity. Innate immune cells, such as antigen-presenting cells (APCs) and other inflammatory cells, may recognize them via different TLRs and produce "help" signals, including alarmins. The recognition of alarmins may lead to the initial overproduction of inflammatory mediators. Thus, the essential pathophysiology of SIRS may be associated with inflammatory cascades that are involved in various inflammatory mediators and other host defense mechanisms. A schematic illustration of the relationships between inflammatory mediators, inflammatory cascades, and neonatal sepsis is shown in Fig. 2. Several cytokines are significantly increased in neonates with sepsis compared with those without sepsis, such as pro-inflammatory cytokines (e.g., IL-1β and TNF-α), anti-inflammatory cytokines (e.g., IL-10 and IL-19), Th1 cytokines (e.g., IL-1ra, IL-2, IL-12, IL-18, and IFN-γ), Th17 cytokines (e.g., IL-6, IL-23, and G-CSF), and chemokines (e.g., IL-8 and MCP-1). However, some cytokines are also decreased, for example, IL-17, transforming growth factor (TGF)-β, and regulated on activation, normal T cell expressed and secreted (RANTES) (Table 4). This chapter focuses on the pathophysiological roles of cytokines in SIRS.

101.4.3 Inflammatory Mediators in Chorioamnionitis (CAM) and Funisitis

Chorioamnionitis and funisitis are representative intrauterine infections and cause various serious neonatal diseases, including sepsis, intraventricular hemorrhage, and bronchopulmonary dysplasia. The pathophysiology of CAM and funisitis is closely associated with the excessive inflammatory responses in the mother and/or neonate (Døllner et al. 2002; Kim et al. 2015). Particularly, inflammatory cytokines, matrix metalloproteinase (MMP) in neutrophil as a toxic substance, and prostaglandins (PG) may be exacerbation factors of these infections (Epstein et al. 2000). Indeed, previous reports showed that

Table 4 Temporal alteration of plasma cytokine levels in neonatal sepsis

Study		
Sood et al. (2012, USA)	Cytokines	TNF-α, IL-1β, IL-4, IL-5, IL-6, IL-10, IL-12, IL-17, IL-18, IFN-γ, and TGF-β
	Subjects	ELBWI [bacterial sepsis, fungal sepsis, no infection]
	Sampling time	0, 3, 7, 14, and 21 days
	Pathogens	*Coagulase-negative staphylococci* (n = 189), *Staphylococcus aureus* (n = 34), *Streptococci* (n = 35; *Group B Streptococcus* n = 4), *Escherichia coli* (n = 20), *Klebsiella* (n = 17)
	Summary	Increased: (post infection) IL-10, I-18, and TNF-α Dcreased: (post infection) TGF-β No significance: IL-1β, IL-12, IL-4, IL-5, IL-6, and IL-17
Schelonka et al. (2011, USA)	Cytokines	IL-2, IL-4, IL-5, IL-6, IL-10, IL-17, IFN-γ, and TNF-α
	Subjects	ELBWI [blood stream infections]
	Sampling time	Within 4 h and 3, 7, 14, and 21 days after birth
	Pathogens	*Coagulase-negative staphylococci* (n = 222), *Staphylococcus aureus* (n = 33), *Enterococcus* sp. and other streptococcal organisms (n = 20), other Gram-positive (n = 24), Gram-negative and enteric organisms (n = 70), *Candida* sp. (n = 45), and polymicrobial infections (n = 25)
	Summary	Increased: IL-6 and IL-10 Dcreased: IL-17 No significance: IL-2, IL-4, IL-5, IFN-γ, TNF-α
Ng PC et al. (2007, Hong Kong)	Cytokines	TNF-α, IL-1β, IL-6, IL-10, IL-12p70, IL-8, MCP-1, RANTES, MIG, and IP-10
	Subjects	Preterm late-onset sepsis
	Sampling time	0 and 24 h from onset
	Pathogens	Gram-positive organisms: *Coagulase-negative staphylococci* (n = 9), *Staphylococcus aureus* (n = 1), *Streptococcus bovis* (n = 1), *Enterococcus* sp. (n = 3); Gram-negative organisms: *Klebsiella* sp. (n = 4), *Enterobacter* sp. (n = 4), *Escherichia coli* (n = 2), *Pseudomonas* sp. (n = 1), *Stenotrophomonas* sp. (n = 2), *Acinetobacter* sp. (n = 1); mixed organisms (n = 3): *Coagulase-negative staphylococci* and *Enterococcus* sp. (n = 1), *Klebsiella* sp. and *Candida parasilosis* (n = 1), *E. coli* and *Enterococcus* sp. (n = 1)
	Summary	Increased: IL-6, IL-10, IL-12p70, IL-8, MCP-1, MIG, IP-10, and TNF-α
Hotoura et al. (2011, Country)	Cytokines	IL-1β, IL-6, and TNF-α
	Subjects	Term neonates sepsis group (early n = 13, late n = 12), suspected infection group healthy neonates
	Sampling time	0, 24, and 48 h from onset
	Pathogens	*Escherichia coli* (n = 7), *Klebsiella* (n = 3), *Staphylococcus aureus* (n = 2), *Streptococcus group* B (n = 2), *Corynobacter* (n = 1), *Listeria* (n = 1), *Streptococcus viridans* (n = 1), *Staphylococcus coagulase-negative* (n = 8)
	Summary	Increased: IL6, TNF-α, and IL-1β

ELBWI extremely low birth weight infants, *MIC* monokine induced by gamma interferon

amniotic fluids in the CAM contained high levels of inflammatory cytokines (e.g., IL-1β, IL-6, and TNF-α) and chemokines (e.g., IL-8, MIP-1α, and MCP-1). Invasive pathogens may also strongly activate the inflammatory cells such as neutrophils and macrophages. Activated inflammatory cells may rapidly migrate to the inflammatory sites and produce/release a large amount of inflammatory mediators. Of them, IL-1β and TNF-α may certainly stimulate to produce not only the PG from amniotic membranes but also release MMP from the infiltrating neutrophils (Romero et al. 2016). Moreover, chorionic infections may downregulate prostaglandin dehydrogenase

Table 5 Summary of the temporal alteration of serum cytokine levels in neonatal sepsis

		Infection		
	Cytokine type	Pre-infection	Onset	Post-infection
Increase	Pro-inflammatory Anti-inflammatory Th1 Th2 Th17 Others	IL-1ra IL-6	IL-1β and TNF-α IL-10 IL-2, IL-12, and IFN-γ IL-4 IL-6, IL-21, IL-23, and G-CSF IL-8, MCP-1, IP-10, MIG, ICAM-1, and E-selectin	TNF-α IL-10 IL-2, IL-18, and IFN-γ IL-4 IL-6
Decrease	Th17 Others		IL-17 RANTES	IL-17 and TGF-β

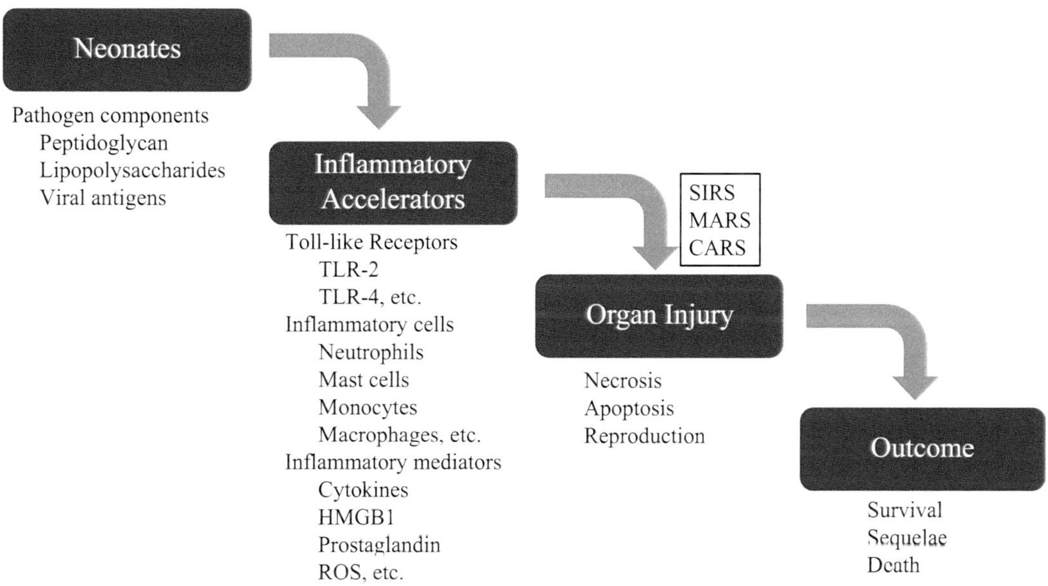

Fig. 2 Inflammatory cascades in neonatal infection

activities. As a result, the PG may not be inactivated, reach myometrium, and stimulate the uterus to contract. The MMP derived from neutrophils may promote the rupture of membrane and cervical ripening, resulting in preterm labor. Indeed, MMP concentrations in amniotic fluids correlate with the severity of acute CAM. On the other hand, pathogenic bacteria in amniotic fluids may increase expression of TLR2 and TLR4 on the fetal epithelium.

In funisitis, significantly increased inflammatory cytokines, such as IL-6, IL-8, and IL-12p55, may be seen (Døllner et al. 2002; Kim et al. 2015). These cytokines may circulate around the body of fetus and stimulate systemic inflammatory responses leading to FIRS (Døllner et al. 2002). FIRS is defined as the cord blood levels of IL-6 greater than 11 pg/mL and may affect many tissues, including the brain, heart, lung, intestine, kidney, and hematopoietic systems (Gantert et al. 2010; Gotsch et al. 2007). For example, in hematopoietic systems, high IL-6 and G-CSF in the fetal plasma with FIRS induce to high-nucleated red blood cell count and neutrophilia, respectively. In the lungs, high levels of IL-1β and IL-6 in amniotic fluids may accelerate lung

maturity but cause abnormal morphology of alveolar, such as decreased number and larger size. Thus, FIRS may affect neonates for the rest of their lives. However, in the present, there is no effective treatment or preventive strategy against FIRS.

101.4.4 Cytokines and Innate Immunity in Neonatal Sepsis

Neonates may be immunocompromised hosts; therefore, they may easily develop a systemic infection, including sepsis, as their immature innate immune system is not sufficient for defending against infections. The innate immune system may play a central role in neonatal sepsis (Wynn et al. 2010). The innate immune system consists mainly of cellular immunity, that is, immune cells, such as neutrophils and APCs (e.g., monocytes, macrophages, and dendritic cells) (Cuenca et al. 2013). Among them, macrophages are the most important APCs, which recognize pathogens via pattern recognition receptors (PRRs) immediately after bacterial invasion. Neonatal macrophages may produce a low amount of some cytokines, such as IL-12p70, IFN-γ, TNF-α, and IL-10 (Belderbos et al. 2013). A key cytokine, IFN-γ, can activate macrophages to kill microbes and promote the activity of other immune cells. Next, neutrophils are an important innate immune cell in the clearance of pathogens. Activated neutrophils kill bacteria by producing various inflammatory mediators, including prostaglandin E, lipid mediators, and ROS. A massive amount of pro-inflammatory cytokines and chemokines are produced promptly by innate immune cells. These mediators play a crucial role in the recruitment of immune cells to the site of inflammation, resulting in a further increase of inflammatory mediators. The responses of neonatal neutrophils are very poor due to decreased lipopolysaccharide-induced signaling via TLR4, resulting in the insufficient production of cytokines, such as TNF-α, IL-12p70, and IFN-γ (Cuenca et al. 2013). In contrast, neonatal neutrophils can produce relatively more of both Th2/Th17 and anti-inflammatory cytokines via other TLR signaling pathways (Cuenca et al. 2013). Moreover, activated primed neutrophils are able to phagocytose microbes and also release small amounts of antimicrobial proteins and peptides (APPs), such as lactoferrin, defensins, and bactericidal/permeability-increasing proteins (BPIs). APPs are important biological defense proteins. The levels of APPs are lower in neonates than in adults. In preterm neonates, there are further decreases of APP levels (Cuenca et al. 2013). APP replacement therapies may be effective for immunostimulation by increasing pro-inflammatory responses (Pammi and Abrams 2015).

TLRs are the most important PRRs, and many cytokines are produced through TLRs. The poor functions of TLRs in preterm and term neonates directly influence the reduction of inflammatory mediators and vulnerability to infections. Each TLR has unique ligands; both lipopolysaccharides of Gram-negative bacteria and the mannan antigen of *Candida* spp. are ligands of TLR4, and double-stranded RNA is a ligand of TLR2. The expression of TLRs in term neonates is similar to that in adults; however, TLR expression by leukocytes in preterm neonates is lower than in term neonates. In addition, neonates have poor TLR function compared with adults. Recognition of ligand via TLRs invokes second messenger signals, for example, MyD88, TIR-domain-containing adaptor protein-inducing IFN-β, and MyD88-adapter-like, and leads to the production of pro-inflammatory cytokines (Cuenca et al. 2013). Impairment of the pathways from ligand recognition to cytokine production results in the reduction of both cytokine levels and inflammatory responses. TLR4 is the most important PRR for the activation of leukocytes during the innate immune response (Cuenca et al. 2013). TLR4 plays a central role in the defense against Gram-negative bacteria and binds to lipopolysaccharides. This difference of TLR function may also lead to the poor production of inflammatory mediators and can be attributed to differences in sensitivity to infections. TLR4 does not mature immediately after birth, resulting in the long-term reduction of pro-inflammatory cytokines, for example, IL-1β

and TNF-α (Levy and Wynn 2014). Conversely, the overexpression of TLR4 may induce systemic inflammatory responses and cause tissue injury. Poor TLR function is favorable for protection of the fetus from inflammation.

101.4.5 Temporal Alteration of Cytokinemia During Sepsis

As mentioned above, in the initial phase of sepsis, the levels of both pro- and anti-inflammatory cytokines increase drastically, as observed in SIRS. Cytokine profiles in sepsis may change over time; therefore, it is important to understand the temporal alteration of cytokines in sepsis. For example, neonatal sepsis due to group B *Streptococcus* showed a temporal alteration of various types of cytokines, including IL-1β, IL-5, IL-6, IL-12, IL-17, IFN-γ, TNF-α, G-CSF, IL-8, and MIP-1, which increased remarkably at 1.5 h after birth. However, the serum levels of each cytokine changed in a time-dependent manner (Okazaki et al. 2008a). In neonates with sepsis, IL-6 and TNF-α in serum are sustained at a high level for a few days. Moreover, fungal sepsis due to *Candida* in an extremely low birth weight infant also showed significantly increased levels of some cytokines (e.g., IL-10 and IL-18) and decreased levels of a few cytokines (e.g., TGF-β) compared with both bacterial sepsis and noninfection. Together, SIRS due to bacterial infection in neonates may show several different cytokine profiles (Tables 4 and 5).

101.4.6 Cytokines as Early Markers of Neonatal Infection

To diagnose and treat various neonatal infections, cytokine profiles may be useful as an early biomarker. Previous studies reported many inflammatory mediators, such as CRP, as markers of bacterial infections. However, the serum concentration of CRP increases at only 6 h or later from infection onset, and it is not necessarily sufficient for use as an early marker of infection. In addition, CRP may be increased in circumstances other than infection, for example, hypoxic-ischemic injury. In contrast, the serum levels of some cytokines may increase earlier than CRP. Thus, these are expected as markers of neonatal infections. Furthermore, IL-6 induces CRP as an acute-phase protein in infection and is one of the most investigated cytokines as a sepsis marker. Other cytokines have also been investigated in neonatal sepsis. For example, IFN-γ-inducible protein 10 may be useful for the early diagnosis of a late-onset bacterial infection (Ng et al. 2007). However, there are currently no inflammatory mediators that can be used as an early marker of neonatal sepsis. It is important to provide a diagnosis by not only one factor but also by some combination of hematologic examination (e.g., number of leukocytes, CRP, and immature to total leukocyte ratio), clinical signs, and maternal or neonatal history. Recently, presepsin (sCD14 subtype) has received attention as a new marker of sepsis in adults and neonates (Shozushima et al. 2011). This is a unique marker of sepsis and reflects the clinical course. In the future, presepsin may be used as a diagnostic marker of neonatal sepsis.

101.5 Clinical Aspects of Neonatal Infections and Inflammatory Mediators

101.5.1 Treatment with Anti-Inflammatory Medications

Although anti-inflammatory therapies are thought to be effective in humans, clinical trials have failed and adverse effects have been reported in some cases (Fisher et al. 1994, 1996). The immune state in sepsis may fluctuate between hyperactivity and immunosuppression, as in SIRS, MARS, and CARS. In an early death group of experimental sepsis, there were increases of both pro-inflammatory (e.g., IL-6, TNF-α, IL-1β, and MCP-1) and anti-inflammatory cytokines (e.g., IL-10 and IL-1 receptor antagonist). However, these pro- and anti-inflammatory cytokines were not elevated in a late death group (Osuchowski et al. 2006). In general, sepsis may be treated with immunosuppressive drugs for

hyperimmune responses. If both pro- and anti-inflammatory cytokines are suppressed, immunosuppressive drugs may be not only ineffective but also worsen sepsis. Thus, the failure of previous clinical trial may have been the result of the immune response state, such as SIRS, MARS, and CARS. The immune state in sepsis starts at SIRS and is followed by MARS and CARS. If the immune state is hyperactive, an immunosuppressive therapy may be effective; conversely, in the immunosuppressive state, an adjuvant therapy may be effective. Thus, individualized immune therapy may be effective as immunotherapy for sepsis. Immunomodulatory or immunostimulatory agents may be effective in CARS.

101.5.2 Non-mediator Treatments

Immunoglobulin G (IgG) therapy is used frequently in various clinical conditions. IgG therapy promotes the activation of opsonic activity or pathogen neutralization. However, preterm neonates may have low serum levels of IgG (100–500 mg/dL). Thus, intravenous IgG may be suitable as therapy for severe infections in preterm neonates. However, recent studies suggested that intravenous IgG therapy for neonatal infections may be ineffective (Brocklehurst et al. 2011; Ohlsson and Lacy 2015).

Next, serum in preterm and term neonates may contain low levels of enhanced immune substances and become unbalanced, such as high adenosine, low mannose-binding protein, and low antimicrobial proteins/peptides, for example, lactoferrin, defensins, and BPIs (Cuenca et al. 2013). Deficiency of these components results in the inability to generate an adequate immune response and clearance of pathogenic microorganisms. Serum component replacements therapies are effective for some diseases with a partial defect of serum components, such as hemophilia, adenosine deaminase deficiency, and lysosomal diseases. Therefore, serum component replacement therapy, for example, fresh frozen plasma, may be effective for neonatal infections.

Hydrocortisone is used widely in many diseases and can suppress cytokine-induced inflammation or increased sensitivity of the cardiovascular system. Cortisol levels increase in neonates with septic shock. However, preterm neonates easily develop hemodynamic instability and hypotension in sepsis because of relative adrenal insufficiency. In neonatal sepsis, hydrocortisone may improve several clinical signs, such as an increase of blood pressure and decrease of heart rate. However, even in adult patients with adrenal insufficiency due to septic shock, hydrocortisone did not improve survival at 28 days and induced a premature reversal of shock (Sprung et al. 2008). This result may be associated with differences in the immune responses states, such as SIRS, MARS, and CARS. The use of hydrocortisone therapy should be monitored closely, even in neonates, due to a lack of studies on its effects.

Probiotics are very important for the control of inflammation. Probiotics can form normal intestinal flora in the gut during the early periods after birth. Normal intestinal flora leads to the production of many cytokines, including IL-10 (Saraiva and O'garra 2010). Well-balanced intestinal flora may contribute to well-balanced cytokine concentrations and confer extreme resistance to pathogen invasion.

101.5.3 Anti-mediator Treatments

Previous studies reported the use of many anti-cytokine or anti-inflammatory medications for sepsis; however, almost all of these treatments were of no benefit, although some did demonstrate a small effect. Triggering receptor expressed on myeloid cells-1 (TREM-1) is an inducer of pro-inflammatory mediators expressed on the surface of monocytes. Recently, it was reported that a TREM-1 inhibitor may suppress pro-inflammatory mediators and break the back of inflammation (Qian et al. 2014). Next, exogenous IFN-γ therapies may be effective as immunostimulators in premature neonates. In neonates, the surface expression levels of innate immune receptors, for example, CD14, TLR2, and TLR4, are remarkably impaired with the decrease in gestational age. However, incubation of neonatal blood with IFN-γ improved the surface expression of

innate immune receptors and the immune function of phagocytes.

VEGF is a potent angiogenic and vascular permeability factor (Leung et al. 1989). Anti-VEGF antibody therapy decreased pro-inflammatory cytokine levels, for example, IL-6, MCP-1, and RANTES, and improved endothelial permeability in a murine sepsis model, resulting in decreased mortality (Jeong et al. 2013).

G-CSF and granulocyte-macrophage colony-stimulating factor (GM-CSF) therapy have also been studied in neonatal sepsis by randomized control trials. These two cytokines increased neutrophil numbers and function in patients with sepsis. However, there is insufficient evidence for the use G-CSF and GM-CSF (Carr et al. 2003). In addition, it is known that G-CSF-primed neutrophils generate ROS in vitro. In particular, under high oxygen tension, systemic neutrophil-activating factors should be used carefully.

Immunosuppressive strategies inhibiting specific pro-inflammatory cytokines have shown controversial effects in patients with severe sepsis. It is important to control Th17 cell and regulatory T-cell differentiation and immunomodulatory functions in such patients. A combination between inhibition of IL-17 and a TNF inhibitor (infliximab and adalimumab) may regulate Th17 cells and repress the excessive production of pro-inflammatory cytokines (Miossec et al. 2009). In future, new therapies may shift to the enhancement of the host defense immune response for inhibition of an excessive inflammatory response (Hotchkiss et al. 2013a).

References

Abraham E, Arcaroli J, Carmody A et al (2000) HMG-1 as a mediator of acute lung inflammation. J Immunol 165:2950–2954

Adib-Conquy M, Cavaillon J-M (2009) Compensatory anti-inflammatory response syndrome. Thromb Haemost 101:36–47

Akdis M, Burgler S, Crameri R et al (2011) Interleukins, from 1 to 37, and interferon-gamma: receptors, functions, and roles in diseases. J Allergy Clin Immunol 127:701–721, e701–770

Ala Y, Palluy O, Favero J et al (1992) Hypoxia/reoxygenation stimulates endothelial cells to promote interleukin-1 and interleukin-6 production. Effects of free radical scavengers. Agents Actions 37:134–139

Aly H, Khashaba MT, El-Ayouty M et al (2006) IL-1β, IL-6 and TNF-α and outcomes of neonatal hypoxic ischemic encephalopathy. Brain Dev 28:178–182

Aly H, Hassanein S, Nada A et al (2009) Vascular endothelial growth factor in neonates with perinatal asphyxia. Brain Dev 31:600–604

Baggiolini M (1998) Chemokines and leukocyte traffic. Nature 392:565–568

Baranova O, Miranda LF, Pichiule P et al (2007) Neuron-specific inactivation of the hypoxia inducible factor 1α increases brain injury in a mouse model of transient focal cerebral ischemia. J Neurosci 27:6320–6332

Belderbos ME, Levy O, Meyaard L et al (2013) Plasma-mediated immune suppression: a neonatal perspective. Pediatr Allergy Immunol 24:102–113

Bianchi ME (2007) DAMPs, PAMPs and alarmins: all we need to know about danger. J Leukoc Biol 81:1–5

Bona E, Andersson AL, Blomgren K et al (1999) Chemokine and inflammatory cell response to hypoxia-ischemia in immature rats. Pediatr Res 45:500–509

Bonizzi G, Karin M (2004) The two NF-κB activation pathways and their role in innate and adaptive immunity. Trends Immunol 25:280–288

Brochu ME, Girard S, Lavoie K et al (2011) Developmental regulation of the neuroinflammatory responses to LPS and/or hypoxia-ischemia between preterm and term neonates: an experimental study. J Neuroinflammation 8:55

Brocklehurst P, Farrell B, King A et al (2011) Treatment of neonatal sepsis with intravenous immune globulin. N Engl J Med 365:1201–1211

Carr R, Modi N, Dore C (2003) G-CSF and GM-CSF for treating or preventing neonatal infections. Cochrane Database Syst Rev Cd003066

Castellheim A, Brekke OL, Espevik T et al (2009) Innate immune responses to danger signals in systemic inflammatory response syndrome and sepsis. Scand J Immunol 69:479–491

Chalak LF, Sanchez PJ, Adams-Huet B et al (2014) Biomarkers for severity of neonatal hypoxic-ischemic encephalopathy and outcomes in newborns receiving hypothermia therapy. J Pediatr 164:468–474.e461

Chapados I, Lee T-F, Chik CL et al (2011) Hydrocortisone administration increases pulmonary artery pressure in asphyxiated newborn piglets reoxygenated with 100% oxygen. Eur J Pharmacol 652:111–116

Chavez-Valdez R, Kovell L, Ahlawat R et al (2013) Opioids and clonidine modulate cytokine production and opioid receptor expression in neonatal immune cells. J Perinatol Off J Calif Perinat Assoc 33:374–382

Chiesa C, Pellegrini G, Panero A et al (2003) Umbilical cord interleukin-6 levels are elevated in term neonates with perinatal asphyxia. Eur J Clin Invest 33:352–358

Chirico V, Lacquaniti A, Salpietro V et al (2014) High-mobility group box 1 (HMGB1) in childhood: from bench to bedside. Eur J Pediatr 173:1123–1136

Cuenca AG, Wynn JL, Moldawer LL et al (2013) Role of innate immunity in neonatal infection. Am J Perinatol 30:105–112

Derugin N, Wendland M, Muramatsu K et al (2000) Evolution of brain injury after transient middle cerebral artery occlusion in neonatal rats. Stroke 31:1752–1761

Dinarello CA (1998) Interleukin-1, interleukin-1 receptors and interleukin-1 receptor antagonist. Int Rev Immunol 16:457–499

Døllner H, Vatten L, Halgunset J et al (2002) Histologic chorioamnionitis and umbilical serum levels of pro-inflammatory cytokines and cytokine inhibitors. BJOG Int J Obstet Gynaecol 109:534–539

Dubovy P, Brazda V, Klusakova I et al (2013) Bilateral elevation of interleukin-6 protein and mRNA in both lumbar and cervical dorsal root ganglia following unilateral chronic compression injury of the sciatic nerve. J Neuroinflammation 10:55

Epstein FHMD, Goldenberg RLMD, Hauth JCMD et al (2000) Intrauterine infection and preterm delivery. N Engl J Med 342:1500–1507

Ergenekon E, Gücüyener K, Erbaş D et al (2004) Cerebrospinal fluid and serum vascular endothelial growth factor and nitric oxide levels in newborns with hypoxic ischemic encephalopathy. Brain Dev 26:283–286

Fan X, Heijnen CJ, Van Der Kooij MA et al (2009) The role and regulation of hypoxia-inducible factor-1α expression in brain development and neonatal hypoxic–ischemic brain injury. Brain Res Rev 62:99–108

Fauchère J-C, Koller BM, Tschopp A et al (2015) Safety of early high-dose recombinant erythropoietin for neuroprotection in very preterm infants. J Pediatr 167:52–57.e53

Felderhoff-Mueser U, Schmidt OI, Oberholzer A et al (2005) IL-18: a key player in neuroinflammation and neurodegeneration? Trends Neurosci 28: 487–493

Fellman V, Raivio KO (1997) Reperfusion injury as the mechanism of brain damage after perinatal asphyxia. Pediatr Res 41:599–606

Feng Y, Rhodes PG, Bhatt AJ (2008) Neuroprotective effects of vascular endothelial growth factor following hypoxic ischemic brain injury in neonatal rats. Pediatr Res 64:370–374

Feng Y, Rhodes PG, Liu H et al (2009) Dexamethasone induces neurodegeneration but also up-regulates vascular endothelial growth factor A in neonatal rat brains. Neuroscience 158:823–832

Fisher CJ Jr, Dhainaut JF, Opal SM et al (1994) Recombinant human interleukin 1 receptor antagonist in the treatment of patients with sepsis syndrome. Results from a randomized, double-blind, placebo-controlled trial. Phase III rhIL-1ra Sepsis Syndrome Study Group. JAMA 271:1836–1843

Fisher CJ Jr, Agosti JM, Opal SM et al (1996) Treatment of septic shock with the tumor necrosis factor receptor: Fc fusion protein. The Soluble TNF Receptor Sepsis Study Group. N Engl J Med 334:1697–1702

Fiuza C, Bustin M, Talwar S et al (2003) Inflammation-promoting activity of HMGB1 on human microvascular endothelial cells. Blood 101:2652–2660

Fotopoulos S, Mouchtouri A, Xanthou G et al (2005) Inflammatory chemokine expression in the peripheral blood of neonates with perinatal asphyxia and perinatal or nosocomial infections. Acta Paediatr 94:800–806

Galasso JM, Liu Y, Szaflarski J et al (2000) Monocyte chemoattractant protein-1 is a mediator of acute excitotoxic injury in neonatal rat brain. Neuroscience 101:737–744

Gantert M, Been JV, Gavilanes AWD et al (2010) Chorioamnionitis: a multiorgan disease of the fetus[quest]. J Perinatol Off J Calif Perinat Assoc 30:S21–S30

Gomez R, Romero R, Ghezzi F et al (1998) The fetal inflammatory response syndrome. Am J Obstet Gynecol 179:194–202

Gotsch F, Romero R, Kusanovic JP et al (2007) The fetal inflammatory response syndrome. Clin Obstet Gynecol 50:652–683

Hedtjarn M, Leverin AL, Eriksson K et al (2002) Interleukin-18 involvement in hypoxic-ischemic brain injury. J Neurosci Off J Soc Neurosci 22:5910–5919

Hedtjärn M, Mallard C, Arvidsson P et al (2004) White matter injury in the immature brain: role of interleukin-18. Neurosci Lett 373:16–20

Hotchkiss RS, Monneret G, Payen D (2013a) Immunosuppression in sepsis: a novel understanding of the disorder and a new therapeutic approach. Lancet Infect Dis 13:260–268

Hotchkiss RS, Monneret G, Payen D (2013b) Sepsis-induced immunosuppression: from cellular dysfunctions to immunotherapy. Nat Rev Immunol 13:862–874

Hotoura E, Giapros V, Kostoula A et al (2011) Tracking changes of lymphocyte subsets and pre-inflammatory mediators in full-term neonates with suspected or documented infection. Scand J Immunol 73:250–255

Irakam A, Miskolci V, Vancurova I et al (2002) Dose-related inhibition of proinflammatory cytokine release from neutrophils of the newborn by dexamethasone, betamethasone, and hydrocortisone. Biol Neonate 82:89–95

Jenkins DD, Rollins LG, Perkel JK et al (2012) Serum cytokines in a clinical trial of hypothermia for neonatal hypoxic-ischemic encephalopathy. J Cereb Blood Flow Metab Off J Int Soc Cereb Blood Flow Metab 32:1888–1896

Jeong SJ, Han SH, Kim CO et al (2013) Anti-vascular endothelial growth factor antibody attenuates inflammation and decreases mortality in an experimental model of severe sepsis. Crit Care 17:R97

Kaandorp JJ, Van Bel F, Veen S et al (2012) Long-term neuroprotective effects of allopurinol after moderate perinatal asphyxia: follow-up of two randomised controlled trials. Arch Dis Child Fetal Neonatal Ed 97: F162–F166

Kelen D, Robertson NJ (2010) Experimental treatments for hypoxic ischaemic encephalopathy. Early Hum Dev 86:369–377

Kim CJ, Romero R, Chaemsaithong P et al (2015) Acute chorioamnionitis and funisitis: definition, pathologic features, and clinical significance. Am J Obstet Gynecol 213:S29–S52

Kollmann TR, Crabtree J, Rein-Weston A et al (2009) Neonatal innate TLR-mediated responses are distinct from those of adults. J Immunol 183:7150–7160

Komine-Kobayashi M, Zhang N, Liu M et al (2006) Neuroprotective effect of recombinant human granulocyte colony-stimulating factor in transient focal ischemia of mice. J Cereb Blood Flow Metab Off J Int Soc Cereb Blood Flow Metab 26:402–413

Kondo M, Itoh S, Isobe K et al (2000) Chemiluminescence because of the production of reactive oxygen species in the lungs of newborn piglets during resuscitation periods after asphyxiation load. Pediatr Res 47: 524–527

Leung DW, Cachianes G, Kuang WJ et al (1989) Vascular endothelial growth factor is a secreted angiogenic mitogen. Science (New York, NY) 246:1306–1309

Levy O, Wynn JL (2014) A prime time for trained immunity: innate immune memory in newborns and infants. Neonatology 105:136–141

Levy MM, Fink MP, Marshall JC et al (2003) 2001 SCCM/ESICM/ACCP/ATS/SIS international sepsis definitions conference. Crit Care Med 31: 1250–1256

Li L, Mbride DW, Doycheva D et al (2015) G-CSF attenuates neuroinflammation and stabilizes the blood–brain barrier via the PI3K/Akt/GSK-3β signaling pathway following neonatal hypoxia-ischemia in rats. Exp Neurol 272:135–144

Liu F, Mccullough LD (2013) Inflammatory responses in hypoxic ischemic encephalopathy. Acta Pharmacol Sin 34:1121–1130

Lv H, Wang Q, Wu S et al (2015) Neonatal hypoxic ischemic encephalopathy-related biomarkers in serum and cerebrospinal fluid. Clin Chim Acta 450:282–297

Marodi L (2001) IL-12 and IFN-gamma deficiencies in human neonates. Pediatr Res 49:316

Maroso M, Balosso S, Ravizza T et al (2011) Interleukin-1 type 1 receptor/toll-like receptor signalling in epilepsy: the importance of IL-1beta and high-mobility group box 1. J Intern Med 270:319–326

Matsui T, Kida H, Iha T et al (2014) Effects of hypothermia on ex vivo microglial production of pro- and anti-inflammatory cytokines and nitric oxide in hypoxic-ischemic brain-injured mice. Folia Neuropathol Assoc Pol Neuropathol Med Res Cent Pol Acad Sci 52:151–158

Mesples B, Plaisant F, Gressens P (2003) Effects of interleukin-10 on neonatal excitotoxic brain lesions in mice. Dev Brain Res 141:25–32

Miossec P, Korn T, Kuchroo VK (2009) Interleukin-17 and type 17 helper T cells. N Engl J Med 361:888–898

Mizuno K, Hida H, Masuda T et al (2008) Pretreatment with low doses of erythropoietin ameliorates brain damage in periventricular leukomalacia by targeting late oligodendrocyte progenitors: a rat model. Neonatology 94:255–266

Murphy BP, Inder TE, Huppi PS et al (2001) Impaired cerebral cortical gray matter growth after treatment with dexamethasone for neonatal chronic lung disease. Pediatrics 107:217–221

Nakamura S, Kusaka T, Koyano K et al (2014) Relationship between early changes in cerebral blood volume and electrocortical activity after hypoxic-ischemic insult in newborn piglets. Brain Dev 36:563–571

Ng PC, Li K, Chui KM et al (2007) IP-10 is an early diagnostic marker for identification of late-onset bacterial infection in preterm infants. Pediatr Res 61:93–98

Ohlsson A, Lacy JB (2015) Intravenous immunoglobulin for suspected or proven infection in neonates. Cochrane Database Syst Rev 3, Cd001239

Okazaki K, Nishida A, Kato M et al (2006) Elevation of cytokine concentrations in asphyxiated neonates. Biol Neonate 89:183–189

Okazaki K, Kondo M, Kato M et al (2008a) Temporal alterations in concentrations of sera cytokines/chemokines in sepsis due to group B streptococcus infection in a neonate. Jpn J Infect Dis 61:382–385

Okazaki K, Kondo M, Kato M et al (2008b) Elevation of high-mobility group box 1 concentration in asphyxiated neonates. Neonatology 94:105–109

Okazaki K, Kusaka T, Kondo M et al (2012) Temporal alteration of serum G-CSF and VEGF levels in perinatal asphyxia treated with head cooling. Cytokine 60:812–814

Okazaki K, Kusaka T, Kondo M, Kimura H (2015) Pathophysiological roles of cytokines in the brain during perinatal asphyxia. Ann Pediatr Child Health 3:1030

Osuchowski MF, Welch K, Siddiqui J et al (2006) Circulating cytokine/inhibitor profiles reshape the understanding of the SIRS/CARS continuum in sepsis and predict mortality. J Immunol 177:1967–1974

Osuchowski MF, Craciun F, Weixelbaumer KM et al (2012) Sepsis chronically in MARS: systemic cytokine responses are always mixed regardless of the outcome, magnitude, or phase of sepsis. J Immunol 189:4648–4656

Pammi M, Abrams SA (2015) Oral lactoferrin for the prevention of sepsis and necrotizing enterocolitis in preterm infants. Cochrane Database Syst Rev 2, Cd007137

Pober JS, Sessa WC (2007) Evolving functions of endothelial cells in inflammation. Nat Rev Immunol 7:803–815

Qian L, Weng XW, Chen W et al (2014) TREM-1 as a potential therapeutic target in neonatal sepsis. Int J Clin Exp Med 7:1650–1658

Rangarajan V, Juul SE (2014) Erythropoietin: emerging role of erythropoietin in neonatal neuroprotection. Pediatr Neurol 51:481–488

Roka A, Beko G, Halasz J et al (2013) Changes in serum cytokine and cortisol levels in normothermic and hypothermic term neonates after perinatal asphyxia. Inflamm Res 62:81–87

Romero R, Chaemsaithong P, Korzeniewski SJ et al (2016) Clinical chorioamnionitis at term II: the intra-amniotic inflammatory response. J Perinat Med 44:5–22

Rosenberg GA (2009) Matrix metalloproteinases and their multiple roles in neurodegenerative diseases. Lancet Neurol 8:205–216

Rossol M, Heine H, Meusch U et al (2011) LPS-induced cytokine production in human monocytes and macrophages. Crit Rev™ Immunol 31:379–446

Sahni R, Sanocka UM (2008) Hypothermia for hypoxic-ischemic encephalopathy. Clin Perinatol 35:717–734, vi

Saraiva M, O'garra A (2010) The regulation of IL-10 production by immune cells. Nat Rev Immunol 10:170–181

Savman K, Blennow M, Gustafson K et al (1998) Cytokine response in cerebrospinal fluid after birth asphyxia. Pediatr Res 43:746–751

Schelonka RL, Maheshwari A, Carlo WA et al (2011) T cell cytokines and the risk of blood stream infection in extremely low birth weight infants. Cytokine 53:249–255

Schlager GW, Griesmaier E, Wegleiter K et al (2011) Systemic G-CSF treatment does not improve long-term outcomes after neonatal hypoxic–ischaemic brain injury. Exp Neurol 230:67–74

Seo JW, Kim JH, Kim JH et al (2012) Time-dependent effects of hypothermia on microglial activation and migration. J Neuroinflammation 9:164

Sharma AA, Jen R, Butler A et al (2012) The developing human preterm neonatal immune system: a case for more research in this area. Clin Immunol 145:61–68

Shozushima T, Takahashi G, Matsumoto N et al (2011) Usefulness of presepsin (sCD14-ST) measurements as a marker for the diagnosis and severity of sepsis that satisfied diagnostic criteria of systemic inflammatory response syndrome. J Infect Chemother Off J Jpn Soc Chemother 17:764–769

Si QS, Nakamura Y, Kataoka K (1997) Hypothermic suppression of microglial activation in culture: inhibition of cell proliferation and production of nitric oxide and superoxide. Neuroscience 81:223–229

Sood BG, Shankaran S, Schelonka RL et al (2012) Cytokine profiles of preterm neonates with fungal and bacterial sepsis. Pediatr Res 72:212–220

Sprung CL, Annane D, Keh D et al (2008) Hydrocortisone therapy for patients with septic shock. N Engl J Med 358:111–124

Verrotti A, Basciani F, Trotta D et al (2001) Effect of anticonvulsant drugs on interleukins-1, -2 and -6 and monocyte chemoattractant protein-1. Clin Exp Med 1:133–136

Volpe JJ (2001) Perinatal brain injury: from pathogenesis to neuroprotection. Ment Retard Dev Disabil Res Rev 7:56–64

Wynn J, Cornell TT, Wong HR et al (2010) The host response to sepsis and developmental impact. Pediatrics 125:1031–1041

Yamaguchi M, Okamoto K, Kusano T et al (2015) The effects of xanthine oxidoreductase inhibitors on oxidative stress markers following global brain ischemia reperfusion injury in C57BL/6 mice. PLoS One 10, e0133980

Yang KD, Liou WY, Lee CS et al (1992) Effects of phenobarbital on leukocyte activation: membrane potential, actin polymerization, chemotaxis, respiratory burst, cytokine production, and lymphocyte proliferation. J Leukoc Biol 52:151–156

Yossuck P, Nightengale BJ, Fortney JE et al (2008) Effect of morphine sulfate on neonatal neutrophil chemotaxis. Clin J Pain 24:76–82

Zhang ZG, Zhang L, Tsang W et al (2002) Correlation of VEGF and angiopoietin expression with disruption of blood–brain barrier and angiogenesis after focal cerebral ischemia. J Cereb Blood Flow Metab 22: 379–392

Zhang J, Takahashi HK, Liu K et al (2011) Anti-high mobility group box-1 monoclonal antibody protects the blood-brain barrier from ischemia-induced disruption in rats. Stroke 42:1420–1428

Neonatal Malignancies

102

Serena Catania, Stefano Chiaravalli, Franca Fossati-Bellani, and Maura Massimino

Contents

Abstract
Neoplastic or tumorlike conditions are rare in the fetus and newborn, but pose important diagnostic and therapeutic problems for pediatricians and oncologists, as well as provoking enormous emotional burdens on parents and caregivers. They also present significant medical and ethical dilemmas.

102.1 Salient Points

- The vast majority of neonatal neoplasms are solid tumors of mesenchymal and embryonic origin, clinically manifest as an abnormal mass located in the abdomen, head and neck, or any soft tissue.
- Surgical ablation is the therapeutic procedure of choice for most solid tumors.

S. Catania (✉) · S. Chiaravalli · F. Fossati-Bellani · M. Massimino
Pediatric Oncology Department, Fondazione IRCCS Istituto Nazionale dei Tumori, Milan, Italy
e-mail: serena.catania@fastwebnet.it; Stefano.Chiaravalli@istitutotumori.mi.it; maura.massimino@istitutotumori.mi.it

G. Buonocore et al. (eds.), *Neonatology*,
https://doi.org/10.1007/978-3-319-29489-6_249

- Chemotherapy for neonates is especially challenging because of their immature renal and hepatic functions.
- Radiation therapy may cause damage to growth, musculoskeletal system, endocrine and cognitive functions, depending on the site and volume of the radiation fields.
- Neuroblastoma is the most common solid, extracranial malignancy of childhood.
- Germinal tumors and teratomas are the most frequent perinatal tumors, more common in females.
- Congenital mesoblastic nephromas are by far the most common renal tumors, followed by Wilms tumor.
- CNS tumors are rare in fetuses and neonates and are characterized by extremely rapid growth and preference for the supratentorial space.
- The most common primary liver tumor is hepatic hemangioma followed by mesenchymal hamartoma and hepatoblastoma.
- Leukemia in the newborn differs from the disease in older children. Acute nonlymphoblastic leukemia is more common than acute lymphoblastic leukemia and has a better prognosis in cases achieving remission.
- Retinoblastoma is the most common intraocular malignancy of childhood and occurs in heritable (25–30%) and nonheritable (70–75%) forms.

102.2 Introduction

Cancer in newborns is rare. Neonatal cancers are defined by their occurrence in an infant in the first 28 days after birth, or up to 44 weeks of gestational age in the case of preterm babies (Moore et al. 2003). Almost all types of pediatric cancer can occur in fetuses and neonates; however, the presentation and behavior of neonatal tumors often differ from that in older children. Although most neonatal neoplasm are considered to have a benign behavior, malignant tumors represent a significant cause of perinatal mortality (Moore et al. 2003; Isaacs 2002a), which may be related to obstetric or postnatal surgical complications or disease progression (Keeling 1993). It is essential to define and distinguish tumorlike conditions (such as hamartomas, hemangiomas, lymphangiomas, and melanocytic nevi) from benign or malignant tumors. Tumors that are benign at histology can still grow aggressively, acquiring a malignant behavior due to their site of onset and local invasiveness. They can cause death, as in the case of extensive lymphangiomas and teratomas of the newborn in the head, neck, or mediastinum. On the other hand, histologically malignant tumors of the newborn, such as neuroblastoma stage Metastatic Special (MS) and neonatal fibrosarcoma, can regress spontaneously and take a benign course even without therapy. Finally there are nonneoplastic conditions (abdominal masses) that can simulate the presence of a tumor and that have to be differentiated by appropriate procedures (Table 1). The vast majority of neonatal neoplasms are solid tumors of mesenchymal and embryonic origin and they can be diagnosed before birth. Because they are so rare, the management of these tumors represents a major challenge for neonatologist, surgeons, and oncologists.

102.2.1 Incidence

Cancer in newborns is rare with an estimated incidence of 365/100,000 live births and comprise 2% of childhood malignancies (Moore et al. 2003). Half of neonatal tumors are found at birth, 20–30% during the first week and the remaining 20–30% within the first month of life. With advances in obstetrical and perinatal care including fetal imaging, an increasing proportion of these tumors can be identified prenatally, thus allowing for proper planning for delivery and postnatal care (Isaacs 1991). The prognosis is related to the tumor behavior, which may differ significantly between the perinatal period and later ages, suggesting a role for developmental biology factors (Moore et al. 2003; Orbach et al. 2013; Raciborska et al. 2016). During the neonatal period, the incidence of a given tumor does not coincide with the related mortality rate because some tumors are rapidly lethal, while others cause

Table 1 Malignant (a), non-malignant (b), tumorlike conditions (c) of the newborn by location

Brain	(a) Teratoma, PNET (medulloblastoma, pinealoblastoma, cerebral neuroblastoma), choroid plexus carcinoma, ependymoma, astrocytoma, atypical teratoid rhabdoid tumor, sarcoma, melanoma
	(b) Teratoma[a], meningioma[a], hamartoma[a], craniopharyngioma[a]
	(c) Vascular malformation, hemorrhage, hydrocephalus
Head and neck	(a) Rhabdomyosarcoma (orbit, nasopharynx, middle ear), neuroblastoma (neck), retinoblastoma, teratoma, melanotic progonoma, Langherans cell histiocytosis
	(b) Teratoma[a], fibromatosis[a], melanotic progonoma[a], hamartoma, brachial cyst, lymphangioma[a]
	(c) Cellulitis, nasopharyngeal brain heterotopia
Trunk	(a) Neuroblastoma, germ cell, soft tissue sarcoma, Langherans cell histiocytosis
	(b) Lymphangioma[a], hamartoma[a], teratoma[a], cardiac rhabdomyoma
	(c) Pulmonary myofibroblastic tumor, massive mesenchymal malformation of lung
Abdomen pelvis	(a) Neuroblastoma, renal tumors, hepatoblastoma, germ cell tumors, soft tissue sarcoma, acute leukemia
	(b) Teratoma, hepatic hamartoma, hemangioma, hemangioendothelioma, congenital mesoblastic nephroma[a]
	(c) Polycystic kidney, hydronephrosis, urinary retention, gastrointestinal duplication, storage disease ovarian cyst, congenital viral infections
Skin and superficial soft tissue	(a) Soft tissue sarcoma, neuroblastoma, acute leukemia, Langherans cell histiocytosis, melanoma
	(b) Hemangioma, fibromatosis, giant nevus
	(c) Infections

[a]Benign tumors potentially life threatening because of size and location or tendency towards malignant transformation

death after the neonatal period, and yet others grow initially and then regress spontaneously. Neuroblastoma and teratomas are the most frequent neonatal neoplastic conditions (accounting for 22% and 23% respectively), followed by soft tissue sarcomas (8%), acute leukemias (6%), central nervous system (CNS) tumors (6%), benign and malignant liver tumors (6%), kidney tumors (7%), and retinoblastomas (5%). Males and females are generally affected equally but retinoblastoma is more common in males, teratoma in females. Leukemias and CNS tumors are the most lethal in this age group.

102.2.2 Etiology

The causes of neonatal cancer are unclear, but genetic factors probably have a key role. Congenital abnormalities are frequently present. Less than 10% of childhood cancers are surely related to a known cancer predisposition syndrome. Any tumor diagnosed in the perinatal period should raise the question of a cancer predisposition syndrome. The other main features suggesting a cancer predisposition syndrome are bilateral or multifocal disease, associated congenital malformation, and cancer in close relatives (Table 2). Several types of perinatal tumors show a strong association with a cancer predisposition syndrome. These tumors can occur sporadically in families because of a high rate of neomutation or autosomal recessive inheritance. If a cancer predisposition syndrome is identified, parents of the affected child should be referred to a genetic clinic for counselling (Orbach et al. 2013).

102.2.3 Clinical Features and Diagnosis

Most tumors are clinically manifest as an abnormal mass located in the abdomen or head and neck or any soft tissue site. They may be detected before birth. Solid malignancies account for approximately 75% of neonatal cancers. For many of these tumors, such as low risk neuroblastoma or sacrococcygeal teratomas,

Table 2 Cancer predisposition syndrome with a risk of tumor during the perinatal period (Orbach et al. 2013, e610)

Syndrome	Identified gene	Tumors possible during perinatal period (risk during infancy, %)	Other tumor risk for children, adolescent, and young adults
Syndromes associated with developmental defects			
Autosomal dominant inheritance			
WAGR	11p13 deletion	Wilms tumor (50%)	–
Denys Drash	Exons 8 and 9 WT 1	Wilms tumor (50%)	Gonadoblastoma
Frasier	Intron 9 WT1	Wilms tumor (10%)	Gonadoblastoma
Beckwith Wiedemann	11p15 telomeric region	Hepatoblastoma	Wilms tumor (10%)
Basal-cell nevus	PTCH1	Medulloblastoma (5%)	Basal cell carcinoma, ovarian fibromas
Down syndrome	Trisomy 21	Transient abnormal myelopoiesis (4–10%) AML7	Seminoma, AML7, LLA
Noonan syndrome	PTPN11, HRAS,KRAS, BRAF,SOS1	Transient abnormal myelopoiesis, juvenile myelomonocytic leukemia, neuroblastoma	Rhabdomyosarcoma, juvenile myelomonocytic leukemia
MEN 2b	RET	Medullary thyroid cancer	Pheochromocytoma
Congenital central hypoventilation	PHOX2B	Neuroblastoma (3%)	–
Autosomal recessive inheritance			
Fanconi anemia	BRCA2, BRIP1, PALB2	Preleukemia, brain tumor, Wilms tumor, neuroblastoma	–
Constitutional mismatch repair deficiency	MLH1,MSH2, MSH6, PMS2	Any malignancy (97%), preleukemia, brain tumor, lymphoma	Early onset gastrointestinal or gynecological cancer
Mosaic variegated aneuploidy	BUB1B, CEP57	Wilms tumor, rhabdomyosarcoma, leukemia (40%)	Gastrointestinal neoplasia
Perlmann	DIS3L2	Wilms tumor (60%)	–
Syndromes not associated with developmental defects			
Li-Fraumeni	TP53	Brain tumor, bone or soft tissue sarcoma, adrenocortical carcinoma	Breast cancer, brain tumor, bone and soft tissue sarcoma, leukemia
Rhabdoid tumors	SMARCB1	Atypical teratoid rhabdoid tumor, renal rhabdoid tumor, extrarenal rhabdoid tumor (around 100%)	Schwannoma
Retinoblastoma	RB1	Retinoblastoma (90%)	Sarcoma, melanoma, glioma, carcinoma
Familial adenomatous polyposis	APC	Hepatoblastoma (1%)	Colorectal cancer, thyroid cancer, medulloblastoma, desmoid tumor
Familial neuroblastoma	ALK	Neuroblastoma (30–70%)	–
Medulloblastoma	SUFU	Medulloblastoma (20%)	–

outcome has been described to be excellent; however, neonatal neoplasm often has a very aggressive clinical presentation that may precipitate rapid clinic deterioration of these vulnerable infants. It is of extreme importance to centralize care in experienced centers where multidisciplinary treatment is available (Raciborska et al. 2016). Advances in diagnostic procedures (ultrasound, US, and magnetic resonance imaging, MR) have facilitated the prenatal

diagnosis of congenital neoplasms such as teratomas, abdominal or intrathoracic masses, with consequent implications for prenatal therapy and the choice of vaginal versus cesarean deliveries and for outcome of the fetus. Diagnostic imaging of perinatal tumors is based on a specific strategy. Since the fetus and neonate have high sensitivity to ionizing radiation, non-irradiating techniques such as ultrasonography and MR should be used rather than techniques based on x-ray or isotopes. Other advantages of ultrasonography include ease of use, real time imaging, high spatial resolution, and possible vascular analysis with Doppler ultrasound. Ultrasonography provides imaging of soft tissues and of anatomical regions not assessable in older patient, e.g., brain and spinal cord. Prenatal imaging of fetus tumors should mainly rely on ultrasonography, but MR might also be helpful. MR provides details of the site and the anatomical extent of a lesion and, in selected cases, it has been instrumental in strategic prenatal therapeutic procedures, such as fetal surgery or fetal rescue at the time of delivery. Postnatally ultrasonography and MRI should be the first-line imaging techniques. MR is more specific for CNS assessment and might be useful antenatally for differential diagnosis of tumor and extensive intracranial hemmorrhage or extra-axial hemangiomas. CT scan is technically easier to do than MR but CT scan is associated with somewhat high radiation doses and should be avoided except in emergency situations or when more detailed lung assessment is needed. Nuclear medicine methods such as 99 m-Tc-medronate bone scintigraphy or 123I- Scintigraphy for neuroblastic tumors might be necessary for staging and must follow specific guidelines. Positron emission tomography (PET) has yet to be validated for use in diagnosing childhood tumors (Orbach et al. 2013).

Imaging data, combined with clinical findings, provide the basis for the histopathological diagnosis of neoplastic lesions that have been totally resected or biopsied. To characterize a neoplasm precisely, the morphological features derived from classic histology must be combined with immunohistochemistry and cytogenetic assessment. For instance, the value of the MYCN oncogene (a molecular marker of NBL) is significant in term of prognosis and treatment.

102.2.4 Principles of Therapy

Interdisciplinary cooperation between all specialists involved at the various stages of the diagnostic and therapeutic process is vital (Moore et al. 2003; Isaacs 1991).

102.2.4.1 Surgery

Surgical ablation is the therapeutic procedure of choice for most solid tumors (such as teratomas, Wilms' tumor, and neuroblastoma).

Pediatric surgeons do not have to undertake aggressive surgery. The timing and strategy of surgical procedures have to consider the newborn's metabolic and physiologic needs, as well as the local extent of the tumor to enable complete excision, and the feasibility of delaying surgery until after shrinking the tumor volume by chemotherapy to avoid mutilating surgery or operations that would interfere with the child's growth or impair any vital functions. In pediatric oncology, the purpose of a multidisciplinary approach is to limit the damage associated with invasive therapies, especially in younger patients, without affecting adversely survival prospects (Azizkhan 2008; Look and Aplan 2006; Reaman and Bleyer 2006).

102.2.4.2 Chemotherapy (CHT)

Use of chemotherapy in neonates is especially challenging because of their immature renal and hepatic functions. There are not enough pharmacologic studies of drug metabolism, clearance and toxicity to organs and functions to support the use of antitumor drugs in the newborn. Data on the pharmacology of antitumor chemotherapy in infants and young children have revealed severe neurotoxicity of vincristine, hepatotoxicity of actinomycin D, myelotoxicity of adriamycin, and ototoxicity of cisplatin (Charles 2007). A study investigating the pharmacokinetic of carboplatin in infant neuroblastoma

patients has been recently completed. The clearance of carboplatin has been shown to change markedly during the first few weeks of life in premature babies, linked with renal function development (Veal and Boddy 2012). Methotrexate (MTX) is used in many pediatric oncology protocols. The main use in neonates is in acute lymphoblastic leukemia (ALL) where high dose regimens are often used to target sanctuary sites and to reduce minimal residual disease (Veal and Boddy 2012; Lucchesi and Guidi 2016). Several data on pharmacokinetics of high dose MTX in infant with ALL are available. In particular, retrospective analysis of Interfant-99 trial confirms the rationale for dose reduction of MTX in infants, since the doses given resulted in comparable steady-state concentrations for infants of all ages. MTX is also an important drug for the treatment of aggressive brain tumors. It has been demonstrated that therapeutically effective concentrations can be achieved in the cerebrospinal fluid at doses of 4 g/m^2. There are some concerns about MTX toxicity, particularly in terms of neurocognitive development and the risk of leukoencephalopathy. Renal clearance is the principal pathway of MTX elimination, and its elimination appears to be related to renal function. On the other hand, nephrotoxicity is one of the most frequently reported side effects of high dose MTX infusion, especially in patients with delayed MTX elimination. Renal function starts to develop in early fetal period and continue to evolve throughout the first years of life until it reaches its complete activity. Overall renal function at birth, both glomerular and tubular, is reduced in comparison with later childhood and adult values. A recently published study has researched correlation between MTX dose and plasma levels, and also between plasma levels and clinical or pharmacokinetic parameters, in infants aged less than 12 months with diagnosis of aggressive brain tumors treated with 8 g/m^2 of MTX. This study shows that the age does not seem to be the determining factor, rather body weight and delayed drug elimination are more determinant, potentially associated with MTX toxicities, in children with a weight less than 4 kg. This analysis confirms that a dose adjustment in infant treated with high dose MTX is required, but a weight-based dose adjustment may not be sufficient in infants weighing less than 4 kg (Lucchesi and Guidi 2016).

In conclusion, traditional cytotoxic drugs, administered at doses adjusted to the infant's weight, enable drug clearance from the patient with fewer global toxic effects and a good therapeutic index. Using a patient's weight to guide dosage has been empirically adopted for the newborn. Drug dosage must be modified in the event of major side effects.

102.2.4.3 Radiation Therapy

The adverse effects of radiation therapy on infants and young children are now well known. They include irreversible damage to growth, the musculoskeletal system, and endocrine and cognitive functions, depending on the site and volume of the radiation fields. Furthermore, the risk of second tumors limits the use of RT in pediatric oncology and makes it contraindicated for the newborn.

102.2.4.4 Supportive Care

In pediatric oncology, good therapeutic results have been achieved (now reaching a 5-year survival rate of 70%) because of improved supportive care. Hydration, antibiotics, blood products, growth factors, antiemetic agents, and nutritional support are all particularly important for the newborn because of their inability to withstand invasive treatments and because of the severe risk of infection and metabolic complications in the short term.

102.3 Tumors

102.3.1 Neuroblastoma

Neuroblastoma is the most common solid, extracranial malignancy of childhood, and the most common malignant tumor in infants under 1 year of age with an overall incidence of 1 case per 100,000 children. Neonatal neuroblastoma accounts for approximately 5% of all cases of the disease. NBL originates from neural crest cells and can occur along the sympathetic chain and in the adrenal medulla. The link identified at

autopsy between infants dying of other causes and a high incidence of NBL in situ might be explained by this tumor's tendency for spontaneous regression.

102.3.1.1 Clinical Findings

Neonatal neuroblastomas can be diagnosed in the prenatal or postnatal period, although more than 70% are first noted in the postnatal period. The most common finding is an abdominal mass originating from the adrenal gland, and, in prenatal period, could be identified as incidental solid or cystic masses on 20-week screening ultrasounds. Approximately 60% of suprarenal masses identified by imaging were localized neuroblastomas, as these tumors can present similarly to adrenal hemorrhage, extrapulmonary sequestration, bronchogenic cyst, and urologic abnormalities during the perinatal period. The primary tumor may be also located in the paravertebral region presenting with spinal cord compression with flaccid leg paralysis and bladder and bowel dysfunction, in the mediastinum and neck, retroperitoneum or pelvis. Abdominal distension with or without respiratory insufficiency is a clinical finding that correlates with massive liver involvement from a small adrenal tumor. Secondary subcutaneous nodules and bone marrow invasion are also observed in this stage, defined as MS. Neonatal patients can also present with paraneoplastic syndromes such as opsoclonus-myoclonus ataxia felt possibly to be secondary to a cross-reactivity of anti-neuroblastoma antibodies and Purkinje cells in the cerebellum. Other symptoms are due to the mass effect of the tumor, according to its location (respiratory insufficiency, or Horner syndrome if it is in the neck or mediastinal region) and/or to any metastasis (Figs. 1 and 2).

102.3.1.2 Staging

The current staging system for neuroblastoma is based on the International Neuroblastoma Staging System (INSS). The INSS is a surgical-pathologic staging system that takes into account several variables including radical resection of primary tumor, ipsilateral and contralateral involvement of lymph nodes, and tumor dimension in relation to the midline.

In order to detect metastatic disease, a metaiodobenzylguanidine (mIBG) scan is performed; this exam measures the uptake of catecholamine precursors in the primary tumor, bone, bone marrow, and lymph nodes. Approximately 90% of neonatal NBLs are MIBG-avid.

The presence of metastatic disease can also be assessed by performing bone marrow aspiration and biopsy, and by assessing lymph nodes through imaging studies, including computed tomography (CT) or magnetic resonance imaging scans (MRI), or surgical exploration.

Catecholamine metabolite levels in the urine and the cytosolic enzyme neuron-specific enolase (NSE) in the blood could be used as a disease marker.

Biology plays a very important role in patient stratification. Most NBLs are associated with chromosomal anomalies, some of the most frequent being amplification of the oncogene N-myc, deletion of chromosome 1p, and aneuploidy.

102.3.1.3 Therapy and Prognosis

The treatment program depends on the stage of the tumor and its biological characteristics. Overall, the 5-year survival for children is 72%, while patients younger than 1 year of age have a 5-year survival of more than 90%. The survival for neonates with neuroblastoma is similar to that of infants. Currently cooperative groups recommend monitoring cystic NBL during the first 3 months by US. Surgical resection is recommended when it neither regresses nor increases in size. Newborns in stages 1 and 2 have a good prognosis with surgery alone even when histology shows microscopic residues but no N-myc amplification in stage 2 cases. NBLs classified as stages 3 and 4 are prevalent in children over 1 year. Chemotherapy (CHT) is performed first to shrink the tumor, delaying surgery until later. For stage 3, the prognosis is excellent while for stage 4 decreases at 50%. If MYCN oncogene is amplified, therapy is usually given in 3 phases: induction, consolidation, and maintenance. Induction consists of cycles of chemotherapy, followed by resection of the primary tumor. The consolidation phase consists of a combination of myeloablative

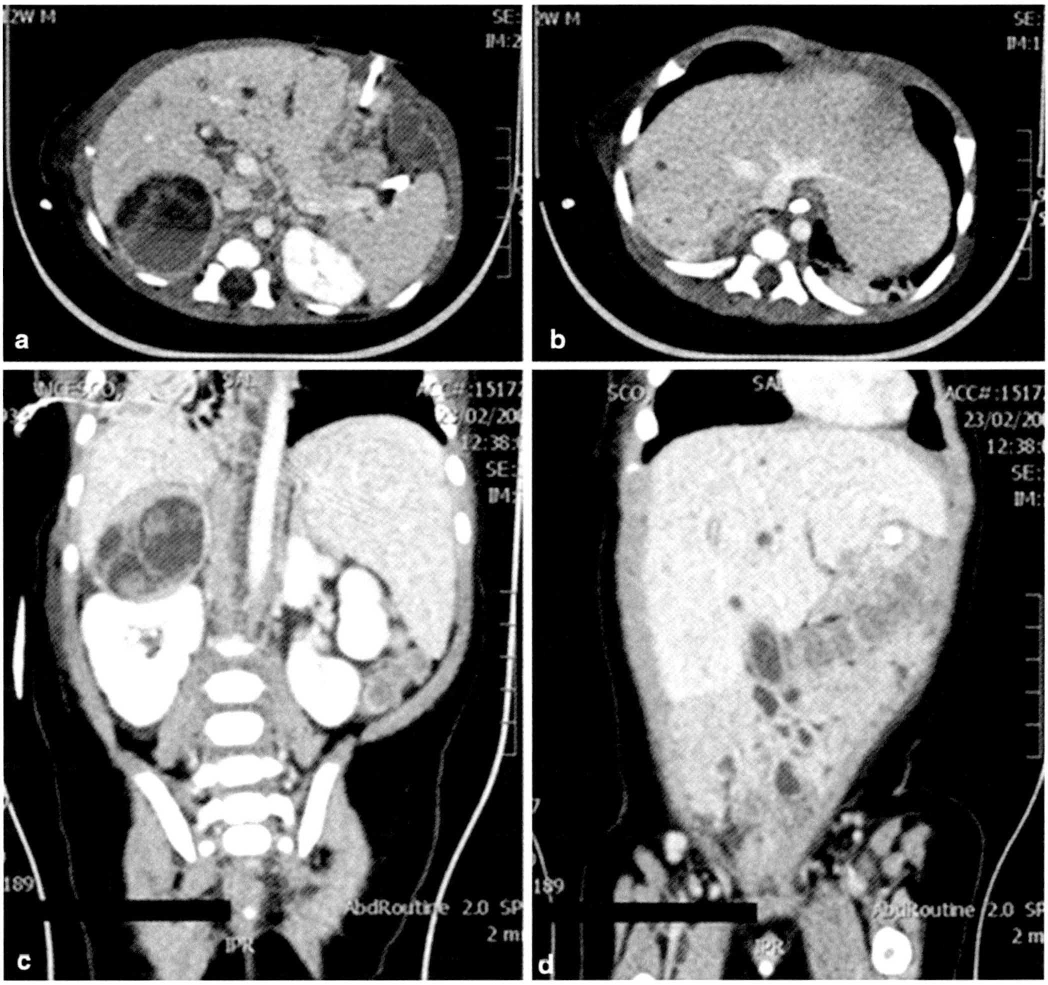

Fig. 1 Neuroblastoma 4S CT imaging. Right adrenal lesion, mostly cystic necrotic (**a–c**) with hematic level. Multiple metastatic little hepatic lesions are present (**b–d**) (Courtesy Dr. Marcello Napolitano)

chemotherapy to clear minimal residual disease and hematopoietic stem cell transplant along with radiation therapy. The maintenance phase consists of the oral agent isotretinoin, used to induce tumor cell differentiation, and immunotherapy with the chimeric anti-GD2 antibody, ch14.18, and interleukin-2.

Newborns with stage MS NBL have a good prognosis in 80% of cases without specific therapy. In cases with hepatic involvement and a risk of respiratory deficiency and/or vena cava compression, CHT can be implemented to accelerate tumor regression; surgery for the primary tumor is considered unnecessary. CHT and surgery are essential, however, in cases with biological markers indicating a poor prognosis (Isaacs 2002a; Azizkhan 2008; Charles 2007; Tsuchida et al. 2003; Nuchtern 2006).

102.3.2 Germinal Tumors (GT) and Teratomas (TRT)

These are the most frequent perinatal tumors. More common in females, they are embryonic tumors that originate from primordial germ cells or germ layers (the ectoderm, mesoderm, and endoderm). The World Health Organization (WHO) classification divides GT into seven categories, but only TRT,

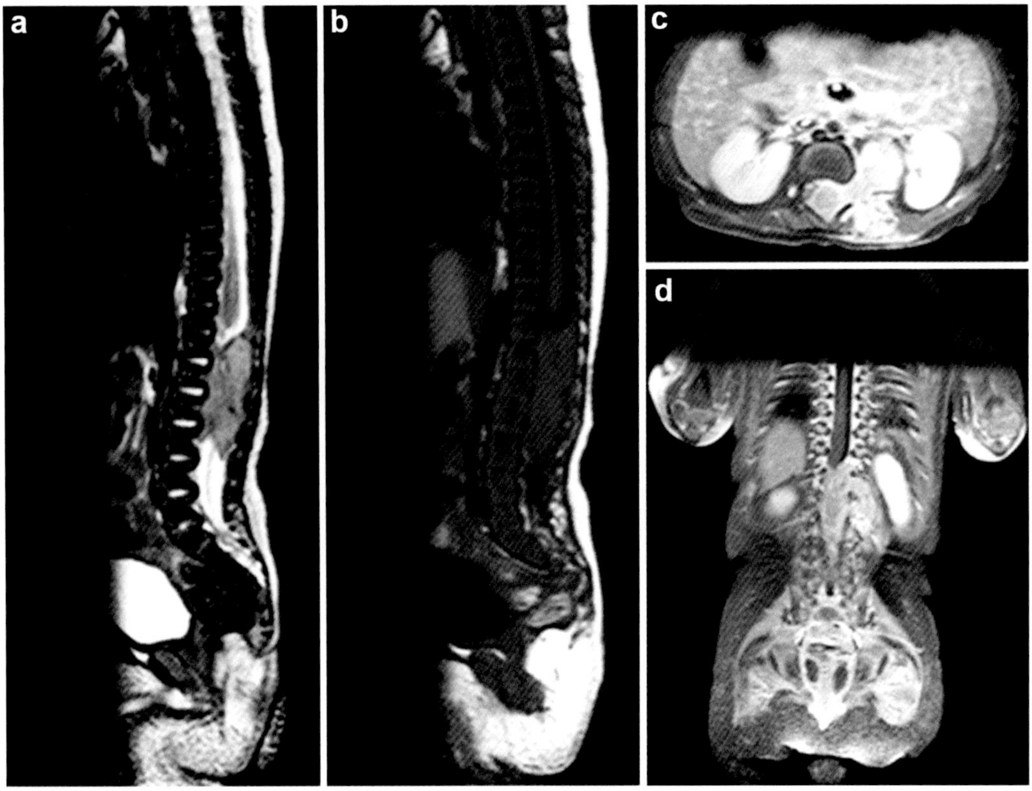

Fig. 2 Paravertebral left neuroblastoma with paraspinal and intrarachideal infiltration through conjugation foramina. MR imaging T2 W (**a**) and T1 W pre (**b**) and after (**c**, **d**) gadolinium (Courtesy Dr. Cecilia Parazzini)

yolk sac tumor, and, more rarely, gonadoblastoma have been described in the perinatal period. More than 50% of TRTs appear at birth in the sacrococcygeal region, but they can occasionally be found in the head and neck, mediastinum, brain, retroperitoneum, and liver. TRTs are classified into three different groups, depending on their histology: (a) mature, consisting mainly of adult tissue; (b) immature, consisting of embryonic tissue; or (c) malignant, consisting of malignant embryonic tissue, which is almost always a yolk sac tumor.

Teratomas are mainly isolated lesion but may form part of the Currarino triad (anorectal malformation, sacral anomaly, and a presacral mass). Other associated anomalies reported are urogenital (hypospadias, vescicoureteral reflux, and vaginal or uterine duplications), congenital dislocation of the hip, central nervous system lesions (anencephaly, trigonocephaly, Dandy-Walker malformations, spina bifida, and myelomeningocele), and Klinefelter's syndrome (strongly associated with mediastinal teratoma). Most teratomas are diagnosed on routine prenatal scanning at 18–20 weeks gestation. Doppler ultrasound is the most useful diagnostic tool although fetal MRI provides better definition of complex lesions. Fetal intervention has been reserved for large teratomas that cause mass effect and hydrops fetalis. Futhermore, large anterior mediastinal and cervical teratomas may cause fetal airway compression requiring strategies for fetal intervention, an EXIT (EX-utero Intrapartum Treatment) procedure or early delivery. Mode of delivery is dictated by the size of the lesion.

Alpha fetal protein has been used as the principal tumor marker and is particularly useful for assessing the presence of residual or recurrent disease. Other markers that may be elevated are

β HCG and LDH (Azizkhan 2008; Charles 2007; Wu et al. 1981; Isaacs 2002b).

102.3.2.1 Sacroccocygeal Teratoma (SCT)

Sacroccocygeal teratoma is the most common congenital tumor and accounts for 35–60% of all teratomas seen in the postnatal period. The presentation is mainly prenatal and easily distinguished from meningomyelocele or other tumors due to ultrasound features of vascularity. Treatment involves complete excision at birth, avoiding tumor rupture and spillage into the operative site, combined with coccygectomy. Large vascularized tumors can cause significant complications including tumor bleeding or cardiac insufficiency, leading to perinatal death in around 25% of cases. Five to ten percent of neonatal sacrococcygeal teratomas relapse; 50% of these relapses are due to a alpha-fetoprotein-secreting yolk sac tumors. The introduction of CHT with cisplatin plus etoposide in metastatic disease or for initially inoperable tumors has achieved complete regression of metastatic deposits and enabled radical surgery by reducing the tumor's initial volume. This strategy allowed a spectacular improvement in survival in both locally advanced and metastatic disease (the prognosis is good in 90% of cases of localized disease and 80% of metastatic cases). Adverse prognostic factors are even minimal presence of yolk sac tumor cells in mature and immature TRT and an incomplete resection (Lakhoo and Sowerbutts 2010).

102.3.2.2 Mediastinal Teratomas

Mediastinal teratomas can be diagnosed antenatally, may present with respiratory distress or an incidental finding on chest radiography. The anterior mediastinum is the most frequent location with occasional lesions noted in the posterior mediastinum, pericardial, intracardiac, or pulmonary area. Imaging and tumor marker values do not differ from those mentioned for sacrococcygeal teratomas. Surgical approaches to mediastinal teratomas vary from thoracotomy to median sternotomy, depending on the anatomical site of the lesion (Lakhoo and Sowerbutts 2010).

102.3.3 Soft Tissue Sarcoma (STS)

Benign and malignant soft tissue tumors are the neoplasms most commonly seen in newborns after neuroblastoma and teratomas. This heterogeneous group of mesenchymal extraskeletal malignant tumors has an incidence rate in the first year of life of 16.0 per million but only 47 cases of STS diagnosed at <1 month of age were registered in the SEER 17 database (1973–2007 period). The family of neonatal STS includes conditions that differ in histology, molecular characteristics, biological behavior, and clinical evolution also if compared both to older children than to adults and, generally, are associated with worse survival. The most common histologies are rhabdomyosarcoma, congenital fibrosarcoma, malignant rhabdoid tumors, hemangiopericytoma, and adult-type sarcomas. These have to be differentiated from benign tumors (that may otherwise exhibit aggressive behavior and cause life-threatening complications) and tumorlike conditions such as fibromatosis and vascular lesions that are the most prevalent soft tissue neoplasms (Azizkhan 2008; Charles 2007; Isaacs 2002c, 2004; Lobe et al. 1994).

102.3.3.1 Rhabdomyosarcoma (RMS)

RMS is an aggressive tumor composed of cells resembling normal fetal skeletal muscle, and it is the most common malignant sarcoma found in the newborn. Even if the peak of incidence in children is between 2 and 6 years of age and 5–10% are diagnosed in children aged <1 year, RMS may be congenital, indeed 1–2% of all RMS are present at birth (but only 14 cases out of 3,217, approximately 4%, were reported in the study of the American IRS – Intergroup Rhabdomyosarcoma Study). RMS is histologically grouped into two main subtypes: embryonal RMS (ERMS), the most common, including botryoid and spindle cell variants, with a better prognosis, and alveolar RMS (ARMS), characterized by the (2;13)(q35; q14) and t(1;13)(p36;q14) chromosomal translocations that is rare and with worse outcome. RMS can occur anywhere in the body where mesenchymal tissue is present, e.g., in the head, neck,

genitourinary area, and extremities. Symptoms may vary, e.g., acute urine retention (when the RMS is located in the pelvis) or cranial nerve palsy (when it affects the head-neck region) and dependent on the effect of the enlarging mass on the surrounding organs. Prenatal sonography can detect a tumor mass that may cause compression of nearby organs. The botryoid variety includes grapelike neoformations, especially in the vulvovaginal area or mouth. Polyhydramnion is likely to be present when the neoplasm is located in the maxillofacial region since it may interfere with swallowing. The tumor may be evident at birth or present as a rapidly growing mass in the first weeks of life. In neonates, RMS can be misdiagnosed as vascular tumors, especially when located on the face and neck. Diagnostic procedures include echography, CT, and MRI (that sometimes are often unable to discriminate between highly vascularized malignant soft-tissue lesions and vascular lesions), while bone marrow aspiration and bone scintigraphy are used to detect distant metastases that are present in about 20% of cases at diagnosis. Neonatal alveolar RMS seems more often associated with the presence of multiple skin nodules and the development of early brain metastases as compared with RMS in older children.

Treatment depends on the stage of the tumor and is the same as for children under 1 year (or infants), as established in cooperative international studies and may be divided into systemic (chemotherapy with drug doses generally calculated based on body weight and not by body surface resulting in a dose reduction of about 30%) and local therapies (surgery and/or radiotherapy). Intensity and timing of treatment needs to be risk-stratified to provide the best chance for cure and to minimize late treatment toxicity.

A combination of CHT and surgery is used, depending on the location and extent of the tumor, and whether it is amenable to surgical resection. Surgery may be the first step for small lesions, since it may be both diagnostic and therapeutic. Where surgery fails to completely remove the tumor, a second-look surgery is recommended after CHT. The prognosis is less favorable in the newborn than in older children, especially in cases with the alveolar histotype, because very young children are more difficult to cure related to different tumor biology, and to the difficulty of delivering appropriate intensity of chemotherapy and radiation therapy.

The overall prognosis of perinatal rhabdomyosarcoma is poor, with expected survival around 40%.

102.3.3.2 Congenital Fibrosarcoma

Congenital fibrosarcoma (CF) is classified in the group of soft part tumors of intermediate prognosis, is a highly vascularized tumor, and generally occurs in deep soft tissues of the distal part of the lower and upper extremities (66% of cases) (Fig. 3), and less frequently in the trunk (20–25%) or head and neck region (10%). It occurs quite exclusively in the first 2 years of life, with 60% of cases diagnosed before the age of 3 months and 30–50% present at birth or diagnosed in utero. The estimated incidence is five new cases per million infants. CF is characterized by the chromosomal translocation t(12:15) with the transcript ETV6-NTRK3, which is shared by cellular mesoblastic nephroma, but the absence of the typical translocation does not exclude congenital fibrosarcoma diagnosis. Tumor growth may be rapid mimicking benign vascular lesions. The radiological appearance may also be similar to that of benign vascular lesions.

Distant metastases are rare and prognosis is typically good, with survival rates of 80–100%. Surgery is done only if initial, nonmutilating complete resection is possible, typically in less than 25% of cases. In view of the high chemosensitivity of fibrosarcoma, conservative resection is often considered as the final step in a multimodal approach that starts with chemotherapy. Because of its efficacy and the absence of any expected long-term toxicity, the VA regimen (vincristine and actinomycin) is the chemotherapy of choice; more intensive regimen chemotherapy (e.g., ifosfamide plus doxorubicin) should only be considered in the event of no response to VA chemotherapy. Radiotherapy is not an option because the patients are so young.

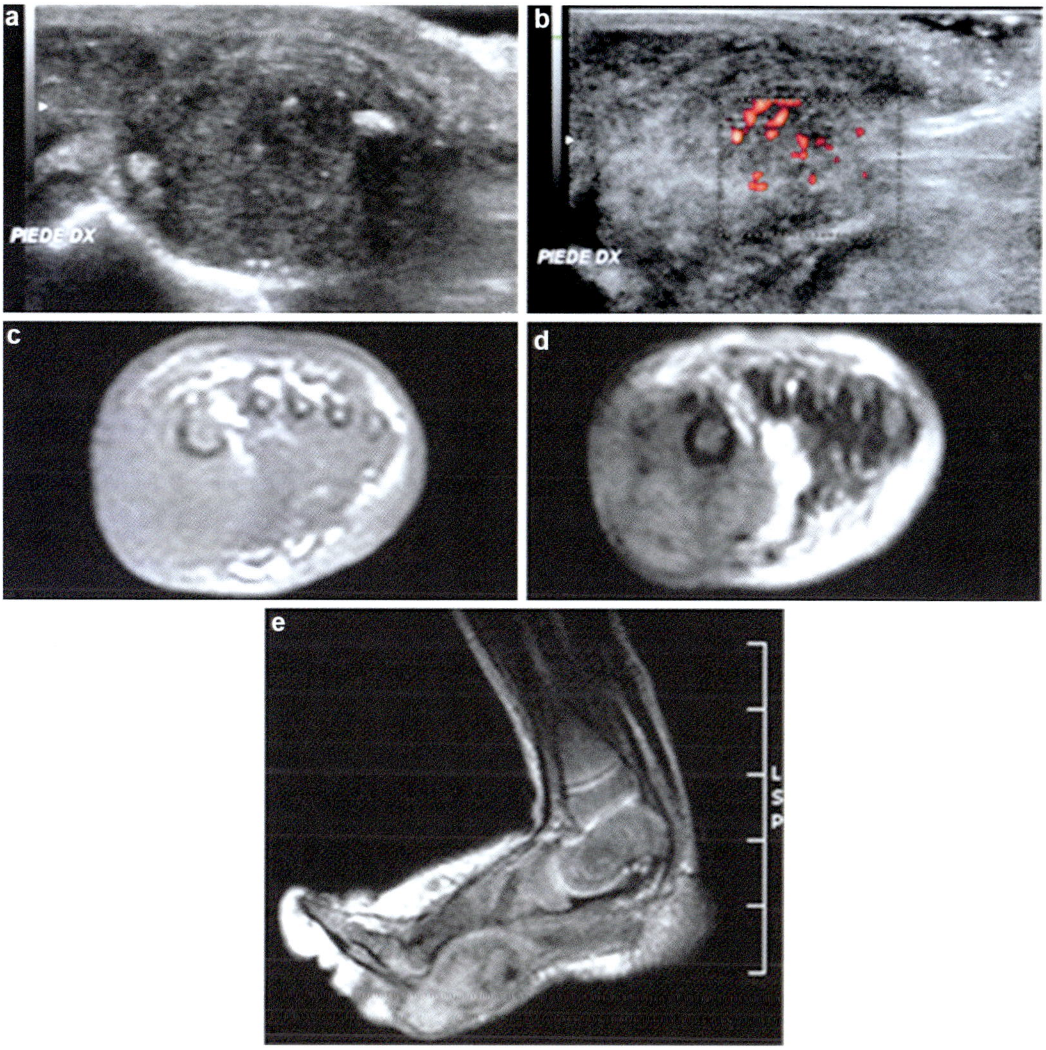

Fig. 3 Foot congenital fibrosarcoma. Ultrasound: hypoechogenic lesion with calcification (**a**), hypervascularization at power Doppler (**b**). MR imaging T1 (**c**) and T2 (**d–e**) (Courtesy Dr. Marcello Napolitano)

102.3.3.3 Other Soft Tissue Sarcomas (STS)

The rhabdoid tumor (RT) of soft tissues (abdomen, pelvis, retroperitoneum, liver, heart, and gastrointestinal tract) is the same malignant tumor arising in the central nervous system and kidney of infants and young children. Typical is the recurrent genetic alteration in the region 11.2 of the long arm of chromosome 22 (22q11.2), characterized by the deletion or mutation of the hSNF5/SMARCB1/INI1 gene resulting in the loss or reduced expression of INI protein. Rhabdoid tumors are very rare and very aggressive and frequently lethal. Individual cases of long-term survivors with the use of intensive chemotherapy regimens have been reported, and currently patients with rhabdoid tumors are treated with multidrug therapy. However, the dismal cure rates of these tumors highlight the need for additional research to cast light on tumor biology and to identify potential new targets for treatment.

There are reports in the literature of other types of STS in the newborn, including peripheral primitive neuroectodermal tumor (pPNET), vascular tumor, and undifferentiated sarcomas.

102.3.3.4 Fibroblastic Tumors of Intermediate Prognosis

Some of the STS of infants are fibroblastic-myofibroblastic tumors of intermediate prognosis (defined as locally aggressive and rarely metastasizing neoplasms). These are tumorlike conditions that need to be distinguished from the abovementioned malignant mesenchymal tumors.

The definition of juvenile fibromatosis includes benign entities such as fibrous hamartoma of infancy which is congenital in 20% of cases and develops in the cutaneous tissue of the shoulders, arms, thighs, armpits, and inguinal areas; infantile solitary myofibroma, which probably forms a morphological continuum with myopericytoma and infantile hemangiopericytoma, or the frequently occurring multicentric myofibromatosis that is more common in males and affects the head and neck, trunk, and skin. The clinical behavior is generally benign, with spontaneous regressions in some instances, but aggressive lethal forms of multicentric myofibromatosis with visceral involvement have been described. A sternomastoid tumor is generally connected with birth trauma. Infant desmoid-type fibromatosis is found in muscles, aponeuroses, shoulders, the head and neck, and the upper limbs. Cranial fasciitis can grow rapidly and infiltrate the skull bone.

Lipofibromatosis is typical of infants (congenital in 25% of cases), arises in the extremities (e.g., feet), and is classified among the intermediate neoplasms for its high risk of recurrence after surgery. It must be differentiated from lipoblastoma and lipoblastomatosis, benign and adipose tissue tumors, respectively.

Historically, surgery had been the mainstay of treatment for these tumors, but treatment strategies are currently evolving from a pure surgical to a multidisciplinary approach incorporating systemic therapies to reduce the functional and cosmetic sequelae of radical surgery.

102.3.4 Kidney Tumors

Roughly 5% of perinatal tumors arise from the kidney. Neonatal kidney masses are benign in more than 40% of cases. Congenital mesoblastic nephromas (CMN) are by far the most common renal tumors, followed by Wilms Tumor. Rhabdoid tumor of the kidney and clear cell sarcoma of the kidney have been also reported in this age group.

102.3.4.1 Congenital Mesoblastic Nephroma (CMN)

Congenital mesoblastic nephroma is a tumor almost exclusively found within the first 6 months of age, with a peak incidence at 3 months of age. It is usually unilateral with a slight male preponderance. Histologically, it is a mesenchymal tumor, predominantly composed of fibroblastic cells. There are two different histological subtypes of mesoblastic nephroma: the classical and the cellular type. The distinction between the two types has no implication for therapy. Complete, wide surgical resection is the only recommended treatment. Local recurence and metastases have been described in a few cases, especially in children older than 6 months. The vast majority of relapses occur within 12 months of nephrectomy, and in about 70% of relapsed cases the tumor is of the cellular type. Overall prognosis is good, with 96–100% survival (Lakhoo and Sowerbutts 2010).

102.3.4.2 Wilms Tumor (WT)

Wilms tumor classically presents in a slightly older age group than CMN. The WT has a more robust link to other congenital anomalies. Common associations include anidridia, genitourinary malformations, the WAGR, and Denys Drash syndrome. Two chromosomal loci have been implicated in the pathogenesis of WT: 11p13 (WT1) and 11P15 (WT2). However, most cases of WT do not have mutations in these genes, and other aetiological factors remain to be elucidated. Neonatal Wilms tumor is often localized with 80% of cases being stage I-II and metastases occurring in less than 1%. Ten percent of cases have a bilateral tumor (stage V). Most WT in neonates have favourable histology. The clinical sign of WT consists of an abdominal mass (Fig. 4), which must be differentiated from other masses using US/CT/MR. Surgery is the therapeutic procedure of choice. In addition to establishing the stage, histopathology

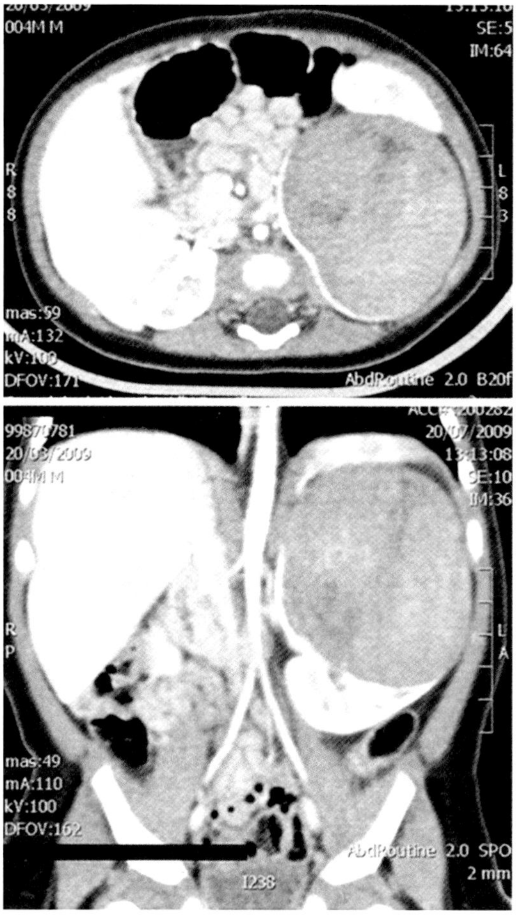

Fig. 4 CT imaging of Wilms' tumor with huge solid mass of left kidney

should give information on the presence of anaplastic areas in tumor specimens, which suggest a poor prognosis. The drugs used postoperatively include vincristine, actinomycin D, and/or adriamycin, depending on the stage of disease. Ifosfamide and carboplatin are used in cases with metastases. The prognosis is extremely good (90%) (Lakhoo and Sowerbutts 2010; Ritchey et al. 1995; Isaacs 2002d, 2008).

102.3.4.3 Rhabdoid Tumor and Clear Cell Sarcoma of the Kidney

Both these diseases demand surgery whenever possible, but metastases often occur. Chemotherapy has no influence on the prognosis, which is poor.

102.3.5 Brain Tumors

CNS tumors in fetuses and neonates are rare. Reports show an annual incidence ranging from 14 to 41 cases per million livebirths. Such tumors account for 0.5–1.9% of all pediatric CNS tumors and less than 10% of all antenatal tumors. Perinatal CNS tumors are characterized by extremely rapid growth and a predilection for the supratentorial space. These tumors are typically detected antenatally on routine ultrasound. Hydrocephalus might be caused by involvement or compression of the ventricular system or by hypersecretion of cerebrospinal fluid in choroid-plexus tumors. Symptoms are unusual, macrocephaly (caused by hydrocephalus or the volume of the tumor) being the most significant clinical sign. The fontanel may pulsate. The tumor may displace normal brain without infiltrating it, which explains the absence of focal symptoms. Vomiting and papilledema are late signs and are due to the increasing size of the neoplasm. Nonspecific symptoms, such as lethargy, fever, and gastrointestinal disorders, are often misinterpreted, causing delay in the correct diagnosis. MR of the brain and spine provides information on the tumor's size and its benign or malignant nature. Hemorrhagic episodes related to the neoplasm may stimulate brain hemorrhage or even cause a massive brain hemorrhage.

All malignant CNS tumor types occurring in infants are seen in the newborn too (teratoma 50%, astrocytoma 16%, medulloblastoma 8%, choroid plexus papilloma 7%, ependymoma 3%, unclassified glioma 22%). Overall survival for perinatal brain tumors is less than 30%.

Teratomas are the most common tumors diagnosed antenatally and intracranial teratomas comprise at least a third of tumor cases in neonates. In most cases, a definitive diagnosis is made after birth. Astrocytoma most often occurs as infant-type malignant anaplastic astrocytoma or glioblastoma multiforme. Embryonal tumors and medulloblastoma are most often diagnosed after birth (Fig. 5).

Treatment options must be discussed on a case-by-case basis and depend on the site and size of the lesion, imaging findings, and the newborn's

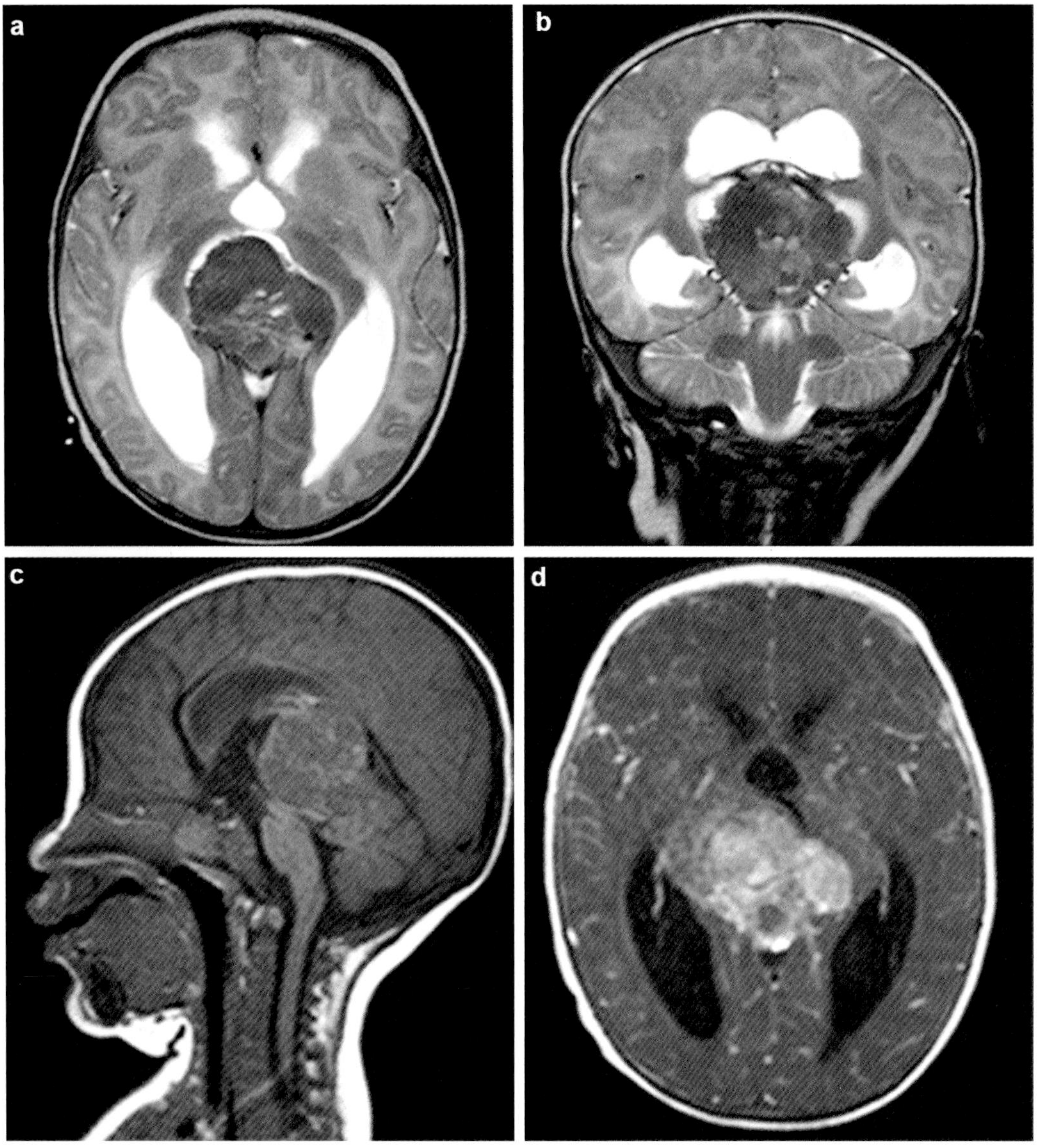

Fig. 5 Pineal gland PNET. MR imaging T2 W (**a**, **b**) and T1 W pre (**c**) and post (**d**) contrast administration (Courtesy Dr. Cecilia Parazzini)

general conditions. Surgery may be curative in patients with benign teratoma and ependymoma. Cases of embryonal tumors and medulloblastoma require pharmacological treatment. Given the poor prognosis (the survival rate is 28% in the most comprehensive case studies in the literature, which include both benign and malignant lesions), nonintervention may often be the best option. An open and frank discussion between caregivers and relatives is essential before any treatment decisions are made (Orbach et al. 2013; Azizkhan 2008; Isaacs 2002e, f).

102.3.6 Liver Tumors

Hepatic tumors comprise around 4% of tumors occurring in the neonatal period. They are a varied

group of benign and malignant neoplasm. The most common primary liver tumor is hepatic hemangioma (HH) followed by mesenchymal hamartoma (HMH) and hepatoblastoma (HB).

102.3.6.1 Hepatic Hemangioma (HH)

The hepatic hemangiomas are benign, mesenchymal derived tumors, composed of masses of blood vessels that are irregular in arrangement and size. Around half of HH are associated with cutaneous hemangiomas, more rarely they are part of more generalized hemangiomatosis syndrome. HH is more common in female infants. Aetiology remains unknown although some studies have suggested a genetic link. Possible link to female hormones have been described.

102.3.6.2 Mesenchymal Hamartoma (HMH)

The mesenchymal hamartoma is a benign hepatic tumor characterized by proliferation of myxomatous mesenchyme and malformed bile ducts. Both solid and cystic forms are seen with cystic tumors being more common in the neonatal period.

102.3.6.3 Hepatoblastoma (HB)

The hepatoblastoma is a rare embryonal tumor. The median age of diagnosis is between 6 months and 3 years. There is a largely unexplained but clearly recognized predominant in white male patients, in premature infants, and those with low birth weight. The incidence of HB in the neonatal period has been increasing over the last two decades, which may reflect the improved survival of preterm infants. There are well recognized links between HB and inherited syndrome, including Beckwith-Wiedemann syndrome and intestinal adenomatous polyposis syndrome. Screening with abdominal ultrasound and AFP levels of these risk population is generally recommended.

The clinical signs are abdominal distension and hepatomegaly. After imaging tests (MR/CT), the diagnosis is confirmed by a liver biopsy and abnormally high levels of alpha-fetoprotein (AFP), which represents a tumor marker. AFP is the major protein produced by fetal liver. AFP levels are markedly elevated in more than 90% of HB. One must relate the AFP values to the physiological AFP levels of premature newborns and infants. The SIOP (Société Internationale d'Oncologie Pédiatrique) protocol relies on primary cisplatin chemotherapy, followed by resection. Hepatoblastomas amenable to surgery have a more than 90% favorable prognosis. Liver transplantation should be considered in cases in which hepatic resection is unfeasible (Azizkhan 2008; Wu et al. 1981; Isaacs 2007).

102.3.7 Leukemia

Neonatal or congenital leukemia is very rare with an estimated incidence of one to five cases per million live-births. It is estimated to be the second most common malignancy in neonates, and leukemia is the most lethal disease of the newborn. It causes fetal hydrops and death, especially in Down syndrome patients. Leukemia in the newborn differs in clinical, hematological, molecular, and biological aspects from the disease in older children.

Acute nonlymphoblastic leukemia (ANLL) is more common (65%) than acute lymphoblastic leukemia (ALL), and the former has a better prognosis in cases achieving remission (the survival rate is 24% for ANLL and 10% for ALL). The clinical findings include hepatosplenomegaly and skin lesions; the CNS is sometimes affected. Bone marrow cytomorphological, immunophenotypic, and cytogenetic investigations are mandatory for diagnostic purposes. Congenital leukemia is CD10-negative and may be positive for markers in both the lymphoid and the myeloid lines. There is a rearrangement of the MLL (mixed linear leukemia) HRX gene on chromosome 11q23 in 50% of cases of congenital leukemia (both ANLL and ALL), and this is an unfavorable prognostic sign at all ages. Despite its unfavorable prognosis, ANLL may sometimes regress, though it may recur later on. It is important to distinguish congenital leukemia from florid neonatal leukemoid reactions, which are benign conditions defined as "transient abnormal myelopoieses," or "transient myeloproliferative

disorders" (TMD), and characterized by hepatosplenomegaly and the presence of myeloid and lymphoid immature cells. The differential diagnosis must also consider fetal erythroblastosis and viral and bacterial infections. TMD differs from congenital leukemia in that the hemoglobin and platelet counts are normal, and blasts in the bone marrow are less than 15%, despite large numbers of white cells and myeloblasts in the peripheral blood. In these benign forms, the newborn's general condition is good and no specific therapy is required. In TMD, hematological indices return to normal over a period of time that may last from a few weeks to 1–2 months. Treatment guidelines for neonatal leukemia are the same as for older children, paying appropriate attention to the dosage of drugs involved, which must be administered in specialized hematological departments. Where feasible, highdose therapeutic programs followed by hematopoietic cell transplants improve the remission and survival rates, which are currently about 20% (Sande et al. 1999; Brester et al. 2002; Isaacs 2002g, 2003).

102.3.8 Retinoblastoma (RB)

Retinoblastoma is the most common intraocular malignancy of childhood and is a tumor that occurs in heritable (25–30%) and nonheritable (70–75%) forms. Heritable disease is defined by the presence of a germline mutation of the RB1 gene. Heritable RB may manifest as unilateral or bilateral disease. Age at presentation correlates with laterality; patients with bilateral disease present at a younger age, usually in the first 12 months of life. Newborn babies with retinoblastoma lack the normal "red reflex" when undergoing ophthalmoscopic examination, which is a part of routine newborn screening. A family history of retinoblastoma mandates a complete ophthalmic investigation because of the risk of bilateral disease. Neonatal retinoblastoma most often presents as small retinal tumors, discovered by ocular fundus on screening of high risk children in the context of familial RB. Therapy is based on the outcome of a complete ophthalmic examination, and MRI can determine the extent of the lesion. The extent of retinal involvement is described as a percentage of the total retinal area. Systemic or intra-arterial chemotherapy (chemoreduction) coupled with aggressive local treatments and very close monitoring is usually the treatment of choice. For localized forms, laser therapy, thermotherapy, and cryotherapy, combined with systemic adjuvant therapy with vincristine, doxorubicin and cyclophosphamide or vincristine, carboplatin, and etoposide are associated with the best prognosis for vision and survival. The delivery of chemotherapy via ophthalmic artery cannulation (intra-arterial melphalan) as initial treatment for advanced unilateral RB appears to be more effective than does systemic chemotherapy for chemoreduction. This treatment has also been shown to be feasible and effective in patients with newly diagnosed bilateral disease and in the salvage setting. Surgery (enucleation) is limited to conditions affecting the extraocular areas, while radiotherapy (which was once used to prevent enucleation) has been abandoned because of the risk of secondary radio-induced tumors in adulthood. Therapy must be coordinated by oncologists and specialized ophthalmologists in an experienced center with a state-of-the-art treatment infrastructure and a dedicated multidisciplinary team (Look and Aplan 2006; Abramson et al. 2002).

102.3.9 Very Rare Congenital Tumors

102.3.9.1 Melanocytic Neuroectodermal Tumor of Infancy (Melanotic Progonoma – MNTI)

MNTI is an extremely rare, pigmented neoplastic entity of neural crest origin characteristically located in the jaw, while other locations include the mediastinum and brain. Histological and immunohistochemical profiles indicate the presence of two components, small rounded neuroblast-like cellular areas and areas with large melanin-containing cells which consists of combination of neural, melanocytic, and epithelial cell types. It may be malignant and produce metastases. Surgery and chemotherapy are used,

depending on the site of the lesion and the mitotic index.

102.3.9.2 Congenital Melanocytic Nevi

This condition is a benign proliferation of cutaneous melanocytes that arises as a result of abnormal growth, development, or migration of melanoblasts. Affecting approximately 1% of newborns, congenital melanocytic nevi form between 5 and 24 weeks of gestation and are present at birth or become apparent within the first year of life. Giant forms are extremely rare and may contain nodular areas with a different mesenchymal cellular component. While they can appear anywhere on the body, the most common anatomic location for a giant congenital melanocytic nevus is the posterior trunk, followed by the legs, arms, head, and neck. They sometimes resemble melanomas. Giant nevi undergo malignant transformation in 2–5% of cases. Fatal cases of congenital melanoma, with an intracranial involvement, can also occur.

102.3.9.3 Langerhans Cell Histiocytosis (LCH)

LCH is a rare disease of the immune system characterized by abnormal proliferation of Langerhans cell, which results in the formation of lesions primarily in the skin, bone, lymph nodes, lungs, liver, spleen, hematopoietic system, and central nervous system. In neonatal age, LCH affects one in a million newborns, and 60% are cases of disseminated disease (with multiple organ involvement) while 40% are only cutaneous conditions. Gastrointestinal disease causes diarrhea, vomiting, and protein-losing enteropathy. The diagnosis of LCH requires a positive outcome of the CD1a immunohistochemical test. Depending on the extent of the disease, treatment may include steroids and vinblastine, with or without 6-Mercaptopurine, as defined by international trial LCH IV.

The survival rate is 50% in cases of multiple-organ involvement, while it is more than 90% in patients with isolated disease (Azizkhan 2008; Isaacs 2006).

References

Abramson DH, Du TT, Beaverson KL (2002) (Neonatal) retinoblastoma in the first month of life. Arch Ophtalmol 120:738–742

Azizkhan RG (2008) Perinatal tumors. In: Carachi R, Grosfeld JL, Azmy AT (eds) The surgery of childhood tumors. Springer, Berlin/Heidelberg, pp 145–170

Brester D, Reus AC, Veerman AJ et al (2002) Congenital leukemia: the Dutch experience and review of literature. Br J Haematol 117:513–524

Charles AK (2007) Congenital tumors. In: Keeling JW, Khong TY (eds) Fetal and neonatal pathology. Springer, London, pp 327–378

Isaacs H Jr (1991) Tumors of the newborn and infants. Mosby-Year Book, St. Louis

Isaacs H Jr (2002a) Neuroblastoma. In: Isaacs H Jr (ed) Tumors of the fetus and infant: an atlas. Springer, New York, pp 137–160

Isaacs H Jr (2002b) Germ cell tumors. In: Isaacs H Jr (ed) Tumors of the fetus and infant: an atlas. Springer, New York, pp 5–36

Isaacs H Jr (2002c) Soft tissue tumors. In: Isaacs H Jr (ed) Tumors of the fetus and infant: an atlas. Springer, New York, pp 37–111

Isaacs H Jr (2002d) Renal tumor. In: Isaacs H Jr (ed) Tumors of the fetus and infant: an atlas. Springer, New York, pp 261–302

Isaacs H Jr (2002e) I. Perinatal brain tumors: a review of 250 cases. Pediatr Neurol 27:249–261

Isaacs H Jr (2002f) II. Perinatal brain tumors: a review of 250 cases. Pediatr Neurol 27:333–342

Isaacs H Jr (2002g) Leukemia. In: Isaacs H Jr (ed) Tumors of the fetus and infant: an atlas. Springer, New York, pp 161–180

Isaacs H Jr (2003) Fetal and neonatal leukemia. J Pediatr Hematol Oncol 25:348–361

Isaacs H Jr (2004) Perinatal (fetal and neonatal) germ cell tumors. J Pediatr Surg 39:1003–1013

Isaacs H Jr (2006) Fetal and neonatal histiocytosis. Pediatr Blood Cancer 47:123

Isaacs H Jr (2007) Fetal and neonatal hepatic tumors. J Pediatr Surg 42:1797–1803

Isaacs H Jr (2008) Fetal and neonatal renal tumors. J Pediatr Surg 43:1587–1595

Keeling JW (1993) Fetal and neonatal pathology, 2nd edn. Springer, Berlin, p 253

Lakhoo K, Sowerbutts H (2010) Neonatal tumours. Pediatr Surg Int 26:1159–1168

Lobe TE, Wiener ES, Hays DM et al (1994) Neonatal rhabdomiosarcoma: the IRS experience. J Pediatr Surg 29:1167–1170

Look AT, Aplan PD (2006) Molecular and genetic basis of childhood cancer. In: Poplak DG, Pizzo PA (eds) Principles and practice of pediatric oncology. Lippincott Williams & Wilkins, Philadelphia, pp 40–85

Lucchesi M, Guidi M (2016) Pharmacokinetics of high-dose methotrexate in infant aged less than 12 months

treated for aggressive brain tumors. Cancer Chemother Pharmacol 77:857–864

Moore SW, Satgé D, Sasco AJ et al (2003) The epidemiology of neonatal tumours. Report of an international working group. Pediatr Surg Int 19:509–519

Nuchtern JG (2006) Perinatal neuroblastoma. Semin Pediatr Surg 15:10–16

Orbach D, Sarnacki S, Brisse HJ (2013) Neonatal cancer. Lancet Oncol 14:e609–e620

Raciborska A, Bilska K et al (2016) Solid cancer in the premature and the newborn: report of three national referral centers. Pediatr Neonatol 57:295–301

Reaman GH, Bleyer WA (2006) Infant and adolescent with cancer: special consideration. In: Pizzo PA, Poplak DG (eds) Principles and practice of pediatric oncology. Lippincott Williams & Wilkins, Philadelphia, pp 452–475

Ritchey ML, Azizkhan RG, Beckwith JB et al (1995) Neonatal Wilms tumor. J Pediatr Surg 30:856–859

Sande JE, Arceci RT, Lampkin BC (1999) Congenital and neonatal leukemia. Semin Perinatol 23:274–285

Tsuchida Y, Ikeda H, Iehara T et al (2003) Neonatal neuroblastoma: incidence and clinical outcome. Med Pediatr Oncol 40:391–393

Veal GJ, Boddy AV (2012) Chemotherapy in newborns and preterm babies. Semin Fetal Neonatal Med 17:243–248

Wu JT, Book L, Sudar K (1981) Serum alphafetoprotein levels in normal infants. Pediatr Res 15:50–52

9783319294872VOL02

Neonatology

Giuseppe Buonocore • Rodolfo Bracci
Michael Weindling
Editors

Neonatology

A Practical Approach to Neonatal Diseases

Second Edition

Volume 3

With 568 Figures and 386 Tables

Springer

Editors
Giuseppe Buonocore
Department of Pediatrics
Obstetrics and Reproductive Medicine
University of Siena
Siena, Italy

Rodolfo Bracci
Department of Pediatrics
Obstetrics and Reproductive Medicine
University of Siena
Siena, Italy

Michael Weindling
Liverpool Women's Hospital Neonatal Unit
Liverpool, UK

ISBN 978-3-319-29487-2 ISBN 978-3-319-29489-6 (eBook)
ISBN 978-3-319-29488-9 (print and electronic bundle)
https://doi.org/10.1007/978-3-319-29489-6

Library of Congress Control Number: 2018940273

Printed on acid-free paper

This Springer imprint is published by the registered company Springer International Publishing AG part of Springer Nature.
The registered company address is: Gewerbestrasse 11, 6330 Cham, Switzerland

Introduction

Neonatology is a science in rapid evolution. The speed of this evolution may cause some to doubt what a traditional textbook is able to achieve in bringing the most up-to-date developments to a reader's attention. Although the interested reader will use other electronic means to access current information, this is not always possible. We firmly believe that, through their own experience, experts are able to bring their own perspective and interest to a subject and act as a guide to the interested and committed reader. We therefore believe that this textbook should act as a conduit of reliable information from the expert to the clinician. We have tried to make this textbook into a genuine guide to the best and most up-to-date answers for neonatologists who are striving to give the best and highest quality care to sick babies.

All practicing clinicians work within their own culture and resources. Each has to make judgments about the best and most appropriate application of available resources to the care of their small sick patients. We hope that this textbook will support the dedicated clinician by providing the best evidence available in the various sub-specialisms of neonatology, particularly when the issue of best treatment continues to be debated. The reader who needs rapid and comprehensive information about a topic requires that the information provided should be synthetized intelligently, exhaustively, and clearly. Subjects should be updated as much as possible. We have endeavored to meet these requirements. We think that the aim of a modern textbook should be to describe the present state of the science, suggesting ways in which this might be improved, and to provide a sound understanding of pathophysiology and diagnostic and therapeutic procedures. Our overall aim is to support and optimize the care of the newborn. In this way, our approach is "practical" and aims to assist neonatologists in their daily work.

In this second edition, the text has been largely revised by experts who contributed to the previous volume. They have added new information, some of it through short- and long-term follow-up, to support the evidence that underpins good clinical practice. Some chapters are completely new.

We are grateful to all the authors for their time and contributions. We would also like to thank Andrew Spencer, Tina Shelton, Vasowati Shome, and the publication team of Springer for their great efforts in publishing this book.

We sincerely hope that this volume has built on the success of its predecessor and continues to support clinicians in a readily accessible and useful way.

Contents

Volume 1

About the Editors

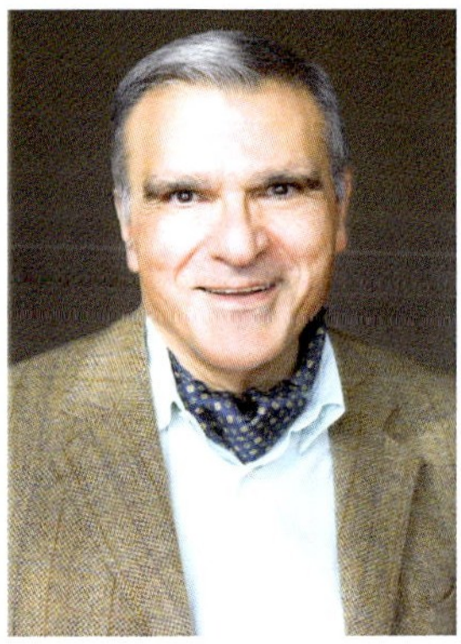

Giuseppe Buonocore is an Italian pediatrician, who is internationally recognized for his research on neonatal diseases, oxidative stress, and early identification of the newborn at high risk of brain damage. He is a full Professor of Pediatrics, Department of Molecular and Developmental Medicine, University of Siena, Italy, and Director of the Division of Pediatric-Neonatology, Azienda Ospedaliera-Universitaria of Siena, Italy. He is Chairman of Pediatrics at the School of Specialization in Pediatrics and Neonatology, University of Siena, Italy.

He is the President and Coordinator of European scientific network EURope Against Infant Brain Injury (EURAIBI). He has been a Visiting Professor at the University of Pennsylvania, the University of Florida, the University Hospitals of New York, as well as at the University of Oulu, Finland, at Taipei Medical University, and at Chang Gung Memorial Hospital at Linkou, Taiwan.

He is also the past President of ESPR and UENPS and currently President of the National College of University Full Professors of Pediatrics. He is involved in the coordination of numerous pan-European clinical trials as well as American and Australian. He has received many scientific awards: including the Seventh annual Dr. Donald V Eitzman lectures "Iron homeostasis metabolism and toxicity," University of Florida (2000), and the "Goccia d'oro 2010" for the efforts and results in the scientific research in the field of

Prenatal, Perinatal, and Neonatal Brain Damage. He also holds the patent of a scientific invention: the "Machine for automatic assessment of pain in neonates."

Dr. Buonocore has supervised more than 200 M.D./Ph.D. students (1994/2018) in Medicine and Surgery, Pediatrics, and Diagnostic Biochemistry. His current research interests are in the mechanisms of cell damage in the neonatal brain, with special reference to hypoxia, and the role of oxidant radicals in neonatal diseases and in babies with birth asphyxia. Additional research interest fields are ethics in perinatology and fetal and neonatal pain prevention. His research team is funded by several agencies including the Italian Ministry of University and Scientific Research as well as the European Community. Prof. Buonocore is author of more than 900 publications: 3 books and 27 book chapters, 300 peer-reviewed articles, and more than 617 presentations at international conferences and national meetings. He is currently Editor-in-Chief of *Current Pediatric Reviews*, Associate Editor of *Journal of Pineal Research*, and on the editorial board of several international scientific journals. He has organized more than 20 European conferences and has been the scientific coordinator or participant in several national and international clinical trials.

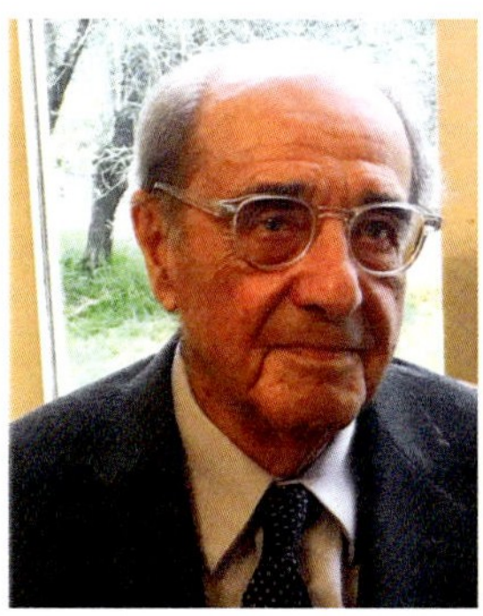

Rodolfo Bracci was born in Siena (Italy) in 1931. After graduating in Medicine and Surgery from the University of Siena Medical School in 1955, he became Assistant Professor of Pediatrics in the University of Siena. He was Post doctoral Trainee at the Albert Einstein College of Medicine, New York (1964–1965). At that time, working under the direction of Professor Ruth Gross, he made the first experiences on the antioxidant properties of the red cells of newborn. After his return to Italy, he became Assistant Professor of Pediatrics at the University of Florence and later at the University of Siena. He continued to be involved in the field of oxygen toxicity of the erythrocyte of newborn, and in 1967, he demonstrated that the red cells of newborn may have not only a low protection against reacting oxygen species but also an increased production of them.

Professor of Neonatology of the University of Siena and Director of the Neonatal Intensive Care Unit of the Siena Hospital, he was leading a staff of researchers involved in the physiopathology of the neonate, particularly in the calcium homeostasis, in the opioids metabolism, and especially in the

problems of oxygen toxicity in the red cells as well as in various organs. More than a hundred papers were published in important international journals by the doctors working under the guidance of Rodolfo Bracci. He was invited speaker in many international congresses and seminars in various cities in Europe and in America.

He has been member of the European Society of Pediatric Hematology and Immunology, the European Society for Pediatric Research, the European Society for Perinatal Medicine, the Neonatal Intensive Care Collegium, the Italian Society of Pediatrics, and the Italian Society of Neonatology.

Retired from University of Siena in 2001, he continued to publish papers, mainly together with Professor G. Buonocore.

Michael Weindling is Emeritus Professor of Perinatal Medicine at the University of Liverpool and Honorary Consultant Neonatologist at Liverpool Women's Hospital, where he was responsible for the care of newborn babies in a tertiary neonatal intensive care unit until he retired from clinical work in 2013. He is an Associate Editor of *Acta Paediatrica*. He continues with his research interest into the maintenance of appropriate brain oxygenation, cerebral hemodynamics, and the prevention of acquired damage of the developing brain.

He studied medicine at Guy's Hospital in London and qualified in 1973. His training in London included a period at the Great Ormond Street Hospital for Sick Children and then as research fellow at the University of Oxford, where he studied the cerebral hemodynamics of the developing brain. Michael Weindling was appointed a Senior Lecturer and consultant in Liverpool in 1985. During his early years as a consultant, he undertook a master's degree in medical ethics at the University of Keele with a dissertation into the changing moral status of the developing human from conceptus to neonate. He was promoted to Professor in 1996 with a personal chair entitled Professor of Perinatal Medicine, a title chosen to reflect his interest into the rapidly changing requirements of the developing brain. He has a considerable interest in medical education and for several years was Head of the School of Paediatrics in Merseyside.

Contributors

Steven H. Abman University of Colorado Denver – Anschutz Medical Campus, Denver, CO, USA

Massimo Agosti Neonatology and NICU – Maternal and Child Department, Ospedale "F del Ponte", Varese, Italy

Rocco Agostino Ethics Committee, Pediatric Hospital Bambino Gesù, Rome, Italy

Carlo Agostoni Pediatric Clinic, Department of Clinical Sciences and Community Health, University of Milan Fondazione, IRCCS Ca Granda, Ospedale Maggiore Policlinico, Milano, Italy

Munir Ahmed Division of Asthma, Allergy and Lung Biology, MRC Centre for Allergic Mechanisms of Asthma, King's College London, London, UK

Uma Sankari Ali Nephrology Division and PICU, BJ Wadia Hospital for Children, Mumbai, India

Karel Allegaert Neonatal Intensive Care Unit, University Hospitals Leuven, Leuven, Belgium

Department of Development and Regeneration, KU Leuven, Leuven, Belgium

Intensive Care and Department of Pediatric Surgery, Erasmus MC – Sophia Children's Hospital, Rotterdam, The Netherlands

Ruben E. Alvaro Department of Pediatrics, WR004 Women's Hospital, University of Manitoba, Winnipeg, MB, Canada

Gina Ancora Neonatology and Neonatal Intensive Care Unit, Ospedale Infermi, Rimini, Italy

Endla K. Anday Department of Pediatrics, Drexel University College of Medicine, St. Christopher's Hospital for Children, Neonatal-Perinatal Medicine, Philadelphia, PA, USA

Generoso Andria Department of Translational Medicine, Section of Pediatrics, Federico II University of Naples, Naples, Italy

Rajesh K. Aneja Departments of Critical Care Medicine and Pediatrics, University of Pittsburgh School of Medicine, Children's Hospital of Pittsburgh, Pittsburgh, PA, USA

Ruby V. Aneja Division of Neonatology, Temple University, West Penn Hospital, Pittsburgh, PA, USA

Molinari Angelo Claudio Thrombosis and Hemostasis Unit, Giannina Gaslini Children's Hospital, Genova, Italy

Rossella Angotti Department of Pediatrics, Obstetrics and Reproductive Medicine, Section of Pediatric Surgery, University of Siena, Siena, Italy

Carmelo Arcidiacono Department of Pediatric Cardiology, IRCCS Policlinico San Donato, San Siro, Milan, Italy

Domenico Arduini Department of Obstetrics and Gynecology, University of Rome Tor Vergata, Rome, Italy

Roberto Aufieri Division of Neonatology and Neonatal Intensive Care, Casilino General Hospital, Rome, Italy

Franco Bagnoli Department of Pediatrics, Obstetrics and Reproductive Medicine, University of Siena, Siena, Italy

Milica Bajcetic Institute of Pharmacology, Clinical Pharmacology and Toxicology, Medical Faculty, University of Belgrade, Belgrade, Serbia

Clinical Pharmacology Unit, University Children's Hospital, Belgrade, Serbia

Sarah Bajorek Department of Pediatrics, Division of Neonatology, University of Florida, College of Medicine, Gainesville, FL, USA

Antonio Balsamo Department of Medical and Surgical Sciences, Pediatric Unit, Center for Rare Endocrine Diseases (CARENDO BO), S.Orsola Malpighi University Hospital, Bologna, Italy

Jane E. Barthell Children's Hospitals and Clinics of Minnesota, Minneapolis, MN, USA

Francesco Bazzini Department of Molecular and Developmental Medicine, University of Siena, Siena, Italy

Roberto Bellù NICU, Ospedale Manzoni, Lecco, Italy

Franca Fossati-Bellani Pediatric Oncology Department, Fondazione IRCCS Istituto Nazionale dei Tumori, Milan, Italy

Carlo V. Bellieni Neonatal Intensive Care Unit, Siena University Hospital, Siena, Italy

Simonetta Bellone Department of Health Sciences, Division of Pediatrics, University of Piemonte Orientale, Novara, Italy

Elisa Belvisi Department of Molecular and Developmental Medicine, University of Siena, Siena, Italy

Britney Benoit School of Nursing, Centre for Pediatric Pain Research, Maternal-Newborn Program, Dalhousie University, IWK Health Centre, Halifax, Canada

Silvano Bertelloni Adolescent Medicine Unit, Division of Pediatrics, S. Chiara Hospital, University of Pisa, Pisa, Italy

Giovanna Bertini Neonatal Intensive Care Unit, Careggi University Hospital, Florence, Italy

Enrico Bertino Neonatal Unit, University of Turin, Turin, Italy

Natascia Bertoncelli Neonatal Intensive Care Unit, Department of Medical and Surgical Sciences of the Mother, Children and Adults, University Hospital of Modena, Modena, Italy

Giulio Bevilacqua Department of Pediatrics and Neonatology, Eastern Liguria Hospital, La Spezia, Italy

Stefania Bezzio Department of Pediatrics, University of Turin, Turin, Italy

Vineet Bhandari Neonatology/Pediatrics, St. Christopher's Hospital for Children/Drexel University College of Medicine, Philadelphia, PA, USA

Drexel University, Philadelphia, PA, USA

Paolo Biban Azienda Ospedaliera Universitaria Integrata Verona, Verona, Italy

Roberta Bilenchi Department of Medical, Surgical and Neurological Sciences, Dermatology Section, University of Siena, Siena, Italy

Caterina Bocchi Obstetrics and Gynecology, Department of Molecular and Developmental Medicine, University of Siena, Siena, Italy

Antonio Boldrini Department of Clinical and Experimental Medicine, Division of Neonatology and Neonatal Intensive Care Unit, Santa Chiara University Hospital, Pisa, Italy

Maria Elena Bolis Neonatology and NICU – Maternal and Child Department, Ospedale "F del Ponte", Varese, Italy

Gianni Bona Department of Health Sciences, Division of Pediatrics, University of Piemonte Orientale, Novara, Italy

Rachele Bonfiglio Department of Anesthesia, Pediatric and Neonatal Intensive Care, Istituto Giannina Gaslini, Genoa, Italy

Alessandro Borghesi Neonatal Intensive Care Unit, Fondazione IRCCS Policlinico 'San Matteo', Pavia, Italy

Giulio Bosco Sapienza Università di Roma, Policlinico Umberto I di Roma, Rome, Italy

Farid Boubred Division of Neonatology, La Conception Hospital, Marseille, France

Rodolfo Bracci University of Siena, Siena, Italy

Nicola Brunetti-Pierri Department of Translational Medicine, Section of Pediatrics, Federico II University of Naples, Naples, Italy

Jenny Bua Division of Neonatology, Institute for Maternal and Child Health IRCCS 'Burlo Garofolo', Trieste, Italy

Wilma Buffolano Heading Coordinating Centre for Perinatal Infection-Campania Region, Translational Medicine Department, Federico II Medical School, Naples, Italy

Giuseppe Buonocore University of Siena, Siena, Italy

Marsha Campbell-Yeo Departments of Pediatrics, Psychology and Neuroscience, Dalhousie University School of Nursing, Halifax, Canada

Letizia Capasso Division of Neonatology, Department of Translational Medical Sciences, Università "Federico II" di Napoli, Naples, Italy

Joseph A. Carcillo Departments of Critical Care Medicine and Pediatrics, University of Pittsburgh School of Medicine, Children's Hospital of Pittsburgh, Pittsburgh, PA, USA

Mario Carminati Department of Pediatric Cardiology, IRCCS Policlinico San Donato, San Siro, Milan, Italy

Virgilio P. Carnielli Division of Neonatology, Salesi Hospital, Polytechnic University of Marche, Ancona, Italy

Elisa della Casa Neonatal Intensive Care Unit, Department of Medical and Surgical Sciences of the Mother, Children and Adults, University Hospital of Modena, Modena, Italy

Alessandra Cassio Department of Medical and Surgical Sciences, Pediatric Endocrinology Unit, S. Orsola-Malpighi University Hospital, Bologna, Italy

Serena Catania Pediatric Oncology Department, Fondazione IRCCS Istituto Nazionale dei Tumori, Milan, Italy

Paolo Cavarzere Pediatric Unit, Department of Mother and Child, University Hospital of Verona, Verona, Italy

Sylvain Chemtob Departments of Pediatrics, Ophthalmology and Pharmacology, Centre Hospitalier, Universitaire Sainte-Justine, Research Center, Montréal, QC, Canada

Department of Ophthalmology, Maisonneuve-Rosemont Hospital Research Center, Montréal, QC, Canada

Stefano Chiaravalli Pediatric Oncology Department, Fondazione IRCCS Istituto Nazionale dei Tumori, Milan, Italy

Gaetano Chirico Neonatology and Intensive Neonatal Therapy Unit, Spedali Civili of Brescia, Brescia, Italy

Robert D. Christensen Divisions of Neonatology and Hematology, Department of Pediatrics, University of Utah School of Medicine, Intermountain Healthcare, Salt Lake City, UT, USA

Massimiliano Ciantelli Department of Clinical and Experimental Medicine, Division of Neonatology and Neonatal Intensive Care Unit, S. Chiara University Hospital, Pisa, Italy

Azienda Ospedaliero-Universitaria Pisana, Pisa, Italy

Elena Ciarmoli Neonatologia e Terapia Intensiva Neonatale, Fondazione MBBM, ASST-Ospedale San Gerardo-Monza, Monza, Italy

Alessandro Cicognani Department of Medical and Surgical Sciences, Pediatric Unit, Center for Rare Endocrine Diseases (CARENDO BO), S.Orsola Malpighi University Hospital, Bologna, Italy

Giovanni Cioni IRCCS Stella Maris, Department of Developmental Neuroscience, Pisa, Italy

University of Pisa, Department of Clinical and Experimental Neuroscience, Pisa, Italy

Olivier Claris Department of Neonatology, Hôpital Femme Mère Enfant, Bron, France

Hospices Civils de Lyon and Université Claude Bernard, Lyon, France

Paola E. Cogo Division of Pediatrics, Department of Medicine, S. Maria della Misericordia University Hospital, University of Udine, Udine, Italy

Richard J. Cooke Department of Pediatrics, University of Tennessee Health Science Center, Memphis, TN, USA

Giovanni Corsello Department of Sciences for Health Promotion and Mother and Child Care, University of Palermo, Palermo, Italy

Alessandra Coscia Neonatal Unit, University of Turin, Turin, Italy

Frans J. C. Cuperus Department of Gastroenterology and Hepatology, University Medical Center Groningen, Groningen, The Netherlands

Tore Curstedt Department of Molecular Medicine and Surgery, Karolinska Institutet, Karolinska University Hospital, Stockholm, Sweden

Mario De Curtis Dipartimento Materno-Infantile, Università "La Sapienza", Rome, Italy

Carlo Dani Neonatal Intensive Care Unit, Careggi University Hospital, Florence, Italy

Università degli Studi di Firenze, Florence, Italy

Riccardo Davanzo Department of Mother and Child Health, Madonna delle Grazie Hospital, Matera, Italy

Franco D'Alberton Department of Medical and Surgical Sciences, Pediatric Unit, Center for Rare Endocrine Diseases (CARENDO BO), S.Orsola Malpighi University Hospital, Bologna, Italy

Andrea De Luca Department of Medical Biotechnologies, University of Siena, Siena, Italy

UOC Malattie Infettive Universitarie, Azienda Ospedaliera Universitaria Senese, Siena, Italy

Linda S. de Vries Department of Neonatology, Wilhelmina Children's Hospital, University Medical Center, Utrecht, The Netherlands

Antonio Del Vecchio Department of Women's and Children's Health, Neonatal Intensive Care Unit, Di Venere Hospital, ASL Bari, Bari, Italy

Maria Delivoria-Papadopoulos Department of Pediatrics, Drexel University College of Medicine, St. Christopher's Hospital for Children, Neonatal-Perinatal Medicine, Philadelphia, PA, USA

Marco Della Monaca Sapienza Università di Roma, Policlinico Umberto I di Roma, Rome, Italy

Paola Di Nicola Neonatal Unit, University of Turin, Turin, Italy

Petr H. Dijk Beatrix Children's Hospital, University Medical Center Groningen, Groningen, The Netherlands

Carmelita D'Ippolito Pediatric Oncohematology and Bone Marrow Transplant, Spedali Civili Hospital, Brescia, Italy

Timothy Disher Centre for Pediatric Pain Research, Dalhousie University School of Nursing and IWK Health Centre, Halifax, Canada

Nicola Disma Department of Anesthesia, Pediatric and Neonatal Intensive Care, Istituto Giannina Gaslini, Genoa, Italy

Marcello Dòmini U.O. di Chirurgia pediatrica – Ospedale S.Orsola, Università degli Studi – Alma Mater Studiorum, di Bologna, Italy

Allison Dorfman Department of Ophthalmology/Neurology, McGill University-Montreal Children's Hospital Research Institute, Montreal, QC, Canada

Elsa Duchemin-Kermorvant INSERM UMRS1138, Centre de Recherche des Cordeliers, Paris, France

Jennifer M. Duchon Division of Neonatology, St. Joseph's Regional Medical Center, Paterson, NJ, USA

Jeroen Dudink Neonatology, Sophia Children's Hospital, Erasmus MC Rotterdam, Rotterdam, Zuid-Holland, The Netherlands

Claudio Fabris Neonatal Unit, University of Turin, Turin, Italy

Maria Teresa Fadda Sapienza Università di Roma, Policlinico Umberto I di Roma, Rome, Italy

Avroy A. Fanaroff Case Western Reserve University School of Medicine Rainbow Babies and Children's Hospital, Cleveland, OH, USA

Jonathan M. Fanaroff Case Western Reserve University School of Medicine Rainbow Babies and Children's Hospital, Cleveland, OH, USA

Vassilios Fanos Department of Surgery, Neonatal Intensive Care Unit, Neonatal Pathology and Neonatal Section, AOU and University of Cagliari, Cagliari, Italy

Maria Grazia Faticato Department of Pediatric Surgery, University of Genoa, Genoa, Italy

Giannina Gaslini Institute, Genoa, Italy

Silvia Ferranti Department of Molecular Medicine and Development, University of Siena, Siena, Italy,

Fabrizio Ferrari Neonatal Intensive Care Unit, Department of Medical and Surgical Sciences of the Mother, Children and Adults, University of Modena and Reggio Emilia, Modena, Italy

Enrico Ferrazzi Prenatal Diagnosis and Fetal Surgery Unit, Dept. of Woman, Mother and Neonate, Buzzi Children's Hospital Department of Clinical Sciences, University of Milan, Milan, Italy

Michele Fimiani Dipartimento di Medicina Clinica e Scienze Immunologiche – Sezione di Dermatologia, Università degli Studi di Siena, Policlinico "Santa Maria alle Scotte", Siena, Italy

Department of Medical, Surgical and Neurological Sciences, Dermatology Section, University of Siena, Siena, Italy

Vittorio Fineschi Department of Anatomical, Histological, Forensic Medicine and Orthopaedic Sciences, "Sapienza" University of Rome, Rome, Italy

Bobbi Fleiss UMR1141, Insem-Paris Diderot University, Hôpital Robert Debré, Paris, France

Centre for the Developing Brain, Department of Perinatal Imaging and Health, Division of Imaging Sciences and Biomedical Engineering, King's College London, King's Health Partners, St. Thomas' Hospital, London, UK

Monica Fumagalli NICU, Department of Clinical Sciences and Community Health, Fondazione IRCCS Ca' Granda Ospedale Maggiore Policlinico Milano, Università degli Studi di Milano, Milan, Italy

Clara Gabiano Department of Pediatrics, University of Turin, Turin, Italy

Silvia Garazzino Department of Pediatrics, University of Turin, Regina Margherita Childrens Hospital, AOU Città della Salute e della Scienza di Torino, Turin, Italy

Elisabetta Garetti Neonatal Intensive Care Unit, Department of Medical and Surgical Sciences of the Mother, Children and Adults, University of Modena and Reggio Emilia, Modena, Italy

Alfredo Garzi Department of Pediatrics, Obstetrics and Reproductive Medicine, Section of Pediatric Surgery, University of Siena, Siena, Italy

Università degli Studi di Salerno, Fisciano, Italy

Diego Gazzolo Neonatal Intensive Care Unit, Department of Maternal, Fetal and Neonatal Medicine, S. Arrigo Children's Hospital, Alessandria, Italy

Giulia Genoni Department of Health Sciences, Division of Pediatrics, University of Piemonte Orientale, Novara, Italy

Maurizio Gente Department of Pediatrics and Infant Neuropsychiatry, Neonatal Emergency Transport Service, Sapienza University of Rome, Rome, Italy

Michael K. Georgieff Division of Neonatology, Department of Pediatrics Center for Neurobehavioral Development, University of Minnesota, Minneapolis, MN, USA

Paolo Ghirri Department of Clinical and Experimental Medicine, Division of Neonatology and Neonatal Intensive Care Unit, Santa Chiara University Hospital, Pisa, Italy

Daniela Gianotti Department of Pediatrics and Neonatology, Eastern Liguria Hospital, La Spezia, Italy

Jason Gien University of Colorado Denver, Denver, CO, USA

Enza Giglione Department of Health Sciences, Division of Pediatrics, University of Piemonte Orientale, Novara, Italy

Mario Giuffrè Department of Sciences for Health Promotion and Mother and Child Care, University of Palermo, Palermo, Italy

Francesca Giuliani Neonatal Unit, University of Turin, Turin, Italy

Kirsten Glaser University Children's Hospital, University of Würzburg, Würzburg, Germany

Peter D. Gluckman Liggins Institute, University of Auckland, Auckland, New Zealand

Sergio Golombek New York Medical College, New York, USA

Misty Good Division of Neonatology, University of Pittsburgh School of Medicine, Children's Hospital of Pittsburgh, Pittsburgh, PA, USA

Glenn R. Gourley Department of Pediatrics, University of Minnesota, Minneapolis, USA

Paul P. Govaert Neonatology, Sophia Children's Hospital, Erasmus MC Rotterdam, Rotterdam, Zuid-Holland, The Netherlands

Anne Greenough Division of Asthma, Allergy and Lung Biology, MRC Centre for Allergic Mechanisms of Asthma, King's College London, London, UK

NIHR Biomedical Centre at Guy's and St Thomas NHS Foundation Trust and King's College London, London, UK

NICU, King's College Hospital, London, UK

Pierre Gressens UMR1141, Insem-Paris Diderot University, Hôpital Robert Debré, Paris, France

Centre for the Developing Brain, Department of Perinatal Imaging and Health, Division of Imaging Sciences and Biomedical Engineering, King's College London, King's Health Partners, St. Thomas' Hospital, London, UK

Floris Groenendaal Department of Neonatology, Wilhelmina Children's Hospital, University Medical Center Utrecht, Utrecht, The Netherlands

Salvatore Grosso Department of Molecular Medicine and Development, University of Siena, Siena, Italy,

Renzo Guerrini Pediatric Neurology and Neurogenetics Unit and Laboratories, Neuroscience Department, A. Meyer Children's Hospital – University of Florence, Florence, Italy

Isotta Guidotti Neonatal Intensive Care Unit, Department of Medical and Surgical Sciences of the Mother, Children and Adults, University Hospital of Modena, Modena, Italy

Jean-Pierre Guignard Lausanne University Medical School, Lausanne, Switzerland

Andrea Guzzetta IRCCS Stella Maris, Department of Developmental Neuroscience, Pisa, Italy

University of Pisa, Department of Clinical and Experimental Neuroscience, Pisa, Italy

Henrik Hagberg Perinatal Center, Department of Obstetrics and Gynecology, Sahlgrenska Academy, University of Gothenburg, Goteborg, Sweden

Centre for the Developing Brain, Division of Imaging Sciences and Biomedical Engineering, King's College London, King's Health Partners, St. Thomas' Hospital, London, UK

Nigel J. Hall University Surgery Unit, Faculty of Medicine, University of Southampton, Southampton, UK

Henry L. Halliday Formerly Regional Neonatal Unit, Royal Maternity Hospital, Belfast, UK

Formerly Department of Child Health, Queen's University Belfast, Belfast, UK

Mikko Hallman Department of Children and Adolescents, Oulu University Hospital, and PEDEGO Research Unit, Medical Research Center Oulu, University of Oulu, Oulu, Finland

Dominique Haumont Department of Neonatology, Saint – Pierre University Hospital, Brussels, Belgium

Axel Heep Department of Neonatology, Southmead Hospital, North Bristol NHS Trust, Bristol, UK

Lena K. Hellström-Westas Department of Women's and Children's Health, Uppsala University and University Hospital, Uppsala, Sweden

Martin J. Herman Department of Orthopaedic Surgery, Drexel University College of Medicine, St. Christopher's Hospital for Children, Philadelphia, PA, USA

Christian V. Hulzebos Beatrix Children's Hospital, University Medical Center Groningen, Groningen, The Netherlands

Petra S. Hüppi Division of Neonatology, Giannina Gaslini Children's Hospital, Genoa, Italy

Giorgio Iannetti Università degli Studi di Siena, Policlinico S. Maria alle Scotte, Siena, Italy

Sapienza Università di Roma, Policlinico Umberto I di Roma, Rome, Italy

Vincenzo Jasonni Department of Pediatric Surgery, University of Genoa, Genoa, Italy

Giannina Gaslini Institute, Genoa, Italy

Kathryn Johnson Centre for Newborn Care, Leeds Teaching Hospitals Trust, Leeds, UK

Celeste Johnston School of Nursing, McGill University, Montreal, Canada

Michael Kaplan Department of Neonatology, Shaare Zedek Medical Center, Jerusalem, Israel

The Faculty of Medicine, Hebrew University, Jerusalem, Israel,

Nandini Kataria Department of Pediatrics, University of Minnesota, Long Beach, California, USA

Tuula Kaukola Department of Children and Adolescents, Oulu University Hospital, and PEDEGO Research Center, MRC Oulu, University of Oulu, Oulu, Finland

Hirokazu Kimura Infectious Diseases Surveillance Center, National Institute of Infectious Diseases, Tokyo, Japan

John P. Kinsella University of Denver, Denver, CO, USA

Panagiotis Kratimenos Neonatologist, Children's National Medical Center, Center for Research in Neuroscience, George Washington University School of Medicine and Health Sciences, Washington, DC, USA

Edmund F. La Gamma Division of Newborn Medicine, Maria Fareri Children's Hospital, Westchester Medical Center – New York Medical College, Valhalla, NY, USA

Arianna Lamberti Department of Medical, Surgical and Neurological Sciences, Dermatology Section, University of Siena, Siena, Italy

Mariano Lanna Prenatal Diagnosis and Fetal Surgery Unit, Dept. of Woman, Mother and Neonate, Buzzi Children's Hospital Department of Clinical Sciences, University of Milan, Milan, Italy

Malcolm Levene Academic Unit of Paediatrics and Child Health, University of Leeds, Leeds, UK

Department of Neonatal Medicine, Leeds Teaching Hospitals Trust, Leeds, UK

Isabelle Ligi Division of Neonatology, La Conception Hospital, Marseille, France

Otwin Linderkamp Division of Neonatology, Department of Pediatrics, University of Heidelberg, Heidelberg, Germany

Gianluca Lista Neonatology and Neonatal Intensive Care Unit, Ospedale dei Bambini V. Buzzi, Milan, Italy

Mariangela Longini Department of Molecular and Developmental Medicine, University of Siena, Siena, Italy

Alessandra Del Longo Department of Pediatric Ophthalmology, Niguarda Ca' Granda Hospital, Milan, Italy

Vassilios Lougaris Pediatrics Clinic, Department of Clinical and Experimental Sciences, University of Brescia and Spedali Civili of Brescia, Brescia, Italy

Felicia M. Low Liggins Institute, University of Auckland, Auckland, New Zealand

Laura Lucaccioni Neonatal Intensive Care Unit, Department of Medical and Surgical Sciences of the Mother, Children and Adults, University Hospital of Modena, Modena, Italy

Licia Lugli Neonatal Intensive Care Unit, Department of Medical and Surgical Sciences of the Mother, Children and Adults, University Hospital of Modena, Modena, Italy

Giuseppe Maggiore Department of Medical Sciences-Pediatrics, University of Ferrara, University Hospital Arcispedale Sant Anna di Cona, CONA (Ferrara), Italy

Francesca Maglietta Department of Legal Medicine, University of Foggia, Foggia, Italy

Akhil Maheshwari Division of Neonatology, University of South Florida, Tampa, FL, USA

Liam Mahoney Academic Department of Paediatrics, Royal Alexandra Children's Hospital, Brighton, UK

M. Jeffrey Maisels Department of Pediatrics, Oakland University William Beaumont School of Medicine, Beaumont Children's Hospital, Royal Oak, MI, USA

Carina Mallard Department of Physiology, Institute of Neuroscience and Physiology, Sahlgrenska Academy, University of Gothenburg, Gothenburg, Sweden

Leila Mameli Department of Anesthesia, Pediatric and Neonatal Intensive Care, Istituto Giannina Gaslini, Genoa, Italy

Filomena Mandato Department of Medical, Surgical and Neurological Sciences, Dermatology Section, University of Siena, Siena, Italy

Paolo Manzoni Division of Neonatology, Department of Obstetrics and Neonatology, AOU Città della Salute e della Scienza, Turin, Italy

Viviana Marchi IRCCS Stella Maris, Department of Developmental Neuroscience, Pisa, Italy

University of Pisa, Department of Clinical and Experimental Neuroscience, Pisa, Italy

Neil Marlow Institute for Women's Health, University College London, London, UK

Richard J. Martin Rainbow Babies and Children's Hospital, Division of Neonatology, Case Western Reserve University School of Medicine, Cleveland, OH, USA

Maura Massimino Pediatric Oncology Department, Fondazione IRCCS Istituto Nazionale dei Tumori, Milan, Italy

Girolamo Mattioli Department of Pediatric Surgery, University of Genoa, Genoa, Italy

Giannina Gaslini Institute, Genoa, Italy

Liz McKechnie Centre for Newborn Care, Leeds Teaching Hospitals Trust, Leeds, UK

Stefania Mei Department of Medical, Surgical and Neurological Sciences, Dermatology Section, University of Siena, Siena, Italy

Mario Messina Department of Pediatrics, Obstetrics and Reproductive Medicine, Section of Pediatric Surgery, Policlinico "Le Scotte", University of Siena, Siena, Italy

Department of Medical, Surgical and Neurological Sciences, Section of Pediatric Surgery, University of Siena, Siena, Italy

Angelo Micheletti Department of Pediatric Cardiology, IRCCS Policlinico San Donato, San Siro, Milan, Italy

Fiorella Migliaro Division of Neonatology, Department of Translational Medical Sciences, Università "Federico II" di Napoli, Naples, Italy

Federica Mignone Department of Pediatrics, University of Turin, Regina Margherita Childrens Hospital, AOU Città della Salute e della Scienza di Torino, Turin, Italy

Francesco Molinaro Department of Pediatrics, Obstetrics and Reproductive Medicine, Section of Pediatric Surgery, Policlinico "Le Scotte", University of Siena, Siena, Italy

Department of Medical, Surgical and Neurological Sciences, Section of Pediatric Surgery, University of Siena, Siena, Italy

Davide Montin Division of Neonatology, Department of Obstetrics and Neonatology, AOU Città della Salute e della Scienza, Turin, Italy

Department of Pediatrics, University of Turin, Turin, Italy

Alice Monzani Department of Health Sciences, Division of Pediatrics, University of Piemonte Orientale, Novara, Italy

Corrado Moretti Università degli Studi di Roma "La Sapienza", Rome, Italy

Colin Morley Dept Obstetrics and Gynecology, University of Cambridge at Rosie Maternity Hospital, Cambridge, UK

Fabio A. Mosca NICU, Department of Clinical Sciences and Community Health, Fondazione IRCCS Ca' Granda Ospedale Maggiore Policlinico Milano, Università degli Studi di Milano, Milan, Italy

Michele Mussap Laboratory Medicine, Ospedale Policlinico San Martino, Genoa, Italy

Niccolò Nami Department of Medical, Surgical and Neurological Sciences, Dermatology Section, University of Siena, Siena, Italy

Diana Negura Department of Pediatric Cardiology, IRCCS Policlinico San Donato, San Siro, Milan, Italy

Josef Neu Department of Pediatrics, Division of Neonatology, University of Florida, College of Medicine, Gainesville, FL, USA

Giovanni Nigro Maternal-Infant Department, University of L'Aquila, L'Aquila, Italy

Akira Nishida Department of Neonatology, Tokyo Metropolitan Children's Medical Center, Tokyo, Japan

Giovanna Oggè Maternal-Fetal Medicine Unit, University of Turin, Turin, Italy

Robin K. Ohls Department of Pediatrics, Division of Neonatology, University of New Mexico, Albuquerque, NM, USA

Kaoru Okazaki Department of Neonatology, Tokyo Metropolitan Children's Medical Center, Tokyo, Japan

Luca Ori Neonatal Intensive Care Unit, Department of Medical and Surgical Sciences of the Mother, Children and Adults, University Hospital of Modena, Modena, Italy

Luis H. Ospina Departments of Pediatrics, Ophthalmology and Pharmacology, Centre Hospitalier, Universitaire Sainte-Justine, Research Center, Montréal, QC, Canada

Erin A. Osterholm Division of Neonatology, Department of Pediatrics Center for Neurobehavioral Development, University of Minnesota, Minneapolis, MN, USA

Roberto Paludetto Translational Medical Sciences, Università "Federico II" di Napoli, Naples, Italy

Niovi Papalexopoulou Division of Asthma, Allergy and Lung Biology, MRC Centre for Allergic Mechanisms of Asthma, King's College London, London, UK

Paola Papoff Pediatric Intensive Care Unit, Sapienza University of Rome, Rome, Italy

Giancarlo Parenti Department of Translational Medicine, Section of Pediatrics, Federico II University of Naples, Naples, Italy

Stefano Parmigiani Department of Pediatrics and Neonatology, Eastern Liguria Hospital, La Spezia, Italy

Elena Parrini Pediatric Neurology and Neurogenetics Unit and Laboratories, Neuroscience Department, A. Meyer Children's Hospital – University of Florence, Florence, Italy

Gaia Pasquali Department of Obstetrics and Gynecology, University of Rome Tor Vergata, Rome, Italy

Mary Elaine Patrinos Case Western Reserve University School of Medicine, Cleveland, OH, USA

Pierluigi Pedersini National Center for Surgical Treatment of Pediatric Hepatobiliary Malformations, Pediatric Surgery, University of Brescia, Brescia, Italy

Serafina Perrone Department of Molecular and Developmental Medicine, University Hospital of Siena, Siena, Italy

Felice Petraglia Obstetrics and Gynecology, Department of Molecular and Developmental Medicine, University of Siena, Siena, Italy

Luciane Piazza Department of Pediatric Cardiology, IRCCS Policlinico San Donato, San Siro, Milan, Italy

Catherine Pieltain Department of Neonatology, University of Liège, CHR de la Citadelle, Liège, Belgium

Agostino Pierro Division of General and Thoracic Surgery, The Hospital for Sick Children, Toronto, Canada

Alessio Pini Prato Giannina Gaslini Institute, Genoa, Italy

Elena Piozzi Department of Pediatric Ophthalmology, Niguarda Ca' Granda Hospital, Milan, Italy

Peter D. Pizzutillo Section of Orthopaedic Surgery, St. Christopher's Hospital for Children, Philadelphia, PA, USA

Tenet Healthcare, Dallas, TX, USA

Alessandro Plebani Pediatrics Clinic, Department of Clinical and Experimental Sciences, University of Brescia and Spedali Civili of Brescia, Brescia, Italy

Francesca R. Pluchinotta Department of Pediatric Cardiology, IRCCS Policlinico San Donato, San Siro, Milan, Italy

Christian F. Poets Department of Neonatology, Tübingen University Hospital, Tübingen, Germany

Simone Pratesi Neonatal Intensive Care Unit, Careggi University Hospital, Florence, Italy

Flavia Prodam Department of Health Sciences, Division of Pediatrics, University of Piemonte Orientale, Novara, Italy

Fabrizio Proietti Department of Molecular and Developmental Medicine, University of Siena, Siena, Italy

Marisa Pugliese Neonatal Intensive Care Unit, Department of Medical and Surgical Sciences of the Mother, Children and Adults, University of Modena and Reggio Emilia, Modena, Italy

Guy Putet Department of Neonatology, Hopital de la Croix-Rousse, Hospices Civils de Lyon and Universite Claude Bernard, Lyon, France

Heike Rabe Academic Department of Paediatrics, Royal Alexandra Children's Hospital, Brighton, UK

Francesco Raimondi Division of Neonatology, Department of Translational Medical Sciences, Università "Federico II" di Napoli, Naples, Italy

Luca A. Ramenghi Division of Neonatology, Giannina Gaslini Children's Hospital, Genoa, Italy

Tara M. Randis Department of Pediatrics, New York University School of Medicine, New York, NY, USA

Roberta Ricotti Department of Health Sciences, Division of Pediatrics, University of Piemonte Orientale, Novara, Italy

Henrique Rigatto Department of Pediatrics, WR004 Women's Hospital, University of Manitoba, Winnipeg, MB, Canada

Jacques Rigo Department of Neonatology, University of Liège, CHR de la Citadelle, Liège, Belgium

Arieh Riskin Department of Neonatology, Bnai Zion Medical Center, Rappaport Faculty of Medicine, Technion, Israel Institute of Technology, Haifa, Israel

Francesco Risso Neonatal Intensive Care Unit, Department of Emergency Medicine, G. Gaslini Children's Hospital, Genoa, Italy

Silvia Riva Pediatric Hepatology and Liver Transplant Unit, IRCCS-ISMETT - University of Pittsburgh Medical Center (UPMC), Palermo, Italy

José Carlos Rivera Departments of Pediatrics, Ophthalmology and Pharmacology, Centre Hospitalier, Universitaire Sainte-Justine, Research Center, Montréal, QC, Canada

Department of Ophthalmology, Maisonneuve-Rosemont Hospital Research Center, Montréal, QC, Canada

Rodney P. A. Rivers Section of Paediatrics, Department of Medicine, Imperial College, London, UK

Hector Rojas-Anaya Academic Department of Paediatrics, Royal Alexandra Children's Hospital, Brighton, UK

Maria Angela Rustico Prenatal Diagnosis and Fetal Surgery Unit, Dept. of Woman, Mother and Neonate, Buzzi Children's Hospital Department of Clinical Sciences, University of Milan, Milan, Italy

Karin Sävman Department of Pediatrics, Sahlgrenska Academy, University of Gothenburg, Gothenburg, Sweden

Timo Saarela Department of Children and Adolescents, Oulu University Hospital, Oulu, Finland

Elie Saliba Department of Neonatology and Pediatric Intensive Care, Université François Rabelais and CHRU de Tours, Tours, France

Inserm U930, France, Université François Rabelais and CHRU de Tours, Tours, France

Janko Samardzic Department of Paediatric Pharmacology, University Children's Hospital Basel, Basel, Switzerland

Institute of Pharmacology, Clinical Pharmacology and Toxicology, Medical Faculty, University of Belgrade, Belgrade, Serbia

Fabrizio Sandri Neonatology and Neonatal Intensive Care Unit, Ospedale Maggiore, Bologna, Italy

Andrea Sannia Neonatal Intensive Care Unit, Department of Emergency Medicine, G. Gaslini Children's Hospital, Genoa, Italy

Javier Fernandez Sarabia Department of Pediatric Cardiology, IRCCS Policlinico San Donato, San Siro, Milan, Italy

Paola Saracco Pediatric Hematology, Department of Pediatrics, University Hospital Città della Salute e della Scienza, Torino, Italy

Antonio Saracino Department of Pediatric Cardiology, IRCCS Policlinico San Donato, San Siro, Milan, Italy

Ola D. Saugstad Department of Pediatric Research, Rikshospitalet, Oslo University Hospital, University of Oslo, Oslo, Norway

Rosa T. Scaramuzzo Neonatology and Neonatal Intensive Care Unit, Santa Chiara University Hospital, Pisa, Italy

Kurt R. Schibler Perinatal Institute, Cincinnati Children's Hospital Medical Center, Cincinnati, OH, USA

Marco Sciveres Pediatric Hepatology and Liver Transplant Unit, IRCCS-ISMETT - University of Pittsburgh Medical Center (UPMC), Palermo, Italy

Carlo Scolfaro Department of Pediatrics, University of Turin, Regina Margherita Childrens Hospital, AOU Città della Salute e della Scienza di Torino, Turin, Italy

Gunnar Sedin Department of Women's and Children's Health, University Children's Hospital, Uppsala, Sweden

Thibault Senterre Department of Neonatology, University of Liège, CHR de la Citadelle, Liège, Belgium

Filiberto Maria Severi Obstetrics and Gynecology, Department of Molecular and Developmental MedicineUniversity of Siena, Siena, Italy

Raanan Shamir Institute of Gastroenterology Nutrition and Liver Diseases, Schneider Children's Medical Center, Sackler Faculty of Medicine, Tel-Aviv University, Petach-Tikva, Israel

Davide Silvagni Azienda Ospedaliera Universitaria Integrata Verona, Verona, Italy

Umberto Simeoni Division of Pediatrics, CHUV and UNIL, Lausanne, Vaud, Switzerland

Adam P. R. Smith Division of Asthma, Allergy and Lung Biology, MRC Centre for Allergic Mechanisms of Asthma, King's College London, London, UK

Augusto Sola Ibero American Society of Neonatology (SIBEN), Wellington, FL, USA

Michael Spear Department of Pediatrics, Drexel University College of Medicine, St. Christopher's Hospital for Children, Philadelphia, PA, USA

Christian P. Speer University Children's Hospital, University of Würzburg, Würzburg, Germany

David K. Stevenson Department of Pediatrics, Stanford University School of Medicine, Medical School Office Building, Stanford, CA, USA

Rosa Maria Strangi Department of Medical, Surgical and Neurological Sciences, Dermatology Section, University of Siena, Siena, Italy

Mauro Stronati Neonatal Intensive Care Unit, Fondazione IRCCS Policlinico 'San Matteo', Pavia, Italy

Veena Supramaniam Perinatal Imaging Group, Robert Steiner MR Unit, MRC Clinical Sciences Centre and Wigglesworth Perinatal Pathology Services, Hammersmith Hospital, Imperial College, London, UK

Paolo Tagliabue Neonatologia e Terapia Intensiva Neonatale, Fondazione MBBM, ASST-Ospedale San Gerardo-Monza, Monza, Italy

Sophie Tardieu Medical Evaluation Department, Public Health Department, La Conception Hospital, Marseille, France

Elena Tavella Division of Neonatology, Department of Obstetrics and Neonatology, AOU Città della Salute e della Scienza, Turin, Italy

Claire Thornton Centre for the Developing Brain, Department of Perinatal Imaging and Health, Division of Imaging Sciences and Biomedical Engineering, King's College London, King's Health Partners, St. Thomas' Hospital, London, UK

Claudio Tiribelli Liver Research Centre, University of Trieste, Trieste, Italy

Tullia Todros Maternal-Fetal Medicine Unit, University of Turin, Turin, Italy

Michela Torricelli Obstetrics and Gynecology, Department of Molecular and Developmental Medicine, University of Siena, Siena, Italy

Pier Angelo Tovo Department of Pediatrics, University of Turin, Regina Margherita Childrens Hospital, AOU Città della Salute e della Scienza di Torino, Turin, Italy

Alberto E. Tozzi Multifactorial and Complex Diseases Research Area, Bambino Gesù Children's Hospital, Rome, Italy

Laura Travan Division of Neonatology, Institute for Maternal and Child Health IRCCS 'Burlo Garofolo', Trieste, Italy

Daniele Trevisanuto Department of Women's and Children's Health, Azienda Ospedaliere di Padova, University of Padua, Padua, Italy

Pietro Tuo Department of Anesthesia, Pediatric and Neonatal Intensive Care, Istituto Giannina Gaslini, Genoa, Italy

Emanuela Turillazzi Department of Legal Medicine, University of Foggia, Foggia, Italy

Alberto G. Ugazio Institute of Child and Adolescent Health, Bambino Gesù Children's Hospital, Rome, Italy

Frank van Bel Department of Neonatology, Wilhelmina Children's Hospital, University Medical Center Utrecht, Utrecht, The Netherlands

John N. van den Anker Division of Pediatric Clinical Pharmacology, Children's National Health System, Washington, DC, USA

Departments of Pediatrics, Integrative Systems Biology, Pharmacology and Physiology, George Washington University, School of Medicine and Health Sciences, Washington, DC, USA

Intensive Care and Department of Pediatric Surgery, Erasmus MC – Sophia Children's Hospital, Rotterdam, The Netherlands

Johannes B. (Hans) van Goudoever Department of Pediatrics, Emma Children's Hospital – AMC and VU University Medical Center, Amsterdam, The Netherlands

Tim van Mieghem Department of Development and Regeneration, KU Leuven, Leuven, Belgium

Obstetrics and Gynecology, University Hospitals Leuven, Leuven, Belgium

Bart Van Overmeire Neonatology Service, Erasmus Hospital Université Libre de Bruxelles, Brussels, Belgium

Silvia Vannuccini Obstetrics and Gynecology, Department of Molecular and Developmental Medicine, University of Siena, Siena, Italy

Maximo Vento Neonatal Research Unit, Health Research Institute Hospital La Fe, University and Polytechnic Hospital La Fe, Valencia, Spain

Gennaro Vetrano U.O.C. Pediatria/Neonatologia/UTIN, Osp. "Sacro Cuore di Gesù", Benevento, Italy

Renaud Viellevoye Department of Neonatology, University of Liège, CHR de la Citadelle, Liège, Belgium

Betty R. Vohr Department of Pediatrics, The Warren Alpert Medical School of Brown University, Providence, RI, USA

Women and Infants Hospital, Providence, RI, USA

Jon F. Watchko Division of Newborn Medicine, Department of Pediatrics, University of Pittsburgh School of Medicine, Pittsburgh, PA, USA

Ronald J. Wong Department of Pediatrics, Stanford University School of Medicine, Stanford, CA, USA

Marco Zaffanello Department of Surgical Sciences, Dentistry, Gynecology and Pediatrics, University of Verona, Verona, Italy

Department of Life and Reproduction Sciences Pediatric Section, University of Verona, Verona, Italy

Department of Surgery, University of Cagliari, Cagliari, Italy

Clelia Zanaboni Department of Anesthesia, Pediatric and Neonatal Intensive Care, Istituto Giannina Gaslini, Genoa, Italy

Giacomo Zanelli Department of Medical Biotechnologies, University of Siena, Siena, Italy

Rinaldo Zanini NICU, Ospedale Manzoni, Lecco, Italy

Tianwei Ellen Zhou Departments of Pediatrics, Ophthalmology and Pharmacology, Centre Hospitalier, Universitaire Sainte-Justine, Research Center, Montréal, QC, Canada

Ekhard E. Ziegler Department of Pediatrics, University of Iowa, Iowa City, IA, USA

Luc J. I. Zimmermann Department of Pediatrics and Neonatology, School for Oncology and Developmental Biology (GROW), Maastricht University Medical Center, Maastricht, The Netherlands

Part X

Fetal and Neonatal Infections

Fetal Infections: Cytomegalovirus, Herpes Simplex, and Varicella

103

Giovanni Nigro

Contents

G. Nigro (✉)
Maternal-Infant Department, University of L'Aquila,
L'Aquila, Italy
e-mail: nigrogio@libero.it

G. Buonocore et al. (eds.), *Neonatology*,
https://doi.org/10.1007/978-3-319-29489-6_250

Abstract

This chapter reviews three herpesviruses that cause infections of the fetus and/or newborn: cytomegalovirus (CMV), herpesvirus (HSV) 1 and 2, and varicella-zoster virus (VZV). CMV and VZV can cause severe fetal disease following a primary maternal infection and subsequent placentitis by viremia. Persistent infection with CMV can cause progressive disease with significant developmental abnormalities which become apparent over the first years of life. Preconceptional immunity generally protects the fetus either from infection or from the severe disease both in utero and after birth for a few months, although symptomatic congenital CMV infection may rarely occur after recurrent maternal infection. The second important factor, which affects both the frequency of transplacental transmission and the severity of disease, is the gestational age when the fetus is infected: the severity is high in the first months; the frequency prevails in the last months of pregnancy. The third factor influencing the severity and the manifestations of an intrauterine infection is the tissue tropism of each virus: many manifestations of intrauterine VZV infection arise from effects upon the developing nervous system.

103.1 Salient Points

- Preconceptional immunity generally protects the fetus and the neonate for a few months, although symptomatic congenital CMV infection and perinatal HSV infection can rarely occur after recurrent maternal infection.
- Persistent CMV infection can cause progressive disease with significant developmental abnormalities over the first years of life.
- After primary maternal infection, severe prenatal diseases can be caused by CMV, VZV, and HSV following viremia by VZV or ascending route by HSV or both viremia and ascending route by CMV.
- The frequency of transplacental transmission and severity of disease are inversely correlated with the gestational age when the fetus is infected: the severity is high in the first months; the frequency prevails in the last months of pregnancy.
- After maternal immunity and gestational age of fetal infection, the third factor influencing the severity and the manifestations of an intrauterine infection is the tissue tropism of each virus.

103.2 Introduction

This chapter reviews three herpesviruses that cause infections of the fetus and/or newborn. These are herpesvirus I and II also called herpes simplex virus 1 and 2 (HSV), herpesvirus III also called varicella-zoster virus (VZV), and herpesvirus V also called cytomegalovirus (CMV). With the exception of HSV, which reaches the fetus by ascending route, CMV and VZV can produce severe fetal disease following a primary maternal infection when, in the absence of maternal immunity, these organisms are carried in the bloodstream to the placenta and then on to the fetus. Primary maternal CMV and VZV infections do not always result in intrauterine infection, and when intrauterine infection does occur, severe fetal disease does not always follow. Most commonly infants infected in utero with CMV appear normal at birth, but persistent infection can cause progressive disease with significant developmental abnormalities which become apparent over the first years of life. In general, infection of the mother with these viruses and the development of immunity prior to conception protect the fetus either from infection or from the severe disease both in utero and after birth for a few months. With CMV, for example, women immune to the virus prior to pregnancy may deliver infants with intrauterine-acquired infection but, with rare exceptions, congenital cytomegalic inclusion disease occurs only as the result of a primary infection during pregnancy.

Along with maternal immunity, another important factor, which affects both the frequency of transplacental transmission and the severity of disease, is the gestational age of the fetus when the woman becomes infected. Infections with HSV 2 are for the most part acquired during delivery from the virus in the maternal cervical-vaginal tract. Maternal immunity to HSV 2 prior to delivery protects the newborn from severe or fatal disease to HSV infection of the newborn. HSV 1 is a virus which is usually orally transmitted but may infect the birth channel and produce severe neonatal disease in the absence of maternal immunity.

Another influence on the severity and the manifestations of an intrauterine infection is the viral tissue tropism, that is, the affinity for specific cell types or tissues. CMV and HSV, like many pathogens causing intrauterine infection, replicate in all organs and tissues, hence causing disease in all or several organs or tissues. On the contrary, many manifestations of severe intrauterine infection with VZV, which is tropic for neural tissue, arise from effects upon the developing nervous system.

103.3 Cytomegalovirus

Human cytomegalovirus (CMV) contains within its capsid a double stranded DNA molecule of 150 million molecular weight. This DNA molecule contains at least several hundred genes and is the largest genome of any known virus. The virus has a 65 nm inner core containing the viral DNA. The inner core is within an icosahedral protein capsid comprised of 162 capsomeres. This is in turn surrounded by a tegument layer and an outer enveloped membrane containing glycoproteins. The envelope glycoproteins are antigenic and are responsible for generating an immune response. The majority of the neutralizing antibodies induced by CMV antigens are directed against the major CMV glycoproteins. Cellular immune responses such as cytotoxic T cells are directed primarily against the major tegument protein, pp65. There is only a single serotype of CMV. Thus antibodies induced by one viral isolate cross-react with most or all epidemiologically unrelated isolates. Genetically, however, there are thousands of different isolates, each of which differs from all other epidemiologically unrelated isolates. CMV infects nearly all humans but causes serious disease mostly in those with impaired immunity associated with immunosuppression due to medical therapy, AIDS, or in the fetus with its immature immune system (Mocarski and Courcelle 2002).

103.3.1 Epidemiology

Cytomegalovirus (CMV) infection is the most frequent congenital infection affecting worldwide approximately 0.5-1% of all live births. In undeveloped areas or among those having low socioeconomic levels, between 1% and 2.5% of all newborns are congenitally infected with CMV, and by 5 years of age the majority of children have acquired the infection. Children with congenital infection will excrete the virus in saliva and urine for several years, depending on the type of maternal infection and the time and severity of prenatal infection. Within the first year of life, for infants not congenitally infected, CMV may be acquired perinatally by contact with maternal cervical-vaginal secretions or postnatally from seropositive mothers via breast milk. Approximately 30% of seropositive mothers shed CMV in breast milk and approximately 70% of infants of mothers excreting CMV in the milk will be infected perinatally. The infection is usually asymptomatic in term neonates, while that in preterm infants may be symptomatic. Heating the milk up to 72 °C for 10 s inactivates the virus saving their immunologic and nutritional properties. After a primary infection, CMV is shed for prolonged periods. Adults may shed the virus for several weeks or months and intermittently thereafter, but infants and young children shed CMV in saliva and urine for many months or years. Thus, those infants not acquiring CMV from maternal sources presumably acquire the infection from frequent contact with other children shedding CMV. In developing areas with infection acquired early in life, CMV rarely causes acute or chronic disease (Kenneson and Cannon 2007; Enright and Prober 2004; Hamprecht et al. 2001).

In developed nations or among those in middle or upper socioeconomic groups, the epidemiology of CMV usually differs from that in undeveloped or poor socioeconomic areas. In the USA, between 40% and 70% of women between 15 and 45 years of age have antibodies to CMV, and seropositivity rates vary by race, being significantly higher among African Americans than Caucasians (Adler and Marshall 2007).

103.3.2 Pathogenesis

Of all congenitally infected infants, approximately 10% of these have signs and symptoms of congenital CMV disease at birth. Of the 90% of congenitally infected infants who are without symptoms at birth, approximately 85% develop normally. Why do only 10% of infants congenitally infected with CMV have symptoms at birth, and why do approximately 15% of infants without disease at birth develop postnatal sequelae such as mental retardation and deafness? With occasional exceptions, the answer is that infants born of women acquiring a primary infection during the first half of pregnancy are those at highest risk for developing congenital disease. In fact the embryo or the fetus in its early stage lack of immune defenses and may be directly damaged by CMV which becomes cytolytic, being usually cytopathic. In addition, CMV transmission and congenital disease expression are enhanced by transient cellular and humoral immunodepression occurring in pregnancy. On the other hand, since the placental functions are more effective than in the last months of pregnancy, maternal-fetal transmission rate of CMV is low in the first months of pregnancy. Therefore the frequency of fetal infection by primary maternal infection increases with gestational age from about 30% to 70%, while the severity of fetal infection decreases. If infection occurs in the 6 months before conception, transmission to the fetus and symptoms at birth will occur at a lower rate. The prevalence of infections following recurrent CMV infection in pregnancy is considered to be lower than 2%, but higher rates have been reported. Pre-existing humoral immunity protects completely seropositive women against reinfection or reactivation at a rate of 75–80%. Neutralizing titers and IgG avidity toward CMV are both inversely correlated with fetal transmission, while the role of cellular immunity is essential in modulating viral transmission and pathogenicity in pregnancy. A major pathogenic site of CMV is the placenta, which may be impaired in its capacity to provide oxygen and nutrients to the developing fetus. CMV has several mechanisms which may contribute to its ability to cause transplacental infection, including direct effects on placental tissue (Boppana et al. 2001; Pereira et al. 2005; Pass et al. 2006; Revello et al. 2006; La Torre et al. 2006; Lanari et al. 2006; Muller et al. 2010).

Of congenitally infected newborns whose mothers acquired a primary CMV infection during early pregnancy, approximately one-third will either have disease at birth or develop significant sequelae (Fig. 1). Although the risk for symptomatic infection is greatest when primary maternal infection occurs in the first half of pregnancy, congenital disease may also occur among infants born of mothers with a primary infection in the second half of pregnancy. Because primary maternal infection is responsible for the majority of congenital CMV diseases, symptomatic infection is most frequent in areas with a high proportion of seronegative women frequently exposed to the virus. However, since primary maternal CMV infections during pregnancy are seldom recognized and many infants who develop neurologic sequelae following a primary maternal infection in early pregnancy are asymptomatic at birth, the precise number of affected infants born annually in any country is unknown. Estimates for the USA

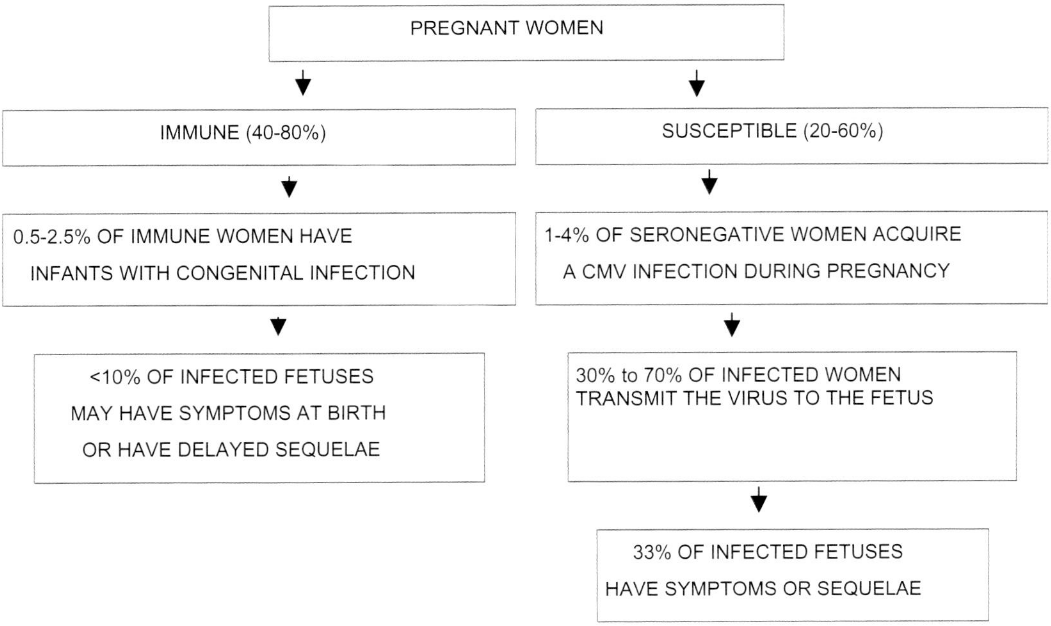

Fig. 1 Relationship of maternal immunity to disease caused by congenital CMV infection

are that between 1% and 4% of four million pregnant women acquire a primary CMV infection in the USA annually and that up to 8,000 newborns annually may develop significant handicaps caused by congenital CMV infection (Enright and Prober 2004; Hamprecht et al. 2001; Adler and Marshall 2007).

103.3.3 Clinical Manifestations

CMV infects the placenta and causes placental dysfunction shown by an enlarged placenta and placental inflammation. Manifestations of placental dysfunction in the newborn include growth retardation and problems of the reticuloendothelial/central nervous systems. Reticuloendothelial problems include hepatosplenomegaly and hepatitis, hemolytic anemia, thrombocytopenia, and direct hyperbilirubinemia. Central nervous system involvement is often manifested by microcephaly and intracranial calcification, typically periventricular. Alterations of the neuronal migration, which occur between the third and fourth month of pregnancy, cause cerebral dysplasia (polymicrogyria, pachygyria, lissencephaly, schizencephaly). CMV is the only congenitally transmitted pathogen capable of causing altered gyral development, the pathogenesis of which include both teratogenic and encephaloclastic mechanisms. Table 1 lists the more common features characteristic of infants who are symptomatic at birth. At birth chorioretinitis or intracranial calcifications or other abnormalities on ultrasound or computerized tomography (CT) or magnetic resonance imaging (MRI) of the head are associated with a poor neurologic prognosis, but none of the other manifestations of congenital infection accurately predict the severity of postnatal mental retardation or hearing deficit (Adler and Marshall 2007; Enders et al. 2001; Manicklal et al. 2013; Nigro et al. 2003; Guerra et al. 2008; Girard et al. 2006).

Approximately 15% of infants asymptomatic at birth will develop significant hearing deficit or mental retardation within the first 5 years of life. This may occur because CMV causes a chronic persistent infection. Symptomatic children are often viremic at birth and viremia may persist for the first few months of life. Both symptomatic and asymptomatic children will excrete CMV in urine and/or saliva at least for up to 5 years postnatally. At birth symptomatic children shed higher titers

Table 1 Common features in children with symptomatic congenital CMV infections

1. Unexplained hepatomegaly associated with abnormal liver function tests
2. Unexplained splenomegaly
3. Unexplained hyperbilirubinemia (usually direct>indirect)
4. Ocular findings, including chorioretinitis, strabismus, optic atrophy, microphthalmia, cataracts, or retinal necrosis
5. Microcephaly
6. Cerebral calcifications
7. Hemolytic anemia

of virus (up to 10^6 PFU/ml of urine) than asymptomatic infants. Hearing deficit, either mild or absent at birth, may develop or progressively worsen over the first several years of life, perhaps as a result of the chronic CMV infection. Therefore, parents of congenitally infected children, including those without symptoms, should not be given a prognosis at birth. When hearing deficit is profound, however, this is not generally reversible. The severity of mental retardation and developmental delay, which are the most serious neurological sequelae of this infection, are difficult to predict at birth. Most children who are symptomatic at birth will have some degree of mental retardation or developmental delay; however, IQ scores may approach 100 or higher in these children. Thus, the level of impairment in these children may be relatively mild or inapparent. Congenital CMV infection should be suspected in any infant with one or more of the manifestations listed in Table 1 (Enright and Prober 2004; Adler and Marshall 2007; Manicklal et al. 2013).

Transmission of CMV within the hospital occurs very infrequently. In numerous studies, CMV transmission from infected patients to hospital personnel has not been observed. Patient-to-patient transmission is rare and may occur when patients are hospitalized in close proximity for prolonged periods. Thus, CMV seronegative women caring for hospitalized young children or for other patients who may be excreting CMV can be reassured that there is minimal risk of acquiring CMV from patients. CMV may be transmitted by transfusion of whole blood and is located in the white cell fraction. For immunocompromised patients requiring transfusion, the risk of CMV acquisition from a blood donor is eliminated either by selecting donors who are CMV seronegative or using blood products with white cells removed (Enright and Prober 2004; Adler and Marshall 2007).

103.3.4 Diagnosis

Without prospective serologic testing of pregnant women, the diagnosis of a primary maternal infection during pregnancy is often difficult and is often only undertaken if signs and symptoms of either maternal infection or fetal disease become apparent. Symptoms of maternal CMV infection may occur in up to 25% of pregnant women infected during pregnancy. Maternal symptoms include a flu-like syndrome, myalgia, and asthenia with or without fever. There may also be a lymphocytosis and/or elevated liver enzymes in about 50% of patients. Signs of fetal infection on maternal ultrasound include growth retardation, microcephaly, echodensities in solid organs or the intestine, or an enlarged placenta (Enders et al. 2001; Manicklal et al. 2013; Nigro et al. 2003; Guerra et al. 2008).

Primary CMV infection in pregnancy is shown by seroconversion of CMV-specific IgG antibodies from negative to positive concomitantly with positive IgM antibody detection. However, this rarely occurs since screening of pregnant women is a standard practice only in particular areas. Since CMV IgM antibody may generally persist up to 6 months after seroconversion, the simultaneous detection of IgM and IgG antibodies at a first screening could represent not only primary infection but also CMV recurrence. Furthermore, a false IgM positive result may be due to polyclonal B-cell activation or to cross-reaction with other herpesviruses or autoantibodies, including rheumatoid factor. IgG avidity, which measures the capacity of antibodies of binding CMV antigen, is very low in the first weeks after a primary infection and allows to exclude a recurrent or falsely active infection (Manicklal et al. 2013; Guerra et al. 2007; Duff 2007).

Prenatal diagnosis of fetal CMV infection, which may be easily and rapidly obtained by CMV DNA detection in the amniotic fluid, does not predict an adverse fetal outcome, even if the viral load is high. Fetal CMV infection should be closely monitored by ultrasound examination for evidence of oligohydramnios or polyhydramnios; intrauterine growth retardation; hyperechogenic bowel, liver, or periventricular area; cerebral ventriculomegaly or atrophy; hydrocephalus; microcephaly; cerebellar atrophy; ascites or hydrops; renal, pleural, or pericardial effusions; hepatosplenomegaly; and necrotic, cystic, or calcified lesions in the brain, liver, or placenta. MRI can reveal cerebral abnormalities caused by migrational disorders, vascular diseases, and genetic factors. Cordocentesis may be a useful adjunct to amniocentesis, since fetal blood can be tested for detection of viral genome and hematologic, immunologic, and enzymatic examinations, but it implies an increased procedural morbidity (Manicklal et al. 2013; Guerra et al. 2008; Girard et al. 2006).

In the newborn the diagnosis of congenital CMV infection is established by CMV DNA detection from urine and/or saliva and blood within 3 weeks from birth, to differentiate congenital from perinatal infection. In neonates with suspected neurological involvement but without a clear clinical or instrumental evidence, this can be confirmed by detection of viral DNA in the cerebrospinal fluid (CSF). CMV infection can also be diagnosed by detecting specific IgM antibodies in cord or neonatal blood specimens, but false positive or, more frequently, negative results may occur (Adler and Marshall 2007; Nigro 2009).

103.3.5 Newborn Evaluation

If a congenital CMV infection is established or suspected, an evaluation should include measurement of transaminases and direct bilirubin. If liver function is abnormal, it should be monitored until near normal, which may take several months. A complete blood count should be obtained as some infants have a hemolytic anemia and many will have low platelets which may be mild or severe. Thrombocytopenia, which is due to reduced platelet production in utero consequent to CMV-induced megakaryocytic lysis and intrauterine hypoxia, usually resolves in 1–2 weeks (Adler and Marshall 2007; Nigro 2009).

Ultrasonography can show abnormalities consisting of periventricular cysts, ventriculomegaly, periventricular echolucencies due to leukomalacia, and thalamic echodensities representing arteries, but precise definition of calcifications and cerebral damage can be obtained by CT scan. MRI is very useful in revealing altered neuronal migration, parenchymal loss, delayed myelination, and cerebral or cerebellar hypoplasia. The possible occurrence of ocular involvement, including microphthalmia, cataract, and chorioretinitis, should be investigated by ophthalmoscopic examination and visual evoked potentials (Manicklal et al. 2013; Nigro 2009).

Hearing deficit is an important consequence of congenital CMV infection and is the main cause of nongenetic sensorineural hearing loss accounting for about 23% of all hearing deficit that occurs before language development. Given this and the fact that hearing loss may be fluctuating and progressive, a complete audiologic examination should be performed soon after diagnosis with frequent subsequent examinations over the first years of life. Most infected infants will develop hearing loss in the first 2 years of life, although hearing deficit may develop as late as 4 years of age. Audio evoked potentials or brainstem evoked potential testing are the most accurate tests (Rosenthal et al. 2009).

103.3.6 Treatment

103.3.6.1 Prenatal Therapy

An effective therapy for fetal CMV disease is not yet available, in spite of relevant advances in the diagnostic procedures of maternal-fetal CMV infection. Pregnancy termination is offered as a management option when injured, or even only infected, fetuses are identified by ultrasonography or amniocentesis, respectively. A few case reports have focused the attention on the safe and useful administration of oral ganciclovir to mothers of

CMV-infected fetuses. One study reported on the reduction of fetal viral load, increase of platelet count and favorable clinical outcome of mildly symptomatic fetuses after administration of valacyclovir to their mothers. The efficacy of CMV immunoglobulins (hyperimmunoglobulins) intravenously to the mother to treat or prevent fetal CMV infection has been reported by several case reports and studies, which evidenced favorable clinical and immunological results. The placenta is probably the key site of activity of hyperimmunoglobulins, as shown by studies in guinea pigs and humans, in which placental enlargement due to CMV infection can be reduced by hyperimmunoglobulins (Nigro et al. 2005; Hamilton et al. 2014; Leruez-Ville et al. 2016).

103.3.6.2 Postnatal Therapy

CMV immunoglobulins were shown to be protective against CMV disease by studies on neonate's transfusions. However, antiviral treatment of neonates or infants with symptomatic congenital CMV infection is based on the use of ganciclovir and its oral prodrug, valganciclovir, which have been given at different endpoints and regimens (both dosage and duration of therapy), and for different clinical manifestations. Ganciclovir is active only after phosphorylation to ganciclovir triphosphate, which substitutes guanosine triphosphate in the viral DNA polymerase with consequent inhibition of the CMV replication. Since the first phosphorylation requires the presence of the CMV-encoded (UL 97 gene) phosphotransferase, ganciclovir can display its activity mostly in the CMV-infected cells. Besides being a possible consequence of CMV infection, neutropenia and increased aminotransferase levels may be associated with ganciclovir therapy, particularly in the immunodepressed patients. A longer duration of antiviral therapy (at a dose of 16 mg per kilogram of body weight, orally twice daily) has been associated with favorable outcome more frequently than shorter courses, probably related to the longer inhibition of CMV. In fact, this virus reactivates soon after stopping therapy, and some of the favorable results obtained during ganciclovir therapy may be lost. Protracted and repeated courses of oral ganciclovir were useful for therapy of several CMV-related diseases, including neurologic and gastrointestinal manifestations (Stronati et al. 2013; Mareri et al. 2015; Kimberlin et al. 2015).

103.3.7 Prevention

Since CMV is a major cause of childhood deafness and neurological handicap, routine antepartum screening should be very useful, but it still appears to be impracticable. To avoid difficulties in differentiating recurrent from primary infections and problematic counseling when positive IgM antibodies are detected, serial examinations of CMV-specific IgG and IgM antibodies at least in the first two trimesters, particularly in women at high risk like daycare workers, may be suggested. In such a way, it is possible to reveal as soon as possible both primary (by seroconversion and high IgM levels) and recurrent (by significant IgG increase concomitantly or not with positive IgM antibodies) infections. To prevent possible viral transmission to the fetus, women with primary infection could receive hyperimmunoglobulins. Appropriate hygienic measures can prevent CMV transmission. The most aggressive preventive approach requires counseling of parents with seropositive children in daycare centers: seronegative parents should be instructed in frequent hand washing after handling diapers and material contaminated with secretions and cautioned about the potential risk of intimate contact, especially mouth-to-mouth. Seronegative women with multiple sexual partners and a history of sexually transmitted diseases should be counseled about the use of condoms (Manicklal et al. 2013; Nigro 2009; Stronati et al. 2013).

Since the detection of CMV DNA in CSF has been associated with developmental delay, in neonates with suspected neurological involvement, this evaluation could be used to identify infants who are at risk for neurodevelopmental problems and who may therefore benefit from antiviral therapy. Vaccines, using both live attenuated virus (Towne 125) and subunit or recombinant proteins, mostly glycoprotein B, have been evaluated for many years. Recent vaccine strategy is based on the use of a poxvirus vector platform to elicit neutralizing antibodies to conformational epitopes of the gH/gL/UL128/UL130/UL131A pentamer complex. However, a suitable CMV vaccine, particularly for women in the childbearing age, has not yet been developed (Pass et al. 2009; Chiuppesi et al. 2015).

103.4 Infection with Herpes Simplex Virus, Serotype 1 and 2

103.4.1 Epidemiology

HSV is a member of the *Herpesviridae* family including two closely related virus types (1 and 2), which are transmitted through mucosal cells or cutaneous lesions and migrate to the nerve tissues, in which they persist in a latent state. HSV-1 predominates in the orofacial manifestations and is typically found in the trigeminal ganglia, whereas HSV-2 is most commonly detected in the lumbosacral ganglia. Nevertheless, these viruses can infect both orofacial areas and the genital tract, where they can reactivate either asymptomatically or with vesicular lesions (Xu et al. 2006; Gantt and Muller 2013) (Table 2).

Vertical transmission is more likely to occur after primary maternal infection, but recurrent genital infections are more frequent and, consequently, they are the most common cause of neonatal herpes infections. The great majority of recurrent genital herpes is due to HSV-2 because this virus reactivates in the genital area more frequently than HSV-1 (7% vs. 2%, respectively). In the asymptomatic period between clinical outbreaks of genital herpes, HSV can reactivate periodically in latently infected cells of sensory ganglia traveling via the neuronal axons back to the genital mucosa, without clinical signs or symptoms ("asymptomatic virus shedding"). The majority of sexual HSV transmission occurs during asymptomatic shedding because the patients are unaware of the viral presence (Gantt and Muller 2013; Cherpes et al. 2012; Sauerbrei and Wutzler 2007a).

Newborns may acquire infections with HSV in utero, peripartum at delivery, or postpartum. Approximately 5% of all neonatal infections with HSV are acquired in utero, 85% are acquired at birth by contact with infected maternal lesions or asymptomatic cervical shedding of HSV, and 10% are acquired postpartum from environmental sources, such as scalp electrodes or individuals with oral HSV infections. Intrauterine infections with HSV occur with a frequency of from 1 in 200,000 to 1 in 300,000 live births as opposed to peripartum infections estimated at 1:5,000. In utero infection during the first 20 weeks of gestation is associated with the highest infant morbidity and mortality, including stillbirths and spontaneous abortions (Xu et al. 2006; Cherpes et al. 2012).

Table 2 Clinical manifestations of congenital or perinatal infection by herpes simplex virus (HSV)

Congenital HSV infection
Cutaneous lesions: scarring, vesicles, bullae, macular erythema, areas of aplastic or denuded skin
Cerebral: hydranencephaly, microcephaly
Ocular: chorioretinitis, microphthalmia
Perinatal HSV infection
Encephalitis
Pneumonia
Esophagitis
Mucocutaneous manifestations
Systemic disease

103.4.2 Pathogenesis

Although the exact route by which infants acquire intrauterine HSV infections is unknown, there is evidence that most infants are infected by virus ascending through the chorioamnionic membrane rather than from a maternal viremia and transplacental passage of HSV to the fetus. The first observation is that during both recurrent and primary maternal HSV infections, maternal viremia does not occur. The second is that HSV is commonly present in the cervical-vaginal tract, and this is the usual site of primary or secondary HSV infection in women who deliver infants with intrauterine HSV infection. Although women with a primary HSV infection deliver infants with the most severe form of intrauterine infection, these primary infections are still in the cervical-vaginal tract and viremia does not occur. The third observation is that even when a woman with viremia develops disseminated HSV disease during pregnancy, the majority of fetuses born of these women die from maternal complications, but not as a consequence of intrauterine HSV. Surviving fetuses of women with widely disseminated maternal disease usually have no evidence of HSV disease at delivery. This suggests that the occurrence of maternal viremia is not necessary for intrauterine infection with HSV (Xu et al. 2006; Cherpes et al. 2012).

The fourth fact is that most infants born with intrauterine HSV infection have cutaneous disease with scarring. The chronicity of the skin infection suggests that, as in postpartum and peripartum acquired infections, the skin or the mucous membranes are the first sites of HSV infection, followed by fetal viremia and subsequent central nervous system infection. The fifth fact suggesting an ascending route of infection is that when HSV is in the placenta, there is an extensive fetal involvement, suggesting passage of virus from fetus to placenta. The sixth fact suggesting an ascending route of infection is that nearly all infants with intrauterine infection are infected with HSV-2, the serotype commonly found in the maternal cervical-vaginal tract. If the route of fetal infection were via the maternal blood stream, one would anticipate frequent fetal infection with HSV-1, since this serotype is common in pregnant women (Cherpes et al. 2012; Sauerbrei and Wutzler 2007a; Anzivino et al. 2009).

Numerous aspects of the innate immune response influence immunity to HSV infection and neonatal susceptibility to disease. Studies in mice and humans suggest that the immunopathology of neonatal HSV infection is related to cytokine production mediated by Toll-like receptor 2. Concerning the adaptive immunity, newborns infected with HSV appear to demonstrate attenuated cellular responses, including both proliferation and cytokine production (Muller et al. 2010).

103.4.3 Clinical Manifestations

Diagnosis of intrauterine HSV infection requires clinical evidence of infection within the first 48 h of life and confirmation by recovery of the virus from the newborn. Symptoms are usually present at birth. The classic symptom triad is skin scarring, hydranencephaly, and chorioretinitis. Skin vesicles and bullae are common. There may also be erythematous maculas that later become vesicles or areas of aplastic or denuded skins or scars. These may occur at sites of trauma, for example, fetal scalp electrode sites. Skin lesions often recur, but do not usually progress to other sites. Dissemination with multi-organ system involvement, if present, includes hepatic (i.e., liver failure), renal (i.e., anuria), and hematologic disorders (i.e., disseminated intravascular coagulopathy). Intrauterine growth retardation and subsequent postnatal growth retardation are also common (Baker 2007).

When hydranencephaly is absent, microcephaly, intracranial calcifications, hydrocephalus, porencephaly, and subdural or epidural cysts may occur with subsequent blindness, deafness, and mental retardation. Involvement of the eye is common, particularly chorioretinitis with strabismus. This occurs more frequently with intrauterine HSV infection than with HSV infection acquired peripartum or postpartum. Disseminated infection in infants with intrauterine disease is much less frequent than in infants with perinatally acquired infection, because those infants who develop disseminated disease usually die in utero (Baker 2007; Enright and Prober 2002).

103.4.4 Peri- and Postnatal HSV Infections

103.4.4.1 Epidemiology

HSV transmission follows a direct contact with oral or genital secretions, even if asymptomatic. HSV-1 infection occurs early in the low economic level populations, while HSV-2 prevalence rapidly increases with sexual activity. Oral recurrences occur in 20–40% of the adult population. The prevalence of neonatal HSV infection is 1/2,500–20,000 infants, being caused by HSV-2 in two thirds of the cases (Xu et al. 2006).

103.4.5 Pathogenesis

After entry at mucosal surfaces or abraded skin, HSV proteins bind to several cell receptors of epidermal and dermal cells, in which the virus replicates. In both clinical and subclinical infections, HSV reaches sensory or autonomic nerve endings and is transported intraxonally to the nerve cell bodies in ganglia, in which initial viral replication takes place. Then, HSV spreads to other mucosal and skin cells by centrifugal migration along peripheral sensory nerves. After primary infection, viral DNA may be found in 10–50% of ganglion cells of the anatomic region initially involved. Ultraviolet light, immunodepression, and trauma are associated with HSV reactivation, but the pathogenic mechanism is unknown (Cherpes et al. 2012; Sauerbrei and Wutzler 2007a; Anzivino et al. 2009).

103.4.6 Clinical Manifestations

103.4.6.1 Neonatal Herpes

Neonatal herpes includes three major clinical features: oculomucocutaneous (50%), encephalic (33%), or systemic manifestations (17%). Mucocutaneous and ocular signs can occur several days after delivery and are generally slight: vesicles, which are often grouped, may be purulent and be considered as bacterial bullae. Encephalitis is shown, 2–3 weeks after birth, by fever and irritability or lethargy in the first 2 weeks, and then by alterated muscular tone and partial or diffuse convulsions. CSF examination shows 50–100 leukocytes, decreased glucose, but increased protein content. EEG reveals signs of disseminated cerebropathy; CT and MRI scans show focal alterations. The systemic infection is shown by fever, lethargy, hepatic dysfunction, pneumonia, disseminated intravascular coagulopathy, and shock. Other signs include seizures, jaundice, and a vesicular exanthema which may be pathognomic. Encephalitis is a common manifestation (60–75%) of the disseminated HSV infection (Enright and Prober 2002, 2004; Whitley 2004).

The rate and severity of neonatal HSV infection are depending on the type of maternal genital infection: the frequency is higher after primary than recurrent maternal infection (50% vs. <3%). However, 70% of neonatal HSV infections result from exposure to asymptomatic maternal HSV shedding during delivery. Prolonged rupture of membranes favors neonatal infection: a cesarean section should be chosen. Invasive obstetrical procedure and fetal scalp monitors can cause lesions which are sites of viral inoculation (Enright and Prober 2002; Whitley 2004).

103.4.7 Gingivostomatitis

Gingivostomatitis is predominantly caused by HSV-1 and typically shown by vesiculoulcerative lesions on the tongue, lips, gingival, labial mucosa, and the hard and soft palate. Fever, painful oropharyngeal mucositis, cervical lymphadenitis, and fetid breath persist for several days and can cause dehydration because of the difficult feeding even with liquids (Enright and Prober 2002; Whitley 2004).

103.4.8 Keratoconjunctivitis

Keratoconjunctivitis is commonly caused by HSV-1 and presents as monolateral follicular conjunctivitis with localized lymphadenomegaly, palpebral vesicles, photofoby, edema e corneal opacity (Enright and Prober 2002).

103.4.9 Encephalitis

Encephalitis is one of the most common acute viral infections of the brain (1/250–500.000 persons every year), caused by HSV-1 in >90% of the cases, predominantly after recurrent infections. If untreated, it is lethal in 60–80% and followed by severe sequelae in >90% of the surviving patients (Anzivino et al. 2009; Whitley 2004).

103.4.10 Cutaneous Herpes

Primary cutaneous infections can be localized in every part of the body, sometimes as an extensive zoster-like manifestation. Recurrences are generally localized on the lips, both mucosal and cutaneous parts. Because the immune system is still developing, then partially immature, in the first and second infancy, herpetic recurrences may be more frequent and extensive than in adults. Occasionally, the children may present recurrent stomatitis or aphthosis with or without an erythema (Cherpes et al. 2012; Whitley 2004).

103.4.11 Herpes in Immunodepressed Children

Herpes in immunodepressed children occurs as an extensive mucocutaneous or multisystem infection, including Kaposi's varicella-like eruption or *eczema herpeticum*, pneumonia, and meningoencephalitis. Children with AIDS may have a rapidly worsening and overwhelming herpetic infection shown by esophagitis, enterocolitis, pneumonia, hepatitis, and neurological manifestations (Enright and Prober 2002, 2004).

103.4.12 Diagnosis

The HSV infection may be identified directly by detection of the virus or one of its components or indirectly by assaying for specific serum antibodies of the viruses. Direct site-specific methods, such as DNA detection by RT-PCR or viral isolation, are the most relevant in patients with active, vesicular lesions at or near a genital site. When lesions have scabbed or are not evident, HSV-1 or HSV-2 infection can be diagnosed indirectly by detection of type-specific IgG against the glycoprotein G of HSV-1 (gG-1) or the glycoprotein G of HSV-2 (gG-2). Indirect testing can provide useful information in symptomatic patients when direct methods have yielded negative results. The detection of HSV-specific IgM antibodies may be negative or nonspecific (Sauerbrei and Wutzler 2007a; Anzivino et al. 2009).

Intrauterine HSV infections are diagnosed by virus detection from the infant's samples within the first 48 h of life. Cultures should not be obtained for HSV this early from asymptomatic infants or infants who have none of the signs or symptoms of intrauterine HSV infection because some infants may only be colonized with HSV at birth. Cultures should be obtained from skin lesions, perianally, mucous membranes, eyes, nose, oral pharynx, and ears. More sensitive than culture is the viral DNA detection from the liquid of vesicles and any other sample, particularly the CSF. A Tzanck preparation or Wright's stain of epithelial cells scrapped from cutaneous lesions may reveal multinucleated giant cells which are associated either with HSV or VZV lesions. After the first 48 h of life, the isolation of HSV from an asymptomatic newborn means an active infection rather than colonization and requires antiviral therapy. Tissue HSV involvement may be also diagnosed using immunohistochemical methods or in situ hybridization. Cerebral imaging and auditory/ophthalmological examination should be performed (Enright and Prober 2002, 2004; Sauerbrei and Wutzler 2007a; Anzivino et al. 2009).

103.4.13 Treatment

Specific antiviral therapy with acyclovir is appropriate for infants with either intrauterine or postnatal HSV infections. To treat encephalitis or systemic HSV infection, intravenous acyclovir (20 mg/kg three times daily) should be started soon after collection of the samples for virologic confirmation. If acyclovir resistance develops, ganciclovir or, preferably, foscarnet should be given. For gingivostomatitis or mucocutaneous lesions, oral acyclovir should be given at a dosage of 15 mg/kg five times daily for 7 days. The starting time of treatment is crucial for prognosis, especially in case of disseminated infections. HSV infections localized to skin, eyes, and mucous membranes are treated for 14 days, whereas CNS or disseminated infections require 21 days of therapy. For recurrent skin lesions, which are frequent after neonatal HSV infection, acyclovir treatment is indicated for weeks to months, at doses of 300 mg/m^2 two to three times daily (Enright and Prober 2002; Whitley 2008).

103.4.14 Prognosis

For both intrauterine and postnatal HSV encephalitis and systemic infections, if untreated, the mortality is about 70%. Treatment with acyclovir reduces mortality until to about 30% and to only 5% for neonates with encephalitis. The effect of antiviral therapy on morbidity is unknown, and some treated infants, particularly those with cerebral manifestations, will be blind, deaf, or profoundly retarded. The outcome is correlated with the virus type and disease expression. Moreover, after a neonatal herpes infection, cutaneous recurrences may occur (Whitley 2004; Kimura et al. 2003).

103.4.15 Prevention

Several antiviral therapies are available to control disease and spread, but these are not completely effective and do not affect latent virus. Therefore, numerous approaches, including subunit or peptide vaccines, live virus vectors, and DNA vaccines, have been used in developing both prophylactic and therapeutic vaccines. Currently, neither active nor passive immunization is available for prevention of HSV infections in the pregnant women and neonates. However, the developing vaccine strategy should take in account the most important features of the herpesvirus family: viral latency, immune escape, and high seroprevalence (Anzivino et al. 2009; Ramachandran and Kinchington 2007).

All pregnant women with genital herpes should be treated with acyclovir or valacyclovir, which were shown not to be associated with teratogenic effects. However, since these drugs are not officially approved for treating pregnant women, patients should give consent about the limited information before the drug is used. The high rate of undiagnosed or asymptomatic HSV infections complicates the prevention. Identification of the pregnant women serostatus during early pregnancy is the first and most important step, to establish their susceptibility to the infection. A history of HSV infection in all pregnant women and their partner should be obtained at the first prenatal visit. Women with a negative personal history of HSV and especially those with a positive history in the male partner should be strongly advised to have no oral and sexual intercourse at the time of recurrence in order to avoid infection, particularly in the third trimester of pregnancy. The use of condoms throughout pregnancy should be recommended to minimize the risk of viral acquisition, although they are not considered to be a complete barrier for the genital region. Prophylactic administration of acyclovir or valacyclovir in the third trimester of pregnancy should be provided to all pregnant women with frequent genital herpes outbreaks and with active genital HSV infection near term or at the time of delivery. A careful examination of the vulva, vagina, and cervix should be performed on any woman who presents signs or symptoms of HSV infection at the onset of labor. Artificial rupture of membranes should be avoided. All pregnant women who have suspected active genital HSV infection should undergo cesarean section, although membranes are intact. PCR testing to rapidly and accurately detect HSV shedding in maternal genital tract swab specimens at the time of all deliveries provide these results approximately 2 h after specimen collection. Neonates, born to women with active genital lesions, with a confirmed or suspected HSV infection should be isolated; managed with precautions to avoid direct contact with skin and mucosal lesions, excretions, and body fluids; and immediately treated with intravenous acyclovir. Since neonatal herpes can also be acquired postnatally, postpartum women, family members, and nursery personnel with active herpetic lesions of the mouth, skin, or breast should take necessary precautionary measures to prevent direct contact with the neonate and/or should be excluded from the neonatal unit until the lesions are fully healed (Enright and Prober 2004; Cherpes et al. 2012; Baker 2007; Ramachandran and Kinchington 2007).

Table 3 Congenital varicella syndrome: principal clinical manifestations

Skin lesions
Microphthalmia, chorioretinitis, cataract, atrophy of the optical nerve
Neurosensorial deafness or hypoacusia
Microcephaly, calcifications, cerebral atrophy, hydrocephalus, mental retardation
Limb hypoplasia or paresis

103.5 Varicella

103.5.1 Epidemiology

VZV is a herpesvirus, which causes chicken pox and shingles. Women who have had chicken pox before pregnancy are immune and their fetuses are not at risk. About 5% of women have not had chicken pox before pregnancy. The average incidence of varicella in pregnancy ranges from 0.7 to 3%. If a woman becomes infected with VZV during pregnancy, infection of the fetus with the development of a varicella syndrome occurs up to the 26th week of gestation. However, the risk for intrauterine disease after a primary maternal VZV chicken pox is low, about 4%, mostly in the first two trimesters. This is much lower than when a woman acquires primary varicella within a few days of delivery, when the risk for the newborn of acquiring postnatal varicella approaches 20%. The rate of spontaneous abortion by varicella does not exceed that of women without varicella. Pregnant women who contract varicella are at risk of severe pneumonia associated with life-threatening ventilatory compromise and death, apparently more often in the third trimester. If a woman develops zoster, also called shingles during pregnancy, there is no risk to the fetus (Enright and Prober 2004; Sanchez et al. 2011; Sauerbrei and Wutzler 2005; Cobelli Kett 2013) (Table 3).

103.5.2 Pathogenesis

VZV causes both primary chicken pox and recurrence within an initially infected dermatome. Recurrence, which occurs months to decades after a primary infection, is called shingles or zoster. VZV infection in a normal person consists of two episodes of viremia. The first episode of viremia follows the replication of the virus at a regional lymph node in the head or neck. This primary viremia results in the seeding and replication of VZV at multiple body sites. After the second stage of viral replication, secondary viremia leads to infection of epithelial cells in the entire body and produces the skin lesions of chicken pox. Various virus-host cell interactions need to occur in the host immune response for the virus to successfully cause disease. Following primary exposure to VZV, there is a prolonged incubation period before emergence of skin lesions, during which time the adaptive immune response is delayed. It has been suggested that VZV encodes functions which benefit the virus by evading the immune response (Abendroth et al. 2010).

Transmission to the fetus occurs with either the primary or secondary viremia. Infection after a primary maternal viremia can cause fetal disease within a day or two after the appearance of skin lesions in the mother. If, however, fetal infection occurs after the secondary maternal viremia, fetal skin lesions do not appear until 10–14 days following the appearance of lesions in the mother.

In the first 20 weeks of gestation, since the fetal organs are embryonic, VZV may cause teratogenic abnormalities. Maternal chicken pox late in gestation may be the cause of high fetal mortality but not structural abnormalities. Spontaneous abortion, fetal demise, and premature delivery can occur at an undetermined but low frequency (Sauerbrei and Wutzler 2005; Abendroth et al. 2010; Schulze and Dietzsch 2000).

103.5.3 Clinical Manifestations

103.5.3.1 Congenital Varicella Syndrome (CVS)

Since VZV has a tropism for peripheral and central neural tissue, the major manifestations of intrauterine varicella infections are those related to the nervous system. The characteristic clinical signs and symptoms, which also include skin lesions in dermatomal distribution, eye diseases, and limb hypoplasia, are zigzag skin lesions and hypopigmented areas; damage to the eye including microphthalmia, cataracts, chorioretinitis, and optic atrophy; damage to the cervical-lumbar spinal cord with hypoplasia of the upper and lower extremities with motor and sensory deficits; absent dependent reflexes; anal dysfunction; and Horner's syndrome. Based on the segmental distribution of some clinical features, related lesions might be not consequent to immediate intrauterine varicella but zoster-like VZV reactivations. Cortical damage includes encephalitis with microcephaly, hydrocephaly, intracranial calcifications, and aplasia of the brain. In spite of the initial poor prognosis, a favorable outcome can occur in children with CVS. In addition to the developing disease, prenatally infected infants may develop VZV infection without symptoms: intrauterine infection is more common than fetal disease. The developmental effects of asymptomatic intrauterine VZV infection are unknown (Schulze and Dietzsch 2000; Smith and Arvin 2009; Enders et al. 1994; Pastuszak et al. 1994; Cobelli Kett 2013).

103.5.4 Neonatal Varicella

Maternal varicella between 4 and 5 days before and 2 days after delivery may be followed by a generalized and severe neonatal varicella, since protective antibodies are not transferred to the infant. The attack rate for the infant ranges 20%. A fatal outcome is more likely if neonatal disease occurs between 5 and 10 days after delivery. Chickenpox occurring after the first 10 days of life is most likely acquired postnatally and is associated with a low morbidity, since most neonates are protected by maternal antibodies. However, premature infants younger than 28 weeks' gestation or weighing below 1,000 g are at an increased risk for severe varicella during the first 6 weeks of life (Sauerbrei and Wutzler 2005; Smith and Arvin 2009; Cobelli Kett 2013).

103.5.5 Complications of Postnatal Varicella

Otherwise healthy children may have secondary bacterial infections, usually caused by *Staphylococcus aureus* and *Streptococcus pyogenes*; meningoencephalitis, which is prevalent under 5 years or over 20 years of age; acute cerebellar ataxia; Reye syndrome, which is significantly reduced by avoidance of salicylates; transverse myelitis; hepatitis; thrombocytopenia; and arthritis. These clinical manifestations may have a vasculitic or immune-mediated pathogenesis. Immunocompromised children, pregnant women, and adults are at high risk of developing a severe and progressive varicella. Varicella pneumonia is the major cause of maternal morbidity and mortality. The risk of progressive disease, including prolonged cutaneous lesions, pneumonia, hepatitis, encephalitis, and disseminated intravascular coagulopathy, is up to 50% for children with lymphoproliferative malignancies or solid tumors, particularly if chemotherapy is given during the incubation of varicella. In children with cancer, disseminated VZV infection may also be associated with esophagitis, enterocolitis, pancreatitis, and necrotizing splenitis. Thrombocytopenia and hepatitis are the major clinical complications in kidney-transplanted patients. Children receiving high doses of corticosteroids, especially during the incubation period, may develop a severe, even fatal varicella (Enright and Prober 2004).

103.5.6 Diagnosis

Maternal varicella may be confirmed by detection of specific IgM and IgG antibodies. Fetal ultrasound and MRI at 16–22 weeks' gestation or

5 weeks after infection can show possible signs of CVS. Fetal infection should be confirmed by detection of VZV DNA in the amniotic fluid. Termination of pregnancy may be suggested if serious fetal abnormalities are shown. The causal relationship between maternal varicella and congenital abnormalities can be verified by detection of viral DNA or antigens in the infant. Contrary to congenital rubella or CMV infection, VZV has not been isolated in cell cultures from any infant with CVS. Serologic diagnosis is mostly based on the detection of VZV-specific IgG beyond 7 months of age, since IgM antibodies are only present in about 25% of infants with CVS. Neonatal varicella is easily diagnosed on the basis of the typical clinical picture but PCR should be used for laboratory diagnosis from skin swabs or biopsies, CSF, and tissue samples (Sauerbrei and Wutzler 2005, 2007b; Benoit et al. 2015).

103.5.7 Treatment

Antiviral therapy with acyclovir or valacyclovir for intrauterine varicella should be started as soon as possible, preferably after contacts with infected children. If a woman develops chicken pox at or within a few days of delivery, prophylactic treatment of infants with acyclovir may be appropriate. If neonates show signs of infection, immediate treatment with acyclovir must be initiated. These newborns are at high risk for death due to chicken pox since they have not maternally acquired antibodies to VZV (Sauerbrei and Wutzler 2005, 2007b; Smith and Arvin 2009).

103.5.8 Prevention

A pregnant woman who does not recall having chicken pox or the vaccine and who is exposed in her household should promptly receive varicella-zoster immune globulin (VZIG) and tested for immunity, to prevent maternal infection or subsequent complications. Although no controlled studies show that VZIG prevents CVS, the biologic plausibility of this treatment comes from favorable results in improving or preventing clinical varicella in immunocompromised or otherwise healthy patients. However, the effectiveness of VZIG has not been evaluated later than 96 h (Enders et al. 1994; Pastuszak et al. 1994; Benoit et al. 2015).

Varicella pneumonia must be regarded as a medical emergency, since pregnant women are at risk of life-threatening ventilatory compromise and death. Neonates exposed to VZV should receive VZIG. Intravenous acyclovir is recommended for maternal pneumonia and severely affected neonates. No controlled study has yet evaluated the effectiveness of acyclovir or valacyclovir for post-exposure prophylaxis to pregnant women or neonates. Most women are immune although they do not recall having had chicken pox, but delaying the administration of VZIG while awaiting a test result is inappropriate. Whereas VZIG is very effective in either preventing or reducing the severity of maternal disease, its effectiveness in preventing intrauterine infection is unknown; nonetheless VZIG is recommended for administration to women during pregnancy (Sauerbrei and Wutzler 2005; Wilson et al. 2008).

Varicella vaccine, which is a live attenuated strain of VZV, is recommended for all adults who have not had chickenpox. Pregnant women should not be immunized because of the potential risk for fetal infection. Women inadvertently immunized 3 months before pregnancy or during pregnancy can be reassured about the low risk and the incident should be reported to the public health authorities and the vaccine manufacturer. However, if a pregnant woman, for whatever reason, received varicella vaccine in the first half of pregnancy, VZIG may be given (Pandolfi et al. 2009; Gershon 2003).

References

Abendroth A, Kinchington PR, Slobedman B (2010) Varicella zoster virus immune evasion strategies. Curr Top Microbiol Immunol 342:155–171

Adler SP, Marshall B (2007) Cytomegalovirus infections. Pediatr Rev 28:92–100

Anzivino E, Fioriti D, Mischitelli M et al (2009) Herpes simplex virus infection in pregnancy and in neonate:

status of art of epidemiology, diagnosis, therapy and prevention. Virol J 6:40–52

Baker DA (2007) Consequences of herpes simplex virus in pregnancy and their prevention. Curr Opin Infect Dis 20:73–76

Benoit G, Etchemendigaray C, Nguyen-Xuan HT, Vauloup-Fellous C, Ayoubi JM, Picone O (2015) Management of varicella-zoster virus primary infection during pregnancy: a national survey of practice. J Clin Virol 72:4–10

Boppana SB, Rivera LB, Fowler KB, Mach M, Britt WJ (2001) Intrauterine transmission of cytomegalovirus to infants of women with preconceptional immunity. N Engl J Med 344:1366–1371

Cherpes TL, Matthews DB, Maryak SA (2012) Neonatal herpes simplex virus infection. Clin Obstet Gynecol 55:938–944

Chiuppesi F, Wussow F, Johnson E et al (2015) Vaccine-derived neutralizing antibodies to the human cytomegalovirus gH/gL pentamer potently block primary cytotrophoblast infection. J Virol. pii: JVI.01701-15

Cobelli Kett J. Perinatal varicella. Pediatr Rev. 2013 Jan;34(1):49-51. https://doi.org/10.1542/pir.34-1-49

Duff P (2007) A thoughtful algorithm for the accurate diagnosis of primary CMV infection in pregnancy. Am J Obstet Gynecol 196:196–197

Enders G, Miller E, Cradock-Watson J, Bolley I, Ridehalgh M (1994) Consequences of varicella and herpes zoster in pregnancy: prospective study of 1,739 cases. Lancet 343:1548–1551

Enders G, Bader U, Lindemann L, Schalasta G, Daiminger A (2001) Diagnosis of congenital cytomegalovirus infection in 189 pregnancies with known outcome. Prenat Diagn 21:362–377

Enright AM, Prober CG (2002) Neonatal herpes infection: diagnosis, treatment and prevention. Semin Neonatol 7:283–291

Enright AM, Prober CG (2004) Herpesviridae infections in newborns: varicella-zoster virus, herpes simplex virus, and cytomegalovirus. Pediatr Clin North Am 51:889–908

Gantt S, Muller WJ (2013) The immunologic basis for severe neonatal herpes disease and potential strategies for therapeutic intervention. Clin Develop Immunol. https://doi.org/10.1155/2013/369172

Gershon AA (2003) Varicella vaccine: rare serious problems – but the benefits still outweigh the risks. J Infect Dis 188:945–947

Girard N, Chaumoitre K, Confort Gouny S, Viola A, Levrier O (2006) Magnetic resonance imaging and the detection of fetal brain anomalies, injury, and physiologic adaptations. Curr Opin Obstet Gynecol 18:164–176

Guerra B, Simonazzi G, Banfi A et al (2007) Impact of diagnostic and confirmatory tests and prenatal counseling on the rate of pregnancy termination among women with positive cytomegalovirus immunoglobulin M antibody titers. Am J Obstet Gynecol 196:221.e1–221.e6

Guerra B, Simonazzi G, Puccetti C et al (2008) Ultrasound prediction of symptomatic congenital cytomegalovirus infection. Am J Obstet Gynecol 198:380.e1–380.e7

Hamilton ST, van Zuylen W, Shand A et al (2014) Prevention of congenital cytomegalovirus complications by maternal and neonatal treatments: a systematic review. Rev Med Virol 24:420–433

Hamprecht K, Maschmann J, Vochem M, Dietz K, Speer CP, Jahn G (2001) Epidemiology of transmission of cytomegalovirus from mother to preterm infant by breastfeeding. Lancet 357:513–518

Kenneson A, Cannon MJ (2007) Review and meta-analysis of the epidemiology of congenital cytomegalovirus (CMV) infection. Rev Med Virol 17:253–276

Kimbelin DW, Jester PM, Sanchez PJ et al (2015) Valganciclovir for symptomatic congenital disease. N Engl J Med 372:933–943

Kimura H, Futamura M, Ito Y et al (2003) Relapse of neonatal herpes simplex virus infection. Arch Dis Child Fetal Neonatal Ed 88:483–486

La Torre R, Nigro G, Best AM, Adler SP (2006) Placental enlargement is predictive of a primary maternal cytomegalovirus infection and fetal disease. Clin Infect Dis 43:994–1000

Lanari M, Lazzarotto T, Venturi V et al (2006) Neonatal cytomegalovirus blood load and risk of sequelae in symptomatic and asymptomatic congenitally infected newborns. Pediatrics 117:e76–e83

Leruez-Ville M, Ghout I, Bussières L, et al (2016) In utero treatment of congenital cytomegalovirus infection with valacyclovir in a multicenter, open-label, phase II study. Am J Obstet Gynecol Apr 13. pii: S0002-9378(16)30044-8. https://doi.org/10.1016/j.ajog.2016.04.003. [Epub ahead of print]

Manicklal S, Emery VC, Lazzarotto T, Boppana SB, Gupta RK (2013) The "silent" global burden of congenital cytomegalovirus. Clin Microbiol Rev 26:86–102

Mareri A, Lasorella S, Iapadre G, Maresca M, Tambucci R, Nigro G (2015) Antiviral therapy for congenital cytomegalovirus infection: pharmacokinetics, efficacy and side effects. J Mat Fet Neon Med. https://doi.org/10.3109/14767058.2015.1058774

Mocarski ES Jr, Courcelle CT (2002) Cytomegaloviruses and their replication. In: Knipe DM, Howley PM, Griffin DE, Lamb RA, Martin MA, Roizman B, Straus SE (eds) Fields virology. Lippincott Williams & Wilkins, Philadelphia, pp 2629–2673

Muller WJ, Jones CA, Koelle DM (2010) Immunobiology of herpes simplex virus and cytomegalovirus infections of the fetus and newborn. Curr Immunol Rev 6:38–55

Nigro G (2009) Maternal-fetal cytomegalovirus infection: from diagnosis to therapy. J Mat Fet Neon Med 22:169–174

Nigro G, Anceschi MM, Cosmi EV, Congenital Cytomegalic Disease Collaborating Group (2003) Clinical manifestations and abnormal laboratory findings in pregnant women with primary cytomegalovirus infection. Brit J Obstet Gynaecol 110:572–577

Nigro G, Adler SP, La Torre R, Best AM, Congenital Cytomegalic Disease Collaborating Group (2005) Passive immunization during pregnancy for congenital cytomegalovirus infection. N Engl J Med 353:1350–1362

Pandolfi E, Chiaradia G, Moncada M, Rava L, Tozzi AE (2009) Prevention of congenital rubella and congenital varicella in Europe. Euro Surveill 14:16–20

Pass RF, Fowler KB, Boppana SB, Britt WJ, Stagno S (2006) Congenital cytomegalovirus infection following first trimester maternal infection: symptoms at birth and outcome. J Clin Virol 35:216–220

Pass RF, Zhang C, Evans A et al (2009) Vaccine prevention of maternal cytomegalovirus infection. N Engl J Med 360:1191–1199

Pastuszak AL, Levy M, Schick B et al (1994) Outcome after maternal varicella infection in the first 20 weeks of pregnancy. N Engl J Med 330:901–905

Pereira L, Maidji E, McDonagh S, Tabata T (2005) Insights into viral transmission at the uterine-placental interface. Trends Microbiol 13:164–174

Ramachandran S, Kinchington PR (2007) Potential prophylactic and therapeutic vaccines for HSV infections. Curr Pharm Des 13:1965–1973

Revello MG, Zavattoni M, Furione M, Fabbri E, Gerna G (2006) Preconceptional primary human cytomegalovirus infection and risk of congenital infection. J Infect Dis 193:783–787

Rosenthal LS, Fowler KB, Boppana S et al (2009) Cytomegalovirus shedding and delayed sensorineural hearing loss. Results from longitudinal follow-up of children with congenital infection. Ped Infect Dis J 28:515–520

Sanchez MA, Bello-Munoz JC, Cebrecos I et al (2011) The prevalence of congenital varicella syndrome after a maternal infection, but before 20 weeks of pregnancy: a prospective cohort study. J Matern Fetal Neonatal Med 24:341–347

Sauerbrei A, Wutzler P (2005) Varicella-zoster virus infections during pregnancy: epidemiology, clinical symptoms, diagnosis, prevention and therapy. Curr Pediatr Rev 1:205–216

Sauerbrei A, Wutzler P (2007a) Herpes simplex and varicella-zoster virus infections during pregnancy: current concepts of prevention, diagnosis and therapy. Part 1: herpes simplex virus infections. Med Microbiol Immunol 196:89–94

Sauerbrei A, Wutzler P (2007b) Herpes simplex and varicella-zoster virus infections during pregnancy: current concepts of prevention, diagnosis and therapy. Part 2: varicella-zoster virus infections. Med Microbiol Immunol 196:95–102

Schulze A, Dietzsch HJ (2000) The natural history of varicella embryopathy: a 25-year follow-up. J Pediatr 137:871–874

Smith CK, Arvin AMV (2009) Varicella in the fetus and newborn. Semin Fet Neon Med 14:209–217

Stronati M, Lombardi G, Garofoli F, Villani P, Regazzi M (2013) Pharmacokinetics, pharmacodynamics and clinical use of valganciclovir in newborns with symptomatic congenital cytomegalovirus infection. Curr Drug Metab 14:208–215

Whitley R (2004) Neonatal herpes simplex virus infection. Curr Opin Infect Dis 17:243–246

Whitley RJ (2008) Therapy of herpes virus infections in children. Adv Exp Med Biol 609:216–232

Wilson E, Goss MA, Marin M et al (2008) Varicella vaccine exposure during pregnancy: data from 10 years of the pregnancy registry. J Infect Dis 197(Suppl 2): S178–S184

Xu F, Sternberg MR, Kottiri BJ et al (2006) Trends in herpes simplex virus type 1 and type 2 seroprevalence in the United States. JAMA 296:964–973

Fetal Infections: Rubella, HIV, HCV, HBV, and Human Parvovirus B19

104

Pier Angelo Tovo, Stefania Bezzio, and Clara Gabiano

Contents

P. A. Tovo (✉)
Department of Pediatrics, University of Turin, Regina Margherita Childrens Hospital, AOU Città della Salute e della Scienza di Torino, Turin, Italy
e-mail: pierangelo.tovo@unito.it

S. Bezzio · C. Gabiano
Department of Pediatrics, University of Turin, Turin, Italy

G. Buonocore et al. (eds.), *Neonatology*,
https://doi.org/10.1007/978-3-319-29489-6_251

Abstract

Congenital rubella (CR) infection leads to damage in over 80% of fetuses during the first trimester of pregnancy, in 25–34% of cases in the second trimester, while no malformations occur in the third trimester CR syndrome is characterized by cardiac, ocular, and hearing defects, although any organ may be affected. All women of child-bearing age should have natural or vaccine-induced immunity to the virus. Mother-to-child transmission (MTCT) of HIV has decreased from 18% down to 1% in bottle-fed infants with adoption of preventive interventions. These include: prenatal antiretroviral (ARV) prophylaxis, administration of ARV during delivery and avoidance of breast feeding. An early combined ARV treatment of HIV-infected infants offers the great benefits of a longer asymptomatic period and of a prolonged survival. No interventions are currently available to prevent MTCT of HCV, that is estimated to be about 5%. The natural history of HCV infection is relatively benign in childhood. More than 90% of HBV exposed infants develop chronic infection. Administration of HBV vaccine and specific immunoglobulins at birth followed by the 3-dose vaccine series has reduced the MTCT rate by about 90%. Primary maternal infection with parvovirus B19 is associated with asymptomatic fetal infection, hydrops fetalis, intrauterine death, and birth defects. In the first and second trimester the MTCT rate is about 30%. In case of hydrops or signs of anemia, intrauterine trasfusions are recommended.

104.1 Salient Points

- Congenital rubella infection is most severe when transmission occurs in the first trimester of pregnancy, and it is characterized by the combination of cardiac, ocular, and hearing defects. To prevent the syndrome, it is important to determine maternal immune status.
- Transmission of HIV during pregnancy may occur in utero, during delivery, and through breast milk. Effective preventive interventions include the administration of prenatal antiretroviral prophylaxis, elective cesarean section, and the avoidance of breastfeeding.
- HCV is transmitted from mother to child in 5% of cases; spontaneous viral clearance occurs in at least one quarter of vertically infected children; the natural history of HCV infection in infancy and childhood is relatively benign.
- More than 90% of children perinatally exposed to HBV develop chronic infection. All term infants born to HbsAg-positive women should receive HBV vaccine and specific immunoglobulins at birth, followed by completion of three-dose vaccine series.
- Maternal infection with parvovirus B19 is associated with asymptomatic fetal infection, nonimmune hydrops fetalis, and intrauterine fetal death. No specific therapy is available; if there is hydrops and/or signs of fetal anemia, intrauterine erythrocyte transfusions are recommended.

104.2 Rubella Virus

104.2.1 Etiology and Pathogenesis

The importance of congenital rubella (CR) was recognized in the 1940s, and the etiological agent was discovered in the 1960s. Rubella epidemics occur at 6- to 9-year intervals and major pandemics every 10–30 years. Theoretically, universal immunization programs should eradicate rubella, but at least 100,000 cases of CRS still occur annually worldwide (Grant et al. 2015; Vynnycky et al. 2016).

The rubella virus, a member of the togavirus family, is composed of an icosahedral nucleocapsid containing a single-stranded RNA genome, surrounded by a lipid envelope. The mechanism by which the virus causes fetal damage is poorly understood. The virus spreads through the bloodstream, it can infect and replicate in the placenta, and it then reaches the fetus, where it persistently infects cells, inducing a decreased growth rate. In the first trimester of gestation, the fetus is unable to mount an adequate immune response, and the passive transfer of maternal antibodies is inefficient; thus the viral replication leads to altered organogenesis. From the second trimester of gestation, the risk of congenital rubella syndrome (CRS) decreases; in fact, changes in the placenta, the appearance of the immune response, and the passive transfer of maternal IgG result in a higher protection from viral damage. The virus can persist for over a year in target organs, where it can undergo recurrent replications. Late-onset CRS manifestations are due to persistent virus-driven tissue damage and scarring.

104.2.2 Transmission

Miscarriage, stillbirth, and a series of birth defects, such as low birth weight, congenital heart disease, and central nervous system damage, are possible sequelae of CRS. Fetal infection may occur at any stage of pregnancy. The outcome of infection depends on the gestational age. Primary maternal infection causes damage in more than 80% of the fetuses during the first trimester of pregnancy, in 25–34% in the second trimester, while no malformations occur in the third trimester. Rubella reinfection may occur both in vaccine-immune and, to a lesser extent, in naturally immune subjects. In these cases, the risk of CRS is estimated to be around 5% in the first trimester of pregnancy (Bouthry et al. 2014).

104.2.3 Clinical Aspects

Rubella infection spreads by droplets, and it is usually subclinical or paucisymptomatic in infants and children. Clinical manifestations (fever, non-confluent maculopapular rash, headache, malaise, lymphadenopathy, usually involving suboccipital, postauricular, and cervical nodes) develop after 14–21 days of incubation.

CRS is typically characterized by the combination of cardiac, ocular, and hearing defects, although the virus can infect any organ (Table 1) (Duszak 2009; Neu et al. 2015).

104.2.4 Diagnosis

Amniotic fluid and fetal blood samples can be used to detect rubella infection by means of nested reverse transcriptase polymerase chain reaction (RT-PCR). Fetal blood, obtained by cordocentesis, can also be tested for specific IgM. Amniocentesis is less invasive than fetal blood sampling. Both tests should be performed 6–8 weeks after maternal infection; the best reliability is when the fetus is 22 weeks old.

Postnatally, CRS is diagnosed by detection of specific IgM, though both false negative and false positive results have been described, or by stable or increased titers of specific IgG over several months. IgG avidity testing may help to differentiate between recent and past infection (Best 2007; Lambert et al. 2015). Identification of the virus in urine, blood, or nasopharyngeal secretions by cultures or by RT-PCR may also confirm the diagnosis.

104.2.5 Prognosis

Children affected by CRS may require medical, surgical, educational, and rehabilitative

Table 1 Congenital rubella syndrome main defects (listed in order of decreasing frequency)

Early-onset manifestations
Deafness
Mental retardation
Cardiovascular defects affecting primarily the left atrium and the heart septa
Ocular defects (nuclear cataracts, microphthalmia, pigmentary retinopathy, glaucoma)
Thrombocytopenia
Hepatitis
Bone lesions
Dental defects
Hypospadias
Cryptorchidism
Inguinal hernia
Interstitial pneumonitis
Meningoencephalitis
Cerebral calcification
Splenic fibrosis
Nephrosclerosis
Nephrocalcinosis
Late-onset manifestations
The delayed manifestations (due to the altered immune system of CRS patients) underscore the importance of careful follow-up of these patients
Insulin-dependent diabetes
Thyroid dysfunction
Neurodegenerative disorders (panencephalitis)
Slow growth rate during preschool years
Smaller head circumference
Ocular defects (secondary glaucoma, strabismus)
Defects in the immune system (transitory hypogammaglobulinemia, especially ipoIgA, defects in cell-mediated immunity)

management. CRS must be managed as a dynamic rather than a static disease, requiring a multidisciplinary approach: for instance, early treatment is critical for hearing defects and psychomotor difficulties.

104.2.6 Therapy and Treatments

The prime strategy for the prevention of CRS is to ensure that all pregnant women are immune to rubella (CDC – Surveillance of congenital rubella syndrome 2014). In developed countries, vaccination programs are based on the universal immunization of infants at 12–15 months of age, plus a second vaccination at 5–6 years of age or before adolescence to achieve immunity in patients who did not receive the first dose or with primary vaccine failure. Furthermore, all women at childbearing age should be tested and vaccinated, if still susceptible. The RA 27/3 strain is used as a rubella vaccine. This is remarkably safe, has high efficacy (over 90%), and induces long-lasting protection. It is used as a component of the measles-mumps-rubella (MMR) vaccine or of the recent tetravalent vaccine (MMR plus varicella).

Vaccination programs have led to marked reduction in morbidity and mortality associated with CRS. Benefits of the vaccine far outweigh the costs of treatment and rehabilitation of affected children and adults.

104.3 Human Immunodeficiency Virus (HIV)

104.3.1 Etiology and Pathogenesis

More than 3.2 million children under 15 years are estimated to be living with human immunodeficiency virus type 1 (HIV-1) infection worldwide in 2013, mostly following mother-to-child transmission (MTCT) (UNAIDS 2016).

HIV is a retrovirus belonging to the subgroup of lentiviruses. The first step of its life cycle is characterized by the integration of the virion envelope glycoproteins (gp120 and gp41) with the cell surface CD4 molecule. After entering the cell, the virus is rapidly uncoated. Then, through reverse transcriptase, its viral RNA is transformed into linear DNA. This is circularized and transferred into the nucleus where it is inserted at random sites as a provirus. The provirus is activated by host cell responses to antigens, cytokines, or products of other viruses. Thousands of infectious particles can originate from a single infected cell, either chronically or as a single burst resulting in cell death. HIV infection leads to a profound qualitative and quantitative attrition of the immune system, particularly of cell-mediated immunity with a decrease in CD4+ cell count.

Immune-mediated damage presumably plays a key role in AIDS pathogenesis.

Two genetically distinct HIV types have been identified: HIV-1 and HIV-2; the latter is localized mainly in Western Africa and causes a less aggressive disease.

HIV infection results in a minimal risk of adverse pregnancy outcomes, such as spontaneous abortion, intrauterine growth restriction, and premature delivery (Sollai et al. 2015).

104.3.2 Transmission

HIV is a sexually transmitted infection that also spreads by contact with contaminated blood. After the screening of blood donors, MTCT has become the most common route of infection in children. MTCT ranges between 15 and 23% in bottle-fed infants. Prolonged breastfeeding may account for an additional 10–15% of infections. With the implementation of effective preventive measures, MTCT rate can be reduced to less than 1% in non-breastfed infants.

Maternal viral load is an independent risk factor for MTCT. Many other viral, maternal, obstetrical, fetal, and infant factors can influence the transmission rate (Table 2). Most children are infected perinatally, though intrauterine transmission may occur. An infant is considered to have been infected in utero when HIV-1 can be detected from peripheral blood within 48 h from birth. In contrast, a non-breastfed child is taken to have had intrapartum infection if he/she becomes viremic subsequently. Transmission due to household contacts is not documented.

Table 2 Maternal, obstetrical, and neonatal factors associated with increased HIV transmission rate

Pregnancy	Labor and delivery	Breastfeeding
High maternal viral load (new infection or advanced AIDS) and/or CD4 cell count <200/mm^3	High maternal viral load (new infection or advanced AIDS) and/or CD4 cell count <200/mm^3 at delivery	High maternal viral load (new infection or advanced AIDS) and/or CD4 cell count <200/mm^3
Viral, bacterial, or parasitic placental infections, such as malaria	Rupture of membranes (>4 h)	Duration of breastfeeding
Sexually transmitted infections	Invasive delivery procedures that increase contact with the mother' s infected blood or body fluids (e.g., episiotomy, artificial rupture of membranes)	Breast abscesses, mastitis, nipple fissures
	Chorioamnionitis (from untreated STI or other infections)	Oral disease in the baby (e.g., thrush or sores)
	Preterm delivery	

104.3.3 Clinical Manifestations

According to the infection status, an infant born to a seropositive mother is classified as exposed (E), infected (I), or seroreverted (SR) (see below). A breastfed infant is at risk of infection in the 6 months after interruption of maternal lactation.

HIV+ children are classified into mutually exclusive, progressive categories according to their clinical and immunological status (Table 3) (Centers for Disease Control and Prevention 1994). Once classified in a more severe category, a child cannot be reclassified in a less severe one, even if the clinical or immunologic situation improves.

HIV progression is more accelerated in children than in adults. HIV-infected newborns are usually asymptomatic, but they can become seriously ill within the first weeks/months of life. Growth delay is an early finding in untreated infected infants. Children more likely than adults have serious bacterial infections, and lymphoid interstitial pneumonia is almost entirely restricted to the pediatric age. P*neumocystis jirovecii* pneumonia (PJP) is the most common opportunistic infection (OI), with the highest incidence at 3–6 months of age.

The use of highly active antiretroviral therapy (HAART) has significantly improved the morbidity and mortality of HIV-infected children, though their rate of severe infections, particularly pneumonias, remains high (Berti et al. 2015).

Table 3 Classification system for HIV infection in children younger than 13 years of age

	Clinical categories			
Immune categories	No symptoms (N)	Mild symptoms (A)	Moderate symptoms (B)	Severe symptoms (C)
(Based on age-specific CD4+ cell count or percentage)				
1 – No suppression	N1	A1	B1	C1
0–11 months → > 1500 cells/μL (≥25%)				
1–5 years → > 1000 cells/μL (≥25%)				
> 6 years → >500 cells/μL (≥25%)				
2 – Moderate suppression	N2	A2	B2	C2
0–11 months → > 750–1499 cells/μL (15–24%)				
1–5 years → 500–999 cells/μL (15–24%)				
> 6 years → 200–499 cells/μL (15–24%)				
3 – Severe suppression	N3	A3	B3	C3
0–11 months → > < 750 cells/μL (<15%)				
1–5 years → > < 500 cells/μL (<15%)				
> 6 years → < 200 cells/μL (<15%)				

Modified from (Centers for Disease Control and Prevention 1994)

104.3.4 Diagnosis

Diagnosis of HIV infection in exposed infants is based on the detection of viremia in two separate determinations. Most uninfected children lose passively acquired maternal antibodies by 12–15 months of age, though in 2% these may persist up to 18 months. Criteria for diagnosis or exclusion of infection (Panel on Antiretroviral Therapy and Medical Management of HIV-Infected Children 2016) through detection of viremia are detailed in Table 4.

104.3.5 Prevention of MTCT

All pregnant women should be tested routinely for HIV during an early prenatal visit (first trimester) in order to adopt effective preventive strategies. These include:

- Administration of combined antiretroviral (cARV) therapy during pregnancy in order to reach a plasma viral load below the limit of detection.
- Prophylaxis with zidovudine (ZDV) during delivery can be considered, even if the additional benefit of intravenous (IV) ZDV in women receiving combination regimens has not been evaluated in randomized clinical trials.
- Elective cesarean section (CS), especially recommended in women with detectable viremia near the time of delivery despite antepartum cARV.
- ARV prophylaxis in the infant.
- Avoidance of breastfeeding.

104.3.5.1 Prenatal ARV Treatment

Prenatal ARV regimens with HAART, regardless of viral load and CD4 cell count, are recommended to all HIV-infected women to prevent MTCT as well as for their own health (Panel on Treatment of HIV-Infected Pregnant Women and Prevention of Perinatal Transmission 2015). In particular, women under ARV treatment should continue their therapy during pregnancy, while those who do not require treatment for their own health should receive a three-drug combination to prevent viral transmission to the offspring. ZDV prophylaxis

Table 4 Diagnosis of HIV infection in exposed children less than 18 months of age (Panel on Antiretroviral Therapy and Medical Management of HIV-Infected Children 2016)

Diagnosis of HIV infection (I)	Exclusion of HIV-1 infection (SR)
1. Positive results on two separate specimens (not including cord blood) from virologic assays that directly detect HIV; HIV antibody tests should not be used HIV RNA and HIV DNA nucleic acid tests are recommended as preferred virologic assays A positive virologic test should be confirmed as soon as possible by a repeat virologic test on a second specimen	1. Definitive exclusion of HIV infection in non-breastfed infants is based on two or more negative virologic tests, with one obtained at age ≥ 1 month and one at age ≥ 4 months
2. Virologic diagnostic testing is recommended for all infants with perinatal HIV exposure at the following ages 14–21 days 1–2 months (preferably, 2–4 weeks after cessation of antiretroviral prophylaxis) 4–6 months	2. At least two negative HIV-1 antibody test results from separate specimens obtained at >6 months of age

alone is no more suggested. After the onset of labor or rupture of membranes (or approximately 3 h before an elective cesarean section), IV ZVD (2 mg/kg over the first hour, then 1 mg/kg per hour until delivery is complete) should be administered. However, IV ZVD is not strictly required in HIV-infected women receiving HAART and with undetectable viral load at delivery (Panel on Treatment of HIV-Infected Pregnant Women and Prevention of Perinatal Transmission 2015).

Although congenital abnormalities have been reported in animals treated with ARV drugs, results from registries and cohort studies do not confirm this association in human beings. Mitochondrial toxicity of clinical relevance has been described, albeit anecdotically, in Europe after in utero exposure to nucleoside analogues, but these findings still remain matter of debate, and the proven efficacy of maternal and infant ARV prophylaxis to prevent perinatal HIV transmission significantly outweighs these concerns. There is no evidence that exposure to antiretroviral drugs in utero or neonatally is associated with an increased risk of childhood cancer (Panel on Treatment of HIV-Infected Pregnant Women and Prevention of Perinatal Transmission 2015).

104.3.5.2 Elective Cesarean Section

The MTCT rate was reported lower in women who delivered by elective cesarean section than in those who delivered by emergency cesarean section or vaginal delivery (CDC – Surveillance of congenital rubella syndrome 2014). Thus, there was general agreement that elective C-section should be recommended at 38 weeks' gestation to all pregnant women with a viral load >1000 RNA copies per mL near the time of delivery.

Recently, several observational studies suggested no additional benefit from scheduled Cesarean delivery in women who received cARV for several weeks and who achieved virologic suppression (Kourtis et al. 2014; Briand et al. 2013). Furthermore, there is a persistently increased risk of maternal complications following CS compared to vaginal delivery (Kourtis et al. 2014). At present, in the great majority of industrialized countries, elective CS is recommended only when the maternal VL is not controlled by ARV therapy (Briand et al. 2013).

104.3.5.3 Infant ARV Prophylaxis

A 4–6-week course of ZDV prophylaxis is recommended for all exposed neonates and should be initiated as soon as possible after birth (Table 5). In certain situations (e.g., treated women with suboptimal viral suppression or only intrapartum ARV therapy or known ZDV-resistant virus), some experts suggest the addition of other ARV drugs (Sollai et al. 2015; Panel on Treatment of HIV-Infected Pregnant Women and Prevention of Perinatal Transmission 2015; Chiappini et al. 2006).

Table 5 Zidovudine prophylaxis in HIV-exposed infants (Panel on Treatment of HIV-Infected Pregnant Women and Prevention of Perinatal Transmission 2015)

Gestational age at birth	Oral dose (mg/kg per dose)	Intravenous dose (mg/kg per dose)	Frequency	Weeks
≥35 weeks	4	3	Every 12 h	4–6
30 > weeks <35	2	1.5	Every 12 h advancing to 3 mg/kg/dose (or 2.3 mg/kg/dose IV) every 12 h at 2 weeks of age	6
<30 weeks	2	1.5	Every 12 h advancing to 3 mg/kg/dose (or 2.3 mg/kg/dose IV) every 12 h at 4 weeks of age	6

104.3.5.4 Breastfeeding

Although the risk of postnatal HIV transmission through maternal milk is well documented, the WHO recommends breastfeeding in the first 6 months of life in some developing countries, because such a risk is lower than that of death from diarrheal diseases and malnutrition. Conversely, in countries where formula feeding is affordable, feasible, acceptable, sustainable, and safe, breastfeeding should be discouraged (Sollai et al. 2015; Panel on Treatment of HIV-Infected Pregnant Women and Prevention of Perinatal Transmission 2015; Chiappini et al. 2006).

104.3.6 Prognosis

The prognosis of perinatally acquired HIV infection was initially poor. Opportunistic infections (OIs), progressive neurological disorders, malignancies, severe bacterial infections, and wasting syndrome were the main causes of death (Tovo et al. 1992). However, morbidity and mortality due to AIDS-defining opportunistic infections have significantly decreased since the introduction of HAART in children. These can grow regularly, remain in good health for many years, and reach adulthood, and pregnant women can give birth to a second generation of HIV-1-exposed infants without additional risk factors for transmission (Calitri et al. 2014). However, severe pneumonia and fungal or bacterial sepsis still represent a problem. Furthermore, several noninfectious conditions related to chronic HIV infection and lifelong treatment, such as metabolic outcomes, renal abnormalities, cardiovascular complications, and non-AIDS-defining malignancies, are progressively emerging (Berti et al. 2015).

104.3.7 Therapy and Treatments

104.3.7.1 Antiretroviral Therapy

Initiation of ARV therapy is recommended in all HIV-infected infants in the first year of life, regardless of clinical and immunological conditions. Subsequently, the therapeutic options should be based on clinical, immunologic, and virologic findings. Whereas all children with severe HIV disease should start prompt treatment, asymptomatic subjects aged ≥1 year and those with mild to moderate clinical manifestations can take more time to fully assess, discuss, and address issues associated with adherence prior to initiating therapy. On the other hand, several studies highlight that initiation of ART at younger ages and higher CD4 values maximizes its potential benefit. The therapeutic regimen should contain at least three ARV drugs, from at least two distinct classes (Panel on Antiretroviral Therapy and Medical Management of HIV-Infected Children 2016).

104.3.7.2 Supportive Care

Every HIV-infected child should be protected from vaccine-preventable diseases (Figs. 1 and 2). In general, all inactivated vaccines can be administered safely, and usual doses and schedules are recommended. Children with HIV infection are at a high risk for complications of varicella zoster and measles. Bearing in mind the limited safety, immunogenicity, and efficacy of varicella and MMR vaccines in HIV-infected children, these

Vaccine ▼ Age ▶	Birth	1 month	2 months	4 months	6 months	9 months	12 months	13 months	15 months	18 months	19-23 months	2-3 years	4-6 years
Hepatitis B[1]	Hep B	HepB		see foot-note1	HepB								
Rotavirus[2]			RV	RV	*RV*[2]								
Diphtheria, Tetanus, Pertussis[2]			DTaP	DTaP	DTaP		see foot-note3		DTaP				DTaP
Haemophilus influenzae type b[4]			Hib	Hib	*Hib*[4]		Hib						
Pneumococcal[5]			PCV	PCV	PCV		PCV					PPSV	
Inactivated Poliovirus			IPV	IPV	IPV								IPV
Influenza[6]					TIV(Yearly)								
Measles, Mumps Rubella[7]							MMR						MMR
				Do not administer to severely immunosupressed children									
Varicella[8]							Varicella		Varicella				
					Do not administer to severely immunosupressed children								
Hepatitis A[9]							Hep A (2 doses)					Hep A Series	
Meningococcal[10]			MCV4										

Fig. 1 Recommendations for routine immunizations in HIV-infected children aged 0–6 years. *HepB* hepatitis B vaccine, *RV* rotavirus vaccine, *DtaP* diphtheria and tetanus toxoids and acellular pertussis vaccine, *Hib Haemophilus influenzae* type B conjugate vaccine, *PCV* pneumococcal conjugate vaccine, *PPSV* pneumococcal polysaccharide vaccine, *IPV* inactivated polio vaccine, *TIV* trivalent inactivated influenza vaccine, *MMR* measles, mumps, and rubella vaccine, *Hep A* hepatitis A vaccine, *MCV4* meningococcal conjugate vaccine (Modified from Panel on Opportunistic Infections in HIV-Exposed and HIV-Infected Children (2013))

should be administered only in subjects without severe immunosuppression (CD4+ cell percentage 15%).

Prophylactic measurements to prevent PJP pneumonia are detailed in Table 6 (Panel on Opportunistic Infections in HIV-Exposed and HIV-Infected Children 2013).

104.4 Hepatitis C Virus (HCV)

104.4.1 Etiology and Pathogenesis

The hepatitis C virus (HCV) is the most common cause of chronic liver disease, with 115 million seropositive subjects (11 million children <15 years) worldwide (Gower et al. 2014). The prevalence of infection in children varies from 0.05–0.4% in developed countries to 2–5% in resource-limited settings. After the screening of blood donors, with consequent disappearance of posttransfusional hepatitis C, MTCT has become the most common route of infection in the pediatric population, at a rate of about 5%

HCV is a small (50 nm in size), enveloped, single-stranded RNA virus. Six major genotypes exist; each genotype comprises hundreds to thousands of subtypes, referred to as quasispecies, resulting from the high viral mutation rates and reflecting the unique ability of the virus to continually alter its immunologically recognizable epitopes. HCV primarily enters hepatocytes, although other cell types, such as dendritic cells and B-cells, can also be infected. The virus is non-cytopathic by itself.

104.4.2 Transmission

Antenatal screening might be useful to identify infected children before the onset of symptoms and to offer post-pregnancy therapy to their

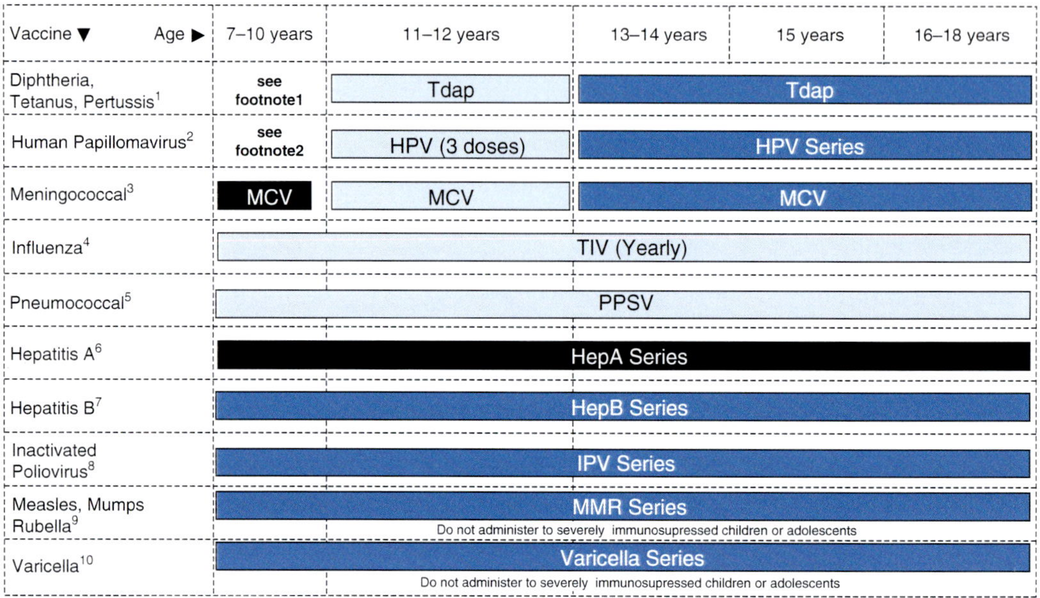

Fig. 2 Recommendations for routine immunizations in HIV-infected children aged 7–18 years. *Tdap* tetanus and diphtheria toxoids and acellular pertussis vaccine, *HPV* human papillomavirus vaccine, *MCV* meningococcal vaccine, *TIV* trivalent inactivated influenza vaccine, *PPSV* pneumococcal polysaccharide vaccine, *HepA* hepatitis A vaccine, *HepB* hepatitis B vaccine, *IPV* inactivated polio vaccine, *MMR* measles, mumps, and rubella vaccine (Modified from Panel on Opportunistic Infections in HIV-Exposed and HIV-Infected Children (2013))

Table 6 Prophylaxis to prevent *Pneumocystis jirovecii* pneumonia in HIV-exposed infants or HIV-infected children

Pathogen	Indication	First choice	Alternative
Pneumocystis jirovecii	Exposed children From 6 weeks until exclusion of infection	TMP-SMX 2,5–5/12,5–25 mg/kg / dose orally twice per day and administered three times weekly on consecutive or alternate days	Dapsone (>1 month of age) 2 mg/kg orally daily or 4 mg/kg once weekly
	Infected children From 6 weeks until 1 year From 1 to 5 years if CD4 < 500 cells/mm^3 From 6 to 12 years if CD4 < 200 cells/mm^3 or percentage < 15%		Atovaquone: children aged 1–3 months and >24 months, 30–40 mg/kg, orally, once daily with food; children aged 4–24 months, 45 mg/kg, orally, once daily; children aged >13 years 1500 mg, orally, once daily
			Aerosolized pentamidine: >5 years, 300 mg every month

TMP trimethoprim, *SMX* sulfamethoxazole, *mon(s)* month(s), *yrs* years (Modified from Panel on Opportunistic Infections in HIV-Exposed and HIV-Infected Children (2013))

mothers. However, because of the absence of effective preventive strategies, universal screening for HCV in pregnant women remains questionable, even if a routine screening and treatment program seem feasible and effective at a cost considered acceptable (Selvapatt et al. 2015). Indeed, antenatal screening is suggested in special circumstances: women positive for HIV or hepatitis B virus, a history of intravenous drug use, transplantation, hemodialysis, blood or blood product transfusion prior to 1992, tattooing, or unexplained elevated liver enzymes (Pembrey et al. 2005).

HCV infection does not impair the course of pregnancy or increase the risk of spontaneous abortion or fetal death (Dunkelberg et al. 2014). The time of transmission remains unclear. The largest studies consistently estimate that 30–50% of HCV infections are acquired in utero, while the remainder occur in the late intrauterine/intrapartum period.

Several risk factors for MTCT have been identified (Table 7) (Tovo et al. 2016). However, none are modifiable and no preventive interventions can be adopted.

High viral load is associated with MTCT (Tovo et al. 2016; Cottrel et al. 2013). Thus, seropositive women with undetectable HCV RNA during pregnancy can be reassured that the risk of transmission to the offspring is very low, though it cannot be excluded. The new direct-acting antiviral agents (DAAs) can dramatically reduce the viral load in few weeks (Barth 2015). However, at present these drugs cannot be used in pregnant women because their effects on the fetus are unknown. An indirect decrease in the global number of vertical infections may derive from a widespread use of these agents in HCV-infected women of childbearing age.

Although the evidence is inconclusive, it is prudent to avoid obstetric procedures that may favor fetal exposure to contaminated maternal blood, such as amniocentesis or internal fetal monitoring. These procedures should only be used when indicated to avoid maternal or infant morbidity.

Most studies highlight that mode of delivery and type of feeding have no significant impact on the MTCT rate. Therefore, elective cesarean section should not be offered to HCV-infected pregnant women, and breastfeeding should not be discouraged.

Table 7 Potential risk factors for HCV mother-to-child transmission

Variable	Risk factor	Strength of the evidence
Maternal HCV/HIV coinfection	Yes	Strong
High maternal viral load	Yes	Strong
Cesarean section	No	Sufficient
Vaginal delivery	No	Sufficient
Breastfeeding	No	Sufficient
Genetic background	Yes	Sufficient
Amniocentesis	?	Insufficient
IV drug users	?	Insufficient
ALT levels during pregnancy	Yes	Insufficient
Internal fetal monitoring	Yes	Insufficient
Forceps deliveries	Yes	Insufficient
Perineal or vaginal lacerations	Yes	Insufficient
Episiotomy	No	Insufficient
Prolonged membrane rupture	Yes	Insufficient
Cigarette smoking	No	Insufficient
Alcohol intake	No	Insufficient
Maternal age	No	Insufficient
HCV genotype	No	Insufficient
Numbers of pregnancies	No	Insufficient
Prematurity	No	Insufficient
Girls gender	Yes	Insufficient

104.4.3 Clinical Aspects

The natural history of vertically acquired HCV infection is ill defined. Spontaneous disappearance of circulating HCV RNA occurs in at least one quarter of cases, mostly in preschool age (Garazzino et al. 2014). IL-28B polymorphisms have been associated with greater chance of viral clearance (Indolfi et al. 2014).

Infected children are asymptomatic at birth, and their general condition usually remains good during childhood with regular growth (England et al. 2005). Only a fraction develop minor abnormalities, such as hepatomegaly, or nonspecific symptoms and signs (European Paediatric Hepatitis C Virus Network 2005).

Alanine aminotransferase (ALT) activity is highest in the first 2 years of life, after which it declines, often assuming a fluctuating pattern. Viremia also fluctuates in a large proportion of infected children (Polywka et al. 2006).

Liver function tests are of little help in assessing the development of aggressive hepatitis and cirrhosis. Necrotic inflammation and fibrosis are usually milder in children than in adults (European Paediatric Hepatitis C Virus Network 2005; Abdel-Hady et al. 2011). Progression of liver damage is not linear; cirrhosis and liver failure are rare in childhood (European Paediatric Hepatitis C Virus Network 2005; Abdel-Hady et al. 2011; Mack et al. 2012). Routine liver biopsy in infected children is not recommended.

HCV-associated extrahepatic manifestations and autoimmune diseases are rare in children with chronic infection, whereas non-organ-specific autoantibodies are frequently detected (Garazzino et al. 2014).

104.4.3.1 Diagnosis

The persistence of anti-HCV antibody beyond 15 months of age represents the "gold standard" for the diagnosis of vertically acquired HCV infection. Earlier diagnosis in an exposed child relies on the detection of HCV RNA by PCR. Children are taken to be infected if PCR is positive in at least two separate determinations. The test is highly specific, but its sensitivity is low at birth (22–33%), whereas it increases up to 85% after the first month of life (Mok et al. 2005).

Since a negative PCR might also reflect fluctuations in viremia, both antibody testing and the detection of serum HCV RNA have been suggested for definition of the infection status in exposed children (Fig. 3).

104.4.4 Therapy and Treatment

There are limited data for the management of children and adolescents with chronic HCV infection. The availability of DAAs with high pan-genotypic effectiveness has displaced the traditional treatments in HCV RNA-positive adults. At present, the combination of pegylated interferon-α and ribavirin remains the standard therapy for pediatric infections (Mack et al. 2012; Lee et al. 2015; Suzuki et al. 2016). However, clinical trials of interferon-free DAA regimens are in progress to verify safety and efficacy of these agents also in children with chronic infection (Ohmer and Honegger 2016). Indeed, since a significant liver damage is rare in preschool age, while during this period about a quarter of infected children show a spontaneous viral clearance, it seems reasonable to postpone any treatment beyond this age in most patients. HCV may however progress to hepatic failure, and liver transplantation has been performed in a few infected children (Mack et al. 2012).

Children with HCV should be immunized against hepatitis A and B.

104.5 Hepatitis B Virus (HBV)

104.5.1 Etiology and Pathogenesis

Two billion people worldwide are estimated to have acquired hepatitis B virus (HBV) and more than 350 million to be chronically infected (Schweitzer et al. 2015). In low-prevalence areas (chronic infection <2%), such as the USA and Western Europe, most new infections occur in young adults and are acquired sexually or through intravenous drug use, while in moderate- or high-prevalence areas (chronic infection 2–7% or >8%, respectively), perinatal and horizontal transmissions are the prevalent routes of infection.

HBV is a member of the Hepadnavirus family. The virus is divided into four major serotypes (adr, adw, ayr, ayw) and into eight genotypes (A–H) (Zhang et al. 2016).

Differences between genotypes affect the disease progression and the response to treatment. Hepatocytes are the primary target of HBV, but the kidney, pancreas, and mononuclear cells can also be infected. HBV is non-cytopathic by itself. The host's immune response causes both viral clearance and hepatocellular injury. The cytotoxic T-cell-mediated lysis of infected hepatocytes is the predominant mechanism of liver damage. Intrauterine exposure to HBV antigens may induce tolerance, accounting for the high rate of carriers among perinatally infected children.

104.5.2 Transmission

Possible routes of HBV transmission include unprotected sexual contact, blood transfusions, reuse of contaminated needles or syringes, and

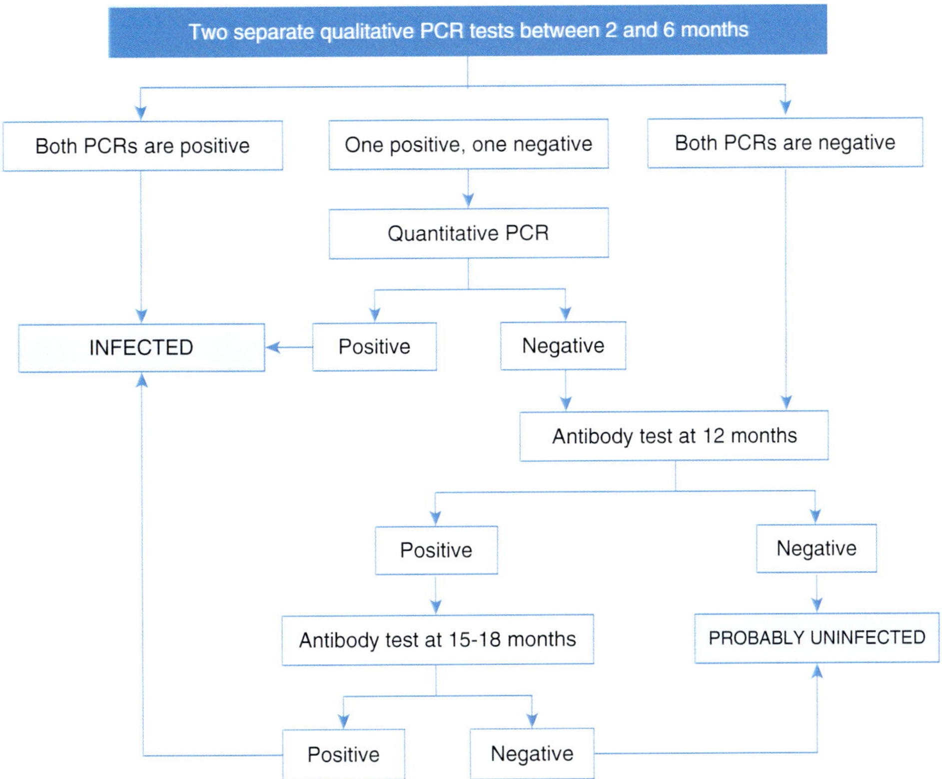

Fig. 3 Recommended follow-up schedule for early diagnosis of infection in infants born to HCV-infected women (Modified from (Pembrey et al. 2005))

MTCT. The vertical transmission rate is 70–90% in untreated infants of HB surface antigen (HbsAg)- and HBe antigen (HbeAg)-positive viremic women, while it decreases to 10–30% in the HBsAg carrier mothers who have anti-e antibody (anti-HBe) and are PCR negative. In utero infection is considered the most important reason for the failure of neonatal immunoprophylaxis in preventing MTCT; the exact mechanism of intrauterine transmission remains to be elucidated. Transmission to the offspring mostly occurs at delivery by microtransfusion or contact with contaminated body fluid. The mode of delivery (cesarean vs. vaginal) does not affect transmission, and breastfeeding is not an additional risk factor in infants treated with proper immunoprophylaxis (Gentile and Borgia 2014; Yi et al. 2016).

Acute HBV hepatitis or exacerbation of chronic disease may occur during pregnancy. However, these conditions increase neither maternal morbidity or mortality nor the risk of fetal complications, though a high number of preterm labors have been reported in women with acute hepatitis B.

104.5.3 Clinical Aspects

The age of HBV acquisition is roughly inversely correlated with the likelihood of developing a persistent infection. Neonates have >90% risk of developing chronic infection, as compared to 25–50% of older children and 5% of adult subjects.

104.5.3.1 Acute Infection

HBV-infected infants and children are usually asymptomatic. However, disease onset may be insidious. Symptoms and signs include anorexia, malaise, nausea, vomiting, abdominal pain, and jaundice. MTCT is the most important route of transmission for acute or fulminating hepatitis in infancy. The incubation period ranges from 6 weeks to 6 months; the mortality rate of fulminating hepatitis is high (around 67%), and this may often require liver transplantation (Abdel-Hady and Kelly 2014).

Extrahepatic manifestations encompass skin rashes, membranous glomerulonephritis, arthralgias, and arthritis.

104.5.3.2 Chronic Infection

Chronic infection is defined as a persistence of HBsAg for >6 months. Affected children are usually asymptomatic with normal growth. In vertically infected children, the spontaneous clearance of HBV (i.e., loss of HBsAg and development of anti-HBs antibody) occurs at a rate of 0.6% per year over the first decade of life (Shah et al. 2009).

Most children who remain infected develop immune tolerance and have normal levels of hepatic transaminases. Chronic hepatitis B may exhibit various degrees of liver inflammation and fibrosis on biopsy. Levels of inflammation and fibrosis correlate with a worse prognosis. Less than 4% of infected children have persistent viral replication (HBeAg+) and elevated HBV DNA levels with ongoing liver inflammation and persistently or intermittently elevated transaminase levels (active hepatitis). Most concerns are focused on the latter patients, because they may develop cirrhosis and hepatocarcinoma (HCC) over a 20–30-year period.

104.5.3.3 Diagnosis

All pregnant women should be tested routinely for HBsAg during an early prenatal visit (first trimester) at each pregnancy, including women previously vaccinated or tested (Vodkin and Patton 2014; Ma et al. 2014).

Antigens and antibodies to be tested include HBsAg and specific antibody (anti-HBs), hepatitis B core antigen (HBcAg) and specific antibody (anti-HBc), and HBeAg and anti-HBe, bearing in mind that at least one serologic marker is present during the various phases of infection (Table 8). The presence of a confirmed HBsAg documents an ongoing infection. The detection of HBeAg and HBV DNA-positive PCR demonstrates viral replication. In general, these markers correlate with high infectivity. The appearance of anti-HBe means a loss of replicating virus, although reversion to HBeAg positivity may occur.

In exposed infants who undergo proper immunoprophylaxis, HBsAg and anti-HBs should be checked at 9–15 months of age or 1–3 months following completion of the primary immunization series to assess whether they are immune or infected.

Table 8 Interpretation of serologic tests for hepatitis B virus infection

Serologic markers				Interpretation
HBsAg	Total anti-HBc	IgM anti-HBc	Anti-HBs	
–	–	–	–	Never infected
+	–	–	–	Early acute infection, transient (up to 18 days) after vaccination
+	+	+	–	Acute infection
–	+	+	–	Acute resolving infection
–	+	–	+	Recovered from past infection and immune
+	+	–	–	Chronic infection
–	+	–	–	False positive (i.e., susceptible), past infection, "low-level " chronic infection, passive transfer to infants born to HBsAg-positive mothers
–	–	–	+	Immune if concentration is >10 mIU/mL, passive transfer after hepatitis B immune globulin administration

HBsAg hepatitis B surface antigen, *anti-HBc* antibody to HBV core antigen, *anti-HBs* antibody to surface antigen

104.5.4 Prevention

Prevention of MTCT of HBV is based on treatments for mothers during pregnancy and efforts for both newborns and their mothers after birth (Thio et al. 2015; Cheung et al. 2013).

Since high HBV DNA level and HBeAg-positive status in pregnant women are the most important risk factors for MTCT of HBV, antiviral therapies in highly viremic mothers can decrease the risk of transmission. Telbivudine, tenofovir, and lamivudine are three oral anti-HBV molecules whose use in pregnant women with chronic HBV infection did not result in increased adverse maternal or fetal outcome. Each drug showed improvement in maternal HBV DNA suppression at delivery and reduced the risk of MTCT (Brown et al. 2016).

All term infants born to HBsAg + women should receive hepatitis B vaccine and hepatitis B immunoglobulin (HBIG) 12–24 h after birth, administered at different injection sites, followed by completion of the three-dose vaccine series.

This schedule prevents infection by 85–95%. Transplacental transmission cannot be interrupted by immunoprophylaxis and may account for the small percentage of unprotected infants.

Hepatitis B immunoprophylaxis for preterm infants differs slightly (Table 9).

104.5.5 Therapy and Treatments

Therapy for HBV infection has not been studied in neonates. Antiviral treatment is contraindicated in children under 1 year of age, given the adverse effects of interferon administered early in life. In general, children with normal ALT levels are not candidates for antiviral treatment.

104.5.5.1 Acute HBV Infection

There is no treatment of proven efficacy for children with acute HBV infection.

104.5.5.2 Chronic HBV Infection

General management of children with chronic infection includes (Ehrhardt et al. 2015; Haber et al. 2009):

Education and counseling of family members (including vaccination with hepatitis B vaccine).
Periodic clinical checks and laboratory investigations for liver disease.
Vaccination with hepatitis A vaccine.
Antiviral therapy, if appropriate.

No limitations in terms of school or other activities should be placed in children with chronic HBV infection.

The goals of chronic hepatitis B treatment are the cessation or reduction of viral replication, the normalization of aminotransferase levels, and the prevention of cirrhosis, hepatic failure, and HCC.

Treatment with two antiviral drugs (i.e., interferon (IFN)-α, adefovir, and lamivudine) (Table 11) is recommended for children over 1 year of age with evidence of chronic infection (i.e., detectable HBsAg for at least 6 months), active viral replication (i.e., presence of HBeAg and/or elevated HBV DNA levels), and increased ALT concentrations. HBV DNA is also essential to monitor response to antiviral therapy (Table 10). Elevated levels ($>$20,000 IU/mL or $>10^5$ copies/mL) after 24 weeks of therapy raise the highest concerns for liver health (Kurbegov and Sokol 2009; Ayoub and Keeffe 2011; Jonas et al. 2016; Jonas et al. 2010).

104.6 Human Parvovirus B19

104.6.1 Etiology and Pathogenesis

Parvovirus B19 (B19) is the only member of the family *Parvoviridae* to be pathogenic in humans. It may cause a wide spectrum of clinical manifestations; its seroprevalence increases with age and infection confers lifelong immunity.

B19 is a single-stranded non-enveloped DNA virus, genetically stable, resistant to heat and detergent inactivation, which can survive in blood products despite elimination procedures. It requires a mitotically active host cell for replication, such as erythroid precursors, fetal liver cells, or cord blood mononuclear cells. B19 infects these cells lytically.

Table 9 Hepatitis B immunization of term and preterm (<2000 g) infants by maternal hepatitis B surface (HBsAg) status

Newborn	Maternal HBsAg status	Drugs	Management dose	Age
Mature infants and preterm infants weighing >2000 g	Positive	Monovalent vaccine	1	Birth (<12 h)
		Monovalent vaccine	2	1 month
		Monovalent/ hexavalent vaccine	3	3 months
		Monovalent/ hexavalent vaccine	4	11–12 months
		HBIG	0.5 mL intramuscularly	Birth (<12 h)
	Unknown	Monovalent vaccine	1	Birth (<12 h)
		Monovalent vaccine	2	1 month
		Monovalent/ hexavalent vaccine	3	2 months
		Monovalent/ hexavalent Vaccine	4	11–12 months
		HBIG[a]	0.5 mL intramuscularly	<1 week of age[b]
Preterm infants weighing <2000 g	Positive	Monovalent vaccine	1	Birth (<12 h)
		Monovalent vaccine	2	1 month
		Monovalent/ hexavalent vaccine	3	2–3 months
		Monovalent/ hexavalent vaccine	4	6–7 months
		HIBG	0.5 mL intramuscularly	
	Unknown	As infants born to HbsAg-positive mother		
	Negative	Delay first dose of vaccine until 1 month of age or hospital discharge. Complete the vaccine series		

[a]If mother tested as soon as possible after admission for delivery is found to be HBsAg positive
[b]As soon as possible if HBsAg-positive status is confirmed

It uses at least three cellular receptors for cell attachment and entry. One of these, the glycolipid globoside (P-ag), is present on the placental trophoblasts, hematopoietic precursors, fetal myocytes, and endothelial cells. The presence of P-ag on these tissues may explain the congenital infection, the hematological disorders, the myocardial disease, and the vasculitis syndromes.

104.6.2 Transmission

Parvovirus B19 is transmitted by respiratory route and blood products and, vertically, from the mother to the offspring. About 30–50% of pregnant women are susceptible to B19 infection (Lamont et al. 2011). In the first and second trimester of pregnancy, the vertical transmission rate reaches 30%. Among vertically infected children, 5–10% presents an abnormal outcome. This risk is higher when maternal infection occurs in the first 20 weeks of pregnancy; about 3% of first trimester spontaneous abortions are estimated to be due to B19 infections. The inflammatory response of the placenta to the virus may lead to adverse fetal outcome even if the fetus is uninfected. Fetal infection is unpredictable, and discordant infections have been reported in twin pregnancies (Bekhit et al. 2009).

104.6.3 Clinical Aspects

Human parvovirus B19 infection may give rise to a large array of clinical manifestations, depending on the patient's immunological and hematologic

Table 10 Algorithm for selection of children for HBV antiviral treatment (Modified from Jonas et al. (2010))

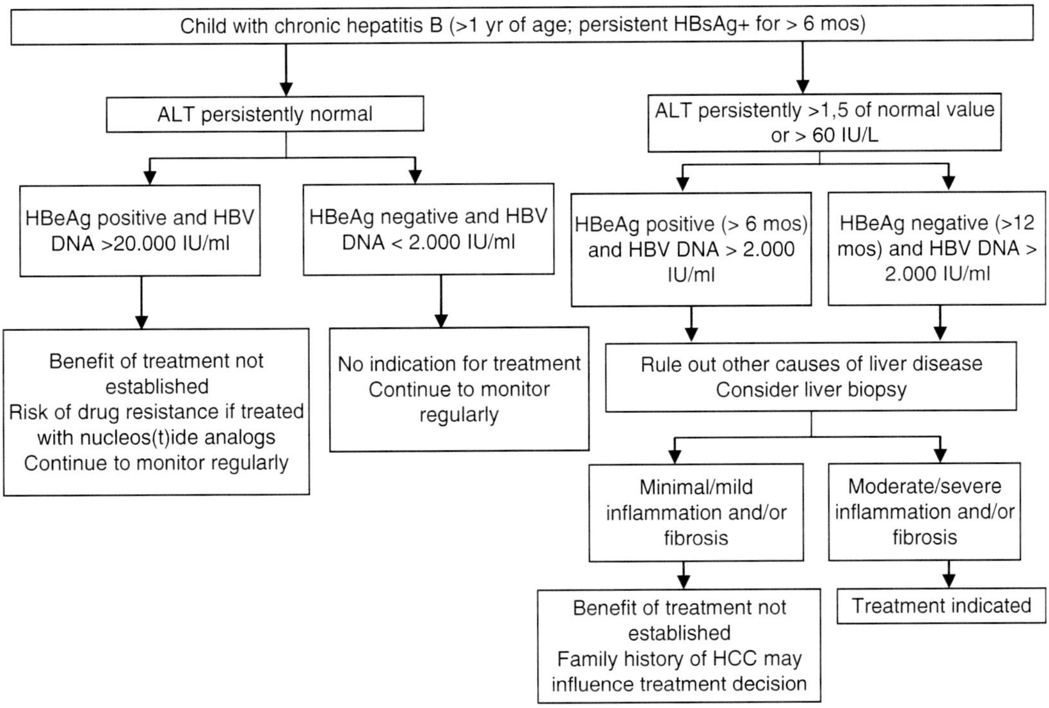

status. In the normal host, the infection may be asymptomatic or give rise to erythema infectiosum (EI) and/or arthropathy. EI, also referred to as fifth disease or slapped cheek syndrome, usually affects school-aged children with low-grade fever, malaise, and the characteristic facial rash, involving the cheeks with relative circumoral pallor, that subsequently spreads to the trunk, back, and extremities. Arthralgia is more frequent in adults.

Patients with underlying hematological or immunological disorders are at risk for transient aplastic crisis, due to the block of erythropoiesis with a profound reticulocytopenia. Other manifestations associated with B19 infection are illustrated in Table 12.

Fetal infection is often asymptomatic, but it may give rise to:

Birth defects, particularly ocular and central nervous system abnormalities (long-term neurologic sequelae in infants with no signs at birth have been described).

Fetal hydrops, occurring in 1 out of 3000 births, with a mean interval of 6 weeks between the onset of maternal infection and fetal symptoms.

Intrauterine fetal death, more common in the first and second trimester, often unassociated with hydrops (de Jong et al. 2011).

Maternal clinical manifestations do not influence the pregnancy outcome.

104.6.3.1 Diagnosis

Diagnosis of B19 infection is based on detecting specific IgG and IgM or viral DNA in blood or tissue samples by PCR (Weiffenbach et al. 2012).

Specific IgM are present 10–12 days after infection; IgG appear shortly afterwards and mediate lifelong immunity. Caution is needed in interpreting serology in immunodeficient individuals or in pregnant women, because they are not always able to mount an adequate antibody response.

PCR analysis of B19 DNA in the serum, bone marrow (BM), and other tissues may integrate serology. In immunocompromised patients, a

Table 11 Treatment for chronic HBV infection

Drugs	Advantage	Disadvantage	Response in children
IFN-α[a]	No drug resistance	Parenteral administration	20–58% HBV DNA or HBeAg loss[b]
	Short duration of treatment	Adverse effects common	
PEG-IFN-2αa[c]	Administration once a week	Parenteral administration	HBV DNA disappearance in 6 out of 13 children without any side effect[c]
		Adverse effects common	
Lamivudine[d]	Minimal adverse effects	Drug resistance common (20%/years)	23–35% HBV DNA and HBeAg loss[e]
	Oral administration		
	Liquid formulation available		16–23% HBV DNA and HBeAg loss[f]
Adefovir[g]	Oral administration	Drug resistance less common than lamivudine	
	Minimal adverse effects		
	Effective in lamivudine resistance		
Entecavir[h]	Oral administration	Side effects in 9–10% of cases	55–82% ALT normalization in 48–52 weeks
	Effective in lamivudine resistance		

[a]Dosage in children >1 year of age: 5–10 MU/m^2 three times a week for 24 weeks
[b]From (Pawlowska and Halota 2007)
[c]In children there is only one preliminary report evaluating the rapid viral response of PEG-INF (100 μg/m^2/week) (Schwarz 2003). Not currently approved in chronic HBV infection in children
[d]Dosage in children >2 years of age: 3 mg/kg/day up to 100 mg/day for 52 weeks (Jonas et al. 2002)
[e]From (Schwarz 2003)
[f]From (Ayoub and Keeffe 2011)
[g]From (Ayoub and Keeffe 2011)
[h]Dosage in children 0.3–1 mg orally once a day. From (Clemente and Vajro 2016)

positive PCR test in blood indicates ongoing acute or persistent infection; in BM it may indicate either acute or previous infection. In cases of fetal complications, PCR analysis of amniotic fluid or cord blood may have a high priority for possible therapeutic interventions. Quantitative PCR allows the viral load concentration in different tissues to be quantified. However, further studies are needed to correlate the viral load with disease progression.

104.6.4 Prognosis

After intrauterine exposure to B19, the risk of fetal death is low (0.1–0.3%). Information on long-term outcomes of congenital infections is limited. However, severe sequelae including neurological disorders in survivors are well documented.

104.6.5 Therapy and Treatments

There is no specific therapy against B19 infection; some alternative interventions are however recommended, such as transfusion therapy to recover from aplastic crisis or intravenous IgG (0.4 g/kg × 5 days or 1 g/kg × 3 days) to facilitate the clearance of the virus in immunocompromised patients.

If maternal B19 infection is confirmed, weekly ultrasound examinations with Doppler

Table 12 Disorders associated with parvovirus B19 infection

Autoimmune disorders
Systemic lupus erythematosus
Systemic vasculitides
Rheumatoid arthritis
Production of autoantibodies to double-stranded DNA, antinuclear soluble antigens, cardiolipin, and rheumatoid factor
Increased bone marrow cell turnover
Transient aplastic crisis with severe anemia, resulting in congestive heart failure, cerebrovascular events, and acute splenic sequestration
Thrombocytopenia
Neutropenia
Pancytopenia
B19 persistence in immunocompetent patients
Persistent infection with potentially severe and chronic anemia, with various long-lasting symptoms such as fatigue, fever, arthralgia, and myalgia
Other associated disorders
Myocarditis and heart failure
Hepatitis
Kawasaki disease
Gloves and socks syndrome
Neurological disease
Fibromyalgia
Infection in immunocompromised individuals
Persistent BM suppression with chronic anemia (predisposing conditions are congenital immunodeficiencies, leukemia, lymphoma, myelodysplastic syndrome, BM and solid organ transplantation, chemotherapy, and infection with human immunodeficiency virus)
Infection-associated hemophagocytosis
Vertical transmission
Nonimmune fetal hydrops
Congenital anemia Thrombocytopenia Myocarditis Generalized edema Perivascular calcifications

measurement of middle cerebral artery flow velocity up to 20 weeks postexposure are appropriate to monitor the fetus (Dijkmans et al. 2012). If hydrops and/or signs of anemia appear, intrauterine erythrocyte transfusions can reduce the mortality rate and improve outcome (Lindenburg et al. 2014), though neurodevelopmental impairment may occur also in children treated with intrauterine transfusions.

References

Abdel-Hady M, Kelly D (2014) Chronic hepatitis B in children and adolescents: epidemiology and management. Paediatr Drugs 15:311–317

Abdel-Hady M, Bunn SK, Sira J et al (2011) Chronic hepatitis C in children – review of natural history at a national Centre. J Viral Hepat 18:e535–e540

Ayoub WS, Keeffe EB (2011) Review article: current antiviral therapy of chronic hepatitis B. Aliment Pharmacol Ther 34:1145–1158

Barth H (2015) Hepatitis C virus: is it time to say goodbye yet? Perspectives and challenges for the next decade. World J Hepatol 7:725–737

Bekhit MT, Greenwood PA, Warren R et al (2009) In utero treatment of severe fetal anaemia due to parvovirus B19 in one fetus in a twin pregnancy-a case report and literature review. Fetal Diagn Ther 25: 153–157

Berti E, Thorne C, Noguera-Julian A et al (2015) The new face of the pediatric HIV epidemic in western countries: demographic characteristics, morbidity and mortality of the pediatric HIV-infected population. Pediatr Infect Dis J 34:S7–S13

Best JM (2007) Rubella. Semin Fetal Neonatal Med 12:182–192

Bouthry E, Picone O, Hamdi G et al (2014) Rubella and pregnancy: diagnosis, management and outcomes. Prenat Diagn 34:1246–1253

Briand N, Jasseron C, Sibiude J et al (2013) Cesarean section for HIV-infected women in the combination antiretroviral therapies era, 2000–2010. Am J Obstet Gynecol 209:335.e1–335.12

Brown RS, McMahon BJ, Lok ASF et al (2016) Antiviral therapy in chronic hepatitis B viral infection during pregnancy: a systematic review and meta-analysis. Hepatology 63:319 333

Calitri C, Gabiano C, Galli L et al (2014) The second generation of HIV-1 vertically exposed infants: a case series from the Italian register for paediatric HIV infection. BMC Infect Dis 14:277. Available at http://www.biomedcentral.com/1471-2334/14/277

CDC – Surveillance of congenital rubella syndrome (2014) Vaccines: congenital rubella syndrome – manual for the surveillance of vaccine-preventable diseases (Chapter 15). www.cdc.gov/vaccines/pubs/surv/chpt15-crs.htm

Centers for Disease Control and Prevention (1994) Revised classification system for human immunodeficiency virus infection in children less than 13 years of age. MMWR Recomm Rep 43:1–20

Cheung KW, Seto MTJ, Wong SF (2013) Towards complete eradication of hepatitis B infection from perinatal transmission: review of the mechanisms of in utero infection and the use of antiviral treatment during pregnancy. Eur J Obstet Gynecol Reprod Biol 169: 17–23

Chiappini E, Galli L, Gabiano C et al (2006) Early triple therapy vs mono or dual therapy for children with perinatal HIV infection. JAMA 295:626–628

Clemente MG, Vajro P (2016) An update on the strategies used for the treatment of chronic hepatitis B in children. Expert Rev Gastroenterol Hepatol 16:1–10

Cottrel EB, Chou R, Wasson N et al (2013) Reducing risk for mother–to-child transmission of hepatitis C virus: a systematic review for the U.S. preventive services task force. Ann Intern Med 158:109–113

de Jong EP, Walther FJ, Kroes AC et al (2011) Parvovirus B19 infection in pregnancy: new insights and management. Prenat Diagn 31:419–425

Dijkmans AC, de Jong EP, Dijkmans BA et al (2012) Parvovirus B19 in pregnancy: prenatal diagnosis and management of fetal complications. Curr Opin Obstet Gynecol 24:95–101

Dunkelberg JC, Berkley EM, Thiel KW et al (2014) Hepatitis B and C in pregnancy: a review and recommendations for care. J Perinatol 34:882–891

Duszak RS (2009) Congenital rubella syndrome-major review. Optometry 80:36–43

Ehrhardt S, Xie C, Guo N et al (2015) Breastfeeding while taking lamivudine or tenofovir disoproxil fumarate: a review of the evidence. Clin Infect Dis 60:275–278

England K, Pembrey L, Tovo PA et al (2005) Growth in the first 5 years of life is unaffected in children with perinatally-acquired hepatitis C infection. J Pediatr 147:227–232

European Paediatric Hepatitis C Virus Network (2005) Three broad modalities in the natural history of vertically acquired hepatitis C virus infection. Clin Infect Dis 41:45–51

Garazzino S, Calitri C, Versace A et al (2014) Natural history of vertically acquired HCV infection and associated autoimmune phenomena. Eur J Pediatr 173:1025–1031

Gentile I, Borgia G (2014) Vertical transmission of hepatitis B virus: challenges and solutions. Int J Womens Health 6:605–611

Gower E, Estes C, Blach S et al (2014) Global epidemiology and genotype distribution of hepatitis C virus infection. J Hepatol 61:S45–S57

Grant GB, Reef SE, Dabbagh A et al (2015) Global progress toward rubella and congenital rubella syndrome control and elimination – 2000-2014. MMWR Morb Mortal Wkly Rep 64:1052–1055

Haber BA, Block JM, Jonas MM et al (2009) Recommendations for screening, monitoring and referral of pediatric chronic hepatitis B. Pediatrics 124:1007–1014

Indolfi G, Mangone G, Bartolini E et al (2014) Interleukin 28B rs12979860 single nucleotide polymorphism predicts spontaneous clearance of hepatitis C virus in children. J Pediatr Gastroenterol Nutr 58:666–668

Jonas M, Mizerski J, Badia IB et al (2002) Clinical trial of lamivudine in children with chronic hepatitis B. N Engl J Med 346:1706–1713

Jonas MM, Block JM, Haber BA et al (2010) Treatment of children with chronic hepatitis B virus infection in the United States: patient selection and therapeutic options. Hepatology 52:2192–2205

Jonas MM, Lok AS, McMahon BJ et al (2016) Antiviral therapy in management of chronic hepatitis B viral infection in children: a systematic review and meta-analysis. Hepatology 63:307–318

Kourtis AP, Ellington S, Pazol K et al (2014) Complications of cesarean deliveries among HIV-infected women in the United States. AIDS 28:2609–2618

Kurbegov AC, Sokol RJ (2009) Hepatitis B therapy in children. Expert Rev Gastroenterol Hepatol 3:39–49

Lambert N, Strebel P, Orenstein W et al (2015) Rubella. Lancet 385:2297–2307

Lamont RF, Sobel JD, Vaisbuch E et al (2011) Parvovirus B19 infection in human pregnancy. BJOG 118:175–186

Lee A, Rajanayagam J, Abdel-Hady M (2015) Chronic hepatitis C infection in children: current treatment and new therapies. J Clin Transl Hepatol 3:36–41

Lindenburg IT, van Kamp IL, Oepkes D (2014) Intrauterine blood transfusion: current indications and associated risks. Fetal Diagn Ther 36:263–271

Ma L, Alla NR, Li X, Mynbaev OA, Shi Z (2014) Mother-to-child transmission of HBV: review of current clinical management and prevention strategies. Rev Med Virol 24:396–406

Mack CL, Gonzales-Peralta RP, Gupta N et al (2012) Diagnosis and management of hepatitis C infection in infants, children and adolescents. J Pediatr Gastroenterol Nutr 54:838–855

Mok J, Pembrey L, Tovo PA et al (2005) When does mother to child transmission of hepatitis C virus occur? Arch Dis Child Fetal Neonatal Ed 90:F156–F160

Neu N, Duchon J, Zachariah P (2015) TORCH infections. Clin Perinatol 42:77–103

Ohmer S, Honegger J (2016) New prospects for the treatment and prevention of hepatitis C in children. Curr Opin Pediatr 28:93–100

Panel on Antiretroviral Therapy and Medical Management of HIV-Infected Children (2016) Guidelines for the use of antiretroviral agents in pediatric HIV infection. Available at http://aidsinfo.nih.gov/contentfiles/lvguidelines/pediatricguidelines.pdf. Accessed 19 Mar 2016

Panel on Opportunistic Infections in HIV-Exposed and HIV-Infected Children (2013) Guidelines for the prevention and treatment of opportunistic infections in HIV-exposed and HIV-infected children. Department of Health and Human Services. Available at http://aidsinfo.nih.gov/contentfiles/lvguidelines/oi_guidelines_pediatrics.pdf. Accessed 26 Mar 2016

Panel on Treatment of HIV-Infected Pregnant Women and Prevention of Perinatal Transmission (2015) Recommendations for use of antiretroviral drugs in pregnant HIV-1-infected women for maternal health and interventions to reduce perinatal HIV transmission in the United States. Available at http://aidsinfo.nih.gov/contentfiles/lvguidelines/PerinatalGL.pdf. Accessed 19 Mar 2016

Pawlowska M, Halota W (2007) Rapid viral response during treatment of chronic hepatitis B with pegylated interferon alfa-2a in children–preliminary report. Przegl Epidemiol 61:427–431

Pembrey L, Newell ML, Tovo PA, EPHN Collaborators (2005) The management of HCV infected pregnant women and their children European paediatric HCV network. J Hepatol 43:515–525

Polywka S, Pembrey L, Tovo PA et al (2006) Accuracy of HCV-RNA PCR tests for diagnosis or exclusion of vertically acquired HCV infection. J Med Virol 78:305–310

Schwarz KB (2003) Pediatric issues in new therapies for hepatitis B and C. Curr Gastroenterol Rep 5:233–239

Schweitzer A, Horn J, Mikolajczyk RT (2015) Estimations of worldwide prevalence of chronic hepatitis B virus infection: a systematic review of data published between 1965 and 2013. Lancet 386:1546–1555

Selvapatt N, Ward T, Bailey H et al (2015) Is antenatal screening for hepatitis C virus cost-effective? A decade's experience at a London Centre. J Hepatol 63:797–804

Shah U, Kelly D, Chang MH et al (2009) Management of chronic hepatitis B in children. J Pediatr Gastroenterol Nutr 48:399–404

Sollai S, Noguera-Julian A, Galli L et al (2015) Strategies for the prevention of mother to child transmission in western countries. An update. Pediatr Infect Dis J 34: S14–S30

Suzuki M, Tajiri H, Tanaka Y et al (2016) Peginterferon therapy in children with chronic hepatitis C: a nation-wide, multi-center study in Japan, 2004–2013. J Pediatr Gastroenterol Nutr 63:88–93

Thio CL, Guo N, Xie C et al (2015) Global elimination of mother-to-child transmission of hepatitis B: revisiting the current strategy. Lancet Infect Dis 1:981–985

Tovo PA, de Martino M, Gabiano C et al (1992) Prognostic factors and survival in children with perinatal HIV-1 infection. The Italian register for HIV infections in children. Lancet 339:1249–1253

Tovo PA, Calitri C, Scolfaro C et al (2016) Vertically acquired hepatitis C virus infection: correlates of transmission and disease progression. World J Gastroenterol 22:1–11

UNAIDS (2016) The GAP report. Available at http://www.unaids.org/sites/default/files/en/media/unaids/contentassets/documents/unaidspublication/2014/UNAIDS_Gap_report_en.pdf. Accessed 9 May 2016

Vodkin I, Patton H (2014) Management of hepatitis B virus infection during pregnancy. Minerva Gastroenterol Dietol 60:205–214

Vynnycky E, Adams EJ, Cutts FT et al (2016) Using seroprevalence and immunisation coverage data to estimate the global burden of congenital rubella syndrome, 1996–2010: a systematic review. PLoS One 11: e0149160

Weiffenbach J, Bald R, Gloning KP et al (2012) Serological and virological analysis of maternal and fetal blood samples in prenatal human parvovirus b19 infection. J Infect Dis 205:782–788

Yi P, Chen R, Huang Y, Zhou RR, Fan XG (2016) Management of mother-to-child transmission of hepatitis B virus: propositions and challenges. J Clin Virol 77:32–39

Zhang ZH, Wu CC, Chen XW et al (2016) Genetic variation of hepatitis B virus and its significance for pathogenesis. World J Gastroenterol 22:126–144

Fetal Infections: Congenital Syphilis and Tuberculosis

105

Pier Angelo Tovo, Carlo Scolfaro, Silvia Garazzino, and Federica Mignone

Contents

Abstract

Syphilis is a major public health problem in developing countries, and it is also resurging in the industrialized world. Congenital tuberculosis (TB) is rare, but it may be fatal if untreated. Infection of the fetus may be the consequence of hematogenous spread, aspiration or ingestion of contaminated amniotic fluid, or contact with maternal genital lesions at delivery. In infants signs and symptoms may be nonspecific, mimicking other disseminated infections. Early recognition is essential for a prompt treatment, as the mortality rate of untreated forms is approximately 50%. Initial therapy consists in the combination of four first-line antituberculous drugs, although the optimal regimen and duration of treatment remain to be established.

P. A. Tovo (✉) · C. Scolfaro · S. Garazzino · F. Mignone
Department of Pediatrics, University of Turin, Regina Margherita Childrens Hospital, AOU Città della Salute e della Scienza di Torino, Turin, Italy
e-mail: pierangelo.tovo@unito.it

105.1 Salient Points

- Syphilis persists worldwide; it is due to *Treponema pallidum* infection.

G. Buonocore et al. (eds.), *Neonatology*,
https://doi.org/10.1007/978-3-319-29489-6_252

- Prevention of congenital syphilis is based on diagnosis and treatment of maternal infection.
- Fetal infection occurs through transplacental passage of *T. pallidum* or contact with genital lesions at delivery.
- Clinical signs are similar to other fetal and perinatal infections.
- Diagnosis is based on newborn serology, to be evaluated in relation with maternal titers.
- Therapy requires parenteral penicillin.
- Follow-up till 15 months of life is suggested to identify children who need re-treatment.

105.2 Syphilis

Although important achievements have been made in the diagnosis and treatment of syphilis since the identification of its causative agent, *Treponema pallidum*, in 1905, syphilis remains a major public health problem in developing countries, and a recrudescence has also been documented in some developed countries over the last decades (Centers for Disease Control and Prevention (CDC) 2009; Doroshenko et al. 2006). Congenital syphilis derives from vertical transmission of the infection (Walker and Walker 2007). A case of congenital infection is a sentinel event that reflects missed opportunities for prevention within health-care systems. Indeed, effective prevention and detection of congenital syphilis are based on adequate antenatal care and proper diagnosis of infection in pregnant women.

105.2.1 Epidemiology

The World Health Organization (WHO) estimates that more than ten million people are infected with syphilis each year (World Health Organization 2008). Untreated early syphilis in pregnant women results in perinatal death in up to 40% of cases if acquired during the four preceding years, and it may lead to fetal infection in 80% of cases.

In sub-Saharan Africa, an estimated two million women with active syphilis become pregnant each year, and in most of them, infection remains undetected during pregnancy. In Latin America and in the Caribbean, the prevalence of syphilis in pregnant women ranges between 5% and 10%, while in Asia it is generally below 5% (Walker and Walker 2007). The rate of primary and secondary syphilis declined in the United States in the 1990s, but in the new millennium, it has increased. The rate of congenital syphilis in the United States rapidly increased during 2012–2014 of about 38%: such an increase coincided with a 22% national increase in the rate of syphilis among women (Centers for Disease Control and Prevention 2015a). A resurgence of syphilis has been reported also in Europe (Doroshenko et al. 2006; Walker and Walker 2007; World Health Organization 2008).

105.2.2 Etiology and Pathogenesis

T. pallidum is a member of the order Spirochaetales, family Spirochaetaceae, and genus *Treponema* (Zeltser and Kurban 2004). If untreated, the infection persists despite evidence of an immune response. *T. pallidum* interacts with vascular endothelium. Its membrane 47 kDa lipoprotein activates vascular endothelial cells to upregulate the expression of intercellular adhesion molecule-1 (ICAM-1) and stimulate procoagulant activity, resulting in fibrin deposition and perivasculitis. Delayed-type hypersensivity to treponemal antigens appears later and may be related to the onset of latency (Ingall et al. 2006).

The newborn can be infected in utero by the transplacental passage of *T. pallidum* from an infected, untreated, or inadequately treated mother or at delivery by contact with an active genital lesion. *T. pallidum* can cross the placenta from about 14 weeks of gestation. Transmission risk increases with gestational age and is inversely related to the duration of maternal infection. The vertical transmission rate in an untreated mother ranges from 70% to 100% during primary syphilis and 40% during early latent syphilis down to 10% during late latent infection (Doroshenko et al. 2006; Walker and Walker 2007). Breastfeeding is not associated with transmission unless cutaneous lesions are present.

105.2.3 Clinical Manifestations

In pregnant women, untreated or inadequately treated syphilis is associated with spontaneous abortion during the second and early third trimesters, perinatal death, premature delivery, low birth weight, and nonimmune hydrops.

Symptoms and signs of congenital syphilis occurring within the first 2 years of life define early congenital syphilis, while clinical manifestations appearing later are referred to as late congenital syphilis (Doroshenko et al. 2006; Follett and Clarke 2011).

Most affected infants are asymptomatic at birth, but two-thirds develop manifestations by 3–8 weeks. Persistent rhinitis (snuffles) can be an early feature, with an infectious discharge that may occasionally be blood-tinged. Other signs include non-tender generalized lymphadenopathy, hepatosplenomegaly, anemia, leukopenia or leukocytosis, thrombocytopenia, and conjugated hyperbilirubinemia. The most common skin lesion is a maculopapular rash or a vesiculobullous eruption than can involve the palms and soles and be associated with desquamation. Nephrotic syndrome with a generalized edema following glomerulonephritis may develop between 2 and 3 months of age. Bone lesions are not unusual, with an involvement of the metaphyses and diaphyses of long bones; radiographic abnormalities can be detected in about 20% of infants with asymptomatic infection. Osteochondritis or Parrot's pseudoparalysis is the most common and earliest manifestation characterized by an asymmetric, painful, flaccid paralysis of the limbs and knees.

Late congenital syphilis can involve many organs, more frequently the bones, teeth, and nervous system. The stigmata of late infection include Hutchinson's triad (notched upper incisors, interstitial keratitis, and eight nerve deafness), saddle nose, palatal erosions, frontal bossing, saber tibia, rhagades, nodules, and gummata.

105.2.4 Diagnosis

Syphilis can be diagnosed by direct and indirect tests (Table 1) (Follett and Clarke 2011; Shahrook et al. 2014). Direct methods can be used for symptomatic patients with primary or secondary syphilis and include:

Table 1 Diagnostic tests for syphilis

Direct tests
Direct examination through dark-field microscopy
Direct fluorescent antibody *T. pallidum* test (DFA-TP)
Polymerase chain reaction (PCR) assay
Indirect tests
Nontreponemal tests
Venereal disease research laboratory (VDRL)
Rapid plasma reagin (RPR)
Treponemal tests
Fluorescent treponemal antibody adsorbed (FTA-ABS)
T. pallidum particle agglutination (TP-PA)
Treponemal enzyme immunoassay (EIA)

> The detection of *T. pallidum* by direct examination of fluid or exudation from lesions immediately after sample collection through dark-field microscopy. The sensitivity of the method (74–86%) is limited by the fact that 10^5 organism/mL are necessary for visualization. However, this method cannot be used for oral lesions because non-pathogenic oral spirochaetes can be confused with *T. pallidum* and systemic antibiotics may result in a false-negative test. Specificity is 77–100% and depends on the experience of the observer;
>
> direct fluorescent antibody *T. pallidum* test (DFA-TP) in smear or tissue section. This does not require motile organisms and is more sensitive and specific than dark-field microscopy, though more expensive;
>
> polymerase chain reaction (PCR) for the identification of treponemal DNA has been developed but not yet standardized. Can detect as few as 10 microorganisms in lesions or tissues. (Ingall et al. 2006; Lautenschlager 2006)

Indirect diagnosis is based on serological tests to detect antibodies. These tests include nontreponemal tests for screening and treponemal ones for confirmation:

> Non-treponemal tests (e.g., Venereal Disease Research Laboratory [VDRL] and Rapid Plasma Reagin [RPR]) measure both IgG and IgM antiphospholipid antibodies against lipoidal material released by damaged host cells and the treponemal cell surface. These tests become positive 6 weeks after exposure and 1–4 weeks after the appearance of the primary lesion. They usually

correlate with disease activity. Results are reported quantitatively and a four-fold titer change is considered significant. Sequential serologyshould be performed using the same test, preferably by the same laboratory. Non-treponemal tests usually become non-reactive over time after treatment, though they may persist at low titer (serofast reaction, which occurs when a nontreponemal test reaction is overwhelmed by antigen-antibody excess) in some patients (Lautenschlager 2006). False-positive results may occur because of cross-reactivity during acute viral infections, autoimmune conditions or pregnancy. False-negative results may be due to prozone reactions.

Treponemal tests (e.g., fluorescent treponemal antibody adsorbed [FTA-ABS], *T. pallidum* particle agglutination [TP-PA]) do not correlate with disease activity and can remain positive regardless of treatment.

Treponemal enzyme immunoassay [EIA] can be useful because it identifies IgG and IgM against *T. pallidum*. (Doroshenko et al. 2006; Walker and Walker 2007; Ingall et al. 2006; Lautenschlager 2006)

Effective prevention and detection of congenital syphilis depends on identifying the infection by routine serological screening at the first antenatal visit and at delivery. Serology should be repeated at the beginning of the third trimester in populations with a high risk of congenital syphilis (e.g., multiple sexual partners, presence of a sexually transmitted disease, drug addiction, lack of antenatal care) or in areas with a high prevalence of syphilis (Table 2). Information about the treatment of the sex partner should be obtained to assess the risk of reinfection. Pregnant women with syphilis should also be tested for HIV infection. No infant should be discharged from the hospital without determining the maternal serological status for syphilis.

Table 2 High risk of congenital syphilis

Symptomatic newborn
Untreated, inadequately treated or non-documented treated maternal syphilis
Non-penicillin treatment of syphilis during pregnancy
Treatment of maternal syphilis for less than 4 weeks before delivery
The absence of at least a fourfold decrease in nontreponemal maternal titers after therapy
Fourfold increase of maternal titers or infant titers at least fourfold greater than maternal titers

Every infant born to a mother with reactive nontreponemal and treponemal test results should be carefully examined for signs and symptoms of congenital syphilis. A quantitative nontreponemal serological test and EIA IgM should be done on infant serum, using the same test as that for the mother to compare titer results. If the EIA IgM test is negative and other tests have titers less than fourfold higher than the mother's, an asymptomatic infant should have repeat serology at 3, 6, and 15 months of age or until seroreversion.

Congenital syphilis is diagnosed if the EIA IgM test is positive and/or the nontreponemal or treponemal titers are fourfold higher than in the mother. Further investigations are mandatory: cerebrospinal fluid (CSF) examination (protein, cell count, and VDRL test), hematology and liver function tests, skeletal X-rays, and ophthalmological assessment. A definitive diagnosis of congenital syphilis is made if PCR and/or dark-field microscopy detects *T. pallidum* in a sample from a lesion, the placenta, or body fluids (Ingall et al. 2006; Lautenschlager 2006; Centers for Disease Control and Prevention 2015b; World Health Organization 2003; Kingston et al. 2015).

105.2.5 Treatment

Several guidelines define the criteria for the correct management of infants born to mothers with syphilis (Follett and Clarke 2011; Centers for Disease Control and Prevention 2015b; World Health Organization 2003; Kingston et al. 2015; Clement et al. 2014). Treatments for infants with suspected congenital syphilis are listed in Table 3. In infants at low risk of congenital syphilis, some specialists recommend a single intramuscular dose of benzyl penicillin G (50,000 U/kg) with follow-up serology.

105.2.6 Follow-Up

Treated infants should receive a careful follow-up at 3, 6, and 12 months of age until serologic nontreponemal tests become nonreactive or the titer has decreased fourfold. In uninfected or

Table 3 Recommended regimens for infants with suspected congenital syphilis

Drug	Route	Dosage	Total duration	Notes
Benzylpenicillin	IV	*Infants < 4 weeks*: 50,000 U/kg/dose every 12 h for the first 7 days of life and every 8 h thereafter	10–14 days	If more than 1 day of therapy is missed, the entire course should be restarted
		Infants > 4 weeks: 200,000–300,000 U/kg/day, administered as 50,000 U/kg every 4–6 h		
Procaine penicillin G IM	IM	50,000 U/kg/dose once daily	10–14 days	

adequately treated children, nontreponemal titers usually decline by 3 months of age and become negative by 6 months of age. If they persist or increase by 6–12 months of age, the infant should be evaluated and treated with a further 10-day course of parenteral penicillin G.

If the newborn's or the mother's situation is unclear, the nontreponemal test should be repeated at 3 and 6 months of age, and a treponemal test should be performed at 15 months of age (Centers for Disease Control and Prevention 2015a, b; World Health Organization 2003; Kingston et al. 2015).

105.3 Tuberculosis

Salient Points

- Tuberculosis (TB) is a worldwide epidemic disease due to *Mycobacterium tuberculosis*.
- Congenital TB is rare in industrialized countries, but fatal if untreated.
- Fetal infection occurs via hematogenous spread and ingestion/aspiration of contaminated amniotic fluid or at delivery.
- Clinical presentation is not typical; it may simulate other congenital or perinatal infections.
- Diagnosis is often difficult: the gold standard is mycobacterial demonstration into tissues or fluids.
- Early treatment is mandatory with a combination of antituberculosis drugs.

Tuberculosis (TB) is a worldwide primary health problem, being the leading cause of death from a single infectious agent. In the last decades, TB has remained a major disease in developing countries, but has also become an emerging infection in industrialized areas, as a consequence of sustained migratory flows and spread of multidrug-resistant strains. The resurgence of TB has raised particular concerns regarding pregnant women and their children: the epidemiology changes of TB have induced significant shifts in at-risk populations, with a dramatic increase of TB incidence among child-bearing age women (World Health Organization 2015).

105.3.1 Etiology and Pathogenesis

The most common form of TB infection in infants is acquired postnatally through exposure to family members with bacillary pulmonary disease. Congenital TB is a rare event – with less than 300 cases available in the scientific literature – deriving from maternal transmission of *Mycobacterium tuberculosis* to the fetus.

Pregnancy per se does not represent a maternal risk factor for TB; however, if the woman develops an active TB during pregnancy, the infection may be transmitted to the offspring. The rate of vertical transmission ranges between 0% and 16%, being lower if the mother has pulmonary TB, rather than miliary or genital forms (Baquero-Artigao et al. 2015). Fetal infection can occur by hematogenous spread of mycobacteria through the placenta, by in utero aspiration or ingestion of infected amniotic fluid, or by direct contact with maternal genital lesions at delivery. The placental involvement may result from the dissemination phase of either a primary maternal infection or a reactivation of a previous infection. Disseminated disease more often complicates an acute infection rather than a reactivation. Therefore, a primary infection during pregnancy implies a higher risk of congenital transmission. This is however unusual if adequate maternal antituberculous treatment is administered. HIV-infected women are at a greater risk of congenitally transmitting the mycobacteria, as they are more frequently affected by miliary or extrapulmonary forms of TB (Baquero-Artigao et al. 2015).

In hematogenous congenital TB, mycobacteria reach the fetus through the umbilical vein, determining a primary pathognomonic lesion with caseating granulomas within the liver and the periportal lymph nodes. The microorganisms may then spread into the main circulation and into the lung. The bacilli generally remain dormant until the increase in pulmonary circulation and oxygenation after birth, when they can determine active pulmonary disease and further systemic dissemination. When congenital TB results from the aspiration or ingestion of infected amniotic fluid, primary complexes develop in the gastrointestinal and/or respiratory tract.

105.3.2 Clinical Patterns

Symptoms and signs of congenital TB are nonspecific, and they often mimic common neonatal diseases, such as sepsis or other congenital or perinatal infections. Clinical manifestations may be evident at birth, but usually appear within 2–3 weeks of age (Table 4); cases of late onset (up to 3 months of life) have also been described (Baquero-Artigao et al. 2015; Starke 2006).

Typically, infected infants are born prematurely with low birth weight for gestational age. Virtually any organ system may be involved, although the lungs, liver, and gut are the most common primary infection sites; dissemination with central nervous system involvement may also occur. A chest X-ray is usually abnormal and often displays a miliary pattern. The natural course of TB in the newborn frequently leads to a disseminated and fatal disease with a mortality rate of about 50% (Starke 2006).

Table 4 Signs and symptoms of congenital tuberculosis

Common	Rare
Hepatosplenomegaly	Vomiting
Respiratory distress	Jaundice
Fever	Cyanosis
Lymphadenopathy	Apnea
Abdominal distension	Seizures
Poor feeding/low weight gain	Petechiae
Lethargy/irritability	
Ear discharge	
Papular skin lesions	

105.3.3 Diagnosis

Diagnosis of congenital TB is often problematic. It should be suspected in newborns with negative tests for other congenital infections and whose mother has risk factors for, or has been diagnosed with TB, even if the physical examination at birth is normal.

Tuberculin skin reaction is poorly reliable in neonates, since it may be initially negative and may turn positive after a few months. However, neonates often yield positive acid-fast bacilli smears and cultures (up to 75%), as disseminated and rapidly progressive diseases lead to high bacillary loads.

Diagnosis relies on the demonstration of *M. tuberculosis* in tissues or fluids. The preferred sample source is the early morning gastric aspirate, which is more easily collectable than sputum in infants. In case of pulmonary TB, mycobacteria may also be demonstrated on the tracheal aspirate, due to high bacillary loads in the lungs. Three consecutive samples of gastric or tracheal aspirate should be obtained, but a single positive smear should be considered indicative of TB.

Data on the accuracy of polymerase chain reaction (PCR) techniques in neonates with congenital TB are limited (Baquero-Artigao et al. 2015; Smith 2002; Whittaker and Kampmann 2008). The development of interferon gamma (IFN-γ) assays has offered new possibilities for the diagnosis of latent TB infection and active disease in adults. Given the depressed IFN-γ production in the first period of life, the reliability of these assays in infants remains to be clarified, particularly in perinatally exposed newborns (Garazzino et al. 2014).

Due to high coinfection rates, all newborns and mothers diagnosed with TB should also be tested for HIV infection.

The diagnostic criteria for distinguishing congenital TB from postnatally acquired disease include documenting tuberculous lesions plus at least one of the following: (1) onset of lesions in the first week of life, (2) primary hepatic complex or caseating granulomas, (3) infection of the placenta or maternal genital tract, and (4) exclusion of TB acquired after birth from mother or other sources.

105.3.4 Therapy and Treatments

Early treatment of congenital TB is mandatory, due to its high mortality rate, although the optimal treatment regimen and its duration have yet to be established. The high mycobacterial loads support the association of several drugs (Table 5). It seems reasonable to start with a combination of four antituberculosis drugs (isoniazid, rifampin, pyrazinamide, and an aminoglycoside or ethambutol) administered for 2 months, followed by a 4-to-6-month regimen with isoniazid (INH) and rifampin (RFP); an alternative 9-month regimen with the two drugs has been suggested (Whittaker and Kampmann 2008; Di Comite et al. 2016; Patel and DeSantis 2008). An extrapulmonary disease requires a longer treatment, with a total duration of 12 months. Indeed, many experts recommend a total duration of 9–12 months, regardless the site of infection, due to the impaired immunologic defenses of neonates and infants.

Table 5 First-line antituberculosis drugs

Drug (generic name)	Daily dose (mg/kg)	Maximal daily dosage	Route
Isoniazid	10–15	300 mg	Oral
Rifampin	10–20	600 mg	Oral
Pyrazinamide	25–40	2 g	Oral
Streptomycin	20	1 g	Intramuscular
Ethambutol	15–25	2.5 g	Oral

Drug-resistant strains are emerging also in childhood (Mignone et al. 2013; National Institute for Health and Care Excellence 2016). In case of drug-resistant TB and/or intolerance to first-line treatment, second-line drugs should be administered. These include fluoroquinolones (i.e., moxifloxacin, levofloxacin, and ciprofloxacin), ethionamide, PAS, cycloserin, aminoglycosides (amikacin, capreomycin, kanamycin), and linezolid (Galli et al. 2016).

During treatment, liver functional tests, serum uric acid levels, and hearing tests (in case of aminoglycosides administration) should be monitored. To prevent INH-induced peripheral neuropathy, the addition of vitamin B6 can be considered. Ethambutol administered in young infants at >15 mg/kg/day can cause optic neuritis and red-green color blindness.

Chest X-rays should be obtained 1–2 months after the start of therapy to evaluate the extent of the pulmonary disease (Baquero-Artigao et al. 2015; Starke 2006; Garazzino et al. 2014; Di Comite et al. 2016), and a gastric aspirate should be repeated with the same timing in previously positive children in order to evaluate the response to specific treatment.

105.3.5 Prevention

The cornerstone for preventing congenital TB is to prevent and treat the active infection in pregnant women (Baquero-Artigao et al. 2015; Starke 2006). The treatment of active disease during pregnancy includes the standard regimen with four active drugs for the first 2 months followed by a consolidation regimen with INH and RFP for a further 4 months. No teratogenic effects have been demonstrated with first-line antituberculosis drugs. Careful monitoring for signs and symptoms of hepatitis and other side effects is strongly recommended. Centers for Disease Control and Prevention recommends treating latent infection during pregnancy at any gestational age if the woman is at high risk of progression to an active disease (i.e., HIV infection, recent TB contact, immunosuppression); in the absence of risk factors, treatment may be delayed after delivery to avoid drug toxicity: this consists in INH administration for 9 months (Centers for Disease Control and Prevention 2016).

The bacille calmette-guérin vaccine is ineffective in preventing congenital tuberculosis. New vaccine development may become a key strategy to prevent future infections.

105.3.6 Prognosis

The early diagnosis and the institution of appropriate therapy have markedly decreased the mortality of congenital TB.

References

Baquero-Artigao F, Mellado Peña MJ, Del Rosal Rabes T et al (2015) Spanish Society for Pediatric Infectious Diseases guidelines on tuberculosis in pregnant women and neonates (I): epidemiology and diagnosis. Congenital tuberculosis. An Pediatr 83:285.e1–285.e8

Centers for Disease Control and Prevention (2015a) Increase in incidence of congenital syphilis – United States, 2012–2014. Morb Mortal Wkly Rep 64:1241–1245

Centers for Disease Control and Prevention (2015b) Sexually transmitted diseases treatment guidelines. Morb Mortal Wkly Rep 64:34–49

Centers for Disease Control and Prevention (2016) Available at http://www.cdc.gov/tb/publications/ltbi/treatment.htm

Centers for Disease Control and Prevention (CDC) (2009) Sexually transmitted disease surveillance 2007 supplement, syphilis surveillance report. U.S. Department of Health and Human Services, Atlanta, Available at http://www.cdc.gov/std/Syphilis2007/

Clement ME, Okeke NL, Hicks CB (2014) Treatment of syphilis: a systematic review. JAMA 312:1905–1917

Di Comite A, Esposito S, Villani A et al (2016) How to manage neonatal tuberculosis. J Perinatol 36:80–85

Doroshenko A, Sherrard J, Pollard AJ (2006) Syphilis in pregnancy and the neonatal period. Int J STD AIDS 17:221–228

Follett T, Clarke DF (2011) Resurgence of congenital syphilis: diagnosis and treatment. Neonatal Netw 30:320–328

Galli L, Lancella L, Garazzino S et al (2016) Recommendations for treating children with drug-resistant tuberculosis. Pharmacol Res 105:176–182

Garazzino S, Galli L, Chiappini E et al (2014) Performance of interferon-γ release assay for the diagnosis of active or latent tuberculosis in children in the first 2 years of age: a multicenter study of the Italian Society of Pediatric Infectious Diseases. Pediatr Infect Dis J 33: e226–e231

Ingall D, Sanchez PJ, Baker CJ (2006) Syphilis. In: Remington JS, Klein JO (eds) Infectious diseases of the fetus and newborn infant, 6th edn. Elsevier Saunders, Philadelphia, pp 545–580

Kingston M, French P, Higgins S et al (2015) UK National guidelines on the management of syphilis 2015. Int J STD AIDS pii: 0956462415624059. [Epub ahead of print]

Lautenschlager S (2006) Diagnosis of syphilis: clinical and laboratory problems. JDDG 12:1058–1072

Mignone F, Codecasa LR, Scolfaro C et al (2013) The spread of drug-resistant tuberculosis in children: an Italian case series. Epidemiol Infect 142:2049–2056

National Institute for Health and Care Excellence (2016) Tuberculosis prevention, diagnosis, management and service organisation NICE guideline, No. 33 Internal Clinical Guidelines Team (UK). National Institute for Health and Care Excellence (UK), London

Patel S, DeSantis ER (2008) Treatment of congenital tuberculosis. Am J Health Syst Pharm 65:2027–2031

Shahrook S, Mori R, Ochirbat T et al (2014) Strategies of testing for syphilis during pregnancy. Cochrane Database Syst Rev 10, CD010385

Smith KC (2002) Congenital tuberculosis: a rare manifestation of a common infection. Curr Opin Infect Dis 15:269–274

Starke J (2006) Tuberculosis. In: Remington S, Baker CJ, Klein JO, Wilson CB (eds) Infectious diseases of the fetus and newborn infant. W B Saunders Co, Philadelphia, pp 581–597

Walker GJ, Walker DG (2007) Congenital syphilis: a continuing but neglected problem. Semin Fetal Neonatal Med 12:198–206

Whittaker E, Kampmann B (2008) Perinatal tuberculosis. New challenges in the diagnosis and treatment of tuberculosis in infants and the newborn. Early Hum Dev 84:795–799

World Health Organisation (2003) Guidelines for the management of sexually transmitted infections (ISBN 92 4 154626 3). World Health Organization, Geneva

World Health Organization (2008) Global incidence and prevalence of selected curable sexually transmitted infections (ISBN: 978 92 4 150383 9). World Health Organization, Geneva

World Health Organization (2015) Global tuberculosis report 2015 (Publication no. WHO/HTM/TB/2015.22). World Health Organization, Geneva

Zeltser R, Kurban AK (2004) Syphilis. Clin Dermatol 22:461–468

Toxoplasmosis in the Fetus and Newborn

106

Wilma Buffolano

Contents

Abstract

Globally, primary toxoplasmosis on gestation generates annually 190,100 new cases of congenital toxoplasmosis with a global burden of 1.20 million DALYs. Although *Toxoplasma gondii* infection is easily diagnosable and effectively treatable on the mother, out of prenatal screening setting, newborn diagnosis and early treatment might be problematic. In fact, the large majority of infected newborn display normal on clinical examination, with positive IgG of maternal origin and possibly negative IgA and IgM, with the consequence of late treatment on subclinical cases who are the ideal target of long-term pharmacological treatment. Moreover, toxoplasmosis is on the list of neglected disease of poverty. As consequence, the interest of manufacturers shows low, and standard of treatment continues to rely on a not curative and toxic medicine combination. Fortunately, research in progress on *Toxoplasma gondii* and host genetics and epigenetic machinery, including unusual histone variants and plantlike transcriptional and

W. Buffolano (✉)
Heading Coordinating Centre for Perinatal Infection-Campania Region, Translational Medicine Department, Federico II Medical School, Naples, Italy
e-mail: wilma@unina.it

G. Buonocore et al. (eds.), *Neonatology*,
https://doi.org/10.1007/978-3-319-29489-6_253

posttranscriptional motifs, could pave the way to potential new drugs and/or to channel the choice to treat or not to treat (and how long) subclinical onset forms. On the chapter, practical sustain on management at birth and on the long term of infant exposed to maternal *Toxoplasma gondii* infection or definitely congenitally infected (text, tables, and figure) is updated on the state of the art.

106.1 Salient Points

- Congenital toxoplasmosis is widespread worldwide and a global burden of 1.20 million DALYs (Disability-adjusted life year) is estimated.
- Consequences on human infection vary according to parasite and host genetic and epigenetic factors, immune status of the host, and route of acquisition.
- Early gestation maternal infection, high parasite load on amniotic fluid, the presence of seizures, and/or neurologic findings and/or brain neuroimaging abnormalities and/or ocular toxoplasmosis near birth are predictors of negative outcomes.
- The large majority of infected newborn are normal on clinical examination, with positive IgG of maternal origin and possibly negative IgA and IgM, making diagnosis and early treatment difficult.
- Pharmacological treatment relies on a few toxic drug combinations (pyrimethamine and sulfonamide) on association with folinic acid to lower the side effect on bone marrow.
- Prompt ventriculoperitoneal shunt placement with frequent assessments of adequate drainage may be necessary. Seizures are treated effectively with levetiracetam, which does not interfere with pyrimethamine and sulfadiazine.
- Compensatory strategies help children compensate for the impact of the disease on cognitive function and quality of life.
- Antibodies against VEGF or focal laser photocoagulation and pars plana vitrectomy, in conjunction with standard antimicrobial therapy, are emerging as effective therapies for complications such as choroidal neovascular membranes.

106.2 Introduction

Toxoplasma gondii infection (TgI) in humans has been considered a benign anthropo-zoonosis harmful for immunocompromised person ("killer no. 3") and unborn child, on which a devastating disease might occur, even when primary maternal TgI is only unveiled by antibody presence (Saadatnia and Golkar 2012).

On the 1980s, focus has concentrated on congenital TgI (CTgI) *See* Toxoplasma gondi infection (TgI) sequelae and prevention and early treatment opportunities and claims for screening. On the EU, monthly or trimestral prenatal testing on antibody-negative pregnant women and fetal damage prophylaxis on seroconverters has been practiced, compulsively on France and Austria and on demand charge-free on Belgium, Germany, and Italy. On Austria and France, case treatment was further facilitated by mother-newborn pair postdelivery testing. On New England and New Hampshire, IgM testing on newborn dried blood spots and sequelae prophylaxis in confirmed positive infant had been launched, since 1986; feasibility of newborn screening had been confirmed in Denmark, Poland, Sweden, Brazil, and Colombia. Furthermore, it had closed on EU countries because of low sensitivity in a low prevalence setting.

Weak proofs of prophylaxis benefits, concerns about infrastructure costs and adverse treatment effects, and differences in test and drug local availability are still contributing to variability in clinical practices. Equipoise considerations in screening countries, lack of funding, and disinterest of manufacturers in developing countries where CTgI has the major impact are yet blocking randomized placebo-controlled trial realization. As consequence, promising new and/or multiplexed assays with potential diagnostic improvement remain not validated and commercialized. Treatment too relies on a few outdated and poorly understood pharmacokinetic/dynamic drugs unable to eradicate tissue cysts and thus to cure toxoplasmosis. TgI has been included in the list of neglected tropical parasitic disease of poverty (Jones et al. 2014).

106.3 Etiology and Pathogenesis

T. gondii is an obligate intracellular protist (*Apicomplexa* phylum). Tachyzoite is the rapidly dividing parasite stage, segregated from host cell apparatus into a parasitophorous vacuole. The *apicoplast* is a complex structure at the apical end, including club-shaped secretory organelles with kinase or pseudokinase signature modulating innate immunity and parasite survival, namely, rhoptries (ROPs) and dense granule bodies (GRA) contributing to the development of microtubules and intra-vacuolar network (IVN), and polar rings sometimes surrounded by rodlike structures, namely, microneme (MIC), which participate on host cell invasion. Certain rhoptry proteins were found to be critical virulence factors that resist innate immunity, while other rhoptry proteins were found to influence chronic infection without affecting virulence (Fox et al. 2016).

Low-level genetic divergence among three major multilocus genotypes (I, II, III), stable in time and space, has been demonstrated on EU (mainly type II strain) isolates, whereas South America, Africa, and Asia isolates display more complex population structure with greater genetic diversity and virulence (atypical strain). On South America, where type II strain is very rare, 88 atypical strains have defined with severe acute course. Genetic diversity reaches the maximum on Amazonian area, where interpenetration of anthropized and wild forest leads to strain hybridization. In French Guiana, high rate fever, systemic disease, and ocular findings have reported on immunocompetent persons with such strains (Carme et al. 2009). In the USA, a fourth clonal type has been recently isolated (type 12) which account for 46.7% of wildlife isolates (Dubey et al. 2011). Genotype I–III crosses identified ROP 18 and ROP16 as key molecules for eye damage on humans (Torres-Morales et al. 2014).

Correlates between host genetic (and epigenetic) markers controlling immune response and outcomes, particularly on ocular toxoplasmosis (OT), are emerging. Linkage disequilibrium on single nucleotide polymorphisms (SNPs) has been shown on NOD2, IFN-γ point mutation (+874 T/A), and parental COL2A1 (Dutra et al. 2013; de Souza et al. 2012; Jamieson et al. 2008). Polymorphism on P2RX7 receptor has been shown in association with eye-brain involvement (Jamieson et al. 2010). More severe ocular lesions have been shown on Brazilian cohorts compared to the EU cohort (Gilbert et al. 2008), and atypical genotypes described in South America have been isolated on severe onset CTgI patient, on France and Tunisia (Delhaes et al. 2010; Boughattas et al. 2011). Type 1 and atypical parasites were associated with clinical problem, regardless of pregnancy period at infection (Rico-Torres et al. 2016).

The wealth of *T. gondii* epigenetic machinery, including unusual histone variants and plantlike transcriptional and posttranscriptional motifs, could open to new chemotherapy approach.

Chemokine release on infected cells leads to an amplification loop activated through direct interaction between dendritic and natural killer (NK) cells, mutually activating and amplifying IL-12 and IFN-γ synthesis and thus tumor necrosis factor alpha (TNF-a) synthesis. The further recognition of parasite antigen by pattern recognition receptors leads to an exacerbation of phagocytic activity with enhanced production of reactive oxygen and nitric oxide species and tryptophan starvation. A strong Th-1 immune response might overwhelm its goal and be responsible for severe inflammation, resulting in tissue damage or even death. Such a deleterious effect of an acute Th-1 immune response in the setting of primary acquired TgI on gestation can result in fetal loss, since IFN-γ destabilizes the Th-2 microenvironment necessary for eye, CNS, and maternal-fetal tolerance.

Transplacental transmission occurs on overall 29% of gestation complicated by primary TGI, conventionally during the temporary parasitemia accompanying early infection. Gestational week of maternal infection (AW), regardless of settings, including parasite genotype, study design, and methods, is the main factor for transmission rate and CTgI severity. More newborns with clinical problems were born from mothers infected during the first half of gestation. Placenta plays a main role in the process as both natural barrier for the fetus protection and target tissue for parasite multiplication. Acute disease acquired ≥6 months before gestation shows a transmission rate approaching zero, and CTgI cases reported on maternal infection in the 2 months before conception are rare. On a recent meta-analysis study, the vertical transmission pooled rate was 20% (95% CI, 15–26%), and the rate by trimesters was 5% (95% CI, 2–16%), 13% (95% CI, 7–23%), and 32% (95% CI, 24–41%), respectively (Li et al. 2014). These values show lower than on EU prospective cohort meta-analysis, on which the odds of transmission increased by 12% per AW after seroconversion time, and the risk of giving birth to a child with clinical signs is greatest (10%) for women acquiring toxoplasmosis between 24 and 30 AW (Systematic Review on Congenital Toxoplasmosis Study Group (SYROCOT) 2007). In fact, the odds of intracranial lesion markedly decrease with older AW at maternal infection, whereas the risk of ocular lesions declines less significantly (Fig. 115.2). Besides pregnancy time at infection, clinical outcome in congenitally infected products depends on parasite burden. A concentration larger than 100 parasites/mL in amniotic fluid was strongly associated with a severe outcome (Romand et al. 2004).

In the fetus, the tachyzoite ability to cross non-permissive biological barriers includes eyes and CNS. Neuron chronic infection underlies *Toxoplasma's* ability to cause devastating neurologic disease and death. Although both astrocytes and neurons might be infected, only IFN-γ-stimulated astrocytes might clear intracellular parasite (Nguyen et al. 2016). Brain microcalcification and ventricular dilation on neuroimaging (Figs. 115.1 and 115.2), retinochoroiditis foci or scars on fundoscopic examination (Fig. 115.3), and/or optical coherence tomography (OCT) reveal tissue damages generated by local Th-1-mediated immune responses. Vasculitis with necrosis gradually sloughing into the ventricles might cause obstructive hydrocephalus (Fig. 115.2).

Four anatomical patterns secondary to CNS involvement have recently categorized (Hutson et al. 2015). The commonest is the aqueduct obstruction with enlargement of the lateral and third ventricles and abnormal fourth ventricle (43% of cases); the second one was Monro foramina obstruction with asymmetric lateral ventricle dilatation and normal third and fourth ventricles (25% of cases). The third pattern shows mixed aqueduct and foramen obstruction (11% of cases). The fourth pattern shows bilateral lateral ventricular dilatation, with normal third and fourth ventricle size, and Monro foramina without peri-foramen calcifications or intraventricular obstructive lesions (21% of cases). This peculiar pattern seems associated with no type II strains. Recurrent and/or progressive ocular damage on the long term has considered the consequence of bradyzoite to tachyzoite reconversion with at times invasion of adjacent cells (recrudescence) and secondary autoimmunity for retinal soluble antigen.

106.4 Epidemiology

T. gondii causes an extremely successful opportunistic infection, and approximately one-third of the human population display TGI serological markers. It is an emerging serious foodborne disease causing millions of disability-adjusted life years (Gangneux and Dardè 2012), depending on CTgI complication, and visual damage, psychosis, change in personality profile, and seizures complicating acquired TgI (Torgerson et al. 2015). OT is the fifth cause of acquired visual loss, with overall 24% of affected eyes becoming legally blind (Bodaghi et al. 2012).

Prevalence increases with age, but the rate of acquisition varies according to climate and anthropogenic factors (hygiene, dietetic habits, sanitation, and quality of water). Transmission occurs by ingestion of oocyst defecated by acutely infected feline on water or soil or of cyst on meat animal with chronic TgI. Sporadically, a Tg-IgG-negative recipient has been infected by organ transplantation or blood transfusion from latent infected subject or laboratory accident. On EU, journey abroad or eating imported exotic food had sporadically reported on severe cases.

TgI is prevalent in socioeconomically disadvantaged groups. On Brazil, most person in the lower socioeconomic level are infected by age 15 years, whereas in the upper are infected after age 20 years, thus having an increased risk for primary TGI on reproductive age (Bahia-Oliveira et al. 2003). On the two last decades, progressive decrease in age-specific prevalence has been reported on economically privileged EU countries as consequence of farming, meat animal breeding, food cleaning and storage improved conditions, and prenatal standards of care, including prenatal screening and health education. In the EU, an incidence updating is in need as an increasing number of women are facing gestation while unprotected.

The global annual CTgI prevalence is estimated to be 190,100 cases, with a global burden of 1.20 million DALYs (Torgerson and Mastroiacovo 2013). In the Northern Hemisphere, gestational toxoplasmosis and CTgI prevalence range from 0.5 to 8 per 1000 susceptible pregnancies and 1 to 10 per 10,000 live newborns, respectively. On Italy, CTgI prevalence had shown 1.38 per 10,000 live newborn (Stagni et al. 2009).

106.5 Laboratory Diagnosis

TgI diagnosis mostly relies on antibody response kinetics (IgG, IgM, IgA isotypes) on blood, instead of direct detection by PCR or culture on placenta (60%–79.5% sensitivity, 92%–97% specificity), cord blood (21.2% sensitivity, 100% specificity), CSF (46% sensitivity), and urine (50% sensitivity) (Gangneux and Dardè 2012). As having a combination of IgM and IgA test results, in addition to IgG, has greater sensitivity than either test alone, IgG, IgM, and IgA should always be tested.

Nowadays, most clinical laboratories use an enzyme immunoassay (EIA) on whole soluble antigen for the routine, whereas further techniques have mostly reserved for pitfall exclusion on expert laboratories.

Maternal Diagnosis

Conversion from a negative postconceptional test to an IgM- and IgG-positive result marks a primary toxoplasmosis on gestation, whereas a negative postdelivery or a positive preconceptional IgG test reasonably rules out offspring risk. On prenatal screening setting, a *short therapeutic window* had shown that a delay of more than 3 weeks on starting treatment increased transmission odds, thus pointing out efficacy of monthly screening (Wallon et al. 2013).

Routinely, a multi-test strategy based on combination of highly sensitive IgM and IgG avidity (or stage specificity) assays has been considered appropriate in confirming or excluding maternal acute TGI (and thus fetal risk) when positive IgG and IgM were found at the first prenatal test ($\leq$12 weeks AW). High IgG avidity results point out residual IgM (Villard et al. 2016). Drug-induced delay on IgG avidity maturation has been reported on spiramycin-treated mother. High-performance low-cost multiplexed assays for IgG, IgM, and IgA on ultra-small blood volume are paving the way to universal prenatal screening implementation (Li et al. 2016).

Fetal diagnosis might carry out at $\geq$18 AW, at least 4 weeks after the estimated infection time, by PCR assay on amniotic fluid (AF) according to laboratory and/or ultrasonographic indications. On France, despite performance variation among systems, PCR has become standard of practice to channel prenatal management. The AF146527 RT-PCR is far more sensitive than B1 gene RT-PCR (Belaz et al. 2015). RT-PCR assay is highly specific, but a negative result does not rule out fetal infection as up to 46% of infected AF contain $<$10 tachyzoites/mL (Filisetti et al. 2015).

Newborn Diagnosis

Postnatal diagnosis is essential because of prenatal diagnosis failure on approximately 15% of cases and late on pregnancy maternal acquisition. Out of prenatal screening, early definition of infant infection status might show problematic. In fact, as most cases show normal on routine clinical examination, cranial findings are not pathognomonic and might go undetected, funduscopic examination could be negative or imprecise even on expert examiner, and sensitivity of serological test is lower when mother acquired their infection early in gestation and/or received treatment during gestation. According to maternal infection AW, IgM sensitivity increases by 29% in the first to 71% in the third trimester, and IgA sensitivity increases by 40% in the first to 64% in the third trimester (EMSCOT- European Multicentre Study on Congenital Toxoplasmosis 2007). The most informative result is a positive IgM result on pairs with second trimester maternal seroconversion (with a pretest probability of 27% and a posttest probability of 79%) and a negative IgM result on pairs with third trimester maternal TgI (with a pretest probability of 59% and a posttest probability of 32%). Better scores have been achieved when the tests have been performed on age 2 weeks.

At birth, high IgG level might reflect transplacental transportation. Sequential specific IgG level monitoring (in parallel with the previous sample) compared to the expected decay on transported IgG (one on half per month) shows between ages 2 and 6 months the infant has been infected according to stabilized or rising IgG level. Beyond age 12 months, IgG persistence or disappearance definitely confirms or rules out CTgI, respectively; unfortunately, the gold standard for diagnosis is useless fore decision about treatment. In some infected infants, treatment can lead to IgG negativization during follow-up, creating the false sense that the infant is not infected. However, in infected infants, treatment discontinuation is followed by a *Toxoplasma* IgG rebound, whereas in uninfected, IgG remains permanently negative.

Demonstration of positive IgM and/or IgA on newborn whole blood or sera sample is highly specific when maternal antibody leak might be ruled out, because neither crosses the placenta. Overall, IgM and IgA sensitivities have shown 52% and 55%, respectively. Immunosorbent agglutination assay (ISAGA) is still preferred, because of better sensitivity (e.g., 81.1% versus 64.8%) and specificity, long-term persistence on infant blood, and few false-positive result (Pinon et al. 2001; Murat et al. 2015). Comparative immunoblot test (IB) for specific IgG and IgM analysis on paired mother-newborn sera (at birth and <3 months follow-up) can confirm CTgI diagnosis and rule out maternal serum contamination on cord blood. In fact, different band patterns on mother-newborn pair indicate antibody neosynthesis. Combination of IB with conventional serological methods has shown to be superior to IB or conventional methods used alone. The IB sensitivity at birth is 48–50% for IgG and 65–79% when combined with IgM detection. A multi-test strategy, including two tests (IgM and IgA) or three tests [IgM, IgA, and immunoblotting (IB)], increases sensitivity up to 73% and 78%, respectively (Rilling et al. 2003). Three-IgM band association at 75, 90, and 100 kDa, called the "IgM triplet," might increase sensitivity to 95.8%, when combined with prenatal and postnatal serological tests (L'Ollivier et al. 2012). The interpretation of IB may be difficult and should not have been performed after age 3 months. On cases with doubtful diagnosis, IFN-γ release after antigen stimulation of fresh resuspended blood pellet might increase diagnostic precision (94% sensitivity and 98% specificity, respectively). Unfortunately, the test is currently not commercially available (Chapey et al. 2015). PCR has more commonly utilized for neonatal diagnosis in regions without screening where higher sensitivity in PCR assays is expected according to the absence of maternal treatment.

On patient with missed diagnosis at birth and suggestive sequelae, retrospective diagnosis might be tempted on cards collected for newborn screening (Marangoni et al. 2014). Since suboptimal storage conditions can seriously affect sensitivity, negative results cannot rule out the diagnosis.

Protein microarray displaying *Toxoplasma* polypeptide products has identified several antigens for IgM antibody detection. Recently, high potential in serological diagnosis has been shown on rROP2186–533 ISAGA assay [100% (48/48) positivity on Toxo-IgM+-IgG– sera and 0% positivity on Toxo-IgG+ sera) (Liu et al. 2012). In the next future, multi-epitope-based antigen approach using software-based prediction tools and molecular techniques may provide a novel and alternative means of acquiring less expensive and more accurate diagnostic kits.

106.6 Clinical Aspects

106.6.1 Acquired Infection

After an incubation period of about 2–3 weeks, lymph node swelling (mostly posterior cervical) and fatigue associated with low fever are the commonest TGI symptoms. Adenopathy can involve other node groups. Hepatosplenomegaly and rash are rarer. Clinical course is usually self-limited, and symptoms resolve on weeks or months. OT might occur in the acute and latent phase and recur by time. Diagnosis is based on clinical feature but may be confirmed by biological tools applied to ocular fluids (Bodaghi et al. 2012). OT has reported on 2% of US population and on 7.7% of 130 mothers delivering a child with CTgI (Noble et al. 2010). In the context of French screening program, clinical signs have been reported only on 5% of mothers and without remarkable prenatal ultrasound (US) findings (Dunn et al. 1999). On HIV-infected patient, on direct parasite inoculation (laboratory accidents), where NE-II strains predominate, and/or small outbreak caused by contaminated water, the incidence of retinochoroiditis seems higher (Bowie et al. 1997). In a no screening setting (US), awareness of TgI compatible clinical signs seems to offer a chance of prompt treatment as 48% of mothers who gave birth to an affected child could recall cervical lymphadenopathy and/or flu-like illness (Boyer et al. 2005).

Although reactivation of chronic TgI in individuals with weakened immune systems causes severe toxoplasmosis, with rare exceptions, reactivation of latent toxoplasmosis poses no threat to the fetus. The potential for overt disease and fetal transmission during the chronic phase has been reported in severely immunocompromised pregnant women (CD4 count <200 cells/mm3) and on a few anecdotic cases (Elbez-Rubinstein et al. 2009; Silveira et al. 2003).

106.6.2 Congenital Infection

The clinical spectrum of fetuses, newborns, and children with CTgI could range widely from complete apparent normality on as much as 80% of cases to severe neurological and ocular disease and even death. Depending on maternal AW of infection and prenatal treatment, parasite genotype, genetic and immunologic status of the mother, and route of acquisition, a huge amount of complications have been reported at a different rate, including miscarriage, stillbirths, prematurity, intrauterine growth restriction (IUGR), purpura, blueberry muffin rash, splenomegaly, hepatomegaly, anemia, leukopenia, thrombocytopenia, abnormal cerebrospinal fluid cells and protein, ocular disease with or without visual loss, strabismus, nystagmus, cataracts, microphthalmus, intracranial calcification, hydrocephalus, microcephalus, electroencephalographic and/or cerebrospinal fluid abnormalities, seizures, intractable epilepsy, cerebral palsy, and neurodevelopmental delay (McLeod et al. 2014). Milder disease has been shown more prevalent in the EU, where overt signs were reported in a minority of infant enrolled in center performing prenatal or neonatal screening, and attributed to differences on *T. gondii* genetics and prenatal care (Gilbert et al. 2008).

Definition of onset severity at birth includes exclusion of systemic involvement by careful physical examination and general laboratory tests and of target organ (eye and CNS) damage.

Eye

The clinical diagnosis of OT on indirect funduscopic examination is usually straightforward. Typically, one or more fluffy white retinal lesion (less than half to four optical disk in diameter, macular, juxta-macular, or peripheral in location) might coexist with pigmented chorioretinal scar and prominent vitreous and anterior chamber cellular reaction. Papillitis, neuroretinitis, and retrobulbar neuritis might be unusual presentations and cataracts, glaucoma, optic atrophy, and microphthalmia late complications.

CNS

Hydrocephalus (approximately 4% of infected infants) is primarily obstructive with third ventricular dilation and associated with high CSF protein levels ($\geq$1 g/dL). Not obstructive hydrocephalus might complicate fibrotic process (loss of brain parenchyma or poor reabsorption). Cerebrospinal fluid (CSF) cells, protein, glucose, and *T. gondii* DNA presence have to investigate on the presence of neurological involvement on expert neurological examination or neuroimaging.

Neuroimaging has aimed to detect primarily ventricular dilation and cranial micro-calcification. Ultrasound (US) examination, via the bregmatic fontanelle before age 6 months, is first-level imaging with high sensitivity (current probes) for ventricular dilation, low cost, large availability, and the absence of irradiation. Scanning (at 3-mm collimation with 5-mm interval and at 10-mm collimation) is second level, with high accuracy on calcification detection, but potential side effect secondary to irradiation. Magnetic resonance imaging (MRI) (1.6 to 4 mm slice thickness, sequence T1-W conventional spin echo or T2-W fast spin echo) is third level to search for parenchymal or cortical anomalies. A 45-s two-sequence MRI study, collectively referred to as "brain shunt hydrocephalus screen" in some US hospitals, which do not require sedation or contrast administration, can be used to follow the progress of ventricular dilatation or the correction of hydrocephalus in a manner that is easy and comfortable for both parent and child. These two sequences are T2 axial and coronal single shots with images at 3-mm intervals.

Ideally, a suspected CTgI should be confirmed on an experienced reference laboratory, and management carried out on (or with the formal support of) a specialized center, where a multidisciplinary expert team working in high-quality standardized conditions and performing valid and reliable measures, reporting in a large database standard format, including retinal photographs and neuroimaging, might minimize potentials (Blankenberg et al. 2000; Hintz et al. 2007). The more clinical onset definition is appropriate based on correct estimation of maternal infection time and interpretation of fetal diagnosis results, and posttest probability measures, the less the misdiagnosis rate, i.e., the number of treated among healthy infants and untreated among congenitally infected ones.

106.7 Differential Diagnosis

A severe TORCH syndrome, including *Cytomegalovirus*, herpes simplex virus, rubella, syphilis, varicella, B19, and West Nile, dengue, chikungunya, malaria, Zika, and Ebola on particular epidemiological conditions, has to rule out in symptomatic newborn infants by a combination of diagnostic tools. Systematic exclusion of congenital cytomegalovirus (cCMV) coinfection within age 2 weeks should channel appropriate onset severity definition/management and outcome measures. A negative postdelivery CMV-IgG test rules out cCMV, whereas a positive CMV-PCR on Guthrie card should allow differentiation between congenital and perinatal infection on case with testing delay. Exclusion of pseudo-TORCH syndrome might be indicated in multisystemic disease simulating TORCH syndrome upon which extensive screening for congenital infectious disease is negative (Knoblauch et al. 2003).

106.8 Therapy and Treatments

Guidelines for prenatal and postnatal treatment have been summarized in Table 115.2.

No safe and curative therapeutic strategy exists against TGI; pharmacological treatment of acquired infection has indicated only on complicated forms, including OT with visual damage, tropical toxoplasmosis (fever, myocarditis, and pneumonitis), and neurotoxoplasmosis. On gestational and periconceptional TGI (or periconceptional symptomatic TGI occurring <6 months before last menstrual data), prompt antibiotic secondary prophylaxis continued until delivery has advocated to reduce transmission rate and short- and long-term severity of fetal infection. Standard regimens rely on spiramycin and on synergistic combination of folate inhibitors, namely, pyrimethamine and sulfonamides, given with folinic acid (PSF) and regular monitoring of complete blood cell counts. The first is the only administrable before 16 AW, absorbed efficiently, well tolerated, and with little side effects to the fetus (Rajapakse et al. 2013). Change to PSF regimen has carried out on confirmed late maternal infection ($\geq$30 AW), positive fetal diagnosis, and the presence of suggestive abnormalities on ultrasonography. On unproven maternal infection, an expert and exhaustive discussion with parents could channel appropriate treatment choices based on presumed AW of infection and offer relief to parental anxiety. Induction of labor or C-section delivery does not prevent CTgI (Wallon et al. 2015). Spiramycin-cotrimoxazole combination displayed comparable result with PSF combination on a single comparative study (Valentini et al. 2015), and should be regarded as an alternative in case of PSF regimen side effect and positive fetal diagnosis.

Although evidences of efficacy of postnatal treatment rely only on observational studies, tertiary prophylaxis has been applied in infected infants on the aim to reduce duration and severity of critical symptoms at birth, neurologic impairment, and new eye lesion. The lack of diffusion into the brain parenchyma and the potential for life-threatening arrhythmias excluded spiramycin from the use in newborns, and PSF combination has yet the standard of treatment (Stramba-Badiale et al. 1997).

Differences in treatment regimens exist among centers, including type of PSF regimen and duration of postnatal treatment. One-year long continuous regimen is the standard, whereas 3-month high-dose continuous and 2-year low-dose discontinuous were the shortest and longest regimens, respectively. On low fixed-dose discontinuous regimen, the potential for early and more severe sulfonamide side effects such as Lyell syndrome has been counterbalanced by potential improvement on adherence to treatment. Dosage adjustment, according to weekly complete blood count, might be necessary on as much as 14–58% of cases because of neutropenia. Precaution: glucose-6-phosphate dehydrogenase (G6PDH) deficiency screening should have been performed before sulfonamide administration. Signs of active infection appear to resolve early (in weeks) during treatment. In case of PSF withholding, depending on severe side effects, alternative treatment includes pyrimethamine combination with clindamycin or azithromycin, with standard dosages according to weight. Steroids (1 mg/kg daily) might have been given for a short time, after loading PSF doses, to shorten the course of vision-threatening retinochoroiditis such as that localized in the proximity of the optic nerve or the macula and/or encephalitis [suggested by protein concentration $\geq$ 1 g/dL on cerebrospinal fluid (CSF)]. When inflammation signs subsid, they are tapered and finally discontinued. Treatment reinstitution after a serological rebound has not been indicated.

OT is characterized by recurrent episodes with potential loss of vision when the macula and optic disk are involved and/or complications such as retinal detachment or neovascularization occur. The timing of recurrences varies between individuals and is unpredictable. If new eye lesions have been detected, standard treatment should have been given for 1–2 weeks after the resolution of acute phase in active lesions though on peripheral location and healed lesions. Four-month intermittent treatment with trimethoprim/sulfamethoxazole (once every 3 days) might have been considered as alternative regimen in children with recurrent eye lesion over age 1 year (Silveira et al. 2002). Treatment with antibiotics probably reduces the risk of recurrent toxoplasma retinochoroiditis, but there is currently no good evidence that this leads to better visual outcomes.

Prompt ventriculoperitoneal shunt placement might be necessary with frequent controls of adequate drainage suitability, as patients usually require repeated shunting procedures. As it is unclear from initial neuroimaging which children will benefit from CSF drainage, shunt placement has to consider in all patterns. Brain lesions can cause seizure secondarily (both the multifocal encephalomalacia and multifocal cerebral calcification). Seizures have been treated effectively with levetiracetam (Keppra) (7 mg/Kg twice a day), which has less sedative hypnotic type effects, does not induce hepatic degradation of pyrimethamine such as phenobarbital, and does not displace sulfadiazine albumin binding such as phenytoin nor does it trigger the bone marrow toxicity associated with carbamazepine.

Compensatory strategies such as large print and "talking" books, camera magnification of materials, and spectacles to maintain best-corrected visual acuity help children compensate for the impact of the disease on cognitive function and quality of life. Plate peripheral neovascularization associated with plaques of cicatricial retinochoroiditis has sometimes been visualized by fluorescein angiography or ocular coherence tomography. The process might have been abrogated by antibodies against VEGF, ranibizumab, in conjunction with standard antiparasitic therapy or by focal laser photocoagulation and pars plana vitrectomy.

Breastfeeding has no contraindication as, even if *T. gondii* has been isolated in many animal species, there is no evidence of transmission on humans (Capobiango et al. 2015).

As neurological or ophthalmological disease might manifest later in life even on subclinical onset patient, psychological and developmental tests, visual evoked potential tests, and audiology tests have to be performed regularly in all cases, probably up to adolescent age.

In the next future, correlations between severity and type of disease and genotype of the infecting strain might be critical to determine appropriate disease treatment and outcome in human cases.

106.9 Prognosis

Maternal AW of infection and parasite load in amniotic fluid are early markers for CT onset severity. Evidences on parasite genotype effect on clinical outcomes are emerging, and an association between serotype II infection and better clinical outcome as compared to non-type II has shown in a large US cohort (Bodaghi et al. 2012).

Long-term evolution of CTgI was not fully documented. In outdated studies, only 11% of asymptomatic untreated patients remained sequelae-free. On the contrary, favorable cognitive, neurological, and auditory outcomes had been found in the group without substantial neurological disease near birth and in over 72% of moderate or severe neurological disease groups after 1-year standard postnatal treatment in the National Collaborative Chicago-based Congenital Toxoplasmosis Study (NCCCTS), recruiting referrals all over the USA (McLeod et al. 2006). New eye lesions remained undetectable in 91% of the children without neurological disease and in 64% of those with moderate or severe neurological disease. Reactivations have reported in as many as 34% of cases with early ocular involvement. More than 70% of patients in the untreated group developed new eye lesion after the first decade of life, whereas new central lesions were uncommon in treated children (Phan et al. 2008a; Phan et al. 2008b) (Table 1).

In the European Multicentre Study on Congenital Toxoplasmosis (EMSCOT), cohorts recruited through screening and treated displayed outcomes milder than anticipated based on historical data. Serious neurological sequelae had been found on 5% of patients on the first 2 years of life, and comparable development and behavior had been reported at 4 years age in treated cases compared to uninfected controls (Freeman et al. 2005). Moreover, 18% of 281 infected children had $\geq$1 retinochoroidal lesions, and 6% had recurrent retinochoroiditis during a median follow-up of 4.1 years. Half of the children who developed OT had already had their first lesion detected before age 4 months. The main determinants were the presence of clinical findings near birth and/or intracranial lesions. The highest risk (80%) had been found in cases with serious neurologic sequelae and the lower (12%) in subclinical cases (European Multicentre Study on Congenital Toxoplasmosis- EMSCOT 2008). On Lyon cohort, only one-fourth of the patients had bilateral ocular lesions, and less than one-sixth had foveal lesions, which probably explains their good performance on visual function assessments and quality-of-life score close to the expected normal range for the general population (74.7 $\pm$ 14.2 vs 73.7$\pm$ 15.3) (Peyron et al. 2011; Wallon et al. 2014). Although at age 12 years, 29.8% of followed cases manifested at least one ocular lesion, and recurrences or new ocular lesions were shown on 33.8% of patient after the appearance of the first lesion, only 2.7% of infected children developed bilateral visual impairment severe enough to affect eligibility for a driving license. Lesions remained unilateral in 69.0% of cases and caused no vision loss in 80.6% (Table 2).

Table 1 Diagnosis of congenital toxoplasmosis

Criteria for diagnostic suspicion		
Toxoplasmosis on gestation	Maternal diagnosis precision	Proven Unproven Unlikely
	Gestational time of infection (weeks)	<13 GW 13–35 ≥36
	PCR on amniotic fluid	Negative Positive
The presence of clinical findings (isolate or on combination) in the first age months	Ocular	Nystagmus or strabismus Posterior segment abnormalities (retinochoroiditis, optic nerve atrophy) External eye abnormalities (microphthalmus, cataract)
	Intracranial	Microcalcifications (particularly spotty distributed) Ventricular dilatation or obstructive hydrocephalus
	Neurological	Seizures, EEG, and/or CSF abnormalities☼ Microcephaly, macrocephaly tone, or motor dysfunction
	Systemic (TORCH syndrome)	rash Hepatosplenomegaly Anemia, thrombocytopenia
Newborn screening	Toxo-IgM and/or IgA positivity	
Onset severity definition		Careful pediatric examination Neurologic evaluation* Expert ophthalmologic examination[*°╥] Brain computed tomography scan[⊥] Brain US or 45-s two-sequence MRI (follow-up) [♣] Auditory brain stem response[#]
Infection status definition	Indirect criteria	Toxo-IgM[♪] and IgA[♫] Toxo-IgG increase or stabilization Toxo-IgG persistence beyond age 12 months Comparative analysis mother/newborn Toxo-IgG/IgM/IgA IB Toxo-IgM triplet IB (75, 90,100 kDa) IFN-γ release after 24-h stimulation with crude Toxo-antigen
	Direct criteria (not routinely)	Parasite isolation or positive inoculation on mice or tissue culture (placenta) Parasite DNA demonstration (PCR on amniotic or cerebrospinal fluid)

Legend: ♪ EIA and ISAGA-IgM; ♫ ELISA-IgA; * data sheets and narrative evaluations for each child at each examination; ° appropriate examination includes cycloplegia and under-sedation indirect fundoscopy to detect both central and peripheral lesions; ╥ fundus photographs and optical coherence tomography (OCT), whenever the patient cooperation allowed; ⊥ without contrast medium enhancement. Brain computed tomography scan sensitivity has reported five times higher than ultrasonography (US) as interobserver agreement. ♣ US is widely practiced to monitor short-term treatment effect; # only on infected infant

Table 2 Treatment of Tg infection in pregnant women and congenital toxoplasmosis (CT)

Mother	Treatment	Dosage	Indication	Comment
	Spiramycin	1 g (3 million U) every 8 h (for a total of 3 g or 9 million U per day)	a. Pregnant women suspected of having acquired the infection <16 AW; b. unproven maternal diagnosis (any AW); c. negative amniotic fluid PCR and negative US at follow-up	Until delivery, not teratogenic
	Pyrimethamine (P), sulfadiazine, and folinic acid	(P) Loading dose: 50 mg each 12 h for 2 days; then 50 mg daily; *sulfadiazine* loading dose: 75 mg/ kg, followed by 50 mg/kg every 12 h (maximum, 4 g daily); *folinic acid*: 10–20 mg daily (during and 1 week after (P) therapy completion)	a. Women with proven infection acquired ≥17 AW; b. women with suspected infection acquired ≥30 AW; c. documented fetal infection (positive result of amniotic fluid PCR or abnormal US)	(P) is teratogenic; half-life is 100 h. Complete blood count twice a week (reversible neutropenia) (a) (b) (d)
	Pyrimethamine (P), sulfadoxine, and folinic acid	2 tablets (50 mg (P) 500 mg *sulfadoxine each tablet*) each 10 days; *folinic acid*: 50 mg weekly	a. Women with proven infection acquired ≥17 AW; b. women with suspected infection acquired ≥30 AW	Sulfadoxine half-life is 200 h. Potential for lethal hepatotoxicity (a) (b) (d)
CT▼	*Gold standard* pyrimethamine (P), sulfadiazine, and folinic acid	(P) Loading dose: 2 mg/kg every 12 h for 2 days; then 1 mg/kg daily for 2 or 6 months; then same dose each alternate day or half dose daily; *sulfadiazine*, 50 mg/kg every 12 h; *folinic acid*, 25 mg twice a week (during and 1 week after completion of (P) therapy)	2-month high-dose regimen on subclinical onset; 6-month high-dose regimen on symptomatic onset	1-year treatment; (P) half-life on infant is 60 h. CSF levels are 10–20% of concomitant serum levels (a) (b) (c)
	Alternative protocol Pyrimethamine (P), sulfadoxine, and folinic acid	(P) 1,25 mg /kg – sulfadoxine 25 mg / kg each 10 days; folinic acid, 50 mg weekly	Pre-regimen with (P) and sulfadiazine for 2 months. Loading dose: 1 mg/kg every 12 h for 2 days; then 1 mg/kg daily; *sulfadiazine*, 50 mg/kg every 12 h for 2 months; then P-sulfadoxine	10–24 months; sulfadoxine half-life on infant is 60 h (a) (b) (c)
	Prednisone	0.5 mg/kg each 12 h	a. CSF protein ≥1 g/dL; b. active chorioretinitis vision threatening; c. systemic findings	Until inflammatory marker subsides (1–2 weeks apart)

Footnotes Before starting sulfonamides, check for G6PDH deficit. Infants have weighed weekly and medications, made fresh each week, and are dosed based on increasing weight each week. Neutrophil counts should have been measured via heel prick once a week while taking (P), and in the week after, this regimen has discontinued. Care is taken to make certain that the baby's teeth are cleaned after medicine administration because of the sugar-suspending agents leading to the development of dental carries. Most children have an absolute neutrophil count 900–1200/mm3 during treatment. When neutrophil count is less than 1000 neutrophils/mm^3, a manual differential counting 500 white blood cells has performed to improve accuracy. (a) Sulfonamide discontinuation if hypersensitivity sign occurs, including rash, Stevens-Johnson, asthma, and micro-hematuria with urolithiasis; continue with (P) alone, (b) urine alkalinization, and diuresis maintenance; (c) on absolute neutrophil count (N) <1500/mm^3, double folinate dosage and repeat count; on N count <1000/mm^3, triple folinate (20 mg/day) and half (P) until N >1000/mm^3; and on N count <500/mm, stop P and S until N >1000/mmc. ▼None is manufactured as pediatric formulation. Seizure can occur on (P) regimen as overdosage consequence. (P) half-life is reduced while phenobarbital is administrated.

More severe OT (frequency, size, and multiplicity of retinochoroidal lesions) was shown in CTgI children in Brazil compared with EU, which might be a consequence of more virulent genotypes predominating there, but rare in Europe (Gilbert et al. 2008).

Sensorineural hearing defect is still associated with CT and neurological impairment.

In conclusion, on countries, performing screening CTgI displays mostly a sight-threatening eye disease in which occurrence of lesions during postnatal treatment contrasts with the regression or even disappearance of cranial lesions and in which long-term follow-up to adolescence is necessary. Ophthalmologic surveillance should be more active in cases with cranial findings. Little has known about the consequence of visual impairment on life quality and comprehension subscale upon which impaired vision might have impact. Further follow-up in recruited cohorts could allow better knowledge of long-term learning disabilities and behavioral problems in congenitally infected patients with and without intracranial lesions, namely, on speech development.

References

Bahia-Oliveira LM, Jones JL, Azevedo-Silva J et al (2003) Highly endemic, waterborne toxoplasmosis in north Rio de Janeiro state, Brazil. Emerg Infect Dis 9(1):55–62

Belaz S, Gangneux JP, Dupretz P et al (2015) A 10-year retrospective comparison of two target sequences, REP-529 and B1, for *Toxoplasma gondii* detection by quantitative PCR. J Clin Microbiol 53:1294–1300

Blankenberg FG, Loh NN, Bracci P et al (2000) Sonography, CT, and MR imaging: a prospective comparison of neonates with suspected intracranial ischemia and hemorrhage. AJNR Am J Neuroradiol 21:213–218

Bodaghi B, Touitou V, Fardeau C et al (2012) Toxoplasmosis: new challenges for an old disease. Eye (Lond) 26(2):241–244

Boughattas S, Abdallah RB, Siala E et al (2011) An atypical strain associated with congenital toxoplasmosis in Tunisia. New Microbiol 34:413–416

Bowie WR, King AS, Werker DH et al (1997) Outbreak of toxoplasmosis associated with municipal drinking water: the BC Toxoplasma Investigation Team. Lancet 350:173–177

Boyer KM, Holfels E, Roizen N et al (2005) Risk factors for Toxoplasma gondii infection in mothers of infants with congenital toxoplasmosis: implications for prenatal management and screening. Am J Obstet Gynaecol 192:564–571

Capobiango JD, Mitsuka-Breganò R, Cabral-Monica T et al (2015) Acute toxoplasmosis in a breastfed infant with possible transmission by water. Rev Inst Med Trop Sao Paulo 57(6):523–526

Carme B, Demar M, Ajzenberg D, Dardé ML (2009) Severe acquired toxoplasmosis caused by wild cycle of Toxoplasma gondii, French Guiana. Emerg Infect Dis 15:656–658

Chapey E, Wallon M, L'Ollivier C et al (2015) Place of interferon-γ assay for diagnosis of congenital toxoplasmosis. Pediatr Infect Dis J 34(12):1407–1409

de Souza NE, Land Curi AL, Cavalcanti de Albuquerque M et al (2012) Genetic polymorphism for IFNγ +874 T/A in patients with acute toxoplasmosis. Rev Soc Bras Med Trop 45:757–760

Delhaes L, Ajzenberg D, Sicot B et al (2010) Severe congenital toxoplasmosis due to a Toxoplasma gondii strain with an atypical genotype: case report and review. Prenat Diagn 30:902–905

Dubey JP, Velmurugan GV, Rajendran C et al (2011) Genetic characterisation of Toxoplasma gondii in wildlife from North America revealed widespread and high prevalence of the fourth clonal type. Int J Parasitol 41:1139–1147

Dunn D, Wallon M, Peyron F et al (1999) Mother to child transmission of toxoplasmosis: risk estimates for clinical counselling. Lancet 353:1829–1833

Dutra MS, Béla ST, Peixoto-Rangel AL et al (2013) Association of a NOD2 gene polymorphism and T-helper 17 cells with presumed ocular toxoplasmosis. JID 207:152–163

Elbez-Rubinstein A, Ajzenberg D, Dardé ML et al (2009) Congenital toxoplasmosis and reinfection during pregnancy: case report, strain characterization, experimental model of reinfection, and review. J Infect Dis 199(2):280–285

EMSCOT- European Multicentre Study on Congenital Toxoplasmosis (2007) Screening for congenital toxoplasmosis: accuracy of immunoglobulin M and immunoglobulin A tests after birth. J Med Screen 14:8–13

European Multicentre Study on Congenital Toxoplasmosis- EMSCOT (2008) Predictors of retinochoroiditis in children with congenital toxoplasmosis: European, prospective cohort study. Pediatrics 121(5):e1215–e1222

Filisetti D, Odile Villard HI, Escande B et al (2015) Contribution of neonatal amniotic fluid testing to diagnosis of congenital toxoplasmosis. J Clin Microbiol 53:1719–1721

Fox BA, Rommereim LM, Guevara RB et al (2016) The Toxoplasma gondii rhoptry kinome is essential for chronic infection. MBio 78(3):e00193–e00116. https://doi.org/10.1128/mBio.00193-16

Freeman K, Salt A, Prusa A et al (2005) Association between congenital toxoplasmosis and parent-reported developmental outcomes, concerns, and impairments, in 3 year old children. BMC Pediatr 5:23

Gangneux F, Dardè ML (2012) Epidemiology and diagnostic strategies for toxoplasmosis. Clin Microbiol Rev 25:264–296

Gilbert RE, Freeman K, Lago EG et al (2008) Ocular sequelae of congenital toxoplasmosis in Brazil compared with Europe. PLoS Negl Trop Dis 2(8):e277

Hintz SR, Slovis T, Bulas D et al (2007) Interobserver reliability and accuracy of cranial ultrasound scanning interpretation in premature infants. J Pediatr 150:592–596

Hutson SL, Wheeler KM, McLone D et al (2015) Patterns of hydrocephalus caused by congenital Toxoplasma gondii infection associate with parasite genetics. Clin Infect Dis 61(12):1831–1834

Jamieson SE, de Roubaix LA, Kuan Tan H et al (2008) COL2A1 and ABCA4 have epigenetically modified and associated with congenital toxoplasmosis. PLoS One 3(6): e2285. https://doi.org/10.1371/journal.pone.0002285

Jamieson SE, Peixoto-Rangel AL, Aubrey AC et al (2010) Evidence for associations between the purinergic receptor P2X7 (P2RX7) and toxoplasmosis. Genes Immun 11(5):374–383

Jones JL, Parise ME, Fiore AE (2014) Neglected parasitic infections in the United States: toxoplasmosis. Am J Trop Med Hyg 90(5):794–799

Knoblauch H, Tennstedt C, Brueck W et al (2003) Two brothers with findings resembling congenital intrauterine infection-like syndrome (pseudo-TORCH syndrome). Am J Med Genet 120A:261–265

L'Ollivier C, Wallon M, Faucher B et al (2012) Comparison of mother and child antibodies that target high-molecular-mass *Toxoplasma gondii* antigens by immunoblotting improves neonatal diagnosis of congenital toxoplasmosis. Clin Vaccine Immunol 19:1326–1328

Li XL, Wei HX, Zhang H et al (2014) A meta analysis on risks of adverse pregnancy outcomes in Toxoplasma gondii infection. PLOS One 9:e97775. https://doi.org/10.1371/journal.pone.0097775

Li X, Pomares C, Gonfrier G et al (2016) Multiplexed anti-toxoplasma IgG, IgM, and IgA assay on plasmonic gold chips: towards making mass screening possible with dye test precision. J Clin Microbiol 54:1726–1733

Liu L, Liu T, Yu L et al (2012) Rrop2(186-533): a novel peptide antigen for detection of IgM antibodies against *Toxoplasma gondii*. Foodborne Pathog Dis 9(1):7–12

Marangoni A, Capretti MG, De Angelis M et al (2014) Evaluation of a new protocol for retrospective diagnosis of congenital toxoplasmosis by use of Guthrie cards. J Clin Microbiol 52:2963–2970

McLeod R, Boyer K, Karrison T et al (2006) Outcome of treatment for congenital toxoplasmosis, 1981-2004: the National Collaborative Chicago-Based, Congenital Toxoplasmosis Study. Clin Infect Dis 42:1383–1394

McLeod R, Lykins J, Noble AG et al (2014) Management of congenital toxoplasmosis. Curr Pediatr Rep 2:166–194

Murat JB, Souvignet A, Fricker-Hidalgo H et al (2015) Assessment of the IgA immunosorbent agglutination assay for the diagnosis of congenital toxoplasmosis on a series of 145 toxoplasmic seroconversions. Clin Vaccine Immunol 22:456–458

Nguyen E, MacDonald WR, Trivedi T et al (2016) Neurons are the primary target cell for the brain- tropic intracellular parasite Toxoplasma gondii. PLoS Pathog 12(2): e1005447. https://doi.org/10.1371/journal. ppat.1005447

Noble AG, Latkany P, Kusmierczyk J et al (2010) Chorioretinal lesions in mothers of children with congenital toxoplasmosis in the National Collaborative Chicago- based Congenital Toxoplasmosis Study. Sci Med (Porto Alegre) 20:20–26

Peyron F, Garweg JG, Wallon M et al (2011) Long-term impact of treated congenital toxoplasmosis on quality of life and visual performance. Pediatr Infect Dis J 30:597–600

Phan L, Kasza K, Jalbrzikowski J et al (2008a) Longitudinal study of new eye lesions in children with toxoplasmosis who were not treated during the first year of life. Am J Ophthalmol 146(3):375–384

Phan L, Kasza K, Jalbrzikowski J et al (2008b) Longitudinal study of new eye lesions in treated congenital toxoplasmosis. Ophthalmology 115(3):553–559

Pinon JM, Dumon H, Chemla C et al (2001) Strategy for diagnosis of congenital toxoplasmosis: evaluation of methods comparing mothers and newborns and standard methods for postnatal detection of immunoglobulin G, M, and A antibodies. J Clin Microbiol 39:2267–2271

Rajapakse S, Shivanthan MC, Samaranayake N et al (2013) Antibiotics for human toxoplasmosis: a systematic review of randomized trials. Pathog Glob Health 107:162–169

Rico-Torres CP, Vargas-Villavicencio JA, Correa D (2016) Is Toxoplasma gondii type related to clinical outcome in human congenital infection? Systematic and critical review. Eur J Clin Microbiol Infect Dis 35:1079–1088

Rilling V, Dietz K, Krczal D et al (2003) Evaluation of a commercial IgG/IgM Western blot assay for early postnatal diagnosis of congenital toxoplasmosis. Eur J Clin Microbiol Infect Dis 22(3):174–180

Romand S, Chosson M, Franck J et al (2004) Usefulness of quantitative polymerase chain reaction in amniotic fluid as early prognostic marker of fetal infection with Toxoplasma gondii. Am J Obstet Gynecol 190(3): 797–802

Saadatnia G, Golkar M (2012) Review on human toxoplasmosis. Scand J Infect Dis 44:805–814

Silveira C, Belfort R Jr, Muccioli C et al (2002) The effect of long-term intermittent trimethoprim/sulfamethoxazole treatment on recurrences of toxoplasmic retinochoroiditis. Am J Ophthalmol 134:41–46

Silveira C, Ferreira R, Muccioli C et al (2003) Toxoplasmosis transmitted to a newborn from the mother infected 20 years earlier. Am J Ophthalmol 136(2): 370–371

Stagni L, Romano MA, Romano A et al (2009) Prenatal screening for congenital toxoplasmosis in Campania: preliminary report on activities and results. Mem Inst Oswaldo Cruz 104(2):374–377

Stramba-Badiale M, Nador F, Porta N et al (1997) QT interval prolongation and risk of life-threatening arrhythmias during toxoplasmosis prophylaxis with spiramycin in neonates. Am Heart J 133(1):108–111

Systematic Review on Congenital Toxoplasmosis Study Group (SYROCOT) (2007) Effectiveness of prenatal treatment for congenital toxoplasmosis: a meta-analysis of individual patients' data. Lancet 369:115–122

Torgerson PR, Mastroiacovo P (2013) The global burden of congenital toxoplasmosis: a systematic review. Bull World Health Organ 91(7):501–508

Torgerson PR, Devleesschauwer B, Praet N et al (2015) World Health Organization estimates of the global and regional disease burden of 11 foodborne parasitic diseases, 2010: a data synthesis. PLoS Med 12(12):e1001940. https://doi.org/10.1371/journal.pmed.1001940

Torres-Morales E, Taborda L, Cardona N et al (2014) Th1 and Th2 immune response to P30 and ROP18 peptides in human toxoplasmosis. Med Microbiol Immunol 203:315–322

Valentini P, Buonsenso D, Barone G et al (2015) Spiramycin/cotrimoxazole versus pyrimethamine/sulfonamide and spiramycin alone for the treatment of toxoplasmosis in pregnancy. J Perinatol 35(2):90–94

Villard O, Cimon B, L'Ollivier C et al (2016) Serological diagnosis of Toxoplasma gondii infection: Recommendations from the French National Reference Center for Toxoplasmosis. Diagn Microbiol Infect Dis 84:22–33

Wallon M, Peyron F, Cornu C et al (2013) Congenital toxoplasma infection: monthly prenatal screening decreases transmission rate and improves clinical outcome at age 3 years. Clin Infect Dis 56(9):1223–1231

Wallon M, Garweg JG, Abrahamowicz M et al (2014) Ophthalmic outcomes of congenital toxoplasmosis followed until adolescence. Pediatrics 133:e601

Wallon M, Kieffer F, Huissoudd C, Peyron F (2015) Cesarean delivery or induction of labor does not prevent vertical transmission of toxoplasmosis in late pregnancy. Int J Gynecol Obstet 129:169–177

Neonatal Bacterial and Fungal Infections

107

Mauro Stronati and Alessandro Borghesi

Contents

Abstract

Neonatal infection is the invasion of the tissue by an infectious organism during the neonatal age. This may be considered early-onset when occurring during the first 72 h of life and late-onset when occurring after the first 72 h of life. Reported rates of neonatal infections range from 6% to 33% and up to 40% in neonates born before 28 weeks' gestational age or with birth weight $<1,000$ g. Septicemia accounts for 45–55% of all infections, followed by lower respiratory tract infections (16–30%) and urinary tract infections (8–18%). The most frequently isolated microorganisms are coagulase-negative *Staphylococci*, group B *Streptococcus*, *Escherichia coli*, other *Enterobacteriaceae* and Gram-negative microorganisms, and, among fungi, *Candida albicans*. Both early-onset and late-onset infections represent a major cause of mortality and morbidity in neonates. Prevention strategies for both early-onset and late-onset infection are available, including prevention of infection

M. Stronati (✉)
Neonatal Intensive Care Unit, Fondazione IRCCS Policlinico 'San Matteo', Pavia, Italy
e-mail: m.stronati@smatteo.pv.it

G. Buonocore et al. (eds.), *Neonatology*,
https://doi.org/10.1007/978-3-319-29489-6_254

associated with premature rupture of membranes and preterm labor, prevention of neonatal group B streptococcal disease, and prevention of neonatal nosocomial infections.

Abbreviations

AAP	American Academy of Pediatrics
ACOG	American College of Obstetricians and Gynecologists
AOM	Acute otitis media
CDC	Centers for Disease Control and Prevention
CFU	Colony-forming unit
CI	Confidence interval
CONS	Coagulase-negative *Staphylococci*
CRP	C-reactive protein
CT	Computerized tomography
CVC	Central venous catheter
DMSA	Dimercaptosuccinic acid
EOS	Early-onset neonatal sepsis
GBS	Group B *Streptococcus*
G-CSF	Granulocyte-colony stimulating factor
HICPAC	Healthcare Infection Control Practices Advisory Committee
IAP	Intrapartum antibiotic prophylaxis
Ig	Immune globulins
IL	Interleukin
IVG	Intravenous immune globulins
LOS	Late-onset neonatal sepsis
MIC	Minimal inhibiting concentration
MRI	Magnetic resonance imaging
MRSA	Methicillin-resistant *Staphylococcus aureus*
NEC	Necrotizing enterocolitis
NICHD	National Institute of Child Health and Human Development
NICU	Neonatal Intensive Care Unit
NTED	Neonatal toxic shock syndrome-like exanthematous disease
OR	Odds ratio
PCR	Polymerase chain reaction
PCT	Procalcitonin
PROM	Premature rupture of membranes
RCOG	Royal College of Obstetricians and Gynaecologists
rRNA	Ribosomal ribonucleic acid
RR	Relative risk
SAA	Serum amyloid A
SSSS	Staphylococcal scalded skin syndrome
TEN	Toxic epidermal necrolysis
TSST-1	Toxic shock syndrome toxin-1
US	Ultrasound
UTI	Urinary tract infection
VAP	Ventilator-associated pneumonia
VLBW	Very low birth weight
VRE	Vancomycin-resistant *Enterococcus*
WHO	World Health Organization

107.1 Salient Points

- Neonatal infections, referred to as the invasion of tissue by an infectious organism, represent a major cause of mortality and morbidity in neonatal intensive care units.
- Neonatal sepsis is the clinical syndrome caused by the host systemic inflammatory response to invading pathogens.
- "Microbiological sepsis" refers to the isolation of a microorganism from a blood culture of a baby with signs of infection and/or abnormal laboratory tests, while the term "clinical sepsis" is used when a neonate with evidence of infection has negative cultures.
- Early-onset sepsis occurs during the first 72 h of life and is usually caused by microorganisms of the maternal genitourinary tract.
- Late-onset sepsis, occurring after the first 72 h of life, is usually caused by nosocomially transmitted or environmental organisms.
- Empirical antibiotic treatment should be started in every neonate with suspected infection, and antibiotics should be stopped after 48–72 h if laboratory and microbiological tests exclude infection, or the spectrum of antibiotics should be narrowed once the microorganism is identified and the antibiogram is available.
- Intrapartum antibiotic prophylaxis is currently the most important preventive measure against early-onset group B streptococcal disease.
- Prevention of late-onset, health care-associated infections is based on strategies that aim at limiting the exposition to pathogens and

interrupting transmission of organisms by health care workers, at reducing susceptibility to pathogens by reducing risk factors while enhancing host defenses and by modulating the host-pathogen interaction, and by promoting the judicious use of antimicrobials.

- The judicious use of antibiotics is the first step in reducing infection and limiting the emergence of resistant strains of microorganisms.

107.2 Introduction

Neonatal infection is the invasion of tissue by an infectious organism during the neonatal age. This may be considered "early-onset" when occurring during the first 72 h of life (very early onset if starting during the first 12 h of life) and "late-onset" when occurring after the first 72 h of life. The two conditions differ in age at the onset, source of infection, route of transmission, clinical presentation, and in terms of prevention possibilities.

Septicemia accounts for 45–55% of all infections, followed by lower respiratory tract infections (16–30%) and urinary tract infections (UTIs, 8–18%) (Clark et al. 2004b; Stolfi et al. 1999).

Infections represent a major cause of mortality and morbidity in the neonatal intensive care units (NICUs), where reported rates range from 6% to 33% (Clark et al. 2004b) and up to 40% in neonates born before 28 weeks' gestational age or with birth weight <1,000 g (extremely low birth weight, ELBW) (Brady 2005).

In the USA, the incidence of early-onset sepsis (EOS) has been estimated to range between 0.77/1,000 and 0.98/1,000 live births (Shane and Stoll 2014). Among very low-birth-weight (weight <1,500 g at birth, VLBW) infants, the rate of EOS has remained stable during the last decades at approximately 1.0% (Kaufman and Fairchild 2004; Hornik et al. 2012; Stoll et al. 2002b; Vergnano et al. 2011). The rates of a first episode of LOS in VLBW infants may vary considerably among centers, ranging from 14% to 36% (Boghossian et al. 2013).

In NICUs, Gram-positive bacteria and particularly coagulase-negative *Staphylococci* (CONS) are the most frequent pathogens associated with nosocomial infections (55–75%), followed by Gram-negative bacteria (18–31%) and fungi (9–13%) (Clark et al. 2004b; Lachassine et al. 2004).

The National Institute of Child Health and Human Development (NICHD) Neonatal Research Network (NRN) reported that 61% of EOS of VLBW infants were caused by Gram-negative microorganisms (*E. coli* in 44% of cases) and 37% by Gram-positive organisms (*S. agalactiae* in 11% of cases), while 70% of LOS of VLBW infants were caused by Gram-positive bacteria, 18% by Gram-negative bacteria, and 12% by fungal organisms (Stoll et al. 2002a, b). CONS were the most frequently isolated late-onset pathogens, accounting for 68% of infections caused by Gram-positive organisms and for 48% of all infections. Other Gram-positive organisms included *S. aureus* (8% of all infections), *Enterococcus* spp., and group B *Streptococcus* (GBS). *Escherichia coli*, *Klebsiella*, *Pseudomonas*, *Enterobacter*, and *Serratia* spp. were the most frequently isolated Gram-negative bacteria. *Candida albicans*, accounting for 6% all infections, was the third most frequently isolated organism.

107.3 Bacterial Infections

107.3.1 Etiology

107.3.1.1 Gram-Positive Bacteria

Coagulase-Negative *Staphylococcus* (CONS)
Colonization and infection by CONS usually occur nosocomially, particularly in VLBW infants with an indwelling intravascular catheter (with higher risk for central venous catheters [CVCs] in place for prolonged times) (Healy et al. 2004); an additional risk factor for CONS sepsis is the use of lipid emulsions in solutions for parenteral nutrition (Freeman et al. 1990; Avila-Figueroa et al. 1998).

Staphylococcus aureus
Infections caused by *S. aureus* are most frequently nosocomial infections and may be superficial,

involving the skin (*impetigo bullosa*, staphylococcal scalded skin syndrome, breast abscess) and the conjunctivae. Deep tissues may be involved (osteomyelitis and septic arthritis, pneumonia, meningitis, infection of ventricular cerebral shunts in neonates with posthemorrhagic hydrocephalus, and endocarditis) with or without associated septicemia (Orscheln et al. 2006) and may induce local pus (cerebral abscesses, empyema, pneumatoceles).

Infants with an indwelling CVC or who have undergone surgical procedures are at increased risk of invasive *S. aureus* infections (Foster 2005).

Enterococci

Enterococci account for a small fraction of nosocomial neonatal sepsis, but in the last two decades an increase in enterococcal infections has been reported, as well as the alarming emergence of vancomycin-resistant *Enterococci* (VRE).

Group B *Streptococcus* (GBS)

GBS (*Streptococcus agalactiae*), the only species belonging to group B of Lancefield classification, is a Gram-positive coccus colonizing the enteric, genital, and urinary tracts of 15–40% of pregnant women (Regan et al. 1996). For GBS sepsis, definitions of EOS and LOS differ from definitions commonly used for other microorganisms, with GBS EOS occurring during the first 6 days of life and GBS LOS occurring at 7 days of life or after (Kaufman and Fairchild 2004).

Approximately 40–70% of infants born to GBS-colonized mothers acquire surface colonization during delivery, and, without *intrapartum* antibiotic prophylaxis, about 1% of colonized full-term infants develop GBS EOS (Kaufman and Fairchild 2004). Maternal vaginal colonization by GBS usually precedes the development of EOS; other risk factors for GBS EOS include maternal fever at delivery (>38 °C), premature rupture of membranes (PROM) if prolonged for more than 18 h before delivery, preterm birth, and GBS urinary tract infection during pregnancy or at delivery (Stronati et al. 2000). Prematurity is the only known risk factor for late-onset invasive streptococcal disease.

107.3.1.2 Gram-Negative Bacteria

Gram-negative sepsis is less frequent than Gram-positive sepsis, but is associated with higher mortality (36% in VLBW neonates) (Stoll et al. 2002a).

Gram-negative pathogens are mainly *Enterobacteriaceae* (*E. coli*, *Klebsiella*, *Serratia* spp.) and *Pseudomonas* (*P. aeruginosa*, *P. mallei*).

Enterobacteriaceae

Enterobacteriaceae colonize the enteric tract soon after birth; invasion of the immature and/or injured mucosa and translocation of organisms to the bloodstream may cause LOS, sometimes associated with necrotizing enterocolitis (NEC).

Among Gram-negative bacteria, *E. coli* is the most frequently isolated organism in term and preterm neonates. In a survey of the *Pediatric Prevention Network* by Sohn et al., *E. coli* was responsible of 8.5% of all NICU infections (Sohn et al. 2001).

Powdered infant formula milk has been implicated as a possible source of Gram-negative pathogens, e.g., a reported association between contamination of powdered milk by *Enterobacter sakazakii* and the occurrence of sepsis and NEC (van Acker et al. 2001; Weir 2002).

Although typically considered a common microorganism responsible for LOS, *E. coli* has emerged, in recent surveillance studies, as an important pathogen associated with EOS, especially among VLBW infants (Shane and Stoll 2014).

Citrobacter

Citrobacter koseri, occasionally causing chorioamnionitis and UTIs in pregnant women, may be vertically transmitted to the neonate causing sepsis and meningitis. Epidemic outbreaks in NICUs and nurseries have been described.

Pseudomonas

Organisms belonging to *Pseudomonas* genus are preferentially transmitted through nosocomial routes of infection in NICUs. *P. aeruginosa* grows in wet environments such as humidified incubators (Harpin and Rutter 1985) and ventilator circuits (Grundmann et al. 1993). Patient-to-patient transmission through the hands of healthcare workers is an important route of transmission (Foca et al. 2000). *P. aeruginosa* may cause focal infections, e.g., pneumonia and severe conjunctivitis. In VLBW infants *P. aeruginosa* is highly virulent: Shah and Gallagher (1998) report a high incidence (39%) of systemic complications (bacteremia, meningitis, cerebral abscess, death) following *Pseudomonas* conjunctivitis. Sepsis by *P. aeruginosa* is associated with a high mortality rate (50–75%) (Leigh et al. 1995).

107.3.1.3 Anaerobic Bacteria

Anaerobic bacteria account for less than 5% of all neonatal sepsis, with premature infants representing a substantial proportion of these cases. Sepsis caused by anaerobic bacteria is almost always associated with preterm maternal chorioamnionitis (Sperling et al. 1988); *Clostridium perfringens* and *Peptostreptococcus* spp. are responsible for the great majority of cases of EOS caused by anaerobic bacteria. LOS caused by Gram-negative anaerobic bacteria (*Bacteroides fragilis*) has been associated with NEC or focal intestinal perforation (FIP). Virulence factors such as pili, fimbriae, and capsular polysaccharide have been reported (Rotimi et al. 1985).

107.3.2 Diagnosis

Diagnosis of infection should be established soon after the onset of clinical signs of infection in order to start effective therapy as soon as possible. Delaying antibiotic treatment may be lethal. Empirical antibiotics therapy (see below) should therefore be started before the results of microbiological investigations are available. The definitive diagnosis of infection is made by appropriate microbiological investigations, but hematological and biochemical investigations are also informative and will determine therapy (Table 1).

107.3.2.1 Microbiological Tests

Isolation of a microorganism from a swab sample or from a body fluid (blood, cerebrospinal fluid [CSF], urines) constitutes the gold standard for the diagnosis of infection and allows for adjustment of antibiotic therapy based on the antibiogram.

Table 1 Diagnostic tests in infants with suspected infection (Modified from Stronati et al. (2000))

Microbiological tests	Cultures (blood, cerebrospinal fluid, urines, swabs)
	Direct identification (*buffy coat*; Gram stain)
	Detection of bacterial antigens (electroimmunophoresis, agglutination, ELISA)
Laboratory tests	Total and differential blood count
	Neutrophils: immature/total
	C-reactive protein
	Fibrinogen, platelet count
	Procalcitonin
	Serum A amyloid
	Cytokines and soluble receptors (IL-6, IL-8, sCD-14, s-TREM)
Molecular diagnostics	Detection and amplification of bacterial DNA (gene coding for 16S RNA) or fungal DNA (gene coding for 18S RNA) by PCR

However, cultures may be falsely negative or positive, making the definitive diagnosis difficult.

False Negative

Blood cultures may be negative despite symptoms and signs of septicemia and even when disseminated bacterial or fungal infection is proven at autopsy. Sensitivity of blood cultures in neonates ranges from 8 to 73% in different studies (Mishra et al. 2006).

Negative blood cultures in infants with sepsis may be due to the administration of antibiotics to the neonate or to the mother during labor, insufficient sample volume, or to a systemic inflammatory response due to noninfectious causes.

Diagnosis of sepsis has become more accurate after the introduction of sensitive and reliable culture tests as "BacTec" or "BacT Alert" that retain high sensitivity even with a small sample size (<0.5 mL) (Buttery 2002).

False Positive

A single positive blood culture from a neonate with clinical signs of infection is considered evidence of sepsis. It has been suggested that two positive cultures may be required to confirm the diagnosis of CONS sepsis because of frequent contamination of samples (Kaufman and Fairchild 2004). Careful disinfection of the skin before taking blood and taking two blood cultures has been effective in reducing the contamination of cultures (Kilbride et al. 2003).

107.3.2.2 Laboratory Tests

Several laboratory tests can make the diagnosis of infection more accurate and timely, including hematologic tests (total and differential blood count) interleukin-6 (IL-6), IL-8, C-reactive protein (CRP), procalcitonin (PCT), and serum A amyloid.

Total white blood cell count (abnormal if <5,000/mL or >20,000/μL) and differential white blood cell count have highly variable degrees of sensitivity (17–90%) and specificity (31–100%) (Weinberg and D'Angio 2006). Serial immature and total neutrophil measurements obtained over 24 h after initiating an evaluation for EOS have been demonstrated to have a high specificity and negative predictive value both in term and preterm neonates and, in conjunction with two blood cultures, could allow early cessation of unnecessary antibiotic therapy (Mikhael et al. 2014).

Thrombocytopenia (<100,000/μL), white blood cell morphology, and single measurements of total neutrophil and immature/total neutrophil ratio have a poor predictive value.

Blood IL-6 and IL-8 concentrations rise 12–24 h before the onset of clinical symptoms and strongly predict infection. However, they are not routinely used by all laboratories because of the rapid fall in blood concentrations after the onset of sepsis and because of expense (Arnon and Litmanovitz 2008).

CRP has a 1,000-fold increase in blood during an acute-phase response (Mishra et al. 2006) and is not influenced by gestational age (Posen and deLemos 1998). Serial measures of CRP seem to have the best predictive value during screening for sepsis, i.e., the sensitivity of a single CRP measurement is about 48–63%, increasing to 90% when the test is repeated 24–48 h after the onset of symptoms (Kaufman and Fairchild 2004). Normal serial CRP measurements may be useful for excluding infection in a neonate with nonspecific symptoms and negative cultures (Ehl et al. 1997) and in guiding the duration of antibiotic therapy.

PCT, a polypeptide precursor of calcitonin, is produced by hepatocytes and monocytes (Mishra et al. 2006), has high sensitivity and specificity (87–100%), and increases during EOS, LOS, and NEC. However, it is not generally available as an emergency diagnostic test and is considered more accurate for LOS than for EOS (Arnon and Litmanovitz 2008; Lopez Sastre et al. 2007).

The diagnostic accuracy of the SAA has been recently evaluated. It is an acute-phase protein induced by IL-6 and IL-8 (Arnon and Litmanovitz 2008), and its diagnostic accuracy is higher than that of CRP in the diagnosis of both EOS and LOS (Arnon et al. 2002, 2007).

Additional biomarkers are not routinely used, but may become valuable tools in the future for either patient stratification according to risk of infection or for early diagnosis. These include additional soluble proteins and cytokines (Srinivasan and Harris 2012); the ApoSAA score computed from plasma apoC2 and SAA (Ng et al. 2010); the heart rate monitoring (Sullivan and Fairchild 2015), cell surface markers (Mazzucchelli et al. 2013), and proteomics and metabolomics (Dessì et al. 2014) for early diagnosis; and the mannose-binding lectin and other proteins of the lectin pathway of complement (Schlapbach et al. 2010; Auriti et al. 2010) and genomics studies (Esposito et al. 2014) for risk stratification.

107.3.2.3 Molecular Diagnostics

The use of molecular techniques (polymerase chain reaction [PCR]) for the diagnosis of neonatal infections is a valuable tool that could reduce the time from the onset of clinical signs to identification of both the pathogen and its virulence and resistance patterns, thus guiding the choice of antimicrobials in the early phases of infection and reducing the use of broad-spectrum antibiotics (van den Brand et al. 2014). The identification of microbial nucleic acids in blood relies on PCR amplification of the gene for the bacterial 16S rRNA or the fungal 18S rRNA, which are not present in humans.

In a study of 548 samples from neonates with suspected sepsis that compared high sensitivity cultural tests (BacTec) with PCR amplification of the gene coding for the 16S rRNA, sensitivity, specificity, and positive and negative predictive values were 96.0%, 99.4%, 88.9%, and 99.8%, respectively. The time to obtain results was 9 h and only 200 μL was required (Jordan and Durso 2000). The high negative predictive value makes this test an important tool to limit the excessive use of antibiotics in neonates with nonspecific symptoms.

107.3.3 Bacterial Sepsis

Sepsis is defined as the clinical syndrome characterized by a host systemic inflammatory response to invading pathogens.

For neonates, "microbiological sepsis" refers to the isolation of a microorganism from a blood culture of a baby with signs of infection and/or abnormal laboratory tests. "Clinical sepsis" is used when a neonate with evidence of infection has negative cultures (Kaufman and Fairchild 2004).

107.3.3.1 Pathogenesis and Routes of Transmission

EOS is associated with maternal complications during pregnancy (preterm birth, premature rupture of membranes, chorioamnionitis). Pathogens associated with EOS are usually organisms of the maternal genitourinary tract. Mortality rates range from 15% to 50% (Stronati et al. 2000).

LOS is usually caused by nosocomially transmitted or environmental organisms. Less commonly, maternal urinary tract organisms colonize the neonate causing later infection. Mortality rates range from 10% to 20% (Stronati et al. 2000).

Very late-onset sepsis (VLOS) are those with the onset after the first 60 days of life in neonates that stay for prolonged times in the NICU.

Neonates may become infected via several routes of transmission. An ascending amniotic infection is thought to be the main route of transmission for EOS. Maternal genital tract organisms (GBS, *E. coli*) ascend through the birth canal and infect the amniotic fluid either through intact amniotic membranes or, more commonly, after the rupture of membranes. Thus, vertically acquired organisms may be aspirated or swallowed by the fetus, penetrate immature mucosae into the bloodstream, and cause sepsis, often with pneumonia.

LOS is generally acquired through horizontal or nosocomial routes of transmission (hands of healthcare workers or parents, water of ventilator circuits and incubators, biomedical instruments such as contaminated stethoscopes). Less commonly, a vertically acquired organism may colonize the neonate and cause LOS later on.

Microorganisms pass into the bloodstream through loss of integrity of the skin and mucosae, and their translocation into deep tissues and bloodstream is increased by repeated trauma due to biomedical devices (endotracheal tubes, nasogastric tubes); alternatively, they may enter the circulation directly through a central venous catheter. Healthcare workers represent the main route of patient-to-patient transmission of microorganisms in the NICU.

Several risk factors predispose the neonate to infection and sepsis: maternal, extrinsic (nosocomial), and intrinsic (the individual susceptibility of the neonate to infection) (Mussi-Pinhata and Rego 2005).

Maternal risk factors include prolonged PROM (>18 h before delivery), intra-amniotic infections, colonization of the maternal genital tract by GBS, maternal infections (UTI, listeriosis), obstetric invasive procedures (amniocentesis, intrauterine transfusions), and low socioeconomic status.

Extrinsic risk factors include:

- *Colonization*. The likelihood of colonization of deep mucosal tissues (respiratory and gastrointestinal tracts) by hospital-acquired organisms is increased by the presence of biomedical devices (endotracheal tubes, nasogastric tubes). Invasive procedures that facilitate the translocation of colonizing organisms into the bloodstream include central venous catheters, total parenteral nutrition, exchange transfusion, chest drainage, prolonged intubation, and frequent tracheal aspirations.
- *CVCs and total parenteral nutrition*. The use of CVCs increases the risk of infection by 3.81- to 7-fold (Lachassine et al. 2004).

Freeman et al. in the early 1990s reported that 14.9 of CONS neonatal infections were associated with the use of CVCs (Freeman et al. 1990 Aug 2), and several subsequent studies have demonstrated a direct correlation between the duration of central venous catheter placement and the incidence of infection (Clark et al. 2004b). In a point prevalence survey by the Pediatric Prevention Network, neonates with a central venous catheter had a relative risk of infection of 3.8 (CI 2.3–6.3, $P < 0.001$) compared to infants without catheters, and the risk was 5.7 (CI 3.5–9.5, $P < 0.001$) for patients receiving total parenteral nutrition (Sohn et al. 2001). See chapter "Prevention of CVC-Related Infections" for the definitions of CVC-related bloodstream infections (CRBSIs).

- *Drugs*. An association between systemic postnatal steroids for chronic lung disease and sepsis has been observed in several studies. Stoll et al. (1999) in a study on 371 VLBW neonates treated with dexamethasone at 14 days of life showed that the incidence of infection was significantly higher in the treated than in the control group (22 vs. 14%).

  The use of antagonists of the histamine type 2 receptor (H2) antagonists for stress gastritis and gastroesophageal reflux increases the risk of both sepsis and NEC in preterm neonates (Stoll et al. 1999; Guillet et al. 2006).

  Prolonged antibiotic therapy selects resistant bacteria and increases the risk of fungal infections (Isaacs 2006). Ampicillin, third-generation cephalosporins, and carbapenems select extended spectrum β-lactamase producing strains of Gram-negative bacteria that are resistant to several antibiotics, not only β-lactams. Similarly, vancomycin selects vancomycin-resistant *Enterococci* and methicillin selects methicillin-resistant *Staphylococci* (Isaacs 2006).
- *Formula milk*. Breast milk is protective for sepsis in both term and preterm neonate. Hylander et al. (1998), in a study of 212 VLBW neonates, showed that the incidence of sepsis was significantly lower in those who were breast-fed compared to those who were formula-fed (19.5% vs. 32.6%; $P = 0.04$).
- *Other risk factors* include overcrowding, prolonged hospital stay, poor attention to good hygiene, and low compliance to hand hygiene (Rondini et al. 1991).

Intrinsic risk factors include:

- *Birth weight and gestational age*. The risk of sepsis increases with decreasing birth weight and gestational age at birth. In a survey conducted by the Neonatal Research Network, the incidence of sepsis was 43% in neonates with birth weight 401–750 g, 28% for 751–1,000 g neonates, 15% for 1,001–1,250 g neonates, and 7% for 1,251–1,500 g neonates. Similarly, the incidence of sepsis was 46% for neonates <25 weeks at birth, 29% for babies born at 25–28 weeks, 10% for babies at 29–32 weeks, and 2% for neonates >32 weeks (Stoll et al. 2002a).
- *Underlying diseases*. Perinatal asphyxia, hyperbilirubinemia, galactosemia, malformations, patent ductus arteriosus, meconium aspiration syndrome, and low Apgar scores increase the risk of infection (Stronati et al. 2000).
- *Immaturity of the immune system*. Neonates have lower IgA levels and lower serum levels of complement factors. Several studies have demonstrated an immaturity in chemotaxis, phagocytosis, and cytotoxicity. Furthermore, maternal-to-fetal transplacental transfer of IgG occurs mainly during the third trimester of pregnancy, and neonates with gestational age <32 weeks have lower IgG levels and an immature humoral immune response (Mussi-Pinhata and Rego 2005). For further details, see Section IX, ▶ Chap. 99, "Fundamentals of Feto-Neonatal Immunology."
- *Gender*. Although many studies have shown that male infants are more likely to develop neonatal infections, particularly by Gram-negative bacteria (Palazzi et al. 2006), studies by the NICHD *Neonatal Research Network* on EOS (Stoll et al. 2002b) and LOS (Stoll et al. 2002a) in VLBW infants failed to confirm this association.

107.3.3.2 Clinical Features

The clinical features of neonatal sepsis are highly variable and depend on the causative organism, the site of the primary infection, neonatal age, and gestation. The lower the gestational age, the more nonspecific the clinical features of sepsis. Thus, clinical features attributable to infection are nonspecific and may also be shown by noninfected neonates. Respiratory distress, disseminated intravascular coagulation, necrotizing enterocolitis, persistent pulmonary hypertension, diminished peripheral perfusion, and septic shock are frequently associated with sepsis (Stronati et al. 2000).

Fanaroff et al. (1998) reported the following clinical signs of sepsis: apnea (55%), gastrointestinal symptoms (43%), dyspnea (29%), lethargy/hypotonia (23%), disturbances in white blood cell count (46%), metabolic acidosis (11%), and hyperglycemia (10%).

Bizzarro et al. reported the following signs in neonates with late-onset sepsis: hypothermia (<36.5 °C, 41%), hyperglycemia (>140 mg/dL, 38%), apnea (38%), bradycardia (30%), hyperthermia (>38 °C, 22%), and hypoglycemia (<40 mg/dL, 7%) (Bizzarro et al. 2005). Organ-specific and systemic signs have been described (Table 2).

Table 2 Clinical signs of neonatal sepsis (Modified from Stronati et al. (2000))

General
Hypothermia, fever, poor feeding
Gastrointestinal tract
Anorexia, vomiting, diarrhea, abdominal distension, hepatomegaly
Respiratory tract
Cyanosis, tachypnea, dyspnea, apnea, respiratory distress
Cardiovascular
Pallor, cold skin, tachycardia, bradycardia, hypotension
Central nervous system
Irritability, lethargy, trembling, seizures, hyporeflexia, hypotonia, bulging fontanelle, irregular breathing, acute crying
Blood
Petechiae, purpura, splenomegaly, pallor, jaundice, bleeding
Urinary tract
Oliguria

107.3.3.3 Prognosis

Both EOS and LOS increase hospital length stay, mortality, and morbidity. Mortality increases with decreasing gestational age and depends on the causative microorganism, ranging between 26% and 42% for Gram-negative sepsis, 8.7–10.1% for Gram-positive sepsis, and 27–28% for fungi (Clark et al. 2004b).

For EOS, the CDC reported a case fatality rate of 10.9% and the NICHD NRN a case fatality rate of 16% (9% for GBS and 33% for *E. coli*) (Shane and Stoll 2014).

For LOS, the NICHD NRN (Stoll et al. 2002a) reported that mortality was significantly higher in VLBW neonates with LOS than in those without LOS (18% vs. 7%, $P < 0.001$) with overall mortality of 10% in VLBW infants. In that study, mortality was 11% in neonates with Gram-positive LOS, 36% in neonates with Gram-negative LOS, and 32% in neonates with fungal sepsis. *Pseudomonas* and *C. albicans* were associated with the highest mortality (44% and 74%, respectively).

The clinical course is usually less severe in Gram-positive compared with Gram-negative sepsis and fungi. In the NICHD NRN study, 76% of deaths due to Gram-negative LOS occurred during the first 7 days from the onset and 24% after day 7. By contrast, only 25% of deaths due to CONS sepsis occurred during the first 7 days and 75% after day 7. Seventy-three percent of deaths due to fungal sepsis occurred during the first 7 days and 27% after day 7 (Stoll et al. 2002a).

107.3.3.4 Therapy

Empirical antibiotic treatment should be started in every neonate (especially preterm neonates) with suspected infection. Antibiotics should be stopped after 48–72 h if laboratory and microbiological tests exclude initial symptoms being due to an infection, or the spectrum of antibiotics should be narrowed once the microorganism is identified and the antibiogram is available (Isaacs 2006; Palazzi et al. 2006; Stronati et al. 2007; Muller-Pebody et al. 2010).

A flowchart for the management of the neonate with suspected sepsis is in Fig. 1. Antibiotic

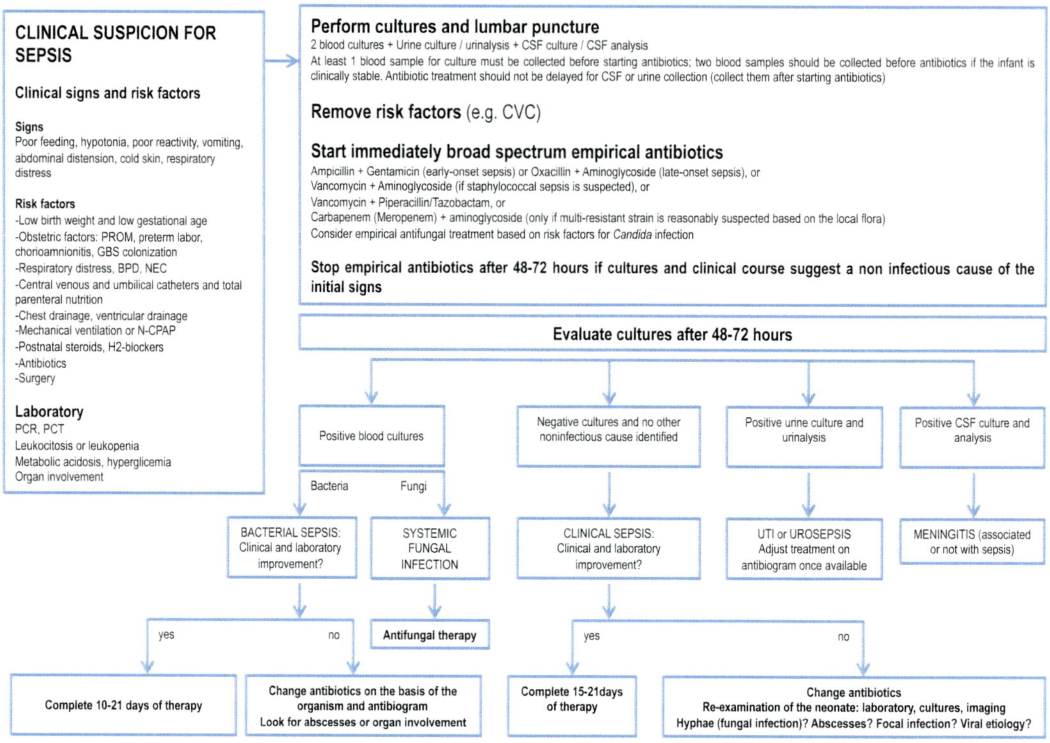

Fig. 1 Flowchart for the management of a newborn infant with suspected sepsis

combinations should be used for empirical treatment. Ampicillin plus gentamicin is still the best antibiotic combination for EOS (Isaacs 2006; Palazzi et al. 2006). Ampicillin is effective against *Enterococci*, some Gram-negative bacteria (*E. coli*, *Proteus*, *Klebsiella*), GBS, and *L. monocytogenes*. Aminoglycosides widen the antimicrobial spectrum, being effective against some ampicillin-resistant *Enterobacteriaceae* (some strains of *E. coli*, *Proteus*, *Klebsiella*) and some ampicillin-resistant *Enterococci*. Gentamicin is the most frequently used aminoglycoside in term and preterm neonates and may be administered in a single daily dose. It is important to note the synergistic effect of ampicillin and gentamicin on several organisms.

Third-generation cephalosporins are effective against many bacterial pathogens and achieve high bactericidal concentrations in the CSF, but they should not be used in the absence of proven bacterial sepsis to reduce the emergence of resistant organisms and fungal infections.

An antistaphylococcal penicillin (oxacillin or nafcillin or flucloxacillin) plus an aminoglycoside is an effective combination for LOS (Isaacs 2006). When a staphylococcal infection by a methicillin-resistant *Staphylococcus* is suspected or proven, vancomycin or teicoplanin should be used in combination with an aminoglycoside. Teicoplanin has fewer side effects (oto- and nephrotoxicity) and a longer half-life than vancomycin, but the emergence of resistant organisms has been described less frequently with vancomycin administration.

Carbapenems may be an option for severe infections by multiresistant organisms. Carbapenems have a very large antimicrobial spectrum (almost all Gram-negative and Gram-positive pathogens) and are resistant to known beta-lactamases. Meropenem is used because of a greater effectiveness against *Haemophilus influenzae*, *Enterobacteriaceae*, and *Pseudomonas*. The incidence of seizures is lower than with imipenem and cilastatin.

The duration of therapy differs for Gram-positive and Gram-negative sepsis. A 10-day antibiotic course seems to be a reasonable option for Gram-positive sepsis; longer courses may be necessary for Gram-negative sepsis and sepsis with organ involvement (2–6 weeks).

Antibiotic dosages are reported in Table 3.

Intravenous immunoglobulins (Ig), once recommended for the treatment of suspected or proven sepsis in neonates, are currently not recommended, according to a Cochrane meta-analysis taking into account nine studies, including the INIS study, which definitely demonstrates no effects on major outcomes of administration of

Table 3 Suggested dosage schedules for systemic antibiotics used in newborns

		Dosage (mg/kg) and interval of administration by weight				
		<1,200 g[b]	1,200–2,000 g		>2,000 g	
Antibiotics	Route	Age 0–4 weeks	Age 0–7 days	Age >7 days	Age 0–7 days	Age >7 days
Amikacin[a] (SDD)	IV, IM	7.5 q12h	7.5 q12h	7.5 q8h	10 q12h	10 q8h
Amikacin[a] (ODD)	IV, IM	18 q48h	15 q36h	15 q24h	15 q24-36h	15 q24h
Ampicillin	IV, IM					
Meningitis		100 q12h	100 q12h	100 q8h	100 q8h	100 q6-8h
Other infections		50 q12h	50 q12h	50 q8h	50 q8h	50 q6-8h
Aztreonam	IV, IM	30 q12h	30 q12h	30 q8h	30 q8-12h	30 q6-8h
Cefazolin	IV, IM	20 q12h	20 q12h	20 q12h	20 q12h	20 q8h
Cefepime	IV, IM	50 q12h	50 q12h	50 q8h	50 q12h	50 q8h
Cefotaxime	IV, IM	50 q12h	50 q12h	50 q8h	50 q12h	50 q8h
Ceftazidime	IV, IM	50 q12h	50 q12h	50 q8h	50 q8h	50 q8h
Clindamycin	IV, IM	5–7.5 q12h	5–7.5 q12h	5–7.5 q8h	5–7.5 q8h	5–7.5 q6h
Gentamicin[a] (SDD)	IV, IM	2.5 q18h	2.5 q12h	2.5 q8h	2.5 q12h	2.5 q8h
Gentamicin[a] (ODD)	IV, IM	5 q48h	4 q36h	4 q24h	4 q24h	4 q24h
Imipenem	IV, IM	20 q12h	20 q12h	20 q12h	20 q12h	20 q8h
Linezolid	IV	10 q8h	10 q12h	10 q8h	10 q12h	10 q8h
Metronidazole	IV	7.5 q48h	7.5 q24h	7.5 q12h	7.5 q12h	15 q12h
Meropenem	IV, IM	20 q12h	20 q12h	20 q8-12h	20 q8-12h	20 q8h
Nafcillin	IV	25 q12h	25 q12h	25 q8h	25 q8h	25–50 q6h
Oxacillin	IV, IM	25 q12h	25 q12h	25 q8h	25 q8h	25–50 q6h
Penicillin G (units)	IV					
Meningitis		50,000 q12h	50,000 q12h	50,000 q8h	50,000 q8h	50,000 q6h
Other infections		25,000 q12h	25,000 q12h	25,000 q8h	25,000 q8h	25,000 q6h
Piperacillin/tazobactam	IV, IM	50–75 q12	50–75 q12h	50–75 q8h	50–75 q8h	50–75 q6h
Rifampin	IV	5–10 q12	5–10 q12h	5–10 q12h	5–10 q12h	5–10 q12h
Ticarcillin-clavulanate		75 q12h	75 q12h	75 q8h	75 q8h	75 q6h
Tobramycin[a] (SDD)	IV, IM	2.5 q18h	2 q12h	2 q8h	2 q12h	2 q8h
Tobramycin (ODD)		5 q48h	4 q36h	4 q24h	4 q24h	4 q24h
Vancomycin[a]	IV	15 q24h	10–15 q12h	10–15 q8-12h	10–15 q8h	10–15 q8h

This table was published as Table 37-11 in Remington & Klein, Wilson, Nizet, Maldonado. Infectious Diseases of the Fetus and Newborn Infant. 2011 Seventh Edition

IM intramuscular, *IV* intravenous, *ODD* once-daily dosing, *PO* oral, *SDD*, standard daily dosing

[a]Adjustments of further dosing intervals should be based on antibiotic half-lives calculated after serum peak and trough concentrations measurements

[b]Dosing for infants <1,200 g is typically based upon limited PK information. The use of most of these drugs remains off-label in neonates due to the need for more pharmacokinetic and safety information. Higher dosing may be indicated for treatment of meningitis or microorganism with higher MIC, such as *Pseudomonas*. In the absence of complete pharmacokinetic information across gestation age and postnatal ages, interhospital variability in dosing guidance is expected

either intravenous IgG or IgM-enriched intravenous IgG (Ohlsson and Lacy 2015).

Exchange transfusion may reduce the severity of sepsis; the volume to be transfused is 160–180 mL/kg, about twice the neonatal blood volume. Benefits depend on the removal of endotoxins, cytokines, and molecules that increase the permeability of vascular endothelium; further advantages depend on the presence in the transfused blood of complement factors, antibodies and coagulation factors, and on the improvement of lung and tissue perfusion. However, there is still little evidence of its effectiveness in reducing morbidity and mortality in patients with sepsis, and its use should be limited to patients with severe sepsis with septic shock and disseminated intravascular coagulation.

Fresh frozen plasma (10–20 mL/kg/day) has been used in the past with the rationale of supplying septic neonates with complement and coagulation factors, but there is no evidence of the benefits of its use in infants with sepsis and is not recommended in the treatment of neonatal sepsis.

The granulocyte-colony stimulating factor (G-CSF) and granulocyte-macrophage-CSF (GM-CSF) are important for differentiation, mobilization, and proliferation of bone marrow white cell precursors. G-CSF, at a dose of 5–10 μg/kg/day subcutaneously or intravenously for 3–10 days, has been shown to improve neutrophil counts in neutropenic neonates and to reduce mortality in neonates with sepsis associated with severe neutropenia and could be considered as an option as adjunctive therapy. Administration should be stopped for neutrophil counts greater than 20,000/μL (El-Ganzoury et al. 2012). However, the authors of a Cochrane review suggest that the limited data on G-CSF to reduce mortality when systemic infection is accompanied by severe neutropenia should be investigated further in adequately powered trials recruiting sufficient infants infected with organisms associated with a significant mortality risk (Carr et al. 2003).

107.3.3.5 Antibiotic Resistance

Data from the Centers for Disease Control and Prevention (CDC) show, in addition to infection caused by methicillin-resistant *S. aureus* (MRSA) and vancomycin-resistant *Enterococcus faecium* (VRE), rapidly increasing rates of infection due to multidrug- or even pandrug-resistant microorganisms. Several highly resistant Gram-negative pathogens, namely, *Acinetobacter* species, multidrug-resistant *P. aeruginosa*, and multidrug-resistant (extended spectrum β-lactamase – ESBL – and carbapenemase-producing) *Klebsiella* species and *Escherichia coli* (carbapenem-resistant *Enterobacteriaceae*), have emerged as significant pathogens worldwide (Boucher et al. 2009). The outbreak caused by those microorganisms may limit our ability to treat infection and may result in high mortality rates inside the NICUs.

Tsai et al. reported 1,106 bacteremia episodes in 8 years in their NICU; 35.5% were caused by Gram-negative organisms and 18.6% by multidrug-resistant strains. The most frequent mechanism of resistance was ESBL production (67.1%), mainly by *K. pneumoniae* (59.6%). Previous antibiotic exposures to third-generation cephalosporin ($P < 0.001$) and carbapenem ($P = 0.017$) were identified as independent risk factors (Tsai et al. 2014).

Datta et al. reported the trend of carbapenem susceptibility in *Enterobacteriaceae* that caused septicemia in their NICU over a 5-year period (2007–2011). One hundred five *Enterobacteriaceae* including *E. coli* ($n = 27$), *K. pneumoniae* ($n = 68$), and *Enterobacter* spp. ($n = 10$) were isolated from the blood of septicemic neonates. In their study, NDM-1 (New Delhi metallo-β-lactamase) was the only carbapenemase identified, detected in 14% of the isolates. NDM-1-producing isolates were resistant to other broad-spectrum antibiotics and possessed other resistance molecules including ESBLs, AmpCs, 16S-rRNA methylases, AAC-Ib-cr (Stoll et al. 2004b), bleomycin-resistant gene, and class 1 integron (Datta et al. 2014).

In another study, Cantey et al. reported an outbreak caused by ESBL-producing *K. pneumoniae* in a III level NICU. The cohort consisted of 61 infants present in the NICU during the outbreak, from April 26, 2011, to May 16, 2011. The index case was an 18-day-old infant born at 25 weeks gestation who developed septicemia from ESBL-producing *K. pneumoniae*. A multidisciplinary team formulated a plan that allowed to control the outbreak and to eradicate the infecting strain. The study well exemplifies how quickly these microorganisms may spread in NICUs: despite the efforts that limited the transmission of the microorganism and allowed quick eradication, 11 infants were either infected or colonized and two infants, in the same room of the index case, developed sepsis from ESBL-producing *Klebsiella* within 48 h and both expired (Cantey et al. 2013).

Novel antibiotics or new compounds able to revert bacterial resistance or virulence by targeting the resistance or virulence genes have been discovered or are under investigation and may be used in the future. The primary goal, however, should be the prevention of the spread of multidrug-resistant microorganisms inside the NICUs, as discussed later in the chapter (see section "Prevention of Early- and Late-Onset Infections").

107.3.4 Meningitis

Isolation of a microorganism from a CSF culture is considered evidence of meningitis.

A national survey of the British Paediatric Surveillance Unit (BPSU) reports an annual incidence of viral and bacterial neonatal meningitis of 0.39/1,000 births (Holt et al. 2001).

Etiology, risk factors, and pathogenesis of neonatal meningitis are similar to those of neonatal sepsis.

Early-onset meningitis (onset during the first 72 h of life, during the first 6 days for GBS) is usually caused by vaginal flora microorganisms transmitted vertically to the fetus (GBS, *E. coli*, *L. monocytogenes*); late onset meningitis (with onset after the first 72 h of life, after the first 6 day of life for GBS) is caused by community or nosocomially acquired organisms (mainly Gram-negative bacteria and *Staphylococci*) (Kaufman and Fairchild 2004).

In the survey by the BPSU of 274 neonates (age <28 days) treated for meningitis during the years 1996–1997, the most frequently isolated organism was GBS (25%), followed by *E. coli* (10%), *L. monocytogenes* (3%), other Gram-positive *Bacilli* (6%), other Gram-negative *Bacilli* (4%), *S. pneumoniae* (3%), and *C. albicans* (2%) (Holt et al. 2001). There was a viral etiology in 7% of cases, and no organism was isolated in 35% of cases.

Stoll et al. (2004b) reported on 9,641 VLBW newborn infants born at centers of the NICHD NRN. Gram-positive bacteria (63%) were most frequently associated with the first episode of late-onset meningitis and CONS accounted for 29% of cases, *Enterococcus* spp. accounted for 13%, *S. aureus* for 8%, and GBS for 7% of cases. Gram-negative bacteria were associated with 19% of cases of late-onset meningitis (*E. coli* accounting for 7%). Fungal organisms were associated with 18% of cases and *C. albicans* accounted for 13% of cases.

Frequently, meningitis is associated with, or is a complication of, neonatal sepsis, but there may be meningitis without bacteremia (Malbon et al. 2006; Garges et al. 2006). In the study of the NICHD NRN, meningitis occurred in 7% VLBW neonates with positive blood cultures compared with 1.5 neonates with negative blood cultures ($P < 0.001$), but about one third of neonates with meningitis (45/134) had negative blood cultures (Stoll et al. 2004b).

Microorganisms may reach the central nervous system and the meninges through breaks in the skin and consequent invasion of soft tissues and cranial sutures, but in many cases organisms reach the choroid plexus by a hematogenous route (Palazzi et al. 2006).

The clinical diagnosis of meningitis in the neonate is often difficult (especially in the preterm neonate) because clinical signs are often nonspecific and subtle. Meningitis can occur without systemic spread of the microorganism, and sometimes it is suspected late during the course of the disease when antibiotic treatment has already been started. Thus, the risk of underestimating the incidence of meningitis and of undertreating an infant with meningitis is very high (Stoll et al. 2004a).

Clinical signs of neonatal meningitis are similar to those of neonatal sepsis: fever, lethargy, vomiting, anorexia, respiratory distress, apnea, seizures, irritability, jaundice, bulging fontanelle, and neck stiffness. Perlman et al. (1992) reported ten cases of late-onset meningitis where the age at the onset was 20 ± 14 days. Clinical signs were nonspecific: apnea and bradycardia in eight neonates, abdominal distension in five, hyponatremia (<130 mEq/L), oliguria, and weight gain (syndrome of inappropriate secretion of antidiuretic hormone) in three. Specific signs were observed in three neonates: seizures in two and third cranial nerve palsy in one. Cranial US abnormalities were found in seven out of ten neonates (70%) and included progressive enlargement of cerebral ventricles (six cases), thalamic echolucency (three cases), ventriculitis (four cases), and cystic leukomalacia (one case). Placement of a ventricular shunt was necessary in all six cases with enlargement of cerebral ventricles.

The diagnosis of meningitis depends on the lumbar puncture for the examination of the CSF (cell count, chemistry, and cultures). Imaging techniques (ultrasonography, magnetic resonance imaging) are mainly useful for prognosis or to establish whether there are complications.

There is debate about whether a lumbar puncture should be always performed in the investigation of an infant with suspected sepsis. Although cardiovascular and respiratory instability may often preclude the immediate performance of the procedure, the risk of undertreatment is very high. Several authors recommend examination of the CSF as a routine during the investigation of suspected sepsis and not only when meningitis is suspected (Malbon et al. 2006).

Garges et al. (2006) evaluated the diagnostic accuracy of cell count and chemistry of the CSF in 9,111 neonates ≥34 weeks: 95 had a microbiological diagnosis of meningitis. In their study, neither white blood cells nor protein or glucose levels in CSF were accurate predictors of neonatal meningitis. Infants with culture-proven meningitis had a mean of 477 white blood cells/mm^3 (0–15,900; interquartile range 38–1,950) in the CSF, higher than infants without meningitis. However, the authors observed that about 5% of infants with bacterial meningitis had 0–1 white blood cells/mm^3 in the CSF, and about 10% of infants with bacterial meningitis had a white blood cell count in the CSF ≤3/mm^3. The sensitivity and specificity for bacterial meningitis of a white blood cell count in the CSF > 0/mm^3 were 97% and 11%, respectively. If a cutoff value of >21/mm^3 was used, sensitivity and specificity were 79% and 81%, respectively. Glucose and protein levels are also very variable and poor predictors of culture-proven meningitis. However, the cell content and biochemical examination of the CSF remains invaluable in the management of an infant with suspected meningitis while culture results are awaited. Suspected bacterial or fungal meningitis should always be confirmed by a positive CSF culture.

The choice of antibiotics is the main tool for the treatment of meningitis, and should take account of potential pathogens (maternal or nosocomial) and their spectrum of sensitivity (based on patterns of sensitivity of previous isolates). To treat all potential pathogens, a combination of three antibiotics should be considered for initial empirical antibiotic therapy (usually ampicillin with a third-generation cephalosporin and an aminoglycoside). Once culture results are available, antibiotic therapy can be modified and one antibiotic can be withdrawn on the basis of the isolated organism and its sensitivity pattern.

Ampicillin is effective against GBS and against *L. monocytogenes*, which is resistant to third-generation cephalosporins.

In GBS meningitis, suggested by Gram stain of the CSF or confirmed by culture, high doses of ampicillin (up to 300–400 mg/kg/day) or penicillin (up to 450,000 U/kg/day) should be used in combination with an aminoglycoside (usually gentamicin) (Heath et al. 2003).

Third-generation cephalosporins are effective against several Gram-negative bacteria and rapidly achieve therapeutic concentrations in the CSF (50–100-fold the MIC). This is in contrast to other antibiotics, such as aminoglycosides (which reach concentrations 2.5-fold the MIC) (Kaufman and Fairchild 2004). Cefotaxime is effective against the great majority of Gram-negative pathogens but not against *P. aeruginosa* (which is sensitive to ceftazidime).

For multiresistant organisms, meropenem together with an aminoglycoside may be a reasonable choice.

Antibiotic therapy should be started as soon as possible and continued for at least 21 days. The effectiveness of the initial empirical antibiotic therapy should be proven by a negative CSF culture, performed 24–48 h after the onset of symptoms and a lumbar puncture for CSF culture before the withdrawal of the antibiotic treatment. If the CSF is not sterile at 24–48 h, a focal infection of the brain (cerebral abscess, subdural empyema, obstructive ventriculitis) should be suspected and excluded by imaging techniques (Heath et al. 2003).

A herpes simplex virus encephalitis should be always considered in a neonate with suspected meningitis. Aciclovir (20–30 mg/kg every 8 h) should be started when Gram staining of the cerebrospinal fluid is negative and should be withdrawn when the herpetic infection has been excluded (Heath et al. 2003).

No consensus has yet been reached on the effectiveness of corticosteroid therapy with dexamethasone to improve the prognosis of infants with meningitis, and no multicenter randomized clinical trials have been performed.

Neonatal meningitis has a high mortality and morbidity. In the BPSU survey (Holt et al. 2001), the mortality rate for neonates with meningitis during 1996–1997 was 6.6%, still high but less than the 19.8% reported by a previous study in 1985–1987.

The neurologic prognosis following neonatal meningitis is generally poor. In a study of 274 babies, who developed meningitis at $\leq$28 days, there were mild-to-moderate neurologic disabilities in 12% of babies with birth weight >2,500 g, 31% for babies with birth weight 1500.2499 g, and 44% for babies with birth weight <1,500 g (Holt et al. 2001). 7.3% had severe disability, 18.2% moderate disability, and 24.1% mild disability (Bedford et al. 2001). Neurologic sequelae following neonatal meningi tis include learning and language defects, motor disorders, seizures, hearing and visual defects, and behavioral disturbances.

107.3.5 Pneumonia

Neonatal pneumonia may be early or late onset. Some authors define early-onset pneumonia as pneumonia during the first 48 h of life and late-onset pneumonia after the first 48 h of life. Other reports define pneumonia as early onset when arising during the first 7 days of life and late onset when the onset as occurring after the first week of life.

Early-onset neonatal pneumonia is caused by pathogens colonizing the birth canal or infect the amniotic fluid (especially after prolonged rupture of membranes or in the presence of chorioamnionitis) and that are inhaled by the fetus during labor. Symptoms may present at birth as neonatal respiratory distress or appear during the first days of life. Neonatal pneumonia is often associated with fetal asphyxia; the mechanism for this association is not certain, but some authors hypothesize that organisms are inhaled during gasping movements caused by asphyxia (Duke 2005; Nissen 2007).

Pathogens may be acquired in utero and localize to the fetal lung causing congenital pneumonia. *Congenital pneumonia* is rarely a focal infection. It presents most often as a part of a systemic congenital infection, acquired transplacentally because of a systemic maternal infection associated with chorioamnionitis or, less frequently, associated with asymptomatic maternal infections, e.g., human immunodeficiency virus, cytomegalovirus, *L. monocytogenes*, *M. tuberculosis*, and *T. pallidum* (Duke 2005).

The term *intrauterine pneumonia* defines an inflammatory disease of the lungs, which is frequently associated with low Apgar scores, respiratory distress syndrome, or even intrauterine death of the fetus. It is usually diagnosed at autopsy in stillbirths or in babies dying during the first days of life; the etiology may be infectious (amniotic infection) or noninfectious (fetal asphyxia) (Barnett and Klein 2006).

Late-onset neonatal pneumonia may be community acquired, nosocomially transmitted in hospitalized neonates, or, rarely, may represent the clinical evolution of an infection acquired in utero.

Pathogens that may cause pneumonia in the neonate are similar to those responsible for sepsis and meningitis (Duke 2005; Nissen 2007). In one study of 261 neonates admitted during the first 4 days of life with respiratory distress, cultures of tracheal aspirates, blood, and CSF demonstrated a prevalence of Gram-positive bacteria (701%) compared with Gram-negative bacteria (29%). GBS (19%) was the most frequently isolated Gram-positive organism, followed by *S. epidermidis* (13%), *S. aureus* (10%), and *S. pneumoniae* (10%). Among Gram-negative bacteria, *E. coli* was the most frequently isolated (13%), followed by *H. influenzae* (6.5%) and *Proteus mirabilis* (6.5%) (Mussi-Pinhata et al. 2004). The WHO young infant study (studying neonates aged 7–29 days) reported *S. pneumoniae* as the most frequent etiologic agent of late-onset community-acquired neonatal pneumonia, followed by *S. aureus*, *Klebsiella*, and *S. epidermidis* (The WHO Young Infants Study Group 1999).

Other causes of neonatal pneumonia are:

- *Treponema pallidum*, frequently associated with poor clinical conditions and severe hypoxemia.
- *Chlamydia trachomatis*, causing a characteristic form of pneumonia with hyperinflation and diffuse bilateral infiltrates of the lungs on chest X-ray, sometimes with a peripheral blood eosinophilia, and the diagnosis is confirmed by an increase in anti-*Chlamydia* IgM.
- *Mycobacterium tuberculosis*, acquired transplacentally or following inhalation of amniotic fluid, and causing pneumonia with a nonspecific clinical course, which may be chronic or acute and which is characterized by multiorgan involvement.
- *L. monocytogenes*, responsible for fulminant sepsis, sometimes associated with pneumonia (Nissen 2007).

The differential diagnosis of neonatal respiratory distress should include viral pneumonia as possible etiology. Viruses causing pneumonia in the neonate include respiratory syncytial virus, metapneumovirus, influenza virus, parainfluenza virus, and adenovirus.

Clinical manifestations of neonatal pneumonia include focal signs (e.g., respiratory distress syndrome) and general signs of infection (poor feeding, lethargy, hypothermia, or hyperthermia) (Mathur et al. 2002). In the three studies of neonates with radiologically confirmed pneumonia, signs included tachypnea (60–89% of cases) and increased respiratory effort (in more than 80% of cases); coughing was not present in about 60% of cases (Shakunthala et al. 1978; Misra et al. 1991; Singhi and Singhi 1990).

The diagnosis of pneumonia is made on the basis of a progressive infiltrate on chest radiography associated with the isolation of a pathogen. However, pulmonary infiltrates on chest radiography may be due to other disease processes: meconium aspiration syndrome, atelectasis, and bronchopulmonary dysplasia (Baltimore 2003). The use of lung ultrasound has been proposed as an adjunctive method to improve the accurateness of the diagnosis of neonatal pneumonia (Cattarossi 2013).

The differential diagnosis of neonatal pneumonia includes diseases associated with respiratory distress syndrome (hyaline membrane disease often not easily distinguishable in the preterm neonate from early-onset pneumonia, transient tachypnea of the neonate, meconium aspiration syndrome, perinatal asphyxia, sepsis, pneumothorax and pneumomediastinum, and congenital defects including congenital heart defects, diaphragmatic hernia, and lung malformations) (Jones et al. 2014). Nonspecific signs of infection are similar to those of other neonatal infections.

Difficulties in the diagnosis of neonatal infections depend on the poor specificity of clinical signs, imaging techniques, and laboratory tests. Guidelines from the CDC and Prevention National Nosocomial Infections Surveillance system included criteria for the diagnosis of pneumonia for infants aged <1 year, but specific criteria for the neonatal age are not provided (Baltimore 2003; Cernada et al. 2014).

In ventilated patients, ventilator-associated pneumonia (VAP) is an extremely difficult diagnosis, particularly in preterm infants. The incidence ranges between 2.7 and 10.9 episodes per 1,000 ventilator days in developed countries and may reach up to 37.2 cases per 1,000 ventilator days in developing countries; the use of different diagnostic criteria in different studies may contribute to this variability (Cernada et al. 2014). Stolfi et al. (1999) define VAP as a pneumonia in a ventilated infant in the presence of the following: (a) onset after at least 24 h of mechanical ventilation and/or (b) onset not later than 48 h after withdrawal of mechanical ventilation. The most common pathogens isolated in the neonatal VAP are *P. aeruginosa* and *S. aureus* (Cernada et al. 2014). Apisarnthanarak et al. (Apisarnthanarak et al. 2003) report 211 newborns ventilated for more than 48 h: signs of VAP included hypothermia (77%), tachypnea >75/min (65%), increase in bronchial secretions (50%), bradycardia <100/min (35%), fever (23%), and apnea (15%). Laboratory findings included purulent tracheal aspirate (>25 leukocytes per high power field) (46%) and thrombocytopenia (15%).

Mechanical ventilation is the most important risk factor for nosocomial pneumonia (Barnett and Klein 2006). Humidification systems and ventilator circuits represent a source of organisms, mainly *P. aeruginosa*. In a study on 170 newborn infants ventilated for more than 48 h, Petdachai (2004) found that the presence of an umbilical catheter ($P = 0.007$), respiratory distress syndrome ($P = 0.03$), and the presence of an orogastric tube ($P = 0.01$) were all independent risk factors for VAP.

Empiric treatment is based on the combination of two antibiotics, ampicillin with an aminoglycoside (usually gentamicin). If a staphylococcal infection is suspected (pneumatoceles, empyema, skin abscesses or pustules, or associated omphalitis), an antistaphylococcal penicillin (cloxacillin, flucloxacillin) or vancomycin should be used instead of ampicillin. Before antibiotic treatment, blood and urine cultures should always be performed to guide treatment in case first-line empiric antibiotic therapy is ineffective. Duration of the antibiotic course depends on the microorganism: Gram-negative or GBS pneumonia should be treated for at least 10 days, but longer courses are needed for staphylococcal pneumonia (3–6 weeks). *C. trachomatis* pneumonia should be treated with a macrolide (erythromycin 50 mg/kg/day in four doses) for 2 weeks.

Treatment of pneumonia should include the treatment of hypoxemia (supplemental oxygen and, if necessary, mechanical ventilation), drainage of pleural purulent effusions, and the maintenance of hydration status and ion balance.

107.3.6 Urinary Tract Infections (UTIs)

UTI is generally defined as the presence of an organism in the urinary tract, which is usually sterile. Urosepsis is the isolation of the same microorganism from urines and blood.

In the neonate, the incidence of UTIs is 0.1–1%, increasing to 14% in febrile neonates (Kanellopoulos et al. 2006). During the first months of life, the incidence is higher in males than in females, and this ratio is reversed after the third month (Larcombe 1999).

Kanellopoulos et al. (2006) evaluated 62 term neonates with UTI (51 males and 11 females). The pathogen most frequently isolated was *E. coli* (73%) followed by *Proteus mirabilis*, *Klebsiella pneumoniae*, *K. oxytoca*, *Proteus vulgaris*, *P. aeruginosa*, *Enterobacter aerogenes*, and *Morganella morganii*. Other potential pathogens for UTIs include GBS, *S. aureus*, and *Enterococcus* spp. (Zorc et al. 2005). *E. coli* is the microorganism most frequently isolated in infants without vesicoureteral reflux, while in the neonates with vesicoureteral reflux, other Gram-negative bacteria are most frequently isolated.

During the first 48–72 h of life, the urine is usually sterile. In a retrospective study of 369 neonates with signs of infection by Tamim et al., blood and urine samples were cultured during the first 24 h of life: no urine culture was positive, while blood culture was positive in eight neonates (2%) (Tamim et al. 2003).

Lower urinary tract colonization after birth is the first step in the pathogenesis of a UTI in a neonate with risk factors for UTIs. Such risk factors include obstructive uropathies (malformations and functional abnormalities of the urinary tract, including urethral valves and phimosis, reported in up to 4% of cases) and vesicoureteral reflux, reported in 25–40% of cases (Kanellopoulos et al. 2006; Larcombe 1999). A UTI is often the first clinical sign of a urinary tract malformation.

During the neonatal period, UTIs are characterized by an elevated incidence of ascending infection and associated sepsis (Zorc et al. 2005); organisms that enter the lower urinary tract may easily reach the upper urinary tract and infect the kidney, leading to a systemic infection (urosepsis), or, less frequently, the kidney may represent the secondary localization of a sepsis (Long and Klein 2006).

Clinical signs of UTIs overlap with those of sepsis; therefore, every neonate with age >3 days with suspected sepsis should undergo diagnostic evaluation for UTIs (Bauer et al. 2003). The presence of fever has been always considered in clinical practice as an indirect sign of upper urinary tract involvement (Zorc et al. 2005).

Kanellopoulos et al. (2006) reported the most common signs of UTI during the neonatal age as fever (77% of cases), poor feeding (48%), lethargy (26%), jaundice (18%), diarrhea (13%), vomiting (8%), and failure to thrive (7%). In their study, the mean age at onset was 20 days for males and 18 days for females. Twenty-four percent of neonates (14/51 males, 1/11 female) had vesicoureteral reflux; there was pyelonephritis in 39% and urinary tract malformations in 8% (including hydronephrosis and ureterohydronephrosis, pyelectasis, double collecting system, posterior urethral valves). UTI should be excluded for every neonate with nonspecific clinical signs, such as poor feeding and failure to thrive.

The diagnosis of UTI should be confirmed by positive urine culture. As urines may be easily contaminated, UTI is defined as the isolation of at least 100 colony-forming units/mL (CFU/mL) from a specimen obtained by suprapubic bladder aspiration or at least 10,000 CFU/mL from a sterile bladder catheterization (Bauer et al. 2003). In preterm infants, lower colony counts may indicate a UTI, especially in the case of Gram-negative bacteria or *Candida* spp. (Kaufman and Fairchild 2004). However, Hoberman et al. (1994) found that 65% of cultures with bacterial counts of 10,000–49,000 CFU/mL yielded Gram-positive bacteria or mixed flora, both indicating contamination rather than infection. The false-positive rate is further increased by using bags for urine specimens (Zorc et al. 2005). Specificity of microbiological diagnosis may be improved by indirect signs of UTI at urinalysis (pyuria, bacteriuria), thus allowing differentiation of infection from contamination. It has been calculated that the positive predictive value of a positive culture obtained by bag may increase from 15% to ~75% in the presence of a positive nitrite test (Newman 2011). Urinary leukocyte esterase, nitrites, and leukocyte count and an increase in blood inflammatory markers suggest upper UTI. Sepsis and meningitis are frequently associated with UTI in the neonate, and a blood culture should be always performed before starting antibiotics. A lumbar puncture should be considered for febrile babies (Long and Klein 2006).

Treatment should be started immediately after taking blood for culture. Sepsis cannot be excluded until blood culture results are available and the initial empirical antibiotic therapy for UTIs is identical to that of sepsis (Long and Klein 2006). The clinician should base the choice of agent on local antimicrobial sensitivity patterns (if available) and should adjust the choice according to sensitivity testing of the isolated uropathogen. A penicillin (ampicillin, piperacillin) and an aminoglycoside (gentamicin, tobramycin) are the first-choice antibiotics. Therapy should last for 10–14 days, but longer courses may be needed for relapses or malformations. A second urine culture should be taken 48 h after starting therapy to assess the effectiveness of treatment (Long and Klein 2006).

About 25–40% of infants with UTI suffer from vesicoureteral reflux, defined as retrograde flow of urine in the ureters and/or the collecting system of the kidney. This is associated with a high risk of pyelonephritis, which, especially when relapsing, is associated with renal scarring, hypertension, and chronic renal insufficiency (McDonald et al. 2000; Bundy 2007).

The American Academy of Pediatrics (AAP) published in 2011 an update of the AAP 1999 UTI practice parameter (Newman 2011; Finnell et al. 2011; Subcommittee on Urinary Tract Infection SCoQI, Management and Roberts 2011). The guideline and technical report address key issues in the management of UTI in children aged 2–24 months, most of which are applicable to neonates:

- Diagnosis is based on the presence of pyuria and at least 50,000 CFUs per mL of a single uropathogen in an appropriately collected specimen of urine (see above for the discussion about the different collection methods); urinalysis alone does not provide a definitive diagnosis.
- After 7–14 days of antimicrobial treatment, close clinical follow-up monitoring should be maintained, with evaluation of the urine during subsequent febrile episodes to permit prompt diagnosis and treatment of recurrent infections.
- Ultrasonography of the kidneys and bladder should be performed to detect anatomic abnormalities requiring further evaluation (e.g., additional imaging or urologic consultation).
- Routine voiding cystourethrogram after the first UTI is not recommended.
- Voiding cystourethrogram is indicated if renal and bladder ultrasounds reveal hydronephrosis, scarring, or other findings that would suggest either high-grade vesicoureteral reflux or obstructive uropathy, as well as in other atypical or complex clinical circumstances. Voiding cystourethrogram also should be performed if there is a recurrence of febrile UTI.

A renal ultrasound should be performed in all neonates with UTI. Although its ability to detect scars in the renal parenchyma is limited, it allows for detection of dilation of the renal collecting system and the exclusion of renal abscesses or obstructive diseases (Johnson 1999).

A voiding cystourethrogram, when indicated, will detect and assess the severity of vesicoureteral reflux (grades I–V, from mildest to severe).

As the risk of recurrent UTI is high in the presence of a vesicoureteral reflux, antibiotic prophylaxis should be started and continued in neonates with confirmed vesicoureteral reflux (Bundy 2007; Darmstadt et al. 2005). Prophylaxis should be performed with a single daily oral antibiotic dose given at night at half of the normal dosage. Cephalosporins and amoxicillin are the most used antibiotics.

Antibiotic prophylaxis may be appropriate for low-grade reflux (grades I–II) which frequently resolves spontaneously during the first year of life, but grade V reflux should be treated surgically. Treatment for grade III, IV, or V reflux should be decided with the involvement of a pediatric urologist and should take into account the probability of spontaneous resolution, the presence of renal scars, and the failure of medical treatment (poor compliance, appearing of resistance to antibiotics, side effects of antibiotics).

Renal scintigraphy (with dimercaptosuccinic acid (DMSA)) is indicated in all infants with grade III, IV, or V reflux or in the presence of renal injury at ultrasound.

The follow-up of a UTI includes urine culture and urinalysis for every unexplained febrile episode. The presence of vesicoureteral reflux should be monitored (annually or less frequently) until resolution or surgical correction.

107.3.7 Osteomyelitis and Septic Arthritis

Osteomyelitis is the infection of the bone and/or the bone marrow. It may be acute or chronic, but in the neonatal age, the course is usually acute. Septic arthritis is the infection of a joint and may present in isolation or as the complication of osteomyelitis (Offiah 2006). Osteomyelitis is infrequent during the neonatal period with a reported incidence of 1–3/1,000 admissions in NICU (Wong et al. 1995).

The pathogen most frequently isolated from infants with osteomyelitis or osteoarthritis is *S. aureus*; other organisms include *C. albicans*, *E. coli*, GBS, and, especially when CVCs are in place, CONS (Offiah 2006; Wong et al. 1995). Wong et al. (1995) studied 94 infants with age 0–3 months who were investigated for osteomyelitis: in 28 out of 94, a microorganism was isolated, including methicillin-sensitive *S. aureus* in 16 cases, methicillin-resistant *S. aureus* in 7 cases, *E. coli* in 3 cases, and GBS in 2 cases.

Organisms may reach the bones by hematogenous spread, which seems to be the most frequent route of infection in neonates, particularly those with vascular catheters. Less often, the skin and tissues surrounding the bones are the site of infection (Offiah 2006).

During the neonatal period, osteomyelitis is frequently associated with arthritis. This association is explained by the vascular supply to the epiphysis and metaphysis in the newborn. In adults and older children, the blood supply for each structure is provided by separate vascular networks, while in the neonate before ossification, epiphyseal cartilage growth depends on metaphyseal vessels. Through these vessels, infection reaches the epiphysis and the joint causing septic arthritis (Offiah 2006).

Risk factors for osteomyelitis include preterm birth, the coexistence of a UTI or neonatal respiratory distress, and the presence of vascular catheters (Offiah 2006; Frederiksen et al. 1993). Wong et al. (1995) reported 30 infants with osteomyelitis, of whom 17 were mechanically ventilated preterm neonates, and four were full-term neonates undergoing intensive care.

Clinical suspicion of osteomyelitis must be confirmed by laboratory and radiological tests. During the early stages, clinical signs may be nonspecific, but swelling or immobility of the limb is common. Physical examination is often characterized by functional limitation of the involved limb, pain during passive movements, joint immobility, swelling, edema, and soft tissue inflammation. General signs of infection include poor feeding and/or irritability; fever and abnormal inflammatory markers are not always present in the early stages.

Narang et al. (1998) reported functional limitation of the involved limb (64%) and local swelling (60%) as the most frequent clinical findings at the time of onset of osteomyelitis; multi-articular involvement was reported in eight cases (32%). Hip (48%) and knee (48%) were most frequently involved. Wong et al. (1995) reported that osteomyelitis was multifocal in 40% of cases and associated with septic arthritis in 47%. In their cohort, fever was present in about 10% of cases.

Septic arthritis is a medical emergency. The destruction of the epiphysis by the infectious process and avascular necrosis caused by compression of the joint by the inflammatory exudate may result in a long-term, severe, functional limitation of the involved joint. The prognosis depends on the rapidity of the diagnosis and institution of appropriate treatment. Osteomyelitis should be suspected in every neonate with local pain, functional limb limitation, or systemic clinical signs without a known source of infection (Offiah 2006).

Microbiological confirmation to guide the choice of antibiotics or to change treatment in the case of lack of therapeutic response is desirable but only available in no more than 50–80% of cases (Gutierrez 2005). Deshpande et al. (2004) reported 15 newborns with positive blood culture in only seven cases (47%) and synovial fluid culture in nine cases (60%). The isolation of a microorganism should be attempted by culture of blood, tip of the central venous catheter, and, if available, synovial fluid, including Gram staining.

X-rays of the involved limb may show nonspecific signs of osteomyelitis and septic arthritis such as edema of soft tissues and an increase of the articular space caused by the presence of purulent exudates. Cortical osteolysis, a sign of bone necrosis, is seen only in the late stages of the disease. The ability of X-rays to detect lesions characteristic of osteomyelitis is limited in neonates because soft tissue edema and enlargement of the articular space are not always evident, and areas of osteolysis are rarely visible in the early phases, appearing as late as 10–21 days after the onset of symptoms (Offiah 2006; Gutierrez 2005). Despite these limitations, X-rays remain an important technique for the confirmation of osteomyelitis (Overturf 2006).

Ultrasound is a highly variable technique that depends on the experience of the physician; a negative result does not exclude osteomyelitis. However, it may be useful during the diagnostic workup of suspected osteomyelitis, showing soft tissue edema, subperiosteal abscesses, or joint effusions (Offiah 2006; Keller 2005).

Bone scintigraphy with 99 m technetium enables diagnosis in 80–100% of cases. It has high sensitivity in detecting single or multiple foci of infection during the first 48–72 h after the onset of signs. These are seen as hyperperfused areas (expression of inflammation) or as "cold spots" (in areas where edema has reduced vascularization) (Gutierrez 2005). However, in the neonatal period, this technique has a lower diagnostic value than in older children, and its use should be limited to neonates with a negative radiograph and clinical evidence of osteomyelitis.

Computerized tomography enables early detection of necrosis and periosteal reaction and may be useful in the diagnosis of osteomyelitis of the bones of the skull (e.g., after infection of a cephalohematoma). MRI may show abscesses and periosteal involvement, but may require sedation of the infant (Overturf 2006).

If a purulent synovial effusion is suspected, puncture should be always performed to reduce pressure within the joint and enable appropriate microbiological investigations.

Success of treatment depends on the appropriateness of antibiotics and the removal of the purulent effusion. The empirical antibiotic combination should take account of known likely etiologic agents: *S. aureus*, GBS, and Gram-negative bacteria. Intravenous vancomycin together with an aminoglycoside or a third-generation cephalosporin (usually cefotaxime) is the suitable option.

Therapy should be modified on the basis of the isolated organism and its sensitivity spectrum. If no microorganism is isolated, the initial empirical treatment should be continued until there is clinical improvement. Lack of response to initial antibiotic therapy should raise the suspicion of antibiotic resistance or the presence of an abscess, to be investigated by appropriate imaging.

Antibiotic therapy should be continued for at least 4–6 weeks or longer and until the clinical condition and radiological and laboratory investigations indicate resolution. Courses shorter than 3 weeks are associated with a high risk of relapse.

Estimates of the frequency of residual complications following osteomyelitis during the neonatal period vary from 6% to 50%. They are due to bone growth abnormalities, asymmetric limb size, gait defects, and pathologic fractures (Gutierrez 2005; Deshpande et al. 2004). Factors affecting prognosis include the delay between the onset of symptoms and start of antibiotic treatment, the duration of antibiotics, and which joint is affected (Gutierrez 2005; Deshpande et al. 2004). The risk for bone deformities is highest for the hip and knee and diagnostic delays longer than 3–4 days (Overturf 2006).

107.3.8 Miscellaneous

107.3.8.1 Ophthalmia Neonatorum

Ophthalmia neonatorum (neonatal conjunctivitis) is the term for any purulent conjunctivitis starting during the first 28 days of life (Amini et al. 2008; Grosskreutz and Smith 1992). It may have infectious and noninfectious etiologies. Noninfectious conjunctivitis is mainly chemical conjunctivitis following prophylaxis of ophthalmia neonatorum with 1–2% silver nitrate.

Infectious causes were identified by Amini et al. (2008), who reported 198 neonates with conjunctivitis. Bacteria included *S. aureus* (31%), *E. coli* (23%), *S. epidermis* (22%), *Klebsiella* (10%), *N. gonorrhoeae* (3%), *C. trachomatis* (2%), and *Pseudomonas aeruginosa* (2%). Viruses have also been implicated (Fransen et al. 1987; Gallardo et al. 2005; Chang et al. 2006). In developed countries, the most frequently isolated pathogen is *C. trachomatis*, with a reported incidence in the USA of 8.2/1,000 live births (Amini et al. 2008; Hammerschlag 2000). In developing countries, the most frequently isolated organisms are *S. aureus* and *C. trachomatis* (Avila-Figueroa et al. 1998; Amini et al. 2008).

The clinical picture, regardless of etiology, is characterized by hyperemia of the conjunctivae, swelling and hyperemia of eyelids, and purulent conjunctival exudate (Foster and Klauss 1995).

Although the disease may be benign if treated promptly, neglected neonatal conjunctivitis may result in blindness.

After the introduction of Credé prophylaxis with 2% silver nitrate solution, first described in 1881 (Credè 1881), there was a reduction in neonatal gonococcal conjunctivitis (the most important cause of blindness in the eighteenth century), and in infantile blindness. Since then, several agents have been proposed to combine wide antimicrobial protection with a reduced incidence of chemical conjunctivitis due to silver nitrate. These agents included 0.5% erythromycin, 1% tetracycline, and gentamicin (Isenberg et al. 2003; Zar 2005). Isenberg et al. (1995), in a clinical trial on 3,117 newborn infants in Kenya, compared the use of 2.5% povidone-iodine with 1% silver nitrate or 0.5% erythromycin. The povidone-iodine solution was more effective than silver nitrate or erythromycin and less toxic. Richter et al. (2006) showed that 1.25% povidone-iodine solutions have no effect on thyroid function.

Although 0.5% erythromycin and 1% Aureomycin are most used, 1% fusidic acid ophthalmic ointment is effective against the most frequent pathogens causing ophthalmia neonatorum (including *N. gonorrhoeae* and *C. trachomatis*), has a prolonged effect (for more than 12 h), and is well tolerated.

107.3.8.2 Acute Otitis Media

Acute otitis media (AOM) is the presence of a purulent exudate in the middle ear, associated with clinical signs of acute disease. It may present as isolated disease or in association with sepsis, meningitis, or pneumonia. Risk factors include the presence of meconium-stained amniotic fluid and the need for neonatal resuscitation, mechanical ventilation, prolonged tracheal intubation, and cleft palate. Breast-fed neonates are less likely to be affected than formula-fed infants (Barnett and Klein 2006).

Turner et al. (2002) studied 137 babies aged <2 months with suspected AOM. At tympanocentesis, the most frequently isolated organism was *S. pneumoniae* (46%), followed by *Haemophilus influenzae* (34%), group A *Streptococcus* (10%), Gram-negative *Bacilli* (7%), *Moraxella catarrhalis* (2%), and *Streptococcus faecalis* (1%). Mixed infections were observed in 20 cases: *S. pneumoniae* + *H. influenzae*, *H. influenzae* + *M. catarrhalis*, *S. pneumoniae* + *H. influenzae* + *M. catarrhalis*, and *Klebsiella* + *Enterobacter*.

Otitis presenting during the first weeks is usually caused by the same organisms as neonatal sepsis (*S. aureus*, GBS, and Gram-negative *Bacilli*). By contrast, otitis presenting after the first 2 weeks in neonates without associated diseases is usually community acquired and frequently caused by *S. pneumoniae* (Barnett and Klein 2006).

The diagnosis of AOM is based on physical examination. Nonspecific signs as poor feeding and irritability may be the first clinical signs, with or without purulent exudate in the external ear. In the study by Turner et al. (2002), the presentation was with fever (70%), conjunctivitis (46%), respiratory distress (27%), lower respiratory tract infections (13%), vomiting (4%), and diarrhea (4%). Both ears were affected in 45% of infants. At otoscopic examination, there is hyperemia and bulging of the tympanic membrane, which is often cloudy with impaired mobility, and an air-fluid level or bubble visible in the middle ear. Tympanocentesis, when indicated, may decompress the middle ear and allows culture of the purulent exudate.

The presence of fever at presentation is not reliably predictive of increased risk of progression to sepsis (Nozicka et al. 1999).

Treatment should take account of the baby's age and possible pathogens. The initial antibiotic treatment should be ampicillin in combination with an aminoglycoside or a third-generation cephalosporin for 10 days for infants aged <2 weeks or those who have clinical signs of systemic infection or who are hospitalized. For nonhospitalized neonates aged >2 weeks and without associated diseases, the most probable infecting agent is *S. pneumoniae*, and the first-line antibiotic is amoxicillin for at least 10 days (Barnett and Klein 2006).

107.3.8.3 Omphalitis

Omphalitis is infection of the umbilical cord. The incidence varies from 0.7% in developed countries to 6.2% in developing countries (Fraser et al. 2006). In a recent study by Mullany et al. in Nepal on 17,198 infants (Mullany et al. 2007), the incidence of omphalitis was 5.5%.

Risk factors include prolonged labor, prolonged rupture of membranes, maternal infections, prematurity, low birth weight at birth, and the presence of umbilical cord catheters (Fraser et al. 2006). Mullany et al. reported an increased risk for infants whose umbilical cord was disinfected with non-hygienic solutions and found that good hand hygiene of healthcare workers was protective (Mullany et al. 2007).

Most frequently isolated organisms include *S. aureus*, *S. epidermidis*, group A and group B *Streptococci*, *E. coli*, *Klebsiella*, *Pseudomonas*, *C. difficile*, and anaerobic bacteria. In developing countries, *C. tetani* remains an important pathogen for omphalitis (Fraser et al. 2006; Mullany et al. 2007).

Omphalitis is characterized by edema and hyperemia of the periumbilical skin, with or without purulent exudate. The infectious process may progress deeper in soft tissues causing cellulitis and lymphangitis of the abdominal wall, sometimes involving the subcutaneous fat and deeper layers (Fraser et al. 2006; Mullany et al. 2007).

Although omphalitis is a localized disease, it may progress to systemic disease if untreated. After infection of the periumbilical skin, dissemination of the infection may occur if there is umbilical vessel involvement. The most frequent complications of omphalitis are sepsis, necrotizing fasciitis, abscesses (of the pelvis, retroperitoneum, skin, liver), peritonitis, and hepatic vein thrombosis.

Prevention of omphalitis using 4% chlorhexidine as first-choice disinfectant has been recently evaluated by Mullany et al. (2006): a randomized clinical trial compared the use of 4% chlorhexidine (4,934 infants) with cleansing with soap and water (5,107 infants) or dry cord care (5,082 infants) and found a reduction of infections and of neonatal mortality in the chlorhexidine group. Severe omphalitis requires urgent intravenous antibiotic treatment effective against *Staphylococci*, *Streptococci*, and Gram-negative bacteria.

107.3.8.4 Impetigo Bullosa and Staphylococcal Scalded Skin Syndrome (SSSS)

Impetigo bullosa is a disease characterized by friable nonerythematous cutaneous vesicles, filled with a yellowish fluid, usually located in the periumbilical skin and the folds of the skin in the axilla or neck. It is caused by *S. aureus* and has a benign course. The skin lesions are focal, but wider skin dissemination has been reported. Treatment is based on topical skin disinfectants, but systemic antibiotics are needed in the case of resistance to local disinfection.

Staphylococcal scalded skin syndrome (SSSS, previously known as Ritter's disease) is a disease characterized by cutaneous desquamation after light rubbing (Nikolsky's sign) that involves extensive areas of the skin. It is an exfoliative process indistinguishable from toxic epidermal necrolysis (TEN). The difference between the two clinical pictures is in the etiology: SSSS is caused by *S. aureus*, while TEN refers to cutaneous exfoliation caused by noninfectious agents or by infectious agents other than *S. aureus*.

The pathogenesis of SSSS is linked to the ability of some strains of *S. aureus* to produce exfoliative toxins A and B, which detach the stratum granulosum from deeper layers of the skin, leading to desquamation and rash, usually without fever, systemic symptoms, or bacteremia (Makhoul et al. 2001).

Pending the results of microbiological tests, the differential diagnosis between SSSS and TEN is by cytology of a smear from a swab of the detached skin: big epithelial cells with small nuclei and lack of inflammatory cells can be observed in SSSS, while cuboidal cells with large nuclei and presence of inflammatory cells can be observed in TEN (Orscheln et al. 2006).

Treatment options for SSSS are β-lactam-resistant penicillins (oxacillin, flucloxacillin) or vancomycin, while corticosteroids, to be considered for TEN, are contraindicated for SSSS.

107.3.8.5 Neonatal Toxic Shock Syndrome-Like Exanthematous Disease

Some strains of *S. aureus* producing the toxic shock syndrome toxin-1 (TSST-1) are responsible, in adult patients, of a fulminant clinical picture characterized by fever, hypotension, and macular cutaneous rash associated with desquamation of the skin and multiorgan dysfunction. Sporadic neonatal cases have been reported.

Takahashi et al., in 1998 (Takahashi et al. 1998), reported on 20 newborn infants with a clinical picture characterized by rash (appearing between 2 and 5 days of life) without desquamation and lasting 2–3 days. Associated thrombocytopenia at the time of the rash is sometimes preceded by fever lasting 1 day. All were colonized by a strain of methicillin-resistant *S. aureus* (MRSA) producing TSST-1. This clinical picture was described as a new nosologic entity and defined neonatal toxic shock syndrome-like exanthematous disease (NTED). The pathogenic mechanism seems to be linked to the ability of TSST-1 to act as a superantigen expanding the T cell compartment. High maternal antibody titers (anti-TSST-1 IgG) appear to be protective for NTED. The same authors performed a case-control study of NTED in Japanese neonatal intensive care units and summarized the clinical findings of 540 patients. The number of NTED patients decreased over the 5-year period from 2000 to 2005 although there were more than 100 patients with NTED in Japan in 2005. Most patients recovered within 5 days of the onset of the exanthematous process without active treatment, but two preterm infants died during the recovery phase (Takahashi et al. 1998).

107.3.8.6 Noma Neonatorum

Noma neonatorum is a gangrenous process, frequently associated with bacteremia, involving the nose, mouth, eyelids, and perineum (Ghosal et al. 1978). It mainly affects low-birth-weight or preterm infants and has a fulminant course and a high mortality within the first 1–3 days after presentation. In most cases reported in the literature, there was an association with the isolation of *P. aeruginosa*. Treatment is based on antibiotics against *P. aeruginosa*.

107.3.8.7 Neonatal Tetanus

Neonatal tetanus is a severe condition, although rare in developed countries. It is caused by *Clostridium tetani*, a Gram-positive, obligate anaerobic, rod-shaped, sporeforming bacterium. Because it is an obligate anaerobe, localization of *C. tetani* in the periumbilical region may be prevented by the disinfection of the umbilical cord with H_2O_2.

Neonates born to vaccinated mothers are protected from the disease by transplacental transfer of specific IgG. Aseptic obstetric and neonatal practices are also vital for prevention.

The time of incubation between inoculation of the spores and onset of symptoms varies from 3 to 21 days. About 90% of neonates with tetanus develop the disease during the first 3–14 days of life (mostly between days 6 and 8). The baby becomes febrile and presents with difficulty in opening the mouth for suction. There is muscle rigidity and spasms extending progressively to the chest wall and limbs and to the diaphragm, leading to respiratory failure. Laryngeal or glottal spasm may lead to airway obstruction or aspiration pneumonia. Episodes of cyanosis and apnea are common in uncontrolled severe disease. Before mechanical ventilation and the availability of effective agents to control muscle spasm, mortality was mainly because of respiratory failure. Autonomic dysfunction may lead to hypertension or hypotension, tachycardia, bradycardia, and arrhythmias that can result in life-threatening hemodynamic instability and cardiac arrest (Roper et al. 2007).

Neonatal tetanus is an emergency. Therapy consists of the use of antibiotics (penicillin), hyperimmune anti-tetanus toxin immunoglobulin (500 UI i.m.), and benzodiazepines (intravenous diazepam, 0.3–0.5 mg/kg/dose, repeatable). Endotracheal intubation and mechanical ventilation may be necessary to treat respiratory failure. The prognosis is characterized by a high mortality, but immediate and effective intensive care may reduce mortality to less than 20% (Roper et al. 2007).

107.4 Fungal Infections

The great majority of fungal infections in the neonate are caused by *Candida* spp. and less frequently by *Malassezia* spp.

Candida is a commensal organism that usually colonizes the skin and mucous membranes of the gastrointestinal tract and respiratory airways. In the immunocompromised host, it behaves as a pathogen, by invading host tissues and entering the circulation.

About 10% of term neonates and 27–63% VLBW neonates admitted to NICUs during the first weeks of life are colonized by fungi (Kaufman and Fairchild 2004). In a study conducted in six NICUs between 1993 and 1995 on 2,847 neonates by Rangel-Frausto et al., the incidence of sepsis caused by *Candida* was 12.3/1,000 admissions (0.64/1,000 patients-days); reported species were *C. albicans* (63%), *C. parapsilosis* (29%), *C. glabrata* (6%), and other species (3%: *C. tropicalis*, *C. kruse*, *C. lusitaniae*, *C. guilliermondii*, *C. dubliniensis*) (Rangel-Frausto et al. 1999).

In a survey conducted in 27 NICUs (20,565 neonates) in Spain, 118 babies (0.57%) had a systemic infection caused by *Candida*. *Candida* spp. were isolated from the blood culture of 79 neonates, from urine cultures of 33, and from the CSF of four. The frequency of infection was significantly higher in VLBW infants (4.8%) than in infants with birth weight >1,500 g (0.2%) ($P < 0.001$) (Lin et al. 2003).

Candida may be acquired by horizontal or, less frequently, vertical transmission. Horizontal transmission occurs mainly through the contaminated hands of healthcare workers. In a multicenter study involving six NICUs (Saiman et al. 2001), *C. albicans* was isolated from the hands of 5% of healthcare workers and *C. parapsilosis* from 19%. Four hundred eighty-six neonates out of 2,157 (23%) were colonized by *Candida*: 299 (14%) by *C. albicans*, 151 (7%) by *C. parapsilosis*, and 74 (3%) by other species. Other sources of infection may be parenteral nutrition solutions or contaminated infusion circuits. Rarely, the reservoir is the environment.

Invasive *Candida* infections are generally preceded by colonization. In a multicenter study of 2,847 neonates (Saiman et al. 2000), candidemia was preceded by colonization in 15/35 (43%) cases.

Both neonatal risk factors and the virulence of the microorganism are implicated in the pathogenesis of invasive *Candida* infections. The most important neonatal risk factors for nosocomial candidiasis are prolonged administration of broad-spectrum antibiotics (courses longer than 21 days), extreme prematurity (gestational age at birth <28 weeks), and the presence of venous catheters (especially if prolonged). Additionally, Saiman et al. (2000) found that total parenteral nutrition and intravenous lipid solutions, administration of H2-blockers, endotracheal intubation, disseminated intravascular coagulation, and prolonged hospital stay were also significant risk factors for invasive *Candida* infections ($P < 0.05$). All types of catheter (vascular, vesical, peritoneal catheters, ventriculoperitoneal and thoracic drains, endotracheal tubes) favor adhesion, growth, and penetration of microorganisms (Bendel 2005). Feja et al. (2005) reported associations between invasive *Candida* infections and gastrointestinal tract diseases (NEC and focal intestinal perforation, OR = 4.57) and previous bacterial sepsis (OR = 8.02). Benjamin et al., studying 4,579 extremely low-birth-weight infants (<1,000 g, ELBW), found that delay in starting enteral nutrition was an added risk factor. Steroid therapy, hyperglycemia, neutropenia, and abdominal or cardiac surgery are additional risk factors (Bendel 2005).

The virulence of the microorganism is linked to its ability to form hyphae (that permit tissue invasion), to the infecting species (*C. albicans* is the most virulent), to the expression of adhesins, and to the ability to form a biofilm that protects the microorganism from the host immune response and from exposure to antifungal drugs. Mixed biofilms (*Candida* together with CONS) are not infrequent. Adam et al. (2002) found that the slime produced in vitro by *S. epidermidis* inhibits the penetration of fluconazole and that the slime produced by *C. albicans* protects *Staphylococci* from the action of vancomycin.

Once the cutaneous and mucous surfaces are colonized, *Candida* may invade tissues locally, leading to parenchymal destruction, sometimes with the formation of abscesses, which are difficult to eradicate. Circulatory involvement may lead to the development of sepsis with end-organ dissemination (endocardium, kidney, central nervous system, bone) (Manzoni et al. 2007a).

There are three clinical pictures: congenital candidiasis, mucocutaneous candidiasis, and fungal sepsis.

Congenital candidiasis is the congenital infection of the fetus by *Candida* species in the presence of *Candida* chorioamnionitis. It is a rare event, accounting for 0.8% of cases of chorioamnionitis (Kaufman and Fairchild 2004; Maudsley et al. 1966). In about 25% of cases, it occurs in women with intrauterine devices and heavily colonized by *Candida* (Kaufman and Fairchild 2004). Affected infants present with pustules, vesicles, skin abscesses, and an erythematous maculopapular rash on the trunk and extremities that sometimes evolves to desquamation (Darmstadt et al. 2000). Histologic evaluation of the umbilical cord and placenta shows microabscesses, hyphae, and granulomas, confirming the diagnosis (Kaufman and Fairchild 2004). Clinical features and evolution of the disease are generally more severe in the preterm infant than in those born at term. Darmstadt et al., reviewing the literature of infants with congenital candidiasis, found that those with birth weight <1,000 g were at higher risk of systemic infection than those >1,000 g (67% vs. 10%) (Darmstadt et al. 2000). Preterm neonates may present with organ involvement (pneumonia, disseminated dermatitis, hyphae in urine, blood, and CSF).

Mucocutaneous candidiasis is the most common manifestation of the disease. It usually presents during the second or third week of life as a diffuse erythematous rash affecting the napkin area and white patches on the oral mucosa, gingivae, and tongues. As the disease progresses, the skin rash becomes more widespread, affecting the abdominal skin and chest. The rash may be papular or pustulous or associated with cutaneous desquamation (Rowen 2003).

Cutaneous involvement may precede systemic spread (Baley and Silverman 1988). The clinical manifestations of fungal sepsis are similar to those of bacterial sepsis. Thrombocytopenia is nonspecific: Guida et al. (2003) found that 84% of infants with fungal sepsis, 75% of infants with Gram-negative sepsis, and 48% of infants with Gram-positive sepsis had platelet counts $<100{,}000/mm^3$.

Frequently, at the time of diagnosis, the infection is already disseminated to organs. *Candida* spp. may cause organ infections as endocarditis, meningitis, endophthalmitis and chorioretinitis, dermatitis, peritonitis, osteomyelitis, and septic arthritis and may form abscesses in the central nervous system, kidneys, liver, spleen, and gut. In a recent meta-analysis, the rate of positive urine cultures was 61% among neonates with candidemia, but ultrasound findings of renal involvement were found in only 5% of cases. The rate of meningitis was 15%, cerebral abscesses or ventriculitis was found in 4% of cases, endocarditis in 5%, and endophthalmitis in 3% (Benjamin et al. 2003).

Urine and CSF cultures, together with blood cultures, should always be performed in infants with suspected *Candida* sepsis. Microscopic examination of the urine may reveal hyphae and ultrasound may show evidence of renal tract involvement. Other imaging studies may include cardiac and cerebral ultrasound and ophthalmologic examination if ophthalmitis is suspected (Bendel 2005).

The identification of the gene coding for 18S rRNA by PCR is under investigation. This gene is present in the genome of almost all clinically relevant fungal species and is absent in the human genome. Löffler et al. (1997) compared the identification of the 18S rRNA gene with traditional culture methods for the diagnosis of fungal infection in 600 samples from febrile and neutropenic adult patients with neoplastic diseases. Compared to traditional cultures, the PCR showed 100% sensitivity and 98% specificity for fungal infections.

Sepsis by *Candida* is associated with increased mortality and morbidity. In a study by the Neonatal Research Network (Stoll et al. 2002a), the mortality rate for VLBW neonates with fungal sepsis was threefold higher than for those without.

Sepsis caused by *C. albicans* is associated with a higher mortality compared to sepsis caused by other *Candida* species. In a study on 45 newborn infants, Faix et al. (1992) found that deaths attributable to infection by *Candida* were 7/29 in infants with infection by *C. albicans* and 0/16 in infants with infection by *C. parapsilosis* ($P = 0.034$). In the study by the Neonatal Research Network, the mortality rate for VLBW infants with *C. albicans* infection was 43.9% compared with 15.9% for *C. parapsilosis* (Stoll et al. 2002a).

In a study conducted between 1988 and 1996 on ELBW neonates with sepsis and/or meningoencephalitis caused by *Candida*, the outcome at 2 years corrected age was compared with a cohort of ELBW neonates without *Candida* infection. Case fatality rate was similar. However, all survivors in the *Candida* group had chronic lung disease at discharge, compared with 33% of the control cases ($P = 0.0001$). There was a high incidence of periventricular leukomalacia (26% vs. 12%, $P = 0.06$) and increased severe retinopathy of prematurity (22% vs. 9%, $P = 0.04$).

Sixty percent of the *Candida* group had adverse neurologic outcomes at 2 years corrected age compared with 35% in the control group, and 41 versus 12% had severe disabilities ($P = 0.005$) (Friedman et al. 2000).

The first-line antifungal drug for the treatment of fungal sepsis is amphotericin B deoxycholate, which is generally well tolerated by the neonate. The dosage is 0.1 mg/kg/day administered intravenously in a single daily dose in 2 h. The dose may be progressively increased to a maximum of 1 mg/kg/day. In some studies on adult patients, levels achieved in the CSF are about 5–10% of plasma levels, but in a small study of 13 preterm infants, CSF levels were 40–90% of plasma levels.

Liposomal amphotericin B is less toxic and can be administered at higher dosages. Amphotericin B deoxycholate is potentially nephrotoxic, and if renal function is compromised, the liposomal formulation of amphotericin B is indicated. Liposomal amphotericin B is prescribed at 1–5 mg/kg/day. The effectiveness and safety of a dose of 5–7 mg/kg/day of liposomal amphotericin B were studied prospectively by Juster-Reicher et al. (2003) in 2003. In 41 cases of systemic candidiasis, the authors found it to be highly effective (recovery in 95% of cases) without side effects except for one infant who had a transient increase in liver enzymes. The time required for eradication was 10.9 ± 4.8 days for infants who had previously received other antifungal drugs and $8.7 + 4.5$ days for infants in whom liposomal amphotericin B was used as the treatment of first choice. The recommended dose for intravenous liposomal amphotericin B is 1 mg/kg/day administered over 2 h, increasing progressively to a maximum of 5 mg/kg/day.

More recently, a study reported higher mortality in infants treated with amphotericin B lipid products compared to amphotericin B deoxycholate (Ascher et al. 2012), possibly because of lower concentrations of the liposomal formulations in the kidneys, which are prime locations for *Candida* end-organ damage (Greenberg and Benjamin 2014).

Fluconazole is the most studied azole in the neonatal age range. Its use for the prevention of fungal infections in high-risk neonates has been evaluated by several studies, but amphotericin B is the first choice for treatment of an infection. Several studies recommend intravenous 5-fluorocytosine in combination with amphotericin B for severe fungal infections. 5-Fluorocytosine achieves high CSF concentrations and is recommended for fungal meningitis. However, it should never be used as a single antifungal because of the frequent emergence of resistant strains. The recommended dose is 50–150 mg/kg/day intravenously over 15 min in four daily doses.

Another class of antifungal agents, echinocandins, act through noncompetitive inhibition of the synthesis of the 1,3-β-glucan in the cellular wall and have been used in adults. Pharmacokinetic studies on neonates are available for micafungin, for which the current recommended dose is 10 mg/kg/day, with no adjustment needed for renal or hepatic impairment (Greenberg and Benjamin 2014). Few data are available for anidulafungin and caspofungin, which are not recommended as first-choice agents. Importantly, echinocandins are able to penetrate the brain tissue but not the CSF, and they do not penetrate the vitreous; this information should be taken in account when using micafungin as first-choice treatment, and a dilated retinal exam is required to exclude endophthalmitis (Greenberg and Benjamin 2014).

The duration of antifungal treatment should be decided on the basis of clinical and microbiological factors: the fungal species, the presence of a central venous catheter, which should always be removed in infants with fungal infections, the number of positive cultures, CSF cell count and chemistry, and imaging (echocardiography, renal ultrasound, ophthalmologic examination, and imaging of the central nervous system). In infants with systemic fungal infections, intravenous treatment should be prolonged for at least 2–4 weeks after the last negative blood culture. Longer courses may be needed for meningitis and end-organ dissemination.

Empirical antifungal therapy should be considered in high-risk infants once *Candida* infection is suspected (Greenberg and Benjamin 2014). Infants who may benefit most from empirical antifungal therapy include high-risk populations, such as ELBW neonates with sepsis and risk factors for fungal infections (presence of a central venous catheter, endotracheal tube, thrombocytopenia, prolonged treatment with third-generation cephalosporins or carbapenems, gestational age <28 weeks). In ELBW infants, empirical therapy has been associated with increased survival without neurodevelopmental impairment (Greenberg et al. 2012).

107.5 Prevention of Early- and Late-Onset Infections

107.5.1 Prevention of Early-Onset Group B Streptococcal Infection

107.5.1.1 Intrapartum Antibiotic Prophylaxis (IAP)

Intrapartum antibiotic prophylaxis (IAP) is currently the most important preventive measure against early-onset group B streptococcal (GBS) disease. There are two strategies. One is based on universal prenatal screening, while the other is based on the presence of *intrapartum* risk factors. The former was proposed by the Centers for Disease Control and Prevention (CDC) (2010). The latter is based on the presence of *intrapartum* risk factors and is recommended by the UK Royal College of Obstetricians and Gynaecologists (RCOG) (2015). Several studies, in particular a case-control study of 5,144 births published by Schrag et al. to compare the two strategies, showed that the screening-based approach was better than the risk-based approach (Schrag et al. 2002). The introduction and the widespread use of IAP and especially the implementation of guidelines issued by the CDC have led to a substantial reduction in the incidence of early-onset GBS disease. A retrospective study demonstrated that screening for GBS before delivery increased from 48 in 1998–1999 to 85% in 2003–2004, and women with an indication for IAP who received prophylaxis increased from 74% to 85% (Van Dyke et al. 2009). This has resulted in a reduction in the incidence of early-onset GBS disease in the USA from 1.7 to 0.35/1,000 live births (Phares et al. 2008). The drug of choice for IAP is penicillin G i.v. (5 million units followed by 2.5 million units every 4 h until birth). This drug is not generally available and an alternative is intravenous ampicillin (2 g followed by 1 g every 4 h until birth) (Committee on Infectious Diseases AAoP et al. 2015).

The screening-based method requires a vaginal-rectal swab to be performed on all pregnant women at 35–37 weeks of gestation and the administration of *intrapartum* antibiotics to colonized women at the time of labor.

The 2010 CDC guidelines provide criteria for identification of candidates to receive IAP to prevent early-onset GBS disease (Table 4). The following are key components of the screening strategy (Centers for Disease Control and Prevention 2010):

- Women with GBS isolated from the urine at any time during the current pregnancy or who had a previous infant with invasive GBS disease should receive IAP and do not need third trimester screening for GBS colonization.
- Women with symptomatic or asymptomatic GBS urinary tract infection detected during pregnancy should be treated according to current standards of care for urinary tract infection during pregnancy and should receive IAP to prevent early-onset GBS disease.
- All other pregnant women should be screened at 35–37 weeks' gestation for vaginal and rectal GBS colonization.
- At the time of labor or rupture of membranes, IAP should be given to all pregnant women who tested positive for GBS colonization, except in the instance of cesarean delivery performed before onset of labor on a woman with intact amniotic membranes.
- For circumstances in which screening results are not available at the time of labor and delivery, IAP should be given to women who are <37 weeks and 0 days' gestation, have a duration of membrane rupture $\geq$18 h, or have a temperature of $\geq$100.4 °F ($\geq$38.0 °C).

Table 4 Indications for intrapartum antimicrobial prophylaxis (IAP) to prevent early-onset GBS disease (Modified from Centers for Disease Control and Prevention (2010))

Intrapartum GBS prophylaxis indicated	Intrapartum GBS prophylaxis not indicated
Previous infant with invasive GBS disease	Colonization with GBS during a previous pregnancy (unless an indication for GBS prophylaxis is present for current pregnancy)
GBS bacteriuria during any trimester of the current pregnancy[a]	GBS bacteriuria during previous pregnancy (unless an indication for GBS prophylaxis is present for current pregnancy)
Positive GBS vaginal-rectal screening culture in late gestation[b] during current pregnancy[a]	Negative GBS vaginal-rectal screening culture in late gestation[b] regardless of intrapartum risk factors
Unknown GBS status at the onset of labor (culture not done, incomplete, or results unknown) and any of the following:	Cesarean delivery performed before the onset of labor on a woman with intact amniotic membranes, regardless of GBS colonization status or gestational age
Delivery at <37 weeks' gestation	
Amniotic membrane rupture ≥18 h	
Intrapartum temperature ≥100.4 °F (≥38.0 °C)[c]	
Intrapartum NAAT[d] positive for GBS	

[a]Intrapartum antibiotic prophylaxis is not indicated in this circumstance if a cesarean delivery is performed before onset of labor on a woman with intact amniotic membranes
[b]Optimal timing for prenatal GBS screening is at 35–37 weeks' gestation
[c]If amnionitis is suspected, broad-spectrum antibiotic therapy that includes an agent known to be active against GBS should replace GBS prophylaxis
[d]Nucleic acid amplification tests (NAAT) testing for GBS is optional and might not be available in all settings. If intrapartum NAAT is negative for GBS but any other intrapartum risk factor (delivery at <37 weeks' gestation, amniotic membrane rupture at ≥18 h, or temperature ≥100.4 °F [≥38.0 °C]) is present, then intrapartum antibiotic prophylaxis is indicated

- In the absence of GBS urinary tract infection, antimicrobial agents should not be used before the intrapartum period to eradicate GBS genitorectal colonization, because such treatment is not effective in eliminating carriage or preventing neonatal disease and can cause adverse consequences.
- IAP to prevent early-onset GBS disease is not recommended as a routine practice for cesarean deliveries performed before labor onset on women with intact amniotic membranes, regardless of the GBS colonization status of the woman or the gestational age of the pregnancy. The use of perioperative prophylactic antibiotics to prevent infectious complications of cesarean delivery should not be altered or affected by GBS status. Women expected to undergo cesarean deliveries should undergo routine vaginal and rectal screening for GBS at 35–37 weeks' gestation because onset of labor or rupture of membranes can occur before the planned cesarean delivery, and under those circumstances GBS-colonized women should receive intrapartum antibiotic prophylaxis.

There are two main limitations to the universal screening-based strategy: (a) the possibility that the woman delivers before vaginal swabs have been taken or before the results are available and (b) the possibility of colonization between obtaining a negative swab and delivery. Yancey et al. (1996) showed that swabs performed 5 weeks before delivery predict colonization at delivery. A retrospective study reported negative screening results in 61% of GBS early-onset disease, an unexpectedly high percentage. The authors suggest several reasons for false-negative results: screening outside the 5-week window before delivery, errors in collecting and processing swabs, and possible errors in the communication of results (Van Dyke et al. 2009). There is debate about the minimum duration of effective IAP. The CDC protocol recommends IAP administration at least 4 h before delivery, but the RCOG recommends at least 2 h.

In a prospective study of 21 women treated with ampicillin before elective cesarean section, Colombo et al. (2006) demonstrated bactericidal levels of ampicillin in the cord blood 30 min after ampicillin administration. The cord blood ampicillin concentration is higher than the maternal blood concentration, and both continue to be above minimal bactericidal concentrations 5–6 h after administration. Ampicillin levels decreased more rapidly in the maternal than the fetal compartments, suggesting decreased clearance of ampicillin by the newborns. Lijoi et al. observed significantly lower colonization in babies of mothers given IAP more than 4 h before delivery (3.7%) than those born to mothers who received IAP closer to the time of birth (12.3%) (Lijoi et al. 2007).

In conclusion, beta-lactam antibiotics for GBS prophylaxis administered $\geq$4 h before delivery have been found to be highly effective at preventing vertical transmission of GBS and early-onset GBS disease. Shorter durations of appropriate antibiotics might provide some protection.

107.5.1.2 Possible Side Effects of IAP

The striking success of this preventive strategy, however, has raised the issue of possible side effects resulting from the adoption of IAP on a large scale.

Van Dyke et al. in a study of 7,691 births found no cases of anaphylaxis after IAP (Van Dyke et al. 2009).

The effect of IAP on neonatal infections by multidrug-resistant microorganisms other than GBS has been considered by Moore et al. (2003) who reviewed 412 articles and explored potential associations between IAP use and changes in the causes of early-onset sepsis. They found (a) a substantial reduction in the incidence of GBS early-onset disease with IAP, both in term and preterm infants, (b) an unvaried number of total early-onset infection, and (c) an increase in non-GBS pathogens and ampicillin-resistant *E. coli* sepsis in preterm, mainly VLBW, neonates but not in term infants. These conclusions led Baltimore to suggest that the risks and benefits of IAP should be monitored in preterm and VLBW infants (Baltimore 2007). GBS resistance to erythromycin and clindamycin has been described but never to date to penicillin, ampicillin, cefazolin, and vancomycin. In a review of 21 studies published between 1996 and 2006, Barcaite et al. (2008) reported no GBS strains resistant to penicillin, ampicillin, cefazolin, and vancomycin. Between 4% and 21% of GBS strains were resistant to erythromycin and between 3% and 20% were resistant to clindamycin.

107.5.1.3 Neonatal Management

Any baby who is unwell with clinical signs compatible with infection must be investigated and treated with antibiotics regardless of any risk factor that may or may not be present. In 2010 the CDC has provided an algorithm for secondary prevention of early-onset GBS disease among newborns (Fig. 2) (Centers for Disease Control and Prevention 2010).

Treatment of a healthy GBS-colonized neonate can create resistant bacteria, does not eliminate colonization, and therefore, does not prevent possible late infection (Berner 2002). Superficial swabs in neonates during the first hours of life have not been found to be useful (Baker 1997; Stronati et al. 2004). Indeed, about 90% of early-onset disease occurs during the first 24 h of life when the results of the cultures are not available (Baker 1997), and 99% of the colonized neonates do not become infected. Guidelines for the prevention of perinatal GBS disease are available at the website www.cdc.gov/groupbstrep/guidelines/guidelines.html.

107.5.2 Prevention of Nosocomial Infections

Neonatal nosocomial infections are late-onset infections (appearing after the first 72 h of life) in hospitalized infants (Clark et al. 2004b). The incidence of infections varies widely among NICUs, depending on environmental factors and on differences in clinical practice. A survey by the World Health Organization (WHO) reported nosocomial infection rates between 7% and 19% in Europe and 14% in the USA (WHO/EIP/SPO/QPS/05.2 2005). Immunological immaturity, frequent invasive

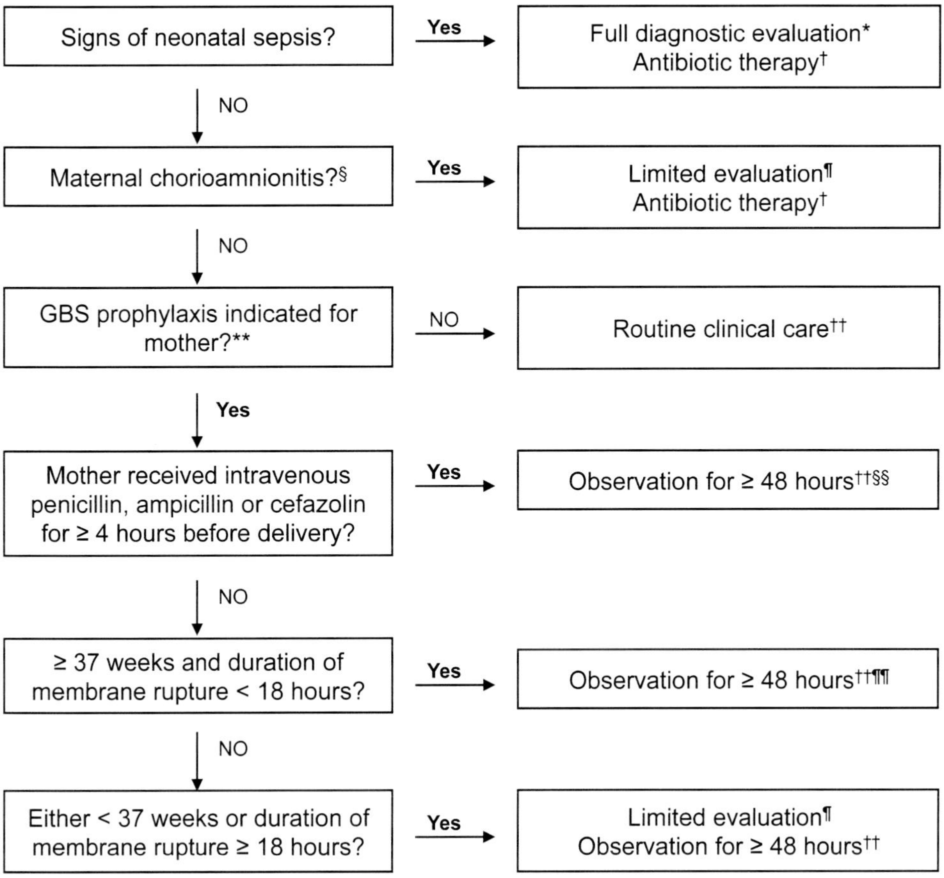

Fig. 2 Algorithm for secondary prevention of early-onset group B streptococcal (GBS) disease among newborns (Modified from Centers for Disease Control and Prevention 2010). * Full diagnostic evaluation includes a blood culture, a complete blood count including white blood cell differential and platelet counts, chest radiograph (if respiratory abnormalities are present), and lumbar puncture (if patient is stable enough to tolerate procedure and sepsis is suspected). † Antibiotic therapy should be directed toward the most common causes of neonatal sepsis, including intravenous ampicillin for GBS and coverage for other organisms (including *Escherichia coli* and other Gram-negative pathogens) and should take into account local antibiotic resistance patterns. § Consultation with obstetric providers is important to determine the level of clinical suspicion for chorioamnionitis. Chorioamnionitis is diagnosed clinically and some of the signs are nonspecific. Limited evaluation includes blood culture (at birth) and complete blood count with differential count and platelets (at birth and/or at 6–12 h of life). ** See Table 4 for indications for intrapartum GBS prophylaxis. †† If signs of sepsis develop, a full diagnostic evaluation should be conducted and antibiotic therapy initiated. §§ If ≥37 weeks' gestation, observation may occur at home after 24 h if other discharge criteria have been met, access to medical care is readily available, and a person who is able to comply fully with instructions for home observation will be present. If any of these conditions is not met, the infant should be observed in the hospital for at least 48 h and until discharge criteria are achieved. ¶¶ Some experts recommend a complete blood count with differential count and platelets at age 6–12 h

procedures, and prolonged hospitalization all account for the high incidence of infection among neonates. Infections may prolong the time of hospitalization and increase mortality and morbidity.

Prevention of healthcare-associated infections is based on strategies that aim at limiting the exposition to pathogens and interrupting transmission of organisms by healthcare workers, at reducing susceptibility to pathogens by reducing risk factors while enhancing host defenses and by modulating the host-pathogen interaction, and at promoting the judicious use of antimicrobials (Jarvis 2004; Borghesi and Stronati 2008).

Strategies for the prevention of nosocomial infections include hand hygiene practices, prevention of CVC-related bloodstream infections (CRBSIs), judicious use of antimicrobials for therapy and chemoprophylaxis, interventions for the modulation of the host-pathogen interaction, and skin care.

107.5.2.1 Hand Hygiene

Since Ignaz Semmelweis demonstrated dramatic reductions in puerperal sepsis after instituting a hand washing regimen in 1847, hand hygiene has been known to reduce healthcare-associated infections and is recommended by the CDC as the single most effective method of preventing the spread of nosocomial infections (Pittet 2001).

Hand washing is a simple, inexpensive procedure that prevents the transmission of infectious pathogens. However, hand hygiene compliance remains low among healthcare workers, with reported adherence rates ranging from 20% to 50% (Cohen et al. 2003).

In a multicenter clinical trial by Pittet et al. (2000), an intense campaign to promote hand hygiene practices led to a significant increase in compliance with protocols (from 48% to 66%, $P < 0.001$) and a concomitant decrease in the overall frequency of nosocomial infections (from 16.9% to 9.9%, $P = 0.04$) and of infections caused by MRSA (from 2.16 to 0.93 cases/10,000 patients-days, $P < 0.001$).

Guidelines for hand hygiene of the CDC Healthcare Infection Control Practices Advisory Committee (HICPAC) (Pittet and Boyce 2003) (http://www.cdc.gov/mmwr/PDF/rr/rr5116.pdf, accessed December 28, 2015) recommend hand washing with antimicrobial or non-antimicrobial soap and water when hands are visibly soiled or contaminated with proteinaceous material and hand decontamination with an alcohol-based hand rub (alcohol-based preparations with 0.5% chlorhexidine) if hands are not visibly soiled and before engaging in direct contact with patients. Additional recommendations include avoiding wearing artificial fingernails and rings, bracelets, and watches when engaging in direct contact with patients and systemic disinfection of stethoscopes after each use (Pittet and Boyce 2003; Longtin et al. 2014).

A recent randomized clinical trial (Kaufman et al. 2014) suggests that the use of nonsterile gloves after hand hygiene prior to patient and line contact is associated with fewer Gram-positive bloodstream infections in preterm infants; however, larger studies are needed to confirm the true beneficial effects of this practice.

107.5.2.2 Prevention of CVC-Related Infections

The definition of CRBSIs may vary among studies. In general, bacteremia can be considered to be CVC related if a catheter has been in place for at least 24 h or if it was removed less than 48 h before the infection (Stolfi et al. 1999). CRBSIs in hospitalized neonates are most frequently caused by CONS, but given that CONS are abundant colonizers of a healthy skin, they frequently contaminate blood culture samples, leading to false-positive results (Garland et al. 2005; Hooven and Polin 2014). In an infant with signs of sepsis, a definite CRBSI can be defined by a positive peripheral blood culture with concordant colonization of the catheter (as demonstrated by drawing blood from the central line or, alternatively, by a positive blood culture of the catheter's tip after aseptic removal) (Garland et al. 2005; Hooven and Polin 2014). When CONS are isolated from cultures, definite CRBSI can be assumed when both the central line and the peripheral blood culture are positive, a presumed colonization when only the central line culture is positive, presumed contamination when only the peripheral culture is positive for CONS, and no bloodstream infection if both are negative. In these latter three cases, the clinical conditions of the patient should guide the therapeutic and further diagnostic decisions as, for instance, performing a lumbar puncture and continuing empiric antibiotic treatment (Hooven and Polin 2014).

Strategies to reduce CRBSIs include (1) precautions during insertion and management of the CVC, (2) reduction of indwelling times for tunneled catheters, and (3) CVC removal after positive blood culture results:

1. Central venous catheter contamination and colonization may occur during insertion and line management (Clark et al. 2004a). Good hand hygiene combined with proper aseptic technique during catheter insertion and manipulation affords protection against infection. Standard aseptic techniques (caps, masks, sterile gowns, sterile gloves, and large sterile drapes) during insertion substantially reduce the incidence of catheter-related bloodstream infections compared with standard precautions (sterile gloves and small drapes) (O'Grady et al. 2002; Raad et al. 1994). Proper management of the central venous catheters should include the establishment of a sterile field and rubbing the hub vigorously with alcohol at the time of hub entry or disconnection (Kilbride et al. 2003), avoiding the use of multilumen catheters, blood withdrawal through the catheter, and daily assessment of the site of insertion and of the integrity of the dressing (Golombek et al. 2002).

   The optimal solution for skin disinfection before aseptic procedures is not well defined for premature infants and infants younger than 2 months of age, and the antiseptic solution to be used before placement of a central catheter may vary according to institution and patient population. In preterm infants, in which the risk of burns associated with chlorhexidine solutions is high due to a thinner or absent stratum corneum, a povidone-iodine solution may be a suitable option (McCay et al. 2014; Anderson et al. 2008). When using a povidone-iodine solution, it should be removed from the patient's skin after it has dried to prevent tissue damage, absorption, and thyroid suppression (McCay et al. 2014).

   Administration sets should be replaced every 48–72 h; when lipid-containing admixtures are given, sets should be replaced every 24 h (O'Grady et al. 2002). Antibiotic lock solutions for the prevention of CRBSIs are currently not recommended in NICU.
2. Reducing the indwelling time of CVCs is the easiest way to reduce the risk of CRBSI. Several studies demonstrated a direct correlation between times of indwelling catheters and incidence of sepsis in newborn infants (Stoll et al. 2002a; Clark et al. 2004a). However, more recently, a retrospective cohort study of 13,327 infants with 15,567 catheters (93% peripherally inserted central catheters [PICCs], 7% tunneled catheters) showed that the increased dwell time was not associated with increased risk of CRBSIs for PICCs (Greenberg et al. 2015). For tunneled catheters, infection incidence was significantly higher in weeks 7 and 9 compared with week 1. While a catheter should be promptly removed when it is not anymore necessary due to possible noninfectious complications, clinicians should not routinely replace uninfected PICCs for fear of infection; instead, should consider removing tunneled catheters before week 7 if no longer needed (Greenberg et al. 2015).
3. Central venous catheters should be promptly removed when blood cultures are positive. Benjamin et al. found that the outcome for patients in whom the central catheter was not removed within 24 h of bacterial organism identification was significantly worse (increased risk of infectious complications defined as the presence of end-organ damage, multiple positive blood cultures drawn at separate times within one episode of sepsis, or death) than for those whose catheters were removed promptly (8% vs. 46%, OR = 9.8) (Benjamin et al. 2001). In a retrospective study by Karlowicz et al., central venous catheter removal within 3 days of the first positive blood culture for *Candida* species was associated with a shorter duration of fungemia (3 vs. 6 days, $P = 0.0002$) and a reduced mortality rate (2 vs. 19%, $P = 0.008$) (Karlowicz et al. 2000). CVCs should be removed as soon as bacteremia and fungemia are detected. When blood cultures are positive for CONS, catheter sterilization may be attempted, but the catheter should be promptly removed if subsequent cultures are positive.

107.5.2.3 Antimicrobial Prophylaxis

Antibiotic prophylaxis. The use of an antibiotic prophylaxis of high-risk infants (extremely preterm infants, infants who undergo endotracheal intubation and mechanical ventilation, chest wall and abdominal drainage, surgical intervention, and immune deficiency, and infants with maternal risk factors as chorioamnionitis and maternal fever) has been evaluated in several studies and is currently not recommended.

In a Cochrane meta-analysis, the antibiotic prophylaxis for infants with CVC was demonstrated to slightly reduce the incidence of sepsis; however, this effect is not associated with a reduction in mortality, and data on the neurodevelopmental outcome and on the emergence of resistant bacterial strains are lacking, and antibiotic prophylaxis cannot be routinely recommended (Jardine et al. 2008).

A Cochrane meta-analysis included five clinical trials studying the use of prophylactic vancomycin for the prevention of CVC-related nosocomial infections (Craft et al. 2000). The use of prophylactic vancomycin in low doses reduces the incidence of nosocomial sepsis, but, given that few clinically important benefits have been demonstrated for VLBW infants and that there is insufficient evidence to ascertain the risk of development of vancomycin-resistant organisms, the authors conclude that routine prophylaxis with vancomycin should not be undertaken at present.

An "antibiotic flush" or "antibiotic lock" prophylaxis has been evaluated in some studies. In a prospective randomized clinical trial (Garland et al. 2005), VLBW infants with a newly placed peripherally inserted CVC were randomized to having the catheter locked two or three times daily for 20 or 60 min with heparinized normal saline or heparinized saline containing vancomycin 25 μg/mL. The incidence of CVC-related bloodstream infections was significantly higher in the control than in the treated group (17.8 vs. 2.3 per 1,000 catheter days); no vancomycin-resistant *Enterococci* or CONS were recovered from any cultures. A heparin/fusidic acid lock solution (fusidic acid, 4 mg/mL; heparin, 10 UI/mL) has been evaluated by Filippi et al. (2007) on 103 newborn infants. In the treated group, the incidence of CRBSIs was significantly lower than in the control group (6.6 vs. 24.9/1,000 catheter-days, $P < 0.01$). However, there are insufficient data to routinely recommend this procedure in NICUs.

Antifungal prophylaxis. The use of prophylactic fluconazole in VLBW infants has shown repeated efficacy in multiple trials in lowering the risk of invasive fungal infection and colonization (Camacho-Gonzalez et al. 2013).

In a large multicenter, randomized trial, Manzoni et al. (2007b) found a statistically significant reduction in *Candida* colonization rate and invasive fungal infection rate in treated infants compared to controls (8.8% vs. 29.2%, $P < 0.0001$ for *Candida* colonization, 3.2% vs. 13.2%, $P = 0.002$ for invasive fungal infections). Another study also demonstrated that fluconazole prophylaxis does not select resistant *C. albicans* strains (Manzoni et al. 2008).

In a Cochrane meta-analysis on ten trials enrolling 1,371 infants comparing the use of systemic antifungal prophylaxis versus placebo or no drug, Cleminson et al. show that prophylactic systemic antifungals reduce the incidence of invasive fungal infection in very preterm or very-low-birth-weight infants (Cleminson et al. 2015). However, the authors further suggest to interpret and apply cautiously this finding as the incidence of invasive fungal infection was very high in the control groups of many of the included trials, and meta-analysis does not demonstrate a statistically significant effect on mortality.

Shane and Stoll report that, based on an annual US preterm birth cohort of ~30,000 VLBW, it has been estimated that fluconazole prophylaxis could prevent ~2,000 to 3,000 cases of invasive candidiasis and ~200 to 300 deaths and adverse neurodevelopmental outcomes of invasive candidiasis in ~400 to 500 infants every year (Shane and Stoll 2014).

However, the risks and benefits of fluconazole prophylaxis must be weighed in each NICU based on the local incidence of *Candida* infection and on the categories of infants that may most benefit from the prophylaxis.

Benjamin et al. in a randomized, blinded, placebo-controlled trial evaluated the efficacy and safety of fluconazole in preventing death or invasive candidiasis in extremely low-birth-weight infants (less than 750 g at birth) assigned to receive either fluconazole 6 mg/kg of body weight or placebo twice weekly for 42 days. Fluconazole prophylaxis compared with placebo did not result in a lower incidence of the composite outcome of death or invasive candidiasis in this cohort, thus not supporting the universal use of prophylactic fluconazole in extremely low-birth-weight infants. The authors further suggest that the routine use of fluconazole prophylaxis should be limited to units with moderate-to-high incidence of invasive candidiasis and that additional research is needed to precisely define the incidence at which the benefits of fluconazole prophylaxis outweigh the risks (Benjamin et al. 2014).

In addition, fluconazole prophylaxis needs continuous monitoring for the emergence of resistant strains and the collection of data on the long-term neurodevelopment after early exposure to fluconazole following preterm birth (Cleminson et al. 2015). Furthermore, the advantages and disadvantages of systemic fluconazole over oral antifungals still need further study.

In a Cochrane meta-analysis (Austin et al. 2015), Austin et al. evaluated four trials (1,800 infants) comparing oral/topical non-absorbed antifungal prophylaxis (nystatin or miconazole) with placebo or no drug and found a reduction in risk of invasive fungal infection in VLBW infants treated with oral/topical non-absorbed antifungals; however, the authors further suggest that these results should be interpreted cautiously because of methodological weaknesses in the included trials. In the same meta-analysis, the authors identified three trials comparing the effect of oral/topical non-absorbed versus systemic antifungal prophylaxis and did not find any statistically significant differences in the incidences of invasive fungal infection or all-cause mortality, suggesting that oral antifungal agents may be as effective as systemic fluconazole (Austin et al. 2015). In a systematic review on the prophylaxis of neonatal fungal infections, Blyth et al. conclude that prophylactic fluconazole and oral nystatin are both highly effective in preventing invasive fungal infections in VLBW infants. Both agents are safe without significant toxicities. Given the paucity of data comparing fluconazole with nystatin, the choice of antifungal agent should be influenced by the incidence of fungal infections, local epidemiology, and relative cost (Blyth et al. 2012).

107.5.2.4 Modulation of the Host-Pathogen Interaction

Antibiotics and antibiotic stewardship. The judicious use of antibiotics is the first step in reducing infection and limiting the emergence of resistant strains. Cotten et al. (2009) found an association between empirical antibiotic therapy for early-onset sepsis given for ≥ 5 days and increased mortality or composite outcome mortality and NEC. Kuppala et al. (2011) showed that antibiotics administered for ≥ 5 in the presence of negative cultures were associated with increased risk of late-onset sepsis, or composite outcome late-onset sepsis, NEC, or death. Alexander et al. (2011) found an association between empirical antibiotics and an increased risk of NEC. This evidence urges to avoid unnecessary antibiotic therapy and to limit empirical treatment with broad-spectrum antibiotics to cases where culture results are pending. Efforts should be put in improving the accuracy of microbiological diagnosis (perform at least two blood cultures and urine and CSF cultures) to identify the pathogen and narrow the spectrum of the antimicrobial agents.

Among other interventions, the CDC recommends that each hospital builds an antibiotic stewardship program, which should rely on infrastructures to provide physicians with the information and tools they need to make the right decisions and on a surveillance program both during and after antibiotic prescription (http://www.cdc.gov/media/releases/2014/p0304-poor-antibiotic-prescribing.html, accessed January 2, 2016) (Kuehn 2014). One of the key elements of the stewardship should be the development of a checklist, allowing to reduce the inappropriate use of antibiotics through a systematic evaluation of all the steps of antibiotic treatment (http://www.cdc.gov/getsmart/healthcare/implementation/checklist.html, accessed January 2, 2016) (Kuehn 2014).

A specific antibiotic stewardship program should be developed for the NICUs (Patel et al. 2012). According to Cantey and Patel

(2014), specific issues of a neonatal antibiotic stewardship program include:

- Diagnostic challenges, due to the often nonspecific signs of sepsis and the frequent occurrence of culture-negative infections (clinical and laboratory signs of sepsis despite negative cultures)
- Duration of treatment, which often varies among NICUs and even in the same unit and that need standardization
- Management of infants born to mothers with chorioamnionitis, which may receive unnecessary yet often unavoidable antibiotics
- Difficulties in dosing and therapeutic drug monitoring
- The optimal regimens for perioperative prophylaxis

Immune prophylaxis. Several studies evaluated the effectiveness of immunoglobulins in preventing nosocomial infections in the preterm infant. A Cochrane meta-analysis by Lacy and Ohlsson found that intravenous pooled polyvalent immunoglobulin administration results in a 3% reduction in sepsis and a 4% reduction in one or more episodes of any serious infection but is not associated with reductions in other clinically important outcomes, including mortality. There are insufficient data to suggest routine use of immunoglobulins to prevent nosocomial sepsis in the preterm infant. The authors conclude that the decision to use prophylactic IVIG will depend on the costs and the values assigned to the clinical outcomes (Ohlsson and Lacy 2013).

Potential benefits can be achieved by the administration of pathogen-specific immunoglobulins.

Studies on two specific anti-staphylococcal immunoglobulins (INH A-21 and Altastaph) (DeJonge et al. 2007; Benjamin et al. 2006) showed no benefit from prophylactic administration, and antistaphylococcal immunoglobulins are currently not recommended for prevention of staphylococcal infections in preterm or VLBW neonates (Shah and Kaufman 2009).

A third specific antistaphylococcal immunoglobulin, pagibaximab, has been evaluated in three studies, demonstrating safety and tolerability of pagibaximab with no observed reduction in sepsis, and is currently not recommended (Patel and Kaufman 2015). The discovery of new antimicrobial-specific and neutralizing immunoglobulins against common pathogens of the neonatal age other than *Staphylococci* may be beneficial (DiGiandomenico et al. 2014). However, despite their potential, there is no demonstration, to date, of the efficacy of any commercially available antimicrobial immunoglobulin for the prevention of infection in the neonatal age.

G-CSF and GM-CSF have been evaluated in a Cochrane review and they are currently not recommended, in neonatal practice, as prophylaxis to prevent systemic infection in high-risk neonates (Carr et al. 2003). In a trial on GM-CSF administered as prophylaxis for reduction of sepsis in extremely preterm, small for gestational age neonates, early postnatal prophylactic GM-CSF corrected neutropenia but did not reduce sepsis or improve survival and short- or long-term outcomes in extremely preterm neonates (Carr et al. 2009; Marlow et al. 2013).

Breast milk. The age of introduction of enteral feeds and the administration of human milk affect the incidence of nosocomial sepsis. The incidence of infection is reduced by human milk compared to formula (Hylander et al. 1998) and early enteral feeding is also beneficial (Flidel-Rimon et al. 2004). Possible mechanisms include (1) prevention of gastrointestinal atrophy, (2) prevention of intestinal bacterial contamination. (3) decreased use of total parenteral nutrition and intravenous devices, and (4) enhancement of mucosal immunity (Flidel-Rimon et al. 2004). Several factors present in breast milk have an anti-infectious activity, including immune globulins, cytokines, complement, fibronectin, enzymes (lysozyme, leukocyte enzymes), macrophages (~60%), neutrophils (~25%), and lymphocytes (~10%).

Lactoferrin. Manzoni et al. established that orally administered bovine lactoferrin, a mammalian milk glycoprotein involved in innate immune host defenses, alone (100 mg/day) or in combination with the probiotic *Lactobacillus rhamnosus* GG (6×10^9 colony-forming units/day) from birth until day 30 of life (day 45 for neonates <1,000 g at birth), significantly reduces the incidence of a first episode of bacterial and fungal LONS in VLBW neonates (risk ratio for lactoferrin vs. control groups: 0.34; 95% CI, 0.17–0.70; $P = 0.002$. Risk ratio for lactoferrin plus *Lactobacillus rhamnosus* vs. control groups: 0.27; 95% CI, 0.12–0.60; $P < 0.001$) (Manzoni et al. 2009). In a Cochrane meta-analysis, Pammi and Abrams point out that evidence of moderate to low quality suggests that oral lactoferrin prophylaxis with or without probiotics decreases late-onset sepsis and NEC stage II or greater in preterm infants without adverse effects (Pammi and Abrams 2015). Clinical trials are currently ongoing to confirm these results and clarify which are the optimum dosing regimens, the best type of lactoferrin (human or bovine), and the long-term outcomes.

Probiotics. In a Cochrane meta-analysis, AlFaleh and Anabrees compared the efficacy and safety of prophylactic enteral probiotics administration versus placebo or no treatment in the prevention of severe NEC or sepsis, or both, in preterm infants and found that enteral supplementation of probiotics prevents severe NEC and all-cause mortality in preterm infants, but there is no evidence of significant reduction of nosocomial sepsis (AlFaleh and Anabrees 2014).

In a recent large multicenter, randomized-controlled phase 3 study (the PiPS trial), infants born between 23 and 30 weeks' gestational age were randomly assigned to probiotic (*Bifidobacterium breve* BBG-001, chosen because when the trial was designed, it was the only probiotic reported to show any benefit) or placebo. The authors found no evidence of benefit for this intervention in this population, thus not supporting the routine use of *B. breve* BBG-001 for prevention of necrotizing enterocolitis and late-onset sepsis in very preterm infants although the authors cannot exclude that the high cross-colonization rate of the placebo group may have masked the benefits of the probiotic intervention (Costeloe et al. 2016).

Use of H2-antagonists. H2-blocker therapy has been found to be associated with higher rates of NEC (Guillet et al. 2006), and its use should be limited to highly selected cases in neonatal practice.

Microbiota. Several studies have been recently published demonstrating that the above described factors, including exposure to antibiotics, the prolonged total parenteral nutrition or the maternal/formula milk, probiotics, lactoferrin, exposure to H2-antagonists, and other interventions may modulate the host-pathogen interaction by, at least in part, modifying the composition of the microbiota (i.e., the totality of the microorganisms in a given niche) in different organs and tissues. In the future, the direct modulation of the microbiota toward a beneficial composition and diversity may become a strategy for the prevention of infection in the neonatal age.

107.5.2.5 Skin Care

The skin barrier, the first line of defense against infection, is compromised in the neonate, particularly in the preterm newborn, because of the thinner stratum corneum (3–16 layers depending on gestational age at birth), which is easily damaged by handling, adhesives, and alcohol and povidone-iodine applications. Hence, several authors have evaluated the effectiveness of skin ointments for the prevention of nosocomial infections.

A Cochrane review by Conner et al. published in 2004 concluded that prophylactic application of topical ointments increases the risk of CONS infection and any nosocomial infection and that this treatment should not be used routinely in preterm infants (Conner et al. 2004).

In 2005, Darmstadt et al. conducted a randomized trial on 497 neonates of gestational age <33 weeks and randomly assigned infants to daily massage with sunflower seed oil or Aquaphor (petrolatum, mineral oil, mineral wax, lanolin alcohol) and compared the incidence of nosocomial infections among infants in these two groups with an untreated control group. In their study Aquaphor did not significantly reduce the risk of infection, while skin applications of sunflower seed oil afforded protection against nosocomial infections (Darmstadt et al. 2005).

The question whether topical skin ointment should be used for VLBW infants is still debatable and further trials are needed.

In a Cochrane meta-analysis, Sinha et al. evaluated the efficacy of neonatal skin or cord care with chlorhexidine versus routine care or no treatment for prevention of infections in late preterm or term newborn infants in hospital and community settings. Among other results, the authors found high-quality evidence that chlorhexidine skin or cord care in the community setting results in a 50% reduction in the incidence of omphalitis and a 12% reduction in neonatal mortality (Sinha et al. 2015).

References

Adam B, Baillie GS, Douglas LJ (2002) Mixed species biofilms of *Candida albicans* and *Staphylococcus epidermidis*. J Med Microbiol 51(4):344–349

Alexander VN, Northrup V, Bizzarro MJ (2011) Antibiotic exposure in the newborn intensive care unit and the risk of necrotizing enterocolitis. J Pediatr 159(3):392–397

AlFaleh K, Anabrees J (2014) Probiotics for prevention of necrotizing enterocolitis in preterm infants. Cochrane Database Syst Rev 4, CD005496

Amini E, Ghasemi M, Daneshjou K (2008) A five-year study in Iran of ophthalmia neonatorum: prevalence and etiology. Med Sci Monit 14(2):CR90–CR96

Anderson J, Leonard D, Braner DA, Lai S, Tegtmeyer K (2008) Videos in clinical medicine. Umbilical vascular catheterization. N Engl J Med 359(15):e18

Apisarnthanarak A, Holzmann-Pazgal G, Hamvas A, Olsen MA, Fraser VJ (2003) Ventilator-associated pneumonia in extremely preterm neonates in a neonatal intensive care unit: characteristics, risk factors, and outcomes. Pediatrics 112(6 Pt 1):1283–1289

Arnon S, Litmanovitz I (2008) Diagnostic tests in neonatal sepsis. Curr Opin Infect Dis 21(3):223–227

Arnon S, Litmanovitz I, Regev R, Lis M, Shainkin-Kestenbaum R, Dolfin T (2002) Serum amyloid A protein in the early detection of late-onset bacterial sepsis in preterm infants. J Perinat Med 30(4): 329–332

Arnon S, Litmanovitz I, Regev RH, Bauer S, Shainkin-Kestenbaum R, Dolfin T (2007) Serum amyloid A: an early and accurate marker of neonatal early-onset sepsis. J Perinatol 27(5):297–302

Ascher SB, Smith PB, Watt K, Benjamin DK, Cohen-Wolkowiez M, Clark RH et al (2012) Antifungal therapy and outcomes in infants with invasive *Candida* infections. Pediatr Infect Dis J 31(5):439–443, Pubmed Central PMCID: 3329577

Auriti C, Prencipe G, Inglese R, Azzari C, Ronchetti MP, Tozzi A et al (2010) Role of mannose-binding lectin in nosocomial sepsis in critically ill neonates. Hum Immunol 71(11):1084–1088

Austin N, Cleminson J, Darlow BA, McGuire W (2015) Prophylactic oral/topical non-absorbed antifungal agents to prevent invasive fungal infection in very low birth weight infants. Cochrane Database Syst Rev 10, CD003478

Avila-Figueroa C, Goldmann DA, Richardson DK, Gray JE, Ferrari A, Freeman J (1998) Intravenous lipid emulsions are the major determinant of coagulase-negative staphylococcal bacteremia in very low birth weight newborns. Pediatr Infect Dis J 17(1):10–17

Baker CJ (1997) Group B, streptococcal infections. Clin Perinatol 24(1):59–70

Baley JE, Silverman RA (1988) Systemic candidiasis: cutaneous manifestations in low birth weight infants. Pediatrics 82(2):211–215

Baltimore RS (2003) The difficulty of diagnosing ventilator-associated pneumonia. Pediatrics 112(6 Pt 1):1420–1421

Baltimore RS (2007) Consequences of prophylaxis for group B streptococcal infections of the neonate. Semin Perinatol 31(1):33–38

Barcaite E, Bartusevicius A, Tameliene R, Kliucinskas M, Maleckiene L, Nadisauskiene R (2008) Prevalence of maternal group B streptococcal colonisation in European countries. Acta Obstet Gynecol Scand 87(3): 260–271

Barnett ED, Klein JO (2006) Bacterial infections of the respiratory tract. In: Remington, Klein, Wilson, Baker (eds) Infectious diseases of the fetus and newborn infant, 6th edn. Elsevier Saunders, Philadelphia, pp 297–317

Bauer S, Eliakim A, Pomeranz A, Regev R, Litmanovits I, Arnon S et al (2003) Urinary tract infection in very low birth weight preterm infants. Pediatr Infect Dis J 22(5): 426–430

Bedford H, de Louvois J, Halket S, Peckham C, Hurley R, Harvey D (2001) Meningitis in infancy in England and Wales: follow up at age 5 years. BMJ 323(7312):533–536

Bendel CM (2005) Nosocomial neonatal candidiasis. Pediatr Infect Dis J 24(9):831–832

Benjamin DK Jr, Miller W, Garges H, Benjamin DK, McKinney RE Jr, Cotton M et al (2001) Bacteremia, central catheters, and neonates: when to pull the line. Pediatrics 107(6):1272–1276

Benjamin DK Jr, Poole C, Steinbach WJ, Rowen JL, Walsh TJ (2003) Neonatal candidemia and end-organ damage: a critical appraisal of the literature using meta-analytic techniques. Pediatrics 112(3 Pt 1):634–640

Benjamin DK, Schelonka R, White R, Holley HP, Bifano E, Cummings J et al (2006) A blinded, randomized, multicenter study of an intravenous *Staphylococcus aureus* immune globulin. J Perinatol 26(5): 290–295

Benjamin DK Jr, Hudak ML, Duara S, Randolph DA, Bidegain M, Mundakel GT et al (2014) Effect of fluconazole prophylaxis on candidiasis and mortality in premature infants: a randomized clinical trial. JAMA 311(17): 1742–1749, Pubmed Central PMCID: 4110724

Berner R (2002) Group B, streptococci during pregnancy and infancy. Curr Opin Infect Dis 15(3):307–313

Bizzarro MJ, Raskind C, Baltimore RS, Gallagher PG (2005) Seventy-five years of neonatal sepsis at Yale: 1928–2003. Pediatrics 116(3):595–602

Blyth CC, Barzi F, Hale K, Isaacs D (2012) Chemoprophylaxis of neonatal fungal infections in very low birthweight infants: efficacy and safety of fluconazole and nystatin. J Paediatr Child Health 48(9):846–851

Boghossian NS, Page GP, Bell EF, Stoll BJ, Murray JC, Cotten CM et al (2013) Late-onset sepsis in very low birth weight infants from singleton and multiple-gestation births. J Pediatr 162(6):1120–1124, 4 e1. Pubmed Central PMCID: 3633723

Borghesi A, Stronati M (2008) Strategies for the prevention of hospital-acquired infections in the neonatal intensive care unit. J Hosp Infect 68(4):293–300

Boucher HW, Talbot GH, Bradley JS, Edwards JE, Gilbert D, Rice LB et al (2009) Bad bugs, no drugs: no ESKAPE! An update from the Infectious Diseases Society of America. Clin Infect Dis 48(1):1–12

Brady MT (2005) Health care-associated infections in the neonatal intensive care unit. Am J Infect Control 33(5): 268–275

Bundy DG (2007) Vesicoureteral reflux. Pediatr Rev 28(2): e6–e8

Buttery JP (2002) Blood cultures in newborns and children: optimising an everyday test. Arch Dis Child Fetal Neonatal Ed 87(1):F25–F28

Camacho-Gonzalez A, Spearman PW, Stoll BJ (2013) Neonatal infectious diseases: evaluation of neonatal sepsis. Pediatr Clin N Am 60(2):367–389, Pubmed Central PMCID: 4405627

Cantey JB, Patel SJ (2014) Antimicrobial stewardship in the NICU. Infect Dis Clin N Am 28(2):247–261

Cantey JB, Sreeramoju P, Jaleel M, Treviño S, Gander R, Hynan LS et al (2013) Prompt control of an outbreak caused by extended-spectrum β-lactamase – producing *Klebsiella pneumoniae* in a neonatal intensive care unit. J Pediatr 163(3):672–679, e3

Carr R, Modi N, Dore C (2003) G-CSF and GM-CSF for treating or preventing neonatal infections. Cochrane Database Syst Rev 3, CD003066

Carr R, Brocklehurst P, Dore CJ, Modi N (2009) Granulocyte-macrophage colony stimulating factor administered as prophylaxis for reduction of sepsis in extremely preterm, small for gestational age neonates (the PROGRAMS trial): a single-blind, multicentre, randomised controlled trial. Lancet 373(9659):226–233

Cattarossi L (2013) Lung ultrasound: its role in neonatology and pediatrics. Early Hum Dev 89(Suppl 1): S17–S19

Centers for Disease Control and Prevention (2010) 2010 guidelines for the prevention of perinatal group B streptococcal disease. MMWR 59(RR-10):1–32

Cernada M, Brugada M, Golombek S, Vento M (2014) Ventilator-associated pneumonia in neonatal patients: an update. Neonatology 105(2):98–107

Chang K, Cheng VY, Kwong NS (2006) Neonatal haemorrhagic conjunctivitis: a specific sign of chlamydial infection. Hong Kong Med J 12(1):27–32

Clark R, Powers R, White R, Bloom B, Sanchez P, Benjamin DK Jr (2004a) Prevention and treatment of nosocomial sepsis in the NICU. J Perinatol 24(7):446–453

Clark R, Powers R, White R, Bloom B, Sanchez P, Benjamin DK Jr (2004b) Nosocomial infection in the NICU: a medical complication or unavoidable problem? J Perinatol 24(6):382–388

Cleminson J, Austin N, McGuire W (2015) Prophylactic systemic antifungal agents to prevent mortality and morbidity in very low birth weight infants. Cochrane Database Syst Rev 10, CD003850

Cohen B, Saiman L, Cimiotti J, Larson E (2003) Factors associated with hand hygiene practices in two neonatal intensive care units. Pediatr Infect Dis J 22 (6):494–499

Colombo DF, Lew JL, Pedersen CA, Johnson JR, Fan-Havard P (2006) Optimal timing of ampicillin administration to pregnant women for establishing bactericidal levels in the prophylaxis of Group B *Streptococcus*. Am J Obstet Gynecol 194(2):466–470

Committee on Infectious Diseases AAoP, Kimberlin DW, Brady MT, Jackson MA, Long SS (2015) Group B streptococcal infections. Red Book 2015; 2015 report of the Committee on Infectious Diseases, 30th edn. pp 745–750. http://ebooks.aappublications.org/content/red-book-30th-edition-2015

Conner JM, Soll RF, Edwards WH (2004) Topical ointment for preventing infection in preterm infants. Cochrane Database Syst Rev 1, CD001150

Costeloe K, Hardy P, Juszczak E, Wilks M, Millar MR, Probiotics in Preterm Infants Study Collaborative Group (2016) Bifidobacterium breve BBG-001 in very preterm infants: a randomised controlled phase 3 trial. Lancet 387(10019):649–60

Cotten CM, Taylor S, Stoll B, Goldberg RN, Hansen NI, Sanchez PJ et al (2009) Prolonged duration of initial empirical antibiotic treatment is associated with increased rates of necrotizing enterocolitis and death for extremely low birth weight infants. Pediatrics 123(1):58–66

Craft AP, Finer NN, Barrington KJ (2000) Vancomycin for prophylaxis against sepsis in preterm neonates. Cochrane Database Syst Rev 2, CD001971

Credè C (1881) Die verhutung der augenentzundung der neugeborenen. Arch Gynaekol 17:50–53

Darmstadt GL, Dinulos JG, Miller Z (2000) Congenital cutaneous candidiasis: clinical presentation, pathogenesis, and management guidelines. Pediatrics 105(2): 438–444

Darmstadt GL, Saha SK, Ahmed AS, Chowdhury MA, Law PA, Ahmed S (2005) Effect of topical treatment with skin barrier-enhancing emollients on nosocomial infections in preterm infants in Bangladesh: a randomised controlled trial. Lancet 365(9464): 1039–1045

Datta S, Roy S, Chatterjee S, Saha A, Sen B, Pal T et al (2014) A five-year experience of carbapenem resistance in Enterobacteriaceae causing neonatal septicaemia: predominance of NDM-1. PLoS One 9, e112101

DeJonge M, Burchfield D, Bloom B, Duenas M, Walker W, Polak M et al (2007) Clinical trial of safety and efficacy of INH-A21 for the prevention of nosocomial staphylococcal bloodstream infection in premature infants. J Pediatr 151(3):260–265, 5 e1

Deshpande SS, Taral N, Modi N, Singrakhia M (2004) Changing epidemiology of neonatal septic arthritis. J Orthop Surg (Hong Kong) 12(1):10–13

Dessì A, Corsello G, Stronati M, Gazzolo D, Caboni P, Carboni R et al (2014) New diagnostic possibilities in systemic neonatal infections: metabolomics. Early Hum Dev 90:S19–S21

DiGiandomenico A, Keller AE, Gao C, Rainey GJ, Warrener P, Camara MM et al (2014) A multifunctional bispecific antibody protects against *Pseudomonas aeruginosa*. Sci Transl Med 6(262):262ra155

Duke T (2005) Neonatal pneumonia in developing countries. Arch Dis Child Fetal Neonatal Ed 90(3):F211–F219

Ehl S, Gering B, Bartmann P, Hogel J, Pohlandt F (1997) C-reactive protein is a useful marker for guiding duration of antibiotic therapy in suspected neonatal bacterial infection. Pediatrics 99(2):216–221

El-Ganzoury MM, El-Farrash RA, Saad AA, Mohamed AG, El-Sherbini IG (2012) In vivo effect of recombinant human granulocyte colony-stimulating factor on neutrophilic expression of CD11b in septic neonates: a randomized controlled trial. Pediatr Hematol Oncol 29(3):272–284

Esposito S, Zampiero A, Pugni L, Tabano S, Pelucchi C, Ghirardi B et al (2014) Genetic polymorphisms and sepsis in premature neonates. PLoS ONE 9(7), e101248, Pubmed Central PMCID: 4085055

Faix RG (1992) Invasive neonatal candidiasis: comparison of albicans and parapsilosis infection. Pediatr Infect Dis J 11(2):88–93

Fanaroff AA, Korones SB, Wright LL, Verter J, Poland RL, Bauer CR et al (1998) Incidence, presenting features, risk factors and significance of late onset septicemia in very low birth weight infants. The National Institute of Child Health and Human Development Neonatal Research Network. Pediatr Infect Dis J 17(7):593–598

Feja KN, Wu F, Roberts K, Loughrey M, Nesin M, Larson E et al (2005) Risk factors for candidemia in critically ill infants: a matched case-control study. J Pediatr 147(2): 156–161

Filippi L, Pezzati M, Di Amario S, Poggi C, Pecile P (2007) Fusidic acid and heparin lock solution for the prevention of catheter-related bloodstream infections in critically ill neonates: a retrospective study and a prospective, randomized trial. Pediatr Crit Care Med 8(6): 556–562

Finnell SM, Carroll AE, Downs SM (2011) Subcommittee on urinary tract I. Technical report-diagnosis and management of an initial UTI in febrile infants and young children. Pediatrics 128(3):e749–e770

Flidel-Rimon O, Friedman S, Lev E, Juster-Reicher A, Amitay M, Shinwell ES (2004) Early enteral feeding and nosocomial sepsis in very low birthweight infants. Arch Dis Child Fetal Neonatal Ed 89(4):F289–F292

Foca M, Jakob K, Whittier S, Della Latta P, Factor S, Rubenstein D et al (2000) Endemic *Pseudomonas aeruginosa* infection in a neonatal intensive care unit. N Engl J Med 343(10):695–700

Foster TJ (2005) Immune evasion by staphylococci. Nat Rev Microbiol 3(12):948–958

Foster A, Klauss V (1995) Ophthalmia neonatorum in developing countries. N Engl J Med 332(9):600–601

Fransen L, Van den Berghe P, Mertens A, Van Brussel K, Clara R, Piot P (1987) Incidence and bacterial aetiology of neonatal conjunctivitis. Eur J Pediatr 146 (2):152–155

Fraser N, Davies BW, Cusack J (2006) Neonatal omphalitis: a review of its serious complications. Acta Paediatr 95(5):519–522

Frederiksen B, Christiansen P, Knudsen FU (1993) Acute osteomyelitis and septic arthritis in the neonate, risk factors and outcome. Eur J Pediatr 152(7):577–580

Freeman J, Goldmann DA, Smith NE, Sidebottom DG, Epstein MF, Platt R (1990) Association of intravenous lipid emulsion and coagulase-negative staphylococcal bacteremia in neonatal intensive care units. N Engl J Med 323(5):301–308

Friedman S, Richardson SE, Jacobs SE, O'Brien K (2000) Systemic *Candida* infection in extremely low birth weight infants: short term morbidity and long term neurodevelopmental outcome. Pediatr Infect Dis J 19 (6):499–504

Gallardo MJ, Johnson DA, Gaviria J, Nguyen L, Melendez R, Connor DA et al (2005) Isolated herpes simplex keratoconjunctivitis in a neonate born by cesarean delivery. J Aapos 9(3):285–287

Garges HP, Moody MA, Cotten CM, Smith PB, Tiffany KF, Lenfestey R et al (2006) Neonatal meningitis: what is the correlation among cerebrospinal fluid cultures, blood cultures, and cerebrospinal fluid parameters? Pediatrics 117(4):1094–1100

Garland JS, Alex CP, Henrickson KJ, McAuliffe TL, Maki DG (2005) A vancomycin-heparin lock solution for prevention of nosocomial bloodstream infection in critically ill neonates with peripherally inserted central venous catheters: a prospective, randomized trial. Pediatrics 116(2):e198–e205

Ghosal SP, Sen Gupta PC, Mukherjee AK, Choudhury M, Dutta N, Sarkar AK (1978) Noma neonatorum: its aetiopathogenesis. Lancet 2(8084):289–291

Golombek SG, Rohan AJ, Parvez B, Salice AL, LaGamma EF (2002) "Proactive" management of percutaneously inserted central catheters results in decreased incidence of infection in the ELBW population. J Perinatol 22(3): 209–213

Greenberg RG, Benjamin DK Jr (2014) Neonatal candidiasis: diagnosis, prevention, and treatment. JInfect 69(Suppl 1):S19–S22, Pubmed Central PMCID: 4252884

Greenberg RG, Benjamin DK Jr, Gantz MG, Cotten CM, Stoll BJ, Walsh MC et al (2012) Empiric antifungal therapy and outcomes in extremely low birth weight infants with invasive candidiasis. J Pediatr

161(2):264–269, Pubmed Central PMCID: 3380169, e2

Greenberg RG, Cochran KM, Smith PB, Edson BS, Schulman J, Lee HC et al (2015) Effect of catheter dwell time on risk of central line-associated bloodstream infection in infants. Pediatrics 136(6): 1080–1086, Pubmed Central PMCID: 4657598

Grosskreutz C, Smith LB (1992) Neonatal conjunctivitis. Int Ophthalmol Clin 32(1):71–79

Grundmann H, Kropec A, Hartung D, Berner R, Daschner F (1993) Pseudomonas aeruginosa in a neonatal intensive care unit: reservoirs and ecology of the nosocomial pathogen. J Infect Dis 168(4):943–947

Guida JD, Kunig AM, Leef KH, McKenzie SE, Paul DA (2003) Platelet count and sepsis in very low birth weight neonates: is there an organism-specific response? Pediatrics 111(6 Pt 1):1411–1415

Guillet R, Stoll BJ, Cotten CM, Gantz M, McDonald S, Poole WK et al (2006) Association of H2-blocker therapy and higher incidence of necrotizing enterocolitis in very low birth weight infants. Pediatrics 117(2): e137–e142

Gutierrez K (2005) Bone and joint infections in children. Pediatr Clin N Am 52(3):779–794

Hammerschlag MR (2000) Treatment of *Chlamydia pneumoniae*. Int J Antimicrob Agents 15(3):239, 41

Harpin VA, Rutter N (1985) Humidification of incubators. Arch Dis Child 60(3):219–224

Healy CM, Palazzi DL, Edwards MS, Campbell JR, Baker CJ (2004) Features of invasive staphylococcal disease in neonates. Pediatrics 114(4):953–961

Heath PT, Nik Yusoff NK, Baker CJ (2003) Neonatal meningitis. Arch Dis Child Fetal Neonatal Ed 88(3): F173–F178

Hoberman A, Wald ER, Reynolds EA, Penchansky L, Charron M (1994) Pyuria and bacteriuria in urine specimens obtained by catheter from young children with fever. J Pediatr 124(4):513–519

Holt DE, Halket S, de Louvois J, Harvey D (2001) Neonatal meningitis in England and Wales: 10 years on. Arch Dis Child Fetal Neonatal Ed 84(2):F85–F89

Hooven TA, Polin RA (2014) Healthcare-associated infections in the hospitalized neonate: a review. Early Hum Dev 90(Suppl 1):S4–S6

Hornik CP, Fort P, Clark RH, Watt K, Benjamin DK Jr, Smith PB et al (2012) Early and late onset sepsis in very-low-birth-weight infants from a large group of neonatal intensive care units. Early Hum Dev 88(Suppl 2):S69–S74, Pubmed Central PMCID: 3513766

Hylander MA, Strobino DM, Dhanireddy R (1998) Human milk feedings and infection among very low birth weight infants. Pediatrics 102(3), E38

Isaacs D (2006) Unnatural selection: reducing antibiotic resistance in neonatal units. Arch Dis Child Fetal Neonatal Ed 91(1):F72–F74

Isenberg SJ, Apt L, Wood M (1995) A controlled trial of povidone-iodine as prophylaxis against ophthalmia neonatorum. N Engl J Med 332(9):562–566

Isenberg SJ, Apt L, Del Signore M, Gichuhi S, Berman NG (2003) A double application approach to ophthalmia neonatorum prophylaxis. Br J Ophthalmol 87(12): 1449–1452

Jardine LA, Inglis GD, Davies MW (2008) Prophylactic systemic antibiotics to reduce morbidity and mortality in neonates with central venous catheters. Cochrane Database Syst Rev 1, CD006179

Jarvis WR (2004) Controlling healthcare-associated infections: the role of infection control and antimicrobial use practices. Semin Pediatr Infect Dis 15(1):30–40

Johnson CE (1999) New advances in childhood urinary tract infections. Pediatr Rev 20(10):335–342

Jones AJ, Starling LD, Keith T, Nicholl R, Seale AN (2014) When pneumonia does not respond to antibiotics: a challenging neonatal diagnosis. Arch Dis Child Educ Pract Ed 99(6):221–230, Pubmed Central PMCID: 4251205

Jordan JA, Durso MB (2000) Comparison of 16S rRNA gene PCR and BACTEC 9240 for detection of neonatal bacteremia. J Clin Microbiol 38(7):2574–2578

Juster-Reicher A, Flidel-Rimon O, Amitay M, Even-Tov S, Shinwell E, Leibovitz E (2003) High-dose liposomal amphotericin B in the therapy of systemic candidiasis in neonates. Eur J Clin Microbiol Infect Dis 22(10): 603–607

Kanellopoulos TA, Salakos C, Spiliopoulou I, Ellina A, Nikolakopoulou NM, Papanastasiou DA (2006) First urinary tract infection in neonates, infants and young children: a comparative study. Pediatr Nephrol 21 (8):1131–1137

Karlowicz MG, Hashimoto LN, Kelly RE Jr, Buescher ES (2000) Should central venous catheters be removed as soon as candidemia is detected in neonates? Pediatrics 106(5), E63

Kaufman D, Fairchild KD (2004) Clinical microbiology of bacterial and fungal sepsis in very-low-birth-weight infants. Clin Microbiol Rev 17(3):638–680

Kaufman DA, Blackman A, Conaway MR, Sinkin RA (2014) Nonsterile glove use in addition to hand hygiene to prevent late-onset infection in preterm infants: randomized clinical trial. JAMA Pediatr 168(10):909–916

Keller MS (2005) Musculoskeletal sonography in the neonate and infant. Pediatr Radiol 35(12):1167–1173

Kilbride HW, Wirtschafter DD, Powers RJ, Sheehan MB (2003) Implementation of evidence-based potentially better practices to decrease nosocomial infections. Pediatrics 111(4 Pt 2):e519–e533

Kuehn BM (2014) CDC: Hospital antibiotic use promotes resistance: checklist can improve practices. JAMA 311(15):1485–1486

Kuppala VS, Meinzen-Derr J, Morrow AL, Schibler KR (2011) Prolonged initial empirical antibiotic treatment is associated with adverse outcomes in premature infants. J Pediatr 159(5):720–725, Pubmed Central PMCID: 3193552, Epub 2011/07/26. eng

Lachassine E, Letamendia-Richard E, Gaudelus E (2004) Epidemiology of nosocomial infections in neonates. Arch Pediatr 11:229–233

Larcombe J (1999) Urinary tract infection in children. BMJ 319(7218):1173–1175

Leigh L, Stoll BJ, Rahman M, McGowan J Jr (1995) Pseudomonas aeruginosa infection in very low birth weight infants: a case-control study. Pediatr Infect Dis J 14(5):367–371

Lijoi D, Di Capua E, Ferrero S, Mistrangelo E, Giannattasio A, Morano S et al (2007) The efficacy of 2002 CDC guidelines in preventing perinatal group B streptococcal vertical transmission: a prospective study. Arch Gynecol Obstet 275(5):373–379

Lin FY, Weisman LE, Troendle J, Adams K (2003) Prematurity is the major risk factor for late-onset group B streptococcus disease. J Infect Dis 188(2):267–271

Loffler J, Hebart H, Schumacher U, Reitze H, Einsele H (1997) Comparison of different methods for extraction of DNA of fungal pathogens from cultures and blood. J Clin Microbiol 35(12):3311–3312

Long SS, Klein JO (2006) Bacterial infections of the urinary tract. In: Remington, Klein, Wilson, Baker (eds) Infectious diseases of the fetus and newborn infant, 6th edn. Elsevier Saunders, Philadelphia, pp 335–346

Longtin Y, Schneider A, Tschopp C, Renzi G, Gayet-Ageron A, Schrenzel J et al (2014) Contamination of stethoscopes and physicians' hands after a physical examination. Mayo Clin Proc 89(3):291–299

Lopez Sastre JB, Solis DP, Serradilla VR, Colomer BF, Cotallo GD (2007) Evaluation of procalcitonin for diagnosis of neonatal sepsis of vertical transmission. BMC Pediatr 7:9

Makhoul IR, Kassis I, Hashman N, Sujov P (2001) Staphylococcal scalded-skin syndrome in a very low birth weight premature infant. Pediatrics 108(1), E16

Malbon K, Mohan R, Nicholl R (2006) Should a neonate with possible late onset infection always have a lumbar puncture? Arch Dis Child 91(1):75–76

Manzoni P, Farina D, Galletto P, Leonessa M, Priolo C, Arisio R et al (2007a) Type and number of sites colonized by fungi and risk of progression to invasive fungal infection in preterm neonates in neonatal intensive care unit. J Perinat Med 35(3):220–226

Manzoni P, Stolfi I, Pugni L, Decembrino L, Magnani C, Vetrano G et al (2007b) A multicenter, randomized trial of prophylactic fluconazole in preterm neonates. N Engl J Med 356(24):2483–2495

Manzoni P, Leonessa M, Galletto P, Latino MA, Arisio R, Maule M et al (2008) Routine use of fluconazole prophylaxis in a neonatal intensive care unit does not select natively fluconazole-resistant *Candida* subspecies. Pediatr Infect Dis J 27(8):731–737

Manzoni P, Rinaldi M, Cattani S, Pugni L, Romeo MG, Messner H et al (2009) Bovine lactoferrin supplementation for prevention of late-onset sepsis in very low-birth-weight neonates: a randomized trial. JAMA 302(13):1421–1428

Marlow N, Morris T, Brocklehurst P, Carr R, Cowan FM, Patel N et al (2013) A randomised trial of granulocyte-macrophage colony-stimulating factor for neonatal sepsis: outcomes at 2 years. Arch Dis Child Fetal Neonatal Ed 98(1):F46–F53, Pubmed Central PMCID: 3533400

Mathur NB, Garg K, Kumar S (2002) Respiratory distress in neonates with special reference to pneumonia. Indian Pediatr 39(6):529–537

Maudsley RF, Brix GA, Hinton NA, Robertson EM, Bryans AM, Haust MD (1966) Placental inflammation and infection. A prospective bacteriologic and histologic study. Am J Obstet Gynecol 95(5):648–659

Mazzucchelli I, Garofoli F, Ciardelli L, Borghesi A, Tzialla C, Di Comite A et al (2013) Diagnostic performance of triggering receptor expressed on myeloid cells-1 and CD64 index as markers of sepsis in preterm newborns. Pediatr Crit Care Med 14(2):178–182

McCay AS, Elliott EC, Walden M (2014) Videos in clinical medicine. PICC placement in the neonate. N Engl J Med 370(11):e17

McDonald A, Scranton M, Gillespie R, Mahajan V, Edwards GA (2000) Voiding cystourethrograms and urinary tract infections: how long to wait? Pediatrics 105(4), E50

Mikhael M, Brown LS, Rosenfeld CR (2014) Serial neutrophil values facilitate predicting the absence of neonatal early-onset sepsis. J Pediatr 164(3):522–528, e1-3

Mishra UK, Jacobs SE, Doyle LW, Garland SM (2006) Newer approaches to the diagnosis of early onset neonatal sepsis. Arch Dis Child Fetal Neonatal Ed 91(3): F208–F212

Misra S, Bhakoo ON, Ayyagiri A, Katariya S (1991) Clinical & bacteriological profile of neonatal pneumonia. Indian J Med Res 93:366–370

Moore MR, Schrag SJ, Schuchat A (2003) Effects of intrapartum antimicrobial prophylaxis for prevention of group-B-streptococcal disease on the incidence and ecology of early-onset neonatal sepsis. Lancet Infect Dis 3(4):201–213

Mullany LC, Darmstadt GL, Khatry SK, Katz J, LeClerq SC, Shrestha S et al (2006) Topical applications of chlorhexidine to the umbilical cord for prevention of omphalitis and neonatal mortality in southern Nepal: a community-based, cluster-randomised trial. Lancet 367 (9514):910–918

Mullany LC, Darmstadt GL, Katz J, Khatry SK, LeClerq SC, Adhikari RK et al (2007) Risk factors for umbilical cord infection among newborns of southern Nepal. Am J Epidemiol 165(2):203–211

Muller-Pebody B, Johnson AP, Heath PT, Gilbert RE, Henderson KL, Sharland M (2010) Empirical treatment of neonatal sepsis: are the current guidelines adequate? Arch Dis Child Fetal Neonatal Ed 96(1):F4–F8

Mussi-Pinhata MM, Rego MA (2005) Immunological peculiarities of extremely preterm infants: a challenge for the prevention of nosocomial sepsis. J Pediatr (Rio J) 81((1 Suppl)):S59–S68, Particularidades imunologicas do pre-termo extremo: um desafio para a prevencao da sepse hospitalar

Mussi-Pinhata MM, Nobre RA, Martinez FE, Jorge SM, Ferlin ML, Goncalves AL (2004) Early-onset bacterial infection in Brazilian neonates with respiratory distress: a hospital-based study. J Trop Pediatr 50(1):6–11

Narang A, Mukhopadhyay K, Kumar P, Bhakoo ON (1998) Bone and joint infection in neonates. Indian J Pediatr 65(3):461–464

Newman TB (2011) The new American Academy of Pediatrics urinary tract infection guideline. Pediatrics 128 (3):572–575

Ng PC, Ang IL, Chiu RW, Li K, Lam HS, Wong RP et al (2010) Host-response biomarkers for diagnosis of late-onset septicemia and necrotizing enterocolitis in preterm infants. J Clin Invest 120(8):2989–3000, Pubmed Central PMCID: 2912182

Nissen MD (2007) Congenital and neonatal pneumonia. Paediatr Respir Rev 8(3):195–203

Nozicka CA, Hanly JG, Beste DJ, Conley SF, Hennes HM (1999) Otitis media in infants aged 0–8 weeks: frequency of associated serious bacterial disease. Pediatr Emerg Care 15(4):252–254

Offiah AC (2006) Acute osteomyelitis, septic arthritis and discitis: differences between neonates and older children. Eur J Radiol 60(2):221–232

O'Grady NP, Alexander M, Dellinger EP, Gerberding JL, Heard SO, Maki DG et al (2002) Guidelines for the prevention of intravascular catheter-related infections. The Hospital Infection Control Practices Advisory Committee, Center for Disese Control and Prevention, U.S. Pediatrics 110(5):e51

Ohlsson A, Lacy JB (2013) Intravenous immunoglobulin for preventing infection in preterm and/or low birth weight infants. Cochrane Database Syst Rev 7, CD000361

Ohlsson A, Lacy JB (2015) Intravenous immunoglobulin for suspected or proven infection in neonates. Cochrane Database Syst Rev 3, CD001239

Orscheln RC, Shinefield HR, Geme JWS III (2006) Staphylococcal infections. In: Remington, Klein, Wilson, Baker (eds) Infectious diseases of the fetus and newborn infant, 6th edn. Elsevier Saunders, Philadelphia, pp 513–543

Overturf GD (2006) Bacterial infections of the bones and joints. In: Remington, Klein, Wilson, Baker (eds) Infectious diseases of the fetus and newborn infant, 6th edn. Elsevier Saunders, Philadelphia, pp 319–333

Palazzi DL, Klein JO, Baker CJ (2006) Bacterial sepsis and meningitis. In: Remington, Klein, Wilson, Baker (eds) Infectious diseases of the fetus and newborn infant, 6th edn. Elsevier Saunders, Philadelphia, pp 247–295

Pammi M, Abrams SA (2015) Oral lactoferrin for the prevention of sepsis and necrotizing enterocolitis in preterm infants. Cochrane Database Syst Rev 2, CD007137

Patel M, Kaufman DA (2015) Anti-lipoteichoic acid monoclonal antibody (pagibaximab) studies for the prevention of staphylococcal bloodstream infections in preterm infants. Expert Opin Biol Ther 15(4): 595–600

Patel SJ, Saiman L (2012) Principles and strategies of antimicrobial stewardship in the neonatal intensive care unit. Semin Perinatol 36(6):431-6

Perlman JM, Rollins N, Sanchez PJ (1992) Late-onset meningitis in sick, very-low-birth-weight infants. Clinical and sonographic observations. Am J Dis Child 146 (11):1297–1301

Petdachai W (2004) Ventilator-associated pneumonia in a newborn intensive care unit. Southeast Asian J Trop Med Public Health 35(3):724–729

Phares CR, Lynfield R, Farley MM, Mohle-Boetani J, Harrison LH, Petit S et al (2008) Epidemiology of invasive group B streptococcal disease in the United States, 1999–2005. JAMA 299(17):2056–2065

Pittet D (2001) Improving adherence to hand hygiene practice: a multidisciplinary approach. Emerg Infect Dis 7(2):234–240

Pittet D, Boyce JM (2003) Revolutionising hand hygiene in health-care settings: guidelines revisited. Lancet Infect Dis 3(5):269–270

Pittet D, Hugonnet S, Harbarth S, Mourouga P, Sauvan V, Touveneau S et al (2000) Effectiveness of a hospital-wide programme to improve compliance with hand hygiene. Infect Control Program Lancet 356(9238): 1307–1312

Posen R, deLemos RA (1998) C-reactive protein levels in the extremely premature infant: case studies and literature review. J Perinatol 18(2):138–141

Raad II, Hohn DC, Gilbreath BJ, Suleiman N, Hill LA, Bruso PA et al (1994) Prevention of central venous catheter-related infections by using maximal sterile barrier precautions during insertion. Infect Control Hosp Epidemiol 15(4 Pt 1):231–238

Rangel-Frausto MS, Wiblin T, Blumberg HM, Saiman L, Patterson J, Rinaldi M et al (1999) National epidemiology of mycoses survey (NEMIS): variations in rates of bloodstream infections due to *Candida* species in seven surgical intensive care units and six neonatal intensive care units. Clin Infect Dis 29(2):253–258

Regan JA, Klebanoff MA, Nugent RP, Eschenbach DA, Blackwelder WC, Lou Y et al (1996) Colonization with group B streptococci in pregnancy and adverse outcome. VIP Study Group. Am J Obstet Gynecol 174(4): 1354–1360

Richter R, Below H, Kadow I, Kramer A, Muller C, Fusch C (2006) Effect of topical 1.25% povidone-iodine eye drops used for prophylaxis of ophthalmia neonatorum on renal iodine excretion and thyroid-stimulating hormone level. J Pediatr 148(3):401–403

Rondini G, Chirico G, Stronati M (1991) Profilassi delle Infezioni nosocomiali nel neonato ed approccio terapeutico. Riv Ital Pediatr 17:420–432

Roper MH, Vandelaer JH, Gasse FL (2007) Maternal and neonatal tetanus. Lancet 370(9603):1947–1959

Rotimi VO, Olowe SA, Ahmed I (1985) The development of bacterial flora of premature neonates. J Hyg (Lond) 94(3):309–318

Rowen JL (2003) Mucocutaneous candidiasis. Semin Perinatol 27(5):406–413

Royal College of Obstetricians and Gynaecologists (2012) Prevention of early onset neonatal group B streptococcal disease. https://www.rcog.org.uk/globalassets/documents/guidelines/gtg36_gbs.pdf. Accessed 27 Dec 2015

Saiman L, Ludington E, Pfaller M, Rangel-Frausto S, Wiblin RT, Dawson J et al (2000) Risk factors for candidemia in neonatal intensive care unit patients. The National Epidemiology of Mycosis Survey study group. Pediatr Infect Dis J 19(4):319–324

Saiman L, Ludington E, Dawson JD, Patterson JE, Rangel-Frausto S, Wiblin RT et al (2001) Risk factors for *Candida* species colonization of neonatal intensive care unit patients. Pediatr Infect Dis J 20(12): 1119–1124

Schlapbach LJ, Mattmann M, Thiel S, Boillat C, Otth M, Nelle M et al (2010) Differential role of the lectin pathway of complement activation in susceptibility to neonatal sepsis. Clin Infect Dis 51(2):153–162

Schrag SJ, Zell ER, Lynfield R, Roome A, Arnold KE, Craig AS et al (2002) A population-based comparison of strategies to prevent early-onset group B streptococcal disease in neonates. N Engl J Med 347(4):233–239

Shah SS, Gallagher PG (1998) Complications of conjunctivitis caused by *Pseudomonas aeruginosa* in a newborn intensive care unit. Pediatr Infect Dis J 17(2): 97–102

Shah PS, Kaufman DA (2009) Antistaphylococcal immunoglobulins to prevent staphylococcal infection in very low birth weight infants. Cochrane Database Syst Rev 2, CD006449

Shakunthala SK, Mallikarjuna Rao G, Urmila S (1978) Diagnostic lung puncture aspiration in acute pneumonia of newborn. Indian Pediatr 15(1):39–44

Shane AL, Stoll BJ (2014) Neonatal sepsis: progress towards improved outcomes. J Infect 68(Suppl 1): S24–S32

Singhi S, Singhi PD (1990) Clinical signs in neonatal pneumonia. Lancet 336(8722):1072–1073

Sinha A, Sazawal S, Pradhan A, Ramji S, Opiyo N (2015) Chlorhexidine skin or cord care for prevention of mortality and infections in neonates. Cochrane Database Syst Rev 3, CD007835

Sohn AH, Garrett DO, Sinkowitz-Cochran RL, Grohskopf LA, Levine GL, Stover BH et al (2001) Prevalence of nosocomial infections in neonatal intensive care unit patients: results from the first national point-prevalence survey. J Pediatr 139(6):821–827

Sperling RS, Newton E, Gibbs RS (1988) Intraamniotic infection in low-birth-weight infants. J Infect Dis 157(1):113–117

Srinivasan L, Harris MC (2012) New technologies for the rapid diagnosis of neonatal sepsis. Curr Opin Pediatr 24(2):165–171

Stolfi I, Moro M, Lana S (1999) Frequenza e variabilità delle infezioni ospedaliere in Terapia Intensiva Neonatale (TIN). Riv Ital Pediatr 25:193–200

Stoll BJ, Temprosa M, Tyson JE, Papile LA, Wright LL, Bauer CR et al (1999) Dexamethasone therapy increases infection in very low birth weight infants. Pediatrics 104(5), e63

Stoll BJ, Hansen N, Fanaroff AA, Wright LL, Carlo WA, Ehrenkranz RA et al (2002a) Late-onset sepsis in very low birth weight neonates: the experience of the NICHD Neonatal Research Network. Pediatrics 110 (2 Pt 1):285–291

Stoll BJ, Hansen N, Fanaroff AA, Wright LL, Carlo WA, Ehrenkranz RA et al (2002b) Changes in pathogens causing early-onset sepsis in very-low-birth-weight infants. N Engl J Med 347(4):240–247

Stoll BJ, Hansen N, Fanaroff AA, Lemons JA (2004a) Enterobacter sakazakii is a rare cause of neonatal septicemia or meningitis in VLBW infants. J Pediatr 144(6):821–823

Stoll BJ, Hansen N, Fanaroff AA, Wright LL, Carlo WA, Ehrenkranz RA et al (2004b) To tap or not to tap: high likelihood of meningitis without sepsis among very low birth weight infants. Pediatrics 113(5):1181–1186

Stronati M, Lombardi G, Chirico G (2000) Le infezioni nel neonato. Prospettive Pediatr 30:201–217

Stronati M, Tzialla C, Lombardi G (2004) Prevention of early-onset neonatal group B streptococcus infection. Ital J Pediatr 30:39–48

Stronati M, Borghesi A, Decembrino L, Bollani L (2007) Antibiotics in neonatal intensive care units (NICUs). J Chemother 19(Suppl 2):52–55

Subcommittee on Urinary Tract Infection SCoQI, Management, Roberts KB (2011) Urinary tract infection: clinical practice guideline for the diagnosis and management of the initial UTI in febrile infants and children 2 to 24 months. Pediatrics 128(3):595–610

Sullivan BA, Fairchild KD (2015) Predictive monitoring for sepsis and necrotizing enterocolitis to prevent shock. Semin Fetal Neonatal Med 20(4):255–261

Takahashi N, Nishida H, Kato H, Imanishi K, Sakata Y, Uchiyama T (1998) Exanthematous disease induced by toxic shock syndrome toxin 1 in the early neonatal period. Lancet 351(9116):1614–1619

Tamim MM, Alesseh H, Aziz H (2003) Analysis of the efficacy of urine culture as part of sepsis evaluation in the premature infant. Pediatr Infect Dis J 22(9): 805–808

The WHO Young Infants Study Group (1999) Bacterial etiology of serious infections in young infants in developing countries: results of a multicenter study. Pediatr Infect Dis J 18(10 Suppl):S17–S22

Tsai M-H, Chu S-M, Hsu J-F, Lien R, Huang H-R, Chiang M-C et al (2014) Risk factors and outcomes for multidrug-resistant Gram-negative bacteremia in the NICU. Pediatrics 133(2):e322–e329

Turner D, Leibovitz E, Aran A, Piglansky L, Raiz S, Leiberman A et al (2002) Acute otitis media in infants younger than two months of age: microbiology, clinical presentation and therapeutic approach. Pediatr Infect Dis J 21(7):669–674 van Acker J, de Smet F, Muyldermans G, Bougatef A, Naessens A, Lauwers S (2001) Outbreak of necrotizing enterocolitis associated with *Enterobacter sakazakii* in powdered milk formula. J Clin Microbiol 39(1): 293–297

van den Brand M, Peters RP, Catsburg A, Rubenjan A, Broeke FJ, van den Dungen FA et al (2014) Development of a multiplex real-time PCR assay for the rapid diagnosis of neonatal late onset sepsis. J Microbiol Methods 106:8–15

Van Dyke MK, Phares CR, Lynfield R, Thomas AR, Arnold KE, Craig AS et al (2009) Evaluation of universal antenatal screening for group B streptococcus. N Engl J Med 360(25):2626–2636

Vergnano S, Menson E, Kennea N, Embleton N, Russell AB, Watts T et al (2011) Neonatal infections in England: the NeonIN surveillance network. Arch Dis Child Fetal Neonatal Ed 96(1):F9–F14

Weinberg GA, D'Angio CT (2006) Laboratory aids for diagnosis of neonatal sepsis. In: Remington, Klein, Wilson, Baker (eds) Infectious diseases of the fetus and newborn infant, 6th edn. Elsevier Saunders, Philadelphia, pp 1207–1222

Weir E (2002) Powdered infant formula and fatal infection with *Enterobacter sakazakii*. CMAJ 166(12):1570

WHO/EIP/SPO/QPS/05.2 (2005) Who guidelines on hand hygiene in health care (advanced draft): a summary. Clean hands are safer hands

Wong M, Isaacs D, Howman-Giles R, Uren R (1995) Clinical and diagnostic features of osteomyelitis occurring in the first three months of life. Pediatr Infect Dis J 14(12):1047–1053

Yancey MK, Schuchat A, Brown LK, Ventura VL, Markenson GR (1996) The accuracy of late antenatal screening cultures in predicting genital group B streptococcal colonization at delivery. Obstet Gynecol 88(5):811–815

Zar HJ (2005) Neonatal chlamydial infections: prevention and treatment. Paediatr Drugs 7(2):103–110

Zorc JJ, Kiddoo DA, Shaw KN (2005) Diagnosis and management of pediatric urinary tract infections. Clin Microbiol Rev 18(2):417–422

Neonatal Septic Shock

108

Rajesh K. Aneja, Ruby V. Aneja, Misty Good, and Joseph A. Carcillo

Contents

R. K. Aneja (✉) · J. A. Carcillo
Departments of Critical Care Medicine and Pediatrics, University of Pittsburgh School of Medicine, Children's Hospital of Pittsburgh, Pittsburgh, PA, USA
e-mail: anejar@upmc.edu; carcilloja@ccm.upmc.edu

R. V. Aneja
Division of Neonatology, Temple University, West Penn Hospital, Pittsburgh, PA, USA
e-mail: rvarughese@pol.net

M. Good
Division of Neonatology, University of Pittsburgh School of Medicine, Children's Hospital of Pittsburgh, Pittsburgh, PA, USA
e-mail: goodml3@upmc.edu

G. Buonocore et al. (eds.), *Neonatology*,
https://doi.org/10.1007/978-3-319-29489-6_255

Abstract
Neonatal sepsis continues to be a major health problem in the world. Over the last decade, there has been an overall decrease in the incidence of neonatal sepsis. The institution of intrapartum Group B *Streptococcus* (GBS) prophylaxis has also led to a decrease in GBS early-onset disease. Early recognition and treatment of sepsis is essential to halt its progression to severe sepsis and septic shock. In this chapter, we compare the essential differences between the hemodynamic response to shock in neonates and older children. We also discuss various factors that make diagnosis and treatment of neonatal shock challenging. The American College of Critical Care Medicine recently published an update to their clinical practice parameters for the management of septic shock. We summarize these guidelines and briefly review thrombocytopenia-associated multiple organ failure in sepsis.

108.1 Salient Points

- Early recognition and treatment/resuscitation improve the outcome in sepsis and septic shock. Thrombotic microangiopathy responds to nonspecific and specific therapies.
- When sepsis is not recognized and treated early, septic shock becomes the predominant predictor of mortality and neurologic morbidity.
- Newborns and premature newborns in particular have a reduced ability to eradicate infection at almost all levels of immunity.
- Septic shock in neonates occurs primarily secondary to cardiac failure which is commonly associated with systemic pulmonary hypertension. Hence therapies that include volume resuscitation, inotropic support, and right ventricle afterload reduction are the mainstays of treatment. ECMO can be lifesaving for term newborns with refractory shock.

108.2 Introduction

Group B *Streptococcus* (GBS) continues to be a leading infectious cause of neonatal morbidity and mortality in the United States (Trends in perinatal group B streptococcal disease – United States 2009). Overall, the incidence of GBS early-onset disease (EOD) over the last three decades has decreased from 1.7 to 0.4 per 1,000 live births, which is a 70% reduction (Nandyal 2008). This success has largely been attributed to the institution of intrapartum prophylaxis. Since the implementation of Group B streptococcal (GBS) prophylaxis, there has been a reduction in GBS EOD from 5.9 to 1.7 per 1,000 live births of infants weighing 401–1,500 g but a concomitant increase in the rate of *Escherichia coli* sepsis from 3.2 to 6.8 per 1,000 live births (Fanaroff et al. 2007).

Investigators used hospital discharge data (from approximately one quarter of the US population) to estimate that 10% of infants and children with severe sepsis (bacterial or fungal infection + organ failure) died in 1995 (Watson et al. 2003; Angus et al. 2001). The incidence of sepsis in the neonatal population was 3.06 per 1,000 children. A decade later, in a follow-up study, the authors noted that the incidence of sepsis in the neonatal population had decreased to 2.22 per 1,000 children. Despite the decline in the overall incidence of sepsis, one cohort that demonstrated a significant increase in the incidence of sepsis was the very-low-birth-weight (VLBW) group, defined as less than 1,500 g (26.5% vs. 9.2% in 1995) (Hartman et al. 2008). Similar observations were made by Stoll and colleagues who published a series of epidemiologic evaluations of newborn sepsis/septicemia/septic shock using US Vital Statistics as well as the National Institute of

Child Health and Human Development sponsored newborn infection registry. Neonatal mortality steadily decreased over the past decade, but remained most prominent in low-birth-weight neonates, defined as less than 2,500 g (Stoll et al. 1998, 2002a, b). Low-birth-weight newborns with EOD are more likely to die than those without infection (37% vs. 13%). Twenty-one percent of low-birth-weight newborns also have one or more episodes of blood culture-positive late-onset disease (LOD) and are also more likely to die (18% vs. 7%). In VLBW newborns with LOD, the common causative organisms were Gram-positive (70%), followed by Gram-negative (17.6%) and fungal (12.2%) organisms. In the same study, mortality was higher in patients with Gram-negative organisms or fungal sepsis (Stoll et al. 2002b).

108.3 Early Recognition and Treatment/Resuscitation Improves Outcome in Sepsis and Septic Shock

Clinical signs of apnea or tachypnea, poor feeding, and temperature instability should be considered as sepsis until proven otherwise, and the clinician should consider antibiotic therapy. In the nursery setting, fetal and neonatal tachycardia remain the most important early clinical predictors of sepsis and septic shock (Graves and Rhodes 1984; Paternoster and Laureti 1996). Prompt fluid and inotrope resuscitation to normalization of heart rate well before hypotension appears prudent in this population. Laboratory tests can also have a role in increasing early suspicion of newborn sepsis. Many investigators have demonstrated that measurement of cord or newborn blood quantitative levels of cytokines and proinflammatory markers including interleukin (IL) -6, procalcitonin, IL-1 receptor antagonist, IL-8,IL-10, tumor necrosis factor (TNF), and C-reactive protein (CRP) can attain over 95% sensitivity in diagnosis of EOD and LOD before blood culture results are available (Kuster et al. 1998; Silveira and Procianoy 1999; Janota et al. 2001; Ng et al. 1997; Rogers et al. 2002; Krueger et al. 2001; Romagnoli et al. 2001; Kashlan et al. 2000; Smulian et al. 1999). These author's believe that universal implementation of these clinical laboratory tests will allow more judicious use of antibiotic therapy than the present standard of care that do not utilize all of these biomarkers.

Shock remains the most prominent risk factor for death in neonatal sepsis (adjusted odds ratio 11.82: confidence interval 5.4–69.4). Best outcomes are attained with early reversal of shock in newborns using NRP/ACCM/PALS guidelines (see below) (Han et al. 2003). Aggressive, timely emergency department fluid and inotrope resuscitation directed to oxygen delivery/consumption goals has also been shown to improve outcome in pediatric septic shock. This preponderance of evidence suggests that early recognition is the key to survival in newborn sepsis and septic shock. Experimental and clinical literature show that early and aggressive fluid resuscitation with antibiotic therapy turns off inflammatory gene expression, prevents thrombosis, and results in 95% or greater survival. Delayed resuscitation on the other hand results in inflammatory gene expression, endothelial activation, thrombosis, the development of thrombocytopenia-associated multiple organ failure, and high mortality rates (Haque and Mohan 2003; Nguyen et al. 2001; Roman et al. 1992, 1993).

108.4 Neonatal Shock

108.4.1 Term Newborn

Term newborns and infants have a remarkably different cardiovascular response to septic shock than older children, and healthy newborns have higher resting heart rates. Therefore, (This change is being requested as there is another hence used one sentence later), in response to shock, newborns compensate by increasing systemic vasoconstriction. This vasoconstriction increases afterload and further impairs cardiac output. Hence, death in majority of newborns and infants with fluid-/dopamine-resistant shock is a result of cardiac failure, not vasoplegia.

Neonatal septic shock is often complicated by lack of the physiologic transition from fetal to neonatal circulation. In utero, 85% of fetal circulation bypasses the lungs through the patent ductus arteriosus and foramen ovale. This flow pattern is maintained by suprasystemic pulmonary artery pressures prenatally. At birth, inhalation of oxygen triggers a cascade of biochemical events that ultimately result in reduction in pulmonary artery pressure and transition from fetal to neonatal circulation with blood flow now being directed through the pulmonary circulation. Closure of the patent ductus arteriosus and foramen ovale completes this transition. Pulmonary artery pressures can remain elevated, and the ductus arteriosus can remain open for the first 6 weeks of life. Sepsis-induced acidosis and hypoxia increase pulmonary vascular resistance, subsequently increasing the pulmonary artery pressure leading to patent ductus arteriosus. This results in persistent pulmonary hypertension (PPHN) and persistent fetal circulation (PFC) in the newborn. Neonatal septic shock with PPHN is associated with increased right ventricle afterload. Despite in utero conditioning, the thickened right ventricle may fail in the presence of systemic pulmonary artery pressures. Decompensated right ventricle failure can be clinically manifested by tricuspid regurgitation and hepatomegaly. Newborn animal models of Group B streptococcal and endotoxin shock have also documented reduced cardiac output and increased pulmonary, mesenteric, and systemic vascular resistance. Therapies directed at reversal of right ventricle failure, through reduction of pulmonary artery pressures, are commonly needed in neonates with fluid refractory shock and PPHN. Newer therapies such as inhaled nitric oxide and ECMO have little to no role in adult septic shock, but are potentially lifesaving in newborns, infants, and children.

108.4.2 Preterm Newborns

The management of neonatal shock is challenging due to many factors outlined below. First, there is lack of consensus about the definition of hypotension in the extremely premature infants (Dempsey and Barrington 2009). The commonly used NICU criteria for mean arterial blood pressure (MAP) is that MAP should be maintained at or greater than the infant's gestational age in weeks (Dempsey and Barrington 2006; Report of working group of the British Association of Perinatal Medicine and Neonatal Nurses Association 1992). In the absence of a precise evidence-based definition, it is difficult to interpret the hemodynamic response to hypotension in preterm newborns. Pediatric data suggest that blood pressure cannot be used as a surrogate for adequate oxygen delivery in critically ill patients. Secondly, there is lack of data about the correlation of CVP with circulating blood volume in VLBW infants. Lastly, there is paucity of data regarding the use of lactate as a surrogate for inadequate tissue oxygen delivery in preterm infants. Serum lactate levels pose a unique challenge as neonates have high blood lactate concentrations at birth, which is normalized by 12 h after birth. Wardle and colleagues examined two groups of ventilated preterm infants with mean gestational age of 27 weeks. They found no difference in median lactate levels between normotensive and hypotensive preterm infants (1.20 vs.1.22 mmol/L). Despite the median lactate levels being similar in the two groups, persistent high lactate levels were associated with an adverse outcome (death or periventricular hemorrhage) (Wardle et al. 1999). Thus, recognition and treatment of shock in low-birth-weight infants should encompass clinical signs (peripheral pulses, perfusion, and urine output) along with biochemical values, i.e., serum lactate levels. Standard practices in resuscitation of premature infants in septic shock employ a more graded approach compared to resuscitation of term neonates and children. This more cautious approach is a response to reports that premature infants at risk for intraventricular hemorrhage (<30 weeks gestation) can develop hemorrhage after rapid shifts in blood pressure (Perry et al. 1990; Miall-Allen et al. 1987); however, some now question whether long-term neurologic outcomes are related to periventricular leukomalacia (a result of prolonged under perfusion) more than to the intraventricular hemorrhage itself. To summarize, while cerebral under perfusion is a setup for periventricular leukomalacia, aggressive resuscitation of critically ill VLBW can predispose them to intraventricular hemorrhages. Hence the resuscitation of a VLBW neonate is challenging and needs to be studied further.

Several other developmental considerations influence therapies for shock. Relative initial deficiencies in the thyroid and parathyroid hormone axes have been appreciated and can result in the need for supplementation with thyroid hormone and/or calcium replacement. Adrenal insufficiency and the need for hydrocortisone have been documented in the preterm infant cohort as well (Soliman et al. 2004). In a double-blind, randomized, controlled study, 48 VLBW infants who had refractory hypotension and required dopamine (>10 μg/kg/min) were assigned to receive stress dose of hydrocortisone (1 mg/kg Q8H) for 5 days or placebo. A significantly higher number of hypotensive VLBW infants treated with hydrocortisone weaned off vasopressor support 72 h after starting treatment. There was decreased use of volume expanders and less cumulative dose of dopamine and dobutamine in steroid-treated patients as compared to control infants (Ng et al. 2006). Other factors that impact the neonate's response to shock include reduced glycogen stores and muscle mass. These are important for gluconeogenesis; hence attention should be paid to the maintenance of serum glucose in a critically ill neonate.

Studies of therapies specifically directed at premature VLBW infants with septic shock are needed. A single-center randomized controlled trial reported improved outcome with use of daily 6 h pentoxifylline infusions (a systemic vasodilator) in very premature infants with sepsis. The Cochrane analysis agrees that the smaller trials are promising but suggests that larger multicenter trials would be helpful (Haque and Mohan 2003; Pammi and Haque 2015).

The American College of Critical Care Medicine (ACCM) sets a priority to establish clinical practice parameters and guidelines for the management of septic shock (Table 1). As a follow-up to their revised guidelines published in 2007 (Brierley et al. 2008; Carcillo and Fields 2002), recently the "2014 update of the 2007 ACCM *Clinical Guidelines for Hemodynamic Support of Neonates and Children with Septic Shock*" was formulated. The major new recommendation is that hemodynamic support of septic shock is addressed at the institutional level rather than only at the practitioner level. The new guidelines recommend that each institution implement their own adopted or homegrown bundles that include the following: (1) *recognition bundle* containing a trigger tool for rapid identification of patients with suspected septic shock at that institution, (2) *resuscitation and stabilization bundle* to drive adherence to consensus best practice at that institution, and (3) *performance bundle* to monitor, improve, and sustain adherence to that best practice. These guidelines should be reviewed by every hospital's expert committee (Fig. 1).

Table 1 Clinical definition of sepsis and septic shock

Sepsis	Clinical suspicion of infection with the following signs: tachycardia, tachypnea or apnea, poor feeding, temperature instability
Septic shock	Clinical suspicion of infection with the following signs: tachycardia or bradycardia, tachypnea or apnea, prolonged capillary refill >2 s, decreased urine output[a] [a]Hypotension is considered a late confirmatory sign

Although the intent was to develop guidelines for the management of premature as well as term newborns, the literature review on septic shock in the premature was relatively sparse. The evidence and expert opinion-based document found age-specific differences in both pathophysiology and response to therapies. Early recognition and rapid fluid resuscitation are the hallmark of therapy. It should be implemented when newborns are in compensated shock and directed to reversal of tachycardia. Newborns with fluid refractory shock can have any hemodynamic state. Some have the classic adult form of septic shock with high cardiac output and low vascular resistance; however, majority have a low cardiac output state commonly associated with elevated, not reduced vascular resistance. If there is heightened concern for a ductal dependent heart lesion, all newborns with shock should be started on prostaglandin E. Newborns have an age-specific resistance to dopamine and dobutamine; hence, epinephrine (cold shock)

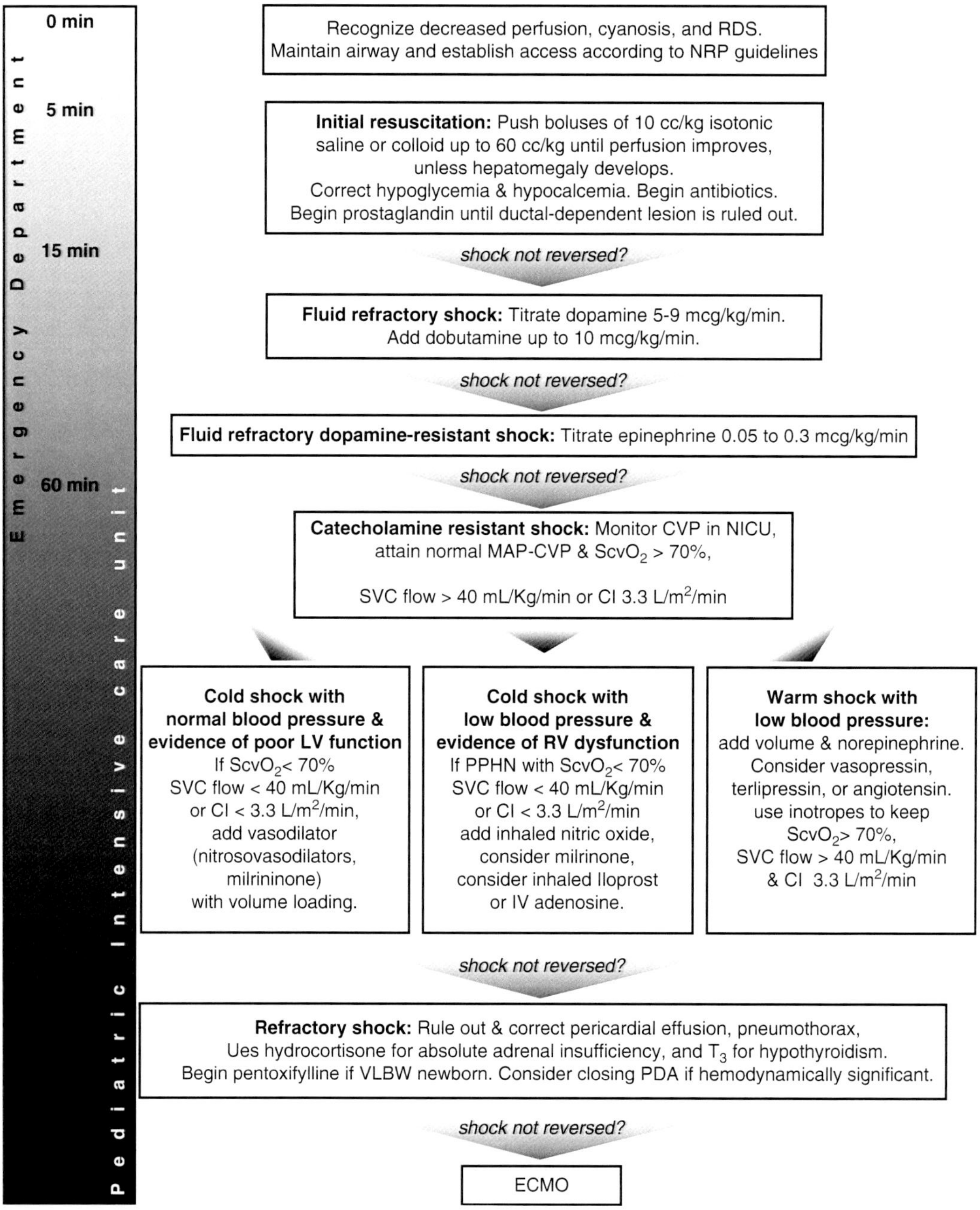

Fig. 1 Algorithm for time-sensitive, goal-directed stepwise management of hemodynamic support in newborns. Proceed to the next step if shock persists. (1) First hour goals – restore and maintain heart rate thresholds, capillary refill ≤ 2 s, and normal blood pressure in the first hour. (2) Subsequent intensive care unit goals – restore normal perfusion pressure (mean arterial pressure [*MAP*]-central venous pressure [*CVP*]), preductal and postductal O_2 saturation difference <5%, and either central venous O_2 saturation (*ScvO2*) >70%, superior vena cava (*SVC*) flow >40 ml/kg/min, or cardiac index (*CI*) >3.3 L/min/m^2 in neonatal intensive care unit (*NICU*). *RDS* respiratory distress syndrome, *NRP* Neonatal Resuscitation Program, *PDA* patent ductus arteriosus, *ECMO* extracorporeal membrane oxygenation

can be more commonly required. Newborns with septic shock have a higher incidence of true adrenal insufficiency cortisol <18 mg/dL when requiring epinephrine, and as such these patients may benefit from hydrocortisone therapy. In patients with low cardiac output and elevated systemic vascular resistance, vasodilators are effective in reversing shock. Additionally, ECMO is lifesaving for refractory newborn septic shock. Inhaled nitric oxide decreases the use of ECMO, but does not improve outcome in ECMO centers. ECMO is recommended for term infants with refractory shock.

108.5 Thrombocytopenia-Associated Multiple Organ Failure; A Thrombotic Microangiopathy Which Responds to Nonspecific and Specific Therapies

Thrombocytopenia, platelet count $<100{,}000\ mm^3$, is an independent risk factor for the development of multiple organ failure and death in critical illness, in part because it is a recognizable clinical sign of endotheliopathy with platelet thrombi (Nguyen et al. 2001). This syndrome is accounted for by variations on two "prototype" thrombotic microangiopathies. The consumptive coagulopathy (reduced fibrinogen levels) occurs when tissue factor complexes with factor VII and initiates coagulation factor consumption cascade. This is commonly called disseminated intravascular coagulation (DIC). Roman and colleagues have documented that newborns with sepsis/septic shock have a prothrombotic/anti-fibrinolytic state with excessive thrombosis – procoagulant (Factors II, VII), and anticoagulant factors (i.e., protein C and antithrombin III) are both consumed. This leads to a paradoxical observation, overwhelming thrombosis (when the anticoagulant factors are depleted), and then overwhelming bleeding (when the procoagulant factors are consumed). Newborns have lower protein C levels than children. Activated protein C (APC) has 40 times the fibrinolytic activity as protein C concentrate, and it is associated with intracranial bleeding. The pediatric arm of the "Extended Evaluation of Recombinant Activated Protein C" (ENHANCE) trial noted increased incidence of significant bleeding in 27% of the patients enrolled, and 3% had a central nervous system bleeding (Goldstein et al. 2006). Due to the adverse risk to benefit ratio associated with use of APC, it is not being used by most practitioners.

The second prototype is a nonconsumptive coagulopathy (normal or increased fibrinogen levels) which is characterized by low ADAM TS 13 activity leading to platelet thrombi. Newborns have lower ADAM TS 13 activity than children and adults. This condition has been named infection-associated thrombotic thrombocytopenic purpura. It responds to daily centrifugation-based plasma exchange therapy for a median of 14 days. Plasma exchange machines are not approved for infants under 5 kg so their use is limited in the newborn period. Nevertheless, newborns have reduced ADAM TS 13 activity and increased circulating ultra large vWF multimers (thrombogenic multimers), which puts the newborn at risk for nonconsumptive coagulopathy. The use of fresh frozen plasma remains a standard approach to both forms of coagulopathy in newborns. Some have reported improved outcome with whole blood exchange, but not blood component exchange therapy (Sadana et al. 1997; Togari et al. 1983).

108.6 Why Do Newborns Have Difficulty Eradicating Infection?

108.6.1 Hypogammaglobulinemia

Newborns and premature newborns in particular have a reduced ability to eradicate infection at almost all levels of immunity. Most notorious is the common deficiency of IgG levels in the VLBW infant. Prophylaxis with IVIG therapy has not reduced late-onset sepsis in this group of patients, but IVIG therapy in newborns with hypogammaglobulinemia and septic shock has been thought to be of benefit. A meta-analysis previously demonstrated that the use of immunoglobulin preparation rich in IgG, IgA, and IgM reduces the mortality in neonatal sepsis or septic shock by 50% (Kreymann et al. 2007). Hence, IVIG therapy should be considered in newborns with

Table 2 Suggested treatments to reverse immune insufficiency and/or to prevent nosocomial infection and sepsis in term infants

Sepsis/MODS	Neutropenia	Prolonged lymphopenia ALC $<1,000/\text{mm}^3$ for 7 days, or IgG <500 mg/dl	Monocyte deactivation HLA-DR $<30\%$ or 8,000 molecules >5 days
Give GM-CSF	Yes		Yes?
Give IVIG		Yes if IgG <500	
Consider empiric and prophylactic antibiotic/protozoal fungal strategies	Yes	Yes	Yes?

hypogammaglobulinemic septic shock or toxic shock (Stiehm 1997; Jenson and Pollock 1998; Cawley et al. 1999; Despond et al. 2001). However, a recent Cochrane meta-analysis demonstrated no reduction in mortality, death, or major disability in infants with infection with IGM-enriched IVIG. Hence, routine IVIG therapy in neonatal sepsis is not recommended {Ohlsson 2015 #243}.

108.6.2 Neutropenia

Neutropenia is commonly seen in newborns with sepsis/septic shock. Some have defined it as an absolute neutrophil count $<1,500/\text{mm}^3$. GM-CSF therapy at 5 μg/kg/day over 12 h for 7 days has been reported to improve outcome in newborns with neutropenic septic shock (Bilgin et al. 2001). G-CSF has also been studied in newborns with non-neutropenic sepsis and was found to be associated with a shortened length of stay (Kucukoduk et al. 2002). In a multicenter trial in United Kingdom, 280 small for gestational age neonates of ≤ 31 weeks gestation were randomized within 72 h of birth to receive GM-CSF 10 μg/kg per day subcutaneously for 5 days or standard management. The primary outcome was sepsis-free survival to 14 days from trial entry. The investigators found that neutrophil counts increased significantly more rapidly in infants treated with GM-CSF than in control infants during the first 11 days; however, there was no significant difference in sepsis-free survival for all infants (Carr et al. 2009). Hence, GM-CSF can be used to increase the neutrophil count but may not provide any survival benefit in septic neonates (Parravicini et al. 2002; Bedford Russell et al. 2001; La Gamma and De Castro 2002; Banerjea and Speer 2002; Goldman et al. 1998) (Table 2).

108.6.3 Prolonged Monocyte Deactivation and Immune Paralysis

Monocyte deactivation ($<30\%$ HLA-DR expression or 8,000 HLA-DR molecules, or ex vivo whole blood TNF response <200 pg/ml for >5 days) is associated with immune paralysis and increased risk of late-onset sepsis from a secondary infection in children (Volk et al. 1996). Hallwirth and colleagues have reported that cord monocyte deactivation is a reliable parameter for predicting EOD in VLBW infants (Hallwirth et al. 2002). The anti-inflammatory cytokine, IL-10, and the reactive oxygen species, nitric oxide, and peroxynitrite radicals both deactivate monocytes. This common response becomes pathogenic when it lasts for more than 5 days. GM-CSF and interferon reverse this process ex vivo (Table 2).

108.6.4 Prolonged Lymphopenia and Lymphoid Depletion Syndrome

Lymphopenia ($<1,000/\text{mm}^3$ for >7 days) is associated with the development of secondary infection, unresolving multiple organ failure, and the finding of lymphoid depletion at autopsy in children (Hotchkiss et al. 2001). Gurevitch et al. examined autopsies from low-birth-weight newborns with sepsis similarly reported lymphoid depletion

(Gurevich et al. 1995). At present prophylactic and empiric antifungal/antiviral strategies may be appropriately considered in these patients as per the clinical experience with patients with low CD4 counts from other immunodeficiency diseases. IVIG therapy should be considered if B-cell numbers are substantially depleted along with hypogammaglobulinemia (IgG level <500 mg/dl) (Table 2).

108.6.5 Antibiotic Prophylaxis, Empiric Therapy, and Antibiotic Resistance

Because EOD is commonly caused by GBS and LOD is commonly caused by *Staphylococcus epidermidis*, antibiotic prophylaxis therapies have been considered. Antepartum and intrapartum antibiotic use has markedly reduced the incidence of GBS EOD, but, not surprisingly, has led to increased incidence of neonatal sepsis caused by resistant organisms. Vancomycin and teicoplanin prophylaxes are both effective in reducing LOD with *Staphylococcus* species (Moller et al. 1997), but routine prophylaxis is not yet recommended because of concern for emergence of resistant organisms (Moller et al. 1997). Fluconazole prophylaxis has been very effective in preventing Candida sepsis in VLBW infants and is recommended (Kaufman 2004). Empirical antifungal therapy should be strongly considered for infants with gestational age <25 weeks, thrombocytopenia, history of third-generation cephalosporin, or carbapenem exposure for 7 days (Benjamin et al. 2003). Empiric use of amphotericin for VLBW babies with risk factors for fungal infection has also been recommended (Brian Smith et al. 2005; Chapman 2003).

108.7 Supporting Organs During Multiple Organ Failure: What's New?

Acute respiratory distress syndrome – Overdistention of alveoli results in systemic inflammation with systemic release of inflammatory cytokines and depression of immunity. Lung protection ventilation strategies which limit volutrauma are prudent (The Acute Respiratory Distress Syndrome 2000).

Acute renal failure – Investigators have demonstrated the efficacy of continuous veno-venous hemofiltration in children with meningococcal septic shock (Smith et al. 1997). A recent randomized controlled adult study showed survival benefit with daily dialysis compared to intermittent dialysis therapy in patients with acute renal failure in the ICU (Schiffl et al. 2002). Peritoneal dialysis/hemofiltration, continuous veno-venous hemofiltration, or continuous arteriovenous hemofiltration can be successfully performed in newborns (Schroder et al. 1992).

Steroid and drug metabolism – Reactive oxygen species impair cytochrome P450 activity. This leads to reduction of cortisol and aldosterone synthesis and reduced drug metabolism during sepsis and multiple organ failure. Newborns have an age-specific reduced cortisol synthesis for a given substrate (17-OH progesterone), as well as reduced drug metabolism due to an immature cytochrome P450 system (Carcillo et al. 2003). Hydrocortisone has reversed epinephrine-resistant septic shock in premature infants with adrenal insufficiency. In a retrospective observational study, 117 infants treated with hydrocortisone for refractory hypotension were reviewed. Refractory hypotension was defined as a mean arterial pressure (MAP) less than the gestational age (GA) despite a total inotrope dose of 20 μg/kg/min. Patients treated with hydrocortisone demonstrated improved hemodynamics and decreased inotropic dose at 6, 12, and 24 h. The incidence of side effects, i.e., intraventricular hemorrhage, periventricular leukomalacia, sepsis, and spontaneous intestinal perforation, was similar to institutional historic controls (Baker et al. 2008).

108.8 Summary

Newborn sepsis remains a major international health-care problem, particularly in low-birth-weight infants. It is a significant cause of mortality and neurologic morbidity including cerebral palsy. As with all major health-care problems, resources should be invested in prevention and early intervention programs. Antepartum GBS prophylaxis has been successful in reducing incidence and mortality. Early clinical signs of sepsis include tachycardia, apnea or tachypnea, poor feeding, and temperature instability. While no one biomarker can diagnose sepsis early, biomarker panel including IL-6, procalcitonin, IL-1 receptor antagonist, IL-8, IL-10, TNF, and CRP might be a better diagnostic tool. Early clinical diagnosis and therapy are the keys to these improved outcomes. However, because antibiotics ultimately are met with the development of resistant organisms, a commitment to the development of specific maternal immunizations (e.g., GBS) in the developed world and the use of heterologous newborn immunizations (e.g., BCG) in the developing world is recommended.

When sepsis is not recognized and treated early, septic shock becomes the predominant predictor of mortality and neurologic morbidity. In contrast to older children, septic shock in neonates occurs primarily secondary to cardiac failure, not vascular failure. This state of cardiac failure is commonly associated with systemic pulmonary hypertension. Hence therapies including volume resuscitation, inotropic support, and right ventricle afterload reduction are the mainstays of treatment. ECMO can be lifesaving for term newborns with refractory shock. At present no specific therapies have been approved for thrombotic complications (DIC or TTP/HUS) in newborns; hence plasma therapies remain the mainstay.

Sepsis is all too common in very-low-birth-weight newborns (20–30% of the neonatal population) with a predominant late (after 72 h) rather than early onset. Development of early diagnostic tests, infection prevention practices, and immunostimulant therapies is urgently needed for this population not only to improve survival but to reduce periventricular leukomalacia.

References

(2009) Trends in perinatal group B streptococcal disease – United States, 2000–2006. MMWR Morb Mortal Wkly Rep 58:109–112

Angus DC, Linde-Zwirble WT, Lidicker J, Clermont G, Carcillo J, Pinsky MR (2001) Epidemiology of severe sepsis in the United States: analysis of incidence, outcome, and associated costs of care. Crit Care Med 29:1303–1310

Baker CF, Barks JD, Engmann C, Vazquez DM, Neal CR Jr, Schumacher RE, Bhatt-Mehta V (2008) Hydrocortisone administration for the treatment of refractory hypotension in critically ill newborns. J Perinatol 28:412–419

Banerjea MC, Speer CP (2002) The current role of colony-stimulating factors in prevention and treatment of neonatal sepsis. Semin Neonatol 7:335–349

Bedford Russell AR, Emmerson AJ, Wilkinson N, Chant T, Sweet DG, Halliday HL, Holland B, Davies EG (2001) A trial of recombinant human granulocyte colony stimulating factor for the treatment of very low birthweight infants with presumed sepsis and neutropenia. Arch Dis Child Fetal Neonatal Ed 84:F172–F176

Benjamin DK Jr, DeLong ER, Steinbach WJ, Cotton CM, Walsh TJ, Clark RH (2003) Empirical therapy for neonatal candidemia in very low birth weight infants. Pediatrics 112:543–547

Bilgin K, Yaramis A, Haspolat K, Tas MA, Gunbey S, Derman O (2001) A randomized trial of granulocyte-macrophage colony-stimulating factor in neonates with sepsis and neutropenia. Pediatrics 107:36–41

Brian Smith P, Steinbach WJ, Benjamin DK Jr (2005) Invasive Candida infections in the neonate. Drug Resist Updat 8:147–162

Brierley J, Carcillo JA, Choong K, Cornell T, Decaen A, Deymann A, Doctor A, Davis A, Duff J, Dugas MA, (2009) Clinical practice parameters for hemodynamic support of pediatric and neonatal septic shock: 2007 update from the American College of Critical Care Medicine. Crit Care Med 37:666–688

Carcillo JA, Fields AI (2002) Clinical practice parameters for hemodynamic support of pediatric and neonatal patients in septic shock. Crit Care Med 30:1365–1378

Carcillo JA, Doughty L, Kofos D, Frye RF, Kaplan SS, Sasser H, Burckart GJ (2003) Cytochrome P450 mediated-drug metabolism is reduced in children with sepsis-induced multiple organ failure. Intensive Care Med 29:980–984

Carr R, Brocklehurst P, Dore CJ, Modi N (2009) Granulocyte-macrophage colony stimulating factor administered as prophylaxis for reduction of sepsis in extremely preterm, small for gestational age neonates (the PROGRAMS trial): a single-blind, multicentre, randomised controlled trial. Lancet 373:226–233

Cawley MJ, Briggs M, Haith LR Jr, Reilly KJ, Guilday RE, Braxton GR, Patton ML (1999) Intravenous immunoglobulin as adjunctive treatment for streptococcal toxic shock syndrome associated with necrotizing fasciitis: case report and review. Pharmacotherapy 19:1094–1098

Chapman RL (2003) Candida infections in the neonate. Curr Opin Pediatr 15:97–102

Cooke RWI (1992) Report of working group of the British Association of Perinatal Medicine and Neonatal Nurses Association on categories of babies requiring neonatal care. Arch Dis Child 67:868–869

Dempsey EM, Barrington KJ (2006) Diagnostic criteria and therapeutic interventions for the hypotensive very low birth weight infant. J Perinatol 26:677–681

Dempsey EM, Barrington KJ (2009) Evaluation and treatment of hypotension in the preterm infant. Clin Perinatol 36:75–85

Despond O, Proulx F, Carcillo JA, Lacroix J (2001) Pediatric sepsis and multiple organ dysfunction syndrome. Curr Opin Pediatr 13:247–253

Fanaroff AA, Stoll BJ, Wright LL, Carlo WA, Ehrenkranz RA, Stark AR, Bauer CR, Donovan EF, Korones SB, Laptook AR et al (2007) Trends in neonatal morbidity and mortality for very low birthweight infants. Am J Obstet Gynecol 196(147):e141–e148

Goldman S, Ellis R, Dhar V, Cairo MS (1998) Rationale and potential use of cytokines in the prevention and treatment of neonatal sepsis. Clin Perinatol 25: 699–710

Goldstein B, Nadel S, Peters M, Barton R, Machado F, Levy H, Haney DJ, Utterback B, Williams MD, Giroir BP (2006) ENHANCE: results of a global open-label trial of drotrecogin alfa (activated) in children with severe sepsis. Pediatr Crit Care Med 7:200–211

Graves GR, Rhodes PG (1984) Tachycardia as a sign of early onset neonatal sepsis. Pediatr Infect Dis 3:404–406

Gurevich P, Ben-Hur H, Czernobilsky B, Nyska A, Zuckerman A, Zusman I (1995) Pathology of lymphoid organs in low birth weight infants subjected to antigen-related diseases: a morphological and morphometric study. Pathology 27:121–126

Hallwirth U, Pomberger G, Zaknun D, Szepfalusi Z, Horcher E, Pollak A, Roth E, Spittler A (2002) Monocyte phagocytosis as a reliable parameter for predicting early-onset sepsis in very low birthweight infants. Early Hum Dev 67:1–9

Han YY, Carcillo JA, Dragotta MA, Bills DM, Watson RS, Westerman ME, Orr RA (2003) Early reversal of pediatric-neonatal septic shock by community physicians is associated with improved outcome. Pediatrics 112:793–799

Haque K, Mohan P (2003) Pentoxifylline for neonatal sepsis. Cochrane Database Syst Rev CD004205

Hartman M, Clermont G, Angus D, Watson R (2008) Pediatric severe sepsis in the US: 1995 vs. 2005. Crit Care Med 36:A76

Hotchkiss RS, Tinsley KW, Swanson PE, Schmieg RE Jr, Hui JJ, Chang KC, Osborne DF, Freeman BD, Cobb JP, Buchman TG et al (2001) Sepsis-induced apoptosis causes progressive profound depletion of B and CD4+ T lymphocytes in humans. J Immunol 166:6952–6963

Janota J, Stranak Z, Belohlavkova S, Mudra K, Simak J (2001) Postnatal increase of procalcitonin in premature newborns is enhanced by chorioamnionitis and neonatal sepsis. Eur J Clin Invest 31:978–983

Jenson HB, Pollock BH (1998) The role of intravenous immunoglobulin for the prevention and treatment of neonatal sepsis. Semin Perinatol 22:50–63

Kashlan F, Smulian J, Shen-Schwarz S, Anwar M, Hiatt M, Hegyi T (2000) Umbilical vein interleukin 6 and tumor necrosis factor alpha plasma concentrations in the very preterm infant. Pediatr Infect Dis J 19:238–243

Kaufman D (2004) Fungal infection in the very low birthweight infant. Curr Opin Infect Dis 17:253–259

Kreymann KG, de Heer G, Nierhaus A, Kluge S (2007) Use of polyclonal immunoglobulins as adjunctive therapy for sepsis or septic shock. Crit Care Med 35:2677–2685

Krueger M, Nauck MS, Sang S, Hentschel R, Wieland H, Berner R (2001) Cord blood levels of interleukin-6 and interleukin-8 for the immediate diagnosis of early-onset infection in premature infants. Biol Neonate 80:118–123

Kucukoduk S, Sezer T, Yildiran A, Albayrak D (2002) Randomized, double-blinded, placebo-controlled trial of early administration of recombinant human granulocyte colony-stimulating factor to non-neutropenic preterm newborns between 33 and 36 weeks with presumed sepsis. Scand J Infect Dis 34:893–897

Kuster H, Weiss M, Willeitner AE, Detlefsen S, Jeremias I, Zbojan J, Geiger R, Lipowsky G, Simbruner G (1998) Interleukin-1 receptor antagonist and interleukin-6 for early diagnosis of neonatal sepsis 2 days before clinical manifestation. Lancet 352:1271–1277

La Gamma EF, De Castro MH (2002) What is the rationale for the use of granulocyte and granulocyte-macrophage colony-stimulating factors in the neonatal intensive care unit? Acta Paediatr Suppl 91:109–116

Miall-Allen VM, de Vries LS, Whitelaw AG (1987) Mean arterial blood pressure and neonatal cerebral lesions. Arch Dis Child 62:1068–1069

Moller JC, Nelskamp I, Jensen R, Reiss I, Kohl M, Gatermann S, Iven H, Gortner L (1997) Comparison of vancomycin and teicoplanin for prophylaxis of sepsis with coagulase negative staphylococci (CONS) in very low birth weight (VLBW) infants. J Perinat Med 25:361–367

Nandyal RR (2008) Update on group B streptococcal infections: perinatal and neonatal periods. J Perinat Neonatal Nurs 22:230–237

Ng PC, Cheng SH, Chui KM, Fok TF, Wong MY, Wong W, Wong RP, Cheung KL (1997) Diagnosis of late onset neonatal sepsis with cytokines, adhesion molecule, and C-reactive protein in preterm very low birthweight infants. Arch Dis Child Fetal Neonatal Ed 77:F221–F227

Ng PC, Lee CH, Bnur FL, Chan IH, Lee AW, Wong E, Chan HB, Lam CW, Lee BS, Fok TF (2006) A double-blind, randomized, controlled study of a "stress dose" of hydrocortisone for rescue treatment of refractory hypotension in preterm infants. Pediatrics 117:367–375

Nguyen T, Hall M, Han Y, Fiedor M, Hasset A, Lopez-Plaza I, Watson S, Lum L, Carcillo JA (2001) Microvascular thrombosis in pediatric multiple organ failure: is it a therapeutic target? Pediatr Crit Care Med 2:187–196

Pammi M, Haque KN (2015) Pentoxifylline for treatment of sepsis and necrotizing enterocolitis in neonates. Cochrane Database Syst Rev 3:CD004205

Parravicini E, van de Ven C, Anderson L, Cairo MS (2002) Myeloid hematopoietic growth factors and their role in prevention and/or treatment of neonatal sepsis. Transfus Med Rev 16:11–24

Paternoster DM, Laureti E (1996) Persistent foetal tachycardia as an early marker of chorion-amnionitis. Description of a clinical case. Minerva Ginecol 48:371–374

Perry EH, Bada HS, Ray JD, Korones SB, Arheart K, Magill HL (1990) Blood pressure increases, birth weight-dependent stability boundary, and intraventricular hemorrhage. Pediatrics 85:727–732

Rogers BB, Alexander JM, Head J, McIntire D, Leveno KJ (2002) Umbilical vein interleukin-6 levels correlate with the severity of placental inflammation and gestational age. Hum Pathol 33:335–340

Romagnoli C, Frezza S, Cingolani A, De Luca A, Puopolo M, De Carolis MP, Vento G, Antinori A, Tortorolo G (2001) Plasma levels of interleukin-6 and interleukin-10 in preterm neonates evaluated for sepsis. Eur J Pediatr 160:345–350

Roman J, Velasco F, Fernandez F, Fernandez M, Villalba R, Rubio V, Torres A (1992) Protein C, protein S and C4b-binding protein in neonatal severe infection and septic shock. J Perinat Med 20:111–116

Roman J, Velasco F, Fernandez F, Fernandez M, Villalba R, Rubio V, Vicente A, Torres A (1993) Coagulation, fibrinolytic and kallikrein systems in neonates with uncomplicated sepsis and septic shock. Haemostasis 23:142–148

Sadana S, Mathur NB, Thakur A (1997) Exchange transfusion in septic neonates with sclerema: effect on immunoglobulin and complement levels. Indian Pediatr 34:20–25

Schiffl H, Lang SM, Fischer R (2002) Daily hemodialysis and the outcome of acute renal failure. N Engl J Med 346:305–310

Schroder CH, Severijnen RS, Potting CM (1992) Continuous arteriovenous hemofiltration (CAVH) in a premature newborn as treatment of overhydration and hyperkalemia due to sepsis. Eur J Pediatr Surg 2:368–369

Silveira RC, Procianoy RS (1999) Evaluation of interleukin-6, tumour necrosis factor-alpha and interleukin-1beta for early diagnosis of neonatal sepsis. Acta Paediatr 88:647–650

Smith OP, White B, Vaughan D, Rafferty M, Claffey L, Lyons B, Casey W (1997) Use of protein-C concentrate, heparin, and haemodiafiltration in meningococcus-induced purpura fulminans. Lancet 350:1590–1593

Smulian JC, Vintzileos AM, Lai YL, Santiago J, Shen-Schwarz S, Campbell WA (1999) Maternal chorioamnionitis and umbilical vein interleukin-6 levels for identifying early neonatal sepsis. J Matern Fetal Med 8:88–94

Soliman AT, Taman KH, Rizk MM, Nasr IS, Alrimawy H, Hamido MS (2004) Circulating adrenocorticotropic hormone (ACTH) and cortisol concentrations in normal, appropriate-for-gestational-age newborns versus those with sepsis and respiratory distress: cortisol response to low-dose and standard-dose ACTH tests. Metabolism 53:209–214

Stiehm ER (1997) Human intravenous immunoglobulin in primary and secondary antibody deficiencies. Pediatr Infect Dis J 16:696–707

Stoll BJ, Holman RC, Schuchat A (1998) Decline in sepsis-associated neonatal and infant deaths in the United States, 1979 through 1994. Pediatrics 102:e18

Stoll BJ, Hansen N, Fanaroff AA, Wright LL, Carlo WA, Ehrenkranz RA, Lemons JA, Donovan EF, Stark AR, Tyson JE et al (2002a) Changes in pathogens causing early-onset sepsis in very-low-birth-weight infants. N Engl J Med 347:240–247

Stoll BJ, Hansen N, Fanaroff AA, Wright LL, Carlo WA, Ehrenkranz RA, Lemons JA, Donovan EF, Stark AR, Tyson JE et al (2002b) Late-onset sepsis in very low birth weight neonates: the experience of the NICHD neonatal research network. Pediatrics 110:285–291

The Acute Respiratory Distress Syndrome, N (2000) Ventilation with lower tidal volumes as compared with traditional tidal volumes for acute lung injury and the acute respiratory distress syndrome. N Engl J Med 342:1301–1308

Togari H, Mikawa M, Iwanaga T, Matsumoto N, Kawase A, Hagisawa M, Ogino T, Goto R, Watanabe I, Kito H et al (1983) Endotoxin clearance by exchange blood transfusion in septic shock neonates. Acta Paediatr Scand 72:87–91

Volk HD, Reinke P, Krausch D, Zuckermann H, Asadullah K, Muller JM, Docke WD, Kox WJ (1996) Monocyte deactivation – rationale for a new therapeutic strategy in sepsis. Intensive Care Med 22(Suppl 4): S474–S481

Wardle SP, Yoxall CW, Weindling AM (1999) Peripheral oxygenation in hypotensive preterm babies. Pediatr Res 45:343–349

Watson RS, Carcillo JA, Linde-Zwirble WT, Clermont G, Lidicker J, Angus DC (2003) The epidemiology of severe sepsis in children in the United States. Am J Respir Crit Care Med 167:695–701

Neonatal Viral Infections: Enteroviruses and Respiratory Syncytial Virus

109

Paolo Manzoni, Davide Montin, Elena Tavella, and Pier Angelo Tovo

Contents

P. Manzoni (✉) · E. Tavella
Division of Neonatology, Department of Obstetrics and Neonatology, AOU Città della Salute e della Scienza, Turin, Italy
e-mail: paolomanzoni@hotmail.com; ele.travella@gmail.com

D. Montin
Division of Neonatology, Department of Obstetrics and Neonatology, AOU Città della Salute e della Scienza, Turin, Italy

Department of Pediatrics, University of Turin, Turin, Italy
e-mail: davide.montin@gmail.com

P. A. Tovo
Department of Pediatrics, University of Turin, Regina Margherita Childrens Hospital, AOU Città della Salute e della Scienza di Torino, Turin, Italy
e-mail: pierangelo.tovo@unito.it

Abstract

The detection and identification of viral infections in newborns have been greatly improved by the recent development of rapid and highly sensitive diagnostic methods, particularly polymerase chain reaction (PCR) techniques. Most common clinical presentations of viral infection are sepsis-like illness, prolonged seizures, respiratory disease, gastrointestinal disease, and NEC-like syndrome. *Enterovirus* and *Parechovirus* (EV/PeV) infections are the most frequently diagnosed infections in newborns and are responsible for the highest

G. Buonocore et al. (eds.), *Neonatology*,
https://doi.org/10.1007/978-3-319-29489-6_256

mortality. These infections can lead to myocarditis, meningitis, and encephalitis and may cause severe cardiac and neurological sequelae. *Respiratory syncytial virus (RSV)* ranks second as incidence, especially during winter. RSV may cause a severe bronchiolitis or pneumonia especially in preterm infants. Palivizumab is a monoclonal antibody which may reduce the burden of RSV-related disease. Palivizumab prophylaxis is recommended in premature infants below 35 weeks of gestational age, in infants with bronchopulmonary dysplasia (BPD), and in infants with severe congenital heart disease in the first year of life.

109.1 Salient Points

- *Enterovirus* and *Parechovirus* (EV/PeV) infections are the most frequently diagnosed infections in newborns and are responsible for the highest mortality.
- EV myocarditis is a rare and life-threatening disease occurring in the first 2 weeks of life; it is frequently caused by Coxsackievirus B.
- EV/PeV may cause meningitis and meningoencephalitis, which are often characterized by white matter changes; especially PeV3 causes severe disturbances, including mild-to-severe white matter injury.
- There is no specific therapy for EV/PeV infection; intravenous immunoglobulins may be considered when there is severe and generalized neonatal infection.
- Respiratory syncytial virus (RSV) may cause a severe bronchiolitis or pneumonia especially in preterm infants.
- Prevention of RSV infection remains paramount, especially in patients at high risk of severe disease.
- Palivizumab prophylaxis is recommended in premature infants below 35 weeks of gestational age, in infants with bronchopulmonary dysplasia (BPD), and in infants with severe congenital heart disease in the first year of life.

109.2 Enteroviruses

109.2.1 Introduction

The detection and identification of viral infections in newborns have been greatly improved by the recent development of rapid and highly sensitive diagnostic methods, particularly polymerase chain reaction (PCR) techniques. Data from a retrospective analysis of neonates admitted to a neonatal intensive care unit (NICU) in the Netherlands during a 12-year period confirmed viral infection in about 1% of cases. *Enterovirus* and *Parechovirus* (EV/PeV) were the most frequently diagnosed infections (39% of cases) and were responsible for the highest mortality and development of serious sequelae (10% and 15%, respectively) (Verboon-Maciolek et al. 2005). Respiratory syncytial virus (RSV) ranked second as incidence (29%), especially during winter when epidemics of respiratory viruses may occur, particularly in preterm infants (Table 1) (Verboon-Maciolek et al. 2005; Civardi et al. 2013). In another study viral pathogens were detected in up to 6–8% of all sepsis evaluations in a NICU (Ronchi et al. 2014).

EVs and PeVs are non-enveloped, single-stranded RNA viruses belonging to the *Picornaviridae* family (pico = small). Until 1999, EVs were divided into five classes, based on their replication properties in tissue culture and animal models: polioviruses, Coxsackieviruses, echoviruses, *Enterovirus*, and human rhinovirus. On the basis of sequence analysis, the EV genus

Table 1 Viral infections in a neonatal intensive care unit over a 12-year period (number of infants, 5396; viral infections, 51) (Verboon-Maciolek et al. 2005)

Virus	Percentage (%)
Enterovirus/Parechovirus	39
Respiratory syncytial virus	29
Rotavirus	10
Cytomegalovirus	6
Adenovirus	4
Parainfluenza virus	4
Herpes simplex virus	4
Rhinovirus	2
Rubella	2

was recently reclassified into four species: *Enteroviruses A*, *B*, *C*, and *D*. Echovirus 22 and echovirus 23 were reclassified as PeV1 and PeV2 types, respectively. Several new PeVs have recently been identified (Abedi et al. 2015).

109.2.2 Epidemiology and Pathogenesis

EV and PeV infections occur throughout the year, but mostly during the summer and autumn in temperate climates (Verboon-Maciolek et al. 2008). EVs spread from person-to-person by fecal-oral or oral-oral (respiratory) routes. Transmission has been documented by the contaminated hands of healthcare personnel and by fomites. Mother-to-child transmission may occur in utero or during or after delivery. Disease severity is greater in neonates than in older children. The pathogenesis and pathology of EV infections depend on virulence, tropism, and inoculum virus concentration, as well as host factors.

The portal of entry is the pharynx and lower alimentary tract. Within 1 day, the infection extends to the regional lymph nodes. On about the third day, minor viremia occurs with subsequent spread to secondary infection sites (e.g., liver, heart, central nervous system) where virus replication causes local damage. Within a week, there is major viremia with associated clinical manifestations. EVs are usually cytolytic. Symptoms and signs are related to the extent and location of cell death. Cessation of viremia correlates with the appearance of serum antibody. Infection may persist in the lower intestinal tract.

109.2.3 Clinical Aspects

In newborns, non-polio EV and PeV infections are common and are characterized by fever, lethargy, irritability, and poor feeding; cutaneous rash may be present (Abzug 2004; Cherry 2006). Occasionally, these infections can lead to sepsis, myocarditis, pneumonia, meningoencephalitis, and multi-organ failure (Abzug 2004; Khetsuriani et al. 2006). Clinical manifestations of EV infections overlap with those associated with PeV, and diseases are often indistinguishable without a specific virological diagnosis (Verboon-Maciolek et al. 2008a). The diagnosis is by virus culture, direct antigen detection, and/or PCR assay.

Sepsis-like illness has been most frequently observed with Coxsackievirus types B-2 to B-5, E-9 and E-1 (Verboon-Maciolek et al. 2008a; Harvala et al. 2011; Piralla et al. 2014), and PeV-3 (Boivin et al. 2005; Piralla et al. 2012). It is characterized by high fever, abdominal distension, irritability, lethargy, and hypotonia. Other clinical features include diarrhea, vomiting, seizures, and shock (Cherry 2006). Skin rash has been linked to PeV-3 infections (Esposito et al. 2014; Khatami et al. 2014).

Most cases of neonatal myocarditis are caused by Coxsackievirus B infections (Freund et al. 2010). EV myocarditis is a rare and life-threatening disease occurring in the first 2 weeks of life. There is often an abrupt onset with listlessness, anorexia, and fever suggesting bacterial sepsis, accompanied by congestive heart failure, cardiogenic shock, and arrhythmias. Progression is rapid and there may be circulatory failure (tachycardia, cardiomegaly, electrocardiographic changes and transitory systolic murmurs, respiratory distress, and cyanosis). The mortality rate is high (Freund et al. 2010).

Respiratory illness associated with non-polio echoviruses is sporadic, except for echoviruses 11 and 22. The clinical presentation includes rhinitis and pharyngitis, and, to a lesser extent, laryngitis or interstitial pneumonitis. Coxsackieviruses A9 and B4 or echoviruses 9, 11, 17, and 31 are more frequently associated with pneumonia (Farzin et al. 2015).

Both EVs and PeVs may cause meningitis and meningoencephalitis (Vollbach et al. 2015), which are often characterized by white matter changes (Wu et al. 2014; Verboon-Maciolek et al. 2008b). Cerebrospinal fluid (CSF) examination may show variations in protein, glucose, and cellular values which may mirror a bacterial disease, but no alterations can also be found (Cilla et al. 2015). Complications have been reported in approximately 10% of cases and include complex seizures, intracranial hypertension, and coma (Rorabaugh et al. 1993). EV 71 has been associated with cases of neurogenic pulmonary edema (Fu et al. 2003); PeV3 causes severe disturbances, including involvement of the CNS with mild-to-severe white matter injury (Verboon-Maciolek et al. 2008b). A unilateral facial paralysis with transitory loss of abdominal reflexes due to Coxsackievirus B2 has been described (Hostetler et al. 2002).

Coxsackieviruses and echoviruses can also cause vomiting, diarrhea, and hepatitis with various degrees of hepatic necrosis. Some EVs serotypes can cause pancreatitis (Zhang et al. 2016). Furthermore, Coxsackieviruses A-4, A-5, A-8, and B-3 and echoviruses 11 and 22 have been related to sudden infant death syndrome (Krous et al. 2009).

Postnatally acquired poliovirus infection may be asymptomatic or cause various symptoms and signs, including paralysis.

Clinical manifestations of *Enterovirus* infection in newborns are summarized in Table 2.

Table 2 Clinical manifestations of enterovirus infection in newborns (Verboon-Maciolek et al. 2005; Cherry 2006)

General symptoms	Specific symptoms
No symptoms	–
Sepsis-like	Fever, poor feeding, abdominal distension, irritability, rash, lethargy and hypotonia, diarrhea, vomiting, seizures, shock, disseminated intravascular coagulation, thrombocytopenia, hepatomegaly, jaundice, and apnea
Respiratory	Rhinitis, pharyngitis, laryngitis, herpangina, coryza, laryngotracheobronchitis, bronchitis, interstitial pneumonitis
Gastrointestinal	Vomiting and diarrhea, hepatitis, hepatic necrosis, pancreatitis, necrotizing enterocolitis
Cardiological	Tachycardia, cardiomegaly, electrocardiographic changes, transitory systolic murmurs, myocarditis, respiratory distress, cyanosis, signs of neurologic involvement
Dermatological	Macular or maculopapular or petechial rash
Neurological	Anorexia, fever, lethargy, jaundice, vomiting, seizures, apnea, tremulousness, general increased tonicity, meningitis, meningoencephalitis, paralysis
Sudden infant death	–

109.2.4 Differential Diagnosis

Hypothermia and hyperthermia in association with other nonspecific signs are common in neonatal enteroviral infections and in bacterial sepsis. An increase in serum C-reactive protein concentrations, considered indicative of bacterial infection, is also seen in infants with EV infections and less frequently in patients with PeV infections. In meningitis, the CSF findings in bacterial and viral illnesses may be similar, and bacterial culture and PCR assays are essential. Skin lesions are common in generalized herpes simplex infections, and scraping a lesion should allow a rapid diagnosis.

Neonatal seizures due to enteroviral meningoencephalitis may be difficult to differentiate from seizures related to hypoxic-ischemic encephalopathy in full-term infants. The differences are that patients with enteroviral infection may have a history of a viral infection in the family and an uneventful pregnancy and delivery, later onset of seizures, and a possible rash. Neonates with PeV infection cannot be distinguished from those with EV infection by clinical signs only. There are similar white matter abnormalities on cranial imaging (Wu et al. 2014; Verboon-Maciolek et al. 2008c). However, the diagnosis may be made by reverse transcription PCR for EV and PeV on blood and/or CSF because of genetic differences between the viruses (Wu et al. 2014; Verboon-Maciolek et al. 2008b).

Fever or hypothermia, lethargy, weakness, and characteristic electrocardiographic changes differentiate neonatal myocarditis from congenital heart disease.

109.2.5 Prognosis

Both EVs and PeVs may lead to severe cerebral disease with associated serious sequelae

(Verboon-Maciolek et al. 2008a). In one study of six infants with CNS involvement, three babies born preterm had abnormal neurodevelopmental outcomes, while the three born at term developed normally; this is likely to be due to the different vulnerability of the white matter during maturation (Verboon-Maciolek et al. 2008b). White matter damage assessed by MRI is frequent in affected newborns, but it is not steadily associated with a poor neurological outcome (Wu et al. 2014).

Myocarditis due to EV or PeV infection causes severe cardiac sequelae, such as chronic heart failure, mitral regurgitation, and aneurysm formation within the left ventricle, requiring long-term cardiac therapy (Freund et al. 2010).

Poliovirus infections in neonates are generally severe, causing persistent paralysis in a consistent number of patients.

109.2.6 Therapy and Treatments

There is no specific therapy for any EV infection. Human immune serum globulin may be considered when there is severe and generalized neonatal infection on the assumption that the infant did not receive protective antibodies from the mother. Early intravenous immunoglobulin therapy may be beneficial for survival (Yen et al. 2015; Schlapbach et al. 2013). However, several pediatric and adult studies reported conflicting results, and so far, no pediatric randomized controlled trial has been performed. The use of corticosteroids in neonatal encephalitis, myocarditis, or other severe illnesses is debated, with some authors taking a view that they should not be used during acute EV infections, with others supporting their use in Coxsackievirus myocarditis, although deleterious effects have been observed in mice (Abzug 2004).

Meningoencephalitis is often associated with convulsions, cerebral edema, and fluid and electrolyte balance disturbances. Serum electrolyte levels and fluids should be closely monitored because inappropriate antidiuretic hormone secretion is common.

In case of serious outbreaks in a nursery, passive protection with immunoglobulins for all exposed infants should be considered. The worldwide use of vaccination with inactivated polio vaccine (IPV) and the oral polio vaccine (OPV) developed by Sabin in the early 1960s made it possible to control the epidemic in most areas. However, logistic problems and the cost of vaccination have meant that poliomyelitis remains endemic in Central Africa and the Indian subcontinent (Hagan et al. 2015). Infants with paralytic poliomyelitis should be observed carefully for evidence of respiratory paralysis with positive-pressure ventilation for respiratory failure. Passive movements of the paralyzed limbs should be started soon after the disappearance of fever.

109.3 Respiratory Syncytial Virus (RSV)

RSV is a ubiquitous paramyxovirus responsible for a huge burden of respiratory morbidity in infants and children <2 years of age. It has a peak during the winter months. Neonates, particularly those born before 35 weeks of gestation, as well as those affected by bronchopulmonary dysplasia and/or critical congenital heart diseases, are the greatest to feature severe RSV infection and respiratory failure often requiring supplemental oxygen, admission to PICU, and mechanical ventilation (Fjaerli et al. 2005).

109.3.1 Epidemiology and Pathogenesis

RSV is extremely contagious. Transmission occurs by inhalation of droplet nuclei from an infected person or from a contaminated surface. Contaminated objects are an important source of infection, and the hand carriage of contaminated secretions by nursery personnel may greatly contribute to spread, thus increasing the risk of nosocomial outbreaks.

109.3.2 Clinical Aspects

RSV may be asymptomatic or cause a disease that varies from a mild afebrile upper respiratory tract infection to severe bronchiolitis or pneumonia with hyperinflated lungs and hypoxemia. The A subtype of RSV appears to be more serious than the B subtype. The risk of severe illness is highest in infants born prematurely and in those with underlying lung disease, significant congenital heart defects, or immune deficiencies (Fjaerli et al. 2005). Infants younger than 1 month have higher viral titers in their secretions than older ones.

After a few days of incubation, the first symptom is usually non-purulent rhinorrhea, followed by cough and wheezing, with or without dyspnea, bronchiolitis, pneumonia, and fever. Irritability, lethargy, and poor feeding may be the initial manifestations in infants. Chest X-ray abnormalities may precede the clinical manifestations of the lower respiratory tract involvement by a few days.

109.3.3 Diagnosis

Rapid diagnosis is made by detecting viral antigens in nasopharyngeal specimens by specific assays, such as immunofluorescence or enzyme immunoassay. These are the so-called rapid antigen-detection tests with an 80–90% sensitivity. Genome detection by real-time polymerase chain reaction (PCR) is the gold standard diagnostic test in consideration of its 93–100% sensitivity and its 64–100% specificity (Baraldi et al. 2014). Viral isolation may be difficult because RSV is a labile virus.

109.3.4 Prognosis

Many infants with severe RSV bronchiolitis experience recurrent wheezing in later childhood. An association between early RSV bronchiolitis and late recurrent wheezing in the first years of life is documented, and palivizumab prophylaxis in infants 33–35 weeks of gestational age during the first months of life has been found protective toward development of recurrent wheezing in infants at risk for severe RSV disease (Blanken et al. 2014). RSV is speculated to be predisposing some infants to the development of childhood asthma, although this association remains poorly understood (Fjaerli et al. 2005).

109.3.5 Therapy and Treatments

As RSV-related bronchiolitis and pneumonia may cause severe disease in high-risk infants, supportive care, such as intravenous hydration, management of bacterial complications, oxygen supplementation, and mechanical ventilation may be needed (Baraldi et al. 2014). The use of 3% saline and aerosolized ribavirin treatment for infants with lower respiratory tract infections caused by RSV remains debatable (Guerguerian et al. 1999). Candidates for ribavirin therapy are infants at risk for complications of RSV due to congenital heart disease, chronic lung disease or immunodeficiency, infants with severe illness and signs of respiratory failure, or those with a prolonged illness because of an underlying medical condition (Chávez-Bueno et al. 2007).

Because of the limitations associated with the management of RSV disease, prevention remains paramount, especially in patients at high risk of severe disease. Palivizumab is a humanized murine monoclonal antibody which has been shown to be safe and efficacious, significantly reducing the burden of RSV-related disease in premature infants below 35 weeks of gestational age. Its use in such high-risk patients is recommended by specific national guidelines in Europe, America, and Asia (Simões et al. 2008; Bollani et al. 2015). Palivizumab prophylaxis is also recommended in infants with bronchopulmonary dysplasia (BPD) and in infants with severe congenital heart disease in the first year of life. Prophylaxis should be prolonged during the second year of life in children with BPD who require medical therapy (Baraldi et al. 2014; Simões et al. 2008; Bollani et al. 2015).

Palivizumab is administered at a dosage of 15 mg/kg in a single monthly intramuscular injection for 5 months courses during the epidemic season.

Important measures for the prevention and control of viral epidemics are careful handwashing by nursery personnel after handling each infant, restricting the nursery area to personnel and visitors free of respiratory illnesses, and barrier nursing sick infants.

References

Abedi GR, Watson JT, Pham H et al (2015) Enterovirus and human parechovirus surveillance – United States, 2009–2013. MMWR Morb Mortal Wkly Rep 64: 940–943

Abzug MJ (2004) Presentation, diagnosis, and management of enterovirus infections in neonates. Paediatr Drugs 6:1–10

Baraldi E, Lanari M, Manzoni P et al (2014) Inter-society consensus document on treatment and prevention of bronchiolitis in newborns and infants. Ital J Pediatr 40:65

Blanken MO, Rovers MM, Bont L, Dutch RSV Neonatal Network (2014) Respiratory syncytial virus and recurrent wheeze. N Engl J Med 369:782–783

Boivin G, Abed Y, Boucher FD (2005) Human parechovirus 3 and neonatal infections. Emerg Infect Dis 11:103–105

Bollani L, Baraldi E, Chirico G et al (2015) Revised recommendations concerning palivizumab prophylaxis for respiratory syncytial virus (RSV). Ital J Pediatr 41:97

Chávez-Bueno S, Mejías A, Merryman RA et al (2007) Intravenous palivizumab and ribavirin combination for respiratory syncytial virus disease in high-risk pediatric patients. Pediatr Infect Dis J 26:1089–1093

Cherry JD (2006) Enterovirus and parechovirus infections in: infectious diseases of the fetus and newborn infant, 6th edn. Elsevier Saunders, Philadelphia, pp 783–822

Cilla A, Arnaez J, Suarez J et al (2015) Human parechovirus and enterovirus in neonates: distinct infections with overlapping features. Early Hum Dev 91:475–478

Civardi E, Tzialla C, Baldanti F et al (2013) Viral outbreaks in neonatal intensive care units: what we do not know. Am J Infect Control 41:854–856

Esposito S, Janette R-L, Beatrice A et al (2014) Pediatric parechovirus infections. J Clin Virol 60:84–89

Farzin A, Saha SK, Baqui AH et al (2015) Population-based incidence and etiology of community-acquired neonatal viral infections in Bangladesh: a community-based and hospital-based surveillance study. Pediatr Infect Dis J 34:706–711

Fjaerli H-O, Farstad T, Rød G et al (2005) Acute bronchiolitis in infancy as risk factor for wheezing and reduced pulmonary function by seven years in Akershus County, Norway. BMC Pediatr 5:31

Freund MW, Kleinveld G, Krediet TG et al (2010) Prognosis for neonates with enterovirus myocarditis. Arch Dis Child Fetal Neonatal Ed 95:F206–F212

Fu Y-C, Chi C-S, Jan S-L et al (2003) Pulmonary edema of enterovirus 71 encephalomyelitis is associated with left ventricular failure: implications for treatment. Pediatr Pulmonol 35:263–268

Guerguerian A-M, Anne-Marie G, Marie G et al (1999) Ribavirin in ventilated respiratory syncytial virus bronchiolitis. Am J Respir Crit Care Med 160: 829–834

Hagan JE, Wassilak SG, Craig AS et al (2015) Progress toward polio eradication – worldwide, 2014–2015. MMWR Morb Mortal Wkly Rep 64: 527–531

Harvala H, Heli H, Nigel M et al (2011) Comparison of human parechovirus and enterovirus detection frequencies in cerebrospinal fluid samples collected over a 5-year period in Edinburgh: HPeV type 3 identified as the most common picornavirus type. J Med Virol 83:889–896

Hostetler MA, Suara RO, Denison MR (2002) Unilateral facial paralysis occurring in an infant with enteroviral otitis media and aseptic meningitis. J Emerg Med 22:267–271

Khatami A, McMullan BJ, Webber M et al (2014) Sepsis-like disease in infants due to human parechovirus type 3 during an outbreak in Australia. Clin Infect Dis 60:228–236

Khetsuriani N, Nino K, Ashley L et al (2006) Neonatal enterovirus infections reported to the national enterovirus surveillance system in the United States, 1983–2003. Pediatr Infect Dis J 25:889–893

Krous HF, Ferandos C, Masoumi H et al (2009) Myocardial inflammation, cellular death, and viral detection in sudden infant death caused by SIDS, suffocation, or myocarditis. Pediatr Res 66:17–21

Piralla A, Furione M, Rovida F et al (2012) Human parechovirus infections in patients admitted to hospital in Northern Italy, 2008–2010. J Med Virol 84: 686–690

Piralla A, Mariani B, Stronati M et al (2014) Human enterovirus and parechovirus infections in newborns with sepsis-like illness and neurological disorders. Early Hum Dev 90(S1):S75–S77

Ronchi A, Michelow IC, Chapin KC et al (2014) Viral respiratory tract infections in the neonatal intensive care unit: the VIRIoN-I study. J Pediatr 165:690–696

Rorabaugh ML, Berlin LE, Heldrich F et al (1993) Aseptic meningitis in infants younger than 2 years of age: acute illness and neurologic complications. Pediatrics 92:206–211

Schlapbach LJ, Joerg E, Christian B et al (2013) Enteroviral myocarditis in neonates. J Paediatr Child Health 49: E451–E454

Simões EAF, Carbonell-Estrany X, Fullarton JR et al (2008) A predictive model for respiratory syncytial virus (RSV) hospitalisation of premature infants born at 33–35 weeks of gestational age, based on data from the Spanish FLIP Study. Respir Res 9:78

Verboon-Maciolek MA, Krediet TG, Gerards LJ et al (2005) Clinical and epidemiologic characteristics of viral infections in a neonatal intensive care unit during a 12-year period. Pediatr Infect Dis J 24:901–904

Verboon-Maciolek MA, Krediet TG, Gerards LJ et al (2008a) Severe neonatal parechovirus infection and similarity with enterovirus infection. Pediatr Infect Dis J 27:241–245

Verboon-Maciolek MA, Utrecht FG, Cowan F et al (2008b) White matter damage in neonatal enterovirus meningoencephalitis. Neurology 71:536

Verboon-Maciolek MA, Floris G, Hahn CD et al (2008c) Human parechovirus causes encephalitis with white matter injury in neonates. Ann Neurol 64:266–273

Vollbach S, Silke V, Andreas M et al (2015) Prevalence, type and concentration of human enterovirus and parechovirus in cerebrospinal fluid samples of pediatric patients over a 10-year period: a retrospective study. Virol J 12:199

Wu T, Fan X-P, Wang et al (2014) Enterovirus infections are associated with white matter damage in neonates. J Paediatr Child Health 50:817–822

Yen M-H, Huang Y-C, Chen M-C et al (2015) Effect of intravenous immunoglobulin for neonates with severe enteroviral infections with emphasis on the timing of administration. J Clin Virol 64:92–96

Zhang Y-F, Deng H-L, Fu J et al (2016) Pancreatitis in hand-foot-and-mouth disease caused by enterovirus 71. World J Gastroenterol 22:2149–2152

Vaccinations and Neonatal Immunity 110

Alberto G. Ugazio and Alberto E. Tozzi

Contents

Abstract

Immune responsiveness quickly matures in both term and preterm neonates after birth, rapidly reaching levels comparable with those observed in children and adults. The duration of this maturation process is variable and also depends on the type of antigen to which immunity is directed. Maternally acquired passive immunity keeps a major protective role during the first months of life, via transplacentally acquired IgG and maternal IgA acquired via breast milk. The safety profile and immunogenicity of routinely administered vaccines are similar in premature neonates to those measured in full-term infants. Preterm and low birth weight infants should be immunized according to their chronological age. Indeed, early and timely immunization of preterm and low birth weight infants is safe and essential for protecting them against diseases to which these infants are particularly susceptible and that may be even fatal. Besides traditional vaccination, maternal immunization during pregnancy is being tested and it is proving quite effective;

A. G. Ugazio (✉)
Institute of Child and Adolescent Health, Bambino Gesù Children's Hospital, Rome, Italy
e-mail: agugazio@gmail.com

A. E. Tozzi
Multifactorial and Complex Diseases Research Area, Bambino Gesù Children's Hospital, Rome, Italy

G. Buonocore et al. (eds.), *Neonatology*,
https://doi.org/10.1007/978-3-319-29489-6_257

new vaccines are therefore being studied in pregnant women. A potential cause of concern is whether vaccines administered to preterm infants induce a good immunological memory, because very preterm infants may develop a weaker immunological long-term response. Another critical aspect regarding neonatal vaccinations is the use of corticosteroids (often used in NICU) since they may decrease the response. In spite of that, their administration should not delay the vaccine schedule. The benefits of early and timely immunization of fragile children far exceed the risk of inducing suboptimal protection.

110.1 Salient Points

- Neonates progressively improve their immune function to respond to infections during infancy;
- Immunologic response to vaccinations progressively increases with gestational age, although preterm infants develop a sufficient response to immunizations to induce protection.
- Since tolerability and safety are not cause for concern in preterm and very preterm infants, all children should receive immunizations according to their chronological age.
- The vaccines that may be administered at birth to induce a more rapid protection are sufficiently safe and immunogenic.
- Immunization of mothers during pregnancy is a safe and efficacious strategy to protect the fetus, and the neonate from infections before immunization in infancy can be completed.
- Immunizations received in infancy safely induce protection even in very preterm infants.
- Waning immunity after primary immunization may be an issue for some vaccines especially in very preterm infants that may develop a weaker immunological memory.
- Although corticosteroids may decrease the response when administered during immunization, their administration should not delay the vaccine schedule.
- Thimerosal, a mercury compound previously used as a preservative in vaccines administrated during infancy, does not affect the neuropsychological development of children.

110.2 Immunological Development of the Neonate

The fetus can be compared to a haploidentical graft, sharing only half of the histocompatibility antigens of the "mother host." As such, the fetus should be rejected by the immune system of the mother. At the same time, since the fetal immune system starts developing around the ninth week of gestation, the fetus should also mount a "graft-versus-host" reaction against those histocompatibility antigens that it has not inherited from the "mother host." It follows that survival of the fetus – indeed of all mammalian species – is strictly dependent on a wide variety of mechanisms preventing graft rejection by the mother and graft-versus-host reaction by the fetus (Koch and Platt 2007). Among the latter, a major role is certainly played by the slow intrauterine maturation of the fetal immune function, ultimately resulting in the physiological immune deficiency of the neonate that involves both innate and adaptive immunity. This immune immaturity – more severe in preterm and in very low birth weight infants – results in a weak immune response to antigen challenge and in the production of a poor immunological memory (Lewis 2004; Basha et al. 2014).

After birth, the immune responsiveness quickly matures in both term and preterm neonates, rapidly reaching levels comparable with those observed in children and adults. The duration of this maturation process is variable and also depends on the type of antigen to which immunity is directed. The optimal period for vaccination is decided therefore on a balance between the need of protecting the newborn as soon as possible against potential infectious threats and the opportunity to trigger protective and durable immune responses. As a result, for at least 1–2 months, exclusively maternal IgG acquired transplacentally and maternal IgA acquired via breast milk protect the neonate/infant from vaccine-preventable infections. Since vaccine-induced protection is very poor following the first vaccine administration, maternally acquired passive immunity keeps a major protective role during the first 4–6 months of life. Unfortunately, over the last decades, the amount of antibodies transferred from the mother is slowly declining: maternal age at reproduction is progressively increasing and antibody titers are inversely related to age, the average titer of vaccine-induced antibodies is lower than that induced by infection and duration of breastfeeding is shortened. Together with the recurrence in the general population of some vaccine-preventable diseases such as pertussis, this window of vulnerability exposes neonates and infants to infections that are particularly severe in this age group.

110.3 General Recommendations

Routine immunizations are often delayed in preterm and low birth weight infants, due to their impaired ability to develop protective immunity and to the perception that they are more susceptible to side effects (Langkamp et al. 2001; Moyes 1999; Tozzi et al. 2014). However, the safety profile and immunogenicity of routinely administered vaccines are similar to those measured in full-term infants. Though immunogenicity might be suboptimal for some vaccines, in most cases, preterm and low birth weight infants should be immunized according to their chronological age (Saari and Committee on Infectious Diseases 2003; Kroger et al. 2006). In addition, vaccine dosage should not be reduced or divided (Saari and Committee on Infectious Diseases 2003).

The site of choice for intramuscular vaccine administration is the anterolateral thigh, and needle length should be chosen on the basis of the available muscle mass (Kroger et al. 2006).

Preterm infants may suffer from cardiorespiratory instability at the time of immunization, and vaccine administration has been suspected to trigger apnea, desaturation, and bradycardia, especially in children with pre-existing cardiorespiratory symptoms (Pfister et al. 2004; Pourcyrous et al. 2007; Klein et al. 2008). Moreover, infants that presented apnea in the 24 h before immunization have been considered more likely to develop postimmunization apnea (Klein et al. 2008); postimmunization apnea has been reported to occur more frequently in the presence of severe illness at birth, younger age, and lower weight (Klein et al. 2008). None of the cardiorespiratory or other adverse events observed in preterm or low birth weight infants had sequelae in the studies published so far, and all of them were transient (Klein et al. 2008; Bonhoeffer et al. 2006). However, based on the data from these observational studies, it has been recommended that infants still hospitalized at the time immunization is due should be monitored in hospital for 48 h after vaccine administration (Bonhoeffer et al. 2006). Severe cardiorespiratory events after the first vaccine dose may occasionally predict similar episodes at the second dose (Flatz-Jequier et al. 2008). More recently, a randomized trial in preterm children immunized with DTaP demonstrated that the rate of prolonged episodes of apnea or bradycardia is similar in immunized infants and controls (Carbone et al. 2008). In essence, though monitoring preterm and very preterm infants after immunization seems prudent, there are no apparent safety concerns that suggest to delay administration of vaccines in this group of infants (Gagneur et al. 2015).

An increase in C reactive protein (CRP) is commonly found in infants after immunization, although such an increase has not been observed with HBV and IPV immunizations (Pourcyrous et al. 2007). The finding of normal CRP values before immunization suggests that high CRP values following immunization are possibly induced by vaccine administration (Pourcyrous et al. 2007).

Early and timely immunization of preterm and low birth weight infants is safe and essential for protecting them against diseases to which these infants are particularly susceptible and that may be even fatal. The benefits of early and timely immunization of fragile children far exceed the risk of inducing suboptimal protection. In addition, immunization of households and contacts of preterm and low birthweight infants, although challenging, may be effective in decreasing the likelihood of exposure before immunization and before full maturation of immune defense mechanisms.

110.4 Vaccines That Can Be Administered at Birth

Since the neonate is not able to mount robust immune responses to most vaccines, immunizations are mostly delayed until the second or third month of age. Nonetheless, in some circumstances where the risk of acquiring some infectious diseases is high, early administration of vaccines, soon or shortly after birth, is crucial for avoiding infections.

BCG BCG is administered to neonates in many countries where the prevalence of tuberculosis is high. Studies in which preterm babies were compared with term infants showed similar responses to the tuberculin reaction after immunization and comparable cellular immune responses (Gaudelus et al. 2007; Negrete-Esqueda and Vargas-Origel 2007). In one study, the authors found a weaker delayed hypersensitivity to tuberculin after BCG in preterm infants compared with full-term neonates and therefore recommended to delay BCG administration in newborns younger than 33 weeks of gestational age (Salious et al. 2002). Other authors found a positive relationship between a positive tuberculin test after BCG and postnatal weight (Okan et al. 2006). Administration of BCG in preterm infants does not result in an increased reactogenicity compared with full-term babies (Gaudelus et al. 2007).

Hepatitis B Virus (HBV) Immunization of newborns against hepatitis B together with hepatitis B immunoglobulin (HBIG) administration within 12 h of birth is recommended in children born to hepatitis B surface antigen (HbsAg)-positive mothers or to those whose HBV status is unknown (American Academy of Pediatrics 2003). It has been shown that HBV vaccine administration in newborns who weigh less than 2,000 g results in decreased seroconversion rates (Lau et al. 1992). These children should be immunized as well within 12 h of birth, although the initial vaccine dose should not be counted towards completion of the HBV series. In some countries as the USA, HBV is administered to all newborns regardless of mother's HBV status (American Academy of Pediatrics 2003). Preterm infants weighing less than 2,000 g and born to HBsAg-negative mothers should receive the first dose of the HepB series at 1 month of chronological age or at hospital discharge in order to take advantage of the increased maturity of the newborn's immune system (Mast et al. 2005; Kim et al. 1997).

110.4.1 Maternal Immunization

The previously mentioned window of susceptibility that exposes neonates and early infants to severe, vaccine-preventable infections has prompted the search and study of alternative protective strategies. The "cocoon strategy" aims to protect neonates and infants from infections, in particular pertussis, by administering a booster Tdap vaccination (tetanus toxoid, diphtheria toxoid, and acellular pertussis) to all close contacts including parents, siblings, grandparents, and child-care providers. Although theoretically well grounded, this strategy has proved very difficult to put into practice due to the need to reach, inform, convince and, ultimately, vaccinate a large number of adults (Forsyth et al. 2015).

Maternal vaccination with Tdap during pregnancy (Fig. 1) – particularly between 28 and 32 weeks of gestation – is proving very effective for preventing pertussis in neonates and infants and is now the strategy of choice for the prevention of neonatal and infant pertussis in several industrialized countries including UK and USA (Forsyth et al. 2015).

Influenza vaccination with the inactivated viruses is highly recommended for all pregnant women due to their high risk of mortality and severe complications of influenza including fetal death with increased rates of stillbirth and prematurity (Swamy and Heine 2015; Chu and Englund 2014). Neonates and infants of influenza-immunized mothers have a more than 60% reduction of laboratory-confirmed influenza and a

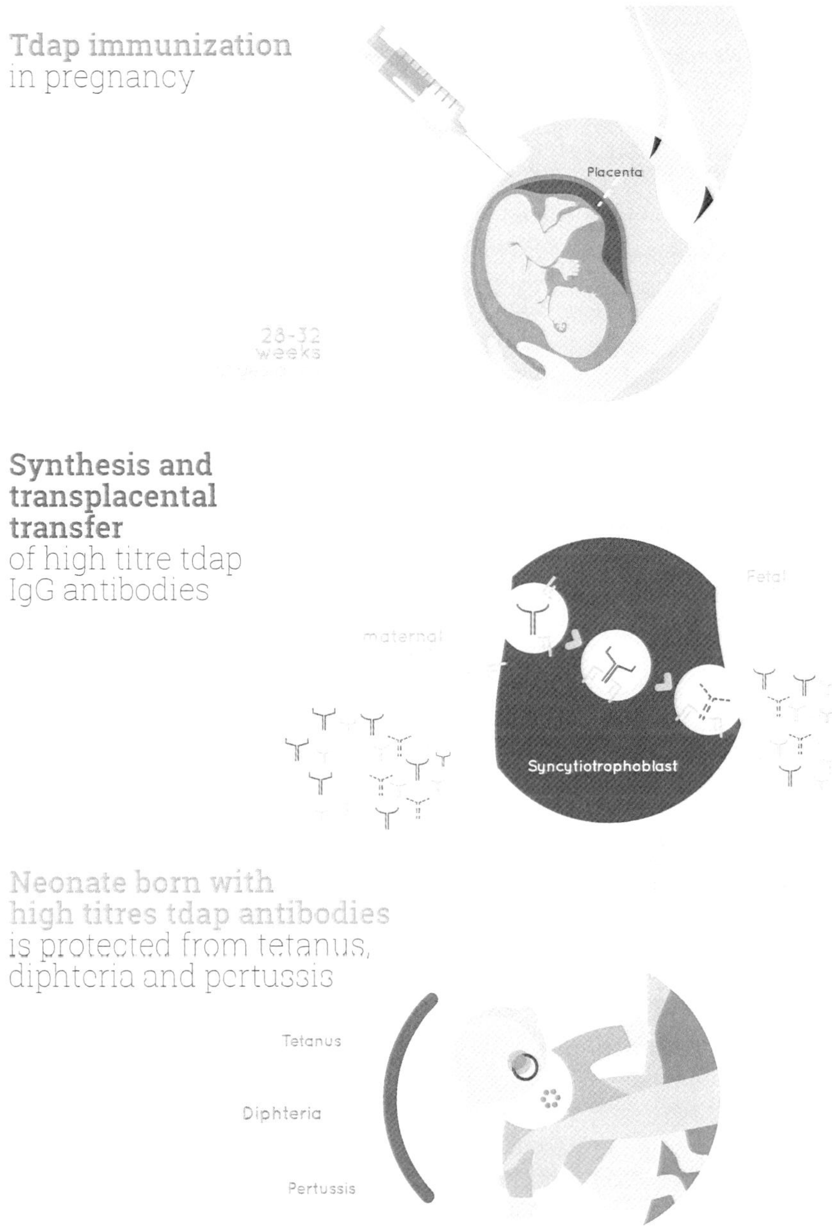

Fig. 1 Maternal immunization aimed at protecting the mother, and infant. (**a**) Pregnant women are immunized with tdap around the 28th–32nd week of gestation. (**b**) The anamnestic response of the maternal immune system generates high titers of IgG antibodies directed against the antigenic determinants of tdap. Placental syncytiotrophoblast cells internalize maternal IgG in endosomes expressing on their internal surface neonatal FcγR (receptors for the Fc fragment of IgG). The endosomes fuse with the membrane on the fetal side of the syncytiotrophoblast where IgG dissociate from FcγR and are released into the fetal circulation. (**c**) The neonate of the immunized mother is protected from tetanus, diphtheria and pertussis by high titers of specific antibodies received from the immunized mother

reduction by one third of febrile respiratory illness (Swamy and Heine 2015; Chu and Englund 2014).

The strategy of maternal immunization during pregnancy to prevent neonatal and infant infections is proving so effective that new vaccines are being directly studied in pregnant women. Group B Streptococcus (GBS) is a prime candidate for prevention by maternal immunization since most "early" GBS infections occur within 48 h from birth. A CRM_{197}, –conjugated capsular polysaccharide vaccine directed against three serotypes (Ia, Ib, and III) responsible for approximately 75% of GBS infections, has been administered between 28 and 35 weeks of gestation (Heyderman et al. 2016; Madhi et al. 2016). Neonates of vaccinated mothers had a serum concentration of specific antibodies much higher than neonates of placebo-treated mothers. A phase 3 study including more than 10,000 mothers and newborns is currently under way (Madhi et al. 2013).

Similarly, a phase 3 study of an RSV nanoparticle vaccine based on a recombinant, near full-length RSV F glycoprotein is currently under way in pregnant women and their children to prevent RSV bronchiolitis during the first 3 months of life (Velasco et al. 2016).

110.5 Vaccines That Can Be Administered in Infancy

As previously mentioned, immunization schedules start as a rule during the second to third month of life and usually include, in industrialized countries, diphtheria, tetanus, pertussis, polio, *Haemophilus* type b and hepatitis B vaccines. Some schedules also include either conjugated pneumococcal vaccine or conjugated meningococcal C vaccine. In developing countries, the schedule may include a more limited number of vaccine components. Unfortunately, good quality efficacy and safety studies have been carried out only for a limited number of vaccines. A synthesis of the available evidence for each specific vaccine is presented below.

Diphtheria-Tetanus-Pertussis Vaccine Diphtheria, tetanus, and pertussis (DTP) immunogenicity has been demonstrated in different studies even when these components are combined with other vaccine antigens (Schloesser et al. 1999; Omeñaca et al. 2005; Slack et al. 2005; Vázquez et al. 2008). Conflicting results have been obtained for the immunogenicity of the pertussis component, with some studies showing low titers in preterm compared with full-term infants (Schloesser et al. 1999; Omeñaca et al. 2005; Slack et al. 2005; Vázquez et al. 2008). To date, a serological correlate of protection from pertussis has not been identified. Therefore, the finding of low titers of antibodies directed against antigenic components of the pertussis vaccine is of doubtful significance. Tolerability of vaccines including DTP antigens in preterm infants is similar to that observed in full-term babies (Schloesser et al. 1999; Omeñaca et al. 2005; Faldella et al. 2007).

Polio Vaccine Inactivated polio vaccine has been shown to be immunogenic and well tolerated in preterm infants even when administered within combined vaccines (Omeñaca et al. 2005; Slack et al. 2005; Linder et al. 1995; Adenyi-Jones et al. 1992). Lower geometric mean titers have been observed for serotypes 2 and 3 in comparison with full-term infants (Omeñaca et al. 2005; D'Angio et al. 1995). Oral polio vaccine, which is still in use in some countries, does not seem to be influenced in its response by gestational age (Conway et al. 1994).

Haemophilus Type b Vaccine (Hib) Tolerability of the Hib component has been shown in several studies carried out with combined vaccines (Vázquez et al. 2008; Faldella et al. 2007). Percentage of responders and antibody titers have been shown to be lower in preterm infants (D'Angio et al. 1995; Berrington et al. 2006; Omeñaca et al. 2007). Available data show an increase in vaccine failures in preterm compared with full-term infants when an accelerated schedule is used (2, 3, and 4 months of age) (Heath et al. 2003).

Hepatitis B Vaccine HBV is well tolerated in preterm and low-birth-weight infants and is fully immunogenic when administered in babies

>2,000 g or older than 60 days (Omeñaca et al. 2005; Faldella et al. 2007; Huang et al. 2007).

Conjugate Pneumococcal Vaccine Heptavalent conjugate pneumococcal vaccine (PCV7) seems to elicit a similar immune response in preterm and full-term infants (Esposito et al. 2005; Shinefield et al. 2002) although one study reported a lower immunogenicity in preterm infants immunized with an accelerated schedule (2, 3, and 4 months of age) (Ruggeberg et al. 2007). Most importantly, efficacy of this vaccine in preterm and low birth weight infants is very high, similarly to what is observed in full-term infants (Shinefield et al. 2002). Local reactions are observed more commonly in preterm and low birth weight than in full-term infants (Shinefield et al. 2002). Results of a recent study of the immune response to 13-valent pneumococcal conjugate vaccine (PCV13) in preterm infants compared with term infants suggest that preterm infants' responses, although lower, exceed the WHO–established threshold of protection (Martinón-Torres et al. 2015).

Conjugate Meningococcal C Vaccine The conjugate meningococcal C vaccine is well tolerated and immunogenic when administered to preterm infants, although the only available studies were performed with an accelerated schedule (2, 3, and 4 months of age) (Slack et al. 2001; Collins et al. 2005).

Conjugate Meningococcal B Vaccine Recently, a meningococcal B vaccine has become available in the market. Although not included in routine schedules in most countries, this vaccine proved to be well tolerated and immunogenic in infancy; though more data are needed to precisely estimate its duration of protection (Watson and Turner 2016).

Measles-Mumps-Rubella and Varicella A single study showed similar geometric mean titers and proportions of responders to measles, mumps, rubella and varicella in severely preterm as compared to full-term infants immunized at 15 months of age (D'Angio et al. 2007). It must be taken into account that preterm infants lose maternal antibodies to measles early after birth (Bonhoeffer et al. 2006). Therefore, preterm infants may be safely immunized during outbreak periods between 6 and 9 months of age (Bonhoeffer et al. 2006).

Rotavirus A pentavalent live attenuated rotavirus vaccine has proved safe and efficacious in preterm babies (Vesikari et al. 2006). Although so far no epidemiological study has investigated the horizontal transmission of vaccine strains, vaccine virus shedding can be observed up to 15 days after administration. Children of appropriate age and still hospitalized may be immunized on the day of discharge.

Influenza One study carried out in infants born prematurely and immunized after 6 months of age with an inactivated influenza vaccine showed greater T-cell proliferative responses to influenza antigen in full-term children than in the preterm children, but similar proportions of responders (Groothuis et al. 1992).

110.6 Immunological Memory in Preterm Infants

A potential cause of concern is whether vaccines administered to preterm infants induce a good immunological memory. DTaP-IPV-Hib-HBV hexavalent vaccine has been shown to induce immunological memory for all the components in most preterm infants primed with this vaccine (Omeñaca et al. 2007). Other studies indicate that the immune response after primary immunization with conjugate meningococcal C or pneumococcal vaccine may be weaker in preterm than in full-term infants, and that it wanes after 1 year if an accelerated schedule is used (2, 3, and 4 months of age) (Ruggeberg et al. 2007; Collins et al. 2005).

110.7 Children Treated with Corticosteroids

Preterm infants are often treated for variable periods with corticosteroids. Dexamethasone-treated preterm infants show significantly reduced antibody levels to diphtheria, tetanus, and pertussis antigens after primary immunization (Robinson et al. 2004). It is not known how much this decreased response reflects on protection, especially for diphtheria and pertussis. A negative effect of dexamethasone treatment has been noted also on immune response to *Haemophilus influenzae* b vaccine (Clarke et al. 2003), whereas it does not seem to decrease the immune response to conjugate meningococcal vaccine given at 12 months of age (Clarke et al. 2006). In general, care should be taken when dexamethasone treated infants travel to endemic areas.

110.8 The Effect of Mercury Additives in Vaccines

Concern has been raised on the potential neurotoxicity of thimerosal-containing vaccines administered early after birth. Since 1999, several international agencies including the European Medicine Agency and the Centers for Diseases Control have recommended that thimerosal be eliminated from vaccines as a precautionary measure (European Agency for the Evaluation of Medicinal Products 2009; Centers for Disease Control and Prevention 1999). Epidemiological studies have shown that administration of thimerosal containing vaccines is not associated with an impaired neuropsychological development or with clear developmental disorders later in life (McCormick et al. 2004; Tozzi et al. 2009).

110.9 The Future of Immunization of Newborns

Advances in immunization have been achieved throughout the last few decades bringing sophisticated means to protect children and the general population from severe transmissible diseases. Still, new approaches to the development of efficacious strategies to prevent some diseases are needed in the perinatal and infancy periods. Incidence of several diseases such as meningococcal and pneumococcal invasive infections, pertussis, and influenza is highest in infancy, and preterm babies often pay the highest toll in terms of morbidity. Moreover, given the relative immaturity of the immunologic system, these children, even when properly vaccinated, may not be optimally protected. Maternal vaccination and subsequent transmission of high titers of specific IgG antibodies to the fetus and neonate is proving quite effective. However, this approach is not applicable to live attenuated vaccines; furthermore, high-risk groups, such as preterm neonates, fail to receive sufficient amounts of antibodies due to the late transplacental passage of maternal IgG, vaccines which stimulate both innate and adaptive immune response may allow induction of better protection of the high risk newborn (Klinman 2004). New routes of immunization may help to achieve the goal of inducing mucosal immunity (Plotkin 2005).

These goals may be achieved within a few years and provide us with new and more efficacious preventive tools for the special category of high-risk newborns.

References

Adenyi-Jones SC, Faden H, Ferdon MB et al (1992) Systemic and local immune responses to enhanced-potency inactivated poliovirus vaccine in premature and term infants. J Pediatr 120:686–689

American Academy of Pediatrics (2003) Hepatitis B. In: Pickering LK (ed) Red book: 2003 report of the committee on infectious diseases, 26th edn. American Academy of Pediatrics, Elk Grove Village, pp 318–336

Basha S, Surendram N, Pichichero M (2014) Immune responses in neonates. Expert Rev Immunol 10 (9):1171–1184

Berrington JE, Cant AJ, Matthews JN et al (2006) Haemophilus influenzae type b immunization in infants in the United Kingdom: effects of diphtheria/tetanus/acellular pertussis/Hib combination vaccine, significant prematurity, and a fourth dose. Pediatrics 117: e717–e724

Bonhoeffer J, Siegrist C-A, Heath PT (2006) Immunisation of premature infants. Arch Dis Child 91:929–935

Carbone T, McEntire B, Kissin D et al (2008) Absence of an increase in cardiorespiratory events after diphtheria-tetanus-acellular pertussis immunization in preterm infants: a randomized, multicenter study. Pediatrics 121:e1085–e1090

Centers for Disease Control and Prevention (1999) Thimerosal in vaccines: a joint statement of the American academy of pediatrics and the public health service. MMWR Morb Mortal Wkly Rep 48:563–565

Chu HY, Englund JA (2014) Maternal immunization. Vaccine 59:560–568

Clarke P, Powell PJ, Goldblatt D, Robinson MJ (2003) Effect of a fourth Haemophilus influenzae type b immunization in preterm infants who received dexamethasone for chronic lung disease. Arch Dis Child Fetal Neonatal Ed 88:F58–F61

Clarke P, Robinson MJ, Ahmad I et al (2006) Response of steroid treated former preterm infants to a single dose of meningococcal C conjugate vaccine. Vaccine 24:3273–3278

ClinicalTrials.gov (2015) A study to determine the safety and efficacy of the RSV F vaccine to protect infants via maternal immunization (NIH: https://clinicaltrials.gov/ct2/show/NCT02624947)

Collins CL, Ruggeberg JU, Balfour G et al (2005) Immunogenicity and immunologic memory of meningococcal C conjugate vaccine in premature infants. Pediatr Infect Dis J 24:966–968

Conway S, James J, Balfour A, Smithells R (1994) Immunisation of the preterm baby. J Infect 28:143–150

D'Angio CT, Maniscalco WM, Pichichero ME (1995) Immunologic response of extremely premature infants to tetanus, Haemophilus influenzae, and polio immunizations. Pediatrics 96:18–22

D'Angio CT, Boohene PA, Mowrer A et al (2007) Measles-mumps-rubella and varicella vaccine responses in extremely preterm infants. Pediatrics 119:e574–e579

Esposito S, Pugni L, Bosis S et al (2005) Immunogenicity, safety and tolerability of heptavalent pneumococcal conjugate vaccine administered at 3, 5 and 11 months post-natally to pre- and full-term infants. Vaccine 23:1703–1708

European Agency for the Evaluation of Medicinal Products (2009) EMEA public statement on thiomersal containing medicinal products, 8 July 1999. www.emea.europa.eu/pdfs/human/press/pus/2096299EN.pdf

Faldella G, Galletti S, Corvaglia L et al (2007) Safety of DTaPIPV- HIb-HBV hexavalent vaccine in very premature infants. Vaccine 25:1036–1042

Flatz-Jequier A, Posfay-Barbe KM, Pfister RE, Siegrist CA (2008) Recurrence of cardiorespiratory events following repeat DTaPbased combined immunization in very low birth weight premature infants. J Pediatr 153:429–431

Forsyth K, Plotkin S, Tan T, Wirsing von König CH (2015) Strategies to decrease pertussis transmission to infants. Pediatrics 135(6):e1475–e1482

Gagneur A, Pinquier D, Quach C (2015) Immunization of preterm infants. Hum Vaccin Immunother 11 (11):2556–2563

Gaudelus J, Lefèvre-Akriche S, Roumegoux C et al (2007) Immunization of the preterm infants. Arch Pediatr 14 (Suppl 1):S24–S30

Groothuis JR, Levin MJ, Lehr MV et al (1992) Immune response to split-product influenza vaccine in preterm and full-term young children. Vaccine 10:221–225

Heath PT, Booy R, McVernon J et al (2003) Hib vaccination in infants born prematurely. Arch Dis Child 88:206–210

Heyderman RS, Madhi SA, Neil F, Clare C, Bagrey N, Doris K, Robert M, Anthonet K, Lisa J, Morounfolu O, Frederik W, Karen S, Dull PM (2016) Group B streptococcus vaccination in pregnant women with or without HIV in AFRICA: a non-randomised phase 2, open-label, multicentre trial. Lancet 16:546–555

Huang FY, Lee PI, Lee CY et al (2007) Hepatitis B vaccination in preterm infants. Arch Dis Child Fetal Neonatal Ed 77:F135–F138

Kim SC, Chung EK, Hodinka RL et al (1997) Immunogenicity of hepatitis B vaccine in preterm infants. Pediatrics 99:534–536

Klein NP, Massolo ML, Greene J et al (2008) Vaccine safety datalink. Risk factors for developing apnea after immunization in the neonatal intensive care unit. Pediatrics 121:463–469

Klinman DM (2004) Immunotherapeutic uses of CpG oligodeoxynucleotides. Nat Rev Immunol 4:249–258

Koch CA, Platt JL (2007) T cell recognition and immunity in the fetus and mother. Cell Immunol 248:12–7

Kroger AT, Atkinson WL, Marcuse EK et al (2006) General recommendations on immunization recommendations of the advisory committee on immunization practices (ACIP). MMWR Recomm Rep 55:1–48

Langkamp DL, Hoshaw-Woodard S, Boye ME, Lemeshow S (2001) Delays in receipt of immunizations in low-birth-weight children: a nationally representative sample. Arch Pediatr Adolesc Med 155:167–172

Lau YL, Tam AY, Ng KW et al (1992) Response of preterm infants to hepatitis B vaccine. J Pediatr 121:962–965

Lewis DB (2004) The physiologic immunodeficiency of immaturity. In: Stiehm ER, Ochs HD, Winkelstein JA (eds) Immunologic disorders in infants and children, 5th edn. Elsevier Saunders, Philadelphia, pp 687–760

Linder N, Yaron M, Handsher R et al (1995) Early immunization with inactivated poliovirus vaccine in premature infants. J Pediatr 127:128–130

Madhi SA, Dangor Z, Heath PT, Schrag S, Izu A, Sobanjo-Ter Meulen A, Dull PM (2013) Considerations for a phase-III trial evaluate a group B Streptococcus polysaccharide-èrptein conjugate vaccine in pregnant women for the prevention of early- and late-onset invasive disease in young-infants. Vaccine 31(Suppl 4):D52–D57

Madhi SA, Cutland CL, Jose L, Koen A, Govender N, Wittke F, Olugbosi M, Meulen AS, Baker S, Dull PM, Narasimhan V, Slobod K (2016) Safety and immunogenicity of an investigational maternal trivalent group B Streptococcus vaccine in healthy women and their infants: a randomized phase 1b/2 trial. Lancet 1–12

Martinón-Torres F, Czajka H, Center KJ, Wysocki J, Ewa M-S, Omeñaca F, Iturbe EB, Gamero DB, Concheiro-Guisán A, Gimenez-Sanchez F, Szenborn L, Giardina PC, Patterson S, Gruber WC, Scott DA, Gurtman A (2015) 13-valent pneumococcal conjugate vaccine (PCV13) in preterm versus term infants. Pediatrics 135:e877–e886

Mast EE, Margolis HS, Fiore AE et al (2005) A comprehensive immunization strategy to eliminate transmission of hepatitis B virus infection in the United States: recommendations of the advisory committee on immunization practices (ACIP); part 1: immunization of infants, children, and adolescents. MMWR Recomm Rep 54:1–31

McCormick M, Bayer R, Berg A (2004) Report of the institute of medicine: immunization safety review–vaccines and autism. National Academy Press, Washington, DC

Moyes C (1999) Immunisation of preterm babies. N Z Med J 112:263–264

Negrete-Esqueda L, Vargas-Origel A (2007) Response to Bacillus Calmette-Guerin vaccine in full term and pre term infants. Am J Perinatol 24:183–189

Okan F, Karagoz S, Nuhoglu A (2006) Bacillus Calmette-Guerin vaccination in preterm infants. Int J Tuberc Lung Dis 10:1337–1341

Omeñaca F, Garcia-Sicilia J, García-Corbeira P et al (2005) Response of preterm newborns to immunization with a hexavalent diphtheria-tetanus-acellular pertussis-hepatitis B virus-inactivated polio and Haemophilus influenzae type b vaccine: first experiences and solutions to a serious and sensitive issue. Pediatrics 116:1292–1298

Omeñaca F, Garcia-Sicilia J, García-Corbeira P et al (2007) Antipolyribosyl ribitol phosphate response of premature infants to primary and booster vaccination with a combined diphtheriatetanus- acellular pertussis-hepatitis B-inactivated polio virus/ Haemophilus influenzae type b vaccine. Pediatrics 119:e179–e185

Pfister RE, Aeschbach V, Niksic-Stuber V et al (2004) Safety of DTaP-based combined immunization in very-low-birth-weight premature infants: frequent but mostly benign cardiorespiratory events. J Pediatr 145:58–66

Plotkin S (2005) Vaccines: past, present, and future. Nat Med 11:S5–S11

Pourcyrous M, Korones SB, Arheart KL, Bada HS (2007) Primary immunization of premature infants with gestational age <35 weeks: cardiorespiratory complications and c-reactive protein responses associated with administration of single and multiple separate vaccines simultaneously. J Pediatr 151:167–172

Robinson MJ, Heal C, Gardener E et al (2004) Antibody response to diphtheria-tetanus-pertussis immunization in preterm infants who receive dexamethasone for chronic lung disease. Pediatrics 113:733–737

Ruggeberg JU, Collins C, Clarke P et al (2007) Immunogenicity and induction of immunological memory of the heptavalent pneumococcal conjugate vaccine in preterm UK infants. Vaccine 25:264–271

Saari TN, Committee on Infectious Diseases (2003) Immunization of preterm and low birth weight infants. Pediatrics 112:193–198

Salious P, Aijan N, Guérin N (2002) Efficacy and tolerance of vaccinations in premature infants. Arch Pediatr 9:629–637

Schloesser RL, Fischer D, Otto W et al (1999) Safety and immunogenicity of an acellular pertussis vaccine in premature infants. Pediatrics 103:e60

Shinefield H, Black S, Ray P et al (2002) Efficacy, immunogenicity and safety of heptavalent pneumococcal conjugate vaccine in low birth weight and preterm infants. Pediatr Infect Dis J 21:182–186

Slack MH, Schapira D, Thwaites RJ et al (2001) Immune response of premature infants to meningococcal serogroup C and combined diphtheria-tetanus toxoids-acellular pertussis-Haemophilus influenzae type b conjugate vaccines. J Infect Dis 184:1617–1620

Slack MH, Cade S, Schapira D et al (2005) DT5aP-Hib-IPV and MCC vaccines: preterm infants' response to accelerated immunisation. Arch Dis Child 90:338–341

Swamy GK, Heine RP (2015) Vaccinations for pregnant women. Clin Expert Ser 125(1):212–226

Tozzi AE, Bisiacchi P, Tarantino V et al (2009) Neuropsychological performance 10 years after immunization in infancy with thimerosal-containing vaccines. Pediatrics 123:475–482

Tozzi AE, Piga S, Corchia C, Di Lallo D, Carnielli V, Chiandotto V, Fertz MC, Miniaci S, Rusconi F, Cuttini M (2014) Timeliness of routine immunization in a population-based Italian cohort of very preterm infants: results of the ACTION follow-up project. Vaccine 32 (7):793–799

Vázquez L, Garcia F, Rüttimann R et al (2008) Immunogenicity and reactogenicity of DTPa-HBV-IPV/Hib vaccine as primary and booster vaccination in low-birth-weight premature infants. Acta Paediatr 97:1243–1249

Velasco C, Helene B, Bipin B, Fallon JT, Alexandra A, Paul G, Galarza JM (2016) A novel respiratory syncytial virus-like particle (VLP) vaccine composed of the postfusion and prefusion conformations of the F glycoprotein. Clin Vaccine Immunol 23:451–459

Vesikari T, Matson DO, Dennehy P et al (2006) Safety and efficacy of a pentavalent human-bovine (WC3) reassortant rotavirus vaccine. N Engl J Med 354:23–33

Watson PS, Turner DP (2016) Clinical experience with the meningococcal B vaccine, Bexsero: prospects for reducing the burden of meningococcal serogroup B disease. Vaccine 34(7):875–880

Part XI

Endocrine, Metabolic, and Renal Diseases

Inborn Errors of Metabolism and Newborns

111

Nicola Brunetti-Pierri, Giancarlo Parenti, and Generoso Andria

Contents

N. Brunetti-Pierri · G. Parenti · G. Andria (✉)
Department of Translational Medicine, Section of Pediatrics, Federico II University of Naples, Naples, Italy
e-mail: generoso.andria@gmail.com

G. Buonocore et al. (eds.), *Neonatology*,
https://doi.org/10.1007/978-3-319-29489-6_258

Abstract
Inborn errors of metabolism are a large group of genetic diseases due to disruption of biochemical reactions. Advances in the understanding of the molecular and biochemical bases of several of these disorders have led to major progress in the diagnosis and treatment. Although individually rare, inborn errors of metabolism are relatively frequent with a collective incidence of up to 1 in 400 births. For several disorders, the patient's outcome in terms of mortality and morbidity is dependent upon a prompt diagnosis and treatment. Unfortunately, neonatal presentations are generally nonspecific and usually include poor feeding, vomiting, breathing difficulties, lethargy, hypotonia, hypothermia, and seizures. Therefore, several patients are often undiagnosed or misdiagnosed. Nevertheless, clues from the history, clinical presentation, or basic biochemical studies should raise the suspicion of a metabolic disease. With a relatively small number of laboratory tests, the neonatologist can initiate appropriate diagnostic investigations and start appropriate therapies. An accurate diagnosis is of primary importance also for parental counseling. The implementation of expanded newborn screening in several countries is allowing detection of a growing number of inborn errors of metabolism in their pre- or early symptomatic phases and is changing their management and treatment which will likely modify also their natural history.

111.1 Salient Points

- Alterations of specific chemical reactions in metabolism result in direct toxicity due to the accumulation of upstream metabolites, deficiency of downstream metabolites, feedback inhibition/activation by the metabolite on the same or on a different pathway, diversion of metabolic flux to secondary pathways, and the buildup of toxic metabolites.
- Early presentations are generally nonspecific: metabolic acidosis, ketosis, hypoglycemia, hyperammonemia, and liver failure. Symptoms include poor feeding, breathing difficulties, lethargy, hypotonia, vomiting, hypothermia, and seizures.
- Measurements of electrolyte concentrations, blood gases, anion gap, ammonia and lactate, neuroimaging studies and plasma amino acid measurement, urine organic analysis, and acylcarnitine profile are essential aids in the diagnosis.
- The conventional approach to the treatment of inborn errors of metabolism involves the following basic principles: restriction of upstream essential nutrients to prevent intoxication, supplementation of downstream nutrients to prevent secondary deficiency, and stimulation of alternative routes for disposal of precursor metabolites.

111.2 Introduction

Inborn errors of metabolism are disorders of great importance to physicians treating newborns because rapid diagnosis and appropriate treatment of these conditions are directly related to the patient's outcome in terms of mortality and morbidity. Although individually rare, as a group these diseases are relatively frequent, and collectively their incidence may approach 1 in 400 births (Chace et al. 2002; Zytkovicz et al. 2001). The presentation of these disorders may occur in any age group, from fetuses and newborns to adulthood. Neonatal onset is common because the newborn period is a time of substantial catabolism. The main problems facing the physician caring for the sick newborn are when to consider an inborn error of metabolism, what test to order to determine quickly and efficiently whether the patient has an inborn error of metabolism, and what therapy to initiate given a specific or a suspected diagnosis. Unfortunately, given the limited repertoire of symptoms of the newborn, early presentations are generally nonspecific and usually include poor feeding, breathing difficulties, lethargy, hypotonia, vomiting, hypothermia, and seizures. Therefore, patients with acute metabolic presentation are often misdiagnosed with other more common conditions such as sepsis, pulmonary disease, pyloric stenosis, and Reye syndrome. However, clues from

Table 1 Clues to the diagnosis of inborn errors of metabolism

History
Consanguinity
Previous neonatal death
Recurrent miscarriages
Siblings with known inborn error of metabolism
Recurrent nonimmune hydrops
Clinical
Unexplained clinical deterioration in infant who was well at birth
Encephalopathy/coma/seizures
Persisting vomiting/feeding difficulties
Major organ failure (heart, liver)
Dysmorphic features, multiple congenital anomalies
Unusual odor
Cataract
Bone marrow suppression
Nonimmune hydrops
Biochemical
Unexplained metabolic acidemia
Unexplained hypoglycemia
Ketosis
Hyperammonemia
Lactic acidemia
Postmortem
Fatty liver
Cardiomyopathy

the history, the clinical presentation, or basic biochemical studies should raise the suspicion of a metabolic disease (Tables 1, 2, 3, 4, 5, 6, and 7). A wide range of tests are required for the diagnosis of inborn errors of metabolism, and the level of clinical and biochemical experience required is often substantial. Nevertheless, the neonatologist can initiate appropriate investigation with a relatively small number of laboratory tests which are readily available in most hospitals (Table 8). In many circumstances, prevention of death or permanent neurologic sequelae is dependent on early diagnosis and institution of appropriate treatments. In addition, an accurate diagnosis is of primary importance for parental counseling.

Intensive efforts are currently ongoing to implement programs of expanded newborn screening using tandem mass spectrometry (MS/MS) with the goal of detecting a large number of inborn errors of metabolism in their presymptomatic early phase and have the potential to significantly change the natural history, the management, and the treatment of these disorders in the near future.

111.3 Etiology and Pathogenesis

Metabolism is regarded as the sum of all chemical reactions that operate in a living cell. Enzymes play an essential role in facilitating each of these reactions serving as catalysts in the conversion of one metabolite to another. Inborn errors of metabolism are genetic disorders caused by alterations of specific chemical reactions in metabolism. The consequences of these alterations can be mediated by (1) direct toxicity of accumulating upstream metabolites, (2) deficiency of downstream metabolites, (3) feedback inhibition/activation by the metabolite on the same or different pathway, and (4) diversion of metabolic flux to secondary pathways and buildup of toxic metabolites (Fig. 1). The majority of the inborn errors of metabolism are autosomal recessive but a few are X-linked. In addition, several of these disorders are included in the group of mitochondrial cytopathies which can exhibit matrilinear, autosomal recessive, autosomal dominant, and X-linked inheritance.

111.4 Clinical Presentations

The clinical presentation of metabolic diseases may include findings in virtually every organ and system. From a clinical standpoint, inborn errors of metabolism can be classified according to the time of onset in prenatal or postnatal onset diseases. It is also useful to separate maternal inborn errors of metabolism affecting the fetus as well as fetal diseases affecting the mother. The postnatal group can be further classified according to the main symptom and laboratory findings at the time of disease onset (Saudubray and Charpentier 2001). On a molecular basis, inborn errors of metabolism can be broadly divided into disorders involving small molecules and those of large molecules. Small molecule diseases involve

Table 2 Inborn errors of metabolism with cardiac presentation in the neonatal period

	Main clinical features	Laboratory abnormalities	Diagnostic test
Fatty acid oxidation disorders	Cardiomyopathy	Hypoketotic hypoglycemia	Plasma acylcarnitine profile
	Arrhythmias	Hyperammonemia	Molecular analysis
	Hypotonia	Elevated creatine kinase	
	Sudden death		
Propionic acidemia and methylmalonic acidemia	Cardiomyopathy	Metabolic acidosis	Urinary organic acid analysis
	Congenital heart defects	Bone marrow suppression	Acylcarnitine profile
	Encephalopathy		Plasma homocysteine
	Vomiting		
Tyrosinemia type I	Liver disease	Increased transaminases	Plasma and urine succinylacetone
	Cardiomyopathy[a]	Elevated tyrosine	
Sugar alcohol disorders	Progressive myocardial hypertrophy	Hypoalbuminemia; decreased coagulation factors	Urinary polyols
Mitochondrial diseases	Cardiomyopathy	Lactic acidosis	Electron transport chain assay/DNA testing
	Arrhythmias	Pancytopenia	
	Hypotonia		
Pompe disease	Cardiomyopathy	Vacuolated lymphocytes	Acid α-glucosidase activity
	Hypotonia	Enlarged QRS complexes; short PR interval	
	Wolff-Parkinson-White syndrome		
Glycogen storage disease type IV	Cardiomyopathy	Elevated creatine kinase	Glycogen branching enzyme activity
Heart-specific phosphorylase kinase deficiency	Cardiac enlargement	Enlarged QRS complexes; short PR interval	Phosphorylase kinase activity
Mucopolysaccharidosis VI (Maroteaux-Lamy disease)	Endocardial fibroelastosis	Increased urinary mucopolysaccharides	Arylsulfatase B activity
	Dysostosis multiplex		
Congenital disorders of glycosylation	Cardiomyopathy	Hypoalbuminemia	Transferrin isoelectrofocusing
	Pericardial effusion	Decreased coagulation factors	
	Hypotonia	Low thyroxine-binding globulin	
	Dysmorphic features	Increased transaminases	

[a]Cardiomyopathy is a common manifestation but has a favorable long-term outcome. Children treated with NTBC are less likely to develop this complication (Arora et al. 2006)

organic acids, amino acids, carbohydrates, fatty acids, nucleotides, and ammonia. Large molecule diseases arise from defects of either synthetic or degradative processing of polymeric molecules, such as glycoproteins and glycolipids. It should be noted that patients with inborn errors of metabolism have often complex and overlapping problems which are a serious limitation of any classification system, including the one used in this chapter.

111.5 Inborn Errors of Metabolism with Prenatal Onset

The fetus with a metabolic disorder is usually protected in utero by the metabolically normal mother through placental exchange of metabolites. Therefore, the majority of inborn errors of metabolism become clinically evident only after birth. The prenatal onset involves a group of

Table 3 Inborn errors of metabolism with neonatal liver involvement

Liver failure
Galactosemia
Tyrosinemia type I
Transaldolase deficiency
Mitochondrial DNA depletion
Cholestasis
Galactosemia
Citrin deficiency
LCHAD deficiency
Niemann-Pick disease type C
Gaucher disease
Wolman disease
Peroxisomal disorders
Congenital disorders of glycosylation
Mitochondrial DNA depletion
Cholesterol biosynthetic defects
Bile acid synthetic disorders

Table 4 Hematological findings in inborn errors of metabolism

Neutropenia
Organic acidemias
Barth syndrome
Lysinuric protein intolerance
Glycogen storage disease type Ib
Megaloblastic anemia
Cobalamin disorders
Transcobalamin II deficiency
Hypoxanthine-guanine-phosphoribosyltransferase (HPRT) deficiency
Pancytopenia
Organic acidemias
Mevalonic aciduria
Pearson syndrome
Tyrosinemia type I
Gaucher disease
Transaldolase deficiency
Acanthocytosis
Abetalipoproteinemia
Wolman disease
Vacuolated lymphocytes
Lysosomal storage disorders

Table 5 Skin and hair findings in inborn errors of metabolism

Thick skin
I-cell disease
GM_1 gangliosidosis
Sialidosis
Galactosialidosis
Mucopolysaccharidosis VII
Cutis laxa
Menkes disease
Congenital disorders of glycosylation
Extensive Mongolian spots
Lysosomal storage diseases
Hypopigmentation
Phenylketonuria
Cystinosis
Homocystinuria
Hyperpigmentation
Glycerol kinase deficiency
Adrenoleukodystrophy
Skin nodules
Farber disease (ceramidase deficiency)
Congenital disorders of glycosylation
Desquamating eczematous or vesiculobullous lesions
Biotinidase deficiency
Multiple carboxylase deficiency
Methylmalonic acidemia
Propionic acidemia
Phenylketonuria
Glutamine synthetase deficiency
Ichthyosis
Gaucher disease type II
Sjögren-Larsson syndrome
Multiple sulfatase deficiency
Multiple carboxylase deficiency
Congenital disorders of glycosylation
Alopecia
Multiple carboxylase deficiency
Kinky hair
Menkes disease
Trichorrhexis nodosa
Argininosuccinic aciduria

disorders in which the maternal-placental unit cannot compensate for the underlying pathogenetic mechanisms, thus resulting in fetal developmental defects.

111.5.1 Small Molecule Diseases

Small molecule diseases with prenatal onset present at birth with complex malformations rather than acute decompensation. However, there is no rigid distinction, and disorders such

Table 6 Eye findings in inborn errors of metabolism

Corneal clouding
Mucopolysaccharidoses
I-cell disease
Peroxisomal disorders
Cataract
Galactosemia
Lowe syndrome
Peroxisomal disorders
Mevalonic aciduria
Mitochondrial diseases
Congenital CPT II deficiency
Dislocated lens
Homocystinuria
Sulfite oxidase deficiency
Macular cherry red spot
GM_1 gangliosidosis
GM_2 gangliosidosis
Sialidosis
Galactosialidosis
Niemann-Pick disease type A
Retinopathy
Mitochondrial diseases
Methylmalonic acidemia
Cobalamin disorders
Sjögren-Larsson syndrome
Peroxisomal disorders
Abetalipoproteinemia
LCHAD deficiency
Optic atrophy
Pyruvate dehydrogenase deficiency
Leigh disease
Peroxisomal disorders

as nonketotic hyperglycinemia, which are associated with acute illness after birth, may also present with brain malformations. Similarly, mitochondrial diseases and fatty acid oxidation defects can exhibit features indicating prenatal onset damage (von Kleist-Retzow et al. 2003; North et al. 1995; Boemer et al. 2016). Accumulation of methylmalonic acid and homocysteine also appears to be involved in various types of congenital heart defects (Table 2) (Profitlich et al. 2009).

Disorders of serine biosynthesis are notable for their severe effects on prenatal development resulting in microcephaly, intractable seizures, and spastic tetraparesis in the affected newborns. Neu-Laxova syndrome, a recognizable human malformation syndrome with fetal growth restriction, microcephaly, distinctive facial appearance, ichthyosis, skeletal anomalies, and prenatal or early postnatal lethality, is caused by mutations in genes encoding enzymes of the serine biosynthesis pathway (Shaheen et al. 2014; Acuna-Hidalgo et al. 2014). These disorders are diagnosed by amino acid analysis in the blood and cerebrospinal fluid (CSF) showing reduced levels of serine and glycine (Table 9). The biochemical abnormalities are more pronounced in CSF rather than plasma, and therefore, CSF amino acid analysis is preferable for the diagnosis. Early recognition of these defects is important because treatment with supplemental serine and glycine has beneficial effects (de Koning et al. 2004; van der Crabben et al. 2013).

Disorders of cholesterol biosynthesis have also significant effects on the fetus as exemplified by Smith-Lemli-Opitz syndrome, a multiple congenital anomaly syndrome caused by deficiency of 7-dehydrocholesterol reductase catalyzing the reduction of 7-dehydrocholesterol to cholesterol in the last step of cholesterol biosynthesis. The clinical presentation of Smith-Lemli-Opitz syndrome is heterogeneous, and severely affected infants have multiple major congenital anomalies of the brain (holoprosencephaly, agenesis of the corpus callosum), heart (atrial and ventricular septal defects, atrioventricular canal defect), lungs (abnormal segmentation), or gastrointestinal tract (pyloric stenosis and colonic aganglionosis). Postnatal growth failure, microcephaly, typical facial features, ambiguous genitalia, and limb anomalies such as postaxial polydactyly and syndactyly of the second and third toes are common findings. Desmosterolosis, lathosterolosis, X-linked chondrodysplasia punctata type II (Conradi-Hunermann syndrome), congenital hemidysplasia with ichthyosiform erythroderma and limb defects (CHILD syndrome), deficiency of sterol-C4-methyl oxidase-like (SC4MOL) enzyme, and a subset of cases with Antley-Bixler syndrome are

Table 7 Clinical and biochemical findings which are characteristic or unique in newborns with inborn errors of metabolism

Microcephaly	Connective tissue abnormalities (cutis laxa, bladder diverticula)
Serine biosynthesis disorders	Menkes disease
Congenital CPT II deficiency	Congenital disorders of glycosylation
Smith-Lemli-Opitz syndrome	Persistent diarrhea
Mitochondrial diseases	Congenital chloride diarrhea
Maternal phenylketonuria embryopathy	Congenital lactase deficiency
Macrocephaly	Glucose/galactose malabsorption
Glutaric aciduria type I	Congenital sucrase-isomaltase deficiency
Canavan disease	Galactosemia
Lysosomal storage disorders	Wolman disease
Seizures	Adrenal calcifications
Biotinidase deficiency	Wolman disease
Pyridoxine-dependent epilepsy	Acute renal failure
Pyridoxamine phosphate oxidase (PNPO) deficiency	HPRT deficiency
GLUT1 deficiency	Renal Fanconi syndrome
Nonketotic hyperglycinemia	Tyrosinemia type I
Methylenetetrahydrofolate reductase (MTHFR) deficiency	Mitochondrial diseases
GABA transaminase deficiency	Congenital disorders of glycosylation
Serine biosynthesis disorders	Cystinosis
Urea cycle disorders	Lowe syndrome
Molybdenum cofactor deficiency	Galactosemia
Sulfite oxidase deficiency	Glycogen storage disease type I
Peroxisomal disorders	Renal cysts
Congenital disorders of glycosylation	Peroxisomal disorders
Coarse facial features	CPT II deficiency
Lysosomal storage disorders	Multiple acyl-CoA dehydrogenase deficiency
Macroglossia	Congenital disorders of glycosylation
Pompe disease	Increased LDH
GM_1 gangliosidosis	Lysinuric protein intolerance
Skeletal abnormalities	Increased triglycerides
Dysostosis multiplex	Glycogen storage disease type I
Lysosomal storage disorders	Glycerol kinase deficiency (pseudo-increase)
Chondrodysplasia punctata	Lipoprotein lipase deficiency
Peroxisomal disorders	Increased uric acid
X-linked chondrodysplasia punctata (ARSE deficiency)	HPRT deficiency
Conradi-Hunermann syndrome	MCAD deficiency
Smith-Lemli-Opitz syndrome	Glycogen storage disease type I
GM_1 gangliosidosis	Decreased uric acid
Galactosialidosis	Molybdenum cofactor deficiency
Combined deficiency of multiple coagulation factors	Increased α-fetoprotein
Rhizomelia	Tyrosinemia type I
Peroxisomal disorders (rhizomelic chondrodysplasia punctata)	Ataxia telangiectasia
Spondyloenchondromatosis	
2-Hydroxyglutaric aciduria	

Table 8 Investigations for suspected inborn errors of metabolism

First-line investigations
Blood
Complete blood counts
Electrolytes
Bilirubin
Glucose
Urea
Blood gases and acid-base analysis
Ammonia
Lactate
Uric acid
Ketones
Urine
Reducing substances
pH
Ketones
Cerebrospinal fluid
Glucose
Lactate
Second-line investigations[a]
Urinary organic acid analysis
Plasma, cerebrospinal fluid, urine amino acid analysis
Plasma acylcarnitine profile
Urine orotic acid
Copper and ceruloplasmin
Specialized investigations[a]
Special biochemical assay (very long-chain fatty acids [VLCFA], bile acid analysis, transferrin isoelectrofocusing, urine purine and pyrimidine, urine sugar alcohols)
Enzyme assays
DNA studies

[a]Before sending samples for second-line specialized investigations, it is recommended to (1) call the laboratory to indicate urgency; (2) give details on drug, diet, and previous blood transfusions; (3) arrange suitable transport of the samples; (4) discuss which tests are indicated with the metabolic consultants; and (5) freeze and save urine of the newborn

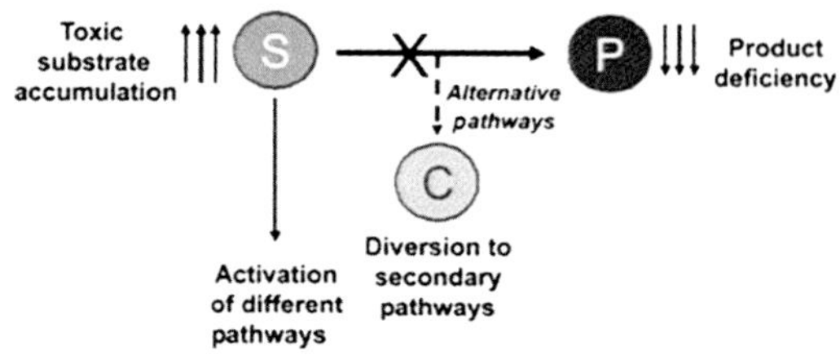

Fig. 1 An enzymatic block results in (1) direct toxicity of accumulating upstream substrate (*S*), (2) deficiency of downstream product (*P*), (3) activation of alternative pathways, and (4) diversion of metabolic flux to secondary pathways and production of alternative metabolite (*C*)

due to defects in other steps of cholesterol biosynthesis, and their clinical presentation partially overlaps with Smith-Lemli-Opitz syndrome. These disorders are diagnosed by analysis of plasma sterols by gas chromatography/mass spectrometry (GC/MS) (Herman and Kratz 2012).

Other examples of inborn errors of metabolism resulting in a complex multisystem involvement include the deficiencies of glutamine synthetase and asparagine synthetase. The deficiency of glutamine synthetase presents with seizures, encephalopathy, and brain malformations (Haberle et al. 2005, 2011), and supplementation with glutamine appears to have some beneficial effect (Haberle et al. 2012). Asparagine synthetase deficiency is a newly recognized disease with severe encephalopathy associated with congenital microcephaly, progressive brain atrophy, intractable seizure, and profound developmental delay (Ruzzo et al. 2013). The identification of these two disorders on the basis of reduced glutamine or asparagine levels is unusual because the interpretation of plasma amino acid profiles and the expanded newborn screening are usually directed toward increased (Table 9), rather than decreased metabolite levels.

111.5.2 Large Molecule Diseases

111.5.2.1 Lysosomal Storage Disorders

Lysosomal storage disorders are due to defects in lysosomal enzymes, cofactors, and transport proteins resulting in progressive accumulation of undegraded products within the lysosomes. These disorders usually present in infancy or early childhood with hepatosplenomegaly, skeletal dysostosis, and cognitive impairment. In the rare neonatal presentation, they manifest as nonimmune hydrops (Bellini et al. 2015; Gimovsky et al. 2015). The presence of dysmorphic features, gum hyperplasia, inguinal and umbilical hernias, extensive Mongolian spots, and corneal clouding (Tables 5, 6, and 7) on physical exam and the presence of placental vacuolization, vacuolated mononuclear cells in the peripheral smear, and bone marrow storage histiocytes are suggestive of these disorders (Staretz-Chacham et al. 2009).

A definitive diagnosis requires enzyme analysis which can be performed either on leukocytes or fibroblasts depending on the specific disease. Among inborn errors of metabolism resulting in nonimmune hydrops, which collectively are responsible for 1.3% of all cases with an established diagnosis (Bellini et al. 2015), lysosomal storage disorders are a major cause (Table 10). Besides hydrops, Gaucher disease may have a perinatal lethal presentation with collodion membrane, hepatosplenomegaly, and arthrogryposis (Mignot et al. 2003). In addition, a significant number of infants with Niemann-Pick type C presents in the newborn period with hypotonia, jaundice, hepatosplenomegaly, and liver failure (Garver et al. 2007).

Cardiomyopathy in the neonatal period has been reported as rare complication of glycogen storage disease type II (Pompe disease) and some mucopolysaccharidoses (Table 2) (Wraith 2002).

111.5.2.2 Peroxisomal Disorders

In contrast to lysosomal storage disorders, several peroxisomal disorders are expressed in the neonatal period. Zellweger syndrome, the prototype of these disorders, classically presents in the newborn period with craniofacial anomalies including a large anterior fontanel with widely spaced sutures, broad forehead and micrognathia, and neurological abnormalities. The presence of hypotonia and the hypo/areflexia in these patients may raise the possibility of spinal muscular atrophy (Baumgartner et al. 1998). Neuronal migration defects, especially pachygyria and polymicrogyria, are observed along with white matter abnormality and are often associated with seizures. The liver is enlarged and fibrotic with micronodular cirrhosis. Renal cysts and chondrodysplasia punctata are also common. Apart from Zellweger syndrome with its neonatal onset and early fatal course, the peroxisomal disorders include neonatal adrenoleukodystrophy and infantile Refsum disease with the least severe course. The clinical features between Zellweger syndrome, neonatal adrenoleukodystrophy, and infantile Refsum disease are overlapping, and it is often difficult to assign a particular patient to one of these clinical subtypes. Most peroxisomal defects can be detected by analysis of very long-chain fatty acids (VLCFA) in plasma. Additional studies such as plasmalogen levels in red blood cells, plasma phytanic acid, and molecular analysis are necessary for further confirmation of the diagnosis (Braverman et al. 2015).

111.5.2.3 Congenital Disorders of Glycosylation

The congenital disorders of glycosylation are highly heterogeneous multisystemic diseases due to a deficiency of carbohydrate residues of glycoproteins and other glycoconjugates (Freeze et al. 2014). In the neonatal period, the neurologic picture comprises reduced spontaneous movements, hypotonia, hyporeflexia, and abnormal slow rolling vertical or horizontal eye movements (Ganetzky et al. 2015). Many patients have dysmorphic features, abnormal adipose tissue distribution, inverted nipples, moderate hepatomegaly, and cerebellum hypoplasia. Some patients develop pericardial effusion and cardiomyopathy (Table 2) or nonimmune hydrops (Table 10). The screening and diagnosis are based on plasma glycosylated transferrin by isoelectrofocusing.

111.6 Maternal Metabolic Diseases Affecting the Fetus

Phenylketonuria is a disorder with increased concentration of phenylalanine in the body fluids resulting from reduced activity of phenylalanine hydroxylase or from defects in the synthesis or recycling of its cofactor, tetrahydrobiopterin. Untreated patients with classic phenylketonuria are normal at birth, but develop microcephaly, seizures, and severe cognitive impairment. In contrast, affected children detected and effectively treated before 3 weeks of age show none of these

Table 9 Interpretation of plasma amino acid profile

Amino acid	Increase	Decrease
Alanine	Energy production defects	Maple syrup urine disease (during acute decompensation)
	Hyperammonemia	
Alloisoleucine	Maple syrup urine disease	Normally not detected
Asparagine	–	Asparagine synthetase deficiency
Arginine	Argininemia	Prematurity
	Citrin deficiency	Urea cycle disorders (deficiency of CPS, OTC, ASS, ASL)
		Δ_1-Pyrroline-5-carboxylate synthase deficiency
Argininosuccinic acid	Argininosuccinic aciduria	Normally not detected
Citrulline	Citrullinemia	OTC deficiency
	Argininosuccinic aciduria	CPS deficiency
	Citrin deficiency	Δ_1-Pyrroline-5-carboxylate synthase deficiency
	Pyruvate carboxylase deficiency	
	Pyruvate dehydrogenase deficiency (E3 deficiency)	
	Lysinuric protein intolerance	
Glutamic acid	Sample mishandling	–
Glutamine	Hyperammonemia	Glutamine synthetase deficiency
	Urea cycle disorders	
Glycine	Nonketotic hyperglycinemia	Disorders of serine biosynthesis
	Organic acidemias	
Histidine	Histidase deficiency[a]	–
Free homocysteine[b]	Homocystinuria[c]	Isolated sulfite oxidase deficiency
	Methylenetetrahydrofolate reductase (MTHFR) deficiency	Molybdenum cofactor deficiency
Branched chain amino acids (isoleucine, leucine, and valine)	Nonfasting	Hepatic dysfunction
	Maple syrup urine disease	Ammonia scavenger treatment
Lysine	Hyperlysinemia[a]	Lysinuric protein intolerance
	Pyruvate carboxylase deficiency	Ornithine aminotransferase I deficiency
Methionine	Homocystinuria	Cobalamin disorders
	Methionine adenosyltransferase deficiency[a]	MTHFR deficiency
	Glycine-*N*-methyltransferase[a]	
	Citrin deficiency	
	Hepatic dysfunction	
Ornithine	Ornithine aminotransferase I deficiency	Lysinuric protein intolerance
	Hyperornithinemia-hyperammonemia-homocitrullinuria (HHH) syndrome	Δ_1-Pyrroline-5-carboxylate synthase deficiency
Phenylalanine	Phenylketonuria	–
	Transient neonatal hyperphenylalaninemia	
	Hepatic dysfunction	
Phosphoethanolamine[d]	Alkaline phosphatase deficiency	–
Proline	Hyperprolinemia types I and II	Δ_1-Pyrroline-5-carboxylate synthase deficiency
	Pyruvate carboxylase deficiency	
Serine	Nonfasting	Disorders of serine biosynthesis
		Homocystinuria

(*continued*)

Table 9 (continued)

Amino acid	Increase	Decrease
S-Sulfocysteine[e]	Isolated sulfite oxidase deficiency	–
	Molybdenum cofactor deficiency	
Threonine	Citrin deficiency	–
	Cholestasis	
	Nonfasting	
Tyrosine	Tyrosinemia type I	Phenylketonuria
	Tyrosinemia type II	
	Tyrosinemia type III	
	Transient tyrosinemia of the newborn	
	Citrin deficiency	
	Hepatic dysfunction	

[a]Clinical relevance of these biochemical abnormalities is not conclusive
[b]Free homocysteine is usually not detected in plasma when standard amino acid analysis is performed
[c]Can be present in cystathionine β-synthase or defects of vitamin B12 synthesis (cobalamin disorders: *cblC*, *cblE*, *cblD*, *cblF*, *cblG*), absorption (hereditary folate malabsorption), and transport (transcobalamin II deficiency)
[d]Phosphoethanolamine is not an amino acid, but it is usually detected in the routine plasma amino acid analysis
[e]Measurement of sulfocysteine requires special sample preparation

abnormalities. Therefore, newborns in developed countries are screened by determination of phenylalanine blood levels. Women with phenylketonuria who have been treated since infancy and become pregnant have an increased risk for fetal malformations such as microcephaly, intellectual disability, and congenital heart disease (Lenke and Levy 1980). These adverse consequences originate in the first trimester and are preventable by a phenylalanine-restricted diet. There is a strong relationship between increasing phenylalanine levels and the severity of neonatal abnormalities. The current recommendation is to maintain the phenylalanine levels <6 mg/dL at least 3 months before conception (National Institutes of Health Consensus Development Panel 2000).

Maternal riboflavin and vitamin B12 deficiency may also affect the newborn. Maternal riboflavin deficiency results in the newborn in transient clinical and biochemical findings of multiple acyl-CoA dehydrogenase deficiency (Chiong et al. 2007; Ho et al. 2011), while maternal vitamin B12 deficiency, often secondary to vegetarian diet, pernicious anemia, and gastric bypass, results in nonspecific clinical presentation with developmental delay, failure to thrive, and irreversible neurologic damage. Early detection and intervention, facilitated by MS/MS newborn screening (Hinton et al. 2010), are critical, and both conditions can be treated by vitamin supplementation.

111.7 Fetal Diseases Affecting the Mother

Mothers who are pregnant with a fetus affected with long-chain 3-hydroxyacyl-coenzyme A dehydrogenase (LCHAD) deficiency have a high risk of developing preeclampsia, HELLP (hemolysis, elevated liver enzymes, low platelets) syndrome, or acute fatty liver of pregnancy (AFLP) (Ibdah et al. 1999). Therefore, screening of offspring of women with AFLP and HELLP syndrome has been proposed, at least when MS/MS screening is not available, because LCHAD is potentially treatable.

111.8 Inborn Errors of Metabolism with Postnatal Onset

The clinical presentations of this group of disorders result from accumulation of toxic compounds proximal to the metabolic defect or from deficiency in energy production. The disorders of the *intoxication* group do not interfere

Table 10 Inborn errors of metabolism with nonimmune hydrops presentation[a]

Disease	Metabolic abnormality
Lysosomal storage diseases	
Oligosaccharidoses	
GM_1 gangliosidosis	β-Galactosidase
Sialidosis	Neuraminidase
Galactosialidosis	Protective protein cathepsin A
Gaucher disease type II	Acid β-glucosidase
Niemann-Pick disease type A	Sphingomyelinase
Niemann-Pick disease type C	NPC1
Farber lipogranulomatosis	Acid ceramidase
Wolman disease	Acid lipase
I-cell disease	Defects affecting mannose-6-phosphate receptor
Infantile sialic acid storage disease	Sialin
Multiple sulfatase deficiency	Sulfatase-modifying factor 1
Mucopolysaccharidoses	
Hurler disease (MPS I)	α-L-Iduronidase
Sly disease (MPS VII)	β-Glucuronidase
Morquio A disease (MPS IVA)	Galactosamine-6-sulfate sulfatase
Others	
Congenital disorders of glycosylation	Several defects
Zellweger disease	Peroxisomal biogenesis defect
Glycogen storage disease type IV	Glycogen branching enzyme
Fatty acid oxidation defects	Several defects
Smith-Lemli-Opitz syndrome	7-Dehydrocholesterol reductase
Pearson syndrome and other respiratory chain defects	Respiratory chain defects
Transaldolase deficiency	Transaldolase
Congenital erythropoietic porphyria	Uroporphyrinogen III synthetase

[a]Based on the following studies (Gimovsky et al. 2015; van de Kamp et al. 2007; Leticee et al. 2010; Dursun et al. 2009; Cox et al. 1999; Oey et al. 2005; Angle et al. 1998; Fayon et al. 1992; Valayannopoulos et al. 2006; Daikha-Dahmane et al. 2001)

with the embryo-fetal development and present with a symptom-free interval ranging from hours to weeks, and indeed even months or years, depending on the severity of the metabolic block and/or the nature of the environmental triggers. The typical clinical features are nonspecific and include poor feeding, vomiting, lethargy, irritability, seizures, and tachypnea if metabolic acidosis is present. Most of these disorders are treatable and require emergency removal of the toxin by special diet, drugs to increase clearance of toxic metabolites, and hemodialysis. The disorders of energy production are less amenable to therapy and affect primarily the liver, myocardium, muscle, and brain. Although there is a significant overlap among the different conditions, from a clinical practice standpoint, it is useful to classify the disorders with postnatal onset on the basis of their main clinical and/or laboratory findings at presentation (Saudubray and Charpentier 2001).

111.8.1 Disorders Presenting with Metabolic Acidosis

Metabolic acidosis is very common in neonates and can be observed in several circumstances such as infections, severe catabolic states, tissue hypoxia, and dehydration. These conditions can also be the trigger for acute decompensation in inborn errors of metabolism. The presence or absence of ketonuria is a major clue for the diagnosis of patients with

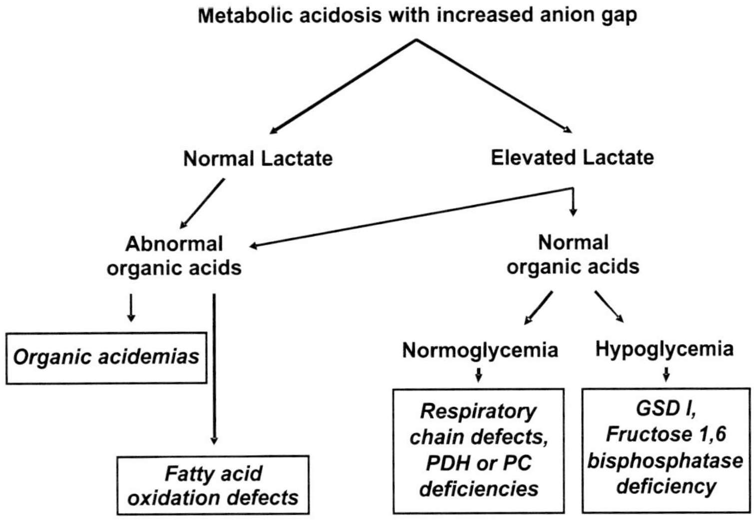

Fig. 2 Diagnostic approach to neonatal metabolic acidosis

metabolic acidosis, particularly in the neonatal period, during which significant ketonuria is highly suspicious of an inborn error of metabolism. An increased anion gap [([Na^+] + [K^+])–([Cl^-] + [HCO_3^-])] greater than 25 mmol/L (normal range, 12–16 mmol/L) resulting from the accumulation of organic anions is observed in several inherited metabolic diseases. Secondary hypoglycemia and hyperammonemia along with accumulation of organic anions result in acute encephalopathy. A number of disorders presenting with acidosis affect the catabolic pathways of branched-chain amino acids or other amino acids and are usually detected by GC/MS or MS/MS on urine specimens. A flowchart for the evaluation of infants with metabolic acidosis is shown in Fig. 2. The number of the disorders of organic acid metabolism and their range of presentations is large. However, some of these conditions merit specific discussion because they are relatively more common.

111.8.1.1 Propionic Acidemia and Methylmalonic Acidemia

Propionic acidemia is caused by deficiency of propionyl-CoA carboxylase which requires biotin as cofactor. Methylmalonic acidemia instead is caused by the deficiency of either the methylmalonyl-CoA mutase or the enzymes involved in the synthesis of its vitamin B12-derived cofactor, 5′-deoxyadenosylcobalamin. Patients with defects in the cofactor synthesis are responsive to vitamin B12 treatment. In most cases of propionic acidemia and methylmalonic acidemia, the onset of the disease is in the neonatal period with nonspecific feeding difficulties, vomiting, neurological manifestations such as hypotonia, lethargy, and seizures, and hematological complications (Table 4). If not promptly and appropriately treated, patients progress into coma with brain edema and die or develop permanent brain damage. Hyperammonemia, which may be as high as in the urea cycle disorders, may complicate the initial episode of decompensation. Elevated glycine in the blood is an important clue to the diagnosis (Table 9) which is based on the presence of characteristic organic acids in urine as detected by GC/MS (Table 11) and elevated propionylcarnitine (C3) in the blood by MS/MS (Table 12). Cell studies on leukocytes or cultured skin fibroblasts and/or DNA studies are used for diagnostic confirmation.

111.8.1.2 Multiple Carboxylase Deficiency

There are two distinct disorders resulting in multiple carboxylase deficiency: biotinidase deficiency and holocarboxylase synthetase deficiency. Biotinidase deficiency is far more frequent and is due to defects in the recycling and release from dietary protein of biotin, a cofactor for the human carboxylases. Whereas patients with partial deficiency (residual activity 10–30% of mean control value) usually do not develop clinical symptoms,

Table 11 Urinary organic acid profiles in organic acidemias[a]

Disease	Metabolites
Propionic acidemia	3-Hydroxypropionic acid, methylcitric acid, tiglylglycine, propionylglycine
Methylmalonic acidemia and cobalamin disorders	Methylmalonic acid, 3-hydroxypropionic acid, methylcitric acid, propionylglycine
Isovaleric acidemia	3-Hydroxyisovaleric acid, isovalerylglycine
Glutaric acidemia type I	Glutaric acid, 3-hydroxyglutaric acid, glutaconic acid
Malonic aciduria	Malonic acid, methylmalonic acid
3-Hydroxy-3-methylglutaryl-CoA lyase deficiency	3-Hydroxy-3-methylglutaric acid, 3-methylglutaconic acid, 3-hydroxyisovaleric acid, 3-methylglutaric acid
3-Methylcrotonyl-CoA carboxylase deficiency	3-Methylcrotonic acid, 3-methylcrotonylglycine acid, tiglylglycine, 3-hydroxyisovaleric acid
β-Ketothiolase deficiency	2-Methyl-3-hydroxybutyric acid, 2-methyl-acetoacetic acid, tiglylglycine
Semialdehyde dehydrogenase deficiency	4-Hydroxybutyric acid, 3-hydroxypropionic acid, 3,4-dihydroxybutyric acid
Glutathione synthetase deficiency	5-Oxoproline
Methylglutaconic aciduria	3-Methylglutaconic acid, 3-methylglutaric acid

[a]Several disorders that are not classified as primary disorders of organic acid metabolism have a characteristic increase in urinary organic acids that suggests the diagnosis: mevalonic acid (mevalonic aciduria); glutaric acid, 2-hydroxyglutaric acid, ethylmalonic acid, dicarboxylic acids, and glycine conjugates of medium-chain dicarboxylic acids (multiple acyl-CoA dehydrogenase deficiency); acyl-CoA-glycine conjugates (fatty acid oxidation defects); 3-hydroxyisovaleric, 3-methylcrotonic, 3-hydroxypropionic, methylcitric, and 3-hydroxybutyric acids, acetoacetate, propionylglycine, and tiglylglycine (biotinidase deficiency); and lactate and 3-methylglutaconic, 2-hydroxybutyric, 3-hydroxybutyric, 2-methyl-3-hydroxybutyric, and ethylmalonic acids (mitochondrial diseases)

untreated patients with profound deficiency (residual activity <10% of mean normal value) may develop various neurological deficits, skin abnormalities (Tables 5 and 7), and metabolic ketoacidosis early in life. Because early recognition and oral biotin supplementation (2–20 mg/day) may completely prevent clinical and neurological deficits in biotinidase deficiency, biotinidase newborn screening has been implemented in various countries (Vallejo-Torres et al. 2015). Patients with holocarboxylase synthetase deficiency present with the characteristic skin manifestations (Tables 5) and an overwhelming illness similar to propionic acidemia. In this condition the activities of all carboxylases in leukocytes or fibroblasts are reduced. Various degrees of response to biotin treatment have been reported (Van Hove et al. 2008).

The increase of metabolites suggestive of multiple carboxylase deficiency associated with lactic acidosis has been recently found in patients with hyperammonemic encephalopathy due to carbonic anhydrase VA deficiency (van Karnebeek et al. 2014) (Table 13).

111.8.2 Disorders Presenting with Ketosis

Maple urine syrup urine disease is one of the most common aminoacidopathies and can present in the newborn period with neurologic deterioration and ketosis. The disease is caused by deficiency of the branched-chain α-keto acid dehydrogenase which is involved in the catabolism of branched-chain amino acids (leucine, isoleucine, and valine). The accumulation of leucine is neurotoxic and results in progressive brain damage. Vomiting, feeding difficulties, and lethargy are common early symptoms. Seizures occur frequently, especially when cerebral edema develops. The characteristic odor may be noted as soon as neurological symptoms develop, but it may be absent in a patient who has not received protein for a prolonged period of time. The diagnostic plasma amino acid pattern shows an increase of branched-chain amino acids and of alloisoleucine which is normally not detected and a reduction of alanine in the acute presentation (Table 9).

Table 12 Plasma acylcarnitine patterns associated with various diseases[a]

Acylcarnitine	Chain length designation	Associated abnormality	Disorder
Free carnitine	C0 (low)		Primary and secondary[b] carnitine deficiency
Free carnitine	C0	C16 (low); C18 (low)	CPT I deficiency
Propionyl	C3		Propionic acidemia
			Methylmalonic acidemia
			Holocarboxylase deficiency
			Biotinidase deficiency
			Succinyl-CoA synthetase deficiency
Malonyl	C3DC		Malonyl-CoA decarboxylase deficiency
Butyryl/isobutyryl	C4		Short-chain acyl-CoA dehydrogenase (SCAD) deficiency[c]
			Ethylmalonic encephalopathy
		C5 and other longer chain species	Multiple acyl-CoA dehydrogenase deficiency
			Isobutyryl-CoA-dehydrogenase deficiency[c]
3-Hydroxybutyryl	C4-OH		3-α-Hydroxyacyl-CoA dehydrogenase deficiency (HADH)
Succinyl/ methylmalonyl	C4-DC		Succinyl-CoA synthetase (SUCLA2) deficiency
Isovaleryl/ methylbutyryl	C5		Isovaleric acidemia
			Methylbutyryl-CoA dehydrogenase deficiency[c]
3-Hydroxyisovaleryl	C5-OH		3-Methylcrotonyl-CoA carboxylase (3-MCC) deficiency[d]
			Holocarboxylase deficiency
		C6-DC	3-Hydroxy-3-methylglutaryl-CoA lyase deficiency
			Biotinidase deficiency
			3-Methylglutaconyl-CoA hydratase deficiency
3-Hydroxy-2-methylbutyryl	C5-OH		2-Methyl-3-hydroxybutyryl-CoA dehydrogenase deficiency
		C5:1	β-Ketothiolase deficiency
Glutaryl	C5-DC		Glutaric acidemia type I
Octanoyl	C8	C6; C10; C10:1	MCAD deficiency
Tetradecenoyl	C14:1	C14; C14:2	VLCAD deficiency
Palmitoyl	C16	C18; C18:1; C18:2	CPT II deficiency
		C18; C18:1; C18:2	CACT deficiency
3-Hydroxy-palmitoyl	C16-OH	C16:1-OH; C18-OH; C18:1-OH	LCHAD deficiency
		C16:1 OH; C18-OH; C18:1-OH	Trifunctional protein deficiency

[a]Acylcarnitine abnormalities include elevations over normal range unless specified otherwise

[b]Secondary carnitine deficiency may occur in organic acidemias, fatty acid oxidation defects, and Fanconi syndrome

[c]The majority of individuals with these biochemical abnormalities are asymptomatic with normal growth and development (Pena et al. 2012; Alfardan et al. 2010)

[d]This enzyme deficiency may lead to a severe clinical phenotype resembling classical organic acidurias. However, a large percentage of patients remain asymptomatic, and thus, the clinical relevance is not conclusive for this biochemical abnormality (Arnold et al. 2012)

Table 13 Causes of neonatal hyperammonemia

Inherited diseases
Urea cycle disorders
Carbamyl phosphate synthetase deficiency
Ornithine transcarbamylase deficiency
Argininosuccinic acid synthetase deficiency
Argininosuccinic acid lyase deficiency
N-Acetylglutamate synthetase deficiency
Citrin deficiency
Lysinuric protein intolerance
Hyperornithinemia-hyperammonemia-homocitrullinuria (HHH) syndrome
Hyperinsulinism with hyperammonemia
Other metabolic disorders
Propionic acidemia
Methylmalonic acidemia
Isovaleric acidemia
β-Ketothiolase deficiency
Multiple carboxylase deficiency
Fatty acid oxidation defects
Pyruvate dehydrogenase deficiency
Mitochondrial cytopathies
Multiple acyl-CoA dehydrogenase deficiency
Carbonic anhydrase VA deficiency
Acquired disorders
Any severe illness
Transient hyperammonemia of prematurity
Perinatal asphyxia
Herpes simplex infection
Total parenteral nutrition
Vascular bypass of the liver

111.8.3 Disorders Presenting with Lactic Acidosis

Increased lactic acid is observed in several inherited metabolic diseases. However, this is also increased in hypoxic-ischemic encephalopathy, sepsis, and other conditions resulting in poor vascular perfusion. Nevertheless, the most common reason for elevated blood lactate is improper sampling technique (the use of tourniquet or struggle in obtaining the sample). The measurement of pyruvate in conjunction with lactate is helpful because an increase in the plasma lactate-pyruvate ratio suggests inadequate oxygen supply. However, to obtain reliable measurements of this ratio, the plasma sample for pyruvate needs to be deproteinized at the bedside which is not practical in most clinical settings. Defects of pyruvate metabolism or respiratory chain result in primary lactic acidosis and should be considered in patients with persistent increase of lactic acid and normal organic acids in urine. Lactic acidosis may result from an increased pyruvate production as in the case of glycogen storage disease type I or from a decreased pyruvate oxidation as a consequence of either pyruvate carboxylase or pyruvate dehydrogenase deficiency (Fig. 3). In addition, it may result from defects in NADH oxidation due to mitochondrial cytopathies caused by defects of the electron transport chain. In the neonatal period, primary lactic acidoses may present with drowsiness, poor sucking, severe hypotonia, abnormal movements, seizures, respiratory distress, liver failure, optic atrophy, and fatal ketoacidotic coma.

111.8.4 Disorders Presenting with Hypoglycemia

Severe and persistent or otherwise unexplained hypoglycemia should be investigated for an underlying metabolic or endocrine cause. Recurrent, unpredictable postprandial hypoglycemia are observed in hyperinsulinism or growth hormone deficiency and related disorders, while organic acidemias or defects of gluconeogenesis (glycogen storage disease type I or fructose 1,6-bisphosphatase deficiency) usually present with associated ketoacidosis. The presence of non-glucose reducing substances in urine is characteristic of classic galactosemia and hereditary fructose intolerance. Both diseases are generally associated with other prominent clinical problems such as liver failure. Hyperinsulinism and fatty acid oxidation disorders are the most frequent causes of hypoketotic hypoglycemia. Hyperinsulinism is rarely part of genetic syndromes Beckwith-Wiedemann syndrome, Perlman syndrome, Sotos syndrome, and Kabuki syndrome (Kapoor et al. 2009). Congenital anomalies and dysmorphic features associated with the hyperinsulinism raise the suspicion for these conditions. Hyperinsulinism due to endocrine causes is

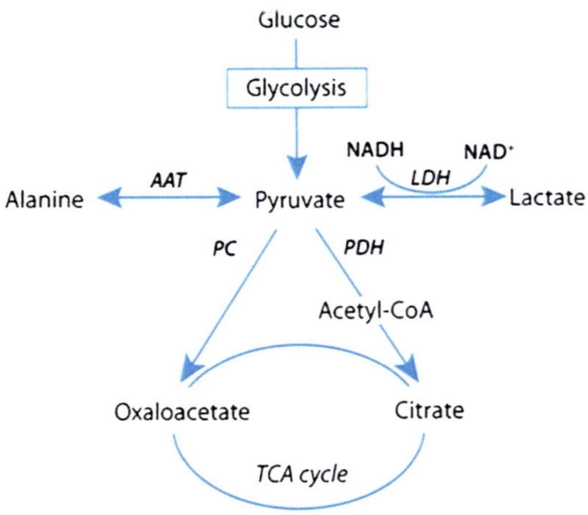

Fig. 3 Pyruvate metabolism. Lactate dehydrogenase (*LDH*), pyruvate dehydrogenase (*PDH*), pyruvate carboxylase (*PC*), alanine aminotransferase (*AAT*), tricarboxylic acid (*TCA*) cycle

described in greater detail in ▶ Chap. 112, "Endocrine Diseases and Disorders of Thyroid Function in Newborns." Nevertheless, it should be noted that congenital hyperinsulinism may also be a feature of inborn errors of metabolism such as hyperinsulinism/hyperammonemia syndrome due to autosomal dominant mutations in the glutamate dehydrogenase (*GDH*) gene (Fig. 4) (Stanley et al. 1998) and defects of the β-oxidation enzyme 3-hydroxyacyl-CoA dehydrogenase (HADH) (Flanagan et al. 2013; Clayton et al. 2001). In hyperinsulinism/hyperammonemia syndrome, the hypoglycemia occurs with fasting but can also be triggered by protein feeding (Hsu et al. 2001). In contrast to urea cycle disorders, the hyperammonemia is mild, stable, and without fluctuations related to fasting or protein feeding. This disorder does not present elevations of plasma glutamine which are typically seen in hyperammonemia (Table 9) (Stanley et al. 1998). The capacity to derive energy from mitochondrial fatty acid oxidation is critically important especially during stress and starvation. Therefore, inherited disorders of fatty acid oxidation are an important and treatable cause of neonatal hypoglycemia.

111.8.4.1 Fatty Acid Oxidation Disorders

Mitochondrial fatty acid oxidation is a complex process involving transport of activated fatty acid molecules into the mitochondria and sequential removal of acetyl-CoA units used as fuel for the tricarboxylic acid cycle or for production of ketone bodies. This process is critical in supplying energy during fasting and metabolic stress, and therefore patients with fatty acid oxidation defects develop hypoketotic hypoglycemia during periods of low glucose intake or intercurrent illnesses. Disorders of fatty acid oxidation may present at any age and have a broad clinical spectrum ranging from severe malformations or sudden death to almost completely asymptomatic adults (Wilcken 2010). They include defects of the uptake and activation of carnitine (primary carnitine deficiency); defects of the carnitine cycle [deficiency of carnitine palmitoyltransferases I (CPT I) and II (CPT II), deficiency of carnitine-acylcarnitine translocase (CACT)], required for mitochondrial entry of fatty acids; and defects of the β-oxidation enzymes. This latter group of disorders is further classified according to the length of the carbon chain of the fatty acids that accumulate and includes medium-chain acyl-CoA dehydrogenase (MCAD) deficiency, very long-chain acyl-CoA dehydrogenase (VLCAD) deficiency, and LCHAD deficiency. Cardiomyopathy, arrhythmias, encephalopathy, and myopathy are frequent findings in these disorders. MCAD deficiency is one of the most common inborn errors of metabolism with an incidence of 1/10,000–20,000 births and might be as high as 1:4,900 live births in some regions (Matern et al. 2015). Up to one quarter of the cases present in the newborn period with fasting hypoketotic hypoglycemia (Wilcken et al. 1993). The treatment of MCAD is based on avoidance of catabolism during fasting or illness (Derks et al. 2007), and neonatal screening is effective in reducing deaths and severe adverse events (Wilcken et al. 2007).

As outlined before, the clinical presentation of fatty acid oxidation defects is highly variable and includes, in the case of the severe lethal neonatal variant of CPT II deficiency, a complex malformation syndrome with dysmorphic features, microcephaly, cataracts, brain and kidney anomalies, periventricular and hepatic calcifications, hypoglycemia, cardiac arrhythmias, seizures, and liver disease (North et al. 1995). Expanded newborn screening has facilitated the detection of neonatal

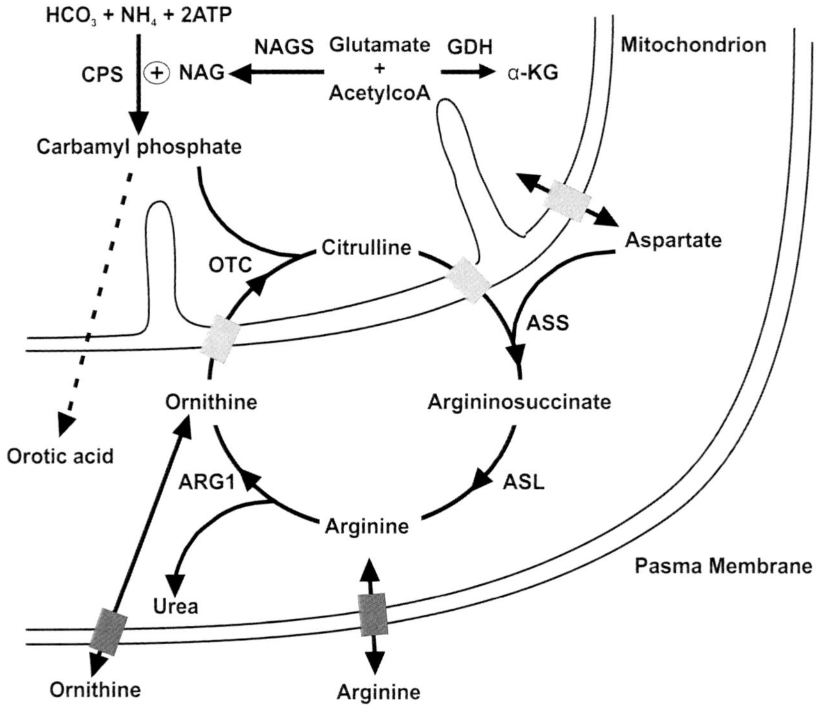

Fig. 4 The urea cycle. The urea cycle converts nitrogen derived from dietary protein intake and breakdown of endogenous protein (catabolism) into urea which can be excreted from the body. The dashed *black arrow* depicts the overflow of excess carbamyl phosphate into pyrimidine synthesis and, hence, to orotic acid, which is excreted in the urine. The *gray cylinders* denote the ornithine and citrulline transporters, the cationic amino acid transporter, and the mitochondrial aspartate and glutamate transporter (citrin). *Abbreviations*: *NAG* *N*-acetylglutamate, *NAGS* *N*-acetylglutamate synthetase, *CPS* carbamyl phosphate synthetase, *OTC* ornithine transcarbamylase, *ASS* argininosuccinic acid synthetase, *ASL* argininosuccinic acid lyase, *ARG1* arginase, *GDH* glutamate dehydrogenase, *α-KG* α-ketoglutarate

CPT II deficiency that, given its presentation, may not raise a high index of suspicion for metabolic diseases (Albers et al. 2001). Multiple acyl-CoA dehydrogenase deficiency (or glutaric aciduria type II) can also present with a malformation phenotype including polycystic kidneys and cerebral cysts and dysplasia (Mitchell et al. 1984).

The expanded newborn screening has also allowed the identification of newborns with primary carnitine deficiency, a treatable disorder characterized by urinary carnitine losses and reduced plasma carnitine levels. The affected newborn is protected by the placental transfer, and therefore, the disease onset typically occurs in infancy or childhood (Magoulas and El-Hattab 2012). A few infants have also been found to have extremely low carnitine levels on newborn screening because they were born to mothers with primary carnitine deficiency who had remained asymptomatic all their lives (Schimmenti et al. 2007).

Acylcarnitine profile analysis by MS/MS helps to establish the diagnosis of these disorders (Table 12). However, intermittent and reversible abnormalities can be missed if the biological specimen is collected outside the critical period. In the context of newborn screening, blood samples taken at age 48–72 h are more likely to be diagnostic because this is a period of substantial catabolism. As for plasma amino acid and urinary organic acid analyses, interpretation of the results of the acylcarnitine profile is based on pattern recognition rather than on individual abnormal values (Table 12). A definitive diagnosis is based on enzyme assays and/or molecular testing.

111.8.5 Disorders Presenting with Hyperammonemia

Hyperammonemia is a clinical emergency which may result in serious derangements of neurological function and structure. The degree of neurological damage is dependent on the duration of the hyperammonemia (Enns et al. 2007), and therefore, prompt recognition and intervention are important. Although the measurement of ammonia levels can be of foremost importance in making the diagnosis of a metabolic disorder, ammonia determination is unfortunately highly susceptible to artifacts resulting in false elevations. Precautions should be followed to avoid incorrect test results: (1) the specimen must be placed on ice at the bedside, and (2) the sample needs to be processed in a timely manner with immediate transfer to the laboratory for instant processing. Elevation of blood ammonia occurs in urea cycle disorders as well as in various other inborn errors of metabolism and in a significant proportion of premature and asphyxiated infants (Table 13).

The urea cycle disorders include defects of the *N*-acetylglutamate synthetase (NAGS), the carbamyl phosphate synthetase (CPS), the ornithine transcarbamylase (OTC), the argininosuccinic acid synthetase (ASS), the argininosuccinic acid lyase (ASL), and arginase (ARG1) (Fig. 4). With the exception of OTC deficiency which is X-linked, all these disorders are inherited as autosomal recessive diseases. Infants with urea cycle disorders appear initially normal but rapidly develop cerebral edema and the related signs of lethargy, anorexia, hypothermia, seizures, neurologic posturing, and coma. Hyperventilation is a common early finding and results in respiratory alkalosis. Hypoventilation and respiratory arrest due to an increased pressure on the brain stem may also occur (Tuchman et al. 2008).

The concentration of citrulline is central in the diagnostic evaluation. If citrulline is markedly elevated, the newborn has citrullinemia (ASS deficiency), and if it is low, a deficiency of OTC, CPS, or NAGS is more likely. Normal or moderately elevated levels of citrulline generally indicate ASL or arginase deficiency (Fig. 5). Enzymatic testing on erythrocytes, fibroblasts, and liver is available along with DNA mutation detection to confirm the diagnosis. Lysinuric protein intolerance, hyperornithinemia-hyperammonemia-homocitrullinuria syndrome, and citrin deficiency are caused by defects in the transporters for the urea cycle intermediates. In these disorders, the deficient transporter activity results in depletion of urea cycle intermediates and decreased urea cycle activity in spite of normal urea cycle enzyme function (Fig. 4).

111.8.6 Disorders Presenting Without Hyperammonemia and Without Ketoacidosis

Hypotonia and/or seizures in the absence of blood pH alteration and hyperammonemia are the main clinical findings in this group of disorders. Hypotonia is rarely isolated in patients with metabolic diseases and is commonly seen in association with other findings. Seizures are the most distinctive sign of neurological disease in the newborn period and can be caused by a broad range of systemic and central nervous system disorders. Among the metabolic defects, it is important to recognize the pyridoxine (vitamin B6)-dependent seizures and glucose transporter type 1 (GLUT1) deficiency syndrome because an effective treatment is available for both disorders. Pyridoxine-dependent seizures have an onset in utero or in the first hours of life (Bejsovec et al. 1967) and are diagnosed empirically by cessation of seizures and normalization of the EEG within minutes after the intravenous injection of 50–100 mg of pyridoxine. Patients affected with pyridoxine-5′-phosphate oxidase deficiency do not respond to pyridoxine but alternatively respond to the administration of pyridoxal phosphate (PLP), the active form of pyridoxine (Mills et al. 2005).

GLUT1 deficiency typically presents with seizures, acquired microcephaly, and complex movement disorders. Several types of seizures (generalized tonic or clonic, focal, myoclonic, atypical absence, atonic) begin before the age of 2 years in approximately 90% and often in the first month of life (Akman et al. 2016). The diagnosis is established by low CSF glucose concentration (<60 mg/dL in all cases reported to date; <40 mg/dL in >90%; 41–52 mg/dL in ~10%).

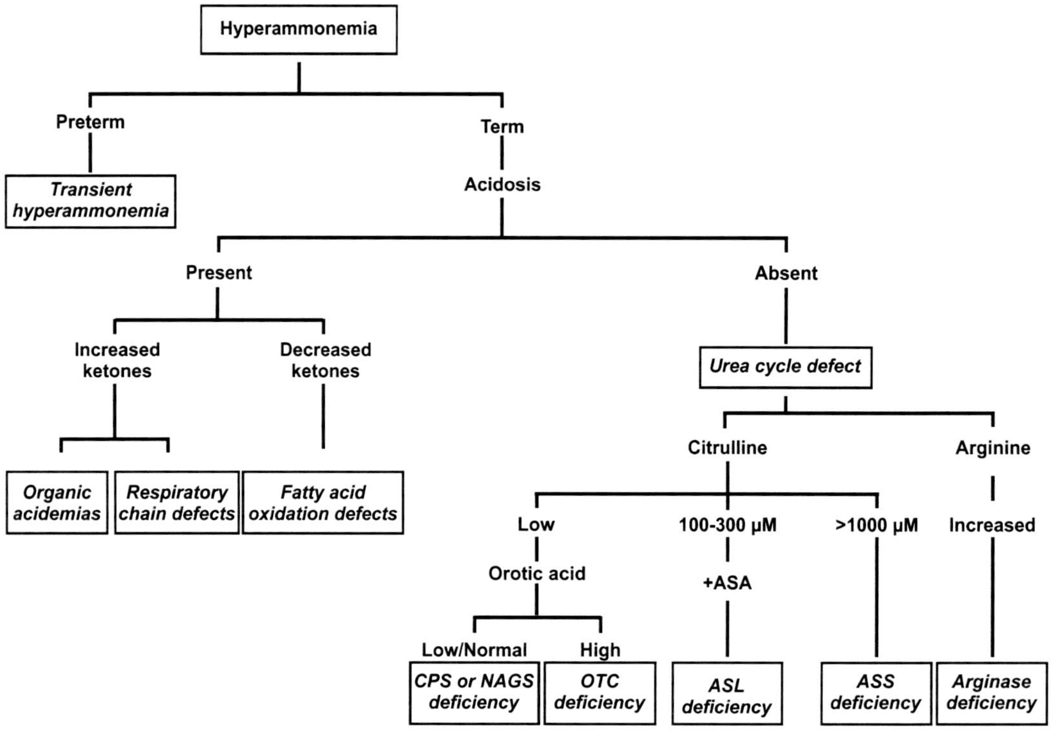

Fig. 5 Diagnostic approach to neonatal hyperammonemia

The ketogenic diet is highly effective in mitigating clinical findings (Akman et al. 2016).

Nonketotic hyperglycinemia (also known as glycine encephalopathy) is caused by defective activity of the glycine cleavage system resulting in the accumulation of glycine in all body tissues and fluids. It typically manifests in the first hours to days of life with progressive lethargy, hypotonia, and myoclonic jerks. Mothers of affected children often report reduced fetal movements and in utero hiccups. Most affected newborns have repeated episodes of severe and prolonged apnea to which they succumb unless ventilatory support is provided until normal spontaneous respiration resumes after several days or weeks. Those infants regaining spontaneous respiration have an extremely poor outcome with profound cognitive impairment and intractable seizures (Hoover-Fong et al. 2004; Swanson et al. 2015). Blood levels of glycine are usually increased although the elevation is occasionally modest. The laboratory diagnosis is based on simultaneous determination of CSF and plasma glycine showing an abnormal CSF-to-plasma glycine ratio (above 0.08). It is important to note that the presence of any blood in the CSF invalidates the results. The differential diagnosis for hyperglycinemia includes disorders resulting in ketotic hyperglycinemia, such as propionic acidemia and methylmalonic acidemia (Table 9). Organic acidemia can be distinguished from glycine encephalopathy by history, determination of urine organic acids (Table 11), and acylcarnitine profile (Table 12). Confirmatory tests include enzymatic analysis in liver tissue and/or mutation analysis (Applegarth and Toone 2001).

Neurologic abnormalities, including seizures with neonatal onset and refractory to treatment, are also prominent features of molybdenum cofactor deficiency and sulfite oxidase deficiency which can be recognized based on elevated urinary sulfocysteine, xanthine, and hypoxanthine, reduced serum levels of uric acid, and nearly undetectable total plasma homocysteine. Seizures and encephalopathy are also features of severe methylenetetrahydrofolate reductase (MTHFR) deficiency and cerebral folate deficiency which are potentially treatable with betaine and folinic acid, respectively. The main biochemical abnormalities are homocystinuria with low or low-normal plasma methionine in MTHFR deficiency and decreased CSF serum folate in cerebral folate deficiency.

In addition, patients with aromatic amino acid decarboxylase (AADC) deficiency present in the first months with motor symptoms of axial hypotonia, hypokinesia, athetosis, dystonia, and limb rigidity. They have ocular symptoms of oculogyric crises and convergence spasms, which can resemble and are often misdiagnosed as seizures. They also have autonomic symptoms of ptosis, nasal congestion, hypothermia, sweating, temperature instability, and blood pressure lability. AADC catalyzes the conversion of L-DOPA to dopamine and of 5-hydroxytryptophan to serotonin, and therefore, its deficiency results in severely reduced dopamine and serotonin and low concentrations of their CSF metabolites homovanillic acid (HVA) and 5-hydroxyindoleacetic acid (5-HIAA). CSF L-DOPA levels are increased and vanillactic acid is present in urine. These patients are treated with dopamine agonists, with monoamine oxidase inhibitors, and with trihexyphenidyl and the AADC cofactor pyridoxal 5′-phosphate. However, the outcome of AADC deficiency tends to be poor with marked neurologic impairment (Brun et al. 2010).

Deficiencies of two enzymes, arginine glycine amidinotransferase (AGAT) and guanidinoacetate methyltransferase (GAMT) involved in synthesis of creatine, and a transporter involved in creatine transport present in infancy with severe to intractable seizures, developmental delay, and hypotonia. The diagnosis is made by assaying creatine and guanidinoacetate in urine and plasma. Creatine in the brain is low by proton magnetic resonance spectroscopy (MRS).

111.8.7 Disorders Presenting with Liver Failure

Severe liver dysfunction in the neonate can occur in a wide variety of metabolic disorders including tyrosinemia type I, galactosemia, hereditary fructose intolerance, mitochondrial hepatopathy, and sugar alcohol defects (Table 3). Neonatal hepatic failure is also a rare presentation of α1-antitrypsin deficiency and of some bile acid synthetic defects which are described in more details in ► Chaps. 77, "Pathology and Treatment of Liver Diseases in Newborns," and ► 78, "Neonatal Cholestasis: Conjugated Hyperbilirubinemia."

Tyrosinemia type I has been rarely described in neonates with severe liver dysfunction. Because elevated tyrosine levels are seen in several conditions with liver dysfunction, the diagnosis of tyrosinemia type I is confirmed by increased succinylacetone in urine or plasma.

Galactosemia will not manifest in an affected newborn until the patient is receiving galactose. Breast milk and most formulas contain lactose (a disaccharide of glucose and galactose); most soy formulas do not. Typical clinical features are hyperbilirubinemia (which may be unconjugated initially but later becomes mainly conjugated), hepatomegaly, liver dysfunction with coagulopathy, hypoalbuminemia, and hypoglycemia. Cataracts may be diagnosed as early as the disease presents in the neonatal period. If undetected the disease may progress into encephalopathy with cerebral edema, metabolic acidosis, and renal dysfunction. Patients with galactosemia have an increased risk for *E. coli* sepsis. Classic galactosemia is diagnosed by measurement of galactose-1-phosphate in serum which is increased and of the defective enzyme, galactose-1-phosphate uridylyltransferase, in red blood cells. Treatment with galactose restriction in the diet results in complete resolution of the acute illness. Therefore, a galactose-free diet is recommended in case of neonatal liver failure until the diagnosis of classical galactosemia has been ruled out.

Hereditary fructose intolerance does not manifest in the newborn period unless fructose or sucrose is added to the diet.

Mitochondrial hepatopathies with deficiency of the respiratory chain enzymes have been recognized in newborns with acute neurologic impairment and liver disease (Al-Hussaini et al. 2014). In some cases, after an initial normal course, a viral infection or some other undefined event triggers hepatic and neurologic deterioration (Cormier-Daire et al. 1997). A fulminant liver failure may also be triggered by sodium valproate, and therefore, this medication should be avoided if there is suspicion of mitochondrial cytopathy (Mindikoglu et al. 2011). The presence of lactic acidosis and hypoglycemia is a useful diagnostic feature, so is the detection of elevated tyrosine. However, these findings are rather nonspecific. Reduced activities of the respiratory chain complexes in the liver or muscle are more specific findings, although secondary defects need to be considered.

Sugar alcohol disorders including transaldolase deficiency and ribose-5-phosphate isomerase deficiency are also responsible for liver disease with neonatal onset (Verhoeven et al. 2005; Huck et al. 2004). Assessment of sugar alcohol in body fluids is usually not a component of the metabolic workup, and therefore, several cases are likely to remain undiagnosed.

111.8.8 Disorders Presenting with Cholestasis

Genetic disorders are an important cause of neonatal cholestasis, and α1-antitrypsin deficiency accounts for a significant portion of these cases. α1-Antitrypsin deficiency and the inborn errors of bile acid synthesis are discussed in ▸ Chaps. 77, "Pathology and Treatment of Liver Diseases in Newborns" and ▸ 78, "Neonatal Cholestasis: Conjugated Hyperbilirubinemia," while this section will focus on other inherited metabolic disorders that can present as isolated cholestasis in newborns. Prolonged neonatal cholestatic jaundice associated with progressive hepatosplenomegaly is the most common sign in Niemann-Pick disease type C. Spontaneously resolving by 2–4 months of age in most patients, it may lead to liver failure in about 10% of cases. Children with this rapidly fatal neonatal cholestatic form die before the age of 6 months, without neurologic symptoms (Kelly et al. 1993).

Patients with neonatal intrahepatic cholestasis caused by citrin deficiency (Fig. 4) have low birth weight, growth retardation, hypoproteinemia, decreased coagulation factors, and increased transaminases. Symptoms disappear by the age of 1 year with fat-soluble vitamin supplementation and lactose-free formulas or formulas containing medium-chain triglycerides. In adulthood, these patients may develop an adult-onset disease with recurring episodes of hyperammonemia. The diagnosis of citrin deficiency is based on biochemical findings, including elevated ammonia, increased concentrations of citrulline and arginine, increased threonine-to-serine ratio (Table 9), and increased serum concentration of pancreatic secretory trypsin inhibitor. Galactose is also elevated in some cases. Conversely, patients with galactosemia can exhibit an amino acid profile resembling the profile seen in citrin deficiency (Feillet et al. 2008).

111.9 Investigations for Inborn Errors of Metabolism

The first line of investigations with relatively rapid and inexpensive evaluations may provide important clues for the diagnosis of metabolic disorders in the newborn (Table 8). Electrolytes, blood gases, anion gap, ammonia, and lactate are useful to discriminate among the different disease groups. Blood ammonia and lactate should be determined in all neonates with unexplained lethargy and neurologic deterioration. Plasma amino acid by HPLC, urine organic analysis by GC/MS, and acylcarnitine profile by MS/MS are essential aid in the diagnosis (Tables 9, 11, and 12). Amino acid analysis of urine is not usually performed in the evaluation of newborns, and there are only a few indications for this test, such as to rule out lysinuric protein intolerance, hyperornithinemia-hyperammonemia-homocitrullinuria syndrome, and cystinuria. Most sick neonates undergo lumbar puncture for CSF collection as part of sepsis evaluation. In the context of a patient with encephalopathy, it is recommended to save an aliquot of CSF for determinations of lactate, amino acid, and neurotransmitters.

Neuroimaging studies can provide important clues for the diagnosis of metabolic disorders. Ultrasound is a reliable, first-line imaging investigation that can be performed at the bedside for early detection of cysts, calcifications, structural brain abnormalities, and edema or altered white matter echogenicity, which can all be suggestive of metabolic disorders (Leijser et al. 2007). MRI is the most sensitive and specific neuroimaging tool for neonatal inborn errors of metabolism. Patterns of brain involvement can be useful in the diagnostic process (van der Knaap and Valk 2005; Poretti et al. 2013). The first important assessment is to establish whether the disease involves primarily gray matter, primarily white matter, both gray and white matters, or cerebellum (Table 14). Moreover, MRS can be helpful for diagnosis and monitoring in a selected number of disorders.

The diagnosis of inborn errors of metabolism should be confirmed by enzyme analysis and/or DNA tests. The choice of one or both of these tests is usually dictated by the availability of laboratory offering these analyses. Enzyme tests can be performed on different tissues (the blood, liver, fibroblasts) depending on the specific disease. DNA tests instead are performed on DNA extracted from the blood. Biochemical methods (detection of metabolites in amniotic fluid and enzyme assays using cultured cells) as well as DNA analysis (mutation detection) are used for prenatal diagnosis. Helpful resources to localize a laboratory for a specific biochemical or molecular test are GeneTests (www.ncbi.nlm.nih.gov/sites/GeneTests/) and Orphanet (www.orpha.net/).

Molecular testing for single genes may not be the best option in several circumstances particularly when there is no indication of which gene may be defective. In these cases, a gene-by-gene approach could lengthen the time to diagnosis and is not cost effective. An alternative to a single-gene approach is to screen many genes simultaneously using next-

Table 14 Pattern of MRI abnormalities in inborn errors of metabolism

Gray matter	White matter	Gray and white matter	Cerebellum
Cortical	*Subcortical*	*Leukodystrophy and striatum*	Pyruvate dehydrogenase deficiency
Lysosomal storage disorders	Mitochondrial diseases	Mitochondrial diseases	Leigh disease
Mucolipidoses	Galactosemia	Propionic acidemia	Congenital disorders of glycosylation
Neuronal ceroid lipofuscinoses	Alexander disease	Glutaric aciduria type I	
Striatum	*Deep white matter*	Molybdenum cofactor deficiency	
Mitochondrial diseases	Krabbe disease	Hypoglycemia	
Propionic acidemia	Metachromatic leukodystrophy	*Leukodystrophy and pallidus*	
Glutaric aciduria type I	GM_2 gangliosidosis	Canavan disease	
Molybdenum cofactor deficiency	Peroxisomal disorders (with neuronal migration defects)	Methylmalonic acidemia	
Hypoglycemia	Lowe syndrome (with small cysts)	2-Hydroxyglutaric aciduria	
Pallidus	Mucolipidosis type IV	Mitochondrial diseases	
Molybdenum cofactor deficiency		Maple syrup urine disease	
Urea cycle disorders			
Methylmalonic acidemia			
Isovaleric acidemia			
Succinic semialdehyde dehydrogenase deficiency			
Pyruvate dehydrogenase deficiency			
Guanidinoacetate methyltransferase (GAMT) deficiency			

Table 15 Specimens to be collected in the event of death when metabolic disease is suspected

Plasma (>2 mL)	Heparinized, separated, and frozen at −80 °C
Blood	Spots on filter paper for MS/MS
Urine	(5–20 mL) deep frozen in a plain tube
CSF	1 mL stored at −80 °C
Sample for DNA	Blood anticoagulated with EDTA and frozen at −80 °C[a]
Skin for fibroblast culture	Taken with sterile precautions into tissue culture medium and stored at 4 °C
Liver	Snap frozen (−80 °C) for histochemistry/enzymology
Muscle	Snap frozen (−80 °C) for histochemistry/enzymology

[a]Skin fibroblasts or other tissues may also be used for DNA extraction

generation sequencing (NGS) technology that is rapidly changing the diagnostic process in inborn errors of metabolism and, more broadly, in genetic disorders. NGS is used to sequence panels of genes providing a comprehensive approach and high diagnostic yields (Pupavac et al. 2016). Gene panels are particularly useful when multiple genes are responsible for a phenotype or when there is extensive clinical overlap between different disorders. Panels are also more cost effective, and results can be obtained more rapidly than a traditional gene-by-gene approach. Another recent advancement in the clinical diagnostic laboratory is the whole-exome sequencing (WES) for identifying the gene defect in patients. WES is a viable option when all previous testing for the patient is negative and there are no additional candidate genes to test. In the future, it is likely that NGS will also dramatically increase the number of disorders identified by newborn screening (Landau et al. 2014).

Inborn errors of metabolism can result in sudden unexplained death. Under these circumstances, it is particularly important to perform a *metabolic autopsy* and skeletal survey and collect appropriate biologic samples to perform further diagnostic tests (Table 15). The findings of these investigations may have important implications for genetic counseling.

111.10 Treatment of the Acute Decompensation

The management of the acutely ill neonate must be initiated early and must be aggressive. It is highly recommended that a neonate who is suspected to have an acute decompensation due to a metabolic disorder is immediately referred to a newborn intensive care unit with expertise in the treatment of metabolic patients. The conventional approach to the treatment of inborn errors of metabolism involves the following basic principles: (1) restriction of upstream essential nutrients to prevent intoxication, (2) supplementation of downstream nutrients to prevent secondary deficiency, and (3) stimulation of alternative routes for disposal of precursor metabolites.

During the acute phase of decompensation, treatment to keep catabolism to a minimum and remove toxic metabolites is required in most disorders. These measures can be started before a precise diagnosis is known. First, any nutrient that may have precipitated the illness, such as galactose or protein, should be halted, and an intravenous high energy intake made up to 10% dextrose (~10 mg/kg/min) with maintenance electrolytes should be started. The need to provide adequate glucose may require the use of concentrated solutions through a central line which can be useful in case extracorporeal dialysis is needed. With high rates of glucose infusion, blood glucose concentrations should be monitored, and if hyperglycemia occurs, insulin may be started. In this context, insulin has the additional advantage of promoting anabolism. Intravenous fluid should be administered with caution to avoid fluid overload and cerebral edema which may occur in maple syrup urine disease and urea cycle disorders. Metabolic acidosis can be corrected by sodium bicarbonate administration, often required in large doses.

Table 16 Medications for acute presentation in selected inborn errors of metabolism

Condition	Medication	Route	Recommended dose
Organic acidurias	L-Carnitine	IV, PO	100 mg/kg bolus followed by maintenance dose of 100 mg/kg/day
Fatty acid oxidation defects			
Methylmalonic acidemia	Hydroxy-cobalamin	IV, IM	1–2 mg/day
Urea cycle disorders	Na benzoate	IV	250 mg/kg bolus in 90–120 min followed by maintenance dose of 250 mg/kg/day
	L-Arginine	IV	200–600 mg/kg followed by maintenance dose of 250 mg/kg/day
	N-Carbamylglutamate	PO/NG tube	100 mg/kg followed by 25–62.5 mg/kg every 6 h
Pyridoxine-responsive seizures	Pyridoxine	IV	100 mg
Pyridoxal phosphate-responsive seizures	Pyridoxal phosphate	PO	10–30 mg/kg/day
MTHFR deficiency	Betaine	PO	100 mg/kg/day
Cerebral folate deficiency	Folinic acid	PO	10–15 mg/kg/day
Biotinidase deficiency	Biotin	PO	1–10 mg/day
Multiple carboxylase deficiency			

Hypoventilation due to cerebral depression is the most common reason for poor tissue oxygenation, and most affected newborns require mechanical ventilation. Many patients with metabolic decompensation may develop sepsis which may aggravate the catabolism and results in therapeutic failure. Therefore, an aggressive search and treatment of infections are crucial for a successful intervention. Sodium benzoate is used to treat the hyperammonemia (Table 16). Carnitine is used for the elimination of some toxic metabolites, and it may be given even before a specific diagnosis is known. In the presence of severe lactic acidosis or unexplained metabolic acidosis, biotin and intramuscular vitamin B12 treatment can be initiated until multiple carboxylase deficiency and methylmalonic acidemia have been excluded (Table 16).

Vitamin B6 can arrest pyridoxine-dependent seizures (Table 16). Sometimes the metabolic derangement cannot be controlled by the approaches outlined above. Given that neurological complications are related to the concentration and duration of the exposure to the toxic metabolites, such as ammonia and leucine, more aggressive therapies such as hemodialysis are required.

References

Acuna-Hidalgo R, Schanze D, Kariminejad A, Nordgren A, Kariminejad MH, Conner P, Grigelioniene G et al (2014) Neu-Laxova syndrome is a heterogeneous metabolic disorder caused by defects in enzymes of the L-serine biosynthesis pathway. Am J Hum Genet 95:285–293

Akman CI, Yu J, Alter A, Engelstad K, De Vivo DC (2016) Diagnosing glucose transporter 1 deficiency at initial presentation facilitates early treatment. J Pediatr 171:220–226

Albers S, Marsden D, Quackenbush E, Stark AR, Levy HL, Irons M (2001) Detection of neonatal carnitine palmitoyltransferase II deficiency by expanded newborn screening with tandem mass spectrometry. Pediatrics 107, E103

Alfardan J, Mohsen AW, Copeland S, Ellison J, Keppen-Davis L, Rohrbach M, Powell BR et al (2010) Characterization of new ACADSB gene sequence mutations and clinical implications in patients with 2-methylbutyrylglycinuria identified by newborn screening. Mol Genet Metab 100:333–338

Al-Hussaini A, Faqeih E, El-Hattab AW, Alfadhel M, Asery A, Alsaleem B, Bakhsh E et al (2014) Clinical and molecular characteristics of mitochondrial DNA depletion syndrome associated with neonatal cholestasis and liver failure. J Pediatr 164:553–559, e551–552

Angle B, Tint GS, Yacoub OA, Clark AL (1998) Atypical case of Smith-Lemli-Opitz syndrome: implications for diagnosis. Am J Med Genet 80:322–326

Applegarth DA, Toone JR (2001) Nonketotic hyperglycinemia (glycine encephalopathy): laboratory diagnosis. Mol Genet Metab 74:139–146

Arnold GL, Salazar D, Neidich JA, Suwannarat P, Graham BH, Lichter-Konecki U, Bosch AM et al (2012) Outcome of infants diagnosed with 3-methyl-crotonyl-CoA-carboxylase deficiency by newborn screening. Mol Genet Metab 106:439–441

Arora N, Stumper O, Wright J, Kelly DA, McKiernan PJ (2006) Cardiomyopathy in tyrosinaemia type I is common but usually benign. J Inherit Metab Dis 29: 54–57

Baumgartner MR, Verhoeven NM, Jakobs C, Roels F, Espeel M, Martinez M, Rabier D et al (1998) Defective peroxisome biogenesis with a neuromuscular disorder resembling Werdnig-Hoffmann disease. Neurology 51:1427–1432

Bejsovec M, Kulenda Z, Ponca E (1967) Familial intrauterine convulsions in pyridoxine dependency. Arch Dis Child 42:201–207

Bellini C, Donarini G, Paladini D, Calevo MG, Bellini T, Ramenghi LA, Hennekam RC (2015) Etiology of non-immune hydrops fetalis: an update. Am J Med Genet A 167A:1082–1088

Boemer F, Deberg M, Schoos R, Caberg JH, Gaillez S, Dugauquier C, Delbecque K et al (2016) Diagnostic pitfall in antenatal manifestations of CPT II deficiency. Clin Genet 89:193–197

Braverman NE, Raymond GV, Rizzo WB, Moser AB, Wilkinson ME, Stone EM, Steinberg SJ et al (2016) Peroxisome biogenesis disorders in the Zellweger spectrum: an overview of current diagnosis, clinical manifestations, and treatment guidelines. Mol Genet Metab 117:313–321

Brun L, Ngu LH, Keng WT, Ch'ng GS, Choy YS, Hwu WL, Lee WT et al (2010) Clinical and biochemical features of aromatic L-amino acid decarboxylase deficiency. Neurology 75:64–71

Chace DH, Kalas TA, Naylor EW (2002) The application of tandem mass spectrometry to neonatal screening for inherited disorders of intermediary metabolism. Annu Rev Genomics Hum Genet 3:17–45

Chiong MA, Sim KG, Carpenter K, Rhead W, Ho G, Olsen RK, Christodoulou J (2007) Transient multiple acyl-CoA dehydrogenation deficiency in a newborn female caused by maternal riboflavin deficiency. Mol Genet Metab 92:109–114

Clayton PT, Eaton S, Aynsley-Green A, Edginton M, Hussain K, Krywawych S, Datta V et al (2001) Hyperinsulinism in short-chain L-3-hydroxyacyl-CoA dehydrogenase deficiency reveals the importance of beta-oxidation in insulin secretion. J Clin Invest 108:457–465

Cormier-Daire V, Chretien D, Rustin P, Rotig A, Dubuisson C, Jacquemin E, Hadchouel M et al (1997) Neonatal and delayed-onset liver involvement in disorders of oxidative phosphorylation. J Pediatr 130:817–822

Cox PM, Brueton LA, Murphy KW, Worthington VC, Bjelogrlic P, Lazda EJ, Sabire NJ et al (1999) Early-onset fetal hydrops and muscle degeneration in siblings due to a novel variant of type IV glycogenosis. Am J Med Genet 86:187–193

Daikha-Dahmane F, Dommergues M, Narcy F, Gubler MC, Dumez Y, Gauthier E, Nordmann Y et al (2001) Congenital erythropoietic porphyria: prenatal diagnosis and autopsy findings in two sibling fetuses. Pediatr Dev Pathol 4:180–184

de Koning TJ, Klomp LW, van Oppen AC, Beemer FA, Dorland L, van den Berg I, Berger R (2004) Prenatal and early postnatal treatment in 3-phosphoglycerate-dehydrogenase deficiency. Lancet 364:2221–2222

Derks TG, van Spronsen FJ, Rake JP, van der Hilst CS, Span MM, Smit GP (2007) Safe and unsafe duration of fasting for children with MCAD deficiency. Eur J Pediatr 166:5–11

Dursun A, Gucer S, Ebberink MS, Yigit S, Wanders RJ, Waterham HR (2009) Zellweger syndrome with unusual findings: non-immune hydrops fetalis, dermal erythropoiesis and hypoplastic toe nails. J Inherit Metab Dis 32(Suppl 1):S345–S348

Enns GM, Berry SA, Berry GT, Rhead WJ, Brusilow SW, Hamosh A (2007) Survival after treatment with phenylacetate and benzoate for urea-cycle disorders. N Engl J Med 356:2282–2292

Fayon M, Lamireau T, Bioulac-Sage P, Letellier T, Moretto B, Parrot-Roulaud F, Coquet M et al (1992) Fatal neonatal liver failure and mitochondrial cytopathy: an observation with antenatal ascites. Gastroenterology 103:1332–1335

Feillet F, Merten M, Battaglia-Hsu SF, Rabier D, Kobayashi K, Straczek J, Brivet M et al (2008) Evidence of cataplerosis in a patient with neonatal classical galactosemia presenting as citrin deficiency. J Hepatol 48:517–522

Flanagan SE, Xie W, Caswell R, Damhuis A, Vianey-Saban C, Akcay T, Darendeliler F et al (2013) Next-generation sequencing reveals deep intronic cryptic ABCC8 and HADH splicing founder mutations causing hyperinsulinism by pseudoexon activation. Am J Hum Genet 92:131–136

Freeze HH, Chong JX, Bamshad MJ, Ng BG (2014) Solving glycosylation disorders: fundamental approaches reveal complicated pathways. Am J Hum Genet 94:161–175

Ganetzky R, Izumi K, Edmondson A, Muraresku CC, Zackai E, Deardorff M, Ganesh J (2015) Fetal akinesia deformation sequence due to a congenital disorder of glycosylation. Am J Med Genet A 167A:2411–2417

Garver WS, Francis GA, Jelinek D, Shepherd G, Flynn J, Castro G, Walsh Vockley C et al (2007) The National Niemann-Pick C1 disease database: report of clinical features and health problems. Am J Med Genet A 143A:1204–1211

Gimovsky AC, Luzi P, Berghella V (2015) Lysosomal storage disease as an etiology of nonimmune hydrops. Am J Obstet Gynecol 212:281–290

Haberle J, Gorg B, Rutsch F, Schmidt E, Toutain A, Benoist JF, Gelot A et al (2005) Congenital glutamine deficiency with glutamine synthetase mutations. N Engl J Med 353:1926–1933

Haberle J, Shahbeck N, Ibrahim K, Hoffmann GF, Ben-Omran T (2011) Natural course of glutamine synthetase deficiency in a 3 year old patient. Mol Genet Metab 103:89–91

Haberle J, Shahbeck N, Ibrahim K, Schmitt B, Scheer I, O'Gorman R, Chaudhry FA et al (2012) Glutamine supplementation in a child with inherited GS deficiency improves the clinical status and partially corrects the peripheral and central amino acid imbalance. Orphanet J Rare Dis 7:48

Herman GE, Kratz L (2012) Disorders of sterol synthesis: beyond Smith-Lemli-Opitz syndrome. Am J Med Genet C Semin Med Genet 160C:301–321

Hinton CF, Ojodu JA, Fernhoff PM, Rasmussen SA, Scanlon KS, Hannon WH (2010) Maternal and neonatal vitamin B12 deficiency detected through expanded newborn screening – United States, 2003–2007. J Pediatr 157:162–163

Ho G, Yonezawa A, Masuda S, Inui K, Sim KG, Carpenter K, Olsen RK et al (2011) Maternal riboflavin deficiency, resulting in transient neonatal-onset glutaric aciduria Type 2, is caused by a microdeletion in the riboflavin transporter gene GPR172B. Hum Mutat 32: E1976–E1984

Hoover-Fong JE, Shah S, Van Hove JL, Applegarth D, Toone J, Hamosh A (2004) Natural history of nonketotic hyperglycinemia in 65 patients. Neurology 63:1847–1853

Hsu BY, Kelly A, Thornton PS, Greenberg CR, Dilling LA, Stanley CA (2001) Protein-sensitive and fasting hypoglycemia in children with the hyperinsulinism/hyperammonemia syndrome. J Pediatr 138:383–389

Huck JH, Verhoeven NM, Struys EA, Salomons GS, Jakobs C, van der Knaap MS (2004) Ribose-5-phosphate isomerase deficiency: new inborn error in the pentose phosphate pathway associated with a slowly progressive leukoencephalopathy. Am J Hum Genet 74:745–751

Ibdah JA, Bennett MJ, Rinaldo P, Zhao Y, Gibson B, Sims HF, Strauss AW (1999) A fetal fatty-acid oxidation disorder as a cause of liver disease in pregnant women. N Engl J Med 340:1723–1731

Kapoor RR, James C, Hussain K (2009) Hyperinsulinism in developmental syndromes. Endocr Dev 14:95–113

Kelly DA, Portmann B, Mowat AP, Sherlock S, Lake BD (1993) Niemann-Pick disease type C: diagnosis and outcome in children, with particular reference to liver disease. J Pediatr 123:242–247

Landau YE, Lichter-Konecki U, Levy HL (2014) Genomics in newborn screening. J Pediatr 164:14–19

Leijser LM, de Vries LS, Rutherford MA, Manzur AY, Groenendaal F, de Koning TJ, van der Heide-Jalving M et al (2007) Cranial ultrasound in metabolic disorders presenting in the neonatal period: characteristic features and comparison with MR imaging. AJNR Am J Neuroradiol 28:1223–1231

Lenke RR, Levy HL (1980) Maternal phenylketonuria and hyperphenylalaninemia. An international survey of the outcome of untreated and treated pregnancies. N Engl J Med 303:1202–1208

Leticee N, Bessieres-Grattagliano B, Dupre T, Vuillaumier-Barrot S, de Lonlay P, Razavi F, El Khartoufi N et al (2010) Should PMM2-deficiency (CDG Ia) be searched in every case of unexplained hydrops fetalis? Mol Genet Metab 101:253–257

Magoulas PL, El-Hattab AW (2012) Systemic primary carnitine deficiency: an overview of clinical manifestations, diagnosis, and management. Orphanet J Rare Dis 7:68

Matern D, Rinaldo P (2015) Medium-chain acyl-coenzyme A dehydrogenase deficiency. In: Pagon RA, Adam MP, Ardinger HH, Wallace SE, Amemiya A, Bean LJH et al eds. GeneReviews(R). Seattle University of Washington, Seattle

Mignot C, Gelot A, Bessieres B, Daffos F, Voyer M, Menez F, Fallet Bianco C et al (2003) Perinatal-lethal Gaucher disease. Am J Med Genet A 120A:338–344

Mills PB, Surtees RA, Champion MP, Beesley CE, Dalton N, Scambler PJ, Heales SJ et al (2005) Neonatal epileptic encephalopathy caused by mutations in the PNPO gene encoding pyridox(am)ine 5′-phosphate oxidase. Hum Mol Genet 14:1077–1086

Mindikoglu AL, King D, Magder LS, Ozolek JA, Mazariegos GV, Shneider BL (2011) Valproic acid-associated acute liver failure in children: case report and analysis of liver transplantation outcomes in the United States. J Pediatr 158:802–807

Mitchell G, Saudubray JM, Gubler MC, Habib R, Ogier H, Frezal J, Boue J (1984) Congenital anomalies in glutaric aciduria type 2. J Pediatr 104:961–962

National Institutes of Health Consensus Development Panel (2001) National Institutes of Health Consensus Development Conference Statement: phenylketonuria: screening and management, October 16–18, 2000. Pediatrics 108:972–982

North KN, Hoppel CL, De Girolami U, Kozakewich HP, Korson MS (1995) Lethal neonatal deficiency of carnitine palmitoyltransferase II associated with dysgenesis of the brain and kidneys. J Pediatr 127: 414–420

Oey NA, den Boer ME, Wijburg FA, Vekemans M, Auge J, Steiner C, Wanders RJ et al (2005) Long-chain fatty acid oxidation during early human development. Pediatr Res 57:755–759

Pena L, Angle B, Burton B, Charrow J (2012) Follow-up of patients with short-chain acyl-CoA dehydrogenase and isobutyryl-CoA dehydrogenase deficiencies identified through newborn screening: one center's experience. Genet Med 14:342–347

Poretti A, Blaser SI, Lequin MH, Fatemi A, Meoded A, Northington FJ, Boltshauser E et al (2013) Neonatal neuroimaging findings in inborn errors of metabolism. J Magn Reson Imaging 37:294–312

Profitlich LE, Kirmse B, Wasserstein MP, Diaz GA, Srivastava S (2009) High prevalence of structural heart disease in children with cblC-type methylmalonic aciduria and homocystinuria. Mol Genet Metab 98:344–348

Pupavac M, Tian X, Chu J, Wang G, Feng Y, Chen S, Fenter R et al (2016) Added value of next generation gene panel analysis for patients with elevated methylmalonic acid and no clinical diagnosis following functional studies of vitamin B metabolism. Mol Genet Metab 117:363–368

Ruzzo EK, Capo-Chichi JM, Ben-Zeev B, Chitayat D, Mao H, Pappas AL, Hitomi Y et al (2013) Deficiency of asparagine synthetase causes congenital microcephaly and a progressive form of encephalopathy. Neuron 80:429–441

Saudubray JM, Charpentier C (2001) Clinical phenotypes: diagnosis/algorithms. In: Scriver CR, Beaudet AL, Sly WS et al eds. The Metabolic & Molecular Bases of Inherited Disease, 8th ed. McGraw-Hill, New York, pp. 1327–1403

Schimmenti LA, Crombez EA, Schwahn BC, Heese BA, Wood TC, Schroer RJ, Bentler K et al (2007) Expanded newborn screening identifies maternal primary carnitine deficiency. Mol Genet Metab 90:441–445

Shaheen R, Rahbeeni Z, Alhashem A, Faqeih E, Zhao Q, Xiong Y, Almoisheer A et al (2014) Neu-Laxova syndrome, an inborn error of serine metabolism, is caused by mutations in PHGDH. Am J Hum Genet 94:898–904

Stanley CA, Lieu YK, Hsu BY, Burlina AB, Greenberg CR, Hopwood NJ, Perlman K et al (1998) Hyperinsulinism and hyperammonemia in infants with regulatory mutations of the glutamate dehydrogenase gene. N Engl J Med 338:1352–1357

Staretz-Chacham O, Lang TC, LaMarca ME, Krasnewich D, Sidransky E (2009) Lysosomal storage disorders in the newborn. Pediatrics 123:1191–1207

Swanson MA, Coughlin CR Jr, Scharer GH, Szerlong HJ, Bjoraker KJ, Spector EB, Creadon-Swindell G et al (2015) Biochemical and molecular predictors for prognosis in nonketotic hyperglycinemia. Ann Neurol 78:606–618

Tuchman M, Lee B, Lichter-Konecki U, Summar ML, Yudkoff M, Cederbaum SD, Kerr DS et al (2008) Cross-sectional multicenter study of patients with urea cycle disorders in the United States. Mol Genet Metab 94:397–402

Valayannopoulos V, Verhoeven NM, Mention K, Salomons GS, Sommelet D, Gonzales M, Touati G et al (2006) Transaldolase deficiency: a new cause of hydrops fetalis and neonatal multi-organ disease. J Pediatr 149:713–717

Vallejo-Torres L, Castilla I, Couce ML, Perez-Cerda C, Martin-Hernandez E, Pineda M, Campistol J et al (2015) Cost-effectiveness analysis of a national newborn screening program for biotinidase deficiency. Pediatrics 136:e424–e432

van de Kamp JM, Lefeber DJ, Ruijter GJ, Steggerda SJ, den Hollander NS, Willems SM, Matthijs G et al (2007) Congenital disorder of glycosylation type Ia presenting with hydrops fetalis. J Med Genet 44:277–280

van der Crabben SN, Verhoeven-Duif NM, Brilstra EH, Van Maldergem L, Coskun T, Rubio-Gozalbo E, Berger R et al (2013) An update on serine deficiency disorders. J Inherit Metab Dis 36:613–619

van der Knaap MS, Valk J (2005) Pattern recognition in white matter disorders. Springer, Berlin, pp 881–904

Van Hove JL, Josefsberg S, Freehauf C, Thomas JA, le Thuy P, Barshop BA, Woontner M et al (2008) Management of a patient with holocarboxylase synthetase deficiency. Mol Genet Metab 95:201–205

van Karnebeek CD, Sly WS, Ross CJ, Salvarinova R, Yaplito-Lee J, Santra S, Shyr C et al (2014) Mitochondrial carbonic anhydrase VA deficiency resulting from CA5A alterations presents with hyperammonemia in early childhood. Am J Hum Genet 94:453–461

Verhoeven NM, Wallot M, Huck JH, Dirsch O, Ballauf A, Neudorf U, Salomons GS et al (2005) A newborn with severe liver failure, cardiomyopathy and transaldolase deficiency. J Inherit Metab Dis 28:169–179

von Kleist-Retzow JC, Cormier-Daire V, Viot G, Goldenberg A, Mardach B, Amiel J, Saada P et al (2003) Antenatal manifestations of mitochondrial respiratory chain deficiency. J Pediatr 143:208–212

Wilcken B (2010) Fatty acid oxidation disorders: outcome and long-term prognosis. J Inherit Metab Dis 33:501–506

Wilcken B, Carpenter KH, Hammond J (1993) Neonatal symptoms in medium chain acyl coenzyme A dehydrogenase deficiency. Arch Dis Child 69:292–294

Wilcken B, Haas M, Joy P, Wiley V, Chaplin M, Black C, Fletcher J et al (2007) Outcome of neonatal screening for medium-chain acyl-CoA dehydrogenase deficiency in Australia: a cohort study. Lancet 369:37–42

Wraith JE (2002) Lysosomal disorders. Semin Neonatol 7:75–83

Zytkovicz TH, Fitzgerald EF, Marsden D, Larson CA, Shih VE, Johnson DM, Strauss AW et al (2001) Tandem mass spectrometric analysis for amino, organic, and fatty acid disorders in newborn dried blood spots: a two-year summary from the New England Newborn Screening Program. Clin Chem 47:1945–1955

Endocrine Diseases and Disorders of Thyroid Function in Newborns 112

Paolo Ghirri, Antonio Balsamo, Massimiliano Ciantelli, Paolo Cavarzere, Alessandro Cicognani, Antonio Boldrini, and Alessandra Cassio

Contents

P. Ghirri (✉) · A. Boldrini (✉)
Department of Clinical and Experimental Medicine, Division of Neonatology and Neonatal Intensive Care Unit, Santa Chiara University Hospital, Pisa, Italy
e-mail: pghirri@med.unipi.it; antonio.boldrini@med.unipi.it

A. Balsamo (✉) · A. Cicognani (✉)
Department of Medical and Surgical Sciences, Pediatric Unit, Center for Rare Endocrine Diseases (CARENDO BO), S.Orsola Malpighi University Hospital, Bologna, Italy
e-mail: antonio.balsamo@unibo.it; alessandro.cicognani@unibo.it

M. Ciantelli (✉)
Department of Clinical and Experimental Medicine, Division of Neonatology and Neonatal Intensive Care Unit, S. Chiara University Hospital, Pisa, Italy

Azienda Ospedaliero-Universitaria Pisana, Pisa, Italy
e-mail: m.ciantelli@ao-pisa.toscana.it

P. Cavarzere
Pediatric Unit, Department of Mother and Child, University Hospital of Verona, Verona, Italy
e-mail: paolocavarzere@yahoo.it

A. Cassio (✉)
Department of Medical and Surgical Sciences, Pediatric Endocrinology Unit, S. Orsola-Malpighi University Hospital, Bologna, Italy
e-mail: alessandra.cassio@unibo.it

G. Buonocore et al. (eds.), *Neonatology*,
https://doi.org/10.1007/978-3-319-29489-6_259

Abstract

Congenital hypopituitarism results from a deficiency of any or all hormones secreted by the anterior pituitary gland or by the posterior pituitary gland. Reduced cortisol and/or aldosterone production may be the consequence of primary cortical adrenal insufficiency or damage; isolated cortisol insufficiency may be caused by pituitary or hypothalamic dysfunction (ACTH or CRF deficiency). Neonatal hypoglycemia is frequent in neonates, especially in those of low birth weights. Hypoglycemia is usually transient and resolves in the first 72 h of life; symptoms are absent or nonspecific. Hyperglycemia may be due to impaired glucose homeostasis, iatrogenic causes, stress, and neonatal diabetes mellitus; it is often asymptomatic and secondary to other severe diseases.

Neonatal hypocalcemia affects 30% of very low birth weight infants. Clinical presentation is nonspecific and therapy may be by oral or intravenous supplementation. Hypercalcemia is defined as an ionized calcium concentration >1.36 mmol/L or total calcium concentration >2.75 mmol/L. Moderate to severe hypercalcemia requires prompt intervention.

Congenital hypothyroidism is the most common endocrine disorder in the neonatal age range, causing significant neurointellectual impairment. Plasma thyroid hormone levels are correlated to gestational age, and preterm infants have lower T3, T4, and FT4 values than term infants.

112.1 Salient Points

- The annual incidence of congenital hypopituitarism ranges from 1 to 42 new cases per million with a prevalence of 300–455 cases per million.
- Reduced cortisol and/ or aldosterone production may be the consequence of primary cortical adrenal insufficiency or damage.
- Antidiuretic hormone (ADH), the renin-angiotensin aldosterone system, norepinephrinec and the thirst mechanism are responsible for the regulation of total body water and osmolality.
- Neonatal hypoglycemia cannot be defined by a single value, and its definition remains debatable.
- Hyperglycemia may be due to different mechanisms: impaired glucose homeostasis, iatrogenic causes, stress, and neonatal diabetes mellitus.
- Neonatal hypocalcemia is relatively common in neonates, affecting 30% of very low birth weight infants.
- Hypercalcemia is defined as an ionized calcium concentration >1.36 mmol/L or total calcium concentration >2.75 mmol/L.
- Congenital hypothyroidism is the most common endocrine disorder in neonatal age with an incidence of primary permanent congenital hypothyroidism of 1:3000 to 1:4000 live births.

112.2 Hypopituitarism

Congenital hypopituitarism results from a deficiency of any or all six hormones secreted by the five different cell types contained into the anterior pituitary gland (adrenocorticotropic hormone [ACTH]; growth hormone [GH]; thyroid-stimulating hormone [TSH]; luteinizing hormone [LH]; and follicle stimulating hormone [FSH]; prolactin [PRL]) or by the posterior pituitary gland (arginine-vasopressin [AVP] and oxytocin). The intermediate lobe secretes pro-opiomelanocortin (POMC), which is a precursor to melanocyte-stimulating hormone (MSH) and endorphins, and involutes in the adult. It is uncommon. The annual incidence ranges from 1 to 42 new cases per million and a prevalence of 300–455 cases per million (Chung and Monson 2015).

112.2.1 Etiology

The incidence variability depends on the heterogeneity of cases. Some cases have a genetic etiology; others with lesions in the sellar region have been attributed to traumatic events or perinatal complications (cesarean section, breech, prolonged or rapid delivery, and low Apgar score) (Mehta et al. 2009). It is, however, difficult to determine whether perinatal insults lead to hypopituitarism because of traumatic disruption of the pituitary stalk, or whether hypopituitarism with structural hypothalamo-pituitary defects (Alatzoglou and Dattani 2009) results in an increased prevalence of perinatal complications.

Congenital hypopituitarism may be due to hypothalamic dysplasia or specific releasing hormone deficiencies (corticotropin- releasing hormone [CRH]; growth-hormone releasing hormone [GHRH]; gonadotropin-releasing hormone [GnRH]; or thyrotropin-releasing hormone [TRH]). Other causes are due to anterior pituitary dysplasia or specific anterior pituitary deficiencies. Posterior pituitary deficiency may be familial (X-linked or autosomal dominant), idiopathic or secondary to inflammatory events (e.g., meningitis), disseminated intravascular coagulation (DIC), intraventricular hemorrhage, trauma/asphyxia, and maternal drugs (e.g., lithium). Congenital rubella and toxoplasmosis have also been implicated.

Recently, mutations in several genes encoding transcription factors that are implicated in normal hypothalamic pituitary (H-P) development have been linked both with hypopituitarism in humans and with structural abnormalities on neuroimaging. Mutations in genes that are implicated in somatotrope proliferation and GH secretion, such as *GH1* and *GHRHR*, are also associated with GH deficiency and with magnetic resonance imaging (MRI) abnormalities. These transcription factors and signaling molecules are expressed either exclusively in the developing pituitary or also in structures such as the hypothalamus and forebrain. A mutation in any one of these can lead to either a pituitary-specific phenotype (Table 1) or a broader clinical presentation such as septo-optic dysplasia, agenesis of the corpus callosum, persistent septum pellucidum, central cleft lip/palate, anencephaly/holoprosencephaly, familial pituitary hypoplasia, and Wolfram syndrome. Congenital hypogonadotropic hypogonadism (CHH) is a rare disorder caused by the deficient production, secretion, or action of gonadotropin-releasing hormone (GnRH), which is the key hormone regulating the reproductive axis. CHH is clinically and genetically heterogeneous, with >25 different causal genes identified to date (Boehm et al. 2015). Isolated gonadotropin deficiency with hyposmia (Kallmann's syndrome) may be inherited as an X-linked disorder, autosomally or occur sporadically. The X-linked disorder occurs in approximately 1/10,000–60,000 live births, and a mutation in the KAL-1 gene is the basis for the disease (Boehm et al. 2015). Mutations in DAX-1, another X chromosome gene, cause hypogonadotropic hypogonadism in association with congenital adrenal hypoplasia in males (see page 9).

Lack of neonatal activation of the HPG axis can provide early diagnostic signals for identifying CHH at birth or during mini-puberty. In male infants, maldescended testes and micropenis can be signs of GnRH deficiency. Penile growth can be assessed using available cross-sectional normative data (Tomova et al. 2010). However, more severe genital anomalies, such as hypospadias, point away from a diagnosis of CHH. No definite clinical signs of CHH present in female neonates. Regardless of sex, when familiarity for CHH exists, it is good practice to monitor reproductive hormones during mini-puberty and to search for mutations previously detected in the parents. Kallman's syndrome usually presents in late adolescence with delayed pubertal initiation or progression and characteristically exhibit hyposmia. Other features which are specific to X-linked Kallmann's syndrome include unilateral renal agenesis and synkinesis (mirror movements), whereas midline facial defects, choanal atresia, short metacarpals, malrotation of the gut, and ocular coloboma are more common in autosomal and sporadic forms of the condition (see appendix) (Boehm et al. 2015). In posterior hypopituitarism, polyhydramnios may be followed by postnatal dehydration, weight loss, irritability, hypernatremia, and seizures. In breast-fed babies, the clinical features are similar but of more gradual onset. In patients with both arginine vasopressin and ACTH deficiency, diabetes insipidus, characterized by polyuria and polydipsia, may be masked by ACTH deficiency given that cortisol is essential for the excretion of a water load. Treatment with hydrocortisone may unmask diabetes insipidus (DI).

112.2.2 Clinical Presentation

Congenital hypopituitarism must be suspected in any child presenting with hypoglycemia and dysmorphic features with midline defects, prolonged jaundice, poor weight gain, hypothermia, cryptorchidism, and/or micropenis in a male infant. Early diagnosis of this condition may prevent impairment of cognition, poor growth, and metabolic abnormalities.

In anterior hypopituitarism, there may be optic nerve hypoplasia/dysplasia. Babies tend to be small, sometimes severely growth restricted.

112.2.3 Investigations

112.2.3.1 Biochemical/Hormonal Measurements

First check blood glucose levels. If there is severe or symptomatic hypoglycemia, the levels of GH, cortisol, and ACTH should be measured. If found to be high because of stress (e.g., difficult venous cannulation), then pituitary function tests may be avoided. Baseline TSH and free thyroxine (fT4) or

LH/FSH levels may also be useful as they should be relatively high in the first days of life.

Tests of pituitary function should be undertaken under the direction of an endocrinologist. A glucagon stimulation test will assess both GH and adrenal axes, but late hypoglycemia may be dangerous. An ACTH stimulation test is safe but only indirectly evaluates ACTH. A CRH test measuring cortisol and ACTH response may be more useful. A gonadotropin-releasing hormone (GnRH) test to stimulate LH and FSH may be helpful for later management of puberty and fertility.

The diagnosis of ADH deficiency is made by monitoring weight, fluid balance, and urine and plasma osmolalities (low urine and high plasma osmolality).

112.2.3.2 Imaging

Cranial ultrasound and MRI scan (hypothalamus and pituitary gland are not visible on ultrasound scan) may reveal associated structural anomalies of the brain, hypothalamic-pituitary axis, and the optic nerves (Table 1).

112.2.3.3 Genetic Analysis

The relevant genetic analysis should be undertaken in patients with multiple pituitary hormone deficiencies, a family history of hypopituitarism or consanguinity, or with associated anatomic abnormalities (Table 1).

112.2.4 Management

112.2.4.1 Acute Interventions

Correction of hypoglycemia is the first step. Substitution therapy with deficient hormones must be undertaken as soon as possible. ACTH, TSH, and ADH deficiencies need replacement with hydrocortisone (8–12 mg/m^2/day orally, in three divided doses), thyroxine (8–12 μg/kg/day, orally once a day), and vasopressin (0.5–2.0 mU/kg/h as a continuous IV infusion) or DDAVP (0.25–10 μg 12 h intranasally, or 0.02–0.2 μg 12 h intravenously, according to response), respectively. When hypoglycemia is caused by GH deficiency, then subcutaneous hGH at 7 mg/m2/weekly dose may be useful.

112.2.4.2 Discharge Instructions

Intramuscular injections to take home (hydrocortisone hemisuccinate, 70 mg/m^2/8 h) need to be prescribed in case of vomiting or profuse diarrhea. In the case of intercurrent illness, instructions from a pediatric endocrinologist should be given to double (nonfebrile illness) or triple (febrile illness) the oral hydrocortisone doses. A steroid card should be provided.

Parents should be instructed in the use of glucose monitoring (sticks) and the management of hypoglycemia (1 μg SC glucagon injections).

In presence of a micropenis, the use of testosterone injections (25 mg/IM monthly, for 3 months) or dihydrotestosterone gel (0.2–0.3 mg/kg topically once a day for 3–4 months) during the first 6 months of life may help further virilization.

Optic nerve involvement mandates ophthalmic referral.

112.2.4.3 Long-Term Follow-Up

Generally, the anterior pituitary deficiencies need a permanent substitution treatment, while the posterior pituitary may recover. Genetic counseling should be provided for inherited causes of hypopituitarism.

112.3 Adrenal Insufficiency

Reduced cortisol and/or aldosterone production may be the consequence of primary cortical adrenal insufficiency (PAI) or damage. Isolated cortisol insufficiency may also be a consequence of pituitary/hypothalamic ACTH/CRF deficiency (secondary/tertiary adrenal insufficiency, respectively). The clinical presentation will differ according to the underlying cause.

112.3.1 Adrenal Development from Fetal to Postnatal Adrenal Gland

Coelomic epithelial cells of mesodermal origin on the urogenital ridge give rise to the kidney, gonadal, and adrenal cortical structures (Fig. 1).

Table 1 Clinical phenotypes, mode of inheritance, and MRI presentation in pituitary hormone deficiencies involving gene alterations (Modified from Alatzoglou and Dattani (2009))

Gene	Inheritance	Deficiency	Anterior hypophysis	Posterior hypophysis	Other abnormalities
HESX1	AR or AD	GH, (TSH, LH, FSH, ACTH, PRL variable)	Hypoplasic	Ectopic	Septo-optic dysplasia
PROP1	AR	GH, TSH, LH, FSH (ACTH variable)	Enlargement with waxing and waning and eventual hypoplasia	Normal	Transient AP hyperplasia
LHX3	AR	GH, TSH, LH, FSH, PRL	Variable	Normal	Abnormalities of head rotation
LHX4	AD	GH, TSH, (LH, FSH, ACTH variable)	Hypoplasic	Variable	Cerebral malformations
POU1F1 (PIT1)	AR or AD	GH, TSH, PRL	Hyperplasia and later hypoplasia	Sometimes ectopic	–
SOX2	AD	HH, variable GHD	Hypoplasic	Normal	An/microphthalmia, esophageal atresia, genital tract abnormalities, hypothalamic hamartoma, sensorineural hearing loss, diplegia
SOX3	XL	IGHD or CPHD	Hypoplasic	Ectopic	Mental retardation
TBX19 (T-PIT)	AR	ACTH	Normal	Normal	Neonatal
KAL-1	X-linked	HH (LH, FSH)	Normal	Normal	Anosmia, unilateral renal agenesis, and synkinesis
DAX-1	X-linked	HH (LH, FSH)	Normal	Normal	Adrenal insufficiency
GH1		GH	Empty sella, hypoplasia	Normal	
IA (del/severe mutations)	AR				IA no GH and GH Ab on treatment
IB (splice site, missense mutations)	AR				IB low detectable GH, no Ab
II (splice site, splice site enhancers, missense muts)	AD				II less severe short stature
GHRHR	AR	High GH	–	Normal	d

AR autosomal recessive, *AD* autosomal dominant, *XL* X-linked, *Ab* antibodies

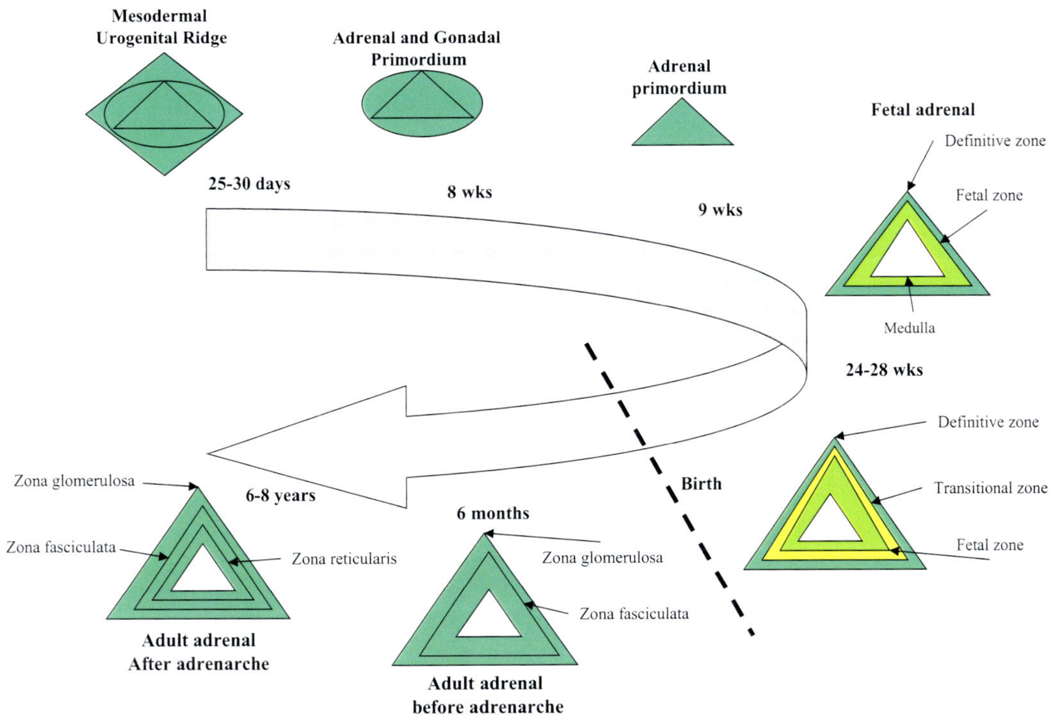

Fig. 1 Scheme of temporal adrenal development in humans (Modified from Kempná and Flück (2008))

The fetal adrenal cortex separates from the other structures and differentiates into a larger inner fetal zone, which produces DHEA and DHEA-S from early gestation, but 3-β-HSD expression is absent after 12 weeks. After 9 weeks' gestation, there is a thinner outer definitive zone, which is quiescent until late gestation. An intermediate transitional zone appears after 24 weeks' gestation and contains the enzymes for cortisol production (expression of 3-β-HSD activity). Shortly after birth, the fetal zone regresses. By 6 months of age, the definitive (adult) adrenal cortex consists of the mineralocorticoid-producing zona glomerulosa and the glucocorticoid-producing zona fasciculata. The zona reticularis does not appear until the end of year 3 and only by around 6 years of age starts to produce adrenal androgens (adrenarche) (Coulter 2004).

Fetal DHEA-S production is important because it is either 16α-hydroxylated in the fetal liver before being converted to estriol (90% of the maternal circulation) or directly converted to estrone and estradiol in the placenta (50% of the maternal circulation) (Fig. 2).

The fetus seems to be protected from high levels of cortisol in utero because cortisol is converted to biologically inactive cortisone through 11β-HSD2 activity in placental and fetal tissues. However, transient expression (weeks 7–12 of gestation) of 3β-HSD2 in the fetal adrenal has been recently demonstrated (Hanley and Arlt 2006) and serves to protect female fetuses from genital virilization. It enables the fetal adrenal to produce cortisol by 8 weeks of gestation and activates the negative feedback on pituitary ACTH which in turn reduces the early production of androgens in the critical time window for genital development (Goto et al. 2006).

112.3.2 Molecular Basis of Adrenal Insufficiency (AI)

The past 20 years has seen substantial advancement in our understanding of the genetic causes

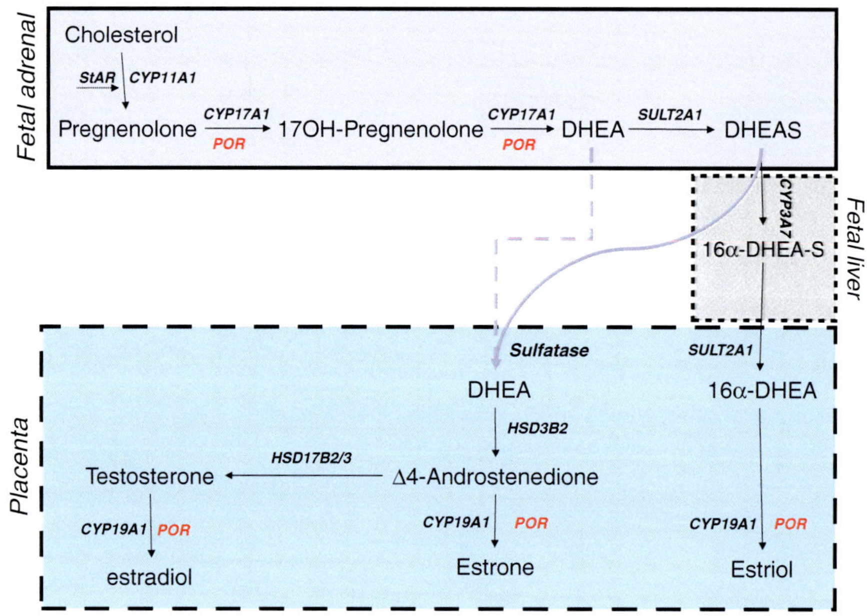

Fig. 2 Steroidogenesis of the fetal-adrenals/-placental unit. DHEA and its sulfate are the main products of the fetal adrenal cortex after 12 weeks' gestation in humans. DHEA-S is produced from the adrenals and converted to estriol in the placenta through previous 16α-hydroxylation in the fetal liver, or converted directly to estrogens in the placenta.

of childhood AI. More than 160 known and candidate genes involved in adrenal development and function are thought to be involved in adrenal development, including genes coding for steroidogenic enzymes, signaling molecules, transcription and growth factors, regulators of cell cycle and angiogenesis, and extracellular matrix proteins (Kempná and Flück 2008). However, the exact role of most of these factors remains unclear (Guran et al. 2016).

Studies of patients with adrenal insufficiency due to gene mutations have revealed that transcription factors such as *GLI3*, *SF1*, and *DAX1* have a central role in the first steps of adrenal formation. Adrenal differentiation requires ACTH stimulation and signaling through biosynthetic steps involving POMC, PCI, TPIT, MC2R, and ALADIN, all of which determine adrenal hypoplasia when mutated. Mutations in some of the steroidogenic enzymes cause congenital adrenal hyperplasia, autosomic recessive inherited diseases impairing both cortisol and/or aldosterone synthesis (Webb and Krone 2015).

112.3.3 Etiology

112.3.3.1 Congenital

Congenital adrenal insufficiency comprises a group of disorders including: (1) impaired steroidogenesis, (2) defects of adrenal development, (3) familial glucocorticoid deficiency (FGD) and FGD-like disorders, (4) adrenal destruction, (5) and disturbed endocrine communication between the pituitary gland and the adrenals. It is significant in the diagnostic work-up to establish if the adrenal insufficiency is of primary or secondary origin. Table 2 summarizes the most frequent inherited conditions associated with neonatal adrenal insufficiency.

Primary Forms

Congenital adrenal hyperplasia (CAH) (CYP21A2, CYP11B1, HSD3B2, CYP17A1, POR deficiencies) constitutes the largest cluster of steroidogenic impairments and the most common cause of PAI in children (Turcu and Auchus 2015). 21-hydroxylase deficiency account for more than 90% of cases and is the most frequent form of cortisol and aldosterone deficiency in

Table 2 Congenital causes of adrenal insufficiency (AI) in the newborn

Condition/deficiency	*Gene*/protein type	Inheritance (OMIM#)	Other associated features
Impaired steroidogenesis			
With congenital adrenal hyperplasia			
Lipoid CAH	**StAR**/shuttle protein,	AR (201710)	46,XY DSD, gonadal insufficiency
3βHSD3 type 2	***HSD3B2/*** enzyme	AR (201810)	46,XX and 46,XY DSD, gonadal insufficiency
P450c21	***CYP21A2***/ enzyme	AR (201910)	46,XX DSD, hyperandrogenism
P450c11	***CYP11B1/*** enzyme	AR (202010)	46,XX DSD, arterial hypertension
POR	***POR*** / *CYP electron donor*	AR (201750)	46,XX and 46,XY DSD, gonadal insufficiency, bone malformation, involvement of all endoplasmic CYP450 enzymes
Without congenital adrenal hyperplasia			
P450scc	***CYP11A1***/ enzyme	AR (118485)	46,XY DSD, gonadal insufficiency
Aldosterone synthase deficiency	**CYP11B2/** enzyme	AR (124080)	Isolated mineralocorticoid deficiency (IMG)
Defects of cholesterol synthesis/metabolism			
Wolman disease	**LIPA**/*enzyme*	AR (278000)	Calcified adrenals, xanthomatous changes in several organs/tissues
Smith-Lemli-Opitz syndrome	***DHCR7***/ enzyme	AR (270400)	46,XY DSD, mental retardation, growth failure, craniofacial malformations, limb abnormalities
Aβ-lipoproteinemia	***MTTP***/TF	AR (200100)	Ataxia, retinopaty, achantocytosis, fat-malabsorption
Familial hypercholesterolemia	***LDLR***/TF (MR)	AR (143890)	Tendinous xanthomas, xanthelasma, corneal arcus
Adrenal dysgenesis			
(without syndromic features)			
X-linked AHC	***DAX1 (NROB1)***/TF (NR)	X linked (300200)	Hypogonadotropic hypogonadism, DMD in contiguous gene syndrome
SF1 linked AHC	***SF1 (NR5A1)***/ TF(NR)	AD / AR (184757)	46,XY DSD, gonadal insufficiency
(with syndromic features)			
IMAGe syndrome	***CDKN1C***/	X linked (300290)	IUGR, metaphyseal dysplasia, genital anomalies (in males: cryptorchidism, micropenis)
Pallister-Hall syndrome	***GLI3***/TF	(165240)	Hypothalamic hamartoblastoma, hypopituitarism, imperforate anus, postaxial polydactilia
Meckel syndrome	***MKS1/***	(249000)	CNS malformations, polycystic kidney with fibrotic liver changes, polydactilia
ACTH resistance			
	MC2R/(MR)	AR (607397)	Isolated glucocorticoid deficiency (IGD), tall stature
Type 2	**MRAP**/(*AP)*	AR (607398)	IGD
Impaired redox homeostasis			
Triple A (Allgrove) syndrome	**AAAS/(***RP)*	AR (231550)	Achalasia, alacrimia; neurologic impairment, deafness, hyperkeratosis, mental retardation

(*continued*)

Table 2 (continued)

Condition/deficiency	*Gene*/protein type	Inheritance (OMIM#)	Other associated features
Mineralocorticoid resistance			
Pseudohypoaldosteronism Type 1	**NR3C2**/*TF (NR)* ***EnaC-α, −β, −γ***	D (177735) AR (600228;600760-1)	Isolated to kidney Extended to kidney, lung, bowels, skin, sudoripare glands
Degenerative metabolic disorders			
Peroxisomal defects			
Adrenoleukodystophy X-ALD Neonatal ALD Zellweger syndrome	**ABCD1**/*TF* *PEX1*/**TF** *PEX1*/**TF**	X linked (300100) AR (601539) AR (214100)	Progressive neurodegeneration, behavioral changes, cognitive and sensorial decline, spasticity, dementia; Craniofacial abnormalities, liver dysfunction; Craniofacial abnormalities, hepatomegalia, severe mental retardation, growth failure, genitourinary abnormalities, stippled epiphyses
Mitochondrial defects			
Deficiency of free radical detoxification	**NNT**/*TF* ***TRXR***/TF ***GPX1, PRDX3***/TF	AR (614736) AR (606448)	IGD IGD Digenic inheritance in 1 pt. with IGD
Kearns-Sayre syndrome	Mitochondrial DNA deletions	VI (530000)	External ophthalmoplegia, retinal degeneration, cardiac conduction defects; other endocrinopathies
CRH deficiency			
Septo-optic dysplasia	**HESX1**/*TR*	VI (182230)	Combined pituitary hormone deficiency, optic-nerve dysplasia, and midline brain defects
ACTH deficiency			
Isolated	**TPIT**	AR (201400)	ACTH deficiency
Combined	**PROP1** **LHX4** ***SOX3***	VI (262600) AD (262700) X linked (312000)	Additional deficiency of GH,TSH, PRL,LH/FSH Additional deficiency of GH and TSH

DSD difference of sex development, *TF* transcription factor, *TR* transcription repressor, *NR* nuclear receptor, *MR* membrane receptor, *AP* accessory protein, *RP* regulatory protein, *VI* various inheritance

the newborn. These forms of CAH can also cause varying degrees of virilization of females (46,XX DSD) and undervirilization of males (46,XY DSD) (Table 2). Patients with P450 oxidoreductase (POR) mutations, a recently described form of CAH, may be at risk of adrenal insufficiency and Addisonian crisis, especially at times of severe febrile illness or major surgery. In these conditions, the hypertrophic adrenals maintain their histological structure. Gene analysis, especially for 21-hydroxylase deficiency, makes it possible to perform prenatal diagnosis and experimentally treat female affected fetuses (see also ▶ Chap. 113, "Disorders of Sexual Development in Newborns").

Adrenal hypoplasia congenita (AHC) due to dysgenetic development can present as two main different clinical forms of PAI without syndromic features:

(a) An X-linked cytomegalic form, in which the normal three zone architecture of the adrenal cortex is absent and has been replaced by large, vacuolated cells resembling fetal adrenocortical cells. It is caused by mutations in the *NR0B1/DAX-1* gene that also cause hypogonadotropic hypogonadism and impaired spermatogenesis (Balsamo et al. 2005). The adrenal insufficiency presents during the first 2 months of life in approximately 40% of affected boys. Typically, boys present with a salt losing adrenal crisis due to mineralocorticoid insufficiency, together with glucocorticoid insufficiency. A basal cortisol value within the normal range does not exclude the diagnosis; however, the response to ACTH-analogue stimulation will usually be impaired (Suntharalingham et al. 2015).

(b) An *NR5A1/SF-1* gene linked form that can be dominantly or recessively inherited. It may be associated with adrenal failure and XY sex-reversal with or without the presence of Mullerian structures. Since the developing adrenals appear less *SF1* dose-dependent than the testes, not all affected patients may have adrenal insufficiency (Suntharalingham et al. 2015).

In isolated hypoaldosteronism (CYP11B2 deficiency) and pseudohypoaldosteronism type 1 (PHA1, affecting the kidney only or where there is multiorgan resistance to mineralocorticoids), the adrenal cortex is normal. Both CYP11B2 deficiency and systemic pseudohypoaldosteronism (PHA) inheritance are autosomal recessive disorders, while the renal PHA form is autosomal dominant (Balsamo et al. 2007; Arai and Chrousos 2013). An acquired form of PHA also exists, and it is important to recognize it during the neonatal period when a urinary tract malformation is detected by prenatal ultrasound. In the case of obstructive uropathy, the risk of salt loss is high when the cause of obstruction is treated by surgery.

Adrenoleucodystrophy is an X-linked (X-ALD) severe neurodegenerative disorder causing progressive demyelinization of the central and peripheral nervous system, adrenal insufficiency, and accumulation of very-long-chain fatty acids in plasma, fibroblasts, and tissues. It is caused by impaired beta-oxidation in peroxisomes due to mutations in the *ABCD1* gene. X-ALD presents with heterogeneous phenotypes ranging from adrenomyeloneuropathy (AMN) to inflammatory demyelinating cerebral ALD (CALD). The onset generally does not occur below 3 years of age, but a contiguous *ABCD1 DXS1357E* deletion syndrome (CADDS) has been described with neonatal onset (Corzo et al. 2002). Its phenotype is similar to that of either peroxisomal biogenesis disorders (PBD) or single-enzyme deficiencies (SED) in the peroxisomal beta-oxidation pathway (acyl CoA oxidase deficiency and bifunctional protein deficiency), which also accumulate very-long-chain fatty acids (VLCFA), but are transmitted in an autosomal recessive manner and present as neonatal onset ALD (Table 2). While previously the lifetime risk for a newborn male X-ALD patient to develop the inflammatory form of X-ALD was estimated to be around 60%, two recent reports suggest an even higher risk to develop CALD. Neonatal screening by tandem mass spectrometry can be used for early diagnosis, reducing morbidity due to these conditions. Preliminary results suggest an incidence rate of around 1:30,000 (Wiesinger et al. 2015; Vogel et al. 2015).

ACTH insensitivity syndromes comprise a group of disorders which all manifest as familial glucocorticoid deficiency (FGD). The type 1 (FGD1) depends on autosomal recessive mutations in the G-protein-coupled ACTH receptor (melanocortin receptor 2, MC2R), while the type 2 (FGD2) is caused by mutations in the gene encoding MC2R accessory protein (MRAP) (Chung et al. 2010). Other forms of FGD and FGD-like conditions have been recently identified (MCM4, NNT, TRXR2 gene defects) that depends by mitochondrial defects. ACTH resistance is one of the three components of the Triple A syndrome (Achalasia-Addisonianism-Alacrima, the Allgrove syndrome), caused by mutations in the *AAAS* gene, encoding a protein named ALADIN, and which manifests itself during the first decade.

Secondary Forms

ACTH deficiency may recur as an isolated feature (IAD) or as part of a multiple pituitary hormone deficiency syndrome (Table 2). IAD is rare and may occur in the neonatal period, but also in later childhood. After consideration of candidate genes (*POMC, PC1, CRH,* and its receptor *CRH-R1*), only mutations in *TPIT* have been found in about 25% of the patients with the isolated, early onset form. Multiple pituitary hormone deficiencies

(MPHD) may result from abnormal hypothalamic-pituitary development caused by anomalous expression of the transcription factors reported in Table 2.

112.3.3.2 Acquired

AIDS, meningococcus, adrenal hemorrhage (Waterhouse-Friderichsen), maternal Cushing's disease/syndrome, adrenal suppression following antenatal steroid therapy to the fetus or to the mother may all cause severe adrenal insufficiency in neonates. The use of dexamethasone postnatally has been largely abandoned because of likely effects on brain growth and more physiological doses of hydrocortisone are currently being used in the context of clinical trial for treatment of the controversial relative adrenal insufficiency (Langer et al. 2006).

112.3.4 Clinical Presentation

Generally, primary congenital adrenal insufficiency may present with hypoglycemia, cardiovascular collapse, hypotension, ambiguous genitalia, skin pigmentation, and hyponatremia/hyperkalemia. Patients with congenital adrenal hypoplasia, steroidogenic defects, or pseudohypoaldosteronism present with clinical signs of salt wasting within the first 20 days after the birth. They may have failure to thrive, anorexia, vomiting, and severe hyponatremic/hyperkalemic dehydration. Skin hyperpigmentation, typical for the forms with reactive ACTH overproduction (congenital adrenal hyperplasia/hypoplasia, familial isolated glucocorticoid deficiency, adrenoleukodystrophy), may color genitalia, umbilicus, nipples, and axillae. Other symptoms at onset, mainly in neonates with severe glucocorticoid deficiency (congenital adrenal hyperplasia, familial isolated glucocorticoid deficiency), may be hypoglycemia with possible ketosis, due to gluconeogenic substrate deficiency. Although most boys present with PAI and classic features of DAX-1 linked AHC, alternative presenting phenotypes have come out. These may include a predominant mineralocorticoid insufficiency and salt loss, similar to other conditions such as aldosterone synthase deficiency or pseudohypoaldosteronism. Infrequently, patients may present with low cortisol and are thought to have familial glucocorticoid deficiency (Suntharalingham et al. 2015).

Hyperpigmentation and salt craving are not observed in patients with secondary adrenal insufficiency. Unless there is a history of recent glucocorticoid therapy, secondary adrenal insufficiency is usually associated with signs of other pituitary hormone deficiencies such as hypoglycemia, growth failure, secondary hypothyroidism, and/or diabetes insipidus (polyuria and polydipsia).

112.3.5 Diagnostic Evaluation

When the adrenal failure is not extremely severe, a pretreatment blood sample for cortisol, electrolyte, glucose, ACTH levels, plasma renin activity, and aldosterone level should be taken. A further diagnostic evaluation under the supervision of a pediatric endocrinologist may need an ACTH test (0–60 mins, half standard dose: 125 μg IV or low dose: 0.5–1 μg/1.73 m^2) to assess the adrenal response. A normal cortisol response is a rise of 200 nmol/L from baseline, although equivocal results may occur during the neonatal period. A peak 17-OH progesterone of more than 150 nmol/L is suggestive of 21-hydroxylase deficiency (for other specific steroidogenic defects see Table 2 and ▶ Chap. 113, "Disorders of Sexual Development in Newborns", Table 113.4). Urine steroid profile may be useful for AHC or CAH differentiation and adrenal ultrasound scan for hemorrhage or hypertrophy. Aldosterone levels are generally low in salt-wasting congenital adrenal hyperplasia/hypoplasia. When isolated aldosterone deficiency is suspected, very high levels of the hormone indicate possible pseudohypoaldosteronism. Plasma renin activity (PRA) or renin levels are elevated when salt wasting is latent or manifest due to aldosterone deficiency or resistance. In aldosterone steroidogenic defects, the PRA/aldosterone ratio is elevated even when mineralocorticoid levels are normal.

Although the indications given above are useful for a diagnostic orientation, there is increasing evidence of nonclassical presentations of various forms of AI. For example, FGD/FGD-like conditions can present with salt loss suggestive of adrenal hypoplasia, and alterations in STAR and CYP11A1 resulting in partial loss of protein function may have a main FGD-like phenotype (Guran et al. 2016). It is likely that improved technologies for molecular genetic analysis using next-generation sequencing (NGS) approaches will become an essential tool to discern these diagnostic pathways (Guran et al. 2016).

112.3.6 Treatment

For the standard treatment of glucocorticoid and/or mineralocorticoid deficiencies, see ▶ Chap. 113, "Disorders of Sexual Development in Newborns" Secondary adrenal insufficiency or familial glucocorticoid deficiency do not need mineralocorticoid substitution. Patients with isolated aldosterone deficiency do not need glucocorticoids and milder forms may be treated by the simple addition of salt to the diet, obviating the need for mineralocorticoid substitution. In patients with pseudohypoaldosteronism, where mineralocorticoid treatment is ineffective, dietary supplementation with sodium chloride is the only possible treatment. No satisfying treatment to prevent the onset or modify the progression of the chronic myelopathy of X-ALD exists. The administration of a mixture of glyceryl trioleate and glyceryl trierucate, also referred as Lorenzo's Oil, has been shown to prevent disease progression in asymptomatic patients with cerebral involvement of X-ALD. Allogeneic hematopoietic stem cell (HSC) transplantation is the treatment of choice for individuals with early stages of the cerebral form of the disease. An alternative option for patients without HLA-matched donors is autologous HSC-gene therapy with lentivirally corrected cells. Once adrenal insufficiency is present, the hormonal replacement therapy is identical to that of autoimmune Addison's disease.

In acute adrenal crisis, an initial hydrocortisone IV bolus of 60–70 mg/m^2 is recommended, followed by 60–70 mg/m^2 per day divided into four IV doses. For restoration of intravascular volume, we recommend an infusion of 5% glucose and 0.9% saline solutions (120–150 mL/kg/24 hrs). The combination of saline and large doses of hydrocortisone maintains mineralocorticoid function during the first hours of treatment. Fludrocortisone (0.05–0.2 mg/day in two divided doses) may be administered orally; intramuscular administration of 1–2 mg/twice a day of corticosterone acetate is a less comfortable way of achieving mineralocorticoid replacement. Additional glucose should be administered parenterally when hypoglycemia is severe (Webb and Krone 2015).

112.4 Hyponatremia, Hypernatremia; Hyperkalemia

Total body water and osmolality is regulated by the renal action of antidiuretic hormone (ADH), the renin-angiotensin aldosterone system, norepinephrine, and by the thirst mechanism. Abnormalities in water balance are manifested as sodium disturbances. Mild to **moderate hyponatremia** (plasma sodium >125–134 < mmol/L) and **severe hyponatremia** (<125 mmol/L) are found in about 15–30% and 1–4% of patients, respectively. It is useful to distinguish between water overload (excessive intake or inadequate excretion) and sodium depletion (excessive salt loss). Common causes of hyponatremia are listed in Table 3. **Hypernatremia** (plasma sodium >145 mmol/L) is caused by primary water deficit (with or without sodium loss) and commonly occurs because of insufficient water intake or impaired thirst mechanism (Table 3).

Hyperkalemia is defined as a potassium (K) level > 6.5 mmol/L. It can be an incidental finding on blood biochemistry; it may be anticipated in the presence of oliguria associated with renal impairment. High levels of K are cardiotoxic and the signs of this condition are a widened QRS complex or tall, tenet T-waves on ECG, and dysrhythmias, such as ventricular tachycardia or fibrillation.

112.4.1 The Renin-Angiotensin-Aldosterone System

Aldosterone secretion is primarily regulated by the renin-angiotensin system and potassium

Table 3 Causes of hyponatremia, hypernatremia, and hyperkalemia in the newborn

Hyponatremia
Water overload
Iatrogenic: excess maternal (prenatal) or neonatal IV fluid administration
Renal failure
Syndrome of inappropriate antidiuretic hormone secretion (SIADH)
Salt depletion
Immaturity
CAH, AHC
Renal impairment: polyuric phase of acute tubular necrosis (ATN), congenital nephrotic syndrome, Bartter syndrome, congenital renal abnormality (previous polyhydramnios)
Gut loss: secretory diarrhea, stoma output following gut resection, congenital chloride diarrhea
Iatrogenic: repeated cerebral spinal fluid removal by ventricular taps
Aldosterone biosynthetic defect or resistance
Hypernatremia
Water depletion
Inadequate fluid intake:
Milk intake: frequent in breastfeeding mothers at first pregnancy
IV fluid infusion: e.g., extreme preterm infant with high insensibile percutaneous or respiratory tract loss
Excessive fluid loss:
Urine: diabetes insipidus (DI), renal concentrating defect, osmotic diuresis secondary to glycosuria
Gut: vomiting or nasogastric aspirates, secondary diarrhea
Skin: cystic fibrosis
Salt excess
Sodium bicarbonate infusion
Malicious salt poisoning
Hyperkalemia
Spurious (hemolyzed blood sample)
Renal impairment (including structural defects such as urethral valves, dysplastic kidneys, and renal vascular accidents)
Renal tubular immaturity in ELBW infants
Acidosis that causes shift of K out of cells into extracellular fluid
Excessive K administration in medication or addition of K to IV fluids (prescribed or inadvertently given) Aldosterone deficiency or resistance
Hemolysis of blood transfusion
Urinary tract infection
Renal tubular acidosis

(Fig. 3), and secondarily by ACTH. Hyponatremia, hypovolemia, low blood pressure, and reduced renal perfusion stimulate the juxtaglomerular apparatus (cells surrounding the renal afferent arteriole, close to the macula densa) to secrete the proteolytic enzyme renin. Renin activates angiotensin I and II through angiotensinogen (liver) and angiotensin converting enzyme (ACE, lung), respectively. Angiotensin II has a potent vasopressor activity and, like potassium, acts directly on the glomerulosa cells in the adrenal cortex to stimulate aldosterone production. The distal tubule and collecting ducts of the kidney respond to increased aldosterone levels by increasing sodium reabsorption and excreting potassium and hydrogen. Aldosterone exerts its effects via the mineralocorticoid receptor (MR) and the resultant activation of specific amiloride-sensitive sodium channels (ENaC) and the Na-K ATPase pump. The mineralocorticoid receptor (MR) is responsive to both cortisol and aldosterone actions, but 11β-hydroxysteroid dehydrogenase (11β-HSD) activity at renal level prevents the conversion of cortisol to cortisone, which has very low mineralocorticoid receptor affinity. Aldosterone increases blood pressure by raising blood volume and by increasing the sensitivity of arterial muscle to vasoconstrictors (Arai and Chrousos 2013).

112.4.2 Antidiuretic Hormone

Antidiuretic hormone (ADH) or arginine vasopressin (AVP) is a nonapeptide that is synthesized as a large prohormone in the paraventricular and supraoptic nuclei of the hypothalamus. The most potent stimuli to ADH release are severe hypovolemia and increased plasma osmolality. ADH acts via vascular V1 receptors and renal tubular V2 receptors. V1 receptor stimulation causes arterial vasoconstriction, and V2 stimulation increases renal free water reabsorption (due to the high interstitial osmolality). Relative or absolute deficiency of ADH causes DI. Central DI may be primary and is usually associated with other

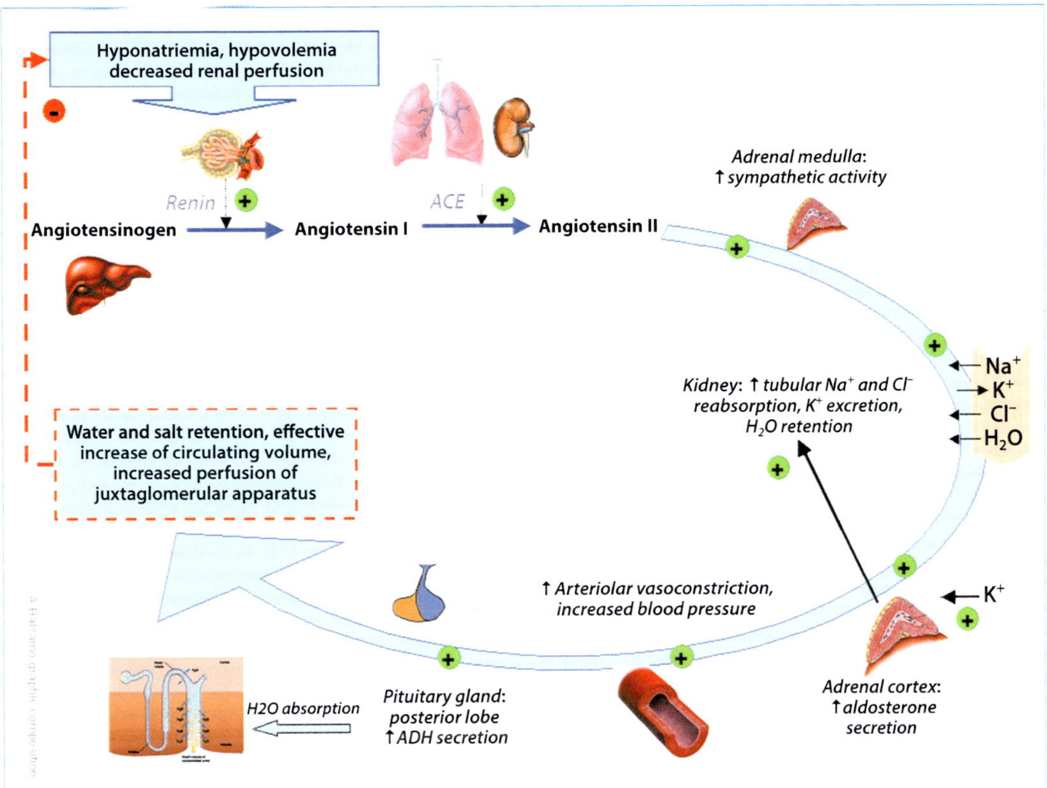

Fig. 3 Renin-angiotensin-aldosterone system

hypothalamo/pituitary gland developmental alterations and multiple hormone deficiencies. DI is rare, with a prevalence estimated at 1:25,000; fewer than 10% of cases are hereditary in nature. Central DI (CDI) accounts for greater than 90% of cases of DI and can present at any age, depending on the cause. No prevalence for hereditary causes of CDI has been established. DI may rarely be caused by renal resistance to ADH (nephrogenic DI, NDI), an X-linked disease (Xq2.8), which is due to mutations in the arginine-vasopressin receptor 2 gene (*AVPR2*). NDI is less frequent than CDI. X-linked NDI (XLNDI) accounts for 90% of cases of male births, and autosomal recessive NDI accounts for the other 10% (Dabrowski et al. 2016; Spanakis et al. 2008).

In ACTH deficiency, reduced cortisol levels may mask the effects of ADH deficiency, and fluid balance should be monitored at the start of hydrocortisone treatment for pituitary deficiency.

In the newborn, ADH excess is more frequent than deficiency and often due to underlying intracranial (e.g., cerebral hypoxic-ischemic) or lung (atrial natriuretic peptide) pathologies. Inappropriate ADH secretion is usually transient. The diagnosis is made by observing urine that is inappropriately concentrated in the presence of a low plasma osmolality. It is treated by fluid restriction (Marcialis et al. 2009).

112.4.3 Investigations

Attention to fluid balance is critical. This is achieved by daily or 12-hourly weighing with serial measurements of the acid-base status, blood concentrations of sodium, potassium, glucose, urea, creatinine, lactate and osmolality, and urine electrolytes and osmolality. Polyuria is defined as urine output (UOP) greater than 2 L/m^2/day, 150 ml/kg/day in neonates.

Urine and blood analysis for reducing substances may be indicated when there is a history of vomiting or jaundice and galactosemia is suspected.

In hyponatremic/hyperkalemic patients, measure plasma 17-OH progesterone (plasma or urine steroid profile with TM spectrometry when available) and karyotype or FISH/PCR for Y fragments in case of genital ambiguity, for the diagnosis of CAH. Plasma renin and aldosterone to exclude deficiency (low aldosterone levels) or resistance (high aldosterone levels).

Ultrasound scans should be performed for the identification of kidney abnormalities (dysplasia, polycystic disease, renal vein thrombosis), adrenal hyperplasia, or hemorrhage. Intracranial abnormalities (e.g., midline defects) in the presence of salt-water imbalance may indicate specific hormonal investigations.

112.4.4 Management

The goal for treating hyponatremia is normalization of the blood sodium concentration by identifying and treating the underlying disease. Patients with mild hyponatremia are almost always asymptomatic. Acute and severe hyponatremia requires prompt and careful administration and monitoring of serum sodium to avoid overcorrection and neurological damage. The long-term treatment depends on the diagnosis. If there is underlying renal disease, involvement by a pediatric nephrologist is indicated.

Management of hypernatremia involves fluid replacement, avoiding neurological complications due to rapid reduction of plasma sodium levels (Marcialis et al. 2009). Fluid balance should be carefully monitored.

When DI is suspected, a vasopressin test may distinguish between central or nephrogenic DI (Ogilvy-Stuart and Midgley 2006). This may be by continuous IV infusion of aqueous vasopressin with a starting dose of 1 mU/kg/h (range 0.5–2.0 mU/kg/h) or DDAVP (IV or SC administration: start with 0.02 mg every 12 h and increase gradually until a suitable response is achieved) or by intranasal solution (start with 0.25 μg every 12 h, increasing gradually according to response; usual maximum dose 5–20 μg every 12 h).

As for Na disturbances, also for hyperkalemia the goal for treatment is normalization of the blood K concentration by identifying and treating the underlying cause. If the cause is likely to be aldosterone deficiency or resistance, it is necessary to replace Na deficit and give Fludrocortisone (see ▶ Chap. 113, "Disorders of Sexual Development in Newborns"). ECG monitoring to see if K needs to be lowered urgently: severe hyperkalemia (K > 8 mmol/L) is life threatening and requires urgent treatment. Calcium resonium (125–250 mg/kg every 6–8 hrs) removes K from the body. Sodium bicarbonate normalizes acid-base balance and will drive K into the cells. Salbutamol infusion (4 mcg/kg over 10 min) facilitates intracellular uptake of K.

If there is evidence of myocardial excitability, calcium gluconate 10% solution (0.5 ml/kg; max 2 ml/kg) will help to prevent arrhythmias. Peritoneal dialysis can be used acutely, under advice from a renal specialist.

112.5 Hypoglycemia and Hyperinsulinism

112.5.1 Hypoglycemia

The definition of the lower normal limit of blood glucose is controversial and cannot be defined by a single value. Normal range should consider many variables such as birth weight, gestational age, clinical conditions, type of sampling, and availability of other energy sources. For a long time, a glucose level <47 mg/dl (2.6 mmol/L) was considered a reliable cut-off to define neonatal hypoglycemia, but this probably led to an overtreatment.

It is important to be aware that the blood glucose concentration usually decreases to 35 mg/dL (1.9 mmol/L) 1–2 h after birth and then rises and about 15% of appropriate for gestational age (AGA) healthy full-term neonates have a blood glucose level <50 mg/dL (2.8 mmol/L) during the first 72 h of life (Committee on Fetus and Newborn and Adamkin 2011; Metzger et al. 2010; Canadian Paediatric Society 2004). Moreover, breastfed term infants have lower concentration of plasma glucose but higher alternative fuels such as ketone bodies and lactate that preserve from brain injury.

In 2000 a concept of "operational threshold" was introduced, identifying cut-off values at which clinicians should consider intervention. For asymptomatic "at risk" newborn, a glucose value <36 mg/dl (2 mmol/L) was adopted, while in case of treatment a target of 47 mg/dl should be aimed. A recent study concluded that neonatal hypoglycemia when treated to maintain a blood glucose level ≥47 mg/dl is not associated with adverse neurological outcomes at 2 years of age despite the number of hypoglycemic events and their severity (McKinlay et al. 2015).

In 2011, the committee on Fetus and Newborn of the American Academy of Pediatrics established new lower intervention limits for asymptomatic late preterm or at-risk term newborns: 25 mg/dl (1.4 mmol/L) in the first 4 h of live and 35 mg/dl from 4 to 24 h of age.

Nevertheless, preterm infants are less able to produce alternative nutrients and are at increased risk of neuroglycopenia; therefore, especially for VLBW infants a blood glucose level above 55 mg/dL (3.1 mmol/L) has been considered safer.

112.5.1.1 Classification and Causes

The overall incidence of hypoglycemia is about 1–5/1000 live births, although it can be as high as 15% among preterm infants and in those with intrauterine growth restriction (IUGR) and 37% of all infants of diabetic mothers.

Low blood glucose levels may be secondary to different mechanisms.

Decreased stores
Placental abnormalities
IUGR
Prematurity
Hyperinsulinemia
Intrapartum glucose
Drug treatment (e.g., propranolol)
Infant of diabetic mother
Severe erythroblastosis fetalis
Other diseases (Table 4)
Other endocrine abnormalities
Panhypopituitarism
Adrenal insufficiency
Hypothyroidism
Increased glucose utilization
Preterms
Severely ill (RDS, sepsis, birth asphyxia)
Hypothermia
Congenital heart disease
Polycythemia
Inadequate production or substrate delivery
Delayed/inadequate feedings
Inborn error of metabolism
Glycogen storage disease

More often hypoglycemia is transient, resolving in the first 72 h of life; when it lasts for many days it is called persistent or recurrent hypoglycemia.

Transient hypoglycemia is mainly due to an impaired or delayed metabolic adaptation after cord clamping or secondary to an increased glucose need:

- IUGR or overgrowth (large for gestational age infants)
- Prematurity or postmaturity
- Maternal diabetes
- Intrapartum administration of glucose
- Perinatal stress (sepsis, birth asphyxia, hypothermia)
- Polycythemia, hyperviscosity
- Maternal drugs (terbutaline, propranolol, oral hypoglycemic agents) (Ghirri et al. 2007)

Persistent or recurrent hypoglycemia is secondary to other diseases:

- Hyperinsulinism: actually 11 genes have been associated with monogenic forms of hyperinsulinism (ABCC8, KCNJ11, GLUD1, GCK, HADH1, UCP2, MCT1, HNF4A, HNF1A, HK1, PGM1); other forms of hyperinsulinism are associates with other syndromes

(e.g., Beckwith-Wiedemann syndrome, Sotos syndrome) (Stanley 2016) see Table 4
- Endocrine disorders: deficiency of GH, glucagon, cortisol, thyroid hormones, epinephrine
- Inborn errors of carbohydrate metabolism: glycogen storage disease, glycogen synthase deficiency, galactosemia, fructose intolerance
- Inborn errors of amino acid metabolism: maple syrup urine disease, propionic acidemia, methylmalonic acidemia, hereditary tyrosinemia, 3-hydroxy-3-methyl glutaric acidemia, glutaric acidemia type II
- Inborn errors of fatty acid metabolism: defects of carnitine metabolism, acyl-coenzyme dehydrogenase defects

112.5.1.2 Clinical Presentation

Usually hypoglycemia is asymptomatic, even at extremely low levels of blood glucose. This suggests that neuroglycopenia and consequent brain injury cannot be defined by a single glucose value.

Symptomatic hypoglycemia may present with nonspecific symptoms:

- Irritability, lethargy, abnormal cry, coma
- Sucking difficulty
- Tremors, seizures
- Pallor, cyanosis, sweating
- Hypothermia
- Hypotonia
- Apnea, irregular respiration
- Tachycardia

Any newborn with unexplained nonspecific signs and symptoms should have their blood glucose levels checked.

112.5.1.3 Screening

Healthy term newborns need no monitoring of blood glucose levels.

All sick infants and newborn with nonspecific unexplained symptoms should undergo blood glucose check.

Infants at risk for compromised adaptation should be monitored:

- SGA (<10th percentile), LGA (>90th percentile), or intrauterine growth restriction
- Infants of diabetic mothers (IDMs)

Table 4 Causes of hyperinsulinism

Condition	Inheritance	Features
Genetic forms		
Recessive K_{ATP} hyperinsulinism	AR	LGA at birth; unresponsive to diazoxide therapy
Focal K_{ATP} hyperinsulinism		Histologically appears as adenomatosis; LGA at birth, unresponsive to diazoxide therapy
Dominant K_{ATP} hyperinsulinism	AD	LGA at birth; responsive to diazoxide therapy; hypoglycemia present at birth or later in infancy
GCK hyperinsulinism	AD	Responsive to diazoxide therapy; hypoglycemia present at birth or later in infancy
GDH hyperinsulinism	AD	Persistent symptomatic hypoglycemia and persistent asymptomatic hyperammonemia; responsive to diazoxide therapy
SCHAD hyperinsulinism	AD	Responsive to diazoxide therapy; severe hypoglycemia
Other		
Beckwith-Wiedemann syndrome	Various	LGA at birth; macroglossia, abdominal wall defects, hypoglycemia
Sotos syndrome		Macrocephaly, large hands and feet, hypertelorism, sometimes hypoglycemia
Pancreatic adenoma		
Oral sulfonylurea drugs		

AR autosomal recessive, *AD* autosomal dominant, *GDH* glutamate dehydrogenase, *SCHAD* short chain 3-hydroxyacyl CoA dehydrogenase

- Preterm infants
- Septic neonates
- Birth weight < 2000 g or >4000 g
- Birth asphyxia, respiratory distress, low Apgar score, shock, polycythemia
- Neonates of mother treated with hypoglycemia-inducing drugs (terbutaline/propranolol/lebatolol/oral hypoglycemic agents)
- Suspected inborn error of metabolism
- Macroglossia or hemihypertrophy (Beckwith-Wiedeman syndrome)

Most of neonatal guidelines suggest evaluating the first blood glucose levels at 1–2 h of life; nevertheless, since blood glucose levels usually fall in the first hours of life, interventions in asymptomatic at risk newborns should be carefully evaluated during this early period.

The duration of glucose levels monitoring varies for different categories of neonates. Large for gestational age infants and infants of diabetic mothers usually have hypoglycemia within 12 h; therefore, glucose monitoring may be discontinued at this time if there is normoglycemia. Small for gestational age infants and preterms may have a later fall in glucose level and hence blood glucose levels should be monitored for 24–36 h.

112.5.1.4 Diagnosis

Semiquantitative measurement of blood glucose levels should be used only as a screening test. To confirm the diagnosis, plasma or serum glucose levels should be measured in the laboratory by chemical analysis. In case of symptomatic hypoglycemia IV treatment should be promptly started without waiting laboratory confirmation.

Plasma glucose levels are about 10–18% higher than blood levels.

In case of persistent or recurrent hypoglycemia, many other investigations may be performed. Samples should be taken during an episode of hypoglycemia.

First stage investigations:

- Insulin and C-peptide
- Ketone bodies in urine
- Insulin/glucose (I/G) ratio
- Ultrasound imaging of pancreas

An I/G ratio > 0.30 suggests a hyperinsulinemic hypoglycemia. The diagnosis of hyperinsulinism in fact is based on inappropriately high insulin levels for blood glucose levels more than the single value of insulin.

Second stage investigations:

- Cortisol, ACTH
- GH
- fT3, fT4, TSH
- Glucagon
- Free fatty acid
- Amino acids (serum and urine)
- Organic acids (urine)
- Lactate, pyruvate, urate, acetoacetate
- Ammonia
- IGF-I, IGF-BPs
- CT scan of the pancreas

112.5.1.5 Prevention

Whenever possible, hypoglycemia should be prevented, especially in at-risk infants.

Skin to skin contact help to prevent hypothermia and to stabilize blood glucose levels; it should be encouraged in all healthy infants, while sick or preterm infants should be placed in incubator.

Moreover, early feeding should be started within 30–60 min after birth with breastmilk, expressed breast milk, or infant formula. Feedings should be as frequent as 8–10 times per day. If the baby is unable to feed, gavage should be considered.

Very low birth weight neonates should have an early initiation of 10% dextrose IV infusion.

112.5.1.6 Management

In case of symptomatic hypoglycemia (BGL <45 mg/dl), urgent IV treatment is required. A bolus of 2 ml/kg of 10% dextrose should be administered quickly, followed by a continuous infusion at 5–7 mg/kg/min (80–100 ml/kg/day of 10% dextrose). If IV access should not be promptly placed, IM glucagon (200 mg/kg) should be administered.

If hypoglycemia persists despite an IV infusion, glucose concentration should be progressively increased up to 20–25%. Concentration greater than 12.5% must be administered using a central line. The glucose concentration target after IV infusion started is above 47 m/dl. In case of refractory hypoglycemia, additional drugs may be used.

Severe hypoglycemia is defined as a blood glucose level < 20–25 mg/dl or <47 mg/dl despite glucose infusion >10–12 mg/kg/min.

Asymptomatic healthy newborns should be managed conservatively as long as possible. If hypoglycemia is detected, the infant should be promptly refed and glucose levels rechecked 30–60 min later; if hypoglycemia persists, IV treatment should be considered.

A recent trial suggests that 40% dextrose oral gel may be more effective than feeding alone to prevent IV treatment (Harris et al. 2013).

After IV infusion has been commenced blood glucose levels should be rechecked after 30 min and adjusted to maintain euglycemia. BGL should be revaluated 30 min after any change of IV infusion rate and prefeed as IV therapy reduces. IV infusion may be decreased once BGL remains stable for 12 h.

Persistent or Recurrent Hypoglycemia In case of persistent or recurrent hypoglycemia, other treatments should be considered in association with IV glucose infusion:

Corticosteroids: hydrocortisone (2.5 mg/kg over 3–5 min bid or tid).

Diazoxide: PO 2–5 mg/kg tid; start with 5 mg/kg tid and reduce to the minimal dose effective. It is useful in hyperinsulinemic hypoglycemia. Concurrent administration of a diuretic (e.g., hydrochlorathiazide 3.5 mg/kg bid) is recommended → reduce fluid retention due to diazoxide use and enhance diazoxide effects on blood sugar levels. Control blood pressure and glucose levels. If hypoglycemia is not responsive to 15 mg/kg/day, start octreotide infusion.

Octreotide: starting dose 1 μg/kg qid IV or SC. Increase according to clinical effect to a maximum of 10 μg/kg qid. Some success in insulinomas and neonatal persistent hypoglycemia (nesidioblastosis). Recently the combination of octreotide with glucagon IV infusion (0.01–0.02 mg/kg/h → max 1 mg/24 h) has been reported for severe hypoglycemia secondary to hyperinsulinism. Monitor ECG and glucose levels during infusion.

Growth hormone: 0.1–0.2 U/day SC; administer only when GH deficiency is confirmed.

Pancreatectomy: subtotal or total pancreatectomy following unsuccessful medical treatment of persistent neonatal hypoglycemia due to hyperinsulinism (Fourtner and Stanley 2004).

112.5.2 Beckwith-Wiedemann Syndrome

Beckwith-Wiedemann syndrome (BWS) is the commonest overgrowth disorder which occurs in about one out of every 13–17,000 live births.

Typical clinical features and their frequency are reported in Table 5.

112.5.2.1 Etiology

Only 15% of cases are familial due to complex inheritance. Chromosomal abnormalities in the highly imprinted region at chromosome 11p15.5 have been reported both in sporadic and familial cases (see Table 6) (Elliott et al. 1994). Several genes in the 11p region have been implicated, e.g., CDKN1C, IGF-2, and H19.

Diagnosis is based on clinical findings and on analysis of the 11p15 region.

Table 5 Main clinical features of BWS

Clinical findings	Frequency
Macrosomia (weight and length)	90%
Macroglossia Visceromegaly (liver, kidney, spleen)	80%
Anterior abdominal wall defects (omphalocele, umbilical hernia, diastasis recti abdominis)	80%
Ear defects (creases or pit)	75%
Craniofacial anomalies (midface hypoplasia, a prominent occiput, and nevus flammeus)	60–70%
Hypoglycemia	50%
Cardiac defects	25%
Hemihypertrophy (↑ risk for cancer)	10–15%
Tumors (Wilms' tumor, hepatoblastoma, adrenal carcinoma, nephroblastoma)	7–20%

Table 6 Genetic alterations in BWS (Ibrahim et al. 2014)

Alterations detected on 11p15.5 region	Frequency[a]
Methylation abnormalities (IC2/IC1 hypermethylation)	55–65%
Paternal uniparental disomy	10–20%
CDKN1C mutations	5–10%
Duplication, translocation, inversion	1–2%

[a]In patients with a "certain" clinical diagnosis of BWS

112.5.2.2 Management and Prognosis

A recent protocol suggests a strict follow-up (Mussa et al. 2016):

At birth:

- Complete blood cell count to assess polycythemia
- Glycemia and insulin
- TSH and fT4 (congenital hypothyroidism)
- Renal function: creatinine, serum electrolytes, and urinary calcium to creatinine excretion ratio to detect and monitor hypercalciuria (one third of patients)
- Abdominal ultrasound: assess organomegaly, in order to estimate Wilms' tumor risk, urinary tract malformations, and abdominal masses
- ECG to exclude rhythm abnormalities (e.g., long QT syndrome)
  Echocardiography (cardiomegaly or cardiac malformations)
- Limbs/spine X-ray (if orthopedic indication)
- Second-level imaging techniques (e.g., tongue magnetic resonance, abdominal organs MR or CT scan)
- Individualized consultations as needed: orthopedic, nephrourologist, odontostomatologist and maxillofacial surgery, general pediatric surgery

Subsequent follow-up:

- Blood alpha fetoprotein (AFP) every 3 months until 4 years of age (hepatoblastoma)
- Abdominal ultrasound should be performed every 3–4 months until the age of 8 years for Wilms' tumor early recognition and treatment. Subsequent follow-up should be performed yearly
- Periodical clinical and auxometric evaluation: every 3 months in the first year of life, every 4 months in the second year, every 6 months until 8 years of age, and then every 12 months
- Yearly blood examination: complete blood count, liver enzymes, creatinine, glycemia, urinalysis, urinary calcium to creatinine excretion

112.6 Hyperglycemia

The definition of the upper normal limit of blood glucose in the newborn remains uncertain. A blood glucose level higher than 125 mg/dL (6.9 mmol/L) or plasma glucose level > 150 mg/dL, regardless of gestational age or postnatal age, is usually considered abnormal (Rozance and Hay 2010). Nevertheless, most neonatologists tolerate blood glucose levels of 180–200 mg/dL (10–11.1 mmol/L) in preterm infants.

Hyperglycemia is relatively common in extremely low birth weight infants (ELBW) and in SGA as a consequence of impaired glucose homeostasis. The incidence is inversely related to birth weight and gestational age. About 80% of neonates <750 g are hyperglycemic during the first days of life. In full-term appropriately grown newborns (AGA), hyperglycemia is rare and mainly affects seriously ill neonates.

Neonatal diabetes mellitus is an extremely rare cause of hyperglycemia that occurs in about 1:400,000 live births (Aguilar-Bryan and Bryan 2008).

112.6.1 Causes

Hyperglycemia may be due to different mechanisms:

- Impaired glucose homeostasis: preterm and SGA infants
- Iatrogenic hyperglycemia: excessive intravenous glucose infusion
- Drugs: corticosteroids, caffeine, theophylline and phenytoin or maternal diazoxide

- Stress: sepsis, intraventricular hemorrhage, birth asphyxia, painful procedures
- Neonatal diabetes mellitus: transient or permanent
- Absence of enteral feeding: diminished "incretin" secretion

Sometimes, more factors may be responsible for high glucose levels: in VLBW infants it is often due to a combination of high glucose IV infusion with parenteral nutrition, low presence of insulin dependent tissues (fat and muscle), reduced ability to inhibit gluconeogenesis in response to intravenous glucose, and high levels of stress hormones (catecholamine, glucocorticoids).

112.6.2 Screening

Screening for hyperglycemia should be performed in "at risk" neonates:

- Preterm infants
- Infants with IV infusion or parenteral infusion
- Sick infants
- Infants who presented glycosuria

112.6.3 Clinical Presentation and Complications

Hyperglycemia is often asymptomatic. More frequent presenting symptoms are polyuria, dehydration with electrolytes imbalance, failure to thrive, and sporadically ketoacidosis.

Rarely, in case of severe and persistent hyperglycemia, seizures, intracranial hemorrhage, and hyperosmolar coma have been reported (each 18 mg/dL rise in blood glucose causes an increase in serum osmolarity of 1 mOsm/L).

Hyperglycemia has been also associated with high sepsis and mortality rates.

112.6.4 Diagnosis

Semiquantitative evaluation of blood glucose levels by reagent strips should only be carried out for screening. To confirm the diagnosis and before starting treatment, plasma or serum glucose concentrations should be measured by quantitative chemical analysis.

Plasma glucose levels are about 15% higher than blood levels because of the presence of erythrocytes which metabolize glucose.

112.6.5 Other Investigations

In case of unexplained hyperglycemia, sepsis should be immediately ruled out.

Other investigations consist of:

- Acid/base status (diabetic ketoacidosis)
- Serum osmolarity
- Urine glucose level (osmotic diuresis)

  In case of persistent unexplained hyperglycemia, other investigations may be carried out:
- Blood insulin concentration
- Blood C-peptide concentration
- Genetic investigations for neonatal diabetes mellitus

112.6.6 Treatment

It is important to remind that hyperglycemia may be secondary to other severe diseases and treatment of the underlying problems is much more important than to correct glucose levels alone.

The cut-off value at which treatment should be started is not universally accepted. Some authors suggest to treat hyperglycemia only in case of significant glucosuria ($\geq$1000 mg/dl) that may lead to dehydration and electrolyte imbalance. Unfortunately, in extremely preterm and sick infants glucosuria may not be so reliable a marker because of decreased renal tubular reabsorptive capacity and consequently glucosuria at normal glucose plasma levels.

Management of hyperglycemia is based on a glucose restriction or exogenous insulin infusion or a combination of both. Insulin infusion allows to maintain an higher glucose provision and an higher caloric intake with a short-term growth improvement. Nevertheless, no improvement of mortality or major morbidity has been reported in the case of insulin infusion compared with glucose restriction.

A possible approach is to initially reduce glucose infusion to reach a glycemic control; in case of failure of this strategy, an IV insulin infusion may be started (Fig. 4). Insulin may even be considered in case of failure to thrive secondary to caloric restriction.

In case of IV insulin infusion, a target of 150–200 mg/dl of blood glucose levels should be targeted; lower levels have been associated with higher risk of hypoglycemia.

112.7 Neonatal Diabetes Mellitus

Neonatal diabetes mellitus (NDM) is a rare monogenic metabolic disorder which presents as uncontrolled hyperglycemia during the first 6 months of life. The estimated incidence is about 1/300,000–500,000 live births. Two different clinical phenotypes have been recognized: transient neonatal diabetes mellitus (TNDM) and permanent diabetes mellitus (PNDM), which differ in the duration of insulin dependence. In TNDM, insulin treatment may be discontinued within 18 months after diagnosis although about 50% relapse during childhood or adulthood. PNDM require treatment for life.

Almost all neonates affected by NDM are SGA, although some with PNDM are not SGA (Aguilar-Bryan and Bryan 2008).

112.7.1 Etiology

About 60–70% of patients affected by TNDM show abnormalities in the 6q24 region. TNDM

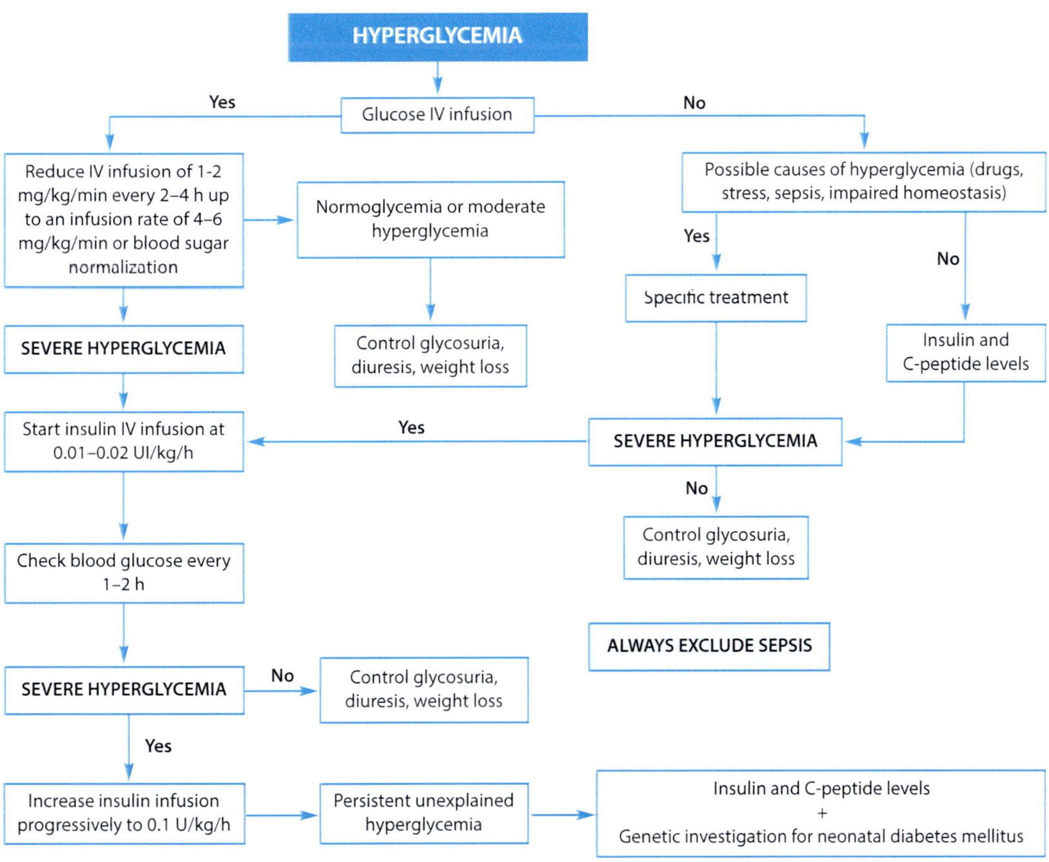

Fig. 4 The management of hyperglycemia. Based on evidence from (Bottino et al. 2009)

is usually sporadic, although about one third of cases have paternal transmission (paternal duplications, paternal isodisomy, methylation defect).

Most patients with PNDM carry mutations of the KATP channel (50–70%). Other genetic defects associated with PNDM are less common (Table 7).

112.7.2 Clinical Presentation

NDM presents as hyperglycemia, failure to thrive, dehydration, and ketoacidosis during the first months of life. TNDM usually onsets early, often in the first week of life, while PNDM onset later, generally within 3 months of life.

PNDM may occur as an isolated abnormality or as a part of a syndrome (Table 7). Patients with mutations of the ATP-sensitive potassium (KATP) channel (*KCNJ11* and *ABCC8* genes) may present with DEND syndrome (delayed development, epilepsy, NDM) or iDEND phenotype (DEND without epilepsy).

112.7.3 Diagnosis

Persistent unexplained hyperglycemia during the first 6 months of life should be investigated for NDM. TNDM patients are usually younger and have lower insulin requirements. PNDM cannot be generally differentiated from TNDM on the basis of clinical features alone. Genetic investigations (chromosome 6, *KCNJ11*, *ABCC8*) allow the diagnosis for the majority of patients affected by NDM (Colombo et al. 2008).

First line examination involves insulin and C-peptide. Second line examination involves genetic investigations.

112.7.4 Prognosis

Prognosis is related to the severity of the disease and to the rapidity of diagnosis and treatment. PNDM associated with other syndromes has a variable prognosis. Patients affected by TNDM should have long-term follow-up because of the risk of later relapse.

112.7.5 Treatment

Insulin therapy and high caloric intake are crucial for good metabolic control. We recommend the initial administration of intravenous insulin at 0.01–0.02 U/kg/h, adjusted according to blood

Table 7 Genes involved and clinical features of neonatal diabetes mellitus

Condition	Chromosome	Inheritance	Neonatal features
β-cell dysfunction			
ABCC8	11p15.1	AD	NDM +/− DEND
KCNJ11	11p15.1	AD	NDM +/− DEND o iDEND
Glucokinase	7p15–13	AR	PNDM
β-cell mass reduction			
FOXP3	Xp11.23-Xq13.3	X-linked	Exfoliative dermatitis, diarrhea, hemolitic anemia, thyreopathy, PNDM (IPEX syndrome)
INS	11p15	AD	PNDM
EIF2AK3	2p12	AR	PNDM, spondyloepiphysel dysplasia, hepatomegaly, renal failure, mental retardation (Wolcott-Rallison syndrome)
Abnormal islet development			
HNF1b	17cen-q21.3	AD	TNDM, renal abnormalities, genital malformation
PTF1 a	10p12.3	AR	PNDM, cerebellar hypoplasia
IPF1	13q21.1	AR	Pancreatic agenesis (PNDM and exocrine failure)
GLIS 3	9p	AR	PNDM, hypothyroidism

AR autosomal recessive, *AD* autosomal dominant

glucose levels, followed by subcutaneous ultralente insulin at 0.4–0.6 U/kg/24 h.

When good metabolic control has been achieved, switching to oral sulfanylurea therapy may be attempted in patients affected by the *KCNJ11* and *ABCC8* gene mutations. The dose of glibenclamide may be as high as 0.8 mg/kg/day (Colombo et al. 2008).

112.8 Hypocalcemia

Neonatal hypocalcemia has not an univocal definition in literature: lower limit of total serum calcium concentration has been variously fixed from 7 mg/dl to 8 mg/dl (1.75–2 mmol/L). Moreover, a distinction between term and preterm infants has been sometimes proposed using 8 mg/dl for term infants and 7 mg/dl for preterms. Lastly, inonized calcium (<1.1 mmol/L) has been used to define hypocalcemia because of a more reliability in certain situations such as preterm birth (see also ► Chap. 41, "Calcium and Phosphorus Homeostasis: Pathophysiology").

This variability is mainly due to frequent lack of clinical findings in large number of neonates even at low calcium concentration.

Physiological hypocalcemia occurs after birth as a consequence of the end of transplacental calcium transfer, of the insufficient supply through feeding, and of the immaturity of the parathyroid glands with consequent reduced secretion of parathyroid hormone (PTH). The nadir in calcium levels occurs during the first 36–48 h of life.

Hypocalcemia is relatively common in neonates, affecting 30% of very low birth weight infants and 80–90% of infants born below 32 weeks (Bringhurst et al. 2008; Ogilvy-Stuart and Midgerly 2006).

112.8.1 Clinical Presentation

Hypocalcemia is often asymptomatic. Clinical presentation includes nonspecific symptoms and signs such as neuromuscular irritability (tremulousness, myoclonic jerks, exaggerated startle responses, seizures), lethargy, apnea, cyanosis, tachypnea, poor feeding, abdominal distension, vomiting, laryngospasm, tachycardia, prolonged QT interval on ECG, decreased myocardial contractility, and heart failure.

112.8.2 Causes and Differential Diagnosis

Neonatal hypocalcemia has been classified by the time of onset in early or late onset forms (Table 8).

To reach a correct diagnosis it is important to collect a medical history focused on specific conditions and to perform a meticulous physical examination.

The history should consider maternal, peripartum, and postnatal events such as maternal diabetes, intrauterine growth restriction, preeclapsia, preterm delivery, perinatal asphyxia, maternal diseases, or drugs assumption. The clinical examination should look for signs and symptoms of hypocalcemia and for dysmorphic features attributable to the 22q deletion syndrome (DiGeorge syndrome: cardiac defect, facial dysmorphisms, thymic aplasia, cleft palate) or to other syndromes.

Early onset hypocalcemia is usually self-limiting although hypocalcemia due to maternal hyperparathyroidism may be prolonged. Late onset hypocalcemia is often iatrogenic but vitamin D deficiency, renal failure, and parathyroid related disorders should be excluded (Tables 8 and 9).

112.8.3 Investigations

In case of persistent or recurrent unexplained hypocalcemia, further investigation should be performed:

- Total and ionized calcium, phosphorus, magnesium, alkaline phosphatase
- pH, blood total protein, creatinine, and electrolyte concentrations
- Blood parathyroid hormone, 25-OH vitamin D, 1,25-OH vitamin D concentrations
- Molecular genetic studies (if indicated)
- Urinary calcium, phosphorus, creatinine, cyclic adenosine monophosphate (cAMP) concentrations – Measure calcium/creatinine ratio, tubular reabsorption of phosphate

Table 8 Causes of hypocalcemia

Timing and causes	Mechanism
Early onset (within 72–96 h)	
Preterm birth	Poor intake, increased calcitonin, decreased responsiveness to vitamin D, hypoalbuminemia (decreased total but normal ionized calcium)
Perinatal asphyxia	Increased calcitonin production and endogenous phosphate load, alkali therapy
Infant of diabetic mother	Hypomagnesemia in the mother and the fetus leading to hypoparathyroidism in the infant
Preeclampsia	
Maternal hyperparathyroidism	Hypercalcemia with suppression of parathyroid activity in the fetus and the newborn (hypocalcemia may be prolonged)
Maternal drugs	Anticonvulsants
Late onset (after 96 h)	
Iatrogenic	Excessive intake of phosphate (phosphate therapy, feeding with phosphate-rich formula or cow's milk), citrated blood products, lipid infusion, bicarbonate therapy, loop diuretics and thiazide diuretics, glucocorticoids, *gentamicin use*
Osteopenia of prematurity	Reduced calcium and phosphorus and increased ALP and PTH
Parathyroid related disorders	See Table 9
Vitamin D deficiency and resistance	Maternal deficiency of vitamin D often associated with use of anticonvulsants, inherited disorders of vitamin D metabolism (impaired 1-α-idroxilation-vitamin D dependent rickets type I and rarely 25-α-idroxilation), resistance to actions of vitamin D (vitamin D dependent rickets type II)
Malabsorption of calcium or vitamin D	
Renal failure	

– Maternal serum calcium and phosphorus concentrations

Maternal hyperparathyroidism is characterized by high calcium, phosphorus, and parathyroid hormone (PTH) levels, whereas calcium and vitamin D levels are low in maternal vitamin D deficiency. Hypocalcemia associated with parathyroid dysfunction is distinguished by low serum calcium, increased serum phosphate, and low or undetectable PTH levels. Inappropriately normal PTH levels may be present if some degree of PTH production is preserved. Serum $1{,}25(OH)_2D_3$ is low because PTH and hypophosphatemia are the main stimuli for the production of renal 25(OH)D 1α-hydroxylase. Elevated levels of PTH are present in syndromes associated with target organ resistance to PTH. Hypomagnesemia and respiratory alkalosis can cause transient abnormality of PTH secretion and target organ resistance to PTH.

Hypocalcemia secondary to vitamin D deficiency, inherited disorders of vitamin D metabolism, or peripheral resistance to the action of vitamin D is differentiated by the presence of hypophosphatemia and elevated PTH levels.

In severe vitamin D deficiency or inherited disorders of vitamin D metabolism, the level of $1{,}25(OH)_2D_3$ is low. In moderate vitamin D deficiency, $1{,}25(OH)_2D_3$ levels may be normal or high due to the stimulation of the renal 1a-hydroxylase by PTH and hypophosphatemia. Levels of $1{,}25(OH)D_3$ may be high when there is peripheral resistance to the action of vitamin D (Table 8).

112.8.4 Congenital Parathyroid Disorders

Among some rare syndromes, hypoparathyroidism is associated with multiple malformations with various inheritance patterns (Table 9). Familial isolated hypoparathyroidism is caused by a mutation in the gene for the transcription factor *GCMB*, which is expressed in the PTH-secreting cells of the developing parathyroid (Ding et al. 2001). An interstitial deletion/insertion at *Xq27.1* near *SOX3* gene is responsible for X-linked

Table 9 Parathyroid related disorders

Classification and mechanism	Diseases
Congenital or inherited parathyroid disorders	
Aplasia or hypoplasia	DiGeorge syndrome, Velocardiofacial syndrome, HDR syndrome, Kenny-Caffey syndrome, Kearns-Sayre syndrome, X-linked or autosomally inherited hypoparathyroidism, Vater association, Charge association, fetal exposure to retinoic acid
Impaired secretion of PTH	PTH gene mutations, activating mutations of the calcium sensing receptor
Target organ resistance	Pseudohypoparathyroidism Type I (IA, IB, IC), Type II, pseudo-pseudohypoparathyroidism
Noncongenital causes of parathyroid disorders	Hypomagnesemia, gestational diabetes mellitus, respiratory alkalosis, neonatal hypoparathyroism secondary to maternal hyperparathyroidism

hypoparathyroidism (Bowl et al. 2005). Specific mutations in the parathyroid hormone gene have been found in families affected by congenital hypoparathyroidism (Sunthornthepvarakul et al. 1999).

Activating mutations in the calcium sensing receptor causes impaired PTH secretion and hypocalcemia with inappropriately normal PTH levels. There is clinical variability with cases affected by hypocalcemia and seizures and cases with asymptomatic hypocalcemia in the same family (Pearce et al. 1996). The term pseudohypoparathyroidism (PHP) refers to congenital forms of PTH resistance when hypocalcemia is associated with increased PTH levels and the administration of PTH fails to increase serum calcium levels and causes a phosphate diuresis. The first cases of PTH resistance were described by Albright. These patients were hypocalcemic and hyperphosphatemic and showed several features (rounded face, foreshortened fourth and other metacarpals, subcutaneous calcifications, short stature, obesity) that are now included in the syndrome, Albright's hereditary osteodystrophy (AHO). The classification of pseudohypoparathyroidism (see Appendix, p. 987) (Farfel et al. 1999) is based on the variable presence of AHO and renal resistance to PTH.

112.8.5 Treatment

Oral treatment with calcium gluconate 10% (3–4 mL/kg/day of (1 mL = 9.4 mg of elemental calcium) in divided doses) should be given to babies with mild to moderate asymptomatic hypocalcemia (<1 mmol/L) or with mild neuromuscular irritability. Oral supplementation should be avoided for neonates at risk of necrotizing enterocolitis.

If there is symptomatic hypocalcemia, especially cardiac arrhythmias or seizures, an IV treatment should be used: 1–2 mL/kg of diluted solution of calcium gluconate 10% slowly over 10 min (risk of bradycardia or cardiac asystole). The use of a central line is preferred. Maintenance IV treatment should be continued at 2–6 mL/kg/day.

The concomitant presence of hypomagnesemia may lead to refractory hypocalcemia: give an initial dose of 100 mg/kg IV over 30 min of magnesium sulfate (0.2 ml/kg of 50% solution) or as an IM injection and then continue with 20–50 mg/kg/h of diluted solution.

Hypoparathyroidism should be treated with alphacalcidiol 0.02–0.05 μg/kg/day.

If vitamin D deficiency is present, it should be treated first with oral supplementation: 5–50 μg/day (200–2000 U/day).

There is a single case report of recombinant PTH therapy in infants: safety and long-term effects are not known (Mannstadt et al. 2013).

112.9 Hypercalcemia

Hypercalcemia can be defined as ionized calcium (iCa) > 1.36 mmol/L (5.44 mg/dL) or total calcium (tCa) concentration > 2.75 mmol/L (11 mg/dL). tCa and iCa usually increase simultaneously, but tCa is not predictive of iCa. Therefore, iCa should be always evaluated for a correct diagnosis. During the neonatal period, hypercalcemia is less common than hypocalcemia.

112.9.1 Clinical Presentation

Mild hypercalcemia is often asymptomatic. Moderate to severe hypercalcemia usually presents with nonspecific signs and symptoms: anorexia, vomiting, constipation, lethargy or irritability, hypotonia, seizures, coma, hypertension, polyuria and dehydration, bradycardia, and shortening of the QT interval on the ECG. In its chronic form, the most common presentation is failure to thrive.

Physical examination is usually normal, except when there are syndromes, subcutaneous fat necrosis, ore bone deformities that may affect patients with severe hyperparathyroidism.

112.9.2 Causes

Hypercalcemia may be due to iatrogenic causes, increased bone turnover, or excessive intestinal or renal absorption.

Iatrogenic hypercalcemia is the most common form and should always be ruled out before investigating other forms (Table 10).

Neonatal hyperparathyroidism may be a rare cause of neonatal hypercalcemia. It can be primary or secondary to maternal pathological conditions, and it may become clinically manifest during the first 6 months of life.

Secondary Hyperparathyroidism It is due to maternal disease. Hypocalcemia, hypoparathyroidism, or pseudohypoparathyroidism during pregnancy may lead to transient neonatal hyperparathyroidism. The prognosis is good and bone disease usually resolves within few months.

Table 10 Causes of hypercalcemia

Causes	Description
Iatrogenic	Excessive intake of calcium or vitamin A (increased bone resorption) or vitamin D (increased intestinal uptake); thiazide diuretics (reduced renal clearance); phosphate deficiency (especially in VLBW infants with low phosphate in parenteral nutrition)
Parathyroid related	Secondary hyperparathyroidism: maternal hypocalcemia, hypoparathyroidism, or pseudohypoparathyroidism. Primary hyperparathyroidism: familial hypocalciuric hypercalcemia, neonatal severe hyperparathyroidism
Syndromic form	Williams syndrome, Jansen's metaphyseal chondrodysplasia, Blue diaper syndrome, idiopathic infantile hypercalcemia; IMAGe syndrome (IUGR, metaphyseal dysplasia, adrenal hypoplasia congenita, and genital anomalies)
Other form Subcutaneous fat necrosis	Excessive intestinal calcium uptake due to increased 1,25$(OH)_2D_3$ production from macrophages infiltrating the lesion
Distal renal tubular acidosis	Acidosis enhance calcium bone resorption; reduced renal excretion is secondary to reduced glomerular filtration rate
Severe infantile hypophosphatasia	Severe hypercalcemia and bone deformity; low ALP
Congenital endocrine diseases (congenital hypothyroidism, adrenal insufficiency)	Unknown mechanism
Metabolic disorders	Congenital carbohydrate malabsorption (disaccharidase deficiency, congenital lactase, glucose-galactose or sucrase-isomaltase deficiency), glycogen storage disease type 1a
Tumor-related hypercalcemia	Increased production of PTH-related protein (hepatic sarcoma, renal adenoma, rhabdoid tumors)

Primary Hyperparathyroidism

- Familial hypocalciuric hypercalcemia is due to an inactivating mutation (autosomal dominant heterozygous) of the CaSR gene. Familial hypocalciuric hypercalcemia usually presents with an asymptomatic hypercalcemia, hypophosphatemia, mild hypermagnesemia, moderate hypocalciuria, and inappropriately normal PTH. Hyperparathyroidism may resolve over several months.
- Neonatal severe hyperparathyroidism is due to homozygous or double heterozygous mutations of the CaSR gene. Neonatal severe hyperparathyroidism presents with severe hypercalcemia, bone demineralization, and hyperparathyroidism. Hypotonia, constipation, and respiratory distress usually occur during the first days of life and may lead to death within a few weeks. Total parathyroidectomy and partial autotransplantation, and, more recently, pamidronate treatment may improve the outcome.

Williams Syndrome It is related to a microdeletion of chromosome 7 (q11.23). It is characterized by inconstant hypercalcemia, elfin facies, cardiovascular disease (80% have supravalvar aortic stenosis), and mental retardation.

Jansen's Metaphyseal Chondrodysplasia It is attributable to a heterozygous mutation in the parathyroid hormone receptor (PTHR) which is situated in the kidney, bone, and growth plate. At birth, these children may have either a normal phenotype or micrognathia, prominent eyes, hypertelorism, and progressive short-limbed dwarfism.

Blue Diaper Syndrome It is a familial disease resulting from a defect in the intestinal transport of tryptophan. Hypercalcemia and nephrocalcinosis are usually manifest a few months after birth. The blue color of the urine is due to a tryptophan metabolite. The clinical presentation is with failure to thrive, gastrointestinal disturbances, recurrent fever, and irritability.

Idiopathic Infantile Hypercalcemia It is often considered part of Williams syndrome. The clinical phenotype is variable, but symptomatic hypercalcemia generally resolves during childhood. Hypercalcemia is secondary to increased intestinal calcium absorption, although the pathogenesis and inheritance are not clear.

Subcutaneous Fat Necrosis (SFN) It may induce hypercalcemia probably due to excessive intestinal calcium uptake because of increased $1,25(OH)_2D_3$ production in the lesion. SFN usually affects large for gestational age term newborns with birth trauma. There have been reports of SFN following hypothermia and birth asphyxia. It presents as indurated plaques or nodules. Hypercalcemia is rarely associated with SFN but is a severe complication which may lead to death if not promptly treated (Ghirri et al. 1999).

Severe Infantile Hypophosphatasia It is an autosomal recessive disorder (chromosome 1) associated with extremely low serum and tissue alkaline phosphatase. These patients have severe bone demineralization. The clinical presentation ranges from a lethal form that presents soon after birth to a milder form that presents later. Laboratory findings include hypercalcemia, low serum alkaline phosphatase, and high urinary pyrophosphate and phosphoethanolamine concentrations.

Tumor Related Hypercalcemia It (paraneoplastic syndrome) is secondary to an elevated level of PTHrP that leads to osteoclast resorption of bone, renal reabsorption of calcium, and renal loss of phosphate.

112.9.3 Diagnostic Evaluation

Hypercalcemia should be evaluated whenever a blood ionized calcium concentration >1.36 mmol/L (5.44 mg/dL) and/or total serum calcium concentration > 2.75 mmol/L (11 mg/dL) is found.

Nevertheless in the presence of acidemia or hypoalbuminemia, total serum calcium concentration may be normal in the presence of high ionized calcium levels.

Calcium, phosphorus, vitamin A, and vitamin D intake of the mother and baby should be assessed. History of birth trauma (subcutaneous fat necrosis), drugs during pregnancy, and inherited disease should be ruled out.

First stage investigations:

- Electrolytes: total and ionized blood calcium, phosphorus, and magnesium concentrations
- Blood: pH, total protein and albumin, creatinine, alkaline phosphatase concentrations
- Urine: calcium, phosphorus, creatinine concentrations
- Other investigations: ECG, chest and limb X-rays, renal ultrasound

Second stage investigations:

- Parathyroid hormone, 25-OH vitamin D, 1,25-OH vitamin D, parathyroid hormone-related protein (PTHrP)
- Molecular genetic studies

112.9.4 Management

Asymptomatic mild hypercalcemia should be managed conservatively.

Hypercalcemia following maternal hypocalcemia is reduced by appropriate intake of Ca/P.

Moderate to severe hypercalcemia requires prompt intervention:

- Limit Ca and vitamin D intake (suspend oral/parenteral supplementation)
- Hyperhydration with normal saline (about twice maintenance requirements)
- Loop diuretics (furosemide 2 mg/kg) to increase calciuria → avoid dehydration and electrolyte imbalance (Fig. 5)

112.9.4.1 Other Specific Interventions

Prednisone (2 mg/kg) → short course may decrease intestinal calcium absorption and bone resorption and increase renal excretion; especially useful in vitamin D excess (avoid long-term use → side effects).

Calcitonin (4–8 IU/kg IV or IM every 12 h) → reduces serum calcium concentration but the effect is short lasting.

Bisphosphonates such as pamidronate (0.5–2.0 mg/kg) are used in the treatment of subcutaneous fat necrosis and may delay parathyroidectomy in neonatal severe hyperparathyroidism (NSHPT) → risk of severe hypocalcemia (Samedi et al. 2014).

Total parathyroidectomy and partial autotransplantation may be necessary in the severe form of NSHPT (Peters and Hindmarsh 2007).

112.10 Disorders of Thyroid Function

112.10.1 Origins of the Thyroid Gland

The thyroid is a bilobed gland located in the neck region, made up of two types of cells: the follicular cells which produce thyroxine and the parafollicular cells which produce calcitonin. The follicular cells are the predominant cell population in the gland and they derive from the endoderm, whereas parafollicular cells are of neuroectodermal origin (Hoyes and Kershaw 1985). These different types of cells migrate from their respective sites of origin to ultimately merge in the definitive thyroid gland. The follicular cells organize into thyroid follicles, whereas the other type of cells scatters into the interfollicular space (De Felice and Di Lauro 2004).

112.10.1.1 Organogenesis

Thyroid embryogenesis begins between the 20th and 22nd days of fetus development with the appearance of the thyroid bud as a thickening in the pharynx floor. It is the first recognizable endocrine structure. On the 26th day of development, the thyroid diverticulum begins its migration toward its definitive pretracheal position which it reaches between the 48th and 50th day of embryonic life. By the 28th day of development, the thyroid is connected to the pharynx by a small pedicle known as the thyroglossal duct (O'Rahilly 1983; De Felice and Di Lauro 2015). This duct disconnects from the pharynx around the 33rd day of development and by the 40th day

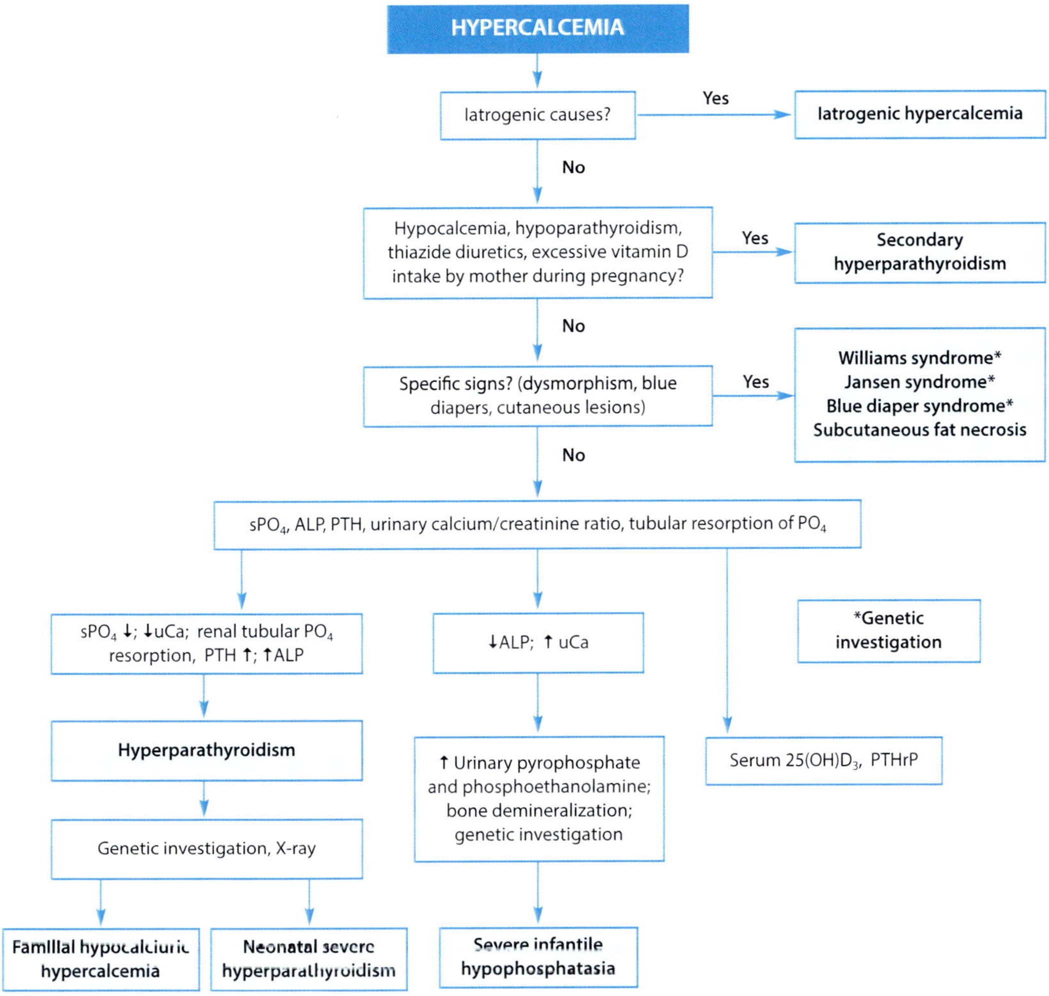

Fig. 5 Differential diagnosis of hypercalcemia

it disappears completely. In some cases, this structure persists and gives origin to thyroglossal duct cysts during infancy (Ellis and van Nostrand 1977). The gland already has a bilobed shape by the 28–30th day of fetal development. Around the 44th day of development, the two cell populations join together and the parafollicular cells are incorporated into the gland. The formation of thyroid follicles and gene expression involved in hormonogenesis begin when migration ends. Hormone synthesis begins during the 10–12th week of development with the incorporation of iodine into the thyroid hormones (O'Rahilly 1983; De Felice and Di Lauro 2015; Fisher et al. 1977).

112.10.1.2 Genetic Regulation

Data from animal models (knockout mice) and insights from patients presenting thyroid dysgenesis (i.e., impaired thyroid development) have allowed to know some genetic mechanisms controlling the development of the thyroid gland (De Felice and Di Lauro 2015; De Felice and Di Lauro 2007; De Felice and Di Lauro 2011; Polak et al. 2004).

Several transcription factors, which are thyroid-specific, are coexpressed in the thyroid anlage, NKX2-1 (formerly called TTF-1), Foxe1 (formerly called TTF-2), Pax8, and Hhex. These genes remain expressed in both precursor and differentiated thyroid follicular cells, but they are also expressed in other tissues.

During embryonic life, NKX2-1 is expressed in the developing brain, lungs, and thyroid and Pax8 is expressed in the kidneys, brain, and thyroid primordium. They are required not for the initial specification of follicular thyroid cells but for the survival and the differentiation of these cells (De Felice and Di Lauro 2011; Kusakabe et al. 2006).

Foxe1 is expressed in tissues which are developed from the pharynx and pharyngeal arches: thyroid, tongue, epiglottis, palate, choanae, and esophagus. Foxe1 has a specific role in controlling the migration of thyroid follicular cell precursors.

Hhex is expressed during embryonic life in several organs derived from the foregut endoderm including the thyroid (Fagman et al. 2011). In absence of this factor, many developmental processes are impaired and *Hhex* knockout embryos die at midgestation; they show severe defects in the liver, forebrain, heart, and thyroid.

These transcription factors are linked in a regulative network during the process of thyroid development (De Felice and Di Lauro 2011). The concurrent presence of NKX2-1, Hhex, and Pax8 is required for the expression of Foxe1. According to this scenario, in the developing human thyroid, the expression of both NKX2–1 and PAX8 precedes the onset of FOXE1 expression (De Felice and Di Lauro 2011; Opitz et al. 2013).

112.10.1.3 Function of the Thyroid Gland

Fetal Thyroid Hormone Production

The main function of the thyroid gland is to produce thyroid hormones. In the early period of gestation, the fetus is entirely dependent on maternal transfer of thyroid hormones; consequently, total serum T4 and T3 levels in early gestation are low, depending entirely on the function of the placenta and maternal thyroid status.

During the first weeks of gestation, the human fetal thyroid gland begins to synthesize only minute amounts of T4 and T3. Around the 20th week of gestation, the fetal hypothalamic-pituitary-thyroid axis begins to function and fetal production of TSH and T4 progressively rises to peak in the month before term (Vulsma et al. 1989). Total T3 levels in fetal blood remain low until the 26–30th week of gestation due to the immature activity of the deiodinase type I enzyme which converts T4 into T3. However, during gestation, both deiodinase types III and II are found to be active. The former, of fetal and placental origin converts T4 into inactive reverse T3 and T3 into di-iodothyronine. The latter mediates the production of T3 from T4 in selected fetal tissues, especially in the brain, where it is actively transferred by MCT8. The maturation of type I occurs gradually in the fetal liver during the last weeks of gestation, although the levels of T3 rise only moderately around term because placental deiodinase III remains at high levels throughout the gestation period (Richard et al. 1998; Santini et al. 1999; Kester et al. 2004). Moreover, plasma thyroid hormone levels are correlated to gestational age; consequently, preterm infants present lower T3, T4, and FT4 values than term infants (Fisher 1998; LaFranchi 1999; van Wassenaer et al. 1997; John and Bamforth 1987).

Finally, it is well known that the limited transplacental passage of thyroid hormones during gestation is sufficient to preserve fetal brain development and its function, in case there is an abnormality in the thyroid ontogenesis (Vulsma et al. 1989; Haddow et al. 1999; de Escobar et al. 2004). On the contrary, when both maternal and fetal hypothyroidism is present, there is significant impairment in neuro-intellectual development despite adequate therapy soon after birth (Haddow et al. 1999). Maternal hypothyroidism can lead to mild but significant cognitive impairment of the offspring (Glinoer 2001; Morreale de Escobar et al. 2000).

Perinatal Thyroid Hormone Modification

At birth, the rapid fall in ambient temperature causes a peak in the newborn TSH level within 30 min after delivery, with a consequential increase in FT4 levels. In term infants, FT4 levels fall within 4–6 weeks of life, whereas in preterm newborns, the increase is blunted and related to gestational age. In infants born after 30–32 weeks of gestation, the FT4 peaks slowly and is comparable to that of term babies; on the contrary, preterm infants born before 30 weeks or with low

(LBW) or very low birth weight (VLBW) present a decline in FT4 with a peak at 1–2 weeks of life, without an increase in TSH (van Wassenaer et al. 1997; Rapaport et al. 2001).

112.10.2 Congenital Hypothyroidism

112.10.2.1 Epidemiology

With the introduction of nationwide newborn screening programs, the incidence of primary permanent CH was reported in the range of 1:3000 to 1:4000 live births, but in the last decades a progressive rise in the incidence rate was reported both in the USA and Europe (range of 1:1660 to 1:2828 live births) (Olivieri 2015; Olivieri et al. 2015). Several factors (changes in screening strategies and TSH cutoffs, increase in preterm survival, demographic changes, and environmental factors) have been proposed to explain this increase. In particular, the impact of lowering TSH cutoff has resulted in a increased detection of milder cases of CH (Olivieri et al. 2015). Different ethnic groups may have a different risk for CH according to the different fertility rate and prevalence of consanguinity among parents in the population.

Nearly all screening programs report a female preponderance among babies with thyroid dysgenesis, with a female-to-male ratio of about 2:1 (Devos et al. 1999). CH may also frequently be associated with an increased risk of congenital extrathyroidal malformations (in particular anomalies of heart, nervous system, and eyes), suggesting a very early impairment in the first stages of embryo development (Olivieri et al. 2002).

112.10.2.2 Etiology

Many different classifications may be proposed for CH. According to the duration of thyroid hormone deficiency, it may be classified into transient and permanent CH. It can be further classified according to the anatomic location of the defect into primary, secondary (or central), and peripheral CH. In addition, some forms of CH are associated with defects in other organs and systems, and they are classified as *syndromic CH* (Cassio et al. 2013a, 2014; Persani 2012) Table 11.

Table 11 Etiologies of congenital hypothyroidism

Central hypothyroidism
Isolated TSH defect (TSH gene β-subunit mutation) TRH defect (isolated, pituitary stalk interruption syndrome, hypothalamic lesion) TRH resistance (TRH receptor gene mutation) Mutations in transcription factors involved in pituitary development (HESX1,LHX3,LHX4,PROP1,PIT1)
Primary hypothyroidism
(A) Permanent forms
Thyroid dysgenesis Ectopy Athyreosis Hypoplasia, hemiagenesia
In situ gland (normal volume or goiter) Iodine transport defect (Na/I symporter defects) Iodine organification defects (TPO,TG,DUOX2-DUOXA-2, DHEAL1 defects) Resistance to TSH binding/signaling (inactivating TSH receptor gene, Gα protein defects)
(B) Transient forms
Maternal factors (transplacental passage of blocking antibodies or antithyroid drugs) Neonatal factors (prematurity,IUGR,NICU) Iodine (deficiency,overload) Genetic factors (DUOX2 heterozygous mutation)
Syndromic hypothyroidism
Mutations in: Pendrin (Pendred syndrome: goiter and sordomutismo) NKX2–1 (Brain-lung-thyroid syndrome) FOXE-1 (Bamforth-Lazarus syndrome:cleft palate, choanal atresia, and athyreosis) PAX8 (renal anomalies, ectopic/hypoplastic thyroid) NKX2–5 (congenital heart defects)
Peripheral hypothyroidism
Thyroid hormone resistance Thyroid hormone transport defect (MCT8 mutation)

Central Congenital Hypothyroidism

Central CH occurs in 1 out of every 50,000 newborns. It is often related to abnormalities during development of the hypothalamus or the pituitary glands and associated with multiple pituitary hormonal deficiencies. Rarer causes of central CH may be ascribed to TRH deficiency, resistance to TRH, isolated TSH deficiency related to mutations in the TSH-β chain, and mutations in transcription factors involved in pituitary development and hormone expression (Persani 2012).

Central CH was also described in babies born from mothers with gestational hyperthyroidism. One cause could be insufficient treatment of the mother during pregnancy and, consequently, the hyperthyroid environment that impairs maturation of the fetal hypothalamic-pituitary-thyroid axis (Kempers et al. 2003).

Thyroid Dysgenesis

Thyroid dysgenesis is the most frequent cause of CH. It includes athyrosis, due to the complete absence of thyroid tissue; ectopic gland, due to an abnormal migration of the embryonic thyroid; and thyroid hypoplasia, due to defective growth of the gland following complete migration. The most frequent type of thyroid dysgenesis is ectopy; the majority of these patients presents a thyroid in the dorsum of the tongue or, less frequently, located in a sublingual position (Cassio et al. 2013a, 2014).

Mutations in transcription factors involved in thyroid development (PAX 8, FOXE1, NKX2–1, NKX2–5), albeit in a minority of cases, have been associated with some forms of thyroid dysgenesis and/or syndromic CH in humans (De Felice and Di Lauro 2011; Krude et al. 2002; Monti et al. 2015; Bamforth et al. 1989; Meeus et al. 2004) (Tables 12 and 13).

In addition, in vivo studies in congenital hypothyroid subjects households showed a frequency of familial forms of thyroid dysgenesis (2%) and minor thyroid morphological abnormalities (7%) markedly higher than that found in the control population (0.9%) and difficult to explain on the basis of chance alone (Castanet et al. 2001; Castanet et al. 2010). Finally, an increased risk of congenital extrathyroidal malformations was found in patients with CH as mentioned above (Olivieri et al. 2002). In conclusion, it appears evident from the recent literature data that the genetics of thyroid dysgenesis is complex and has likely polygenic and multifactorial bases that do not follow, in most cases, the pattern of Mendelian inheritance (De Felice and Di Lauro 2004; De Filippis et al. 2017).

Table 12 Symptoms of congenital hypothyroidism

Prolonged jaundice
Skin mottling
Large anterior and/or posterior fontanel
Abdominal distension
Umbilical hernia
Hypotonia
Constipation
Poor feeding
Failure to thrive
Hoarse cry
Hearing impairment
Neurodevelopmental delay
Irreversible mental retardation (in absence of precocious diagnosis)
Goiter (rare at birth)

Thyroid Dyshormonogenesis

These genetic defects in each step of synthesis of thyroid hormones (TH) are inherited as autosomal recessive traits. Clinical manifestations

Table 13 Signs and symptoms of congenital hyperthyroidism

Fetal signs
Growth restriction
Fetal tachycardia
Goiter
Hydrops
Premature births (frequent)
Increased fetal motility
Neonatal signs
Tachycardia
Hyperexcitability
Increased appetite with poor weight gain
Vomiting
Diarrhea
Fever with sweating or erythema
Tachypnea
Goiter (50% of newborns)
Thyrotoxic signs
Heart failure
Jaundice
Cholestasis
Thrombocytopenia
Hepatomegaly
Splenomegaly
Liver function abnormalities (also in absence of heart failure)
Stare and eyelid retraction
Exophthalmia
Small fontanels
Craniosynostosis
Advanced bone maturation

comprise a variable degree of congenital hypothyroidism (CH), with increased secretion of TSH and goiter.

Occasionally, these disorders can be identified prenatally, when a fetus with goitrous nonimmune hypothyroidism is diagnosed in a euthyroid mother. Intra-amniotic injections of L-thyroxine have been reported to decrease the size of the fetal thyroid gland. However, experience with this procedure is limited, and the risk of provoking premature labor or infections should be evaluated with care by multidisciplinary specialist teams (Cassio et al. 2015). When thyroid gland is in situ, the disorder may be related to inborn errors of metabolism during one of the several steps required for normal thyroid hormone synthesis (thyroid dyshormonogenesis). Different mutations were reported in the genes encoding the thyroglobulin protein, the sodium iodide symporter and the pendrin channel, as well as in the thyroid peroxidase (TPO), and more recently in the dual oxidases 2 (DUOX2) enzyme and its maturation factor DUOXA2 (Szinnai et al. 2006; Palos et al. 2008; Bakker et al. 2000; Moreno et al. 2002; Moreno and Visser 2007; Zamproni et al. 2008).

Transient Congenital Hypothyroidism

CH is sometimes transient and often has an environmental or iatrogenic origin. Transient CH may be related to a deficiency of iodide or to exposure to an excess of iodine, usually due to the application of iodinated disinfectants on the skin (Weber et al. 1998; Chanoine et al. 1988; Matsuura et al. 1980; Rovelli et al. 2010). Other causes are treatment with antithyroid drugs and, more seldom, the trans-placental crossing of antibodies blocking the action of TSH (Matsuura et al. 1980; Rovelli et al. 2010). Recently, heterozygous mutations in the DUOX2 gene have been found in patients with transient CH (Zamproni et al. 2008; Muzza et al. 2014).

Resistance to TSH

In this rare condition, the response to bioactive TSH may be impaired at the thyroid follicular cell level and the cause could be found in mutations that inactivate the TSHR (Rovelli et al. 2010). Total insensitivity to TSH leads to a small orthotopic gland with a phenotype ranging from CH to euthyroid hyperthyrotropinemia (Nicoletti et al. 2009; Cassio et al. 2013b; Abramowicz et al. 1997).

Peripheric Hypothyroidism

This rare form of CH can be due to tissue resistance to the action of thyroid hormones, caused by inactivating mutations of the β-receptor of triiodothyronine or to abnormalities in thyroid hormone transport across the cell membrane, as in MCT8 mutations (Refetoff et al. 1993). In the first condition, free thyroid hormones increase and TSH is inappropriately normal or higher; in the second case, FT3 is higher, whereas FT4 is low and TSH is normal or increased. Clinically, children affected by the first condition show a variable phenotype ranging from isolated biochemical abnormalities to variable features of hypothyroidism; those affected by the second condition present severe neurological symptoms with major hypotonia and delay of acquisitions (Friesema et al. 2004).

112.10.2.3 Clinical Signs

The transplacental passage of maternal thyroid hormone protects newborns with CH for about 2 weeks (LaFranchi and Austin 2007); consequently, at birth, only 1–4% of newborns with CH are detected by clinical examination (Carranza et al. 2006). Infants with CH are usually overdue and have a high birth weight for their gestational age (Van Vliet et al. 2003). Other signs of CH are represented in Table 12.

Children with central CH often have clinical manifestations of other associated hormonal deficiencies such as hypoglycemia, micropenis, and cryptorchidism (Persani 2012; Carranza et al. 2006).

112.10.2.4 Neonatal Screening

Screening programs have led to the successful early detection and treatment of infants with CH and have eliminated the severe mental retardation resulting from late diagnosis. As a screening method, the most sensitive test to detect primary CH is the measurement of TSH on dried blood spot at 48–72 h of age. Primary T4 screening with confirmatory TSH testing entails a risk of missing some cases of mild forms of primary CH but can detect some cases of central CH (Cassio et al. 2013a; Leger et al. 2014; Van Vliet and Czernichow 2004; American Academy of Pediatrics et al. 2006; Grüters and Krude 2007). There is a subgroup of neonates at risk (preterm newborns, babies with very low birth weight, twins and critically ill babies admitted to Neonatal Intensive Care Unit) in which CH may be masked by normal TSH levels at the initial screening test. These can be due to hypothalamic-pituitary immaturity, fetal blood mixing in multiple birth, serious neonatal illnesses, and some medications such as dopamine and glucocorticoids. For these special categories of neonates, the screening procedure should routinely include a repeat TSH test at 2 and/or 4 weeks of life (Olivieri et al. 2007; Goldsmit et al. 2011; Filippi et al. 2007).

112.10.2.5 Procedures to Confirm Diagnosis

All newborns with abnormal results at screening for CH must undergo FT4, and TSH serum measurements to confirm the diagnosis; newborns with hypothyroidism typically present low FT4 and high TSH concentrations (Olivieri et al. 2007; Goldsmit et al. 2011; Filippi et al. 2007). In addition, it is imperative to make TSH and FT4 measurements as quickly as possible in all cases of clinical suspicion of hypothyroidism, regardless of screening results (Cassio et al. 2013a; Leger et al. 2014).

Etiological diagnosis of CH is based on scintigraphy, ultrasound analysis, and measurements of thyroglobulin serum. High thyroglobulin levels may suggest dyshormonogenesis, absent levels an athyreosis (Leger et al. 2014; Olivieri et al. 2007; Daneman and Daneman 2005). In addition urinary iodide, as well as tests for thyroid autoimmunity (anti-peroxidase, anti-TSH receptor, and anti-thyroglobulin antibodies), are helpful in making a complete etiologic diagnosis (Cassio et al. 2013a; Leger et al. 2014; Olivieri et al. 2007; Delange et al. 2002; Etling et al. 1984).

Thyroid Scintigraphy

Iodine-123 scintigraphy of the thyroid gland is helpful in obtaining information about the function of the thyroid gland. More frequently scintigraphy is performed with Technetium, which is easily available (Leger et al. 2014; Schoen et al. 2004). Thyroid scintigraphy allows diagnosis of an ectopic gland enabled the identification of the exact area of the contrast, of athyreosis or, in the presence of high doses of thyroglobulin, the diagnosis of mutations that inactivate the TSHR, NIS mutation, or maternal antibodies against TSH (Djemli et al. 2004). When scintigraphy shows a normally located thyroid gland, a positive perchlorate discharge test will enable the diagnosis of iodine organification defects (Schoen et al. 2004; Meller et al. 1997).

Thyroid Ultrasonography

Thyroid ultrasonography is helpful in defining the structure of a normally positioned gland. It is less useful in making a diagnosis because it does not allow the diagnosis of an ectopic gland (Bubuteishvili et al. 2003). On the other hand, fetal ultrasound can make a prenatal diagnosis of dysgenesis or fetal goiter (Ranzini et al. 2001). At present, the best approach for a postnatal diagnosis of CH is to do both an ultrasound, to determine thyroid-gland size and morphology, and scintigraphy, to detect functional thyroid tissue (Leger et al. 2014; Perry et al. 2006; Karakoc-Aydiner et al. 2012).

Further Diagnostic Tools

At diagnosis of CH, the absence of one knee's epiphyses at radiography is a marker of fetal origin of the disease and therefore an indication that the infant is at a higher risk of developmental retardation. Urinary iodide measurements aid in determining iodide deficiency or excess. Tests for thyroid autoimmunity allow the physician to associate CH with transplacental passage of maternal antibodies (Mengreli et al. 2003; Chiovato et al. 1994; Wasniewska et al. 2003).

112.10.2.6 Therapy

Treatment with L-thyroxine must be initiated as soon as possible (Cassio et al. 2013a; Leger et al. 2014; Bongers-Schokking and de Muinck Keizer-Schrama 2005). The goal of the therapy is to normalize T4 levels within 2 weeks and TSH values within 1 month. This way, it is possible to assure the normal growth and development of babies with neurocognitive outcome similar to the child's genetic potential. An initial dosage of 10–15 μg/kg/day is recommended (Cassio et al. 2013a; Leger et al. 2014; Olivieri et al. 2007). In general, patients with athyreosis require higher doses compared to patients with ectopy, and these require higher doses compared to children with CH due to dyshormonogenesis (Hanukoglu et al. 2001). In children with preexisting cardiac insufficiency, the L-thyroxine dose must be introduced at 50% of the target replacement dose and increasing in accordance with FT4 levels (Leger et al. 2014).

The drug must be taken in the morning at least 30 min before breakfast. L-thyroxine tablets should be crushed and mixed with a few milliliters of liquid to prepare the daily dose. Several substances such as soy protein, iron, and calcium are reported to interfere with thyroxine. There have been no proven advantages so far to the association of L-thyroxine with triiodothyronine treatment (Cassio et al. 2003).

If permanent hypothyroidism has not been confirmed, it is advisable to stop the therapy after 3 years and to wait 4 weeks and reassess thyroid function (Eugster et al. 2004). If it is normal, transient hypothyroidism is presumed and treatment can be permanently interrupted. However, the interruption of treatment must be limited to infants with a normally developed or enlarged thyroid gland that shows, during replacement therapy, TSH levels in the normal range. Moreover reevaluation is essential in subjects who were preterm or sick during the neonatal period. Finally, because iodine deficiency may mimic dyshormonogenesis, retesting is indicated in children who appear to have mild dyshormonogenesis (Cassio et al. 2013a; Leger et al. 2014; Rabbiosi et al. 2013).

112.10.2.7 Follow-Up

Newborns with CH must be assessed after 1–2 weeks from the start of therapy, then every 2 weeks until TSH levels are completely normalized and successively every 1–3 months until the first year of life (Cassio et al. 2013a; Leger et al. 2014). After that age, a follow-up checkup must be done every 2–4 months until 3 years of life, then every 6–12 months (Leger et al. 2014; Olivieri et al. 2007). During follow-up, the dosage of the drug must be changed in relation to TSH and FT4 levels, especially during the first 3 years of life when growth is most rapid. Serum FT4 and TSH should be monitored every 4–6 weeks after any change in L-thyroxine dosage. FT3 measurements are not helpful in monitoring the treatment because this test may be normal despite low FT4 and high TSH levels (Van Vliet et al. 2003).

In the first months of life, it is essential to be aware of possible prolonged hyperthyroidism that can be associated with premature craniosynostosis. Four or more episodes of insufficiently suppressed TSH after the age of 6 months is the most important variable associated with poor school performance. At follow-up visits, regular height and weight must be observed. Delayed bone age usually becomes compatible with the actual age within the third year of life (Leger et al. 2014).

Neurodevelopmental delay is not common in patients with CH in therapy from the first month of life (Bongers-Schokking and de Muinck Keizer-Schrama 2005; Simoneau-Roy et al. 2004). Nevertheless, it is possible to notice slight difficulties in motor skills and impairment of visuospatial processes and selective memory, presumable signs of poorly compensated fetal hypothyroidism (Rovet 2002; Van Vliet 2001). However, children with properly treated CH do not show differences in school performance compared with healthy children (Léger et al. 2001; Rochiccioli et al. 1992).

112.10.3 Thyroid Dysfunctions in Preterm Infants

112.10.3.1 Thyroid Function in Preterm Infants

Alterations of thyroid function in preterm infants are often transient and, in most cases, do not require any treatment. The function of the hypothalamic-pituitary-thyroid axis in preterm newborns is attenuated at birth for an unknown postnatal duration. In preterm babies, there is reduced hypothalamic TRH production, an immature response of the thyroid gland to TSH, an inefficient capacity of the thyroid follicular cells to organify iodine, and a low capacity to convert T4 into active T3. The responses of TSH and T4 to TRH are normal, so the site of immaturity seems to be the hypothalamus (Ogilvy-Stuart 2002). Moreover, neonatal health conditions related to preterm delivery, such as respiratory distress, can influence serum thyroid hormone levels (Murphy et al. 2004).

112.10.3.2 Hypothyroxinemia of Prematurity

Approximately 12% of preterm infants present low T4 and FT4 with normal TSH values. This condition is known as transient hypothyroxinemia of prematurity (Williams et al. 2006). In particular, the correct definition is the presence of a normal or low TSH concentration in conjunction with a concentration of total T4, that is, $\leq$10th percentile of cord total T4 of the equivalent gestational age had the infant remained in utero (Williams and Hume 2011). The cause is not clear; we can hypothesize an immaturity of the hypothalamic axis, the withdrawal of maternal-placental T4 transfer, developmental constraints on the synthesis, immature peripheral metabolism of iodothyronines, iodide deficiency, and nonthyroidal illness. Associations have been shown between transient hypothyroxinemia and prolonged oxygen supplementation, mechanical ventilation, intraventricular hemorragia, and cerebral white matter damage (Williams and Hume 2011; Ares et al. 1997; Paul et al. 1998). Bacteremia, persistent ductus arteriosus, necrotizing enterocolitis, and the use of drugs such as aminophylline, caffeine, glucocorticoids, and dopamine have also been found to be significantly associated with transient hypothyroxinemia (Williams et al. 2005). This condition is present in the majority of infants born under 30 weeks of gestation and can be associated with later neurodevelopmental deficits (Lucas et al. 1988). However, it remains unclear whether morbidity and developmental disabilities are caused by, or simply associated with, hypothyroxinemia of prematurity (Rapaport et al. 2001; Osborn and Hunt 2007). Treatment with L-thyroxine has not been shown to be beneficial; on the contrary, it may be detrimental. Presently, in the absence of high TSH, the evidence does not support a cognitive benefit of L-thyroxine treatment for this condition in premature infants (Rapaport et al. 2001; Biswas et al. 2003).

112.10.3.3 Hypothyroidism with Delayed TSH Elevation

Some LBW or VLBW newborns or critical ill neonates frequently present CH characterized by low FT4 and delayed TSH elevation. On the basis of one recent Italian study, the incidence of this condition is 1:400 for VLBW babies and 1:1384 for LBW newborns (Cavarzere et al. 2016). Serum TSH in these babies increases during the first few weeks of life until concentration levels are typical of primary hypothyroidism. It is not known if this type of CH is transient or permanent, or whether it depends on an abnormality of pituitary-thyroid feedback regulation. If TSH is still high at 6 weeks of age, the infant must begin therapy (American Academy of Pediatrics et al. 2006).

112.10.3.4 Transient Congenital Hypothyroidism

Approximately 5% of preterm infants admitted to neonatal intensive care present a transient form of CH with low FT4 and increased TSH. Causes vary from maternal exposure to antithyroid drugs to maternal TRB antibody status. There is evidence suggesting a relationship between this clinical finding and the exposure to iodine-containing antiseptics used in neonatal units. The therapy should begin immediately just as it is for permanent CH; an attempt should be made later in life to suspend treatment. On the contrary, the hormone levels in babies born from mothers in treatment with antithyroid drugs usually return to the normal range within 1–3 weeks without therapy (Cassio et al. 2013a; American Academy of Pediatrics et al. 2006).

112.10.4 Asymptomatic Neonatal Hyperthyrotropinemia

Asymptomatic hyperthyrotropinemia is defined as a high serum TSH level associated with normal T4, FT4, and T3 values (American Academy of Pediatrics et al. 2006; Salerno et al. 2016). This subclinical condition, transient or permanent, is relatively frequent with a prevalence of 1:8000 newborns in Europe, and it is more frequent in infants with Down syndrome (Calaciura et al. 2002).

112.10.4.1 Diagnosis

Affected newborns are detected by neonatal screening. About 60–70% of infants with increased TSH levels at neonatal screening present nearly normal serum TSH values with normal FT4 levels and require follow-up during childhood (Calaciura et al. 2002; Leonardi et al. 2008).

112.10.4.2 Etiologies

The cause is not known, though it is possible that the same factors involved in the origins of CH, when they are less severe, are responsible for subclinical hypothyroidism. Some studies have identified genetic abnormalities, thyroid gland malformations, and autoantibodies in children with hyperthyrotropinemia (Leonardi et al. 2008). These defects often present different degrees of severity and therefore could increase TSH concentrations moderately and intermittently (Leonardi et al. 2008). This clinical finding appears more evident at birth because the thyroid gland is less mature and there is a greater thyroid hormone requirement during neonatal life. Other causes of asymptomatic hyperthyrotropinemia are defects in the biological activity of TSH or of its receptor, subtle developmental defects such as hemithyroid, and a disturbance in the TSH feedback control system (Filippi et al. 2007).

112.10.4.3 Evolution

Repeated thyroid function evaluation is essential because TSH values in the same individual can spontaneously fluctuate around the upper normal range. With age this condition can become clinically evident as the disease progresses, as in overt hypothyroidism. In other cases, high TSH values in very young children may subsequently normalize; perhaps, the cause is due to reduced thyroid hormone requirements in more advanced childhood (Calaciura et al. 2002; Leonardi et al. 2008). In any case, hyperthytotropinemia requires periodic follow-up visits to assess thyroid gland function and to monitor possible metabolic complications (Cerbone et al. 2014, 2016).

112.10.4.4 Treatment

Whether subclinical hypothyroidism requires treatment or not is still a matter of debate also because only few studies have investigated the effect of L-thyroxine therapy in children with subclinical hypothyroidism. Nevertheless, there is a general consensus to treat all subjects with TSH levels over 20 mU/L and normal FT4 (Leger et al. 2014). Over-treating must be avoided and the therapy discontinued after 3 years of age in order to reassess thyroid function (Olivieri et al. 2007; Gharib et al. 2005).

112.10.5 Neonatal Hyperthyroidism

Neonatal hyperthyroidism is a relatively rare condition (incidence varying between 1:4000 and 1:40,000) that could be due to maternal thyroid autoimmune disorders, to continually activated TSH receptor or to McCune-Albright syndrome.

112.10.5.1 Graves' Disease

The most frequent cause of neonatal hyperthyroidism is the mother suffering from Graves' disease, which occurs in 0.1–0.4% of pregnant women. However, only 1–2% of neonates born to these affected women presents hyperthyroidism, and in all cases this form of disease is transient (Léger 2016).

Etiology

The transplacental passage of maternal immunoglobulin stimulates the fetal thyroid by activating the TSH receptor. Consequently, thyroid hormone secretion in the uterus is already increased by thyrotoxicosis that continues after birth until the maternal antibodies have disappeared from the infant's circulation. This fetal condition begins in the second trimester of gestation when fetal TSH receptor begins to respond to TSH stimulation; it is related to the severity of the mother's disease and goes away within 4 months of postnatal life (Léger 2016).

Clinical Signs

Thyrotoxic fetus may present growth restriction, fetal tachycardia, increased fetal motility, goiter, and hydrops (Ogilvy-Stuart 2002; Léger 2016; Besancon et al. 2014; Polak et al. 2006; Spiegel 2000). These are frequently premature births (Davis et al. 1989). In other cases, the symptoms are only noticed at birth or several days afterward when the effect of maternal drugs have disappeared, and the maternal immunoglobulins, which have a longer halflife, have increased thyroid hormone production allowing the clinical signs of the disease to become evident (Zakarija et al. 1983). The neonatal symptoms vary from tachycardia and hyperexcitability to increased appetite with poor weight gain, vomiting or diarrhea, fever with sweating or erythema, tachypnea in some cases, and goiter in 50% of newborns (Ogilvy-Stuart 2002; Léger 2016; Polak et al. 2006) (Table 14). Often, the goiter is the first sign of thyroid dysfunction and already appears during fetal life (Luton et al. 2005). Mortality has been reported to be between 12 and 20% (Krude et al. 1997). Heart failure is one of the major risks; consequently, early diagnosis and treatment are necessary for a good prognosis (Polak et al. 2006). In thyrotoxic newborns, jaundice, cholestasis, and thrombocytopenia are also indicated as signs of the disease. Hepatomegaly and splenomegaly can be present, and liver function abnormalities can occur even in the absence of heart failure (Ogilvy-Stuart 2002; Polak et al. 2006). Stare and eyelid retraction are present, whereas exophthalmia is related to the autoimmune process. The fontanels are small and some infants show craniosynostosis; bone maturation is often advanced as a result of fetal hyperthyroidism (Ogilvy-Stuart 2002; Polak et al. 2006), Table 13.

Diagnosis of Fetal Hyperthyroidism

Diagnosis of prenatal hyperthyroidism is based on high maternal TSH receptor binding antibody titers, accelerated fetal bone maturation, and a fetal heart rate over 160 bpm, in the last part of gestation (Besancon et al. 2014). A threshold value for a maternal second-generation thyroid binding inhibitory immunoglobulin assay of 5 IU/L during the second half of gestation and delivery has recently been identified for defining risk situations for fetal and neonatal hyperthyroidism (Abeillon-du Payrat et al. 2014). Scans should be performed monthly, from 20 weeks of gestation onwards (Léger 2016). If a fetal goiter is present, it is necessary to determine whether the cause is hyperthyroidism related to maternal Graves' disease or hypothyroidism related to maternal antithyroid drugs. To make a correct diagnosis, it is helpful to use a Doppler of the fetal thyroid which indicates hypothyroidism when it shows a flash confined to the periphery of the gland (Luton et al. 1997). A combination of maternal criteria (TRAb titers, ATD use, and dose) and fetal criteria (thyroid Doppler signal, fetal heart rate, and bone maturation) is used to distinguish between fetal hypothyroidism and hyperthyroidism (Luton et al. 2005). Finally, a fetal blood sample is the gold standard to differentiate fetal hypothyroidism from fetal hyperthyroidism, but it is not easy to obtain and can be risky for abortion and fetal infection (Polak et al. 2006; van der Kaay et al. 2016). Assessment of fetal thyroid hormones during pregnancy must be done only in cases when the status of the fetus is in doubt, the mother has positive TSH receptor binding antibody titers and takes antithyroid drugs, and when intraamniotic L-thyroxine therapy may be necessary to resolve the fetal clinical condition (Spiegel 2000). Fetal FT4 levels are related to maternal FT4 values: a fetal euthyroidism can be achieved by maintaining maternal FT4 in the upper normal-to-mild thyrotoxic range during treatment with antithyroid drugs (Polak et al. 2006).

Diagnosis of Neonatal Hyperthyroidism

The diagnosis of neonatal hyperthyroidism is confirmed by high FT4 and FT3 levels with low values of TSH. Since a delayed appearance of hyperthyroidism is possible, these tests should be performed at day 3–5 of life, repeated at day 10–14 of life, and followed clinically until 2–3 months of life (Ogilvy-Stuart 2002; Polak et al. 2006; van der Kaay et al. 2016). The determination of antibodies is a useful marker of the etiology of the disease (Abeillon-du Payrat et al. 2014).

Treatment

It is essential to treat newborns for hyperthyroidism soon after birth in order to avoid short-term and long-term morbidity (Léger 2016). Methimazole is the drug preferred at a dosage of 0.5–1 mg/kg/day, depending on the initial severity of the disease, in 3 divided doses. It blocks thyroid hormone secretion. Alternatively, propylthiouracil, which promptly restores a normal heart rate, may be administered orally at a dosage of 5–10 mg/kg/day divided into three doses (Ogilvy-Stuart 2002; Léger 2016; Polak et al. 2006). Currently, however, the use of propylthiouracil is not recommended in children for the high risk of severe hepatotoxicity reported by Food and Drug Administration (Rivkees and Szarfarm 2010). The dose of these drugs can be progressively reduced, according to the TH levels. In some cases, it might be helpful to treat the newborns with fixed doses of antithyroid drugs and to add L-thyroxine when plasma FT4 levels reach the hypothyroid range. This combined treatment is usually required for 1 month (Léger 2016). However, dose titration should be preferred over "block-and-replace" approaches (Léger 2016).

Propranolol, which inhibits deiodination of T4 to T3 and controls symptoms caused by adrenergic stimulation, may be given at a dosage of 2 mg/kg/day, in two divided doses when tachycardia is present during the first 1–2 weeks of treatment (Léger 2016; Pearce 2006). In the most severe cases of the disease, a saturated solution of potassium iodide (1 drop/day) or Lugol's solution (1–3 drops/day) can be added in order to decrease thyroglobulin proteolysis and thyroid hormone production. Sodium iopanoate (iopanic acid, 500 mg orally once every third day) and glucocorticoids (prednisone 2 mg/kg/day) are rarely used to decrease thyroid hormone production and to inhibit T4 conversion to T3 (Transue et al. 1992).

Other helpful measures such as high liquid and calorie intake and sedatives are also useful in the treatment of these newborns (Ogilvy-Stuart 2002; Polak et al. 2006). The therapy should be continued until maternal antibodies are no longer present. During treatment, the patients must be seen weekly until they are stable and then every 1–2 weeks, reducing the dosage as soon as possible.

Treating the mother with propylthiouracil or methimazole, at a dosage under 150 mg/day and 30 mg/day, respectively, does not mean breastfeeding should be discontinued since the quantity of drugs that the newborn would ingest is minimal; however, it is necessary to do periodic assessments of neonatal thyroid function.

Although the lower milk concentration of propylthiouracil compared to methimazole, considering the potential harmful effects of first drug, the second drug should be preferred during lactation (Karras et al. 2010; Karras and Krassas 2012).

112.10.6 Mutations of TSH Receptors

Activating mutations of the TSH receptor cause constitutive activation of the receptor, which is not related to an autoimmune mechanism and is dominantly transmitted (DuPrez et al. 1994). The phenotype appears with neonatal hyperthyroidism. This permanent condition is often associated with a severe course with moderate or diffuse goiter due to the mitogenic effects of cyclic AMP on thyroid follicular cells, possible developmental delay, absence of extrathyroidal signs of Graves' disease, and recurrence after treatment. Sporadic congenital nonautoimmune hyperthyroidism may be also caused by de novo mutation of the TSH receptor gene. Definitive treatment with thyroidectomy and radioiodine therapy is possible at older ages (Krude et al. 1997).

112.10.6.1 McCune-Albright Syndrome

McCune-Albright syndrome results from an activating mutation in the gene encoding the α-subunit of the stimulatory G proteins; in some cases, its symptoms are similar to neonatal hyperthyroidism. Clinically besides symptoms of hyperthyroidism, cafe-au-lait spots are present with irregular borders, polyostotic fibrous dysplasia, and other endocrinological alterations. The medical treatment is the same as Graves' disease, but it must be prolonged during postnatal life. Once euthyroidism has been restored, an ablative approach is possible (Shenker et al. 1993).

112.10.6.2 Hashimoto's Thyroiditis

Maternal Hashimoto's thyroiditis may cause hyperthyroidism in the newborn but usually there are no consequences in the fetus, even though antibodies against TPO or thyroglobulin can cross the placenta and be found in the fetus. However, cases of fetal and neonatal hyperthyroidism have been found in the offspring of affected mothers (Kohn et al. 1997).

112.10.6.3 Resistance to Thyroid Hormones

Resistance to thyroid hormones is a rare condition characterized by decreased responsiveness to thyroid hormones. High FT3 and FT4 are present with inappropriately normal or elevated TSH concentrations (Sunthornthepvarakui et al. 1995). Clinically, the affected patients show a variable phenotype ranging from isolated biochemical abnormalities to variable features of hypo- or hyperthyroidism in the rare case of pituitary resistance (Refetoff et al. 2001). Asymptomatic patients do not require any treatment, whereas therapy must be initiated to resolve the symptoms of hypo- or hyperthyroidism.

Take Home Messages

Hypopituitarism

- Suspect of congenital hypopituitarism in any child presenting with hypoglycemia and dysmorphic features with midline defects, prolonged jaundice, poor weight gain, hypothermia, cryptorchidism, and/or micropenis in a male infant.
- Early diagnosis of this condition may prevent impairment of cognition, poor growth, and metabolic abnormalities.
- Parents should be instructed in the use of glucose monitoring (sticks) and the management of hypoglycemia (1 μg SC glucagon injections).

Adrenal Insufficiency

- CAH constitutes the largest cluster of steroidogenic impairments and the most common cause of PAI in children.
- In the case of obstructive uropathy, the risk of salt loss is high when the cause of obstruction

is treated by surgery.

- Neonatal screening by tandem mass spectrometry can be used for early diagnosis of X-ALD, reducing morbidity due to this condition.
- Intramuscular injections of hydrocortisone hemisuccinate need to be prescribed in case of vomiting or profuse diarrhea. In the case of intercurrent illness, instructions from a pediatric endocrinologist should be given to double (nonfebrile illness) or treble (febrile illness) the oral hydrocortisone doses. A steroid card should be provided both to ADI and panhypopituitaric patients with ACTH deficiency.

Hyponatremia, Hypernatremia and Aldosterone Disturbances

- Attention to fluid balance is critical. Polyuria is defined as urine output (UOP) greater than 2 L/m^2/day, 150 ml/kg/day in neonates.
- In hyponatremic/hyperkalemic patients, measure plasma 17-OH-progesterone (plasma or urine steroid profile with TM spectrometry when available) and karyotype or FISH/PCR for Y fragments in case of genital ambiguity, for the diagnosis of CAH.
- Plasma renin and aldosterone to exclude deficiency (low aldosterone levels) or resistance (high aldosterone levels).

Hypoglycemia

- Neonatal hypoglycemia cannot be defined by a single value.
- Usually hypoglycemia is transient, resolving in the first 72 h of life.
- Persistent hypoglycemia needs investigations.
- Whenever possible hypoglycemia should be managed by feeding.

Hyperglycemia

- Hyperglycemia definition in the newborn remains uncertain.
- Frequently hyperglycemia is secondary to other severe diseases and may be resolved by treating the underlying problems.
- The cut-off value at which treatment should be started is not universally accepted.
- Management of hyperglycemia is based on a glucose restriction or exogenous insulin infusion or a combination of both.

Hypocalcemia

- Neonatal hypocalcemia has not a univocal definition.
- Clinical presentation includes nonspecific symptoms and signs.
- Treatment may be managed orally or IV.

Hypercalcemia

- Hypercalcemia can be defined as ionized calcium >1.36 mmol/L or total calcium concentration > 2.75 mmol/L.
- Asymptomatic mild hypercalcemia should be managed conservatively.
- Moderate to severe hypercalcemia requires prompt intervention.

Thyroid Diseases

- The introduction of newborn screening programs changed the approach to the diagnosis and the treatment of congenital hypothyroidism, the most frequent endocrine disorder in neonatal age.
- Transient hypothyroxinemia of the prematurity and hypothyroidism with delayed TSH elevation are rare dysfunctions of thyroid in preterm infants.
- The conditions of asymptomatic hyperthyrotropinemia of newborns in which a treatment is suggested must be identified.
- Neonatal hyperthyroidism, a relatively rare condition, is in most cases due to maternal Graves' disease.

Appendix

See Table Appendix A1.

Appendix A1 "Rare diseases" with associated hormone abnormalities (*On behalf of A. Balsamo, P. Ghirri, A. Cicognani and A. Boldrini*)

Disease/OMIM	Gene/OMIM/map gene locus	Clinical and diagnostic features	Possible specific treatment
Aarskog-Scott S./305400 and 100050	*FGD1*/300546 Xp11.21	Aarskog syndrome affects mainly males, but females may have a milder form. *Short stature*, hypertelorism, and *shawl scrotum* are the main clinical features. Facial dysmorphisms may include rounded face, widow's peak hairline, hypertelorism, blepharoptosis, downslanting eye slits, small nose with anteverted nostrils, broad philtrum, and ear anomalies	–
		Other signs described: "simian crease" in the palm of hand, clinodactyly of the 5th finger, brachydactyly, *delayed sexual maturation, cryptorchidism*, pectus excavatum. Mild to moderate mental problems are usually present	
Antley-Bixler S./207410	*FGFR2*/176943 10q26	There is evidence that the ABS can be caused by mutation in a fibroblast growth factor receptor gene (FGFR2) and is characterized by craniosynostosis (trapezoidocephaly, midface hypoplasia, proptosis, choanal stenosis, or hypoplasia), humeroradial synostosis, bowing of the femora and ulnas, long bone fractures, long slender fingers with camptodactyly, cardiac and renal malformations. ABS-like phenotype with *ambiguous genitalia and disordered steroidogenesis* is a distinct disorder caused by mutations in the cytochrome P450 oxidoreductase (POR) gene (see ► Chap. 113, "Disorders of Sexual Development in Newborns"). *Steroid profile between 21-OHase and 17-OHase deficiency*	–
	POR/124015 7q11.2		Hydrocortisone
Beckwith-Wiedemann S./130650	*CDKN1C*/600856 H19/103280 IGF2/147470 11p15.5, 11p15.5, 11p15.5, 5q35	See section "Beckwith-Wiedemann Syndrome"	See section "Beckwith-Wiedemann Syndrome"
CHARGE association/214800	*SEMA3E*/608166 CHD7/608892 8q12.1 7q21.11	Patients affected present with various association of: Coloboma, heart defects, choanal atresia, renal and *genital anomalies*, and ear abnormalities. Frequently reported features include: facial palsy, cleft palate, dysphagia, and *growth retardation*. May be associated with *hypocalcemia*	Support therapy, correction of choanal atresia and heart defects
Denis Drash S./194080	*WT1*/607102 11p13	*Genital ambiguity*, congenital nephropathy, and Wilms' tumor. *Proteinuria, renal impairment*. Frasier syndrome and Meacham syndrome are allelic disorders with similar clinical features	Surgery for Wilms' T.

Frasier S./136680 11p13	*WT1*/607102	*Genital ambiguity, streak gonads*, and XY karyotype; frequently develop gonadoblastoma; progressive glomerulopathy; Wilms' tumor is not a usual feature. Often the diagnosis is during adolescence or adulthood	Prophylactic bilateral gonadectomy; dialysis; and renal transplantation
		No mutant protein is produced by the mutations in WT1 causing Frasier syndrome. Instead, the mutation results in an altered ratio of the two splice isoforms of the protein, those with and those without the extra three amino acids (KTS)	
Meacham S./608978 11p13	*WT1*/607102	*46,XY karyotype, with complex sex reversal or ambiguous genitalia* (retention of Müllerian annexes, double vagina), and congenital diaphragmatic hernia. Other symptoms, including heart, pulmonary, and genital defects, are variable. All patients die early in life. None has renal mesangial sclerosis or Wilms' tumor. Heterozygous mutations in the WT1 gene were identified in some cases	Surgical correction of malformations
DiGeorge S. (DGS)/188400	*TBX1*/602054 22q11.2	A deletion on Cr 22 alters the migration of *neural crest*-derived tissues, affecting development of the pharyngeal pouches and arches. The main clinical features of Digeorge syndrome are cardiac abnormality (mainly tetralogy of Fallot, interrupted aortic arch, ventricular septal defect, and persistent truncus arteriosus), abnormal facies (hypertelorism), T-cell deficit secondary to thymic hypoplasia, cleft palate, and hypocalcemia due to *hypoparathyroidism*. The acronym "CATCH phenotype" has been used to describe this association. Recurrent infections are due to T-cell deficit; seizures secondary to *hypocalcemia* are common. Renal anomalies, hearing loss, skeletal anomalies, autoimmune diseases, feeding difficulties, and developmental delay have been frequently reported. DGS is overlapped with other two syndromes: conotruncal anomalies face (CTAF) and velocardiofacial syndrome (VCFS)	Cardiac surgery, antibiotics and Vitamin D and calcium supplementation
Dubowitz S./223370	? / – AR inheritance	Developmental disorder involving IUGR, short stature, microcephaly, mild mental retardation. Behavior problems, eczema, and unusual and distinctive facies are constant features. Various minor malformations, such as pilonidal dimples, submucous clefts, hypospadias, cryptorchidism, ptosis, high-pitched voice and sparse hair, were also seen	–
		Persistent low serum lipid levels and an arachnoid cyst have been recently associated	

(continued)

Appendix A1 (continued)

Disease/OMIM	Gene/OMIM/map gene locus	Clinical and diagnostic features	Possible specific treatment
EEC1 S./129900	? / – 7q11.2-q21.3	Ectrodactyly, ectodermal dysplasia with severe keratitis, and cleft lip palate (EEC type 1); EEC1 can be associated with GH *deficiency and/or genital anomalies* secondary to developmental defects of the hypothalamus	GH treatment
		Another form of the disorder, designated EEC3 is caused by mutation in the *TP63* gene, but without apparent endocrine disorders	
Fanconi anemia/227650	*FANCA*/607139 16q24.3	FA-A is the most common complementation group, accounting for approximately 65% of all affected individuals. All marrow elements are usually affected, resulting in anemia, leukopenia, and thrombocytopenia (may not manifest in the neonatal period). Pigmentary changes in the skin (cafè-au-lait spots) and malformations of the heart, kidney, and limbs (aplasia of the radius, thumb deformity) are associated congenital features. *Abnormal sexual development* (especially in males) may be present and represents *hypergonadotropic hypogonadism*	Stem cell transplantation
		The *gold-standard screening test for FA is based on the characteristic hypersensitivity of FA cells to the crosslinking agents, such as mitomicin C or diepoxybutane.This is usually a reliable technique to identify FA homozygotes but could not be able to identify individual FA heterozygotes*	
Fanconi-Bickel S./227810	*SLC2A2, GLUT2*/138160 3q26.1-q26.3	Is a metabolic syndrome secondary to impaired utilization of glucose and galactose. Glycogen is accumulated in the liver and kidney. The proximal renal tubular dysfunction leads to polyuria and dehydration. The impaired utilization of glucose and galactose induces fasting hypoglycemia and postprandial hyperglycemia and hypergalactosemia	Diet (low galactose intake, vitamin D, phosphate, water, and electrolytes supplementation)
		Growth is compromised and rickets and osteoporosis later in life were constant	
IMAGe syndrome/614732	*CDKN1C*/600856 11p15.4	See section "Hypercalcemia"	–

Kallmann S.: KS1 308700/ ***KS2*** 147950/ ***KS3*** 244200/ ***KS4*** 610628/ ***KS5*** 612370/ ***KS6*** 600483	*KAL1*/308700 Xp22.3 *FGFR1*/136350 8p11.2-p11.1 *PROKR2*/607123 20p13 *PROK2*/607002 3p21. *CHD7*/608892 8q12.1 *FGF8*/600483 10q24	KS1: hypogonadotropic hypogonadism and anosmia (constantly); sometimes: midline cranial anomalies (choanal atresia and cleft lip or palate), optic nerve atrophy, deafness, cryptorchidism, renal agenesis Loss-of-function mutations in KAL1 and FGFR1 account for approximately 20% of all cases of Kallmann syndrome and mutations in the PROKR2 and PROK2 genes account for an additional 10%. No postnatal increase of LH and testosterone; blunted response to GnRH and hCG tests	Since therapeutic success with substitution therapy is probably age dependent, early diagnosis is important
Kearns-Sayre S./530000	Various mitochondrial deletions	The main features reported for KSS are: ophthalmoplegia, pigmentary degeneration of the retina, and cardiomyopathy. Other signs and symptoms are: muscle weakness, ptosis, CNS dysfunction (cerebellar ataxia and mental retardation), cataracts, cardiac involvement (bradycardia or congestive cardiac failure), endocrine dysfunction (hypogonadism, *diabetes mellitus, growth hormone deficiency, and hypoparathyroidism*). Diagnosis is confirmed with muscle biopsy of the orbicularis muscle. Blood lactate and pyruvate levels are usually elevated. CSF analysis shows elevated proteins (>100 mg/dL) and lactate levels	Coenzyme Q10 administration and vitamin supplements
Kenny-Caffey S. type 1/244460 ***Kenny-Caffey S. type 2***/127000	*TBCE*/604934 1q42-q43	KCS is a skeletal disorder characterized by growth retardation, craniofacial anomalies, and small hands and feet. Bone X-rays show cortical thickening of long bones with medullary stenosis and absent diploic space in the skull. Hypocalcemia consequent to *hypoparathyroidism* may lead to convulsions. *Blood examinations reveal low levels of calcium, phosphorus, and PTH*. In type 2, hypocalcemia may be transient	Prevent severe hypocalcemia
Laron S./262500 5p13-p12	*GHR*/600946	A GH receptor mutation leads to a *GH insensitivity*. Neonatal birthweight and length are usually normal. Postnatal growth is severely compromised. Developmental milestones are delayed and mental retardation may be present. Facial dysmorphism may be present at birth (frontal bossing, hypoplastic nasal bridge, shallows orbits, blue sclera, and decreased vertical dimension of face). Musculoskeletal involvement includes hip dysplasia, hypotrophic musculature, and osteopenia. Obesity is usually present. Sexual development is impaired with *micropenis in childhood* but normal genital growth during adolescence. The puberty is delayed but the reproductive function is conserved. Blood investigations may reveal hypoglycemia and hyercholesterolemia. IGF-1 levels are low despite serum levels of GH normal or elevated. X-ray investigations show bone age delay	Treatment with synthetic IGF1

(*continued*)

Appendix A1 (continued)

Disease/OMIM	Gene/OMIM/map gene locus	Clinical and diagnostic features	Possible specific treatment
Laurence-Moon S./245800 & ***Bardet-Biedl S.***/209900	*BBS1-14*/ 209901-606151-608845-600374-603650-604896-607590-608132-607968-610148-602290-610683-609883-61014211q13/;16q21;3p12-q13; 15q22.3;2q31; 20p12; 4q27;14q32.11; 7p14;12q; 9q33.1; 4q27;17q23; 12q21.3	BBS is a genetically heterogeneous disorder. Polydactyly, *obesity*, retinitis pigmentosa, renal anomalies, mental retardation with progressive ataxia, and spastic diplegia. These patients have *hypogonadism* There has been longstanding uncertainty as to the relationship between the Laurence-Moon syndrome and the Bardet-Biedl syndrome	Support therapy (physiotherapy, rehabilitation, etc.)
Majewski S./263520	*NEK1*/604588 4q33	Malformations included median cleft lip, pre- and postaxial polysyndactyly, short ribs and limbs (typically dysproportionate shortening of the tibia), *ambiguous genitalia,* and anomalies of epiglottis, kidney, CNS, and lung	–
Mitochondrial trifunctional protein deficiency/609015	*HADHA*/600890 HADHB/ 143450 2p23, 2p23	Trifunctional protein deficiency leads to decreased activity of three enzymes. Clinically, it may present with SIDS, a Reye-like syndrome, cardiomyopathy, and/or skeletal myopathy. Early onset symptoms are *hypotonia*, feeding difficulties, *lethargy*, and hypoketotic *hypoglycemia*. Liver, heart, and respiratory system may be involved and may lead to sudden death. The late-onset form is usually milder	Dietary treatment
Müllerian duct aplasia, unilateral renal agenesis, and cervicothoracic somite anomalies (MURCS)/601076	–	MURCS is probably the second most frequent cause of *primary amenorrhoea* after Turner syndrome. It is an association of: Müllerian duct aplasia, unilateral renal aplasia, and cervicothoracic somite dysplasia. Other features reported in literature are: *absent vagina*, Klippel-Feil deformity of the cervical spine, short stature, and conductive deafness	–
Noonan S.: NS1 163950/NS2 605275/NFNS 601321/ NS3 609942/NS4 610733/ NS5 611553 /	*PTPN11*/176876 NF1/162200 *KRAS*/190070 SOS1/182530 *RAF1*/164760 12q24.1, 17q11.2, 12p12.1, 2p22-p21, 3p25	The estimated incidence is of 1 in 1000–2500 live births. Mutations in the *PTPN11* gene accounted for about half the patients reported (NS1). Mutations in the *NF1* (site of mutations causing classic neurofibromatosis type I) have been found in neurofibromatosis – Noonan syndrome (NFNS). De novo germline mutations of the KRAS gene account for less than 5% of NS3 cases. Other forms of Noonan syndrome, such as NS2, NS4, and NS5, have been identified. The syndrome is characterized by hypertelorism, a downward eye slant, and low-set posteriorly rotated ears. Other features include *short stature*, a short neck with webbing or redundancy of skin, cardiac anomalies, epicanthic folds, deafness,	GH treatment may be usefull in some cases

		motor delay, and a bleeding diathesis. *Metacarpophalangeal pattern profile (MCPP) analysis may be useful as a diagnostic tool in screening subjects for Noonan syndrome (PubMed ID: 10797437)*	
Pallister-Hall S./146510	*GLI3*/165240 7p13	Hypothalamic hamartoblastoma (may be lethal in neonatal period), postaxial polydactyly, and imperforate anus. Sometimes had laryngeal cleft, abnormal lung lobation, renal agenesis or dysplasia, short 4th metacarpals, nail dysplasia, multiple buccal frenula, *hypoadrenalism, genital anomalies (microphallus or hypospadia)*, congenital heart defect, and *IUGR*	–
Pendred S./274600	*SLC26A4*/605646 7q21	PDS is the most common syndromal form of deafness; typical features are: bilateral sensorineural hearing loss and *goitre* (usually associated with compensated hypothyroidism) with occasional overt *hypothyroidism*. Mental retardation has been reported	Cochlear implants, speech support, and sometimes L-thyroxine substitutive treatment
Permanent and transient neonatal diabetes mellitus/ 606176/601410/610374/ 610582/610199/609069/ 304790/226980/137920/ 260370	*ABCC8*/600509 KCNJ11/600937 GCK/138079 ZFP57/612192 PLAGL1/603044 ABCC8/ 600509 GLIS3/610192 PTF1A/ 607194 FOXP3/300292 EIF2AK3/604032 HNF1B/ 189907 IPF1/600733 See section 5.4 for chromosome mapping	See section "Hyperglycemia"	See section "Hyperglycemia"
Prader-Willi S./176270	*NDN*/602117 D15S227E/60016 D15S226E/600161 SNRPN/ 182279 15q11-q13	Muscular hypotonia, respiratory distress, and feeding difficulties may be present at birth. Later in life: obesity and hyperphagia, mental retardation, *short stature, hypogonadotropic hypogonadism*, and small hands and feet. It can be considered an autosomal dominant disorder caused in 75% of the patients by deletion of the 15q11-q13 and in 24% by maternal uniparental disomy of the proximal arm of chromosome 15	GH treatment may improve growth management
Robinow S./AD 180700; AR 268310	*WNT5A* /164975 3p14.3 (AD) *ROR2*/602337 9q22 (AR)	Is a genetically heterogeneous disorder characterized by shortlimbed *dwarfism* and abnormal face (fetal face with short, upturned nose, prominent forehead, and flat nasal bridge) and *external genitalia* (micropenis, hypospadia, reduced size clitoris, and underdeveloped labia minora). Adult fertility in females seems to be normal which may explain a lack of male to male transmission in the AD form. The AR form tends to be more severe	–
Sanjad-Sakati S. or Hypoparathyroidism-retardation-dysmorphism S. (HRD)/241410	*TBCE*/604934 1q42-q43	HRD is a rare form of congenital *hypoparathyroidism* associated with growth and mental retardation and seizures. Facial dysmorphism are typical: deep-set eyes, abnormal external ears, depressed nasal bridge with beaked nose, long philtrum, thin upper	–

(*continued*)

Appendix A1 (continued)

Disease/OMIM	Gene/OMIM/map gene locus	Clinical and diagnostic features	Possible specific treatment
		lip, and micrognathia. *Hypocalcemia is associated with hyperphosphatemia and very low concentrations of PTH*	
Septo-optic dysplasia/182230	*HESX1*/601802 3p21.2-p21.1	Clinically heterogeneous disorder defined by any combination of optic nerve hypoplasia, pituitary gland hypoplasia, and midline abnormalities of the brain, including absence of the corpus callosum and septum pellucidum. See section "Hypopituitarism"	Hormone deficient substitutive treatment
Silver-Russel S./180860	*H19*/103280 and *IGF2*/147470 11p15.5, *RSS*/180860 7p11.2	SRS is caused by the epigenetic changes of DNA hypomethylation at the telomeric imprinting control region (ICR1). SRS can also be caused by maternal uniparental disomy of chromosome 7. Severe IUGR, poor postnatal growth, craniofacial features such as a triangular shaped face and a broad forehead, body asymmetry, and a variety of minor malformations	GH treatment; GnRH analogues
Smith-Lemli-Opitz S./270400	*DHCR7*/602858	See ► Chap. 113, "Disorders of Sexual Development in Newborns"	–
Sotos S./117550	NSD1/606681 5q35	Also known as cerebral gigantism; is characterized by excessive growth during the first 2–3 years, *mental retardation*, delayed developmental milestones, and *hypotonia*. Birth length is increased (90–97th centiles), as well as skull dimension. Facial dysmorphism included protrusive forehead, *hypertelorism*, downslanting eyes, highly arched palate, prognathism, pointed chin, and large ears. *Scoliosis*, seizures, heart and kidney defects, hearing loss, and problems with vision are less common features. An increased risk of developing tumors is associates with Sotos syndrome. *X-ray investigations show an advanced bone age*	
Urioste S./235255 (Müllerian derivatives, persistence of, with lymphangiectasia and postaxial polydactyly)	? / – AR or X-linked	*Genital ambiguity* (46,XY with Müllerian duct remnants), IUGR, lung anomalies, redundant nuchal skin, postaxial polydactyly, and lymphangiectasia are constant. Hepatic failure and hypoproteinemia are frequent	Usually early death
VATER association/192350	*PTEN*/601728 10q23.31	The acronym means: vertebral defects, anal atresia, tracheoesophageal fistula associated with esophageal atresia, radial, and renal abnormalities. VACTERL association includes cardiac malformations and limb anomalies. May be associated with *hypocalcemia*	Surgical correction of malformation

Very long-chain acyl-coenzyme A dehydrogenase deficiency (VLCAD)/201475	*ACADVL*/609575 17p13	VLCAD: usually presents with nonketotic *hypoglycemia, lethargy,* and *muscle* weakness. High prevalence of liver dysfunction and life-threatening events (heart disease) has been reported. Diagnosis is confirmed by VLCAD protein in skeletal muscle biopsies	
Long-chain acyl-coenzyme A dehydrogenase deficiency (LCAD)/201460	*ACADL*/609576 2q34-q35	LCAD: nonketotic hypoglycemia, hepatomegaly, cardiomegaly, and hypotonia are the main clinical features. Total plasma carnitine concentration is low. As in ACADM, dicarboxylic acids in the urine are relatively low	
Medium-chain acyl-coenzyme A dehydrogenase deficiency (ACADM)/201450	*ACADM*/607008 1p31	ACADM: may present with intolerance to prolonged fasting and recurrent episodes of hypoglycemic coma. Laboratory findings include medium-chain dicarboxylic aciduria, impaired ketogenesis, and low plasma and tissue carnitine levels	
Vitamin D-dependent rickets, type I (VDDRI)/264700	*CYP27B1*/609506 12q13.1-q13.3	VDDR I is an hereditary selective enzymatic deficiency that leads to lack of the active form of vitamin D (1,25-dihydroxyvitamin D3). Usually presents with defective bone mineralization and clinical features of rickets (hypotonia, tetany, hypocalcemic seizures, irritability, motor retardation, deformations, and growth failure). Laboratory findings include hypocalcemia, increased phosphaturia, markedly decreased serum 1,25-dihydroxyvitamin D3, normal serum 25-hydroxyvitamin D3, aminoaciduria, hyperparathyroidism, and absence of 1-a-hydroxylase activity	VDDR I: large doses of vitamin D2 and physiologic doses of 1-α-hydroxyvitamin D_3
Vitamin D-dependent rickets type II (VDDRII)/277440	*VDR*/601769 12q12-q14	VDDR II is caused by autosomal recessive mutations of the vitamin D receptor. Most patients have total alopecia in addition to rickets. Patients display rapidly progressing rachitic bone changes, hypocalcemia, and secondary hyperparathyroidism. *Serum levels of* $1,25(OH)_2D_3$ *are very high*	VDDR II: limited success to high doses of oral calcium and supraphysiologic doses of 1,25 $(OH)_2D_3$ (1058)
Hypophosphatemic rickets X-linked dominant (XLH)/307800	*PHEX*/300550 Xp22.2-p22.1 1 $(OH)D_3$ or $1,25(OH)_2D_3$	XLH is the most common disease associated with hyperphosphaturia in infancy. Clinical features include growth retardation with rachitic and osteomalacic bone disease. Renal defects in phosphate reabsorption and vitamin D metabolism. Vitamin D treatment does not prevent growth failure. The bone disease is much less severe in females	X-linked: oral phosphate supplementation and physiologic doses Vitamin 1,25 $(OH)_2D_3$
Hypophosphatemic rickets autosomal dominant (ADHR)/193100	*FGF23*/605380 12p13	ADHR: patients frequently present with bone pain, rickets, and tooth abscesses. The penetrance is incomplete and the age at onset is variable (childhood to adult). Resolution of the phosphate-wasting defect has been described in rare cases	This therapy improves but does not cure the bone disease, causes nephrocalcinosis in 60% of the patients and may cause renal failure or hyperparathyroidism

(*continued*)

Appendix A1 (continued)

Disease/OMIM	Gene/OMIM/map gene locus	Clinical and diagnostic features	Possible specific treatment
Hypophosphatemic rickets autosomal recessive (ARHR)/241520	*DMP1*/600980 4q21	ARHP: clinical features very similar to those observed in ADHR, but the inheritance is recessive	Thiazide diuretics decrease urinary calcium excretion and prevent progression of nephrocalcinosis
Hypophosphatemic rickets X-linked recessive/300554	*CLCN5*/300008 Xp11.22	X-recessive form presents with rickets, osteomalacia, and early onset lower extremity deformities. It may progress in renal insufficiency during adulthood	ADHR: phosphate and high doses of vit. D
Hypophosphatemic rickets with hypercalciuria/241530	*SLC34A3*/609826 9q34	Hypophosphatemic rickets with hypercalciuria: presents with rickets, bone pain, muscle weakness, and failure to thrive. XLH: *hypophosphatemia and increased alkaline phosphatase, normal or low serum levels of 1,25-dihydroxyvitamin D_3*. ADHR: hypophosphatemia and inappropriately normal 1,25-dihydroxyvitamin D_3 (calcitriol) levels. X-recessive: hypercalciuria, hypophosphatemia, nephrocalcinosis, and proteinuria. Hypophosphatemic rickets with hypercalciuria: hypophosphatemia with hyperphosphaturia, normocalcemia with hypercalciuria, high plasma $1,25(OH)_2D_3$ concentration, low PTH concentration, and elevated plasma alkaline phosphatase activity	Hypercalciuric form: supplemental phosphate
Pseudohypoparathyroidism type IA (PHP IA)/103580	*GNAS*/139320 20q13.2	PHP is a heterogeneous group of disorders characterized by resistance to the parathyroid hormone. Its pathogenesis has been linked to dysfunctional *G Proteins* (*Gs alpha subunit* (GNAS)) **PHP IA**: presents with a constellation of developmental and skeletal defects, collectively termed Albright hereditary osteodystrophy (AHO). These features include short stature, rounded face, shortened fourth metacarpals and other bones of the hands, obesity, dental hypoplasia, and soft-tissue calcifications. Mental retardation has been reported in some patients. PHP1A is also associated with resistance to TSH, glucagon, and gonadotropins. Alterations may even affect ADH, ACTH, and GH-releasing hormone. GNAS1 mutation is in the maternally derived allele	Symptomatic hypocalcemia needs intravenous calcium administration. Oral calcium and calcitriol should be initiated in every patient with a diagnosis of PHP

Pseudopseudohypo parathyroidism (PPHP)/ 612463	*STX*/603666 20q13.32, 20q13.2, 20q13.2	**PPHP**: AHO phenotype without endocrine abnormalities. GNAS1 mutation is in the paternally inherited allele	The goals of therapy are to maintain serum total and ionized calcium levels within the reference range to avoid hypercalciuria and to maintain PTH levels to normal
Pseudohypoparathyroidism type IB (PHP IB)/603233		**PHP IB**: renal PTH resistance without AHO features; the Gs activity is normal but an imprinting/methylation defects at the GNAS locus results in lack of expression of the maternal allele in renal tissue. Classically, patients do not have features of AHO. TSH resistance has been reported	
Pseudohypoparathyroidism type IC (PHP1C)/612462		**PHP IC**: probably is a variant of PHPIA; the only difference is a normal GNAS activity	
Pseudohypoparathyroidism type II (PHP II)/203330		**PHP II**: isolated renal PTH resistance in patients without AHO phenotype. The resistance may be transient. The Gs activity is normal. The disease seems to be a heterogeneous clinical disorder secondary to a defect in PTH responsiveness distal to cAMP. *Laboratory findings: hypocalcemia, hyperphosphatemia, inappropriately high PTH.* ***PHP1A, PHPIB, PHP IC****: decreased urinary cAMP response to PTH infusion and decreased urinary PO4 response to PTH.* ***PPHP****: normal urinary cAMP response to PTH infusion and normal urinary PO4 response to PTH.* ***PPH II****: normal urinary cAMP response to PTH infusion and decreased urinary PO4 response to PTH*	
WAGR S./194072	*WT1*/607102 PAX6/607108 *BDNF*/113505 11p13 *WBSCR26*/ 612545 *WBSCR27*/612546 *WBSCR28*/612547 7q11.23	Wilms' tumor, aniridia, genitourinary anomalies (ambiguous genitalia or gonadoblastoma of testes or avaries), and mental retardation. Obesity is present in the subtype WAGRO (mutation of the *BDNF* gene)	–
Williams S./194050	*WBS*/194050	See section "Hypercalcemia"	See section "Hypercalcemia"

References

Abeillon-du Payrat J, Chikh K, Bossard N et al (2014) Predictive value of maternal second-generation thyroid-binfing inhibitory immunoglobulin assay for neonatal autoimmune hyperthyroidism. Eur J Endocrinol 171:451–460

Abramowicz MJ, Duprez L, Parma J et al (1997) Familial congenital hypothyroidism due to inactivating mutation of the thyrotropin receptor causing profound hypoplasia of the thyroid gland. J Clin Invest 99:3018–3024

Aguilar-Bryan L, Bryan J (2008) Neonatal diabetes mellitus. Endocr Rev 29:265–291

Alatzoglou KS, Dattani MT (2009) Genetic forms of hypopituitarism and their manifestation in the neonatal period. Early Hum Dev 85:705–712

American Academy of Pediatrics, Rose SR, Section on Endocrinology and Committee on Genetics et al (2006) Update of newborn screening and therapy for congenital hypothyroidism. Pediatrics 117:2290–2303

Arai K, Chrousos G (2013) Aldosterone deficiency and resistance. In: De Groot LJ, Beck-Peccoz P, Chrousos G, Dungan K, Grossman A, Hershman JM, Koch C, McLachlan R, New M, Rebar R, Singer F, Vinik A, Weickert MO (eds) Endotext [Internet], South Dartmouth. http://www.ncbi.nlm.nih.gov/pubmed/25905305

Ares S, Escobar-Morreale HF, Quero J et al (1997) Neonatal hypothyroxinemia: effects of iodine intake and premature birth. J Clin Endocrinol Metab 82:1704–1712

Bakker B, Bikker H, Vulsma T et al (2000) Two decades of screening for congenital hypothyroidism in the Netherlands: TPO gene mutations in total iodide organification defects (an update). J Clin Endocrinol Metab 85:3708–3712

Balsamo A, Antelli A, Baldazzi L et al (2005) A new DAX1 gene mutation associated with congenital adrenal hypoplasia and hypogonadotropic hypogonadism. Am J Med Genet A 135:292–296

Balsamo A, Cicognani A, Gennari M et al (2007) Functional characterization of naturally occurring NR3C2 gene mutations in Italian patients suffering from pseudohypoaldosteronism type 1. Eur J Endocrinol 156:249–256

Bamforth JS, Hughes IA, Lazarus JH et al (1989) Congenital hypothyroidism, spiky hair, and cleft palate. J Med Genet 26:49–51

Besancon A, Beltrand J, Le Gac I et al (2014) Management of neonates born to women with Graves' disease: a color study. Eur J Endocrinol 170:855–862

Biswas S, Buffery J, Enoch H et al (2003) Pulmonary effects of triiodothyronine (T3) and hydrocortisone (HC) supplementation in preterm infants less than 30 weeks gestation: results of the THORN trial–thyroid hormone replacement in neonates. Pediatr Res 53:48–56

Boehm U, Bouloux PM, Dattani MT, de Roux N, Dodé C, Dunkel L, Dwyer AA, Giacobini P, Hardelin JP, Juul A, Maghnie M, Pitteloud N, Prevot V, Raivio T, Tena-Sempere M, Quinton R, Young J (2015) Expert consensus document: European consensus statement on congenital hypogonadotropic hypogonadism – pathogenesis, diagnosis and treatment. Nat Rev Endocrinol 11(9):547–564. http://www.ncbi.nlm.nih.gov/pubmed/26194704

Bongers-Schokking JJ, de Muinck Keizer-Schrama S (2005) Influence of timing and dose of thyroid hormone replacement on mental, psychomotor, and behavioral development in children with congenital hypothyroidism. J Pediatr 147:768–774

Bottino M, Cowett RM, Sinclair JC (2009) Interventions for treatment of neonatal hyperglycemia in very low birth weight infants. Cochrane Database Syst Rev 1: CD007453

Bowl MR, Nesbit MA, Harding B et al (2005) An interstitial deletion- insertion involving chromosomes 2p25.3 and Xq27.1, near SOX3, causes X-linked recessive hypoparathyroidism. J Clin Invest 115:2822–2831

Bringhurst ER, Demay MB, Kronenberg HM (2008) Hormones and disorders of mineral metabolism. In: Kronenberg HM, Melmed S, Polonsky KS et al (eds) Williams textbook of endocrinology, 11th edn. Saunders, Philadelphia, pp 1241–1249

Bubuteishvili L, Garel C, Czernichow P, Léger J (2003) Thyroid abnormalities by ultrasonography in neonates with congenital hypothyroidism. J Pediatr 143:759–764

Calaciura F, Motta RM, Miscio G et al (2002) Subclinical hypothyroidism in early childhood: a frequent outcome of transient neonatal hyperthyrotropinemia. J Clin Endocrinol Metab 87:3209–3214

Canadian Paediatric Society (2004) Screening guidelines for newborns at risk for low blood glucose. Paediatr Child Health 9:723–740

Carranza D, Van Vliet G, Polak M (2006) Congenital hypothyroidism. Ann Endocrinol (Paris) 67:295–302

Cassio A, Cacciari E, Cicognani A et al (2003) Treatment for congenital hypothyroidism: thyroxine alone or thyroxine plus triiodothyronine? Pediatrics 111:1055–1060

Cassio A, Corbetta C, Antonozzi I et al (2013a) The Italian screening program for primary congenital hypothyroidism: actions to improve screening, diagnosis, follow-up, and surveillance. J Endocrinol Investig 36:195–203

Cassio A, Nicoletti A, Rizzello A et al (2013b) Current loss-of-function mutations in the thyrotropin receptor gene: when to investigate, clinical effects, and treatment. J Clin Res Pediatr Endocrinol 5(Suppl 1):XX

Cassio A, Cantasano A, Bal MO (2014) Ipotiroidismo congenito. Prospect Pediatr 44:2–7

Cassio A, Bal MO, Bettocchi I et al (2015) Thyroid enlargement from newborn to adolescent. In: Bona G et al (eds) Thyroid diseases in childhood: recent advances from basic science to clinical practice. Springer International Publishing, Swithzerland

Castanet M, Polak M, Bonaiti-Pellié C et al (2001) Nineteen years of national screening for congenital hypothyroidism: familial cases with thyroid dysgenesis suggest the involvement of genetic factors. J Clin Endocrinol Metab 86:2009–2014

Castanet M, Marinovic D, Polak M, Léger J (2010) Epidemiology of thyroid dysgenesis: the familial component. Horm Res Paediatr 73(4):231–237

Cavarzere P, Camilot M, Popa FI et al (2016) Congenital hypothyroidism with delayed TSH elevation in low-birth-weight infants. Incidence, diagnosis and mangement. Eur J Endocrinol 175:395–402

Cerbone M, Capalbo D, Wasniewska M et al (2014) Cardiovascular risk factors in children with long-standing untreated idiopathic subclinical hypothyroidism. J Clin Endocrinol Metab 99:2697–2703

Cerbone M, Capalbo D, Wasniewska M et al (2016) Effect of L-thyroxine treatment on early markers of atherosclerotic disease in childrenwith subclinical hypothyroidism. Eur J Endocrinol 175:11–19

Chanoine JP, Pardou A, Bourdoux P, Delange F (1988) Withdrawal of iodinated disinfectants at delivery decreases the recall rate at neonatal screening for congenital hypothyroidism. Arch Dis Child 63:1297–1298

Chiovato L, Lapi P, Santini F et al (1994) Thyroid autoimmunity and congenital hypothyroidism. Ann Ist Super Sanita 30:317–323

Chung TT, Monson JP (2015) Hypopituitarism. In: De Groot LJ, Beck-Peccoz P, Chrousos G, Dungan K, Grossman A, Hershman JM, Koch C, McLachlan R, New M, Rebar R, Singer F, Vinik A, Weickert MO (eds) Endotext [Internet], South Dartmouth. http://www.ncbi.nlm.nih.gov/pubmed/25905222

Chung TT, Chan LF, Metherell LA, Clark AJ (2010) Phenotypic characteristics of familial glucocorticoid deficiency (FGD) type 1 and 2. Clin Endocrinol 72(5):589–594. http://www.ncbi.nlm.nih.gov/pubmed/19558534

Colombo C, Porzio O, Liu M et al (2008) Early Onset Diabetes Study Group of the Italian Society of Pediatric Endocrinology and Diabetes (SIEDP). Seven mutations in the human insulin gene linked to permanent neonatal/infancy-onset diabetes mellitus. J Clin Invest 118:2148–2156

Committee on Fetus and Newborn, Adamkin DH (2011) Postnatal glucose homeostasis in late-preterm and term infants. Pediatrics 127:575–579

Corzo D, Gibson W, Johnson K et al (2002) Contiguous deletion of the X-linked adrenoleukodystrophy gene (ABCD1) and DXS1357E: a novel neonatal phenotype similar to peroxisomal biogenesis disorders. Am J Hum Genet 70:1520–1531

Coulter CL (2004) Functional biology of the primate fetal adrenal gland: advances in technology provide new insight. Clin Exp Pharmacol Physiol 31:475–484

Dabrowski E, Kadakia R, Zimmerman D (2016) Diabetes insipidus in infants and children. Best Pract Res Clin Endocrinol Metab 30(2):317–328. http://www.ncbi.nlm.nih.gov/pubmed/27156767

Daneman D, Daneman A (2005) Diagnostic imaging of the thyroid and adrenal glands in childhood. Endocrinol Metab Clin N Am 34:745–768

Davis LE, Lucas MJ, Hankins GD et al (1989) Thyrotoxicosis complicating pregnancy. Am J Obstet Gynecol 160:63–70

De Felice M, Di Lauro R (2004) Thyroid development and its disorders: genetics and molecular mechanisms. Endocr Rev 25:722–746

De Felice M, Di Lauro R (2007) Murine models for the study of thyroid gland development. Endocr Dev 10:1–14

De Felice M, Di Lauro R (2011) Intrinsic and extrinsic factors in thyroid gland development: an update. Endocrinology 152:163

De Felice M, Di Lauro R (2015) Thyroid embryogenesis. In: Bona G et al (eds) Thyroid diseases in childhood: recent advances from basic science to clinical practice. Springer International Publishing, Switzerland

De Filippis T, Gelmini G, Paraboschi E, Vigone MC, Di Frenna M, Marelli F, Bonomi M, Cassio A, Larizza D, Moro M, Radetti G, Salerno M, Ardissino D, Weber G, Gentilini D, Guizzardi F, Duga S, Persani L (2017) A frequent oligogenic involvement in congenital hypothyroidism. Hum Mol Genet 26(13):2507–2514. https://doi.org/10.1093/hmg/ddx145. https://www.ncbi.nlm.nih.gov/pubmed/28444304

Delange F, Bürgi H, Chen ZP, Dunn JT (2002) World status of monitoring iodine deficiency disorders control programs. Thyroid 12:915–924

Devos H, Rodd C, Gagne N et al (1999) A search for the possible molecular mechanisms of thyroid dysgenesis: sex ratios and associated malformations. J Clin Endocrinol Metab 84:2502–2506

Ding C, Buckingham B, Levine MA (2001) Familial isolated hypoparathyroidism caused by a mutation in the gene for the transcription factor GCMB. J Clin Invest 108:1215–1220

Djemli A, Fillion M, Belgoudi J et al (2004) Twenty years later: a reevaluation of the contribution of plasma thyroglobulin to the diagnosis of thyroid dysgenesis in infants with congenital hypothyroidism. Clin Biochem 37:818–822

DuPrez L, Parma J, Van Sande J et al (1994) Germline mutations in the thyrotropin receptor gene cause non-autoimmune autosomal dominant hyprthyroidism. Nat Genet 7:396–401

Elliott M, Bayly R, Cole T et al (1994) Clinical features and natural history of Beckwith-Wiedemann syndrome: presentation of 74 new cases. Clin Genet 46:168–174

Ellis PD, van Nostrand AW (1977) The applied anatomy of thyroglossal tract remnants. Laryngoscope 87:765–770

de Escobar GM, Obregón MJ, del Rey FE (2004) Maternal thyroid hormones early in pregnancy and fetal brain development. Best Pract Res Clin Endocrinol Metab 18:225–248

Etling N, Padovani E, Gehin-Fouque F, Tato L (1984) Serum and urine thyroid hormone levels in healthy preterm and small for date infants on the first and fifth day of life. Hely Paediatr Acta 39:223–230

Eugster EA, LeMay D, Zerin JM, Pescovitz OH (2004) Definitive diagnosis in children with congenital hypothyroidism. J Pediatr 144:643–647

Fagman H, Amendola E, Parrillo L et al (2011) Gene expression profi ling at early organogenesis reveals both common and diverse mechanisms in foregut patterning. Dev Biol 359:163

Farfel Z, Bourne H, Iiri T (1999) The expanding spectrum of G protein disease. N Engl J Med 340:1012–1020

Filippi L, Pezzati M, Poggi C et al (2007) Dopamine versus dobutamine in very low birthweight infants: endocrine effects. Arch Dis Child Fetal Neonatal Ed 92:F367–F371

Fisher DA (1998) Thyroid function in premature infants. The hypothyroxinemia of prematurity. Clin Perinatol 25:999–1014

Fisher DA, Dussault JH, Sack J, Chopra J (1977) Ontogenesis of hypothalamic-pituitary-thyroid function and metabolism in man, sheep and rat. Recent Prog Horm Res 33:59–116

Fourtner SH, Stanley CA (2004) Genetic and nongenetic forms of hyperinsulinism in neonates. NeoReviews 5: e370–e376

Friesema EC, Grueters A, Biebermann H et al (2004) Association between mutations in a thyroid hormone transporter and severe Xlinked psychomotor retardation. Lancet 364:1435–1437

Gharib H, Tuttle RM, Baskin HJ et al (2005) Subclinical thyroid dysfunction: a joint statement on management from the American Association of Clinical Endocrinologists, the American Thyroid Association, and the Endocrine Society. J Clin Endocrinol Metab 90:581–587

Ghirri P, Bottone U, Coccoli L et al (1999) Symptomatic hypercalcemia in the first months of life: calcium-regulating hormones and treatment. J Endocrinol Investig 22:349–353

Ghirri P, Ladaki C, Bartoli A et al (2007) Low birth weight for gestational age associates with reduced glucose concentrations at birth, infancy and childhood. Horm Res 67:123–131

Glinoer D (2001) Potential consequences of maternal hypothyroidism on the offspring: evidence and implications. Horm Res 55:109–114

Goldsmit GS, Valdes M, Herzovich V et al (2011) Evaluation and clinical application of changes in thyroid hormone and TSH levels in critically ill full-term newborns. J Perinat Med 39:59–64

Goto M, Piper Hanley K et al (2006) In humans, early cortisol biosynthesis provides a mechanism to safeguard female sexual development. J Clin Invest 116:953–960

Grüters A, Krude H (2007) Update on the management of congenital hypothyroidism. Horm Res 68(Suppl 5):107–111

Guran T, Buonocore F, Saka N et al (2016) Rare causes of primary adrenal insufficiency: genetic and clinical characterization of a large nationwide cohort. J Clin Endocrinol Metab 101(1):284–292. http://www.ncbi.nlm.nih.gov/pmc/articles/PMC4701852/

Haddow JE, Palomaki GE, Allan WC et al (1999) Maternal thyroid deficiency during pregnancy and subsequent neuropsychological development of the child. N Engl J Med 341:549–555

Hanley NA, Arlt W (2006) The human fetal adrenal cortex and the window of sexual differentiation. Trends Endocrinol Metab 17:391–397

Hanukoglu A, Perlman K, Shamis I et al (2001) Relationship of etiology to treatment in congenital hypothyroidism. J Clin Endocrinol Metab 86:186–191

Harris D, Weston P, Battin M, Harding JE (2013) Dextrose gel for treating neonatal hypoglycemia: a randomized placebo-controlled trial (The sugar babies study). Lancet 382:2077–2083

Hoyes AD, Kershaw DR (1985) Anatomy and development of the thyroid gland. Ear Nose Throat J 64:318–333

Ibrahim A, Kirby G et al (2014) Methylation analysis and diagnostics of Beckwith-Wiedemann syndrome in 1,000 subjects. Clin Epigenetics 6(1):11

John R, Bamforth FJ (1987) Serum free thyroxine and free triiodothyronine concentrations in healthy fullterm, preterm and sick preterm neonates. Ann Clin Biochem 24:461–465

van der Kaay DC, Wasserman JD, Palmert MR (2016) Management of neonates born to mothers with Graves' diease. Pediatrics 137:e20151878

Karakoc-Aydiner E, Turan S, Akpinar I et al (2012) Pitfalls in the diagnosis of thyroid dysgenesis by thyroid ultrasography and scintigraphy. Eur J Endocrinol 166:43–48

Karras S, Krassas GE (2012) Breastfeeding and antithyroid drugs: a view from within. Eur Thyroid J 1:30–33

Karras S, Tzotzas T, Kaltsas T et al (2010) Pharmacological treatment of hyperthyroidism during lactation: review of the literature and novel data. Pediatr Endocrinol Rev 8:25–33

Kempers MJ, van Tijn DA, van Trotsenburg AS et al (2003) Central congenital hypothyroidism due to gestational hyperthyroidism: detection where prevention failed. J Clin Endocrinol Metab 88:5851–5857

Kempná P, Flück CE (2008) Adrenal gland development and defects. Best Pract Res Clin Endocrinol Metab 22:77–93

Kester MH, Martinez de Mena R, Obregon MJ et al (2004) Iodothyronine levels in the human developing brain: major regulatory roles of iodothyronine deiodinases in different areas. J Clin Endocrinol Metab 89:3117–3128

Kohn LD, Suzuki K, Hoffman WH et al (1997) Characterization of monoclonal thyroid-stimulating and thyrotropin bindinginhibiting autoantibodies from a Hashimoto's patient whose children had intrauterine and neonatal thyroid disease. J Clin Endocrinol Metab 82:3998–4009

Krude H, Biebermann H, Kroh HP et al (1997) Congenital hyperthyroidism. Exp Clin Endocrinol Diabetes 1o5 (Suppl 4):6–11

Krude H, Schütz B, Biebermann H et al (2002) Choreoathetosis, hypothyroidism and pulmonary alterations due to human NKX2-1 haploinsufficiency. J Clin Invest 109:475–480

Kusakabe T, Kawaguchi A, Hoshi N et al (2006) Thyroid-specifi c enhancer-binding protein/NKX2.1 is required for the maintenance of ordered architecture and function of the differentiated thyroid. Mol Endocrinol 20:1796–1809

LaFranchi S (1999) Thyroid function in the preterm infant. Thyroid 9:71–78

LaFranchi SH, Austin J (2007) How should we be treating children with congenital hypothyroidism? J Pediatr Endocrinol Metab 20:559–578

Langer M, Modi BP, Agus M (2006) Adrenal insufficiency in the critically ill neonate and child. Curr Opin Pediatr 18:448–453

Léger J (2016) Management of fetal and neonatal Graves disease. Horm Res Paediatr 87:1–6

Léger J, Larroque B, Norton J, Association Française pour le Dépistage et la Prévetion des Handicaps de l'Enfant (2001) Influence of severity of congenital hypothyroidism and adequacy of treatment on school achievement in young adolescents: a population-based cohort study. Acta Paediatr 90:1249–1256

Leger J, Olivieri A, Donaldson M et al (2014) European society for paediatric endocrinology consensus guidelines on screening, diagnosis, and management of congenital hypothyroidism. J Clin Endocrinol Metab 99:363–384

Leonardi D, Polizzotti N, Carta A et al (2008) Longitudinal study of thyroid function in children with mild hyperthyrotropinemia at neonatal screening for congenital hypothyroidism. J Clin Endocrinol Metab 93:2679–2685

Lucas A, Rennie J, Baker BA, Morley R (1988) Low plasma triiodo- thyronine concentrations and outcome in preterm infants. Arch Dis Child 63:1201–1206

Luton D, Fried D, Sibony O et al (1997) Assessment of fetal thyroid function by colored Doppler echography. Fetal Diagn Ther 12:24–27

Luton D, Le Gac I, Vuillard E et al (2005) Management of Graves' disease during pregnancy: the key role of fetal thyroid gland monitoring. J Clin Endocrinol Metab 90:6093–6098

Mannstadt M, Clarke BL et al (2013) Efficacy and safety of recombinant human parathyroid hormone (1–84) in hypoparathyroidism (REPLACE): a double-blind, placebo-controlled, randomised, phase 3 study. Lancet Diabetes Endocrinol 1(4):275–283

Marcialis MA, Dessì A, Contu S, Vassilios F (2009) Nephrogenic syndrome of inappropriate antidiuresis: a novel cause of euvolemic hypotonic hyponatremia in newborns. Diagnosis and practical management. J Matern Fetal Neonatal Med 22(sup 3):67–71. https://doi.org/10.1080/14767050903196037

Matsuura N, Yamada Y, Nohara Y et al (1980) Familial neonatal transient hypothyroidism due to maternal TSH-binding inhibitor immunoglobulins. N Engl J Med 303:738–741

McKinlay CJ, Alsweiler JM, Ansell JM, Anstice NS, Chase JG, Gamble GD, Harris DL, Jacobs RJ, Jiang Y, Paudel N, Signal M, Thompson B, Wouldes TA, Yu TY, Harding JE, CHYLD Study Group (2015) Neonatal glycemia and neurodevelopmental outcomes at 2 years. N Engl J Med 373(16):1507–1518

Meeus L, Gilbert B, Rydlewski C et al (2004) Characterization of a novel loss of function mutation of PAX8 in a familial case of congenital hypothyroidism with in place, normalsized thyroid. J Clin Endocrinol Metab 89:4285–4291

Mehta A, Hindmarsh PC, Mehta H, Turton JP, Russell-Eggitt I, Taylor D, Chong WK, Dattani MT (2009) Congenital hypopituitarism: clinical, molecular and neuroradiological correlates. Clin Endocrinol 71 (3):376–382. http://www.ncbi.nlm.nih.gov/pubmed/19320653

Meller J, Zappel H, Conrad M et al (1997) Diagnostic value of 123- iodine scintigraphy and perchlorate discharge test in the diagnosis of congenital hypothyroidism. Exp Clin Endocrinol Diabetes 105(Suppl 4):24–27

Mengreli C, Maniati-Christidi M, Kanaka-Gantenbein C et al (2003) Transient congenital hypothyroidism due to maternal autoimmune thyroid disease. Hormones 2:113–119

Metzger BE, Persson B, HAPO Study Cooperative Research Group et al (2010) Hyperglycemia and adverse pregnancy outcome study: neonatal glycemia. Pediatrics 126:e1545–e1552

Monti S, Nicoletti A, Cantasano A et al (2015) NKX2.1-related disorders: a novel mutation with mild clinical presentation. Ital J Pediatr 41:45–49

Moreno JC, Visser TJ (2007) New phenotypes in thyroid dyshormonogenesis: hypothyroidism due to DUOX2 mutations. Endocr Dev 10:99–117

Moreno JC, Bikker H, Kempers MI et al (2002) Inactivating mutations in the gene for thyroid oxidaxe 2 (DUOX2) and congenital hypothyroidism. N Engl J Med 347:95–102

Morreale de Escobar G, Obregón MJ, Escobar del Rey F (2000) Is neuropsychological development related to maternal hypothyroidism or to maternal hypothyroxinemia? J Clin Endocrinol Metab 85:3975–3987

Murphy N, Hume R, van Toor H et al (2004) The hypothalamic-pituitary-thyroid axis in preterm infants; changes in the first 24 hours of postnatal life. J Clin Endocrinol Metab 89:2824–2831

Mussa A et al (2016) Recommendations of the Scientific Committee of the Italian Beckwith-Wiedemann Syndrome Association on the diagnosis, management and follow-up of the syndrome. Eur J Med Genet 59 (1):52–64

Muzza M, Rabbiosi S, Vigone MC et al (2014) The clinical and molecular characterization of patients with dyshormonogenic congenital hypothyroidism reveals specific diagnostic clues for DUOX2 defects. J Clin Endocrinol Metab 99(3):E544–E553

Nicoletti A, Bal M, De Marco G et al (2009) Thyrotropin-stimulating hormone receptor gene analysis in pediatric patients with non-autoimmune subclinical hypothyroidism. J Clin Endocrinol Metab 94:4187–4194

O'Rahilly R (1983) The timing and sequence of events in the development of the human endocrine system during the embryonic period proper. Anat Embryol 166:439–451

Ogilvy-Stuart AL (2002) Neonatal thyroid disorders. Arch Dis Child Fetal Neonatal Ed 87:165–171

Ogilvy-Stuart A, Midgerly P (2006) Hypocalcemia. In: Practical neonatal endocrinology. Cambridge University Press, New York, pp 133–142

Ogilvy-Stuart A, Midgley P (2006) Hypernatraemia. In: Practical neonatal endocrinology. Cambridge University Press, New York, p 115

Olivieri A (2015) Epidemiology of congenital hypothyroidism. In: Bona G et al (eds) Thyroid diseases in childhood: recent advances from basic science to clinical practice. Springer International Publishing, Swithzerland

Olivieri A, Stazi MA, Mastroiacovo P et al (2002) A population-based study on the frequency of additional congenital malformations in infants with congenital hypothyroidism: data from the Italian registry for congenital hypothyroidism (1991–1998). J Clin Endocrinol Metab 87:557–562

Olivieri A, Medda E, De Angelis S et al (2007) High risk of congenital hypothyroidism in multiple pregnancies. J Clin Endocrinol Metab 92:3141–3147

Olivieri A, Fazzini C, Medda E et al (2015) Multiple factors influencing the incidence of congenital hypothyroidism detected by neonatal screening. Horm Res Paediatr 83:86–93

Opitz R, Antonica F, Costagliola S (2013) New model systems to illuminate thyroid organogenesis. Part I: an update on the zebrafi sh toolbox. Eur Thyroid J 2:229

Osborn DA, Hunt RW (2007) Postnatal thyroid hormones for preterm infants with transient hypothyroxinaemia. Cochrane Database Syst Rev 1:CD005945

Palos F, García-Rendueles ME, Araujo-Vilar D et al (2008) Pendred syndrome in two Galiacian families: insights into clinical phenotypes through cellular, genetic, and molecular studies. J Clin Endocrinol Metab 93:267–277

Paul DA, Leef KH, Stefano JL, Bartoshesky L (1998) Low serum thyroxine on initial newborn screening is associated with intraventricular hemorrhage and death in very low birth weight infants. Pediatrics 101:903–907

Pearce EN (2006) Diagnosis and management of thyrotoxicosis. BMJ 332:1369–1373

Pearce SH, Williamson C, Kifor O et al (1996) A familial syndrome of hypocalcemia with hypercalciuria due to mutations in the calcium- sensing receptor. N Engl J Med 335:1115–1122

Perry RJ, Maroo S, Maclennan AC et al (2006) Combined ultrasound and isotope scanning is more informative in the diagnosis of congenital hypothyroidism than single scanning. Arch Dis Child 91:972–976

Persani L (2012) Central hypothyroidism: pathogenetic, diagnostic, and therapeuticchallanges. J Clin Endocrinol Metab 97:3068–3078

Peters CJ, Hindmarsh PC (2007) Management of neonatal endocrinopathies – best practice guidelines. Early Hum Dev 83:553–561

Polak M, Sura-Trueba S, Chauty A et al (2004) Molecular mechanisms of thyroid dysgenesis. Horm Res 62(Supp 13):14–21

Polak M, Legac I, Vuillard E et al (2006) Congenital hyperthyroidism: the fetus as a patient. Horm Res 65:235–242

Rabbiosi S, Vigone MC, Cortinovis F et al (2013) Congenital hypothyroidism with eutopic thyroid gland. Analysis of clinical and biochemical features at diagnosis and after re-evaluation. J Clin Endocrinol Metab 98:1395–1402

Ranzini AC, Ananth CV, Smulian JC et al (2001) Ultrasonography of the fetal thyroid: nomograms based on biparietal diameter and gestational age. J Ultrasound Med 20:613–617

Rapaport R, Rose SR, Freemark M (2001) Hypothyroxinemia in the preterm infants: the benefits and risks of thyroxine treatment. J Pediatr 139:182–188

Refetoff S, Weiss RE, Usala SJ (1993) The syndromes of resistance to thyroid hormone. Endocr Rev 14:348–399

Refetoff S, Dumont J, Vassart G (2001) Thyroid disorders. In: Scriver CR, Beaudet AL, Sly WS, Valle D (eds) The metabolic and molecular basis of inherited disease. McGraw-Hill, New York

Richard K, Hume R, Kaptein E et al (1998) Ontogeny of iodothyronine deiodinases in human liver. J Clin Endocrinol Metab 83:2868–2874

Rochiccioli P, Rogé B, Alexandre F, Tauber MT (1992) School achievement in children with hypothyroidism detected at birth and search for predictive factors. Horm Res 38:236–240

Rovelli R, Vigone MC, Giovanettoni C et al (2010) Newborn of mothers affected by autoimmune thyroiditis: the importance of thyroid function monitoring in the fi rst months of life. Ital J Pediatr 36:24

Rovet JF (2002) Congenital hypothyroidism: an analysis of persisting deficits and associated factors. Child Neuropsychol 8:150–162

Rozance PJ, Hay WW Jr (2010) Neonatal hyperglycemia. NeoReviews 11:632–639

Rivkees SA, Szarfarm A (2010) Dissimilar hepatotoxicity profiles of propylthiouracil and methimazole in children. J Clin Endocrinol Metab 95(7):3260–7. https://doi.org/10.1210/jc.2009-2546. Epub 2010 Apr 28

Salerno M, Capalbo D, Cerbone M et al (2016) Subclinical hypothyroidism in childhood-current knowledge and open issues. Nat Rev Endocrinol 12:734–746

Samedi VM, Yusuf K, Yee W, Obaid H, Al Awad EH (2014) Neonatal hypercalcemia secondary to subcutaneous fat necrosis successfully treated with pamidronate: a case series and literature review. AJP Rep 4(2):e93–e96

Santini F, Chiovato L, Ghirri P et al (1999) Serum iodothyronines in the human fetus and the newborn: evidence for an important role of placenta in fetal thyroid hormone homeostasis. J Clin Endocrinol Metab 84:493–498

Schoen EJ, Clapp W, To TT, Fireman BH (2004) The key role of newborn thyroid scintigraphy with isotopic iodide (123I) in defining and managing congenital hypothyroidism. Pediatrics 114:e683–e688

Shenker A, Weinstein LS, Moran A et al (1993) Severe endocrine and non-endocrine manifestations of the McCune-Albright syndrome associated with activating mutations of stimulatory G protein GS. J Pediatr 123:509–518

Simoneau-Roy J, Marti S, Deal C et al (2004) Cognition and behavior at school entry in children with congenital hypothyroidism treated early with high-dose levothyroxine. J Pediatr 144:747–752

Spanakis E, Milord E, Gragnoli C (2008) AVPR2 variants and mutations in nephrogenic diabetes insipidus: review and missense mutation significance. J Cell Physiol 217:605–617

Spiegel AM (2000) G protein defects in signal transduction. Horm Res 53(Supp 13):17–22

Stanley CA (2016) Perspective on the genetics and diagnosis of congenital hyperinsulinism disorders. J Clin Endocrinol Metab 101(3):815–826

Suntharalingham JP, Buonocore F, Duncan AJ, Achermann JC (2015) DAX-1 (NR0B1) and steroidogenic factor-1 (SF-1, NR5A1) in human disease. Best Pract Res Clin Endocrinol Metab 29(4):607–619. http://www.ncbi.nlm.nih.gov/pubmed/26303087

Sunthornthepvarakui T, Gottschalk ME, Hayashi Y, Refetoff S (1995) Brief report: resistance to thyrotropin caused by mutations in the thyrotropin-receptor gene. N Engl J Med 332:155–160

Sunthornthepvarakul T, Churesigaew S, Ngowngarmratana S (1999) A novel mutation of the signal peptide of the preproparathyroid hormone gene associated with autosomal recessive familial isolated hypoparathyroidism. J Clin Endocrinol Metab 84:3792–3796

Szinnai G, Kosugi S, Derrien C et al (2006) Extending the clinical heterogeneity of iodide transport defect (ITD): a novel mutation R124H of the sodium/iodide symporter gene and review of genotype-phenotype correlations in ITD. J Clin Endocrinol Metab 91:1199–1204

Tomova A, Deepinder F, Robeva R, Lalabonova H, Kumanov P, Agarwal A et al (2010) Growth and development of male external genitalia: a cross-sectional study of 6200 males aged 0 to 19 years. Arch Pediatr Adolesc Med 164:1152–1157. http://www.ncbi.nlm.nih.gov/pubmed/21135345

Transue D, Chan J, Kaplan M (1992) Management of neonatal Graves disease with iopanoic acid. J Pediatr 121:472–474

Turcu AF, Auchus RJ (2015) The next 150 years of congenital adrenal hyperplasia. J Steroid Biochem Mol Biol 153:63–71. http://www.ncbi.nlm.nih.gov/pubmed/26047556

Van Vliet G (2001) Treatment of congenital hypothyroidism. Lancet 358:86–87

Van Vliet G, Czernichow P (2004) Screening for neonatal endocrinopathies: rationale, methods and results. Semin Neonatol 9:75–85

Van Vliet G, Larroque B, Bubuteishvili L et al (2003) Sex-specific impact of congenital hypothyroidism due to thyroid dysgenesis on skeletal maturation in term newborns. J Clin Endocrinol Metab 88:2009–2013

van Wassenaer AG, Kok JH, Dekker FW, de Vijlder JJ (1997) Thyroid function in very preterm infants: influences of gestational age and disease. Pediatr Res 42:604–609

Vogel BH, Bradley SE, Adams DJ, D'Aco K, Erbe RW, Fong C, Iglesias A, Kronn D, Levy P, Morrissey M, Orsini J, Parton P, Pellegrino J, Saavedra-Matiz CA, Shur N, Wasserstein M, Raymond GV, Caggana M (2015) Newborn screening for X-linked adrenoleukodystrophy in New York State: diagnostic protocol, surveillance protocol and treatment guidelines. Mol Genet Metab 114(4):599–603. http://www.ncbi.nlm.nih.gov/pubmed/25724074

Vulsma T, Gons MH, de Vijlder JJ (1989) Maternal-fetal transfer of thyroxine in congenital hypothyroidism due to a total organification defect or thyroid agenesis. N Engl J Med 321:13–16

Wasniewska M, De Luca F, Cassio A et al (2003) In congenital hypothyroidism bone maturation at birth may be a predictive factor of psychomotor development during the first year of life irrespective of other variables related to treatment. Eur J Endocrinol 149:1–6

Webb EA, Krone N (2015) Current and novel approaches to children and young people with congenital adrenal hyperplasia and adrenal insufficiency. Best Pract Res Clin Endocrinol Metab 29(3):449–468. http://www.ncbi.nlm.nih.gov/pubmed/?term=current+and+novel+approaches+to+children+and+young+people+with+CAH+and+adrenal#

Weber G, Vigone MC, Rapa A et al (1998) Neonatal transient hypothyroidism: aetiological study. Arch Dis Child Fetal Neonatal Ed 79:F70–FF7

Weksberg R, Shuman C, Beckwith JB (2009) Beckwith–Wiedemann syndrome. Eur J Hum Genet 18:8–14

Wiesinger C, Eichler FS, Berger J (2015) The genetic landscape of X-linked adrenoleukodystrophy: inheritance, mutations, modifier genes, and diagnosis. Appl Clin Genet 8:109–121

Williams F, Hume R (2011) The measuremenet, definition, etiology and clinical consequences of neonatal transient hypothyroxinemia. Ann Clin Biochem 48:7–22

Williams FL, Ogston SA, van Toor H et al (2005) Serum thyroid hormones in preterm infants: associations with postnatal illnesses and drug usage. J Clin Endocrinol Metab 90:5954–5963

Williams FL, Visser TJ, Hume R (2006) Transient hypothyroxinaemia in preterm infants. Early Hum Dev 82:797–802

Zakarija M, McKenzie JM, Munro DS (1983) Immunoglobulin G inhibitor of thyroid-stimulating antibody is a cause of delay in the onset of neonatal Graves' disease. J Clin Invest 72:1352–1356

Zamproni I, Grasberger H, Cortinovis F et al (2008) Biallelic inactivation of the dual oxidase maturation factor 2 (DUOXA2) gene as a novel cause of congenital hypothyroidism. J Clin Endocrinol Metab 93:605–610

Disorders of Sexual Development in Newborns

113

Antonio Balsamo, Paolo Ghirri, Silvano Bertelloni, Rosa T. Scaramuzzo, Franco D'Alberton, Alessandro Cicognani, and Antonio Boldrini

Contents

A. Balsamo · F. D'Alberton (✉) · A. Cicognani (✉)
Department of Medical and Surgical Sciences, Pediatric Unit, Center for Rare Endocrine Diseases (CARENDO BO), S.Orsola Malpighi University Hospital, Bologna, Italy
e-mail: antonio.balsamo@unibo.it; franco.dalberton@gmail.com; alessandro.cicognani@unibo.it

P. Ghirri (✉) · A. Boldrini (✉)
Department of Clinical and Experimental Medicine, Division of Neonatology and Neonatal Intensive Care Unit, Santa Chiara University Hospital, Pisa, Italy
e-mail: pghirri@med.unipi.it; antonio.boldrini@med.unipi.it

S. Bertelloni (✉)
Adolescent Medicine Unit, Division of Pediatrics, S. Chiara Hospital, University of Pisa, Pisa, Italy
e-mail: s.bertelloni@ao-pisa.toscana.it

R. T. Scaramuzzo (✉)
Neonatology and Neonatal Intensive Care Unit, Santa Chiara University Hospital, Pisa, Italy
e-mail: r.scaramuzzo@ao-pisa.toscana.it

G. Buonocore et al. (eds.), *Neonatology*,
https://doi.org/10.1007/978-3-319-29489-6_260

Abstract
The understanding, care, and treatment of newborns born with disorders of sex development conditions have evolved considerably over the last few decades. Biological assessment of atypical genitalia is based on a structured sequence of endocrine and genetic investigations, starting from a suitable history and a complete examination of the external genital anatomy. Investigations are particularly relevant in the 46,XY DSD where the diagnostic yield is less successful than in the 46,XX conditions. The era of next-generation sequencing is increasingly being applied to investigate complex medical diseases of unknown cause, including DSD. The challenge for health professionals will lie in integrating vast amounts of genetic information with phenotypes and counseling families appropriately. Regarding those who require evaluation before gender assignment is made, each "generation" of approach reflects the contemporary biological, social, and psychological understanding. The most recent generation needs to consider the significantly changed societal viewpoints regarding the acceptance and expansion beyond a binary perception of sexuality. This together with advances in genetic etiologies, surgical refinements, and psychological support should result in better care and quality of life (QoL) outcomes for patients with these conditions.

113.1 Salient Points

- Differences of the external genitalia that need further investigation may occur in about 1 in 4,000 births.
- Phenotypic sex is the result of a coordinated and sequential series of developmental events.
- Evidence now shows that biological sex, gender identity, gender role, and choice of sexual partner are a combination of each individual's personal experience in a "bimodal continuum rather than a binary-categorical system."
- Disorders of ovarian development are not usually manifest until puberty when a failure of estrogenization becomes apparent.
- Congenital adrenal hyperplasia (CAH) due to 21-hydroxylase deficiency is the commonest cause of ambiguous genitalia of the newborn. CAH are genetic disorders with autosomal recessive inheritance.
- In families at risk for a virilized female baby, prenatal diagnosis and treatment may be undertaken with early administration of dexamethasone to the mother to prevent genital virilization.
- Endocrine disruptors with androgenic or anti-androgenic action or estrogenic chemicals may interfere with normal sexual differentiation.
- The evaluation and management of a newborn with abnormalities of genitalia should be carried out by an experienced multidisciplinary team.
- Cancer risk in a dysgenetic gonad should be considered along a medical spectrum as well as the sum of genetic factors and environmental factors, which act as epigenetic determinants on the germ cell's maturational process.
- Cryptorchidism is the failure of the testis to descend from an intra-abdominal location into the scrotum; it is more frequent in preterms.

113.2 Sex Determination and Differentiation

113.2.1 Sex Development

It is rare to be unable at birth to differentiate a male from a female newborn because of the presence of atypical genitalia, but differences of the external genitalia that need further investigation may occur in about 1 in 4000 births (Sax 2002). Antenatal ultrasound scanning has improved our ability to predict these conditions.

Sexual development is a genetically and hormonally controlled process, which in humans starts at fertilization by the establishment of the chromosomal sex (XX or XY). According to the classical "binary" physiology, this is the first step of the process of sex determination which continues with the formation of the gonad (testis or ovary). Gender determination depends on the sex chromosome complement of the embryo and is established by multiple genetic and molecular events that direct the development of germ cells, their migration to the urogenital ridge, and the formation of either a testis in the presence of the Y chromosome (46,XY) or an ovary in the absence of the Y chromosome and the presence of a second X chromosome (46,XX). Recent discoveries have indicated that the identity of the gonad emerges from a contest between two opposing networks of gene activity. Changes in the activity or amounts of molecules (such as WNT4 or SOX9) in the networks can tip the balance toward or away from the sex expected on the basis of the chromosomes (Ainsworth 2015).

The second step in sex development is sex differentiation, which refers to the formation of the phenotypic sex (appearance of the external genitalia and internal annexes) and the subsequent acquisition at puberty of secondary sexual characteristics and reactivation of reproductive axis.

This process depends on the sex-specific secretion of hormones produced by the gonads during intrauterine life and the response of their target tissues.

At birth, phenotypic sex is the result of a coordinated and sequential series of developmental events controlled by a complex system of temporally expressed genes, transcription factors, and optimal hormone secretion during critical developmental windows. Any condition affecting this complex pathway may result in disorders or differences in sex differentiation and a child with an atypical genetic, gonadal, or phenotypic sex.

113.2.2 Gonads

In humans, bipotential gonads begin their development at around 4–5 weeks' gestation, separating from the adrenal primordium. They arise as paired condensations of the coelomic epithelium at the medioventral region of the mesonephros on either side of the dorsal aorta. The gonad contains both somatic and germ cells. The primordial germ cells, which migrated into the gonads from the yolk sac, generate the gametes (spermatocytes or ova). Until about 40 days' gestation, the primitive gonads remain bipotential. The presence, or absence, of testicular determining genes depends on chromosomal sex and determines whether the gonads differentiate into testes or ovaries.

Four major cell types are present in the indifferent gonads: supporting, steroidogenetic, germ lineage, and connective cells that will differentiate in the testes as Sertoli cells, Leydig cells, spermatogonia, and peritubular myoid cells, respectively. The Sertoli cell is the first cell type that differentiates to produce the antimullerian hormone (AMH) and its role is essential for the nutrition of germ cells; the Leydig cells are steroidogenic cells that produce testosterone. Both hormones serve as an essential step for the normal progression versus male phenotypic development of the fetus.

In the ovary as granulose/follicular cells, steroid-producing cells (theca cells produce androgens, that are converted to estrogens in the granulose cells, that also produce progesterone), oocytes, and stromal cells, respectively. Ovarian differentiation starts about 1 week later than testis differentiation, and its steroidogenic function before puberty is poor defined and likely of little clinical relevance.

113.2.3 Internal Ducts

At 6 weeks' gestation, both the Wolffian ducts (from which arises the seminal vesicles, the vas deferens, and the epididymis) and the Müllerian ducts (from which arise the fallopian tubes, the upper vagina, and the uterus) are present. In normal male differentiation, the regression of the Müllerian structures and the inhibition of FSH are dependent on AMH and inhibin B (InB) production through Sertoli cell activity. Neonatal pituitary luteinizing hormone (LH) and placental human chorionic gonadotropin (hCG) stimulate Leydig cells to produce testosterone, indispensable to stabilize the Wolffian derivates, while dihydrotestosterone (DHT), deriving from peripheral conversion of testosterone by 5-α-reductase, acts to complete virilization of the external genitalia and the scrotal migration of testes. The other protein hormone produced by fetal Leydig cells (INSL3) is also involved in the testicular descent into the scrotum.

In normal female differentiation, the lack of testosterone and AMH leads to regression of the Wolffian structures and development of Müllerian derivatives. However, the recent studies of gene expression have shown that there is a series of specific genes actively implicated in ovarian development and integrity, rendering the latter process more active than previously hypothesized. In fact, WNT4, one of a few factors with a demonstrated function in the ovarian determination pathway, has been found to be involved in sexual differentiation by suppressing male sexual differentiation, promoting Müllerian duct differentiation and maintaining oocyte health. WNT4 expression in the ovary seems to be regulated by R-spondin 1 (RSPO1), a thrombospondin family member protein. The role and interactions of WNT4, RSPO1, and other factors, such as FOXL2, as well as the possible role of chromatin modifiers (CBX2) in ovarian development and function, shed new light in these processes (Biason-Lauber 2010; Biason-Lauber and Chaboissier 2015).

113.2.4 External Genitalia

The external genitalia are initially identical, regardless of the genetic or gonadal sex, and consist of a genital tubercle, urogenital folds, and the genital swellings. Male differentiation occurs when sufficient amounts of testosterone and DHT are produced from the 7–8th weeks of gestation and when the fetus has developed sensitivity to androgens. In this case, the genital tubercle develops as a penis, the urethral folds fuse to create a tubular penile urethra with the meatus located at the tip of the penis, and the genital swellings join to form a scrotum.

If androgenic effects are lacking, the genital tubercle forms a clitoris, and the urethral folds and the genital swellings develop into the labia minora and majora, respectively. Finally, in the absence of AMH production, a normal vagina is formed (Yamada et al. 2003).

113.2.5 Psychosexual Development

Psychosexual development refers to a number of distinct components that determine whether a person views themselves as a man or woman (gender identity), whether that person is viewed by other members of society as masculine or feminine (gender role), and their choice of sexual partner and erotic interest (heterosexual, bisexual, homosexual) including behavior, fantasies, and attractions (sexual orientation). Gender identity, gender role, and sexual orientation have been conceived in a strictly homogeneous binary construct for a long time. In biology (Ainsworth 2015), sex is now considered to be a spectrum of possibilities between female and male bodily expression, rather than variants of a distinct, binary male/female code. The same happens in psychosexual development, where more evidence now shows that biological sex, gender identity, gender role, and choice of sexual partner are a combination of each individual's personal experience in a "bimodal continuum rather than a binary-categorical system" (Meyer-Bahlburg et al. 2016). When the strictly binary sex construct was the mainstream, early sex attribution had to be made as quickly as possible in disordered sexual development (DSD) babies, but now a more open approach is needed in cases where the sex of rearing is not easily defined and more time is needed in order for the individual to follow their natural inclination. Of the experiences reported by people living with a disorder of sexual development (DSD), in many situations people are satisfied with their gender allocation (D'Alberton et al. 2015) whereas others, when interviewed, expressed uncertainty about belonging to a specific gender (Schweizer et al. 2014).

113.2.6 Understanding Normal Sex Development by Genetic Advancements

Sex development requires the interaction of several factors together with the production of hormones and their consequent signaling action. It is therefore not surprising that an increasing number of genes have been discovered that contribute both early and late to the process of sex determination and differentiation, and there will undoubtedly be more. Knowledge of the molecular basis of these pathways will influence the diagnosis and management of these conditions. Transcription factors and signaling molecules play an important role in the formation and differentiation of the gonad, processes which are genetically determined. In contrast, genes that cause postgonadal 46,XY or 46, XX DSD often encode enzymes or factors necessary for sex steroid biosynthesis or action.

113.3 Nomenclature and Classification

Terms like intersex, hermaphroditism, or pseudohermaphroditism have been considered unacceptable by the medical community, affected individuals, and support groups. Thus, a new nomenclature has been proposed (Hughes and Deeb 2006; Hughes et al. 2007). The inclusion of congenital in the definition of DSD excludes disorders of pubertal development as well as conditions of gender dysphoria. Table 1 outlines the nomenclature and the classification system based on causes, workable in clinical practice. According to karyotype, DSD is divided into disorders with normal or abnormal sex chromosomes. In the two groups with normal karyotype, the causes of DSD are subdivided into disorders of gonadal development or postgonadal disorders (hormonal or receptor defects, syndromic forms, etc.). In 2008, a European

Table 1 DSD classification (Chicago Consensus Conference 2006)

Sex chromosome DSD	46,XY DSD		46,XX DSD	
A: 47,XXY (Klinefter syndrome and variants)	A: Disorders of gonadal (testicular) development	1. Complete or partial gonadal dysgenesis (SRY, SOX9, SF1, WT1, DHH, etc.) (Swyer syndrome)	A: Disorders of gonadal (ovarian) development	1. Testicular dysgenesis (SRY+, dup SOX9)
		2. Testis regression		2. Gonadal dysgenesis
		3. Ovotesticular DSD		3. Ovotesticular DSD
B: 45,X0 (Turner syndrome and variants)	B: Disorders of androgen synthesis or action	1. Androgen biosynthesis/metabolism defect (17-OH-steroid-dehydrogenase deficiency, 5α-reductase deficiency, StAR mutations, etc.)	B: Androgen excess	1. Fetal (21α-hydroxylase deficiency, 11a-hydroxylase deficiency, glucocorticoid receptor mutations)
		2. Androgen action defect (CAIS, PAIS, drugs, and environmental modulators)		2. Feto-placentar (aromatase deficiency)
		3. LH-receptor defect (Leydig cell hypoplasia or aplasia)		3. Maternal (luteoma, androgenic drugs, etc.)
		4. AMH or AMH-receptor defect (persistent Müllerian duct syndrome)		
C: 45,X0/46,XY (mixed gonadal dysgenesis, ovotesticular DSD)	C: Other	Syndromic associations, hypospadias, cloacal extrophy, cryptorchidism, vanishing testis syndrome, etc.	C: Other	Syndromic associations, MURCS (Müllerian aplasia, renal aplasia, and cervico thoracic somite dysplasia), cloacal extrophy, vaginal atresia, etc.

consortium on DSD was created (EuroDSD, changed to I-DSD on 2012: www.i-dsd.org) based on a research project supported by the EU Commission within the 7th Framework Programme. The I-DSD Registry project provides a means of connecting clinical and research centers around the world within a virtual environment and allows experts to enter standardized information that will improve clinical practice, research, and understanding of these challenging conditions with respects to security and ethics (Ahmed et al. 2014). The project links patient data collection and analysis tools with research on the development of novel diagnostic strategies to identify new causes of DSD, in conjunction with a program to study the functional molecular biology of the androgen receptor, thereby allowing for an in-depth analysis of key factors in the pathogenesis of DSD. The COST arm of the DSD net aims to obtain new knowledge about biological pathways of sex development in human and to provide information about clinical management for physicians and psychologists caring for people with DSD (www.dsdnet.eu) (Polizzi et al. 2014).

113.4 DSD with Karyotype Abnormalities

These DSD include diseases in which the number of sex chromosome is impaired (Table 2). The first two of these conditions will generally escape neonatal diagnosis and will be diagnosed later in childhood or adulthood due to specific features (Simm et al. 2008), e.g., impaired puberty or infertility. However, a recent paper by Lee et al. (2007) reported seven Klinefelter patients (KS) (47,XXY and variants; incidence between 1:500 and 1:1000 live births (Nielsen and Wohlert 1991)) with abnormalities of genitalia ranging from mild anomalies (chordee) to moderate undervirilization (bifid scrotum and perineal hypospadias). In the same paper, a review of other cases revealed a range of mild to severe abnormalities that underline the importance of recognizing this condition as one of the causes of abnormal genitalia at birth. Early diagnosis and treatment might improve the quality of life of men with KS since they are born with spermatogonia and lose large numbers of germ cells during puberty. The classic form of Turners' syndrome (TS) (about 1:2,500 live births (Elsheikh et al. 2002)) is characterized by a 45,X0 karyotype and occurs in about 50% of cases; mosaic forms (45,X/46,XX) and forms with structural anomalies of the X chromosome are each found in 25% of cases. None of these show genital ambiguity. However, a prenatal diagnosis of TS may be made incidentally (advanced maternal age, detection of increased occipital translucency on fetal ultrasound scan) following amniocentesis (AC) or chorionic villous sampling (CVS). During the neonatal period, the diagnosis may be suspected in female neonates with lymphoedema, occipital folds, low hairline,

Table 2 Sex chromosome DSD (Modified from Achermann and Hughes 2007)

Condition	Karyotype	Gonad	Müllerian structures	External genitalia	Possible neonatal features
Klinefelter's S.	47,XXY and variants	Hyalinized testes[a]	–	Male	Micropenis, hypospadias, cryptorchidism
Turner's S.	46,X and variants	Streak gonad or immature ovary	Uterus	Female	Lymphedema, web neck, cardiac defect, and coartation of the aorta, renal, and urinary abnormalities
Mixed gonadal dysgenesis	45,X/46,XY and variants	Testis or dysgenetic gonad	+/–	Female, ambiguous, male	Possible presence of some features of Turner's syndrome; increased risk of gonad tumors
Ovotesticular DSD	46,XX/46,XY chimerism Africa 46,XX; rare 46,XY	Dysgenetic testis	+/–	Ambiguous	Possible increased risk of gonad tumors

[a]Mainly from puberty onward

or left-sided heart defects. Girls with classic TS have ovarian dysgenesis, an observation which underlines the need for two copies of the X chromosome for regular ovarian development. Gonadectomy is indicated for TS patients when the karyotype contains a Y fragment with the *TSPY* locus because of the increased risk of developing gonadoblastoma.

The true prevalence of classic mixed gonadal dysgenesis (MGD) (45,X/46,XY mosaicism) is unknown. The clinical phenotype of this condition is highly variable ranging from normal male to normal female phenotype; cases described in the literature are mainly the most severe forms showing various degrees of ambiguous genitalia. The genital phenotypes vary from normal female external genitalia or mild clitoromegaly to all stages of ambiguous genitalia including hypospadias or a normal penis (Telvi et al. 1999). Gonadal phenotypes vary from streak gonads, through dysgenetic testes to testes with normal histological structure. The position of the gonad reflects the level of structural differentiation with streak-like gonads being more likely to be found intra-abdominally and well-formed testes in the inguinal or scrotal region. Müllerian structures may be present in the most severely affected cases due to impaired AMH production by Sertoli cells. Gonadal development may be different between the right and the left side or even within a single gonad; the more the gonad is affected on one side, the less the Müllerian structures are inhibited on the same side (paracrine action of AMH). Somatic features may vary from a Turner syndrome-like appearance (occipital folds, cardiac and renal anomalies) to normal male newborn. Recent amniocentesis data report that up to 90% of fetuses diagnosed as having a 45,X/46,XY mosaic karyotype with the condition confirmed postnatally have a normal male phenotype and apparently normal testis development (Hsu and Benn 1999). The correlation between the level of mosaicism in peripheral blood sampling and gonad, or somatic phenotype seems to be poor. Several karyotype variants have been reported in MGD, e.g., 45,X/47, XYY or 45,X/46,XY/47,XYY.

Ovotesticular DSD (OT DSD) (46,XX/46,XY chimerism and variants; the old definition of true hermaphroditism) has been described in about 500 individuals worldwide and is likely due to different etiologies. Both ovarian and testicular tissues are present either in the same or in a controlateral gonad. The finding of pure 46,XX/46,XY chimerism is quite rare and has occasionally been described in North American or European patients. By contrast, OT DSD with a 46,XX karyotype is quite common in Africa and the Middle East (Mac Laughlin and Danahoe 2004). The molecular basis of this disorder still needs elucidation; transmission in familial cases is reported by autosomal recessive or sex-limited autosomal dominant transmission. OT DSD with a 46,XY karyotype is rare and may be explained either by cryptic gonadal mosaicism with a Y chromosome deletion or by an early sex-determining gene mutation (Biason-Lauber 2010).

Asymmetry of the gonads and therefore of reproductive ducts and external genitalia is common, with testes, ovaries, and ovotestes present in various combinations. In 50% of unilateral cases, there is an ovotestis on one side and an ovary or testis on the other. In 30% of bilateral cases, testicular and ovarian tissues are present bilaterally, usually as an ovotestis. In 20% of cases, there is a testis on one side, mostly the right, and an ovary on the other side. The ovary tends to maintain its normal anatomical position; the testis, by contrast, may be found anywhere along the pathway of testicular descent, most often in the right inguinal region. Generally, in this disorder, gonadal dysgenesis is less severe than in patients with mixed gonadal dysgenesis (Nihoul-Fekete et al. 1984). A prevalence of 3–4% of gonadoblastoma and/or germinoma has been estimated in the testicular tissue of patients with 46,XX OT DSD; since the ovotesticular tissue is usually dysgenetic, the removal of this testicular tissue has been recommended (Cools et al. 2006).

113.5 46,XX DSD

In this section, three different groups of disorders will be described: (1) disorders of ovarian development, (2) disorders of androgen excess, and (3) other conditions affecting sex development.

The first group (ovarian dysgenesis or resistance) are not usually manifest until puberty, when a failure of estrogenization becomes apparent. However, a number of nonmetabolic causes of premature ovarian failure (POF) have recently been described (FMR1, Xq26-q28; DIAPH2, Xq22; POF1B, Xq21; FOXL2, 3q22; BMP15, Xp11.2; NOBOX, 7q35; FIGLA, 2p12; SF1/NR5A1, 9q33) as well as mitochondrial disorders affecting ovarian development (mutant mitochondrial DNA polymerase gamma) (Biason-Lauber 2010). It is possible that more severe forms of these disorders might interfere with earlier aspects of ovarian development and that a prenatal or neonatal ultrasound examination might reveal some anatomic dysgenetic features. Other conditions that can be included in this group are 46,XX OT DSD or 46,XX testicular DSD (XX males). 46,XX OT DSD commonly presents at birth with ambiguous genitalia and progressive virilization during puberty. On the contrary, individuals with 46,XX testicular DSD usually have a male phenotype and absent Müllerian structures and are often diagnosed after karyotype analysis during work up for infertility (Ahmed et al. 2016). In these cases, there should be sufficient testicular tissue in the gonad to produce androgenization of the phenotype and regression of Müllerian structures (Table 3). In 46,XX testicular DSD, about 80–90% of patients will have Y chromosomal material including a translocated SRY gene, which is only rarely detected in 46,XX ovotesticular DSD. In other cases of 46,XX testicular DSD, duplications of the SOX9 gene and mutations of the RSPO1 gene have been described. Hypergonadotropic ovarian dysgenesis with 46,XX karyotype can be caused by mutations in the gene encoding follicle-stimulating hormone receptor (FSHR, 2p21–p26) (Biason-Lauber 2010).

The second group is characterized by fetal androgen excess in 46,XX individuals. Congenital adrenal hyperplasia (CAH) due to 21-hydroxylase deficiency (21-OHD) is the commonest cause of ambiguous genitalia of the newborn (Speiser and White 2003). It may be also caused by 11-hydroxylase (11-OHD), 3β-hydroxysteroid dehydrogenase (3β- HSD2), and P450 oxidoreductase (POR) deficiencies (Fig. 1, Table 4). The clinical presentation is characterized by various degree of genital virilization (Prader staging) with possible genital pigmentation (expression of excessive ACTH production). A salt-losing crisis may be the first presentation in neonates with 21-OHD misdiagnosed as males or in the patients with severe 3β-HSD2 and only mild clitoromegaly (due to the peripheral conversion of DHEA to T by 3β-HSD1). 11-OHD can cause marked virilization because of excess testosterone production (Menabò et al. 2014). Deoxycortocosterone (DOC) is also produced in excess and acts as a mineralocorticoid able to prevent a salt-losing crisis, which has been reported as a rare transient manifestation when starting glucocorticoid treatment. Hypertension due to DOC excess is very rare in the neonatal period.

Table 3 Genes involved in 46,XX gonadal DSD, with testicular development (Modified from Achermann and Hughes 2007)

Gene/ protein type	Chrom. location	Inheritance	Gonad	Müllerian structures	External genitalia	Other associated features
SRY/TF	Yp11.3	Translocation	Testis or ovotestis	–	Male or ambiguous	Infertility
SOX9/TF	17q24	Dup17q24	Not investigated	–	Male or ambiguous	
RSPO1/ sign. molecule	1p34.3	AR	Testis or ovotestis	–	Male	+ Palmoplantar hyperkeratosis and predisposition to squamous cell carcinoma of the skin, +/– congenital bilateral corneal opacities, onychodystrophy, hearing impairment

TF transcription factor, *AR* autosomal recessive, +/– present or absent

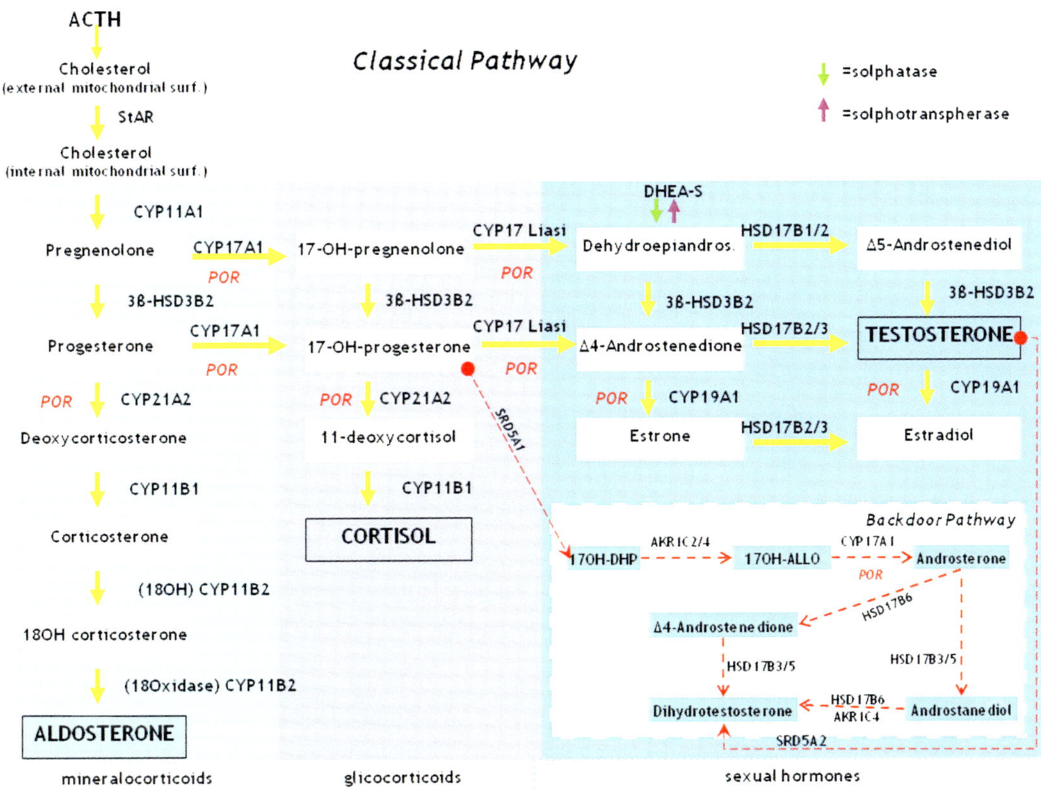

Fig. 1 Adrenal and gonadal steroidogenesis (classical and backdoor pathways)

Mutations in the gene encoding the steroidogenetic acute regulatory protein (StAR protein) can also cause CAH (lipoid CAH), as can P450 oxidoreductase deficiency. The latter conditions cause a complex set of disorders combining deficiencies of multiple steroid metabolizing enzymes (CYP17A1, CYP21A2, CYP19A1, and many other targets). The POR deficiency (PORD) was first reported in patients with symptoms of defects in steroidogenic cytochrome P450 enzymes and ambiguous genitalia, and bone malformation features resembling Antley-Bixler syndrome. POR is now classified as a separate and rare form of congenital adrenal hyperplasia (CAH), which may cause disorder of sexual development (DSD). Since the initial description of PORD in 2004, a large number of POR mutations and polymorphisms have been described. The mutations in POR that were identified in patients with disruption of steroidogenesis also have severe effects on cytochrome P450 proteins involved in metabolism of drugs. Mutation analysis shows that Japanese (R457H), Caucasian (A287P), and Turkish (399–401) populations can be linked to unique founder mutations. Other mutations recognized so far were identified as rare alleles or in single isolated reports (Burkhard et al. 2016).

Table 4 summarizes clinical and hormonal data that are helpful in making a differential diagnosis of the adrenal steroid enzyme defects and lipoid CAH. Diagnosis is based on increased levels of basal and/or ACTH stimulated steroid precursor(s) that accumulate above the enzymatic block, with the exceptions of StAR and P450scc deficiencies in which almost no steroids are produced (Table 4).

All CAH are genetic disorders with autosomal recessive inheritance. The genes involved in all the defects have been isolated and characterized, and specific mutations have been identified

Table 4 Clinical and hormonal data helpful for a differential etiologic diagnosis of the adrenal/gonadal steroid enzyme defects and lipoid CAH

Enzyme deficiency	Sexual ambiguity		Symptoms		Hormonal findings (plasma levels)								
Classical forms	46,XX	46,XY	Salt loss	Hypertension	17-Preg	17OHP	Δ4-A	DHEA	T	Aldo	Renin	11-D	DOC
StAR	No	Yes	Yes	No	↓↓↓↓	↓↓↓↓	↓↓↓↓	↓↓↓↓	↓↓↓↓	↓↓↓↓	↑↑↑↑	↓↓↓↓	↓↓↓↓
P450 scc [a]	No	Yes	Yes	No	↓↓↓↓	↓↓↓↓	–	↓↓↓↓	↓↓↓↓	↓↓↓↓	↑↑↑↑	–	–
3β-HSD2	±	Yes	Yes	No	↑↑↑↑	↑	±	↑↑↑	↑↓ [b]	↓↓↓	↑↑↑	↓↓	↑↑
P450c21 SW	Yes	No	Yes	No	↑	↑↑↑↑	↑↑↑	N or ↑	↑	↓	↑↑	N	N
P450c21 SV	Yes	No	No	No	↑	↑↑↑	↑↑	N or ↑	↑	N	N (±↑)	N	N
P450c11	Yes	No	No	Yes [c]	N	N or ↑	↑↑↑	↑	↑	↓↓	↓↓	↑↑↑↑	↑↑↑
P450c17	No	Yes	No	Yes [c]	↓↓	↓↓	↓↓	↓↓	↓↓	↓↓	↓↓	↓	↑↑↑
P450c17 lyase	No	Yes	No	No	N	N	↓↓	↓↓	↓↓	N	N	±	N
P450OR	±	Yes	No	±	↑	↑↑	↑↑	↓↓	↓↓	↓↓	N(±↑)	↓↓	↑↑

[a]Severe forms were thought to be incompatible with survival due to placental failure to produce progesterone. The recent report of several cases demonstrated that severe disruption of P450scc could be compatible with survival in rare instances. Furthermore, heterozygote carriers were healthy and fertile. The possibility of P450scc-independent pathways of steroid synthesis in addition to the current concept of luteo-placental shift of progesterone synthesis in humans has to be questioned

[b]Normal or elevated for normal girls, or decreased in boys

[c]Almost never in newborn period

P450c21 21-hydroxylase, *P450c11* 11-hydroxylase, *3β-HSD* 3beta-hydroxysteroid dehydrogenase, *P450c17* 17-hydroxylase, *P450c17 lyase* 17–20 lyase, *P450 scc* side chain cleavage enzyme, *StAR* steroidogenetic acute regulatory protein, *POR* P450 oxidoreductase, *17-Preg* 17-OH-pregnenolone, *17OHP* 17-OH-progesterone, *Δ4-A* androstenedione, *DHEA* dehydroepiandrosterone, *T* testosterone, *Aldo* aldosterone, *11-D* 11-deoxycortisol, *DOC* deoxycorticosterone, *N* normal level

(Table 5) (Turcu and Auchus 2015). Genetic analysis for the identification of mutations of the genes involved is informative for the index case and for future prenatal diagnosis (Balsamo et al. 2010). Figure 2 describes the allelic frequencies of the most common *CYP21A2* gene mutations found in a sample of Italian patients affected by 21-OHD and followed at the Bologna Center for Rare Endocrinological Diseases (CARENDO BO). This center is also able to provide neonatal screening for patients of the Emilia-Romagna Region with classical presentation and to prevent salt losing crises of affected males who are most likely to miss early diagnosis (Balsamo et al. 1996). Preterm babies have higher 17-OHP levels than those born at term and specific gestational age and/or weight related data are required (Speiser 2007). The use of steroid profiling (LC-MS MS) as a second-tier test on the original heel prick sample will reduce the false positive rates of this specific neonatal screening (Seo et al. 2014).

In families at risk for a virilized female baby because of an index case affected by classical

Table 5 Genes involved in 46,XX DSD due to androgen excess (Modified from Achermann and Hughes 2007)

Gene/protein type	Chrom. location	Inheritance	Gonad	Müllerian structures	External genitalia	Other associated features
HSD3B2/enzyme	1p13.1	AR	Ovary	+	Female or ambiguous	CAH, primitive adrenal insufficiency, partial androgenization
CYP21A2/enzyme	6p21.23	AR	Ovary	+	Female, ambiguous or male	CAH, +/− adrenal insufficiency
CYP11B1/enzyme	8q21.22	AR	Ovary	+	Female, ambiguous or male	CAH, +/− hypertension
POR/CYP electron donor	7q11.2	AR	Ovary	+	Female or ambiguous	Mixed features of 21-OH Def, 17-OH Def/17–20-lyase Def, aromatase Def; +/− Antley-Bixler S
CYP19/enzyme	15q21	AR	Ovary	+	Ambiguous	Maternal androgenization during pregnancy, absent breast development at puberty, except partial cases

AR autosomal recessive, +/− present or absent

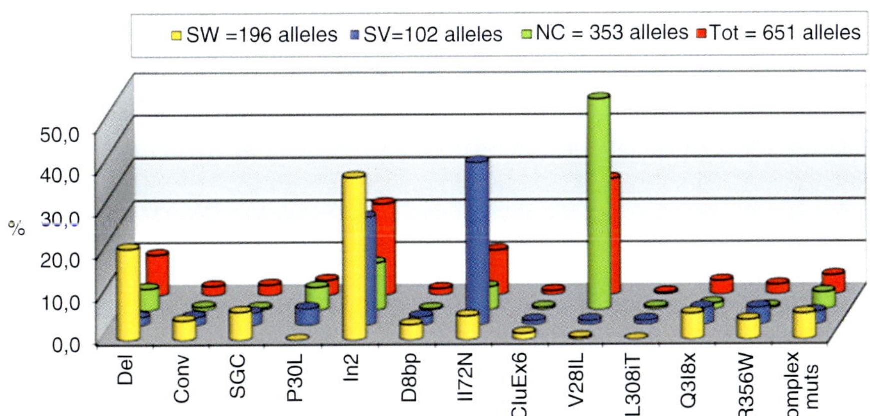

Fig. 2 Allelic frequencies of deletions, conversions, and mutations present in *CYP21A1P* (651 alleles – Italian Population – Bologna cases 2015)

21-OHD or 11-OHD, prenatal diagnosis and treatment may be undertaken. Early administration (before 8 weeks' gestation) of dexamethasone to the mother (20 mcg/kg/prepregnancy) prevents genital virilization in most affected females. Treatment has to be started before chorionic villus sampling (CVS) for sex, and genetic analyses can be performed at 10–11 weeks' gestation and only female affected fetuses need to be treated throughout the pregnancy. To reduce the number of fetuses exposed to dexamethasone unnecessarily, polymerase chain reaction (PCR) testing for cell-free Y DNA in maternal blood at 5–6 weeks of gestation for prenatal sex determination is now available as an experimental technique (Shearer et al. 2007; Zimmermann et al. 2007). Due to possible maternal side effects (Cushing syndrome) and lack of long-term trials for its safety, antenatal dexamethasone treatment should be carried out in specialized centers using approved protocols (Lajic et al. 2008).

Aromatase deficiency is a recent, well-characterized disorder of steroidogenesis in which there is exposure of the mother and a female fetus to fetal androgens that are normally aromatized by the fetally derived placenta. The lack of aromatase action has a virilizing effect on the mother and on her female newborn (Jones et al. 2007).

Maternal causes of androgen excess that may virilize a female fetus are either endogenous because of secretion by adrenal and ovarian tumors or exogenous because of maternal ingestion of androgenic compounds (Danazol).

The third group of disorders refer to some syndromic associations that can cause developmental genital abnormalities in 46,XX girls. Abnormalities of uterine development can result in a bicornuate uterus, uterine hemiagenesis or hypoplasia, or uterine agenesis.

These conditions can be associated with renal, cardiac, and cervical spinal abnormalities as part of the Mayer-Rokitansky-Kuster-Hauser syndrome. Uterine anomalies have also been associated with maturity-onset diabetes of the young type 5 (MODY 5, mutations in *HNF1β*) and with vaginal abnormalities with hand-foot-genital syndrome (mutations in *HOXA13*) and McKusick-Kaufman syndrome (mutations in *BBS6*). Relative clitoral hypertrophy can be associated with conditions such as Frasier syndrome or neurofibromatosis, and careful assessment is necessary before a hyperandrogenic cause is diagnosed. Apparent clitoromegaly may be a common finding in premature babies or when there is little labial adipose tissue present, assessment by a physician with experience of normal variability in clitoral size is important.

113.6 46,XY DSD

46,XY DSD are divided into: (1) disorders of gonadal development; (2) disorders of testosterone biosynthesis, metabolism, or action; and (3) other conditions (Table 1).

113.6.1 Disorders of Gonadal Development

Total gonadal agenesis or bilateral gonadal streak (Swyer syndrome) is rare and has been described in 46,XY subjects. There are both internal and external female genitalia, due to the complete absence of testicular determination, with persistent Müllerian structures due to insufficient AMH production. The origin of this disorder remains uncertain but may be due to a defect in genes critical to bipotential gonad development (Mendonca et al. 2009).

Partial gonadal dysgenesis has been reported in some clinical conditions, characterized by impaired testicular development and ambiguous external genitalia with or without Müllerian structures (similarly to 45,X0/46,XY conditions). Mutations in the SRY gene have been related to this phenotype in about 20% cases (mostly as de novo mutations). Heterozygous mutations in SF1 gene have also been recently found to be causative of XY DSD without apparent adrenal involvement (Ferraz-de Souza et al. 2011).

Other genes acting on testicular determinations (e.g., DHH gene) may be rarely involved.

Testicular regression syndrome is a condition in which a testis is thought to have once existed but has atrophied and disappeared during early development. The timing of the regression process is critical. If this process occurs before differentiation of the male external genitalia is completed, the newborn will have an undervirilized appearance (DSD), while if it happens late during gestation, the male newborn will have cryptorchidism with undetectable testis (vanishing testis). In some boys with such a condition, mutations of SF1 or WT1 have been described. The identification of these mutations should assure adequate follow-up, since affected individuals may develop adrenal insufficiency or renal dysfunction respectively later in life.

Genetic mutations and chromosomal changes involved primarily in 46,XY gonadal DSD may be associated with other clinical features (Tables 6 and 7).

113.6.2 Disorders of Testosterone Biosynthesis

During intrauterine male development, both maternal hCG and fetal LH act on Leydig cells by a hCG/LH common-G-protein coupled receptor, stimulating testosterone production. An inactivating mutation in the gene coding for this

Table 6 Genes involved in 46,XY gonadal DSD (Modified from Achermann and Hughes 2007)

Gene/ protein type	Chrom. location	Inheritance	Gonad	Müllerian structures	External genitalia	Other associated features
SRY/TF	Yp11.3	Y	Dysgenetic testis or ovotestis	+/−	Female or ambiguous	−
SOX9/TF	17q24–25	AD	Dysgenetic testis or ovotestis	+/−	Female or ambiguous	Camptomelic dysplasia
SF1 (NR5A1)/ TF (NR)	9q33	AD/AR	Dysgenetic testis	+/−	Female or ambiguous	+/− Primitive adrenal insufficiency
DHH/sign. molecule	12q13.1	AD/AR	Dysgenetic testis	+	Female	+/− Minifascicular neuropathy (1 case)
ATRX/ Helicase	Xq13.3	X	Dysgenetic testis		Female, ambiguous or male	α-Thalassemia, mental retardation
ARX/TF	Xp22.13	X	Dysgenetic testis	−	Ambiguous	+ Lissencephaly, epilepsy, temperature instability

TF transcription factor, *NR* nuclear receptor, +/− present or absent, *AD* autosomal dominant (or de novo mutation), *AR* autosomal recessive, *Y* Y-linked, *X* X-linked

Table 7 Chromosomal changes involved in 46,XY gonadal DSD (Modified from Achermann and Hughes (2007))

Candidate gene/protein type	Chrom. location	Inheritance structures	Gonad	Müllerian	External genitalia	Other associated features
DAX1 (NROB1)/TF (NR)	Xp21	Dupl Xp21	Dysgenetic testis or ovary	+/−	Female or ambiguous	
DMRTs/TF	9p24.3	Del 9p24.3 red. penetrance	Dysgenetic testis or normal testis	+/−	Female or ambiguous	Mental retardation, somatic dismorphisms
WNT4/sign. molecule	1p35	Dupl 1p35	Dysgenetic testis	+	Ambiguous	Mental retardation

TF transcription factor, *NR* nuclear receptor, +/− present or absent receptor may cause Leydig cell hypoplasia with complete or partial impairment of hormone secretion, so that an undervirilized variable phenotype arises at birth (Latronico and Arnhold 2006).

Testosterone biosynthesis, like all steroidal hormones, starts from cholesterol as a precursor.

7-Dehydrocholesterol reductase (DHCR7) deficiency is a disorder affecting the cholesterol biosynthesis pathway and causes Smith-Lemli-Opitz syndrome (which includes microcephaly, mental retardation, facial dysmorphism, polydactyly genital anomalies; renal hypoplasia and unilobar lung are also commonly associated).

Lipoid adrenal hyperplasia due to deficiency of StAR protein, which facilitates the rapid movement of cholesterol from the outer to the inner mitochondrial membrane, is rare in Europe and America but more common in Japan. Patients are phenotypic females (despite having a testis) with enlarged adrenal cortex, engorged by cholesterol and cholesterol esters. Severe adrenal insufficiency is the main potentially lethal consequence, since virtually no steroids are made (Manna and Stocco 2005).

Enzymatic defects altering the normal testosterone biosynthesis, cholesterol side-chain cleavage (CYP11A1), 3β-hydroxysteroid dehydrogenase (3β *-HSD2*), 17α-hydroxylase/17–20-lyase (CYP17), and P450 oxidoreductase (POR) enzyme deficiencies are inherited as autosomal recessive conditions. The clinical presentation of this group of DSD is characterized by various degree of genital under-masculinization with possible genital pigmentation due to excessive ACTH production in cases associated with antenatal insufficiency. A salt-losing crisis and hypoglycemia may be the first clinical sign. Babies with severe deficiency are often misdiagnosed as females.

P450scc (CYP11A1) is the mitochondrial enzyme that converts cholesterol to pregnenolone and is therefore responsible for the first rate-limiting step in steroid synthesis, which is required for pregnenolone production by the placenta as well as for mineralcorticoid, glucocorticoid, and androgen production by the adrenal glands and gonads.

P450c17 or *CYP17* (gene locus in 10q24.3) are expressed both in the zona fasciculata and in the zona reticularis of the adrenal cortex and in gonadal tissues as a steroidogenic enzyme with dual functions, hydroxylation and as a lyase. The first activity results in hydroxylation of pregnenolone and progesterone at the C17 position to generate 17α-hydroxypregnenolone and 17α-hydroxyprogesterone. The latter enzyme activity cleaves the C17–C20 bond of 17α-hydroxypregnenolone and 17α-hydroxyprogesterone to form dehydroepiandrosterone and androstenedione, respectively.

Patients with *3β-HSD2* usually show some degree of virilization (due to peripheral conversion of DHEA to T by 3β-HSD1) or hypospadias, which suggests the diagnosis. In 17-OHD deficiency, the genital phenotype may vary from that of a complete female to severe hypospadias; corticosterone (C) and deoxycortocosterone (DOC) are produced in excess and have glucocorticoid and mineralocorticoid functions, respectively. Hypertension due to DOC excess is very rare during the neonatal period. In 17–20 lyase deficiency, the genital phenotype is similar, but there is no cortisol deficiency and no mineralocorticoid excess.

As in 46XX patients, P450 oxidoreductase deficiency may cause mild virilization of a male fetus, with the biochemical features of both 21-OHD and 17-OHD (Burkhard et al. 2016). Recently, mutations in two aldo-keto reductase enzymes the AKR1C2 and its homolog AKR1C4 have been reported. This discovery has suggested two different pathways (classical and backdoor, respectively) for androgen production in the fetal adrenals to regulate the process of male/female sexual differentiation. POR is involved in both pathways (Biason-Lauber et al. 2013) (Fig. 1). Table 4 summarizes the clinical and hormonal data for the differential etiologic diagnosis of adrenal steroid enzyme defects and lipoid CAH. For the enzymatic diagnosis see discussion of congenital adrenal hyperplasia in section on "46,XX DSD."

46XY DSD due to mutations in the *HSD17B3* gene (encoding the 17β-HSD3 isoenzyme) is characterized by a female phenotype or various degrees of ambiguous genitalia at birth, with the presence of a blind vaginal pouch and intra-abdominal or inguinal testes. Impaired conversion of androstenedione into testosterone explains the virilization defect. Virilization occurs at puberty likely due to increased activity of mutated enzyme under LH stimulation or androstenedione conversion by the other 17B-HSD isoenzymes. Changes from female to male gender role behavior at puberty have been reported in about 50% of affected individuals, providing that gonads are not removed (Bertelloni et al. 2009).

113.6.3 Disorders in Testosterone Metabolism: 5-Alpha-Reductase Deficiency

SRD5A2 gene (2p23) encodes the steroid 5-alpha-reductase 2 isoenzyme, which converts testosterone into dihydrotestosterone (DHT) mainly in target tissues.

Affected 46,XY individuals have normal or increased testosterone plasmatic levels but decreased DHT levels and an elevated testosterone/DHT ratio in basal blood samples or after HCG stimulation. Newborns present with ambiguous undervirilized or almost female external genitalia. However, Wolffian differentiation normally occurs, since its differentiation is driven by testosterone itself as well as male imprinting of brain. The testes are usually located in the abdomen or in the inguinal region. As in 17BHSD3 deficiency, virilization occurs at puberty and the majority of adolescents raised as females, who were not submitted to orchidectomy in childhood, undergo a male social sex change (Table 8). Spontaneous or assisted fertility has been reported when male sex was assigned and orchidopexy has been properly performed. In adulthood, gender dysphoria may develop in patients raised as females. Thus correct early diagnosis is mandatory and male gender should be assigned.

The main differential diagnoses are described in Table 1 and molecular analysis of the *SRD5A2* gene is indicated during the newborn period before assigning female sex and performing gonadectomy (Imperato-McGinley and Zhu 2002; Bertelloni et al. 2007).

Extensive research has revealed a tendency for specific *SRD5A2* gene mutations to be passed along certain racial, ethnic, and geographically isolated groups, which suggests population specificity of these mutations (Samtani et al. 2010). Generally, this specific DSD has a high incidence in Caribbean areas (especially the Dominican Republic), while in Europe it has probably been long underestimated (Bertelloni et al. 2016).

113.6.4 Disorders in Testosterone Action

Androgen receptor (AR) mediates the pleiotropic effects of testosterone. The phenotype of androgen insensitivity, an X-linked recessive disorder, depends on the degree of AR disruption. The phenotype of complete androgen insensitivity syndrome (CAIS) is that of a normal female, with an XY karyotype and developed testis secreting adequate testosterone concentrations for normal male range. Data on prevalence are scarce, ranging from 1:20,400 to 1:99,000 genetic males.

Presentation may vary from the perinatal period to adulthood. In pregnancy, the diagnosis may be suspected because of a male fetal karyotype and female phenotype ultrasound scanning of the fetus or at birth. During the perinatal period and childhood, the main presentation of CAIS is as a bilateral inguinal or labial hernia in normal phenotypic female. Thus all girls with this type of hernia must undergo karyotyping.

In partial androgen insensitivity syndrome (PAIS) , the external genitalia may be ambiguous at birth, thus making immediate sex assignment difficult. The phenotype varies, depending on the degree of hormonal resistance, from perineoscrotal hypospadias, micropenis, and a bifid scrotum with undescended testes to isolated clitoridomegaly, marginally different from CAIS. The milder end of the spectrum of PAIS includes isolated hypospadias in the newborn and infertility in adulthood (minimal androgen insensitivity syndrome [MAIS]).

PAIS should be differentiated from sex chromosome DSD with 45,X0/46,XY or 46,XX/46, XY karyotype, defects in gonadal development, or a defect in androgen biosynthesis. Dynamic endocrine investigations (hCG stimulating test

Table 8 Comparison of main clinical and laboratory findings among Leydig cell hypoplasia/aplasia, 17β-HSD3 deficiency, 5α-reductase deficiency, and complete androgen insensitivity syndrome (AIS) (Bertelloni et al. 2009)

	Leydig cell hypoplasia	17β-HSD3 deficiency	5α.Reductase deficiency	Complete AIS
Eponymous	–	17-Ketosteroid reductase deficiency	Pesudovaginal perinoscrotal hypoplasia	Morris syndrome
Karyotype	46,XY	46,XY	46,XY	46,XY
Inheritance	Autosomal recessive	Autosomal recessive	Autosomal recessive	X-linked recessive
External phenotype	Female or ambiguous	Female or ambiguous	Ambiguous or female	Female
Blind ending vagina	Present (70–80%)	Present (80%)	Present (50%)	Present (100%)
Internal phenotype				
Wolffian structures	Male (hypoplasic)	Male	Male	Absent or male (hypoplasic)
Prostate	–	Absent/highly hypoplasic	Absent or hypoplasic	Absent
Müllerian structures	Absent	Absent	Absent	Absent or rudimental (~30%)
Testes	Intra- or extra-abdominal	Extra-abdominal	Extra-abdominal	Intra-abdominal
(% of patients)	–	(~90%)	(~100%)	(70%)
Hormone profile	↓↓ All androgens T/DHT N, Estrogens N or ↓	Δ^4-A↑;T↓T/Δ^4-A↓ T/DHT↑, T/Δ4-AN, Estrogens N	Δ^4-AN;TN or ↑, DHT ↓, T/DHT N or ↓, Estrogens ↑	Δ^4-AN;TN or ↑, T/Δ^4-AN
Gender assignment at birth	Female or ambiguous	Mainly female	Female or male	Female
Puberty	Sexual infantilism/ virilization	Virilization	Virilization	Feminization
Breast development	Absent	Variable	Absent	Normal female
Androgen hair	Variable	Normal male	Normal male	Absent or scanty
Gender role change	Not present	Present	Present	Not present
(% of patients)		(30–50%)[a]	(~75%)[b]	
Brain androgenization	Dependent on impairment of androgen production	Dependent on prenatal and postanatal T production	Likely male	Absent
Genetics, mutation of	*LHGCR*	*17β-HSD3* gene	*SRD5A2*	*AR* gene
Chromosomal gene map	2p21	9q22	2p23	Xq11–12

[a]Mainly in Israel and Eastern countries
[b]mainly in the areas with high prevalence, but also in Western countries
N normal, ↑ increased, ↓ decreased, Δ^4-A Δ^4-Androstenedione, *T* testosterone, *DHT* dihydrotestosterone

and/or tests to assess androgen sensitivity) should be performed to select patients for genetic investigation. Some individuals previously misclassified as PAIS without demonstrated AR mutations have been recently diagnosed as heterozygous carriers of *SF1* (NR5A1) gene mutations. In the majority of these cases, the adrenal function was apparently normal (Ferraz-de Souza et al. 2011). Anyway, a large number of subjects with suspected PAIS do not show any mutations in *AR* gene and CGH-array or NGS (next generation sequencing) DNA studies are indicated for such individuals.

113.6.5 Persistent Müllerian Duct Syndrome

Anti-Müllerian hormone (AMH), a member of the transforming growth factor beta (TGF-beta) family, is produced by gonadal somatic cells and is mainly responsible for the regression of müllerian ducts during male sex differentiation with signaling through two serine/threonine kinase receptors. A defect of AMH production or action causes the persistence of Müllerian derivates in otherwise normally virilized males. Its inheritance is as a recessive autosomal and is due, in 84% of cases, to mutations of *AMH* and *AMH* receptor type II genes. Serum AMH is normal for age in males with mutations in the *AMH* type II receptor gene and low or undetectable in those with mutations in AMH gene, although some exceptions have been recently described (Menabò et al. 2008). In 14% of cases, the origin of the condition is unknown (di Clemente and Belville 2006).

113.6.6 Endocrine Disruptors in Pregnancy

The timing of intrauterine hormone secretion is critical for normal organogenesis, and any external disruption may cause time-dependent alterations of male genitalia development. Androgen action is most critical, since it causes masculinization of the genitalia early in pregnancy (from week 7–8). Androgen exposure of the female fetus during this period will cause masculinization, whereas impaired androgen action in a male fetus will result in undermasculinization (Hughes et al. 2001).

Endocrine disruptors with androgenic or antiandrogenic action or estrogenic chemicals (i.e., diethylstilbestrol) may, therefore, interfere with normal sexual differentiation. Hypospadias and cryptorchidism can be caused by antiandrogens. Phthalate esters, ubiquitous in the past and still widely used as plasticizers, disturb androgen biosynthesis, and exposure to these chemicals causing antiandrogenic effects has been related to altered Leydig cell function (Toppari 2008). Exposure to phthalates occurs via skin, airways, intravenous transfusion, food, and drink (Wittassek and Angerer 2008) and absorption through the skin is very rapid (Janjua et al. 2008).

The first step to prevent environmental causes of disorders of sexual differentiation is the effective recognition of endocrine disrupting properties of chemicals in developing fetuses and children. However, although great effort has been put into the development of robust testing methods of endocrine disruptors in industrialized countries, progress is slow.

113.7 Ethics and Sex Assignment

Optimal management of DSD depends on establishing an exact diagnosis as early as possible. However, a precise diagnosis may be difficult and is actually made in more than 50% of children with 46XY DSD. There are also legal reasons for assigning a gender to all newborns with ambiguous genitalia, even though it is possible to postpone assignment when expert assessment is needed. At this critical early stage, discussion with the parents must be open, and parents' participation in decision-making should be encouraged.

A multidisciplinary team should be established at the time of the first communication of the diagnosis of DSD with the aim of helping professionals and parents to evaluate the pros and the cons of any decisions regarding management. The multidisciplinary team should help with anxieties both in physicians and parents that may lead to premature and irreversible decisions (Austin et al. 2011; D'Alberton 2010; Brain et al. 2010). According to the 5th World Congress on Family Law and Children Rights (Halifax, August 2009), the principles of ethical guidelines for the management of infants with DSD should be: (1) minimizing physical risk to child, (2) minimizing psychosocial risk to child, (3) preserving potential for fertility, (4) preserving or promoting capacity to have satisfying sexual relations, (5) leaving options open for the future if necessary, and (6) respecting the parents' wishes and beliefs if possible (Gillam et al. 2010).

There is general agreement that 46XY DSD due to complete testicular dysgenesis, severe testosterone biosynthesis defect, or Leydig cell aplasia should be assigned to the female sex.

In CAIS, gender assignment and sex of rearing is female. Inguinal hernias need repair. There is no uniformity of practice for early versus late gonadectomy: parents require appropriate information to enable them to reach a joint decision with the professional healthcare team. Two important points for discussion are the merits of spontaneous puberty with gonads in situ versus induction of puberty by estrogen replacement therapy and the possible risk of gonadal tumor development (usually seminoma) if gonadectomy is delayed until adulthood.

In 46XX CAH with genital virilization, gender assignment is female, even when there is complete virilization at birth. Steroid replacement is mandatory. In salt-wasting forms, it is necessary to start this therapy as soon as possible in order to prevent electrolytes imbalance or to treat hypovolemic shock.

In 5-α-reductase deficiency, male assignment is the first choice. Possible assignment to the male sex should be seriously discussed in cases of 17-α-OH-steroid-dehydrogenase deficiency and 46,XY DSD due to PAIS or partial testicular dysgenesis. Many authors suggest that gender assignment should also be based on presumptive prenatal androgen brain exposure (McCarty 2008; Jurgensen et al. 2010). In the next years, functional imaging studies of the brain may give more informative data about male/female brain imprinting.

Social and cultural factors appear to influence gender role and gender role change. DSD may carry a stigma. In some societies, female infertility precludes marriage, which also affects employment prospects and creates economic dependence. Religious and philosophical views may influence how parents respond to the birth of an infant affected by this medical condition. There may also be fatalism and guilt feelings related to congenital malformations or genetic conditions, and poverty and illiteracy impair access to health care (Warne 2008). Support groups integrate the work of the health care team. Peer and parent support groups may provide a context in which intimate issues of concern can be approached safely with someone who has been there, even though parents may be more amenable to these discussions than adolescent patients. Support groups can also help families and consumers to find the best quality care (www.dsd.guidelines.org). However, concerns have been expressed by some stakeholders (Cools et al. 2016) about the authority of LGBT (lesbian, gay, bisexual, and trans) movement to represent the community of people with variant sex development as published in an issue paper edited in 2015 by the Council of Europe (COE) on human rights and intersex people.

Long-term outcome should be studied in every treatment center, with special attention to different cultural settings (Jurgensen et al. 2010; Kleinemeier et al. 2010). So far, studies have shown that while many patients fare well and are leading productive lives, gender dysphoria has been underestimated in the past and gender counseling as well as sexual counseling should be part of the multidisciplinary service concerning DSD patients. More emphasis is also needed on strategies to prevent the development of germ cell cancers (i.e., seminoma in CAIS and dysgerminoma in gonadal dysgenesis DSD) or unnecessary gonadectomy. Urological problems in both males and females with DSD should not be underestimated (Warne and Raza 2008).

In cases of genetic defects carried by both parents as heterozygous, genetic counseling should be planned and offered to families (risk of recurrence). The use of I-DSD registry for research purposes has recently shown a changing tendency in sex assignment from female to male (Kolesinska et al. 2014).

113.8 Medical Management of DSD in the Newborn

The evaluation and management of a newborn with abnormalities of genitalia should be carried out by an experienced multidisciplinary team, avoiding the cure by professionals with poor experience in the field. A careful familial, gestational, and neonatal history must be done exploring unexplained neonatal death, siblings with virilization or precocious puberty or female sexual infantilism, maternal drug assumption, or androgen changes during pregnancy. There should also be a complete physical examination (external genitalia appearance including the presence or absence of palpable gonads, measurement of phallus length, urethral opening identification, presence or absence of a vagina), laboratory, and radiological investigations (Ghirri et al. 2015).

A diagnostic schedule is proposed in Fig. 3. At 24–48 h and 72–96 h of life, blood samples should be collected and a serum sample should be stored to decide on the most appropriate diagnostic test after the results of karyotyping.

Timing is important because of the physiological changes which occur in the hormonal profile shortly after birth (Migeon et al. 1994). If hormonal tests (i.e., hCG stimulation test) and imaging investigations do not lead to a definite diagnosis, laparoscopy should be performed. Skin biopsy may be used for functional studies

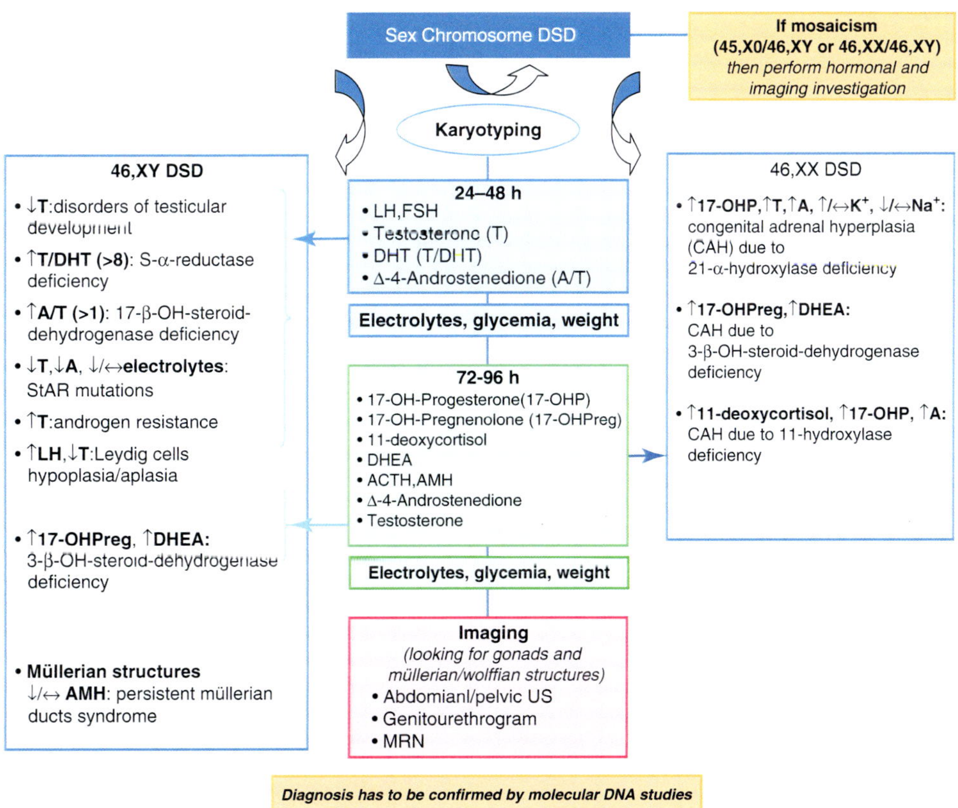

Fig. 3 A diagnostic schedule for early diagnosis of DSD in the newborn

on intracellular mechanisms induced by androgen receptor activation. New technologies as tandem-mass steroid profiling and new generation sequencing may allow a better diagnostic process.

The standard treatment of CAH is hydrocortisone 10–20 mg/m ^{2}/day (3.0–5.0 mg/day) usually in three divided doses (10 mg tablets can be dissolved in 2.5 ml water). For sick infants, 2 mg/kg of hydrocortisone hemisuccinate by i.v. bolus, followed by 20–30 mg/m ^{2}/day by constant i.v. infusion may be a more appropriate initial treatment. Blood electrolytes should be monitored daily from day 3, and if K^+ raises or Na + falls (salt loss may occur between 6 and 21 days of life), 9α-fludrocortisone should be started at 0.05 mg/day in two divided doses. The latter dose may be increased to 0.2 mg/day in two divided doses in resistant cases. Salt supplementation (5 mEq/kg/day; 5 mL sol 20% NaCl =1 g = 17 mEq) complements mineralocorticoid treatment during the first 6 months of life. Kidney sensitivity to mineralocorticoid increases at approximately 3 months' age, and the fludrocortisone dose can be reduced at this time to 0.05–0.1 mg/day. During childhood, the hydrocortisone dose should be titrated to maintain a 17 hydroxyprogesterone level below 70 nmol/L. This permissively elevated value maintains androgen suppression while minimizing side effects associated with glucocorticoid over-replacement, and serum androstenedione can be monitored simultaneously to ensure androgen suppression. Fludrocortisone replacement should be titrated to maintain plasma renin activity in the normal range. Following cessation of longitudinal growth, glucocorticoid replacement may be achieved through the use of longer acting formulations such as prednisolone or dexamethasone, which may improve oligomenorrhoea and reduced fertility in affected females. Parents should be educated regarding the requirement to increase the glucocorticoid replacement dose by a factor of two to three during periods of physiological stress such as febrile illness. The risk of adrenal crisis is greater in children aged below 4 years and requires intramuscular or intravenous glucocorticoid, e.g., hydrocortisone 2–3 mg/kg. This acute stress dose should also be administered at the time of elective anaesthetic induction (Hewitt and Zacharin 2015).

For the management of acute adrenal insufficiency, see section on "46,XX DSD."

113.9 Surgical Management of DSD: An Approach

There is an increasing tendency to recommend that any decision about genital surgery should be made by the parents and, when appropriate, the patient, in discussion with the medical team (Nabhan and Lee 2007). Of course, patient involvement in decision-making implies the delay of all the interventions not primarily directed to functional repair or to remove malignant tissue.

The goal is genitalia that are compatible with the assigned gender sex, prevention of urinary infections or incontinence, and provision of good adult sexual and reproductive function (Joint LWPES/ESPE CAH Working Group 2002). Surgeons with expertise in DSD management, together with the DSD team, need to explain the surgical sequences and the transition from infancy to adulthood.

There is controversy about the timing of feminizing genitoplasty (FG) in girls with virilizing CAH. Many pediatric urologists and endocrinologists continue to recommend early FG in agreement with the guidelines of American Academy of Pediatrics (recommended period between 2 and 6 months of age). However, intersex advocacy groups would delay genital surgery. When possible, FG should be a one-stage repair. Clitoroplasty should only be considered in cases of severe virilization (Prader III–V) with emphasis on functional outcome rather than cosmetic appearance. Vaginoplasty should be performed in infancy only if the persistence of a urogenital sinus causes complications. Generally, surgical refinement needs to be done at puberty. Vaginal dilation is not recommended during childhood, while its use during young adulthood may be useful in avoiding the need for bowel vaginoplasty, especially in women with CAH or CAIS.

In patients raised as males, the repair of hypospadias with correction of chordee, urethral construction, and orchidopexy for undescended testes are recommended. Because of limitations in penile reconstruction, the complexity of phalloplasty should be explained to the parents during initial counseling, especially if gender assignment depends on it.

The risk of gonadal malignancy should inform the timing of gonadectomy, although there is some controversy about this. Newborns affected by partial gonadal dysgenesis or partial androgen insensivity syndrome are believed to have a high likelihood (15–35% risk) for developing germ cell tumors if their gonads are located in the abdomen; thus, prophylactic bilateral early gonadectomy was widely recommended in newborns with this type of 46XY DSD. However, according to the current approach, the risk of cancer can be more realistically estimated basing on molecular analysis, which therefore constitutes the main instrument for defining the adequate conditions and timing for gonads removal. The current pathophysiological hypothesis holds that cancer risk in a dysgenetic gonad should be considered along a medical spectrum: the ultimate risk is derived from the sum of genetic factors (i.e., molecular factors that regulate hormonal balance, endogenous androgen, and estrogen) and environmental factors (exogenous estrogen), which act as epigenetic determinants on the germ cell's maturational process. The decision on surgical opportunities has to be ultimately based on the analysis of the overall clinical picture and the family context: if dysgenetic gonads are not removed in childhood, the patient will require close and careful follow-up, possibly including biopsy and histopathological analysis. The position of the gonads is critical because of the possibility of access during the clinical examination or instrumental evaluations; however, the risk of malignant transformation in itself is not affected by the shift in the scrotum (Abacı et al. 2015; Cools et al. 2011; Slowikowska-Hilczer et al. 2015).

In 5aRD patients, while male sex rearing is recommended, the risk for germ cell malignancy in affected individuals is unknown. However, gonadectomy is not currently supported by the literature. For female patients with ovotesticular DSD and functional ovarian tissue, separation and removal of the testicular component in early life is advised in an attempt to preserve fertility.

113.10 Cryptorchidism and Hypospadias

Cryptorchidism, failure of the testis to descend from its intra-abdominal location into the scrotum, has a prevalence of approximately 3% in newborns at term but is 10 times higher in preterms. If there is late spontaneous descent during the first 6–9 months of life, the prevalence of cryptochidism declines to 1% in infants born at term but it is still threefold higher in infants born preterm or low birth weight (Ghirri et al. 2002).

The so-called vanishing testis syndrome (VTS) is a clinical condition characterized by the absence or the incomplete development of a testicle in patients with 46XY karyotype and generally normal male external genitalia. It is considered that it is generally due to the atrophy and subsequent disappearance, during fetal life, of a testicle initially normal and is characterized by the presence of a rudimentary spermatic cord without macroscopically visible testicular tissue. It affects less than 5% of cases of cryptorchidism but was diagnosed in 35–60% of patients with nonpalpable testicles.

VTS seems to be mainly caused by mechanical factors such as testicular torsion local ischemia that occurred during fetal or perinatal life; less frequently it seems to be due to genetic or endocrine disorders. Indeed, testicular tissue of the controlateral testis in patients with unilateral vanishing testis generally has no abnormality and a normal number of germ cells. Risk factors include incomplete testicular descent and twisting in utero, localized trauma affecting testicles in the scrotum, and ischemic damage. This would justify the increased involvement of the left testicle in VTS, for its earlier descent than the right one. Testicular regression was also observed in association with genetic abnormalities such as Y chromosome microdeletions and persistence of Müllerian ducts. In addition, a testicular regression can be a part of the clinical spectrum of 46XY partial gonadal dysgenesis. However, in most cases, VTS appears as a sporadic condition and the patients are otherwise normal, with silent family history (Ghirri et al. 2002).

Using a two-handed technique, testes may be palpable (inguinal or prescrotal) or impalpable (abdominal). If cryptorchidism is unilateral, the consistency and size of the undescended testis should be noted, in comparison with the opposite one.

A family history should be investigated in cases where there is doubt about the diagnosis of DSD and for other cases of undescended testes. If cryptorchidism is bilateral (impalpable testes in an otherwise normal boy), urgent karyotype is mandatory as well as in cases of cryptorchidism associated with an ambiguous appearance of external genitalia (see section "Medical Management of DSD in the Newborn").

The testosterone response to hCG stimulation can clarify normal Leydig cell function, and elevated gonadotropin levels suggest primary gonadal failure. The measurement of AMH and inhibin B levels, secreted by Sertoli cells, may be sensitive markers for the presence of functioning testicular tissue. Imaging (ultrasound [US], magnetic resonance imaging [MRI]) may be useful for identifying inguinal or abdominal testes, but there is a high false-negative rate.

If one or both testes are palpable and the genitalia are normal male, the newborn should be referred to a pediatric surgeon. Hormonal treatment (intramuscular hCG or intranasal GnRH) was widely used in the past with many different protocols. Since hormonal therapy induced permanent testicular descent in a minority of young cryptorchid boys with either unilateral or bilateral palpable testis (Saggese et al. 1989; Bertelloni et al. 2001), actual guidelines indicate surgical orchiopexy as the gold standard for the treatment. It should be performed between 6–12 months of age and no later than 24 months to preserve fertility and to allow a better monitoring of testicular cancer lesions (20–48-fold increased risk in undescended testes); the incidence of malignant transformation related to testicular dysgenesis syndrome is also increased in the unaffected testis (Wohlfahrt-Veje et al. 2009; Massart and Saggese 2009). Presence of testicular microcalcifications at ultrasound may be a sign of increased cancer risk and requires stricter follow-up.

Hypospadias is a congenital displacement of the urethral meatus in male newborns. The exact position of the meatus determines whether the form of hypospadias is glandular or coronal (mild), penile (moderate), scrotal or perineal (severe). While most cases of mild forms usually occur as isolated defects, severe forms may be a sign of DSD. The prevalence is about 3–4 per 1000 live births. The pathogenesis of isolated hypospadias is multifactorial (genetic, endocrine, and environmental factors) (Kalfa et al. 2011); however, the prevalence of hypospadias is higher in infants born small for gestational age than in newborns of normal birth weight.

Patients need surgical repair, since they may have urological disorders and subfertility (Ghirri et al. 2009).

Cryptorchidism and hypospadias may be part of the clinical spectrum of complex genetic syndromes, e.g., Opitz GBB syndrome, Robinow syndrome, and CHARGE association.

Opitz syndrome (22q11.2 del) is marked by hypertelorism or telecanthus; laryngotracheoesophageal cleft; clefts of lip, palate, and uvula; swallowing difficulty and hoarse cry; genitourinary defects (hypospadias in males and splayed labia majora in females); mental retardation; developmental delay; and congenital heart defects.

Robinow syndrome (autosomal dominant or autosomal recessive due to a mutation of receptor tyrosine kinase-like orphan receptor gene-2, ROR2 in 9q22) may present with mesomelic limb shortening and facial and genital anomalies.

The CHARGE association, possibly due to a mutation of 7q21.11 (semaphorin-3E gene, *SEMA3E*) or 8q12.1 (chromodomain helicase DNA-binding protein-7, CHD7), is characterized by coloboma of the eye, heart anomalies, choanal atresia, delayed mental and somatic development, microphallus, ear abnormalities, and/or deafness. Facial palsy, cleft palate, and dysphagia are commonly associated.

References

Abacı A, Çatlı G, Berberoğlu M (2015) Gonadal malignancy risk and prophylactic gonadectomy in disorders of sexual development. J Pediatr Endocrinol Metab 28(9–10):1019–1027. https://doi.org/10.1515/jpem-2014-0522

Achermann JC, Hughes IA (2007) Disorders of sex development. In: Kronenberg H, Melmed S, Polonsky K,

Larsen PR (eds) Williams textbook of endocrinology, 11th edn. Saunders Elsevier, Philadelphia

Ahmed SF, Bryce J, Hiort O (2014) International networks for supporting research and clinical care in the field of disorders of sex development. In: Understanding differences and disorders of sex development (DSD). Endocrine development, vol 27. pp 284–292. Karger, Basel. https://www.karger.com/Article/Abstract/363676

Ahmed SF, Achermann JC, Arlt W et al (2016) Society for endocrinology UK guidance on the initial evaluation of an infant or an adolescent with a suspected disorder of sex development (revised 2015). Clin Endocrinol 84:771–788

Ainsworth C (2015) Sex redefined. Nature 518(7539): 288–291. http://www.ncbi.nlm.nih.gov/pubmed/25693544

Austin J, Tamar-Mattis A, Mazur T et al (2011) DSD: when and how to tell the patient. Pediatr Endocrinol Rev 8:213–217

Balsamo A, Cacciari E, Piazzi S et al (1996) Congenital adrenal hyperplasia: neonatal mass screening compared to clinical diagnosis only in the Emilia-Romagna region of Italy (1980–1995). Pediatrics 98:362–367

Balsamo A, Baldazzi L, Menabò S, Cicognani A (2010) Impact of molecular genetics on congenital adrenal hyperplasia management. Sex Dev 4:233–248

Bertelloni S, Baroncelli GI, Ghirri P et al (2001) Hormonal treatment for unilateral inguinal testis: comparison of four different treatments. Horm Res 55:236–239

Bertelloni S, Scaramuzzo RT, Parrini D et al (2007) Early diagnosis of 5-alpha-reductase deficiency in newborns. Sex Dev 1:147–151

Bertelloni S, Balsamo A, Giordani L et al (2009) 17beta-Hydroxysteroid dehydrogenase-3 deficiency: from pregnancy to adolescence. J Endocrinol Investig 32:666–670

Bertelloni S, Baldinotti F, Russo G, Ghirri P, Dati E, Michelucci A, Moscuzza F, Meroni S, Colombo I, Sessa MR, Baroncelli GI (2016) 5α-reductase-2 deficiency: clinical findings, endocrine pitfalls, and genetic features in a large Italian cohort. Sex Dev 10:28–36

Biason-Lauber A (2010) Control of sex development. Best Pract Res Clin Endocrinol Metab 24:163–186

Biason-Lauber A, Chaboissier MC (2015) Ovarian development and disease: the known and the unespected. Semin Cell Dev Biol 45:59–67

Biason-Lauber A, Miller WL, Pandey AV, Flück CE (2013) Of marsupials and men: backdoor dihydrotestosterone synthesis in male sexual differentiation. Mol Cell Endocrinol 371:124–132. http://www.ncbi.nlm.nih.gov/pubmed/3376007

Brain CE, Creighton SM, Mushtaq I et al (2010) Holistic management of DSD. Best Pract Res Clin Endocrinol Metab 24:335–354

Burkhard FZ, Parween S, Udhane SS, Fluck CE, Pandey AV (2016) P450 oxidoreductase deficiency: analysis of mutations and polymorphisms. J Steroid Biochem Mol Biol. https://doi.org/10.1016/j.jsbmb.2016.04.003

Cools M, Drop SL, Wolffenbuttel KP et al (2006) Germ cell tumors in the intersex gonad: old paths, new directions, moving frontiers. Endocr Rev 27:468–484

Cools M, Wolffenbuttel KP, Drop SLS, Oosterhuis JW, Looijenga LH (2011) Gonadal development and tumor formation at the crossroads of male and female sex determination. Sex Dev 5:167–180

Cools M, Simmonds M, Elford S, Gorter J, Ahmed SF, D'Alberton F, Springer A, Hiort O, Management Committee of the European Cooperation in Science and Technology Action BM1303 (2016) Response to the council of Europe human rights commissioner's issue paper on human rights and intersex people. Eur Urol. https://doi.org/10.1016/j.eururo.2016.05.015. pii: S0302–2838(16): 30179-8 [Epub ahead of print]. http://www.ncbi.nlm.nih.gov/pubmed/27210458

D'Alberton F (2010) Disclosing DSD and opening the doors. Sex Dev 4:304–309

D'Alberton F et al (2015) Quality of life and psychological adjustment of women living with 46, XY differences of sex development. J Sex Med 12(6):1440–1449

di Clemente N, Belville C (2006) Anti-Müllerian hormone receptor defect. Best Pract Res Clin Endocrinol Metab 20:599–610

Elsheikh M, Dunger DB, Conway GS, Wass JA (2002) Turner's syndrome in adulthood. Endocr Rev 23:120–140

Ferraz-de Souza B, Lin L, Acherman JC (2011) Steroidogenic factor 1 (SF1, NR5A1) and human diseases. Mol Cell Endocrinol 336:198–205

Ghirri P, Ciulli C, Vuerich M et al (2002) Incidence at birth and natural history of cryptorchidism: a study of 10,730 consecutive male infants. J Endocrinol Investig 25:709–715

Ghirri P, Scaramuzzo RT, Bertelloni S et al (2009) Prevalence of hypospadias in Italy according to severity, gestational age and birthweight: an epidemiological study. Riv Ital Pediatr 35:18

Ghirri P, Scaramuzzo MR, Greggio N, Salerno MC (2015) (Italian) Protocollo diagnostico e management in età neonatale. In: http://www.gruppodistudio-it-dsd.org/diffsvilup/32_protoc_neonatale_dsd.pdf

Gillam LH, Hewitt JK, Warne GL (2010) Ethical principles for the management of infants with DSD. Horm Res Paediatr 74:412–418

Hewitt J, Zacharin M (2015) Hormone replacement in disorders of sex development: current thinking. Best Pract Res Clin Endocrinol Metab 29:437e447

Hsu LY, Benn PA (1999) Revised guidelines for the diagnosis of mosaicism in amniocytes. Prenat Diagn 19:1081–1082

Hughes IA, Deeb A (2006) Androgen resistance. Best Pract Res Clin Endocrinol Metab 20:577–598

Hughes IA, Lim HN, Martin H et al (2001) Developmental aspects of androgen action. Mol Cell Endocrinol 185:33–41

Hughes IA, Nihoul-Fékété C, Thomas B, Cohen-Kettenis PT (2007) Consequences of the ESPE/LWPES guidelines for diagnosis and treatment of disorders of sex development. Best Pract Res Clin Endocrinol Metab 21:351–365

Imperato-McGinley J, Zhu YS (2002) Androgens and male physiology the syndrome of 5-alpha-reductase-2 deficiency. Mol Cell Endocrinol 198:51–59

Janjua NR, Frederiksen H, Skakkebaek NE et al (2008) Urinary excretion of phthalates and paraben after repeated whole-body topical application in humans. Int J Androl 31:118–130

Joint LWPES/ESPE CAH Working Group (2002) Consensus statement on 21-hydroxylase deficiency from the Lawson Wilkins pediatric endocrine society and the European society for paediatric endocrinology. J Clin Endocrinol Metab 87:4048–4053

Jones ME, Boon WC, McInnes K et al (2007) Recognizing rare disorders: aromatase deficiency. Nat Clin Pract Endocrinol Metab 3:414–421

Jurgensen M, Kleinemeier E, Lux A et al (2010) Psychosexual development in children with DSD: results from the German clinical evaluation study. J Pediatr Endocrinol Metab 23:565–578

Kalfa N, Philibert P, Baskin LS, Sultan C (2011) Hypospadias: interactions between environment and genetics. Mol Cell Endocrinol 335:89–95

Kleinemeier E, Jurgensen M, Lux A et al (2010) Psychological adjustment and sexual development of adolescents with DSD. J Adolesc Health 47:463–471

Kolesinska Z, Ahmed SF, Niedziela M, Bryce J, Molinska-Glura M, Rodie M, Jiang J, Sinnott RO, Hughes IA, Darendeliler F, Hiort O, van der Zwan Y, Cools M, Guran T, Holterhus PM, Bertelloni S, Lisa L, Arlt W, Krone N, Ellaithi M, Balsamo A, Mazen I, Nordenstrom A, Lachlan K, Alkhawari M, Chatelain P, Weintrob N (2014) Changes over time in sex assignment for disorders of sex development. Pediatrics 134(3):e710–e715. https://doi.org/10.1542/peds.2014-1088. Epub 4 Aug 2014. http://www.ncbi.nlm.nih.gov/pubmed/25092939

Lajic S, Nordenström A, Hirvikoski T (2008) Long-term outcome of prenatal treatment of congenital adrenal hyperplasia. Endocr Dev 13:82–98

Latronico AC, Arnhold IJ (2006) Inactivating mutations of LH and FSH receptors–from genotype to phenotype. Pediatr Endocrinol Rev 4:28–31

Lee YS, Cheng AW, Ahmed SF (2007) Genital anomalies in Klinefelter's syndrome. Horm Res 68:150–155

Mac Laughlin DT, Danahoe PK (2004) Sex determination and differentiation. N Engl J Med 350:367–378

Manna PR, Stocco DM (2005) Regulation of the steroidogenic acute regulatory protein expression: functional and physiological consequences. Curr Drug Targets Immune Endocr Metabol Disord 5:93–108

Massart F, Saggese G (2009) Sex steroidal targets & genetic susceptibility to idiopathic cryptorchidism. Pediatr Endocrinol Rev 6:481–490

McCarty MM (2008) Estradiol and the developing brain. Physiol Rev 88:91–124

Menabò S, Balsamo A, Nicoletti A et al (2008) Three novel AMH gene mutations in a patient with persistent müllerian duct syndrome and normal AMH serum dosage. Horm Res 70:124–128

Menabò S, Polat S, Baldazzi L, Kulle AE, Holterhus PM, Grötzinger J, Fanelli F, Balsamo A, Riepe FG (2014) Congenital adrenal hyperplasia due to 11-beta-hydroxylase deficiency: functional consequences of four CYP11B1 mutations. Eur J Hum Genet 22(5): 610–616. https://doi.org/10.1038/ejhg.2013.197. Epub 11 Sep 2013. PubMed PMID: 24022297; PubMed Central PMCID: PMC3992560. http://www.ncbi.nlm.nih.gov/pubmed/24022297

Mendonca BB, Domenice S, Arnhold IJP, Costa EMF (2009) 46, XY disorders of sex development (DSD). Clin Endocrinol 70:173–187

Meyer-Bahlburg HFL et al (2016) Gender assignment, reassignment and outcome in disorders of sex development: update of the 2005 consensus conference. Horm Res Paediatr 85(2):112–118

Migeon CJ, Berkovitz DG, Brown TR (1994) Sexual differentiation and ambiguity. In: Kappy MS, Blizzard RM, Migeon CJ (eds) The diagnosis and treatment of endocrine disorders in childhood and adolescence, 4th edn. Thomas, Springfield

Nabhan ZM, Lee PA (2007) Disorder of sex development. Curr Opin Obstet Gynecol 19:440–445

Nielsen J, Wohlert M (1991) Chromosome abnormalities found among 34,910 newborn children: results from a 13-year incidence study in Arhus, Denmark. Hum Genet 87:81–83

Nihoul-Fekete C, Lortat-Jacob S, Cachin O, Josso N (1984) Preservation of gonadal function in true hermaphroditism. J Pediatr Surg 19:50–55

Polizzi A, Balsamo A, Bal MO, Taruscio D (2014) Rare diseases research and practice. Endocr Dev 27:234–256. http://www.ncbi.nlm.nih.gov/pubmed/25247660

Saggese G, Ghirri P, Gabrielli S, Cosenza GC (1989) Hormonal therapy for cryptorchidism with a combination of human chorionic gonadotropin and follicle-stimulating hormone. Success and relapse rate. Am J Dis Child 143:980–982

Samtani R, Bajpai M, Ghosh PK, Saraswathy KN (2010) SRD5A2 gene mutations – a population-based review. Pediatr Endocrinol Rev 8(1):34–40

Sax L (2002) How common is intersex? A response to Anne Fausto- Sterling. J Sex Res 39:174–178

Schweizer K et al (2014) Gender experience and satisfaction with gender allocation in adults with diverse intersex conditions (divergences of sex development, DSD). Psychol Sex 5(1):56–82

Seo JY, Park HD, Kim JW, Oh HJ, Yang JS, Chang YS, Park WS, Lee SY (2014) Steroid profiling for congenital adrenal hyperplasia by tandem mass spectrometry as a second-tier test reduces follow-up burdens in a tertiary care hospital: a retrospective and prospective evaluation. J Perinat Med 42(1):121–127. http://www.ncbi.nlm.nih.gov/pubmed/23989111

Shearer BM, Thorland EC, Gonzales PR, Ketterling RP (2007) Evaluation of a commercially available focused aCGH platform for the detection of constitutional chromosome anomalies. Am J Med Genet A 143:2357–2370

Simm D, Degenhardt K, Gerdemann C et al (2008) Chronological age of patients with Turner syndrome at diagnosis. Klin Padiatr 220:16–20

Slowikowska-Hilczer J, Szarras-Czapnik M, Wolski JK, Oszukowska E, Hilczer M, Jakubowski L, Walczak-Jedrzejowska R, Marchlewska K, Filipiak E, Kaluzewski B, Baka-Ostrowska M, Niedzielski J, Kula K (2015) The risk of neoplasm associated with dysgenetic testes in prepubertal and pubertal/adult patients. Folia Histochem Cytobiol 53(3): 218–226

Speiser PW (2007) Prenatal and neonatal diagnosis and treatment of congenital adrenal hyperplasia. Horm Res 68(Suppl 5):90–92

Speiser PW, White PC (2003) Congenital adrenal hyperplasia. N Engl J Med 349:776–788

Telvi L, Lebbar A, Del Pino O (1999) 45,X/46,XY mosaicism: report of 27 cases. Pediatrics 104(2 Part 1): 304–308

Toppari J (2008) Environmental endocrine disrupters. Sex Dev 2:260–267

Turcu AF, Auchus RJ (2015) The next 150 years of congenital adrenal hyperplasia. J Steroid Biochem Mol Biol 153:63–71

Warne GL (2008) Long-term outcome of disorders of sex development. Sex Dev 2:268–277

Warne G, Raza J (2008) Disorders of sex development (DSDs), their presentation and management in different cultures. Rev Endocr Metab Disord 9:227–236

Wittassek M, Angerer J (2008) Phthalates: metabolism and exposure. Int J Androl 31:131–138

Wohlfahrt-Veje C, Main KM, Skakkebæk NE (2009) Testicular dysgenesis syndrome; fetal origin of adult reproductive problems. Clin Endocrinol 71:459–465

Yamada G, Satoh Y, Baskin LS, Cunha GR (2003) Cellular and molecular mechanisms of development of external genitalia. Differentiation 71:445–470

Zimmermann B, Zhong XY, Holzgreve W et al (2007) Real-time quantitative polymerse chain reaction measurement of male fetal DNA in maternal plasma. Methods Mol Med 132:43–49

Pathophysiology of Fetal and Neonatal Kidneys

114

Farid Boubred and Umberto Simeoni

Contents

Abstract

Fetal renal development is a complex phenomenon. The ureteric bud and metanephric mesenchyme interaction is essential for nephrogenesis which results from the expression of specific genes, the fetal environment, or the interaction of both factors. IUGR, maternal diabetes, maternal undernutrition, micronutrient deficiency, and fetal or neonatal exposure to drugs (NSAIDS, ACE-Is, glucocorticoids, aminoglycosides) or to toxic (alcohol) are known to affect nephrogenesis. After a brief review of fetal and neonatal renal physiology, pathologic situations including preterm birth, congenital anomalies of the kidney and urinary tract, kidney diseases, and kidney-pharmacology interactions will be developed. Renal maldevelopment and exposure to factors that can alter the fetal and neonatal renal functions and structure increase the risk of hypertension and chronic renal disease in adulthood. Long-term follow-up is thus required and early markers of nephron

F. Boubred
Division of Neonatology, La Conception Hospital, Marseille, France
e-mail: farid.boubred@ap-hm.fr

U. Simeoni (✉)
Division of Pediatrics, CHUV and UNIL, Lausanne, Vaud, Switzerland
e-mail: Umberto.simeoni@chuv.ch

G. Buonocore et al. (eds.), *Neonatology*,
https://doi.org/10.1007/978-3-319-29489-6_261

dosing and renal injury should be developed with the aim to implement preventive strategies.

114.1 Salient Points

- Fetal renal development starts with an interaction between the ureteric bud and metanephric mesenchyme.
- During intrauterine life, the placenta is responsible for fetal homeostasis. Glomerular filtration rate, renal blood flow, and tubular functions increase with renal growth and nephrogenesis.
- Serum creatinine is used to assess glomerular filtration rate in neonates.
- Nephrogenesis is affected by intrauterine growth restriction, maternal diabetes, maternal undernutrition, micronutrient deficiency, and fetal or neonatal exposure to drugs or toxins.
- In preterm infants, nephrogenesis is incomplete and may be altered at birth.
- Congenital abnormalities of the kidney and urinary tract are a range of anomalies including malformations of ureteropelvic junction, vesicoureteric junction, or vesicourethral area and dysplastic kidneys.
- Renal maldevelopment and exposure to factors that can alter fetal and neonatal renal function and structure increase the risks of hypertension and chronic renal disease in adulthood.
- Long-term follow-up is required and early markers of nephron dosing and renal injury should be developed with the aim of implementing preventive strategies.

114.2 Kidney Development

The definitive kidney, the metanephros, is formed by two processes: nephrogenesis (formation of glomerulus and tubules) and branching morphogenesis (formation of collecting ducts, calyces, pelvis, and ureter). The metanephric kidney takes place after the formation and involution of two embryonic kidneys, the pronephros (nonfunctional organ) and mesonephros (first functional kidney), that in turn evolves into the ureteric bud (UB). The metanephros appears in the fifth gestational week and develops from the specific interaction of the epithelial UB and the undifferentiated metanephric mesenchyme (MM). This interaction is crucial for the differentiation of mesenchyme and the induction of UB branching division (Fig. 1). The UB undergoes branching morphogenesis and invades the MM in response to signals elaborated by the mesenchymal cells. This process gives a 15 branch generation. At 20–22 weeks of gestation, branching morphogenesis is completed and will result in the collecting system. Mesenchymal cells that are in close contact with the invading UB undergo an epithelial transformation. The induced MM gives the nephrons through the consecutive stages of condensation, renal vesicle, vascular cleft, and S-shaped body. The nephrons develop in successive stages from the inner to the outer area of the kidney in parallel with the vascular system. The glomerular capillary tuft is formed via recruitment and proliferation of endothelial and mesangial cell precursors. In human, the primitive glomerulus appears at approximately 9–10 weeks of gestation. Nephrogenesis is completed by 34–36th weeks of gestation with about 60% of the nephrons being formed during the third trimester of pregnancy (Saxen 1987; Merlet-Benichou et al. 1999). Once nephrogenesis is complete, stroma cells differentiate into fibroblast-, pericyte-, and lymphocyte-like cells. At birth the final nephron varies from 500,000 to 1 million per kidney. Such variation in nephron number is due to genetic factors, to the fetal environment, or to a combination of both (Chevalier 1996). Several genes and molecular pathways control the formation of the renal collecting system and nephrogenesis, such as transcriptional factors (PAX-2, WT1), growth factors (IGF, EGF, TGF, GDNF, FGF), oncogenes, extracellular matrix, and vascular factors (Table 1) (Burrow 2000). These factors act at a specific time of kidney development especially when the UB interacts with the adjacent MM. For instance, blockade of VEGF receptor, inhibition of the renin-angiotensin system (RAS), and knockout mice for COX-2 gene expression are associated with impaired nephrogenesis including glomerular cysts, dysplastic tubules,

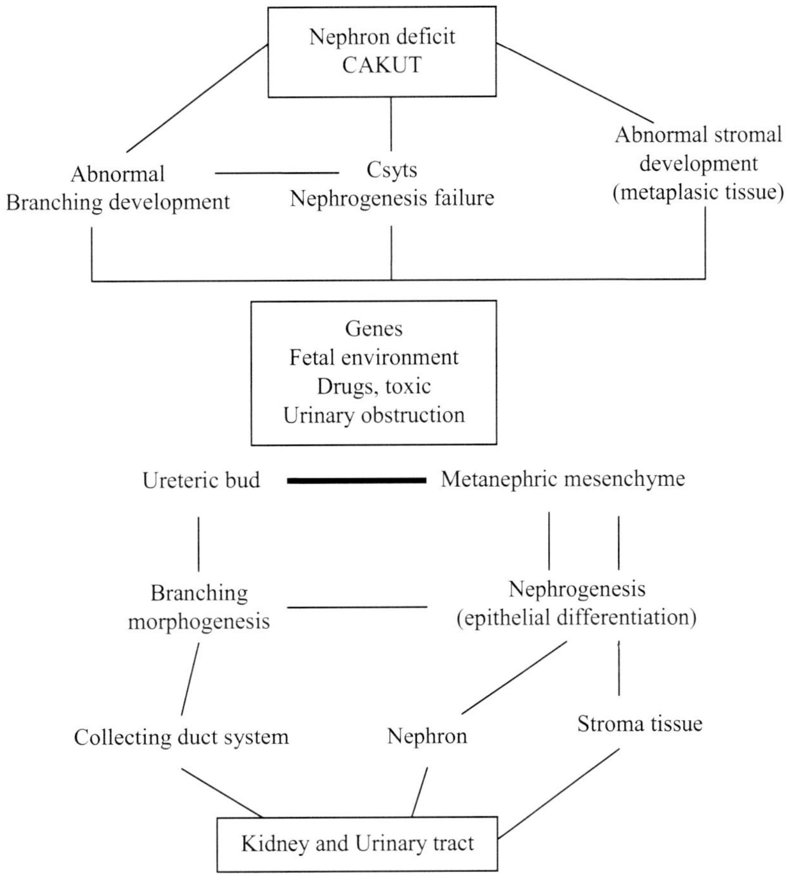

Fig. 1 Kidney development: simplified schematic process of normal and pathologic kidney development

and tubular dysgenesis (Dinchuk et al. 1995; McGrath-Morrow et al. 2006; Pryde et al. 1993).

114.3 Renal Physiology

114.3.1 The Fetus

During intrauterine life, the homeostasis of the fetus is assigned to the placenta. Glomerular filtration rate, renal blood flow, and tubular functions progress with renal growth and nephrogenesis. The kidney is involved in urine production which is essential in fetal well-being and in hormonal production (1.25 OH vitD_3 and erythropoietin). The formation of the urine, the main component of amniotic fluid in the third trimester, begins by 12 weeks of gestation. The urinary flow rate increases tenfold from 6 ml/h at 20 weeks to 60 ml/h at 40 weeks of gestation, which expresses an optimal structural and functional renal development. In the near-term period, the fetal kidney shows sufficient glomerular and tubular development to allow the adaptation to extrauterine life (Brophy and Robillard 2004).

114.3.2 Glomerular Function

During fetal life, the glomerular filtration rate (GFR) increases progressively, while renal vascular resistances (RVRs) remain elevated. The fetal GFR is mainly driven by nephrogenesis. Systemic blood pressure, around 40–60 mmHg, and renal blood flow are low in comparison with the newborn or the adult. For instance, in sheep, the fetal kidneys receive 3% of cardiac output compared to 15% in the neonatal period. Low RBF is associated with elevated RVRs. This state is due to a subtle equilibrium between vasoconstrictive

Table 1 Syndromes and gene defects associated with abnormal kidney development (CAKUT)

Syndrome	Gene defects	Kidney malformations
Renal-coloboma syndrome	*PAX 2*	Hypoplasia, VUR
Renal cysts and diabetes syndrome	*HNF1b*	Dysplasia, hypoplasia
Branchio-oto-renal syndrome	*EYA1, SIX1*	Unilateral or bilateral agenesia/ dysplasia
Renal tubular dysgenesis	*RAS components*	Tubular dysplasia/dysgenesis
Campomelic dysplasia	*SOX9*	Dysplasia, hydronephrosis
Townes-Brocks syndrome	*SALL1*	Dysplasia, hypoplasia, VUR
Simpson-Golabi-Behmel syndrome	*GPC3*	Medullary dysplasia
Kallmann syndrome	*KAL1,FGFR1, PROK*	Renal agenesis
Fraser syndrome	*FRAS1*	Dysplasia, renal agenesis
Alpert syndrome	*FGRG2*	Hydronephrosis
Alagille syndrome	*JAGGED1*	Cystic dysplasia
Meckel-Gruber syndrome	*MKS1,MKS3*	Cystic renal dysplasia
Hypoparathyroidism, deafness, and renal anomaly syndrome (HDR)	*GATA3*	Dysplasia, VUR
DiGeorge syndrome	*22q11*	Agenesia, dysplasia, VUR
Beckwith-Wiedemann syndrome	*P57*	Dysplasia
Pallister-Hall syndrome	*GLI3*	Dysplasia
Nail-patella syndrome	*LMX1B*	Agenesia, glomerular anomalies
Smith-Lemli-Opitz syndrome	*7 hydroxy-cholesterol reductase*	Agenesia, dysplasia
Zellweger syndrome	*PEX1*	Cystic dysplasia, VUR
Glutaric aciduria type II	*Glutaryl CoA dehydrogenase*	Cystic dysplasia
STAR syndrome	*FAM58A*	CAKUT
Hypothyroidism	*PAX8*	Renal agenesis
–	*SOX17, DSTYK, BMP4*	CAKUT

factors including the renin-angiotensin system (RAS) and renal sympathetic nervous system and vasorelaxing factors such the prostaglandins, nitric oxide, and other factors (Fig. 2). Highly expressed during the active development of the kidney, these vasoactive factors participate to nephrogenesis and in the regulation of intrarenal vascular blood flow (essential for the development as well).

In the fetal kidney, the RAS is the principal vasoconstrictive factor; it is upregulated during active nephrogenesis and downregulated at the end of this process. The RAS maintains renal blood flow and renal pressure perfusion. The fetus is able to release renin into the fetal circulation. Renin does not cross the placenta and the fetal plasma renin levels are higher than maternal levels. Angiotensin II increases mainly the glomerular efferent tone which is highly sensitive to angiotensin. Renal sympathetic nervous system increases renal vascular tone, in afferent and efferent arteriole. The fetal renal vasculature is more sensitive to alpha2-adrenoreceptor stimulation than the neonatal one. Upregulation of alpha2-receptors is associated with down-regulation of beta2-adrenoreceptors. Adenosine vasodilates glomerular arterioles in physiologic state but increases tone of afferent glomerular arterioles in stress conditions, responsible for reduced GFR.

Vasoconstrictive forces are counterbalanced by vasodilating factors that principally act on the glomerular afferent arteriole to maintain a sufficient renal blood flow. Prostaglandins, nitric oxide (NO), and kallikrein-kinin system are principal factors. Prostaglandins, in particular E2 and I2,

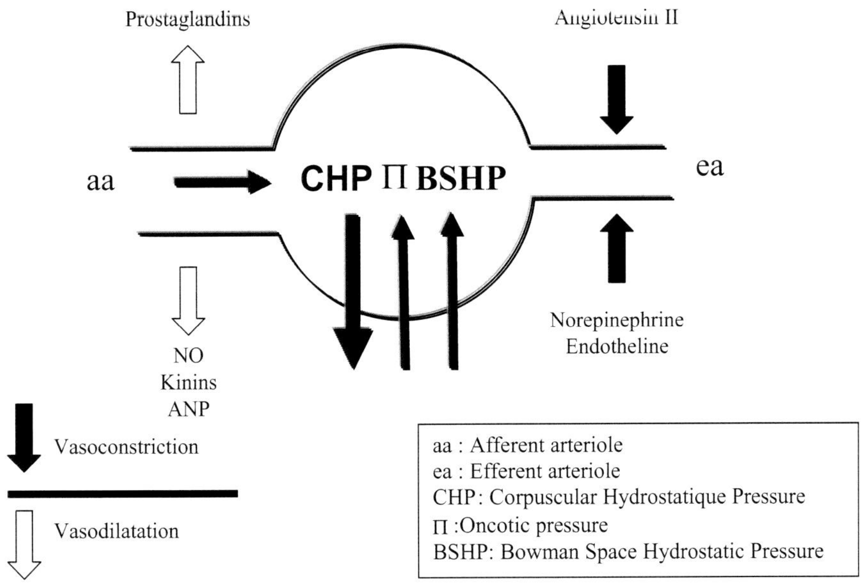

Fig. 2 Determinants of glomerular filtration with preglomerular and postglomerular vasoactive forces

are of major importance. These prostaglandins are produced by the placenta, membranes, and the fetus, from the action of two enzyme isoforms, the cyclooxygenase types 1 and 2 (COX-1 and COX-2), and their production is stimulated by angiotensin II (34). COX-2 is constitutive in fetal kidney and appears essential for the development and function of the kidney (Khan et al. 2001). Administration of COX inhibitors during pregnancy decreases renal blood flow, impairs renal function, and induces oligohydramnios. Nitric oxide is synthetized by endothelial cells and vasodilates the afferent arteriole. In sheep, inhibition of NO increases renal vascular resistance, impairs renal function, and reduces sodium excretion. Other factors including endothelin and atrial natriuretic factors modulate renal hemodynamic as well.

114.3.3 Tubular Function

The tubular system has different secretion and reabsorption activities depending on the tubular segment. For example, the proximal tubule is principally involved in regulation of fluid, electrolytes, amino acids, glucose, and the distal tubules and collecting system in fluid and tonicity regulation. Tubular transporters mature differently during the development of the nephrons. Distal tubular phosphorus and potassium channels mature early to make them available for cellular functions. These features are responsible in part for higher fetal plasma potassium and phosphorus levels than in the mother. Renal tubules are the target of hormones including RAS, aldosterone, prostaglandins, atrial natriuretic peptide, and cortisol (maturational effect). The sensitivity of renal tubules to such hormones matures progressively along gestation. Finally the relative tubular immaturity associated with hypotonic urines (100–250 mOsm/kg H_2O) allows the production of amniotic fluid at a sufficient rate which is essential for fetal well-being (Brophy and Robillard 2004).

The excretion of sodium is high during fetal life but decreases with renal development. This state is related to various factors including high circulating sodium concentrations and high sensitivity to natriuretic factors, large extracellular fluid volume, relative insensitivity to hormonal factors, and dysmaturity of tubular sodium reabsorption. In opposition with adult physiology, the sodium is mainly reabsorbed in the distal portion of the immature tubules. The sodium/hydrogen exchangers (NHE, four different isoforms) play an important role. These exchangers mediate the exchange of one sodium for one hydrogen and contribute to the acidification of urine. The NHE three channel, located at the apical or luminal membrane of tubular cells, is thought to be responsible for the bulk of tubular reabsorption of sodium. It is downregulated in the proximal portion of the immature tubules when it is markedly upregulated after birth. Its expression and activity are dependent on tubular Na+, K+-ATPase which is downregulated in immature kidney (Hoster 2000).

The balance of potassium is positive in the fetus, due to active transplacental transfer and renal immaturity. They both make potassium available for cell growth and cell functions. Renal secretion is low and tends to increase toward term. Potassium excretion increases with glomerular and tubular surface area, with maturation of tubular Na+, K+-ATPase activity, and with the progressive tubular sensitivity to aldosterone.

As for potassium, the fetus is characterized by a positive phosphorus balance resulting from a transplacental transport against a concentration gradient, a high rate of tubular reabsorption via a sodium-phosphorus co-transporter, and a relative parathyroid insufficiency. Calcium is important for the adequate mineralization, growth, and fetal skeleton. Vitamin D-dependent calcium-binding proteins, involved in transepithelial calcium transfer, are present in fetal kidney. However, the major role of the kidney in fetal calcium homeostasis is the production of $1.25(OH)_2D_3$ rather than renal regulation of calcium excretion.

During fetal development, the placenta regulates the fetal acid-base balance. The reabsorption of bicarbonates and chloride in the proximal tubule increases with gestational age, which allows the fetus to participate to acid-base homeostasis, near term. This function is mainly related to the maturation of the carbonic anhydrase activity.

The fetus produced hypotonic urine at an elevated rate of 1.5 l every day. The urine concentration capacity is blunted in the immature kidney. This defect is related to various factors including a low sensitivity of the collecting duct to arginine vasopressin (AVP), a structural immaturity of the loop of Henle with preferential distribution of blood flow to the inner cortex, a low gradient concentration in the medulla due to limited protein intake to generate significant amounts of urea, and a low expression of aquaporin 2 (AQ2). AQ2, a water channel, is located in the apical membrane of collecting duct cells and is involved in water reabsorption. Humans who lack aquaporins (AQs) have a urinary concentrating defect. Expression of AQs is regulated by the AVP via the V2 receptor. AVP is highly synthesized during the last trimester in pregnancy (Nielsen and Frokaier 2002). The immaturity of tubular functions and its maturation explain the high rate of amniotic fluid production which decreases at the end of gestation.

114.3.4 The Newborn

114.3.4.1 Glomerular Function

After birth hemodynamic changes (increased blood pressure and renal blood flow) and structural changes contribute to postnatal maturation of GFR. As nephrogenesis is terminated at birth, postnatal structural change is based on the maturation of preexisting renal structures. This process includes increase in glomerular membrane permeability, in corpuscular glomerular diameter (especially of glomeruli from the outer area of cortex), in filtration surface area, and in intrarenal redistribution of blood flow. Glomerular size reaches adult values at the age of 3 years. These structural changes result in enhanced filtration surface area.

Transition of fetal circulation to extrauterine life is characterized by a rapid increase in systemic blood pressure and renal blood flow. The rapid change in RBF is associated with postnatal decrease in renal vascular resistances (decrease in glomerular vasoconstriction). Glomerular capillary hydrostatic pressures increase as well but remain lower than in the adult (Solbaug and Jose 2004).

After birth GFR rapidly increases (2.5- to threefold increase) from 20 ml/min/1.73 m^2 to half of adult values at the end of the neonatal period (Guignard 1975). In preterm infants GFR correlates with gestational and is at birth less than 15 ml/min/1.73 m^2. Postnatal maturation depends on gestational age with a delayed maturation being possibly observed in very low birth weight infants (Gubhaju et al. 2014). In term infants, plasma creatinine concentrations are elevated at birth (60–70 mcmol/l) and stabilize at the end of the first week (30–40 mcmol/l). In preterm infants, creatinine levels are elevated on the first day (90–110 mcmol/l), increasing transiently within days 3–5 (reaching 130–150 mcmol/l) and then decrease progressively (Gallini et al. 2000). Neonates and especially preterm infants are in a state of physiologically renal insufficiency. A delicate balance of vasoconstrictor and vasodilator forces which maintains GFR and immature renal structure makes newborn and especially preterm infants at high risk to develop renal dysfunction in specific conditions (hypotension, hypovolemia, perinatal asphyxia, and nephrotoxic drugs).

Serum creatinine is widely used to assess glomerular filtration rate (GFR) in neonates. Clearance of endogenous creatinine can be used in clinical practice and needs strict 12–24-h urine collection which can be difficult in preterm infants. Creatinine is a metabolite of creatine located in skeletal muscle and is filtered and secreted in part by renal tubular cells. Muscle mass influences serum creatinine levels. Other markers of GFR including inulin, cystatin C, and beta trace protein are not used routinely in neonates. Clearance of inulin is the gold standard to evaluate GFR. Inulin is inert, being not metabolized and neither reabsorbed nor secreted by the renal tubules; however, it has limited applications in clinical practice. Cystatin C is produced by all nucleated cells and is independent of muscle mass. It is freely filtered and reabsorbed but catabolized in the kidney, which prevents clearance measurement. Serum levels are high during the neonatal period and stabilize at 12 months of age. Cystatin C and beta trace protein are being evaluated in newborn and preterm infants. Current data consider cystatin C as a valuable tool to assess GFR in newborn and preterm infants (Filler et al. 2016).

114.3.4.2 Tubular Function

The postnatal maturation of renal tubules follows the maturation of GFR. Postnatal maturation is characterized by a tenfold increase in proximal tubular length and diameter within the weaning period.

After birth, the regulation of homeostasis is transferred from the placenta to the kidney. Postnatal fluid and electrolytic adaptation is characterized by a transient increase in diuresis during the first week of life due to the contraction of the extracellular volume. Commonly neonates lose around 5–10% of their birth weight. Very low birth weight may undergo a higher weight loss of up to 15% of their birth weight. Fractional excretion of sodium in neonates is around 1% and decreases progressively in relation to a rapid maturation of proximal tubules. Fetal exposure to glucocorticoids at the end of gestation accelerates the maturation of tubular transporters (NHE, Na+, K+-ATPase, etc.) (Brophy and Robillard 2004).

The neonate is able to achieve maximal dilution with urine osmolarity as low as 40–60 mOsm/l. Diluting capacity tends to mature rapidly in the newborn and in the preterm infant who at 36th postconceptional age have the same dilution capacity than adult. Within the limits allowed by of GFR, neonates, even preterm infants, tolerate a large range of fluid intakes (150 ml/kg/day) without major alterations in water and electrolyte parameters. Diluting capacity is greater than concentrating capacity, which is limited to 400–600 mOsm/l. Children reach the adult maximal urine concentration ability (1300–1400 mOsm/kg) by 2 years of age. This characteristic may be explained by reduced tonicity of the medullary interstitium, low expression of water channels (aquaporins), and relative tubular insensitivity to ADH. Higher production of prostaglandin E2 in neonate may inhibit the tubular effect of ADH. Low neonatal concentrating capacity is of limited importance in healthy neonates. However, neonates and especially preterm infants are more vulnerable to insufficient water intakes and extrarenal water loss (skin losses, diarrhea, etc.) with the risk of hypernatremic dehydration and osmotic diuresis and

Fig. 3 Renal mechanism of systemic hypertension and renal damage, the "Brenner hypothesis"

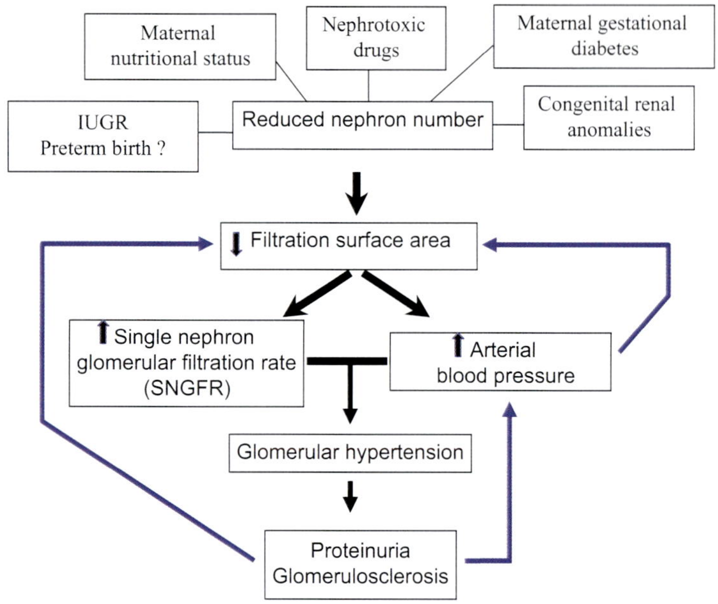

favored by a lower threshold for renal glucose excretion.

The newborn has a diminished threshold for bicarbonates. The large extracellular fluid (ECF) volume expansion may result in depressed proximal tubular bicarbonate reabsorption. When ECF is contracted, renal reabsorption increases and urinary pH becomes more acidic. In preterm infants, immaturity of carbonic anhydrase may prolong the depressed tubular bicarbonate reabsorption. The normal range for plasma bicarbonate concentration is lower in preterm infants (16–20 mmol/l) than term infants (21–24 mmol/l).

114.4 Pathophysiology

114.4.1 The Immature Kidney

In the preterm infants, nephrogenesis is incomplete at birth and has to continue in an unfit environment. Nephrogenesis may be altered in preterm infants (Rodriguez et al. 2004; Sutherland et al. 2011). Experimental studies show discordant findings (Stelloh et al. 2012; Gubhaju et al. 2009). In rodents only one study has shown reduced nephron endowment in pups born preterm (Stelloh et al. 2012). Such a finding has not been found in preterm baboon (Gubhaju et al. 2009). The degree of immaturity may explain such discordant findings. In contrast with the baboon model, preterm birth occurred during the early stage of nephrogenesis in the rodent models. These findings suggest that extremely preterm infants are at high risk of reduced nephron endowment. Data are limited in preterm infants; autopsy findings have shown an alteration of glomerular structure and acceleration of nephron maturation with a possibly reduced nephron endowment (Rodriguez et al. 2004; Sutherland et al. 2011). Impairment of mesenchymal cell differentiation has been suggested. Moreover it is not excluded that environment factors to which preterm infants face up during the neonatal period including infection/inflammation, oxidative stress, nephrotoxic drug use, or undernutrition can influence nephrogenesis and thus nephron endowment. For instance, neonatal undernutrition has been shown to be associated with reduced kidney volume (a surrogate of nephron mass) in infants born preterm (Bacchetta et al. 2009). Collectively the current findings suggest that the extremely preterm infants and preterm infants exposed to adverse neonatal complications have a high risk of nephron deficit.

In comparison with term neonates, GFR is lower in preterm infants and increases

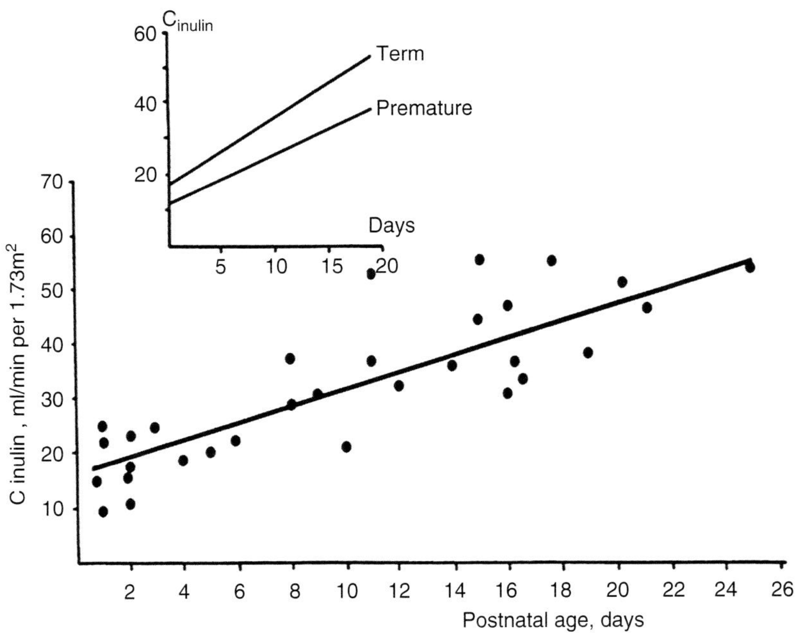

Fig. 4 Postnatal glomerular filtration rate in neonates (C inulin: inulin clearance) (From Guignard et al. 1981)

progressively after birth (Gubhaju et al. 2014; Bueva and Guignard 1994) (Figs. 4, 5 and 6). Structural maturation drives the progressive maturation of GFR in very preterm infants in whom postnatal nephrogenesis continues after birth. Blood pressure and renal blood flow are low in preterm infants. The RVRs are high and the RAS upregulated. The immature kidney is particularly dependent on vasodilator forces to maintain a sufficient GFR. Administration of prostaglandin inhibitors (indomethacin) for closure of a patent ductus arteriosus impairs renal function, leads to oliguria, and reduces RBF and GFR. Ibuprofen, another COX inhibitor, has moderate renal effects. However, these adverse renal effects can be prolonged up to 1 month and can limit renal excretion of some medications (Giniger et al. 2007; Vieux et al. 2011). In animal, neonatal indomethacin administration results in reduced nephron number in adult rats unlike ibuprofen (Kent et al. 2014).

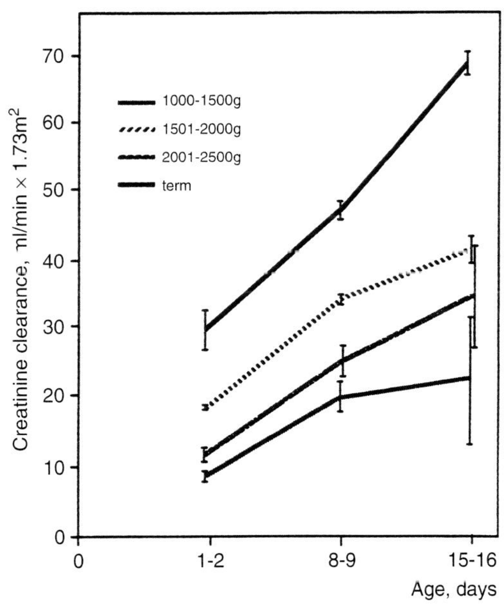

Fig. 5 Postnatal maturation of glomerular filtration rate in term and preterm infants (Bueva and Guignard 1994)

Postnatal hydro-electrolytic adaptation is characterized by an excessive water and sodium losses during the first 10 days after birth. Preterm infants are prone to water and salt wasting with high risk of early hypernatremia and late hyponatremia. Fractional excretion of sodium is elevated in preterm infants (5% vs <1% in term infants) and reaches term values progressively after days 15–21. A postnatal contraction of the extracellular fluid volume occurs during the first postnatal days

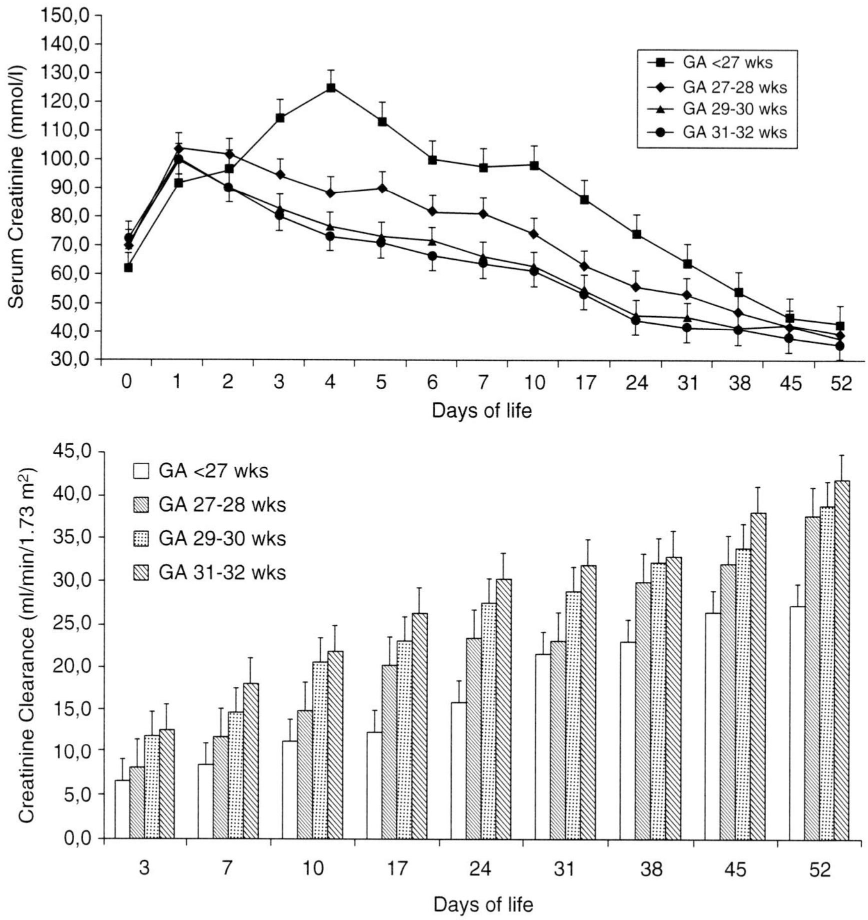

Fig. 6 Postnatal maturation of glomerular filtration rate in extremely low gestational age neonates (Gallini F et al. Pediatre Nephrol 15:119–124)

and translates into a 2–3% daily weight loss. The optimal maximum weight loss is unknown; a maximum limit of 10–15% total weight loss is common especially in extremely preterm infants and should be not exceeded. Fluid and electrolyte balance has to be thus closely followed up and adapted. Moreover, the kidney of preterm infants cannot efficiently excrete excessive water and sodium loads which increase the risk of bronchopulmonary dysplasia, intracerebral hemorrhage, and necrotizing enterocolitis. It is common to introduce sodium, potassium, and phosphorus by postnatal day 2 and to adapt individually electrolyte intake (especially sodium). However, nutritional practices have recently changed with early introduction of high protein and caloric intakes, which stimulates anabolism and prevents early catabolism. This new nutritional strategy enhances cellular use of potassium and phosphorus and increases the risk of early hypokalemia and hypophosphatemia especially in intrauterine growth restricted preterm infants (Boubred et al. 2015). Potassium and phosphorus intake can be thus introduced early from birth onwards for some infants. Rapid growth induces sodium cell utilization and together with sodium wasting favors the occurrence of late hyponatremia. Fluid, minerals, and electrolyte balances should be adapted tightly and individualized to promote optimal growth and deficiency (Boubred et al. 2015; Sweet D and the working group on prematurity 2007).

Table 2 Glomerular and tubular consequences of immature kidney

Fluid-electrolytes therapy in preterm infants[a]	Glomerular immaturity: consequences	Tubular immaturity: consequences
D1–D2: Volume: 80–100 ml/kg/d Na: 0 K: 0 (except if <3.5 mmol/l)	Reduced ability to salt/water overload excretion	Sodium wasting
	Hyperkalemia	Metabolic acidosis
		Reduced urine concentration capacity with conservative urine dilution capacity
D3–D5: Volume: 120–140 ml/kg/d Na: 2–4 mmol/kg/d K: 1–2 mmol/kg/d	High sensitivity to vasoactive drugs	Glycosuria
	Increased risk of renal failure	Elevated urinary calcium excretion
≥D5: Volume: 140–170 ml/kg/d Na: 4–6 mmol/kg/d K: 1–3 mmol/kg/d	Reduced clearance of drugs	High sensitivity to diuretics

[a]Fluid, micronutrient, and electrolyte intakes are individually adapted

Glomerular and tubular consequences of immaturity are shown in Table 2.

Preterm infants are more likely to receive drugs in neonatal intensive care unit. Most drugs are eliminated by the kidney and undergo glomerular filtration or tubular metabolism both being immature in preterm infants. Circulating levels of drugs such as vancomycin or aminoglycosides need to be monitored to optimize dosage and to reduce toxicity.

Glomerular and tubular consequences of prematurity are blunted by maternal administration of synthetic glucocorticoids (GCs) (betamethasone and dexamethasone). Prenatal administration of GC improves systemic blood pressure, RBF, and GFR and accelerates the maturation of tubular functions with enhanced proximal reabsorption of sodium and excretion of potassium. This treatment limits dysnatremia and hyperkalemia events in preterm infants. Increased expression and activity of sodium exchanger, Na+, K+-ATPase activity, and renal sympathetic nerve activity are involved (Catarelli et al. (2002).

114.4.2 Congenital Tubulopathies

Congenital tubular diseases are rare and include various diseases according to defect in epithelial tubular channels (Rodriguez-Soriano 2000). Bartter syndrome is a group of tubulopathies involving the regulation and expression of various tubular transporters located in the ascending limb of Henle and the corresponding gene (upregulation of NKCC2 and ROMK and downregulation of Barttin and ClC-Kb). Bartter syndrome is characterized by salt wasting, by hypovolemia with a low or conserved blood pressure, by hyper-reninism, and by metabolic alkalosis. Polyhydramnios and hypercalciuria are often observed in fetal and neonatal forms. Treatment consists of salt adaptation, water and potassium intake, and amiloride and/or indomethacin use.

Primary pseudo-hypoaldosteronism is an autosomal recessive disease due to defective epithelial ENaC channel (in collecting ducts). This syndrome is characterized by life-threatening salt wasting, risk of dehydration and arterial hypotension, severe hyperkalemia, distal tubular acidosis, and hyperaldosteronism. This disease is treated by sodium supplementation. When ENaC activity is increased, sodium reabsorption is exaggerated with hypertension and metabolic hypokalemia. Renin activity and aldosterone levels are decreased. Liddle syndrome, an autosomal dominant disease, displays such features. Treatment consists in salt restriction and amiloride.

Nephrogenic diabetes insipidus, an X-linked or autosomal transmitted disease, is characterized by polyuria-polydipsia, dehydration, irritability, and failure to thrive. These symptoms are due to a defect in the arginine vasopressin-V2 receptor or in AQ2.

114.4.3 Parenchymal Consequences of Urinary Tract Anomalies

Congenital abnormalities of the kidney and urinary tract (CAKUT) are a wide range of anomalies including malformations of ureteropelvic junction, of vesicoureteric junction, or of vesicourethral area and dysplastic kidneys.

114.4.3.1 Renal Structure Changes

The pathophysiological mechanism of CAKUT remains unknown. One can postulate that urinary obstruction affects the interaction UB-MM with failure in the induction of metanephrogenic blastema. After an early compliance stage, obstruction of the collecting system induces urinary hyper-pressure and muscular hypertrophy. In fetal lamb, early and complete ureteral obstruction impairs renal architecture with abnormal tubular differentiation, inflammation, and reduced nephron endowment. Changes in renal expression of transcription factors (Pax2, Wnt) involved in early stage of nephrogenesis have been demonstrated in such a situation. In human, congenital ureteropelvic junction obstruction is associated with renal histologic changes including decreased glomerular density, interstitial fibrosis, and tubular dilatation (Peters et al. 1992).

A genetic and developmental mechanism has been proposed for CAKUT. Various defects in specific genes involved in renal development affect kidney parenchyma and urinary tract development (few examples in Table 1). However, the pathogenesis of this syndrome is multifactorial and involves single nucleotide variants and epigenetic mechanism through which environment can impair the development of the kidney and urinary tract (Nicolaou et al. 2015). The quality of the ureteric bud-mesenchymal interaction, the position at which arises the UB from the pronephros, and the number of branching morphogenesis are critical for the kidney development. Failure of induced ureteric bud outgrowth leads to renal agenesis. An aberrant outgrowth of more than one UB may result in double collecting system and duplication of the ureter. An ectopic positioning of the UB is associated with renal tissue malformation, abnormalities of the ureterovesical junction, and a nephron deficit related to reduced branching morphogenesis (Fig. 1).

114.4.3.2 Renal Function Changes

The outcome of CAKUT depends on the importance of urinary obstruction, on the kidney structure, on fetal renal functions (oligohydramnios, urinary sodium concentrations, fetal beta2-microglobulin), and on defects in other organs. Early occurrence of urinary tract obstruction, bilateral renal dysplasia, reduction of the kidney size, and oligohydramnios (a surrogate of severe fetal renal insufficiency) is associated with poor renal prognosis. Infants with severe pathology often die in the perinatal period as a consequence of Potter's sequence (pulmonary hypoplasia resulting from oligohydramnios and fetal renal function insufficiency). Survivors may develop renal failure during childhood. Dialysis during neonatal period should be discussed with parents and the multidisciplinary nephrology team before and after birth.

Infants with severe obstructive nephropathy are prone to acid-base and hydro-electrolytic balance abnormalities and to impaired GFR. Complete and prolonged fetal ureteral obstruction is associated with decrease RBF and GFR proportional to loss of parenchyma. The RAS is upregulated in such situations. Renal dysfunctions lead to type IV renal tubular acidosis (hyperchloremic metabolic acidosis) with hyperkalemia, salt wasting, and defect in urine concentration responsible for water wasting and nephrogenic diabetes insipidus. Various changes in tubular channel exchanger, decreased NA+, K+-ATPase activity, unresponsiveness of the damaged distal nephron to aldosterone with secondary hyperaldosteronisme, loss of H+ ATPase on the surface of intercalated cells, and downregulation of aquaporins have been described. Treating and preventing renal infection, adapting protein intake, and limiting the use of or close monitoring of nephrotoxic drugs aim to preserve renal functions.

114.4.4 Pharmacological Interactions

The number of pregnant women and women of childbearing age receiving drugs is constantly increasing. These drugs can cross the placenta and can impair potentially the function and structure of the fetal kidney. The newborn may in turn express renal failure with various severities up to neonatal death. Selective COX-2 inhibitors and nonselective nonsteroidal anti-inflammatory drugs (NSAIDs), ACE-Is, and AT1R antagonists are the main drugs affecting the development and the function of perinatal kidney [review 32].

Nonsteroidal anti-inflammatory drugs (NSAIDs) can be used as antalgic or as tocolytic agent in pregnant woman (indomethacin). The renal side effects of in utero exposure to NSAIDs vary from transient fetal oligohydramnios to severe and lethal renal failure in babies. Quickly after the initiation of indomethacin therapy, a significant reduction of fetal urine production occurs. This effect, frequent and transient in many cases, is the basis of treatment of polyhydramnios. The available information originates principally from retrospective studies and indicates a rate of incidence from 1.5% to 20%. Experimental and human studies show that NSAIDs decrease fetal GFR (consequence of renal blood flow reduction) and increase urine osmolality (enhanced activity of arginine vasopressin). The risk of neonatal renal failure seems increasing with prolonged and cumulate doses, short time period between treatment and delivery, preexisting fetal distress, and low birth weight. In addition to the changes of renal functions, a singular renal nephrotoxicity dysplasia attributable to NSAIDs has been described: various degrees of ischemic injuries and fibrosis of medullary area, cortical necrosis, focal tubular and glomerular microcysts of developing nephron, loss of differentiation between proximal and distal tubules, and decreased renal mass. These lesions are associated with increased expression of renin in the juxtaglomerular apparatus. The severity of renal hypoperfusion induced by NSAIDs may lead to irreversible glomerular and tubular injuries. Such effects have been noted recently after prenatal exposure to the selective inhibitors of COX-2, new generations of NSAIDs, proposed as an alternative to nonspecific NSAIDs with the aim of preventing adverse side effects.

When administered during pregnancy, inhibitors of the RAS (ACE-Is and AT1R antagonists) can induce a variety of serious fetal complications, with a high degree of mortality rate. These complications named angiotensin-converting enzyme inhibitor fetopathy include intrauterine growth retardation, profound fetal and neonatal hypotension refractory to any treatment, renal failure, oligohydramnios with limb deformities and pulmonary hypoplasia, hypocalvaria, and increased rate fetal loss. Renal histology shows typically proximal tubular dysgenesis. Numerous cases have been reported with a wide range of adverse fetal and neonatal renal effects varying from transient oligohydramnios (when treatment was arrested rapidly) to severe (requiring peritoneal dialysis) and lethal renal failure. The magnitude of these adverse renal effects cannot be quantifiable precisely, but the risk increases by chronic administration and the stage of fetal exposure, especially during the second and third trimester. In contrast, elective exposure in the first trimester of gestation is not associated with an enhanced risk of teratogenicity. When therapy is interrupted rapidly before 2nd trimester, poor or no adverse renal effects are noted.

Experimental studies have shown that maternal antenatal administration of various drugs can affect nephrogenesis in the absence of renal dysfunctions in the fetus and newborn infants. In rodents and sheep, antenatal maternal administration of glucocorticoids (GCs) at a specific time of pregnancy reduces nephron number and induces hypertension in adult offspring. The mechanism by which GCs alter the fetal kidney structure is unclear. Several pathways are suspected. In utero exposure to GC may (1) disturb cell differentiation/proliferation ratio at the expense of reduced proliferation, (2) reduce ureteric bud branching, (3) alter gene expression of specific genes involved in kidney development (GNDF), (4) decrease renal AT1R and renin gene expression, or (5) alter epigenetic marks.

Maternal administration of cyclosporine A (CsA) during gestation (E14–18, and E20–24) affects fetal growth and nephrogenesis leading to a permanent nephron deficit in rat offspring (average of 25–30%). CsA may block epithelial transformation of the metanephric mesenchyme. In human, outcome of infants exposed in utero to CsA has not shown any changes of renal function and morphology in childhood. But data are too scarce, and long-term follow-up (the maximal age of follow-up was 7 years) is insufficient to conclude definitely on the side effects at adulthood.

Antenatal maternal administration of ampicillin and aminoglycosides reduces nephron number (20–30%) and induces hypertension in adult rat offspring. Reduced nephron number results from a defect in UB branching morphogenesis affecting the first branching division. Administration during the late stage of nephrogenesis does not induce a nephron deficit. Other aminoglycosides, such amikacin and netilmicin, have less adverse renal effects. Antenatal maternal administration of ampicillin is associated with 20% reduction of nephron number in rat offspring; apoptosis mechanism of MM is the suspected. Such experimental observations have not been found in human. Other drugs, such as chlorambucil and antineoplastic drugs, can impair renal development with urinary tract malformation and renal agenesis.

In summary, in most cases, newborn do not express clinical renal failure postnatally. However, experimental studies suggest that prenatal exposure to certain drugs may decrease nephron endowment. One must be careful in extrapolating data from animal to human, since major interspecies differences in renal sensitivity to drugs exist. However, long-term follow-up of infants exposed in utero to drugs is needed.

114.4.5 Long-Term Consequences of Nephron Number Reduction

It is suspected for a long date, since the works of Brenner et al. in the 1980s, that a reduced nephron number increases the risk of hypertension and chronic renal insufficiency in adulthood (Brenner et al. 1988). Reduced nephron number is associated with renal changes including single nephron glomerular filtration hyperfiltration (SNGHF) and glomerular and tubular hypertrophy. Such hemodynamic changes are responsible for glomerular injury through increase in glomerular capillary hypertension. Over a long time, a vicious cycle takes place leading to glomerular sclerosis, chronic renal insufficiency, and hypertension (cf Fig. 3). In human, an inverse relationship has been established between nephron number and hypertension (Keller et al. 2003). However, this relationship is complex and involves various factors such as nephron dosing and postnatal factors. For instance, congenital agenesis, a situation of severe nephron deficit, is associated with early development of systemic hypertension and early chronic renal insufficiency during infancy of adolescent. It is postulated that a moderate nephron deficit at birth is insufficient to induce long-term cardiovascular and chronic renal diseases but constitutes a factor of vulnerability when other postnatal factors including early catch-up growth or overfeeding accelerate the development of these diseases (Boubred et al. 2013).

At birth the final nephron number varies from 500,000 to 1 million per kidney. Such variation in nephron number is due to genetic factors, to the fetal environment, or to a combination of both. Various perinatal factors have been shown to induce nephron deficit including intrauterine growth restriction (IUGR), maternal nutrient deficiency (vitamin A, iron depletion, zinc deficiency), maternal protein or global nutrition deficit, exposure to drugs (see above) or toxic (alcohol), maternal and fetal stress, and maternal gestational diabetes (Merlet-Benichou et al. 1999). Preterm birth with postnatal adverse environment (postnatal denutrition, stress, exposure to nephrotoxic drugs) and renal and urinary tract malformations are associated with impaired nephrogenesis which may lead to reduced nephron endowment.

Such perinatal events are less likely to affect renal functions during the neonatal period but increase the susceptibility of hypertension and chronic renal disease in adulthood. Long-term follow-up is needed, with close assessment of blood pressure and renal parameters (creatinine, proteinuria) to prevent such adverse evolutive cardiovascular and renal diseases. Future studies may focus on the development of markers of nephron number endowment and of early biomarkers of SNGHF and renal injury with the aim to implement preventive strategies).

References

Bacchetta J, Harambat J, Dubourg L et al (2009) Both extrauterine and intrauterine growth restriction impair renal function in children born very preterm. Kidney Int 76(4):445–452

Boubred F, Vendemia M, Garcia-Meric P et al (2006) Effects of maternally administered drugs on the fetal and neonatal kidney. Drug Saf 29:397–419

Boubred F, Saint-Faust M, Buffat C et al (2013) Developmental origins of chronic renal disease: an integrative hypothesis. Int J Nephrol 2013:346067. https://doi.org/10.1155/2013/346067

Boubred F, Herlenius E, Bartocci M et al (2015) Extremely preterm infants who are small for gestational age have a high risk of early hypophosphatemia and hypokalemia. Acta Paediatr 104:1077–1083

Brenner BM, Garcia DL, Anderson S (1988) Glomeruli and blood pressure. Less of one, more the other. Am J Hypertens 1:335–347

Brophy PD, Robillard JE (2004) Functional development of the kidney *in utero*. In: Polin A, Fox W (eds) Fetal and neonatal physiology, 3rd edn. W.B. Saunders Company, Philadelphia, pp 1229–1239

Bueva A, Guignard JP (1994) Renal function in preterm neonates. Pediatr Res 36:572–577

Burrow CR (2000) Regulatory molecules in kidney development. Pediatr Nephrol 14:240–253

Catarelli D, Chirico G, Simoni U (2002) Renal effects of antenally and postnatally administered steroids. Pediatr Med Chir 24:157–162

Chevalier RL (1996) Developmental renal physiology of the low birth weight preterm newborn. J Urol 156:714–719

Dinchuk JE, Car BD, Focht RJ et al (1995) Renal abnormalities and an altered inflammatory response in mice lacking cyclooxygenase 2. Nature 378:406–409

Filler G, Guerrero-Kanan R, Alvarez-Elias AC (2016) Assessment of glomerular filtration rate in the neonate: is creatinine the best tool? Curr Opin Pediatr 28 (2):173–179

Gallini F, Maggio L, Romagnoli C et al (2000) Progression of renal function in preterm neonates with gestational age ≤ 32 weeks. Pediatr Nephrol 15:119–112

Giniger RP, Buffat C, Millet V et al (2007) Renal effects of ibuprofen for the treatment of patent ductus arteriosus in premature infants. J Matern Fetal Neonatal Med 20:275–283

Gubhaju L, Sutherland MR, Yoder BA et al (2009) Is nephrogenesis affected by preterm birth? Studies in a non-human primate model. Am J Physiol Renal Physiol 297:F1668–F1677

Gubhaju L, Sutherland MR, Horne RS, Medhurst A, Kent AL, Ramsden A, Moore L, Singh G, Hoy WE, Black MJ (2014) Assessment of renal functional maturation and injury in preterm neonates during the first month of life. Am J Physiol Renal Physiol 307(2):F149–F158

Guignard JP (1975) Glomerular filtration rate in the first three weeks of life. J Pediatr 87:268–272

Guignard JP, Gruskin AB, Norman ME (eds) (1981) Pediatric nephrology. Martinus Nijhoff, The Hague

Hoster M (2000) Embryonic epithelial membranes transporters. Am J Phys 279:F74–F52

Keller G, Zimmer G, Gerhard M et al (2003) Nephron number in patients with primary hypertension. N Engl J Med 348:101–108

Kent AL, Koina ME, Gubhaju L et al (2014) Indomethacin administered early in the postnatal period results in reduced glomerular number in the adult rat. Am J Physiol Renal Physiol 307:F1105–F1110

Khan KNM, Stanfield KM, Dannenberg A et al (2001) Cyclooxygenase-2 expression in the developing human kidney. Pediatr Dev Pathol 4:461–466

McGrath-Morrow S, Choc C, Molls R et al (2006) VEGF receptor 2 blockade leads to renal cyst formation in mice. Kidney Int 69:1741–1748

Merlet-Benichou C, Gilbert T, Vilar J et al (1999) Nephron number: variability is the rule. Causes and consequences. Lab Investig 79:515–526

Nicolaou N, Renkema KY, Bongers EM et al (2015) Genetic, environmental, and epigenetic factors involved in CAKUT. Nat Rev Nephrol 11:720–731

Nielsen S, Frokaier J, Marples D et al (2002) Aquaporins in the kidney: from molecule to medicine. Physiol Rev 82:205–244

Peters CA, Carr MC, Lais A et al (1992) The response of the fetal kidney to obstruction. J Urol 148:503–509

Pryde PG, Sedman AB, Nugent CE et al (1993) Angiotensin-converting enzyme inhibitor fetopathy. J Am Soc Nephrol 3:1575–1582

Rodriguez MM, Gomez AH, Abitbol CL (2004) Histomorphometric analysis of postnatal glomerulogenesis on extremely preterm infants. Pediatr Dev Pathol 7:17–25

Rodriguez-Soriano J (2000) New insight into the pathogenesis of renal tubular acidosis-from functional to molecular studies. Pediatr Nephrol 14:1121–1136

Saxen L (1987) Organogenesis of the kidney. Cambridge University Press, Cambridge

Solbaug MJ, Jose PA (2004) Postnatal maturation of renal blood flow. In: Polin A, Fox W (eds) Fetal and neonatal physiology, 3rd edn. W.B. Saunders Company, Philadelphia, pp 1243–1249

Stelloh C, Allen KP, Mattson DL et al (2012) Prematurity in mice leads to reduction in nephron number, hypertension, and proteinuria. Transl Res 159:80–89

Sutherland MR, Gubhaju L, Moore L, Kent AL, Dahlstrom JE, Horne RS, Hoy WE, Bertram JF, Black MJ (2011) Accelerated maturation and abnormal morphology in the preterm neonatal kidney. J Am Soc Nephrol 22 (7):1365–1374

Sweet D, the working group on prematurity (2007) European consensus guidelines on the management of neonatal respiratory distress syndrome. J Perinat Med 35:175–186

Vieux R, Fresson J, Guillemin F et al (2011) Perinatal drug exposure and renal function in very preterm infants. Arch Dis Child Fetal Neonatal Ed 96: F290–F295

Acute and Chronic Renal Failure in the Newborn Infant

115

Jean-Pierre Guignard and Uma Sankari Ali

Contents

J.-P. Guignard (✉)
Lausanne University Medical School, Lausanne, Switzerland
e-mail: jean-pierre.guignard@unil.ch

U. S. Ali
Nephrology Division and PICU, BJ Wadia Hospital for Children, Mumbai, India
e-mail: dr_usali@yahoo.com

G. Buonocore et al. (eds.), *Neonatology*,
https://doi.org/10.1007/978-3-319-29489-6_262

Abstract

Acute renal failure (ARF) is one of the most common renal disorders of the newborn. For diagnostic and therapeutic purposes, ARF is divided into three categories: prerenal (functional), renal (intrinsic), and postrenal (obstructive). ARF may be oliguric or non-oliguric, the latter having a better prognosis. Risk factors for ARF include prematurity, respiratory and vascular disorders, heart failure, congenital uropathies, and administration of nephrotoxic drugs. Chemical analysis of urine and ultrasounds help to differentiate the different forms of ARF. Conservative management of prerenal forms of ARF consists in carefully maintaining fluid and electrolyte balances. Early relief of obstruction is mandatory in severe postrenal forms. Renal replacement therapy is necessary when ARF is secondary to intrinsic renal damage: peritoneal dialysis is the treatment of choice. In newborn infants with chronic renal failure, strict control of electrolyte disorders and anemia as well as adequate nutrition is essential. Overall prognosis of ARF and outcome of CRF are still a source of concern.

Abbreviations

ARF	Acute renal failure
CRF	Chronic renal failure
GRF	Glomerular filtration rate
RRT	Renal replacement therapy
ELBW	Extremely low birth weight

115.1 Salient Points

- Acute renal failure (ARF) is the consequence of a sudden decrease in glomerular filtration rate with consequent retention of nitrogen waste products and disturbances in water, electrolyte, and acid–base balance.
- Premature birth increases renal vulnerability. In healthy premature neonates, nephrogenesis continues after birth, but for only 40 days.
- Risk factors for the development of acute renal failure include perinatal asphyxia, antepartum hemorrhage, sepsis, hyaline membrane disease, administration

of NSAIDs pre- or post-natally, and hypernatremic dehydration.

- The renin-angiotensin system is highly activated in fetal and neonatal life, and the maintenance of a normal GFR in the face of physiologically low arterial pressures is dependent on efferent arteriolar vasoconstriction mediated by angiotensin II.
- The occurrence of oligohydramnios may suggest fetal oliguria and the presence of severely affected kidneys in utero.
- The presence of external features such as Potter's facies, preauricular tags, polydactyly, single umbilical artery, or sacral abnormalities may indicate the presence of an underlying developmental renal anomaly.
- Laboratory evaluation consists of urinanalysis, blood count, plasma urea and creatinine concentration measurements, and plasma cystatin C determination.
- Imaging of the genitourinary tract by ultrasound is useful for assessing the size, shape, and echogenicity of the kidneys, for diagnosing pelvicalyceal dilatation, and for examining the ureters and the bladder.
- In the prerenal types of ARF, restoration of volume by the administration of 20 ml/kg of normal saline over 1–2 h usually improves urine output.
- When urine output fails to improve after fluid repletion, a trial of diuretics can be given. Intravenous furosemide at 1–3 mg/kg may improve diuresis.
- Acute renal replacement therapy is indicated when renal failure produces serious derangements; in neonates and infants peritoneal dialysis is the treatment of choice.
- Congenital abnormalities of the kidneys and urinary tract are the most common causes of chronic renal failure (CRF).
- Vascular disorders such as thrombosis of the renal vein or artery, prolonged ischemia with subsequent irreversible tubular or cortical necrosis, disseminated intravascular coagulation, and hemolytic disease with massive myoglobinuria constitute acquired causes of CRF.
- Congenital forms (Finnish type) of nephrotic syndrome can induce early onset CRF.

115.2 Introduction

Acute renal failure (ARF), often coined as acute kidney injury, is the consequence of a sudden decrease in glomerular filtration rate with consequent retention of nitrogen waste products and disturbances in water, electrolyte, and acid-base balance. Because of its physiological specifics, the premature fetal and neonatal kidneys are particularly vulnerable to common endogenous and exogenous stresses occurring before birth, during delivery, or after birth. Clinical studies have shown that 8–24% of all neonates hospitalized in intensive neonatal care units may present with ARF (Andreoli 2012; Gouyon and Guignard 2000; Guignard and John 1986; Toth-Heyn et al. 2000). The causes of ARF (Table 1) are divided into prerenal (functional), renal (intrinsic), and postrenal (obstructive) causes. Functional prerenal insufficiency is the most frequent form of ARF. It is preventable if treated early and adequately.

115.2.1 The Fetal Kidney

The fetal kidney lives in a protected environment without real homeostatic responsibilities. Perfusion is limited, the fetal kidney receiving only 3–4% of the cardiac output. GFR is also extremely low in the fetus. Nephrogenesis is complete by 35 weeks of gestation. At birth, the immature kidney is abruptly thrust into an independent extrauterine existence where it has to assume the responsibility of safeguarding the life and well-being of the neonate by providing the moment-to-moment fine-tuning required for body homeostasis (Drukker and Guignard 2002).

115.2.2 The Neonatal Kidney

GFR at birth is close to 20 ml/min per 1.73 m^2 in term neonates. It doubles within 2 weeks and reaches 50 ml/min per 1.73 m^2 at 4 weeks of life (Fig. 1) (Guignard and John 1986; Drukker and

Table 1 Etiology of acute renal failure

Prerenal
Hypovolemia or renal hypoperfusion
Asphyxia
Respiratory distress syndrome (RDS)
Dehydration
Hemorrhage (maternal antepartum, twin-to-twin transfusion, intraventricular bleeding, hemolytic disease)
Sepsis
Cardiac disease (patent ductus arteriosus, aortic coarctation)
Polycythemia (hyperviscosity)
Renal
Acute tubular necrosis (ATN)
Persistent prerenal disturbances
Nephrotoxins (nephrotoxic antibiotics, e.g., aminoglycosides, contrast agents, angiotensin-converting enzyme [ACE] inhibitors and angiotensin II AT1 receptor blockers)
Myoglobinuria, hemoglobinuria, hyperuricemia
Vascular disorders (renal vein thrombosis, renal artery thrombosis, aortic thrombosis, disseminated intravascular coagulation)
Congenital renal anomaly (dysplasia, hypoplasia, polycystic kidney, agenesis)
Pyelonephritis
Transient acute renal failure of the neonate
Maternal etiology (gentamicin, indomethacin, ACE inhibitors, paraproteinemia)
Postrenal
Congenital anomaly (ureteral or urethral obstruction, neurogenic bladder, magacystis-megaureter)
Obstruction secondary to circumcision
Renal candidiasis
Calculi
Neurogenic bladder

Guignard 2002). The neonatal kidney is thus in a state of relative physiological renal insufficiency during the first postnatal month and is ill-equipped to handle major homeostatic challenges. The driving force for producing the glomerular filtrate is the systemic arterial pressure which is quite low in the newborn period (Table 1). The two major vasoactive forces that optimize the driving force for filtration are the prostaglandins that relax the afferent arteriolar tone and angiotensin II (ATII) that constricts the efferent arteriole, thus increasing the effective transglomerular pressure gradient (Fig. 2). This hydrostatic pressure is opposed by the intratubular pressure as well as by the oncotic pressure, resulting in a net driving force of only a few mm Hg (Toth-Heyn et al. 2000). GFR shows a progressive direct correlation with both gestational and postnatal ages (Guignard and John 1986; Vieux et al. 2010).

Premature birth increases the renal vulnerability. In healthy premature neonates, nephrogenesis continues after birth, but for only 40 days (Rodriguez et al. 2004). Nephrogenesis stops at birth in growth-retarded neonates. Low birth weight infants have consequently a lower number of nephrons as compared to term infants. GFR is lower in low birth weight infants and increases more gradually than in full-term neonates.

115.2.3 Definition

Acute renal failure can be oliguric or non-oliguric, so that urine flow rate cannot define ARF, the diagnosis of which is based on the follow-up of plasma creatinine concentration. ARF is suspected when the plasma creatinine is above 130 umol/l (15 mg/l) for at least 24–48 h, while maternal renal function is normal. In very premature neonates, the elevated plasma creatinine present at birth increases in the first 3–4 days of life because of tubular reabsorption of creatinine across leaky tubules (Guignard and Drukker 1999). In clinical practice, repeated measurements of plasma creatinine are used to confirm the presence of ARF.

Oliguria is defined by a urine output less than 1.0 ml/ kg per h in preterm and less than 0.5 ml/kg per h in term neonates.

115.3 Etiology and Pathogenesis

115.3.1 Etiology

Risk factors for the development of acute renal failure include perinatal asphyxia, antepartum hemorrhage, sepsis, hyaline membrane disease,

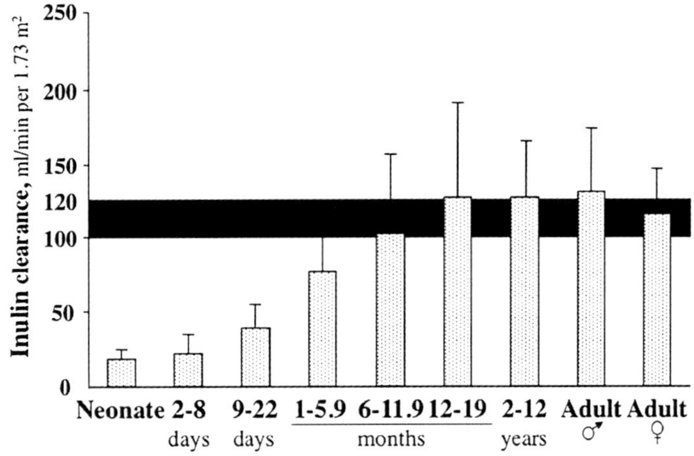

Fig. 1 Development of glomerular filtration rate

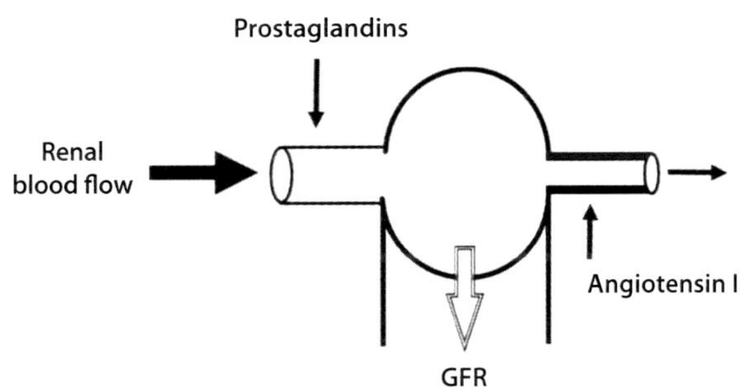

Fig. 2 The glomerulus: intrarenal regulation of GFR

Table 2 Blood pressure in the neonate[a]

Age	<1.0 kg	1.0–1.5 kg	>2.5 kg
Birth	33 ± 15	39 ± 18	49 ± 19
1 Week	41 ± 15	47 ± 18	60 ± 19
2 Weeks	45 ± 15	50 ± 18	64 ± 19
4 weeks	48 ± 15	53 ± 18	68 ± 19

[a]Mean ± 95 % confidence limits for single measurements; measurement via umbilical artery catheterization or by Dynamap (Adapted from Ong et al. (1998))

administration of NSAIDs pre- or postnatally, and hypernatremic dehydration (Choker and Gouyon 2004; Table 1). The primary disease may manifest clinically as respiratory distress in hyaline membrane disease or as lethargy, apnea, poor feeding, prolonged capillary refill, and hypotension in sepsis (Table 2). More than 75% of cases of neonatal renal failure are prerenal in nature. Intrinsic renal failure accounts for less than 10% of the cases and may occur due to drug-induced nephrotoxicity or when the hypoxic-ischemic insults are prolonged or severe (Guignard and John 1986).

115.3.1.1 Prerenal Causes

All factors that decrease cardiac output can lead to ARF. Some insults to the kidney begin in prenatal life. Fetal hypovolemia as a result of feto-fetal transfusions, feto-maternal transfusions, and antepartum hemorrhage can lead to renal ischemia in utero with or without fetal hypotension resulting in fetal oliguria, oligohydramnios, and postnatal renal failure. Hypotension, hypoxemia, metabolic acidosis, metabolic alkalosis, small changes in body temperature, and the administration of vasoconstrictive agents are common stresses that increase the renal vascular resistance (Toth-Heyn et al. 2000). Cardiac diseases, the persistence of patent ductus arteriosus, and hyperviscosity states can also impair cardiac output (Guignard and John 1986).

115.3.1.2 Intrinsic Causes

Persistent prerenal disturbances can lead to acute renal necrosis and severely impair renal function (Toth-Heyn et al. 2000; Andreoli 2012). The renal parenchyma can also be injured by vascular disorders, renal thrombosis, nephrotoxins, acute pyelonephritis, myoglobinuria, and hemoglobinuria. Cortical necrosis may result from severe ischemia and microthrombi formation. Congenital renal anomalies, including hypodysplasia, and cystic diseases can favor the occurrence of both ARF and chronic renal failure.

115.3.1.3 Postrenal Causes

Obstruction on the urinary tract, whatever the cause, can lead to ARF. The obstruction can occur at the level of the ureters, the bladder, or the urethra. When not relieved immediately, the obstruction can induce permanent damage to the kidney (Chevalier 2012).

115.3.1.4 Nephrotoxic Drugs

Nephrotoxicity of drugs may play an important role in producing renal injury (Guignard and Gouyon 1988). They can affect the fetus when administered to the pregnant mother or the neonate when administered postnatally. Aminoglycosides may cause renal injury even with normal blood levels due to the high tissue concentrations of the drugs that can be achieved. All cephalosporins are potentially nephrotoxic though clinically the third-generation cephalosporins appear to be reasonably safe. Vancomycin needs to be used in appropriate dosages and monitored closely. The use of two simultaneous nephrotoxic drugs should preferably be avoided. Vasoactive drugs interfering with the synthesis of prostaglandins as well as with the renin-angiotensin system are particularly deleterious to the immature kidney (Andreoli 2012; Guignard and John 1986; Toth-Heyn et al. 2000).

Nonsteroidal Anti-Inflammatory Drugs (NSAIDs)

The maintenance of prenatal as well as postnatal GFR is highly dependent upon prostaglandin-mediated afferent arteriolar dilatation (Toth-Heyn et al. 2000). Inhibition of prostaglandins can decrease renal perfusion and GFR (Allegaert et al. 2005; Pacifici 2014) and even lead to severe fetal or neonatal failure that can even be irreversible (Pacifici 2014). In utero exposure to the nonselective NSAID inhibitors such as aspirin, indomethacin and ibuprofen have indeed been associated with adverse fetal outcomes such as fetal oliguria and neonatal renal failure. Administration of NSAIDs early in pregnancy carries a high risk of inducing renal tubular dysgenesis in the fetus, with fetal oliguria and oligohydramnios. COX-2 is indeed also expressed in the proximal tubular cells and is believed to play an important role in the differentiation of the renal tubules.

The NSAIDs are cyclooxygenase (COX) inhibitors, some of which nonselectively inhibit COX-1 and COX-2, while others selectively inhibit COX-2. Because COX-1 is constitutively expressed in several cell types in the gastrointestinal tract, liver, platelets, and kidney, toxicities are fairly commonly encountered when it is inhibited. COX-2 is an inducible enzyme and is not expressed in the gastrointestinal tract and liver. COX-2 inhibitors were thus expected to have a better safety profile. Experimental and clinical studies on nimesulide, a COX-2 selective inhibitor, have shown that the drug can also produce renal dysgenesis and failure when administered pre- or postnatally (Ali et al. 2006). When really needed, all NSAIDs must be used with great caution, be it before or after birth (Toth-Heyn et al. 2000; Andreoli 2012).

Angiotensin Inhibitors Converting Enzyme Inhibitors (ACEIs) and Angiotensin II AT1 Receptor Blockers (ARBs)

The renin-angiotensin system is highly activated in fetal and neonatal life, and the maintenance of a normal GFR in the face of physiologically low arterial pressures is dependent on efferent arteriolar vasoconstriction mediated by angiotensin II (Toth-Heyn et al. 2000). Interfering with the action of angiotensin II by maternal ingestion of ACEIs or ARBs can result in a dramatic fall in GFR leading to fetal oliguria, oligohydramnios, and postnatal oliguric renal failure that can be irreversible. Angiotensin II receptors type 2 are expressed prominently during fetal life in the proximal tubules and play an important role in

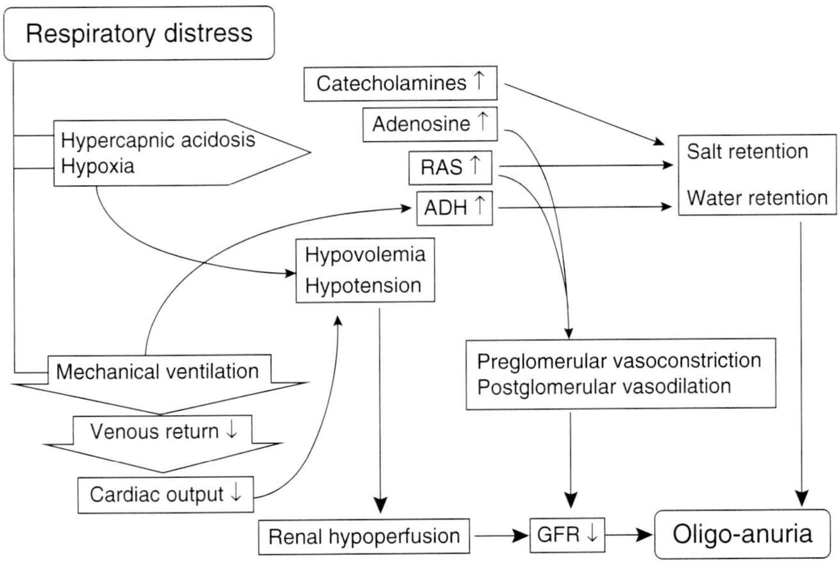

Fig. 3 Pathogenesis of hypoxic renal failure

the tubular differentiation. Maternal ingestion of ACEIs and ARBs produces a classical fetopathy with renal tubular dysgenesis (Mason 1994). Postnatal administration of drugs interfering with the action of angiotensin II can also depress GFR and lead to renal failure. Drugs interfering with angiotensin II must definitively be avoided during pregnancy and used with great caution after birth.

Miscellaneous Drugs and Iatrogenic Intervention

Tolazoline, an alpha-adrenergic blocking agent used in the past as a pulmonary vasodilator, as well as D-tubocurarine or pancuronium can all increase the renal vascular resistance (Toth-Heyn et al. 2000).

Ventilation with continuous positive airway pressure has deleterious effects on renal function due to decreased venous return and low cardiac output, increased renal sympathetic nervous activity, and elevated serum vasopressin levels (Toth-Heyn et al. 2000).

115.3.2 Specific Pathogenesis

The hemodynamic effects of stresses such as preterm birth, respiratory distress, asphyxia, and sepsis lead to decreased systemic arterial pressure, diminished renal blood flow, and a marked increase in the renovascular resistance (Fig. 3). These changes further reduce the already small net effective filtration pressure, leading to a clinically deleterious fall in GFR (Toth-Heyn et al. 2000).

115.3.2.1 Hypoxemic-Hypoxic Insults

Hypoxia is one of the commonest stresses faced by the neonate, and it leads to the activation of various potent intrarenal vasoactive factors such as the catecholamines, angiotensin II, adenosine, and endothelin that play a role in the pathogenesis of ARF. Hypoxic-ischemic insults also activate the intracellular hydrolysis of ATP that generates adenosine. Studies in newborn rabbits have shown that adenosine causes constriction of the afferent arterioles and relaxation of the efferent arterioles leading to a profound drop in GFR. Pretreatment with theophylline, a nonspecific adenosine antagonist, prevents the development of ARF in hypoxic animals and asphyxic neonates (Gouyon and Guignard 1988). Endothelin is a potent vasoconstrictor, but its role in the pathogenesis of vasomotor nephropathy is still inconclusive (Pacifici 2014). The occurrence of renal failure in severely asphyxiated neonates is extremely frequent, in up to two-thirds of the patients (Andreoli 2012; Drukker and

Guignard 2002; Gouyon and Guignard 2000; Guignard and John 1986; Toth-Heyn et al. 2000).

115.3.2.2 Sepsis

ARF in sepsis is part of multiorgan dysfunction and is mediated by both hemodynamic and non-hemodynamic factors. Sepsis-mediated cardiorespiratory depression results in renal hypoperfusion and a decline in GFR that is sustained by various vasoactive substances such as angiotensin II, the catecholamines, adenosine, endothelin, and thromboxane A2 (Thijs and Thijs 1998). Renal failure can occur in septic states in the absence of altered global hemodynamics. Bacterial lipopolysaccharides (LPS) along with pro-inflammatory cytokines, free oxygen radicals, and procoagulant and immunological factors generated by the host both intra- and extrarenally contribute to the development of ARF.

Platelet-activating factor (PAF) produced by LPS-stimulated resident renal cells as well as by polymorphonuclear leucocytes plays an important role in the pathogenesis of ARF producing a fall in renal blood flow and GFR when infused in animals. Intrarenal production of endothelin-1 (ET-1) stimulated by tumor necrosis factor produces a marked fall in renal blood flow and GFR that is ameliorated by administration of ET-1 antibodies or receptor blockers. Endotoxemia also increases the renal expression of inducible nitric oxide synthase mRNA that leads to a fall in blood pressure and decrease in GFR (Camussi et al. 1998; Hunley and Kon 2001). The intermediate host response to the inciting agent thus results in the sequential production of several inflammatory cytokines and chemical mediators that facilitate the progression of the inflammatory cascade resulting in multiorgan dysfunction and renal failure.

115.4 Clinical Events

Clues to the presence of renal dysfunction may manifest in prenatal life as oligohydramnios. As fetal urine is the major contributor to the amniotic fluid volume, the occurrence of oligohydramnios may suggest fetal oliguria and the presence of severely affected kidneys in utero. Bilateral renal agenesis, multicystic dysplastic kidneys, autosomal recessive polycystic kidneys (ARPKD), and obstructive uropathies can all lead to oligohydramnios. Late onset oligohydramnios is a characteristic finding in renal tubular dysgenesis and warrants a thorough evaluation for exposure to drugs such as NSAIDs, ACEIs, and ARBs. The technological and pharmacological interventions used to improve the outcome of sick neonates may themselves contribute to the occurrence of ARF.

Mechanical ventilation reduces the preload by increasing the intrathoracic pressure and results in decreased cardiac output and renal perfusion. Mechanical ventilation per se may generate cytokines and chemical mediators that lead to multiorgan dysfunction (Kruper et al. 2005). Vasoactive infusions used to maintain normotension may lead to excessive splanchnic vasoconstriction, renal ischemia, and ARF. Umbilical artery and vein catheterization can lead to renal artery or renal vein thrombosis. Indwelling urinary catheters favor the occurrence of urinary tract infections, and the use of broad-spectrum antibiotics may result in the development of fungal UTIs and fungal bezoars (Gouyon and Guignard 2000).

115.4.1 Physical Features

The presence of external features such as Potter's facies, preauricular tags, polydactyly, single umbilical artery, or sacral abnormalities may indicate the presence of an underlying developmental renal anomaly. Enlarged kidneys may indicate autosomal polycystic renal disease or obstructive uropathy. Palpable bladder and a poor stream of urine in a male child suggest the presence of posterior urethral valves. Although these congenital uropathies may present as acute renal failure, they are chronic problems that tend to be persistent or progressive in nature (Sanna-Cherchi et al. 2009).

Edema due to fluid overload, hypoproteinemia, or capillary leak may complicate the clinical course. Hypotension due to hypovolemia, sepsis, or cardiac dysfunction may coexist. Hypertension due to renal failure may be encountered during the course of illness as a result of volume overload or a high renin state. Recognition of hypertension requires reference to appropriate charts as the normal range of blood pressure in neonates would vary depending on gestational age, weight, and postnatal age (Flynn 2012).

115.4.2 Oliguric ARF

Thirty percent of normal newborns void soon after birth; 92% will void within the first 24 h and 99% by 48 h. Oliguria is observed in the majority of neonates presenting with ARF. Oliguria can also result from poor fluid intake or be due to inappropriate ADH secretion in sick neonates.

115.4.3 Non-oliguric ARF

One fourth to one third of neonates with ARF may have non-oliguric failure, and the renal failure can only be recognized by the finding of elevated urea and serum creatinine concentrations. Birth asphyxia, aminoglycoside therapy, and methoxyflurane anesthesia are some of the conditions leading to non-oliguric renal failure (Karlowicz and Adelman 1995).

115.5 Laboratory Evaluation

115.5.1 Urinalysis

Urinalysis in vasomotor nephropathy may show normal urine, epithelial cells and coarse granular casts, mild proteinuria, and microscopic hematuria. Gross or microscopic hematuria is usually seen in renal vein thrombosis and sometimes in urinary tract infections. Pus cells or pus cell casts reflect severe UTIs.

115.5.2 Blood Count

Anemia is present in neonates with ARF, in whom it may also reflect bleeding or dilution by fluid retention. Eosinophilia suggests an allergic reaction to drugs.

115.5.3 Plasma Urea

Azotemia refers to the retention of nitrogenous waste products and is detected by the finding of elevated levels of plasma urea and creatinine. Plasma urea is a poor marker of renal function as it is influenced by multiple factors such as protein intake, urine output, gastrointestinal bleeding, and a hypercatabolic state. It may be deceptively low in sick neonates as a result of poor protein intake.

115.5.4 Plasma Creatinine

Creatinine is the most widely used surrogate marker for GFR albeit not a perfect one as it is not only filtered by the glomeruli but also secreted by the renal tubules in term neonates. The serum creatinine in the first few days of life reflects maternal creatinine levels and gradually comes down to normal neonatal levels close to 4 mg/l (35 umol/l) by 1 week of age in term infants. In preterm babies, the creatinine may actually rise further before falling slowly to normal neonatal levels over 2–3 weeks (Fig. 4 and Table 3) (Gallini et al. 2000; Miall et al. 1999). This increase occurs because of back-leak of filtered creatinine through leaky immature tubules (Guignard and Drukker 1999). Failure of plasma creatinine to decrease below the maternal level after the first few days of life or a rise in serum creatinine greater than 25–30 umol/l (3 mg/l) per day is indicative of acute renal failure (Choker and Gouyon 2004).

Creatinine levels may also be artifactually elevated depending on the associated comorbid conditions as well as the methodology employed for its estimation. In the commonly used Jaffe's method that also measures non-creatinine chromogens, creatinine levels may be spuriously high in the presence of hyperbilirubinemia or treatment with cephalosporins. However, the use of newer techniques such as the kinetic or enzymatic assays does not measure these chromogens and give truer values of creatinine. Further improvement in measuring creatinine has recently been achieved by the use of newer techniques such as the high-performance liquid

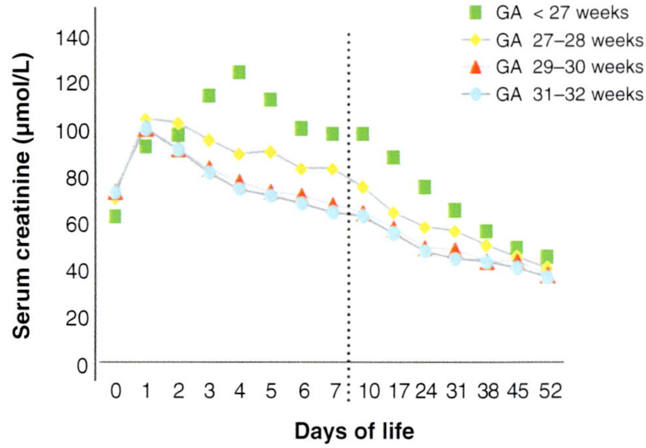

Fig. 4 Plasma creatinine in the first weeks of life of premature neonates

Table 3 Peak increases in plasma creatinine in premature neonates

Group gestation age (wk)	Birth Creatinine (μmol/l)[a]	Peak plasma Creatinine (μmol/l)[a]	Time to peak plasma Creatinine (h)[a]
23–26	67–92	195–247	40–78
27–29	65–89	158–200	28–51
30–32	60–69	120–158	25–40
33–45	67–79	99–140	8–23

[a]Mean ± 95 % confidence intervals (Adapted from Miall 1999)

chromatography and the gas chromatography-isotope dilution mass spectrometry (Guignard 2012a).

115.5.5 Plasma Cystatin C

Cystatin C, a non-glycosylated 13-kDa basic protein produced by all nucleated cells, has been claimed to be a better glomerular marker than creatinine. Cystatin C is freely filtered, almost completely reabsorbed and catabolized by proximal tubular cells. The clinical use of this marker suffers however important drawbacks: (a) the handling of this product by the immature tubular cells, in particular when they are injured, is not known; (b) its production and concentration are influenced by factors independent of GFR, such as rises in serum protein C-reactive levels, thyroid dysfunction, or corticosteroid administration; and (c) its measurement is considerably more expensive than that of creatinine, by a factor of at least 12 (Guignard 2012a).

115.5.6 Urinary Indices

Chemical analysis of urine may help in distinguishing prerenal from intrinsic ARF. Previously healthy kidneys respond to acute hypoperfusion by maximally conserving water and electrolyte, thus excreting concentrated urine with low sodium concentration (U_{Na}). By contrast an intrinsically damaged kidney is not able to concentrate urine and retain sodium. A urinary osmolality (U_{osm}) above 400 mosm per kg H_20, a U_{Na} below 40 mmol/l, and a fractional excretion of sodium (FE_{Na}) below 2% therefore suggest the presence of hypoperfusion of the kidney. The assessment of FE_{Na} is more reliable than the U_{Na} only. It should be noted that these urinary indices are only valid when measured before the administration of volume expanders or diuretics and that they cannot be used in very premature salt-wasting neonates who may "normally" present with FE_{Na} above 5% (Andreoli 2012; Gouyon and Guignard 2000; Guignard and John 1986; Toth-Heyn et al. 2000).

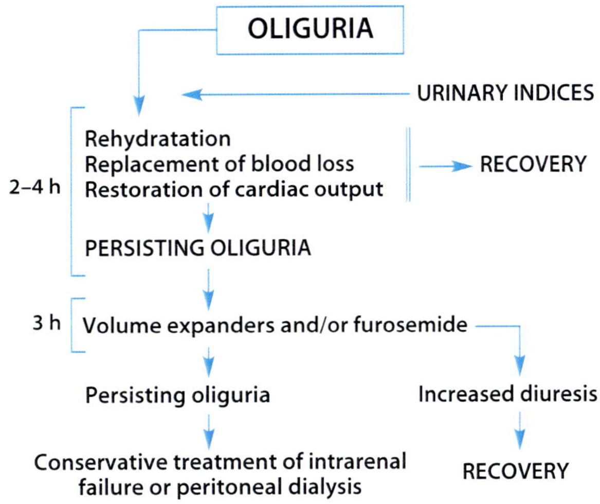

Fig. 5 Management of acute renal failure

115.5.7 Imaging

Imaging of the genitourinary tract by ultrasound is useful for assessing the size, the shape, and the echogenicity of the kidneys, for diagnosing pelvicalyceal dilatation, and for examining the ureters and the bladder. Imaging is almost an extension of the clinical examination and gives highly valuable diagnostic information. Evaluation of the renal vessels by color Doppler gives important information regarding the presence of renal vein or renal arterial thrombosis. Radionuclear scan utilizing various isotopes may help to differentiate the causes of ARF.

115.6 Conservative Management

115.6.1 Management of Suspected Prerenal Oliguric ARF

A schema for the conservative management of acute oliguric ARF is given in Fig. 5. ARF should be proactively detected in the neonatal intensive care unit by regular monitoring of urine output and serial measurements of serum creatinine. As the cause of ARF is generally multifactorial, reassessment of both the primary problem and all the therapeutic interventions needs to be done in order to identify the contributory factors. When feasible nephrotoxic drugs should be substituted by non-nephrotoxic agents. Drug dosages should be adjusted to the presupposed level of GFR (Daschner 2005).

115.6.1.1 Fluid Challenge and Rehydration

In the prerenal types of ARF, restoration of volume by the administration of 20 ml/kg of normal saline over 1–2 h usually improves urine output. Such an administration should not be given when there is clinical evidence of fluid overload or strong suspicion of a cardiac cause for the prerenal failure. In neonates with fluid refractory hypotension, dopamine infusion should be started to improve blood pressure and renal perfusion. Low-dose hydrocortisone may be useful in fluid and dopamine refractory hypotension (Seri 2006).

115.6.1.2 Low-Dose Dopamine

The use of low, non-pressor doses of dopamine in preterm babies with hyaline membrane disease has sometimes been claimed to improve renal blood flow, glomerular filtration rate, natriuresis, and diuresis. The renal vasodilatory and diuretic responses presumably result from stimulation of dopaminergic receptors that occurs with low-dose dopamine. Higher doses lead to alpha-receptor stimulation that causes systemic vasoconstriction as well as an increase in renal vascular resistance. What constitutes a renal vasodilator dose in a given patient is not always clear and has varied from 2.5 ug to 6 ug/kg per min. Variations in the dopaminergic receptor density, increase in half-life of dopamine, decreased adrenoreceptor sensitivity mediated by extreme prematurity, systemic hypoperfusion, and other pathological states may be responsible for the variations in the renal vasodilatory dose. What may be a vasodilator dose in one baby may be a pressor dose in another. Dopamine can have several adverse effects such as tachycardia, cardiac arrhythmia, and increase in pulmonary vascular resistance (Subhedar 2000). The modest benefits that may be obtained in some babies with low-dose dopamine have to be weighed against the possible adverse effects of the drug. Noteworthy is the fact that all neonatal studies in favor of the "renal" doses of dopamine were uncontrolled and that a placebo-controlled randomized study in adult patients failed to demonstrate that low-dose dopamine could protect the stressed kidney (Australian and New Zealand Intensive Care Society Clinical Trials Group 2000).

115.6.1.3 Furosemide

When urine output fails to improve after fluid repletion, a trial of diuretics can be given. Intravenous furosemide at 1–3 mg/kg may improve the diuresis. The natriuretic and diuretic responses to furosemide are highly variable and depend on the level of GFR (Dubourg et al. 2000). When a diuretic response is present, it carries the risk of inducing hyponatremia, with consequent vasoconstriction of the kidney. Torasemide, a loop diuretic with close similarities to furosemide, is sometimes used instead of furosemide. When given to immature rabbits undergoing hypoxemic vasomotor nephropathy, torasemide has been shown to increase sodium excretion and urine output without improving renal perfusion and GFR (Guignard 2012b). Clearly, loop diuretics should basically not be used to treat oliguric neonates but primarily those presenting with edematous states and congestive heart failure.

When given together, dopamine and furosemide have been claimed to have a synergetic effect in increasing urine output. That this would also improve renal function remains questionable.

115.6.1.4 Mannitol

Mannitol is best avoided in the neonate as it can increase intravascular volume and produce fluid overload in the absence of diuresis. Being hyperosmolar it should be specially avoided in premature babies as it may give rise to intracranial hemorrhage. Mannitol itself can cause or exacerbate acute renal failure.

115.6.2 Fluid Management in Neonates with Intrinsic ARF

Oliguric neonates who fail to respond to the above maneuvers (Fig. 5) should be considered to have intrinsic renal failure and would require additional measures to prevent major homeostatic disturbances (Rees 2008). In those neonates responding to the above measures by an increase in urine output, a progressive fall in the serum creatinine is observed. Persistence of elevated creatinine, or increases in creatinine levels in the face of a good urine output, suggests the presence of non-oliguric renal failure.

In a normal neonate with intact renal function, urine output contributes to 50–80% of the total fluids administered and varies with the amount of solute to be excreted. In oliguric neonates, fluid administration should be restricted to insensible water losses plus the ongoing renal and extrarenal losses. The insensible water losses in full-term neonates amount to 35 ml/kg per day whereas in preterms this may vary from 60 to 70 ml/kg per day. The fluid administered should be electrolyte-free and the concentration of glucose adjusted to deliver the adequate amount of glucose. Daily weight is the best parameters to judge adequacy of fluid management. In oligo-anuric neonates, a daily weight loss of 0.5% is expected and reflects appropriate fluid balance.

115.6.3 Electrolyte Disorders

115.6.3.1 Hyponatremia

Hyponatremia when present is usually dilutional in nature and should not be treated by giving sodium chloride. Free-water administration should be restricted instead to produce a gradual increase in the serum sodium concentration. However, when serum sodium level is less than 120 mmol/l, it can give rise to cerebral edema that may manifest as lethargy, seizures, and apnea. In such situations, 3% NaCl may be given iv at a slow rate of 5–6 ml/kg over 2–4 h. The amount of sodium required to correct the hyponatremia can also be estimated by the formula Na (mmol) = (desired Na-actual Na (mmol/l)) × 0.8 × BW (kg), where BW represents body weight and 0.8 × BW represents total body water.

115.6.3.2 Hyperkalemia

Elevated potassium levels are fairly common in ARF. Care should be taken to confirm that potassium has been eliminated from the iv infusions and that medications containing potassium are not administered. Mild hyperkalemia of 6–6.5 mmol/l without ECG changes may require nothing more than the correction of coexisting metabolic acidosis. Higher levels of potassium or the presence of electrocardiographic (ECG) changes requires active cardioprotective measures that include intravenous calcium administration (0.5–1.0 ml/kg of 10% calcium gluconate, over 5 min under ECG surveillance), inhaled or parenteral salbutamol (4 mg/kg over 20 min), and glucose-insulin infusions. When the neonate is still passing urine, diuretics such as furosemide (1 mg/kg) can be tried. The use of potassium-binding resins is not without risk in infants. It may cause gastric erosions when given orally and colonic ulcerations and impaction when given rectally (Ohlsson and Hosking 1987). They are best avoided in a sick neonate (Warady and Bunchman 2000). Severe hyperkalemia (>7.5 mmol/l) and/or major ECG changes represent an indication for dialysis.

115.6.3.3 Hypocalcemia

Hypocalcemia is common but the ionic fraction may not be very low because of concomitant hypoalbuminemia and metabolic acidosis. When the hypocalcemia is symptomatic, intravenous calcium gluconate (10% calcium gluconate at a dose of 0.5–1.0 ml/kg in 5 min under cardiac monitoring) needs to be given and repeated every 6–8 h. Caution is required in the administration of iv calcium in the presence of hyperphosphatemia, as it may lead to soft tissue calcification and nephrocalcinosis.

115.6.3.4 Hyperphosphatemia

Hyperphosphatemia is common in neonates with renal failure. Calcium-containing phosphate binders such as calcium carbonate may be used although severe hyperphosphatemia is best treated with dialysis. Aluminum-containing phosphate binders are best avoided.

115.6.3.5 Acidosis

Mild metabolic acidosis is common in renal failure. When the plasma bicarbonate concentration falls below 12 mmol/l and/or the plasma pH below 7.20, correction of the acidosis is best achieved by adding sodium bicarbonate to the maintenance fluid.

115.6.4 Convulsions

Convulsions are the consequence of electrolyte imbalance or arterial hypertension. Symptomatic therapy is achieved by giving diazepam (0.5 mg/kg iv or rectally), iv clonazepam (0.1 mg/kg), or iv phenobarbital (15–20 mg/kg).

115.6.5 Hypertension

Hypertension may occur as a result of volume overload as well as hyperreninemia. Severe or symptomatic hypertension is best treated with continuous iv infusion of nicardipine. Esmolol, enalaprilat, or sodium nitroprusside can be used with caution (Table 4) (Gouyon and Guignard 2000; Guignard and John 1986; Flynn 2012). The optimal oral therapy of hypertension in newborn infants is not clearly known. ACE inhibitors notably captopril has been used in neonatal hypertension. However, its use in the context of neonatal renal failure is risky. If necessary, it should be used cautiously in small doses. Calcium channel blockers can be used as first-line drugs. Beta-blockers should be used with caution and are best avoided in babies with coexisting respiratory problems. In these babies diuretics may form a good adjunct.

Table 4 Hypotensive agents in the neonate

Agent	Starting dosage	Intervals	Maximum recommended	Route of administration
Furosemide	1 mg/kg	q 4–6 h	5 mg/kg/day	O/IV
Hydrochlorothiazide	1 mg/kg	q 8 h	3 mg/kg/day	O
Propranolol	0.25 mg/kg/dose	q 6–8 h	5 mg/kg/day	O/IV
Atenolol	0.5 mg/kg/dose	q 12–24 h	4 mg/kg/day	O
Labetalol	0.5 mg/kg/dose	q 1–4 h	2 mg/kg/day	IV
Sodium nitroprusside	0.5 μg/kg/min	–	6 μg/kg/min	IV
Captopril	0.1 mg/kg/dose	q 8–12 h	0.5 mg/kg/day	O
Enalapril	5 μg/kg/dose	q 8–24 h	20 μg/kg/day	IV
Nifedipine	0.5 mg/kg/dose	q 4–6 h	2 mg/kg/day	O

115.6.6 Sepsis

Severe infection is a common cause of death in neonates with ARF. Adequate intravenous antibiotherapy is essential. The dosage of drugs excreted mainly by the kidney (aminoglycosides, vancomycin) must be adapted to the severity of renal failure. When possible, monitoring of plasma concentrations is recommended (Table 5).

Table 5 Drugs requiring dose adjustment when GFR is compromised

Antibiotics
Aminoglycoides (amikacin, gentamicin, totramycin)
Amoxycillin, amoxycillin-clavulanic acid
Cephalosporin (cefixime, cefotaxime, ceftazidime)
Cotrimoxazole
Ticarcillin
Vancomycin
Antifungial agents
Cardiac drugs
Digoxin

115.6.7 Nutrition

Unless aggressively managed, neonatal renal failure invariably results in nutritional deficiency. Nutritional inadequacy is an important contributor to neonatal mortality. Enteral nutrition when feasible should consist of appropriate formulae that are calorically dense with a low electrolyte content. Neonates require 120 cal/kg per day. Protein restriction should be avoided in these neonates. When enteral nutrition is not feasible, parenteral nutrition may have to be resorted to. High concentrations of glucose need to be given to provide the required nonprotein calories in the limited permissible volume necessitating central venous access.

115.7 Acute Renal Replacement Therapy (RRT)

RRT is indicated when the renal failure produces serious derangements such as fluid overload, severe hyperkalemia, uncontrolled metabolic acidosis, hyperphosphatemia, or hyponatremia unresponsive to fluid restriction (Andreoli 2012; Gouyon and Guignard 2000; Guignard and John 1986; Toth-Heyn et al. 2000). Even in the absence of these indications, RRT may be required to create enough fluid space by ultrafiltration to enable administration of the necessary medications, blood products, and nutrition that the infant may need.

115.7.1 Peritoneal Dialysis

Peritoneal dialysis is the most common and widely used option for RRT in this age group (Andreoli 2012). It is easily instituted even in the very low birth weight infant with either percutaneous bedside placement of a stiff catheter or surgical placement of a soft Tenckhoff catheter. Acutely ill babies on ventilator may not tolerate large intraperitoneal volumes. Small volumes with short dwelling times may suffice to tackle the acute life-threatening problems. Bicarbonate dialysis is needed in children with liver dysfunction or advanced sepsis as the use of lactate-based dialysis fluid may lead to worsening of acidosis in these babies. The presence of intra-abdominal pathology may preclude the use of the peritoneum for dialysis.

115.7.2 Hemodialysis

Hemodialysis is infrequently used in this age group and can be considered only in hemodynamically stable babies. In neonates it requires the availability of suitably small dialyzers and tubings. Blood or albumin priming of the lines and filter is usually needed. It can be only done in units where sufficient technical expertise is available.

115.7.3 Continuous Venovenous Hemofiltration

Continuous venovenous hemofiltration is a modality that can be used in sick neonates requiring renal replacement. It allows greater fluid removal, better hemodynamic stability, and better nutrition. Its use in critically ill children with renal failure is increasing steadily, and 30% of centers surveyed in North America considered it as the preferential mode of treatment irrespective of age (Warady and Bunchman 2000).

115.8 Outcome

Despite major advances in both neonatology and nephrology, the mortality in neonates with ARF is fairly high and ranges from 45% to 60% (Warady and Bunchman 2000). Neonates with prerenal failure have a much better outcome than those with intrinsic renal failure. The worst outcome is seen in babies with intrinsic renal failure in the context of multiple organ dysfunction. As the development of renal failure is a reflection of the severity of illness, it is not surprising that the mortality is so high. Babies with non-oliguric renal failure have a much better outcome than those with oligo-anuric renal failure (Otukesh et al. 2006).

Following recovery from the acute renal failure, residual renal dysfunction may be seen in more than half the babies without an underlying congenital uropathy (Sanna-Cherchi et al. 2009). Incomplete recovery is invariable in those neonates who have suffered cortical necrosis. Although numerically not a large group, babies with in utero exposure to NSAIDs, ACEIs, or ARB have a poor renal outcome and are likely to have persistent irreversible renal failure. Long-term follow-up of ELBW infants with neonatal renal failure has shown that nearly 45% of the children show a decrease in GFR over time. Urine proteins/creatinine ratio >70 g/mol creat (0.6 mg/mg creat) and serum creatinine >55 umol/l (6 mg/l) at 1 year of age were predictors of a poor prognosis for long-term renal function (Abitbol et al. 2003).

115.9 Present and Future Challenge

The challenges that lie before us are the following: (a) to find markers that could detect renal injury much before it develops into renal failure, (b) to find pharmacological measures that could prevent the development of renal failure in babies faced with stressful renal situations, and (c) to identify measures that would ameliorate renal failure and hasten renal recovery.

115.9.1 Early Diagnosis

Creatinine is an insensitive biomarker for GFR, especially in the neonatal period and is blind to an early fall in GFR. More sensitive biomarkers are required that will facilitate early identification of renal injury. The hope that cystatin C could play such a role appears illusory (Guignard 2012a).

The appearance of markers of renal tubular injury in the urine may precede the changes in GFR and may aid in the diagnosis of acute kidney injury even before failure sets in. Screening for tubular injury in high-risk neonates rather than for a fall in GFR could become valuable if/when reliable tubular markers are discovered.

115.9.2 Prevention and Amelioration of Renal Failure

115.9.2.1 Animal Studies

Several pharmacological measures have shown varying degrees of success in preventing or ameliorating renal failure in experimental animals. Agents that favorably modulate renal hemodynamics as well as agents that counteract the mechanisms mediating cellular injury have been studied.

Protection of the renal hemodynamics has been attempted by the use of selective antagonists to endogenously produced vasoconstrictors or by the use of renal vasodilators. Selective antagonists that have been used with success include theophylline in hypoxia-induced renal failure and endothelin antagonists in sepsis. Atrial natriuretic peptide, a potent renal vasodilator, has also shown some promising results. Hypoxic-ischemic insults to the kidney lead to renal tubular injury by cellular depletion of ATP as well as intracellular accumulations of calcium. Measures to restore cellular ATP by administration of ATP-MgCl2 appear to ameliorate the hypoxemia-induced ARF in animals. Thyroxine also hastens cellular repair and renal recovery by restoration of cellular ATP and may prevent reoxygenation injury (Guignard and John 1986; Toth-Heyn et al. 2000) Pretreatment with calcium channel blockers prevents the intracellular accumulation of calcium and the intense vasoconstriction that occurs with various renal insults such as ischemia and cyclosporine administration.

115.9.2.2 Human Studies

Many of the vasoactive agents have pronounced systemic effects or could potentially affect extrarenal organs and systems that preclude their routine clinical use until validated by human studies. Low-dose theophylline has shown promising results when used to prevent renal failure in neonates undergoing perinatal asphyxia or respiratory distress syndrome (Al-Wassia et al. 2013; Bhat et al. 2006; Cattarelli et al. 2006; Guignard and John 1986; Guignard 2012a; Jenik et al. 2000). In two small studies, thyroxine has been used in neonates with hypoxemic renal failure with recovery of renal function. The possibility of using pharmacological measures to prevent renal failure needs to be systematically studied in humans before it can translate into standard clinical practice.

The most important measures to prevent acute neonatal renal failure is to pay attention to general measures that include adequate hydration and maintenance of electrolyte and acid-base balance and to limit the use of nephrotoxic drugs including NSAIDs in the hemodynamically vulnerable perinatal period.

115.10 Chronic Renal Failure

115.10.1 Causes of Chronic Renal Failure in Newborn Infants

In certain circumstances, infants presenting with ARF do not recover completely and enter a state of chronic renal failure (CRF). Other babies present from the start with a state of chronic renal failure. The main neonatal causes leading to CRF are listed in Table 6. Prolonged ischemia can lead to irreversible tubular necrosis and cortical necrosis. Congenital abnormalities of the kidneys and urinary tract are the most common

Table 6 Causes of chronic renal failure in the first year of life[a]

Cause	No of patients
Renal dysplasia	18 (37 %)
Obstructive uropathy	16 (33 %)
Polycystic kidney disease	5 (10 %)
Congenital nephrotic syndrome	5 (10 %)
VACTERL association	3 (6 %)
Denys-Drash syndrome	1 (2 %)
Unknown origin	1 (2 %)
Antifungal agents (Fluconazole)	–
Cardiac drugs (Digoxin)	–

[a]Data from 49 infants (Reproduced from Wedekin et al. (2008) with permission)

causes of CRF and include renal hypoplasia and cystic dysplasia, polycystic disease of the kidney, severe obstructive uropathy or reflux nephropathy, and posterior urethral valves (Chevalier 2012; Sanna-Cherchi et al. 2009). Vascular disorders such as renal vein or artery thrombosis, prolonged ischemia with subsequent irreversible tubular or cortical necrosis, disseminated intravascular coagulation, and hemolytic disease with massive myoglobinuria represent acquired causes of CRF. Congenital forms (finnish type) of nephrotic syndrome can also induce early onset CRF.

115.10.2 Presentation

115.10.2.1 Malformative Uropathies

Antenatal ultrasound may reveal anomalies of the kidney, bladder, and urinary tract that can permanently compromise postnatal renal function. Obstruction to urine flow by posterior urethral valves results in bilateral hydronephrosis and hydroureter, distended thick-walled bladder, dilated urethra, and renal dysplasia (Kousidis et al. 2008). The associated oligo-anuria and oligohydramnios may be the cause of marked pulmonary hypoplasia. Optimal management of posterior urethral valves requires a multidisciplinary approach by obstetricians, neonatologists, pediatric nephrologists, and urologists.

After birth, the presence of a palpable abdominal mass or bladder may be the first clue to underlying CRF. Ultrasound examination usually leads to the diagnosis. The occurrence of urinary tract infection is often the first clinical manifestation of congenital uropathies (Chevalier 2012).

115.10.2.2 Failure to Thrive and Anemia

Failure to thrive usually associated with poor and difficult feeding is almost always present in infants with chronic renal failure (Cano et al. 2007). Normochromic-normocytic anemia, secondary to the uremic state, is a manifestation of a decrease in erythropoietin formation by the sick kidneys.

115.10.2.3 Hypertension and Congestive Heart Failure

Arterial hypertension may have a renovascular origin or be secondary to salt and water overload with or without congestive heart failure. Loop diuretics are indicated.

115.10.2.4 Nephrotic Syndrome

The presence of edema, heavy proteinuria, and hypoalbuminemia at birth indicates the presence of a nephrotic syndrome, usually of the finnish type. The prognosis is extremely poor, the infants dying from sepsis or developing chronic renal failure in the first weeks of life.

115.10.3 Management of Chronic Renal Failure

115.10.3.1 Nutrition

Adequate nutritional therapy is essential to preserve the growth of the infant (Hanna et al. 1996). An energy intake of 115 kcal/kg is necessary to sustain growth during the first 3 months of life, with appropriate calcium, phosphorus, and sodium intakes. Many anorexic infants require calorie supplements (glucose polymers or fat emulsions) that often can only be administered by nasogastric or gastrostomy tubings. The help of a skilled pediatric dietitian is mandatory to provide optimal nutrition in infants with CRF. When nutritional intervention fails to improve growth, treatment with growth hormone must be considered (Haffner and Fischer 2009).

115.10.3.2 Fluid, Electrolyte, and Acid-Base Balance

Most infants with CRF present with metabolic acidosis, hypocalcemia, and hyperphosphatemia. These factors all inhibit growth. The acidosis must thus be compensated by the administration of sodium bicarbonate (2–3 mmol/kg per day), with the risk of inducing arterial hypertension, and the hypocalcemia and the hyperphosphatemia by the administration of calcium carbonate (starting dose: 100 mg/kg per day). The levels of parathormone (PTH) may be increased in response to both the hypocalcemia and the hyperphosphatemia, the administration of calcium not being sufficient to prevent the occurrence of hyperparathyroidism and renal osteodystrophy. In this case, the administration of calcitriol (1,25-dihydroxycholecalciferol), orally or intraperitoneally, may be necessary (Cano et al. 2007).

115.10.3.3 Anemia

The anemia associated with CRF is due to inadequate production of erythropoietin by the kidney. Recombinant alpha or beta erythropoietin, or continuous erythropoietin receptor activator, given weekly or twice monthly by sc or iv injection, will correct the anemia.

115.10.3.4 Arterial Hypertension

When hypervolemia contributes to the hypertension, loop diuretics (furosemide, torasemide) or metolazone can be administered. ACE inhibitors or ARBs are particularly effective in renin-dependent hypertension. But drugs interfering with angiotensin II can induce a sharp decrease in GFR in volume-depleted patients because of an acute decrease in intraglomerular pressure. Calcium channel blockers are usually well tolerated. The use of beta-blockers is limited because of the risk of symptomatic bradycardia (Flynn 2012).

115.10.4 Renal Replacement Therapy

115.10.4.1 Dialysis

Failure to normalize growth or to control the electrolyte disturbances is an indication to start dialysis. In neonates and infants, peritoneal dialysis is the method of choice (Hijazi et al. 2009). It is easy to perform and has been shown to be effective. It can be used until the child can undergo renal transplantation. Peritoneal dialysis can be performed manually with four to five dialysis fluid exchanges a day. When available it is best performed using an automated cycling machine that can deliver eight to ten exchanges over 8–10 h.

Although providing effective renal replacement therapy (Rheault et al. 2009), peritoneal dialysis in infants carries a significant risk of infection and death, with repeated episodes of peritonitis. For parents, the burden of long-term peritoneal treatment in infants is substantial (Guignard 2012b; Wedekin et al. 2008).

115.10.4.2 Renal Transplantation

No neonate with CRF should be started on RRT unless there is a hope for later kidney transplantation. Full immunization should be completed before considering transplantation, usually only after a body weight of 8–10 kg and an age of 2–3 years are attained.

115.11 Conclusion

The morbidity rate of ARF in newborn infants is elevated. In those developing CRF, RRT is possible with relative success. Decisions concerning RRT must be discussed with the family and an expert ethical committee, keeping in mind the long-term outcome of severe CRF in very young children. In developed countries, this outcome is globally as follows: one third of the infants die, half have a functioning renal graft, and the rest will have returned to dialysis in the first years of life (Rees 2008).

References

Abitbol CL, Bauer CR, Montane B, Chandar J (2003) Long term followup of ELBW infants with neonatal renal failure. Pediatr Nephrol 18:887–895

Ali U, Khubchandani S, Andankar P, Parekhji S et al (2006) Renal tubular dysgenesis associated with in utero exposure to nimuselide. Pediatr Nephrol 26:274–276

Allegaert K, Vanbole C, DeHoon J, Guignard JP et al (2005) Non-selective cyclooxygenase inhibitors and glomerular filtration rate in preterm neonates. Pediatr Nephrol 20:1557–1561

Al-Wassia H, Alshaikh B, Sauve R (2013) Prophylactic theophylline for the prevention of severe renal dysfunction in term and post-term neonates with perinatal asphyxia: a systematic review and meta analysis of randomized controlled trials. J Perinatol 33:271–277

Andreoli SP (2012) Kidney injury in the neonate. In: Oh W, Guignard JP, Baumgart S (eds) Nephrology and fluid/electrolyte physiology: neonatology questions and controversies. Saunders Elsevier, Philadelphia, pp 285–303

Australian and New Zealand Intensive Care Society Clinical Trials Group (2000) Low dose dopamine in patients with early renal dysfunction: a placebo controlled trial. Lancet 356:2139–2143

Bhat MA, Shah ZA, Makhdoomi MS, Mufti MH (2006) Theophylline for renal function in term neonates with perinatal asphyxia: a randomized placebo controlled trial. J Pediatr 149:180–184

Camussi G, Ronco C, Montrucchio G, Picolli G (1998) Role of soluble mediators in sepsis and renal failure. Kidney Int 3:S38–S42

Cano FJ, Azocar MA, Guerrero JL, Delucchi MA et al (2007) Intraperitoneal calcitriol in infants on peritoneal dialysis. Perit Dial Int 27:651–653

Cattarelli D, Spandrio M, Gasparoni A, Bottini R, Offer C, Chirico G et al (2006) A randomized double blind placebo trial of the effect of theophylline in prevention of vasomotor nephropathy in very preterm neonates with respiratory distress syndrome. Arch Dis Child Fetal Neonatal Ed 91(F):80–84

Chevalier RL (2012) Obstructive uropathy: assessment of renal function in the fetus. In: Oh W, Guignard JP, Baumgart S (eds) Nephrology and fluid/electrolyte physiology: neonatology questions and controversies. Saunders Elsevier, Philadelphia, pp 335–359

Choker G, Gouyon JB (2004) Diagnosis of acute renal failure in very preterm infants. Biol Neonate 86:212–216

Daschner M (2005) Drug dosage in children with reduced renal function. Pediatr Nephrol 20:1675–1686

Drukker A, Guignard JP (2002) Renal aspects of the term and preterm infant: a selective update. Curr Opin Pediatr 14:175–182

Dubourg L, Drukker A, Guignard JP (2000) Failure of the loop diuretic torasemide to improve renal function of hypoxemic vasomotor nephropathy in the newborn rabbit. Pediatr Res 47:504–508

Flynn JT (2012) Neonatal hypertension: diagnosis and management. In: Oh W, Guignard JP, Baumgart S (eds) Nephrology and fluid/electrolyte physiology: neonatology questions and controversies. Saunders Elsevier, Philadelphia, pp 251–265

Gallini F, Maggio L, Romagnoli C, Marroco G et al (2000) Progression of renal function in preterm neonates with gestational aged <32 weeks. Pediatr Nephrol 15:119–124

Gouyon JB, Guignard JP (1988) Theophylline prevents the hypoxemia induced renal hemodynamic changes in rabbits. Kidney Int 33:1078–1083

Gouyon JB, Guignard JP (2000) Management of acute renal failure in the newborn. Pediatr Nephrol 14:1037–1044

Guignard JP (2012a) Glomerular filtration rate in neonates. In: Oh W, Guignard JP, Baumgart S (eds) Nephrology and fluid/electrolyte physiology: neonatology questions and controversies. Saunders Elsevier, Philadelphia, pp 117–135

Guignard JP (2012b) Use of diuretics in the newborn. In: Oh W, Guignard JP, Baumgart S (eds) Nephrology and fluid/electrolyte physiology: neonatology questions and controversies. Saunders Elsevier, Philadelphia, pp 233–250

Guignard JP, Drukker A (1999) Why do newborns have elevated plasma creatinine levels? Pediatrics 103 (4/e):49

Guignard JP, Gouyon JB (1988) Adverse effects of drugs on the immature kidney. Biol Neonate 53:243–252

Guignard JP, John G (1986) Renal function in tiny premature infant. Clin Perinatol 13:377–401

Haffner D, Fischer DC (2009) Growth hormone treatment of infants with chronic kidney disease: requirement, efficacy, and safety. Pediatr Nephrol 24:1097–1100

Hanna JD, Krieg RJ Jr, Scheinman JI, Chan JC (1996) Effects of uremia on growth in children. Semin Nephrol 16:230–241

Hijazi R, Abitbol CL, Chandar J, Seeherunvong W et al (2009) Twenty-five years of infant dialysis: a single center experience. J Pediatr 155:111–117

Hunley TE, Kon V (2001) Updates on endothelins-biology and clinical implications. Pediatr Nephrol 16:752–762

Jenik AG, Cernadas JMC, Gorenstein A, Ramirez JA et al (2000) A randomized, double blind, placebo controlled trial of the effects of prophylactic theophylline on renal function in term neonates with perinatal asphyxia. Pediatrics 105(4):e-45

Karlowicz MG, Adelman RD (1995) Non-oliguric and oliguric acute renal failure in asphyxiated newborns. Pediatr Nephrol 9:718–722

Kousidis G, Thomas DF, Morgan H, Haider N et al (2008) The long-term outcome of prenatally detected posterior urethral valves: a 10 to 23-year follow-up study. BJU Int 102:1020–1024

Kruper JN, Groenweld AB, Slutsky AS, Plotz FB (2005) Mechanical ventilation and acute renal failure. Crit Care Med 33:1408–1415

Mason B (1994) Teratogen update. Angiotensin converting enzyme inhibitors. Teratology 50:399–409

Miall LS, Henderson MJ, Turner AJ, Brownlee KJ et al (1999) Plasma creatinine rises dramatically in the first 48 hours of life in preterm infants. Pediatrics 104: e76

Ohlsson A, Hosking M (1987) Complications following oral administration of exchange resins in extremely low birth weight infants. Eur J Pediatr 146:571–574

Ong WH, Guignard JP, Sharma A, Aranda JV (1998) Pharmacological approach to the management of neonatal hypertension. Semin Neonatol 3:149–163

Otukesh H, Hoseini R, Hooman N, Chalian M et al (2006) Prognosis of acute renal failure in children. Pediatr Nephrol 21:1873–1878

Pacifici GM (2014) Differential renal adverse effects of ibuprofen and indomethacin in preterm infants: a review. Clin Pharmacol Adv Appl 6:111–116

Rees L (2008) Management of the neonate with chronic renal failure. Semin Fetal Neonatal Med 13:181–188

Rheault MN, Rajpal J, Chavers B, Nevins TE (2009) Outcomes of infants <28 days old treated with peritoneal dialysis for end-stage renal disease. Pediatr Nephrol 24:2035–2039

Rodriguez MM, Gomez A, Abitbol C, Chandar J (2004) Comparative renal histomorphometry: a case study of oligonephropathy of prematurity. Pediatr Nephrol 20:945–949

Sanna-Cherchi S, Ravani P, Corbani V, Parodi S et al (2009) Renal outcome in patients with congenital anomalies of the kidney and urinary tract. Kidney Int 76:528–533

Seri I (2006) Hydrocortisone is effective in treatment of vasopressin-resistant hypotension in very low birth weight neonates. J Pediatr 149:422–423

Subhedar NV, Shaw NJ (2000) Dopamine versus dobutamide for hypotensive preterm infants. Cochrane Database Syst Rev. (2):CD001242

Thijs A, Thijs LG (1998) Pathogenesis of renal failure in sepsis. Kidney Int 53(Suppl 66):534–537

Toth-Heyn P, Drukker A, Guignard JP (2000) The stressed neonatal kidney: from pathophysiology to clinical management of neonatal vasomotor nephropathy. Pediatr Nephrol 14:227–239

Vieux R, Hascoet JM, Mendariu D, Guillemin F (2010) Glomerular filtration rate reference values in very preterm infants. Pediatrics 125(5):e1186–e1192

Warady BA, Bunchman T (2000) Dialysis therapy for children with acute renal failure: survey results. Pediatr Nephrol 15:11–13

Wedekin M, Ehrich JH, Offner G, Pape L (2008) Aetiology and outcome of acute and chronic renal failure in infants. Nephrol Dial Transplant 23: 1575–1580

Diagnosis and Treatment of Renal and Urinary Tract Malformations in Newborns

116

Vassilios Fanos, Marco Zaffanello, and Michele Mussap

Contents

V. Fanos (✉)
Department of Surgery, Neonatal Intensive Care Unit, Neonatal Pathology and Neonatal Section, AOU and University of Cagliari, Cagliari, Italy
e-mail: vafanos@tin.it

M. Zaffanello
Department of Surgical Sciences, Dentistry, Gynecology and Pediatrics, University of Verona, Verona, Italy

Department of Life and Reproduction Sciences Pediatric Section, University of Verona, Verona, Italy

Department of Surgery, University of Cagliari, Cagliari, Italy

M. Mussap
Laboratory Medicine, Ospedale Policlinico San Martino, Genoa, Italy

G. Buonocore et al. (eds.), *Neonatology*,
https://doi.org/10.1007/978-3-319-29489-6_263

Abstract

Renal and urinary tract malformations in newborns are mostly congenital anomalies with genetic causes and can be classified according to location. Renal agenesis can be detected by ultrasound, and it can be isolated or part of a syndrome. Abnormal migration and positioning of the kidney during embryogenesis can result in malrotation or malpositioning. Polycystic kidney disease (PKD) is a genetic disorder presenting different pattern of inheritance: autosomal recessive polycystic kidney disease (ARPKD), autosomal dominant polycystic kidney disease (ADPKD), and nephronophthisis/ medullary cystic kidney disease. ARPKD is associated with congenital hepatic fibrosis leading to the development of portal hypertension. Obstructive uropathy is also common in the newborn and can be divided as high and low tract obstruction, among which pelvic-ureteric junction obstruction and posterior urethral valves (PUVs) are respectively the most common causes. Obstructive hydrouretero-nephrosis may include primary or congenital vesicoureteric junction obstruction (VUJO) and a secondary form of VUJO (i.e., ureterocele, retroperitoneal fibrosis, calculus). Vescico-ureteric reflux (VUR) is the retrograde flow of urine into the upper urinary tract, often primary or associated with dysplastic kidneys. Moreover, VUR can be a result of ureteral duplications, ectopia, and ureterocele. Hypospadias is one of the most frequent genital malformations and results from abnormal penile and urethral development. Ultrasound (US) screening for fetal anomalies is the major imaging tool. For postnatal causes, imaging investigations include US, computerized-tomography, and magnetic resonance imaging. The usual recommendation is that renography should be delayed until the age of 4 weeks, because of the immaturity of nephrons in newborns.

116.1 Salient Points

- Anomalies that affect the renal system may be classified according to the renal and urinary tract region involved.
- In the kidney, these anomalies include hypoplasia, dysplasia, or a complete lack of kidney formation (agenesis) and ectopies.
- The proximal ureter can be obstructed or grossly dilated (mega ureter). Distally the ureter can be blocked at its insertion into the bladder (vesicoureteric junction obstruction). Alternatively, the ureter may be incompetent or be inserted outside the bladder.
- Prenatal diagnosis can identify either specific pathologies (i.e., multicystic dysplastic kidney (MDK), renal agenesis) or nonspecific pathologies (hydronephrosis, ureteral dilatation, bladder enlargement, and oligohydramnios). US screening for fetal anomalies is the major imaging modality.
- Compared with the normal population, children with any degree of antenatal hydronephrosis are at greater risk of postnatal pathology. A favorable prognosis is related to monolateral pathology, late obstruction, and renal pelvis dilation.

116.2 Introduction

Renal and urinary tract malformations in newborns are mostly congenital anomalies with genetic bases. The routine of antenatal ultrasound (US) scans has resulted in the early detection of these conditions and in selected cases has led to the development of prenatal management strategies including fetal intervention and/or the organization of the diagnostic procedures, postnatal surgical intervention, and/or clinical follow-up. In minor cases, where diagnosis is not allowed during prenatal life, it may be obtained after a postnatal routine follow-up or subsequently a clinical complication, generally urinary tract infection (UTI).

116.3 Etiology and Pathogenesis

The development of the kidney results from the interaction between the ureteric bud and the metanephrogenic mesoderm in the intermediate mesodermal layer. At the fifth week of embryonic development, the ureteric bud grows and comes in close contact with mesodermal elements. The ureteric bud undergoes a series of divisions, which give rise to the pelvicalyceal system. At the same time, mesoderm differentiates to form the nephrons, a process that is completed by 36 weeks of gestation. During intrauterine life, the placenta provides the main source of fluid and electrolyte regulation. Therefore, urine secreted by the fetal kidney provides the main volume of the amniotic fluid (Joseph 2006).

Several genes may have roles in multiple stages of kidney and lower urinary tract morphogenesis. Specific mutations of genes involved in renal tract development have been found in individuals with familial occurrence. Several recessive mutations in the genes FRAS1, FREM2, GRIP1, FREM1, ITGA8, and GREM1 may be involved, all of which function in the interaction of the ureteric bud and the metanephric mesenchyme (Kohl et al. 2014). Pax2 and Pax8 have emerged as crucial players at multiple steps of kidney and urinary tract development (Sharma et al. 2015).

116.3.1 Genetic Factors

A spectrum of renal tract malformations is part of the genetically defined syndromes with Mendelian distribution of inheritance that could be classified as syndromic and nonsyndromic urinary tract malformations.

116.3.1.1 Syndromic Renal and Urinary Tract Malformations

Edith Potter subdivided cystic dysplastic kidney (CDKs) into those with little normal tissue, which she considered to arise from a primary defect in interaction and induction between the ureteric bud and metanephric mesenchyme versus others, in which nephrogenesis had begun, but then become

Table 1 Syndromes associated with renal and urinary tract malformations

Autosomal dominant syndromes
1. Branchio-oto-renal (Kochhar et al. 2007)
2. Hypoparathyroidism, sensorineural deafness, and renal dysplasia (Muroya et al. 2001)
3. Mayer-Rokitansky-Küster-Hauser (Biason-Lauber et al. 2004)
4. Renal coloboma (Salomon et al. 2001)
5. Renal cysts and diabetes (Edghill et al. 2006)
6. Townes-Brocks (Reardon et al. 2007)
Autosomal recessive syndromes
1. Bardet-Biedl (Tobin and Beales 2007; Sharifian et al. 2007)
2. Fraser (McGregor et al. 2003; Jadeja et al. 2005)
3. Jeune (Beales et al. 2007)
4. Meckel-Gruber (Consugar et al. 2007)
5. Prune belly syndrome (Ramasamy et al. 2005)
X-linked syndromes
1. Kallmann (Duke et al. 1998)
2. Simpson-Golabi-Behmel (Grisaru and Rosenblum 2001)

interrupted. Many corresponding genes are known to be expressed in development of the human renal tract, with some of these genes recently found to be mutated in individuals with either isolated (nonsyndromic) kidney malformations or renal tract malformations associated (syndromic) with defects in other organ systems (Woolf 2008). Thus, multiorgan syndromes associating with a renal tract malformation may be autosomal dominant, autosomal recessive, or X-linked (Kerecuk et al. 2008). Each syndrome may associate a large spectrum of renal tract malformations with the involvement of different organs (Table 1).

116.3.1.2 Nonsyndromic Renal and Urinary Tract Malformations

Common renal malformations encountered in the fetal period are hydronephrosis associated with primary vesicoureteral reflux (VUR) and duplex kidneys. These malformations may have genetic bases because they sometimes affect more than one family member, perhaps with two or more abnormal genes necessary in any one person to produce the anatomical change (Lu et al. 2007). Analysis of data from humans and mice suggests that some of the renal damage associated with VUR is congenital and is due to a kidney malformation, not to secondary VUR/UTI related damage (Murawski and Gupta 2006). Human nonsyndromic renal tract malformations may be of both sporadic pattern and inherited fashion, dominant and recessive inheritance.

Half a decade ago the key anatomical differences between cystic dysplastic kidney (CDK) malformations and congenital polycystic kidney disease (PKD) were defined for the first time, with the identification of genes inherited with dominant (ADPKD) or recessive (ARPKD) fashion. However, dominant inheritance has been described for primary vesicoureteral reflux (VUR) (Feather et al. 2000), dysplastic or hypoplastic kidneys (Sanna-Cherchi et al. 2007), and pyeloureteral junction obstruction (PUJO) (Sanna-Cherchi et al. 2007). Primary VUR and nephropathy have been described in few patients with *UPKIIIA* (Jenkins et al. 2005) and *ROBO2* genes mutations (Lu et al. 2007).

Dominant mutations of the paired box 2 (*PAX2*) gene, which is expressed in developing fetal kidney tubules, should be considered in individuals with renal hypoplasia or dysplasia, who have either visual impairment, from associated optic nerve coloboma, and/or a similarly affected first degree relative (Salomon et al. 2001; Weber et al. 2006). Apolymorphism of the transcription factor *PAX2* is associated with reduced neonatal kidney size (Stahl et al. 2006; Quinlan et al. 2007). Moreover, the *PAX2* gene, which is expressed in developing fetal kidney tubules, should be considered in individuals with renal hypoplasia or dysplasia, who have either visual impairment (from associated optic nerve coloboma) and/or a similarly affected first-degree relative in renal-coloboma syndrome (RCS), an autosomal dominant disorder (Woolf 2008).

The main cause of fetal bilateral hyperechogenic kidneys is associated with hepatocyte nuclear factor 1-β (*HNF1B*) gene mutations (Decramer et al. 2007). Mutations of the gene that encodes the transcription factor *HNF1B* are associated with renal cysts and diabetes (RCAD) syndrome. Moreover, *HNF1B* mutations lead to different types of renal tract malformations, including multicystic dysplastic kidney (MDK), congenital solitary functioning kidneys (CSFK), cystic dysplastic kidneys, hypoplastic kidneys, and glomerulocystic kidneys

(Edghill et al. 2006; Weber et al. 2006; Decramer et al. 2007; Ulinski et al. 2006). *HNF1B* mutations or variants may be found in 8% of children who have dysplastic/hypoplastic kidneys and renal failure and in 22% who have cysts (Weber et al. 2006; Ulinski et al. 2006; Zaffanello et al. 2008a). However, intronic regulatory expression sequences have been identified in the *HNF1B* gene (Pouilhe et al. 2007) named retinoic acid regulatory element (*RARE*) and *T-MARE* (MafB responsive element) which links retinoic acid (RA) and *MafB* pathways with *HNF1B* gene regulation. Both *MafB*, a member of the large Maf family of transcription factors, and the RA signaling pathway have been implicated in renal development. In particular, *MafB* is specifically expressed in glomerular epithelial cells (podocytes) and is essential for podocyte differentiation and renal tubule survival (Moriguchi et al. 2006). However, RA signaling modulates the expression of renal transcription factors and components of signaling pathways that are known to direct segment fates during mammalian nephrogenesis.

Several other genes are identified since involved in aberrant renal and urinary tract morphogenesis. The *c-ret* gene encodes an epithelial cell, transmembrane tyrosine kinase receptor protein. In *c-ret* mutants, renal agenesis, severe hypodysplasia, and blind-ending ureters are observed (Stahl et al. 2006). Two X-linked gene mutations, angiotensin type II receptor gene (*Agtr2*) (Nishimura et al. 1999; Hohenfellner et al. 2001) and L1-cell adhesion molecule (*L1-CAM*) are involved in PUJO or MDK and in the process of kidney and urogenital tract organogenesis (Stahl et al. 2006). Bone morphogenic protein 4 (BMP4) has also been shown to interact with proteins in systems outside of the kidney and urinary tract that have been identified as regulators of kidney and urinary tract organogenesis. WNT11 is a target molecule of glial cell line derived neurotrophic factor (GDNF) and downregulation by BMP4 results in the inhibition of ectopic ureteric bud formation from the Wolffian duct. The *Foxc1 C*/ *Foxc2* C compound heterozygotes have hypoplastic kidneys and single ureters. However, *Uroplakin* genes may be critical for development of both the upper and lower urinary tract in humans. De novo heterozygous mutations in *Uroplakin IIIA* are associated with severe renal adysplasia and hypodysplasia with kidney failure in childhood (Winyard and Chitty 2008). Furthermore, mutations of genes encoding renin-angiotensin system (RAS) components are associated with perinatal kidney disease. The renal phenotype usually comprises slightly large kidneys, appearing bright on fetal ultrasound, together with a profound decrease in amniotic fluid volume (Lacoste et al. 2006). Finally, evidence is emerging that posterior urethral valves (PUVs) may have a genetic basis, possibly a male-limited autosomal recessive condition (Woolf 2008). Recently, a potential role of copy number variants (CNVs) has been found in up to 57% of cases examined (Boghossian et al. 2016).

Considerable recent progress has been made in unraveling the rather complex genetic bases of the spectrum of diseases known as the Bardet-Biedl, Meckel-Gruber, and Joubert syndromes. These syndromes show considerable phenotypic overlap, with all featuring perinatal kidney disease with dysplasia and cysts (Woolf 2008).

116.3.2 Environmental Factors

Some observational studies linked the environmental factors with the development of malformation in renal and urinary tract in the fetus and newborn. Renal tract malformations are more common in fetuses of mothers with high alcohol intake or diabetes mellitus (Kerecuk et al. 2008). However, gross gestational insults, such as twin–twin transfusion syndrome and heavy prematurity, may perturb human kidney differentiation (Mahieu-Caputo et al. 2000; Rodríguez et al. 2004). Moreover, the discovery of mutations in genes coding for the RAS cascade in patients with renal tubular dysgenesis (Lacoste et al. 2006) is associated with the increased incidence of renal anomalies in fetuses exposed to drugs that block angiotensin II signaling (Quan 2006). Renal tubular dysgenesis is usually observed in fetuses exposed to angiotensin-converting enzyme inhibitors or angiotensin receptor antagonists during the second and/or third trimesters of gestation (Plazanet et al. 2014).

116.4 Clinical Aspects

116.4.1 Prevalence and Prognosis

Prenatal ultrasound (US) screening programs assessing the diagnostic prevalence of renal anomalies in 20 registries of 12 European countries identified unilateral MDK in 1:7100 of fetuses, unilateral renal agenesis in 1:12,500, bilateral renal agenesis or dysplastic kidneys in 1:7700, and PUVs in 1:33,300. Terminations of pregnancies were performed in 67% of the detected bilateral renal agenesis/dysgenesis but only 4% of the unilateral MDK malformations (Wiesel et al. 2005). The US screening of fetuses in the last trimester showed that 7.7% had transient upper renal tract dilatation (Gunn et al. 1995; Mendelsohn 2004). From a multicenter study, prenatal hydronephrosis had an overall prevalence of 11.5 cases per 10,000 births. The large majority of cases were live births (96% of total), only a minority were terminations of pregnancy or fetal deaths. Boys accounted for 72% of all cases. A high proportion of the cases (86%) had an isolated renal tract malformation (Garne et al. 2009). Hydronephrosis may be bilateral in 37–57% of cases (Boubaker et al. 2006). Among hydronephrosis, PUJO was the most common cause of prenatal pelvis dilatation, accounting for 33% of infant cases, followed by primary VUR (28%), megaureter (18%), and complicated renal duplex kidney (12%). Less frequent conditions of prenatal renal pelvis dilatation were MDK, PUVs, hydronephrotic horseshoe kidneys, and hereditary renal adysplasia (Ismaili et al. 2004a). MDK, although not classified as hydronephrosis, may be mistaken for hydronephrosis (Piepsz 2007). Postnatal hydronephrosis in antenatally detected urinary tract abnormalities showed more commonly were UJO (44.8%), VUR (30%), and megaureter (9.5%). Moreover, MDK (43.5%), renal agenesis (19.4%), and VUR (19.4) were mostly encountered in patients without postnatal hydronephrosis (Gokce et al. 2012).

Sometimes the hyperechogenic kidney, detected with prenatal US, may pose problems of differential diagnosis. The prevalence of renal pathology associated with kidney hyperechogenicity at US detected after 17 weeks' gestation has been assessed in a retrospective multicenter study. The conditions more frequently associated with fetal hyperechogenic kidneys were ADPKD and ARPKD. Less frequent conditions were Bardet-Biedl syndrome, Meckel-Gruber syndrome, and Ivemark II syndrome. Jarcho-Levin syndrome, Beemer syndrome, and Meckel-like syndrome were rare. Lastly, one third of the fetuses with hyperechogenic kidneys had renal cysts (Chaumoitre et al. 2006).

Mild isolated antenatal hydronephrosis (5–15 mm) at third trimester of gestation had total resolution in 73% of renal unit during the first year (Alconcher and Tombesi 2012). Primary megaureter in newborns resolved in 52.8%, persisted in 25% and require surgical procedure in the follow-up period; predictive factors for surgery were poor drainage on (99 m)Tc-DTPA scan, grade IV-V hydronephrosis, and ureteric diameter more than 15 mm (Arena et al. 2012).

116.4.2 Classification of Renal Anomalies

An abnormal human renal tract may develop from the beginning of the metanephros to the end of nephron formation, which occurs at about 34 weeks of gestation (Alam-Faruque et al. 2014). The acronym CAKUT means congenital anomalies of the kidney and urinary tract, a syndrome that includes a wide spectrum of anomalies affecting the formation of the kidney and bladder. CAKUT is an important group of human disorders characterized by a combination of renal hypoplasia with congenital abnormalities of the urinary tract. In the kidney, these anomalies include hypoplasia, dysplasia, or a complete lack of kidney formation (agenesis). Proximally the ureter can be obstructed (PUJO) or grossly dilated (megaureter). Distally the ureter can be blocked at its insertion into the bladder (vesicoureteral junction obstruction [VUJO]). Alternatively, the ureter may be incompetent (VUR) or insert outside the bladder (ectopic). Bladder and urethral anomalies include abnormal hemitrigone formation as well as urethral valves (PUVs) and urethral atresia (Stahl et al. 2006). A deregulation of microRNAs is addressed as etiological factor of CAKUT in culture (Bartram et al. 2013). Moreover, a significant proportion of patients with CAKUT harbour submicroscopic chromosomal imbalances since CNV was detected in 10.1% of patients investigated (Caruana et al. 2015).

The anomalies that affect the renal system may be classified according to the renal and urinary tract district involved (Table 2) (Joseph 2006).

Table 2 Classification of main anomalies affecting the renal system

Renal agenesis
Unilateral
Bilateral (Potter's syndrome)
Abnormalities of position (ectopia)
Kidney fusion
Horseshoe kidney
Crossed fused ectopia
Dysplasia/cystic renal disease
Aplastic or tiny dysplastic remnant kidney
Hypoplastic kidney
Simple renal cysts
Multilocular cysts
Multicystic dysplastic kidney (MDK)
Polycystic kidney disease (ADPKD and ARPKD)
Obstructive uropathy
Posterior urethral valves (PUVs)
Pelviureteric junction obstruction (PUJO)
Vesicoureteric junction obstruction (VUJO)
Vesicoureteral reflux (VUR)
Ureteral alterations, duplications, and ectopia
Ectopic ureter
Ureterocele
Ureteral duplications
Anomalies of the bladder
Epispadias
Classical bladder exstrophy
Bladder exstrophy complex
Anomalies of the penis

Modified from (Joseph 2006)

116.4.3 Renal Agenesis

Embryologically, renal agenesis occurs because the ureteric bud has not interacted with the metanephric mesenchyme. The bud fails to form the ureter, renal pelvis, and collecting ducts. The mesenchyme fails to form nephrons. On occasion, unilateral renal agenesis is accompanied by genital tract anomalies on the same side (Mishra 2007). The most profound and severe renal tract malformation is the complete bilateral kidney development, called renal agenesis, oligohydramnios sequence, or Potter's syndrome, often accompanied by absent ureters. Prenatal diagnosis of oligohydramnios in the second trimester is dependent on US scanning, and often a full postmortem examination is necessary to identify any underlying fetal cause (Stahl et al. 2006). Bilateral renal agenesis or hypoplasia was associated with a mother's risk factors such as adiposity prior to pregnancy, smoking during the periconceptional period, and binge drinking during the second month of pregnancy (Slickers et al. 2008). In Fraser syndrome, data provided by the European Surveillance of Congenital Anomalies (EUROCAT) network of birth defect registries showed bilateral renal agenesis in 50% and unilateral in 17% cases (Barisic et al. 2013).

116.4.3.1 Diagnosis

Renal agenesis is suspected when US does not identify the renal parenchyma, and a postnatal scintigraphic scan does not show any renal function in a given side of the body. A nonfunctional kidney is diagnosed when US identifies residual renal parenchyma, without valuable scintigraphic renal function (Fig. 1).

116.4.3.2 Management of Bilateral Renal Agenesis

The diagnosis of bilateral renal agenesis is made during pregnancy by US scan, which shows the absence of the kidneys and nonvisualization of the bladder. Since this syndrome (Potter's syndrome) is frequently associated with poorer life expectancy, termination of the pregnancy is the most frequent outcome. A case of bilateral renal agenesis was treated with serial amnioinfusion in which the newborn survived the newborn period and was able to undergo peritoneal dialysis as a bridge to planned renal transplantation (Bienstock et al. 2014).

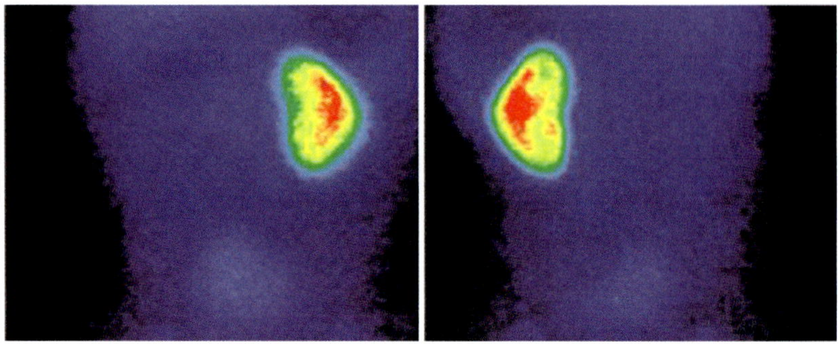

Fig. 1 Renal DMSA scintigraphy performed in a male baby with left solitary hypertrophic functioning kidney and right iliac-sided ectopic not functioning kidney (Reproduced from Zaffanello et al. 2009a with permission)

116.4.3.3 Management of Unilateral Renal Agenesis

Diagnosis of unilateral renal agenesis is generally performed by prenatal US. Controlateral compensatory renal hypertrophy can be detected in the third trimester and occasionally in the latter part of second trimester (Hill et al. 2000).

Postnatal radionuclide scan (DMSA) may confirm the diagnosis and establish the functional state of the congenital solitary functioning kidney (CSFK). After the diagnosis of unilateral renal agenesis, postnatal screening is mandatory to rule out other associated renal anomalies. Early diagnosis and treatment of urological anomalies associated with CSFK is imperative to decrease the long-term risk of renal damage (Cascio et al. 1999). The early identification of risk factors for renal damage is essential because CSFK may further exhibit growth failure even if it was initially normal (Zaffanello et al. 2009a). The management of VUR in CSFK follows the same strategies used to manage unilateral VUR in children with two normally functioning kidneys (Palmer et al. 1997). On the other hand, infants with PUJO in CSFK who have severe pelvis dilatation and decreased renal function require early surgical therapy or selective internal ureteric stenting (Choo and Borzi 2001). Severe renal hypodysplasia, mistaken for renal aplasia, may evolve into renal malignancy and may cause hypertension.

116.4.3.4 Prognosis

CSFK may progressively lead to persistent hyperfiltration, microalbuminuria, and increasing proteinuria, with focal and segmentary hyalinization of the renal glomeruli requiring periodical long-term follow-up. At follow-up, the majority of patients with solitary kidney showed renal damage in adulthood (Basturk et al. 2015).

116.4.4 Abnormalities of Position

During embryological development, the kidney undergoes rotation as well as cranial migration taking its blood supply from the middle sacral artery, iliac artery, and the aorta. Malrotation may occur as a result of incomplete, excessive, or reversed rotation. In these situations, the renal hilum faces in an abnormal direction and gives rise to obstruction. Anomalies of ascent may result in abnormal positions of the kidney of which the most common is the pelvic kidney. The abnormal location frequently predisposes to UTI and VUR (Joseph 2006).

116.4.4.1 Management

Asymptomatic patients, with adequate renal function, require inclusion into follow-up protocols. Imaging with US and radionuclide scan (DMSA) is required to identify location and associated abnormalities. Overall, a radionuclide scans is advisable when the pelvic position makes the kidney difficult to identify by US. Computed tomography/magnetic resonance imaging (CT/MRI) scan is advisable in cases where renal function is poor. Voiding cystoureterogram (VCUG) or scintigraphic screening may rule out a concomitant VUR.

Adequate renal function associated with clinical and radiological evidence of obstruction or

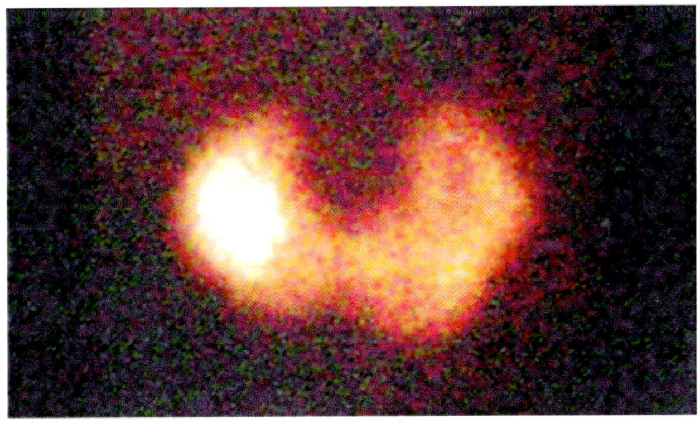

Fig. 2 Anterior view of DMSA scintigraphy in a baby with horseshoe kidney

VUR may require surgical consideration. Not functioning, poorly functioning, and MDK associating obstruction or recurrent infections are normally treated by nephrectomy.

116.4.5 Kidney Fusion

In crossed fused ectopia, the upper pole of one kidney is fused with the lower pole of the opposite kidney. Crossed renal ectopia is most frequently associated with VUR and UTI. Fusion of renal elements may occur across the midline to produce a horseshoe kidney (Fig. 2), which is one of the most frequent genitourinary abnormalities with an overall incidence of 1/666 (Weizer et al. 2003). Renal fusion anomalies may be asymptomatic but are frequently associated with obstruction and infection. In a horseshoe kidney, the most common clinical problem is obstruction at the pelviureteric junction. Horseshoe kidney may be part of the spectrum of well-known syndromes associated anomalies affecting multiple organs such as Turner's, Frasier's, renal coloboma, and Mayer-Rokitansky.

A recent survey reports that concomitant urogenital and nonurogenital malformations were equally frequent for horseshoe kidney and crossed fused ectopia. Severe anomalies or malformations were found in 23% of patients, less frequent than previously reported (Glodny et al. 2009). Half of children with horseshoe kidney have renal complications (pelvocaliectasis, VUR) or extrarenal diseases (gastrointestinal and vertebral) or syndromes (Turner syndrome) (Je et al. 2015).

116.4.5.1 Management

The diagnosis of fusion abnormalities can be made with the commonly used imaging modalities, such as US and scintigraphy. In cases of obstruction confirmed by radionuclide scan (MAG3), a pyeloplasty is commonly required. Patients with VUR, demonstrated by VCUG, require surgery if UTIs are frequent. Individual cases of complex anatomical situations require special examination strategies, and CT appears to be the most reliable imaging method (Glodny et al. 2009). Finally, parenchyma with poor renal function or dysplasia associated with recurrent infections may need partial nephroureterectomy.

116.4.6 Renal Dysplasia

Dysplastic kidneys are so-called because both organs are present but development is abnormal and incomplete. These organs contain incompletely branched ducts derived from cells of the ureteric bud and collecting duct line, surrounded by undifferentiated and metaplastic stroma. The classic antenatal presentation of dysplastic kidneys is of large bright kidneys, with or without cystic spaces, occurring within the cortex at the routine 20-week scan (Winyard and Chitty 2008).

116.4.6.1 Aplastic or Dysplastic Kidney

The dysplastic kidney may be either aplastic (a few millimeters long) or large and distended by multiple cysts. Ureters attached to MDKs are scarcely formed and with nonpatent sections.

These severe types of dysplastic kidneys generally have no excretory function.

116.4.6.2 Hypoplastic Kidney

Hypoplastic kidneys contain fully formed nephrons but have a deficit in nephron number. Kidney hypoplasia is defined as kidney mass below 2 standard deviations of that of age matched normal individuals or a combined estimated kidney mass of less than half of normal for the patient's age. Oligomeganephronia represents a severe variant of hypoplasia in which both kidneys are one eighth to one half normal weight. Nephron number is reduced by 80% and nephrons are markedly hypertrophied, with glomerular diameter more than twice normal. Premature babies and/or infants small for gestational age due to intrauterine malnutrition will be born with relatively small kidneys and a certain nephron deficit, a condition called congenital oligonephropathy (Puddu et al. 2009).

116.4.6.3 Cystic Dysplastic Kidney

In dysplastic kidneys, cysts arise in the context of abnormal renal development. Cystic dysplastic kidney contains primitive tubules and cysts alongside normal nephrons and generally may have excretory function. Renal tubular dysgenesis is related to incomplete differentiation of proximal tubular nephron segments, often associated with fetal anuria and oligohydramnios. In the variant of kidney malformation associated with obstruction, the first filtering nephrons develop normally, but nephrogenesis subsequently halts developing subcapsular cysts from nephron precursors (Vujic et al. 2007; Daïkha-Dahmane et al. 1997). Moreover, dysplasia is sometimes limited to the medulla and, in the presence of a duplex ureter, only the upper moiety is generally dysplastic.

116.4.6.4 Multicystic Dysplastic Kidney

Histology of fetal MDK showed that few nephrons, containing relatively normal glomeruli and proximal tubules, are present in these kidneys (Matsell et al. 1996). MDK results from complete obstruction early in embryonic development. Abnormal structures seem to be destroyed later in gestation or postnatally (Hiraoka et al. 2002). In unilateral MDK, the presence of minimal function is rare (3–7%), occurring in 4% cases of patients (Damen-Elias et al. 2005). The overall prevalence of MDK is 4.12 per 10,000 births. Cases with unilateral MDK are mainly liveborn, and only 16% have associated major malformations or a syndrome (Winding et al. 2014).

Management and Prognosis

In asymptomatic patients, a follow-up with serial US scans is mandatory. In healthy infants with US diagnosis of unilateral MDK and normal bladder US, nuclear medicine scan may be unnecessary to confirm the diagnosis (Whittam et al. 2014). US screening may detect spontaneous involution in the most severely affected kidney. All MDK patients on conservative management will need regular scans until at least 5 years of age.

Symptomatic patients with increasing abdominal distension and poor feeding may require nephrectomy (Narchi 2005). Surgeons advocated prophylactic removal of these asymptomatic lesions for possible risks of hypertension and malignancy. The risk of hypertension is less than 1%. If severe hypertension is detected it will be necessary to carry out curative nephrectomy (Thomas 2008). However, malignancy has not been found (Narchi 2005). Involution rate was 53.6% for right-sided and only 16.7% for left-sided kidneys (Tiryaki et al. 2013). If neoplasms occur, they usually present as Wilms tumor. If any increase in size or unusual features appears, this will be an indication to proceed to nephrectomy.

Bilateral involvement leads to lethal pulmonary hypoplasia from anhydramnios.

116.4.6.5 Polycystic Kidney Disease

Polycystic kidney disease (PKD) is a genetic disorder presenting diverse forms:

Autosomal recessive polycystic kidney disease (ARPKD)
Autosomal dominant polycystic kidney disease (ADPKD)
Nephronophthisis/medullary cystic kidney disease

PKD is a disease of the nephron with multiple renal tubular cysts that leads ultimately to end stage renal failure (ESRF) (Wilson 2004). It has been estimated that there are approximately 6.5 million people in the world with inherited PKD (Bissler and Dixon 2005). Inherited PKD may have either dominant or recessive inherited fashion. The dominant form (ADPKD) is due to mutations in two different genes, *PKD1* or *PKD2*. The protein products of the PKD genes, polycystin-1 and polycystin-2, regulate renal tubule epithelial cell division and differentiation. The recessive form (ARPKD) and nephronophthisis/medullary cystic kidney disease are associated with the *PKHD1* and *NPH1* genes and their protein products are fibrocystin and nephrocystin, respectively.

Nephronophthisis or medullary cystic kidney disease was associated in one fourth of cases with Joubert syndrome, an autosomal recessive disorder that is described in patients with cerebellar ataxia, mental retardation, hypotonia, and neonatal respiratory dysregulation (Valente et al. 2006).

ARPKD is an inherited recessive disorder in which both kidneys are affected by cysts developing from dilated collecting ducts. The condition is associated with congenital hepatic fibrosis leading to the development of portal hypertension. The renal cystic changes appear in utero and are associated with poor renal function leading to oligohydramnios. Severe kidney disease tends to be associated with milder liver involvement, whereas milder renal disease applies when liver manifestations are predominant. Differential diagnosis is made on the history, clinical examination, and prenatal and postnatal imaging by US. In some cases, biopsy of the kidney and liver may be necessary to confirm the diagnosis. Many families who lost a child with severe ARPKD desire an early and reliable prenatal diagnosis. Given the limitations of antenatal US, this is only feasible by molecular genetics that became possible from 1994 when *PKHD1* was mapped (Bergmann et al. 2004). More than 300 different mutations in the PKHD1 gene (ARPKD) have been described. More than 60% of neonates with pulmonary hypoplasia may survive; about 25% need postnatal dialysis. After 10 years, 60% require renal replacement therapy (Hoyer 2015).

Management

Patients require evaluation of renal function providing appropriate supportive measures if renal failure occurs, treating hypertension and metabolic disturbances. If kidneys are massively enlarged causing respiratory difficulty, a nephrectomy may be required with either unilateral or bilateral and dialysis.

116.4.7 Obstructive Uropathy

Prenatal suspicious of obstructive uropathy at US may be made as marked dilatation of the urinary tract. Antenatal pelvicalyceal dilatation has been reported in ~0.6% of pregnancies. Fetal lower urinary tract obstruction affects 2.2 per 10,000 births (Lissauer et al. 2007).

Many different causes are involved in the pelvicalyceal dilatation, including transient hydronephrosis, physiological hydronephrosis, PUJO, and PUVs (Woodward and Frank 2002). Obstructive uropathy can be classified as lower or higher urinary tract obstruction. High urinary tract obstruction is suggested when there is hydronephrosis or pelvicalyceal dilatation in the absence of visible ureteral bladder pathology, either at prenatal or postnatal assessment. The most common lower anomaly is PUVs, which account for approximately half of cases, followed by urethral obstruction/atresia (Lissauer et al. 2007). Congenital megaloureter is a poorly defined entity in which ureterectasis is associated with no reflux and normal bladder (Pates and Dashe 2006). Many newborns with pelvicalyceal dilatation can be safely treated nonoperatively, and obstruction occurs in only small number of patients. In a series of patients, 54% of cases the hydronephrosis improved or resolved spontaneously during the first 3 years of life (Onen 2007).

116.4.7.1 Posterior Urethral Valves

PUVs are congenital disease of high mortality and morbidity, starting in the uterus and leading to progressive renal dysfunction. PUVs are recognized as the most common cause of bladder outlet obstruction in boys with an incidence of 1 in 2000–4000 live male births (Joseph 2006).

Commonly, PUVs consist of two folds arising from the urethra at the level of the veru montanum and fusing anteriorly in the midline. A much rarer form is a diaphragm extending across the lumen of the urethra just beyond the veru montanum. The degree of obstruction can vary from minimal with associated symptoms of dysfunctional voiding to severe with dilated posterior urethra, trabeculated bladder, and severely hydronephrotic kidneys.

Antenatal Diagnosis

The antenatal diagnosis is made on the finding of dilated upper tracts associated with a thick-walled bladder and oligohydramnios. The bladder appears thick-walled and tense in cases of obstruction whereas in prune belly syndrome the bladder appears floppy (Agarwal and Fisk 2001). A detailed sonographic evaluation of the fetus is carried out to exclude extrarenal abnormalities. MRI is reported of benefit when used in addition to US if the resolution of US is impaired by oligohydramnios (Poutamo et al. 2000).

Antenatal Management

Prenatal diagnosis provides the opportunity to improve functional outcome by either decompression of the obstructed bladder in intrauterine life or prompt postnatal intervention to relieve obstruction, minimize the risk of sepsis, and optimize management of the valves (Thomas 2008). Fetal intervention is not without risk of complications and should be avoided where renal function is poor with little possibility of survival. However, fetal intervention is not indicated in patients detected prior to 24 weeks because the renal changes are not reversible. Where the diagnosis is made after 24 weeks, the outcome in terms of renal function is generally favorable (Crombleholme et al. 1990). Thus, fetal intervention should not be performed if the US indicates marked renal dysplasia or in cases with adequate renal function with stable amniotic fluid volume. Fetal intervention has conventionally been restricted to male fetuses with suspected PUVs, good renal prognosis, and oligohydramnios. The procedure most commonly performed is percutaneous vesicoamniotic shunt (Agarwal and Fisk 2001). In utero percutaneous vesicoamniotic drainage possibly improves overall perinatal survival as compared to the nondrainage group (Clark et al. 2003). On the other hand, open fetal vesicostomy has a high risk of complications since risk for preterm labor, maternal morbidity, premature ruptures of the membranes, and fetal death. Fetoscopic laser ablation for PUV can achieve bladder decompression and amniotic fluid normalization with a single procedure in selected cases with anyhydramnios (Martínez et al. 2015).

Postnatal Management

Open or endoscopic procedures would provide a definitive treatment of obstruction, although limitations are the uncertainty whether renal function can be significantly improved (Quintero et al. 2000). Anyway, some cases of PUVs may benefit from timely identification and surgical intervention, although prenatal diagnosis has little impact on mortality or ESRF in the first 10 years of life, reflecting the crucial role of renal dysplasia as a determinant of early renal impairment (Thomas 2008).

Surgical Treatment

The initial management is to pass a urethral catheter into the bladder and establish drainage. If a urethral catheter cannot be passed because the bladder may contract around the urethral catheter, suprapubic drainage is required. Moreover, if contrast study of bladder and urethra visualizes the urethra adequately, the diagnosis of PUV will be confirmed and VUR if present will also be identified.

Primary valve ablation is performed transurethrally with miniature endoscopes and under direct vision; the coagulating electrode fulgurates the valve leaflets. There is good evidence that early valve ablation can lead to recovery of bladder function and improvement in the upper tracts (Mitchell and Close 1996). Vesicostomy is generally reserved for neonates with severe upper tract changes and poor renal function especially if associated VUR. The temporary decompression of the bladder may help to improve upper tract function. Closure of the vesicostomy is carried out after valve ablation and when upper tract surgical intervention has been completed (Jaureguizar et al. 2000; Bajpai et al. 2001). Use of double-J stents in neonates with PUV was a safe and effective alternative method for lower urinary tract decompression (Penna et al. 2015).

In a long-term study, primary valve ablation gave the best results with good capacity, compliant bladders similar to those with ureterostomy, while the vesicostomy group had small capacity and hyperreflexic bladders (Puri et al. 2002). From another study, the long-term results of prenatally detected PUVs confirm that early valve ablation can be considered as the primary treatment in the majority of patients, without the need for preoperative drainage or diversion (Sarhan et al. 2008).

Prognosis

Cases where the US features of PUVs appear early (before 20 weeks of gestational age) and upper tract dilatation is moderate to severe have a poor prognosis (Hutton et al. 1997). The kidneys are often dysplastic and have poor function. Many of these fetuses would either abort or be stillborn. In appropriately selected fetuses, intervention may improve perinatal survival, but long-term renal morbidity among survivors remains problematic. An important prognostic feature on US is the presence of significant oligohydramnios, which if present prior to 24 weeks is associated with a higher prevalence of pulmonary hypoplasia (Crombleholme et al. 1990). Moreover, both gestational age at diagnosis and oligohydramnios were statistically significant predictors of final renal outcome (Sarhan et al. 2008). Finally, poor renal function associated with renal dysplasia could not improve even after relief of obstruction. Thus, a high percentage of cases progress to renal failure regardless of prenatal diagnosis (Thomas 2008). Urinary TGF-beta1, TNF-alpha-, and microalbumin can be used as biomarkers for an early recognition of ongoing renal damage in these patients (Mandelia et al. 2013).

116.4.7.2 Pelviureteric Junction Obstruction

Hydronephrosis secondary to PUJO is the commonest anomaly affecting the renal collecting system. On total of the antenatally diagnosed renal pelvis dilatation, PUJO occurred in 13% of cases (Ismaili et al. 2004a). Of total fetal hydronephrosis, PUJO accounted for 0.2–0.4% of cases, of which 20–25% of cases were bilateral (Woodward and Frank 2002).

Pathogenesis

The condition results from an intrinsic stenosis of the ureter at the point where it joins the pelvis. PUJO is characterized by aberrant pyeloureteric smooth muscle, which typically exhibits hypertrophy and perifascicular fibrosis and abnormal innervation (Zhang et al. 2000). The abnormal ureteric segment has decreased peristaltic activity resulting in failure of transport of urine from pelvis down to the ureter.

Clinical Presentation

Renal pelvis dilatations are frequently detected with prenatal US. Pelvicalyceal dilatation in the fetus must be interpreted with caution as many of these resolve spontaneously in the postnatal period. A system of grading based on the anteroposterior diameter (APD) of the renal pelvis is used to evaluate the severity of the hydronephrosis. Measurements of 3 mm or less are considered normal at any gestational age. Beyond 30 weeks' gestation, thresholds for diagnosis of mild, moderate, and severe hydronephrosis were defined as 5–8 mm, 9–15 mm, and greater than 15 mm, respectively. Most agree that postnatal evaluation is prudent if the renal pelvis APD reaches 10 mm at any point in gestation, or if calyceal dilation is noted. Recent prospective studies have found that even mild hydronephrosis that is stable or resolves over a pregnancy may redevelop, progress, and necessitate surgery after birth (Pates and Dashe 2006).

Management

The management of hydronephrosis secondary to PUJO is aimed at preserving long-term renal function. In infants, asymptomatic unilateral hydronephrosis with stable differential renal function can be managed conservatively, while obstructive dilatation requires serial assessments and early surgical correction (Riccabona 2004). Ensuring a sufficient follow-up interval, especially during the first 3 years of life, is essential to prevent permanent loss of renal function in kidneys that do develop signs of obstruction (Onen 2007).

All patients with prenatally detected hydronephrosis should have US scans, MAG-3 renograms, and VCUG (to rule out VUR). On the US scan, APD of the renal pelvis, degree of caliectasis, renal length, thickness of the renal cortex, echogenicity, and corticomedullary differentiation should be assessed.

The concept of measuring renal pelvic dilatation on US allows children to be categorized into a conservatively managed group (APD below 12 mm) and an early surgical intervention group (APDN 40 mm). If APD is below 12 mm, these patients are not at risk and are followed up with US scans at 3 months and 1 year. When APD is from 12 to 20 mm these patients require US scans at 3 months and 1 year and MAG-3 scan at 3 months. If APD is from 20 to 40 mm, these patients requires MAG-3 scan at age 1 month (Dhillon 1998). MAG-3 renogram provides a more accurate assessment of obstruction. On diuretic MAG3 scintigraphy, infants show renal pelvis dilatation with delayed drainage and relatively reduced renal function (Dudley et al. 1997).

Table 3 Treatment and follow-up protocol for ureteropelvic junction hydronephrosis

Grade 1
Follow-up with serial ultrasound starting at 1 month
No prophylactic antimicrobial
No renal scintigraphy
Follow-up for development of urinary symptoms
Grade 2
Follow-up with ultrasound plus renal scintigraphy starting at 1 month
Antibacterial prophylaxis may be beneficial
Renal scintigraphy at every other control
Grade 3
Close follow-up with ultrasound plus scintigraphy
Antibacterial prophylaxis could be necessary
Renal scintigraphy at every other control as far as renal function >35%
Surgical (pyelography) indications if significant increase[a] in hydronephrosis, decrease in renal function
Grade 4
Early intervention, after short period of follow-up, is safe for prevention of renal function. Delay in prompt treatment may cause irreversible renal deterioration

[a]Control if the echography is comparable (i.e., empty or full bladder) (Modified from Onen 2007)

Fetal Intervention

Hydronephrosis with normal renal parenchyma is generally associated with good renal function and hence does not require fetal intervention. Fetal intervention should be considered in cases of severe bilateral hydronephrosis associated with oligohydramnios, bilateral hydronephrosis with dysplastic renal parenchyma, and solitary kidney with severe hydronephrosis. Therefore, the risk of chronic or ESRF posed by upper tract obstruction is exceptionally low, except in the rare instances when it affects a solitary kidney (Thomas 2008).

Postnatal Management and Prognosis

Close follow-up is required in the first 2 years of life to identify the subgroup (35%) of children with obstruction that requires prompt surgery. Nonoperative management with close follow-up during the first 2 years is a safe and recommended approach for neonates with primary bilateral PUJO type hydronephrosis (Onen 2007). Large numbers of children have been submitted to an unnecessary pyeloplasty for asymptomatic PUJO, which was otherwise destined to resolve spontaneously (Thomas 2008). However, from 20 to 40 mm with function near 40% these patients need close follow-up, by US and MAG-3 scan at 3 months, 6 months, and 1 year. If the APD is near 40 mm, surgical intervention is required. Treatment and follow-up protocol for UPJO hydronephrosis was proposed by Onen et al. (2007) (Table 3).

Pyeloplasty of renal units with PUJO and decline of kidney function is widely suggested to improve renal outcome or delay long-term morbidity (Sheu et al. 2006). Such an approach prevented permanent loss of renal function. Actually, unilateral PUJO is less indicated for surgery, especially if renal function is unaffected. During follow-up, the main indications for surgery are deterioration of renal function of 5% or more, glomerular filtration rate drop to 40% or less, bilateral hydronephrosis, or solitary kidney (Chertin et al. 2002). Generally, amelioration has been related to kidney maturation rather than a result of surgery (Capolicchio et al. 1999). If renal function is already reduced, the operation is made even if there is no proof of improving final renal outcome, as usually split renal function does not change. When renal function is poor at the beginning despite the pyeloplasty, the functional amelioration of the operated kidney is frequently absent or minimal (Ylinen et al. 2004a). In terms of relieving obstruction, a pyeloplasty has a success rate in excess of 95%. In the small percentage of patients requiring repeat pyeloplasty, the failure of the original procedure is usually apparent within a year or two of the original procedure (Thomas 2008).

PUJO in a duplex kidney is a rare but challenging anomaly that requires careful evaluation. Surgery was performed in 14/21 patients, including pyelopyelostomy or ureteropyelostomy, dismembered pyeloplasty, and heminephrectomy (Rubenwolf et al. 2015).

Prenatal diagnosis and surgical intervention have contributed to a reduction in long-term morbidity in children with PUJO. Therefore, many children have almost certainly undergone unnecessary early pyeloplasty for an obstruction that would have resolved spontaneously (Thomas 2008). The long-term follow-up of dismembered pyeloplasty for congenital midline-crossing giant hydronephrosis caused by UPJO was satisfactory (Baek et al. 2010).

Differential Diagnosis

The less common mid-ureteral stricture accounts for 4% of prenatal hydronephrosis (Ismaili et al. 2004b).

116.4.7.3 Vesicoureteric Junction Obstruction

Causes of pediatric obstructive hydroureteronephrosis may include primary or congenital vesicoureteric junction obstruction (VUJO) and a secondary form of VUJO (i.e., ureterocele, retroperitoneal fibrosis, calculus).

Diagnosis

An US screening during pregnancy enables the physician to make an early diagnosis of primary VUJO, which involves 4% of the total fetal hydronephrosis (Lim et al. 2003). Prenatal diagnosis of VUJO requires postnatal US confirmation and follow-up. Most series have reported an operation rate, predominantly performed because of reduced renal function, in the range 10–20%. Prenatally detected VUJO follows an even more benign course than PUJO with a high tendency to spontaneous resolution (Shukla et al. 2005). However, MRI techniques make it possible to see the anatomical details of the obstruction level from the third trimester of pregnancy to postnatal life (Cassart et al. 2004). Primary obstruction may become symptomatic late in infancy, especially in patients with normal prenatal US screening (Zaffanello et al. 2009b).

Management

Surgical treatment consists of excision of the distal ureteric segment, tapering of the ureter, and reimplantation or insertion of a JJ stent (Shenoy and Rance 1999).

116.4.8 Vesicoureteral Reflux

VUR is the retrograde flow of urine into the upper urinary tract. The estimated prevalence of VUR affects about 1% of the general infant population (Marra et al. 1994). Mild fetal renal dilatation (fetal renal pelvis 4–10 mm) was associated with VUR ranges between 13% and 30% (Marra et al. 1994), with an increasing risk in children of parents with VUR. Infants with a family history of VUR, persistent fetal renal dilatation after 30 weeks of gestation should be investigated (Anderson et al. 2003).

Generally, in newborns a reflux is primary. Primary reflux can be associated with dysplastic kidneys, especially in boys (Risdon et al. 1993). There is growing evidence that congenital renal dysplasia rather than acquired infective scarring is the most important determinant of reflux nephropathy in males with high-grade VUR, who are the infants most commonly identified by prenatal US (Thomas 2008). The mean overall relative risk of kidney damage is higher in renal units with VUR, particularly in those carrying high-grade VUR, than in not-refluxing kidney (Zaffanello et al. 2009b).

Some cases of VUR are associated with duplicated renal tracts: the lower ureter may be refluxing since it inserts laterally into the bladder. The upper moiety might be associated with an obstructed ureter that inserts into the bladder in a more distal position than normal, or inserts ectopically, for example into the urethra. Finally, some cases of VUR are secondary to other conditions, such as fetal bladder outflow obstruction from PUVs (Krishnan et al. 2006).

116.4.8.1 Postnatal Management

Three methods are currently used to identify VUR in children: X-ray voiding cystourethrography (VCUG), radionuclide voiding cystography, and echo-enhanced voiding urosonography (Novljan et al. 2003). Diagnosis of VUR is traditionally performed with serial VCUG scans. In young patients, US showed higher diagnostic accuracy than radionuclide cystography in assessing the grade of VUR (Ascenti et al. 2003). Normal US is rare with grade IV-V reflux, and moderate to severe hydronephrosis is rare with reflux grades <IV (Kovanlikaya et al. 2014).

Treatment goals include the prevention of pyelonephritis, reflux nephropathy, and other complications of reflux. Treatment alternatives include antibiotic prophylaxis and surgical correction (open, injection therapy, or laparoscopic) performed after the neonatal period (Fanos and Cataldi 2004), although the additional benefit of surgery over antibiotics alone is small at best (Hodson et al. 2007). The treatment of choice, with antibiotic prophylaxis and/or with surgery, needs to be discussed on an individual basis.

116.4.8.2 Prognosis

Surgery procedure (ureteral reimplantation or endoscopic correction) leads to similar renal outcomes as medical or supportive treatment. Generally, a congenitally damaged kidney does not ameliorate after each treatment. However, prenatal detection of VUR does not seem to modify the outcome of the kidney significantly (Zaffanello et al. 2008a). Despite treatment of affected children for the past 40 years, the incidence of end-stage renal disease secondary to VUR has not decreased (Craig et al. 2000). Thus, the association of VUR and renal failure may be caused by a genetic defect affecting both the formation of the kidney and the urinary tract (Murawski and Gupta 2006). High-grade (IV or V) vesicoureteral reflux presentation after urinary tract infection and female gender were important risk factors for breakthrough UTI (Hidas et al. 2015).

116.4.9 Ureteral Duplications and Ectopia

Ureteral duplications arise from one of two embryological anomalies: a single ureteric bud branching into two before reaching the metanephric mesoderm or two ureteric bud arising from the mesonephric duct and each individually reaching the metanephros to induce formation of two renal moieties.

Ectopia occurs when the ureteric bud arises from an abnormal position on the mesonephric duct. The site of origin of the ureteric bud determines whether the ectopic ureter opens into or outside the bladder. The latter occurs in females and the ectopic orifice is frequently associated with the genital tract.

Ureteroceles represent cystic dilatation of the submucosal part of the ureter. Ureteroceles may be associated with single systems but are more commonly seen in duplex systems (Joseph 2006).

116.4.9.1 Clinical Presentation

Prenatal US scans are capable of identifying most urinary tract abnormalities including duplications, ectopic ureters, and ureteroceles. Postnatally many infants may be completely asymptomatic and the diagnosis may be missed in the perinatal period if routine US scans are not available. They may also be associated with obstruction of the upper tracts causing hydronephrosis.

The common postnatal presentation includes UTIs, bladder outlet obstruction, and incontinence. Ureteroceles may prolapse through the urethra and present as a mass causing obstruction. Such cases may present with abdominal distension and palpable masses due to the dilated ureter and pelvicalyceal system. Ectopic ureters in males always insert proximal to the sphincter.

116.4.9.2 Diagnosis

US scan is usually the first line of investigation and will show up hydronephrosis, renal dysplasia, dilated ureters, ureteroceles, and indicate duplex systems. VCUG will demonstrate the presence of ureteroceles. Moreover, it will show reflux and dilated ureter or part of the duplex system. Radionuclide scan (DMSA) is the most useful for detecting duplex systems and providing an assessment of renal function. Endoscopy provides direct visualization of ureteroceles and some ectopic ureters. Contrast studies in retrograde fashion improve the delineation of the anatomy.

116.4.9.3 Management

Ectopic Ureters

If renal function is adequate, the procedure of choice is reimplantation of the ureter with single system ureters. In duplex systems, either reimplantation of both ureters or anastomosis to the lower moiety ureter as an uretero-ureterostomy may be required. Nephroureterectomy is advisable with absent or poor renal function in duplex system. Removal of the ureteric remnant can be mandatory when there is reflux into the ectopic ureter (Plaire et al. 1997).

Ureterocele

The initial management in the neonate is cystoscopic incision to provide drainage. Subsequently, the renal morphology and function can be assessed with follow-up US and DMSA scans. If these remain satisfactory and no UTIs occur, the patients do not require further surgical intervention (Merlini and Lelli 2004). Incomplete excision can leave a cuff of ureterocele at the bladder outlet that acts as a valve obstruction when the patient voids. Finally, complications are infections, obstruction, and nonfunction of the renal moiety requiring treatment by nephrectomy with complete excision of the ureterocele.

Ureteral Duplication

The most common congenital abnormality of the urinary tract is ureteric duplication. Many children with renal tract duplications remain asymptomatic and do not require surgical intervention. Therefore, ureteric duplication is frequently associated with other urinary tract anomalies. Duplex systems are prone to UTIs because of VUR or obstruction. Hydronephrosis in complete duplicated systems usually affects the upper pole and is mostly secondary to obstruction at the lower end of its ureter by an ureterocele or due to an ectopic ureteric insertion. Hydronephrosis of the lower segment is most often a result of VUR. Low-grade VUR in duplex system has an outcome similar to that of VUR in single system cases. Females with moderate or high-grade VUR and a duplex system should be treated differently because they present more often with complications (Afshar et al. 2005).

Obstruction at the level of the PUJ in duplex kidneys is rare (Horst and Smith 2008).

When symptoms occur in duplex system, surgical management is required (Whitten and Wilcox 2001). Duplications associated with poorly functioning renal moiety and complicated by UTIs should be treated by heminephroureterectomy. Duplications with preserved renal function but complicated by obstruction or infection should be treated by reimplantation of the ureter/ureters. All of the surgical procedures can be done laparoscopically with equally good results compared to open surgery. The ultimate goal of surgical intervention remains the elimination of complications associated with urinary tract abnormalities in the perinatal period and the preservation of renal function.

116.4.10 Anomalies of the Bladder

Bladder exstrophy is a complex anomaly involving the urinary, genital, and intestinal tracts and the musculoskeletal system. The severity ranges from simple epispadias to complete exstrophy of the cloaca involving exposure of the entire hindgut and the bladder. The diagnosis is made typically at the newborn examination or on fetal US that is performed by an experienced observer (Mourtzinos and Borer 2004). Exstrophy of the urinary bladder occurs about once in every 30,000–50,000 births, with male preponderance (Ben-Chaim et al. 1996).

116.4.10.1 Clinical Manifestations

Anomalies of the bladder are hypothesized to result when the mesoderm fails to invade the cephalad extension of the cloacal membrane; the extent of this failure determines the degree of the anomaly. In classic bladder exstrophy, the bladder protrudes from the abdominal wall and its mucosa is exposed. The umbilicus is displaced downward, the pubic rami are widely separated in the midline, and the rectus muscles are separated. In males, there is complete epispadias with dorsal chordee, and the overall penile length is approximately half that of unaffected boys (Ludwig et al. 2009). Undescended testes and inguinal hernias are common. Females also have epispadias, with separation of the two halves of the clitoris and wide separation of the labia. The anus is displaced anteriorly in both sexes, and there may be rectal prolapse. The pubic rami are widely separated.

Children with more complex cases of cloacal exstrophy associating with omphalocele, exstrophy of the cloaca, and imperforate anus had a prevalence of 1:200,000 live births. The real incidence is unknown since many cases are incorrectly diagnosed prenatally or these pregnancies are prematurely terminated (Martínez-Frías et al. 2001). However, other severe abnormalities of the colon and the rectum are present such as short bowel syndrome (Nepple et al. 2009), upper urinary tract anomaly, and spina bifida. Current reconstructive techniques result in a satisfactory outcome in most patients.

Epispadias is in the spectrum of exstrophy anomalies, affecting approximately 1 in 117,000 boys and 1 in 480,000 girls. Epispadias, classic bladder exstrophy, and cloacal exstrophy are causally related, representing a spectrum of the same developmental defect, with a small risk of recurrence within families (Gambhir et al. 2008). In boys, the diagnosis is obvious because the prepuce is distributed primarily on the ventral aspect of the penile shaft and the urethral meatus is on the dorsum of the penis. In girls, the clitoris is bifid and the urethra is split dorsally.

116.4.10.2 Treatment and Prognosis

Initially, the bladder should be covered with plastic wrap to keep the bladder mucosa moist. These individuals are prone to latex allergy, so latex precautions should be practiced in their care. Early bladder closure with reconstructive surgery can be applied to almost all neonates with classic bladder exstrophy. Conventional therapy has included a series of staged reconstructive procedures, but a single-stage complete reconstruction in the neonatal infant has gained popularity (Gargollo et al. 2008). Treatment should be deferred in selected situations when surgical therapy would be excessively risky or complex, such as in a premature baby or when it would have to be performed by inexperienced surgeons. Postoperatively, the infant's upper urinary tract is monitored closely for the possible development of hydronephrosis and infection. Most infants with bladder exstrophy have VUR and should receive antibiotic prophylaxis.

Children who undergo reconstructive surgery as newborns have a greater chance of obtaining a normally functioning bladder.

116.4.11 Anomalies of the Penis

Hypospadias is one of the most frequent genital malformations in the male newborn and results from an abnormal penile and urethral development; estimates of its prevalence range from 3–8 cases per 1000 male births (Carmichael et al. 2003). Hypospadias referring to an incomplete development of the prepuce, called a dorsal hood, in which the foreskin is on the sides and dorsal aspect of the penile shaft and absent ventrally. Hypospadias shows a genetic pattern especially in familial and syndromic forms and in forms due to abnormal genital development or associated with a defect of the androgens pathway (Kalfa et al. 2009).

116.4.11.1 Clinical Manifestations

Hypospadias is classified according to the position of the urethral meatus after taking into account whether chordee is present. The deformity is described as glanular (on the glans penis), coronal, subcoronal, midpenile, penoscrotal, scrotal, or perineal. In the most severe cases, the scrotum is bifid and sometimes extends to the dorsal base of the penis (Soomro and Neal 1998). Approximately 10% of boys with hypospadias have an undescended testis; inguinal hernias also are common (Leung and Robson 2004). In the newborn, the differential diagnosis of proximal hypospadias associated with an undescended testis should include forms of ambiguous genitalia, particularly female virilization (congenital adrenal hyperplasia) and mixed gonadal dysgenesis. A karyotype should be obtained in patients with midpenile or proximal hypospadias and cryptorchidism.

116.4.11.2 Treatment

Management begins in the newborn period. This malformation is usually corrected surgically when the infant is between 6 and 24 months. Whereas hypospadias repair is recommended for boys with midpenile and proximal hypospadias, some boys with distal hypospadias will have no functional abnormality and do not need any surgical correction.

116.5 Differential Diagnosis

Although histology provides the purest way of classifying renal tract malformations, renal biopsies are rarely performed in suspected cases of dysplastic or hypoplastic kidneys. Consequently, in clinical practice, most diagnoses of renal tract malformations are made on the basis of radiological investigations (Zagar et al. 2002).

116.5.1 Fetal Radiology

Prenatal diagnosis can identify either specific pathologies (MDK, duplex collecting system, renal agenesis, PKD) or nonspecific pathologies (hydronephrosis, ureteral dilatation, bladder enlargement and oligohydramnios, hyperechogenicity, enlarged kidneys, hypoplastic kidneys). US screening for fetal anomalies is becoming routine and abnormally shaped bladders from midway through gestation (Wiesel et al. 2005). The finding of a renal tract malformation during antenatal screening leads to careful evaluation of the rest of the fetus. In some cases, other organ systems are found to be malformed, which can indicate the presence of a particular syndrome (Ickowicz et al. 2006).

MRI contribution to the analysis of urinary tract abnormalities is far less well-developed, although this method has proven useful in small series (Poutamo et al. 2000; Cassart et al. 2004; Hawkins et al. 2008). With regard to nephropathy, the potential contribution of MRI is not currently well-defined and US examination is still the major imaging tool, despite its usefulness in cases with inconclusive sonographic findings (maternal obesity and/or oligohydramnios).

116.5.1.1 Fetal Renal Pelvis Dilatation

Fetal renal pelvis dilatation is a frequent abnormality that has been observed in 4.5% of pregnancies (Ismaili et al. 2003). The fetal kidneys can be easily visualized on US scans at 12 weeks. After 16 weeks, fetal urine production becomes the primary source of amniotic fluid (Pates and Dashe 2006). US provides the opportunity to diagnose upper tract obstruction based on measurements of the renal pelvic APD. Measurements of 3 mm or less are considered normal at any gestational age. It is generally accepted that a fetal renal pelvic diameter greater than 10 mm at 26 weeks gestation is indicative of significant dilatation. In particular, fetal renal dilatation after 23 weeks can be used to predict obstructive uropathy, especially if the renal pelvic diameter continues to increase throughout pregnancy (Anderson et al. 1997). The threshold for the diagnosis of abnormal fetal renal pelvis dilatation is significantly higher among pediatric urologists than nephrologists.

Postnatal renal pelvis dilatation is considered abnormal if the APD was 11 ± 1.9 mm by the pediatric urologists and 9 ± 2.9 mm by the pediatric nephrologists (Ismaili et al. 2004b). The third trimester threshold value for renal pelvis APD of 7 mm is beyond any doubt the best prenatal criterion both for the screening of urinary tract dilatation and for the selection of patients needing postnatal investigation. In cases where only a second-trimester fetal examination is performed, a 4 mm threshold value for pelvis APD should be used as a warning sign because this finding may reveal a significant urologic abnormality in 12% of cases (Ismaili et al. 2004a). Hydronephrosis has an association with aneuploidy and is a component of several well-described syndromes if associated with other organ system (VACTERL association).

The risk for trisomy 21 is approximately 1.5 times the patient's background risk (Wickstrom et al. 1996).

VUR is diagnosed in 9–15% of infants with prenatally detected hydronephrosis and persistent postnatal hydronephrosis with VCUG performed during the first week of life. Prenatally detected VUR is more frequent in boys and is associated with poorly functioning kidneys in 15–30% of infants without a previous history of UTI (Penido Silva et al. 2006).

116.5.1.2 Renal Agenesis

Diagnosis of renal agenesis can be complicated when the fetal adrenal gland occupies the empty renal bed, since the adrenal gland can mimic a kidney in US scans.

116.5.1.3 Dysplastic Kidney

MDK and severely hydronephrotic kidneys appear as collections of hypoechogenic spaces. These spaces are noncommunicating with the renal pelvis in multicystic disease and communicate in hydronephrotic ones. Moreover, increased echogenicity in variably enlarged fetal or neonatal kidneys is a nonspecific finding associated with polycystic and cystic dysplastic kidneys (Tsatsaris et al. 2002).

116.5.1.4 Posterior Urethral Valves

PUVs are characterized by variably enlarged, thick-walled urinary bladders and a dilated anterior urethra, both of which findings are highly variable and not specific for the condition (Abbott et al. 1998). Other entities, such as urethral atresia and prune belly syndrome, can mimic the radiological appearance of PUVs. Prune belly syndrome involves severe dilatation of the lower renal tract in the absence of overt anatomical obstruction, in association with deficiency of the abdominal wall musculature and cryptorchidism (Bogart et al. 2006).

116.5.1.5 Polycystic Kidney Disease

In PKD, the US prenatal screening report unspecific hyperechogenic kidneys. Therefore, fetal MRI is not disadvantaged by a lack of amniotic fluid and, in addition to renal analysis, can be used to look for pulmonary hypoplasia or associated brain malformations. Fetal MRI images with high resolution allow the visualization of cysts in cases of ARPKD (Cassart et al. 2004; Liu et al. 2006). In particular, fetal MRI appearance of ARPKD has been described as increased renal signal intensity on T2-weighted images (Nishi 1995), whereas low renal signal intensity is observed on T1-weighted images because of high water content in the renal parenchyma, consistent with tiny renal cysts. RAREMR urography can be used to show directly the microcystic dilatation of collecting ducts (Kern et al. 2000).

116.5.2 Postnatal Radiology

Generally, postnatal neonatal radiology includes US, CT, and MRI. Considering the immaturity of nephrons in newborns, the usual recommendation is that renography would be delayed until the age of 4 weeks (Boubaker et al. 2006).

Scintigraphy helps establish correct and accurate diagnosis in most congenital renal anomalies, indicates the current functional state of the individual kidneys, provides prognostic information, and can be used for decisions about intervention (Sfakianakis and Sfakianaki 2001).

116.5.2.1 Hydronephrosis

The objectives of postnatal evaluation are to confirm hydronephrosis and then to determine its cause and to assess renal function. Neonatal urine generation can take a few days to be fully established. Hydronephrosis can be missed in cases of urinary flow obstruction if US scanning is performed too soon. Remarkably, the first postnatal US study is usually performed during the first week after birth, depending on the severity of the prenatal findings, but not during the first 72 h because of reduced urine output after delivery. Hydronephrosis does not generally represent a surgical emergency in the newborn. Most infants probably do not need surgery. The decision should be taken only on the basis of at least two evaluations demonstrating either a progressive increase in dilatation or a progressive reduction in glomerular filtrate. Normal appearing urinary tracts on two successive neonatal US rarely coexist with abnormal findings at VCUG (Ismaili et al. 2005). Unilateral hydronephrosis is generally considered a benign condition that rarely leads to renal failure. Follow-up would appear to be mandatory in all patients, even over lengthy periods. Prenatal renal pelvic dilatation correlates with obstruction, and 15 mm maximum dilatation appears to be the most accurate predictor of postnatal obstruction (Coplen et al. 2006). Severe renal pelvic dilatation was defined as an APD of 15 mm, mild and moderate dilatation was defined as 6 to <10 mm and 10 to <15 mm, respectively (Kumar et al. 2012). Bilateral hydronephrosis requires prompt evaluation by US and VCUG, especially in boys, in order not to miss PUVs (Woodward and Frank 2002; de Bruyn and Marks 2008).

116.5.2.2 Dysplastic Kidneys

MDKs often regress at US in the first few postnatal years (Belk et al. 2002). Therefore, it is infrequent that kidney remnant remains below the limit of radiological detection. Moreover, involution of noncystic dysplastic kidneys can also occur (Hiraoka et al. 2002; Winyard et al. 1996). In a child with a CSFK, it is difficult to distinguish either unilateral renal agenesis or aplasia from a regressed dysplastic kidney unless prenatal data are available. Large cysts replacing kidney parenchyma and lack of central pelvis or tiny remnant kidney characterize MDK. Cystic dysplastic kidneys have echobright kidney, echobright kidney with cysts, and poor corticomedullary differentiation (González Celedón et al. 2007). Renal agenesis and MDK commonly affect only one renal tract, although the contralateral tracts have an increased incidence of PUJO and primary VUR (Woolf and Hillman 2007; Woolf 2006). ARPKD have bright kidney, echobright, large kidney with small cysts. ADPKD have large, bright kidney, sometimes with cysts that increase in size and number with age.

116.5.2.3 Renal Agenesis and Hypoplasia

Renal agenesis or aplasia is characterized by absent kidney at fetal US (adrenal gland might be mistaken for kidney). In CSFK, the kidney might be larger than normal, whereas it is hypoplastic when small kidney at US (Heymans et al. 1998). Some excretory functional compensation occurs postnatally in humans with bilateral dysplastic or hypoplastic kidneys. Distinguishing between dysplastic remnants and aplastic kidneys can be clinically relevant, because dysplastic remnants can sometimes drive hypertension (Webb et al. 1997). Not all small kidneys, detectable by US and DMSA scintigraphy, may be caused by developmental malformations. Moreover, neonatal renal vein thrombosis (Winyard et al. 2006) or severe renal artery stenosis can all damage a normal kidney, resulting in a small organ (Gandy et al. 2007).

116.5.2.4 Vesicoureteral Reflux

VUR is the main risk factor for nephropathy (Lambert et al. 2011). The histological finding of dysplastic changes was reported in some poorly functioning kidneys attached to ureters with primary VUR (Risdon et al. 1993). Some of the babies with VUR, especially the boys, showed parenchymal defects, without history of UTIs (Yeung et al. 1997). In these subjects, the scarring associated with primary VUR was related as congenital kidney malformations. On the other hand, in girls, renal parenchymal changes associated with primary VUR were more commonly associated with a history of UTIs (Chen et al. 2004).

Scintigraphy with DMSA scan is currently used to detect nephropathy from VUR since concentrates only in functioning tubules. The DMSA scintigraphy may detect focal parenchymal defects that in most cases occur transiently after acute pyelonephritis but that resolve over 3–12 months (Hoberman et al. 2003). To screen high-grade VUR in young infants with febrile UTI, US and acute DMSA scan could be performed first. VCUG is only indicating when abnormalities are apparent on either US or DMSA scan or both (Tsai et al. 2012).

116.5.2.5 Posterior Urethral Valves

PUVs are diagnosed by VCUG or cystoscopy revealing an obstruction at the urethral level in males (Fig. 3). VCUG can reveal the presence, grade, and position of the VUR. In addition, dynamic radioisotope renography MAG3 can

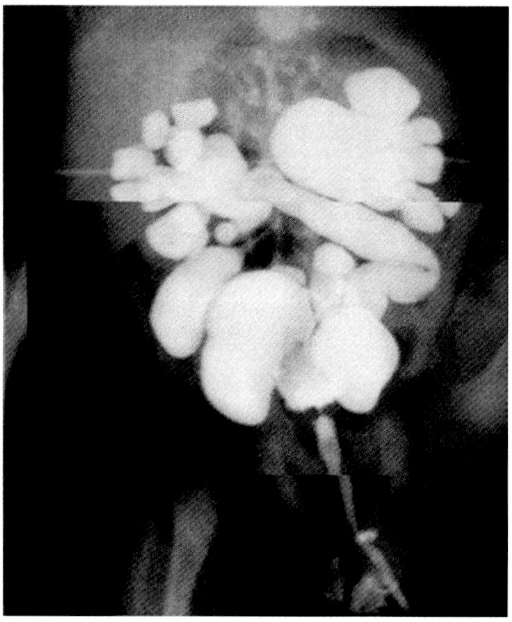

Fig. 3 Voiding cystoureterogram in a baby with posterior urethral valves

provide information about the flow of urine. Drainage from a very-dilated upper tract might be slower than normal even if there is no anatomical obstruction.

116.6 Prognosis

116.6.1 Antenatal Hydronephrosis

Children with any degree of antenatal hydronephrosis are at greater risk of postnatal pathology as compared with the normal population. Favorable prognosis in children with antenatal hydronephrosis is related with monolateral pathology, such as renal agenesis or MDK, late obstruction, and renal pelvis dilation. These forms are associated with normal amniotic fluid and normal lung development and the risk of renal failure in childhood is minimal (Woolf and Hillman 2007; Woolf and Jenkins 2006). Although prenatal hydronephrosis has good prognosis, it raises the risk of hospitalization for pyelonephritis in infancy (Walsh et al. 2007). There was a significant increase in risk of pathology per increasing degree of hydronephrosis. The risk of any postnatal pathology per degree of antenatal hydronephrosis was 11.9% for mild, 45.1% for moderate, and 88.3% for severe (Lee et al. 2006). Spontaneous resolution of idiopathic prenatal hydronephrosis occurs in most cases when the renal pelvic APD is less than 12 mm but is less frequent when dilatation is greater than 12 mm (Sidhu et al. 2006). Low-grade hydronephrosis diagnosed within the first year of life remains stable or improves in 97.4% of renal units (Madden-Fuentes et al. 2014). Of the mild/moderate cases of RPD, 5% progressed to severe dilatation. An obstructive cause is usually present in severe cases, which are more likely to require surgery if there is PUJO (Kumar et al. 2012).

116.6.2 Renal Agenesis and Dysplasia

Nonfavorable renal prognosis is related to bilateral pathology, such as bilateral agenesis, bilateral MDK, early urethral obstruction (PUVs). Generally, these forms are associated with oligohydramnios and abnormal lung development. The renal functional outcomes in children with bilateral renal pathology are worse than those in children with uncomplicated unilateral disease (Feldenberg and Siegel 2000), and decreased glomerular filtration rate (GFR) at presentation predicts progression to renal failure during childhood (González Celedón et al. 2007). On follow-up, unobstructed and obstructed dysplastic or hypoplastic kidneys together account for about 40% of all children on renal replacement therapy. Dysplastic or hypoplastic kidneys are 10 times more common than PKD in children with renal replacement therapy (Kerecuk et al. 2008).

116.6.3 Vesicoureteral Reflux

The risk of VUR was similar for all degrees of antenatal hydronephrosis (Lee et al. 2006). In most infants with VUR, the reflux is of low grade and resolves rapidly. Reflux resolved spontaneously in 56% of cases at the 12-month follow-up and 72% at the 24-month follow-up. In those children with high-grade VUR, spontaneous resolution is rare at age 2 years. High-grade VUR had complete resolution of reflux in 9% at 12 months and 18% at 24 months (Ismaili et al. 2006). The outcome of severely refluxing renal units was similar after medical treatment or surgical correction. Finally, prenatal and postnatal diagnosis of hydronephrosis from VUR did not seem to modify the renal outcome at follow-up (Zaffanello et al. 2008a).

116.6.4 Pyeloureteral Junction Obstruction

A prospective study on unilateral congenital PUJO showed that in kidneys with good function, followed conservatively, about a quarter underwent pyeloplasty because of an observed decrease in function (Ransley et al. 1990). Obstructed kidneys may undergo stabilization or a relative reduction of the scintigraphic renal function than the unaffected contralateral kidney (Zaffanello et al. 2008b). In this latter case, failure of the pyeloplasty could be due to underlying concomitant congenital renal dysplasia.

116.6.5 Posterior Urethral Valves

For several decades in newborns with PUVs, it has been technically feasible to decompress fetal bladders affected by outflow obstruction by use of vesicoamniotic shunts. Unfortunately, no clear improvement in renal outcomes with such interventions has been shown, but only weak evidence that perinatal survival increased (Clark et al. 2003). Although fetal intervention has the capacity to reduce neonatal mortality from pulmonary hypoplasia, increased survival of infants with severe renal dysplasia is destined to progress rapidly into ESRF.

116.7 Overview of Treatment Options

The most severe types of malformations, such as bilateral renal agenesis or dysplasia, although rare, lead to renal failure. With advances in dialysis and transplantation for young children, it is now possible to prevent the early death of at least some individuals with severe malformations. Now intervention could be either prenatal or postnatal for some disease. Treatment options for specific diseases are discussed in the related sections.

116.7.1 Fetal Intervention

Therapeutic termination of pregnancy is often undertaken if a fetus has severe renal tract malformations (Wiesel et al. 2005). The main factor that leads to the decision to terminate is poor renal function and/or severe bladder outflow obstruction, which is manifested by reduced amniotic fluid, sometimes leading to impaired lung growth (oligohydramnios sequence or Potter's syndrome). However, some fetuses are found to have anomalies in other organ systems (e.g., brain, heart, or gut), which are sometimes accompanied by gross chromosomal aberrations, such as trisomies (Ariel et al. 1991). With advances in dialysis for young babies and renal transplantation for young children (Kari et al. 2000), termination might not always be necessary (Klaassen et al. 2007). In a case report, serial amnioinfusion appears to have mitigated the severe pulmonary compromise that has, in the past, led to the death of newborns with bilateral renal agenesis (Bienstock et al. 2014).

The long-term outcomes for children born with PUVs remain poor, with some dying perinatally of lung hypoplasia and respiratory failure, and a significant subset of survivors going into severe renal failure within the next two decades of life (Clark et al. 2003; Ylinen et al. 2004b). Even if infants with PUVs undergo bladder decompression, the risk of developing ESRF rises with increasing age (Neild et al. 2004). The long-term protection of kidney function from PUVs with prenatal surgical decompression aimed to slow the progression of renal failure needs to be established as well (Woolf 2008).

Therefore, prenatal diagnosis may have made an important, although numerically small, contribution to reducing the risk of renal failure in significant obstruction or high-grade reflux in a solitary functioning kidney.

116.7.2 Postnatal Therapies

The association between chronic pyelonephritis and VUR in childhood suggested an active treatment of individuals born with primary VUR to minimize kidney damage. The treatment options for specific disease are discussed in each section. The postnatal therapeutic options include surgery for obstructed kidneys and severely refluxing kidneys that are rarely performed before the first month of life and antimicrobial prophylaxis to treat and prevent infective complications.

116.7.3 Nonobstructed Hydronephrosis

Early correction of VUR in neonatal period is not performed since most of VUR resolve spontaneously. Few data support the primacy of either long-term antibiotic therapy or antireflux surgery for renoprotection (Fanos and Cataldi 2004; Wheeler et al. 2004). The era of active therapy has not reduced the incidence of end-stage renal disease (ESRD) that occurs as a result of reflux nephropathy, which accords with the concept that reflux nephropathy is often caused by dysplasia or hypoplasia rather than by pyelonephritic damage (Hodson et al. 2007). Finally, after postnatal ages the initiation of therapies such as with prophylactic antibiotics, to prevent UTIs (Montini et al. 2008) or angiotensin blockade for reflux nephropathy (Zaffanello et al. 2008c), may be indicated in selected cases to improve the long-term renal outcomes.

116.7.4 Urinary Tract Obstruction

Rapid decline of the renal function related to severe obstruction, such as in newborns with solitary kidney, needs to be discussed for early surgical intervention with an expert pediatric urologist, as well as for early postnatal ablation of the urethral valves in newborns since early ablation and bladder management gave a better outcome (Sudarsanan et al. 2009). Long-term results of prenatally detected PUVs confirm that early valve ablation can be considered as the primary treatment in the majority of patients, without the need for preoperative drainage or diversion. Gestational age at diagnosis and volume of amniotic fluid are significant predictors of postnatal renal outcome (Sarhan et al. 2008). Moreover, in low birth weight neonates, primary valve ablation by a visually guided Fogarty catheter gave effective disruption of the valvular obstructive mechanism (Soliman 2009).

116.8 Laboratory Management of Kidney Diseases

Laboratory management of renal function is usually performed by urinalysis as well as by determining blood urea nitrogen (BUN) and serum creatinine for the estimation of the glomerular filtration rate (GFR). This traditional strategy, which has existed for more than 100 years, seems no longer to meet the demands to detect and exclude renal lesions in early and treatable states, especially in the neonatal age (Hofmann et al. 1994). The most important factor appears to be the renal functional reserve that masks renal degeneration, as assessed by GFR, BUN, and creatinine, up to the point where over 75% of the functioning nephrons have been lost. It should be stressed that these factors measure incipient renal failure and in most cases, the finding of normal results does not mean the absence of renal dysfunction. In addition, tubular proteinuria, which reflects tubulotoxic and tubulointerstitial diseases, is likewise not detected by the protein test strip. Therefore, there is a growing demand for clinically convenient and reliable markers of renal function.

116.8.1 Biomarkers in Pediatric and Neonatal Nephrology

The widespread availability of enabling technologies such as functional genomics and proteomics has accelerated the rate of novel biomarker discovery and therapeutic targets for kidney diseases (Hortin and Sviridov 2007). The advent of the microarray, or cDNA chip, allows investigators to search through thousands of genes simultaneously, making the process very efficient. Such gene expression profiling studies have identified several genes whose protein products have emerged as chronic kidney disease (CKD) and acute kidney injury (AKI) biomarkers. However, microarray-based methods cannot be used for the direct analysis of biological fluids and usually require downstream confirmation by proteomic techniques prior to clinical use. Proteomics is the study of both the structure and function of proteins by a variety of methods, such as gel electrophoresis, immunoblotting, mass spectrometry, and enzymatic or metabolic assays. Each method is used to determine different types of information and has its own set of strengths and limitations. Advancing technologies have radically improved the speed and precision of identifying and measuring proteins in biological fluids, and proteomic approaches are also beginning to yield novel and noninvasive biomarkers for assessing kidney damage. Urinary proteins include soluble proteins and protein components of solid phase elements of urine (Table 4). Solid phase elements consist of sediments that can be precipitated at low centrifugation speeds and exosomes that are of very low density and sediment only with ultracentrifugation. Prefractionation of these components can be useful as a means of enriching for markers of particular types of disease. A study of urine collected from normal human adult subjects indicated that, of the total urinary protein excreted, ~48% was in sediments, 49% was soluble, and the remaining 3% was in exosomes (Zhou et al. 2006).

Table 4 Sources of urinary proteins

Sources of urinary proteins	Comments
1. Soluble proteins	
a. Glomerular filtration of plasma proteins	Normally present (< 150 mg/day)
	Defects in glomerular filter increase high molecular weight protein (e.g., albumin) excretion
	Defects in proximal tubule reabsorption or abnormal production of low molecular weight plasma proteins increase low molecular weight protein (e.g., 2-microglobulin, immunoglobulin light chains, retinol-binding protein, and amino acids) excretion
b. Epithelial cell secretion of soluble proteins	Via exocytosis (e.g., epidermal growth factor) or glycosylphosphatidylinositol-anchored protein detachment (e.g., Tamm-Horsfall protein)
2. Solid phase components	
a. Epithelial cells	
Whole cell shedding	Increased cell number compatible with several diseases including acute tubular necrosis (e.g., renal tubule cell shedding) and glomerular diseases (e.g., podocyte shedding)
Plasma membrane and intracellular component shedding	Could be due to nonspecific, nephrotoxic, or apoptotic processes
Exosome secretion	Normal process
b. Other cells	In certain diseases, red blood cells, white blood cells, or tumor cells (e.g., bladder cancer and lymphoma) can be present in urine

Modified from (Pisitkun et al. 2006)

Some of the soluble proteins in urine originate as membrane-bound proteins that are proteolytically cleaved from their membrane attachments. One of these is Tamm-Horsfall protein (uromodulin), an abundant soluble urinary protein that is secreted by the thick ascending limb of Henle loop, a nephron segment downstream from the proximal tubule (Serafini-Cessi et al. 2003). It originates as a glycosylphosphatidylinositol-linked protein present in the apical plasma membrane that can be cleaved from its cell attachment proteolytically.

116.8.2 Markers for Assessing Glomerular Filtration Rate

Serum creatinine concentration and endogenous creatinine clearance have been used for such a long time to assess glomerular filtration rate (GFR); nevertheless, serum creatinine has a limited diagnostic value, because this marker shows no response until the GFR is reduced by approximately 40% (Rule et al. 2004). Creatinine clearance is affected by inaccuracies in quantitatively collecting urine and by the renal tubular secretion of creatinine, which would falsely elevate the apparent GFR (National Kidney Foundation 2002). Moreover, proteins and substances with a ketone group are known to interfere in the Jaffe (alkaline picrate) reaction for the measurement of creatinine in serum and urine; this prevents the measurement of the true concentration of creatinine (Miller et al. 2005). Finally there is a lack of availability of pediatric creatinine serum standards referenced to an isotope dilution mass spectrometry method (Panteghini and Division 2008).

Because serum creatinine concentration is influenced by both the production rate and the excretion rate, the nephrology community concluded that results should be interpreted in light of the expected rate of production of creatinine. Thus, equations based on serum creatinine are more accurate and precise than serum creatinine alone for estimating GFR (*e*GFR), as recommended by the clinical practice guidelines for CKD in children (Hogg et al. 2003). Estimating equations include variables such as sex, age, body size, and ethnicity in addition to serum creatinine, as surrogates for muscle mass. Equations have the advantage of providing an estimate of GFR which empirically combines all of these average effects while allowing for the marked differences in creatinine production between individuals (Stevens et al. 2006). Clinical laboratories should report an estimate of GFR using a prediction equation, in addition to reporting the serum creatinine measurement (Levey et al. 2006). Two of the common formulas used for adults are the Cockcroft Gault and the Modification of Diet in Renal Disease (MDRD) formulas, but these are not appropriate for use in children and babies (Levey et al. 1999). In the newborn and in the early infancy, the most widely used estimate of GFR is the original Schwartz equation (Schwartz et al. 1976); based on serum creatinine (SCr), height, and an empirical age-related constant k, this equation was firstly devised in the mid-1970s. It has been successful because it relates GFR to (patient's height)/(SCr) rather than to 1/(SCr). Although simple to use, the Schwartz formula may give biased and imprecise eGFR, unless the values of k are derived from local estimates of mean height, GFR, and SCr. When locally derived estimates of k are used, the bias decreases substantially but the precision of *e*GFR remains poor. In addition, the Schwartz equation assumes that there is no intercept associated with the relationship of GFR versus height/SCr which, if incorrect, could lead to more biased *e*GFR and to incorrect values for the slope, k. It remains unknown whether a less biased and more precise estimation of GFR can be achieved using regression to determine the relation between GFR and height/SCr in a local population, rather than substituting variables and computing mean k (Zappitelli et al. 2007). Finally, pediatricians need to recognize that the formula requires updating when analytically specific methods of measuring serum creatinine, such as enzymatic assays, are used in their institutions (Panteghini et al. 2006).

The accuracy of the *e*GFR is important for the early detection of CKD in adults, children, and newborns, as has been recognized in the recent awareness campaigns in the European Union and in the United States (www.NKDEP.nih.gov). An early detection of changes in GFR leads to an early appropriate treatment options, such as weight loss, exercise, or blood pressure control, especially with angiotensin-converting enzyme (ACE) inhibitors, slowing or even halting progression of renal injury and/or dysfunction. Because serum creatinine concentration and the *e*GFR are interrelated, the performance of the creatinine analysis affects GFR estimates (Levey et al. 2007). The Laboratory Working Group of the National Kidney Disease Education Program (NKDEP), in collaboration with international professional organizations, has developed a plan that enables standardization and improved accuracy (trueness) of serum creatinine measurements in clinical laboratories worldwide. The Working Group developed a report in the United States, reviewing the information on the nonspecificity of routine creatinine methods and recommended that manufacturers of in vitro diagnostics address and reduce the influence of interfering substances in patient samples (Myers et al. 2006). Two serum pools with creatinine concentrations within the pediatric reference interval were spiked with albumin, IgG, unconjugated bilirubin, adult hemoglobin (HbA), and fetal hemoglobin (HbF) to produce one unspiked and five spiked samples per pool. Albumin, IgG, and fetal hemoglobin (HbF) interfered with Jaffe creatinine assays, leading to inaccuracies in *e*GFRs that are clinically important, especially in children and neonates. In particular, albumin interference leads to a GFR underestimation ranging from 17% to 27%, while HbF interference to a GFR overestimation ranging from 24% to 60%. Because protein error and HbF interference do not occur with any of the enzymatic methods tested, the authors conclude that enzymatic creatinine methods are preferred for evaluation of kidney function in pediatric cases. The more recent enzymatic creatinine method results in lower determinations compared with the older Jaffe method, even when the latter was improved with a dialysis step and elimination of interfering samples (Ceriotti et al. 2008).

In 2009, Schwartz proposed a new formula for calculating *e*GFR in children with CKD (Schwartz et al. 2009). The new equation includes serum creatinine, measured by an enzymatic analytical method, cystatin C, and BUN together with an accurate height measurement. Based on a carefully described, prospectively recruited cohort of children with various types of kidney diseases that have compromised function, the results seem to provide a more accurate, noninvasive method of estimating the GFR in the pediatric and neonatal age. This formula yielded 87.7% of *e*GFR within 30% of the GFR assessed by iohexol plasma disappearance and 45.6% within 10%. This new equation permits to improve the adjustment of drug dosing and can be used as a research tool. But it can also be used clinically as a confirmatory screening tool for children with impaired renal function and to determine whether CKD in children is stable or progressing. Unfortunately, it cannot yet be used as a general screening tool, since it has not yet been verified in a cohort of children with normal renal function.

Taking into account the extreme importance of the accuracy in the measurement of serum creatinine when creatinine-based equation is used to estimate GFR (Harmon 2009), the National Disease Education Program (NKDEP) has developed several recommendations for the improvement and development of creatinine assays (Myers et al. 2006). These recommendations include optimizing creatinine assays to provide accurate (traceable to MS-IDMS) and precise measurements (imprecision goal of approximately 8% to meet the maximum 10% impact on *e*GFR) particularly at a concentration of 1.00 mg/dL, revising GFR-estimating equations based on more accurate methods, and introducing proficiency testing programs that use commutable serum materials with target values traceable to Mass Spectrometry Isotope Dilution (MS-IDMS) procedure (Dodder et al. 2007). The National Institute for Standards and Technology has developed a reference material at concentrations of approximately 0.80 and 4.00 mg/dL to help manufacturers in the standardization of creatinine assays (Bunk 2007).

116.8.3 Low Molecular Mass Proteins

Over the past 20 years, interest has been shown in the diagnostic power of low molecular mass proteins (low-M_r proteins) in serum and urine for the evaluation of renal function. These proteins are freely filtered through the capillary wall, then reabsorbed and catabolized in the proximal tubular cells. Thus, if the GFR in the kidney is reduced, the serum concentrations of low-M_r proteins increase and may be taken as suitable markers of GFR (Tomlinson et al. 1997). On the other hand, if the tubular reabsorption capacity is reduced, or if tubular cells have been damaged by nephrotoxic drugs or agents, the urinary excretion of these proteins increase and may be taken as suitable index of renal tubular impairment and dysfunction (Guder and Hofmann 1992). In the normal kidney, the reabsorption of low-M_r proteins by proximal tubular cells is nearly complete so that only trace amounts of these proteins are excreted in urine (approximately 0.1 mg/24 h). As a corollary, low-M_r proteins in urine are very sensitive markers of impaired proximal tubular function. The urinary excretion of low-M_r proteins reflects the reabsorptive capacity of proximal tubules when the GFR is normal or only slightly abnormal. Herget-Rosenthal has measured urinary excretion of a number of candidate low-M_r proteins, such as α_1-microglobulin (protein HC), β_2-microglobulin, cystatin C, retinol-binding protein, α-glutathione *S*-transferase, lactate dehydrogenase, and *N*-acetyl-β-(D)-glucosaminidase, early in the course of nonoliguric acute renal failure in humans (Herget-Rosenthal et al. 2004). In this cohort of patients with established acute renal failure (ARF) from a variety of causes, urinary excretion of α_1-microglobulin and cystatin C were found to be predictive of severe ARF requiring renal replacement therapy, with an area under characteristic curve (AUC) of 0.86 and 0.92, respectively. α_1-Microglobulin is a tubular protein that belongs to the lipocalin superfamily, while cystatin C is a cysteine protease inhibitor that is synthesized and released into the blood at a relatively constant rate by all nucleated cells. Both α_1-microglobulin and cystatin C are stable in the urine (Donaldson et al. 1989) and can be easily measured by immunonephelometric methods in most standard clinical chemistry laboratories. The predictive role of these urinary proteins in early AKI remains to be determined.

116.8.4 Cystatin C

Cystatin C is a nonglycosylated 13 kDa basic protein that acts as a cysteine proteinase inhibitor and is produced at a relatively constant rate. This constancy is apparently not influenced by the presence of inflammatory conditions, muscle mass, gender, body composition, and age after 12 months (Bökenkamp et al. 1998). Blood cystatin C level is approximately 1 mg/L in healthy individuals of age > 1 year, while in the neonatal age and in the early infancy, blood cystatin C is significantly higher (Harmoinen et al. 2000). Cystatin C is catabolized and almost completely reabsorbed by renal proximal tubular cells, so that a very small amount is excreted in the urine (Tenstad et al. 1996) and cannot be used to calculate a clearance GFR. Interindividual variation of cystatin C level is significantly less (25%) than that of creatinine (93%) (Keevil et al. 1998). The upper limit of the population reference interval for cystatin C is seldom more than 3–4 standard deviations (SD) from the mean value of any healthy individual (compared with 13 SD for creatinine). These findings suggest that cystatin C is potentially a better marker than creatinine for detecting impaired renal function. From a number of clinical studies on cystatin C, two key findings are evident. First, the concentration of serum cystatin C correlated better with directly measured values for GFR than did serum creatinine. Second, subtle decrements in GFR are more readily detected by the determination of serum cystatin C than by creatinine concentration (Mussap and Plebani 2004). Thus, while cystatin C is not a conventional marker of GFR, reciprocal values of serum cystatin C levels are reasonably well correlated with GFR in adults (Christensson et al. 2003) and in children (Filler and Lepage 2003). Some studies have suggested that the serum concentration of cystatin C might be superior to serum creatinine in distinguishing normal from abnormal GFR (Laterza et al. 2002). However, because it is metabolized and not excreted, cystatin C cannot be used to measure GFR by standard urinary clearance techniques (Schwartz and Furth 2007). Nevertheless, serum cystatin can be used to estimate GFR in milliliters per minute per 1.73 square meters according to the following formula: $\log_{10}(\text{GFR}) = 1.962 + [1.123 * \log_{10}(1/\text{cysC})]$, where cysC is cystatin C (Filler et al. 1999). Additional formulae using both cystatin C and creatinine to estimate GFR have recently been reported. Such studies have shown that plasma cystatin C is slightly better than plasma creatinine in diagnosing renal insufficiency but is less sensitive than creatinine clearance or *e*GFR (from *k* * L/Pcr) (Martini et al. 2003).

116.8.5 Albumin in Urine and Kidney Disease

The appearance of albumin in the urine has long been recognized as a cardinal feature of kidney disease and more recently has been shown to also be an independent cardiovascular risk factor associated with insulin resistance. Normal human urine contains only very small quantities of albumin, less than 30 mg/d. In a position statement published in 2003, the National Kidney Foundation and the National Institute of Diabetes and Digestive and Kidney Diseases recommend a spot, untimed urine specimen be used for measurement of urinary albumin (Eknoyan et al. 2003). Using the ratio of urine albumin to urine creatinine, microalbuminuria is defined as a level of 30–300 mg albumin/g creatinine (Assadi 2002).

Urine albumin has traditionally been screened in the office setting by use of a variety of semiquantitative dipsticks. These tests involve wetting a chemically impregnated test strip with urine. Some commercial dipsticks detect microalbuminuria by albumin binding to a sulfonephthalein dye, which produces a color reaction that is read reflectometrically in a portable urine chemistry analyzer. Comparisons of this dipstick to reference laboratory tests have shown that the sensitivity ranges from 79% to 95.4% and that the specificity ranges from 73% to 81% (Meinhardt et al. 2003). Other commercial dipsticks detect albumin by a different chemical method: albumin passes via a wick fleece into a conjugate fleece, where it binds to specific, gold-labeled antibodies, and then flows to a detection pad (Parsons et al. 1999). A chemical reaction in the detection pad produces a color that is compared visually with color blocks. Comparisons of this test to reference laboratory results have shown that the sensitivity ranges from 93% to 97.1% and the specificity ranges from 33.3% to 81% (Mogensen et al. 1997).

Quantitative measurement of urine albumin is traditionally based on three laboratory methods: immunonephelometry, immunoturbidimetry, and radioimmunoassay (RIA). The performance characteristics of these methods are listed in Table 5. Conventional immunoassays suggest that normal humans would only excrete less than 30 mg/d of albumin, whereas the amount of albumin-derived material excreted may range from 1 to 3 g/d (Greive et al. 2001). These studies demonstrate that a considerable amount of peptide-derived low molecular weight fragments is commonly excreted in urine of healthy subjects. The degradation process occurs in tubular epithelial cells, where albumin is endocytosed and trafficked to lysosomes. Once degraded, albumin is exocytosed into the tubular lumen and excreted in urine. The degradation products are exclusively found in urine and they never return in blood stream. This technique is likely to provide new information as a diagnostic tool because changes in the peptide profile, or fingerprint, can reflect renal disease and possibly other diseases, such as cancer.

Table 5 Performances of the most common analytical methods for the measurement of microalbuminuria

Analytical method reproducibility (CV, %)	Interassay	Detection limit
Radioimmunoassay (RIA)	9.2% at 12.2 mg/L	16 μg/L
	4.8% at 33.0 mg/L	(0.016 mg/L)
Immunonephelometry	4.2% at 12.1 mg/L	2 mg/L
(Beckman Array Analyzer)	5.3% at 45.0 mg/L	
Immunoturbidimetry	4.1% at 10.6 mg/L	6 mg/L
(Siemens Turbitimer)	2.2% at 43.2 mg/L	
	4.2% at 77.9 mg/L	
Immunoturbidimetry	8.5% at 8.0 mg/L	6 mg/L
(Siemens Dimension RxL)	3.4% at 35.0 mg/L	
HPLC	2.4% at 95.8 mg/L	2 mg/L

Modified from (Comper and Osicka 2005)

116.8.6 Novel Markers for Kidney Ischemia, Hypoxia, and Drug-Induced Toxicity

Proteomic approaches have recently yielded additional biomarkers for acute kidney injury (AKI). AKI is a term proposed to reflect the entire spectrum of acute renal failure, a complex disorder that occurs in a wide variety of settings with clinical manifestations ranging from a minimal elevation in serum creatinine to anuric renal failure (Mehta et al. 2007). In current clinical practice, AKI is typically diagnosed by measuring serum creatinine. Unfortunately, during acute changes in glomerular filtration, serum creatinine does not accurately depict kidney function until steady state equilibrium has been reached, which may require several days.

Conventional urinary biomarkers such as casts and fractional excretion of sodium have been insensitive and nonspecific for the early recognition of AKI. Other traditional urinary biomarkers such as filtered high molecular weight proteins and tubular proteins or enzymes have also suffered from lack of specificity and dearth of standardized assays.

Identification of novel AKI biomarkers has been designated as a top priority by the American Society of Nephrology (2005). The concept of developing a new toolbox for earlier diagnosis of disease states is also prominently featured in the NIH Road Map for biomedical research (Zerhouni 2003). The application of innovative technologies such as functional genomics and proteomics to human and animal models of kidney disease has uncovered several novel candidates that are emerging as biomarkers and therapeutic targets (O'Riordan et al. 2006). Several human models of AKI have consistently demonstrated the presence of apoptotic changes in tubule cells (Schwarz et al. 2002). Importantly, proteomic studies have now identified a multitude of apoptotic pathways, including the intrinsic (Bcl-2 family, cytochrome c, caspase 9), extrinsic (Fas, FADD, caspase 8), and regulatory (p53) factors, that are activated in tubule cells following human AKI (Hauser et al. 2004). As a consequence of these studies, inhibition of apoptosis has emerged as a promising approach in human AKI (Fleischer et al. 2006). Cell-permeable caspase inhibitors have provided particularly attractive targets for study. In this regard, an orally active small molecule pan-caspase inhibitor (IDN-6556, Pfizer) has been shown to be effective in preventing injury after lung and liver transplantation in animals (Quadri et al. 2005).

116.8.7 Neutrophil Gelatinase-Associated Lipocalin (NGAL)

Supavekin also identified neutrophil gelatinase-associated lipocalin (NGAL, also known as *lcn2*) as one of the most upregulated transcripts in the early postischemic mouse kidney [*222*], a finding that has now been confirmed in several other transcriptome profiling studies. Downstream proteomic studies have also revealed NGAL to be one of the earliest and most robustly induced proteins in the kidney after ischemic or nephrotoxic AKI in animal models, and NGALprotein is easily detected in the blood and urine soon after AKI (Mori et al. 2005). These findings have spawned a number of translational proteomic studies to evaluate NGAL as a novel biomarker in human AKI.

In a cross-sectional study, subjects in the intensive care unit with established ARF displayed a greater than 10-fold increase in plasma NGAL and more than a 100-fold increase in urine NGAL by Western blotting when compared to normal controls (Mori et al. 2005). Both plasma and urine NGAL correlated highly with serum creatinine levels. Kidney biopsies in these patients showed intense accumulation of immunoreactive NGAL in 50% of the cortical tubules. These results identified NGAL as a widespread and sensitive response to established AKI in humans. Urine NGAL has been shown to predict the severity of AKI and dialysis requirement in a multicenter study of children with diarrhea-associated hemolytic uremic syndrome (Trachtman et al. 2006). Preliminary results also suggest that plasma and urine NGAL measurements represent predictive biomarkers of AKI following contrast administration (Hirsch et al. 2007) and in the intensive care setting (Wheeler et al. 2008). In summary, NGAL is emerging as a center-stage player in the AKI field, as a novel predictive biomarker. However, it is acknowledged that the studies published thus far are small, in which NGAL appears to be most sensitive and specific in relatively uncomplicated patient populations with AKI. NGAL measurements may be influenced by a number of coexisting variables such as preexisting renal disease (Hinze et al. 2009) and systemic or urinary tract infections (Lavery et al. 2008). Large multicenter studies to further define the predictive role of plasma and urine NGAL as a member of the putative AKI panel have been initiated; simultaneously, a new chemiluminescent microparticle method, optimized on a fully automated analytical platform (ARCHITECT, Abbott Diagnostics Inc., Abbott Park, IL, USA) has been developed for the measurement of urine NGAL in the clinical practice and, specifically, in the emergency setting (Grenier et al. 2010). This new simple method permits to measure urine NGAL in all the clinical laboratories in a time closely comparable with that occurring for measuring creatinine. Thus, both NGAL and cystatin C may represent promising tandem biomarker candidates for inclusion in the blood AKI panel (Haase-Fielitz et al. 2009).

116.8.8 Kidney Injury Molecule 1 (KIM-1)

Kidney injury molecule 1 (KIM-1) is a type-1 transmembrane protein with glycosylated mucin and IgG-like domains in the ectodomain of the protein and a relatively short intracellular domain that is tyrosine phosphorylated. Downstream proteomic studies have also shown KIM-1 to be one of the most highly induced proteins in the kidney after AKI in animal models, and a proteolytically processed domain of KIM-1 is easily detected in the urine soon after AKI. In a small human cross-sectional study, KIM-1 was found to be markedly induced in proximal tubules in kidney biopsies from patients with established AKI (primarily ischemic), and urinary KIM-1 measured by ELISA distinguished ischemic AKI from prerenal azotemia and chronic renal disease (Ichimura et al. 2004). Patients with AKI induced by contrast did not have increased urinary KIM-1.

Recent preliminary studies have expanded the potential clinical utility of KIM-1 as a predictive AKI biomarker (Bonventre 2009). KIM-1 represents a promising candidate for inclusion in the urinary AKI panel. An advantage of KIM-1 over NGAL is that it appears to be more specific to ischemic or nephrotoxic AKI and not significantly affected by prerenal azotemia, urinary tract infections, or chronic kidney disease. It is likely that NGAL and KIM-1 will emerge as tandem biomarkers of AKI, with NGAL being most sensitive at the earliest time points and KIM-1 adding significant specificity at slightly later time points.

116.8.9 Additional Protein Markers: CYR61, SSAT, Zf9, TSP-1, IL-18

Gene expression studies have provided several additional clues regarding the AKI proteome, but human data are hitherto lacking. For example, Muramatsu et al. have utilized a subtractive hybridization approach to identify *Cyr61* (also known as *CCN1*) as a markedly upregulated gene in the rat kidney very early after ischemic injury (Muramatsu et al. 2002). CYR61 protein was induced in the kidney within 1 h and detectable in the urine at 3–6 h after ischemic injury, but not after volume depletion. However, this detection required a complex bioaffinity purification step with heparin-Sepharose beads, and even after such purification, several cross-reacting peptides were apparent. A more convenient platform for the evaluation of CYR61 as a urinary biomarker in humans has not been available to date. Zahedi et al. described spermidine/spermine N1-acetyltransferase (SSAT), the rate-limiting enzyme in polyamine catabolism, as a novel early biomarker of tubular cell damage after ischemic injury in rats (Zahedi et al. 2003). SSAT protein appears to play a role in the initiation of oxidant-mediated injury to tubules, raising the possibility of inhibition of polyamine catabolism as a future therapeutic approach (Wang et al. 2004).

Tarabishi et al. showed that another maximally induced gene identified very early after ischemic injury in animal models is Zf9, a Kruppel-like transcription factor involved in the regulation of a number of downstream targets (Tarabishi et al. 2005). Zf9 protein is markedly upregulated in the postischemic tubule cells, along with its major trans-activating factor, TGF-β1. Gene silencing of Zf9 abrogated TGF-β1 protein expression and mitigated the apoptotic response to ischemic injury in vitro (Tarabishi et al. 2005). These studies have thus identified a novel pathway that may play a critical role in the early tubule cell death that accompanies ischemic renal injury. Thakar et al. have employed transcriptome profiling in rat models to identify thrombospondin 1 (TSP-1), a previously known p53-dependent proapoptotic and antiangiogenic molecule, as another maximally induced gene early after ischemic AKI (Thakar et al. 2005). The TSP-1 protein product is upregulated in the postischemic proximal tubule cells, where it colocalizes with activated caspase- 3. TSP-1 null mice were partially protected from ischemic injury, with striking structural preservation of kidney tissue (Thakar et al. 2005). These results have thus identified yet another previously unknown apoptotic protein that is activated in proximal tubule cells early after ischemic AKI in animals. Transcripts that have been consistently reported to be either upregulated or downregulated in animal models of AKI are listed in Tables 4 and 5, respectively. While many of them have now been confirmed by downstream proteomic analysis, the majority of these studies remain in the preclinical research realm, and convincing data attesting to their utility in human AKI are currently unavailable.

IL-18 is a proinflammatory cytokine that is known to be induced and cleaved in the proximal tubule and subsequently easily detected in the urine following ischemic AKI in animal models (Molitoris et al. 2008). In a cross-sectional study, urine IL-18 levels measured by ELISA were markedly increased in patients with established AKI but not in subjects with urinary tract infection, chronic kidney disease, nephritic syndrome, or prerenal failure (Parikh et al. 2004). Urinary IL-18 was significantly upregulated up to 48 h prior to the increase in serum creatinine in patients with acute respiratory distress syndrome who develop AKI, with an AUC of 0.73, and represented an independent predictor of mortality in this cohort (Parikh et al. 2005). Both urinary IL-18 and NGAL were recently shown to represent early, predictive, sequential AKI biomarkers in children undergoing cardiac surgery (Parikh et al. 2006a). In patients who developed AKI 2–3 days after surgery, urinary NGAL was induced within 2 h and peaked at 6 h whereas urine IL-18 levels increased around 6 h and peaked at over 25-fold at 12 h post surgery (AUC 0.75). Both IL-18 and NGAL were independently associated with duration of AKI among cases.

Urine NGAL and IL-18 have also emerged as predictive biomarkers for delayed graft function following kidney transplantation (Parikh et al. 2006b). In a prospective multicenter study of children and adults, both NGAL and IL-18 in urine samples collected on the day of transplant predicted delayed graft function and dialysis requirement with AUC of 0.9. Thus, IL-18 may also represent a promising candidate for inclusion in the urinary "AKI panel." IL-18 is more specific to ischemic AKI, and not affected by nephrotoxins, chronic kidney disease or urinary tract infections. It is likely that NGAL, IL-18, and KIM-1 will emerge as sequential urinary biomarkers of AKI (Pisitkun et al. 2006; Comper and Osicka 2005; Vaidya et al. 2008).

116.8.10 Metabolomics

In the immediate future, specific studies performed in neonatology, with the application of reliable predictive biomarkers, among which metabolomics applied to the urine in particular, will contribute to a better understanding what takes place in critical stages of postnatal kidney development (Fanos et al. 2012).

By studying the urinary metabolomics both in experimental animals and neonates, it has emerged that the capacity to respond to and survive a strong, acute stimulus appears as an intrinsic property of the subject, independent of the application of suitable protocols: some patients

Table 6 Main urinary metabolites found in kidney diseases in humans (From Fanos et al. 2016 with permission)

Metabolomics biomarker	Kidney disease in humans
P-aminohippuric acid Scyllo inositol	Urinary tract infection
Fenyl acetyl glutamine	Interstitial cystitis
Methanol	ADPKD
3-indoxyl sulfate	Renal dysfunction (acute kidney injury, chronic kidney injury, diabetes)
P-cresol sulfate	Renal dysfunction (acute kidney injury, chronic kidney injury)
Kynurenate, kynurenine, 3-indole-lactate	Acute kidney injury

Table 7 Geography of damage and metabolomics markers (From Fanos et al. 2016 with permission)

Geography of damage	Metabolomics markers
Medullary injury	↑TMAO (trimethylamino oxide)
Papillary damage	↑ Dimethyl amine, sorbitol, myo-inositol
Tubular proximal cells mitochondrial dysfunction	↓ Citrate, αketoglutarate, succinate a

are fragile whereas others are resilient and overcome the critical moment, some with and some without insufficiency of one or more organs, namely the kidney. This takes place because there is a marked basal individual variability from the metabolic and energy standpoints. This increases following a strong stimulus such as severe asphyxia, sepsis. It depends on the metabolism of the individual: the basal metabolome of each organism differs greatly from that of the others (Fanos 2016).

Some experimental and clinical studies have been performed in pediatric nephrology. Main results are presented in Tables 6 and 7, regarding the main metabolites found in kidney diseases and the geography of damage (Fanos 2016).

The involvement of indoxyl sulfate and kynurenine, together with xanthurenic acid, suggests a complex dialogue between the gut microbiome. At the moment there is a need to improve the number of studied patients as well as the standardization of methods. In amniotic fluid, high glutamine level, glutamine/glutamate ratios, increase in glycoprotein P1, and lower urea level reflect kidney disorders/underdevelopment.

Metabolomics was able to discriminate newborns with and without acute renal injury (Atzori et al. 2011a) and acute kidney injury (Mercier et al. 2017).

Today, we apply the same treatment protocol to all patients, but these protocols pay very little attention to the individuality of each patient. Metabolomics will contribute to the assessment of phenomena in a more precise and personalized way, even taking into account perinatal programming (Atzori et al. 2011b). The final goal of metabolomics could be to find specific metabolites for common and rare nephropathies and to prepare easy, quick, and reliable tools, like "dipsticks for urine," able to differentiate patients from controls, or a patient before and after a nutritional or pharmacologic intervention (Mussap et al. 2014; Fanos et al. 2014).

References

Abbott JF, Levine D, Wapner R (1998) Posterior urethral valves: inaccuracy of prenatal diagnosis. Fetal Diagn Ther 13:179 183

Afshar K, Papanikolaou F, Malek R, Bagli D, Pippi-Salle JL, Khoury A (2005) Vesicoureteral reflux and complete ureteral duplication. Conservative or surgical management? J Urol 173:1725–1727

Agarwal SK, Fisk NM (2001) In utero therapy for lower urinary tract obstruction. Prenat Diagn 21:970–976

Alam-Faruque Y, Hill DP, Dimmer EC, Harris MA, Foulger RE, Tweedie S et al (2014) Representing kidney development using the gene ontology. PLoS One 9:e99864

Alconcher LF, Tombesi MM (2012) Natural history of bilateral mild isolated antenatal hydronephrosis conservatively managed. Pediatr Nephrol 27:1119–1123

American Society of Nephrology (2005) American Society of Nephrology Renal Research Report. J Am Soc Nephrol 16:1886–1903

Anderson NG, Abbott GD, Mogridge N, Allan RB, Maling TM, Wells JE (1997) Vesicoureteric reflux in the newborn: relationship to fetal renal pelvic diameter. Pediatr Nephrol 11:610–616

Anderson NG, Wright S, Abbott GD, Wells JE, Mogridge N (2003) Fetal renal pelvic dilatation – poor predictor of familial vesicoureteral reflux. Pediatr Nephrol 18:902–905

Arena S, Magno C, Montalto AS, Russo T, Mami C, Baldari S et al (2012) Long-term follow-up of neonatally diagnosed primary megaureter: rate and predictors of spontaneous resolution. Scand J Urol Nephrol 46:201–207

Ariel I, Wells TR, Landing BH, Singer DB (1991) The urinary system in down syndrome: a study of 124 autopsy cases. Pediatr Pathol 11:879–888

Ascenti G, Zimbaro G, Mazziotti S, Chimenz R, Baldari S, Fede C (2003) Vesicoureteral reflux: comparison between urosonography and radionuclide cystography. Pediatr Nephrol 18:768–771

Assadi FK (2002) Quantitation of microalbuminuria using random urine samples. Pediatr Nephrol 17:107–110

Atzori L, Antonucci R, Barberini L, Locci E, Marincola FC, Scano P et al (2011a) 1H NMR-based metabolomic analysis of urine from preterm and term neonates. Front Biosci (Elite Ed) 3:1005–1012

Atzori L, Mussap M, Noto A, Barberini L, Puddu M, Coni E et al (2011b) Clinical metabolomics and urinary NGAL for the early prediction of chronic kidney disease in healthy adults born ELBW. J Matern Fetal Neonatal Med 24(Suppl 2):40–43

Baek M, Park K, Choi H (2010) Long-term outcomes of dismembered pyeloplasty for midline-crossing giant hydronephrosis caused by ureteropelvic junction obstruction in children. Urology 76:1463–1467

Bajpai M, Dave S, Gupta DK (2001) Factors affecting outcome in the management of posterior urethral valves. Pediatr Surg Int 17:11–15

Barisic I, Odak L, Loane M, Garne E, Wellesley D, Calzolari E et al (2013) Fraser syndrome: epidemiological study in a European population. Am J Med Genet A 161A:1012–1018

Bartram MP, Höhne M, Dafinger C, Völker LA, Albersmeyer M, Heiss J et al (2013) Conditional loss of kidney microRNAs results in congenital anomalies of the kidney and urinary tract (CAKUT). J Mol Med (Berl) 91:739–748

Basturk T, Koc Y, Ucar Z, Sakaci T, Ahbap E, Kara E et al (2015) Renal damage frequency in patients with solitary kidney and factors that affect progression. Int J Nephrol 2015:876907

Beales PL, Bland E, Tobin JL, Bacchelli C, Tuysuz B, Hill J et al (2007) IFT80, which encodes a conserved intraflagellar transport protein, is mutated in Jeune asphyxiating thoracic dystrophy. Nat Genet 39:727–729

Belk RA, Thomas DF, Mueller RF, Godbole P, Markham AF, Weston MJ (2002) A family study and the natural history of prenatally detected unilateral multicystic dysplastic kidney. J Urol 167:666–669

Ben-Chaim J, Docimo SG, Jeffs RD, Gearhart JP (1996) Bladder exstrophy from childhood into adult life. J R Soc Med 89:39P–46P

Bergmann C, Senderek J, Schneider F, Dornia C, Küpper F, Eggermann T et al (2004) PKHD1 mutations in families requesting prenatal diagnosis for autosomal recessive polycystic kidney disease (ARPKD). Hum Mutat 23:487–495

Biason-Lauber A, Konrad D, Navratil F, Schoenle EJ (2004) A WNT4 mutation associated with Müllerian-duct regression and virilization in a 46,XX woman. N Engl J Med 351:792–798

Bienstock JL, Birsner ML, Coleman F, Hueppchen NA (2014) Successful in utero intervention for bilateral renal agenesis. Obstet Gynecol 124:413–415

Bissler JJ, Dixon BP (2005) A mechanistic approach to inherited polycystic kidney disease. Pediatr Nephrol 20:558–566

Bogart MM, Arnold HE, Greer KE (2006) Prune-belly syndrome in two children and review of the literature. Pediatr Dermatol 23:342–345

Boghossian NS, Sicko RJ, Kay DM, Rigler SL, Caggana M, Tsai MY et al (2016) Rare copy number variants implicated in posterior urethral valves. Am J Med Genet A 170:622–633

Bökenkamp A, Domanetzki M, Zinck R, Schumann G, Brodehl J (1998) Reference values for cystatin C serum concentrations in children. Pediatr Nephrol 12:125–129

Bonventre JV (2009) Kidney injury molecule-1 (KIM-1): a urinary biomarker and much more. Nephrol Dial Transplant 24:3265–3268

Boubaker A, Prior JO, Meuwly JY, Bischof-Delaloye A (2006) Radionuclide investigations of the urinary tract in the era of multimodality imaging. J Nucl Med 47:1819–1836

de Bruyn R, Marks SD (2008) Postnatal investigation of fetal renal disease. Semin Fetal Neonatal Med 13:133–141

Bunk DM (2007) Reference materials and reference measurement procedures: an overview from a national metrology institute. Clin Biochem Rev 28:131–137

Capolicchio G, Leonard MP, Wong C, Jednak R, Brzezinski A, Salle JL (1999) Prenatal diagnosis of hydronephrosis: impact on renal function and its recovery after pyeloplasty. J Urol 162:1029–1032

Carmichael SL, Shaw GM, Nelson V, Selvin S, Torfs CP, Curry CJ (2003) Hypospadias in California: trends and descriptive epidemiology. Epidemiology 14:701–706

Caruana G, Wong MN, Walker A, Heloury Y, Webb N, Johnstone L et al (2015) Copy-number variation associated with congenital anomalies of the kidney and urinary tract. Pediatr Nephrol 30:487–495

Cascio S, Paran S, Puri P (1999) Associated urological anomalies in children with unilateral renal agenesis. J Urol 162:1081–1083

Cassart M, Massez A, Metens T, Rypens F, Lambot MA, Hall M et al (2004) Complementary role of MRI after sonography in assessing bilateral urinary tract anomalies in the fetus. AJR Am J Roentgenol 182:689–695

Ceriotti F, Boyd JC, Klein G, Henny J, Queraltó J, Kairisto V et al (2008) Reference intervals for serum creatinine concentrations: assessment of available data for global application. Clin Chem 54:559–566

Chaumoitre K, Brun M, Cassart M, Maugey-Laulom B, Eurin D, Didier F et al (2006) Differential diagnosis of fetal hyperechogenic cystic kidneys unrelated to renal tract anomalies: a multicenter study. Ultrasound Obstet Gynecol 28:911–917

Chen JJ, Mao W, Homayoon K, Steinhardt GF (2004) A multivariate analysis of dysfunctional elimination syndrome, and its relationships with gender, urinary tract infection and vesicoureteral reflux in children. J Urol 171:1907–1910

Chertin B, Rolle U, Farkas A, Puri P (2002) Does delaying pyeloplasty affect renal function in children with a prenatal diagnosis of pelvi-ureteric junction obstruction? BJU Int 90:72–75

Choo KL, Borzi PA (2001) Surgical correction of pelviureteric junction obstruction in childhood – dorsal lumbotomy approach and selective internal ureteric stenting. Pediatr Surg Int 17:152–156

Christensson A, Ekberg J, Grubb A, Ekberg H, Lindström V, Lilja H (2003) Serum cystatin C is a more sensitive and more accurate marker of glomerular filtration rate than enzymatic measurements of creatinine in renal transplantation. Nephron Physiol 94:p19–p27

Clark TJ, Martin WL, Divakaran TG, Whittle MJ, Kilby MD, Khan KS (2003) Prenatal bladder drainage in the management of fetal lower urinary tract obstruction: a systematic review and meta-analysis. Obstet Gynecol 102:367–382

Comper WD, Osicka TM (2005) Detection of urinary albumin. Adv Chronic Kidney Dis 12:170–176

Consugar MB, Kubly VJ, Lager DJ, Hommerding CJ, Wong WC, Bakker E et al (2007) Molecular diagnostics of Meckel-Gruber syndrome highlights phenotypic differences between MKS1 and MKS3. Hum Genet 121:591–599

Coplen DE, Austin PF, Yan Y, Blanco VM, Dicke JM (2006) The magnitude of fetal renal pelvic dilatation can identify obstructive postnatal hydronephrosis, and direct postnatal evaluation and management. J Urol 176:724–727. discussion 727

Craig JC, Irwig LM, Knight JF, Roy LP (2000) Does treatment of vesicoureteric reflux in childhood prevent end-stage renal disease attributable to reflux nephropathy? Pediatrics 105:1236–1241

Crombleholme TM, Harrison MR, Golbus MS, Longaker MT, Langer JC, Callen PW et al (1990) Fetal intervention in obstructive uropathy: prognostic indicators and efficacy of intervention. Am J Obstet Gynecol 162:1239–1244

Daïkha-Dahmane F, Dommergues M, Muller F, Narcy F, Lacoste M, Beziau A et al (1997) Development of human fetal kidney in obstructive uropathy: correlations with ultrasonography and urine biochemistry. Kidney Int 52:21–32

Damen-Elias HA, Stoutenbeek PH, Visser GH, Nikkels PG, de Jong TP (2005) Concomitant anomalies in 100 children with unilateral multicystic kidney. Ultrasound Obstet Gynecol 25:384–388

Decramer S, Parant O, Beaufils S, Clauin S, Guillou C, Kessler S et al (2007) Anomalies of the TCF2 gene are the main cause of fetal bilateral hyperechogenic kidneys. J Am Soc Nephrol 18:923–933

Dhillon HK (1998) Prenatally diagnosed hydronephrosis: the Great Ormond Street experience. Br J Urol 81(Suppl 2):39–44

Dodder NG, Tai SS, Sniegoski LT, Zhang NF, Welch MJ (2007) Certification of creatinine in a human serum reference material by GC-MS and LC-MS. Clin Chem 53:1694–1699

Donaldson MD, Chambers RE, Woolridge MW, Whicher JT (1989) Stability of alpha 1-microglobulin, beta 2-microglobulin and retinol binding protein in urine. Clin Chim Acta 179:73–77

Dudley JA, Haworth JM, McGraw ME, Frank JD, Tizard EJ (1997) Clinical relevance and implications of antenatal hydronephrosis. Arch Dis Child Fetal Neonatal Ed 76:F31–F34

Duke V, Quinton R, Gordon I, Bouloux PM, Woolf AS (1998) Proteinuria, hypertension and chronic renal failure in X-linked Kallmann's syndrome, a defined genetic cause of solitary functioning kidney. Nephrol Dial Transplant 13:1998–2003

Edghill EL, Bingham C, Ellard S, Hattersley AT (2006) Mutations in hepatocyte nuclear factor-1beta and their related phenotypes. J Med Genet 43:84–90

Eknoyan G, Hostetter T, Bakris GL, Hebert L, Levey AS, Parving HH et al (2003) Proteinuria and other markers of chronic kidney disease: a position statement of the national kidney foundation (NKF) and the national institute of diabetes and digestive and kidney diseases (NIDDK). Am J Kidney Dis 42: 617–622

Fanos V (2016) Metabolomics and microbiomics: personalized medicine from the fetus to the adult. Academic Press/Elsevier, London

Fanos V, Cataldi L (2004) Antibiotics or surgery for vesicoureteric reflux in children. Lancet 364:1720–1722

Fanos V, Chevalier R, Faa G, Cataldi L (2012) Developmental nephrology: from embryology to metabolomics. Hygeia Press, Quartu S. Elena

Fanos V, Noto A, Caboni P, Pintus MC, Liori B, Dessì A et al (2014) Urine metabolomic profiling in neonatal nephrology. Clin Biochem 47:708–710

Fanos V, Puddu M, Ottonello G (2016) Metabolomics in nephrology: from the fetus to the adult. Selected Lectures of the 12th International Workshop on Neonatology. J Pediatr Neonatal Individual Med 5: e050246

Feather SA, Malcolm S, Woolf AS, Wright V, Blaydon D, Reid CJ et al (2000) Primary, nonsyndromic vesicoureteric reflux and its nephropathy is genetically heterogeneous, with a locus on chromosome 1. Am J Hum Genet 66:1420–1425

Feldenberg LR, Siegel NJ (2000) Clinical course and outcome for children with multicystic dysplastic kidneys. Pediatr Nephrol 14:1098–1101

Filler G, Lepage N (2003) Should the Schwartz formula for estimation of GFR be replaced by cystatin C formula? Pediatr Nephrol 18:981–985

Filler G, Priem F, Vollmer I, Gellermann J, Jung K (1999) Diagnostic sensitivity of serum cystatin for impaired glomerular filtration rate. Pediatr Nephrol 13:501–505

Fleischer A, Ghadiri A, Dessauge F, Duhamel M, Rebollo MP, Alvarez-Franco F et al (2006) Modulating apoptosis as a target for effective therapy. Mol Immunol 43:1065–1079

Gambhir L, Höller T, Müller M, Schott G, Vogt H, Detlefsen B et al (2008) Epidemiological survey of 214 families with bladder exstrophy-epispadias complex. J Urol 179:1539–1543

Gandy SJ, Armoogum K, Nicholas RS, McLeay TB, Houston JG (2007) A clinical MRI investigation of the relationship between kidney volume measurements and renal function in patients with renovascular disease. Br J Radiol 80:12–20

Gargollo PC, Borer JG, Diamond DA, Hendren WH, Rosoklija I, Grant R et al (2008) Prospective followup in patients after complete primary repair of bladder exstrophy. J Urol 180:1665–1670. discussion 1670

Garne E, Loane M, Wellesley D, Barisic I, EUROCAT Working Group (2009) Congenital hydronephrosis: prenatal diagnosis and epidemiology in Europe. J Pediatr Urol 5:47–52

Glodny B, Petersen J, Hofmann KJ, Schenk C, Herwig R, Trieb T et al (2009) Kidney fusion anomalies revisited: clinical and radiological analysis of 209 cases of crossed fused ectopia and horseshoe kidney. BJU Int 103:224–235

Gokce I, Biyikli N, Tugtepe H, Tarcan T, Alpay H (2012) Clinical spectrum of antenatally detected urinary tract abnormalities with respect to hydronephrosis at postnatal ultrasound scan. Pediatr Surg Int 28:543–552

González Celedón C, Bitsori M, Tullus K (2007) Progression of chronic renal failure in children with dysplastic kidneys. Pediatr Nephrol 22:1014–1020

Greive KA, Balazs ND, Comper WD (2001) Protein fragments in urine have been considerably underestimated by various protein assays. Clin Chem 47:1717–1719

Grenier FC, Ali S, Syed H, Workman R, Martens F, Liao M et al (2010) Evaluation of the ARCHITECT urine NGAL assay: assay performance, specimen handling requirements and biological variability. Clin Biochem 43:615–620

Grisaru S, Rosenblum ND (2001) Glypicans and the biology of renal malformations. Pediatr Nephrol 16: 302–306

Guder WG, Hofmann W (1992) Markers for the diagnosis and monitoring of renal tubular lesions. Clin Nephrol 38(Suppl 1):S3–S7

Gunn TR, Mora JD, Pease P (1995) Antenatal diagnosis of urinary tract abnormalities by ultrasonography after 28 weeks' gestation: incidence and outcome. Am J Obstet Gynecol 172:479–486

Haase-Fielitz A, Bellomo R, Devarajan P, Story D, Matalanis G, Dragun D et al (2009) Novel and conventional serum biomarkers predicting acute kidney injury in adult cardiac surgery – a prospective cohort study. Crit Care Med 37:553–560

Harmoinen A, Ylinen E, Ala-Houhala M, Janas M, Kaila M, Kouri T (2000) Reference intervals for cystatin C in pre- and full-term infants and children. Pediatr Nephrol 15:105–108

Harmon WE (2009) Glomerular filtration rate in children with chronic kidney disease. Clin Chem 55:400–401

Hauser P, Schwarz C, Mitterbauer C, Regele HM, Mühlbacher F, Mayer G et al (2004) Genome-wide gene-expression patterns of donor kidney biopsies distinguish primary allograft function. Lab Invest 84:353–361

Hawkins JS, Dashe JS, Twickler DM (2008) Magnetic resonance imaging diagnosis of severe fetal renal anomalies. Am J Obstet Gynecol 198:328.e321–328.e325

Herget-Rosenthal S, Poppen D, Hüsing J, Marggraf G, Pietruck F, Jakob HG et al (2004) Prognostic value of tubular proteinuria and enzymuria in nonoliguric acute tubular necrosis. Clin Chem 50:552–558

Heymans C, Breysem L, Proesmans W (1998) Multicystic kidney dysplasia: a prospective study on the natural history of the affected and the contralateral kidney. Eur J Pediatr 157:673–675

Hidas G, Billimek J, Nam A, Soltani T, Kelly MS, Selby B et al (2015) Predicting the risk of breakthrough urinary tract infections: primary vesicoureteral reflux. J Urol 194:1396–1401

Hill LM, Nowak A, Hartle R, Tush B (2000) Fetal compensatory renal hypertrophy with a unilateral functioning kidney. Ultrasound Obstet Gynecol 15:191–193

Hinze CH, Suzuki M, Klein-Gitelman M, Passo MH, Olson J, Singer NG et al (2009) Neutrophil gelatinase-associated lipocalin is a predictor of the course of global and renal childhood-onset systemic lupus erythematosus disease activity. Arthritis Rheum 60:2772–2781

Hiraoka M, Tsukahara H, Ohshima Y, Kasuga K, Ishihara Y, Mayumi M (2002) Renal aplasia is the predominant cause of congenital solitary kidneys. Kidney Int 61:1840–1844

Hirsch R, Dent C, Pfriem H, Allen J, Beekman RH, Ma Q et al (2007) NGAL is an early predictive biomarker of contrast-induced nephropathy in children. Pediatr Nephrol 22:2089–2095

Hoberman A, Charron M, Hickey RW, Baskin M, Kearney DH, Wald ER (2003) Imaging studies after a first febrile urinary tract infection in young children. N Engl J Med 348:195–202

Hodson EM, Wheeler DM, Vimalchandra D, Smith GH, Craig JC (2007) Interventions for primary vesicoureteric reflux. Cochrane Database Syst Rev 18:CD001532

Hofmann W, Regenbogen C, Edel H, Guder WG (1994) Diagnostic strategies in urinalysis. Kidney Int Suppl 47:S111–S114

Hogg RJ, Furth S, Lemley KV, Portman R, Schwartz GJ, Coresh J et al (2003) National Kidney Foundation's Kidney Disease Outcomes Quality Initiative clinical practice guidelines for chronic kidney disease in children and adolescents: evaluation, classification, and stratification. Pediatrics 111:1416–1421

Hohenfellner K, Wingen AM, Nauroth O, Wühl E, Mehls O, Schaefer F (2001) Impact of ACE I/D gene polymorphism on congenital renal malformations. Pediatr Nephrol 16:356–361

Horst M, Smith GH (2008) Pelvi-ureteric junction obstruction in duplex kidneys. BJU Int 101:1580–1584

Hortin GL, Sviridov D (2007) Diagnostic potential for urinary proteomics. Pharmacogenomics 8:237–255

Hoyer PF (2015) Clinical manifestations of autosomal recessive polycystic kidney disease. Curr Opin Pediatr 27:186–192

Hutton KA, Thomas DF, Davies BW (1997) Prenatally detected posterior urethral valves: qualitative assessment of second trimester scans and prediction of outcome. J Urol 158:1022–1025

Ichimura T, Hung CC, Yang SA, Stevens JL, Bonventre JV (2004) Kidney injury molecule-1: a tissue and urinary biomarker for nephrotoxicant-induced renal injury. Am J Physiol Renal Physiol 286:F552–F563

Ickowicz V, Eurin D, Maugey-Laulom B, Didier F, Garel C, Gubler MC et al (2006) Meckel-Grüber syndrome: sonography and pathology. Ultrasound Obstet Gynecol 27:296–300

Ismaili K, Hall M, Donner C, Thomas D, Vermeylen D, Avni FE et al (2003) Results of systematic screening for minor degrees of fetal renal pelvis dilatation in an unselected population. Am J Obstet Gynecol 188:242–246

Ismaili K, Avni FE, Wissing KM, Hall M, Brussels Free University Perinatal Nephrology Study Group (2004a) Long-term clinical outcome of infants with mild and moderate fetal pyelectasis: validation of neonatal ultrasound as a screening tool to detect significant nephrouropathies. J Pediatr 144:759–765

Ismaili K, Avni FE, Piepsz A, Wissing KM, Cochat P, Aubert D et al (2004b) Current management of infants with fetal renal pelvis dilation: a survey by French-speaking pediatric nephrologists and urologists. Pediatr Nephrol 19:966–971

Ismaili K, Hall M, Piepsz A, Alexander M, Schulman C, Avni FE (2005) Insights into the pathogenesis and natural history of fetuses with renal pelvis dilatation. Eur Urol 48:207–214

Ismaili K, Hall M, Piepsz A, Wissing KM, Collier F, Schulman C et al (2006) Primary vesicoureteral reflux detected in neonates with a history of fetal renal pelvis dilatation: a prospective clinical and imaging study. J Pediatr 148:222–227

Jadeja S, Smyth I, Pitera JE, Taylor MS, van Haelst M, Bentley E et al (2005) Identification of a new gene mutated in Fraser syndrome and mouse myelencephalic blebs. Nat Genet 37:520–525

Jaureguizar E, Lopez Pereira P, Martinez Urrutia MJ, Espinosa L, Lobato R (2000) Does neonatal pyeloureterostomy worsen bladder function in children with posterior urethral valves? J Urol 164:1031–1033. discussion 1033–1034

Je BK, Kim HK, Horn PS (2015) Incidence and spectrum of renal complications and extrarenal diseases and syndromes in 380 children and young adults with horseshoe kidney. AJR Am J Roentgenol 205:1306–1314

Jenkins D, Bitner-Glindzicz M, Malcolm S, Hu CC, Allison J, Winyard PJ et al (2005) De novo Uroplakin IIIa heterozygous mutations cause human renal adysplasia leading to severe kidney failure. J Am Soc Nephrol 16:2141–2149

Joseph VT (2006) The management of renal conditions in the perinatal period. Early Hum Dev 82:313–324

Kalfa N, Philibert P, Sultan C (2009) Is hypospadias a genetic, endocrine or environmental disease, or still an unexplained malformation? Int J Androl 32:187–197

Kari JA, Gonzalez C, Ledermann SE, Shaw V, Rees L (2000) Outcome and growth of infants with severe chronic renal failure. Kidney Int 57:1681–1687

Keevil BG, Kilpatrick ES, Nichols SP, Maylor PW (1998) Biological variation of cystatin C: implications for the assessment of glomerular filtration rate. Clin Chem 44:1535–1539

Kerecuk L, Schreuder MF, Woolf AS (2008) Renal tract malformations: perspectives for nephrologists. Nat Clin Pract Nephrol 4:312–325

Kern S, Zimmerhackl LB, Hildebrandt F, Ermisch-Omran B, Uhl M (2000) Appearance of autosomal recessive polycystic kidney disease in magnetic resonance imaging and RARE-MR-urography. Pediatr Radiol 30:156–160

Klaassen I, Neuhaus TJ, Mueller-Wiefel DE, Kemper MJ (2007) Antenatal oligohydramnios of renal origin: long-term outcome. Nephrol Dial Transplant 22:432–439

Kochhar A, Fischer SM, Kimberling WJ, Smith RJ (2007) Branchio-oto-renal syndrome. Am J Med Genet A 143A:1671–1678

Kohl S, Hwang DY, Dworschak GC, Hilger AC, Saisawat P, Vivante A et al (2014) Mild recessive mutations in six Fraser syndrome-related genes cause isolated congenital anomalies of the kidney and urinary tract. J Am Soc Nephrol 25:1917–1922

Kovanlikaya A, Kazam J, Dunning A, Poppas D, Johnson V, Medina C et al (2014) The role of ultrasonography in predicting vesicoureteral reflux. Urology 84:1205–1210

Krishnan A, de Souza A, Konijeti R, Baskin LS (2006) The anatomy and embryology of posterior urethral valves. J Urol 175:1214–1220

Kumar S, Walia S, Ikpeme O, Zhang E, Paramasivam G, Agarwal S et al (2012) Postnatal outcome of prenatally diagnosed severe fetal renal pelvic dilatation. Prenat Diagn 32:519–522

Lacoste M, Cai Y, Guicharnaud L, Mounier F, Dumez Y, Bouvier R et al (2006) Renal tubular dysgenesis, a not uncommon autosomal recessive disorder leading to oligohydramnios: role of the Renin-Angiotensin system. J Am Soc Nephrol 17:2253–2263

Lambert HJ, Stewart A, Gullett AM, Cordell HJ, Malcolm S, Feather SA et al (2011) Primary, nonsyndromic vesicoureteric reflux and nephropathy in sibling pairs: a United Kingdom cohort for a DNA bank. Clin J Am Soc Nephrol 6:760–766

Laterza OF, Price CP, Scott MG (2002) Cystatin C: an improved estimator of glomerular filtration rate? Clin Chem 48:699–707

Lavery AP, Meinzen-Derr JK, Anderson E, Ma Q, Bennett MR, Devarajan P et al (2008) Urinary NGAL in premature infants. Pediatr Res 64:423–428

Lee RS, Cendron M, Kinnamon DD, Nguyen HT (2006) Antenatal hydronephrosis as a predictor of postnatal outcome: a meta-analysis. Pediatrics 118:586–593

Leung AK, Robson WL (2004) Current status of cryptorchidism. Adv Pediatr 51:351–377

Levey AS, Bosch JP, Lewis JB, Greene T, Rogers N, Roth D (1999) A more accurate method to estimate glomerular filtration rate from serum creatinine: a new prediction equation. Modification of Diet in Renal Disease Study Group. Ann Intern Med 130:461–470

Levey AS, Stevens LA, Hostetter T (2006) Automatic reporting of estimated glomerular filtration rate – just what the doctor ordered. Clin Chem 52:2188–2193

Levey AS, Coresh J, Greene T, Marsh J, Stevens LA, Kusek JW et al (2007) Expressing the Modification of Diet in Renal Disease Study equation for estimating glomerular filtration rate with standardized serum creatinine values. Clin Chem 53:766–772

Lim DJ, Park JY, Kim JH, Paick SH, Oh SJ, Choi H (2003) Clinical characteristics and outcome of hydronephrosis detected by prenatal ultrasonography. J Korean Med Sci 18:859–862

Lissauer D, Morris RK, Kilby MD (2007) Fetal lower urinary tract obstruction. Semin Fetal Neonatal Med 12:464–470

Liu YP, Cheng SJ, Shih SL, Huang JK (2006) Autosomal recessive polycystic kidney disease: appearance on fetal MRI. Pediatr Radiol 36:169

Lu W, van Eerde AM, Fan X, Quintero-Rivera F, Kulkarni S, Ferguson H et al (2007) Disruption of ROBO2 is associated with urinary tract anomalies and confers risk of vesicoureteral reflux. Am J Hum Genet 80:616–632

Ludwig M, Ching B, Reutter H, Boyadjiev SA (2009) Bladder exstrophy-epispadias complex. Birth Defects Res A Clin Mol Teratol 85:509–522

Madden-Fuentes RJ, McNamara ER, Nseyo U, Wiener JS, Routh JC, Ross SS (2014) Resolution rate of isolated low-grade hydronephrosis diagnosed within the first year of life. J Pediatr Urol 10:639–644

Mahieu-Caputo D, Dommergues M, Delezoide AL, Lacoste M, Cai Y, Narcy F et al (2000) Twin-to-twin transfusion syndrome. Role of the fetal renin-angiotensin system. Am J Pathol 156:629–636

Mandelia A, Bajpai M, Agarwala S, Gupta AK, Kumar R, Ali A (2013) The role of urinary TGF-β_1, TNF-α, IL-6 and microalbuminuria for monitoring therapy in posterior urethral valves. Pediatr Nephrol 28: 1991–2001

Marra G, Barbieri G, Moioli C, Assael BM, Grumieri G, Caccamo ML (1994) Mild fetal hydronephrosis indicating vesicoureteric reflux. Arch Dis Child Fetal Neonatal Ed 70:F147–F149. discussion 149–150

Martínez JM, Masoller N, Devlieger R, Passchyn E, Gómez O, Rodo J et al (2015) Laser ablation of posterior urethral valves by fetal cystoscopy. Fetal Diagn Ther 37:267–273

Martínez-Frías ML, Bermejo E, Rodríguez-Pinilla E, Frías JL (2001) Exstrophy of the cloaca and exstrophy of the bladder: two different expressions of a primary developmental field defect. Am J Med Genet 99:261–269

Martini S, Prévot A, Mosig D, Werner D, van Melle G, Guignard JP (2003) Glomerular filtration rate: measure creatinine and height rather than cystatin C! Acta Paediatr 92:1052–1057

Matsell DG, Bennett T, Goodyer P, Goodyer C, Han VK (1996) The pathogenesis of multicystic dysplastic kidney disease: insights from the study of fetal kidneys. Lab Invest 74:883–893

McGregor L, Makela V, Darling SM, Vrontou S, Chalepakis G, Roberts C et al (2003) Fraser syndrome and mouse blebbed phenotype caused by mutations in FRAS1/Fras1 encoding a putative extracellular matrix protein. Nat Genet 34:203–208

Mehta RL, Kellum JA, Shah SV, Molitoris BA, Ronco C, Warnock DG et al (2007) Acute kidney injury network: report of an initiative to improve outcomes in acute kidney injury. Crit Care 11:R31

Meinhardt U, Ammann RA, Flück C, Diem P, Mullis PE (2003) Microalbuminuria in diabetes mellitus: efficacy of a new screening method in comparison with timed overnight urine collection. J Diabetes Complications 17:254–257

Mendelsohn C (2004) Functional obstruction: the renal pelvis rules. J Clin Invest 113:957–959

Mercier K, McRitchie S, Pathmasiri W, Novokhatny A, Koralkar R, Askenazi D et al (2017) Preterm neonatal urinary renal developmental and acute kidney injury metabolomic profiling: an exploratory study. Pediatr Nephrol 32:151–161

Merlini E, Lelli CP (2004) Obstructive ureterocele-an ongoing challenge. World J Urol 22:107–114

Miller WG, Myers GL, Ashwood ER, Killeen AA, Wang E, Thienpont LM et al (2005) Creatinine measurement: state of the art in accuracy and interlaboratory harmonization. Arch Pathol Lab Med 129:297–304

Mishra A (2007) Renal agenesis: report of an interesting case. Br J Radiol 80:e167–e169

Mitchell ME, Close CE (1996) Early primary valve ablation for posterior urethral valves. Semin Pediatr Surg 5:66–71

Mogensen CE, Viberti GC, Peheim E, Kutter D, Hasslacher C, Hofmann W et al (1997) Multicenter evaluation of the Micral-test II test strip, an immunologic rapid test for the detection of microalbuminuria. Diabetes Care 20:1642–1646

Molitoris BA, Melnikov VY, Okusa MD, Himmelfarb J (2008) Technology insight: biomarker development in

acute kidney injury – what can we anticipate? Nat Clin Pract Nephrol 4:154–165
Montini G, Rigon L, Zucchetta P, Fregonese F, Toffolo A, Gobber D et al (2008) Prophylaxis after first febrile urinary tract infection in children? A multicenter, randomized, controlled, noninferiority trial. Pediatrics 122:1064–1071
Mori K, Lee HT, Rapoport D, Drexler IR, Foster K, Yang J et al (2005) Endocytic delivery of lipocalin-siderophore-iron complex rescues the kidney from ischemia-reperfusion injury. J Clin Invest 115:610–621
Moriguchi T, Hamada M, Morito N, Terunuma T, Hasegawa K, Zhang C et al (2006) MafB is essential for renal development and F4/80 expression in macrophages. Mol Cell Biol 26:5715–5727
Mourtzinos A, Borer JG (2004) Current management of bladder exstrophy. Curr Urol Rep 5:137–141
Muramatsu Y, Tsujie M, Kohda Y, Pham B, Perantoni AO, Zhao H et al (2002) Early detection of cysteine rich protein 61 (CYR61, CCN1) in urine following renal ischemic reperfusion injury. Kidney Int 62:1601–1610
Murawski IJ, Gupta IR (2006) Vesicoureteric reflux and renal malformations: a developmental problem. Clin Genet 69:105–117
Muroya K, Hasegawa T, Ito Y, Nagai T, Isotani H, Iwata Y et al (2001) GATA3 abnormalities and the phenotypic spectrum of HDR syndrome. J Med Genet 38:374–380
Mussap M, Plebani M (2004) Biochemistry and clinical role of human cystatin C. Crit Rev Clin Lab Sci 41:467–550
Mussap M, Noto A, Fanos V, Van Den Anker JN (2014) Emerging biomarkers and metabolomics for assessing toxic nephropathy and acute kidney injury (AKI) in neonatology. Biomed Res Int 2014:602526
Myers GL, Miller WG, Coresh J, Fleming J, Greenberg N, Greene T et al (2006) Recommendations for improving serum creatinine measurement: a report from the Laboratory Working Group of the National Kidney Disease Education Program. Clin Chem 52:5–18
Narchi H (2005) Risk of hypertension with multicystic kidney disease: a systematic review. Arch Dis Child 90:921–924
National Kidney Foundation (2002) K/DOQI clinical practice guidelines for chronic kidney disease: evaluation, classification, and stratification. Am J Kidney Dis 39:S1–266
Neild GH, Dakmish A, Wood S, Nauth-Misir R, Woodhouse CR (2004) Renal transplantation in adults with abnormal bladders. Transplantation 77:1123–1127
Nepple KG, Cooper CS, Austin JC (2009) Rare variant of bladder exstrophy associated with urethral, bladder, and colonic duplication. Urology 73:928.e921–928.e923
Nishi T (1995) Magnetic resonance imaging of autosomal recessive polycystic kidney disease in utero. J Obstet Gynaecol (Tokyo 1995) 21:471–474
Nishimura H, Yerkes E, Hohenfellner K, Miyazaki Y, Ma J, Hunley TE et al (1999) Role of the angiotensin type 2 receptor gene in congenital anomalies of the kidney and urinary tract, CAKUT, of mice and men. Mol Cell 3:1–10
Novljan G, Kenig A, Rus R, Kenda RB (2003) Cyclic voiding urosonography in detecting vesicoureteral reflux in children. Pediatr Nephrol 18:992–995
Onen A (2007) Treatment and outcome of prenatally detected newborn hydronephrosis. J Pediatr Urol 3:469–476
O'Riordan E, Gross SS, Goligorsky MS (2006) Technology insight: renal proteomics – at the crossroads between promise and problems. Nat Clin Pract Nephrol 2:445–458
Palmer LS, Andros GJ, Maizels M, Kaplan WE, Firlit CF (1997) Management considerations for treating vesicoureteral reflux in children with solitary kidneys. Urology 49:604–608
Panteghini M, Division IS (2008) Enzymatic assays for creatinine: time for action. Clin Chem Lab Med 46:567–572
Panteghini M, Myers GL, Miller WG, Greenberg N, International Federation of Clinical Chemistry and Laboratory Medicine, Working Group on Standardization of Glomerular Filtration Rate Assessment (WG-GFRA) (2006) The importance of metrological traceability on the validity of creatinine measurement as an index of renal function. Clin Chem Lab Med 44:1287–1292
Parikh CR, Jani A, Melnikov VY, Faubel S, Edelstein CL (2004) Urinary interleukin-18 is a marker of human acute tubular necrosis. Am J Kidney Dis 43:405–414
Parikh CR, Abraham E, Ancukiewicz M, Edelstein CL (2005) Urine IL-18 is an early diagnostic marker for acute kidney injury and predicts mortality in the intensive care unit. J Am Soc Nephrol 16:3046–3052
Parikh CR, Mishra J, Thiessen-Philbrook H, Dursun B, Ma Q, Kelly C et al (2006a) Urinary IL-18 is an early predictive biomarker of acute kidney injury after cardiac surgery. Kidney Int 70:199–203
Parikh CR, Jani A, Mishra J, Ma Q, Kelly C, Barasch J et al (2006b) Urine NGAL and IL-18 are predictive biomarkers for delayed graft function following kidney transplantation. Am J Transplant 6:1639–1645
Parsons M, Newman DJ, Pugia M, Newall RG, Price CP (1999) Performance of a reagent strip device for quantitation of the urine albumin: creatinine ratio in a point of care setting. Clin Nephrol 51:220–227
Pates JA, Dashe JS (2006) Prenatal diagnosis and management of hydronephrosis. Early Hum Dev 82:3–8
Penido Silva JM, Oliveira EA, Diniz JS, Bouzada MC, Vergara RM, Souza BC (2006) Clinical course of prenatally detected primary vesicoureteral reflux. Pediatr Nephrol 21:86–91
Penna FJ, Bowlin P, Alyami F, Bägli DJ, Koyle MA, Lorenzo AJ (2015) Novel strategy for temporary decompression of the lower urinary tract in neonates using a ureteral stent. J Urol 194:1086–1090
Piepsz A (2007) Antenatally detected hydronephrosis. Semin Nucl Med 37:249–260
Pisitkun T, Johnstone R, Knepper MA (2006) Discovery of urinary biomarkers. Mol Cell Proteomics 5:1760–1771

Plaire JC, Pope JC, Kropp BP, Adams MC, Keating MA, Rink RC et al (1997) Management of ectopic ureters: experience with the upper tract approach. J Urol 158:1245–1247

Plazanet C, Arrondel C, Chavant F, Gubler MC (2014) Fetal renin-angiotensin-system blockade syndrome: renal lesions. Pediatr Nephrol 29:1221–1230

Pouilhe M, Gilardi-Hebenstreit P, Desmarquet-Trin Dinh C, Charnay P (2007) Direct regulation of vHnf1 by retinoic acid signaling and MAF-related factors in the neural tube. Dev Biol 309:344–357

Poutamo J, Vanninen R, Partanen K, Kirkinen P (2000) Diagnosing fetal urinary tract abnormalities: benefits of MRI compared to ultrasonography. Acta Obstet Gynecol Scand 79:65–71

Puddu M, Fanos V, Podda F, Zaffanello M (2009) The kidney from prenatal to adult life: perinatal programming and reduction of number of nephrons during development. Am J Nephrol 30:162–170

Puri A, Grover VP, Agarwala S, Mitra DK, Bhatnagar V (2002) Initial surgical treatment as a determinant of bladder dysfunction in posterior urethral valves. Pediatr Surg Int 18:438–443

Quadri SM, Segall L, de Perrot M, Han B, Edwards V, Jones N et al (2005) Caspase inhibition improves ischemia-reperfusion injury after lung transplantation. Am J Transplant 5:292–299

Quan A (2006) Fetopathy associated with exposure to angiotensin converting enzyme inhibitors and angiotensin receptor antagonists. Early Hum Dev 82:23–28

Quinlan J, Lemire M, Hudson T, Qu H, Benjamin A, Roy A et al (2007) A common variant of the PAX2 gene is associated with reduced newborn kidney size. J Am Soc Nephrol 18:1915–1921

Quintero RA, Shukla AR, Homsy YL, Bukkapatnam R (2000) Successful in utero endoscopic ablation of posterior urethral valves: a new dimension in fetal urology. Urology 55:774

Ramasamy R, Haviland M, Woodard JR, Barone JG (2005) Patterns of inheritance in familial prune belly syndrome. Urology 65:1227

Ransley PG, Dhillon HK, Gordon I, Duffy PG, Dillon MJ, Barratt TM (1990) The postnatal management of hydronephrosis diagnosed by prenatal ultrasound. J Urol 144:584–587. discussion 593–584

Reardon W, Casserly LF, Birkenhäger R, Kohlhase J (2007) Kidney failure in Townes-Brocks syndrome: an under recognized phenomenon? Am J Med Genet A 143A:2588–2591

Riccabona M (2004) Assessment and management of newborn hydronephrosis. World J Urol 22:73–78

Risdon RA, Yeung CK, Ransley PG (1993) Reflux nephropathy in children submitted to unilateral nephrectomy: a clinicopathological study. Clin Nephrol 40:308–314

Rodríguez MM, Gómez AH, Abitbol CL, Chandar JJ, Duara S, Zilleruelo GE (2004) Histomorphometric analysis of postnatal glomerulogenesis in extremely preterm infants. Pediatr Dev Pathol 7:17–25

Rubenwolf P, Ziesel C, Beetz R, Kamal MM, Thüroff JW, Stein R (2015) Presentation, management and long-term outcome of ureteropelvic junction obstruction in duplex kidneys. J Urol 194:427–432

Rule AD, Larson TS, Bergstralh EJ, Slezak JM, Jacobsen SJ, Cosio FG (2004) Using serum creatinine to estimate glomerular filtration rate: accuracy in good health and in chronic kidney disease. Ann Intern Med 141:929–937

Salomon R, Tellier AL, Attie-Bitach T, Amiel J, Vekemans M, Lyonnet S et al (2001) PAX2 mutations in oligomeganephronia. Kidney Int 59:457–462

Sanna-Cherchi S, Caridi G, Weng PL, Dagnino M, Seri M, Konka A et al (2007) Localization of a gene for non-syndromic renal hypodysplasia to chromosome 1p32-33. Am J Hum Genet 80:539–549

Sarhan O, Zaccaria I, Macher MA, Muller F, Vuillard E, Delezoide AL et al (2008) Long-term outcome of prenatally detected posterior urethral valves: single center study of 65 cases managed by primary valve ablation. J Urol 179:307–312. discussion 312–303

Schwartz GJ, Furth SL (2007) Glomerular filtration rate measurement and estimation in chronic kidney disease. Pediatr Nephrol 22:1839–1848

Schwartz GJ, Haycock GB, Edelmann CM, Spitzer A (1976) A simple estimate of glomerular filtration rate in children derived from body length and plasma creatinine. Pediatrics 58:259–263

Schwartz GJ, Muñoz A, Schneider MF, Mak RH, Kaskel F, Warady BA et al (2009) New equations to estimate GFR in children with CKD. J Am Soc Nephrol 20:629–637

Schwarz C, Hauser P, Steininger R, Regele H, Heinze G, Mayer G et al (2002) Failure of BCL-2 up-regulation in proximal tubular epithelial cells of donor kidney biopsy specimens is associated with apoptosis and delayed graft function. Lab Invest 82:941–948

Serafini-Cessi F, Malagolini N, Cavallone D (2003) Tamm-Horsfall glycoprotein: biology and clinical relevance. Am J Kidney Dis 42:658–676

Sfakianakis GN, Sfakianaki E (2001) Renal scintigraphy in infants and children. Urology 57:1167–1177

Sharifian M, Dadkhah-Chimeh M, Einollahi B, Nafar M, Simforoush N, Basiri A et al (2007) Renal transplantation in patients with Bardet-Biedl syndrome. Arch Iran Med 10:339–342

Sharma R, Sanchez-Ferras O, Bouchard M (2015) Pax genes in renal development, disease and regeneration. Semin Cell Dev Biol 44:97–106

Shenoy MU, Rance CH (1999) Is there a place for the insertion of a JJ stent as a temporizing procedure for symptomatic partial congenital vesico-ureteric junction obstruction in infancy? BJU Int 84:524–525

Sheu JC, Koh CC, Chang PY, Wang NL, Tsai JD, Tsai TC (2006) Ureteropelvic junction obstruction in children: 10 years' experience in one institution. Pediatr Surg Int 22:519–523

Shukla AR, Cooper J, Patel RP, Carr MC, Canning DA, Zderic SA et al (2005) Prenatally detected primary

megaureter: a role for extended followup. J Urol 173:1353–1356
Sidhu G, Beyene J, Rosenblum ND (2006) Outcome of isolated antenatal hydronephrosis: a systematic review and meta-analysis. Pediatr Nephrol 21:218–224
Slickers JE, Olshan AF, Siega-Riz AM, Honein MA, Aylsworth AS, National Birth Defects Prevention Study (2008) Maternal body mass index and lifestyle exposures and the risk of bilateral renal agenesis or hypoplasia: the National Birth Defects Prevention Study. Am J Epidemiol 168:1259–1267
Soliman SM (2009) Primary ablation of posterior urethral valves in low birth weight neonates by a visually guided fogarty embolectomy catheter. J Urol 181:2284–2289. discussion 2289–2290
Soomro NA, Neal DE (1998) Treatment of hypospadias: an update of current practice. Hosp Med 59:553–556
Stahl DA, Koul HK, Chacko JK, Mingin GC (2006) Congenital anomalies of the kidney and urinary tract (CAKUT): a current review of cell signaling processes in ureteral development. J Pediatr Urol 2:2–9
Stevens LA, Coresh J, Greene T, Levey AS (2006) Assessing kidney function – measured and estimated glomerular filtration rate. N Engl J Med 354:2473–2483
Sudarsanan B, Nasir AA, Puzhankara R, Kedari PM, Unnithan GR, Damisetti KR (2009) Posterior urethral valves: a single center experience over 7 years. Pediatr Surg Int 25:283–287
Tarabishi R, Zahedi K, Mishra J, Ma Q, Kelly C, Tehrani K et al (2005) Induction of Zf9 in the kidney following early ischemia/reperfusion. Kidney Int 68:1511–1519
Tenstad O, Roald AB, Grubb A, Aukland K (1996) Renal handling of radiolabelled human cystatin C in the rat. Scand J Clin Lab Invest 56:409–414
Thakar CV, Zahedi K, Revelo MP, Wang Z, Burnham CE, Barone S et al (2005) Identification of thrombospondin 1 (TSP-1) as a novel mediator of cell injury in kidney ischemia. J Clin Invest 115:3451–3459
Thomas DF (2008) Prenatally diagnosed urinary tract abnormalities: long-term outcome. Semin Fetal Neonatal Med 13:189–195
Tiryaki S, Alkac AY, Serdaroglu E, Bak M, Avanoglu A, Ulman I (2013) Involution of multicystic dysplastic kidney: is it predictable? J Pediatr Urol 9:344–347
Tobin JL, Beales PL (2007) Bardet-Biedl syndrome: beyond the cilium. Pediatr Nephrol 22:926–936
Tomlinson PA, Dalton RN, Hartley B, Haycock GB, Chantler C (1997) Low molecular weight protein excretion in glomerular disease: a comparative analysis. Pediatr Nephrol 11:285–290
Trachtman H, Christen E, Cnaan A, Patrick J, Mai V, Mishra J et al (2006) Urinary neutrophil gelatinase-associated lipocalcin in D+HUS: a novel marker of renal injury. Pediatr Nephrol 21:989–994
Tsai JD, Huang CT, Lin PY, Chang JH, Lee MD, Huang FY et al (2012) Screening high-grade vesicoureteral reflux in young infants with a febrile urinary tract infection. Pediatr Nephrol 27:955–963
Tsatsaris V, Gagnadoux MF, Aubry MC, Gubler MC, Dumez Y, Dommergues M (2002) Prenatal diagnosis of bilateral isolated fetal hyperechogenic kidneys. Is it possible to predict long term outcome? BJOG 109:1388–1393
Ulinski T, Lescure S, Beaufils S, Guigonis V, Decramer S, Morin D et al (2006) Renal phenotypes related to hepatocyte nuclear factor-1beta (TCF2) mutations in a pediatric cohort. J Am Soc Nephrol 17:497–503
Vaidya VS, Waikar SS, Ferguson MA, Collings FB, Sunderland K, Gioules C et al (2008) Urinary biomarkers for sensitive and specific detection of acute kidney injury in humans. Clin Transl Sci 1:200–208
Valente EM, Brancati F, Silhavy JL, Castori M, Marsh SE, Barrano G et al (2006) AHI1 gene mutations cause specific forms of Joubert syndrome-related disorders. Ann Neurol 59:527–534
Vujic A, Kosutic J, Bogdanovic R, Prijic S, Milicic B, Igrutinovic Z (2007) Sonographic assessment of normal kidney dimensions in the first year of life – a study of 992 healthy infants. Pediatr Nephrol 22: 1143–1150
Walsh TJ, Hsieh S, Grady R, Mueller BA (2007) Antenatal hydronephrosis and the risk of pyelonephritis hospitalization during the first year of life. Urology 69:970–974
Wang Z, Zahedi K, Barone S, Tehrani K, Rabb H, Matlin K et al (2004) Overexpression of SSAT in kidney cells recapitulates various phenotypic aspects of kidney ischemia-reperfusion injury. J Am Soc Nephrol 15:1844–1852
Webb NJ, Lewis MA, Bruce J, Gough DC, Ladusans EJ, Thomson AP et al (1997) Unilateral multicystic dysplastic kidney: the case for nephrectomy. Arch Dis Child 76:31–34
Weber S, Moriniere V, Knüppel T, Charbit M, Dusek J, Ghiggeri GM et al (2006) Prevalence of mutations in renal developmental genes in children with renal hypodysplasia: results of the ESCAPE study. J Am Soc Nephrol 17:2864–2870
Weizer AZ, Silverstein AD, Auge BK, Delvecchio FC, Raj G, Albala DM et al (2003) Determining the incidence of horseshoe kidney from radiographic data at a single institution. J Urol 170:1722–1726
Wheeler DM, Vimalachandra D, Hodson EM, Roy LP, Smith GH, Craig JC (2004) Interventions for primary vesicoureteric reflux. Cochrane Database Syst Rev 15: CD001532
Wheeler DS, Devarajan P, Ma Q, Harmon K, Monaco M, Cvijanovich N et al (2008) Serum neutrophil gelatinase-associated lipocalin (NGAL) as a marker of acute kidney injury in critically ill children with septic shock. Crit Care Med 36:1297–1303
Whittam BM, Calaway A, Szymanski KM, Carroll AE, Misseri R, Kaefer M et al (2014) Ultrasound diagnosis of multicystic dysplastic kidney: is a confirmatory nuclear medicine scan necessary? J Pediatr Urol 10:1059–1062
Whitten SM, Wilcox DT (2001) Duplex systems. Prenat Diagn 21:952–957

Wickstrom EA, Thangavelu M, Parilla BV, Tamura RK, Sabbagha RE (1996) A prospective study of the association between isolated fetal pyelectasis and chromosomal abnormality. Obstet Gynecol 88:379–382

Wiesel A, Queisser-Luft A, Clementi M, Bianca S, Stoll C, EUROSCAN Study Group (2005) Prenatal detection of congenital renal malformations by fetal ultrasonographic examination: an analysis of 709,030 births in 12 European countries. Eur J Med Genet 48:131–144

Wilson PD (2004) Polycystic kidney disease: new understanding in the pathogenesis. Int J Biochem Cell Biol 36:1868–1873

Winding L, Loane M, Wellesley D, Addor MC, Arriola L, Bakker MK et al (2014) Prenatal diagnosis and epidemiology of multicystic kidney dysplasia in Europe. Prenat Diagn 34:1093–1098

Winyard P, Chitty LS (2008) Dysplastic kidneys. Semin Fetal Neonatal Med 13:142–151

Winyard PJ, Nauta J, Lirenman DS, Hardman P, Sams VR, Risdon RA et al (1996) Deregulation of cell survival in cystic and dysplastic renal development. Kidney Int 49:135–146

Winyard PJ, Bharucha T, De Bruyn R, Dillon MJ, van't Hoff W, Trompeter RS et al (2006) Perinatal renal venous thrombosis: presenting renal length predicts outcome. Arch Dis Child Fetal Neonatal Ed 91: F273–F278

Woodward M, Frank D (2002) Postnatal management of antenatal hydronephrosis. BJU Int 89:149–156

Woolf AS (2006) Unilateral multicystic dysplastic kidney. Kidney Int 69:190–193

Woolf AS (2008) Perspectives on human perinatal renal tract disease. Semin Fetal Neonatal Med 13:196–201

Woolf AS, Hillman KA (2007) Unilateral renal agenesis and the congenital solitary functioning kidney: developmental, genetic and clinical perspectives. BJU Int 99:17–21

Woolf A, Jenkins D (2006) Development of the kidney. In: Jennette JCOJ, Schwartz MM, Silva FG (eds) Heptinstall's pathology of the kidney. Lippincott Williams & Wilkins, Philadelphia, pp 71–95

Yeung CK, Godley ML, Dhillon HK, Gordon I, Duffy PG, Ransley PG (1997) The characteristics of primary vesico-ureteric reflux in male and female infants with pre-natal hydronephrosis. Br J Urol 80:319–327

Ylinen E, Ala-Houhala M, Wikström S (2004a) Outcome of patients with antenatally detected pelviureteric junction obstruction. Pediatr Nephrol 19:880–887

Ylinen E, Ala-Houhala M, Wikström S (2004b) Prognostic factors of posterior urethral valves and the role of antenatal detection. Pediatr Nephrol 19:874–879

Zaffanello M, Brugnara M, Cecchetto M, Fedrizzi M, Fanos V (2008a) Renal involvement in children with vesicoureteral reflux: are prenatal detection and surgical approaches preventive? Scand J Urol Nephrol 42:330–336

Zaffanello M, Cecchetto M, Brugnara M, Martone E, Zuffante M, Fedrizzi M et al (2008b) Pelvi-ureteric junction obstruction and renal function after pyeloplasty: a retrospective study in 29 children. Minerva Urol Nefrol 60:1–6

Zaffanello M, Franchini M, Fanos V (2008c) New therapeutic strategies with combined renin-angiotensin system inhibitors for pediatric nephropathy. Pharmacotherapy 28:125–130

Zaffanello M, Brugnara M, Zuffante M, Franchini M, Fanos V (2009a) Are children with congenital solitary kidney at risk for lifelong complications? A lack of prediction demands caution. Int Urol Nephrol 41:127–135

Zaffanello M, Brugnara M, Cecchetto M, Manfredi R, Zuffante M, Fanos V (2009b) Paediatric unilateral giant hydroureteronephrosis from idiopathic ureterovesical stricture: a case report. BMJ Case Rep 2009

Zagar I, Anderson PJ, Gordon I (2002) The value of radionuclide studies in children with autosomal recessive polycystic kidney disease. Clin Nucl Med 27:339–344

Zahedi K, Wang Z, Barone S, Prada AE, Kelly CN, Casero RA et al (2003) Expression of SSAT, a novel biomarker of tubular cell damage, increases in kidney ischemia-reperfusion injury. Am J Physiol Renal Physiol 284: F1046–F1055

Zappitelli M, Joseph L, Gupta IR, Bell L, Paradis G (2007) Validation of child serum creatinine-based prediction equations for glomerular filtration rate. Pediatr Nephrol 22:272–281

Zerhouni E (2003) Medicine. The NIH roadmap. Science 302:63–72

Zhang PL, Peters CA, Rosen S (2000) Ureteropelvic junction obstruction: morphological and clinical studies. Pediatr Nephrol 14:820–826

Zhou H, Yuen PS, Pisitkun T, Gonzales PA, Yasuda H, Dear JW et al (2006) Collection, storage, preservation, and normalization of human urinary exosomes for biomarker discovery. Kidney Int 69:1471–1476

Part XII

Neurology

Brain Development and Perinatal Vulnerability to Cerebral Damage

117

Luca A. Ramenghi, Monica Fumagalli, and
Veena Supramaniam

Contents

L. A. Ramenghi (✉)
Division of Neonatology, Giannina Gaslini Children's Hospital, Genoa, Italy

M. Fumagalli
NICU, Department of Clinical Sciences and Community Health, Fondazione IRCCS Ca' Granda Ospedale Maggiore Policlinico Milano, Università degli Studi di Milano, Milan, Italy

V. Supramaniam
Perinatal Imaging Group, Robert Steiner MR Unit, MRC Clinical Sciences Centre and Wigglesworth Perinatal Pathology Services, Hammersmith Hospital, Imperial College, London, UK

G. Buonocore et al. (eds.), *Neonatology*,
https://doi.org/10.1007/978-3-319-29489-6_264

Abstract
The recent exponential rise in detailed magnetic resonance (MR) imaging studies has emphasized the concept of gestationally determined regional vulnerability in the brain. The site and nature of the injury is determined by a combination of the characteristics of the insult, the specific tissue and cell vulnerability, and the gestational age. Acute perinatal hypoxic ischemic events, previously considered characteristic for the term newborn presenting with hypoxic-ischemic encephalopathy, may occur at earlier points in gestation. White matter lesions, which are considered the hallmark of injury to the preterm brain, may also occur in a small percentage of term neonates. The regional tissue vulnerability at a given gestational age will be determined by the local metabolic requirements in combination with specific cell characteristics, such as the expression of different glutamatergic receptor subtypes and endogenous antioxidant mechanisms. In addition, neonatal neurons are programmed for cell death to allow for essential pruning and optimal connectivity, but this characteristic increases the vulnerability of such cells to injury. The nature of the insult is also important in dictating lesion site. In this chapter we will discuss the vulnerability of tissue and cell types in relation to gestational age and examine how these relate to patterns of injury seen on brain MR imaging and the clinical history and presentation of the infant.

117.1 Salient Points

- Gestational age is an important determinant of the lesion site, making white matter (WM) more vulnerable in preterm infants and gray matter more vulnerable in term infants, but the nature of the insult is also an important factor.
- The first half of gestation is characterized by neuronal proliferation and migration. During the second half, glial cell proliferation and programmed cell death predominate.
- Neuronal migration continues during a period when an infant born preterm may be exposed to a variety of potentially damaging factors. Acquired injuries to the immature brain may target replicating neuroblasts and disrupt neuronal migration.
- The subplate is a structure present at all phases of intrauterine brain development; it reaches its maximum width between 25 and 29 weeks, when WM is highly vulnerable to injury, before gradually decreasing in size.
- There are many factors responsible for WM vulnerability in preterms, ranging from the anatomy of the cerebrovasculature and low baseline blood flow to the inherent susceptibility of pre-oligodentrocytes to injury.
- Microglia are the main cell type implicated in injuries to the developing WM.
- Early migrating neurons and pre-oligodentrocytes are vulnerable to injury as well as the germinal matrix in the preterm brain.
- Cortex, central gray matter, and brainstem are common targets for perinatal injury complicating an acute hypoxic ischemic event.
- A predisposition to programmed cell death may be induced after injury, resulting in an increase in cellular apoptosis in injured regions and consequent disturbed and disrupted connectivity.

117.2 Introduction

The recent exponential rise in detailed magnetic resonance (MR) imaging studies has emphasized the concept of gestationally determined regional vulnerability in the brain: the site and nature of the injury sustained being determined by a combination of the characteristics of the insult, the specific

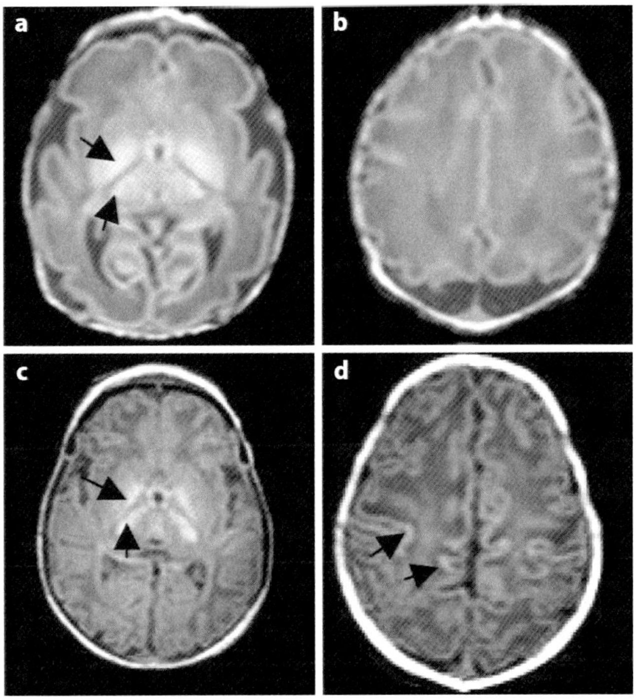

Fig. 1 Basal ganglia and thalamic (BGT) injury. BGT lesions are the hallmark of an acute hypoxic-ischemic event regardless of gestational age. (**a**, **b**) Preterm infant born at 32 weeks gestation by emergency cesarean section (EMCS) for abnormal fetal heart rate. There is abnormal high signal intensity (SI) either side (*arrows*) of the low SI posterior limb of the internal capsule (PLIC) (unmyelinated at this age). There is no obvious abnormality in or adjacent to the developing central sulcus or interhemispheric fissure (**b**). (**c**, **d**) Term born neonate born by EMCS for fetal distress. There is bilateral abnormal high signal intensity in the globus pallidus and thalamus (*arrows*). There is no myelin in the PLIC, which is abnormal at this age (**c**). Superiorly there is some increased SI in the central sulci and cortex along the interhemispheric fissure (*arrows*). The subcortical white matter adjacent to these regions is abnormally low SI (**d**)

tissue and cell vulnerability and the gestation of the infant. The type of insult may also be partly dependent on gestation. However, it is now known that acute perinatal hypoxic ischemic events, previously considered characteristic for the term born neonate presenting with hypoxic-ischemic encephalopathy (HIE), may occur at earlier points in gestation (Barkovich and Sargent 1995; Logitharajah et al. 2009). Nevertheless, such events occur less often in the infant born preterm where lesions develop in similar brain regions and in other areas characteristically more vulnerable in more premature babies (Fig. 1). Similarly, white matter (WM) lesions, which are considered the hallmark of injury to the preterm brain because they are characteristic of perinatal injury relating to inflammation, infection or hypoglycemia in the term brain, may also occur in a small percentage of neonates with an encephalopathy (Fig. 2) (Rutherford et al. 2010).

The regional tissue vulnerability at a given gestation will be determined by the local metabolic requirements in combination with specific cell characteristics, e.g., density of glutamate receptors (Patel et al. 2005). Regional tissue vulnerability at different gestational ages has been demonstrated by numerous *in vivo* brain imaging studies, as well as by conventional postmortem examinations. However, animal studies have highlighted the concept of a specific vulnerability by certain cell types, e.g. the subplate neurons (McQuillen et al. 2003) and oligodendrocyte precursors (Volpe 2009) are most vulnerable in the preterm brain. In the term brain, excitatory pyramidal projection neurons especially in the deep grey nuclei are at greatest risk during ischemic insults (Fig. 1). The vulnerability of a

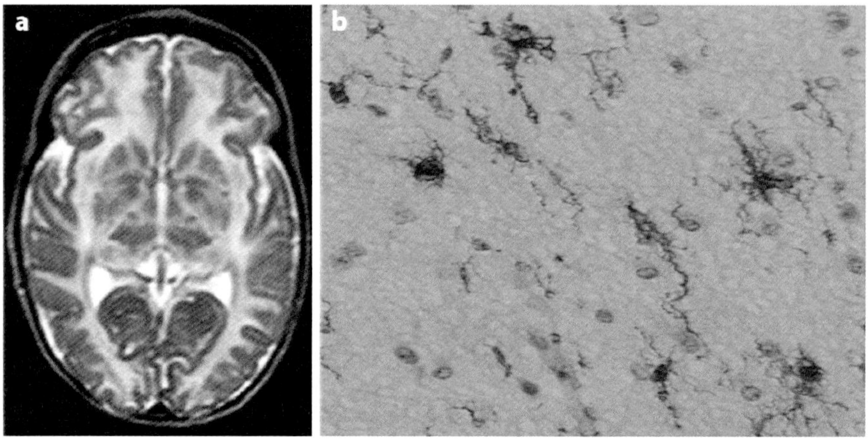

Fig. 2 T2 weighted scan (**a**) obtained at 9 days of age in a neonate with severe perinatal basal ganglia and thalamic injury showing diffuse high signal intensity in the white matter. Marked microglial activation (**b**) was seen in the white matter at post mortem ten weeks later

specific cell type at a given gestation relates to characteristics such as the expression of different glutamatergic receptor subtypes that favor calcium entry and excitability, and endogenous antioxidant mechanisms (Kjellmer 1991). In addition, the neonatal neuron is programmed for cell death to allow for essential pruning and optimal connectivity, but this characteristic increases the vulnerability of such cells to injury. However, while research has focussed on WM vulnerability in preterm infants and gray matter vulnerability in term infants, the nature of the insult is also important in dictating lesion site.

In this chapter we will discuss the vulnerability of tissue and cell types in relation to gestational age and examine how these relate to patterns of injury seen on brain MR imaging and the clinical history and presentation of the infant.

117.3 Brain Development

In order to understand the vulnerability of the immature brain to injury, it is essential to consider the stages of brain development from early fetal life until term at around 40 weeks' postmenstrual age (PMA). A full description of brain development is beyond the scope of this chapter so we will concentrate on regions of the preterm brain that are known to be particularly vulnerable; the immature white matter and the germinal matrix. In the more mature term brain we will focus on the deep gray matter and myelinating white matter with different cell types that may contribute to this changing vulnerability.

The first half of gestation is characterized by neuronal proliferation and migration. During the second half, glial cell proliferation and programmed cell death predominate (Rakic 1978; Skoff 1980; Rakic and Zecevic 2000). The last trimester of gestation is characterized by developing connectivity. There is axonal and dendritic sprouting and synapse formation. These processes, which involve programmed cell death, continue throughout childhood and into adolescence. Whilst early myelination in central brain structures, such as the brainstem and thalami, is present by 26 weeks, further myelination in the posterior limb of the internal capsule is then not detected until the end of gestation (Counsell et al. 2002). The majority of brain myelination occurs in the first 2 years after birth (Fig. 3). There is, however, extensive premyelination occurring within hemispheric white matter during late gestation and the abundance of oligodendrocyte precursors are particularly vulnerable to damage (Volpe 2009). This pre-myelination is in part responsible for the anisotropy of WM tracts documented in diffusion tensor images of the preterm brain before the appearance of myelination. Measures of anisotropy can therefore be used as an indirect measure of oligodendrocyte injury in

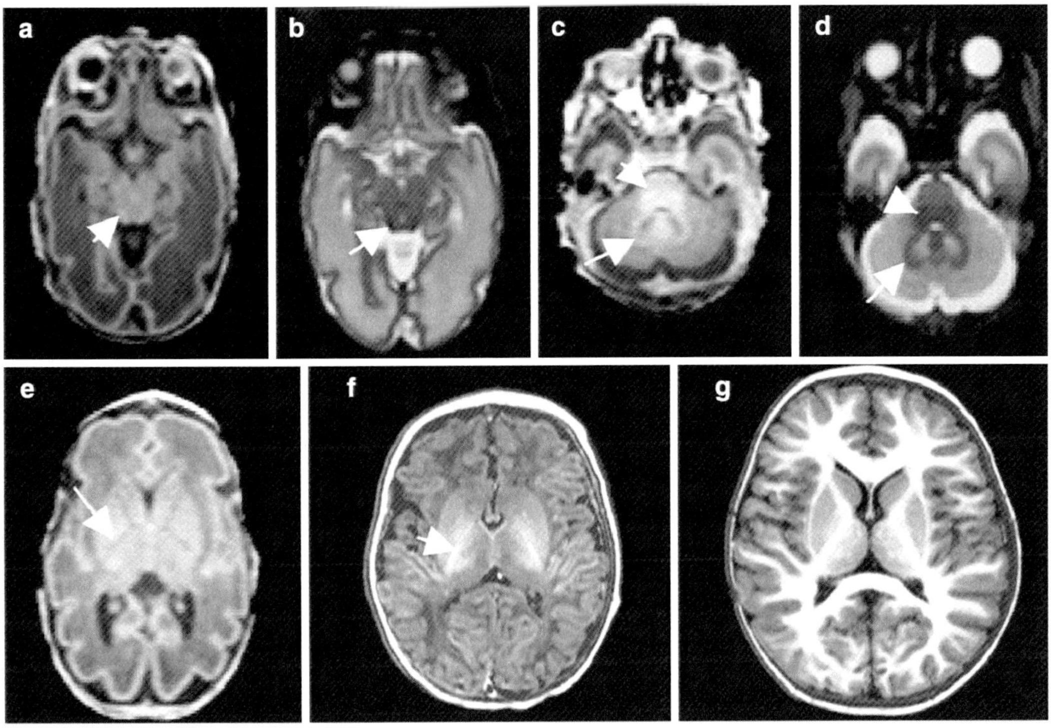

Fig. 3 Myelination. Preterm infant born at 26 + 5 weeks gestation and imaged at 29 weeks (**a**–**e**). Term born neonate (**f**). Two year old child (**g**). Myelination is seen as high signal intensity on T1 weighted images (**a**, **c**, **e**, **f**, **g**) and low signal intensity on T2 weighted images (**b**, **d**). At 29 weeks postmenstrual age myelination is detected in many central brain areas such as in brainstem regions e.g., lateral lemnisci (*arrows*) (**a**, **b**) and the medial lemnisci (*short arrows*) (**c**, **d**) and in the dentate nuclei (*long arrow*) (**c**, **d**). Myelination is easier to detect on T2 weighted images in the preterm brain. Myelination in the PLIC is visible from around 37 weeks postmenstrual age (*arrow*) (**f**). Prior to myelination the PLIC may look low signal intensity on T1 weighted images (*arrow*) (**e**). The majority of brain myelination occurs during the first 2 years of postnatal life (**g**)

the immature brain prior to myelination (Counsell et al. 2002; Hüppi and Dubois 2006).

Knowledge of the timing of events, such as myelination, allows us to understand the vulnerability of tissue types. *In vivo* methodology to assess such injuring processes provides an insight into the neurological sequelae that may result from lesions sustained at a given gestation.

117.4 Regional Vulnerability

117.4.1 Neuronal Migration

From the fifth week PMA, the neural tube starts to develop and differentiate. Specific proliferation areas can be identified in the ventricular and subventricular zones from where excitatory pyramidal neurons migrate to their final destination, mostly following specialized radial glial fibers. This radial migration process is closely regulated by complex molecular interactions between neurons and glial cells mediated by glycoproteins, membrane lipids and neurotransmitters (Métin et al. 2008).

More recently it has been appreciated that, in addition to this radial migration, there are two further modes of migration, tangential and multipolar migration (Nadarajah and Parnavelas 2002; Tabata and Nakajima 2003). The latter occurs independently of radial glia. It was originally thought that all neuronal migration ceased by 20 weeks PMA, but this referred to radially migrating pyramidal neurons. Gabaminergic inhibitory interneurons generated in the ganglionic eminences migrate in a tangential manner initially and then along the radial glia into the cortex in an inside-out manner. This process continues until past term (Rakic 1978; Zhang et al. 2009). Later, the medial and lateral ganglionic eminences appear and give rise to different populations of interneuron; those from the lateral or caudal eminence migrate and occupy superficial layers of the cortex (Miyoshi et al. 2010). Thus neuronal migration continues during a period when an infant born preterm may be exposed to a variety of potentially damaging factors. Many recognized disturbances in neuronal migration result from genetic defects (Marcorelles et al. 2010), giving rise to profound abnormalities of cortical development such as the lissencephalies. Acquired injuries to the immature brain such as ischemia, viral infection (Barkovich and Lindan 1994; Luo et al. 2010) or maternal drug abuse (Lee et al. 2010) may target replicating neuroblasts and disrupt neuronal migration. Acquired injuries result in more focal cortical dysplasias such as polymicrogyria, which is frequently associated with cytomegalovirus infection (Fig. 4) (Luo et al. 2010; Barkovich and Lindan 1994). Earlier insults (Fig. 4) cause more severe disruption of cortical development, and later insults may result in subtle abnormalities in cortical development that may not be visually obvious but that could be investigated using more advanced imaging techniques such as diffusion tensor imaging.

117.4.2 The Cortical Subplate

The cortical subplate is an important anatomical and functional structure, which is present at all phases of intrauterine brain development from early gestation to near term. The first populations of migrating neurons occupy the transient cortical subplate from approximately 7–8 weeks post conception. The subplate is essential for normal cortical development and subplate neurons develop both intracortical and subcortical projections (Allendoerfer and Shatz 1994). The subplate zone becomes visible in the human brain at around 14–15 post-conceptional weeks (PCW),

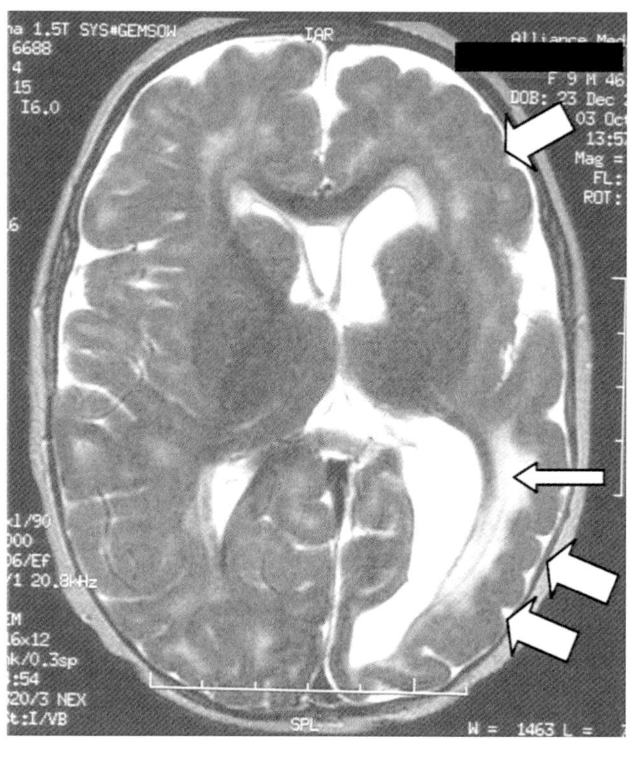

Fig. 4 Congenital CMV. Axial T2 scan of a term baby with CMV infection acquired around the 12th week of intrauterine life. The early fetal infection has determined cortical malformations such as polymicrogyria (*white arrows*) more evident in the right hemisphere and diffuse and severe white matter abnormalities (*thin arrow*)

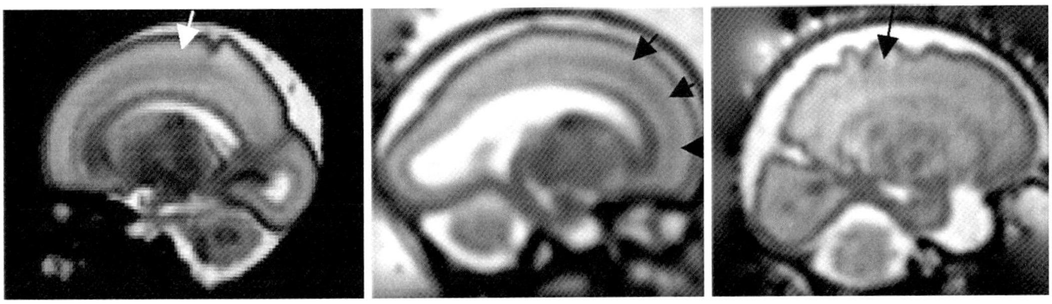

Fig. 5 Subplate visualization. T2 weighted images. Preterm infant 26 + 2 imaged at 28 + 1 weeks post-menstrual age. The subplate can be seen as a band of high signal intensity adjacent to the cortex (*arrows*)

the beginning of the second trimester of human gestation. This coincides with the invasion of the subplate region by thalamocortical afferents as well as basal forebrain afferents, leading to rapid expansion of the subplate so that it comprises 35% of the cerebral wall by 16 PCW. From 14 to 25 PCW in the human, a large number neurons are continuously added to the subplate compartment, which increases in width concurrent with the growth of the cortical plate. The highest density of cells is always found at the border between cortical plate and subplate. At its peak of development, the human subplate zone is four times the width of the cortical plate (Kostovic and Rakic 1990), reaching its maximum thickness in the late second and early third trimester, more or less between 25 and 29 weeks. This is a period of high vulnerability for WM injury. Thereafter it gradually decreases in size and becomes unrecognizable by the sixth month post-term (Kostovic and Rakic 1990).

Early thalamo-cortical afferents remain within the subplate until approximately 28 weeks when they progress into the cortex to form the earliest functional neurocircuits of the neocortex. The subplate layer contains a hydrophilic extracellular matrix that enables visualization of the subplate *in vivo* using MR imaging of the fetal or preterm infant brain. It can be quantified using volumetric scanning or diffusion tensor imaging (Dudink et al. 2010; Widjaja et al. 2010). On MR imaging the subplate layer is thicker than the cortex until approximately 24 weeks, equivalent to the cortex until about 28 weeks, and then starts to involute, being visible only at the tops of gyri throughout the third trimester (Figs. 5 and 6). A normal term infant usually only displays a few regions of residual subplate on imaging, and, in infants with overt lesions, the subplate may disappear prematurely. In contrast, in preterm infants imaged at term equivalence, the subplate may persist abnormally when compared to term born controls. This alteration in subplate involution associated with preterm birth may be due to more subtle forms of injury. The consequences of these alterations in subplate evolution on cortical development are unknown. However cortical gyration is reduced in the preterm brain at term equivalence, in comparison with normal term born control brains. However, MR cortical maturation at term corrected age is delayed in preterm babies with mild white matter abnormalities compared to those without (Fig. 7) (Ajayi-Obe et al. 2000; Kapellou et al. 2006; Ramenghi et al. 2007).

In a rodent animal model of perinatal HI, the subplate neurons appear to be selectively vulnerable and their loss corresponds to the severity of the insult (McQuillen et al. 2003). Investigators speculated that the glutamate receptor played a role in the pathogenesis, although the problem seems further complicated by more recent observations, suggesting a novel mechanism for subplate vulnerability.

It is, however, well known that selective ablation of subplate neurons at critical time periods in development may cause altered cortical organisation (McQuillen et al. 2003; Ghosh and Shatz 1992). Thus, isolated injury to the subplate neurons, which play a fundamental role in axonal

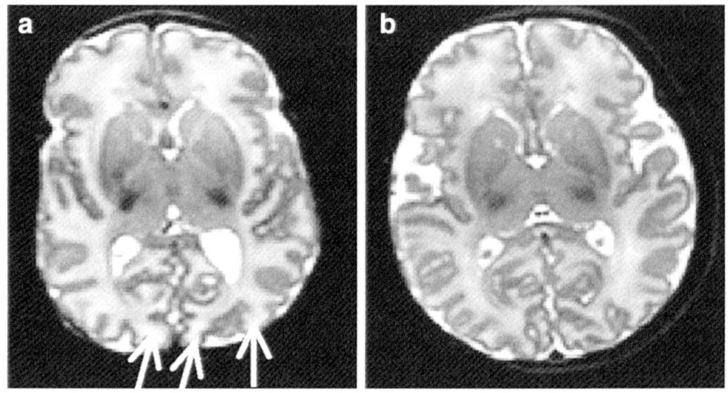

Fig. 6 Subplate involution. Preterm infant born at 26 + 3 and imaged at term (**a**). Term born control infant (**b**). Preterm infants at term have more subplate remnants, seen as regions of high SI adjacent to the gyral cortex (*arrows*) than term born controls, suggesting abnormal or delayed involution of the subplate layer

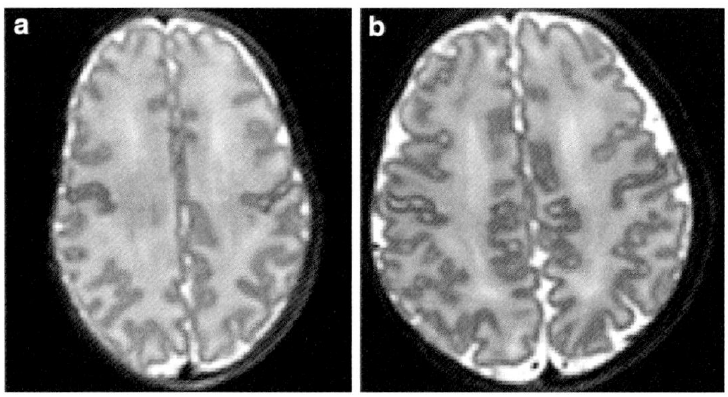

Fig. 7 Cortical development in the preterm. (**a**) Preterm infant born at 26 + 3 weeks gestation and imaged at term age. (**b**) Term born control infant T2 weighted images acquired in the transverse plane, at the level of the centrum semiovale. Preterm infants imaged at term age have less complex cortical folding than the term born controls (Ajayi-Obe et al. 2000; Kapellou et al. 2006)

routing to and from the developing cortex, may result in abnormal thalamocortical connectivity. It has been speculated that this may explain the visual and somatosensory impairment seen in prematurely born humans (Kostovic and Judas 2006). Seventy-one percent of premature infants with moderate periventricular leukomalacia (PVL) during the neonatal period were found to have at least one abnormality of visual testing at 1 year of age, and yet 66% of these children had normal optic radiations, and all had a visual cortex that appeared normal (Cioni et al. 1997). Primary abnormalities within the visual cortex of subcortical white matter have not generally been demonstrated by imaging studies of infants with PVL, although the accelerated disappearance of the subplate may be a sign of injury. Cortical abnormalities in terms of loss of volume have been documented following PVL (Inder et al. 1999), but no studies to date have looked specifically at the visual cortex. The neurobiological basis for their visual impairment is therefore not well understood and abnormalities in the visual cortical function may occur as a secondary phenomenon due to injury elsewhere. In more recent studies, Ricci (Ricci et al. 2006) and colleagues reported an association with poor visual function and thalamic atrophy. However, others (Bassi et al. 2008) have suggested a plausible explanation for failing visual test during the neonatal age period is that an unspecific parenchymal lesion may damage the complex connectivity network as (Ricci et al. 2006; Bassi et al. 2008; Ramenghi et al. 2010).

The cortical subplate continues to be related to brain development even late in gestation. In newborn babies at term with HIE, potential WM involvement may occur due to subcortical laminar necrosis in the subcortical subplate, as shown by highlighting in areas close to the cortex, which is particularly evident at the depths of sulci. The predilection of cortical necrosis at the bottom of sulci remains unexplained, although the fact that the subplate first disappears at the depths of sulci as the cortex folds may indicate an increasing vulnerability of the local resident neurons as they are more mature than those at the tops of gyri.

The role of subplate neuronal injury as a neurological basis for later impairments needs to be further investigated. A more sophisticated *in vivo* imaging approach such as serial diffusion tensor imaging studies is needed (Dudink et al. 2010; Widjaja et al. 2010).

117.4.3 The Developing White Matter

The association of preterm delivery and white matter injury in the form of periventricular leukomalacia (PVL) has been recognised since the 1960s (Banker and Larroche 1962). Imaging studies have emphasised that injury to the developing white matter is associated with secondary abnormalities involving the entire thalamo-cortical circuit, giving rise to thalamic atrophy and a decrease in cortical volume (Inder et al. 1999). Recent MR studies have also identified a spectrum of WM abnormalities in the preterm brain. PVL represents the most severe, with new findings of punctuate WM lesions and the diffuse appearance of DEHSI being reported more recently (Rutherford et al. 2010).

117.4.4 Oligodendrocytes

The vulnerability of preterm white matter appears to be multifactorial, relating to vessel anatomy with arterial end and border zone regions of relatively poor perfusion, low baseline blood flow, impaired regulation of blood flow in the sick infant and inherent susceptibilities of pre-oligodendrocytes (preOLs) to injury (Volpe 2009; Khwaja and Volpe 2008). The current theory is that both hypoxia-ischemia and infection lead to microglia activation that in turn leads to cytokine release, production of free radicals with both reactive oxygen and reactive nitrogen species and glutamate release, all of which contribute to death of the immature oligodendrocyte which demonstrate a vulnerability to oxidative stress (Haynes et al. 2003) and glutamate receptor immaturity (Deng et al. 2004).

The ultimate result of either event would be a deficit of mature oligodendroglia, and a consequent impairment of myelination, the hallmark of PVL. Early white matter injury may result in a combination of delayed preOL degeneration and preOL maturation arrest. The persistence of susceptible populations of preOLs renders chronic white matter lesions markedly more vulnerable to recurrent hypoxia-ischemia. PreOL maturation arrest may predispose to more severe white matter injury in preterm survivors that sustain recurrent hypoxia- ischemia (Segovia et al. 2008).

117.4.5 Axons

Axonal injury has been recognized for many years to be a feature of the focal necrotic component of PVL. Perhaps more important quantitatively, axonal degeneration, detected by the apoptotic marker fractin, has been recently found to be a feature of the diffuse component of human PVL. Whether the axonal degeneration observed in diffuse PVL is a primary injury or a secondary effect remains unclear. However, if primary axonal injury did occur, the expected results would be hypomyelination via failure of axonal-oligodendroglial interactions and decreased cortical (Inder et al. 1999) and thalamic/basal ganglia volumes (Boardman et al. 2006; Srinivasan et al. 2006).

117.4.6 Thalami

We have included thalami in this section due to direct links with white matter. Recent human neuropathological data have demonstrated a high incidence of damage to specifically mediodorsal and reticular nuclei of the thalami in infants with PVL. Four patterns may be considered: diffuse gliosis, status marmoratus, micro-infarcts, and macro-infarcts. Irrespective of the pattern and/or mechanism, it has been suggested that the reduced thalamic volumes revealed by neuroimaging are caused by neuronal loss (Ligam et al. 2009). Thalamic neuronal loss would be consistent with either primary injury and/or secondary anterograde and retrograde trophic effects. If there is primary neuronal injury, secondary effects would involve white matter axons, with subsequent hypomyelination and impaired development of the cerebral cortex, and such changes would be expected to compound the effects of the initial WM injury characteristic of PVL.

The role of the cerebral cortex in the cognitive deficits in preterm survivors is poorly understood. Periventricular leukomalacia (PVL), the key feature of the encephalopathy of prematurity, is characterized by periventricular necrotic foci and diffuse gliosis in the surrounding cerebral white matter. A recent study tested the hypothesis that reductions in the density of layer I neurons and/or pyramidal neurons in layers III and/or V are associated with PVL, indicating cortical pathology potentially associated with cognitive deficits in long-term survivors. In 15 controls (23 gestational weeks to 18 postnatal months), there was no difference in pyramidal density among incipient Brodmann areas, suggesting that cytoarchitectonic differences across functional areas are not fully mature during the fetal and infant periods. There was a marked reduction (38%) in the density of layer V neurons in all areas sampled in children with PVL cases compared with controls, in whom the six-layer cortex was visually distinct ($P < 0.024$). This may reflect a dying-back loss of somata complicating transection of layer V axons projecting through the necrosis in the underlying white matter. This study emphasised the potential role of secondary cortical injury in the encephalopathy of prematurity (Andiman et al. 2010).

117.4.7 The Role of Microglia in WM Injury

Microglia are the main cell type implicated in injuries to the developing WM. Microglia are hemopoietic in origin and migrate into the brain from approximately 6 weeks' gestation. There are at least three morphological forms (amoeboidal, activated and ramified), which are distinguished by staining with markers such as tomato lectin and Iba. In the normal adult brain, the majority of microglia are ramified or resting, and activated microglia are assumed to be pathological. The normal immature brain contains all recognized morphological forms of microglia (ramified, activated and amoeboidal), although the exact site and numbers of the different forms alters with increasing gestation. Normal developmental or resident microglia perform many essential roles. These include the phagocytosis of unwanted tissue from programmed cell death as shown by labelling of microglia and apoptotic cells in regions of synaptogenesis and neuronal differentiation (Rezaie and Male 1999). Resident activated microglia are also involved in brain modelling by secreting growth factors such as nerve growth factor (NGF), basic fibroblast growth factor (bFGF) and neurotrophin-3 (Elkabes et al. 1998), which provide trophic support for neurons and glia cells.

There is a maturation dependent concentration of microglia in apparently normal cerebral white matter during the third trimester of human gestation (Billiard et al. 2006). A few of these microglia are MHC II immunopositive cells, further evidence that they are developmentally activated resident cells and not immune induced. It has been suggested that the presence of numerous resident microglia in the immature brain increases its susceptibility to WM injury. Microglia co-exist during this developmental period with pre-oligodendrocytes which, as discussed, are also particularly susceptible to ischemic and inflammatory injury. Microglia are known to play a pivotal role in diffuse white matter injuries in the immature brain such as PVL.

Microglia are a potent source of both inflammatory cytokines and free radicals. Reactive oxygen and nitrogen species (ROS/RNS) release is mediated via Toll-like receptors known to be present on microglia. Interferon γ expression has been demonstrated in astrocytes in diffuse PVL. Interferon g toxicity is greater for pre-OLs than for mature cells and is potentiated by tumor necrosis factor alpha (TNFα), which is produced by microglia. Evidence

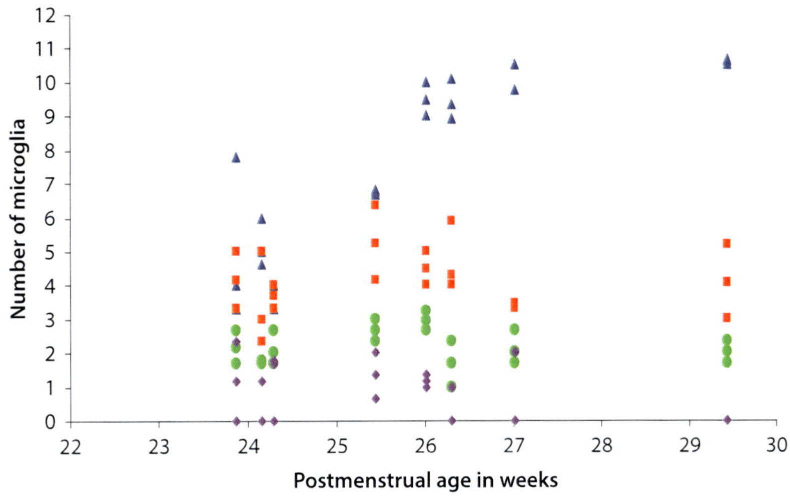

Fig. 8 Distribution of Iba 1 immunopositive microglia in the frontal, occipital and parietal lobes of the extremely preterm normal brain. Microglia numbers at the PVWM (*blue*) were significantly higher than deep white matter ($p = 0.0251$; *red*), subplate ($p < 0.0001$; *green*) and cortex ($p < 0.0001$; *purple*). This difference was most marked over the gestational age range in which PVL is most common

for the contribution of inflammation to preterm white matter injury emanates from studies of pregnant and neonatal animal models, where responses to exogenous lipopolysaccharide (LPS) are particularly involved. These studies have identified striking upregulation of inflammatory cytokines and microglial activation. LPS activates the innate immune system through an interaction with a specific toll-like receptor (TLR4) on immune cells, including microglia. Further evidence supporting the role of microglia in WM injury is provided by many studies using animal models of WM injury which demonstrate a decrease in injury in the presence of inhibitors of microglial activation such as chloroquine, minocycline and melatonin. Strategies for decreasing immune activated microglial activity in response to injurious processes should ideally not interfere with the function of normal developmentally active resident microglia.

In vivo and *in vitro* imaging studies of the immature brain have attributed regions of altered signal intensity within the developing white matter to the presence of dense clusters of microglia (Judas et al. 2005). An increase in activated microglia in all periventricular white matter areas (sometimes called WM crossroads) compared to the deep white matter and subplate has been demonstrated in a cohort of 23 human brains with gestational ages of 22–40 weeks (Fig. 8). In addition, these authors demonstrated increased numbers of periventricular microglia in association with germinal matrix/intraventricular hemorrhage (Supramaniam et al. 2010). Although the morphological appearances of Iba positive cells do not differentiate normal developmentally activated microglia from abnormal immunoactivated microglia, some differentiation between developmentally activated microglia and immune/injury activated microglia may be made based on their site and number and the presence of overt tissue injury. However, functional differentiation may require more specific immunological markers. For example, mouse models have shown that in response to ibotenate, early microglial activation was CD45 negative, i.e., these cells are likely to have originated from the normal resident population (Dommergues et al. 2003).

In vitro studies of animal models have shown that the LPS-induced inflammatory response initiated by microglia was mediated via the TLR4 *My*D88-dependent pathway (Dean et al. 2009; Wang et al. 2009). This activation of microglia causes neuronal death, whilst *My*D88-deficient microglia do not. Manipulation of this activation may provide an opportunity for neuroprotective intervention. In a separate rodent model, LPS preconditioning was shown to have an altered protective response to subsequent ischemic injury via the TRIF-IRF3-IFNβ TLR4 cascade (Marsh et al. 2009), which may have a beneficial effect on microglia. Investigation of these TLR4 activation pathways would enable functional characterization of different microglial phenotypes in the immature human brain, especially in association with lesions detected by MR imaging. In addition, co-labelling for apoptosis and for axonal injury would determine any deleterious effect by immune activated microglia.

117.4.8 The Germinal Matrix

The term germinal matrix is used by neonatologists to describe dense regions of tissue seen primarily within the caudothalamic notch on cranial ultrasound. On MR imaging scans of younger babies similar areas are also seen in the roof of the temporal horn and in the frontal areas externally adjacent to the frontal horns. These areas correspond to the ganglionic eminences referred to by neurobiologists. The germinal layer lining the entire ventricle may be identified on MR imaging of the fetal or very preterm brain but is not seen on ultrasound. In the fetal brain this layer is very prominent, but in infants born preterm, involution is already evident. On MR imaging of postmortem specimens, the germinal layer increases exponentially; it reaches a maximum at around 23 weeks' PMA and then decreases dramatically (Kinoshita et al. 2001).

The germinal and subventricular layers are sites of neuronal and glial cell proliferation and migration. The characteristic vulnerabilities of early migrating neurons and preoligodendrocytes to injury have already been discussed, but their site of origin, the germinal matrix itself, is a common site of injury in the preterm brain. It is vulnerable to both hemorrhagic injury, as a result of the dense vascular network, and to injury from infection, e.g. by cytomegalovirus, which results in necrosis and cyst formation.

Germinal matrix intraventricular hemorrhage (GMH/IVH) has decreased in incidence because of improvements in intensive care, specifically in respiratory morbidity with the introduction of antenatal steroids for threatened preterm labor and artificial surfactant at the time of delivery. However, with the survival of the most extremely preterm infants who remain very vulnerable, germinal matrix hemorrhage remains a major cause of morbidity and mortality. The incidence in those born at 24–26 weeks' gestation or below 750 g birthweight is approximately 20–30%. The inverse relationship with gestational age indicates that the larger the matrix, the more susceptible it is to hemorrhage. In the term born neonate in contrast, intraventricular hemorrhage is thought to originate from the choroid plexus and is recognized as being a complication of sinus thrombosis particularly when associated with thalamic hemorrhage (Wu et al. 2003). A germinal matrix hemorrhage can also derive from sinus thrombosis in latepreterm babies (Ramenghi et al. 2002). The site of hemorrhage in the preterm is usually from the ganglionic eminence of the caudothalamic notch or less frequently in the temporal horn (Hambleton and Wigglesworth 1976). These regions have a rich capillary network, which is vulnerable to rupture and hemorrhage because of the poor vascular integrity of involuting immature vessels and inadequate connective tissue support with a deficiency in mesenchymal and glial elements. Furthermore, a pressure passive circulation, compliant skull and disturbances in coagulation in the sick preterm exacerbate the fragility of the matrix. Hemorrhagic lesions are thought to be secondary to venous congestion with distortion and tearing of local small venous tributaries by the presence of blood in the perivenous space (Ghazi-Birry et al. 1997; Towbin 1968; Leech and Kohnen 1974). The hemorrhage originates and destroys the germinal matrix and this may impair proliferation and late migration of GABAergic interneurons to upper cortical layers, and the thalamus could contribute to defective cortical and thalamic development. There is some neuropathological data to support this (Marin Padilla 1999), although it is difficult to determine the independent effect of progenitor cell loss on subsequent brain development because infants that die are likely to have additional brain lesions. Such complications of GMH/IVH include venous infarction and ventricular dilation, both of which will additionally injure developing white matter and possibly thalamic tissue and therefore disrupt thalamo-cortical connectivity and cortical development. So, whilst there is likely to be a disturbance of the late GABAergic neuronal proliferation and migration from the subventricular zone (SVZ) and the ganglionic eminence (GE) to upper layers of the cerebral cortex and from the GE to the thalamus, venous infarction will cause additional destruction of both axons and pre-OLs, resulting in the formation of a porencephalic cyst. Thalamocortical connections will be disrupted, resulting in thalamic atrophy and overlying cortical development may be impaired. Thalamo-cortical disconnection may be demonstrated at a distance from the site of infarction.

The neurodevelopmental consequences of this are evident in follow-up studies such as the DRIFT trial, which enrolled neonates with marked ventricular dilation complicating GMH/IVH. The majority also had evidence of venous infarction. While the trial demonstrated some improvement in neurodevelopmental outcome following specific intervention, as a study group these infants with complications showed severe neurodevelopmental impairments at 2 years corrected age (Whitelaw et al. 2010). A secondary imaging study of total brain tissue volume and cerebellar volume highlighted the need to preserve supratentorial tissue and avoid cerebellar compression by a dilated fourth ventricle (Carli et al. 2010). Reduced cerebellar size following GMH/IVH may be multifactorial and related to a primary cerebellar hemorrhage or to secondary atrophy as a consequence of supratentorial lesions (Boardman et al. 2006; Srinivasan et al. 2006).

117.4.9 The Cerebellum in Extremely Preterm Babies

Primary cerebellar hemorrhage arising from the external granular layer and associated tissue infarction is relatively common in very preterm infants. There is a well documented association between intraventricular and cerebellar hemorrhage. In one large ultrasound study of 1242 preterm infants with intraventricular hemorrhage, 77% of infants also had cerebellar hemorrhages (Limperopoulos et al. 2005). MR imaging studies seem to confirm this high vulnerability of the most premature babies to develop cerebellar hemorrhage (Fumagalli et al. 2009).

A study using the mastoid window for better visualization of the posterior fossa demonstrated an incidence of cerebellar hemorrhage in 3% of preterm infants <1500 g, with nearly 60% of these occurring in infants less than 750 g (Limperopoulos et al. 2005). In the very preterm infant, the hemorrhage originates within the hemisphere with involvement initially of the subpial and subependymal layers sites of the germinal matrices and subventricular zones respectively. The more extensive lesions extend and involve both the cerebellar cortex and white matter. In contrast, in the term infant the site of origin is more frequently the vermis. Pathogenesis in the preterm infant shares many similarities with the causes of intraventricular hemorrhage. In the term infant, trauma is a more important factor. Injury to the developing cerebellum will result in disruption of neuronal migration, which continues into infancy in the cerebellum with consequent cerebellar disconnectivity.

The role of the cerebellum in cognitive function is being increasingly recognized. It is not surprising therefore that 40% survivors of preterm cerebellar hemorrhage demonstrate cognitive deficits and 37% have autistic spectrum disorders (Limperopoulos et al. 2007). In term infants, subsequent motor impairments are described more frequently, particularly in association with larger lesions (Limperopoulos et al. 2009; Takashima 1982).

117.4.10 Effects of Germinal Matrix Intraventricular Hemorrhage

There is evidence to suggest that less severe forms of GMH/IVH may be associated with periventricular WM injury. This may result in milder degrees of ventricular dilation and studies have reported an association with later cognitive function in such infants (Ment et al. 2005; Miller et al. 2005). In addition, two studies have reported worse outcomes in survivors of preterm birth where subsequent ventricular dilation was associated with an original GMH/IVH (Vollmer et al. 2006; Dyet et al. 2006). In the rabbit kit, IVH was associated with an increase in periventricular white matter (PVWM) microglial activation and axonal disruption and apoptosis (Dommergues

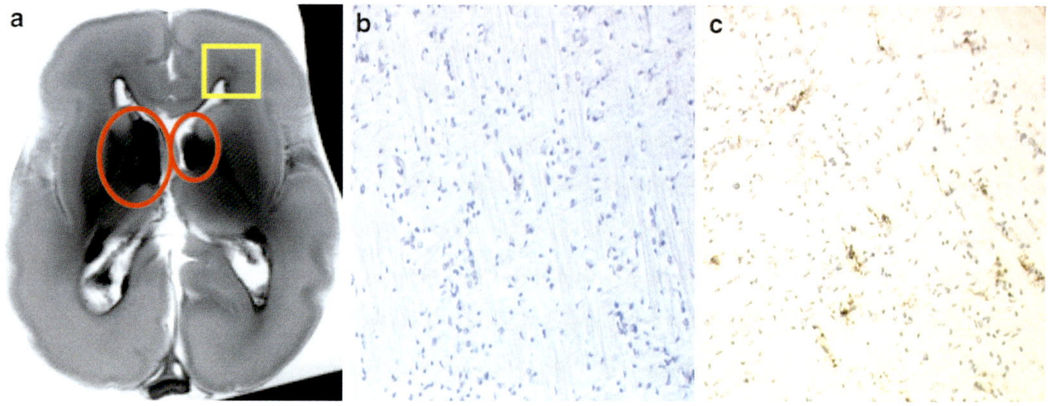

Fig. 9 T2 weighted MRI image (**a**) of a preterm infant born at 26 weeks and imaged postmortem at 28 weeks. There is bilateral germinal matrix/intraventricular hemorrhage seen as foci of low signal intensity (red circles). PAS (**b**) and Iba (**c**) staining through anterior periventricular white matter, (in the region of the yellow rectangle) showing intersecting axons, so called WM crossroads (**b**). Many of the cells in this region are microglia (**c**), which have roles associated with axonal guidance and WM modeling. Their presence may enhance the susceptibility of these regions to injury

et al. 2003). An increase in activated microglia has also been demonstrated in human PVWM in the presence of uncomplicated IVH (Fig. 9). Tissue injury may occur secondary to free radical release, secondary to the presence of free iron from the blood and the presence of resident activated microglia may exacerbate this process.

It is unclear whether as the germinal matrix involutes it becomes less susceptible to the effects of infection. The development of subependymal cysts in the persisting germinal matrix of the caudothalamic groove postnatally suggests that the tissue remains vulnerable to viral infection in more mature infants, but the consequences for progenitor cell destruction may be less severe as the infant matures.

117.5 The Late Preterm Infant

In recent years the vulnerability of late preterm infants of gestation between 34 and 37 weeks has become recognized. Reports demonstrate increased short-term neonatal morbidity in low risk late preterm pregnancies (Mateus et al. 2010; Melamed et al. 2009) with a 12-fold increase in mortality compared with term born controls and a mortality rate of 0.8% (Kitsommart et al. 2009). Studies of surviving late preterm infants have conflicting results, with no significant differences in childhood outcome (Gurka et al. 2010). A study at school entry showed that the risk for developmental delay or disability was 36% higher among late preterm infants compared with term infants (Morse et al. 2009). However, outcome studies at 12 and 18 months stress the importance of correcting for gestational age when interpreting results (Romeo et al. 2010).

Neuromorbidity in this group has been attributed to many factors. The cellular pathology of PVL and the developmental characteristics of oligodendrocytes and neurons put the late preterm brain at risk of injury. The cortical volume in the very preterm infant at 28 gestational weeks is 13% of term volume (Counsell et al. 2002). The cortical volume in the late preterm infant is only 53% of the term volume, with approximately half the volume being attained in the last 6 weeks before 40 gestational weeks. In addition, minimal myelinated white matter is present in the very preterm infant (around 29 weeks), but increases dramatically in volume as term is approached, with a fivefold increase between 35 and 41 weeks (Hüppi et al. 1996).

Studies of HIE in the preterm usually only include mature preterms and demonstrate that whilst mature preterms sustain injury to the central gray matter, the sites may differ to the more mature term brain. Mature preterm infants are more likely to show thalamic and globus pallidum lesions. In addition, they are more likely to sustain brainstem lesions (Logitharajah et al. 2009). This may because of more severe injury or indicate a particular susceptibility of the brain stem at these slightly younger gestations (Jiang et al. 2009).

It is of interest that the late preterm infant does not demonstrate cortical abnormalities around the central sulcus, which is a frequent abnormality n the term infant. This region is probably vulnerable due to the presence of myelination, which does not occur until approximately term (Logitharajah et al. 2009).

117.6 The Term Brain

Studies of injury to the more mature term brain have concentrated on the vulnerability of the neuronal population. Imaging studies of neonates with perinatal injury complicating an acute hypoxic ischemic event demonstrate involvement of the cortex, central gray matter and brainstem. Vulnerability to specific neuronal populations in the term brain is due to multiple factors but, like white matter vulnerability in the preterm brain, excitotoxicity and oxidative stress play major roles in term injury. Vulnerability may be related to the maturational state of the neurons. There is over-expression of certain glutamate receptors in selective regions like the basal ganglia.

The N-methyl-D-aspartate (NMDA) glutamate receptor subtype is the predominant mediator of this type of injury because of its coupling to neuronal nitric oxide synthase-containing neurons in the postsynaptic density complex. The NMDA receptor can change subunit compositions with development of the NR2B subunit predominating early, followed by increasing expression of NR2A. NMDA receptors with NR2B seem to have a slower deactivation and higher conductance. Following an hypoxic insult, there are differential effects on NMDA receptor subunit composition and these effects differ by age. This interaction may result in the production of both nitrogen and oxygen free radicals that in turn injure nearby cells (McQuillen and Ferriero 2004). The vulnerability to neurons in the basal nuclei also appears to be related also to the local environment as neuronal nitric oxide synthase-containing neurons make neurons relatively resistant to severe hypoxic ischemia (Ferriero et al. 1988). There is also an overabundance of NMDA receptors in this region at term allowing for the robust glutamatergic synapses necessary for long-term potentiation and connectivity but also allowing the neuron to be more vulnerable to glutamate attack. It has been suggested that these neurons may be protected either pharmacologically or by gene knockout to render the region less vulnerable and prevent neuronal loss (Ferriero et al. 1995, 1996).

Regions of vulnerability following acute hypoxic ischemia at term are recognized as being those that are metabolically active with increased energy requirements such as the basal ganglia and thalami (Chugani et al. 1993). Regions that are actively myelinating also appear to be more vulnerable. In the term infant, regions around the myelinating corticospinal tracts arising from the cortex at the central sulcus are frequently involved. However, in less mature infants these areas are often spared the metabolic demands of myelination, which may compound the additional vulnerability of cortical neurons, which express a high number of Ca^{2+} permeable glutamate receptors at term. This contrasts with the peak period for overexpression of these receptors in oligodendrocytes and subplate neurons, which is in the late second and early third trimesters.

117.7 Focal Infarction

White matter injury is often seen in the mature term brain, presumed either to be due to a vascular event relating to vessel obstruction by an embolus or by vessel spasm. Affected areas are as middle cerebral artery infarction or more global hypoperfusion such as in parasagittal or watershed injury. Bilateral injury is often associated with a history that suggests chronic hypoxia, e.g. decreased fetal movements, infection or hypoglycemia. Injury usually involves both the

WM and the cortex. Thalamic involvement is common but may occur as a secondary phenomenon. Posterior WM may be involved more frequently than anterior WM regions, particularly in association with hypoglycemia. This may be explained in terms of watershed injury, with posterior regions representing the watershed areas for all three cerebral arteries. However posterior involvement with hypoglycemia does not always selectively involve borderzones between arterial territories.

The hypothesis of a chronic or repeated event priming the WM suggests that the WM is made progressively more vulnerable so that it can be injured by a relatively mild hypoxicischemic event. The additional role for infection in such term infants may again relate to a cascade of injurious events precipitated by a fetal inflammatory response. The underlying mechanism for this acquired increased vulnerability remains unclear, but it may involve altered mitochondrial function. When mature oligodendrocytes die after exposure to kainate, (1) AMPA receptors are the most important mediators, (2) kainate receptors play a smaller role, and (3) death occurs predominantly by necrosis, not apoptosis (Leuchtmann et al. 2003).

117.8 Programmed Cell Death

Apoptosis is a critical component of normal brain development but, as the brain is poised to initiate programmed cell death around human birth, it becomes more susceptible to the initiation of a cell death pathway. Although necrosis plays a major role in early neuronal death in both the immature and mature brains after injury, there is a spectrum of cell death that includes apoptosis within the first 24 h following perinatal hypoxic ischemia (Northington et al. 2005). Programmed cell death is a crucial mechanism in the control of the final number of neurons and glial cells. This process, commonly referred to as apoptosis, can be observed from the earliest gestational ages with different times of cell death peaks in different brain regions (Graaf-Peters and Hadders-Algra 2006). In addition to refining normal brain development and connectivity, the plasticity it provides may be important in repair mechanisms following injury. However, a predisposition to programmed cell death may be exploited following injury and result in an increase in cellular apoptosis in injured regions as a consequence of disturbances disrupted connectivity.

The concept of priming of a brain region to injury is an important one, although a region such as the white matter is not traditionally considered to be vulnerable. There is, however, animal evidence to suggest that such priming occurs with preinjury insults (i.e., delivery related events) such as hypoglycemia, intrauterine growth restriction (IUGR) and infection. The biological mechanisms by which such events increase the susceptibility of WM to injury are poorly understood but investigations of preconditioning may explain the acceleration of such events due to birth.

References

Ajayi-Obe M, Saeed N, Cowan FM et al (2000) Reduced development of cerebral cortex in extremely preterm infants. Lancet 356:1162–1163

Allendoerfer KL, Shatz CJ (1994) The subplate, a transient neocortical structure: its role in the development of connections between thalamus and cortex. Annu Rev Neurosci 17:185–218

Andiman SE, Haynes RL, Trachtenberg FL et al (2010) The cerebral cortex overlying periventricular leukomalacia: analysis of pyramidal neurons. Brain Pathol 20:803–814

Banker BQ, Larroche JC (1962) Periventricular leukomalacia of infancy. A form of neonatal anoxic encephalopathy. Arch Neurol 7:386–410

Barkovich AJ, Lindan CE (1994) Congenital cytomegalovirus infection of the brain: imaging analysis and embryologic consideration. AJNR Am J Neuroradiol 15:703–715

Barkovich AJ, Sargent SK (1995) Profound asphyxia in the premature infant: imaging findings. AJNR Am J Neuroradiol 16:1837–1846

Bassi L, Ricci D, Volzone A et al (2008) Probabilistic diffusion tractography of the optic radiations and visual function in preterm infants at term equivalent age. Brain 131:573–582

Billiard SS, Haynes RL, Folkerth RD et al (2006) Development of microglia in the cerebral white matter of the human fetus and infant. J Comp Neurol 497:199–208

Boardman JP, Counsell SJ, Rueckert D et al (2006) Abnormal deep grey matter development following preterm birth detected using deformation-based morphometry. NeuroImage 32:70–78

Chugani HT, Shewmon DA, Shields WD et al (1993) Surgery for intractable infantile spasms: neuroimaging perspectives. Epilepsia 34:764–771

Cioni G, Fazzi B, Coluccini M et al (1997) Cerebral visual impairment in preterm infants with periventricular leukomalacia. Pediatr Neurol 17:331–338

Counsell SJ, Maalouf EF, Fletcher AM et al (2002) MR imaging assessment of myelination in the very preterm brain. AJNR Am J Neuroradiol 23:872–881

De Carli A, Jary S, Ramenghi LA et al (2010) Magnetic resonance imaging (MRI) at term equivalent age correlates with neurodevelopment at 2 years in preterm infants with post-hemorrhagic ventricular dilatation. PAS Meeting Abstract 3746

de Graaf-Peters V, Hadders-Algra M (2006) Ontogeny of the human central nervous system: what is happening when? Early Hum Dev 82:257–266

Dean JM, Wang X, Kaindl AM et al (2009) Microglial MyD88 signaling regulates acute neuronal toxicity of LPS-stimulated microglia *in vitro*. Brain, Behaviour and Immunity. J Neurosci 16:2508–2521

Deng W, Wang H, Rosenberg PA et al (2004) Role of metabotropic glutamate receptors in oligodendrocytes excitotoxicity and oxidative stress. Proc Natl Acad Sci U S A 101:7751–7756

Dommergues MA, Plaisant F, Verney C, Gressens P (2003) Early microglial activation following neonatal excitotoxic brain damage in mice: a potential target for neuroprotection. Neuroscience 121:619–628

Dudink J, Buijs J, Govaert P et al (2010) Diffusion tensor imaging of the cortical plate and subplate in very-low-birth-weight infants. Pediatr Radiol 40:1397–1404

Dyet LE, Kennea N, Counsell SJ et al (2006) Natural history of brain lesions in extremely preterm infants studied with serial magnetic resonance imaging from birth and neurodevelopmental assessment. Pediatrics 118:536–548

Elkabes S, Peng L, Black IB (1998) Lipopolysaccharide differentially regulates microglial trk receptor and neurotrophin expression. J Neurosci Res 54:117–122

Ferriero DM, Arcavi LJ, Sagar SM et al (1988) Selective sparing of NADPH-diaphorase neurons in neonatal hypoxia-ischemia. Ann Neurol 24:670–676

Ferriero DM, Sheldon RA, Black SM, Chuai J (1995) Selective destruction of nitric oxide synthase neurons with quisqualate reduces damage after hypoxia-ischemia in the neonatal rat. Pediatr Res 38:912–918

Ferriero DM, Holtzman DM, Black SM, Sheldon RA (1996) Neonatal mice lacking neuronal nitric oxide synthase are less vulnerable to hypoxic-ischemic injury. Neurobiol Dis 3:64–71

Fumagalli M, Ramenghi LA, Righini A et al (2009) Cerebellar haemorrhages and pons development in extremely low birth weight infants. Front Biosci 1:537–541

Ghazi-Birry HS, Brown WR, Moody DM et al (1997) Human germinal matrix: venous origin of hemorrhage and vascular characteristics. AJNR Am J Neuroradiol 18:219–239

Ghosh A, Shatz CJ (1992) Involvement of subplate neurons in the formation of ocular dominance columns. Science 255:1441–1443

Gurka MJ, LoCasale-Crouch J, Blackman JA (2010) Long-term cognition, achievement, socioemotional, and behavioral development of healthy late-preterm infants. Arch Pediatr Adolesc Med 164:525–532

Hambleton G, Wigglesworth JS (1976) Origin of intraventricular haemorrhage in the preterm infant. Arch Dis Child 51:651–659

Haynes RL, Folkerth RD, Keefe RJ et al (2003) Nitrosative and oxidative injury to premyelinating oligodendrocytes in periventricular leukomalacia. J Neuropathol Exp Neurol 62:441–450

Hüppi PS, Dubois J (2006) Diffusion tensor imaging of brain development. Semin Fetal Neonatal Med 11:489–497

Hüppi PS, Schuknecht B, Boesch C et al (1996) Structural and neurobehavioral delay in postnatal brain development of preterm infants. Pediatr Res 39:895–901

Inder TE, Huppi PS, Warfield S et al (1999) Periventricular white matter injury in the premature infant is followed by reduced cerebral cortical gray matter volume at term. Ann Neurol 46:755–760

Jiang ZD, Brosi DM, Wu YY, Wilkinson AR (2009) Relative maturation of peripheral and central regions of the human brainstem from preterm to term and the influence of preterm birth. Pediatr Res 65:657–662

Judas M, Rados M, Jovanov-Milosevic N et al (2005) Structural, immunocytochemical, and MR imaging properties of periventricular crossroads of growing cortical pathways in preterm infants. AJNR Am J Neuroradiol 26:2671–2684

Kapellou O, Counsell SJ, Kennea N et al (2006) Abnormal cortical development after premature birth shown by altered allometric scaling of brain growth. PLoS Med 3: e265

Khwaja O, Volpe JJ (2008) Pathogenesis of cerebral white matter injury of prematurity. Arch Dis Child Fetal Neonatal Ed 93:F153–F161

Kinoshita Y, Okudera T, Tsuru E, Yokota A (2001) Volumetric analysis of the germinal matrix and lateral ventricles performed using MR images of postmortem fetuses. AJNR Am J Neuroradiol 22:382–388

Kitsommart R, Janes M, Mahajan V et al (2009) Outcomes of latepreterm infants: a retrospective, single-center, Canadian study. Clin Pediatr (Phila) 48:844–850

Kjellmer I (1991) Mechanism of perinatal brain damage. Ann Med 23:675–679

Kostovic I, Judas M (2006) Prolonged coexistence of transient and permanent circuitry elements in the developing cerebral cortex of fetuses and preterm infants. Dev Med Child Neurol 48:388–393

Kostovic I, Rakic P (1990) Developmental history of the transient subplate zone in the visual and somatosensory cortex of the macaque monkey and human brain. J Comp Neurol 297:441–470

Lee CT, Chen J, Worden LT, Freed WJ (2010) Cocaine causes deficits in radial migration and alters the distribution of glutamate and GABA neurons in the developing rat cerebral cortex. Synapse 65:21–34

Leech RW, Kohnen P (1974) Subependymal and intraventricular hemorrhage in the newborn. Am J Pathol 77:465–475

Leuchtmann EA, Ratner AE, Vijitruth R et al (2003) AMPA receptors are the major mediators of excitotoxic death in mature oligodendrocytes. Neurobiol Dis 14:336–348

Ligam P, Haynes RL, Folkerth RD et al (2009) Thalamic damage in periventricular leukomalacia: novel pathologic observations relevant to cognitive deficits in survivors of prematurity. Pediatr Res 65:524–529

Limperopoulos C, Benson CB, Bassan H et al (2005) Cerebellar hemorrhage in the preterm infant: ultrasonographic findings and risk factors. Pediatrics 116:717–724

Limperopoulos C, Bassan H, Gauvreau K et al (2007) Does cerebellar injury in premature infants contribute to the high prevalence of long-term cognitive, learning, and behavioral disability in survivors? Pediatrics 120:584–593

Limperopoulos C, Robertson RL, Sullivan NR et al (2009) Cerebellar injury in term infants: clinical characteristics, magnetic resonance imaging findings, and outcome. Pediatr Neurol 41:1–8

Logitharajah P, Rutherford MA, Cowan FM (2009) Hypoxic-ischemic encephalopathy in preterm infants: antecedent factors, brain imaging and outcome. Pediatr Res 66:222–229

Luo MH, Hannemann H, Kulkarni AS et al (2010) Human cytomegalovirus infection causes premature and abnormal differentiation of human neural progenitor cells. J Virol 84:3528–3541

Marcorelles P, Laquerrière A, Adde-Michel C et al (2010) Evidence for tangential migration disturbances in human lissencephaly resulting from a defect in LIS1, DCX and ARX genes. Acta Neuropathol 120:503–515

Marin Padilla M (1999) Developmental neuropathology and impact of perinatal brain damage. III: gray matter lesions of the neocortex. J Neuropathol Exp Neurol 58:407–429

Marsh B, Stevens SL, Packard AE et al (2009) Systemic lipopolysaccharide protects the brain from Ischemic Injury by reprogramming the response of the brain to stroke: a critical role for IRF3. J Neurosci 29:9839–9849

Mateus J, Fox K, Jain S et al (2010) Preterm premature rupture of membranes: clinical outcomes of late-preterm infants. Clin Pediatr (Phila) 49:60–65

McQuillen PS, Ferriero DM (2004) Selective vulnerability in the developing central nervous system. Pediatr Neurol 30:227–235

McQuillen PS, Sheldon RA, Shatz CJ, Ferriero DM (2003) Selective vulnerability of subplate neurons after early neonatal hypoxiaischemia. J Neurosci 23:3308–3315

Melamed N, Klinger G, Tenenbaum-Gavish K et al (2009) Shortterm neonatal outcome in low-risk, spontaneous, singleton, late preterm deliveries. Obstet Gynecol 114 (2 Part 1):253–260

Ment LR, Allan WC, Makuch RW et al (2005) Grade 3 to 4 intraventricular hemorrhage and Bayley scores predict outcome. Pediatrics 116:1597–1598

Métin C, Vallee RB, Rakic P, Bhide PG (2008) Modes and mishaps of neuronal migration in the mammalian brain. J Neurosci 28:11746–11752

Miller SP, Ferriero DM, Leonard C et al (2005) Early brain injury in premature newborns detected with magnetic resonance imaging is associated with adverse early neurodevelopmental outcome. J Pediatr 147: 609–616

Miyoshi G, Hjerling-Leffler J, Karayannis T et al (2010) Genetic fate mapping reveals that the caudal ganglionic eminence produces a large and diverse population of superficial cortical interneurons. J Neurosci 30:1582–1594

Morse SB, Zheng H, Tang Y, Roth J (2009) Early school-age outcomes of late preterm infants. Pediatrics 123: e622–e629

Nadarajah B, Parnavelas JG (2002) Modes of neuronal migration in the developing cerebral cortex. Nat Rev Neurosci 3:423–432

Northington FJ, Graham EM, Martin LJ (2005) Apoptosis in perinatal hypoxic-ischemic brain injury: how important is it and should it be inhibited? Brain Res Brain Res Rev 50:244–257

Patel AB, de Graaf RA, Mason GF et al (2005) The contribution of GABA to glutamate/glutamine cycling and energy metabolism in the rat cortex *in vivo*. Proc Natl Acad Sci U S A 15:5588–1593

Rakic P (1978) Neuronal migration and contact guidance in the primate telencephalon. Postgrad Med J 54:25–40

Rakic S, Zecevic N (2000) Programmed cell death in the developing human telencephalon. Eur J Neurosci 12:2721–2734

Ramenghi LA, Gill BJ, Tanner SF et al (2002) Cerebral venous thrombosis, intraventricular haemorrhage and white matter lesions in a preterm newborn with factor V (Leiden) mutation. Neuropediatrics 33:97–99

Ramenghi LA, Fumagalli M, Righini A et al (2007) Magnetic resonance imaging assessment of brain maturation in preterm neonates with punctate white matter lesions. Neuroradiology 49:161–167

Ramenghi LA, Ricci D, Mercuri E et al (2010) Visual performance and brain structure in the developing brain of preterm infants. Early Hum Dev 86(Suppl 1):73–75

Rezaie P, Male D (1999) Colonisation of the developing human brain and spinal cord by microglia: a review. Microsc Res Tech 45:359–382

Ricci D, Anker S, Cowan F et al (2006) Thalamic atrophy in infants with PVL and cerebral visual impairment. Early Hum Dev 82:591–595

Romeo DM, Di Stefano A, Conversano M et al (2010) Neurodevelopmental outcome at 12 and 18 months in late preterm infants. Eur J Paediatr Neurol 14:503–507

Rutherford MA, Supramaniam V, Ederise A et al (2010) Magnetic resonance imaging of white matter diseases of prematurity. Neuroradiology 52:505–521

Segovia KN, McClure M, Moravec M et al (2008) Arrested oligodendrocyte lineage maturation in chronic perinatal white matter injury. Ann Neurol 63:520–530

Skoff RP (1980) Neuroglia: a reevaluation of their origin and development. Pathol Res Pract 168:279–300

Srinivasan L, Allsop J, Counsell SJ et al (2006) Smaller cerebellar volumes in very preterm infants at term equivalent age are associated with the presence of supratentorial lesions. AJNR Am J Neuroradiol 117:376–386

Supramaniam V, Srinivasan L, Doherty K et al (2010) The distribution and morphology of microglial (MG) cells in the periventricular white matter (PVWM) of immature human brain. PAS Meeting Abstract 3105

Tabata H, Nakajima K (2003) Multipolar migration: the third mode of radial neuronal migration in the developing cerebral cortex. J Neurosci 23:9996–10001

Takashima S (1982) Olivocerebellar lesions in infants born prematurely. Brain and Development 4:361–366

Towbin A (1968) Cerebral intraventricular hemorrhage and subependymal matrix infarction in the fetus and premature newborn. Am J Pathol 52:121–140

Vollmer B, Roth S, Riley K et al (2006) Neurodevelopmental outcome of preterm infants with ventricular dilatation with and without associated haemorrhage. Dev Med Child Neurol 48:348–352

Volpe JJ (2009) Brain injury in premature infants: a complex amalgam of destructive and developmental disturbances. Lancet Neurol 8:110–124

Wang X, Stridh L, Li W et al (2009) Lipopolysaccharide sensitizes neonatal hypoxic-ischemic brain injury in a MyD88-dependent manner. J Immunol 183:7471–7477

Whitelaw A, Jary S, Kmita G et al (2010) Randomized trial of drainage, irrigation and fibrinolytic therapy for premature infants with posthemorrhagic ventricular dilatation: developmental outcome at 2 years. Pediatrics 125:e852–e858

Widjaja E, Geibprasert S, Mahmoodabadi SZ et al (2010) Alteration of human fetal subplate layer and intermediate zone during normal development on MR and diffusion tensor imaging. AJNR Am J Neuroradiol 31:1091–1099

Wu YW, Hamrick SE, Miller SP et al (2003) Intraventricular hemorrhage in term neonates caused by sinovenous thrombosis. Ann Neurol 54:123–126

Zhang Y, Allodi S, Sandeman DC, Beltz BS (2009) Adult neurogenesis in the crayfish brain: proliferation, migration, and possible origin of precursor cells. Dev Neurobiol 69:415–436

Inflammation and Perinatal Brain Injury

118

Henrik Hagberg, Carina Mallard, and Karin Sävman

Contents

H. Hagberg (✉)
Perinatal Center, Department of Obstetrics and Gynecology, Sahlgrenska Academy, University of Gothenburg, Goteborg, Sweden

Centre for the Developing Brain, Division of Imaging Sciences and Biomedical Engineering, King's College London, King's Health Partners, St. Thomas' Hospital, London, UK
e-mail: henrik.hagberg@obgyn.gu.se

C. Mallard
Department of Physiology, Institute of Neuroscience and Physiology, Sahlgrenska Academy, University of Gothenburg, Gothenburg, Sweden

K. Sävman
Department of Pediatrics, Sahlgrenska Academy, University of Gothenburg, Gothenburg, Sweden

Abstract

Inflammation is a critical contributor to both normal development and injury outcome in the immature brain. The consequences of immune activation in brain injury will be entirely different depending on context and stage of central nervous system (CNS) maturity. The immature brain can be exposed to inflammation in connection with viral or bacterial infection during pregnancy or as a result of sterile CNS insults such as hypoxia-ischemia and neonatal stroke. Through efficient anti-inflammatory and reparative processes, inflammation may resolve without any harmful effects on the brain. Alternatively, inflammation contributes to injury or enhances CNS vulnerability. Acute inflammation can also be shifted to a chronic inflammatory state and/or

G. Buonocore et al. (eds.), *Neonatology*,
https://doi.org/10.1007/978-3-319-29489-6_265

adversely affect brain development resulting in neurologic disease in children or adults.

118.1 Salient Points

- Inflammation is a critical contributor to outcome in the immature brain.
- The immature brain can be exposed to inflammation in connection with viral or bacterial infection during pregnancy. Brain injury may also be the result of sterile CNS insults such as hypoxia-ischemia and neonatal shock.
- There is a potential for neuroprotective immune-modulatory therapies to be developed, but we still need more detailed knowledge about the basic mechanism.

118.2 Introduction

Inflammation is a systemic and local immune reaction to injury secondary to microbial invasion or other damaging events like trauma and hypoxia-ischemia (Fig. 1). This response aids in identifying extrinsic pathogens and kills microbes (and affected cells) if the injury is caused by infection (Hagberg et al. 2015). Irrespective of the primary triggering event, inflammation often causes brain damage during its acute stage (collateral damage) followed by secondary and tertiary phases that in most cases promotes tissue repair and regeneration (Fleiss and Gressens 2012).

Historically, several findings support a link between brain injury and antenatal/postnatal inflammation (Dammann and O'Shea 2008). In the 1970s, it was discovered that postnatal sepsis was strongly associated with brain injury in spite of the lack of microbial invasion in the brain parenchyma (Leviton et al. 1976). Induction of systemic inflammation in newborn kittens with lipopolysaccharide (LPS, fragment of the gram-negative bacterial cell wall) induced white matter injury (Gilles et al. 1977). These studies suggested that infection triggers a systemic inflammatory response that inflicts brain injury under some conditions. During the 1960s–1970s, it was discovered that cytokines, a family of ubiquitous and pleiotropic immune molecules with pro-, anti-, or immunomodulatory properties, orchestrate the inflammatory response (Vilcek 1998). Indeed, cytokines were shown to play a critical role in preterm delivery (Romero et al. 2014; Gomez et al. 1998) and initiation of a fetal inflammatory response with subsequent development of brain injury and cerebral palsy (Gomez et al. 1998; Yoon et al. 2000).

In parallel, experimental work demonstrated that noninfectious insults like hypoxia-ischemia and excitotoxicity elicited cytokine expression (Szaflarski et al. 1995) and activation of immunoinflammatory microglia/macrophages (McRae et al. 1995; Tahraoui et al. 2001) in the immature brain that seemed to play a role for the development of brain injury (Giulian and Vaca 1993; Hagberg et al. 1996; Dommergues et al. 2000). Epidemiological studies found that chorioamnionitis was associated with cerebral palsy in term infants (Grether and Nelson 1997), and there was a remarkable correlation between cytokine levels 2.5 days after birth and cerebral palsy, particularly in term infants (Nelson et al. 1998).

These early studies indicated that cytokine-mediated inflammation is an important factor for the development of brain injury irrespective of whether the inflammatory response was caused by infection, hypoxia-ischemia, or excitotoxicity. However, since these early reports, the complexity, diversity, and sometimes contradictory (Jekyll-Hyde) properties of the inflammatory reaction have become increasingly clear. Furthermore, cytokines have been discovered to have other roles, e.g., in brain development and in the setting of CNS vulnerability as well as in neuronal and oligodendroglial regeneration (Hagberg and Mallard 2005). In this short review, we will summarize some of the recent pertinent experimental and clinical findings.

118.3 Immune Molecules and Brain Development

Molecules classically involved in immune responses are pleiotropic and have critical nonimmune functions during normal CNS

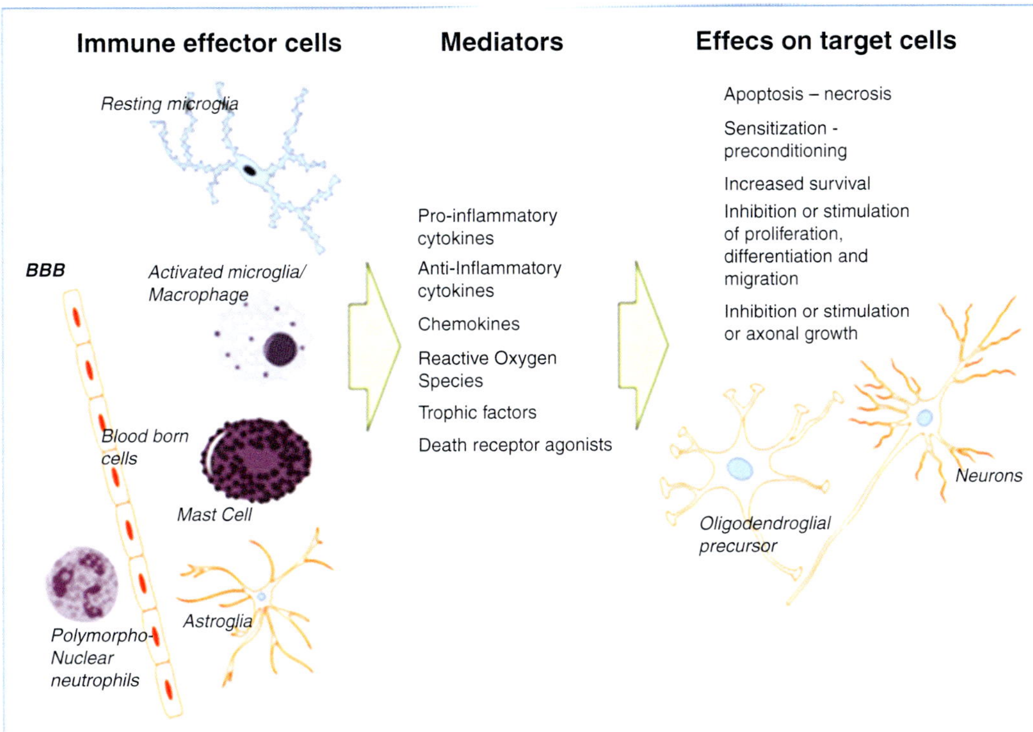

Fig. 1 Inflammation and perinatal brain injury. Infection, hypoxia-ischemia, or other insults activate immune effector cells in the vascular compartment as well as in the brain parenchyma. These cells produce a plethora of mediators that exert protective as well as toxic effects in the immature CNS

development, including neuronal and glial cell migration, cell differentiation, axonal path finding, and synaptic plasticity. These molecules include classical pro-inflammatory cytokines and chemokines as well as proteins of both the innate and adaptive immune system.

Cytokines are of importance during all stages of neural development. Members of the transforming growth factor beta (TGFβ) cytokine superfamily, including bone morphogenetic proteins (BMPs), are critical for neural induction, and normal CNS development requires active inhibition of BMPs (Gaulden and Reiter 2008). Later in CNS development, maintenance of the progenitor cell population is dependent on several members of the gp130 cytokine family, including leukemia inhibitory factor (LIF) and ciliary neurotrophic factor (CNTF) (Shimazaki et al. 2001). Also classical pro-inflammatory cytokines, such as interleukin-1 beta (IL-1β), have been reported to modulate neuronal and glial cell survival during development (Giulian et al. 1988) and to regulate progenitor proliferation (de la Mano et al. 2007). There is also evidence to suggest that IL-1β promotes differentiation of oligodendrocyte progenitors as well as maturation and survival of differentiating oligodendrocytes (Vela et al. 2002) (see Hagberg et al. 2015 for a more comprehensive update).

Chemokines are traditionally considered as secreted leukocyte chemoattractants. However, several chemokines and their respective receptors are constitutively expressed in the CNS, and significant evidence supports chemokines, such as CXCL12, as key regulators of early brain development, including survival and migration of neural and oligodendrocyte precursors (Dziembowska et al. 2005; Tran et al. 2007; Zou et al. 1998). CXCL12, via activation of its receptor CXCR4, is also crucial for tangential migration of Cajal-Retzius cells and thereby the normal development of the cerebral cortex (Borrell and Marin 2006).

Innate immune responses have been implicated in normal CNS development. Both C1q and C3, components of the classical complement cascade, are expressed in neurons in the developing brain and play an important role in synapse pruning in the visual system during development (Stephan et al. 2012), and complement-derived C3a regulates differentiation and migration of neural progenitor cells (Shinjyo et al. 2009). Toll-like receptors (TLRs) belong to a recently discovered family of innate immune receptors (Mallard et al. 2009). TLRs are expressed in the developing brain, and stimulation of TLR3 negatively regulates both axonal growth in sensory neurons (Cameron et al. 2007) and embryonic neural progenitor cell proliferation (Lathia et al. 2008). Furthermore, TLR8 is expressed in neurons and axons during mouse development, and stimulation of TLR8 in cultured cortical neurons causes inhibition of neurite outgrowth and induces apoptosis (Ma et al. 2006). In addition, TLRs are expressed in adult neural progenitor cells and may influence their proliferation and differentiation as TLR2 deficiency impaired hippocampal neurogenesis, whereas the absence of TLR4 resulted in enhanced proliferation and neuronal differentiation (Rolls et al. 2007). Also the adaptive immune system, including the class I MHC molecules, has been shown to play a role during normal development and plasticity (Huh et al. 2000).

118.4 Inflammation and Brain Injury in Preterm Infants

Infection/inflammation is strongly associated with preterm delivery and accounts for 20–40% of all cases with preterm birth (Goldenberg et al. 2008) including the majority of cases with spontaneous preterm birth before 30 weeks of gestation, i.e., those at highest risk of neurological morbidity (Hagberg et al. 2015; Goldenberg et al. 2008; Hagberg et al. 2012). Hypothetically, ascending microbes activate TLRs leading to increased accumulation of polymorphonuclear neutrophils and expression of pro-inflammatory cytokines (IL-6, IL-8, IL-1β, TNF-α) in the decidual and chorioamniotic membranes, i.e., histological chorioamnionitis (HCA). The inflammatory response elicits myometrial contractions, cervical ripening, and preterm prelabor rupture of the membranes (PPROM) subsequently resulting in preterm delivery (Patni et al. 2007). In most cases, chorioamnionitis (CA) is subclinical and manifests rarely as clinical chorioamnionitis (CCA) (maternal fever, tachycardia, uterine tenderness, malodorous amniotic fluid, and leukocytosis/raised C-reactive protein). CA is a predominately fetal infection, and spread of the inflammation and/or microbial invasion from the membranes to amniotic fluid to umbilical cord to fetal blood (fetal inflammatory response syndrome) increases, not unexpectedly, the risks of fetal morbidity and mortality (see below) (Goldenberg et al. 2008; Yoon et al. 2001). The degree of fetal inflammation (defined as, e.g., IL-6 elevation in amniotic fluid or blood) determines at least acute neonatal morbidity.

Some data indicate that intrauterine inflammation is associated with neurological injury. Severe brain lesions were 10 times more common after spontaneous onset of labor (with high occurrence of CA) than in physician-initiated delivery (with a low occurrence of CA) at a comparable gestational age offering support of the inflammatory hypothesis (Verma et al. 1997). A similar, but not as marked, correlation was found between diplegic cerebral palsy (CP) and type of delivery onset (Dammann et al. 1998), whereas no such association was found by Jacobsson et al. (Jacobsson et al. 2002). In a very important study, the presence of umbilical cord inflammation (funisitis) or high amniotic IL-6 and IL-8 levels conferred an increased risk of CP in the offspring at 3 years of age even after adjustment for differences in gestational age (Yoon et al. 2000). The proposal that fetal rather than maternal involvement predicts neurological outcome is supported also by a large study (1078 infants, 500–1500 g, 47 with sonographic echolucency) showing that fetal vasculitis was associated with an increased risk of late echolucent white matter injury in cases born shortly after PPROM (OR 10.1, CI 1.03–114) (Leviton et al. 1999). Furthermore, cytokines and CD45RO

(+) T lymphocytes in fetal blood predicted cerebral white matter injury detected by magnetic resonance imaging soon after birth (Duggan et al. 2001).

According to a meta-analysis, CCA is associated with CP (RR 1.9, CI 1.4–2.5) and cystic periventricular leukomalacia (PVL) (3.0; 2.2–4.0), whereas CA constitutes a risk factor for PVL (2.1; 1.5–2.9) but not CP (1.6; 0.9–2.7) (Wu and Colford 2000). However, a strong association was found between polymicrogyria (a migratory disturbance of the cortical plate/cerebral cortex) and CA (Toti et al. 1998). The brains of fetuses at gestational age 15–26 weeks in the context of CA were compared with those aborted for other reasons. Polymicrogyria was found in 25/32 cases (78%) with infection compared with none in the control group. These remarkable results suggest that inflammation inflicts on brain development (see above), which agree with experimental studies in adult rodents (Monje et al. 2003) and with a recently published review suggesting that microglial activation may disturb cortical migration and stem cell survival (Leviton and Gressens 2007).

Moreover, several investigators have shown that intravenous administration of LPS to fetal sheep (Duncan et al. 2002; Mallard et al. 2003; Yan et al. 2004; Dean et al. 2009a) or into the amniotic fluid (Nitsos et al. 2006; Gavilanes et al. 2009) results in white matter damage. Early studies suggested that LPS caused brain damage by reducing cerebral blood flow (Young et al. 1982; Ando et al. 1988); however, more recent evidence, using lower doses of LPS, does not find that perfusion deficits contribute to injury (Dalitz et al. 2003; Duncan et al. 2006).

It is important to mention that not all studies support the inflammatory hypothesis. For example, no association between white matter injury/neurological outcome and HCA or umbilical blood IL-6 was found by Kaukola et al. (2006). Reiman et al. (2008) found no correlation between fetal or maternal HCA and brain injury defined by ultrasound or magnetic resonance imaging (MRI), which agrees with Chau et al. (2009), who found no association between fetal or maternal HCA and MRI-defined brain abnormalities in preterm infants at 24–32 weeks of gestation. Furthermore, Kumazaki et al. (2002) detected no difference in ultrasound-defined PVL in cases with versus without fetal or maternal HCA.

These discrepancies cannot easily be explained, but generally there is a lack of statistical power in many studies (both those pro and con the inflammatory hypothesis), inconsistencies in the definition of CA (see above), differences in cases included and study design, or the fact that inflammation has many different phenotypes (toxic, beneficial, no effect) depending on context, timing, and other circumstances (Fig. 1).

There are several clinical and experimental studies indicating that CA may be a stronger risk factor if combined with another exposure, the so-called multiple-hit hypothesis (Stanley 1994). For example, HCA alone was not a risk factor, but if combined with signs of a placental perfusion defect, the risk of abnormal neurological outcome was increased (3/10 with HCA vs. 3/43 without HCA) (Kaukola et al. 2006). In another study, culture positive postnatal infection increased the risk of MRI-defined brain injury if occurring in combination with hypotension (Chau et al. 2009). Indeed, chorioamnionitis (with or without funisitis) increases the risk of hypotension in very low birth infants (Lee et al. 2006).

118.5 Inflammation in Term Brain Injury

Inflammation has been extensively studied as part of the secondary response to experimental hypoxic-ischemic (HI) injury, and the presence of an inflammatory response has been demonstrated also after clinical HI. There are, however, also studies that suggest that infection/inflammation may precede brain injury or sensitize to subsequent HI. In addition, the inflammatory response and its involvement in injury and repair in the immature brain are dependent on timing as well as context and differ substantially from that seen in the adult brain.

118.5.1 Clinical Findings of Inflammatory Factors in Term Brain Injury

Several studies demonstrate that an inflammatory response is elicited in CSF from term infants fulfilling criteria for acute intrapartum asphyxia. Elevated levels of pro-inflammatory cytokines IL-6 and IL-8 in CSF are correlated with severity of encephalopathy as well as neurodevelopmental outcome (Martin-Ancel et al. 1997; Savman et al. 1998). In samples obtained within 24 h after birth, IL-1β and TNF-α show similar correlations (Oygur et al. 1998; Aly et al. 2006), and comparisons with serum levels suggest that the cytokines are produced within the brain (Aly et al. 2006; Silveira and Procianoy 2003). Support of cytokines contributing to brain injury rather than just being biomarkers of inflammation is presented in a study showing increased risk for CP in infants with specific IL-6 genotype (Wu et al. 2009).

The correlation between brain injury and systemic inflammation is less well documented, but at least one study shows that asphyxiated infants with adverse outcome had elevated pro-inflammatory cytokines in serum (Bartha et al. 2004). An intriguing study of dried blood spots from term infants who later developed spastic CP demonstrates, however, elevated levels of multiple cytokines in virtually all affected infants in comparison with term matched controls even if HI is likely to be the cause of only a minor fraction of the CP cases in that study (Nelson et al. 1998).

The suggestion that exposure to infection or inflammation in itself or together with HI may lead to term brain injury is further supported by individual studies (Grether and Nelson 1997) as well as a large meta-analysis showing that clinical chorioamnionitis is an independent risk factor (OR 4.1) for term/near-term CP (Wu et al. 2003). In the same analysis, chorioamnionitis in the mother was also associated (OR around 5) with signs of neonatal depression (APGAR at 5 min <7, clinical diagnosis of birth asphyxia) as well as signs of neonatal encephalopathy (seizures) (Wu et al. 2003). Since data on metabolic acidosis and from neuroimaging were not available, it cannot be excluded that these findings were secondary to exposure to chorioamnionitis only. Extensive MRI studies show, however, that a large majority of term infants with the combination of neonatal depression and neonatal encephalopathy have acutely evolving injuries suggesting intrapartum asphyxia (Cowan et al. 2003). It is thus likely that at least some of the infants with subsequent CP were exposed to chorioamnionitis as well as HI, giving additional support to the multiple-hit hypothesis. Further evidence of the detrimental effect of fetal inflammation in combination with HI is provided by a study of term spastic CP showing relatively low OR for exposure to chorioamnionitis as well as potentially asphyxiating factors (placental and cord complication), while the combination of both increased the risk for severe spastic CP 100-fold (Nelson and Grether 1998). In addition, neonatal serum cytokines are elevated after exposure to chorioamnionitis, but the increase is most pronounced in infants who also fulfill very strict criteria for hypoxic-ischemic encephalopathy (including metabolic acidosis, moderate-severe encephalopathy, and multiorgan failure), illustrating the close relationship between exposure to infection and clinical HI (Shalak et al. 2002).

118.5.2 Experimental Studies Supporting Inflammatory Factors in Post-HI Injury

The inflammatory response after experimental HI includes an early but restricted accumulation of neutrophil cells, mainly in blood vessels adjacent to injury (Hudome et al. 1997; Bona et al. 1999). Resident microglia and/or invading macrophages are, however, the predominant inflammatory cell type after neonatal HI, and infiltration of activated cells is detected as early as 2–3 h after injury, followed by a marked increase in the following days that persists for weeks (McRae et al. 1995; Bona et al. 1999). Inflammatory cells may contribute to injury by release of excitatory amino acids, pro-inflammatory cytokines, degrading enzymes, and reactive oxygen species (ROS), but microglia can also produce neurotrophic or neuronal survival factors upon activation (Kim and de Vellis 2005). In the neonatal setting, HI is accompanied by a massive change in the expression of inflammation-related genes with close to 150 genes differentially regulated at 2–72 h after the insult including upregulation of cytokines, chemokines, proteases, and ROS-forming enzymes (Hedtjarn et al. 2004).

A number of experimental studies show that inflammatory cells and inflammatory mediators may contribute to injury, but the complexity of the inflammatory response is illustrated by conflicting data or results limited to certain contexts. In addition, several studies indicate that the inflammatory mechanisms related to the development of brain injury are substantially different in the immature compared with the adult brain and that inflammatory cells may also have protective properties.

Factors that may influence the results of anti-inflammatory interventions include means and timing of inhibition and degree of injury. As an example, the pro-inflammatory cytokine IL-1β is upregulated at the mRNA as well as protein level after HI, and soluble IL-1 receptor antagonist protects newborn rats from HI injury (Hagberg et al. 1996; Martin et al. 1994), while genetic inhibition of IL- 1β or IL-1α/β combined confers no protection in newborn mice (Hedtjarn et al. 2005). IL-18 is another cytokine that is upregulated after HI in newborn mice, and transgenic mice lacking functional IL-18 are protected from injury (Hedtjarn et al. 2002). Genetic inhibition of interleukin-1 converting enzyme (ICE) that converts IL-1β as well as IL-18 to their active forms is, however, protective only after moderate but not severe HI (Liu et al. 1999). A similar restriction is found for matrix metalloproteinase-9 (MMP-9), a tissue degrading enzyme expressed by activated microglia, where genetic knockout attenuates injury after moderate HI only (Svedin et al. 2007).

The difference between the adult and immature brain is illustrated by findings after neutrophil depletion and inhibition of the enzyme NADPH oxidase that is responsible for ROS formation in inflammatory cells. Neutrophil inhibition is protective after adult (Matsuo et al. 1994) as well as neonatal HI injury (Hudome et al. 1997), but neutrophil infiltration is limited in the immature brain (Bona et al. 1999), and protection is only seen if the depletion is induced well before injury suggesting early effects on brain microcirculation (Palmer et al. 2004). Neutrophil depletion also results in reduced free radical formation in the adult brain (Matsuo et al. 1995), and mice lacking functional NADPH oxidase have 40% reduction of infarction volume after adult stroke (Walder et al. 1997). This is in stark contrast to the immature brain, where genetic or pharmacological inhibition of NADPH oxidase results in unaltered or even aggravated brain injury (Doverhag et al. 2008). These findings imply maturity-related differences in the inflammatory response to injury and suggest that ROS may have protective properties in the developing brain.

Recently, the possible protective properties of inflammation and in particular microglia cells have come into focus. Exogenous microglia cells are protective in adult models of ischemic injury (Kitamura et al. 2004; Imai et al. 2007), but studies of microglia inhibition with minocycline after neonatal HI are contradictory with reports of strong protective effect after HI in neonatal rats (Arvin et al. 2002), worsening of injury after HI in newborn mice (Tsuji et al. 2004), and transient protection after neonatal stroke (Fox et al. 2005). It has thus been suggested that intervention aimed at protecting the brain from inflammatory injury should modulate microglia phenotype rather than merely inhibit the inflammatory response or single inflammatory mediators. Such a concept is supported by a recent study demonstrating protective effect of an immunomodulatory peptide in neonatal HI preceded by LPS administration (Bolouri et al. 2014).

In adult brain, different microglia populations have been identified after stroke, and resident proliferating microglia expressing insulin-like growth factor-1 (IGF-1) and galectin-3 are protective (Lalancette-Hebert et al. 2007). Such subpopulations of microglia are yet to be identified in the neonatal brain, but a recent study of the inflammatory marker galectin-3 illustrates the possibility of modulating the inflammatory response after HI (Doverhag et al. 2010). Previous studies show that galectin-3 activates NADPH oxidase (Almkvist et al. 2001) and augments inflammation by increased chemotaxis and decreased apoptosis in inflammatory cells (Colnot et al. 1998; Hsu et al. 2000). In the neonatal setting, genetic inhibition of galectin-3 resulted in attenuated HI injury with no effect on apoptosis or growth factor expression. Instead, galectin-3-deficient mice had increased microglia infiltration but decreased oxidative stress and MMP-9 expression, suggesting changes in microglia phenotype (Doverhag et al. 2010).

In addition, the protection and the changes in inflammatory response in galectin-3-deficient mice were more pronounced in male pups, suggesting that gender may also influence the immune response in the immature brain (Doverhag et al. 2010). The gender differences at this early age are more likely to depend on genetic differences than hormonal factors (Johnston and Hagberg 2007) and open new intriguing avenues of research.

118.6 Inflammation and CNS Vulnerability

As pointed out above, there is strong experimental evidence to show that infection/inflammation may act in synergy with other insults and aggravate brain injury. Studies in both rats and mice have shown that exposure to LPS sensitizes the immature brain to subsequent HI (Eklind et al. 2001; Coumans et al. 2003; Yang et al. 2004; Wang et al. 2007a) and results in extended cerebral damage and long-lasting memory and learning impairment (Ikeda et al. 2004). Recently, it was demonstrated that also the TLR3 agonist poly I:C sensitizes the immature brain to HI in a TLR3-dependent way Stridh et al. (2013). Similar sensitizing effects are seen with excitotoxicity (Dommergues et al. 2000), where pro-inflammatory cytokines and IL-9 exacerbate excitotoxic lesions of the newborn murine neopallium (Dommergues et al. 2000). The underlying mechanisms of sensitization are not well understood; however, at least LPS-induced aggravation of injury is known to act in a TLR-4- and MyD88-dependent manner (Lehnardt et al. 2003; Wang et al. 2009). Microglia cells appear to play an important role in the injury process as LPS-stimulated microglia are able to kill neurons and oligodendrocytes, at least when grown in culture (Lehnardt et al. 2002; Dean et al. 2009b). Oxidative stress may also be involved in LPS-induced sensitization as the free radical scavenger *N*-acetylcysteine (NAC) provided marked neuroprotection following LPS/HI insult in neonatal rats (Wang et al. 2007b). As mentioned above, inflammatory stimuli can under certain circumstances also protect the brain from further events, so-called preconditioning or tolerance (Mallard and Hagberg 2007). Although the mechanisms that are responsible for the switch from protection to injury are not well understood, it has been suggested that endotoxin-induced tolerance may be mediated by upregulation of corticosterone in neonatal rats (Ikeda et al. 2006), and interestingly, the synthetic corticosteroid anti-inflammatory drug dexamethasone was able to prevent both structural brain damage and subsequent learning and memory deficits in neonatal rats exposed to LPS-induced HI injury (Ikeda et al. 2005).

118.7 Conclusions

There is today ample support to show that inflammation is involved in perinatal brain injury. Early studies provided support for the hypothesis that inflammation can aggravate brain injury during the acute phase both in the setting of infection and sterile insults like hypoxia-ischemia. Subsequent clinical and experimental work supports the concept that the immunoinflammatory molecular network is complex and multifaceted with important roles in brain development as well as setting of CNS vulnerability and during the acute and repair phases of injury. There is potential for neuroprotective immunomodulatory therapies to be developed, but we still need a more detailed knowledge about the basic mechanisms. Hence, the net effect of immune responses – protective versus beneficial – is often difficult to predict and depends on many factors, for example, which cells and mediators are activated, time point in relation to insult, molecular context, gender, and developmental age.

References

Almkvist J, Fäldt J, Dahlgren C et al (2001) Lipopolysaccharide induced gelatinase granule mobilization primes neutrophils for activation by galectin-3 and formylmethionyl-Leu-Phe. Infect Immun 69: 832–837

Aly H, Khashaba MT, El-Ayouty M et al (2006) IL-1beta, IL-6 and TNF-alpha and outcomes of neonatal hypoxic ischemic encephalopathy. Brain Dev 28:178–182

Ando M, Takashima S, Mito T (1988) Endotoxin, cerebral blood flow, amino acids and brain damage in young rabbits. Brain Dev 10:365–370

Arvin KL, Han BH, Du Y et al (2002) Minocycline markedly protects the neonatal brain against hypoxic-ischemic injury. Ann Neurol 52:54–61

Bartha AI, Foster-Barber A, Miller SP et al (2004) Neonatal encephalopathy: association of cytokines with MR spectroscopy and outcome. Pediatr Res 56:960–966

Bolouri H, Sävman K, Wang W et al (2014) Innate defense regulator peptide 1018 protects against perinatal brain injury. Ann Neurol 75(3):395–410

Bona E, Andersson AL, Blomgren K et al (1999) Chemokine and inflammatory cell response to hypoxia-ischemia in immature rats. Pediatr Res 45:500–509

Borrell V, Marin O (2006) Meninges control tangential migration of hem-derived Cajal-Retzius cells via CXCL12/CXCR4 signaling. Nat Neurosci 9: 1284–1293

Cameron JS, Alexopoulou L, Sloane JA et al (2007) Toll-like receptor 3 is a potent negative regulator of axonal growth in mammals. J Neurosci 27: 13033–13041

Chau V, Poskitt KJ, McFadden DE et al (2009) Effect of chorioamnionitis on brain development and injury in premature newborns. Ann Neurol 66:155–164

Colnot C, Ripoche MA, Milon G et al (1998) Maintenance of granulocyte numbers during acute peritonitis is defective in galectin-3- null mutant mice. Immunology 94:290–296

Coumans AB, Middelanis JS, Garnier Y et al (2003) Intracisternal application of endotoxin enhances the susceptibility to subsequent hypoxic-ischemic-brain damage in neonatal rats. Pediatr Res 53: 770–775

Cowan F, Rutherford M, Groenendaal F et al (2003) Origin and timing of brain lesions in term infants with neonatal encephalopathy. Lancet 361:736–742

Dalitz P, Harding R, Rees SM et al (2003) Prolonged reductions in placental blood flow and cerebral oxygen delivery in preterm fetal sheep exposed to endotoxin: possible factors in white matter injury after acute infection. J Soc Gynecol Investig 10:283–290

Dammann O, O'Shea TM (2008) Cytokines and perinatal brain damage. Clin Perinatol 35:643–663

Dammann O, Allred EN, Veelken N (1998) Increased risk of spastic diplegia among very low birth weight children after preterm labor or prelabor rupture of membranes. J Pediatr 132:531–535

de la Mano A, Gato A, Alonso MI et al (2007) Role of interleukin- 1beta in the control of neuroepithelial proliferation and differentiation of the spinal cord during development. Cytokine 37:128–137

Dean JM, Farrag D, Zahkouk SA et al (2009a) Cerebellar white matter injury following systemic endotoxemia in preterm fetal sheep. Neuroscience 160:606–615

Dean JM, Wang X, Kaindl AM et al (2009b) Microglial MyD88 signaling regulates acute neuronal toxicity of LPS-stimulated microglia in vitro. Brain Behav Immun 24:776–783

Dommergues MA, Patkai J, Renauld JC et al (2000) Proinflammatory cytokines and interleukin-9 exacerbate excitotoxic lesions of the newborn murine neopallium. Ann Neurol 47:54–63

Doverhag C, Keller M, Karlsson A et al (2008) Pharmacological and genetic inhibition of NADPH oxidase does not reduce brain damage in different models of perinatal brain injury in newborn mice. Neurobiol Dis 31:133–144

Doverhag C, Hedtjärn M, Poirier F et al (2010) Galectin-3 contributes to neonatal hypoxic-ischemic brain injury. Neurobiol Dis 38:36–46

Duggan PJ, Maalouf EF, Watts TL et al (2001) Intrauterine T-cell activation and increased proinflammatory cytokine concentrations in preterm infants with cerebral lesions. Lancet 358:1699–1700

Duncan JR, Cock ML, Scheerlinck JP et al (2002) White matter injury after repeated endotoxin exposure in the preterm ovine fetus. Pediatr Res 52:941–949

Duncan JR, Cock ML, Suzuki K et al (2006) Chronic endotoxin exposure causes brain injury in the ovine fetus in the absence of hypoxemia. J Soc Gynecol Investig 13:87–96

Dziembowska M, Tham TN, Lau P et al (2005) A role for CXCR4 signaling in survival and migration of neural and oligodendrocyte precursors. Glia 50: 258–269

Eklind S, Mallard C, Leverin AL et al (2001) Bacterial endotoxin sensitizes the immature brain to hypoxic – ischaemic injury. Eur J Neurosci 13:1101–1106

Fleiss B, Gressens P (2012) Tertiary mechanisms of brain damage: a new hope for treatment of cerebral palsy? Lancet Neurol 11:556–566

Fox C, Dingman A, Derugin N et al (2005) Minocycline confers early but transient protection in the immature brain following focal cerebral ischemia-reperfusion. J Cereb Blood Flow Metab 25:1138–1149

Gaulden J, Reiter JF (2008) Neur-ons and neur-offs: regulators of neural induction in vertebrate embryos and embryonic stem cells. Hum Mol Genet 17:R60–R66

Gavilanes AW, Strackx E, Kramer BW et al (2009) Chorioamnionitis induced by intra-amniotic lipopolysaccharide resulted in an interval- dependent increase in central nervous system injury in the fetal sheep. Am J Obstet Gynecol 200(437):e431–e438

Gilles FH, Averill DR Jr, Kerr CS (1977) Neonatal endotoxin encephalopathy. Ann Neurol 2:49–56

Giulian D, Vaca K (1993) Inflammatory glia mediate delayed neuronal damage after ischemia in the central nervous system. Stroke 24:I84–I90

Giulian D, Young DG, Woodward J et al (1988) Interleukin-1 is an astroglial growth factor in the developing brain. J Neurosci 8:709–714

Goldenberg RL, Culhane JF, Iams JD et al (2008) Epidemiology and causes of preterm birth. Lancet 371:75–84

Gomez R, Romero R, Ghezzi F et al (1998) The fetal inflammatory response syndrome. Am J Obstet Gynecol 179:194–202

Grether JK, Nelson KB (1997) Maternal infection and cerebral palsy in infants of normal birth weight. JAMA 278:207–211

Hagberg H, Mallard C (2005) Effect of inflammation on central nervous system development and vulnerability. Curr Opin Neurol 18:117–123

Hagberg H, Gilland E, Bona E et al (1996) Enhanced expression of interleukin (IL)-1 and IL-6 messenger RNA and bioactive protein after hypoxia-ischemia in neonatal rats. Pediatr Res 40:603–609

Hagberg H, Gressens P, Mallard C (2012) Inflammation during fetal and neonatal life: implications for neurologic and neuropsychiatric disease in children and adults. Ann Neurol 71(4):444–457

Hagberg H, Mallard C, Ferriero DM et al (2015) The role of inflammation in perinatal brain injury. Nat Rev Neurol 11:192–208

Hedtjarn M, Leverin AL, Eriksson K et al (2002) Interleukin-18 involvement in hypoxic-ischemic brain injury. J Neurosci 22:5910–5919

Hedtjarn M, Mallard C, Hagberg H (2004) Inflammatory gene profiling in the developing mouse brain after hypoxia-ischemia. J Cereb Blood Flow Metab 24:1333–1351

Hedtjarn M, Mallard C, Iwakura Y et al (2005) Combined deficiency of IL-1beta18, but not IL-1alphabeta, reduces susceptibility to hypoxia- ischemia in the immature brain. Dev Neurosci 27:143–148

Hsu DK, Yang RY, Pan Z et al (2000) Targeted disruption of the galectin-3 gene results in attenuated peritoneal inflammatory responses. Am J Pathol 156:1073–1083

Hudome S, Palmer C, Roberts RL et al (1997) The role of neutrophils in the production of hypoxic-ischemic brain injury in the neonatal rat. Pediatr Res 41:607–616

Huh GS, Boulanger LM, Du H et al (2000) Functional requirement for class I MHC in CNS development and plasticity. Science 290:2155–2159

Ikeda T, Mishima K, Aoo N et al (2004) Combination treatment of neonatal rats with hypoxia-ischemia and endotoxin induces long-lasting memory and learning impairment that is associated with extended cerebral damage. Am J Obstet Gynecol 191:2132–2141

Ikeda T, Mishima K, Aoo N et al (2005) Dexamethasone prevents long-lasting learning impairment following a combination of lipopolysaccharide and hypoxia-ischemia in neonatal rats. Am J Obstet Gynecol 192:719–726

Ikeda T, Yang L, Ikenoue T et al (2006) Endotoxin-induced hypoxic- ischemic tolerance is mediated by up-regulation of corticosterone in neonatal rat. Pediatr Res 59:56–60

Imai F, Suzuki H, Oda J et al (2007) Neuroprotective effect of exogenous microglia in global brain ischemia. J Cereb Blood Flow Metab 27:488–500

Jacobsson B, Hagberg G, Hagberg B et al (2002) Cerebral palsy in preterm infants: a population-based case–control study of antenatal and intrapartal risk factors. Acta Paediatr 91:946–951

Johnston MV, Hagberg H (2007) Sex and the pathogenesis of cerebral palsy. Dev Med Child Neurol 49:74–78

Kaukola T, Herva R, Perhomaa M et al (2006) Population cohort associating chorioamnionitis, cord inflammatory cytokines and neurologic outcome in very preterm, extremely low birth weight infants. Pediatr Res 59: 478–483

Kim SU, de Vellis J (2005) Microglia in health and disease. J Neurosci Res 81:302–313

Kitamura Y, Takata K, Inden M et al (2004) Intracerebroventricular injection of microglia protects against focal brain ischemia. J Pharmacol Sci 94:203–206

Kumazaki K, Nakayama M, Sumida Y et al (2002) Placental features in preterm infants with periventricular leukomalacia. Pediatrics 109:650–655

Lalancette-Hebert M, Gowing G, Simard A et al (2007) Selective ablation of proliferating microglial cells exacerbates ischemic injury in the brain. J Neurosci 27:2596–2605

Lathia JD, Okun E, Tang SC et al (2008) Toll-like receptor 3 is a negative regulator of embryonic neural progenitor cell proliferation. J Neurosci 28:13978–13984

Lee R, Ng D, Fung G et al (2006) Chorioamnionitis with or without funisitis increases the risk of hypotension in very low birthweight infants on the first postnatal day but not later. Arch Dis Child 91: F346–F348

Lehnardt S, Lachance C, Patrizi S et al (2002) The toll-like receptor TLR4 is necessary for lipopolysaccharide-induced oligodendrocyte injury in the CNS. J Neurosci 22:2478–2486

Lehnardt S, Massillon L, Follett P et al (2003) Activation of innate immunity in the CNS triggers neurodegeneration through a Toll-like receptor 4-dependent pathway. Proc Natl Acad Sci U S A 100:8514–8519

Leviton A, Gressens P (2007) Neuronal damage accompanies perinatal white-matter damage. Trends Neurosci 30:473–478

Leviton A, Gilles F, Neff R et al (1976) Multivariate analysis of risk of perinatal telencephalic leucoencephalopathy. Am J Epidemiol 104:621–626

Leviton A, Paneth N, Reuss ML et al (1999) Maternal infection, fetal inflammatory response, and brain damage in very low birth weight infants. Developmental epidemiology network investigators. Pediatr Res 46:566–575

Liu XH, Kwon D, Schielke GP et al (1999) Mice deficient in interleukin- 1 converting enzyme are resistant to neonatal hypoxic-ischemic brain damage. J Cereb Blood Flow Metab 19:1099–1108

Ma Y, Li J, Chiu I et al (2006) Toll-like receptor 8 functions as a negative regulator of neurite outgrowth and inducer of neuronal apoptosis. J Cell Biol 175:209–215

Mallard C, Hagberg H (2007) Inflammation-induced preconditioning in the immature brain. Semin Fetal Neonatal Med 12:280–286

Mallard C, Welin AK, Peebles D et al (2003) White matter injury following systemic endotoxemia or asphyxia in the fetal sheep. Neurochem Res 28:215–223

Mallard C, Wang X, Hagberg H (2009) The role of toll-like receptors in perinatal brain injury. Clin Perinatol 36:763–772, v–vi

Martin D, Chinookoswong N, Miller G (1994) The interleukin-1 receptor antagonist (rhIL-1ra) protects against cerebral infarction in a rat model of hypoxia-ischemia. Exp Neurol 130:362–367

Martin-Ancel A, Garcia-Alix A, Pascual-Salcedo D et al (1997) Interleukin- 6 in the cerebrospinal fluid after perinatal asphyxia is related to early and late neurological manifestations. Pediatrics 100:789–794

Matsuo Y, Onodera H, Shiga Y et al (1994) Correlation between myeloperoxidase-quantified neutrophil accumulation and ischemic brain injury in the rat. Effects of neutrophil depletion. Stroke 25:1469–1475

Matsuo Y, Kihara T, Ikeda M et al (1995) Role of neutrophils in radical production during ischemia and reperfusion of the rat brain: effect of neutrophil depletion on extracellular ascorbyl radical formation. J Cereb Blood Flow Metab 15:941–947

McRae A, Gilland E, Bona E, Hagberg H (1995) Microglia activation after neonatal hypoxic-ischemia. Brain Res Dev Brain Res 84:245–252

Monje ML, Toda H, Palmer TD (2003) Inflammatory blockade restores adult hippocampal neurogenesis. Science 302:1760–1765

Nelson KB, Grether JK (1998) Potentially asphyxiating conditions and spastic cerebral palsy in infants of normal birth weight. Am J Obstet Gynecol 179:507–513

Nelson KB, Dambrosia JM, Grether JK et al (1998) Neonatal cytokines and coagulation factors in children with cerebral palsy. Ann Neurol 44:665–675

Nitsos I, Rees SM, Duncan J et al (2006) Chronic exposure to intra-amniotic lipopolysaccharide affects the ovine fetal brain. J Soc Gynecol Investig 13:239–247

Oygur N, Sonmez O, Saka O et al (1998) Predictive value of plasma and cerebrospinal fluid tumour necrosis factor-alpha and interleukin-1 beta concentrations on outcome of full term infants with hypoxic-ischaemic encephalopathy. Arch Dis Child Fetal Neonatal Ed 79: F190–F193

Palmer C, Roberts RL, Young PI (2004) Timing of neutrophil depletion influences long-term neuroprotection in neonatal rat hypoxic- ischemic brain injury. Pediatr Res 55:549–556

Patni S, Flynn P, Wynen LP et al (2007) An introduction to Toll-like receptors and their possible role in the initiation of labour. BJOG 114:326–1334

Reiman M, Kujari H, Maunu J et al (2008) Does placental inflammation relate to brain lesions and volume in preterm infants? J Pediatr 152:642–647

Rolls A, Shechter R, London A et al (2007) Toll-like receptors modulate adult hippocampal neurogenesis. Nat Cell Biol 9:1081–1088

Romero R, Dey SK, Fisher SJ (2014) Preterm labor: one syndrome, many causes. Science 345(6198): 760–765

Savman K, Blennow M, Gustafson K et al (1998) Cytokine response in cerebrospinal fluid after birth asphyxia. Pediatr Res 43:746–751

Shalak LF, Laptook AR, Jafri HS et al (2002) Clinical chorioamnionitis, elevated cytokines, and brain injury in term infants. Pediatrics 110:673–680

Shimazaki T, Shingo T, Weiss S (2001) The ciliary neurotrophic factor/leukemia inhibitory factor/gp130 receptor complex operates in the maintenance of mammalian forebrain neural stem cells. J Neurosci 21:7642–7653

Shinjyo N, Stahlberg A, Dragunow M et al (2009) Complement-derived anaphylatoxin C3a regulates in vitro differentiation and migration of neural progenitor cells. Stem Cells 27:2824–2832

Silveira RC, Procianoy RS (2003) Interleukin-6 and tumor necrosis factor-alpha levels in plasma and cerebrospinal fluid of term newborn infants with hypoxic-ischemic encephalopathy. J Pediatr 143:625–629

Stanley FJ (1994) The aetiology of cerebral palsy. Early Hum Dev 36:81–88

Stephan AH, Barres BA, Stevens B (2012) The complement system: an unexpected role in synaptic pruning during development and disease. Annu Rev Neurosci 35:369–389

Stridh L, Mottahedin A, Johansson ME et al (2013) Toll-like receptor-3 activation increases the vulnerability of the neonatal brain to hypoxia-ischemia. J Neurosci 33 (29):12041–12051

Svedin P, Hagberg H, Savman K et al (2007) Matrix metalloproteinase- 9 gene knock-out protects the immature brain after cerebral hypoxia-ischemia. J Neurosci 27:1511–1518

Szaflarski J, Burtrum D, Silverstein FS (1995) Cerebral hypoxia- ischemia stimulates cytokine gene expression in perinatal rats. Stroke 26:1093–1100

Tahraoui SL, Marret S, Bodenant C et al (2001) Central role of microglia in neonatal excitotoxic lesions of the murine periventricular white matter. Brain Pathol 11:56–71

Toti P, De Felice C, Palmeri ML et al (1998) Inflammatory pathogenesis of cortical polymicrogyria: an autopsy study. Pediatr Res 44:291–296

Tran PB, Banisadr G, Ren D et al (2007) Chemokine receptor expression by neural progenitor cells in neurogenic regions of mouse brain. J Comp Neurol 500:1007–1033

Tsuji M, Wilson MA, Lange MS et al (2004) Minocycline worsens hypoxic-ischemic brain injury in a neonatal mouse model. Exp Neurol 189:58–65

Vela JM, Molina-Holgado E, Arevalo-Martin A et al (2002) Interleukin- 1 regulates proliferation and differentiation of oligodendrocyte progenitor cells. Mol Cell Neurosci 20:489–502

Verma U, Tejani N, Klein S et al (1997) Obstetric antecedents of intraventricular hemorrhage and periventricular leukomalacia in the low-birth-weight neonate. Am J Obstet Gynecol 176:275–281

Vilcek J (1998) The cytokines: an overview. In: Thomson AW (ed) The cytokine handbook, 3rd edn. Academic, San Diego, pp 1–21

Walder CE, Green SP, Darbonne WC et al (1997) Ischemic stroke injury is reduced in mice lacking a functional NADPH oxidase. Stroke 28:2252–2258

Wang X, Hagberg H, Nie C et al (2007a) Dual role of intrauterine immune challenge on neonatal and adult brain vulnerability to hypoxia- ischemia. J Neuropathol Exp Neurol 66:552–561

Wang X, Svedin P, Nie C et al (2007b) *N*-acetylcysteine reduces lipopolysaccharide-sensitized hypoxic-ischemic brain injury. Ann Neurol 61:263–271

Wang X, Stridh L, Li W et al (2009) Lipopolysaccharide sensitizes neonatal hypoxic-ischemic brain injury in a MyD88-dependent manner. J Immunol 183: 7471–7477

Wu YW, Colford JM Jr (2000) Chorioamnionitis as a risk factor for cerebral palsy: a meta-analysis. JAMA 284:1417–1424

Wu YW, Escobar GJ, Grether JK et al (2003) Chorioamnionitis and cerebral palsy in term and near-term infants. JAMA 290:2677–2684

Wu YW, Croen LA, Torres AR et al (2009) Interleukin-6 genotype and risk for cerebral palsy in term and near-term infants. Ann Neurol 66:663–670

Yan E, Castillo-Melendez M, Nicholls T et al (2004) Cerebrovascular responses in the fetal sheep brain to low-dose endotoxin. Pediatr Res 55:855–863

Yang L, Sameshima H, Ikeda T et al (2004) Lipopolysaccharide administration enhances hypoxic-ischemic brain damage in newborn rats. J Obstet Gynaecol Res 30:142–147

Yoon BH, Romero R, Park JS et al (2000) Fetal exposure to an intra-amniotic inflammation and the development of cerebral palsy at the age of three years. Am J Obstet Gynecol 182:675–681

Yoon BH, Romero R, Moon JB et al (2001) Clinical significance of intra-amniotic inflammation in patients with preterm labor and intact membranes. Am J Obstet Gynecol 185:1130–1136

Young RS, Hernandez MJ, Yagel SK (1982) Selective reduction of blood flow to white matter during hypotension in newborn dogs: a possible mechanism of periventricular leukomalacia. Ann Neurol 12:445–448

Zou YR, Kottmann AH, Kuroda M et al (1998) Function of the chemokine receptor CXCR4 in haematopoiesis and in cerebellar development. Nature 393:595–599

Normal and Abnormal Neurodevelopmental and Behavioral Outcomes of Very Low-Birth Weight (VLBW) Infants

119

Betty R. Vohr

Contents

Abstract

Advances in perinatal and neonatal management of very low-birth weight (VLBW) infants (<1500 g) have resulted in increased survival of fragile "high-risk" infants, including those with extremely low birth weight (<1000 g). These high-risk preterm survivors have increased post-discharge morbidities including

B. R. Vohr (✉)
Department of Pediatrics, The Warren Alpert Medical School of Brown University, Providence, RI, USA

Women and Infants Hospital, Providence, RI, USA
e-mail: bvohr@wihri.org

G. Buonocore et al. (eds.), *Neonatology*,
https://doi.org/10.1007/978-3-319-29489-6_266

neurologic/neurosensory, cognitive, visual motor/fine motor, speech and language, motor function/coordination, functional skills for daily living, and behavior sequelae. Most tertiary care programs in the United States and all neonatal training programs have a structured follow-up program whose primary areas of responsibility are surveillance and research. Multiple assessment tools are used by these follow-up programs to identify the neurodevelopmental sequelae of preterm birth. Assessments in the first 3 years of life reliably identify major neurosensory morbidities and major neurodevelopmental sequelae. The majority of major abnormalities can be identified by 18–24 months of age. These early childhood assessments are often the primary outcome for clinical trials and also facilitate referral to appropriate intervention services. Although there are data demonstrating neurodevelopmental recovery with increasing age, there is also evidence of sustained adverse outcomes of executive functions, atypical behavior, and psychological problems into school age and adolescence. Assessments at school age rather than early childhood are felt to provide a more reliable prediction of long-term outcomes.

Abbreviations

ABR	Auditory brainstem response
ASD	Autism spectrum disorder
Bayley II	Bayley Scales of Infant Development II
BDI	Battelle Developmental Inventory
Beery VMI	Beery Developmental Test of Visual Motor Integration 4th Ed
BPD	Bronchopulmonary dysplasia
BSID-III	Bayley Scales of Infant Development III
CBCL	Child Behavior Checklist
CP	Cerebral palsy
DCD	Developmental coordination disorder
ELBW	Extremely low birth weight
ELM2	Early Language Milestone Scale2
ESP	Early Screening Profiles
GMFCS	Gross Motor Function Classification System
HL	Hearing loss
IVH	Intraventricular hemorrhage
MABC	Movement Assessment Battery for Children
M-CHAT	Modified Checklist for Autism in Toddlers
MDI	Mental Developmental Index
NDI	Neurodevelopmental impairment
NICHD	National Institute of Child Health and Human Development
NICU	Neonatal intensive care unit
PDDST II	Pervasive Developmental Disorders Screening Test II
PDI	Psychomotor Developmental Index
PDMS	Peabody Developmental Motor Scales
PLS	Preschool Language Score
PPVT-R	Peabody Picture Vocabulary Test
PVL	Periventricular leukomalacia
SB-4	Stanford-Binet Intelligence Scale, 4th edition
SICDR	Sequenced Inventory of Communication Development Revised
VABS	Vineland Adaptive Behavior Scale
VLBW	Very low birth weight
WeeFIM	Functional Independence Measure for Children
WISC-III	Wechsler Intelligence Scale for Children
WPPSI	Wechsler Preschool and Primary Scales of Intelligence

119.1 Salient Points

- Primary areas of responsibility for follow-up programs are surveillance and research.
- Major neurodevelopmental sequelae can be identified by 18–24 months of age.
- Multiple assessment tools can be used to identify neurodevelopmental sequelae of preterm birth.
- Assessments in the first 3 years of life reliably identify major neurosensory morbidities.
- Assessments at school age provide the most reliable long-term outcomes including executive functions and academic success.

119.2 Introduction

Advances over the past 10–20 years in perinatal and neonatal management of very low-birth weight (VLBW) infants (<1500 g and <30 weeks' gestation) have resulted in a significant increase in survival of fragile "high-risk" infants, including those with extremely low birth weight (ELBW) (<1000 g) (El-Metwally et al. 2000; Fanaroff et al. 2003; Hintz et al. 2005a, b, c; National Institutes of Health (NIH) 1995; Costeloe et al. 2012; Stoll et al. 2010, 2015; Patel et al. 2015). Therapeutic advances including the use of antenatal steroids (Crowley et al. 1990; McCormick 1993), surfactant for respiratory distress syndrome (Schwartz et al. 1994; Ware et al. 1990), prophylactic indomethacin for prevention of intraventricular hemorrhage (Ment et al. 1994; Schmidt et al. 2001), improved nutritional management, and new ventilatory techniques (Barrington and Finer 2007; Ballard et al. 2015; Vaucher et al. 2012; Finer et al. 2010) have all contributed to improved survival especially for infants with birth weights less than 1000 g (El-Metwally et al. 2000; Fanaroff et al. 2003; Hintz et al. 2005a, b, c, 2011). These high-risk preterm survivors have increased complex neonatal medical morbidities affecting all organ systems including the lungs, gastrointestinal tract, kidneys, and brain and post-discharge morbidities including increased growth failure, neurologic, developmental, cognitive, neuropsychological, functional, and behavioral sequelae (Hintz et al. 2011, 2015; Blakely et al. 2005; Ehrenkranz et al. 2006; Laptook et al. 2005; Schmidt et al. 2003; Shankaran et al. 2004; Walsh et al. 2005; Vohr et al. 2005a, 2012).

Most tertiary care programs in the United States and all neonatal training programs currently include a requirement for fellow participation in the care and evaluation of discharged infants in a structured follow-up program. A workshop on the Follow-up Care of high-risk infants sponsored by the National Institute of Child Health and Human Development (NICHD), the National Institute of Neurologic Disorders and Stroke, and the Centers for Disease Control and Prevention held in 2002 established guidelines for the provision of Follow-up Services (Vohr et al. 2004a). The workshop concluded that two primary areas of responsibility for Neonatal Follow-up Programs are surveillance and research.

Surveillance is indicated so that centers can systematically monitor and report on the care of high-risk infants during their hospitalization and their outcomes after discharge from the neonatal intensive care unit (NICU). The availability of a data management surveillance system for the NICU facilitates the ability to annually audit the safety and efficacy of interventions, monitor identified quality indicators for the individual NICU, summarize annual data on neonatal morbidities, and summarize annual post-discharge outcomes such as rates of cerebral palsy (CP), mental retardation, developmental delay, blindness, hearing impairment, behavioral abnormalities, autism, learning disabilities, growth failure, and medical morbidities. Information about center outcomes for specific conditions and by gestational age categories also allows staff caring for high-risk infants to counsel parents with regard to prognosis (American Academy of Pediatrics. Committee on Fetus and Newborn 1995). A follow-up clinic may also provide a mechanism for the provision of seamless comprehensive medical, psychosocial, and intervention services to NICU graduates (Broyles et al. 2000). Outcome data can be shared with the Departments of Health and Education to aid in planning for adequate service provision for high-risk NICU graduates.

Research is an integral part of academic neonatal programs. An advantage of having a structured follow-up program is that it provides a mechanism to carry out research ranging from observational studies to randomized control trials that include post-discharge outcomes. Currently, post-discharge neurodevelopmental impairment (NDI) is a common primary outcome for randomized control trials of NICU infants. With the introduction of the Bayley Scales of Infant and Toddler Development III (Bayley 2006), the NDI definition was modified by the NICHD NRN. It is currently considered to reflect moderate/severe neurologic disability and is defined as one or more of the following: moderate to severe

CP, neurologic exam abnormal, non-CP with associated GMFCS ≥Level 2, BSID-III cognitive score <70, bilateral blindness with vision <20/200, or permanent hearing loss which interferes with ability to understand or communicate with or without amplification. In addition, the cutpoints of the Bayley III cognitive composite cutpoints used by the NICHD Network have been modified to moderate delay 80–84 and severe to profound delay <70. Language delay can be reported separately. The use of post-discharge NDI as a standard outcome for intervention trials evolved with the recognition of the frequent disconnect between perinatal outcomes and long-term outcomes. Examples include (1) the aggressive administration of oxygen for relief of respiratory distress syndrome and subsequent retinopathy of prematurity/blind infants and (2) the administration of postnatal steroids for weaning infants with bronchopulmonary dysplasia from a ventilator and subsequent CP (Barrington 2001; Kinsey et al. 1977; Msall et al. 2000; Thebaud et al. 2001). The combined outcome of NDI or death is often a choice for primary outcome since it is well recognized that death is a competing outcome with NDI. Utilization of the same definition for outcome among studies allows one to more readily compare the findings.

119.2.1 Methodological Issues and Follow-Up Techniques

Differences in the reported incidence of neonatal morbidities (i.e., bronchopulmonary dysplasia (BPD)) or post-discharge outcomes (i.e., CP) may not be secondary to a specific intervention, but may be related to the specific characteristics of the center's NICU population (race, health insurance, poverty rates) and differences in management style. Examples of medical management confounders include a center's policies for antenatal and obstetric care; variability of use of ventilators, medications, and enteral and parenteral nutrition; and approaches to care for infants at the limits of viability (Rysavy et al. 2015). Neonatal factors affecting outcome include multiple versus singleton, inborn versus out-born, gestational age at birth and male versus female (Tyson et al. 2008). Social and environmental characteristics with significant heterogeneity include poverty level, public versus private insurance, level of parent education, single parent, English speaking versus bilingual or non-English speaking, cultural and religious differences, and availability of post-discharge medical, therapeutic, early intervention and educational services (Watson et al. 1996). One of the challenges of follow-up studies which can contribute to bias in interpreting NDI rates is that poor and less educated families are less likely to return for follow-up (Aylward et al. 1985).

119.2.1.1 Assessment in the Follow-Up Program

Age of follow-up assessment impacts on the findings that can be reliably identified. In the first 2–3 years of life, valid primary outcomes include moderate to severe CP, mental retardation, bilateral blindness, and bilateral hearing impairment. Current studies in the first 3 years often use the composite outcome of (NDI) as the primary outcome. At school age, however, a broad spectrum of subtle cognitive and neuropsychological deficits including impaired language skills, perceptual-motor skills, executive function, memory skills, and attention problems become apparent and can be identified with standardized test administration.

The question that is often raised is at what age one can identify the "real" impact of a neonatal intervention. It is clear that neurologic status at the time of discharge has limited predictive value. There is consensus that major neurologic and sensory impairments can be identified at 18–24 months of age. Do the findings at 18–24 months predict school-age findings? Longitudinal studies of preterm children have demonstrated variability in the progression of neurologic and developmental findings and include stability (Hintz et al. 2011; Rickards et al. 1988), improvement (Vohr et al. 2012; Wilson-Costello et al. 2007; Luu et al. 2009a), and worsening (McCormick et al. 1990; Taylor et al. 2000a) of neuropsychological findings. Limitations in the predictive value of early assessments (Aylward 2002) may be secondary to differences in the follow-up rates, the inclusion or exclusion of children with major neurologic or sensory impairments, and the post-discharge environment (Aylward 1992). To minimize bias a follow-up rate of 90% is optimal. The validity of outcome data is always enhanced by the utilization of a gender and age-matched comparison group. Because of the exorbitant costs of tracking families to school age, the majority of trials and observational studies report outcomes at 18–24 months, an age at which major sequelae can be identified.

119.3 Assessments

One approach of outcome studies is to report comprehensive neurological, developmental, functional, and health-care status, which permits a total view of the child within the context of the family. Table 1 lists assessments suitable for follow-up studies of children up to 36 months of age divided into seven major categories: neurologic/neurosensory, cognitive, visual motor/fine motor, speech and language,

Table 1 Assessments

Tests		Ages
1. Neurologic and sensory		
Vision	Ophthalmologic examination	All ages
Hearing	Auditory brainstem test	All ages
	Otoacoustic emissions	All ages
	Tympanometry	>6 months
	Visual reinforcement audiometry	>6 months
Neurologic	Standard neurologic examination	All ages
	Categorize child as normal/suspect/abnormal	
	Cerebral palsy: mild, moderate, severe	
2. Developmental/intelligence and developmental tests		
Bayley Scales of Infant Development II (BSID II) (Bayley 1993)		1–42 months
Bayley III Scales of Infant and Toddler Development (Bayley 2006)		1–42 months
Stanford-Binet Intelligence Test, 4th edition (SB-4) (Thorndike et al. 1986)		2–18 years
Differential Ability Scales (Elliott 1990)		2.5–18 years
McCarthy Scales (Mc Carthy 1972)		2.5–8.5 years
3. Vision motor		
Beery Developmental Test of Vision Motor Integration (VMI), (Beery 1989)		Short form 3–8
4. Speech/language/vocabulary		
Preschool Language Scale 3 (Zimmerman et al. 1992)		Birth–6 years
Peabody Picture Vocabulary Test-Revised (PPVT-R) (Dunn and Dunn 1997)		2 years 6 months–adult
Early Language Milestone 2 (ELM2) (Coplan 1993)		Birth–36 months
Sequenced Inventory of Communicative Development-Revise (SICDR) (Hendrick et al. 1984)		4 months–4 years
5. Motor function		
Peabody Developmental Motor Scales (Folio and Fewell 1983)		0–7 years
AGS Early Screening – Motor Profile (Harrison et al. 1990)		2–11 year
Palisano Gross Motor Classification Scale (Palisano et al. 1997)		2–18 years
Movement Assessment Battery of Children (M ABC) (Barnett et al. 2007)		3 years – 16:11
6. Functional status		
WeeFim (Msall et al. 1994)		6 months–8 years
Vineland Adaptive Behavior Scale (VABS) (Sparrow et al. 1984)		Birth–18 years 11 month
Battelle Developmental Inventory (BDI) (Newborg et al. 1984)		Birth–8 years
Pediatric Evaluation of Disability Inventory (PEDI) (Haley et al. 1992)		6 months–7.5 years
7. Behavioral outcomes		
Child Behavior Checklist (CBCL 1.5–5) (Achenbach 1991b)		1.5–5 years

motor function/coordination, functional skills for daily living, and behavior.

119.3.1 Neurologic/Neurosensory

Because of its significant impact on the child and family, neurologic status, especially CP, is an important quality indicator for a NICU. A diagnosis of CP is obtained by performing a systematic neurologic assessment (Amiel-Tison 1987). CP is defined as a nonprogressive central nervous system disorder with abnormal muscle tone in at least one extremity and abnormal control of movement and posture which interfere with age-appropriate activities (Amiel-Tison 1987). CP is a challenging diagnosis to make on infants less than a year of age because of the prevalence of hypertonicity among premature infants in the first year of life (Drillien 1972). A definitive diagnosis of moderate to severe CP can be made by 18 months of age. CP is classified as "moderate" if the child can sit independently or with support, but an assistive device is required for ambulation and "severe" if the child is unable to sit or walk even with support. The Gross Motor Function Classification System (GMFCS) categorizes children ages 2–18 with CP into five levels of severity and is frequently used to classify severity of motor impairment (Russell et al. 2002; Palisano et al. 2006). Other neurologic findings identified in preterm children include hypertonicity, hypotonicity, seizures, dyspraxia, absent pincer, or facial palsy without a specific diagnosis of CP. Explicit criteria for describing hand function, sitting ability, and self-mobility have also been developed (Msall et al. 1997). Moderate to severe CP is a component of NDI.

Vision abnormalities are common among former preterm infants (Msall et al. 2004). The standard of care within tertiary care centers determines that VLBW infants have ophthalmologic examinations for retinopathy of prematurity prior to discharge with appropriate follow-up and intervention where appropriate. This has facilitated the identification of both severe and milder degrees of vision impairment. In addition, ongoing monitoring for the detection of strabismus and myopia is indicated. Bilateral blindness is included in the composite outcome of NDI.

Since NICU infants are at increased risk of all types of permanent hearing loss (HL) including neural (auditory neuropathy/auditory dyssynchrony) HL, the Joint Committee on Infant Hearing (JCIH) 2007 (Year 2007) has recommended automated auditory brainstem response (ABR) screening for all infants that require NICU care for >5 days. Infants who fail the screen should have a comprehensive audiology assessment by 3 months of age. An audiology diagnostic assessment for infants less than 6 months at a minimum consists of a diagnostic auditory brainstem response (ABR) and otoacoustic emissions. Children who are at least 6 months of developmental age should also have a behavioral assessment, visual reinforcement audiometry, completed. Bilateral HL that requires amplification is included in the composite outcome of NDI.

119.3.2 Cognitive

The Bayley Scales of Infant Development (Bayley II) (Bayley 1993) was previously the most commonly reported assessment of development from 4 to 36 months of age and provides information for both cognitive (the Mental Developmental Index (MDI)) and motor (the Psychomotor Developmental Index (PDI)) domains. Bayley scores of 100 $\pm$ 15 represent the mean $\pm$ 1 standard deviation (SD) of a population of normal infants born at term. A score <70 (2 SDs below the mean) is interpreted as evidence of developmental delay. The Bayley Scales of Infant Development III (BSID-III) is currently available for assessments from 1 to 42 months of age (Bayley 2006). The Bayley III was developed, in part, to separate cognitive from language domains to eliminate the bias imposed for children residing in a bilingual or non-English-speaking household. In contrast to the Bayley II, the BSID-III consists of three domains: the Cognitive, Language, and Motor Composite scores. In addition there are subscores for receptive communication, expressive communication, and fine motor and gross motor skills.

The Stanford-Binet Intelligence Scale, 4th edition (SB-4) (Thorndike et al. 1986), the Differential Ability Scales (Elliott 1990), and the McCarthy Scales of Children's Abilities (Mc Carthy 1972) are all tests of early cognitive/developmental ability. For studying populations of children, outcome data can be used to compare groups with one another (intervention vs. control) or with normative data. Children's overall performance is often evaluated on a battery of tests which include visual-perceptual skills (Beery 1989; Colarusso and Hammill 2003), speech and language skills (Coplan 1993; Hendrick et al. 1984; Zimmerman et al. 1992; Dunn and Dunn 1997), cognition (Thorndike et al. 1986; Elliott 1990; Mc Carthy 1972; Wechsler 1989; Woodcock and Johnson 1989), fine and gross motor function (Bruininks 1978; Folio and Fewell 1983; Harrison et al. 1990; Palisano 1993) behavior (Ireton 1992; Larson and Vitali 1988; Miller 1988; Nehring et al. 1992), functional skills, and health-care status (Msall et al. 1994; Newborg et al. 1984; Sparrow et al. 1984).

For an individual child, early test results have limited predictive validity of cognitive status. First, tests administered at younger ages may not tap into the same psychological capacities as those present in older children, and the child resides within a changing environment with a spectrum of influences on development. School-age outcomes have the most validity for final status of cognitive function.

At school age, cognitive functioning is assessed using a variety of different measures including the Stanford-Binet Intelligence Scale, 4th edition; the Wechsler Preschool and Primary Scales of Intelligence, 3rd edition (WPPSI); the Wechsler Intelligence Scale for Children (WISC-III), the Woodcock-Johnson Psycho-Educational Battery, Revised; the Differential Abilities Scales; the McCarthy Scales of Children's Abilities; the British Abilities Scale; and the Kaufman Assessment Battery of Childhood. Each of these assessments provides an intelligence quotient (IQ) and subtest scores that allow for a limited assessment of specific areas of strengths and weaknesses. These tests, like the Bayley, have a mean of 100 with a standard deviation of 15 in the general population.

119.3.3 Visual Motor/Fine Motor Skills

The third category is visual motor and fine motor skills (Beery 1989; Colarusso and Hammill 2003). The most commonly used test for visual motor skills is the Beery Developmental Test of Visual Motor Integration 4th Ed. (Beery VMI) (Beery 1989). The VMI assesses the degree to which visual perception and motor behavior are integrated. It can help identify visual motor problems before they develop into more serious difficulties. The VMI consists of geometric figures arranged in order of increasing difficulty. The child copies the figures as accurately as possible with pencil and paper. Fine motor skills can be assessed using the Peabody Developmental Motor Scales (PDMS) (Folio and Fewell 1983). This test presents the child with a variety of fine motor tasks including block design and shape copying, cutting, folding, and manual dexterity tasks. A developmental motor quotient is calculated for each child's performance based on age. Mean developmental quotient is 100 ± 15.

119.3.4 Speech and Language

Speech language delays are common among preterms and a variety of tests are available (Vohr et al. 2014). The Preschool Language Scale, 3rd edition (PLS-3) (Zimmerman et al. 1992) is a standardized assessment which includes two subscales – auditory comprehension and expressive communication – to assess attention, vocal development, social communication, semantics, language structure, and integrative thinking skills. The Peabody Picture Vocabulary Test (PPVT-R) (Dunn and Dunn 1997) is a nonverbal, multiple-choice test that measures receptive vocabulary. The Early Language Milestone Scale, Second Edition (ELM Scale-2) (Coplan 1993) assesses speech and language development in three areas: auditory expressive, auditory receptive, and visual. The Sequenced Inventory of Communication Development Revised edition (SICDR) (Hendrick et al. 1984) is a diagnostic test that evaluates the communication abilities of children who are between 4 months and 4 years of age. It has been used successfully with children with sensory impairments and varying degrees of retardation (Wagner et al. 1999a, b; Semel et al. 1995; Peterson et al. 2002).

119.3.5 Motor Function/Coordination

The PDMS (Folio and Fewell 1983) are a test of gross and fine motor skills of children ages birth through 83 months. The Early Screening Profiles (ESP) (Harrison et al. 1990) measure motor, cognitive/language, and developmental skills in children. The ESP consists of three profiles: motor profile, cognitive/language profile, and self-help/social profile. A Gross Motor Function Classification System (GMFCS) skill level derived from the work of Russell et al. and Palisano et al. (Russell et al. 1989, 2000, 2002; Palisano et al. 1997) is used in outcome studies to assess gross motor function. A scoring system consisting of skill levels ranging from 0 to 5 was developed by Palisano and colleagues (Russell et al. 1989, 2000, 2002; Palisano et al. 1997). This system was developed as a method for assessment of a child's motor function by direct observation of the child's gross motor performance. It describes a child's function, not the fluidity of their movements. Palisano's system classifies gross motor function on a 5-point scale. Normal function at 18–24 months is defined as Level 0 and involves the ability to walk at least ten steps independently. An infant at Level 1 can sit with hands free, creep or crawl on hands and knees, pull to stand, and cruise or walk with hands held. Those at Level 2 use their hands for sitting support, creep on their stomach, and may pull to stand; those at Level 3 require external support to sit, roll, and may creep; those at Level 4 maintain head control in a supported sitting position and can roll prone to supine. Level 5 is the inability to maintain antigravity movements of the head and trunk (Palisano et al. 1997; Vohr et al. 2005b). The GMFCS does not assess fine motor skills. The Movement Assessment Battery for Children, Second Edition (Movement ABC-2) (Barnett et al. 2007; Johnson et al. 2005) provides objective, quantitative data on movement competence. The test is divided into three age bands and evaluates manual dexterity, aiming and catching, and balance.

119.3.6 Functional Measures

The sixth area of assessment includes functional measures of daily living skills. Functional assessment is the process of determining as accurately as possible an individual's ability to perform the tasks of daily living and to fulfill the social roles expected of a physically and emotionally healthy person of the same age and culture (Msall 1996, 2005; Duffner et al. 2012). In children, the key tasks include feeding, dressing, bathing, maintaining consistency, mobility, communication, play, and social interaction (Granger et al. 1987). The social roles expected include involvement with peers and attending school. Four functional outcome measures are currently available (Msall et al. 1994; Sparrow et al. 1984; Haley et al. 1991, 1992). The Pediatric Evaluation of Disability Inventory (PEDI) assesses developmental skills in self-care, mobility, and social function, care giver assistance, and modification of environment in children 6 months to 7.5 years (Haley et al. 1992). The Vineland Adaptive Behavior Scale (VABS) measures communication, daily living, socialization, and motor skills in children from birth to 18 years (Sparrow et al. 1984). The Vineland has been used with children with motor, cognitive, and sensory disabilities. Rosenbaum et al. have advocated its use for describing degrees of disability in children who were very low birth weight (Rosenbaum et al. 1995). The Battelle Developmental Inventory (BDI) is a developmental educational assessment battery for children age 0–8 years with or without developmental delays (Newborg et al. 1984). The Battelle consists of five domains: personal-social, adaptive, motor, communicative, and cognitive. It is widely used in early intervention. The Functional Independence Measure for Children (WeeFIM) (Msall et al. 1994) can be used in children with and without disabilities through age 8 years. After age 8 years, individuals with developmental skills less than 8 years can continue to be assessed with the WeeFIM (Granger et al. 1993) through adolescence.

119.3.7 Behavior and Psychology

Evaluations of behavior are routinely obtained in infancy and childhood by parent, teacher, or subject interviews with standardized measures of behavior, attention, adaptive skills, and depression. The Child Behavior Checklist (Achenbach 1991a) is a parent report questionnaire designed to describe social competencies and emotional/behavioral issues of children and is commonly used in follow-up studies. It has a version for 1.5–5-year-olds and a version for ages 4–18. It provides scores for internalizing (i.e., anxious, depressive, and overcontrolled) and externalizing (i.e., aggressive, hyperactive, noncompliant, and under-controlled) behaviors and has scores that were derived for withdrawn, somatic complaints, anxious/depressed, social problems, thought problems, attention problems, delinquent behavior, aggressive behavior, and the presence of any behavior problem. The Conners Rating Scales (Conners 1996; Gianarris et al. 2001) are questionnaires designed for parents or teachers to describe symptoms of inattention, hyperactivity, and oppositionality in school-age children (Scott et al. 2012). Increasing reports have identified a spectrum of mental health challenges at older ages (Farooqi et al. 2007; McLaughlin et al. 2011; Hack 2006; Lindstrom et al. 2009). Multiple different measures of childhood depression exist and have been studied in this population. The Modified Checklist for Autism in Toddlers (M-CHAT) (Robins et al. 2001; Kleinman et al. 2008) and the Pervasive Developmental Disorders Screening Test II (PDDST II) (Siegel 2004) are currently available as screeners for autism spectrum disorder.

119.3.8 Definitions of Normal and Abnormal Outcome

Although the traditional outcome described for infants is an abnormal outcome defined as NDI, more recent investigators have attempted to define a normal outcome. A study by Gargus et al. (Gargus et al. 2009) defined a normal outcome at 18–22 months corrected age as infants who were "unimpaired"; they had both Bayley II (Bayley 1993) MDI and PDI scores within 1 standard deviation of the mean, normal neurologic findings, normal vision, hearing, normal functional ability for swallowing by parent report, and normal ambulation. In addition, infants were classified as having mild impairments if they had any of the following: Bayley MDI or PDI between 70 and 84, CP, mild other neurologic findings, or minor sensory impairments (glasses, transient conductive hearing loss, unilateral hearing loss, or unilateral blindness). "Normal" outcome has been evaluated at 30 months of age in extremely low-birth weight infants (Kumar et al. 2013). Severe NDI with the Bayley II was defined as any of the following: Bayley MDI <70, Bayley PDI<70, moderate to severe CP, bilateral blindness, or bilateral hearing loss requiring amplification. The NICHD definition of degree of cognitive impairment was modified after the introduction of the Bayley Scales of Infant and Toddler Development III (Bayley 2006). And the definition is described in the cognitive subsection.

119.3.9 VLBW Outcomes

The majority of published reports of neurodevelopmental outcome in infancy focus primarily on the incidence of moderate to severe disability (Hack and Fanaroff 2000; Vohr 2013). This has been the neurodevelopmental outcome of interest due to the severity of the developmental impact of these severe and often combined morbidities. Unlike mortality rates which have dramatically improved (Fanaroff et al. 2003; Hintz et al. 2005b; Blaymore-Bier et al. 1994; Hack et al. 1996; O'Shea et al. 1997; Piecuch et al. 1997; Wilson-Costello et al. 2005), the incidence of moderate to severe disabilities have not changed significantly over the past 20 years (Hintz et al. 2005b; Wilson-Costello et al. 2005, 2007; Blaymore-Bier et al. 1994; Hack et al. 1996, 2000a; Piecuch et al. 1997; Lorenz et al. 1998;

Vohr and Msall 1997). Rates are highest in ELBW populations, and like mortality rates, rates of disability generally increase with decreasing gestational age and birth weight (Hack and Fanaroff 2000; O'Shea et al. 1997; Wilson-Costello et al. 2005; Emsley et al. 1998; Vohr et al. 2000a). Worldwide rates of severe disability in infants of 24–25 weeks gestation range from 22% to 45% in infants born at 24 weeks, 12–35% in infants born at 25 week, and 9–37% in infants born <800 g birth weight (Hack and Fanaroff 2000; Lorenz et al. 1998).

In the NICHD Neonatal Research Network, rates of NDI in the 1990s ranged from 28% to 40% in infants born 27–32 weeks and 45–50% in infants born 22–26 weeks (Vohr et al. 2005a). Only 21% of all ELBW infants were unimpaired (no CP, normal cognitive and motor scores, no visual or hearing impairment) at 18 months (Hintz et al. 2005b). Regional and local studies in the 1990s report similar wide ranges of major NDI rates, from 20% to 48% (Wilson-Costello et al. 2005, 2007; Blaymore-Bier et al. 1994; Hack et al. 1996; O'Shea et al. 1997; Msall et al. 1992) (Table 2).

119.3.10 Neurologic/Neurosensory

Extremely preterm infants are born during a period of active brain development and maturation, placing them at extremely high risk for brain injury from hypoxia, ischemia, undernutrition, and infection, which are associated with both intraventricular hemorrhage (IVH) and periventricular leukomalacia (PVL). PVL is injury to the periventricular white matter as a result of hypoperfusion and infarction. It is visualized radiographically as echolucency, echodensity, or cystic degeneration. Although IVH, ventriculomegaly at term, and cystic PVL are all associated with CP, cystic PVL is the strongest predictor (Vohr et al. 2005b).

Rates of CP in ELBW vary from 5% to 30% (Hintz et al. 2005b; Shankaran et al. 2004; Vohr et al. 2005a, b; Wilson-Costello et al. 2005, 2007; Hack and Fanaroff 2000; O'Shea et al. 1997; Lorenz et al. 1998; Vohr and Msall 1997; Emsley et al. 1998; Marlow et al. 2005; Doyle and Anderson 2005; Wood et al. 2000, 2005) but are most commonly cited at 15–23% (Hintz et al. 2005b, 2011; Vohr et al. 2005b; Marlow et al. 2005; Doyle and Anderson 2005; Wood et al. 2000). The most common form of CP in this population is spastic diplegia, accounting for 40–50% of all cases, followed by spastic quadriplegia and hemiplegia (Vohr et al. 2005b; Wood et al. 2000). This is not surprising as PVL lesions involve injury to the white matter that contains the descending motor tracts for the lower extremities. More extensive lesions also involve upper extremity motor tracts.

While CP is the most well-known and potentially most disabling motor abnormality associated with prematurity, infants born preterm often demonstrate less severe differences in their neurologic development. During the first year of life transient dystonia is a common deviation in the motor development of VLBW infants (Drillien 1972; Bracewell and Marlow 2002; Pedersen et al. 2000). Transient dystonia was first described in 1972 by Drillien as transient abnormalities on neurologic examination in close to half of all low-birth weight infants (<2000 g) in the first year of life. More recently, these transient findings have been redescribed as occurring in 21–36% of preterm infants with a peak incidence at 7 months corrected age (Bracewell and Marlow 2002; Pedersen et al. 2000; De Vries et al. 2004a, b). The motor features described include increased extensor tone of the trunk and lower extremities and increased adductor tone in the lower extremities leading to shoulder retraction and hip rotation, persistent primitive reflexes, head lag on pull to sit, and delayed supportive responses (Drillien 1972). The presence of findings consistent with dystonia increases the risk of later cognitive and motor problems including CP but have a low specificity as they are transient in 80% of the infants in which they occur, disappearing gradually between 8 and 12 months of age. The other 20% often go on to be diagnosed with CP.

Table 2 Cognitive Outcomes at 12–36 Months Corrected Age for ELBW Infants

Year of birth	Sample size	BW (grams)/GA (weeks)	Subgroups	Mean MDI	MDI <70	Age months	Location	Author
1982–1992	88	<750 g	1982–88 1990–92	83 89	26% 20%	20 m	Local center, USA	Hack et al. (1996)
1993–1999	246	<750 g	N/A	N/A	46%	18–22 m	NICHD, USA	Shankaran et al. (2004)
1987–1995	Review	<800 g	N/A	N/A	13–48%	12–36 m	Worldwide review	Hack et al. (2000)
1977–1994	Review	<800 g <27 weeks	N/A	N/A	14%	Variable	Worldwide review	Lorenz et al. (1998)
1979–1994	216	<800 g	1979–84 1984–89 1989–94	96 96 93	13% 20% 13%	12 m	Regional, USA	O'Shea et al. (1997)
1982–1998	623	<1,000 g	1982–89 500–749 g 750–999 g 1990–98 500–749 g 750–999 g	86 81 88 84 80 85	20% 28% 18% 26% 34% 22%	20 m	Local center, USA	Wilson-Costello et al. (2005)
1982–2002	872	<1,000 g	1982–89 1990–99 2000–02	86 84 86	20% 24% 21%	20 m	Local center, USA	Wilson-Costello et al. (2007)
1992–1995	221	<1,000 g	N/A	75	42%	20 m	Local center, USA	Hack et al. (2000)
1993–1994	1,151	<1,000 g	<500 g 501–600 g 601–700 g 701–800 g 801–900 g 901–1,000 g	78 73 74 74 77 79	31% 45% 41% 42% 35% 31%	18–22 m	NICHD, USA	Vohr et al. (2000)
1993–1994	1,151	<1,000 g	12 centers	70–83	17–62%	18–22 m	NICHD, USA	Vohr et al. (2004)
1993–1999	777	<25 weeks	1993–96 ≤23 weeks 24 weeks 1996–99 ≤23 weeks 24 weeks	75 72	40% 38% 40% 47% 52% 44%	18–22 m	NICHD, USA	Hintz et al. (2005)

(*continued*)

Table 2 (continued)

Year of birth	Sample size	BW (grams)/GA (weeks)	Subgroups	Mean MDI	MDI <70	Age months	Location	Author
1995	251	≤25 weeks	≤23 weeks 24 weeks 25 weeks	84	27% 30% 30%	30 m	UK and Ireland	Wood et al. (2000)
1993–1998	3,785	22–32 weeks	1993–94 22–26 weeks 27–32 weeks 1995–96 22–26 weeks 27–32 weeks 1997–98 22–26 weeks 27–32 weeks	N/A	1993–94 42% 30% 1995–96 39% 26% 1997–98 37% 23%	18–22 m	NICHD, USA	Vohr et al. (2005)
2006–2007 2008–2011	1,012 1,616	<27 weeks	400–1,000 g	BSID II 77 BSID III 88	37% 10%	18–22 m	NICHD, USA	Vohr et al. (2012)
2005	221	<28 weeks	<1,000	BSID III 97	< −1 SD 13% < −2 SD 3%	24 m	Victoria, Australia	Anderson et al. (2010)

While much less common than motor disabilities, rates of neurosensory disabilities are higher in ELBW infants than the general population. Unilateral or bilateral blindness occurs in 1–10% of ELBW infants (Hintz et al. 2005b; Shankaran et al. 2004; Wilson-Costello et al. 2005, 2007; Hack and Fanaroff 2000; O'Shea et al. 1997; Vohr et al. 2000a, 2004b; Wood et al. 2000). Milder visual impairments including myopia, strabismus, and lack of stereopsis (depth perception) occur at rates of 9–25% (Wood et al. 2000; Vohr et al. 2004b; Cooke et al. 2004).

Hearing impairment requiring amplification is reported in 1–9% of ELBW infants (Hintz et al. 2005b; Shankaran et al. 2004; Wilson-Costello et al. 2005, 2007; Hack and Fanaroff 2000; Hack et al. 1996; Emsley et al. 1998; Wood et al. 2000; Vohr et al. 2004b). Milder hearing impairment has been reported in 11–13% (Wood et al. 2000; Vohr et al. 2000b). When transient conductive or unilateral hearing loss is included, rates of milder impairment are as high as 28% (Vohr et al. 2004b). These rates of neurosensory impairment persist at school age (Marlow et al. 2005; Doyle and Anderson 2005; Hack et al. 2000b, 2005).

119.3.11 Cognitive

The most common severe impairment seen in VLBW and ELBW infants at 18 and 30 months is developmental delay. In the era of the Bayley Scales of Infant Development II (Bayley II) (Bayley 1993), impairment was defined as scores more than 2 standard deviations below the mean on standardized cognitive testing. Most follow-up studies of ELBW infants prior to 2008 used the Bayley II. Average score for ELBW infants at 18–22 months corrected age on the Bayley II in the NICHD was ~76 but varied from center to center with a range of 70–83 (Vohr et al. 2004b). In a cohort of <1000 g infants born from 1982 to 2002, Wilson-Costello and Hack report average MDIs of 84–86 (and 83–89 in a subset of <750 g infants) at 20-month follow-up (Wilson-Costello et al. 2005, 2007; Hack et al. 1996). Wood et al. reported similar results at 30 months corrected age in a cohort of 20–25 week infants in the United Kingdom whose average MDI was 84 (Wood et al. 2000).

A limitation of the Bayley II is its inclusion of only two developmental scores, the Mental Developmental Index (MDI), a composite of cognitive, receptive, and expressive language tasks, and the Psychomotor Developmental Index (PDI), a composite of fine and gross motor skills. This limitation contributed to the development of the Bayley Scales of Infant and Toddler Development, Third Edition (Bayley III) (Bayley 2006). The majority of users made the switch to the Bayley III and the NRN converted to the Bayley III in January 2008.

The Bayley III contains three individual developmental scores: a cognitive composite score, a language composite score (with receptive and expressive subscores), and a motor composite score (with gross and fine motor subscores), in addition to social-emotional and adaptive behavior, and this facilitates evaluating more specific areas of development including language.

Bayley III cognitive and motor scores have been shown by many investigators to be higher than Bayley II scores (Vohr et al. 2012). The reasons for this difference are not clear. The Bayley III separation of language and cognitive scores was done to minimize effects of language delay on the cognitive assessment. Intelligence tests invariably separate verbal IQ from performance IQ. The Bayley II has not been a stellar predictor of school-age outcomes. It is known that preterm children have evidence of recovery with increasing age (Luu et al. 2011a). One perspective regarding the higher scores is that Bayley III cognitive scores may be more predictive since the test eliminates the bias of language delay. There is also evidence that the new Bayley III underestimates delay of both preterm and term infants (Anderson et al. 2010). This has resulted in modification of the cutpoints of the Bayley III cognitive composite score. Current categories used by NICHD are moderate delay 70–84, severe delay <70, and profound delay ≤54.

Like rates of NDI and CP, rates of cognitive impairment, defined as a score <70 on cognitive assessment, vary worldwide and are inversely proportional to gestational age and birth weight. Rates of cognitive impairment range from 14% to 39% at 24 weeks, 10–30% at 25 weeks (Hack and Fanaroff 2000), 4–24% at <26 weeks, and 11–18% at < 29 weeks worldwide. In infants born <800 g, rates of cognitive impairment range from 13% to 50% (Shankaran et al. 2004; Hack and Fanaroff 2000; O'Shea et al. 1997; Lorenz et al. 1998; Vohr and Msall 1997) and at <1250 g 26% (Vohr and Msall 1997). Rates of cognitive impairment are reported at 37–47% in 22–26-week infants (Hintz et al. 2005b, 2011), 23–30% in 27–32-week infants, and 34–37% in all infants <1000 g in the NICHD (Vohr et al. 2000a). Wilson-Costello and Hack cite 20–26% rates of cognitive impairment in their cohort of ELBW infants at 18 months (Wilson-Costello et al. 2005, 2007; Hack et al. 1996), and at 30 months, 30% of Wood's cohort had cognitive impairment (Wood et al. 2000).

While cognitive functioning can be measured in infancy, it may not be predictive of cognitive functioning later in life. The assessment of an infant's cognitive function is highly dependent on their motor, language, and social-emotional development. Hack et al. found that MDI at 20 months corrected age was not predictive of cognitive functioning at 8 years of age. In their cohort of ELBW infants, MDI at 20 months was 76 compared to a cognitive score of 88 at 8 years, and rate of cognitive impairment dropped from 39% at 20 months to 16% at 8 years. The positive predictive value of having a low cognitive score at 8 years (<70) given a low cognitive score at 20 months (<70) was only 0.37 (Hack et al. 2005). Ment et al. reported recovery of test scores in a cohort of VLBW infants (Ment et al. 2003). Mean expressive language scores increased from 88 at 3 years to 99 at 8 years of age and full scale IQ increased from 90 to 96.

Mean IQ for VLBW and ELBW infants at school age (5–14 years) ranges from 82 to 105 (Doyle and Anderson 2005; Hack et al. 2005; Ment et al. 2003; Anderson and Doyle 2003; Bhutta et al. 2002; Botting et al. 1998; Halsey et al. 1996; Rickards et al. 2001; Taylor et al. 2000b; Whitfield et al. 1997). Although the mean IQ is within the average or low average range for children born ELBW or VLBW, they have significantly lower IQ scores than their normal birth weight peers (0.5–1.0 SD lower) (Marlow et al. 2005; Anderson and Doyle 2003; Bhutta et al. 2002; Botting et al. 1998; Rickards et al. 2001; Taylor et al. 2000b; Whitfield et al. 1997; Litt et al. 2005) and significantly higher rates of cognitive impairment (Marlow et al. 2005; Doyle and Anderson 2005; Horwood et al. 1998). Cognitive scores at school age remain significantly correlated with gestational age and birth weight (Taylor et al. 2000a, b; Anderson and Doyle 2003; Bhutta et al. 2002). While environmental factors such as type of health insurance, bilingual household, income level, single parent, teenage mother, and level of maternal education are known to impact on intelligence, differences in IQ between preterm and term controls persist after adjustment for these confounders (Breslau et al. 2001; Luu et al. 2011b). In the Indomethacin trial (Luu et al. 2011a), significant catch-up in receptive vocabulary is observed by the age of 16 years among very preterm children compared to term peers. The absence of neurosensory impairment and residing in a favorable socioeconomic milieu are associated with the most optimal developmental trajectories.

In addition to impairments in global cognitive functioning, more subtle cognitive impairments are often detected in school age. These higher prevalence, lower severity dysfunctions reportedly occur in 50–70% of children born VLBW (Msall et al. 1992). Children born VLBW or ELBW have relative impairments of executive functioning (Taylor et al. 2000b, 2006; Luu et al. 2011b; Anderson and Doyle 2004; Marlow et al. 2007), visual motor skills (Marlow et al. 2007), and memory (Taylor et al. 2006), especially verbal memory (Taylor et al. 2000c). They score lower on tests of academic achievement (Hack et al. 2005; Botting et al. 1998; Taylor et al. 2006), perceptual-organizational skills (Taylor et al. 2000b; Litt et al. 2005), visual processing tasks (Taylor et al. 2000b; Litt et al. 2005), and adaptive functioning (Taylor et al. 2000c) compared to their normal birth weight peers. Even ELBW infants without neurosensory or cognitive impairment have higher rates of learning disabilities (Anderson and Doyle 2003), especially in math (Rickards et al. 2001; Taylor et al. 2000b; Litt et al. 2005), ranging from 25% to 40% (Anderson and Doyle 2003; Litt et al. 2005).

So it is not surprising that ELBW infants have higher rates of academic underachievement and need for special education services (Anderson and Doyle 2003; Halsey et al. 1996; Horwood et al. 1998). Like their cognitive scores, mean scores on formal tests of academic achievement fall within the normal range (94–105), but are lower than scores of normal birth weight peers (Anderson and Doyle 2003; Halsey et al. 1996). Teachers of VLBW infants report rates of below average school performance in all academic areas, ranging from 24% to 41% (Anderson and Doyle 2003; Botting et al. 1998; Horwood et al. 1998; O'Callaghan et al. 1996). Approximately 25% of VLBW infants and up to 62% of ELBW infants receive special education service (Hack et al. 2000b; Halsey et al. 1996; Taylor et al. 2000b; Horwood et al. 1998; Lefebvre et al. 2005; Saigal et al. 2003). Between 15% and 34% required grade repetition (Taylor et al. 2000b; Saigal et al. 2003; Klebanov et al. 1994).

An increasing number of investigators have reported on cognitive and academic abilities of former VLBW and ELBW teenagers and young adults (Taylor et al. 2000a, b,c, 2006; Doyle and Anderson 2005; Marlow et al. 2007; Saigal et al. 2000, 2003). ELBW teens continue to have mean cognitive scores in the average to low average range but persist in having significantly lower cognitive and academic scores than teens born normal birth weight (Lefebvre et al. 2005; Grunau et al. 2004; Hack et al. 2002) and significantly higher rates of cognitive impairment (Lefebvre et al. 2005; Hack et al. 2002). Cognitive differences are greatest in areas of visual-perceptual tasks (Grunau et al. 2004). Academic differences are seen in reading and mathematics (Grunau et al. 2004). As a result, only 56–74% of preterm children, significantly fewer than normal birth weight teens, graduate from high school (Lefebvre et al. 2005; Hack et al. 2002). Hack's report on a single center cohort of VLBW infants showed significant gender differences in graduation rates: 66% of VLBW males compared to 75% for term males and 81% for VLBW females compared to 90% for term females (Hack et al. 2002).

119.3.12 Visual Motor/Fine Motor

Difficulties with fine motor skills and with visual motor skills, described as problems with visual perception, visual motor control, hand-eye coordination, or visual motor integration, are common in children born VLBW or ELBW. These difficulties can impact on academic performance and functional abilities. Fine motor difficulties have been described in as many as 70% and fine motor difficulties resulting in impairment in 23% at 5 years of age (Goyen et al. 1998). Average scores on the Beery VMI are significantly lower in ELBW infants than term controls at age 7–8 (91 vs. 97, $p < 0.001$) (Foulder-Hughes and Cooke 2003) and age 12 (82 vs. 92) (Luu et al. 2009a), and visual motor integration deficits (VMI <70) are found in 16–24% of ELBW infants at school age (Foulder-Hughes and Cooke 2003; Luu et al. 2009b).

119.3.13 Speech and Language

Speech and language develop atypically during early childhood in previously ELBW infants, with delays in the acquisition of expressive language, receptive language, and articulation (Vohr et al. 1988, 1989; Ortiz-Mantilla et al. 2008). Children born at or before 25 weeks' gestation have significantly lower total scores on the PLS (90 vs. 104) and significantly higher rates of language impairment (16% vs. 2%) at 6 years of age. Scores on auditory comprehension, expressive communication, and articulation subtests of the PLS are uniformly lower (Wolke et al. 2008). In addition, rates of language impairment, defined as standard scores of <70 on language assessment, are higher. Former ELBW infants have significantly lower scores (92 vs. 105) and higher rates of impairment (13% vs. 4%) on the PPVT, as well as lower expressive, receptive, and total scores (85–87 vs. 100–103) and higher rates of impairment

(22–24% vs. 3–4%) on the CELF at age 12 (Luu et al. 2009a). While language development in infancy and early childhood is often an early proxy for overall cognitive development, specific language deficits have been described including phonological short-term memory (Briscoe et al. 1998) and prosodic processing (Herold et al. 2008). At 12 years of age, children who were born <1250 g have less pronounced differences on tests of lower-level language skills (phonological processing, phonemic decoding, and sight word reading) compared to term controls, but exhibit significantly more difficulty with higher-level skills (syntax, semantics, verbal language memory, and reading comprehension) (Luu et al. 2009a, b). In addition, when given a semantic processing task, preterm children have abnormal patterns of brain activity on functional MRI, resembling the brain activity of term controls during phonologic processing (Peterson et al. 2002).

119.3.14 Motor Function/Coordination

Arguably more important than the type or location of impairment is the functional level of the affected infant. Level of gross motor function is most commonly assessed and categorized using Palisano's GMFCS (Palisano et al. 1997). In an NICHD Neonatal Network study, though 27% of a cohort of ELBW infants diagnosed with CP at 18–22 months had moderate to severe gross motor function (Levels 3–5), 28% had gross motor function consistent with Level 0 or 1 and were ambulatory (Vohr et al. 2005b). It is important to remember that a diagnosis of CP includes a wide spectrum of motor performance.

More subtle motor abnormalities are also seen more commonly in former preterm infants, and children born preterm are more likely to have difficulty with motor coordination. In the past these children were often labeled as "clumsy," but in recent years the diagnosis of developmental coordination disorder (DCD) has been used. DCD is defined as impairment in motor performance sufficient to produce functional impairment that cannot be otherwise explained by the child's age, cognitive ability, or neurologic or psychiatric diagnosis. Scores of less than the 5th–10th% on the Movement Assessment Battery for Children (MABC) are considered diagnostic. DCD is found in 31–34% of VLBW and 50% of ELBW infants (Foulder-Hughes and Cooke 2003; Hall et al. 1995; Edwards et al. 2011).

119.3.15 Functional Outcomes

As a result of the high rates of associated cognitive, motor, neurosensory, and behavioral difficulties seen in children who were born preterm, these children have higher rates of functional limitations than children who were born at term (Hack et al. 2000b). These functional delays are observed in VLBW infants with and without severe impairments. While 93% of ELBW infants achieve sitting balance, 83% walk, and 86% feed themselves independently by 18–22 months corrected age, more subtle functional deficits become apparent later in life (Vohr et al. 2000a). At 10–14 years of age, 27% of children who were VLBW and 32% of those who were ELBW report restricted physical activity, and 24% of VLBW and 29% of ELBW report they are unable to participate in sports (Hack et al. 2000b). Functional outcomes are considered particularly important by parents.

119.3.16 Behavioral and Psychological

Very low birth weight has been associated with a wide variety of behavioral and psychological diagnoses and disabilities. Recent concern has arisen that rates of autism spectrum disorder (ASD) may be higher in ELBW infants than previously thought. Though low birth weight (<2500 g) may result in a two- to threefold increase in the risk of ASD (Kolevzon et al. 2007; Schendel and Bhasin 2008), true risk of ASD in very preterm infants is unknown. Two prior studies have investigated rates of autistic characteristics in children born very low birth weight (VLBW, <1500 g). Indredavik et al. (2004) demonstrated a trend toward higher scores on the Autism

Spectrum Screening Questionnaire in a population of 56 VLBWs at 14 years of age compared to full-term controls. Limperopoulos et al. (2008) recently reported that 25% of VLBW infants screen positive on the M-CHAT at 18 months. However, the M-CHAT was developed for use in the general population and not for a high-risk population such as VLBW infants where false-positive screening rates are likely high due to associated cognitive, language, and motor delays. In addition no diagnostic confirmation was performed (Limperopoulos et al. 2008). Further studies are needed to determine the true risk of autism in this population. In one study (Stephens et al. 2012) screening extremely preterm infants for autism with a three-component screen of the Pervasive Developmental Disorders Screening Test, response to name, and joint attention had a 20% positive screen at 18 months corrected age. Follow-up to older ages and diagnostic testing is needed.

At school age (8–12 years old), parents and teachers of VLBW/ELBW infants report higher rates of inattention and hyperactivity (Anderson and Doyle 2003; Bhutta et al. 2002; Taylor et al. 2000b; Horwood et al. 1998; Klebanov et al. 1994; Indredavik et al. 2004; Botting et al. 1997; Breslau and Chilcoat 2000), with rates of 23–27% in VLBW and 33–37% in ELBW infants (Horwood et al. 1998; Indredavik et al. 2004). At 12–14 years of age, one quarter to one half of VLBW/ELBW infants have symptoms of anxiety and/or social withdrawal (Horwood et al. 1998), 8–14% meet criteria for generalized anxiety disorder (compared to 1–4% of peers) (Indredavik et al. 2004; Botting et al. 1997), and 25–28% meet criteria for a psychiatric disorder (compared to 7–10% of peers) (Indredavik et al. 2004; Botting et al. 1997). At 17 and 20 years of age, ELBWs score higher on measures of inattention, anxiety/depression, withdrawn behavior, and social problems (Grunau et al. 2004; Hack et al. 2004). In addition, VLBW teens score significantly lower on measures of self-esteem (Rickards et al. 2001; Grunau et al. 2004). They report less confidence in their athletic-, school-, romantic-, and job-related abilities (Grunau et al. 2004). In contrast, VLBW adults report lower rates of alcohol and drug use, sexual activity, and pregnancy than adults born normal birth weight (Hack et al. 2002; 2004).

119.3.17 Late Preterm

While the majority of neonatal outcomes research has focused on the ELBW infant, more recent studies have brought a long neglected population of infants to our attention, the late preterm population. Recent data indicate that increased risks associated with prematurity extend to moderate and late preterm infants (Ananth et al. 2013; Kuzniewicz et al. 2013; Jain and Cheng 2006). During the 1990s the rates of delivery at 40 or more weeks' gestation decreased, while rates of deliveries between 34 and 36 weeks increased steadily (Davidoff et al. 2006). From 1990 to 2005 the rate of late preterm births increased from 7.3% to 9.1% of all births (Engle et al. 2007). Compared to term infants, these "late preterm infants" have higher mortality rates (Khashu et al. 2009; McIntire and Leveno 2008; Tomashek et al. 2007). They also have higher rates of neonatal morbidities such as respiratory distress, temperature instability, hypoglycemia, kernicterus, apnea seizures, infection, and feeding problems (Ananth et al. 2008, 2013; Engle et al. 2007; Khashu et al. 2009; McIntire and Leveno 2008; Bastek et al. 2008; Raju et al. 2006). All of these morbidities have the potential to increase the risk of long-term neurodevelopmental sequelae. In addition, the brain of the late preterm infant is more immature than the term infants' brain. At 34 weeks there are significantly fewer gyri and sulci, and the brain weighs an estimated 60% of that of a term infant (Raju et al. 2006). While there is a large body of literature that addresses the neurodevelopmental outcome of VLBW and ELBW infants, there is a paucity of information published about the neurodevelopmental sequelae of late preterm birth. Infants born 34–36 weeks are 3.39 times as likely as term infants to develop CP and 1.25 times as likely to have cognitive impairment (Petrini et al. 2009). They are more likely to qualify for special needs' preschool and are more likely to have problems with school readiness (Adams-Chapman 2006). In kindergarten and first grade, they have lower reading scores, teachers report math skills below those of their full-term peers, and they are more likely to qualify for special education services (Chyi et al. 2008).

119.4 Summary

In summary, preterm infant survivors remain at increased risk of adverse neurodevelopmental outcomes. Longitudinal assessment of outcomes is indicated to identify neurosensory, developmental, and behavioral sequelae and to ensure appropriate supports and interventions are provided. Continued surveillance of center outcomes is needed to meet clinical and research goals and improve program performance. In addition, randomized trials are needed to identify key risk factors and identify effective perinatal interventions that optimize outcomes.

Acknowledgments We gratefully acknowledge the contribution of Bonnie E. Stephens MD to the 2009 edition of *Normal and Abnormal Neurodevelopmental and Behavioral Outcomes of Very Low Birth Weight Infants*.

References

Achenbach TM (1991a) Integrative guide for the 1991 CBCL/4-18 YSR and TRF profiles. University of Vermont, Department of Psychiatry, Burlington

Achenbach T (1991b) Child behavior checklist. Department of Psychiatry, Burlington

Adams-Chapman I (2006) Neurodevelopmental outcome of the late preterm infant. Clin Perinatol 33(4): 947–964; abstract xi

American Academy of Pediatrics. Committee on Fetus and Newborn (1995) The initiation or withdrawal of treatment for high-risk newborns. Pediatrics 96:362–363

Amiel-Tison C (1987) Neuromotor status. In: Taeusch HW, Yogman MW (eds) Follow-up management of the high-risk infant. Little, Brown & Company, Boston

Ananth CV, Gyamfi C, Jain L (2008) Characterizing risk profiles of infants who are delivered at late preterm gestations: does it matter? Am J Obstet Gynecol 199 (4):329–331

Ananth CV, Friedman AM, Gyamfi-Bannerman C (2013) Epidemiology of moderate preterm, late preterm and early term delivery. Clin Perinatol 40(4):601–610

Anderson P, Doyle LW (2003) Neurobehavioral outcomes of school-age children born extremely low birth weight or very preterm in the 1990s. JAMA 289(24):3264–3272

Anderson PJ, Doyle LW (2004) Executive functioning in school-aged children who were born very preterm or with extremely low birth weight in the 1990s. Pediatrics 114(1):50–57

Anderson PJ, De Luca CR, Hutchinson E, Roberts G, Doyle LW (2010) Underestimation of developmental delay by the new Bayley-III scale. Arch Pediatr Adolesc Med 164(4):352–356

Aylward GP (1992) The relationship between environmental risk and developmental outcome. J Dev Behav Pediatr 13(3):222–229

Aylward GP (2002) Methodological issues in outcome studies of at-risk infants. J Pediatr Psychol 27(1):37–45

Aylward GP, Hatcher RP, Stripp B, Gustafson NF, Leavitt LA (1985) Who goes and who stays: subject loss in a multicenter, longitudinal follow-up study. J Dev Behav Pediatr 6(1):3–8

Ballard PL, Keller RL, Black DM, Durand DJ, Merrill JD, Eichenwald EC et al (2015) Inhaled nitric oxide increases urinary nitric oxide metabolites and cyclic guanosine monophosphate in premature infants: relationship to pulmonary outcome. Am J Perinatol 32(3): 225–232

Barnett A, Henderson S, Sugden D (2007) The movement assessment battery for children-2. Pearson Assessment, London, United Kingdom

Barrington KJ (2001) The adverse neuro-developmental effects of postnatal steroids in the preterm infant: a systematic review of RCTs. BMC Pediatr 1(1):1

Barrington KJ, Finer NN (2007) Inhaled nitric oxide for respiratory failure in preterm infants. Cochrane Database Syst Rev 3:CD000509

Bastek JA, Sammel MD, Pare E, Srinivas SK, Posencheg MA, Elovitz MA (2008) Adverse neonatal outcomes: examining the risks between preterm, late preterm, and term infants. Am J Obstet Gynecol 199(4):367 e361–368

Bayley N (1993) Bayley scales of infant development-II. Psychological Corporation, San Antonio

Bayley N (2006) Bayley scales of infant and toddler development – third edition. Harcourt Assessment, San Antonio

Beery K (1989) Developmental test of visual-motor integration, 3rd edn. Western Psychological Services, Los Angeles

Bhutta AT, Cleves MA, Casey PH, Cradock MM, Anand KJ (2002) Cognitive and behavioral outcomes of school-aged children who were born preterm: a meta-analysis. JAMA 288(6):728–737

Blakely ML, Lally KP, McDonald S, Brown RL, Barnhart DC, Ricketts RR et al (2005) Postoperative outcomes of extremely low birth-weight infants with necrotizing enterocolitis or isolated intestinal perforation: a prospective cohort study by the NICHD Neonatal Research Network. Ann Surg 241(6):984–989; discussion 989–994

Blaymore-Bier J, Pezzullo J, Kim E, Oh W, Garcia-Coll C, Vohr BR (1994) Outcome of extremely low-birth-weight infants: 1980–1990. Acta Paediatr 83(12): 1244–1248

Botting N, Powls A, Cooke RW, Marlow N (1997) Attention deficit hyperactivity disorders and other psychiatric outcomes in very low birthweight children at 12 years. J Child Psychol Psychiatry 38 (8):931–941
Botting N, Powls A, Cooke RW, Marlow N (1998) Cognitive and educational outcome of very-low-birthweight children in early adolescence. Dev Med Child Neurol 40(10):652–660
Bracewell M, Marlow N (2002) Patterns of motor disability in very preterm children. Ment Retard Dev Disabil Res Rev 8(4):241–248
Breslau N, Chilcoat HD (2000) Psychiatric sequelae of low birth weight at 11 years of age. Biol Psychiatry 47 (11):1005–1011
Breslau N, Johnson EO, Lucia VC (2001) Academic achievement of low birthweight children at age 11: the role of cognitive abilities at school entry. J Abnorm Child Psychol 29(4):273–279
Briscoe J, Gathercole SE, Marlow N (1998) Short-term memory and language outcomes after extreme prematurity at birth. J Speech Lang Hear Res 41(3):654–666
Broyles RS, Tyson JE, Heyne ET, Heyne RJ, Hickman JF, Swint M et al (2000) Comprehensive follow-up care and life-threatening illnesses among high-risk infants: a randomized controlled trial. JAMA 284(16): 2070–2076
Bruininks R (1978) Bruininks-Oseretsky test of motor proficiency. American Guidance Service, Circle Pines
Chyi LJ, Lee HC, Hintz SR, Gould JB, Sutcliffe TL (2008) School outcomes of late preterm infants: special needs and challenges for infants born at 32 to 36 weeks gestation. J Pediatr 153(1):25–31
Colarusso R, Hammill DD (2003) Motor-free visual perception test manual. Western Psychological Services, Los Angeles
Conners CK (1996) Connors parent rating scales revised. Psychological Corporation, San Antonio
Cooke RW, Foulder-Hughes L, Newsham D, Clarke D (2004) Ophthalmic impairment at 7 years of age in children born very preterm. Arch Dis Child Fetal Neonatal Ed 89(3):F249–F253
Coplan J (1993) Early language milestone scale-second edition. Pro-ed, Austin
Costeloe KL, Hennessy EM, Haider S, Stacey F, Marlow N, Draper ES (2012) Short term outcomes after extreme preterm birth in England: comparison of two birth cohorts in 1995 and 2006 (the EPICure studies). BMJ 345:e7976
Crowley P, Chalmers I, Keirse MJ (1990) The effects of corticosteroid administration before preterm delivery: an overview of the evidence from controlled trials. Br J Obstet Gynaecol 97(1):11–25
Davidoff MJ, Dias T, Damus K, Russell R, Bettegowda VR, Dolan S et al (2006) Changes in the gestational age distribution among U.S. singleton births: impact on rates of late preterm birth, 1992 to 2002. Semin Perinatol 30(1):8–15
De Vries LS, Van Haastert IL, Rademaker KJ, Koopman C, Groenendaal F (2004a) Ultrasound abnormalities preceding cerebral palsy in high-risk preterm infants. J Pediatr 144(6):815–820
de Vries LS, Gunardi H, Barth PG, Bok LA, Verboon-Maciolek MA, Groenendaal F (2004b) The spectrum of cranial ultrasound and magnetic resonance imaging abnormalities in congenital cytomegalovirus infection. Neuropediatrics 35(2):113–119
Doyle LW, Anderson PJ (2005) Improved neurosensory outcome at 8 years of age of extremely low birthweight children born in Victoria over three distinct eras. Arch Dis Child Fetal Neonatal Ed 90(6):F484–F488
Drillien CM (1972) Abnormal neurologic signs in the first year of life in low-birthweight infants: possible prognostic significance. Dev Med Child Neurol 14(5): 575–584
Duffner PK, Granger C, Lyon N, Niewczyk P, Barczykowski A, Bauer S et al (2012) Developmental and functional outcomes in children with a positive newborn screen for Krabbe disease: a pilot study of a phone-based interview surveillance technique. J Pediatr 161(2):258–263, e251
Dunn LM, Dunn L (1997) Peabody picture vocabulary test, 3rd edn. American Guidance Service, Circle Pines
Edwards J, Berube M, Erlandson K, Haug S, Johnstone H, Meagher M et al (2011) Developmental coordination disorder in school-aged children born very preterm and/or at very low birth weight: a systematic review. J Dev Behav Pediatr 32(9):678–687
Ehrenkranz RA, Dusick AM, Vohr BR, Wright LL, Wrage LA, Poole WK (2006) Growth in the neonatal intensive care unit influences neurodevelopmental and growth outcomes of extremely low birth weight infants. Pediatrics 117(4):1253–1261
Elliott CD (1990) Differential ability scales. Introductory and technical handbook. The Psychological Corp., New York
El-Metwally D, Vohr B, Tucker R (2000) Survival and neonatal morbidity at the limits of viability in the mid 1990s: 22 to 25 weeks. J Pediatr 137(5):616–622
Emsley HC, Wardle SP, Sims DG, Chiswick ML, D' Souza SW (1998) Increased survival and deteriorating developmental outcome in 23 to 25 week old gestation infants, 1990-4 compared with 1984-9. Arch Dis Child Fetal Neonatal Ed 78(2):F99–F104
Engle WA, Tomashek KM, Wallman C (2007) "Late-preterm" infants: a population at risk. Pediatrics 120(6): 1390–1401
Fanaroff AA, Hack M, Walsh MC (2003) The NICHD neonatal research network: changes in practice and outcomes during the first 15 years. Semin Perinatol 27(4): 281–287
Farooqi A, Hagglof B, Sedin G, Gothefors L, Serenius F (2007) Mental health and social competencies of 10- to 12-year-old children born at 23 to 25 weeks of gestation in the 1990s: a Swedish national prospective follow-up study. Pediatrics 120(1):118–133
Finer NN, Carlo WA, Walsh MC, Rich W, Gantz MG, Laptook AR et al (2010) Early CPAP versus surfactant in extremely preterm infants. N Engl J Med 362(21): 1970–1979

Folio MR, Fewell RR (1983) Peabody developmental motor scales and activity cards. Developmental Learning Materials Resource, Allen

Foulder-Hughes LA, Cooke RW (2003) Motor, cognitive, and behavioural disorders in children born very preterm. Dev Med Child Neurol 45(2):97–103

Gargus RA, Vohr BR, Tyson JE, High P, Higgins RD, Wrage LA et al (2009) Unimpaired outcomes for extremely low birth weight infants at 18 to 22 months. Pediatrics 124(1):112–121

Gianarris WJ, Golden CJ, Greene L (2001) The Conners' parent rating scales: a critical review of the literature. Clin Psychol Rev 21(7):1061–1093

Goyen TA, Lui K, Woods R (1998) Visual-motor, visual-perceptual, and fine motor outcomes in very-low-birthweight children at 5 years. Dev Med Child Neurol 40(2):76–81

Granger CV, Seltzer GB, Fishbein CF (eds) (1987) Primary care of the functionally disabled: assessment and management. Lippincott, Philadelphia

Granger CV, Hamilton BB, Linacre JM, Heinemann AW, Wright BD (1993) Performance profiles of the functional independence measure. Am J Phys Med Rehabil 72(2):84–89

Grunau RE, Whitfield MF, Fay TB (2004) Psychosocial and academic characteristics of extremely low birth weight (< or =800 g) adolescents who are free of major impairment compared with term-born control subjects. Pediatrics 114(6):e725–e732

Hack M (2006) Young adult outcomes of very-low-birth-weight children. Semin Fetal Neonatal Med 11(2): 127–137

Hack M, Fanaroff AA (2000) Outcomes of children of extremely low birthweight and gestational age in the 1990s. Semin Neonatol 5(2):89–106

Hack M, Friedman H, Fanaroff AA (1996) Outcomes of extremely low birth weight infants. Pediatrics 98(5): 931–937

Hack M, Wilson-Costello D, Friedman H, Taylor GH, Schluchter M, Fanaroff AA (2000a) Neurodevelopment and predictors of outcomes of children with birth weights of less than 1000 g: 1992–1995. Arch Pediatr Adolesc Med 154(7):725–731

Hack M, Taylor HG, Klein N, Mercuri-Minich N (2000b) Functional limitations and special health care needs of 10- to 14-year-old children weighing less than 750 grams at birth. Pediatrics 106(3):554–560

Hack M, Flannery DJ, Schluchter M, Cartar L, Borawski E, Klein N (2002) Outcomes in young adulthood for very-low-birth-weight infants. N Engl J Med 346(3): 149–157

Hack M, Youngstrom EA, Cartar L, Schluchter M, Taylor HG, Flannery D et al (2004) Behavioral outcomes and evidence of psychopathology among very low birth weight infants at age 20 years. Pediatrics 114 (4):932–940

Hack M, Taylor HG, Drotar D, Schluchter M, Cartar L, Wilson-Costello D et al (2005) Poor predictive validity of the Bayley Scales of Infant Development for cognitive function of extremely low birth weight children at school age. Pediatrics 116(2):333–341

Haley SM, Coster WJ, Ludlow LH (1991) Pediatric functional outcome measures. Phys Med Rehabil Clin N Am 2:689–723

Haley SM, Coster WJ, Ludlow LH et al (1992) Pediatric Evaluation of Disability Inventory (PEDI), version I, development, standardization and administration manual. New England Medical Center-PEDI Research Group, Boston

Hall A, McLeod A, Counsell C, Thomson L, Mutch L (1995) School attainment, cognitive ability and motor function in a total Scottish very-low-birthweight population at eight years: a controlled study. Dev Med Child Neurol 37(12):1037–1050

Halsey CL, Collin MF, Anderson CL (1996) Extremely low-birth-weight children and their peers. A comparison of school-age outcomes. Arch Pediatr Adolesc Med 150(8):790–794

Harrison P, Kaufman AS, Kaufman NL et al (1990) Early Screening Profiles (ESP). American Guidance Service

Hendrick DL, Prather M, Tobin AR (1984) Sequenced Inventory of Communication Development (SICD)-revised edition. Pro-ed, Austin

Herold B, Hohle B, Walch E, Weber T, Obladen M (2008) Impaired word stress pattern discrimination in very-low-birthweight infants during the first 6 months of life. Dev Med Child Neurol 50(9):678–683

Hintz SR, Kendrick DE, Stoll BJ, Vohr BR, Fanaroff AA, Donovan EF et al (2005a) Neurodevelopmental and growth outcomes of extremely low birth weight infants after necrotizing enterocolitis. Pediatrics 115(3):696–703

Hintz SR, Kendrick DE, Vohr BR, Poole WK, Higgins RD (2005b) Changes in neurodevelopmental outcomes at 18 to 22 months' corrected age among infants of less than 25 weeks' gestational age born in 1993–1999. Pediatrics 115(6):1645–1651

Hintz SR, Poole WK, Wright LL, Fanaroff AA, Kendrick DE, Laptook AR et al (2005c) Changes in mortality and morbidities among infants born at less than 25 weeks during the post-surfactant era. Arch Dis Child Fetal Neonatal Ed 90(2):F128–F133

Hintz SR, Kendrick DE, Wilson-Costello DE, Das A, Bell EF, Vohr BR et al (2011) Early-childhood neurodevelopmental outcomes are not improving for infants born at <25 weeks' gestational age. Pediatrics 127(1): 62–70

Hintz SR, Barnes PD, Bulas D, Slovis TL, Finer NN, Wrage LA et al (2015) Neuroimaging and neurodevelopmental outcome in extremely preterm infants. Pediatrics 135(1):e32–e42

Horwood LJ, Mogridge N, Darlow BA (1998) Cognitive, educational, and behavioural outcomes at 7 to 8 years in a national very low birthweight cohort. Arch Dis Child Fetal Neonatal Ed 79(1):F12–F20

Indredavik MS, Vik T, Heyerdahl S, Kulseng S, Fayers P, Brubakk AM (2004) Psychiatric symptoms and disorders in adolescents with low birth weight. Arch Dis Child Fetal Neonatal Ed 89(5):F445–F450

Ireton H (1992) Child development inventory. Behavior Science Systems, Minneapolis

Jain S, Cheng J (2006) Emergency department visits and rehospitalizations in late preterm infants. Clin Perinatol 33(4):935–945; abstract xi

Johnson S, Ring W, Anderson P, Marlow N (2005) Randomised trial of parental support for families with very preterm children: outcome at 5 years. Arch Dis Child 90(9):909–915

Joint Committee on Infant Hearing (2007) Year 2007 position statement: principles and guidelines for early hearing detection and intervention programs. Pediatrics 120:898–921

Khashu M, Narayanan M, Bhargava S, Osiovich H (2009) Perinatal outcomes associated with preterm birth at 33 to 36 weeks' gestation: a population-based cohort study. Pediatrics 123(1):109–113

Kinsey VE, Arnold HJ, Kalina RE, Stern L, Stahlman M, Odell G et al (1977) PaO2 levels and retrolental fibroplasia: a report of the cooperative study. Pediatrics 60(5):655–668

Klebanov PK, Brooks-Gunn J, McCormick MC (1994) Classroom behavior of very low birth weight elementary school children. Pediatrics 94(5):700–708

Kleinman JM, Robins DL, Ventola PE, Pandey J, Boorstein HC, Esser EL et al (2008) The modified checklist for autism in toddlers: a follow-up study investigating the early detection of autism spectrum disorders. J Autism Dev Disord 38(5):827–839

Kolevzon A, Gross R, Reichenberg A (2007) Prenatal and perinatal risk factors for autism: a review and integration of findings. Arch Pediatr Adolesc Med 161(4): 326–333

Kumar P, Shankaran S, Ambalavanan N, Kendrick DE, Pappas A, Vohr BR et al (2013) Characteristics of extremely low-birth-weight infant survivors with unimpaired outcomes at 30 months of age. J Perinatol 33(10):800–805

Kuzniewicz MW, Parker SJ, Schnake-Mahl A, Escobar GJ (2013) Hospital readmissions and emergency department visits in moderate preterm, late preterm, and early term infants. Clin Perinatol 40(4):753–775

Laptook AR, O' Shea TM, Shankaran S, Bhaskar B (2005) Adverse neurodevelopmental outcomes among extremely low birth weight infants with a normal head ultrasound: prevalence and antecedents. Pediatrics 115 (3):673–680

Larson SL, Vitali GJ (1988) Kindergarten Readiness Test (KRT). Slosson Educational Publication, East Aura

Lefebvre F, Mazurier E, Tessier R (2005) Cognitive and educational outcomes in early adulthood for infants weighing 1000 grams or less at birth. Acta Paediatr 94 (6):733–740

Limperopoulos C, Bassan H, Sullivan NR, Soul JS, Robertson RL Jr, Moore M et al (2008) Positive screening for autism in ex-preterm infants: prevalence and risk factors. Pediatrics 121(4):758–765

Lindstrom K, Lindblad F, Hjern A (2009) Psychiatric morbidity in adolescents and young adults born preterm: a Swedish national cohort study. Pediatrics 123(1): e47–e53

Litt J, Taylor HG, Klein N, Hack M (2005) Learning disabilities in children with very low birthweight: prevalence, neuropsychological correlates, and educational interventions. J Learn Disabil 38(2): 130–141

Lorenz JM, Wooliever DE, Jetton JR, Paneth N (1998) A quantitative review of mortality and developmental disability in extremely premature newborns. Arch Pediatr Adolesc Med 152(5):425–435

Luu TM, Vohr BR, Schneider KC, Katz KH, Tucker R, Allan WC et al (2009a) Trajectories of receptive language development from 3 to 12 years of age for very preterm children. Pediatrics 124(1):333–341

Luu TM, Ment LR, Schneider KC, Katz KH, Allan WC, Vohr BR (2009b) Lasting effects of preterm birth and neonatal brain hemorrhage at 12 years of age. Pediatrics 123(3):1037–1044

Luu TM, Vohr BR, Allan W, Schneider KC, Ment LR (2011a) Evidence for catch-up in cognition and receptive vocabulary among adolescents born very preterm. Pediatrics 128(2):313–322

Luu TM, Ment L, Allan W, Schneider K, Vohr BR (2011b) Executive and memory function in adolescents born very preterm. Pediatrics 127(3):e639–e646

Marlow N, Wolke D, Bracewell MA, Samara M (2005) Neurologic and developmental disability at six years of age after extremely preterm birth. N Engl J Med 352(1):9–19

Marlow N, Hennessy EM, Bracewell MA, Wolke D (2007) Motor and executive function at 6 years of age after extremely preterm birth. Pediatrics 120(4):793–804

Mc Carthy DA (1972) Manual for the McCarthy scales of children's abilities. The Psychological Corp., New York

McCormick MC (1993) Has the prevalence of handicapped infants increased with improved survival of the very low birth weight infant? Clin Perinatol 20(1):263–277

McCormick MC, Gortmaker SL, Sobol AM (1990) Very low birth weight children: behavior problems and school difficulty in a national sample. J Pediatr 117(5):687–693

McIntire DD, Leveno KJ (2008) Neonatal mortality and morbidity rates in late preterm births compared with births at term. Obstet Gynecol 111(1):35–41

McLaughlin KA, Breslau J, Green JG, Lakoma MD, Sampson NA, Zaslavsky AM et al (2011) Childhood socio-economic status and the onset, persistence, and severity of DSM-IV mental disorders in a US national sample. Soc Sci Med 73(7):1088–1096

Ment LR, Oh W, Ehrenkranz RA, Philip AG, Vohr B, Allan W et al (1994) Low-dose indomethacin and prevention of intraventricular hemorrhage: a multicenter randomized trial. Pediatrics 93(4):543–550

Ment LR, Vohr B, Allan W, Katz KH, Schneider KC, Westerveld M et al (2003) Change in cognitive function over time in very low-birth-weight infants. JAMA 289(6):705–711

Miller LJ (1988) Miller Assessment for Preschoolers (MAP). The Psychological Corporation, San Antonio

Msall ME (1996) Functional assessment in neurodevelopmental disabilities. In: Capute AJ, Accardo PJ (eds) Developmental disabilities in infancy and children, 2nd edn. Paul Brookes Publishing, Baltimore, pp 371–392

Msall ME (2005) Measuring functional skills in preschool children at risk for neurodevelopmental disabilities. Ment Retard Dev Disabil Res Rev 11(3):263–273

Msall ME, Buck GM, Rogers BT, Catanzaro NL (1992) Kindergarten readiness after extreme prematurity. Am J Dis Child 146(11):1371–1375

Msall ME, DiGaudio K, Duffy LC, LaForest S, Braun S, Granger CV, Wee FIM (1994) Normative sample of an instrument for tracking functional independence in children. Clin Pediatr (Phila) 33(7):431–438

Msall ME, Rogers B, Ripstein H et al (1997) Measurements of functional outcomes in children with cerebral palsy. Mental Retard Dev Disabil Res Rev 3:431

Msall ME, Phelps DL, DiGaudio KM, Dobson V, Tung B, McClead RE et al (2000) Severity of neonatal retinopathy of prematurity is predictive of neurodevelopmental functional outcome at age 5.5 years. Behalf of the Cryotherapy for Retinopathy of Prematurity Cooperative Group. Pediatrics 106(5):998–1005

Msall ME, Phelps DL, Hardy RJ, Dobson V, Quinn GE, Summers CG et al (2004) Educational and social competencies at 8 years in children with threshold retinopathy of prematurity in the CRYO-ROP multicenter study. Pediatrics 113(4):790–799

National Institutes of Health (NIH) (1995) Consensus development conference: effects of corticosteroids for fetal maturation on perinatal outcomes. Am J Obstet 173:246–248

Nehring AD, Nehring EM, Bruni JR et al (1992) Learning Accomplishment Profile – Diagnostic (LAP-D) standardized assessment – 1992 revision and standardization. Kaplan Press, Examiner's Manual, Lewisville

Newborg J, Jock JR, Wnek L et al (1984) Battelle development inventory and recalibrated technical data and morns: examiner's manual. DLG, LINC Associates. Teaching Resources, Allen

O'Callaghan MJ, Burns YR, Gray PH, Harvey JM, Mohay H, Rogers YM et al (1996) School performance of ELBW children: a controlled study. Dev Med Child Neurol 38(10):917–926

O'Shea TM, Klinepeter KL, Goldstein DJ, Jackson BW, Dillard RG (1997) Survival and developmental disability in infants with birth weights of 501 to 800 grams, born between 1979 and 1994. Pediatrics 100(6): 982–986

Ortiz-Mantilla S, Choudhury N, Leevers H, Benasich AA (2008) Understanding language and cognitive deficits in very low birth weight children. Dev Psychobiol 50 (2):107–126

Palisano RJ (1993) Validity of goal attainment scaling in infants with motor delays. Phys Ther 73(10):651–658; discussion 658–660

Palisano R, Rosenbaum P, Walter S, Russell D, Wood E, Galuppi B (1997) Development and reliability of a system to classify gross motor function in children with cerebral palsy. Dev Med Child Neurol 39(4):214–223

Palisano RJ, Cameron D, Rosenbaum PL, Walter SD, Russell D (2006) Stability of the gross motor function classification system. Dev Med Child Neurol 48 (6):424–428

Patel RM, Kandefer S, Walsh MC, Bell EF, Carlo WA, Laptook AR et al (2015) Causes and timing of death in extremely premature infants from 2000 through 2011. N Engl J Med 372(4):331–340

Pedersen SJ, Sommerfelt K, Markestad T (2000) Early motor development of premature infants with birthweight less than 2000 grams. Acta Paediatr 89(12):1456–1461

Peterson BS, Vohr B, Kane MJ, Whalen DH, Schneider KC, Katz KH et al (2002) A functional magnetic resonance imaging study of language processing and its cognitive correlates in prematurely born children. Pediatrics 110(6):1153–1162

Petrini JR, Dias T, McCormick MC, Massolo ML, Green NS, Escobar GJ (2009) Increased risk of adverse neurological development for late preterm infants. J Pediatr 154(2):169–176

Piecuch RE, Leonard CH, Cooper BA, Sehring SA (1997) Outcome of extremely low birth weight infants (500 to 999 grams) over a 12-year period. Pediatrics 100(4): 633–639

Raju TN, Higgins RD, Stark AR, Leveno KJ (2006) Optimizing care and outcome for late-preterm (near-term) infants: a summary of the workshop sponsored by the National Institute of Child Health and Human Development. Pediatrics 118(3):1207–1214

Rickards AL, Ryan MM, Kitchen WH (1988) Longitudinal study of very low birthweight infants: intelligence and aspects of school progress at 14 years of age. Aust Paediatr J 24(1):19–23

Rickards AL, Kelly EA, Doyle LW, Callanan C (2001) Cognition, academic progress, behavior and self-concept at 14 years of very low birth weight children. J Dev Behav Pediatr 22(1):11–18

Robins DL, Fein D, Barton ML, Green JA (2001) The modified checklist for autism in toddlers: an initial study investigating the early detection of autism and pervasive developmental disorders. J Autism Dev Disord 31(2):131–144

Rosenbaum P, Saigal S, Szatmari P, Hoult L (1995) Vineland adaptive behavior scales as a summary of functional outcome of extremely low-birthweight children. Dev Med Child Neurol 37(7):577–586

Russell DJ, Rosenbaum PL, Cadman DT, Gowland C, Hardy S, Jarvis S (1989) The gross motor function measure: a means to evaluate the effects of physical therapy. Dev Med Child Neurol 31(3):341–352

Russell DJ, Avery LM, Rosenbaum P, Raina PS, Walter SD, Palisano R (2000) Improved scaling of the gross motor function measure for children with cerebral palsy: evidence of reliability and validity. Phys Ther 80:873–885

Russell DJ, Avery LM, Rosenbaum PL, Raina PS, Walter SD, Palisano RJ (2002) Gross motor function measure (GMFM-66 & GMFM-88) user's manual. Mackeith Press, London

Rysavy MA, Li L, Bell EF, Das A, Hintz SR, Stoll BJ et al (2015) Between-hospital variation in treatment and outcomes in extremely preterm infants. N Engl J Med 372(19):1801–1811

Saigal S, Hoult LA, Streiner DL, Stoskopf BL, Rosenbaum PL (2000) School difficulties at adolescence in a regional cohort of children who were extremely low birth weight. Pediatrics 105(2):325–331

Saigal S, den Ouden L, Wolke D, Hoult L, Paneth N, Streiner DL et al (2003) School-age outcomes in children who were extremely low birth weight from four international population-based cohorts. Pediatrics 112 (4):943–950

Schendel D, Bhasin TK (2008) Birth weight and gestational age characteristics of children with autism, including a comparison with other developmental disabilities. Pediatrics 121(6):1155–1164

Schmidt B, Davis P, Moddemann D, Ohlsson A, Roberts RS, Saigal S et al (2001) Long-term effects of indomethacin prophylaxis in extremely-low-birth-weight infants. N Engl J Med 344(26):1966–1972

Schmidt B, Asztalos EV, Roberts RS, Robertson CM, Sauve RS, Whitfield MF (2003) Impact of bronchopulmonary dysplasia, brain injury, and severe retinopathy on the outcome of extremely low-birth-weight infants at 18 months: results from the trial of indomethacin prophylaxis in preterms. JAMA 289 (9):1124–1129

Schwartz RM, Luby AM, Scanlon JW, Kellogg RJ (1994) Effect of surfactant on morbidity, mortality, and resource use in newborn infants weighing 500 to 1500 g. N Engl J Med 330(21):1476–1480

Scott MN, Taylor HG, Fristad MA, Klein N, Espy KA, Minich N et al (2012) Behavior disorders in extremely preterm/extremely low birth weight children in kindergarten. J Dev Behav Pediatr 33(3):202–213

Semel E, Wiig EH, Secord WA (1995) Clinical evaluation of language fundamentals, 3rd edn. The Psychological Corporation Harcourt Base Co., San Antonio

Shankaran S, Johnson Y, Langer JC, Vohr BR, Fanaroff AA, Wright LL et al (2004) Outcome of extremely-low-birth-weight infants at highest risk: gestational age < or =24 weeks, birth weight < or =750 g, and 1-minute Apgar < or =3. Am J Obstet Gynecol 191 (4):1084–1091

Siegel B (2004) Pervasive developmental disorders screening test-II. Psych Corp, San Antonio

Sparrow S, Balla D, Cicchetti D (1984) Vineland adaptive behavior scales: interview edition, survey form manual. A revision of the Vineland Social Maturity Scale by E.A. Doll. American Guidance Service, Circle Pines

Stephens BE, Bann CM, Watson VE, Sheinkopf SJ, Peralta-Carcelen M, Bodnar A et al (2012) Screening for autism spectrum disorders in extremely preterm infants. J Dev Behav Pediatr 33(7):535–541

Stoll BJ, Hansen NI, Bell EF, Shankaran S, Laptook AR, Walsh MC et al (2010) Neonatal outcomes of extremely preterm infants from the NICHD Neonatal Research Network. Pediatrics 126(3):443–456

Stoll BJ, Hansen NI, Bell EF, Walsh MC, Carlo WA, Shankaran S et al (2015) Trends in care practices, morbidity, and mortality of extremely preterm neonates, 1993–2012. JAMA 314(10):1039–1051

Taylor HG, Klein N, Hack M (2000a) School-age consequences of birth weight less than 750 g: a review and update. Dev Neuropsychol 17(3):289–321

Taylor HG, Klein N, Minich NM, Hack M (2000b) Middle-school-age outcomes in children with very low birthweight. Child Dev 71(6):1495–1511

Taylor GH, Klein NM, Minich NM, Hack M (2000c) Verbal memory deficits in children with less than 750 g birth weight. Child Neuropsychol 6(1):49–63

Taylor HG, Klein N, Drotar D, Schluchter M, Hack M (2006) Consequences and risks of <1000-g birth weight for neuropsychological skills, achievement, and adaptive functioning. J Dev Behav Pediatr 27(6):459–469

Thebaud B, Lacaze-Masmonteil T, Watterberg K (2001) Postnatal glucocorticoids in very preterm infants: "the good, the bad, and the ugly"? Pediatrics 107(2):413–415

Thorndike RI, Hagan EP, Sattler JM (1986) Stanford-Binet intelligence scale, 4th edn. Riverside, Chicago

Tomashek KM, Shapiro-Mendoza CK, Davidoff MJ, Petrini JR (2007) Differences in mortality between late-preterm and term singleton infants in the United States, 1995-2002. J Pediatr 151(5):450–456, 456 e451

Tyson JE, Parikh NA, Langer J, Green C, Higgins RD (2008) Intensive care for extreme prematurity – moving beyond gestational age. N Engl J Med 358(16): 1672–1681

Vaucher YE, Peralta-Carcelen M, Finer NN, Carlo WA, Gantz MG, Walsh MC et al (2012) Neurodevelopmental outcomes in the early CPAP and pulse oximetry trial. N Engl J Med 367(26):2495–2504

Vohr B (2013) Long-term outcomes of moderately preterm, late preterm, and early term infants. Clin Perinatol 40(4):739–751

Vohr BR, Msall ME (1997) Neuropsychological and functional outcomes of very low birth weight infants. Semin Perinatol 21(3):202–220

Vohr BR, Garcia Coll C, Oh W (1988) Language development of low-birthweight infants at two years. Dev Med Child Neurol 30(5):608–615

Vohr BR, Garcia-Coll C, Oh W (1989) Language and neurodevelopmental outcome of low-birthweight infants at three years. Dev Med Child Neurol 31(5): 582–590

Vohr BR, Wright LL, Dusick AM, Mele L, Verter J, Steichen JJ (2000a) Neurodevelopmental and functional outcomes of extremely low birth weight infants in the National Institute of Child Health and Human Developmental Neonatal Research Network, 1993–1994. Pediatrics 105(6):1216–1226

Vohr BR, Widen JE, Cone-Wesson B, Sininger YS, Gorga MP, Folsom RC et al (2000b) Identification of neonatal hearing impairment: characteristics of infants in the neonatal intensive care unit and well-baby nursery. Ear Hear 21(5):373–382

Vohr B, Wright LL, Hack M, Aylward G, Hirtz D (2004a) Follow-up care of high-risk infants. Pediatr Suppl 114:1377–1397

Vohr BR, Wright LL, Dusick AM, Perritt R, Poole WK, Tyson JE et al (2004b) Center differences and outcomes of extremely low birth weight infants. Pediatrics 113 (4):781–789

Vohr BR, Wright LL, Poole WK, Mc Donald SA (2005a) Neurodevelopmental outcomes of extremely low birth weight infants <32 weeks' gestation between 1993 and 1998. Pediatrics 116(3):635–643

Vohr BR, Msall ME, Wilson D, Wright LL, Mc Donald S, Poole WK (2005b) Spectrum of gross motor function in extremely low birth weight children with cerebral palsy at 18 months of age. Pediatrics 116(1):123–129

Vohr BR, Stephens BE, Higgins RD, Bann CM, Hintz SR, Das A et al (2012) Are outcomes of extremely preterm infants improving? Impact of Bayley assessment on outcomes. J Pediatr 161(2):222-228.e3–222-228.e223

Vohr BR, Topol D, Watson V, St Pierre L, Tucker R (2014) The importance of language in the home for school-age children with permanent hearing loss. Acta Paediatr 103(1):62–69

Wagner RK, Torgesen JK, Rashotte CA (1999a) Comprehensive test of phonological processing. PRO-ED, Austin

Wagner RK, Torgesen JK, Rashotte CA (1999b) Test of word reading efficiency. PRO-ED, Austin

Walsh MC, Morris BH, Wrage LA, Vohr BR, Poole WK, Tyson JE et al (2005) Extremely low birthweight neonates with protracted ventilation: mortality and 18-month neurodevelopmental outcomes. J Pediatr 146(6):798–804

Ware J, Taeusch HW, Soll RF, McCormick MC (1990) Health and developmental outcomes of a surfactant controlled trial: follow-up at 2 years. Pediatrics 85(6): 1103–1107

Watson JE, Kirby RS, Kelleher KJ, Bradley RH (1996) Effects of poverty on home environment: an analysis of three-year outcome data for low birth weight premature infants. J Pediatr Psychol 21(3):419–431

Wechsler D (1989) Manual for the Wechsler preschool and primary scale of intelligence-revised. Psychological Corporation, San Antonio

Whitfield MF, Eckstein Grunau RV, Holsti L (1997) Extremely premature (≤800 g) school children: multiple areas of hidden disability. Arch Dis Child 77: F85–F90

Wilson-Costello D, Friedman H, Minich N, Fanaroff AA, Hack M (2005) Improved survival rates with increased neurodevelopmental disability for extremely low birth weight infants in the 1990s. Pediatrics 115 (4):997–1003

Wilson-Costello D, Friedman H, Minich N, Siner B, Taylor G, Schluchter M et al (2007) Improved neurodevelopmental outcomes for extremely low birth weight infants in 2000–2002. Pediatrics 119(1):37–45

Wolke D, Samara M, Bracewell M, Marlow N (2008) Specific language difficulties and school achievement in children born at 25 weeks of gestation or less. J Pediatr 152(2):256–262

Wood NS, Marlow N, Costeloe K, Gibson AT, Wilkinson AR (2000) Neurologic and developmental disability after extremely preterm birth. EPICure Study Group. N Engl J Med 343(6):378–384

Wood NS, Costeloe K, Gibson AT, Hennessy EM, Marlow N, Wilkinson AR (2005) The EPICure study: associations and antecedents of neurological and developmental disability at 30 months of age following extremely preterm birth. Arch Dis Child Fetal Neonatal Ed 90(2):F134–F140

Woodcock RW, Johnson MB (1989) Woodcock Johnson psycho-educational. Battery revised. DLM Teaching Resources, Allen

Zimmerman IL, Steiner VG, Pond RE (1992) Preschool language scale, 3rd edn. The Psychological Corporation, San Antonio

Neurological Examination of the Newborn Infant 120

Fabrizio Ferrari, Licia Lugli, Luca Ori, Elisa della Casa, Isotta Guidotti, Natascia Bertoncelli, and Laura Lucaccioni

Contents

F. Ferrari (✉)
Neonatal Intensive Care Unit, Department of Medical and Surgical Sciences of the Mother, Children and Adults, University of Modena and Reggio Emilia, Modena, Italy
e-mail: fabrizio.ferrari@unimore.it

L. Lugli · L. Ori · E. della Casa · I. Guidotti · N. Bertoncelli · L. Lucaccioni
Neonatal Intensive Care Unit, Department of Medical and Surgical Sciences of the Mother, Children and Adults, University Hospital of Modena, Modena, Italy

Abstract

A simple neurological screening examination should be performed on all term and preterm newborn infants, as part of the general medical examination. A full comprehensive neurological examination (NE) of the newborn infant should fulfill diagnostic and prognostic aims. As far as diagnosis is concerned, the NE needs

G. Buonocore et al. (eds.), *Neonatology*,
https://doi.org/10.1007/978-3-319-29489-6_267

to assess the severity of the acute (or subacute) brain dysfunction and to select those babies who may benefit from therapeutic hypothermia; the cooled newborn babies need to be assessed with serial NE during the first days after birth. As to the prognostic power of NE, repeated longitudinal assessment is needed in order to depict a developmental trajectory that better predicts the developmental outcome. The NE available for preterm and term newborn infants are discussed in relation to their peculiarities and strengths.

120.1 Salient Points

- A simple neurological screening examination should be performed on all newborn infants as part of the general medical examination.
- A full and comprehensive neurological examination should be performed to assess at-risk or sick newborn infants.
- Several schemes of examinations have been developed during the last decades to document clinical neurological signs with three major aims: to evaluate the age appropriateness of newborn neurological performances, to test the severity of the neurological dysfunction, and to predict the outcome of the infant.

120.2 Aims of the Neurological Examination and Basic Requirements

A simple neurological **screening examination** should be performed on all newborn infants as part of the general medical examination. It should consist of an assessment of state of consciousness reactivity; spontaneous motor activity; neck, trunk, and limb muscle tone and some primitive reflexes (e.g., suck and grasp). Not all experts include the Moro reflex in the general examination on the basis that it is cruel to startle a person (Volpe 2008).

A more comprehensive neurological examination is needed for assessing at-risk or sick newborn infants. Several **schemes of examinations** have been developed during the last decades to document clinical neurological signs and their evolution or their disappearance (Amiel-Tison and Grenier 1980; Brazelton 1973; Dubowitz et al. 1998a; Sarnat and Sarnat 1976). The number and type of clinical neurological signs included in the various schemes are very heterogeneous. Some more detailed schemes are designed essentially for research purposes; others are simpler clinical tools that aim to assess the integrity of the central nervous system (CNS).

Three **major aims** of the NE are stressed by the literature: first, to test whether the neurological performances of the baby are age appropriate; second, to test the severity of the neurological dysfunction and its correlation with the type and severity of the concomitant brain abnormality seen at the neuroimaging investigations; and third, to predict the outcome of the infant.

Extra questions such as the presence of an acute or a chronic brain disorder and the central or peripheral nature of the problem need also to be addressed.

All these questions cannot be all answered by one single protocol; each NE protocol, with its own peculiarities and strengths, has also limitations in it. Therefore in view of choosing the most appropriate scheme, it is crucial to know the primary aim to be pursued in the study group.

As to the first aim, i.e., age appropriateness of the neurological performances, the Dubowitz and Dubowitz scheme (Fig. 3) displays graphically posture and muscle tone as expected for the postconceptional age. Moreover the authors have provided some general guidelines on the most common findings at each gestational age.

As to the second aim, i.e., the need to assess the severity of brain dysfunction, few schemes address this issue. Still there is a lack of consensus on the items to be adopted in the presence of specific encephalopathy, and more data are needed to valid one or the other scheme. The specific schemes are mentioned later on this chapter.

As to the third aim, the prognostic value of the neurological examination, many contributions are available from the literature. All of them agree on the need of repeated longitudinal assessments that contribute to build a developmental trajectory and to provide information on the effects of intervention.

Despite advances in the care of full-term and preterm infants, it is still difficult to predict adverse neurodevelopmental outcome and subsequent disability (see also the chapter on Early Marker of Poor Outcome). The early use of structural magnetic resonance imaging (MRI), combined with neurodevelopmental assessment, leads to the early detection of brain lesions, particularly for subtle injury in the periventricular white matter and in cerebellum and to a good prediction of future motor dysfunction.

120.3 The Single Neurological Protocols in the Preterm Newborn Infant

The neurological examination of a preterm infants must be very concerned with the fragility of these babies; handling and manipulation must be minimal, and maneuvers that could stress the baby (for instance, the Moro response or the pull-to-sit maneuver) should be avoided.

There have been several reviews describing newborn or neonatal assessments, using different instruments of evaluation: Assessment of Preterm Infants' Behavior (APIB), Neonatal Intensive Care Unit Network Neurobehavioral Scale (NNNS), Test of Infant Motor Performance (TIMP), Prechtl's Assessment of General Movements (GMs), Neurobehavioral Assessment of the Preterm Infant (NAPI), Dubowitz Neurological Assessment of the Preterm and Full-Term Infant (Dubowitz), and Neuromotor Behavioral Assessment (NMBA).

The primary purposes included prediction (TIMP, GMs, Dubowitz), discrimination (all assessments), and evaluation of change (TIMP, NAPI) (See Table 1).

Properties of longitudinal neonatal neurobehavioral and neuromotor assessments for preterm infants have been systematically reviewed in a recent article by Noble et al. (Noble and Boyd 2012). In the absence of standardized criteria for neonatal neuromotor assessments, the NNNS and APIB seem to have strong psychometric qualities with better utility for research. Similarly, the GMs, TIMP, and NAPI have strong psychometric qualities but better utility for clinical settings. The GMs has also best prediction of future outcome and the TIMP has best evaluative validity (Noble and Boyd 2012).

The recognition of an acute neonatal encephalopathy in full-term (or near-term preterm) infants requires an examination specifically designed for acutely ill babies. The recognition of emotional and temperamental characteristics, as well as the response to stressors, requires the use of behaviorally oriented protocols (Brazelton 1973; Als and Brazelton 1981).

120.3.1 The Main Requisite of the Neurological Examination

The neurological examination to be used depends on the study group and the purpose of the examination. According to Prechtl, there are a few basic requirements for the neurological assessment and for its successful use in clinical practice (Cioni et al. 1997; Prechtl 1977). It should include items related to the age-specific repertoire of the CNS, which changes very rapidly during the pre- and early postnatal period.

The diagnostic procedure must be non-invasive and relatively quick to perform, as the neurological examination should be included within the routine clinical assessment and should be repeated to document the evolution of neurological abnormalities and to facilitate prognostic accuracy. One single evaluation of the infant's repertoire may be misleading.

Reliability and prognostic capability are two critical requirements. There should also be good inter-observer agreement. Multiple variables, especially clinical conditions, may be taken into account as they may reflect reactivity and well-being of the baby. This is also true for the drugs assumed by the baby such as analgesic, antiepileptic, vasoactive, caffeine, and corticosteroids that, among the others, may have an influence on the neurobehavior of the infants.

This chapter describes the different approaches to the neurological examination of the newborn

Table 1 Characteristics of the different newborn and neonatal assessments (Table from Noble and Boyd 2012)

Assessment tool	Age range (min weeks PMA: max post-term)	Primary purposes	Expanded purpose	Subsystems/components tested	Type of test	Normative sample
APIB	28 weeks–1 month	Discriminative	Documents spectrum of preterm and term infants' neurobehavioral functioning/ competence	Autonomic, motor, state, attention/interaction, self-regulation	Criterion	n/a
Dubowitz	30 weeks–4 months	Discriminative/ predictive	Provides a detailed profile of neurological status and identifies infants with neurological abnormalities	Posture and tone, reflexes, movements, neurobehavioral responses	Criterion/ norm	224 low-risk term infants, 37–42 weeks gestation only (optimality score), from UK
GMs	Preterm–4 months	Discriminative/ predictive	Documents spontaneous movements to identify early CNS dysfunction	Movement patterns	Criterion	n/a
NAPI	32 weeks–term	Discriminative/ evaluative	Measures the progression of neurobehavioral performance	Motor development and vigor, scarf sign, popliteal angle, attention / orientation,% asleep, irritability, vigor of cry	Criterion/ norm	521 infants from 32–37 weeks gestation from USA
NBAS	36 weeks–6 weeks post-term	Discriminative/ Predictive	Identifies full range of individual neurobehavioral functioning and identifies areas of difficulty	Autonomic, motor and reflexes, state, social/attention	Criterion	n/a
NMBA	30–36 weeks	Discriminative	Identifies preterm infants developmentally at risk	Neurological (e.g., tone, reflexes), behavioral, autonomic, motor functions	Criterion	n/a
NNNS	30 weeks–4 months (46/48 weeks post-term)	Discriminative	Assesses at-risk infants (particularly substance exposed), documenting neurological integrity and broad range of behavioral functioning	Neurological (tone, reflexes), behavioral, stress/abstinence items	Criterion/ norm	125 term infants (38–41 weeks gestation) from USA
TIMP	32 weeks-4 months	Discriminative/ evaluative/ predictive	Evaluates motor control and organization of posture and movement for functional activities	Orientation head in space, response to auditory and visual stimuli, body alignment, limb movements	Criterion/ norm	990 infants at risk of poor neurological outcome from 11 geographic locations across the USA

infant and neurological protocols that best fulfill the above criteria.

120.4 Available Neurological Examinations

Because each method represented an improved approach to understanding the neonatal nervous system, the methods will be considered according to the chronological order they were elaborated. Few studies have compared the different protocols, and it cannot be claimed that one is better than another. The French school (André Thomas and Saint-Anne Dargassies, Amiel-Tison) highlighted spontaneous posture, some neonatal reflexes, and various aspects of muscle tone. Active tone considers "fonctions de redressement" and is associated with spontaneous movements. Passive tone is the capacity of muscle to be lengthened when the joints are moved passively and the tone that can be seen by allowing the extremity to swing at each joint. Saint-Anne Dargassies described the ontogenesis of muscle tone in premature infants, outlining the progressive maturation of muscle tone, with development of flexor predominance in caudal-cephalic direction (Brazelton 1973; Saint-Anne Dargassies 1955).

The Amiel-Tison neurologic assessment at term (ATNAT) has recently been updated for clinical application. The complete procedure takes a few minutes. A simple 0, 1, and 2 scoring system is proposed. The ATNAT is part of a set of three different instruments based on a neuro-maturative framework. By sharing a similar methodology and scoring system, the use of these three assessments allows for the follow-up of high-risk children from 32 weeks postconception to 6 years of age (Brazelton 1973; Gosselin et al. 2005).

Prechtl and co-workers (Gosselin et al. 2005; Cioni et al. 1989) developed a comprehensive examination, based on the assessment of spontaneous and elicited responses. They studied the various neurological responses of normal healthy term infants and documented any abnormality in the responses. They analyzed and documented trunk and limb posture, spontaneous movements of the various parts of the body and of the eyes, the power and the resistance to passive movements, involuntary activities such as skin color and respiration, skin reflexes (abdominal, cremasteric, anal reflex), osteo-tendon reflexes, evoked responses such as palmar and plantar reflex, Babinski, Moro, tonic neck asymmetric reflex, rooting, sucking, placing, Bauer reflex, crawling, automatic stepping, abnormal movements (athetoid, tremors), and crying. Each single response and behavior was evaluated in its optimal state. They demonstrated the dependency of these patterns on an infant's behavioral state. When the behavioral state was considered, normal infants responded consistently to the elicited stimuli. Non-responsiveness, despite being in the right behavioral state, was considered an abnormal neurological sign (Prechtl 1974, 1990; Prechtl and Dijkstra 1960).

120.4.1 Behavioral State

Recognition of behavioral states was a major advance in the field of neonatal neurology. Behavioral states are an expression of the complexity of the nervous system; they are relatively stable over time (ranging from a few minutes to half an hour or more) and occur in particular sequential patterns. They are recognized on the basis of three to four essential physiological parameters (respiration, eyes open or closed, eye movements, body movements) that remain stable over time for at least a few minutes. Prechtl identified two states of sleep (state 1 or quiet sleep, state 2 or active sleep) and three states of wakefulness (state 3 or quiet wakefulness, state 4 or active wakefulness, state 5 or crying) (Prechtl 1974). Evoked reflexes and responses as well as spontaneous activity (such as body and eye movement and respiratory patterns) change according to the behavioral states.

The Groningen school showed that two sleep states are recognizable from the 36th week of gestation, while before 34 weeks' gestation, indeterminate sleep is predominant. Before 28 weeks, the newborn states of wakefulness and sleep are difficult to distinguish (Prechtl 1974).

The recognition of different behavioral states is fundamental for the diagnosis of neurological integrity in the newborn. One of the earliest and most sensitive sign of cerebral dysfunction is the disorganization of the behavioral states. Such disorganization of states can be a loose state cycle, a qualitative alteration of a single state or a physiological parameter defining states or the presence of an unstable sleep pattern (Prechtl 1974; Prechtl and Dijkstra 1960).

A useful and major innovation by Prechtl was the clustering of neurological signs into diagnostic syndromes. Using the computerized analysis of individual neurological deviations, he recognized four main syndromes: the hyper-excitable syndrome with increased responsiveness to various stimuli, the apathetic syndrome with decreased responsiveness, the hemi-syndrome with asymmetry of response, and the comatose syndrome (Prechtl and Dijkstra 1960; Prechtl 1990).

Up to this point, the Prechtl examination was the most detailed and comprehensive examination: it gave reliable information about the newborn infant neurological status and was able to differentiate central from peripheral involvement. The shortcomings of the Prechtl examination are the long time to perform the examination (about 30 min) and its complexity: a fairly large number of items are explored and each has to be observed in its optimal state. Furthermore, it is restricted to the full-term infant in good physical health, because the degree of handling required may be unsuitable for the ill and fragile baby (Prechtl 1977).

Prechtl also developed a shorter version of the protocol, suitable for neurological screening. It includes evaluation of head, trunk, and limb posture; eye coordination; normal and abnormal limb movements; head, trunk, and limb resistance to passive movement; traction test and the Moro response. The neurological screening examination cannot replace a full neurological examination: it gives more false-positive results and, if abnormalities are suspected, a full examination is required. The short version of Prechtl examination is illustrated in Fig. 1.

Brazelton (Dubowitz et al. 1998a) developed the Neonatal Behavioral Assessment Scale (NBAS), a structured scheme for term infants which combined 27 items of behavior and 20 reflex items derived from the neurological examination by Prechtl. The behavioral and neurological items can be grouped into seven major clusters of items (Fig. 2). The NBAS was designed to score the babies' behavioral repertoire and to document the organized responses to various environmental events. It was not originally conceived as a neurological examination but as a tool to evaluate the behavioral characteristics of the single baby. The intention was to predict temperament and emotional control, allowing the parents to perceive the baby as a person from the very first. The author suggested performing the test in front of the mother who would then recognize how bright and talented her baby was. In this context, the Brazelton scale aims to reinforce early mother-infant interaction. It has also the power to evaluate cultural and ethnic differences in neonatal behavior in different settings. Despite this premise, the examination has often been used as a neurological evaluation. The Brazelton test had a great impact on pediatricians: its major contribution was toward abandoning the idea of the newborn infant as incompetent, immature, and disorganized. Attention was drawn to the amazing capacities of the newborn infant for attention, with very predictable behaviors and the capacity to respond and interact with the environment. Attention was drawn to the baby's sensory capacities and visual and auditory responses: visual orientation to an inanimate stimulus (a red ball) and to the human face and auditory orientation to the sound of a rattle, bell, and the human voice were introduced as integral part of the assessment. Some of these items were later adopted in other neurological schemes (Dubowitz et al. 1998a).

Based on the NBAS of Brazelton's assessment of term infant, Als et al. (1982) developed the Assessment of Preterm Infant Behavior (APIB). This is a strategy to document systematically behavioral ingredients of the premature infant, from the stage when the baby can first be handled in room temperature and room air, without technological aids, to the stage when the infant's attention span is relatively independent from other subsystems and the baby can use it to regulate and control investigation of the environment, i.e., by approximately 1-month post-term for a healthy,

Name ________________ Date of birth ________________ Gestational age ________________

Date of examination ________________ Gestational age at examination ________________

Behavioral state:

	Posture(head in the midline)		
Superior limbs	Semi-flexion	Flexion	Extension
Inferior limbs	Semi-flexion	Flexion	Extension
Symmetrical posture	Yes		No
Opisthotonus	Yes		No
Frog posture	Yes		No
Head turned to one side	Yes		No
	Eyes		
In the middle	Yes		No
Constant deviation to one side	Yes		No
Constant strabismus	Yes		No
	Spontaneous movements		
Arm and leg alternative movements	Yes		No
Symmetrical movements	Yes		No
Normal strength and length movements	Yes		No
Tremor	Yes		No
Exaggerated fast movements	Yes		No
Starties	Yes		No
Seizures	Yes		No
	Resistance to passive mobilisation (passive tone)		
Neck	Scarce	Normal	High
Trunk	Scarce	Normal	High
Arms	Scarce	Normal	High
Arms	Symmetrical	Asymmetrical	Right/Left
Legs	Scarce	Normal	High
Legs	Symmetrical	Asymmetrical	Right/Left
	Traction test		
Arm resistance	Scarce	Normal	High
Head control	Less than 3 sec	3-10 sec	More than 10 sec
Sucking	Absent	Weak	Present and strong
	Moro reflex		
Abduction and extensions	Yes		No
Flexion absent, only abduction	Yes		No
Asymmetrical	Yes		No
Tremor	Yes		No
Diagnosis	Normal	Suspect	Abnormal

Fig. 1 Prechtl screening neurological examination

full-term infant (Als and Brazelton 1981; Als et al. 2005). The assessment is used as a starting point to plan individualized and family-focused intervention strategies. The Neonatal Individualized Developmental Care Assessment Program (NIDCAP) is at present the most comprehensive and advanced method to promote individualized developmental supportive and family-centered care in neonatal intensive care units (Als et al. 1982, 2005).

Dubowitz and Dubowitz (Dubowitz et al. 1998b) and Dubowitz et al. (Sarnat and Sarnat 1976; Dubowitz and Dubowitz 1981) developed an examination that included the assessment of

Name ------------------------- Date of birth ----------------- Gestational Age -----------------
Weight --------------------- Length --------------------- Head circumference ------------------
Date -------------------------- Examiner ---

INFANT BEHAVIOUR										
HABITUATION	9	8	7	6	5	4	3	2	1	Commet
Response Dec.-Light										
Response Dec.-Rattle										
Response Dec.-Bell										
Response Dec.-Foot										
SOCIAL-INTERACTIVE	9	8	7	6	5	4	3	2	1	
Animate Visual										
Animate Visual+Auditory										
Inanimate Visual										
Inanimate Visual+Auditory										
Animate Auditory										
Inanimate Auditory										
Alertness										
MOTOR SYSTEM	9	8	7	6	5	4	3	2	1	
General Tone										
Motor Maturity										
Pull to sit										
Defensive										
Activity Level										
STATE ORGANIZATION	9	8	7	6	5	4	3	2	1	
Peak of Excitement										
Rapidity of Build-up										
Irritability										
Lability of States										
STATE REGULATION	9	8	7	6	5	4	3	2	1	
Cuddliness										
Consolability										
Self-Quieting										
Hand to Mouth										
AUTONOMIC SYSTEM	9	8	7	6	5	4	3	2	1	
Tremoulousness										
Starties										
Lability of Skin Color										
SMILES										

Fig. 2 NBAS scoring form

neurological and behavioral items, taking into account behavioral states (Sarnat and Sarnat 1976; Dubowitz et al. 1998b; Dubowitz and Dubowitz 1981). The authors stated that "ideally, a meaningful neurological assessment should be part of the routine clinical examination of every newborn infant." One of the strengths of this examination is that it is suitable for preterm infants as well as for full-term infants and for both ill and healthy infants. It is a simple, objective recording system, based on drawings and diagrams, recorded on a pro forma that includes definitions. The diagrams are easy to tick and are suitable for staff with no particular expertise or experience in neonatal neurology. The examination does not take more than 15 min to perform and can be used as part of the routine clinical assessment of newborn infant. It is also suitable for repeated examinations. It is therefore possible to document the normal or abnormal evolution of neurological behavior in the preterm infant after birth, to compare this behavior with that expected in newborn infants of corresponding postmenstrual age, and to detect features of a neonatal encephalopathy. The examination includes assessment of behavioral states, tone, and primitive reflexes and also motility and some aspects of behavior. One advantage of this method has been the development of an optimality score that allows quantification of the deviant scores and use in different settings.

Another advantage is that authors have updated the examination and have provided some general guidelines on the most common findings at each gestational age (Fig. 3). The examination has been validated in full-term and preterm

Hammersmith Neonatal Neurological Examination CODE ________ D.O.E. ________

NAME ______________________ SEX ___ RACE _____ D.O.B. ______ AGE _____ G.A. ______ BW _____

Posture and tone

						STATE	ASYMM
POSTURE Infant supine_ Look mainly at position of legs but also note arms. *Score predominant posture.*	arms & legs extended or very slightly flexed	Legs slightly flexed	legs well flexed but not adducted	legs well flexed & adducted near abdomen	abnormal posture: a) opisthotonus b) marked leg extension, strong arm flexion		
ARM RECOIL Take both hands, quickly extend arms parallel to the body, Count to three. Release, Repeat 3 times.	arms do not flex	arms flex slowly. not always not completely	arms flex slowly, more completely	arms flex quickly and completely	arms difficult to extend: snap back forcefully		
ARM TRACTION Hold wrist and pull arm upwards. Note flexion at elbow and resistance while shoulder lifts off table. *Test each side separately.*	arms remain straight: no resistance felt R L	arms flex slightly or some resistance felt R L	arms flex well till shoulder lifts, then straighten R L	arms flex at approx 100° & maintained as shoulder lifts R L	flexion of arms <100°: maintained when body lifts up R L		
LEG RECOIL Take *both* anides in one hand, flex hips + knees. Quickly extend. Release Repeat 3 times.	No flexion	incomplete or variable flexion	complete but slow flexion	complete fast flexion	legs difficult to extend; snap back forcefully		
LEG TRACTION Grasp ankie and slowly pull leg upwards. Note flexion at knees and resistance as buttocks lift/ *Test each side separately.*	legs straight - no resistance felt R L	legs flex slightly or some resistance felt R L	legs flex well till bottom lifts up R L	knee flexes remains flexed when bottom up R L	flexion stays when back+bottom up R L		
POPLITEAL ANGLE Fix knee on abdomen, extend leg by gentle, pressure with index finger behind the ankle. Note angle at knee. *Test each side separately.*	180° R L	−150° R L	−110° R L	−90° R L	<90° R L		
HEAD CONTROL(1) ***(extensor tone)*** Infant setting upright. Encircle chest with both hands holding shoulders. Let head drop forward.	no attempt to raise head	infant tries: effort better felt than seen	raises head but drops forward or back	raises head: remains vertical; it may wobble			
HEAD CONTROL (2) ***(flexor tone)*** Infant sitting upright. Encircle chest with both hands holding shoulders. Let head drop backward.	no attempt to raise head	infant tries; effort better felt than seen	raises head but drops forward or back	raises head: remains vertical; it may wobble	head upright or extended; cannot be passively flexed		
HEAD LAG Pull infant towards sitting posture by traction on both wrists & support head slightly. Also note arm flexion.	head drops & stays back	tries to lift head but it drops back	able so lift head slightly	lifts head in line with body	head in front of body		
VENTRAL SUSPENSION Hold infant in ventral suspension, Oberve back, flexion of limbs and relation of head to trunk. If it looks different, DRAW.	back curved, head & limbs hang straight	back curved, head ↓ limbs Slightly flexed	back slightly curved, limbs flexed	back straight, head in line, limbs flexed	back straight, head above body		

Fig. 3 (continued)

Tone patterns

FLEXOR TONE(1) **(on traction: arm versus leg)** Compare scores of arm traction with leg traction.		score for arm flexion less than leg flexion	score for arm flexion equal to leg flexion	score for arm flexion more than leg flexion but difference 1 column or less	score for arm flexion more than leg flexion but difference more than 1 column		
FLEXOR TONE(2) **(arm versus leg)** Posture in supine.			arms and legs flexed	strong arm flexion with strong leg extension *intermittent*	strong arm flexion with strong leg extension *continuous*		
LEG EXTENSOR TONE Compare scores of leg traction and popliteal angle.		score for leg traction more than score for popliteal angle	score for leg traction equal to score for popliteal angle	score for leg traction less than score for popliteal angle, by 1 column only	score for leg traction less than score for popliteal angle, by more than 1 column		
NECK EXTENSOR TONE (SITTING) Compare scores of head control 1 and 2.		score for head extension less than head flexion	score for head extension equal to head flexion	score for head extension more than head flexion. but difference 1 column or less	score for head extension more than head flexion but difference more than 1 column		
INCREASED ENTENSOR TONE (HORIZONTAL) Compare scores of head lag and ventral suspension.		score for ventral suspension less than head lag	score for ventral suspension equal to head lag	score for ventral suspension more than head lag but difference 1 column or less	score for ventral suspension more than head lag but difference more than 1 column		

Reflexes

TENDON REFLEX Test biceps, knee, and ankle jerks.	absent	felt, not seen	seen	"exaggerated" (very brisk)	clonus		
SUCK / GAG Little finger into mouth with pulp of finger upwards.	no gag/ no suck	weak irregular suck only No stripping	weak regular suck Some stripping	strong suck: (a) irregular (b) regular Good stripping	no suck but strong clenching		
PALMAR GRASP Put index finger into the hand and gently press palmar surface. Do not touch dorsal surface. *Test each side separately.*	no response R L	short weak flexion of fingers R L	strong flexion of fingers R L	strong finger flexion shoulder 1 R L	very strong grasp: infant can be lifted off couch R L		
PLANTAR GRASP Press thumb on the sole below the toes. *Test each side separately.*	no response R L	partial plantar flexion of toes R L	toes curve around the examiner's finger R L				
PLACING Lift infant in an upright position and stroke the dorsum of the foot against a protruding edge of a flat surface. *Test each side separately.*	no response R L	dorsiflexion of ankle only R L	full placing response with flexion of hip and knee & placing sole on surface R L				
MORO REFLEX One hand supports infant's head in midline, the other the back. Raise infant to 45° and when infant is relaxed let head fall through 10°. Note if jerky. Repeat 3 times.	no response, or opening of hands only	full abduction at shoulder and extension of the arms: no adduction 	full abduction, but only delayed or partial adduction 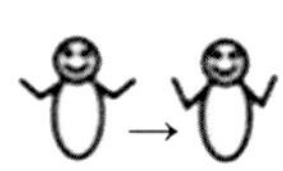	partial abduction at shoulder,and extension of arms followed by smooth adduction 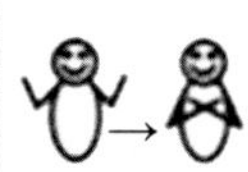	• minimal abduction or adduction • no abduction or adduction; only forward extension of arms • marked adduction only 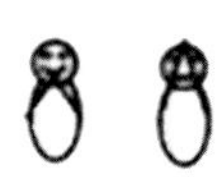 or		

Fig. 3 (continued)

Movements

SPONTANEOUS MOVEMENT (quantity) Watch infant lying supine.	no movement	sporadic and short isolated movements	frequent isolated movements	frequent generalized movements	continuous exaggerated movements
SPONTANEOUS MOVEMENT (quantity) Watch infant lying supine.	only stretches	stretches and random abrupt movements; some smooth movements	fluent movements but monotonous	fluent alternating movements of arms + legs; good variability	• cramped, synchronized • mouthing • jerky or other abnormal movements
HEAD RAISING PRONE Infant in prone, head in midline.	no response	infant rolls head over, chin not raised	infant raises cin, rolls head over	infant brings head and chin up	infant brings head up and keeps it up

Abnormal signs/patterns

ABNORMAL HAND OR TOE POSTURES		hands open, toes straight most of the time	intermittent fisting or thumb adduction	continuous fisting or thumb adduction; index finger flexion, thumb opposition	continuous big toe extension or flexion of all toes
TREMOR		no tremor, or tremor only when crying or only after sudden noise	tremor occasionally when awake	frequent tremors when awake	continuous tremors
STARTLE	no startle even to sudden noise	no spontaneous startle but reacts to sudden noise	2-3 spontaneous starties	more than 3 spontaneous starties	continuous starties

Orientation and behaviour

EYE APPEARANCES	does not open eyes		full conjugated eye movements	*transient* • nystagmus • strabismus • reving eye movements • sunset sign	*presistent* • nystagmus • strabismus • reving eye movements abnormal pupils
AUDITORY ORIENTATION Infant awake. Wrap infatn, Hold rattle 10 to 15 cm from ear.	no reaction	auditory startie; brightens and stills; no true orientation	shifting of eyes head might turn towards source	prolonged head turn to stimulus; search with eyes; smooth	turns head (jerkly, abruptly) & eyes towards noise every time
VISUAL ORIENTATION Wrap infant, wake up with rattle if needed or rock gently. Note if baby can see and follow red ball (B) or target (T).	does not follow or focus on stimuli B T	stills, focuses, follows briefly to the side but loses stimuli B T	follows horizontally and vertically; no head turn B T	follows horizontally and vertically; turns head B T	follows in a circle B T
ALERTNESS *Tested as response to visual stimuli (B or T).*	will not respond to stimuli	when awake, looks only briefly	when awake, looks at stimuli but loses them	keeps interest in stimuli	does not tire (hyper-reactive)
IRRITABILITY In response to stimuli.	quiet all the time, not irritable to any stimuli	awakes, cries sometimes when handled	cries often when handled	cries always when handled	cries even when not handled
CONSOLABILITY Ease to quiet infant.	not crying; consoling not needed	cries briefly; consoling not needed	cries; becomes quiet when talked to	cries; needs picking up to be consoled	cries; cannot be consoled
CRY	no cry at all	whimpering cry only	cries to stimuli but normal pitch		High-pitched cry; often continuous

SUMMARY OF EXAMINATION:

HEAD AND TRUNK TONE: LIMB TONE:

MOTILITY: REFLEXES:

ORIENTATION AND ALERTNESS: IRRITABILITY:

CONSOLABILITY: LIST DEVIANT SIGNS:

Fig. 3 Hammersmith Neurological examination. Reproduced from (Dubowitz et al. 1998a) with permission infants (Sarnat and Sarnat 1976; Dubowitz and Dubowitz 1981).

120.5 Spontaneous Movement Patterns and General Movements

The general movements (GMs) method was the last scheme of assessment of the nervous system to be standardized and validated. It was conceived by Prechtl and co-workers during the late 1980s (Cioni et al. 1989; Ferrari et al. 1990; Roodenburg et al. 1991; Prechtl and Hopkins 1986). It is based on the observation of spontaneous movements of the fetus and of the newborn infant, either preterm or full-term. Since the 1970s, Prechtl and co-worker had focused their attention on the spontaneous movements of the fetus observed using ultrasound scans: they recognized that spontaneous movements could be distinguished as movements clearly constant in form and therefore easily recognizable. Prechtl defined these sequences as "movement patterns." With the aid of ultrasound, he was able to recognize several fetal movements patterns such as startles, GMs, isolated limb movements, twitches, stretches, breathing movements, hiccups, yawns, head rotations, head flexion, sucking, swallowing, and others (Roodenburg et al. 1991). They emerge as early as 9–12 weeks postmenstrual age (Table 1). It is striking that they look complex and differentiated from their first appearance. They hardly show any change in form in the first weeks after birth, despite the profound changes in the environmental conditions; thus, an intrauterine or extrauterine environment seems to influence them very little. Two of these movement patterns (stretches and yawns) are maintained throughout life without changing form. Surprisingly, local and isolated movements of the limbs appear 1–2 weeks sooner than GMs. They continue to be present during the whole preterm period and are seen until the age of 5–6 months post-term. The immature nervous system of the fetus generates these movement patterns without being stimulated: they are generated endogenously and reflect spontaneous activity of the brain (Table 2).

The chance to observe, record and eventually measure endogenously generated brain activity is one of the dreams of neurobiologists. Prechtl's idea was that spontaneous movements were markers of brain impairment and dysfunction (Prechtl 1990).

It is likely that GMs are produced by complex nervous networks, the so-called central pattern generators (CPG) that are located in different parts of the brain and at different brain levels, especially in the higher parts of medulla and the brain stem. Breathing, sucking, chewing, eye

Table 2 Fetal motor repertoire age is given in postmenstrual age. Reproduced from Roodenburg et al. (1991), with permission

10 weeks	12 weeks	14 weeks	20 weeks
Startles	Startles	Startles	Startles
GMs	GMs	GMs	GMs
Isolated arm movements	Isolated arm movements	Isolated arm movements	Isolated arm movements
Isolated leg movements	Isolated leg movements	Isolated leg movements	Isolated leg movements
Hiccup	Hiccup	Hiccup	Hiccup
	Breathing movements	Breathing movements	Breathing movements
	Hand-face	Hand-face	Hand-face
	Head retroflexion	Head retroflexion	Head retroflexion
	Head anteflexion	Head anteflexion	Head anteflexion
	Head rotation	Head rotation	Head rotation
	Stretch	Stretch	Stretch
	Yawn	Yawn	Yawn
		Sucking and swallowing	Sucking and swallowing
			Eye movements

movements, swimming, crawling, and walking are other spontaneous motor activities that appear to be endogenously generated, i.e., generated without any recognizable external stimulus. The combination of these motor activities varies depending on the ongoing behavioral state. During state 2 (irregular breathing), slow and rapid eyes movements and body movements are fired by CPG (termed "active" or "agitated" sleep). During state 1 (quiet sleep), there is regular breathing with no eye and no body movements, reflecting the different neural mechanisms that actively inhibit (or modulate in the case of respiration) these motor activities from higher cortical and subcortical structures. GMs as well as the other movement patterns are typical of states 2, 4, and 5. Startling, which appears in state 1, is an exception (Ferrari et al. 1990; Prechtl and Hopkins 1986).

120.6 What Are General Movements?

General movements (GMs) consist of movements that involve the whole body in a variable sequence of arm, leg, neck, and trunk movements. They wax and wane in intensity, force, and speed, with a gradual beginning and end. Rotation along the axis of the limbs and continuous changes in the direction of movement make them fluent and elegant and create an impression of complexity and variability. Minor changes can be seen during early development: preterm, GMs are of large amplitude and often accompanied by lifting of the pelvis; at term, GMs are smaller in amplitude and show a writhing character that gradually disappears; at 6–9 weeks post-term, fidgety GMs start to appear (Cioni et al. 1989; Einspieler et al. 2004).

GMs are the most frequent of the various movement patterns exhibited by newborn babies and also the most complex. It is likely that their complexity makes them vulnerable to brain dysfunction and therefore a sensitive indicator of brain injury.

Brain lesions affect the quality rather than the quantity of GMs. The only exception to this rule is that severe perinatal asphyxia is accompanied by a transient phase of hypokinesia. Other brain lesions are associated with preterm and writhing GMs changing in character with loss of fluency, variability, and complexity, with a poor repertoire and becoming cramped synchronized or chaotic. Abnormal fidgety GMs may be either exaggerated or absent (Einspieler et al. 2004; De Vries and Cowan 2009).

Poor repertoire GMs are the most common abnormality, and variability in sequence is lost or poor. When abnormal GMs are followed by normal fidgety movements, recovery from brain lesions and a normal outcome are expected. However, absence of fidgety movements is likely to herald cerebral palsy (Ferrari et al. 2002). Cramped synchronized GMs also represent a severe GM abnormality and are recognized when all limbs and trunks muscle contract and relax almost simultaneously (Fig. 4) (De Vries and Cowan 2009). If this abnormal character of GMs persists for weeks and is accompanied and/or followed by no fidgety movements, the development of a spastic form of cerebral palsy is predictable (Fig. 5) (Einspieler et al. 2004; De Vries and Cowan 2009; Ferrari et al. 2002).

120.7 The Neurological Examination in the Sick Newborn Infant

Sick infants should have a daily neurological examination. This should be with minimal handling if there is cardiorespiratory instability. The neurological examination is hampered by long lines, monitoring, and sedation, in which case the examination may be curtailed to a few items that can be assessed reasonably quickly. The baby's level of consciousness should be assessed. The general use of cerebral ultrasound and MRI scans enables documentation of the presence, evolution, and severity of brain lesions.

Neuroprotective strategies such as brain cooling require the recognition of a severe neonatal encephalopathy (NE) soon after birth. A neurological scheme for assessing the severity and evolution of acute brain dysfunction is described in Fig. 6. It is based on nine items, mostly requiring observation of spontaneous

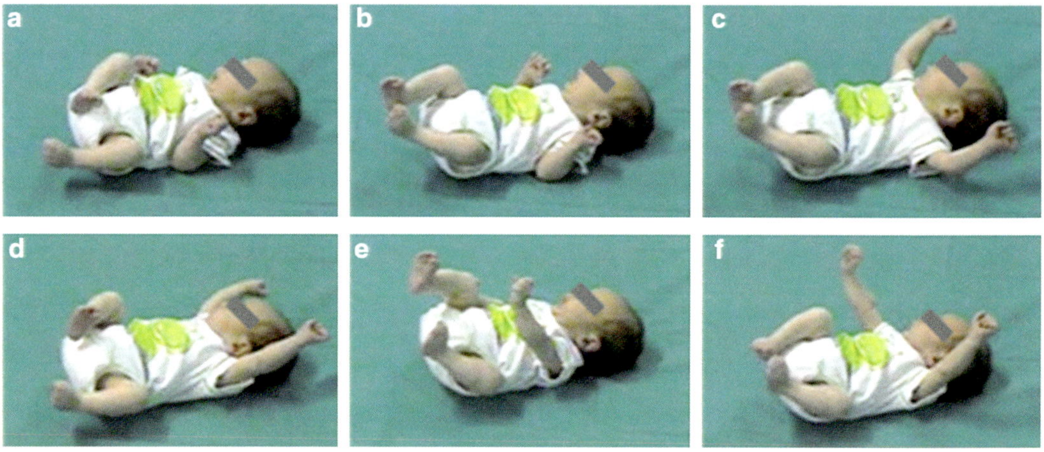

Fig. 4 A cramped synchronized GMs: the six pictures show synchronous lifting of the four limbs in sequence, followed by extension and adduction

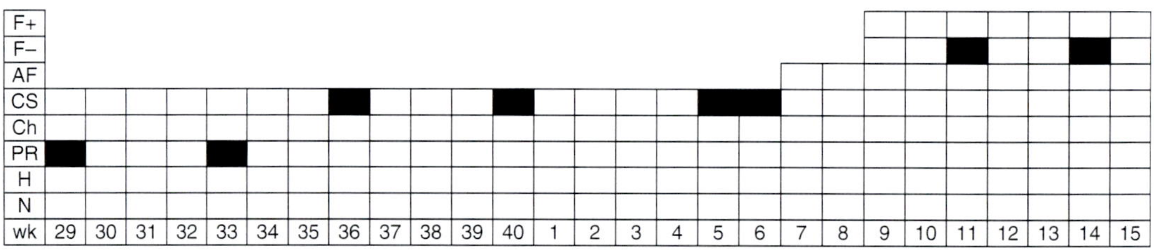

Fig. 5 Individual developmental trajectory. Trajectory of a preterm infant, born at 27 weeks postmenstrual age. PR GMs in the preterm age and CS at term and early post-term age are followed by absent fidgety movements and subsequent cerebral palsy. Poor repertoire (*PR*), cramped synchronized (*CS*), hypokinesia (*H*), chaotic movements (*Ch*), abnormal fidgety movements (*AF*), fidgety movements (*F*), absent fidgety (*F–*)

movements. It includes assessing the level of consciousness (motor response to pinch of the skin of the leg, pupillary size, and reaction to light); respiration; posture, spontaneous general movements and eye movements; brain stem reflexes (corneal and oculocephalic); resistance of the trunk, neck, and limbs to passive movement; and abnormal movements (seizures and/or limb automatisms, such brain stem release phenomena, BSRP).

120.8 Hypoxic Ischemic Events and NE in the Full-Term Infant

NE is a clinical syndrome of disturbed neurological function. It is manifested by difficulty in the initiation and maintenance of respiration, depression of tone and reflexes, abnormal level of consciousness, and often seizures (Levene et al. 1985). NE may be caused by perinatal asphyxia, as well as other conditions such as stroke, infection, mitochondrial disease, brain malformation, and metabolic disorders.

Volpe has provided an accurate description of the development of NE due to perinatal asphyxia (HIE) in full-term infants (Volpe 2008). From birth to 12 h, severely affected infants are stuporose or comatose (i.e., not arousable and with minimal or no response to sensation) and have periodic breathing or respiratory irregularity, intact pupillary responses, and spontaneous eye movements. Infants are hypotonic and have minimal spontaneous or elicited movements, and hypokinesia is common. Very few babies show signs of brain stem injury, such as pupils that are

Name .... Date of birth .... Gestational age ....
Number of the assessment .... Date .... Hours/days of life ....
Examiner ....

N	ITEMS	SCORE 0	SCORE 1	SCORE 2
1	**Respiration**	Normal	Ataxic/periodic Polipnea Apneas	Absent
2	**Posture**	Variable	No variable posture Exaggerated flexion/extension	Decerebrated/decorticated Stiff in flexion Flat on the mattress
3	**General Movements**	Present	Hypokinesis/poor repertoire GMs	Absent/cramped synchronized/chaotic GMs
4	**Eye movements**	Present	Rare	Absent/eye deviation
5	**Resistance to passive movs:**			
	Neck	Normal	Poor/exaggerated	Severely reduced/increased
	Trunk	Normal	Poor/exaggerated	Severely reduced/increased
	Limbs	Normal	Poor/exaggerated	Severely reduced/increased
6	**Motor response to pain**	Present	Reduced	Absent
7	**Pupils**	Normal	Mydriasis or myosis, reactive to light	No response to light
8	**Brainstem reflexes:**			
	Sucking	Present	Poor	Absent
	Corneal	Present	Poor	Absent
	Oculocephalic	Present	Poor	Absent
9	**Seizures** (clonic jerks, tonic, subtle) **or motor automatisms** (rowing, pedalling)	Absent	Isolated	Frequent

Annotations: ....

Fig. 6 Neurological assessment of the sick newborn infant

fixed and in the midposition and dilated, and eye movements, which are fixed when the doll's eye maneuver is performed.

50–60% of NE infants who ultimately convulse have seizures, which are mostly subtle, by 6–12 h after birth. By 12–24 h, the infant's level of consciousness may appear to improve, and there are severe seizures with overt status epilepticus, apneic spells, jitteriness, and weakness in a hip-shoulder distribution. Babies with basal ganglia (BG) injury may have spontaneous or evoked hypertonus. Between 24 and 72 h, the baby with NE may be in deep stupor or coma, with irregular ataxic respirations (and even respiratory arrest) and brain stem oculomotor and papillary disturbances (i.e., constricted hyporeactive pupils, fixed to light dilated pupils) (Volpe 2008).

Sarnat and Sarnat in 1976 (Noble and Boyd 2012) developed a clinical grading system for the severity and the progression of the neurological signs in HIE. Stage 1 lasted less than 24 h, characterized by hyperalertness, uninhibited Moro and stretch reflexes, sympathetic effects, and a normal electroencephalogram. Stage 2 is characterized by obtundation, hypotonia, strong distal flexion, and multifocal seizures. The electroencephalogram (EEG) shows a periodic pattern, sometimes preceded by continuous delta activity. Infants in stage 3 are stuporous and flaccid, with suppressed brain stem and autonomic functions. The EEG is isoelectric or with infrequent periodic discharges. Amiel-Tison (1978), Finer (Finer et al. 1981), Fenichel (1983), Levene (Levene et al. 1985), and others developed alternative scoring systems along similar lines.

Clinical encephalopathy has been examined over the past three decades as an early predictor of neurologic and developmental outcome. The Sarnat evaluation correlates with subsequent neurodevelopmental impairment in infancy and childhood and other scoring systems adapted from the Sarnat evaluation are also used to predict outcome (Thompson et al. 1997; Miller et al. 2004).

Hypothermia to a target temperature of 33–34 °C for 72 h has currently been shown to reduce death or disability at 18 months or increase the rate of survivors without disabilities.

Table 3 reports the main trials that have all included moderate/severe stage of encephalopathy as eligibility criteria at study random assignment at <6 h of age with three trials having the additional criteria for abnormal amplitude integrated electroencephalography. Main trials have established a relationship between the stage of hypoxic-ischemic encephalopathy (HIE) at <6 h of life and early childhood outcome (Jacobs et al. 2011; Simbruner et al. 2010; Shankaran et al. 2005; Eicher et al. 2005a; Eicher et al. 2005b; Azzopardi et al. 2009; Gluckman et al. 2005; Zhou et al. 2010).

The National Institute of Child Health and Human Development (NICHD) Neonatal Research Network (NRN) randomized controlled trial (RCT) data of serial neurologic examinations provided an opportunity to examine the evolution of encephalopathy as a clinical biomarker and its relationship with outcome. Neurologic examinations over the first few days may serve as a marker of brain injury after hypoxia-ischemia as well as response to treatment. Stage of encephalopathy was evaluated at <6 h of age, during study intervention, and at discharge among 204 participants in the NICHD-NRN-RCT of whole-body hypothermia for HIE. HIE was examined as a predictor of outcome by regression models. On serial neurologic examinations, improvement in stage of HIE was associated with cooling. Persistence of severe HIE at 72 h and an abnormal neurologic exam at discharge were associated with a greater risk of death or disability (Shankaran et al. 2012a).

Recent MRI studies have demonstrated that in acute severe global hypoxic ischemia, the basal ganglia (BG) and thalami (T) are mainly affected. Lesions in these areas are often associated with abnormal signal intensity in the posterior limb of the internal capsule (PLIC). Concomitant injury to the cortex (C) of the central sulcus and the adjacent subcortical white matter (WM) is common. In severe cases, the brain stem may also be involved. When the predominant lesion involves WM and cortex but spares the BGT and PLIC, the likely cause is prolonged partial hypoxia-ischemia (Volpe 2008; Ferrari et al. 1990; De Vries and Cowan 2009). The clinical correlates of these lesions during the first hours of life are not known. Future studies based on early diffusion-weighted imaging and early serial neurological examinations may provide an answer. Some signs are markers of specific brain structure involvement. Seizures with clonic focal or multifocal jerks are likely to rise from damage to the cortex and white matter. Akinesia (no eye and body movements), divergent eye position, unresponsive pupils, monotonous respiration, and brain stem release phenomena are markers of brain stem involvement and/or BGT and PLIC lesions. Coma or severe stupor, accompanied by tonic seizures, BSRP, and lack of body and eye movements indicate a more severe and diffuse brain involvement as in the most serious MRI pattern seen after perinatal asphyxia with lesions in the BGT, PLIC, WM, and C (Volpe 2008; De Vries and Cowan 2009).

The difficulties relating to the use of neurological examination depend on the fact that the neurological evaluation should be done in the first hour of life: the neurological condition of the asphyxiated newborn changes constantly during the first hours of life, as well as during the following days. There are at least two conditions that can explain such behavior: on one hand, the presence of particular anatomical and pathological lesions (the multicystic encephalomalacia is one of the major neuropathological frameworks,

Table 3 The table reports the main trials that have all included moderate/severe stage of encephalopathy as eligibility criteria at study random assignment at <6 h of age (Jacobs et al. 2011; Simbruner et al. 2010; Shankaran et al. 2005; Eicher et al. 2005a, b; Azzopardi et al. 2009; Gluckman et al. 2005; Zhou et al. 2010)

Author	Jacobs 2011 (ICE Trial)	Simbruner 2010 (neo.nEURO Trial)	Shankaran 2005 (NICHD)	Eicher 2005	Azzopardi 2009 (TOBY Trial)	Gluckman 2005 (CoolCap Trial)	Zhou 2010
Gestational age	$\geq$35 weeks' gestation	$\geq$36 weeks' gestation	$\geq$36 weeks' gestation	$\geq$35 weeks' gestation $\geq$2000 g birth weight	$\geq$36 weeks' gestation	$\geq$36 weeks' gestation	$\geq$37 weeks and birth weight $\geq$ 2500 g
Age	<6 h of birth	<5.5 h of age	$\leq$6 h of age	$\leq$6 h after birth or hypoxic-ischemic insult	$\leq$6 h of age	$\leq$6 h of age	$\leq$6 h of age
Neurological assessment	Moderate or severe encephalopathy (lethargy, stupor, coma, abnormal tone, and/or seizures)	Encephalopathy (lethargy, stupor, or coma) and $\geq$1 of: 1. Hypotonia 2. Abnormal reflexes, including oculomotor or pupillary abnormalities 3. Absent or weak suck 4. Clinical seizures	Either diagnosis of encephalopathy or seizures: Encephalopathy: presence of $\geq$1 signs in $\geq$3 of the 6 categories: 1. Level of consciousness 2. Spontaneous activity 3. Posture 4. Tone 5. Primitive reflexes (suck or Moro) 6. Autonomic nervous system (pupils, heart rate, or respiration)	$\geq$2 Neurologic findings of hypoxia-ischemia: 1. Posturing 2. Seizures 3. Autonomic dysfunction 4. Increased/decreased abnormalities of tone 5. Increased/decreased abnormalities of reflexes 6. Increased/decreased abnormalities of state of consciousness	Moderate-to-severe encephalopathy: altered state of consciousness (lethargy, stupor, or coma) and $\geq$1 of: 1. Hypotonia 2. Abnormal reflexes (including oculomotor or pupillary abnormalities) 3. Absent/weak suck 4. Clinical seizures	Acute moderate-severe encephalopathy and abnormal neurological examination: lethargy, stupor, or coma and $\geq$1 between: 1. Hypotonia 2. Abnormal reflexes (including oculomotor or pupillary abnormalities) 3. Absent/weak suck 4. Clinical evidence of seizures	Diagnosis of encephalopathy (mild, moderate and severe) lethargy, stupor, or coma, with $\geq$1 of the following: 1. Hypotonia 2. Abnormal reflexes 3. Clinical seizure

(continued)

Table 3 (continued)

Author	Jacobs 2011 (ICE Trial)	Simbruner 2010 (neo.nEURO Trial)	Shankaran 2005 (NICHD)	Eicher 2005	Azzopardi 2009 (TOBY Trial)	Gluckman 2005 (CoolCap Trial)	Zhou 2010
Clinical indicators of peripartum hypoxia-ischemia	At least two of the following clinical characteristics: 1. An Apgar score ≤ 5 at 10 min 2. Continued need for mechanical ventilation at 10 min 3. Metabolic acidosis: cord pH <7.00; arterial, venous, or capillary pH < 7.00; base deficit of >12 within 60 min of birth	≥1 of: 1. Apgar score < 5 at 10 min after birth 2. Continued need for resuscitation (including ET intubation/mask ventilation) at 10 min after birth 3. Umbilical cord pH or any arterial pH of <7.00 within 60 min after birth 4. Base deficit >16 mmol/L within 60 min after birth	Poor respiratory effort at birth and need for resuscitation: 1. pH ≤7.0 or base deficit ≥16 mmol/l in a sample of umbilical-cord blood or any blood during the first hours after birth 2. pH 7.01–7.15 or base deficit 10–15.9 mmol/l or blood gas not available + 2a. Acute perinatal event (late/variable decelerations, cord prolapse, cord rupture, uterine rupture, maternal trauma, hemorrhage, or cardiorespiratory arrest) + 2b. 10-min Apgar score ≤ 5 or assisted	≥1 Clinical sign hypoxia-ischemia: 1. Cord gas pH ≤7.0 or base deficit ≥13 2. Initial infant gas pH <7.1 3. Apgar score ≤ 5 at 10 min 4. Continued resuscitation after 5 min 5. Fetal bradycardia with heart rate < 80 beats/min lasting ≥15 min 6. Postnatal hypoxic-ischemic event with O2 desaturation <70% or arterial O2 tension <35 mmHg for 20 min with evidence of ischemia (chest compressions, hypotension, hemorrhage)	≥1 Clinical sign hypoxia-ischemia: 1. Apgar score ≤ 5 at 10 min 2. Continued need for resuscitation (ET/mask ventilation) at 10 min 3. Acidosis within 60 min after birth = umbilical-cord, arterial, or capillary pH <7.00 4. Base deficit ≥16 mmol/l in umbilical cord or any blood sample (arterial, venous, or capillary) within 60 min after birth	Clinical evidence of exposure to perinatal hypoxia-ischemia: 1. Apgar score ≤ 5 at 10 min after birth 2. A continued need for resuscitation (ET/mask ventilation) at 10 min after birth 3. Severe acidosis = pH <7.00 or base deficit ≥16 mmol/L in an umbilical cord blood sample or arterial/venous blood sample obtained within 60 min of birth or clinical evidence of seizures	Clinical evidence of exposure to perinatal hypoxia-ischemia: 1. Apgar score ≤ 3 at 1 min and ≤5 at 5 min 2. Cord blood gas pH <7.0 or base deficit ≤16 mmol/L 3. Need for resuscitation or ventilation at 5 min of age

			ventilation initiated at birth and continued for at least 10 min				
pEEG/aEEG	/	Abnormal standard EEG or aEEG findings: 1. Moderately abnormal aEEG/EEG findings + mild/moderate encephalopathy 2. Suppressed aEEG/EEG findings + severe encephalopathy	/	/	Abnormal standard aEEG findings: 1. Abnormal background activity of at least 30-min duration 2. Seizures a) Normal background with some seizure activity b) Moderately abnormal activity c) Suppressed activity d) Continuous seizure activity	1 Abnormal aEEG recording (≥1 h of age): 1. Background voltage moderately abnormal: upper margin >10 mV and lower margin <5 **m**V) 2. Background voltage severely abnormal: upper margin <10 mV) 3. Seizures: sudden increase in voltage + narrowing band + brief period of suppression	/
Treatment	Whole-body hypothermia to 33.5 °C	33.5 °C (range: 33.0–34.0 °C) for 72 h	Whole-body hypothermia to 33.5 °C for 72 h	33 ± 0.5 °C for 48 h	Total-body cooling at	Selective head-cooling	

(continued)

Table 3 (continued)

Author	Jacobs 2011 (ICE Trial)	Simbruner 2010 (neo.nEURO Trial)	Shankaran 2005 (NICHD)	Eicher 2005	Azzopardi 2009 (TOBY Trial)	Gluckman 2005 (CoolCap Trial)	Zhou 2010
					33.5 + 0.5 °C for 72 h		
Exclusion criteria	a) >6 h of birth b) Birth weight < 2000 g c) Major congenital abnormalities suspected d) Overt bleeding e) Infant requiring >80% inspired oxygen f) Imminent death (refractory hypotension/unresponsive acidosis) g) Therapeutic hypothermia commenced < assessment	a) Infants >5.5 h of age at time of random assignment b) Administration of high-dose AEDs (PB >20 mg/kg) c) Birth weight < 1800 g or GA <36 weeks. d) Head circumference > 3° p for GA if birth weight and length > 3°p e) Major congenital malformations with poor developmental prognosis f) Imperforate anus g) Gross hemorrhage h) Infant "in extremis"	a) Inability to enroll by 6 h of age b) Major congenital abnormality c) Severe growth restriction (birth weight of ≤1800 g) d) Refusal of consent by a parent/attending neonatologist e) Moribund infants for whom no further aggressive treatment was planned	a) Neonates with clinical sepsis b) Maternal chorioamnionitis c) Weight or head circumference < 10th percentile for gestation age d) Congenital abnormalities	1. ≥6 h of age at the time of randomization 2. Major congenital abnormalities that required surgery (diaphragmatic hernia) or were suggestive of chromosomal anomaly or syndromes that involve brain dysgenesis	1. >5.5 h of age 2. Prophylactic administration of high-dose AED 3. Major congenital abnormalities 4. Head trauma causing major intracranial hemorrhage 5. Severe growth restriction, with birthweight <1800 g 6. Head circumference < −2 SD for gestation if birth weight and length > −2 SD 7. Infants judged critically ill and unlikely to benefit from neonatal intensive care by the attending neonatologist 8. Unavailability of essential equipment 9. Planned concurrent participation in other experimental treatments	1. Major congenital abnormalities 2. Infection (ROM >18 h or maternal fever >38 °C or amniotic fluid foul smell) 3. Other encephalopathy (neonatal stroke, CNS abnormality, intracranial hemorrhage diagnosed by CT/cUS 4. Severe anemia (Hb <120 g/L).

Withdrawn of treatment				1. Sepsis/meningitis by positive blood or cerebrospinal fluid culture obtained at birth 2. Pneumonia by chest radiograph in the first 36 h of life 3. Uncontrolled disseminated intravascular coagulopathy 4. Sustained bradycardia <70 beats/min with hypotension and acidosis on inotropic medications, which did not respond to rewarming to 34 °C 5. Parental request	1. parents request withdrawal 2. Attending clinician withdraws cooling because of clinical, EEG, and imaging evidence of severe, irreversible brain injury or continued inability to maintain rectal temperature in the desired range 3. Baby receives extra-corporeal membrane oxygenation Apparent improvement on continuous aEEG recording, after trial entry, is not an indication for discontinuing cooling		
Enrollment period	February 14, 2001 - July 27, 2007	January 2001–April 2006	July 2000–May 2003	January 1998–January 2001 (+12-month follow-up period)	December 2002–30 November 2006	July 1999 - January, 2002	
Patients	221 randomizzati Australia, New Zealand, Canada, USA	125 randomizzati (Austria, Germania, Francia - 24 centers)	208 randomizzati (15 centers)	65	325	218	

although missing in the early hours of severe clinical neurological signs); on the other, the "physiological" delay between the beginning of the typical metabolic processes of HIE and appearance of corresponding neurological signs.

In many cases, after resuscitation, there is a transitional apparent normalization of the neurological picture, and only later the appearance of neurological signs of distress happens. In such cases, the early neurological observation can be misleading: this is why the observation of the first hour should always be repeated at least twice during the first 6 h of life in order to identify the onset of initial signs of encephalopathy between 3 and 6 h of life. A striking example of this delayed manifestation of clinical signs consist on neonatal seizures that are present in the first 3–5 h after birth only in few cases, usually they appear later. Clinical seizures are considered one of the most typical signs of HIE and are included as neurological signs for the selection of cases to be cooled. Seizures often appear at 10–15 or even 20 h after asphyxia and cannot be considered as an early clinical sign.

It is mandatory to bear in mind that the neurological examination performed 1 or 2 h from birth, although essential for the decision of cooling, may not identify the severity of the neurological signs; a neurological examination performed few hours later may correlate better with the severity of the neurological damage (Ferrari et al. 2011).

Brain injury findings on MRI in encephalopathic newborns who have undergone whole-body hypothermia have been described in two large multicenter randomized controlled trials (*NICHD and TOBY trials*) (Shankaran et al. 2012b; Rutherford et al. 2010). However, data about the post-hypothermia functional-anatomical correlation between neonatal neurobehavioral abnormalities and brain injury findings on MRI were not published. A reason for this deficiency may lie in the fact that the neurological evaluation is further complicated by the effect of the sedative drugs used during the hypothermia that can affect the neonatal neurobehavior.

Early assessment of infants at risk for functional impairment after perinatal asphyxia is mandatory to plan a developmentally supportive care and guide referrals to early intervention services. The NICU network neurobehavioral scale (NNNS) is a strong candidate for documenting neurobehavioral status post-therapeutic hypothermia.

The NNNS is a comprehensive standardized assessment of neurological integrity and behavioral functioning in high-risk infants: the examination consists of 45 administration items and 70 observational items that are scored and transformed into 13 summary scores based on conceptual and statistical grouping of items.

These scores offer quantitative measures of individual neurobehavioral domains including habituation, attention, handling, quality of movement, regulation, nonoptimal reflexes, asymmetrical reflexes, stress/abstinence, arousal, hypertonicity, hypotonicity, excitability, and lethargy. The NNNS has been related to a later developmental outcome in other high-risk neonatal populations as neonates exposed to substances during pregnancy or preterm infants. Neonatal neurobehavioral abnormalities identified by the NNNS have been demonstrated to be associated with MRI brain injury in encephalopathic newborns post-hypothermia. In this perspective, the NNNS can provide an early functional assessment of structural brain injury in newborns, which may guide rehabilitative therapies (Coleman et al. 2013).

120.9 Other Brain Injuries

120.9.1 Periventricular Leukomalacia (PVL)

The initial neurological correlates of PVL are not established: cystic or noncystic PVL takes 2–4 weeks to become manifest after the USA has demonstrated increased periventricular echogenicity, which is clinically silent. Other hemorrhagic, metabolic, or infective disorders may be associated. Several clinical signs have been described: in preterm infants, who later develop cerebral palsy, signs such as irritability, abnormal posture of fingers, spontaneous Babinski reflex, popliteal angle reduction, increased extensor tone, inferior limbs weakness, and marked hypotonia have been observed. Long-term correlates of PVL include spastic diplegia and intellectual deficits (Volpe 2008; Dubowitz and Dubowitz 1981).

120.9.2 Intraventricular Hemorrhage (IVH) in Preterm Infants

Three clinical syndromes are associated with IVH:

Catastrophic clinical deterioration, which is a dramatic presentation usually in the most severe degrees of IVH. It is characterized by deep stupor and coma, respiratory abnormalities (hypoventilation and apneas), seizures, decerebrate posturing, pupils fixed to light, and eyes fixed to vestibular stimulation, and by a flaccid quadriparesis.

Saltatory syndrome, which is most subtle in presentation and evolves over many hours. Signs are altered consciousness, decreased quantity and quality of spontaneous movement, altered ocular position, and motility.

A clinically silent syndrome, when neurological signs are so subtle that they are not seen (Volpe 2008; Prechtl and Dijkstra 1960).

120.9.3 Bilirubin Encephalopathy

The clinical features in infants with bilirubin injury depend on the damage topography and on the infant age. Acute bilirubin encephalopathy is characterized by three phases:

In the first phase, stupor and hypotonia are prominent, often accompanied by poor sucking. Seizures occur in a minority of cases.

In the second phase, the principal signs are hypertonia, particularly in the extensor muscles with backward arching of the neck (retrocollis) or of the back (opisthotonus). The increase in tone is probably of extrapyramidal origin, and newborns, who show these signs, later develop features of chronic bilirubin encephalopathy.

In the third phase, hypertonia evolves into hypotonia, usually after the first week of life (Volpe 2008).

120.9.4 Metabolic Disease

Metabolic disorders during the neonatal period are generally associated with altered level of consciousness, seizures, hypotonia or hypertonia, impaired feeding, and delayed neurological development. Stupor, coma and seizures, and urine with the odor of maple syrup occur in maple syrup disease. Seizures, stupor, or coma associated with myoclonus and hiccups are typical of nonketotic hyperglycinemia. Hyperammonemic states are accompanied by vomiting, poor feeding, stupor, and coma. There are dysmorphic facial features in some metabolic diseases such as the mitochondriopathies, which may manifest in the neonatal period with seizures, hypotonia, stupor, coma, and tachypnea due to a metabolic acidosis (Volpe 2008).

120.9.5 Jitteriness

Jitteriness is a disorder of movement frequently observed during the neonatal period. Movements are generalized and symmetrical, have the quality of a coarse tremor, are stimulus sensitive, and can be diminished by gentle flexion of the limbs. It is frequently accompanied by brisk tendon reflex and an easily elicited Moro reflex (hyperexcitability syndrome). Jitteriness is often related to neurological hyperirritability, as in HIE, hypoglycemia, hypocalcemia, and drug withdrawal syndrome. In some cases, no cause can be found (Volpe 2008; Prechtl and Dijkstra 1960).

120.9.6 Stiff Baby Syndrome

Stiff baby syndrome or hyperekplexia is a familiar disorder (autosomal dominant). It is characterized by marked hypertonia, which is accentuated by minor sensory stimulation. An episode of hypertonia may involve respiratory muscles, causing apnea. Hypertonia is accompanied by an exaggerated startle response, which may mimic seizures (Volpe 2008).

120.9.7 Neuromuscular Disorders or Spinal Cord Disease: The Floppy Infant

The term floppy baby or infant is used to denote an infant with poor muscle tone affecting the limbs, trunk, and the craniofacial musculature. Hypotonia may be caused by congenital or acquired disorders, as a consequence of central or peripheral nervous system involvement. Lower motor neuron lesions result in a loss of muscle tone and flaccidity. Lesions affecting the upper motor neurons result in reduced supraspinal inhibitory influences, leading during early infancy to flaccidity and diminished muscle tone with preserved or hyperactive reflexes and later evolving into spasticity. Thus hypotonia with no obvious weakness and normal or increased reflexes suggests CNS involvement. In neuromuscular disorders, hypotonia is usually associated with weakness and/or contractures. Contractures, skin dimpling, and poor dermatoglyphic patterns are indicators of poor fetal movements and are highly suggestive of a neuromuscular disorder. In myasthenia gravis and infantile botulism, diffuse hypotonia and weakness are present, often in conjunction with CNS involvement. In congenital myopathies, proximal extremity weakness is prominent, and there are limb deformities if the onset was in utero.

Spinal cord trauma with a tear in the cervical dura can be caused by a difficult breech delivery. This results in symmetric lower extremity paralysis with sparing of the face and cranial nerves and involvement of the sphincters. The most common injury involving the peripheral nerves is the proximal cervical roots of C5, C6, and C7, usually caused by a traumatic delivery with shoulder dystocia. In Erb's palsy, there is paralysis of shoulder abduction, elbow flexion, and finger extension, so that the arm is held extended, externally rotated with flexion at the wrist. There is no biceps reflex, although the triceps reflex may be present (Volpe 2008).

120.10 Conclusions

Advances in neuroimaging and other diagnostic techniques do not reduce the importance of performing a neurological examination, which may highlight the presence of neurological abnormalities and help to select those infants who need investigation, neuroprotection, and follow-up.

A full neurological examination will show if the development of the baby is appropriate for postmenstrual age.

Sick newborn infants require a simple noninvasive test to evaluate the state of consciousness and the severity of the brain damage. If there is coma or stupor, brain stem involvement should be considered, and the neurological test should be repeated every few hours.

Seizures are the most important sign of an acute brain disorder. They may be difficult to recognize without concomitant EEG recording. Only clonic jerks are easily recognizable, indicating acute cortical involvement. Spontaneous movements and GMs in particular are reliable and effective tools for the diagnosis of brain dysfunction and may predict the motor outcome.

References

Als H, Brazelton TB (1981) A new model of assessing the behavioral organization in preterm and fullterm infants: two case studies. J Am Acad Child Psychiatry 20:239–263

Als H, Lester BM, Tronick Z, Brazelton T (1982) Manual for the assessment of preterm infants' behavior (APIB). In: Fitzgerald HE, Lester BM, Yogman MW (eds) Theory and research in behavioral pediatrics, vol 1. Plenum Press, New York, pp 65–132

Als H, Butler S, Kosta S, McAnulty G (2005) The Assessment of Preterm Infants' Behavior (APIB): furthering the understanding and measurement of neurodevelopmental competence in preterm and full-term infants. Ment Retard Dev Disabil Res Rev 11:94–102

Amiel-Tison C (1978) A method for neurological evaluation within the first year of life: experience with full-term newborn infants with birth injury. Ciba Found Symp 59:107–137

Amiel-Tison C, Grenier A (1980) Évaluation neurologique du nouveau – né et du nourrisson. Masson, Paris
Azzopardi DV, Strohm B, Edwards AD, Dyet L, Halliday HL, Juszczak E et al (2009) Moderate hypothermia to treat perinatal asphyxial encephalopathy. N Engl J Med 361:1349–1358
Brazelton TB (1973) Neonatal behavioural assessment scale. In: Clinics in developmental medicine, no. 50. Spastics International Medical Publication/William Medical Books/JB Lippincott, London/Philadelphia
Cioni G, Ferrari F, Prechtl HF (1989) Posture and spontaneous motility in fullterm infants. Early Hum Dev 18:247–262
Cioni G, Ferrari F, Einspieler C et al (1997) Comparison between observation of spontaneous movements and neurologic examination in preterm infants. J Pediatr 130:704–711
Coleman MB, Glass P, Brown J, Kadom N, Tsuchida T, Scafidi J et al (2013) Neonatal neurobehavioral abnormalities and MRI brain injury in encephalopathic newborns treated with hypothermia. Early Hum Dev 89:733–737
De Vries LS, Cowan FM (2009) Evolving understanding of hypoxic-ischemic encephalopathy in the term infant. Semin Pediatr Neurol 16:216–225
Dubowitz LM, Dubowitz V (1981) The neurological assessment of the preterm and full-term newborn infant. Spastic International Medical Publications/William Heinemann Medical Books, London
Dubowitz LMS, Dubowitz V, Mercuri E (1998a) The neurological assessment of the preterm and full-term newborn infant. Textbook of clinics in developmental medicine. Mc Keith Press, Cambridge
Dubowitz LM, Mercuri E, Dubowitz V (1998b) An optimality score for the neurologic examination of the term newborn. J Pediatr 133:406–416
Eicher DJ, Wagner CL, Katikaneni LP, Hulsey TC, Bass WT, Kaufman DA et al (2005a) Moderate hypothermia in neonatal encephalopathy: safety outcomes. Pediatr Neurol 32:18–24
Eicher DJ, Wagner CL, Katikaneni LP, Hulsey TC, Bass WT, Kaufman DA et al (2005b) Moderate hypothermia in neonatal encephalopathy: efficacy outcomes. Pediatr Neurol 32:11–17
Einspieler C, Prechtl HF, Bos A et al (2004) Prechtl's method on the qualitative assessment of general movements in preterm, term and young infants. Mac Keith Press, London
Fenichel GM (1983) Hypoxic-ischemic encephalopathy in the newborn. Arch Neurol 40:261–266
Ferrari F, Cioni G, Prechtl HF (1990) Qualitative changes of general movements in preterm infants with brain lesions. Early Hum Dev 23:193–231
Ferrari F, Cioni G, Einspieler C et al (2002) Cramped synchronized general movements in preterm infants as an early marker for cerebral palsy. Arch Pediatr Adolesc Med 156:460–467
Ferrari F, Todeschini A, Guidotti I, Martinez-Biarge M, Roversi MF, Berardi A et al (2011) General movements in full-term infants with perinatal asphyxia are related to basal ganglia and thalamic lesions. J Pediatr 158:904–911
Finer NN, Robertson CM, Richards RT et al (1981) Hypoxic-ischemic encephalopathy in term neonates: perinatal factors and outcome. J Pediatr 98:112–117
Gluckman PD, Wyatt JS, Azzopardi D, Ballard R, Edwards AD, Ferriero DM et al (2005) Selective head cooling with mild systemic hypothermia after neonatal encephalopathy: multicentre randomised trial. Lancet 365:663–670
Gosselin J, Gahagan S, Amiel-Tison C (2005) The Amiel-Tison neurological assessment at term: conceptual and methodological continuity in the course of follow-up. Ment Retard Dev Disabil Res Rev 11:34–51
Jacobs SE, Morley CJ, Inder TE, Stewart MJ, Smith KR, McNamara PJ et al (2011) Whole-body hypothermia for term and near-term newborns with hypoxic-ischemic encephalopathy: a randomized controlled trial. Arch Pediatr Adolesc Med 165:692–700
Levene ML, Kornberg J, Williams TH (1985) The incidence and severity of post-asphyxial encephalopathy in full-term infants. Early Hum Dev 11:21–26
Miller SP, Latal B, Clark H, Barnwell A, Glidden D, Barkovich AJ et al (2004) Clinical signs predict 30-month neurodevelopmental outcome after neonatal encephalopathy. Am J Obstet Gynecol 190:93–99
Noble Y, Boyd R (2012) Neonatal assessments for the preterm infant up to 4 months corrected age: a systematic review. Develop Med Child Neur 54: 129–139
Prechtl HF (1974) The behavioural states of the newborn infant. Brain Res 76:185–212
Prechtl HFR (1977) The neurological examination of the full-term newborn infant, 2nd revised edn. Heinemann, London
Prechtl HFR (1990) Qualitative changes of spontaneous movements in fetus and preterm infants are a marker of neurological dysfunction. Early Hum Dev 23: 151–158
Prechtl HFR, Dijkstra J (1960) Neurological diagnosis of cerebral injury in the newborn. In: ten Berge BS (ed) Prenatal care. Noordhof, Groningen
Prechtl HF, Hopkins B (1986) Developmental transformations of spontaneous movements in early infancy. Early Hum Dev 14:233–238
Roodenburg PJ, Wladimiroff JW, van Es A, Prechtl HF (1991) Classification and quantitative aspects of fetal movements during the second half of normal pregnancy. Early Hum Dev 25:19–35
Rutherford M, Ramenghi LA, Edwards AD, Brocklehurst P, Halliday H, Levene M et al (2010) Assessment of brain tissue injury after moderate hypothermia in neonates with hypoxic-ischaemic encephalopathy: a nested

substudy of a randomised controlled trial. Lancet Neurol 9:39–45

Saint-Anne Dargassies S (1955) Méthode d'examen neurologique du nouveau-né. Études Néonatales 3:101–123

Sarnat HB, Sarnat MS (1976) Neonatal encephalopathy following fetal distress. A clinical and electroencephalographic study. Arch Neurol 33:696–705

Shankaran S, Laptook AR, Ehrenkranz RA, Tyson JE, McDonald SA, Donovan EF et al (2005) Whole body hypothermia for neonates with hypoxic ischemic encephalopathy. N Engl J Med 353 (1574):1584

Shankaran S, Laptook AR, Tyson JE, Ehrenkranz RA, Bann CM, Das A et al (2012a) Evolution of encephalopathy during whole body hypothermia for neonatal hypoxic-ischemic encephalopathy. J Pediatr 160:567–572

Shankaran S, Barnes PD, Hintz SR, Laptook AR, Zaterka-Baxter KM, McDonald SA et al (2012b) Brain injury following trial of hypothermia for neonatal hypoxic-ischaemic encephalopathy. Arch Dis Child Fetal Neonatal Ed 97:F398–F404

Simbruner G, Mittal RA, Rohlmann F, Muche R, neo.nEURO.network Trial Participants (2010) Systemic hypothermia after neonatal encephalopathy: outcomes of neo.nEURO.Network RCT. Pediatrics 126:e771–e778

Thompson CM, Puterman AS, Linley LL, Hann FM, van der Elst CW, Molteno CD et al (1997) The value of a scoring system for hypoxic ischaemic encephalopathy in predicting neurodevelopmental outcome. Acta Paediatr 86:757–761

Volpe JJ (2008) Neurological evaluation. In: Volpe JJ (ed) Neurology of the newborn, 5th edn. WB Saunders, Philadelphia

Zhou WH, Cheng GQ, Shao XM, Liu XZ, Shan RB, Zhuang DY et al (2010) Selective head cooling with mild systemic hypothermia after neonatal hypoxic-ischemic encephalopathy: a multicenter randomized controlled trial in China. J Pediatr 157: 367–372

Neonatal Electroencephalography 121

Lena K. Hellström-Westas

Contents

Abstract
The electroencephalogram (EEG) records electrocortical activity and is a sensitive method for assessing brain function. Neurological symptoms may be very vague or entirely absent in infants requiring neonatal intensive care. The EEG is an important tool for detecting abnormal brain activity in both term and preterm infants and can be used for diagnosing epileptic seizures and following effects of antiepileptic treatment; the EEG can also contribute with predictive information on later neurodevelopmental prognosis.

- The EEG is sensitive for assessing brain function and for detecting brain dysfunction.
- The amplitude-integrated EEG trend (aEEG) can be used for monitoring high risk infants.
- The aEEG gives prolonged information on trends in brain activity, while the EEG gives detailed information and confirms findings in the aEEG.
- The aEEG and EEG can be used for prediction of outcome, diagnosis of seizures, and evaluation of effects of antiepileptic treatment

121.1 The Neonatal Electroencephalogram

The electroencephalogram (EEG) records electrocortical activity from the brain's surface. The EEG activity is also influenced by subcortical activity;

L. K. Hellström-Westas (✉)
Department of Women's and Children's Health, Uppsala University and University Hospital, Uppsala, Sweden
e-mail: lena.westas@kbh.uu.se

G. Buonocore et al. (eds.), *Neonatology*,
https://doi.org/10.1007/978-3-319-29489-6_268

a dissociation of thalamocortical connection is associated with the discontinuous burst-suppression activity. Consequently, the EEG reflects brain function and can be used for early detection of both general and focal brain dysfunction.

The EEG is usually recorded from electrodes placed over the scalp according to the International 10–20 system which uses the nasion and the inion as anatomical landmarks on the skull to identify electrode positions (Jasper 1958). The inter-electrode distance is usually 10% or 20% of the total distance between these positions. The electrode positions are defined by capital letters followed by a number, for example, F for frontal, C for central, T for temporal, O for occipital, with even numbers indicating the right side and odd numbers the left side (Fig. 1). Additionally, respiration, electrocardiogram, eye movement, and electromyogram are recorded, which together with the EEG give supplementary information such as sleep states, movements, seizures, and possible artifacts. The EEG changes with the infant's maturation. The terms postconceptional age (PCA) and postmenstrual age (PMA) represent a summary of gestational age and postnatal age and are used when assessing EEG maturation.

121.1.1 Normal EEG Maturation

Waveforms and background activity in the EEG can be described according to amplitude, frequency, topographic distribution of activity, and temporal (time) evolution. The normal EEG background in very preterm infants is mainly discontinuous, a pattern that is called *tracé discontinu* which is characterized by high-amplitude bursts of activity alternating with periods of low-voltage activity, interburst intervals (IBI). With increasing maturation, the duration of the bursts increases, while their amplitude decreases, and simultaneously the IBIs become shorter, resulting in an increasingly continuous EEG background. The mean IBI duration is around 18–26 s at 21–24 weeks PCA and decreases to 10–12 s at 25–30 weeks PCA and down to 6–8 s at 34–36 weeks (Fig. 2). The topographic organization of the developing EEG occurs in an occipitalfrontal direction. Interhemispheric synchrony of electrocortical activity changes during maturation: at extremely low PCA the EEG activity is usually synchronous, and between 26 and 30 weeks' PCA there is increased desynchronization, which again is followed by increasing synchronization at PCAs above 30 weeks (André et al. 2010; Mizrahi et al. 2004).

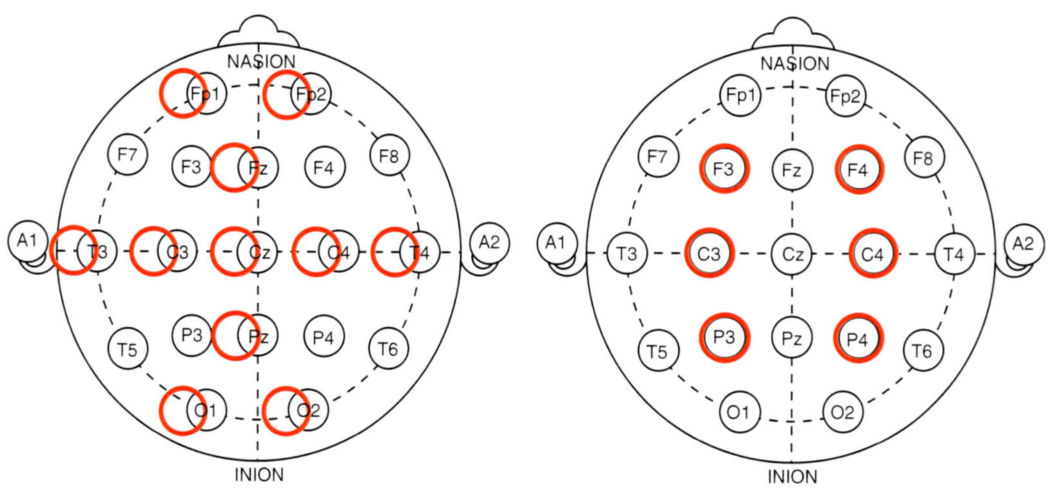

Fig. 1 Electroencephalogram electrode positions according to the International 10–20 system (Jasper 1958). The *red circles* mark electrode positions that are commonly used in newborn infants, on the left side for neonatal EEG and on the right side long-term monitoring of aEEG/EEG

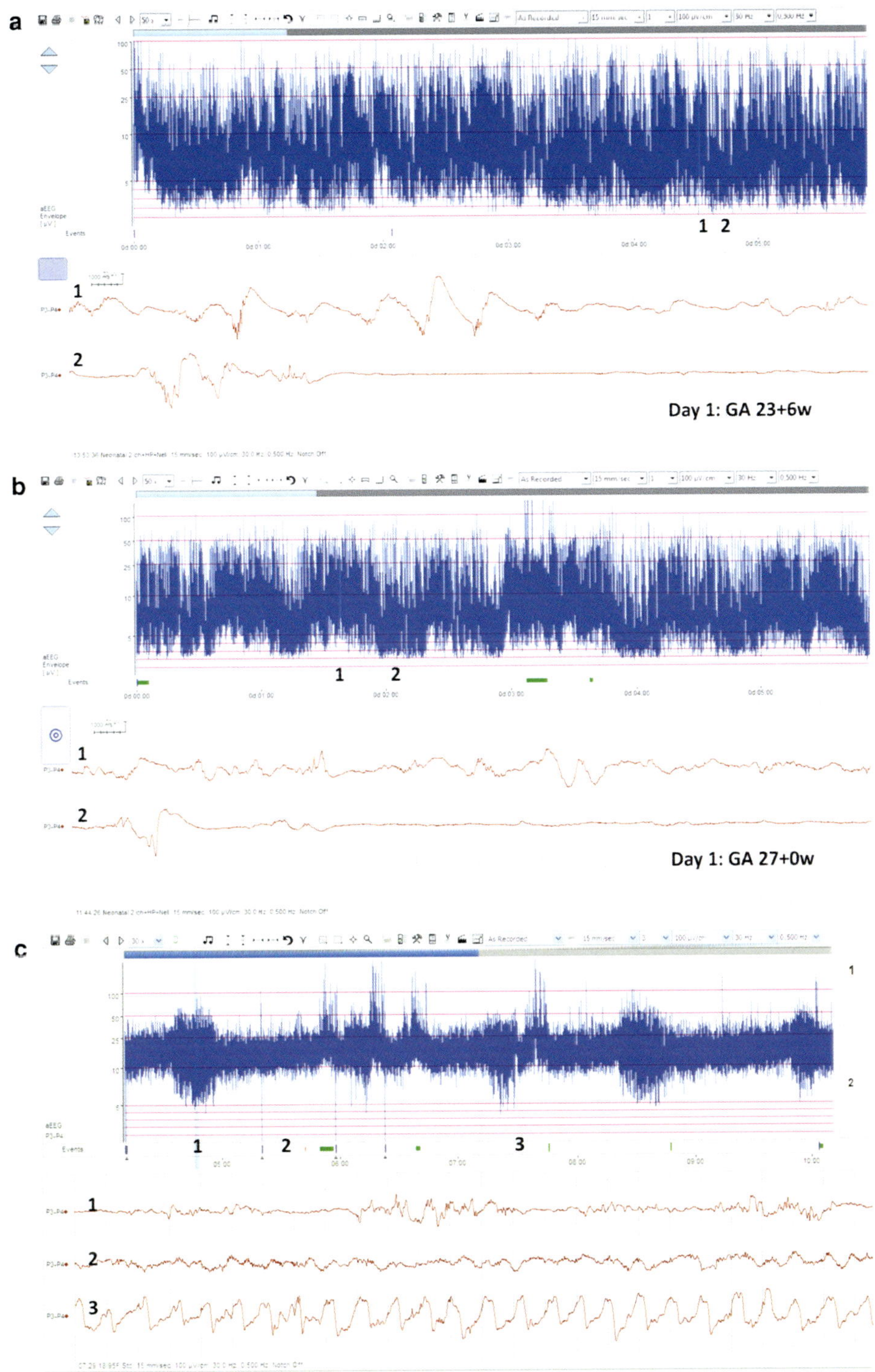

Fig. 2 Examples of aEEG trends (duration 6 h) with corresponding raw EEG (25 s). (**a**) Single-channel aEEG/EEG (P3-P4) from the first day of life in a GA 23+6 w stable infant. The aEEG/EEG activity dominated by discontinuous activity although short periods of more continuous activity can be seen (*1*). (**b**) Single-channel aEEG/

Sleep wake cycling can be identified in the EEG from around 30 weeks' PCA, but immature cycling can be seen already from around 24–25 weeks PCA although specific sleep states cannot be distinguished. Active sleep, or rapid eye movement (REM) sleep, can usually not be distinguished from wakefulness in the EEG without other measures, that is, direct observation or evaluation of eye movements, respiration, and muscular activity. Quiet sleep, or non-REM, sleep is characterized by increased discontinuity. The EEG during quiet sleep in term infants is either discontinuous (*tracé alternant*) or contains high voltage slow activity (HVS) (Fig. 2).

The distribution of the main EEG frequencies, that is, delta (< 4 Hz), theta (4–8 Hz), alpha (8–12 Hz), beta (13–20 Hz), also change with maturation, although there is usually a mix of frequencies at all PCA. In preterm infants, high voltage delta activity and, to some extent, theta activity is predominant, while more theta and alpha activity can be identified in term infants (André et al. 2010; Mizrahi et al. 2004). Very slow EEG activity (<0.5 Hz) has also been demonstrated both in term and preterm infants. Experimental data indicate that this activity may be essential for the development of brain wiring processes (Vanhatalo and Kaila 2006). The EEG signal is weak (measured in microvolts) and can easily be disturbed by movements, electrical interferences in the neonatal intensive care unit (NICU), and respiration. Especially when the EEG activity is very depressed, the recording may pick up the signal from the electrocardiogram (ECG), which is measured in millivolt and consequently has a magnitude of 1000 times that of the EEG. High frequency oscillation ventilation (HFOV) in the NICU is often performed with frequencies between 10 and 15 Hz, that is, frequencies that are parts of the normal EEG activity. Care has to be taken to avoid such interference by avoiding contact between the electrodes and the bedding and to evaluate the raw-EEG signal for this artifact when using amplitude-integrated EEG (aEEG) monitoring.

During normal EEG maturation, several distinctive waveforms and patterns are expected to appear and disappear at certain PCA: these features can be used for evaluation of the infant's brain maturation, but their functional and anatomical correlates are not known (Vanhatalo and Kaila 2006). Delta brush pattern is characterized by runs of fast activity (alpha-beta) superimposed on delta waves; this pattern is typical of the very preterm EEG. Temporal theta bursts (temporal saw-tooth) are brief, rhythmic, 4–6 Hz transients that first appear around 26 weeks' PCA and reach a maximum at 30–32 weeks before they disappear. Temporal sharp waves may appear during the first weeks of life in infants born at 31–32 weeks' gestation. However, if abundant, or persisting, they are associated with brain injury. Frontal sharp wave transients appear from 34 to 35 weeks' PCA and disappear around 10 weeks later (André et al. 2010; Mizrahi et al. 2004).

The accuracy of estimation of PCA from various EEG measures is usually 2 weeks. An interesting observation in a few publications is that the EEG activity in very preterm infants seems to exhibit a progressive increase during the first days of life: whether this is due to postnatal adaptation or recovery after the delivery is not known (Victor et al. 2005).

121.1.2 Abnormal EEG

When a hypoxic-ischemic, hemorrhagic, or metabolic insult occurs, for example, perinatal asphyxia, intracranial hemorrhage, or severe hypoglycemia, the EEG activity is immediately affected. The response, a transient depression, is very similar in humans of all ages and animals. The magnitude of

Fig. 2 (continued) EEG (P3-P4) from the first day of life in a stable infant with GA 27+0 weeks demonstrating alternating periods with continuous (*1*) and more discontinuous (*2*) activity, which may represent crude sleep wake cycling. (**c**) Two-day-old full-term infant with a suspected stroke. Continuous aEEG/EEG background with sleep wake cycling, including (*1*) tracé alternant sleep, (*2*) continuous activity representing wakefulness or rapid eye movement (REM) sleep, and (*3*) a brief seizure the EEG depression and the time to recovery of the EEG background activity correlates with the severity of the insult. The electrocortical activity usually recovers after a time-period that may last from minutes to weeks. Seizures of varying intensity often develop during the recovery phase (Watanabe et al. 1999). Sleep-wake cycling is usually depressed or entirely absent during the acute stage. Chronic EEG changes, such as abnormal waveforms or poor synchronization of activity, may persist as markers of permanent damage. The consistent way by which the electrocortical activity behaves after an insult, and the relation between the severity of the EEG activity and the brain damage, makes EEG sensitive for diagnosis of brain damage and for early prediction of outcome.

A severe insult may result in an entirely flat (inactive, isoelectric) EEG, while milder insults may only result in subtle slowing of the EEG or increased discontinuity. Burst-suppression (BS) and undifferentiated extremely low voltage patterns may also be present after severe insults. These EEG patterns are associated with increased risk for adverse outcome in asphyxiated term infants.

In the preterm infant, milder insults may cause prolonged IBIs, and more severe insults may also change the background activity to a BS pattern. Burst suppression is characterized by bursts of activity with a flat (inactive) or very low-amplitude IBIs, as compared to the normal discontinuous background of the preterm infant in which the IBIs contain more activity. The BS pattern is abnormal at all maturational stages; it is associated with the presence of brain damage, administration of sedative medications, and some rare encephalopathies (mainly nonketotic hyperglycinemia and Ohtahara syndrome). In term infants, a recording with predominant IBI duration of more than 30 s is highly predictive of death or poor neurological outcome (Menache et al. 2002).

Chronic stage EEG changes may appear within a few weeks after an insult and are markers of persisting brain injury. Chronic stage background abnormalities can be categorized as being either dysmature or disorganized. Dysmature EEG patterns are characterized by delayed development (> 2 weeks) and are associated with cognitive impairment. Disorganized EEG patterns develop after severe acute insults and are characterized by deformity of delta waves and brushes, as well as presence of abnormal sharp waves; they are closely associated with white matter damage and development of cerebral palsy (Okumura et al. 2002). Some waveforms, especially positive rolandic sharp waves (PRSW), are markers of white matter damage. PRSW are predictive of later cerebral palsy when appearing with a frequency of more than two per minute in the neonatal EEG (Marret et al. 1992).

121.1.3 Effects of Medications

Administration of antiepileptic or sedative medications such as benzodiazepines (diazepam, midazolam), phenobarbital, opioids (morphine, fentanyl), and lidocaine is associated with transient depression of the EEG background that may last for minutes to hours. The most common response to a loading dose of sedative or anticonvulsant medication in a term infant with normal continuous EEG background is a change of the background activity to a moderately discontinuous pattern. Preterm infants and term infants with already compromised brain function tend to respond with more profound discontinuity, including burst-suppression pattern. The EEG background usually recovers within 2–2.5 h after a single dose of sedative medications in term infants, but in preterm infants the EEG depression may last longer (Norman et al. 2013; Shany et al. 2008) (Fig. 3). Repeated doses and continuous infusion of such medications may, of course, be associated with prolonged and more marked discontinuity. In several studies, it has been demonstrated that surfactant treatment is associated with a profound aEEG depression that occurs immediately after administration and has a duration of up to 10 min in some infants, the reason for this response is not known (Hellström-Westas et al. 1992).

121.1.4 Seizures

The electrographic appearance of neonatal seizures can be very variable as regards waveform

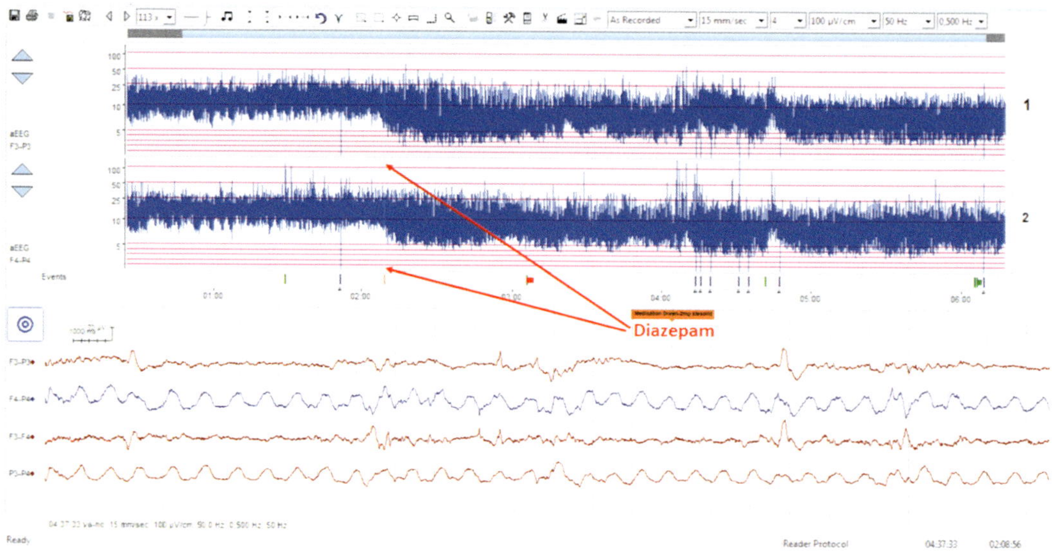

Fig. 3 Two-channel aEEG-recording showing 6 h of aEEG and 25 s of EEG in a full-term asphyxiated infant treated with hypothermia. The aEEG/EEG background was continuous when the infant received diazepam due to a suspected right-sided electroclinical seizure (seen as rhythmic activity in F4-P4 and P3-P4). After diazepam, the aEEG trend was moderately depressed for 6 h before recovery (not shown). The traces are from *top* to *bottom*: aEEG: *left side* (F3-P3), aEEG: *right side* (F4-P4), EEG: *left side* (F3-P3), EEG: *right side* (F4-P4), EEG: cross-cerebral frontal (F3-F4), EEG: cross-cerebral parietal (P3-P4)

morphology, frequency, localization, and temporal evolution. A seizure pattern in the EEG is often defined as "a sudden, repetitive, evolving and stereotyped ictal pattern with a clear beginning middle and ending and a minimum duration of 10 seconds" (Shellhaas and Clancy 2007). However, also ictal patterns with shorter duration than 10 s, and more prolonged epileptiform activity, for example, periodic lateralized epileptiform discharges (PLED), are associated with adverse outcomes (Oliveira et al. 2000).

Status epilepticus is usually defined as continuously ongoing epileptic activity or repetitive seizures with a duration of more than 30 min. Seizures are most frequently seen in temporal and central areas and are less commonly detected in frontal and occipital EEG leads (Shellhaas and Clancy 2007; Patrizi et al. 2003). Term infants tend to have a focal onset of seizures, while seizures in a preterm more often are regional (Patrizi et al. 2003). Clinical seizure identification can be difficult, since ill newborn infants may have seizure-like movements without corresponding seizure activity in the EEG. However, several studies have demonstrated that a majority of neonatal seizures actually are entirely subclinical and these seizures can consequently only be diagnosed with EEG.

In babies with electroclinical seizures (clinical and EEG seizures), administration of antiepileptic drugs is associated with a phenomenon called electroclinical dissociation, that is, the clinical seizures stop while subclinical seizures in the EEG persist or even increase in numbers (Boylan et al. 2002).

121.2 EEG-Monitoring

Video-EEG monitoring is the gold standard of EEG-monitoring. However, multiple channel EEG and video is not available in all NICUs, and it is often too complicated for the neonatal staff to interpret the EEG bedside on a 24 h/7 day basis unless continuous service is provided from an EEG department. This limitation has, so far, confined the use of video-EEG to complicated cases and research studies. In contrast, continuous EEG-monitoring with limited numbers of channels, usually one to three (cross-cerebral and fronto-central or fronto-parietal leads), and including compressed EEG trends such as the amplitude integrated EEG (aEEG), is increasingly used in many NICUs. These monitors are easy to apply and to interpret by the neonatal staff and can be used 24/7. The first analogue aEEG monitor was created in the 1960s by Prior and Maynard and was called Cerebral Function Monitor (CFM) (Maynard et al. 1969). Modern digital monitors display and store the raw EEG, which is also necessary to assess – at least intermittently – for correct evaluation of the activity in the aEEG/EEG and for excluding potential artifacts.

The aEEG trend is derived from the raw EEG; first the EEG signal is passed through an asymmetric filter which strongly attenuates low (<2 Hz) and high (>15 Hz) EEG frequencies, then the signal undergoes rectification, semi-logarithmic display (to give better resolution within very low voltage activity), and time-compression. The resulting aEEG trend gives a good overview of changes in minimum and maximum electrocortical activity over hours and days (Fig. 2). Maturational aEEG changes parallels the EEG development, which is expected since it is derived from the EEG. A main developmental feature in the aEEG trend is the progressive rise of the lower border (during the more discontinuous quiet sleep) reflecting the increasing EEG continuity with increasing gestational age (Zhang et al. 2011a).

The usefulness of the aEEG has been demonstrated in a large number of studies in both term and preterm infants. Several studies have shown that the findings in aEEG recorded within the first 3–6 h after birth asphyxia are highly predictive of neurodevelopmental outcome (Spitzmiller et al. 2007). Abnormal background patterns (BS, extremely low voltage, flat) are predictive of adverse outcome, while normal continuous or slightly discontinuous patterns are associated with normal outcome. Sleep wake cycling appearing before 36 postnatal hours is associated with better outcome in infants with moderate hypoxic-ischemic encephalopathy (HIE). These studies were all performed in asphyxiated infants who did not receive treatment with therapeutic hypothermia. However, postasphyctic intervention with moderate hypothermia is associated with an altered predictive value of the aEEG/EEG (Thoresen et al. 2010). This is expected, since hypothermia is an intervention that aims to change and improve outcome. In hypothermia-treated infants, an early normalization of the aEEG/ EEG is associated with good outcome, while a delayed recovery of an abnormal aEEG/EEG background until 36–48 h may still be associated with a healthy recovery. It is recommended to monitor brain function during the whole hypothermia treatment since seizures may appear during the rewarming. A full EEG should always be recorded in these infants.

Also in late preterm infants the aEEG/EEG is predictive of outcome after perinatal asphyxia (Jiang et al. 2015). Several studies have also shown that the early electrocortical background activity is predictive of outcome in very preterm infants, including infants with intraventricular hemorrhages (IVH) and white matter damage (West et al. 2011; Wikström et al. 2012; Song et al. 2015; Iyer et al. 2015). The highest number of bursts for a specified time and the lowest interburst intervals, that is, the best electrocortical activity, are sensitive measures when the electrocortical background is discontinuous. Seizures, mainly subclinical, may also be prevalent in infants developing both IVH and periventricular leukomalacia (PVL). As in more mature infants, presence of sleep-wake cycling during the first week of life is usually an indicator of good recovery. However, also extra-cranial factors, such as cardiac output and blood pressure, and carbon dioxide levels seem to affect the aEEG/EEG background in preterm infants.

121.2.1 Seizure Management with aEEG/EEG

Continuous aEEG/EEG-monitoring can be very useful for early detection of seizures in high-risk

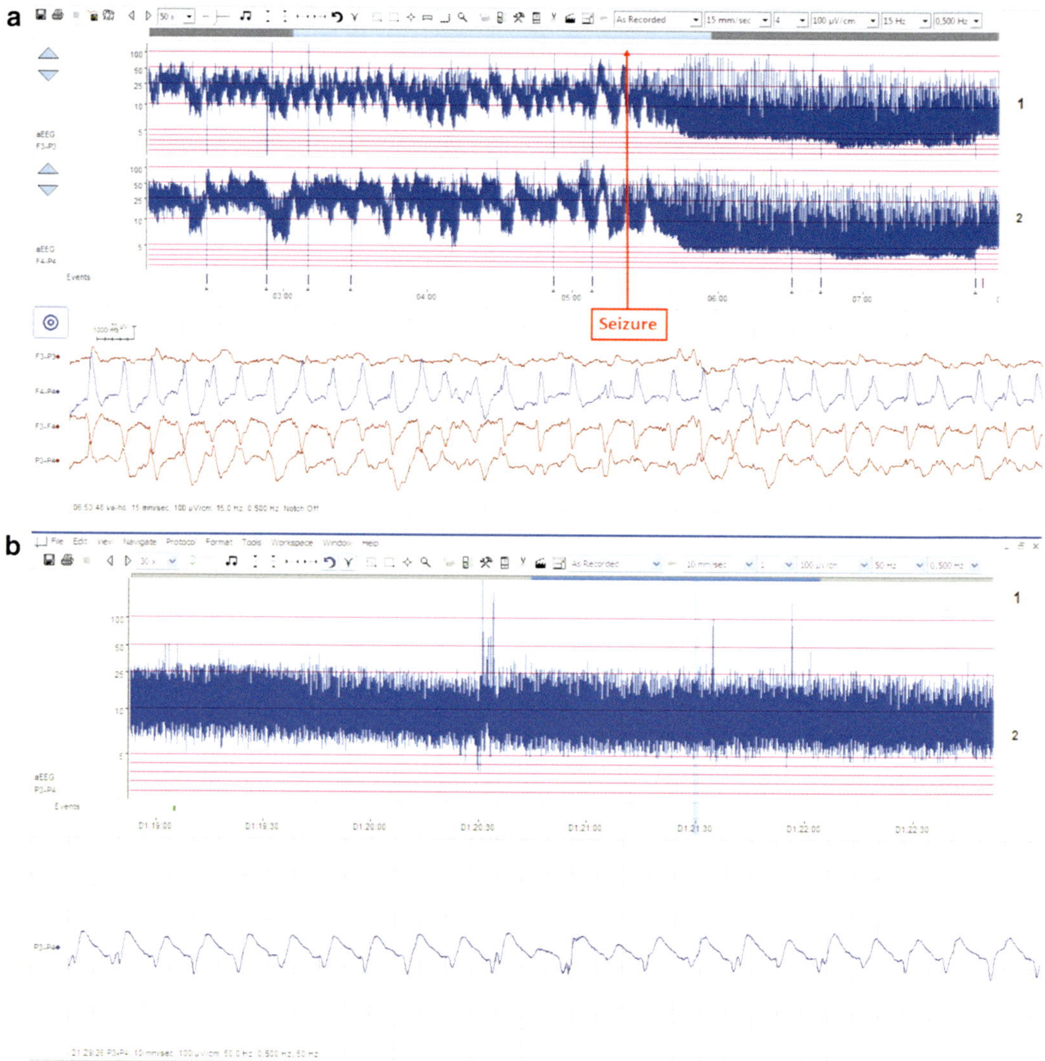

Fig. 4 Subclinical status epileptics in two full-term infants treated with moderate hypothermia for perinatal asphyxia. (**a**) This figure shows 6 h of aEEG and 25 s of EEG and a clearly visible saw-tooth pattern indicating repeated seizures. The seizure pattern disappears after administration of effective antiepileptic treatment, changing the background pattern to discontinuous. The seizure displayed in the EEG started 2 min earlier on the left side (F3-P3), not shown in the EEG but can be seen in the aEEG trace. The seizure activity in the EEG is right-sided and can also be seen in frontal (F3-F4) and parietal (P3-P4) leads. (**b**) A single-channel recording with aEEG duration 4 h, and 38 s of EEG below. The seizures are continuously on-going during the whole aEEG recording, and therefore, there is no saw-tooth pattern in the aEEG. Inspection of the raw EEG should identify the seizures, and a seizure detection alarm would probably also detect the seizures. The aEEG background looks continuous without any variability, but due to the seizures the background activity cannot be assessed

infants. However, the reduced number of EEG electrodes will record fewer seizures than a full EEG. Nevertheless, it has been demonstrated that a single-channel EEG from bilateral central leads, or a two-channel aEEG/EEG, can record around 75–85% of all seizures in a full EEG (Shellhaas and Clancy 2007; Zhang et al. 2011b). A reason for this is that at least 60–70% of neonatal seizures appear in the central, temporal, and parietal areas (Patrizi et al. 2003). A high detection rate of seizures in the aEEG/EEG requires that the full raw EEG is inspected. If just the aEEG trend is inspected, only 20–40% of seizures in the EEG will be detected (Shellhaas et al. 2007). Seizure identification in the aEEG trend requires the electrographic features of the seizure to be clearly distinguishable from the overall background activity since this will produce a transient change (often a rise, rarely a brief decrease) in the aEEG pattern. Repeated seizures and status epilepticus will result in a pattern similar to a saw-tooth, while ongoing epileptic seizure activity may be difficult to distinguish since there is no major change in the aEEG trend (Figs. 1c and 4). Brief seizures (< 30 s) may be very difficult to identify in the compressed aEEG trend, and for this reason it is also important to review the raw-EEG for seizure activity. Some of the newer aEEG/EEG monitors have seizure alerts which can be useful for identification of brief seizures, although no seizure alarms have a 100% sensitivity.

121.3 Conclusions

The EEG and the aEEG/EEG gives clinically important information on brain function and can be used for diagnosing seizures and for evaluation of brain function through assessment of electrocortical background abnormalities. The background activity shortly after an insult is highly predictive of neurological injury and outcome. Metabolic diseases are frequently associated with background abnormalities and seizures (Olischar et al. 2012). For continuous monitoring in the NICU, video-EEG is the gold standard, but this method is not available for daily use in many hospitals. Other EEG trends such as IBI or frequency-based trends may also prove to be of value for evaluation of brain function. When aEEG/EEG is recorded with a reduced number of electrodes, it is necessary to perform repeated EEGs and perform the monitoring in close collaboration with clinical neurophysiologists or neurologists.

References

André M, Lamblin MD, d'Allest AM et al (2010) Electroencephalography in premature and full-term infants. Developmental features and glossary. Neurophysiol Clin 40:59–124

Boylan GB, Rennie JM, Pressler RM, Wilson G, Morton M, Binnie CD (2002) Phenobarbitone, neonatal seizures, and video-EEG. Arch Dis Child Fetal Neonatal Ed 86:F165–F170

Hellström-Westas L, Bell AH, Skov L, Greisen G, Svenningsen NW (1992) Cerebroelectrical depression following surfactant treatment in preterm neonates. Pediatrics 89:643–647

Iyer KK, Roberts JA, Hellström-Westas L et al (2015) Cortical burst dynamics predict clinical outcome early in extremely preterm infants. Brain 138:2206–2218

Jasper HH (1958) The ten-twenty electrode system of the International Federation. Electroencephalogr Clin Neurophysiol 10:371–373

Jiang CM, Yang YH, Chen LQ et al (2015) Early amplitude-integrated EEG monitoring 6 h after birth predicts long-term neurodevelopment of asphyxiated late preterm infants. Eur J Pediatr 174:1043–1052

Marret S, Parain D, Jeannot E et al (1992) Positive rolandic sharp waves in the EEG of the premature newborn: a five year prospective study. Arch Dis Child 67:948–951

Maynard D, Prior PF, Scott DF (1969) Device for continuous monitoring of cerebral activity in resuscitated patients. Br Med J 29:545–546

Menache CC, Bourgeois BF, Volpe JJ (2002) Prognostic value of neonatal discontinuous EEG. Pediatr Neurol 27:93–101

Mizrahi EM, Hrachovy RA, Kellaway P (2004) Atlas of neonatal encephalography, 3rd edn. Lippincott Williams & Wilkins, Philadelphia

Norman E, Wikström S, Rosén I, Fellman V, Hellström-Westas L (2013) Premedication for intubation with morphine causes prolonged depression of electrocortical background activity in preterm infants. Pediatr Res 73:87–94

Okumura A, Hayakawa F, Kato T et al (2002) Developmental outcome and types of chronic-stage EEG abnormalities in preterm infants. Dev Med Child Neurol 44:729–734

Olischar M, Shany E, Aygün C et al (2012) Amplitude-integrated electroencephalography in newborns with inborn errors of metabolism. Neoplasma 102:203–211

Oliveira AJ, Nunes ML, Haertel LM, Reis FM, da Costa JC (2000) Duration of rhythmic EEG patterns in neonates: new evidence for clinical and prognostic significance of brief rhythmic discharges. Clin Neurophysiol 111:1646–1653

Patrizi S, Holmes GL, Orzalesi M, Allemand F (2003) Neonatal seizures: characteristics of EEG ictal activity in preterm and fullterm infants. Brain Dev 25:427–437

Shany E, Benzaquen O, Friger M et al (2008) Influence of antiepileptic drugs on amplitude-integrated electroencephalography. Pediatr Neurol 39:387–391

Shellhaas RA, Clancy RR (2007) Characterization of neonatal seizures by conventional EEG and single-channel EEG. Clin Neurophysiol 118:2156–2161

Shellhaas RA, Soaita AI, Clancy RR (2007) Sensitivity of amplitude-integrated electroencephalography for neonatal seizure detection. Pediatrics 120:770–777

Song J, Xu F, Wang L et al (2015) Early amplitude-integrated electroencephalography predicts brain injury and neurological outcome in very preterm infants. Sci Rep 5:13810

Spitzmiller RE, Phillips T, Meinzen-Derr J, Hoath SB (2007) Amplitude- integrated EEG is useful in predicting neurodevelopmental outcome in full-term infants with hypoxic-ischemic encephalopathy: a meta-analysis. J Child Neurol 22:1069–1078

Thoresen M, Hellström-Westas L, Liu X, de Vries LS (2010) Effect of hypothermia on amplitude-integrated electroencephalogram in infants with asphyxia. Pediatrics 126:e131–e139

Vanhatalo S, Kaila K (2006) Development of neonatal EEG activity: from phenomenology to physiology. Semin Fetal Neonatal Med 11:471–478

Victor S, Appleton RE, Beirne M et al (2005) Spectral analysis of electroencephalography in premature newborn infants: normal ranges. Pediatr Res 57:336–341

Watanabe K, Hayakawa F, Okumura A (1999) Neonatal EEG: a powerful tool in the assessment of brain damage in preterm infants. Brain Dev 21:361–372

West CR, Harding JE, Williams CE, Nolan M, Battin MR (2011) Cot-side electroencephalography for outcome prediction in preterm infants: observational study. Arch Dis Child Fetal Neonatal Ed 96:F108–F113

Wikström S, Pupp IH, Rosén I et al (2012) Early single-channel aEEG/EEG predicts outcome in very preterm infants. Acta Paediatr 101:719–726

Zhang D, Liu Y, Hou X et al (2011a) Reference values for amplitude-integrated EEGs in infants from preterm to 3.5 months of age. Pediatrics 127: e1280–e1287

Zhang L, Zhou YX, Chang LW, Luo XP (2011b) Diagnostic value of amplitude-integrated electroencephalogram in neonatal seizures. Neurosci Bull 27:251–257

Neuroimaging Studies

122

Luca A. Ramenghi and Petra S. Hüppi

Contents

Abstract

Combining different neuroimaging modalities like cranial transfontanellar ultrasound (CUS) and MRI techniques remains the key point to optimize the diagnostic approach to investigate late-preterm and term newborn babies with neurological symptoms. In addition, CUS and MRI are used also to screen very preterm babies at high risk for developing perinatally acquired lesions like hemorrhages (germinal matrix hemorrhage-intraventricular hemorrhage and cerebellar hemorrhage) and hypoxic/inflammatory abnormalities of white matter. CUS can be used in very preterm babies from the first hours of life, while MRI is utilized more often at term equivalent age. Despite the American Academy of Pediatrics recently included "routine MRI a term-corrected age" of very premature babies among the five things not to do, we believe it is nowadays a common prac-

L. A. Ramenghi (✉) · P. S. Hüppi
Division of Neonatology, Giannina Gaslini Children's Hospital, Genoa, Italy
e-mail: lucaramenghi@ospedale-gaslini.ge.it

G. Buonocore et al. (eds.), *Neonatology*,
https://doi.org/10.1007/978-3-319-29489-6_269

tice in the western world NICUs and, perhaps, it is justified practice for a special medicine like neonatal intensive care, a modern medicine always so deeply linked with the most modern research.

Magnetic resonance imaging (MRI) is the modality that allows assessment of the developing brain in great detail because of its resolving power and noninvasiveness. MR techniques are unique in that they provide the best sensitivity in detecting also metabolic and functional information without the use of ionizing radiation. Conventional MRI is therefore now widely used for identifying normal and pathologic brain morphology and giving objective information about the structure of the neonatal brain during development and injury.

122.1 Salient Points

- The combined use of cranial transfontanellar ultrasound (CUS) and magnetic resonance imaging (MRI) is becoming more common in the daily routine of a modern neonatal intensive care unit.
- Initial investigation with CUS in newborn babies born after the 34–35 weeks of gestation and presenting with neurological symptoms is always justified since it can diagnose directly specific pathologies, such as arterial stroke, or it can help identify an intraventricular bleed or a posterior fossa hemorrhage.
- In the case of seizures affecting late preterm and term newborns, MRI is the ideal diagnostic neuroimaging tool.
- MRI is indicated when there is a clinical suspicion of central sinus venous thrombosis, asphyxia, symptomatic hypoglycemia, arterial and venous stroke, and metabolic disorders.
- In preterm babies, both US and MRI should be performed in order to evaluate the presence of germinal matrix-intraventricular hemorrhage, hydrocephalus, pseudocysts, cerebellar hemorrhages, and punctate white matter lesions.
- In very preterm babies, CUS is used for initial screening during the first hours of life followed by a later, more accurate MRI, usually at term-corrected age.

122.2 Introduction

Many years have passed since the introduction of cranial transfontanellar ultrasound (CUS) to diagnose acquired brain lesions in neonates. CUS remains an important technique in the daily practice of neonatal units, but major improvements have been obtained by combining different imaging modalities. Magnetic resonance imaging (MRI) is the modality that allows assessment of the developing brain in great detail because of its resolving power and noninvasiveness. MR techniques are unique in that they provide not only detailed structural but also metabolic and functional information without the use of ionizing radiation. Conventional MRI is therefore now widely used for identifying normal and pathologic brain morphology and giving objective information about the structure of the neonatal brain during injury and the following developmental phase.

Technical advances in MRI have revealed hitherto unknown aspects of brain development and have characterized patterns of injury to the developing brain. Fast diffusion-weighted imaging has provided understanding about brain white matter (WM) connectivity in health and disease. It also allows correlation of the structural development of the brain with the functional development of the child, even in the absence of overt brain lesions. This technique, together with new image postprocessing tools to assess quantitative brain volume and surface changes, has produced more accurate neuroimaging correlates for later neurocognitive disorders.

MR spectroscopy has also provided new insights into metabolic processes in response to acute and chronic brain injury. Functional MR imaging, although still limited in the newborn, has the potential to throw light on the early functional organization of the brain and the origins of sensory, motor, and cognitive functions in the newborn (Ramenghi and Hüppi 2009; Ramenghi et al. 2005).

122.3 The Combined Use of Cranial Transfontanellar Ultrasound and Magnetic Resonance Imaging

The combined use of cranial transfontanellar ultrasound (CUS) and magnetic resonance imaging (MRI) is progressively more common in the daily life of a modern neonatal intensive care unit. Timing of use of both techniques tends to be different in cases of term and late-preterm babies in which we need to investigate the nature of a symptoms (encephalopathy) compared to very preterm babies when we aim to screen babies in order to exclude the presence of typical lesions of prematurity (intraventricular-cerebellar hemorrhage and white matter lesions). In the encephalopathic late-preterm or term babies, both techniques should be used very soon, at the same time of the arousal of symptoms, compared to very preterm babies in which CUS is used for the initial screening from the first hours of life followed by a later, more accurate MRI, usually at term-corrected age.

Improving the knowledge and the clinical skills of neonatologists to identify newborn babies suspected for an underlying neurological abnormality remains very important. Efforts to categorize babies are also really justified (Ramenghi and Hüppi 2009; Ramenghi et al. 2005). Accordingly, a clear definition of encephalopathy in the newborn age helps to recognize those babies at higher risks. Neonatal encephalopathy is a clinical syndrome of disordered neurological function occurring in the first days of life in term-born and late-preterm neonates and is characterized by difficulty initiating and maintaining respiration, an abnormal level of consciousness, depression of tone and reflex responses, and often seizures. This symptom complex affects about 3–5 in every 1000 births and is an important predictor of perinatal death and a major contributor to long-term adverse neurological outcomes, particularly cerebral palsy. The presence of seizures gives more often a feeling of real emergency. Accordingly, we believe that an encephalopathic baby even with a normal CUS should undergo MRI as soon as possible for a number of reasons. First of all, we believe it is mandatory to exclude the presence of the very rare but underdiagnosed cerebral sinus venous thrombosis (CSVT) which is amenable to treatment that, unique condition in perinatal medicine, can otherwise move to a further and more severe development of the lesion (propagation). This suspicion of CSVT is even more plausible in case there is a thalamic hemorrhage in a term baby or a late-appearing intraventricular hemorrhage in a late-preterm baby at CUS; in these cases chances to diagnose venous thrombosis are extremely high (Fig. 1). Many other conditions showing encephalopathy at birth will benefit of this combined use of CUS-MRI for cases of congenital (malformations, infections like CMV, etc.) and acquired lesions (arterial stroke, hypoglycemia, etc.).

In the very preterm baby, CUS remains a corner point of the neuroimaging screening as in the first days of life, it is crucial to exclude the presence of intraventricular and cerebellar hemorrhage, while in the following days and weeks, CUS is used to diagnose white matter lesions. MRI, often performed at term-equivalent age, discloses more subtle hemorrhagic and white matter lesions and also the so-called incidental findings (Parodi et al. 2015a, 2015b; Malova and Rossi 2017).

The skills to perform an ultrasound examination are still in the hands of neonatologists and more rarely of radiologists; more and more often neonatologists deeply interact with neuroradiologists who perform magnetic resonance imaging (MRI). Many neuroradiologists are nowadays fully skilled not only to adjust MRI sequence for the neonatal brain with higher content of water but also to interpret not only images but also those key points in the perinatal history of the baby, crucial to understand the nature of acquired perinatal lesions. The role of neonatologists remains fundamental in sensitizing neuroradiologists to the changing world (i.e., incidence of certain pathologies, latest hypothesis on pathogenesis) of perinatally acquired lesions of neonates, while neuroradiologists remain magisterial experts in recognizing and studying malformations and the effects of the lesions in the developing brain.

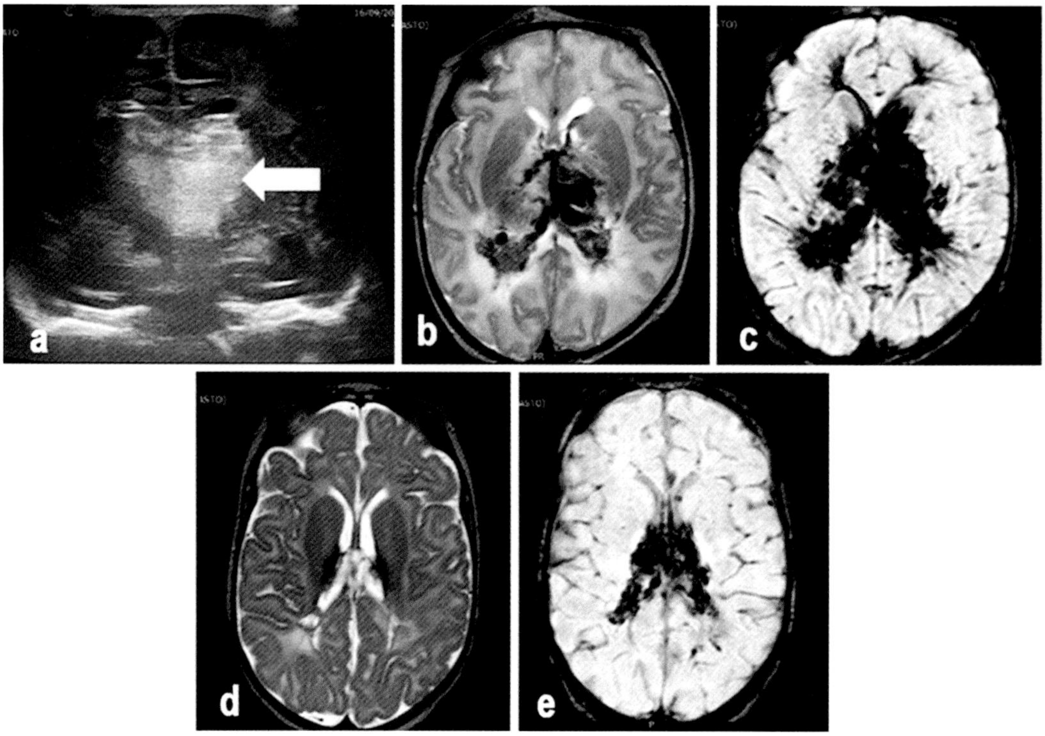

Fig. 1 Term baby with clonic seizures at day 6 of life. (**a**) CUS showing what we would name intraventricular and thalamic hemorrhage, more obvious on the left (arrow). (**b**) and (**c**) are T2 and SWI sequence at day 6 confirming the important presence of a bleed. (**d**) and (**e**) are T2 and SWI sequences showing at 29 days of life and almost complete resolution. The baby was started on e.v. heparin for a week and LMWH up to 3 months of life

122.4 Ultrasound

Initial investigation with CUS in newborn babies born after the 34–35 weeks of gestation and presenting neurological symptoms is always justified. The likelihood of CUS showing a perinatally acquired brain lesion in late-preterm and term babies is not high, especially during the acute phase of the disease. CUS can diagnose directly specific pathology like an arterial stroke if the lesion is large, or it can help to identify a brain lesion caused by underlying disease, such as an intraventricular bleed or a posterior fossa hemorrhage caused by traumatic birth or by venous thrombosis. The value of CUS during the acute phase of a hypoxic-ischemic encephalopathy is limited since it relies on the exclusion of other lesions which may mimic the clinical features of asphyxia (i.e., malformations, major subarachnoid or subdural hemorrhages, and, more rarely, stroke). CUS is also useful for the identification of severe basal ganglia lesions that become visible only a few days after the asphyxic event (Ramenghi and Hüppi 2009; Ramenghi et al. 2005) (Fig. 2).

122.5 The Role of MRI in the Symptomatic Late-Preterm or Term Newborn Baby

Seizure is a striking clinical feature of the neurologically abnormal neonate. It is useful to differentiate fitting babies born with normal Apgar scores from those who are born in a very depressed state because of perinatal asphyxia. The most common causes in the non-asphyxic group are focal brain injury due to arterial infarction and also hemorrhages. In addition, neonatal

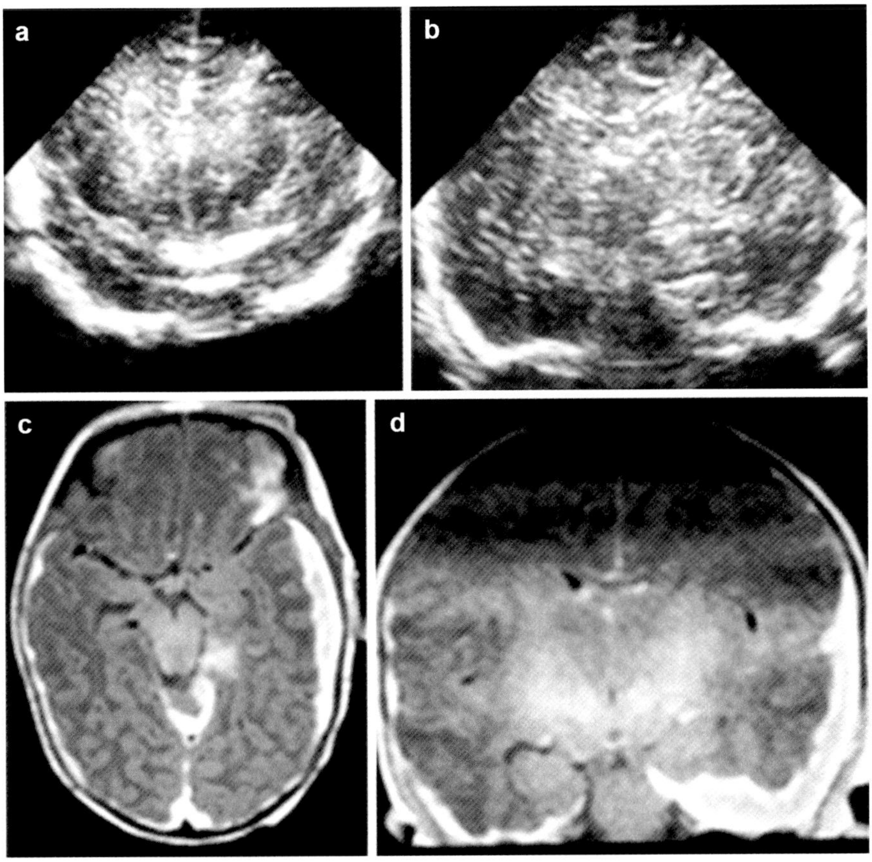

Fig. 2 A term baby born after ventouse application and mimicking perinatal asphyxia syndrome, with acidosis at birth and seizures at 6 h of life: CUS coronal scans (**a**, **b**), MR axial T1 (**c**), and coronal T1 (**d**) scans. Neuroimaging was performed at 24 h of life. CUS showed midline shift and left increased echogenicity, highly suspicious for arterial infarction. MRI clearly showed a subarachnoid hemorrhage probably related to dystocia. At 5 years of age, the baby was neurologically normal (Fig. 3)

seizures may be caused by central nervous system infections, transient metabolic disturbances like hypoglycemia, congenital abnormalities of the brain including those due to chromosomal anomalies, cytomegalovirus infection, inborn errors of metabolism, and benign neonatal convulsions, which may be familial or non-familial, and detailed neuroimaging is an important tool in the diagnostic work-up. Brain malformations range from highly localized focal dysplasia not diagnosable by CUS to catastrophic defects, which are partially diagnosable by CUS.

In all instances of seizures in later preterm and term newborns, MRI is the ideal diagnostic neuroimaging tool. A clinical diagnosis has to rely on a careful medical history and on consideration of the most likely causes, for instance, if seizures occur unexpectedly in a perfectly normal newborn, stroke and hemorrhage have to be the first disorders to be excluded together with CSVT (Ramenghi and Hüppi 2009; Ramenghi et al. 2005; Govaert et al. 2009; Rutherford et al. 2012; Ramenghi et al. 2009).

122.5.1 Arterial and Venous Neonatal Stroke

Perinatal stroke is an area of damaged cerebral tissue resulting either from disruption to blood flow in a major cerebral artery from thrombosis or embolism or from thrombosis in a major cerebral vein (cerebral sinus venous thrombosis,

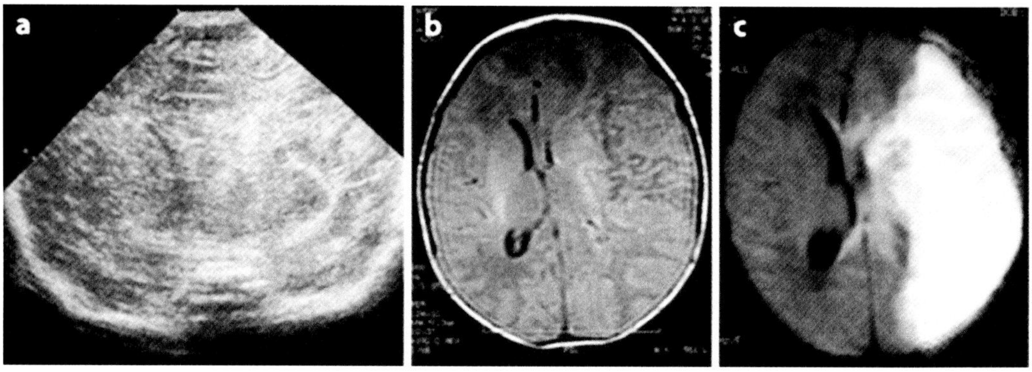

Fig. 3 A large perinatal arterial infarct of the left middle cerebral artery is shown on all the scans: (**a**) CUS with area of increased echogenicity, (**b**) conventional MR axial T1 scan with evident midline shift and (**c**) even better from the huge area of restriction (*white*) at DWI. The baby was macrosomic, born by vaginal delivery and depressed at birth needing resuscitation and mechanical ventilation for few hours

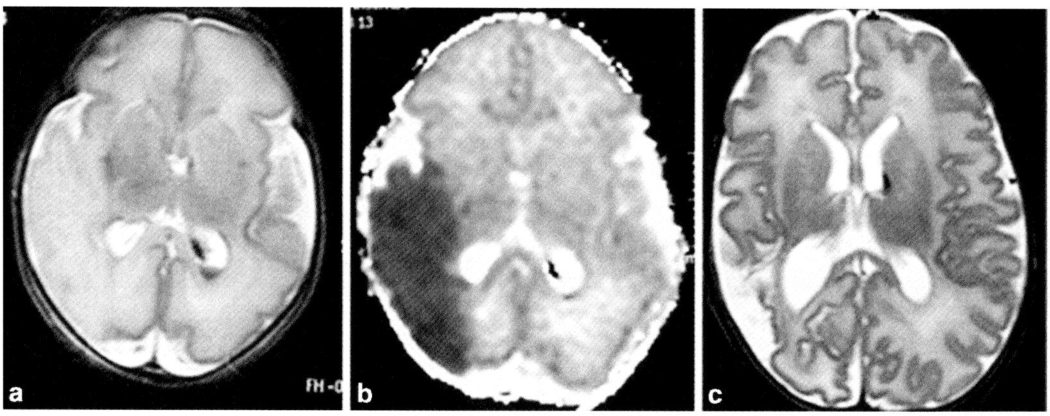

Fig. 4 A 30-week preterm baby showing at 4 days of life abnormal neuroimaging by MR axial T2 scan (**a**) and MR axial ADC map (**b**), highly suggestive of a right arterial infarct: loss of cortical details on T2, more obvious reduction in apparent diffusion coefficient values. At term equivalence MR axial T2 scan (**c**) showed that the resulting infarcted area was smaller. At 2 years of age, the child was treated for recurrent seizures but 18 months later was off medications. At 5 years of age, the child presented with a left hemiplegia and good independent walking

CSVT), which occurs between 20 weeks of fetal life and the 28th postnatal day, and confirmed by neuroimaging or neuropathologic studies. An acute neurological syndrome is not essential for the diagnosis of neonatal stroke (Govaert et al. 2009; Rutherford et al. 2012; Ramenghi et al. 2009) (Fig. 3). As a bedside method, CUS is useful when it may show areas of asymmetrical echogenicity, usually during the first 12–36 h following the onset of seizures. Nevertheless, MRI is the standard neuroimaging tool for the diagnosis of neonatal stroke. Conventional MRI shows loss of cortico-subcortical differentiation in both T1- and T2-weighted imaging. This is due to increased T2 signal intensity in the edematous cortex, which approaches the signal intensity of the unmyelinated white matter. This is also called the disappeared cortex sign (Fig. 4).

The best modality to identify a focal ischemic infarct is diffusion-weighted imaging (DWI). DWI shows a striking reduction of water molecule movement (Fig. 3), corresponding to a decrease in the apparent diffusion coefficient (ADC) in the acute phase. There is normalization by 6–10 days followed by tissue dissolution, which results in a porencephalic cyst with T2 characteristics of cerebrospinal fluid (CSF). Areas of decreased values can be observed acutely, even a few hours after the beginning of a stroke, when conventional MR imaging remains normal until at least day 4 (Govaert et al. 2009; Rutherford et al. 2012; Ramenghi et al. 2009). The cavitational phase of the infarction is recognizable using all techniques, and it occurs at a variable time after the initial insult. The pattern of signal intensity changes seems to be remarkably consistent among patients, suggesting that perinatal arterial ischemic stroke in symptomatic term infants occurs within a very limited timeframe around birth (Cowan et al. 1994; Bouza et al. 1994; D'Arceuil et al. 1998; Tuor et al. 1998; Dudnik et al. 2009).

The majority of these focal lesions affect term babies and seem to be less common after birth by cesarean section performed in the absence of labor (Cheong and Cowan 2009). Premature infants seem to be less vulnerable to this disease, although the incidence has been reported as particularly high in certain studies (Benders et al. 2007) not confirmed by other authors.

122.5.1.1 Cerebral Sinus Venous Thrombosis (CSVT)

A spectrum of neurological signs, appearing early, within 48 h of birth, or later, has been described. An early presentation may be confounded by many other comorbidities (maternal preeclampsia/hypertension, fetal distress) and acute illness (asphyxia, respiratory problems), whereas a later presentation is more often associated with neurological symptoms such as seizures, lethargy, apnea, and poor feeding. An acute illness, e.g., dehydration, may also be associated with delayed presentation. Seizures occur in about two thirds of cases and can be subtle, focal, or generalized, irrespective of time of presentation. The diversity in clinical presentation may derive from a different velocity in clot formation, known to be a slow process in adults. Part of the beauty and the challenge of such a disease rely on the correlation of symptoms with clot formation. A venous clot, fully developed, will induce occlusion of cerebral venous vessels and a consequent rise in cerebral venous pressure. The velocity with which venous vessels become occluded is likely to play a role in modulating the intensity of symptoms; a sudden and severe occlusion may be more readily related to a clear change in the clinical scenario. The increased intracranial pressure can be diffuse or regional in the territory drained by the thrombosed veins. Local tissue pressure elevation can result in permanent insult causing tissue infarction results from a persistent regional increase of the venous pressure exceeding the regional arterial perfusion pressure. Such reduction of local perfusion impairment adds an ischemic arterial insult to the primary venous event. Almost all instances of infarction due to sinus thrombosis are of hemorrhagic nature (red infarction, ramollissement rouge) (Ramenghi et al. 2009).

The most fascinating aspect of this disease remains the possibility to receive anticoagulation therapy. Despite anticoagulation is controversial, the very convincing rationale is to stop thrombus extension at first and recurrence, to favor and accelerate spontaneous thrombus resolution, and to prevent further brain damage due to the potential progression into hemorrhagic infarction. There are no randomized clinical trials in neonates and children, and it will remain very difficult to run such studies in this heterogeneous groups of patients. Of course the risk of heparin-induced intracerebral hemorrhage has to be weighed against the risk of hemorrhage caused by progressive thrombosis. Despite evidence-based clinical practice guidelines on antithrombotic therapy in neonates suggest its use in CSVT without significant intracranial hemorrhage, the word "significant" remains very enigmatic and ambiguous. When anticoagulation is undertaken, initially it should be performed with unfractionated heparin and subsequently with LMWH for a minimum of 6 weeks and no longer than 3 months. It is very tempting to stop the thrombus even in case of the presence of a hemorrhage such as in the case shown in Fig. 1. We recommend to perform a control MRI 2 or 3 days after the beginning of anticoagulation therapy especially if this treatment was initiated when a hemorrhage accompanied the diagnosis of cerebral sinus venous thrombosis in late-preterm and term newborn infants. More cautiousness should be used in starting anticoagulation in premature infants more prone to develop hemorrhage. We confirm that a late-preterm baby with an expectedly late GMH-IVH appearance should indicate the possible presence of CSVT (Fig. 9) (Ramenghi et al. 2002).

122.5.2 Asphyxia

Although antenatal factors have been implicated in the etiology of hypoxic-ischemic encephalopathy (HIE), evidence of antenatal injury (i.e., isolated white matter lesions) is rarely seen on early MRI scans in neonates who present with HIE. MRI remains the best technique to detect perinatally acquired cerebral lesions, and the pattern and severity of the lesions are a reliable guide to prognosis. In the presence of a sentinel event consistent with a severe acute hypoxic-ischemic insult, lesions in the basal ganglia and thalami can be associated with abnormalities in specific cortical regions and in the adjacent subcortical white matter. Abnormal signal intensity in the posterior limb of the internal capsule coexists with lesions in the basal ganglia and thalami (BGT) and is a powerful predictor of abnormal motor outcome (Fig. 5). Moderate and severe lesions in the basal ganglia and thalami and severe white matter lesions are associated with cerebral palsy

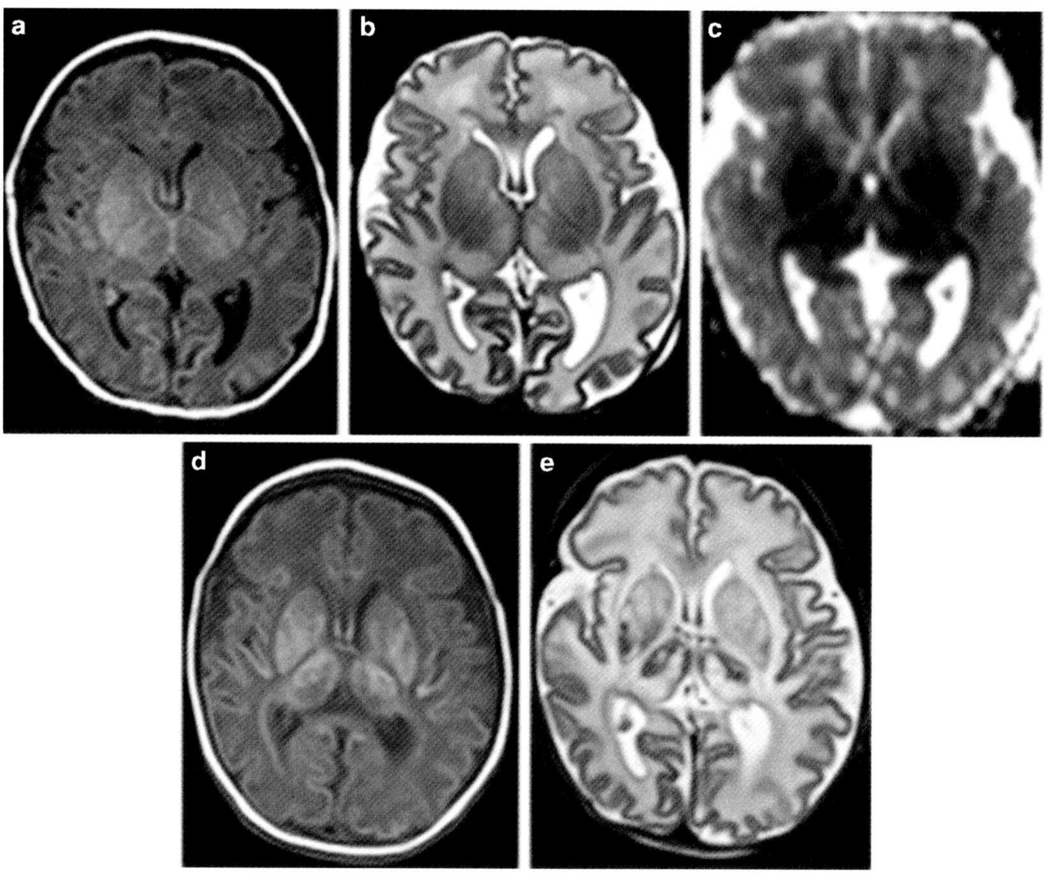

Fig. 5 A severe asphyxiated baby born by emergency cesarean section due to maternal rupture of the uterus. (**a–c**) MR axial T1 and T2 scans and ADC map. There is a markedly abnormal reduction in ADC values at the level of all basal ganglia and thalami on day 4 of life after being treated with hypothermia. (**d–e**) MR axial T1 and T2 scans. Two weeks later, the severity of lesions at the basal ganglia and thalami is obvious. At 15 months, the baby developed severe developmental delay and epilepsy (West syndrome)

(Rutherford et al. 1998). In approximately 50% of neonates with BGT lesions, there will be more extensive WM abnormalities. The motor outcome for these children is still dictated by the BGT lesions, but WM involvement may exacerbate any cognitive deficit. However, infants with severe BGT lesions have severe cognitive impairment regardless of the severity of additional WM involvement. Later there is often white matter atrophy due to the original lesions in the basal ganglia.

DWI seems to underestimate the severity of brain lesions during perinatal asphyxia at early scans, particularly at the level of basal ganglia. Nevertheless, if DWI of the basal ganglia is abnormal, the developing lesions are very likely to be severe, like in the shown case (Fig. 5).

The ability of MRI to predict neurological outcomes up to 18 months of age in babies who have undergone therapeutic hypothermia seems to be unaffected. In a large cohort of infants who had an MRI after HIE and had previously undergone hypothermia, there were no unusual patterns of lesions and no increase in hemorrhagic or thrombotic lesions (Rutherford et al. 2010a). A common question concerns the optimal timing of an MRI in perinatal asphyxia. The answer relates to the reason for the scan. If it is being done for a differential diagnosis (Fig. 2), the scan should be done as soon as possible. On the other hand, if the MRI is being done to predict prognosis, it is better to wait until the 7–10 days of life. A repeat scan is particularly useful in the case of an asphyxiated baby born before the 37th week of gestation to look at the posterior limb of internal capsule (PLIC), which is such an important marker of the normal development.

Proton magnetic resonance spectroscopy (^{1}H–MRS) permits the noninvasive study of metabolic alterations in the brain tissue. It is trying also to enter the clinical arena of MR techniques used routinely for the evaluation of the brain. When oxidative phosphorylation is impaired, energy metabolism follows the alternative route of anaerobic glycolysis and produces lactic acid. Lactate has a chemical shift of 1.3 ppm and presents as a doublet peak in the in vivo ^{1}H–MRS due to coupling effects. Groenendal et al. (1994) first described markedly elevated lactate levels in five infants with severe perinatal asphyxia. Early spectroscopy (<18 h after the event) and measurement of high Lac/Cr ratios in 1H–MRS correlate well with neurodevelopment at 1 year (Hanrahan et al. 1999). MRS performed in the first 24 h after an insult is sensitive to the presence of hypoxic-ischemic brain injury in the specific regions of interest (i.e., thalami) and seems to be suitable for the detection of brain injury on the first day when conventional MR imaging and DWI might not yet detect the injury (Fig. 6) (Hüppi 2001).

122.5.3 Hypoglycemia

Unexpected neurological signs may be due to hypoglycemia (Parodi et al. 2015a). An MRI brain scan is justified in the case of symptomatic hypoglycemia even in the absence of abnormalities at CUS. Infarction following hypoglycemia has been reported in the newborn, and specific imaging patterns have been attributed to neonatal hypoglycemic injury (Ramenghi and Hüppi 2009), e.g., bilateral, fairly symmetrical evidence of injury to the occipital and posterior parietal cortices and underlying white matter. The cortical ribbon may be lost on T2 as well as T1 MRI, and there may be infarction with subsequent cavitation. Injury beyond the area covered by the posterior cerebral artery is too extensive to be classified as watershed, but the appearance on imaging is similar. The lesion should not be regarded as a stroke (Fig. 7). Another less frequent post-hypoglycemic paradigm is unilateral complete hemispheric neocortical necrosis. The most frequent abnormalities affect occipital white matter and cortex, although there can be other lesions mimicking asphyxia and there is an overlap of symptoms between perinatal asphyxia and hypoglycemia (Burns et al. 2008).

122.5.4 Metabolic Disorders

Occasionally infants with an apparent global hypoxic-ischemic injury have a metabolic disorder which either masquerades as an acute insult or coexists with one. This is important to recognize

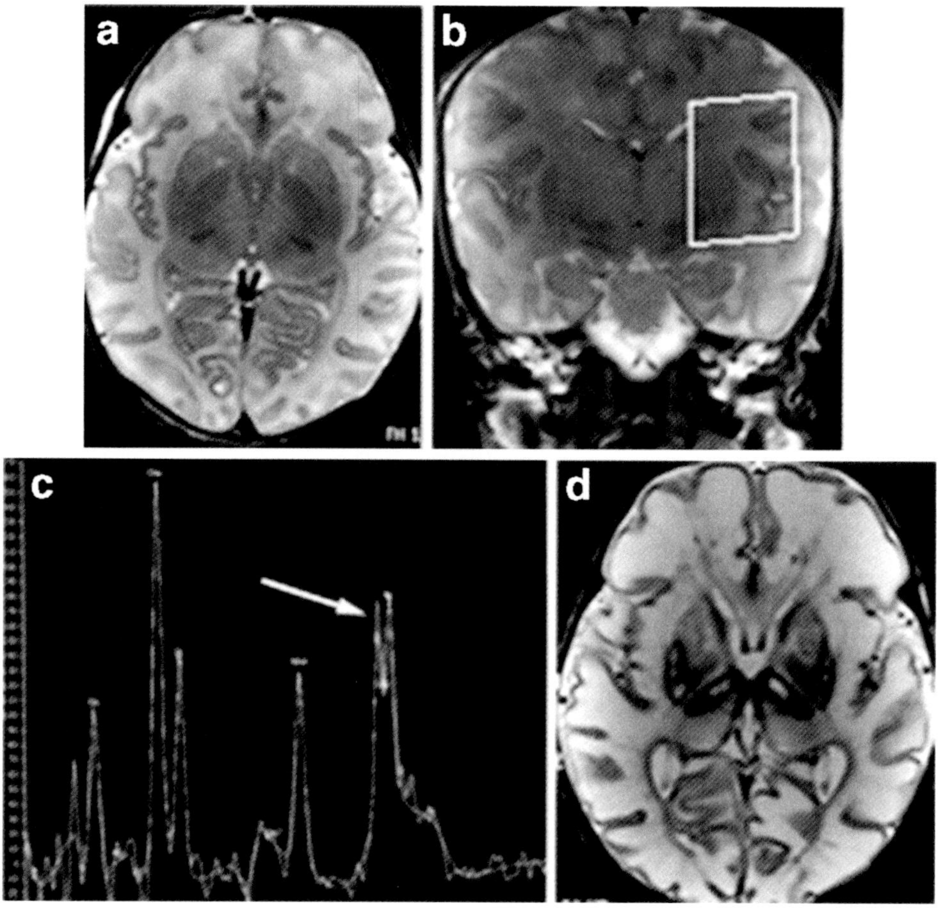

Fig. 6 A very severely asphyxiated baby with early scan at 36 h of life. MR axial and coronal T2 scans (**a**, **b**) show uncertain signs at this stage (diffuse increased signal), while MR spectroscopy (**c**) in the region of interest (highlighted) shows a severely abnormal peak of lactate (*arrow*). Three weeks later, an axial T2 scan (**d**) showed dramatic evolution in a pre-multicystic encephalomalacia damage. The baby was born by emergency cesarean section following severe abruptio placentae

because the implications for allegations of medical negligence and for genetic counseling are considerable. Conventional MRI is able to identify brain malformations that may accompany some metabolic disorders, such as callosal agenesis in nonketotic hyperglycinemia or cortical migration defects in peroxisomal disorders such as Zellweger's syndrome (Ramenghi and Hüppi 2009). White matter in these infants may have long T1 and long T2 times, and this may be reflected in increased ADC values (Tanner et al. 2000). Occasionally the results from DWI are more informative. In infants with maple syrup urine disease, DWI is pathognomonic, showing actively myelinating areas (Fig. 8) (Righini et al. 2003). DWI may also allow differentiation between cytotoxic (reduced ADC) and vasogenic (increased ADC) edema. However, areas showing reduced ADC values may normalize with treatment, and therefore DWI has the potential to be used to monitor therapy. Reversible ADC reduction has also been documented in other metabolic conditions such as hypoglycemia and hypernatremia (Righini et al. 2005). A suspicious pattern of diffusion should alert the clinician to the possibility of a metabolic disorder. Abnormalities, e.g., affecting the cerebral peduncles and internal capsule, may mimic those found with more

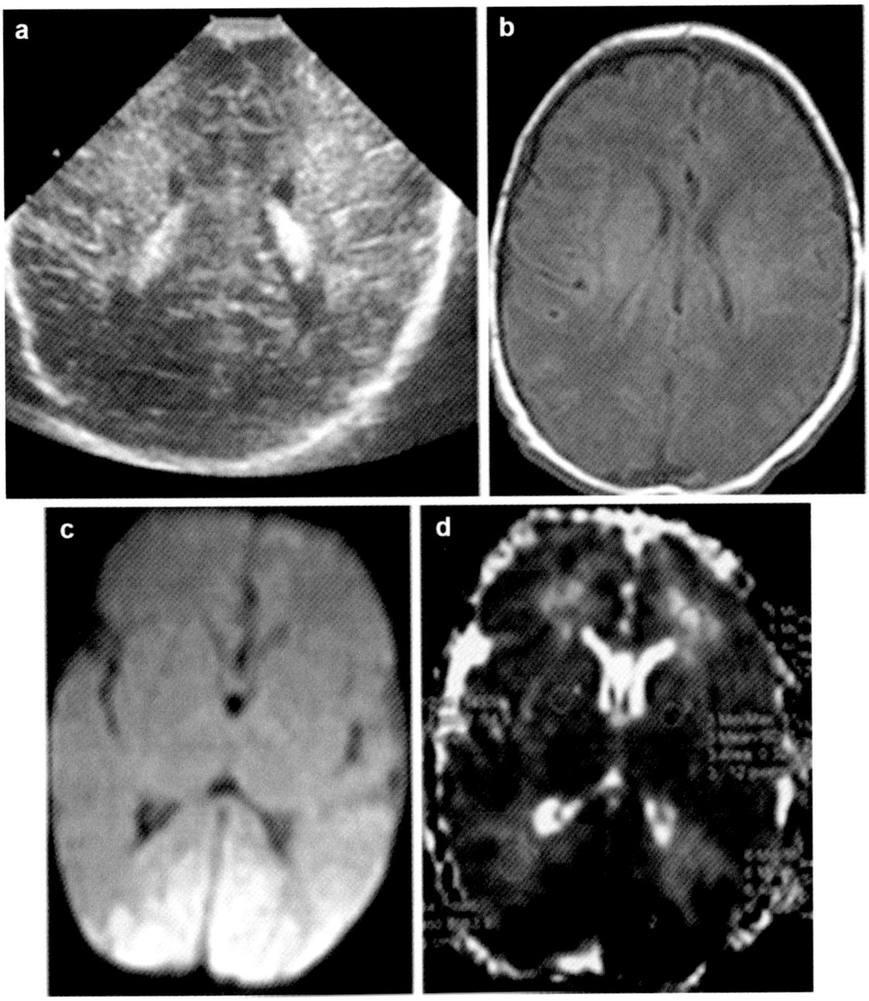

Fig. 7 Neuroimaging performed 2 h after the onset of a severe hypoglycemic event: coronal CUS (**a**) and MR axial T1 (**b**) scans showed no obvious abnormality, which was different to MR axial DWI (**c**) and the axial ADC map (**d**), which showed respectively reduction and pathologically low ADC values in the posterior areas of the brain

straightforward HIE, and an underlying metabolic disorder may be missed. This is particularly likely if a neonate dies in the first few days, as the characteristic clinical evolution of the metabolic disorder has not yet developed. This emphasizes further the need to investigate fully any infant presenting with neonatal seizures, not only by a careful history and examination but also with metabolic investigations and neuroimaging. The latter should be MRI and include DWI and 1H–MRS if possible. If an infant dies before imaging is possible, postmortem MRI should be considered as an adjunct to autopsy, especially if the parents are unlikely to agree to a conventional postmortem examination (Fig. 9).

122.6 Imaging the Preterm Newborn Brain

Several different aspects have to be considered when considering brain lesions affecting the developing brain of premature babies, particularly very premature babies, like the different developmental stages and vulnerability for injury. Typical brain lesions less frequently affect the relatively

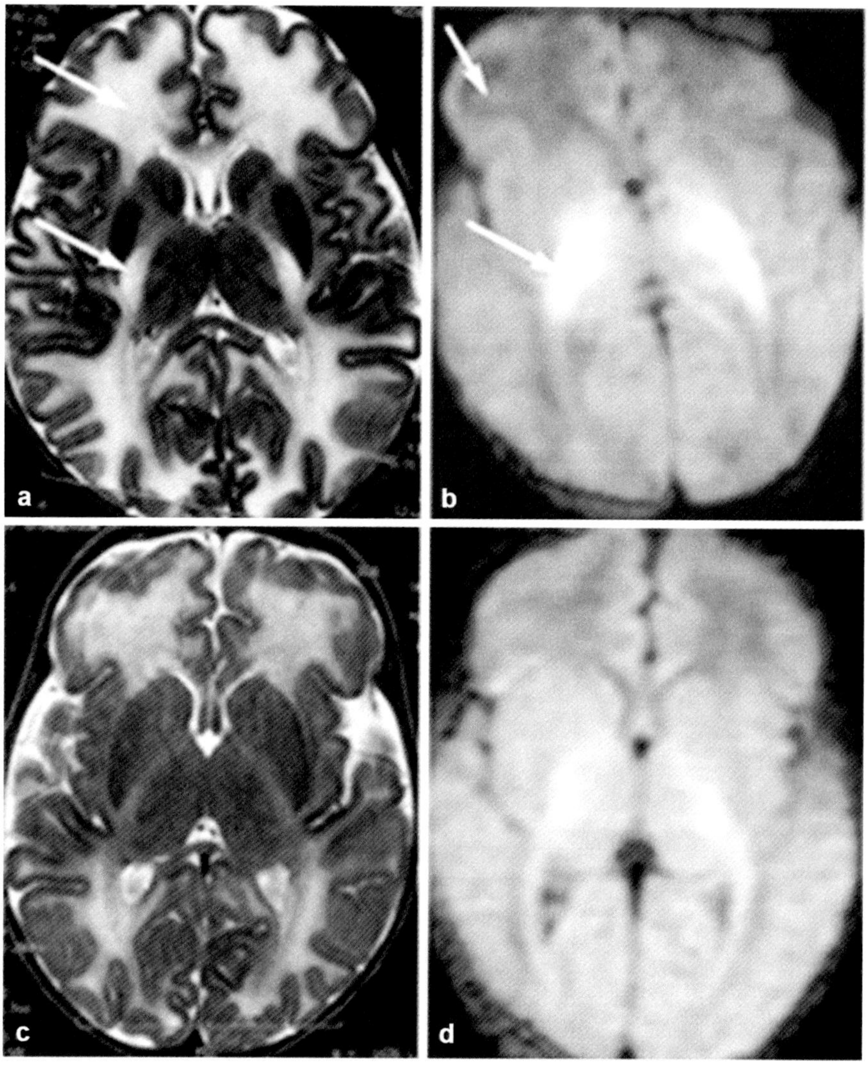

Fig. 8 A baby with maple syrup urine disease showing at the first MR (**a**, **b**) severe abnormalities of the signal (arrows). On axial T2 scan (**a**) increased signal (arrows) in the frontal white matter and at the level of posterior limbs of internal capsule (PLIC) are observed. Interestingly the DWI scan (**b**) shows a completely different pathogenesis; PLIC are represented by a restriction signal on DWI, signs of reduced movements of water molecules, while in the frontal areas DWI shows an opposite signal (increased water molecules movement) very likely expression of vasogenic oedema. **c**, **d** A week after renal dyalisis performed to reduce the amount of the toxic levels of leucine a dramatic improvement of the signal abnormalities is observed

large number of late-preterm babies and are much more frequent in the extremely low birth weight (ELBW) babies, who are fewer in number but very vulnerable (Ramenghi et al. 2005). In the late-preterm group, brain injury comprises multiple lesions, principally germinal matrix intraventricular hemorrhage, venous hemorrhagic infarction, posthemorrhagic hydrocephalus, periventricular leukomalacia, and cerebellar lesions although in these babies symptoms may guide in the timing of neuroimaging. However, many preterm infants have neurodevelopmental delay without having been diagnosed with any of these typical perinatal brain injuries. In these babies, abnormal development of the brain is possible even in the absence of common brain lesions (i.e., there may

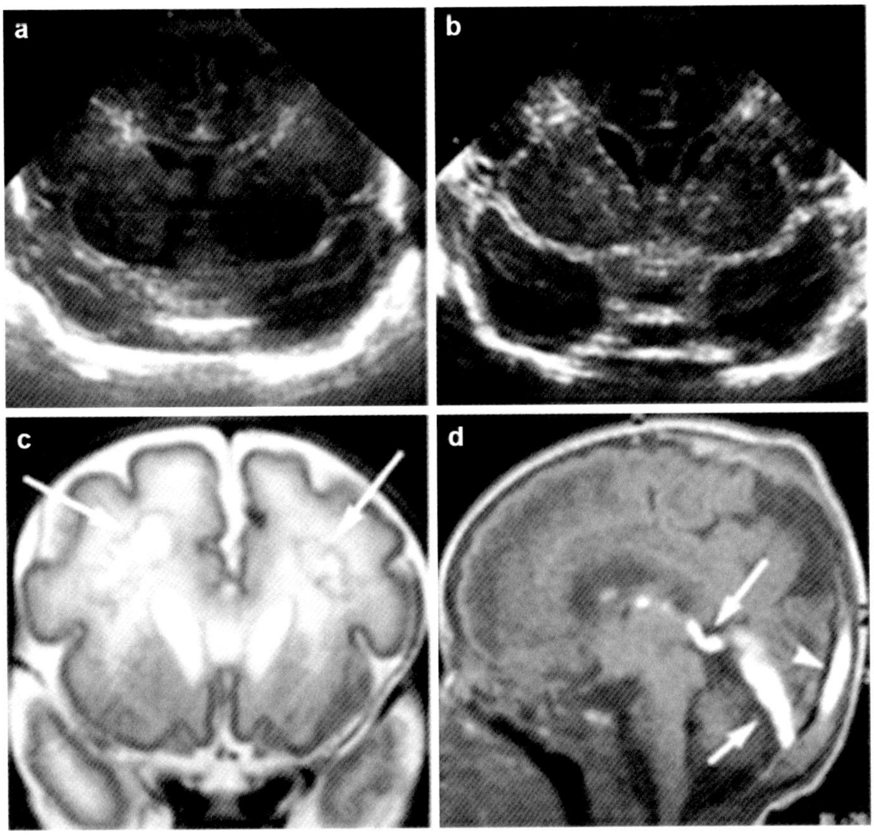

Fig. 9 CUS and MR scans at different times in a 35-week baby. The first US scan at 4 days of life (**a**) shows normal periventricular echogenicity, progressively increasing at day 9 (**b**). Later, MR T2 scans at 3 weeks of age show (**c**) cavitations in periventricular area (*arrows*) and (**d**) thrombi in the deep venous system (*arrows*) and partially in the sagittal sinus (*arrowhead*)

be loss of WM, even in the absence of periventricular leukomalacia). Early exposure to a challenging postnatal environment and removal from a protective milieu are factors that interfere profoundly with normal development, especially in the most vulnerable babies (Ment et al. 2009; Volpe 2009).

122.6.1 Specific Lesions in the most Premature Babies

122.6.1.1 Germinal Matrix-Intraventricular Hemorrhage (GMH-IVH)

The lower the gestational age, the higher the risk of developing germinal matrix-intraventricular hemorrhage (GMH-IVH), which is the most frequent cause of intracranial hemorrhage in the neonate (Sannia et al.). Ultrasound is now accepted as the primary modality for the diagnosis of GMH-IVH, and there have been full descriptions of the ultrasonic findings. GMH is seen as an area of intense increased echogenicity beneath the floor of the lateral ventricle, just anterior to the caudothalamic notch. The abnormality should be seen in two planes and should be distinguished from other normal echogenic structures, such as the normal choroid plexus. Larger hemorrhages may rupture into the lateral ventricle and, when acute, appear as an echogenic clot within the ventricle which may distend the ventricular lumen.

The most commonly used grading system for GMH-IVH was first reported by Papile et al., who

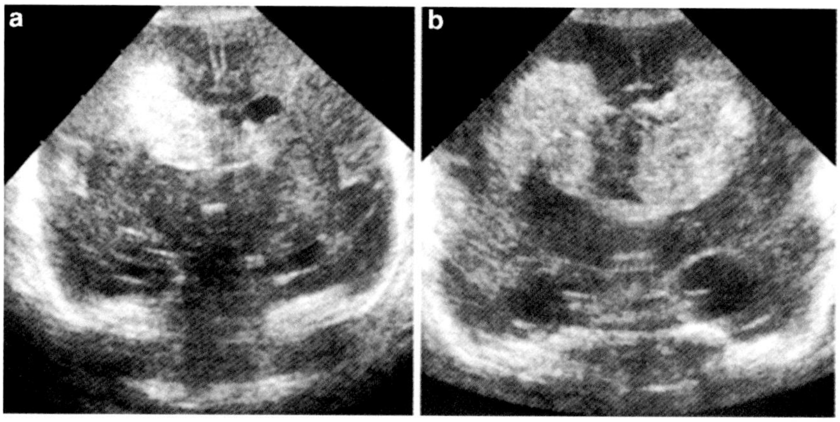

Fig. 10 CUS coronal scans. (**a**) A 24-week baby scanned at 8 h of life and showing severe intraventricular hemorrhage on the right with adjacent venous infarct. (**b**) The same baby scanned 12 h later showing a further deterioration with a bilateral intraventricular hemorrhage and very rare double venous infarct. The baby died aged 36 h

classified hemorrhages into grades from I to IV. Grade III–IV GMH-IVH is known to be associated with adverse neurodevelopmental outcomes, including cerebral palsy and cognitive impairment. Interestingly, previous studies investigating the effects of grade I–II GMH-IVH (also referred to as low-grade GMHIVH) on neurodevelopment showed conflicting results. Conversely, more recent studies demonstrated that even low-grade GMH-IVH can determine a significant impact on neurodevelopmental outcome of preterm infants.

The appearance of GMH-IVH and venous infarction change with time (Fig. 10). GMHs resolve leaving a small subependymal cyst or a linear echodense line. The margins of a clot within the lateral ventricles remain echogenic, while the more central region gradually becomes increasingly echopoor and smaller until the hemorrhage finally resolves by approximately 12 weeks of age.

We mentioned already that several grading systems have been proposed to classify GMH-IVH. The majority are based on the extent of bleeding into the germinal matrix and lateral ventricle, the development of venous infarction, and the presence of ventricular dilatation.

The accuracy of ultrasound imaging in the diagnosis of GMH-IVH depends on the level of severity, and concerns arise for minor degrees. The use of susceptibility-weighted imaging (SWI) has allowed major precision in comparing CUS with MRI data. SWI is a recently developed MRI sequence and is based on high-resolution, three-dimensional, fully velocity-compensated gradient-echo sequences using both magnitude and phase images (Parodi et al. 2015a; Parodi and Rossi 2015b). SWI is very sensitive to detect magnetic susceptibility changes in tissues such as blood, iron, and calcification. Moreover, it has been shown to be more sensitive than conventional gradient-echo sequence or CT in detecting small-sized cerebral hemorrhages.

We have recently shown that CUS sensitivity in detecting grade I–II GMH-IVH proved surprisingly low, in contrast with specificity when compared to SWI-MRI technique (Fig. 11). We think that low-grade GMH-IVH may be underdiagnosed in VLBW infants when assessed with CUS exclusively.

The role and potential prognostic meaning of minor forms of GMH-IVH remain controversial. Unlike previously reported in the literature, recent investigations showed a detrimental effect of low-grade GMH-IVH on neurodevelopmental outcome in premature infants. These studies were based on ultrasonographic assessment, and therefore a bias in patient recruitment may have contributed to this discrepancy in neurological outcome. In particular, patients with undiagnosed small subependymal or intraventricular bleedings may have been included in controls and newborn infants with ultrasound scans were classified as normal.

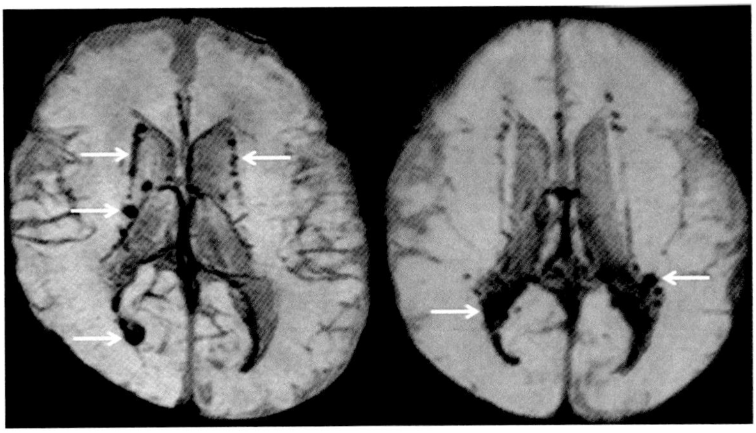

Fig. 11 Two different very premature babies at term-corrected age with SWI-positive findings showing the presence of hemosiderin. T1 and T2 MRI scans were normal. Ultrasound in the first weeks of life was negative for GMH-IVH

122.6.1.2 Parenchymal Hemorrhage/Venous Infarction

In general, ultrasound scanning should be the first imaging modality, but if the ultrasound scan is nonconclusive and there is a strong clinical suspicion of acute hemorrhage, an MRI should be considered. Hemorrhage occurring peripherally in the brain or in the cerebellum may not be easy to visualize by ultrasound, particularly if the anterior fontanelle is relatively small. MRI scanning is the most sensitive technique and should be substituted for CT at all times.

GMH-IVH can present with unilateral parenchymal hemorrhage, better known as venous infarction at the first scan or more commonly within a few hours in a later scan. The region involved can be quite large and just dorsal and lateral to the external angle of the lateral ventricle, usually sparing the cortical mantle, although location and size can vary (Ramenghi and Hüppi 2009; Ramenghi et al. 2005). Less often, the lesion develops in more posterior parts of the brain, in the temporal lobe or around the atrium. In these cases, the inferior ventricular veins or lateral atrial veins are involved. It is still possible to have bilateral venous infarction, but this condition is extremely rare and well differentiated from PVL. At first, the lesion appears as a triangular density often not touching the ventricle, but later the lesion grows and extends to the ventricle, merging the area of increased density due to matrix hemorrhage (Ramenghi and Hüppi 2009; Ramenghi et al. 2005). Sometimes there is no progression to this stage, and the lesion remains as a triangular density. The hyperdense area tends to decrease in size during the second week, and the real infarcted area bends up being smaller than expected. Cystic degeneration is the most common evolution of severe cases with a smooth-walled cavity in the parenchyma communicating with the ventricle (unlike in periventricular leukomalacia) .

122.6.1.3 Hydrocephalus

Ultrasound imaging is the most appropriate modality for the initial assessment of ventricular size. The slightly rounded shape of the frontal horns can represent the initial appearance of dilatation, while balloon-shaped frontal horns are a sign of severe dilatation. Latero-lateral and diagonal measurements of the diameter are a well-established modality by which to monitor ventricular dilatation. Absence of widening of the frontal horns may be falsely reassuring as neonates tend to have dilated occipital horns (colpocephaly). Many units have their own guidelines for measuring frontal horns but very often not for measuring the posterior horns (Ramenghi and Hüppi 2009; Ramenghi et al. 2005).

MRI can be useful as detailed imaging is often required prior to shunting and also after surgery to verify the functioning of the shunt, provided the intraventricular device is MRI compatible.

122.6.1.4 Pseudocysts

Cavitation in the germinal matrix represents a phenomenon called germinolysis. There is a lack of proper epithelium, and it occurs typically at the caudothalamic notch, causing a pseudocyst (Larroche 1972). During the postnatal period, pseudocysts occur mainly following small to moderate GMH-IVH, although a mechanism based on pure infarction of the germinal matrix has been hypothesized. Pseudocysts are sometimes detected at the caudothalamic notch a few weeks after birth in normal preterm babies with no obvious reason (Ramenghi et al. 1997).

122.6.1.5 Cerebellar Hemorrhages

Few in vivo studies have focused on cerebellar hemorrhagic lesions. Cerebellar hemorrhages (CH) are known to be highly represented in postmortem studies, varying from 10% to 25% in very low birth weight infants. However, an in vivo diagnosis, even with MRI, seems to be around only 10% in preterm infants less than 32 weeks of gestation (Parodi and Rossi 2015b). Ultrasound studies performed through the posterior fontanelle, which is more sensitive for visualizing the cerebellum than the more conventional view through the anterior fontanelle, show a low incidence of about 3%, especially in extremely low birth weight babies. Ultrasound using the occipital window appears to be a better approach, and the incidence is probably higher although mastoid fontanelle appears to be the most sensitive one (Ramenghi and Hüppi 2009). In some cases, cerebellar hemorrhages can be severe and associated with flattening of the pons (Fig. 12). A degree of pontine atrophy has been observed in preterm babies with PVL, and a flattened anterior curvature of the pons has been detected by MRI in 28 premature infants born before the 30th week of gestation (Fumagalli et al. 2009).

Acquired pontocerebellar atrophy should be differentiated from congenital pontocerebellar hypoplasia (an association of pontine, vermis, and cerebellar hemisphere hypoplasia) and marks a neurodegenerative disorder. Acquired forms of pontocerebellar atrophy have been described in association with fetal drug exposure, sepsis in premature babies, twin-to-twin transfusion syndrome, and vascular undersupply.

The causes of the association between impaired pontine development and cerebellar hemorrhage remain unknown. The cerebellum receives excitatory input from the frontoparietal cortex via the corticopontocerebellar tracts; an interruption, with secondary degeneration of corticopontocerebellar tracts, could explain pontine atrophy linked to supratentorial lesions, which has been reported in premature babies with little or no PVL. In the same way, primary cerebellar lesions can cause degeneration of pontine fibers through the presence of pontocerebellar tracts. However, a sequence beginning with cerebellar hemorrhage and ending with pontine atrophy has not been demonstrated. The diagnosis of pontine flattening is often made by MRI at term equivalence. This intrinsic vulnerability of the myelinating posterior fossa at low gestation may partly explain impaired development of the pons.

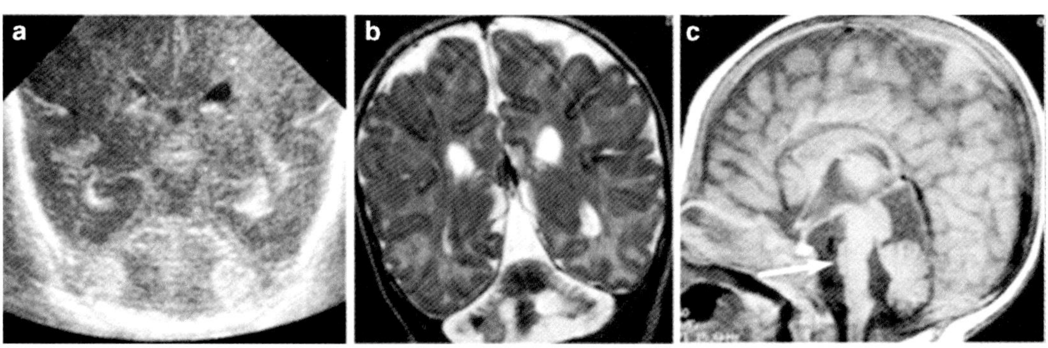

Fig. 12 Coronal CUS scan (**a**) of a 24-week baby scanned at 10 days and showing bilateral cerebellar hemorrhages. MR scans at term equivalence: coronal T2 (**b**) showing cerebellar atrophy at the hemispheres; axial T1 (**c**) showing flattening of the pons (*arrow*)

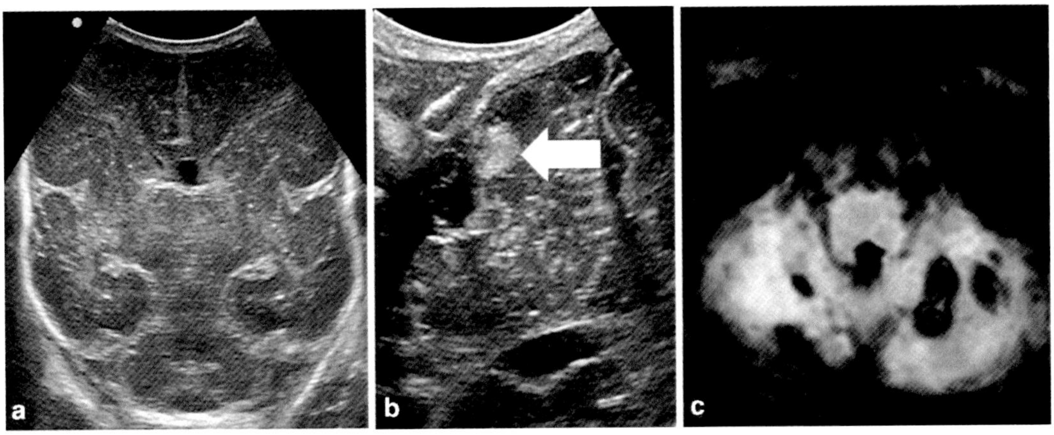

Fig. 13 (**a**) Normal coronal ultrasound scan from anterior fontanelle. (**b**) Ultrasound scan from mastoid fontanelle showing the cerebellar hemorrhage (white arrow). (**c**) SWI-MRI sequence showing more foci of cerebellar hemorrhage

Clinical follow-up studies are needed to investigate whether or not pontine lesions worsen the outcome of babies with isolated cerebellar lesions. The prognostic role of cerebellar hemorrhage is further compounded in case of minor forms of cerebellar hemorrhage, and the accuracy in diagnosis is far to be high in such cases when based on ultrasound only.

Despite the widespread use of high-resolution cranial ultrasound, detection of minor forms of hemorrhage may be challenging even when mastoid fontanelle is used. In fact, diagnostic accuracy of cranial ultrasound in detecting cerebellar hemorrhages depends on the choice of the acoustic window (anterior fontanelle vs mastoid fontanelle) and on the size of the bleeding (Fig. 13). We have recently shown that limited hemorrhages are better identified when the mastoid approach is used although the overall sensitivity of CUS in detecting cerebellar hemorrhages is confirmed to be very low when cerebellar microhemorrhages are included (Parodi and Rossi 2015b). In other words, microhemorrhages proved to be undetectable by ultrasound in spite of the routine use of mastoid fontanelle, as shown by previous studies. The impact of this mild form of CBH on neurodevelopmental outcomes of preterm infants is still controversial, since two previous small studies (10 and 16 cases, respectively) showed conflicting results (Zayek et al. 2012; Steggerda et al. 2013). Interestingly, most lesions in patients with microhemorrhages were detected within the most external portion of cerebellar parenchyma, suggesting an origin from the cerebellar cortex or the subcortical white matter. However, since intraventricular blood resulting from GMH-IVH was detected in most patients with cerebellar microhemorrhages (65%), we speculate that, in some cases, peripheral SWI hypointensities might actually represent hemosiderin depositions on the cerebellar surface originating from a supratentorial bleeding and conveyed by the cerebrospinal fluid to the subarachnoid space of the posterior fossa rather than primary cerebellar hemorrhages.

The possible extracerebellar origin of some of these hemosiderin depositions contributes to the heterogeneity of this group of patients. For these reasons, we believe that precisely assessing the contribution of these minor lesions to the neurodevelopmental disabilities affecting ex-preterm children remains challenging even with the use of MRI. MRI-based studies focusing on the prognostic significance of cerebellar microhemorrhages should be performed on very large populations, in order to minimize the impact of confounding factors, such as associated GMH-IVH, and to better clarify the impact of microhemorrhages on the neurological outcome of the very premature infants.

122.6.2 Premature Babies: The Importance of White Matter

Periventricular leukomalacia (PVL) is described in detail in other chapters. In clinical practice, at least in the older preterm infant, a white matter disease is ascertained by MRI technique more than conventional use of CUS. The increased periventricular echogenicity that in the past has generated numbers of false positive for a very prudent approach of some neonatologists is not any more a problem in the current practice thanks to the role of MRI (Rutherford et al. 2010b).

The predilection of injury to the periventricular white matter is shared by the newer WM diseases identified by MRI in vivo studies. White matter injury in preterm neonates is accompanied by diffuse neuronal and axonal disease, affecting not only cerebral white matter but also deep gray, cortex, and cerebellum. The vulnerability of the periventricular WM has been extensively studied in the context of PVL and is thought to be due less to the presence of a vascular watershed (very popular explanation until the late 1980s) and much more to an inherent susceptibility of preoligodendrocytes to injury (Rutherford et al. 2010b). In addition, there are populations of resident microglia at these sites of periventricular white matter. It is possible that these microglia, which are essential for axonal guidance and white matter tract modeling, are activated abnormally in the presence of injury.

MR imaging of chronic white matter injury in the immature brain is characterized by the presence of cysts and, more importantly, by a persistent punctuate T1-weighted hyperintensities in the periventricular white matter. Similar abnormalities without cystic generation characterize minor forms of the periventricular white matter lesions observed together with cavitational cysts. PVL is a pathological term that does not imply a particular etiology. Punctate lesions are imaging terms and therefore do not imply either etiology or pathology although they are potentially a minor form of white matter mimicking minor PVL (Childs et al. 2001; Cornette et al. 2002).

122.6.2.1 Punctate White Matter Lesions of Premature Babies at Term-Corrected Age

With the decline of frequency of cystic periventricular leukomalacia, milder forms of brain damage connected with prematurity, like punctate white matter lesions affecting about 10–20% of preterm infants, are gaining increasing interest. Punctate white matter lesions are often considered ischemic or inflammatory in origin, although a hemorrhagic nature was also postulated. In the absence of wide pathology studies, pathophysiology of punctate white matter lesions remains a matter of debate, and their controversial prognostic meaning could be also explained by their observed heterogeneity.

Advanced MRI techniques, such as susceptibility-weighted imaging (SWI), sensitive in detecting blood products, can be also used to evidence subgroups of punctate white matter lesions (Fig. 14). Preliminary non-published data shows that in our population of 464 very preterm infants ($\leq$32 weeks of GA) scanned in our unit (birth weight, mean1146 $\pm$ 364) with MRI at term-corrected age, punctate white matter lesions are identifiable in about 20% of patients and in 25% of cases these lesions were visible on SWI.

We believe the prevalence of punctate white matter lesions can be also correlated with gestational age-dependent brain vulnerability. In our population prevalence of punctate white matter lesions is twice as high in infants born at 28–32 gestational weeks compared to those born before 28 weeks of gestational age. This finding may be explained by selective vulnerability of preoligodendrocytes to ischemic or inflammatory insults in this specific developmental period.

In few cases, cystic periventricular leukomalacia was observed together with SWI-PWML, reinforcing the idea of their possible common substrate.

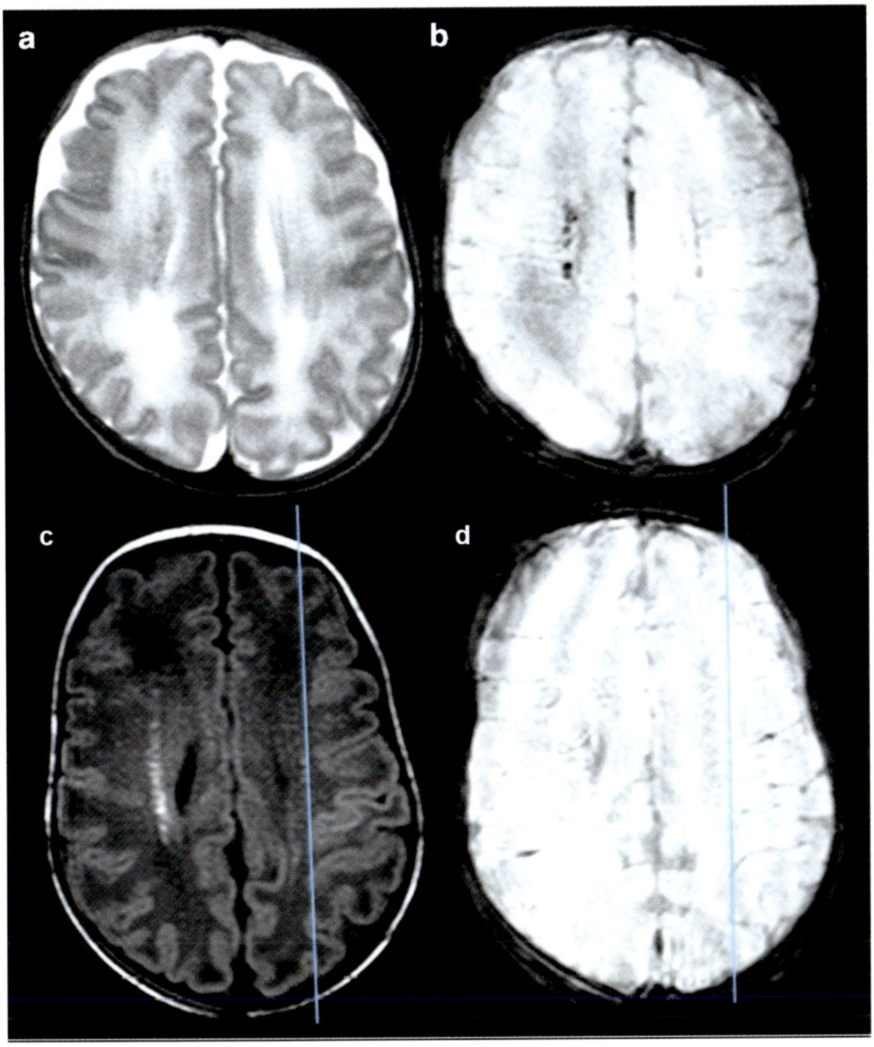

Fig. 14 SWI-positive punctate white matter lesions are visible on axial T2 (**a**) and SWI (**b**) and SWI-negative punctate white matter lesions are visible on axial T1 (**c**) but not on SWI (**d**)

On the other hand, about one fourth of all punctate white matter lesions present a hypointense signal on SWI, consistent with hemorrhagic/petechial nature of lesions. These punctate white matter lesions with a positive signal on SWI seem to be more often associated with GMH/IVH and are often located along the course of medullary veins, corroborating the hypothesis of their venous hemorrhagic origin, as reported in the literature (Kersbergen et al. 2014; Wagenaar et al. 2017) (Fig. 15).

Brain maturation is very rapid during the third trimester of pregnancy and for the preterm infant in the early weeks of life prior to term age. Assessment of brain maturation at term-equivalent age has therefore become an important indicator of brain development with potential implications for future functional outcome. When preterm infants are imaged at term-equivalent age with MRI, the secondary effects of white matter disease on various brain structures can be visualized and quantified.

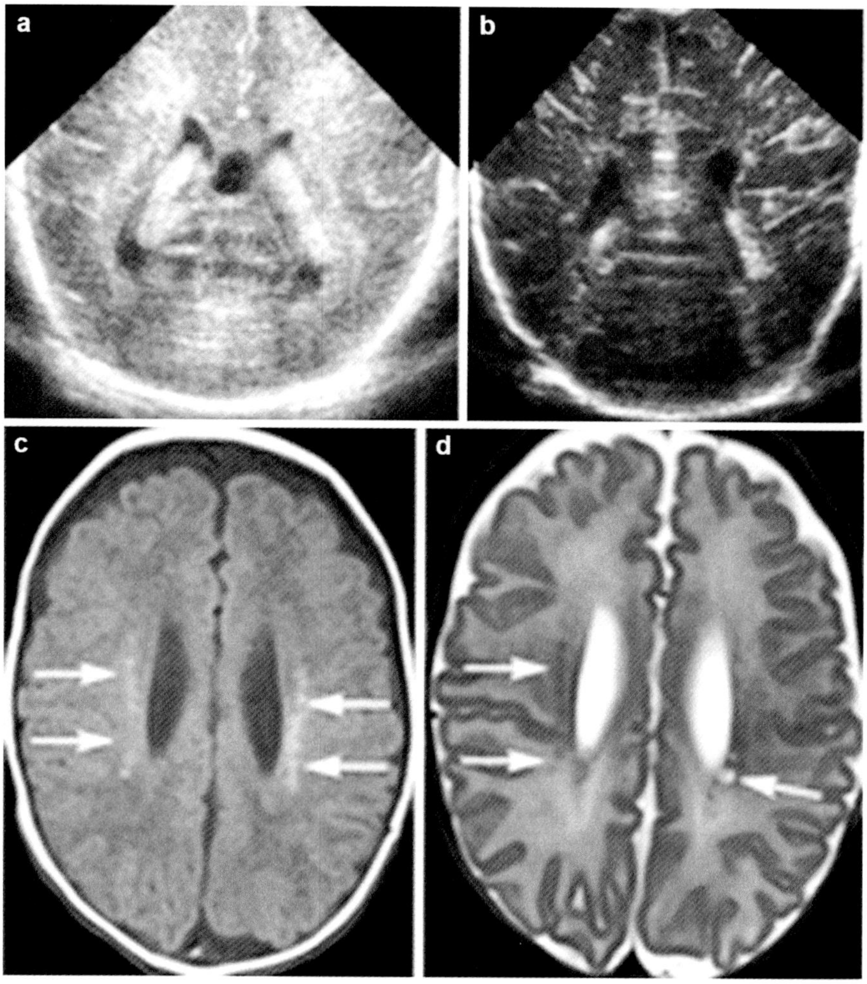

Fig. 15 (**a**) Coronal CUS scan showing a transient increased periventricular echogenicity at 10 days of a 29-week baby. (**b**) CUS scan at term equivalence showing normal echogenicity, while MR axial scans (**c** T1, **d** T2) highlight periventricular abnormalities (*white arrows*) usually called punctate lesions. On T1-weighted images, these abnormalities at term equivalence may also represent mild glial scars

References

Benders MJ, Groenendaal F, Uiterwaal CS et al (2007) Maternal and infant characteristics associated with perinatal arterial stroke in the preterm infant. Stroke 38:1759–1765

Bouza H, Dubowitz LM, Rutherford M et al (1994) Late magnetic resonance imaging and clinical findings in neonates with unilateral lesions on cranial ultrasound. Dev Med Child Neurol 36:951–964

Burns CM, Rutherford MA, Boardman JP, Cowan FM (2008) Patterns of cerebral injury and neurodevelopmental outcomes after symptomatic neonatal hypoglycemia. Pediatrics 122:65–74

Cheong JL, Cowan FM (2009) Neonatal arterial ischaemic stroke: obstetric issues. Semin Fetal Neonatal Med 14:267–271

Childs AM, Cornette L, Ramenghi LA et al (2001) Magnetic resonance and cranial ultrasound characteristics of periventricular white matter abnormalities in newborn infants. Clin Radiol 56:647–655

Cornette LG, Tanner SF, Ramenghi LA (2002) Magnetic resonance imaging of the infant brain: anatomical characteristics and clinical significance of punctate lesions. Arch Dis Child Fetal Neonatal 86:F171–F177

Cowan FM, Pennock JM, Hanrahan JD et al (1994) Early detection of cerebral infarction and hypoxic ischemic encephalopathy in neonates using diffusion-weighted magnetic resonance imaging. Neuropediatrics 25:172–175

D'Arceuil HE, de Crespigny AJ, Röther J et al (1998) Diffusion and perfusion magnetic resonance imaging of the evolution of hypoxic ischemic encephalopathy in the neonatal rabbit. J Magn Reson Imaging 8:820–828
Dudnik J, Mercuri E, Al-Nakib L et al (2009) Evolution of unilateral arterial ischemic stroke on conventional and diffusion-weighted MR imaging. AJNR Am J Neuroradiol 30:998–1004
Fumagalli M, Ramenghi LA, Righini A et al (2009) Cerebellar haemorrhages and pons development in extremely low birth weight infants. Front Biosci 1: 537–541
Govaert P, Ramenghi L, Taal R et al (2009) Diagnosis of perinatal stroke I: definitions, differential diagnosis and registration. Acta Paediatr 98:1556–1567
Groenendaal F, Veenhoven RH, van der Grond J et al (1994) Cerebral lactate and N-acetyl-aspartate/choline ratios in asphyxiated full-term neonates demonstrated in vivo using proton magnetic resonance spectroscopy. Pediatr Res 35:148–151
Hanrahan JD, Cox IJ, Azzopardi D et al (1999) Relation between proton magnetic resonance spectroscopy within 18 hours of birth asphyxia and neurodevelopment at 1 year of age. Dev Med Child Neurol 41:76–82
Hüppi PS (2001) MR imaging and spectroscopy of brain development. Magn Reson Imaging Clin N Am 9:1–17
Kersbergen KJ, Benders MJ, Groenendaal F et al (2014) Different patterns of punctate white matter lesions in serially scanned preterm infants. PLoS One 9(10): e108904
Larroche JC (1972) Sub-ependymal pseudo-cysts in the newborn. Biol Neonate 21:170–183
Malova M, Rossi A, Severino M et al (2017) Incidental findings on routine brain MRI scans in preterm infants. Arch Dis Child Fetal Neonatal Ed 102:F73–F78
Ment LR, Hintz D, Hüppi PS (2009) Imaging biomarkers of outcome in the developing preterm brain. Lancet Neurol 8:1042–1055
Parodi A, Morana G, Severino MS et al (2015a) Low-grade intraventricular hemorrhage: is ultrasound good enough? J Matern Fetal Neonatal Med 28(Suppl 1):2261–2264
Parodi A, Rossi A, Severino M et al (2015b) Accuracy of ultrasound in assessing cerebellar haemorrhages in very low birthweight babies. Arch Dis Child Fetal Neonatal Ed 100:F289–F292
Ramenghi LA, Hüppi PS (2009) Imaging of the neonatal brain. In: Levene MI, Chevernak FA (eds) Fetal and neonatal neurology and neurosurgery. Churchill Livingstone, London, Edinburgh, pp 68–103
Ramenghi LA, Domizio S, Quartulli L, Sabatino G (1997) Prenatal pseudocysts of the germinal matrix in preterm infants. J Clin Ultrasound 25:169–173
Ramenghi LA, Gill BJ, Tanner SF et al (2002) Cerebral venous thrombosis, intraventricular haemorrhage and white matter lesions in a preterm newborn with factor V (Leiden) mutation. Neuropediatrics 33:97–99
Ramenghi LA, Mosca F, Counsell S, Rutherford M (2005) Magnetic resonance imaging of the brain in preterm infants. In: Tortori Donati P (ed) Pediatric neuroradiology. Springer, Berlin, pp 199–234
Ramenghi LA, Govaert P, Fumagalli M et al (2009) Neonatal cerebral sinovenous thrombosis. Semin Fetal Neonatal Med 14:278–283
Righini A, Ramenghi LA, Parini R et al (2003) Water apparent diffusion coefficient and T2 changes in the acute stage of maple syrup urine disease: evidence of intramyelinic and vasogenic-interstitial edema. J Neuroimaging 13:162–165
Righini A, Ramenghi L, Zirpoli S et al (2005) Brain apparent diffusion coefficient decrease during correction of severe hypernatremic dehydration. AJNR Am J Neuroradiol 26:1690–1694
Rutherford MA, Pennock JM, Counsell SJ et al (1998) Abnormal magnetic resonance signal in the internal capsule predicts poor neurodevelopmental outcome in infants with hypoxic-ischemic encephalopathy. Pediatrics 102:323–328
Rutherford M, Ramenghi LA, Edwards AD et al (2010a) Assessment of brain tissue injury after moderate hypothermia in neonates with hypoxic-ischaemic encephalopathy: a nested substudy of a randomised controlled trial. Lancet Neurol 9:39–45
Rutherford MA, Supramaniam V, Ederies A et al (2010b) Magnetic resonance imaging of white matter diseases of prematurity. Neuroradiology 52(6):505–521
Rutherford MA, Ramenghi LA, Cowan FM (2012) Arch Dis Child Fetal Neonatal Ed 97:F377–F384
Steggerda SJ, De Bruïne FT, van den Berg-Huysmans AA et al (2013) Small cerebellar hemorrhage in preterm infants: perinatal and postnatal factors and outcome. Cerebellum 12:794–801
Tanner SF, Ramenghi LA, Ridgway JP et al (2000) Quantitative comparison of intrabrain diffusion in adults and preterm and term neonates and infants. AJR Am J Roentgenol 174:1643–1649
Tuor UI, Kozlowski P, Del Bigio MR (1998) Diffusion- and T2- weighted increases in magnetic resonance images of immature brain during hypoxia-ischemia: transient reversal posthypoxia. Exp Neurol 150: 321–328
Volpe JJ (2009) Brain injury in premature infants: a complex amalgam of destructive and developmental disturbances. Lancet Neurol 8:110–124
Wagenaar N, Chau V, Groenendaal F et al (2017) Clinical risk factors for punctate white matter lesions on early magnetic resonance imaging in preterm newborns. J Pediatr 182:34–40
Zayek MM, Benjamin JT, Maertens P et al (2012) Cerebellar hemorrhage: a major morbidity in extremely preterm infants. J Perinatol 32:699–704

Malformations of Cortical Development in Newborns: Genetic Aspects

123

Renzo Guerrini and Elena Parrini

Contents

Abstract

The malformations of cortical development (MCD) represent a major cause of developmental disabilities, severe epilepsy, and reproductive disadvantage. Genes that have been associated to MCD are mainly involved in cell proliferation and specification, neuronal migration, and late cortical organization. Lissencephaly-pachygyria-severe band heterotopia are diffuse neuronal migration disorders (NMDs) causing severe, global neurological impairment. Abnormalities of the *LIS1*, *DCX*, *ARX*, and *RELN* genes have been associated with these malformations. Recent work has also established a relationship of lissencephaly, with or without associated microcephaly, corpus

R. Guerrini (✉) · E. Parrini
Pediatric Neurology and Neurogenetics Unit and Laboratories, Neuroscience Department, A. Meyer Children's Hospital – University of Florence, Florence, Italy
e-mail: renzo.guerrini@meyer.it; elena.parrini@meyer.it

G. Buonocore et al. (eds.), *Neonatology*,
https://doi.org/10.1007/978-3-319-29489-6_270

callosum dysgenesis, and cerebellar hypoplasia and, at times, a morphological pattern consistent with polymicrogyria with mutations of several genes (*KIF2A, KIF5C, TUBA1A, TUBA8, TUBB, TUBB2B, TUBB3, TUBG1,* and *DYNC1H1)* regulating the synthesis and function of microtubule and centrosome key components and hence defined as tubilinopathies. MCDs only affecting subsets of neurons, such as mild subcortical band heterotopia and periventricular heterotopia, cause neurological and cognitive impairment that vary from severe to mild deficits. They have been associated with abnormalities of the *DCX, FLN1A,* and *ARFGEF2* genes. Polymicrogyria results from abnormal late cortical organization and is inconstantly associated with abnormal neuronal migration. Localized polymicrogyria has been associated with anatomo-specific deficits, including disorders of language and higher cognition. Polymicrogyria is genetically heterogeneous and only in a small minority of patients has a definite genetic cause been identified. Megalencephaly with normal cortex by imaging, megalencephaly with polymicrogyria, dysplastic megalencephaly (including hemimegalencephaly), and focal cortical dysplasia can all result from mutations of the same genes in the PI3K-AKT-mTOR pathway which are often postzygotic and can be limited to the dysplastic tissue in the less diffuse forms.

List of Abbreviations

a > p	Anterior > posterior
BFPP	Bilateral frontoparietal PMG
BPP	Bilateral perisylvian PMG
CNV	Copy number variants
EEG	Electroencephalogram
ILS	Isolated LIS
LIS	Lissencephaly
MCD	Malformations of cortical development
MDS	Miller-Dieker syndrome
MLPA	Multiplex ligation-dependent probe amplification
MRI	Magnetic resonance imaging
p > a	Posterior > anterior
PMG	Polymicrogyria

123.1 Salient Points

- Malformations of cortical development (MCD) represent major causes of developmental disabilities, severe epilepsy, and reproductive disadvantage.
- Genes associated with MCD are mainly involved in cell proliferation and specification, neuronal migration, and late cortical organization.
- Lissencephaly is characterized by absent (agyria) or decreased (pachygyria) convolutions, cortical thickening, and a smooth cerebral surface. Patients with severe lissencephaly have early developmental delay, hypotonia and later spastic quadriplegia, and eventual severe or profound mental retardation.
- Lissencephaly-pachygyria-severe band heterotopia are diffuse neuronal migration disorders causing severe, global neurological impairment.
- MCDs affecting only subsets of neurons, such as mild subcortical band heterotopia and periventricular heterotopia, cause neurological and cognitive impairment.
- Polymicrogyria results from abnormal late cortical organization and is inconstantly associated with abnormal neuronal migration; it is genetically heterogeneous and only in a small minority of patients has a definite genetic cause been identified.
- Megalencephaly with a normal cortex on imaging, megalencephaly with polymicrogyria, dysplastic megalencephaly, and focal cortical dysplasia can all result from mutations of the same genes in the PI3K-AKT-mTOR pathway.

123.2 Introduction

The development of the human cerebral cortex is a complex dynamic process that occurs during several gestational weeks (Gleeson and Walsh 2000). During the first stage, stem cells proliferate and differentiate into young neurons or glial cells deep in the forebrain, in the ventricular and subventricular zones lining the cerebral cavity. During the second stage, cortical neurons migrate away from their place of origin: most cells migrate along the radial glial fibers from the periventricular region towards the pial surface, where each successive generation passes one another and settles in an inside-out pattern within the cortical plate. When neurons reach their destination, they stop migrating and order themselves into specific "architectonic" patterns guiding cells to the correct location in the cerebral cortex. This third phase involves final organization within the typical six layers of cortex, associated with synaptogenesis and apoptosis.

Abnormal cortical development is increasingly recognized as a cause of developmental disabilities and epilepsy. This recognition is due, in part, to the improved use of magnetic resonance imaging (MRI), which makes it possible to assess the distribution and depth of cortical sulci, cortical thickness, the boundaries between gray and white matter, and variations in signal intensity. Abnormalities of any or all of these features may be observed in different malformations of cortical development (MCD), which may be restricted to discrete cortical areas or may, alternatively, be diffuse (Guerrini et al. 2008; Guerrini and Dobyns 2014).

So far, more than 100 genes are reported to be associated with one or more types of MCD. The biological pathways include cell-cycle regulation at many steps (especially mitosis and cell division), apoptosis, cell-fate specification, cytoskeletal structure and function, neuronal migration and basement-membrane function, and many inborn errors of metabolism. Importantly, a subset of MCD genes – especially those associated with megalencephaly – are associated with postzygotic (i.e., mosaic) mutations (Lee et al. 2012).

Genetic testing needs accurate assessment of imaging features, and familial distribution, if any, and can be straightforward in some disorders but requires a complex diagnostic algorithm in others. Because of substantial genotypic and phenotypic heterogeneity for most of these genes, a comprehensive analysis of clinical, imaging, and genetic data is needed to properly define these disorders. Exome sequencing and high-field MRI are rapidly modifying the classification of these disorders.

In the following sections we will discuss the most frequent MCD.

123.3 Lissencephaly and Subcortical Band Heterotopia

Lissencephaly (LIS) is characterized by absent (agyria) or decreased (pachygyria) convolutions, cortical thickening, and a smooth cerebral surface (Guerrini and Dobyns 2014; Barkovich et al. 2012). Several types of LIS have been recognized. The most common, classical LIS, features a very thick cortex (10–20 mm vs. the normal 4 mm) and no other major brain malformations.

Subcortical band heterotopia (SBH) is a related disorder in which bands of gray matter are interposed in the white matter between the cortex and the lateral ventricles (Guerrini and Parrini 2010). Histopathology demonstrates that heterotopic neurons settle close to the "true" cortex in a pattern suggestive of laminar organization.

On the basis of findings from genetic studies, the full range of lissencephaly now extends from severe lissencephaly with cerebellar hypoplasia to classic lissencephaly to subcortical band heterotopia and also includes a polymicrogyria-like cortical malformation that can be distinguished from both lissencephaly and typical polymicrogyria by high-resolution brain imaging.

123.3.1 Genetic Basis and Diagnosis

Lissencephaly, subcortical band heterotopia, and lissencephaly with cerebellar hypoplasia are always genetic. Studies to date have identified 12 lissencephaly genes (Table 1), which account for roughly 90% of patients. However, two major genes have been associated with classical LIS and SBH. The *LIS1* gene is responsible for the autosomal form of LIS (Cardoso et al. 2002), while the *DCX* gene is X-linked (Matsumoto et al. 2001). Although either gene can result in either LIS or SBH, most cases of classical LIS are due to deletions or mutations of *LIS1* (Cardoso et al. 2002), whereas most cases of SBH are due to mutations of *DCX* (Matsumoto et al. 2001). *LIS1*-related LIS is more severe in the posterior brain regions ($p > a$ gradient) (Fig. 1a), whereas *DCX*-related

Table 1 Genes and chromosomal loci associated with MCD

Cortical malformation	Pattern of inheritance	Gene	Locus	OMIM
Lissencephaly (LIS)				
MDS	AD	*LIS1*	17p13.3	*601545
ILS or SBH	AD	*LIS1*	17p13.3	*601545
ILS or SBH	X-linked	*DCX*	Xq22.3-q23	*300121
ILS or SBH	AD	*TUBA1A*	12q12-q14	*602529
XLAG	X-linked	*ARX*	Xp22.13	*300382
LIS cerebellar hypoplasia	AR	*RELN*	7q22	*600514
LIS cerebellar hypoplasia	AR	*VLDR*	9p24.2	*192977
ILS	AD	*DYNC1H1*	14q32.31	*600112
ILS	AD	*KIF2A*	5q12.1	*602591
ILS	AD	*TUBA1A*	17q13.12	*602529
ILS	AD	*TUBB2B*	6p25.2	*612850
ILS	AD	*TUBG1*	17q21.2	*191135
Periventricular nodular heterotopia (PNH)				
Classical bilateral PNH	X-linked	*FLNA*	Xq28	*300017
Ehlers-Danlos syndrome and PNH	X-linked	*FLNA*	Xq28	*300017
Facial dysmorphisms, severe constipation, and PNH	X-linked	*FLNA*	Xq28	*300017
Fragile-X syndrome and PNH	X-linked	*FMR1*	Xq27.3	*309550
Microcephaly and PNH	AR	*ARFGEF2*	20q13.13	*605371
Donnai-Barrow syndrome and PNH	AR	*LRP2*	2q24-q31	*600073
PNH with limb abnormalities (limb reduction abnormality or syndactyly)	X-linked	...	Xq28	
Williams syndrome and PH	AD	...	7q11.23	
PH	AD	...	5p15.1	
PH	AD	...	5p15.33	
Agenesis of the corpus callosum, polymicrogyria, and PNH	AD	...	6q27 (C6orf70)	
PH	AD	...	6p25	
PH	AD	...	4p15	
PH	AD	...	5q14.3-q15	
PH	AD	...	22q11	
PH and steroid sulfatase deficiency	AD	...	Xp22.3	
PH	AD	...	Xp22.11	
PH and Smith-Magenis syndrome	AD	...	17p11.2	
Agenesis of the corpus callosum and PNH	AD	...	1p36.22-pter	
Polymicrogyria (PMG)				
Bilateral frontoparietal PMG	AR	*GPR56*	16q13	*604110
Asymmetric PMG	AD	*TUBB2B*	6p25.2	*612850
PMG and rolandic seizures, oromotor dyspraxia	X-linked	*SRPX2*	Xq21.33-q23	*300642
PMG and agenesis of the corpus callosum (ACC), microcephaly	AD	*TBR2*	3p21.3-p21.2	*604615
PMG and aniridia	AD	*PAX6*	11p13	*607108
PMG and microcephaly	AR	*NDE1*	16p13.11	*609449
PMG and microcephaly	AR	*WDR62*	19q13.12	*613583

(*continued*)

Table 1 (continued)

Cortical malformation	Pattern of inheritance	Gene	Locus	OMIM
PMG and fumaric aciduria	AR	*FH*	1q43	*136850
PMG and "band-like calcifications"	AR	*OCLN*	5q13.2	*602876
Perysilvian PMG and CHARGE syndrome	AD	*CHD7*	8q12.1-q12.2	*608892
PMG and Warburg micro syndrome	AR	*RAB3GAP1*	2q21.3	*602536
PMG and Warburg micro syndrome	AR	*RAB3GAP2*	1q41	*609275
PMG and Warburg micro syndrome	AR	*RAB18*	10p12.1	*602207
PMG-like, microcephaly, ACC	AD	*DYNC1H1*	14q32.31	*600112
PMG-like, microcephaly, ACC	AD	*KIF5C*	2q23.1	*604593
PMG-like, microcephaly, ACC, CBLH	AD	*TUBA1A*	17q13.12	*602529
PMG-like, microcephaly, ACC, CBLH	AR	*TUBA8*	22q11.21	*605742
PMG-like, microcephaly, ACC, CBLH	AD	*TUBB3*	16q24.3	*602661
PMG-like, microcephaly, ACC, CBLH	AD	*TUBB*	6p21.33	*191130
PMG-like, microcephaly, ACC	AR	*EOMES*	3p24.1	*604615
PMG and Goldberg-Shprintzen syndrome	AR	*KIAA1279*	10q21.3	*609367
PMG	AD	...	1p36.3-pter	
PMG and microcephaly	AD	...	1q44-qter	
PMG and facial dysmorphisms	AD	...	2p16.1-p23	
PMG and microcephaly, hydrocephalus	AD	...	4q21-q22	
PMG	AD	...	21q2	
PMG	AD	...	6q26-27	
PMG	AD	...	13q3	
PMG	AD	...	18p11	
PMG and Di George syndrome	AD	...	22q11.2	
Bilateral perysilvian PMG	AD	*PIK3R2*	19p13.11	*603157
Megalencephaly-polymicrogyria and dysplastic megalencephaly				
MPPH, DMEG	AD	*AKT3*	1q43q44	*611223
Weaver syndrome	AD	*EZH2*	7q36.1	*601573
MCAP	AD	*PIK3CA*	3q26.32	*171834
MPPH	AD	*PIK3R2*	19p13.11	*603157

AD autosomal dominant, *AR* autosomal recessive, *ACC* agenesis of the corpus callosum, *CBLH* diffuse cerebellar hypoplasia, *MPPH* megalencephaly-polymicrogyria-polydactyly-hydrocephalus syndrome, *DMEG* dysplastic megalencephaly, *MCAP* megalencephaly-capillary malformation syndrome
*=gene/locus MIM number

LIS is more severe in the anterior brain (a > p gradient) (Fig. 1b).

About 60% of patients with p > a isolated LIS (ILS) carry genomic alterations or mutations involving *LIS1* (Mei et al. 2008). A simplified gyral pattern in the posterior brain, with underlying SBH, has been associated with mosaic mutations of *LIS1* (Cardoso et al. 2002). Miller-Dieker syndrome (MDS) is caused by deletion of *LIS1* and contiguous genes and features severe p > a LIS, accompanied by distinct dysmorphic facial features and additional malformations (Fig. 1c) (Cardoso et al. 2002).

Most *DCX* mutations cause a > p SBH/pachygyria. Mutations of *DCX* have been found in all reported pedigrees and in 80% of sporadic females and 25% of sporadic males with SBH (Matsumoto et al. 2001). Genomic

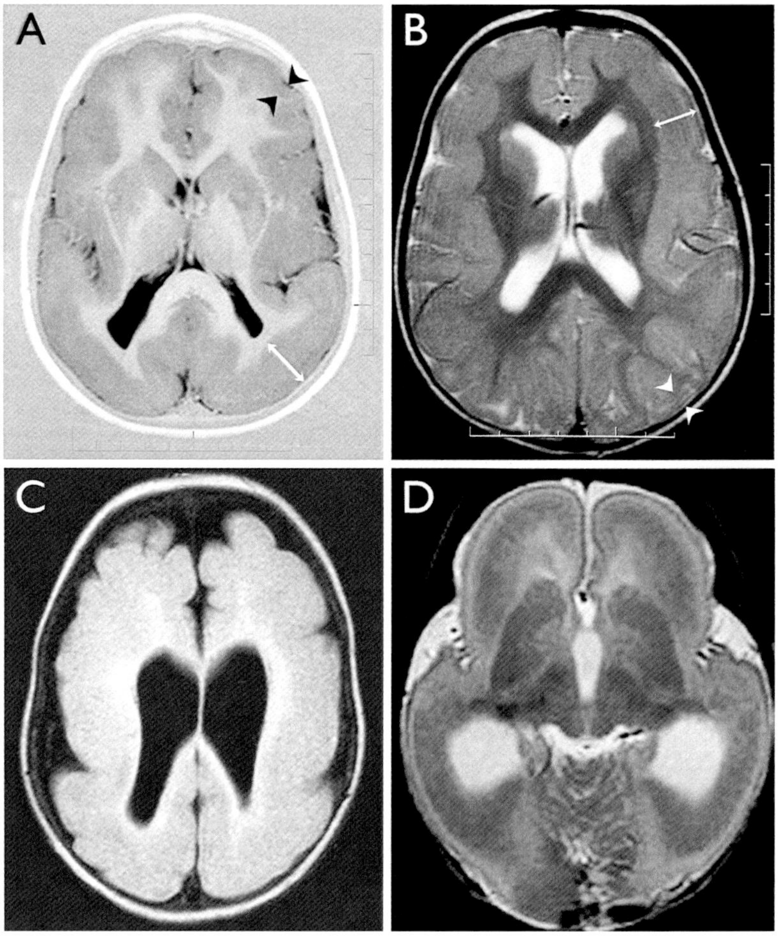

Fig. 1 Brain MRI of four different patients; axial sections: (**a**) classical LIS in a boy with *LIS1* gene mutation; (**b**) LIS in a girl with *DCX* mutation. In (**a**), there is a p > a gradient, cortical thickness is around 6 mm in the frontal lobes (*two black arrowheads*) and around 3 cm in the posterior brain (*white arrow*). In (**b**), there is a typical ar > p pattern; cortical thickness is around 2 cm in the frontal lobes (*white arrow*) and around 4 mm in the posterior brain (*two white arrowheads*). (**c**) LIS in a patient with MDS. (**d**) Severe diffuse LIS with relatively small frontal lobes in a boy with *DCX* mutation

deletions of *DCX* are rarely observed (Guerrini and Parrini 2010). Maternal germline or mosaic *DCX* mutations may occur in about 10% of cases of either SBH or XLIS (Gleeson et al. 2000). Hemizygous males with *DCX* mutations have classical LIS (Fig.1d), but rare boys with missense mutations and SBH have been described (Guerrini et al. 2003).

123.3.2 Phenotype

Classical LIS is rare, with a prevalence of about 12 per million births. Patients with severe LIS have early developmental delay, early diffuse hypotonia, later spastic quadriplegia, and eventual severe or profound mental retardation. Seizures occur in over 90% of LIS children, with onset before 6 months in about 75% of cases. Between 35% and 85% of children with classic lissencephaly develop infantile spasms, often without classic hypsarrhythmia. Most LIS children subsequently have multiple seizure types. In patients with MDS, classical LIS is accompanied by distinct dysmorphic facial features (Cardoso et al. 2002). The main clinical manifestations of SBH are mental retardation and epilepsy. Epilepsy is present in almost all patients and is intractable in about 65% of cases. About 50% of these epilepsy patients have focal seizures, and the remaining 50% have generalized epilepsy, often within the spectrum of Lennox-Gastaut syndrome (Guerrini and Parrini 2010).

Children with some lissencephaly syndromes (especially Miller-Dieker syndrome, and severe forms of lissencephaly with cerebellar hypoplasia or the X-linked syndrome of lissencephaly with abnormal genitalia) have a severe course and high mortality rates. However, these data do not apply to children with less severe forms of lissencephaly, subcortical band heterotopia, or lissencephaly with cerebellar hypoplasia, because all of these disorders are associated with better motor and cognitive function and longer survival (Dobyns et al. 2012).

123.3.3 Laboratory Investigations

In patients with classical LIS, the cytogenetic and molecular investigations are part of the diagnostic process. When MDS is suspected, a standard karyotype and FISH for the 17pl3.3 region is indicated. When isolated LIS is diagnosed, careful assessment of the antero-posterior gradient of cortical pattern abnormality will be suggestive of the involvement of either the *LIS1* or the *DCX* gene. When LIS is more severe posteriorly, it is worth performing first MLPA in order to rule out *LIS1* deletions/duplications. If a deletion/duplication is not found, *LIS1* sequencing should then be performed. In boys whose MRI shows more severe pachygyria in the frontal lobes, sequencing of the *DCX* gene is indicated. In patients with SBH direct sequencing of *DCX* should be performed. If a *DCX* mutation is not found, MLPA analysis should then be performed. Direct sequencing is also indicated in the mothers of patients harbouring a *DCX* mutation or other female relatives.

123.3.4 Genetic Counseling

All reported *LIS1* alterations are *de novo*. Given the theoretical risk of germline mosaicism in either parent (which has never been demonstrated for *LIS1*), a couple with a child with lissencephaly is usually given a 1% recurrence risk.

When a *DCX* mutation is found in a boy with LIS, mutation analysis of *DCX* should be extended to the proband's mother, even if her brain MRI is normal. If the mother is a mutation carrier, the mutation will be transmitted according to Mendelian inheritance. If the mother is not a carrier, she can still be at risk of germline mosaicism; the risk of transmitting the mutation might roughly be estimated at around 5%.

123.4 Heterotopia

There are three main groups of heterotopia: periventricular (usually nodular: PNH), subcortical, and leptomeningeal, of which only the first two can be detected by imaging. PNH is by far the most frequent. SBH is a mild form of LIS and classified in that group.

123.4.1 Periventricular Nodular Heterotopia (PNH)

PNH consists of nodules of gray matter located along the lateral ventricles with a total failure of migration of some neurons (Guerrini and Dobyns 2014; Barkovich et al. 2012); it ranges from isolated, single, to confluent bilateral nodules (Fig. 2). The overlying cortex may show an abnormal organization. When the nodules are bilateral and numerous, a genetic basis is probable and other brain malformations are often reported (Parrini et al. 2006).

123.4.2 Genetic Basis and Diagnosis

PNH is a clinically and genetically heterogeneous disorder occurring most frequently in women as an X-linked trait (classical bilateral PNH), associated with high rates of prenatal lethality in male fetuses and 50% recurrence risk in the female offspring. Almost 100% of families and 26% of sporadic patients harbor mutations of the *FLNA* gene (Parrini et al. 2006), which also causes cardiovascular abnormalities in some patients of both sexes and gut malformations in boys. Only a few living male patients with PNH owing to *FLNA* mutations have been reported (Guerrini et al. 2004).

A rare recessive form of PNH owing to mutations of the *ARFGEF2* gene was described in two

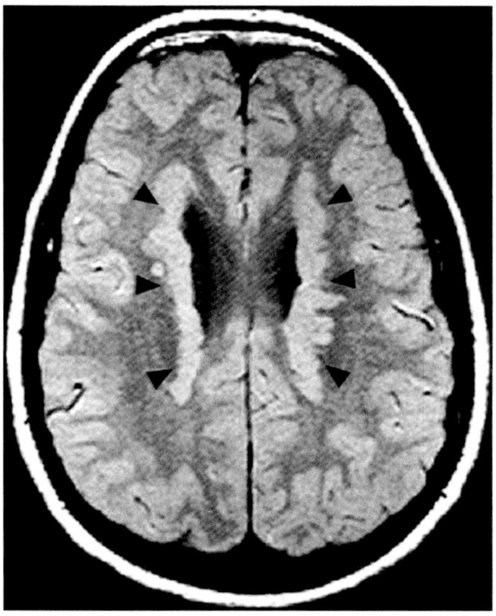

Fig. 2 Brain MRI: Axial section. Typical, classical bilateral PNH in a woman with a missense FLNA mutation. Bilateral nodules of subependymal heterotopia are contiguous and rather symmetric, extensively lining the ventricular walls (*black arrows*)

consanguineous pedigrees (Sheen et al. 2004) in which affected children had microcephaly, severe delay, and early-onset seizures.

Other genetic forms of periventricular nodular heterotopia have been mapped to several chromosomal loci (Table 1), but a putative causal gene has only been identified for the 6q27-related form (Conti et al. 2013).

123.4.3 Phenotype

Although most patients with PNH come to medical attention because they have focal epilepsy of variable severity, there is a wide spectrum of clinical presentations, including several syndromes with mental retardation and dysmorphic facial features. There is some correlation between the size of PNH and the likelihood of concomitant structural abnormality of the cortex and clinical severity (Parrini et al. 2006) but there seem to be no correlation between the size and number of heterotopic nodules and cognitive outcome. Most female patients with PNH due to *FLNA* mutations have epileptic seizures, with normal or borderline cognitive level. However, patients with even small isolated nodules caused by unknown genetic abnormalities or by copy number variations and severe cognitive impairment have been reported.

123.4.4 Laboratory Investigations

FLNA mutation analysis should be performed in patients with "classical" bilateral PNH. When autosomal recessive PH associated with microcephaly is suspected, *ARFGEF2* mutation analysis should be performed. Patients with PH associated with other brain malformations or extraneurological defects should be studied with array-CGH as genomic deletions/duplications have often been associated to PH.

123.4.5 Genetic Counseling

Classical PNH is much more frequent in women and likely to be due to *FLNA* mutations. Among carrier women, about half have *de novo FLNA* mutations, whereas the remaining half have inherited mutations. Although maternal transmission is much more likely, father-to-daughter transmission is possible. Given that germline mosaicism of *FLNA* has never been reported, the recurrence risk (for other children) seems to be very low when a mutation is found in the proband but neither parent is a carrier. Counseling is very difficult when PNH is not related to either *FLNA* or *ARFGEF2;* array-CGH study for the search of copy number variations is advised. The number of known cases of familial PNH unrelated to these genes is extremely low.

123.5 Polymicrogyria Phenotypes and Genetics

The term "polymicrogyria" (PMG) defines an excessive number of abnormally small gyri that produce an irregular cortical surface with lumpy aspect (Lee et al. 2012). Polymicrogyria can be localized to a single gyrus, involve a portion of one hemisphere, be bilateral and asymmetrical, bilateral and symmetrical or diffuse. The imaging appearance of polymicrogyria varies with the patient's age. In newborns and young infants, the malformed cortex is very thin with multiple, very small undulations. After myelination, polymicrogyria appears as thickened cortex with irregular cortex-white matter junction (Guerrini et al. 2008; Guerrini and Dobyns 2014).

The clinical manifestations of polymicrogyria vary widely and depend on several factors. The most severe outcomes occur in children with severe microcephaly (−3SD or smaller), abnormal neurological examination (especially spasticity), widespread distribution of polymicrogyria, and additional brain malformations (especially cerebellar hypoplasia). The best outcomes are in individuals who have localized unilateral polymicrogyria without other malformations. Polymicrogyria can affect eloquent cortical areas representing language or primary motor functions, yet these functions can be retained with little or no disability (Guerrini and Barba 2010).

Polymicrogyria is associated with a wide number of patterns and syndromes and with mutations in several genes (Table 1). Various PMG syndromes have been described, which have been designated according to their lobar topography (Barkovich et al. 2012).

Bilateral perisylvian polymicrogyria (BPP) (Fig. 3a, b) is the most frequent form. It is associated with mild to moderate mental retardation, epilepsy, and impaired oromotor skills. Most cases are sporadic but genetic heterogeneity is suggested (Barkovich et al. 2012). BPP, frequently asymmetric and with a striking predisposition for the right hemisphere, has also been reported in children with 22q11.2 deletion (Barkovich et al. 2012). Recently, mutations in *PIK3R2*, a regulatory subunit of the PI3K-AKT-

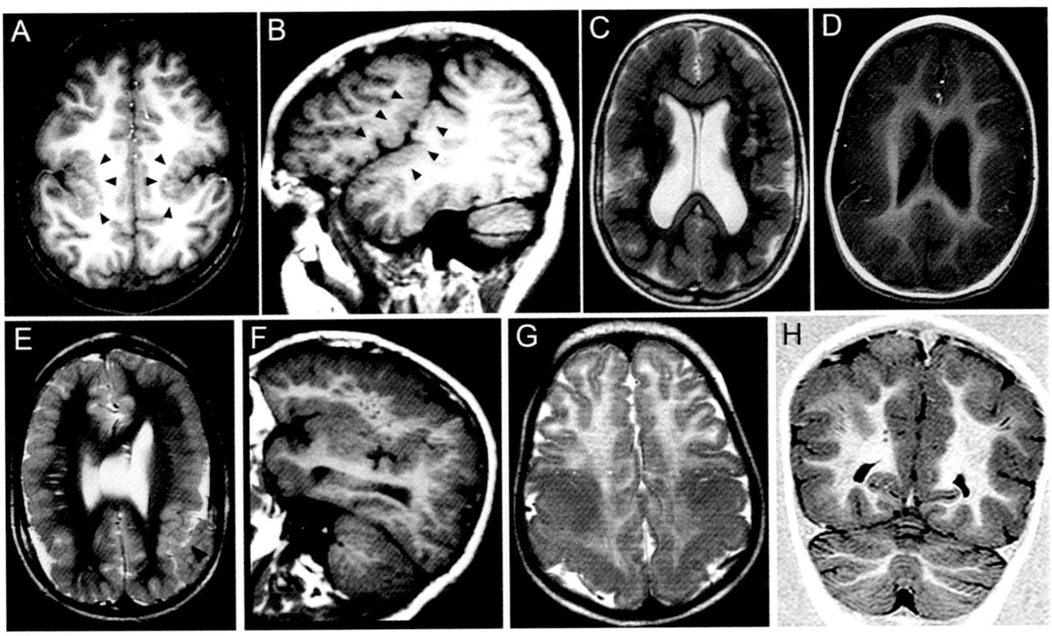

Fig. 3 Brain MRI scan in patients with PMG or tubulinophaties. (**a**) Axial section and (**b**) Sagittal section in a patient with BPP. The sylvian fissures are open and the perisylvian cortex is thickened and irregular (*black arrows*). Note the abnormally vertical orientation of the sylvian fissure, which appears to be fused with the rolandic fissure. (**c**) Axial section. BFPP in a girl with a *GPR56* mutation and Lennox-Gastaut syndrome. (**d**) Axial section in a patient with a symplified gyral pattern and *TUBA1A* mutation. (**e**) Axial and (**f**) sagittal section in a patient with cortical thickening, diffuse polymicrogyira, and *TUBB2B* mutation. (**g**) Axial section in a patient with posterior pachygyria and *DYNC1H1* mutation. (**h**) Coronal section in a patient with posterior pachygyria, cortical thickening, and *DYNC1H1* mutation

mTOR pathway, have been associated with BPP (Mirzaa et al. 2015).

Bilateral frontoparietal polymicrogyria (BFPP) (Fig. 3c) has been reported in families with recessive pedigrees and has been associated with mutations of the *GPR56* gene (Piao et al. 2004). The imaging characteristics of BFPP resemble those of the cobblestone malformative spectrum (muscle-eye-brain disease and Fukuyama congenital muscular dystrophy) (Barkovich et al. 2012).

Some copy-number variants have been associated with polymicrogyria (Table 1), but only deletions in 1p36.3 and 22q11.2 are common (Dobyns et al. 2008; Robin et al. 2006). Indeed, when these two loci are excluded, copy number variants seem to be rare. The causal gene has not been identified for any of these loci (Robin et al. 2006).

123.6 Tubulinopathies and Related Disorders

Classic lissencephaly and polymicrogyria have long been thought of as distinct disorders, but they have been associated with mutations of the same genes (tubulin or tubulin-related genes) that function during the early stages of neuronal proliferation, migration, differentiation, and axonal guidance (i.e., much earlier than the genes usually associated with polymicrogyria and schizencephaly) (Jaglin et al. 2009; Poirier et al. 2013; Cushion et al. 2013). The full range of these malformations vary from extreme lissencephaly with completely absent gyri, total agenesis of the corpus callosum, and severe cerebellar hypoplasia, to less severe lissencephaly with moderate-to-severe cerebellar hypoplasia, to classic lissencephaly, to an atypical polymicrogyria-like cortical malformation with cerebellar hypoplasia (Fig. 3d–h). By definition, tubulinopathies are always genetic. Investigators have identified nine genes (*KIF2A, KIF5C, TUBA1A, TUBA8, TUBB, TUBB2B, TUBB3, TUBG1,* and *DYNC1H1*; Table 1), but we expect additional genes to be reported in the near future. Findings from functional studies suggest that abnormal brain development in tubulinopathies results from a dominant negative effect of heterozygous missense mutations (in the absence of loss-of-function mutations) on the regulation of microtubule-dependent mitotic processes in progenitor cells and on the traffcking activities of the microtubule-dependent molecular motors KIF2A, KIF5C, and DYNC1H1 in postmitotic neuronal cells (Poirier et al. 2013).

AICARDI SYNDROME is exclusively observed in females, with the exception of two reported males with two X-chromosomes and is thought to be caused by an X-linked gene with lethality in the hemizygous male. However, the genetic basis is still unknown. Clinical features include severe mental retardation, infantile spasms, and chorioretinal lacunae. Neuropathological findings are consistent with a neuronal migration disorder and include diffuse unlayered polymicrogyria with fused molecular layers, agenesis of the corpus callosum, and nodular heterotopias in the periventricular or subcortical region. Microgyri are packed and usually not visible at MRI (Fig. 4) (Sutton and Van den Veyver 2006). The specific cause of Aicardi syndrome has not yet been identified.

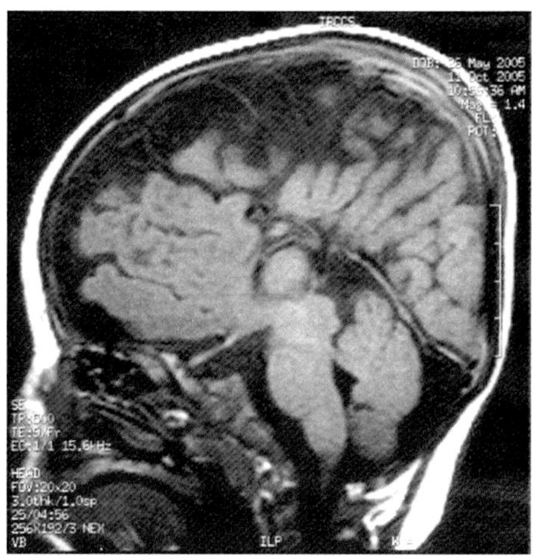

Fig. 4 T1 weighted sagittal MRI scan of the brain of a 5-months-old girl with Aicardi syndrome and intractable infantile spasms. Note the extremely hypoplastic corpus callosum with an extensive area of polymicrogyria involving the frontal lobe. There is a posterior fossa cyst

123.7 Megalencephaly, Dysplastic Megalencephaly, and FCD Type 2

The term megalencephaly refers to an abnormally large brain that exceeds the mean for age and gender by 2 SD (DeMyer 1986). Megalencephaly has most often been classified simply as a disorder of brain size, but recent studies have shown that megalencephaly with normal cortex by imaging, megalencephaly with polymicrogyria, and dysplastic megalencephaly (including classic hemimegalencephaly), and FCD can all result from mutations of the same genes in the PI3K-AKT-mTOR pathway (Lee et al. 2012; Poduri et al. 2012; Rivière et al. 2012). Dysplastic megalencephaly includes all forms of segmental brain overgrowth with cortical dysplasia. The developmental and health complications of megalencephaly differ widely. The most common problems include developmental delay, intellectual disability, and seizures that can start early in life and become intractable. The histological changes are similar if not identical to those in FCD type 2, which is characterized by cortical dyslamination and dysmorphic neurons without (type 2a) or with (type 2b) balloon cells, blurred junctions between grey and white matter, and increased heterotopic neurons in white matter (Blümcke et al. 2011). The highly focal and variable nature of FCD type 2b, and the pathological resemblance to tubers in tuberous sclerosis, led to the hypothesis that somatic mosaic mutations of genes that encode proteins in the mTOR pathway, which includes *TSC1* and *TSC2* that cause tuberous sclerosis, were implicated in FCD (Crino 2009). This hypothesis has been in part confirmed by recent studies documenting pathogenic germline and somatic mosaic mutations in the *MTOR* gene or in other genes belonging to the PI3K-AKT-mTOR pathway in the dysplasic tissue of FCD type 2a and 2b (D'Gama et al. 2015; Lim et al. 2015). In almost all patients with FCD type 2, the lesion is detected after onset of focal epilepsy. A growing number of syndromes and genes have been associated with megalencephaly, especially with more severe phenotypes (Mirzaa et al. 2012a). Megalencephaly without cortical malformations occurs in benign autosomal dominant macrocephaly, a poorly defined disorder. Megalencephaly with polymicrogyria occurs in megalencephaly-capillary malformation syndrome (with mutations of *PIK3CA*) and megalencephaly-polymicrogyria-polydactyly-hydrocephalus syndrome (with mutations of *PIK3R2* or *AKT3*) (Mirzaa et al. 2015; Mirzaa et al. 2012b). Dysplastic megalencephaly most often occurs without syndromic features and has recently been associated with mosaic mutations of *PIK3CA*, *AKT3*, and *MTOR* (Lee et al. 2012).

References

Barkovich AJ, Guerrini R, Kuzniecky RI et al (2012) A developmental and genetic classification for malformations of cortical development: update 2012. Brain 135:1348–1369

Blümcke I, Thom M, Aronica E et al (2011) The clinicopathologic spectrum of focal cortical dysplasias: a consensus classifi cation proposed by an ad hoc Task Force of the ILAE Diagnostic Methods Commission. Epilepsia 52:158–174

Cardoso C, Leventer RJ, Dowling JJ et al (2002) Clinical and molecular basis of classical lissencephaly: mutations in the LIS1 gene (PAFAH1B1). Hum Mutat 19:4–15

Conti V, Carabalona A, Pallesi-Pocachard E et al (2013) Periventricular heterotopia in 6q terminal deletion syndrome: role of the C6orf70 gene. Brain 136: 3378–3394

Crino PB (2009) Focal brain malformations: seizures, signaling, sequencing. Epilepsia 50(Suppl 9):3–8

Cushion TD, Dobyns WB, Mullins JG et al (2013) Overlapping cortical malformations and mutations in TUBB2B and TUBA1A. Brain 136:536–548

DeMyer W (1986) Megalencephaly: types, clinical syndromes, and management. Pediatr Neurol 2:321–328

D'Gama AM, Geng Y, Couto JA et al (2015) Mammalian target of rapamycin pathway mutations cause hemimegalencephaly and focal cortical dysplasia. Ann Neurol 77:720–725

Dobyns WB, Mirzaa G, Christian SL et al (2008) Consistent chromosome abnormalities identify novel polymicrogyria loci in 1p36.3, 2p16.1-p23.1, 4q21.21-q22.1, 6q26-q27, and 21q2. Am J Med Genet A 146A:1637–1654

Dobyns WB, Guerrini R, Leventer RL (2012) Malformations of cortical development. In: Swaiman KF, Ashwal S, Ferriero DM, Schor NF (eds) Swaiman's pediatric neurology: principles and practice, 5th edn. Elsevier Saunders, Edinburgh, pp 202–231

Gleeson JG, Walsh CA (2000) Neuronal migration disorders: from genetic diseases to developmental mechanisms. Trends Neurosci 23:352–359

Gleeson JG, Minnerath S, Kuzniecky RI et al (2000) Somatic and germline mosaic mutations in the doublecortin gene are associated with variable phenotypes. Am J Hum Genet 67:574–581

Guerrini R, Barba C (2010) Malformations of cortical development and aberrant cortical networks: epileptogenesis and functional organization. J Clin Neurophysiol 27:372–379

Guerrini R, Dobyns WB (2014) Malformations of cortical development: clinical features and genetic causes. Lancet Neurol 13:710–726

Guerrini R, Parrini E (2010) Neuronal migration disorders. Neurobiol Dis 38:154–166

Guerrini R, Moro F, Andermann E et al (2003) Nonsyndromic mental retardation and cryptogenic epilepsy in women with doublecortin gene mutations. Ann Neurol 54:30–37

Guerrini R, Mei D, Sisodiya S et al (2004) Germline and mosaic mutations of FLN1 in men with periventricular heterotopia. Neurology 63:51–56

Guerrini R, Dobyns W, Barkovich A (2008) Abnormal development of the human cerebral cortex: genetics, functional consequences and treatment options. Trends Neurosci 31:154–162

Jaglin XH, Poirier K, Saillour Y et al (2009) Mutations in the beta-tubulin gene TUBB2B result in asymmetrical polymicrogyria. Nat Genet 41:746–752

Lee JH, Huynh M, Silhavy JL et al (2012) De novo somatic mutations in components of the PI3K-AKT3-MTOR pathway cause hemimegalencephaly. Nat Genet 44: 941–945

Lim JS, Kim WI, Kang HC et al (2015) Brain somatic mutations in MTOR cause focal cortical dysplasia type II leading to intractable epilepsy. Nat Med 21:395–400

Matsumoto N, Leventer RJ, Kuc JA et al (2001) Mutation analysis of the DCX gene and genotype/phenotype correlation in subcortical band heterotopia. Eur J Hum Genet 9:5–12

Mei D, Lewis R, Parrini E et al (2008) High frequency of genomic deletions and duplication in the LIS1 gene in lissencephaly: implications for molecular diagnosis. J Med Genet 45:355–361

Mirzaa G, Ashwal S, Dobyns WB (2012a) Disorders of brain size. In: Swaiman KF, Ashwal S, Ferriero DF, Schor NF (eds) Swaiman's pediatric neurology: principles and practice, 5th edn. Elsevier Saunders, Edinburgh, pp 173–201

Mirzaa GM, Conway RL, Gripp KW et al (2012b) Megalencephaly-capillary malformation (MCAP) and megalencephaly-polydactyly-polymicrogyria-hydrocephalus (MPPH) syndromes: two closely related disorders of brain overgrowth and abnormal brain and body morphogenesis. Am J Med Genet A 158A:269–291

Mirzaa GM, Conti V, Timms AE et al (2015) Characterisation of mutations of the phosphoinositide-3-kinase regulatory subunit, PIK3R2, in perisylvian polymicrogyria: a next-generation sequencing study. Lancet Neurol 14:1182–1195

Parrini E, Ramazzotti A, Dobyns WB et al (2006) Periventricular heterotopia: phenotypic heterogeneity and correlation with Filamin A mutations. Brain 129:1892–1906

Piao X, Hill RS, Bodell A et al (2004) G protein-coupled receptor-dependent development of human frontal cortex. Science 303:2033–2036

Poduri A, Evrony GD, Cai X et al (2012) Somatic activation of AKT3 causes hemispheric developmental brain malformations. Neuron 74:41–48

Poirier K, Lebrun N, Broix L et al (2013) Mutations in TUBG1, DYNC1H1, KIF5C and KIF2A cause malformations of cortical development and microcephaly. Nat Genet 45:639–647

Rivière JB, Mirzaa GM, O'Roak BJ, Finding of Rare Disease Genes (FORGE) Canada Consortium et al (2012) De novo germline and postzygotic mutations in AKT3, PIK3R2 and PIK3CA cause a spectrum of related megalencephaly syndromes. Nat Genet 44:934–940

Robin NH, Taylor CJ, McDonald-McGinn DM et al (2006) Polymicrogyria and deletion 22q11.2 syndrome: window to the etiology of a common cortical malformation. Am J Med Genet A 140:2416–2425

Sheen VL, Ganesh VS, Topcu M et al (2004) Mutations in ARFGEF2 implicate vesicle trafficking in neural progenitor proliferation and migration in the human cerebral cortex. Nat Genet 36:69–76

Sutton VR, Van den Veyver IB (2006) Aicardi syndrome. In: Pagon RA, Adam MP, Ardinger HH, Wallace SE et al (eds) GeneReviews® [Internet]. University of Washington, Seattle, pp 1993–2015

Congenital Malformations of the Brain: Spectrum and Causes

124

Elie Saliba

Contents

Abstract

Defective nervous system development results in a diverse group of diseases, ranging from major malformations that are incompatible with postnatal life to moderate or severe disabilities. Congenital malformations of the brain refer to any structural abnormality of the central nervous system (CNS), present at birth, and due to interrupted or modified CNS development

E. Saliba (✉)
Department of Neonatology and Pediatric Intensive Care, Université François Rabelais and CHRU de Tours, Tours, France

Inserm U930, France, Université François Rabelais and CHRU de Tours, Tours, France
e-mail: elie.saliba@univ-tours.fr

G. Buonocore et al. (eds.), *Neonatology*,
https://doi.org/10.1007/978-3-319-29489-6_271

during intrauterine life, whatever the etiology. The frequency of CNS malformations has been estimated to be 5–10/1000 births, found in 5–10% of stillborn infants, or early deceased neonates.

124.1 Salient Points

- Defective nervous system development results in a diverse group of diseases, ranging from major malformations that are incompatible with postnatal life to moderate or severe disabilities.
- In holoprosencephaly, there is defective subdivision of the early embryonic forebrain to form the bilateral telencephalic vesicles, the precursors of the cerebral hemispheres.
- Failure of neural tube closure results in malformations termed neural tube defects (NTDs).
- Brain herniation yields a defect called encephalocele, while herniation of the spinal cord is termed meningocele.
- Agenesis or hypoplasia of the vermis may be found in a large number of malformations of the brain, including the Dandy–Walker malformation and syndromes with agenesis of the vermis as a constant feature, such as the Joubert syndrome and Walker–Warburg syndrome, and a large group of syndromes in which absence of the vermis may occur, such as Meckel–Gruber and Smith–Lemli–Opitz syndromes.
- Ponto-cerebellar hypoplasias are autosomal recessive disorders.
- Malformations of cortical development include three major groups that recapitulate the main developmental steps: malformations due to abnormal cell proliferation, neuronal migration or postmigrational cortical organization and connectivity.
- Human microcephaly comprises a heterogeneous group of conditions that are characterized by a failure of normal brain growth.
- The etiology of microcephaly can be broadly divided into environmental (as congenital infections, intrauterine exposure to teratogenic agents, and hypoxic–ischemic injury) and genetic causes.
- Decreased neuronal proliferation may lead to microcephaly with a normal to thin cortex, microlissencephaly, and microcephaly with polymicrogyria or other cortical dysplasia.
- Agenesis of the corpus callosum has been associated with numerous syndromes (Aicardi syndrome) and several inborn errors of metabolism, including non-ketonic hyperglycinemia and fetal alcohol syndrome. It may be observed in various malformations of cortical development, including the lissencephalies, polymicrogyria, and schizencephaly, and in chromosomal disorders.
- Intracranial arachnoid cysts are benign, non-genetic developmental cysts that contain spinal fluid and occur within the arachnoid membrane.
- Hydrocephalus signifies dilated lateral ventricles resulting from an increased amount of CSF inside the ventricles and increased intracranial pressure, while ventriculomegaly is a dilatation of the lateral ventricles without increased intracranial pressure. Ventriculomegaly may be due to cerebral hypoplasia or a CNS anomaly such as agenesis of the corpus callosum.
- Genetic hydrocephalus is rare, but it is important in counseling couples about subsequent pregnancies. It is now well recognized that a small proportion of all cases of hydrocephalus show X-linked inheritance.

124.2 Introduction

The development of the brain is a complex and tightly organized process. It involves a complex cascade of genetic material signaling the formation of intricate structures at critical periods of time. This process can be influenced and disrupted by environmental factors or by inherited or de novo genetic mutations. The type of disruptive insult (e.g., hemorrhage or infection) is not as important as the timing (in regard to structural development) and the genetic susceptibility of the fetus. Congenital brain malformation can result in a wide range of developmental disorders according to the timing of their occurrence

Table 1 Cerebral development and major disorders

Developmental stage	Disorders
Primary neurulation (3–4 weeks' gestation)	Neural tube defects
Prosencephalic development (23 months' gestation)	Holoprosencephaly; agenesis of the corpus callosum
Neuronal proliferation (34 months' gestation)	Microcephaly
Neuronal migration (35 months' gestation)	Lissencephaly; polymicrogyria; schizencephaly. Other migration disorders
Myelination (mainly after birth)	White matter hypoplasia

during CNS development (Table 1). The following pages review the main categories of central brain malformations. A detailed description of the clinical and neuropathological aspects of these defects is beyond the scope of the present chapter.

124.3 Prenatal Diagnosis

Suspicion of a congenital brain malformation may arise on clinical grounds or because of an abnormal result from a routine prenatal investigation. A pregnancy may be at high risk of abnormality because of a particular family history, the advanced age of the mother, or some acquired etiologies (Table 2). Higher-risk groups for chromosome abnormalities include older mothers, those with a previous chromosomally abnormal child, and when one parent is a translocation carrier. Usually, these women are offered chorionic villus sampling or amniocentesis. Ultrasonography is the method of choice for prenatal scanning of fetal anomalies. High-frequency ultrasonography allows visualization of the normal and abnormal development of the embryo or fetus. However, there remain circumstances in which ultrasound data obtained are limited or technically difficult, for example, in oligohydramnios and unfavorable position of the fetus. Moreover, some subtle parenchymal abnormalities cannot be seen on ultrasound. Magnetic resonance imaging (MRI) may be a useful adjuvant when ultrasound is indeterminate. MRI is also especially useful in cases in which fetal ventriculomegaly is associated with other CNS malformations. Other anomalies such as lissencephaly and schizencephaly and also more subtle parenchymal migration disorders such as heterotopia and polymicrogyria have been visualized with MRI.

Table 2 Example of acquired etiologies of human nervous malformations, neural tube defects (NTDs), and intrauterine growth restriction (IUGR)

Agent	Most common congenital anomalies
Drugs	
Alcohol	Neuronal migration disorders; fetal alcohol syndrome; IUGR; facial anomalies
Cocaine	Microcephaly; IUGR
Isotretinoin (Accutane)	NTD; craniofacial malformations
Methotrexate	Hydrocephalus; myelomeningocele; skeletal anomalies
Phenytoin (Dilantin)	Microcephaly; cleft lip/palate; facial anomalies
Valproic acid	NTD; facial anomalies
Infectious agents	
Cytomegalovirus	Microcephaly; hydrocephalus; brain calcifications
Herpes virus type 1 and 2	Hydranencephaly
Human immune-deficiency virus	Microcephaly; IUGR
Rubella virus	Microcephaly; IUGR; heart abnormalities
Toxoplasma gondii	Microcephaly; ventriculomegaly; brain calcifications
Varicella virus	Hydrocephalus

124.4 Major Congenital Brain Malformations

124.4.1 Holoprosencephaly

Subdivision of the early embryonic forebrain to form the bilateral telencephalic vesicles, the precursors of the cerebral hemispheres, is defective in holoprosencephaly. At its most severe, the forebrain is completely undivided (alobar holoprosencephaly) leading to a monoventricle and non-separation of

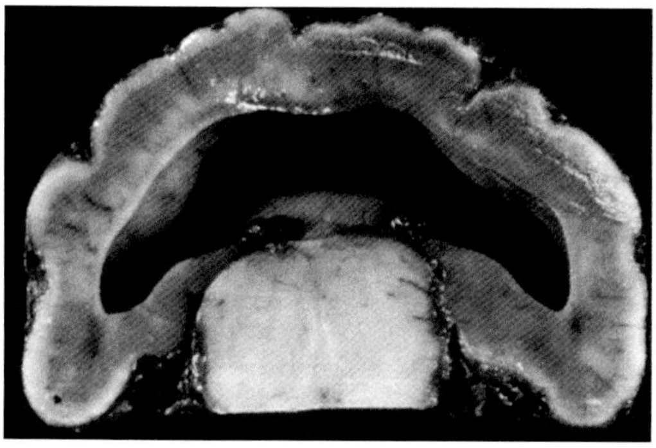

Fig. 1 Alobar holoprosencephaly

Table 3 Facial defects in holoprosencephaly

Cyclopia	Single eye or single orbit. Arrhinia with proboscis
Ethmocephaly	Extreme hypotelorism arrhinia with proboscis
Cebocephaly	Orbital hypotelorism proboscis-like nose, no cleft
Median cleft	Orbital hypotelorism. Flat nose
Agnathia-astomia	Hypoplasia or absence of the mandible. Small or absent mouth. Abnormal position of the ears

the thalami (Fig. 1). Non-separation of these structures declines in less severe forms (e.g., semilobar holoprosencephaly). Holoprosencephaly is usually associated with craniofacial malformations such as brachycephaly, microcephaly, and abnormal facial development (Table 3). In the most severe form, holoprosencephaly may be accompanied by failure of separation of the optic vesicles and eye primordia, yielding the birth defect cyclopia. In less severe forms, the most noticeable abnormalities are often a reduction of midline craniofacial features, with close-set eyes (hypotelorism) or a single central incisor tooth. The detection rate by routine fetal anomaly scan is high for both the lobar and semilobar forms of holoprosencephaly, even in the first trimester (Blaas et al. 2002). Several chromosomal regions have been linked to holoprosencephaly. The genetic basis of most of the chromosomal linkages in holoprosencephaly has now been elucidated. Several of the causative genes are transcription factors (*ZIC2*, *SIX3*, and *TGIF*) (Ming and Muenke 2002). These genes are known to be expressed in the embryonic brain.

124.4.2 Neural Tube Defects

Failure of neural tube closure results in malformations termed neural tube defects (NTDs). In craniorachischisis, the most severe type of NTD, the neural tube fails to close along most of the body axis, although the forebrain usually closes normally. If the neural tube fails to close specifically in the future brain, exencephaly results, which is concerted to anencephaly owing to neurodegeneration in later gestation. In contrast, if the low spine is primarily affected, this leads to open spina bifida. Related to these open CNS defects are a series of closed defects in which the neural tube and/or meninges herniate through an opening in the skull or in the neural arches of the vertebral column (Fig. 2).

Brain herniation yields a defect called encephalocele, while herniation of the spinal cord is termed meningocele. A further category of neural tube defect is so-called occult spina bifida, which mainly affect the low spinal region and are skin-covered lesions in which the spinal cord may be split or tethered to the surrounding tissues, often in association with a bony spur or a fatty mass (lipoma). While covered lesions are protected from the potentially toxic amniotic environment, open neural tube defect lesions undergo erosion of the exposed neuroepithelium so that, by the late stages of gestation, the region of affected nervous system is largely degenerate, leading to severe disability or death after birth. Surgery of the human fetus during pregnancy, with the aim of covering the neural tube defect lesion with muscle and skin, has shown that this process of degeneration can be halted (Pedreira et al. 2016), minimizing damage to the exposed CNS but not recovering full function.

Neural tube defects (NTDs) are not only very heterogeneous in morphology but also in etiology (Padmanabhan 2006; Leduc et al. 2016). Causes include chromosome abnormalities, single mutant genes, teratogens, maternal predisposing factors, and multifactorial inheritance. The high recurrence in siblings and in close relatives of individual with NTD suggests a strong genetic basis, although there is a

Fig. 2 Neural tube defects. (**a**) Meningocele, covered with full-thickness skin. (**b**) Myelomeningocele, failure of primary neurulation that results in an open neural tube that is still attached peripherally to the adjacent skin. (**c**) Lipomyelomeningocele (spinal lipoma)

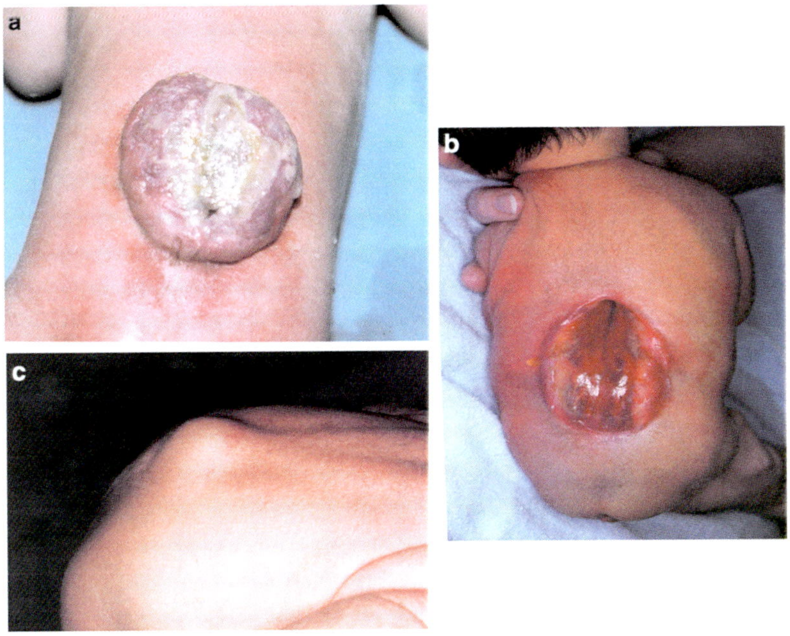

marked lack of large families with NTD, arguing against causation based on single genes. It has been suggested, therefore, that NTDs have a multifactorial causation, with many variants interacting to determine individual. Despite the many genetic loci that have been implicated in mouse NTD, few human genes have so far been definitively shown to predispose to human NTD. The best known of these is the gene encoding 5, 10-methylene tetrahydrofolate reductase (MTHFR), an enzyme of folic acid metabolism. A polymorphic, variant of the MTHFR gene (the C677T variant) exhibits a higher frequency among NTD cases and their families than among normal controls in several populations and seems responsible for imparting an increased risk of NTDs, especially in combination with a low folate and/or vitamin B_{12} level during pregnancy (Yadav et al. 2015).

Many environmental factors have been suggested to play a role in NTD etiology (Sarmah et al. 2016). Nutritional deficiency, maternal diabetes, and the use of certain therapeutic drugs such as anticonvulsants and insulin are known risk factors. Periconceptional supplementation of folic acid lowers the occurrence and recurrence risks of human NTD. The mechanisms involved in NTD due to a lower maternal folate status may be defective folic acid mechanism in the mother (Yadav et al. 2015; Sarmah et al. 2016). A list of recognized cause of NTD in human is presented (Table 4).

Table 4 Examples of recognized cause of NTD in human

Causes	Examples
Chromosome abnormalities	Trisomy 13
	Trisomy 18
	Various unbalanced chromosome rearrangements, ring chromosomes, triploidy
Single mutant genes: autosomal recessive	Walker–Warburg syndrome Jarcho Levin syndrome Meckel–Gruber syndrome Robert syndrome
Teratogens	Valproic acid carbamazepine (possible) hyperthermia (possible)
Maternal predisposing factors	Diabetes mellitus: anencephaly more frequent than spina bifida

124.4.2.1 Neural Tube Defects: Prenatal Diagnosis

NTD can be detected by ultrasound and by analyzing the alpha fetoprotein (AFP) level in amniotic fluid or maternal serum. Increased levels of AFP are also found in other fetal anomalies such as gastroschisis and esophageal and intestinal atresia, in sacrococcygeal teratoma, and in Turner syndrome, but decreased levels are found in trisomies 21 and 18. Moreover, the AFP method has a high false-positive rate and a relatively poor sensitivity. Ultrasound is the main method for detection of NTD. Prenatal diagnosis of a myelomeningocele is usually prompted by the recognition of the associated Chiari II malformation. The most efficient sonographic findings, indicating a Chiari II malformation, are the diagnostic "lemon" and "banana" signs (Fig. 3) (Nicolaides et al. 1986). The lemon sign of the head has become the diagnostic key for detecting spina bifida in the second trimester. The banana sign represents the cerebellum surrounding stem in a small posterior fossa. The lemon sign is transient and usually not present anymore by the end of the second trimester. It represents an abnormal cranial vault that is narrowed rostrally and results from low pressure in the ventricular cavity due to loss of CSF through the open NTD to the amniotic cavity. With the introduction of transvaginal ultrasound, detailed diagnosis became possible in the early fetal period and even around the end of the embryonic period (Blass et al. 2000).

124.4.3 Developmental Disorders of the Cerebellum

Anatomically, cerebellar malformations may be classified into unilateral and bilateral abnormalities. Unilateral cerebellar malformations are most likely due to acquired insults, such as intracerebellar bleeding associated with prematurity. Depending on the part of the cerebellum involved, bilateral cerebellar malformations may be further classified into midline or vermis malformations and malformations affecting both the vermis and the cerebellar hemispheres (Ramaekers 2000). The combination of pontine hypoplasia with cerebellar malformation is considered as a separate group, i.e., the pontocerebellar hypoplasia.

124.4.3.1 Midline or Vermis Malformations

Agenesis or hypoplasia of the vermis may be found in a large number of malformations of the brain (Aicardi 1998), including the Dandy–Walker malformation and syndromes with agenesis of the vermis as a constant feature, such as the Joubert syndrome and Walker–Warburg syndrome, and a large group of syndromes in which absence of the vermis may occur, such as Meckel–Gruber and Smith–Lemli–Opitz syndromes.

The Dandy–Walker malformation is characterized by the following triad: cystic dilatation of the fourth ventricle and an enlarged posterior fossa, varying degrees of vermian aplasia or hypoplasia, and hydrocephalus (Fig. 4). Hydrocephalus, associated with a bulging occiput, is unusual at birth but is present by 3 months of age in about 75% of patients (Bordarier and Aicardi 1990; Barkovich 2000). Mental retardation and seizures have been reported in up to 50% of cases with a Dandy–Walker malformation (Pascual-Castroviejo et al. 1991a). Associated CNS malformations are present in up to 68% of the cases, the most common of which is agenesis or hypogenesis of the

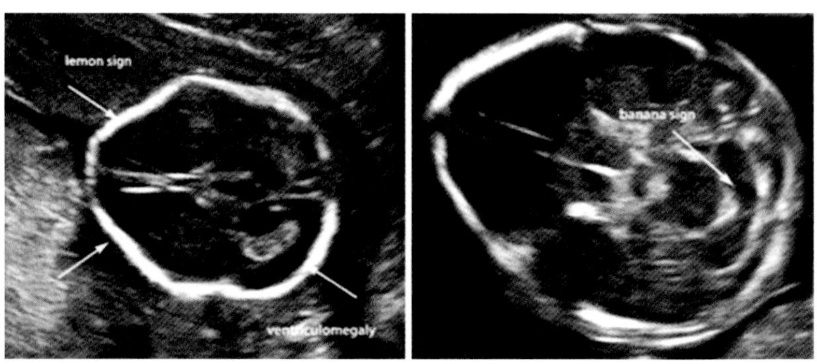

Fig. 3 The cranial signs: The cranial signs ("lemon" and "banana") associated with open spina bifida

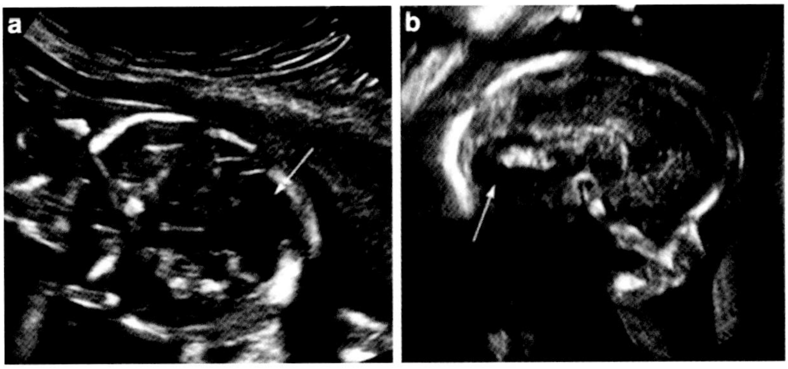

Fig. 4 Dandy–Walker malformation: (**a**) axial plane demonstrating a large cisterna communicating with the area of the fourth ventricle (*white arrow*); (**b**) sagittal view demonstrating a large cisterna magna

corpus callosum (Barkovich 2003). Other CNS malformations include neuronal heterotopias, polymicrogyria, schizencephaly, occipital encephaloceles, and lumbosacral meningoceles (Bordarier and Aicardi 1990).

Most cases of Dandy–Walker malformation are sporadic. The etiology remains unknown. Distinguishing inheritable syndromes from isolated cases of vermian–cerebellar hypoplasia is important for genetic counseling. Bordarier and Aicardi classified the genetically heritable syndromes with complex vermian–cerebellar hypoplasia into two groups: (1) those in which vermis aplasia is a constant feature, the most common entities being Joubert syndrome, Walker–Warburg syndrome, and related cerebro-oculomuscular syndromes, and (2) those in which vermis aplasia is an occasional component, such as Meckel–Gruber syndrome, Coffin–Siris syndrome, Smith–Lemli–Opitz syndrome, and Ellis–van Creveld syndrome, all autosomal-recessive traits (Bordarier and Aicardi 1990). Dandy–Walker syndrome has recently been shown to be related in some cases to genetic disorders of two members of the *ZIC* gene family, which encode zinc finger transcription factors (Grinberg et al. 2004). Joubert syndrome is a relatively rare, autosomal-recessive disorder defined by vermis hypoplasia, hypotonia, developmental delay, and at least one of two additional manifestations: abnormal breathing pattern (hyperpnea intermixed with central apnea in the neonatal period) or abnormal eye movements (Joubert et al. 1969). In Joubert syndrome, ataxia, mental retardation, and behavioral disorders become manifest in late infancy and childhood (Aicardi 1998). The prognosis of Joubert syndrome is poor; a causative gene was recently identified (Ferland et al. 2004).

124.4.3.2 Cerebellar Hypoplasia

In cerebellar hypoplasia, the cerebellum does not reach its normal size. Global cerebellar hypoplasia may result from a variety of exogenous or endogenous factors. It is found as a result of intrauterine exposure to drugs (e.g., phenytoin) or irradiation and as an autosomal-recessive trait in a variety of chromosomal disorders such as trisomies 13, 18, and 21 (Norman et al. 1995; Ramaekers et al. 1997). Cerebellar hypoplasia may also be found in various complex malformations involving the brain and other systems. Primary degeneration of the granular layer of the cerebellum or granular layer aplasia (GLA) occurs as an autosomal regressive disorder (Pascual-Castroviejo et al. 1994). Patients with features consistent with GLA have been found to have elevated levels of serum asialotransferrin and heterozygous deficiency of phosphomannomutase type 2 (PMM2). This deficit is involved in the congenital disorders of glycosylation (CDGs) (Pascual-Castroviejo 2002).

124.4.3.3 Pontocerebellar Hypoplasia

The pontocerebellar hypoplasia forms a large group of disorders characterized by a smaller volume of the pons and varying degrees of cerebellar hypoplasia up to near-total absence of the cerebellum. Most types of pontocerebellar hypoplasia arise in the fetal period, suggesting a rhombic lip defect and the *MATH1* gene as candidate for this disorder. Most pontocerebellar hypoplasias are autosomal-recessive disorders (Gardner et al. 2001).

124.5 Malformations of Cortical Development

The development of the human cerebral cortex is a complex and tightly organized process. Disruption of any of the overlapping steps that contribute to this process can result in a wide range of malformations. These defects are grouped under the term of malformations of cortical development (MCD). MCD includes three major groups that recapitulate the main developmental steps as malformations of cell proliferation, neuronal migration, or postmigrational cortical organization and connectivity. Many of these disorders are recognized as malformations in studies of brain imaging and include lissencephaly, polymicrogyria, schizencephaly, focal cortical dysplasia (FCD), and periventricular nodular heterotopia.

Knowledge of the main morphological features of the normal pattern of cortical development has helped the prenatal diagnosis of some MCD, including regional polymicrogyria at an early sulcation stage with the use of either neurosonography or fetal MRI. Diagnoses can sometimes be made before 24 weeks of gestation and can help select the most appropriate genetic testing and counseling. For these reasons, detailed neurosonographic examination or fetal brain MRI is recommended even when minor CNS anomalies, or even non-CNS anomalies, are detected by previous ultrasound. However, these imaging techniques also have serious limitations, because of the risk of detection of non-pathological variants, very little association with neuropathological findings, and complexities in provision of appropriate counseling.

Neuronal migration consists of nerve cells moving from their original site in the ventricular and subventricular zones to their final location. Regulation of timing and direction of these simultaneous migrations is carried out with extreme precision. Neurons originating in the cortical ventricular zone migrate radially to form the cortical plate and mainly become projection neurons (Kanatani et al. 2005). Migration of neocortical neurons occurs mostly between the fifth gestational week, when the telencephalic vesicle appears, and 22 weeks of gestation in the human (Bielas et al. 2004). The neurons that migrate first will stop in the deepest cortical layers; those which migrate afterward pass through the layers formed previously to form the outer cortical layers, according to a migration scheme defined as "inside-out." Neocortical migration neurons can adopt different types of trajectories: a large proportion of neurons migrate radially along radial glial guides, from the germinative zone to the cortical plate. Another important group of neurons adopt a tangential trajectory at the level of the ventricular or subventricular germinative zones before adopting a classic radial migrating pathway along glial guides. Tangentially migrating neurons have also been located at intermediate zone level (prospective white matter). Three large classes of genes underlie the vast majority of neuronal migration disorders that are seen clinically: (1) those involving the formation of the extracellular environment encountered by migrating neurons and axons, (2) those encoding for intracellular signaling mechanisms, and (3) those encoding the intracellular system that mediates cellular and axonal physical movements (Gressens 2005; Meyer 2007). Another group of genes is involved in encoding for the enzymatic regulator of glycosylation, which, in turn, seems to provide stop signs for migrating neurons (Guerrini and Dobyns 2014). A list of genes implicated in neuronal migration disorders is presented in Table 5.

124.5.1 Lissencephaly

Lissencephaly (LIS), which literally means smooth brain, consists of a set of rare brain disorders characterized by the lack of normal cortical convolutions (Fig. 5). The severity ranges from absence (agyria) to reduction (pachygyria) of normal gyral

Table 5 Genes implicated in neuronal migration disorders

Neuronal migration disorder	Gene	Gene function	Location
Lissencephaly (Miller–Dieker and isolated lissencephaly sequence)	*LIS1*	Microtubule activating protein	17p13.3
X-linked lissencephaly	*DCX* (doublecortin)	Microtubule stabilizing protein	Xq22.3-q23
X-linked lissencephaly with ambiguous genitalia	ARX	Homeobox transcription factor	Xp22.13
Autosomal-recessive lissencephaly	*RELN* (reelin)	Extracellular matrix signaling protein	7q22
Cobblestone (Type 2) lissencephaly (Fukuyama muscular dystrophy)	*FCMD* (fukutin)		
Cobblestone (type 2) lissencephaly (Walker–Warburg syndrome)	*POMT1*	αOMT1estone (type 2) lissencephaly	9q34.1
	FLNA (filamin-A)	Actin-binding protein	Xq2

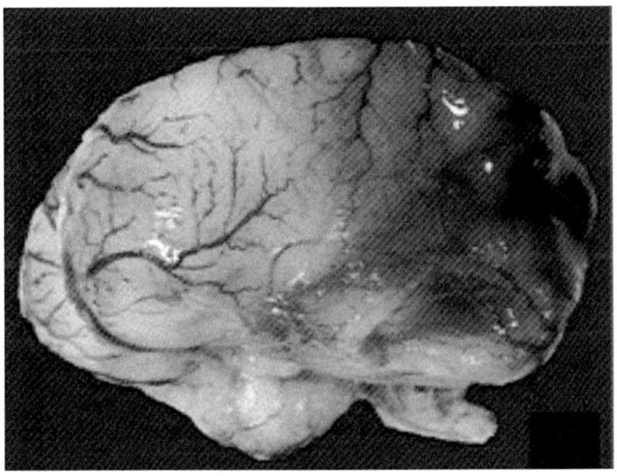

Fig. 5 View of the brain of a fetus with lissencephaly. Note the absence of Sylvian fissure of normal gyral pattern and of cortical convolutions

pattern. On the basis of etiologies and associated malformations, five groups of lissencephaly can be identified: classical lissencephaly, cobblestone lissencephaly, X-linked lissencephaly with agenesis of the corpus callosum, lissencephaly with cerebellar hypoplasia, and microlissencephaly (Verrotti et al. 2010). The onset of lissencephaly is considered to occur no later than the 12th–16th week of gestation (Diamandis et al. 2016). Different subtypes of LIS are readily distinguished based on the number of cortical layers affected and include two-layered, three-layered, and four-layered forms. The most common, classical LIS (four-layered form) features a very thick cortex (10–20 mm vs. the normal 4 mm) and no other major brain malformations. The cytoarchitecture consists of 4 primitive layers, including an outer marginal layer, which contains Cajal–Retzius neurons (layer 1); a superficial cellular layer, which contains numerous large and disorganized pyramidal neurons (layer 2) corresponding to the true cortex; a variable cell-sparse layer (layer 3); and a deep cellular layer (composed of medium and small neurons), which extends more than half the width of the mantle (layer 4) (Fig. 6). On brain imaging, for all forms of lissencephaly, the brain surface appears smooth with areas of absent (agyria) and abnormally wide (pachygyria) gyri (Fig. 7). The cerebral cortex is abnormally thick 8–15 mm compared with 2·5–4 mm for normal cortex—except when the cerebral wall is thin, as can occur with two-layered and occasionally four-layered lissencephaly. The various clinical subtypes of lissencephaly have different risks of recurrence in siblings. Isolated lissencephaly is causally heterogeneous. Genetic counseling is always indicated for families with children with lissencephaly (Diamandis et al. 2016). The main causative genes are *LIS1, YWHAE, DCX*, and *TUBA1A*.

Patients with severe LIS have early developmental delay, early diffuse hypotonia, later spastic quadriplegia, and eventual severe or profound mental retardation. Seizures occur in over 90% of LIS children, with onset before 6 months in about 75% of the cases.

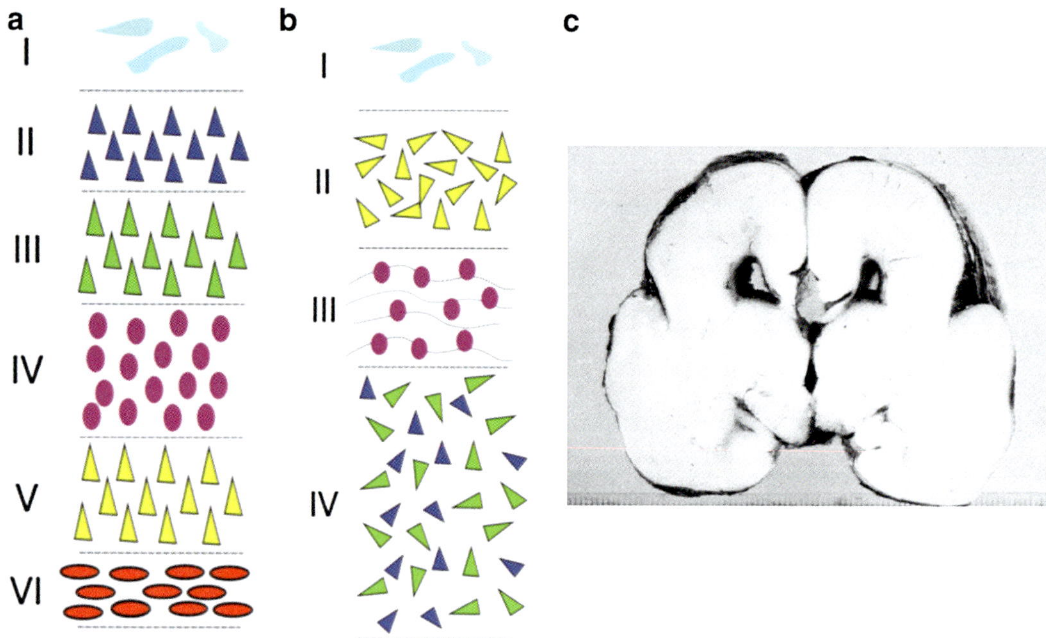

Fig. 6 (**a**) Normal cortical laminar organization (6 layers). (**b**) Cortical layering in classical lissencephaly (four non-organized layers). (**c**) Type I lissencephaly

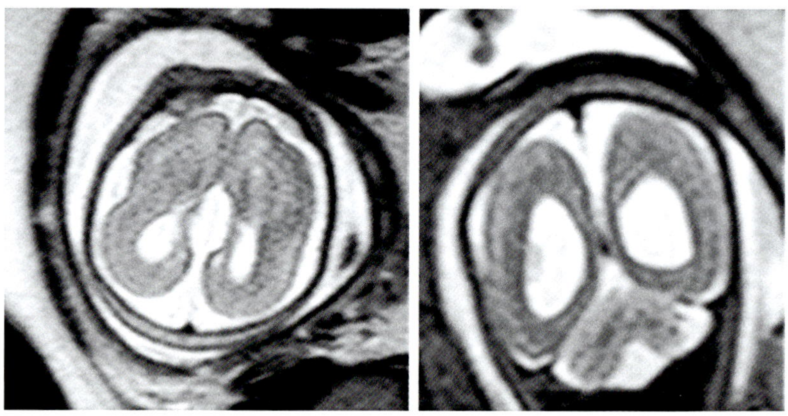

Fig. 7 Fetus at 32 weeks' gestation with complete agyria and virtually no sulci

124.5.2 Polymicrogyria

Polymicrogyria (PMG) is a cortical malformation characterized by an irregular brain surface with many excessively small convolutions, which might or might not be visible on gross inspection of the brain surface.

PMG can be focal or diffused or unilateral or bilateral. It can be an isolated lesion or associated with other brain malformations such as heterotopia, white matter lesions. Two types of polymicrogyria can be identified by histology: a simplified four-layered form and an unlayered form (Barth 1992). One specific pattern of polymicrogyria occurs in schizencephaly. Although PMG most often occurs as an isolated cortical malformation, it may be associated with other brain malformations including agenesis of the corpus callosum, microcephaly or megalencephaly, periventricular nodular heterotopia, cerebellar vermis hypoplasia, or more diffuse cerebellar hypoplasia.

Little is known about the factors that contribute to the development of polymicrogyria. PMG appears to be a highly heterogeneous disorder in terms of pathogenesis, topographic distribution, pathological appearance, imaging features, and clinical presentation. Evidence for both genetic and nongenetic etiologies exists (Diamandis et al. 2016; Jansen and Andermann 2005). Polymicrogyria occurs at the periphery of ischemic insults, and in association with congenital infections, particularly cytomegalovirus, fetal cerebral ischemia from placental perfusion failure, twin–twin transfusion, loss of a twin in utero, and maternal drug ingestion can be involved in its pathogenesis. The association of polymicrogyria with several genetically determined syndromes such as Zellweger, Aicardi, and Walker–Warburg syndromes, its presence in patients with chromosomal abnormalities, and the occurrence of familial cases, all strongly indicate a genetic component in its development.

On brain imaging, polymicrogyric cortices often appear mildly thickened (usually 6–10 mm) because of cortical overfolding. Diffusely abnormal signal in white matter should suggest in utero infection (e.g., by cytomegalovirus). Polymicrogyria has been described in several topographic patterns. The most common by far is bilateral perisylvian polymicrogyria (Fig. 8).

The clinical manifestations of polymicrogyria vary widely and depend on several factors. The most severe outcomes occur in children with severe microcephaly (−3 SD or smaller), abnormal neurological examination, widespread anatomic abnormality, and additional brain malformations such as heterotopia or cerebellar hypoplasia. The best outcomes are in individuals who have localized unilateral polymicrogyria without other malformations.

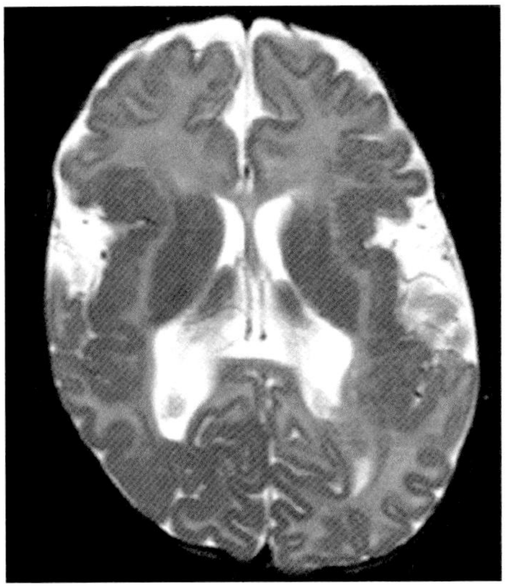

Fig. 8 Cerebral MRI at the age of 3 months. Extended symmetric polymicrogyria

124.5.3 Schizencephaly

Schizencephaly is a structural abnormality of the brain, characterized by congenital clefts spanning the cerebral hemisphere from the pial surface to the lateral ventricle and lined by cortical gray matter (Fig. 9) (Packard et al. 1997). The gray matter lining the cleft has the imaging appearance of polymicrogyria with an irregular surface, deep infolding (the cleft), mildly thick cortex, and stippling of the interface between gray and white matter. Schizencephaly is often bilateral but frequently asymmetrical. Cleft localization varies widely, but perisylvian region is more often involved. Causes including genetic, vascular, toxic, metabolic, and infectious factors might be involved. Exposure in utero to toxins and CMV infections has been incriminated (Barkovich et al. 2001).

Patients with closed-lip unilateral schizencephaly typically present with hemiparesis or motor delay, whereas patients with open-lip schizencephaly typically present with hydrocephalus or seizures. Outcomes are worst for patients with bilateral open-lip schizencephaly and best for those with unilateral closed-lip schizencephaly.

124.5.4 Tubulinopathies (Synonym: Tubulin-Related Cortical Dysgenesis)

The tubulinopathies are a wide and overlapping range of brain malformations caused by mutation

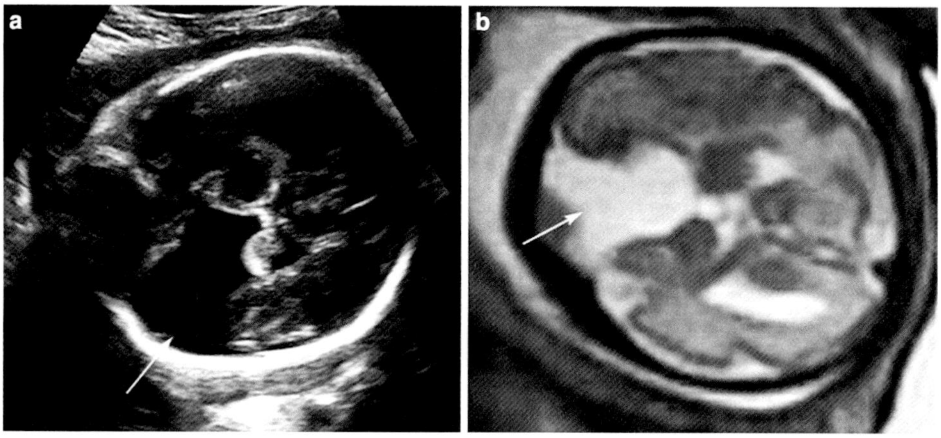

Fig. 9 Schizencephaly: Fetus of 32 weeks. (**a**) Ultrasound image: axial view (*arrow*); (**b**) magnetic resonance image (*arrow*)

of one of seven genes encoding different isotypes of tubulin. Tubulinopathies include a range of brain malformations: lissencephalies (classic lissencephaly, lissencephaly with cerebellar hypoplasia, lissencephaly with agenesis of the corpus callosum, and centrally predominant pachygyria), polymicrogyria-like cortical dysplasia, simplified gyral pattern, and microlissencephaly often in combination with dysplastic basal ganglia, corpus callosum abnormalities, and hypoplasia or dysplasia of the brain stem and cerebellum. The diagnosis of a tubulinopathy (regardless of the gene involved) is based on the presence of characteristic complex brain malformations. Establishing the genetic cause requires molecular genetic testing to identify a heterozygous pathogenic variant in one of six genes (*TUBA1A, TUBB2A, TUBB2B, TUBB3, TUBB* [*TUBB5*], or *TUBG1*) or biallelic pathogenic variants in *TUBA8*.

124.5.4.1 Prenatal Testing and Preimplantation Genetic Diagnosis

Once the tubulinopathy-related pathogenic variant has been identified in an affected family member, prenatal testing and preimplantation genetic diagnosis for a pregnancy at increased risk are possible options. Clinical features include motor and intellectual disabilities, epilepsy, and ocular findings of varying severity.

Table 6 Classification of heterotopia from Barkovich et al. (2001)

1. Periventricular heterotopia
(a) Periventricular nodular heterotopia (PNH)
(i) Bilateral PNH with FLN1 mutations
(ii) PNH with mutations of chromosome 5
(iii) PNH with bilateral polymicrogyria-perisylvian and posterior subtypes
(b) Periventricular linear heterotopia (unilateral or bilateral)
2. Subcortical heterotopia
(a) Large subcortical heterotopia with cortical infolding, abnormal cortex, hypogenetic corpus callosum
(b) Pure subcortical heterotopia nodules
(c) Columnar heterotopia
(d) Excessive single neurons in white matter
3. Marginal glioneuronal heterotopia

124.5.5 Neuronal Heterotopia

Neuronal heterotopia is a neuronal migration disorder characterized by a cluster of disorganized neurons in abnormal locations, and it includes three main groups: periventricular nodular heterotopia (PNH), subcortical heterotopia (SBH), and marginal glioneuronal heterotopia. The most frequent form is the PNH. A classification of neuronal heterotopia is presented Table 6.

Periventricular nodular heterotopia (PNH) is a malformation in which group of neurons are abnormally positioned close to the ventricular cavities. This form may be associated with hypoplasia of corpus callosum and cerebellum. PNH can be caused by genetic mutations or extrinsic factors such as infections or prenatal injuries (Pang et al. 2008). X-linked periventricular heterotopia results mainly from mutation in the gene encoding filamin 1 (FLNA1), an actin-cross-linking phosphoprotein that interacts with filamin-B- and filamin-A-interacting protein (FILIP) to regulate the actin reorganization necessary for neuronal migration (Nagano et al. 2004). When the function of this protein complex is disturbed, neuroblasts are unable to initiate migration. Mutation of the FLNA gene (Xq28) causes bilateral PNH in the majority of patients; this form is often fatal for males, therefore explaining the female preponderance. Other gene mutation can cause PNH in both genders like the *ARFGEF2* gene mutation (Battaglia et al. 2006). MRI in patients with X-linked dominant mutation shows bilateral symmetric nodules adjacent to the lateral ventricular walls. Unilateral PNH is commonly located in the posterior paratrigonal zone of the lateral ventricles. Subcortical band heterotopia (SBH) is caused by alterations in two genes: *LIS1* at 17p13.32 and *DCX* at Xq22.3–q23.3. MRI of the brain in SBH demonstrates two parallel layers of gray matter, a thin outer ribbon and a thick inner band, separated by a very thin layer of white matter (Guerrini and Carrozzo 2001; D'Agostino et al. 2002). Although most patients with PNH come to medical attention because they have focal epilepsy of variable severity, there is a wide spectrum of clinical presentations, including several syndromes with intellectual disability and dysmorphic facial features. Patients with SBH may have mild–moderate cognitive abnormalities and, frequently, seizures (Guerrini and Carrozzo 2001). The brain malformation is often detected after onset of seizures in childhood. In the remaining patients, referral is prompted by developmental delay, behavioral, or learning problems, alone or in association. Seizures often start in the first decade and vary from partial to generalized attacks. SBH may progress to multiple seizure types and result in Lennox–Gastaut syndrome. It often produces drug-resistant symptomatic generalized epilepsy.

124.5.6 Disorders of CNS Cell Number: Microcephaly

Human microcephaly comprises a heterogeneous group of conditions that are characterized by a failure of normal brain growth. Microcephaly is usually defined as a condition in which the size of the head, measured by the occipitofrontal circumference (OFC), is greater than two standard deviations below the mean for gestational age and gender. The etiology of microcephaly can be broadly divided into environmental and genetic cause. Common environmental causes are congenital infections such as cytomegalovirus (CMV), intrauterine exposure to teratogen agents, and hypoxic–ischemic injury in the fetal period (Fig. 10). The genetic causes of congenital microcephaly can be further subdivided, based on the presence of normal versus abnormal brain architecture as found on MRI examination and its combination with non-CNS abnormalities (Mochida and Walsh 2001). Microcephaly is a characteristic feature in holoprosencephaly and lissencephaly. Decreased neuronal proliferation may lead to microcephaly with a normal to thin cortex (primary microcephaly or microcephaly vera, and extreme forms of microcephaly with a simplified gyral pattern), microlissencephaly (extreme microcephaly with thick cortex), and microcephaly with polymicrogyria or other cortical dysplasia.

Investigation of patients with microcephaly includes evaluation for prenatal exposure to teratogens, especially alcohol, drugs, and isotretinoin (a vitamin A analog), and assessment of the family history, birth history, and associated dysmorphic conditions. Laboratory studies should include toxoplasmosis, rubella virus, CMV, and herpes simplex; evaluation of maternal metabolic disorders; and chromosome analysis (Table 7).

124.6 Disorders of Cortical Connectivity: Malformations of the Corpus Callosum

Malformation of the corpus callosum, the large white matter tract that connects the cerebral hemispheres, is a common congenital anomaly

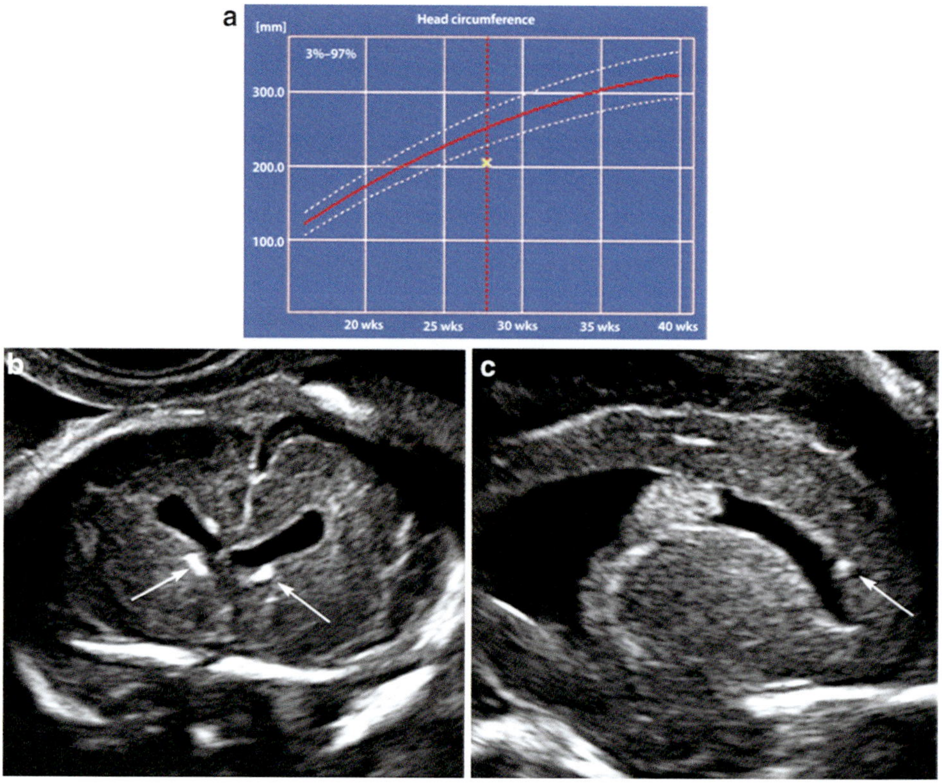

Fig. 10 Microcephaly in a 28 weeks' fetus with CMV infection. (**a**) Head circumference: 203 mm (−2 SD); (**b**) coronal view showing mild ventriculomegaly and calcifications (*white arrows*); (**c**) parasagittal view showing calcification (*white arrow*)

(Chouchane et al. 1999). If normal development of the corpus callosum is disturbed, it may be completely absent (agenetic), partially formed (hypogenetic), formed in a defective way (dysgenetic), or contain too few axons (hypoplastic).

Agenesis of the corpus callosum (ACC) occurs in about one to three per 1000 births, is usually sporadic, and may be transmitted as a sex-linked, autosomal-dominant, or autosomal-recessive trait (Shevell 2002; Pascual-Castroviejo et al. 1991b). Prenatal diagnosis of ACC can be established by 20 weeks' gestation with ultrasonography (Fig. 11). In about half of the reported fetal US studies, ACC is an isolated finding; in the remaining studies, other abnormalities or findings suggestive of specific syndromes are found. Male fetuses are more likely to have isolated agenesis that is considered benign. The etiology of ACC has been associated with numerous syndromes (Aicardi syndrome) and several inborn error of metabolism, including non-ketonic hyperglycinemia and fetal alcohol syndrome. ACC may be observed in various malformations of cortical

Table 7 Assessment of a newborn with microcephaly

Family history	Parental consanguinity, family history, antenatal exposure to teratogens including alcohol
Parental consanguinity	Parental OFC
Child examination	Dysmorphic features
Special investigations	Chromosome analysis, congenital infection screening, metabolic screening, eye examination, brain MRI

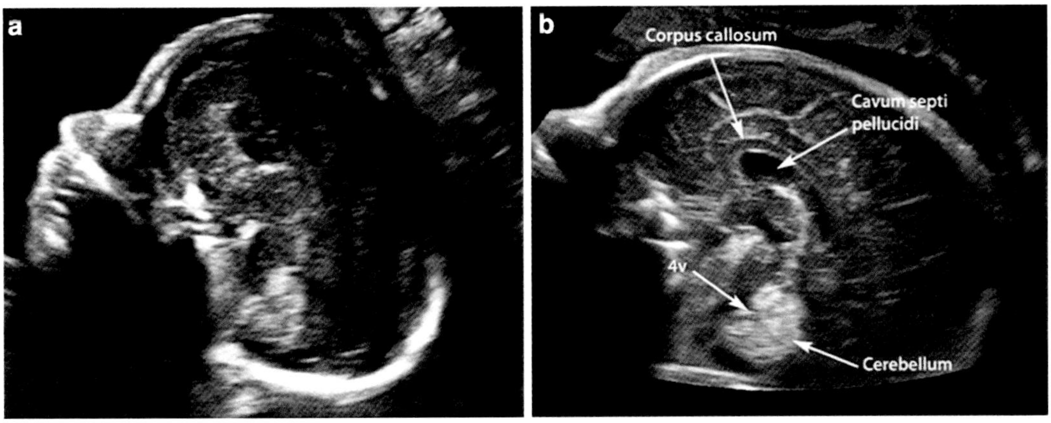

Fig. 11 Sagittal planes at 32 weeks: (**a**) complete agenesis of the corpus callosum; (**b**) normal sagittal plane

development, including the lissencephalies, polymicrogyria, and schizencephaly. Chromosomal disorders, particularly trisomies 8, 13, and 18, are also associated with ACC. Clinically, the extent and nature of neurologic compromise result from the congenital absence of the corpus callosum and the associated brain abnormalities.

124.7 Intracranial Arachnoid Cysts

Intracranial arachnoid cysts are benign, nongenetic developmental cysts that contain spinal fluid and occur within the arachnoid membrane (Pooh et al. 2003). The walls of the cyst result from splitting of the arachnoid membrane. There is no epithelium lining the cystic place, and the fluid it contains is translucent (Fig. 12). The cysts occur in proximity to arachnoid cisterns, most often in the Sylvian fissure. Arachnoid cysts occur most often in males and in patients with Marfan syndrome, and there are few reports of familial middle and posterior fossa arachnoid cysts. The mechanism of formation during embryogenesis is uncertain. Macrocephaly is the major presenting symptom, and associated features include the following: cranial asymmetry, aqueductal stenosis, and agenesis of the corpus callosum (Pooh et al. 2003).

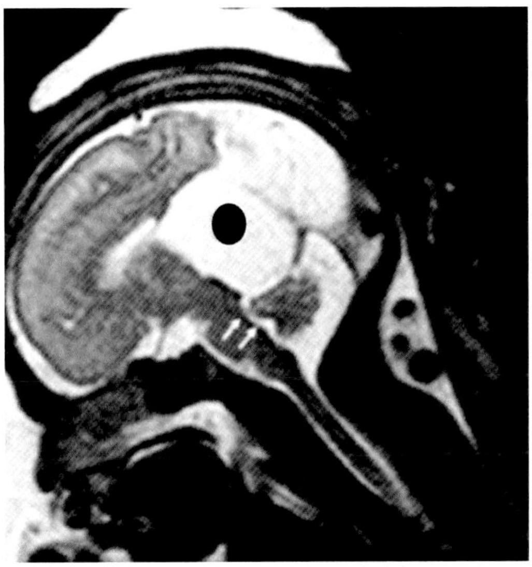

Fig. 12 T2-weighted axial MR image demonstrating a large arachnoid cyst at quadrigeminal cistern (*circle*)

124.8 Hydrocephalus and Ventriculomegaly

Hydrocephalus signifies dilated lateral ventricles resulting from an increased amount of CSF inside the ventricles and increased intracranial pressure, while ventriculomegaly is a dilatation of lateral ventricles without increased intracranial pressure, due to cerebral hypoplasia or CNS anomaly such as agenesis of the corpus callosum (Cardoza et al. 1988). Ventriculomegaly is defined as an enlargement of the lateral cerebral ventricles. It can be regarded as a nonspecific marker of abnormal brain development and is encountered with many different cerebral anomalies. Evaluation of the integrity of the cerebral lateral ventricles is therefore of particular importance while screening for fetal cerebral anomalies. Although many different approaches to the evaluation of the integrity of lateral ventricles have been proposed, measurement of the internal width of the atrium of the lateral ventricle at the level of the glomus of the choroid plexus is currently favored (Almog et al. 2003; Signorelli et al. 2004). Under normal conditions, the measurement is less than 10 mm, while a value of more than 15 mm indicates severe ventriculomegaly, which is almost always associated with an intracranial malformation at birth. The outcome of these fetuses is variable and depends largely upon the underlying etiology of the ventricular dilatation. The available studies suggest that fetuses with isolated severe ventriculomegaly have an increased risk of perinatal death and a probability of severe neurologic sequelae in the range of 50% of survivors (Pilu et al. 1999). An intermediate value for the atrial width, 10–15 mm, is commonly referred as to as mild ventriculomegaly and is associated with a much increased probability of cerebral and extracerebral malformations, aneuploidies, and infections and therefore should be carefully evaluated in an expert center. Fetuses with isolated mild ventriculomegaly usually have a good outcome, and, in most infants, the ventricles return to normal size during pregnancy. However, these infants also run an increased risk of neurologic compromise and, in some cases, develop severe cerebral anomalies in the last of the gestation or after birth, including hydrocephalus, white matter injury, and cortical plate abnormalities (Gaglioti et al. 2005). The risk is particularly increased when the atria width is greater than 12 mm, when the dilatation affects both ventricles and in females (Gupta et al. 1994). It has been suggested that the term mild ventriculomegaly should be limited only to cases with atrial measurements of 10–12 mm, while values of 12.1–15 mm should be referred to as moderate ventriculomegaly, as they tend to have, in general, a worse outcome (Serville et al. 1993).

Congenital hydrocephalus is classified into three categories by causes that disturb the CSF circulation pathway: simple hydrocephalus, dysgenetic hydrocephalus, and secondary hydrocephalus:

- Simple hydrocephalus caused by developmental abnormality, which is localized within the CSF circulation pathway, includes aqueductal stenosis, atresia of Monro foramen and maldevelopment of arachnoid granulation.
- Dysgenetic hydrocephalus indicates hydrocephalus as a result of cerebral development disorder and includes hydranencephaly, holoprosencephaly, porencephaly, schizencephaly, Dandy–Walker malformation, dysraphism, and Chiari malformation.
- Secondary hydrocephalus is caused by an intracranial pathology such as brain tumor, intracranial infection, and intracranial hemorrhage.

Genetic hydrocephalus is rare, but it is important in counseling couples on subsequent pregnancies. It is now well recognized that a small proportion of all cases of hydrocephalus show X-linked inheritance. Most of these X-linked cases are known to be caused by mutations in the *L1CAM* gene which is located at Xq28 (Serville et al. 1993). The *L1CAM* gene encodes a neuronal cell adhesion molecule, known as L1, which is involved in neuronal migration and axonal extension. Mutation in *L1CAM* can result in several different phenotypes such as X-linked hydrocephalus, hydrocephalus due to stenosis of the aqueduct of Sylvius, the MASA syndrome (mental retardation aphasia, shuffling gait, adducted thumbs), X-linked complicated spastic paresis, and X-linked corpus callosum agenesis.

124.8.1 Conclusions

Congenital brain malformations are a significant cause of morbidity and mortality. In recent years, significant advances in basic neuroscience research have improved our understanding of the molecular and genetic underpinnings of brain development. Continued advances in genomics research will move us toward an even better understanding of these developmental processes, with the hope of one day being able to provide parents and clinicians with the information they so desperately need to make informed decisions.

References

Aicardi J (1998) Diseases of the nervous system in childhood, 2nd edn. Cambridge University Press, Cambridge

Almog B, Gamzu R, Achiron R et al (2003) Fetal lateral ventricular width: what should be its upper limit? A prospective cohort study and reanalysis of the current and previous data. J Ultrasound Med 22:39–43

Barkovich AJ (2000) Pediatric neuroimaging, 3rd edn. Lippincott Williams & Wilkins, Philadelphia

Barkovich AJ (2003) Anomalies of the corpus callosum and cortical malformations. In: Barth PG (ed) Disorders of neuronal migration. MacKeith Press, London, pp 83–103

Barkovich AJ, Kuzniecky RI, Jackson GD et al (2001) Classification system for malformations of cortical development: update 2001. Neurology 57: 2168–2178

Barth PG (1992) Schizencephaly and non-lissencephalic cortical dysplasias. Am J Neuroradiol 13:104–106

Battaglia G, Chiapparini L, Franceschetti S et al (2006) Periventricular nodular heterotopia: classification, epileptic history, and genesis of epileptic discharges. Epilepsia 47:86–97

Bielas S, Higginbotham H, Koizumi H (2004) Cortical neuronal migration mutants suggest separate but intersecting pathways. Annu Rev Cell Dev Biol 20: 593–618

Blaas HGK, Eriksson AG, Salvesen KA et al (2002) Brains and faces in holoprosencephaly: pre- and postnatal description of 30 cases. Ultrasound Obstet Gynecol 19:24–38

Blass HGK, Eik-Nes SH, Isaksen CV (2000) The detection of spina bifida before 10 gestational weeks using two- and three-dimensional ultrasound. Ultrasound Obstet Gynecol 16:25–29

Bordarier C, Aicardi J (1990) Dandy-Walker syndrome and agenesis of the cerebellar vermis: diagnostic problems and gebetic counseling. Dev Med Child Neurol 32:285–294

Cardoza JD, Goldstein RB, Filly RA (1988) Exclusion of fetal ventriculomegaly with a single measurement: the width of the lateral ventricular atrium. Radiology 169:711–774

Chouchane M, Benouachkou-Debuche V, Giroud M et al (1999) Agenesis of the corpus callosum: etiological and clinical aspects, diagnostic methods and prognosis. Arch Pediatr 6:1306–1311

D'Agostino MD, Bernasconi A, Das S et al (2002) Subcortical band heterotopia (SBH) in males: clinical, imaging and genetic findings in comparison with females. Brain 125:2507–2522

Diamandis P, Chitayat D, Toi A, Blaser S, Shannon P. The pathology of incipient polymicrogyria. Brain and Development. 2016. pii: S0387-7604(16)30067-5

Ferland RJ, Eyaid W, Collura RV, Tully LD (2004) Abnormal cerebellar development and axonal decussation due to mutations in AHI1 in Joubert syndrome. Nat Genet 36:1008–1013

Gaglioti P, Danelon D, Bontempo S et al (2005) Fetal cerebral ventriculomegaly: outcome in 176 case. Ultrasound Obstet Gynecol 25:372–377

Gardner RJM, Coleman LT, Mitchell LA et al (2001) Near-total absence of the cerebellum. Neuropediatrics 32:62–68

Gressens P (2005) Neuronal migration disorders. J Child Neurol 20:968–971

Grinberg I, Northrup H, Ardinger H, Prasad C (2004) Heterozygous deletion of the linked genes ZIC1 and ZIC4 is involved in Dandy-Walker malformation. Nat Genet 36:1053–1055

Guerrini R, Carrozzo R (2001) Epiletogenic brain malformations: clinical presentation, mal formative patterns and indications for genetic testing. Seizure 10:532–547

Guerrini R, Dobyns WB (2014) Malformations of cortical development: clinical features and genetic causes. Lancet Neurol 13:710–726

Gupta JK, Bryce FC, Lilford RJ (1994) Management of apparently isolated fetal ventriculomegaly. Obstet Gynecol Surv 49:716–721

Jansen A, Andermann E (2005) Genetics of the polymicrogyria syndromes. J Med Genet 42:369–378

Joubert M, Eisenring JJ, Robb JP, Andermann F (1969) Familial agenesis of the cerebellar vermis. A syndrome of episodic hyperpnea abnormal eye movements, ataxia, and retardation. Neurology 19:813–825

Kanatani S, Tabata H, Nakajima K (2005) Neuronal migration in cortical development. J Child Neurol 20: 274–279

Leduc RY, Singh P, McDermid HE (2016) Genetic backgrounds and modifier genes of NTD mouse models: an opportunity for greater understanding of the multifactorial etiology of neural tube defects. Birth Defects Res A Clin Mol Teratol:109(2):140–52

Meyer G (2007) Genetic control of neuronal migrations in human cortical development. Adv Anat Embryol Cell Biol 189:1–111

Ming JE, Muenke M (2002) Multiple hits during early embryonic development: digemic diseases and holoprosencephaly. Am J Hum Genet 71:1017–1032

Mochida GH, Walsh CA (2001) Molecular genetics of human microcephaly. Curr Opin Neurobiol 14:151–156

Nagano T, Morikubo S, Sato M (2004) Filamin A and FILIP (Filamin A-interacting protein) regulate cell polarity and motility in neocortical subventricular and intermediate zones during radial migration. J Neurosci 24:9648–9657

Nicolaides KH, Gabbe SG, Campbell S, Guidetti R (1986) Ultrasound screening for spina bifida: cranial and cerebellar signs. Lancet 2:72–74

Norman MG, McGillivray BC, Kalousek DK et al (1995) Congenital malformations of the brain. Pathological, embryological, clinical, radiological and genetic aspects. Oxford University Press, New York

Packard AM, Miller VS, Delgado MR (1997) Schizencephaly: correlations of clinical and radiologic features. Neurology 48:1427–1434

Padmanabhan R (2006) Etiology, pathogenesis and prevention of neural tube defects. Congenit Anom (Kyoto) 46(2):55–67

Pang T, Atefy R, Sheen V (2008) Malformations of cortical development. Neurologist 14:181–191

Pascual-Castroviejo I (2002) Congenital disorders of glycosylation syndromes. Dev Med Child Neurol 44:357–358

Pascual-Castroviejo I, Velez A, Pascual-Pascual SI et al (1991a) Dandy-Walker malformation: an analysis of 38 cases. Childs Nerv Syst 7:88–97

Pascual-Castroviejo I, Roche MC, Martinez Bermejo A et al (1991b) Primary intracranial arachnoidal cysts: a study of 67 childhood cases. Childs Nerv Syst 7: 257–263

Pascual-Castroviejo I, Gutierrez M, Morales C et al (1994) Primary degeneration of the granular layer of the cerebellum. A study of 14 patients and review of the literature. Neuropediatrics 25:183–190

Pedreira DA, Zanon N, Nishikuni K, Moreira de Sá RA, Acacio GL, Chmait RH, Kontopoulos EV, Quintero RA (2016) Endoscopic surgery for the antenatal treatment of myelomeningocele: the CECAM trial. Am J Obstet Gynecol 214:111.e1–111.11

Pilu G, Falco P, Gabrielli S et al (1999) The clinical significance of fetal isolated cerebral borderline ventriculomegaly: report of 31 cases and review of the literature. Ultrasound Obstet Gynecol 14:320–326

Pooh RK, Maeda K, Pooh KH (2003) An atlas of fetal central nervous system disease. Diagnosis and management. Parthenon CRC, London

Ramaekers VT (2000) Cerebellar malformations. In: Klockgether T (ed) Handbook of ataxia disorders. Dekker, New York, pp 115–150

Ramaekers VT, Heinman G, Reul J et al (1997) Genetic disorders and cerebellar structural abnormalities in childhood. Brain 120:1739–1751

Sarmah S, Muralidharan P, Marrs JA (2016) Common congenital anomalies: environmental causes and prevention with folic acid containing multivitamins. Birth Defects ReC Embryo Today 108(3):274–286

Serville F, Benit P, Saugier P et al (1993) Prenatal exclusion of Xlinked hydrocephalus-stenosis of the aqueduct of Sylvius sequence using closely linked DNA markers. Prenat Diagn 3:269–272

Shevell MI (2002) Clinical and diagnostic profile of agenesis of the corpus callosum. J Child Neurol 17:896–900

Signorelli M, Tiberti A, Valseriati D et al (2004) Width of the fetal lateral ventricular atrium between 10 and 12 mm: a simple variation of the norm? Ultrasound Obstet Gynecol 23:14–18

Verrotti A, Spalice A, Ursitti F et al (2010) New trends in neuronal migration disorders. Eur J Paediatr Neurol 14:1–12

Yadav U, Kumar P, Yadav SK, Mishra OP, Rai V (2015) Polymorphisms in folate metabolism genes as maternal risk factor for neural tube defects: an updatedmeta-analysis. Metab Brain Dis 30(1):7–24

Biochemical Basis of Hypoxic-Ischemic Encephalopathy

125

Maria Delivoria-Papadopoulos, Panagiotis Kratimenos, and Endla K. Anday

Contents

M. Delivoria-Papadopoulos (✉) · E. K. Anday
Department of Pediatrics, Drexel University College of Medicine, St. Christopher's Hospital for Children, Neonatal-Perinatal Medicine, Philadelphia, PA, USA
e-mail: delivoria@drexelmed.edu; mdelivor@gmail.com; endla.anday@drexelmed.edu

P. Kratimenos
Neonatologist, Children's National Medical Center, Center for Research in Neuroscience, George Washington University School of Medicine and Health Sciences, Washington, DC, USA
e-mail: panagiotis.kratimenos@childrensnational.org

G. Buonocore et al. (eds.), *Neonatology*,
https://doi.org/10.1007/978-3-319-29489-6_272

Abstract

Hypoxic-ischemic encephalopathy (HIE), the most common cause of neurologic disease during the perinatal period, is associated with a high mortality and morbidity rate and also has long-term consequences like cerebral palsy, mental retardation, and seizures. Perinatal HIE is caused by processes that alter the cerebral blood flow (CBF) in the fetus and newborn compromising the supply of oxygen to the brain. They may develop antepartum (20%), intrapartum (30%), antepartum and intrapartum (35%), or postpartum (10%). Acute or long-term consequences of HIE are related either to necrosis or to apoptosis of neuronal cells. Cell necrosis will lead to generalized disruption of internal homeostasis and eventually to the lysis of the cells, which give rise to an inflammatory response with the release of oxygen free radicals and activation of the microglial cells. Apoptosis is programmed cell death, not associated with the lysis of the plasma membrane and inflammation, which can be triggered by hypoxia. It is crucial to restore any failures in the respiratory and circulatory systems, in order to prevent neuronal cell death. However, neonatologists should also be aware of the hazards of medically induced hyperoxia (high FIO_2) because this condition may increase the production of oxygen free radicals thus worsening the neuronal insult. Elucidating basic cellular mechanisms in response to hypoxia of the developing brain will enable the development of novel strategies for preventing or attenuating the deleterious effects of hypoxia in the human newborn.

125.1 Salient Points

- Acute- or long-term consequences of hypoxic-ischemic encephalopathy are related to necrosis or apoptosis of neuronal cells.
- During hypoxia, the fall of ATP levels includes cell membrane depolarization and disruption of voltage-dependent ion channels allowing excessive amounts of Ca^{++} to enter the cytosol and initiating the release of glutamate with consequent activation of N-methyl-D-aspartate (NMDA).
- Excessive activation of NMDA and non-NMDA receptors may initiate a number of biochemical events that lead to free radical generation and cell death. In addition to Ca^{++} mediation, there are other potential mechanisms for free radical generation during hypoxia.
- Hypoxic brain injury is associated with the formation of nitric oxide, which has been reported to cause neuronal damage though various mechanisms.
- The ratio of proapoptotic protein Bax to antiapoptotic protein Bcl-2 increases in all compartments of the cell during hypoxia. This may lead to activation of a hypoxia induced cascade resulting in neuronal death.
- Neuroprotective treatments that may be effective in humans include the administration of magnesium sulfate, allopurinol, opioids, and hypothermia.

125.2 Introduction

Perinatal hypoxia-ischemia is the most common cause of neurologic disease during the neonatal period. Hypoxic-ischemic encephalopathy (HIE) is associated with a high mortality and morbidity rate, also cerebral palsy, mental retardation, and seizures (Volpe 2001). The incidence of perinatal asphyxia is about 1.0–1.5% in most centers and is usually related to gestational age and birth weight. It occurs in 9.0% of infants less than 36 weeks of gestation and in 0.5% of infants more than 36 weeks of gestation (Legido 1994; Hill and Volpe 1999). The etiology of perinatal HIE includes those circumstances that can affect the cerebral blood flow in the fetus and newborn compromising the supply of oxygen to the brain. They may develop antepartum (20%), intrapartum (30%), antepartum and intrapartum (35%), or postpartum (10%) (Raichle 1983).

HIE develops in the setting of perinatal asphyxia, which is a multiorgan system disease (Legido 1994). Assessment and management of these complications is an integral part of the treatment of perinatal asphyxia/HIE (Legido 1994). The present chapter primarily focuses on cellular and molecular mechanisms of the hypoxic neuronal injury in the newborn brain.

A large amount of information has been collected on the fetal cardiovascular and respiratory response to oxygen limitations, giving rise to a better understanding and management of neonatal deterioration induced by hypoxia. Besides these physiologic studies, cellular and biochemical mechanisms that result in brain cell death are being increasingly explored, particularly in the adult with respect to focal (stroke) and global (cardiac arrest) hypoxia-ischemia (Raichle 1983). These studies have shown that complex and interrelated biochemical alterations are triggered during hypoxia-ischemia in mature subjects that ultimately result in neuronal death. Studies are in progress to investigate mechanisms of hypoxic brain injury in the fetus and newborn brain (Legido et al. 2001). To focus on cellular and molecular mechanisms of hypoxic injury in the developing brain, it is important to recognize the factors that may determine the susceptibility of the developing brain to neonatal and perinatal hypoxia.

The determinants of the susceptibility of the developing brain to hypoxia include the lipid composition of the brain cell membrane, the rate of lipid peroxidation, the presence of antioxidant defenses, the development and modulation of the excitatory neurotransmitter receptors such as the *N*-methyl-D-aspartate (NMDA) receptor, and the intracellular Ca^{++} influx mechanisms. In addition to the developmental status of these cellular components, the response of these potential mechanisms to hypoxia determines the fate of the hypoxic brain cell in the developing brain in the fetus and the newborn. Elucidating basic cellular mechanisms in response to hypoxia of the developing brain will enable the development of novel strategies for preventing or attenuating the deleterious effects of hypoxia in the human newborn. Several excellent reviews on different aspects of hypoxic-ischemic cell injury in the developing brain have been published recently (Delivoria-Papadopoulos and Mishra 1998; Fritz and Delivoria-Papadopoulos 2006; Davidson et al. 2015).

125.3 Steps of Posthypoxic Brain Injury

Acute or long-term consequences of hypoxic-ischemic encephalopathy are related either to necrosis or to apoptosis of neuronal cells. Necrosis is characterized by passive cell swelling; rapid energy loss; generalized disruption of internal homeostasis leading to eventual lysis of the nucleus, organelles, and plasma cell membranes; and the release of intracellular components that induce a local inflammatory response, resulting in edema and injury to the neighboring cells. This inflammatory response results in the expression of the cytokines interleukin-1-beta (IL-beta) and tumor necrosis factor-alpha (TNF-alpha) stimulating oxygen free radical release from neutrophils, activating microglial cells.

Necrosis is only one of the mechanisms of cell death following hypoxia or ischemia to the brain. Programmed cell death, or apoptosis, also appears to contribute to cell death following hypoxia-ischemia, especially cell death that occurs days to weeks following the insult (Linnik et al. 1993; Ferrer et al. 1994). Apoptosis is an active process that requires the activation of a genetic program and specific endonucleolytic digestion of nuclear DNA. In contrast to necrosis, programmed cell death is characterized by cell shrinkage, coarse chromatin aggregation with extensive nuclear DNA fragmentation, nuclear pyknosis, and extrusion of membrane-bound cytoplasmic fragments or apoptotic bodies, but is not associated with the lysis of the plasma membrane (Wylie et al. 1980; Columbano 1995).

Studies in cell culture models have demonstrated that hypoxia can trigger programmed cell death (Rosenbaum et al. 1994). Programmed cell death as assessed by the cleavage of genomic DNA has also been shown to occur in the brain following focal (Linnik et al. 1993; Dragunow et al. 1994; Gillardon et al. 1996) and global ischemia (Ferrer et al. 1994; Kitada et al. 1996).

The mechanism by which hypoxia causes DNA fragmentation has been extensively studied but is not well understood.

125.3.1 Energy Breakdown

Under normal conditions, the oxidative phosphorylation and the synthesis of high-energy phosphates like adenosine 5-triphosphate or ATP need adequate oxygen supply. Under anaerobic conditions, the metabolic cost of ATP production is critically increased leading to a breakdown of energy balance depleting the brain cells of high-energy compounds, necessary for energy-dependent metabolic processes in neurons and glial cells.

125.3.2 Excitotoxic Mechanisms

The fall of ATP levels includes a cell membrane depolarization and a disruption of voltage-dependent ion channels allowing excessive amounts of Ca^{++} to enter the cytosol, initiating the release of glutamate consequently activating *N*-methyl-D-aspartate (NMDA) receptors. The increased expression/activation of NMDA receptors further enhances cellular calcium influx. This whole mechanism is further accelerated by the dysfunction of the energy-dependent reuptake of glutamate both in neurons and in astrocytes in a vicious circle manner.

125.4 NMDA Receptors

Glutamate is the major excitatory amino acid neurotransmitter that contributes to a number of developmental processes such as synaptogenesis, synaptic plasticity, long-term potentiation (LTP), learning and memory, as well as neurodegeneration and hypoxia-induced injury (Choi 1990; Rothman and Olney 1986). The physiological and pathological effects of glutamate in the central nervous system (CNS) are mediated through its interaction with specific cell membrane receptors, of which the *N*-methyl-D-aspartate (NMDA), kainate, and AMPA subtypes are the best characterized (Monaghan et al. 1989). The use of specific antagonists (Monaghan et al. 1989; Bashir et al. 1991; Tacconi et al. 1993; Hoffman et al. 1994a) of the NMDA receptor supports the role of receptor activation in long-term potentiation and hypoxic-ischemic cerebral injury. The NMDA-type glutamate receptor is a predominant mediator of excitotoxicity in the immature as compared to the adult brain due to overexpression of the receptor in the developing immature brain (Johnston 1995). Within the developmental period, however, the extent of NMDA receptor-mediated processes such as LTP and hypoxia-induced excitotoxicity may depend on the ontogeny of the NMDA receptor sites and subunits leading to altered function of the ion-channel complex. In addition, the function of the receptor may be modified by intracellular mechanisms such as phosphorylation/dephosphorylation, nitration, and pathways of free radical generation.

125.4.1 Structure and Function of the NMDA Receptor

The activity of the NMDA receptor ion-channel complex is regulated by a number of pharmacologically distinct binding sites. The NMDA receptor possesses a neurotransmitter binding site, or recognition site, which binds glutamate or NMDA, a coactivator site which binds glycine, a channel site that binds MK-801 in its open state, a voltage-dependent Mg^{++} binding site, a polyamine site that binds spermine and spermidine, an ifenprodil site, and an inhibitory divalent cation site that binds Zn^{++} (Monaghan et al. 1989). The activity of the receptor ion channel can also be modified by redox agents (Aizenman et al. 1989; Lipton 1999). Ligand binding studies indicate that there are two distinct binding sites or states associated with the glutamate recognition site, one that preferentially binds agonists and one that preferentially binds antagonists (Monaghan et al. 1988).

The NMDA receptor is associated with a cation-selective ion channel that gates Na^{+}, K^{+}, and Ca^{++} ions, and, in the resting state, when blocked by Mg++ in a voltage-dependent manner (Nowak et al. 1984; Mayer et al. 1984), the blockade of the ion-channel complex by glutamate or NMDA is allowed, and the agonist-dependent Ca^{++} influx occurs. The influx of Ca^{++} ions is thought to initiate biochemical processes responsible for both NMDA receptor-induced plasticity in the developing brain and NMDA receptor-mediated excitotoxic cell death (Rothman and Olney 1986; Collingridge 1987; Tang et al. 1999).

Each of the regulatory sites of the NMDA receptor ion-channel complex is modified during brain development and may alter the site-dependent influx of NMDA receptor-mediated Ca^{++} and site-specific responses of the receptor during development and during hypoxia.

125.4.2 Mechanism of NMDA Receptor Modification During Hypoxia

Brain tissue hypoxia modifies the NMDA receptor recognition, coactivator, and the ion-channel sites. A decrease in the apparent number of NMDA receptors and an increase in receptor affinity for MK-801 were observed in hypoxic fetal guinea pig and newborn piglet brain (Mishra and Delivoria-Papadopoulos 1992; Hoffman et al. 1994b). In these same studies, glutamate and glycine-dependent activation of the NMDA receptor was decreased, and spermine-dependent and basal-state receptor activation was increased during hypoxia. In brains of hypoxic newborn piglets, it was noted that hypoxia modified the recognition, coactivator, and modulatory sites of the NMDA receptor ion-channel complex, probably through NO-mediated nitration (Hoffman et al. 1994b; Fritz et al. 1996). Several lines of evidence support this conclusion.

First, in neurons of the central nervous system, neuronal nitric oxide synthase (nNOS) is colocalized with the NMDA receptor (Bhat et al. 1997; Aoki et al. 1997), thereby favoring nitration of the receptor. Second, nNOS activity is decreased by phosphorylation and increased by dephosphorylation (Bredt et al. 1992; Dawson et al. 1993), a condition that may be achieved during hypoxia.

Furthermore, dephosphorylation of the receptor will make tyrosine sites available for nitration by peroxynitrite, which is produced by NO and superoxide radicals, both of which are produced during hypoxia. Peroxynitrite-dependent nitration inhibits phosphorylation of proteins (Gow et al. 1996), indicating possible steric hindrance between the phospho- and nitro groups on the same tyrosine residue. Thus, dephosphorylation during hypoxia may facilitate peroxynitrite-mediated nitration on the 3-position of tyrosine. In view of these considerations, a critical role of the nitric oxide synthase (NOS) pathway in NO-mediated mechanism of hypoxia-induced modification of the NMDA receptor in newborn brain is strongly suggested.

In neurons of the central nervous system, nNOS is colocalized with NMDA receptors (Bhat et al. 1997; Aoki et al. 1997). In addition, neuronal NOS is activated by Ca^{++} influx through the NMDA receptor ion channel; however, nNOS is not efficiently stimulated by activation of non-NMDA receptors that also induce Ca^{++} influx (Kiedrowski et al. 1992). In synaptic plasma membranes, the nNOS immunoreactivity is associated with the NMDA receptor (Aoki et al. 1993). The synaptic localization of nNOS in the brain may be mediated by the postsynaptic density protein, PSD-95. Recently, it was demonstrated that nNOS, PSD-95, and NMDA receptor subunit NR2B from the brain coimmunoprecipitate and that the PSD-95 is sufficient to assemble a tight ternary complex with nNOS and the NR2B subunit of the NMDA receptor (Christopherson et al. 1999).

In summary, results of these studies indicate that NO production in the brain is preferentially activated by Ca^{++} influx through the NMDA receptor ion channel and that there is a specific structural and functional link between the NMDA receptor and nNOS.

125.5 Free Radicals

Free radicals are molecular species with unpaired electrons in the outer orbit with a strong tendency to initiate chain reactions that result in membrane peroxidation, protein oxidation, nucleic acid oxidation, and cell damage. Normally, more than 80% of the oxygen consumed by the cell is completely reduced by cytochrome oxidase to water without production of oxygen free radicals. The remaining 10–20% undergoes other oxidation reduction reactions in the cytoplasm and mitochondria that produce a superoxide anion radical.

125.5.1 Free Radical Generation in Cerebral Cortex of Newborn Piglets

The production of free radicals during hypoxia was documented by measuring the signal of spin adducts with electron spin resonance spectroscopy. Newborn piglets of 3–5 days were assigned to either normoxia (PaO_2 – 120 mmHg) or hypoxia (PaO_2 <20 mmHg) for 1 h. Cortical samples were obtained by biopsy from anesthetized, ventilated piglets.

The data provided direct evidence of increased free radical generation during hypoxia in the newborn model. On the basis of the characteristics of the spin adduct signal, the free radical species present in the hypoxic tissue was identified to be an alkoxyl radical.

These studies demonstrate increased free radical generation during hypoxia in the cerebral cortex of the fetus and the newborn, and intervening with the inhibitors of pathways of free radical generation reduced the hypoxia-induced production of free radical species. Alkoxyl radical appears to be the predominant free radical species identified during hypoxia, indicating that free radical-mediated lipid peroxidation is an ongoing event during cerebral hypoxia, a mechanism of hypoxic neuronal injury.

125.5.2 Mechanisms of Free Radical Generation During Hypoxia

There are a number of potential mechanisms of free radical generation under hypoxic conditions. During hypoxia, the increased accumulation intracellular Ca^{++} due to excessive activation of NMDA (Zanelli 1999) and non-NMDA receptors is crucial in hypoxia-induced excitotoxicity. Increased intracellular Ca^{++} can initiate a number of biochemical events that could lead to free radical generation and cell death such as (1) activation of phospholipase A2 leading to increased generation of oxygen free radicals from cyclooxygenase and lipoxygenase pathways; (2) activation of NOS, leading to peroxynitrite formation and generation of free radicals; (3) activation of proteases, leading to conversion of xanthine dehydrogenase to xanthine oxidase and resulting in increased free radical generation; (4) activation of phospholipase C_1 leading to IP3 formation and resulting in the release of Ca^{++} from intracellular stores; and (5) free radical generation further triggering the release of additional excitatory amino acid neurotransmitters as well as influencing the activation of the NMDA receptor ion-channel activity through the redox site.

In addition to Ca^{++} mediation, there are other potential mechanisms of free radical generation during hypoxia such as (1) reduction of electron transport chain components including ubiquinone (a component that undergoes auto-oxidation to produce free radicals), (2) increased release of ferritin under the conditions of decreased cellular high-energy compounds, and (3) increased degradation of ATP during hypoxia, increasing the substrate for the xanthine oxidase reaction and leading to increased free radical generation.

125.5.3 Nitric Oxide Free Radicals and Neuronal Injury

The role of nitric oxide (NO) in neuronal injury, both in vitro and in vivo, has been controversial (Dawson 1994a, b). This controversy may be due to the use of nonspecific NOS inhibitors. Three major isoforms of NOS have been identified: constitutive neuronal, constitutive endothelial, and inducible macrophage isoforms. Following ischemia, NO produced from neuronal NOS has toxic effects, but NO produced from endothelial NOS has protective effects in the brain (Huang 1994).

Hypoxic brain injury is associated with the formation of NO, a gaseous free radical (Beckman 1991; Cazevielle 1993). Although under normal conditions NO physiologically mediates cerebral vasodilatation (Faraci 1991), recent studies suggest that NO may react with superoxide anion to form peroxynitrite and cause neurotoxicity (Beckman 1990; Dawson 1991; Delivoria-Papadopoulos and Mishra 1998; Hamada 1994). Furthermore, *Nw*-nitro-L-arginine (NNLA), an NOS inhibitor, administration in a middle cerebral artery occlusion model reduced the volume of cortical infarct in the mouse, indicating the role of NO in neurotoxicity (Nowicki 1991).

Nitric oxide is reported to cause neuronal damage through various mechanisms. We tested the hypothesis that NO synthase inhibition by NNLA will result in decreased oxygen-derived free radical production, leading to the preservation of cell membrane structure and function during cerebral hypoxia (Numagami 1997). Results demonstrated that free radicals, corresponding to alkoxyl radicals, were induced by hypoxia but were inhibited by pretreatment with NNLA before inducing hypoxia. NNLA also inhibited hypoxia-induced generation of conjugated dienes, products of lipid peroxidation. Na^{+}-/K^{+}-ATPase activity, an index of cellular membrane function, decreased following hypoxia but was preserved by pretreatment with NNLA. This data demonstrated that during hypoxia NOS generates free radicals via peroxynitrite production, presumably causing lipid peroxidation and membrane dysfunction.

The appearance of primary free radicals, such as superoxide anion or hydroxyl radical, may not indicate oxidative injury. The reactivity of superoxide radicals is limited (Baum 1984; Sawyer 1981), but hydroxyl radicals are highly reactive to almost all molecules (Mishra and Delivoria-Papadopoulos 1999) so that they can target even noncritical molecules. Therefore, their concentration does not necessarily correlate with the degree of oxidative damage, particularly when assessing lipid peroxidation. Furthermore, these radicals damage cells in cooperation with other radical species or oxidants (Beckman 1990, 1991; Cazevielle 1993; Faraci 1991). In contrast, the production of secondarily formed lipid free radicals provides strong evidence of peroxidative injury. This is particularly true for alkoxyl radicals, which are generated from lipid peroxide by either iron or copper ions and can abstract hydrogen atoms from polyunsaturated fatty acids, leading to further lipid peroxidation (Mishra and Delivoria-Papadopoulos 1999). Our results suggested that NO has an in vivo role in the generation of alkoxyl radicals, leading to free radical-mediated lipid peroxidation.

The exact molecular mechanism of hypoxic membrane damage is not clear. An appealing hypothesis is that when peroxynitrite (formed by the reaction between superoxide anions and NO) is protonated, it decomposes rapidly to form nitrogen dioxide and hydroxyl radicals, both of which are strong oxidants and can initiate oxidative reactions (Beckman 1990, 1991; Radi 1991). It has been shown that peroxynitrite can cause lipid peroxidation in vitro (Radi 1991). Therefore, high concentration of NO during may result in an increased production of peroxynitrite, causing lipid peroxidation.

125.5.4 Inhaled Nitric Oxide and Neuroprotection

Nitric oxide is known to be involved in several critical processes in the developing brain. Recent studies have shown that exposure to inhaled nitric oxide (iNO) during the first week of postnatal life improves myelination in the developing brain and significantly reduced the size of excitotoxic lesion in the neonatal rat brain (Delivoria-Papadopoulos et al. 2011a). iNO also significantly improves cerebral blood flow during ischemia and reduced the infarct volume (Delivoria-Papadopoulos et al. 2011b). In P7 rat model, exposure to 20 ppm iNO was associated with progressive and significant increase in cortical nitric oxide concentration of up to 140% of the basal nitric oxide concentration. Infarct volumes were significantly decreased in the 20 ppm iNO. Nitric oxide is known to react with oxygen free radicals to generate peroxynitrite that leads to nitration of cellular proteins, an index of cell damage. Exposure to 20 ppm iNO during ischemia decreased the density of nitrotyrosine-positive cells by 43% in the cortex. In neonatal rats subjected to postnatal hyperoxia following gestational hypoxia, iNO exposure during the first postnatal week significantly attenuated the cerebral white matter damage in neonatal rats (Lawn et al. 2005). iNO was associated with decreased astrogliosis, microglial activation, and apoptotic cell death through both caspase-dependent and caspase-independent pathways.

iNO has been demonstrated to be effective in various animal models (Kurinczuk et al. 2010). The iNO was protective in a well-characterized model of murine perinatal hypoxia-ischemia. Tissue loss and pathological scores were significantly attenuated by 50 ppm iNO 3 days after the insult. iNO, in an ovine model of ischemic stroke, selectively increased CBF in the ischemic penumbra as compared to a control animal not receiving iNO. These findings substantiate the view that inhalation of nitric oxide causes selective vasodilation of vessels in lowly perfused brain tissue. Recent studies have investigated whether the acute beneficial effects of iNO also translate into long-term neurological improvement; functional outcome was assessed over a period of 7 days after MCA occlusion. Mice treated with iNO (50 ppm) for 24 h after onset of ischemia performed significantly in neurological tests analyzing motor function, agility, and coordination. Furthermore, iNO-treated mice recovered significantly better from postischemic weight loss and showed an improved survival. These studies suggest the need for further preclinical and clinical investigations into the beneficial effects of iNO in neonates at high risk of brain damage.

125.6 Neuronal Nuclear Ca^{++} Influx

A number of critical nuclear functions including regulation of transcription factors, cell cycle regulation transcription, DNA replication, and nuclear envelope breakdown are controlled by intracellular Ca^{++} (Mishra and Delivoria-Papadopoulos 1999; Delivoria-Papadopoulos et al. 2003). Furthermore, nuclear Ca^{++} signals potentially control a number of events leading to hypoxia-induced programmed cell death. Nuclear and cytosolic Ca^{++} signals are differently regulated, and the extranuclear Ca^{++} concentration determines the mode of Ca^{++} entry into the nucleus.

The increased intracellular Ca^{++} is a primary mediator of activity-dependent gene transcription under a number of experimental conditions (Ghosh and Greenberg 1995; Hardingham and Bading 1998; Chawla and Bading 2001). The patterns of neuronal impulse and the specific properties of the stimulus-induced calcium transients determine the nature and amplitude of the genomic response (Hardingham and Bading 1998; Fields et al. 1997). Several factors including the site of calcium entry and the amplitude and the spatial properties of the calcium signals determine the calcium-regulated gene expression (Lerea and McNamara 1993; Hardingham et al. 1999; Dolmetsch et al. 2001). Furthermore, the duration of calcium signal also contributes to the specificity of the transcription induction. In cells of the immune system, only a continuous rise in intracellular Ca^{++} concentration, but not a brief spike, induced translocation of transcription factors, NF-ATc (Dolmetsch et al. 1997). Gene expression in neurons is also determined by the duration of calcium transients and the activity-dependent transcription is regulated by the duration of calcium transients (Chawla and Bading 2001).

In previous studies, we have shown that cerebral hypoxia results in increased nuclear Ca^{++} influx in neuronal nuclei of the cerebral cortex of newborn piglets (Delivoria-Papadopoulos et al. 2003; Mishra and Delivoria-Papadopoulos 2000). The nuclear Ca^{++} influx increased as a function of increase in cerebral tissue hypoxia, as measured by decrease in high-energy phosphates, ATP, and phosphocreatine (PCr). Cerebral hypoxia results in increased Ca^{++}/calmodulin kinase (CaM kinase) IV activity and CREB protein phosphorylation in neuronal nuclei of newborn piglets (Vannucci 1990). NO donors increased neuronal nuclear Ca^{++} influx (Mishra and Delivoria-Papadopoulos 2002) and hypoxia resulted in generation of NO free radicals and increased high-affinity Ca^{++}-ATPase activity in neuronal nuclei. The high-affinity Ca^{++}-ATPase activity increased as a function of increase in cerebral tissue hypoxia (Mishra and Delivoria-Papadopoulos 2001). In addition, IP3-dependent Ca^{++} influx is increased in neuronal nuclei of hypoxic animals as compared to normoxic ones, and this increase was a function of cerebral tissue hypoxia.

During hypoxia, NO-mediated modification of the nuclear membrane high-affinity Ca^{++}-ATPase and IP3 receptor is a potential mechanism of increased intranuclear Ca^{++} that leads to activation of Ca^{++}-dependent nuclear mechanisms and activates cascades of hypoxic programmed cell death.

125.7 Expression and Posttranslational Modification of Apoptotic Proteins

Bcl-2 family of proteins (including Bcl-2 and Bax) control cell proliferation, differentiation, and programmed cell death during normal brain development (Oltvai et al. 1993). Bax and Bcl-2 are inducible genes found in the developing and adult central and peripheral nervous systems (Chen et al. 1996; Reed 1996). Bcl-2 prevents apoptosis by forming a heterodimer with the proapoptotic protein Bax and protects cells from programmed cell death following hypoxia (Oltvai et al. 1993).

Prolonged cerebral hypoxia may lead to a state of primary energy failure, depletion of cellular reserves of high-energy compounds (ATP and phosphocreatine (PCr)), and mitochondrial dysfunction. Failure of the ability of the neuronal membrane to maintain its electrochemical homeostasis results in lipid peroxidation and subsequent modification of the NMDA receptor, influx of calcium into the cytosol, and free radical formation (Oltvai et al. 1993; Reed 1996). Following the calcium influx and the deactivation of the phosphatases located in the cytosol, there is activation of a protein complex that extends from the membrane to the nucleus and the mitochondria, the system of focal adhesions (FAs). The FAs include a number of proteins maintaining a dynamic state while activating each other and changing morphology thus contributing to the signal transduction the nucleus. The proteins of FAs play a crucial role to the cell migration and motility and are very important regulatory factors of the apoptotic cascade as they enter in the nucleus mediating phosphorylation of calmodulin, activation of CaM kinase IV, and CREB protein-mediated transcription of Bax. Subsequently, there is increased expression of caspases leading to DNA fragmentation and cell death (Kratimenos et al. 2018; Oltvai et al. 1993).

In the mitochondrial level, we know that hypoxia leads to mitochondrial outer membrane permeabilization (MOMP) and opening of the mitochondrial permeability transition pores (mPTP) leading to the leakage of the proapoptotic proteins into the cytosol. We also know that during hypoxia, two of the major mitochondrial proteins, second mitochondria-derived activator of caspases (Smac, direct inhibitor of apoptosis-binding protein with a low isoelectric point) and cytochrome c, are translocated into the cytosol. Smac/DIABLO, discovered in 2000, is a small-sized protein (27 kDa) initially formed in a premature form localized in mitochondria and is subsequently released into the cytosol as a bigger mature protein along with cytochrome c, maintaining a dynamic interaction. Cytochrome c protein (12 kDa) is a crucial element of the electron transport chain in mitochondria, and it is also involved in the initiation of apoptosis. It is released to the cytoplasm and binds apoptotic protease activating factor-1 (Apaf-1). Smac is released concurrently with cytochrome c from mitochondria into the cytosol during apoptosis and deactivates the inhibitor of apoptosis protein (IAP)-mediated inhibition leading to the activation of the caspases and cell death (Kratimenos et al. 2017; Oltvai et al. 1993).

Concentrating on focal adhesions, our previous data in guinea pigs show that hypoxia leads to decreased concentration of Smac and cytochrome c in mitochondria, while their expression increases in the cytosol. These findings indicate that there is probably translocation of Smac and cytochrome c from the mitochondria to the cytosol during hypoxia.

We have also shown that hypoxia increases the activation of several proteins of the focal adhesions, including the Src kinase. Since the mitochondria are located in the area of FAs, one of the generated questions is whether the proteins of the FAs contribute to the trafficking of the mitochondrial proteins in the cytosol.

Cerebral hypoxia results in increased expression of Bax protein in neuronal nuclei of the cerebral cortex of newborn piglets. The Bax protein increased as a function of increase in degree of cerebral tissue hypoxia as measured by decrease in high-energy phosphates, ATP, and phosphocreatine (Ravishankar et al. 2001). The expression of Bax protein increases in the mitochondrial, cytosolic, as well as neuronal nuclear fractions indicating increased expression of the protein rather than its translocation, e.g., from mitochondria to cytosol. The expression of anti-apoptotic protein Bax to anti-apoptotic protein Bcl-2 did not increase during hypoxia. Therefore, the ratio of proapoptotic protein Bax to anti-apoptotic protein Bcl-2 increases in all compartments of the cell during hypoxia that may lead to activation of hypoxia-induced cascade of neuronal death.

Administration of NOS inhibitor prevented the hypoxia-induced increased expression of proapoptotic protein Bax indicating that the hypoxia-induced increased expression of Bax is NO-mediated (Zanelli et al. 2002).

125.7.1 Posthypoxic Expression and Activation of Caspase-3, Caspase-8, and Caspase-9 in the Newborn Brain

Caspases are a unique family of proteases that play an important role in the initiation and execution of apoptosis (Delivoria-Papadopoulos et al. 2008). All caspases contain a cysteine residue at their active site and specifically cleave substrate proteins at an aspartic acid residue. These cysteine proteases reside predominantly in the cytosolic compartment of animal cells as inactive zymogens and become activated by proteolytic cleavage at internal aspartate residues on apoptotic stimulation (Mishra et al. 2001). These are divided into two main classes: those with long prodomain are the class I caspases and those with short prodomain are the class II caspases.

Class I caspases such as 8, 9, and 10 can autocatalyze their own activation and are activated in the early phase of apoptosis. These are called the initiator caspases. Class II caspases, such as 3, 6, and 7, require cleavage by another protease and are responsible for the breakdown of cells (Delivoria-Papadopoulos et al. 2008). These are called the effector or the executioner caspases. The upstream caspases activated during apoptosis lead to the activation of downstream caspases in a self-amplifying cascade (Delivoria-Papadopoulos et al. 2008).

Two well-studied pathways of caspase activation are the cell surface death receptor-mediated pathway and the mitochondria-initiated pathways. The recruitment and the cleavage of procaspase-8 to produce the active form of caspase-8 is a critical biochemical event in the death receptor-mediated apoptosis (Delivoria-Papadopoulos et al. 2008). Following its activation, caspase-8 can activate downstream caspase by direct cleavage or indirectly by cleaving the proapoptotic protein and inducing cytochrome c (cyt c) release from the mitochondria (Delivoria-Papadopoulos et al. 2008). In the proposed mitochondria-initiated pathway, caspase activation is triggered by formation of an oligomeric apoptotic protease activation factor (Apaf-1)/cyt c complex, which leads to recruiting and activating procaspase-9, an upstream caspase in this pathway (Mishra and Delivoria-Papadopoulos 2010). The complex formed by the combination of Apaf-1, cyt c, Bax/Bcl-2, and procaspase-9 is referred to as the apoptosome (Mishra and Delivoria-Papadopoulos 2010; Ashraf et al. 2007).

Two other less defined pathways of apoptotic caspase activation are the ceramide pathway that may act predominantly through the initiator caspase-8 or caspase-9, depending on the stimulus that induces ceramide synthesis, and the granzyme B-perforin pathway, which may be directly initiated by the effector caspase-3 and caspase-7. All these pathways, with the exception of the granzyme pathway, are known to be active in neurons.

Studies were conducted to investigate the role of caspase cascade-mediated programmed cell death. Using our 3- to 5-day-old newborn piglet model, we investigated the hypoxia-induced alterations in the activity and expression of caspase-3, caspase-8, and caspase-9. Results of these studies after 1 h of severe hypoxia in newborn piglets demonstrated that following hypoxia, there is an increase in the activity of the initiator caspase-8 and caspase-9 in the cytosolic fraction of the cerebral cortex. The activity of caspase-3 also increased in the cytosolic fraction of the cerebral cortex. In addition, the expression of caspase-8, caspase-9, and caspase-3 protein increased following hypoxia (Delivoria-Papadopoulos et al. 2008; Mishra and Delivoria-Papadopoulos 2010; Ashraf et al. 2007).

125.7.2 Mechanisms of Caspase Activation During Hypoxia in the Newborn Brain

To investigate the mechanism of caspase activation, we used selective inhibitors such as clonidine, an inhibitor of high-affinity Ca^{++}-ATPase; 7-nitroindazole sodium salt (7-NINA), an inhibitor of neuronal NO synthase; and z-Leu-Glu(OMe)-His-Asp(OMe)-fluoromethylketone (z-LEHD-FMK), a selective caspase inhibitor.

125.7.2.1 The Role of Nuclear Ca^{++} Influx in Caspase-9 and Caspase-3 Activation

Studies performed in newborn piglets were specifically designed to investigate the role of nuclear Ca++ influx in caspase activation during hypoxia by administration of a Ca^{++}-ATPase inhibitor (clonidine) to block the nuclear Ca^{++} influx. It was shown that the increased activity of caspase-9 and caspase-3 during hypoxia is mediated by nuclear Ca^{++} influx. The levels of tissue high-energy phosphates (ATP and PCr) in the cerebral cortex of normoxic, hypoxic, and hypoxic pretreated with clonidine piglets were comparably decreased. The determination of caspase-9 activity in the normoxic, hypoxic, and hypoxic pretreated with clonidine groups of piglets showed that cerebral tissue hypoxia results in increased caspase-9 activity and that the pretreatment with high-affinity Ca^{++}-ATPase inhibitor prevents this hypoxia-induced increase in caspase-9 activity.

Assessment of the activity of caspase-3 in the normoxic, hypoxic, and hypoxic pretreated with clonidine groups of piglets demonstrated that cerebral tissue hypoxia resulted in increased caspase-3 activity, a consequence of caspase-9 activation, and that the pretreatment with clonidine prevented this increase in caspase-3 activity. These results demonstrate that hypoxia-induced increase in caspase-3 activity is mediated by nuclear Ca^{++} influx.

125.7.2.2 The Role of NO in Caspase-9 and Caspase-3 Activation

These studies in newborn piglets were specifically designed to investigate the role of NO derived from nNOS in caspase activation during hypoxia by administration of a relatively selective inhibitor of nNOS, 7-NINA (Mishra and Delivoria-Papadopoulos 2006). After having confirmed that cerebral tissue hypoxia achieved in the hypoxic and hypoxic pretreated with 7-NINA groups was comparable, the activity of caspase-9 in the normoxic, hypoxic, and hypoxic pretreated with 7-NINA groups of piglets was determined, and the results demonstrated that cerebral tissue hypoxia results in increased caspase-9 activity and that the pretreatment with the nNOS inhibitor prevents the hypoxia-induced increase in caspase-9 activity.

Cerebral tissue hypoxia resulted in increased caspase-3 activity, a consequence of caspase-9 activation, and the pretreatment with the nNOS inhibitor prevented this hypoxia-induced increase in caspase-3 activity. It demonstrates that the hypoxia-induced increase in caspase-9 is mediated by nNOS-derived NO.

125.7.2.3 The Effect of Caspase-9 Inhibition During Hypoxia on Prevention of Downstream Events Including Caspase-3 Activation

To demonstrate that caspase-3 activation is a downstream event of caspase-9 activation during hypoxia, we used its selective inhibitor z-LEHD-FMK (Chiang et al. 2007, 2008).

The activity of caspase-9 was determined in the cytosolic fraction of the cerebral cortex of newborn piglets. Cerebral tissue hypoxia resulted in increased caspase-9 activity and the pretreatment with the caspase-9 inhibitor prevented the hypoxia-induced increase in caspase-9 activity.

The activity of caspase-3 in the cytosolic fraction of the cerebral cortex increased as a consequence of caspase-9 activation, and the pretreatment with a caspase-9 inhibitor prevented this hypoxia-induced increase. The same study showed that pretreatment with caspase-9 inhibitor prevents the hypoxia-induced increase in the expression of active caspase-9 and active caspase-3 (protein levels).

These studies demonstrate that caspase-9 can be activated during hypoxia by multiple mechanisms that are dependent on generation of nNOS-derived NO and neuronal nuclear Ca^{++} influx. The increase in nuclear Ca^{++} influx leading to Ca^{++}-dependent activation of Ca/calmodulin-dependent protein kinase IV may result in increased phosphorylation or cyclic AMP response element binding protein at serine 133 and transcription of caspases as well as proapoptotic proteins. NO-mediated phosphorylation of anti-apoptotic proteins may alter their anti-apoptotic potential due to a defect in dimerization and increased caspase-9 activation.

We have shown that NO increases Ca^{++} influx in synaptosomes as well as neuronal nuclei. By increasing nuclear Ca^{++} influx, NO can increase expression of caspase-9 as well as proapoptotic proteins. NO-mediated modification of caspase protein may alter its activation.

Thus, caspase activation during hypoxia in the newborn brain is mediated by transcription-dependent and transcription-independent mechanisms.

Studies using z-LEHD-FMK, a selective inhibitor of caspase-9, indicate that the role of caspase-9, the inhibitor caspase, is highly significant in the hypoxia-induced programmed cell death in the newborn brain.

125.8 DNA Fragmentation

It has been proposed that the cleavage of DNA at its intranucleosomal linkage region is produced by specific endonucleases that are Ca^{++} dependent (Ishida et al. 1974).

Caspase-3 acting as cysteine protease cleaves and inactivates a chain reaction by nuclear enzymes like PARP, a DNA repair enzyme, and ICAD, the inhibitor of caspase-activated DNase. Then, the caspase-activated DNase enters the nucleus and cleaves genomic chromosomal DNA (Hameed et al. 1989; Tominaga et al. 1993). This nuclear genomic DNA fragmentation correlates exponentially with the degree of cerebral tissue hypoxia in newborn piglets (Waseem et al. 2001) and is characteristic of cellular apoptosis. However, in our study, there was no significant increase in fragmentation until the ATP and phosphocreatine levels decreased by more than 50%, compared with baseline levels.

125.9 Temporal Biochemical Changes

The steps of posthypoxic neuronal injury are evolving within hours in the necrotic process and within days in the apoptotic process. Temporal biochemical changes and associated nuclear fragmentation have been assessed in the cerebral cortex of newborn guinea pigs following hypoxia. Initial cellular injury may be followed by a failure of cellular repair mechanisms leading to further delayed brain injury. Neuronal nuclear Ca^{++} influx increases immediately following hypoxia and remains elevated through 7 days of age. Similar nuclear Bax protein expression increases immediately following hypoxia and remains elevated through 7 days where Bcl-2 protein remains similar to control during hypoxia.

All these temporal (biphasic) changes may reflect not only the primary hypoxic insult but also a secondary cellular damage due to a recurrent (continuing) free radical release during the reperfusion-reoxygenation phase.

125.10 Clinical Implications

The understanding of the very complex and interrelated mechanisms of cell death after a hypoxic-ischemic result may serve as background in critical care of the newborn.

Hypoxia at the cellular level is the consequence of failure in oxygen transport from the lung alveolar space to the mitochondria. In order to prevent neuronal cell death, to restore any insufficiency or failure in the respiratory and circulatory systems is an emergency in terms of minutes.

Among the hazards in restoring oxygen supply, medically induced hyperoxia (high FIO2) may worsen the neuronal insult by the production of additional oxygen free radicals.

The temporal evolution of the posthypoxic biochemical disturbances may alter the opportunity of pharmacologic interventions at key steps of the biochemical events, like magnesium sulfate, a NMDA receptor antagonist, or allopurinol, an inhibitor of the enzyme xanthine oxidase.

125.11 Neuroprotective Treatments with Suggested Efficacy in Humans

125.11.1 Magnesium Sulfate

In the clinical setting, $MgSO_4$ has been widely used in obstetrics practice for more than 60 years. Its indications include suppression of preterm labor and management of pregnancy-induced hypertension (Levene et al. 1999). A retrospective epidemiologic study by Nelson and Grether (1995) suggested that premature fetuses whose mothers received $MgSO_4$ for the treatment of preeclampsia or as a tocolytic agent are less likely to develop cerebral palsy compared to a gestational age-matched group of fetuses not exposed to the drug. The Collaborative Eclampsia Trial (1995) reported that babies of women who had been given $MgSO_4$ before delivery were significantly less likely to be intubated at the place of delivery or to be admitted to a special care nursery than the babies of mothers who had been given phenytoin. These studies suggested that $MgSO_4$ might provide a protective effect against brain damage in immature fetuses and newborn infants. Randomized, controlled, double-blind trials were established to examine this hypothesis. One was discontinued after interim analysis showed that administration of $MgSO_4$ to mothers in preterm labor before 34 weeks of gestation was associated with significant increase in infants' mortality (Mittendorf et al. 1997). However, other trials have not shown any difference in the mortality rates between the placebo and treatment groups (Benichou et al. 1997).

A multicenter randomized, controlled trial of $MgSO_4$ vs. placebo, for the prevention of cerebral palsy, in 2,241 women at risk of imminent premature delivery at 24–31 weeks of gestation carried out in the USA was published in 2008 (Rouse et al. 2008). The primary outcome was the composite of stillbirth or infant death by 1 year of corrected age or moderate or severe cerebral palsy at or beyond 2 years of corrected age. The primary outcome was not significantly different in the $MgSO_4$ group and the placebo group. However, in a prespecified secondary analysis, moderate or severe cerebral palsy occurred significantly less frequently in the $MgSO_4$ group (1.9% vs. 3.5%). A similar study in France followed up 606 infants of less than 33 weeks of gestation, whose mothers were treated with $MgSO_4$. Compared to placebo, treated infants showed a decrease of all primary end points (total mortality, severe white matter injury, and their combined outcome) and of all secondary end points (motor dysfunction, cerebral palsy, cognitive dysfunction, and their combined outcomes at 2 years of age). The decrease was nearly significant or significant for gross motor dysfunction and combined criteria: death and cerebral palsy, death and gross motor dysfunction, and death, cerebral palsy, and cognitive dysfunction (Moriette et al. 2008). Doyle et al. (2009) reviewed the evidence of the neuroprotective effects of $MgSO_4$ given to women considered at risk of preterm birth. The authors concluded that the neuroprotective role for antenatal $MgSO_4$ therapy given to mothers at such risk is now established. The number of women needed to treat to benefit one baby by avoiding cerebral palsy is 63 (95% confidence interval 43–87). Given the beneficial effects of $MgSO_4$ on substantial gross motor function in early childhood, outcomes later in childhood should be evaluated to determine the presence or absence of later potentially important neurologic effects, particularly on motor or cognitive function.

125.11.2 Allopurinol

In experimental animal models, administration of allopurinol to immature rats 30 min before inducing focal hypoxia-ischemia reduced the severity of the secondary edema and the extent of the neuropathologic lesions in the treated compared with a control group (Palmer et al. 1990). Similarly, pretreatment with allopurinol preserved cerebral energy metabolism of the 7-day postnatal rat during hypoxia-ischemia (Williams et al. 1992). The same group of researchers found that oxypurinol, the active metabolite of allopurinol, administered at the same dose and at the same time as allopurinol after hypoxia-ischemia reduced brain injury in the immature rat (Palmer and Roberts 1991). Administration of allopurinol in newborn piglets prevented the hypoxia-induced modification of NMDA receptor as well as cell membrane preoxidation and neuronal dysfunction (Marro et al. 1994; Maro et al. 1998).

In the clinical setting, a 7-day course of enteral allopurinol (20 mg per kg) given after birth to 400 infants between 24 and 32 weeks of gestation did not change the incidence of periventricular leukomalacia (Russell and Cooke 1995). In a study of 22 asphyxiated newborn infants, intravenous allopurinol in a dose of 40 mg per kg given 4 h after birth resulted in a decreased mortality (2/11 vs. 6/11 in the control group) and in a beneficial effect on free radical formation, cerebral blood flow, and electrical brain activity, without toxic side effects (Van Bel et al. 1998). Clancy et al. (2001) conducted a clinical trial to test the hypothesis that allopurinol could reduce death, seizures, coma, and cardiac events in infants who underwent heart surgery using deep hypothermic circulatory arrest. They studied a total of 318 infants, 131 hypoplastic left heart syndrome (HLHS) and 187 non-HLHS. In HLHS surgical survivors, 40 of 47 (85%) allopurinol-treated infants did not experience any end point event, compared to 27 of 49 (55%) controls ($p = 0.002$). There were fewer seizure-only ($p = 0.05$) and cardiac-only ($p = 0.03$) events in the allopurinol versus placebo groups. Allopurinol did not reduce efficacy end point events in non-HLHS infants. Treated and control infants did not differ in adverse events. Recently, Bender et al. (2006) investigated whether postnatal allopurinol would reduce free radical-induced reperfusion/reoxygenation injury of the brain in severely asphyxiated neonates. In an interim analysis of a randomized, double-blind, placebo-controlled study, 32 severely asphyxiated infants were given allopurinol or a vehicle within 4 h of birth. The analysis showed an unaltered (high) mortality and morbidity in infants treated with allopurinol. The authors concluded that allopurinol treatment started postnatally was too late to reduce the early reperfusion-induced free radical surge. Allopurinol administration to the fetus with (imminent) hypoxia via the mother during labor may be more effective in reducing free radical-induced post-asphyxial brain damage.

Chaudhari and McGuire (2008) performed a meta-analysis to evaluate the evidence of the effect of allopurinol on mortality or morbidity in newborn infants with suspected hypoxic-ischemic encephalopathy. The authors concluded that the available data are not sufficient to determine whether allopurinol has clinically important benefits for newborn infants with hypoxic-ischemic encephalopathy, and, therefore, larger trials are needed. Such trials could assess allopurinol as an adjunct to therapeutic hypothermia in infants with moderate and severe encephalopathy and should be designed to exclude clinically important effects on mortality and adverse long-term neurodevelopmental outcomes.

125.11.3 Opioids

The antinociceptive effects of opioids are mediated through a combination of pre- and postsynaptic hyperpolarization, which produces a decrease in the release of and the sensitivity to endogenous mediators like glutamate (Lee et al. 2004; Yamakura et al. 1999). This suggests that they may have a neuroprotective effect. Indeed, studies in cell cultures have demonstrated that endogenous and exogenous opioids may protect cortical neurons from hypoxia-induced cell death (Zhang et al. 2000, 2002). Similarly, opioids may induce ischemic tolerance in cerebellar Purkinje cells subject to ischemia-reperfusion (Lim et al. 2004). Antagonists of opioid receptors increase the survival time during severe hypoxia in intact animals (Mayfield and D'Alecy 1992, 1994) and enhance tissue preservation and survival time of organs used for transplants (Chein et al. 1994).

In 2005, Angeles et al. (2005) published the results of a retrospective study of 52 term newborns with perinatal asphyxia, in which they analyzed the relationship between treatment with opioid analgesics (morphine or fentanyl) and neurological damage. A total of 33% of them received opioids; in spite of having a more severe degree of asphyxia (higher levels of lactate, lower 5 min Apgar scores), this group of patients had less severe signs of brain damage on the MRI performed after 7 days of life. Moreover, their neurologic outcome at a mean follow-up of 13 months was better than the group of newborns who did not receive opioids. The same group of researchers also performed a follow-up study with magnetic resonance (MR) spectroscopy of 28 term newborns treated with opioids and 20 controls (Angeles et al. 2007). The results showed that occipital gray matter NAA/Cr was significantly decreased and lactate was present in a significantly higher amount in non-opioid-treated neonates compared with opioid-treated neonates. Also, compared with controls, untreated neonates showed large changes in more metabolites in the basal ganglia, thalami, and occipital gray matter with greater significance than treated neonates. The authors concluded that the use of opioids during the first week following perinatal asphyxia has no long-term adverse effects and may increase brain resistance to hypoxia-ischemia. The authors speculated that the neuroprotective effect of opioids may be mediated by increasing the levels of adenosine, and endogenous nucleoside with neuroprotective activity, or by inducing neuronal hyperpolarization, which results in diminishing intracellular penetration of calcium.

Despite the potential benefit of opioids on asphyxiated term neonates as indicated in these studies, caution must be exercised in the use of this class of medications. Available literature suggests that the routine use of opioid analgesics can be complicated by problems such as tolerance, withdrawal symptoms, and ventilator dependence. Very few studies have examined the long-term effects of exposure to opioids in the neonatal period. In addition, previous reports indicate that endogenous opioids can suppress DNA synthesis in vivo in mature cerebellar and glial cells (opioid receptors are widely distributed in the CNS with functions that include pain modulation, cardiorespiratory regulation), whereas exogenous opioids can exacerbate neurotoxicity in animal models of cerebral ischemia. Future prospective randomized trials are warranted to determine whether there is truly an immediate neuroprotective effect on hypoxic-ischemic brain injury and whether these agents can play a role in improving long-term outcome.

125.11.4 Hypothermia

Hypothermia has developed during the past few years as an alternative for treating perinatal asphyxia/HIE (Gunn and Gunn 1998; Wagner et al. 1999). Hypothermia during experimental cerebral ischemia is associated with potent dose-related, long-lasting neuroprotection. Conversely, hyperthermia of only 1–2 °C extends and markedly worsens damage and in particular tends to promote pannecrosis (Gunn and Gunn 1998).

Although the majority of such studies involved global ischemia in adult rodents (Coimbria and Wielock 1994), similar results were reported from studies on hypoxia-ischemia in 7-day-old rats (Trescher et al. 1997) and newborn piglets (Thorensen et al. 1995), kittens, rabbits, and puppies (Miller 1971).

The study of the mechanisms of action of hypothermic neuroprotection suggests that cooling affects many or all of the pathways leading to delayed cell death (Gunn and Gunn 1998). Hypothermia reduces the rate of oxygen-requiring enzymatic reactions and cerebral oxygen consumption, slows the fall of phosphocreatine/inorganic phosphate (PCr/Pi), and confers a protective effect of the brain after ATP exhaustion. In addition, hypothermia decreases oxygen consumption of the brain by 6–7% and cerebral energy utilization rate by 5.3% per degree. Additional experimental evidence suggests that hypothermia suppresses cytotoxic excitatory amino acid accumulation, inhibits nitric oxide synthase activity, decreases interleukin-1 levels, decreases the release of other cytotoxic cytokines by microglial cells, and suppresses free radical activity and delayed cell death by apoptosis. Hypothermia also decreases blood-brain barrier permeability and intracranial pressure and facilitates recovery of electrophysiologic function after cerebral ischemia.

The efficacy of hypothermia is dependent on a number of factors, such as the timing of initiation of cooling, its duration, and the depth of cooling attained. Mild hypothermia is defined as a reduction in core temperature of 1–3 °C, moderate as 4–6 °C, severe as 8–10 °C, and profound as 15–20 °C. Brief (0.5–3 h); mild-to-moderate hypothermia immediately after hypoxia-ischemic injury may be most effective after relatively mild insults. Protection appears to be lost if brief hypothermia is delayed by as little as 15–45 min after the primary insult. A more recent approach has been to try to suppress the secondary encephalopathic processes by maintaining hypothermia throughout the course of the secondary phase. An extended period of cooling (between 5 and 72 h) appears to be more consistently effective and remains effective after significant delays (possibly up to 6 h) between the primary insult and the start of cooling; however, the degree of neuroprotection progressively declines if cooling is initiated more than a few hours post-insult (Gunn and Gunn 1998). In addition, cerebral hypothermia seems to be less effective when started after postischemic seizures occur (Gunn et al. 1999).

Potential adverse effects of induced hypothermia (the risk increasing with depth of hypothermia) include increased blood viscosity, mild metabolic acidosis, decreased oxygen availability, intracellular shift of potassium, cardiac arrhythmias, coagulation abnormalities and platelet dysfunction, and choreic syndrome (Wagner et al. 1999).

125.11.5 Selective Head Cooling

The first study on neuroprotection of perinatal HIE with selective head cooling was published in 1998 by (Gunn et al. 1998), who basically proved the safety of this procedure. Later on, the same group of researchers published the results of other studies in a small number of patients, which confirmed the lack of side effects and a tendency to a better neurologic prognosis in those newborns with moderate or severe HIE treated with this hypothermia technique (Battin et al. 2001, 2003).

In 2005 Gluckman et al. (2005) published the results of the most important study that has produced reliable and significant data about the neuroprotective effect of selective head cooling hypothermia. It was a multicenter investigation that included 234 newborns with HIE and expected gestational age (EGA) above 36 weeks. Patients were randomized before 5.5 h of life into two groups: body normothermia or hypothermia of 34.5 °C, induced through selective head cooling during 72 h. Patients treated with hypothermia had a significantly higher incidence of arrhythmia (mostly sinus bradycardia). A total of 218 infants were followed up until 18 months of age. The presence of death or neurological disability was found in 66% of patients in the control group and 55% in the hypothermia group ($p < 0.1$). However, when newborns with severe neurological depression or those who had seizures on the aEEG were excluded, 66% of infants in the control group and 48% in the hypothermia group died or had neurological disability ($p < 0.2$). Moreover, the presence of severe neurological disability was 28% and 12% in each group, respectively. The authors concluded that, except in newborns with the most severe forms of HIE, selective head cooling applied immediately following delivery may be a feasible therapeutic technique to decrease neurological sequelae of perinatal HIE.

125.11.6 Generalized Body Hypothermia

The first study with generalized body hypothermia in perinatal HIE was published in 2000 by Azzopardi et al. (2000), who found that prolonged hypothermia of 33–34 °C was associated with minimal physiological changes (e.g., decreased heart rate, increased blood pressure), but was well tolerated. During the next 3 years, other research protocols in a limited number of patients corroborated that generalized body hypothermia was a feasible and clinically safe technique (Shankaran et al. 2002; Debillon et al. 2003).

In 2005, Eicher et al. (2005) published the results of a pilot multicenter study about the safety and efficacy of generalized body hypothermia in the treatment of 32 newborns with perinatal HIE. Adverse effects included bradycardia, hypotension, decreased platelets, increased prothrombin time, and higher incidence of seizures, but none of them was severe, and they all responded to treatment (Eicher et al. 2005). The efficacy results showed a higher incidence of death or severe neurological motor involvement in the control group (82%) compared to the group of hypothermia-treated newborns (52%) ($p = 0.019$). A severe psychomotor developmental delay (less than 70%) was seen in 64% of infants in the control group and in 24% of those subjected to hypothermia ($p = 0.053$).

Also in 2005, Shankaran et al. (2005) published a large multicenter study on the use of body hypothermia to treat perinatal HIE. A total of 208 newborns with HIE and EGA more than 36 weeks were included and randomized before 6 h of life into two groups: body normothermia or hypothermia of 33.5 °C, induced by body cooling, during 72 h. Patients were followed up until 18–22 months. The incidence of mild complications was similar in both groups. The incidence of death or moderate or severe neurological disability was 62% in the control group and 44% in the hypothermia-treated group ($p = 0.01$). The incidence of cerebral palsy was 30% in the control newborns and 19% in those treated with hypothermia ($p = 0.20$). The authors concluded that generalized body hypothermia reduces the risk of death and neurological disability in newborns with moderate or severe HIE.

A magnetic resonance imaging (MRI) follow-up study of infants enrolled in the abovementioned trial (Shankaran et al. 2005) aimed to measure relative volumes of subcortical white matter. They were significantly large in hypothermia-treated than in control infants. Furthermore, relative total brain volumes correlated significantly with death or neurosensory impairments. Relative volumes of the cortical gray and subcortical white matter also correlated significantly with Bayley Scales psychomotor development index (Parikh et al. 2009). There is growing body of evidence supporting that total body hypothermia improves significantly survival and disability in full-term neonates with HIE with better neurodevelopmental outcomes in infancy and early childhood (Jacobs et al. 2013; Azzopardi et al. 2014; Shankaran et al. 2012).

Hypothermia has already translated from the clinical research experience to direct clinical application and has already become the standard of care to treat newborns with perinatal asphyxia (Zanelli et al. 2008; Kapetanakis et al. 2008; Tan and Parks 1999; Gunn et al. 2005; Sahni and Sanocka 2008; Wagner et al. 2002; Hoeger et al. 2006; Talati et al. 2005; Van Bel and Groenendaal 2008; Higgins et al. 2006; Jacobs et al. 2013; Azzopardi et al. 2014; Shankaran et al. 2012). However, the clinical trials with hypothermia in premature newborns and/or in combination with neuroprotective agents such as xenon, erythropoietin, melatonin, and allopurinol have also addressed many questions, which need to be answered before they are implemented in routine clinical practice.

References

Aizenman E, Lipton SA, Loring RH (1989) Selective modulation of NMDA responses by reduction and oxidation. Neuron 2:1257–1263

Angeles DM, Wycliffe N, Michelson D et al (2005) Use of opioids in asphyxiated term neonates: effects of neuroimaging and clinical outcome. Pediatr Res 57:873–878

Angeles DM, Ashwal S, Wycliffe ND et al (2007) Relationship between opioid therapy, tissue damaging procedures, and brain metabolites as measured by proton MRS in asphyxiated term neonates. Pediatr Res 60:614–621

Aoki C, Fenstemaker S, Lubin M et al (1993) Nitric oxide synthase in the visual cortex of monocular monkeys as revealed by light and electron microscopic immunocytochemistry. Brain Res 620:97–113

Aoki C, Rhee J, Lubin M et al (1997) NMDA-R1 subunit of the cerebral cortex co-localizes with neuronal nitric oxide synthase at pre and postsynaptic sites and in spines. Brain Res 750:25–140

Ashraf QM, Mishra OP, Delivoria-Papadopoulos M (2007) Mechanisms of expression of apoptotic protease activating factor-1 (Apaf-1) in nuclear, mitochondrial and cytosolic fractions of the cerebral cortex of newborn piglets. Neurosci Lett 415:253–258

Azzopardi D, Robertson NJ, Cowan FM et al (2000) Pilot study of treatment with whole body hypothermia for neonatal encephalopathy. Pediatrics 106:684–694

Azzopardi D, Strohm B, Marlow N, Brocklehurst P, Deierl A, Eddama O et al (2014) Effects of hypothermia for perinatal asphyxia on childhood outcomes. N Engl J Med 371:140–149. https://doi.org/10.1056/NEJMoa1315788

Bashir ZI, Alford S, Davies SN et al (1991) Long-term potentiation of NMDA receptor-mediated synaptic transmission in the hippocampus. Nature 349:156–158

Battin MR, Dezoete JA, Gunn TR et al (2001) Neurodevelopmental outcome of infants treated with head cooling and mild hypothermia after perinatal asphyxia. Pediatrics 107:480–484

Battin MR, Penrice J, Gunn TR, Gunn AJ (2003) Treatment of term infants with head cooling and systematic hypothermia (35.0 degrees and 34.5 degrees C) after perinatal asphyxia. Pediatrics 111:244–251

Baum RM (1984) Superoxide theory of oxygen toxicity is center of heated debate. Chem Eng News 9:20–28

Beckman JS (1990) Apparent hydroxyl radical production by peroxynitrite: implications for endothelial injury from nitric oxide and superoxide. Proc Natl Acad Sci U S A 87:1620–1624

Beckman JS (1991) The double-edged role of nitric oxide in brain function and superoxide-mediated injury. J Dev Physiol 15:53–59

Bender MJ, Bos AF, Rademaker CM et al (2006) Early postnatal allopurinol does not improve short term outcome after severe birth asphyxia. Arch Dis Child Fetal Neonatal Ed 91:F163–F165

Benichou J, Zupan V, Fernandez H et al (1997) Tocolytic magnesium sulphate and pediatric mortality. Lancet 351:290–291

Bhat GK, Mahesh VB, Lamar CA et al (1997) Histochemical localization of nitric oxide neurons in the hypothalamus: association with gonadotropin-releasing hormone neurons and co-localization with N-methyl-D-aspartate receptors. Neuroendocrinol Lett 62:187–197

Bredt DS, Ferris CD, Snyder SH (1992) Nitric oxide synthase regulatory sites. Phosphorylation by cyclic AMP-dependent protein kinase, protein kinase C, and calcium/calmodulin protein kinase, identification of flavin and calmodulin sites. J Biol Chem 267: 10976–10981

Cazevielle C (1993) Superoxide and nitric oxide cooperation in hypoxia/reoxygenation-induced neuron injury. Free Radic Biol Med 14:359–395

Chaudhari T, McGuire W (2008) Allopurinol for preventing mortality and morbidity in newborn infants with suspected hypoxic-ischemic encephalopathy. Cochrane Database Syst Rev 2:CD006817

Chawla S, Bading H (2001) CREB/CBP and SRE-interacting transcriptional regulators are fast on-off switches: duration of calcium transients specifies the magnitude of transcriptional responses. J Neurochem 79:849–858

Chein S, Oeltgen PR, Diana JN et al (1994) Extension of tissue survival time in multiorgan block preparation with a delta DADLE (D-Ala2, D-leu5)-enkephalin). J Thorac Cardiovasc Surg 107:964–967

Chen J, Zhu RL, Nakayama M et al (1996) Expression of the apoptosis- effector gene, Bax, is up-regulated in vulnerable hippocampal CA1 neurons following global ischemia. J Neurochem 67:64–71

Chiang MC, Ashraf QM, Ara J et al (2007) Mechanism of caspase-3 activation during hypoxia in the cerebral cortex of newborn piglets. Neurosci Lett 421:67–71

Chiang MC, Ashraf QM, Mishra OP, Delivoria-Papadopoulos M (2008) Mechanism of DNA fragmentation during hypoxia in the cerebral cortex of newborn piglets. Neurochem Res 33:1232–1237

Choi DW (1990) Cerebral hypoxia: some new approaches and unanswered questions. J Neurosci 10:2493–2501

Christopherson KS, Hillier BJ, Lim WAS et al (1999) PSD-95 assembles a ternary complex with the N-Methyl-D-Aspartic acid receptor and bivalent neuronal NO synthase PDX domain. J Boi Chem 274:27467–27473

Clancy RR, McGaurn SA, Goin JE et al (2001) Allopurinol neurocardiac protection trial in infants undergoing heart surgery using deep hypothermic circulatory arrest. Pediatrics 108:61–70

Coimbria C, Wielock T (1994) Moderate hypothermia mitigates neuronal damage in the rat brain when initiated several hours following transient cerebral ischemia. Acta Neuropathol (Berlin) 87:325–331

Collingridge G (1987) Synaptic plasticity. The role of NMDA receptors in learning and memory. Nature 330:604–605

Columbano A (1995) Cell death: current difficulties in discriminating apoptosis and necrosis in the context of pathological processes in vivo. J Cell Biochem 58:181–190

Davidson JO, Wassink G, van den Heuij LG et al (2015) Therapeutic hypothermia for neonatal hypoxic-ischemic encephalopathy – where to from here? Front Neurol 14:6–198

Dawson VL (1991) Nitric oxide mediates glutamate neurotoxicity in primary cortical cultures. Proc Natl Acad Sci U S A 88:6368–6371

Dawson DA (1994a) Nitric oxide and focal cerebral ischemia: multiplicity of actions and diverse outcome. Cerebrovasc Brain Metab 64:299–324

Dawson TM (1994b) Gases as biological messengers: nitric oxide and carbon monoxide in the brain. J Neurosci 14:5147–5159

Dawson TM, Steiner JP, Dawson VL et al (1993) Immunosuppressant FK506 enhances phosphorylation of nitric oxide synthase and protects against glutamate neurotoxicity. Proc Natl Acad Sci U S A 90:9808–9812

Debillon T, Daoud P, Durand P et al (2003) Whole-body cooling after perinatal asphyxia: a study in term neonates. Dev Med Child Neurol 45:17–23

Delivoria-Papadopoulos M, Mishra OP (1998) Mechanisms of cerebral injury in perinatal asphyxia and strategies for prevention. J Pediatr 132:S30–S34

Delivoria-Papadopoulos M, Akhter W, Mishra OP (2003) Hypoxia-induced Ca2+ -influx in cerebral cortical neuronal nuclei of newborn piglets. Neurosci Lett 342:119–123

Delivoria-Papadopoulos M, Ashraf QM, Ara J, Mishra OP (2008) Nuclear mechanisms of hypoxic cerebral injury in the newborn: the role of caspases. Semin Perinatol 32:334–343

Delivoria-Papadopoulos M, Ashraf QM, Mishra OP (2001a) Brain tissue energy dependence of CaM kinase IV cascade activation during hypoxia in the cerebral cortex of newborn piglets. Neurosci Lett 491(2):113–117

Delivoria-Papadopoulos M, Ashraf QM, Mishra OP (2001b) Mechanism of CaM kinase IV activation during hypoxia in neuronal nuclei of the cerebral cortex of newborn piglets: the role of Src kinase. Neurochem Res 36(8):1512–1519

Dolmetsch RE, Lewis RS, Goodnow CC (1997) Differential activation of transcription factors induced by Ca2+ response amplitude and duration. Nature 386:855–858

Dolmetsch RE, Pajvani U, Fife K et al (2001) Signaling to the nucleus by an L-type calcium channel-calmodulin complex through the MAP kinase pathway. Science 294:333–339

Doyle LW, Crowther CA, Middleton P et al (2009) Magnesium bias sulphate for women at risk of preterm birth for neuroprotection of the fetus. Cochrane Database Syst Rev 1:CD004661

Dragunow M, Beiharz E, Sirimanne E et al (1994) Immediately early gene protein expression in neurons undergoing delayed death, but not necrosis following hypoxic-ischemic injury to the young rat brain. Brain Res Mol Brain Res 25:1933

Eicher DJ, Wagner CL, Katikaneni LP et al (2005) Moderate hypothermia in neonatal encephalopathy: safety outcomes. Pediatr Neurol 32:18–24

Faraci FM (1991) Role of endothelium-derived relaxing factor in cerebral circulation: large arteries vs. microcirculation. Am J Physiol 261:H1038–H1042

Ferrer I, Tortosa A, Macaya A et al (1994) Evidence of nuclear DNA fragmentation following hypoxia-ischemia in the infant rat brain, and transient forebrain ischemia in the adult gerbil. Brain Pathol 4:115–122

Fields RD, Esthete F, Stevens B et al (1997) Action potential-dependent regulation of gene expression: temporal specificity in Ca2+, cAMP-responsive element binding proteins, and mitogen-activated protein kinase signaling. J Neurosci 17:7252–7266

Fritz K, Delivoria-Papadopoulos M (2006) Mechanisms of injury to the newborn brain. Clin Perinatol 33:573–591

Fritz KI, Groenenedaal F, McGowan JE et al (1996) Effects of 3- (2-carboxy-piperzine-4-yl) propyl-1-phosphonic acid (CPP) on NMDA receptor binding characteristics and brain cell membrane function during cerebral hypoxia in newborn piglets. Brain Res 729:66–74

Ghosh A, Greenberg ME (1995) Calcium signaling in neurons: molecular mechanisms and cellular consequences. Science 268:239–247

Gillardon F, Lenz C, Waschke KF (1996) Altered expression of Bcl- 2, Bcl-X, Bax and c-Fos colocalizes with DNA fragmentation and ischemic cell damage following middle cerebral artery occlusion in rats. Brain Res Mol Brain Res 40:254–260

Gluckman PD, Wyatt JS, Azzopardi D et al (2005) Selective head cooling with mild systemic hypothermia after neonatal encephalopathy: multicenter randomized trial. Lancet 365:663–670

Gow AJ, Duran D, Malcom S et al (1996) Effect of peroxynitrite-induced protein modification on tyrosine phosphorylation and degradation. FEBS Lett 385:63–66

Gunn AJ, Gunn TR (1998) The 'pharmacology' of neuronal rescue with cerebral hypothermia. Early Hum Dev 53:19–35

Gunn AJ, Gluckman PD, Gunn TR (1998) Selective head cooling in newborn infants after perinatal asphyxia: a safety study. Pediatrics 102:885–892

Gunn AJ, Bennet L, Gunning MI et al (1999) Cerebral hypothermia is not neuroprotective when started after postischemic seizures in fetal sheep. Pediatr Res 46:274–280

Gunn AJ, Battin M, Gluckman PD et al (2005) Therapeutic hypothermia: from lab to NICU. J Perinat Med 33:340–346

Hamada Y (1994) Inhibitors of nitric oxide synthesis reduce hypoxic-ischemic brain damage in the neonatal rat. Pediatr Res 35:10–14

Hameed A, Olsen KJ, Lee MK et al (1989) Cytolysis by Ca-permeable transmembrane channels: pore formation causes extensive DNA degradation and cell lysis. J Exp Med 169:765–777

Hardingham GE, Bading H (1998) Nuclear calcium: a key regulator of gene expression. Biometals 11:345–358

Hardingham GE, Chawla S, Cruzalegui FH, Bading H (1999) Control of recruitment and transcription-activating function of CBP determines gene regulation by NMDA receptors and L-type calcium channels. Neuron 22:789–798

Higgins RD, Rahu TN, Perlman J et al (2006) Hypothermia and perinatal asphyxia: executive summary of the national institute of child health and human development workshop. J Pediatr 148:170–175

Hill A, Volpe J (1999) Hypoxic-ischemic cerebral injury in the newborn. In: Swaiman KF, Ashwal S (eds) Pediatric neurology, principles and practice. Mosby, St. Louis, pp 191–204

Hoeger H, Engidawork E, Stolzlechner D et al (2006) Long-term effect of moderate and profound hypothermia on morphology, neurological, cognitive and behavioural functions in a rat model of perinatal asphyxia. Amino Acids 31:385–396

Hoffman DJ, Marro PJ, McGowan JE et al (1994a) Protective effect of MgSO4 infusion on NMDA receptor binding characteristics during cerebral cortical hypoxia in newborn piglets. Brain Res 644:144–149

Hoffman DJ, McGowan JE, Marro PJ et al (1994b) Hypoxia-induced modification of the N-methyl-D-aspartate (NMDA) receptor in the brain of newborn piglets. Neurosci Lett 167:156–160

Huang Z (1994) Effects of cerebral ischemia in mice deficient neuronal nitric oxide. Science 265:1883–1885

Ishida R, Akiyoshi H, Takahashi T (1974) Isolation and purification of calcium and magnesium dependent endonuclease from rat liver nuclei. Biochem Biophys Res Commun 56:703–710

Jacobs SE, Berg M, Hunt R, Tarnow-Mordi WO, Inder TE, Davis PG (2013) Cooling for newborns with hypoxic ischaemic encephalopathy. Cochrane Database Syst Rev 1:CD003311.10.1002/14651858.CD003311.pub3

Johnston MV (1995) Neurotransmitters and vulnerability of the developing brain. Brain Dev 17:301–306

Kapetanakis A, Azzopardi D, Wyatt J et al (2008) Therapeutic hypothermia for neonatal encephalopathy: a UK survey of opinion, practice and neuron-investigation at the end of 2007. Acta Paediatr 98:631–635

Kiedrowski I, Costa E, Wroblewski JT (1992) Glutamate receptor agonist stimulate nitric oxide synthase in primary cultures of cerebellar granule cells. J Neuroch 58:335–341

Kitada S, Krajewski S, Miyashita T (1996) Gamma-radiation induces upregulation of Bax protein and apoptosis in radiosensitive cells in vivo. Oncogene 12:187–192

Kratimenos P, Koutroulis I, Marconi D et al (2014) Multi-targeted molecular therapeutic approach in aggressive neuroblastoma: the effect of Focal Adhesion Kinase–Src–Paxillin system. Expert Opin Ther Targets 18(12):1395–1406

Kratimenos P, Koutroulis I, Agarwal B, Theocharis S, Delivoria-Papadopoulos M (2017) Effect of concurrent Src kinase inhibition with short-duration hypothermia on Ca2+/calmodulin kinase IV activity and neuropathology after hypoxia-ischemia in the newborn swine brain. Sci Rep 7(1):16664. https://doi.org/10.1038/s41598-017-16983-1

Kratimenos P, Koutroulis I, Jain A, Malaeb S, Delivoria-Papadopoulos M (2018) Effect of Src kinase inhibition on cytochrome c, Smac/DIABLO and apoptosis inducing factor (AIF) following cerebral hypoxia-ischemia in newborn piglets. Neonatology 113(1):37–43. https://doi.org/10.1159/000480067

Kurinczuk JJ, White-Koning M, Badawi N (2010) Epidemiology of neonatal encephalopathy and hypoxic-ischaemic encephalopathy. Early Hum Dev 86(6):329–338

Lawn JE, Cousens S, Zupan J (2005) 4 million neonatal deaths: when? Where? Why? Lancet 365(9462):891–900

Lee J, Kim MS, Park C et al (2004) Morphine prevents glutamate-induced death of primary rat neonatal astrocytes through modulation of intracellular redox. Immunopharmacol Immunotoxicol 26:17–28

Legido A (1994) Perinatal hypoxic-ischemic encephalopathy: current advances in diagnosis and treatment. Int Pediatr 9:114–136

Legido A, Katsetos CD, Mishra OP et al (2001) Perinatal hypoxia-ischemia encephalopathy: current and future treatments. Int Pediatr 15:143–151

Lerea L, McNamara JO (1993) Ionotropic glutamate receptor subtypes activate c-fos transcription by distinct calcium-requiring intracellular signaling pathways. Neuron 10:31–41

Levene MI, Evans DJ, Mason S et al (1999) An international network for evaluation neuroprotective therapy after severe birth asphyxia. Sem Perinatol 23:226–233

Lim YJ, Zheng S, Zuo Z (2004) Morphine preconditions Purkinje cells against cell death under in vitro simulated ischemia- reperfusion conditions. Anesthesiology 100:562–568

Linnik MD, Zobirst RH, Hatfield MD (1993) Evidence supporting a role for programmed cell death in focal cerebral ischemia in rats. Strokes 24:2002–2008

Lipton S (1999) Redox sensitivity of NMDA receptor. Meth Mol Biol 128:121–130

Maro PJ, Hoffman D, Schneiderman R et al (1998) Effect of allopurinol on NMDA receptor modification following recurrent asphyxia in newborn piglets. Brain Res 787:71–77

Marro PJ, McGowan JE, Razdan B et al (1994) Effect of allopurinol on uric acid levels and brain cell membrane Na+, K+-ATPase activity during hypoxia in newborn piglets. Brain Res 650:9–15

Mayer ML, Westbrook GL, Guthric PB (1984) Voltage-dependent block by Mg++ of NMDA responses in spinal cord neurons. Nature 309:261–263
Mayfield KP, D'Alecy LG (1992) Role of endogenous opioid peptides in the acute adaptation to hypoxia. Brain Res 582:226–231
Mayfield KP, D'Alecy LG (1994) Delta-1 opioid agonist acutely increases hypoxic tolerance. J Pharmacol Exp Ther 268:683–688
Miller JA (1971) New approaches to preventing brain damage during asphyxia. Am J Obstet Gynecol 110:125–132
Mishra OP, Delivoria-Papadopoulos M (1992) NMDA receptor modification of the fetal guinea pig brain during hypoxia. Neurochem Res 17:1211–1216
Mishra OP, Delivoria-Papadopoulos M (1999) Cellular mechanisms of hypoxic injury in the developing brain. Brain Res Bull 48:233–238
Mishra OP, Delivoria-Papadopoulos M (2000) Hypoxia-induced generation of nitric oxide free radicals in cerebral cortex of newborn guinea pigs. Neurochem Res 25:1559–1565
Mishra OP, Delivoria-Papadopoulos M (2001) Effect of graded hypoxia on high-affinity Ca2+-ATPase activity in cortical neuronal nuclei of newborn piglets. Neurochem Res 26:1335–1341
Mishra OP, Delivoria-Papadopoulos M (2002) Nitric oxide-mediated Ca++-influx in neuronal nuclei and cortical synaptosomes of normoxic and hypoxic newborn piglets. Neurosci Lett 318:93–97
Mishra OP, Delivoria-Papadopoulos M (2006) Effect of neuronal nitric oxide synthase inhibition on caspase-9 activity during hypoxia in the cerebral cortex of newborn piglets. Neurosci Lett 401:81–85
Mishra OP, Delivoria-Papadopoulos M (2010) Mechanism of tyrosine phosphorylation of procaspase-9 and Apaf-1 in cytosolic fractions of the cerebral cortex of newborn piglets during hypoxia. Neurosci Lett 480:35–39
Mishra OP, Fritz KI, Delivoria-Papadopoulos M (2001) NMDA receptor and neonatal hypoxic brain injury. Ment Retard Dev Disabil Res Rev 7:249–253
Mittendorf R, Covert R, Boman J et al (1997) Is tocolytic magnesium sulphate associated with increased total pediatric mortality? Lancet 350:1517–1519
Monaghan DT, Olvenman HJ, Nguyen L et al (1988) Two classes of N-methyl-D-aspartate recognition sites: differential distribution and differential regulation by glycine. Proc Natl Acad Sci U S A 85:9836–9840
Monaghan DT, Bridges RJ, Cotman CW (1989) The excitatory amino acid receptors: their classes, pharmacology, and distinct properties in the function of the central nervous system. Annu Rev Pharmacol Toxicol 29:365–402
Moriette G, Barrat J, Truffert P et al (2008) Effect of magnesium sulphate on mortality and neurologic morbidity of the very preterm newborn (of less than 33 weeks) with two-year neurological outcome: results of the prospective PREMAG trial. Gynecol Obstet Fertil 36:278–288
Nelson KB, Grether JK (1995) Can magnesium sulphate reduce the risk of cerebral palsy in very low birth weight infants? Pediatrics 95:263–269
Nowak L, Bregetovski P, Ascher P et al (1984) Magnesium gates glutamate-activated channels in mouse central neurons. Nature 307:462–465
Nowicki JP (1991) Nitric oxide mediates neuronal death after focal cerebral ischemia in the mouse. Eur J Pharmacol 204:339–340
Numagami Y (1997) Lipid free radical generation and brain cell membrane alteration following nitric oxide synthase inhibition during cerebral hypoxia in the newborn piglet. J Neurochem 69:1542–1547
Oltvai ZN, Milliman CL, Korsmeyer SJ (1993) Bcl-2 heterodimerizes in vivo with a conserved homolog, Bax, that accelerates programmed cell death. Cell 74:609–619
Palmer C, Roberts RL (1991) Reduction of perinatal brain damage with oxypurinol treatment after hypoxic-ischemic injury. Pediatr Res 29:362–368
Palmer C, Vanucci RC, Towfighi J (1990) Reduction of perinatal hypoxic-ischemic brain damage with allopurinol. Res Pediatr 27:332–336
Parikh NA, Lasky RE, Garza CN et al (2009) Volumetric and anatomical MRI hypoxic-ischemic encephalopathy: relationship to hypothermia therapy and neurosensory impairments. J Perinatol 29:143–149
Radi R (1991) Peroxynitrite-induced membrane lipid peroxidation: the cytotoxic potential of superoxide and nitric oxide. Arch Biochem Biophys 288:481–487
Raichle ME (1983) The pathophysiology of brain ischemia. Ann Neurol 13:2–10
Ravishankar S, Ashraf QM, Mishra OP et al (2001) Expression of Bax and Bcl-2 proteins during hypoxia in cerebral cortical neuronal nuclei of newborn piglets: effect of administration of magnesium sulfate. Brain Res 901:23–29
Reed JC (1996) Mechanisms of Bcl-2 family protein function and dysfunction in health and disease. Behring Inst Mitt 97:72–100
Rosenbaum DM, Michaelson M, Batter DK et al (1994) Evidence for hypoxia induced programmed cell death of cultured neurons. Ann Neurol 25:19–33
Rothman SM, Olney JW (1986) Glutamate and the pathophysiology of hypoxic-ischemic brain damage. Ann Neurol 19:105–111
Rouse D, Hirtz DG, Thom E et al (2008) A randomized controlled trial of magnesium sulfate for the prevention of cerebral palsy. N Engl J Med 359:895–905
Russell GA, Cooke RW (1995) Randomized controlled trial of allopurinol prophylaxis in very preterm infants. Arch Dis Child Fetal Neonatal Ed 73:F27–F31
Sahni R, Sanocka UM (2008) Hypothermia for hypoxic-ischemic encephalopathy. Clin Perinatol 35:717–734
Sawyer DT (1981) How super is superoxide? Acc Chem Res 14:393–400
Shankaran S, Laptook A, Wright LL et al (2002) Whole-body hypothermia for neonatal encephalopathy: animal observations as a basis for randomized, controlled pilot study in term infants. Pediatrics 110:377–385

Shankaran S, Laptook AR, Ehrenkranz RA et al (2005) Whole-body hypothermia for neonates with hypoxic-ischemic encephalopathy. N Engl J Med 353:1574–1584

Shankaran S, Pappas A, McDonald SA, Vohr BR, Hintz SR, Yolton K et al (2012) Childhood outcomes after hypothermia for neonatal encephalopathy. N Engl J Med 366:2085–2092. https://doi.org/10.1056/NEJMoa1112066

Tacconi S, Ratti E, Marien MR et al (1993) Inhibition of (3H)- (+)-MK-801 binding to rat brain sections by CPP and 7-chlorokynurenic acid: an autoradiographic analysis. Br J Pharmacol 108:668–674

Talati AJ, Yang W, Yolton K et al (2005) Combination of early perinatal factors to identify near-term and term neonates for neuroprotection. J Perinatol 25: 245–250

Tan S, Parks DA (1999) Preserving brain function during neonatal asphyxia. Clin Perinatol 26:733–747

Tang YP, Shimizu E, Dube GR et al (1999) Genetic enhancement of learning and memory in mice. Nature 401:63–69

The Eclampsia Trial Collaborative Group (1995) Which anticonvulsant for eclampsia? Evidence from the Collaborative Eclampsia Trial. Lancet 345: 1455–1463

Thorensen M, Penrice J, Lorek A (1995) Mild hypothermia after severe transient hypoxia-ischemia ameliorates delayed cerebral energy failure in the newborn piglet. Pediatr Res 37:667–670

Tominaga T, Kagure S, Narisawa K et al (1993) Endonuclease activation following focal ischemic injury in the rat brain. Brain Res 608:21–26

Trescher WH, Ishiwa S, Johnston MV (1997) Brief post-HI hypothermia markedly delays neonatal brain injury. Brain Dev 19:326–328

Van Bel F, Groenendaal F (2008) Long-term pharmalogic neuroprotection after birth asphyxia: where do we stand? Neonatology 94:203–210

Van Bel F, Shadid M, Moison RM et al (1998) Effect of allopurinol on postasphyxial free radical formation, cerebral hemodynamics, and electrical brain activity. Pediatrics 101:185–193

Vannucci RC (1990) Experimental biology of cerebral hypoxia-ischemia: relation to perinatal brain damage. Pediatr Res 27:317–326

Volpe J (2001) Neurology of the newborn, 3rd edn. WB Saunders, Philadelphia

Wagner CL, Eicher DJ, Katikkaneni LD et al (1999) The use of hypothermia: a role in the treatment of neonatal asphyxia? Pediatr Neurol 21:429–443

Wagner BP, Nedelcu J, Martin E (2002) Delayed postischemic hypothermia improves long-term behavioral outcome after cerebral hypoxia-ischemia in neonatal rats. Pediatr Res 51:182–193

Waseem W, Ashraf QM, Zanelli SA et al (2001) Effect of graded hypoxia on cerebral cortical genomic DNA fragmentation in newborn piglet. Biol Neonate 79:187–193

Williams GD, Palmer C, Heitjan DF et al (1992) Allopurinol preserves cerebral energy metabolism during perinatal hypoxic-ischemia: a 31P NMR study in anaesthetized immature rats. Neurosci Lett 144:104–106

Wylie AH, Kerr JFR, Currie AR (1980) Cell Death, the significance of apoptosis. Int Rev Cytol 68:251–306

Yamakura T, Sakimura K, Shimoji K (1999) Direct inhibition of the N-methyl-D-aspartate receptor channel by high concentration of opioids. Anesthesiology 91:1053–1063

Zanelli SA (1999) NMDA receptor-mediated calcium influx in cerebral cortical synaptosomes of the hypoxic guinea pig fetus. Neurochem Res 24:434–446

Zanelli SA, Ashraf QM, Mishra OP (2002) Nitration is a mechanism of regulation of the NMDA receptor function during hypoxia. Neuroscience 112:869–877

Zanelli SA, Naylor M, Dobbins N et al (2008) Implementation of a "hypothermia for HIE" program: 2-year experience in a single NICU. J Perinatol 28:171–175

Zhang J, Haddad GG, Xia Y (2000) Delta-, but not mu- and kappa, opioid receptor activation protects neocortical neurons from glutamate- induced excitotoxic injury. Brain Res 885:143–153

Zhang J, Gibney GT, Zhao P (2002) Neuroprotective role of delta opioid receptors in cortical neurons. Am J Physiol 282:C1225–C1234

Clinical Aspects and Treatment of the Hypoxic-Ischemic Syndrome

126

Floris Groenendaal and Frank van Bel

Contents

Abstract

In the Western world, perinatal asphyxia is still a relatively common phenomenon in perinatal care. Since differences in causes and patterns of brain injury following perinatal asphyxia exist between full-term and preterm neonates, this chapter will focus on full-term neonates.

126.1 Salient Points

- Antenatal diagnosis of (severe) hypoxia with the STAN method opens the possibility for maternal (pharmacological) treatment of the compromised fetus.
- The development of more specific biochemical markers of neuronal damage is important for

F. Groenendaal (✉) · F. van Bel
Department of Neonatology, Wilhelmina Children's Hospital, University Medical Center Utrecht, Utrecht, The Netherlands
e-mail: f.groenendaal@umcutrecht.nl; F.vanBel@umcutrecht.nl

G. Buonocore et al. (eds.), *Neonatology*,
https://doi.org/10.1007/978-3-319-29489-6_273

the selection and allocation of neuroprotective strategies.

- Early advanced MRI techniques can be developed further as biomarkers of long-term neurodevelopmental outcome.
- Monitoring of the pattern of brain background activity and the presence of seizures using aEEG and cerebral oxygenation assessed with near-infrared spectroscopy (NIRS) can be used to assess efficacy of (neuroprotective) treatment.
- Add-on therapy during moderate hypothermia has the potential to improve outcome after (severe) perinatal asphyxia even further.
- Lidocaine is a very effective second-line anticonvulsant in neonates with hypoxia-ischemia-induced seizures.

126.2 Epidemiology

In the Western world, perinatal asphyxia is still a relatively common phenomenon in perinatal care. Since differences in causes and patterns of brain injury following perinatal asphyxia exist between full-term and preterm neonates, this chapter will focus on full-term neonates.

Generally, it has been assumed that in the Western world, 0.1–0.4% of all full-term neonates need resuscitation at birth because of perinatal asphyxia (Hull and Dodd 1992; Smith et al. 2000). Recent studies indicated that at least 0.5% of full-term neonates needed some degree of resuscitation at birth because of a 5-min Apgar score of 6 or less (Casey et al. 2001). Of all full-term neonates, 0.07% had a 5-min Apgar score of 3 or less. Mortality in these severely depressed neonates was 24%. Data from the Netherlands Perinatal Registry show that in 2013 at least 0.2% of all full-term neonates have a 5-min Apgar score of 3 or less.

Although the concept of perinatal asphyxia has been challenged by some, combined magnetic resonance imaging (MRI) and pathology studies showed acute hypoxic-ischemic changes in brain tissue in the vast majority of full-term neonates with perinatal asphyxia and encephalopathy (Cowan et al. 2003; Alderliesten et al. 2013).

Perinatal asphyxia may be caused by antenatal factors, such as severe maternal diseases or shock; perinatal factors such as a difficult delivery with compromised blood flow through the umbilical cord, placental abruption, or uterine rupture; or postnatal factors such as respiratory difficulties as in congenital diaphragmatic hernia or muscle diseases. The presence of intrapartum factors is essential for the presence of hypoxic-ischemic encephalopathy (Martinez-Biarge et al. 2013).

126.3 Pathology and Outcome

During perinatal asphyxia, two different processes contribute to brain injury: hypoxia (lack of oxygen) and ischemia (lack of blood flow due to bradycardia, thereby reducing flow of, e.g., glucose) contribute to cellular compromise. This is even further aggravated by reperfusion with production of a large amount of oxygen and nitrogen-free radicals and nonprotein-bound iron. Brain injury is the resultant of hypoxia-ischemia, reperfusion, and inflammation.

Different patterns of cerebral involvement after perinatal asphyxia have been described in post-mortem studies and have been confirmed in experimental animals and in vivo in the human neonate using MRI (Alderliesten et al. 2013; Myers 1975; de Vries and Groenendaal 2010):

1. (Near-) Total brain necrosis
2. Injury of the basal ganglia and thalamus
3. Watershed lesions

Total brain necrosis is the most serious form of brain injury. Most infants with this lesion will not survive, since the brain stem is involved. Pathology studies have described this pattern in detail. In the rare neonate who survives, multicystic encephalomalacia or ulegyria can be seen (Squier 2002). These children will show major and multiple handicaps, including cerebral visual impairment.

Injury of the basal ganglia and thalamus is seen in neonates with an acute and severe insult with no previous signs of fetal compromise. This pattern has been demonstrated in vivo in neonates using cranial ultrasound and using MRI, especially with diffusion-weighted MRI (Alderliesten et al. 2011) (Fig. 1). In surviving neonates, this pattern of brain injury leads to gliosis of the basal ganglia and thalamus. On postmortem examination, this pattern has been referred to as status marmoratus because of the marble-like appearance (Squier 2002). Children with this type of cerebral injury display the dyskinetic type of cerebral palsy. Epilepsy has been described, possibly due to injury of the hippocampus.

Watershed lesions were described in the late 1970s using technetium scans (Volpe et al. 1985). Reduced perfusion of cerebral border zones between anterior and middle cerebral arteries and middle and posterior cerebral arteries is the most important aspect of this type of lesion (Fig. 1b). A more chronic, intrauterine form of perinatal asphyxia has been suggested as the causative factor of this type of lesion.

In more severe cases, long-term effects are volume loss of the frontal and parieto-occipital parts of the cerebrum, but in milder cases, we have observed normal development without long-term effects up to 2 years of age (Harteman et al. 2013). In more severe cases, disturbances of mental development are the most important long-term effects.

In the present chapter, we will not discuss focal infarcts. Focal infarcts have been increasingly demonstrated in full-term as well as preterm neonates (van der Aa et al. 2014). However, since they occur often in neonates without signs of perinatal asphyxia, these types of brain lesions are beyond the scope of this chapter.

126.4 Clinical Picture of Hypoxic-Ischemic Syndrome

As can be extracted from the former section discussing the etiology of the hypoxic-ischemic syndrome, the basis of this syndrome is mostly (±70%) a disturbance in gas exchange between the fetus and mother in the direct antepartum and intrapartum period, at least when referring to the full-term infant. Although there is no ideal measure to assess, from the clinical point of view, the severity of perinatal hypoxia-ischemia during the initial clinical presentation of the infant immediately after birth, the most used instrument here is the Apgar score, introduced in 1953 by the anesthesiologist Virginia Apgar (1953). The Apgar score is usually recorded at 1 and 5 min after birth and

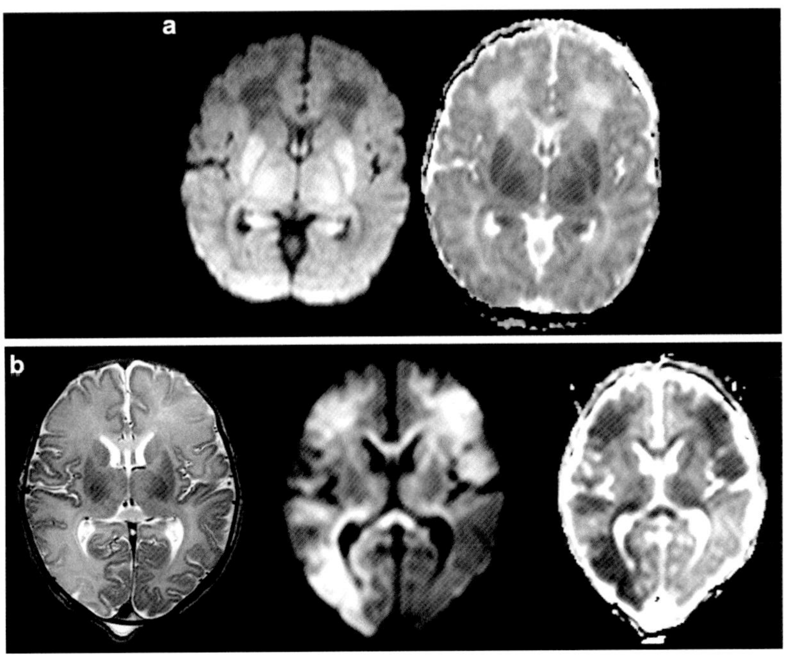

Fig. 1 MRI of two full-term neonates with perinatal asphyxia. (**a**) Abnormalities of the basal ganglia and thalamus on the 4th day of life in a full-term neonate with perinatal asphyxia: DWI (*left*) and ADC map (*right*). ADC values of the basal ganglia were 770×10^{-6} mm^2/s. The patient died 5 days after birth. (**b**) Abnormalities of gray and white matter in a full-term neonate with watershed infarcts. MRI on day 3 after birth. T2-weighted (*left*) and diffusion-weighted (*middle*) images and ADC map (*right*). This infant showed normal development at 1 year of age

includes an assessment of heart, pulmonary, and neurological functions by an assessment of color, heart rate, respiration, and tone (see also below). In 2014 the American College of Obstetricians and Gynecologists' Task Force on Neonatal Encephalopathy defined the following criteria for the presence of perinatal asphyxia (the American College of Obstetricians and Gynecologists' Task Force on Neonatal Encephalopathy 2014):

a metabolic parameter (arterial umbilical cord pH < 7.00 or base deficit greater thanor equal to 12 mmol/L, or both)
a persistence of an Apgar score of 0-to-3 at 5-minutes of extrauterine life
clinical and neurological sequelae in the immediate neonatal period
clinical and chemical evidence of multi-organ failure in the early neonatal period.

Lactate levels and lactate/pyruvate ratios in arterial umbilical cord blood or neonatal arterial blood in the first hour of life are also indicators of preexisting substantial perinatal asphyxia (Chou et al. 1998). Heavy meconium staining of amniotic fluid before delivery is associated with perinatal asphyxia and a poor clinical condition at birth and related to early death (Meis et al. 1978). We will discuss these issues in more detail under the section dealing with diagnosis and prognosis.

The persistence of clinical symptoms after antepartum and perinatal hypoxia-ischemia differ and are related to the severity and duration of the actual hypoxic-ischemic insult (Low et al. 1984). Symptoms can range from subtle neurological symptoms such as a transient drowsiness without involvement of other organ systems to overt involvement of important organ systems with renal, cardiac, and pulmonary abnormalities in association with a full-blown neurological syndrome (Perlman et al. 1989). We will discuss here those conditions where perinatal hypoxia leads to dysfunctions of the central nervous system and other important organ systems.

During the first 12–24 h of life after moderate-to-severe perinatal fetal hypoxia-ischemia, infants show abnormal neurological behavior which ranges from relatively mild to an overt abnormal neurological picture (Sarnat and Sarnat 1976). Mildly affected infants show increased restlessness and moderate hypertonia often accompanied by periodic breathing and feeding difficulties, which subside in the first days of life. Part of these symptoms may be related to an abnormal stimulation or transient malfunction of certain regions of the central nervous system. Amplitude-integrated EEG is extremely useful to diagnose background abnormalities and the presence of seizures (Toet et al. 2008).

Severely asphyxiated infants show a variety of neurological symptoms such as a lowered level of consciousness, hypotonia, gazing with abnormal papillary size, and eventually with subtle signs of seizure activity (sucking, odd movements of the mouth with smacking etcetera). The most severely affected infants are often profound lethargic or even stuporous and show already in an early phase overt convulsive activity as indicated by apneic spells and abnormal (clonic or tonic) movements. In full-term infants, these seizures are mostly multifocal with clonic characteristics, whereas less mature infants show often tonic seizures which are often generalized (Volpe 2008). Systemic symptoms may be lacking in the mildly affected infants, but mostly there is a decrease or even a lack of urinary production because of a mostly transient hypoxic damage to the kidneys. In the more severely affected babies, there is almost always respiratory insufficiency with prolonged apnea, probably related to malfunction of the central nervous system, sometimes giving rise for the need of artificial ventilation, often somewhat later in life, after 48–72 h of life. A hypoxia-induced myocardiopathy is a prominent feature and its severity mirrors the severity of the perinatal hypoxic-ischemic insult (Van Bel and Walther 1990). In most cases, however, there are no or only mild clinical signs, although relatively often inotropes are needed to prevent hypotension. In most infants recovery of myocardial contractility occurs in the first 24–48 h after birth (Van Bel and Walther 1990). In a minority of cases, massive cardiac failure occurs, but in such situations, there is invariably severe irreversible brain damage.

From 24 h onward, those infants with initially mild-to-moderate neurological symptoms can exhibit an improvement of their clinical and neurological condition with normalization of consciousness and neurological behavior and start to drink their feedings. In these infants also urine production starts or increases and no further support of blood pressure is necessary. This is accompanied by normalization of their plasma parameters of renal (creatinine, urea) and liver functions and of echocardiographically determined cardiac function. Infants who are neurologically normal at 1 week of life have mostly a normal developmental outcome (Sarnat and Sarnat 1976). Those infants with more severe neurological symptoms, often accompanied with renal and cardiac failure, will often deteriorate. The level of consciousness decreases, and in this particular time frame, respiratory insufficiency becomes manifest and intubation and assisted ventilation is necessary, probably on a neurological basis. Derailment of brain stem functions become manifest now with further loss of responsiveness, overt and increasing frequency of clinical and subclinical seizure activity, and abnormal movements of the eyes and dilated pupils (Volpe 2008). An explanation for this delayed deterioration is probably related to secondary energy failure of the brain which occurs typically between 24 and 72 h after birth or the hypoxic-ischemic insult (Hope et al. 1984; Lorek et al. 1994). In this particular time frame, the most severely affected children die and autopsy invariably shows cytotoxic brain swelling and major and extensive neuronal damage (Alderliesten et al. 2013). When these severely asphyxiated infants survive, their physical condition shows a sustained improvement, but they will continue to have abnormal neurological features with (slight) disturbances in consciousness, feeding difficulties because of decreased sucking, and swallow abnormalities. Dependent of the site of cerebral damage, the infants show overt hypotonia or hypertonia (in particular during involvement of the basal ganglia). Also here it is important to realize that the stage of development of the nervous system gives rise to a different clinical symptom complex after perinatal hypoxia-ischemia especially in relation to tone and the occurrence of hemiparesis.

It was already decades ago suggested that the neurological condition in the first few days of life was a more specific predictor of subsequent neurological outcome than signs of fetal distress or the Apgar score (Brown et al. 1974).

In 1976 Sarnat and Sarnat developed a scoring system which was a combination of neurological symptoms as described above and the accompanying electroencephalographic (EEG) features (Sarnat and Sarnat 1976). This score was in fact a grading of the severity of the encephalopathy caused by the perinatal hypoxia-ischemia. It contains three stages, mild hypoxic-ischemic encephalopathy (HIE), stage 1, moderate HIE: stage 2, and severe HIE: stage 3 (Table 1). In 1983 Fenichel modified this score to a score solely on clinical symptoms, which distinguishes a mild, moderate, and severe encephalopathy which could be linked to later neurodevelopmental outcome (Table 1) (Fenichel 1983; Levene et al. 1986).

The Thompson score (Thompson et al. 1997) has been developed more recently and has the advantage of quantifying the severity of encephalopathy in more detail. These scores correlate directly with the incidence of neurological sequelae. Follow-up studies suggested that infants with mild hypoxic-ischemic encephalopathy (Sarnat HIE stage 1) did not have subsequent deficits, whereas in infants with moderate encephalopathy, 5% died (Sarnat HIE stage 3), 24% had neurological sequelae, and 71% were apparently normal. All infants with severe encephalopathy had an adverse outcome (Volpe 2008). In particular the Sarnat score is widely used to assess the severity of hypoxia-ischemia-induced encephalopathy and subsequent outcome and has been used to select infants for inclusion in trials of neuroprotection, such as hypothermia and other means of neuroprotection (Shankaran et al. 2005; Kaandorp et al. 2012).

126.5 Treatment of Hypoxic-Ischemic Syndrome

126.5.1 Reduction or Prevention of Fetal Hypoxia

Prevention may be the most important issue when discussing treatment modalities with respect to perinatal hypoxic-ischemic syndrome. Since the primary insult is in a vast majority of cases of

Table 1 Hypoxic-ischemic encephalopathy (HIE) according to Sarnat and Sarnat (1976) (a) and Fenichel (1983) (b)

(a) Symptoms	Stage 1	Stage 2	Stage 3
Consciousness	Hyperalert	Lethargic or obtunded	Stuporous
Neuromuscular control	Normal	Mild hypotonia	Flaccid
Suck/Moro reflex	Normal	Weak	Absent
OV/TN reflex	Normal	Strong	Absent
Autonomic function	In general sympathetic	In general parasympathetic	Both depressed
Seizures	None	(Multi)focal	Decerebrated
EEG findings	Normal	Low voltage (δ/0 waves)	Isoelectric
Duration	<24 h	2–14 days	Hours to weeks
(b) Symptoms	**Mild**	**Moderate**	**Severe**
Consciousness	Irritable/hyperalert	Lethargic	Comatose
Tone	Mildly abnormal	Moderately abnormal	Severely abnormal
Suck reflex	Abnormal	Poor	Absent
Primitive reflexes	Exaggerated	Depressed	Absent
Seizures	Absent	Present	Present
Brain stem reflexes	Normal	Normal	Impaired
Respiration	Tachypneic	Occasional apnea	Severe apnea

OV oculo-vestibular, *TN* tonic neck

intrauterine hypoxia, early identification may alter long-term consequences of hypoxic-ischemic syndrome. Unfortunately, extensive ante- and intrapartum monitoring of heart rate of the high-risk fetus has led to increased obstetrical interventions without improving neonatal outcome (Grant et al. 1989), although the combination with fetal blood gas assessment and the introduction of the fetal electrocardiography technique may contribute to a reduction of fetal hypoxia-related long-term adverse outcome (Low et al. 2001; Westerhuis et al. 2012). Adequate interventions such as emergency cesarean section may prevent progression from mild fetal hypoxia to a moderate or severe perinatal hypoxic-ischemic syndrome. Although beyond the scope of this chapter, antenatal drug treatment via the mother with free radical scavengers or other neuroprotective agents may be an option to reduce or prevent hypoxic brain damage of the fetus (Kaandorp et al. 2012; Torrance et al. 2009).

126.5.2 General Supportive Care

The baby born after substantial perinatal hypoxia-ischemia shows, in addition to nervous system damage, mostly dysfunction of several other important organ systems. In order of occurrence and importance, one should mention here: pulmonary dysfunction with insufficient ventilation and oxygenation and cardiac dysfunction with suboptimal or overtly low blood pressure (Van Bel and Walther 1990; Shankaran et al. 1991). Later on renal and liver function disturbances and clotting abnormalities and hyperviscosity can occur which need treatment. Details are presented in Table 2.

126.5.2.1 Ventilation and Oxygenation

Especially non-adequate ventilation and persistence of hypoxia can further aggravate nervous system damage and should be treated promptly. Although oxygen supplementation is an issue nowadays and hyperoxia during the resuscitation phase has been reported to contribute to additional reperfusion injury to neuronal cells, adequate oxygenation of the compromised newborn is crucial.

The current guideline is to start resuscitation with room air, since resuscitation with 100% oxygen is not desirable and potentially damaging (Saugstad 2003; Vento and Saugstad 2010; Sola et al. 2007). As soon as possible, the high-risk infant should be connected to a pulse oximeter to monitor systemic arterial saturation in order to

Table 2 General supportive care

During resuscitation phase
Establish heart rate monitoring
Establish adequate ventilation (if needed: intubation and artificial ventilation)
Connect infant with pulse oximeter for appropriate oxygenation
Avoid hyperoxygenation (to avoid free radical production and ROP [preterm baby])
Avoid hyper-/hypocapnia (preterm baby)
Correct metabolic acidosis (after normalization of $PaCO_2$)
Insert intravenous line for fluid and glucose administration
Subacute phase
Cardiac support, if necessary, with positive inotropes (hypotension) and/or fluid (blood loss)
Aim for normoglycemic plasma levels
After stabilization
Ensure appropriate caloric intake by intravenous route
First 48 h no enteral feeding
Monitor urine production
Monitor coagulation and thrombocytes
Treat convulsive activity (see also Table 3)

avoid hyperoxia or hypoxia during resuscitation (Hay et al. 1991). It is further important to realize that hypoxia and hypercapnia negatively influence the infant's capability to autoregulate the cerebral vascular bed with, as a consequence, blood pressure passive cerebral perfusion. Therefore, assisted ventilation with bag and mask after endotracheal intubation and artificial ventilation may be an important option to stabilize the newborn and to correct in a quick and appropriate way the blood gases and metabolic demands. In particular the effects of hypocapnia are pronounced and have important metabolic and vascular effects (Klinger et al. 2005).

126.5.2.2 Cardiac Dysfunction

Adequate perfusion of the brain is mandatory to prevent additional cerebral damage. Perinatal hypoxia-ischemia has been known to cause hypoxia-induced myocardiopathy which can lead to transient hypotension and hypoperfusion of important organs such as the brain (Van Bel and Walther 1990). Especially during severe perinatal hypoxia-ischemia, inotropes may be needed to prevent hypotension, although myocardiopathy subsides mostly within the first 24–48 h of life. Dobutamine is preferred above dopamine because of its positive inotropic effect on the myocardium without the peripheral effects such as peripheral vasoconstriction which may further compromise cardiac function. This is also the reason to avoid volume expanders, although in a number of conditions circulating blood volume can be too low, such as in cases with fetal and neonatal blood loss during the perinatal period.

126.5.2.3 Additional Measures

Normoglycemic levels should be maintained, and adequate protein and caloric intake should be provided as soon as possible. Furthermore, it is important to realize that early enteral feeding may carry the risk of necrotizing enterocolitis, because the gut may be already affected by hypoxic-ischemic damage (Caplan et al. 1994). In general up to 48 h of life, only minimal enteral feeding is provided, and parenteral feeding is given. Birth asphyxia-related disseminated intravascular coagulation reduces levels of coagulation factors and thrombocytes, which can result in prolonged bleeding times (Castle et al. 1986). Renal dysfunction accompanied by acute necrosis of the tubules is often a temporary problem that resolves over the first week of life and needs rarely more specific therapy such as hemodilution (Luciano et al. 1998). Table 2 summarizes the general care measures to be undertaken in the perinatally hypoxic-ischemic infant. Therapeutic hypothermia did not affect any of these complications of asphyxia, although thrombocytopenia with counts below 150 * 10^9/L was reported in some studies.

126.5.3 Treatment of Seizures

Since seizure activity has been recognized to be related to add substantially to additional neuronal damage (Van Rooij et al. 2010), early recognition of seizure activity is extremely important. It therefore is recommended to connect the neonate at risk for birth asphyxia-related brain damage to a one- or two-channel continuous amplitude-integrated electroencephalography (aEEG)

Table 3 Dosing scheme of anticonvulsive drugs used for full-term neonates

Full-term infant		
First choice: phenobarbital, 20 mg/kg iv; if necessary 2nd dose of 10–20 mg/kg iv (van den Broek et al. 2012)		
Second choice: lidocaine (van den Broek et al. 2013)		
	≥2.0–2.5 kg	≥2.5 kg
Normothermia		
Loading dose	2 mg/kg in 10 min	2 mg/kg in 10 min
Phase 1 (4 h)	6 mg/kg/h	7 mg/kg/h
Phase 2 (12 h)	3 mg/kg/h	3.5 mg/kg/h
Phase 3 (12 h)	1.5 mg/kg/h	1.75 mg/kg/h
Therapeutic hypothermia		
Loading dose	2 mg/kg in 10 min	2 mg/kg in 10 min
Phase 1 (3.5 h)	6 mg/kg/h	7 mg/kg/h
Phase 2 (12 h)	3 mg/kg/h	3.5 mg/kg/h
Phase 3 (12 h)	1.5 mg/kg/h	1.75 mg/kg/h
Third choice: midazolam (van den Broek et al. 2015)		
Loading dose	0.05 mg/kg	
Maintenance	0.1–0.15 mg/kg/h[a]	
Alternative for midazolam Levetiracetam (Ramantani et al. 2011)	10 mg/kg iv twice daily, increasing over 3 days to 20 mg/kg twice daily	
Preterm infant		
First choice: phenobarbital, 20 mg/kg iv; if necessary 2nd dose of 10–20 mg/kg iv (van den Broek et al. 2012)		
Second choice: lidocaine (van den Broek et al. 2011)		
	≥0.8–1.5 kg	≥1.5–2.5 kg
Loading dose	2 mg/kg in 10 min	2 mg/kg in 10 min
Phase 1 (4 h)	5 mg/kg/h	6 mg/kg/h
Phase 2 (6 h)	2.5 mg/kg/h	3 mg/kg/h
Phase 3 (12 h)	1.25 mg/kg/h	1.5 mg/kg/h
Third choice: clonazepam 0.1 mg/kg/day (Andre et al. 1986)		

[a]Risk of hypotension when using higher doses

monitor, which facilitates detection of subclinical seizures which frequently occur during the first days after perinatal hypoxia-ischemia (Toet et al. 1999, 2008). Furthermore, seizures can cause sudden increase of blood pressure and changes in blood glucose, further aggravating asphyxia-related brain damage (Cataltepe et al. 1995).

Commonly, phenobarbital is used as a first-line anticonvulsive with a total dose not exceeding 30 mg/kg iv (van den Broek et al. 2012). If necessary, phenobarbital can be given as maintenance, starting a few days after the loading dose. When seizure activity continues or reappears, we use a tapering continuous iv infusion of lidocaine (van den Broek et al. 2011, 2013). Although the effect of lidocaine can be sustained (after 1–1.5 h), it has a very good antiepileptic activity. During lidocaine treatment, the ECG should be monitored because lidocaine can cause cardiac arrhythmia although in our hands and dosing regimen it is extremely rare. The dosing should be adjusted during therapeutic hypothermia, since it is known that hypothermia influences pharmacokinetics (van den Broek et al. 2013). If a third antiepileptic drug is necessary, we use midazolam starting with a loading dose followed by a maintenance dose as a continuous infusion (up to 0.5 mg/kg iv) (van den Broek et al. 2015). Table 3 provides a detailed dosing scheme of mostly used anticonvulsive drugs in our institution. Although newer anticonvulsive drugs such as topiramate or levetiracetam may be useful, little is known about the pharmacokinetics after perinatal asphyxia

(Filippi et al. 2012; Pressler and Mangum 2013; Ramantani et al. 2011).

In all infants with persisting seizures, administration of pyridoxine (loading dose 50 mg/kg, maintenance 15–30 mg/kg/day with a maximum of 200 mg/day) should be considered.

126.5.4 Specific Treatment of Perinatal Hypoxic-Ischemic Syndrome

During perinatal hypoxia and concomitant ischemia and especially during reoxygenation and reperfusion at birth, potentially destructive molecular pathways are activated in the fetal and neonatal brain that ultimately leads to brain damage (Fellman and Raivio 1997). Animal and clinical studies demonstrated excessive influx of calcium into the neuronal cells through ion-regulated and N-methyl-D-aspartic acid (NMDA)-receptor-regulated channels. This intracellular calcium gives rise to enzyme activation and production of reactive oxygen and nitrogen species which damages neuronal cell membranes and DNA and initiates apoptosis (Hagberg et al. 2015). Experimental and human studies have shown that the energy metabolism of the perinatal hypoxic-ischemic brain recovers upon reperfusion/reoxygenation, but that after 6–12 h the energy metabolism of the brain becomes increasingly disturbed ("secondary energy failure") and irreversible brain damage occurs (Hope et al. 1984; Lorek et al. 1994; Vannucci et al. 2004). It is likely that full development of destructive molecular pathways as mentioned above occurs in this time frame and that in the first 6 h after recovery of brain perfusion and oxygenation (also called the therapeutic window), therapies aimed to prevent activation of these destructive molecular pathways may have a neuroprotective effect. This assumption was indeed supported by evidence from experimental studies in several newborn animal species (Robertson et al. 2012). A more detailed review is beyond the aim of this chapter, but we will briefly summarize those therapies already established in daily practice, such as moderate hypothermia, and those which may be suitable for clinical use in the near future. Moderate hypothermia for 72 h and starting within 6 h after birth, either selective head cooling (Gluckman et al. 2005) or total body cooling (33–34 °C) (Shankaran et al. 2005; Azzopardi et al. 2009), has been proven to be neuroprotective after moderate-to-severe perinatal hypoxia-ischemia. A meta-analysis of cooling studies showed that especially the infants eventually developing moderate birth-related encephalopathy benefit from this approach (Jacobs et al. 2013). Although hypothermia seems to be a rather safe therapy, adverse effects may occur. In particular sinus bradycardia, thrombocytopenia, and hypokalemia are reported (Jacobs et al. 2013). Drug metabolism may be altered (Roka et al. 2008; van den Broek et al. 2010). We suggest therefore to confine hypothermia for treatment of neonatal posthypoxic-ischemic encephalopathy to neonatal intensive care units (Groenendaal and Brouwer 2009).

It is conceivable that combining moderate hypothermia with a pharmacological means of treatment may further improve outcome after perinatal hypoxia-ischemia (Robertson et al. 2012).

126.6 Diagnosis of the Severity of Perinatal Asphyxia and Prediction of Long-Term Outcome

Animal experiments have demonstrated that perinatal asphyxia can lead to brain injury and cerebral palsy comparable to patterns seen in the human neonate (Ranck and Windle 1959; Myers 1977). During the last decade, many studies have focused on early detection of brain injury in neonates following perinatal asphyxia. Meanwhile, research has focused on neuroprotective strategies aiming at a reduction of permanent brain injury. In this section both assessment of the severity of the hypoxic-ischemic event and prediction of the long-term outcome will be discussed.

126.6.1 Prenatal Assessment of Fetal Hypoxia

Abnormal fetal heart rate patterns (Arduini et al. 1989; Schifrin 1994), changes in umbilical and cerebral blood flow observed using antenatal

Table 4 Indications of fetal hypoxia

Indications of fetal hypoxia	References
Fetal heart rate patterns	(Arduini et al. 1989; Schifrin 1994)
Fetal behavior	(Herrmann et al. 1989; Maeda et al. 1991)
Scalp blood gases	(Boenisch and Saling 1976)
Meconium production	(Fujikura and Klionsky 1975)
Fetal ECG changes	(Westerhuis et al. 2012; Amer-Wahlin et al. 2001)

Doppler examinations (Arduini et al. 1989; Arabin et al. 1995), altered fetal behavior (Herrmann et al. 1989; Maeda et al. 1991), abnormal scalp blood gas values (Boenisch and Saling 1976), or the intrauterine passage of meconium (Fujikura and Klionsky 1975) may indicate fetal hypoxia. However, they do not predict the development of neonatal encephalopathy and are poor predictors of the development of cerebral palsy (Nelson et al. 1996). Recently, changes in the fetal electrocardiogram (ECG) have been reported to correlate well with fetal hypoxia. This so-called STAN method needs further study, but appears a promising tool for better evaluation of the fetus (Table 4) (Westerhuis et al. 2012; Amer-Wahlin et al. 2001).

126.6.2 Postnatal Assessment of the Neonate

126.6.2.1 Apgar Score

Virginia Apgar has published a scoring system for clinical assessment of the neonate (Apgar 1953). This scoring system has been designed to help in the decision whether or not to resuscitate the neonate, but has been wrongfully used to make the diagnosis of perinatal asphyxia (American Academy of Pediatrics et al. 2006).

Since the Apgar score can be low due to transplacentally obtained drugs that depress the central nervous system (like anesthesia), trauma during delivery or reflex inhibition of breathing due to frequent suctioning, clinicians debated whether a low Apgar score always reflects perinatal asphyxia and predicts neonatal encephalopathy and cerebral palsy. Nevertheless, a 10 min Apgar score of 5 or less had a sensitivity of 43% and a specificity of 95% toward an adverse outcome (Levene et al. 1986). A good Apgar score does not guarantee the absence of cerebral palsy (CP) in later life, since neonates with antenatally acquired brain lesions may have normal Apgar scores (de Vries et al. 1998). Apgar scores of 0–3 at 1 min were found in 31% of full-term neonates with encephalopathy compared to 1% of control infants (Adamson et al. 1995). In neonates with seizures, Apgar scores were significantly lower at 1–20 min after birth compared to control neonates (Holden et al. 1982).

In preterm infants, the Apgar score may be influenced by prematurity (Catlin et al. 1986). Respiratory efforts, muscle tone, and reflex activity were significantly lower at declining gestational ages. The Apgar score alone is not enough to ascertain perinatal asphyxia and predict neonatal encephalopathy.

126.6.2.2 Blood Gas Values

In the years following the use of the Apgar score, insight was obtained in the values of pH, oxygen, and carbon dioxide in fetal scalp blood (Boenisch and Saling 1976) and umbilical cord blood (Daniel et al. 1966). It was shown that severely depressed neonates had lower pH values, larger base deficits, and elevated levels of lactate compared to vigorous and moderately depressed neonates, reflecting anaerobic glycolysis (Daniel et al. 1966). Sykes et al. demonstrated that Apgar scores do not reflect the degree of acidosis at delivery (Sykes et al. 1982), as only 19% of the neonates with a 5 min Apgar score <7 had a pH ≤ 7.10 and a base deficit ≥ 13 mmol/L and 86% of the neonates with a pH ≤ 7.10 and a base deficit ≥ 13 mmol/L had a 5 min Apgar score ≥ 7. Similar findings were reported thereafter (Ruth and Raivio 1988). A pH value below 7.0 seems to have a better predictive value toward a poor outcome than higher cutoff values (Goodwin et al. 1992; Winkler et al. 1991; van den Berg et al. 1996). In the study by Goodwin et al., 31% of the term neonates with a pH of the umbilical artery below 7.0 developed neonatal encephalopathy. Neonates with more severe forms of acidosis

Table 5 Postnatal evidence of asphyxia

Mode of assessment	References
Apgar score	(Apgar 1953; American Academy of Pediatrics et al. 2006)
(Cord) Blood gas values	(Boenisch and Saling 1976; Daniel et al. 1966; Ruth and Raivio 1988; Goodwin et al. 1992; Winkler et al. 1991; van den Berg et al. 1996; Lavrijsen et al. 2005; Low et al. 1985; King et al. 1998)
Lactate, hypoxanthine	(Chou et al. 1998; Ruth and Raivio 1988; Mathew et al. 1980; Huang et al. 1999; Pourcyrous et al. 1999; Buonocore et al. 1998)
Brain-specific proteins	(Niklinski et al. 1987; Thornberg et al. 1995; Nagdyman et al. 2003)
Cytokines	(Gazzolo et al. 2004; Savman et al. 1998; Oygur et al. 1998; Foster-Barber et al. 2001; Xanthou et al. 2002; Chiesa et al. 2003)
Clinical scoring systems	(Sarnat and Sarnat 1976; Thompson et al. 1997; Wayenberg et al. 1994)
Neurophysiology	
Evoked potentials	(Eken et al. 1995; Taylor et al. 1992; Mercuri et al. 1994; Muttitt et al. 1991; de Vries 1993; Gibson et al. 1992)
aEEG	(Toet et al. 2002; Connell et al. 1989; Bjerre et al. 1983; Archbald et al. 1984; Hellstrom-Westas et al. 1995)
Neuroimaging	
CBF	(Archer et al. 1986; Van Bel et al. 1987)
NIRS	(Wyatt 1993; Toet et al. 2006; Lemmers et al. 2013)
Ultrasound	(Eken et al. 1994)
MRI	(Cowan et al. 2003; de Vries and Groenendaal 2010; Baenziger et al. 1993; Barkovich et al. 1995; Rutherford et al. 1996, 1998, 2004; L'Abee et al. 2005; Sie et al. 2000; Okereafor et al. 2008)
MRS	(Roth et al. 1992; Groenendaal et al. 1994; Robertson et al. 2002)

had a much higher chance of seizures and more severe forms of neonatal encephalopathy (Goodwin et al. 1992). Recently, this was confirmed in our institute. In addition, the good outcome in the encephalopathic neonates suggests that an adverse long-term outcome could be prevented with adequate neonatal care (Lavrijsen et al. 2005) (Table 5).

Others have used a low buffer base in the umbilical artery as a sign of fetal hypoxia. Of the 25 neonates with a buffer base <30 mmol/L, 14 (56%) developed neonatal encephalopathy, and only six (2%) severe neonatal encephalopathy (Low et al. 1985). Nevertheless, unexpectedly low pH values in vigorous neonates do not seem to result in neonatal encephalopathy (King et al. 1998). Elevated levels of (nor)adrenalin may play a role in these hypoxic but vigorous neonates (Nylund et al. 1987).

Belai studied umbilical arteriovenous PCO_2 differences in neonates with an umbilical artery pH <7.00 in relation to neonatal encephalopathy (Belai et al. 1998). Cutoff value of the AV-PCO_2 difference was 25 mmHg or more (sensitivity 89%, specificity 56%).

Scoring systems combining Apgar scores, or the need for resuscitation, blood gas values, and fetal monitoring have claimed to be of a better predictive value toward the development of severe clinical complications, including neonatal encephalopathy (Portman et al. 1990; Perlman and Risser 1996; Ekert et al. 1997; Carter et al. 1998; Bonifacio et al. 2015). These systems, however, have not yet been used widely.

In a group of term and preterm neonates with a pH <7.0, a high arterial base deficit (>16 mmol/L) and a 5-min Apgar score <7 predicted neonatal morbidity, including cerebral complications (Sehdev et al. 1997).

Blood gas values cannot be used for prediction of long-term outcome. This may be caused in part by the reflection of total body metabolism with blood gases, whereas specific CNS measurements would render more specific information.

126.6.2.3 Other Biochemical Markers of Perinatal Asphyxia

Umbilical cord blood lactate levels and lactate/pyruvate ratios were found to be elevated in all full-term neonates with neonatal encephalopathy (Chou et al. 1998), and these may be more accurate than blood gases, although this has been questioned in an earlier study (Ruth and Raivio 1988). Cerebrospinal fluid (CSF) lactate was elevated in a small sample of asphyxiated infants within 8 h after birth (Mathew et al. 1980). Urine lactate/creatine ratios identified newborn infants at risk for hypoxic-ischemic encephalopathy (Huang et al. 1999). Decreased cAMP levels were described in neonates with severe neonatal encephalopathy and a poor outcome (Pourcyrous et al. 1999). Hypoxanthine has also been used as a biochemical marker of birth asphyxia (Saugstad 1976; Ruth et al. 1988). Hypoxanthine correlated well with plasma malondialdehyde levels of cord blood, indicating free radical-induced oxidative stress (Buonocore et al. 1998). Also nonprotein-bound iron and nucleated red blood cells count at birth reflect fetal hypoxia (Table 5) (Buonocore et al. 1999. 2003).

All the aforementioned biochemical methods were used to determine the severity of hypoxia, but were not specific in predicting neonatal encephalopathy.

It was hoped that more specific markers of brain injury could be used for early prediction. CK-BB, the brain fraction of creatine kinase, was elevated in cord blood of term neonates with asphyxia (Niklinski et al. 1987). However, the time course of CK-BB rise in peripheral blood following neonatal encephalopathy is unknown. Neuron-specific enolase (NSE) in serum was significantly increased in neonates with neonatal encephalopathy, but levels of brain-specific proteins (S-100B, NSE, and CK-BB) on the first day of life were of limited value in predicting a poor outcome (Thornberg et al. 1995; Nagdyman et al. 2003). Brain-specific proteins (neurofilament protein, glial fibrillary acidic protein, S 100B, NSE) in the CSF of asphyxiated neonates correlated with outcome at 1 year (Gazzolo et al. 2004; Blennow et al. 2001).

Production of cytokines has been demonstrated in plasma and CSF and correlated with severity of encephalopathy and long-term outcome (Savman et al. 1998; Oygur et al. 1998; Foster-Barber et al. 2001; Xanthou et al. 2002; Chiesa et al. 2003; Martin-Ancel et al. 1997).

126.6.2.4 Clinical Scoring Systems

As described above the Sarnat score consists of a combined clinical and electrophysiological (EEG) score (Sarnat and Sarnat 1976). The Sarnat score has been used to predict long-term outcome. Whereas neonates with a score of I mostly showed a normal development and neonates with grade III were almost uniformly abnormal (Levene et al. 1985, 1986; Holden et al. 1982; Mellits et al. 1982), prediction of development in neonates with grade II neonatal encephalopathy was very difficult, as 25% had an abnormal outcome. As the Sarnat score is performed at 24 h, its value in selection of neonates for intervention is very limited.

Wayenberg et al. developed an early neurological score which was assigned at 30 min of life based on consciousness, respiratory pattern, Moro, and grasp reflexes (Wayenberg et al. 1994). The predictive value toward the development of neonatal encephalopathy was not better than measurement of an arterial base deficit.

Thompson et al. designed a clinical scoring system to quantify encephalopathy during the first few hours after birth (Thompson et al. 1997). Larger studies are needed to verify the usefulness of this system.

126.6.2.5 Neuroimaging

Cerebral Blood Flow and Oxygen Consumption

Studies in term neonates with severe neonatal encephalopathy using Doppler ultrasound or near-infrared spectroscopy (NIRS) demonstrated changes in cerebral blood flow (CBF) and blood volume predicting an adverse outcome (Archer et al. 1986; Van Bel et al. 1987; Wyatt 1993; Toet et al. 2006; Lemmers et al. 2013). Further studies are needed to assess the clinical value of NIRS and CBF measurements.

Cranial Ultrasound Imaging

Cranial ultrasound abnormalities, such as lesions in the thalami and basal ganglia, are usually first seen after the first day of life (Eken et al. 1994). The presence of the abnormalities mentioned above on the first day of life would therefore strongly suggest an antenatal onset of the insult.

Cranial Magnetic Resonance Imaging

Cranial magnetic resonance imaging (MRI) is increasingly being used during the immediate neonatal period (de Vries and Groenendaal 2010; Baenziger et al. 1993; Barkovich et al. 1995; Rutherford et al. 1996). Using MRI we have demonstrated that acute insults were common in neonates with neonatal encephalopathy (Cowan et al. 2003). MRI on the first day of life may still be normal (Rutherford et al. 1996). Diffusion-weighted MRI has been extremely useful to detect early changes in hypoxic-ischemic brain tissue. By creating maps of the apparent diffusion coefficient (ADC) of water, values of individual areas can be calculated (Alderliesten et al. 2011). These ADC changes reflect cytotoxic edema and are dependent on the time after the insult, since cytotoxic edema will subside and be replaced by vasogenic edema which has a different ADC value (Rutherford et al. 2004). This is called pseudo-normalization of the ADC (Rutherford et al. 2004; Bednarek et al. 2012).

When MRI is performed before the second day of life, images may still be normal since full secondary energy failure has not yet developed (L'Abee et al. 2005). We advise to perform MRI between days 4 and 7 in asphyxiated full-term neonates (Alderliesten et al. 2011). MRI is a good predictor of long-term motor development (de Vries and Groenendaal 2010).

Different patterns of cerebral involvement after perinatal asphyxia have been described using MRI (de Vries and Groenendaal 2010; Sie et al. 2000; Okereafor et al. 2008). In brief, abnormalities of the basal ganglia and thalamus are seen after an acute hypoxic-ischemic event such as placental abruption or uterine rupture. In the most severe cases, abnormalities of the white matter can be seen. In more chronic hypoxic-ischemic events, abnormalities of the white matter are encountered, sometimes in a watershed-like distribution (Harteman et al. 2013). Neonates with these abnormalities do not show any changes in the basal ganglia or thalamus.

These different patterns are similar to those in animal experiments in the 1970s and in human postmortem studies (Alderliesten et al. 2013; Myers 1977).

Cranial Magnetic Resonance Spectroscopy

Cerebral metabolism will change during and following asphyxia. High-energy phosphates will decrease, and lactate will be increased. Changes in energy metabolism can be visualized by $^{31-}$phosphorus magnetic resonance spectroscopy (MRS). Decreased phosphocreatine and ATP levels in the first week of life correlated with an abnormal outcome (Hope et al. 1984; Lorek et al. 1994). In addition, the presence of a secondary energy failure could be identified in experiments and human neonates (Lorek et al. 1994). Elevated cellular pH levels could be demonstrated in neonates with perinatal asphyxia and a poor long-term outcome (Robertson et al. 2002).

With ^{1}H-MRS, increased lactate levels could be seen in the brain tissue of asphyxiated neonates with a poor neurodevelopmental outcome. In addition, decreased levels of N-acetylaspartate, a neuronal marker, could be identified (Fig. 2) (Groenendaal et al. 1994). These abnormalities may persist for a prolonged period.

Neurophysiology

The electroencephalogram (EEG) has been used during the last few decades in asphyxiated neonates and is recognized to be of predictive value with regard to neurodevelopmental outcome (Holmes et al. 1982; Watanabe et al. 1980; Monod et al. 1972; Grigg-Damberger et al. 1989). These studies showed that the electrical background activity was more predictive than the presence or absence of seizure activity.

The use of conventional multichannel recordings has practical limitations. Recordings usually last 30–45 min, making it difficult to follow changes over a longer period of time and recognition of prolonged subclinical seizures (Connell

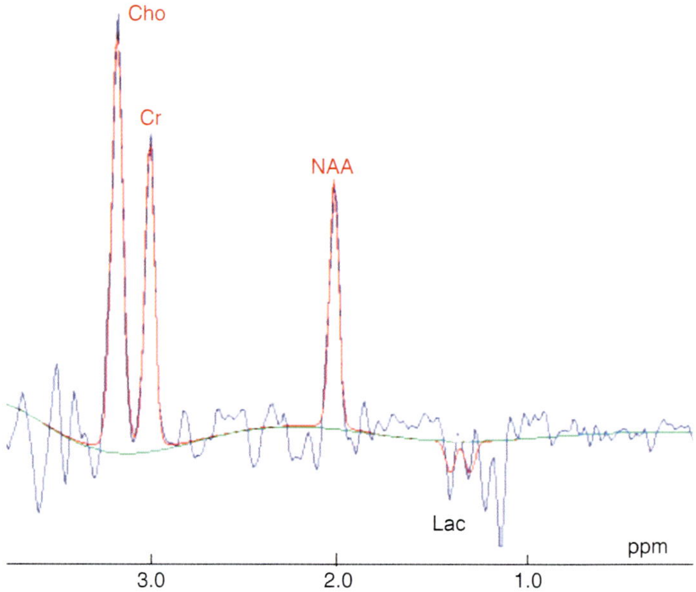

Fig. 2 Proton magnetic resonance spectroscopy of the basal ganglia of patient A in Fig. 1, demonstrating a low *N*-acetyl-aspartate/choline ratio and elevated lactate (inverted doublet at 1.33 ppm). At 1.1 ppm the inverted doublet of propan-1,2-diol (component of phenobarbital solution) is visible (not fitted)

et al. 1989). Smaller systems have been used in neonatal intensive care units. The cerebral function monitor (CFM) was first introduced in the neonatal intensive care unit by Bjerre. Since then, many studies have been performed in newborn infants using this technique (Bjerre et al. 1983). It records one or two EEG channels from biparietal electrodes. The filtered signal is rectified, smoothed, and amplitude integrated before it is written out on a semilogarithmic scale at slow speed (6 cm/h). The CFM, usually referred to as the amplitude-integrated EEG (aEEG) is easy to apply and has a high concordance with the standard EEG (Toet et al. 2002). Continuous recordings can be made, allowing us to assess the background pattern and the presence or absence of sleep-wake cycling. Seizure activity can be recognized as a sawtooth pattern. In the newer types of the devices, the raw EEG is stored on hard disk and available for evaluation. Several groups have now used the aEEG in infants with neonatal encephalopathy (Toet et al. 1999; al Naqeeb et al. 1999). Recovery of the aEEG background pattern within 24 h after birth resulted in a good outcome in 61%, whereas all infants with a suppressed background pattern after 24 h showed a poor outcome (Van Rooij et al. 2005).

Several studies have shown that aEEG and EEG performed before 6 h of age can be used to reliably select infants at risk of subsequent neurological handicap. Hellström-Westas et al. (1995) were the first to report infants, in whom aEEG registration was started before 6 h of age. A continuous aEEG background pattern was almost a guarantee of a normal outcome. A flat or CLV pattern predicted death or a severe handicap. Very similar data were obtained by Eken et al. (1995). Techniques such as aEEG are extremely useful to select neonates who may benefit from an intervention after perinatal asphyxia (Fig. 3) (Azzopardi et al. 2009).

Evoked potentials (EPs) are averaged clinical responses, occurring in the EEG in response to repetitive stimuli (auditory, visual, somatosensory) and can examine the functional integrity of the sensory pathways within the nervous system in a non-invasive way (Eken et al. 1995; Taylor et al. 1992; Mercuri et al. 1994; Muttitt et al. 1991). The EEG is of higher amplitude than the EP, but is random to the applied stimulus. The EP is of small amplitude, but constant relative to the applied stimulus and will gradually emerge from the EEG, when an adequate number of stimuli are averaged.

Both visual potential (VEP) and somatosensory potential (SEP) have a very strong predictive value with regard to neurodevelopmental outcome, when

Fig. 3 Different aEEG patterns in asphyxiated full-term neonates written on a semilogarithmic scale (Courtesy Dr. Mona C. Toet). *Upper panel*: continuous normal voltage. *Lower panel*: repetitive seizures on a very suppressed background pattern

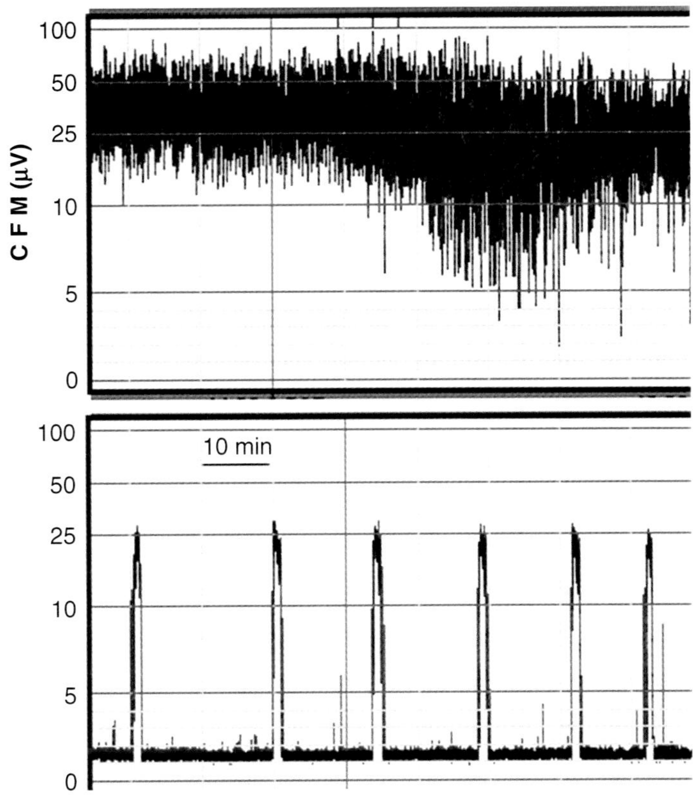

performed during the first week of life (Eken et al. 1995; van Laerhoven et al. 2013). SEPs are more likely to be abnormal on the initial test, but normalization within the first 3–4 days of life is still compatible with a normal neurological outcome (de Vries 1993; Gibson et al. 1992). Abnormal VEPs during the first week of life were always predictive of death or cerebral palsy according to Taylor, but this was not supported by our own data.

During the last decade, aEEG has replaced VEP and SEP as a bedside tool to assess the severity of neonatal encephalopathy after perinatal asphyxia.

126.7 Summary

At present, acidosis of cord blood and clinical observations such as the Sarnat or Thompson scores in combination with continuous aEEG monitoring are the best ways to detect neonatal encephalopathy after perinatal asphyxia. Well-documented perinatal asphyxia, including need for resuscitation, and neonatal encephalopathy are good predictors of an adverse outcome and could be used to select neonates for neuroprotective strategies. Patterns of brain injury can be visualized with MRI, especially diffusion-weighted MRI and ADC maps, preferably performed between days 4 and 7.

Abnormal NIRS and aEEG parameters, abnormal evoked potentials, the presence of lactate in the basal ganglia and thalamus on (Hull and Dodd 1992) H-MRS, and diffusion-weighted changes on MRI in the basal ganglia and thalamus all have an excellent predictive value toward and adverse outcome and could be used to select infants for treatments aimed at neuronal recovery.

References

Adamson SJ, Alessandri LM, Badawi N, Burton PR, Pemberton PJ, Stanley F (1995) Predictors of neonatal encephalopathy in full-term infants. BMJ 311:598–602

al Naqeeb N, Edwards AD, Cowan FM, Azzopardi D (1999) Assessment of neonatal encephalopathy by amplitude-integrated electroencephalography. Pediatrics 103:1263–1271

Alderliesten T, de Vries LS, Benders MJ, Koopman C, Groenendaal F (2011) MR imaging and outcome of term neonates with perinatal asphyxia: value of diffusion-weighted MR imaging and ^{1}H MR spectroscopy. Radiology 261:235–242

Alderliesten T, Nikkels PG, Benders MJ, de Vries LS, Groenendaal F (2013) Antemortem cranial MRI compared with postmortem histopathologic examination of the brain in term infants with neonatal encephalopathy following perinatal asphyxia. Arch Dis Child Fetal Neonatal Ed 98:F304–F309

American College of Obstetricians and Gynecologists' Task Force on Neonatal Encephalopathy (2014) Executive summary: neonatal encephalopathy and neurologic outcome, second edition. Report of the American College of Obstetricians and Gynecologists' Task Force on Neonatal Encephalopathy. Obstet Gynecol 123:896–901

American Academy of Pediatrics, Committee on Fetus and Newborn, American College of Obstetricians and Gynecologists and Committee on Obstetric Practice (2006) The Apgar score. Pediatrics 117:1444–1447

Amer-Wahlin I, Hellsten C, Noren H et al (2001) Cardiotocography only versus cardiotocography plus ST analysis of fetal electrocardiogram for intrapartum fetal monitoring: a Swedish randomised controlled trial. Lancet 358:534–538

Andre M, Boutroy MJ, Dubruc C et al (1986) Clonazepam pharmacokinetics and therapeutic efficacy in neonatal seizures. Eur J Clin Pharmacol 30:585–589

Apgar V (1953) A proposal for a new method of evaluation of the newborn infant. Curr Res Anesth Analg 32: 260–267

Arabin B, Ragosch V, Mohnhaupt A (1995) From biochemical to biophysical placental function tests in fetal surveillance. Am J Perinatol 12:168–171

Archbald F, Verma UL, Tejani NA, Handwerker SM (1984) Cerebral function monitor in the neonate. II: Birth asphyxia. Dev Med Child Neurol 26:162–168

Archer LN, Levene MI, Evans DH (1986) Cerebral artery Doppler ultrasonography for prediction of outcome after perinatal asphyxia. Lancet 2:1116–1118

Arduini D, Rizzo G, Romanini C, Mancuso S (1989) Are blood flow velocity waveforms related to umbilical cord acid- base status in the human fetus? Gynecol Obstet Invest 27:183–187

Azzopardi DV, Strohm B, Edwards AD et al (2009) Moderate hypothermia to treat perinatal asphyxial encephalopathy. N Engl J Med 361:1349–1358

Baenziger O, Martin E, Steinlin M et al (1993) Early pattern recognition in severe perinatal asphyxia: a prospective MRI study. Neuroradiology 35:437–442

Barkovich AJ, Westmark K, Partridge C, Sola A, Ferriero DM (1995) Perinatal asphyxia: MR findings in the first 10 days. AJNR Am J Neuroradiol 16:427–438

Bednarek N, Mathur A, Inder T, Wilkinson J, Neil J, Shimony J (2012) Impact of therapeutic hypothermia on MRI diffusion changes in neonatal encephalopathy. Neurology 78:1420–1427

Belai Y, Goodwin TM, Durand M, Greenspoon JS, Paul RH, Walther FJ (1998) Umbilical arteriovenous PO2 and PCO2 differences and neonatal morbidity in term infants with severe acidosis. Am J Obstet Gynecol 178:13–19

Bjerre I, Hellstro"m-Westas L, Rosen I, Svenningsen N (1983) Monitoring of cerebral function after severe asphyxia in infancy. Arch Dis Child 58:997–1002

Blennow M, Savman K, Ilves P, Thoresen M, Rosengren L (2001) Brain-specific proteins in the cerebrospinal fluid of severely asphyxiated newborn infants. Acta Paediatr 90:1171–1175

Boenisch H, Saling E (1976) The reliability of pH values in fetal blood samples: a study of the second stage. J Perinat Med 4:45

Bonifacio SL, deVries LS, Groenendaal F (2015) Impact of hypothermia on predictors of poor outcome: how do we decide to redirect care? Semin Fetal Neonatal Med 20:122–127

Brown JK, Purvis RJ, Forfar JO, Cockburn F (1974) Neurological aspects of perinatal asphyxia. Dev Med Child Neurol 16:567–580

Buonocore G, Zani S, Perrone S, Caciotti B, Bracci R (1998) Intraerythrocyte nonprotein-bound iron and plasma malondialdehyde in the hypoxic newborn. Free Radic Biol Med 25:766–770

Buonocore G, Perrone S, Gioia D et al (1999) Nucleated red blood cell count at birth as an index of perinatal brain damage. Am J Obstet Gynecol 181:1500–1505

Buonocore G, Perrone S, Longini M et al (2003) Non protein bound iron as early predictive marker of neonatal brain damage. Brain 126:1224–1230

Caplan MS, Hedlund E, Adler L, Hsueh W (1994) Role of asphyxia and feeding in a neonatal rat model of necrotizing enterocolitis. Pediatr Pathol 14:1017–1028

Carter BS, McNabb F, Merenstein GB (1998) Prospective validation of a scoring system for predicting neonatal morbidity after acute perinatal asphyxia. J Pediatr 132:619–623

Casey BM, McIntire DD, Leveno KJ (2001) The continuing value of the Apgar score for the assessment of newborn infants. N Engl J Med 344:467–471

Castle V, Andrew M, Kelton J, Giron D, Johnston M, Carter C (1986) Frequency and mechanism of neonatal thrombocytopenia. J Pediatr 108:749–755

Cataltepe O, Vannucci RC, Heitjan DF, Towfighi J (1995) Effect of status epilepticus on hypoxic-ischemic brain damage in the immature rat. Pediatr Res 38:251–257

Catlin EA, Carpenter MW, Brann BS, Mayfield SR, Shaul PW, Goldstein M (1986) The Apgar score revisited: influence of gestational age. J Pediatr 109:865–868

Chiesa C, Pellegrini G, Panero A et al (2003) Umbilical cord interleukin-6 levels are elevated in term neonates with perinatal asphyxia. Eur J Clin Invest 33:352–358

Chou YH, Tsou Yau KI, Wang PJ (1998) Clinical application of the measurement of cord plasma lactate and pyruvate in the assessment of high-risk neonates. Acta Paediatr 87:764–768

Connell J, Oozeer R, de Vries L, Dubowitz LM, Dubowitz V (1989) Clinical and EEG response to anticonvulsants in neonatal seizures. Arch Dis Child 64:459–464

Cowan F, Rutherford M, Groenendaal F et al (2003) Origin and timing of brain lesions in term infants with neonatal encephalopathy. Lancet 361:736–742

Daniel SS, Adamsons K Jr, James LS (1966) Lactate and pyruvate as an index of prenatal oxygen deprivation. Pediatrics 37:942–953

de Vries LS (1993) Somatosensory-evoked potentials in term neonates with postasphyxial encephalopathy. Clin Perinatol 20:463–482

de Vries LS, Groenendaal F (2010) Patterns of neonatal hypoxic-ischaemic brain injury. Neuroradiology 52:555–566

de Vries LS, Eken P, Groenendaal F, Rademaker KJ, Hoogervorst B, Bruinse HW (1998) Antenatal onset of haemorrhagic and/or ischaemic lesions in preterm infants: prevalence and associated obstetric variables. Arch Dis Child Fetal Neonatal Ed 78:F51–F56

Eken P, Jansen GH, Groenendaal F, Rademaker KJ, de Vries LS (1994) Intracranial lesions in the fullterm infant with hypoxic ischaemic encephalopathy: ultrasound and autopsy correlation. Neuropediatrics 25:301–307

Eken P, Toet MC, Groenendaal F, de Vries LS (1995) Predictive value of early neuroimaging, pulsed Doppler and neurophysiology in full term infants with hypoxic-ischaemic encephalopathy. Arch Dis Child Fetal Neonatal Ed 73:F75–F80

Ekert P, Perlman M, Steinlin M, Hao Y (1997) Predicting the outcome of postasphyxial hypoxic-ischemic encephalopathy within 4 hours of birth. J Pediatr 131:613–617

Fellman V, Raivio KO (1997) Reperfusion injury as the mechanism of brain damage after perinatal asphyxia. Pediatr Res 41:599–606

Fenichel GM (1983) Hypoxic-ischemic encephalopathy in the newborn. Arch Neurol 40:261–266

Filippi L, Fiorini P, Daniotti M et al (2012) Safety and efficacy of topiramate in neonates with hypoxic ischemic encephalopathy treated with hypothermia (NeoNATI). BMC Pediatr 12:144

Foster-Barber A, Dickens B, Ferriero DM (2001) Human perinatal asphyxia: correlation of neonatal cytokines with MRI and outcome. Dev Neurosci 23: 213–218

Fujikura T, Klionsky B (1975) The significance of meconium staining. Am J Obstet Gynecol 121:45–50

Gazzolo D, Marinoni E, Di Iorio R et al (2004) Urinary S100B protein measurements: a tool for the early identification of hypoxic-ischemic encephalopathy in asphyxiated full-term infants. Crit Care Med 32: 131–136

Gibson NA, Graham M, Levene MI (1992) Somatosensory evoked potentials and outcome in perinatal asphyxia. Arch Dis Child 67:393–398

Gluckman PD, Wyatt JS, Azzopardi D et al (2005) Selective head cooling with mild systemic hypothermia after neonatal encephalopathy: multicentre randomised trial. Lancet 365:663–670

Goodwin TM, Belai I, Hernandez P, Durand M, Paul RH (1992) Asphyxial complications in the term newborn with severe umbilical acidemia. Am J Obstet Gynecol 167:1506–1512

Grant A, O'Brien N, Joy MT, Hennessy E, MacDonald D (1989) Cerebral palsy among children born during the Dublin randomised trial of intrapartum monitoring. Lancet 2:1233–1236

Grigg-Damberger MM, Coker SB, Halsey CL, Anderson CL (1989) Neonatal burst suppression: its developmental significance. Pediatr Neurol 5:84–92

Groenendaal F, Brouwer AJ (2009) Clinical aspects of induced hypothermia in full term neonates with perinatal asphyxia. Early Hum Dev 85:73–76

Groenendaal F, Veenhoven RH, van der Grond J, Jansen GH, Witkamp TD, de Vries LS (1994) Cerebral lactate and N-acetyl-aspartate/choline ratios in asphyxiated full-term neonates demonstrated in vivo using proton magnetic resonance spectroscopy. Pediatr Res 35:148–151

Hagberg H, Edwards AD, Groenendaal F (2015) Perinatal brain damage: the term infant. Neurobiol Dis

Harteman JC, Groenendaal F, Toet MC et al (2013) Diffusion-weighted imaging changes in cerebral watershed distribution following neonatal encephalopathy are not invariably associated with an adverse outcome. Dev Med Child Neurol 55:642–653

Hay WW Jr, Thilo E, Curlander JB (1991) Pulse oximetry in neonatal medicine. Clin Perinatol 18:441–472

Hellstrom-Westas L, Rosen I, Svenningsen NW (1995) Predictive value of early continuous amplitude integrated EEG recordings on outcome after severe birth asphyxia in full term infants. Arch Dis Child Fetal Neonatal Ed 72:F34–F38

Herrmann U Jr, Durig P, Amato M, Sidiropoulos D, Schneider H (1989) Outcome of fetuses with abnormal biophysical profile. Gynecol Obstet Invest 27:122–125

Holden KR, Mellits ED, Freeman JM (1982) Neonatal seizures. I. Correlation of prenatal and perinatal events with outcomes. Pediatrics 70:165–176

Holmes G, Rowe J, Hafford J, Schmidt R, Testa M, Zimmerman A (1982) Prognostic value of the electroencephalogram in neonatal asphyxia. Electroencephalogr Clin Neurophysiol 53:60–72

Hope PL, Costello AML, Cady EB et al (1984) Cerebral energy metabolism studied with phosphorous NMR spectroscopy in normal and birth asphyxiated infants. Lancet 8399:366–370

Huang CC, Wang ST, Chang YC, Lin KP, Wu PL (1999) Measurement of the urinary lactate: creatinine ratio for the early identification of newborn infants at risk for hypoxic-ischemic encephalopathy. N Engl J Med 341:328–335

Hull J, Dodd KL (1992) Falling incidence of hypoxic-ischaemic encephalopathy in term infants. Br J Obstet Gynaecol 99:386–391

Jacobs SE, Berg M, Hunt R, Tarnow-Mordi WO, Inder TE, Davis PG (2013) Cooling for newborns with hypoxic ischaemic encephalopathy. Cochrane Database Syst Rev 1, CD003311

Kaandorp JJ, van Bel F, Veen S et al (2012) Long-term neuroprotective effects of allopurinol after moderate perinatal asphyxia: follow-up of two randomised controlled trials. Arch Dis Child Fetal Neonatal Ed 97: F162–F166

King TA, Jackson GL, Josey AS et al (1998) The effect of profound umbilical artery acidemia in term neonates admitted to a newborn nursery. J Pediatr 132:624–629

Klinger G, Beyene J, Shah P, Perlman M (2005) Do hyperoxaemia and hypocapnia add to the risk of brain injury after intrapartum asphyxia? Arch Dis Child Fetal Neonatal Ed 90:F49–F52

L'Abee C, de Vries LS, van der Grond J, Groenendaal F (2005) Early diffusion-weighted MRI and 1H-magnetic resonance spectroscopy in asphyxiated full-term neonates. Biol Neonate 88:306–312

Lavrijsen SW, Uiterwaal CSPM, Stigter RH, de Vries LS, Visser GHA, Groenendaal F (2005) Severe umbilical cord acidemia and neurological outcome in preterm and full-term neonates. Biol Neonate 88:27–34

Lemmers PM, Zwanenburg RJ, Benders MJ et al (2013) Cerebral oxygenation and brain activity after perinatal asphyxia: does hypothermia change their prognostic value? Pediatr Res 74:180–185

Levene MI, Kornberg J, Williams THC (1985) The incidence and severity of postasphyxial encephalopathy in full-term infants. Early Hum Dev 11:21–28

Levene MI, Sands C, Grindulis H, Moore JR (1986) Comparison of two methods of predicting outcome in perinatal asphyxia. Lancet 1:67–69

Lorek A, Takei Y, Cady EB et al (1994) Delayed ("secondary") cerebral energy failure after acute hypoxia-ischemia in the newborn piglet: continuous 48-hour studies by phosphorus magnetic resonance spectroscopy. Pediatr Res 36:699–706

Low JA, Galbraith RS, Muir DW, Killen HL, Pater EA, Karchmar EJ (1984) Factors associated with motor and cognitive deficits in children after intrapartum fetal hypoxia. Am J Obstet Gynecol 148:533–539

Low JA, Galbraith RS, Muir DW, Killen HL, Pater EA, Karchmar EJ (1985) The relationship between perinatal hypoxia and newborn encephalopathy. Am J Obstet Gynecol 152:256–260

Low JA, Pickersgill H, Killen H, Derrick EJ (2001) The prediction and prevention of intrapartum fetal asphyxia in term pregnancies. Am J Obstet Gynecol 184: 724–730

Luciano R, Gallini F, Romagnoli C, Papacci P, Tortorolo G (1998) Doppler evaluation of renal blood flow velocity as a predictive index of acute renal failure in perinatal asphyxia. Eur J Pediatr 157:656–660

Maeda K, Tatsumura M, Nakajima K (1991) Objective and quantitative evaluation of fetal movement with ultrasonic Doppler actocardiogram. Biol Neonate 60(Suppl 1):41–51

Martin-Ancel A, Garcia-Alix A, Pascual-Salcedo D, Cabanas F, Valcarce M, Quero J (1997) Interleukin-6 in the cerebrospinal fluid after perinatal asphyxia is related to early and late neurological manifestations. Pediatrics 100:789–794

Martinez-Biarge M, Diez-Sebastian J, Wusthoff CJ, Mercuri E, Cowan FM (2013) Antepartum and intrapartum factors preceding neonatal hypoxic-ischemic encephalopathy. Pediatrics 132:e952–e959

Mathew OP, Bland H, Boxerman SB, James E (1980) CSF lactate levels in high risk neonates with and without asphyxia. Pediatrics 66:224–227

Meis PJ, Hall M III, Marshall JR, Hobel CJ (1978) Meconium passage: a new classification for risk assessment during labor. Am J Obstet Gynecol 131:509–513

Mellits ED, Holden KR, Freeman JM (1982) Neonatal seizures. II. A multivariate analysis of factors associated with outcome. Pediatrics 70:177–185

Mercuri E, von Siebenthal K, Daniels H, Guzzetta F, Casaer P (1994) Multimodality evoked responses in the neurological assessment of the newborn. Eur J Pediatr 153:622–631

Monod N, Pajot N, Guidasci S (1972) The neonatal EEG: statistical studies and prognostic value in full-term and preterm babies. Electroencephalogr Clin Neurophysiol 32:529–544

Muttitt SC, Taylor MJ, Kobayashi JS, MacMillan L, Whyte HE (1991) Serial visual evoked potentials and outcome in term birth asphyxia. Pediatr Neurol 7:86–90

Myers RE (1975) Four patterns of perinatal brain damage and their conditions of occurrence in primates. Adv Neurol 10:223–234

Myers RE (1977) Experimental models of perinatal brain damage: relevance to human pathology. In: Gluck L (ed) Intrauterine asphyxia and the developing fetal brain. Year Book Medical Publ, Chicago, pp 37–97

Nagdyman N, Grimmer I, Scholz T, Muller C, Obladen M (2003) Predictive value of brain-specific proteins in serum for neurodevelopmental outcome after birth asphyxia. Pediatr Res 54:270–275

Nelson KB, Dambrosia JM, Ting TY, Grether JK (1996) Uncertain value of electronic fetal monitoring in predicting cerebral palsy. N Engl J Med 334: 613–618

Niklinski W, Palynyczko Z, Jozwik M, Sledziewski A (1987) Cord blood serum creatine kinase isoenzymes with placental dysfunction. J Perinatol Med 15: 350–354

Nylund L, Dahlin I, Lagercrantz H (1987) Fetal catecholamines and the Apgar score. J Perinat Med 15:340–344

Okereafor A, Allsop J, Counsell SJ et al (2008) Patterns of brain injury in neonates exposed to perinatal sentinel events. Pediatrics 121:906–914

Oygur N, Sonmez O, Saka O, Yegin O (1998) Predictive value of plasma and cerebrospinal fluid tumour necrosis factor-alpha and interleukin-1 beta concentrations on outcome of full term infants with hypoxic-ischaemic encephalopathy. Arch Dis Child Fetal Neonatal Ed 79: F190–F193

Perlman JM, Risser R (1996) Can asphyxiated infants at risk for neonatal seizures be rapidly identified by current high-risk markers? Pediatrics 97:456–462

Perlman JM, Tack ED, Martin T, Shackelford G, Amon E (1989) Acute systemic organ injury in term infants after asphyxia. Am J Dis Child 143:617–620

Portman RJ, Carter BS, Gaylord MS, Murphy MG, Thieme RE, Merenstein GB (1990) Predicting neonatal morbidity after perinatal asphyxia: a scoring system. Am J Obstet Gynecol 162:174–182

Pourcyrous M, Bada HS, Yang W et al (1999) Prognostic significance of cerebrospinal fluid cyclic adenosine monophosphate in neonatal asphyxia. J Pediatr 134:90–96

Pressler RM, Mangum B (2013) Newly emerging therapies for neonatal seizures. Semin Fetal Neonatal Med 18:216–223

Ramantani G, Ikonomidou C, Walter B, Rating D, Dinger J (2011) Levetiracetam: safety and efficacy in neonatal seizures. Eur J Paediatr Neurol 15:1–7

Ranck JB, Windle WF (1959) Brain damage in the monkey, Macaca mulatta, by asphyxia neonatorum. Exp Neurol 1:130–154

Robertson NJ, Cowan FM, Cox IJ, Edwards AD (2002) Brain alkaline intracellular pH after neonatal encephalopathy. Ann Neurol 52:732–742

Robertson NJ, Tan S, Groenendaal F et al (2012) Which neuroprotective agents are ready for bench to bedside translation in the newborn infant? J Pediatr 160:544–552

Roka A, Melinda KT, Vasarhelyi B, Machay T, Azzopardi D, Szabo M (2008) Elevated morphine concentrations in neonates treated with morphine and prolonged hypothermia for hypoxic ischemic encephalopathy. Pediatrics 121:e844–e849

Roth SC, Edwards AD, Cady EB et al (1992) Relation between cerebral oxidative metabolism following birth asphyxia, and neurodevelopmental outcome and brain growth at one year. Dev Med Child Neurol 34:285–295

Ruth VJ, Raivio KO (1988) Perinatal brain damage: predictive value of metabolic acidosis and the Apgar score. BMJ 297:24–27

Ruth V, Fyhrquist F, Clemons G, Raivio KO (1988) Cord plasma vasopressin, erythropoietin, and hypoxanthine as indices of asphyxia at birth. Pediatr Res 24:490–494

Rutherford M, Pennock J, Schwieso J, Cowan F, Dubowitz L (1996) Hypoxic-ischaemic encephalopathy: early and late magnetic resonance imaging findings in relation to outcome. Arch Dis Child Fetal Neonatal Ed 75:F145–F151

Rutherford MA, Pennock JM, Counsell SJ et al (1998) Abnormal magnetic resonance signal in the internal capsule predicts poor neurodevelopmental outcome in infants with hypoxic- ischemic encephalopathy. Pediatrics 102:323–328

Rutherford M, Counsell S, Allsop J et al (2004) Diffusion-weighted magnetic resonance imaging in term perinatal brain injury: a comparison with site of lesion and time from birth. Pediatrics 114:1004–1014

Sarnat HB, Sarnat MS (1976) Neonatal encephalopathy following fetal distress; a clinical and electroencephalographic study. Arch Neurol 33:696–705

Saugstad OD (1976) Hypoxanthine as a measurement of hypoxia. Pediatr Res 9:575

Saugstad OD (2003) Oxygen toxicity at birth: the pieces are put together. Pediatr Res 54:798

Savman K, Blennow M, Gustafson K, Tarkowski E, Hagberg H (1998) Cytokine response in cerebrospinal fluid after birth asphyxia. Pediatr Res 43:746–751

Schifrin BS (1994) The ABCs of electronic fetal monitoring. J Perinatol 14:396–402

Sehdev HM, Stamilio DM, Macones GA, Graham E, Morgan MA (1997) Predictive factors for neonatal morbidity in neonates with an umbilical arterial cord pH less than 7.00. Am J Obstet Gynecol 177:1030–1034

Shankaran S, Woldt E, Koepke T, Bedard MP, Nandyal R (1991) Acute neonatal morbidity and long-term central nervous system sequelae of perinatal asphyxia in term infants. Early Hum Dev 25:135–148

Shankaran S, Laptook AR, Ehrenkranz RA et al (2005) Whole-body hypothermia for neonates with hypoxic-ischemic encephalopathy. N Engl J Med 353:1574–1584

Sie LT, van der Knaap MS, Oosting J, de Vries LS, Lafeber HN, Valk J (2000) MR patterns of hypoxic-ischemic brain damage after prenatal, perinatal or postnatal asphyxia. Neuropediatrics 31:128–136

Smith J, Wells L, Dodd K (2000) The continuing fall in incidence of hypoxic-ischaemic encephalopathy in term infants. BJOG 107:461–466

Sola A, Rogido MR, Deulofeut R (2007) Oxygen as a neonatal health hazard: call for detente in clinical practice. Acta Paediatr 96:801–812

Squier W (2002) Acquired damage to the developing brain: timing and causation. Acquired damage to the developing brain: timing and causation. Oxford University Press, London

Sykes GS, Molloy PM, Johnson P et al (1982) Do Apgar scores indicate asphyxia? Lancet 1:494–496

Taylor MJ, Murphy WJ, Whyte HE (1992) Prognostic reliability of somatosensory and visual evoked potentials of asphyxiated term infants. Dev Med Child Neurol 34:507–515

Thompson CM, Puterman AS, Linley LL et al (1997) The value of a scoring system for hypoxic ischaemic encephalopathy in predicting neurodevelopmental outcome. Acta Paediatr 86:757–761

Thornberg E, Thiringer K, Hagberg H, Kjellmer I (1995) Neuron specific enolase in asphyxiated newborns: association with encephalopathy and cerebral function monitor trace. Arch Dis Child Fetal Neonatal Ed 72:F39–F42

Toet MC, Hellstrom-Westas L, Groenendaal F, Eken P, de Vries LS (1999) Amplitude integrated EEG at 3 and 6 hours after birth in full term neonates with hypoxic-ischaemic encephalopathy. Arch Dis Child Fetal Neonatal Ed 81:F19–F23

Toet MC, van der Meij W, de Vries LS, Uiterwaal CS, van Huffelen KC (2002) Comparison between simultaneously recorded amplitude integrated electroencephalogram (cerebral function monitor) and standard electroencephalogram in neonates. Pediatrics 109: 772–779

Toet MC, Lemmers PM, van Schelven LJ, Van Bel F (2006) Cerebral oxygenation and electrical activity after birth asphyxia: their relation to outcome. Pediatrics 117:333–339

Toet MC, Van Rooij LG, de Vries LS (2008) The use of amplitude integrated electroencephalography for assessing neonatal neurologic injury. Clin Perinatol 35:665–678, v

Torrance HL, Benders MJ, Derks JB et al (2009) Maternal allopurinol treatment during fetal hypoxia lowers cord blood levels of the brain injury marker protein S-100B. Pediatrics 124:350–357

Van Bel F, Walther FJ (1990) Myocardial dysfunction and cerebral blood flow velocity following birth asphyxia. Acta Paediatr Scand 79:756–762

Van Bel F, Van de Bor M, Stijnen T, Baan J, Ruys JH (1987) Cerebral blood flow velocity pattern in healthy and asphyxiated newborns: a controlled study. Eur J Pediatr 146:461–467

van den Berg PP, Nelen WL, Jongsma HW et al (1996) Neonatal complications in newborns with an umbilical artery pH < 7.00. Am J Obstet Gynecol 175:1152–1157

van den Broek MP, Groenendaal F, Egberts AC, Rademaker CM (2010) Effects of hypothermia on pharmacokinetics and pharmacodynamics: a systematic review of preclinical and clinical studies. Clin Pharmacokinet 49:277–294

van den Broek MP, Huitema AD, van Hasselt JG et al (2011) Lidocaine (lignocaine) dosing regimen based upon a population pharmacokinetic model for preterm and term neonates with seizures. Clin Pharmacokinet 50:461–469

van den Broek MP, Groenendaal F, Toet MC et al (2012) Pharmacokinetics and clinical efficacy of phenobarbital in asphyxiated newborns treated with hypothermia: a thermopharmacological approach. Clin Pharmacokinet 51:671–679

van den Broek MP, Rademaker CM, van Straaten HL et al (2013) Anticonvulsant treatment of asphyxiated newborns under hypothermia with lidocaine: efficacy, safety and dosing. Arch Dis Child Fetal Neonatal Ed 98:F341–F345

van den Broek MP, van Straaten HL, Huitema AD et al (2015) Anticonvulsant effectiveness and hemodynamic safety of midazolam in full-term infants treated with hypothermia. Neonatology 107:150–156

van der Aa NE, Benders MJ, Groenendaal F, de Vries LS (2014) Neonatal stroke: a review of the current evidence on epidemiology, pathogenesis, diagnostics and therapeutic options. Acta Paediatr 103:356–364

van Laerhoven H, de Haan TR, Offringa M, Post B, van der Lee JH (2013) Prognostic tests in term neonates with hypoxic-ischemic encephalopathy: a systematic review. Pediatrics 131:88–98

Van Rooij LG, Toet MC, Osredkar D, van Huffelen AC, Groenendaal F, de Vries LS (2005) Recovery of amplitude integrated electroencephalographic background patterns within 24 hours of perinatal asphyxia. Arch Dis Child Fetal Neonatal Ed 90:F245–F251

Van Rooij LG, Toet MC, van Huffelen AC et al (2010) Effect of treatment of subclinical neonatal seizures detected with aEEG: randomized, controlled trial. Pediatrics 125:e358–e366

Vannucci RC, Towfighi J, Vannucci SJ (2004) Secondary energy failure after cerebral hypoxia-ischemia in the immature rat. J Cereb Blood Flow Metab 24:1090–1097

Vento M, Saugstad OD (2010) Resuscitation of the term and preterm infant. Semin Fetal Neonatal Med 15:216–222

Volpe JJ (2008) Neurology of the newborn. Saunders Book Company, Philadelphia

Volpe JJ, Herscovitch P, Perlman JM, Kreusser KL, Raichle ME (1985) Positron emission tomography in the asphyxiated term newborn: parasagittal impairment of cerebral blood flow. Ann Neurol 17:287–296

Watanabe K, Miyazaki S, Hara K, Hakamada S (1980) Behavioral state cycles, background EEGs and prognosis of newborns with perinatal hypoxia. Electroencephalogr Clin Neurophysiol 49:618–625

Wayenberg JL, Vermeylen D, Bormans J, Magrez P, Muller MF, Pardou A (1994) Diagnosis of severe birth asphyxia and early prediction of neonatal neurological outcome in term asphyxiated newborns. J Perinat Med 22:129–136

Westerhuis ME, Porath MM, Becker JH et al (2012) Identification of cases with adverse neonatal outcome monitored by cardiotocography versus ST analysis: secondary analysis of a randomized trial. Acta Obstet Gynecol Scand 91:830–837

Winkler CL, Hauth JC, Tucker JM, Owen J, Brumfield CG (1991) Neonatal complications at term as related to the degree of umbilical artery acidemia. Am J Obstet Gynecol 164:637–641

Wyatt JS (1993) Near-infrared spectroscopy in asphyxial brain injury. Clin Perinatol 20:369–378

Xanthou M, Fotopoulos S, Mouchtouri A, Lipsou N, Zika I, Sarafidou J (2002) Inflammatory mediators in perinatal asphyxia and infection. Acta Paediatr Suppl 91:92–97

Neuroprotective Strategies for Newborns

127

Bobbi Fleiss, Claire Thornton, and Pierre Gressens

Contents

B. Fleiss (✉) · P. Gressens
UMR1141, Insem-Paris Diderot University, Hôpital Robert Debré, Paris, France

Centre for the Developing Brain, Department of Perinatal Imaging and Health, Division of Imaging Sciences and Biomedical Engineering, King's College London, King's Health Partners, St. Thomas' Hospital, London, UK
e-mail: bobbi.fleiss@inserm.fr; pierre.gressens@inserm.fr

C. Thornton
Centre for the Developing Brain, Department of Perinatal Imaging and Health, Division of Imaging Sciences and Biomedical Engineering, King's College London, King's Health Partners, St. Thomas' Hospital, London, UK
e-mail: claire.thornton@kcl.ac.uk

Abstract

Perinatal brain injury is the leading cause of death and disability in children. Such damage can be induced by multiple factors, varies in severity between individuals, affects infants of different genetic backgrounds, and occurs at various stages of the physiological developmental program. This complexity creates innumerable difficulties in creating therapeutic agents. A wealth of experimental studies has engaged in the understanding of brain injury pathophysiology and in the development of strategies that may be beneficial for the

G. Buonocore et al. (eds.), *Neonatology*,
https://doi.org/10.1007/978-3-319-29489-6_274

neurological outcome of infants. Clinical trials have demonstrated the partial neuroprotective effects of hypothermia and magnesium sulfate in human neonates. Trials for the neuroprotective effects of the pluripotent hormone melatonin are ongoing. In the following chapter we review the experimental and clinical data on neuroprotective strategies.

Abbreviations

AMPA	Alpha-3-amino-hydroxy-5-methyl-4-isoxazole propionic acid
ATP	Adenosine triphosphate
BBB	Blood brain barrier
CNS	Central nervous system
COX	Cyclooxygenase
EPO	Erythropoietin
iNOS	Inducible form of nitric oxide synthase
KA	Kainate
MMPs	Matrix metalloproteases
NAC	*N*-Acetylcysteine
NMDA	*N*-Methyl-D-aspartate
NO	Nitric oxide
NSAIDS	Nonsteroidal anti-inflammatory drugs
rEPO	Recombinant form of erythropoietin
RNS	Reactive nitrogen species
ROS	Reactive oxygen species
TBI	Traumatic brain injury

127.1 Salient Points

- Neuroprotective strategies applied currently in the clinical practice are limited and often do not take into account the diversity of perinatal brain lesions as well as of affected infants.
- Neuroprotective strategies consist mainly in preventing aggravating situations such as pain, cardiovascular instability, and hyperthermia.
- Within the last few years, hypothermia in newborns diagnosed with stage II and III hypoxic-ischemic encephalopathy as well as administration of magnesium to mothers in the context of imminent premature birth have been shown to be efficient as therapeutic strategies. The benefits gained by these measures, however, remain partial, highlighting the need for additional therapies.
- Clinical trials regarding the neuroprotective effect of erythropoietin in term infants have been put on hold due to adverse effects. In preterm infants, a large clinical trial has shown beneficial effects on MRI parameters but no significant effect on neurobehavior at 2 years of age.
- Clinical trials regarding the neuroprotective effect of xenon have just recently reported no additional beneficial effect as an adjunct with hypothermia. The trial was a robust clinical trial incorporating early assessment via MRI and considering clinical outcomes at discharge.
- Further potential neuroprotective strategies identified in animal models have emerged. Some of them, such as allopurinol, are currently being tested in clinical trials. However, the translation of potential protective strategies from animal studies to clinical trials faces the variable quality of the animal studies, the ethical problem of studying drug effects in newborns, the uncertainty of the innoxiousness of these molecules for the developing human brain, and the lack of clear predictors of infant brain damage.

127.2 Introduction

Despite the mortality of infants, especially premature infants, decreasing remarkably throughout the last decades due to improved antenatal care their rates of morbidity have not improved at the same pace. Furthermore, although rates of neonatal encephalopathy in term infants remaining relatively constant in the developed world (at around 1/1000 births), the rates of preterm births in the same setting are increasing steadily. Perinatal brain injury is the largest contributor to disability adjusted life years (DALYs) in children and thus,

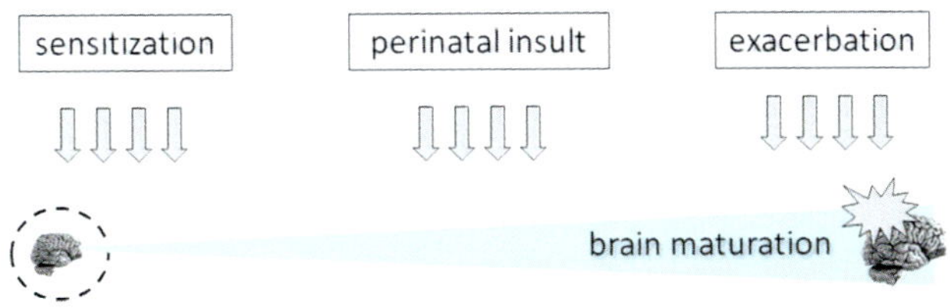

Fig. 1 Multiple-hit hypothesis for the development of perinatal brain damage. Schematic representation illustrates the multiple-hit hypothesis including pre-, peri-, and postnatal factors. Several risk factors are implicated and are frequently associated with the pathogenesis of perinatal brain damage in animal models. These comprise prenatal risk factors such as inflammation/cytokine release and maternal stress, perinatal factors such as hypoxic-ischemic stimuli, and postnatal factors such as growth factor deprivation, inflammation/cytokine release, drug side effects, and pain (see Table 1). Furthermore, a combination of such factors in experimental models has resulted in the emergence of a multiple-hit hypothesis, which consists of a sensitization state created by a mild first event, leading to an increased susceptibility to a second injury. These factors may cause various lesions depending also on the developmental stage of the brain

treatments for neurocognitive morbidity is an important health care issue. Despite this, currently available intervention strategies are limited but novel drugs are demonstrating great promise.

Perinatal brain damage is a term that encompasses injuries that are multifactorial, multihit processes that vary in severity between individuals, affects infants of different genetic backgrounds, and occurs at various stages of the physiological developmental program (Fig. 1). Very broadly, we define perinatal brain injury relative to the stage of development of the infant based on the differing vulnerability of the gray versus white matter at extremes of preterm and term infants. For instance, periventricular leukomalacia is particularly frequent in the premature infant, while a diagnosis of hypoxic-ischemic encephalopathy is made predominantly in the term infant. The development of novel neuroprotective strategies thereby demands a clear understanding of the pathophysiology of each of the disorders in order to identify readouts or targets/pathways to test for the efficacy of candidate molecules. In addition, as developmental processes are also targets for injury and therapies, careful attention needs to be paid to acute and long-term toxic effects. It remains to be elucidated, for example, across what time and dose response that a decrease of apoptotic cell death is beneficial or detrimental.

127.3 Pathophysiology of Brain Diseases and Definition of targets

The development of neuroprotective strategies is based on fundamental knowledge on the causes and mechanism induced subsequent to injury. For this, brain pathology has been studied in postmortem tissues from patients as well as in animal models that mimic human pathology. Such approaches have allowed to distinguish various intertwined causes and mechanisms that induce white and/or gray matter damage of the central nervous system (Table 1; for review, see (Perlman 2006)). Critically, however, it must be noted that both cause and downstream injurious processes must be understood to adequately model injury. For example, blood–brain barrier disruption, neuronal loss, and inflammation are observed in the brain of infants who had been diagnosed with HIE, but this injury can also be induced by blunt force trauma. No one would advocate for modeling HIE using traumatic brain injury, but it remains incompletely understood in term infants in particular whether the brain of the infants suffers from a lack of oxygen in all cases of HIE and what the depth of this could be and/or the relative sensitizing effects of any prior occult inflammatory processes.

Table 1 Risk factors for the development of encephalopathy of prematurity

Antenatal factors	Perinatal factors	Postnatal factors
Inflammation	Hypoxia-ischemia	Oxidative stress
Hypoxia-ischemia	Excitotoxicity	Inflammation
Toxins	Oxidative stress	Pain
Malnutrition	Loss of maternal GF	Excitotoxicity
Maternal stress	Drugs	Drugs
Genetic factors	Genetic factors	Loss of maternal GF
		Genetic factors

GF growth factor

Using approaches variously encompassing epidemiologic and experimental studies, the susceptibility of infants at various stages of development to perinatal insults is increasingly understood. Periventricular white matter damage (PWMD) affects preterm neonates born between 23 and 32 weeks of gestation and involves a blockage of maturation of oligodendrocytes and subsequent hypomyelination. Subtle deficits in gray matter, such as interneuron and synapse density, are increasingly hypothesized to be involved (Boardman et al. 2006; Roumier et al. 2008; Lazarini et al. 2012). The presence of underlying inflammation/infection is the major contributor to this injury type. In parallel, brain lesions proceeding from established acute hypoxia-ischemia (i.e., placental abruption, cord occlusion/prolapse) in at term neonates involve an apoptotic/necrotic process leading to early and delayed neuronal cell death in the gray matter, mainly at thalamic level. Pathophysiologic events in conditions of perinatal brain damage that represent targets for neuroprotective therapy are summarized in Table 2 (see also Figs. 2 and 3).

127.4 Neuroprotective Strategies: Experimental Results

In general, neuroprotective approaches can include mechanisms such as an inhibition of sensitizing factors, preconditioning against damage, a pharmacological blockage of mechanisms involved in primary or secondary damage, or treatment that increases endogenous reparation processes or cause reparation by themselves (Fig. 4). Various therapeutic strategies have been tested in vitro and in vivo in animal models. Principal limiting factors of these pharmacologic approaches are: (i) the passage of molecules via the BBB, (ii) the potential toxicity of applied molecules, (iii) the therapeutic window and thus the existence of a beneficial effect even when a molecule is applied relatively late after a brain damage, and (iv) the persistence of a long-term protective effect. Several therapies have been shown to be efficient in the reduction of lesion sizes and their consequences and the most efficient of these target multiple pathophysiological pathways (i.e., hypothermia, melatonin, and erythropoietin). Even though drugs often act on several levels of a damage cascade, we will classify them below according to their most prominent (or most studied) effect.

127.4.1 Anti-inflammatory Agents

127.4.1.1 Minocycline

Minocycline is a second-generation semisynthetic tetracycline that is best known for reducing proinflammatory responses via effects on microglia (Homsi et al. 2010; Kobayashi et al. 2013; Ng et al. 2012; Sriram et al. 2006). Minocycline has been used successfully to reduce brain damage across a diverse range of models of injury, such as multiple sclerosis (EAE), term and preterm brain injury (excitotoxicity and hypoxia-ischemia), and Alzheimer's disease (for review Garrido-Mesa et al. 2013). Minocycline decreases the activation of MMPs (Koistinaho et al. 2005) and caspase-1 and caspase-3 (Sanchez Mejia et al. 2001), increases levels of the antiapoptotic protein Bcl-2 (Wang et al. 2004), and chelates magnesium and calcium (Gonzalez et al. 2007). In contrast, studies also demonstrate that minocycline fails to improve outcome in models of adult and perinatal brain injury (Sriram et al. 2006; Fernandez-Gomez et al. 2005; Fox et al. 2005). Outstanding questions remain on the target cell of minocycline, importance of timing and dose, and the necessity of

Table 2 Pathophysiologic events in conditions of perinatal brain damage that represents targets for neuroprotective therapy

Primary and secondary energy failure	In situations of reduced oxygen supply the metabolism is redirected towards anaerobic glycolysis to reduce the requirement for oxygen
	This leads to a decreased production of ATP and primary energy metabolites and thus to a secondary energy failure
Excitotoxicity	Energetic breakdown induces a surge of glutamate that accumulates in the synaptic gap due to cell damage and the inability of astrocytes to recycle these high levels of the neurotransmitter at an adequate pace
	Excitotoxicity refers to the deleterious effects of such high glutamate levels on brain tissue: over activation of glutamate receptors, massive influx of calcium, secondary cell damage, etc.
Oxidative stress	Oxidative stress, i.e., an increase of free radicals, results from activation of multiple pathways such as excitotoxicity or microglia activation
	This can lead to fragmentation of DNA and of membranes and thereby trigger necrotic cell death
	During the fetal and neonatal phase recycling of such free radicals by scavengers is limited, and this renders the developing brain particularly vulnerable to oxidative stress
Mitochondrial failure and cell death	Mitochondria are central organelles implicated in physiological energy supply but also in the process of cell death following initial brain injury through mitochondrial outer membrane permeabilization
	Leakage of proapoptotic proteins from the mitochondrion (apoptosis-inducing factor, cytochrome c, etc.) results in caspase-dependent and independent cell death
	Disturbances in mitochondrial dynamics (fission, fusion) coupled with impaired mitochondrial quality control may contribute to neuronal death
Microglia activation	Microglia, the resident macrophages of the central nervous system (CNS), constantly screen the CNS and can be activated rapidly through various environmental changes. In the activation process, microglia change their phenotype, proliferate, migrate to the site of damage, and secrete proinflammatory factors and participate in the generation of oxidative stress (of note, a protective role of microglia is also known)
	Microglia are critical in the processes of normal development, including proliferation and synaptogenesis. Activation of microglia disrupts their participation in these important processes and is thought to be a contributing factor in brain injury
Increase in brain–blood barrier (BBB) permeability	Brain damage increases the permeability of the BBB (which is functional even in preterm infants) and thereby facilitates the infiltration of immune cells (e.g., macrophages, lymphocytes), toxic molecules, and of water from the circulating blood pool
	One reason for the dysfunction of the BBB is the degradation of tight junctions within this barrier by increased activation of matrix metalloproteases (MMPs) in the extracellular matrix
Neuroplasticity	Neuroplasticity refers to changes that occur in the organization of the CNS throughout brain development and also within the mature brain
	Following lesions, various phenomena of plasticity and reparation can appear such as increased rates of stem cell proliferation and differentiation

allowing glial activation to facilitate repair and regeneration. Although being well tolerated by adults, minocycline is contraindicated in children below an age of 8 years due to discoloration of dental enamel.

127.4.1.2 Nonsteriodal Anti-inflammatory Drugs (NSAIDs)

Cyclooxygenases are essential for the formation of prostaglandins and thromboxan from membranous arachidonic acid. Two types of cyclooxygenase are

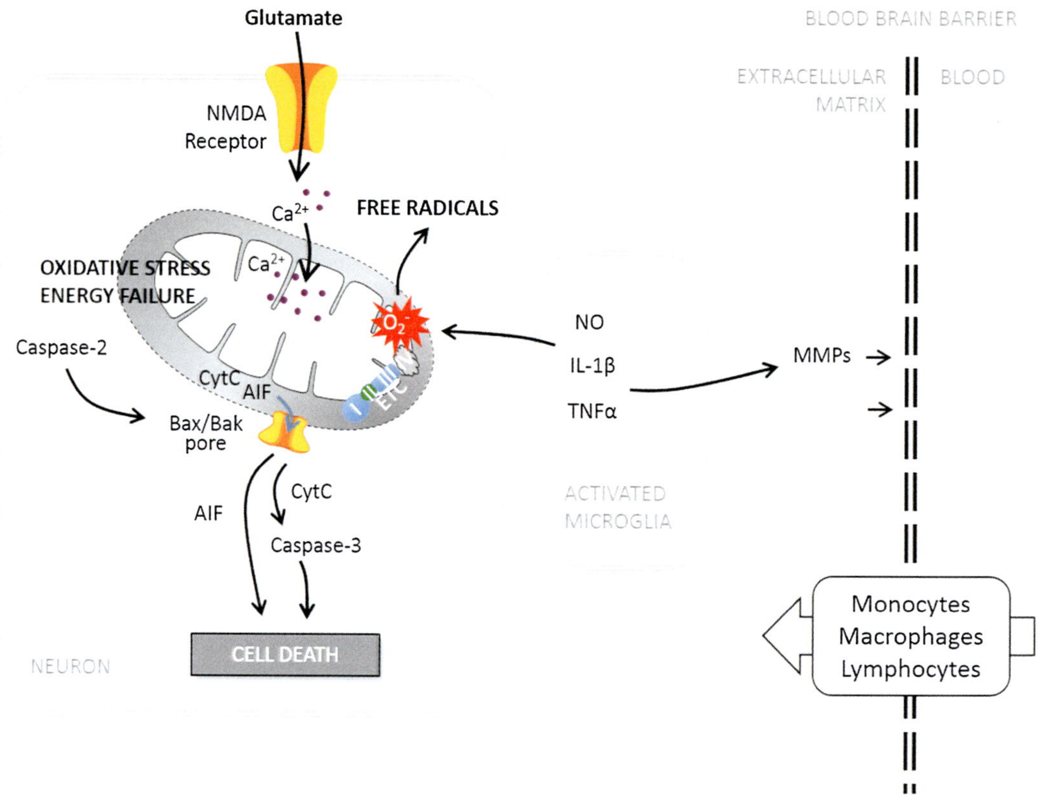

Fig. 2 Pathophysiologic mechanisms implicated in cell death following a brain lesion. Activation of microglia and abberant neuronal energy metabolism mediate cell death mechanisms contributing to the development of the injury. Abbreviations: *CytC* cytochrome C, *AIF* apoptosis-inducing factor, *MMPs* metalloproteinases, *NO* nitric oxide, *NMDAR* *N*-methyl-D-aspartate receptor

distinguished: the cyclooxygenase type 1 (COX-1) or constitutive type and the cyclooxygenase type 2 (COX-2) or inflammation inducible type. NSAIDs that block selectively COX-2 such as nimesulide are preferably applied, even though positive results have been obtained with indomethacin and ibuprofen. Nimesulide has been shown to have a neuroprotective effect in models of focal and diffuse ischemia and systemic inflammation in a sustained manner despite a late application up to 6 h after the acute incident. Neuroprotective mechanisms include an inhibition of TNFα expression while increasing that of IL-10, a prevention of BBB dysfunction, and a reduction of oxidative stress (Candelario-Jalil et al. 2007; Favrais et al. 2007; Candelario-Jalil 2008). These promising results have not been confirmed in humans so far. Thus, their administration needs to be seen with caution in the context of inflammatory brain diseases, also because of potentially toxic effects in the newborn in which the hepatic metabolism for NSAIDs is reduced.

127.4.2 Excitotoxicity Reducing Agents

Strategies developed to limit excitotoxicity are based on an inhibition of postsynaptic glutamate receptors. Thereby, the principal difficulty is to block toxic/ overstimulated receptors without inhibiting the physiologic function of these receptors essential for normal brain development and function. It has been demonstrated that an unselective inhibition of the NMDA receptor in critical periods of brain development triggers apoptosis, inhibits cell proliferation, and causes

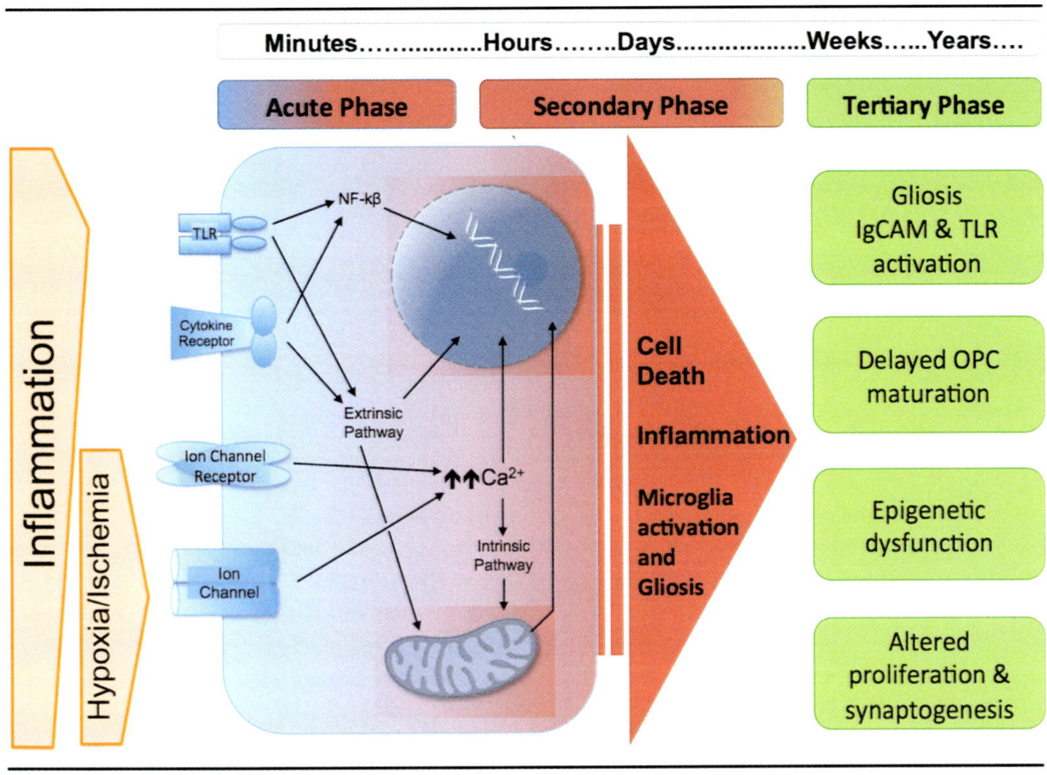

Fig. 3 Schematic of the stages of injury and pathophysiological processes following brain lesion. The discovery of the period of secondary energy failure was critical in the design and implementation of hypothermia as a therapeutic for term infants. Increased understanding of the processes at each stage and in particular of the tertiary phase holds promise for novel therapy development (Adapted from Fleiss and Gressens 2012)

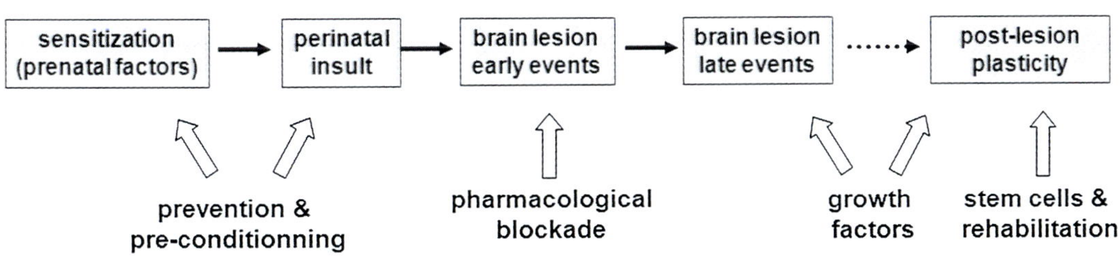

Fig. 4 Schematic representation of the potential strategies for neuroprotection against perinatal brain damage

neurobehavioral deficits in rodents. Still, blockage of NMDA receptors, especially of certain subunits, can be neuroprotective, as has been shown in various animal models for example using memantine. This paradox illustrates the difficulty in the balance between beneficial and harmful effects of neuroprotective strategies in the course of brain development.

127.4.2.1 Magnesium

Magnesium binds NMDA receptors and inhibits their activation; this block is removed by membrane depolarization. Thereby, magnesium possesses a modulatory role and inhibits excitotoxic stress. An antiapoptotic effect has been demonstrated in animal models. The administration of magnesium to pregnant women presenting with threatening premature birth has shown to be beneficial with regard to the incidence of cerebral palsy and motor dysfunction in the infant born prematurely (Doyle et al. 2009) with a good tolerance of the protocols administrated (Marret et al. 2007). In adult victims of traumatic brain injury, epidemiologic studies have identified low magnesium levels <1.3 mmol/l as a negative prognostic factor (Stippler et al. 2007). Still, a prolonged intravenous supplementation of high doses of magnesium was not beneficial, and the passage of magnesium across the BBB in the adult is uncertain (Temkin et al. 2007; McKee et al. 2005). Of interest, magnesium sulfate has also recently been shown to be able to modulate inflammation, this adding a potential new target (Sugimoto et al. 2012).

127.4.2.2 Topiramate

The antagonism of AMPA and kainate receptors, for example through topiramate, has not shown effects as deleterious on neuronal survival as those acknowledged for NMDA receptor antagonists in the developing brain. In addition, a protective effect of topiramate on preoligodendrocytes, cells that have been shown to be severely affected after an excitotoxic stress or hypoxic-ischemic stress in the neonatal period, has been demonstrated (Sfaello et al. 2005). Topiramate has been approved for use as an antiepileptic drug in children older than 2 years. So far, topiramate is not used as a neuroprotective agent but its good tolerance and further experimental data argue for further analysis of this application.

127.4.3 Antioxidants

Two approaches have been developed to limit oxidative stress. The first consists in a reduction of free radical production through xanthine oxidase inhibition, of lipid peroxidation, and of iNOS. The second approach consists in increasing antioxidant defense mechanisms through an increase of ROS and RNS scavengers.

127.4.3.1 Allopurinol

Allopurinol is an inhibitor of the xanthine oxidase. Its neuroprotective action is particularly through the reduction of oxidative stress and of cerebral edema, and its good tolerance has been shown in various animal models; this supports the realization of clinical studies in humans. It has been employed in therapeutic essays in infants with hypoxic-ischemic encephalopathy. In a first study, a reduction of the NO concentrations at 72–96 h of life was measured in the serum of newborns suffering moderate to severe hypoxic-ischemic encephalopathy following allopurinol treatment. This was associated with an amelioration of the poor neurologic outcome at 12 months of life (Gunes et al. 2007). Nevertheless, a meta-analysis of various therapeutic essays realized for this indication has not been able to show a beneficial effect of allopurinol on mortality or on progression of neonatal convulsions (Chaudhari and McGuire 2012). More recently, clinical trials have been initiated to test the therapeutic potential of allopurinol in perinatal brain damage (Kaandorp et al. 2015).

127.4.3.2 *N*-Acetylcysteine

N-Acetylcysteine (NAC) induces the production of glutathione which permits the clearance of free radicals. In various animal models, especially those of maternal-fetal infection, a robust neuroprotective effect has been found which is accompanied by a reduction of oxidative stress, of proinflammatory cytokine production, and of apoptosis (Paintlia et al. 2004; Wang et al. 2007). No secondary effects were observed when NAC was administered to humans in the framework of clinical studies. In the premature infant, systemic parenteral nutritional supplementation neither modified the mean mortality at 36 weeks of gestation nor the frequency of retinopathy, periventricular leukomalacia, or intraventricular hemorrhage (Soghier and Brion 2006). A randomized controlled clinical study is currently being performed in children. Recently, in a rabbit model of perinatal white matter damage induced by systemic inflammation, it has been shown that low doses of NAC bound to nanoparticle dendrimers specifically target activated microglia leading to significant neuroprotection (Kannan et al. 2012).

127.4.3.3 Melatonin

Melatonin is a hormone that participates in sleep regulation and that is secreted physiologically by the pineal gland. Its role as a neuroprotector has been shown in several animal models in the framework of degenerative diseases such as acute brain lesions. Melatonin is well tolerated and crosses the BBB passively. Two of the implicated mechanisms seem to dominate its neuroprotective effects. First, its antioxidant effect can inhibit the NO synthase and lipid peroxidation as well as RNA degradation favoring the transcription of other antioxidant enzymes. Further, in acute lesion rodent models, melatonin favors axonal outgrowth with a long-term improvement of neurocognitive function in comparison to the control animals (Husson et al. 2002; Bouslama et al. 2007; Gonzalez-Burgos et al. 2007). In addition, in a preclinical pig model of term encephalopathy, melatonin was shown to enhance protection afforded by hypothermia (Robertson et al. 2013). Clinical trials are ongoing to test protective effects of melatonin in preterm infants, and it is very likely that similar trials will be set up in the future for term infants.

127.4.4 Prevention of Protracted Cell Death and Modulation of Plasticity

Possible strategies against apoptotic cell death or those that favor mechanisms of reparation are particularly interesting because the treatment window relative to the initial damage is particularly large.

127.4.4.1 Erythropoietin

Erythropoietin (EPO) is a hematopoietic growth factor whose secretion is induced by hypoxia. It is also a ubiquitous cytokine for which receptors exist on cells of the central nervous system. Moreover, it is currently applied in its recombinant form (rEPO) in neonatal medicine for treatment of anemia of prematurity and because of that has also been tested in experimental animal models regarding its effect on lesions of the developing brain. Experimental data have demonstrated an antiapoptotic effect and this effect is accompanied by a reduction of proinflammatory cytokines, a reduction of oxidative stress, a recuperation of the energetic level, and an increase of trophic factors involved in reparative processes (Kumral et al. 2004; Kumral et al. 2007; Kaindl et al. 2008; Xiong et al. 2009). In animal models, often, high doses of rEPO are applied (higher than those currently used in the human newborns), and the beneficial effects are dose-dependent (Xiong et al. 2009). Using the currently applied doses, no study has been able yet to show a beneficial effect on brain development (Ohls et al. 2004). Due to concern regarding increased side effects, a clinical trial in term neonates with encephalopathy has been placed on hold. Additional trials might be necessary to establish risks and benefits of such a treatment in addition to hypothermia. In preterm neonates, a large clinical trial has shown significant benefit on early brain imaging but unfortunately the follow-up at 2 years of age did not confirm the benefit on neurodevelopmental scores (O'Gorman et al. 2015; Natalucci et al. 2016).

127.4.4.2 Hypothermia

Beginning in the early 1990s, hypothermia has been the focus of several animal studies regarding its neuroprotective effect following hypoxia-ischemia or traumatic brain injury. Results of these studies have indicated that hypothermia reduces secondary energy breakdown, oxidative stress, BBB rupture extent, and apoptotic cell death (for review see Thoresen 2000). These studies have allowed us to determine the window for effective therapy initiation (within 6 h of life), the duration of therapy (72 h), and the ideal cooling temperatures (33–35 °C). Clinical studies have allowed us to establish the relative innoxiousness of moderate hypothermia in the term newborn and have only shown individual cases of sinus bradycardia and thrombopenia without hemorrhage. Two cooling procedures have been applied in these clinical studies with the indication of hypoxic-ischemic encephalopathy stage II or III: (1) selective head cooling using a cooling cap with a maintenance of the body temperature at 34.5 °C and a gradient between the scalp (25 °C) and the deep brain structures (35 °C) and (2) a cooling of the entire body to 33.5 °C leading to a homogenous cooling of the cerebral structures. So far, clinical studies have not demonstrated convincingly a difference between the two currently available protocols. Several clinical studies in the newborn suffering from a stage II or III encephalopathy have been reviewed in a meta-analysis (Edwards et al. 2010). The latter strongly supported the notion that moderate hypothermia has a benefit on mean mortality and severe handicap at 18 months of age (Jacobs et al. 2007). However, the benefit is partial with about eight kids to treat for one child without disability, pointing to the need for additional therapies to be combined with hypothermia. In addition, in a rodent model of combined systemic inflammation and hypoxic-ischemic insult, it was shown that hypothermia was not efficient (Osredkar et al. 2015; Osredkar et al. 2014), suggesting that the etiology of brain damage in neonates influences the efficacy of neuroprotective strategies. The importance of infection/inflammation in term infants is being increasingly understood and may be a key for better patient stratification and application of therapies (discussed in Fleiss et al. 2015).

127.4.4.3 Xenon

Xenon is an odorless noble gas that acts to block the NMDA subtype of the glutamate receptor, and in doing so xenon inhibits a key step in the neurotoxic cascade (Franks et al. 1998). In addition, xenon activates the 2-pore K^+ channel, inhibits the calcium/calmodulin-dependent protein kinase II, activates antiapoptotic effectors Bcl-xl and Bcl-2 (Ma et al. 2005; Ma et al. 2006), and induces expression of hypoxia-inducible factor 1a and its downstream effectors erythropoietin and vascular endothelial growth factor, which can interrupt the apoptotic pathway (Ma et al. 2009). Xenon has been shown to reduce injury in small and large animals of perinatal hypoxia-ischemia with and without co-application of hypothermia (Ma et al. 2005; Hobbs et al. 2008; Dingley et al. 2006; Martin et al. 2007; Thoresen et al. 2009). Of note, in a preclinical model of HI in the piglet, xenon plus hypothermia demonstrates robust neuroprotection (Faulkner et al. 2011). Xenon is an attractive neurotherapeutic agent as it has positive effects on cardiovascular stability (Coburn et al. 2005), myocardial protective properties (Preckel et al. 2002), and ability to rapidly cross the blood–brain barrier due to its very low blood–gas partition coefficient (Goto et al. 1997). Unfortunately, xenon is expensive and must be used with a closed-circuit delivery and recycling systems.

Clinical trials for xenon augmented hypothermia have recently reported their first data (Toby Xenon trial), unfortunately, with no improvement in early brain integrity via MRI and it is unknown if further trials will be performed.

127.4.4.4 Argon

Argon is another inert noble gas that is available at a cost 200 times lower than Xenon. *In vitro* and in vivo models of cerebral ischemia demonstrate robust neuroprotection, for which the therapeutic window lasts up to 3 h (Loetscher et al. 2009; Ryang et al. 2011; Zhuang et al. 2012). Argon is capable of increasing gamma-aminobutyric acid (GABA) neurotransmission by acting at the benzodiazepine binding site of the $GABA_A$ receptor under hyperbaric conditions (Abraini et al. 2003). Argon has also been seen to have oxygen-like properties (Soldatov et al. 2008), to increase antiapoptotic signaling via increased expression of Bcl-2 (Zhuang et al. 2012), and enhancement of the ERK 1/2 activity in astrocytes, neurons, and microglia by direct activation of the MEK/ERK 1/2 pathway (Fahlenkamp et al. 2012). A recent study of the adjunct neuroprotection by argon together with hypothermia in the piglet model of HIE has demonstrated even greater protection than that using xenon in this model (Hassell et al. 2014).

127.4.4.5 Postischemic Conditioning

Ischemic preconditioning describes brief non-cell-lethal episodes of ischemia which confer protection against a subsequent sustained period of severe ischemia in the same organ and was first described in the myocardium in 1986 (Murry et al. 1986). Ischemic postconditioning (IPostC) was developed following its discovery (Vinten-Johansen et al. 2005a, b) and is defined as intermittent interruptions in blood flow at the time of reperfusion *after* the severe ischemia in the same organ (Zhao and Vinten-Johansen 2006). IPostC has an obvious therapeutic advantage over preconditioning regarding timing. The benefits of IPostC appear to be mediated by similar molecular pathways (Pignataro et al. 2008), namely the reperfusion injury salvage (RISK) signaling pathway (made up of several survival kinases such as P13-kinase/Akt and ERK1/2). The neuroprotective effects of activation of this cascade are the inhibition of the mitochondrial permeability transition pore (MPTP) opening via inhibition of glycogen synthase kinase-3ß (GSK-3ß) through ERK activation, increased NO through Akt activation, and reduced intracellular Ca^{2+} levels (Barrere-Lemaire et al. 2012). Of particular interest is that IPostC has been shown to be effective even if performed on a nonvital organ such as a limb remote to the affected organ – remote IPostC (RIPostC) (Ren et al. 2009). Use of a remote limb makes IPostC a feasible clinical treatment strategy. In addition, RIPostC provides long-term neuroprotection if initiated 3 or 6 h after the initial ischemia in small animal adult (Ren et al. 2009; Sun et al. 2012) and neonatal (Zhou et al. 2011) experimental stroke models. This makes it likely that RIPostC could be implemented clinically. In a preclinical piglet model of HIE, five bursts of RIPostC on the hind limb were able to reduce cell death and improve mitochondrial function (Ezzati et al. 2016).

127.4.4.6 Future Directions

Behind the drugs rapidly approaching clinical trials are a battery of novel neurotherapeutic targets for which therapies are being designed and validated in animal models. Mitochondrial dysfunction is a key cellular event in the development of brain injury following hypoxic-ischemic encephalopathy (Hagberg et al. 2014) and thus interventions designed to protect mitochondrial integrity in the hours following hypoxia-ischemia should thus safeguard neuronal survival providing additional neuroprotection for infants where hypothermia alone is inadequate. Although there are currently no mitoprotective therapies in clinical trial, treatments reducing mitochondrial permeabilization post injury show promising results in in vivo models (Wang et al. 2010; Nijboer et al. 2013; Nijboer et al. 2011). However, intervention earlier in the cascade would prevent the initiation of mitochondrial damage. Caspase-2 is an early responder in the apoptotic cell death pathway and is highly expressed at birth. Genetic inhibition offers significant protection after both HI injury and ibotenate-induced excitotoxicity in neonatal rodents (Carlsson et al. 2011). Furthermore, after HI injury, caspase-2 knockout mice showed enhanced neuroprotection when subjected to hypothermia (Carlsson et al. 2012). Intravenous injection of a caspase-2-derived pentapeptide inhibitor provided significant neural protection in three rodent models of immature brain injury models. Importantly for translation, the inhibitor crossed the blood brain barrier, had negligible toxicity, did not alter physiological parameters, or affect developmental apoptosis when tested in rodents and larger animals (Chauvier et al. 2011; Sifringer et al. 2012).

In addition to the well-characterized mitochondrial permeabilization, disruptions in mitochondrial dynamics are emerging as a consequence of hypoxic-ischemic insult in mice and in vitro. Alterations in cristae, distribution, and increases in mitochondrial fission have been reported (Puka-Sundvall et al. 2000; Northington et al. 2007; Baburamani et al. 2015; Sanderson et al. 2015) although whether these changes are detrimental per se or an attempt at survival through enhancing quality control mechanisms (e.g., mitophagy) is, as yet, unknown.

A novel concept in the treatment of perinatal brain injury is that of delayed injurious processes, lasting in weeks, months, and years after injury.

These processes include glial reactivity, and it is increasingly considered that targeted immunomodulatory therapies might be applied in this delayed window to improve outcome (for review see Fleiss and Gressens 2012). A delayed and wide therapeutic window creates opportunities for using drugs with toxicity profiles that are unsuitable in the acute period or that may have incremental benefits hidden from view in normal acute therapy trials.

127.4.5 Stem Cell Therapy

The development of an adequate protocol for stem cell culturing and application has permitted envisaging the use of these cells for the reparation of cerebral lesions. While some studies but not all have shown a positive effect of stem cell therapy on the lesion size/extent and/or outcome following brain lesions, it is not clear yet whether the stem cells themselves or factors secreted by stem cells mediate the positive effect. If stem cells integration is important for their effect, these cells need to proliferate, find the site of lesion and differentiate into an adequate cell type (e.g., neuron, oligodendrocyte), and integrate into the tissue to be functional. The ethical problem associated with the use of human stem cells is less evident in mesenchymal stem cells that can be taken from cord blood or when induced pluripotent stem cells (iPS) are used. Such cells permit an autologous transplant and do not entail the problem of immune tolerance of the transplanted cells. Several clinical studies using cord blood-derived stem cells are currently being performed in children with perinatal brain insults. However, in our view, the preclinical studies do not seem sufficient to design the optimum clinical trial (see, Fleiss et al. 2014).

A further intriguing alternative to treatment with stem cells is to stimulate the production of endogenous neuronal stem cells. It has already been shown that stem cells accumulate in the subventricular zone following an acute brain lesion. These results open a new perspective: the stimulation of this stem cell population to support the physiological reparation processes of a lesion. Still, these cells will need to integrate and function correctly in the damaged tissue (for review, see Vawda et al. 2007). Moreover, stimulation of stem cell proliferation bears the potential risk, even if mitigated, of cancer induction.

127.5 Neuroprotective Strategies and the Reality

The field of perinatal brain injury is fortunate to currently have numerous trials of neurotherapeutic underway (including for melatonin and magnesium). Each of these trials is logistically and economically challenging but holds great promise to improve the lives of many thousands of children and their families. To justify a clinical trial, a therapy must display robust protection across species and variations in models of injury. Failures in clinical trials where there is a wealth of robust animal data (such as the failed Toby Xenon trials) remind translational neurobiologists of two critical points. Firstly, that any animal model has striking genetic and physiological differences to human infants, and secondly that animal models lack the heterogeneous injury observed in human infants, for whom we know very little in real terms regarding the severity, duration, and specific nature of their brain injury. The first issue cannot be fully abrogated, although it is surprising (even with their ethical concerns) that more drugs are not validated in primate models prior to clinical trials. The second issue is being approached via work on biomarkers – molecules in the fluids and tissues accessible to the clinician from which a robust indicator of the severity/type/progression of an injury could be ascertained. Biomarkers will allow for patient identification and stratification and we believe could facilitate the reevaluation of previously failed neurotherapeutic (such as thyroid hormones for preterm infants; see Schang et al. 2014) based on patient tailored application.

127.6 Conclusion

The neuroprotective concept and protocols for neuroprotective strategies have been largely developed through experimental studies. Despite the success of hypothermia and magnesium sulfate, application in humans is still limited due to the difficulties of performing clinical studies in infants with drugs that have for the most part not been FDA or EMA approved at that age in their primary indication, due to the heterogeneity of the population and the mostly moderate results in animal models. Moreover, a worldwide systematization of clinical studies on neuroprotective strategies is needed. Since the pathologies are inhomogeneous, several molecules or techniques may need to be combined to further ameliorate the neurologic prognosis.

References

Abraini J et al (2003) Gamma-aminobutyric acid neuropharmacological investigations on narcosis produced by nitrogen, argon, or nitrous oxide. Anesth Analg 96 (3):746–749

Baburamani AA et al (2015) Mitochondrial Optic Atrophy (OPA) 1 processing is altered in response to neonatal hypoxic-ischemic brain injury. Int J Mol Sci 16 (9):22509–22526

Barrere-Lemaire S, Nargeot J, Piot C (2012) Delayed postconditioning: not too late? Trends Cardiovasc Med 22(7):173–179

Boardman JP et al (2006) Abnormal deep grey matter development following preterm birth detected using deformation-based morphometry. Neuroimage 32 (1):70–78

Bouslama M et al (2007) Melatonin prevents learning disorders in brain-lesioned newborn mice. Neuroscience 150(3):712–719

Candelario-Jalil E (2008) Nimesulide as a promising neuroprotectant in brain ischemia: new experimental evidences. Pharmacol Res 57(4):266–273

Candelario-Jalil E et al (2007) Cyclooxygenase inhibition limits blood–brain barrier disruption following intracerebral injection of tumor necrosis factor-alpha in the rat. J Pharmacol Exp Ther 323(2):488–498

Carlsson Y et al (2011) Genetic inhibition of caspase-2 reduces hypoxic-ischemic and excitotoxic neonatal brain injury. Ann Neurol 70(5):781–789

Carlsson Y et al (2012) Combined effect of hypothermia and caspase-2 gene deficiency on neonatal hypoxic-ischemic brain injury. Pediatr Res 71(5):566–572

Chaudhari T, McGuire W (2012) Allopurinol for preventing mortality and morbidity in newborn infants with hypoxic-ischaemic encephalopathy. Cochrane Database Syst Rev 7:CD006817

Chauvier D et al (2011) Targeting neonatal ischemic brain injury with a pentapeptide-based irreversible caspase inhibitor. Cell Death Dis 2:e203

Coburn M et al (2005) Randomized controlled trial of the haemodynamic and recovery effects of xenon or propofol anaesthesia. Br J Anaesth 94(2):198–202

Dingley J et al (2006) Xenon provides short-term neuroprotection in neonatal rats when administered after hypoxia-ischemia. Stroke 37(2):501–506

Doyle LW et al (2009) Antenatal magnesium sulfate and neurologic outcome in preterm infants: a systematic review. Obstet Gynecol 113(6):1327–1333

Edwards AD et al (2010) Neurological outcomes at 18 months of age after moderate hypothermia for perinatal hypoxic ischaemic encephalopathy: synthesis and meta-analysis of trial data. BMJ 340:c363

Ezzati M et al (2016) Immediate remote ischemic postconditioning after hypoxia ischemia in piglets protects cerebral white matter but not grey matter. J Cereb Blood Flow Metab 36(8):1396–1411

Fahlenkamp A et al (2012) The noble gas argon modifies extracellular signal-regulated kinase 1/2 signaling in neurons and glial cells. Eur J Pharmacol 674(2–3):104–111

Faulkner S et al (2011) Xenon augmented hypothermia reduces early lactate/*N*-acetylaspartate and cell death in perinatal asphyxia. Ann Neurol 70(1):133–150

Favrais G et al (2007) Cyclooxygenase-2 mediates the sensitizing effects of systemic IL-1-beta on excitotoxic brain lesions in newborn mice. Neurobiol Dis 25 (3):496–505

Fernandez-Gomez FJ et al (2005) Minocycline fails to protect cerebellar granular cell cultures against malonate-induced cell death. Neurobiol Dis 20 (2):384–391

Fleiss B, Gressens P (2012) Tertiary mechanisms of brain damage: a new hope for treatment of cerebral palsy? Lancet Neurol 11(6):556–566

Fleiss B et al (2014) Stem cell therapy for neonatal brain injury. Clin Perinatol 41:133–148

Fleiss B et al (2015) Inflammation-induced sensitization of the brain in term infants. Dev Med Child Neurol 57 (Suppl 3):17–28

Fox C et al (2005) Minocycline confers early but transient protection in the immature brain following focal cerebral ischemia-reperfusion. J Cereb Blood Flow Metab 25(9):1138–1149

Franks NP et al (1998) How does xenon produce anaesthesia? Nature 396(6709):324

Garrido-Mesa N, Zarzuelo A, Galvez J (2013) Minocycline: far beyond an antibiotic. Br J Pharmacol 169(2):337–352

Gonzalez JC et al (2007) Neuroprotectant minocycline depresses glutamatergic neurotransmission and Ca (2+) signalling in hippocampal neurons. Eur J Neurosci 26(9):2481–2495

Gonzalez-Burgos I et al (2007) Long-term study of dendritic spines from hippocampal CA1 pyramidal cells, after neuroprotective melatonin treatment following global cerebral ischemia in rats. Neurosci Lett 423 (2):162–166

Goto T et al (1997) Xenon provides faster emergence from anesthesia than does nitrous oxide-sevoflurane or nitrous oxide-isoflurane. Anesthesiology 86(6): 1273–1278

Gunes T et al (2007) Effect of allopurinol supplementation on nitric oxide levels in asphyxiated newborns. Pediatr Neurol 36(1):17–24

Hagberg H et al (2014) Mitochondria: hub of injury responses in the developing brain. Lancet Neurol 13 (2):217–232

Hassell JK et al (2014) Argon augments hypothermic neuroprotection in a piglet model of perinatal asphyxia. In: Pediatric academic society meeting. Vancouver, Canada

Hobbs C et al (2008) Xenon and hypothermia combine additively, offering long-term functional and histopathologic neuroprotection after neonatal hypoxia/ischemia. Stroke 39(4):1307–1313

Homsi S et al (2010) Blockade of acute microglial activation by minocycline promotes neuroprotection and reduces locomotor hyperactivity after closed head injury in mice: a twelve-week follow-up study. J Neurotrauma 27(5):911–921

Husson I et al (2002) Melatoninergic neuroprotection of the murine periventricular white matter against neonatal excitotoxic challenge. Ann Neurol 51(1):82–92

Jacobs S et al (2007) Cooling for newborns with hypoxic ischaemic encephalopathy. Cochrane Database Syst Rev 4:CD003311

Kaandorp JJ et al (2015) Maternal allopurinol administration during suspected fetal hypoxia: a novel neuroprotective intervention? A multicentre randomised placebo controlled trial. Arch Dis Child Fetal Neonatal Ed 100(3):F216–F223

Kaindl AM et al (2008) Erythropoietin protects the developing brain from hyperoxia-induced cell death and proteome changes. Ann Neurol 64(5):523–534

Kannan S et al (2012) Dendrimer-based postnatal therapy for neuroinflammation and cerebral palsy in a rabbit model. Sci Transl Med 4(130):130ra46

Kobayashi K et al (2013) Minocycline selectively inhibits M1 polarization of microglia. Cell Death Dis 4:e525

Koistinaho M et al (2005) Minocycline protects against permanent cerebral ischemia in wild type but not in matrix metalloprotease-9-deficient mice. J Cereb Blood Flow Metab 25(4):460–467

Kumral A et al (2004) Selective inhibition of nitric oxide in hypoxic-ischemic brain model in newborn rats: is it an explanation for the protective role of erythropoietin? Biol Neonate 85(1):51–54

Kumral A et al (2007) Erythropoietin attenuates lipopolysaccharide-induced white matter injury in the neonatal rat brain. Neonatology 92(4):269–278

Lazarini F et al (2012) Early activation of microglia triggers long-lasting impairment of adult neurogenesis in the olfactory bulb. J Neurosci 32(11):3652–3664

Loetscher P et al (2009) Argon: neuroprotection in in vitro models of cerebral ischemia and traumatic brain injury. Crit Care 13(6):R206

Ma D et al (2005) Xenon and hypothermia combine to provide neuroprotection from neonatal asphyxia. Ann Neurol 58(2):182–193

Ma D et al (2006) Xenon preconditioning reduces brain damage from neonatal asphyxia in rats. J Cereb Blood Flow Metab 26(2):199–208

Ma D et al (2009) Xenon preconditioning protects against renal ischemic-reperfusion injury via HIF-1alpha activation. J Am Soc Nephrol 20(4):713–720

Marret S et al (2007) Magnesium sulphate given before very-preterm birth to protect infant brain: the randomised controlled PREMAG trial*. BJOG 114 (3):310–318

Martin JL et al (2007) Asynchronous administration of xenon and hypothermia significantly reduces brain infarction in the neonatal rat. Br J Anaesth 98 (2):236–240

McKee JA et al (2005) Analysis of the brain bioavailability of peripherally administered magnesium sulfate: a study in humans with acute brain injury undergoing prolonged induced hypermagnesemia. Crit Care Med 33(3):661–666

Murry CE, Jennings RB, Reimer KA (1986) Preconditioning with ischemia: a delay of lethal cell injury in ischemic myocardium. Circulation 74 (5):1124–1136

Natalucci G, Latal B, Koller B, Rüegger C, Sick B, Held L, Bucher HU, Fauchère JC, Swiss EPO Neuroprotection Trial Group (2016) Effect of early prophylactic high-dose recombinant human erythropoietin in very preterm infants on neurodevelopmental outcome at 2 years: a randomized clinical trial. JAMA 315(19):2079–2085. https://doi.org/10.1001/jama.2016.5504

Ng SY et al (2012) Attenuation of microglial activation with minocycline is not associated with changes in neurogenesis after focal traumatic brain injury in adult mice. J Neurotrauma 29(7):1410–1425

Nijboer CH et al (2011) Targeting the p53 pathway to protect the neonatal ischemic brain. Ann Neurol 70 (2):255–264

Nijboer CH et al (2013) Mitochondrial JNK phosphorylation as a novel therapeutic target to inhibit neuroinflammation and apoptosis after neonatal ischemic brain damage. Neurobiol Dis 54:432–444

Northington FJ et al (2007) Failure to complete apoptosis following neonatal hypoxia-ischemia manifests as :"continuum" phenotype of cell death and occurs with multiple manifestations of mitochondrial dysfunction in rodent forebrain. Neuroscience 149 (4):822–833

O'Gorman RL et al (2015) Tract-based spatial statistics to assess the neuroprotective effect of early erythropoietin on white matter development in preterm infants. Brain 138(Pt 2):388–397

Ohls RK et al (2004) Neurodevelopmental outcome and growth at 18 to 22 months' corrected age in extremely low birth weight infants treated with early erythropoietin and iron. Pediatrics 114(5):1287–1291

Osredkar D et al (2014) Hypothermia is not neuroprotective after infection-sensitized neonatal hypoxic-ischemic brain injury. Resuscitation 85(4):567–572

Osredkar D et al (2015) Hypothermia does not reverse cellular responses caused by lipopolysaccharide in

neonatal hypoxic-ischaemic brain injury. Dev Neurosci 37(4–5):390–397
Paintlia MK et al (2004) *N*-acetylcysteine prevents endotoxin-induced degeneration of oligodendrocyte progenitors and hypomyelination in developing rat brain. J Neurosci Res 78(3):347–361
Perlman JM (2006) Intervention strategies for neonatal hypoxic-ischemic cerebral injury. Clin Ther 28 (9):1353–1365
Pignataro G et al (2008) In vivo and in vitro characterization of a novel neuroprotective strategy for stroke: ischemic postconditioning. J Cereb Blood Flow Metab 28(2):232–241
Preckel B et al (2002) Xenon produces minimal haemodynamic effects in rabbits with chronically compromised left ventricular function. Br J Anaesth 88(2):264–269
Puka-Sundvall M et al (2000) Subcellular distribution of calcium and ultrastructural changes after cerebral hypoxia-ischemia in immature rats. Brain Res Dev Brain Res 125(1–2):31–41
Ren C et al (2009) Limb remote ischemic postconditioning protects against focal ischemia in rats. Brain Res 1288:88–94
Robertson NJ et al (2013) Melatonin augments hypothermic neuroprotection in a perinatal asphyxia model. Brain 136(Pt 1):90–105
Roumier A et al (2008) Prenatal activation of microglia induces delayed impairment of glutamatergic synaptic function. PLoS One 3(7):e2595
Ryang Y et al (2011) Neuroprotective effects of argon in an in vivo model of transient middle cerebral artery occlusion in rats. Crit Care Med 39(6):1448–1453
Sanchez Mejia RO et al (2001) Minocycline reduces traumatic brain injury-mediated caspase-1 activation, tissue damage, and neurological dysfunction. Neurosurgery 48(6):1393–1399; discussion 1399–1401
Sanderson TH, Raghunayakula S, Kumar R (2015) Neuronal hypoxia disrupts mitochondrial fusion. Neuroscience 301:71–78
Schang AL, Gressens P, Fleiss B (2014) Revisiting thyroid hormone treatment to prevent brain damage of prematurity. J Neurosci Res 92:1609–1610
Sfaello I et al (2005) Topiramate prevents excitotoxic damage in the newborn rodent brain. Neurobiol Dis 20 (3):837–848
Sifringer M et al (2012) Prevention of neonatal oxygen-induced brain damage by reduction of intrinsic apoptosis. Cell Death Dis 3:e250
Soghier LM, Brion LP (2006) Cysteine, cystine or *N*-acetylcysteine supplementation in parenterally fed neonates. Cochrane Database Syst Rev 4:CD004869
Soldatov P et al (2008) Physiologically active argon-based gas mixtures as a means of creating fire-safe gaseous environments in pressurized modules of varying purpose. Aviakosm Ekolog Med 42(2):45–52
Sriram K, Miller DB, O'Callaghan JP (2006) Minocycline attenuates microglial activation but fails to mitigate striatal dopaminergic neurotoxicity: role of tumor necrosis factor-alpha. J Neurochem 96(3):706–718
Stippler M et al (2007) Serum and cerebrospinal fluid magnesium in severe traumatic brain injury outcome. J Neurotrauma 24(8):1347–1354
Sugimoto J et al (2012) Magnesium decreases inflammatory cytokine production: a novel innate immunomodulatory mechanism. J Immunol 188(12):6338–6346
Sun J et al (2012) Protective effect of delayed remote limb ischemic postconditioning: role of mitochondrial K (ATP) channels in a rat model of focal cerebral ischemic reperfusion injury. J Cereb Blood Flow Metab 32 (5):851–859
Temkin NR et al (2007) Magnesium sulfate for neuroprotection after traumatic brain injury: a randomised controlled trial. Lancet Neurol 6(1):29–38
Thoresen M (2000) Cooling the newborn after asphyxia – physiological and experimental background and its clinical use. Semin Neonatol 5(1):61–73
Thoresen M et al (2009) Cooling combined with immediate or delayed xenon inhalation provides equivalent long-term neuroprotection after neonatal hypoxia-ischemia. J Cereb Blood Flow Metab 29(4):707–714
Vawda R et al (2007) Stem cell therapies for perinatal brain injuries. Semin Fetal Neonatal Med 12(4):259–272
Vinten-Johansen J, Yellon DM, Opie LH (2005a) Postconditioning: a simple, clinically applicable procedure to improve revascularization in acute myocardial infarction. Circulation 112(14):2085–2088
Vinten-Johansen J et al (2005b) Postconditioning – a new link in nature's armor against myocardial ischemia-reperfusion injury. Basic Res Cardiol 100(4):295–310
Wang J et al (2004) Minocycline up-regulates Bcl-2 and protects against cell death in mitochondria. J Biol Chem 279(19):19948–19954
Wang X et al (2007) *N*-acetylcysteine reduces lipopolysaccharide-sensitized hypoxic-ischemic brain injury. Ann Neurol 61(3):263–271
Wang X et al (2010) Neuroprotective effect of Bax-inhibiting peptide on neonatal brain injury. Stroke 41(9):2050–2055
Xiong Y, Chopp M, Lee CP (2009) Erythropoietin improves brain mitochondrial function in rats after traumatic brain injury. Neurol Res 31(5):496–502
Zhao ZQ, Vinten-Johansen J (2006) Postconditioning: reduction of reperfusion-induced injury. Cardiovasc Res 70(2):200–211
Zhou Y et al (2011) Remote limb ischemic postconditioning protects against neonatal hypoxic-ischemic brain injury in rat pups by the opioid receptor/Akt pathway. Stroke 42(2):439–444
Zhuang L et al (2012) The protective profile of argon, helium, and xenon in a model of neonatal asphyxia in rats. Crit Care Med 40(6):1724–1730

Cerebral Hemorrhage in Newborns 128

Linda S. de Vries and Axel Heep

Contents

Abstract

Hemorrhagic lesions of the central nervous system (CNS) occur during the fetal, perinatal, and postnatal period. Due to the timing of the hemorrhage and the vulnerability of the developing brain, hemorrhagic lesions are associated with specific morbidity and mortality.

Germinal matrix hemorrhage-intraventricular hemorrhage (GMH-IVH) is still a common and serious condition in premature infants. Especially a large GMH-IVH, often complicated by posthemorrhagic ventricular dilation or associated with a unilateral parenchymal hemorrhage, is associated with an increased risk of adverse neurologic sequelae.

The widespread use of cranial ultrasonography since the early 1980s has shown a gradual

L. S. de Vries (✉)
Department of Neonatology, Wilhelmina Children's Hospital, University Medical Center, Utrecht, The Netherlands
e-mail: l.s.devries@umcutrecht.nl

A. Heep
Department of Neonatology, Southmead Hospital, North Bristol NHS Trust, Bristol, UK
e-mail: axel.heep@nbt.nhs.uk

G. Buonocore et al. (eds.), *Neonatology*,
https://doi.org/10.1007/978-3-319-29489-6_275

decrease in the incidence of GMH-IVH and has helped with the identification of risk factors and timing of the lesion. The increased use of magnetic resonance imaging (MRI) has contributed to better define the site and extent of the lesion and to visualize associated white matter (WM) damage as well as associated cerebellar hemorrhages.

Hemorrhagic lesions of the CNS in the fetal period are associated with vascular malformation, thrombophilic disorders, and rarely brain malignancies. Perinatally acquired hemorrhagic CNS lesions in the full-term infant are associated with sinovenous thrombosis or traumatic parenchymal hemorrhage related to assisted vaginal deliveries.

Abbreviations

CSF	Cerebrospinal fluid
CSVT	Cerebral sinovenous thrombosis
CT	Computed tomography
cUS	Cranial ultrasound
DQ	Developmental quotient
DRIFT	Drainage intervention fibrinolytic therapy
ECMO	Extracorporeal membrane oxygenation
GMH-IVH	Germinal matrix hemorrhage-intraventricular hemorrhage
HPI	Hemorrhagic parenchymal infarction
iNO	Inhaled nitric oxide
IPL	Intraparenchymal Lesion
MRI	Magnetic resonance imaging
NIRS	Near-infrared spectroscopy
NAITP	Neonatal alloimmune thrombocytopenia
PVHI	Periventricular hemorrhagic infarction
PVL	Periventricular leukomalacia
PLAI	Platelet surface antigen
PLIC	Posterior limb of the internal capsule
PHVD	Posthemorrhagic ventricular dilatation
VI	Venous infarction
VM	Ventriculomegaly

128.1 Salient Points

- A large GMH-IVH is still seen in 5–10% of VLBW infants.
- Unilateral parenchymal hemorrhage is due to impaired venous drainage and is often associated with the development of hemiparesis.
- Hemiparesis following PVHI can be predicted with conventional MRI performed at term-equivalent age or with DTI-MRI performed at 30 weeks of postmenstrual age showing asymmetry of the PLIC.
- PHVD is especially common following a large GMH-IVH.
- Best timing for intervention of PHVD is still to be determined.
- Impaired neurodevelopmental outcome is also more common following small GMH-IVH and is related to reduced cerebral and cerebellar volumes.
- IVH-PVHI and subdural hemorrhages also occur in full-term infants.
- Unilateral thalamic hemorrhage in the full-term infant is often associated with a sinovenous thrombosis.

128.2 Neonatal Intracranial Hemorrhage in Preterm Infants

In the late 1970s, computed tomography (CT) and shortly afterward cranial ultrasound (cUS) could be used for the first time to visualize intracranial lesions (Burstein et al. 1979). cUS initially used the temporal bone, but soon the anterior fontanelle was preferably used as an acoustic window. The first cUS studies used a low-resolution linear mechanical sector transducer, limiting the field of view to the lateral ventricles. The adjacent white matter was poorly visualized, until a mechanical sector scanner was introduced with a wider angle of insonation. Data collected in the early years is therefore very different from the data that can be obtained today, using high-resolution cUS and color Doppler studies as well as magnetic resonance imaging (MRI). Since the more routine use of neonatal MRI, it has become clear that injurious processes to the vulnerable white matter of the preterm infant are of more importance than the hemorrhages in the germinal matrix and the ventricles (GMH-IVH). Lesions that were in the past visualized as GMH-IVH are often associated with subtle injury to the white matter, which can either be entirely overlooked using cUS or underestimated. Associated hemorrhages in the cerebellum are common, and punctate hemorrhages will not be diagnosed with cUS even when using the mastoid window (Parodi et al. 2015a). Long-term outcome data of preterm infants studied in the 1980s with cUS therefore need to be interpreted with care. A decline in the incidence in severe white matter lesions, referred to as cystic periventricular leukomalacia (PVL), has been reported (Hamrick et al. 2004; Khwaja and Volpe 2008), but although a decline in the overall incidence of GMH-IVH has been reported as well, no decline has been noted by several groups for the more severe grades of GMH-IVH, and these severe hemorrhagic lesions will still have a major impact on neurodevelopmental outcome (Hamrick et al. 2004; Khwaja and Volpe 2008; Batton et al. 1994). Using more acoustic windows than the anterior fontanelle, for example, the mastoid window, hemorrhagic lesions of the cerebellum have increasingly been recognized, especially in the very immature and extremely low birth weight infant (Parodi et al. 2015a; Limperopoulos et al. 2005; Steggerda et al. 2009a).

128.3 Neuropathology and Pathogenesis

The germinal matrix area is highly vascularized and is described as an "immature vascular rete" as the vessels within the germinal matrix are primitive and cannot be classified as arterioles, venules, or capillaries. It is a transient structure and is initially the site where neuroblast and glioblast mitotic activity occurs, before cells migrate to other parts of the brain. Once cell division and migration is complete, the germinal matrix progressively decreases in size with regression being almost complete by term-equivalent age. The subventricular zone (SVZ) becomes the predominant site of cell generation after around 15 weeks, when it starts to expand rapidly in some sites, forming prominent ganglionic eminences along the lateral walls of the frontal (and to a lesser extent the temporal) horns of the lateral ventricles. The ganglionic eminence (GE) is the source of neocortical GABAergic inhibitory interneurons. The dorsal telencephalic SVZ, which gives rise to projection neurons early in gestation, previously has been considered to be principally gliogenic after 20 weeks of gestation. In contrast to some years back, it is now generally accepted that the SVZ actively generates neurons until at least 25–27 weeks. Approximately 35% of these later arriving neurons are generated from the ventral GE (Volpe 2009). The germinal matrix area is most abundant over the head and body of the caudate nucleus but is also seen in the roof of the temporal horn. It regresses gradually in a site-specific manner with final gross involution of the GE by 34–36 weeks of gestation.

MRI has recently confirmed the abundance of the germinal matrix and has shown that smaller GMHs are often seen on MRI in the temporal horn, which were not identified on cUS (Parodi et al. 2015b; Plaisier et al. 2015). More than a third of cases from a large autopsy series from New Jersey with a germinal matrix hemorrhage had involvement of the temporal or occipital germinal matrix (Paneth et al. 1994). The arterial supply of the germinal matrix is from the recurrent artery of Heubner (a branch of the anterior cerebral artery), as well as terminal branches of the lateral striate arteries. Venous drainage of the deep white matter occurs through a fan-shaped leash of short and long medullary veins through which blood flows into the germinal matrix and subsequently into the terminal vein which lies below the germinal matrix (Takashima et al. 1986). This has led to the understanding of a unilateral parenchymal hemorrhage, which is now considered to be due to venous infarction (Gould et al. 1987) or to a reperfusion injury following an ischemic insult.

It is most often considered that hemorrhage arises from the thin-walled veins (Volpe 1989; Moody et al. 1994; Ghazi-Birry et al. 1997), although Pape and Wigglesworth (1979) suggested from their injection studies that capillary bleeding was more common than terminal vein rupture. Developmental anomalies of the cerebral venous system are known to predispose to intracranial hemorhage. MR imaging venography studies

(Tortora et al. 2016, 2018) have demonstrated an increased variability in subependymal vein anatomy in preterm infants. Preterm infants presenting with a narrower curvature of the terminal proportion of subependymal veins were found to have significantly increased incidence of GMH-IVH (Tortora et al. 2018). Serial cUS studies describe the onset of GMH-IVH at a mean of 24–48 h following delivery. However, approximately 10% of GMH-IVH cases are already present at first cUS examination within the first 12 h of life. This *early GMH-IVH* might be related to a different underlying pathogenesis related to the multifactorial etiology of GMH-IVH. Ment et al. (1995a) have suggested that the germinal matrix vessels change significantly over the first days of life to greater continuity of the basement membrane. Rapid maturation of the germinal matrix vessels, presumably as a consequence of early birth, may be one of the reasons why GMH-IVH usually occurs during the first few days of life.

GMH-IVH causes mechanical disruption of the ventricular lining facilitating the release of blood and neural cells populating the periventricular subependymal germinal matrix into the cerebrospinal fluid. Evidence from neuropathology studies, and animal models of neonatal hydrocephalus, demonstrates disruption of the germinal matrix and migration of neural progenitor cells into the CSF (Jiménez et al. 2009; Rodríguez et al. 2012; Krueger et al. 2006).

Animal studies have recently demonstrated that the increased metHb formation in the intraventricular space following GMH-IVH is associated with periventricular inflammation (Gram et al. 2013). Microglial and astrocytic activation following IVH and subsequent inflammation has been shown to be a primary event leading to white matter brain damage in preterm infants (Khwaja and Volpe 2008; Volpe et al. 2011).

128.4 Risk Factors Related to the Pre- and Perinatal Period

In the *antenatal* period, histological signs of amniotic infection have been shown to increase the risk of GMH-IVH (Thorp et al. 2001). A correlation was shown between raised blood cytokine concentrations and altered hemodynamic function (Yanowitz et al. 2002).

In another study, the presence of clinical maternal chorioamnionitis was associated with an increased risk of early sepsis (OR, 5.54; 95% [CI] 2.87–10.69) and severe intraventricular hemorrhage (OR, 1.62; 95% [CI] 1.17–2.24), adjusting in a multivariate regression analysis for illness severity (Soraisham et al. 2009).

Increased interleukin-6 serum concentrations, a surrogate of early sepsis, measured within the first 12 h postpartum, were found to be associated with the development and extent of GMH-IVH in preterm infants born $<$ 28 weeks of gestation (Heep et al. 2003).

Several clinical studies have implicated that the reduced coagulation profile in preterm infants, in particular the diminished vitamin K-dependent prothrombin activity, is involved in the pathogenesis of GMH-IVH in preterm infants (Salonvaara et al. 2005; Poralla et al. 2011; Neary et al. 2013; Duppre et al. 2015). In addition to the immaturity of hemostasis, coexisting perinatal risk factors adversely affect the vitamin K-dependent coagulation pathway (Poralla et al. 2012). So far, prophylactic substitution of plasmatic coagulation components or fresh frozen plasma has failed to reduce the incidence of GMH-IVH in preterm infants (Waltl et al. 1973; Beverley et al. 1985; Northern Neonatal Nursing Initiative Trial Group 1996; Veldman et al. 2006; Dani et al. 2009).

First small trials looking at the efficacy of antenatal maternal vitamin K substitution and the incidence of GMH-IVH were initially promising (Liu et al. 2006; El-Ganzoury et al. 2014), but a review on this topic concludes that "Vitamin K administered to woman prior to very preterm birth has not been shown to significantly prevent periventricular haemorrhage in preterm infants or to improve neurodevelopmental outcomes in childhood" (Crowther et al. 2010).

There is no evidence that cesarean section protects the premature infant against GMH-IVH. In a hospital-based study in preterm infants with a birth weight of $\leq$1,250 g, no beneficial effect was shown of an elective cesarean section on either reduced mortality or neuro-disability at 2 years of age (Haque et al. 2008). Breech delivery is in some studies associated with a higher risk of large GMH-IVH, but this effect was lost in a multivariate analysis (Herbst and Källén 2007). In another study, a positive effect was shown for the most immature infants with a gestation <27 weeks (Thorp et al. 2001). A reduced mortality, but not a reduced risk of a GMH-IVH, was recently reported in a Swedish population-based study for preterm infants with a gestation of 25–36 weeks (Herbst and Källén 2007).

The importance of delayed cord clamping was suggested by Mercer et al., showing a reduction in GMH-IVH, with 5 [14%] in the delayed clamping group versus 13 [36%] in the non-delayed group ($P = 0.03$) (Mercer et al. 2006). The impact of delayed cord clamping on IVH was evaluated adjusting for gestational age and cesarean section. The final model indicated that the IVH rate was >3 times higher in the immediate cord clamping group ([OR]: 3.5, 95% [CI] 1.1–11.1). In a systematic review by Rabe et al., there were no significant differences for infant deaths, but a significant difference in the incidence of all grades IVH, but not grade III or IV, in 10 of the 15 published studies enrolling 539 infants (RR 0.59, 95% CI 0.41–0.85) (Rabe et al. 2008). It was suggested that this could be due to a higher flow in the superior vena cava following delayed cord clamping (Heuchan et al. 2002).

It has also been suggested that infants born outside a perinatal center and transported in have a higher incidence of GMH-IVH (Thorp et al. 2001; Palmer et al. 2005). Data from the NEOPAIN trial did show that outborn babies were more likely to have severe IVH ($p = 0.0005$), and this increased risk persisted after controlling for severity of illness, but when adjustments were made for use of antenatal steroids, the effect of birth center was no longer significant (Palmer et al. 2005). It has been suggested that underlying clinical variables rather than the transport explain the increased risk of GMH-IVH (Osborn et al. 2003).

Cardiovascular and respiratory problems have always been considered to play a major role in the development of a GMH-IVH in the immediate *neonatal* period. Fluctuations of the intravascular pressure or blood flow may lead to the rupture of the "immature vascular rete" in the germinal matrix, and occurrence of a hemorrhage is known to occur during reperfusion following a period of hypotension.

Early assessment of the superior vena cava flow (SVCF), within the first few hours after birth, has been used as surrogate parameter of cerebral perfusion (Drayton and Skidmore 1987; Sirc et al. 2013). Early studies have shown that repetitive measure of low SVCF within the first 24 h was preceding a GMH-IVH (Kluckow and Evans 2000). However, recent studies performing single assessment of SVCF within the first 24 h of life did not confirm SVCF measured at the first day of life as an independent risk factor for GMH-IVH (Holberton et al. 2012; Bates et al. 2015).

Although the possible lack of cerebral autoregulation, rendering the cerebral circulation "pressure-passive," is still considered important, it is not present in all preterm infants (Tsuji et al. 2000). Continuous monitoring with near-infrared spectroscopy may be a useful tool in the identification of infants at risk (Soul et al. 2007). Two recent studies looked at the value of NIRS. In one, using continuous NIRS and MABP measurements, MABP-rScO2 correlation suggested more blood pressure-passive brain perfusion in infants with an IVH (Alderliesten et al. 2013). In the other study, a lower systemic perfusion and cerebral blood flow (CBF) followed by an increase in these variables were found to precede the development of GMH-IVH (Noori et al. 2014).

Respiratory risk factors can occur with complications during mechanical ventilation, such as vasodilatation secondary to hypercapnia, for instance, following a pneumothorax (Fabres et al. 2007). Improvement in ventilatory techniques and increased use of noninvasive ventilatory support such as CPAP and even BIPAP are likely to further reduce the incidence of GMH-IVH. A recent clinical multicenter study confirmed a significant reduction in the incidence of pneumothorax (4.8% vs. 12.6%; $P = 0.04$) and severe intraventricular hemorrhage (10.3% vs. 22.1%; $p = 0.02$) studying early postnatal surfactant application using a less invasive surfactant application (LISA) strategy without invasive ventilation in preterm infants less than 27 weeks of gestational age (Kribs et al. 2015).

The role of hypernatremia (>150 mmol/L) has also been identified as an independent risk factor in the development of a GMH-IVH. High sodium levels are especially common in extremely preterm infants, the group also especially at risk to develop GMH-IVH (Dalton et al. 2015; Barnette et al. 2010).

128.4.1 Genetic Factors

More recently, there has been an interest in the role of thrombophilic disorders in the development of GMH-IVH. These factors included heterozygosity for factor V Leiden mutation, which renders factor V resistant to cleavage by activated protein C, methylenetetrahydrofolate (MTHFR) mutation, and heterozygosity for prothrombin G20210A mutation, which was found to be associated with raised plasma concentrations of prothrombin. A large prospective study was unable to confirm previously reported associations of abovementioned gene variants and development of intraventricular hemorrhage in very low birth weight infants (Härtel et al. 2006). Interleukin-6 CC genotype increased the risk of the development of severe hemorrhagic lesions ([OR]: 3.5; 95% [CI]: 1.0–12.2; *P* 0.038) (Harding et al. 2004). This observation could however not be confirmed in a considerably larger sample size (Göpel et al. 2006).

The impact of genetic variants in the vitamin K-dependent coagulation system on the development of GMH-IVH has been looked at studying polymorphisms in the genes encoding vitamin K epoxide reductase complex 1 (VKORC1 – 1639G>A) and coagulation factor 7 (F7 -323Ins10) in a cohort of 90 preterm infants <32 weeks of gestational age (Schreiner et al. 2014). In this small study, F7-323Ins10 genotype was associated with lower factor VII levels, however not with individual GMH-IVH risk. A logistic regression analysis described a higher GMH-IVH risk in VKORC1 wild type, compared to carriers of the -1639A allele, supporting the assumption that genetic variants influence the vitamin K-dependent coagulation profile and thereby the IVH risk in preterm infants.

Antenatal porencephaly can be associated with a mutation in the collagen 4A1 or 4A2 gene (*COL4A1 and COLAA2*) encoding procollagen type 4 α1 and 4 α2, a basement membrane protein (de Vries et al. 2009; Meuwissen et al. 2015).

A *reduced risk* of GMH-IVH was found with maternal preeclampsia, which appears to be due to enhanced in utero maturation of the fetus, associated with a reduced risk of postnatal development of respiratory distress (Spinillo et al. 2007).

In a systematic review, inhaled nitric oxide (iNO) in intubated preterm infants did not show a clear effect of iNO on the frequency of all grades of IVH or of severe IVH. Early rescue treatment was associated with a nonsignificant 20% increase in severe IVH. There was no effect on the incidence of neurodevelopmental impairment (Barrington and Finer 2010).

128.5 Incidence of GMH-IVH

The incidence of GMH-IVH is directly related to the maturity of the infant (Thorp et al. 2001). Initial studies in the late 1970s and early 1980s showed an incidence as high as 40–50% in those weighing <1,500 g (Burstein et al. 1979; Dolfin et al. 1983), but these numbers have come down to 20% in the 1990s according to some studies (Batton et al. 1994; Heuchan et al. 2002) but not according to others (Gleissner et al. 2000). The average incidence of a unilateral parenchymal hemorrhage varies from 3% to 11% with the lowest incidence coming from a French population-based study (de Vries et al. 2001; Lemons et al. 2001; Larroque et al. 2003). No decrease in this type of lesion was seen by Hamrick et al. (2004) in contrast to their decrease in cystic white matter disease and in a recent study by Sarkar (Sarkar et al. 2009).

128.6 Diagnosis

Even though MRI is increasingly being used, GMH-IVH is still more likely to be diagnosed during routine bedside cUS. Performing ultrasound as part of the admission procedure, and several times during the first week, will allow the most accurate timing and identification of antenatal onset of the lesion. Almost all hemorrhages will have developed by the end of the first week after birth and most within the first 24–28 hours after birth. Only about 10% of the GMH-IVH occurs beyond the end of the first week, in contrast to white matter injury, where late onset is not uncommon (Andre et al. 2001). Progression from a small GMH-IVH to a parenchymal hemorrhage can occur, and this is most likely related to impaired venous drainage of the medullary veins in the white matter with obstruction at the site of the germinal matrix (de Vries et al. 2001).

Clinical diagnosis does not play a major role, as most of the GMH-IVH will be silent. Three clinical syndromes have been described in the past (Volpe 2008a), the first one being associated with a *catastrophic* deterioration, with a sudden deterioration of the clinical state of the infant, such as a sudden fall in blood pressure and/or metabolic acidosis. It is however more common to find a sudden fall in hemoglobin without a clear change in the condition of the child. The second clinical syndrome is the *salutatory* one, with a more gradual onset, presenting with a change in general movements. Most commonly the *silent*, asymptomatic syndrome is seen, and this can even occur in infants who show a parenchymal hemorrhage on a routine repeat ultrasound examination.

The classification system suggested by Volpe (2008a) is suitable to describe early and late ultrasound appearances (Table 1). The use of grade IV is avoided and a separate description of the size, site, and appearance of a parenchymal lesion is preferred, and a hemorrhage in the parenchyma is usually referred to as periventricular hemorrhagic infarction (PVHI). Making a distinction between a small hemorrhage restricted to the germinal matrix or a GMH with some blood ruptured through the ependyma into the ventricular lumen is not always possible. An improvement in the diagnosis of a small IVH by using the posterior fontanelle as an alternative acoustic window has been advocated by Correa et al. (2004) (Fig. 1). GMHs at sites, other than the head of the caudate nucleus, like the roof of the temporal horn, often remain undiagnosed and will only be diagnosed when an MRI is also performed (Parodi et al. 2015a; Plaisier et al. 2015; Maalouf et al. 2001).

Table 1 Ultrasound description of GMH-IVH, adapted from Volpe (2008)

Description	Generic term
Grade I: Germinal matrix hemorrhage	GMH
Grade II: Intraventricular hemorrhage without ventricular dilatation	GMH-IVH
Grade III: Intraventricular hemorrhage with acute ventricular dilatation (clot fills >50 % of the ventricle)	GMH-IVH and ventriculomegaly
Intraparenchymal lesion – describe size, location	IPL

The diagnosis of a large IVH can be confidently made with US, although associated white matter damage and/or associated cerebellar hemorrhages may be more reliably diagnosed with early MRI (Figs. 2 and 3). Distinction of a large, bulky choroid plexus, which is common in very immature infants, from a large IVH is not always easy, and sequential examinations and an examination through the posterior fontanelle and high-resolution color Doppler studies may aid in making this distinction. Blood can acutely dilate the ventricle or can lead to posthemorrhagic ventricular dilatation (PHVD) a few weeks later, and the larger the amount of blood, the more likely this will subsequently occur. Blood will rapidly spread through the foramen of Monro into the third ventricle, the aqueduct of Sylvius, the fourth ventricle, and the foramina of Magendie and Luschka to eventually spread into the posterior fossa. Clot formation can occur at any level and lead to outflow obstruction, but it is most commonly seen at the level of the aqueduct or more diffusely in the posterior fossa. Using the mastoid view and color

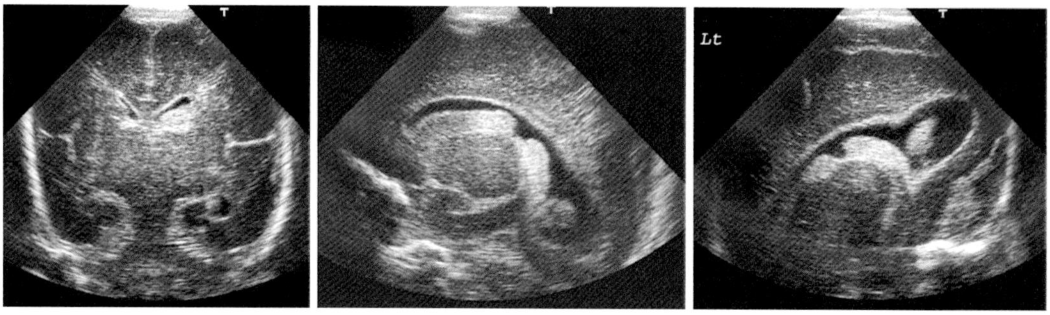

Fig. 1 Cranial ultrasound of a preterm infant born at 29 weeks of GA, coronal and parasagittal views, taken through the anterior (*left*, *middle*) and posterior (*right*) fontanelle, showing an intraventricular clot and a dilated occipital horn

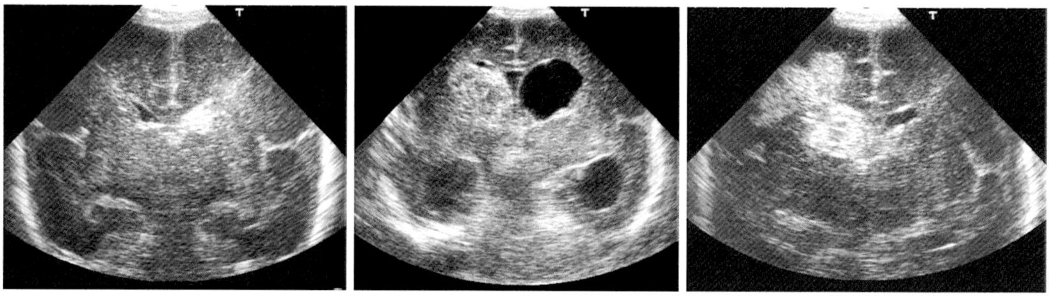

Fig. 2 Cranial ultrasound, coronal views, of three preterm infants, showing a small IVH with focal ipsilateral periventricular echogenicity (*left*), a large right-sided intraventricular hemorrhage with acute ventricular dilatation (*middle*), and a parenchymal hemorrhage and large IVH on the right

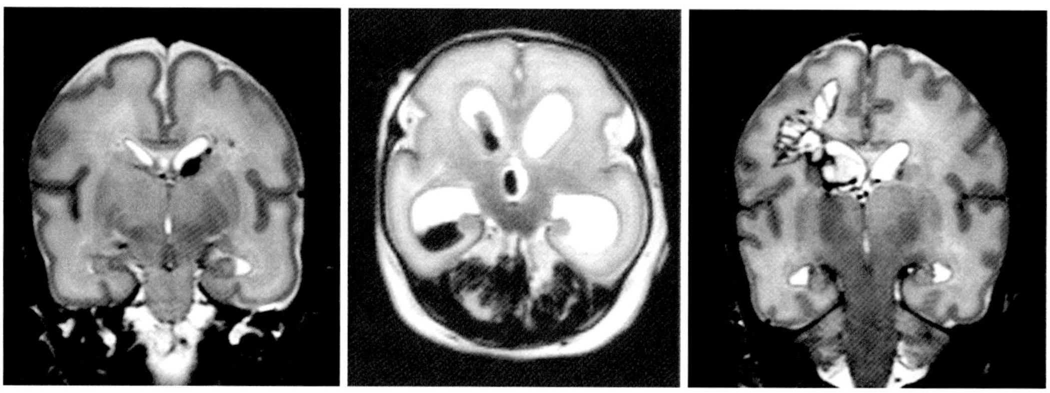

Fig. 3 MRI (T2-weighted sequence) of the three preterm infants shown in Fig. 2; IVH associated with petechial hemorrhage in the left periventricular white matter (*left*); besides large IVH, bilateral cerebellar hemorrhages are seen (*middle*); IVH and PHI, similar to cUS (*right*)

Doppler studies in patients developing progressive PHVD, one can assess the aqueduct, which usually appears patent within the first 2–3 weeks following a GMH-IVH, providing an opportunity for CSF drainage via lumbar tap. A sudden change of dynamics including progressive dilatation of the third ventricle and the absence of cellular components or clot particles reflecting the

Doppler signal likely indicates obstruction of CSF flow. Depending on the degree of blood and the site of obstruction, PHVD can be rapidly progressive and noncommunicating, usually due to obstruction at the level of the aqueduct of Sylvius, or be of more gradual in onset, communicating and considered to be due to obliterative arachnoiditis (Larroche 1972; Robinson 2012).

A unilateral parenchymal hemorrhage, referred to in the literature as periventricular hemorrhagic infarction (PVHI) or venous infarction (VI), accounts for 3–15% of all GMH-IVH (de Vries et al. 2001; Lemons et al. 2001; Larroque et al. 2003). It is usually unilateral, triangular in shape, with the apex at the outer border of the lateral ventricle and associated with a moderate to large ipsilateral GMH-IVH. It has been thought in the past that parenchymal hemorrhage was due to direct extension of hemorrhage into the periventricular white matter, but this is no longer considered to be the most likely explanation for this type of parenchymal lesion. Most would now agree that this type of lesion is caused by the presence of GMH-IVH which can lead to impaired venous drainage and subsequent venous infarction of the medullary veins of the white matter. This sequence of events can sometimes be followed by sequential ultrasound examinations, changing from a normal image to a stage of simple GMH-IVH and involvement of the parenchyma on the following day. While this type of lesion used to be globular and would usually communicate with the lateral ventricle with subsequent evolution into a porencephalic cyst, more recently this pattern has been shown to be more variable, with a more discrete parenchymal lesion, which does not necessarily communicate with the lateral ventricle and can evolve into few small cysts in the white matter that may resolve with eventual ex vacuo dilatation on the affected side. These white matter cysts can be misinterpreted as unilateral cystic leukomalacia, but seeing the evolution of this unilateral lesion with sequential ultrasound examinations would not be in favor for leukomalacia, which is almost invariably bilateral and not often associated with a large IVH. MRI performed later in infancy or early childhood will also help to make a distinction between the two conditions, showing more focal injury in those with a unilateral parenchymal hemorrhage. Detailed studies by Dudink et al. (2008) have made it possible to identify the veins that were involved in the parenchymal injury. A proposal was made by Bassan et al. (2006) to grade the severity of this parenchymal lesion, taking the extent of the lesion, the presence of a contralateral parenchymal lesion, and also the presence of a midline shift due to this lesion into account. The grading system also helped to predict neurodevelopmental outcome at 2 years of age (Bassan et al. 2007).

128.6.1 Intracerebellar Hemorrhage

One of the important and recent changes, when discussing GMH-IVH in the preterm infants, is the improved recognition of intracerebellar hemorrhages. This type of lesion is most often associated with a GMH-IVH and is especially common in those with a birth weight <750 g and a gestational age below 27 weeks (Limperopoulos et al. 2005; Steggerda et al. 2009b). Twenty-five of the 35 infants studied by Limperopoulos et al. (2005) had a unilateral hemispheric hemorrhage. Of the 35 infants, 27 also had supratentorial lesions. Apnea, bradycardia, and a falling hematocrit may be associated with this type of lesion (Steggerda et al. 2009b). Ultrasonography can be diagnostic when the lesion is larger than 4 mm and provided the posterolateral fontanelle is used as the acoustic window (Limperopoulos et al. 2005; Steggerda et al. 2009b). Ecury-Goossen et al. describe six presentations of cerebellar hemorrhage in their clinical cohort: subarachnoid, folial, lobar, bilateral lobar, giant lobar including vermis, and contusional cerebellar hemorrhage (Ecury-Goossen et al. 2010). MRI will give better definition of the extent of the lesion and will also identify punctate lesions in the cerebellar hemisphere (Steggerda et al. 2009b). Follow-up at a mean age of 32 months showed neurologic abnormalities in 66% of the infants with isolated cerebellar hemorrhagic injury compared with 5% of the control preterm infants (Limperopoulos et al. 2007). Infants with isolated cerebellar hemorrhagic injury versus controls had severe motor disabilities (48% vs. 0%), expressive language (42% vs. 0%), delayed receptive language (37% vs. 0%), and cognitive deficits (40% vs. 0%). Preterm infants with cerebellar hemorrhagic injury and supratentorial parenchymal injury were not at overall greater risk for neurodevelopmental disabilities, although neuromotor impairment was more severe. Cerebellar atrophy without apparent cerebellar hemorrhage has also been reported as a common sequel of severe immaturity (Messerschmidt et al. 2005). Srinivasan et al. (2006) only showed reduced cerebellar volume in preterm infants at term-equivalent age in association with supratentorial pathology such as hemorrhagic parenchymal infarction, intraventricular hemorrhage with dilation, and periventricular leukomalacia. Quantitative MRI using tractography showed reduced fractional anisotropy (FA) values in the superior cerebellar peduncle in extremely preterm infants with a low-grade GMH-IVH compared with controls (Morita et al. 2015). They suggest that this is due to hemosiderin disposition in the proximity to the SCP, the most vulnerable WM tract in the cerebellum. In another study, low-grade IVH led to disturbed cerebellar development, with cerebellar volume reduction shown by volumetric analysis (Tam et al. 2011).

128.7 Management

Once the diagnosis of a GMH-IVH is made, immediate clinical management will not be different from other at-risk preterm infants. Optimizing of any coagulopathy, minimal handling, prevention of fluctuations in blood pressure or CO_2 levels, and prevention of breathing against the ventilator may be used trying to prevent extension of the initial hemorrhage. Continuous (a) EEG registration may help to detect subclinical seizures, which will often be subclinical and may require treatment (Olischar et al. 2007). The presence of aEEG seizures is significantly associated with the presence of an IVH. The aEEG background pattern was adversely affected by the presence of a severe hemorrhage. Among 92 infants with a GA <32 weeks, a low-voltage aEEG was present in 4 out of 14 (28.6%) infants with a severe grade III hemorrhage or a PVHI, and a significant relationship was noted between the presence of low-voltage tracings and death ($p = 0.015$) and the combined neurological lesion/death outcome ($p = 0.01$) (Benavente-Fernández et al. 2015). Similar findings were reported in another study by Soubasi et al. (Soubasi et al. 2012). Pathological tracings (burst suppression, continuous low voltage, flat trace) or discontinuous low voltage (DLV), the absence of cyclicity, and lower border <3 μV in the initial aEEG had a sensitivity of 88.9%, 63%, and 51.9%, respectively, for severe brain injury (grade III/PVHI as well as c-PVL). In a study enrolling 30 extremely preterm infants, a burst suppression pattern with low voltage was identified in 57% of the infants with severe intracranial hemorrhage (grade III/PVHI), whereas no infant without a hemorrhage showed this aEEG background pattern ($P = 0.014$) (Chalak et al. 2011). Among 92 preterm infants with a GA <30 weeks, a high seizure burden, diagnosed on the aEEG, was found to be associated with an increased risk of a severe GMH-IVH on day 3 (RR 4.0, 95% CI 1.5–10.8) (Vesoulis et al. 2014).

128.7.1 Posthemorrhagic Ventricular Dilatation (PHVD)

Especially in those infants with a large IVH with or without associated parenchymal hemorrhage, posthemorrhagic ventricular dilatation (PHVD) may develop over the next 10–14 days. Repeat US scans are therefore indicated to timely diagnose this complication. PHVD can progress either slowly or rapidly. In the majority of cases (65%), slowly progressive PHVD is followed by spontaneous arrest. In the remaining 30–35% of infants with PHVD, ventricular size increases rapidly over the course of days to weeks (Murphy et al. 2002).

There is no agreement whether treatment of progressive PHVD before the occurrence of clinical symptoms is beneficial to the child. Increase in ventricular size, as assessed with repeated ultrasound examinations, will precede any clinical symptoms, such as a rapid increase in head circumference (>2 cm/week), diastasis of the sutures, a full fontanelle, vomiting, irritability, bradycardias, and apneas, by several weeks, due to the large extracerebral space and the high water content of the white matter (Ingram et al. 2014). Sun setting will only be seen at a late stage. Measurements are usually taken in the coronal view at the foramen of Monro, using the "ventricular width," according to Levene and Starte (1981). The "ventricular index" is the distance between the midline and the lateral border of the ventricle. Most intervention studies have taken the p97+ 4 mm as a starting point for randomization. Another useful measurement is the so-called anterior horn width, taken just anterior of the thalamic notch (Davies et al. 2001). This anterior horn width measurement does not change much with increasing maturation and should be <3 mm and measurements >6 mm suggest PHVD. Measuring the occipital horn in a sagittal plane can also be useful, as there can be a discrepancy between dilatation of the anterior and posterior horn. Although the angle of insonation may be more variable in the sagittal plane, any measurement of the occipital horn ≥25 mm also does suggest severe PHVD (Whitelaw and Aquilina 2012). As there were no infants included in the dataset from Levene and Starte (1981) with a gestational age below 26 weeks, new cross-sectional and longitudinal reference data for the VI, AHW and TOD were published, with an age range between 24 and 42 weeks (Brouwer et al. 2012). Obtaining a midsagittal view allows the assessment of the third and fourth ventricle. A discrepancy between a large third and a small fourth ventricle would suggest an obstruction at the level of the aqueduct, while a dilatation of an outflow obstruction due to obstruction of the foramen of Luschka and Magendie. In both situations, it is not recommended to perform a lumbar puncture. Assessing the shape of the lateral ventricles may be useful, when making a distinction between pressure-driven PHVD and ex vacuo dilatation following white matter injury. Measuring the cerebrospinal fluid pressure may also aid in making a distinction, but reliable measurements can be hard to obtain (Kaiser and Whitelaw 1985).

Adverse short-term effects of PHVD on the central nervous system have been shown using different techniques, including evoked potentials, aEEG, Doppler ultrasonography, and near-infrared spectroscopy (NIRS) (Soul et al. 2004; van Alfen-van der Velden et al. 2007; Klebermass-Schrehof et al. 2013). Cerebrospinal fluid (CSF) measurements of cytokines, nonprotein-bound iron, hypoxanthine, and sFas were all noted to be raised in infants with PHVD and especially so in those with associated periventricular leukomalacia (Sävman et al. 2002; Felderhoff-Mueser et al. 2003; Heep et al. 2004a; Schmitz et al. 2007). In spite of all these data, there is no direct evidence that early drainage of CSF alters the natural and long-term outcome of children with PHVD. In the two largest RCT so far, randomization was done once the 97th centile + 4 mm line was crossed and 60% of the infants in both arms subsequently required shunt placement (Ventriculomegaly Trial Group 1994; Kennedy et al. 2001). The RCT for DRIFT (drainage intervention fibrinolytic therapy) also used this measurement as an entry point for the study (Whitelaw et al. 2003). The initial data were promising with shunt requirement in 22%, but the RCT was stopped early, due to a high risk (33%) of secondary bleeding in the DRIFT group, without an apparent positive effect on the need for a ventriculoperitoneal shunt (Whitelaw et al. 2007). Severe cognitive disability in survivors and overall death or severe disability was significantly reduced in the DRIFT group. Of 39 infants assigned to DRIFT, 21 (54%) died or were severely disabled versus 27 of 38 (71%) in the standard group (adjusted odds ratio 0.25 [95% confidence interval: 0.08–0.82]). Among the survivors, 11 of 35 (31%) in the DRIFT group had severe cognitive disability versus 19 of 32 (59%) in the standard group (adjusted odds ratio: 0.17 [95% confidence interval: 0.05–0.57]). Median Mental Development Index was 68 with DRIFT and <50 with standard care (Whitelaw et al. 2010).

A recently performed RCT enrolled 126 preterm infants ≤34 weeks gestation with progressive PHVD following a severe IVH. Treatment was either started at a low threshold (LT) with VI >p97 and AHW >6 mm or at a higher threshold (HT) with VI>p97+4 mm and AHW>10 mm.

There was no significant difference between the two groups for the primary outcome, being death and / or VP shunt placement (30% LT and 37% for HT infants). A VP shunt was inserted in 12/64 (19%) in the LT and 14/62 (23%) infants in the HT group, the lowest rate reported so far in the literature. More neurosurgical interventions were required in the LT group. Neurodevelopmental outcome will determine whether very early intervention is required or whether using effective intervention started as soon as the VI has crossed the 97th centile +4mm line is sufficient. (de Vries et al. 2018).

In two retrospective observational studies, a significant reduction in the need for shunt placement was noted, when intervention was started before this line was crossed and when the threshold for inserting a subcutaneous reservoir was low (de Vries et al. 2002; Brouwer et al. 2008). In another retrospective study performed in 32 preterm infants, with ten infants receiving early external ventricular drainage (≤25 days of life) and 22 infants late intervention (>25 days of life), early intervention was associated with better scores for adaptive, personal social, communication, and cognitive functions. The incidences of cerebral palsy and neurosurgical complications were equal for the two groups. The beneficial effect was only seen in infants with a grade III IVH and not in those with parenchymal injury (Bassan et al. 2012). In another study 18-24 month neurodevelopmental outcome was compared between preterm infants with and without intervention within cohorts undergoing either an early approach in Dutch centres or late approach in a Canadian centre. The study showed that infants undergoing intervention at an early stage, even when eventually requiring a VP shunt, had outcomes indistinguishable from infants without intervention, all being within the normal range. In contrast, later intervention for progressive PHVD was associated with an increased risk of unfavorable outcome and intervention-related complications (Leijser et al. 2018).

128.7.1.1 Outcome Following GMH-IVH

There is at present no agreement about the effect of low-grade GMH-IVH on neurodevelopmental outcome. In most studies reported so far, the diagnosis of a grade I or II GMH-IVH was based on an ultrasound diagnosis and associated more subtle lesions in the periventricular white matter, or lesions in the cerebellum may have been missed, which could explain why some infants in these studies have shown a less favorable outcome (van de Bor et al. 1984; Patra et al. 2006; Vavasseur et al. 2007; Beaino et al. 2011; Bolisetty et al. 2014; Vohr et al. 2014). In the EPIPAGE study, 6.8% and 8.1% of infants with a grade I and II GMH-IVH, respectively, developed cerebral palsy (CP) based on cUS rather than MRI data (Beaino et al. 2011). A third study reported outcome on an Australian cohort consisting of more than 2,000 preterm infants, with 515 (21.3%) infants with a grade I–II GMH-IVH diagnosed with cUS. The authors reported increased rates of neurosensory impairment, developmental delay, CP (10.4%), and deafness at 2–3 years of corrected age in those with a grade I–II GMH-IVH. The CP rate was quite high (6.8%) in those without cUS abnormalities (Bolisetty et al. 2014). Other studies of infants with mild grades of GMH-IVH (hemorrhage restricted to the germinal matrix or small amount of ventricular blood) suggest that these infants were performing as well in cognitive and motor developmental outcome as preterm infants with no GMH-IVH, although a lower score was found with regard to their visual-motor integration (Vohr et al. 1992; Payne et al. 2013; Ross et al. 1996). In a large cohort, no difference was found between those without a hemorrhage and those with a grade I–II GMH-IVH (Payne et al. 2013). In this study, there was quite a high percentage of infants who developed CP, 8% and 9% of infants without or with a grade I and grade II GMH-IVH, respectively, which might be explained by associated white matter injury not recognized with cUS. In a recent large cohort study, similar neurodevelopmental outcomes were noted for infants with grade I, II, and III GMH-IVH compared with infants without GMH-IVH, but they did find an increased risk of mild CP in infants with grade II (13%) and III (18%) GMH-IVH compared to those without a GMH-IVH (7%) (Radic et al. 2015). Neonatal 3D volumetric imaging studies, however, have shown reduced gray matter volumes at term-equivalent age (Vasileiadis et al. 2004) associated with a reduced MDI on the BSID-II, but this was only seen in the most immature infants with gestation below 30 weeks. Whether associated mild white matter abnormalities were present and could have played a role is not discussed in these studies. This association was previously suggested by Kuban et al. (1999).

The term ventriculomegaly (VM) has been used for infants with ventricular enlargement following a GMH-IVH but also for those without apparent preceding hemorrhage and are then more likely to be occurring due to white matter loss. It is therefore preferable to use VM in those without an apparent preceding large GMH-IVH and use the term posthemorrhagic ventricular dilatation (PHVD) when ventricular enlargement follows a large hemorrhage (Kuban et al. 1999; Ment et al. 1999). Having access to sequential ultrasound examinations and looking at the shape of the ventricles will enable us in most cases to make this important distinction.

The risk of a poor outcome has been reported to increase significantly with the presence of PHVD following a large GMH-IVH (40–60%) and even further in those who require shunt insertion (75–88%) (Ventriculomegaly Trial Group 1994; Fernell et al. 1993; Persson et al. 2006). In a cohort from Sweden, associated problems (cerebral visual impairment, epilepsy, and especially cognitive problems) were very common (Persson et al. 2006). In a retrospective hospital-based population study, outcome was considerably better than reported previously with cerebral palsy occurring in only 7.4% of the infants with a large IVH (grade III according to Papile) compared to 37 (48.7%) of the 76 infants with a parenchymal hemorrhage ($p < 0.001$). The mean developmental quotient (DQ) in the grade III group was 99 and in the grade IV group 95 at 24-month corrected age (Brouwer et al. 2008). Whether this better outcome was related to earlier treatment of PHVD or due to a cohort with more localized lesions and of higher GA needs to be confirmed and follow-up of a prospective randomized controlled trial is now underway (de Vries et al. 2018).

While the infants without apparent parenchymal involvement are more likely to develop diplegia, those with a venous infarction are more at risk of developing a hemiparesis. Outcome with unilateral parenchymal hemorrhage varies and depends on the extent and site of the lesion (Bassan et al. 2007; Rademaker et al. 1994) although others did not find the site of the lesion to be predictive (Roze et al. 2008). A recent score reported by Bassan et al. showed an association between a higher score, based on the presence of a more extensive lesion, a midline shift, or a bilateral parenchymal involvement and mortality and outcome at 2 years of age (Bassan et al. 2007). Long-term outcome into childhood and adolescence showed that most of the children with a parenchymal hemorrhage and subsequent porencephaly were ambulatory but required learning assistance in school and had social challenges (Sherlock et al. 2008; Roze et al. 2009).

Early prediction of development of a hemiparesis is now possible, using MRI at 40–42 weeks. Myelination of the posterior limb of the internal capsule (PLIC) should be present at term-equivalent age. In infants who go on to develop a hemiparesis asymmetry and even lack of myelination of the PLIC was noted (De Vries et al. 1999; Cowan and de Vries 2005). Using diffusion tensor imaging, visualization of the tracts can be possible at an earlier stage, and data were initially available in preterm-born children studied in childhood looking at thalamocortical connectivity, but similar observations could be made in preterm infants who had an MRI 3–4 weeks following the development of the PVHI (Counsell et al. 2007; Staudt et al. 2006; Roze et al. 2015).

128.7.1.2 Prevention of GMH-IVH in the Preterm Infant

Most studies have shown a reduction in the incidence of GMH-IVH over time. Both prenatal and postnatal pharmacologic prophylaxes have been used to reduce the incidence of GMH-IVH. Many different drugs have been used, such as phenobarbital, tranexamic acid, pancuronium, ethamsylate, vitamin E, and indomethacin. Only a few of these will be discussed here in more detail.

128.7.1.3 Antenatal Prevention

Antenatal Steroids

Antenatal administration of corticosteroids has been shown in several studies to be the most important protective factor for development of GMH-IVH (Ment et al. 1995b; Roberts et al. 2017). A systematic review of 16 randomized controlled trials involving over 6,000 babies has shown that corticosteroid administration is associated with a significant reduction in the risk of GMH-IVH (OR 0.55; CI 0.40, 0.76) and with a strong trend toward improving long-term neurologic outcome in survivors (OR 0.64; CI 0.14, 2.98) (Roberts et al. 2017). The effect of steroid administration could be due to a reduction in risk and severity of respiratory distress syndrome, postnatal stabilization of blood pressure, or maybe even a direct cerebral protective effect. Repeated courses of antenatal corticosteroids are not recommended as a negative effect on brain growth has been shown (Modi et al. 2001) without a further reduction on GMH-IVH or leukomalacia (Crowther and Harding 2007). Betamethasone instead of dexamethasone is recommended, as the latter was associated with an increased incidence of PVL (Baud et al. 1999).

Magnesium Sulfate

Antenatal administration of magnesium sulfate was not associated with a reduction in the incidence of either a small or a large GMH-IVH in a recent large randomized multicenter study (Crowther et al. 2003). A recent meta-analysis showed that antenatal magnesium sulfate therapy given to women at risk of preterm birth substantially reduced the risk of cerebral palsy in their children (relative risk [RR] 0.69; 95% confidence interval [CI] 0.54–0.87). The number needed to treat to prevent one case of cerebral palsy was 63 (95% CI 43–155). Moreover, there was a significant reduction in the rate of substantial gross motor dysfunction (RR 0.61; 95% CI 0.44–0.85) (Doyle et al. 2009).

Vitamin K

Antenatal, maternal Vitamin K administration has been used to prevent neonatal GMH-IVH, as vitamin K-dependent factors are deficient in preterm infants. Although the initial reports were promising, this was not supported by a recent systemic review comparing nine randomized studies involving 1,750 women to evaluate the role of vitamin K in the prevention of GMH-IVH, given to women in labor or very likely to deliver a premature infant. Only two trials were of sufficient quality to be used for the final analysis (Crowther et al. 2010; Morales et al. 1988; Pomerance et al. 1987).

128.7.1.4 Postnatal Prevention

Phenobarbital

The rationale for phenobarbital use was sedation of the preterm infant to prevent the fluctuations of blood pressure that occurs with clinical care of high-risk infants. Phenobarbital was the first drug that was used postnatally in the prevention of GMH-IVH. A meta-analysis of 12 trials showed no difference between the phenobarbital-treated group and the control group in either all IVH (typical risk ratio (RR) 0.91; 95% CI 0.77–1.08), severe IVH (typical RR 0.77; 95% CI 0.58–1.04), posthemorrhagic ventricular dilation (typical RR 0.89; 95% CI 0.38–2.08), severe neurodevelopmental impairment (typical RR 1.44; 95% CI 0.41–5.04), or death before hospital discharge (typical RR 0.88; 95% CI 0.64–1.21). There was a consistent trend in the trials toward increased use of mechanical ventilation in the phenobarbital-treated group, which was supported by the meta-analysis (typical RR 1.18; 95% CI 1.06–1.32; typical risk difference 0.129; 95% CI 0.04–0.21) (Smit et al. 2013).

Indomethacin

A meta-analysis on the postnatal use of indomethacin in the prevention of GMH-IVH and subsequent brain injury showed a significant reduction in the incidence of severe intraventricular hemorrhage (typical RR 0.66, 95% CI 0.53–0.82) (Fowlie and Davis 2010).

Outcome measures of death or severe neurosensory impairment were reported in four studies, but no significant effect of indomethacin could be found (RR 1.02; CI 0.90, 1.15) (Schmidt et al. 2001). A recent post hoc analysis of the original indomethacin trial suggested that boys exposed to indomethacin had significantly better outcome in verbal test scores than females, suggesting a gender-specific effect (Ment et al. 2006).

Ibuprofen

Ibuprofen is used as an alternative to indomethacin for use in the medical management of patent ductus arteriosus and acts in a similar manner by prostaglandin synthase inhibition. A recent RCT has evaluated whether ibuprofen when given shortly after birth to a group of premature infants (<28 weeks gestation) reduces the incidence of GMH-IVH (Dani et al. 2005). Ibuprofen did not reduce the incidence of any degree of GMH-IVH when compared to controls (OR 0.96 CI 0.48, 2.03) or more severe GMH-IVH (grade 2–4) (OR 0.87 CI 0.25, 3.05) compared with controls.

General Measurements

Paying closer attention to blood pressure, gentle handling, synchronous ventilation, and less severe respiratory distress syndrome due to antenatal corticosteroids and postnatal surfactant therapy was associated with a reduction in GMH-IVH (Wells and Ment 1995). Data from the Canadian network also showed that the incidence and severity of GMH-IVH are affected by NICU characteristics. A high patient volume and a high neonatologist/staff ratio were associated with a lower rate of severe IVH (Synnes et al. 2006).

128.7.1.5 Rare Intracranial Hemorrhage of the Preterm Infant

Traumatic Subdural Hemorrhage

Following assisted vaginal delivery of the preterm infant, cUS may present with increased extracerebral spaces indicating the development of subdural effusions, followed by a subdural hemorrhage. In most cases, this is a clinically inapparent finding not requiring neurosurgical management; however, coagulation profile and cUS examination including posterior fontanelle and lateral mastoid view should be performed to exclude parenchymal injury and cerebellar involvement.

Necrotizing Intracranial Hemorrhage in the Preterm Infant

Nosocomial infections particularly involving serratia marcescens, bacillus cereus, and proteus mirabilis in preterm infants are characterized by endotoxin secretion including specific hemolysins (Braun et al. 1992; Beecher 2002). These toxins are known to increase vascular permeability, causing extensive inflammation and hemolysis leading to tissue necrosis, hemorrhagic necrotizing encephalitis, and the development of brain abscess in bacillus cereus cases (Heep et al. 2004b).

In line with the clinical picture of the acute onset septic shock and coagulation derangement, cUS demonstrates the development of bilateral parenchymal hyperechogenicity and subacute cystic evolution of the parenchyma including intraventricular and parenchymal hemorrhage.

128.7.1.6 Intraventricular Hemorrhage in the Full-Term Infant

Intraventricular hemorrhage (IVH) is an uncommon problem in full term as compared to preterm neonates. Origins of the IVH can be the germinal matrix, choroid plexus, or parenchyma. The latter was recently reported as hemorrhagic parenchymal infarction (Armstrong-Wells et al. 2009). In term infants, only remnants of the germinal matrix remain. The incidence of germinal matrix hemorrhage is therefore considered to be low, but the true incidence is not really known, as infants are usually asymptomatic. The mechanism of IVH in term infants has been attributed to trauma at birth (precipitous delivery) or hypoxia; however, no etiology is detected in many cases. Recently, thalamic hemorrhage associated with an intraventricular hemorrhage was recognized to be related to cerebral sinovenous thrombosis (CSVT) involving the straight sinus (Wu et al. 2003; Kersbergen et al. 2009). The pathogenesis of thalamic hemorrhage is a hemorrhagic venous infarction of the large venous channels that are in close proximity to the ventricular walls. In the majority of infants, none of the previously associated risk factors for thalamic hemorrhage were noted, such as coagulation disorders or hypoxic-ischemic birth injury. Predisposing factors noted by Roland et al. (1990) included sepsis, cyanotic heart disease, and polycythemia.

Clinical symptoms (irritability, seizures, apnea, bulging fontanelle) occurred later than that seen in infants with IVH from choroid plexus or germinal matrix hemorrhage. Anticoagulation therapy can be considered to prevent propagation of the thrombosis (Kersbergen et al. 2009).

Management of IVH in term infants is supportive. Prognosis depends on the location and extent of the underlying insult. As a rule, among infants for whom no etiology of the IVH is detected, outcome appears to be good. Neurodevelopmental sequelae are seen in infants with IVH with parenchymal involvement (Jocelyn and Casiro 1992). When bilateral thalamic hemorrhage is associated with birth asphyxia, mortality is high and sequelae in survivors are high. Thalamic hemorrhage with IVH seen in infants with an uneventful birth history is associated with a greater risk for cerebral palsy than IVH from other sites.

Subdural Hemorrhage in Term Infants

Subdural and subarachnoid hemorrhages are probably under diagnosed, as they are difficult to recognize using cranial ultrasound. Subdural hemorrhage usually occurs secondary to birth trauma. These hemorrhages are relatively uncommon currently because of improvements in obstetric care. Vaginal breech deliveries, for instance, have become less common since recent multicenter-randomized studies (Hofmeyr and Hannah 2003). Occipital diastasis can occur during a vaginal breech delivery with excessive extension of the neck of the infant. The pathogenesis is secondary to mechanical injury to the cranium associated with instrumental delivery with forceps or ventouse extraction of the head, abnormal presentation (face or brow), precipitous delivery, and a large infant resulting in a difficult delivery, although others did not find an increased risk with assisted vaginal delivery and showed a prevalence of 26% following vaginal birth using MRI in a total of 97 infants (Volpe 2008b; Hanigan et al. 1995; Looney et al. 2007). There are shearing forces on the tentorium and the deep venous system. Children are usually born at term and present with a full fontanelle, lethargy, apneas, and/or seizures. Hydrocephalus can develop due to outflow obstruction and temporary external drainage, sometimes followed by permanent drainage, due to difficulties of CSF reabsorption at the level of the arachnoid granulations. Secondary cerebral infarction has also been reported and has been related to prolonged arterial compression (Govaert et al. 1992). The majority of the subdural hemorrhages are infratentorial, but a supratentorial location can also be noted and is then sometimes associated with a lobar hemorrhage, which can be large and associated with a shift of the midline, requiring neurosurgical intervention (Fig. 4). Short-term outcome in children with an isolated infratentorial subdural hemorrhage but also in those with a lobar hemorrhage has often been reported to be more favorable than expected, but the groups studied tend to be small (Hanigan et al. 1995; Chamnanvanakij et al. 2002).

Subgaleal Hemorrhage in Term Infants

Subgaleal hemorrhage is a rare and potentially fatal condition of the neonate often associated with instrumental delivery. It is caused by rupture of the emissary veins, which are connections between the dural sinuses and the scalp veins. Blood accumulates between the epicranial aponeurosis of the scalp and the periosteum. Most cases of subgaleal hemorrhage reported have been associated with the use of the vacuum extractor. The incidence of subgaleal hemorrhage is estimated to occur in 4–6 of 10,000 spontaneous vaginal deliveries and in 46–59 of 10,000 vacuum-assisted deliveries (Uchil and Arulkumaran 2003; Chadwick et al. 1996). The children will present with diffuse swelling of the head and evidence of hypovolemic shock. In a study by Kilani et al. (Kilani and Wetmore 2006), associated intracranial hemorrhage was present in half of the 34 infants studied and four (11.8%) infants died. In another study, 31% had a poor outcome (five died, four had epilepsy, three with severe auditory dysfunction, two with cerebral palsy, and one with renal vein thrombosis) (Chang et al. 2007). The group with the poor outcome had significantly more patients who had been transferred from other hospitals ($P < 0.001$). Those with a poor outcome had significantly more hypotension ($P < 0.001$) and

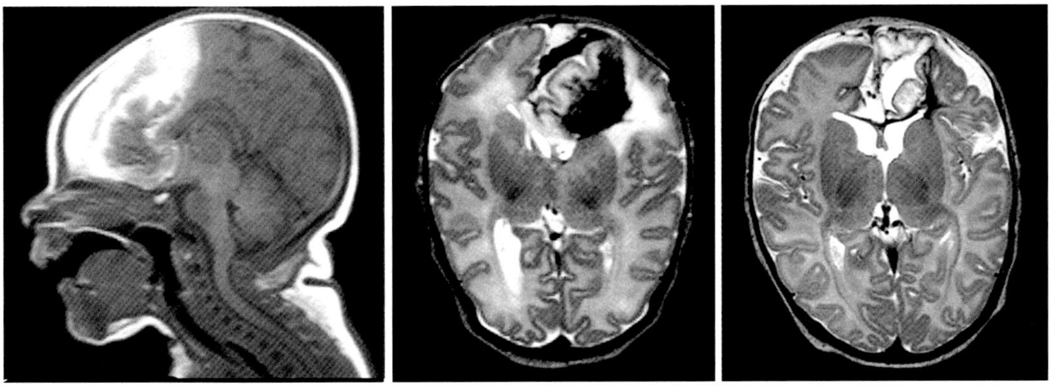

Fig. 4 Full-term infant, easy vaginal delivery, admitted with neonatal seizures. MRI on day 7 (*left* and *middle*) and at 3 months (*right*), showing a supratentorial subdural hemorrhage and a large frontal intraparenchymal hemorrhage, with a shift of the midline. A repeat scan at 3 months shows resolution of the hemorrhage and associated loss of brain tissue

seizures ($P < 0.05$). Prompt and aggressive administration of blood products and treatment of associated coagulopathy are recommended to improve outcome.

128.7.1.7 ICH in Other Specific Conditions in Full-Term Infants

Hypoxic Ischemic Encephalopathy

Newborn infants presenting with severe hypoxic-ischemic encephalopathy, in particular following placental abruption involving fetal blood loss requiring mass transfusion or GBS septicemia, may present with severe hypocoagulopathy and are likely to develop post-ischemic cerebral hemorrhage including subgaleal, subdural, and parenchymal hemorrhage (Forman 2014).

Neonatal Alloimmune Thrombocytopenia

In neonatal alloimmune thrombocytopenia (NAITP), fetal and neonatal thrombocytopenia results from the formation of a maternal antiplatelet antibody to a paternally derived platelet antigen, usually platelet surface antigen (PLAI), expressed on the surface of the fetal platelets. Neonatal alloimmune thrombocytopenia occurs in 1 in 2,000 to 1 in 5,000 fetuses. ICH occurs in as many as 10–30% of the infants with alloimmune thrombocytopenia, 25–50% of which occur in utero (Dale and Coleman 2002; Kamphuis et al. 2014). NAITP has an estimated mortality rate of 15%, with ICH accounting for most deaths. Fetal and neonatal platelet counts less than 20×10^9 are common even before 24 weeks' gestation, and repeated episodes of antenatal hemorrhage have been reported (Bussel et al. 1997). Management in the antenatal period includes administration of intravenous gamma globulin to the mother with or without corticosteroids prior to delivery (van der Lugt et al. 2015). Transfusion of matched compatible platelets to the fetus may protect against ICH during the birthing process. Abdominal delivery is suggested if cordocentesis reveals fetal thrombocytopenia. After birth, transfusion with antigen-negative platelets (maternal platelets) is recommended (Bussel and Sola-Visner 2009). Hemispheric porencephalic cyst, following a hemorrhage which is most commonly located within a temporal lobe, is usually present at birth, but extra-axial hemorrhages, intraventricular hemorrhage, acute parenchymal hemorrhage, and neuronal migrational disorder have also been reported (Dale and Coleman 2002).

Extracorporeal Membrane Oxygenation (ECMO)

ECMO is the treatment of choice in infants with persistent pulmonary hypertension and cardiorespiratory failure unresponsive to inhaled nitric oxide. In term infants, ICH following ECMO occurs in 10–13% of infants (Hardart and Fackler 1999; de Mol et al. 2008). The lesions are hemorrhagic with ischemia (60%) or hemorrhage alone (40%). The pathogenesis of ICH following ECMO is multifactorial and has been attributed to reperfusion injury, hemodynamic and cerebrovascular instability, systemic heparinization, and increased central venous pressure. Initially, gestational age (GA) <34 weeks, acidosis, sepsis, coagulopathy, and treatment with epinephrine are major independent factors associated with ICH in neonates treated with ECMO (Hardart and Fackler 1999). Intravascular volume administration (>8 infusions or >300 mL of volume infusion in the first 8 h and >10 infusions in the first 24 h of treatment) was also shown to be a contributing risk factor for intracranial hemorrhage during ECMO (de Mol et al. 2008). In ECMO-treated infants, the combination of a normal bedside US and an EEG without marked abnormalities is highly predictive of normal post-ECMO CT and MRI neuroimaging studies (Gannon et al. 2001). Among 152 ECMO survivors, 26 infants had moderate to severe neuroimaging abnormalities. There was an increased risk for being disabled at 5 years both following moderate abnormalities (OR 26.00; 95% CI 2.57–263.06) and severe imaging abnormalities (OR 69.33; 95% CI 7.351–653.91) (Bulas and Glass 2005). The same group previously showed that survivors with non-hemorrhagic abnormalities had a higher risk of delayed development than did those with isolated hemorrhagic abnormalities (39% vs. 21%) (Bulas et al. 1995). Attempts at decreasing risk of ICH with ECMO include venovenous (VV) ECMO where integrity of blood flow to the brain is maintained and cannulation and sacrifice of only the internal jugular vein occur.

References

Alderliesten T, Lemmers PM, Smarius JJ et al (2013) Cerebral oxygenation, extraction, and autoregulation in very preterm infants who develop peri-intraventricular hemorrhage. J Pediatr 162(4):698–704

Andre P, Thebaud B, Delavaucoupet J et al (2001) Late-onset cystic periventricular leukomalacia in premature infants: a threat until term. Am J Perinatol 18:79–86

Armstrong-Wells J, Johnston SC, Wu YW et al (2009) Prevalence and predictors of perinatal hemorrhagic stroke: results from the Kaiser pediatric stroke study. Pediatrics 123:823–828

Barnette AR, Myers BJ, Berg CS, Inder TE (2010) Sodium intake and intraventricular hemorrhage in the preterm infant. Ann Neurol 67(6):817–823

Barrington KJ, Finer NN (2010) Inhaled nitric oxide for respiratory failure in preterm infants. Cochrane Database Syst Rev CD000509

Bassan H, Benson CB, Limperopoulos C et al (2006) Ultrasonographic features and severity scoring of periventricular hemorrhagic infarction in relation to risk factors and outcome. Pediatrics 117:2111–2118

Bassan H, Limperopoulos C, Visconti K et al (2007) Neurodevelopmental outcome in survivors of periventricular hemorrhagic infarction. Pediatrics 120:785–792

Bassan H, Eshel R, Golan I, External Ventricular Drainage Study Investigators et al (2012) Timing of external ventricular drainage and neurodevelopmental outcome in preterm infants with posthemorrhagic hydrocephalus. Eur J Paediatr Neurol 16(6):662–670

Bates S, Odd D, Luyt K et al (2015) Superior vena cava flow and intraventricular haemorrhage in extremely preterm infants. J Matern Fetal Neonatal Med 30:1–7

Batton DG, Holtrop P, Dewitte D et al (1994) Current gestational age-related incidence of major intraventricular hemorrhage. J Pediatr 125:623–625

Baud O, Foix-L'Helias L, Kaminski M et al (1999) Antenatal glucocorticoid treatment and cystic periventricular leukomalacia in very premature infants. N Engl J Med 341:1190–1196

Beaino G, Khoshnood B, Kaminski M et al (2011) Predictors of the risk of cognitive deficiency in very preterm infants: the EPIPAGE prospective cohort. Acta Paediatr 100:370–378

Beecher DJ (2002) The *Bacillus cereus* group. In: Sussman M (ed) Molecular medical microbiology. Academic, San Diego, pp 1161–1181

Benavente-Fernández I, Lubián-López SP, Jiménez-Gómez G et al (2015) Low-voltage pattern and absence of sleep-wake cycles are associated with severe hemorrhage and death in very preterm infants. Eur J Pediatr 174(1):85–90

Beverley D, Pitts-Tucker T, Congdon P et al (1985) Prevention of intraventricular haemorrhage by fresh frozen plasma. Arch Dis Child 60(8):710–713

Bolisetty S, Dhawan A, Abdel-Latif M, New South Wales and Australian Capital Territory Neonatal Intensive Care Units' Data Collection et al (2014) Intraventricular hemorrhage and neurodevelopmental outcomes in extreme preterm infants. Pediatrics 133:55–62

Braun V, Hobbie S, Ondraczek R (1992) Serratia marcescens forms a new type of cytolysin. FEMS Microbiol Lett 100(1–3):299–305

Brouwer AJ, Groenendaal F, van Haastert IC et al (2008) Neurodevelopmental outcome of preterm infants with severe intraventricular hemorrhage and therapy for post-hemorrhagic ventricular dilatation. J Pediatr 152:648–654

Brouwer MJ, de Vries LS, Groenendaal F et al (2012) New reference values for the neonatal cerebral ventricles. Radiology 262(1):224–233

Bulas D, Glass P (2005) Neonatal ECMO: neuroimaging and neurodevelopmental outcome. Semin Perinatol 29:58–65

Bulas DI, Glass P, O'Donnell RM (1995) Neonates treated with ECMO: predictive value of early CT and US neuroimaging findings on short-term neurodevelopmental outcome. Radiology 195:407–412

Burstein J, Papile L, Burstein R (1979) Intraventricular hemorrhage in premature newborns: a prospective study with CT. Am J Radiol 132:631–635

Bussel JB, Sola-Visner M (2009) Current approaches to the evaluation and management of the fetus and neonate with immune thrombocytopenia. Semin Perinatol 33:35–42

Bussel JB, Zavusky MR, Berkowitz RL, McFarland JG (1997) Fetal alloimmune thrombocytopenia. N Engl J Med 337:22–26

Chadwick LM, Pemberton PJ, Kurinczuk JJ (1996) Neonatal subgaleal haematoma: associated risk factors, complications and outcome. J Paediatr Child Health 32:228–232

Chalak LF, Sikes NC, Mason MJ, Kaiser JR (2011) Low-voltage aEEG as predictor of intracranial hemorrhage in preterm infants. Pediatr Neurol 44(5):364–369

Chamnanvanakij S, Rollins N, Perlman JM (2002) Subdural hematoma in term infants. Pediatr Neurol 26:301–314

Chang HY, Peng CC, Kao HA et al (2007) Neonatal subgaleal hemorrhage: clinical presentation, treatment, and predictors of poor prognosis. Pediatr Int 49:903–907

Correa F, Enríquez G, Rosselló J et al (2004) Posterior fontanelle sonography: an acoustic window into the neonatal brain. AJNR Am J Neuroradiol 25:1274–1282

Counsell SJ, Dyet LE, Larkman DJ et al (2007) Thalamo-cortical connectivity in children born preterm mapped using probabilistic magnetic resonance tractography. Neuroimage 34:896–904

Cowan FM, de Vries LS (2005) The internal capsule in neonatal imaging. Semin Fetal Neonatal Med 10:461–474

Crowther CA, Harding JE (2007) Repeat doses of prenatal corticosteroids for women at risk of preterm birth for preventing neonatal respiratory disease. Cochrane Database Syst Rev 18(3):CD003935

Crowther CA, Hiller JE, Doyle LW et al (2003) Effect of magnesium sulfate given for neuroprotection before preterm birth. JAMA 290:2669–2676

Crowther CA, Crosby DD, Henderson-Smart DJ (2010) Cochrane Database Syst Rev 20(1), CD000229. https://doi.org/10.1002/14651858.CD000229.pub2

Dale ST, Coleman LT (2002) Neonatal alloimmune thrombocytopenia: antenatal and postnatal imaging findings in the pediatric brain. AJNR Am J Neuroradiol 23:1457–1465

Dalton J, Dechert RE, Sarkar S (2015) Assessment of association between rapid fluctuations in serum sodium and intraventricular hemorrhage in hypernatremic preterm infants. Am J Perinatol 32 (8):795–802

Dani C, Bertini G, Pezzati M, IntraVentricular Ibuprofen Study Group et al (2005) Prophylactic ibuprofen for the prevention of intraventricular hemorrhage among preterm infants: a multicenter, randomized study. Pediatrics 115:1529–1535

Dani C, Poggi C, Ceciarini F et al (2009) Coagulopathy screening and early plasma treatment for the prevention of intraventricular hemorrhage in preterm infants. Transfusion 49(12):2637–2644

Davies MW, Swaminathan M, Chuang SI, Betheras FR (2001) Reference ranges for the linear dimensions of the intracranial ventricles in preterm neonates. Arch Dis Child Fetal Neonatol Ed 82:F219–F223

de Mol AC, Gerrits LC, van Heijst AF, Straatman H (2008) Intravascular volume administration: a contributing risk factor for intracranial hemorrhage during extracorporeal membrane oxygenation? Pediatrics 121:e1599–e1603

De Vries LS, Groenendaal F, Eken P et al (1999) Asymmetrical myelination of the posterior limb of the internal capsule: an early predictor of hemiplegia. Neuropediatrics 30:314–319

de Vries LS, Rademaker KJ, Roelants-van Rijn AM (2001) Unilateral haemorrhagic parenchymal infarction in the preterm infant. Eur J Pediatr Neurol 5:139–149

de Vries LS, Liem KD, van Dijk K et al (2002) Early versus late treatment of posthaemorrhagic ventricular dilatation: results of a retrospective study from five neonatal intensive care units in the Netherlands. Acta Paediatr 91:212–217

de Vries LS, Koopman C, Groenendaal F et al (2009) COL4A1 mutation in two preterm siblings with antenatal onset of parenchymal hemorrhage. Ann Neurol 65.12–18

de Vries LS, Groenendaal F, Liem KD, Heep A, Brouwer AJ, van 't Verlaat E, Benavente-Fernández I, van Straaten HL, van Wezel-Meijler G, Smit BJ, Govaert P, Woerdeman PA, Whitelaw A, ELVIS study group (ed) (2018) Treatment thresholds for intervention in posthaemorrhagic ventricular dilation: a randomised controlled trial. Arch Dis Child Fetal Neonatal. https://doi.org/10.1136/archdischild-2017-314206. pii: fetalneonatal-2017-314206 [Epub ahead of print]

Dolfin T, Skidmore MB, Fong KW et al (1983) Incidence, severity and timing of subependymal and intraventricular hemorrhages in preterm infants born in a perinatal unit as detected by serial real-time ultrasound. Pediatrics 71:541–546

Doyle LW, Crowther CA, Middleton P (2009) Magnesium sulphate for women at risk of preterm birth for neuroprotection of the fetus. Cochrane Database Syst Rev 21(1), CD004661

Drayton MR, Skidmore R (1987) Vasoactivity of the major intracranial arteries in newborn infants. Arch Dis Child 62:236–240

Dudink J, Lequin M, Weisglas-Kuperus N et al (2008) Venous subtypes of preterm periventricular haemorrhagic infarction. Arch Dis Child Fetal Neonatal Ed 93:F201–F206

Duppre P, Sauer H, Giannopoulou EZ et al (2015) Cellular and humoral coagulation profiles and occurrence of IVH in VLBW and ELBW infants. Early Hum Dev 91:695–700

Ecury-Goossen GM, Dudink J, Lequin M et al (2010) The clinical presentation of preterm cerebellar haemorrhage. Eur J Pediatr 169(10):1249–1253

El-Ganzoury MM, El-Farrash RA, Saad AA et al (2014) Antenatal administration of vitamin K1: relationship to vitamin K-dependent coagulation factors and incidence rate of periventricular-intraventricular hemorrhage in preterm infants; Egyptian randomized controlled trial. J Matern Fetal Neonatal Med 27(8):816–820

Fabres J, Carlo WA, Phillips V et al (2007) Both extremes of arterial carbon dioxide pressure and the magnitude of fluctuations in arterial carbon dioxide pressure are associated with severe intraventricular hemorrhage in preterm infants. Pediatrics 119:299–305

Felderhoff-Mueser U, Buhrer C, Groneck P et al (2003) Soluble Fas (CD95/Apo-1), soluble Fas ligand and activated Capspase 3 in the cerebrospinal fluid of infants with posthemorrhagic and nonhemorrhagic hydrocephalus. Pediatr Res 54:659–664

Fernell E, Hagberg G, Hagberg B (1993) Infantile hydrocephalus in preterm, low-birth-weight infants: a nationwide Swedish cohort study 1979–1988. Acta Paediatr 82:45–48

Forman K (2014) Coagulopathy in newborns with hypoxic ischemic encephalopathy (HIE) treated with therapeutic hypothermia: a retrospective case-control study. BMC Pediatr 14:277

Fowlie PW, Davis PG (2010) Prophylactic intravenous indomethacin for preventing mortality and morbidity in preterm infants. Cochrane Database Syst Rev 7(7): CD000174

Gannon CM, Kornhauser MS, Gross GW et al (2001) When combined, early bedside head ultrasound and electroencephalography predict abnormal computerized tomography or magnetic resonance brain images obtained after extracorporeal membrane oxygenation treatment. J Perinatol 21:451–455

Ghazi-Birry HS, Brown WR, Moody DM et al (1997) Human germinal matrix: venous origin of hemorrhage and vascular characteristics. AJNR Am J Neuroradiol 18:219–229

Gleissner M, Jorch G, Avenarius S (2000) Risk factors for intraventricular hemorrhage in a birth cohort of 3721 premature infants. J Perinat Med 28:104–110

Göpel W, Härtel C, Ahrens P et al (2006) Interleukin-6-174-genotype, sepsis and cerebral injury in very low birth weight infants. Genes Immun 7:65–68

Gould SJ, Howard S, Hope PL, Reynolds EO (1987) Periventricular intraparenchymal cerebral haemorrhage in preterm infants: the role of venous infarction. J Pathol 151:197–202

Govaert P, Vanhaesebrouck P, de Praeter C (1992) Traumatic neonatal intracranial bleeding and stroke. Arch Dis Child 67:840–845

Gram M, Sveinsdottir S, Ruscher K, Hansson SR, Cinthio M, Akerström B, Ley D (2013) Hemoglobin induces inflammation after preterm intraventricular hemorrhage by methemoglobin formation. J Neuroinflammation 10:100. https://doi.org/10.1186/1742-2094-10-100

Hamrick SE, Miller SP, Leonard C et al (2004) Trends in severe brain injury and neurodevelopmental outcome in premature newborn infants: the role of cystic periventricular leukomalacia. J Pediatr 145:593–599

Hanigan WC, Powell FC, Miller TC, Wright RM (1995) Symptomatic intracranial hemorrhage in full-term infants. Childs Nerv Syst 11:698–707

Haque KN, Hayes AM, Ahmed Z et al (2008) Caesarean or vaginal delivery for preterm very-low-birth weight (</=1,250 g) infant: experience from a district general hospital in UK. Arch Gynecol Obstet 277:207–212

Hardart GE, Fackler JC (1999) Predictors of intracranial hemorrhage during neonatal extracorporeal membrane oxygenation. J Pediatr 134:156–159

Harding DR, Dhamrait S, Whitelaw A et al (2004) Does interleukin-6 genotype influence cerebral injury or developmental progress after preterm birth? Pediatrics 114:941–947

Härtel C, König I, Köster S et al (2006) Genetic polymorphisms of hemostasis genes and primary outcome of very low birth weight infants. Pediatrics 118:683–689

Heep A, Behrendt D, Nitsch P et al (2003) Increased interleukin-6 serum levels are associated with severe intraventricular hemorrhage in extremely premature infants. Arch Dis Child 88:F501–F504

Heep A, Stoffel-Wagner B, Bartmann P et al (2004a) Vascular endothelial growth factor and transforming growth factor-beta1 are highly expressed in the cerebrospinal fluid of premature infants with posthemorrhagic hydrocephalus. Pediatr Res 56:768–774

Heep A, Schaller K, Rittmann N et al (2004b) Multiple brain abscesses in an extremely preterm infant: treatment surveillance with interleukin-6 in the CSF. Eur J Pediatr 163:44–45

Herbst A, Källén K (2007) Influence of mode of delivery on neonatal mortality and morbidity in spontaneous preterm breech delivery. Eur J Obstet Gynecol Reprod Biol 133:25–29

Heuchan AM, Evans N, Henderson Smart DJ, Simpson JM (2002) Perinatal risk factors for major intraventricular haemorrhage in the Australian and New Zealand Neonatal Network, 1995–97. Arch Dis Child Fetal Neonatal Ed 86(2):F86–F90

Hofmeyr GJ, Hannah ME (2003) Planned caesarean section for term breech delivery. Cochrane Database Syst Rev 3, CD000166

Holberton JR, Drew SM, Mori R, Konig K (2012) The diagnostic value of a single measurement of superior vena cava flow in the first 24 h of life in very preterm infants. Eur J Pediatr 171:1489–1495

Ingram MC, Huguenard AL, Miller BA, Chern JJ (2014) Poor correlation between head circumference and cranial ultrasound findings in premature infants with intraventricular hemorrhage. J Neurosurg Pediatr 14:184–189

Jiménez AJ, García-Verdugo JM, González CA et al (2009) Disruption of the neurogenic niche in the subventricular zone of postnatal hydrocephalic hyh mice. J Neuropathol Exp Neurol 68(9):1006–1020. https://doi.org/10.1097/NEN.0b013e3181b44a5a

Jocelyn LJ, Casiro OG (1992) Neurodevelopmental outcome of term infants with intraventricular hemorrhage. Am J Dis Child 146:194–197

Kaiser A, Whitelaw A (1985) Cerebrospinal fluid pressure during posthaemorrhagic ventricular dilatation in newborn. Arch Dis Child 60:920–924

Kamphuis MM, Paridaans NP, Porcelijn L, Lopriore E, Oepkes D (2014) Incidence and consequences of neonatal alloimmune thrombocytopenia: a systematic review. Pediatrics 133:715–721

Kennedy CR, Ayers S, Campbell MJ et al (2001) Randomized, controlled trial of acetazolamide and furosemide in posthemorrhagic ventricular dilation in infancy: follow-up at 1 year. Pediatrics 108:597–607

Kersbergen K, de Vries LS, van Straaten HLM et al (2009) Anticoagulation therapy and imaging in neonates with a unilateral thalamic hemorrhage due to cerebral sinovenous thrombosis. Stroke 40(8):2754–2760

Khwaja O, Volpe JJ (2008) Pathogenesis of cerebral white matter injury of prematurity. Arch Dis Child Fetal Neonatal Ed 93:F153–F161

Kilani RA, Wetmore J (2006) Neonatal subgaleal hematoma: presentation and outcome – radiological findings and factors associated with mortality. Am J Perinatol 23:41–48

Klebermass-Schrehof K, Rona Z, Waldhör T et al (2013) Can neurophysiological assessment improve timing of intervention in posthaemorrhagic ventricular dilatation? Arch Dis Child Fetal Neonatal Ed 98(4):F291–F297

Kluckow M, Evans N (2000) Low superior vena cava flow and intraventricular haemorrhage in preterm infants. Arch Dis Child Fetal Neonatal Ed 82:F188–F194

Kribs A, Roll C, Göpel W et al (2015) Nonintubated surfactant application vs conventional therapy in extremely preterm infants: a randomized clinical trial. JAMA Pediatr 169(8):723–730

Krueger RC, Wu H, Zandian M et al (2006) Neural progenitors populate the cerebrospinal fluid of preterm patients with hydrocephalus. J Pediatr 148(3):337–340. e3. https://doi.org/10.1016/j.jpeds.2005.09.035

Kuban K, Sanocka U, Leviton A et al (1999) White matter disorders of prematurity: association with intraventricular hemorrhage and ventriculomegaly. The Developmental Epidemiology Network. J Pediatr 134:539–546

Larroche JC (1972) Post-haemorrhagic hydrocephalus in infancy. Anatomical study. Biol Neonate 20(3):287–299

Larroque B, Marret S, Ancel P-Y et al (2003) White matter damage and intraventricular hemorrhage in very preterm infants: the EPIPAGE study. J Pediatr 143:477–483

Leijser LM, Miller SP, van Wezel-Meijler G, Brouwer AJ, Traubici J, van Haastert IC, Whyte HE, Groenendaal F, Kulkarni AV, Han KS, Woerdeman PA, Church PT, Kelly EN, van Straaten HLM, Ly LG, de Vries LS (2018) Posthemorrhagic ventricular dilatation in preterm infants: When best to intervene? Neurology. 90 (8):e698–e706. https://doi.org/10.1212/WNL.0000000000004984

Lemons JA, Bauer CR, Oh W et al (2001) Very low birth weight outcomes of the National Institute of Child Health and Human Development Neonatal Research Network, January 1995 through December 1996. NICD Neonatal Research Network. Pediatrics 107(1), E1

Levene MI, Starte DR (1981) A longitudinal study of posthaemorrhagic ventricular dilatation in the newborn. Arch Dis Child 56:905–910

Limperopoulos C, Benson CB, Bassan H et al (2005) Cerebellar hemorrhage in the preterm infant: ultrasonographic findings and risk factors. Pediatrics 116:717–724

Limperopoulos C, Bassan H, Gauvreau K et al (2007) Does cerebellar injury in premature infants contribute to the high prevalence of long-term cognitive, learning, and behavioral disability in survivors? Pediatrics 120:584–593

Liu J, Wang Q, Gao F et al (2006) Maternal antenatal administration of vitamin K1 results in increasing the activities of vitamin K-dependent coagulation factors in umbilical blood and in decreasing the incidence rate of periventricular-intraventricular hemorrhage in premature infants. J Perinatal Med 34(2):173–176

Looney CB, Smith JK, Merck LH (2007) Intracranial hemorrhage in asymptomatic neonates: prevalence on MR images and relationship to obstetric and neonatal risk factors. Radiology 242:535–541

Maalouf EF, Duggan PJ, Counsell SJ et al (2001) Comparison of findings on cranial ultrasound and magnetic resonance imaging in preterm infants. Pediatrics 107:719–727

Ment LR, Stewart WB, Ardito TA, Madri JA (1995a) Germinal matrix microvascular maturation correlates inversely with the risk period for neonatal intraventricular hemorrhage. Brain Res Dev Brain Res 84:142–149

Ment LR, Oh W, Ehrenkranz RA, Philip AG et al (1995b) Antenatal steroids, delivery mode, and intraventricular hemorrhage in preterm infants. Am J Obstet Gynecol 172:795–800

Ment LR, Vohr B, Allan W et al (1999) The etiology and outcome of ventriculomegaly at term in very low birth weight infants. Pediatrics 104:243–248

Ment LR, Peterson BS, Meltzer JA et al (2006) A functional magnetic resonance imaging study of the long-term influences of early indomethacin exposure on language processing in the brains of prematurely born children. Pediatrics 118:961–970

Mercer JS, Vohr BR, McGrath MM et al (2006) Delayed cord clamping in very preterm infants reduces the incidence of intraventricular hemorrhage and late-onset sepsis: a randomized, controlled trial. Pediatrics 117:1235–1242

Messerschmidt A, Brugger PC, Boltshauser E et al (2005) Disruption of cerebellar development: potential complication of extreme prematurity. AJNR Am J Neuroradiol 26:1659–1667

Meuwissen ME, Halley DJ, Smit LS et al (2015) The expanding phenotype of COL4A1 and COL4A2 mutations: clinical data on 13 newly identified families and a review of the literature. Genet Med. https://doi.org/10.1038/gim.2014.210

Modi N, Lewis H, Al-Naqeeb N et al (2001) The effects of repeated antenatal glucocorticoid therapy on the brain. Pediatr Res 50:581–585

Moody DM, Brown WR, Challa VR et al (1994) Alkaline phosphatase histochemical staining in the study of germinal matrix hemorrhage and brain vascular morphology in a very-low-birth-weight neonate. Pediatr Res 35:424–430

Morales WJ, Angel JL, O'Brien WF et al (1988) The use of antenatal vitamin K in the prevention of early neonatal intraventricular hemorrhage. Am J Obstet Gynecol 159:774–779

Morita T, Morimoto M, Yamada K et al (2015) Low-grade intraventricular hemorrhage disrupts cerebellar white matter in preterm infants: evidence from diffusion tensor imaging. Neuroradiology 57(5):507–514

Murphy BP, Inder TE, Rooks V, Taylor GA et al (2002) Posthaemorrhagic ventricular dilatation in the premature infant: natural history and predictors of outcome. Arch Dis Child Fetal Neonatal Ed 87:F37–F41

Neary E, Okafor I, Al-Awaysheh F et al (2013) Laboratory coagulation parameters in extremely premature infants born earlier than 27 gestational weeks upon admission to a neonatal intensive care unit. Neonatology 104 (3):222–227

Noori S, McCoy M, Anderson MP et al (2014) Changes in cardiac function and cerebral blood flow in relation to peri/intraventricular hemorrhage in extremely preterm infants. J Pediatr 164(2):264–70.e1-3. https://doi.org/10.1016/j.jpeds.2013.09.045

Northern Neonatal Nursing Initiative Trial Group (1996) Randomised trial of prophylactic early fresh-frozen plasma or gelatin or glucose in preterm babies: outcome at 2 years. Lancet 348:229–232

Olischar M, Klebermass K, Waldhoer T et al (2007) Background patterns and sleep-wake cycles on amplitude-integrated electroencephalography in preterms younger than 30 weeks gestational age with peri-/intraventricular haemorrhage. Acta Paediatr 96:1743–1750

Osborn DA, Evans N, Kluckow M (2003) Hemodynamic and antecedent risk factors of early and late periventricular/intraventricular hemorrhage in premature infants. Pediatrics 112:33–39

Palmer KG, Kronsberg SS, Barton BA (2005) Effect of inborn versus outborn delivery on clinical outcomes in ventilated preterm neonates: secondary results from the NEOPAIN trial. J Perinatol 25:270–275

Paneth N, Rudelli R, Kazam E, Monte W (1994) Brain damage in the preterm infant, Clinics in developmental medicine no. 131. MacKeith Press, London

Pape KE, Wigglesworth JS (1979) Haemorrhage, ischaemia and perinatal brain, Clinics in developmental medicine no. 69/70. SIMP/Heinemann, London, pp 133–148

Parodi A, Rossi A, Severino M et al (2015a) Accuracy of ultrasound in assessing cerebellar haemorrhages in very low birthweight babies. Arch Dis Child Fetal Neonatal Ed 100(4):F289–F292

Parodi A, Morana G, Severino MS et al (2015b) Low-grade intraventricular hemorrhage: is ultrasound good enough? J Matern Fetal Neonatal Med 28(Suppl 1):2261–2264

Patra K, Wilson-Costello D, Taylor HG et al (2006) Grades I-II intraventricular hemorrhage in extremely low birth weight infants: effects on neurodevelopment. J Pediatr 149(2):169–173

Payne AH, Hintz SR, Hibbs AM et al (2013) Eunice Kennedy Shriver National Institute of Child Health and Human Development Neonatal Research Network: neurodevelopmental outcomes of extremely low-gestational age neonates with low-grade periventricular-intraventricular hemorrhage. JAMA Pediatr 167:451–459

Persson EK, Hagberg G, Uvebrant P (2006) Disabilities in children with hydrocephalus – a population-based study of children aged between four and twelve years. Neuropediatrics 37:330–336

Plaisier A, Raets MM, Ecury-Goossen GM et al (2015) Serial cranial ultrasonography or early MRI for detecting preterm brain injury? Arch Dis Child Fetal Neonatal Ed 100(4):F293–F300

Pomerance JJ, Teal JG, Gogolok JF et al (1987) Maternally administered antenatal vitamin K1: effect on neonatal prothrombin activity, partial thromboplastin time, and intraventricular hemorrhage. Obstet Gynecol 70:235–241

Poralla C, Hertfelder H, Oldenburg J et al (2011) Elevated interleukin-6 concentration and alterations of the coagulation system are associated with the development of intraventricular hemorrhage in extremely preterm infants. Neonatology 102(4):270–275

Poralla C, Traut C, Hertfelder HJ (2012) The coagulation system of extremely preterm infants: influence of perinatal risk factors on coagulation. J Perinatol 32:869–873

Rabe H, Reynolds G, Diaz-Rossello J (2008) A systematic review and meta-analysis of a brief delay in clamping the umbilical cord of preterm infants. Neonatology 93:138–144

Rademaker KJ, Groenendaal F, Jansen GH et al (1994) Unilateral haemorrhagic parenchymal lesions in the preterm infant: shape, site and prognosis. Acta Paediatr 83:602–628

Radic JA, Vincer M, McNeely PD (2015) Outcomes of intraventricular hemorrhage and posthemorrhagic hydrocephalus in a population-based cohort of very preterm infants born to residents of Nova Scotia from 1993 to 2010. J Neurosurg Pediatr 15(6):580–588

Roberts D, Dalziel S (2006) Antenatal corticosteroids for accelerating fetal lung maturation for women at risk of preterm birth. Cochrane Database Syst Rev 19(3), CD004454

Roberts D, Brown J, Medley N, Dalziel SR (2017) Antenatal corticosteroids for accelerating fetal lung maturation for women at risk of preterm birth. Cochrane Database Syst Rev 3:CD004454

Robinson S (2012) Neonatal posthemorrhagic hydrocephalus from prematurity: pathophysiology and current treatment concepts. J Neurosurg Pediatrics 9(3):242–258. https://doi.org/10.3171/2011.12.PEDS11136

Rodríguez EM, Guerra MM, Vío K et al (2012) A cell junction pathology of neural stem cells leads to abnormal neurogenesis and hydrocephalus. Biol Res 45(3):231–241. https://doi.org/10.4067/S0716-976020 12000300005

Roland EH, Flodmark O, Hill A (1990) Thalamic hemorrhagic with intraventricular hemorrhage in the full term newborn. Pediatrics 85:737–742

Ross G, Boatright S, Auld PA, Nass R (1996) Specific cognitive abilities in 2-year-old children with subependymal and mild intraventricular hemorrhage. Brain Cogn 32(1):1–13

Roze E, Kerstjens JM, Maathuis CG et al (2008) Risk factors for adverse outcome in preterm infants with periventricular hemorrhagic infarction. Pediatrics 122: e46–e52

Roze E, Van Braeckel KN, van der Veere CN (2009) Functional outcome at school age of preterm infants with periventricular hemorrhagic infarction. Pediatrics 123:1493–1500

Roze E, Benders MJ, Kersbergen KJ et al (2015) Neonatal DTI early after birth predicts motor outcome in preterm infants with periventricular hemorrhagic infarction. Pediatr Res 78(3):298–303

Salonvaara M, Riikonen P, Kekomäki R et al (2005) Intraventricular haemorrhage in very-low-birthweight preterm infants: association with low prothrombin activity at birth. Acta Paediatr 94(6):807–811

Sarkar S, Bhagat I, Dechert R et al (2009) Severe intraventricular hemorrhage in preterm infants: comparison of risk factors and short-term neonatal morbidities between grade 3 and grade 4 intraventricular hemorrhage. Am J Perinatol 26:419–424

Sävman K, Blennow M, Hagberg H et al (2002) Cytokine response in cerebrospinal fluid from preterm infants with posthaemorrhagic ventricular dilatation. Acta Paediatr 91:1357–1363

Schmidt B, Davis P, Moddeman D et al (2001) Trial of indomethacin prophylaxis in preterm investigators. Long-term effects of indomethacin prophylaxis in extremely-low-birth-weight infants. N Eng J Med 344:1966–1972

Schmitz T, Heep A, Groenendaal F et al (2007) Interleukin-1beta, interleukin-18, and interferon-gamma expression in the cerebrospinal fluid of premature infants with posthemorrhagic hydrocephalus-markers of white matter damage? Pediatr Res 61:722–726

Schreiner C, Suter C, Watzka M et al (2014) Genetic variants of the vitamin K dependent coagulation system and intraventricular hemorrhage in preterm infants. BMC Pediatr 14:219

Sherlock RL, Synnes AR, Grunau RE et al (2008) Long term outcome after neonatal intraparenchymal echodensities with porencephaly. Arch Dis Child Fetal Neon Ed 93:F127–F131

Sirc J, Dempsey EM, Miletin J (2013) Cerebral tissue oxygenation index, cardiac output and superior vena cava flow in infants with birth weight less than 1250 grams in the first 48 hours of life. Early Hum Dev 89:449–452

Smit E, Odd D, Whitelaw A (2013) Postnatal phenobarbital for the prevention of intraventricular hemorrhage in preterm infants. Cochrane Database Syst Rev 8, CD001691

Soraisham AS, Singhal N, McMillan DD, Canadian Neonatal Network et al (2009) A multicenter study on the clinical outcome of chorioamnionitis in preterm infants. Am J Obstet Gynecol 372:e1–e6

Soubasi V, Mitsakis K, Sarafidis K et al (2012) Early abnormal amplitude-integrated electroencephalography (aEEG) is associated with adverse short-term outcome in premature infants. Eur J Paediatr Neurol 16 (6):625–630

Soul JS, Eichenwald E, Walter G et al (2004) CSF removal in infantile posthemorrhagic hydrocephalus results in significant improvement in cerebral hemodynamics. Pediatr Res 55:872–876

Soul JS, Hammer PE, Tsuji M et al (2007) Fluctuating pressure-passivity is common in the cerebral circulation of sick premature infants. Pediatr Res 61:467–473

Spinillo A, Gardella B, Preti E (2007) Preeclampsia and brain damage among preterm infants: a changed panorama in a 20-year analysis. Am J Perinatol 24:101–106

Srinivasan L, Allsop J, Counsell SJ et al (2006) Smaller cerebellar volumes in very preterm infants at term-equivalent age are associated with the presence of supratentorial lesions. AJNR Am J Neuroradiol 27:573–579

Staudt M, Braun C, Gerloff C, Erb M, Grodd W, Krägeloh-Mann I (2006) Developing somatosensory projections bypass periventricular brain lesions. Neurology 67: 522–525

Steggerda SJ, Leijser LM, Wiggers-de Bruïne FT et al (2009a) Cerebellar injury in preterm infants: incidence and findings on US and MR images. Radiology 252(1):190–199. https://doi.org/10.1148/radiol.2521081525

Steggerda SJ, Leijser LM, Wiggers-de Bruïne FT et al (2009b) Cerebellar injury in preterm infants: incidence and findings on US and MR images. Radiology 252(1):190–199

Synnes AR, Macnab YC, Qiu Z et al (2006) Neonatal intensive care unit characteristics affect the incidence of severe intraventricular hemorrhage. Med Care 44 (8):754–759

Takashima S, Takashi M, Ando Y (1986) Pathogenesis of periventricular white matter haemorrhage in preterm infants. Brain Dev 8:25–30

Tam EW, Miller SP, Studholme C et al (2011) Differential effects of intraventricular hemorrhage and white matter

injury on preterm cerebellar growth. J Pediatr 158 (3):366–371
Thorp JA, Jones PG, Clark RH et al (2001) Perinatal factors associated with severe intracranial hemorrhage. Am J Obstet Gynecol 185:859–862
Tortora D, Severino M, Malova M, Parodi A, Morana G, Ramenghi LA, Rossi A (2016) Variability of cerebral deep venous system in preterm and term neonates evaluated on MR SWI venography. AJNR Am J Neuroradiol. https://doi.org/10.3174/ajnr.A4877
Tortora D, Severino M, Malova M, Parodi A, Morana G, Sedlacik J, Govaert P, Volpe JJ, Rossi A, Ramenghi LA (2018) Differences in subependymal vein anatomy may predispose preterm infants to GMH-IVH. Arch Dis Child Fetal Neonatal Ed 103(1):F59–F65. https://doi.org/10.1136/archdischild-2017-312710
Tsuji M, Saul JP, du Plessis A et al (2000) Cerebral intravascular oxygenation correlates with mean arterial pressure in critically ill premature infants. Pediatrics 106(4):625–632
Uchil D, Arulkumaran S (2003) Neonatal subgaleal hemorrhage and its relationship to delivery by vacuum extraction. Obstet Gynecol Surv 58:687–693
van Alfen-van der Velden AA, Hopman JC, Klaessens JH, Feuth T et al (2007) Cerebral hemodynamics and oxygenation after serial CSF drainage in infants with PHVD. Brain Dev 29:623–629
van de Bor M, Verloove-Vanhorick SP, Baerts W, Brand R, Ruys JH (1984) Outcome of periventricular-intraventricular hemorrhage at 2 years of age in 484 very preterm infants admitted to 6 neonatal intensive care units in The Netherlands. Neuropediatrics 19(4):183–185
Van Der Lugt NM, Kamphuis MM, Paridaans NP et al (2015) Neonatal outcome in alloimmune thrombocytopenia after maternal treatment with intravenous immunoglobulin. Blood Transfus 13:66–71
Vasileiadis GT, Gelman N, Han VK et al (2004) Uncomplicated intraventricular hemorrhage is followed by reduced cortical volume at near-term age. Pediatrics 114:e367–e372
Vavasseur C, Slevin M, Donoghue V, Murphy JF (2007) Effect of low grade intraventricular hemorrhage on developmental outcome of preterm infants. J Pediatr 151(2), e6
Veldman A, Josef J, Fischer D et al (2006) A prospective pilot study of prophylactic treatment of preterm neonates with recombinant activated factor VII during the first 72 hours of life. Pediatr Crit Care Med 7(1):34–39
Ventriculomegaly Trial Group (1994) Randomised trial of early tapping in neonatal posthaemorrhagic ventricular dilatation: results at 30 months. Arch Dis Child 70: F129–F136
Vesoulis ZA, Inder TE, Woodward LJ et al (2014) Early electrographic seizures, brain injury, and neurodevelopmental risk in the very preterm infant. Pediatr Res 75(4):564–569
Vohr BR, Garcia-Coll C, Flanagan P, Oh W (1992) Effects of intraventricular hemorrhage and socioeconomic status on perceptual, cognitive, and neurologic status of low birth weight infants at 5 years of age. J Pediatr 121:280–285
Vohr BR, Allan W, Katz KH et al (2014) Adolescents born prematurely with isolated grade 2 haemorrhage in the early 1990s face increased risks of learning challenges. Acta Paediatr 103(10):1066–1071
Volpe JJ (1989) Intraventricular hemorrhage in the premature infant-current concepts. Part I. Ann Neurol 25:3–11
Volpe JJ (2008a) Neonatal neurology, 4th edn. Saunders, Philadelphia
Volpe JJ (2008b) Intracranial hemorrhage: subdural, primary subarachnoid, intracerebellar, intraventricular (term infant), and miscellaneous. In: Neurology of the newborn. Saunders, Philadelphia, pp 483–516
Volpe JJ (2009) Brain injury in premature infants: a complex amalgam of destructive and developmental disturbances. Lancet Neurol 8(1):110–124. https://doi.org/10.1016/S1474-4422(08)70294-1
Volpe JJ, Kinney HC, Jensen FE, Rosenberg PA (2011) The developing oligodendrocyte: key cellular target in brain injury in the premature infant. Int J Dev Neurosci 29(4):423–440. https://doi.org/10.1016/j.ijdevneu.2011.02.012
Waltl H, Födisch HJ, Kurz R et al (1973) Intracranial haemorrhage in low-birth-weight infants and prophylactic administration of coagulation-factor concentrate. Lancet 1:1284–1286
Wells JT, Ment LR (1995) Prevention of intraventricular haemorrhage in preterm infants. Early Hum Dev 42:209–233
Whitelaw A, Aquilina K (2012) Management of posthaemorrhagic ventricular dilatation. Arch Dis Child Fetal Neonatal Ed 97:F229–F233
Whitelaw A, Pople I, Cherian S et al (2003) Phase 1 trial of prevention of hydrocephalus after intraventricular hemorrhage in newborn infants by drainage, irrigation and fibrinolytic therapy. Pediatrics 111:759–765
Whitelaw A, Evans D, Carter M et al (2007) Randomized clinical trial of prevention of hydrocephalus after intraventricular hemorrhage in preterm infants: brain-washing versus tapping fluid. Pediatrics 119:e1071–e1078
Whitelaw A, Jary S, Kmita G et al (2010) Randomized trial of drainage, irrigation and fibrinolytic therapy for premature infants with posthemorrhagic ventricular dilatation: developmental outcome at 2 years. Pediatrics 125(4):e852–e858
Wu YW, Hamrick SEG, Miller SP et al (2003) Intraventricular hemorrhage in term neonates caused by sinovenous thrombosis. Ann Neurol 54:123–126
Yanowitz TD, Jordan JA, Gilmour CH et al (2002) Hemodynamic disturbances in premature infants born after chorioamnionitis: association with cord blood cytokine concentrations. Pediatr Res 51:310–316

Neonatal Stroke: Mechanisms

129

Paul P. Govaert and Jeroen Dudink

Contents

Abstract

Thrombosis plays a role in many instances of neonatal ischemic stroke, be it arterial or venous. Apart from limb or visceral embolism and from intravascular manipulations, the clinical context is not specific of thrombotic stroke. To arrive at the diagnosis of primary thrombosis, a sequential diagnostic scheme has to be processed. First of all, entities that mimic stroke have to be appropriately excluded, which may not be straightforward in case of hypoglycemia or vascular malformation within the brain. Secondly, hemorrhagic stroke types, mainly lobar hematoma and subarachnoid hematoma, of cerebrum or cerebellum have to

P. P. Govaert (✉) · J. Dudink
Neonatology, Sophia Children's Hospital, Erasmus MC Rotterdam, Rotterdam, Zuid-Holland, The Netherlands
e-mail: govaert@icloud.com; j.dudink@erasmusmc.nl

G. Buonocore et al. (eds.), *Neonatology*,
https://doi.org/10.1007/978-3-319-29489-6_279

be recognized, sometimes because of a typical hemostatic context. Thirdly, apparent arterial or venous infarctions can be linked to obvious cranial birth trauma or to brain inflammation. Fourthly, vascular imaging of the cervical great vessels and of brain vessels may be needed to document congenital vascular malformations or arterio-/venopathy. Fifthly, a diligent search for primary thrombi outside the brain (in aorta or carotid arteries, in systemic veins, in the heart, or in the placental-umbilical system) may be warranted. Treatment of thrombotic events in the newborn brain is at the moment limited to heparinization in cardio-embolic stroke and in progressive sinovenous thrombosis, both in the absence of major brain hemorrhage.

Abbreviations

DW	Diffusion weighted
ECMO	Extracorporeal membrane oxygenation
HS	Hemorrhagic stroke
MRI	Magnetic resonance imaging
NAIS	Neonatal arterial ischemic stroke
NCSVT	Neonatal cerebral sinovenous thrombosis
PVI	Periventricular venous infarction
US	Ultrasound

129.1 Salient Points

- There are three types of neonatal stroke: ischemic arterial, ischemic sinovenous, and hemorrhagic.
- Thrombosis plays a role in ischemic stroke types.
- Not all focal brain lesions are stroke.
- Lobar and subarachnoid hematomas are hemorrhagic stroke types that can mimic ischemic stroke.
- Recognizable mechanisms include trauma and inflammation.
- Imaging techniques may indicate vessel malformation or disease.
- Embolism is an important, sometimes preventable, cause of arterial ischemic stroke.
- Primary arterial or venous thrombosis may be associated with prothrombotic conditions, often in association with a clinical risk factor.
- There are no evidence-based treatment guidelines for neonatal brain thrombosis.

129.2 Introduction

Neonatal stroke is defined as "a group of heterogeneous conditions in which there is focal disruption of cerebral blood flow secondary to arterial or cerebral venous thrombosis or embolization, between 20 weeks of fetal life through 28th postnatal day, and confirmed by neuroimaging or neuropathological studies" (Raju et al. 2007). Two types of ischemic neonatal strokes are arterial ischemic stroke (NAIS) and cerebral sinovenous thrombosis (CSVT). The third stroke type is primary bleeding (hemorrhagic stroke, HS). Additional forms of ischemic stroke unique to the perinatal period include periventricular venous infarction (PVI) and presumed perinatal stroke detected in infancy or childhood (both not discussed in this chapter). Vessels are occluded by thrombosis, embolism, direct trauma, compression, spasm, or obliteration by an inflammatory process. Open vessel ischemia, e.g., during hypovolemia, arrhythmia, or asphyxia, is not included in the definition of stroke.

Neonatal arterial ischemic stroke (*NAIS*) can be defined by either of the two methods: (i) document partial or complete occlusion of the artery related to a focal brain lesion or (ii) document a lesion pattern with imaging that cannot be otherwise explained than by occlusion of a specific brain artery. Precise vascular designation (Govaert et al. 2009a) and site description are important in reporting perinatal stroke, because outcome correlates with them. MCA stroke covers more than 50% of pial strokes, complete and posterior truncal stroke being most common. Templates for the diagnosis of neonatal perforator stroke have been published [with ultrasound and MRI for MCA stroke types (de Vries et al. 1997) and with ultrasound for the other perforator stroke types (Abels et al. 2006); see preceding chapter]. Multiple separate strokes in the same infant can be due to infarction with meningitis, embolism (including air), thrombophilia, arteriopathy, breakdown of a large thrombus into several emboli, and triggered arterial spasm.

Neonatal cerebral sinovenous thrombosis (*NCSVT*) is defined as the presence of thrombus in a sinus, a large deep brain vein, or a smaller pial vein, with partial or complete occlusion. Complete occlusion, depending on tempo of thrombosis, hemostatic dysfunction, and collateral potential, may or may not cause venous infarction (red softening) in brain areas draining into the vessel. In a minority, such infarcts remain purely ischemic, suggesting that arterial occlusion in response to venous ischemia occurs prior to vein rupture. Specific hemorrhagic lesions have been reported in this context: thalamoventricular hemorrhage with occlusion of the internal cerebral vein (bilateral with great vein of Galen occlusion) (Govaert et al. 1992a), striato-hippocampal bleeding with basal vein thrombosis (Govaert et al. 2001), parasagittal subcortical bleeding with superior sagittal sinus thrombosis (Bailey and Hass 1958), temporal lobe or cerebellar hemorrhage with transverse sinus thrombosis (Baram et al. 1988), temporal lobe anterolateral hemorrhage with tentorial sinus or temporal diploic vein rupture (Huang and Robertson 2004), and temporal lobe hemorrhage with vein of Labbé thrombosis (Kalpatthi et al. 2005). Large veins and sinuses usually recanalize following thrombosis, over a period of weeks to months (Moharir et al. 2006).

Hemorrhagic stroke (brain hemorrhage, HS) results from rupture of an (ab)normal intracranial blood vessel, but it is difficult to document damage of a vessel in such instances. In the newborn, intracranial hemorrhage is usually described under the heading of the brain compartment affected: intraventricular (bleeding in choroid plexus and ventricle), thalamoventricular (related to internal cerebral vein occlusion), lobar cerebral (bleeding in the parenchyma of a cerebral lobe), cerebellar, subarachnoid, and sub-/epidural. Because sub-/epidural bleeding is often due to trauma or hemostatic failure, and because intraventricular hemorrhage cannot be confused with arterial stroke, it seems appropriate to register only lobar (including subarachnoid) hematoma as stroke (Hayashi et al. 1987; Hanigan et al. 1995; Sandberg et al. 2001). Specific types of frank hemorrhage are due to venous thrombosis (see above).

This chapter is a guide to the diagnosis of primary thrombosis in the newborn brain, be it arterial or venous. The likelihood of finding a prothrombotic condition and/or a dysfunctional platelet-endothelium interaction is probably greater in such instances. A systematic exclusion of mechanisms other than primary thrombosis is therefore clinically relevant. The clinical presentation and treatment of neonatal stroke are subject of another chapter in this volume.

129.3 Etiology, Pathogenesis, and Differential Diagnosis

129.3.1 Step 1: Exclude Entities Mimicking Stroke

Several focal lesions have to be differentiated from NAIS and NCSVT: kernicterus, encephalitis (bacterial and viral), metabolic disorders (including hypoglycemia, pyridoxine dependent epilepsy, and mitochondrial disorders) (Mercimek-Mahmutoglu et al. 2012), posterior reversible encephalopathy, phakomatous change, and tumor.

Consistent lesion and imaging patterns of neonatal hypoglycemic injury have been reported (Liu et al. 2013). Bilateral, rather symmetrical, injury of occipital and posterior parietal cortex and underlying white matter was well documented in a postmortem study of three patients (Anderson et al. 1967) and subsequently in many in vivo studies (Burns et al. 2008). Injury spreads beyond the area covered by the posterior cerebral artery and is too extensive to be classified as watershed infarction. Infarction with cavitation, not a feature in adults, has been reported in the newborn (Barkovich et al. 1998). This lesion type is specific of newborns and young infants (Gataullina et al. 2015). A second post-hypoglycemic paradigm seems to be unilateral hemispheric necrosis (Yager 2002; Fig. 1).

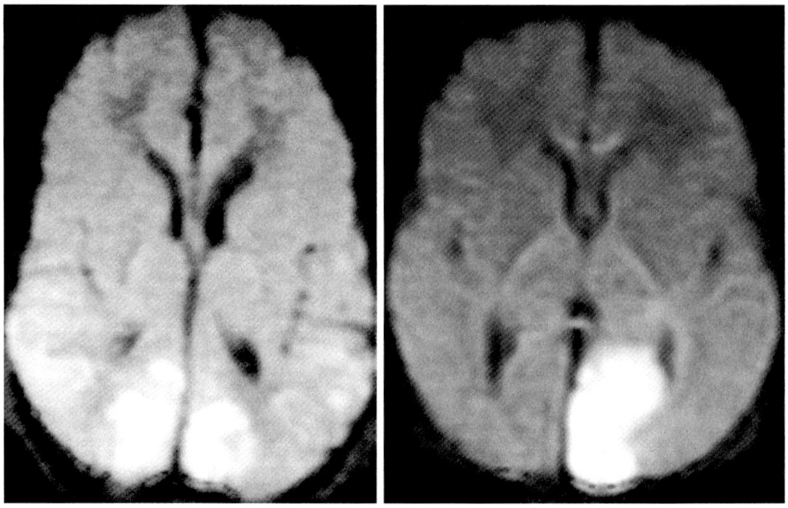

Fig. 1 DW axial MRI in a term infant with profound hypoglycemia and seizures: focal bilateral occipital subcortical cell injury may mimic PCA stroke (compare with DWI on the right of infant with tip of the basilar artery stroke leading to cerebellar infarction and left PCA pial stroke)

Bleeding from a vascular anomaly (aneurysm, AVM, cavernous hemangioma, or developmental venous anomaly) should be distinguished from stroke. It is advised to repeat targeted ultrasound Doppler exams and/or MRA 4–6 weeks after hemorrhagic stroke, if the cause of the insult is not obvious (no source of embolism, no infection, no trauma, normal hemostasis) (Lasjaunias et al. 1995; Alvarez et al. 2007). A genetic (familial) context is possible for such vascular malformations. The same applies to moyamoya sequence that has led to presentation with perinatal stroke in an infant with trisomy 21 (Pysden et al. 2010). Developmental venous anomalies may resemble focal pial/deep gray matter stroke or periventricular venous infarction in some infants (Horsch et al. 2014). Watershed injury resulting from partial asphyxia, hypocapnia, or hypotension (e.g., due to acute blood loss) does not fit under the stroke umbrella (McCann et al. 2014; Harteman et al. 2013). One must be aware though that signal intensity change in parasagittal areas can be due to interarterial watershed injury but also to superior sagittal sinus thrombosis or even venous watershed injury. It is important not to confuse with "stroke" different degrees of bilateral white matter injury typical of the preterm (former leukomalacia, often with petechial, linear, or nodular hemorrhage in affected areas) (Ramenghi et al. 2007; Arrigoni et al. 2011; Raybaud et al. 2013; Kersbergen et al. 2014). Similar white matter damage has also been reported in term infants with congenital heart disease (Block et al. 2010).

Matters are more complicated concerning PVI (periventricular venous infarction), regularly seen in the preterm infant, but also at term (Takanashi et al. 2003). Such (almost invariably) unilateral white matter hemorrhage in preterm infants is in fact consequent to venous obstruction following ipsilateral germinal matrix hemorrhage or IVH and can be classified as stroke, but the clinical context is different from NAIS or NCSVT. In addition routine serial sonographic screening reliably offers recognition of PVI in the acute stage (Bassan et al. 2006; Dudink et al. 2007). Some instances are not due to compression of a medullary collector vein by germinal matrix hemorrhage but are due to primary thrombosis. For this reason, clinicians, certainly against a positive family history of thrombosis, may opt to screen for prothrombotic conditions in infants where venous infarction is not obviously explained by primary germinal matrix hemorrhage (Ramenghi et al. 2002).

129.3.2 Step 2: Recognize Hemorrhagic Stroke

Lobar hematoma. Figures 2 and 3 in a limited number of newborn infants, often in the absence

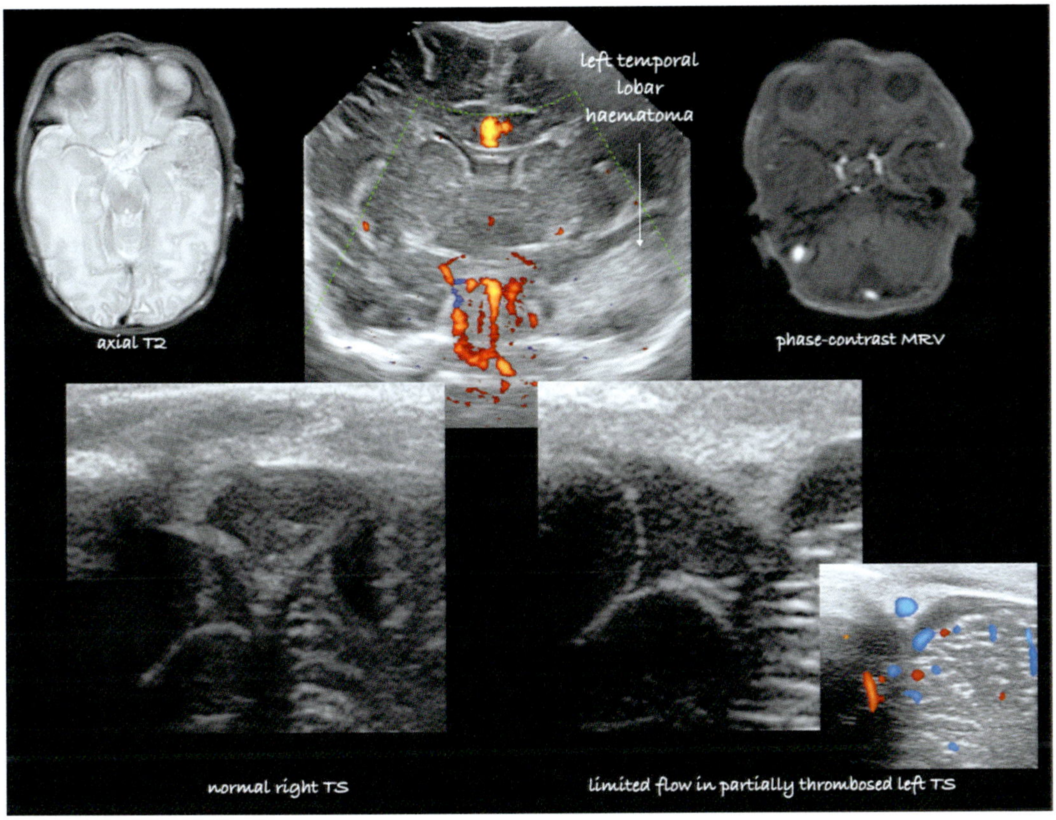

Fig. 2 Composite image of a term infant with first-day apnea and left temporal lobar hematoma. The ipsilateral transverse sinus is partially thrombosed, with limited residual flow. Notice non-visualization of the left transverse sinus on uncontrasted MRV

of IVH, one may find hemorrhage in one or more brain lobes, outside the basal ganglia and thalamus (Hanigan et al. 1995; Sandberg et al. 2001; Bergman et al. 1985; Armstrong-Wells et al. 2009). Lesions in every lobe of the cerebrum have been described. It is common for lobar hematomas to be associated with a subdural or subarachnoid extra-axial component: this raises the question whether the primary focus is in parenchyma or in the extracerebral space. The presenting sign has often been apnea (Hoogstraate et al. 2008; Tramonte and Goodkin 2004) or (multi)focal convulsive activity, but some lobar hematomas are asymptomatic (Wang et al. 2004). In most instances, the mechanism is elusive (Hayashi et al. 1987). Rarely sinus thrombosis has been documented in relation to large lobar hemorrhage in the absence of a hemostatic deficiency, encouraging a search for prothrombotic tendencies (Baram et al. 1988; Huang and Robertson 2004; Singh and Chakera 2002).

The association of lobar hematoma with focal arterial ischemia in another additional brain area is suggestive of embolism with hemorrhagic conversion of arterial ischemic stroke.

Lobar lesions also warrant a diligent search for evidence of trauma, hemostatic failure (Ries et al. 1995), and vascular malformation. Recognition and prevention of vitamin K deficiency or resistance are important in this context. Saccular arterial aneurysms can present with seizures and meningeal signs in infancy: the MCA is commonly affected, but location can be within the posterior fossa or in other supratentorial arteries. Most aneurysms exceed 1 cm in diameter and should be MRA present. Arteriovenous malformations (other than vein of Galen malformation) present with congestive heart failure

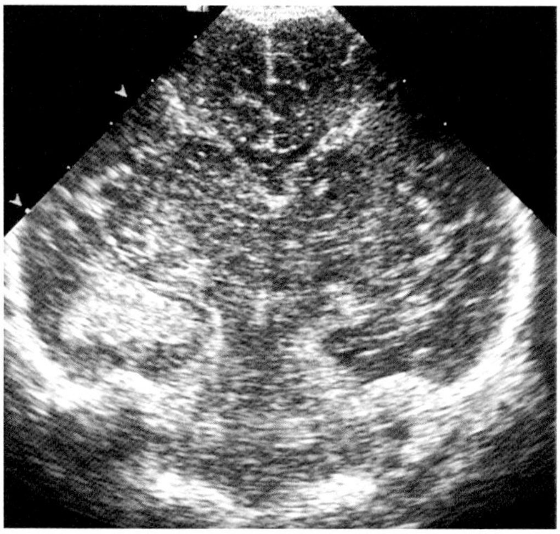

Fig. 3 Coronal US 6 h after birth of a term infant presenting with apnea and cyanosis: hyperechoic right temporal lobe lesion, later demonstrated to be a hematoma; tumor and vascular malformation excluded by MRA and serial (Doppler) imaging

(usually large fistulae), hemorrhage, or hydrocephalus of the communicating type. Most are supratentorial (9/10). Spontaneous thrombosis of an AVM is exceptional. A family history may point to hereditary hemorrhagic telangiectasia (Nishida et al. 2012). Cavernous angiomata are associated with hemorrhage as a rule, from mild to extensive. One must be aware of an underlying tumor facing lobar, subdural, or intraventricular hemorrhage: astrocytoma is a rare cause of neonatal lobar hematoma.

Subarachnoid hematoma. Figure 4 refers to a space-occupying hemorrhage on the brain surface, located under the arachnoid membranes (Chessells and Wigglesworth 1970; Govaert et al. 1992b). The primary lesion is a fast-growing subarachnoid or subpial hemorrhage (Govaert et al. 1995), mostly along and under the temporal and parietal lobes, more often on the left. There is usually a context of hemorrhagic diathesis, frequently intravascular coagulation (or thrombocytopenia of any cause) during sepsis. On any imaging technique, the borders of the hematoma irregularly penetrate the parenchyma because sulci and fissures are filled with clot and the displaced parenchyma is edematous. Subdural hemorrhage displaces but does not penetrate the adjacent parenchyma. The midline may be shifted and the ipsilateral ventricle can be closed under pressure. Rupture of an arterial aneurysm or AVM is another cause of subarachnoid hematoma (McLellan et al. 1986; Hayashi et al. 1994; Tan et al. 1998). Subarachnoid hemorrhage was one of the components of a strange and often fatal pattern of hemorrhagic necrosis in both parietal lobes of extremely preterm infants (Cross et al. 1992). These lesions are cavitated in the parenchyma. Vigorous chest physiotherapy was recognized as the underlying mechanism, and the situation is thereafter discussed as shaken newborn syndrome (Williams and Sunderland 2002; Rushton 2003).

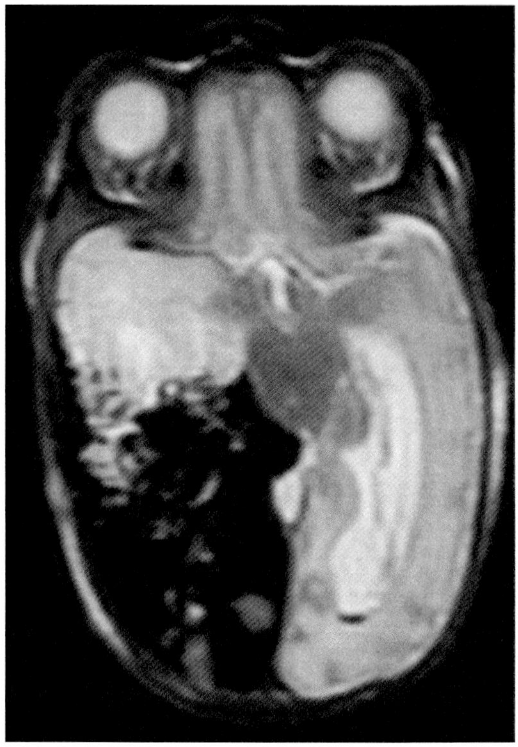

Fig. 4 Axial T2 MRI: subarachnoid hematoma associated with gram-negative septicemia in a preterm infant

Cerebellar hematoma. Preterm primary cerebellar hemorrhage probably develops in germinative cortical and periventricular areas under the same clinical circumstances as GMH (Wigglesworth and Pape 1980; Limperopoulos et al. 2005; Muller et al. 2007; Johnsen et al. 2002; Pape and Wigglesworth 1979;

Ecury-Goossen et al. 2010). The lower the gestational age, the higher the risk, in viable preterm infants. The extensive lobar nature of some hematomas argues against a primary pial arterial occlusion, although extensive subarachnoid hemorrhage might occlude adjacent pial arteries due to spasm and lead to secondary cerebellar infarction. A strong case was made for venous injury leading to large hemispheric cerebellar bleeding associated with face-mask ventilation of preterm infants (Pape et al. 1976), and a similar mechanism may well be operative in many preterms. The site of bleeding can be in the pial plexus related to the external granular layer, in the core of a folium, or in the vascular plexus around the deep cerebellar nuclei. Alternatively, secondary subarachnoid bleeding may mimic primary cerebellar parenchymal hemorrhage: clot is scattered across folia in case of lateral ventricle IVH, following passage of fragments through the outlet foramina of the fourth ventricle, first into Blake's pouch remnant and subsequently into retrocerebellar arachnoid spaces. To think of preventive strategies, we need to study the microcirculation and veins of the cerebellum both before and after birth (Gveric-Ahmetasevic et al. 2011). In adults, cerebellar hematoma, also uncommon, may follow transverse sinus thrombosis (Ushiwata et al. 1989). This suggests a possible role for venous thrombosis in perinatal cerebellar hematoma, to be studied in more detail (Fumagalli et al. 2009). Fetal cerebellar hemorrhage has been linked to vascular malformations and dysplasias, but also to fetopathy by CMV or parvovirus.

129.3.3 Step 3: Link Stroke to (Birth) Trauma

There are several possibilities for mechanically difficult delivery to cause vessel occlusion. Direct injury to the vertebro-basilar arterial system is possible (Krauland 1952; Hamida et al. 2014). Several reports are associated with difficult instrumental traction with intimal damage to the internal carotid or middle cerebral artery resulting in local occlusion from thrombosis and stroke (Roessmann and Miller 1980; Hill et al. 1983; Turnpenny et al. 1992; Choy et al. 2001; Lequin et al. 2004; Kumar et al. 2004; Onate Vergara et al. 2006; Ng et al. 2010). Focal brain damage in the sense of contusion can be observed with bone fracture or dehiscence (Mannino and Trauner 1983; Govaert et al. 1992c). Both PCA and superior cerebellar artery can be compressed and occluded during uncal herniation induced by lobar parenchymal, epidural, or subdural hematoma (Remillard et al. 1974; Deonna and Prod'hom 1978; Feske et al. 1992; Hanigan et al. 1993; Steinbok et al. 1995). It may well be that herniation of tissue at the level of the tentorial notch – either up- or downward – not only leads to arterial but also to venous ischemia. In the vicinity of subdural or subarachnoid bleeding, stroke has been tentatively (because never angiographically documented in the newborn) linked to spasm (Lequin et al. 2004; Govaert et al. 1992c; Steinbok et al. 1995; Jan and Camfield 1998; Koelfen et al. 1995; Mazumdar et al. 2003; Talvik et al. 2010). Trauma may predispose to arterial infarction outside the context of difficult delivery. During ECMO, embolism from the cannulated (traumatized) carotid artery or hypoperfusion on that part of the circle of Willis can cause stroke (de Vries et al. 1997).

There have been several reports on focal spinal cord infarction before birth, associated with neck hyperextension in utero and subsequent spinal ischemia (anterior spinal artery kinking, traction, and/or compression) in the lower cervical to higher thoracic cord (Bhagwanani et al. 1973; Bresnan and Abroms 1974; Maekawa et al. 1976). Most children were quadriplegic from birth, often delivered with cesarean section. Some had paraplegia or paralysis of the arms (Fig. 5).

CSVT of traumatic origin has been reported as infected cephalhematoma, osteitis, and transverse sinus thrombosis (Chan et al. 2002), superior sagittal sinus thrombosis due to impression of the occipital squama (Cowan and Thoresen 1985; Govaert et al. 1992d; Fig. 6), propagated thrombosis from superior sagittal sinus into deep veins (Govaert et al. 1992a), and transverse sinus thrombosis (Baram et al. 1988). Venous congestion associated with thrombosis at the torcular

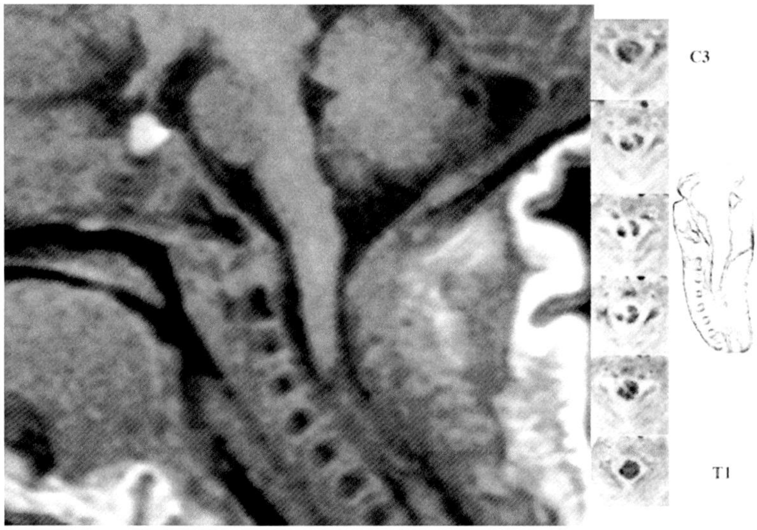

Fig. 5 Term boy with quadriparesis from birth (hyperextended breech for which elective cesarean deceased due to respiratory insufficiency in early infancy). MRI (sagittal T1 with assorted T2 axial scans at different cervical levels) pointed to a lesion from C3 to T1 that divided the cervical cord into a smaller right and larger left portion

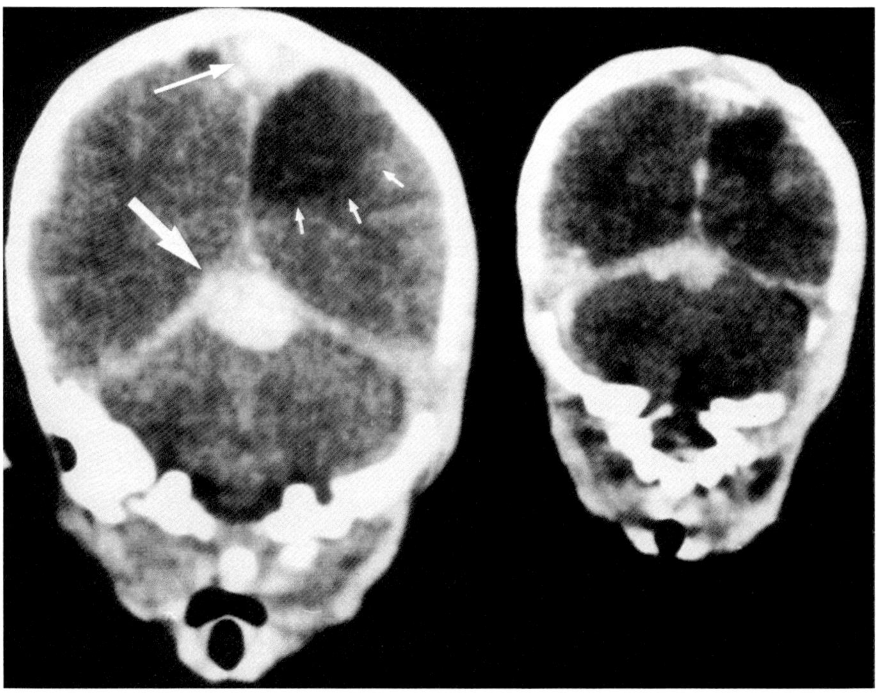

Fig. 6 Coronal CT sections in a term infant with sinus thrombosis (*left*) due to impressed occipital squama (*right*). Also observe tentorial subdural hematoma (*large arrow*) and area of ischemia on the left convexity (*small arrows*)

may lead to deep vein thrombosis without propagation of the clot directly. Intrapartum and postpartum neck rotation may sufficiently impede jugular venous flow (occlusion on the side to which the head is turned) to contribute to thrombosis. Direct sinus trauma from a penetrating scalp electrode can also induce thrombosis (McGregor and McFarren 1989).

Cranial compression encephalopathy is the term recently put forward by obstetricians to

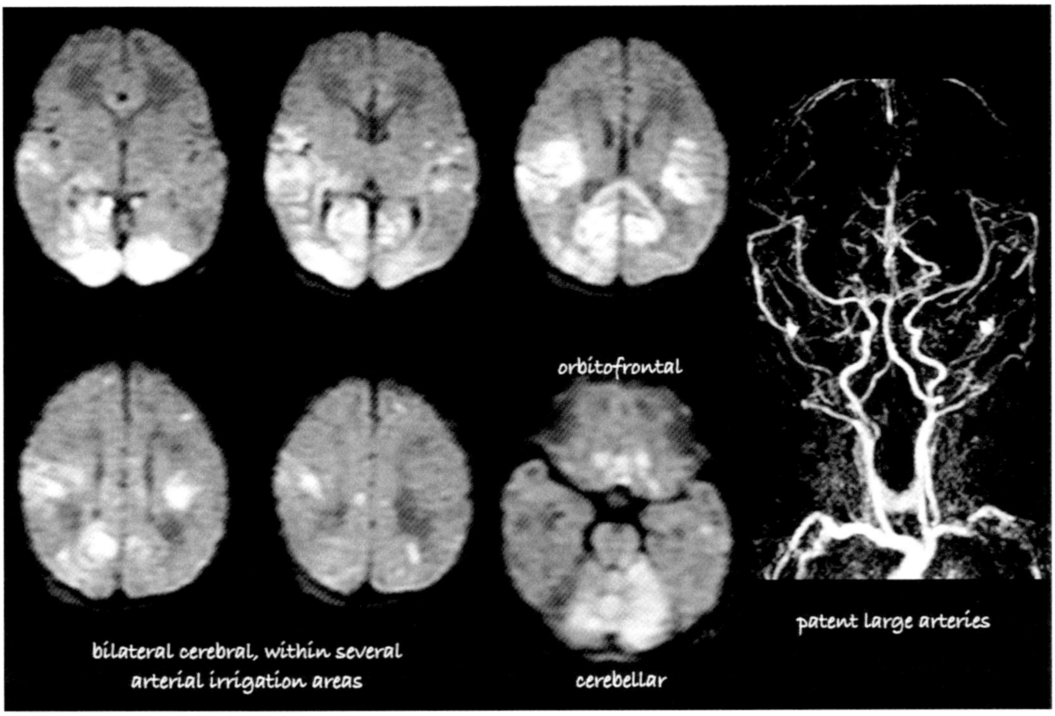

Fig. 7 Personal observation (medicolegal case) of multiple ischemic lesions most likely associated with prolonged excessive skull pressure during delivery. Notice normal MRA. Both epi- and intracranial hemorrhage were minimal

denominate ischemic injury to the brain due to very high and/or prolonged and/or relentless pressure on the term skull during delivery (Schifrin and Ater 2006). On rare occasions, one may indeed notice multiple, mainly non-hemorrhagic brain infarcts defying easy explanation by arterial thrombosis or embolism. Pressures in the cranium are higher than amniotic pressures, which often reach up to 100 mmHg for minutes. The pressure distribution will depend on the position of the head in the pelvis, most pressure probably exerted on brain parts facing the pubic bone. Venous ischemia by pressure is probably the first lesional mechanism before pressure compresses arteries. Although this concept has been reported and described in the literature, it would be helpful to a better understanding of this type of injury where it is pure and unassociated with other bone injury than mere molding and without extensive intracranial hemorrhage, if more such cases were reported (Fig. 7).

We have recently observed a pattern of mechanical neonatal brain injury, mainly in term infants, not clearly described before (paper submitted). The novelty is not the pattern but the context of mechanical injury during birth. A similar pattern has been reported with the term contusional tearing, under the umbrella of non-accidental injury during infancy. The hallmark is focal, unilateral, or (if bilateral) asymmetrical hyperechoic change in the core of the superior frontal gyri, in some leading to cavitation within days, and the lesions do not fit with a global hypoxic-ischemic or focal macrovascular venous or arterial template of injury. Because shearing forces – as with acute acceleration or deceleration following shaking or blunt head trauma – are unlikely to be present during birth, the existence of this lesional pattern raises the question of which is the intermediary mechanism. A stage of selective subcortical venous ischemia by bone displacement is a candidate. Because the superior frontal gyri are readily accessible to high-resolution ultrasound, this may be the method

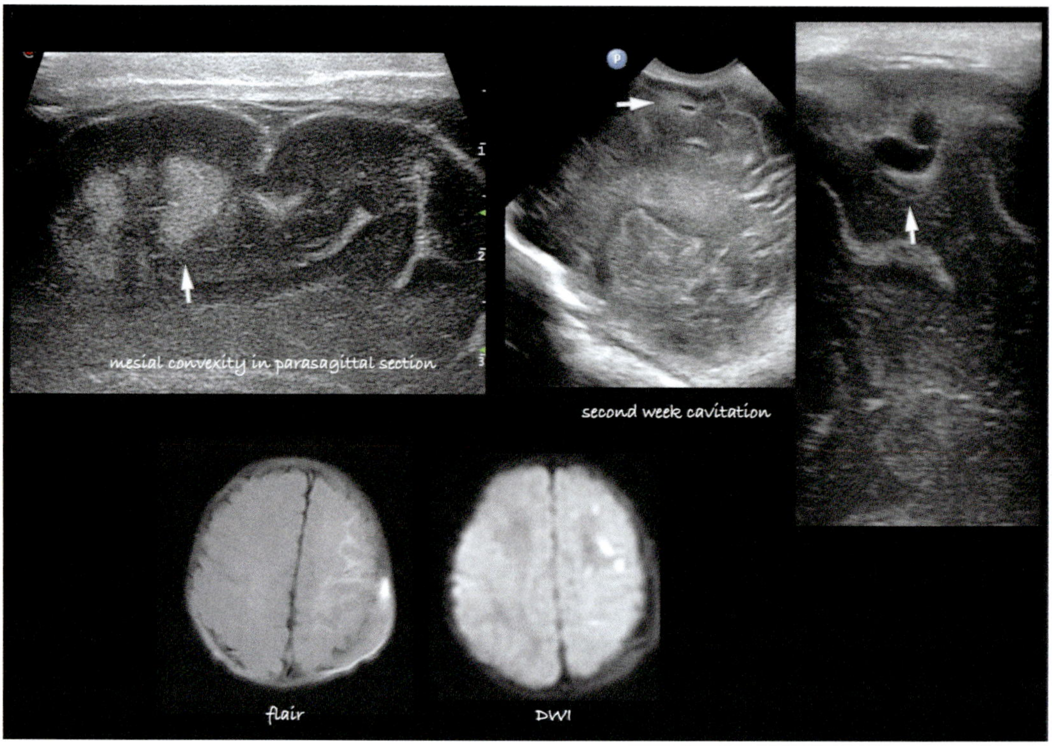

Fig. 8 Composite image of a hyperechoic lesion in the left superior frontal gyral core associated with difficult vaginal delivery (prolonged second stage, persistent occiput posterior, secondary cesarean section) of a term infant with left frontal epileptic activity. The second week sonogram top right is from another infant with similar lesions but with cavitation documented by serial scanning

of screening for this lesion pattern shortly after admission following mechanically difficult delivery (Fig. 8).

129.3.4 Step 4: Link Brain Infection to Stroke

Both meningitis and ventriculitis can lead to inflammation and occlusion of arteries and veins with focal or diffuse subcortical and/or periventricular infarction (Berman and Banker 1966; Chang et al. 2003) (Fig. 9). Large vessel NAIS has been reported infrequently, sometimes with exotic organisms [syphilis (Snyder et al. 1981; Ment et al. 1986), enterobacter (Ries et al. 1994), meningococcus (Chiu et al. 1995), listeria (Harris 1997), pasteurella multocida (Wade et al. 1999), salmonella (Kay's Kayemba

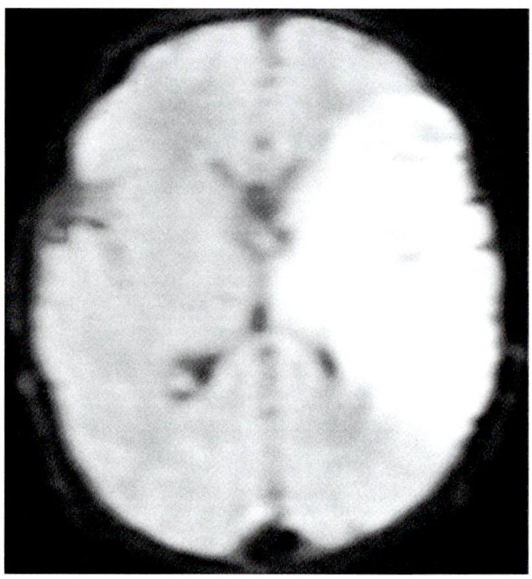

Fig. 9 DW MRI: focal large artery stroke (MCA) associated with listeria meningitis in a term infant

et al. 2000; Harteman et al. 2012a)]. Sinus thrombosis similarly can follow bacterial meningitis (Krebs et al. 1998; Farstad et al. 2003; Fitzgerald and Golomb 2007). Local infection may be a portal of entry for thrombophlebitis of a sinus: from scalp infection via emissary veins to a sinus (Bailey and Hass 1958; Byers and Hass 1933), infection in aplasia cutis invading superior sagittal sinus (Lavine et al. 1978; Kantor et al. 2005), or from orbital cellulitis into the cavernous sinus (Jackson and Baker 1986).

Acute chorioamnionitis is recently suggested as a possible cause of first umbilical venous and later cardiac or brain thromboembolism (Redline et al. 2008). There is no evidence for direct cerebral arteritis in this situation. Fetal infections like rubella, CMV, and toxoplasmosis can be associated with brain arteritis.

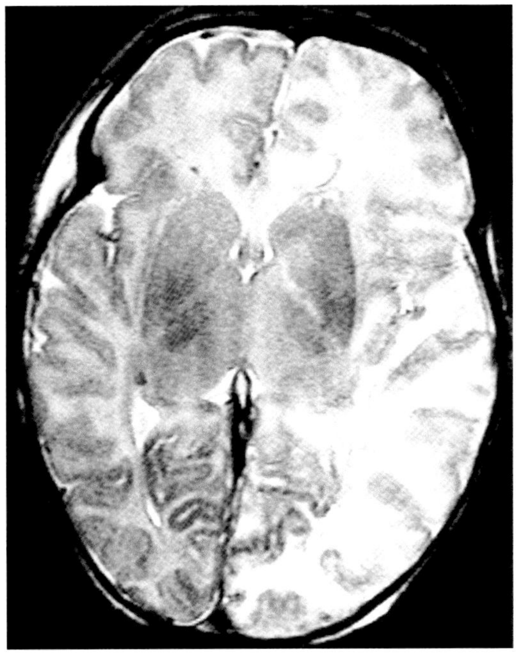

Fig. 10 T1 MRI: multifocal ischemic infarction of the left side of the brain in incontinentia pigmenti

129.3.5 Step 5: Recognize an Arteriopathy (Venopathy) or Arterial (Venous) Malformation

Noninfectious inflammatory conditions can predispose to arterial stroke, some grouped under the umbrella of pseudo-TORCH conditions. Incontinentia pigmenti probably causes obliteration of small- and medium-sized arteries in the neonatal period (Maingay-de Groof et al. 2008 Fig. 10), Aicardi-Goutieres syndrome can lead to focal arterial ischemia (Barth et al. 1999), and infantile arterial calcinosis can induce focal infarction in the basal ganglia and watershed injury at cortical level (Juul et al. 1990; van der Sluis et al. 2006).

Hemorrhagic destruction of the brain, subependymal calcification, and cataracts (AR) (junctional adhesion molecule 3): subependymal calcifications, cataracts, microphthalmia, hepatomegaly, renal cystic dysplasia, and ectopic kidney.

Aicardi-Goutieres syndrome (AR)(three prime repair exonuclease 1, ribonuclease H2 subunit B, ribonuclease H2 subunit C, ribonuclease H2 subunit A, SAM domain and HD domain 1, adenosine deaminase RNA specific): progressive microcephaly, intracranial calcification, white matter destruction, brain atrophy, thrombocytopenia, hepatosplenomegaly, elevated liver transaminases, intermittent fever, glaucoma, cataract, chilblain lupus, and arthropathy.

Band-like calcification with simplified gyration and polymicrogyria (AR) (occludin): band-like intracranial calcifications, simplified gyral pattern, and progressive microcephaly.

Incontinentia pigmenti (X-L) (NF-kappaB essential modulator): corpus callosum hypoplasia; cerebral atrophy; hair, nail, and dental abnormalities; ophthalmological abnormalities; and pathognomonic skin inflammation/ hyper- and hypopigmentation.

Cerebroretinal microangiopathy with calcifications and cysts (AR) (CTS telomere maintenance complex component 1): intracranial calcification, retinal telangiectasia and exudates, osteopenia, vasculature ectasias in stomach, small intestine and liver, anemia, and thrombocytopenia.

Leukoencephalopathy, cystic, and without megalencephaly (AR) (ribonuclease T2): intracranial calcification, microcephaly, and hearing loss.

Other hereditary conditions associated with arterial occlusion presenting in the neonatal period or early infancy: inborn errors of metabolism (hyperhomocysteinemia, primary hyperoxaluria, galactosialidosis, molybdenum cofactor deficiency, mitochondrial disorders) and anomalies of karyotype (Miller-Dieker lissencephaly, trisomy 13, 22q11 deletion). Hypoplastic or absent (malformed) arteries can be associated with congenital or postnatal brain tissue loss (Lie 1968) (Fig. 11). Such malformations are seen in PHACE syndrome (Rossi and Tortori-Donati 2006; Drolet et al. 2006; Judd et al. 2007) and in Goldenhar syndrome (Ottaviano et al. 2007). Carotid hypoplasia may lack an obvious cause (Lee et al. 2003) or be associated with maternal drug abuse, toxins, or infectious agents (Guajardo et al. 1994; Afifi et al. 1987; Lien et al. 1995). Other neonatal arterial anomalies have been linked to fibromuscular dysplasia, to carotid elastin hyperplasia (Thompson et al. 1975), or to Ehlers-Danlos I or Stickler syndrome (Curry et al. 2007). Although neonatal stroke has not yet been reported yet, it is expected that arterial tortuosity syndromes may cause either focal infarction or bleeding (Meuwissen et al. 2013). We have observed perinatal MCA stroke associated with altered shape and thrombosis of the aortic arch, without any of the above diagnoses. All these observations warrant documentation of the structure and patency of large intracranial arteries in diverse instances of NAIS. Interruption or coarctation of the aorta can lead to subclavian steal syndrome, which may thus become a rare cause of neonatal stroke (Beattie et al. 2006).

Scarce case reports of sinus thrombosis associated with jugular vein hypoplasia (N'Diaye et al. 2004) or with abnormal superior vena cava anatomy (Smilari et al. 2005) suggest it may be informative to search for such venous anomalies in instances where neonatal sinus thrombosis is without obvious cause. Jugular bulb anomalies have been reported in CHARGE association (Friedmann et al. 2012). A map of venous brain drainage may have practical consequences before starting neonatal ECMO (Cassady et al. 2011).

129.3.6 Step 6: Find an Embolic Source for Arterial Ischemic Stroke

Emboli find brain arteries in many situations (review in Govaert et al. 2009b; Fig. 12). The source may be in the left heart (following exchange transfusion, balloon atrial septostomy, cardiac surgery, due to tumor or arrhythmia), in the carotid or vertebral artery or in the aortic arch, or anywhere in the body because of paradoxical embolism through a patent foramen ovale: right heart, umbilical vein, ductus venosus, portal vein, renal vein, or inferior caval vein (Amlie-Lefond et al. 2008). To assume a placental origin needs exclusion of other sources and preferably confirmation of a placental histopathological change, possibilities are extensive infarction, fetal thrombotic vasculopathy, chronic villitis with obliterative fetal vasculopathy, and meconium-stained vascular necrosis (Redline 2005; Ghidini and Locatelli 2006; Das et al. 2008; Amlie-Lefond

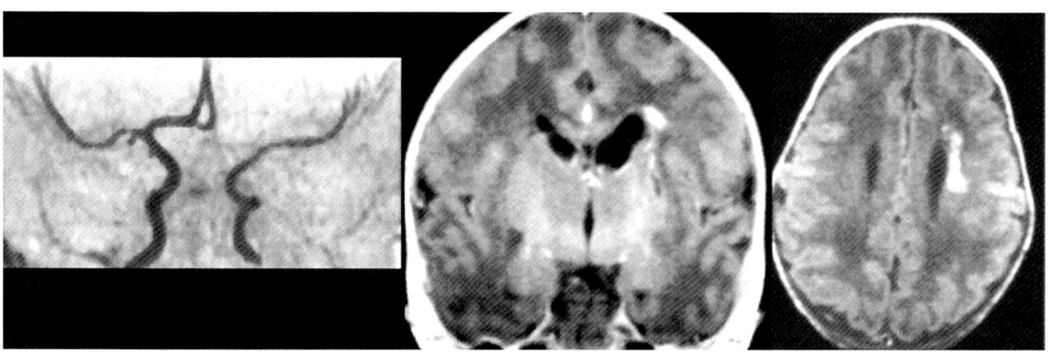

Fig. 11 Absence of the left ACA A1 part, attenuated left MCA, and ipsilateral periventricular injury, in a term infant with one episode of neonatal convulsions (*left* MRA, *middle* coronal, and *right* axial T1 MRI)

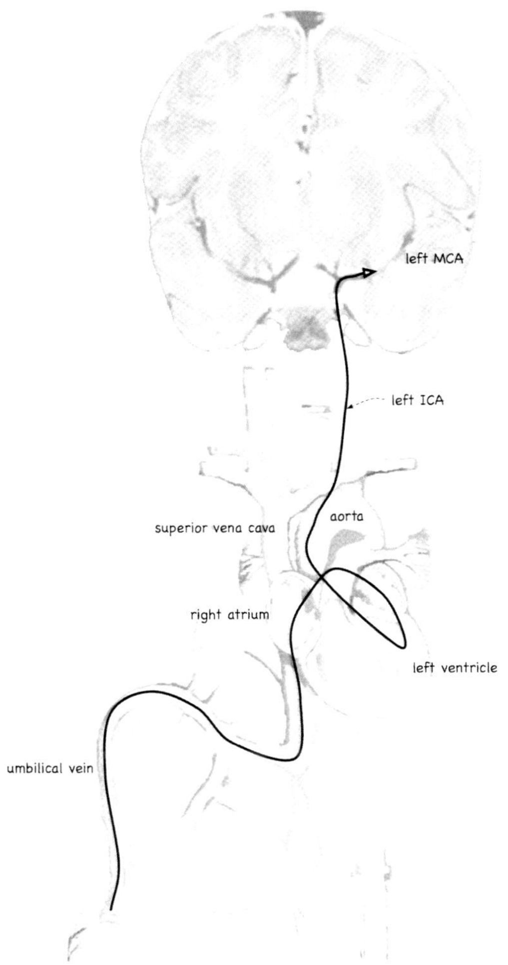

Fig. 12 Schematic presentation of paradoxical embolism from inferior vena cava into the left MCA (*IVC* inferior vena cava, *Ao* aorta, *UV* umbilical vein, *ICA* internal carotid artery)

et al. 2011; Chabrier et al. 2011). Placental exam seems to be more rewarding in arterial ischemic stroke than in sinovenous thrombosis (Elbers et al. 2011). Recent data emphasize the relation with intravascular manipulation in neonates with congenital heart defect (McQuillen et al. 2006). Atrial septal aneurysm and persistent Eustachian valve remnants may increase the risk of thrombus formation in the heart (Aypar et al. 2013). The existence of a central venous line with thrombus around the tip must be excluded. An embolic mechanism can underlie stroke in twin-twin transfusion. Inadvertent injection of embolism-prone material and air embolism are other possibilities. Flushing a temporal artery catheter (Prian et al. 1978; Bull et al. 1980) and instrumentation of the carotid artery for an ECMO procedure (Luisiri et al. 1988; Campbell et al. 1988) can both cause NAIS. It is important to document associated limb (see clinical presentation above) or visceral (heart, gut) infarction: concurrent independent infarction inside and outside the brain probably increases the likelihood of detecting a prothrombotic condition, an arteriopathy, or embolism (Bednarek et al. 2007).

129.3.7 Step 7: Diagnose Primary Thrombotic Arterial Ischemic Stroke

Spasm and primary thrombosis are two conditions where vessel occlusion is intrinsic. The balance of hemostasis can be disturbed in the direction of thrombosis, even in the absence of all extrinsic conditions mentioned above (Golomb 2003). Hypotension (due to infection, heart tamponade, or acute blood loss), septicemia, and asphyxia probably contribute to thrombosis through endothelial injury (Mittendorf et al. 2003). Intrinsic prothrombotic conditions, detailed in the hematological chapters of this book, manifest along several pathways, probably more readily causing venous than arterial thrombosis: reduced fibrinolytic activity, enhanced generation or function of thrombin, enhanced platelet aggregation, and endothelial dysfunction promoting platelet adhesion.

The extent of testing for genetic prothrombotic risk factors needed in clinical practice is not determined, but extensive screening is often recommended, largely based on experience with older children (Thornburg and Pipe 2006; Beardsley 2007; Young et al. 2008; Roach et al. 2008; Mineyko and Kirton 2011; Kirton et al. 2011). Prothrombotic risk factors readily find partners in the perinatal period to cause NAIS, as reported in many small cohort and a few case-control studies. Familial activated protein C resistance due to factor V Leiden mutation was mentioned first (Pellicer et al. 1992; Thorarensen et al. 1997; Debus et al. 1998). A modest state of thrombophilia can also be induced by hyperhomocysteinemia above 10 μmol/L. One multicenter case-control study of stroke at term found that none of 91 instances were associated with protein S deficiency (Kurnik et al. 2003). Other factors enhancing the risk of thrombosis detected included increased serum lipoprotein A, homozygous C677T polymorphism in methylenetetrahydrofolate reductase (MTHFR), protein C deficiency, and prothrombin (factor II) mutation. Antithrombin deficiency is exceptionally part of the list (Brenner et al. 1988). Plasminogen activator inhibitor-1 polymorphism may be a candidate to add as well (Baumeister et al. 2000). We have recently observed familial dysfibrinogenemia as a cause of fetal internal cerebral vein thrombosis presenting with posthemorrhagic hydrocephalus within days of birth (unpublished). Multiple heterozygosity or other risk combinations enhance the prothrombotic tendency (Abdelhamid 2012).

At present, there is not enough evidence to force clinicians into an exhaustive search for thrombophilia faced with every first and recent perinatal stroke, mainly because of the very low recurrence rate, but many clinicians start a prothrombotic screen when the family history is positive for early thrombosis and vascular disease, or when the clinical context of the newborn does not readily explain the stroke at hand (Cnossen et al. 2009). Even typical preterm GMH may need to be revisited in this context (Ramenghi et al. 2011). The detection of a combination of genetic prothrombotic risk factors may necessitate secondary prevention with use of anticoagulants during periods of increased risk (surgery, immobilization, puberty, pregnancy). A prothrombotic screen may be warranted before some types of surgery for congenital heart disease (Emani et al. 2014).

Maternal antiphospholipid antibodies (detected as lupus anticoagulants or anticardiolipin IgG antibodies) may induce thrombosis within the fetoplacental vasculature resulting in paradoxical embolism from the umbilical vein; IgG antibodies may also cross the placenta and potentially cause thrombosis directly within fetal organs (Boffa and Lachassinne 2007; Rego Sousa et al. 2012; Peixoto et al. 2014). The true significance of fetal thrombotic vasculopathy in relation to NAIS is not yet clear, but screening the mother for prothrombotic conditions may elucidate a possible mechanism in some infants with arterial ischemic stroke (Kraus and Acheen 1999; Simchen et al. 2009). A hypothetical sequence from amnionitis to fetal vasculitis (and systemic inflammation) to intracardiac thrombosis to embolic stroke was recently discussed (Redline et al. 2008). Amnionitis in preterm deliveries is not reported to contribute to stroke in that population, except for possibly increasing the risk of PVI (Harteman et al. 2012b).

The possible link between arterial ischemic stroke and hyperviscosity (in practice polycythemia) – long ago referred to as a risk factor for lateral striate infarction (Amit and Camfield 1980) – is not recently confirmed. Congenital nephrotic syndrome can present in the neonatal period with both arterial and venous cerebral thrombosis (Fofah and Roth 1997; Horsch et al. 2007). Congenital disorders of glycosylation (CDG) balance the clotting equilibrium toward thrombosis (Arnoux et al. 2008). Clotting factor suppletion could be a risk factor for NAIS (Barmada et al. 1979).

Prolonged *arterial spasm* with subsequent infarction has been linked to endogenous constrictors like subarachnoid hemorrhage and to exogenous constrictors like cocaine and others (amphetamines, blue cohosh, codeine) (Chan and Nelson 2004; Reynolds et al. 2007; Robinson et al. 2000). This mechanism is of course difficult to really prove. Spasm in a brain artery by "blunt" skull trauma is common in children but has not been reported in the newborn. Although acute hypocapnia can lead to brain ischemia, this mechanism has not been linked to unilateral focal arterial infarction so far.

129.3.8 Step 8: Diagnose Primary Sinovenous Thrombosis With(out) Infarction

As described above, both trauma and inflammation are associated with NCSVT (Fig. 13). Venous malformations rarely induce sinus thrombosis. Embolism is not a cause of sinus thrombosis, but the reverse may exist in the newborn: fragmentation of clot in a thrombosed sinus, migration along

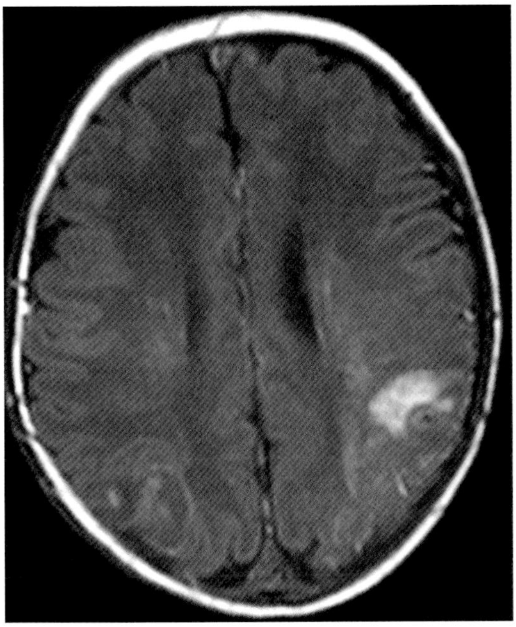

Fig. 13 Term infant with first-day thrombocytopenia and focal seizures: T1-MR showing superior sagittal sinus thrombosis with hemorrhagic parasagittal infarction

the jugular vein into the heart and paradoxically into the brain. Hyperviscosity was on occasion mentioned as a risk factor for NCSVT, e.g., in infants of a diabetic mother (Schubiger et al. 1982; Konishi et al. 1987). The limited number of descriptions of thrombophilia associated with NCSVT does not permit conclusions about the differential sensitivity with arterial thrombosis. Predispositions implicated are deficiency in antithrombin III, homozygous deficiency of protein C (or S), fV Leiden mutation, f II mutation, the presence of antiphospholipid antibodies, tPAI1 polymorphism, high lipoprotein A, factor VII replacement, congenital nephrotic syndrome, and the presence of (post hepatitis B vaccination) antinuclear antibodies (Brenner et al. 1988; Tarras et al. 1988; Tabbutt et al. 1994; Pohl et al. 1998; Worth and Hoots 1998; Ibrahim et al. 2000; Kapogiannis et al. 2001; Abrantes et al. 2002; Heineking et al. 2003; Friese et al. 2003; Swarte et al. 2004; Fitzgerald et al. 2006). The combination of neonatal brain hemorrhage and sinus thrombosis has been recently found with von Willebrand type 3 disease (Wetzstein et al. 2006). A contribution of cooling to postasphyxial NCSVT was suggested in a pilot study, but not confirmed later (Azzopardi et al. 2000). Dehydration, i.e., by insufficient breast feeding, is a risk factor specific of venous thrombosis, decades ago referred to as marantic thrombosis (Bailey and Hass 1958; Aicardi and Goutieres 1973; Hilliard et al. 1988; Gebara and Everett 2001). Sinus thrombosis can follow endovascular treatment of a vein of Galen malformation (Meyers et al. 2000). A relation between preeclampsia and sinus thrombosis remains to be confirmed (Hunt et al. 2001).

129.3.9 Step 9: No Obvious Cause, Just a Context of Obstetric Difficulties

Clinical experience, recently reiterated in a meta-analysis of case-control studies, has suggested that AIS is often consequent to obstetric problems. Abnormal cardiotocography, instrumental deliveries, and emergency cesarean sections are reported risk factors in term infants (Cheong and Cowan 2009). Uncomplicated vaginal delivery and prelabor cesarean section are uncommon in cases of PAIS. The presence of multiple risk factors increases the odds of developing PAIS. For preterm babies, fetal heart abnormalities, twin-twin transfusion, and hypoglycemia are possible risk factors.

In a case-control study, the population prevalence of PAS was 20 per 100,000 live births (Lee et al. 2005). The majority (85%) of infants with PAS were delivered at term. Factors more common among case than control infants were primiparity (73% vs. 44%), fetal heart rate abnormality (46% vs. 14%), emergency cesarean delivery (35% vs. 13%), chorioamnionitis (27% vs. 11%), prolonged rupture of membranes (26% vs. 7%), prolonged second stage of labor (25% vs. 4%), vacuum extraction (24% vs. 11%), cord abnormality (22% vs. 6%), preeclampsia (19% vs. 5%), and oligohydramnios (14% vs. 3%). Risk factors independently associated with PAS on multivariate analysis were preeclampsia (OR 5.3), prolonged rupture of membranes (OR 3.8), and chorioamnionitis (OR 3.4). The rate of PAS increased dramatically when multiple risk factors were present.

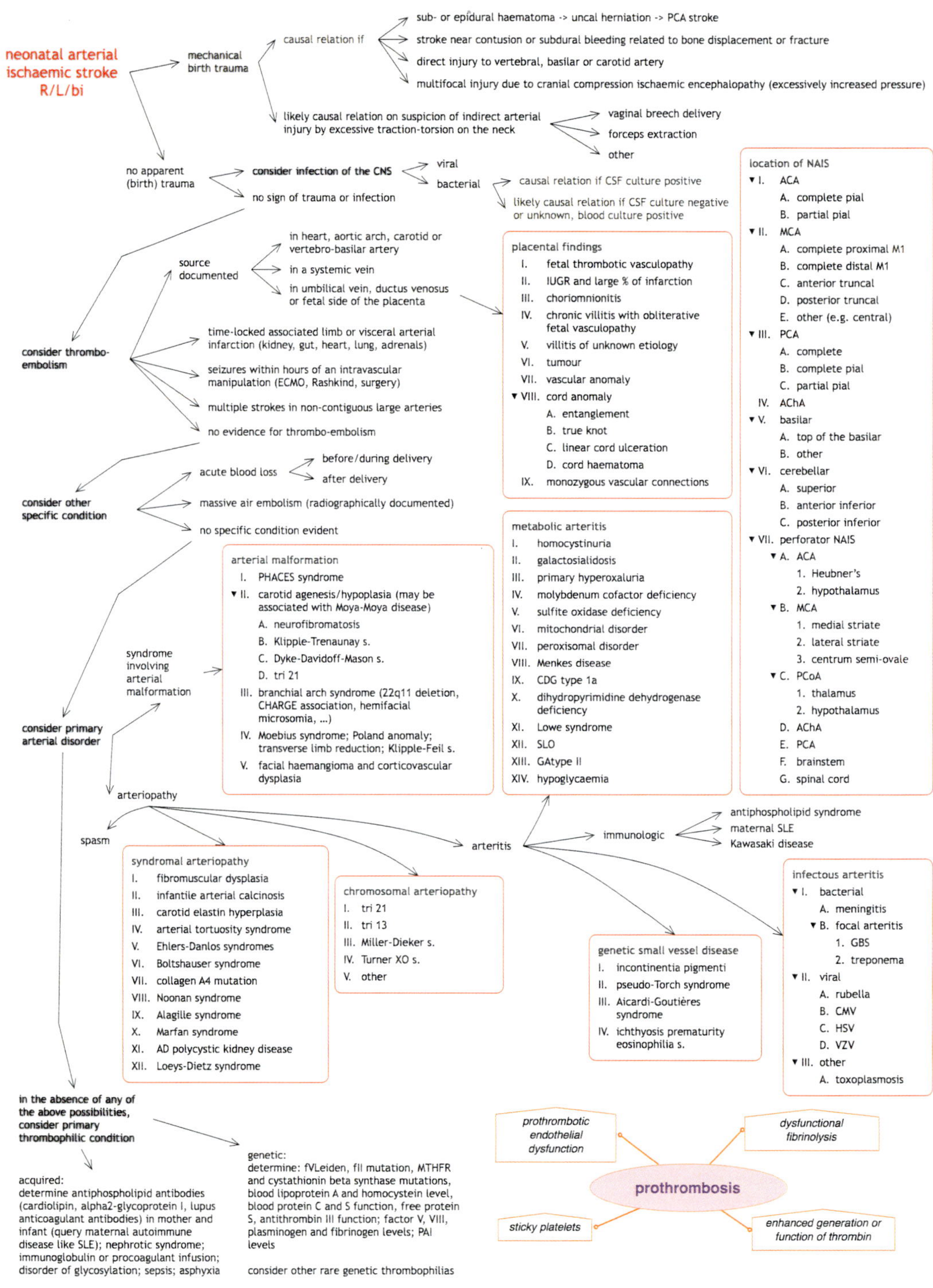

Fig. 14 Algorithm for arterial ischemic stroke

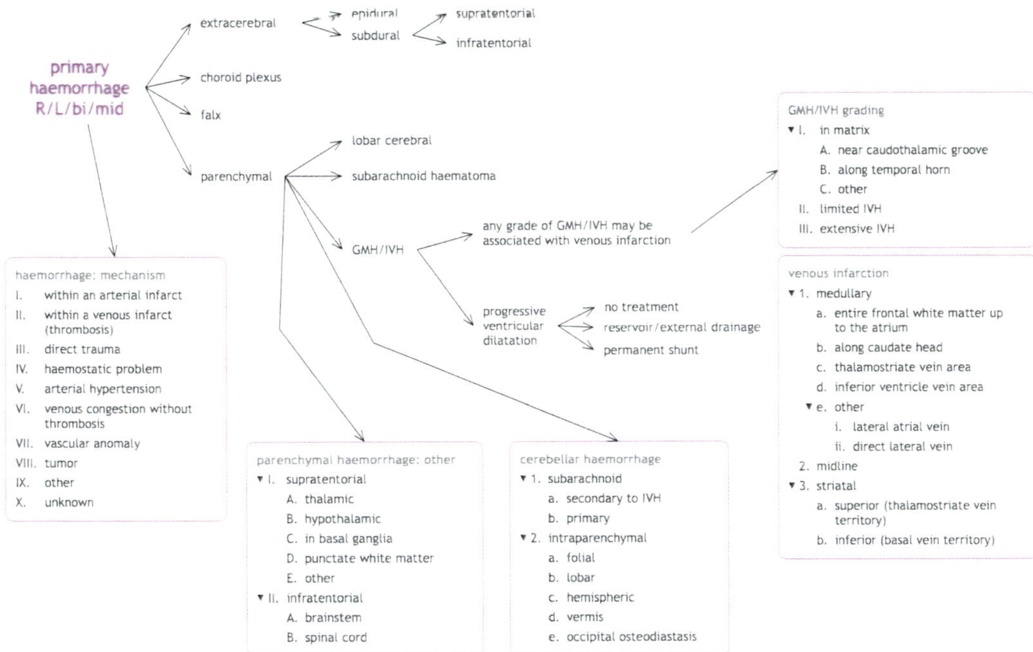

Fig. 15 Algorithm for hemorrhage

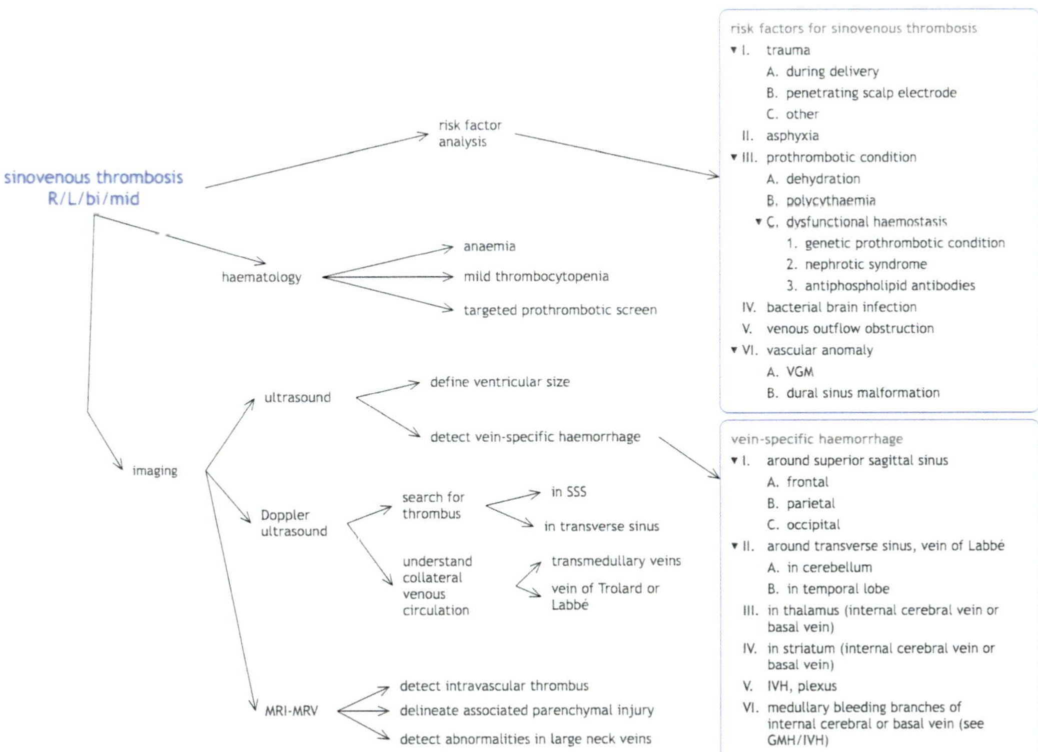

Fig. 16 Algorithm for sinovenous thrombosis

In the Luo et al.'s meta-analysis (Luo et al. 2014), significant high ORs were observed for (in order of magnitude) fetal heart rate abnormalities, a low Apgar score, reduced fetal movements, resuscitation at birth, meconium staining of the amniotic fluid, ventouse delivery, and pre-eclampsia. In spite of these findings, controlled cohort studies are required to further study mechanisms behind the obstetric pathway(s) to perinatal arterial stroke. Astute observation of fetal behavior during difficult labor will be needed to sort this question out, of significant medicolegal importance. Components may be embolism from an abnormally burdened umbilical vascular network, traction and/or torsion of neck vessels, increased thrombus formation in the ductus venosus or the heart, compression of the skull, and repetitive hypoperfusion (hypoxemia and low glucose delivery) of the fetal body and head.

129.4 Summary

The diagnostic work-up of a focal brain lesion, suspect of stroke, is summarized in three algorithms, related to the three main subtypes (Figs. 14, 15, and 16).

129.5 Cross-References

▶ Neonatal Stroke: Clinical Presentation, Imaging, Treatment, and Prognosis

References

Abdelhamid AE (2012) Preterm infant with a catastrophic hemorrhagic-thromboembolic incident. Neonatology 102:293–299

Abels L, Lequin M, Govaert P (2006) Sonographic templates of newborn perforator stroke. Pediatr Radiol 36 (7):663–669

Abrantes M, Lacerda AF, Abreu CR, Levy A, Azevedo A, Da SL (2002) Cerebral venous sinus thrombosis in a neonate due to factor V Leiden deficiency. Acta Paediatr 91(2):243–245

Afifi AK, Godersky JC, Menezes A, Smoker WR, Bell WE, Jacoby CG (1987) Cerebral hemiatrophy, hypoplasia of internal carotid artery, and intracranial aneurysm. A rare association occurring in an infant. Arch Neurol 44(2):232–235

Aicardi J, Goutieres F (1973) Intracranial venous thromboses. Complication of acute dehydration in infants. Arch Fr Pediatr 30(8):809–829

Alvarez H, Garcia Monaco R, Rodesch G, Sachet M, Krings T, Lasjaunias P (2007) Vein of galen aneurysmal malformations. Neuroimaging Clin N Am 17 (2):189–206

Amit M, Camfield PR (1980) Neonatal polycythemia causing multiple cerebral infarcts. Arch Neurol 37:109–110

Amlie-Lefond CM, Basir MA, Franciosi RA (2008) Fatal neonatal stroke from a prenatal cardiac thrombus. Pediatr Neurol 38:140–142

Amlie-Lefond CM, Basir MA, Franciosi RA (2011) Placental pathology in neonatal stroke. Pediatrics 127: e722–e729

Anderson JM, Milner RD, Strich SJ (1967) Effects of neonatal hypoglycaemia on the nervous system: a pathological study. J Neurol Neurosurg Psychiatry 30 (4):295–310

Armstrong-Wells J, Johnston J, Wu YW (2009) Prevalence and predictors of perinatal hemorrhagic stroke: results from the Kaiser pediatric stroke study. Pediatrics 123:823–828

Arnoux JB, Boddaert N, Valayannopoulos V, Romano S, Bahi-Buisson N, Desguerre I, de Keyzer Y, Munnich A, Brunelle F, Seta N, Dautzenberg MD, de Lonlay P (2008) Risk assessment of acute vascular events in congenital disorder of glycosylation type Ia. Mol Genet Metab 93:444–449, Epub 2008 Feb 21

Arrigoni F, Parazzini C, Righini A, Doneda C, Ramenghi LA, Lista G, Triulzi F (2011) Deep medullary vein involvement in neonates with brain damage: an MR imaging study. AJNR Am J Neuroradiol 32:2030–2036

Aypar E, Sert A, Odabas D (2013) Unusually prominent Chiari's network prolapsing into the right ventricle in an asymptomatic newborn. Pediatr Cardiol 34:1017–1019

Azzopardi D, Robertson NJ, Cowan FM, Rutherford MA, Rampling M, Edwards AD (2000) Pilot study of treatment with whole body hypothermia for neonatal encephalopathy. Pediatrics 106(4):684–694

Bailey OT, Hass GM (1958) Dural sinus thrombosis in early life. J Pediatr 11:755–772

Baram TZ, Butler IJ, Nelson MD Jr, McArdle CB (1988) Transverse sinus thrombosis in newborns: clinical and magnetic resonance imaging findings. Ann Neurol 24 (6):792–794

Barkovich AJ, Ali FA, Rowley HA, Bass N (1998) Imaging patterns of neonatal hypoglycemia. AJNR Am J Neuroradiol 19(3):523–528

Barmada MA, Moossy J, Shuman RM (1979) Cerebral infarcts with arterial occlusion in neonates. Ann Neurol 6:495–502

Barth PG, Walter A, van Gelderen I (1999) Aicardi-Goutières syndrome: a genetic microangiopathy? Acta Neuropathol 98(2):212–216

Bassan H, Benson CB, Limperopoulos C, Feldman HA, Ringer SA, Veracruz E, Stewart JE, Soul JS, Disalvo DN, Volpe JJ, du Plessis AJ (2006) Ultrasonographic features and severity scoring of periventricular hemorrhagic infarction in relation to risk factors and outcome. Pediatrics 117:2111–2118

Baumeister FA, Auberger K, Schneider K (2000) Thrombosis of the deep cerebral veins with excessive bilateral infarction in a premature infant with the thrombogenic 4G/4G genotype of the plasminogen activator inhibitor-1. Eur J Pediatr 159:239–242

Beardsley DS (2007) Venous thromboembolism in the neonatal period. Semin Perinatol 31:250–253

Beattie LM, Butler SJ, Goudie DE (2006) Pathways of neonatal stroke and subclavian steal syndrome. Arch Dis Child Fetal Neonatal Ed 91:F204–F207

Bednarek N, Morville P, Delebarre G, Akhavi A, Sommer C (2007) Necrotic skin lesions and cerebral infarction in the newborn: two case reports. J Child Neurol 22 (3):354–357

Bergman I, Bauer RE, Barmada MA, Latchaw RE, Taylor HG, David R, Painter MJ (1985) Intracerebral hemorrhage in the full-term neonatal infant. Pediatrics 75:488–496

Berman PH, Banker BQ (1966) Neonatal meningitis. A clinical and pathological study of 29 cases. Pediatrics 38:6–24

Bhagwanani SG, Price HV, Laurence KM, Ginz B (1973) Risks and prevention of cervical cord injury in the management of breech presentation with hyperextension of the fetal head. Am J Obstet Gynecol 115 (8):1159–1161

Block AJ, McQuillen PS, Chau V, Glass H, Poskitt KJ, Barkovich AJ, Esch M, Soulikias W, Azakie A, Campbell A, Miller SP (2010) Clinically silent preoperative brain injuries do not worsen with surgery in neonates with congenital heart disease. J Thorac Cardiovasc Surg 140:550–557

Boffa MC, Lachassinne E (2007) Infant perinatal thrombosis and antiphospholipid antibodies: a review. Lupus 16(8):634–641

Brenner B, Fishman A, Goldsher D, Schreibman D, Tavory S (1988) Cerebral thrombosis in a newborn with a congenital deficiency of antithrombin III. Am J Hematol 27 (3):209–211

Bresnan MJ, Abroms IF (1974) Neonatal spinal cord transection secondary to intrauterine hyperextension of the neck in breech presentation. J Pediatr 84(5):734–737

Bull MJ, Schreiner RL, Garg BP, Hutton NM, Lemons JA, Gresham EL (1980) Neurologic complications following temporal artery catheterization. J Pediatr 96 (6):1071–1073

Burns CM, Rutherford MA, Boardman JP, Cowan FM (2008) Patterns of cerebral injury and neurodevelopmental outcomes after symptomatic neonatal hypoglycemia. Pediatrics 122(1):65–74

Byers RK, Hass GM (1933) Thrombosis of the dural venous sinuses in infancy and childhood. Am J Dis Child 45:1161–1183

Campbell LR, Bunyapen C, Holmes GL, Howell CG Jr, Kanto WP Jr (1988) Right common carotid artery ligation in extracorporeal membrane oxygenation. J Pediatr 113(1 Pt 1):110–113

Cassady CI, Mehollin-Ray AR, Olutoye OO, Cass DL (2011) Jugular vein hypoplasia can preclude extracorporeal membrane oxygenation cannulation in the neonate with congenital diaphragmatic hernia: potential identification of the neonate at risk by fetal magnetic resonance imaging. Fetal Diagn Ther 30:225–228

Chabrier S, Husson B, Dinomais M, Landrieu P, Nguyen The Tich S (2011) New insights (and new interrogations) in perinatal arterial ischemic stroke. Thromb Res 127:13–22

Chan GM, Nelson LS (2004) More on blue cohosh and perinatal stroke. N Engl J Med 351:2239–2241, author reply 2239–2241

Chan MS, Wong YC, Lau SP, Lau KY, Ou Y (2002) MRI and CT findings of infected cephalhaematoma complicated by skull vault osteomyelitis, transverse venous sinus thrombosis and cerebellar haemorrhage. Pediatr Radiol 32(5):376–379

Chang CJ, Chang WN, Huang LT, Chang YC, Huang SC, Hung PL, Ho HH, Chang CS, Wang KW, Cheng BC, Lui CC, Chang HW, Lu CH (2003) Cerebral infarction in perinatal and childhood bacterial meningitis. QJM 96:755–762

Cheong JL, Cowan FM (2009) Neonatal arterial ischaemic stroke: obstetric issues. Semin Fetal Neonatal Med 14:267–271

Chessells JM, Wigglesworth JSW (1970) Secondary haemorrhagic disease of the newborn. Arch Dis Child 45:539–543

Chiu CH, Lin TY, Huang YC (1995) Cranial nerve palsies and cerebral infarction in a young infant with meningococcal meningitis. Scand J Infect Dis 27(1):75–76

Choy CM, Tam WH, Ng PC (2001) Skull fracture and contralateral cerebral infarction after ventouse extraction. BJOG 108(12):1298–1299

Cnossen MH, van Ommen CH, Appel IM (2009) Etiology and treatment of perinatal stroke; a role for prothrombotic coagulation factors? Semin Fetal Neonatal Med 14:311–317

Cowan F, Thoresen M (1985) Changes in superior sagittal sinus blood velocities due to postural alterations and pressure on the head of the newborn infant. Pediatrics 75:1038–1047

Cross JH, Harrison CJ, Preston PR, Rushton DI, Newell SJ, Morgan MEI, Durbin GM (1992) Postnatal encephaloclastic porencephaly—a new lesion? Arch Dis Child 67:307–311

Curry CJ, Bhullar S, Holmes J, Delozier CD, Roeder ER, Hutchison HT (2007) Risk factors for perinatal arterial stroke: a study of 60 mother-child pairs. Pediatr Neurol 37:99–107

Das S, Ankola P, Chiechi M, Sandhu J (2008) Perinatal cerebral arterial infarction associated with a placental chorioangioma. Am J Perinatol 25:381–383 de Vries LS, Groenendaal F, Eken P, van Haastert IC, Rademaker KJ, Meiners LC (1997) Infarcts in the vascular distribution of the middle cerebral artery in preterm and full term infants. Neuropediatrics 28 (2):88–96

Debus O, Koch HG, Kurlemann G, Strater R, Vielhaber H, Weber P, Nowak-Gottl U (1998) Factor V Leiden and genetic defects of thrombophilia in childhood porencephaly. Arch Dis Child Fetal Neonatal Ed 78: F121–F124

Deonna T, Prod'hom L-S (1978) Temporal lobe epilepsy and hemianopsia in childhood of perinatal origin. Neuropadiatrie 11:85–90

Drolet BA, Dohil M, Golomb MR, Wells R, Murowski L, Tamburro J, Sty J, Friedlander SF (2006) Early stroke and cerebral vasculopathy in children with facial hemangiomas and PHACE association. Pediatrics 117:959–964

Dudink J, Lequin M, Weisglas-Kuperus N, Conneman N, Goudoever JV, Govaert P (2007) Venous subtypes of preterm periventricular haemorrhagic infarction. Arch Dis Child Fet Neonatal Ed 93(3):F201–F206

Ecury-Goossen GM, Dudink J, Lequin M, Feijen-Roon M, Horsch S, Govaert P (2010) The clinical presentation of preterm cerebellar haemorrhage. Eur J Pediatr 169:1249–1253

Elbers J, Viero S, MacGregor D, DeVeber G, Moore AM (2011) Placental pathology in neonatal stroke. Pediatrics 127:e722–e729

Emani S, Zurakowski D, Baird CW, Pigula FA, Trenor C 3rd, Emani SM (2014) Hypercoagulability panel testing predicts thrombosis in neonates undergoing cardiac surgery. Am J Hematol 89:151–155

Farstad H, Gaustad P, Kristiansen P, Perminov G, Abrahamsen TG (2003) Cerebral venous thrombosis and Escherichia coli infection in neonates. Acta Paediatr 92(2):254–257

Feske SK, Carrazana EJ, Kupsky WJ, Volpe JJ (1992) Uncal herniation secondary to bacterial meningitis in a newborn. Pediatr Neurol 8(2):142–144

Fitzgerald KC, Golomb MR (2007) Neonatal arterial ischemic stroke and sinovenous thrombosis associated with meningitis. J Child Neurol 22(7):818–822

Fitzgerald KC, Williams LS, Garg BP, Carvalho KS, Golomb MR (2006) Cerebral sinovenous thrombosis in the neonate. Arch Neurol 63(3):405–409

Fofah O, Roth P (1997) Congenital nephrotic syndrome presenting with cerebral venous thrombosis, hypocalcemia, and seizures in the neonatal period. J Perinatol 17(6):492–494

Friedmann DR, Amoils M, Germiller JA, Lustig LR, Glastonbury CM, Pramanik BK, Lalwani AK (2012) Venous malformations of the temporal bone are a common feature in CHARGE syndrome. Laryngoscope 122:895–900

Friese S, Muller-Hansen I, Schoning M, Nowak-Gottl U, Kuker W (2003) Isolated internal cerebral venous thrombosis in a neonate with increased lipoprotein (a) level: diagnostic and therapeutic considerations. Neuropediatrics 34(1):36–39

Fumagalli M, Ramenghi LA, Righini A, Groppo M, Bassi L, De Carli A, Parazzini C, Triulzi F, Mosca F (2009) Cerebellar haemorrhages and pons development in extremely low birth weight infants. Front Biosci (Elite Ed) 1:537–541

Gataullina S, Delonlay P, Lemaire E, Boddaert N, Bulteau C, Soufflet C, Lain GA, Nabbout R, Chiron C, Dulac O (2015) Seizures and epilepsy in hypoglycaemia caused by inborn errors of metabolism. Dev Med Child Neurol 57:194–199

Gebara BM, Everett KO (2001) Dural sinus thrombosis complicating hypernatremic dehydration in a breastfed neonate. Clin Pediatr (Phila) 40(1):45–48

Ghidini A, Locatelli A (2006) Diffuse placental chorioangiomatosis causing multiple fetal cerebral embolism: a case report. J Reprod Med 51:321–324

Golomb MR (2003) The contribution of prothrombotic disorders to peri- and neonatal ischemic stroke. Semin Thromb Hemost 29:415–424

Govaert P, Achten E, Vanhaesebrouck P, De Praeter C, Van Damme J (1992a) Deep cerebral venous thrombosis in thalamo-ventricular haemorrhage of the term newborn. Pediatr Radiol 22(2):123–127

Govaert P, Leroy J, Caemaert J, Wood BP (1992b) Radiological case of the month. Extensive neonatal subarachnoid hematoma. Am J Dis Child 146:635–636

Govaert P, Vanhaesebrouck P, de Praeter C (1992c) Traumatic neonatal intracranial bleeding and stroke. Arch Dis Child 67:840–845

Govaert P, Voet D, Achten E, Vanhaesebrouck P, van Rostenberghe H, van Gysel D, Afschrift M (1992d) Noninvasive diagnosis of superior sagittal sinus thrombosis in a neonate. Am J Perinatol 9(3):201–204

Govaert P, Bridger J, Wigglesworth J (1995) Nature of the brain lesion in fetal allo-immune thrombocytopenia. Dev Med Child Neurol 37:485–495

Govaert P, Swarte R, Oostra A, Zecic A, Vanzieleghem B, Van Langenhove P (2001) Neonatal infarction within basal cerebral vein territory. Dev Med Child Neurol 43 (8):559–562

Govaert P, Ramenghi L, Taal R, Dudink J, Lequin M (2009a) Classification issues in perinatal stroke. II: mechanisms and clinical phenotypes. Acta Paediatr 98:1720–1726

Govaert P, Ramenghi L, Taal R, de Vries L, deVeber G (2009a) Classification issues in perinatal stroke. I: definitions, differential diagnosis and classification. Acta Paediatr 98:1556-1567

Guajardo L, Strauss A, Amster J (1994) Idiopathic cerebral infarction and upper limb ischemia in neonates. Am J Perinatol 11(2):119–122

Gveric-Ahmetasevic S, Colic A, Gveric T, Gasparovic VE, Pavlisa G, Ozretic D (2011) Coexistence of cerebral sinovenous thrombosis and Dandy Walker malformation in newborn. Coll Antropol 35(Suppl 1):303–307

Hamida N, Hakim A, Fourati H, Ben Thabet A, Walha L, Bouraoui A, Mnif Z, Gargouri A (2014) Neonatal cervical artery dissection secondary to birth trauma. Arch Pediatr 21:201–205
Hanigan WC, Olivero WC, Miller TC (1993) Traumatic neonatal intracranial bleeding and stroke. Arch Dis Child 68(3 Spec No):339–340
Hanigan WC, Powell FC, Palagallo G, Miller TC (1995) Lobar haemorrhages in full-term neonates. Child's Nerv Syst 11:276–280
Harris NL (1997) Case records of the Massachusetts General Hospital. Weekly clinicopathological exercises. Case 15–1997. Respiratory distress and seizure in a neonate. N Engl J Med 336:1439–1446
Harteman JC, Groenendaal F, Kwee A, Welsing PM, Benders MJ, de Vries LS (2012a) Risk factors for perinatal arterial ischaemic stroke in full-term infants: a case-control study. Arch Dis Child Fetal Neonatal Ed 97:F411–F416
Harteman JC, Nikkels PG, Kwee A, Groenendaal F, de Vries LS (2012b) Patterns of placental pathology in preterm infants with a periventricular haemorrhagic infarction: association with time of onset and clinical presentation. Placenta 33:839–844
Harteman JC, Groenendaal F, Toet MC, Benders MJ, Van Haastert IC, Nievelstein RA, Koopman-Esseboom C, de Vries LS (2013) Diffusion-weighted imaging changes in cerebral watershed distribution following neonatal encephalopathy are not invariably associated with an adverse outcome. Dev Med Child Neurol 55:642–653
Hayashi T, Harada K, Honda E, Utsunomiya H, Hashimoto T (1987) Rare neonatal intracerebral haemorrhage. Two cases in full-term infants. Child's Nerv Syst 3:161–164
Hayashi N, Endo S, Oka N, Takeda S, Takaku A (1994) Intracranial hemorrhage due to rupture of an arteriovenous malformation in a full-term neonate. Child's Nerv Syst 10:344–346
Heineking B, Riebel T, Scheer I, Kulozik A, Hoehn T, Buhrer C (2003) Intraventricular hemorrhage in a full-term neonate associated with sinus venous thrombosis and homozygosity for the plasminogen activator inhibitor-1 4G/4G polymorphism. Pediatr Int 45 (1):93–96
Hill A, Martin DJ, Daneman A, Fitz CR (1983) Focal ischemic cerebral injury in the newborn: diagnosis by ultrasound and correlation with computed tomographic scan. Pediatrics 71(5):790–793
Hilliard TN, Marsh MJ, Malcolm P, Murdoch IA, Wood BP (1988) Radiological case of the month. Sagittal sinus thrombosis in hypernatremic dehydration. Arch Pediatr Adolesc Med 152(11):1147
Hoogstraate SR, Lequin ML, Ahmed S, Govaert P (2008) Apnoea in relation to neonatal temporal lobe haemorrhage. Eur J Paediatr Neurol 13:356–361
Horsch S, Schaper J, Roll C (2007) Lesions in congenital nephrotic syndrome. J Pediatr 151(2):221
Horsch S, Govaert P, Cowan FM, Benders MJ, Groenendaal F, Lequin MH, Saliou G, de Vries LS (2014) Developmental venous anomaly in the newborn brain. Neuroradiology 56:579–588
Huang AH, Robertson RL (2004) Spontaneous superficial parenchymal and leptomeningeal hemorrhage in term neonates. AJNR Am J Neuroradiol 25(3):469–475
Hunt RW, Badawi N, Laing S, Lam A (2001) Pre-eclampsia: a predisposing factor for neonatal venous sinus thrombosis? Pediatr Neurol 25 (3):242–246
Ibrahim A, Damon G, Teyssier G, Billiemaz K, Rayet I, Tardy B (2000) Heterozygous protein C deficiency: apropos of 2 cases with cerebral venous thrombosis in the neonatal period. Arch Pediatr 7(2):158–162
Jackson K, Baker SR (1986) Clinical implications of orbital cellulitis. Laryngoscope 96(5):568–574
Jan MM, Camfield PR (1998) Outcome of neonatal stroke in full-term infants without significant birth asphyxia. Eur J Pediatr 157:846–848
Johnsen SD, Tarby TJ, Lewis KS, Bird R, Prenger E (2002) Cerebellar infarction: an unrecognized complication of very low birthweight. J Child Neurol 17:320–324
Judd CD, Chapman PR, Koch B, Shea CJ (2007) Intracranial infantile hemangiomas associated with PHACE syndrome. AJNR Am J Neuroradiol 28(1):25–29
Juul S, Ledbetter D, Wight TN, Woodrum D (1990) New insights into idiopathic infantile arterial calcinosis. Three patient reports. Am J Dis Child 144(2):229–233
Kalpatthi R, Coley BD, Rusin JA, Blanchong CA (2005) Neonatal temporal lobar hemorrhage secondary to thrombosis of the vein of Labbe. J Perinatol 25 (9):605–607
Kantor J, Yan AC, Hivnor CM, Honig PJ, Kirschner R (2005) Extensive aplasia cutis congenita and the risk of sagittal sinus thrombosis. Arch Dermatol 141 (5):554–556
Kapogiannis BG, Gussin HA, Teodorescu M (2001) De novo production of IgG antinuclear antibodies in a neonate. J Rheumatol 28(12):2744–2747
Kay's Kayemba S, Raobijoana H, Francois P, Croize J, Bost-Bru C (2000) Acute Salmonella typhi meningitis in a 25-day-old newborn infant complicated by obstruction of the sylvian artery. Arch Pediatr 7(2):154–157
Kersbergen KJ, Benders MJ, Groenendaal F, Koopman-Esseboom C, Nievelstein RA, van Haastert IC, de Vries LS (2014) Different patterns of punctate white matter lesions in serially scanned preterm infants. PLoS One 9:e108904
Kirton A, Armstrong-Wells J, Chang T, Deveber G, Rivkin MJ, Hernandez M, Carpenter J, Yager JY, Lynch JK, Ferriero DM (2011) Symptomatic neonatal arterial ischemic stroke: the International Pediatric Stroke Study. Pediatrics 128:e1402–e1410
Koelfen W, Freund M, Varnholt V (1995) Neonatal stroke involving the middle cerebral artery in term infants: clinical presentation, EEG and imaging studies, and outcome. Dev Med Child Neurol 37(3):204–212

Konishi Y, Kuriyama M, Sudo M, Konishi K, Hayakawa K, Ishii Y (1987) Superior sagittal sinus thrombosis in neonates. Pediatr Neurol 3(4):222–225

Krauland W (1952) Riss der art. basilaris als geburtzverletzung. Beitr Gerichtl Med 19:82

Kraus FT, Acheen VI (1999) Fetal thrombotic vasculopathy in the placenta: cerebral thrombi and infarcts, coagulopathies, and cerebral palsy. Hum Pathol 30:759–769

Krebs VL, Chieffi LN, Jurfest ME, Ceccon R, Diniz EM, Feferbaum R, Takeuchi CA, Marques-Dias MJ, Carneiro JD, Vaz FA (1998) Neonatal Streptococcus pyogenes meningitis and sagittal sinus thrombosis: case report. Arq Neuropsiquiatr 56(4):829–832

Kumar M, Avdic S, Paes B (2004) Contralateral cerebral infarction following vacuum extraction. Am J Perinatol 21:15–17

Kurnik K, Kosch A, Strater R, Schobess R, Heller C, Nowak-Gottl U (2003) Recurrent thromboembolism in infants and children suffering from symptomatic neonatal arterial stroke: a prospective follow-up study. Stroke 34:2887–2892

Lasjaunias P, Hui F, Zerah M, Garcia-Monaco R, Malherbe V, Rodesch G, Tanaka A, Alvarez H (1995) Cerebral arteriovenous malformations in children. Management of 179 consecutive cases and review of the literature. Childs Nerv Syst 11(2):66–79

Lavine D, Lehman JA Jr, Thomas R (1978) Congenital scalp defect with thrombosis of the sagittal sinus. Case report. Plast Reconstr Surg 61(4):599–602

Lee JH, Oh CW, Lee SH, Han DH (2003) Aplasia of the internal carotid artery. Acta Neurochir 145(2):117–125, discussion 125

Lee J, Croen LA, Backstrand KH, Yoshida CK, Henning LH, Lindan C, Ferriero DM, Fullerton HJ, Barkovich AJ, Wu YW (2005) Maternal and infant characteristics associated with perinatal arterial stroke in the infant. JAMA 293:723–729

Lequin MH, Peeters EA, Holscher HC, de Krijger R, Govaert P (2004) Arterial infarction caused by carotid artery dissection in the neonate. Eur J Paediatr Neurol 8:155–160

Lie TA (1968) Congenital anomalies of the carotid arteries. Excerpta Medica, Amsterdam, pp 35–51

Lien JM, Towers CV, Quilligan EJ, de Veciana M, Toohey JS, Morgan MA (1995) Term early-onset neonatal seizures: obstetric characteristics, etiologic classifications, and perinatal care. Obstet Gynecol 85(2): 163–169

Limperopoulos C, Benson CB, Bassan H, Disalvo DN, Kinnamon DD, Moore M, Ringer SA, Volpe JJ, du Plessis AJ (2005) Cerebellar hemorrhage in the preterm infant: ultrasonographic findings and risk factors. Pediatrics 116:717–724

Liu K, Ye XJ, Hu WY, Zhang GY, Bai GH, Zhao LC, He JW, Zhu H, Shao JB, Yan ZH, Gao HC (2013) Neurochemical changes in the rat occipital cortex and hippocampus after repetitive and profound hypoglycemia during the neonatal period: an ex vivo ^{1}H magnetic resonance spectroscopy study. Mol Neurobiol 48 (3):729–736

Luisiri A, Graviss ER, Weber T, Silberstein MJ, Tantana S, Connors R, Brodeur AE (1988) Neurosonographic changes in newborns treated with extracorporeal membrane oxygenation. J Ultrasound Med 7(8):429–438

Luo L, Chen D, Qu Y, Wu J, Li X, Mu D (2014) Association between hypoxia and perinatal arterial ischemic stroke: a meta-analysis. PLoS One 9:e90106

Maekawa K, Masaki T, Kokubun Y (1976) Fetal spinal-cord injury secondary to hyperextension of the neck: no effect of caesarean section. Dev Med Child Neurol 18 (2):228–232

Maingay-de Groof F, Lequin M, Roofthooft DW, Oranje A, de Coo IF, Bok LA, Mancini GM, Govaert PP (2008) Extensive cerebral infarction in the newborn due to incontinentia pigmenti. Eur J Paediatr Neurol 12 (4):284–289

Mannino FL, Trauner DA (1983) Stroke in neonates. J Pediatr 102(4):605–610

Mazumdar A, Mukherjee P, Miller JH, Malde H, McKinstry RC (2003) Diffusion-weighted imaging of acute corticospinal tract injury preceding Wallerian degeneration in the maturing human brain. AJNR Am J Neuroradiol 24(6):1057–1066

McCann ME, Schouten AN, Dobija N, Munoz C, Stephenson L, Poussaint TY, Kalkman CJ, Hickey PR, de Vries LS, Tasker RC (2014) Infantile postoperative encephalopathy: perioperative factors as a cause for concern. Pediatrics 133:e751–e757

McGregor JA, McFarren T (1989) Neonatal cranial osteomyelitis: a complication of fetal monitoring. Obstet Gynecol 73:490–492

McLellan NJ, Prasad R, Punt J (1986) Spontaneous subhyaloid and retinal haemorrhages in an infant. Arch Dis Child 61:1130–1132

McQuillen PS, Hamrick SE, Perez MJ, Barkovich AJ, Glidden DV, Karl TR, Teitel D, Miller SP (2006) Balloon atrial septostomy is associated with preoperative stroke in neonates with transposition of the great arteries. Circulation 113:280–285

Ment LR, Ehrenkranz RA, Duncan CC (1986) Bacterial meningitis as an etiology of perinatal cerebral infarction. Pediatr Neurol 2(5):276–279

Mercimek-Mahmutoglu S, Horvath GA, Coulter-Mackie-M, Nelson T, Waters PJ, Sargent M, Struys E, Jakobs C, Stockler-Ipsiroglu S, Connolly MB (2012) Profound neonatal hypoglycemia and lactic acidosis caused by pyridoxine-dependent epilepsy. Pediatrics 129(5): e1368–e1372

Meuwissen ME, Lequin MH, Bindels-de Heus K, Bruggenwirth HT, Knapen MF, Dalinghaus M, de Coo R, van Bever Y, Winkelman BH, Mancini GM (2013) ACTA2 mutation with childhood

cardiovascular, autonomic and brain anomalies and severe outcome. Am J Med Genet A 161A:1376–1380
Meyers PM, Halbach VV, Phatouros CP, Dowd CF, Malek AM, Lempert TE, Lefler JE, Higashida RT (2000) Hemorrhagic complications in vein of Galen malformations. Ann Neurol 47(6):748–755
Mineyko A, Kirton A (2011) The black box of perinatal ischemic stroke pathogenesis. J Child Neurol 26:1154–1162
Mittendorf R, Montag AG, MacMillan W, Janeczek S, Pryde PG, Besinger RE, Gianopoulos JG, Roizen N (2003) Components of the systemic fetal inflammatory response syndrome as predictors of impaired neurologic outcomes in children. Am J Obstet Gynecol 188 (6):1438-4–1444-6
Moharir M, Shroff M, MacGregor D (2006) Clinical and radiographic features of thrombosis propagation in neonatal and childhood cerebral sinovenous thrombosis. Ann Neurol 60(Suppl):S141
Muller H, Beedgen B, Schenk JP, Troger J, Linderkamp O (2007) Intracerebellar hemorrhage in premature infants: sonographic detection and outcome. J Perinat Med 35:67–70
N'Diaye M, Lasjaunias P, Husson B, Seibel N, Landrieu P (2004) Neonatal thrombosis of the jugular veins: long-term repercussions on cerebral development (two cases). Rev Neurol (Paris) 160(3):342–346
Ng YY, Su PH, Chen JY, Lee IC (2010) Do vacuum-assisted deliveries cause intracranial vessel injuries? J Child Neurol 25:222–226
Nishida T, Faughnan ME, Krings T, Chakinala M, Gossage JR, Young WL, Kim H, Pourmohamad T, Henderson KJ, Schrum SD, James M, Quinnine N, Bharatha A, Terbrugge KG, White RI Jr (2012) Brain arteriovenous malformations associated with hereditary hemorrhagic telangiectasia: gene-phenotype correlations. Am J Med Genet A 158A:2829–2834
Onate Vergara E, Sota Busselo I, Cortajarena Altuna M, Collado Espiga V, Echeverria Lecuona J, Gaztanaga Exposito R, Nogues Perez A, Paisan Grisolia I (2006) Arterial stroke after birth trauma. An Pediatr (Barc) 64:379–384
Ottaviano G, Calzolari F, Martini A (2007) Goldenhar syndrome in association with agenesia of the internal carotid artery. Int J Pediatr Otorhinolaryngol 71 (3):509–512
Pape KE, Wigglesworth J (1979) Haemorrhage, ischaemia and the perinatal brain. Clinics in developmental medicine. Spastics International Medical Publications, London
Pape KE, Armstrong DL, Fitzhardinge PM (1976) Central nervous system pathology associated with mask ventilation in the very low birthweight infant: a new etiology for intracerebellar hemorrhages. Pediatrics 58:473–483
Peixoto MV, de Carvalho JF, Rodrigues CE (2014) Clinical, laboratory, and therapeutic analyses of 21 patients with neonatal thrombosis and antiphospholipid antibodies: a literature review. J Immunol Res 2014:672603
Pellicer A, Cabanas F, Garcia-Alix A, Perez-Higueras A, Quero J (1992) Stroke in neonates with cardiac right-to-left shunt. Brain Dev 14:381–385
Pohl M, Zimmerhackl LB, Heinen F, Sutor AH, Schneppenheim R, Brandis M (1998) Bilateral renal vein thrombosis and venous sinus thrombosis in a neonate with factor V mutation (FV Leiden). J Pediatr 132(1):159–161
Prian GW, Wright GB, Rumack CM, O'Meara OP (1978) Apparent cerebral embolization after temporal artery catheterization. J Pediatr 93(1):115–118
Pysden K, Fallon P, Moorthy B, Ganesan V (2010) Presumed perinatal stroke in a child with Down syndrome and moyamoya disease. Dev Med Child Neurol 52:212–214
Raju TNK, Nelson KB, Ferriero D, Lynch J, the NICHD-NINDS Perinatal Stroke Workshop Participants (2007) Perinatal haemorrhagic stroke: summary of a workshop sponsored by NICHD and NINDS on classification, challenges and opportunities. Pediatrics 120 (3):609–616
Ramenghi LA, Gill BJ, Tanner SF, Martinez D, Arthur R, Levene MI (2002) Cerebral venous thrombosis, intraventricular haemorrhage and white matter lesions in a preterm newborn with factor V (Leiden) mutation. Neuropediatrics 33:97–99
Ramenghi LA, Fumagalli M, Righini A, Bassi L, Groppo M, Parazzini C, Bianchini E, Triulzi F, Mosca F (2007) Magnetic resonance imaging assessment of brain maturation in preterm neonates with punctate white matter lesions. Neuroradiology 49:161–167
Ramenghi LA, Fumagalli M, Groppo M, Consonni D, Gatti L, Bertazzi PA, Mannucci PM, Mosca F (2011) Germinal matrix hemorrhage: intraventricular hemorrhage in very-low-birth-weight infants: the independent role of inherited thrombophilia. Stroke 42:1889–1893
Raybaud C, Ahmad T, Rastegar N, Shroff M, Al Nassar M (2013) The premature brain: developmental and lesional anatomy. Neuroradiology 55(Suppl 2):23–40
Redline RW (2005) Severe fetal placental vascular lesions in term infants with neurologic impairment. Am J Obstet Gynecol 192:452–457
Redline RW, Sagar P, King ME, Krishnmoorthy KS, Grabowski EF, Roberts DJ (2008) Case 12–2008: a newborn infant with intermittent apnea and seizures. N Engl J Med 358(16):1713–1723
Rego Sousa P, Figueira R, Vasconcellos R (2012) Neonatal stroke associated with de novo antiphospholipid antibody and homozygous 1298C/C methylenetetrahydrofolate reductase mutation. BMJ Case Rep. pii: bcr2012006451. https://doi.org/10.1136/bcr-2012-006451
Remillard GM, Ethier R, Andermann F (1974) Temporal lobe epilepsy and perinatal occlusion of the posterior cerebral artery. A syndrome analogous to infantile

hemiplegia and a demonstrable etiology in some patients with temporal lobe epilepsy. Neurology 24 (11):1001–1009

Reynolds EW, Riel-Romero RM, Bada HS (2007) Neonatal abstinence syndrome and cerebral infarction following maternal codeine use during pregnancy. Clin Pediatr (Phila) 46(7):639–645

Ries M, Harms D, Scharf J (1994) Multiple cerebral infarcts with resulting multicystic encephalomalacia in a premature infant with Enterobacter sakazakii meningitis. Klin Padiatr 206:184–186

Ries M, Wölfel D, Maier-Brandt B (1995) Severe intracranial hemorrhage in a newborn infant with transplacental transfer of an acquired factor VIII:C inhibitor. J Pediatr 127:649–650

Roach ES, Golomb MR, Adams R, Biller J, Daniels S, deVeber G, Ferriero D, Jones BV, Kirkham FJ, Scott RM, Smith ER (2008) Management of stroke in infants and children: a scientific statement from a Special Writing Group of the American Heart Association Stroke Council and the Council on Cardiovascular Disease in the Young. Stroke 39:2644–2691

Robinson R, Iida H, O'Brien TP, Pane MA, Traystman RJ, Gleason CA (2000) Comparison of cerebrovascular effects of intravenous cocaine injection in fetal, newborn, and adult sheep. Am J Physiol Heart Circ Physiol 279:H1–H6

Roessmann U, Miller RT (1980) Thrombosis of the middle cerebral artery associated with birth trauma. Neurology 30:889–892

Rossi A, Tortori-Donati P (2006) Agenesis of bilateral internal carotid arteries in the PHACE syndrome. Am J Neuroradiol 27:1602

Rushton DI (2003) Neonatal shaken baby syndrome – historical inexactitudes. Arch Dis Child Fetal Neonatal Ed 88:F161, author reply F161–2

Sandberg DI, Lamberti-Pasculli M, Drake JM, Humphreys RP, Rutka JT (2001) Spontaneous intraparenchymal haemorrhage in full-term neonates. Neurosurgery 48:1042–1049

Schifrin BS, Ater S (2006) Fetal hypoxic and ischemic injuries. Curr Opin Obstet Gynecol 18:112–122

Schubiger G, Schubiger O, Tonz O (1982) Superior sagittal sinus thrombosis is the newborn – diagnosis by computerized tomography. Helv Paediatr Acta 37(2):193–199

Simchen MJ, Goldstein G, Lubetsky A, Strauss T, Schiff E, Kenet G (2009) Factor V Leiden and antiphospholipid antibodies in either mothers or infants increase the risk for perinatal arterial ischemic stroke. Stroke 40:65–70

Singh T, Chakera T (2002) Dural sinus thrombosis presenting as unilateral lobar haematomas with mass effect: an easily misdiagnosed cause of cerebral haemorrhage. Australas Radiol 46:351–365

Smilari P, Romeo MG, Sciacca P, Scalzo G, Gallo C, Mattia C, Manfre L, Distefano G (2005) Cerebral venous sinuses thrombosis in an infant with supramitral obstructive membrane associated with partial anomalous pulmonary venous return. Minerva Pediatr 57(2): 111–116

Snyder RD, Stovring J, Cushing AH, Davis LE, Hardy TL (1981) Cerebral infarction in childhood bacterial meningitis. J Neurol Neurosurg Psychiatry 44:581–585

Steinbok P, Haw CS, Cochrane DD, Kestle JR (1995) Acute subdural hematoma associated with cerebral infarction in the full-term neonate. Pediatr Neurosurg 23(4):206–215

Swarte R, Appel I, Lequin M, van Mol C, Govaert P (2004) Factor II gene (prothrombin G20210A) mutation and neonatal cerebrovenous thrombosis. Thromb Haemost 92:719–721

Tabbutt S, Griswold WR, Ogino MT, Mendoza AE, Allen JB, Reznik VM (1994) Multiple thromboses in a premature infant associated with maternal phospholipid antibody syndrome. J Perinatol 14(1):66–70

Takanashi J, Barkovich AJ, Ferriero DM, Suzuki H, Kohno Y (2003) Widening spectrum of congenital hemiplegia: periventricular venous infarction in term neonates. Neurology 61:531–533

Talvik I, Peet A, Laugesaar R, Lintrop M, Talvik T (2010) Vehicle-associated closed trauma-induced stroke in a 27-day-old girl. Medicina (Kaunas) 46:624–627

Tan MP, McConachie NS, Vloeberghs M (1998) Ruptured fusiform cerebral aneurysm in a neonate. Child's Nerv Syst 14:467–469

Tarras S, Gadia C, Meister L, Roldan E, Gregorios JB (1988) Homozygous protein C deficiency in a newborn. Clinicopathologic correlation. Arch Neurol 45 (2):214–216

Thompson JA, Grunnet ML, Anderson RE (1975) Carotid arterial elastic hyperplasia in a newborn. Stroke 6:391–394

Thorarensen O, Ryan S, Hunter J, Younkin DP (1997) Factor V Leiden mutation: an unrecognized cause of hemiplegic cerebral palsy, neonatal stroke, and placental thrombosis. Ann Neurol 42:372–375

Thornburg C, Pipe S (2006) Neonatal thromboembolic emergencies. Semin Fetal Neonatal Med 11:198–206

Tramonte JJ, Goodkin HP (2004) Temporal lobe hemorrhage in the full-term neonate presenting as apneic seizures. J Perinatol 24:726–729

Turnpenny PD, Stahl S, Bowers D, Bingham P (1992) Peripheral ischaemia and gangrene presenting at birth. Eur J Pediatr 151:550–554

Ushiwata I, Saiki I, Murakami T, Kanaya H, Konno J, Wada S (1989) Transverse sinus thrombosis accompanied by intracerebellar hemorrhage: a case report. No Shinkei Geka 17:51–55

van der Sluis IM, Boot AM, Vernooij M, Meradji M, Kroon AA (2006) Idiopathic infantile arterial calcification: clinical presentation, therapy and long-term follow-up. Eur J Pediatr 165:590–593

Wade T, Booy R, Teare EL, Kroll S (1999) Pasteurella multocida meningitis in infancy – (a lick may be as bad as a bite). Eur J Pediatr 158(11):875–878

Wang LW, Huang CC, Yeh TF (2004) Major brain lesions detected on sonographic screening of apparently normal term neonates. Neuroradiology 46:368–373

Wetzstein V, Budde U, Oyen F, Ding X, Herrmann J, Liebig B, Schneppenheim R (2006) Intracranial hemorrhage in a term newborn with severe von Willebrand disease type 3 associated with sinus venous thrombosis. Haematologica 91(12 Suppl):ECR60

Wigglesworth JS, Pape KE (1980) Pathophysiology of intracranial haemorrhage in the newborn. J Perinat Med 8:119–133

Williams AN, Sunderland R (2002) Neonatal shaken baby syndrome: an aetiological view from Down Under. Arch Dis Child Fetal Neonatal Ed 87:F29–F30, discussion F30

Worth LL, Hoots WK (1998) Development of a subdural vein thrombosis following aggressive factor VII replacement for postnatal intracranial haemorrhage in a homozygous factor VII-deficient infant. Haemophilia 4(5):757–761

Yager JY (2002) Hypoglycemic injury to the immature brain. Clin Perinatol 29:651–674

Young G, Albisetti M, Bonduel M, Brandao L, Chan A, Friedrichs F, Goldenberg NA, Grabowski E, Heller C, Journeycake J, Kenet G, Krümpel A, Kurnik K, Lubetsky A, Male C, Manco-Johnson M, Mathew P, Monagle P, van Ommen H, Simioni P, Svirin P, Tormene D, Nowak-Göttl U (2008) Impact of inherited thrombophilia on venous thromboembolism in children. A systematic review and meta-analysis of observational studies. Circulation 118(13):1373–82

Neonatal Stroke: Clinical Presentation, Imaging, Treatment, and Prognosis

130

Paul P. Govaert and Jeroen Dudink

Contents

P. P. Govaert (✉) · J. Dudink
Neonatology, Sophia Children's Hospital, Erasmus MC Rotterdam, Rotterdam, Zuid-Holland, The Netherlands
e-mail: govaert@icloud.com

Abstract

Stroke comprises acute focal brain injury due to arterial or venous occlusion, or due to primary hemorrhage. In the perinatal context its

G. Buonocore et al. (eds.), *Neonatology*,
https://doi.org/10.1007/978-3-319-29489-6_276

onset can be in utero, during delivery or at any time in the neonatal period. Although seizures and apnea are characteristic presentations, other signs and chance imaging finding are common. Staging with imaging, be it ultrasound or MRI, proceeds from acute lesional swelling with cell invasion, over frank necrosis in the core, to organization and tissue loss. The flow of diagnosis is often suspicion on ultrasound followed by clear definition of the lesion with diffusion weighted MRI in the acute stage. Knowledge of the developmental anatomy of brain vessels is indispensible because the recognition of the vessel signature (the template: for cerebral pial and perforator as well as brainstem and cord arteries, and for superficial as well as deep brain veins) is often the only manner to define the stroke type; it is only in a minority that description with imaging of arterial occlusion or venous thrombosis will confirm the fact the injury is due to stroke. Focal changes on the EEG guide diagnosis but especially management. Anticoagulants or antiplatelet agents may play a role in the (sub)acute stage. Pharmacological neuroprotection and cooling are subject of research and will find their place in the near future. Any stroke where the mechanism is elusive is open to a query of genetic causes, including prothrombotic conditions, mutations of collagen A4 and of brain-barrier junctional molecules. Genetic inflammatory conditions may be complicated by vascular lesions mimicking stroke.

130.1 Salient Points

- Perinatal stroke affects at least 1 in 2,000 newborn infants. At least 10% of neonatal seizures are stroke-related.
- Vigilant ultrasound imaging and EEG monitoring increase the chance of early detection.
- Immediate MR confirmation is the only way to prepare for (pending) neuroprotective strategies. Volumetric studies will be needed to prove the efficacy of such strategies. The differentiation by any imaging technique between infarct core and penumbra is an urgent research issue.
- Detailed knowledge of vascular developmental anatomy is crucial to the definition of perinatal stroke and required the examination of a panel of perinatal stroke genes.
- Anticoagulation plays a role in the prevention of recurrent arterial stroke in certain contexts and of the progression of venous thrombosis. There is no evidence to support the use of thrombolysis.

130.2 Epidemiology and Definitions

Ischemic perinatal stroke is defined as "a group of heterogeneous conditions in which there is a (multi)focal disruption of blood flow secondary to arterial or venous thrombosis or embolization, between 20 weeks of fetal life through the twenty-eighth postnatal day confirmed by neuroimaging or neuropathology" (Raju et al. 2007). Many authors also include specific types of parenchymal hemorrhage under the designation stroke. Neonatal stroke can be further categorized as a term or preterm clinical event depending on the gestational age of the infant. Preterm neonatal stroke is defined as occurring in a preterm infant variably defined as less than 35–37 weeks of gestational age (de Vries et al. 1997). The incidence of NAIS (neonatal arterial ischemic stroke) is reported as 1 in 2,300–4,000 deliveries and that of CSVT 1–2.69 per 100,000 newborns (reviews in (Chabrier et al. 2011; Lehman and Rivkin 2014; Rutherford et al. 2012)). These are likely to be underestimations, because incidences in hospital-based studies are invariably higher than population-based ones. A population study in Estonia arrived at 63 perinatal strokes per 100,000 live births (Laugesaar et al. 2007). Arterial ischemic stroke is the diagnosis in 10–15% of neonates with seizures (which affect 1–3.5/1,000 live-born infants) and for approximately 30% of childhood hemiplegia cases (affecting around 0.6/1,000 live births). AIS occurs even more frequently among preterm newborns. A male predominance (ratio around 1.3) occurs in term neonatal AIS but has not been observed in preterm neonatal AIS.

Whatever the exact prevalence, it is clear that the perinatal period leads to a high risk of stroke.

For AIS clinical chronological definitions have been defined. Fetal AIS is diagnosed before birth through the use of fetal imaging methods or in stillbirth on the basis of neuropathologic examination that reveals a pattern of ischemic brain injury in an arterial distribution. Neonatal AIS constitutes an acute presentation of encephalopathy manifesting as seizure, altered mental status, and/or neurological deficit between birth and the 29th postnatal day for which a pattern of ischemic brain injury in an arterial distribution is evident by neuroimaging. Presumed perinatal AIS is diagnosed in individuals >28 days of age with focal neurological deficits (hemisyndrome with early handedness, ophtalmoplegia) or epilepsy and a corresponding chronic infarct in arterial distribution in whom it is presumed that injury occurred between the 28th week of fetal life through the 28th postnatal day but was not detected during that period.

Sinovenous thrombosis is suspected when a parenchymal lesion (three-fourth hemorrhagic, one-fourth purely ischemic) is near a partial or completely occluded sinus or large vein. Pure sinus thrombosis without parenchymal injury is rare but can be included.

Primary hemorrhage is diagnosed when a parenchymal bleeding is not compatible with an arterial template and when regional veins and sinuses are patent. The most common venous infarct is parenchymal white matter injury of the preterm infant. The involvement of a vein is possible in many instances of lobar cerebral hematoma, often difficult to prove however.

Focal brain lesions due to vessel occlusion are inherent to the definition of stroke. Lesions due to infection and watershed injury can mimic stroke to such extent that their inclusion is warranted in any neonatal stroke register (Fig. 1).

130.3 Clinical Presentation

Seizures are the usual (at least 70% of the time) presentation of NAIS (Sreenan et al. 2000). Onset is fifty-fifty divided between day 1 and later in the first week, rarely beyond day 3 (Jan and Camfield 1998). Focal seizures are a more common first sign of NAIS than general seizures. Because the interval insult to seizures may be short (less than an hour) but also add up to several hours, the timing in hours of an arterial insult in relation to labor stages is impossible. Acute embolic stroke may cause seizures within the hour of the event (Pellicer et al. 1992) or onset of seizures may be delayed for several hours (Fischer et al. 1988). Seizures tend to occur earlier in HIE associated with intrapartum asphyxia than in relation to stroke (Rafay et al. 2009). Many newborns with stroke present with apneic spells or cyanotic attacks, often of epileptic nature (Hoogstraate et al. 2008; Chabrier et al. 2010). Seizures can be repetitive and lead to status epilepticus, typically projected on one hemisphere against a normal or only mildly altered EEG background. Most children seem to be alert between seizures and even accept oral feeding. Some present with temperature instability (Roodhooft et al. 1987), others with bouts of hyper- or hypotension due to hypothalamic injury. In some infants hemiplegia can be predicted from neonatal appreciation of asymmetrical general movements (Guzzetta et al. 2003), but most often future hemiplegia is inconspicuous in the neonatal period. Abnormal tone or altered level of consciousness has on occasion been the presenting sign, as have feeding problems. Neurologic alarm signs, except occasional clinical seizures, are usually lacking in perforator stroke and in the preterm, where stroke is often a surprise finding at brain US scanning.

In the context of NAIS, an alarming event may be acute pallor and loss of pulsation of (part of) a limb due to arterial embolism (or spasm ?), as reported by several authors ((Asindi et al. 1988; Raine et al. 1989; Gudinchet et al. 1991; Silver et al. 1992; Guajardo et al. 1994), one personal observation). Most of these limb-brain strokes present with limb pallor within minutes of delivery, strongly suggesting that embolic stroke preceded delivery for hours. In some cases, antiphospholipid antibodies in newborn serum were associated, and aortic thrombosis has been documented in this context (Raine et al. 1989; Gudinchet et al. 1991), personal observation], as

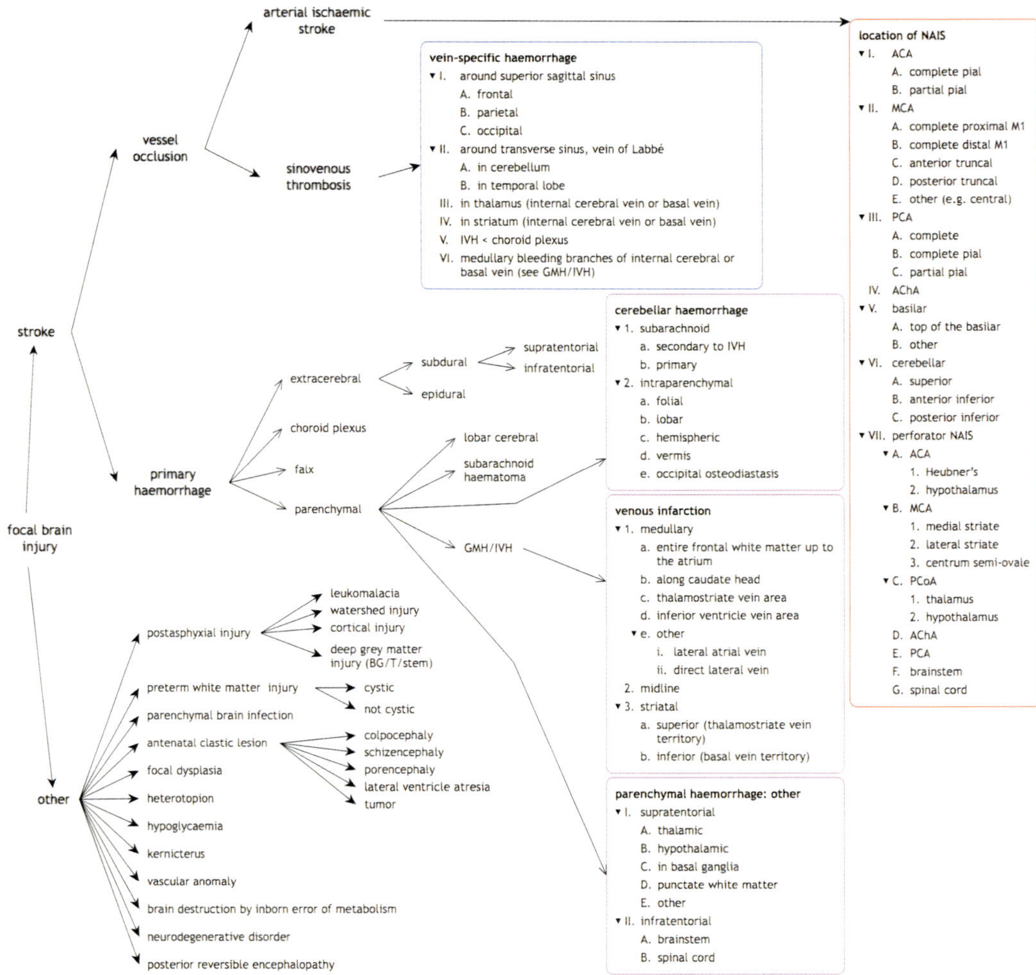

Fig. 1 Algorithm for focal lesions in the neonatal brain

has subclavian steal from the vertebrobasilar circulation documented with MRI (Broxterman et al. 2000; Beattie et al. 2006) (Fig. 2).

Clinical signs due to CSVT suggest that parenchymal destruction around veins followed an increase of venous tension above the arterial pressure level (hemorrhagic lesions) or an arterial ischemic response to venous occlusion. Neonates with NCSVT present either with seizures in the majority or with focal neurological signs like hemimotor paresis or cranial nerve palsies (Berfelo et al. 2010; Fitzgerald et al. 2006; Nwosu et al. 2008). Most often this is within the first days of life, not necessarily so in infants with congenital heart disease and dehydration or in preterms. A context of mechanical cranial trauma is possible. Fever, altered level of consciousness, or jitteriness is possible but not typical. The underlying cause may dominate the picture as with asphyxia, congenital heart disease or dehydration. Thrombosis without infarction is asymptomatic and thus an incidental finding (for instance, in a search for the cause of a low platelet count or during ECMO). Platelet consumption is seen with extensive NCSVT, with or without venous

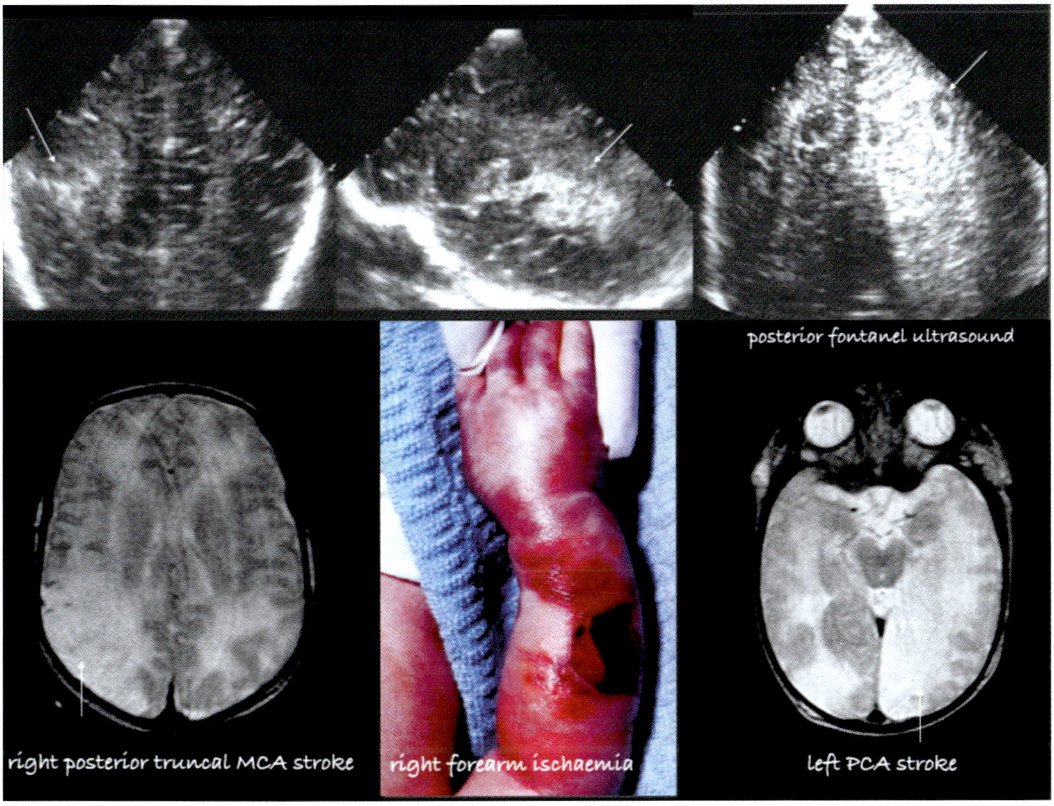

Fig. 2 Limb-brain arterial ischemia on day 1 of life

infarction, ant it can be observed with NAIS if the arterial process causes organ or limb necrosis (Berfelo et al. 2010). Propagation of thrombosis is possible in the first week, perhaps explaining evolving clinical signs.

A recent report referred to ALTE following acute thalamic unilateral stroke in infancy (Gupta et al. 2009). This finding adds to the description of apnea following temporal lobe lesions, such that a work-up of supratentorial injury is warranted in unexplained apnea. Extensive stroke lesions (mainly hemorrhagic) in cerebellum can lead to hypertension in the posterior fossa with Cushing response (bradycardia, hypertension) and several types of respiratory problems (sighing, apnea). Cranial nerve palsy is a rare presentation of posterior fossa stroke. Some of the more specific clinical signs of hindbrain infarction are mentioned in the section on "stroke templates" (Fig. 3).

130.4 Imaging

130.4.1 Staging with Any Type of Imaging

130.4.1.1 Swelling

From 30 min to a few hours cytotoxic edema increases water content. Changes in water diffusion occur within minutes on DWI; nadir ADC is on average around 33 h after the insult and it takes 4–10 days before ADC normalizes and overshoots the normal (Pellicer et al. 1992; Hill et al. 1983; Raybaud et al. 1985; Bode

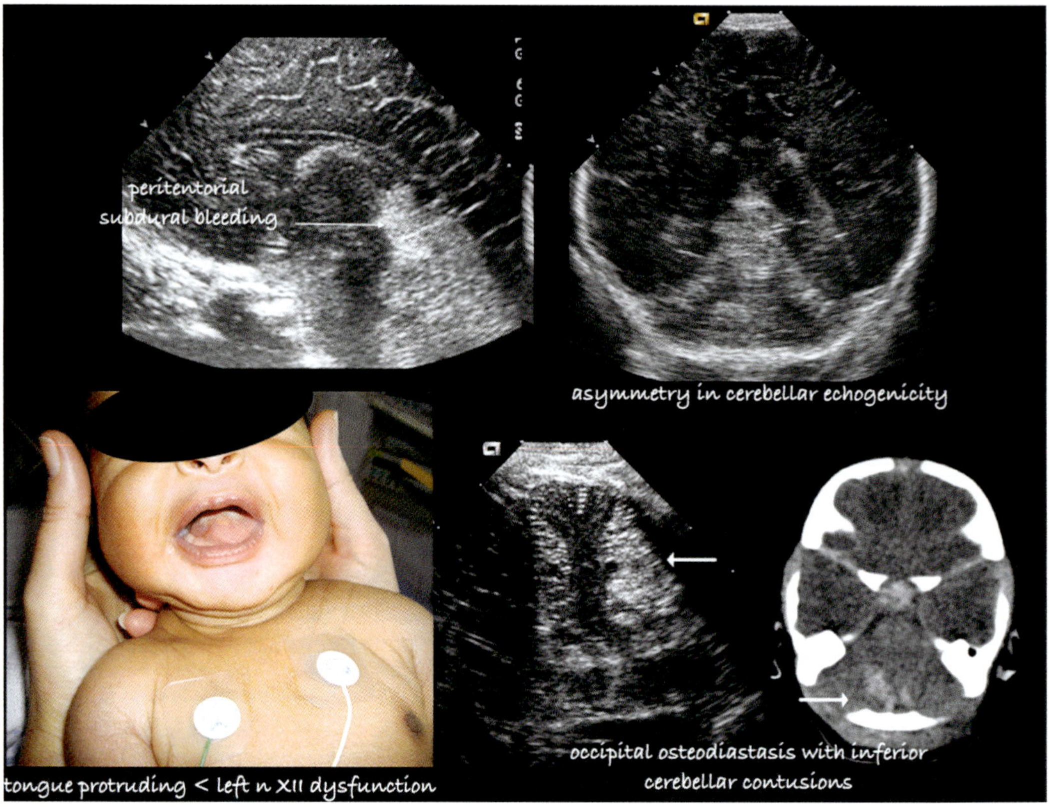

Fig. 3 Term vaginal breech delivery leading to occipital osteodiastasis, contusion of the inferomesial cerebellar hemispheres, and left cranial nerve XII compression`

et al. 1986; Hernanz-Schulman et al. 1988; Taylor et al. 1993; Koelfen et al. 1995; Mader et al. 2002; Cowan et al. 2005) (Fig. 4). In the vessel, flow void is lost in the affected artery for hours: this dampening disappears within 24 h (d'Orey et al. 1999). Most neonatal strokes present with reopened vessel at clinical detection.

130.4.1.2 Necrosis

From 6 h to about 6 days, edema and coagulation necrosis are associated with breakdown of the blood-brain barrier. Maturation of the infarct follows reperfusion of a pressure-passive vascular bed, through recanalized or anastomotic arteries. The peak of events is 2–4 days following acute infarction. Invading macrophages and glial cells visualize the infarct at postmortem and on images between 24 and 72 h after onset. If very large, swelling produces mass effect for about a week. As measured on DWI, large strokes reach a maximal size around 70 h after onset. In adults the penumbra shows restricted diffusion: consequently the final T2 lesion is smaller than the volume of diffusion restriction. Changes on T2 and PD images likely represent definitive damage. Disappearance of the cortical ribbon in the affected pial area is typical.

130.4.1.3 Organization

From 3 days to 6 weeks, this involves gliosis, breakdown of myelin, microcyst formation, and neovascularization. Disappearance of edema accounts for the loss of mass effect. Total necrosis may lead to central liquefaction with ensuing cyst formation. Microscopically it is represented by petechial (capillary) hemorrhage in cortex and

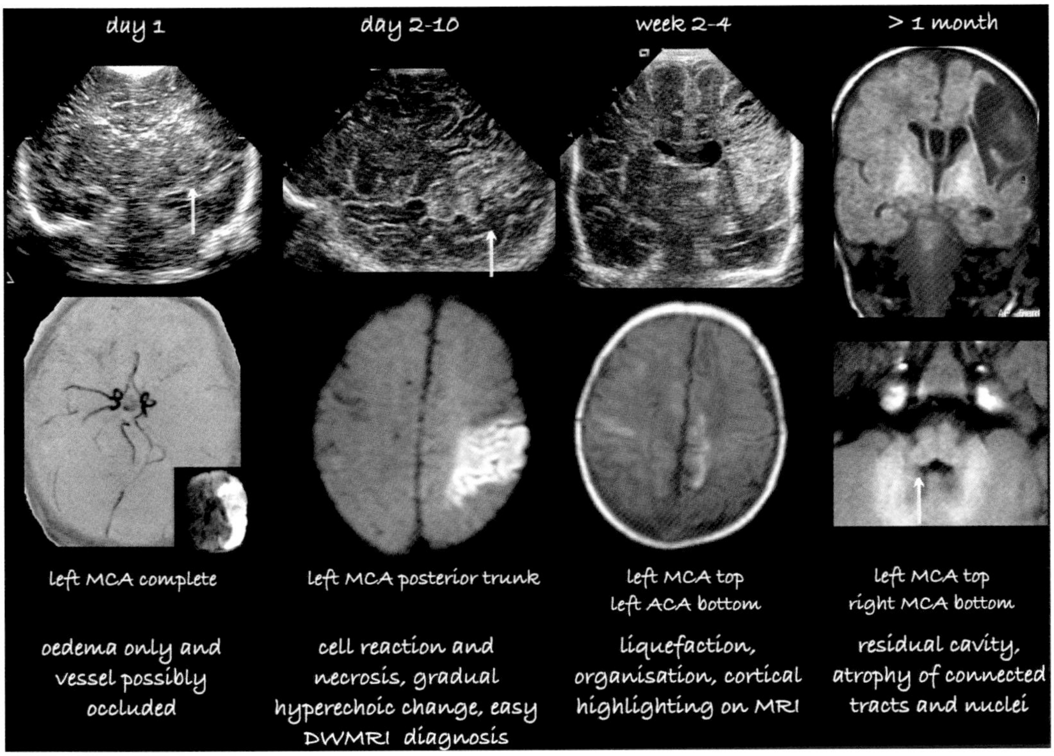

Fig. 4 Mixed image panel to illustrate stages of arterial ischemic stroke

basal ganglia: starting at about 3–6 days, this event peaks at 9–14 days when up to 90% of the infarcts are affected, and it regresses in half of the instances near the end of the first month.

130.4.1.4 Tissue Loss

From the second month onward infarction within a major cerebral artery will be recognized as an area of cortico-subcortical tissue loss, based against the skull bone. Because all tissue has disappeared, including cortex, this cystic remnant opens into the subarachnoid space. Infarction close to the occlusion site or central in the arterial territory may not present with the typical triangular tissue distribution. Wallerian degeneration of the ipsilateral pyramidal tract and transsynaptic degeneration of ipsilateral thalamus and contralateral cerebellar hemisphere will proceed for several months after the initial injury. Thalamus on the side of extensive frontoparietal (sub)cortical tissue loss will shrink by 20–40% in 3–6 months.

130.4.2 Ultrasound in NAIS

NAIS can nearly always be visualized with US, except for small cortical infarcts far away from the transducer. It may, however, take several days before hyperechoic change is apparent beyond doubt (de Vries et al. 1997; Pellicer et al. 1992; Hill et al. 1983; Bode et al. 1986; Hernanz-Schulman et al. 1988; Cowan et al. 2005; d'Orey et al. 1999; Pape and Wigglesworth 1979; Donaldson 1987; Govaert et al. 2000; Sreenan et al. 2000). Even in cases of temporal or occipital infarction targeted insonation from asterion or posterior fontanelle can detect the lesion. Perforator stroke in thalamus and striatum is particularly sensitive to detection with ultrasound. Pial strokes gradually become sharply demarcated within arterial template confines.

On recuperation, discrepant high flow velocities may be recorded up to 160 cm/s; this is regional luxury perfusion and may persist for

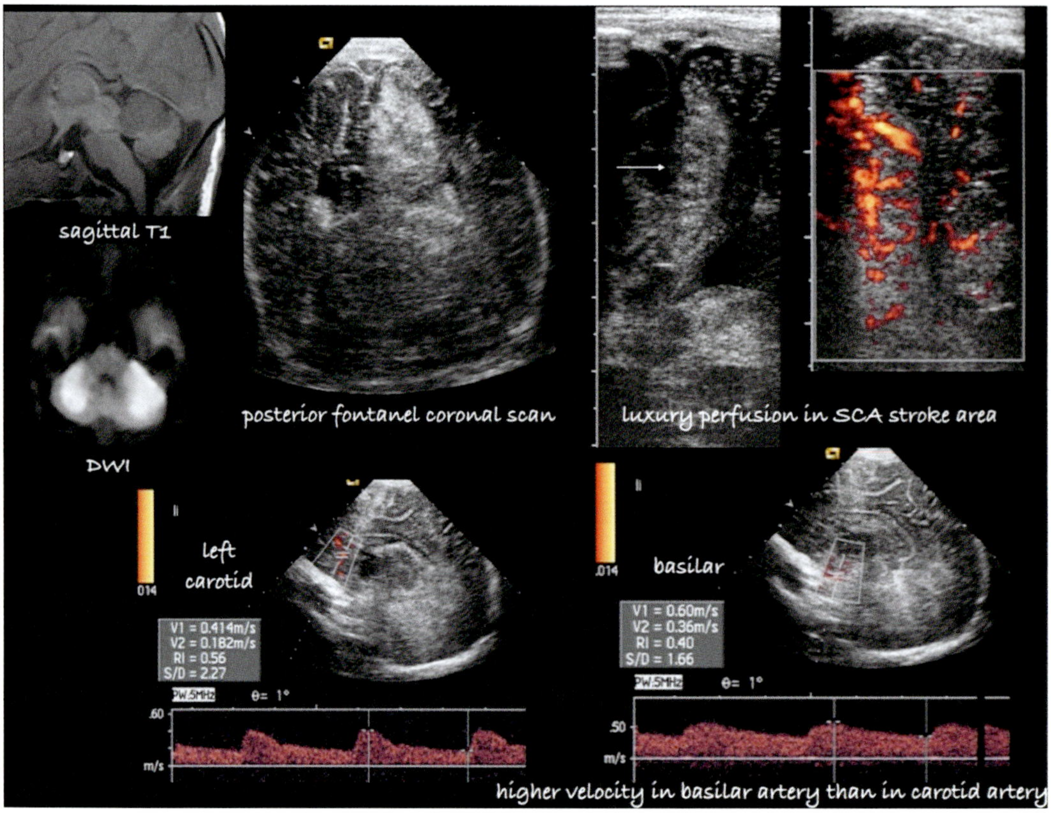

Fig. 5 *Top* of the basilar artery stroke with luxury perfusion in the infarct area, also confirmed by high velocities in the basilar artery (Govaert et al. 2009)

over a week (Steventon and John 1997; Taylor et al. 1993; Taylor 1994). Systolic but even more diastolic velocity increases, with a reduction of the resistance index compared with the healthy contralateral vessel. In this subacute stage, power Doppler imaging may suggest an increase in size and number of visible vessels in the periphery of large infarcts. Deep venous blood flow velocity about doubles on the affected side (measured in the internal cerebral vein) during the stage of hyperperfusion (Fig. 5).

Ultrasound staging is as follows:

- Day 1: decreased pulsatility of affected vessel and mild, inconspicuous hyperechogenicity.
- Over the next few days, increase of echogenicity in core and penumbra, due to the increasing presence of cell nuclei from neutrophils and macrophages; associated hemorrhage increases inhomogeneity; the hyperechoic stage persists for 3–4 weeks; cavitation follows an intermediate checkerboard pattern.
- Swelling for about a week, with effaced sulci and mass effect in case of complete MCA infarction.
- A CSF cavity is fully developed after 6–10 weeks; compensatory neuropil growth around the infarct may create the impression that the defect shrinks over the ensuing months; some have interpreted this as compensatory growth of the area adjacent to the infarct (Fig. 6).

130.4.3 MRI in NAIS

See Raybaud et al. (1985), Mader et al. (2002), Bouza et al. (1994a), Krishnamoorthy

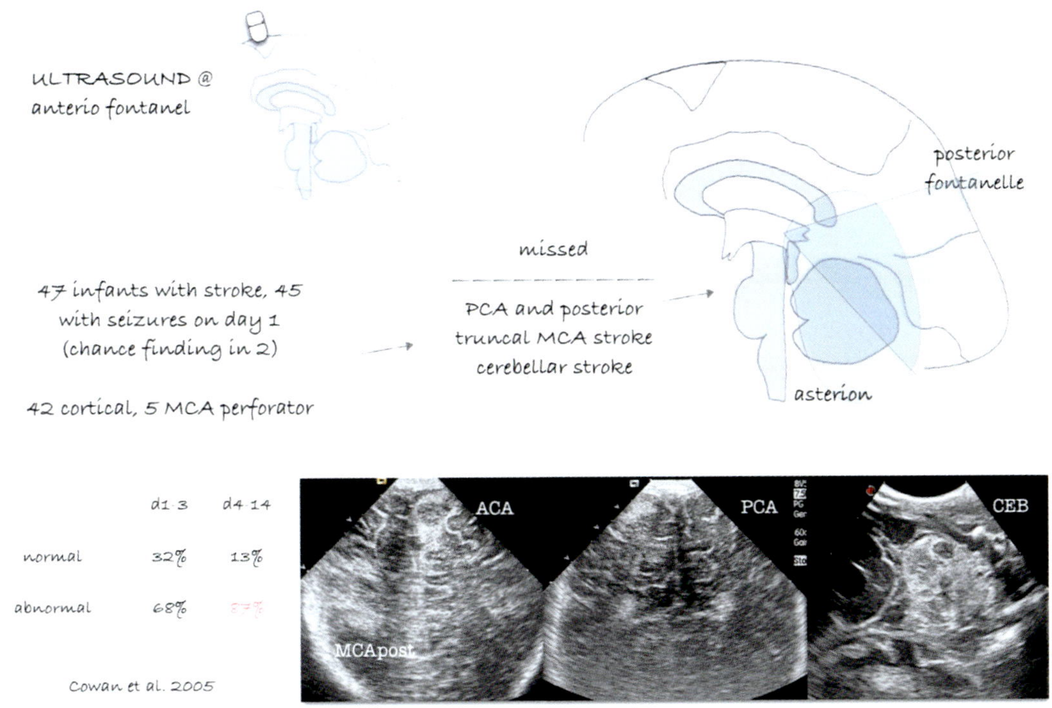

Fig. 6 The possibilities and limitations of detecting NAIS with ultrasound (Cowan et al. 2005)

et al. (2000), Mercuri (2001), Seghier et al. (2004), Dudink et al. (2009), de Vries et al. (2011), and Gunny and Lin (2012)

Technical background of advanced MRI modalities is a complex matter, and imaging accuracy depends on many aspects, including acquisition and processing methodology. MRI provides the highest anatomic resolution and the best sensitivity to detect acute ischemia. Specific sequences to obtain include diffusion-weighted imaging (DWI, from insult to about 7 days later), T1- and T2- weighted imaging (T1W and T2W), and susceptibility weighted imaging. A magnetic resonance angiography (MRA) of the head and neck should be considered because it can easily be added to the initial MR evaluation. Contrast MRA/V is not needed. MRA may detect arterial variation, carotid dissection or asymmetry between the MCAs. Advanced MRI techniques such as diffusion tensor (DTI), functional MRI, volumetric MRI, and proton magnetic resonance spectroscopy are used in research to better determine the full spectrum of brain injury. From DTI diffusion anisotropy measures such as fractional anisotropy (FA) can be computed.

DWI is used to depict cytotoxic edema and in neonates is sensitive enough to provide image alterations within hours of the initial injury, similar to adults. Visualization of the lesion using DWI is best observed within the first 2–4 days from the moment of the initial injury. As measured on DWI large strokes reach a maximal size around 70 h after onset. In adults the penumbra shows restricted diffusion: consequently the final T2 lesion is smaller than the volume of diffusion restriction. Changes on T2 (and PD, proton density) images likely represent definitive damage. On conventional MRI sequences term infants with neonatal stroke in the first postnatal weeks have on T2W images a high signal intensity in affected cortical gray matter and white matter during the first week of life, whereas T1W imaging reveals a low signal intensity in the involved cortical gray matter (missing cortex). From

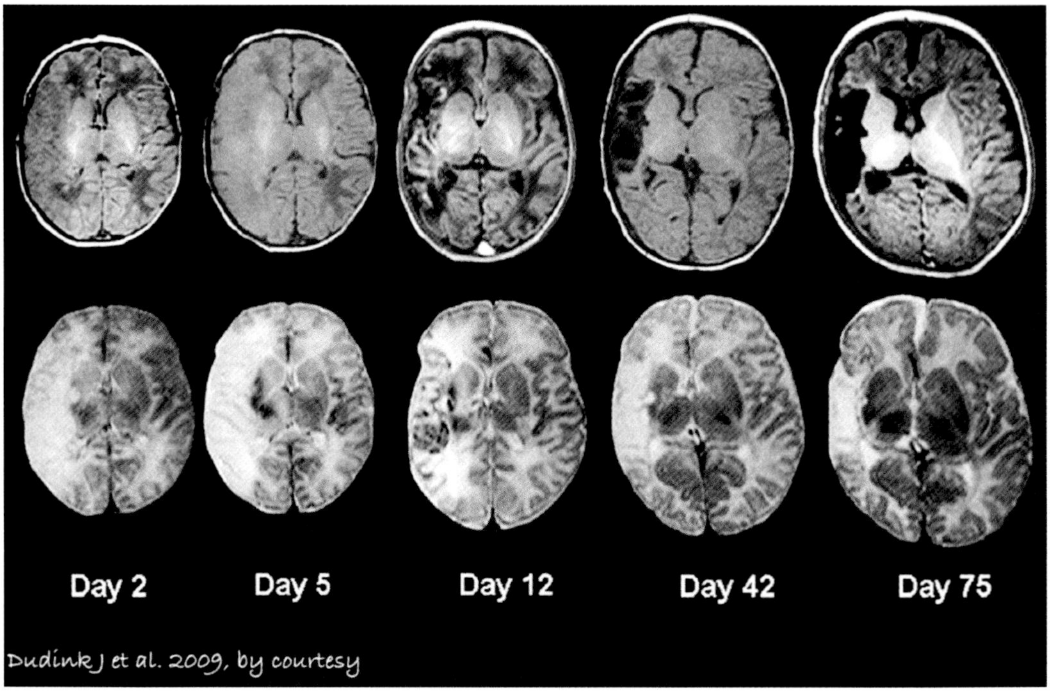

Fig. 7 Sequential aspects of T1 and T2 appearances in NAIS (Dudink et al. 2009)

1 week to 1 month after birth, cortical gray matter signal intensity is high on T1W and low on T2W imaging (cortical highlighting). Serial MRI studies confirm that in neonates with AIS, the onset of injury is around the time of delivery. Tissue breakdown is maximal around 6 weeks. Three-site involvement of the hemisphere (cortex and/ or white matter), the basal ganglia, and the posterior limb of the internal capsule is strongly associated with later contralateral hemiplegia irrespective of the size of the infarct (Fig. 7).

In the acute stage intensity changes are seen on DWI along the pyramidal tract; this phenomenon has prognostic value especially at mesencephalic and pontine level and is referred to as pre-Wallerian degeneration (Fig. 8). The extent of such acute corticospinal changes may predict severity of the hemisyndrome and also of recruitment of ipsilateral tracts for maintaining function in the affected limbs (Mazumdar et al. 2003; de Vries et al. 2005; Kirton et al. 2007; Lama et al. 2011; van der Aa et al. 2013). Advanced postacquisition quantification of diffusion tensor imaging data allows mapping of white matter connections, so-called tractography. Tractography is able to refine subjective prediction of motor dysfunction (Roze et al. 2012).

The presence of a penumbra has been demonstrated with ASL sequences, showing hyperperfusion compared to healthy tissue in the acute stage (5–6 days after birth); in some the whole infarct area can be hyperperfused (Wintermark and Warfield 2012; De Vis et al. 2013) (Fig. 9). This type of early visualization may in the future guide immediate postlesional treatment with neuroprotective agents.

Connected nuclei – like pulvinar – may also secondarily suffer from cell injury with restriction of water diffusion in the acute phase, referred to as network injury (Govaert et al. 2008; Dudink et al. 2012; Okabe et al. 2014) (Fig. 10). Response to injury in a developing brain may be faster than that in a mature one. Acute callosal changes reflect

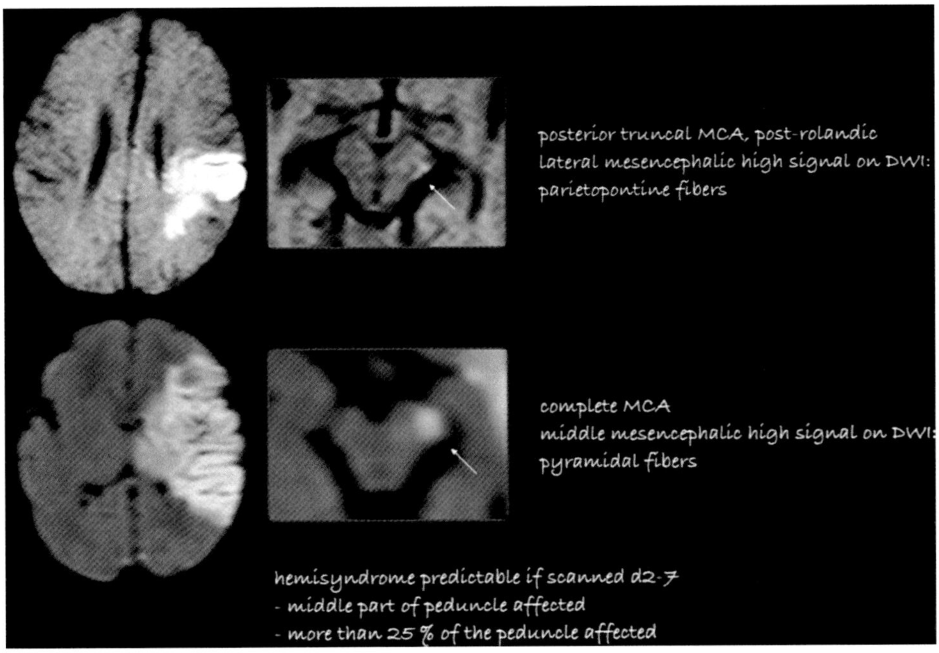

Fig. 8 Differences in hypersignal on DWI at the level of the cerebral peduncles relate to differences in cortical involvement

network injury to connected tracts, similar to the corticospinal tract (Righini et al. 2010). Crossed cerebellar atrophy (diaschizis) related to supratentorial stroke has recently been demonstrated in children (Mah et al. 2013).

Susceptibility-weighted imaging (SWI) is useful, improving the differentiation between small ischemic and hemorrhagic lesions. Recent evidence suggests that SWI may depict changes in the veins involved in an arterial infarct, and a mismatch with DWI may be helpful to define windows of opportunity for intervention (Meoded et al. 2014; Kidwell et al. 2003; Lequin et al. 2009). Hypoxemia and stasis in veins draining an infarct make the vessels stand out on SWI, of course dependent on the timing of imaging after the insult. Hemorrhagic conversion of any focal lesions is also well seen with SWI.

Functional MRI and transcranial magnetic stimulation will certainly help to study how the brain adapts to focal neonatal lesions; these methods will be needed to document the effect of targeted rehabilitation (Staudt et al. 2005; Fair et al. 2006; Walther et al. 2009).

130.4.4 Stroke Templates (Focus on Sonographic Aspects)

General references (Vander 1959; Stephens and Stilwell 1969; Govaert 2009; Lee 1995; Bogousslavsky and Caplan 1995)

Multiple strokes on either side of the brain occur often; a case of hydranencephaly would be classified as bilateral ACA plus MCA stroke; multicystic encephalopathy could be classified as bilateral ACA, MCA plus cortical PCA stroke; infarction within the ICA can be scored as ipsilateral ACA + MCA stroke; complete MCA stroke is different from combined ipsilateral anterior and posterior truncal MCA stroke (the latter with intact striatum). It is advised to visualize the carotid arteries and the circle of Willis in some conditions mentioned; withering of large cerebral

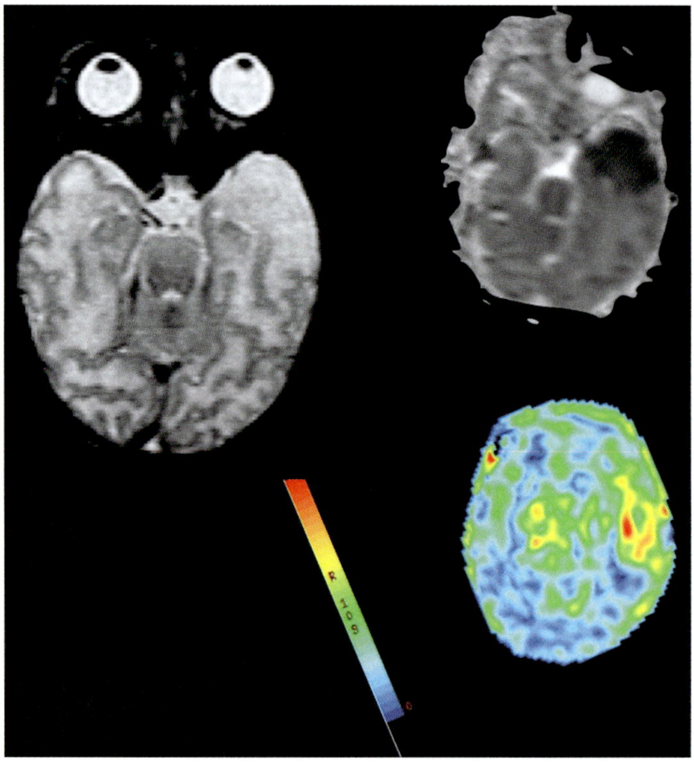

Fig. 9 Near-term infant with second day apnea due to partial left MCA stroke: low ADC values (on day 3 of life) in the ischemic area but high perfusion on the ASL image in the area around the infarct core. This was presumed embolism from partial internal carotid artery thrombosis

arteries involved in the cavitation may be secondary to stroke.

130.5 Pial Arteries

See Fig. 11

130.5.1 MCA Stroke

M1 (origin to limen insulae): medial parts of striatum including anterior commissure and ventral striatum, genu capsulae internae in its lower part, anterior pallidum internum; lateral parts of striatum (aa putamino-capsulo-caudate) including lateral and dorsal caudate head and corpus, crus anterius lateral part, entire putamen except for a ventral posterior portion, pallidum externum; thalamus is perfused from anterior choroidal, posterior communicating and posterior cerebral artery

M2-4: entire convex cortical and immediate subcortical area except for a margin of 1–2 cm perfused by either anterior or posterior cerebral artery pial branches; insular gyri and lateral orbital gyri (de Vries et al. 1997; Bode et al. 1986; Hernanz-Schulman et al. 1988; Koelfen et al. 1995; Govaert et al. 2000; Steventon and John 1997; Govaert 2009; Ramenghi et al. 2010)

MCA complete infarction. Hyperechoic change in caudate or pallidum can be the first indicator of complete MCA stroke. Hyperechoic change spreads in neostriatum as well as lateral pallidum and in white matter, from the ventricular border to the (sub)cortex, in and around the insula. A true linear medial margin appears from near the cranial midline to the midtemporal base; the only condition with comparable linear hyperechoic margination is bacterial encephalitis. Complete purely cortical infarction of the MCA, without involvement of striatum, is rare, as is infarction within the

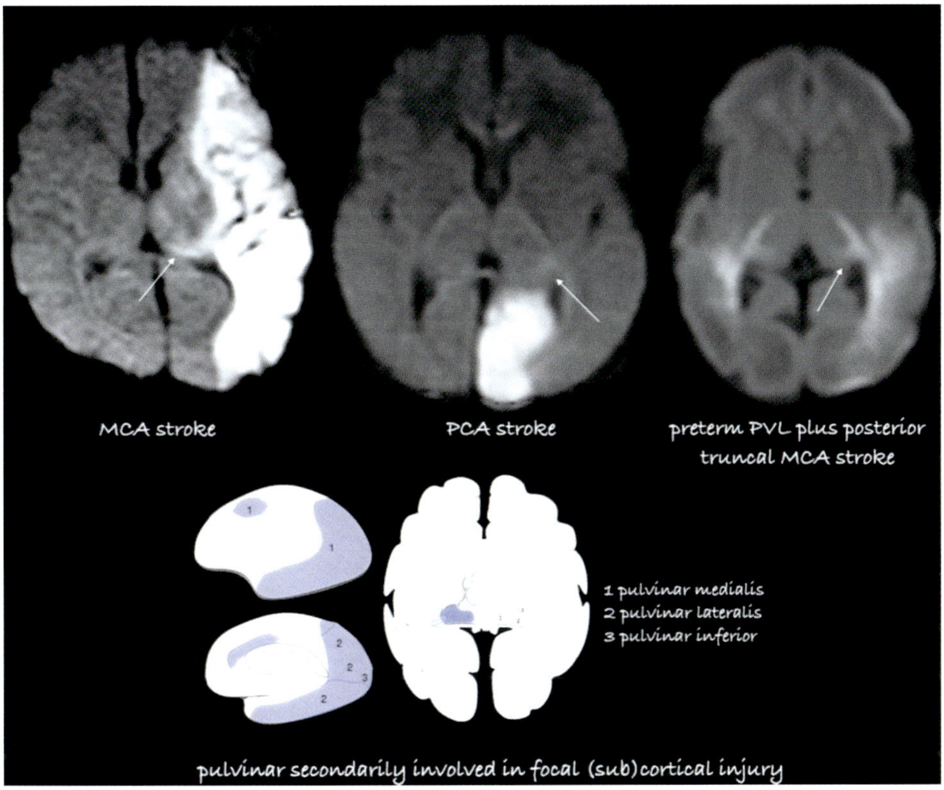

Fig. 10 Examples of network injury to pulvinar

striatal nuclei plus partial pial infarction, in the MCA anterior or posterior cortical field. Variation in vascular anatomy and anastomoses influencing the size of the penumbra may explain such unusual infarcts; multifocal arterial occlusion is the alternative, for example, distal migration of a thrombus wedged temporarily in the M1 part.

MCA anterior truncal infarction. The anterior trunk splits into several arteries: prefrontal, precentral, central, and anterior parietal. These vessels irrigate the cortex on the cerebral convexity up to the level of the postcentral gyrus. Complete infarction of the anterior trunk would often involve motor cortex, whereas partial infarction limited to the premotor and/or supplementary motor area could lead to contralateral disturbances in motor coordination without hemiplegia. The hyperechoic focus is a triangle with its point at the insular limen and its base spread across the parasagittal sector from frontal bone to central groove. The anterior part of the insular gyri is involved as well. Lobar frontal hematoma at term may sometimes represent hemorrhagic conversion of anterior truncal MCA stroke.

MCA posterior truncal infarction. The posterior trunk perfuses temporal and occipital lobe convexity and a variable portion of posterior parietal lobe. Its terminal, the angular artery, runs a course prolonging the horizontal lower border of the insula behind the postcentral gyrus. Extension of this truncus as far anterior as the motor cortex is uncommon. Infarction within this territory affects the posterior temporal and occipital lobe on the convexity. Recognition can be difficult if the insula is not inspected. The hyperechoic focus points towards the posterior insula on parasagittal section and has a triangular extension with fuzzy base against the occiput. On coronal view a blurred hyperechoic area is seen behind and underneath the circular groove of the insula.

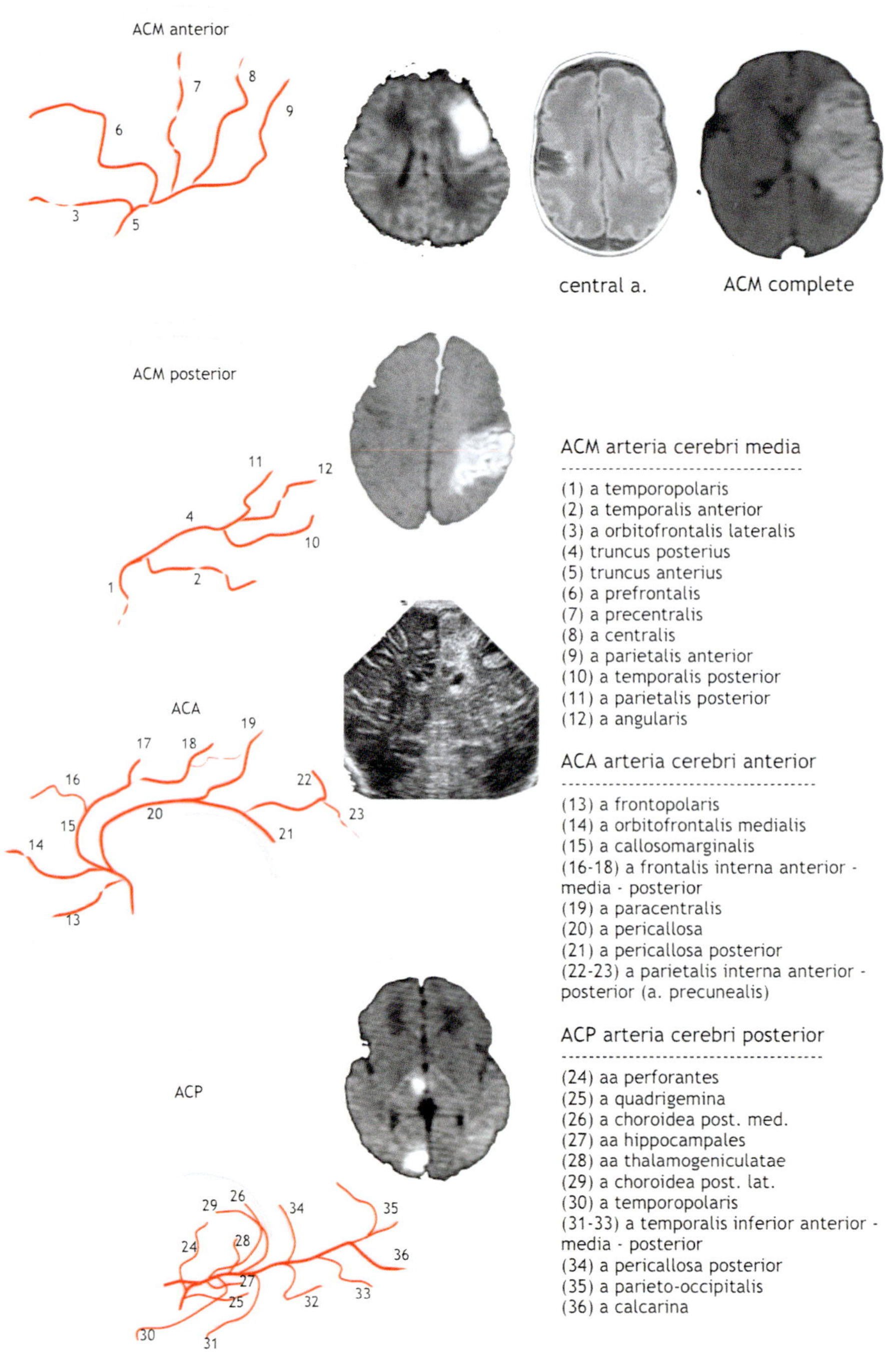

Fig. 11 Pial arterial templates

130.5.2 ICA Stroke

Some MCA strokes are part of a larger event, including ACA (ipsi- or contralateral) or PCA stroke (Campbell et al. 1988; Bergevin et al. 1991; Alfonso et al. 2001; Lequin et al. 2004; Hamida et al. 2014). This suggests occlusion of the ICA, for instance, due to embolism or to local thrombosis following trauma. In those cases it is important to exclude dissection of the carotid artery as the mechanism. Arterial dissection results from disruption of the intima, resulting in intramural hematoma; hematoma narrows the lumen, and impedes flow, which predisposes to thrombus formation and distal embolization. Dissection is demonstrable with noninvasive techniques, like MRI, MRA, and US. It may not be possible to recognize dissection of the wall in vivo facing complete thrombotic occlusion, although crescentic hyperintensity on T1 in the carotid wall is strongly suggestive of intramural changes. Segments of the ICA are defined as follows: C1, cervical (bifurcation of common carotid artery to carotid canal); C2, petrous; C3, cavernous; and C4, supraclinoid. Only a few cases of neonatal carotid artery dissection have been reported. The most common site of dissection is at C1 or C4. Neck rotation may be the cause of the dissection below the skull base, due to an intimal tear by compression of the vessel against the transverse processes of the upper cervical vertebra. Both carotid and vertebral artery dissection in one patient is possible (Hamida et al. 2014). The enlarged artery may compress lower cranial nerves. Carotid ligation during ECMO is another risk factor for ICA stroke.

130.5.3 ACA Stroke

A1 (pars precommunicalis): chiasma, fasciculus and tractus opticus, hypothalamus anterior, septum pellucidum, columna fornicis, commissura anterior medialis, anterior and inferior striatum and crus anterius; a communicans anterior: chiasma opticum, rostrum corporis callosi, lamina terminalis, area pre-optica hypothalami, commissura anterior

A2-4: cortical areas between falx and the area perfused by the arteria cerebri media, including gyrus cinguli; corpus callosum and septum pellucidum in front of the splenium (Billard et al. 1982; Huang et al. 1987; Sashikumar et al. 2014)

Infarction within pial branches of the ACA may present with seizures limited to one limb. If occluded close to the anterior communicating artery, the hyperechoic focus should involve gyrus cinguli, mesial frontal cortex against the falx, a 1–2 cm broad cortical area on the cerebral convexity near the superior sagittal sinus (extending caudally up to the parieto-occipital sulcus), and part of corpus callosum. In case of occlusion of A1, due to the very common existence of an anterior communicating artery with perfusion of the distal portions from the other side, simultaneous necrosis in caudate head and cortical areas is rare. Partial infarction can be seen along the midline in the premotor cortical area due to occlusion of a branch of the internal frontal artery. Association with ipsilateral MCA stroke suggests either ICA involvement or compression of the ACA by swelling from the MCA area.

130.5.4 PCA Stroke

Posterior hypothalamus, medial subthalamus, all but the polar thalamic area, posterior part of lateral geniculate, medial geniculate, splenium of the corpus callosum, middle part of posterior limb and of cerebral peduncle, quadrigeminal plate, choroid plexus of third and lateral ventricle, mesial cortical area of cuneus (visual cortex) and posterior precuneus, posterior temporal cortex, optic radiation caudal to the lateral ventricle. (Anderson et al. 1995; de Vries et al. 1996; Correa et al. 2004)

Cortical PCA stroke is recognized by insonation from the posterior fontanelle. One hardly spots the area of ischemia from the anterior fontanelle: upon scrutiny subcortical white matter may be hyperechoic at the far caudal end of the sector.

Brain swelling or the presence of a space-occupying process in the supratentorial compartment can shift the temporal lobe towards the tentorial edge (uncal herniation), endangering perfusion of the visual cortex through compression of the ambient segment of the PCA and of the ipsilateral basal vein. The triad following such lesion, in its typical form, consists of: temporal lobe epilepsy, homonymous hemi- or quadrantanopia and enlargement of the occipital horn. Oculomotor palsy may be part of this spectrum.

130.5.5 Interarterial Watershed Injury

Watershed injury, or cell loss in border zones between the major cerebral and cerebellar arteries, is best known in the context of global peripartum forebrain ischemia or against a background of hypotension, due to endotoxin mediated shock or blood loss for instance (Swarte et al. 2009; Harteman et al. 2013). This type of injury can be asymmetrical and can be mixed rostral or caudal. It can mimic distal partial AIS. Hyperechoic change is present in periventricular and subcortical white matter and is not maximal in the cingular area and in the corpus callosum. This type of injury is not always confidently visualized with US. It can be hemorrhagic or not and lead to cavitation or not.

130.5.6 Anterior Choroidal Artery Stroke

> *1 proximal branches to optic tract, crus posterius and pallidum mediale; 2 medial branches to pedunculus cerebri, nu. ruber, su. nigra, subthalamus, anterolateral thalamus; 3 lateral branches to uncus, parahippocampal gyrus, dentate gyrus, amygdaloid nuclei, caudate tail; 4 distal branches to optic radiation and lateral geniculate; 5 plexus segment for plexus of temporal horn]* (Takahashi et al. 1994, details in (Abels et al. 2006)

Abbie's syndrome due to AChA infarction (hemiparesis, hemihypoesthesia, homonymous hemianopia) is reported in the newborn. A hyperechoic lesion is seen between pallidum and thalamus, covering the middle and lower part of the posterior limb of the internal capsule (PLIC). Because lower limb corticospinal fibers course more posteriorly through PLIC, leg monoplegia can be the sequel. Extensive infarction involves pial areas near the optic tract.

130.5.7 Perforator Stroke

Templates for perforator stroke (the artery occluded is not a cortical branch but a perforator artery stemming from the proximal parts of the circle of Willis arteries) are available (Abels et al. 2006; De Vries et al. 1992; Garg and DeMyer 1995; Donzelli et al. 1998; van Wezel-Meijler et al. 1999; Miller et al. 2000; Roitberg et al. 2002; Feekes et al. 2005; Marinkovic et al. 2005; Bain et al. 2009) (Fig. 12). Perforator has to be differentiated from hemorrhage due to limited thrombosis in one of the veins drained by the internal cerebral or basal vein.

130.5.7.1 MCA Perforator Stroke

Many striate perforators arise from the MCA. The term giant lacunar infarction is used to describe the wedge of infarcted striatal tissue within lateral lenticulostriate M1 branches. This hyperechoic triangular focus is sufficiently typical in US: it has curved regular margins, the inner one through pallidum and the outer one just beneath the insular cortex. The base of the triangle is the posterior and superior part of the head of caudate. The infarct does not reach far into white matter, sustaining the angiographic finding that perforators from the MCA do not end in long ventriculofugal terminals.

130.5.7.2 ACA Perforator Stroke

The basilar side branches of the anterior cerebral artery (ACA) are the aa. striatae mediales, three or four very thin branches perforating directly the substantia perforata. One of them stands out by a wider caliber: the a. recurrens of Heubner. The

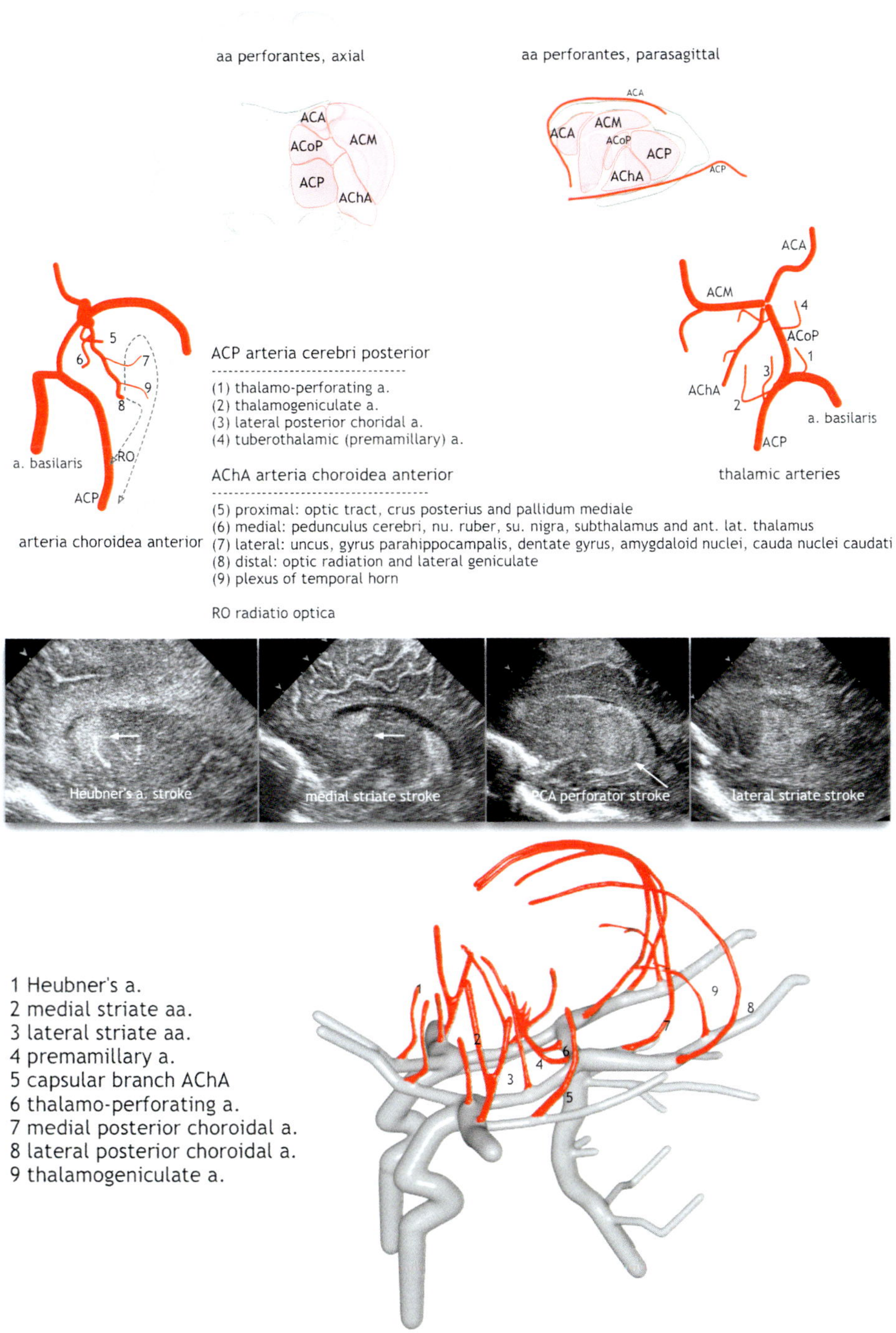

Fig. 12 Perforator arterial templates

level of its origin varies in relation to the anterior communicating artery. This recurrent artery runs in a lateral and dorsal direction, gives off a fine branch for the tuber olfactorium, and finally penetrates into the lateral part of the anterior substantia perforata. Heubner's artery stroke is recognized as a focal lesion in the lateral, anterior caudate head in front of the foramen of Monro.

Heubner's artery, large in the late fetal and perinatal period because of its contribution to matrix perfusion, seems to be a common route for emboli. In children with this type of stroke, contralateral upper limb dystonia has been reported. An important perforator from the anterior communicating artery, the subcallosal artery, perfuses columna fornicis and anterior commissure, leading to basal forebrain amnesia when this territory is infarcted in the adult (no neonatal reports).

130.5.7.3 PCA Perforator Stroke

Around the brain stem the PCA gives off a series of side branches subdivided into two groups, branches from the crural part (of interest here) and those from the distal cortical part. The branches from the crural part are deep penetrating vessels (perforating or choroidal). First, there are the arteriolae retromammilares which are divided in an anteromedial and a posteromedial group. The anteromedial (thalamostriate) group supplies the median-posterior part of the mammillary bodies; to them belong the aa. perforantes thalami which vascularize the median anterior part of thalamus, the superior part of nucleus ruber, the median part of subthalamic nucleus, the posterior part of hypothalamus, and the superior part of the brachia conjunctiva. In adults the presence of an unpaired median thalamic perforator artery (Percheron's artery) has led, if obstructed, to bilateral paramedian thalamic infarction. The posteromedial group supplies the middle part of the crus cerebri after having perforated the intercrural substantia perforata. The a. quadrigemina arises close to the origin of the PCA, just medial to the point where the posterior communicating artery joins the latter. It forms a pericrural arc. The aa. choroideae posteriores are usually double and originate separately or via a common stem. They also curve around the crus cerebri. The first, the a. chorioidea posterior medialis, takes a posteroanterior course towards the pineal body, to which it gives off some small branches; it diminishes in size in the choroid plexus of the third ventricle. The second, the a. chorioidea posterior lateralis gives two end branches. One follows the median part of the upper side of the thalamus, the supero-median part of which it irrigates. The other reaches the choroid plexus of the lateral ventricle opposite the lateral part of the pulvinar. It also vascularizes the posterior part of the caudate nucleus. During their ascending course the posterior choroidal arteries give off small branches entering the median part of the pulvinar. The aa. thalamogeniculatae usually arise just beyond the point where the posterior communicating artery joins the posterior cerebral artery. Thalamogeniculate arteries are five or six thin branches penetrating into posterior thalamus, to supply corpus geniculatum mediale and laterale, the lower half of the lateral thalamus, the lateral part of the pulvinar, and also the median part of the crus occipitale of the internal capsule.

130.5.7.4 PCoA Perforator Stroke

The posterior communicating artery (PCoA) runs beneath the optic tract and above the oculomotor nerve and joins the PCA at a small distance from the division of the basilar artery. Five to six small arteries arise from the PoCA, participating in the vascularization of the floor of the third ventricle (hypothalamic nuclei), and of the supero-anterior part of the medial thalamic nuclei. A lateral branch, the premamillary artery, irrigates the caudal hypothalamus, the medial subthalamus (the substantia nigra, Forel's field, and the zona incerta), and a rostral portion of the thalamus (the ventral part of the anterior group of nuclei, the ventral anterior nucleus, the rostral part of the midline and reticular thalamic nuclei, as well as the rostral part of the mediodorsal nucleus). Finally, peduncular branches nourish the ventromedial part of the rostral crus cerebri.

A focal, lentiform lesion in thalamus, anteriorly and slightly laterally, is not uncommon in sick newborn infants of any gestational age. One type with a focus in thalamus superior and anterior, next to the genu capsulae internae and with a free bridge of unaffected tissue between infarct and midline, may be due to premamillary artery stroke. An up- and outward oblique direction accords with perforator trajectories from MCA or circle of Willis. The other with a lower and more mesial location, abutting on the midline, may be one of the variants of PCA perforator stroke. Outcome of unilateral thalamic focal infarction can appear normal in infancy and early childhood.

The PLIC (posterior limb of the internal capsule) containing the corticospinal tract can be involved in stroke within: (1) lateral striatal perforator from MCA, (2) premamillary a., (3) anterior choroidal artery, (4) thalamogeniculate a., and (5) medial posterior choroidal a.

130.5.7.5 Centrum Semiovale Stroke

An echodense nodule is occasionally encountered within the centrum semiovale immediately next to the lateral ventricle. Context and imaging are often indicative of an embolic ischemic lesion. Infarction in a terminal lateral striatal MCA branch is a likely possibility. The alternative explanation would be stroke of one ventriculopetal cortical arterial branch of the ACA, MCA, or PCA; depending on the site of occlusion this mechanism might also lead to focal subcortical infarction, e.g., in the pericentral area. If hemorrhagic, one must also consider isolated paraventricular venous thrombosis to explain these lesions, an associated germinal matrix hemorrhage would sustain that hypothesis.

130.5.8 Hindbrain Arterial Ischemic Stroke

There are a limited number of neonatal descriptions of cerebellar or brainstem stroke (Govaert et al. 2009; Norman 1974; Pollack et al. 1983) (Fig. 13). As for the forebrain, hindbrain arteries are well formed early in fetal life (details beyond this discussion), so recognizable patterns of infarction in superior, anterior inferior, and posterior inferior cerebellar arteries are present in the perinatal period. Because of a similar endstage for hemorrhage and infarction of the cerebellar hemisphere, i.e., a permanent cleft disrupting foliation around it, the existing literature on purely ischemic cerebellar stroke is limited. The posterior spinal artery usually originates from the posterior inferior cerebellar artery, but it may arise from the vertebral artery. Although the labyrinthine artery may occasionally branch from the basilar, it most frequently originates from the anterior inferior cerebellar artery. Many vessels that arise ventrally course around the brainstem to serve dorsal structures (circumferential branches); others perforate near the midline (paramedian branches). Pontine anterior strokes have been linked to neonatal GBS meningitis with arteritis around the circle of Willis.

130.5.9 Spinal Cord Arterial Ischemic Stroke

The spinal cord is irrigated by: (i) a single median anterior spinal artery derived from both vertebral arteries, extending down to the cauda equina; neck hyperextension may lead to occlusion/spasm in this vessel at low cervical level and cause the central cord syndrome; (ii) a posterior spinal artery on each side from the inf. post. cerebellar arteries, extending medial to the posterior root; (iii) segmental arteries from vertebral, subclavian, intercostal, and hypogastric arteries or from the aorta; the post (Young et al. 1983; de Vries et al. 1995; Ruggieri et al. 1999; Carrascosa-Romero et al. 2002; Simanovsky et al. 2004). radicular and spinal arteries are provided along the cord in 12 unpaired vessels and form a rich posterior spinal collateral network; there are 7–10 unpaired anterior radicular and spinal feeders, with a much less efficient collateral circulation; there is usually a large (70% on the left) anterior segmental artery from the aorta at T9 to L2 level (high or low position) called the Adamkiewicz artery; this vessel is vulnerable to hypoperfusion of the aorta (coarctation, aortic surgery) or to aortic catheter-induced emboli or vasospastic agents (UAC in high position, above T9–L2). Most of the lateral and the entire anterior column, including spinal gray matter, are perfused from central branches of the anterior spinal artery. These branches alternate sides; hypoperfusion within the anterior spinal artery may cause necrosis on both sides (central cord syndrome) or on one side (partial Brown-Séquard syndrome), facilitated by the

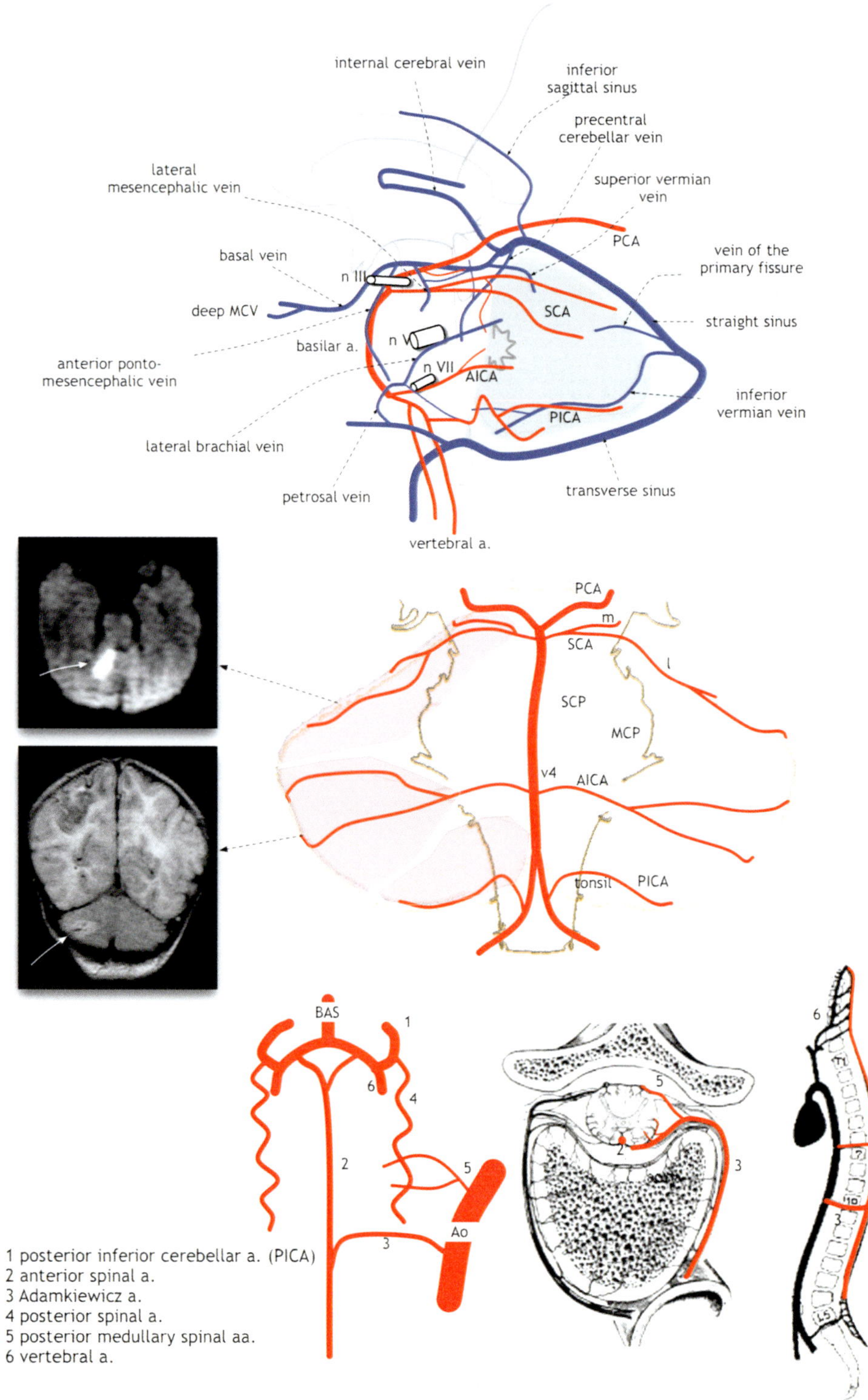

Fig. 13 Hindbrain and cord vessel templates

absence of important anastomoses between anterior and posterior spinal circulation. The clinical features of spinal cord infarction in children include: initial radicular pain; flaccid para- or quadriplegia later evolving into spasticity (lesions of corticospinal and rubrospinal tract); loss of pain and temperature sensitivity below the upper level of the infarct with preserved touch and vibration sensitivity; bowel and bladder paralysis. Patients with posterior spinal artery syndrome have back pain and leg paresthesias together with loss of touch, vibration sensitivity, and position sense below the lesion; due to partial damage to the lateral corticospinal tract a milder degree of flaccid paralysis may be associated. Interarterial watershed injury will cause centrospinal infarction syndrome (pencil shaped on sagittal MRI, en crayon); this may be seen above and below a genuine anterior spinal infarct. To differentiate cord stroke from cervical spinal cord, birth trauma is important.

130.5.10 Venous Thrombosis Templates (Fig. 14)

130.5.10.1 Superior Sagittal Sinus

Almost all infarctions due to venous thrombosis are hemorrhagic (Review Raets et al. 2015). Typical SSS thrombosis can lead to parasagittal hemorrhagic infarction particularly in the arm area of the motor homunculus, explaining hemimotor sequelae in some children. Thrombosis within the SSS usually starts in the vicinity of the parietal lobe, probably due to the peculiar forward course – against sinus flow direction – of the posterior frontal, parietal, and occipital bridging veins as they drain the convexity. Underneath the anterior fontanelle and further distally under the tip of the occipital squame, the sinus is exposed to mechanical forces during (difficult) delivery. It is long known that about half of SSS thromboses are associated with TS thrombosis and that about a third of sinus thromboses are associated with deep involvement (Berfelo et al. 2010; Bailey 1959; Bailey and Hass 1958; Byers and Hass 1933; Ehlers 1936). Sinus thrombosis can propagate into the deep venous system, and probably the reverse exists as well. There have been anecdotal reports of neonatal cavernous sinus thrombosis with eyelid chemosis, facial swelling, and external ophtalmoplegia (Fumagalli et al. 2004). Exceptionally an infarct is purely ischemic but clearly related to sinus thrombosis, which is possibly due to reactive arteriospasm. For unknown reasons hemorrhagic infarction associated with SSS thrombosis is within the parasagittal cerebral (sub)cortex and not within parenchyma bordering the interhemispheric fissure or deeper down along the convexity. The existence of transmedullary, transnuclear (through basal ganglia), and meningeal collaterals is of importance in avoiding infarction, depending on probably many factors such as the speed of occlusion, rheology of blood, and presence of prothrombotic risk factors. A typical red infarct leaves hemosiderin and gliosis in the residual scar, sometimes with figured calcification along the vein. Over a period of weeks to months a sinus usually gradually recanalizes (Moharir et al. 2011; Moharir 2006).

130.5.10.2 Internal Cerebral Vein or Straight Sinus

Thrombosis of the GCV and/or the ICV puts fragile veins under pressure in the vicinity of germinal matrix or choroid plexus. This may lead to deep venous infarction (Govaert et al. 1992). The phenomenon is nearly always associated with IVH. An infarct related to ICV thrombosis may stretch as far as corpus callosum and periventricular white matter, sparing subcortical areas. When a single branch of the ICV is thrombosed, the most striking phenomenon may be unilateral hemorrhagic infarction in thalamus or caudate nucleus: thalamoventricular hemorrhage. Collaterals mitigate injury when occlusion of the deep venous system is not abrupt. At the moment of diagnosis the affected vein may not be without flow due to recanalization. Besides propagation from thrombosis in the superior sagittal sinus along the straight sinus to the deep venous system, risk factors of primary deep venous thrombosis are similar to sinus thrombosis.

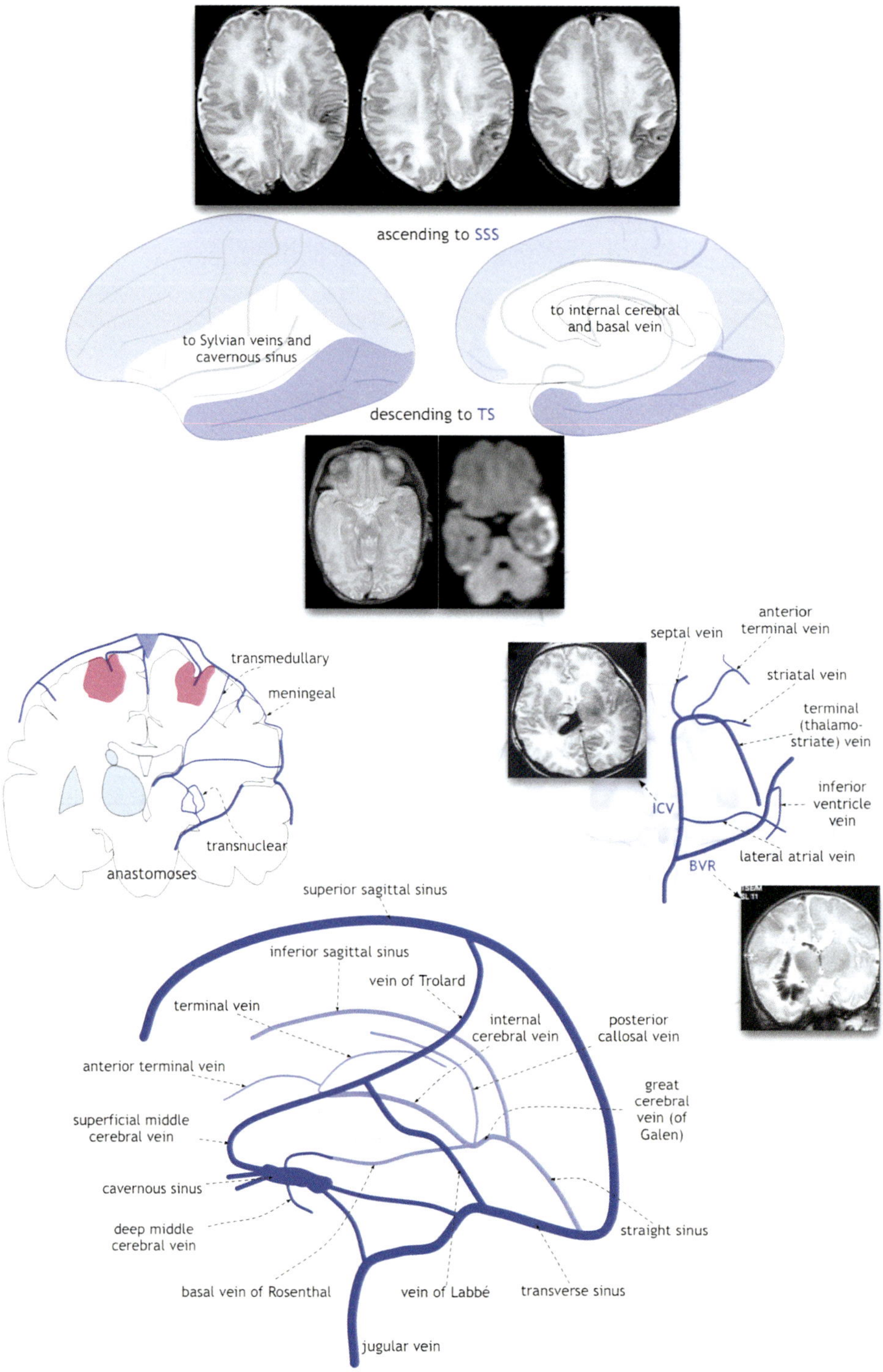

Fig. 14 Sinovenous templates

130.5.10.3 Basal Vein of Rosenthal

Basal vein thrombosis can induce hemorrhage with feathered margins in the center of the temporal lobe and extending upward into inferolateral hemistriatum (Govaert et al. 2001). The hematoma does not reach the temporal lobe convexity. The typical ends-tage BVR runs around the brainstem and drains posteriorly into the Galenic system, in three segments: striate, peduncular, and mesencephalic. The BVR is derived around the 11th fetal week from the formation of longitudinal anastomoses between embryonic precursors. Its formation is sensitive to anatomic variation (Chung and Weon 2005). Prospective tributaries may drain almost independently of each other into various sinuses. In about 10% the BVR does not even connect to the GCV. The sonographic study of the BVR is possible with high-quality Doppler technique, but its horizontal course and variability present sources of difficulty.

130.5.10.4 Transverse Sinus

Hemorrhage into the temporal lobe (basal and temporal parts) or around the tentorium and in cerebellum may be associated with TS thrombosis (Baram et al. 1988; Eichler et al. 2007a). In adults several patterns of TS bridging veins have been described. Tentorial lakes of type I mainly drain to straight sinus, torcular and mesial/middle TS, of type II to lateral TS and transverse-petrosal junction (Guppy et al. 1997; Muthukumar and Palaniappan 1998). A large draining vein of the cerebral convexity into the TS, the vein of Labbé, is connecting the SMCVs to the vein of Trolard and indirectly to the SSS, but this vein can also be absent, such that its absence alone does not seem robust enough to name its thrombosis as the cause of underlying temporal lobe hematoma. Young infants are more vulnerable to subdural hematoma because of relatively large venous lakes in the dura around the posterior fossa (Browder et al. 1975). Smooth muscle layers at bridging vein orifices suggest that they are sphincters (Dagain et al. 2009). Variation in end-stage anatomy and maturation of these sphincters will codetermine what type of temporal lobe hematoma follows thrombosis of affected veins. Ultrasound can confirm or refute flow gaps observed with MR venography (Miller et al. 2012). That ultrasound, including color Doppler, can depict sinovenous thrombosis at an early stage, presents therapeutic options prior to parenchymal injury. The transverse to sigmoid transmission may be a developmental, neonatal venous Achilles heel because of: (i) relative jugular obstruction in the fetal period; (ii) asymmetrical development of the transverse sinus; (iii) dwindling of the tentorial sinus (summarized in Raets et al. (2015)).

130.5.10.5 Sinovenous Thrombosis and Its Relation to Hemorrhage

SSS. As stated above, thrombosis of a brain sinus may lead to hemorrhage in the newborn period (Raets et al. 2015; Nwosu et al. 2008). The parasagittal location of injury in SSS thrombosis induces lesions similar to hemorrhagic watershed injury. Thrombosis of cortical veins is often, but not obligatory observed in situations where thrombosis of a sinus led to brain injury. In the newborn about three-fourth sinus thrombosis are associated with brain injury, itself hemorrhagic in about 80%) (Nwosu et al. 2008; Eichler et al. 2007b).

TS. In adults cerebellar bleeding has been associated with TS thrombosis (Ushiwata et al. 1989). Temporal lobar hematoma is linked to TS thrombosis (Nwosu et al. 2008; Baram et al. 1988; Huang and Robertson 2004; Miller et al. 2012), not unexpected given drainage of temporal veins via bridging veins and the vein of Labbé into TS. Helpful diagnostic sign may be subarachnoid hemorrhage (SAH) near the thrombosis (Kato et al. 2010). With perfusion CT congestion may present as low perfusion hyperemia, associated with subsequent vessel rupture into the subarachnoid space. This phase, vasogenic edema and SAH, may present with increased ADC values on MRI. Be it from trauma or thrombosis, the tentorial sinus, vein of Labbé, and the temporal diploic vein are candidates for temporal lobe/fossa bleeding. Peritentorial subdural bleeding has been linked to neonatal transverse sinus thrombosis (Eichler et al. 2007b). An infected cephalhematoma may also lead to TS thrombosis (Chan et al. 2002). Recanalization of the affected sinus is the rule (Nwosu et al. 2008).

Deep veins. Deep thrombosis in the galenic venous system causes thalamoventricular hemorrhage (Govaert et al. 1992; Wu et al. 2003), in the basal vein territory hemorrhage in striatum and mesial temporal lobe (Govaert et al. 2001). Reversible dilatation of the vein of Galen and sinuses following difficult delivery may be one way of documenting the link between trauma and IVH (Komiyama et al. 2001; Hunt et al. 2002). Dilatation may mimic vein of Galen malformation on superficial inspection. Purely ischemic damage due to this mechanism has not yet been described. Tables 1 and 2 summarize some morphological lesion patterns.

130.5.11 EEG Findings in the Acute Stage

The area of infarction is the focus of epileptic discharge (Jan and Camfield 1998; Mercuri et al. 1999), but exceptions of epileptic focalization contralateral to the infarct confirm the rule. Clinical status epilepticus is always correlated with abnormal EEG (van Rooij et al. 2007). EEG monitoring may be an aid in detecting stroke in ventilated and sedated infants, e.g., with pulmonary hypertension (Clancy et al. 1985; Klesh et al. 1987; Scher and Beggarly 1989; Koelfen et al. 1995; Evans and Levene 1998; Clancy 2006; Plouin and Kaminska 2013). Stroke types with subclinical seizures, escaping detection with routine serial US, like NAIS due to PCA occlusion, can be suspected through EEG monitoring. Ischemic stroke is associated with early (though often beyond 12 h after birth) and focal seizures (Rafay et al. 2009). Interictal EEG is asymmetrical, with focal or unilateral patterns. The best EEG predictor of hemiplegia is not neonatal epileptic activity but a disturbed background (Mercuri et al. 1999; Mercuri 2001), a finding not shared by all authors (Sreenan et al. 2000). Children with later cerebral palsy may keep numerous unilateral postictal positive rolandic slow sharp waves (Selton et al. 2003). Anticonvulsants have a different effect on the neonatal brain than on adults (Jennekens et al. 2012). Midazolam induces immediate suppression of the aEEG background pattern for 30–60 min, with a decrease of total and absolute frequency band powers; relative delta power decreases, theta power increases while alpha and beta powers remain constant. Lidocaine induces no aEEG background pattern suppression; total and absolute EEG band powers remain unchanged; relative delta power decreases, theta and alpha power increases, and beta power remains constant. Effects of lidocaine are pronounced in the stroke-affected hemisphere.

In a term infant with left MCA infarction, before the onset of seizures, monitoring of the EEG from birth permitted observation at 3 h after delivery of occasional focal sharp waves over the stroke region (Walsh et al. 2011). After electroclinical seizures, focal sharp waves became more frequent, complex, and of higher amplitude, particularly in "quiet sleep". In "active sleep," sharp waves often disappeared. Diffuse optical tomography has potential as a valuable clinical tool for the early detection of functional deficits and for providing prognostic information in newborns with brain injury (White et al. 2012).

130.5.12 Genetic Aspects

Although the classification of cerebrovascular disorder in the categories AIS, CVT, and primary hemorrhagic stroke is essential for perinatal management, this subclassification is of less use for neurogeneticists. Several genetic factors underlying infantile cerebrovacular disorders have been identified. However, mutations in the same gene may underly a broad spectrum of cerebrovascular disorders, presenting as either ischemic or hemorrhagic stroke. In addition, in

Table 1 Arterial lesions

Arteries	Vessel	Vessel	Lesion description	Resulting cavity
Arterial cortical	ACA	Complete pial	Mesial orbitofrontal and supracallosal cortex	–*Transmantle porencephaly*: triangular cortical and subcortical defect extending from ventricle to pia limitans, often not communicating with ventricle; with time defects may appear to be covered by surrounding healthy tissue in partial pial stroke; bordered by polymicrogyria if insult at or before 25 weeks –*Schizencephaly*: some instances are due to bleeding or vascular insufficiency, leading to transmantle necrosis (a cleft bordered by grey matter) with communication from ventricle to pia; always prenatal onset (before 20 weeks) –*Hydranencephaly, cerebral hemiatrophy (hemihydranencephaly)*: complete destruction with expansive cavitation of ICA territories, atrophic separated thalami and atrophic basal ganglia, intact posterior fossa; may be associated with hypoplasia of the carotid canal; hemiatrophy follows destruction of an area perfused by ICA on one side; basket brain with uni- or bilateral tissue remnants in ACA *Multicystic encephalopathy*: is an intermediate stage before hydranencephaly, arterial occlusion often not documented
		Partial pial		
	MCA	Complete, begin M1	Includes putamen, PLIC adjacent to thalamus, part of caudate, entire MCA cortical area	
		Anterior trunk	MCA cortical area from insula on rostrally	
		Posterior trunk	MCA cortical area from insula on caudally	
		Pial other	Focal cortical lesion within anterior or posterior trunk, or within a central artery between these trunks	
	PCA	Complete pial	Mesial occipital cortex and occipital pole	
		Partial pial		
	Basilar a.	Top of basilar	PCA pial stroke plus superior cerebellar a. Stroke	
	Cerebellara.	Superior	Superior cerebellar surface	
		Anterior inferior	Inferolateral surface and dentate region	
		Posterior inferior	Inferomedial surface	
Arterial perforator	ACA	Heubner's a.	Caudate head rostral and lateral, lateral ALIC	*Ventral porencephaly*: orbitofrontal arteries from the ACA, MCA, or circle of Willis; cavity from lateral or third ventricle near the midline towards the orbita
	MCA	Lenticulostriate	Up to lateral ventricle, including posterior caudate head; pointing to MCA origin near limen insulae; medial striate arteries around caudothalamic groove and to pallidum, lateral striate arteries to putamen; vary variable size	*Porencephaly due to arterial perforator stroke*: cavity in striatum or thalamus, not communicating with ventricle, sparing most of the white matter except for a small area above the line between caudate and lateral fissure; the cavity may be a triangle with point towards the circle of Willis except for PCA perforator stroke
		Centrum-semiovale	Nodule lateral to and above lateral ventricle, isolated white matter damage, without GMH	Simple *paraventricular white matter cyst* in the middle of healthy centrum semiovale
	PCA		Lesion in any part of thalamus except for anterolateral parts perfused by AChA or from circle of Willis	
	AChA		Caudal end of PLIC with surrounding parts of thalamus and pallidum/putamen, parts of temporal lobe near optic radiation	
	Circle of Willis	Hypothalamus		
		Thalamus	Superolateral parts	
Arterial other	Brainstem		Basilar a, PCA, circle of Willis branches	Absence of pons, midbrain disconnection: focal brainstem infarction presenting as segmental cavitation and distortion of the brainstem or cord; to be differentiated from genetic causes of brainstem malformation
	Spinal cord		Anterior spinal a., posterior spinal aa., Adamkiewicz a.	

Table 2 Venous lesions

Veins	Vessel	Subclass	Vessel	Resulting cavity
Venous	Sinus	SSS	SSS anterior	
			SSS complete	
		Other	Transverse sinus L/R	
			Straight sinus, great cerebral vein of Galen	
			Cavernous sinus	
	Deep vein	Internal cerebral vein	Complete: anterior and posterior terminal vein PVI	–*Thalamostriatal porencephaly*: periventricular cavity extending into caudate and thalamus; can communicate with ventricle, spares putamen and white matter; hemosiderin in cavity walls –*Periventricular porencephaly*: periventricular cavity, communicating with ventricle, sparing subcortex; may contain hemosiderin in cavity walls; may be expansive; some infarcts only cause mild ventricular dilatation
			Posterior terminal (thalamostriate) vein PVI	
			Anterior terminal (caudate) vein PVI	
			Septocallosal vein PVI	
			Striatal vein PVI	
			Para-atrial vein PVI	
			Other PVI	
		Basal vein	Basolateral striatal vein PVI	
			Temporal vein PVI	
	Other	Pial vein, sinus patent	Cerebral	
			Cerebellar	

the perinatal period, developmental defects often intermingle with vascular disorders. Examples of known pathophysiological processes for genetic cerebrovascular disorders are: (i) structural changes of blood-brain barrier integrity: mutations in genes coding for basement membrane components (i.e., COL4A1 and COL4A2), tight junction proteins (i.e., JAM3 and OCLN), and components of the cytoskeleton involved in the anchoring of tight junction proteins in the cell membrane (i.e., ACTA2); (ii) dysregulation of innate immune response/cerebrovascular inflammation: dysregulation of the type I interferon (IFN) signaling has been demonstrated to underly a broad range of cerebrovascular disorders (such as Aicardi-Goutières syndrome and mutations in the recently identified USP18 gene); another example of dysregulated inflammation in cerebrovascular disease is incontinentia pigmenti, due to aberrant NF-kB activation. Methods to study genetic causes of stroke in the newborn include a targeted gene panel, whole exome sequencing and RNA-profiling (Barr et al. 2010; Vandeweyer et al. 2014). Of course genetic patterns exist in certain presentations of arteriovenous malformation, brain cavernous hemangioma, arterial aneurysm, moya-moya sequence, and hemostatic and prothrombotic disorders: they are not discussed here. Genetic mechanisms are elucidated further in the chapter on stroke mechanisms, elsewhere in this book.

130.5.13 Medical Treatment

There are guidelines for the treatment of pediatric arterial ischemic childhood stroke: outside proactive transfusion policy in sickle cell disease the suggested treatment schedules are mainly based on cohort studies and extrapolation from adult stroke insights (reviews Bernard et al. 2008; Monagle et al. 2008; Roach et al. 2008: summarized in table). There are, therefore, no evidence-based treatment options.

In the acute phase of NAIS, supportive measures such as hydration and anticonvulsants are part of standard care. Thrombolysis is not recommended as neither effectiveness nor safety has been demonstrated in neonates. Recommendations propose heparinization (for a period of months in some cases) in instances with ongoing thrombosis in the heart or a large systemic vein or with carotid artery dissection (Nowak-Gottl et al. 2003; Chalmers 2005). For the remainder, anticoagulation or antiplatelet therapy is not recommended as the risk of recurrent stroke is low (Fullerton et al. 2007). A study of 215 neonates with AIS followed for a median of 3.5 years, documented symptomatic recurrence in seven (AIS in four, CVST in two, and deep venous thrombosis in one patient). Factors associated with an increased recurrence rate include thrombophilia and the presence of comorbidities such as complex congenital heart disease or dehydration. Only when AIS reoccurs, therapy is suggested. A heparinization protocol following cardiac catheterization may be useful (Weissman et al. 1985). It seems obvious that efforts be undertaken to maintain and salvage tissue, particularly within the ischemic penumbra. The synthesis of suggestions for pharmacological intervention from animal stroke experiments is beyond the scope of this chapter (Ashwal and Pearce 2001; Ashwal et al. 2007; Ginsberg 2008). Easily applicable candidates could be albumin or hypothermia (Fehlings et al. 2000). Insight has to be gained in many areas of NAIS to arrive at treatment options. Theoretically this may facilitate intervention at five levels: (i) prevention of risk factors (like vaginal breech delivery or difficult instrumental traction, like catheter-related embolism), (ii) reopening of an occluded vessel with fibrinolytics and/or maintaining collateral patency, (iii) protection of cells in the penumbra from secondary excitotoxic or apoptotic death (by maintaining perfusion and metabolic homeostasis), (iv) prevention of recurrence (in children with important risk factors), and finally (v) specific rehabilitation strategies. Some of these will have to be tested in trials including identical strokes, e.g., complete MCA stroke, to avoid the confounding influence of stroke type on outcome (Boyd et al. 2001; Eliasson et al. 2003; Kenet et al. 2007).

Experimental data suggest that subventricular zone neural progenitor cells proliferate and migrate to the site of injury after neonatal stroke and multiple doses of EPO, with a shift in cell fate toward neurogenesis and oligodendrogliosis at both early and late time points (Gonzalez et al. 2013). rhEPO in neonates with perinatal arterial ischemic stroke had no adverse effects on red blood cells, white blood cells, platelets counts, or coagulation. rhEPO, 3,000 IU/kg in total, given during a 3-day period, thus appears to be safe. The beneficial effects remain to be demonstrated in a randomized, double-blind, placebo-controlled trial (Benders et al. 2014). Melatonin and stem cell injections are also in the stage of promising animal research for mitigation of injury in focal ischemic insults.

The role of anticoagulants in NCSVT is controversial as recurrency is also rare. Recurrent thrombotic episodes occurred in 6% of children during a mean follow-up period of 36 months (Kenet et al. 2007). Strikingly, children younger than 2 years of age did not develop recurrent thrombosis at all. However, extension of the initial thrombus 1 week after diagnosis has been reported in a cohort study of 68 neonates: in 10 out of 40 neonates without anticoagulation (25%), in comparison to one of 28 neonates on anticoagulants (3%). Extension of the thrombus was asymptomatic in all but one neonate, who presented with a novel venous infarction (Moharir et al. 2011). Although randomized controlled trials were not performed, safety of anticoagulation in NSVT has been monitored (deVeber et al. 2001; Fitzgerald et al. 2006). In the Canadian Stroke Registry no patients died or showed signs of neurologic deterioration due to bleeding during heparin treatment (deVeber et al. 2001). Consequently, the ACCP guidelines recommend treatment of neonates with SVT without significant intracranial hemorrhage, with UFH or LMWH initially, followed by LMWH or vitamin K antagonists for 6–12 weeks. For neonates with SVT and significant hemorrhage, radiological monitoring is recommended and anticoagulation warranted if extension of the thrombus occurs, 5–7 days after the onset of the initial hemorrhage (Monagle et al. 2008). There may be a place for use of heparin to prevent (recurrent) infarction in bacterial meningitis (Boelman et al. 2014). "Regional attitudes of treatment" should be replaced by

Table 3 Guidelines for treatment of neonatal stroke

		RCP (UK)	ACCP (USA)
Acute AIS	Acute systemic thrombolysis	No evidence to support use of thrombolytic agents such as tissue plasminogen activator (tPA)	Use of thrombolytic agents in children with AIS has been rare, and the risk/benefit ratio is unknown
	Acute intraarterial thrombolysis	Not recommended	Not recommended
	Acute heparinization	Not recommended, except in case of dissection or cardioembolic stroke	UFHeparin or LMWHeparin for 5–7 days and until cardioembolic stroke and vascular dissection have been excluded
Secondary prevention of AIS	Dissection	Anticoagulation for $\leq$6 months	Anticoagulation with heparin for 3–6 months
	Cardioembolic stroke	Anticoagulation in consultation with cardiologist	Anticoagulation with heparin for 3–6 months
	APL antibodies or inherited thrombophilia	No recommendations	No recommendations
Sinovenous thrombosis		Consider anticoagulation (LMWH or UFH) in selected neonates with	Heparin (first unfractionated, later fractionated) is recommended if no significant intracranial hemorrhage is associated, for 6 (if early recanalization is observed) up to 12 weeks (if recanalization is incomplete at 6 weeks)
		Severe thrombophilic disorders	
		Multiple cerebral or systemic emboli	
		Propagating SVT despite supportive therapy	
		Thrombolytic agents are not recommended	

AIS arterial ischemic stroke, *SVT* sinovenous thrombosis, *RCP* Royal College of Physicians, *ACCP* American College of Chest Physicians, *LMWH* low molecular weight heparin, *UFH* unfractionated heparin

evidence in the near future (Jordan et al. 2010; Greenway and Massicotte 2004) (Table 3).

130.5.14 Prognosis

Corticospinal axons reach the spinal cord before 24 weeks postmenstrual age and innervate spinal gray matter prior to birth. Monosynaptic corticomotoneuronal connections are probably present in human term newborns (Eyre et al. 2000). Since development of fine *motor* control occurs at 6–12 months after birth, there seems to be a window for cortical influence on spinal motor centers in the fetal third trimester and in the early months of life. In the perinatal period the corticospinal tract still has bilateral representations from one cortical area to both sides of the cord; the same was observed for somatosensory lateralization, emerging in this period. There is research going on about the options of a perinatal brain to adapt to injury in an attempt to preserve function. Digital and manual dexterity may also be altered in the nonparetic hand because of bilateral effects of the lesion at spinal motor centers. Many (around 50%) strokes lead to hemiplegia or contralateral motor dysfunction (Koelfen et al. 1995; Bouza et al. 1994a; Neville and Goodman 2001; Golomb et al. 2007), but most hemiplegic children walk alone at 2 years of age. CP is predicted by large stroke size, but specific regional injury (to Broca's or Wernicke's areas and to PLIC) is also important. Spasticity develops when at cortical level both the primary and premotor/supplementary motor cortices are affected, not with pure M1 lesions. Only large strokes would involve damage to basal nuclei, PLIC, and cortex and thus predict hemiplegia. Besides plasticity, the extent of infarction does influence outcome. Upper limb corticospinal fibers are injured more by lesions lateral and anterior to sites where lower limb fibers are injured (Staudt et al. 2000). Asymmetry of tone in the neonatal period is not helpful to predict hemiplegia: tone can be postictally altered and the focus of seizures is not the lesion core. Hemimotor symptoms are subtle before 6 months of age: a tight popliteal angle and asymmetrical kicking in vertical suspension are early signs (Bouza et al. 1994b). By 6 months of age hand preference is obvious. This timing agrees with transition from bimanual skills to single hand preference in normal infants. In some deterioration may seem present due to loss of preexisting skills, without explanation from seizure onset.

Thalamic shrinkage from transneuronal atrophy is associated with a reduction in SSEP amplitude, suggesting a clinical effect on *sensory* perception. Following venous white matter infarction in preterm infants, MRI around term of myelination in the PLIC may aid to predict hemiplegia. DWI provides quantitative data of acute corticospinal tract injury at an early time point after the insult. The presence of increased SI on DW-MRI at the level of the PLIC and the cerebral peduncles in newborn infants with NAIS is followed by Wallerian degeneration and subsequent development of hemiplegia (Mazumdar et al. 2003; de Vries et al. 2005; Kirton et al. 2007; Lama et al. 2011; van der Aa et al. 2013).

Visual dysfunction originating in cortex injured by NAIS is more common in children with complete than truncal MCA stroke; visual dysfunction is often but not always associated with the involvement of optic radiations or occipital primary visual cortex (Mercuri et al. 1996, 2003). The recuperation of visual function following stroke can be followed with fMRI in combination with diffusion weighted imaging (Seghier et al. 2004).

The relation between neonatal stroke and mental, motor, and *language* development was investigated in detail. Motor is as a rule worse than mental performance. The psychomotor development index is below 90 in many children with severe or moderate hemiplegia (Kolk et al. 2001). Epilepsy in congenital hemiplegia affects cognition in children with normal IQ; *cognitive* dysfunction is more severe in contralateral to lesion handedness (absence of interhemispheric transfer). Persistent dysphasia develops with left-sided lesion, expressive more than receptive; not all left hemiplegics have a language deficit (Vargha-Khadem et al. 1985). Language delay already presents in the earliest communicative efforts (babbling) (Wulfeck et al. 1991). Cortical language areas may differ transiently from normal in perinatal posterior truncal MCA stroke (Fair et al. 2006).

Epilepsy following stroke may be of late onset (after 2 years or more) and weigh on cognitive function (Kolk et al. 2001). The contrasting low incidence of epilepsy in cohorts gathered from the neonatal period on could be due to short follow-up. In the long run epilepsy affects 25–50% of the affected (Gaggero et al. 2001): severe epilepsy correlates with cortical lesions and onset before 2 years; mental retardation develops in 14/34 hemiplegic children with epilepsy; the first epileptic insult is after 3 years in about half of the affected children. Pharmacoresistance (epilepsy failing response to treatment with at least three first choice antiepileptics) is expected in cases with mixed and frequent seizures in infancy and early childhood. Hippocampal sclerosis is uncommon in children with early onset strokes but develops in many children whose strokes are of later origin (Squier et al. 2003). Cognitive dysfunction is worse in children with partial epilepsy and hemiplegia than in children with partial epilepsy only. The association of stroke with neonatal presentation and later infantile spasms carries a bad prognosis (Golomb et al. 2006). Children with cerebral palsy after perinatal stroke who had neonatal presentation are more likely to have severe cognitive impairment or severe epilepsy than children with presentation in infancy.

An early developmental insult can cause later sleep induced epilepsy. Patients with prominent sleep-potentiated epileptiform activity have a higher frequency of early developmental lesions and thalamic lesions than a comparable population of patients without sleep epilepsy (Sanchez Fernandez et al. 2012). Vascular lesions are the type of early developmental lesions most related. Neonates with thalamic hemorrhage associated with straight sinus thrombosis, without evidence of more widespread cerebral damage, are at high risk of developing electrical status epilepticus in slow wave sleep (35%), sleep-induced epileptic activity (14%), or focal epilepsy (14%) (Kersbergen et al. 2013). Electrographic abnormalities may already be present prior to recognition of cognitive deficits.

Plasticity by reorganization of cortical maps and tracts can be studied at several levels. Small lesions permit ipsilateral use of cortex as primary motor area, premotor reorganization happens in unaffected cortex; severe lesions do not permit ipsilateral cortical use, primary motor reorganization occurs in unaffected contralateral cortex (Staudt et al. 2005). Axonal sprouting can be shown from unlesioned CST to ipsilateral proximal and distal arm muscles of the hemiplegic side (Maegaki et al. 1995). Competition in unaffected cortex leads to impaired dexterity of the unaffected hand; dysfunction of the paretic hand is a.o. due to differences in fingertip force and time shifts between muscle activations (Thonnard et al. 2003). In young children with hemispherectomy because of unilateral clastic lesions leading to refractory epilepsy, paradoxical lateralization of the EEG to the "good" hemisphere was sustained by recording prominent ictal rhythms with either 3–7 Hz spike and wave complexes or beta frequency sharp waves (paroxysmal fast) over the unaffected (contralesional) hemisphere (Garzon et al. 2009). This EEG pattern was compatible with seizure free outcome after surgery, provided other clinical findings and tests were concordant with origin from the abnormal hemisphere. Ongoing research on plasticity, combined with early rehabilitation sustained by evidence from controlled trials, will be very interesting in the near future (Golomb 2009).

References

Abels L, Lequin M, Govaert P (2006) Sonographic templates of newborn perforator stroke. Pediatr Radiol 36 (7):663–669

Alfonso I, Prieto G, Vasconcellos E, Aref K, Pacheco E, Yelin K (2001) Internal carotid artery thrombus: an underdiagnosed source of brain emboli in neonates? J Child Neurol 16(6):446–447

Anderson NG, Hay R, Hutchings M, Whitehead M, Darlow B (1995) Posterior fontanelle cranial ultrasound: anatomic and sonographic correlation. Early Hum Dev 42(2):141–152

Ashwal S, Pearce WJ (2001) Animal models of neonatal stroke. Curr Opin Pediatr 13:506–516

Ashwal S, Tone B, Tian HR, Chong S, Obenaus A (2007) Comparison of two neonatal ischemic injury models using magnetic resonance imaging. Pediatr Res 61:9–14

Asindi AA, Stephenson JB, Young DG (1988) Spastic hemiparesis and presumed prenatal embolisation. Arch Dis Child 63:68–69

Bailey OT (1959) Results of long survival after thrombosis of the superior sagittal sinus. Neurology 9:741–746

Bailey OT, Hass GM (1958) Dural sinus thrombosis in early life. J Pediatr 11:755–772

Bain SE, Hsieh DT, Vezina LG, Chang T (2009) Bilateral paramedian thalamic and mesencephalic infarcts in a newborn due to occlusion of the artery of percheron. J Child Neurol 24:219–223

Baram TZ, Butler IJ, Nelson MD Jr, McArdle CB (1988) Transverse sinus thrombosis in newborns: clinical and magnetic resonance imaging findings. Ann Neurol 24 (6):792–794

Barr TL, Conley Y, Ding J, Dillman A, Warach S, Singleton A, Matarin M (2010) Genomic biomarkers and cellular pathways of ischemic stroke by RNA gene expression profiling. Neurology 75:1009–1014

Beattie LM, Butler SJ, Goudie DE (2006) Pathways of neonatal stroke and subclavian steal syndrome. Arch Dis Child Fetal Neonatal Ed 91(3):F204–F207

Benders MJ, van der Aa NE, Roks M, van Straaten HL, Isgum I, Viergever MA, Groenendaal F, de Vries LS, van Bel F (2014) Feasibility and safety of erythropoietin for neuroprotection after perinatal arterial ischemic stroke. J Pediatr 164:481–486, e1–2

Berfelo FJ, Kersbergen KJ, van Ommen CH, Govaert P, van Straaten HL, Poll-The BT et al (2010) Neonatal cerebral sinovenous thrombosis from symptom to outcome. Stroke 41(7):1382–1388

Bergevin MA, Daugherty CC, Bove KE, McAdams AJ (1991) The internal carotid artery siphon in children and adolescents. Hum Pathol 22(6):603–606

Bernard TJ, Goldenberg NA, Armstrong-Wells J, Amlie-Lefond C, Fullerton HJ (2008) Treatment of childhood arterial ischemic stroke. Ann Neurol 63(6):679–696

Billard C, Dulac O, Diebler C (1982) Ischemic cerebral softening in newborn infants. Possible etiology of neonatal convulsive states. Arch Fr Pediatr 39(9): 677–683

Bode H, Strassburg HM, Pringsheim W, Kunzer W (1986) Cerebral infarction in term neonates: diagnosis by cerebral ultrasound. Childs Nerv Syst 2:195–199

Boelman C, Shroff M, Yau I, Bjornson B, Richrdson S, deVeber G, MacGregor D, Moharir M, Askalan R (2014) Antithrombotic therapy for secondary stroke prevention in bacterial meningitis in children. J Pediatr 165:799–806

Bogousslavsky J, Caplan C (1995) Stroke syndromes. Part II: arterial and topographic syndromes. Cambridge University Press, Cambridge, pp 233–402

Bouza H, Dubowitz LM, Rutherford M, Pennock JM (1994a) Prediction of outcome in children with congenital hemiplegia: a magnetic resonance imaging study. Neuropediatrics 25:60–66

Bouza H, Rutherford M, Acolet D, Pennock JM, Dubowitz LM (1994b) Evolution of early hemiplegic signs in full-term infants with unilateral brain lesions in the neonatal period: a prospective study. Neuropediatrics 25:201–207

Boyd RN, Morris ME, Graham HK (2001) Management of upper limb dysfunction in children with cerebral palsy: a systematic review. Eur J Neurol 8(Suppl 5):150–166

Browder J, Kaplan HA, Krieger AJ (1975) Venous lakes in the suboccipital dura mater and falx cerebelli of infants: surgical significance. Surg Neurol 4(1):53–55

Broxterman KJ, Mathew P, Chicoine L (2000) Left brachial artery thrombus, left axillary vein thrombus, and stroke in a neonate with factor V Leiden mutation. J Pediatr Hematol Oncol 22(5):472–475

Byers RK, Hass GM (1933) Thrombosis of the dural venous sinuses in infancy and childhood. Am J Dis Child 45:1161–1183

Campbell LR, Bunyapen C, Holmes GL, Howell CG Jr, Kanto WP Jr (1988) Right common carotid artery ligation in extracorporeal membrane oxygenation. J Pediatr 113:110–113

Carrascosa-Romero MC, Ruiz-Cano R, Abad-Ortiz L, Calatayud-Perez V, Martinez-Gutierrez A, Tebar-Gil R (2002) Intrauterine spinal cord injury resulting from a transverse lie. Magnetic resonance imaging. Rev Neurol 35:398–399

Chabrier S, Saliba E, Nguyen The Tich S, Charollais A, Varlet MN, Tardy B, Presles E, Renaud C, Allard D, Husson B, Landrieu P (2010) Obstetrical and neonatal characteristics vary with birthweight in a cohort of 100 term newborns with symptomatic arterial ischemic stroke. Eur J Paediatr Neurol 14:206–213

Chabrier S, Husson B, Dinomais M, Landrieu P, Nguyen The Tich S (2011) New insights (and new interrogations) in perinatal arterial ischemic stroke. Thromb Res 127:13–22

Chalmers EA (2005) Perinatal stroke – risk factors and management. Br J Haematol 130:333–343

Chan MS, Wong YC, Lau SP, Lau KY, Ou Y (2002) MRI and CT findings of infected cephalhaematoma complicated by skull vault osteomyelitis, transverse venous sinus thrombosis and cerebellar haemorrhage. Pediatr Radiol 32(5):376–379

Chung JI, Weon YC (2005) Anatomic variations of the deep cerebral veins, tributaries of basal vein of Rosenthal: embryologic aspects of the regressed embryonic tentorial sinus. Interv Neuroradiol 11 (2):123–130

Clancy RR (2006) Summary proceedings from the neurology group on neonatal seizures. Pediatrics 117: S23–S27

Clancy R, Malin S, Laraque D, Baumgart S, Younkin D (1985) Focal motor seizures heralding stroke in full-term neonates. Am J Dis Child 139:601–606

Correa F, Enríquez G, Rosselló J, Lucaya J, Piqueras J, Aso C, Vázquez E, Ortega A, Gallart A (2004) Posterior fontanelle sonography: an acoustic window into the neonatal brain. Am J Neuroradiol 25(7):1274–1282

Cowan F, Mercuri E, Groenendaal F, Bassi L, Ricci D, Rutherford M, de Vries L (2005) Does cranial ultrasound imaging identify arterial cerebral infarction in term neonates? Arch Dis Child Fetal Neonatal Ed 90: F252–F256

d'Orey MC, Melo MJ, Ramos I, Guimaraes H, Alves AR, Silva JS, Vasconcelos G, Costa A, Silva G, Santos NT (1999) Cerebral ischemic infarction in newborn infants. Diagnosis using pulsed and color Doppler imaging. Arch Pediatr 6:457–459

Dagain A, Vignes R, Dulou R, Delmas JM, Riem T, Guerin J et al (2009) (Study of the junction between the cortical bridging veins and basal cranial venous sinus) Etude anatomique du drainage des veines corticales inferieures dans le sinus transverse. Neurochirurgie 55 (1):19–24

De Vis JB, Petersen ET, Kersbergen KJ, Alderliesten T, de Vries LS, van Bel F, Groenendaal F, Lemmers PM, Hendrikse J, Benders MJ (2013) Evaluation of perinatal arterial ischemic stroke using noninvasive arterial spin labeling perfusion MRI. Pediatr Res 74:307–313

De Vries LS, Smet M, Goemans N, Wilms G, Devlieger H, Casaer P (1992) Unilateral thalamic haemorrhage in the pre-term and full-term newborn. Neuropediatrics 23 (3):153–156

de Vries E, Robben SG, van den Anker JN (1995) Radiologic imaging of severe cervical spinal cord birth trauma. Eur J Pediatr 154:230–232

de Vries LS, Eken P, Beek E, Groenendaal F, Meiners LC (1996) The posterior fontanelle: a neglected acoustic window. Neuropediatrics 27(2):101–104

de Vries LS, Groenendaal F, Eken P, van Haastert IC, Rademaker KJ, Meiners LC (1997) Infarcts in the vascular distribution of the middle cerebral artery in preterm and fullterm infants. Neuropediatrics 28(2):88–96

de Vries LS, Van der Grond J, Van Haastert IC, Groenendaal F (2005) Prediction of outcome in newborn infants with arterial ischaemic stroke using diffusion-weighted magnetic resonance imaging. Neuropediatrics 36:12–20

de Vries LS, van Haastert IC, Benders MJ, Groenendaal F (2011) Myth: cerebral palsy cannot be predicted by neonatal brain imaging. Semin Fetal Neonatal Med 16:279–287

deVeber G, Andrew M, Adams C, Bjornson B, Booth F, Buckley DJ (2001) Cerebral sinovenous thrombosis in children. N Engl J Med 345(6):417–423

Donaldson B (1987) Real time ultrasound, arterial pulsation and neonatal cerebral infarction. Postgrad Med J 63:263–265

Donzelli R, Marinkovic S, Brigante L, de Divitiis O, Nikodijevic I, Schonauer C, Maiuri F (1998) Territories of the perforating (lenticulostriate) branches of the middle cerebral artery. Surg Radiol Anat 20 (6):393–398

Dudink J, Mercuri E, Al-Nakib L, Govaert P, Counsell SJ, Rutherford MA, Cowan FM (2009) Evolution of unilateral perinatal arterial ischemic stroke on conventional and diffusion-weighted MR imaging. AJNR Am J Neuroradiol 30:998–1004

Dudink J, Counsell SJ, Lequin MH, Govaert PP (2012) DTI reveals network injury in perinatal stroke. Arch Dis Child Fetal Neonatal Ed 97:F362–F364

Duque J, Thonnard J-L, Vandermeeren Y, Sébire G, Cosnard G, Olivier E (2003) Correlation between impaired dexterity and corticospinal tract dysgenesis in congenital hemiplegia. Brain 126:732–747

Ehlers H, Courville C (1936) Thrombosis of internal cerebral veins in infancy and childhood. J Pediatr 8:600–623

Eichler F, Krishnamoorthy K, Grant PE (2007) Magnetic resonance imaging evaluation of possible neonatal sinovenous thrombosis. Pediatr Neurol 37(5):317–323

Eliasson AC, Bonnier B, Krumlinde-Sundholm L (2003) Clinical experience of constraint induced movement therapy in adolescents with hemiplegic cerebral palsy – a day camp model. Dev Med Child Neurol 45:357–359

Evans D, Levene M (1998) Neonatal seizures. Arch Dis Child Fetal Neonatal Ed 78:F70–F75

Eyre JA, Miller S, Clowry GJ, Conway EA, Watts C (2000) Functional corticospinal projections are established prenatally in the human foetus permitting involvement in the development of spinal motor centres. Brain 123:51–64

Fair DA, Brown TT, Petersen SE, Schlaggar BL (2006) fMRI reveals novel functional neuroanatomy in a child with perinatal stroke. Neurology 67:2246–2249

Feekes JA, Hsu SW, Chaloupka JC, Cassell MD (2005) Tertiary microvascular territories define lacunar infarcts in the basal ganglia. Ann Neurol 58(1): 18–30

Fehlings D, Rang M, Glazier J, Steele C (2000) An evaluation of botulinum-A toxin injections to improve upper extremity function in children with hemiplegic cerebral palsy. J Pediatr 137:331–337

Fischer AQ, Anderson JC, Shuman RM (1988) The evolution of ischemic cerebral infarction in infancy: a sonographic evaluation. J Child Neurol 3(2): 105–109

Fitzgerald KC, Williams LS, Garg BP, Carvalho KS, Golomb MR (2006) Cerebral sinovenous thrombosis in the neonate. Arch Neurol 63(3):405–409

Fullerton HJ, Wu YW, Sidney S, Johnston SC (2007) Risk of recurrent childhood arterial ischemic stroke in a population-based cohort: the importance of cerebrovascular imaging. Pediatrics 119(3):495–501

Fumagalli M, Ramenghi LA, Mosca F (2004) Palpebral ecchymosis and cerebral venous thrombosis in a near term infant. Arch Dis Child Fetal Neonatal Ed 89(6): F530

Gaggero R, Devescovi R, Zaccone A, Ravera G (2001) Epilepsy associated with infantile hemiparesis: predictors of long-term evolution. Brain Dev 23:12–17

Garg BP, DeMyer WE (1995) Ischemic thalamic infarction in children: clinical presentation, etiology, and outcome. Pediatr Neurol 13(1):46–49

Garzon E, Gupta A, Bingaman W, Sakamoto AC, Luders H (2009) Paradoxical ictal EEG lateralization in children with unilateral encephaloclastic lesions. Epileptic Disord 11:215–221

Ginsberg MD (2008) Neuroprotection for ischemic stroke: past, present and future. Neuropharmacology 55 (3):363–389

Golomb MR (2009) Outcomes of perinatal arterial ischemic stroke and cerebral sinovenous thrombosis. Semin Fetal Neonatal Med 14:318–322

Golomb MR, Garg BP, Williams LS (2006) Outcomes of children with infantile spasms after perinatal stroke. Pediatr Neurol 34:291–295

Golomb MR, Saha C, Garg BP, Azzouz F, Williams LS (2007) Association of cerebral palsy with other disabilities in children with perinatal arterial ischemic stroke. Pediatr Neurol 37(4):245–249

Gonzalez FF, Larpthaveesarp A, McQuillen P, Derugin N, Wendland M, Spadafora R, Ferriero DM (2013) Erythropoietin increases neurogenesis and oligodendrogliosis of subventricular zone precursor cells after neonatal stroke. Stroke 44:753–758

Govaert P (2009) Sonographic stroke templates. Semin Fetal Neonatal Med 14:284–298

Govaert P, Achten E, Vanhaesebrouck P, De Praeter C, Van Damme J (1992) Deep cerebral venous thrombosis in thalamo-ventricular hemorrhage of the term newborn. Pediatr Radiol 22(2):123–127

Govaert P, Matthys E, Zecic A, Roelens F, Oostra A, Vanzieleghem B (2000) Perinatal cortical infarction within middle cerebral artery trunks. Arch Dis Child Fetal Neonatal Ed 82:F59–F63

Govaert P, Swarte R, Oostra A, Zecic A, Vanzieleghem B, Van Langenhove P (2001) Neonatal infarction within basal cerebral vein territory. Dev Med Child Neurol 43 (8):559–562

Govaert P et al (2008) Network injury to pulvinar with neonatal arterial ischemic stroke. Neuroimage 39:1850–1857

Govaert P, Dudink J, Visser G, Breukhoven P, Vanhatalo S, Lequin M (2009) Top of the basilar artery embolic stroke and neonatal myoclonus. Dev Med Child Neurol 51(4):324–327

Greenway A, Massicotte MP, Monagle P (2004) Neonatal thrombosis and its treatment. Blood Rev 18(2):75–84

Guajardo L, Strauss A, Amster J (1994) Idiopathic cerebral infarction and upper limb ischemia in neonates. Am J Perinatol 11(2):119–122

Gudinchet F, Dreyer JL, Payot M, Duvoisin B, Laurini R (1991) Imaging of neonatal arterial thrombosis. Arch Dis Child 66(10 Spec No):1158–1159

Gunny RS, Lin D (2012) Imaging of perinatal stroke. Magn Reson Imaging Clin N Am 20:1–33

Guppy KH, Origitano TC, Reichman OH, Segal S (1997) Venous drainage of the inferolateral temporal lobe in relationship to transtemporal/transtentorial approaches to the cranial base. Neurosurgery 41(3):615–619, discussion 9–20

Gupta S, Fernandez D, Siddiqui A, Lin JP, Garside L, Lim M (2009) Thalamic infarct presenting as apparent life-threatening event in infants. Acta Paediatr 98:2002–2005

Guzzetta A, Mercuri E, Rapisardi G, Ferrari F, Roversi MF, Cowan F, Rutherford M, Paolicelli PB, Einspieler C, Boldrini A, Dubowitz L, Prechtl HF, Cioni G (2003) General movements detect early signs of hemiplegia in term infants with neonatal cerebral infarction. Neuropediatrics 34:61–66

Hamida N, Hakim A, Fourati H, Thabet AB, Walha L, Bouraoui A, Mnif Z, Gargouri A (2014) Dissection artérielle cervicale néonatale secondaire à un traumatisme obstétrical. Arch Pediatr 21:201–205

Harteman JC, Groenendaal F, Toet MC, Benders MJ, Van Haastert IC, Nievelstein RA, Koopman-Esseboom C, de Vries LS (2013) Diffusion-weighted imaging changes in cerebral watershed distribution following neonatal encephalopathy are not invariably associated with an adverse outcome. Dev Med Child Neurol 55:642–653

Hernanz-Schulman M, Cohen W, Genieser NB (1988) Sonography of cerebral infarction in infancy. Am J Roentgenol 150:897–902

Hill A, Martin DJ, Daneman A, Fitz CR (1983) Focal ischemic cerebral injury in the newborn: diagnosis by ultrasound and correlation with computed tomographic scan. Pediatrics 71:790–793

Hoogstraate SR, Lequin ML, Ahmed S, Govaert PP (2008) Apnoea in relation to neonatal temporal lobe haemorrhage. Eur J Paediatr Neurol (epub 29 Aug) 13; 356–361

Huang AH, Robertson RL (2004) Spontaneous superficial parenchymal and leptomeningeal hemorrhage in term neonates. AJNR Am J Neuroradiol 25:469–475

Huang C-C, Ho M-Y, Shen E-Y (1987) Sonographic changes in a parasagittal cerebral lesion in an asphyxiated newborn. J Clin Ultrasound 15:68–70

Hunt RW, Loughnan P, Fink AM, Volpe JJ, Inder TE (2002) Magnetic resonance demonstration in the newborn of generalized cerebral venous dilation with spontaneous resolution. Eur J Paediatr Neurol 6(5):289–292

Jan MM, Camfield PR (1998) Outcome of neonatal stroke in full-term infants without significant birth asphyxia. Eur J Pediatr 157:846–848

Jennekens W, Dankers F, Janssen F, Toet M, van der Aa N, Niemarkt H, van Pul C, de Vries L, Andriessen P (2012) Effects of midazolam and lidocaine on spectral properties of the EEG in full-term neonates with stroke. Eur J Paediatr Neurol 16:642–652

Jordan LC, Rafay MF, Smith SE, Askalan R, Zamel KM, de Veber G, Ashwal S (2010) Antithrombotic treatment in neonatal cerebral sinovenous thrombosis: results of the international pediatric stroke study. J Pediatr 156:704–710, 710.e1–710.e2

Kato Y, Takeda H, Furuya D, Nagoya H, Deguchi I, Fukuoka T, Tanahashi N (2010) Subarachnoid hemorrhage as the initial presentation of cerebral venous thrombosis. Intern Med 49:467–470

Kenet G, Kirkham F, Niederstadt T, Heinecke A, Saunders D, Stoll M, Brenner B, Bidlingmaier C, Heller C, Knöfler R, Schobess R, Zieger B, Sébire G, Nowak-Göttl U (2007) European Thromboses Study Group. Risk factors for recurrent venous thromboembolism in the European collaborative paediatric database on cerebral venous thrombosis: a multicentre cohort study. Lancet Neurol 6(7):595–603

Kersbergen KJ, de Vries LS, Leijten FS, Braun KP, Nievelstein RA, Groenendaal F, Benders MJ, Jansen FE (2013) Neonatal thalamic hemorrhage is strongly associated with electrical status epilepticus in slow wave sleep. Epilepsia 54:733–740

Kidwell CS, Alger JR, Saver JL (2003) Beyond mismatch. Evolving paradigms in imaging the ischemic penumbra with multimodal magnetic resonance imaging. Stroke 34:2729–2735

Kirton A, Shroff M, Visvanathan T, deVeber G (2007) Quantified corticospinal tract diffusion restriction predicts neonatal stroke outcome. Stroke 38:974–980

Klesh KW, Murphy TF, Scher MS, Buchanan DE, Maxwell EP, Guthrie RD (1987) Cerebral infarction in persistent pulmonary hypertension of the newborn. Am J Dis Child 141:852–857

Koelfen W, Freund M, Varnholt V (1995) Neonatal stroke involving the middle cerebral artery in term infants: clinical presentation, EEG and imaging studies, and outcome. Dev Med Child Neurol 37(3): 204–212

Kolk A, Beilmann A, Tomberg T, Napa A, Talvik T (2001) Neurocognitive development of children with congenital unilateral brain lesion and epilepsy. Brain Dev 23:88–96

Komiyama M, Kitano S, Sakamoto H, Ehara E, Miyagi N, Kusuda S (2001) Rapid normalization of marked dilatation of the cerebral duro-venous system in a newborn infant mimicking a great vein of Galen varix. Pediatr Neurosurg 35:149–152

Krishnamoorthy KS, Soman TB, Takeoka M, Schaefer PW (2000) Diffusion-weighted imaging in neonatal cerebral infarction: clinical utility and follow-up. J Child Neurol 15:592–602

Lama S, Qiao M, Kirton A, Sun S, Cheng E, Foniok T, Tuor UI (2011) Imaging corticospinal degeneration in neonatal rats with unilateral cerebral infarction. Exp Neurol 228:192–199

Laugesaar R, Kolk A, Tomberg T, Metsvaht T, Lintrop M, Varendi H, Talvik T (2007) Acutely and retrospectively diagnosed perinatal stroke: a population-based study. Stroke 38:2234–2240

Lee RM (1995) Morphology of cerebral arteries. Pharmacol Ther 66:149–173

Lehman LL, Rivkin MJ (2014) Perinatal arterial ischemic stroke: presentation, risk factors, evaluation, and outcome. Pediatr Neurol 51:760–768

Lequin MH, Peeters EA, Holscher HC, de Krijger R, Govaert P (2004) Arterial infarction caused by carotid artery dissection in the neonate. Eur J Paediatr Neurol 8 (3):155–160

Lequin MH, Dudink J, Tong KA et al (2009) Magnetic resonance imaging in neonatal stroke. Semin Fetal Neonatal Med 14:299–310

Mader I, Schoning M, Klose U, Kuker W (2002) Neonatal cerebral infarction diagnosed by diffusion-weighted MRI: pseudonormalization occurs early. Stroke 33: 1142–1145

Maegaki Y, Yamamoto T, Takeshita K (1995) Plasticity of central motor and sensory pathways in a case of unilateral extensive cortical dysplasia: investigation of magnetic resonance imaging, transcranial magnetic stimulation, and short-latency somatosensory evoked potentials. Neurology 45:2255–2261

Mah S, deVeber G, Wei XC, Liapounova N, Kirton A (2013) Cerebellar atrophy in childhood arterial ischemic stroke: acute diffusion MRI biomarkers. Stroke 44:2468–2474

Marinkovic S, Gibo H, Filipovic B, Dulejic V, Piscevic I (2005) Microanatomy of the subependymal arteries of the lateral ventricle. Surg Neurol 63(5):451–458

Mazumdar A, Mukherjee P, Miller JH, Malde H, McKinstry RC (2003) Diffusion-weighted imaging of acute corticospinal tract injury preceding Wallerian degeneration in the maturing human brain. Am J Neuroradiol 24:1057–1066

Meoded A, Poretti A, Benson JE, Tekes A, Huisman TA (2014) Evaluation of the ischemic penumbra focusing on the venous drainage: the role of susceptibility weighted imaging (SWI) in pediatric ischemic cerebral stroke. J Neuroradiol 41:108–116

Mercuri E (2001) Early diagnostic and prognostic indicators in full term infants with neonatal cerebral infarction: an integrated clinical, neuroradiological and EEG approach. Minerva Pediatr 53:305–311

Mercuri E, Atkinson J, Braddick O, Anker S, Nokes L, Cowan F, Rutherford M, Pennock J, Dubowitz L (1996) Visual function and perinatal focal cerebral infarction. Arch Dis Child Fetal Neonatal Ed 75: F76–F81

Mercuri E, Rutherford M, Cowan F, Pennock J, Counsell S, Papadimitriou M, Azzopardi D, Bydder G, Dubowitz L (1999) Early prognostic indicators of outcome in infants with neonatal cerebral infarction: a clinical, electroencephalogram, and magnetic resonance imaging study. Pediatrics 103:39–46

Mercuri E, Anker S, Guzzetta A, Barnett A, Haataja L, Rutherford M, Cowan F, Dubowitz L, Braddick O, Atkinson J (2003) Neonatal cerebral infarction and visual function at school age. Arch Dis Child Fetal Neonatal Ed 88:F487–F491

Miller SP, O'Gorman AM, Shevell MI (2000) Recurrent artery of Heubner infarction in infancy. Dev Med Child Neurol 42(5):344–346

Miller E, Daneman A, Doria AS, Blaser S, Traubici J, Jarrin J et al (2012) Color Doppler US of normal cerebral venous sinuses in neonates: a comparison with MR venography. Pediatr Radiol 42(9):1070–1079

Moharir MDSM, MacGregor D (2006) Clinical and radiographic features of thrombosis propagation in neonatal and childhood cerebral sinovenous thrombosis. Ann Neurol 60(suppl):S141

Moharir MD, Shroff M, Pontigon AM, Askalan R, Yau I, Macgregor D et al (2011) A prospective outcome study of neonatal cerebral sinovenous thrombosis. J Child Neurol 26(9):1137–1144

Monagle P, Chalmers E, Chan A, de Veber G, Kirkham F, Massicotte P, Michelson AD (2008) Antithrombotic therapy in neonates and children. Chest 133 (6, supplement):887s–968s

Muthukumar N, Palaniappan P (1998) Tentorial venous sinuses: an anatomic study. Neurosurgery 42 (2):363–371

Neville B, Goodman R (2001) Congenital hemiplegia. McKeith Press, London en Cambridge University Press, Cambridge, UK as Clinics in Developmental Medicine, nr 150

Norman MG (1974) Unilateral encephalomalacia in cranial nerve nuclei in neonates: report of two cases. Neurology 24:424–427 [one preterm with basilar artery thrombosis and infarction of one oculomotor nucleus]

Nowak-Gottl U, Gunther G, Kurnik K, Strater R, Kirkham F (2003) Arterial ischemic stroke in neonates, infants, and children: an overview of underlying conditions, imaging methods, and treatment modalities. Semin Thromb Hemost 29:405–414

Nwosu ME, Williams LS, Edwards-Brown M, Eckert GJ, Golomb MR (2008) Neonatal sinovenous thrombosis: presentation and association with imaging. Pediatr Neurol 39:155–161

Okabe T, Aida N, Niwa T, Nozawa K, Shibasaki J, Osaka H (2014) Early magnetic resonance detection of cortical necrosis and acute network injury associated with neonatal and infantile cerebral infarction. Pediatr Radiol 44:597–604

Pape K, Wigglesworth J (1979) Haemorrhage, ischaemia and the perinatal brain. McKeith Press, London en Cambridge University Press, Cambridge, UK as Clinics in Developmental Medicine, nrs 69/70

Pellicer A, Cabanas F, Garcia-Alix A, Perez-Higueras A, Quero J (1992) Stroke in neonates with cardiac right-to-left shunt. Brain Dev 14:381–385

Plouin P, Kaminska A (2013) Neonatal seizures. Handb Clin Neurol 111:467–476

Pollack MA, Llena JL, Fleischman A, Fish B (1983) Neonatal brainstem infarction. Arch Neurol 40:52–53 (cystic necrosis in pons and right cerebellar hemisphere following coarctectomy on day 17, together with right arm gangrene due to brachial artery catheter-related thrombosis; also extensive cerebral grey and white matter infarction)

Raets M, Dudink J, Raybaud C, Ramenghi L, Lequin M, Govaert P (2015) Brain vein disorders in newborn infants. Dev Med Child Neurol 57:229–240

Rafay MF, Cortez MA, de Veber GA, Tan-Dy C, Al-Futaisi A, Yoon W, Fallah S, Moore AM (2009) Predictive value of clinical and EEG features in the diagnosis of stroke and hypoxic ischemic encephalopathy in neonates with seizures. Stroke 40:2402–2407

Raine J, Davies H, Gamsu HR (1989) Multiple idiopathic emboli in a full term neonate. Acta Paediatr Scand 78 (4):644–646

Raju TNK, Nelson KB, Ferriero D, Lynch J, NICHD-NINDS Perinatal Stroke Workshop Participants (2007) Perinatal haemorrhagic stroke: summary of a workshop sponsored by NICHD and NINDS on classification, challenges and opportunities. Pediatrics 120(3):609–616

Ramenghi LA, Bassi L, Fumagalli M, Ometto A, Groppo M, De Carli A, Pisoni S, Dessimone F, Fare P, Mosca F (2010) Neonatal stroke. Minerva Pediatr 62:177–179

Raybaud CA, Livet MO, Jiddane M, Pinsard N (1985) Radiology of ischemic strokes in children. Neuroradiology 27:567–578

Righini A, Doneda C, Parazzini C, Arrigoni F, Matta U, Triulzi F (2010) Diffusion tensor imaging of early changes in corpus callosum after acute cerebral hemisphere lesions in newborns. Neuroradiology 52:1025–1035

Roach ES, Golomb MR, Adams R, Biller J, Daniels S, deVeber G, Ferriero D, Jones BV, Kirkham FJ, Scott RM, Smith ER (2008) Management of stroke in infants and children: a scientific statement from a special writing group of the American Heart Association Stroke Council and the council on cardiovascular disease in the young. Stroke 39:2644–2691

Roitberg BZ, Tuccar E, Alp MS (2002) Bilateral paramedian thalamic infarct in the presence of an unpaired thalamic perforating artery. Acta Neurochir (Wien) 144(3):301–304

Roodhooft AM, Parizel PM, Van Acker KJ, Deprettere AJ, Van Reempts PJ (1987) Idiopathic cerebral arterial infarction with paucity of symptoms in the full-term neonate. Pediatrics 80:381–385

Roze E, Harris PA, Ball G, Elorza LZ, Braga RM, Allsop JM, Merchant N, Porter E, Arichi T, Edwards AD, Rutherford MA, Cowan FM, Counsell SJ (2012) Tractography of the corticospinal tracts in infants with focal perinatal injury: comparison with normal controls and to motor development. Neuroradiology 54:507–516

Ruggieri M, Smarason AK, Pike M (1999) Spinal cord insults in the prenatal, perinatal, and neonatal periods. Dev Med Child Neurol 41:311–317

Rutherford MA, Ramenghi LA, Cowan FM (2012) Neonatal stroke. Arch Dis Child Fetal Neonatal Ed 97: F377–F384

Sanchez Fernandez I, Takeoka M, Tas E, Peters JM, Prabhu SP, Stannard KM, Gregas M, Eksioglu Y, Rotenberg A, Riviello JJ Jr, Kothare SV, Loddenkemper T (2012) Early thalamic lesions in patients with sleep-potentiated epileptiform activity. Neurology 78:1721–1727

Sashikumar P et al. (2014) Bilateral perinatal arterial stroke in a neonate. BMJ Case Rep 2014

Scher MS, Beggarly M (1989) Clinical significance of focal periodic discharges in neonates. J Child Neurol 4:175–185

Seghier ML, Lazeyras F, Zimine S, Maier SE, Hanquinet S, Delavelle J, Volpe JJ, Huppi PS (2004) Combination of event-related fMRI and diffusion tensor imaging in an infant with perinatal stroke. Neuroimage 21:463–472

Selton D, Andre M, Hascoet JM (2003) EEG and ischemic stroke in full-term newborns. Neurophysiol Clin 33:120–129

Silver RK, MacGregor SN, Pasternak JF, Neely SE (1992) Fetal stroke associated with elevated maternal anticardiolipin antibodies. Obstet Gynecol 80(3 Pt 2):497–499

Simanovsky N, Stepensky P, Hiller N (2004) The use of ultrasound for the diagnosis of spinal hemorrhage in a newborn. Pediatr Neurol 31:295–297

Squier W, Salisbury H, Sisodiya S (2003) Stroke in the developing brain and intractable epilepsy: effect of timing on hippocampal sclerosis. Dev Med Child Neurol 45:580–585

Sreenan C, Bhargava R, Robertson CM (2000) Cerebral infarction in the term newborn: clinical presentation and long-term outcome. J Pediatr 137(3):351–355

Staudt M, Niemann G, Grodd W, Krageloh-Mann I (2000) The pyramidal tract in congenital hemiparesis: relationship between morphology and function in periventricular lesions. Neuropediatrics 31:257–264

Staudt M, Krageloh-Mann I, Grodd W (2005) Ipsilateral corticospinal pathways in congenital hemiparesis on routine magnetic resonance imaging. Pediatr Neurol 32:37–39

Stephens RB, Stilwell DL (1969) Arteries and veins of the human brain. Charles C. Thomas, Springfield

Steventon DM, John PR (1997) Power Doppler ultrasound appearances of neonatal ischaemic brain injury. Pediatr Radiol 27:147–149

Swarte R, Lequin M, Cherian P, Zecic A, van Goudoever J, Govaert P (2009) Imaging patterns of brain injury in term-birth asphyxia. Acta Paediatr 98:586–592

Takahashi S, Ishii K, Matsumoto K, Higano S, Ishibashi T, Suzuki M (1994) The anterior choroidal artery syndrome. II. CT and/or MR in angiographically verified cases. Neuroradiology 36(5):340–345

Taylor GA (1994) Alterations in regional cerebral blood flow in neonatal stroke: preliminary findings with color Doppler sonography. Pediatr Radiol 24:111–115

Taylor GA, Trescher WA, Traystman RJ, Johnston MV (1993) Acute experimental neuronal injury in the newborn lamb: US characterization and demonstration of hemodynamic effects. Pediatr Radiol 23:268–275

Ushiwata I, Saiki I, Murakami T, Kanaya H, Konno J, Wada S (1989) Transverse sinus thrombosis accompanied by intracerebellar hemorrhage: a case report. No Shinkei Geka 17:51–55

van der Aa NE, Verhage CH, Groenendaal F, Vermeulen RJ, de Bode S, van Nieuwenhuizen O, de Vries LS (2013) Neonatal neuroimaging predicts recruitment of contralesional corticospinal tracts following perinatal brain injury. Dev Med Child Neurol 55:707–712

van Rooij LG, de Vries LS, Handryastuti S, Hawani D, Groenendaal F, van Huffelen AC, Toet MC (2007) Neurodevelopmental outcome in term infants with status epilepticus detected with amplitude-integrated electroencephalography. Pediatrics 120:e354–e363

van Wezel-Meijler G, Hummel TZ, Oosting J, de Groot L, Sie LT, Huisman J, Lafeber HN, van der Knaap MS (1999) Unilateral thalamic lesions in premature infants: risk factors and short-term prognosis. Neuropediatrics 30(6): 300–306

Vander Eecken (1959) Normal cerebral arterial anatomy. In: The anastomoses between the leptomeningeal arteries of the brain. Thomas C.C., Springfield

Vandeweyer G, Van Laer L, Loeys B, Van den Bulcke T, Kooy RF (2014) VariantDB: a flexible annotation and filtering portal for next generation sequencing data. Genome Med 6:74

Vargha-Khadem F, O'Gorman AM, Watters GV (1985) Aphasia and handedness in relation to hemispheric side, age at injury and severity of cerebral lesion during childhood. Brain 108:677–696

Walsh BH, Low E, Bogue CO, Murray DM, Boylan GB (2011) Early continuous video electroencephalography in neonatal stroke. Dev Med Child Neurol 53:89–92

Walther M, Juenger H, Kuhnke N, Wilke M, Brodbeck V, Berweck S, Staudt M, Mall V (2009) Motor cortex plasticity in ischemic perinatal stroke: a transcranial magnetic stimulation and functional MRI study. Pediatr Neurol 41:171–178

Weissman BM, Aram DM, Levinsohn MW, Ben-Shachar G (1985) Neurologic sequelae of cardiac catheterization. Cathet Cardiovasc Diagn 11: 577–583

White BR, Liao SM, Ferradal SL, Inder TE, Culver JP (2012) Bedside optical imaging of occipital resting-state functional connectivity in neonates. Neuroimage 59:2529–2538

Wintermark P, Warfield SK (2012) New insights in perinatal arterial ischemic stroke by assessing brain perfusion. Transl Stroke Res 3:255–262

Wu YW, Hamrick SE, Miller SP, Haward MF, Lai MC, Callen PW, Barkovich AJ, Ferriero DM (2003) Intraventricular hemorrhage in term neonates caused by sinovenous thrombosis. Ann Neurol 54(1): 123–126

Wulfeck BB, Trauner DA, Tallal PA (1991) Neurologic, cognitive, and linguistic features of infants after early stroke. Pediatr Neurol 7:266–269

Young RS, Towfighi J, Marks KH (1983) Focal necrosis of the spinal cord in utero. Arch Neurol 40:654–655

Neonatal Seizures

131

Lena K. Hellström-Westas and Malcolm Levene

Contents

Abstract

Neonatal seizures affect 1–3 infants per 1000 newborns in the general population. The incidence of neonatal seizures is higher in preterm infants than in term infants. The most common etiologies of neonatal seizures are perinatal hypoxic-ischemic and hemorrhagic insults, resulting in hypoxic-ischemic encephalopathy, stroke, and intracranial hemorrhages. Since most neonatal seizures occur as a result of perinatal insults, a majority of neonatal seizures emerge during the first 3 days of life. Infants with suspected seizures should be evaluated immediately. EEG and aEEG/EEG should be recorded early since several studies have shown that clinical recognition of neonatal seizures is not reliable. The prognosis is usually dependent on the underlying condition; the overall mortality is 10–30%, and 30–40% of survivors develop neurodevelopmental sequels with less than 20% developing postnatal epilepsy.

L. K. Hellström-Westas (✉)
Department of Women's and Children's Health, Uppsala University and University Hospital, Uppsala, Sweden
e-mail: lena.westas@kbh.uu.se

M. Levene
Academic Unit of Paediatrics and Child Health, University of Leeds, Leeds, UK

Department of Neonatal Medicine, Leeds Teaching Hospitals Trust, Leeds, UK

131.1 Salient Points

- Neonatal seizures are mainly due to previous hypoxic-ischemic, hemorrhagic, or metabolic insults, while seizures due to epileptic

G. Buonocore et al. (eds.), *Neonatology*,
https://doi.org/10.1007/978-3-319-29489-6_277

syndromes and congenital conditions are rare in newborns.

- The most common causes of neonatal seizures are hypoxic-ischemic brain injury, intracranial hemorrhages, and stroke.
- Clinical recognition of neonatal seizures is unreliable since a majority of neonatal seizures are subclinical, or have only subtle clinical expression, and also since clinically observed seizure-suspected motor activity may not have an epileptic origin.
- EEG or aEEG/EEG is necessary for correct identification of neonatal seizures and is associated with earlier detection of seizures, more precise treatment of seizures, and less use of antiepileptic medications.
- Clinically important questions that need to be addressed include: Do all neonatal seizures require antiepileptic treatment? Is antiepileptic treatment associated with less brain injury and better outcome? Which medications should be used? For how long should antiepileptic treatment be administered?

131.2 Incidence

Neonatal seizures affect 1–3 infants per 1000 newborns in the general population (Ronen et al. 1999; Sheth et al. 1999). The incidence in different populations varies according to differences in diagnostic criteria (clinical seizures or EEG required for diagnosis) and the studied time period, but may also be associated with differences in maternal characteristics (parity, smoking, obesity), living conditions, and standard of perinatal care. The incidence of neonatal seizures is higher in preterm infants than in term infants (Ronen et al. 1999; Sheth et al. 1999; Scher et al. 1993). Seizures are more prevalent in high-risk populations such as infants requiring neonatal intensive care (NICU); older studies indicate that 3–5% of infants may be affected but the exact numbers are difficult to establish (Scher et al. 1993; Hellström-Westas et al. 1995). Recent studies indicate that the seizure incidence may be quite high in extremely preterm infants and associated with intraventricular hemorrhages and mortality (Vesoulis et al. 2014). A majority of these seizures are brief and subclinical and only possible to detect with EEG or aEEG/EEG.

The most common etiologies of neonatal seizures are perinatal hypoxic-ischemic and hemorrhagic insults, resulting in hypoxic-ischemic encephalopathy, stroke, and intracranial hemorrhages (Scher et al. 1993; Weeke et al. 2015; Glass et al. 2016). Other relatively common causes of seizures include infections and metabolic disturbances such as hypoglycemia and metabolic diseases. Seizures are prevalent in metabolic diseases, and intense seizures (mainly subclinical) can be seen in infants with disorders of energy metabolism, hyperammonemia, peroxisomal disorders, and organic/amino acidopathies (Olischar et al. 2012). Pyridoxine (vitamin B6) dependent seizures are rare but should always be considered in infants with therapy-resistant seizures. Hereditary familial seizures are caused by various mutations, including genes coding for voltage-gated sodium and potassium channels. They usually have a variable clinical course and outcome. So-called fifth day fits were previously described as being relatively prevalent but they are now rarely seen. Othahara syndrome, or early infantile epileptic encephalopathy (EIEE), and early myoclonic epileptic encephalopathy (EMEE) are severe conditions caused by a variety of disorders including cerebral malformations and various mutations. They are characterized by burst-suppression pattern in the EEG (constant in EIEE and during sleep in EMEE) and severe outcomes (Hart et al. 2015) (Table 1).

Since most neonatal seizures occur as a result of perinatal insults, a majority of neonatal seizures emerge during the first 3 days of life. This is a strong argument for using routine aEEG/EEG or EEG monitoring of high-risk infants during the first 3 days of life in order to enhance epileptic seizure detection and cerebral compromise in these infants. Only in moderately preterm infants, the peak of incidence is somewhat later, because seizures in these

Table 1 Etiologies of neonatal seizures (Ronen et al. 1999; Weeke et al. 2015; Glass et al. 2016; Tekgul et al. 2006; Yildiz et al. 2012)

Etiology	Prevalence (%)
Hypoxic-ischemic encephalopathy	29–46
Intracranial hemorrhage	12–18
Perinatal stroke	13–18
Infections, including sepsis	7–20
Metabolic, including hypoglycemia	9–19
Cerebral dysgenesis	3–5
Epileptic syndromes, other	1–2

infants are more often caused by infections (Sheth et al. 1999).

Table 2 Suggested initial management of infants with suspected seizures

Prompt clinical evaluation should include perinatal medical history and physical examination.
Blood glucose should be checked immediately since hypoglycemia is a treatable condition.
A decision should be taken regarding administration of antiepileptic treatment.
Further observation and evaluation in a NICU should include a standard EEG or video EEG, continuous monitoring with aEEG/EEG, and cranial ultrasound.
Biochemical evaluation should include hemoglobin, blood gas, glucose, lactate, electrolytes (Na, K, Mg, Ca), bilirubin, CRP, white blood cell count, and platelets.
Decision should be taken on further investigations, e.g., lumbar puncture, MRI, other biochemical tests.

131.3 Diagnosing Seizures

Observation of clinically suspected seizures in newborn infants is the most common way of diagnosing neonatal seizures. Suspected clinical seizures in a newborn infant in the NICU, maternity unit, or at home, if the baby was already discharged from the hospital, should be given prompt attention. These infants should immediately be examined clinically: blood glucose should be checked, a decision should be taken whether antiepileptic treatment should be administered, and the baby should be referred to a NICU for further observation and evaluation (Table 2).

The first strategy should be to identify the potential etiology and to rule out disorders that could be treatable with a timely intervention, e.g., hypoglycemia, infection, and intracranial hemorrhages requiring surgery.

Clinical description of suspected neonatal seizures can give important clues to the etiology. Clinical seizures are clinically observed events suspected of being electroclinical seizures. Electroclinical seizures are clinical seizures with simultaneous epileptic activity in the EEG, while electrographical seizures denote presence of epileptic seizure activity in the EEG but no clinical symptoms (often called subclinical seizures).

Clinical seizures were traditionally classified by Volpe as subtle, clonic (focal or multifocal), tonic (focal or generalized), or myoclonic (focal, multifocal, or generalized) (Volpe 1989). More recently, Nagarajan et al. classified clinical features of electroclinical seizures (seizure semiology) with brief and for neonatologist's clinically very useful definitions as: (1) clonic (repetitive clonic jerking of the limbs, head, or trunk), (2) tonic (stiffening of limbs or trunk), (3) myoclonic (single jerk or slow serial jerking of the limbs, head, or trunk), (4) ocular (features around eyes, e. g., blinking, wide opening, eye deviation, nystagmus), (5) orolingual (mouthing/chewing type movements, tongue thrusting/ movements, crying/grimacing type of movements, noises/ vocalizations, dry retching), (6) autonomic (color change, change in breathing pattern, oxygen desaturation, apneas, blood pressure changes, changes in heart rate), (7) hypomotor (obvious decrease or cessation of behavioral activity, staring), and (8) other (Nagarajan et al. 2012).

Several studies have shown that clinical recognition of neonatal seizures is not reliable and that many clinically suspected seizures do not have corresponding EEG seizure activity. Furthermore, a majority of neonatal seizures are actually subclinical. Mizrahi and Kellaway demonstrated that some clinical seizure types are more closely associated with EEG seizures: focal clonic, generalized myoclonic, and focal tonic seizures, including tonic eye deviation. Other clinical seizures types were more inconsistently associated with electrographic seizure activity, including generalized tonic and myoclonic seizures, motor automatisms including oral-buccal and ocular movements, progression movements including pedaling, stepping and rotatory arm movements (Mizrahi and Kellaway 1987). Term and preterm infant seem to exhibit similar types of clinical seizures, although subclinical seizures are more prevalent in preterm infants (Scher et al. 1993). In a video-EEG study of term asphyxiated infants less than 10% of all seizures were correctly identified by clinical observation in the NICU due to the fact that a majority of seizures were subclinical and many clinically suspected events could not be confirmed as seizures in the EEG (Murray et al. 2008).

Although some clinical manifestations of seizures are very typical for specific etiologies, e.g., unilateral clonic seizures in babies with stroke, many electroclinical seizures contain different clinical seizure types. Orolingual and autonomic symptoms are common at the onset of seizures, while ocular events more often appear during seizures (Nagarajan et al. 2012).

It has been suggested that clinical differentiation between epileptic and nonepileptic movements could be enhanced by applying mild restraint to the active limb or part of the body since nonepileptic movements are expected to stop. However, it may still be difficult to differentiate epileptic from nonepileptic movements clinically, and recording of EEG or aEEG/EEG is best way to increase the certainty of the epileptic nature of such movements.

In spite of the nonconsistent association between clinically suspected seizures and epileptic activity in the EEG, abnormal movements suspected to be clinical seizures are still conditions associated with increased risk for adverse outcome both in term and preterm infants (Davis et al. 2010; Glass et al. 2009). Seizure-suspected movements may be caused by immaturity, jitteriness, tremors, or other abnormal movements in compromised infants (Facini et al. 2016). Some of these infants (usually with severe cerebral compromise) may also display subcortical epileptic seizures that are not possible to recognize in the EEG or aEEG/EEG.

131.4 Treatment of Neonatal Seizures

Treatment of neonatal seizures is very much based on traditions and old studies assessing efficacy on clinical seizures. However, newer data demonstrates how administration of antiepileptic medications can abolish clinical seizures while electrographical (subclinical) seizures persist or even increase (Boylan et al. 2002). There is a lack of evidence as regards best treatment of neonatal studies, since only a few randomized studies compared antiepileptic medications while assessing electrographical seizures with EEG and none included structured follow-up and long-term outcome. Two small randomized studies evaluated whether the use of aEEG/EEG monitoring was associated with decreased seizure burden. In both studies, there was a decrease in seizure burden when using aEEG/EEG, but the differences were only border-line significant (Lawrence et al. 2009; van Rooij et al. 2010). One interesting observation in one of the studies was that there was a correlation between seizure burden and the severity of brain injury (scored by MRI); higher seizure burden was associated with more severe brain injury. This correlation was, however, not present in the group allocated to aEEG/EEG with the option of treating also electrographical seizures. The results indicate that treatment of subclinical seizures can limit brain injury in newborns. Other studies have demonstrated that use of EEG monitoring or aEEG/EEG is associated with more precise management, i.e., earlier identification of seizures which is associated with similar number or fewer administered antiepileptic drugs (Shellhaas and Barks 2012; Wietstock et al. 2015). Consequently, EEG monitoring or aEEG/EEG should be standard of care for infants with neonatal seizures. The benefits and limitations of aEEG/EEG as compared to standard EEG are discussed in ▶ Chap. 121, "Neonatal Electroencephalography".

Phenobarbital (or phenobarbitone) is the first drug of choice in many centers and countries, and bensodiazepines (diazepam, midazolam, clonazepam) are also commonly used. Lidocaine (or lignocaine) is frequently used in northern Europe, while phenytoin or fosphenytoin is more commonly used in southern Europe, in the UK, and the USA as presented in a number of surveys on treatment strategies. Phenobarbital and fenytoin seem to be equally efficient as first-line medications and abolish seizures in around 45% of term infants receiving these drugs, when adding the two drugs efficacy is seen in around 60% of infants (Painter et al. 1999). There are only observational studies regarding the efficacy of bensodiazepines (e.g., diazepam, lidocaine, clonazepam). Care should be taken when administering bensodiazepines to preterm infants, since these drugs may cause arterial hypotension. The GABA receptor is excitatory in early life and seizure-like events have been observed after midazolam although even more worrying is recent data indicating abnormal hippocampal growth and neurodevelopmental outcome in preterm infants related to midazolam (Duerden et al. 2016).

Lidocaine was previously considered an efficient second-line medication after phenobarbital (lidocaine should not be combined with phenytoin or fosphenytoin), but a large evaluation demonstrated that it was actually only efficient as a third-line drug after administration of phenobarbital and bensodiazepines (Weeke et al. 2016). Levetiracetam is a drug that has gained increased use in many countries, but so far there are no randomized trials published on this drug. Topiramate is another promising drug that has been used off-label, but so far no controlled neonatal studies have been conducted (Glass et al. 2011). When neonatal seizures become difficult to treat, it is usually advisable to consult with neurologists, both for evaluation of the potential etiology of the seizures and for more effective management. The possibility of pyridoxine-dependent seizures should always be considered. Administration of pyridoxine should be done when the infant is monitored with EEG or aEEG/EEG and when the infant is in the NICU, since hypotone reactions with EEG depression and apnea have occurred in pyridoxine-dependent infants after administration of pyridoxine (Hellström-Westas et al. 2002). Table 3 summarizes suggested doses of some commonly used antiepileptic medications (van Rooij et al. 2013; Painter et al. 1999).

Table 3 Commonly used antiepileptic medications

Drug	Loading dose	Maintenance
Phenobarbital	20–40 mg/kg in 20 min i.v.	5 mg/kg/day (target level: 40–60 μg/mL)
Midazolam	0.05 mg/kg in 10 min i.v.	0.15 mg/kg/h (max. dose: 0.5 mg/kg/h)
Lorazepam	0.05–0.1 mg/kg i.v.	
Clonazepam	0.01 mg/kg i.v.	0.1–0.5 mg/kg per 24 h
Phenytoin/fosphenytoin	20 mg/kg in 30 min i.v.	5 mg/kg/day (target level: 10–20 μg/mL)
Lidocaine[a]	2 mg/kg in 10 min i.v.	Body weight 2.5–4.5 kg: 7 mg/kg/h for 4 h (3.5 h during hypothermia) 3.5 mg/kg/h for 12 h 1.75 mg/kg/h for 12 h
Pyridoxine	100 mg i.v.	

[a]Lidocaine should not be combined with phenytoin/fosphenytoin. Please note that lidocaine metabolism is affected by hypothermia treatment and that the initial dosage reduction should be faster than in non-cooled babies. For dosage recommendations of infants below 2.5 kg, please see van Rooij et al. (2013)

131.5 Prophylactic Treatment

Prophylactic long-term antiepileptic treatment is frequently administered to infants with neonatal seizures. A recent meta-analysis included data from more than 4538 children in 44 studies and demonstrated that the average risk of epilepsy after neonatal seizures was 17.9% (Pisani et al. 2015). Of the children developing epilepsy, 68.5% had seizure recurrence during the first year of life and 80.7% had neurological impairments (Pisani et al. 2015). There is little data to guide which infants could benefit from prophylactic treatment. In a NICU cohort of infants, in which aEEG/EEG and EEG was used for diagnosis and treatment of neonatal seizures, antiepileptic treatment was discontinued after a median of 4.5 days. Recurrence rate during the first year of life was 8.3% and two of the three children developing epilepsy were already receiving prophylactic phenobarbital due to recurring neonatal seizures and persisting abnormalities in the EEG (Hellström-Westas et al. 1995).

131.6 Prognosis

The overall mortality in infants with neonatal seizures is around 10–30%, but the prognosis is usually dependent on the underlying condition (Ronen et al. 1999; Sheth et al. 1999; Scher et al. 1993; Weeke et al. 2015; Glass et al. 2016; Tekgul et al. 2006; Yildiz et al. 2012; van Rooij et al. 2013). Neurodevelopmental sequels develop in 30–40% of survivors, while less than 20% develop postnatal epilepsy.

131.7 Conclusion

There are many unsolved question as regards optimal management of neonatal seizures. Clinically important questions that need to be addressed in the future include: Do all neonatal seizures require antiepileptic treatment? Is antiepileptic treatment associated with less brain injury and better outcome? Which medications should be used? For how long should antiepileptic treatment be administered?

References

Boylan GB, Rennie JM, Pressler RM, Wilson G, Morton M, Binnie CD (2002) Phenobarbitone, neonatal seizures, and video-EEG. Arch Dis Child Fetal Neonatal Ed 86:F165–F170

Davis AS, Hintz SR, Van Meurs KP et al (2010) Seizures in extremely low birth weight infants are associated with adverse outcome. J Pediatr 157:720–725

Duerden EG, Guo T, Dodbiba L et al (2016) Midazolam dose correlates with abnormal hippocampal growth and neurodevelopmental outcome in preterm infants. Ann Neurol 79:548–559

Facini C, Spagnoli C, Pisani F (2016) Epileptic and non-epileptic paroxysmal motor phenomena in newborns. J Matern Fetal Neonatal Med 29:3652–3659

Glass HC, Glidden D, Jeremy RJ, Barkovich AJ, Ferriero DM, Miller SP (2009) Clinical neonatal seizures are independently associated with outcome in infants at risk for hypoxic-ischemic brain injury. J Pediatr 155:318–323

Glass HC, Poulin C, Shevell MI (2011) Topiramate for the treatment of neonatal seizures. Pediatr Neurol 44:4439–4442

Glass HC, Shellhaas RA, Wusthoff CJ et al (2016) Contemporary profile of seizures in neonates: a prospective cohort study. J Pediatr 174:98–103

Hart AR, Pilling EL, Alix JJ (2015) Neonatal seizures – part 2: aetiology of acute symptomatic seizures, treatments and the neonatal epilepsy syndromes. Arch Dis Child Educ Pract Ed 100:226–232

Hellström-Westas L, Blennow G, Lindroth M, Rosén I, Svenningsen NW (1995) Low risk of seizure recurrence after early withdrawal of antiepileptic treatment in the neonatal period. Arch Dis Child Fetal Neonatal Ed 72:F97–F101

Hellström-Westas L, Blennow G, Rosén I (2002) Amplitude-integrated encephalography in pyridoxine-dependent seizures and pyridoxine-responsive seizures. Acta Paediatr 91:977–980

Lawrence R, Mathur A, Nguyen The Tich S, Zempel J, Inder T (2009) A pilot study of continuous limited-channel aEEG in term infants with encephalopathy. J Pediatr 154:835–841

Mizrahi EM, Kellaway P (1987) Characterization and classification of neonatal seizures. Neurology 37:1837–1844

Murray DM, Boylan GB, Ali I, Ryan CA, Murphy BP, Connolly S (2008) Defining the gap between electrographic seizure burden, clinical expression and staff recognition of neonatal seizures. Arch Dis Child Fetal Neonatal Ed 93:F187–F191

Nagarajan L, Palumbo L, Ghosh S (2012) Classification of clinical semiology in epileptic seizures in neonates. Eur J Paediatr Neurol 16:118–125

Olischar M, Shany E, Aygün C et al (2012) Amplitude-integrated electroencephalography in newborns with inborn errors of metabolism. Neonatology 102:203–211

Painter MJ, Scher MS, Stein AD et al (1999) Phenobarbital compared with phenytoin for the treatment of neonatal seizures. N Engl J Med 341:485–489

Pisani F, Facini C, Pavlidis E, Spagnoli C, Boylan G (2015) Epilepsy after neonatal seizures: literature review. Eur J Paediatr Neurol 19:6–14

Ronen GM, Penney S, Andrews W (1999) The epidemiology of clinical neonatal seizures in Newfoundland: a population-based study. J Pediatr 134:71–75

Scher MS, Aso K, Beggarly ME, Hamid MY, Steppe DA, Painter MJ (1993) Electrographic seizures in preterm and full-term neonates: clinical correlates, associated brain lesions, and risk for neurologic sequelae. Pediatrics 91:128–134

Shellhaas RA, Barks AK (2012) Impact of amplitude-integrated electroencephalograms on clinical care for neonates with seizures. Pediatr Neurol 46:32–35

Sheth RD, Hobbs GR, Mullett M (1999) Neonatal seizures: incidence, onset, and etiology by gestational age. J Perinatol 19:40–43

Tekgul H, Gauvreau K, Soul J et al (2006) The current etiologic profile and neurodevelopmental outcome of seizures in term newborn infants. Pediatrics 117:1270–1280

van Rooij LG, Toet MC, van Huffelen AC et al (2010) Effect of treatment of subclinical neonatal seizures detected with aEEG: randomized, controlled trial. Pediatrics 125:e358–e366

van Rooij LG, Hellström-Westas L, de Vries LS (2013) Treatment of neonatal seizures. Semin Fetal Neonatal Med 18:209–215

Vesoulis ZA, Inder TE, Woodward LJ, Buse B, Vavasseur C, Mathur AM (2014) Early electrographic seizures, brain injury, and neurodevelopmental risk in the very preterm infant. Pediatr Res 75:564–569

Volpe JJ (1989) Neonatal seizures: current concepts and revised classification. Pediatrics 84:422–428

Weeke LC, Groenendaal F, Toet MC et al (2015) The aetiology of neonatal seizures and the diagnostic contribution of neonatal cerebral magnetic resonance imaging. Dev Med Child Neurol 57:248–256

Weeke LC, Toet MC, van Rooij LG et al (2016) Lidocaine response rate in aEEG-confirmed neonatal seizures: retrospective study of 413 full-term and preterm infants. Epilepsia 57:233–242

Wietstock SO, Bonifacio SL, McCulloch CE, Kuzniewicz MW, Glass HC (2015) Neonatal neurocritical care service is associated with decreased administration of seizure medication. J Child Neurol 30:1135–1141

Yildiz EP, Tatli B, Ekici B et al (2012) Evaluation of etiologic and prognostic factors in neonatal convulsions. Pediatr Neurol 47:186–192

The Timing of Neonatal Brain Damage

132

Serafina Perrone and Giuseppe Buonocore

Contents

Abstract

Brain injury in newborns is a complex process involving multiple pathways, which may complicate the determination of timing of the injury and the early identification of infants at risk for neonatal encephalopathy. Much of the injury occurs before birth and may be the result of more than a single injury. An abnormal insult applied to a critical point in intrauterine life determines permanent changes in phenotype disrupting the normal fetal development and leading to fetal programming of diseases. Additionally, brain development, including maturation and structure, may render the baby more or less susceptible to perinatal injury. At present there is no universal agreement on objective laboratory biomarkers as a gold standard to

S. Perrone (✉)
Department of Molecular and Developmental Medicine, University Hospital of Siena, Siena, Italy
e-mail: saraspv@yahoo.it

G. Buonocore
University of Siena, Siena, Italy
e-mail: giuseppe.buonocore@unisi.it

G. Buonocore et al. (eds.), *Neonatology*,
https://doi.org/10.1007/978-3-319-29489-6_278

support the diagnosis of perinatal asphyxia. Placental findings can serve as markers for processes occurring in the mother or fetus. An expert assessment of the placental pathology can provide temporally and mechanistically specific data not available from any other source. Magnetic resonance imaging (MRI) of the infants with neonatal encephalopathy is very contributive to elucidate the mechanism and timing of asphyxia in conjunction with the clinical examination.

Evidence of multi-organ failure in infants with severe encephalopathy is helpful and used as an additional diagnostic criterion in the recognition of the hypoxic–ischemic insult; however, it is not specific or essential. Several tissue biomarkers suggestive of brain injury in newborns with neonatal encephalopathy have been identified; however, they are not still validated as useful in clinical practice.

In the event of newborn with clinical signs of perinatal hypoxia at birth, it is necessary to have access to a readable cardiotocography, a well-documented partogram, a complete analysis of umbilical cord gases, a placental pathology, and an extensive clinical work-up of the newborn infant including cerebral MRI. Placental histologic examination should be required in order to confirm sudden catastrophic events occurring before or during labor or to detect occult thrombotic processes affecting the fetal circulation, patterns of decreased placental reserve, and adaptive responses to chronic hypoxia.

132.1 Salient Points

- Timing of neonatal brain damage is fundamental for exact diagnosis and prevention, in addition to being a key element in the legal arena.
- A thorough placental examination in all potential cases of adverse neurological outcomes is recommended, since placental pathology might play a pivotal role in perinatal asphyxia.
- Fetal Doppler studies and cardiotocography, especially if combined with pulse oximetry, fetal blood pH analysis, and fetal ECG help the clinician in the recognition of situations of inadequate intrapartum fetal oxygenation, which may lead to relevant complications.
- Neuroimaging remains the gold standard for identification, characterization, and prevention of brain injury in infants with neonatal encephalopathy: combined use of serial cranial ultrasound and magnetic resonance imaging improves detection of common patterns of brain injury. Advanced MR techniques provide perspectives on neonatal brain metabolism, microstructure, and connectivity.
- Neurodiagnostic tests, such as standard EEG and amplitude-integrated EEG, identify the presence of brain injury and may determine the severity of outcome.
- Raised nucleated red blood cell counts in newborns may indicate perinatal hypoxia and can predict brain injury and neurological outcomes in asphyxiated infants.
- Clinical assessment of newborns with perinatal encephalopathy could be difficult due to the variable clinical presentation: health-care providers need to carefully investigate causes of neonatal brain injury.
- Although most evidence to date emanate from small single-centered studies in research settings, the use of a panel of biomarkers seems to be very promising in the setting of neonatal brain injury evaluation.

132.2 Introduction

Early abnormalities of brain development and underlying genetic factors can affect brain susceptibility to the injury (Ambalavanan et al. 2006; Fily et al. 2006; Yager and Miller 2009). Some infants may inherit a predisposition to have significant injury in the event of a normally sublethal insult (Nelson 2005). These newly identified risk factors for brain damage in different periods make the timing of lesions important for exact diagnosis and prevention.

Incidence of neonatal encephalopathy is estimated as 3.0 per 1000 live births (95%CI 2.7–3.3) and for hypoxic–ischemic encephalopathy is 1.5 (95%CI 1.3–1.7) (Kurinczuk et al. 2010). Hypoxic–ischemic encephalopathy ranges from about 1.0 to 8.0 per 1000 live births. Epidemiological data shows that 30% of cases of neonatal encephalopathy in developed populations and 60% in developing populations have some evidence of intrapartum hypoxic ischemia.

Perinatal hypoxic–ischemic brain injury was demonstrated to be a major contributor to developmental disabilities in children, accounting for 25% of all cases (Shevell 2001). Of the antepartum events that contribute significantly to the development of neonatal encephalopathy, fetal growth restriction ranks high. Increasingly, a strong role for fetal inflammation as one of the most frequent causes of acquired brain damage in perinatal period is being recognized.

132.3 Fetal Programming Hypothesis

Fetal development may be influenced by inherited genetic profile as well as external stimuli. Early intrauterine life is particularly vulnerable to perturbations. Perturbation of fetal environment implies both short-term complications, including altered fetal growth and increased perinatal morbidity, and long-lasting consequences on offspring's subsequent health. The concept of *fetal programming* focuses on the processes of developmental plasticity, which in normal situations provide the settings for homeostatic mechanisms to ensure proper growth and development (Perrone et al. 2016a, b). Fetal programming of later diseases occurs when the normal pattern of fetal development is disrupted by an abnormal stimulus or an "insult" during intrauterine life, which leads to adaptations by the fetus to allow its survival, but could finally result in permanent structural and physiological changes with consequences to short- and long-term outcome. Permanent changes in fetal phenotype can generate a mismatch with extrauterine environment. In sight of this theory, impaired neonatal transition and cardiovascular or metabolic diseases in adult life can be traced back to their intrauterine origins (Fig. 1).

132.4 Placental Pathology

The placenta has been described as a diary of intrauterine life, and placental pathology assists in characterizing the antenatal environment. Dramatic, but at least common, are sentinel lesions, each of which can cause hypoxia sufficient to result in brain injury (Redline 2006). There are three mechanisms for sudden catastrophic injury: (1) the placenta becomes prematurely separated from the underlying maternal uterine vascular supply: abruptio placenta or uterine rupture; (2) fetal placental blood vessels rupture; or (3) prolonged umbilical venous blood flow interruption. Placental findings that support a diagnosis of massive feto-maternal hemorrhage include a profound increase in the number of circulating nucleated red blood cells in the villous circulation, the finding of a large intervillous hematoma, villous edema, fetal arterial constriction, and villous capillary-venous dilatation. Large vessel hemorrhages generally affect vessels that are not protected by Wharton's jelly or the chorionic plate. Pathologic lesions associated with complete umbilical vessel occlusion include tight true umbilical cord knots, occlusive umbilical vein thrombi, tightly twisted (hypercoiled) umbilical cords, prolapse, or tight entanglements around body parts. When this occurs, there may be an abrupt change in umbilical cord color, shape, or diameter that suggests chronicity. Other pathologic umbilical cord lesions, such as an excessively long cord length, lesser degrees of hypercoiling, abnormal cord insertion sites, and paucity of Wharton's jelly, are significantly more common in infants with cerebral palsy (Redline 2006; Machin et al. 2000; Nasiell et al. 2016; McDonald et al. 2004). The mechanisms by which feto-placental large vessel lesions act on the vascular wall include toxic damage (meconium-associated vascular necrosis), maternal antifetal vasculitis (obliterative fetal vasculopathy), infiltration by activated fetal neutrophils (chorioamnionitis with intense fetal inflammatory response), and thrombosis (fetal thrombotic vasculopathy) (Nasiell et al. 2016; McDonald et al. 2004; Chau et al. 2013). Fetal thrombotic vasculopathy and chronic villitis with obliterative fetal vasculopathy begin weeks

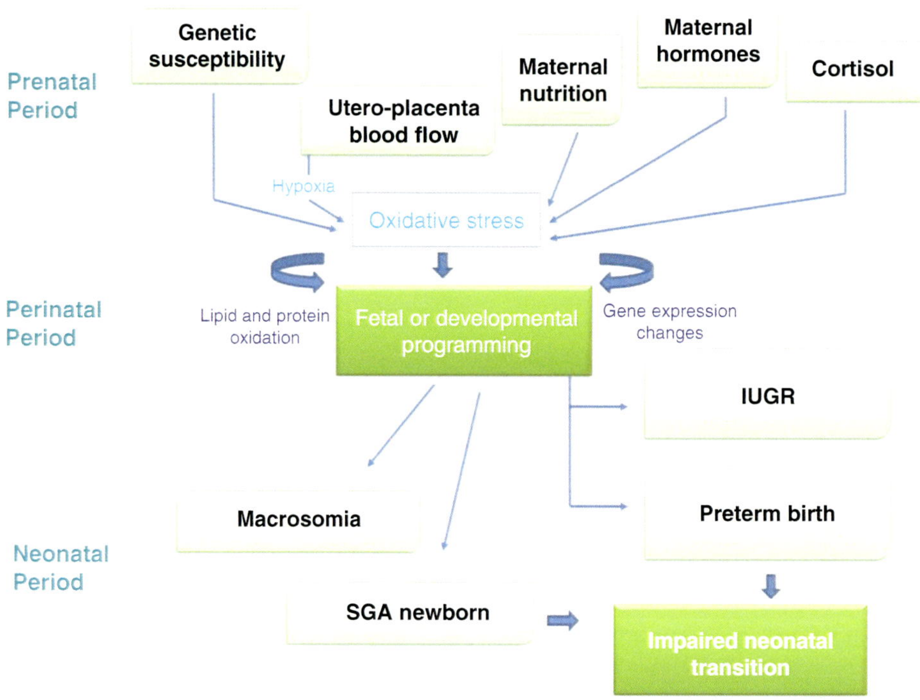

Fig. 1 The peculiar susceptibility of fetal period of development to environmental cues. Oxidative stress may be the link between adverse insults (associated with preterm birth or adverse fetal growth) and developmental programming. Oxidative stress acts indirectly by lipid and protein oxidation or modifying gene expression

before delivery and continue to evolve and progress until parturition (Perrone et al. 2016c). Vascular occlusion is the result of an inflammatory vasodestructive process that develops when maternal leukocytes inappropriately cross the trophoblastic barrier to enter fetal tissue. Chorioamnionitis with a severe fetal inflammatory response (intense chorionic vasculitis) and meconium-associated necrosis of vascular smooth muscle cells develop as a consequence of subacute processes beginning days before delivery (Chau et al. 2013; Perrone et al. 2016c; Redline et al. 2003; Altshuler et al. 1992).

An increased time of exposure to meconium-stained amniotic fluid leads to a gradual progression of pigment through the amnion into the chorionic plate and eventually into contact with large fetal vessels. Placentas can be abnormally small and have a decreased total gas-exchanging surface area. Alternatively, they may have decreased efficiency owing to diffuse chronic injury. Other placental findings are markers for processes affecting either mother or fetus. In some cases, they may represent attempts to ameliorate an adverse environment; in others, they may be maladaptive consequences of it. Perhaps the most controversial of these findings is a significant increase in the number of circulating nucleated red blood cells to more than 2500/cm^3 in the fetal placental capillary circulation (Hermansen 2001; Naeye and Lin 2001). An increase of this magnitude represents a fetal bone marrow response to hypoxia that takes 6–12 h or more to mount (Blackwell et al. 2004). A second adaptive response is a generalized increase in the number of fetal capillaries per terminal villous cross section or chorangiosis (Ogino and Redline 2000; Stanek 1999). Placental pathology assists in characterizing the antenatal environment. Histological examination of the placenta is a sensitive and accurate diagnostic system for identifying lesions that can either directly cause or decrease the threshold for brain injury. Less than 10% of placentas from term infants that later develop cerebral palsy lack any evidence of placental abnormalities potentially related to adverse outcome, supporting the importance of a thorough placental examination in all potential cases of adverse neurologic outcomes.

132.5 Cardiotocography and Fetal Doppler Studies

Cardiotocography (CTG) is an indirect sign of fetal well-being with various technical pitfalls and a high incidence of false positives. Currently the technique is improved in the determination of the risk and timing of brain injury. In particular, the evaluation of trends and the speed of CTG changes in deceleration patterns make it possible to distinguish harmful ischemic events from other forms of hypoxia which do not necessarily injure the fetal brain (Ugwumadu 2013). A newly defined CTG pattern, the "conversion" pattern, appears to be a specific marker of ischemic injury and could help to redefine the role of CTG monitoring.

The majority of infants with HIE have normal CTG traces on admission but develop pathological CTG patterns within hours of delivery. More severe encephalopathy was associated with normal admission CTG and acute sentinel events shortly before deliver.

CTG combined with pulse oximetry, fetal blood pH, and ECG provides further advantages (Murray et al. 2009). Fetal electrocardiography (ECG) wave form analysis indicates the ability of the fetal heart to respond to the stress of labor. An increased T/QRS ratio identifies a fetal heart muscle that responds to hypoxia by increased utilization of heart glycogen (Brand-Niebelschutz and Saling 1994). ST segment depression may indicate a situation in which the heart does not respond fully and a negative ST may signify cardiac dysfunction and hypotension. It has been suggested that an increase in T/QRS ratio maintained for more than 10 min is associated with aggravation of fetal condition when intrapartum hypoxia may progress to asphyxia. Automatic analysis of CTG and ECG has been reported to enable a reduction in the incidence of newborns with severe neurological symptoms (Rosèn et al. 2004). Doppler ultrasound of the blood flow in the umbilical artery (UA), descending fetal aorta (DAo), and middle cerebral artery (MCA) gives insight into fetal cardiovascular responses to intrauterine growth restriction, fetal anemia, and fetal hypoxia (Graves 2007). Blood flow is classified as abnormal when pulsatility index (PI) values of MCA falling below the 5th percentile or PI value of UA, DAo, UA/MCA ratio, and Dao/MCA ratio above the 95th (Arduini and Rizzo 1990). Absent or reversed end diastolic flow of the UA, absent or retrograde net blood flow of the aortic isthmus, and absent or retrograde end-diastolic flow of the ductus venosus are also classified as abnormal. The presence of a notch, as signal of increased perinatal vascular impedance and of brain sparing, is also highly significantly related to maternal blood serum concentration of tumor necrosis factor-alpha (TNF-alpha) and interleukin-6 (IL-6) level (Dubiel et al. 2005). Severe abnormalities in fetal blood flow might result in neuroanatomical or functional changes that correlate to later cognitive capacity (Maunu et al. 2007).

132.6 Neuroimaging

Cranial ultrasound (US) has been used for many years to determine the type and evolution of brain damage. The ultrasound criteria of cerebral cavitation have been selected in order to give assurance that the damage may have occurred before delivery. US and postmortem studies of the evolution of brain abnormalities suggest that cystic lesions develop over 14 days (Weindling et al. 1985; Levene 1988). Serial US images have been used to study the timing of hypoxic–ischemic injury, though the reliability of US is limited by poor visualization of the subarachnoid space, cerebral cortex, and posterior fossa. It is also difficult to distinguish between hemorrhagic and non-hemorrhagic ischemic damage. Traditionally, CUS is used to detect germinal matrix hemorrhage and intraventricular hemorrhage (GMH-IVH) and periventricular leukomalacia (PVL). Its value in detecting other lesions as well is increasing owing to technical developments such as high-resolution ultrasound

(<200 m), quantitative measurements, and use of supplemental acoustic windows (mastoid and posterior fontanel). CUS seems sensitive for recognizing stroke and sinovenous thrombosis, but may miss small posterior fossa abnormalities (Leijser et al. 2006; Govaert and De Vries 2010; Ciambra et al. 2013; Graca et al. 2013; van Wezel-Meijler et al. 2010; Steggerda and van Wezel-Meijler 2016).

Conventional magnetic resonance imaging (MRI), volumetric analysis, diffusion tensor imaging (DTI) methods, and surface-based morphometry (SBM) methods have recently been used to detect antenatal, perinatal, and neonatal abnormalities and timing on the basis of standardized assessment of brain maturation (Mathur et al. 2008; Hüppi and Dubois 2006). MR imaging allows reliable assessment of myelination and establishment of a timetable for maturation and myelination of the developing brain in vivo. The peak of subplate formation and function that are required for normal cortical development correlates with the peak period of vulnerability to injury in preterm infants. Injury to subplate cells has been implicated in the causation of cortical deficits in preterm infants (McQuillen and Ferriero 2004; Volpe 1996). If lesions or delayed maturation of white matter (WM) disrupts specific subsets of cortico-cortical, long-distance connections, these altered connectivity patterns could in turn give rise to specific abnormalities in cortical folding patterns. Thus, WM injury resulting in a secondary disruption of cortical gray matter (GM) development may be a major mediator of cognitive deficits faced by preterm infants. Cortical development may be also altered in the absence of WM or subplate injury in preterm infants. The high sensitivity of MR is important to detect early damage occurring before reliable US imaging, particularly for WM lesions in the preterm infants. Accurate measurement of specific cerebral tissue volumes is achieved by segmentation of the imaged volume into tissue types, followed by 3D reconstructions. Volume changes during normal maturation of cerebral tissue between 29 and 41 weeks gestation have been defined in vivo using MR tissue segmentation of the brain. Segmentation is the process wherein contours are constructed that divide the brain into the representative structures of interest depending on their signal intensity (e.g., gray matter, myelinated white matter, cerebrospinal fluid [CFS]) determined using mathematic algorithms (Zacharia et al. 2006). Preterm infants with WM lesions have a 17% reduction in absolute cortical GM volume as well as a 25% reduction in absolute myelinated WM volume compared with preterm infants without WM lesions (Inder et al. 2005). Volumetric MRI studies conducted in school-aged preterm children have reported shorter corpus callosum (Nosarti et al. 2004; Peterson et al. 2000), hippocampus (Nosarti et al. 2002), basal ganglia, and amygdala (Peterson et al. 2000) as well as enlarged lateral ventricles (Nosarti et al. 2002). All have been shown to be associated with neuropsychological impairment.

Diffusion tensor imaging and diffusion anisotropy are based on measurement of physical characteristics of water molecules in tissue. One parameter describing these displacements is the apparent diffusion coefficient (ADC). ADC values are commonly used clinically for the detection of acute cerebral injury. Diffusion anisotropy provides information about the local environment. Anisotropy values for WM show a steady increase during development, particularly when fiber tracts undergo myelination (Neil et al. 1998). Anisotropy can also be applied to GM maturation. The loss of anisotropy associated with maturation can be used to assess cortical development and reflects varying rates of development among different cortical areas (Deipolyi et al. 2005). The developing cortex showed lower ACD values and anisotropy with increasing maturation, likely related to the increasing complexity in tissue organization in the mature cortex (Kroenke et al. 2006). Diffusion-based MR images may be normal on the first day after injury, decrease between 2 and 4 days after injury, and return to normal after approximately 7 days (Neil and Inder 2004). MR images illustrate the natural history of acquired fetal brain lesions in relation to stage of development (Girard et al. 2003). The detection of a single type of damage in the developing fetus is evidence of acute or chronic lesions, which can be seen alone or in combination. Patterns can indicate infection or hypoxia–ischemia at various stages of intrauterine life.

Phosphorus magnetic resonance spectroscopy studies changes of cerebral oxidative metabolism during and following asphyxia (Miller et al. 2002). Infants with neonatal encephalopathy often have normal cerebral oxidative metabolism on magnetic resonance spectroscopy shortly after birth, but many then develop delayed energy failure 6–15 h later. In survivors, the degree of secondary energy failure after 24–48 h was closely associated with neurodevelopmental impairments at 18 months and 4 years of age (Roth et al. 1997). Sequential MRI allows demonstration that the acute brain injury associated with encephalopathy in term infants evolves progressively over time to involve initially unaffected regions (Barkovich 2006).

Proton MR-spectroscopy (H-MR spectroscopy) has also been used in neonates and studies the changes in concentrations of metabolites such as choline (Cho), creatine, and phosphocreatine as a single peak (Cr), *N*-acetylaspartate (NAA), and, when present, lactate (Lac). It is an accurate quantitative biomarker for the prediction of neurodevelopmental outcome after hypoxic–ischemic encephalopathy in term infants. The cerebellar NAA/Cho ratio at term is suggested to correlate with cognitive outcome at 24 months (Bapat et al. 2014).

The increased use of neuroimaging techniques and MRI, in particular, has been a tremendous help in timing of brain injury and recognizing patterns of injury. These findings may be important for medicolegal issues. MRI and magnetic resonance spectroscopy are the most sensitive neuroimaging modalities to assist with the timing of cerebral injury. MRI, combining conventional, diffusion, and spectroscopy, between 24 and 96 h of life provides the most useful guide on the potential timing of a cerebral insult. There are several well-defined patterns of brain injury and their evolution on MRI that are typical of hypoxic–ischemic cerebral injury in the newborn. If a different pattern of brain injury or evolution of injury exists on MRI, then alternative diagnoses should be actively pursued (e.g., metabolic and genetic investigations) (Task Force on Neonatal Encephalopathy 2014). In the term newborn, these patterns associated with neonatal asphyxia are the following:

1. The basal ganglia thalamus pattern (BGT) predominantly affecting bilaterally the central gray nuclei (ventrolateral thalami and posterior putamina) and perirolandic cortex. It suggests a near total asphyxia and often follows an acute sentinel event.
2. The watershed predominant pattern of injury (WS), also referred to as a pattern seen following "prolonged partial asphyxia." It involves the parasagittal white matter, in the vascular watershed, and may extend to the cortical gray matter if the insult is severe enough (Miller et al. 2005; Sie et al. 2000).

If a different pattern of brain injury or evolution of injury exists on MRI, then alternative diagnoses should be considered.

132.7 Electroencephalography

The timing of brain insult can be assessed by considering serial EEG recording findings in relation to the time of birth (Shellhaas 2015). The timing can be considered prenatal if an EEG immediately after birth already shows chronic stage abnormalities, perinatal if it shows acute stage abnormalities, and postnatal if it is normal, and a later EEG shows acute stage abnormalities. The detection of even mild seizures is an important indication of timing since prolonged seizures exacerbate hypoxic brain damage (Yager et al. 2002). Routine serial EEG studies in preterm infants demonstrated that one fourth of cerebral palsies in these infants were of antenatal origin and two thirds of perinatal origin and postnatal injuries played the smallest role. Periventricular leukomalacia (PVL) manifesting itself on the ultrasound in the late neonatal period and suggesting postnatal origin was often found to be of antenatal origin with an EEG soon after birth (Okumara et al. 1999). PVL without apparent causes was often associated with abnormal fetal heart rate patterns and early neonatal EEG abnormalities and considered to have originated in the antepartum period. Documentation of the time of the first suspected seizure is also important, as seizures occurring close to the time of birth may be reflective of an earlier insult Recently, the cerebral function monitor, a single- or double-channel amplitude-integrated EEG (aEEG), has been introduced for the brain monitoring of neonates with suspected encephalopathy and used primarily to define selection criteria for hypothermia therapy among infants with neonatal encephalopathy. The aEEG provides the clinician with a method to identify the presence of brain injury and determine the severity of encephalopathy and outcome (Hellstrom-Westas et al. 2008). Continuous monitoring with cerebral function monitor/aEEG has become helpful to monitor for seizure activity during the 72 h of the cooling process, to monitor responses to antiepileptic drugs, and to identify changes in brain function over time. EEG and aEEG abnormalities (seizures and a suppressed background pattern) have high predictive values toward an adverse outcome after perinatal asphyxia, both in normothermic infants and during therapeutic hypothermia (Toet et al. 1999; van Laerhoven et al. 2013).

132.8 Hematology

Nucleated red blood cell (NRBC) count indicates fetal hypoxia in term and preterm newborns. Since NRBC is physiological in cord blood of preterm neonates, single NRBC counts need to be compared with standard values for the baby's gestational age (Buonocore et al. 1999). Use of NRBC as a marker of timing of asphyxia is justified by information about fetal response to hypoxia, namely, increased erythropoietin (EPO) secretion due to decreased fetal PO_2 (Widness et al. 1986). A relationship between asphyxia, high levels of circulating EPO, and high NRBC has been demonstrated (Vatansever et al. 2002). Although the exact time elapsing between hypoxia and appearance of NRBC is not known, experimental studies showed a complex mechanism of EPO-induced late erythroid differentiation, and there is evidence that a period of more than 24 h is necessary between decreased fetal PO_2 and appearance of NRBC in blood (Bondurant et al. 1985). The concept that increased NRBC in cord blood may be regarded as a marker of hypoxia for a period of more than 24 h before birth has also been accepted on the basis of clinical observations (Blackwell et al. 2000; Naeye and Russell Localio 1995).

Increased lymphocyte count is considered a reliable index of brain damage and makes it possible to establish timing since the increase seems to occur approximately 25 min after fetal bradycardia and hypoxia (Naeye and Lin 2001). Thrombocytopenia can also help to determine the timing of brain damage since it appears 20–28 h after bradycardia. Thrombocytopenia has been confirmed to occur after fetal hypoxia although the cause is unknown (Saxonhouse et al. 2003). Although it may be misleading in certain conditions, the number of circulating lymphocytes together with other markers such as bradycardia, time of correcting acidosis, thrombocytopenia, and clinical condition may be useful in determining the time of brain lesions.

132.9 Clinical Assessment

Challenges remain in early identification of high-risk infants with neonatal encephalopathy. Badawi et al. in a West Australian case–control study demonstrated that almost 70% of cases had no clear evidence of adverse intrapartum events, 24% had antepartum and intrapartum risk factors, and 5% of cases had only intrapartum risk factors (Badawi et al. 1998a, b). The severity of a perinatal hypoxic–ischemic insult is difficult to quantitate, and many infants may only have transitory neurologic signs of neonatal encephalopathy at the time of birth and complete recovery after stabilization. Clinical presentation of infants with neonatal encephalopathy of varying etiologies can overlap and therefore make it difficult to identify etiology through the use of neurological examination alone. Thus, it is very important to exclude other causes of neonatal encephalopathy in symptomatic patients with unclear perinatal history risk factors (Wachtel and Hendricks-Muñoz 2011).

Clinical presentation of infants with neonatal encephalopathy after perinatal asphyxia can range from subtle, with a hyperalert state or mild hypotonia, to severe, consisting of stupor, coma, profound hypotonia, and absent reflexes. Importantly, clinical subtle signs and symptoms of neonatal encephalopathy as well as difficulties in neonatal seizure recognition may lead to a delay in the diagnosis and proper neuroprotective intervention. Neonatal seizures affect 1.5–3.5 per 1000 live term births in the US and are more common in the neonatal period than at any other time in life (Wachtel and Hendricks-Muñoz 2011). Furthermore, seizures are very common among infants with neonatal encephalopathy because of hypoxia–ischemia. The widely accepted classification of clinical seizures proposed by Volpe (2008) includes subtle, clonic, tonic, and myoclonic seizures, which can be focal, multifocal, or generalized. They are often classified as being either electroclinical, when electrographic changes and clinical symptoms occur, or electrographic and clinically silent (Hellstrom-Westas et al. 2008). It can be challenging for the clinician to diagnose neonatal seizures. In fact, only approximately 20–30% of electrographic neonatal seizures provoke obvious clinical signs (Murray et al. 2008). Electrographic seizures in neonates have also been correlated with the subsequent development of cerebral palsy and microcephaly. When prolonged, seizures may also exacerbate brain injury initiated by the precipitating acute hypoxic–ischemic injury (Abend and Wusthoff 2012).

There is no ideal measure to assess the severity of perinatal hypoxia–ischemia during the initial clinical presentation of the infant immediately after birth. At present the Apgar score is no longer considered to be a marker of perinatal asphyxia and encephalopathy, although the score still predicts outcomes at a population level and the prognosis of term neonates with a very low Apgar score at 5 or 10 min after birth remains poor. Clinical scoring systems have been used widely to assess the severity of neonatal encephalopathy. The most commonly used is the Sarnat score (Sarnat and Sarnat 1976) that combines information of clinical examinations and EEG and grades encephalopathy as mild (grade I), moderate (grade II), or severe (grade III).

During the first 12–24 h of life, after moderate to severe perinatal fetal hypoxia–ischemia, signs of neonatal encephalopathy include poor tone and feeding, difficulty maintaining respiration seizures, and lethargy or coma.

132.10 Biomarkers

The term biomarker can refer to any entity that occurs in the body and can be measured to predict the diagnosis, onset, or progression of disease process. Laboratory studies generally use cord blood or amniotic fluid. They provide much information about conditions jeopardizing the central nervous system. Cord blood pH was the most widely used test for additional information on the severity of intrauterine asphyxia. The criteria promulgated by ACOG and AAP (American College of Obstetricians and Gynecologists and American Academy of Pediatricians 2003) to attribute intrapartum hypoxia as a cause of neonatal encephalopathy and later cerebral palsy include (1) an umbilical arterial PH of 7.0, (2) early onset of moderate-to-severe neonatal encephalopathy, (3) a diagnosis of cerebral palsy with quadriparesis of the spastic or dyskinetic type, and (4) the absence of other possible causes. When using an umbilical arterial pH at the time of birth to define intrapartum asphyxia, the incidence of umbilical arterial pH <7.0 is 3.7 of 1000 term live births. Of neonates with this degree of acidosis, 17.2% survived with neonatal neurologic morbidity, 16.3% had seizures, and 5.9% died during the neonatal period. In developed countries the incidence of hypoxic–ischemic encephalopathy (HIE) at term is 2.5 of 1000 live births, and the proportion of cases of cerebral palsy associated with intrapartum asphyxia is 14.5% (Graham et al. 2008). Since pH is influenced by both respiratory and metabolic factors, it represents an inverse log of the hydrogen ion concentration; before it does not change linearly with hydrogen ion concentration or with the use of base. If one assumes that organ and cellular response to hypoxia–ischemia result in accumulation of acid in a relatively linear proportion to the degree and duration of the insult, the exponential function pH has limited usefulness in the prediction of hypoxia timing. On the contrary, the base excess represents a linear correlate and thus a potentially valuable index of the degree and duration of metabolic acidosis. It has been proposed that a base excess of −12 mmol/L is a threshold of a metabolic acidosis associated with newborn complication (Low et al. 1997), while a base excess of −22 has been reported to be associated with minor or major deficit in 80% of infants with intrapartum asphyxia (Low et al. 1984). Following Hagelin and Leyon (Hagelin and Leyon 1998) on average, the second-stage labor decreases base excess by approximately 1 mmol/L per hour in the normal fetus. Studies carried out with the comparison between base excess and prolonged heart deceleration suggest a loss of 1 mmol/L per 2 min of severe compromise, while subacute fetal compromise may reduce the buffer base by 1 mmol/L per 6–15 min.

Measurement of the degree of acidosis should be associated with heart rate and blood pressure recording. In particular, unremitting bradycardia has been observed to coincide with the development of ischemic basal ganglia brain damage (Meyer 1975). Studies on timing have been carried out with heart rate and pH recording at birth together with lymphocyte and thrombocyte count (Naeye 1991). Neonates may have severe metabolic acidosis and disorders responsible for hypoxia–ischemia, unremitting until birth. A hypoxia-induced myocardiopathy mirrors the severity of perinatal hypoxic–ischemic insult. Myocardiopathy can lead to hypotension and hypoperfusion of important organs, such as the brain. In most infants recovery of myocardial contractility occurs in the first 24–48 h after birth (Van Bel and Walther 1990).

The availability of rapid methods for measuring lactate in cord blood and blood of neonates suggests their extensive use for the detection of severe metabolic acidosis which reflects asphyxia and is a signal of brain damage (Boog 2004). Da Silva et al. (2000) showed that blood lactate concentrations over 9 mmol/L at 30 min of life have 84% sensitivity and 67% specificity in the prediction of moderate-to-severe brain damage. Values less than 5 mmol/L indicate absence of risk (Chou et al. 1998).

132.10.1 Oxidative Stress Biomarkers

The occurrence of oxidative stress in cord blood appears to be a good index of severe prenatal hypoxia/asphyxia. During hypoxia, increased production of free radicals and/or decreased detoxification leads to mitochondrial dysfunction, inhibition of protein synthesis, inhibition of adenosine-5-triphosphate synthesis, inner mitochondrial membrane damage, activation of pro-caspase and other mechanisms of apoptosis, generation of nitro peroxide, and increased oxidative stress (Delivoria-Papadopoulos and Misbra 1998). Free radicals affect glial cells, consequently decreasing glutamate uptake, and *N*-methyl-D-aspartate receptor dysfunction, increasing intracellular calcium and further increasing brain cell damage (Mishra and Delivoria-Papadopoulus 1998). Free radical excess may also be responsible for endothelial dysfunction, coagulation disorders, and vasoconstriction. The central nervous system is vulnerable to free radical damage due to its high content of metals which may catalyze formation of free radicals, especially hydroxyl radicals and nitro peroxide. Antioxidant defenses, which are even low in the central nervous system of adults, are particularly low in fetal and neonatal oligodendroglia. Increased oxidative stress in hypoxic fetuses and neonates can be detected by assaying serum isoprostanes, serum total hydroperoxides, advanced oxidative protein products, and increased nonprotein-bound iron (NPBI) in serum. These markers can be used for the early prediction of the risk for oxidative stress-related diseases (Perrone and Tataranno 2010). Plasma NPBI has been found to be the best early predictive marker of neurodevelopmental outcome, with 100% sensitivity and 100% specificity for good outcome at 0–1.16 μmol/L and for poor outcome at >15.2 μmol/L (Buonocore et al. 2003). Postmortem assessment of oxidative stress has been proposed in order to clarify the origin of brain lesions. Assessment is currently made by measuring advanced glycation end products from oxidation of proteins, carbohydrates, and lipids in cytoplasm, nucleus, and membranes (Yamamoto et al. 2002). The results of studies using these methods may help to determine the timing of brain injury, since oxidation products appear to vary in relation to gestational age. By measuring isoprostanes in amniotic fluid, it is possible to distinguish fetal growth restriction pregnancies from normal ones (Longini et al. 2005). Oxidative stress in pregnancy is also associated with preterm premature rupture of membranes (PROM), and amniotic fluid isoprostanes may be a reliable predictive index of risk of preterm PROM (Longini et al. 2007).

132.10.2 Inflammatory Biomarkers

Perinatal infection and the fetal inflammatory response syndrome (FIRS) are another entity that is slowly being unraveled, but is clearly capable of producing long-term neurologic sequelae (Kuypers et al. 2012). Intrauterine infection may be followed by brain damage due to the direct effects of bacterial toxins and lipopolysaccharides on glial cells, due to astrocyte deregulation and due to the effects of phagocyte activation, particularly on coagulation and the endothelium (Dammann and Leviton 2004). The many observations of poor outcome in babies whose gestations were complicated by chorioamnionitis, and of high cytokines such as IL-6, IL-1β, IL-8, IL-9, TNF-α in serum of premature and full-term newborns with placental lesions typical of chorioamnionitis, suggest that it may at least be worthwhile assaying IL-6 as a marker of brain damage in utero (Kotiranta-Ainamo et al. 2004; Jun et al. 2000). A meta-analysis of chorioamnionitis and cerebral palsy indicated a positive association among preterm and full-term infants, with a relative risk of 4.7 for the full-term infants (Wu and Colford 2000). Similarly, maternal fever was linked with an increased incidence of neonatal encephalopathy (Impey et al. 2001). Cord blood concentrations of B-lymphocyte chemoattractants, ciliary neutrophil factor, epidermal growth factor, IL-5, IL-12, IL-13, IL-15, macrophage migration inhibitory factor, monocyte chemoattractant protein-3, monokine induced by interferon-γ, and tumor necrosis factor-related apoptosis-inducing ligands have been found significantly high in preterm and full-term newborns who develop cerebral palsy. Preterm infants with cerebral palsy have higher epidermal growth factor and lower levels of granulocyte macrophage colony-stimulating factor, IL-23, macrophage-derived chemokine, as well as pulmonary and activation-regulated chemokine than matched controls (Kaukola et al. 2004). IL-18 has also been identified as a marker of brain damage risk (Minagawa et al. 2002). Matrix metalloproteinases (MMPs) and their inhibitors, the tissue inhibitors of metalloproteinases (TIMPs), are microglial-secreted proteins, making them easily measurable in fluids, including the peripheral blood (Lorenzl et al. 2003; Leonardo and Pennypacker 2009). MMP-9 has been demonstrated to be upregulated in peripheral cortex at 24–48 h after ischemic and hemorrhagic stroke in human brain tissue after ischemic and hemorrhagic stroke (Rosell et al. 2006). Plasmatic levels of MMP-9 and TIMP-1 were explored in perinatal asphyxia: MMP-9 levels were significantly higher in the group of patients with unfavorable outcomes (Sunugawa et al. 2009).

132.10.2.1 Ubiquitin Carboxyl-Terminal Esterase L1 (UCH-L1)

UCH-L1 is a cytoplasmic enzyme, component of the ubiquitin proteasome system. Because of its high expression in the neurons, elevated levels of serum UCH-L1 have been suggested as marker of neuronal apoptosis (Thompson et al. 1983; Schofield et al. 1995; Day and Thompson 2010; Zhang et al. 2013). Recent studies showed high levels of UCH-L1 in the umbilical cord of neonates with hypoxic–ischemic encephalopathy. Serum concentrations of about 131 ng/ml had a specificity of 100% for the diagnosis of hypoxic–ischemic encephalopathy and concentrations of about 28 ng/ml a specificity of 95% (Douglas-Escobar et al. 2014).

132.10.2.2 PS100B

Protein S100 is brain specific and is a very promising marker of brain damage in newborn, also providing information about timing (Blennow et al. 2001). The glial protein S100 belongs to a family of calcium-binding proteins found as homo- or hetero-dimers of two different subunits (α and β). Different combinations of the subunits make up the heterodimeric forms α-α, α-β, and β-β; types α-β and β-β are described as S100B protein and are shown to be highly specific for nervous tissue (Fujii et al. 2004).

S100B can be measured in several biological fluids such as CSF, blood, amniotic fluid, and urine. During active brain injury, at least some of the S100B released from the damaged tissue could spread into the systemic circulation as a result of hemodynamic rearrangement of the blood–brain barrier. In preterm infants with intraventricular hemorrhage (IVH), concentrations of S100 in blood were elevated before a radiological diagnosis could be made (Gazzolo et al. 1999). S100B blood concentrations also correlated with abnormal cerebral hemodynamic patterns (increased cerebrovascular resistance) and with the extent of IVH both in preterm and in full-term asphyxiated infants (Gazzolo et al. 1999; Gazzolo et al. 2002). In asphyxiated full-term infants, an early increase in S100B was found to be predictive of HIE and subsequent adverse neurological outcomes (Nagdyman et al. 2001). Longitudinal S100B protein monitoring in peripheral blood demonstrated a peak concentration of the protein 6 h after birth with a progressive decrease in S100B at 24 h. The positive predictive value of S100B for HIE with a protein cutoff of 8.5 μg/L at 2 h from birth was 71%, the negative predictive value was 90%, the sensitivity was 71%, and the specificity was 90% (Nagdyman et al. 2001). In intrauterine growth restriction (IUGR) fetuses, a significant correlation between protein S100 and cerebral hemodynamics was observed, and high values of this protein were detected in the maternal bloodstream of pregnant women complicated by IUGR whose newborns developed IVH (Gazzolo et al. 2006). S100B is also measurable in the urine fluid, and its concentrations at birth are significantly higher in preterm newborns who later developed cerebral bleeding and/or brain damage at a stage when all routine clinical, laboratory, and ultrasound investigations were still silent (Gazzolo et al. 2001). The very fast increase in S100 protein after hypoxic insult may be useful in determining the timing of brain injury occurring independently of enduring CTG abnormalities. Serial urine determinations of S100 protein showed increasing values from birth to 72 h in newborns with abnormal outcome and were higher than in babies with normal outcome. The values were reported in relation to time and severity of brain insult.

132.10.2.3 Glial Fibrillary Acidic Protein (GFAP)

GFAP, a cytoskeleton intermediate filament protein of the astrocytes, is a marker of physiological and pathological state of astrocytes. It is released into the blood when astrocytes die and has been correlated with brain injury. The changes of its concentrations can reflect the state of astrocytes but also of blood–brain barrier. It has been used as a predictor of mortality and poor neurological outcomes in children requiring ECMO (Pelinka et al. 2004a, b; Lumpkins et al. 2008; Kaneko et al. 2009; Vos et al. 2004). The GFAP level is related with severity on HIE. A threshold of 0.08 ng/ml at admission distinguished neonates with moderate/severe NE who underwent SHT from controls without NE. GFAP levels equal to or greater than 0.15 ng/mL upon NICU admission were predictive of an abnormal brain MRI despite hypothermia therapy. Ennen et al. detected serum GFAP levels in neonates with HIE and with HIE and abnormal MRI and healthy newborns and showed that its serum concentrations were higher in the neonates with HIE despite healthy newborns and were higher in the neonates with HIE and abnormal MRI despite neonates with HIE and normal MRI. So GFAP appears as promising biomarker of brain damage and above all a good biomarker for the prognosis of HIE. Elevated GFAP, along with other biomarkers such as IL-1, IL-6, and IL-8, tumor necrosis factor, and interferon at 6–24 h were associated with abnormal neurological outcomes (Ennen et al. 2011).

132.10.2.4 Neuron-Specific Enolase (NSE)

NSE belongs to the family of glycolytic enzyme enolases, present in the cytoplasm of all tissues and organisms capable of glycolysis, but with high specificity for cell with neuroendocrine differentiation and neurons of brain tissue. High levels of NSE in CSF and serum have been correlated with poor outcome in patients with cardiac arrest (Roine et al. 1989; Rundgren et al. 2009), in patients with cerebrovascular accident (Hay et al. 1984), and in pediatric patients with traumatic brain injury (Berger et al. 2005). Elevated serum NSE concentrations in neonates undergoing cardiac surgery were also correlated with poor prognosis (Schmitt et al. 1998). Serum NSE concentrations have also been associated in a small neonatal study with severity of NE. A serum cutoff concentration of 45.4 μg/l could distinguish infants with poor outcomes from infants with normal outcomes (Celtik et al. 2004).

132.10.2.5 Myelin Basic Protein (MBP)

MBP is a proteic component of the myelin sheath, fundamental for the integrity of the myelin structure and for its function (Barbrese et al. 1988). MBP can be detected in the cerebrospinal fluid in normal conditions, but only a small amount is released into the blood. If a brain damage involves white matter (myelin sheath), the level of MBP in the blood or cerebrospinal fluid increases rapidly, reflecting the severity of myelin injury. So it can be used as a biomarker of white matter lesions or nerve fiber demyelination (Waigt and Górny 1983; Davies et al. 1987; Petersson et al. 2002; Hu et al. 2009; Sun et al. 2007).

132.10.2.6 Brain-Derived Neurotrophic Factor (BDNF)

BDNF is secreted by neurons and astrocytes of brain tissue to promote growth, differentiation, regeneration, and repair of neurons. There are few studies investigating the relationship between BDNF and neonatal HIE. Chouthai et al. showed that its concentration in the cord blood of premature neonates with severe cerebral hemorrhage was significantly lower than healthy newborns (Chouthai et al. 2003). Imam et al. studied its role as diagnostic and prognostic marker in neonates with perinatal asphyxia and showed that its levels were significantly higher than in the control group (Imam et al. 2009).

132.10.2.7 Tau Protein

Tau protein is a neuronal scaffolding protein that participates in actin filaments composed of neurons. There is no study that investigates about the relationship between tau protein levels and HIE, but Nurullah et al. showed that its concentration in blood and cerebrospinal fluid was higher in term neonates with encephalopathy bilirubin linked. So they suggested a possible use as biomarker of brain damage (Nurullah et al. 2008).

132.10.2.8 MicroRNA (miRNA)

miRNA belongs to a family of small, genome-encoded endogenous RNas that are transcribed but not translated into proteins. In recent years, miRNA has been shown to be essential in many aspect of brain function. It is involved also in the pathophysiology of neurodegeneration and neurological disorders in responses to hypoxic–ischemic injury. miRNA in brain tissues was closely related to the occurrence and development of hypoxic–ischemic encephalopathy (Filipowicz et al. 2008; Zhang and Guo 2012). The study of 49 cases of neonates with HIE showed the serum miRNA and hypoxia-induced factor 1a mRNA concentration was significantly higher than in the healthy control group, and increased concentrations of serum miRNA-21 indicated neonatal HIE (Chen and Yang 2015).

132.10.2.9 Activin A

Hypoxemia is a specific trigger for an increase in activin A in the circulation of fetal lambs. Activin A is a dimeric protein belonging to the transforming growth factor (TGF) superfamily, mainly produced by the placenta, decidua, and fetal membranes and secreted in large amounts in the maternal circulation (Debieve et al. 2000). Activin A is involved in cell growth and differentiation, neuronal survival, early embryonic development, and erythropoiesis. Activin A concentrations significantly increase in maternal serum with advancing gestation (Florio et al. 2001). Disorders of pregnancy due to reduced placental perfusion and various degrees of feto-placental hypoxemia, such as preeclampsia and fetal growth restriction, are characterized by increased levels of maternal and umbilical cord activin A (Roberts and Copper 2001). Feto-placental or maternal isocapnic hypoxemia is a specific trigger for an increase in activin A. Cord blood activin A levels increase in sheep after induction of hypoxia, remain elevated throughout hypoxia, and return to control values when normal

Fig. 2 Reliable markers in biological fluids associated with abnormal outcomes or death in newborns with clinical sign of encephalopathy at birth

Predictors of death or abnormal outcomes in single reports:

→ Cord blood:	Interleukin-6
	Nucleated red blood cells
	Nonprotein-bound iron
	Advanced oxidative protein products
→ Urine:	Lactate
→ Urine:	S100 protein
→ Serum:	Nonprotein-bound iron
→ Serum:	CD14 cell, NFkB activation
→ Serum:	Interleukin-8
→ Serum:	Ionized calcium

in meta-analysis:

→ Serum:	Interleukin-1b
→ Serum:	Interleukin-6
→ Cerebrospinal fluid:	Neuron-specific enolase
→ Cerebrospinal fluid:	Interleukin-1b

blood flow is restored (Jenkin et al. 2001). Neonates with clinical signs of perinatal hypoxia have higher activin A levels, which are correlated with biochemical features of hypoxia, such as higher nucleated red blood cell counts, plasma hypoxanthine, xanthine, base deficit levels, and lower pH (Florio et al. 2003). Activin A concentration at birth is increased in preterm newborns who later develop IVH and is useful for the early identification of infants with hypoxic–ischemic brain insults who are at high risk for IVH (Florio et al. 2006) (Fig. 2).

132.11 Conclusions

The actual knowledge gaps still preclude a definitive test or set of markers that accurately identifies an infant in whom neonatal encephalopathy is attributable to an acute intrapartum event. At least until reliable biomarkers of brain damage timing detection would not be available, the documentation of the status of the baby at birth, including a thorough neurologic exam, can be extremely helpful to provide the best and safest patient care. The recent task force convened by the ACOG and the AAP suggested a checklist that needs to be fulfilled in order to establish a reasonable causal link between an intrapartum event and subsequent long-term neurologic impairment.

1. Does the baby meet the clinical criteria of neonatal encephalopathy?
2. Are the neonatal signs consistent with an acute peri- or intrapartum event? Is the Apgar score < 5 at 5 and 10 min? Is metabolic acidemia (pH <7.0 or base deficit _12 mmol/L) present in the umbilical arterial blood gas analysis? Is there a compatible pattern seen on magnetic resonance brain imaging or magnetic resonance spectroscopy? Is there evidence of multisystem organ failure, as feature of prolonged asphyxia?
3. Are contributing factors present, which help to time or categorize an acute peri- or intrapartum event, such as a uterine rupture, a severe placental abruption, or an umbilical cord prolapse? Was the electronic fetal heart rate monitor pattern indicative of such an event? Is there dissuasive evidence of other factors that could account for the baby's condition,

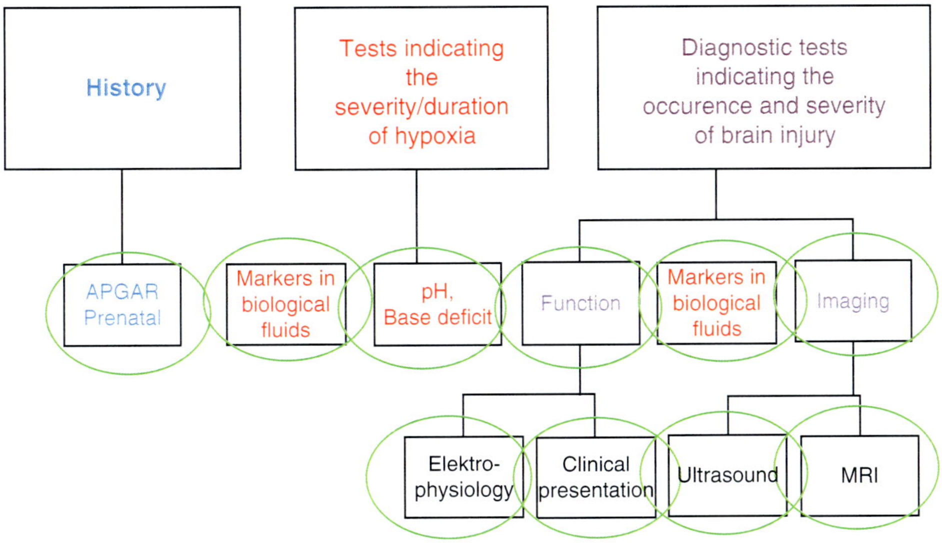

Fig. 3 The need of integration of biomarkers in the current tools for timing, diagnosis, and prognosis of neonatal encephalopathy

such as intrauterine growth restriction, maternal infection, neonatal infection, or placental dysfunction?

4. Is the child's ultimate neurological condition compatible with that which is known to follow peri- or intrapartum HIE, namely, spastic quadriplegic or dyskinetic CP?

Biomarkers are needed to determine the timing of the injury in HIE. This is important, because the insult often begins in utero and there is a limited therapeutic window to achieve benefit from treatment with hypothermia (Fig. 3).

The timing of injury also has major medicolegal ramifications for the obstetric and neonatal team taking care of the infant.

Using a panel rather than a single biomarker seems most likely to yield results but is still mostly research based.

While nonprotein-bound iron, cytokines, and neuroprostanes appear as the most promising brain-specific biomarkers, there is no currently available biomarker to be recommended for immediate use in clinical settings. Development of a panel of biomarkers could allow for more individualized care of neonates with HIE.

References

Abend NS, Wusthoff CJ (2012) Neonatal seizures and status epilepticus. J Clin Neirophysiol 29(5):441–448

Altshuler G, Arizawa M, Molnar-Nadasdy G (1992) Meconium induced umbilical cord vascular necrosis and ulceration: a potential link between the placenta and poor pregnancy outcome. Obstet Gynecol 79:760–766

Ambalavanan N, Carlo WA, Shankaran S et al (2006) Predicting outcomes of neonates diagnosed with hypoxemic-ischemic encephalopathy. Pediatrics 118:2084–2093

American College of Obstetricians and Gynecologists, American Academy of Pediatricians (2003) Criteria required to define an acute intrapartum hypoxic event as sufficient to cause cerebral palsy. In: Van Eerden P, Bernstein PS (eds) Neonatal encephalopathy and cerebral palsy. ACOG, Washington, DC, pp 73–80

Arduini D, Rizzo G (1990) Normal values of Pulsatility index from fetal vessels: a cross-sectional study on 1556 healthy fetuses. J Perinat Med 18:165–172

Badawi N, Kurinczuk JJ, Keogh JM et al (1998a) Intrapartum risk factors for newborn encephalopathy: the western Australian case-control stdy. BMJ 317:1554–1558

Badawi N, Kurinczuk JJ, Keogh JM et al (1998b) Antepartum risk factors for newborn encephalopathy: the western Australian case-control study. BMJ 317:1549–1553

Bapat R, Narayana PA, Zhou Y, Parikh NA (2014) Magnetic resonance spectroscopy at term-equivalent age in

extremely preterm infants: association with cognitive and language development. Pediatr Neurol 51(1):53–59
Barbrese E, Barry C, Chou CH et al (1988) Expression and localization of myelin basic protein in oligodendrocytes and transfected fibroblasts. J Neurochem 51:1737–1745
Barkovich AJ (2006) A magnetic resonance approach to metabolic disorders in childhood. Rev Neurol 43: S5–S16
Berger RP, Adelson PD, Pierce MC, Dulani T, Cassidy LD, Kochanek PM (2005) Serum neuron-specific enolase, S100B, and myelin basic protein concentrations after inflicted and noninflicted traumatic brain injury in children. J Neurosurg 103(1 Suppl):61–68. [PubMed PMID: 16122007. Epub 2005/08/27. eng]
Blackwell SC, Refuerzo JS, Wolfe HM et al (2000) The relationship between nucleated red blood cell counts and early-onset neonatal seizures. Am J Obstet Gynecol 182:1452–1457
Blackwell SC, Hallak M, Hotra JW et al (2004) Timing of fetal nucleated red blood cell count elevation in response to acute hypoxia. Biol Neonate 85: 217–220
Blennow M, Savman K, Ilves P et al (2001) Brain-specific proteins in the cerebrospinal fluid of severely asphyxiated newborn infants. Acta Paediatr 90:1171–1175
Bondurant MC, Lind RN, Koury MJ, Ferguson ME (1985) Control of globin gene transcription by erythropoietin in erythroblasts from fried virus-infected mice. Mol Cell Biol 5:675–683
Boog G (2004) Microdosage rapide des lactates au sang du cordon et au scalp foetal. Gynecol Obstet Fertil 32:241–244
Brand-Niebelschutz S, Saling E (1994) Indication for operative termination of labor on cardiotocography and fetal blood analysis: the reliability of these methods. J Perinat Med 22:19–27
Buonocore G, Perrone S, Gioia D et al (1999) Nucleated red blood cell count at birth as an index of perinatal brain damage. Am J Obstet Gynecol 181:1500–1505
Buonocore G, Perrone S, Longini M et al (2003) Non protein bound iron as predictive marker of neonatal brain damage. Brain 126:1–7
Celtik C, Acunas B, Oner N, Pala O (2004) Neuron-specific enolase as a marker of the severity and outcome of hypoxic ischemic encephalopathy. Brain Dev 26 (6):398–402. [PubMed PMID: 15275704. Epub 2004/07/28. eng]
Chau V, McFadden DE, Poskitt KJ, Miller SP (2013) Chorioamnionitis in the pathogenesis of brain injury in preterm infants. Clin Perinatol 41(1):83–103
Chen H, Yang TT (2015) Expression and significance of serum miRNA-21 control HIF-1a in newborn with asphyxia, chin. J Child Health Care 23:32–34
Chou YH, Tsou Yau KI, Wang PJ (1998) Clinical application of the measurement of cord plasma lactate and pyruvate in the assessment of high-risk neonates. Acta Paediatr 87:764–768
Chouthai N, Sampers N, Desai N et al (2003) Changes in neurotrophin levels in umbilical cord blood from infant with different gestational age and clinical conditions. Pediatr Res 53:965–969
Ciambra G, Arachi S, Protano C et al (2013) Accuracy of transcranial ultrasound in the detection of mild white matter lesions in newborns. Neuroradiol J 26:284–289
Da Silva S, Hennerbert N, Denis R, Wayenberg JL (2000) Clinical value of a single postnatal lactate measurement after intrapartum asphyxia. Acta Paediatr 89:320–322
Dammann O, Leviton A (2004) Biomarker epidemiology of cerebral palsy. Ann Neurol 55:158–161
Davies L, McLeod JG, Muir A et al (1987) Diagnostic value of cerebrospinal fluid myelin basic protein in patients with neurological illness. Clin Exp Neurol 24:5–7
Day IN, Thompson RJ (2010) UCHL1 (PGP 9.5): neuronal biomarker and ubiquitin system protein. Prog Neurobiol 90:327–362
Debieve F, Beerlandt S, Hubinont C, Thomas K (2000) Gonadotropins, prolactin, inhibin a, inhibin B, and activin a in human fetal serum from midpregnancy and term pregnancy. J Clin Endocrinol Metab 85:270–274
Deipolyi AR, Mukherjee P, Gill K et al (2005) Comparing microstructural and macrostructural development of the cerebral cortex in premature newborns: diffusion tensor imaging versus cortical gyration. NeuroImage 27:579–586
Delivoria-Papadopoulos M, Misbra OP (1998) Mechanisms of cerebral injury perinatal asphyxia and strategies for prevention. J Pediatr 132:S30–S34
Douglas-Escobar MV, Heaton SC, Bennett J et al (2014) UCH-L1 and GFAP serum levels in neonates with hypoxic-ischemic encephalopathy: a single center pilot study. Front Neurol 5:273
Dubiel M, Seremak-Mrozikiewicz A, Breborowicz GH et al (2005) Fetal and maternal Doppler velocimetry and cytokines in high-risk pregnancy. J Perinat Med 33:17–21
Ennen CS, Huisman TA, Savage WJ, Northington FJ, Jennings JM, Everett AD et al (2011) Glial fibrillary acidic protein as a biomarker for neonatal hypoxic-ischemic encephalopathy treated with whole-body cooling. Am J Obstet Gynecol 205(3):251 e1–251 e7. [PubMed PMID: 21784396. Epub 2011/07/26. eng.]
Filipowicz W, Bhattacharyya SN, Sonenberg N (2008) Mechanisms of post- transcriptional regulation by microRNA: are the answers in sight? Nat Rev Genet 9:102–114
Fily A, Pierrat V, Delporte V et al (2006) Factors associated with neurodevelopmental outcome at 2 years after very preterm birth: the population-based Nord-pas-de-Calais EPIPAGE cohort. Pediatrics 117:357–366
Florio P, Cobellis L, Luisi S et al (2001) Changes in inhibins and activin secretion in healthy and pathological pregnancies. Mol Cell Endocrinol 180:123–130
Florio P, Perrone S, Luisi S et al (2003) Activin a plasma levels at birth: an index of fetal hypoxia in preterm newborn. Pediatr Res 54:696–700
Florio P, Perrone S, Luisi S et al (2006) Increased plasma concentrations of activin a predict intraventricular

hemorrhage in preterm newborns. Clin Chem 52:1516–1521

Fujii EY, Kozuki M, Mu J et al (2004) Correlation of neuron-specific enolase and S100B with histological cerebral damage in fetal sheep after severe asphyxia. Brain Res 1018:136–140

Gazzolo D, Vinesi P, Bartocci M et al (1999) Elevated S100 blood level as an early indicator of intraventricular hemorrhage in preterm infants. Correlation with cerebral Doppler velocimetry. J Neurol Sci 170:32–35

Gazzolo D, Bruschettini M, Lituania M et al (2001) Increased urinary S100B protein as an early indicator of intraventricular hemorrhage in preterm infants: correlation with the grade of hemorrhage. Clin Chem 47:1836–1838

Gazzolo D, di Iorio R, Marinoni E et al (2002) S100B protein is increased in asphyxiated term infants developing intraventricular hemorrhage. Crit Care Med 30:1356–1360

Gazzolo D, Marinoni E, Di Lorio R et al (2006) High maternal blood S100B concentrations in pregnancies complicated by intrauterine growth restriction and intraventricular hemorrhage. Clin Chem 52:819–826

Girard N, Gire C, Sigandy S, Porcu G et al (2003) MR imaging of acquired fetal brain disorders. Childs Nerv Syst 19:490–500

Govaert P, De Vries LS (2010) An atlas of neonatal brain sonography, 2nd edn. Mac Keith Press, London

Graca AM, Cardoso KR, da Costa JM et al (2013) Cerebral volume at term age: comparison between preterm and term-born infants using cranial ultrasound. Early Hum Dev 89:643–648

Graham EM, Ruis KA, Hartman AL et al (2008) A systematic review of the role of intrapartum hypoxia-ischemia in the causation of neonatal encephalopathy. Am J Obstet Gynecol 199:587–595

Graves CR (2007) Antepartum fetal surveillance and timing of delivery in the pregnancy complicated by diabetes mellitus. Clin Obstet Gynecol 50:1007–1013

Hagelin A, Leyon J (1998) The effect of labor on the acid-base status of the newborn. Acta Obstet Gynecol Scand 158:356–361

Hay E, Royds JA, Davies-Jones GA, Lewtas NA, Timperley WR, Taylor CB (1984) Cerebrospinal fluid enolase in stroke. J Neurol Neurosurg Psychiatry 47 (7):724–729. [PubMed PMID: 6747647. Pubmed Central PMCID: 1027902. Epub 1984/07/01. eng]

Hellstrom-Westas L, de Vries LS, Rosen I (2008) Atlas of amplitude-integrated EEGs in the newborn, 2nd edn. Informa Healthcare, London

Hermansen MC (2001) Nucleated red blood cells in the fetus and newborn. Arch Dis Child Fetal Neonatal Ed 84:F211–F215

Hu SJ, Cheng YW, Han ZL et al (2009) Serum level of mylin basic protein in hypoxic-ischemic encephalopathy neonates. Acta Acad med Qingdao Univ 45:63–64

Hüppi PS, Dubois J (2006) Diffusion tensor imaging of brain development. Semin Fetal Neonatal Med 11:489–497

Imam SS, Gad GI, Aterf SH et al (2009) Gord blood brain derived neurotrophic factor: diagnostic and prognostic marker in full-term newborns with perinatal asphyxia. Pak J Biol Sci 12:1498–1504

Impey L, Greenwood C, MacQuillan K et al (2001) Fever in labour and neonatal encephalopathy: a prospective cohort study. Br J Obstet Gynecol 108:594–597

Inder TE, Warfield SK, Wang H et al (2005) Abnormal cerebral structure is present at term in premature infants. Pediatrics 115:286–294

Jenkin G, Ward J, Hooper S et al (2001) Feto-placental hypoxemia regulates the release of fetal activin a and prostaglandin E (2). Endocrinology 142:963–966

Jun JK, Yoon BH, Romero R et al (2000) Interleukin 6 determinations in cervical fluid have diagnostic and prognostic value in preterm premature rupture of membranes. Am J Obstet Gynecol 183:868–873

Kaneko T, Kasaoka S, Miyauchi T, Fujita M, Oda Y, Tsuruta R et al (2009) Serum glial fibrillary acidic protein as a predictive biomarker of neurological outcome after cardiac arrest. Resuscitation 80(7):790–794. [PubMed PMID: 19411130. Epub 2009/05/05. eng]

Kaukola T, Satyaraj E, Patel DD (2004) Cerebral palsy is characterized by protein mediators in cord serum. Ann Neurol 55:186–194

Kotiranta-Ainamo A, Rautonen J, Rautonen N (2004) Imbalanced cytokine secretion in newborn. Biol Neonate 85:55–60

Kroenke CD, Bretthorst GL, Inder TE, Neil JJ (2006) Modeling water diffusion anisotropy within fixed newborn primate brain using Bayesian probability theory. Magn Reson Med 55:187–197

Kurinczuk JJ, White-Koning M, Badawi N (2010) Epidemiology of neonatal encephalopathy and hypoxic–ischaemic encephalopathy. Early Hum Dev 86:329–338

Kuypers E, Ophelders D, Jellema RK et al (2012) White matter injury following fetal inflammatory response syndrome induced by chorioamnionitis and fetal sepsis: lessons from experimental ovine models. Early Hum Dev 88(12):931–936

van Laerhoven H, de Haan TR, Offringa M, Post B, van der Lee JH (2013) Prognostic tests in term neonates with hypoxic-ischemic encephalopathy: a systematic review. Pediatrics 131(1):88–98

Leijser LM, de Vries LS, Cowan FM (2006) Using cerebral ultrasound effectively in the newborn infant. Early Hum Dev 82:827–835

Leonardo CC, Pennypacker KR (2009) Neuroinflammation and MMPs: potential therapeutic targets in neonatal hypoxic-ischemic injury. J Neuroinflammation 6:13

Levene MI (1988) Cerebral ultrasound and neurological impairment: telling the future. Arch Dis Child 63:17–22

Longini M, Perrone S, Kenanidis A et al (2005) Isoprostanes in amniotic fluid: a predictive marker for fetal growth restriction in pregnancy. Free Radic Biol Med 38:1537–1541

Longini M, Perrone S, Vezzosi P et al (2007) Association between oxidative stress in pregnancy and preterm premature rupture of membranes. Clin Biochem 40:793–797

Lorenzl S, De Pasquale G, Segal AZ, Beal MF (2003) Dysregulation of the levels of matrix metalloproteinases and tissue inhibitors of matrix metalloproteinases in the early phase of cerebral ischemia. Stroke 34:37–38

Low JA, Galbraith RS, Muir DW et al (1984) Factors associated with motor and cognitive deficits in children after intrapartum fetal hypoxiam. J Obstet Gynaecol 148:533–539

Low JA, Lindasay BG, Derrick EJ (1997) Threshold of metabolic acidosis associated with newborn complications. Am J Obstet Gynecol 177:1391–1394

Lumpkins KM, Bochicchio GV, Keledjian K, Simard JM, McCunn M, Scalea T (2008) Glial fi- brillary acidic protein is highly correlated with brain injury. J Trauma 65(4):778–782. [discussion 82–4; PubMed PMID: 18849790. Epub 2008/10/14. eng]

Machin GA, Ackerman J, Gilbert-Barness E (2000) Abnormal umbilical cord coiling is associated with adverse perinatal outcomes. Pediatr Dev Pathol 3:462–471

Mathur AM, Neil JJ, McKinstry RC, Inder TE (2008) Transport, monitoring, and successful brain MR imaging in unsedated neonates. Pediatr Radiol 38:260–264

Maunu J, Ekholm E, Parkkola R et al (2007) Antenatal Doppler measurements and early brain injury in very low birth weight infants. J Pediatr 150:51–56

McDonald DG, Kelehan P, McMenamin JB et al (2004) Placental fetal thrombotic vasculopathy is associated with neonatal encephalopathy. Hum Pathol 35:875–880

McQuillen PS, Ferriero DM (2004) Selective vulnerability in the developing central nervous system. Pediatr Neurol 30:227–235

Meyer RS (1975) Four patterns of perinatal brain damage and their conditions of occurrence in primates. Adv Neurol 10:223–234

Miller SP, Newton N, Ferriero DM et al (2002) Predictors of 30- month outcome after perinatal depression: role of proton MRS and socioeconomic factors. Pediatr Res 52:71–77

Miller SP, Ramaswamy V, Michelson D et al (2005) Patterns of brain injury in term neonatal encephalopathy. J Pediatr 146:453–460

Minagawa K, Tsuji Y, Ueda H et al (2002) Possible correlation between high levels of IL-18 in the cord blood of preterm infants and neonatal development of periventricular leukomalacia and cerebral palsy. Cytokine 17:164–170

Mishra OP, Delivoria-Papadopoulus M (1998) Cellular mechanisms of hypoxic in the developing brain. Brain Res Bull 48:233–238

Murray DM, Boylan GB, Ali I, Ryan CA, Murphy BP, Connolly S (2008) Defining the gap between electrographic seizure burden, clinical expression and staff recognition of neonatal seizures. Arch Dis Child Fetal Neonatal Ed 93:F187–F191

Murray DM, O'Riordan MN, Horgan R, Boylan G, Higgins JR, Ryan CA (2009) Fetal heart rate patterns in neonatal hypoxic-ischemic encephalopathy: relationship with early cerebral activity and neurodevelopmental outcome. Am J Perinatol 26(8):605–612

Naeye RL (1991) Acute chorioamnionitis and the disorders that produce placental insufficiency. Monogr Pathol 33:286–307

Naeye RL, Lin HM (2001) Determination of the timing of fetal brain damage from hypoxemia-ischemia. Am J Obstet Gynecol 184:217–224

Naeye RL, Russell Localio A (1995) Determining the time before birth when ischemia and hypoxemia initiated cerebral palsy. Obstet Gynecol 86:713–719

Nagdyman N, Komen W, Ko HK et al (2001) Early biochemical indicators of hypoxic-ischemic encephalopathy after birth asphyxia. Pediatr Res 49:502–506

Nasiell J, Papadogiannakis N, Löf E, Elofsson F, Hallberg B (2016) Hypoxic ischemic encephalopathy in newborns linked to placental and umbilical cord abnormalities. J Matern Fetal Neonatal Med 29(5):721–726

Neil JJ, Inder TE (2004) Imaging perinatal brain injury in premature infants. Semin Perinatol 28:433–443

Neil JJ, Shiran SI, McKinstry RC et al (1998) Normal brain in human newborns: apparent diffusion coefficient and diffusion anisotropy measured by using diffusion tensor MR imaging. Radiology 209:57–66

Nelson KB (2005) Neonatal encephalopathy: etiology and outcome. Dev Med Child Neurol 47:292

Nosarti C, Al-Asady MH, Frangou S et al (2002) Adolescents who were born very preterm have decreased brain volumes. Brain 125(Pt 7):1616–1623

Nosarti C, Rushe TM, Woodruff PW et al (2004) Corpus Callosum size and very preterm birth: relationship to neuropsychological outcome. Brain 127(Pt 9):2080–2089

Nurullah O, Canan T, Eray EO et al (2008) Tau and s-100B proteins as biochemical markers of bilirubin-induced neurotoxicity in term neonates. Pediatr Neurol 39:245–250

Ogino S, Redline RW (2000) Villous capillary lesions of the placenta: distinctions between chorangioma, chorangiomatosis, and chorangiosis. Hum Pathol 31:945–954

Okumara A, Hayakawa F, Okumura A (1999) Neonatal EEG: a powerful tool in the assessment of brain damage in preterm infants. Brain Dev 21:361–372

Pelinka LE, Kroepfl A, Leixnering M, Buchinger W, Raabe A, Redl H (2004a) GFAP versus S100B in serum after traumatic brain injury: relationship to brain damage and out- come. J Neurotrauma 21 (11):1553–1561. [PubMed PMID: 15684648. Epub 2005/02/03. eng]

Pelinka LE, Kroepfl A, Schmidhammer R, Krenn M, Buchinger W, Redl H et al (2004b) Glial fibrillary acidic protein in serum after traumatic brain injury and multiple trauma. J Trauma 57(5):1006–1012. [PubMed PMID: 15580024. Epub 2004/12/08. eng]

Perrone S, Tataranno ML, Negro S et al (2010) Early identification of the risk for free radical related diseases in preterm newborns. Early Hum Dev 86:241–244

Perrone S, Tataranno ML, Santacroce A et al (2016a) Fetal programming, maternal nutrition and oxidative stress hypothesis. J Pediatr Biochem 6:96–102

Perrone S, Santacroce A, Picardi A, Buonocore G (2016b) Fetal programming and early identification of newborn at high risk of free-radical mediated diseases. World J Clin Pediatr 5:172–181

Perrone S, Tataranno ML, Longini M et al (2016c) Placental histological examination and the relationship with oxidative stress in preterm infants. Placenta 46:72–78

Peterson BS, Vohr B, Staib LH et al (2000) Regional brain volume abnormalities and long-term cognitive outcome in preterm infants. JAMA 284:1939–1947

Petersson KH, Pinar H, Stopa EG et al (2002) White matter injury after cerebral ischemia in ovine fetuses. Pediatr Res 51:768–778

Redline RW (2006) Placental pathology and cerebral palsy. Clin Perinatol 33:503–516

Redline RW, Faye-Petersen O, Heller D et al (2003) Amniotic infection syndrome: nosology and reproducibility of placental reaction patterns. Pediatr Dev Pathol 6:435–448

Roberts JM, Copper DW (2001) Pathogenesis and genetics of preeclampsia. Lancet 357:53–56

Roine RO, Somer H, Kaste M, Viinikka L, Karonen SL (1989) Neurological outcome after out-of-hospital cardiac arrest. Prediction by cerebrospinal fluid enzyme analysis. Arch Neurol 46(7):753–756. [PubMed PMID: 2742544. Epub 1989/07/01. eng]

Rosell A, Ortega-Aznar A, Alvarez-Sabin J et al (2006) Increased brain expression of matrix metalloproteinase- 9 after ischemic and hemorrhagic human stroke. Stroke 37:1399–1406

Rosèn KG, Amer-Wahlin I, Luzietti R, Noren H (2004) Fetal ECG waveform analysis. Best Pract Res Clin Obstet Gynaecol 18:485–514

Roth SC, Baudin J, Cady E et al (1997) Relation of deranged neonatal cerebral oxidative metabolism with neurodevelopmental outcome and head circumference at 4 years. Dev Med Child Neurol 39:718–725

Rundgren M, Karlsson T, Nielsen N, Cronberg T, Johnsson P, Friberg H (2009) Neuron specific enolase and S-100B as predictors of outcome after cardiac arrest and induced hypothermia. Resuscitation 80(7):784–789. [PubMed PMID: 19467754. Epub 2009/05/27. eng]

Sarnat HB, Sarnat MS (1976) Neonatal encephalopathy following fetal distress. A clinical and electroencephalographic study. Arch Neurol 33:696–705

Saxonhouse MA, Rimsza LM, Christensen RD et al (2003) Effects of anoxia on megakaryocyte progenitors derived from cord blood CD34pos cells. Eur J Haematol 71:359–365

Schmitt B, Bauersfeld U, Schmid ER, Tuchschmid P, Molinari L, Fanconi S et al (1998) Serum and CSF levels of neuron-specific enolase (NSE) in cardiac surgery with cardiopulmonary bypass: a marker of brain injury? Brain Dev 20(7):536–539. [PubMed PMID: 9840675. Epub 1998/12/05. eng]

Schofield JN, Dayl N, Thompson RJ et al (1995) PGP 9.5, a ubiquitin C-terminal hydro- lase: pauem of mRNA and protein expression during neural development in the mouse. Brain Res Dev Brain Res 85:224–228

Shellhaas RA (2015) Continuous long-term electroencephalography: the gold standard for neonatal seizures diagnosis. Semin Fetal Neonatal Med 20(3):149–153

Shevell MI (2001) The pediatric neurologist as expert witness with particular reference to perinatal asphyxia. Can J Neurol Sci 28:107–112

Sie LT, van der Knaap MS, Oosting J, de Vries LS, Lafeber HN, Valk J (2000) MR patterns of hypoxic-ischemic brain damage after prenatal, perinatal or postnatal asphyxia. Neuropediatrics 31:128–136

Stanek J (1999) Numerical criteria for the diagnosis of placental chorangiosis using CD34 immunostaining. Trophoblast res 13:443–452

Steggerda SJ, van Wezel-Meijler G (2016) Cranial ultrasonography of the immature cerebellum: role and limitations. Semin Fetal Neonatal Med 21(5):295–304

Sun YL, Meng L, Guo JL et al (2007) Relationship between serum myelin basic protein and neonatal hypoxic ischemic encephalopathy. Chin J Birth Health Hered 15:16–17

Sunugawa S, Ichiyama T, Honda R et al (2009) Matrix metalloproteinase- 9 and tissue inhibitor of metalloproteinase-1 in perinatal asphyxia. Brain Dev 31:588–593

Task Force on Neonatal Encephalopathy (2014) Neonatal encephalopathy and neurologic outcome, second edition report of the American College of Obstetricians and Gynecologists. Obstet Gynecol 123(4): 896–901

Thompson RJ, Doran JF, Jackson P et al (1983) PGP 9.5-a new marker for vertebrate neurons and neuroendocrine cells. Brain Res 278:224–228

Toet MC, Hellstrom-Westas L, Groenedal F, Eken P, de Vries LS (1999) Amplitude integrated EEG 3 and 6 hours after birth in full term neonates with hypoxic-ischaemic encephalopathy. Arch Dis Child Fetal Neonatal Ed 81(1):F19–F23

Ugwumadu A (2013) Understanding cardiotocographic patterns associated with intrapartum fetal hypoxia and neurologic injury. Best Pract Res Clin Obstet Gynaecol 27(4):509–536

Van Bel F, Walther FJ (1990) Myocardial dysfunction and cerebral blood flow velocity following birth asphyxia. Acta Paediatr Scand 79:756–762

Vatansever U, Acuna B, Demin AM et al (2002) Nucleated red blood cell counts and erythropoietin levels in high-risk neonates. Pediatr Int 44:590–595

Volpe JJ (1996) Subplate neurons – missing link in brain injury of the premature infant? Pediatrics 97:112–113

Volpe J (ed) (2008) Neurology of the newborn, 5th edn. W.B. Saunders, Philadelphia

Vos PE, Lamers KJ, Hendriks JC, van Haaren M, Beems T, Zimmerman C et al (2004) Glial and neuronal proteins in serum predict outcome after severe traumatic brain injury. Neurology 62(8):1303–1310. [PubMed PMID: 15111666. Epub 2004/04/28. eng]

Wachtel EV, Hendricks-Muñoz KD (2011) Current management of the infants who presents with neonatal encephalopathy. Curr Probl Pediatr Adolesc Health Care 41(5):132–153

Waigt A, Górny M (1983) CSF antibodies to myelin basic protein and to myelin- associated glycoprotein in multiple sclerosis. Evidence of the intrathecal production of antibodies. Acta Neurol Scand 68:337–345

Weindling AM, Rochefort MJ, Calcert SA, Fok TF (1985) Developed of cerebral palsy after ultrasonographic detection of periventricular cysts in the newborn. Dev Med Child Neurol 27:800–806

van Wezel-Meijler G, Steggerda SJ, Leijser LM (2010) Cranial ultrasonography in neonates: role and limitations. Semin Perinatol 34:28–38

Widness JA, Teramo KA, Clemons GK et al (1986) Temporal response of immunoreactive erythropoietin to acute hypoxemia in fetal sheep. Pediatr Res 20:15–19

Wu YW, Colford JM Jr (2000) Chorioamnionitis as a risk factor for cerebral palsy: a meta-analysis. JAMA 284:1417–1424

Yager JY, Miller SP (2009) Controversies and advances in neonatal neurology: overview. Introduction. Pediatr Neurol 40:143–144

Yager JY, Armstrong EA, Miyashita H, Wirrell EC (2002) Prolonged neonatal seizures exacerbate hypoxic-ischemic brain damage: correlation with cerebral energy metabolism and excitatory amino acid release. Dev Neurosci 24:367–381

Yamamoto T, Shibata N, Maramatsu F et al (2002) Oxidative stress in the human fetal brain: an immunohistochemical study. Pediatr Neurol 26:116–122

Zacharia A, Zimine S, Lovblad KO et al (2006) Early assessment of brain maturation by MR imaging segmentation in neonates and premature infants. AJNR Am J Neuroradiol 27:972–977

Zhang Y, Guo J (2012) MicroRNA and cerebral ischemic injury. Acta Acad Med Sci 34:418–421

Zhang W, Su P, Kuang ZZ (2013) Application value – li in early identification of acute is- chemic cerebrovascular disease. Shandong Med J 53:15–17

Epidemiology of Adverse Cerebral Outcome of Newborns

133

Neil Marlow

Contents

Abstract

Continuing improvement in perinatal and neonatal care has emphasized the importance of adverse childhood outcomes as the most important sequelae of care. Major disabling conditions such as cerebral palsy are related to the occurrence of brain injury and appear to be reducing in prevalence and severity among the very preterm group. However, the most common problems found after preterm birth relate to intellectual disability, defined in early childhood as low developmental test scores. Severe visual and hearing impairments are much less prevalent but nonetheless important impairments. In this chapter I will discuss time trends in outcomes and short-term prevalences up to 3 years of age.

133.1 Salient Points

- Neonatal intensive care has brought about significant increases in survival at very low gestational age and birth weight. It is of great importance to monitor the development of adverse cerebral outcomes for such children.
- The prevalence of cerebral palsy increases with both decreasing gestational age and birthweight. However, it appears to be reducing in prevalence and severity among the very preterm group over the last years.

N. Marlow (✉)
Institute for Women's Health, University College London, London, UK
e-mail: n.marlow@ucl.ac.uk

G. Buonocore et al. (eds.), *Neonatology*,
https://doi.org/10.1007/978-3-319-29489-6_280

- Developmental outcome at 2 years has become an international standard for reporting outcomes.
- Intellectual disability is a common problem found after preterm birth. Cognitive scores are related to gestational age at birth.
- The prevalence of hearing and visual impairment among very preterm group, although an important source of morbidity, remains very low.

133.2 Introduction

Since the beginnings of neonatal intensive care, in particular the recognition that mechanical ventilation could improve survival, there has been debate and discussion as to whether the steady advancement of survival rates comes at the cost of an increased risk of adverse outcomes. This was addressed in 1981 by Stewart, Reynolds, and Lipscomb in a review of the world literature on outcomes for very low birth weight (VLBW) births (Stewart et al. 1981). Since the mid-1940s, survival across a range of reports had steadily improved and despite increasing numbers of survivors the proportion of all births surviving with handicaps had remained constant at 6–8%. Indeed, the rate of impaired outcome as a proportion of survivors had progressively increased.

Since then improvements in survival have continued and the reported lowest birthweight and gestational ages of survivors have fallen progressively so that now it is not unusual for babies to survive birth as early as 22 weeks of gestation or weighing significantly less than 500 g at birth. Much interest is now focused on this group, because extremely preterm infants (sometimes referred to as previable, which is not strictly accurate) excite much the same debate as raged in the 1970s over instituting invasive intensive care. It is therefore of great importance to monitor and record the outcomes for such children so that accurate prognostic data can be provided.

One problem is that the numbers of such children cared for by individual institutions over any year is very small – for example, in England during 2006 there were only four survivors after birth at 22 weeks and the number of babies surviving at 23 weeks equates to an average of under one per NICU (Moore et al. 2012). Hence, reliable evidence of the proportion surviving with adverse outcome, including reasonably narrow confidence intervals, can only be achieved by averaging over many years, encompassing changing care practices, or by performing large population studies. Population studies are often compared to studies from centers of excellence, something which is really not feasible unless there is 100% referral into such centers, as it is well described that children survive more frequently in such settings and it is likely that morbidities will be reduced. Thus all reports of comparisons have to come with caveats because of a range of rarely matched issues (Table 1). It is possible to make careful comparisons of outcomes between epidemiological studies – for example, there are remarkable similarities in outcomes between the EPICure (UK and Ireland) and EPIPAGE (regional study, France) in terms of prevalence of both cerebral palsy and cognitive impairment (Bodeau-Livinec et al. 2007), and in 2–3 year outcomes between EPICure2 and EXPRESS, despite large differences in survival rates (Marlow 2014).

Morbidity following extremely preterm birth must be considered with reference to survival as the "profit and loss" for care at such low gestations is key information for parents. Indeed whereas the outcome for many studies of perinatal care has been traditionally a composite of death of moderate/severe neurodevelopmental impairment, increasingly unimpaired outcome is being preferred, as that is the goal of our care (Lees et al. 2015). However, for parents the guide still remains the risk of death or serious disability.

Although the bulk of babies born preterm are delivered at more mature gestations, most reports include very preterm (<32 weeks) or extremely preterm (<28 weeks) births. This is because mortality and morbidity are inversely related to gestational age.

133.3 Mortality

Neonatal intensive care has brought about significant increases in survival at very low gestations, mortality being rare at more mature gestational

Table 1 Pitfalls in the comparison of data from different studies of adverse outcomes

Problem		Suggested solution for reports
Gestational ages and birth weights	*No agreed definition of "extremely low GA," more consensus over birthweight categories*	Report in fixed categories by Single completed gestational weeks (to 30 weeks) 250 g weight intervals (to 1,500 g) Always use confidence intervals
Population bases	*Some report hospital-based outcomes other community or population*	Population data preferred for comparative data as circumvents issues of referral bias
Perinatal baseline	*Some units report outcomes only for admissions, others live births, others for babies alive at the onset of labor; often babies receiving nonactive care are included*	Report all statistics if possible; important as parents need updated risk information depending upon their pathway though labor and delivery; including babies who have not been offered active care worsens the prognosis (see below)
Assessment ages	*Most authorities agree that more accurate data come from later acquisition of information*	24 months is the most common age of initial assessment and should be adhered to
Outcome measures	Variation in definition, cutoffs, and tests used	Use standard published definitions of outcome and ensure contemporary developmental tests, where not possible collect reference or comparator data for term infants
Population	Immigration and social disadvantage important contributors to rate of preterm birth and morbidity	Evaluate and report population mix in terms of ethnicity, social advantage, and baseline prematurity rate
Health systems	No clarity on policy at extremely low GA in terms of options for parents and for babies	State policy (even if cannot be agreed, estimate variation) and proportion of children at each GA week in whom resuscitation is attempted

ages. Figures reported from national studies or large datasets show variability at extremely low gestations commensurate with local policy. Studies reporting outcomes 2000–2010 are shown in Fig. 1.

Survival varies widely among different regions at extremely low gestations in Sweden and may be related to the level of active care provided in the antenatal and neonatal period (Serenius et al. 2014). Among the 24 NICHD network hospitals, there is similar variation in active intervention immediately after birth, from 0–100% at 22 weeks, 25–100% at 23 weeks to 65–100% at 24 weeks. Nonactive intervention explains 78% variation in survival and 71% variation in survival without 2 year morbidity between hospitals (Rysavy et al. 2015). Furthermore, survival rates differ between hospitals with different categories of neonatal service, being lowest in more expert hospitals and in those with highest throughput (Marlow et al. 2014; Watson et al. 2014). Mortality rates at low gestations are not static and change over time with evolving attitudes and expertise, for example, in England mortality <26 weeks fell by 15% between 1995 and 2006.

133.4 Determining Later Morbidity

Developmental outcome at 2 years has become an international standard for reporting outcomes. Two years was chosen because all but the mildest forms of cerebral palsy are detectable at this age and developmental tests are thought to be reliable indicators of later development at this age. High follow-up rates can be obtained over this short period although dropouts can be troublesome, representing children with more severe impairments (Wolke et al. 1995; Tin et al. 1997) and more with social disadvantage (Moore et al. 2012). Definitions of morbidity vary between studies in detail but rarely in content. Recent recommendations from the British Association

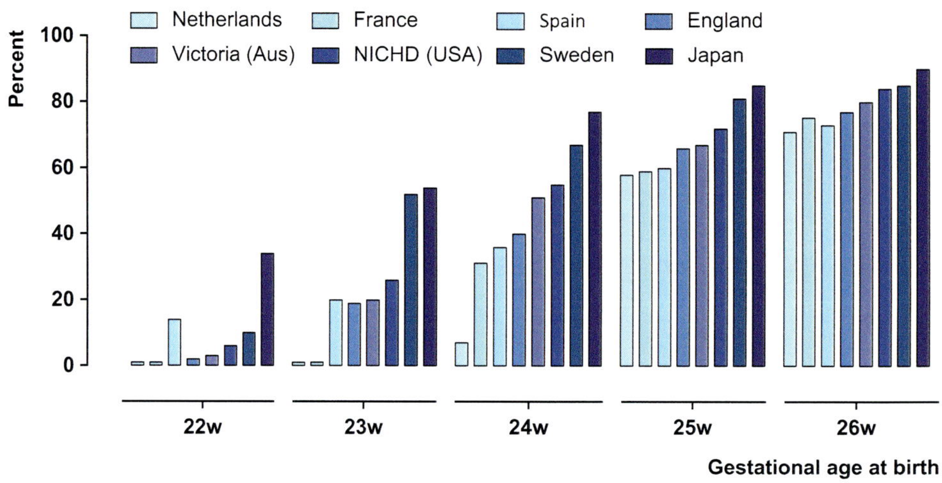

Fig. 1 Survival of livebirths in large populations 2003–2011

of Perinatal Medicine are shown in Table 2. Wherever possible data should be compared to those from a control population of children born at full term. A discussion of the practicalities of follow-up assessment is described elsewhere (Marlow 2007).

133.5 Cerebral Palsy

The prevalence of cerebral palsy (CP) increases with both decreasing gestational age and birthweight. The rate of CP in the individual populations varies between 10 and 20% with all the caveats mentioned above. Better data come from the reports of population studies, such of those of Hagberg and colleagues from southern Sweden (Himmelmann et al. 2005), or broader register collaborations such as SCPE (Krageloh-Mann and Cans 2009). In these studies, care has been taken to use a geographically based approach and careful case definition to produce consistent trends.

The rise in prevalence of all types of CP seen from the late 1960s has now been replaced by a steady decline during the 1990s, which has continued to 2003 (Fig. 2). Initially the prevalence among ELBW liveborn children rose up to the mid-1990s probably paralleling survival for a group of babies with the highest risk of CP but reassuringly over the past 10 years the prevalence appears to have declined. In particular, there has been a parallel decrease in the prevalence of moderate-severe cerebral palsy in very and extremely low birthweight births (Sellier et al. 2016) and of diplegia (Marlow 2014) itself associated with preterm birth, and a small increase in dyskinetic types of CP – more associated with acute intrapartum hypoxia at full term. Furthermore, CP associated with preterm or very low birthweight births tends to have less associated disability (Moore et al. 2012; Surman et al. 2009). Most studies report outcomes for CP in functional grades using the Gross Motor Function Classification System. Grade 1 representing mild functional loss and Grade 5 the severest outcomes. In population based data, the rate of moderate to severe CP (Grades 3–5) among survivors is now less than 6% at gestational ages above 24 weeks (Fig. 3).

It seems clear that the prevalence is falling in keeping with the reduction seen in ultrasound diagnosed brain injury from hemorrhagic parenchymal infarction and cystic periventricular leukomalacia (PVL). This mirrors the observation of Pharoah and colleagues that birthweight-specific prevalence of CP first increased in line with survival (a possible practice effect) before falling as practice improves further (Pharoah et al. 1987). CP is also more common among children who are small-for-gestational age at birth. For some time, it has been considered that the effect of prematurity swamped any relationship at gestational ages below 34 weeks. In fact

Table 2 Categorization of outcome at 2 years in preterm populations (Report of a BAPM/RCPCH working group 2008)

Criteria for	Severe neurodevelopmental disability	Moderate neurodevelopmental disability
Domain	*Any one of the below:*	*Any one of the below:*
Motor	Cerebral palsy with GMFCS level 3, 4, or 5	Cerebral palsy with GMFCS level 2
Cognitive function	Score < -3 standard deviations below norm (DQ < 55)	Score -2SD to -3SD below norm (DQ 55–70)
Hearing	No useful hearing even with aids (profound >90 dBHL)	Hearing loss corrected with aids (usually moderate 40–70 dBHL) *or*
		Some hearing but loss not corrected by aids (usually severe 70–90 dBHL)
Speech and language	No meaningful words/signs	Some but fewer than five words or signs
	or	*or*
	Unable to comprehend cued command (i.e., commands only understood in a familiar situation or with visual cues, e.g., gestures).	Unable to comprehend un-cued command but able to comprehend a cued command
Vision	Blind	Seems to have moderately reduced vision but better than severe visual impairment
	or	*or*
	Can only perceive light or light reflecting objects	Blind in one eye with good vision in the contralateral eye
Other disabilities (included as additional impairments to SND or NDI)		
Respiratory	Requires continued respiratory support or oxygen	Limited exercise tolerance
Gastrointestinal	Requires TPN, NG, or PEG feeding	On special diet or has stoma
Renal	Requires dialysis or awaiting organ transplant	Renal impairment requiring treatment or special diet

most preterm children are small at birth compared to well fetuses of a similar gestational age. When estimated fetal weight standards are used this relationship is clearly seen (Jarvis et al. 2006). Interestingly, it is seen that being large-for gestational age also increases risk across the gestational range. More recent studies have indicated a very low rate of CP among 2-year-old children born after closely monitored pregnancies with fetal growth restriction (Lees et al. 2015), emphasizing the differences between a population defined by being small for gestational age and the more dynamic description of failing fetal growth.

133.6 Developmental or Cognitive Outcomes

There are fewer systematic studies associating cognitive outcomes over time. Partly this is due to the difficulty of drifting test norms and evolving developmental or psychometric test development, making it very difficult to compare changes over time.

Cognitive scores are related to gestational age at birth. In a whole population study in Bavaria a clear relationship is seen with no significant correlation at gestations above 33 weeks whereas below 33 weeks there is a steady fall off with gestational age of around 2 IQ points per gestational week (Wolke et al. 2001). The EPICure data are consistent with this trend (Marlow et al. 2005), which has been confirmed by systematic review (Kerr-Wilson et al. 2012). This is also reflected in educational outcomes, such as special educational needs (MacKay et al. 2010) and attainment (Mathiasen et al. 2010). Data comparing the two EPICure studies using adjusted scores to reflect the difference in editions of the Bayley Scales seem to indicate an improving trend in scores between 1995 and 2006 (Fig. 4).

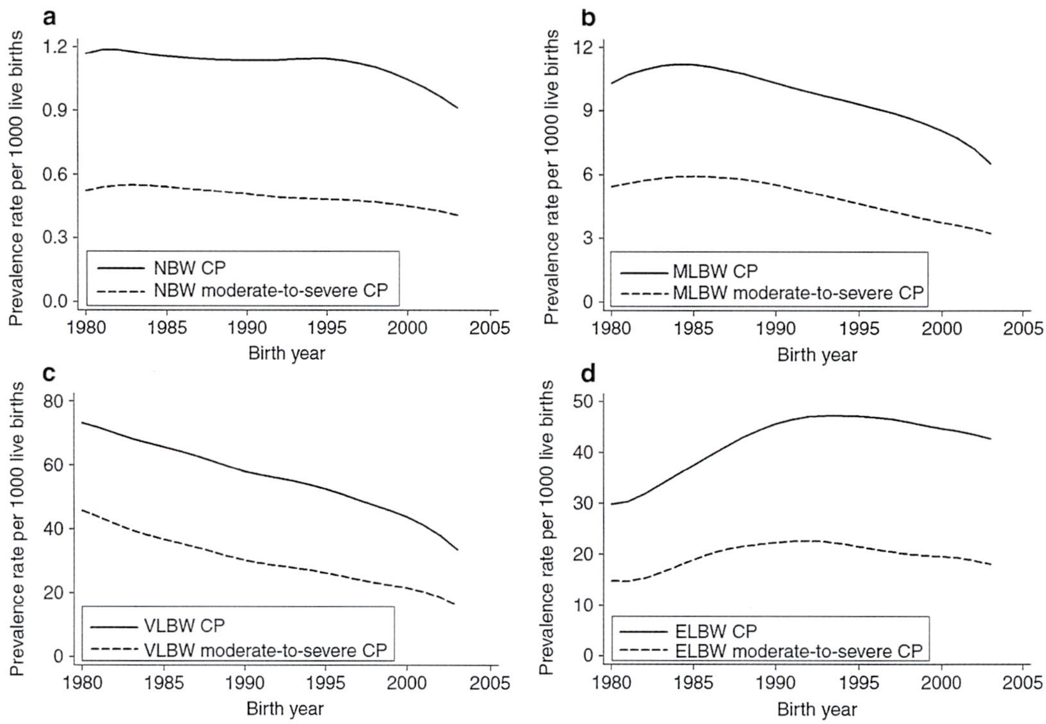

Fig. 2 Changing prevalence of cerebral palsy by birthweight (**a**) ≥2,500 g, (**b**) 1,500–2,499 g, (**c**) 1,000–1,499 g, (**d**) <1,000 g (Sellier et al. 2016)

Fig. 3 Prevalence of cerebral palsy among 3-year-old children born at <27 weeks of gestation, categorized by Gross Motor Function Classification Scale. Percentages are the proportion with GMFCS grade 3 through 5 (Moore et al. 2012)

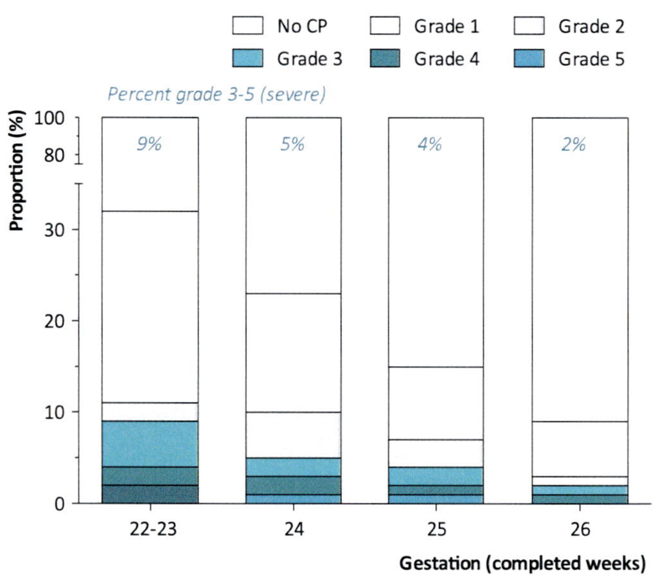

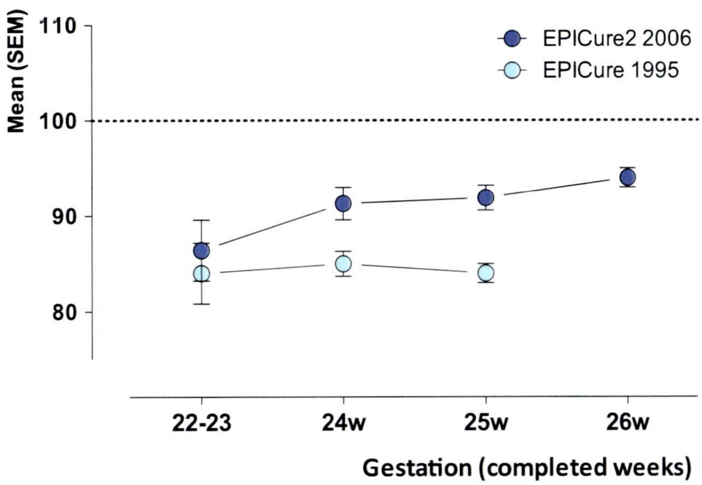

Fig. 4 Mean (SEM) mental developmental indices (MDI) in two English cohorts by gestational age <27 weeks (Data from Moore et al. 2012; Wood et al. 2000). The difference in means for births 22–25 weeks was 8 points (95%CI 5–10)

Further discussion of the detail of cognitive deficits is found in ▶ Chap. 14, "Follow-Up Outcomes of High-Risk Infants".

The relationship with size at birth in epidemiological studies is less clear. Where there is evidence of failing fetal growth, cognitive scores are reduced (Morsing et al. 2011). Systematic reviews indicate that an effect by gestational age using size at birth is difficult to determine, but in some recent large studies, scores tend to be lower than appropriately grown babies and births at the extreme of <−3SD are at much greater risk.

Further discussion of these areas is outside the remit of this chapter but may be found in ▶ Chap. 14, "Follow-Up Outcomes of High-Risk Infants".

133.7 Sensory Outcomes

There are fewer epidemiological studies of sensory outcomes. Retinopathy of prematurity is common at extremely low gestations but blindness is rare. Furthermore, little distinction is made of the aetiology of visual impairment in preterm populations. For example, in the BOOST-II studies, 151 children developed retinopathy that received laser treatment (BOOST-II UK Group et al. 2013) but only 23 (1.6%) had later severe visual impairment (BOOST-II Australia Group et al. 2016). Within the UK group, the large majority of these had central visual impairment consequent on brain injury, in contrast to late sequelae of retinopathy.

Similarly, there are few epidemiological studies of hearing loss among preterm populations and the aetiology is poorly understood. The prevalence of hearing and visual impairment among very or extremely low gestational age survivors, although an important source of morbidity, remains very low.

References

Bodeau-Livinec F, Ancel P, Marlow N et al (2007) Care and early childhood outcome of extremely preterm infants in the British Isles and in France. Am J Epidemiol 165(11):S19–S19

BOOST-II Australia Group et al (2016) Outcomes of two trials of oxygen-saturation targets in preterm infants. N Engl J Med 374(8):749–760

BOOST-II UK Group et al (2013) Oxygen saturation and outcomes in preterm infants. N Engl J Med 368 (22):2094–2104

Himmelmann K, Hagberg G, Beckung E et al (2005) The changing panorama of cerebral palsy in Sweden. IX. Prevalence and origin in the birth-year period 1995–1998. Acta Paediatr 94(3):287–294

Jarvis S, Glinianaia SV, Blair E (2006) Cerebral palsy and intrauterine growth. Clin Perinatol 33(2):285–300

Kerr-Wilson CO, Mackay DF, Smith GC et al (2012) Meta-analysis of the association between preterm delivery and intelligence. J Public Health 34(2):209–216

Krageloh-Mann I, Cans C (2009) Cerebral palsy update. [Review] [47 refs]. Brain Dev 31(7):537–544

Lees CC, Marlow N, van Wassenaer-Leemhuis A et al (2015) 2 year neurodevelopmental and intermediate perinatal outcomes in infants with very preterm fetal growth restriction (TRUFFLE): a randomised trial. Lancet

MacKay DF, Smith GC, Dobbie R et al (2010) Gestational age at delivery and special educational need: retrospective cohort study of 407,503 schoolchildren. PLoS Med 7(6), e1000289

Marlow N (2007) Neurodevelopmental follow-up – what tests, when and why. Acta Paediatr 96:242–243

Marlow N (2014) Interpreting regional differences in neonatal outcomes for extremely preterm babies. Acta Paediatr 103(1):4–5

Marlow N, Wolke D, Bracewell MA et al (2005) Neurologic and developmental disability at six years of age after extremely preterm birth. N Engl J Med 352 (1):9–19

Marlow N, Bennett C, Draper ES et al (2014) Perinatal outcomes for extremely preterm babies in relation to place of birth in England: the EPICure 2 study. Arch Dis Child Fetal Neonatal Ed 99(3): F181–F188

Mathiasen R, Hansen BM, Andersen AM et al (2010) Gestational age and basic school achievements: a national follow-up study in Denmark. Pediatrics 126(6):e1553–e1561

Moore T, Hennessy EM, Myles J et al (2012) Neurological and developmental outcome in extremely preterm children born in England in 1995 and 2006: the EPICure studies. BMJ 345, e7961

Morsing E, Asard M, Ley D et al (2011) Cognitive function after intrauterine growth restriction and very preterm birth. Pediatrics 127(4):e874–e882

Pharoah PO, Cooke T, Rosenbloom I et al (1987) Trends in birth prevalence of cerebral palsy. Arch Dis Child 62(4):379–384

Report of a BAPM/RCPCH Working Group (2008) Classification of Health Status at 2 years as a perinatal outcome. BAPM, London

Rysavy MA, Li L, Bell EF et al (2015) Between-hospital variation in treatment and outcomes in extremely preterm infants. N Engl J Med 372 (19):1801–1811

Sellier E, Platt MJ, Andersen GL et al (2016) Decreasing prevalence in cerebral palsy: a multi-site European population-based study, 1980 to 2003. Dev Med Child Neurol 58(1):85–92

Serenius F, Sjors G, Blennow M et al (2014) EXPRESS study shows significant regional differences in 1-year outcome of extremely preterm infants in Sweden. Acta Paediatr 103(1):27–37

Stewart AL, Reynolds EO, Lipscomb AP (1981) Outcome for infants of very low birthweight: survey of world literature. Lancet 1(8228):1038–1040

Surman G, Hemming K, Platt MJ et al (2009) Children with cerebral palsy: severity and trends over time. Paediatr Perinat Epidemiol 23(6):513–521

Tin W, Wariyar UK, Hey EN (1997) Selection biases invalidate current low birthweight weight-for-gestation standards. The Northern Neonatal Network. Br J Obstet Gynaecol 104(2):180–185

Watson SI, Arulampalam W, Petrou S et al (2014) The effects of designation and volume of neonatal care on mortality and morbidity outcomes of very preterm infants in England: retrospective population-based cohort study. BMJ Open 4(7), e004856

Wolke D, Sohne B, Ohrt B et al (1995) Follow-up of preterm children: important to document dropouts. Lancet 345(8947):447

Wolke D, Schulz J, Meyer R (2001) Entwicklungslangzeitfolgen bei ehemaligen, sehr unreifen Frühgeborenen. Monatsschr Kinderheilkd 149(Suppl 1):53–61

Wood NS, Marlow N, Costeloe K et al (2000) Neurologic and developmental disability after extremely preterm birth. EPICure Study Group. N Engl J Med 343(6):378–384

Neuromuscular Disorders in Newborns

134

Salvatore Grosso and Silvia Ferranti

Contents

S. Grosso (✉) · S. Ferranti
Department of Molecular Medicine and Development,
University of Siena, Siena, Italy,
e-mail: salvatore.grosso@unisi.it; grosso@unisi.it;
silvia.ferranti@hotmail.it

G. Buonocore et al. (eds.), *Neonatology*,
https://doi.org/10.1007/978-3-319-29489-6_281

Abstract
Neuromuscular disorders (NDs) are important causes of neonatal weakness and hypotonia. They are pathogenetically related to primitive disorders of the motor unit. They can be acquired or genetically determined, and inherited according to various models of inheritance. NDs with neonatal onset have great clinical variability in severity ranging from fatal to mild pictures. Weakness, generalized or localized to a peculiar district (i.e., facial muscles), and hypotonia are cardinal features. Diagnostic workup includes serum creatine kinase level analysis, motor nerve conduction investigation, electromyography, and muscle biopsy. In neonates indications for muscle biopsy should be carefully evaluated as several limitations there exist. It could be considered in those patients in whom diagnosis is still lacking in spite of several laboratory investigations.

134.1 Salient Points

- Neuromuscular disorders are important causes of neonatal weakness and hypotonia; they are caused by pathological changes affecting the motor unit.
- Congenital myopathies are a heterogeneous group of genetic muscle disorders characterized by generalized weakness manifesting at birth or during the first months of life, hypotonia, hypoactive deep tendon reflexes, reduced muscle bulk, intact sensation, absence of cardiac involvement, and normal cognitive development.
- Congenital muscular dystrophies are a group of genetically and clinically heterogeneous hereditary muscular diseases. These are characterized by weakness with a dystrophic pattern on muscle biopsy and are present at birth or become manifest during the first months of life.
- Metabolic myopathies (e.g., Pompe disease and mitochondrial myopathies) are disorders with prominent involvement of muscle and with neonatal onset.
- Diagnosis is commonly reached through integration of the clinical examination and biochemical data, motor nerve conduction studies, electromyography, and muscle biopsy.

134.2 Introduction

Neuromuscular disorders (NDs) are important causes of neonatal weakness and hypotonia. They are caused by pathological changes affecting the motor unit, which anatomically includes a motor neuron, its axon, the neuromuscular junction, and all the muscle fibers innervated by that single neuron (Dubowitz 1995). They can be acquired or genetically determined and inherited according to various models of inheritance (Volpe 2008a, b). Chief laboratory investigations include: (i) serum creatine kinase (CK) levels, which can be normal in some congenital dystrophies or myopathies-moreover high CK levels are commonly observed during the first few days of life after vaginal delivery, reflecting muscle damage during labor; (ii) motor nerve conduction studies, which may detect a disorder of the peripheral nerve; (iii) electromyography, which provides information about every level of motor unit, is generally obtained with the muscle at rest and with spontaneous or elicited contractions, but it may be difficult to be interpreted as severely hypotonic neonates make few spontaneous movements; (iv) muscle biopsy is often a crucial diagnostic procedure; indications for muscle biopsy should be carefully considered in patients in whom the diagnosis remains uncertain in spite of laboratory, electrophysiological, and DNA analysis investigations (Volpe 2008a, b).

134.3 Congenital Myopathies (CM)

Congenital myopathies are a heterogeneous group of genetic muscle disorders characterized by distinctive and specific morphological abnormalities of muscle fiber architecture on light and/or electron microscopy. Pathological changes are located within the myofiber (North 2008). Histological classification was previously based on the major morphological features seen on muscle biopsy (rods, cores, central nuclei, selective hypotrophy of type I fibers). Nowadays, the genetic basis of many of these forms has been identified. The relationship between each congenital myopathy, defined on histological grounds, and the genetic cause, is complex because (i) many of the CMs can be caused by mutations in more than one gene (genetic heterogeneity), (ii) mutation of the same gene can cause different CMs, (iii) the same genetic mutation can lead to different pathological features in members of the same family or in the same individual at different ages (North et al. 2014).

Main clinical features include generalized weakness manifesting at birth or in the first months of life, hypotonia, hypoactive deep tendon reflexes, reduced muscle bulk, intact sensation, absence of cardiac involvement and normal cognitive development. Prominent facial weakness with or without ptosis, long narrow face and high-arched palate are frequent findings; clinical course is slowly progressive (Romero and Clarke 2013; North et al. 2014). A common histological feature is predominance of type I fibers that are however smaller than type II fibers (Fenichel 2009). Serum CK levels are commonly normal and the EMG is typically normal or mildly myopathic.

134.3.1 Central Core Disease (CCD)

Etiology and Pathogenesis AD and rarely AR mutation of RYR1 gene (19q12-13.2) that encodes the transmembrane domain of the skeletal muscle ryanodine receptor. This calcium channel is located in the sarcoplasmic reticulum and is involved in the excitation-contraction mechanism (Laing et al. 2007). Three main clinical patterns can be identified: congenital form, juvenile form, and malignant hyperthermia triggered by anesthetics administration (Fenichel 2009; Zuccotti and Giovannini 2012).

Clinical Picture Decreased fetal movements during pregnancy, breech presentation, early-onset hypotonia, weakness mainly affecting proximal limb muscles, more pronounced in the upper than in the lower extremities, delayed motor development mainly involving walking acquisition, hip dislocation, contractures, and kyphoscoliosis (Zhou et al. 2006, 2007).

Investigations Muscular biopsy shows cores, i.e., single or multiple well-defined rounded unstained lesions on oxidative stains, classically located in the central portion of the sarcomeres or under the sarcolemma. They are immunohistochemically characterized by increased RYR-1 protein, desmin, vimentin, tubulin, and developmental myosin heavy chain (Sharma et al. 2009). These areas of oxidative enzyme deficiency may be rimmed by a darker staining zone that may also be positive for desmin. Cores may be more than one per fiber and they extend down an appreciable length of the fibers (North et al. 2014).

The role of muscle MR imaging in the diagnosis of CCD has been emphasized (Jungbluth et al. 2004).

Differential Diagnosis In the neonatal period, classical histopathological anomalies may be lacking, and differential diagnosis with multiminicore disease may be difficult. Peculiar clinical features such as external ophthalmoplegia and respiratory impairment, commonly lacking in CCD, may help in differentiation (Sharma et al. 2009, Zhou et al. 2007). Nemaline myopathy (NM) with mutations in the ACTA1 gene has also been associated with both central cores and minicores (Kaindl et al. 2004).

134.3.2 Nemaline Myopathy (NM)

Nemaline myopathy is the most common form of CM.

Etiology and Pathogenesis Heterogeneous inheritance: 50% sporadic, 20% AD, and 30% AR. Mutations can involve eight different genes: NEM1 (TPM3: slow α-tropomyosin), NEM2 (NEB: nebulin), NEM3 (ACTA1: α-actin), NEM4 (TPM2: β-tropomyosin), NEM5 (TNNT1: slow skeletal muscle troponin T), NEM6 (KBTBD13: Kelch repeat and BTB domain containing 13), NEM7 (CFL2: skeletal muscle cofilin-2), NEM8 (KLHL40: Kelch-like family member 40); the most common forms are NEM2 and NEM3 (North et al. 2014; Laing et al. 2007; Sharma et al. 2009; Wallgren-Pettersson and Laing 2006; Wallgren-Pettersson et al. 2004, 2011 Wallgren-Pettersson and Laing 1996; Ravenscroft et al. 2013).

Clinical Picture Six different clinical forms, with three of them presenting in the neonatal period:

(i) *Typical Congenital NM:* characterized by hypotonia and weakness, ogival palate, pectus carinatum, and micrognathia.
(ii) *Severe Congenital NM:* characterized by rapid respiratory insufficiency, lack of muscular movements, arthrogryposis multiplex and sometimes fractures. Polyhydramnios, decreased fetal movements and abnormal fetal presentation or fetal distress can occur.
(iii) *Intermediate Congenital NM:* similar to the severe form, but the neonate is able to perform spontaneous movements and does not develop severe contractures or respiratory insufficiency (Volpe 2008b; Wallgren-Pettersson and Laing 1996; Ryan et al. 2001).

The severe and intermediate forms have a poor prognosis; mortality within the first year of life is directly related to respiratory insufficiency at delivery and the presence of arthrogryposis multiplex congenita (Volpe 2008b; Wallgren-Pettersson and Laing 1996; Ryan et al. 2001).

Investigations Muscular biopsy shows dense red-purple threadlike inclusions on modified Gomori trichrome stain and dense bodies on EM (Figs. 1 and 2). The greatest concentration of particles is under the sarcolemma; in a rare subtype of nemaline myopathy called intranuclear rod myopathy (IRM), nemaline bodies are present inside myonuclei. They may be restricted to type I fibers and occur in peripheral clusters, in lines, or scattered through fibers. Their shape can be rod-like or ovoid and filaments may be attached to them. Type I fibers predominance is a prominent feature (Volpe 2008b; North et al. 2014; Buonocore et al. 1993; Tanner et al. 1998).

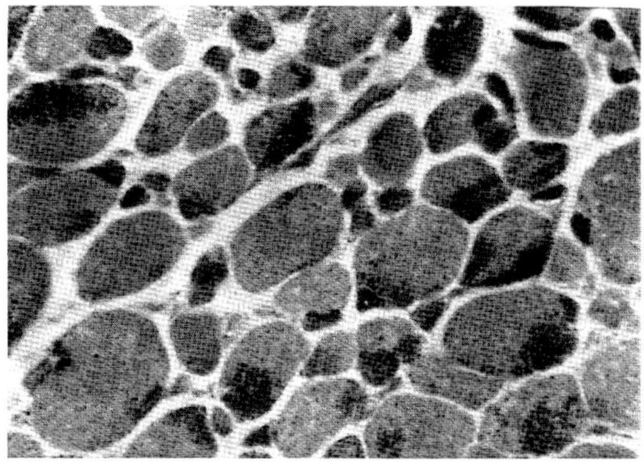

Fig. 1 900X. Gomori's trichrome reaction, transverse section. Presence of numerous typical rod-shaped bodies (Kaindl et al. 2004)

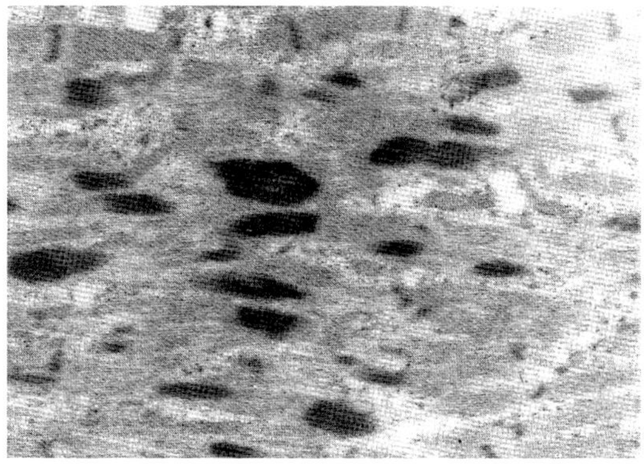

Fig. 2 14,000X. Longitudinal view of a fiber with several nemaline bodies measuring 3–5 μm in length and 1–2 μm in width

CK is normal or mildly elevated and EMG is myopathic.

134.3.3 Myotubular Myopathy (MM)

Etiology and Pathogenesis AD, AR, X-linked inheritance. Neonatal form is caused by X-linked recessive mutations in MTM1 gene encoding myotubularin (XLMTM), which belongs to the family of tyrosine phosphatases (Volpe 2008b; Laing et al. 2007; Jungbluth et al. 2008). It is involved in signal transduction between nucleus and cytoplasm and likely has a role in the cellular differentiation and development. More than 300 MTM1 mutations have been identified to date.

Clinical Picture Males show a severe phenotype with frequent antenatal onset (reduced fetal movements and polyhydramnios), profound hypotonia and weakness at birth, and respiratory and bulbar involvement requiring invasive ventilation and nasogastric tube feeding. Marked facial weakness, extraocular muscle involvement including ptosis and ophthalmoplegia, high-arched palate, micrognathia, clubfeet, joint contractures, arthrogryposis multiplex, and cryptorchidism are typical. Macrosomia suggesting overgrowth syndrome is frequently observed. Thinning of the ribs on chest X-rays has been reported. It is usually fatal within the first year. Only a proportion of affected males survive into their teens or beyond; however, motor outcome is poor as many of them are bedridden or wheelchair-bound (Jungbluth et al. 2011).

Investigations Muscular biopsy shows type I fibers predominance and hypotrophy. There is an apparent arrest in the morphogenesis of the muscle fiber at the myotube stage (8–15 weeks' gestation). The central areas of the fibers surrounding the nuclei display an increased glycogen staining and a decreased myofibrillar ATPase reaction. Electron microscopy shows central areas of fibers occupied by aggregated mitochondria and glycogen particles whereas myofilaments are reduced within these areas and confined to the periphery of the myofiber. Immunohistochemical studies demonstrate increased signal from myofibers with antibodies to proteins such as vimentin, desmin, neural cell adhesion molecule, and utrophin, probably related to the immaturity of myofibers (Wallgren-Pettersson 2000; Mercuri and Dubowitz 2008).

CK is normal or mildly increased and EMG is myopathic.

134.3.4 Congenital Fiber-Type Disproportion (CFTD)

Etiology and Pathogenesis Sporadic or familial inheritance, due to mutations of genes TPM3, RYR1, ACTA1, TPM2 and SEPN1.

Clinical Picture The onset is at birth or within the first year of life and is defined by hypotonia and mild-to-severe generalized muscle weakness of limbs, neck and face. Bulbar signs, extraocular muscle involvement, and respiratory failure can occur at any age. Neonatal disability may be severe with contractures of the hips, knees, ankles, elbows, and fingers. The course of the disorder is variable, and some individuals may be able to walk.

Investigations Muscular biopsy shows type I fibers predominance and hypoplasia – they are at least 12% smaller than type IIA and IIB muscle fibers diameter in the absence of other structural abnormalities. Fiber-type disproportion can occur in a variety of diseases such as neurogenic atrophy, other congenital myopathies, muscular dystrophies, Lowe's syndrome, polymyositis, rigid spine syndrome, Cockayne's syndrome. Its existence as an independent entity has therefore been questioned.

CK is mildly increased (Volpe 2008b; North 2008; North et al. 2014; Laing et al. 2007; Mercuri and Dubowitz 2008; Kissiedu and Prayson 2016).

134.3.5 Multi-Minicore Disease (MmD)

MmD has a wide clinical spectrum with four distinct phenotypes: a classic form, a form with external ophthalmoplegia, a moderate form with hand involvement, and a severe neonatal form. Recent studies have shown a significant overlap between the last three forms, due to common RYR1 involvement compared to a more prominent SEPN1 mutation in the classic subtype.

Etiology and Pathogenesis Sporadic and AR mutations of both SEPN1 (selenoprotein) and RYR1 (ryanodine receptor) genes.

Clinical Picture The classic form is characterized by onset during the neonatal period or within the first year of life with a peculiar slow course. Typical features include hypotonia, subtle or only slowly progressive generalized weakness mostly affecting proximal muscles, particularly of the shoulder girdle, early spinal rigidity, scoliosis, and respiratory impairment. Feeding difficulties with failure to thrive, high-pitched voice, and myopathic facial features are common. Respiratory failure may lead to secondary right ventricular failure and is often grossly out of proportion to the overall degree of weakness.

Investigations Muscular biopsy shows focal, poorly delimited small zones of sarcomeric disorganization lacking mitochondria in muscle fibers, affecting both types I and II fibers. On electron microscopy, they consist of small areas of Z-line streaming and myofibrillar disruption extending a small number of sarcomeres. There is type I fibers predominance (Volpe 2008b; North 2008; Laing et al. 2007; Jungbluth et al. 2011; Mercuri and Dubowitz 2008).

134.4 Congenital Muscular Dystrophies

Congenital muscular dystrophies (CMDs) are a group of genetically and clinically heterogeneous hereditary muscular diseases with a predominantly AR model of inheritance. Weakness and dystrophic pattern on muscle biopsy are present at birth or emerge during the first months of life. Muscular biopsy shows great variability in size of muscle fibers, marked endomysial and perimysial proliferation, and later increase of adipose tissue; internal nuclei and necrotic as well as regenerating fibers are seen. In comparison with muscular dystrophies with later onset, muscle weakness tends to be more stable overall. Patients may have CNS and ocular changes. A classification of CMDs based on biochemical and genetic defects has been proposed and is continuously updated. While disorders with normal mental development are mostly caused by genetic defects of extracellular matrix proteins or proteins of the endoplasmic reticulum, CMDs with brain involvement are commonly due to defects of glycosylation of α-dystroglycan. It may be practical to define CMDs according to the involvement of the CNS and the presence or absence of merosin (Mercuri and Dubowitz 2008; Muntoni et al. 2008; Reed 2009a, b; Kirschner 2013).

134.4.1 Merosin-Negative CMD (MDC1A)

MDC1A accounts for 22–30% of the CMDs.

Etiology and Pathogenesis The disease is due to mutations of the LAMA2 gene that codes for merosin, also called laminin α-2. It is a critical α-dystroglycan binding, basement membrane protein of the muscle extracellular matrix. It is also expressed in the basal lamina of the cerebral blood vessels and Schwann cells, explaining the pathological changes seen in muscle, heart, and central and peripheral nervous systems. The clinical manifestations of LAMA2-related muscular dystrophy are highly variable, ranging from severe early-onset CMD (referred to as MDC1A) to mild, later childhood-onset limb-girdle-type muscular dystrophy.

Clinical Picture Patients with complete deficiency present with marked hypotonia and weakness of the extremities, with possible worsening in the first weeks of life precluding independent ambulation. Muscle atrophy, facial weakness and dysmorphism, impaired chewing and swallowing are typically observed; arthrogryposis may be present. In one third of patients, death supervenes during the first year due to cardiopulmonary complications. Cognitive impairment, neuronal migration defects, mainly in the occipital cortex, and seizures (30% of patients) have been reported. A peripheral demyelinating neuropathy affecting predominantly motor fibers has been described. Patients with partial deficiency present a later onset and a slowly progressive disease that does not preclude the achievement of independent walking.

Investigations Muscular biopsy shows a dystrophic process with fiber necrosis and regeneration. Complete absence of laminin α-2 staining on muscle or skin biopsy is common, and, in general, is associated with a more severe phenotype compared to partial deficiency.

CK is markedly raised and EMG shows a myopathy. Brain MRI shows periventricular and subcortical high signals in white matter on T2-weighted and FLAIR images; these findings are most obvious in patients greater than 6 months of age (Volpe 2008b; Mercuri and Dubowitz 2008; Kissiedu and Prayson 2016; Muntoni et al. 2008; Reed 2009a, b; Beytía Mde et al. 2014; Bönnemann et al. 2014).

134.4.2 Congenital Muscular Dystrophies with Structural Anomalies of the Central Nervous System (α-Dystroglycanopathies)

They are a heterogeneous group of muscular dystrophies associated with central nervous system (disorders of neural migration, cerebral white matter abnormalities, and hindbrain anomalies) and more rarely eye pathology.

Etiology and Pathogenesis AR, due to eight genes (DPM3, DPM2, POMT1, POMT2, POMGNT1, LARGE, FKTN, FKRP), which encode specific or putative glycosyltransferases involved in the glycosylation of the α-dystroglycan. Its reduced glycosylation is associated with a decreased binding capacity.

Clinical Picture

(i) *Fukuyama Congenital Muscular Dystrophy (FCMD)*

FCMD mostly occurs in Japan, and it represents the most common AR disorder in the Japanese population. Clinical picture includes poor fetal movements, impaired respiration, generalized weakness, hypotonia, facial weakness, joint contractures, hypertrophy of the calves, quadriceps, and tongue muscles. Profound delay of motor development, mostly precluding independent ambulation, is typical. Dilative cardiomyopathy may develop later. Severe mental retardation and seizures are present. CNS abnormalities are represented by cerebral and cerebellar micropolygyria, obstructive hydrocephalus, occipital cobblestone cortex, hypoplasia of the pons and cerebellar vermis, cerebellar cysts, fibroglial proliferation of the leptomeninx, focal interhemispheric fusion, and hypoplasia of the corticospinal tracts. Ocular changes include retinal anomalies with folding, fusion, focal dysplasia and detachment, abnormal eye movements, myopia, and microphthalmia (Volpe 2008b; Mercuri and Dubowitz 2008; Reed 2009a; Kirschner 2013; Yoshioka et al. 1991).

(ii) *Walker-Warburg Syndrome (WWS)*

Walker-Warburg Syndrome is the most severe of CMDs; it shows an AR inheritance. Neonatal generalized weakness and hypotonia are associated with brain malformations (lissencephaly type II, prenatal obstructive hydrocephalus, neuronal band heterotopias, corpus callosum agenesis, pontocerebellar hypoplasia, intraventricular hemorrhage, cerebellar polymicrogyria, collicular fusion, fusion of occipital poles, and sporadically occipital encephalocele and Dandy-Walker cyst). Ocular changes involve both anterior and posterior chamber (retinal detachment, blindness, microphthalmia, optic nerves heterotopia, colobomas, congenital glaucoma, cataract, and megalocornea). Genital anomalies in males, macrocephaly or microcephaly and facial dysmorphisms with cleft lip or palate, have been reported. Affected children do not reach any motor or mental milestones and commonly present seizures and need gastric tube feeding. Death usually supervenes before 3 years of age (Volpe 2008b; Mercuri and Dubowitz 2008; Reed 2009a; Muntoni and Voit 2005; Voit 1998; Lee 2014).

(iii) *Muscle-Eye-Brain Disease (MEB)*

Initially reported in Finland, MEB is now recognized worldwide. Although it is less severe than WWS, the spectrum of clinical severity is broad, including patients with a WWS-like phenotype. Ocular defects include high myopia, congenital glaucoma, optic nerve hypoplasia, retinal dysplasia, coloboma of the optic nerve, and cataracts. CNS abnormalities are represented by cortical malformations including pachygyria, polymicrogyria, agyria, cobblestone dysplasia, associated with flat and kinking brainstem, cerebellar hypoplasia and cysts, and white matter abnormalities. Hydrocephalus, seizures, and facial dysmorphisms (short nasal bridge, micrognathia, and midface hypoplasia) have been reported. The clinical course is variable, ranging from patients being able to walk and speak to others presenting with severe motor and cognitive delay (Reed 2009a, b; Yiş et al. 2014).

Investigations CK is increased, but normal values do not exclude the diagnosis. EMG shows a myopathy (Volpe 2008b; Mercuri and Dubowitz 2008; Muntoni et al. 2008; Reed 2009a, b; Muntoni and Voit 2005; Godfrey et al. 2011).

134.4.3 Congenital Myotonic Dystrophy

Myotonic dystrophies are AD, multisystem diseases characterized by progressive myopathy, myotonia and multiorgan involvement. Two distinct forms caused by similar mutations have been described: DM1 (that can be divided into four main categories, including the congenital form) and DM2 (Meola and Cardani 2015).

Etiology and Pathogenesis Congenital myotonic dystrophy is caused by mutations in DMPK gene (19q13) which encodes for myotonin protein kinase and contains an unstable CTG trinucleotide. In normal people CTG repeats range from 5 to 34; these patients have larger, up to several thousands, CTG repeats. The mother is usually the parent who transmits the larger repeat, but transmission by the father has been reported (Zeesman et al. 2002). There is genetic anticipation. Repeat expansion length is predictive of clinical severity and age of onset. However, due to somatic mosaicism, CTG size correlates more significantly with age of onset and disease severity below 400 CTG repeats (Mercuri and Longman 2005).

Clinical Picture CMT includes a severe and a mild form.

(i) *Cmt1 Severe Form*

The clinical picture includes polyhydramnios, reduced fetal movements, preterm delivery, severe generalized weakness, hypotonia, arthrogryposis, especially of lower extremities, feeding difficulties and respiratory insufficiency requiring mechanical ventilatory support. Facial diplegia, with tent-shaped upper lip and carp mouth, is constant. Areflexia and atrophy are common. In neonates percussion myotonia, where percussion of a muscle evokes a myotonic phenomenon, is elicited only sporadically. Severity of the clinical course is consistent with the clinical picture at onset. Neonatal mortality is high, up to 40%, and mainly due to respiratory failure. Surviving patients experience gradual improvement in motor function; almost all CMD children are able to walk after the age of 2 years. Cognitive and motor milestones are however delayed and all patients develop learning difficulties (Mercuri and Longman 2005).

(ii) *Cmt1 Mild Form*

Gestational age is normal and polyhydramnios is infrequent. Feeding and swallowing difficulties, generalized hypotonia, and arthrogryposis are present. No respiratory distress is seen.

A careful examination of the mother may show typical myotonic facies with ptosis, atrophy of the masseter and temporalis muscle, and percussion myotonia. Presenile cataract, frontal baldness, and gonadal atrophy may also be seen in affected family members (Mercuri and Dubowitz 2008; Reed 2009a; Meola and Cardani 2015).

134.4.4 Collagen VI-Related Disorders

Mutations in each of the three collagen VI genes COL6A1, COL6A2, COL6A3 – that encode, respectively, the α1, α2, and α3 chains of collagen VI – cause two types of muscle disorders that probably form a clinical spectrum: (i) Bethlem myopathy, with a mild or moderate phenotype and (ii) Ullrich CMD, with a severe phenotype.

(i) *Bethlem Myopathy:*

Etiology and Pathogenesis AD inheritance; COL6A1 is the most commonly involved gene.

Clinical Picture The onset may be in the neonatal period, childhood, or adolescence; disease is slowly progressive. Early contractures of the interphalangeal joints of the fingers, elbows, and ankles represent a hallmark. Follicular hyperkeratosis and keloid formation can be present.

Investigations Histopathological findings on muscle biopsy are nonspecific and compatible with dystrophic changes. Immunohistochemistry with Col VI antibodies can be normal in the muscle; only the fibroblast culture offers conclusive results for the diagnosis. CK levels are normal or mildly elevated.

(ii) *Ullrich CMD:*

Etiology and Pathogenesis AR or AD inheritance.

Clinical Picture Majority of patients have the classic severe form that includes neonatal weakness, proximal joint contractures, hyperlaxity of the distal joints, failure to thrive, lack of independent ambulation, and severe respiratory impairment by the end of the first decade of life. Intelligence is normal. Follicular hyperkeratosis, "sandpaper" papular rash, hyperhidrosis, keloids, congenital hip dislocation, torticollis, prominent ears, facial weakness, high-arched palate, prominent heels, and scoliosis can be present.

Investigations Muscular biopsy shows typical, generally marked, dystrophic pattern. The immunohistochemical analysis of collagen VI in muscle biopsies shows decreased immunolabelling, but the most secure and helpful immunohistochemical analysis of collagen VI is in skin fibroblasts cultures. CK levels can be normal or increased (Reed 2009a).

134.5 Metabolic Myopathies

Disorders with prominent involvement of muscle and neonatal onset mainly include defects of glycogen metabolism and respiratory chain.

134.5.1 Pompe Disease (PD)

Etiology and Pathogenesis It is a lysosomal storage disease (glycogen storage disease type II) caused by the absence or deficiency of the acid α-glucosidase (GAA, also called acid maltase), an enzyme that is responsible for the cleavage of the α-1,4- and α-1,6-glycosidic bonds of glycogen to glucose.

Clinical Picture Accumulation of glycogen occurs in several tissues but cardiac and skeletal muscle manifestations are predominant. The classic infantile form manifests at birth with severe muscle weakness, hypotonia, and hypertrophic cardiomyopathy. Macroglossia, hepatomegaly, feeding difficulties, and significant delay in motor milestones are typically seen in the rapidly progressive form. Respiratory muscle weakness and cardiomegaly frequently lead to death before the end of the first year. In the nonclassical infantile form clinical manifestations are milder and do not include respiratory insufficiency and cardiac involvement, allowing longer survival. The clinical phenotype may mimic SMA1.

The disease is detectable by newborn screening. It is the first metabolic myopathy for which corrective targeted enzyme replacement therapy with recombinant human precursor (acid α-glucosidase) has become available (Volpe 2008a, b; Lim et al. 2014).

134.5.2 Mitochondrial Myopathies (MM)

Etiology and Pathogenesis MM are highly heterogeneous conditions related to mitochondrial DNA or nuclear DNA mutations with defects of oxidative phosphorylation. They are generally multisystem and affect highly aerobic postmitotic tissues, such as muscle and nerve.

Clinical Picture Autosomal recessive inherited defects of cytochrome C oxidase may present with a neonatal myopathy syndrome. Cardinal clinical features are axial and facial weakness, hypotonia, and hypo/areflexia. Systemic involvement is also common with hepatomegaly, cardiomyopathy, and renal dysfunctions.

Investigations Lactic acidosis and the presence on muscle biopsy of ragged red fibers with cytochrome C deficiency are diagnostic (Volpe 2008b).

134.6 Myasthenia

134.6.1 Neonatal Myasthenia Gravis (NMG)

Etiology and Pathogenesis Neonatal myasthenia gravis is a transient disorder of neuromuscular transmission that occurs in 10–15% of newborns born to women with myasthenia gravis due to antibodies against acetylcholine receptor (AChR) and less frequently against muscle-specific kinase (MuSK) (Nogajski et al. 2009). NMG is related to the passive transfer of antibodies against AChR across the placenta, which is thought to be followed by decreasing AChR at the postsynaptic muscle membrane. Due to degradation of the maternally derived IgG, the effect upon the infant will usually be transient. Rarely the disorder persists, causing permanent disability. No correlation to maternal disease severity or absolute maternal Ab titers has been found, but transient NMG tends to recur in further pregnancies. Why NMG develops only 10–15% of infants born to MG mothers is unclear. The antibody epitope specificity of the mother has been suggested to be a major factor. There are two forms of AChR Ab that differ in one subunit: one is mainly directed at the fetal AChR, and the other is directed at the adult AChR found in mature end plates (Hacohen et al. 2014; Midelfart Hoff and Midelfart 2015).

Clinical Picture Clinical onset usually occurs within a few hours of birth or during the first 72 h. There may be facial diplegia with feeding, sucking and swallowing difficulties, generalized weakness, hypotonia, respiratory insufficiency, and inability to handle pharyngeal secretions. Symptoms are usually mild or moderate; respiratory support and tube feeding are only necessary in a few cases. Ptosis and oculomotor dysfunctions occur in a minority of patients. The most severely affected infants show arthrogryposis, polyhydramnios, pulmonary hypoplasia, and death (Midelfart Hoff and Midelfart 2015).

Investigations Repetitive nerve stimulation at 5–20 Hz typically shows a decrement in the amplitude of the motor action potential.

Treatment Neostigmine, an anticholinesterase, is the drug of choice. Initial doses of 0.04 mg/kg intramuscularly are followed by 0.4 mg/kg given by gastric tube. Exchange transfusion is ineffective. Few data are available on the efficacy of intravenous immunoglobulins (Volpe 2008a; Mercuri and Dubowitz 2008).

134.6.2 Non-Autoimmune Congenital Myasthenic Syndromes (CMSs)

Etiology and Pathogenesis These syndromes are inherited heterogeneous disorders affecting the neuromuscular junction. In most patients clinical onset is at birth or in early childhood. Classification is based on the site of neuromuscular transmission defect (presynaptic, synaptic, or postsynaptic), but accurate identification of the defect is not always possible. The most common causes of CMS are:

(i) Defects in the acetylcholine receptor (mainly primary AChR deficiency)
(ii) Mutations that affect end plate development and maintenance (mainly deficiency of rapsyn, a protein that concentrates and anchors the AChR in the postsynaptic membrane and is needed for the development of the junctional folds.)
(iii) Synaptic basal lamina associated
(iv) Presynaptic (mainly deficiency of choline acetyltransferase ChAT, which catalyzes the synthesis of Ach from acetyl coenzyme A and choline in cholinergic neurons. A diagnosis of this deficiency can be suggested by sudden episodes of apnea provoked by stress.)

Clinical Picture Although phenotypic variability exists among CMSs, several clinical features are shared by these disorders. Ptosis, ophthalmoplegia, early facial and bulbar involvement with feeding difficulties and respiratory failure, hypotonia, and weakness are common. Reduced fetal movements, arthrogryposis, and polyhydramnios may be observed. Peculiar clinical findings may occur in specific CMS syndromes (i.e., pupillary dysfunction is typical of end plate AChE deficiency).

Investigations They include single-fiber EMG, specific staining for AChR, electron microscopy or motor end plate, and molecular genetic studies.

Treatment Anticholinesterase drugs are crucial in the therapeutic strategy. 3,4-Diaminopyridine is effective in combination with anticholinesterase. Steroids and thymectomy are ineffective. Medication should be protracted since an interruption may lead to apnea and sudden death (Volpe 2008a; Mercuri and Dubowitz 2008; Nogajski et al. 2009; Middleton 1995; Ohno et al. 1999; Deymeer et al. 1999; Engel et al. 2015).

134.7 Spinal Muscular Atrophy (SMA)

Etiology and Pathogenesis Spinal muscular atrophies comprise a group of AR disorders characterized by loss of lower motor neurons in the anterior horn cells of the spinal cord and cranial nerve nuclei (Rudnick-Schoneborn et al. 1996). Consequent weakness is usually symmetrical and more proximal than distal, with lower limbs generally more affected than upper limbs (D'Amico et al. 2011). The gene for the SMA1 is located in 5q11-q13 and termed survival motor neuron (SMN). Each individual has two SMN genes, SMN1 and SMN2. More than 95% of patients with SMA1 have a homozygous mutation in the SMN1 gene (Lefebvre et al. 1995). SMN1 gene should be screened for mutation. Muscle biopsy should be considered in the diagnostic workup when genetic analysis is normal.

Clinical Picture It may include poor weight gain, sleep difficulties, scoliosis, joint contractures, restrictive lung disease, and constipation, with intelligence being unaffected. Five SMA subtypes exist with classification dependent upon milestones achieved (Carré and Empey 2016).

Type 0 (Prenatal) Presents in utero with lack of fetal movements, arthrogryposis, joint contractures, possible congenital bone fractures, and extremely thin ribs. It is the most severe form, fatal at birth unless treated (Carré and Empey 2016; MacLeod et al. 1999).

Type I (Werdnig-Hoffman Disease) The most common subtype of SMA (60–70% of SMA cases). It presents with axial and limb weakness and hypotonia at birth or in the first weeks of life. There is little spontaneous activity, which is limited to the feet and hands. Facial muscles are spared and the infant shows a normal bright expression; the extraocular muscles are not involved. Deep tendon reflexes are absent or diminished but sensitivity is preserved. Combination of diaphragm sparing with weakened intercostal muscles results in paradoxical breathing. The extensive paralysis of the limbs and distinctive breathing pattern are associated with the characteristic jug-handle posturing of the upper limbs with internal rotation of the shoulders and pronation of the forearms. The involvement of bulbar motor neurons is responsible for tongue fasciculations, poor sucking, and swallowing difficulty. Death from respiratory failure can occur before 18 months. With the use of respiratory support, life expectancy can be extended. (D'Amico et al. 2011; Carré and Empey 2016).

134.7.1 SMA Variants

Among variants of SMA, those with a potential neonatal onset include (i) SMA with respiratory distress type I (SMARD1) and (ii) SMA with pontocerebellar hypoplasia (PCH1).

(i) *SMARD1:* very rare AR motor neuron disease due to mutation of the gene coding for the immunoglobulin-binding protein 2 (IGHMBP2) located on chromosome 11q13 and implicated in transcription and pre-mRNA processing. Distinctive clinical features include low birth weight, diaphragmatic palsy, symmetrical distal muscular weakness, muscle atrophy, peripheral sensory neuropathy, autonomic nerve dysfunction, foot deformities, and limb contractures. The vast majority of patients die within the first 13 months of life. Peculiarly, respiratory distress in SMARD1 is the consequence of severe diaphragmatic paralysis with elevation of both hemidiaphragms on chest X-ray rather than the severe intercostal muscle impairment of SMA1 (MacLeod et al. 1999; Kaindl et al. 2008; Messina et al. 2012).

(ii) *PCH1:* extremely rare AR disease characterized by central and peripheral motor dysfunctions from birth; life span is short and ranges from a few hours to several months. Pontocerebellar hypoplasia and gliosis are seen in association with anterior horn cell degeneration. Severe respiratory complications, dysmorphism, hypotonia, deep tendon areflexia, nystagmus, microcephaly, and arthrogryposis multiplex congenita are described (Barth 1993; Rudnik-Schöneborn et al. 2003; Guillot et al. 2008).

References

Barth PG (1993) Pontocerebellar hypoplasia. An overview of a group of inherited neurodegenerative disorders with fetal onset. Brain Dev 15:411–422

Beytía Mde L, Dekomien G, Hoffjan S, Haug V, Anastasopoulos C, Kirschner J (2014) High creatine kinase levels and white matter changes: clinical and genetic spectrum of congenital muscular dystrophies with laminin alpha-2 deficiency. Mol Cell Probes 28(4):118–122

Bönnemann CG, Wang CH, Quijano-Roy S, Deconinck N, Bertini E, Ferreiro A, Muntoni F, Sewry C, Béroud C, Mathews KD, Moore SA, Bellini J, Rutkowski A, North KN (2014) Members of international standard of care committee for congenital muscular dystrophies. Diagnostic approach to the congenital muscular dystrophies. Neuromuscul Disord 24(4): 289–311

Buonocore G, Balestri P, Toti P et al (1993) A new case of severe congenital nemaline myopathy. Acta Paediatr 82:1082–1084

Carré A, Empey C (2016) Review of Spinal Muscular Atrophy (SMA) for prenatal and pediatric genetic counselors. J Genet Couns 25(1):32–43

D'Amico A, Mercuri E, Tiziano FD, Bertini E (2011) Spinal muscular atrophy. Orphanet J Rare Dis 6:71

Deymeer F, Serdaroglu R, Ozdemir C (1999) Familial infantile myasthenia: confusion in terminology. Neuromuscul Disord 9:129–130

Dubowitz V (1995) Muscle disorders in childhood. Saunders, London

Engel AG, Shen XM, Selcen D, Sine SM (2015) Congenital myasthenic syndromes: pathogenesis, diagnosis, and treatment. Lancet Neurol 14(4):420–434

Fenichel GM (2009) Clinical pediatric neurology. A signs and symptoms approach, Chapter 6. Saunder Elservier, Philadelphia

Godfrey C, Foley AR, Clement E, Muntoni F (2011) Dystroglycanopathies: coming into focus. Curr Opin Genet Dev 21(3):278–285

Guillot N, Cuisset JM, Cuvellier JC, Hurtevent JF, Joriot S, Vallee L (2008) Unusual clinical features in infantile Spinal Muscular Atrophies. Brain Dev 30 (3):169–178

Hacohen Y, Jacobson LW, Byrne S, Norwood F, Lall A, Robb S, Dilena R, Fumagalli M, Born AP, Clarke D, Lim M, Vincent A, Jungbluth H (2014) Fetal acetylcholine receptor inactivation syndrome: a myopathy due to maternal antibodies. Neurol Neuroimmunol Neuroinflamm 2(1):e57

Jungbluth H, Davis MR, Muller C et al (2004) Magnetic resonance imaging of muscle in congenital myopathies associated with *RYR1* mutations. Neuromuscul Disord 14:785–790

Jungbluth H, Wallgren-Pettersson C, Laporte J (2008) Centronuclear (myotubular) myopathy. Orphanet J Rare Dis 3:26

Jungbluth H, Sewry CA, Muntoni F (2011) Core myopathies. Semin Pediatr Neurol 18(4):239–249. Review

Kaindl AM, Ruschendorf F, Krause S et al (2004) Missense mutations of ACTA1 cause dominant congenital myopathy with cores. J Med Genet 41:842–848

Kaindl AM, Guenther UP, Rudnik-Schöneborn S et al (2008) Spinal muscular atrophy with respiratory distress type 1 (SMARD1). J Child Neurol 23:199–204

Kirschner J (2013) Congenital muscular dystrophies. Handb Clin Neurol 113:1377–1385

Kissiedu J, Prayson RA (2016) Congenital fiber type disproportion. J Clin Neurosci 26:136–7

Laing NG, Sewry CA, Lamont P (2007) Congenital myopathies. Handb Clin Neurol 86:1–33

Lee CY (2014) Walker-Warburg syndrome: rare congenital muscular dystrophy associated with brain and eye abnormalities. Hong Kong Med J 20(6):556.e4–556.e5

Lefebvre S, Biirglen L, Reboullet S et al (1995) Identification and characterization of a spinal muscular atrophy-determining gene. Cell 13(80):1–5

Lim JA, Li L, Raben N (2014) Pompe disease: from pathophysiology to therapy and back again. Front Aging Neurosci 6:177

MacLeod MJ, Taylor JE, Lunt PW et al (1999) Prenatal onset spinal muscular atrophy. Eur J Paediatr Neurol 3:65–72

Meola G, Cardani R (2015) Myotonic dystrophies: an update on clinical aspects, genetic, pathology, and molecular pathomechanisms. Biochim Biophys Acta 1852(4):594–606

Mercuri E, Dubowitz V (2008) Neuromuscular disorders. In: Levine MI, Chervenak FA (eds) Fetal and neonatal neurology and neurosurgery. Churchill Livingston Elsevier, Philadelphia, pp 792–809

Mercuri E, Longman C (2005) Congenital muscular dystrophy. Pediatr Ann 34:564–568

Messina MF, Messina S, Gaeta M, Rodolico C, Salpietro Damiano AM, Lombardo F, Crisafulli G, De Luca F (2012) Infantile spinal muscular atrophy with respiratory distress type I (SMARD 1): an atypical phenotype and review of the literature. Eur J Paediatr Neurol 16(1):90–94

Middleton LT (1995) Report on the 34th ENMC international workshop – congenital myasthenia syndromes. Neuromuscul Disord 6:133–136

Midelfart Hoff J, Midelfart A (2015) Maternal myasthenia gravis: a cause for arthrogryposis multiplex congenita. J Child Orthop 9(6):433–5

Muntoni F, Voit T (2005) 133rd ENMC international workshop on congenital muscular dystrophy (IXth international CMD workshop) 21–23 January 2005, Naarden. The Netherlands. Neuromuscul Disord 15:794–801

Muntoni F, Torelli S, Brockington M (2008) Muscular dystrophies due to glycosylation defects. Neurotherapeutics 5:627–632

Nogajski JH, Kiernan MC, Ouvrier RA, Andrews PI et al (2009) Congenital myasthenic syndromes. J Clin Neurosci 16:1–11

North K (2008) What's new in congenital myopathies? Neuromuscul Disord 18:433–442

North KN, Wang CH, Clarke N, Jungbluth H, Vainzof M, Dowling JJ, Amburgey K, Quijano-Roy S, Beggs AH, Sewry C, Laing NG, Bönnemann CG (2014) International standard of care committee for congenital myopathies. Approach to the diagnosis of congenital myopathies. Neuromuscul Disord 24(2):97–116

Ohno K, Anlar B, Engel AG (1999) Congenital myasthenic syndrome caused by a mutation in the Ets binding site of the promoter region of the acetylcoline receptor e subunit gene. Neuromuscul Disord 9:131–135

Ravenscroft G, Miyatake S, Lehtokari VL et al (2013) Mutations in KLHL40 are a frequent cause of severe autosomal-recessive nemaline myopathy. Am J Hum Genet 93(1):6–18

Reed UC (2009a) Congenital muscular dystrophy. Part I: a review of phenotypical and diagnostic aspects. Arq Neuropsiquiatr 67:144–168

Reed UC (2009b) Congenital muscular dystrophy. Part II: a review of pathogenesis and therapeutic perspectives. Arq Neuropsiquiatr 67:343–362

Romero NB, Clarke NF (2013) Congenital myopathies. Handb Clin Neurol 113:1321–1336. Review

Rudnick-Schoneborn FR, Hahnen E et al (1996) Clinical spectrum and diagnostic criteria of infantile spinal muscular atrophy: further delineation on the basis of 5MN deletion findings. Neuropediatrics 27:8–15

Rudnik-Schöneborn S, Sztriha L, Aithala GR, Houge G, Laegreid LM, Seeger J, Huppke M, Wirth B, Zerres K (2003) Extended phenotype of pontocerebellar hypoplasia with infantile spinal muscular atrophy. Am J Med Genet A 117A(1):10–17

Ryan MM, Schnell C, Strickland CD et al (2001) Nemaline myopathy: a clinical study of 143 cases. Ann Neurol 50:312–320

Sharma MC, Jain D, Sarkar C et al (2009) Congenital myopathies-a comprehensive update of recent advancements. Acta Neurol Scand 119:281–292

Tanner SM, Laporte J, Guiraurd-Chaumeil C et al (1998) Confirmation of prenatal diagnosis results of X-linked recessive myotubular myopathy by mutational screening and description of three new mutations in the *MTM1* gene. Hum Mutat 11:62–68

Voit T (1998) Congenital muscular dystrophies: 1997 update. Brain Dev 20:65–74

Volpe J (2008a) Neuromuscular disorders: levels above the lower motor neuron to the neuromuscular junction. In: Volpe J (ed) Neurology of the newborn. Saunders Elsevier, Philadelphia, pp 767–800

Volpe J (2008b) Neuromuscular disorders: muscle involvement and restricted disorders. In: Volpe J (ed) Neurology of the newborn. Saunders Elsevier, Philadelphia, pp 801–840

Wallgren-Pettersson C, Laing NG (1996) Nemaline myopathy. Neuromuscul Disord 6:389–391

Wallgren-Pettersson C (2000) 72nd ENMC international workshop: myotubular myopathy 1–3 October 1999, Hilversum, The Netherlands. Neuromuscul Disord 10:525–529

Wallgren-Pettersson C, Laing NG (2006) 138th ENMC workshop: nemaline myopathy, 20–22 May 2005, Naarden. The Netherlands. Neuromuscul Disord 16:54–60

Wallgren-Pettersson C, Pelin K, Nowack KJ et al (2004) ENMC international consortium on Nemaline myopathy. Genotype-phenotype correlations in nemaline myopathy caused by mutations in the genes for nebulin and skeletal muscle alpha-actin. Neuromuscul Disord 14:461–470

Wallgren-Pettersson C, Sewry CA, Nowak KJ, Laing NG (2011) Nemaline myopathies. Semin Pediatr Neurol 18(4):230–238

Yiş U, Uyanik G, Rosendahl DM, Carman KB, Bayram E, Heise M, Cömertpay G, Kurul SH (2014) Clinical, radiological, and genetic survey of patients with muscle-eye-brain disease caused by mutations in POMGNT1. Pediatr Neurol 50(5):491–497

Yoshioka M, Saiwai S, Kuroki S (1991) MR imaging of the brain in Fukuyama-type congenital muscular dystrophy. AJNR Am J Neuroradiol 12:63–65

Zeesman S, Carson N, Whelan DT (2002) Paternal transmission of the congenital form of myotonic dystrophy type 1: a new case and review of the literature. Am J Med Genet 107:222–226

Zhou H, Yamaguchi N, Xu L et al (2006) Characterization of recessiveRYR1mutations in core myopathies. Hum Mol Genet 15:2791–2803

Zhou H, Jungbluth H, Sewry CA et al (2007) Molecular mechanisms and phenotypic variation in RYR1-related congenital myopathies. Brain 130:2024–2036

Zuccotti GV, Giovannini M (2012) Manuale di Pediatria- la pratica clinica, Chapter 22. Societa' editrice Esculapio, Bologna

Part XIII

Ophthalmology, Orthopedics, and Skin Diseases

Ocular Malformations

135

Elena Piozzi and Alessandra Del Longo

Contents

E. Piozzi (✉) · A. Del Longo
Department of Pediatric Ophthalmology, Niguarda Ca' Granda Hospital, Milan, Italy
e-mail: elena.piozzi@ospedaleniguarda.it

Abstract

Ocular malformations are numerous: some are already evident at birth or during the first few months of life, while others show themselves at a later stage.

G. Buonocore et al. (eds.), *Neonatology*,
https://doi.org/10.1007/978-3-319-29489-6_282

Ocular malformations can be a sign of more complex and general pathologies, and the importance of early recognition should not be underestimated for those which can cause a damage to the vision and/or amblyopia (interruption of the development of the visual function).

Ocular malformations of the anterior segment are easily recognizable during examination, the ones of the posterior segment either are associated with the former or, more frequently, have as first symptom a constant or intermittent strabismus.

Differences in size, asymmetry, opening, and color between the two eyes should never be underestimated as they could be a sign of possible malformations.

The pediatrician is crucial and can help in a timely diagnosis of congenital eye pathologies and will recommend that the patient sees a specialist for further examination.

135.1 Salient Points

- Some ocular malformations are already evident at birth or become apparent during the first few months of life, others show themselves a later stage.
- Ocular malformations can be a sign of more complex and general pathologies.
- Differences in size, asymmetry, opening, and color between two eyes should never be underestimated as they could be signs of possible malformations.

135.2 Introduction

There are multiple ocular malformations: some are evident at birth or during the first few months of life, while others are revealed at a later stage.

Ocular malformations can be a sign of more complex and general pathology. The importance of early recognition is particularly important for those that can damage vision and/or cause amblyopia (interruption of the development of visual function).

Ocular malformations of the anterior segment are recognized at examination. Malformations of the posterior segment may present either because of their frequent association with anterior malformations or, more often, as a constant or intermittent strabismus.

It is important to be aware that possible serious ocular malformations may be indicated by asymmetry of the eyes, as well as by differences in their color and the sizes of the globes, irises, and palpebral fissures. Thus, the role of the pediatrician is crucial in the timely diagnosis of congenital eye pathologies and an appropriate specialist referral (Ricci 2006; Taylor 1990).

135.3 Eyelid Malformations

Eyelid development occurs in the second month of fetal life. Eyelid opening occurs during the fifth month of pregnancy as the development of the eyelid is completed. During the embryogenesis of these tissues, a series of pathological events may occur which cause development of eyelid position and lid margin anomalies.

135.3.1 Developmental Anomalies

135.3.1.1 Coloboma

Lack of tissue which causes a defect of the lid margin whose severity is proportional to the extension of the defect itself (Fig. 1).

It can be uni- or bilateral, symmetrical or asymmetrical, and isolated or associated with other alterations (Tawfik et al. 2015). Particularly, it can present itself with corneo-palpebral adhesion, dermoids, or syndromic forms (S. Tessier, S. Goldhenar and Fraser).

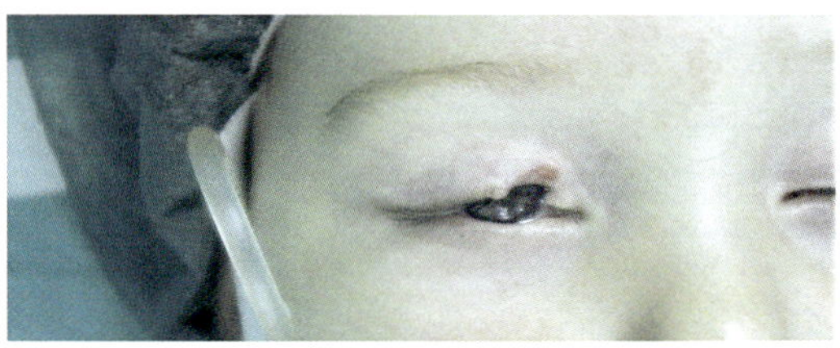

Fig. 1 Eyelid coloboma

It may affect the nasal half of the superior eyelid.

The lack of protection from the eyelid can cause a keratitis from being exposed.

The therapy can be medical or surgical.

In the presence of mild coloboma, it is sufficient to use lubricating ointments or eyedrops.

The severe forms need treatment from an oculoplastic surgeon to prevent corneal ulcers that can produce scar tissue with visual damage.

135.3.1.2 Epicanthus

Semilunar skinfold with a down-orientation toward the inner corner (canthus) that simulates a convergent strabismus (Fig. 2).

It is always present in Down syndrome.

This condition can simulate convergent squinting especially in lateral versions when the eye in adduction disappears behind the fold.

Extra attention must be given to those cases in which a strabismus could be disguised.

The surgical treatment is complex and needs multiple operations over various time periods.

135.3.2 Anomalies of the Rima (Palpebral Fissure)

135.3.2.1 Distichiasis

The condition is characterized by the growth a second row of eyelashes.

It affects more frequently the lower lid.

It can be isolated or hereditary (autosomal dominant).

If it affects the inner part of the lid margin, it causes corneal ulcers, lachrymation, and photophobia.

The therapy, in the presence of corneal involvement, is surgical.

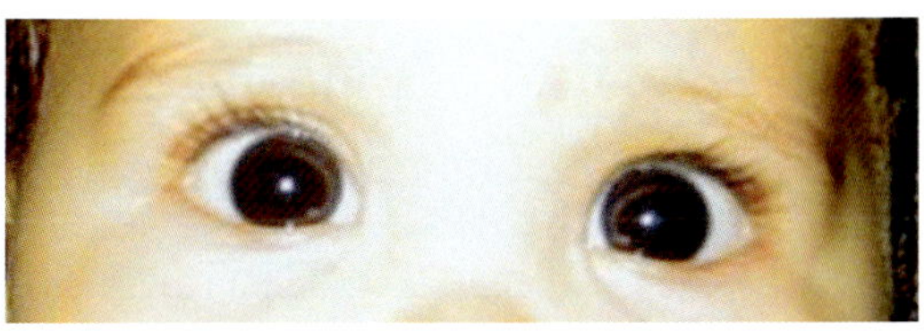

Fig. 2 Epicanthus

135.3.2.2 Blepharophimosis

This is a complex syndrome autosomal dominant characterized by multiple characteristic ocular abnormalities (Allen and Rubin 2008): telecanthus, epicanthus inversus, and horizontal shortening of the palpebral fissure (Fig. 3).

Two forms:

- Type 1 associated with early ovaric atrophy responsible for precocious menopause and infertility
- Type 2 without the association of ovaric atrophy

It can be connected with different ocular alterations: strabismus, microphthalmia, and optic disk coloboma.

The therapy is complex and multidisciplined:

Ophthalmologist, plastic surgeon endocrinologist, and geneticist (Allen and Rubin 2008).

135.3.2.3 Angiomas

Benign vascular growth which shows up few days after the birth and which depending on the extension and on the location can be a cause of total or of partial palpebral ptosis with a consequent possible amblyopia if the visual axis is involved (Fig. 4).

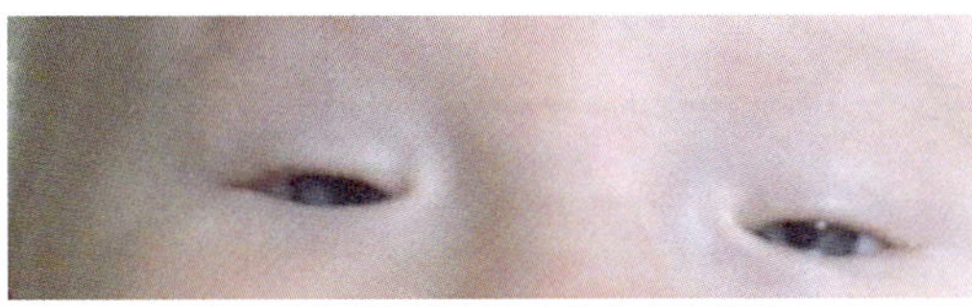

Fig. 3 Blepharophimosis

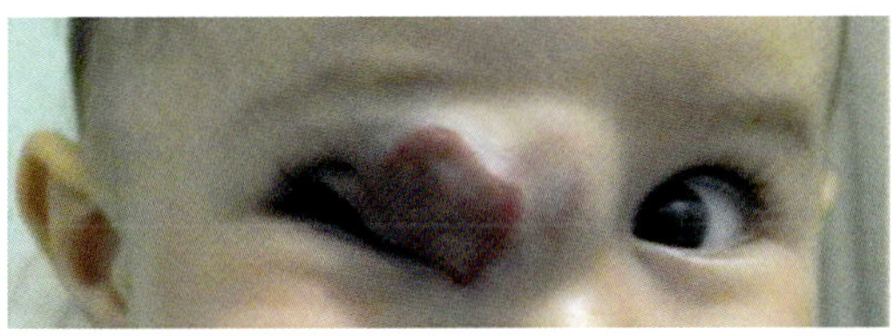

Fig. 4 Angiomas

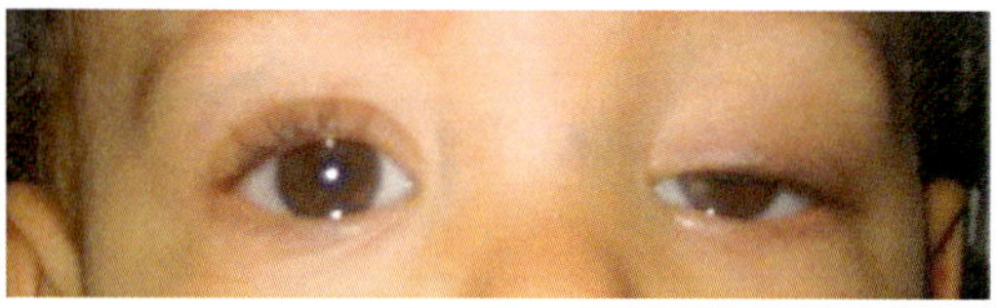

Fig. 5 Eyelid ptosis

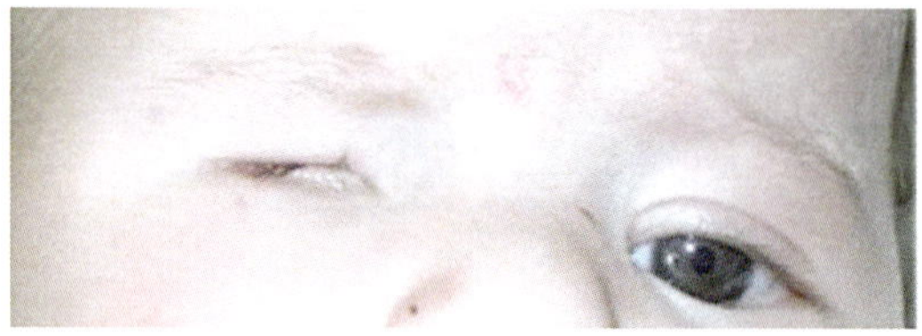

Fig. 6 Anophthalmia

In some cases, the palpebral angioma is part of the syndromic malformation as Sturge-Weber syndrome.

An echography is useful to establish the extension within the orbit.

The therapy for the angioma is medical (cortisone, beta-blockers) and surgical.

In selective cases, the laser therapy can be considered.

135.3.3 Position Anomalies

135.3.3.1 Palpebral Ptosis

A drooping eyelid which can be of a different entity (Fig. 5).

In the most severe cases, it can cause a visual disturbance (amblyopia) and an anomalous head position. Uni- or bilateral, it manifests itself with a difficulty of the newborn in opening the eyelid from the first days of life.

The causes are different:

- Muscle elevator superior lid agenesis
- 3° cranial nerve palsy
- Neoformations as neurofibromatosis
- Syndromic etiologies

The patient examination is very important: static and dynamic (Baroody et al. 2005; Clauser et al. 2006).

Timely surgery is reserved for the total ptosis, whereas in other cases the therapy is normally directed to the cure of the amblyopia, postponing the surgery (esthetical) for children over 5 years old.

The surgical techniques are generally:

- Elevator muscle resection
- Frontal muscle suspension (Gazzola et al. 2011)

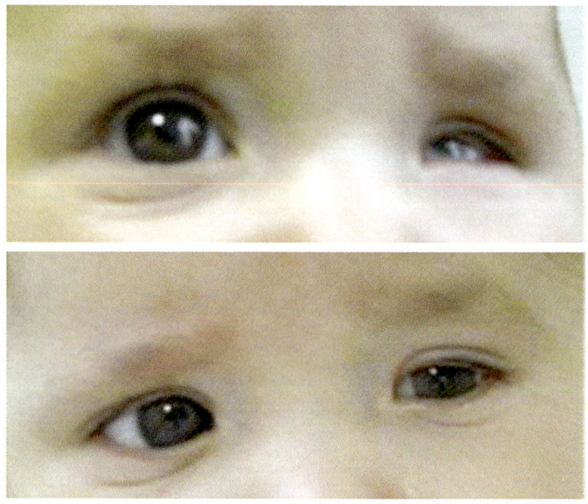

Fig. 7 Left eye microphthalmia without and with prosthesis

135.4 Ocular Bulb Malformations

135.4.1 Anophthalmia

Total absence of the eye (Schittkowski and Guthoff 2010) (Fig. 6).

When diagnosed, a systemic assessment is mandatory since there can be associated chromosomal or systemic abnormalities.

MRI may be considered since significant maldevelopment of the eye can be associated with midline brain abnormalities.

135.4.2 Microphthalmia

Reduced volume of the eye (the normal length of the eye at birth being approx. 17 mm) (Fig. 7).

The diagnosis is simple in monolateral forms due to the interocular difference, while more complicated in bi-ocular forms.

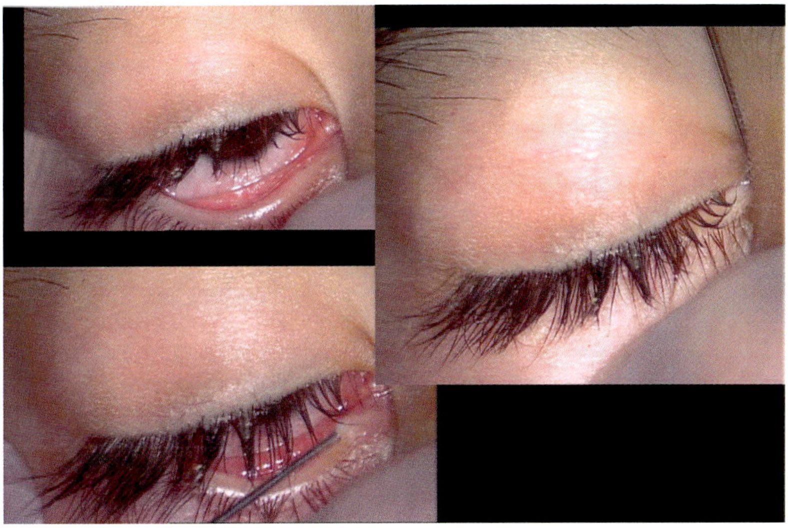

Fig. 8 Congenital nasolacrimal-duct obstruction

Microphthalmia is associated with reduction of the lid margin, drooping of the lid, and enophthalmos (sunken eye).

It can be isolated or associated with multi-organ alterations.

An MRI is necessary to exclude orbital malformations as cysts and to evaluate cerebral optic pathways.

The examination in sedation is useful for orbital cavity evaluation.

In presence of anophthalmia and microphthalmia, an eye prosthesis must be inserted to consent the orbital growth.

135.5 Nasolacrimal-Duct Malformation

135.5.1 Congenital Nasolacrimal-Duct Obstruction

Epiphora since the first days of life. Weeping can be associated with the presence of abundant mucous material. By applying pressure near the lacrimal sac, mucous and purulent material from the inferior lacrimal point is discharged.

Children with congenital nasolacrimal-duct obstruction had a higher prevalence of amblyopia risk factors than children in the general population (Kim et al. 2013).

Therapy: massage of the lacrimal sac region, cleaning the nose with physiological solution, and local antibiotics as and when needed.

Surgical therapy: for cases not soved by medical therapy (Fig. 8).

135.6 Corneal Malformations

135.6.1 Size Anomalies

135.6.1.1 Megalocornea

- Simple, isolated, A.D.
- Associated (megalophthalmos) X-linked
- Associated to congenital glaucoma (buphthalmos)

If a bigger eye is suspected, it is very important to have the corneal diameter and the eye pressure measured by an ophthalmologist for the differential diagnosis with the congenital glaucoma.

Possible symptoms are watering and photophobia, which can manifest themselves at a later stage as a consequence of the eye pressure imbalance.

135.6.1.2 Microcornea

Corneal diameter inferior to the average (normal value 9.5–10 mm in newborn) (Fig. 9).

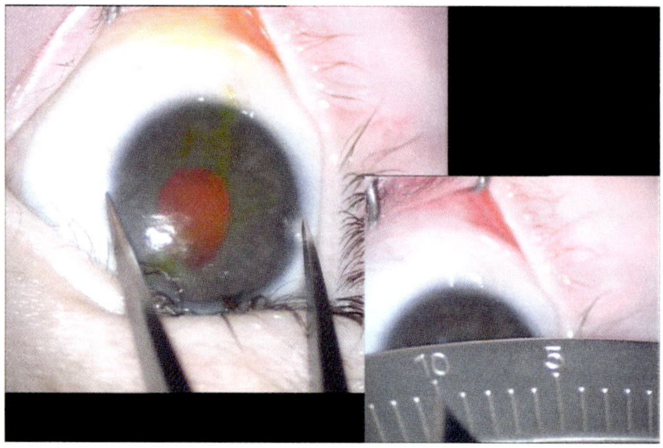

Fig. 9 Microcornea

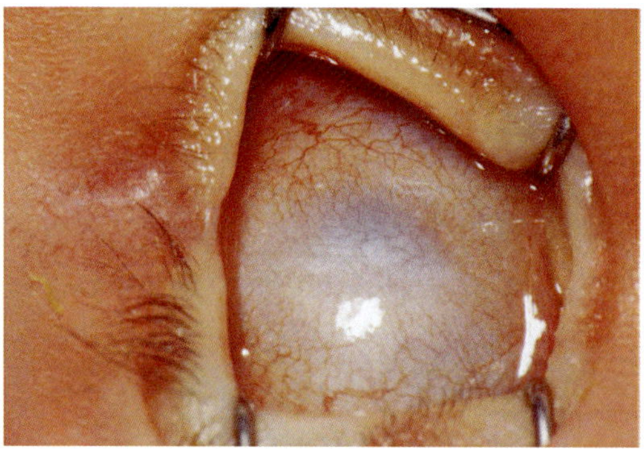

Fig. 10 Sclerocornea

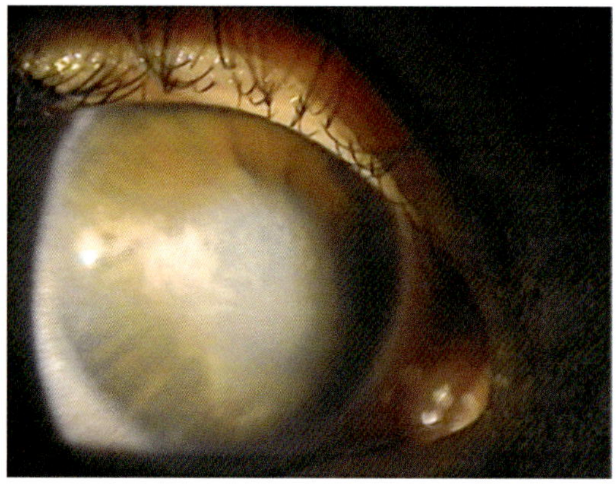

Fig. 11 Peter's anomaly

It can be associated with microphthalmos and with other pathologies of the anterior segment.

The examination must be done under sedation for the correct evaluation of the other possible associated anomalies.

135.6.2 Anomalies of Transparency

Anomalies in the transparency (congenital corneal opacity, sclerocornea (Kraker et al. 2005) (Fig. 10), Peter's anomaly (Fig. 11), corneal dystrophy, corneal opacity associated with metabolic illnesses or congenital infections). They alter the normal corneal aspect which is by definition mirroring and transparent, in order to allow a good look at the iris and at the pupil.

They can be isolated or widespread, they are often associated with the impossibility in opening the eye, and they have to be considered as an indication of serious metabolic illnesses.

In metabolic disease it is extremely rare for the cornea to be cloudy at birth.

135.6.3 Epibulbar Dermoids

With an appearance similar to a solid white mass, present in the limbus and more frequently in the inferior-temporal location.

They can affect the entire thickness of the cornea or only some layers.

They are often associated with the Goldenhar syndrome.

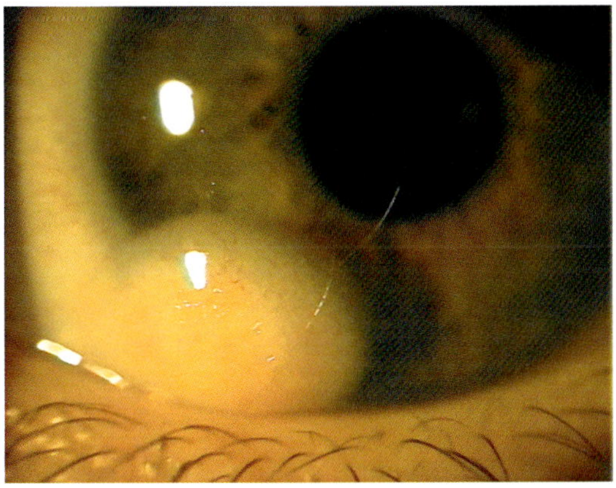

Fig. 12 Epibulbar dermoid

Generally, the opacification is situated at limbus sparing the visual axis (Fig. 12).

They tend to involve the cornea causing astigmatismus, and in the more evolved phases, they involve the optic axis with consequent visual damage.

The therapy is conservative in mild opacification, while surgical if the corneal dermoid reduces the visual acuity.

135.7 Crystalline Lens Anomalies

135.7.1 Epipupillary Membrane Persistence

Failure to reabsorb the epipupillary membrane due to atrophy during normal fetal development.

It is the cause of a net formed by thin vases and residual mesodermic tissue which partially or totally occlude the pupil leading to difficulties in pupil dilatation and interfering with the visual axis.

The therapy is medical through mydriatics; in cases of a thicker membrane, the treatment is surgery.

135.7.2 Position Anomalies

Dislocation of the crystalline lens from its physiological position as a consequence of a malformation of the zonule (suspensory ligament of the lens) is a pathology associated with general syndromes such as Marfan syndrome and Marchesani syndrome.

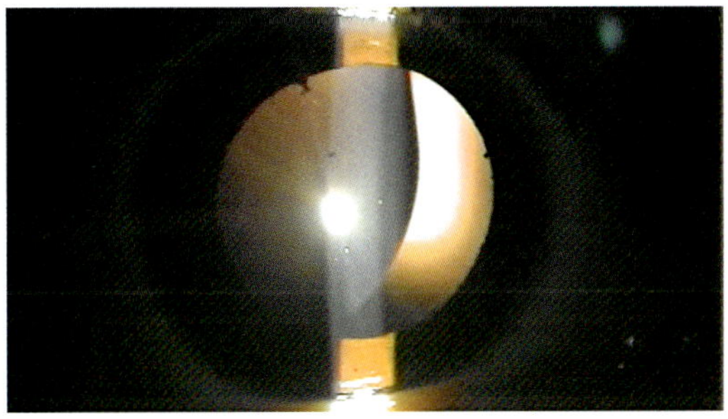

Fig. 13 Sub-dislocation of lens

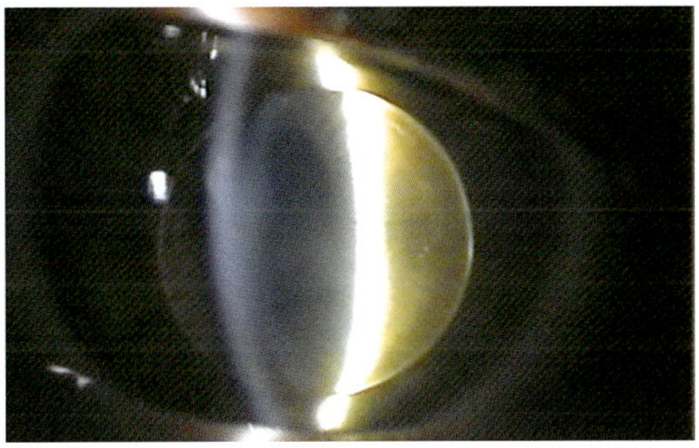

Fig. 14 Complete dislocation of lens

The dislocation can be incomplete (sub-dislocation) (Fig. 13) or complete (dislocation) (Fig. 14).

Since the lens is not in the correct position with respect to the pupil, it can cause a serious refractive defect and amblyopia as a consequence.

The luxation can cause the fall of the crystalline lens to the back of the eye (in the vitreous) which results in retinal damage or to the front (toward the cornea) with endothelial damage.

The therapy is surgical.

135.7.3 Transparency Anomalies

Congenital cataracts can be unilateral or bilateral or isolated or associated with general pathologies, including intrauterine infections (rubella, cytomegalovirus, toxoplasmosis) or metabolic diseases (galactosemia). The lens can be more or

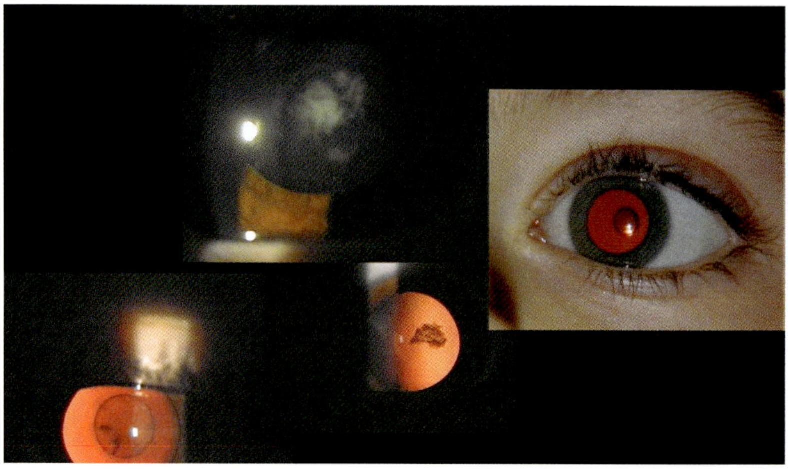

Fig. 15 Congenital cataracts

less opaque (Fig. 15). In those cases where it is total opaque, it gives a characteristic white color of the pupil (leukokoria).

The therapy depends on the density with a consequent obstacle to vision.

In cases with a dense cataract, especially if unilateral, an operation must be performed as soon as possible.

The surgery is aimed at the removal of the opaque lens with an implant of intraocular lens given suitable anatomical conditions.

In the case where the intraocular lens cannot be inserted, the ideal optical correction is contact lenses.

Anti-amblyopic treatment is important after the surgery.

135.7.4 Malformative Glaucoma

An anomaly in the development of drainage causes an increase in the ocular pressure which results in a peculiar big eye effect (buphthalmos) in a child (Faiq et al. 2013) (Fig. 16).

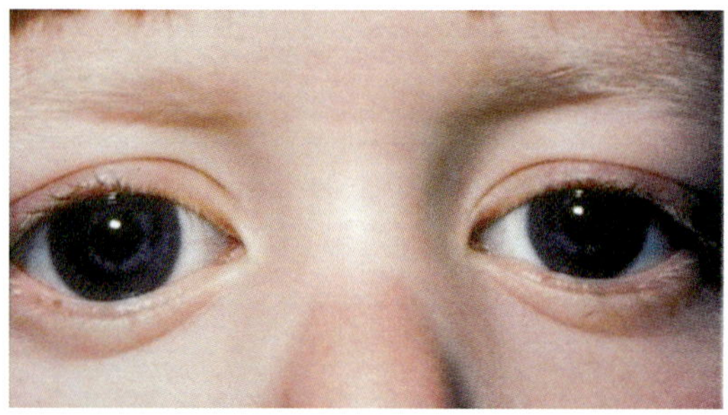

Fig. 16 Buphthalmos

The alterations of the anterior segment (corneal edema, striated lines) can be present at birth or can manifest at a later stage.

Subjective signs are high levels of photophobia and watering.

An early acknowledgement of the pathology is at the basis of a good visual prognosis.

The glaucoma is a hereditary disease. Nowadays, a genetic study in finding the mutated gene is being carried out (CYP1B1, MIOC) in all the children affected by congenital glaucoma.

The therapy is surgical with or without medical therapy.

The choice of surgery depends on the corneal condition and the morphological characteristics of drainage angle structures.

135.8 Congenital Anomalies of the Iris and Pupil

135.8.1 Aniridia

Total or partial absence of the iris, normally bilateral (Fig. 17) (Shiple et al. 2015; Lee 2010).

Symptoms and signs: nystagmus and photophobia.

Aniridia may be associated with glaucoma, cataract, and corneal abnormalities with pannus formation due to stem cell deficiency.

It can be hereditary with dominant autosomal transmission.

In aniridia eye examination includes regular measure of eye pressure and corneal evaluation at the slit lamp.

In isolated forms it is frequently associated with nephroblastoma or Wilms tumor (always carry out an abdominal echography).

Vision correction and the use of tinted lenses (better if contact lenses as they reconstruct the pupillar foramen) can increase the visual quality for those patients.

The use of single-dose eyedrops to reduce the toxicity on the ocular surface is recommended.

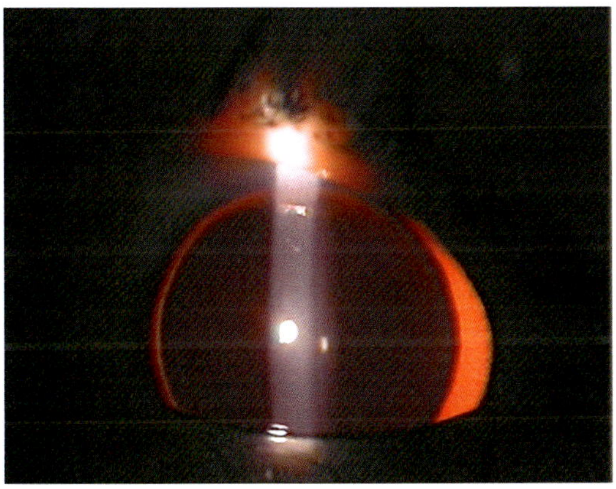

Fig. 17 Aniridia

135.8.2 Iris Coloboma

The coloboma of the iris can be identified as lack of a part of the iris (normally of the inferior sector) (Fig. 18) due to an anomalous closure of the fetal fissure.

Therefore, near the coloboma, the pupil appears irregular and has an elongated oval aspect.

Such a malformation is normally reported by the mother who notices that "the pupil looks strange" while she is breastfeeding.

Such anomaly can be associated with colobomas of the posterior segment (choroid, retina).

It is important to evaluate the fundus.

It can be isolated or associated with syndromes.

135.8.3 Leukokoria

The presence of a white pupil reflex signalizes a cataract or malformatives and congenital vitreoretinal pathologies.

Fig. 18 Iris coloboma

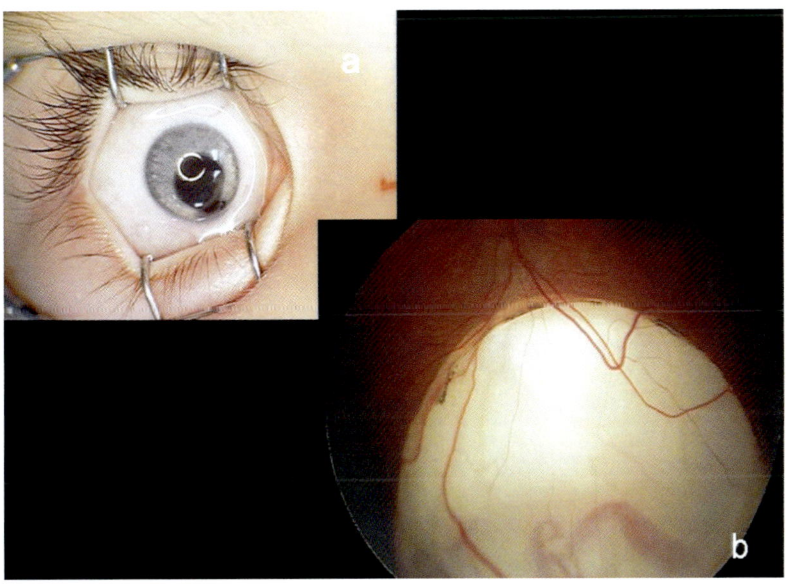

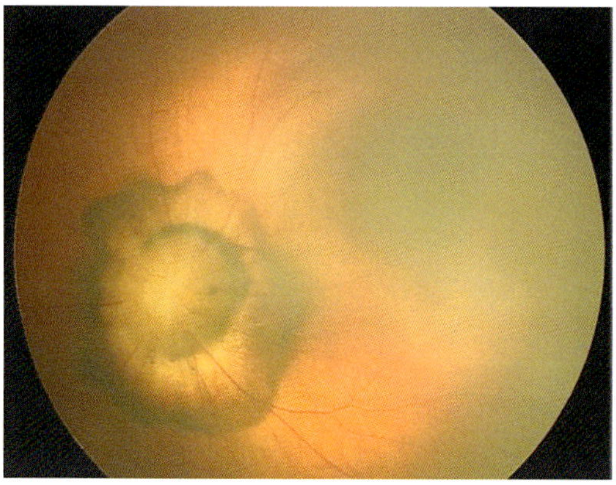

Fig. 19 Photo Ret-Cam our patient

In presence of leukokoria exclude first retinoblastoma an ocular tumor that can be present at birth.

Examination under sedation is crucial (American Academy of Pediatrics 2008).

135.8.4 Malformations of the Posterior Segment

The malformations of the posterior segment are:

- Chorioretinal coloboma interesting or not the optic nerve (Uhumwangho and Jalali 2014)
- Congenital malformation of the optic nerve (morning glory, myelinic aberrant fibers)
- Vitreoretinal changes (dragging disk, Coats' disease, hamartomas)

It can be evident mainly through various forms of constant or intermittent strabismus.

It is appropriate that the pediatrician, in these cases of repeated strabismus reported by the parents, refers the patient for an ophthalmology check.

The ophthalmologic evaluation also involves examining sedation possibly with fluorescein angiography.

Treatment depends on the diagnosis (Fig. 19).

References

Allen CE, Rubin PA (2008 Spring) Blepharophimosis-ptosis-epicanthus inversus syndrome (BPES): clinical manifestation and treatment. Int Ophthalmol Clin 48(2):15–23

American Academy of Pediatrics (2008) Reflex examination in neonates, infants, and children. Pediatrics 122:1401–1404

Baroody M, Holds JB, Vick VL (2005) Advances in the diagnosis and treatment of ptosis. Curr Opin Ophthalmol 16:351–355

Clauser L, Tieghi R, Galiè M (2006) Palpebral ptosis: clinical classification, differential diagnosis, and surgical guidelines: an overview. J Craniofac Surg 17:246–254

Faiq M, Sharma R, Dada R, Mohanty K, Saluja D, Dada T (2013) Biochemical and clinical insights into primary congenital glaucoma. J Curr Glaucoma Pract 7(2):66–84

Gazzola R, Piozzi E, Lanfranchi AL, Baruffaldi Preis FW (2011) Congenital ptosis and blefarophimosis: retrospective analysis of the effectiveness of correction with levator resection and frontalis suspension. Pediatr Med Chir 33(3):129–133

Kim JW, Lee H et al (2013) Amblyopia risk factors in infants with congenital naso-lacrimal duct obstruction. J Craniofac Surg 24(4):1123–1125

Kraker JH, Mannis MJ, Holland EJ (2005) Cornea: fundamentals, diagnosis and management, 2nd edn. Elsevier Mosby, Philadelphia

Lee H (2010) Complication and visual prognosis in children with aniridia. J Pediatr Ophthalmol Strabismus 47:205–210

Ricci B (2006) Oftalmologia Pediatrica. Trattati Mattioli, Roma

Schittkowski MP, Guthoff RF (2010) Systemic and ophthalmological anomalies in congenital anophthalmic or microphthalmic patients. Br J Ophthalmol 94:487–493

Shiple D, Finklea B, Lauderdale JD, Netland PA (2015) Keratopathy, cataract, and dry eye in a survey of aniridia subjects. Clin Ophthalmol 9:291–295 . Published online 2015 February 10

Tawfik HA, Abdulhafez MH, Fouad YA (2015) Congenital upper eyelid coloboma: embryologic, nomenclatorial, nosologic, etiologic, pathogenetic, epidemiologic, clinical, and management perspectives. Ophthal Plast Reconstr Surg 31(1):1–12

Taylor D (1990) Pediatric ophthalmology, 1st edn. Blackwell Scientific Publications, London

Uhumwangho OM, Jalali S (2014) Chorioretinal coloboma in a paediatric population. Eye (Lond) 28(6):728–733

Retinopathy of Prematurity

136

José Carlos Rivera, Elsa Duchemin-Kermorvant, Allison Dorfman, Tianwei Ellen Zhou, Luis H. Ospina, and Sylvain Chemtob

Contents

J. C. Rivera · S. Chemtob (✉)
Departments of Pediatrics, Ophthalmology and Pharmacology, Centre Hospitalier, Universitaire Sainte-Justine, Research Center, Montréal, QC, Canada

Department of Ophthalmology, Maisonneuve-Rosemont Hospital Research Center, Montréal, QC, Canada
e-mail: jc.rivera@umontreal.ca; sylvain.chemtob@umontreal.ca

E. Duchemin-Kermorvant
INSERM UMRS1138, Centre de Recherche des Cordeliers, Paris, France

A. Dorfman
Department of Ophthalmology/Neurology, McGill University-Montreal Children's Hospital Research Institute, Montreal, QC, Canada

T. E. Zhou · L. H. Ospina
Departments of Pediatrics, Ophthalmology and Pharmacology, Centre Hospitalier, Universitaire Sainte-Justine, Research Center, Montréal, QC, Canada

G. Buonocore et al. (eds.), *Neonatology*,
https://doi.org/10.1007/978-3-319-29489-6_283

Abstract

Retinopathy of prematurity (ROP) is an ocular disorder that affects the integrity and function of the immature vasculature and neurons of the developing retina. ROP is considered the major cause of visual impairment and blindness in premature infants. This chapter includes a general review of the current knowledge about this disorder including demographic incidence, risk factors, recent observations regarding neurovascular dysfunctions in both the inner and outer immature retina, mechanisms and factors implicated in the pathophysiology of ROP. Finally, recommendations for surveillance and follow-up for ROP, as well as current and future preventive therapeutic strategies to preserve retinal structure and function are discussed.

136.1 Salient Points

- Retinopathy of prematurity (ROP) is an ocular disorder that affects the integrity and function of the immature vasculature and neurons of the developing retina.
- ROP is considered the major cause of visual impairment and blindness in premature infants. In the USA, the incidence of ROP increased from 0.12% in 1997 to 0.17% in 2005.
- The vasculature of the human retina begins to develop by approximately 16 weeks gestation and reaches the periphery at near-term gestation.
- Causative factors contributing to the development of ROP include low birth weight, low gestational age, and supplemental oxygen therapy, as well as a genetic component.
- Several factors are involved in the vaso-obliteration that precedes the preretinal neovascular phase. There is O_2-dependent suppression of the important endothelial growth factor vascular endothelial growth factor (VEGF). Expression of the nutrition-dependent factor insulin-like growth factor (IGF-1) is decreased. Furthermore, the newborn has a diminished ability to autoregulate oxygen delivery compared to the adult. There is also increased generation of reactive species of oxygen and their products and increased vulnerability of the neuroretinal endothelium to oxidant stress.The ocular vasculature of the newborn is also particularly vulnerable to oxidative damage.
- ROP develops initially within the peripheral retina and is divided into five stages. Stages 4 and 5 of ROP will usually require surgical treatment.
- When there is abnormal dilatation of retinal veins with florid abnormal new vessels, the condition is called "plus disease," which has a very poor prognosis.
- The disease can advance very quickly and rapidly progressing ROP is called Rush disease, which is usually associated with very extensive or aggressive growth of abnormal blood vessels and requires urgent therapy.
- Apart from retinal detachment, the main retinal and vitreal complications of ROP include retinal folds, foveal heterotopia, preretinal membranes, and hemorrhages. Long-term effects are refractive errors, astigmatism, loss of visual field, strabismus, and blindness.
- The first examination for ROP screening is between 4 and 6 weeks of life or between 31 and 33 weeks postmenstrual age, whichever is later.
- Cryotherapy has been mostly replaced by laser photocoagulation, which is easier to administer and has fewer adverse effects.
- The most effective means of reducing the incidence of ROP appears to be limitation of oxygenation.

136.2 Introduction

Retinopathy of prematurity (ROP) is an ocular disease that occurs in premature infants and affects the immature blood vessels of the developing retina. It is characterized by the onset of visible vascular abnormalities in the second or third month after birth. The pathogenesis of ROP is related to many causative factors, like low birth weight, low gestational age, and supplemental oxygen therapy, and some lines of evidence suggest the role of a genetic component. ROP is mild and undergoes spontaneous regression with no visual sequels in the majority of affected infants. However, progression to advanced ROP does occur in a significant number of infants and can lead to severe visual impairment and even complete unilateral or bilateral blindness in some cases. In general, more than 50% of premature infants weighing less than 1250 g at birth show evidence of ROP, and in approximately 3% of children undergo abnormal retinal vascular development, neovascularization, and, in its more severe forms, traction retinal detachment (Csak et al. 2006). These injuries may occur despite the interventions currently available, such as cryotherapy, laser photocoagulation, or even by using the new anti-VEGF therapies recently used for this sight-threatening disease.

ROP has been recognized since 1942 as a blinding disease of the very premature infants (Terry 1942), and the incidence of blinding forms of retinopathy has varied greatly over the intervening decades. Over more than half a century of intense clinical and laboratory research, great efforts have been made in developing effective therapies for severe stages of ROP, and the understanding of the nature of this disease has improved tremendously. But modest progress has been made in truly understanding the cellular and molecular mechanisms causing this pathology and even less in developing effective prophylactic treatments. At present, the problem increases worldwide with the technological advances in neonatology leading not only to an increased survival rate of very low birth weight infants but also to a correspondingly increased incidence of ROP. This, in turn, has provided a major challenge to all physicians treating the premature infant and has created renewed interest in the pathogenesis, prevention, and treatment of ROP. However, the central mysteries of this disease have not been adequately unraveled to effectively eradicate unfavorable visual outcomes and the efforts continue. The purpose of this chapter is to present current knowledge about ROP, demographic incidence, risk factors and its more recent treatment strategies, as well as the possible promising future therapies against this serious disease.

136.3 Historical Background

Prior to the 1940s, ROP was an unknown disease because severe prematurity was often fatal. The first case of ROP was described in Boston by Dr. T.L Terry in 1942 (Terry 1942). His initial report referred to this new disease as possible fibroblastic overgrowth of the persistent tunica vasculosa lentis. In a second report (Terry 1943), and containing several pathological specimens in the cicatricial end stages of the disease with multiples complications, Terry clearly misinterpreted the involved pathophysiology. He did not recognize the retina as the source of the problem and still linked it to the rare congenital birth defect of persistence of hyaloid artery and tunica vasculosa lentis. However, he did recognize the salient epidemiology and showed that the disease occurred much more frequently in infants born extremely prematurely (Terry 1943). In this same report Dr. Harry K. Messenger, colleague of Terry suggested the term "retrolental fibroplasia" that was used for about 40 years and that described the end stage of the disease in which a white, vascularized plaque could be seen behind the lens in an eye that was often completely blind. At that time, there was inadequate technology to carefully monitor oxygen levels in neonatal intensive care units, and high doses of oxygen were being administered to premature infants without monitoring; the pulse oximeter was not yet available. In fact, during the next 12 years following the first report, more than 10,000 premature infants in North America were blinded before it became appreciated that the outbreak was related to the use of supplemental oxygen (Jacobson and Feinstein 1992). Much of our understanding of ROP can be credited to Kate Campbell from Melbourne, Australia, who compared the incidence of ROP at hospitals that charged for oxygen use and hospitals that did not (Campbell 1951). This investigator found that the incidence of ROP was higher at those hospitals where the use of the oxygen was free and unrestricted. Furthermore, with the advent of pulse oximetry in the 1970s and beyond, oxygen administration became more controlled, and it was thought that ROP would disappear. Unfortunately, this proved to be untrue.

As neonatologists got better at saving tinier and sicker babies, the rate of ROP rose again to frighteningly high levels. Soon, small gestational age and very low birth weight correlated more strongly with occurrence of ROP than did oxygen administration. During the 1980s and early 1990s a major understanding in the physiopathology disease progressed with the use of animal models (Penn et al. 1994; Smith et al. 1994), suggesting that the degree of prematurity of the eye at birth was the critical and necessary risk factor for the disorder and that ROP goes through several well-defined stages before getting to the irreversible retrolental fibroplasia. During the early 1980s, the term of retrolental fibroplasia was renamed to retinopathy of prematurity, and with all new knowledge about of ROP pediatrics, ophthalmologists and neonatologists united to find a treatment. The first step was the development of a common nomenclature, followed by a natural history study and a treatment protocol. In 1984, the International Classification of Retinopathy of Prematurity (ICROP) was developed (The International Classification of Retinopathy of Prematurity 1984). Despite the efforts, no treatment for ROP was available during several years. Major advances in ROP treatment came in the 1980s and 1990s, when cryotherapy and laser photocoagulation – that consist of destroying the portion of the retina that is unvascularized in order to preserve the rest of it – showed to be partially effective in preventing blindness in ROP infants. However, these surgical procedures are sometimes uncomfortable or painful and can only reduce the incidence of blindness by 25% in infants with late-stage disease, besides these patients often still have poor visual acuity after treatment (Chen and Smith 2007). Nowadays, the fight against ROP continues generating new information including possible genetic predisposition (Shastry et al. 1997), the role of angiogenic growth factors such as insulin-like growth factor (IGF-1; Hellstrom et al. 2001) or vascular endothelial growth factor (VEGF; Penn et al. 2008), as well as the potential contribution of circulating endothelial progenitor cells to the development of pathologic retinal neovascularization in preterm infants (Machalinska et al. 2013). Over this decade, new agents targeting VEGF have become commercially available for intraocular use (Klufas and Chan 2015). Development of pharmacological strategies for treating ocular neovascularization has revolutionized the care of some neovascular ocular diseases and has great potential for ROP. Cellular therapy provides an attractive therapeutic approach in treating ROP and thereby restoring vision (Lai 2013). The use of preventive and less destructive therapies for this pathology such as nutritional supplements, including forms of vitamin E (Johnson et al. 1982), amino acids (Darlow et al. 2005), or omega 3 fatty acids (SanGiovanni and Chew 2005), would be much more desirable; however, understanding the molecular basis of the disease is important to the development of new medical interventions or therapeutic treatments.

136.4 Epidemiology

It is estimated that of the 45 million people who are blind worldwide in the 2000s, 1.4 million are children from middle-income and low-income countries, the majority of whom live in the poorest regions of Africa and Asia (Maida et al. 2008). In 1995, ROP accounted for 10.6% of cases of blindness in children in schools for the blind in South Africa (Varughese et al. 2008). However, ROP is not considered a significant cause of childhood blindness in very poor countries due to the low survival rate of premature infants (Wheatley et al. 2002). Yet, ROP is emerging as a major cause of childhood blindness in middle-income countries (Gilbert et al. 1997). For example, a study from 1997 through 2005 showed that of the 34 million live births analyzed in the United States, 58,722 newborns were identified with ROP. This study showed that the incidence of ROP has increased from 0.12% to 0.17% and that the patient population at risk for ROP has doubled from 7.35% to 15% (Lad et al. 2009). Furthermore, almost half of the world's 50,000 children who are blind from ROP live in Latin America (Vision for Children). The World Health Organization estimates that 24,000 of the 100,000 visually impaired infants in Latin America are attributed to ROP (Gilbert 2008; Haddad et al. 2007). An observational study (Gilbert et al. 2005) comparing characteristics of infants who develop severe ROP from countries with low, moderate, and high levels of development showed that larger, more mature infants are at risk in the less developed countries. In the developing countries, the mean birth weight of infants with severe ROP ranged from 903 to 1527 g, compared with 737 to 763 g in the highly developed countries. The mean gestational age of infants with severe ROP from the developing countries was 26.3–33.5 weeks, compared with 25.3–25.6 weeks in highly developed countries. In nearly all of the middle-income countries, infants who developed severe ROP had gestational age of more than 32 weeks and weighed more than 1500 g. This fact demonstrates the inadequacy of the current screening guidelines used in developed countries when evaluating infants from middle-income countries (Wilkinson et al. 2008; Screening examination of premature infants for retinopathy of prematurity 2006).

While exposure to an oxygen-rich extrauterine environment is clearly identified as a major factor in the genesis of ROP (see below), it is not the only predisposing factor. Interestingly, there are many premature infants that are treated with supplemental oxygen who will never end up developing ROP, while other children that are nearly full term who receive little or no treatment will eventually present with the disease (Brown et al. 1998). In fact, an attempt was made in a recent study to identify the presence of cytokines or growth factors in cord blood, which could serve as biomarkers for more accurately predicting the development of ROP (Woo et al. 2013). Not only are low birth weight and low gestational age correlated with the incidence of ROP, but ethnicity is also a factor that has been reported to significantly influence its epidemiology (Saunders et al. 1997). Furthermore, maternal ethnicity has been shown to be an important predictor for the development of ROP, with an even greater predictive power than early weight gain (Husain et al. 2013). Findings by some have suggested that fundus pigmentation might play a protective role against the progression to severe ROP given the greater incidence of threshold ROP in Caucasian infants as compared to African American infants (Saunders et al. 1997; Tadesse et al. 2002). Underlying genetics might explain the latter differential susceptibility, as demonstrated with gene frequencies of single nucleotide polymorphisms in eNOS that differed in Caucasians and African Americans (Yanamandra et al. 2010). In contrast, however, others have reported that an even greater incidence in the onset of threshold ROP exists in Alaskan natives, a darkly pigmented race, when compared to other racial subgroups (Lang et al. 2005; Arnold et al. 1994). There are also many indications that the patient's genetic makeup plays a role in whether ROP develops and how severe it will be. Although ROP occurs in all populations, it long has been noted to occur in its most severe form less frequently in blacks than in whites. In the CRYO-ROP study, 3.2% of black infants developed threshold ROP compared with 7.4% of white infants. In black South African infants, a similar rate of 3.2% in infants born at less than 1251 g was found (Delport et al. 2002). This is unlikely to be caused by the environment, because it is constant across continents. It could be a protective effect of increased retinal pigment, but it also could be because of differential genetic effects, more common in one population than another. Males also were found to have a higher risk than females in the CRYO-ROP study. And in several studies, variations in the Norrie disease gene, a gene responsible for an X-linked form of congenital retinal detachment or dysgenesis, were more common in infants with severe ROP than in those in whom the disease resolved on its own (Shastry et al. 1997; Hiraoka et al. 2001). Each person carries genetic predispositions to certain disorders, but less widely understood are genetic proclivities toward outside effects – trauma, hypoxia, and premature birth, among them. Further investigation into the potential factors that might contribute to these discrepancies, including genetics, socioeconomic status, and dietary intake, is warranted.

136.5 General Definition

Retinopathy of prematurity (ROP) is a blinding eye disease of premature infants that affects more than 80% of babies born with birth weight less than 1000 g. It is a disease confined to the immature retinal vascular system, and it is characterized by disorganized growth of retinal blood vessels which may result in scarring and retinal detachment. ROP can be mild and undergoes spontaneous regression with no visual sequels in the majority of affected infants. However, progression to advanced ROP does occur in a significant number of infants and can lead to severe visual impairment and even complete unilateral or bilateral blindness in some cases. Many causative factors can contribute to the development of ROP including low birth weight, low gestational age, and supplemental oxygen therapy, and some lines of evidence suggest the role of a genetic component.

136.5.1 Progression of ROP

Retinal blood vessel development commences around 16 weeks of gestation. The nasal retina is vascularized by 36 weeks gestation and the temporal retina by 40–45 weeks (Michaelson 1948). Therefore, the retinas of premature infants are incompletely vascularized. Two phases of ROP are characterized (Smith 2004). The first phase begins when retinal vascular growth ceases after premature birth. The relative hyperoxic environment causes downregulation of the major hypoxia-triggered vascular endothelial growth factor (VEGF) resulting in vaso-obliteration of the developing retinal capillaries. The ensued relatively vascular-depleted retina becomes increasingly hypoxic, and a second phase begins. In this phase, VEGF and other growth factors are upregulated, leading to a proliferation of abnormal neovascularization that ensues with the development of stage 3 ROP. VEGF is an important hypoxia-regulated factor in the development of ROP. Studies have shown that serum levels of VEGF are higher in infants with stage 3 and threshold ROP compared to those with less severe disease (Alon et al. 1995).

The time of the appearance of ROP is determined both by the immaturity of the child at birth and by perinatal events that are associated with increased incidence of ROP. In full-term infants, ROP almost never develops when oxygen is delivered in high concentration. Also, when oxygen is monitored carefully and controlled in mildly preterm infants with zone II or III disease, the retinal vasculopathy is usually mild; this inference has been corroborated by a number of human studies wherein lower O_2 saturation revealed decreased rates of ROP, without causing increased neurologic complications (see section "Pathogenesis"). Conversely, the risk of ROP rises in very premature infants whose eyes have large areas of avascular retina.

136.6 Pathogenesis

The vasculature of the human retina begins to develop by approximately 16 weeks gestation and reaches the periphery at near-term gestation; accordingly, in the premature infant, retinal vascularization is incomplete. The endothelial cells committed from angioblasts lead the way in response to increasing metabolic demands of the developing retina (Cringle et al. 2006). Pericytes develop later, and their absence facilitates angiogenic stimuli to induce endothelial cell proliferation (Antonelli-Orlidge et al. 1989). This process of angiogenesis occurs as expected in part through expression and actions of VEGF (Provis et al. 1997; Stone et al. 1995).

Increased retinal oxygenation is an important factor in the pathogenesis of ROP (Arroe and Peitersen 1994; Gallo et al. 1993; Sola et al. 2007); in utero, the immature subject is exposed to much lower levels of O_2 than postnatally. Some studies (Tin et al. 2001; Chow et al. 2003; Wright et al. 2006; Vanderveen et al. 2006a; Deulofeut et al. 2006; Wallace et al. 2007) have concluded that the rate of ROP can be reduced by limiting O_2 administration; this of course needs to be done cautiously. A recent meta-analysis and systematic review named NEOPROM (Neonatal Oxygenation Prospective Meta-analysis) (Saugstad and Aune 2014), which

Table 1 Summary meta-analysis of severe ROP in infants in low versus high oxygen saturation target. Relative risks (RRs) and 95 % CIs are shown in the table. RR exceeding 1 favors a high oxygen saturation target. The table was elaborated based in the data collected by Saugstad and Aune (2014)

	SUPPORT (Surfactant, Positive Pressure, and Pulse Oximetry Randomized Trial)		BOOST II (Benefits of Oxygen Saturation Targeting)		COT (Canadian Oxygen Trial)	
Oxygen saturation (SpO_2)	**Low SpO_2** 91–94 %	**High SpO_2** 96–99 %	**Low SpO_2** 91–94 %	**High SpO_2** 96–99 %	**Low SpO_2** 91–94 %	**High SpO_2** 96–99 %
Gestational age (weeks)	26.0±1	26.0±1	26.0±1.2	26.0±1	25.6±1.2	25.6±1.2
Birth weight (grams)	836.0±193	825.0±193	826.0±184	837.0±189	827.0±190	844.0±199
Number of infants	654	662	1224	1224	578	569
Severe ROP	**8.6 %**	**17.9 %**	**10.6 %**	**13.5 %**	**12.8 %**	**13.1 %**
Relative risk (RR; 95 % CIs)	**0.52 (0.37–0.73)** $p < 0.05$		**0.79 (0.63–1.39)** $p < 0.05$		**0.95 (0.65–1.39)** $p < 0.05$	

include five multicenter trials [SUPPORT trial (Surfactant, Positive Pressure and Pulse Oximetry Randomized), the three BOOST II trials from the United Kingdom, Australia, and New Zealand, and the Canadian Oxygen Trial (COT)], was performed including a total of 4911 infants with gestational age <28 weeks and randomized to either a low (85–89%) or high (91–95%) functional oxygen saturation (SpO_2). In this meta-analysis study, severe ROP was significantly reduced in the low saturation arm in the SUPPORT trial 8.6 versus 17.9%, relative risks (RR; 95% CIs); 0.52 (0.37–0.73). When combining the three BOOST II trials, severe ROP was found in 10.6% and 13.5% (RR 0.79, 0.63–1.00) in the low and high saturation groups and in COT 12.8% in the low versus 13.1% in the high saturation groups, RR 0.95 (0.65–1.39) (Table 1). These findings confirm other meta-analyses performed prior to this one on efficacy of restricting O_2 to prevent ROP (Chen et al. 2010; Askie et al. 2011).

In contrast to the adult (Pournaras et al. 1989; Yu et al. 1998), the immature newborn is unable to regulate O_2 delivery (principally from the highly perfused choroid) to the inner retina (Chemtob et al. 1991; Hardy et al. 1994, 1996a, b). In response to the ensued retinal hyperoxia, not only the particularly vulnerable endothelial cells at the vascular front degenerate but also a marked involution of the choriocapillaris in the central choroid was recently reported as an important contribution to central photoreceptor compromise in the OIR/ROP (Alon et al. 1995; Ashton 1957; Shao et al. 2011). This endothelial cytotoxicity embodies the vaso-obliterative phase of ROP (Gu et al. 2002) and impacts on neovascularization [as well as on retinal function secondary to the ensued ischemia (Dorfman et al. 2008; Dorfman et al. 2009)].

A number of factors participate in the vaso-obliteration that precedes the preretinal neovascular phase: (a) O_2-dependent suppression of the important endothelial growth/survival factor VEGF through stabilization of hypoxia-inducible factor (HIF) (Neufeld et al. 1999; Ozaki et al. 1999); (b) decreased expression of the nutrition-dependent factor insulin-like growth factor (IGF-1); (c) inability of the newborn to autoregulate oxygen delivery compared to the adult; (d) increased generation of reactive species of oxygen and their products, notably thromboxane A_2, platelet-activating factor (PAF), lysophosphatidic acid (LPA), and trans-arachidonic acids (Shao et al. 2011); (e) increased vulnerability of the neuroretinal endothelium to oxidant stress (more so than neurons and glia).

The increased generation of reactive oxygen species is the result of an incompletely developed antioxidant potential in the immature subject and a tissue (the retina) highly prone to peroxidation due to high content of polyunsaturated fatty acids; in fact the retina contains the highest concentration of long-chain fatty acids in the organism. Antioxidants are molecules that can safely interact with ROS and terminate the chain reaction before vital molecules are damaged. The concentrations of all the major components of the antioxidant systems in neonates, which include heme oxygenase-1, metallothionein, Cu-Zn superoxide dismutase, catalase, vitamins C and E, and glutathione peroxidase, are reduced in retinal tissues. Hence, a limited ability of the newborn to autoregulate oxygen delivery, the abundant unsaturated fatty acids in retina, and the reduced antioxidant systems, renders the ocular vasculature of the newborn more vulnerable to oxidative damage.

136.6.1 Oxygen-Independent Factors and ROP

136.6.1.1 Hypercapnia

In addition to hyperoxia, other factors regularly encountered in neonates with bronchopulmonary dysplasia, such as high carbon dioxide (CO_2) tension (hypercapnia) and associated acidosis, have also been shown to play a role in the development of ROP (Holmes et al. 1998). Interestingly, ischemia also results in a concomitant elevation in CO_2 (Johnson and Weil 1991). This local tissue hypercapnia arises as a consequence of (1) decreased waste removal, (2) continued aerobic CO_2 production until O_2 stores are depleted, and (3) increased anaerobic CO_2 generation from the bicarbonate buffering of hydrogen ions (derived from lactic acid breakdown and high-energy phosphate hydrolysis). The specific consequences of hypercapnia have generally been overlooked with respect to neovascularization.

Exposure of endothelial cells to hypercapnia has been shown to inhibit their proliferation, migration, and differentiation into capillary-like structures and to decrease their viability apparently through cytotoxic nitration (Checchin et al. 2006). Hypercapnia also attenuates developmental retinal neovascularization with acute and prolonged exposure. Likewise, in a mouse model of O_2-induced retinopathy, retinas are unable to revascularize as efficiently when CO_2 levels are concomitantly elevated (Checchin et al. 2006).

136.6.1.2 Insulin-Like Growth Factor-1 (IGF-1)

Of all contributors, prematurity remains the greatest risk for ROP, suggesting that certain key factors present in utero that partake in normal fetal development are lacking in preterm infants. This hypothesis was explored in the seminal works of Lois Smith (Hellstrom et al. 2001) on the role of deficiency of the major growth factor, IGF-1 in premature subjects. Plasma levels of IGF-1 rise with gestational age and considerably augment during the third trimester of pregnancy (when premature infants predisposed to ROP are born). Importantly, IGF-1 decreases postnatally, thus underscoring the placental and amniotic source of the factor. In human subjects, low IGF-1 serum levels directly correlate with the severity of ROP and interestingly may also account for abnormal brain development where retinal vessel growth was retarded, akin to patterns noted in premature babies with ROP (Hack et al. 1994); interestingly, IGF-1 binding protein IGFB3 was also found to be decreased in premature infants and may also contribute to retinal vessel depletion. It was also found that IGF-1 modulates VEGF actions. On the one hand, IGF-1 curtails protective actions of VEGF during the vaso-obliterative phase. Subsequently, when retinal ischemia develops and VEGF levels rise, IGF-1 plays an essential role as a permissive factor allowing VEGF to exert its vasoproliferative actions. Hence, early on IGF-1 depletion participates in vaso-obliteration, and later IGF-1 repletion contributes to the aberrant preretinal neovascularization. Accordingly, clinical trials are being undertaken to address the merits of treatment with IGF-1 at an early stage to prevent the vaso-obliteration in the premature infants (Chen and Smith 2007). Based on these and animal observations, the question of poor weight gain in premature infants at risk of ROP has been raised. In this context, it was recently found that inadequate weight gain during the first few weeks of postnatal life is associated with more severe ROP. Accordingly, an algorithm based on weight gain and IGF-1 was developed as a predictor of ROP (WINROP). Using serial weight and IGF-1 measurements in a cohort of

50 premature babies, WINROP predicted all infants who later developed ROP by a mean age of 10 weeks (Lofqvist et al. 2006). Moreover, measurements of weight gain (and exclusion of IGF-1) were sufficient to demonstrate in a cohort of 351 patients that insufficient weight gain could predict all infants who required treatment and 75% of babies who did not develop ROP (Hellstrom et al. 2009).

136.6.1.3 Circulating Endothelial Progenitor Cells (EPCs)

There is a growing interest in the identification of markers that may facilitate prediction and prevention of premature birth complications. In recent years much attention has particularly focused in clarifying the function of human endothelial progenitor cells (EPCs) on vascular diseases. Described in 1997 (Asahara et al. 1997), EPCs are able to differentiate into mature endothelial cells and repair damaged endothelium (Asahara et al. 1997, 1999). To date, multiple techniques have developed to isolate and characterize human EPCs. In parallel, a number of studies have applied these methodologies to investigate the functions of circulating EPCs in neonatal diseases. EPCs have been implicated in postnatal vasculogenesis during physiological and pathological conditions; however, their role in ROP is not clear. Initial evidences support the hypothesis that circulating EPCs might play an important role in the development of pathologic neovascularization in ROP. Some studies have demonstrated that early EPCs in the peripheral blood are significantly greater in the preterm infants with ROP than in the preterm infants without ROP (Machalinska et al. 2010, 2011, 2013). It was also shown that the number of endothelial progenitor cell in peripheral blood was significantly decreased during the regression of abnormal vasculature in the retina of the same ROP neonates (Machalinska et al. 2013). This may indicate that pathological blood vessel formation during the proliferative phase of ROP results not only from local endothelial proliferation but also from the systemic endothelial progenitor cell mobilization. The mechanism of action of EPCs is still controversial; however, a growing number of studies indicate that EPCs do not engraft into blood vessels, but that such circulating cells may regulate vascular repair via paracrine mechanisms (Zhang et al. 2014).

136.7 Classification

Prior to the early 1980s, most ophthalmologists recorded observations about the natural course of ROP using different classification systems (Reese and Owens 1953). Though these systems were similar in the extreme degrees of ROP, moderately severe grades of retinopathy had different emphases that made the discussion of ocular findings and comparison of treatment effects difficult. This situation was radically altered with the introduction of the International Classification of Retinopathy of Prematurity (ICROP) in 1984 (The International Classification of Retinopathy of Prematurity 1984). This classification was a group effort of 23 ophthalmologists and ophthalmic pathologists from 11 countries. The ICROP group suggested four major components for an international classification, including: (1) localization (zones I, II, and III) of the retinopathy between the ora serrata and the optic disk, (2) severity (stages 0–5) of disease at the junction between the vascularized and non-vascularized retina, (3) extent of involvement of disease (given in clock hours 0 through 12) at the junction, and (4) presence or absence of plus disease, defined as abnormal dilatation and tortuosity of the vessels of the posterior pole of the eye. The major theme of the classification was that the more posterior, more severe, and more extensive retinopathy was, the most likely to have the worst long-term outcome for the child. All these components until now have greatly enhanced the study of the course and the treatment of both the acute and cicatricial phases of the disease.

136.7.1 Zones in ROP

The area of the retina affected by ROP is divided into three zones (Fig. 1). Zone I, the most posterior, is the area bound by a circle that has the disk at its

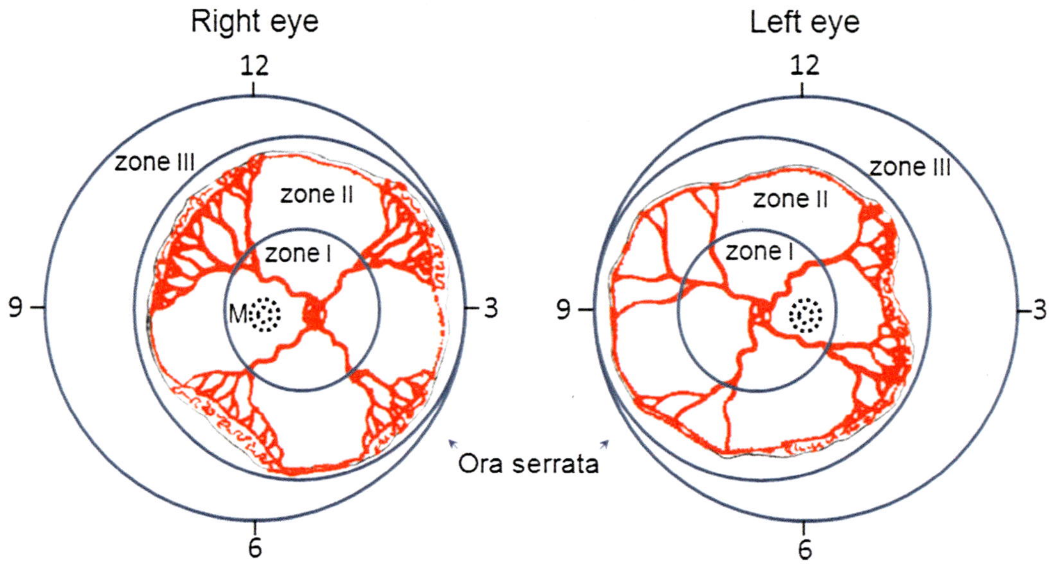

Fig. 1 The International Classification of Retinopathy of Prematurity zones and stages. This figure shows threshold disease in both eyes, with dilation and tortuosity of the posterior pole vessels (Modified from reference (The international classification of retinopathy of prematurity revisited 2005))

center and a radius of twice the disk to foveal region distance. ROP develops in this zone if the retina in this area is most underdeveloped. Zone II is concentric around zone I and having a radius defined from the disk to the nasal ora serrata. Zone III is the crescent of peripheral retina from the edge of zone II to the ora serrata. Thus, ROP that extends for 12 clocks hours (360°) must occur in zone I or II. Disease in zone I is more severe compared with disease limited to zones II or III.

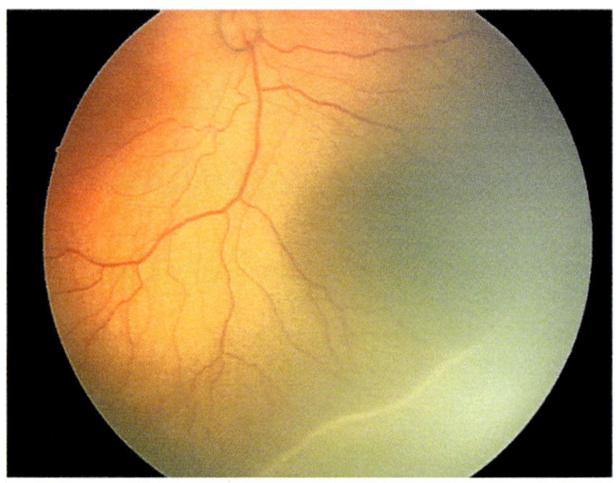

Fig. 2 ROP stage 2, the vascular and avascular retina are separated by thick ridge

136.7.2 Stages in ROP

ROP is divided into stages 0 to 5.

- **Stage 0** is the first stage of this disease characterized by an incomplete vascularization of the retina, leaving avascular tissue in a doughnut shape, or a temporal ellipse, around the optic nerve.
- **Stage 1** is uniformly recognizable as a white line develops at the junction between the vascularized and non-neovascularized retina.
- **Stage 2** occurs when the line develops height and width. Stages 1 and 2 do not usually require treatment in the majority of the cases (Fig. 2).
- **Stage 3** is characterized by extension of fibrovascular proliferation into the vitreous cavity (Fig. 3). The presence of neovascular tufts, called "popcorn" were described as being present in active disease (Wallace et al. 1998). Some cases can present an ominous sign called plus, in which the retinal vessels around the optic nerve and in severe cases on the iris also become engorged and tortuous. The

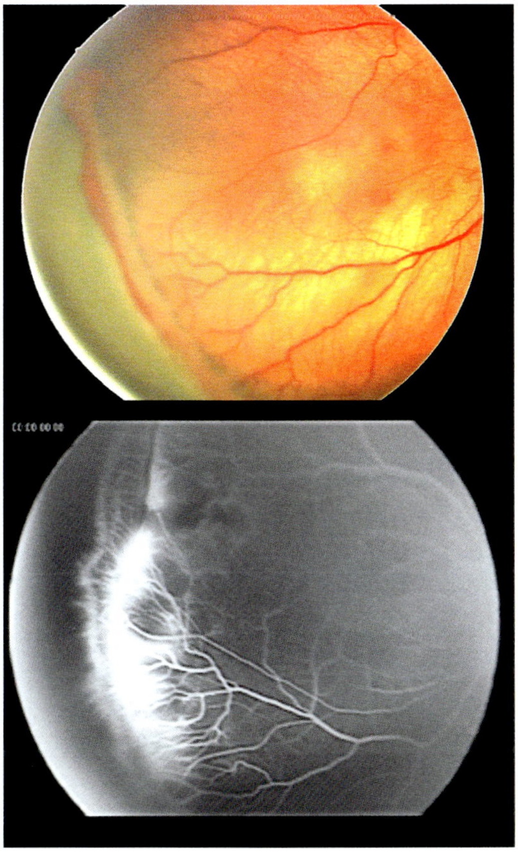

Fig. 3 Funduscopy (**a**) and fluoroangiography (**b**) show how the neovessels grow toward the vitreous posterior to the white line (Fluoroangiography courtesy APEC, Association to Prevent Blindness in Mexico)

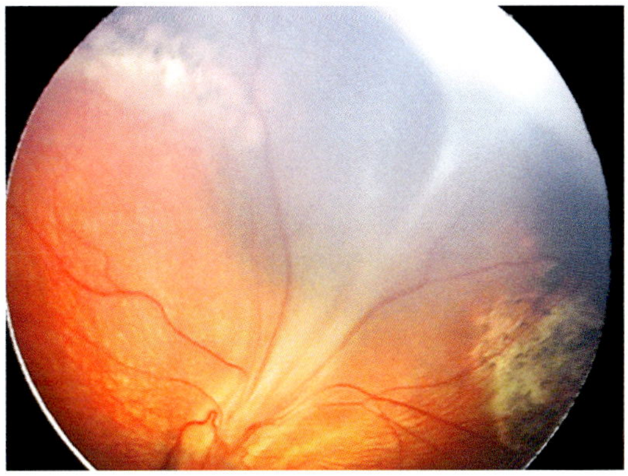

Fig. 4 ROP in stage 4B, the fovea becomes involve in a partial retinal detachment (Courtesy APEC, Association to Prevent Blindness in Mexico)

natural history study showed that if an eye developed five contiguous or eight cumulative clock hours of stage 3 in zones I or II in the presence of plus, there is a 50% chance of retinal detachment with a poor visual outcome (Drack 2006). This point in the disease was termed "threshold." Approximately, 95% of the babies who require laser or cryotherapy develop threshold disease between 32 and 42 weeks after conception. Lower zone and higher stage correlate in general with younger and smaller premature birth and higher risk (e.g., zone I stage 3 is more ominous than zone III stage 1).

- **Stage 4 ROP** is the beginning of the blinding consequences of ROP. The neovascular ridge contracts, pulling the retina up with it and causing partial retinal detachment. This stage is divided in stage 4A if there is a partial retinal detachment not involving the macular region or stage 4B (Fig. 4) if the partial retinal detachment involves the macula. At this stage, the retina may sometimes reattach spontaneously; however, in many cases the retinal detachment which is unlikely to regress requires treatment. Treatment modalities are cryopexy for shallow retinal detachment or scleral buckling for more advanced cases. Stage 4 may progress quickly in some babies, and its treatment has frequently been unsuccessful leading to stage 5 ROP.
- **Stage 5 ROP** shows a total retinal detachment and is the end stage of the disease. Stage 5 in its most severe form shows a dense white membrane or scar behind the lens of the eye. The detached retina is adherent to this scar tissue. The condition was previously called retrolental fibroplasia (RLF), because the scar is white and visible through the pupil (Terry 1943). Spontaneous reattachment of the retina rarely happens in stage 5 ROP. If the eye is left alone at this stage, the baby becomes permanently and often totally blind in both eyes. In addition, some babies develop high intraocular pressure, causing glaucoma. Others develop problems leading to clouding of the cornea.

136.7.3 Severe ROP

136.7.3.1 Plus Disease

Abnormal dilatation of retinal veins with florid abnormal new vessels is called "plus disease," a sign of very poor prognosis in ROP. It is characterized by progressive vascular incompetence with increasing dilatation and tortuosity of veins and arteries of the posterior pole, as shown in Fig. 5. Also, frequently seen in moderate to severe plus disease are iris vascular engorgement, pupillary rigidity, vitreous haze, and increasing dilatation and tortuosity of the peripheral retinal vessels (Davitt and Wallace 2009).

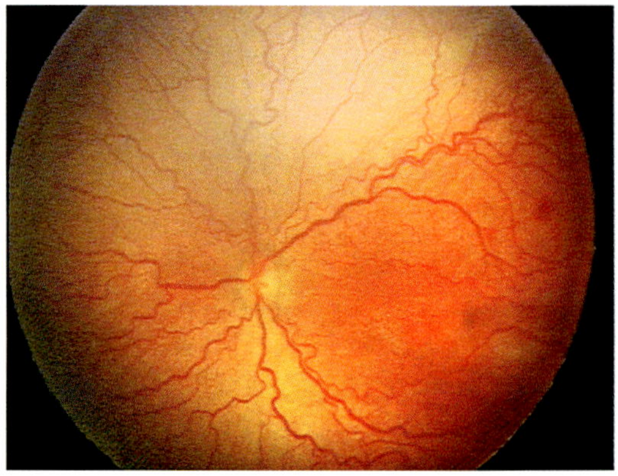

Fig. 5 Plus disease, increasing dilatation and tortuosity of veins and arteries of the posterior pole

136.7.3.2 Rush Disease

Timing is one of the important factors that make the treatment successful in ROP, because the disease can advance very quickly and delayed treatment often reduces the chances of success. The rapidly progressing ROP is called *Rush disease*, and it is usually associated with very extensive or aggressive growth of abnormal blood vessels (Sylvester 2008).

136.7.4 New Classification

The Revised International Classification (The international classification of retinopathy of prematurity revisited 2005) introduced the new form which concerns premature infants with extremely low GA, defined as aggressive posterior ROP (AP-ROP) and a description of an intermediate level of plus disease: pre-plus.

The criteria that characterize AP-ROP are the same: posterior location (zone I), increasing dilatation and tortuosity of the posterior arteries and veins in all four quadrants and shunting from vessel to vessel, within the retina and not solely at the junction between the vascularized and non-vascularized retina, and a flat network of neovascularization. Timing is one of the important factors that make the treatment successful in ROP, because the disease can advance very quickly and delayed treatment often reduces the chances of success. The rapidly progressing ROP is usually associated with very extensive or aggressive growth of abnormal blood vessels (Multicenter Trial of Cryotherapy for Retinopathy of Prematurity 1988).

136.7.5 Diagnostic Examination

Indirect ophthalmoscopy with 25–28 D lens is the correct modality to observe the premature retina. This examination is fundamental, and it needs papillary dilatation with eye drops which combines 2.5% phenylephrine and 1% tropicamid, three times in each eye 1 h before examination.

In the last years, RETCAM is a new device, which permits the taking of pictures of the retina and allows comparisons between experts.

The fluorescein angiography is important to complete the ROP valuation especially in forms that need treatment. After treatment RETCAM examination and fluorescein angiography help to determine if treatment is complete or not.

136.7.6 Clinical Presentation

Much of our knowledge regarding the clinical presentation of ROP has been obtained from follow-up data from infants enrolled in the no-treatment arm of prospective randomized trials (natural history cohorts), mainly the CRYO-ROP and ET-ROP studies. The CRYO-ROP study was a multicenter randomized blinded trial designed to evaluate the risks and benefits of trans-scleral cryotherapy (The Multicenter Trial of Cryotherapy for Retinopathy of Prematurity 1988). It enrolled 4099 infants weighing less than 1250 g at birth who were born between January 1986 and November 1987. The ET-ROP study was a multicenter, randomized trial conducted 15 years later and designed to investigate the potential benefits of early (prethreshold) treatment versus conventional (threshold) treatment in high-risk prethreshold eyes (Early Treatment for Retinopathy of Prematurity Cooperative Group 2003), during which 6998 infants born between October 2000 and September 2002 with a birth weight of less than 1251 g were screened for ROP.

136.8 Onset

136.8.1 Age at Onset

While the risk of developing ROP is influenced by several factors including gestational age and neonatal events, the time at which ROP develops appears to be rather constant and closely related to postmenstrual age (Palmer et al. 1991; Fielder et al. 1992; Subhani et al. 2001). Data from the CRYO-ROP study showed that retinal conditions indicating a risk of poor outcome are not observed before 31 weeks' postmenstrual age (PMA) or 4 weeks' chronologic age in 99% of infants (Reynolds et al. 2002). In the ET-ROP study and in the CRYO-ROP study, the median postmenstrual age at first identification of any ROP was 34.1 and 34.3 weeks, respectively (Good et al. 2005). However, a study by Subhani et al. suggests that ROP onset is slightly accelerated in the most immature infants thus occurring at a slightly earlier postmenstrual age (Subhani et al. 2001). ROP can also develop after 37 weeks; it is then most unlikely to develop into disease requiring treatment (Reynolds et al. 2002).

136.8.2 Site of Onset

ROP develops initially within the peripheral retina, more frequently in the nasal retina in the most immature infants (Fielder et al. 1992). However, over time location of disease can change (Repka et al. 2000), maybe due to ocular growth. The risk of developing significant ROP depends on the location of incomplete vascularization by zone. Zone I ROP is high-risk disease, while zone III has very low risk and zone II is intermediate.

136.9 Natural Evolution

Despite advances in neonatal care, the CRYO-ROP and the ET-ROP natural history studies have shown little change in the natural evolution of ROP (Good et al. 2005).

136.9.1 Regression

In the CRYO-ROP study, ROP was found to regress with vascularization of the retina growing into zone III in 80% of cases (Cryotherapy for Retinopathy of Prematurity Cooperative Group 1988). The mean age at which ROP began to involute was 38.6 weeks postmenstrual age (Repka et al. 2000). Involution was observed in 90% of infants before 44 weeks PMA, but in 3% of eyes, regression had still not occurred by 3 months' corrected age (Repka et al. 2000). In the conventional treatment arm of the ET-ROP study, ROP regressed without reaching threshold in 33.6% of high-risk eyes. The other 66.4% underwent peripheral retinal ablation for progression to threshold (Good 2004).

136.9.2 Timing and Rate of Progression

The median age at onset of prethreshold ROP was 36.1 PMA in the CRYO-ROP as well as in the ET-ROP study (Good et al. 2005), occurring before 32.1 weeks PMA in 5% of infants enrolled in the ET-ROP trial (Good et al. 2005) and before 30.9 weeks PMA in 1% of babies in the CRYO-ROP study (Reynolds et al. 2002). In the ET-ROP trial, 95% of babies developed prethreshold at 7 postnatal weeks or more (Good et al. 2005), and in the CRYO-ROP study 99% of eyes were free of prethreshold ROP of before 4.7 weeks postnatal age (Reynolds et al. 2002). Subhani et al. (2001) reported earlier onset of prethreshold disease with 3.2% of babies developing prethreshold before 30 weeks PMA in the most premature infants, but the definition of prethreshold in this study differed from that used in the ET-ROP trial and CRYO-ROP studies.

The earliest onset of threshold ROP is reported between 31.0–32.6 weeks PMA and 6.6–8.0 weeks postnatal age (Reynolds et al. 2002; Good 2004). The earliest age of onset of stage 3 disease is reported between 30.3–35.6 weeks PMA and 3.8–6.7 weeks postnatal age (Palmer et al. 1991; Fielder et al. 1992; Good et al. 2005; Ells et al. 2005).

In the CRYO-ROP study, threshold ROP developed in 6% of infants, at a mean PMA of 37.7 weeks. The median time from prethreshold to threshold disease did not exceed 1 week (Palmer et al. 1991). Of note, aggressive posterior ROP progressing from onset to stage 4 in less than a week has also been reported (Goggin and O'Keefe 1993).

136.9.3 Risk Factors for Progression and Unfavorable Outcome

Lower birth weights and younger gestational age carry an increased risk of reaching threshold ROP (Schaffer et al. 1993). Eyes in which vascularization has grown only into zone I before 35 weeks PMA have a 30% risk of developing threshold ROP compared to eyes in which vascularization have reached zone III. At fundus examination, risk factors for progression and unfavorable structural outcome include the presence of plus disease, zone I or posterior zone II ROP, increased circumferential involvement, and stage 3 ROP (Early Treatment for Retinopathy of Prematurity Cooperative Group 2003; Cryotherapy for Retinopathy of Prematurity Cooperative Group 1994). A faster rate of progression to prethreshold disease is also associated with an unfavorable outcome (Schaffer et al. 1993). Conversely, infants with zone II ROP without plus disease or with zone III ROP are at very low risk (<1%) of developing sight-threatening ROP and unfavorable outcome (Reynolds et al. 2002; Repka et al. 2000; Cryotherapy for Retinopathy of Prematurity Cooperative Group 1994). The risk to the baby's sight appears to be minimal in infants with acute ROP that demonstrated involution by moving from zone II to zone III with moderate ROP (Reynolds et al. 2002; Repka et al. 2000).

136.10 Complications

Unfavorable visual outcome may be observed in up to 40% to 50% of severe ROP at 1-year follow-up compared to less than 1% in infants with no or less severe ROP (Cryotherapy for Retinopathy of Prematurity Cooperative Group 1994). Prior to the introduction of retinal ablation to stop the progression of ROP, infants with prethreshold disease were predicted to have a 50% risk of blindness (Cryotherapy for Retinopathy of Prematurity Cooperative Group 1988).

136.10.1 Anatomical Abnormalities

Apart from retinal detachment (stage 4 ROP), the main retinal and vitreal complications of ROP include retinal folds, foveal heterotopia, preretinal membranes, and hemorrhages. In the CRYO-ROP study, eyes with zone I ROP or with zone II, stage 3+ were reported to have a higher risk of retinal and vitreous damage than eyes with less severe ROP (Cryotherapy for Retinopathy of Prematurity Cooperative Group 1994).

Serious anatomical damage of the anterior segment can also occur in infants with severe ROP. Synechiae were observed in 37.4% of eyes with stage 3 to 5 ROP, and cataract was diagnosed in 6.3% of cases in the CRYO-ROP study (Cryotherapy for Retinopathy of Prematurity Cooperative Group 1994).

136.10.2 Refractive Errors

136.10.2.1 Myopia

While regressed mild ROP confers no additional risk for refractive errors (O'Connor et al. 2002; Wang et al. 2013), prevalence of myopia increases dramatically following treatment for severe ROP. Twenty percent of children enrolled in the CRYO-ROP study were found to be myopic at 1 year of age (Quinn et al. 1992). Approximately 70% of eyes with high-risk prethreshold ROP during the neonatal period were myopic in early childhood as well as in early school years in a follow-up report from the ET-ROP Study Group (Davitt et al. 2005; Quinn et al. 2008). The proportion of eyes with high myopia (>5 diopters) increased steadily between 6 months and 3 years (Quinn et al. 2008), but became relatively stable beyond, affecting 35–39% of eyes at 6 years of age, with no significant difference between earlier treated and conventionally managed eyes (Quinn et al. 2013). A retrospective observational study for adult patients (45 ~ 56 years old) who had various degrees of ROP reported a remarkably high rate (90.7%) of myopia (Smith and Tasman 2005), compared to 42.9% in adults aged 43 ~ 54 years and 25.1% in those of 55 ~ 64 years (Foster and Jiang 2014).

136.10.2.2 Astigmatism

Prevalence of astigmatism in preterm children who participated in the ET-ROP study was similar in either arm of treatment (early or conservative). By 3 years of age, astigmatism $\geq$ 1.00 diopters occurred in 43% of eyes treated at high-risk prethreshold ROP; 20% of eyes had astigmatism $\geq$ 2.00 diopters (Davitt et al. 2009). By 6 years of age, over 50% of such eyes developed astigmatism $\geq$ 1.00 diopters, and nearly 25% them had high astigmatism ($\geq$2.00 D) (Davitt et al. 2011). A cross-sectional study that compared 9-year-old children with threshold ROP and aged-matched term-born controls found the former had a mean astigmatism of 3.47 D with 98% of eyes showed astigmatism $\geq$0.5 D and 50% had high astigmatism (>3.0 D) (Yang et al. 2013).

136.10.3 Loss of Visual Field

Visual field was shown to be reduced by approximately 30% in children with ROP, whether they underwent retinal ablation or not, compared with infants without ROP (Cryotherapy for Retinopathy of Prematurity Cooperative Group 2001a). In the ET-ROP study, earlier laser ablative treatment for high-risk prethreshold ROP did not adversely affect visual field extent, compared to conventional management (Quinn et al. 2011).

136.10.4 Strabismus

The prevalence of strabismus in the first year of life was 14.7% and was correlated with ROP severity in the CRYO-ROP study (Bremer et al. 1998). At 6 years, cumulative prevalence of strabismus reached 60% in children with high-risk prethreshold ROP in the ET-ROP study (VanderVeen et al. 2011).

136.10.5 Late Sequelae

The percentage of eyes with unfavorable outcome increases over time. In the CRYO-ROP study, nearly half of eyes developed unfavorable outcomes at 10 years (Cryotherapy for Retinopathy of Prematurity Cooperative Group 2001b). Unfavorable visual outcome (vision $\leq$ 20/200) and unfavorable structural outcome (posterior retinal folds or worse) were reported in 62.1% and 47.9% of untreated eyes, respectively (Cryotherapy for Retinopathy of Prematurity Cooperative Group 2001b). Compared to outcome at 5 years, total retinal detachments had continued to occur in control eyes, increasing from 38.6% to 41.4% at 10 years (Cryotherapy for Retinopathy of Prematurity Cooperative Group 2001b). Unfavorable visual acuity outcomes were reported in 64.3% of untreated eyes at 15 years, along with new retinal detachments in 0,51% of untreated eyes each year (Palmer et al. 2005).

Although surgical treatment of severe ROP is associated with better long-term visual and structural outcomes, it still carries a risk of both short- and long-term ophthalmic morbidities, including retinal detachment and blindness. Laser-treated severe ROP remained associated with unfavorable visual outcome in 11% of cases at 3 months of age (Laser ROP Study Group 1994). Total retinal detachment was observed in 22% of treated eyes in the CRYO-ROP 10-year follow-up study (Cryotherapy for Retinopathy of Prematurity Cooperative Group 2001b). At 15 years, unfavorable visual acuity outcomes were as high as 44.7% of cryotherapy-treated eyes (Palmer et al. 2005). After early laser treatment, only 35% of high-risk prethreshold eyes achieved a normal vision at 6 years (visual acuity of 20/40 or better) in the ET-ROP study (Good et al. 2010). Iris atrophy and cataracts have also been reported following peripheral retinal ablation (Kaiser and Trese 2001).

136.10.6 Choroidal Involution

Choroid vasculature is vital for the proper function of the outer retina, most notably, retinal pigment epithelium and photoreceptors (Linsenmeier and Padnick-Silver 2000). Accordingly, the choroid exhibits the highest perfusion rate within the human body (1200 ~ 2000 μl/min) (Alm and Bill 1973), and a small drop in total vasculature radius can lead to a drastic decrement in volumetric flow rate that cause deleterious effects in the outer retinal function.

Choroidal atrophy in ROP was first described in a rodent model of oxygen-induced retinopathy (Shao et al. 2011) and then confirmed by two clinical studies in older children and young adults using optical coherence tomography (Table 2). For instance, at 10 years children with former threshold ROP had significantly thinner subfoveal choroid (210.0 μm) compared to those with spontaneously regressed ROP (261.1 μm) (Wu et al. 2013a). Unlike retinal vessels that undergo revascularization, choroidal atrophy persists into late teens (15 ~ 17 years old) in which ROP adolescence continued to have thinner choroid (257.2 μm) than their healthy, termed-born counterparts (320.5 μm) (Anderson et al. 2014). In both cases, choroidal radii in the ROP group were 17 ~ 19% less, therefore reducing blood flow by 53% ~ 57% in affected eyes based on Hagen-Poiseuille's law (Caccavale et al. 2011).

Table 2 Clinical reports from ROP patients with choroidal involution

Article	Major findings	Patient age at examination (years old)
Wu et al. (2013a)	"Patients in the treated group had a significantly thinner choroidal thickness than the patients in the nontreated group after adjusting for age, axial length, and spherical power"	Threshold ROP (treated): 9.5 +/ − 2.9; Spontaneous regressed ROP (untreated): 10.1 +/- 2.9
Anderson et al. (2014)	Mean subfoveal choroidal thickness, adjusted for refraction, was 271.1 μm in the ex-ROP group, which was significantly thinner than 327.4 μm in controls ($p = 0.008$). Similarly, mean adjusted temporal choroidal thickness was 257.2 μm in ex-ROP's vs. 320.5 μm in controls ($p = 0.001$).	Former ROP: 15.2 +/−2.84; Controls: 17.3 +/ −3.21

136.10.7 Functional Changes

The vasculopathy associated with ROP has long been considered the hallmark of the disease, and it is therefore not surprising that many efforts have been aimed at better understanding it and limiting it over the years (Kong et al. 2015; Hellgren et al. 2016; Yalin Imamoglu et al. 2014; Sato et al. 2012). However, it has been shown that

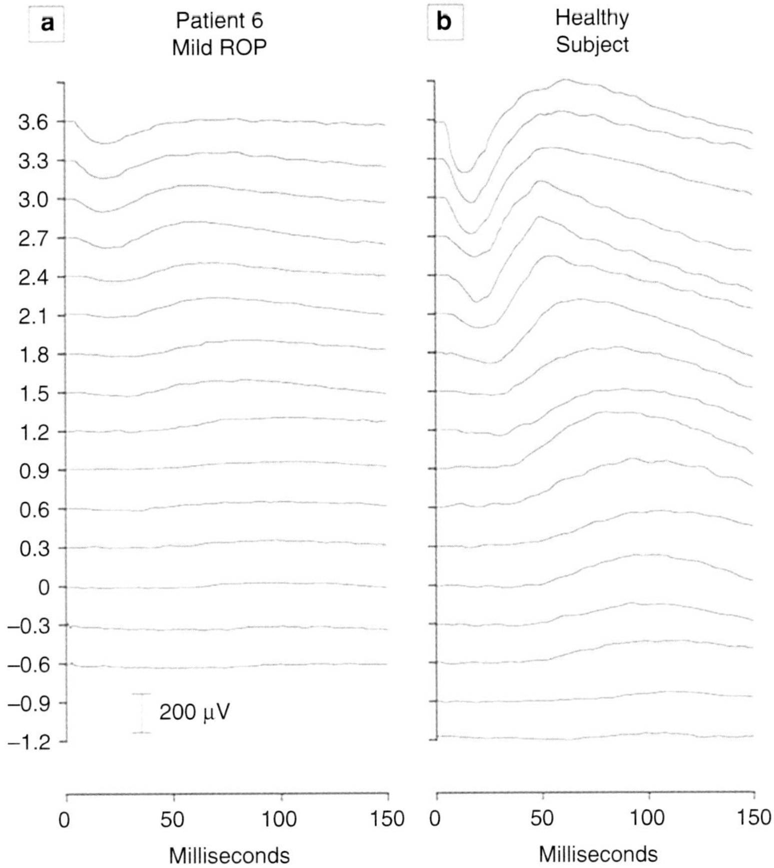

Fig. 6 (**a**) Sample electroretinographic record at 2.5 months' post-term in patient 6 with mild retinopathy of prematurity (ROP). (**b**) Electroretinographic record of a healthy, term-born infant. The numbers to the *left* of each trace indicate the stimulus in log scotopic troland seconds (Adapted from Fulton et al. (2001))

while the vascular sequels of ROP can ultimately regress in some cases (Hammer et al. 2008), lasting functional consequences can nonetheless ensue. In fact, ROP has previously been referred to as a "lifetime disease" for which lifelong follow-up is required (Tasman et al. 2006). Flash and multifocal electroretinography (fERG and mfERG, respectively) have been instrumental in the evaluation of the functional integrity of the retina in ROP both in infants and adults alike. For example, patients with a history of ROP reveal significant abnormalities in the a- and b-waves of the fERG (Fig. 6), findings that have been shown to persist in the absence of any abnormal retinal vasculature (Fulton et al. 2001; Fulton and Hansen 1996). Furthermore, elevations of the scotopic visual thresholds in children with a history of resolved mild ROP in addition to the slower maturation of the rod-mediated thresholds in the central retina are also suggestive of photoreceptor involvement (Fulton et al. 2009; Hansen and Fulton 2000; Reisner et al. 1997). In fact, increasing severity of the disease resulted in an even greater decrease in rod sensitivity in most cases (Fulton et al. 2009). Similarly, a subsequent study undertaken by Hansen et al. (2010) revealed that the kinetics of deactivation of the rod response were abnormally slow in older subjects with a history of ROP with use of the paired flash technique. The latter could suggest that either a halt in maturation occurs in the latter process or that the functional impairment becomes increasingly worse with age (Hansen et al. 2010). In parallel with the above, while patients with a history of mild ROP reveal some improvement in post-receptoral sensitivity with age, those with severe ROP do not (Harris et al. 2011). Collectively, findings above suggest that despite the resolution of the early clinical features of ROP, lasting functional deficits can remain.

Interestingly, a differential susceptibility between cone and rod function has been suggested in subjects with a history of preterm birth, where higher cone sensitivity and minimal cone dysfunction could be observed compared to that of rods (Fulton et al. 2008). While this discrepancy requires further elucidation, it has been postulated that the earlier maturation of the cones might carry out a beneficial protective effect with respect to their function in comparison with the relative immaturity of the rods that might render them more susceptible to oxidative stress (Fulton et al. 2008). However, a recent study by Ecsedy et al. (2011) revealed the presence of cone dysfunction in adults with a history of laser-treated ROP. The latter was demonstrated with attenuated cone-mediated ERG b-wave amplitudes obtained using both a standard photopic ERG protocol as well as an S-cone protocol (blue light stimuli on amber background). Future studies aimed at uncovering the mechanisms behind rod and cone function susceptibility in ROP are warranted.

In addition to findings obtained with the full-field flash ERG, the mfERG, a central retinal response, also reveals significant deficits in amplitude and implicit time in subjects whose clinical features of ROP had completely resolved more than 10–20 years earlier (Fulton et al. 2005). These findings suggest that a history of ROP can carry out lasting consequences on central retinal development as revealed with the mfERG. ON- and OFF-bipolar cells contribute to this central response, and therefore amplitude attenuation might occur should ROP specifically target these cells, thereby resulting in an altered summation of depolarization and hyperpolarization in these subjects (Fulton et al. 2005). More recently, the morphologic changes of the macular structure have also been studied in formerly preterm children with mild or no sequelae of regressed ROP using optical coherence tomography (OCT). Findings in formerly preterm infants revealed a larger central retinal region in addition to a decreased foveal depression compared to children born at full term, which was suggested to result from problematic centrifugal movement of foveal cones as well as inner retinal cells throughout retinal maturation (Ecsedy et al. 2007). Overall, despite the resolution of vascular abnormalities, which is commonly reported in ROP patients, careful consideration and monitoring of structural changes and neural dysfunction in the retina that can carry on throughout adulthood are necessary.

Several other types of visual manifestations, in addition to ROP, have been thought to result from the challenges of premature birth on the developing ocular system. For example, an increased incidence in refractive errors such as myopia, astigmatism, and anisometropia has been noted, in addition to an increased incidence in strabismus (O'Connor et al. 2004, 2007; VanderVeen et al. 2006b). Similar to the manifestations of ROP on eye growth and movement, visual functions including visual acuity, contrast sensitivity, color vision, and visual fields may also be significantly altered and can consequently impact psychological and educational development (O'Connor et al. 2004, 2007).

An association between the oscillatory potentials (OPs) of the ERG and ametropias has also been reported in patients with a history of ROP. For example, while a stronger ON signal and lower OFF signal (as revealed by an increase in OP_3 and a decrease in OP_4, respectively) were found in myopic patients, the reverse was documented in hyperopic patients, and thus it could be concluded that the ON and OFF pathways might play a role in determining refractive development in these patients (Fulton and Hansen 1995, 1996). Interestingly, OPs have previously been shown to be particularly susceptible to disease processes wherein the retinal vasculature is compromised, including diabetic retinopathy and central retinal vein occlusion (Kizawa et al. 2006; Yonemura et al. 1962), and ROP is no exception. In fact, a study of the dark-adapted electroretinogram in ROP showed that while the OPs of ROP infants contained greater energy than in infants born at term, adults with a history of ROP had lower energy in their OPs than that found in the control population (Akula et al. 2007). More recently, another study aimed to explore the development of dark-adapted OPs in premature infants with and without ROP (Mactier et al. 2013). Results therein revealed a low incidence of OP1 in infants with severe ROP, findings supportive of the notion that suppression of early OPs could be considered as a marker for developing ROP (Mactier et al. 2013).

136.11 Surveillance of ROP and Follow-Up

136.11.1 Screening

Based on published data regarding evolution of ROP, screening guidelines to identify infants requiring treatment for ROP while minimizing the number of stressful examinations have been established in many countries (Fierson 2013; Wilkinson et al. 2009). In industrialized countries, they vary little, with respect to the gestational age and birth weight of screened infants, timing of first examination, and frequency of subsequent examinations. Screened infants are born between 1250 and 1500 g and between 30 and 32 weeks PMA. Screening recommendations also generally include selected larger or more mature infants with unstable clinical course who are considered at high risk by the attending neonatologist (Fierson 2013). In countries with low/moderate level of development, where larger and more mature infants develop severe ROP (Gilbert et al. 2005; Ells et al. 2005), ROP screening programs include infants up to 1750 g and 33 weeks PMA (Ells et al. 2005). Timing of first examination ranges between 4 and 6 weeks of life or 31 and 33 weeks postmenstrual age, whichever is later (Ells et al. 2005). Subsequent follow-up examinations are recommended biweekly when examination is normal or at least once a week in other cases. In the absence of any ROP, screening can be stopped when the retinal vascularization is completed, i.e., when retinal capillaries have grown into zone III. Screening by an experienced ophthalmologist is recommended, using binocular indirect ophthalmoscopy after pupillary dilation (Box 1).

As an example, the recently updated screening recommendations for ROP published jointly by the American Academy of Pediatrics (AAP), the American Academy of Ophthalmology (AAO), and the American Academy for Pediatric Ophthalmology and Strabismus (AAPOS) are summarized in Box 2 (Fierson 2013).

Box 1 Pain Prevention During Screening for ROP

Screening examination is performed using indirect ophthalmoscopy after pupils' dilation. In some cases, an eyelid speculum and a scleral depressor are used to rotate the eye in the appropriate position, making the examination stressful and painful for the baby. ROP screening examinations can have short-term effects on blood pressure, heart rate, and respiratory function in the premature baby. The baby should therefore be clinically stable at the time of the examination, which should be kept as short as possible. Nesting, use of oral sucrose, and use of a topical anesthetic are recommended prior to screening of babies for ROP.

Box 2 Screening Guidelines from the AAP/AAPOS and AAO (Fierson 2013)

Infants to be screened:

- Infants with a birth weight < 1500 g
- Or with a gestational age < 30 weeks
- Selected infants with a birth weight between 1500 and 2000 g or gestational age of more than 30 weeks with an unstable clinical course, including those requiring cardiorespiratory support and who are believed by their attending pediatrician or neonatologist to be at high risk

(continued)

Timing of initial examination:

Gestational age (weeks)	Postmenstrual age at first examination (weeks)	Chronologic age (weeks)
22	31	9
23	31	8
24	31	7
25	31	6
26	31	5
27	31	4
28	32	4
29	33	4
30	34	4
Older gestational age, high-risk factors (consider timing based on severity of comorbidities)		4

Frequency of subsequent examinations:

- One-week or less follow-up:
  - Immature vascularization: zone 1 – no ROP
  - Immature retina extends into posterior zone II, near the boundary of zone I
  - Stage 1 or 2 ROP: zone I
  - Stage 3 ROP: zone II
  - Presence or suspected presence of aggressive posterior ROP
- One– to 2-week follow-up
  - Immature vascularization; posterior zone II
  - Stage 2 ROP: zone II
  - Unequivocally regressing ROP: zone I
- Two-week follow-up
  - Stage 1 ROP: zone II
  - Immature vascularization: zone II – no ROP
  - Unequivocally regressing ROP: zone II
- Two- to three-week follow-up
  - Stage 1 or 2 ROP: zone III
  - Regressing ROP: zone III

Termination of screening criteria:

- Zone III retinal vascularization attained without previous zone I or II ROP (if there is examiner doubt about the zone or if the postmenstrual age is less than 35 weeks, confirmatory examinations may be warranted)
- Full retinal vascularization in the close proximity to the ora serrata for 360°
- Postmenstrual age of 50 weeks and no prethreshold disease (defined as stage 3 ROP in zone II, any ROP in zone I) or worse ROP is present
- Regression of ROP (care must be taken to be sure that there is no abnormal vascular tissue present that is capable of reactivation and progression in zone II or III)

136.11.2 Telemedicine Approach to Screening for ROP

While clinical examinations by an experienced ophthalmologist using binocular indirect ophthalmoscopy remain the gold standard for identifying ROP (Fierson 2013; Fierson and Capone 2015), technical advances have permitted an innovative approach to remote ROP evaluation, using digital retinal imaging systems (Fierson and Capone 2015; Wu et al. 2006). The role of telemedicine as a useful adjunct to (but not a replacement of) binocular indirect ophthalmoscopy for evaluation of ROP was recently underlined in a joint report from the AAP/AAPOS and AACO (Fierson and Capone 2015). Wide-field digital fundus photography has demonstrated high diagnostic accuracy to detect clinically significant ROP (Fierson and Capone 2015; Wang et al. 2015), even in systems consisting of trained nonphysician imagers and readers (Quinn et al. 2014). Advantages of this technique therefore include, in areas with limited availability of experienced ophthalmologists, a decrease in the number of eye examinations that would require an evaluation by an ophthalmologist. Digital retinal imaging also allows for remote retrospective interpretation of images by experts as well as automatic image analysis and ROP education and fellowship training. Further studies, though, are still needed to address cost-effectiveness issues due to high implementation costs.

136.11.3 Predictive Statistical Models for ROP Risk Assessment

Because detection of ROP requires repeated uncomfortable eye examinations, while less than 10% of at-risk infants ultimately require treatment, several predictive statistical models based on gestational age, birth weight, postnatal weight gain, and/or neonatal morbidity have been developed to identify extremely preterm infants at risk for ROP requiring treatment at an early stage and to reduce the number of eye examinations in low risk infants. These models include WINROP, a computer-based ROP risk algorithm that identifies slowdowns in postnatal growth based on weekly cumulative deviations from expected weight gain (Wu et al. 2012), and two logistic regression-based models named ROPScore (Eckert et al. 2012) and CHOP ROP (Binenbaum et al. 2012). The main limitations of these models include their poor sensitivity and generalizability in middle-income countries, where poorly controlled oxygen use plays a more important role than weight gain in the pathogenesis of the disease and where more mature and bigger babies are at risk. Despite their promising performances in highly developed neonatal care settings, it is suggested that these models be used as "an adjunct to and not a replacement for standard ophthalmological screening" (Wu et al. 2012), since most studies published so far have limited sample size and larger studies are needed to achieve a more precise estimate of sensitivity prior to generalized clinical use.

136.11.4 Ophthalmologic Follow-Up Beyond the Neonatal Period

Although the risk of long-term visual disorders, such as refractive errors, strabismus, or amblyopia, is well recognized in ROP, there is little consensus regarding when, how frequent, and how long ophthalmologic follow-up should take place (O'Connor et al. 2006). Eye examination is indicated after discharge (Fierson 2013), even in case of ROP regression. An early first post-discharge examination – for example, within 6 months of expected full-term birth – could help detect amblyogenic factors and reduce the risk of later visual impairment.

136.12 Treatments

136.12.1 Cryotherapy

Cryotherapy to the vascular peripheral retina of the eyes with severe forms of active ROP had been used in Japan since the early 1970s (Yamashita 1972) and gradually gained advocates in several countries. Many ophthalmologists were reluctant to employ this treatment modality because of untoward or unexpected results. In the CRYO-ROP study, the method used to ablate avascular retina was cryotherapy. This treatment is still used in some hospitals, but it largely has been supplanted by diode laser in many countries. The cryotherapy probe is a long, thin, curved metal hand piece with a slightly rounded tip. It is applied to the external eyeball using enough force to indent the wall of the eye. This indentation can be seen using the indirect ophthalmoscope. A foot pedal attached to the probe is depressed when it is seen to be in proper position. The retina blanches as it freezes and leaves a treated spot. The probe is removed and moved to the next spot, either contiguous with or leaving a small space next to the previous treatment. The process is repeated over and over until the entire unvascularized retina has been treated. Cryotherapy is a painful and inflammatory procedure. Adverse effects include conjunctivitis, eyelid swelling, hypotony, infection, retinal detachment, and glaucoma. Pressing on the eye with the cryoprobe may elicit the oculocardiac reflex, a sudden bradycardia. Infants are usually put on topical antibiotics and steroids for a week or so after cryotherapy (Drack 2006).

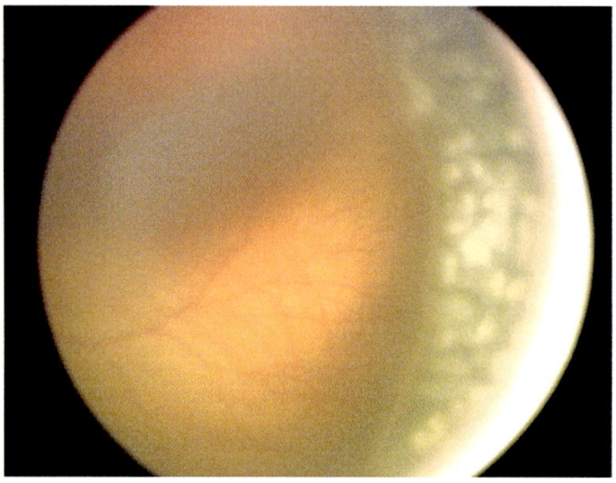

Fig. 7 Diode laser photocoagulation of the peripheral avascular retina

Table 3 Treatment strategies based on stage and location (zone) of ROP

Consider early treatment of eyes with prethreshold-type 1 disease: Zone 1, any stage of ROP with plus disease Zone 1, stage 3 with or without plus disease or Zone 2, stage 2 or 3 with plus disease
Observe closely eyes with prethreshold-type 2 disease (consider treating when progression to type 1 or threshold ROP): Zone 1, stage 1 or 2 with no plus disease or Zone 2, stage 3 with no plus disease

136.12.2 Photocoagulation

The benefit of ablating the peripheral avascular retina in ROP derived from the CRYO-ROP study (The Multicenter Trial of Cryotherapy for Retinopathy of Prematurity 1988). Easier to administrate and with less adverse effects than cryotherapy, laser photocoagulation soon became the standard of care to treat ROP. Ablation of the peripheral retina (Fig. 7) causes the stimulus for neovascularization to decrease, probably through decline of angiogenic factors. Laser photocoagulation was used for years following CRYO-ROP recommendation: to treat "threshold" ROP, a point in the progression of the disease at which the risk of retinal detachment approached 50% (The Multicenter Trial of Cryotherapy for Retinopathy of Prematurity 1988). Nonetheless, poor visual results remained common, and the ET-ROP (early treatment for retinopathy of prematurity) study demonstrated better outcomes with laser ablation performed earlier (Early Treatment for Retinopathy of Prematurity Cooperative Group 2003; Table 3). In that trial, infants with high-risk prethreshold ROP had one eye randomized to early intervention and the contralateral-control eye to conventional treatment. Unfavorable visual and structural outcomes were reduced from 19.8% to 14.3% and 15.6% to 9%, respectively (Early Treatment for Retinopathy of Prematurity Cooperative Group 2003). Other laser treatment long-term outcome studies report best mean corrected visual acuities between 20/46 and 20/98 (McLoone et al. 2006; Ospina et al. 2005; Yang et al. 2010). Over 65% of the eyes from those series had vision of 20/40 or better.

Unfortunately, in spite of early laser intervention, there remains a clear suboptimal outcome for zone 1 ROP-treated eyes: Kychental et al. found unfavorable anatomic results in 35% of eyes treated with anterior zone 1 ROP and in all laser-treated eyes with posterior zone 1 ROP (Kychenthal et al. 2006). In 2011 the BEAT-ROP study showed improved outcomes with intravitreal injection of bevacizumab compared with laser for eyes with zone I ROP (Mintz-Hittner et al. 2011). The off-label use of the same medication has become common for posterior ROP needing treatment, but most centers continue to use laser in cases of zone II ROP, for which the same trial did not show bevacizumab superiority over laser (Mintz-Hittner et al. 2011). Further prospective controlled studies comparing laser with the use of anti-VEGF medications and addressing safety concerns of the latter are necessary. A recent retrospective case series found no difference in outcomes for eyes with type 1 ROP treated with intravitreal bevacizumab versus laser (Hwang et al. 2015).

Laser photocoagulation, applied transpupillary through an indirect ophthalmoscope can be performed in the nursery under intravenous sedation in spontaneous respiration or in the operating room under general anesthesia. Argon laser was used initially used but is now widely replaced by diode laser, which requires less power. Many studies describe placement of laser burns 0.5–1 burn width apart, on the avascular retina extending from the ridge to the ora serrata for 360°. A more confluent pattern of burns may not only reduce the rate of progression (Rezai et al. 2005; Banach et al. 2000) but also the need for retreatment (Rezai et al. 2005). Generally, regression can be seen 5–7 days after treatment. Retreatment must be considered when retinopathy continues to progress and there are “skipped areas” that can be treated.

Complications from indirect laser photocoagulation include cataract, corneal or iris burns, choroidal or vitreous hemorrhage, hyphema, phthisis bulbi, and choroidal rupture (Clark and Mandal 2008; McNamara 1993). Even though visual field reduction has been demonstrated not to have a significant impact on visual function (McLoone et al. 2006; Quinn et al. 2011), the extensive ablations that sometimes are necessary continue to be a concern.

The refractive status of treated eyes deserves special mention, since myopia remains a significant and very common finding in all series of patients treated with laser. In a randomized bilateral treatment study, Connolly et al. found that laser-treated eyes were less myopic than those treated with cryotherapy (mean spherical equivalent −4.48 and −7.65 diopters, respectively) (Connolly et al. 2002). Other authors have found similar results (Shalev et al. 2001; Knight-Nanan and O’Keefe 1996; Laws et al. 1997). The problem of myopia is compounded by the fact that prematurity, ROP itself, and the treatment predispose to this refractive error (Varughese et al. 2008; O’Connor et al. 2002; Quinn et al. 1998; Choi et al. 2000).

136.12.3 Anti-VEGF

VEGF is a dominant factor that contributes to the neovascular phase of ROP. Accordingly the potential use of anti-VEGF therapy during this phase has been proposed. Some advantages of anti-VEGF therapy over the use of laser include:

(a) Easier administration under topical anesthesia and possibly reduction in the incidence of myopia (Mintz-Hittner et al. 2011; Chen et al. 2014; Geloneck et al. 2014; Harder et al. 2013), although, refractive errors may depend on other factors like duration of follow-up and the location of the disease. For instance, zone I disease appears to associate with higher myopia, even in the eyes treated with anti-VEGF (Hwang et al. 2015).

(b) Preservation of the peripheral retina that allows continuous vascularization of the retina and prevents the peripheral visual field defects of laser ablation (Pertl et al. 2015). Nevertheless, persistent avascularity of the periphery can occur, and even though it is not necessarily seen as a sign of treatment failure, the appropriate management is not yet established.

Until 2014, 55 clinical studies (predominantly in the form of case reports and small case series) have documented the use of bevacizumab (Avastin®), ranibizumab (Lucentis®), pegaptanib (Macugen®), and aflibercept (Eylea®) as anti-VEGF therapy for the treatment of ROP (Fig. 8 and Table 4). A generally favorable outcome was detected in the majority of the reports; however, in some of the studies, adverse effects were also reported (Klufas and Chan 2015; Micieli et al. 2009).

136.12.3.1 Bevacizumab (Avastin®)

Bevacizumab is a monoclonal antibody against VEGF that has been approved for use in colorectal, breast, and lung cancer; this antibody has also been widely used for proliferative macular degeneration and diabetic retinopathy. Since the cryotherapy and the early treatment ROP trials detected an unfavorable visual outcome in relatively advanced proliferative retinopathy in 78% and 55% of infants, respectively, it was reasonable for practitioners to attempt using anti-VEGF therapy with the hope of improving outcome. Forty-nine studies have been reported on the use of bevacizumab until 2014 (Klufas and Chan 2015), and there are some possible reasons to understand why bevacizumab is the most commonly reported agent to treat ROP. First, bevacizumab provides complete blockage of VEGF-A activity, whereas the activity of pegaptanib is only partial. Second, bevacizumab is a full-length antibody (149 kDa) that may have less tissue penetration and therefore less systemic

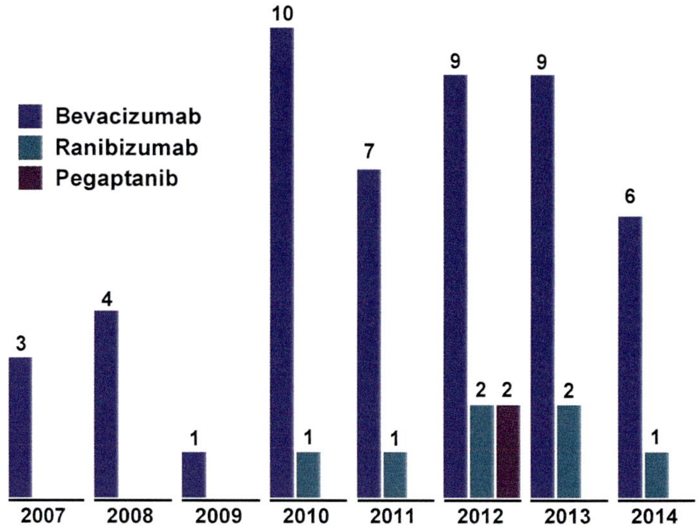

Fig. 8 Clinical studies report on use of intravitreal anti-VEGF therapy for the treatment of ROP in recent years

Table 4 Summary of clinical studies using anti-VEGF therapy for the treatment of ROP. The table was elaborated based on the data collected by Kuflas and Chan (2015)

Anti-VEGF agent	Number of studies	Study Type(s)	Dose	General outcome	Follow-up
Bevacizumab	**55**	Predominantly case reports and small case series, with one randomized controlled trial	*Range* 0.25–1.25 mg	A generally favorable outcome was detected in 39 of the 49 reports. However, retinal detachment, contraction of proliferative membrane, optic atrophy, vitreous or preretinal hemorrhages, choroidal rupture, and cataract were detected as ocular complications in some studies	*Range* 1 week–5 years
Ranibizumab vs. Bevacizumab	1	Retrospective	Ranibizumab 0.25 mg Bevacizumab 0.625 mg	No major ocular complications including cataract, tractional, or rhegmatogenous retinal detachment or endophthalmitis	1 year
Ranibizumab	7		*Range* 0.2–0.3 mg	No ocular or systemic adverse effects were reported in ROP patients	*Range* 1 week–3 years
Pegaptanib	2	Prospective, randomized controlled trials	0.3 mg	No systemic or significant ocular complications from intravitreal injections	Mean 19.3–23.5 mo

absorption compared to antibody fragments (40 kDa). However, this has resulted partly true because preliminary studies in neonates have showed that intravitreal bevacizumab causes systemic VEGF level suppression for up to 7 weeks after injection (Hong et al. 2015), whereas intravitreal ranibizumab suppresses systemic VEGF levels for about 2–3 weeks postinjection (Hoerster et al. 2013). Systemic VEGF suppression can be explained at least in part by an impaired blood-retina barrier of the immature retina of the neonates but also due to the prolonged half-life of bevacizumab (20 days) compared with ranibizumab (2 h). Another important reason to use bevacizumab in ROP is its cost. Bevacizumab is a more cost-effective option (up to 100 times less) compared to other more expensive anti-VEGF drugs.

A generally favorable outcome (controlled progressive neovascularization) was detected in 39 of the 49 reports using bevacizumab for ROP treatment (Klufas and Chan 2015). Despite a postmortem histopathological analysis of pediatric eyes treated for ROP with bevacizumab showing normal retinal development and morphology (Kong et al. 2008), some doubts about possible interference with normal ocular formation derive from ROP animal models revealing delayed vascular (Lutty et al. 2011) and neurovascular (Tokunaga et al. 2014) and retinal development after intravitreal anti-VEGF. Compared to laser, the need for long-term surveillance constitutes an additional drawback of anti-VEGF use, because disease reactivation has been reported as late as 69 weeks (Hu et al. 2012). Moreover, in some clinical studies, retinal detachment, contraction of proliferative membrane, optic atrophy, vitreous or preretinal hemorrhages, choroidal rupture, and cataract were detected as ocular adverse effects (Hu et al. 2012; Jalali et al. 2013; Atchaneeyasakul and Trinavarat 2010; Wu et al. 2013b). Furthermore, timing (stage/zone of ROP), dose (range: 0.25–1.25 mg iv), and frequency of administration of bevacizumab, as well as co-treatment with photocoagulation, varied tremendously between reports.

136.12.3.2 Ranibizumab (Lucentis®)

Ranibizumab is a recombinant humanized monoclonal antibody fragment that binds and inhibits all isoforms of VEGF (Ferrara et al. 2006). Ranibizumab was specifically developed for intraocular use based in part by preliminary studies suggesting that full-length monoclonal antibodies would not distribute across all retinal layers (Mordenti et al. 1999). Furthermore, the relatively long systemic half-life of full-length antibodies (versus antibody fragments) raised concerns about systemic toxicity in patients requiring long-term anti-VEGF blockade (Ferrara et al. 2006). Ranibizumab was approved for intravitreal use in clinic to treat neovascular (wet) age-related macular degeneration. At date, seven studies using ranibizumab alone or in combinations with bevacizumab or laser therapy have been reported in ROP patients (Klufas and Chan 2015). The dose used in all these studies did not vary considerably (range between 0.2–0.3 mg iv). No ocular or systemic adverse effects were reported in ROP patients (Klufas and Chan 2015); however, due to the biological similarity to bevacizumab, systemic unfavorable outcomes have been detected in neovascular age-related macular degeneration patients between these two anti-VEGF therapies (Moja et al. 2014).

136.12.3.3 Pegaptanib (Macugen®)

Pegaptanib sodium is an RNA aptamer that binds to the heparin-binding domain of VEGF and, thus, prevents the predominant $VEGF_{165}$ isoform from binding to VEGF receptors (Ng et al. 2006). Pegaptanib was approved in 2004 for the treatment of all the types of neovascular age-related macular degeneration (Ng et al. 2006). However, there is an interest in the use of pegaptanib in ROP given its selective suppression of the principal isoform ($VEGF_{165}$) involved in retinal pathologic neovascularization. Up to now, two clinical studies using pegaptanib have been reported (Autrata et al. 2012a, b). The dose used was 0.3 mg, and no systemic or significant ocular complications from intravitreal injections were reported.

136.12.3.4 Aflibercept (Eylea®)

Aflibercept (VEGF Trap-Eye) is a pharmacologically engineered protein that blocks the effects of all VEGF isoforms by acting as a decoy receptor (Dixon et al. 2009). In 2011, the FDA approved VEGF Trap-Eye for the treatment of patients with neovascular AMD. However, currently there are no published reports on the use of aflibercept in neonates with ROP.

To date, the interest in the use of anti-VEGF therapy in ROP continues to grow. Despite initial evidence of their efficacy, specialists who treat ROP remain cautious about the use of intravitreal anti-VEGF medications. The unknown possible deleterious effects that blocking VEGF may have on the developing brain constitute the principal concern over the incorporation of a new promising treatment for ROP (Hard and Hellstrom 2011). Moreover, systemic adverse effects are difficult to evaluate in preterm infants, who often suffer from neurological and developmental sequelae, pulmonary bronchodysplasia, and other comorbidities related to prematurity. A number of issues still need to be addressed in future well-conducted randomized trials: (a) adjunct photocoagulation therapy with anti-VEGF treatment; (b) impact on retinal ganglion cell integrity, since this neuron expresses the receptor for VEGF and is cytoprotected by VEGF; (c) timing of anti-VEGF therapy; (d) systemic effects of larger doses (1.25 mg) of bevacizumab, notably on cerebral vasculature; (e) long-term impact on visual acuity and visual fields; (f) cost-benefit versus currently available treatment.

136.12.4 Scleral Buckling and Vitrectomy

Almost one in 10 infants will develop unfavorable structural outcomes despite timely appropriate laser treatment (Hubbard 2008). Stages 4 and 5 of ROP will often require surgical treatment. It is possible to observe a small, localized, and shallow retinal detachment which may not progress or can even reattach, especially in the absence of active neovascularization and plus disease (Rubaltelli and Hirose 2008). Nonetheless, examinations and treatment decisions under those circumstances should not be delayed to prevent macular retinal detachment (Capone et al. 2014).

Acute retinal detachments result from contraction of neovascularization along the ridge and growth of vessels into the overlying vitreous leading to traction on the retina. Exudation causing subretinal accumulation of fluid is a much less common mechanism. Available techniques to treat retinal detachments from ROP include scleral buckling and different modalities of vitrectomy. The latter is now favored by vitreoretinal surgeons who feel that it addresses more thoroughly all the involved transvitreal traction forces. In a comparative nonrandomized study, Hartnett et al. found it superior to scleral buckling to treat stage 4 retinal detachment (Hartnett et al. 2004). The use of scleral buckling is reserved for cases of traction located near the equator of the eye or anterior to it (Rubaltelli and Hirose 2008; Roohipoor et al. 2009; Sears and Sonnie 2007).

Scleral buckling (encircling the eye at the equator or anteriorly with a silicone band) intends to correct the retinal detachment mechanically by moving the wall of the eye closer to the detached retina, thus counteracting the forces that exert traction on it. In a study using fundus fluorescein angiography, Yokoi et al. suggested that scleral buckling may also reduce the neovascular activity in the eyes with peripheral proliferation (Yokoi et al. 2009). They speculated that retinal reattachment may improve the vascular supply from the choroid to the retina, therefore decreasing the stimulus for VEGF expression. Buckling has a success rate of retinal reattachment in stage 4A ROP of around 70% (Tasman et al. 2006; Trese 1994). Nonetheless, the technique is not useful to treat posterior detachments in zone 1 or posterior zone 2, in which the ridge is located behind the equator and there is a large attached retina anteriorly. A major disadvantage of buckling is that the indentation caused by the silicone band elongates the eye inducing myopia of up to -9 or -11 diopters (Smiddy et al. 1989; Chow et al. 1998), thus increasing the risk of amblyopia, a significant concern given the age group. Furthermore, a second operation is required later to divide or remove the buckle to promote normal growth of the eye, improve its anterior circulation, and correct the refractive error.

Vitrectomy works through direct release of multi-vectorial vitreoretinal traction forces, and the removal of angiogenic factors like VEGF and vasodilators may constitute an additional mechanism of action (Sears and Sonnie 2007). Lens removal to access the vitreous cavity is no longer necessary for most of cases. Lens sparing vitrectomy has become the preferred technique to treat stage 4A and B ROP and even certain cases of stage 5 ROP (Hubbard 2008; Capone et al. 2014). Lens preservation reduces the risk of amblyopia. Vitreous access through the pars plicata allows treatment of retinal detachments resulting from posterior zone ROP, in which operating posterior to the equator is necessary (Rubaltelli and Hirose 2008). When more anterior disease causes retrolental membranes, removal of the lens may be necessary (vitrectomy and lensectomy) (Rubaltelli and Hirose 2008). The outcome is better when vitrectomy is performed after neovascularization and plus disease have resolved (Hubbard 2008). Unfortunately, sometimes surgery under those circumstances is necessary because a retinal detachment can progress rapidly in an eye that is still vascularly active; bleeding, continued proliferation, and contraction can occur with the procedure (Rubaltelli and Hirose 2008; Hartnett et al. 2004). Other complications of lens sparing vitrectomy are cataract, infection, and retinal breaks (Hartnett et al. 2004; Ferrone et al. 1997). Combining buckling was not found to add any benefit to lens sparing vitrectomy (Sears and Sonnie 2007). Nudleman et al. found a retinal reattachment rate of 82.1% for stage 4A, 69.5% for stage 4B, and 42.6% for stage 5 ROP, following lens sparing vitrectomy (Nudleman et al. 2015). In the same study close to 20% of patients needed additional retinal surgery after a mean follow-up time of 4.8 years. Performing lensectomy remains necessary for many stage 5 cases (Capone et al. 2014).

Some of the strategies to improve the outcome of vitrectomy aim at improving visualization during the procedure and dissolving the vitreous to facilitate it. Accordingly, the use of intravitreal triamcinolone has been advocated as a means to better view vitreal traction, the vitreous, and the posterior hyaloid (Lakhanpal et al. 2006; Shah et al. 2007). Similarly, performing vitrectomy following fluorescein angiography would have the double advantage of providing diagnostic information and also allowing for a safer and more complete vitrectomy of the dye-stained vitreous (Kobayashi et al. 2011). Enzymatic vitreolysis with autologous plasmin has been reported to improve the anatomic results of vitrectomy for ROP stage 5 (Tsukahara et al. 2007). More recently, ocriplasmin was used successfully in a controlled pediatric trial, but the small number of patients evaluated failed to demonstrate superiority over placebo (Drenser et al. 2016).

Unfortunately, despite improved anatomic results, the visual outcomes of surgery for ROP-related retinal detachment remain disappointing. At 6-year follow-up, information was available for 70 eyes with retinal detachment from the ETROP, although treatment of retinal detachment was not specifically addressed in the same study. Only 6 eyes (8.6%) retained vision over 20/200. Five of those had stage 4A, the other was not classified. Among 10 eyes with stage 5 in the same study, only one retained light perception (Repka et al. 2006). Comparably, Cusick et al. found vision better than 5/200 in only 8 of 183 eyes treated for stage 5 ROP (Cusick et al. 2006). Therefore, further developments are still needed in order to improve the very modest successes of surgery for ROP retinal detachment.

136.12.5 Prevention

The development of preventive and less destructive therapies for ROP such as nutritional supplements, including forms of vitamin E, vitamin C, and omega 3 fatty acids, would be much more desirable; however, despite numerous trials, prophylactic supplementation with this component remains controversial. Limitation of oxygenation has already been addressed above as an effective means of reducing ROP incidence and will not be repeated in this section.

136.12.5.1 Vitamin E

The most extensively studied medical treatment of ROP is the use of antioxidant vitamin E (alpha tocopherol). Vitamin E is a naturally occurring potent, free radical scavenger that decreases lipid peroxidation and helps maintain membrane integrity (Engin 2009). The retinal cells of the premature infant who has these clinical complications have their antioxidant defense system severely compromised, and they may be particularly vulnerable to the deleterious effects of oxygen-derived free radicals. It is known that premature infants are born with only 10% of adult levels of retinal vitamin E (Nielsen et al. 1988). The rationale for using vitamin E as treatment for ROP stems from the idea that peroxidative damage to cells is a causal factor and that vitamin E supplements may prevent this damage. The first reports of its use in the 1940s (Owens and Owens 1949) provide encouraging preliminary results of possible benefits of vitamin E prophylaxis in preventing ROP. However, this study was soon followed by the observation that oxygen therapy had a close link with ROP (Kinsey 1956; Lanman et al. 1954), and investigations into the effect of vitamin E were abandoned until the 1970s. In 1974 Johnson et al. (Johnson et al. 1974) reported a randomized clinical trial using oral and parenteral alpha tocopherol acetate supplements to achieve physiologic serum levels (1–3 mg/dl) in premature infants. Subsequent works showed a beneficial effect on incidence and severity of ROP associated with vitamin E prophylaxis that yielded physiologic serum levels of the antioxidants (Johnson et al. 1982). Three clinical trials enrolling 418 infants (less than or equal to 1500 g birth weight) elucidated the efficacy of vitamin E in suppressing the development of severe ROP. In this study only continuous vitamin E supplementation to adult physiologic levels from the first hours of life suppressed the development of severe ROP (Hittner et al. 1984). Other randomized clinical trials increasing serum concentrations of vitamin E at physiologic range reduced in a 52% the incidence of severe threshold (stage 3 +) ROP in the very low birth weight infant (Raju et al. 1997). Besides that several clinical trials have shown to determine the effectiveness of vitamin E in preventing ROP, prophylactic supplementation with vitamin E remains controversial (Muller 1992). Subsequent trials have shown no effect, and questions revolve around the route of administration (oral versus intramuscular versus intravenous), dose, timing of therapy, appropriate plasma levels, and trends toward higher plasma tocopherol levels in control groups (Schaffer et al. 1985; Phelps et al. 1987). A study in 2003 showed that extra vitamin E supplementation on preterm babies (born before 37 weeks) reduces the chances of some complications including ROP; however, the risk of life-threatening infections was increased (Brion et al. 2003). Furthermore, the risk of bleeding in the brain was increased when extra vitamin E is given by vein but decreased when the extra vitamin E is given by other routes (Brion et al. 2003). The protection mechanism of vitamin E in suppressing the development of severe ROP is not well known. A report proposes that spindle cells, mesenchymal precursors of the inner retinal capillaries, are the primary inducers of the neovascularization associated with ROP and the exposure of spindle cells to elevated oxygen tension increases their gap junction area. This early morphologic event immediately halts the normal vasoformative process and eventually triggers the neovascularization that is observed clinically 8–12 weeks later. Vitamin E supplementation above the deficient plasma levels of these infants suppresses gap junction formation and clinically reduces the severity without altering the total incidence of ROP (Kretzer et al. 1984).

136.12.5.2 Vitamin C

Vitamin C (ascorbic acid) is an important aqueous phase antioxidant in cells and plasma (Halliwell 1996). Vitamin C has a number of important metabolic functions and is actively transported across the placenta (Streeter and Rosso 1981). Vitamin C concentrations in cord plasma are higher than the mother's, and, in term infants, plasma concentrations fall considerably over the first 24 h of life (Hamil et al. 1947). Preterm infants generally have higher cord vitamin C concentrations than term infants, and concentrations then decline over a few days (Berger et al. 1996). Most preterm infants receive vitamin C as part of a multivitamin supplement, but there are few data on which to base optimum concentrations (Nutrient needs and feeding of premature infants 1995). One recommendation derives from the concentrations found in healthy breast-fed-term infants, with an adequate vitamin C concentration stated in approximately 34 mmol/l (Greene et al. 1992). Breast milk contains 3.5–5.5 mg vitamin C per 100 ml (Ingalls et al. 1938; Buss et al. 2001), so that an average infant having 150 ml/kg/day of milk will receive 5.2–8 mg/kg/day. The alternative view is that preterm infants should receive higher doses of vitamin C (25–31 mg/kg/day), to achieve concentrations closer to those in utero in the third trimester (Greene et al. 1992).

Vitamin C also has shown to have pro-oxidant activity (Carr and Frei 1999; Proteggente et al. 2001), and few studies of the relation between vitamin C concentration and morbidity in very preterm infants remain controversial. Silvers et al. (Silvers et al. 1994) reported that plasma vitamin C concentrations within 2 h of birth were significantly higher in infants who died compared with survivors. These researchers also observed that higher vitamin C concentrations on day 2 were associated with a greater risk of developing bronchopulmonary dysplasia (Silvers et al. 1998). In contrast, Moison et al. (1995) reported lower plasma vitamin C concentrations on day 10 in preterm infants who developed bronchopulmonary dysplasia compared with those who did not. In a pilot observational study of very low birth weight infants, an increased risk of retinopathy of prematurity (ROP) with higher plasma vitamin C concentrations at day 7 and an increased risk of bronchopulmonary dysplasia with lower concentrations at 28 days were found (Sluis et al. 1996). In another study, Darlow et al. (2005) hypothesized that maintaining a lower plasma vitamin C concentration (target 35–50 mmol/l) in the first week of life and a higher concentration (target 90 mmol/l) in weeks 3–4 would be accompanied by improved clinical outcome and least morbidity (chronic lung disease and ROP) in very low birth weight infants.

136.12.5.3 Omega-3 Fatty Acids

In 2007, Connor et al. demonstrated that dietary omega-3 fatty acids (PUFAs) protect against pathologic neovascularization in a mouse model of ROP (Connor et al. 2007). These findings suggest the possibility that omega-3 fatty acids act as protective factors in diseases that affect retinal blood vessels. Importantly, Western diets are often deficient in omega-3 PUFAs, and premature infants lack the important transfer of omega-3 PUFAs from their mother in the third trimester. Therefore, supplementing omega-3 PUFAs' intake to premature infants may be of benefit in preventing retinopathy. In this regard, a recent meta-analysis was conducted to evaluate whether LCPUFA supplementation of infant formulas improves infants' visual acuity (Qawasmi et al. 2013). The study demonstrated a significant benefit of LCPUFA supplementation on infants' visual acuity at 2, 4, and 12 months of age when visual acuity was assessed by using visual evoked potential and at 2 months of age by using behavioral methods (Qawasmi et al. 2013). However, in a secondary subgroup analyses and meta-regression examining the effects of LCPUFA dose and timing, preterm versus term birth status, the study failed to show any moderating effects on the association between LCPUFA supplementation and visual acuity (Qawasmi et al. 2013). These findings suggest that LCPUFA supplementation of infant formulas improves infants' visual acuity up to 12 months of age. The impact of fortification of infant formula or supplementation with omega-3 fatty acids to breast-feeding mothers on phase I or phase II ROP in low birth weight infants needs further study. Currently a trial conducted by the University of California is in the planning stage to supplement very low birth weight infants with omega-3 PUFAs for the prevention of ROP (http://clinicaltrials.gov/show/NCT02486042).

136.13 Future Directions

Some advances have been made in reducing severe retinal damage due to aberrant preretinal neovascularization with the use of cryo- and photocoagulation therapy. Likewise, preventive measures to diminish adverse consequences of relative hyperoxia have also started to be tackled by reducing oxygen administration to premature infants. Yet, a number of issues require future investigations. These can be divided along the following lines: (a) genetic predisposition, (b) improved inhibition of preretinal neovascularization, and (c) most importantly, preservation of retinal microvasculature (and parenchyma).

136.13.1 Genetic Predisposition

Despite the widespread exposure of premature infants to adverse risk factors, notably hyperoxia, relatively few babies develop severe forms of ROP; this infers genetic predisposition to advanced forms of ROP. So far only the Norrin gene and Frizzled-4 have been clearly associated with an increased risk for ROP (Shastry et al. 1997; Ells et al. 2010). There is a need to identify other genetic susceptibility determinants.

136.13.2 Inhibition of Preretinal Neovascularization

In addition to anti-VEGF therapy, other solutions to neovascularization can be envisaged to affect vascular development and factors that trigger expression of angiogenic factors; along these lines, the role of anti-inflammatory agents and modulators of carbohydrate metabolite receptors (Sapieha et al. 2008) is also worthy to explore.

136.13.3 Preservation of Retinal Microvasculature

Finally, it is paramount to preserve retinal microvasculature (Rivera et al. 2013) since its integrity prevents not only aberrant preretinal neovascularization but also retinal function. Hence, strategies suggested above regarding growth infer that IGF-1 may be an interesting potential avenue to pursue. Along the same lines, countering pro-inflammatory lipids using ω-3 fatty acids may also turn out to be effective (Connor et al. 2007). In addition, acceleration of normal revascularization may also be a worthy approach. Finally, prevention of prematurity is a long-term goal.

Acknowledgments We thank Drs. Maria Ana Martinez, Daniel Moreno, and Hugo Quiroz of the Association to Prevent Blindness in Mexico (APEC) for the contribution of the pictures in Figs. 3 and 4.

References

Akula JD, Mocko JA, Moskowitz A, Hansen RM, Fulton AB (2007) The oscillatory potentials of the dark-adapted electroretinogram in retinopathy of prematurity. Invest Ophthalmol Vis Sci 48:5788–5797

Alm A, Bill A (1973) Ocular and optic nerve blood flow at normal and increased intraocular pressures in monkeys (macaca irus): a study with radioactively labelled microspheres including flow determinations in brain and some other tissues. Exp Eye Res 15:15–29

Alon T, Hemo I, Itin A, Pe'er J, Stone J, Keshet E (1995) Vascular endothelial growth factor acts as a survival factor for newly formed retinal vessels and has implications for retinopathy of prematurity. Nat Med 1:1024–1028

An international classification of retinopathy of prematurity (1984) The committee for the classification of retinopathy of prematurity. Arch Ophthalmol 102:1130–1134

Anderson MF, Ramasamy B, Lythgoe DT, Clark D (2014) Choroidal thickness in regressed retinopathy of prematurity. Eye (Lond) 28:1461–1468

Antonelli-Orlidge A, Saunders KB, Smith SR, D'Amore PA (1989) An activated form of transforming growth factor beta is produced by cocultures of endothelial cells and pericytes. Proc Natl Acad Sci U S A 86:4544–4548

Arnold RW, Kesler K, Avila E (1994) Susceptibility to retinopathy of prematurity in alaskan natives. J Pediatr Ophthalmol Strabismus 31:192–194

Arroe M, Peitersen B (1994) Retinopathy of prematurity: review of a seven-year period in a Danish neonatal intensive care unit. Acta Paediatr 83:501–505

Asahara T, Murohara T, Sullivan A, Silver M, van der Zee R, Li T, Witzenbichler B, Schatteman G, Isner JM (1997) Isolation of putative progenitor endothelial cells for angiogenesis. Science 275:964–967

Asahara T, Masuda H, Takahashi T, Kalka C, Pastore C, Silver M, Kearne M, Magner M, Isner JM (1999) Bone marrow origin of endothelial progenitor cells responsible for postnatal vasculogenesis in physiological and pathological neovascularization. Circ Res 85:221–228

Ashton N (1957) Experimental retrolental fibroplasia. Annu Rev Med 8:441–454

Askie LM, Brocklehurst P, Darlow BA, Finer N, Schmidt B, Tarnow-Mordi W (2011) Neoprom: neonatal oxygenation prospective meta-analysis collaboration study protocol. BMC Pediatr 11:6

Atchaneeyasakul LO, Trinavarat A (2010) Choroidal ruptures after adjuvant intravitreal injection of bevacizumab for aggressive posterior retinopathy of prematurity. J Perinatol 30:497–499

Autrata R, Krejcirova I, Senkova K, Holousova M, Dolezel Z, Borek I (2012a) Intravitreal pegaptanib combined with diode laser therapy for stage 3+ retinopathy of prematurity in zone i and posterior zone ii. Eur J Ophthalmol 22:687–694

Autrata R, Senkova K, Holousova M, Krejcirova I, Dolezel Z, Borek I (2012b) Effects of intravitreal pegaptanib or bevacizumab and laser in treatment of threshold retinopathy of prematurity in zone i and posterior zone ii--four years results. Cesk Slov Oftalmol 68:29–36

Banach MJ, Ferrone PJ, Trese MT (2000) A comparison of dense versus less dense diode laser photocoagulation

patterns for threshold retinopathy of prematurity. Ophthalmology 107:324–327, discussion 328
Berger TM, Rifai N, Avery ME, Frei B (1996) Vitamin c in premature and full-term human neonates. Redox Rep 257–262
Binenbaum G, Ying GS, Quinn GE, Huang J, Dreiseitl S, Antigua J, Foroughi N, Abbasi S (2012) The chop postnatal weight gain, birth weight, and gestational age retinopathy of prematurity risk model. Arch Ophthalmol 130:1560–1565
Bremer DL, Palmer EA, Fellows RR, Baker JD, Hardy RJ, Tung B, Rogers GL (1998) Strabismus in premature infants in the first year of life. Cryotherapy for retinopathy of prematurity cooperative group. Arch Ophthalmol 116:329–333
Brion LP, Bell EF, Raghuveer TS (2003) Vitamin e supplementation for prevention of morbidity and mortality in preterm infants. Cochrane Database Syst Rev CD003665
Brown BA, Thach AB, Song JC, Marx JL, Kwun RC, Frambach DA (1998) Retinopathy of prematurity: evaluation of risk factors. Int Ophthalmol 22:279–283
Buss IH, McGill F, Darlow BA, Winterbourn CC (2001) Vitamin c is reduced in human milk after storage. Acta Paediatr 90:813–815
Caccavale A, Romanazzi F, Imparato M, Negri A, Morano A, Ferentini F (2011) Central serous chorioretinopathy: a pathogenetic model. Clin Ophthalmol 5:239–243
Campbell K (1951) Intensive oxygen therapy as a possible cause of retrolental fibroplasia; a clinical approach. Med J Aust 2:48–50
Capone AJ, Trese MT, Hartnett ME (2014) Treatment of stages 4 and 5 retinopathy of prematurity. In: Hartnett ME (ed) Pediatric retina, 2nd edn. Lippincott Williams & Wilkins, a Wolters Kluwer Health, Philadelphia, pp 597–603
Carr A, Frei B (1999) Does vitamin c act as a pro oxidant under physiological conditions? Faseb J 13:1007–1024
Checchin D, Sennlaub F, Sirinyan M, Brault S, Zhu T, Kermorvant-Duchemin E, Hardy P, Balazy M, Chemtob S (2006) Hypercapnia prevents neovascularization via nitrative stress. Free Radic Biol Med 40:543–553
Chemtob S, Beharry K, Rex J, Chatterjee T, Varma DR, Aranda JV (1991) Ibuprofen enhances retinal and choroidal blood flow autoregulation in newborn piglets. Invest Ophthalmol Vis Sci 32:1799–1807
Chen J, Smith LE (2007) Retinopathy of prematurity. Angiogenesis 10:133–140
Chen ML, Guo L, Smith LE, Dammann CE, Dammann O (2010) High or low oxygen saturation and severe retinopathy of prematurity: a meta-analysis. Pediatrics 125:e1483–e1492
Chen YH, Chen SN, Lien RI, Shih CP, Chao AN, Chen KJ, Hwang YS, Wang NK, Chen YP, Lee KH, Chuang CC, Chen TL, Lai CC, Wu WC (2014) Refractive errors after the use of bevacizumab for the treatment of retinopathy of prematurity: 2-year outcomes. Eye (Lond) 28:1080–1086, quiz 1087
Choi MY, Park IK, Yu YS (2000) Long term refractive outcome in eyes of preterm infants with and without retinopathy of prematurity: comparison of keratometric value, axial length, anterior chamber depth, and lens thickness. Br J Ophthalmol 84:138–143
Chow DR, Ferrone PJ, Trese MT (1998) Refractive changes associated with scleral buckling and division in retinopathy of prematurity. Arch Ophthalmol 116:1446–1448
Chow LC, Wright KW, Sola A (2003) Can changes in clinical practice decrease the incidence of severe retinopathy of prematurity in very low birth weight infants? Pediatrics 111:339–345
Clark D, Mandal K (2008) Treatment of retinopathy of prematurity. Early Hum Dev 84:95–99
Connolly BP, Ng EY, McNamara JA, Regillo CD, Vander JF, Tasman W (2002) A comparison of laser photocoagulation with cryotherapy for threshold retinopathy of prematurity at 10 years: part 2. Refractive outcome. Ophthalmology 109:936–941
Connor KM, SanGiovanni JP, Lofqvist C, Aderman CM, Chen J, Higuchi A, Hong S, Pravda EA, Majchrzak S, Carper D, Hellstrom A, Kang JX, Chew EY, Salem N Jr, Serhan CN, Smith LE (2007) Increased dietary intake of omega-3-polyunsaturated fatty acids reduces pathological retinal angiogenesis. Nat Med 13:868–873
Cringle SJ, Yu PK, Su EN, Yu DY (2006) Oxygen distribution and consumption in the developing rat retina. Invest Ophthalmol Vis Sci 47:4072–4076
Cryotherapy for Retinopathy of Prematurity Cooperative Group (1988) Multicenter trial of cryotherapy for retinopathy of prematurity. Preliminary results. Arch Ophthalmol 106:471–479
Cryotherapy for Retinopathy of Prematurity Cooperative Group (1994) The natural ocular outcome of premature birth and retinopathy. Status at 1 year. Arch Ophthalmol 112:903–912
Cryotherapy for Retinopathy of Prematurity Cooperative Group (2001a) Effect of retinal ablative therapy for threshold retinopathy of prematurity: results of goldmann perimetry at the age of 10 years. Arch Ophthalmol 119:1120–1125
Cryotherapy for Retinopathy of Prematurity Cooperative Group (2001b) Multicenter trial of cryotherapy for retinopathy of prematurity: ophthalmological outcomes at 10 years. Arch Ophthalmol 119:1110–1118
Csak K, Szabo V, Szabo A, Vannay A (2006) Pathogenesis and genetic basis for retinopathy of prematurity. Front Biosci 11:908–920
Cusick M, Charles MK, Agron E, Sangiovanni JP, Ferris FL 3rd, Charles S (2006) Anatomical and visual results of vitreoretinal surgery for stage 5 retinopathy of prematurity. Retina 26:729–735
Darlow BA, Buss H, McGill F, Fletcher L, Graham P, Winterbourn CC (2005) Vitamin c supplementation in very preterm infants: a randomised controlled trial. Arch Dis Child Fetal Neonatal Ed 90:F117–F122
Davitt BV, Wallace DK (2009) Plus disease. Surv Ophthalmol 54:663–670

Davitt BV, Dobson V, Good WV, Hardy RJ, Quinn GE, Siatkowski RM, Summers CG, Tung B (2005) Prevalence of myopia at 9 months in infants with high-risk prethreshold retinopathy of prematurity. Ophthalmology 112:1564–1568

Davitt BV, Dobson V, Quinn GE, Hardy RJ, Tung B, Good WV (2009) Astigmatism in the early treatment for retinopathy of prematurity study: findings to 3 years of age. Ophthalmology 116:332–339

Davitt BV, Quinn GE, Wallace DK, Dobson V, Hardy RJ, Tung B, Lai D, Good WV (2011) Astigmatism progression in the early treatment for retinopathy of prematurity study to 6 years of age. Ophthalmology 118:2326–2329

Delport SD, Swanepoel JC, Odendaal PJ, Roux P (2002) Incidence of retinopathy of prematurity in very-low-birth-weight infants born at kalafong hospital, pretoria. S Afr Med J 92:986–990

Deulofeut R, Critz A, Adams-Chapman I, Sola A (2006) Avoiding hyperoxia in infants < or = 1250 g is associated with improved short- and long-term outcomes. J Perinatol 26:700–705

Dixon JA, Oliver SC, Olson JL, Mandava N (2009) Vegf trap-eye for the treatment of neovascular age-related macular degeneration. Expert Opin Investig Drugs 18:1573–1580

Dorfman A, Dembinska O, Chemtob S, Lachapelle P (2008) Early manifestations of postnatal hyperoxia on the retinal structure and function of the neonatal rat. Invest Ophthalmol Vis Sci 49:458–466

Dorfman AL, Polosa A, Joly S, Chemtob S, Lachapelle P (2009) Functional and structural changes resulting from strain differences in the rat model of oxygen-induced retinopathy. Invest Ophthalmol Vis Sci 50:2436–2450

Drack A (2006) Retinopathy of prematurity. Adv Pediatr 53:211–226

Drenser K, Girach A, Capone A (2016) A randomized, placebo-controlled study of intravitreal ocriplasmin in pediatric patients scheduled for vitrectomy. Retina 36:565–575

Early Treatment for Retinopathy of Prematurity Cooperative Group (2003) Revised indications for the treatment of retinopathy of prematurity: results of the early treatment for retinopathy of prematurity randomized trial. Arch Ophthalmol 121:1684–1694

Eckert GU, Fortes Filho JB, Maia M, Procianoy RS (2012) A predictive score for retinopathy of prematurity in very low birth weight preterm infants. Eye (Lond) 26:400–406

Ecsedy M, Szamosi A, Karko C, Zubovics L, Varsanyi B, Nemeth J, Recsan Z (2007) A comparison of macular structure imaged by optical coherence tomography in preterm and full-term children. Invest Ophthalmol Vis Sci 48:5207–5211

Ecsedy M, Varsanyi B, Szigeti A, Szrnka G, Nemeth J, Recsan Z (2011) Cone function in children with a history of preterm birth. Doc Ophthalmol 122:141–148

Ells A, Hicks M, Fielden M, Ingram A (2005) Severe retinopathy of prematurity: longitudinal observation of disease and screening implications. Eye (Lond) 19:138–144

Ells A, Guernsey DL, Wallace K, Zheng B, Vincer M, Allen A, Ingram A, DaSilva O, Siebert L, Sheidow T, Beis J, Robitaille JM (2010) Severe retinopathy of prematurity associated with fzd4 mutations. Ophthalmic Genet 31:37–43

Engin KN (2009) Alpha-tocopherol: looking beyond an antioxidant. Mol Vis 15:855–860

Ferrara N, Damico L, Shams N, Lowman H, Kim R (2006) Development of ranibizumab, an anti-vascular endothelial growth factor antigen binding fragment, as therapy for neovascular age-related macular degeneration. Retina 26:859–870

Ferrone PJ, Harrison C, Trese MT (1997) Lens clarity after lens-sparing vitrectomy in a pediatric population. Ophthalmology 104:273–278

Fielder AR, Shaw DE, Robinson J, Ng YK (1992) Natural history of retinopathy of prematurity: a prospective study. Eye (Lond) 6(Pt 3):233–242

Fierson WM (2013) Screening examination of premature infants for retinopathy of prematurity. Pediatrics 131:189–195

Fierson WM, Capone A Jr (2015) Telemedicine for evaluation of retinopathy of prematurity. Pediatrics 135:e238–e254

Foster PJ, Jiang Y (2014) Epidemiology of myopia. Eye (Lond) 28:202–208

Fulton AB, Hansen RM (1995) Electroretinogram responses and refractive errors in patients with a history of retinopathy prematurity. Doc Ophthalmol 91:87–100

Fulton AB, Hansen RM (1996) Photoreceptor function in infants and children with a history of mild retinopathy of prematurity. J Opt Soc Am A Opt Image Sci Vis 13:566–571

Fulton AB, Hansen RM, Petersen RA, Vanderveen DK (2001) The rod photoreceptors in retinopathy of prematurity: an electroretinographic study. Arch Ophthalmol 119:499–505

Fulton AB, Hansen RM, Moskowitz A, Barnaby AM (2005) Multifocal erg in subjects with a history of retinopathy of prematurity. Doc Ophthalmol 111:7–13

Fulton AB, Hansen RM, Moskowitz A (2008) The cone electroretinogram in retinopathy of prematurity. Invest Ophthalmol Vis Sci 49:814–819

Fulton AB, Hansen RM, Moskowitz A (2009) Development of rod function in term born and former preterm subjects. Optom Vis Sci 86:E653–E658

Gallo JE, Jacobson L, Broberger U (1993) Perinatal factors associated with retinopathy of prematurity. Acta Paediatr 82:829–834

Geloneck MM, Chuang AZ, Clark WL, Hunt MG, Norman AA, Packwood EA, Tawansy KA, Mintz-Hittner HA (2014) Refractive outcomes following bevacizumab monotherapy compared with conventional laser treatment: a randomized clinical trial. JAMA Ophthalmol 132:1327–1333

Gilbert C (2008) Retinopathy of prematurity: a global perspective of the epidemics, population of babies at risk and implications for control. Early Hum Dev 84:77–82

Gilbert C, Rahi J, Eckstein M, O'Sullivan J, Foster A (1997) Retinopathy of prematurity in middle-income countries. Lancet 350:12–14

Gilbert C, Fielder A, Gordillo L, Quinn G, Semiglia R, Visintin P, Zin A (2005) Characteristics of infants with severe retinopathy of prematurity in countries with low, moderate, and high levels of development: implications for screening programs. Pediatrics 115:e518–e525

Goggin M, O'Keefe M (1993) Diode laser for retinopathy of prematurity–early outcome. Br J Ophthalmol 77:559–562

Good WV (2004) Final results of the early treatment for retinopathy of prematurity (etrop) randomized trial. Trans Am Ophthalmol Soc 102:233–248, discussion 248–250

Good WV, Hardy RJ, Dobson V, Palmer EA, Phelps DL, Quintos M, Tung B (2005) The incidence and course of retinopathy of prematurity: findings from the early treatment for retinopathy of prematurity study. Pediatrics 116:15–23

Good WV, Hardy RJ, Dobson V, Palmer EA, Phelps DL, Tung B, Redford M (2010) Final visual acuity results in the early treatment for retinopathy of prematurity study. Arch Ophthalmol 128:663–671

Greene HL, Porchelli P, Adcock E, Swift L (1992) Vitamins for newborn infant formulas: a review of recommendations with emphasis on data from low birth-weight infants. Eur J Clin Nutr 46(Suppl 4):S1–S8

Gu X, Samuel S, El-Shabrawey M, Caldwell RB, Bartoli M, Marcus DM, Brooks SE (2002) Effects of sustained hyperoxia on revascularization in experimental retinopathy of prematurity. Invest Ophthalmol Vis Sci 43:496–502

Hack M, Taylor HG, Klein N, Eiben R, Schatschneider C, Mercuri-Minich N (1994) School-age outcomes in children with birth weights under 750 g. N Engl J Med 331:753–759

Haddad MA, Sei M, Sampaio MW, Kara-Jose N (2007) Causes of visual impairment in children: a study of 3,210 cases. J Pediatr Ophthalmol Strabismus 44:232–240

Halliwell B (1996) Vitamin c: antioxidant or pro-oxidant in vivo? Free Radic Res 25:439–454

Hamil BM, Munks B et al (1947) Vitamin c in the blood and urine of the newborn and in the cord and maternal blood. Am J Dis Child 74:417–433

Hammer DX, Iftimia NV, Ferguson RD, Bigelow CE, Ustun TE, Barnaby AM, Fulton AB (2008) Foveal fine structure in retinopathy of prematurity: an adaptive optics fourier domain optical coherence tomography study. Invest Ophthalmol Vis Sci 49:2061–2070

Hansen RM, Fulton AB (2000) Background adaptation in children with a history of mild retinopathy of prematurity. Invest Ophthalmol Vis Sci 41:320–324

Hansen RM, Harris ME, Moskowitz A, Fulton AB (2010) Deactivation of the rod response in retinopathy of prematurity. Doc Ophthalmol 121:29–35

Hard AL, Hellstrom A (2011) On the use of antiangiogenetic medications for retinopathy of prematurity. Acta Paediatr 100:1063–1065

Harder BC, Schlichtenbrede FC, von Baltz S, Jendritza W, Jendritza B, Jonas JB (2013) Intravitreal bevacizumab for retinopathy of prematurity: refractive error results. Am J Ophthalmol 155:1119–1124 e1111

Hardy P, Abran D, Li DY, Fernandez H, Varma DR, Chemtob S (1994) Free radicals in retinal and choroidal blood flow autoregulation in the piglet: interaction with prostaglandins. Invest Ophthalmol Vis Sci 35:580–591

Hardy P, Nuyt AM, Abran D, St-Louis J, Varma DR, Chemtob S (1996a) Nitric oxide in retinal and choroidal blood flow autoregulation in newborn pigs: Interactions with prostaglandins. Pediatr Res 39:487–493

Hardy P, Peri KG, Lahaie I, Varma DR, Chemtob S (1996b) Increased nitric oxide synthesis and action preclude choroidal vasoconstriction to hyperoxia in newborn pigs. Circ Res 79:504–511

Harris ME, Moskowitz A, Fulton AB, Hansen RM (2011) Long-term effects of retinopathy of prematurity (rop) on rod and rod-driven function. Doc Ophthalmol 122:19–27

Hartnett ME, Maguluri S, Thompson HW, McColm JR (2004) Comparison of retinal outcomes after scleral buckle or lens-sparing vitrectomy for stage 4 retinopathy of prematurity. Retina 24:753–757

Hellgren G, Lofqvist C, Hard AL, Hansen-Pupp I, Gram M, Ley D, Smith LE, Hellstrom A (2016) Serum concentrations of vascular endothelial growth factor in relation to retinopathy of prematurity. Pediatr Res 79:70–75

Hellstrom A, Perruzzi C, Ju M, Engstrom E, Hard AL, Liu JL, Albertsson-Wikland K, Carlsson B, Niklasson A, Sjodell L, LeRoith D, Senger DR, Smith LE (2001) Low igf-i suppresses vegf-survival signaling in retinal endothelial cells: direct correlation with clinical retinopathy of prematurity. Proc Natl Acad Sci U S A 98:5804–5808

Hellstrom A, Hard AL, Engstrom E, Niklasson A, Andersson E, Smith L, Lofqvist C (2009) Early weight gain predicts retinopathy in preterm infants: new, simple, efficient approach to screening. Pediatrics 123: e638–e645

Hiraoka M, Berinstein DM, Trese MT, Shastry BS (2001) Insertion and deletion mutations in the dinucleotide repeat region of the norrie disease gene in patients with advanced retinopathy of prematurity. J Hum Genet 46:178–181

Hittner HM, Rudolph AJ, Kretzer FL (1984) Suppression of severe retinopathy of prematurity with vitamin e supplementation ultrastructural mechanism of clinical efficacy. Ophthalmology 91:1512–1523

Hoerster R, Muether P, Dahlke C, Mehler K, Oberthur A, Kirchhof B, Fauser S (2013) Serum concentrations of vascular endothelial growth factor in an infant treated with ranibizumab for retinopathy of prematurity. Acta Ophthalmol 91:e74–e75

Holmes JM, Zhang S, Leske DA, Lanier WL (1998) Carbon dioxide-induced retinopathy in the neonatal rat. Curr Eye Res 17:608–616

Hong YR, Kim YH, Kim SY, Nam GY, Cheon HJ, Lee SJ (2015) Plasma concentrations of vascular endothelial growth factor in retinopathy of prematurity after intravitreal bevacizumab injection. Retina 35:1772–1777

Hu J, Blair MP, Shapiro MJ, Lichtenstein SJ, Galasso JM, Kapur R (2012) Reactivation of retinopathy of prematurity after bevacizumab injection. Arch Ophthalmol 130:1000–1006

Hubbard GB 3rd (2008) Surgical management of retinopathy of prematurity. Curr Opin Ophthalmol 19:384–390

Husain SM, Sinha AK, Bunce C, Arora P, Lopez W, Mun KS, Reddy MA, Adams GG (2013) Relationships between maternal ethnicity, gestational age, birth weight, weight gain, and severe retinopathy of prematurity. J Pediatr 163:67–72

Hwang CK, Hubbard GB, Hutchinson AK, Lambert SR (2015) Outcomes after intravitreal bevacizumab versus laser photocoagulation for retinopathy of prematurity: a 5-year retrospective analysis. Ophthalmology 122:1008–1015

Ingalls TH, Draper R, Teel HM (1938) Vitamin c in human pregnancy and lactation. II. Studies during lactation. Am J Dis Child 56:1011–1019

Jacobson RM, Feinstein AR (1992) Oxygen as a cause of blindness in premature infants: "autopsy" of a decade of errors in clinical epidemiologic research. J Clin Epidemiol 45:1265–1287

Jalali S, Balakrishnan D, Zeynalova Z, Padhi TR, Rani PK (2013) Serious adverse events and visual outcomes of rescue therapy using adjunct bevacizumab to laser and surgery for retinopathy of prematurity. The Indian twin cities retinopathy of prematurity screening database report number 5. Arch Dis Child Fetal Neonatal Ed 98:F327–F333

Johnson BA, Weil MH (1991) Redefining ischemia due to circulatory failure as dual defects of oxygen deficits and of carbon dioxide excesses. Crit Care Med 19:1432–1438

Johnson L, Schaffer D, Boggs TR Jr (1974) The premature infant, vitamin e deficiency and retrolental fibroplasia. Am J Clin Nutr 27:1158–1173

Johnson L, Schaffer D, Quinn G, Goldstein D, Mathis MJ, Otis C, Boggs TR Jr (1982) Vitamin e supplementation and the retinopathy of prematurity. Ann N Y Acad Sci 393:473–495

Kaiser RS, Trese MT (2001) Iris atrophy, cataracts, and hypotony following peripheral ablation for threshold retinopathy of prematurity. Arch Ophthalmol 119:615–617

Kinsey VE (1956) Retrolental fibroplasia; cooperative study of retrolental fibroplasia and the use of oxygen. AMA Arch Ophthalmol 56:481–543

Kizawa J, Machida S, Kobayashi T, Gotoh Y, Kurosaka D (2006) Changes of oscillatory potentials and photopic negative response in patients with early diabetic retinopathy. Jpn J Ophthalmol 50:367–373

Klufas MA, Chan RV (2015) Intravitreal anti-vegf therapy as a treatment for retinopathy of prematurity: what we know after 7 years. J Pediatr Ophthalmol Strabismus 52:77–84

Knight-Nanan DM, O'Keefe M (1996) Refractive outcome in eyes with retinopathy of prematurity treated with cryotherapy or diode laser: 3 year follow up. Br J Ophthalmol 80:998–1001

Kobayashi Y, Yokoi T, Yokoi T, Hiraoka M, Nishina S, Azuma N (2011) Fluorescein staining of the vitreous during vitrectomy for retinopathy of prematurity. Retina 31:1717–1719

Kong L, Mintz-Hittner HA, Penland RL, Kretzer FL, Chevez-Barrios P (2008) Intravitreous bevacizumab as anti-vascular endothelial growth factor therapy for retinopathy of prematurity: a morphologic study. Arch Ophthalmol 126:1161–1163

Kong L, Bhatt AR, Demny AB, Coats DK, Li A, Rahman EZ, Smith OE, Steinkuller PG (2015) Pharmacokinetics of bevacizumab and its effects on serum vegf and igf-1 in infants with retinopathy of prematurity. Invest Ophthalmol Vis Sci 56:956–961

Kretzer FL, Mehta RS, Johnson AT, Hunter DG, Brown ES, Hittner HM (1984) Vitamin e protects against retinopathy of prematurity through action on spindle cells. Nature 309:793–795

Kychenthal A, Dorta P, Katz X (2006) Zone i retinopathy of prematurity: clinical characteristics and treatment outcomes. Retina 26:S11–S15

Lad EM, Hernandez-Boussard T, Morton JM, Moshfeghi DM (2009) Incidence of retinopathy of prematurity in the united states: 1997 through 2005. Am J Ophthalmol 148:451–458

Lai AKW, Fu ZJ, Lo AC (2013) Stem cell therapy for retinopathy of prematurity. Anat Physiol 3:126

Lakhanpal RR, Fortun JA, Chan-Kai B, Holz ER (2006) Lensectomy and vitrectomy with and without intravitreal triamcinolone acetonide for vascularly active stage 5 retinal detachments in retinopathy of prematurity. Retina 26:736–740

Lang DM, Blackledge J, Arnold RW (2005) Is pacific race a retinopathy of prematurity risk factor? Arch Pediatr Adolesc Med 159:771–773

Lanman JT, Guy LP, Dancis J (1954) Retrolental fibroplasia and oxygen therapy. J Am Med Assoc 155:223–226

Laser ROP Study Group (1994) Laser therapy for retinopathy of prematurity. Arch Ophthalmol 112:154–156

Laws F, Laws D, Clark D (1997) Cryotherapy and laser treatment for acute retinopathy of prematurity: refractive outcomes, a longitudinal study. Br J Ophthalmol 81:12–15

Linsenmeier RA, Padnick-Silver L (2000) Metabolic dependence of photoreceptors on the choroid in the normal and detached retina. Invest Ophthalmol Vis Sci 41:3117–3123

Lofqvist C, Andersson E, Sigurdsson J, Engstrom E, Hard AL, Niklasson A, Smith LE, Hellstrom A (2006) Longitudinal postnatal weight and insulin-like growth factor i measurements in the prediction of retinopathy of prematurity. Arch Ophthalmol 124:1711–1718

Lutty GA, McLeod DS, Bhutto I, Wiegand SJ (2011) Effect of vegf trap on normal retinal vascular development and oxygen-induced retinopathy in the dog. Invest Ophthalmol Vis Sci 52:4039–4047

Machalinska A, Modrzejewska M, Kotowski M, Dziedziejko V, Kucia M, Kawa M, Safranow K, Baskiewicz-Masiuk M, Modrzejewska A, Karczewicz D, Rudnicki J, Machalinski B (2010) Circulating stem cell populations in preterm infants: implications for the development of retinopathy of prematurity. Arch Ophthalmol 128:1311–1319

Machalinska A, Kotowski M, Safranow K, Lewandowska J, Modrzejewska M, Rudnicki J, Czajka R, Machalinski B (2011) The role of circulating endothelial progenitor cells in the progression of retinopathy of prematurity–a prospective study. Klin Oczna 113:223–227

Machalinska A, Modrzejewska M, Kawa M, Paczkowska E, Dziedziejko V, Safranow K, Lubinski W, Machalinski B (2013) Potential contribution of mobilized circulating endothelial progenitor cells to development of retinal neovascularization in preterm infants with rop. Klin Oczna 115:194–198

Mactier H, Bradnam MS, Hamilton R (2013) Dark-adapted oscillatory potentials in preterm infants with and without retinopathy of prematurity. Doc Ophthalmol 127:33–40

Maida JM, Mathers K, Alley CL (2008) Pediatric ophthalmology in the developing world. Curr Opin Ophthalmol 19:403–408

McLoone E, O'Keefe M, McLoone S, Lanigan B (2006) Long term functional and structural outcomes of laser therapy for retinopathy of prematurity. Br J Ophthalmol 90:754–759

McNamara JA (1993) Laser treatment for retinopathy of prematurity. Curr Opin Ophthalmol 4:76–80

Michaelson I (1948) The mode of development of the vascular system of the retina, with some observations on its significance for certain retinal diseases. Trans Ophthalmol Soc UK 68:137–180

Micieli JA, Surkont M, Smith AF (2009) A systematic analysis of the off-label use of bevacizumab for severe retinopathy of prematurity. Am J Ophthalmol 148:536–543 e532

Mintz-Hittner HA, Kennedy KA, Chuang AZ (2011) Efficacy of intravitreal bevacizumab for stage 3+ retinopathy of prematurity. N Engl J Med 364:603–615

Moison RM, van Zoeren-Grobben D, Haasnoot AA et al (1995) Early biochemical detection of bronchopulmonary dysplasia (bpd) in preterm babies [abstract]. Pediatr Res 37:43A

Moja L, Lucenteforte E, Kwag KH, Bertele V, Campomori A, Chakravarthy U, D'Amico R, Dickersin K, Kodjikian L, Lindsley K, Loke Y, Maguire M, Martin DF, Mugelli A, Muhlbauer B, Puntmann I, Reeves B, Rogers C, Schmucker C, Subramanian ML, Virgili G (2014) Systemic safety of bevacizumab versus ranibizumab for neovascular age-related macular degeneration. Cochrane Database Syst Rev 9:CD011230

Mordenti J, Cuthbertson RA, Ferrara N, Thomsen K, Berleau L, Licko V, Allen PC, Valverde CR, Meng YG, Fei DT, Fourre KM, Ryan AM (1999) Comparisons of the intraocular tissue distribution, pharmacokinetics, and safety of 125i-labeled full-length and fab antibodies in rhesus monkeys following intravitreal administration. Toxicol Pathol 27:536–544

Muller DP (1992) Vitamin e therapy in retinopathy of prematurity. Eye (Lond) 6(Pt 2):221–225

Multicenter trial of cryotherapy for retinopathy of prematurity (1998) Preliminary results. Cryotherapy for retinopathy of prematurity cooperative group. Arch Ophthalmol 106:471–479

Neufeld G, Cohen T, Gengrinovitch S, Poltorak Z (1999) Vascular endothelial growth factor (vegf) and its receptors. Faseb J 13:9–22

Ng EW, Shima DT, Calias P, Cunningham ET Jr, Guyer DR, Adamis AP (2006) Pegaptanib, a targeted anti-vegf aptamer for ocular vascular disease. Nat Rev Drug Discov 5:123–132

Nielsen JC, Naash MI, Anderson RE (1988) The regional distribution of vitamins e and c in mature and premature human retinas. Invest Ophthalmol Vis Sci 29:22–26

Nudleman E, Robinson J, Rao P, Drenser KA, Capone A, Trese MT (2015) Long-term outcomes on lens clarity after lens-sparing vitrectomy for retinopathy of prematurity. Ophthalmology 122:755–759

Nutrient needs and feeding of premature infants. Nutrition committee, Canadian Paediatric Society. CMAJ 152:1765–1785 (1995)

O'Connor AR, Stephenson T, Johnson A, Tobin MJ, Moseley MJ, Ratib S, Ng Y, Fielder AR (2002) Long-term ophthalmic outcome of low birth weight children with and without retinopathy of prematurity. Pediatrics 109:12–18

O'Connor AR, Stephenson TJ, Johnson A, Tobin MJ, Ratib S, Moseley M, Fielder AR (2004) Visual function in low birthweight children. Br J Ophthalmol 88:1149–1153

O'Connor AR, Stewart CE, Singh J, Fielder AR (2006) Do infants of birth weight less than 1500 g require additional long term ophthalmic follow up? Br J Ophthalmol 90:451–455

O'Connor AR, Wilson CM, Fielder AR (2007) Ophthalmological problems associated with preterm birth. Eye (Lond) 21:1254–1260

Ospina LH, Lyons CJ, Matsuba C, Jan J, McCormick AQ (2005) Argon laser photocoagulation for retinopathy of prematurity: long-term outcome. Eye (Lond) 19:1213–1218

Owens WC, Owens EU (1949) Retrolental fibroplasia in premature infants; studies on the prophylaxis of the disease; the use of alpha tocopheryl acetate. Am J Ophthalmol 32:1631–1637

Ozaki H, Yu AY, Della N, Ozaki K, Luna JD, Yamada H, Hackett SF, Okamoto N, Zack DJ, Semenza GL, Campochiaro PA (1999) Hypoxia inducible factor-1 alpha is increased in ischemic retina: temporal and spatial correlation with vegf expression. Invest Ophthalmol Vis Sci 40:182–189

Palmer EA, Flynn JT, Hardy RJ, Phelps DL, Phillips CL, Schaffer DB, Tung B (1991) Incidence and early course of retinopathy of prematurity. The cryotherapy for retinopathy of prematurity cooperative group. Ophthalmology 98:1628–1640

Palmer EA, Hardy RJ, Dobson V, Phelps DL, Quinn GE, Summers CG, Krom CP, Tung B (2005) 15-year outcomes following threshold retinopathy of prematurity: final results from the multicenter trial of cryotherapy for retinopathy of prematurity. Arch Ophthalmol 123:311–318

Penn JS, Tolman BL, Henry MM (1994) Oxygen-induced retinopathy in the rat: relationship of retinal nonperfusion to subsequent neovascularization. Invest Ophthalmol Vis Sci 35:3429–3435

Penn JS, Madan A, Caldwell RB, Bartoli M, Caldwell RW, Hartnett ME (2008) Vascular endothelial growth factor in eye disease. Prog Retin Eye Res 27:331–371

Pertl L, Steinwender G, Mayer C, Hausberger S, Poschl EM, Wackernagel W, Wedrich A, El-Shabrawi Y, Haas A (2015) A systematic review and meta-analysis on the safety of vascular endothelial growth factor (vegf) inhibitors for the treatment of retinopathy of prematurity. PLoS One 10:e0129383

Phelps DL, Rosenbaum AL, Isenberg SJ, Leake RD, Dorey FJ (1987) Tocopherol efficacy and safety for preventing retinopathy of prematurity: a randomized, controlled, double-masked trial. Pediatrics 79:489–500

Pournaras CJ, Riva CE, Tsacopoulos M, Strommer K (1989) Diffusion of o2 in the retina of anesthetized miniature pigs in normoxia and hyperoxia. Exp Eye Res 49:347–360

Proteggente AR, England TG, Rice-Evans CA, Halliwell B (2001) Iron supplementation and oxidative damage to DNA in healthy individuals with high plasma ascorbate. Biochem Biophys Res Commun 288:245–251

Provis JM, Leech J, Diaz CM, Penfold PL, Stone J, Keshet E (1997) Development of the human retinal vasculature: cellular relations and vegf expression. Exp Eye Res 65:555–568

Qawasmi A, Landeros-Weisenberger A, Bloch MH (2013) Meta-analysis of lcpufa supplementation of infant formula and visual acuity. Pediatrics 131:e262–e272

Quinn GE, Dobson V, Repka MX, Reynolds J, Kivlin J, Davis B, Buckley E, Flynn JT, Palmer EA (1992) Development of myopia in infants with birth weights less than 1251 grams. The cryotherapy for retinopathy of prematurity cooperative group. Ophthalmology 99:329–340

Quinn GE, Dobson V, Kivlin J, Kaufman LM, Repka MX, Reynolds JD, Gordon RA, Hardy RJ, Tung B, Stone RA (1998) Prevalence of myopia between 3 months and 5 1/2 years in preterm infants with and without retinopathy of prematurity. Cryotherapy for retinopathy of prematurity cooperative group. Ophthalmology 105:1292–1300

Quinn GE, Dobson V, Davitt BV, Hardy RJ, Tung B, Pedroza C, Good WV (2008) Progression of myopia and high myopia in the early treatment for retinopathy of prematurity study: findings to 3 years of age. Ophthalmology 115:1058–1064 e1051

Quinn GE, Dobson V, Hardy RJ, Tung B, Palmer EA, Good WV (2011) Visual field extent at 6 years of age in children who had high-risk prethreshold retinopathy of prematurity. Arch Ophthalmol 129:127–132

Quinn GE, Dobson V, Davitt BV, Wallace DK, Hardy RJ, Tung B, Lai D, Good WV (2013) Progression of myopia and high myopia in the early treatment for retinopathy of prematurity study: findings at 4 to 6 years of age. J AAPOS 17:124–128

Quinn GE, Ying GS, Daniel E, Hildebrand PL, Ells A, Baumritter A, Kemper AR, Schron EB, Wade K (2014) Validity of a telemedicine system for the evaluation of acute-phase retinopathy of prematurity. JAMA Ophthalmol 132:1178–1184

Raju TN, Langenberg P, Bhutani V, Quinn GE (1997) Vitamin e prophylaxis to reduce retinopathy of prematurity: a reappraisal of published trials. J Pediatr 131:844–850

Reese ABKM, Owens WC (1953) A classification of retrolental fibroplasia. Am J Ophthalmol 36:1333–1335

Reisner DS, Hansen RM, Findl O, Petersen RA, Fulton AB (1997) Dark-adapted thresholds in children with histories of mild retinopathy of prematurity. Invest Ophthalmol Vis Sci 38:1175–1183

Repka MX, Palmer EA, Tung B (2000) Involution of retinopathy of prematurity. Cryotherapy for retinopathy of prematurity cooperative group. Arch Ophthalmol 118:645–649

Repka MX, Tung B, Good WV, Shapiro M, Capone A Jr, Baker JD, Barr CC, Phelps DL, van Heuven WA (2006) Outcome of eyes developing retinal detachment during the early treatment for retinopathy of prematurity study (etrop). Arch Ophthalmol 124:24–30

Reynolds JD, Dobson V, Quinn GE, Fielder AR, Palmer EA, Saunders RA, Hardy RJ, Phelps DL, Baker JD, Trese MT, Schaffer D, Tung B (2002) Evidence-based screening criteria for retinopathy of prematurity: natural history data from the cryo-rop and light-rop studies. Arch Ophthalmol 120:1470–1476

Rezai KA, Eliott D, Ferrone PJ, Kim RW (2005) Near confluent laser photocoagulation for the treatment of threshold retinopathy of prematurity. Arch Ophthalmol 123:621–626

Rivera JC, Sitaras N, Noueihed B, Hamel D, Madaan A, Zhou T, Honore JC, Quiniou C, Joyal JS, Hardy P, Sennlaub F, Lubell W, Chemtob S (2013) Microglia and interleukin-1beta in ischemic retinopathy elicit microvascular degeneration through neuronal semaphorin-3a. Arterioscler Thromb Vasc Biol 33:1881–1891

Roohipoor R, Karkhaneh R, Riazi-Esfahani M, Ghasemi F, Nili-Ahmadabadi M (2009) Surgical management in advanced stages of retinopathy of prematurity; our experience. J Ophthalmic Vis Res 4:185–190

Rubaltelli DM, Hirose T (2008) Retinopathy of prematurity update. Int Ophthalmol Clin 48:225–235

SanGiovanni JP, Chew EY (2005) The role of omega-3 long-chain polyunsaturated fatty acids in health and disease of the retina. Prog Retin Eye Res 24:87–138

Sapieha P, Sirinyan M, Hamel D, Zaniolo K, Joyal JS, Cho JH, Honore JC, Kermorvant-Duchemin E, Varma DR, Tremblay S, Leduc M, Rihakova L, Hardy P, Klein WH, Mu X, Mamer O, Lachapelle P, Di Polo A, Beausejour C, Andelfinger G, Mitchell G, Sennlaub F, Chemtob S (2008) The succinate receptor gpr91 in neurons has a major role in retinal angiogenesis. Nat Med 14:1067–1076

Sato T, Wada K, Arahori H, Kuno N, Imoto K, Iwahashi-Shima C, Kusaka S (2012) Serum concentrations of bevacizumab (avastin) and vascular endothelial growth factor in infants with retinopathy of prematurity. Am J Ophthalmol 153:327–333 e321

Saugstad OD, Aune D (2014) Optimal oxygenation of extremely low birth weight infants: a meta-analysis and systematic review of the oxygen saturation target studies. Neonatology 105:55–63

Saunders RA, Donahue ML, Christmann LM, Pakalnis AV, Tung B, Hardy RJ, Phelps DL (1997) Racial variation in retinopathy of prematurity. The cryotherapy for retinopathy of prematurity cooperative group. Arch Ophthalmol 115:604–608

Schaffer DB, Johnson L, Quinn GE, Weston M, Bowen FW Jr (1985) Vitamin e and retinopathy of prematurity. Follow-up at one year. Ophthalmology 92:1005–1011

Schaffer DB, Palmer EA, Plotsky DF, Metz HS, Flynn JT, Tung B, Hardy RJ (1993) Prognostic factors in the natural course of retinopathy of prematurity. The cryotherapy for retinopathy of prematurity cooperative group. Ophthalmology 100:230–237

Screening examination of premature infants for retinopathy of prematurity. Pediatrics 117:572–576 (2006)

Sears JE, Sonnie C (2007) Anatomic success of lens-sparing vitrectomy with and without scleral buckle for stage 4 retinopathy of prematurity. Am J Ophthalmol 143:810–813

Shah PK, Narendran V, Tawansy KA, Raghuram A, Narendran K (2007) Intravitreal bevacizumab (avastin) for post laser anterior segment ischemia in aggressive posterior retinopathy of prematurity. Indian J Ophthalmol 55:75–76

Shalev B, Farr AK, Repka MX (2001) Randomized comparison of diode laser photocoagulation versus cryotherapy for threshold retinopathy of prematurity: seven-year outcome. Am J Ophthalmol 132:76–80

Shao Z, Dorfman AL, Seshadri S, Djavari M, Kermorvant-Duchemin E, Sennlaub F, Blais M, Polosa A, Varma DR, Joyal JS, Lachapelle P, Hardy P, Sitaras N, Picard E, Mancini J, Sapieha P, Chemtob S (2011) Choroidal involution is a key component of oxygen-induced retinopathy. Invest Ophthalmol Vis Sci 52:6238–6248

Shastry BS, Pendergast SD, Hartzer MK, Liu X, Trese MT (1997) Identification of missense mutations in the norrie disease gene associated with advanced retinopathy of prematurity. Arch Ophthalmol 115:651–655

Silvers KM, Gibson AT, Powers HJ (1994) High plasma vitamin c concentrations at birth associated with low antioxidant status and poor outcome in premature infants. Arch Dis Child Fetal Neonatal Ed 71:F40–F44

Silvers KM, Gibson AT, Russell JM, Powers HJ (1998) Antioxidant activity, packed cell transfusions, and outcome in premature infants. Arch Dis Child Fetal Neonatal Ed 78:F214–F219

Sluis KB, Inder T, Wilkinson A et al (1996) Plasma and endotracheal vitamin c concentrations in premature infants: relationship to outcome measures. In: Proceedings of the 14th annual congress of the Australian Perinatal Society [abstract]

Smiddy WE, Loupe DN, Michels RG, Enger C, Glaser BM, de Bustros S (1989) Refractive changes after scleral buckling surgery. Arch Ophthalmol 107:1469–1471

Smith LE (2004) Pathogenesis of retinopathy of prematurity. Growth Horm IGF Res 14(Suppl A):S140–S144

Smith BT, Tasman WS (2005) Retinopathy of prematurity: late complications in the baby boomer generation (1946–1964). Trans Am Ophthalmol Soc 103:225–234, discussion 234–226

Smith LE, Wesolowski E, McLellan A, Kostyk SK, D'Amato R, Sullivan R, D'Amore PA (1994) Oxygen-induced retinopathy in the mouse. Invest Ophthalmol Vis Sci 35:101–111

Sola A, Rogido MR, Deulofeut R (2007) Oxygen as a neonatal health hazard: call for detente in clinical practice. Acta Paediatr 96:801–812

Stone J, Itin A, Alon T, Pe'er J, Gnessin H, Chan-Ling T, Keshet E (1995) Development of retinal vasculature is mediated by hypoxia-induced vascular endothelial growth factor (vegf) expression by neuroglia. J Neurosci 15:4738–4747

Streeter ML, Rosso P (1981) Transport mechanisms for ascorbic acid in the human placenta. Am J Clin Nutr 34:1706–1711

Subhani M, Combs A, Weber P, Gerontis C, DeCristofaro JD (2001) Screening guidelines for retinopathy of prematurity: the need for revision in extremely low birth weight infants. Pediatrics 107:656–659

Sylvester CL (2008) Retinopathy of prematurity. Semin Ophthalmol 23:318–323

Tadesse M, Dhanireddy R, Mittal M, Higgins RD (2002) Race, Candida sepsis, and retinopathy of prematurity. Biol Neonate 81:86–90

Tasman W, Patz A, McNamara JA, Kaiser RS, Trese MT, Smith BT (2006) Retinopathy of prematurity: the life of a lifetime disease. Am J Ophthalmol 141:167–174

Terry T (1942) Extreme prematurity and fibroplastic overgrowth of persistent vascular sheath behind each crystalline lens. I. Preliminary report. Am J Ophthalmol 25:203–204

Terry T (1943) Fibroblastic overgrowth of persistent tunica vasculosa lentis in premature infants. II. Report of cases–clinical aspects. Arch Ophthalmol 29:36–53

The international classification of retinopathy of prematurity revisited (2005) Arch Ophthalmol 123:991–999

Tin W, Milligan DW, Pennefather P, Hey E (2001) Pulse oximetry, severe retinopathy, and outcome at one year in babies of less than 28 weeks gestation. Arch Dis Child Fetal Neonatal Ed 84:F106–F110

Tokunaga CC, Mitton KP, Dailey W, Massoll C, Roumayah K, Guzman E, Tarabishy N, Cheng M, Drenser KA (2014) Effects of anti-vegf treatment on the recovery of the developing retina following oxygen-induced retinopathy. Invest Ophthalmol Vis Sci 55:1884–1892

Trese MT (1994) Scleral buckling for retinopathy of prematurity. Ophthalmology 101:23–26

Tsukahara Y, Honda S, Imai H, Kondo N, Fujii S, Yokoyama N, Hirata A, Kawaji T, Fukushima M, Tanihara H, Negi A (2007) Autologous plasmin-assisted vitrectomy for stage 5 retinopathy of prematurity: a preliminary trial. Am J Ophthalmol 144:139–141

Vanderveen DK, Mansfield TA, Eichenwald EC (2006a) Lower oxygen saturation alarm limits decrease the severity of retinopathy of prematurity. J AAPOS 10:445–448

VanderVeen DK, Coats DK, Dobson V, Fredrick D, Gordon RA, Hardy RJ, Neely DE, Palmer EA, Steidl SM, Tung B, Good WV (2006b) Prevalence and course of strabismus in the first year of life for infants with prethreshold retinopathy of prematurity: findings from the early treatment for retinopathy of prematurity study. Arch Ophthalmol 124:766–773

VanderVeen DK, Bremer DL, Fellows RR, Hardy RJ, Neely DE, Palmer EA, Rogers DL, Tung B, Good WV (2011) Prevalence and course of strabismus through age 6 years in participants of the early treatment for retinopathy of prematurity randomized trial. J AAPOS 15:536–540

Varughese S, Gilbert C, Pieper C, Cook C (2008) Retinopathy of prematurity in South Africa: an assessment of needs, resources and requirements for screening programmes. Br J Ophthalmol 92:879–882

Vision for children. A global overview of blindness, childhood and vision 2020: The right to sight. World health organization (who) and the international agency for the prevention of blindness (iapb). www.V2020.Org

Wallace DK, Kylstra JA, Greenman DB, Freedman SF (1998) Significance of isolated neovascular tufts ("popcorn") in retinopathy of prematurity. J AAPOS 2:52–56

Wallace DK, Veness-Meehan KA, Miller WC (2007) Incidence of severe retinopathy of prematurity before and after a modest reduction in target oxygen saturation levels. J AAPOS 11:170–174

Wang J, Ren X, Shen L, Yanni SE, Leffler JN, Birch EE (2013) Development of refractive error in individual children with regressed retinopathy of prematurity. Invest Ophthalmol Vis Sci 54:6018–6024

Wang SK, Callaway NF, Wallenstein MB, Henderson MT, Leng T, Moshfeghi DM (2015) Sundrop: six years of screening for retinopathy of prematurity with telemedicine. Can J Ophthalmol 50:101–106

Wheatley CM, Dickinson JL, Mackey DA, Craig JE, Sale MM (2002) Retinopathy of prematurity: recent advances in our understanding. Br J Ophthalmol 86:696–700

Wilkinson AR, Haines L, Head K, Fielder AR (2008) Uk retinopathy of prematurity guideline. Early Hum Dev 84:71–74

Wilkinson AR, Haines L, Head K, Fielder AR (2009) Uk retinopathy of prematurity guideline. Eye (Lond) 23:2137–2139

Woo SJ, Park KH, Lee SY, Ahn SJ, Ahn J, Oh KJ, Ryu A (2013) The relationship between cord blood cytokine levels and perinatal factors and retinopathy of prematurity: a gestational age-matched case-control study. Invest Ophthalmol Vis Sci 54: 3434–3439

Wright KW, Sami D, Thompson L, Ramanathan R, Joseph R, Farzavandi S (2006) A physiologic reduced oxygen protocol decreases the incidence of threshold retinopathy of prematurity. Trans Am Ophthalmol Soc 104:78–84

Wu C, Petersen RA, VanderVeen DK (2006) Retcam imaging for retinopathy of prematurity screening. J AAPOS 10:107–111

Wu C, Lofqvist C, Smith LE, VanderVeen DK, Hellstrom A (2012) Importance of early postnatal weight gain for normal retinal angiogenesis in very preterm infants: a multicenter study analyzing weight velocity deviations for the prediction of retinopathy of prematurity. Arch Ophthalmol 130:992–999

Wu WC, Shih CP, Wang NK, Lien R, Chen YP, Chao AN, Chen KJ, Chen TL, Hwang YS, Lai CC, Huang CY, Tsai S (2013a) Choroidal thickness in patients with a history of retinopathy of prematurity. JAMA Ophthalmol 131:1451–1458

Wu WC, Kuo HK, Yeh PT, Yang CM, Lai CC, Chen SN (2013b) An updated study of the use of bevacizumab in the treatment of patients with prethreshold retinopathy of prematurity in taiwan. Am J Ophthalmol 155:150–158 e151

Yalin Imamoglu E, Gunay M, Gursoy T, Imamoglu S, Balci Ekmekci O, Celik G, Karatekin G, Ovali F (2014) Effect of laser photocoagulation on plasma levels of vegf-a, vegfr-2, and tie2 in infants with retinopathy of prematurity. J AAPOS 18:466–470

Yamashita Y (1972) Studies on retinopathy of prematurity. III. Cryocautery for retinopathy of prematurity. Jpn J Clin Ophthalmol 26:385–393

Yanamandra K, Napper D, Pramanik A, Bocchini JA Jr, Dhanireddy R (2010) Endothelial nitric oxide synthase genotypes in the etiology of retinopathy of prematurity in premature infants. Ophthalmic Genet 31:173–177

Yang CS, Wang AG, Sung CS, Hsu WM, Lee FL, Lee SM (2010) Long-term visual outcomes of laser-treated threshold retinopathy of prematurity: a study of refractive status at 7 years. Eye (Lond) 24:14–20

Yang CS, Wang AG, Shih YF, Hsu WM (2013) Astigmatism and biometric optic components of diode laser-treated threshold retinopathy of prematurity at 9 years of age. Eye (Lond) 27:374–381

Yokoi T, Yokoi T, Kobayashi Y, Hiraoka M, Nishina S, Azuma N (2009) Evaluation of scleral buckling for stage 4a retinopathy of prematurity by fluorescein angiography. Am J Ophthalmol 148:544–550 e541

Yonemura D, Aoki T, Tsuzuki K (1962) Electroretinogram in diabetic retinopathy. Arch Ophthalmol 68:19–24

Yu DY, Alder VA, Cringle SJ, Su EN, Burns M (1998) Intraretinal oxygen distribution in urethane-induced retinopathy in rats. Am J Physiol 274:H2009–H2017

Zhang M, Malik AB, Rehman J (2014) Endothelial progenitor cells and vascular repair. Curr Opin Hematol 21:224–228

Neonatal Orthopedic Surgery

137

Peter D. Pizzutillo and Martin J. Herman

Contents

Abstract

The physical examination of neonates is unique and reflects stages of development. It may reveal musculoskeletal deformities which have to be differentiated from physiological anatomical variants. The presence of congenital anomalies of the spine and of the limbs, although not requiring urgent intervention, prompts investigations for associated anomalies in spinal cord and in the renal and cardiovascular systems. Other common muscoloskeletal problems in neonates are limb fractures and cervical injuries, as consequences of a difficult delivery, infections (arthritis with osteomyelitis, generally in multiple sites), and developmental dysplasia of the hip. Early diagnosis of these conditions is of paramount importance to ensure specific treatment and normal limb growth and function.

P. D. Pizzutillo (✉)
Section of Orthopaedic Surgery, St. Christopher's Hospital for Children, Philadelphia, PA, USA

Tenet Healthcare, Dallas, TX, USA
e-mail: peter.pizzutillo@tenethealth.com

M. J. Herman
Department of Orthopaedic Surgery, Drexel University College of Medicine, St. Christopher's Hospital for Children, Philadelphia, PA, USA

137.1 Salient Points

- The musculoskeletal deformities revealed by physical examination may be physiological anatomical variants or pathologies.
- Congenital anomalies of the spine and of the limbs may be associated with anomalies of the spinal cord, renal, and cardiovascular systems.
- Early diagnosis and treatment of common neonatal musculoskeletal problems (fractures, infections, and developmental dysplasia of the hip) is essential to improve functional outcome.

G. Buonocore et al. (eds.), *Neonatology*,
https://doi.org/10.1007/978-3-319-29489-6_284

137.2 Introduction

The physical examination of the neonate is unique and reflects stages of development. While the examination may suggest deformities of the spine and extremities, it is important to recognize physiologic variations of anatomy and growth that are characteristic of the neonate and distinguish them from pathologic anatomy. Timely recognition of clinical problems is especially important for prompt and appropriate interventions in this population. Delay in treatment of acute problems may interfere with normal limb growth and function or survival of the neonate.

137.3 Clinical Findings

While congenital anomalies of the spine or limb may not require urgent attention, they are associated with a host of anomalies involving other organ systems, such as renal, cardiovascular, or spinal cord, which may require immediate evaluation and interventions. Fractures and infections are the most common clinical problems that demand early diagnosis and treatment.

In the absence of bone dysplasias, such as osteogenesis imperfecta, vaginal delivery or difficult cesarean section is associated with fractures of the clavicle, humerus, femur, and injury of the cervical spine. When the infant presents with a flail upper limb, fracture of the clavicle, fracture of the proximal or distal humeral physes, brachial plexus injury, or septic arthritis of the shoulder must be considered. Radiographs of the injured area may or may not confirm injury due to skeletal immaturity and incomplete ossification. Ultrasonographic evaluation of the proximal or distal humerus or proximal femur may document pathologic motion of the unossified epiphysis to confirm the diagnosis of a transphyseal fracture. Radiographs of long bones may reveal periosteal reaction that is a normal finding in 35% of infants older than 1 month and younger than 4 months of age. The periosteal reaction is characterized as regular and less than 2 mm in thickness. In the neonate, a periosteal reaction thicker than 2 mm may be associated with infection, syphilis, prostaglandin infusion, ECMO, or Caffey disease. In infants older than 4 months of age, child abuse must be considered.

When more than one limb is flaccid, neonatal cervical spinal cord injury may be responsible. Injury of the cord may occur with distraction forces applied to the head. Due to the differential in plasticity of the vertebral column and the spinal cord, neurologic injury may occur without injury to the vertebral column. Radiographs of the cervical spine may appear normal and MRI would be required to diagnose injury of the cord. Complete or incomplete injury of the cervical spinal cord may present as a stillborn infant or an infant with significant neurologic deficits and delays that suggest the diagnosis of cerebral palsy. Early diagnosis is important since incomplete injury of the cord requires immobilization of the spine to prevent increasing injury.

Infection of the musculoskeletal system is of special concern in the neonate since the immature immune system may not express the expected findings of fever or abnormal laboratory studies, such as white blood cell count, ESR, and CRP. Early examination of an infected joint may not reveal any signs of inflammation and may create a false sense of security that will delay diagnosis. A more common presentation of infection in the neonate includes diminished interest in feeding, irritability, and decreased motion of an affected limb. Common sites of infection involve the hip, knee, and shoulder joints with associated osteomyelitis. Ultrasonographic evaluation of suspected joints will confirm the presence of fluid and can guide aspiration of the joint. MRI of an infected joint is helpful to determine the coexistence of osteomyelitis. Multiple sites of infection are the rule in the neonate, and effective treatment includes not only appropriate antibiotic coverage of *Staphylococcus aureus* and Gram negative organisms but also surgical drainage of septic joints.

Table 1 Common musculoskeletal findings and diagnoses

Neck	Congenital muscular torticollis
	Limited neck motion, short neck (Klippel-Feil syndrome)
Arm	Swelling, tenderness clavicle (fracture)
	Flail arm (brachial plexus injury) swelling, diminished movement (infection, fracture), radial deviation of hand (TAR syndrome), polydactyly, syndactyly
	Swelling, diminished movement (infection, fracture)
	Radial deviation of hand (TAR syndrome)
	Polydactyly, syndactyly
Spine	Curvature (scoliosis)
	Rib abnormalities (congenital scoliosis, spondylocostal dysplasia)
	Midline defects (myelomeningocele, spinal cord anomalies)
Hip	Positive Ortolani/Barlow (DDH)
	Short femur (DDH, congenital anomalies of the femur, skeletal dysplasia)
Leg	Tibial bowing
	Posterior apex (calcaneovalgus foot)
	Anterolateral apex (congenital pseudoarthrosis of tibia, fibular hemimelia)
	Hyperextended knee (congenital knee dislocation)
Foot	Medial midfoot crease, forefoot inward (metatarsus adductus)
	Fixed ankle equinus with forefoot down and inward, heel inward (clubfoot)
	Rocker bottom foot (congenital vertical talus), foot dorsiflexed and touching shin (calcaneovalgus foot)

Table 2 Common traumatic birth injuries and their associated physical findings

Fractures	
Clavicle	Tenderness and swelling over mid-clavicle, diminished spontaneous arm movement (pseudoparalysis) Consider congenital pseudarthrosis if right-sided
Humerus	Upper arm swelling, crepitus, diminished spontaneous arm movement (pseudoparalysis)
Elbow	Elbow swelling, deformity, painful, and limited elbow ROM
Femur	Thigh swelling, pain with diaper changes, limited hip ROM
Brachial plexus	
Erb's palsy	Shoulder internal rotation, elbow extension, wrist flexion
	Diminished spontaneous arm movement proximal to hand
Complete plexus injury	Flail arm without spontaneous movement Ptosis of the ipsilateral eye (Horner's syndrome)
Spinal cord injury	
Apnea	
No spontaneous bilateral extremity movement	
Progressive increase in extremity tone with truncal hypotonia	
Cephalohematoma	
Focal area of head swelling, ecchymosis	

Repeated daily aspiration of the septic hip joint is not capable of complete evacuation of harmful inflammatory elements and is painful. Repeated aspiration of the knee or ankle may be effective, but surgical drainage of the involved hip joint is the standard of care.

137.4 Diagnosis and Syndromes

Delay in diagnosis and treatment of septic arthritis of the hip results in impaired physeal function, progressive angular deformity of the limb, limb length discrepancy, and permanent destruction of the hip joint.

Developmental dysplasia of the hip (DDH) joint responds well to nonoperative intervention when treatment is initiated in infancy. Fixed dislocation of the hip, the so-called teratologic dislocation, is rare and associated with more generalized disorders, such as arthrogryposis and Larsen syndrome. DDH is associated with breech presentation and delivery, congenital muscular torticollis, foot deformities, and congenital dislocation of the knee.

There are a host of musculoskeletal conditions that may be diagnosed in the neonate. Tables 1, 2, 3, and 4 provide a menu of commonly occurring problems. A high index of suspicion for occult acute clinical problems will serve the clinician

Table 3 Important orthopedic diagnoses and syndromes in the NICU

Achondroplasia
Frontal bossing, depressed nasal bridge, midface hypoplasia
Global hypotonia
Joint laxity
Apnea, foramen magnum stenosis
Thoracolumbar kyphosis
Hip flexion contracture
Rhizomelic short limbs
Spondylocostal Dysplasia (Jarcot-Levin syndrome)
Prominent occiput
Short neck
Thoracic hypoplasia and insufficiency
Chest wall defects, rib fusions
Congenital scoliosis
Down syndrome
Depressed nasal bridge, medial epicanthal folds, hypertelorism
Simian crease
Global hypotonia
Joint hyperlaxity
Hip dysplasia
Arthrogryposis
Severe joint stiffness
Elbow extension, wrist flexed and in ulnar deviation, fingers flexed with thumb in palm deformity
No skin creases in antecubital fossa or palm
Hip and knee flexion contractures
Hip dislocations
Severe, rigid clubfeet
Myelomeningocele
Midline low thoracic or lumbar spine skin defects with exposed meninges
Limited or no spontaneous movement of lower extremities
Exaggerated reflex response in lower extremities
Hip dislocation
Clubfeet or congenital vertical talus
Caffey's Disease
Diminished spontaneous arm movement (pseudoparalysis)
Swelling of mandible or extremity, especially the ulna
Exuberant periosteal reaction by radiographs
Evaluation inconsistent with infection or trauma

Table 4 Hallmarks of musculoskeletal infection in the newborn

Irritability, poor feeding, focal limb swelling and diminished spontaneous limb movement (pseudoparalysis)
Most common sites: hip, knee, and shoulder
Most common diagnoses: osteoarticular infections and cellulitis with soft tissue abscesses of the extremities
Most common infectious agents: *Staphylococcus aureus* and gram negative bacteria
Most common complication: joint and angular deformities and leg-length inequality
Pitfalls
1. Immature immune response may delay diagnosis and treatment
2. Osteomyelitis and septic arthritis often occur concurrently and at multiple sites
3. Bone scan is less sensitive than other imaging modalities for identifying infection; ultrasound and MRI most useful

well in the care of these unique patients. Specific information of each of these conditions may be readily found in textbooks of pediatric orthopedics.

References

Herring JA (ed) (2002) Tachdjian's pediatric orthopaedics from the Texas Scottish Rite Hospital for Children, 3rd edn. WB Saunders Company, Philadelphia

Morrissy RT, Weinstein SL (eds) (2006) Lovell and Winter's pediatric orthopaedics, 6th edn. Williams and Wilkins, Lippincott

Sankar WN, Weiss J, Skaggs DL (2009) Orthopaedic conditions in the newborn. J Am Acad Orthop Surg 17:112–122

Neonatal Skin Disorders

138

Michele Fimiani, Roberta Bilenchi, Filomena Mandato, Stefania Mei, Niccolò Nami, Rosa Maria Strangi, and Arianna Lamberti

Contents

M. Fimiani (✉)
Dipartimento di Medicina Clinica e Scienze Immunologiche – Sezione di Dermatologia, Università degli Studi di Siena, Policlinico "Santa Maria alle Scotte", Siena, Italy

Department of Medical, Surgical and Neurological Sciences, Dermatology Section, University of Siena, Siena, Italy
e-mail: fimiani@unisi.it

R. Bilenchi · F. Mandato · S. Mei · N. Nami · R. M. Strangi · A. Lamberti
Department of Medical, Surgical and Neurological Sciences, Dermatology Section, University of Siena, Siena, Italy

G. Buonocore et al. (eds.), *Neonatology*,
https://doi.org/10.1007/978-3-319-29489-6_285

Abstract

Skin is a dynamic complex organ, which accomplishes versatile functions and thus plays a key role in the maintenance of the homeostasis of the organism. At birth, the development of the skin is not fully complete. The beginning of the postnatal life is a period for active adaptation and maturation of the cutaneous structure and functions. The environment around the skin changes drastically after birth: a newborn infant goes from the warm, wet, sterile, and safe womb to a cooler, dry, bacteria-laden nursery; concurrently the baby begins the journey to self-sufficiency by breathing air, taking nutrition, and maintaining body temperature. Newborn skin is critical to this transition and performs many functions (barrier to water loss, light, and irritants; infection control and immunosurveillance; resilience to mechanical trauma; sensation and tactile discrimination; thermal regulation; and acid mantle formation).

A variety of normal and abnormal lesions may be present on newborn skin surface (including adnexa, oral mucosa, and genito-anal area). Although these findings are often benign, it is important to distinguish them and to be aware about the nature of the disease, to manage them properly.

138.1 Salient Points

- The primary functions of neonatal skin are mechanical protection, thermoregulation, prevention of insensible fluid loss, and immune surveillance.
- Normal physiological characteristics of newborns that reflect immaturity and transition from intrauterine to extrauterine life should be recognized and differentiated from true disease.
- Most neonatal disorders are benign and often transient, but several serious diseases can present in neonates.
- Vesicular and pustular disorders are common during the first months of life.

138.2 Neonatal Skin Structure and Functions

By the end of pregnancy, fetal skin anatomy and composition are similar to those of adults. By 22–24 weeks all anatomical elements are present,

Table 1 Structural differences between preterm neonate, term neonate, and adult skin

	Adult	Term infant	Preterm infant (30–32 weeks)
Skin surface	Dry	Vernix	Vernix (gelatinous)
Skin thickness	2.1 mm (media)	1.2 mm	0.9 mm
Epidermal thickness	50 μm	50 μm	27.4 μm
Stratum corneum thickness	9–15 μm	9–10 μm	4–5 μm
Melanocytes	Number decreases with aging	Number as in young adults, fewer melanosomes, and low melanin production	Number as in term infants, few mature melanosomes
Dermal epidermal junction	Rigid	Flat but rigid	Flat but rigid antigen expressed
	Antigen expressed	Antigen expressed	
Anchoring filaments, fibrils and hemidesmosomes	All normal	All normal	All fewer and smaller
Papillary dermal collagen	Normal	Normal	Edematous
Reticular dermal collagen	Normal	Smaller-intermediate boundless with the hypodermis	Much smaller boundless with the hypodermis
Reticular dermal elastic fibers	Normal	Smaller in size and immature in structure	Finer than in term infants, immature in structure
Reticular dermal cell count	Fibroblasts ±	Fibroblasts ++	Fibroblasts +++
Hypodermis	Well developed	Well developed	Well developed

while functional and biochemical maturity is delayed for years (Table 1). There are structural differences between the skin of the preterm neonate, term neonate, and adult that have significant physiological and clinical consequences (Mancini et al. 1994).

The primary functions of neonatal skin are mechanical protection, thermoregulation, prevention of insensible fluid loss, and immunosurveillance. The skin of premature infants is thinner and much less effective in these functions. It is subject to fissuring from use of adhesives and their removal. Chemical burns from topical alcohol swabs or disinfectants and thermal burns from transcutaneous oxygen monitoring are well-recognized problems in neonatal intensive care settings. Neonatal skin has increased permeability that reflects the reduced water-holding capacity of the stratum corneum. Transcutaneous absorption is increased in neonates, especially premature infants, and may lead to local and systemic side effects from many topical agents such as iodine soap, hexachlorophene, benzyl alcohol, and steroids (Table 2 and Fig. 1) (Visscher et al. 2015). The increased permeability of neonatal skin can also be an alternative method of drug administration. Other structural parameters that affect neonatal skin permeability are low surface lipid production, epidermal and dermal thickness due to incomplete development, and underdeveloped basement membrane and papillar vasculature. Altered permeability of neonatal skin also permits transepidermal water loss from the internal environment, which can lead to extreme dehydration, and poor autonomic control of skin vessels and reduced sweating contribute to poor thermal regulation in preterm infants.

138.3 The Physical Dermatological Examination of the Newborn

It is important in the newborn to evaluate the total skin surface including the adnexa, the oral mucosa, and the genito-anal region. Dermatological examination is primarily morphologically and descriptively oriented. A good knowledge of

Table 2 Potential dermatological and/or side/untoward effects from topical application of some skin care applied substances in newborns

Agent	Vehicle/use	Neurologic side/ untoward effect(s)	Dermatologic side/untoward effect(s)
Adhesives	Adhesives removes		Toxic epidermal necrolysis
Adhesives monitoring leads	Adhesives devices		Anetoderma of prematurity, skin breakdown
Alcohols	Topical antiseptic		Skin necrosis (especially in immature occluded skin)
Boric acid	Diaper powder	Seizures	Erythroderma
Corticosteroids	Topical anti-inflammatory agent		Skin atrophy, striae distensae
Glycerin	Emollient	Seizures	
Hexachlorophene	Antiseptic cleanser	Vacuolar encephalopathy, seizures	
Lidocaine	Local anesthetic	Seizures	
Lindane	Scabicide lotion	Seizures	Rash
Neomycin	Local antibiotic	Ototoxicity, neural deafness	Contact dermatitis
Pentachlorophenol	Laundry detergent		Sweating
Propylene glycol	Excipient	Seizures	
Salicylates	Keratolytic ointment	Encephalopathy	
Silver sulfadiazine	Topical antibacterial	Kernicterus	Argyria
Tincture of benzoin	Antiseptic		Skin breakdown
Triclosan	Topical antibacterial		Contact dermatitis

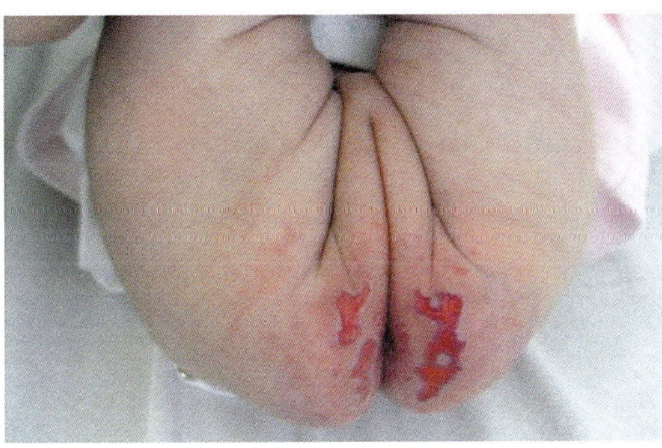

Fig. 1 Severe acute irritant dermatitis in a newborn, with erosive lesions of the perianal zone

elementary skin lesions is essential for a reliable description of dermatoses (Table 3).

138.4 Transient Physiologic Disorders in the Newborn

Normal physiological characteristics of newborns that reflect immaturity and transition from life in utero should be recognized and differentiated from true diseases.

138.4.1 Vernix Caseosa (VC)

VC is a white waxy or cheese-like substance coating the skin of newborns. It is composed of sebum, shed lanugo, and sloughed-off fetal skin cells. VC is secreted by sebaceous glands around the 20th week of gestation and decreases in amount toward the end of gestation. It is thought to protect the baby's skin from dehydration in the womb. Vernix color and odor can reflect intrauterine problems as in hemolytic diseases (yellow-brown discoloration) or infections.

138.4.2 Rubor and Acrocyanosis (RaA)

RaA are manifestations of vasomotor instability, frequent in neonatal life. Generalized redness, reflecting vasodilatation, is often present at the birth, associated with peripheral acrocyanosis. Acrocyanosis has no pathologic significance and gradually disappears after several weeks. It presents as bilateral, symmetric, intermittent bluish discoloration of the hands and feet.

Table 3 Elementary lesions in dermatological semiology

Type primary (P)/ secondary (S)	Description or definition
Erythema P	Redness of the skin caused by dilatation and congestion of the capillaries
Wheal P	Skin elevation caused by swelling that can be itchy and usually disappears soon after erupting
Papule P	Circumscribed solid, raised lesion less than in 1 cm across
	A patch of closely grouped papules more than in 1 cm across is called a plaque
Nodule P	Circumscribed solid lesion with distinct edges usually more deeply rooted than a papule
Vesicle P	Circumscribed raised lesion less than in 5 mm across filled with a clear fluid
Bulla P	Circumscribed raised lesion are more than in 5 mm across and filled with a clear fluid
Pustule P/S	Circumscribed raised lesion filled with purulent fluid
Macule P/S	Not palpable small, circumscribed usually brown, white, or red flat spot less than in 1 cm in diameter
Erosion S	Lesion that involves loss of the epidermis healing without scarring
Ulcer S	Lesion that involves loss of the upper portion of the skin (epidermis) and part of the lower portion (dermis) healing with scarring
Crust S	Dried collection of blood, serum, or pus overlying an impaired epidermis
Fissure S	Linear painful loss of the skin
Lichenification P/S	Rough, thick epidermis with exaggerated skin lines
Atrophy/S	Area of very thin and wrinkled skin
Scar/S	Discolored, permanent fibrous tissue that replaces normal skin after destruction of the dermis

138.4.3 Cutis Marmorata (CM)

CM is a transient benign reticulate bluish discoloration of the skin occurring in preterm and full-term infants, due to an exaggerated vasomotor response to hypothermic stress. It disappears after warming the infant and resolves after a few weeks. Profound or persistent CM has been reported in trisomy 21, trisomy 18, hypothyroidism, Cornelia de Lange syndrome, and neonatal lupus. Differential diagnosis includes cutis marmorata telangiectatica congenita, a persistent vascular anomaly that presents at birth with marked purple reticular discoloration that may be segmental or diffuse. Associated features are skin atrophy, telangiectasias, phlebectasias, and ulcerations (Fig. 2).

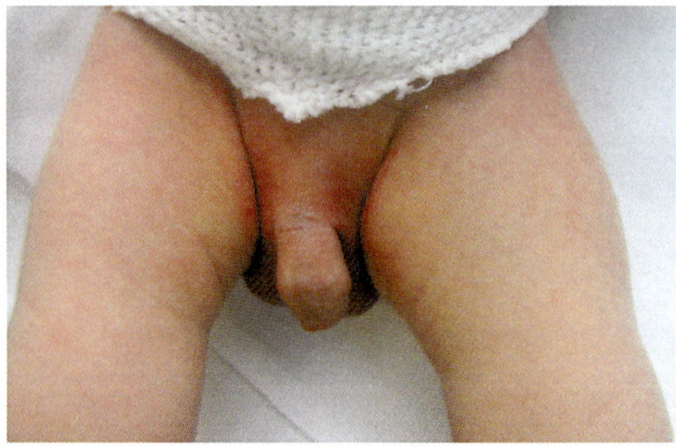

Fig. 2 Cutis marmorata of the lower limbs

138.4.4 Harlequin Color Change (HCC)

HCC is a harmless vascular phenomenon characterized by a transient pink to reddish discoloration that occurs in a symmetric half of an infant's body shortly after birth. Due to immaturity of the hypothalamus and inconsistent regulation of peripheral vessels, it affects 10% of newborns. It is most common in low-birthweight infants. It appears as an episodic skin color change after lying on the side: a sharp line from the forehead to the pubis divides the neonate body into two vertical halves. One side turns dark red (dependent side), the other quite pale (Januário and Salgado 2011). Episodes last for up to 20 min and disappear with movement or crying. No intervention or investigation is required.

138.4.5 Linea Nigra and Genital Hyperpigmentation (LNGH)

LNGH is a common finding in newborns, especially those with pigmented skin. The presence of linea nigra seems to be influenced by maternal hormone levels. It disappears gradually over several weeks.

138.4.6 Physiological Lanugo

Lanugo is the first body hair formed in the embryo. It is fine and soft without pigment and is usually shed in utero at 28–32 weeks of gestation. Preterm infants may show profuse lanugo on the face, limbs, and trunk that is shed in the first few months of life. **Congenital hypertrichosis lanuginosa** (**ChL**) is a very rare inherited syndrome characterized by confluent, generalized overgrowth of silvery blonde to gray lanugo at birth or in early infancy. ChL continues to grow and persists throughout life. Differential diagnosis of increased neonatal hair includes several rare genetically determined disorders.

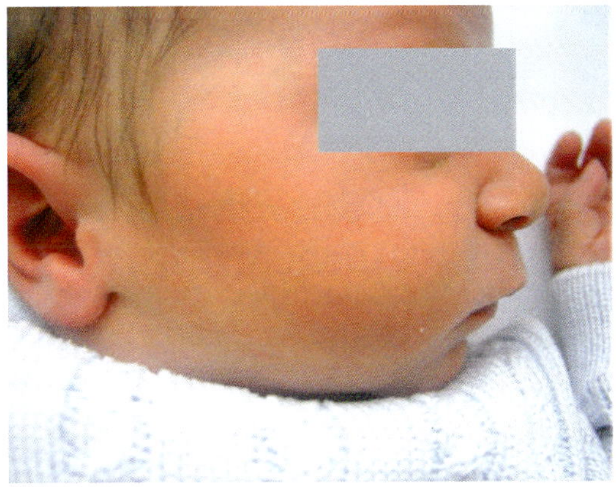

Fig. 3 Milia on the cheek of a newborn

138.4.7 Transient Neonatal Conditions (Miscellaneous)

138.4.7.1 Milia

Milia are tiny keratin-filled lesions due to retention cysts of pilosebaceous follicles. Common in newborn babies, they manifest as uniform, superficial, pearly white to yellowish domed lesions measuring 1–2 mm in diameter, usually situated around the nose and eyes and sometimes on the genitalia. Milia may also be a feature of a number of very rare genodermatoses (e.g., Bazex-Dupré Christol syndrome). In neonates, milia often disappear within 2–4 weeks. Persistent milia have been reported as familial disorders with autosomal dominant inheritance (Fig. 3).

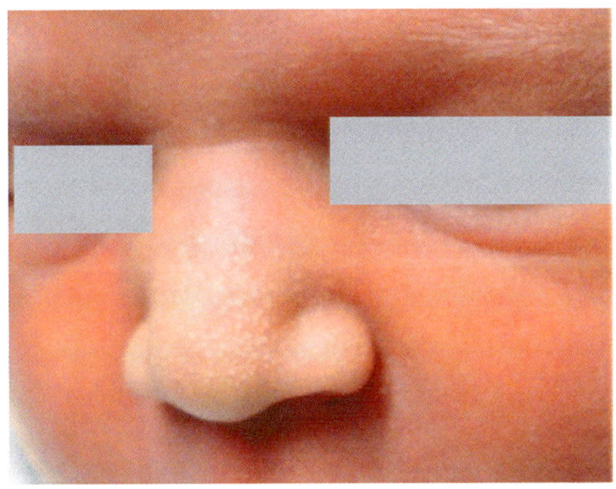

Fig. 4 Sebaceous hyperplasia of the nose

138.4.7.2 Sebaceous Hyperplasia (SH)

SH is a common, transient, benign condition of the sebaceous glands, caused by exposure to maternal androgen in uterus. The lesions may appear as small (1–3 mm), superficial yellow-pink papules with a central pore almost always located on the tip of the nose (Fig. 4).

138.4.7.3 Sucking Blisters (SB)

Neonatal SB appear as unilateral or symmetrical bullae or erosions involving the upper extremities. They are self-inflicted trauma due to intrauterine sucking. The lesions are present at birth, most often on the dorsal and lateral aspect of the wrist or forearm. The infant exhibits excessive sucking. The number and the location of the lesions are diagnostic.

138.4.7.4 Subcutaneous Fat Necrosis of the Newborn (SCFN)

SCFN is an uncommon disorder characterized by firm, erythematous, painless nodules and plaques over the trunk, arms, buttocks, thighs, and cheeks, manifest in full-term newborns in the first few weeks of life. SCFN is usually self-limiting, but may be complicated by hypercalcemia and other metabolic abnormalities. The pathogenesis is not known. Cold- or stress-induced injury to immature fat is thought to lead to solidification and necrosis.

No other organ systems are involved, unless hypercalcemia develops. Differential diagnosis is from a deep hemangioma, lipogranulomatosis, plexiform neurofibroma, and sarcomas.

138.5 Neonatal Disorders with Pustules, Blisters, Erosions, and Scaly Crusts

Vesicular and pustular disorders are common during the first months of life. Most are benign conditions, often transient, but several serious infectious and noninfectious diseases can present in neonates. They can be diagnosed clinically because of their distinctive appearances; some cases may require simple investigations including microscopic examination of the pustule content, culture, and skin biopsy.

138.5.1 Transient Sterile Pustular Disorders in Newborns

138.5.1.1 Toxic Erythema of the Newborn

This is a benign, asymptomatic skin condition occurring within 24–48 h after birth and disappearing spontaneously after several days. It affects 30–70% of newborns. The eruption, generally starting on the trunk, is characterized by small erythematous papules, vesicles, and occasionally pustules, usually surrounded by a distinctive, diffuse, blotchy, erythematous halo (Fig. 5).

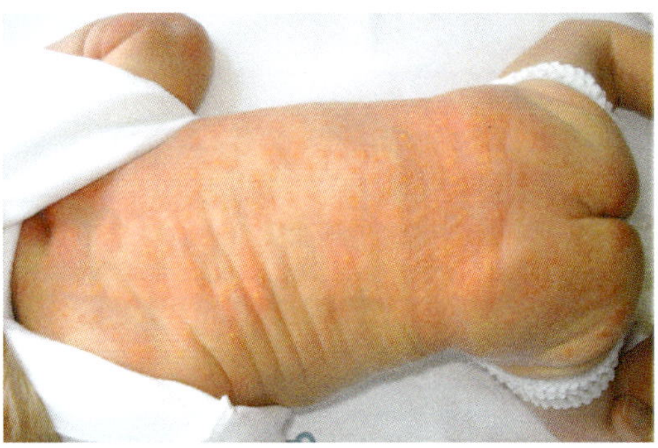

Fig. 5 Erythema patches and small pustular lesions of the trunk in a 3-day-old newborn affected by toxic erythema

Individual lesions disappear within hours and then appear elsewhere on the body. Wright-Giemsa (WG) staining of the pustular smear reveals eosinophils. The etiology is unknown (Monteagudo et al. 2012).

138.5.1.2 Transient Neonatal Pustular Melanosis (TNPM)

TNPM is a benign, asymptomatic, self-limiting skin condition with distinctive features characterized by vesicles, superficial pustules, and pigmented macules. The lesions are generally present at birth on the chin, neck, forehead, chest, and back especially in black neonates. The palms and soles are seldom involved. No systemic signs are associated with the skin eruptions. The vesicles and pustules clear up within 48 h, while the brown macules persist for several months. Etiology is unknown. WG staining of a smear reveals many neutrophils without evidence of changes due to bacteria, yeast, or virus.

138.5.1.3 Infantile Acropustulosis (IA)

IA is a rare benign idiopathic disorder characterized by recurrent crops of 1–2 mm intensely itchy vesiculopustules found on the distal extremities of newborns or early infants. It is more common in black infants. Permanent recovery occurs around 2–3 years. WG staining of smear reveals polymorphonuclear and eosinophilic leukocytes. The duration of recurrent crops is shortened by topical steroids.

138.5.1.4 Eosinophilic Pustulosis

This relatively rare disorder is characterized by recurrent crops of itchy follicular papulopustules located primarily on the scalp but also on the face, trunk, and extremities. The pustules may be present at birth or may occur during the first few months of life and show peripheral extension with crusts and central clearing. The disorder may last days to weeks or relapse over years. WG staining of a pustular smear shows polymorphonuclear and eosinophilic leukocytes without evidence of changes due to bacteria, yeast, or viruses. There may be a peripheral leukocytosis and eosinophilia. Most cases respond to topical corticosteroids.

138.5.1.5 Miliaria (M)

M is a disorder of the eccrine sweat glands that often occurs under hot humid conditions. Although it affects people of all ages, it is especially common in children and infants due to their underdeveloped sweat glands. M is caused by blockage of the sweat glands and can be classified according to the level at which obstruction occurs: M cristallina, M rubra, and M profunda. The most common form in newborns is M rubra provoking a local inflammatory reaction and the typical redness and blister-like lesions. When pustules develop in lesions of M rubra, the term miliaria pustulosa is used. M usually affects neonates aged 1–3 weeks. Superficial clear vesicles of M cristallina occur in often confluent crops, without any surrounding erythema. Lesions tend to occur on the head, neck, and upper trunk. The disorder clears up spontaneously in few days with superficial branny desquamation.

138.5.1.6 Neonatal Cephalic Pustulosis (NCP) and Neonatal Acne (NA)

NA is a true comedonal and papulopustular acne induced by maternal hormones that cause excessive facial sebum production in infants (Serna-Tamayo et al. 2014). NCP is a newer entity, consisting of a pustular condition of the head (face and/or scalp) without comedones, often occurring during the third week of life, thought to be caused by overgrowth of various *Malassezia*. NCP usually clears up without treatment in a few weeks (Ghosh 2015).

138.6 Infective Diseases Characterized by Pustules, Blisters, Erosions, and Crusts

138.6.1 Varicella (Chickenpox)

The infections due to varicella-zoster virus (VZV) are rare before 6 months of age. Varicella of newborns is serious and potentially fatal, manifesting with disseminated red spots developing into papules and then rapidly into vesicles and pustules that finally form a scab after a few days. Congenital varicella can present with erosive lesions, but often typical depressed, pigmented or hypopigmented, cicatrized lesions are evident (Table 4). When varicella occurs from 8 days before delivery to 2 days after delivery, the baby may develop diffuse skin eruptions with necrotic ulcerated or hemorrhagic lesions (Smith and Arvin 2009).

138.6.2 Herpes Simplex

Neonatal herpes simplex virus (HSV) infection occurs in 0.1–0.5% of live births. HSV-2 is responsible for about 70% of cases and the rest are caused by HSV-1. HSV-2 infections generally result from contact with maternal genital secretions during delivery and are mostly due to primary genital infection acquired by the mother in late pregnancy. Transplacental transmission of the virus has been documented less

Table 4 Clinical manifestations of congenital varicella syndrome

Skin (76%)	Nervous system (60%)	Eyes (51%)	Musculoskeletal (49%)	Other
Dermatomal scarring	Intrauterine encephalitis	Chorioretinitis	Limb/muscle hypoplasia	Intrauterine growth retardation
Cutaneous defects	Cortical atrophy/ porencephaly	Cataracts		Developmental delay
Hypopigmentation	Seizures	Microphthalmia		Cardiovascular defects
	Mental retardation	Horner syndrome		Gastrointestinal reflux
	Autonomic instability	Nystagmus		Hydroureter
		Anisocoria		Hydronephrosis
				Neurogenic bladder
				Early death

Table 5 Herpes simplex virus infection in neonates: clinical presentation, mortality, and morbidity

Neonatal disease	Cutaneous lesions	Visceral involvement	Vesicles at onset	Age of onset	Mortality	Disability
Skin-eye-mouth disease	Vesicles in the skin, mouth, or conjunctive, cornea	None	All cases	5–11 days	0%	0%
Disseminated disease	Vesicles	Sepsis-like jaundice, clotting disorders, pneumonia, hepatomegaly, DIC (meningoencephalitis)	20%	5–11 days	29%	13%
CNS disease	Vesicles	Seizures Lethargy Fever	50%	2–4 weeks	4%	70%
Congenital	Vesicles, scarring of skin	Brain damage, microcephaly, low birthweight	Vesicles or scars	At delivery	?	100%
Asymptomatic infection	–	–	–	–	–	–

Modified from Malm (James and Kimberlin 2015) a mortality and morbidity data in children treated with 21 days of high-dose acyclovir: modified from Kimberlin et al. (Neylon et al. 2010)

often and may result in miscarriage or premature birth of a severely ill baby (James and Kimberlin 2015).

The symptoms in neonates have been classified into three forms. The classification has predictive value for outcome.

1. Skin-eye-mouth (SEM) manifestations without visceral or CNS involvement
2. Disseminated form (DISS) with sepsis-like symptoms, DIC, and visceral involvement with or without CNS symptoms
3. CNS form without involvement of other visceral organs

A fourth form, asymptomatic infection, can be added. The various forms are summarized in Table 5.

Skin lesions manifest at birth or within 24 h in the case of infection in utero and appear at about 7–14 days in babies who contracted the infection during delivery. Initially lesions are usually manifest on the head. Sometimes they become pustular but soon transform into erosions, which may be deep and hemorrhagic. On the palm or sole, vesicles or pustules tend to remain integral.

Table 6 Differential diagnosis of herpes simplex virus infections in newborns

Staphylococcal scalded skin syndrome
Toxic epidermal necrolysis
Aplasia cutis congenita
Bullous epidermolysis
Pemphigus
Incontinentia pigmenti
Neonatal Behçet disease
Neonatal lupus
Erythema annulare centrifugum
Infantile annular erythema
Mechanobullous disease

Prognosis of disseminated forms is poor. Neurological sequelae are also frequent.

Differential diagnosis is seldom necessary (Table 6). The diagnosis can be confirmed by cytodiagnosis, immunofluorescence, or viral culture. The treatment of choice is high-dose, prolonged acyclovir therapy.

138.6.3 Staphylococcal Scalded Skin Syndrome (SSSS)

Staphylococcus aureus can cause a spectrum of exfoliative skin conditions ranging from localized bullous impetigo to generalized cutaneous involvement with systemic illness. SSSS generally affects neonates, infants, and children under 5 years of age (Neylon et al. 2010). Skin manifestations appear several days after a local and often unapparent staphylococcus infection. Macular erythema first appears in periorificial patches, spreading to the whole skin surface in 12–24 h. The body becomes covered in large flaccid blisters that are easily ruptured. There is widespread epidermal lifting revealing large areas of red, shiny, exudative skin, resembling burns. The mucous membranes are spared. The child has edema, fever, weakness, and altered general state and may die if antibiotic therapy (penicillinase-resistant semisynthetic penicillin) and fluid and electrolyte replacement are not begun immediately. When patients respond to treatment, recovery is achieved in 1–2 weeks without scarring. Pathogenesis is linked to entry of epidermolytic toxins (ET-A and ET-B) of *S. aureus* into the bloodstream (Neylon et al. 2010; Courjon et al. 2013). Diagnosis is generally helped by the typical appearance of the syndrome, but in newborns it is necessary to distinguish scaly and eczematous erythrodermal syndromes.

138.6.4 Cutaneous Fungal Infection

Cutaneous fungal infections are quite common in newborns. The more premature the newborn, the greater the risk (Kucinskiene et al. 2014). Clinical manifestations can be the result of infection with *Candida* species or of skin colonization with *Malassezia* species; cutaneous infection with other fungal pathogens is rare (Table 7). Immunocompromised and premature neonates, however, are susceptible to infection with opportunistic pathogens such as *Mucor* and *Aspergillus* species and are at higher risk of invasive infection by common pathogens such as *Candida*.

Table 7 Clinical presentation of uncommon fungal infections in neonates

Dermatophytes (*Trichophyton rubrum*, *T. tonsurans*, *T. mentagrophytes*, *Microsporum canis*, *Epidermophyton floccosum*)	Tinea corporis (scaly erythematous annular patches, with papulopustular component), tinea faciei, tinea capitis (scaling erythematous scalp eruption with or without alopecia), tinea diaper dermatitis
Malassezia species (*M. furfur*, *M. sympodialis*)	Neonatal cephalic pustulosis (self-limiting eruption characterized by scattered erythematous papules and pustules on the face, scalp, and neck, without comedones or follicular localization) or invasive fungal disease (septicemia and pneumonia)
Aspergillus species	Primary cutaneous infection (erythematous papules or plaques, evolving to necrotic skin lesions) or systemic infection (often fatal, may involve gastrointestinal, pulmonary, and central nervous system), especially in VLBW and immunocompromised neonates
Zygomycetes (*Rhizopus*, *Mucor*, *Rhizomucor*, *Absidia*)	Primary cutaneous infection (erythematous papules, nodules, or plaques, progressing to necrosis and crusted eschars) or systemic infection (often fatal, may involve gastrointestinal, pulmonary, and central nervous system), especially in VLBW and immunocompromised neonates

138.6.4.1 *Candida* Species

Candida albicans accounts for the majority of *Candida* infections in neonates.

Congenital candidiasis is acquired in utero from previous candida chorioamnionitis and generally presents at birth or in the first 2 days of life with a variety of clinical features, ranging from monilial diaper dermatitis and diffuse eruption of pustules and papulovesicles on an erythematous and scaling base with widespread erosions to a burn-like dermatitis followed by peeling. It is not generally accompanied by thrush. The palms and soles may be involved, and onychomycosis and paronychia have been reported. In healthy full-term infants, congenital candidiasis is a benign condition that can be treated with topical antifungal agents or no therapy at all. Premature infants may present with systemic infections and widespread dermatitis. In such cases, systemic therapy is required (amphotericin B, fluconazole, or itraconazole) (Sket et al. 2013; Greenberg and Benjamin 2014).

Neonatal candidiasis is acquired during delivery or later from nursery contacts. It usually appears after the fifth day of life and commonly manifests as oral thrush or diaper dermatitis. The typical presentation is erythematous patches with satellite papules and pustules and scaling in intertriginous areas. Invasive fungal dermatitis is seen predominantly in very low-birthweight infants as diffuse erosive, crusted, and sometimes necrotic dermatitis. This condition is often fatal (Greenberg and Benjamin 2014).

138.6.5 Scabies

The pathognomonic skin lesion of scabies is the burrow, a white-grayish linear or tortuous ridge, with a small vesicle at the end. Several non-pathognomonic lesions can also be observed: 1–2 mm inflammatory papules, vesicles, pustules, crusts, and, if the patient is not treated, red-brown nodules. These last lesions may persist for several weeks after successful therapy and represent a hypersensitivity reaction to the mite and its products. Neonatal scabies is often characterized by a more or less diffuse and polymorphic eruption of inflammatory papules, vesicles, pustules, crusts, and nodules also involving areas normally spared in adults and older children, such as the face, scalp, palms, and soles (Boralevi et al. 2014). Pruritus is usually absent. The nails may be involved. A frequent complication is impetiginization of lesions. The demonstration of *Sarcoptes scabiei* mites, eggs, or fecal pellets is diagnostic. A superficial scraping followed by microscopic observation of the skin samples after application of potassium hydroxide preparation seems to be the most sensible method. Dermoscopy, a new noninvasive technique, is very useful in newborns, because it allows, if well performed, rapid identification of the burrows and the mite at the end of it (Fig. 6).

Permethrin 5% cream is regarded as a safe drug and is recommended in scabies therapy of newborn and preterm infants (Bethel 2014). The parents must be treated too.

138.6.6 Bullous Impetigo

This is the most superficial form of pyoderma. In newborns and nursing babies, staphylococcus infection is common, manifesting with vesiculobullous lesions containing serum, germs, and polymorphonuclear neutrophils, which soon become pustules that erode and form yellowish-brown crusts. Lesions generally start from the periumbilical regions, spreading to the trunk, scalp, and exposed skin due to frequent self-inoculation from the hands. Diagnosis is generally straightforward, though in newborns various diagnoses must be considered (Table 8).

138.6.7 Congenital Syphilis (CS)

Syphilis is a sexually transmitted infection (STI), caused by the bacterium *Treponema pallidum*. Vertical transmission is usually transplacental and can occur at any time during pregnancy and at any stage of disease. It is particularly likely during the first 2 years of the mother's infection. Pregnancies complicated by syphilis may result in intrauterine growth restriction, nonimmune hydrops fetalis, stillbirth, preterm delivery, and CS.

CS occurs in over 60% of infants born to untreated infected mothers. The timing of infection in utero impacts whether early signs are present at birth. For live-born infants, CS is divided into early or late disease depending on whether it presents before or after 2 years of age. Two-thirds

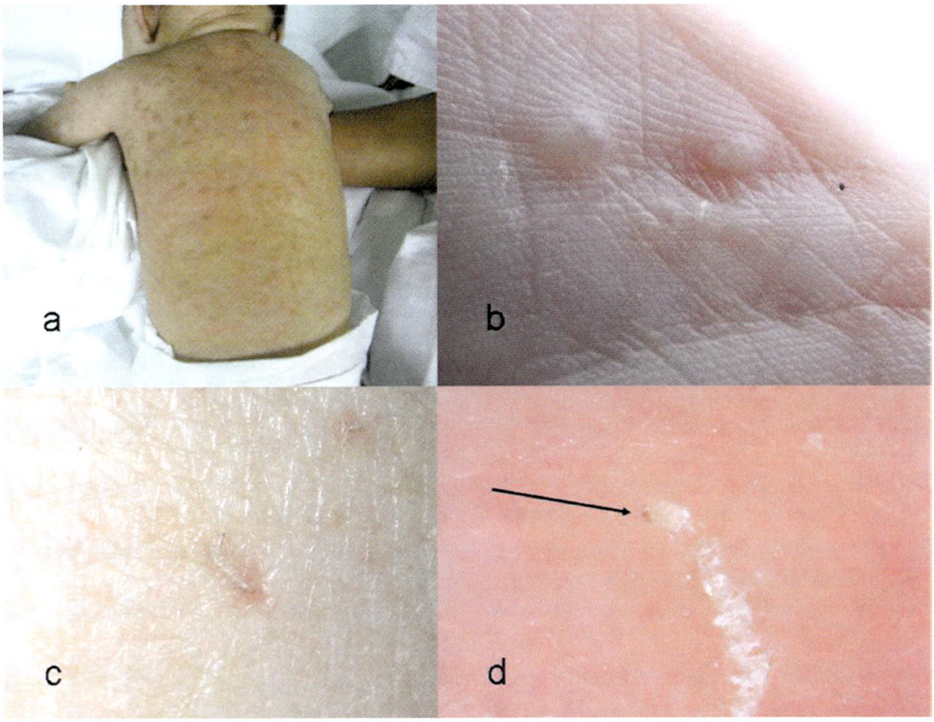

Fig. 6 Neonatal scabies diffuse to the trunk. (**a**) Vesicles and scales of the palm. (**b**) A detail of a burrow. (**c**) Dermoscopic features of burrow; (**d**) note the mite at the end of the burrow (*arrow*)

Table 8 Differential diagnosis of impetigo in newborns

Neonatal syphilis
Bullous epidermolysis
Incontinentia pigmenti
Neonatal pustolosis (congenital candidiasis, toxic erythema, transient pustular melanosis)
Infantile acropustolosis
Profuse scabies of unweaned babies
Sweat retention syndromes

Table 9 Clinical manifestations in early congenital syphilis (presentation before 2 years of age)

Manifestations	Incidence%
Prematurity	Depend on whether vertical transmission happened
Jaundice	15
Hepatosplenomegaly	33–100
Generalized lymphadenopathy	20–50
Skeletal involvement (osteochondritis, epiphysitis, and periostitis)	70
Neurological symptoms and signs (hydrocephalous, cranial nerve palsies)	40–60
Meningitis	10
Mucocutaneous lesions	30–60

of infants with CS are asymptomatic at birth, but signs appear within the 3–8 weeks after birth. Neonates born with overt manifestations of infection at delivery are usually severely affected and with a poor prognosis. Lesions are usually inflammatory and exudative. Early manifestations of CS involving multiple organ systems are described in Tables 9 and 10. Neonates show irritability, failure to gain weight or failure to thrive, and nonspecific fever. The most striking lesions affect the mucocutaneous tissues and bones (Kwak and Lamprecht 2015). Dermatological findings are quite variable, although palmar/plantar, perioral, and anogenital regions are classically involved. Mucous patches, rhinitis, and warty lesions are

Table 10 Cutaneous lesions in early congenital syphilis (presentation before 2 years of age)

Lesions	Distribution
Ragadized mucous patches	Mouth and perianal area
Snuffles	Nose
Condylomata lata	Intertriginous and periorificial areas
Maculopapular desquamative rash	First palms and soles, then extremities, face, diaper area, and trunk
Vesicular-bullous rash	Palms and soles

highly characteristic features of tegumental involvement in early CS. Smooth, round, moist mucous patches involve the mouth and perianal area. Rhinitis with profuse and occasionally bloody rhinorrhea is invariably present in symptomatic babies. The infant may have a characteristic "old man" look with fissured lesions around the mouth. Moist, flat warty lesions (*condylomata lata*) may develop in intertriginous and periorificial areas. Mucocutaneous lesions usually appear between 2 and 6 weeks of age. Snuffles are followed quickly by a diffuse maculopapular desquamative rash that involves extensive sloughing of the epithelium and begins on the palms and soles and spreads over the extremities, face, diaper area, and trunk. In contrast to acquired syphilis, a vesicular rash and bullae may develop. All these lesions are highly infective. The rash appears over 7 days and may remain for several months as copper-colored lesions. Screening of neonates at risk of syphilis includes specific treponemal and non-treponemal studies. Serological tests that detect IgG may be positive due to passive transfer of maternal antibodies. A positive anti-treponemal EIA IgM is indicative of congenital infection. Diagnosis of CS is made when the mother of an infant has a reactive treponemal and non-treponemal serologic test with characteristic clinical findings in the infant or when *T. pallidum* is demonstrated by dark-field microscopy or immunofluorescence from placental, skin, or umbilical lesions. Infants with clinical signs of illness or suggestive serologic test results also should have lumbar puncture with CSF-specific analysis and long bone x-rays. Serological tests may be negative in infants infected in late pregnancy and should be repeated. Early diagnosis and treatment with high-dose penicillin prevents late complications of syphilis.

138.7 Noninfective Blistering and Pustular Conditions

138.7.1 Inherited Blistering Diseases

138.7.1.1 Epidermolysis Bullosa (EB)

This is a group of rare inherited disorders characterized by blister formation caused by minor frictional trauma (Fine et al. 2014). These diseases are the result of various genetic defects in essential dermal-epidermal adhesion molecules, which anchor basal keratinocytes to the underlying papillary dermis. Thirty subtypes of EB are described and have been divided into four major forms, simplex (EBS), junctional (JEB), dystrophic (DEB), and Kindler syndrome, based on clinical findings, pattern of inheritance, presence or absence of scarring, and particularly the level within which blisters arise (Table 11) (Fine et al. 2014; Has and Kiritsi 2015).

In all 12 subtypes of EBS, blistering, often congenital from passage through the birth canal, is superficial and heals without scarring. The most common subtypes are inherited in an autosomal dominant pattern. In newborns, blistering and large erosions primarily affect the feet, hands, neck, and lower legs (Fig. 7). The severity of phenotypes varies greatly.

Junctional EB is an autosomal recessive disorder with seven subtypes, the most common of which is called Herlitz JEB. This very severe variant of EB is associated with a 50–80% mortality in the first 2 years of life. These infants have massive erosions that heal very slowly, often forming thick granulation tissue. The nail plates are often absent at birth, replaced by abundant granulation tissue. These infants are prone to infection, electrolyte imbalance, temperature instability, and high metabolic demand. Airway disease, growth retardation, eye problems, and gastrointestinal diseases are often associated (Fine et al. 2014).

Table 11 Major EB types and subtypes

Histopathology	Major EB type	Major EB subtypes	Targeted protein(s)
Intraepidermal cleavage	EBS	Suprabasal EBS	Plakophilin-1, desmoplakin, others
		Basal EBS	Keratins 5,14, plectin, α6β4 integrin
Intra-lamina lucida cleavage	JEB	Herlitz JEB	Laminin-332 (laminin-5)
		JEB, other	Laminin-332, type XVII collagen, α6β4 integrin
Sub-lamina densa cleavage	DEB	Dominant DEB	Type VII collagen
		Recessive DEB	Type VII collagen
Mixed	Kindler syndrome	–	Kindlin-1

EB epidermolysis bullosa, *EBS* epidermolysis bullosa simplex, *JEB* junctional epidermolysis bullosa, *DEB* dystrophic epidermolysis bullosa

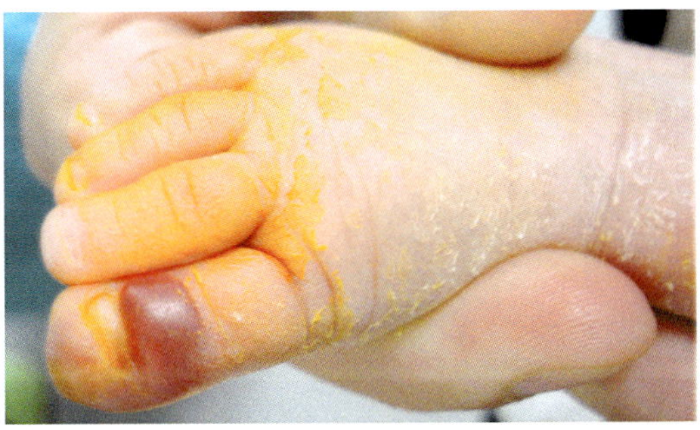

Fig. 7 A blister of the big toe in a newborn affected by epidermolysis bullosa. *Orange* color is due to topical antiseptics

Dystrophic EB is inherited, autosomal, dominant, and recessive. In the latter form, much more severe, widespread blistering begins at birth and results in contractures with severe scarring and milia formation due to split trough pilosebaceous or sweat ducts. Fusion of digits and autoamputations lead to classic "mitten deformities." Systemic involvement may be severe, with gastrointestinal complications being the most common. Nail changes are a rule in all forms of DEB.

Diagnosis may be established by electron microscope examination of a new blister, immunofluorescence mapping, and mutational analysis. Management of all forms of EB consists of good wound care with antibacterial creams and non-adherent dressings, prevention of trauma, and prevention and treatment of infection. In severe forms, newborns should initially be nursed naked in a humidified crib on non-adherent material and with barrier nursing. Nasogastric tubes, tourniquets, adhesive urine collection bags, identification bands, and pacifiers should all be avoided. Some evidences of phenotypic reversion of JEB keratinocytes by somatic gene therapy have been reported recently.

138.7.1.2 Mastocytosis

The term mastocytosis denotes a heterogeneous group of disorders characterized by abnormal growth and accumulation of mast cells in one or more organ systems (Akin and Valent 2014). The diagnosis of cutaneous mastocytosis (CM) is based on typical clinical and histological skin lesions and absence of definitive criteria of systemic involvement. Most patients with CM are children and have maculopapular cutaneous mastocytosis/urticaria pigmentosa (UP) (Méni et al. 2015; Wiechers et al. 2015). In UP, rarely present at birth, the skin shows a maculopapular rash, often with pigmented lesions, a wheal and flare phenomenon with stroking, and a positive "Darier's sign" (Fig. 7) (Tables 12 and 13) (Cohn and Mahon 1994). Other less frequent forms of CM, diffuse cutaneous mastocytosis (DCM) and mastocytoma of the skin, are usually congenital (Requena 1992; Scheck et al. 1987). Mastocytomas appear as one or several, isolated, skin-colored to light yellow-brown, 1–5 cm macules, nodules, or plaques, typically on the trunk or extremities (Fig. 8). Spontaneous or friction-induced blistering is common and bullous lesions may also develop. In diffuse cutaneous

Table 12 Classification of cutaneous mastocytosis

Variants	Criteria	MC burden	Grade	Typical findings
Urticaria pigmentosa (UP)	Maculopapular lesions	Low	Low	–
Maculopapular cutaneous mastocytosis (MPCM)				
Subvariants:				
Typical UP	Maculopapular	Low	Low	Vast majority of cases
Plaque-form	Plaques	Low	Low	Often found in infants
Nodular	Mastocytoma-like lesions (≥2)	Low (rarely	Low	Rare
Telangiectasia macularis eruptiva perstans (TEMP)	Telangiectasias, macules	High	Low	Rare
Diffuse cutaneous mastocytosis (DCM)	Erythrodermic rash	Low or high	Low	More diffuse patterns
Mastocytoma of skin	Unifocal (local) tumor	Low	Low	–

Table 13 Clinical characteristics of hyper IgE syndrome

Pustular and eczematoid rash
Blisters
"Cold" abscesses
Pyogenic pneumonia
Pneumatocele
Bronchiectasis
Eczema
Mucocutaneous candidiasis, disseminated *Cryptococcus* and *Histoplasma* infection
Peak serum IgE >2,000 IU/mL
Eosinophilia
Increased incidence of lymphoma (both Hodgkin and non-Hodgkin)
Scoliosis, osteopenia, minimal trauma fractures, hyperextensibility
Craniosynostosis
Arterial aneurisms
Facial asymmetry, deep-set eyes, prominent forehead
Retained primary dentition
High arched palate
Alteration of oral mucosa and tongue

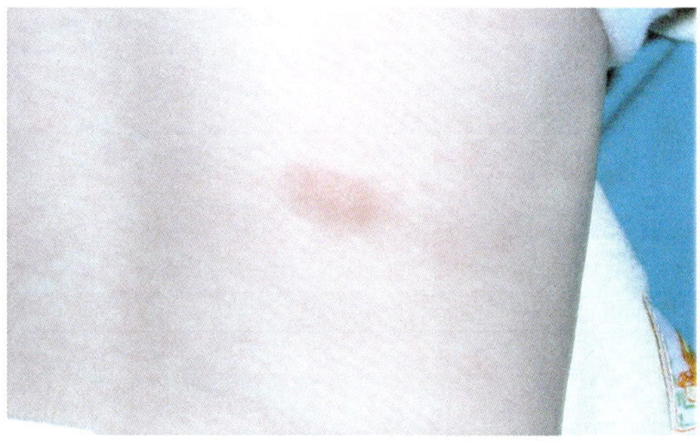

Fig. 8 Solitary mastocytoma of the trunk

mastocytosis, a more diffuse erythrodermic rash is found, and some patients may show generalized thickening of the skin, often described as "doughy" or additional nodular lesions (Fig. 9). Sometimes, rubbing, bullous lesions may develop. All forms of cutaneous mastocytosis improve with time, sometimes healing completely at puberty. The major mediators secreted by mast cells are histamine, heparin, and prostaglandins, the effects of which account for many of the clinical features of mastocytosis. The predominant symptom in all is pruritus. Additional mediator-related symptoms include flushing, hypotension, fatigue, diarrhea, vomiting, and abdominal pain.

138.7.1.3 Incontinentia Pigmenti (IP)

IP is a rare, X-linked dominant genodermatosis, usually lethal in males. It affects the skin and its appendages, bones, eyes, and central nervous system (Minić et al. 2014; Nelson 2006). Cutaneous lesions usually appear at birth or in the first days of life and have three distinct morphological stages

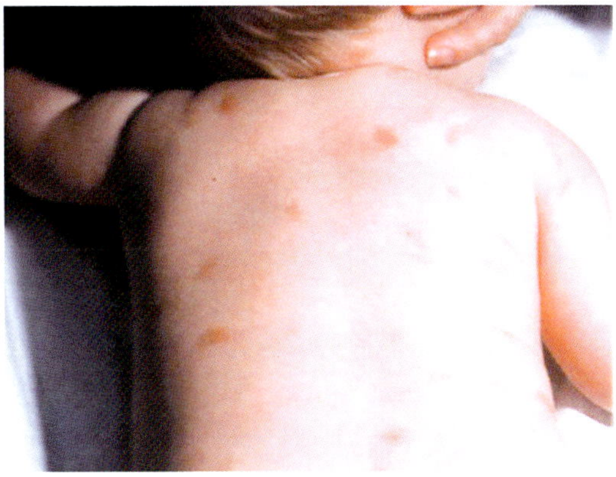

Fig. 9 Diffuse cutaneous mastocytosis

(vesiculopustular, verrucous, and pigmented) with stage one occurring in the neonatal period (Hull et al. 2015). Initially there are clear-to-yellow vesicles, measuring 2–4 mm, clustered in a linear configuration, mostly on the trunk and distal limbs. They may sometimes be pustular or crusted. At this stage, peripheral blood eosinophilia is often associated. Vesicular and pustular lesions are replaced within several weeks by gray to brown, linear and swirled verrucous papules and plaques, the second stage of the disease, and after years by brown to gray macular hyperpigmentation in streaks and whorls.

The diagnosis of IP is based on clinical findings (Babu et al. 2015). It should be considered when inflammatory linear groups of vesicles are seen in a newborn female infant. Biopsy of a blister reveals a subcorneal vesicle filled with eosinophils. Lyonization accounts for the linear pattern of this disease, typical of mosaic disorders (Happle 2006). Ocular, skin appendage, dental, and skeletal abnormalities may also occur (Chang et al. 2008). No specific treatment is required for the skin lesions, as spontaneous healing usually occurs.

138.7.1.4 Neonatal Pemphigus Vulgaris (NPV)

The term "pemphigus" refers to a group of diseases characterized by cutaneous or mucosal blisters and erosions and antiepidermal autoantibodies against desmoglein 1 and desmoglein 3 (Gushi et al. 2008). NPV is caused by passive transfer of maternal IgG antibodies across the placenta in pregnancy from mothers with PV or pemphigus foliaceus (Lorente Lavirgen et al. 2012; Meurer 2009). Lesions are usually present at birth, ranging from flaccid bullae and/or vesicles to large erosions on the whole body. The mucous membranes are rarely involved. Histopathology findings include intraepithelial blisters and acantholytic cells. Direct immunofluorescence is always positive and indirect immunofluoresence, almost always positive. Neonatal prognosis is excellent: non-corticosteroid ointments usually produce prompt epithelialization of the erosive lesions, and skin eruptions generally disappear within 3 weeks.

138.7.1.5 Herpes Gestationis (HG)

HG is an uncommon, autoimmune, bullous disease that appears during the second or third trimester of pregnancy (Bedocs et al. 2009). It almost invariably recurs in subsequent pregnancies. Anti-180-kDa bullous pemphigoid autoantibody is the cause. The disorder may be evident at birth or within several hours in neonates from mothers affected by HG. The skin eruption consists of red macules or papules, often progressing to vesicles or bullae. The typical rash usually starts around the umbilicus and spreads over the trunk and extremities. Rapid improvement occurs over few days with spontaneous recovery by 1 month of age (Panko et al. 2009).

138.8 Disease with Systemic Involvement Presenting with Pustulas, Blistering, and Erosions

138.8.1 Acrodermatitis Enteropathica (AE)

This rare autosomal recessive disease is caused by the impaired absorption of zinc in the gastrointestinal tract. Signs and symptoms of AE may be neurological-behavioral, gastrointestinal (diarrhea),

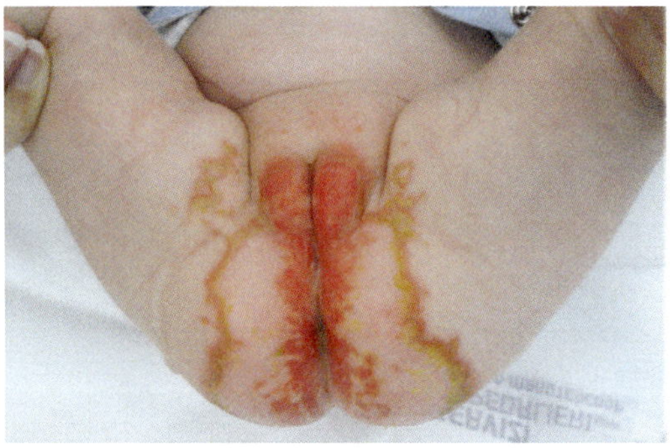

Fig. 10 Acrodermatitis enteropathica with perianal and genital lesions

ophthalmologic, infectious, or dermatological. Cutaneous manifestations of zinc deficiency are obligatory and diagnostic. Skin lesions are erythematous with peripheral crusting. Margins are well-defined, progressing to vesiculobullous, erosive, or pustular lesions. Typical distribution is periorificial and acral (Fig. 10) (Lakdawala and Grant-Kels 2015). AE patients need zinc supplementation for life. The main differential diagnoses are diaper dermatitis, chronic mucocutaneous candidiasis, atopic dermatitis, impetigo, epidermolysis bullosa, psoriasis, and seborrheic dermatitis.

138.8.2 Hyper-immunoglobulin E Syndrome (HIES)

Hyper-immunoglobulin E syndrome, also called Job's syndrome, is a very rare primary immunodeficiency, characterized by chronic eczematous dermatitis, recurrent skin and respiratory tract infections, markedly elevated serum IgE (>2,000 IU/ml), and a variety of connective tissue and skeletal abnormalities (Table 14) (Freeman et al. 2009). In almost all cases, an eczematoid rash, first affecting the face, scalp, and upper trunk and later progressing over the whole body, with papules or pustules, usually due to *S. aureus* infection, manifests in the first month of life (Freeman and Holland 2009). Blistering is a classic finding in this disease. To control the rash antibiotic prophylaxis is indicated.

138.8.3 Langerhans Cell Histiocytosis (LCH)

LCH is a rare group of disorders of the monophagocytic system, with a peak of incidence at 1–4 years of age, characterized by proliferation of a distinct cell type that is CD1a, S100, CD207 positive and contains Birbeck granules, in various organs. Cutaneous involvement is encountered in 50% of the cases. It includes four main clinical forms: Letterer-Siwe disease, Hand-Schuller-Christian disease, eosinophilic granuloma, and congenital self-healing Langerhans cell histiocytosis (CSHLCH) (Kilborn et al. 2003). CSHLCH is most frequently found in newborns. It presents at birth or in the neonatal period with papulonodules or less commonly with vesiculopustules and blisters. It usually affects otherwise healthy infants. Systemic involvement must be excluded anyway (Simko et al. 2014).

138.8.4 Porphyrias

Porphyrias are a group of metabolic disorders of heme biosynthesis that may present with acute neurovisceral symptoms, skin lesions, or both (Karim et al. 2015). Of the cutaneous porphyrias, erythropoietic protoporphyria (EPP), congenital erythropoietic porphyria (CEP), hepatoerythropoietic porphyria (HEP), and the hereditary form of porphyria cutanea tarda can present in infancy.

138.8.4.1 Erythropoietic Protoporphyria (EPP)

EPP is characterized by acute photosensitivity, with rare subepidermal bullae in exposed areas. It may occur in neonates during phototherapy. Liver disease is an uncommon, potentially fatal complication of EPP.

138.8.4.2 Congenital Erythropoietic Porphyria (CEP)

CEP presents soon after birth with typical reddish urine, severe photosensitivity, hypertrichosis of the face and extremities, mechanical fragility leading to formation of bullae, erythrodontia, and hemolytic anemia. The blisters cause scarring, dyschromia, and deformations (Katugampola et al. 2012).

Table 14 Neonatal erythroderma: more common causes and management

Disease	Clinical features	Etiology	Treatment
Infections			
SSSS	Preceding purulent infection, skin tenderness, superficial blisters, positive Nikolsky sign	Bacterial infection	Antibiotic, contact tracing
Toxic shock syndrome	Concomitant maternal infection, skin tenderness hypotension/shock	Bacterial infection	Antibiotic, intravenous Ig
Congenital cutaneous Candidiasis	Maternal vaginal candida infection, oral cavity spared, may have paronychia and nail dystrophy	Mycological infection	Antimycotics
Ichthyoses			
Nonbullous ichthyosiform erythroderma	Collodion baby; when shed leaves disseminated ichthyosiform scaling	Transglutaminase 1 gene defect and other genetic defects	Emollients, bland keratolytic creams
Bullous ichthyosiform erythroderma	Superficial blistering and erosions, ichthyosiform erythroderma, family history, linear epidermal nevus parents or sibling	Keratine gene 1,2,10 defects	Emollients, bland keratolytic creams
Netherton's syndrome	Diarrhea, failure to thrive atopy, sparse hair, trichorrhexis invaginata (bamboo hair)	Genetic defects	Emollients, adequate hydration
Conradi-Hunermann syndrome	Linear and swirled patterns	Genetic defects	Emollients
Drugs			
Ceftriaxone	Infection for which it was prescribed	Allergic reaction	Reversible on discontinuation
Vancomycin	"The red man syndrome," sudden hypotension, and erythema	Allergic reaction	Reversible on discontinuation
Others			
Seborrheic dermatitis	Cradle cap, accentuation in skin folds of neck, axilla, and nappy area	Multifactorial	Moisturizing agents, miconazole-hydrocortisone ointment, protective cream nappy area
Atopic dermatitis	Encrusted eczema on the scalp and face, generalized eczematous skin, family history for atopy	Allergy	Weak topical steroid, systemic antibiotics if the skin is infected
Psoriasis	Erythematosquamous patches, can be pustular, may have positive family history	Multifactorial	Bland emollient creams, wet dressing is helpful
Pityriasis rubra pilaris	Similar to psoriasis, follicular accentuation, skin thickening of palms and soles, may have positive family history	Cornification disorder	Along same lines as psoriasis
Diffuse mastocytosis	Darier's sign often with blistering	Abnormal proliferation of mastocytes	H1 and H2 antagonists, oral sodium cromoglycate, avoidance of substances with potential for mast cell degranulation

Modified from Hoeger and Harper (1998)

138.8.4.3 Hepatoerythropoietic Porphyria (HEP)

HEP appears at birth or in the first years of life. It is characterized by early severe photosensitivity resulting in bullae, erosions, crusts in sun areas, and severe hypertrichosis. Patients must be protected from light by clothing, sunscreen, and beta-carotene.

Whenever photosensitivity is observed in a neonate, porphyrin levels in red cells, plasma, urine, and feces should be measured (Gross et al. 2000).

138.8.5 Skin Manifestation in Down Syndrome

Skin manifestations are rare but characteristic. There have been few reports in the literature describing crusted, erythematous, vesiculopustular eruptions associated with trisomy 21 concentrated in the face and spreading to the trunk and extremities.

138.9 Red Scaly Skin in the Newborn

The term neonatal or infantile erythroderma denotes diffuse erythema with variable scaliness affecting more than 90% of the body surface. A number of major conditions can present with erythroderma in the neonate or young baby (Table 15) (Ott et al. 2008; Dhar et al. 2012). Prognosis is poor, especially in babies with immune deficiency or chronic disease (mortality 26.2%). Severe skin diseases persist in 60% of survivors (Dhar et al. 2012).

138.9.1 Immunodeficiencies (ID)

Because of the protective effect of maternal immunity, congenital ID syndromes are rarely symptomatic at birth. It is now clear that what was described in the past as Leiner's disease is a phenotype of non-congenital early-onset erythroderma, diarrhea, and failure to thrive.

138.9.1.1 Omenn's Syndrome

Omenn's syndrome is an autosomal recessive form of severe combined ID characterized by exfoliative erythroderma that occurs at birth or in the early neonatal period in association with diffuse alopecia, lymphadenopathy, hepatosplenomegaly, recurrent infections, and failure to thrive.

138.9.1.2 Graft Versus Host Reaction

Graft versus host reaction from maternal engraftment can occur as a result of transplacental passage of maternal lymphocytes during intrauterine or postnatal transfusions. In immunocompetent newborns, clinical manifestations are minimal, often resulting in only a transient macular rash. In contrast, in newborns with congenital ID, GVH reaction occurs within the first 2 or 3 weeks of life with fever, eosinophilia, lymphocytosis, lymphadenopathy, and hepatosplenomegaly, but may be present at birth as a morbilliform rash which evolves into erythroderma (Mallory 1991).

In the first weeks of life, ID should be suspected in cases in which the presenting features include pruritic erythroderma combined with skin induration; nondysplastic alopecia of hair, eyelashes, and eyebrows; widespread lymphadenopathy; and deep systemic infection. Skin infiltration is strongly indicative of Omenn's syndrome or ID, although true atopic dermatitis with marked lichenification can have a similar appearance. An association with diarrhea and extreme failure to thrive should also suggest the diagnosis. Histological findings in these cases are helpful.

Table 15 Common versus rare forms of non-syndromic ichthyosis

	X-linked ichthyosis	Lamellar ichthyosis (or CIE)	Bullous ichthyosis (or EHK)
Inheritance	XR	AR	AD
First appearance	Infancy (not at birth)	At birth	At birth
Affected gene(s)	STS	TGM1, Ichthyin, ALOXE3/12B, etc.	KRT 1,2,10
Histopathology	Retention hyperkeratosis	Hyperproliferative hyperkeratosis	Hyperproliferative hyperkeratosis
Cutaneous clinical features	Brown scales also on the trunk	Collodion baby; dry, scaly skin; ectropion; hypohidrosis, erythema	Intense blistering at birth, verrucous hyperkeratosis, and erythema

CIE congenital ichthyosiform erythroderma, *EHK* epidermolytic hyperkeratosis, *STS* steroid sulfatase gene, *TGM1* transglutaminase 1 gene, *ALOX* lipoxygenase gene, *KRT* keratin gene

138.9.2 Ichthyoses

Congenital ichthyoses are a large and heterogeneous group of monogenic disorders of cornification, sometimes associated with systemic symptoms (Table 16). A common feature is rough, dry scaly skin. Some patients have complex ichthyoses, with systemic manifestations, mainly involving the CNS, immune system, and skeleton. The two most common forms of ichthyosis, autosomal dominant ichthyosis vulgaris (IVU) and X-linked recessive ichthyosis (XRI), start early in life, but are not present at birth. Lamellar ichthyosis, with its variants nonbullous ichthyosiform erythroderma and bullous ichthyosiform erythroderma, is invariably present at birth with variable degrees of erythroderma (Alper 1986).

Table 16 Clinical manifestations of neonatal lupus erythematosus

Organ	Clinical manifestations
Skin	Annular-polycyclic erythematous plaques
	Persistent telangiectasias, atrophy, or pigmentation (less frequent)
	Confluent erythema around the eyes, giving an "owl eye" or "eye mask" appearance
Heart	Congenital heart block with or without NLE. Cardiac blocks usually develop in utero between weeks 18 and 20 of pregnancy. Once established it is irreversible. Most surviving children require permanent pacemaker implantation
	Cardiomyopathy, present in some cases usually in association with heart block, is evident at or prior to birth, and is often life threatening
Blood	Thrombocytopenia
	Pancytopenia
	Anemia
	Neutropenia
	Hypocomplementemia
Liver	Hepatomegaly with mild elevation of aminotransferase levels
	Neonatal hemochromatosis
	Cholestasis with conjugated hyperbilirubinemia and minimal elevation of transaminase
Others	Macrocephaly
	Hydrocephalus
	Gastrointestinal bleeding

138.9.2.1 Nonbullous Ichthyosiform Erythroderma

Nonbullous ichthyosiform erythroderma, an autosomal recessive congenital ichthyosis, is characterized by fine white-grayish scales and erythroderma. Many patients suffer from deep skin fissures, and some develop flexion contractures. About 90% of patients with nonbullous ichthyosiform erythroderma present as "collodion babies" enveloped in a glistening membrane resembling sausage skin that may produce ectropion, lip eversion, nasal obstruction, temperature instability, and fluid loss. The membrane peels off in days or weeks, and this may be a presentation of various forms of ichthyosis besides congenital ichthyosiform erythroderma. The most severe phenotype of autosomal recessive congenital ichthyosis is "harlequin ichthyosis," in which neonates are covered with platelike scales and massive hyperkeratosis, leading to severe disfigurement, particularly of the face. The skin soon splits forming bleeding fissures and then peels off leaving red scaly skin.

138.9.2.2 Bullous Ichthyosiform Erythroderma

Bullous ichthyosiform erythroderma presents with generalized erythema and superficial blisters. Bullous lesions become less prominent as the infant grows and may eventually disappear completely. These children later develop typical ichthyosiform hyperkeratosis, with hyperkeratosis more pronounced in the flexural areas, in which the dark, warty scales often acquire a ridged pattern with frequent maceration that causes a strong unpleasant odor.

138.9.2.3 Netherton's Syndrome

Netherton's syndrome is a complex ichthyosis with high mortality (30–40%) characterized by a triad of generalized exfoliative dermatitis, sparse hair with trichorrhexis invaginata (bamboo hair), and atopic features. It usually presents at birth as erythroderma. Patients are atopic and suffer from recurrent angio-edema and urticaria.

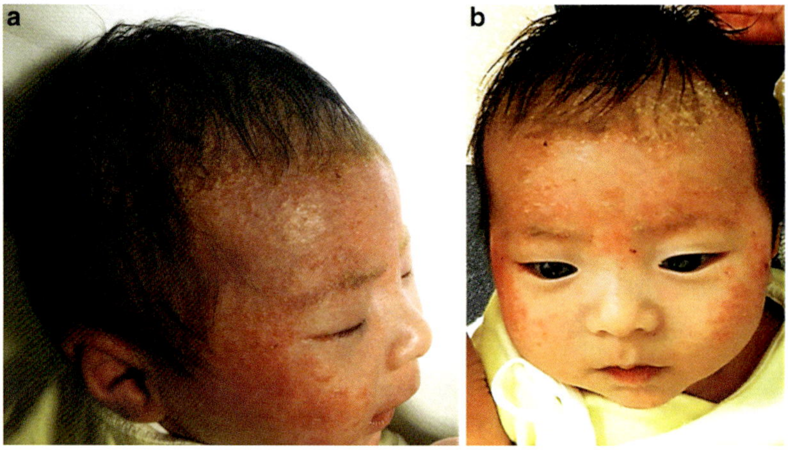

Fig. 11 Seborrheic dermatitis of the scalp (**a**) and forehead (**b**) in a 40-day-old baby

138.9.3 Drugs

Although many drugs can determine an erythematous maculopapular rash, erythroderma has only been described in neonates treated with ceftriaxone and vancomycin.

138.9.4 Seborrheic Dermatitis (SB)

Infantile SB is a papulosquamous eruption that typically develops in the first 12 weeks of life. The characteristic feature is yellowish, inflammatory scaling of the scalp (cradle cap) which spreads over the face, including the forehead, eyebrows, ear, and nose (Fig. 11a, b). Lesions often involve skin folds of the neck, postauricular regions, midtrunk, umbilicus, axilla, and groin. The scales may be absent in the flexures, and secondary candidiasis is common. Other forms of presentation include a psoriasiform variant or rarely erythroderma. Pityrosporum ovale is usually found in this disorder. SD is often asymptomatic and self-limiting after the early months of life. Scales on the scalp may be treated with mild baby shampoo and a soft-bristled toothbrush.

138.9.5 Atopic Dermatitis

Although about 18% of all children develop skin symptoms within the first 4 weeks of life, this condition rarely presents in the neonatal period with an erythrodermic rash. These patients are likely to go on to difficult long-term disease. In young infants, the primary lesion of atopic eczema is frequently vesicular and exudation is common. Atopic dermatitis more often involves the face, especially the cheeks, and flexural creases of the limbs and usually spares the nappy area (Fig. 12). In atopic dermatitis, itching is usually not apparent until 2–3 months of age. Total IgE and eosinophil count, usually considered to be markers of atopy, are neither constant nor specific. Management involves emollients and careful use of weak topical steroids, sometimes with wet dressing.

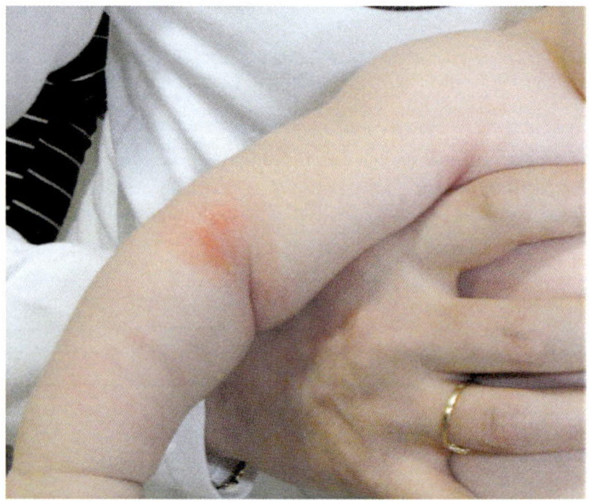

Fig. 12 Flexural lesion of the upper limb in a 30-day-old boy affected by atopic dermatitis

138.9.6 Psoriasis

Psoriasis may rarely present at birth or shortly after as generalized erythroderma, sometimes evolving into pustular psoriasis. A dramatic form of psoriasis seen in babies is napkin (diaper) psoriasis with dissemination. Starting with a bright-red napkin rash, this form of the disease later develops with small scaly patches beyond the margins. An explosive psoriasic eruption develops on the scalp and face and all over the trunk, self-limiting in a few weeks.

138.9.7 Pityriasis Rubra Pilaris (PRP)

This disease is characterized by scaly erythematous plaques similar to psoriasis and follicular hyperkeratosis. They may coalesce to larger plaques and become generalized as erythroderma. Palmoplantar keratoderma is frequently associated. Congenital erythrodermic PRP is inherited as an autosomal dominant trait and, unlike the acquired forms of PRP, tends to last a lifetime.

138.10 Neonatal Lupus Erythematosus (NLE)

NLE is a rare condition caused by transplacental passage of maternal antibodies against SS-A/Ro and SS-B/La (Inzinger et al. 2012). Only 1% of infants with positive maternal autoantibodies develop NLE, when the mothers have clinical or subclinical LES, LECS, or Sjogren syndrome. Most infants have heart and skin manifestations, but some may also have blood and liver involvement (Table 17). Skin lesions occur in the first month of life or may be present at birth. Cutaneous findings usually disappear at about the sixth month of life. Lesions resemble those of subacute cutaneous lupus erythematosus (SCLE): mild scaling erythematous plaques with well-defined margins, often annular, predominately affecting the scalp, neck, and face (Singalavanija et al. 2014). The plaques are typically periorbital, but may appear on the trunk or extremities. In male babies they are more often crusted. Solar exposure can precipitate the eruption. In some cases, erythema spreads over the entire body. Thrombocytopenia and hepatic disease may also be common. Healing tends to be associated with mild cutaneous atrophy, with or without telangiectasia. The histologic aspect of the cutaneous lesions is similar to that of SCL. NLE is the most common cause of congenital complete heart block and is associated with significant morbidity and mortality. Treatment of the mother with corticosteroids early in pregnancy may prevent heart block.

Table 17 Epidermal nevi

Verrucous epidermal nevus	Consists of hyperplasia of the surface epidermis and typically appears as verrucous papules that coalesce to form well-demarcated, skin-colored to brown, papillomatous plaques
Sebaceous nevus	Includes many of the surface findings of verrucous epidermal nevus, but also contains malformations of the dermis, most prominently hyperplasia and malpositioning of the sebaceous glands
Nevus comedonicus	Manifests as groups of closely set, dilated follicular openings with dark keratin plugs resembling comedones
Eccrine nevus	Is a rare cutaneous condition histologically characterized by an increase in size or number of eccrine secretory coils
Apocrine nevus	Is an extremely rare cutaneous condition found more often on the upper chest and axilla histologically composed of hyperplastic mature apocrine glands
Becker's nevus	First appears as an irregular pigmentation (melanosis or hyperpigmentation) on the trunk or upper arm and gradually enlarges irregularly, becoming thickened and often hairy
White sponge nevus	Consists of bilateral white keratotic macules and plaques found especially on the buccal mucosae, but labial, lingual, vaginal, and rectal mucosa may be involved

138.11 Congenital Disorders of Melanin Pigmentation

Depigmented nevi simplex type 1 (DNS type 1) is the most frequently found white spot on newborns and infants (Ruiz-Maldonado 2007). Up to 1 in 130 otherwise healthy newborns have at least one depigmented nevus present at birth, more commonly on the trunk, usually measuring 2–3 cm. The lesions are well circumscribed with irregular borders, nonprogressive, lighter than the surrounding skin but seldom white. Depigmented nevi simplex type 2 (DNS type 2) is larger than 10 cm, blocklike or linear lesions, with or without whorls. They may or may not follow Blaschko lines, are usually present at birth, and involve one or several body segments. There is no associated pathology. Metameric or segmental nevi have also been described. In such cases, the main differential diagnosis is metameric or segmental vitiligo, but this condition does not occur at birth. Rarely depigmented maculae are a part of multisystemic disorders (e.g., hypomelanosis of Ito (HI) or neurocutaneous melanosis).

138.11.1 Nevus Anemicus

Nevus anemicus resembles an achromic nevus, 1–3 cm in diameter, round, slightly hypochromic, and with a ragged outline. If pressure is applied with a convex glass, the nevus disappears, and if stroked, no flare is elicited.

138.11.2 Neurofibromatosis

Neurofibromatosis 1 (NF1) is a common neurocutaneous condition with autosomal dominant inheritance (Hersh 2008). Some cutaneous features of NF are present at birth, others are age related. Café au lait spots are usually the initial clinical manifestation of NF1 and may be present at birth or appear in infancy. They may be found anywhere on the skin but rarely on the face and scalp. They tend to increase in number and size throughout early childhood. Plexiform neurofibromas, found in at least 25% of patients with NF1, are also congenital. They feel like a bag of worms and cause gross disfigurement. They may also affect deep structures and cause pulmonary or vascular involvement. Early in life, the lesions may only be recognized as soft tissue enlargement or a patch of cutaneous hyperpigmentation with or without hypertrichosis. The other typical cutaneous findings of NF appear later.

138.11.3 Tuberous Sclerosis (TS)

The TS complex is an autosomal dominant multisystem neurocutaneous disorder characterized by widespread hamartomas in several organs, including the brain, heart, skin, eyes, kidney, lung, and liver (Curatolo et al. 2008). Most features of tuberous sclerosis only become evident after 3 years of age. The earliest cutaneous lesion to appear in TS is the hypopigmented macule, also called "ash leaf" macule, frequently present at birth. These lesions often come in other shapes: they may be round but most are polygonal, usually 0.5–2.0 cm in diameter, resembling a thumbprint. Another manifestation of TS that may be seen at birth is a hypopigmented tuft of hair. However, these findings are not pathognomonic of TS. Any newborn with a hypopigmented macule or white tuft of hair should be followed for development of other manifestations of TS.

138.11.4 Hypomelanosis of Ito (HI)

Initially described as incontinentia pigmenti achromians, IH is a congenital multisystemic neurocutaneous disorder often characterized by neurological, musculoskeletal, and eye abnormalities (Gómez-Lado et al. 2004). The disease is characterized by depigmented maculae disposed on the limbs, where they appear as lines and on the trunk where they appear as whorls or have a mottled appearance. These maculae appear at birth or during the first year of life. They may be asymmetric, unilateral, or bilateral and may occur anywhere, except on the palms, soles, and mucous membranes. No bullous or verrucous stages are seen. The skin returns to its normal color late in childhood or early adulthood. The most severe complications concern the central nervous system (CNS), causing mental retardation and epilepsy, which are both present in more than 50% of cases and are the two most severe and frequent disorders.

138.11.5 Piebaldism

Piebaldism is a rare autosomal dominant disorder. It is due to a defect in migration and maturation of melanoblasts from the neural crest. It is characterized by congenital, extensive, and symmetrically white patches on the forehead, anterior thorax, and limbs and a tuft of white hair on the forehead. Small patches of normally pigmented skin are characteristically observed inside depigmented areas. In stable piebaldism, cutaneous depigmentation remains unchanged through life (Sa et al. 2007).

138.11.6 Albinism

Genetic abnormalities of the melanin pigment system in which the synthesis of melanin is reduced or absent are called albinism. Oculocutaneous albinism (OCA) is a group of inherited disorders of melanin biosynthesis characterized by a generalized reduction in pigmentation of the hair, skin, and eyes (Summers 2009). The reduction in melanin synthesis can also be localized primarily to the eye, resulting in ocular albinism. The clinical spectrum of OCA ranges with OCA1A being the most severe type with a complete lack of melanin production throughout life. Foveal hypoplasia is invariably present and individuals with albinism often have other characteristic ocular symptoms. The degree of skin and hair hypopigmentation varies with the type of OCA, but is in general reduced. The incidence of skin cancer may be increased. All four types of OCA are inherited as autosomal recessive disorders. The diagnosis is based on findings of hypopigmentation of the skin and hair, in addition to ocular symptoms. Strabismus and nystagmus should be corrected and sunscreens are recommended. Regular skin checks for early detection of skin cancer should be offered. Persons with OCA have normal lifespan, development, intelligence, and fertility.

138.11.7 Waardenburg Syndrome (WS)

WS is an autosomal dominant disorder classified into four types. WS type 1 is clinically characterized by dystopia canthorum, sensorineural hearing loss, congenital patches of achromic skin, white forelock, broad nasal root, synophrys, and heterochromia of irides.

138.11.8 Chediak-Higashi Syndrome (CHS)

This autosomal recessive condition is due to a gene defect localized in chromosome 1q. CHS is clinically characterized by lighter skin than parents and siblings in sun-protected skin areas, slate-gray hair, and periodic, life-threatening "accelerated phase" of systemic involvement, with fever and hepatic, splenic, and lymph node enlargement. Epstein-Barr induced malignant lymphoma is usually fatal.

138.11.9 Xeroderma Pigmentosum (XP)

XP is a rare, recessive disorder based on a deficiency in nucleotide excision repair (NER) or postreplication repair (PRR) (Lichon and Khachemoune 2007). The earliest manifestation of the disease is recognized as acute sun sensitivity. This is noted as irritability followed by prolonged erythema, edema, and blistering. The severe actinic changes lead to early onset of skin cancers. Most patients do not reach adulthood, but die from metastatic cutaneous malignancies. Diagnosis can be confirmed by unscheduled DNA synthesis. XP must be distinguished from other so-called DNA repair deficiency syndromes, including Cockayne syndrome and trichothiodystrophy.

138.11.10 Neurocutaneous Melanosis (NCM)

NCM is a rare congenital phakomatosis characterized by a focal or diffuse proliferation of melanin-producing cells in both the skin and the leptomeninges (Burstein et al. 2005). This syndrome is believed to result from an error in the morphogenesis of embryonal neuroectoderm. Two-thirds of patients with NCM have giant congenital melanocytic nevi, and the remaining one-third have numerous lesions but no giant lesions. Patients may present with neurologic manifestations early in life secondary to intracranial hemorrhages, impairment of cerebrospinal fluid circulation, or malignant transformation of the melanocytes. The prognosis of patients with symptomatic NCM is poor. In their follow-up of patients with large or multiple congenital melanocytic nevi, physicians should be aware of this condition, to aid in prompt diagnosis and treatment.

138.12 Birthmarks

138.12.1 Pigmented Birthmarks

138.12.1.1 Congenital Melanocytic Nevi (CMN)

CMN are thought to arise from disrupted migration of melanocyte precursors in the neural crest and occur in 0.2–2.1% of infants at birth. CMN have been arbitrarily divided into three size ranges: small, intermediate, and giant with diameters of less than 1.5 cm (Fig. 13), 1.5–20 cm (Figs. 14 and 15), and over 20 cm, respectively. Colors range from brown to black and the commonest site is the lower back and thigh area. At birth they are often flat and pink or pale brown and most are small. Giant CMN are immediately obvious at birth. They are extremely rare and darken as the infant grows, the surface often becoming rugose or warty with nodules developing within it. The hairy component, typical of 95% of lesions, tends to become more prominent at puberty. Giant CMN of the head, neck, or posterior midline area may be associated with underlying neurocutaneous melanosis. Malignant potential increases with the size of lesion and the numbers of satellite nevi near the large lesion (Krengel et al. 2006). Smaller nevi are not well studied, but malignant changes in lesions projected to grow to less than 1.5 cm in adulthood and appear to occur rarely and only after puberty. There are various treatment options for the management of giant CMN: surgical excision (total or staged), exploiting grafts, tissue expanders, dermabrasion, and curettage. Curettage is best performed before 2 weeks of age (Batta 2000).

138.12.1.2 Use of Dermoscopy in Management of Congenital Melanocytic Nevi

Dermoscopy is a noninvasive technique that allows visualization of structures that are not visible by clinical examination. If expertly performed, it has been shown to increase diagnostic accuracy for pigmented skin lesions, especially for malignant melanoma. Dermoscopic features of congenital nevi are equally distributed between reticular, globular (Fig. 13), and homogeneous patterns (Fig. 14).

138.12.1.3 Dermal Melanocytosis (DM)

DM includes Mongolian spots, nevi of Ota and Ito, and the blue nevi. Mongolian spots are flat, blue-gray, or brown lesions with poorly defined margins that arise when melanocytes are trapped

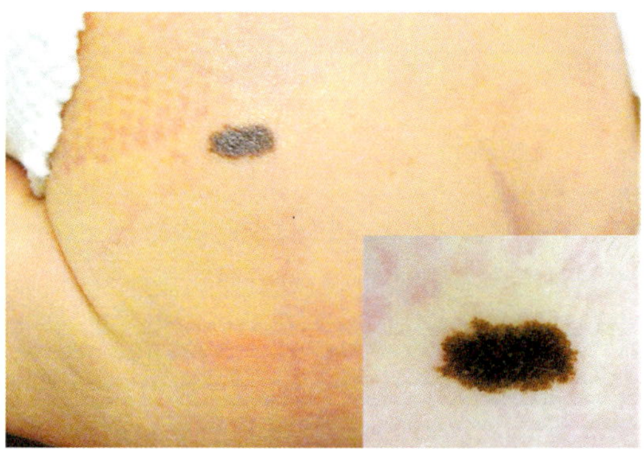

Fig. 13 A small (less than 1.5 cm) congenital nevus of the buttock, showing on dermoscopic evaluation a homogeneous distribution of globules (globular pattern)

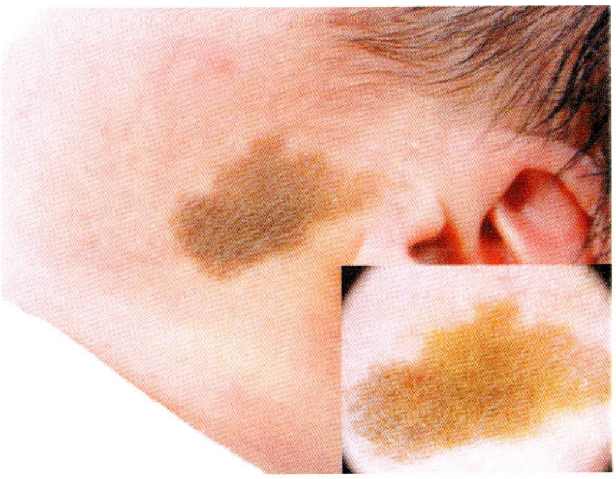

Fig. 14 An intermediate (1.5–20 cm) congenital nevus of the cheek, showing on dermoscopic evaluation a diffuse homogeneous pattern

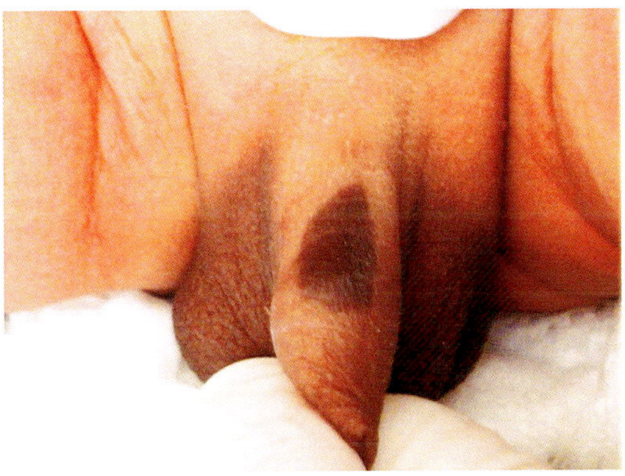

Fig. 15 An intermediate congenital nevus of the penis

deep in the skin. These lesions may be single or multiple and generally occur on the back or buttocks, although other areas may be involved. They may easily be mistaken for bruises. They are more common in black, Native American, Asian, and Hispanic populations. Most lesions fade by 2 years of age and do not require treatment. Nevus of Ota, a persistent patchy blue-gray discoloration of the face, is usually unilateral and often accompanied by an ipsilateral patchy blue discoloration of sclera, conjunctiva, cornea, retina, or oral mucosa. It is most common in Orientals and is present at birth in more than 50% of cases of associated glaucoma. Very rarely melanoma may occur in adult life (Sinha et al. 2008). Nevi of Ito are distinguished from those of Ota for

Table 18 Types of epidermal nevus syndromes

Well-defined syndromes, based on histopathology, extracutaneous manifestations, and genetic features	Sebaceous nevus syndrome (SNS)
	Nevus comedonicus syndrome (NCS)
	Becker nevus syndrome (BNS)
	Phacomatosis pigmentokeratotica (PPK)
	Proteus syndrome
	Congenital hemidysplasia with ichthyosiform nevus and limb defects (CHILD)

their location in the supraclavicular, scapular, or deltoid regions. It may be associated with an Ota nevus with ipsilateral or bilateral distribution. Common blue nevi are acquired dome-shaped blue-black papules measuring less than 1 cm in diameter. They are often located on the backs of the hands or feet or nearly.

138.12.1.4 Epidermal Nevi (EN)

EN are hamartomas characterized by epidermal and adnexal hyperplasia. They may be classified into distinct variants (Table 18). The lesions may be deeply or slightly pigmented, have unilateral or bilateral distribution, and involve any area of the skin, though they are usually located on the extremities along Blaschko lines. On the face and scalp, EN are yellowish due to prominent sebaceous glands and devoid of hair. They often have a linear distribution. In infancy they are flat, tending to become warty and papillomatous in puberty in response to androgens. Most EN remain stable. However, benign or malignant tumors can arise within them. Sebaceous nevi of Jadassohn (SNJ) are a well-known congenitally hamartoma of the skin and its adnexa. They can present as isolated lesions or as rare, more complex syndrome. Sebaceous nevus syndrome (SNS) is characterized by a sebaceous nevus and extracutaneous abnormalities, usually involving organs derived from the neuroectoderm. Today at least six different types of epidermal nevus syndromes (ENS) are known (Table 19) (Harrison-Balestra et al. 2007).

Table 19 Nail disorders in newborns

Nail disorder	Description
Anonychia	Absence of nails; rare; may be the result of a congenital ectodermal defect or anomalies like epidermolysis bullosa, severe exfoliative diseases, or infections
Micronychia	Small nail plate, shorter or narrower than normal; unusual; it is associated with syndromes or toxin exposure
Onychoschizia	Splitting of the distal nail plate into layers of the free edge. It is most noted on the big toes and thumbs, with thumb-sucking being an exacerbating factor
Infantile ingrowing toenails	The thin, sharp edge of the big toenail implants into the hypertrophic lateral nail folds of the hallux. Often bilaterally, this condition improves spontaneously with age
Racket nails or brachyonychia	Nails are broad and shortened and reflect an underlying disturbance in the formation of distal phalanx
Polyonychia	Rare; several nails on the same digit due to bifurcation of the distal phalanx. A history of maternal teratogen exposure should be searched
Congenital malalignment of the great toenail	Lateral deviation of the nail plate from the longitudinal axis of the distal phalanx. Spontaneous improvement occurs in approximately 50% of patients

138.12.2 Vascular Birthmarks

Vascular birthmarks are divided in vascular tumors and vascular malformations on the basis of their cellular features, clinical characteristics, and natural history. Vascular tumors, also called hemangioma, are associated to vascular proliferation and can be infantile or congenital. Vascular malformations have an initial rapid proliferative phase followed by an involutional phase, and they

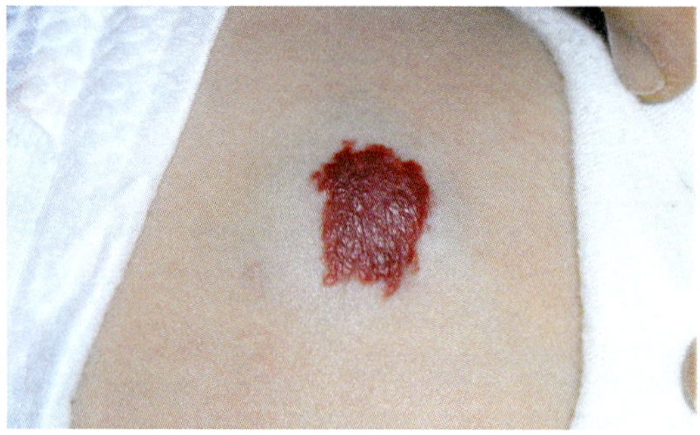

Fig. 16 A bright strawberry-*red* color hemangioma of the abdomen

are developmental anomalies classified according to the type of vessel involved: capillary, vein, lymphatic vessel, artery, or mixed malformations. They are present at birth, grow proportionally with the child, and do not spontaneously involute (Krengel et al. 2006).

138.13 Vascular Tumors

138.13.1 Hemangiomas (Strawberry Nevi)

Hemangiomas are the most common benign vascular tumors of infancy, occurring in 1.1–2.6% of newborns (Fig. 16). Females are three times more likely to have hemangiomas than male infants, and prematurity increases the risk. At birth, the lesions may vary from bright strawberry-red-colored lesions to pale patches or telangiectasias surrounded by blanched halo maculae. Hemangiomas may proliferate for 18 months and then begin to involute. Approximately 50% of hemangiomas disappear by 5 years of age and 90% by 10 years of age. After spontaneous disappearing, there may be residual epidermal atrophy, telangiectasia, hypopigmentation, or scarring (Moure et al. 2007). Despite their benign nature, hemangiomas can be complicated by ulceration, pain, infections, hemorrhage, and scarring (Fig. 17). Hemangiomas that compress the eye, nose, mouth, auditory canal, or vital organs require

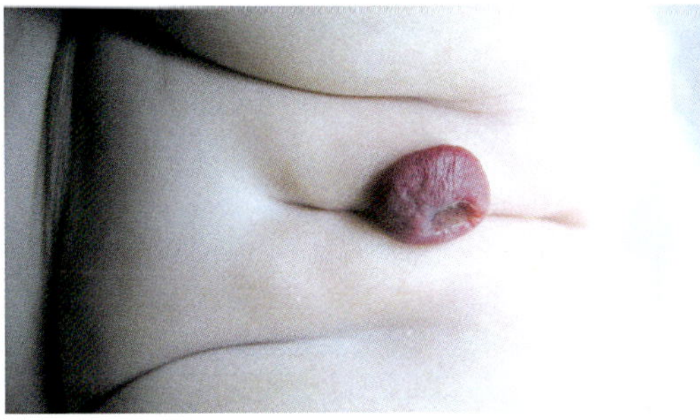

Fig. 17 Ulceration of a genital hemangioma

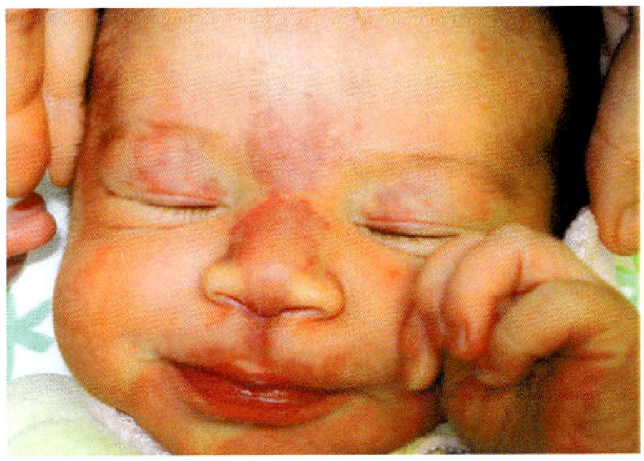

Fig. 18 Capillary malformation (port-wine stains or nevus flammeus) of the face in a newborn

immediate referral in the neonatal period. Uncomplicated hemangiomas should be observed with reassurance. Systemic steroids are the elective treatment for problematic proliferating hemangiomas. Laser treatment is an option if the lesion threatens to interfere with the airway or the ocular axis. Propranolol is also a treatment for life-threatening hemangiomas (Smolinski and Yan 2005; Denoyelle et al. 2009). The high efficacy rate and low adverse event rates reported with propranolol explain why this treatment is now widely considered a first-line treatment for complicated hemangiomas (Yang et al. 2015).

138.13.2 Kasabach-Merritt Syndrome (KMS)

KMS is a form of consumptive coagulopathy in patients with rapidly spreading hemangiomas, vascular tumors, and other malformations. It consists of thrombocytopenia which is secondary to platelet trapping within the lesions, microangiopathic hemolytic anemia, and localized consumptive coagulopathy. In some cases there is true disseminated intravascular coagulation (DIC) (Abass et al. 2008). KMS is not associated with classical hemangiomas, but rather kaposiform hemangioendotheliomas or tufted hemangiomas. They are usually deep red/blue and firm and have an equal male/female distribution. If untreated, KMS can be life threatening. It requires aggressive therapy including corticosteroids, interferon alpha, vincristine, radiation therapy, and surgery. Antiplatelet drugs and transfusion of blood products can be required too.

138.14 Vascular Malformations

138.14.1 Capillary Malformation (Port-Wine Stains or Nevus Flammeus)

Capillary malformation is a vascular birthmark, occurring in 0.3% of newborns, composed of mature dilated capillaries in the dermis that appear as variably sized pink to dark red maculae. The face is most frequently affected, often unilaterally (Fig. 18) (Ch'ng and Tan 2008). The lesions grow proportionally with the child and tend to darken with age. Port-wine stains in the ophthalmic distribution of the trigeminal nerve are associated with ipsilateral glaucoma.

138.14.2 The Sturge-Weber Syndrome

The syndrome is classically defined by the triad of glaucoma, convulsions, and port-wine stain and involves angiomas of the brain and meninges. Port-wine stains in the ophthalmic branch of the trigeminal nerve distribution (V1) are a strong indication of underlying neurological and/or ocular disorders that require ongoing ophthalmologic surveillance and/or neurological or neurosurgical management (Hennedige et al. 2008).

138.14.3 Nevus Simplex

Nevus simplex is a vascular birthmark that occurs in 33% of newborns. These flat, salmon-colored lesions are caused by telangiectasias in the dermis. They occur over the eyes, scalp, and neck, with a symmetric pattern and fade when compressed.

138.14.4 Venous Malformations (VM)

VM are always present at birth, but they may manifest clinically later in life depending on their location. Appearance varies from a vague blue patch to a soft blue mass. When venous pressure increases, for example, during crying, they usually swell, though some may remain asymptomatic throughout life. Episodic thromboses are common in VM, even in infants under 2 years of age.

138.14.5 Arteriovenous Malformation (AVM)

AVM is a congenital defect in which arteries and veins are tangled and not connected by capillaries. In early developmental stages, large shunts exist between future arteries and veins, and a defect or arrest occurring at this stage may allow some of these connections to persist. AVM manifests as a skin-colored mass with warm overlying skin that pulsates on auscultation. It is often asymptomatic, but symptoms depend on site. Localization in the CNS is not rare and may be associated with major neurological symptoms.

138.14.6 Lymphatic Malformations (LM)

LM are considered rare. There are two main types: lymphangioma and cystic hygroma. The former manifest as a group of lymphatic vessels forming a mass or lump, the latter as a large cyst or pocket of lymphatic fluid resulting from blocked lymphatic vessels. Both usually present as slowly enlarging, non-tender masses. Frequent sites are the head and neck followed by the trunk, axilla, and extremities. There is a predominance of right-sided lesions. Laryngeal and oral involvement is not uncommon. In such cases and when other vital structures are involved, surgical extirpation is usually the treatment of choice (Bloom et al. 2004).

138.15 Adnexal Congenital Disorders

138.15.1 Congenital Nail Disorders

The most common nail disorders in newborns and infants are listed in Table 20. A number of genodermatoses primarily involving the skin and mucosa are associated with more or less characteristic nail changes (Fistarol and Itin 2002). In epidermolysis bullosa nail changes are seen especially in junctional and dystrophic types. In X-linked dyskeratosis congenita, the nail plate is completely absent or hypoplastic. A pterygium formation may also be present. Pachyonychia congenita (PC) is a rare, autosomal dominant genodermatosis, characterized by symmetrical thickening and discoloration of the nails with a wedge-shaped, pinched-up, or claw-like appearance. Cutaneous cysts, hair abnormalities, and presence of teeth at birth can be observed (Das et al. 2009). Nail-patella syndrome is a genodermatosis with autosomal dominant transmission associated with bone and renal disorders.

Table 20 Congenital alopecia

Circumscribed alopecia	Diffuse alopecia
Neonatal telogen effluvium	Alopecia areata
Neonatal occipital alopecia	Marie Unna hypotrichosis
Tinea capitis	Rothmund-Thomson syndrome
Alopecia areata	Ectodermal dysplasia
Congenital triangular alopecia	Epidermolysis bullosa
Congenital aplasia cutis	
Underlying meningocele or cystic lesion	
Congenital nevi	

Table 21 Systemic distribution of associated findings of aplasia cutis congenita

Central nervous system	Hydrocephaly
	Meningocele
	Spastic paralysis and mental retardation
	Occult spinal dysraphism
Cardiovascular system	Arterovenous malformation
	Coarctation of aorta
	Congenital heart defects
Gastrointestinal system	Cleft lip-palate
	Intestinal lymphangiectasia
	Omphalocele
Eyes	Myopia and cone-rod dysfunction
	Oculo-ectodermal syndrome
Miscellaneous	Ventral body wall and/or neural tube Closure defects
	Cutis marmorata
	Piebaldism

The nail abnormalities recognized at birth include micronychia or anonychia, especially on the thumbs. The lunula can be triangular or V shaped.

138.16 Main Causes of Alopecia in Newborns

Alopecia in newborn can be classified as circumscribed and diffuse as shown in Table 21. Some manifestations as neonatal occipital alopecia and telogen effluvium may be observed frequently and are considered as physiological skin changes, others are rare.

138.16.1 Alopecia Areata (AA)

AA is a form of nonscarring hair loss, rarely reported in the neonatal period (Lenane et al. 2005).

138.16.2 Congenital Triangular Alopecia (CTA)

CTA is a triangular, lancet, or oval-shaped area of hair loss usually behind the frontotemporal hairline (Fig. 19). It may be congenital but usually appears in childhood. The hair loss may be uni- or bilateral, and complete or fine vellus hairs may remain. CTA may occur as a paradominant trait.

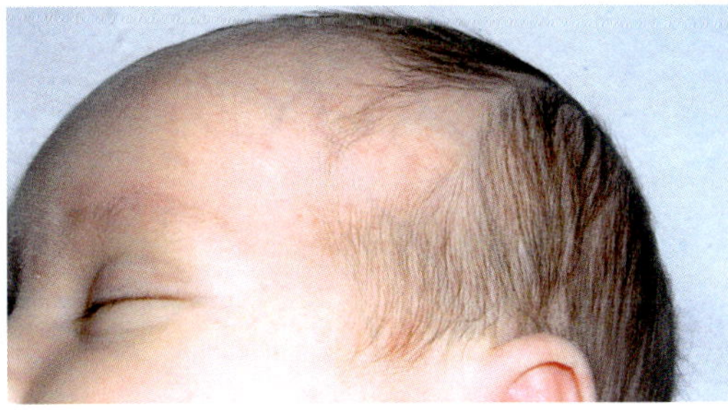

Fig. 19 Congenital triangular alopecia of the temporal zone

138.16.3 Marie Unna Hypotrichosis (MUH)

MUH is a rare autosomal dominant pilar dysplasia which can be seen at birth as a progressive hair loss.

138.17 More Common Congenital Tumors

138.17.1 Dermoid Cyst (DC)

DC is a benign, congenital, solitary or occasionally multiple, hamartomatous tumor. It is covered in a thick dermis-like wall that contains multiple sebaceous glands and almost all skin adnexa. Hair and abundant fatty masses cover poorly to fully differentiated structures derived from the ectoderm. These growths are usually located at the midline and commonly have a deep sinus that connects to the epidermis. Common sites include the forehead, lateral eye, and neck (Rosa et al. 2008). A superficial DC on the dorsal nose is referred to as a fistula and is characterized by a central tuft of hair or intracranial communication. DC can be located deep in the subcutaneous tissue, intracranially or intraorbitally. Infections, rupture, and abscess formation from manipulation of DC are possible serious complications. Surgical excision is the treatment of choice in any localization.

138.17.2 Congenital Leukemia (CL)

CL associated with skin infiltration in 25–30% of patients and usually presents as firm blue, red, or purple nodules in a generalized distribution. CL cutis may precede other manifestations of leukemia by as much as 4 months.

138.17.3 Meningocele

Meningocele is a developmental defect related to abnormal attachment and closure of the neural tube during embryogenesis. It typically presents as a skin-colored nodule on the scalp over the midline or along the spine. The treatment of choice is surgical excision.

138.17.4 Granuloma Gluteale Infantum (GGI)

GGI is a benign granulomatous eruption involving the gluteal region that may simulate a neoplastic process. It arises as a complication of primary irritant diaper dermatitis and typically resolves without treatment.

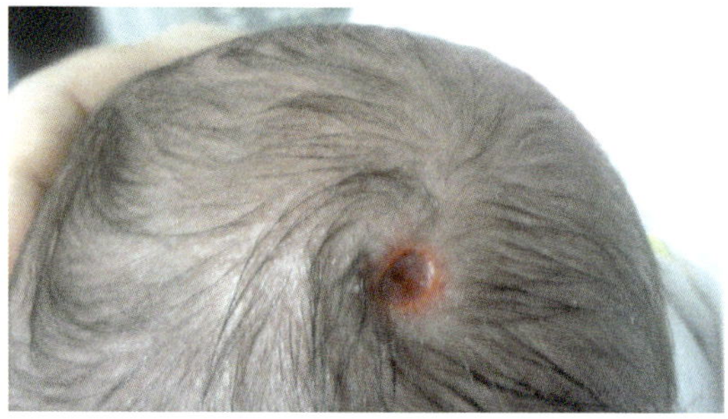

Fig. 20 Congenital aplasia cutis

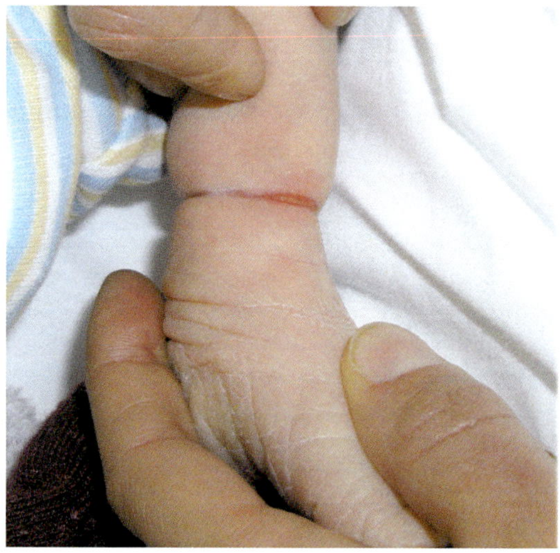

Fig. 21 Amniotic band syndrome (*ABS*) caused by entrapment of lower limb in fibrous amniotic bands during intrauterine life

138.18 Other Skin Malformations

138.18.1 Congenital Aplasia Cutis (CAC)

CAC is a rare anomaly presenting with localized or widespread absence of the skin at birth (Fig. 20). Lesions are commonly present as noninflammatory ulcerated or membranous defects with well-defined borders of variable size, near the midline of the scalp vertex. Absent hair is a constant feature. Most single defects are oval shaped and small (0.5–3 cm) and heal gradually during the first week after birth, leaving a residual atrophic or hypertrophic scars with alopecia (Aloulou et al. 2008).

Extensive scalp defects may extend to and involve the dura mater. Differential diagnoses include scalp infection, small meningocele, heterotopic brain or glial tissue, traumatic lesions, “en coup de sabre” morphea, sebaceous nevus, herpes simplex type 2, incontinentia pigmenti, and epidermolysis bullosa. The condition may be associated with specific teratogens, intrauterine infections, epidermolysis bullosa, chromosomal abnormalities, ectodermal dysplasia, or other syndrome of malformation (Table 21) (Burkhead et al. 2009).

138.18.2 Supernumerary Nipples (SN)

SN are a common congenital malformation with male predominance, consisting of extra nipples and/or related tissue besides the two nipples normally appearing on the chest. They are usually located along the embryonic milk line. Sometimes pigmented, they may be mistaken for congenital melanocytic nevi.

138.18.3 Accessory Tragus (AT)

AT is a common congenital defect linked to maldevelopment of the first and second branchial arches, which appears as a small skin-colored tag or nodule arising near the tragus. It is composed of normal epidermis with dermal adipose tissue, pilosebaceous units, eccrine glands, elastic fibers, and cartilage.

138.18.4 Branchial Cleft Cysts (BCC)

BCC are congenital epithelial cysts, which arise on the lateral part of the neck, usually near the front edge of the sternocleidomastoid muscle, from a failure of obliteration of branchial cleft in embryonic development (Koch 2005). BCC are the most common of congenital neck masses, and they are bilateral in about 2–3% of the cases. Usually asymptomatic, but, if infected, they may form a deep neck abscess or a draining fistula. Depending on the size and the anatomical extension of the mass, dysphagia, dysphonia, dyspnea, and stridor may occur.

Surgery is indicated for branchial anomalies because of the lack of spontaneous regression, a high rate of recurrent infection and rare malignant degeneration.

138.18.5 Amniotic Band Syndrome (ABS)

ABS is a rare congenital disorder caused by entrapment of fetal parts (usually a limb or digits) in fibrous amniotic bands during intrauterine life (Goldfarb et al. 2009). Prognosis depends on the location and severity of the constricting bands. In mild cases, a band may result in amputations of the fingers or toes or syndactyly (Fig. 21). In more severe cases, an amniotic band can become extremely constrictive leading to decreased blood supply and possible amputation of the limb. The most severe and life-threatening complication of amniotic band syndrome is fetal death, if a band becomes wrapped around vital areas such as the head or umbilical cord.

References

Abass K, Saad H, Kherala M, Abd-Elsayed AA (2008) Successful treatment of Kasabach-Merritt syndrome with vincristine and surgery: a case report and review of literature. Cases J 1:9

Akin C, Valent P (2014) Diagnostic criteria and classification of mastocytosis in 2014. Immunol Allergy Clin N Am 34(2):207–218

Aloulou H, Chaari W, Khanfir S et al (2008) Aplasia cutis congenita of the scalp (5 observations). Arch Pediatr 15:382–387

Alper JC (1986) The genodermatoses and their significance in pediatric dermatology. Pediatr Dermatol Clin 4:45–54

Babu NA, Rajesh E, Krupaa J, Gnananandar G (2015) Genodermatoses. J Pharm Bioallied Sci 7(1): S203–S206

Batta K (2000) Management of large birthmarks. Semin Neonatol 5:325–332

Bedocs PM, Kumar V, Mahon MJ (2009) Pemphigoid gestationis: a rare case and review. Arch Gynecol Obstet 279:235–238

Bethel J (2014) Identification and treatment of scabies in infants. Emerg Nurse 22(4):24–27

Bloom DC, Perkins JA, Manning SC (2004) Management of lymphatic malformations. Curr Opin Otolaryngol Head Neck Surg 12:500–504

Boralevi F, Diallo A, Miquel J, Guerin-Moreau M, Bessis D, Chiavérini C, Plantin P, Hubiche T, Maruani A, Lassalle M, Boursault L, Ezzedine K, Groupe de Recherche Clinique en Dermatologie Pédiatrique (2014) Clinical phenotype of scabies by age. Pediatrics 133(4):e910–e916

Burkhead A, Poindexter G, Morrell DS (2009) A case of extensive aplasia cutis congenita with underlying skull defect and central nervous system malformation: discussion of large skin defects, complications, treatment and outcome. J Perinatol 29:582–584

Burstein F, Seier H, Hudgins PA, Zapiach L (2005) Neurocutaneous melanosis. J Craniofac Surg 16:874–876
Ch'ng S, Tan ST (2008) Facial port-wine stains – clinical stratification and risks of neuro-ocular involvement. J Plast Reconstr Aesthet Surg 61:889–893
Chang JT, Chiu PC, Chen YY et al (2008) Multiple clinical manifestations and diagnostic challenges of incontinentia pigmenti-12 years' experience in a medical center. J Chin Med Assoc 71:455–460
Cohn MS, Mahon MJ (1994) Telangiectasia macularis eruptiva perstans. J Am Osteopath Assoc 94:246–248
Courjon J, Hubiche T, Phan A, Tristan A, Bès M, Vandenesch F, Etienne J, Del Giudice P, Gillet Y (2013) Skin findings of Staphylococcus aureus toxin-mediated infection in relation to toxin encoding genes. Pediatr Infect Dis J 32(7):727–730
Curatolo P, Bombardieri R, Jozwiak S (2008) Tuberous sclerosis. Lancet 372:657–668
Das JK, Sengupta S, Gangopadhyay A (2009) Pachyonychia congenita type 2. Indian J Adv Dermatol Venereol Leprol 75:321–322
Denoyelle F, Leboulanger N, Enjolras O et al (2009) Role of propranolol in the therapeutic strategy of infantile laryngotracheal hemangioma. Int J Pediatr Otorhinolaryngol 73:1168–1172
Dhar S, Banerjee R, Malakar R (2012) Neonatal erythroderma: diagnostic and therapeutic challenges. Indian J Dermatol 57(6):475–478
Fine JD, Bruckner-Tuderman L, Eady RA et al (2014) Inherited epidermolysis bullosa: updated recommendations on diagnosis and classification. J Am Acad Dermatol 70(6):1103–1126
Fistarol SK, Itin PH (2002) Nail changes in genodermatoses. Eur J Dermatol 12:119–128
Freeman AF, Holland SM (2009) Clinical manifestations, etiology, and pathogenesis of the hyper-IgE syndromes. Pediatr Res 65:32R–37R
Freeman AF, Domingo DL, Holland SM (2009) Hyper IgE (Job's) syndrome: a primary immune deficiency with oral manifestations. Oral Dis 15:2–7
Ghosh S (2015) Neonatal pustular dermatosis: an overview. Indian J Dermatol 60(2):211
Goldfarb CA, Sathienkijkanchai A, Robin NH (2009) Amniotic constriction band: a multidisciplinary assessment of etiology and clinical presentation. J Bone Joint Surg Am 91:S68–S75
Gómez-Lado C, Eirís-Puñal J, Blanco-Barca O et al (2004) Hypomelanosis of Ito. A possibly under-diagnosed heterogeneous neurocutaneous syndrome. Rev Neurol 38:223–228
Greenberg RG, Benjamin DK Jr (2014) Neonatal candidiasis: diagnosis, prevention, and treatment. J Infect 69 (Suppl (1)):S19–S22
Gross U, Hoffmann GF, Doss MO (2000) Erythropoietic and hepatic porphyrias. J Inherit Metab Dis 23:641–661
Gushi M, Yamamoto Y, Mine Y et al (2008) Neonatal pemphigus vulgaris. J Dermatol 35:529–535
Happle R (2006) X-chromosome inactivation: role in skin disease expression. Acta Paediatr Suppl 95:16–23
Harrison-Balestra C, Gugic D, Vincek V et al (2007) Clinically distinct form of acquired dermal melanocytosis with review of published work. J Dermatol 34:178–182
Has C, Kiritsi D (2015) Therapies for inherited skin fragility disorders. Exp Dermatol 24(5):325–331
Hennedige AA, Quaba AA, Al-Nakib K (2008) Sturge-Weber syndrome and dermatomal facial port-wine stains: incidence, association with glaucoma, and pulsed tunable dye laser treatment effectiveness. Plast Reconstr Surg 121:1173–1180
Hersh JH (2008) Health supervision for children with neurofibromatosis. American Academy of pediatrics committee on genetics. Pediatrics 121:633–642
Hoeger PH, Harper JI (1998) Neonatal erythroderma: differential diagnosis and management of the "red baby". Arch Dis Child 79:186–191
Hull S, Arno G, Thomson P et al (2015) Somatic mosaicism of a novel IKBKG mutation in a male patient with incontinentia pigmenti. Am J Med Genet A 167 (7):1601–1604
Inzinger M, Salmhofer W, Binder B (2012) Neonatal lupus erythematosus and its clinical variability. J Dtsch Dermatol Ges 10(6):407–411
James SH, Kimberlin DW (2015) Neonatal herpes simplex virus infection: epidemiology and treatment. Clin Perinatol 42(1):47–59
Januário G, Salgado M (2011) The Harlequin phenomenon. J Eur Acad Dermatol Venereol 25(12):1381–1384
Karim Z, Lyoumi S, Nicolas G et al (2015) Porphyrias: a 2015 update. Clin Res Hepatol Gastroenterol 39(4):412–425
Katugampola RP, Anstey AV, Finlay AY et al (2012) A management algorithm for congenital erythropoietic porphyria derived from a study of 29 cases. Br J Dermatol 167(4):888–900
Kilborn TN, Teh J, Goodman TR (2003) Paediatric manifestation of Langerhans cell histiocytosis: a review of clinical and radiological findings. Clin Radiol 58:269–278
Koch BL (2005) Cystic malformations of the neck in children. Pediatr Radiol 35:463–477
Krengel S, Hauschild A, Schäfer T (2006) Melanoma risk in congenital melanocytic naevi: a systematic review. Br J Dermatol 155:1–8
Kucinskiene V, Sutkute A, Valiukeviciene S (2014) Cutaneous fungal infection in a neonatal intensive care unit patient: a case report and literature review. Pediatr Dermatol 31(3):267–270
Kwak J, Lamprecht C (2015) A review of the guidelines for the evaluation and treatment of congenital syphilis. Pediatr Ann 44(5):e108–e114
Lakdawala N, Grant-Kels JM (2015) Acrodermatitis enteropathica and other nutritional diseases of the folds (intertriginous areas). Clin Dermatol 33(4): 414–419
Lenane P, Pope E, Krafchik B (2005) Congenital alopecia areata. J Am Acad Dermatol 52:S8–S11
Lichon V, Khachemoune A (2007) Xeroderma pigmentosum: beyond skin cancer. J Drugs Dermatol 6:281–288
Lorente Lavirgen AI, Bernabeu-Wittel J, Dominguez-Cruz J, Conejo-Mir J (2012) Neonatal pemphigus foliaceus. J Pediatr 161(4):768

Mallory SB (1991) Neonatal skin disorders. Pediatr Clin N Am 38:745–761

Mancini AJ, Sookdeo-Drost S, Madison KC et al (1994) Semipermeable dressings improve epidermal barrier function in premature infants. Pediatr Res 36:306–314

Méni C, Bruneau J, Georgin-Lavialle S et al (2015) Paediatric mastocytosis: a systematic review of 1747 cases. Br J Dermatol 172(3):642–651

Meurer M (2009) Pemphigus diseases in children and adolescents. Hautarzt 60:208–216

Minić S, Trpinac D, Obradović M (2014) Incontinentia pigmenti diagnostic criteria update. Clin Genet 85 (6):536–542

Monteagudo B, Labandeira J, Cabanillas M, Acevedo A, Toribio J (2012) Prospective study of erythema toxicum neonatorum: epidemiology and predisposing factors. Pediatr Dermatol 29(2):166–168

Moure C, Reynaert G, Lehmman P et al (2007) Classification of vascular tumors and malformations: basis for classification and clinical purpose. Rev Stomatol Chir Maxillofac 108:201–209

Nelson DL (2006) NEMO, NFkappaB signaling and incontinentia pigmenti. Curr Opin Genet Dev 16: 282–288

Neylon O, O'Connell NH, Slevin B, Powell J, Monahan R, Boyle L, Whyte D, Mannix M, McElligott F, Kearns AM, Philip RK (2010) Neonatal staphylococcal scalded skin syndrome: clinical and outbreak containment review. Eur J Pediatr 169(12):1503–1509

Ott H, Hütten M, Baron JM et al (2008) Neonatal and infantile erythrodermas. J Dtsch Dermatol Ges 6(12): 1070–1085

Panko J, Florell SR, Hadley J et al (2009) Neonatal pemphigus in an infant born to a mother with serologic evidence of both pemphigus vulgaris and gestational pemphigoid. J Am Acad Dermatol 60(6):1057–1062

Requena L (1992) Erythrodermic mastocytosis. Cutis 49:189–192

Rosa PA, Hirsch DL, Dierks EJ (2008) Congenital neck masses. Oral Maxillofac Surg Clin N Am 20:339–352

Ruiz-Maldonado R (2007) Hypomelanotic conditions of the newborn and infant. Dermatol Clin 25:373–382

Sa J, Khachemoune A, Guldbakke KK (2007) Piebaldism: a case report and a concise review of the literature. Cutis 80:411–414

Scheck O, Horny HP, Ruck P et al (1987) Solitary mastocytoma of the eyelid. A case report with special reference to the immunocytology of human tissue mast cells, and a review of the literature. Virchows Arch 412:31–36

Serna-Tamayo C, Janniger CK, Micali G, Schwartz RA (2014) Neonatal and infantile acne vulgaris: an update. Cutis 94(1):13–16

Simko SJ, Garmezy B, Abhyankar H et al (2014) Differentiating skin-limited and multisystem langerhans cell histiocytosis. J Pediatr 165(5):990–996

Singalavanija S, Limpongsanurak W, Aoongern S (2014) Neonatal lupus erythematosus: a 20-year retrospective study. J Med Assoc Thai 97(6):S74–S82

Sinha S, Cohen PJ, Schwartz RA (2008) Nevus of Ota in children. Cutis 82:25–29

Sket KV, Giachetti A, Sojo M, Garrido D, Lupo E, Brener P (2013) Congenital cutaneous candidiasis. Arch Argent Pediatr 111(6):556–558

Smith CK, Arvin AM (2009) Varicella in the fetus and newborn. Semin Fetal Neonatal Med 14:209–217

Smolinski KN, Yan AC (2005) Hemangiomas of infancy: clinical and biological characteristics. Clin Pediatr (Phila) 44:747–766

Summers CG (2009) Albinism: classification, clinical characteristics, and recent findings. Optom Vis Sci 86:659–662

Visscher MO, Adam R, Brink S, Odio M (2015) Newborn infant skin: physiology, development, and care. Clin Dermatol 33(3):271–280

Wiechers T, Rabenhorst A, Schick T et al (2015) Large maculopapular cutaneous lesions are associated with favorable outcome in childhood-onset mastocytosis. J Allergy Clin Immunol 136(6):1581–1590

Yang B, Li L, Zhang LX et al (2015) Clinical characteristics and treatment options of infantile. Medicine 94 (40):1–9

Part XIV

Appendices

Laboratory Medicine: Reference Values and Evidence-Based Medicine 139

Mariangela Longini, Fabrizio Proietti, Francesco Bazzini, and Elisa Belvisi

Contents

Abstract

Accurate and reliable laboratory tests are essential for appropriate clinical management. Individual variability means that there are wide ranges in laboratory test results that are non-pathological and it is necessary for reference intervals to be defined in statistical terms. Rational interpretation of laboratory tests is a critical part of the clinical decision-making process and must take account of not only the test value but also the clinical condition. Evidence-based medicine is the conscientious, explicit, and judicious use of current best evidence in making decisions about the care of individual patients; it means avoiding doing laboratory investigations without a specific clinical suspicion.

M. Longini (✉) · F. Proietti · F. Bazzini · E. Belvisi
Department of Molecular and Developmental Medicine, University of Siena, Siena, Italy
e-mail: mariangela.longini@unisi.it; proiettifabrizio3@gmail.com; francesco_bazzini@hotmail.it; elybel87@hotmail.it

139.1 Salient Points

- Analytical procedures should provide results with appropriate reference ranges.
- Interpretation of laboratory results should take into account not only the test value but also the patient's clinical condition.
- An appropriate test is a test that is able to give a clear answer to a clear clinical question.
- The application of diagnostic tests without specific clinical suspicion is an important cause of increased cost and a source of anxiety for the patient (Ulysses syndrome).

The accuracy and reliability of laboratory test results is essential for appropriate clinical management decisions. Use of appropriate analytical procedures providing results traceable to an appropriate reference measurement system may allow one to minimized errors. The use of adequate reference intervals may further minimize variations caused by the presence of physiological changes and by analytical or biological variation.

Because there are wide ranges in the non-pathological values of laboratory tests, linked to the fact of enormous individual variability (age, gender, race, lifestyle, work, physical training,

G. Buonocore et al. (eds.), *Neonatology*,
https://doi.org/10.1007/978-3-319-29489-6_286

hormonal activity), some individuals, while presenting values within those reference, may have a disease not yet diagnosed or may belong to a population at high risk of developing a disease, or they may be sick, but for various reasons do not have values altered in that specific test. Moreover, in a pediatric population it is difficult to establish these conditions.

The range of reference values for a specific test can be evaluated and defined in statistical terms. Considering, as typically occurs, a symmetric Gaussian distribution in the distribution values of the results of a test applied to a given population (reference) the reference values are with 95% interval, so the 5% of nonpathological values of laboratory tests are outside to reference values.

Test values outside of the reference range are a sign for the laboratory that indicates the probability of the presence of the disease. The more narrow are the limits of these intervals, the higher will be the percentage of individuals that the ranking indicates are sick but for which there is no presence of the disease (false positive, low specificity of the test). On the other hand a wider range of reference values leads to an increase in the percentage of sick individuals with normal values tests (false negatives, low sensitivity of the test). On the other hand a wider range of the reference values implies the increase in the percentage of diseased individuals who have normal values (false negatives, low sensitivity of the test) (Geffré et al. 2009).

Careful interpretation of laboratory results must consider not only the test value but also the clinical valutation. A rational clinical interpretation of the data is crucial. Hence the concept of "evidence-based medicine" (EBM).

The term EBM was coined at McMaster Medical School in Canada in the 1980s to label the clinical learning strategy, which people at the school had been developing for over a decade (Rosenberg and Donald 1995).

EBM is the conscientious, explicit, and judicious use of current best evidence in making decisions about the care of individual patients. The practice of EBM means integrating individual clinical expertise with the best available external clinical evidence from systematic research (Sackett et al. 1996).

The principles of EBM were developed in the early 1990s (Guyatt 1991) and slowly began to be put into practice soon after. At the beginning of the next decade, the impact of the principles of EBM in laboratory medicine was recognized (Price 2000). EBM embraces the diagnostic modalities while evidence-based laboratory medicine (EBML) focuses on the use of diagnostic tests and the goal of improving patient outcomes. A definition of EBLM, developed from the definition of EBM given by Sackett et al. (Sackett et al. 1996), is "the conscientious, judicious and explicit use of best evidence in the use of laboratory medicine investigations for assisting in making decisions about the care of individual patients."

Laboratory medicine is an integral part of the practice of medicine and so any analysis of the impact of EBLM on the practice of laboratory medicine has to look at the quality of evidence that can be used to inform clinical decision-making and the success with which this evidence is adopted.

Laboratory testing significantly contributes to the clinical decision-making, and the number of tests that a modern clinical laboratory can now perform is considerable. The impact of Laboratory Medicine in Neonatology has substantially evolved and increased over the past years.

Today many new diagnostic techniques and laboratory tests have been introduced as a result of both research on the fundamental pathogenesis of diseases and the development of new methods in themselves. Laboratory tests provide from two thirds to three fourths of the information used for making medical decisions. The age-old "truth standard" for the quality of evidence describes three dimensions that are important – a test should tell the truth, the whole truth, and nothing but the truth. This three-dimensional model can be used to characterize the clinical and analytical reliability of laboratory tests and guide the translation of outcome criteria, or quality goals, into practical specifications for method performance (Westgard and Darcy 2004).

An appropriate test is a test that is able to give a clear answer to a clear clinical question. This will enable the clinician to make a decision and initiate some form of action leading to a benefit for the patient. An appropriate test may also be one in which there is an operational or economic benefit, without any adverse health benefit detriment to the patient (Price 2003).

The application of diagnostic tests without a specific clinical suspicion is the main cause of cost increase and a source of apprehension for the patient. This is the well-known "Ulysses syndrome" which is caused by unnecessary and inappropriate investigations or wrong interpretation of results. Patients with Ulysses syndrome find themselves caught in a web of further investigations, referrals, and sometimes treatment before finally being recognized as healthy, which they were in the first place. It was first described 40 years ago (Rang 1972) and the number of tests available is now much greater. With greater choice comes greater responsibility and the need for greater discernment.

In this age of evidence-based medicine, nothing is more important than the quality of laboratory tests. Advising on the optimal use of laboratory tests is, and has always been, a fundamental part of the clinical biochemists remit. Many difficulties faced by pathology have their origin in a relentless increase in activity in the face of diminishing budgets rather than in the efficiency or inefficiency of service delivery. (Waine 2002) Besides this, there are the potential benefits of improved practice, reducing the number, particularly and in particular the unnecessary repetitions, of tests, greatly decreases costs not only of the general practitioner, but also of the laboratory nonreagent materials (forms, bottles, collection materials, etc.).

Changing the list of tests which make up a given profile can quickly effect change, for example: the profiles of routine electrolyte and liver function tests, those for diagnosing and monitoring thyroid dysfunction, for diagnosing the acute coronary syndrome, and for urine analysis and microscopy. These changes, whether made on the initiative of an individual laboratory or as a result of changing national trends, produce large changes in test numbers (Van Walraven et al. 1998). This type of intervention is possible only when there is a widespread consensus on benefits. Several studies have demonstrated the power of the laboratory request form to effect change, usually in combination with other behavioral changes (Van Walraven et al. 1998; Solomon et al. 1998; Novich et al. 1985; Zaat et al. 1992). The move away from test profile requests towards more diagnosis-based requesting undoubtedly enables the laboratory to optimize analyses.

Changes in health service structure and funding make it possible for more active interaction between laboratories and primary care trusts in addressing encouraging best practices in the use of pathology tests.

This requires ongoing dialogue between the laboratory and clinicians and must be seen in a context of mutual help and not one of criticism or prescriptive testing practice. These initiatives will succeed only with the active support of both of laboratories and of users and will require the composition of best-practice advice across the range of pathology tests, supported by the professional bodies. Although excellent work has been done already, there is a need to bring the matter of appropriateness of testing up on top of the pathology agenda, not just with the production of guidelines but with the design of suitable systems to help improve appropriateness.

On the subject of how to bring about change, Lundberg in 1998 wrote both pessimistically and optimistically: know the literature; set up an appropriate group; agree terms of reference; implement change; educate; accept positive (and negative) criticism; respond to valid complaints; enjoy a better service (Lundberg 1998a; Lundberg 1998b).

The advent of "omics" science has had a massive impact in the clinic, for better understanding of the function of genes, proteins, metabolites, and their interactions with the environment. The omics sciences would be able to identify many physiological and pathophysiological mechanisms of many diseases. The future application of these techniques could have an enormous potential in the clinical practice as with regards to the diagnosis, prognosis, and follow-up (Rinaudo et al. 2016).

References

Geffré A, Friedrichs K, Harr K et al (2009) Reference values: a review. Vet Clin Pathol 38(3):288–298

Guyatt GH (1991) Evidence-based medicine. ACP J Club 114:A16

Lundberg GD (1998a) The need for an outcomes research agenda for clinical laboratory testing. JAMA 280:565–566

Lundberg GD (1998b) Changing physician behaviour in ordering tests. JAMA 280:2036–2037

Novich M, Gillis L, Tauber AI (1985) The laboratory test justified: an effective means to reduce routine laboratory testing. Am J Clin Pathol 84:756–759

Price PC (2000) Evidence-based laboratory medicine: supporting decision-making. Clin Chem 46:1041–1050

Price CP (2003) Application of the principles of evidence-based medicine to laboratory medicine. Clin Chim Acta 333(2):147–154

Rang M (1972) The Ulysses syndrome. Can Med Assoc J 106:122–123

Rinaudo P, Boudah S, Junot C et al (2016) Biosigner: a new method for the discovery of significant molecular signatures from omics data. Front Mol Biosci 3:26

Rosenberg W, Donald A (1995) Evidence based medicine: an approach to clinical problem-solving. BMJ 310 (6987):1122–1126

Sackett DL, Rosenberg WMC, Muir Gray JA et al (1996) Evidence based medicine: what it is and what it isn't. BMJ 312:71–72

Solomon DH, Hideki H, Daltroy L et al (1998) Techniques to improve physicians' use of diagnostic tests. JAMA 280:2020–2027

Van Walraven C, Goel V, Chan B (1998) Effect of population-based interventions on laboratory utilization. JAMA 280:2028–2033

Waine C (2002) Pathology in primary care. Address to the opportunities in UK pathology meeting. Laing and Buisson (organizers), London

Westgard JO, Darcy T (2004) The truth about quality: medical usefulness and analytical reliability of laboratory tests. Clin Chim Acta 346(1):3–11

Zaat JOM, van Eijk JTM, Bonte HA (1992) Laboratory test form design in•uences testordering by general practitioners in The Netherlands. Med Care 30:189–9839

140 Laboratory Medicine: Reference Intervals for Laboratory Tests and Procedures

Mariangela Longini, Fabrizio Proietti, Francesco Bazzini, and Elisa Belvisi

M. Longini (✉) · F. Proietti · F. Bazzini · E. Belvisi
Department of Molecular and Developmental Medicine, University of Siena, Siena, Italy
e-mail: mariangela.longini@unisi.it; proiettifabrizio3@gmail.com; francesco_bazzini@hotmail.it; elybel87@hotmail.it

G. Buonocore et al. (eds.), *Neonatology*,
https://doi.org/10.1007/978-3-319-29489-6_288

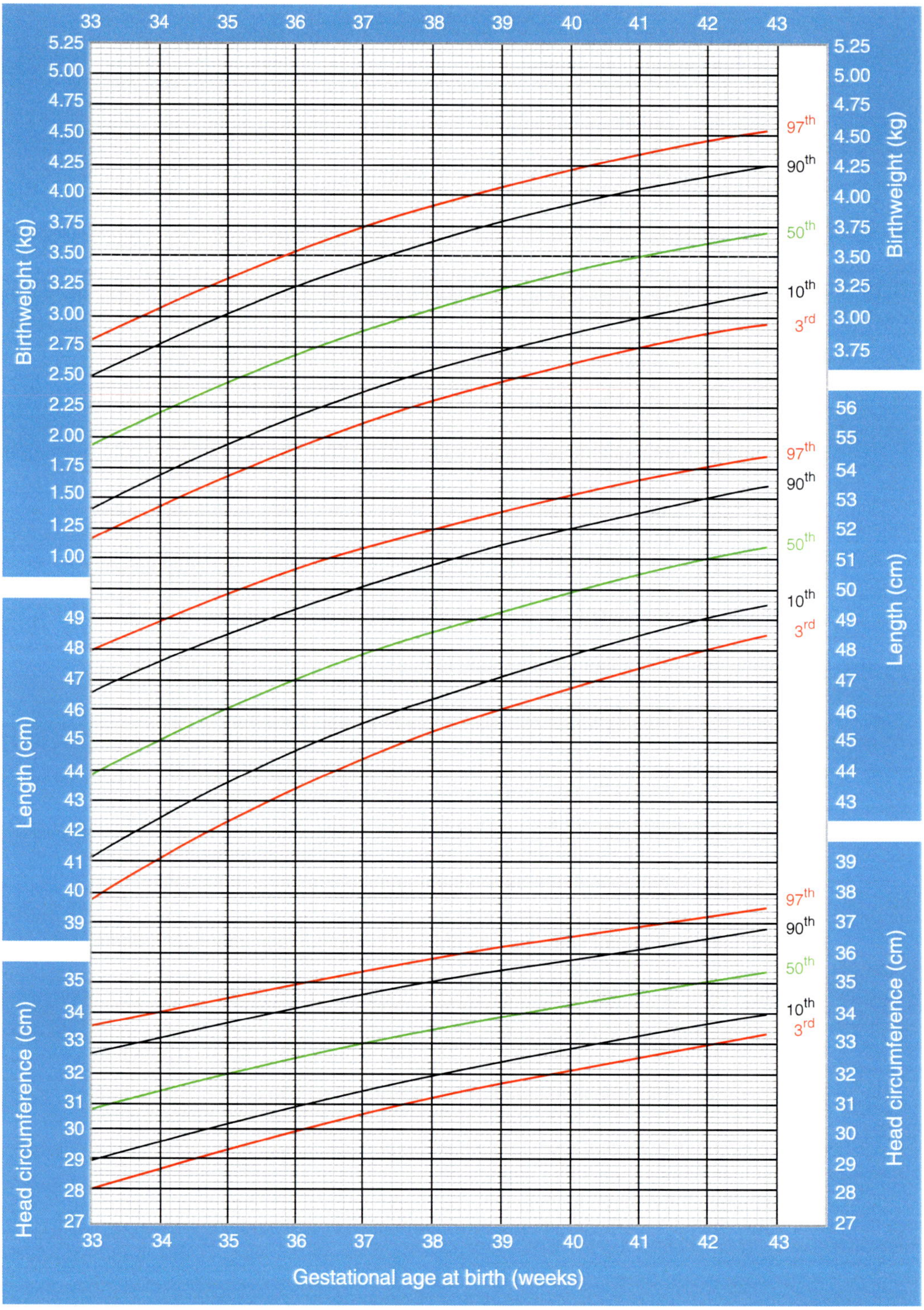

Fig. 1 International standards for size at birth (boys)

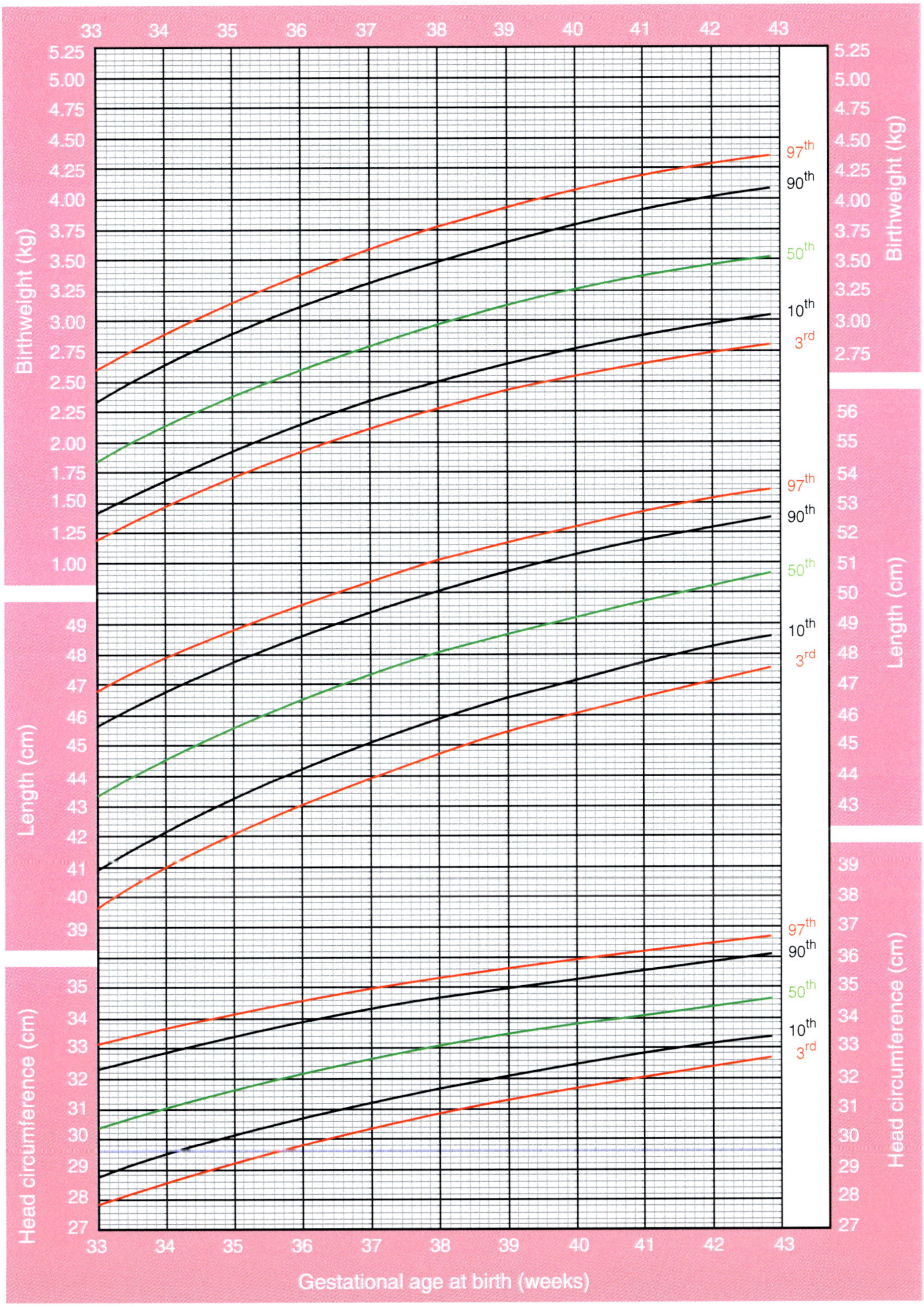

Fig. 2 International standards for size at birth (girls) (Villar J, Cheikh Ismail L, Victora CG et al (2014) International standards for newborn weight, length, and head circumference by gestational age and sex: the Newborn Cross-Sectional Study of the INTERGROWTH-21st Project. Lancet 384(9946):857–868. PMID: 25209487)

Table 1 Hematologic values in normal fetuses at different gestational ages in cord blood

Week of gestation	Hemoglobin (g/dL)	RBCs ($\times 10^6$ mL)	Hematocrit (%)	Mean corpuscular volume (fL)	Total WBCs ($\times 10^6$ μL)	Corrected WBCs ($\times 10^6$ μL)	Platelets ($\times 10^6$ μL)
18–21 (N = 760)	11.69 ± 1.27	2.85 ± 0.36	37.3 ± 4.32	131.1 ± 11.0	4.68 ± 2.96	2.57 ± 0.42	234 ± 57
22–25 (N = 1200)	12.2 ± 1.6	3.09 ± 0.34	38.59 ± 3.94	125.1 ± 7.8	4.72 ± 2.82	3.73 ± 2117	247 ± 59
26–29 (N = 460)	12.91 ± 1.38	3.46 ± 0.41	40.88 ± 4.4	118.5 ± 8.0	5.16 ± 2.53	4.08 ± 0.84	242 ± 69
>30 (N = 440)	13.64 ± 2.21	3.82 ± 0.64	43.55 ± 7.2	114.4 ± 9.3	7.71 ± 4.99	6.4 ± 2.99	232 ± 87

Partially modified from Forestier P, Daffos F, Catherine N et al (1991) Developmental hematopoiesis in normal human fetal blood. Blood 77:2360

RBCs Red blood cells, *WBCs* white blood cells

Hematologic data obtained with a Coulter S plus II instrument. Total WBC count included nucleated red blood cells. Corrected WBC count included only WBCs, after subtracting the nucleated red cell component, based on a 100-cell manual differential

Table 2 WBC manual differential counts in normal fetuses at different gestational ages in cord blood

Week of gestation	Lymphocytes (%)	Neutrophils (%)	Eosinophils (%)	Basophils (%)	Monocytes (%)	Nucleated RBCs (% of WBCs)
18–21 (N = 186)	88 ± 7	6 ± 4	2 ± 3	0.5 ± 1	3.5 ± 2	45 ± 86
22–25 (N = 230)	87 ± 6	6.5 ± 3.5	3 ± 3	0.5 ± 1	3.5 ± 2.5	21 ± 23
26–29 (N = 144)	85 ± 6	8.5 ± 4	4 ± 3	0.5 ± 1	3.5 ± 2.5	21 ± 67
>30 (N = 172)	68.5 ± 15	23 ± 15	5 ± 3	0.5 ± 1	3.5 ± 2	17 ± 40

From Forestier F, Daffos F, Catherine N et al (1991) Developmental hematopoiesis in normal human fetal blood. Blood 77:2360
RBCs Red blood cells, *WBCs* white blood cells

Table 3 Hematologic values for cord blood (vaginal delivery and cesarean section)

	Vaginal delivery (N = 63)		Cesarean section (N = 104)	
Characteristic	Mean	Range	Mean	Range
WBC ($\times 10^9$ per l)	18.4	12.0–34.1	13.6	8.54–39.7
RBC ($\times 10^{12}$ per l)	4.78	3.89–6.30	4.62	3.46–6.62
Hb (g/dL)	17.6	14.0–23.0	17.1	13.0–23.4
Hct (%)	54.7	41.9–73.1	52.6	40.1–72.2
MCV (fl)	114	105–127	112	97.7–125
MCH (pg)	36.5	31.4–41	36.6	32–39.9
MCHC (g/dL)	32.3	30.8–35.9	32.4	30.3–34.4
RDW (%)	17.4	14.9–23.6	17.4	14.2–23.3
PLT ($\times 10^9$ per l)	297	169–607	254	161–424
MPV (fl)	8.7	7.7–11.4	8.8	7.5–11.5
Plateletcrit (%)	0.26	0.15–0.48	0.23	0.15–0.36
CD34+ cells ($\times 10^6$ per l)	47.7	15.9–253	39.9	7.14–120

Partially modified from Eskola M, Juutistenaho S, Aranko K et al (2011) J Perinatol 258–262. Data obtained with Sysmex K-1000 analyzer (Sysmex, Kobe Japan)

Hb Hemoglobin, *Hct* hematocrit, *MCH* mean corpuscular hemoglobin, *MCHC* mean corpuscular hemoglobin concentration, *MCV* mean corpuscular volume, *MPV* mean platelet volume, plateletcrit MPV × PLT, *PLT* platelet, *RBC* red blood cell, *RDW* red blood cell distribution width, *WBC* white blood cell

Table 4 Red cell and reticulocyte indices and serum marker of iron status in cord blood

Parameter	Mean	SD	Reference range
Cellular indices			
Hb, g/dL	15.9	1.5	14.6–18.9
HCT,%	49	0.5	44–58
MCV, fL	109	4	102–118
MCVr, fL	124	6	115–136
MCH, pg	35	1	33–38
MCHC, g/dL	32.5	1.0	30.6–34.2
%Retic, %	4.0	0.8	2.6–5.4
IRF-H, %	24.1	7.8	10.2–40.0
CI-Im, pg	34.9	1.3	32.5–37.2
CHr, pg	35.6	1.3	33.1–38.6
%HYP0m, %	3.0	3.0	0.4–9.9
%HYPOr, %	42.0	15.6	18.3–76.8
Serum measurements			
TFR, mg/L	2.0	0.7	1.2–4.0
Ferritin, µg/L	198	137	45–636
TfR-F index	0.95	0.43	0.49–2.1
Iron, µmol/L	27.4	7.7	12.2–42.1
Transferrin, g/L	2.0	0.4	1.2–2.9
TfSat, %	55	19	21–111

From Ervasti M, Kotisaari S, Sankilampi U et al (2007) The relationship between red blood cell and reticulocyte indices and serum markers of iron status in the cord blood of newborns. Clin Chem Lab Med 45:1000–1003
CHm Cellular hemoglobin in red blood cells, *CHr* cellular hemoglobin in reticulocytes, *Hb* hemoglobin, *HCT* hematocrit, *%HYPOm* percentage of hypochromic red blood cells, *%HYPOr* percentage of hypochromic reticulocytes, *IRF-H* high immature reticulocyte fraction, *MCH* mean cell hemoglobin, *MCHC* mean cell hemoglobin concentration, *MCV* mean cell volume of red blood cells, *MCV* mean cell volume of reticulocytes, *%Retic* proportion of reticulocytes, *TfR* transferrin receptor, *TfR-F index* transferrin receptor/log (ferritin), *TfSar* transferrin saturation
Hematologic data obtained in 199 full-term newborn infants with a ADVIA 120 analyzer (Siemens Diagnostic Solutions)

Table 5 Reference ranges for NRBC at birth in cord blood

Week of gestation	Birth weight (g)	Upper reference value of NRBC	90% CI
26–28 (N = 120)	780–1105	22583	14080–31709
29–31 (N = 128)	1100–1720	11420	8348–14002
34–36 (N = 215)	1940–2520	3748	3200–4182
38–40 (N = 232)	2905–3590	2329	1806–2580

Partially modified from Perrone S, Vezzosi P, Longini M et al (2005) Nucleated red blood cell count in term and preterm newborns: reference values at birth. Arch Dis Child Fetal Neonatal 90:174–175
NRBC was expressed as absolute count (NRBC/mm^3), calculated by light microscope examination of May–Grunwald–Giemsa stained blood smears

Table 6 Reference ranges for HCt, Retic. Parameters, S-TfR during the first 15 weeks of life

	Hb, g/dL			Hct, %			Reticulocyte, $\times 10^9$/L		
	Reference			Reference			Reference		
Age, week	Mean	Lower	Upper	Mean	Lower	Upper	Mean	Lower	Upper
0.5	15.0	10.2	22.2	45	30	65			
1.5	13.8	9.8	19.6	41	29	58	59.5	20.2	175.6
2.5	12.8	9.4	17.6	38	28	52	66.8	24.7	181.1
3.5	12.0	9.0	16.1	36	27	47	74.1	29.2	187.9
4.5	11.3	8.6	15.0	34	26	44	81.2	33.7	195.8
5.5	10.8	8.2	14.2	32	25	42	87.9	37.8	204.3
7.0	10.2	7.8	13.3	30	23	39	96.7	43.1	216.7
9.0	9.7	7.3	12.7	29	22	38	105.2	48.4	228.8
11.0	9.5	7.1	12.5	28	21	37	109.0	51.3	231.9
13.0	9.6	7.2	12.7	28	21	37	107.6	51.4	225.2
15.0	10.0	7.6	13.3	30	22	39	101.2	48.1	212.9
	CHr, pg			IRF			S-TfR, mg/L		
	Reference			Reference			Reference		
Age, week	Mean	Lower	Upper	Mean	Lower	Upper	Mean	Lower	Upper
0.5	35.7	31.5	39.9	36.6	13.5	59.7			
1.5	35.0	31.1	38.9	35.5	13.7	57.2	1.4	0.9	2.4
2.5	34.3	30.6	38.1	34.3	13.6	55.1	1.3	0.8	2.3
3.5	33.7	30.1	37.4	33.3	13.1	53.4	1.3	0.8	2.1
4.5	33.1	29.5	36.7	32.2	12.4	52.1	1.2	0.7	2.0
5.5	32.6	29.0	36.2	31.3	11.6	50.9	1.2	0.7	1.9
7.0	31.9	28.3	35.5	29.9	10.3	49.6	1.1	0.7	1.8
9.0	31.2	27.5	34.8	28.4	8.6	48.1	1.1	0.7	1.8
11.0	30.6	26.9	34.3	27.0	7.4	46.7	1.1	0.7	1.9
13.0	30.2	26.5	33.9	25.9	6.7	45.0	1.2	0.7	2.0
15.0	30.0	26.4	33.6	24.9	6.7	43.3	1.3	0.8	2.2

Proni Mäkelä E, Takal TI, Suomine P et al (2008) Hematological parameters in preterm infants from birth to 16 weeks of age with reference to iron balance. Clin Chem Lab Med 46:551–557

CHr Reticulocyte hemoglobin content, *Hb* hemoglobin, *Hct* hematocrit, *IRF* immature reticulocyte fraction, *S-Tfr* soluble transferrin receptor

Hematologic data obtained with ADVIA 120, Siemens Medical Solutions, Tarrytown, NY. S-TfR measured with an automated immunoturbidimetric methods (IDeA sTfR-IT, Orion Diagnostica), Espoo, Finland. Ferritin assayed with Elecsys ferritin electrochemiluminescence immunoassay on a Modular E analyzer (Roche Diagnostics)

Table 7 Reference ranges for ferritin during the first 15 weeks of life

	Ferritin[a], µg/L			Ferritin, No Transfusions[b], µg/L		
	Reference interval			Reference interval		
Age, week	Mean	Lower	Upper	Mean	Lower	Upper
1.5	221.4	77	636.8	215.5	73.5	631.6
2.5	199.9	65.6	609.2	178.5	56.9	559.8
3.5	180.4	52.8	616.5	149.2	43.9	507.2
4.5	162.8	41.4	640.2	125.9	34.1	465.4
5.5	147.0	32.3	668.4	107.2	26.8	429.7
7.0	126.0	22.6	702.3	85.7	19.2	382.1
9.0	102.6	14.9	708.7	65.7	13.3	324.6
11.0	83.5	10.6	659.1	52.3	10.1	271.7
13.0	68.0	8.2	563.0	43.2	8.3	224.0
15.0	55.3	6.9	444.8	37.0	7.5	182.9

Proni Mäkelä E, Takal TI, Suomine P et al (2008) Hematological parameters in preterm infants from birth to 16 weeks of age with reference to iron balance. Clin Chem Lab Med 46:551–557

[a]The information under the column "Ferritin" shows the values calculated for the neonates who had not been transfused at least 2 weeks of measurements

[b]The information under the column "Ferritin, no transfusions" shows the values calculated for those neonates who had not been transfused at all (indicating ferritin level development in the most stable preterm neonates)

Ferritin assayed with Elecsys ferritin electrochemiluminescence immunoassay on a Modular E analyzer (Roche Diagnostics)

Table 8 Reference ranges for CBC, retieulocytes, ferritin, and S-TfR during the first year of life in preterm and term infants

	Hb, g/dL		Hct%		RBC count, × 10^{12}/L		MCV, fL	
Age, weeks	Mean	95% RI	Mean	95% RI	Mean	95% RI	Mean	95% RI
Preterm								
20	11.2	9.2–13.7	32.7	27.1–39.5	4.03	3.15–4.92	81.6	73.2–90.0
25	11.6	9.8–13.8	34.0	28.7–40.1	4.27	3.48–5.07	80.1	72.3–88.0
30	12.0	10.3–14.1	35.1	30.0–41.1	4.47	3.70–5.25	79.0	71.2–86.7
35	12.4	10.6–14.4	36	30.9–42.1	4.64	3.83–5.44	78.1	70.1–86.0
40	12.7	10.8–14.8	36.8	31.5–43.1	4.76	3.92–5.60	77.5	69.3–85.7
45	12.9	10.9–15.2	37.4	31.9–43.8	4.85	3.98–5.71	77.3	68.9–85.6
50	13.0	11.0–15.3	37.8	32.3–44.2	4.89	4.03–5.75	77.3	69.0–85.6
55	13.1	11.1–15.3	38	32.6–44.2	4.90	4.07–5.73	77.6	69.6–85.7
60	13.0	11.2–15.1	37.9	32.9–43.7	4.87	4.11–5.62	78.2	70.7–85.8
Term								
20	12.0	10.2–14.1	34.5	29.3–40.7	4.32	3.76–4.87	80.3	74.2–86.4
25	11.9	10.2–13.8	34.5	29.6–40.2	4.38	3.84–4.92	79.0	73.1–84.9
30	11.8	10.1–13.7	34.5	29.8–40.0	4.44	3.90–4.98	78.1	72.3–83.9
35	11.8	10.1–13.7	34.6	30.0–40.0	4.48	3.93–5.03	77.6	71.8–83.4
40	11.8	10.2–13.7	34.8	30.3–40.0	4.51	3.96–5.06	77.4	71.6–83.2
45	11.9	10.3–13.7	35.1	30.7–40.1	4.54	3.99–5.08	77.6	71.7–83.5
50	12.0	10.4–13.8	35.4	31.3–40.2	4.55	4.01–5.08	78.2	72.2–84.1
55	12.1	10.5–14.0	35.9	31.9–40.3	4.55	4.04–5.06	79.1	73.1–85.1

	MCH, pg		Retie, × 109/L		Ferritin, μg/L		S-TfR, mg/L	
Age, weeks	Mean	95% RI	Mean	95% RI	Mean	95% RI	Mean	95% RI
Preterm								
20	28.1	25.2–31.0	77.4	39.0–153.5	37.8	7.37–193.9	1.52	1.07–2.16
25	27.7	24.8–30.5	69.7	36.7–132.5	30.1	7.48–120.8	1.54	1.10–2.15
30	27.3	24.4–30.3	64.1	34.3–119.6	24.7	7.06–86.6	1.56	1.12–2.16
35	27.1	24.0–30.2	60.1	32.4–111.8	21.1	6.41–69.5	1.57	1.14–2.17
40	26.9	23.7–30.1	57.6	30.9–107.2	18.6	5.80–59.9	1.59	1.16–2.19
45	26.8	23.5–30.0	56.3	30.1–105.1	17.1	5.41–53.8	1.61	1.17–2.21
50	26.7	23.6–29.9	56.1	30.0–105.2	16.2	5.25–49.8	1.63	1.18–2.25
55	26.8	23.7–29.8	57.2	30.3–107.7	15.9	5.31–47.5	1.65	1.18–2.30
60	26.9	24.0–29.7	59.4	31.1–113.5	16.2	5.44–47.9	1.67	1.18–2.36
Term								
20	27.9	25.6–30.2	45.5	25.3–82.2	71.7	21.5–239.7	1.49	1.06–2.08
25	27.3	24.9–29.6	45.2	25.1–81.5	51.1	16.1–162.2	1.52	1.08–2.12
30	26.8	24.3–29.2	45.4	26.1–78.9	38.5	11.5–128.7	1.54	1.09–2.19
35	26.5	23.9–29.0	46.0	27.6–76.6	30.6	8.76–107.0	1.57	1.09–2.27
40	26.3	23.7–28.9	47.1	28.8–76.8	25.8	7.46–89.1	1.60	1.08–2.37
45	26.3	23.6–29.0	48.7	28.7–82.5	22.9	7.01–75.0	1.63	1.07–2.48

(*continued*)

Table 8 (continued)

	MCH, pg		Retie, × 109/L		Ferritin, μg/L		S-TIR, mg/L	
Age, weeks	Mean	95% RI	Mean	95% RI	Mean	95% RI	Mean	95% RI
Preterm								
50	26.5	23.8–29.2	50.9	26.9–96.3	21.6	6.78–68.6	1.66	1.05–2.62
55	26.9	24.2–29.6	53.7	23.9–121.0	21.5	5.90–78.0	1.69	1.04–2.76

	CHr, pg		WBC count, × 10^9/L		Platelet count, × 10^9/L	
Age, weeks	Mean	95% RI	Mean	95% RI	Mean	95% RI
Preterm						
20	29.8	26.6–33.1	9.48	5.63–16.0	478	294–777
25	29.6	26.4–32.8	9.60	5.73–16.1	465	290–744
30	29.4	26.2–32.7	9.71	5.82–16.2	452	286–714
35	29.3	26.0–32.6	9.83	5.92–16.3	439	280–687
40	29.2	25.9–32.6	9.94	6.01–16.5	427	274–663
45	29.2	25.8–32.6	10.1	6.09–16.6	415	268–642
50	29.3	25.8–32.7	10.2	6.17–16.8	403	260–623
55	29.4	25.8–32.9	10.3	6.24–17.0	391	252–607
60	29.5	25.9–33.2	10.4	6.31–17.2	380	244–593
Term						
20	29.8	27.4–32.1	9.36	5.84–15.0	426	282–646
25	29.2	25.7–32.6	9.19	5.73–14.7	415	269–640
30	28.8	24.7–32.9	9.02	5.57–14.6	404	258–634
35	28.7	24.5–32.9	8.85	5.37–14.6	394	247–628
40	28.9	25.1–32.6	8.68	5.14–14.7	383	237–621
45	29.2	26.4–32.1	8.52	4.88–14.9	373	227–614
50	29.9	27.6–32.2	8.36	4.61–15.2	363	218–607
55	30.8	27.0–34.5	8.21	4.33–15.5	354	209–599

From Takale TI, Mäkelä E, Suomine P et al (2010) Blood cell and iron status analytes of preterm and full-term infants from 20 weeks onward during the first year of life. Clin Chem Lab Med 48:1295–1301

CBC complete blood count, *CHr* reticulocyte hemoglobin content, *Hb* hemoglobin, *Hct* hematocrit, *MCH* mean corpuscular hemoglobin, *MCV* mean corpuscular volume, *RBC* red blood cell, *Retic* reticulocyte, *RI* reference interval, *S-Tfr* soluble transferrin receptor, *WBC* white blood cell

Hematologic data obtained with ADVIA 120, Siemens Medical Solutions, Tarrytowrz, NY. S-TfR measured with an automated immunoturbidimetric methods (IDeA sTfR-IT, Orion Diagnostica), Espoo, Finland. Ferritin assayed with Elecsys ferritin electrochemiluminescence immunoassay on a Modular E analyzer (Roche Diagnostics)

Table 9 Circulating platelet counts at different ages

Age categories	Platelet count (10^9/L)
Core blood	288 ± 53
2 days	303 ± 48
5 days	338 ± 59
1 month	343 ± 72
2–11 months	365 ± 49
1–2 years	314 ± 78
3–4 years	304 ± 66
5–6 years	303 ± 65
7–10 years	295 ± 58
11–15 years	251 ± 40

Partially modified from Ishiguro A, Nakahata T, Matsubara K et al (1999) Age-related changes in thrombopoietin in children: reference interval for serum thrombopoietin levels. Br J Haematol 106(4):884–888

Table 10 Comparison of selected coagulation factor values in newborns[a]

Age	Fibrinogen (mg/dL)	F II (U/mL)	F VIII (U/mL)	F IX (U/mL)	F XII (U/mL)	Antithrombin (U/mL)	Protein C (U/mL)
Term							
Hathaway and Bonnar (1987) and Manco-Johnson et al. (1988)	240 (150)	0.52 (0.25)	1.5 (0.55)	0.35 (0.15)	0.44 (0.16)	0.56 (0.32)	0.32 (0.16)
Andrew et al. (1987, 1988)	283 (177)	0.48 (0.26)	1.0 (0.50)	0.53 (0.25)	0.53 (0.20)	0.63 (0.25)	0.35 (0.17)
Corrigan (1992)[5]	246 (150)	0.45 (0.22)	168 (0.50)	0.40 (0.20)	0.44 (0.16)	0.52 (0.20)	0.31 (0.17)
Preterm							
Hathaway and Bonnar (1987) and Manco-Johnson et al. (1988)	300 (120)	0.45 (0.26)	0.93 (0.54)	0.41 (0.20)	0.33 (0.23)	0.40 (0.25)	0.24 (0.18)
Andrew et al. (1987, 1988)[a]	243 (150)	0.45 (0.25)	1.1 (0.50)	0.35 (0.19)	0.38 (0.10)	0.38 (0.14)	0.28 (0.12)
Corrigan (1992)s	240 (150)	0.35 (0.21)	1.36 (0.21)	0.35 (0.10)	0.22 (0.09)	0.35 (0.10)	0.28 (0.12)

Hathaway W, Bonnar J (1987) Hemostatic disorders of the pregnant woman and newborn infant. Elsevier, New York; Manco-Johnson M, Marlar R et al (1988) Severe protein C deficiency in newborn infants. J Pediatr 113:359

Andrew M, Paes B, Milner R et al (1987) Development of the human coagulation system in the full-term infant. Blood 70:165; Andrew M, Paes B, Milner R et al (1988) Development of the human coagulation system in the healthy premature infant. Blood 72:1651

Corrigan JJ Jr (1992) Normal hemostasis in fetus and newborn: coagulation. In: Polin RA, Fox WW (eds) Fetal and neonatal physiology. Saunders, Philadelphia, pp 1368–1371

[a]Data are expressed as mean and lower limits of normal. Preterm = 30–36-weeks' gestational age

Table 11 Reference ranges for coagulation parameters[a], inhibitors and fibrinolysis in preterm newborns

	Premature SGA newborns (N = 68) (mean ± SD and 2.5th–97.5th percentile)	Premature AGA newborns (N = 71) (mean ± SD and 2.5th–97.5th percentile)
[1]INR	1.35 ± 0.22 (1.02–2.09)	1.32 ± 0.20 (1.02–1.85)
[1]PT (s)	16.6 ± 2.1 (13.2–23.1)	16.4 ± 1.98 (13.3–21.4)
[2]APTT (s)	51 ± 11 (35.4–97.6)	51 ± 12(34.2–102.9)
[1]Fibrinogen (mg/dL)	158 ± 46 (65–243)	183 ± 80 (64–478)
[1]IIc (%)	37.6 ± 6.5 (23.4–53)	37.2 ± 9 (20.5–58)
[1]Vc (%)	61 ± 22 (23–128)	62 ± 20.4 (22.6–120)
[1]VIIc (%)	61.2 ± 20.5 (17.9–116.5)	68.8 ± 23.7 (27.8–124.2)
[1]VIIIc (%)	142 ± 80 (26–389)	116 ± 57 (28–276)
[2]IXc (%)	32 ± 22 (11.8–107.5)	28 ± 11 (11.6–60.5)
[1]Xc (%)	41.2 ± 9.7 (18.2–65.5)	41.5 ± 10 (27.0–68.7)
[1]XIc (%)	33.5 ± 14.2 (11.3–76.9)	30.5 ± 11.0(13.2–60.4)
[1]XIIc (%)	50 ± 22 (16–110.7)	47 ± 24 (12.7–119.6)
[1]AT Act (%)	37.2 ± 11.0 (19.5–67.8)	39.0 ± 13.7(16.7–80.3)
[2]PC Act (%)	24 ± 8 (11.0–50.3)	24 ± 9 (10.4–52)
[1]FREE PS Act (%)	31.5 ± 9.0 (17–57)	31.1 ± 5.9 (20–47.6)
[2]APCR	2.3 ± 0.30 (1.32–3.13)	2.2 ± 0.34 (1.43–3.16)
[2]tPA (ng/ml)	13.8 ± 8.2 (4.5–44.1)	11.4 ± 7.0 (3.2–34.6)
[2]PAI-1 (ng/ml)	55.3 ± 24.4 (14.9–102.6)	46 ± 24 (16.5–122)
[1]VWF Ag (%)	202 ± 64 (105–355)	193 ± 59 (95–339)

Partially modified from Mitsiako G, Giougi E, Chatziioannidis I et al (2010) Haemostatic profile of healthy premature small for gestational age neonates. Thromb Res 126:103–106. 1: T test; 2: Mann–Whitney U test; *Act* activity, *Ag* antigenic value, *c* coagulant activity

[a]All parameters were determined utilizing a STA Compact Analyzer and reagents from Diagnostica Stago (Asnières sur Seine, France)

Table 12 Reference ranges for coagulation tests in healthy, term newborns

Test	Newborns
PT (s)	13.1 ± 0.9
aPTT (s)	35 ± 4.5
Platelets (×109/L)	214 ± 55
Fibrinogen (mg/dL)	251 ± 51
Factor II (%)	73 ± 7
Factor V (%)	93 ± 13
Factor VII (%)	88 ± 12
Factor VIII (%)	113 ± 38
Factor IX (%)	86 ± 18
Factor X (%)	72 ± 10
Hematocrit (%)	59 ± 3.0

Partially modified from Cerneca F, de Vonderweid U, Simeone R et al (1994) The importance of hematocrit in the interpretation of coagulation tests in the term newborn infant. Hematologica 79:25

[a]Data were obtained in 71 newborns and expressed as mean ± standard deviation. Samples were collected with a constant anticoagulant-to-blood ratio, based on a previous determination of hematocrit level

Table 13 Template bleeding time in neonate according to gestational age

	≤28 Weeks			29–32 Weeks			33–37 Weeks (N = 104)			≥38 Weeks (N = 104)		
DOL	BT	PL	MPV	BT	PL	MPV	BT	PL	MPV	BT	PL	MPV
1	204 ± 80	255.5 ± 69.4	8.9 ± 1.02	207 ± 105	286.6 ± 81.0	10.8 ± 1.0	157 ± 68	307.0 ± 106.1	10.6 ± 0.8	107 ± 38	315.9 ± 80.9	10.5 ± 1.4
10	152 ± 59	286.0 ± 81.1	9.7 ± 1.3	146 ± 79	300.9 ± 124.3	10.4 ± 1.4	163 ± 92	347.6 ± 93.9	10.7 ± 1.1	88 ± 31	344.2 ± 99.4	10.5 ± 1.6
30	104 ± 45	277.5 ± 99.8	9.9 ± 1.4	173 ± 86	306.1 ± 125.0	10.5 ± 1.4	146 ± 92	314.1 ± 120.9	10.3 ± 1.3	82 ± 39	352.3 ± 139.3	11.3 ± 1.2

Partially modified from Del Vecchio A, Latini G, Henry E et al (2008) Template bleeding times of 240 neonates born at 24–41 weeks gestation. J Perinatol 28:427–431

BT bleeding time, *DOL* day of life, *MPV* mean platelet volume, *PL* platelets

[a]Patients were tested on either day of life 1 (N 1/420 in each gestational age group), day of life 10 (N 1/420 per group), or day of life 30 (N 1/420 per group)

Table 14 Coagulation screening tests and factor levels in fetuses and term newborns

	Fetuses (weeks' gestation)			
Parameter	19–23 (N = 20)	24–29 (N = 22)	30–38 (N = 22)	Newborns (N = 60)
PT (s)	32.5 (19–45)	32.3 (19–44)	22.6 (16–30)	16.7 (12.0–23.5)
PT (INR)	6.4 (1.7–11.1)	6.2 (2.1–10.6)	3.0 (1.5–5.0)	1.7 (0.9–2.7)
APTT (s)	168.6 (83–250)	154.0 (87–210)	104.8 (76–128)	44.3 (35–52)
TCT (s)	34.2 (24–44)	26.2 (24–28)	21.4 (17.0–23.3)	20.4 (15.2–25.0)
Factor				
I (g/L Von Clauss)	0.85 (0.57–1.50)	1.12 (0.65–1.65)	1.35 (1.25–1.65)	1.68 (0.95–2.45)
I Ag (g/L)	1.08 (0.75–1.50)	1.93 (1.56–2.40)	1.94 (1.30–2.40)	2.65 (1.68–3.60)
IIc (%)	16.9 (10–24)	19.9 (11–30)	27.9 (15–50)	43.5 (27–64)
VIIc (%)	27.4 (17–37)	33.8 (18–48)	45.9 (31–62)	52.5 (28–78)
IXc (%)	10.1 (6–14)	9.9 (5–15)	12.3 (5–24)	31.8 (15–50)
Xc (%)	20.5 (14–29)	24.9 (16–35)	28.0 (16–36)	39.6 (21–65)
Vc (%)	32.1 (21–44)	36.8 (25–50)	48.9 (23–70)	89.9 (50–140)
VIIIc (%)	34.5 (18–50)	35.5 (20–52)	50.1 (27–78)	94.3 (38–150)
XIc (%)	13.2 (8–19)	12.1 (6–22)	14.8 (6–26)	37.2 (13–62)
XIIc (%)	14.9 (6–25)	22.7 (6–40)	25.8 (11–50)	69.8 (25–105)
PK (%)	12.8 (8–19)	15.4 (8–26)	18.1 (8–28)	35.4 (21–53)
HMWK (%)	15.4 (10–22)	19.3 (10–26)	23.6 (12–34)	38.9 (28–53)

Partially modified from Reverdiau Moalic P, Delahouse B, Body G et al (1996) Evaluation of blood coagulation activators and inhibitors in the healthy human fetus. Blood 88:900
Ag antigenic value, *c* coagulant activity
Values are the mean, followed in parentheses by the lower and upper boundaries including 95% of the population

Table 15 Coagulation inhibitors in fetuses and term newborns

	Fetuses (weeks' gestation			
Parameter	19–23 (N = 20)	24–29 (N = 22)	30–38 (N = 22)	Newborns (N = 60)
AT (%)	20.0 (12–31)[a]	30.0 (20–39)	37.1 (24–55)	59.4 (42–80)
HCII (%)	10.3 (6–16)	12.9 (5.5–20)	21.2 (11–33)	52.1 (19–99)
TFPI (ng/ML)	21.0 (16.0–29.2)	20.6 (13.4–33.2)	20.7 (10.4–31.5)	38.1 (22.7–55.8)
PC Ag (%)	9.5 (6–14)	12.1 (8–16)	15.9 (8–30)	32.5 (21–47)
PC Act (%)	9.6 (7–13)	10.4 (8–13)	14.1 (8–18)	28.2 (14–42)
Total PS (%)	15.1 (11–21)	17.4 (14–25)	21.0 (15–30)	38.5 (22–55)
Free PS (%)	21.7 (13–32)	27.9 (19–40)	27.1 (18–40)	49.3 (33–67)
Ratio of free PS to total PS	0.82 (0.75–0.92)	0.83 (0.76–0.95)	0.79 (0.70–0.89)	0.64 (0.59–0.98)
C4b-BP (%)	1.8 (0.6)	6.1 (1–12.5)	9.3 (5–14)	18.6 (3–40)

Partially modified from Reverdiau Moalic P, Delahouse B, Body G et al (1996) Evaluation of blood coagulation activators and inhibitors in the healthy human fetus. Blood 88:900
Values are the mean, followed in parentheses by the lower and upper boundaries including 95% of the population
Ag antigenic value, *AT* antithrombin, *c* coagulant activity, *HCII* heparin cofactor II, *TFPI* tissue factor pathway inhibitor, *PC* protein C, *PS* protein S, *C4b-BP* C4b-binding protein

Table 16 Neonatal biochemical reference ranges – PLASMA/SERUM

		Preterm			Term			
Analyte	Unit	Gestational age (weeks)	Age	Reference range	Age	Reference range		Comment
Alanine aminotransferase (ALT) (p, s) (Soldin et al. 1997)	IU/L				1–7 d 8–30 d	M 6–40 10–40	F 7–40 8–32	Method: Vitro 500 (ortho-clinical Diagnostics Raritan, NJ)
Albumin (p, s) (Ghoshal and Soldin 2003)	g/L	27 29 31 33 35		21–33 23–34 22–35 22–35 22–36	1–7 d 8–30 d	M 24–39 21–45	F 19–40 19–44	
Alkaline phosphatase (ALP) (p, s) (Ghoshal and Soldin 2003)	IU/L				1–7 d 8–30 d	M 121–351 138–486	F 107–357 107–474	Method: Dade Behring Dimension RxL analyzer (Dade Behring Inc., Newark, De)
α1-antitrypsin (s) (Davis et al. 1996)	g/L				0–30 d	0.79–2.23		Method: Beckman Array 360 (Beckman Instruments, Brea CA)
α-fetoprotein (AFP) (s) (Dugaw KA et al. 2001)	ng/mL				0–30 d 50,	0–100,000		Method: Chemiluminescent Immunoassay, Vitros Eci (ortho-clinical Diagnostics Raritan, NJ)
Aldosterone (s) (Soldin et al. 1999)	ng/dL	26–28 31–35	4 d 4 d	5–635 19–141	3 d 1 w 1 m	7–18 45–175 5–90		
Aluminium (p, s) (NHS Supraregional Assay Service Handbook 1998)	μmol/L					0.07–0.80		
Ammonia (p) (Diaz et al. 1995)	μmol/L				0–30 d	21–95		Preterm and/or sick babies may have concentrations up to 200 μmol/l
Amylase (p) (Soldin et al. 1995)	U/L				0–30 d	0–6		Method: Hitachi 717 using Boehringer Mannheim reagents (Boehringer Mannheim Diagnostic, Indianapolis, IN)
Androstenedione (p) (Garagorri et al. 2008)	nmol/L				0 d 15 d 30 d	M 1.47–13 1.0–8.7 0.6–5.9	F 0.8–12 0.7–7.9 0.5–5.3	

Aspartate transaminase (AST) (p, s) (Ghoshal and Soldin 2003)	U/L				1–7 d 8–30 d	M 26–98 16–67	F 20–93 20–69	Method: Dade Behring Dimension RxL analyzer (Dade Behring Inc., Newark, De)
Bilirubin(s) (Soldin et al. 1999a)					Birth-1 d	<100		
Total	μmol/L				1–2 d 3–5 d	<140 <200		
Conjugated					0–30 d	<10		
Caeruloplasmin (p, s) (Soldin et al. 1997a)	mg/L				1–30 d	M 77–253	F 33–275	Increases from birth throughout first year
Calcium (p, s)								
Total (Thaime 1962; Ghoshal and Soldin 2003)	mmoL/L	21–28	2.14–2.65		0–7 d 8–30 d	1.83–2.85 2.10–2.98		Results should be interpreted in conjunction with serum albumin concentration
Ionised (Wandrup et al. 1988; Nelson et al. 1989)	mmoL/L	25–36	1 d 2 d 3 d	0.81–1.41 0.72–1.44 1.04–1.52	1 d 3 d 5 d	1.05–1.37 1.10–1.44 1.20–1.48		
Chloride (p, s) (Ghoshal and Soldin 2003)	mmoL/L				0–30 d	97–108		
Cholesterol (p, s) (Hicks et al. 1996)	mmoL/L				1–30 d	M 1.4–3.9	F 1.6–4.0	Gradual increase from birth
Copper (s) (Lockitch et al. 1988)	μmoL/L	28–34	3.0–8.3		0–5 d 5–28 d	1.4–7.2 4.0–11.0		Rapid increase during first week
Cortisol (p) (Heckmann et al. 1991; Garagorri et al. 2008)	mmoL/L	24	0–4 d	73–562	0 d 3 d 15 d 30 d	54–839 54–814 54–728 55–645		If there is doubt about the integrity of the hypothalamopituitary adrenal axis, a short Synacthen test should be performed
C-reactive protein (CRP) (p, s) (Soldin et al. 2004)	mg/L					<16		
Creatine kinase (CK) (s) (Jedeikin et al. 1982)	IU/L				Cord blood 5–8 h 24–33 h 72–100 h	70–380 214–1175 130–1200 87–725		Method: GEMSAEC analyzer (Electro-Nucleonics Inc., Fairfield, NJ)

(*continued*)

Table 16 (continued)

Analyte	Unit	Preterm Gestational age (weeks)	Preterm Age	Preterm Reference range	Term Age	Term Reference range		Comment
Creatinine (p) (Rudd et al. 1983; Sonntag et al. 1996; Finney et al. 2000)	pmoL/L	24–28	1 d	35–136	2 d	37–113		Creatinine rises in the first 48 h, especially in infants <30 weeks' gestation (Mieli et al. 1999)
Cystatin C (p) (Finney et al. 2000)	mg/L	24–28 29–36		0.65–3.37 0.62–4.42	0–28 d	0.81–2.32		
Dehydroepiandrosterone sulphate (DHEAS) (p) (Garagoni et al. 2008)	μmoL/L				0 d 3 d 15 d 30 d	M 0.7–8.9 0.7–8.4 0.6–6.6 0.5–4.8	F 0.8–10 0.9–9.6 0.7–8.1 0.6–6.3	
Ferritin (s) (Murthy et al. 1995)	μg/L				1–30 d	M 36–381	F 36–483	
Glucose (p, s) (Ghoshal and Soldin 2003)	mmoL/L				1–7 d 8–30 d	2.71–6.11 3.00–6.49		
γ-Glutamyttransferase (GGT) (p, s) (Ghoshal and Soldin 2003)	IU/L				1–7 d 8–30 d	18–14 815–140		Method: Dade Behring Dimension RxL analyzer (Dade Behring Inc., Newark, De)
17α-Hydroxyprogesterone (17-OHP) (p) (Garagorri et al. 2008)	nmoL/L				0 d 3 d 15 d 30 d	17.2–252 9.9–33.1 8.8–29.2 7.4–24.5		Premature and/or sick infants may have concentrations two- to threefold higher
Immunoglobulins (s) (Soldin et al. 1995b, 1999a)						M	F	Lower in premature infants
IgG	g/L				1–30 d	1.21–8.38	1.88–8.76	
IgA	g/L					0.01–0.17	0.01–0.16	
IgM	g/L					0.08–0.17	0.13–0.70	
IgD	mg/L					None		
IgE	kIU/L				0–12 m	2–24	0–20	
Immunoreactive trypsin (Heeley and Bangert 1992)	μg/L					<60		Blood spot
Insulin								Should be measured during documented hypoglycemia. There

									may be cross-reactivity with proinsulins and values may be higher in premature infant, hence results should always be interpreted in light of clinical features and intravenous glucose requirements
Insulin-like growth factor-1 (IGF-1) (s) (Soldin et al. 1997b)	ng/mL					0 d 1–30 d	22.8–10 0.97–92		
Insulin-like growth factor binding protein-3 (IGFBP-3) (s) (Blum et al. 1990)	mg/L					0–1 w 1–4 w	0.42–1.39 0.77–2.09		
Iron (p, s) (Soldin et al. 1999b)	μmoL/L						M 5.7–20	F 5.2–22.7	
Lactate (p, s) (Ghoshal and Soldin 2003)	mmoL/L					0–90 d	1.0–3.5		
Lactate dehydrogenase (LDH) (p, s) (Ghoshal and Soldin 2003)	U/L					1–30 d 1–3 m	M 178–629 158–373	F 167–600 152–353	
Magnesium (p, s) (Meites 1989; Nelson et al. 1989)	mmoL/L	25–36	1 d 3 d 5 d 7–28 d	0.62–1.02 0.66–1.10 0.68–1.24 0.75–1.00		1 d 3 d 5 d 7–28 d	0.72–1.00 0.81–1.05 0.78–1.02 0.65–1.00		
Manganese (p, s) (NHS Supraregional Assay Service Handbook 1998)	nmoL/L						>360		Risk of toxicity
Nonesterified fatty acids (s) (Hawdon et al. 1992)	mmoL/L	26–36	3 d	0.01–1.04		3 d	0.04–1.34		
Osmolality (Davies 1973)	mOsmoL/kg		Birth 7 d 28 d	275–300 276–305 274–305			275–295		
Phenylalanine (Hommes 1991)	μmoL/L			98–213			38–137		
Phosphate (s) (Thalme 1962)	mmoL/L					2–3 d 3–4 d 4–6 d 6–12 d 21 d	1.81–3.00 1.74–2.76 1.64–2.70 1.39–3.03 1.74–2.66		Tend to be higher in babies fed formula milk

(continued)

Table 16 (continued)

Analyte	Unit	Preterm: Gestational age (weeks)	Preterm: Age	Preterm: Reference range	Term: Age	Term: Reference range	Comment
Potassium (p, s) (Greeley et al. 1993; Ghoshal and Soldin 2003)	mmoL/L		7 d	4.6–6.7	0–1 w 1 w–1 m	3.2–5.7 3.4–6.2	Results from capillary blood tend to be higher. Serum potassium concentrations are higher than those of plasma due to potassium released from platelets during clotting
Prolactin (s) (Cook et al. 1992)	mU/L				0–30 d	9–2850	May be considerably higher in the first 2 weeks
Protein (total) (s) (Zlotkin and Casselman 1987; Hicks et al. 1995)	g/L	22–36		36–63	1–30 d	41–63	
Pyruvate (s) (Soldin et al. 1999a)	µmoL/L				1–30 d	80–150	
Selenium (s) (Muntau et al. 2002)	µmoL/L				0–4 w	0.19–1.35	
Sodium (s) (Ghoshal and Soldin 2003)	mmoL/L				0–7 d 7–31 d	131–144 132–142	
Testosterone (s)(Soldin et al. 1999a)	nmoL/L	26–28 31–35	4 d 4 d	M: 2.1–4.4, 1.3–6.9 F: 0.18–0.6, 0.18–0.8		M: 2.6–14 F: 0.7–2.2	
Thyroid-stimulating hormone (TSH) (s) (Cuestas 1978; Clark et al. 2001; Dugaw et al. 2001)	mU/L	28–40	>7 d	0.8–12.0	1 d 2 d 3–30 d	3.0–120 3.0–30 0.5–6.0	Rapid increase during the first 24 h
Thyroxine free (FT4) (s) (Adams et al. 1995; Dugaw et al. 2001)	pmoL/L	25–30 31–36	0–7 0–7	6.4–42.5 16.7–60.6	1–3 d 1–4 w	25.7–68.2	
Triiodothyronine free (FT3) (s) (Cuestas 1978; John and Bamforth, 1987; Adams et al. 1995)	pmoL/L	29–36	1–3 d 4–10 d	l.2–7.3 1.2–4.9	1–3 d 4–10 d	2.5–9.3 2.8–5.7	Lower in small sick infants
Triglyceride (p, s) (Soldin and Morse 1998)	mmoL/L				0–7 d 8–30 d	M: 0.24–2.06, 0.34–2.08 F: 0.32–1.88, 0.34–1.86	

Urate (s) (Soldin et al. 1997d)	µmoL/L					0–1 d 1–2 d 2–3 d 3–7 d	300–505 200–490 190–395 150–290	
Urea (s) (Soldin et al. 1997e)	mmoL/L					1–7 d 8–30 d	0.7–4.6 0.7–5.7	May be higher in infants fed formula milk
Zinc (s) (Riikgauer et al. 1997; Lockitch et al. 1998)	µmoL/L	28–34		10–24		0–5 d	9.9–21.4	Higher in preterms. Concentration decreases during first week

h hour(s), *d* day(s), *w* week(s), *m* month(s)
p plasma, *s* serum

Davis ML, Austin C, Messmer BL et al (1996) IFCC-standardized pediatric reference intervals for ten serum proteins using Beckman Array 360 system. Clin Biochem 29:489–492
Diaz I, Tornei PL, Martinez P (1995) Reference intervals for blood ammonia in healthy subjects, determined by microdiffusion. Clin Chem 41:1048
Dugaw KA, Jack RM, Rutledge J (2001) Pediatric reference ranges for TSH, free T4, total T4, total T3 and T3 uptake on the Vitros ECi analyzer. Clin Chem 47:A108
Finney H, Newman DJ, Thakkar H et al (2000) Reference ranges for plasma cystatin C and creatinine measurements in premature infants, neonates and older children. Arch Dis Child 82:71–75
Garagorri JM, Rodríguez G, Lario-Elboj AJ et al (2008) Reference levels for 17-hydroxyprogesterone, 11-desoxycortisol, cortisol, testosterone, dehydroepiandrosterone sulfate and androstenedione in infants from birth to 6 months of age. Eur J Pediatr 167:647–653
Ghoshal AK, Soldin SJ (2003) Evaluation of the Dade Behring Dimension RxL: integrated chemistry system – pediatric reference ranges. Clin Chim Acta 331:135–146
Greeley C, Snell J, Colaco A et al (1993) Pediatric reference ranges for electrolytes and creatinine. Clin Chem 39:1172
Hawdon JM, Ward Platt MP, Aynsley-Green A (1992) Patterns of metabolic adaptation for preterm and term infants in the first week of life. Arch Dis Child 68:274–279
Heeley AF, Bangert SK (1992) The neonatal detection of cystic fibrosis by measurement of immunoreactive trypsin in blood. Ann Clin Biochem 29:464–467
Hicks JM, Bjom S, Beatey J (1995) Pediatric reference ranges for albumin, globulin and total protein on the Hitachi 747. Clin Chem 41:S93
Hicks JM, Bailey J, Beatey J (1996) Pediatric reference ranges for cholesterol. Clin Chem 42:S307
Hommes FA (ed) (1991) Techniques in diagnostic human biochemical genetics – a laboratory manual. Wiley Liss, New York
Jedeikin R, Makela SK, Shennan AT et al (1982) Creatine kinase isoenzymes in serum from cord blood and the blood of healthy full-term infants during the first three postnatal days. Clin Chem 28:317–322
John R, Bamforth FJ (1987) Serum free thyroxine and free triiodothyronine concentrations in healthy full term, pre-term and sick pre-term neonates. Ann Clin Biochem 24:461–465
Lockitch G, Halstead AC, Wadsworth L et al (1988) Age and sex specific pediatric reference intervals and correlations for zinc, copper, selenium, iron, vitamins A and E and related proteins. Clin Chem 34:1625–1628
Muntau AC, Streiter M, Kappler M et al (2002) Age-related reference ranges for serum selenium concentrations in infants and children. Clin Chem 48:555–560
Murthy JN, Hicks JM, Soldin SJ (1995) Evaluation of the Technicon Immuno I random access immunoassay analyzer and calculation of pediatric reference ranges for endocrine tests, T-uptake, and ferritin. Clin Biochem 28(2):181–185
Nelson N, Finnstrom O, Larsson L (1989) Plasma ionised calcium, phosphate and magnesium in preterm and small for gestational age infants. Acta Paediatr Scand 78:351–357
NHS (1998) Supraregional assay service handbook, 3rd edn
Rudd PT, Hughes EA, Placzek MM et al (1983) Reference ranges for plasma creatinine during the first month of life. Arch Dis Child 58:212–215
Rükgauer M, Klein J, Kruse-Jarres JD (1997) Reference values for the trace elements copper, manganese, selenium and zinc in the serum/plasma of children, adolescents and adults. J Trace Elem Med Biol 11:92–98
Soldin SJ, Hickson JM, Bailey J et al (1995a) Pediatric reference ranges for amylase. Clin Chem 41:594

(continued)

Table 16 (continued)

Analyte	Unit	Preterm			Term		Comment
		Gestational age (weeks)	Age	Reference range	Age	Reference range	

Soldin SJ, Morales A, Albalos F et al (1995b) Pediatric reference ranges on the Abbott Imx for FSH, LH, prolactin, TSH, T4, T3, free T4, free T3, T-uptake, IgE and ferritin. Clin Biochem 28:603–606

Soldin SJ, Hicks JM, Bailey J (1997a) Pediatric reference ranges for β2-microglobulin and ceruloplasmin. Clin Chem 43:S199

Soldin SJ, Hicks JM, Bailey J (1997b) Pediatric reference ranges for creatinine kinase and insulin-like growth factor J. Clin Chem 43:S199

Soldin SJ, Savwoir TV, Guo Y (1997c) Pediatric reference ranges for alkaline phosphatase, aspartate aminotransferase and alanine aminotransferase in children less than 1 year old on the Vitros 500. Clin Chem 43:S199

Soldin SJ, Savwoir TV, Guo Y (1997d) Pediatric reference ranges for lactate dehydrogenase and uric acid during the first year of life on the Vitros 500 analyzer. Clin Chem 43:S199

Soldin SJ, Savwoir TV, Guo Y (1997e) Pediatric reference ranges for gamma-glutamyltransferase and urea nitrogen during the first year of life on the Vitros 500 analyzer. Clin Chem 43:SI99

Soldin SJ, Morse AS (1998) Pediatric reference ranges for calcium and triglycerides in children <1 year old using the Vitros 500 analyzer. Clin Chem 44:A16

Soldin SJ, Brugnara C, Hichs JM (eds) (1999a) Pediatric reference ranges, 3rd edn. AACC Press, Washington, DC

Soldin SJ, Bailey J, Bjom J (1999b) Pediatric reference ranges for iron on the Hitachi 747 with Boehringer Mannheim reagents. Clin Chem 45:A22

Soldin OP, Bierbower LH, Choi JJ et al (2004) Serum iron, ferritin, transferrin, total iron binding capacity, hs-CRP, LDL, cholesterol and magnesium in children; new reference intervals using the Dade dimension clinical chemistry system. Clin Chim Acta 342:211–217

Sonntag J, Prankel B, Waltz S (1996) Serum creatinine concentration, urinary creatinine excretion and creatinine clearance during the first 9 weeks in preterm infants with a birth weight below 1500 g. Eur J Paediatr 155:815–819

Thalme B (1962) Calcium, chloride, cholesterol, inorganic phosphorus and total protein in blood plasma during the early neonatal period studied with ultramicrochemical methods. Acta Paediatr Scand 51:649–660

Wandrup J, Kroner J, Pryds O et al (1988) Age related reference values for ionized calcium in the first week of life in premature and full term neonates. Scand J Clin Lab Invest 48:255–260

Zlotkin SH, Casselman CW (1987) Percentile estimates of reference values for total protein and albumin in sera of premature infants (<37 weeks of gestation). Clin Chem 33:411–413

Table 17 Neonatal biochemical reference ranges – URINE

		Reference range				
		Preterm		Term		
Analyte	Unit	Age	Reference range	Age	Reference range	Comment
Calcium (Karlen et al. 1985)	mmol/l	0–7 d	0.2–1.6	0–1 w	<0.6	
Calcium:creatinine ratio (Sargent et al. 1993)	mmol/mmol			1–4 w	<2.4	
Creatinine clearance (Sonntag et al. 1996)	ml/min/ 1.73 m^2	1 w 2 w 2–4 w	7–22 10–28 11–34			
Fractional sodium excretion (Rossi et al. 1994)	%			0–3 d	<0.72	$\frac{\text{Urinary[Sodium]} \times \text{Serum[Creatinine]}}{\text{Serum[Sodium]} \times \text{Urinary[Creatinine]}}$
Phosphate (Rossi et al. 1994)	mmol/24 h	1–2 w 3–4 w	<0.5–9.9 0.5–12	0–7 d	<18	
Potassium (Wilkins 1992)	mmol/l mmol/kg/24 h	0–30 d	228 0.2–1.2		<5	Dependent upon intake
Sodium (Wilkins 1992)	mmol/l	0–30 d	1–15		<1	Dependent upon intake
Transport maximum of phosphate in relation to GFR (TmP/GFR) (Bistarakis et al. 1986; Rossi et al. 1994)	μmol/ml			0–30 d	1.89–2.37	Tubular phosphate reabsorption/ml GFF1: Pphos-(Uphos × P[Creat]/ Ur[Creat])
Urate:creatinine ratio (Kaufman et al. 1968)	mmol/mmol				0.1–2.0	The ratio is generally elevated in Lesch-Nyhan syndrome and <0.03 mmol/mmol in sulphite oxidase deficiency

Bistarakis L, Voskaki I, Lambadaridis J et al (1986) Renal handling of phosphate in the first 6 months of life. Arch Dis Child 61:677–681

Karlen J, Aperia A, Zetterstrom R (1985) Renal excretion of calcium and phosphate in preterm and term infants. J Pediatr 106:814–819

Kaufman JM, Greene ML, Seegmiller JE (1968) Urine uric acid:creatinine ratio – a screening test for inherited disorders of purine metabolism. J Pediatr 73:583–592

Rossi R, Danzebrink S, Linnenburger K et al (1994) Assessment of tubular reabsorption on sodium, glucose phosphate and amino acid based on spot urine samples. Acta Paediatr 83:1282–1286

Sargent JD, Strukel TA, Kresel J et al (1993) Normal values for random urinary calcium to creatinine ratios in infancy. J Paediatr 123:393–397

Sonntag J, Prankel B, Waltz S (1996) Serum creatinine concentration, urinary creatinine excretion and creatinine clearance during the first 9 weeks in preterm infants with a birth weight below 1500 g. Eur J Paediatr 155:815–819

Table 18 Normal blood gas values

	PaO_2				$PaCO_2$				H^+			
	Full-term		Preterm		Full-term		Preterm		Full-term		Preterm	
	kPa	mmHg	kPa	mmHg	kPa	mmHg	kPa	mmHg	nmol/l	pH	nmol/l	pH
15 min	11.6	87			3.7	28			48	7.32		
30 min	11.4	86			4.3	32			43	7.37		
60 min	10.8	81			4.1	31			40	7.40		
1–6 h	8.0–10.6	60–80	8.0–9.3	60–70	4.7–6.0	35–45	4.7–6.0	35–45	46–49	7.31–7.34	42–48	7.32–7.38
6–24 h	9.3–10	70–75	8.0–9.3	60–70	4.4–4.8	33–36	3.6–5.3	27–40	37–43	7.37–7.43	35–45	7.36–7.45
48 h–1 week	9.3–11.3	70–85	10.0–10.6	75–80	4.4–4.8	33–36	4.3–4.5	32–36	42–44	7.36–7.38	40–48	7.32–7.40
2 weeks					4.8–5.2	36–39	5.1	38	43	7.37	48	7.32
3 weeks					5.3	40	5.1	38	42	7.38	49	7.31
1 month					5.2	39	4.9	37	41	7.39	49	7.31

Reproduced from Rennie J, Roberton R (2002) Manual of neonatal intensive care, NRC 4th edn. Edward Amold, London
Data from 1 h to 1 week are drawn from the literature on arteria' samples
Data beyond 1 week are on capillary samples

Table 19 Conversion table from conventional unit to standard international unit

Component	Conventional unit	Conversion factor (multiply by)	SI unit
Adrenocorticotropic hormone	pg/mL	0.22	pmol/L
Alanina amino transferase (ALT)	U/L	0.0167	mkat/L
Albumin	g/dL	10	g/L
Aldosterone	ng/dL	27.74	pmol/L
Alkaline phosphatase	U/L	0.0167	mkat/L
Ammonia	mg/dL	0.714	mmol/L
Amylase	U/L	0.0167	mkat/L
Androstenedione	ng/dL	0.0349	nmol/L
Antidiuretic hormone	pg/mL	0.923	pmol/L
Alpha-I-antitrypsin	mg/dL	0.184	mmol/L
Aspartate aminotransferase (AST)	U/L	0.0167	mkat/L
Bicarbonate	mEq/L	1	mmol/L
Bilirubin	mg/dL	17.104	mmol/L
Blood gases			
Carbon dioxide (PCo_2)	mm Hg	0.133	kPa
Oxygen (PO2)	mm Hg	0.133	kPa
Brain natriuretic peptide (BNP)	pg/mL	1	ng/L
C-reactive protein (PCR)	mg/L	9524	nmol/L
Caffeine	mg/L	0.515	mmol/L
Calcium, ionized	mg/dL	0.25	mmol/L
Calcium, total	mg/dL	0.5	mmol/L
Chloride	mEq/L	1	mmol/L
Copper	mg/dL	0.157	mmol/L
Cortisol	mg/dL	27.59	nmol/L
Creatinine	mg/dL	88.4	mmol/L
D-dimer	mg/mL	5476	nmol/L
Dehydroepiandrosterone (DHEA)	ng/mL	3.47	nmol/L
Dehydroepiandrosterone sulfate (DHEA)	mg/dL	0.027	mmol/L
Digoxin	ng/mL	1.281	nmol/L
Estradiol	pg/mL	3671	pmol/L
Ferritin	ng/mL	2.247	pmol/L
Fibrinogen	mg/dL	0.0294	mmol/L
Follicle-stimulating hormone (FSH)	mIU/mL	1	IU/L
Gamma-glutamyltransferase (GGT)	U/L	0.0167	mkat/L
Gentamicin	mg/mL	20.9	mmol/L
Glucose	mg/dL	0.555	mmol/L
(G6PD)	U/g hemoglobin	0.0167	hemoglobin
Growth hormone	ng/mL	1	mg/L
Hematocrit	%	0.01	Proportion of 1.0
Hemoglobin	g/dL	10	g/L
Insulin	mUI/mL	6.945	pmol/L
Iron	mg/dL	0.179	mmol/L
Iron-binding capacity	mg/dL	0.179	mmol/L
Lactate	mg/dL	0.111	mmol/L
Lactate dehydrogenase (LDH)	U/L	0.0167	mkat/L
Lead	mg/dL	0.0483	mmol/L

(continued)

Table 19 (continued)

Component	Conventional unit	Conversion factor (multiply by)	SI unit
Lipase	U/L	0.0167	mkat/L
Luteinizing hormone (LH)	mIU/mL	1	IU/L
Magnesium	mEq/L	0.5	mmol/L
Methemoglobin	g/dL	155	mmol/L
	% of total hemoglobin	0.01	Proportion of total
Osmolarity	mOsmol/kg	1	mmol/kg
Phenobarbital	mg/mL	4.31	mmol/L
Phenytoin	mg/L	3.968	mmol/L
Phosphate	mg/dL	0.323	mmol/L
Platelet count	$\times 10^3$/mL	1	$\times 10^9$/L
Potassium	mEq/L	1	mmol/L
Prealbumin	mg/dL	10	mg/L
Progesterone	ng/mL	3.18	nmol/L
Pyruvate	mg/dL	113.56	mmol/L
Red blood cell count	$\times 10^6$/mL	1	$\times 10^{12}$/L
Reticulocyte count	$\times 10^3$/mL	1	$\times 10^9$/L
	% of red blood cells	0.01	Proportion of red blood cells
Sodium	mEq/L	1	mmol/L
Testosterone	ng/dL	0.347	nmol/L
Theophylline	mg/mL	5.55	mmol/L
Thyroglobulin	ng/mL	1	mg/L
Thyroid-stimulating hormone (TSH)	mIU/L	1	mIU/L
Thyroxine, free (FT_4)	ng/dL	12871	pmol/L
Thyroxine, total (T_4)	mg/dL	12871	nmol/L
Thyroxine-binding globulin	mg/mL	17094	nmol/L
Triglycerides	mg/dL	0.0113	mmol/L
Triiodothyronine, free (FT_3)	pg/mL	0.0154	pmol/L
Triiodothyronine, total (T_3)	ng/dL	0.0154	nmol/L
Urea nitrogen	mg/dL	0.357	mmol/L
Vancomycin	mg/mL	0.69	mmol/L
Vitamin A (retinol)	mg/dL	0.349	mmol/L
Vitamin B_1 (Thiamine)	mg/dL	29.6	nmol/L
Vitamin B_2 (riboflavine)	mg/dL	26.6	nmol/L
Vitamin B_3	mg/mL	4.56	mmol/L
Vitamin B_6 (Pyridoxine)	ng/mL	4046	nmol/L
Vitamin B_{12}	pg/mL	0.7378	pmol/L
Vitamin C (ascorbic acid)	mg/dL	56.78	mmol/L
Vitamin D (1,25-dihydroxyvitamin D)	pg/dL	2.6	pmol/L
Vitamin D (25-hydroxyvitamin D)	ng/mL	2496	nmol/L
Vitamin E (alpha-tocopherol)	mg/mL	23.22	mmol/L
Vitamin K	ng/mL	2.22	nmol/L
White blood cell (WBC) count	/mL	0.001	$\times 10^9$/L
WBC differential counts			
Neutrophils, segmented	/mL	0.001	$\times 10^9$/L

(*continued*)

Table 19 (continued)

Component	Conventional unit	Conversion factor (multiply by)	SI unit
Neutrophils, bands	/mL	0.001	$\times 10^9$/L
Lymphocytes	/mL	0.001	$\times 10^9$/L
Monocytes	/mL	0.001	$\times 10^9$/L
Eosinophils	/mL	0.001	$\times 10^9$/L
Basophils	/mL	0.001	$\times 10^9$/L
WBC differential counts (number fractions)			
Neutrophils, segmented	%	0.01	Proportion of 1.0
Neutrophils, bands	%	0.01	Proportion of 1.0
Lynphocytes	%	0.01	Proportion of 1.0
Monocytes	%	0.01	Proportion of 1.0
Eosinophils	%	0.01	Proportion of 1.0
Basophils	%	0.01	Proportion of 1.0
Zinc	ug/dL	0.153	mmol/L

Modified from Iverson C et al (2007) Table 2. Selected laboratory tests, with reference ranges and conversion factors. In: AMA manual of style: a guide for authors and editors. Oxford University Press, New York

Index

G. Buonocore et al. (eds.), *Neonatology*,
https://doi.org/10.1007/978-3-319-29489-6

B

H

N

P

Y

Z

9783319294872VOL03